CURRENT SURGICAL THERAPY

CURRENT SURGICAL THERAPY

12th EDITION

JOHN L. CAMERON

MD, FACS, FRCS (Eng) (hon), FRCS (Ed) (hon), FRCSI (hon)

The Alfred Blalock Distinguished Service Professor
Department of Surgery
The Johns Hopkins University School of Medicine
Baltimore, Maryland

ANDREW M. CAMERON

MD, PhD, FACS

Chief, Division of Transplantation
Surgical Director, Liver Transplantation
Department of Surgery
The Johns Hopkins University School of Medicine
Baltimore, Maryland

ELSEVIER

ELSEVIER

1600 John F. Kennedy Blvd.
Ste 1800
Philadelphia, PA 19103-2899

CURRENT SURGICAL THERAPY, TWELFTH EDITION

ISBN: 978-0-323-37691-4

Notices

Previous editions copyrighted 2014, 2011, 2008, 2004, 2001, 1998, 1995, 1992, 1989, 1986, 1984 by Saunders, an imprint of Elsevier Inc.

ISBN: 978-0-323-37691-4

Publishing Manager: Michael Houston
Senior Content Development Specialist: Kathryn DeFrancesco
Publishing Services Manager: Patricia Tannian
Senior Project Manager: Claire Kramer
Design Direction: Brian Salisbury

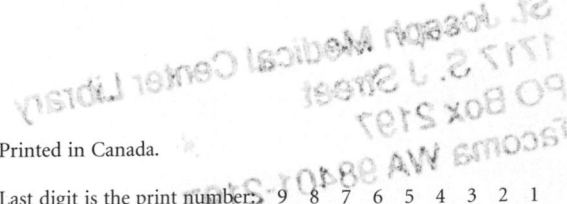

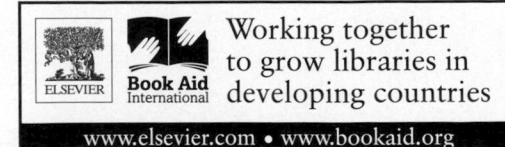

Working together to grow libraries in developing countries

www.elsevier.com • www.bookaid.org

CONTRIBUTORS

Abbas El-Sayed Abbas, MD, MS, FACS
Associate Professor and Chief of Division of
Thoracic Surgery
Director of Thoracic and Foregut Surgery
Thoracic Medicine and Surgery
Temple University School of Medicine
Philadelphia, Pennsylvania

*THE MANAGEMENT OF
GASTROESOPHAGEAL REFLUX DISEASE*

Fizan Abdullah, MD, PhD
Vice-Chair, Department of Surgery
Head, Division of Pediatric Surgery
Program Director, Fellowship in
Pediatric Surgery
Ann & Robert H. Lurie Children's Hospital
of Chicago
Professor of Surgery
Northwestern University
Chicago, Illinois

*EXTRACORPOREAL LIFE SUPPORT FOR
RESPIRATORY FAILURE*

Gerard J. Abood, MD
Director of Thoracic and Foregut Surgery
Thoracic Medicine and Surgery
Temple University School of Medicine
Philadelphia, Pennsylvania

*IS A NASOGASTRIC TUBE NECESSARY AFTER
ALIMENTARY TRACT SURGERY?*

Christopher J. Abularrage, MD
Assistant Professor
Division of Vascular Surgery and
Endovascular Therapy
The Johns Hopkins Hospital
Baltimore, Maryland

*THE MANAGEMENT OF RECURRENT
CAROTID ARTERY STENOSIS*

Ali F. AbuRahma, MD
Professor of Surgery
Chief, Vascular and Endovascular Surgery
Director, Vascular Fellowship Program
Department of Surgery
Robert C. Byrd Health Sciences Center
West Virginia University
Charleston, West Virginia

BRACHIOCEPHALIC RECONSTRUCTION

Zachary T. AbuRahma, DO
Vascular Surgery Resident
Charleston Area Medical Center
West Virginia University
Charleston, West Virginia

BRACHIOCEPHALIC RECONSTRUCTION

David B. Adams, MD
Professor of Surgery
Department of Surgery
Co-Director
Digestive Disease Center
Medical University of South Carolina
Charleston, South Carolina

*PANCREAS DIVISUM AND OTHER VARIANTS
OF DOMINANT DORSAL DUCT ANATOMY*

Cheguevara Afaneh, MD
Assistant Professor of Surgery
Department of Surgery
New York Presbyterian Hospital–Weill
Cornell Medicine
New York, New York

*LAPAROSCOPIC TREATMENT OF
ESOPHAGEAL MOTILITY DISORDERS*

Vatche G. Agopian, MD
Assistant Professor
Department of Surgery
David Geffen School of Medicine at
University of California, Los Angeles
Los Angeles, California

*THE MANAGEMENT OF ECHINOCOCCAL
CYST DISEASE OF THE LIVER*

Ali Karim Ahmed, BS
Medical Student
The Johns Hopkins University
Baltimore, Maryland

*NECROTIZING SKIN AND SOFT TISSUE
INFECTIONS*

Steven A. Ahrendt, MD
Associate Professor
Division of Surgical Oncology
Department of Surgery
University of Pittsburgh Medical Center
Pittsburgh, Pennsylvania

*THE MANAGEMENT OF CYSTIC DISORDERS
OF THE BILE DUCTS*

Nita Ahuja, MD, FACS
Associate Professor
Department of Surgery
The Johns Hopkins Medical Institution
Baltimore, Maryland

*THE MANAGEMENT OF TUMORS OF
THE ANAL REGION*

Nitin K. Ahuja, MD
Gastroenterology Fellow
Division of Gastroenterology and
Hepatology
Johns Hopkins Medicine
Baltimore, Maryland

*THE MANAGEMENT OF ACUTE COLONIC
PSEUDO-OBSTRUCTION (OGILVIE'S
SYNDROME)*

Louis H. Alarcon, MD
Associate Professor
Departments of Surgery and Critical
Care Medicine
University of Pittsburgh School of Medicine
Pittsburgh, Pennsylvania

INJURY TO THE SPLEEN

Maria B. Albuja-Cruz, MD
Department of Surgery
University of Colorado Anschutz Medical
Campus
Aurora, Colorado

LAPAROSCOPIC ADRENALECTOMY

Alison R. Althans, BA
Medical Student/Research Assistant
University Hospitals Cleveland Medical
Center/Case Western Reserve University
School of Medicine
Cleveland, Ohio

*LAPAROSCOPIC COLON AND RECTAL
SURGERY*

Azah A. Althumairi, MD
Postdoctoral Fellow
Colorectal Surgery
Department of Surgery
The Johns Hopkins University School
of Medicine
Baltimore, Maryland

*THE MANAGEMENT OF DIVERTICULAR
DISEASE OF THE COLON*

*THE MANAGEMENT OF TOXIC
MEGACOLON*

John C. Alverdy, MD, FACS
Sara and Harold Lincoln Thompson
Professor of Surgery
Executive Vice-Chair
Department of Surgery
Pritzker School of Medicine
University of Chicago
Chicago, Illinois
*THE MANAGEMENT OF PANCREATIC
NECROSIS*

Joselin L. Anandam, MD
Assistant Professor
Department of Surgery
University of Texas Southwestern
Medical Center
Dallas, Texas
THE MANAGEMENT OF COLON CANCER

Mark P. Androes, MD
Chief, Division of Vascular Surgery
Greenville Health System
Greenville, South Carolina
FEMOROPOPLITEAL OCCLUSIVE DISEASE

Amir Mehdi Ansari, MD
Surgical Research Fellow
The Johns Hopkins University School
of Medicine
Baltimore, Maryland
*NECROTIZING SKIN AND SOFT TISSUE
INFECTIONS*

Dean J. Arnaoutakis, MD
Fellow
Division of Vascular and Endovascular
Surgery
Brigham and Women's Hospital
Boston, Massachusetts
AORTOILIAC OCCLUSIVE DISEASE

Meghan A. Arnold, MD
Assistant Professor
Department of Surgery
Division of Pediatric Surgery
University of Michigan
Ann Arbor, MI
THE MANAGEMENT OF VASCULAR INJURIES

Chady I. Atallah, MD
PGY-IV General Surgery Resident
Department of Surgery
The Johns Hopkins University
Baltimore, Maryland
*THE MANAGEMENT OF CHRONIC
ULCERATIVE COLITIS*

Hugh G. Auchincloss, MD, MPH
Cardiothoracic Fellow
Massachusetts General Hospital
Boston, Massachusetts
PRIMARY TUMORS OF THE THYMUS

Andrea L. Axtell, MD
Department of Surgery
Massachusetts General Hospital
Boston, Massachusetts
*THE MANAGEMENT OF TRACHEAL
STENOSIS*

Patricia Ayoung-Chee, MD, MPH
Assistant Professor
Department of Surgery
New York University School of Medicine
New York, New York
PENETRATING ABDOMINAL TRAUMA

Nilofer Azad, MD
Associate Professor
Department of Gastrointestinal Oncology
The Johns Hopkins University School
of Medicine
Baltimore, Maryland
*NEOADJUVANT AND ADJUVANT TREATMENT
FOR COLORECTAL CANCER*

Faris K. Azar, MD
Halsted Surgery Resident
Johns Hopkins Hospital
Baltimore, Maryland
PRIMARY HYPERPARATHYROIDISM

Saïd C. Azoury, MD
Halsted Surgery Resident
Department of Surgery
The Johns Hopkins Hospital
Baltimore, Maryland
*INCISIONAL, EPIGASTRIC, AND UMBILICAL
HERNIAS*

Christina E. Bailey, MD, MSCI
Assistant Professor
Department of Surgery
Vanderbilt University Medical Center
Nashville, Tennessee
*THE MANAGEMENT OF SMALL BOWEL
TUMORS*

Ian B. Bailey, BA
Department of Surgery
State University of New York Upstate
Medical University
Syracuse, New York
*BUERGER'S DISEASE (THROMBOANGIITIS
OBLITERANS)*

Charles M. Balch, MD
Professor of Surgery
Department of Surgical Oncology
University of Texas MD Anderson
Cancer Center
Houston, Texas
*THE MANAGEMENT OF CUTANEOUS
MELANOMA*

Glen C. Balch, MD
Associate Professor of Surgery
Department of Surgery
Emory University Medical School
Atlanta, Georgia
*THE MANAGEMENT OF CUTANEOUS
MELANOMA*

Chad G. Ball, MD
Associate Professor
Department of Surgery
University of Calgary
Foothills Medical Center
Calgary, Alberta, Canada
*THE MANAGEMENT OF BENIGN BILIARY
STRICTURES*

Dennis F. Bandyk, MD
Section Chief
Department of Vascular and Endovascular
Surgery
University of California, San Diego
San Diego, California
*THE MANAGEMENT OF CHRONIC
MESENTERIC ISCHEMIA*

**Philip S. Barie, MD, MBA, Master
CCM, FIDSA, FACS**
Professor
Department of Surgery
Weill Cornell Medical College
New York, New York
BURN WOUND MANAGEMENT

Andrew Bates, MD
Clinical Instructor
Department of Surgery
Stony Brook University Hospital
Stony Brooke, New York
LAPAROSCOPIC INGUINAL HERNIORRHAPHY

Richard Battafarano, MD, PhD
Associate Professor and Chief
Division of Thoracic Surgery
Johns Hopkins Medicine
Baltimore, Maryland
*THE MANAGEMENT OF ZENKER'S
DIVERTICULUM*

Kristin Wilson Beard, MD
Surgeon-in-Chief
UConn Health
Farmington, Connecticut
*THE MANAGEMENT OF DISORDERS OF
ESOPHAGEAL MOTILITY*

Peter Beaulieu, DO, MPH
Vascular Surgery Resident
Grand Rapids Medical Education Partners
Michigan State University College of
Human Medicine
Grand Rapids, Michigan
GANGRENE OF THE FOOT

Robert J. Beaulieu, MD
Resident
Department of Surgery
John Hopkins Medicine
Baltimore, Maryland

THE DIABETIC FOOT

Marshall S. Bedine, MD
Assistant Professor of Medicine
Department of Medicine
Division of Gastroenterology and
Hepatology
Johns Hopkins Medicine
Baltimore, Maryland

*THE MANAGEMENT OF ACUTE COLONIC
PSEUDO-OBSTRUCTION (OGILVIE'S
SYNDROME)*

Edo K. S. Bedzra, MD
Cardiothoracic Fellow
University of Washington
Seattle, Washington

MEDIASTINAL MASSES

Susan E. Beekmann, RN, MPH
Department of Internal Medicine
Carver College of Medicine
University of Iowa
Iowa City, Iowa

*OCCUPATIONAL EXPOSURE TO HUMAN
IMMUNODEFICIENCY VIRUS AND OTHER
BLOODBORNE PATHOGENS*

Kevin E. Behrns, MD
Professor and Chairman
Department of Surgery
University of Florida
Gainesville, Florida

*THE MANAGEMENT OF GALLSTONE
PANCREATITIS, PART A*

John-Paul Bellistri, MD
Resident
Department of Surgery
Montefiore Medical Center
Bronx, New York

*SPLENECTOMY FOR HEMATOLOGIC
DISORDERS*

Ricardo J. Bello, MD, MPH
Postdoctoral Research Fellow
Department of Plastic and Reconstructive
Surgery
The Johns Hopkins University School
of Medicine
Baltimore, Maryland

LYMPHEDEMA

Ehsan Benrashid, MD
Resident, Department of Surgery
Duke University Medical Center
Durham, North Carolina

*VENOUS THROMBOEMBOLISM:
PREVENTION, DIAGNOSIS, AND TREATMENT*

David L. Berger, MD
Associate Professor of Surgery
Harvard Medical School
Massachusetts General Hospital
Boston, Massachusetts

*THE MANAGEMENT OF ASYMPTOMATIC
(SILENT) GALLSTONES*

Julia R. Berian, MD
General Surgery Resident
Department of Surgery
University of Chicago Medicine
Chicago, Illinois

*PREOPERATIVE BOWEL PREPARATION: IS IT
NECESSARY?*

Karl Y. Bilimoria, MD, MS
Director of Surgical Outcomes and Quality
Improvement Center (SOQIC)
Department of Surgery
Northwestern Hospital
Northwestern University
Chicago, Illinois

*COMPARATIVE EFFECTIVENESS RESEARCH
IN SURGERY*

Marc A. Bjurlin, DO, MSc, FACOS
Director of Urologic Oncology
New York University Lutheran
Medical Center
Clinical Assistant Professor
Department of Urology
New York University School of Medicine
New York University Langone Health
System
New York, New York

*RETROPERITONEAL INJURIES: KIDNEY AND
URETER*

James H. Black III, MD
David Goldfarb, MD Associate Professor
of Surgery
The Johns Hopkins University School
of Medicine
Baltimore, Maryland

*ENDOVASCULAR TREATMENT OF
ABDOMINAL AORTIC ANEURYSM*

Kirby Bland, MD
Professor of Surgery
Department of Surgery
University of Alabama at Birmingham
Birmingham, Alabama

*THE ROLE OF STEREOTACTIC BREAST
BIOPSY IN THE MANAGEMENT OF
BREAST DISEASE*

Joseph-Vincent V. Blas, MD
Division of Vascular Surgery
Greenville Health System
Greenville, South Carolina

FEMOROPOPLITEAL OCCLUSIVE DISEASE

Joshua I. Bleier, MD
Associate Professor of Clinical Surgery
Department of Surgery
University of Pennsylvania
Philadelphia, Pennsylvania

*THE MANAGEMENT OF RECTOVAGINAL
FISTULA*

Jennifer Blumetti, MD
Program Director
Colon and Rectal Surgery Residency
Program
Division of Colon and Rectal Surgery
John H. Stroger Hospital of Cook County
Chicago, Illinois

THE MANAGEMENT OF HEMORRHOIDS

Adam Bodzin, MD
Clinical Associate
Department of Surgery
Section of Transplantation
University of Chicago
Chicago, Illinois

*HEPATIC MALIGNANCY: RESECTION VERSUS
TRANSPLANTATION*

Brian A. Boone, MD
Fellow
Surgical Oncology
University of Pittsburgh
Pittsburgh, Pennsylvania

MINIMALLY INVASIVE PANCREATIC SURGERY

Louis J. Born, BS
Postbaccalaureate Research Assistant
The Johns Hopkins University
Baltimore, Maryland

*NECROTIZING SKIN AND SOFT TISSUE
INFECTIONS*

Judy C. Boughey, MD, FACS
Professor of Surgery
Department of Surgery
Mayo Clinic
Rochester, Minnesota

*THE MANAGEMENT OF RECURRENT AND
METASTATIC BREAST CANCER*

Daniel Boyett, MD
Assistant Professor of Surgery
Department of Surgery
The Johns Hopkins University
Baltimore, Maryland

*METABOLIC CHANGES FOLLOWING
BARIATRIC SURGERY*

*LAPAROSCOPIC 360-DEGREE
FUNDOPLICATION*

Justin T. Brady, MD
Resident in General Surgery
Department of Surgery
University Hospitals Cleveland Medical
Center/Case Western Reserve University
Cleveland, Ohio

*LAPAROSCOPIC COLON AND RECTAL
SURGERY*

Murray F. Brennan, MD
Benno C. Schmidt Chair in Clinical
Oncology
Department of Surgery
Memorial Sloan Kettering Cancer Center
New York, New York

*THE MANAGEMENT OF SOFT TISSUE
SARCOMA*

Bruce M. Brenner, MD
Associate Professor
Department of Surgery
University of Connecticut
Farmington, Connecticut

*THE MANAGEMENT OF GASTRIC
ADENOCARCINOMA*

L. D. Britt, MD, MPH, FACS, FCCM
Brickhouse Professor and Chairman
Department of Surgery
Eastern Virginia Medical School
Norfolk, Virginia

*INITIAL ASSESSMENT AND RESUSCITATION
OF THE TRAUMA PATIENT*

Malcolm Brock, MD
Professor of Surgery
Division of Thoracic Surgery
The Johns Hopkins Medical Institutions
Baltimore, Maryland

ESOPHAGEAL FUNCTION TESTS

Evan R. Brownie, MD
Chief Resident in General Surgery
Vanderbilt University Medical Center
Nashville, Tennessee

*BALLOON ANGIOPLASTY AND STENTS IN
CAROTID ARTERY OCCLUSIVE DISEASE*

F. Charles Brunicardi, MD
Moss Foundation Professor and
Vice-Chairman
Department of Surgery
University of California, Los Angeles
Los Angeles, California

*THE MANAGEMENT OF BENIGN GASTRIC
ULCERS*

L. Michael Brunt, MD
Professor of Surgery
Section Chief Minimally Invasive Surgery
Department of Surgery
Washington University School of Medicine
St. Louis, Missouri

ADRENAL INCIDENTALOMA

Jessica Burgess, MD
Assistant Professor of Surgery
Eastern Virginia Medical School
Norfolk, Virginia

*INITIAL ASSESSMENT AND RESUSCITATION
OF THE TRAUMA PATIENT*

Mark S. Burke, MD, FACS
Department of Plastic and Reconstructive
Surgery
ECMC Hospital
Buffalo, New York

*BREAST RECONSTRUCTION AFTER BREAST
CANCER TREATMENT: GOALS, OPTIONS,
AND REASONING*

Clay Cothren Burlew, MD, FACS
Director, Surgical Intensive Care Unit
Department of Surgery
Denver Health Medical Center
Denver, Colorado
Professor of Surgery
University of Colorado
Aurora, Colorado

*ABDOMINAL COMPARTMENT SYNDROME
AND MANAGEMENT OF THE OPEN
ABDOMEN*

Errol Bush, MD
Assistant Professor of Surgery
Surgical Director
Advanced Lung Disease and Lung
Transplant Program
Division of Thoracic Surgery
The Johns Hopkins Medical Institutions
Baltimore, Maryland

ESOPHAGEAL FUNCTION TESTS

Ronald W. Busuttil, MD, PhD
Distinguished Professor and Executive
Chairman
Dumont Professor of Transplantation
Surgery and Chief of the Division of Liver
and Pancreas Transplant
Department of Surgery
David Geffen School of Medicine at
University of California, Los Angeles
Los Angeles, California

*HEPATIC MALIGNANCY: RESECTION VERSUS
TRANSPLANTATION*

Julie Caffrey, DO, MS
Assistant Professor
Plastic and Reconstructive Surgery
The Johns Hopkins University School
of Medicine
Baltimore, Maryland

*MEDICAL MANAGEMENT OF THE BURN
PATIENT*

Glenda G. Callender, MD
Associate Professor of Surgery
Section of Endocrine Surgery
Department of Surgery
Yale University School of Medicine
New Haven, Connecticut

SURGICAL APPROACH TO THYROID CANCER

Richard P. Cambria, MD
Chief, Division of Vascular and
Endovascular Surgery
Department of Surgery
Massachusetts General Hospital
Boston, Massachusetts

*OPEN REPAIR OF ABDOMINAL AORTIC
ANEURYSMS*

Andrew M. Cameron, MD, PhD, FACS
Chief, Division of Transplantation
Surgical Director, Liver Transplantation
Department of Surgery
The Johns Hopkins University School
of Medicine
Baltimore, Maryland

*PORTAL HYPERTENSION AND THE ROLE OF
SHUNTING PROCEDURES*

Melissa S. Camp, MD, MPH
Assistant Professor
Department of Surgery
The Johns Hopkins Hospital
Baltimore, Maryland

*DUCTAL AND LOBULAR CARCINOMA IN
SITU OF THE BREAST*

Kurtis A. Campbell, MD
Department of Surgical Oncology
Mercy Medical Center
Baltimore, Maryland

*INCISIONAL, EPIGASTRIC, AND UMBILICAL
HERNIAS*

Shamus R. Carr, MD
Assistant Professor of Surgery
Division of Thoracic Surgery
University of Maryland School of Medicine
Baltimore, Maryland

MINIMALLY INVASIVE ESOPHAGECTOMY

Michael J. Cavnar, MD
Complex Surgical Oncology Fellow
Department of Surgery
Memorial Sloan Kettering Cancer Center
New York, New York

*THE MANAGEMENT OF GASTROINTESTINAL
STROMAL TUMORS*

Elliot L. Chaikof, MD, PhD
Johnson and Johnson Professor of Surgery
Harvard Medical School
Chairman, Roberta and Stephen R. Weiner
Department of Surgery
Surgeon-in-Chief
Beth Israel Deaconess Medical Center
Boston, Massachusetts

PERIPHERAL ARTERIAL EMBOLISM

Bradley J. Champagne, MD, FACS, FASCRS
Professor of Surgery
Cleveland Clinic Lerner School of Medicine
Chairman
Department of Surgery
Fairview Hospital
Medical Director
Fairview Ambulatory Surgery Center
Cleveland, Ohio

THE MANAGEMENT OF RADIATION INJURY TO THE SMALL AND LARGE BOWEL

Yamile Haito Chavez, MD
Gastrointestinal Endoscopy Advanced
Therapeutic Fellow
Internal Medicine—Gastroenterology and
Hepatology
The Johns Hopkins University
Baltimore, Maryland

OBSTRUCTIVE JAUNDICE: ENDOSCOPIC THERAPY

Herbert Chen, MD, FACS
Chairman, Department of Surgery
Fay Fletcher Kerner Endowed Chair
University of Alabama at Birmingham
Birmingham, Alabama

THE MANAGEMENT OF PANCREATIC ISLET CELL TUMORS EXCLUDING GASTRINOMAS

Yen-I Chen, MD
McGovern Medical School
University of Texas Health Science Center
Houston, Texas

ENDOSCOPIC THERAPY FOR ESOPHAGEAL VARICEAL HEMORRHAGE

Albert Chi, MD, MSE
Associate Professor
Division of Trauma, Critical Care, and
Acute Care Surgery
Oregon Health and Science University
Portland, Oregon

THE MANAGEMENT OF INTRA-ABDOMINAL INFECTIONS

Arun Chockalingam, BS
Division of Interventional Radiology
The Johns Hopkins University
Baltimore, Maryland

TRANSJUGULAR INTRAHEPATIC PORTOSYSTEMIC SHUNT

TRANSHEPATIC INTERVENTIONS FOR OBSTRUCTIVE JAUNDICE

Walter Cholewczynski, MD
Associate Chairman of Surgery
Director, Surgical Critical Care
Department of Surgery
Yale New Haven Health
Bridgeport Hospital
Bridgeport, Connecticut
Clinical Assistant Professor of Surgery
Yale University School of Medicine
New Haven, Connecticut

ANTIBIOTICS FOR CRITICALLY ILL PATIENTS

Michael A. Choti, MD
Professor and Chair
Department of Surgery
University of Texas Southwestern
Medical Center
Dallas, Texas

THE MANAGEMENT OF COLON CANCER

Ioannis A. Christakis, MD, MSc, MSc(surg), PhD, FRCS(eng)
Postdoctoral Fellow
Surgical Oncology
MD Anderson Cancer Center
Houston, Texas

EVALUATION AND MANAGEMENT OF PERSISTENT OR RECURRENT HYPERPARATHYROIDISM

Dara H. Christante, MD
Fellow, Colon and Rectal Surgery
Department of Surgery
University of Minnesota
Minneapolis, Minnesota

THE MANAGEMENT OF ANORECTAL ABSCESS AND FISTULA

Jose R. Cintron, MD
Chairman, Division of Colon and
Rectal Surgery
Department of Surgery
John H. Stroger Hospital of Cook County
Associate Professor of Surgery
Department of Surgery
University of Illinois College of Medicine
at Chicago
Chicago, Illinois

THE MANAGEMENT OF HEMORRHOIDS

Jeffrey A. Claridge, MD, MS, FACS
Professor of Surgery
Case Western Reserve University
Department of Surgery
MetroHealth Medical Center
Cleveland, Ohio

ANTIFUNGAL THERAPY IN THE SURGICAL PATIENT

Damon Clark, MD
Assistant Professor of Surgery
Acute Care Surgery
University of Southern California
Los Angeles, California

MULTIPLE ORGAN DYSFUNCTION AND FAILURE

Hiram S. Cody III, MD
Attending Surgeon
Breast Service, Department of Surgery
Memorial Sloan Kettering Cancer Center
Professor of Clinical Surgery
Weill Cornell Medical College
New York, New York

THE MANAGEMENT OF MALE BREAST CANCER

Thomas H. Cogbill, MD, FACS
Attending Surgeon
Department of General and Vascular
Surgery
Gundersen Health System
La Crosse, Wisconsin

ATHEROSCLEROTIC RENAL ARTERY STENOSIS

Jessica N. Cohan, MD
Resident
Department of Surgery
University of California, San Francisco
San Francisco, California

THE MANAGEMENT OF ANORECTAL STRICTURE

Damon S. Cooney, MD, PhD
Assistant Professor
Department of Plastic and Reconstructive
Surgery
The Johns Hopkins University
Baltimore, Maryland

LYMPHEDEMA

Zara Cooper, MD, MSc
Associate Surgeon
Division of Trauma, Burns, and Surgical
Critical Care
Brigham and Women's Hospital
Associate Professor of Surgery
Harvard Medical School
Boston, Massachusetts

SURGICAL PALLIATIVE CARE

Britney L. Corey, MD
Assistant Professor of Surgery
Department of Surgery
University of Alabama at Birmingham
Birmingham, Alabama

GLYCEMIC CONTROL AND CARDIOVASCULAR DISEASE RISK REDUCTION AFTER BARIATRIC SURGERY

Gregory A. Coté, MD, MS
Associate Professor of Medicine
Department of Medicine
Division of Gastroenterology and
Hepatology
Medical University of South Carolina
Charleston, South Carolina

PANCREAS DIVISUM AND OTHER VARIANTS OF DOMINANT DORSAL DUCT ANATOMY

Morgan L. Cox, MD
Surgical Resident
Department of Surgery
Duke University
Durham, North Carolina

THE MANAGEMENT OF ACUTE CHOLANGITIS

Todd C. Crawford, MD
General Surgery Resident
Department of Surgery
The Johns Hopkins University School
of Medicine
Baltimore, Maryland

THE USE OF ESOPHAGEAL STENTS

Martin A. Croce, MD, FACS
Professor and Chief, Trauma and Surgical
Critical Care
Department of Surgery
University of Tennessee Health Science
Center
Memphis, Tennessee

THE MANAGEMENT OF RECTAL INJURIES

H. Gill Cryer, MD, PhD
Professor of Surgery
Chief, Trauma and Critical Care
Director, Trauma and Emergency
Surgery Service
University of California, Los Angeles
Los, Angeles

*UROLOGIC COMPLICATIONS OF PELVIC
FRACTURE*

Robert F. Cuff, MD, FACS
Vascular Surgeon
Division of Vascular Surgery
Spectrum Health Medical Group
Assistant Professor of Surgery
Department of Surgery
Michigan State University—College of
Human Medicine
Grand Rapids, Michigan

*THE MANAGEMENT OF LOWER EXTREMITY
AMPUTATIONS*

Steven C. Cunningham, MD, FACS
Director of Pancreatic and Hepatobiliary
Surgery
Saint Agnes Hospital and Cancer Institute
Baltimore, Maryland

*THE MANAGEMENT OF BILE DUCT
CANCER*

*THE MANAGEMENT OF GALLSTONE
PANCREATITIS, PART B*

Alan P. B. Dackiw, MD, PhD, MBA
Professor of Surgery
University of Texas
Southwestern Medical Center
Dallas, Texas

*THE MANAGEMENT OF ADRENAL
CORTICAL TUMORS*

Nabil N. Dagher, MD
Associate Professor
Chief of Transplant
NYU Langone Transplant Institute
New York, New York

LAPAROSCOPIC DONOR NEPHRECTOMY

Benjamin W. Dart IV, MD, FACS
Assistant Professor
Department of Surgery
University of Tennessee College of Medicine
Chattanooga, Tennessee

*THE MANAGEMENT OF CLOSTRIDIUM
DIFFICILE COLITIS*

Jashodeep Datta, MD
Chief Resident in General Surgery
Department of Surgery
University of Pennsylvania Perelman School
of Medicine,
Philadelphia, Pennsylvania

UNUSUAL PANCREATIC TUMORS

Jeffery B. Dattilo, MD
Associate Professor and Program Director
Surgical Residency Program
University of Tennessee Health Science
Center
College of Medicine
Nashville, Tennessee

*BALLOON ANGIOPLASTY AND STENTS IN
CAROTID ARTERY OCCLUSIVE DISEASE*

Bradley Davis, MD
Vice-Chair, Surgical Education
Department of Surgery
University of Cincinnati
Cincinnati, Ohio

THE MANAGEMENT OF PRURITUS ANI

Donald Davis, MD
Department of Surgery
University of South Florida
Tampa, Florida

*THE MANAGEMENT OF ACUTE
PANCREATITIS*

Conor P. Delaney, MD, MCh, PhD
Chairman
Digestive Disease and Surgical Institute
Professor of Surgery
Cleveland Clinic Lerner School of Medicine
Cleveland Clinic
Cleveland, Ohio

*LAPAROSCOPIC COLON AND RECTAL
SURGERY*

Keith Delman, MD
Associate Professor of Surgery
Carlos Professor of Surgery
Division of Surgical Oncology
Department of Surgery
Emory University School of Medicine
Atlanta, Georgia

*THE MANAGEMENT OF CUTANEOUS
MELANOMA*

Ronald P. DeMatteo, MD, FACS
Vice-Chair
Department of Surgery
Memorial Sloan Kettering Cancer Center
New York, New York

*THE MANAGEMENT OF GASTROINTESTINAL
STROMAL TUMORS*

Steven R. DeMeester, MD
Professor of Surgery
University of Southern California
Los Angeles, California

*THE MANAGEMENT OF BARRETT'S
ESOPHAGUS*

Tom R. DeMeester, MD
Professor and Chairman, Emeritus
Department of Surgery
University of Southern California
Los Angeles, California

*NEW APPROACHES TO
GASTROESOPHAGEAL REFLUX
DISEASE (LINX)*

Daniel T. Dempsey, MD, MBA
Professor
Department of Surgery
University of Pennsylvania
Philadelphia, Pennsylvania

*THE MANAGEMENT OF DUODENAL
ULCERS*

Sandra R. DiBrito, MD
Resident
Department of Surgery
The Johns Hopkins University School
of Medicine
Baltimore, Maryland

*MANAGEMENT OF SMALL BOWEL
OBSTRUCTION*

Justin B. Dimick, MD, MPH
George Zuidema Professor of Surgery
Chief, Division of Minimally Invasive
Surgery
Director, Center for Healthcare Outcomes
and Policy
Department of Surgery
University of Michigan
Ann Arbor, Michigan

MEASURING OUTCOMES OF SURGERY

Francesca M. Dimou, MD
Department of Surgery
University of South Florida
Tampa, Florida
Department of Surgery
University of Texas Medical Branch
Galveston, Texas

*INTRADUCTAL PAPILLARY MUCINOUS
NEOPLASMS OF THE PANCREAS*

Peter Dixon, MD
Surgical Resident
Department of Surgery
Saint Agnes Hospital
Baltimore, Maryland

*THE MANAGEMENT OF GALLSTONE
PANCREATITIS, PART B*

James Donahue, MD
Assistant Professor of Surgery
Division of Thoracic Surgery
University of Maryland School of Medicine
Baltimore, Maryland

MINIMALLY INVASIVE ESOPHAGECTOMY

Quan-Yang Duh, MD
Chief, Section of Endocrine Surgery
Department of Surgery
University of California
Attending Surgeon
Department of Surgery
VA Medical Center
San Francisco, California

THE MANAGEMENT OF THYROID NODULES

Mark Duncan, MD
Vice-Chair
Associate Professor of Surgery and
Oncology
Department of Surgery
The Johns Hopkins University
Baltimore, Maryland

*MANAGEMENT OF SMALL BOWEL
OBSTRUCTION*

Christine M. Durand, MD
Assistant Professor
Department of Medicine
The Johns Hopkins University School
of Medicine
Baltimore, Maryland

THE MANAGEMENT OF HEPATIC ABSCESS

Francisco A. Durazo, MD
Associate Clinical Professor of Medicine
and Surgery
Digestive and Liver Diseases, Dumont—
UCLA Liver Transplant Program
University of California, Los Angeles
Los Angeles, California

*THE MANAGEMENT OF REFRACTORY
ASCITES*

David Earle, MD, FACS
Attending Surgeon
Lowell Surgical Associates
Lowell General Hospital
Lowell, Massachusetts

LAPAROSCOPIC APPENDECTOMY

Barish H. Edil, MD
Associate Professor of Surgery
Department of Surgery
University of Colorado Anschutz Medical
Campus
Aurora, Colorado

*THE MANAGEMENT OF CHRONIC
PANCREATITIS*

David T. Efron, MD
Professor of Surgery
Department of Surgery
The Johns Hopkins University School
of Medicine
Director of Adult Trauma Services
Chief, Division of Acute Care Surgery
Department of Surgery
The Johns Hopkins Hospital
Baltimore, Maryland

THE MANAGEMENT OF LIVER INJURIES

Jonathan E. Efron, MD
Professor of Surgery and Urology
Department of Surgery
The Johns Hopkins University School
of Medicine
Baltimore, Maryland

*THE MANAGEMENT OF CHRONIC
ULCERATIVE COLITIS*

*THE MANAGEMENT OF TOXIC
MEGACOLON*

Bryan A. Ehlert, MD
Vascular Surgery Fellow
The Johns Hopkins Hospital
Baltimore, Maryland

*THE MANAGEMENT OF THORACIC AND
THORACOABDOMINAL AORTIC ANEURYSMS*

David W. Eisele, MD, FACS
Andelot Professor and Director
Department of Otolaryngology—Head and
Neck Surgery
The Johns Hopkins University School
of Medicine
Baltimore, Maryland

*MANAGEMENT OF THE SOLITARY NECK
MASS*

David Elliott, MD
Colonel (Retired), US Army Medical Corps
General and Trauma Surgeon
Médecins Sans Frontières (Doctors
WITHOUT BORDERS)

DAMAGE CONTROL OPERATION

Sean J. English, MD
Conrad Jobst Vascular Research Laboratory
Department of Surgery
University of Michigan
Ann Arbor, Michigan

*AXILLOBIFEMORAL BYPASS GRAFTING IN
THE TWENTY-FIRST CENTURY*

Calvin Eriksen, MD
Clinical Instructor
Department of Surgery
David Geffen School of Medicine at
University of California, Los Angeles
Los Angeles, California

*THE MANAGEMENT OF ECHINOCOCCAL
CYST DISEASE OF THE LIVER*

**Mohammad H. Eslami, MD, FACS,
FACC**
Professor of Surgery
Division of Vascular Surgery
University of Pittsburgh Medical School
Pittsburgh, Pennsylvania

ACUTE MESENTERIC ISCHEMIA

Jesus Esquivel, MD
Department of Surgery
Frederick Memorial Hospital
Frederick, Maryland

*MANAGEMENT OF PERITONEAL SURFACE
MALIGNANCIES OF APPENDICEAL OR
COLORECTAL ORIGIN*

David M. Euhus, MD
Professor
Department of Surgery
The Johns Hopkins University
Baltimore, Maryland

BREAST CANCER: SURGICAL THERAPY

John C. Eun, MD
Assistant Professor of Surgery
VA Eastern Colorado Healthcare System
Denver, Colorado
Section of Vascular and Endovascular
Surgery
University of Colorado Denver
Aurora, Colorado

*TIBIOPERONEAL ARTERIAL OCCLUSIVE
DISEASE*

Douglas B. Evans, MD
Professor and Chair
Department of Surgery
Medical College of Wisconsin
Milwaukee, Wisconsin

*NEOADJUVANT AND ADJUVANT THERAPY
FOR LOCALIZED PANCREATIC CANCER*

Heather L. Evans, MD, MS, FACS
Associate Professor
Department of Surgery
University of Washington
Seattle, Washington

*CATHETER SEPSIS IN THE INTENSIVE
CARE UNIT*

Timothy C. Fabian, MD
Harwell Wilson Alumni Professor
Department of Surgery
University of Tennessee Health Science
Center
Memphis, Tennessee

*INJURIES TO THE SMALL AND LARGE
BOWEL*

Peter J. Fabri, MD, PhD, FACS
Professor Emeritus
Surgery and Industrial and Management
Systems Engineering
University of South Florida
Tampa, Florida

*THE MANAGEMENT OF DIVERTICULOSIS OF
THE SMALL BOWEL*

Anne C. Fabrizio, MD
Research Fellow
Department of Surgery
The Johns Hopkins Medical Institutions
Baltimore, Maryland

*THE MANAGEMENT OF LARGE BOWEL
OBSTRUCTION*

Peter J. Fagenholz, MD
Division of Trauma, Emergency Surgery,
and Critical Care
Massachusetts General Hospital
Assistant Professor of Surgery
Harvard Medical School
Boston, Massachusetts

*THE MANAGEMENT OF ACUTE
CHOLECYSTITIS*

Carole Fakhry, MD, MPH, FACS
Associate Professor of Otolaryngology—
Head and Neck Surgery
The Johns Hopkins University School of
Medicine
Baltimore, Maryland

*MANAGEMENT OF THE SOLITARY NECK
MASS*

Sandy H. Fang, MD
Assistant Professor
Department of Surgery
The Johns Hopkins Hospital
Baltimore, Maryland

*THE MANAGEMENT OF CHRONIC
ULCERATIVE COLITIS*

Richard J. Fantus, MD, FACS
Vice-Chairman
Department of Surgery
Trauma Medical Director
Chief, Section of Surgical Critical Care
Advocate Illinois Masonic Medical Center
Clinical Professor
Department of Surgery
University of Illinois College of Medicine
Chicago, Illinois

*RETROPERITONEAL INJURIES: KIDNEY AND
URETER*

Liane S. Feldman, MD, FACS, FRCS
Professor
Department of Surgery
Director of General Surgery
McGill University
Montreal, Quebec, Canada

*ENHANCED RECOVERY AFTER SURGERY:
COLON SURGERY*

David V. Feliciano, MD
Battersby Professor and Chief
Division of General Surgery
Department of Surgery
Indiana University Medical Center
Indianapolis, Indiana

*THE MANAGEMENT OF DIAPHRAGMATIC
INJURIES*

David Feller-Kopman, MD
Director, Bronchoscopy and Interventional
Pulmonology
Associate Professor of Medicine,
Otolaryngology—Head and Neck Surgery
The Johns Hopkins Hospital
Baltimore, Maryland

TRACHEOSTOMY, PART ONE

Paula A. Ferrada, MD, FACS
Associate Professor of Surgery
Medical Director, Surgical and Trauma
Intensive Care Unit
Director, Surgical Critical Care Fellowship
Virginia Commonwealth University
Richmond, Virginia

*THE SURGEON'S USE OF ULTRASOUND IN
THORACOABDOMINAL TRAUMA*

Linda Ferrari, MD
Department of Surgery
University of Washington Medical Center
Seattle, Washington

*THE USE OF PET SCANNING IN THE
MANAGEMENT OF COLORECTAL CANCER*

Peter F. Ferson, MD
Professor of Cardiothoracic Surgery
Charles Gray Watson Professor of Surgical
Education
Department f Cardiothoracic Surgery
University of Pittsburgh
Pittsburgh, Pennsylvania

VIDEO-ASSISTED THORACOSCOPIC SURGERY

**Alessandro Fichera, MD, FACS,
FASCRS**
Professor and Section Chief,
Gastrointestinal Surgery
Department of Surgery
University of Washington Medical Center
Seattle, Washington

*THE USE OF PET SCANNING IN THE
MANAGEMENT OF COLORECTAL CANCER*

Amy G. Fiedler, MD
General Surgery Resident
Massachusetts General Hospital
Boston, Massachusetts

*THE MANAGEMENT OF ASYMPTOMATIC
(SILENT) GALLSTONES*

Brendan M. Finnerty, MD
General Surgery Resident
Department of Surgery
New York Presbyterian Hospital—Weill
Cornell Medicine
New York, New York

*LAPAROSCOPIC TREATMENT OF
ESOPHAGEAL MOTILITY DISORDERS*

Josef E. Fischer, MD
William V. McDermott Distinguished
Professor of Surgery
Department of Surgery
Harvard Medical School
Boston, Massachusetts

*THE MANAGEMENT OF
ENTEROCUTANEOUS FISTULAS*

P. Marco Fisichella, MD
Associate Professor of Surgery
Department of Surgery
Harvard Medical School
Associate Chief of Surgery
Department of Surgery
West Roxbury VA
Boston, Massachusetts

*THE MANAGEMENT OF CYSTS, TUMORS,
AND ABSCESSES OF THE SPLEEN*

James W. Fleshman, MD
Seeger Professor and Chairman
Department of Surgery
Baylor University Medical Center
Dallas, Texas

THE MANAGEMENT OF CROHN'S COLITIS

Zhi Ven Fong, MD
General Surgery Resident
Department of Surgery
Massachusetts General Hospital
Boston, Massachusetts

*ABLATION OF COLORECTAL CARCINOMA
LIVER METASTASES*

Christopher L. Forthman, MD
Consultant
Curtis National Hand Center
Medstar Union Memorial Hospital
Baltimore, Maryland

HAND INFECTIONS

**Todd D. Francone, MD, FACS,
FASCRS**
Staff Surgeon
Department of Colon and Rectal Surgery
Lahey Hospital and Medical Center
Burlington, Massachusetts

THE MANAGEMENT OF ANAL FISSURES

Heidi Frankel, MD, FACS, FCCM
Acute Care Surgery
University of Southern California
Los Angeles, California

*MULTIPLE ORGAN DYSFUNCTION AND
FAILURE*

David P. Franklin, MD
Chairman of Surgery
Chief of Vascular Surgery
Division of Vascular Surgery
Geisinger Medical Center
Danville, Pennsylvania

*FEMORAL AND POPLITEAL ARTERY
ANEURYSMS*

Vivian Gahtan, MD
Chief, Vascular Surgery and Endovascular
Services
Department of Surgery
State University of New York Upstate
Medical University
Department of Surgery
VA Medical Center
Syracuse, New York

*BUERGER'S DISEASE (THROMBOANGIITIS
OBLITERANS)*

Susan Galandiuk, MD
Professor of Surgery
Program Director, Section of Colon and
Rectal Surgery
Hiram C. Polk, Jr., MD, Department
of Surgery
Director, Price Institute of Surgical Research
University of Louisville
Louisville, Kentucky

THE MANAGEMENT OF ISCHEMIC COLITIS

James J. Gallagher, MD, FACS
Weill Cornell Medical College
Department of Surgery
New York Presbyterian Hospital
New York, New York

BURN WOUND MANAGEMENT

Alexandra Gangi, MD
Instructor in Surgery
H. Lee Moffitt Cancer Center
Tampa, Florida

*LYMPHATIC MAPPING AND SENTINEL
LYMPHADENECTOMY*

Erin M. Garvey, MD
Chief Resident
Department of Surgery
Mayo Clinic Arizona
Phoenix, Arizona

LAPAROSCOPIC GASTRIC SURGERY

Susan L. Gearhart, MD
Associate Professor of Colorectal Surgery
Director, Colorectal Surgery Fellowship
Program
The Johns Hopkins University School
of Medicine
Baltimore, Maryland

*THE MANAGEMENT OF DIVERTICULAR
DISEASE OF THE COLON*

Timothy M. Geiger, MD
Chief
Division of General Surgery
Director of Colon and Rectal Surgery
Vanderbilt University Medical Center
Nashville, Tennessee

*THE MANAGEMENT OF COLONIC
VOLVULUS*

Mary L. Gemignani, MD
Breast Service
Department of Surgery
Memorial Sloan Kettering Cancer Center
New York, New York

*THE MANAGEMENT OF THE AXILLA IN
BREAST CANCER*

**Christos Georgiades, MD, PhD, FSIR,
FCIRSE**
Associate Professor and Vice-Chairman
Radiology and Radiological Sciences
The Johns Hopkins University
Baltimore, Maryland

*TRANSHEPATIC INTERVENTIONS FOR
OBSTRUCTIVE JAUNDICE*

VENA CAVA FILTERS

Patrick E. Georgoff, MD
Surgery Resident
Surgical Critical Care Fellow
University of Michigan
Ann Arbor, Michigan

THE MANAGEMENT OF VASCULAR INJURIES

Jean-Francois H. Geschwind, MD
Chairman and Chief
Department of Radiology and Biomedical
Imaging
Yale University School of Medicine
New Haven, Connecticut

*TRANSARTERIAL CHEMOEMBOLIZATION
FOR LIVER METASTASES*

Mark L. Gestring, MD, FACS
Medical Director, Kessler Trauma Center
Associate Professor of Surgery
Emergency Medicine and Pediatrics
Division of Acute Care Surgery
Department of Surgery
University of Rochester School of Medicine
Rochester, New York

PANCREATIC AND DUODENAL INJURIES

Iman Ghaderi, MD, MSc
Assistant Professor of Surgery
Department of Surgery
University of Arizona
Tucson, Arizona

*THE MANAGEMENT OF RECURRENT
INGUINAL HERNIA*

Joseph S. Giglia, MD
Associate Professor
Department of Surgery
University of Cincinnati College
of Medicine
Cincinnati, Ohio

RAYNAUD'S PHENOMENON

Armando E. Giuliano, MD
Executive Vice-Chair, Surgery
Chief, Surgical Oncology
Cedars-Sinai Medical Center
Los Angeles, California

*LYMPHATIC MAPPING AND SENTINEL
LYMPHADENECTOMY*

Natalia O. Glebova, MD, PhD
Assistant Professor of Surgery
Section of Vascular and Endovascular
Surgery
University of Colorado Denver
Aurora, Colorado

*TIBIOPERONEAL ARTERIAL OCCLUSIVE
DISEASE*

Ana L. Gleisner, MD
Assistant Professor of Surgery
University of Colorado School of Medicine
Aurora, Colorado

*THE MANAGEMENT OF MALIGNANT LIVER
TUMORS*

Steven B. Goldin, MD
Chief of Hepatobiliary and Pancreatic
Surgery for Charlotte County
Twenty-First Century Oncology
Port Charlotte, Florida

THE MANAGEMENT OF GALLSTONE ILEUS

Seth Goldstein, MD, MPhil
Pediatric Surgery Fellow
The Johns Hopkins Hospital
Baltimore, Maryland

*EXTRACORPOREAL LIFE SUPPORT FOR
RESPIRATORY FAILURE*

Christopher J. Goodenough, MD, MPH
Department of Surgery
University of Texas Health Center
at Houston
Houston, Texas

ENDOCRINE CHANGES IN CRITICAL ILLNESS

Naeem Goussous, MD
Department of Surgery
Saint Agnes Hospital
Baltimore, Maryland

*THE MANAGEMENT OF BILE DUCT
CANCER*

Jay A. Graham, MD
Attending Surgeon
Department of Surgery
Montefiore Medical Center
Assistant Professor
Department of Surgery
Albert Einstein Medical College
Bronx, New York

TRANSPLANTATION OF THE PANCREAS

LAPAROSCOPIC LIVER RESECTION

Miral Sadaria Grandhi, MD
Assistant Professor of Surgery
Division of Surgical Oncology
Rutgers Cancer Institute of New Jersey/
Rutgers Robert Wood Johnson Medical
School
New Brunswick, New Jersey

LAPAROSCOPIC DISTAL PANCREATECTOMY

Clive S. Grant, MD
Professor of Surgery, Emeritus
Department of Surgery
Mayo Clinic
Rochester, Minnesota

HYPERTHYROIDISM

Richard J. Gray, MD, FACS
Professor of Surgery
Section of Surgical Oncology
Department of Surgery
Mayo Clinic,
Scottsdale, Arizona

MARGINS: HOW TO AND HOW BIG?

Shea C. Gregg, MD, FACS
Chief, Section of Trauma, Burns, and
Surgical Critical Care
Department of Surgery
Yale New Haven Health
Bridgeport Hospital
Bridgeport, Connecticut
Clinical Assistant Professor of Surgery
Yale University School of Medicine
New Haven, Connecticut

ANTIBIOTICS FOR CRITICALLY ILL PATIENTS

Irena Gribovskaja-Rupp, MD
Clinical Assistant Professor
Department of Surgery
University of Iowa Hospitals and Clinics
Iowa City, Iowa

*SURGICAL MANAGEMENT OF FECAL
INCONTINENCE*

Margaret M. Griffen, MD, FACS
Chief of the Division of Trauma and Acute
Care Surgery
Inova Fairfax Medical Campus
Falls Church, Virginia

SPINE AND SPINAL CORD INJURIES

James F. Griffin, MD
Surgical Resident
Department of Surgery
The Johns Hopkins Hospital
Baltimore, Maryland

*THE MANAGEMENT OF PERIAMPULLARY
CANCER*

Joshua C. Grimm, MD
Resident
Department of Surgery
Johns Hopkins Medicine
Baltimore, Maryland

THE DIABETIC FOOT

Jose G. Guillem, MD, MPH
Department of Surgery
Colorectal Service
Memorial Sloan-Kettering Cancer Center
New York, New York

THE MANAGEMENT OF RECTAL CANCER

Jinny Ha, MD
Cardiothoracic Surgery Fellow
Division of Thoracic Surgery
The Johns Hopkins University School
of Medicine
Baltimore, Maryland

*THE MANAGEMENT OF ZENKER'S
DIVERTICULUM*

THE USE OF ESOPHAGEAL STENTS

Fahim Habib, MD, MPH, FACS
Fellow
Advanced Minimally Invasive and Robotic
Esophageal Surgery
Esophageal and Lung Institute
Allegheny Health Network
Pittsburgh, Pennsylvania

*THE MANAGEMENT OF ACHALASIA OF
THE ESOPHAGUS*

*THE MANAGEMENT OF ESOPHAGEAL
CANCER*

David Hackam, MD, PhD
Chief of Pediatric Surgery
The Johns Hopkins University
Pediatric Surgeon-in-Chief
The Johns Hopkins Children's Center
Baltimore, Maryland

CONGENITAL CHEST WALL DEFORMITIES

James P. Hamilton, MD
Assistant Professor
Department of Medicine
Division of Gastroenterology and
Hepatology
The Johns Hopkins University School
of Medicine
Baltimore, Maryland

*THE MANAGEMENT OF BUDD-CHIARI
SYNDROME*

Alden H. Harken, MD, FACS
Professor and Chair
Department of Surgery
University of California, San Francisco—
East Bay
Oakland, California

CARDIOVASCULAR PHARMACOLOGY

John W. Harmon, MD, FACS
Professor of Surgery
The Johns Hopkins University
Baltimore, Maryland

*NECROTIZING SKIN AND SOFT TISSUE
INFECTIONS*

Mark Hartney, MD, MS
Associate Professor of Surgery
Department of Surgery
University of South Florida
Tampa, Florida

*THE MANAGEMENT OF DIVERTICULOSIS OF
THE SMALL BOWEL*

Heitham T. Hassoun, MD
Associate Professor
Department of Surgery
The Johns Hopkins Medicine
Baltimore, Maryland

THE DIABETIC FOOT

Christine E. Haugen, MD
The Johns Hopkins Hospital
Baltimore, Maryland

*PORTAL HYPERTENSION AND THE ROLE OF
SHUNTING PROCEDURES*

Elliott R. Haut, MD, PhD
Associate Professor of Surgery,
Anesthesiology/Critical Care Medicine
(ACCM), and Emergency Medicine
Division of Acute Care Surgery
Department of Surgery
The Johns Hopkins University School
of Medicine
Baltimore, Maryland

THE ABDOMEN THAT WILL NOT CLOSE

Jin He, MD, PhD
Assistant Professor of Surgery and
Oncology
The Johns Hopkins University School
of Medicine
Baltimore, Maryland

LAPAROSCOPIC CHOLECYSTECTOMY

Marie-Noëlle Hébert-Blouin, MD
Assistant Professor
Division of Neurology and Neurosurgery
McGill University
Montreal, Quebec, Canada

NERVE INJURY AND REPAIR

Beth A. Helmink, MD, PhD
General Surgeon
Vanderbilt University Medical Center
Nashville, Tennessee

*THE MANAGEMENT OF SMALL BOWEL
TUMORS*

David K. Henderson, MD
Deputy Director for Clinical Care
Clinical Center
National Institutes of Health
Bethesda, Maryland

*OCCUPATIONAL EXPOSURE TO HUMAN
IMMUNODEFICIENCY VIRUS AND OTHER
BLOODBORNE PATHOGENS*

B. Todd Heniford, MD
Professor and Chief
Division of Gastrointestinal and Minimally
Invasive Surgery
Department of Surgery
Carolinas Medical Center
Charlotte, North Carolina

LAPAROSCOPIC GASTRIC SURGERY

Alan Herline, MD
Vice-Chair
Department of Surgery
J. Harold Harrison Distinguished University
Chair in Surgery
Augusta University Health
Augusta, Georgia

*THE MANAGEMENT OF COLONIC
VOLVULUS*

Joseph M. Herman, MD
Department of Radiation Oncology and
Molecular Radiation Sciences
The Johns Hopkins University School
of Medicine
Baltimore, Maryland

*THE MANAGEMENT OF TUMORS OF
THE ANAL REGION*

Caitlin W. Hicks, MD, MS
Vascular Surgery Fellow
Division of Vascular Surgery and
Endovascular Therapy
The Johns Hopkins Hospital
Baltimore, Maryland

THORACIC OUTLET SYNDROME

O. Joe Hines, MD
Professor and Chief
Department of Surgery
David Geffen School of Medicine at
University of California, Los Angeles
Los Angeles, California

*PALLIATIVE THERAPY FOR PANCREATIC
CANCER*

Melissa E. Hogg, MD, MS
Assistant Professor of Surgery
Department of Surgical Oncology
University of Pittsburgh
Pittsburgh, Pennsylvania

MINIMALLY INVASIVE PANCREATIC SURGERY

*MINIMALLY INVASIVE MANAGEMENT OF
PERIPANCREATIC FLUID COLLECTIONS*

Brian P. Holly, MD
Assistant Professor of Radiology and
Radiological Science
The Johns Hopkins School of Medicine
Baltimore, Maryland

*TRANSJUGULAR INTRAHEPATIC
PORTOSYSTEMIC SHUNT*

Kelvin Hong, MD
Division Chief
Interventional Radiology
The Johns Hopkins University
Baltimore, Maryland

*TRANSJUGULAR INTRAHEPATIC
PORTOSYSTEMIC SHUNT*

*TRANSHEPATIC INTERVENTIONS FOR
OBSTRUCTIVE JAUNDICE*

Isaac W. Howley, MD
Resident
Department of Surgery
The Johns Hopkins Hospital
Baltimore, Maryland

SPLENIC SALVAGE PROCEDURES

Margo Hoyler, MD
Resident Physician
Department of Surgery
New York Presbyterian Hospital—Columbia
University Medical Center
New York, New York

THE TREATMENT OF CLAUDICATION

Kevin S. Hughes, MD, FACS
Co-Director, Avon Comprehensive Breast
Evaluation Center
Division of Surgical Oncology
Massachusetts General Hospital
Associate Professor
Department of Surgery
Harvard Medical School
Boston, Massachusetts
Medical Director
Bermuda Cancer Genetics and Risk
Assessment Clinic
Hamilton, Paget, Bermuda

GENETIC COUNSELING AND TESTING

Steven J. Hughes, MD
Professor and Chief, General Surgery
Department of Surgery
University of Florida
Gainesville, Florida

*THE MANAGEMENT OF GALLSTONE
PANCREATITIS, PART A*

Eric S. Hungness, MD
Associate Professor
Department of Surgery
Northwestern University
Chicago, Illinois

*LAPAROSCOPIC COMMON BILE DUCT
EXPLORATION*

**John G. Hunter, MD, FACS, FRCS
Edin (hon)**
Mackenzie Professor and Dean (Interim)
Oregon Health and Science University
Editor-in-Chief
World Journal of Surgery
Portland, Oregon

LAPAROSCOPIC SPLENECTOMY

David F. Hutcheon, MD
Assistant Professor of Medicine
Department of Medicine
The Johns Hopkins Medical Institutions
Baltimore, Maryland

*ENTERAL STENTS IN THE TREATMENT OF
COLONIC OBSTRUCTION*

Matthew M. Hutter, MD, MPH
Associate Professor of Surgery
Harvard Medical School
Director, Codman Center for Clinical
Effectiveness in Surgery
Director, Massachusetts General Hospital
Hernia Center
Department of Surgery
Massachusetts General Hospital
Boston, Massachusetts

*LAPAROSCOPIC REPAIR OF RECURRENT
INGUINAL HERNIAS*

Neil H. Hyman, MD
Chief, Section of Colon and Rectal Surgery
Co-Director, Digestive Diseases Center
University of Chicago Medicine
Chicago, Illinois

*PREOPERATIVE BOWEL PREPARATION: IS IT
NECESSARY?*

Elizabeth Ann Ignacio, MD
Associate Professor of Interventional
Radiology
George Washington University Medical
Center
Washington, District of Columbia

*ACUTE PERIPHERAL ARTERIAL AND BYPASS
GRAFT OCCLUSION: THROMBOLYTIC
THERAPY*

Nadia Ijaz, MD
Primary Care Center Resident Preceptor
Division of Internal Medicine
Medstar Franklin Square Hospital
Baltimore, Maryland

*COAGULATION ISSUES AND THE TRAUMA
PATIENT*

Lisa K. Jacobs, MD, MSPH
Associate Professor of Surgery
Associate Professor of Oncology
Johns Hopkins Bayview Medical Center
Baltimore, Maryland

*THE MANAGEMENT OF BENIGN BREAST
DISEASE*

Neha Jakhete, MD
Division of Gastroenterology and
Hepatology
Department of Medicine
The Johns Hopkins School of Medicine
Baltimore, Maryland

*THE MANAGEMENT OF HEPATIC
ENCEPHALOPATHY*

Donald H. Jenkins, MD
Consultant
Division of Trauma, Critical Care, and
General Surgery
Trauma Center
Mayo Clinic
Rochester, Minnesota

THE SEPTIC RESPONSE AND MANAGEMENT

Robert T. Jensen, MD
Chief
Cell Biology Section
Digestive Diseases Branch
National Institute of Diabetes and Digestive
Kidney Diseases
National Institutes of Health
Bethesda, Maryland

*THE MANAGEMENT OF THE ZOLLINGER-
ELLISON SYNDROME*

Reena Jha, MD
Director of Magnetic Resonance Imaging
Professor of Radiology
Department of Radiology
Medstar Georgetown University Hospital
Washington, District of Columbia

LAPAROSCOPIC LIVER RESECTION

Blair A. Jobe, MD, FACS
Director
Esophageal and Lung Institute
Allegheny Health Network
Pittsburgh, Pennsylvania

*THE MANAGEMENT OF ACHALASIA OF
THE ESOPHAGUS*

*THE MANAGEMENT OF ESOPHAGEAL
CANCER*

Eric K. Johnson, MD, FACS, FASCRS
Associate Professor of Surgery
Uniformed Services University of the
Health Sciences
MultiCare Colorectal Surgery
Tacoma, Washington

THE MANAGEMENT OF PILONIDAL DISEASE

Lynt B. Johnson, MD, MBA
Robert J. Coffey Professor and Chairman
Department of Surgery
Medstar Georgetown University Hospital
Washington, District of Columbia

LAPAROSCOPIC LIVER RESECTION

Bellal Joseph, MD, FACS
Department of Surgery
Banner University Medical Center
Tucson, Arizona

*COAGULOPATHY IN THE CRITICALLY ILL
PATIENT*

Gregory J. Jurkovich, MD
Professor and Vice-Chairman
Department of Surgery
University of California, Davis
Sacramento, California

*CHEST WALL, PNEUMOTHORAX, AND
HEMOTHORAX*

Brian Kadera, MD
Department of Surgery
David Geffen School of Medicine at
University of California, Los Angeles
Los Angeles, California

*PALLIATIVE THERAPY FOR PANCREATIC
CANCER*

Stacie A. Kahan, MD
General and Endocrine Surgeon
Department of Surgery
White Plains Hospital—A Member of the
Montefiore Health System
White Plains, New York

NONTOXIC GOITER

Fady M. Kaldas, MD, FACS
Assistant Professor
Department of Surgery
University of California, Los Angeles
Los Angeles, California

*THE MANAGEMENT OF CYSTIC DISEASE OF
THE LIVER*

Anthony N. Kalloo, MD
The Moses and Helen Golden Paulson
Professor of Gastroenterology
Director, Division of Gastroenterology
and Hepatology
The Johns Hopkins Hospital
Baltimore, Maryland

*OBSTRUCTIVE JAUNDICE: ENDOSCOPIC
THERAPY*

Lillian S. Kao, MD, MS, FACS
Professor
Department of Surgery
University of Texas Health Science Center at
Houston
Houston, Texas

ENDOCRINE CHANGES IN CRITICAL ILLNESS

Muneera R. Kapadia, MD
Clinical Associate Professor
Department of Surgery
University of Iowa Hospitals and Clinics
Iowa City, Iowa

*SURGICAL MANAGEMENT OF FECAL
INCONTINENCE*

Lewis J. Kaplan, MD
Section Chief, Surgical Critical Care
Department of Surgery
Philadelphia VA Medical Center
Associate Professor of Surgery
Department of Surgery
Division of Trauma, Surgical Critical Care,
and Emergency Surgery
Perelman School of Medicine
University of Pennsylvania
Philadelphia, Pennsylvania

*ACUTE KIDNEY INJURY IN THE INJURED
AND CRITICALLY ILL*

Krista L. Kaups, MD, MSc
Professor of Clinical Surgery
Department of Surgery
University of California, San Francisco
Fresno, California

*GLUCOSE CONTROL IN THE POSTOPERATIVE
PERIOD*

Electron Kebebew, MD
Chief and Senior Investigator
Endocrine Oncology Branch
National Cancer Institute
Bethesda, Maryland
Professor
Department of Surgery
The George Washington University School
of Medicine and Health Sciences
Washington, District of Columbia

*THE MANAGEMENT OF
PHEOCHROMOCYTOMA*

Scott R. Kelley, MD, FACS, FASCRS
Assistant Professor Surgery
Colon and Rectal Surgery
Mayo Clinic
Rochester, Minnesota

SURGERY FOR THE POLYPOSIS SYNDROMES

Ronan Kelly, MD
Associate Professor
Department of Oncology
John Hopkins Medicine
Baltimore, Maryland

*NEOADJUVANT AND ADJUVANT THERAPY
OF ESOPHAGEAL CANCER*

K. Craig Kent, MD
Dean, College of Medicine
Professor, Vascular Surgery
Department of Surgery
The Ohio State University College
of Medicine
Columbus, Ohio

*THE MANAGEMENT OF RUPTURED
ABDOMINAL AORTIC ANEURYSM*

Mouen A. Khashab, MD
Associate Professor of Medicine
Director of Therapeutic Endoscopy
Gastroenterology and Hepatology
The Johns Hopkins Hospital
Baltimore, Maryland

THE MANAGEMENT OF THE MALLORY-WEISS SYNDROME

Nagi Khouri, MD
Carol Ann Flanagan Professor in Breast Imaging
Associate Professor of Radiology and Oncology
The Johns Hopkins Hospital
Baltimore, Maryland

BREAST IMAGING

Amy K. Kim, MD
Assistant Professor of Medicine
Division of Gastroenterology and Hepatology/Department of Medicine
The Johns Hopkins School of Medicine
Baltimore, Maryland

THE MANAGEMENT OF HEPATIC ENCEPHALOPATHY

Karen M. Kim, MD
Assistant Professor of Cardiac Surgery
Department of Cardiac Surgery
University of Michigan
Ann Arbor, Michigan

THE MANAGEMENT OF ACUTE AORTIC DISSECTIONS

Laszlo Kiraly, MD
Associate Professor of Surgery
Division of Trauma, Critical Care, and Acute Care Surgery
Oregon Health Sciences University
Portland, Oregon

NUTRITION THERAPY IN CRITICAL ILLNESS

Amanda Kirane, MD
Complex General Surgical Oncology Fellow
Department of Surgery
Memorial Sloan Kettering Cancer Center
New York, New York

THE MANAGEMENT OF SOFT TISSUE SARCOMA

David A. Kleiman, MD, MSc
Department of Surgery
Memorial Sloan-Kettering Cancer Center
Department of Surgery
Weill Cornell Medicine
New York, New York

THE MANAGEMENT OF RECTAL CANCER

V. Suzanne Klimberg, MD, FACS
Professor and Director of Breast Cancer Program
Department of Surgery
Winthrop P. Rockefeller Cancer Institute
Little Rock, Arkansas

ABLATIVE TECHNIQUES IN THE TREATMENT OF BENIGN AND MALIGNANT BREAST DISEASE

Kerry Klinger, MD
Assistant Professor of Anesthesia and Perioperative Care
Department of Anesthesia and Perioperative Care
University of California, San Francisco, School of Medicine
Clinical Director of Anesthesia and Perioperative Care
Zuckerberg San Francisco General Hospital
San Francisco, California

AIRWAY MANAGEMENT IN THE TRAUMA PATIENT

L. Mark Knab, MD
Research
Department of Surgery
Northwestern University Feinberg School of Medicine
Chicago, Illinois

CONTRALATERAL PROPHYLACTIC MASTECTOMY

Gopal C. Kowdley, MD, PhD, FACS
Program Director
General Surgery Residency
Department of Surgery
Saint Agnes Hospital
Baltimore, Maryland

THE MANAGEMENT OF GALLSTONE PANCREATITIS, PART B

Richard A. Kozarek, MD
Department of Gastroenterology
Virginia Mason Medical Center
Seattle, Washington

PANCREATIC DUCTAL DISRUPTIONS LEADING TO PANCREATIC FISTULA, PANCREATIC ASCITES, OR PANCREATIC PLEURAL EFFUSION

Geoffrey W. Krampitz, MD
Department of Surgery
Stanford University School of Medicine
Stanford, California

THE MANAGEMENT OF THE ZOLLINGER-ELLISON SYNDROME

Monika A. Krezalek, MD
Resident
Department of Surgery
Pritzker School of Medicine
University of Chicago
Chicago, Illinois

THE MANAGEMENT OF PANCREATIC NECROSIS

Helen Krontiras, MD
Professor of Surgery
Department of Surgery
Division of Surgical Oncology
University of Alabama at Birmingham
Birmingham, Alabama

MOLECULAR TARGETS IN BREAST CANCER

David M. Krpata, MD
Assistant Professor
General Surgery
Cleveland Clinic
Cleveland, Ohio

ABDOMINAL WALL RECONSTRUCTION

Nathan Kugler, MD
Department of Surgery
Medical College of Wisconsin
Milwaukee, Wisconsin

FLUID AND ELECTROLYTE THERAPY

Swati A. Kulkarni, MD
Associate Professor of Surgery
Department of Surgery
Northwestern University Feinberg School of Medicine
Chicago, Illinois

CONTRALATERAL PROPHYLACTIC MASTECTOMY

Vivek Kumbhari, MD
Assistant Professor of Medicine
Directory of Endoscopy
Bayview Medical Center
Director of Bariatric Endoscopy
Johns Hopkins Medicine
Baltimore, Maryland

THE MANAGEMENT OF THE MALLORY-WEISS SYNDROME

Timothy Kuwada, MD
Program Director
Bariatric Surgery Fellowship
Department of Surgery
Carolinas Healthcare Systems
Charlotte, North Carolina

THE MANAGEMENT OF INGUINAL HERNIA

David Kuwayama, MD, MPA
Assistant Professor
Department of Vascular Surgery
University of Colorado Denver
Denver, Colorado

ABDOMINAL AORTIC ANEURYSM AND UNEXPECTED ABDOMINAL PATHOLOGY

Angela LaFace, MD
Department of Surgery
University of South Florida
Tampa, Florida

THE MANAGEMENT OF ACUTE PANCREATITIS

Glenn M. LaMuraglia, MD
Division of Vascular and Endovascular
Surgery
Massachusetts General Hospital
Professor of Surgery
Harvard Medical School
Boston, Massachusetts

THE TREATMENT OF CLAUDICATION

R. Todd Lancaster, MD, MPH
Division of Vascular and Endovascular
Surgery
Department of Surery
Massachusetts General Hospital
Boston, Massachusetts

*OPEN REPAIR OF ABDOMINAL AORTIC
ANEURYSMS*

Rodney J. Landreneau, MD
Landreneau Thoracic Surgical Associates
Kittanning, Pennsylvania

*THE MANAGEMENT OF ACHALASIA OF
THE ESOPHAGUS*

*THE MANAGEMENT OF ESOPHAGEAL
CANCER*

Russell C. Langan, MD
Fellow in Surgical Oncology
Department of Surgery
Memorial Sloan Kettering Cancer Center
New York, New York

LAPAROSCOPIC LIVER RESECTION

Julie R. Lange, MD, ScM
Associate Professor of Surgery
The Johns Hopkins University School
of Medicine
Baltimore, Maryland

SCREENING FOR BREAST CANCER

Frank Lay, BS,
Research Technician
The Johns Hopkins University
Baltimore, Maryland

*NECROTIZING SKIN AND SOFT TISSUE
INFECTIONS*

Anna M. Ledgerwood, MD
Professor
Michael and Marian Ilitch Department
of Surgery
Wayne State University
Trauma Medical Director
Trauma Services
Detroit Receiving Hospital
Detroit, Michigan

PENETRATING NECK TRAUMA

BLUNT ABDOMINAL TRAUMA

Andrew J. Lee, MD, PhD
Chief Resident
Department of Surgery
University of Chicago
Chicago, Illinois

*TOTAL PANCREATECTOMY AND
AUTOLOGOUS ISLET TRANSPLANTATION FOR
CHRONIC PANCREATITIS*

**W. Robert Leeper, MD, BSc, FRCSC,
FACS**
Assistant Professor of Surgery, Trauma, and
Critical Care Medicine
Division of General Surgery
Department of Surgery
The Schulich School of Medicine and
Dentistry
London, Ontario, Canada

THE ABDOMEN THAT WILL NOT CLOSE

David Lehenbauer, MD
Division of Cardiac Surgery
Department of Surgery
The Johns Hopkins Hospital
Baltimore, Maryland

BLUNT CARDIAC INJURY

Robert P. Liddell, MD
Assistant Professor of Radiology
and Surgery
The Johns Hopkins School of Medicine
Baltimore, MD

*ACUTE PERIPHERAL ARTERIAL AND BYPASS
GRAFT OCCLUSION: THROMBOLYTIC
THERAPY*

Anne Lidor, MD, MPH
Professor
Department of Surgery
University of Wisconsin
Madison, Wisconsin

*LAPAROSCOPIC 360-DEGREE
FUNDOPLICATION*

Amy L. Lightner, MD
Fellow
Colon and Rectal Surgery
Mayo Clinic
Rochester, Minnesota

*THE MANAGEMENT OF BENIGN GASTRIC
ULCERS*

THE MANAGEMENT OF COLONIC POLYPS

Keith D. Lillemoe, MD
W. Gerald Austen Professor of Surgery
Harvard Medical School
Chief of Surgery
Department of Surgery
Massachusetts General Hospital
Boston, Massachusetts

*THE MANAGEMENT OF BENIGN BILIARY
STRICTURES*

Elizabeth J. Lilley, MD, MPH
The Center for Surgery and Public Health
Brigham and Women's Hospital
Boston, Massachusetts

SURGICAL PALLIATIVE CARE

Jieqiong Liu, MD
Guangdong Provincial Key Laboratory
of Malignant Tumor Epigenetics and
Gene Regulation
Breast Tumor Center
Sun Yat-sen Memorial Hospital
Sun Yat-sen University
Guangzhou, China
Department of Surgery
The Johns Hopkins University School
of Medicine
Baltimore, Maryland

*THE MANAGEMENT OF BENIGN BREAST
DISEASE*

Yuk Ming Liu, MD, MPH
Acute Burn and Critical Care Fellow
Department of Surgery
Massachusetts General Hospital
Boston, Massachusetts

EXTREMITY GAS GANGRENE

Laurie A. Loiacono, MD, FCCP
Associate, Critical Care Medicine
Geisinger Clinics
Wilkes-Barre, Pennsylvania

ELECTRICAL AND LIGHTNING INJURY

KMarie Reid Lombardo, MD
General Surgery Specialist
Mayo Clinic
Rochester, Minnesota

*THE MANAGEMENT OF MOTILITY
DISORDERS OF THE STOMACH AND SMALL
BOWEL*

Bonnie E. Lonze, MD, PhD
Assistant Professor
Department of Surgery
The Johns Hopkins University School
of Medicine
Baltimore, Maryland

HEMODIALYSIS ACCESS SURGERY

LAPAROSCOPIC DONOR NEPHRECTOMY

Erica A. Loomis, MD
Consultant
Division of Trauma, Critical Care, and
General Surgery
Department of Surgery
Mayo Clinic
Rochester, Minnesota

THE SEPTIC RESPONSE AND MANAGEMENT

Irene Lou, MD
General Surgery Resident
University of Rochester
Rochester, New York

*THE MANAGEMENT OF PANCREATIC ISLET
CELL TUMORS EXCLUDING GASTRINOMAS*

Charles E. Lucas, MD
Professor
Michael and Marian Ilitch Department
of Surgery
Wayne State University
Surgeon
Department of Surgery
Detroit Receiving Hospital
Detroit, Michigan

BLUNT ABDOMINAL TRAUMA

PENETRATING NECK TRAUMA

James D. Luketich, MD
Henry T. Bahnson Professor of
Cardiothoracic Surgery
Department of Cardiothoracic Surgery
Chief of the Division of Thoracic and
Foregut Surgery
University of Pittsburgh School of Medicine
Pittsburgh, Pennsylvania

*THE ENDOSCOPIC TREATMENT OF
BARRETT'S ESOPHAGUS*

VIDEO-ASSISTED THORACOSCOPIC SURGERY

Ying Wei Lum, MD
Assistant Professor
Division of Vascular Surgery and
Endovascular Therapy
The Johns Hopkins Hospital
Baltimore, Maryland

*PSEUDOANEURYSMS AND ARTERIOVENOUS
FISTULAS*

THORACIC OUTLET SYNDROME

Keri E. Lunsford, MD, PhD
Clinical Instructor
Department of Surgery
Division of Liver and Pancreas
Transplantation
David Geffen School of Medicine at
University of California, Los Angeles
Los Angeles, California

*THE MANAGEMENT OF CYSTIC DISEASE OF
THE LIVER*

Kevin Lynch, MS
West Virginia University
School of Medicine
Morgantown, West Virginia

*THE MANAGEMENT OF LOWER
GASTROINTESTINAL BLEEDING*

Thomas E. MacGillivray, MD
Chief of Cardiac Surgery and Thoracic
Transplant Surgery
Jimmy Howell Endowed Chair of
Cardiovascular Surgery
Department of Cardiovascular Surgery
Houston Methodist
Houston, Texas

*THE MANAGEMENT OF ACUTE AORTIC
DISSECTIONS*

Robert C. Mackersie, MD, FACS
Professor of Surgery
University of California, San Francisco
Medical Director, Trauma Services
Zuckerberg San Francisco General Hospital
San Francisco, California

*AIRWAY MANAGEMENT IN THE TRAUMA
PATIENT*

Thomas Magnuson, MD
Chair, Department of Surgery
Johns Hopkins Bayview Medical Center
The Johns Hopkins University School
of Medicine
Baltimore, Maryland

THE MANAGEMENT OF MORBID OBESITY

*METABOLIC CHANGES FOLLOWING
BARIATRIC SURGERY*

*LAPAROSCOPIC SURGERY FOR MORBID
OBESITY*

**Ronald V. Maier, MD, FACS,
FRCS Ed (Hon)**
Jane and Donald D. Trunkey Professor and
Vice-Chair of Surgery
University of Washington
Surgeon-in-Chief
Department of Surgery
Harborview Medical Center
Seattle, Washington

ACID-BASE PROBLEMS

Martin A. Makary, MD, MPH
Professor of Surgery and Health Policy
and Management
Chief, The Johns Hopkins Islet
Transplantation Center
Director, Minimally Invasive Pancreas
Surgery
The Johns Hopkins Hospital
Baltimore, Maryland

LAPAROSCOPIC DISTAL PANCREATECTOMY

Konstantinos Makris, MD
Assistant Professor of Surgery
Division of General Surgery
Baylor College of Medicine
Houston, Texas

*THE MANAGEMENT OF ADRENAL
CORTICAL TUMORS*

Mark A. Malangoni, MD
Associate Executive Director
American Board of Surgery
Philadelphia, Pennsylvania

*ANTIFUNGAL THERAPY IN THE SURGICAL
PATIENT*

Mahmoud B. Malas, MD, MHS
Director of Endovascular Surgery
Johns Hopkins Bayview Medical Center
Baltimore, Maryland

AORTOILIAC OCCLUSIVE DISEASE

Warren R. Maley, MD
Professor of Surgery
Department of Surgery
Sidney Kimmel Medical College at Thomas
Jefferson University
Philadelphia, Pennsylvania

*VASCULAR RECONSTRUCTION DURING THE
WHIPPLE PROCEDURE*

Paul N. Manson, MD
Distinguished Service Professor
Department of Plastic Surgery
The Johns Hopkins University
Baltimore, Maryland

*THE MANAGEMENT OF FROSTBITE,
HYPOTHERMIA, AND COLD INJURIES*

M. Ashraf Mansour, MD, FACS
Professor and Chairman
Department of Surgery
Michigan State University College of
Human Medicine
Academic Chair
Surgical Specialties
Spectrum Health Medical Group
Grand Rapids, Michigan

GANGRENE OF THE FOOT

Rebecca A. Marmor, MD
Department of Surgery
University of California, San Diego
San Diego, California

*THE MANAGEMENT OF GALLBLADDER
CANCER*

Guy P. Marti, MD
Assistant Surgical Research Professor
The Johns Hopkins University
Baltimore, Maryland

*NECROTIZING SKIN AND SOFT TISSUE
INFECTIONS*

Laura Martin, MD
Department of Surgery
The Johns Hopkins Hospital
Baltimore, Maryland

CONGENITAL CHEST WALL DEFORMITIES

Robert G. Martindale, MD, PhD
Professor and Chief
Division of General Surgery
Department of Surgery
Oregon Health and Science University
Portland, Oregon

NUTRITIONAL THERAPY IN CRITICAL ILLNESS

Leonard L. Mason III, MD
Assistant Professor
Department of Surgery
Division of Acute Care Surgery
Temple University
Philadelphia, Pennsylvania

INJURIES TO THE SMALL AND LARGE BOWEL

Sarah Jean Mathew, MD, BA
Fellow
Trauma and Surgical Critical Care
University of Pennsylvania
Philadelphia, Pennsylvania

THE MANAGEMENT OF TRAUMATIC BRAIN INJURY

Kellie L. Mathis, MD, MSc
Assistant Professor of Surgery
Mayo Clinic College of Medicine
Division of Colon and Rectal Surgery
Mayo Clinic
Rochester, Minnesota

THE MANAGEMENT OF COLONIC POLYPS

Douglas J. Mathisen, MD
Chief of Thoracic Surgery
Department of Surgery
Massachusetts General Hospital
Boston, Massachusetts

THE MANAGEMENT OF TRACHEAL STENOSIS

Aerielle E. Matsangos, BS
Postbaccalaureate Research Assistant
The Johns Hopkins University
Baltimore, Maryland

NECROTIZING SKIN AND SOFT TISSUE INFECTIONS

Jeffrey B. Matthews, MD, FACS
Dallas B. Phemister Professor and
Chairman
Department of Surgery
University of Chicago
Chicago, Illinois

TOTAL PANCREATECTOMY AND AUTOLOGOUS ISLET TRANSPLANTATION FOR CHRONIC PANCREATITIS

Robert Maxwell, MD, FACS
Professor
Department of Surgery
University of Tennessee College of Medicine
Chattanooga, Tennessee

THE MANAGEMENT OF ESOPHAGEAL PERFORATION

Damian McCartan, MD
Breast Service
Department of Surgery
Memorial Sloan Kettering Cancer Center
New York, New York

THE MANAGEMENT OF THE AXILLA IN BREAST CANCER

David W. McFadden, MD
Chairman
Department of Surgery
University of Connecticut
Farmington, Connecticut

THE MANAGEMENT OF GASTRIC ADENOCARCINOMA

Christopher R. McHenry, MD, FACS
Vice-Chairman, Department of Surgery
Metro Health Medical Center
Professor of Surgery
Case Western Reserve University
Cleveland, Ohio

THE MANAGEMENT OF THYROIDITIS

Robert C. McIntyre, Jr., MD
Department of Surgery
University of Colorado Anschutz Medical
Campus
Aurora, Colorado

LAPAROSCOPIC ADRENALECTOMY

Nathaniel McQuay, Jr., MD
Assistant Professor of Surgery
Department of Surgery
Johns Hopkins Bayview Medical Center
Baltimore, Maryland

MULTIPLE ORGAN DYSFUNCTION SYNDROME

Joseph K. Melancon, MD
Department of Surgery
George Washington Medical Center
Washington, District of Columbia

TRANSPLANTATION OF THE PANCREAS

Jay Menaker, MD
Associate Professor
Department of Surgery
R Adams Cowley Shock Trauma Center
University of Maryland School of Medicine
Baltimore, Maryland

EMERGENCY DEPARTMENT THORACOTOMY

Avedis Meneshian, MD
Assistant Professor of Surgery
The Johns Hopkins University School
of Medicine
Baltimore, Maryland
Thoracic Surgeon
Anne Arundel Medical Center
Annapolis, Maryland

THE MANAGEMENT OF PARAESOPHAGEAL HIATAL HERNIA

Raman Menon, MD
Swedish Colon and Rectal Clinic
Department of Surgery
Swedish Medical Center
Seattle, Washington

THE MANAGEMENT OF ANAL CONDYLOMA

Anthony A. Meyer, MD
Colin G. Thomas Jr., Distinguished
Professor and Chair Emeritus of Surgery
The University of North Carolina School
of Medicine
Chapel Hill, North Carolina

ELECTROLYTE DISORDERS

William C. Meyers, MD
President
Vincera Institute
Philadelphia, Pennsylvania

CORE MUSCLE INJURIES (ATHLETIC PUBALGIA, SPORTS HERNIA)

Fabrizio Michelassi, MD
Lewis Atterbury Stimson Professor
and Chairman
Department of Surgery
Weill Cornell Medical College
New York, New York

STRICTUREPLASTY IN CROHN'S DISEASE

Fernando Mier, MD, PhD
Advanced Laparoscopic and
Gastrointestinal Surgery Fellow
Department of General and Gastrointestinal
Surgery
Oregon Health and Science University
Portland, Oregon

LAPAROSCOPIC SPLENECTOMY

Stephen M. Milner, MS, BS, BDS, DSc, FRCS(Ed)
Professor
Plastic and Reconstructive Surgery
The Johns Hopkins University School
of Medicine
Baltimore, Maryland

NECROTIZING SKIN AND SOFT TISSUE INFECTIONS

MEDICAL MANAGEMENT OF THE BURN PATIENT

Emily Miraflor, MD
Assistant Professor of Surgery
University of California, San Francisco—
East Bay
Oakland, California

CARDIOVASCULAR PHARMACOLOGY

Jonathan B. Mitchem, MD
Department of Colon and Rectal Surgery
Lahey Hospital and Medical Center
Burlington, Massachusetts

THE MANAGEMENT OF ANAL FISSUES

Jacob Moalem, MD, FACS
Associate Professor
Department of Surgery
University of Rochester
Rochester, New York

MINIMALLY INVASIVE PARATHYROIDECTOMY

Rushabh Modi, MD, MPH
Assistant Professor of Clinical Medicine
Division of Gastroenterology
Department of Medicine
Keck Medical Center of USC
Los Angeles, California

THE MANAGEMENT OF REFRACTORY ASCITES

Daniela Molena, MD
Director
Esophageal Surgery Program
Thoracic Surgery Service
Memorial Sloan Kettering Cancer Center
New York, New York

THE USE OF ESOPHAGEAL STENTS

Forrest O'dell Moore, MD
Medical Director and Section Chief
of Trauma
Chandler Regional Medical Center
Associate Program Director
William Beaumont Army Medical Center
General Surgery Residency
Clinical Associate Professor of Surgery
University of Arizona College of
Medicine—Phoenix
Phoenix, Arizona

VENTILATOR-ASSOCIATED PNEUMONIA

Scott M. Moore, MD
Trauma and Acute Care Surgery Fellow
Denver Health Medical Center
University of Colorado, Denver
Denver, Colorado

CHEST WALL, PNEUMOTHORAX, AND HEMOTHORAX

ELECTROLYTE DISORDERS

Christopher R. Morse, MD
Cardiothoracic Fellow
Massachusetts General Hospital
Boston, Massachusetts

PRIMARY TUMORS OF THE THYMUS

John Mullinax, MD
Surgical Oncology
Sarcoma Department
H. Lee Moffitt Cancer Center
Tampa, Florida

THE MANAGEMENT OF GALLSTONE ILEUS

Leila Mureebe, MD, MPH, FACS
Associate Professor of Surgery
Division of Vascular Surgery
Duke University Medical Center
Section Chief
Division of Vascular Surgery
Durham VA Medical Center
Durham, North Carolina

VENOUS THROMBOEMBOLISM: PREVENTION, DIAGNOSIS, AND TREATMENT

Adrian Murphy, MD
Clinical Fellow
Department of Medical Oncology
The Johns Hopkins Hospital
Baltimore, Maryland

NEOADJUVANT AND ADJUVANT THERAPY OF ESOPHAGEAL CANCER

Peter Muscarella II, MD
Associate Professor
Department of Surgery
Montefiore Einstein Comprehensive
Cancer Center
Bronx, New York

SPLENECTOMY FOR HEMATOLOGIC DISORDERS

W. Conan Mustain, MD
Assistant Professor of Surgery
Division of Colon and Rectal Surgery
University of Arkansas for Medical Sciences
Little Rock, Arkansas

THE MANAGEMENT OF RADIATION INJURY TO THE SMALL AND LARGE BOWEL

Melinda Cherie Myzak, MD, PhD
Medical Oncology Fellow
Department of Oncology
The Johns Hopkins University
Baltimore, Maryland

NEOADJUVANT AND ADJUVANT TREATMENT FOR COLORECTAL CANCER

Lena M. Napolitano, MD, FACS, FCCP, FCCM
Professor of Surgery
Division Chief, Acute Care Surgery
Director, Trauma and Surgical Critical Care
Associate Chair, Department of Surgery
University of Michigan Health System
Ann Arbor, Michigan

TRACHEOSTOMY, PART TWO

William Hawe Nealon, MD
Northwell University School of Medicine/
North Shore/LIJ Hospital
Professor and Vice-Chairman of Surgery
Chief, Division of Gastrointestinal and
Colorectal Surgery for the Northwell System
of Hospitals
Co-Director of the Pancreas Center/
Director of Pancreatic Surgery North Shore/
LIJ Hospital
Manhasset, New York

THE MANAGEMENT OF PANCREATIC PSEUDOCYST

Uri Netz, MD
Division of Colorectal Surgery
Department of Surgery
University of Louisville
Louisville, Kentucky

THE MANAGEMENT OF ISCHEMIC COLITIS

Leigh Neumayer, MD, MS
Professor and Chair of Surgery
Department of Surgery
University of Arizona College of Medicine
Tucson, Arizona

THE MANAGEMENT OF RECURRENT INGUINAL HERNIA

Lisa Newman, MD, MPH, FACS, FASCO
Director, Breast Oncology Program
Henry Ford Health System
Medical Director
Henry Ford Health System International
Center for Study of Breast Cancer Subtypes
Detroit, Michigan

ADVANCES IN NEOADJUVANT AND ADJUVANT THERAPY FOR BREAST CANCER

Christopher Ng, BS
Postbaccalaureate Research Assistant
The Johns Hopkins University
Baltimore, Maryland

NECROTIZING SKIN AND SOFT TISSUE INFECTIONS

Gladys Ng, MD, MPH
Assistant Professor of Urology
Department of Urology
David Geffen School of Medicine at
University of California, Los Angeles
Los Angeles, California

UROLOGIC COMPLICATIONS OF PELVIC FRACTURE

Hien T. Nguyen, MD, FACS
Director of the Comprehensive
Hernia Center
Assistant Professor of Surgery
Department of Surgery
The Johns Hopkins University School
of Medicine
Baltimore, Maryland

THE MANAGEMENT OF SEMILUNAR, LUMBAR, AND OBTURATOR HERNIAS

Naris Nilubol, MD
Associate Research Physician
National Cancer Institute
Bethesda, Maryland

THE MANAGEMENT OF PHEOCHROMOCYTOMA

Jeffrey A. Norton, MD
Professor of Surgery
Stanford University School of Medicine
Stanford, California

THE MANAGEMENT OF THE ZOLLINGER-ELLISON SYNDROME

Kathleen M. O'Connell, MD
Surgical Critical Care Fellow
University of Washington
Harborview Medical Center
Seattle, Washington

ACID-BASE PROBLEMS

CATHETER SEPSIS IN THE INTENSIVE CARE UNIT

Terence O'Keeffe, MBChB, FACS, FCCM
Associate Professor
Department of Surgery
Banner University Medical Center
Tucson, Arizona

COAGULOPATHY IN THE CRITICALLY ILL PATIENT

Patrick I. Okolo III, MD, MPH, FASGE
Chief of Endoscopy
Department of Medicine
The Johns Hopkins Hospital
Associate Professor
Department of Medicine
The Johns Hopkins University School of Medicine
Baltimore, Maryland

ENDOSCOPIC THERAPY FOR ESOPHAGEAL VARICEAL HEMORRHAGE

Charles S. O'Mara, MD, MBA
Professor and Associate Vice-Chancellor for Clinical Affairs
Department of Surgery
University of Mississippi Medical Center
Jackson, Mississippi

THE MANAGEMENT OF ANEURYSMS OF THE EXTRACRANIAL CAROTID AND VERTEBRAL

Greg Osgood, MD
Assistant Professor of Orthopaedic Surgery
Chief, Orthopaedic Trauma
Department of Orthopaedic Surgery
The Johns Hopkins School of Medicine
Baltimore, Maryland

THE MANAGEMENT OF EXTREMITY COMPARTMENT SYNDROME

Michael J. Osgood, MD
Vascular Surgery Fellow
Vascular Surgery and Endovascular Therapy
The Johns Hopkins Hospital
Baltimore, Maryland

ENDOVASCULAR TREATMENT OF ABDOMINAL AORTIC ANEURYSM

THE MANAGEMENT OF RECURRENT CAROTID ARTERY STENOSIS

H. Leon Pachter, MD, FACS
The George David Stewart Professor
Chairman of the Department of Surgery
New York University School of Medicine
New York, New York

PENETRATING ABDOMINAL TRAUMA

Alessandro Paniccia, MD
General Surgery Resident
Department of Surgery
University of Colorado Anschutz Medical Campus
Aurora, Colorado

THE MANAGEMENT OF CHRONIC PANCREATITITS

Sam G. Pappas, MD
Department of Surgical Oncology
Loyola Medicine
Maywood, Illinois

IS A NASOGASTRIC TUBE NECESSARY AFTER ALIMENTARY TRACT SURGERY?

Theodore N. Pappas, MD
Professor
Department of Surgery
Duke University
Durham, North Carolina

THE MANAGEMENT OF ACUTE CHOLANGITIS

Pauline K. Park, MD
Professor of Surgery
Department of Surgery
Division of Acute Care Surgery
University of Michigan
Ann Arbor, Michigan

POSTOPERATIVE RESPIRATORY FAILURE

Catherine Parker, MD
Assistant Professor of Surgery
Department of Surgery
Division of Surgical Oncology
University of Alabama at Birmingham
Birmingham, Alabama

THE ROLE OF STEREOTACTIC BREAST BIOPSY IN THE MANAGEMENT OF BREAST DISEASE

MOLECULAR TARGETS IN BREAST CANCER

Madhumithaa Parthasarathy, MBBS
Research Fellow
Department of General Surgery
Saint Agnes Hospital
Baltimore, Maryland

THE MANAGEMENT OF GALLSTONE PANCREATITIS, PART B

Jesse D. Pasternak, MD
University Health Network
Toronto General Hospital
Department of General Surgery
Division of General Surgery
Toronto, Ontario, Canada

THE MANAGEMENT OF THYROID NODULES

Dhaval Patel, MD
Endocrine Oncology Branch
National Cancer Institute
Bethesda, Maryland

THE MANAGEMENT OF PHEOCHROMOCYTOMA

Jayshil J. Patel, MD
Associate Professor of Medicine
Division of Pulmonary and Critical Care Medicine
Medical College of Wisconsin
Milwaukee, Wisconsin

NUTRITION THERAPY IN CRITICAL ILLNESS

Madhukar S. Patel, MD, MBA, ScM
Resident in General Surgery
Massachusetts General Hospital
Boston, Massachusetts

PERIPHERAL ARTERIAL EMBOLISM

Nishant Patel, MD
Division of Cardiac Surgery
Department of Surgery
The Johns Hopkins Hospital
Baltimore, Maryland

BLUNT CARDIAC INJURY

Shirali T. Patel, MD
General Surgery
Saint Agnes Hospital
Baltimore, Maryland

THE MANAGEMENT OF BILE DUCT CANCER

Jasmeet Singh Paul, MD, FACS
Associate Professor
Department of Surgery
University of New Mexico
Albuquerque, New Mexico

FLUID AND ELECTROLYTE THERAPY

Timothy M. Pawlik, MD, MPH, PhD
Professor and Chair
Department of Surgery
The Urban Meyer III and Shelley Meyer Chair for Cancer Research
Wexner Medical Center at the Ohio State University
Columbus, Ohio

THE MANAGEMENT OF LIVER HEMANGIOMA

Walter Pegoli, Jr., MD
Joseph M. Lobozzo II Professor in Pediatric Surgery
Department of Surgery
University of Rochester
Rochester, New York

THE MANAGEMENT OF ACUTE APPENDICITIS

Andrew B. Peitzman, MD
Mark M. Ravitch Professor of Surgery
Department of Surgery
University of Pittsburgh
Pittsburgh, Pennsylvania

INJURY TO THE SPLEEN

Arjun Pennathur, MD, FACS
Sampson Endowed Chair in Thoracic
Surgical Oncology
Department of Cardiothoracic Surgery
University of Pittsburgh School of Medicine
University of Pittsburgh Medical Center
Pittsburgh, Pennsylvania

VIDEO-ASSISTED THORACOSCOPIC SURGERY

Bruce A. Perler, MD, MBA
Julius H. Jacobson, II Professor
Vice-Chair for Clinical Operations and
Financial Affairs
Department of Surgery
The Johns Hopkins University School
of Medicine
Baltimore, Maryland

CAROTID ENDARTERECTOMY

Jennifer A. Perone, MD
Department of Surgery
University of Texas Medical Branch
Galveston, Texas

*INTRADUCTAL PAPILLARY MUCINOUS
NEOPLASMS OF THE PANCREAS*

Nancy D. Perrier, MD, FACS
Walter and Ruth Sterling Endowed
Professor of Surgery
Surgical Oncology
MD Anderson Cancer Center
Houston, Texas

*EVALUATION AND MANAGEMENT OF
PERSISTENT OR RECURRENT
HYPERPARATHYROIDISM*

Walter R. Peters, MD
Chief
Division of Colon and Rectal Surgery
Baylor University Medical Center
Dallas, Texas

THE MANAGEMENT OF CROHN'S COLITIS

Patrick J. Phelan, MD
Fellow
Vascular Surgery
University of Wisconsin School of Medicine
and Public Health
Madison, Wisconsin

*THE MANAGEMENT OF RUPTURED
ABDOMINAL AORTIC ANEURYSM*

Benjamin Philosophe, MD, PhD
Surgical Director, Comprehensive
Transplant Center
Johns Hopkins University
Baltimore, Maryland

LIVER TRANSPLANTATION

Fredric M. Pieracci, MD, MPH, FACS
Trauma Medical Director, Denver Health
Medical Center
Associate Professor of Surgery
University of Colorado Denver School
of Medicine
Denver, Colorado

*CHEST WALL, PNEUMOTHORAX, AND
HEMOTHORAX*

Henry A. Pitt, MD
Professor of Surgery
Lewis Katz School of Medicine at
Temple University
Philadelphia, Pennsylvania

*THE MANAGEMENT OF PRIMARY
SCLEROSING CHOLANGITIS*

Jennifer K. Plichta, MD, MS
Assistant Professor of Surgery
Duke University School of Medicine
Durham, North Carolina

INFLAMMATORY BREAST CANCER

Jeffrey L. Ponsky, MD
Professor of Surgery
Department of General Surgery
Cleveland Clinic Lerner College
of Medicine
Professor of Surgery
School of Medicine
Case Western Reserve University
Cleveland, Ohio

NOTES: WHAT IS CURRENTLY POSSIBLE?

Alexander E. Poor, MD
Surgeon, Director of Research
Vincera Institute
Philadelphia, Pennsylvania
Director of Adult Trauma Services
Chief, Division of Acute Care Surgery
Department of Surgery
The Johns Hopkins Hospital
Baltimore, Maryland

*CORE MUSCLE INJURIES (ATHLETIC
PUBALGIA, SPORTS HERNIA)*

Katherine E. Poruk, MD
Surgical Resident
Department of Surgery
The Johns Hopkins Hospital
Baltimore, Maryland

*THE MANAGEMENT OF BENIGN LIVER
LESIONS*

*THE MANAGEMENT OF PERIAMPULLARY
CANCER*

Priya Prakash, MD
Trauma and Surgical Critical Care Fellow
Department of Surgery
Division of Trauma, Surgical Critical Care,
and Emergency Surgery
Perelman School of Medicine
University of Pennsylvania
Philadelphia, Pennsylvania

*ACUTE KIDNEY INJURY IN THE INJURED
AND CRITICALLY ILL*

Jason D. Prescott, MD, PhD
Assistant Professor
Department of Surgery
The Johns Hopkins School of Medicine
Baltimore, Maryland

PRIMARY HYPERPARATHYROIDISM

Leigh Ann Price, MD
Director, National Burn Reconstructive
Center
Department of Surgery
Medstar Good Samaritan Hospital
Assistant Professor
Plastic and Reconstructive Surgery
The Johns Hopkins University School
of Medicine
Baltimore, Maryland

ELECTRICAL AND LIGHTNING INJURY

Aurora D. Pryor, MD
Professor of Surgery
Department of Surgery
Stony Brook University
Stony Brook, New York

LAPAROSCOPIC INGUINAL HERNIORRHAPHY

Carlos A. Puig, MD
Department of General Surgery
Mayo Clinic
Rochester, Minnesota

*THE MANAGEMENT OF RECURRENT AND
METASTATIC BREAST CANCER*

Christopher D. Raeburn, MD
Associate Professor
Department of Surgery
University of Colorado Anschutz Medical
Campus
Aurora, Colorado

LAPAROSCOPIC ADRENALECTOMY

Siavash Raigani, MD
General Surgery Resident
Massachusetts General Hospital
Boston, Massachusetts

*THE MANAGEMENT OF ASYMPTOMATIC
(SILENT) GALLSTONES*

Philip T. Ramsay, MD
General Surgery and Trauma/Critical
Care Surgery
Atlanta Medical Center
Atlanta, Georgia

*THE MANAGEMENT OF DIAPHRAGMATIC
INJURIES*

Laila Rashidi, MD
Colon and Rectal Surgery
Swedish Colon and Rectal Clinic
Seattle, Washington

THE MANAGEMENT OF ANAL CONDYLOMA

David Rattner, MD
Chief, Division of General and
Gastrointestinal Surgery
Massachusetts General Hospital
Professor of Surgery
Harvard Medical School
Boston, Massachusetts

*LAPAROENDOSCOPIC SINGLE-SITE SURGERY
AS AN EVOLVING SURGICAL APPROACH*

Trista Reid, MD
Assistant Professor of Surgery
Division of General and Acute Care Surgery
Department of Surgery
University of North Carolina School
of Medicine
Chapel Hill, North Carolina

*PREHOSPITAL MANAGEMENT OF THE
TRAUMA PATIENT*

Thomas Reifsnyder, MD
Department of Surgery
The Johns Hopkins University
Baltimore, Maryland

HEMODIALYSIS ACCESS SURGERY

Jessica K. Reynolds, MD
Department of Surgery
University of Tennessee College of Medicine
Chattanooga, Tennessee

*THE MANAGEMENT OF ESOPHAGEAL
PERFORATION*

Taylor S. Riall, MD, PhD
Professor
Department of Surgery
University of Arizona
Tucson, Arizona

*INTRADUCTAL PAPILLARY MUCINOUS
NEOPLASMS OF THE PANCREAS*

Amy Rivere, MD
Instructor in Surgery
Ochsner Medical Center
New Orleans, Louisiana

*ABLATIVE TECHNIQUES IN THE TREATMENT
OF BENIGN AND MALIGNANT BREAST
DISEASE*

Addi Z. Rizvi, MD
Vascular and Endovascular Surgeon
Providence Vascular Institute
Sacred Heart Medical Center
Spokane, Washington

PROFUNDA FEMORIS RECONSTRUCTION

**Bryce R. H. Robinson, MD, MS, FACS,
FCCM**
Associate Professor of Surgery
Associate Medical Director
Critical Care Services
Department of Surgery
Harborview Medical Center
University of Washington
Seattle, Washington

BLOOD TRANSFUSION THERAPY IN TRAUMA

Thomas N. Robinson, MD, MS
Professor
Department of Surgery
University of Colorado
Aurora, Colorado

*FRAILTY AND THE SURGICAL CARE OF THE
OLDER ADULT*

Aurelio Rodriguez, MD, FACS
Professor of Surgery (Retired)
University of Maryland School of Medicine,
Baltimore
Drexel University College of Medicine
Philadelphia, Pennsylvania

DAMAGE CONTROL OPERATION

John H. Rodriguez, MD
General Surgery
Cleveland Clinic Lerner College
of Medicine
Cleveland, Ohio

NOTES: WHAT IS CURRENTLY POSSIBLE?

Alexander S. Rosemurgy II, MD
Director of Hepatopancreaticobiliary
Surgery
Florida Hospital Tampa
Tampa, Florida

PARAESOPHAGEAL HERNIA

Michael J. Rosen, MD
Professor of Surgery
Lerner College of Medicine
Cleveland Clinic Foundation
Cleveland, Ohio

ABDOMINAL WALL RECONSTRUCTION

*LAPAROSCOPIC VENTRAL AND INCISIONAL
HERNIA REPAIR*

Kelly J. Rosso, MD, MS
Henry Ford Health System
Detroit, Michigan

*ADVANCES IN NEOADJUVANT AND
ADJUVANT THERAPY FOR BREAST CANCER*

Gedge D. Rosson, MD
Associate Professor
Department of Plastic and Reconstructive
Surgery
The Johns Hopkins University School
of Medicine
Baltimore, Maryland

LYMPHEDEMA

Michael F. Rotondo, MD, FACS
Chief Executive Officer
University of Rochester Medical Faculty
Group
Vice-Dean for Clinical Affairs
School of Medicine
Professor of Surgery
Division of Acute Care Surgery
Vice-President of Administration
Strong Memorial Hospital
University of Rochester School of Medicine
Rochester, New York

PANCREATIC AND DUODENAL INJURIES

Mario Rueda, MD
Assistant of Surgery
Department of Surgery
The Johns Hopkins University School
of Medicine
Baltimore, Maryland

THE MANAGEMENT OF LIVER INJURIES

*THE MANAGEMENT OF INTRA-ABDOMINAL
INFECTIONS*

Mark L. Ryan, MD, MSPH
Clinical Instructor
Department of Surgery
University of Tennessee Health
Science Center
Memphis, Tennessee

THE MANAGEMENT OF RECTAL INJURIES

Justin M. Sacks, MD, MBA, FACS
Director of Oncological Reconstruction and
Assistant Professor of Plastic Surgery
The Johns Hopkins University School
of Medicine
Baltimore, Maryland

*EVALUATION AND MANAGEMENT OF THE
PATIENT WITH CRANIOMAXILLOFACIAL
TRAUMA*

Arghavan Salles, MD, PhD
Instructor of Surgery
Department of Surgery
Washington University School of Medicine
St. Louis, Missouri

ADRENAL INCIDENTALOMA

Byron F. Santos, MD
Assistant Professor of Surgery
Department of Surgery
Geisel School of Medicine at Dartmouth
College
Hanover, New Hampshire
Staff Surgeon
Veterans Affairs Medical Center
White River Junction, Vermont

*MANAGEMENT OF COMMON BILE DUCT
STONES: LAPAROSCOPIC COMMON BILE
DUCT EXPLORATION*

Michael G. Sarr, MD
James C. Masson Professor of Surgery
Department of Surgery
Mayo Clinic
Rochester, Minnesota

*THE MANAGEMENT OF MOTILITY
DISORDERS OF THE STOMACH AND SMALL
BOWEL*

Nicole M. Saur, MD
Assistant Professor of Clinical Surgery
Colon and Rectal Surgery
University of Pennsylvania
Philadelphia, Pennsylvania

THE MANAGEMENT OF RECTAL PROLAPSE

*THE MANAGEMENT OF RECTOVAGINAL
FISTULA*

Thomas M. Scalea, MD, FACS, MCCM
Francis X. Kelly Professor of Trauma
Surgery
Director of Program in Trauma
Physician-in-Chief, R Adams Cowley Shock
Trauma Center
The University of Maryland School of
Medicine
R Adams Cowley Shock Trauma Center
Baltimore, Maryland
Assistant Profess or Plastic Surgery
Department of Surgery
Virginia Commonwealth University
Richmond, Virginia

EMERGENCY DEPARTMENT THORACOTOMY

Shaina Schaetzel, MD
Fellow
Acute Care Surgery
University of California, San Francisco
Fresno, California

*GLUCOSE CONTROL IN THE POSTOPERATIVE
PERIOD*

Lara Schaheen, MD
Cardiothoracic Surgery Resident
Department of Cardiothoracic Surgery
University of Pittsburgh
Pittsburgh, Pennsylvania

*THE ENDOSCOPIC TREATMENT OF
BARRETT'S ESOPHAGUS*

Dennis K. Schimpf, MD, FACS
Plastic Surgery Trident Health
Summerville, South Carolina

*BREAST RECONSTRUCTION AFTER BREAST
CANCER TREATMENT: GOALS, OPTIONS, AND
REASONING*

Todd Schlachter, MD
Assistant Professor
Department of Radiology and Biomedical
Imaging
Yale University School of Medicine
New Haven, Connecticut

*TRANSARTERIAL CHEMOEMBOLIZATION
FOR LIVER METASTASES*

Richard D. Schulick, MD
Professor and Chair
Department of Surgery
University of Colorado School of Medicine
Aurora, Colorado

*THE MANAGEMENT OF MALIGNANT LIVER
TUMORS*

Diane A. Schwartz, MD
Assistant Professor of Surgery
The Johns Hopkins University
Baltimore, Maryland

*NECROTIZING SKIN AND SOFT TISSUE
INFECTIONS*

Michael A. Schweitzer, MD
Associate Professor of Surgery
Department of Surgery
The Johns Hopkins University
Baltimore, Maryland

THE MANAGEMENT OF MORBID OBESITY

*METABOLIC CHANGES FOLLOWING
BARIATRIC SURGERY*

*LAPAROSCOPIC SURGERY FOR MORBID
OBESITY*

Christopher Sciortino, MD, PhD
Assistant Professor
Division of Cardiac Surgery
Department of Surgery
The Johns Hopkins Hospital
Baltimore, Maryland

BLUNT CARDIAC INJURY

Roy Semaan, MD
Fellow
Section of Interventional Pulmonology
The Johns Hopkins Hospital
Baltimore, Maryland

TRACHEOSTOMY, PART ONE

Anthony J. Senagore, MD, MS, MBA
University of Texas Medical Branch
at Galveston
Department of Surgery
Galveston, Texas

*THE MANAGEMENT OF SOLITARY RECTAL
ULCER SYNDROME*

Amar Shah, MD
General Surgery Resident
Virginia Commonwealth University
Richmond, Virginia

*THE SURGEON'S USE OF ULTRASOUND IN
THORACOABDOMINAL TRAUMA*

Aqsa Shakoor, MD
Senior Resident in Surgery
Department of Surgery
University of Rochester
Rochester, New York

*THE MANAGEMENT OF ACUTE
APPENDICITIS*

A. M. James Shapiro, MD, PhD, FRCS
Director, Clinical Islet Transplant Program
Professor of Surgery, Medicine, and Surgical
Oncology
University of Alberta
Edmonton, Alberta, Canada

*ISLET ALLOTRANSPLANTATION FOR
DIABETES*

Palma Shaw, MD
Associate Professor of Surgery
Department of General Surgery
Upstate Medical Center
Syracuse, New York

*BUERGER'S DISEASE (THROMBOANGIITIS
OBLITERANS)*

Alexander D. Shepard, MD
Head, Division of Vascular Surgery
Department of Surgery
Henry Ford Hospital
Professor of Surgery

*UPPER EXTREMITY ARTERIAL OCCLUSIVE
DISEASE*

Robert Sheridan, MD
Department of Surgery
Massachusetts General Hospital
Boston, Massachusetts

EXTREMITY GAS GANGRENE

Michele A. Shermak, MD
Associate Professor
Department of Plastic Surgery
The Johns Hopkins University School
of Medicine
Baltimore, Maryland

NONMELANOMA SKIN CANCERS

Jason K. Sicklick, MD, FACS
Associate Professor of Surgery
Division of Surgical Oncology
Moores University of California San Diego
Cancer Center
University of California San Diego Health
System
La Jolla, California

*THE MANAGEMENT OF GALLBLADDER
CANCER*

Melvin Silverstein, MD
Medical Director, Hoag Breast Center
Newport Beach, California

*INTRAOPERATIVE RADIATION FOR BREAST
CANCER*

Justin M. Simmons, DO
Vascular Surgeon
Division of Vascular Surgery
Spectrum Health Medical Group
Grand Rapids, Michigan

*THE MANAGEMENT OF LOWER EXTREMITY
AMPUTATIONS*

Carrie Sims, MD, MS, FACS
Associate Professor of Surgery
Director of Research
Division of Trauma, Surgical Critical Care,
and Emergency Surgery
University of Pennsylvania
Philadelphia, Pennsylvania

*THE MANAGEMENT OF TRAUMATIC BRAIN
INJURY*

Michael Sise, MD
Clinical Professor
Department of Surgery
University of California, San Diego,
Medical Center
Medical Director
Division of Trauma
Scripps Mercy Hospital
San Diego, California

*ENDOVASCULAR MANAGEMENT OF
ARTERIAL INJURY*

Barbara L. Smith, MD, PhD
Director, Breast Program
Division of Surgical Oncology
Massachusetts General Hospital
Boston, Massachusetts
Chief of Surgery
Alameda Health System
Oakland, California

INFLAMMATORY BREAST CANCER

Kevin C. Soares, MD
Resident in General Surgery
Department of Surgery
The Johns Hopkins Hospital
Baltimore, Maryland

*THE MANAGEMENT OF LIVER
HEMANGIOMA*

David Sonntag, MD
Department of Radiology
Saint Luke's Health Care System
Boise, Idaho

*PANCREATIC DUCTAL DISRUPTIONS
LEADING TO PANCREATIC FISTULA,
PANCREATIC ASCITES, OR PANCREATIC
PLEURAL EFFUSION*

Julie A. Sosa, MD, MA
Professor of Surgery and Medicine
(Oncology)
Chief, Section of Endocrine Surgery
Duke University School of Medicine
Durham, North Carolina

*SECONDARY AND TERTIARY
HYPERPARATHYROIDISM*

David A. Spain, MD
Ned and Carol Spieker Professor and Chief
of Acute Care Surgery
Department of Surgery
Stanford University
Stanford, California

*PREHOSPITAL MANAGEMENT OF THE
TRAUMA PATIENT*

Robert J. Spinner, MD
Professor
Departments of Anatomy, Neurologic
Surgery, and Orthopedic Surgery
Mayo Clinic
Rochester, Minnesota

NERVE INJURY AND REPAIR

Richard D. Stahl, MD
Associate Professor of Surgery
Department of Surgery
University of Alabama at Birmingham
Birmingham, Alabama

*GLYCEMIC CONTROL AND
CARDIOVASCULAR DISEASE RISK
REDUCTION AFTER BARIATRIC SURGERY*

Gregory A. Stanley, MD
Assistant Professor of Surgery
Department of Surgery
University of Mississippi Medical Center
Jackson, Mississippi

*THE MANAGEMENT OF EXTRACRANIAL
CAROTID AND VERTEBRAL ARTERY
ANEURYSMS*

J. Daniel Stanley, MD, FACS, FASCRS
Associate Professor
Department of Surgery
University of Tennessee College of Medicine
Chattanooga, Tennessee

*THE MANAGEMENT OF CLOSTRIDIUM
DIFFICILE COLITIS*

Scott R. Steele, MD, FACS, FASCRS
Chief
Division of Colorectal Surgery
University Hospitals Case Medical Center
Professor of Surgery
Case Western Reserve University School
of Medicine
Cleveland, Ohio

THE MANAGEMENT OF PILONIDAL DISEASE

**Dimitrios Stefanidis, MD, PhD, FACS,
FASMBS**
Chief, MIS and Bariatric Surgery
Vice-Chair of Education
Department of Surgery
Indiana University School of Medicine
Indianapolis, Indiana

THE MANAGEMENT OF INGUINAL HERNIA

*LAPAROSCOPIC REPAIR OF PARASTOMAL
HERNIAS*

Sharon Stein, MD
Department of Surgery
Case Western Reserve University Hospital
Cleveland, Ohio

*LAPAROSCOPIC TREATMENT OF CROHN'S
DISEASE*

Marc P. Steurer, MD, DESA
President, Trauma Anesthesiology Society
Associate Professor of Anesthesia and
Perioperative Care
Department of Anesthesia and Perioperative
Care
University of California, San Francisco,
School of Medicine
Vice-Chief of Anesthesia and Perioperative
Care
Zuckerberg San Francisco General Hospital
San Francisco, California

*AIRWAY MANAGEMENT IN THE TRAUMA
PATIENT*

Kent A. Stevens, MD
Assistant Professor
Department of Surgery
The Johns Hopkins Medical Institutions
Baltimore, Maryland

SPLENIC SALVAGE PROCEDURES

Patrick A. Stone, MD
Associate Professor of Surgery
Division of Vascular and Endovascular
Surgery
Department of Surgery
West Virginia University
Charleston, West Virginia

BRACHIOCEPHALIC RECONSTRUCTION

Jerry Stonemetz, MD
Vice-Chairman, Clinical Operations
Medical Director, Center for Perioperative
Optimization
Anesthesia and Critical Care Medicine
The Johns Hopkins University
Baltimore, Maryland

*PREOPERATIVE PREPARATION OF THE
SURGICAL PATIENT*

Steven M. Strasberg, MD
Pruett Professor of Surgery
Section of Hepato-Pancreato-Biliary
Surgery
Washington University in Saint Louis
St. Louis, Missouri

*MANAGEMENT OF COMMON BILE DUCT
STONES: LAPAROSCOPIC COMMON BILE
DUCT EXPLORATION*

Michael B. Streiff, MD
Associate Professor of Medicine
Department of Medicine (Hematology)
The Johns Hopkins Medical Institutions
Baltimore, Maryland

*COAGULATION ISSUES AND THE TRAUMA
PATIENT*

Jonah J. Stulberg, MD, PhD, MPH
Assistant Professor of Surgery
Department of Surgery
Northwestern University
Chicago, Illinois

*COMPARATIVE EFFECTIVENESS RESEARCH
IN SURGERY*

Motokazu Sugimoto, MD
Center for Pancreatic Disease
Saint Luke's Health Care System
Boise, Idaho

*PANCREATIC DUCTAL DISRUPTIONS
LEADING TO PANCREATIC FISTULA,
PANCREATIC ASCITES, OR PANCREATIC
PLEURAL EFFUSION*

Srinivas M. Susarla, MD, DMD, MPH
Acting Instructor
Department of Surgery
Division of Plastic Surgery and Department
of Oral and Maxillofacial Surgery
University of Washington Medical Center
Acting Staff, Craniofacial Center
Seattle Children's Hospital
Seattle, Washington

*EVALUATION AND MANAGEMENT OF THE
PATIENT WITH CRANIOMAXILLOFACIAL
TRAUMA*

Jacob Swann, MD
General Surgery Resident
William Beaumont Army Medical Center
El Paso, Texas

VENTILATOR-ASSOCIATED PNEUMONIA

Lee L. Swanstrom, MD
IHU-Strasbourg
Institut de Chirurgie Guidée par l'image
University of Strasbourg
Strasbourg, Alsace, France

*THE MANAGEMENT OF DISORDERS OF
ESOPHAGEAL MOTILITY*

Mark A. Talamini, MD
Chairman
Department of Surgery
Stony Brook Medicine
Stony Brook, New York

*THE MANAGEMENT OF CROHN'S DISEASE
OF THE SMALL BOWEL*

Vernissia Tam, MD
General Surgery Resident
Department of General Surgery
University of Pittsburgh
Pittsburgh, Pennsylvania

*MINIMALLY INVASIVE MANAGEMENT OF
PERIPANCREATIC FLUID COLLECTIONS*

Kenneth K. Tanabe, MD
Professor
Department of Surgery
Massachusetts General Hospital
Boston, Massachusetts

*ABLATION OF COLORECTAL CARCINOMA
LIVER METASTASES*

John L. Tarpley, MD
Professor Emeritus of Surgery and
Anesthesiology
Department of Surgery
Vanderbilt University School of Medicine
Nashville, Tennessee

*THE MANAGEMENT OF SMALL BOWEL
TUMORS*

Spence M. Taylor, MD
President, Greenville Health System
Professor of Surgery
University of South Carolina School
of Medicine
Greenville, South Carolina

FEMOROPOPLITEAL OCCLUSIVE DISEASE

Erik J. Teicher, MD, FACS
Division of Trauma and Acute Care Surgery
Inova Fairfax Medical Campus
Falls Church, Virginia

SPINE AND SPINAL CORD INJURIES

Ezra N. Teitelbaum, MD
General Surgery Resident
Department of Surgery
Northwestern University
Chicago, Illinois

*LAPAROSCOPIC COMMON BILE DUCT
EXPLORATION*

*LAPAROSCOPIC BYPASS FOR PANCREATIC
CANCER*

Jon S. Thompson, MD
Professor of Surgery
Department of Surgery
University of Nebraska Medical Center
Omaha, Nebraska

*THE MANAGEMENT OF SHORT BOWEL
SYNDROME*

Amy J. Thorsen, MD
Clinical Assistant Professor
Department of Surgery
University of Minnesota
Minneapolis, Minnesota

*THE MANAGEMENT OF ANORECTAL
ABSCESS AND FISTULA*

Alan H. Tieu, MD
Fellow at Johns Hopkins Medicine
Baltimore, Maryland

*THE MANAGEMENT OF THE MALLORY-
WEISS SYNDROME*

L. William Traverso, MD
Center for Pancreatic Disease
Saint Luke's Health Care System
Boise, Idaho

*PANCREATIC DUCTAL DISRUPTIONS
LEADING TO PANCREATIC FISTULA,
PANCREATIC ASCITES, OR PANCREATIC
PLEURAL EFFUSION*

Susan Tsai, MD, MHS
Assistant Professor of Surgical Oncology
Department of Surgery
Medical College of Wisconsin
Milwaukee, Wisconsin

*NEOADJUVANT AND ADJUVANT THERAPY
FOR LOCALIZED PANCREATIC CANCER*

Maria Tsitskari, MD
Vascular and Interventional Radiology
American Medical Center
Nicosia, Cyprus

VENA CAVA FILTERS

Anthony P. Tufaro, DDS, MD, FACS
Associate Professor
Plastic and Reconstructive Surgery
The Johns Hopkins Hospital
Baltimore, Maryland

*INCISIONAL, EPIGASTRIC, AND UMBILICAL
HERNIAS*

Ryan S. Turley, MD
Fellow, Division of Vascular Surgery
Duke University Medical Center
Durham, North Carolina

*VENOUS THROMBOEMBOLISM:
PREVENTION, DIAGNOSIS, AND TREATMENT*

Robert Udelsman, MD, MBA
William H. Carmalt Professor of Surgery
and Oncology
Chairman of Surgery
Department of Surgery
Yale University School of Medicine
New Haven, Connecticut

SURGICAL APPROACH TO THYROID CANCER

Heidi Umphrey, MD
Associate Professor
Department of Radiology
University of Alabama at Birmingham
Birmingham, Alabama

*THE ROLE OF STEREOTACTIC BREAST
BIOPSY IN THE MANAGEMENT OF BREAST
DISEASE*

Marshall Urist, MD
Professor of Surgery
Department of Surgery
Division of Surgical Oncology
University of Alabama at Birmingham
Birmingham, Alabama

MOLECULAR TARGETS IN BREAST CANCER

Madhulika G. Varma, MD
Chief, Section of Colorectal Surgery
Department of General Surgery
University of California, San Francisco
San Francisco, California

*THE MANAGEMENT OF ANORECTAL
STRICTURE*

Vic Velanovich, MD
Professor of Surgery
Department of Surgery
University of South Florida
Tampa, Florida

*THE MANAGEMENT OF ACUTE
PANCREATITIS*

George Velmahos, MD, PhD, MSEd
Chief, Division of Trauma, Emergency
Surgery, and Critical Care
Massachusetts General Hospital
John F. Burke Professor or Surgery
Harvard Medical School
Boston, Massachusetts

*THE MANAGEMENT OF ACUTE
CHOLECYSTITIS*

Anthony M. Villano, MD
Resident Physician
General Surgery
Medstar Georgetown University Hospital
Washington, District of Columbia

LAPAROSCOPIC LIVER RESECTION

Courtney A. Vito, MD
Assistant Clinical Professor
Department of Surgery
City of Hope
Duarte, California

INTRAOPERATIVE RADIATION FOR BREAST CANCER

Charles M. Vollmer, Jr., MD
Professor of Surgery
Department of Surgery
University of Pennsylvania
Philadelphia, Pennsylvania

UNUSUAL PANCREATIC TUMORS

Nilesh A. Vyas, MD, FAANS
Director of Cerebrovascular and Skull
Base Surgery
Department of Neuroscience
Inova Fairfax Medical Campus
Falls Church, Virginia

SPINE AND SPINAL CORD INJURIES

Matthew J. Wall, Jr., MD
Professor of Surgery
ME Debakey Department of Surgery
Baylor College of Medicine
Deputy Chief of Surgery
Ben Taub General Hospital
Houston, Texas

ENDOVASCULAR MANAGEMENT OF ARTERIAL INJURY

Paul Waltz, MD
Resident
General Surgery Residency Program
University of Pittsburgh
Pittsburgh, Pennsylvania

INJURY TO THE SPLEEN

Tracy S. Wang, MD, MPH
Associate Professor
Chief, Section of Endocrine Surgery
Department of Surgery
Medical College of Wisconsin
Milwaukee, Wisconsin

SECONDARY AND TERTIARY HYPERPARATHYROIDISM

Michael T. Watkins, MD
Associate Professor of Surgery
Surgery-Vascular and Endovascular
Massachusetts General Hospital
Boston, Massachusetts

AXILLOBIFEMORAL BYPASS GRAFTING IN THE TWENTY-FIRST CENTURY

Ryan S. Watson, MD
General Surgery Residency
Department of Medical Education
Gundersen Medical Foundation
La Crosse, Wisconsin

ATHEROSCLEROTIC RENAL ARTERY STENOSIS

M. Libby Weaver, MD
Halsted General Surgery Resident
Department of Surgery
The Johns Hopkins Hospital
Baltimore, Maryland

PSEUDOANEURYSMS AND ARTERIOVENOUS FISTULAS

Mitchell R. Weaver, MD
Senior Staff Surgeon
Division of Vascular Surgery
Henry Ford Hospital
Detroit, Michigan

UPPER EXTREMITY ARTERIAL OCCLUSIVE DISEASE

Travis P. Webb, MD, MHPE
Professor
Department of Surgery
Medical College of Wisconsin
Milwaukee, Wisconsin

SURGICAL SITE INFECTIONS

Cynthia E. Weber, MD
Department of Surgical Oncology
Loyola Medicine
Maywood, Illinois

IS A NASOGASTRIC TUBE NECESSARY AFTER ALIMENTARY TRACT SURGERY?

Eric G. Weiss, MD
Education Center Director
Cleveland Clinic Florida
Weston, Florida

THE SURGICAL MANAGEMENT OF CONSTIPATION

Matthew J. Weiss, MD
Assistant Professor of Surgery and
Oncology
Department of Surgery
The Johns Hopkins Hospital
Baltimore, Maryland

THE MANAGEMENT OF BENIGN LIVER LESIONS

Nicole L. Werner, MD, MS
Surgical Fellow
Department of Surgery
University of Michigan
Ann Arbor, Michigan

POSTOPERATIVE RESPIRATORY FAILURE

Steven D. Wexner, MD, PhD(Hon)
Director, Digestive Disease Center
Chair, Department of Colorectal Surgery
Cleveland Clinic Florida
Weston, Florida

THE MANAGEMENT OF RECTAL PROLAPSE

Richard Whyte, MD, MBA
Professor of Surgery
Harvard Medical School
Vice-Chair for Clinical Affairs
Department of Surgery
Beth Israel Deaconess Medical Center
Boston, Massachusetts

THE MANAGEMENT OF PRIMARY CHEST WALL TUMORS

Elizabeth C. Wick, MD
Associate Professor
Department of Surgery
The Johns Hopkins University
Baltimore, Maryland

THE MANAGEMENT OF LARGE BOWEL OBSTRUCTION

Ory Wiesel, MD
Division of Thoracic Surgery
Brigham and Women's Hospital
Harvard Medical School
Boston, Massachusetts

THE MANAGEMENT OF CYSTS, TUMORS, AND ABSCESSES OF THE SPLEEN

Alison M. Wilson, MD
Professor
Department of Surgery
West Virginia University School
of Medicine
Morgantown, West Virginia

THE MANAGEMENT OF LOWER GASTROINTESTINAL BLEEDING

Jennifer L. Wilson, MD
Instructor of Surgery
Harvard Medical School
Division of Thoracic Surgery and
Interventional Pulmonology
Beth Israel Deaconess Medical Center
Boston, Massachusetts
Cambridge Health Alliance
Cambridge Massachusetts

THE MANAGEMENT OF PRIMARY CHEST WALL TUMORS

Megan Winner, MD
Fellow in Surgical Oncology
Department of Surgery
The Johns Hopkins University School
of Medicine
Baltimore, Maryland
Mineola, New York

THE MANAGEMENT OF TUMORS OF THE ANAL REGION

SCREENING FOR BREAST CANCER

Elan R. Witkowski, MD, MS
Instructor of Medicine
Harvard Medical School
Department of Surgery
Massachusetts General Hospital
Boston, Massachusetts

*LAPAROSCOPIC REPAIR OF RECURRENT
INGUINAL HERNIAS*

*LAPAROENDOSCOPIC SINGLE-SITE SURGERY
AS AN EVOLVING SURGICAL APPROACH*

Piotr Witkowski, MD, PhD
Associate Professor
Director, Pancreatic and Islet Transplant
Program
Department of Surgery
University of Chicago
Chicago, Illinois

*TOTAL PANCREATECTOMY AND
AUTOLOGOUS ISLET TRANSPLANTATION FOR
CHRONIC PANCREATITIS*

Joshua H. Wolf, MD
Fellow
Colon and Rectal Surgery
Cleveland Clinic Florida
Weston, Florida

*THE SURGICAL MANAGEMENT OF
CONSTIPATION*

Christopher L. Wolfgang, MD
Chief, Hepatobiliary and Pancreatic Surgery
Professor of Surgery, Pathology, and
Oncology
Department of Surgery
The Johns Hopkins Hospital
Baltimore, Maryland

*THE MANAGEMENT OF PERIAMPULLARY
CANCER*

Douglas E. Wood, MD
Professor and Chief, Endowed Chair in
Lung Cancer Research
Division of Cardiothoracic Surgery
University of Washington
Seattle, Washington

MEDIASTINAL MASSES

Cameron D. Wright, MD
Professor of Surgery
Division of Thoracic Surgery
Massachusetts General Hospital
Boston, Massachusetts

*THE MANAGEMENT OF ACQUIRED
ESOPHAGEAL RESPIRATORY TRACT FISTULA*

Charles J. Yeo, MD
Samuel D. Gross Professor and Chair
Department of Surgery
Sidney Kimmel Medical College at Thomas
Jefferson University
Philadelphia, Pennsylvania

*VASCULAR RECONSTRUCTION DURING THE
WHIPPLE PROCEDURE*

Heather Yeo, MD, MHS
Assistant Professor of Surgery
Department of Surgery
New York Presbyterian—Weill Cornell
Medical Center
New York, New York

STRICTUREPLASTY IN CROHN'S DISEASE

Jeniann Yi, MD, MS
Department of Surgery
University of Colorado Anschutz Medical
Campus
Aurora, Colorado

*ABDOMINAL AORTIC ANEURYSM AND
UNEXPECTED ABDOMINAL PATHOLOGY*

Linda M. Youngwirth, MD
Resident, Department of Surgery
Duke University Medical Center
Durham, North Carolina

*VENOUS THROMBOEMBOLISM:
PREVENTION, DIAGNOSIS, AND TREATMENT*

Rasa Zarnegar, MD
Associate Professor of Surgery
Department of Surgery
New York-Presbyterian Hospital—Weill
Cornell Medicine
New York, New York

*LAPAROSCOPIC TREATMENT OF
ESOPHAGEAL MOTILITY DISORDERS*

Herbert J. Zeh III, MD
Professor of Surgery
Department of Surgical Oncology
University of Pittsburgh
Pittsburgh, Pennsylvania

MINIMALLY INVASIVE PANCREATIC SURGERY

Martha A. Zeiger, MD, FACS
Professor of Surgery, Oncology, Cellular
and Molecular Medicine
Department of Surgery
The Johns Hopkins University School
of Medicine
Baltimore, Maryland

NONTOXIC GOITER

Michael E. Zenilman, MD
Professor of Surgery
Weill Cornell Medicine
Chair, Department of Surgery
New York Methodist Hospital
Brooklyn, New York

*FRAILTY AND THE SURGICAL CARE OF THE
OLDER ADULT*

Luke X. Zhan, MD, PhD
Vascular and Endovascular Surgeon
Providence Vascular Institute
Sacred Heart Medical Center
Spokane, Washington

PROFUNDA FEMORIS RECONSTRUCTION

Brenda M. Zosa, MD
Resident
Case Western Reserve University
Department of Surgery
MetroHealth Medical Center
Cleveland, Ohio

*ANTIFUNGAL THERAPY IN THE SURGICAL
PATIENT*

Melissa Silva Zoumberos, MD
General Surgery Resident
Department of Surgery
University of South Florida
Tampa, Florida

*THE MANAGEMENT OF DIVERTICULOSIS OF
THE SMALL BOWEL*

Kashif A. Zuberi, MD
Fellow
Johns Hopkins Bayview Medical Center
Baltimore, Maryland

*LAPAROSCOPIC SURGERY FOR MORBID
OBESITY*

Amer H. Zureikat, MD, FACS
Assistant Professor of Surgery
Department of Surgical Oncology
University of Pittsburgh
Pittsburgh, Pennsylvania

MINIMALLY INVASIVE PANCREATIC SURGERY

Nicholas J. Zyromski, MD
Associate Professor
Department of Surgery
Indiana University School of Medicine
Indianapolis, Indiana

*THE MANAGEMENT OF PRIMARY
SCLEROSING CHOLANGITIS*

The first edition of *Current Surgical Therapy* was published in 1984. The textbook has thus been in existence for more than 33 years, and this is the twelfth edition. In each edition, we have updated the material to reflect the continuing evolution of the field of general surgery. The textbook continues to be perhaps the most popular surgical book in the country, and as long as it fulfills a need, we plan to continue the publication every 3 years. It has been a special privilege and honor for the two editors to be able to review contributions from surgeons around the country and, indeed, from around the world, on what they believe is the current surgical therapy for virtually all general surgical topics. It is an enjoyable task and keeps two surgeons, who care for surgical patients, current on all general surgical topics.

The twelfth edition contains more than 280 chapters. This is twice the number of chapters in the first edition of *Current Surgical Therapy*. The length, however, has been held constant through the last few editions in an effort to keep the text at a manageable size. As with prior editions, nearly every chapter is new and has been written by a new author. All authors have contributed their specific and personal thoughts on the current surgical therapy of the disease about which they are experts. Therefore, to obtain a broad view of the topic, the reader should review the contributions of other experts in the last two or three editions of *Current Surgical Therapy*.

As with the past editions, disease presentation, pathophysiology, and diagnosis are discussed only briefly, with the emphasis on current surgical therapy. When an operative procedure is discussed, an effort has been made to contain brief and concise descriptions, with figures and diagrams, when possible. *Current Surgical Therapy* is written for surgical residents, fellows, and fully trained surgeons in private practice or in an academic setting. Many have told us that it is an excellent textbook to review before taking the general surgical boards or recertifying. In addition, medical students have given us feedback that they believe the text is of value to them. However, *Current Surgical Therapy* is not written principally for medical students. We believe a more classic surgical textbook with substantial sections on disease presentation, diagnosis, and pathophysiology is more appropriate for medical students.

We remain grateful to the many surgeons throughout the country, as well as to the international surgeons, who participated in creating this textbook. Most of the potential authors whom we solicit respond enthusiastically to the opportunity to present their expert views. Their efforts obviously are what make this textbook a success. In addition, Andrew and I could not have compiled this textbook without the herculean efforts of Ms. Irma Silkworth, who has been involved with virtually all of these editions. Ms. Katie DeFrancesco at Elsevier has also been a terrific help and stands out in the publishing industry.

Both editors continue to enjoy and thrive in our chosen profession of general surgery. In recruiting medical students into our specialty over the last 40 years, I have used the statement, "If you pick a profession you love, you never have to work the rest of your life." In our view, that profession is surgery.

Finally, we would like to dedicate this edition, as with the others, to the surgical house staff and fellows at the Johns Hopkins Hospital, who are "the best of the best."

ANDREW M. CAMERON, MD
JOHN L. CAMERON, MD

CONTENTS

The Liver

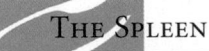

THE SPLEEN

HERNIA

THE BREAST

ENDOCRINE GLANDS

TRAUMA AND EMERGENCY CARE

MINIMALLY INVASIVE SURGERY

VIDEO CONTENTS

CURRENT SURGICAL THERAPY

ESOPHAGEAL FUNCTION TESTS

Errol Bush, MD, and Malcolm Brock, MD

The function of the esophagus is to facilitate the passage of food and drink to the stomach and to ensure that enteric secretions remain there. Esophageal dysfunction is complex, caused by a variety of anatomically distinct variables that can be measured and diagnosed with esophageal function tests. Esophageal dysfunction can exist at any level of the esophagus, although most patients evaluated by surgeons have issues with lower esophageal sphincter (LES) function. In these patients, common symptoms such as dysphagia, regurgitation, reflux, and pain prompt a diagnostic workup, and the concomitant history of certain comorbidities engenders a high index of suspicion for esophageal dysfunction. A detailed history from patients with dysphagia is imperative because many patients suffer unnecessarily because the natural history of the disease is unappreciated by their physicians. Finally, esophageal function tests are essential for confirmatory diagnosis and for planning optimal surgical intervention. This chapter provides a brief overview of commonly encountered esophageal function disorders and a review of the primary esophageal function tests used in their diagnosis.

■ DISORDERS OF ESOPHAGEAL FUNCTION

Gastroesophageal Reflux

Gastroesophageal reflux disease (GERD) is the symptomatic presentation of the reflux of gastric contents into the esophagus. There is a degree of physiologic reflux that is considered normal and usually is limited and not nocturnal. Pathologic reflux outside of these parameters results in GERD, a common disorder that often brings patients to medical attention for acid-suppressing medication. It is reported to affect 20% of the U.S. population. A subset of these patients has concomitant esophageal inflammation, which then is referred to as *reflux esophagitis.* Chronic reflux, Barrett's esophagus, stricture, and regurgitation of stomach contents into the mouth or pharynx are common indications for surgical referral. The cause of the reflux or regurgitation can be complex and may be related to the amount and type of dietary consumption or to an anatomic problem, usually a hiatal hernia that alters the geometry of the gastroesophageal junction (GEJ). Certain systemic illnesses, for example, autoimmune diseases such as scleroderma, or isolated pulmonary conditions, such as emphysema and interstitial lung diseases, have been associated with a high prevalence of GERD and can even hasten the need for lung transplantation. A mechanically defective LES is diagnosed when any one of three anatomic components is abnormal (pressure <6 mm Hg; total length <2 cm; abdominal length <1 cm). Invariably, the risk of GERD increases as the number of defective components rises and reaches more than 90% when all three LES components are abnormal. The etiology and severity of reflux varies by patient but can usually be determined with pH studies, impedance testing, motility or manometry studies, or a combination of each. There are even data that indicate interpretation of these results should be gender based because there are known gender-specific differences in esophageal function, anatomic position of sphincters, tone, and physiologic reflux. Physiologic reflux may account for increased episodes of acid exposure in men in the upright position, especially after meals, as well as a higher incidence in men of pulsion diverticula.

Achalasia

Achalasia is the most common esophageal motility disorder and is defined as relaxation failure or incomplete relaxation of the LES accompanied by an absence of peristalsis in the esophageal body. The LES is hypertensive in about 50% of cases and almost always shows a failure of normal relaxation in patients with achalasia. Patients need to know that although swallowing is improved after surgery or pneumatic dilation of the LES, esophageal function never recovers fully to normal because of abnormal esophageal peristalsis. The primary cause of achalasia remains unknown, but a decreased number of inhibitory ganglion cells is present on pathologic review. An esophagram is a good screening test for a patient with dysphagia; the classic finding being a dilated esophagus with smooth tapering at the GEJ, the "bird's beak" appearance (Figure 1). Pseudoachalasia, or any condition that can masquerade as achalasia, should always be ruled out. Pseudoachalasia is caused most often by malignant disease with adenocarcinoma infiltrating the myenteric plexus or the LES itself. Endoscopic examination is an imperative part of the pseudoachalasia evaluation and usually shows some resistance at the GEJ, with a classic "popping" feeling as the scope passes into the stomach. Endoscopy also can include the placement of a wire to facilitate the passage of a manometric catheter, whenever blind passage proves difficult. Both traditional water-perfused and now solid-state manometry are the gold standards for confirmation of achalasia and classically show aperistalsis as well as incomplete relaxation of the LES after a swallow (Figure 2, see Figure 10).

Traditional indiscriminate treatments of achalasia comprise a combination of medical, endoscopic, and surgical techniques with various degrees of efficacy. The recent development and use of high resolution, solid-state catheters (see Figure 9) (high-resolution manometry, HRM), has led to a greater understanding and improved application of treatments of achalasia. By allowing simultaneous evaluation of both the LES and the length of the esophagus with HRM as compared to 5 cm interval with traditional manometry, we are now able to discern three main types of achalasia, referred to as the *Chicago classification system.* Type I achalasia (Figure 3, *A*) occurs in 25% to 40% of patients and is characterized by low pressure contractions and minimal esophageal function often appearing as a dilated esophagus on esophagrams. Type II achalasia, (Figure 3, *B*) is the most common type of achalasia, occurring in 50% to 65% of patients, and is characterized as more normal amplitude propulsion waves with maintenance of esophageal body function. It typically appears as a bird's beak appearance on esophagram. Type III

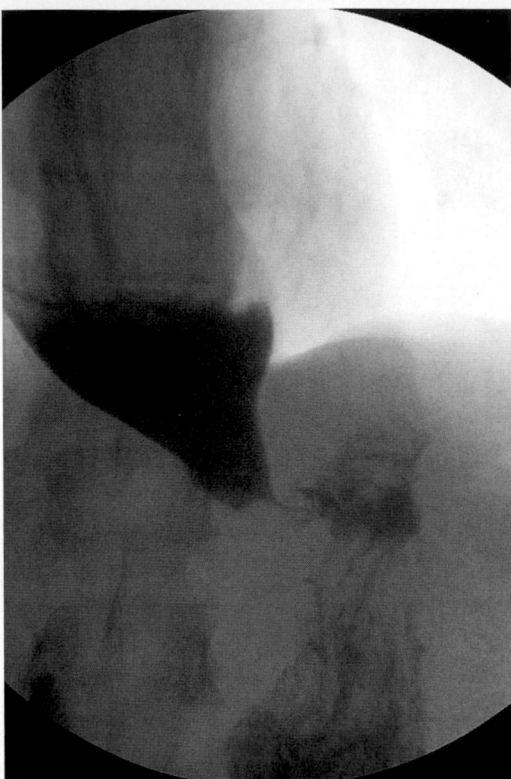

FIGURE 1 Classic bird's-beak appearance of achalasia on upper gastrointestinal series.

achalasia, (Figure 3, *C*) is the least common type, representing approximately 10% of patients. It is noted by uncoordinated spastic activity in the distal two thirds of the esophagus without relaxation of the LES, resulting in a corkscrew appearance on esophagram. Previously, techniques such as myotomy or pneumatic dilation of the LES, especially in type III achalasia, resulted in poor and unsustained results, often requiring multiple reinterventions. Short-term results for endoscopic myotomy, for example, are similar to traditional surgical treatment, but long-term outcomes differ usually because of the inability of the former to address chronic reflux, which can result after the procedure. The new classification of achalasia made possible by high-resolution manometry has allowed more discriminate application of surgical and nonsurgical techniques to give the best potential patient outcomes and avoid some treatment failures. In type III achalasia, for example, success with traditional surgical treatment is known to be around 50%, compared with 85% and 95% for types I and II, respectively. However, type III achalasia, which typically has poor success after traditional interventions, is now favored by endoscopic myotomy, where comparatively it has been demonstrated to be more durable and with a higher success rate. Its 96% rate of successful outcomes is likely secondary to the ability to perform a longer intrathoracic myotomy endoscopically.

Hypertensive Lower Esophageal Sphincter

Hypertensive LES is diagnosed when a patient has an LES pressure above the 95th percentile of normal and has symptoms of dysphagia or noncardiac chest pain. The exact value that determines LES hypertension differs according to the method used for measurement, but this condition can be diagnosed only with manometry. High-resolution manometry has become the gold standard for this diagnosis, although the use of video esophagram and upper endoscopy often are used concomitantly as diagnostic adjuncts. In hypertensive LES, relaxation of the LES and peristalsis are present, unlike in achalasia.

Diffuse Esophageal Spasm

Diffuse esophageal spasm (DES) is an uncommon condition that accounts for less than 10% of esophageal motility abnormalities. DES is characterized by uncoordinated contractions of the esophagus that typically result in symptoms of chest pain, dysphagia, or both. The esophagram may be abnormal, but manometry is usually necessary for the diagnosis. As with achalasia, the introduction of HRM changed the diagnostic criteria for DES. Initially, the Chicago Classification based both high-resolution manometry and conventional manometry on the same criteria of rapid or simultaneous contractions but modified this to a parameter known as *distal latency*, which is only apparent with HRM and is a more reliable indicator of DES. Distal latency is more than likely associated with the onset of inhibitory myenteric neuron activity after contractions and seems shorter in patients with DES with a resultant increased state of contractions in the distal esophagus. Current guidelines define DES by HRM as patients who have a normal integrated relaxation pressure at the LES but who have a distal latency less than 0.4 seconds in 20% of wet swallows.

Medical treatment options include nitrates and sildenafil and tricyclic antidepressants, which help with noncardiac chest pain. Valium and Ativan are also frequently effective if they fail to control symptoms. Use of proton pump inhibitors (PPIs) for treatment of concomitant GERD also may be helpful. A long myotomy can be effective in many patients with refractory DES but has a very high morbidity rate.

Hypercontractile "Nutcracker" Esophagus

Hypercontractile, or "nutcracker," esophagus is a manometric diagnosis defined by high pressure (>180 mm Hg) or long duration of swallow responses (>7 seconds) in patients who have either chest pain or dysphagia (Figures 4 and 5). The peristaltic contractions propagate normally, and the LES relaxes appropriately. Diltiazem has been shown to lower distal peristaltic pressures and may reduce chest pain; however, these results are not reliably reproducible. As in DES, nitrates, sildenafil, PPIs, and tricyclic antidepressants may be useful in the treatment of noncardiac chest pain. Interestingly, with HRM, the clinical significance of this diagnosis is now somewhat controversial, and "nutcracker esophagus" is not present in the latest edition of the Chicago Classification.

Ineffective Esophageal Motility

Ineffective esophageal motility is characterized by decreased distal esophageal peristaltic wave pressures (amplitudes <30 mm Hg) or an absence of esophageal contractions in more than 30% of wet swallows. A distinguishing feature between ineffective esophageal motility and achalasia is that resting LES pressure typically is decreased in ineffective esophageal motility. Systemic conditions, such as scleroderma, can be associated with ineffective esophageal motility. Unfortunately, no standard treatment options exist, besides PPIs and lifestyle modifications. Patients are advised to eat small meals, remain upright after eating, chew food well, and take acid-suppressing medication.

Nonspecific Esophageal Motility

Nonspecific esophageal motility disorder is an esophageal motility disorder that does not have features of a named motility disorder. These abnormalities often are not associated with dysphagia and are nonspecific. Examples of frequently encountered nonspecific esophageal motility disorders are triple-peaked and retrograde contractions. Systemic diseases such as diabetes mellitus, hypothyroidism, eosinophilic esophagitis, and amyloidosis can be associated with nonspecific esophageal motor abnormalities. These abnormalities also may be seen in patients with paraesophageal hernia who have a shortened esophagus.

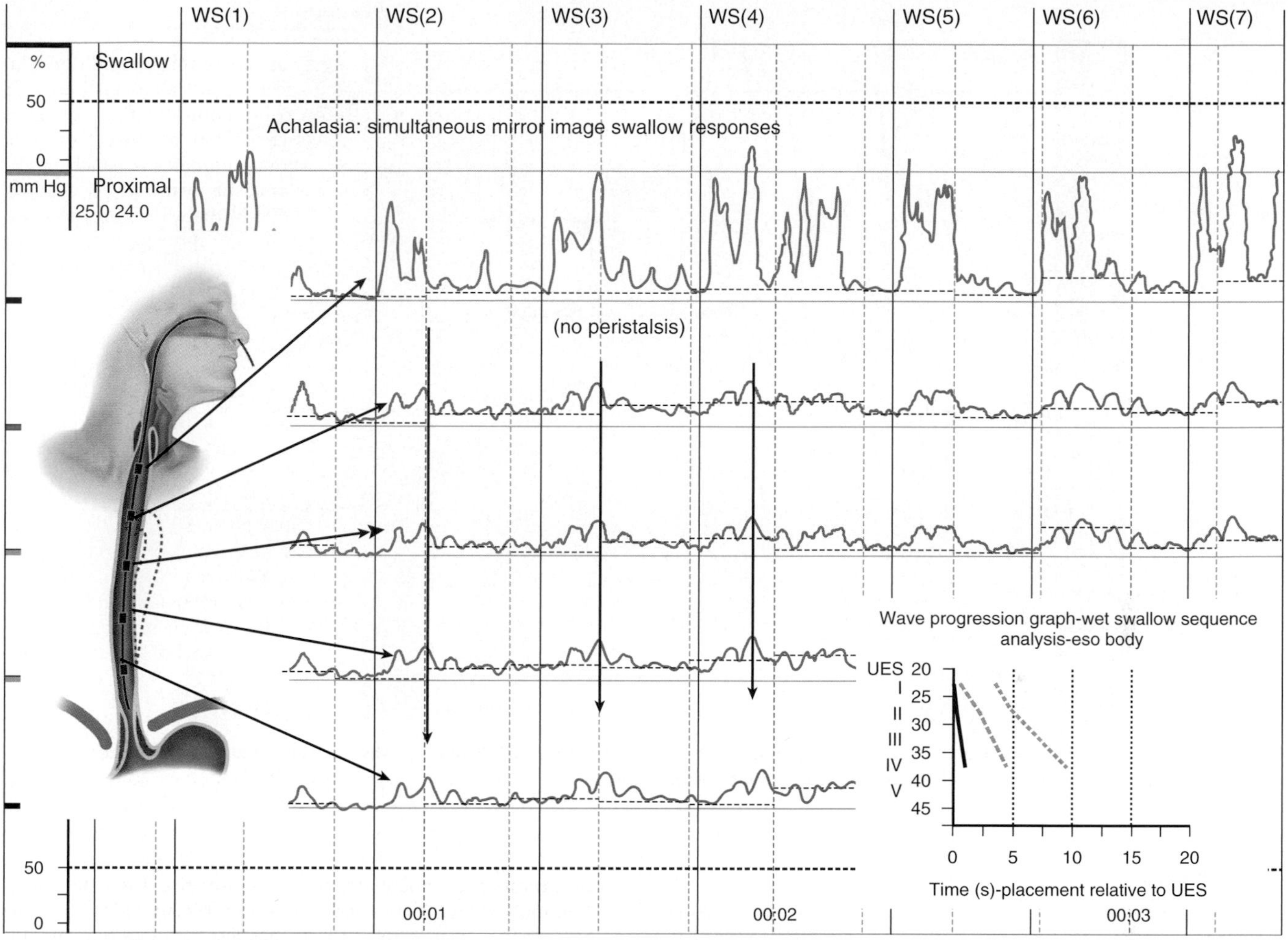

		WS(1)	WS(2)	WS(3)	WS(4)	WS(5)	WS(6)	WS(7)

%   Swallow

50

0

mm Hg   Proximal
25.0 24.0

Achalasia: simultaneous mirror image swallow responses

(no peristalsis)

Wave progression graph-wet swallow sequence
analysis-eso body

UES 20
I   25
II   30
III 35
IV   40
V   45

0   5   10   15   20

Time (s)-placement relative to UES

50

0

00:01   00:02   00:03

FIGURE 2 Manometry tracing of achalasia. The swallow study shows mirror-image swallow responses in the esophageal body.

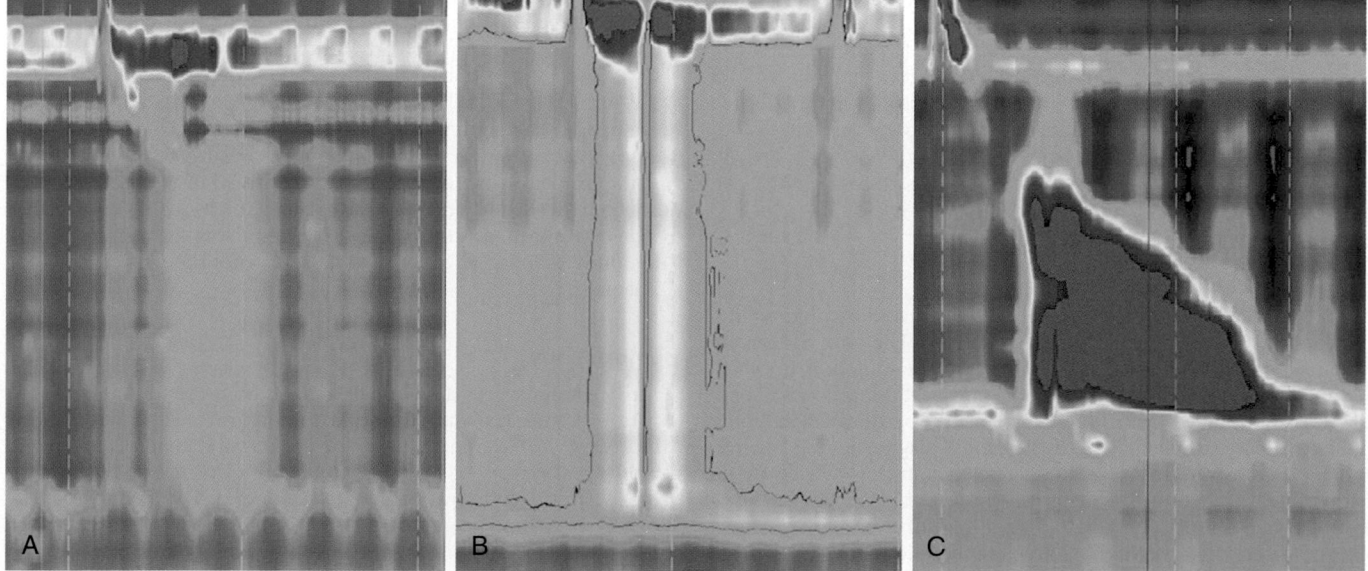

FIGURE 3 High-resolution manometry demonstrating achalasia subtypes. Type I (*a*) characterized by minimal esophageal pressurizations, type II (*b*) with panesophageal pressurization wave (black line demarcates 30-mm Hg contour), and type III (*c*) with premature spastic contractions.

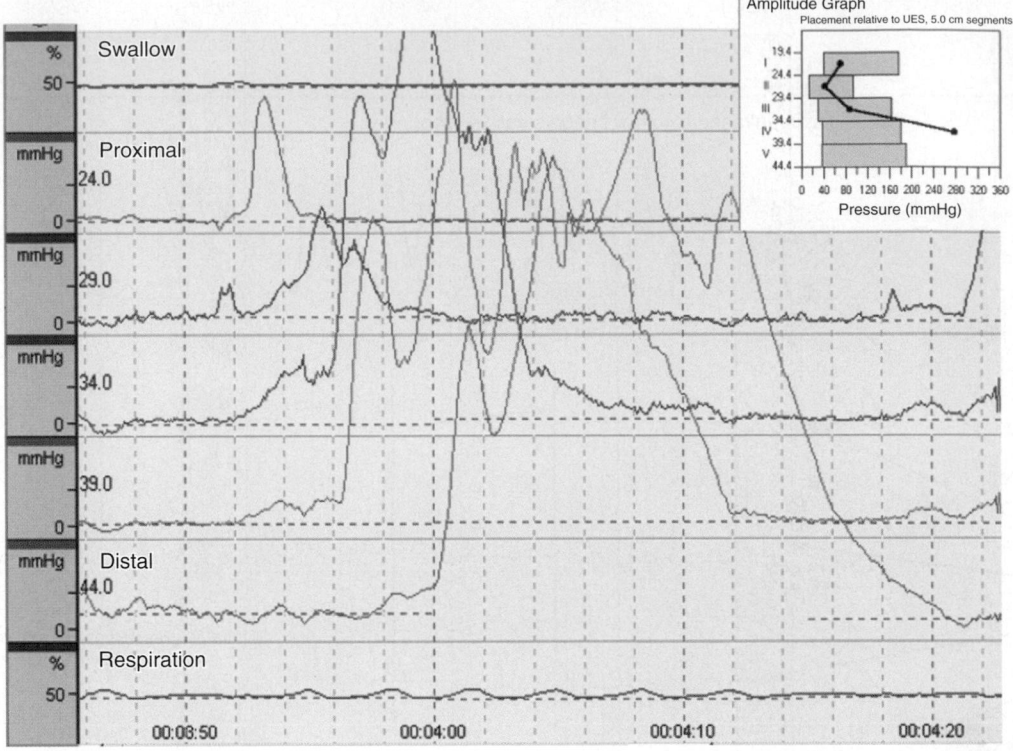

FIGURE 4 Manometry showing hypercontractile esophageal body with pressures more than 180 mm Hg, which is designated as a "nutcracker" esophagus, with these high pressures and symptoms of chest pain or dysphagia.

Hiatal Hernia

The presence of a hiatal hernia alters the usual location and structure of the LES, displacing it into the negatively pressured thorax and disrupting the reinforcement offered by the diaphragmatic crura. The manometric profile often shows the LES and the crura and intra-abdominal stomach as having increased pressure, a "double hump." High resolution manometry makes the diagnosis of hiatal hernia by manometry relatively easy. Manometry in paraesophageal hernias can be unpredictable depending on the anatomy of the hernia and the stomach because the esophagus may be shortened or of normal length. Manometry guides surgeons in repair of the hiatal hernia and helps them to choose the type of fundoplication to perform. Although a paucity of evidence is found, most esophageal surgeons avoid a complete wrap for patients with abnormal peristalsis and perform a partial, 180-degree or 270-degree, fundoplication to prevent postoperative dysphagia.

◼ DIAGNOSTIC TESTS FOR ESOPHAGEAL DISEASES

Radiographic Imaging

Radiographic tests of the esophagus include the fluoroscopic esophagram and cross-sectional imaging. An esophagram, or barium swallow, often is performed as a biphasic examination in which double- or single-contrast techniques are used and always should have a solid bolus administered as a 13-mm barium tablet. Liquid and solid-contrast agents are used in most diagnostic tests for dysphagia. Because the act of swallowing is a dynamic process, the inclusion of video or cine recording is imperative for better assessment of oropharyngeal function and esophageal motility.

A properly conducted videoesophagram allows the physician to comment on oropharyngeal function, morphology of the esophagus, esophageal motility, appearance of the mucosal surface, evaluation of the GEJ, presence and degree of reflux, and efficiency of secondary wave clearance. A videoesophagram is sensitive for detection of certain motility disorders, such as achalasia (94%) and scleroderma (100%); however, it is relatively insensitive for detection of most other motility disorders. The decision of whether to obtain radiographic imaging before endoscopic examination or to proceed directly to esophagogastroduodenoscopy (EGD) can be difficult. We recommend a videoesophagram as the initial diagnostic test in conditions such as a suspected cricopharyngeal bar, esophageal web, diverticulum, Schatzki's ring, early achalasia, or complex stricture, where an esophagram may provide the endoscopist a "road map."

Cross-sectional imaging with computed tomographic (CT) scan is helpful for evaluation of extraluminal esophageal disease, including staging for esophageal cancer and evaluation of esophageal trauma. However, the videoesophagram is still the gold standard in evaluation for esophageal leak. CT scan is used in evaluation of esophageal changes of the wall, such as thickening, but is not accurate in the evaluation of esophageal mucosal disease or motility disorders. Magnetic resonance imaging can produce high-quality multiplanar images without use of ionizing radiation but has limited utility for most esophageal diseases because of motion artifact and long imaging times.

Endoscopy

Although not strictly an esophageal function test, endoscopic examination is often necessary for evaluation or treatment for esophageal disorders. We routinely perform an on-table endoscopy before esophageal surgery because the surgeon is ultimately responsible for the diagnosis and treatment option selected. For example, endoscopic evaluation in achalasia rules out pseudoachalasia and can confirm the diagnosis with the characteristic "pop" on passing through the LES. For hiatal hernia surgery, it can identify Barrett's esophagus, rule out early malignant disease of the stomach or esophagus that has been missed, and help identify the presence of a short

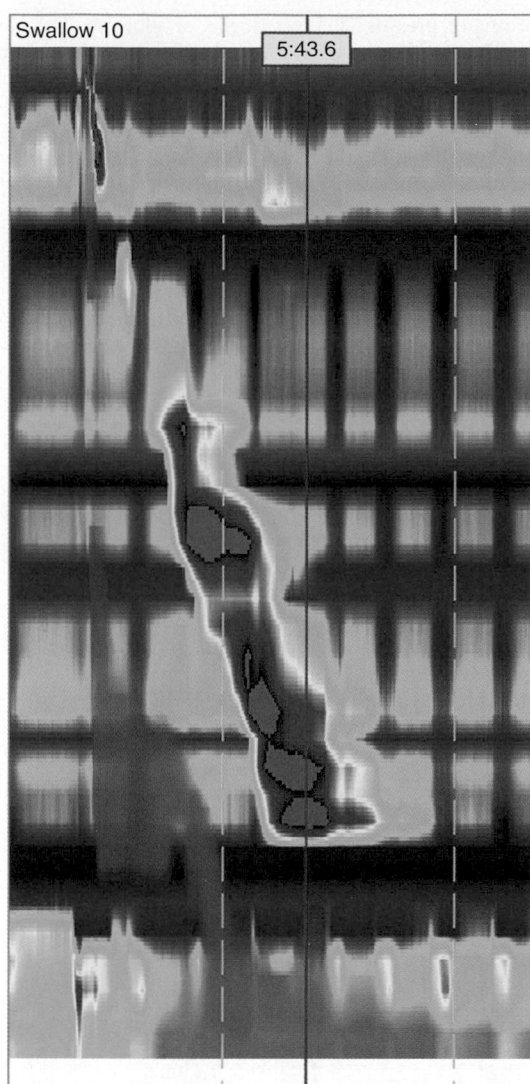

Swallow 10

5:43.6

FIGURE 5 High-resolution manometry showing "nutcracker" esophagus and relaxation after the swallow.

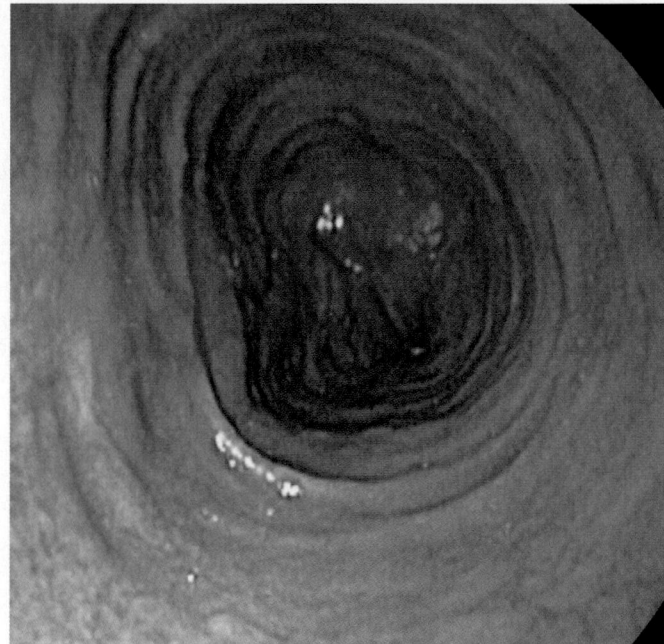

FIGURE 6 Eosinophilic esophagitis. Mucosal rings consistent with "trachealization" of the esophagus.

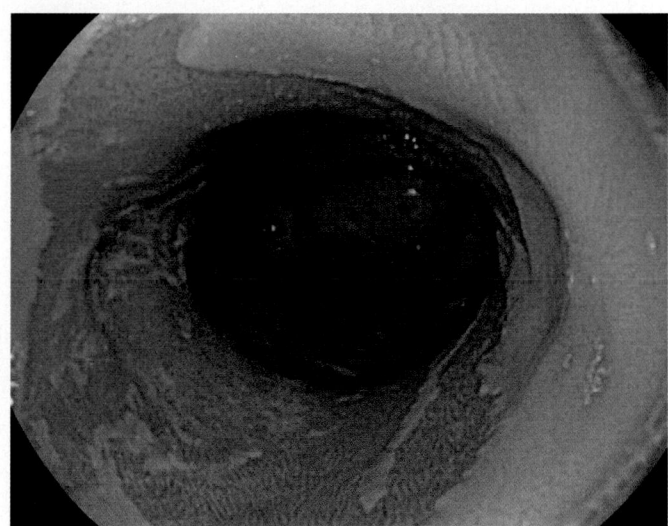

FIGURE 7 Salmon-colored mucosal changes seen in Barrett's esophagus.

esophagus that may need an esophageal lengthening procedure as part of the hernia repair.

Endoscopic evaluation for esophageal disorders begins with a good view of the vocal cords and aryepiglottic folds, which can appear inflamed in patients with chronic GERD. The upper esophageal sphincter (UES) consists of the cricopharyngeal muscle and is best seen on the final withdrawal of the endoscope. As the esophagus is entered, the mucosa can be inspected carefully for signs of mucosal inflammation or luminal irregularities, such as esophageal webs, rings, strictures, or esophagitis. Evaluation of the esophagus for distension or tonicity is also important because an atonic or patulous appearance may indicate the presence of a motility disorder.

At the level of the aortic arch, the striated muscle of the upper esophagus transitions to smooth muscle in the distal half of the esophagus. Patients with dysphagia should have random biopsies sampled from the distal and proximal esophagus for evaluation for eosinophilic esophagitis, particularly if the endoscopic examination shows the corrugated "feline" esophagus, with multiple concentric rings and linear furrows (Figure 6). In patients with long-standing GERD, the squamocolumnar junction proximal to the LES should be inspected carefully for signs of Barrett's esophagus (Figure 7), which appears as intestinal mucosa, with a pinker or salmon-colored appearance. The length of the Barrett's mucosa should be quantified, and multiple biopsies should be taken for assessment for dysplasia or malignancy.

The LES should really be called the LES complex because it is not one discrete muscle but rather a combination of esophageal muscle, phrenoesophageal ligament, and diaphragm. On endoscopy, it appears as a flap valve. Once the endoscope has entered the stomach, the endoscopist notes whether the gastric wall is poorly distensible and uses retroflex to examine the cardia and GEJ. The flap valve of the GEJ may be seen and assessed for competence under air pressure or for whether a hiatal hernia has expanded this area and allowed reflux and regurgitation.

Endoscopy offers multiple therapeutic maneuvers, from dilation to biopsy to botulinum toxin injection. Mucosal ablative techniques are also used for Barrett's esophagus, and endoscopic ultrasound scan has become the gold standard for the local and regional lymph node staging of esophageal cancer.

Esophageal Manometry

Esophageal manometry is the gold standard for assessment of esophageal motor function. It is the only modality that can define the pressure profile of peristalsis and measure LES pressure. Conventional manometry uses eight sensors, placed at various points of the esophagus, typically four in the esophageal body and four at the level of the GEJ. High-resolution manometry, specifically the ManoScan (Sierra Scientific Instruments, LLC, Los Angeles, CA), is vastly superior and will replace older manometry equipment. High-resolution manometry provides a much clearer picture of esophageal pressure changes during swallowing and includes pressure monitors every centimeter along the catheter. This new technology offers the ability to simplify the procedural setup, eliminate motion artifact, simplify the ability to interpret data, and allow for a more sophisticated interpretation of esophageal motility. Indications for esophageal manometry are summarized in Box 1.

Technical Considerations

For conventional manometry, a solid-state or water-perfused catheter is used. The manometry catheter is swallowed until all of the sensors are in the stomach, and the catheter then is pulled back in increments of 0.5 to 1 cm for measurement of the resting pressure of the LES, esophageal body, and UES (Figure 8). Once the resting pressures have been calibrated, the catheter is positioned across the entire esophagus

for recording of pressure changes during swallowing. The contraction and relaxation of the UES, the body of the esophagus, and the LES are recorded with 10 consecutive swallows of a 5-mL bolus of water. These pressure values are compared with standardized normal values (Figure 9; Table 1). Plotting of the pressure values with the passage of the water bolus down the esophagus allows for the detection of abnormal peristalsis and sphincter dysfunction. These patterns form the basis of esophageal dysmotility conditions.

The high-resolution manometry catheters have sensors every 1 cm. These catheters are able to span from the pharynx to the stomach, which obviates the need to retract the catheter to measure resting pressures. Pressure measurements are recorded in the resting phase and for 10 swallows in a similar fashion to the older equipment.

BOX 1: Indications for Esophageal Manometry

1. Dysphagia: For the assessment of functional disorders after structural causes have been ruled out
2. Noncardiac chest pain: For assessment for esophageal dysmotility as a cause of symptoms
3. Diagnosis or confirmation of a suspected motility disorder
4. Preoperative assessment of esophageal motility before planned esophageal surgery
5. Postoperative assessment: For detection of response to surgery or confirmation of response to treatment or for assessment of the cause of persistent symptoms after surgery

---

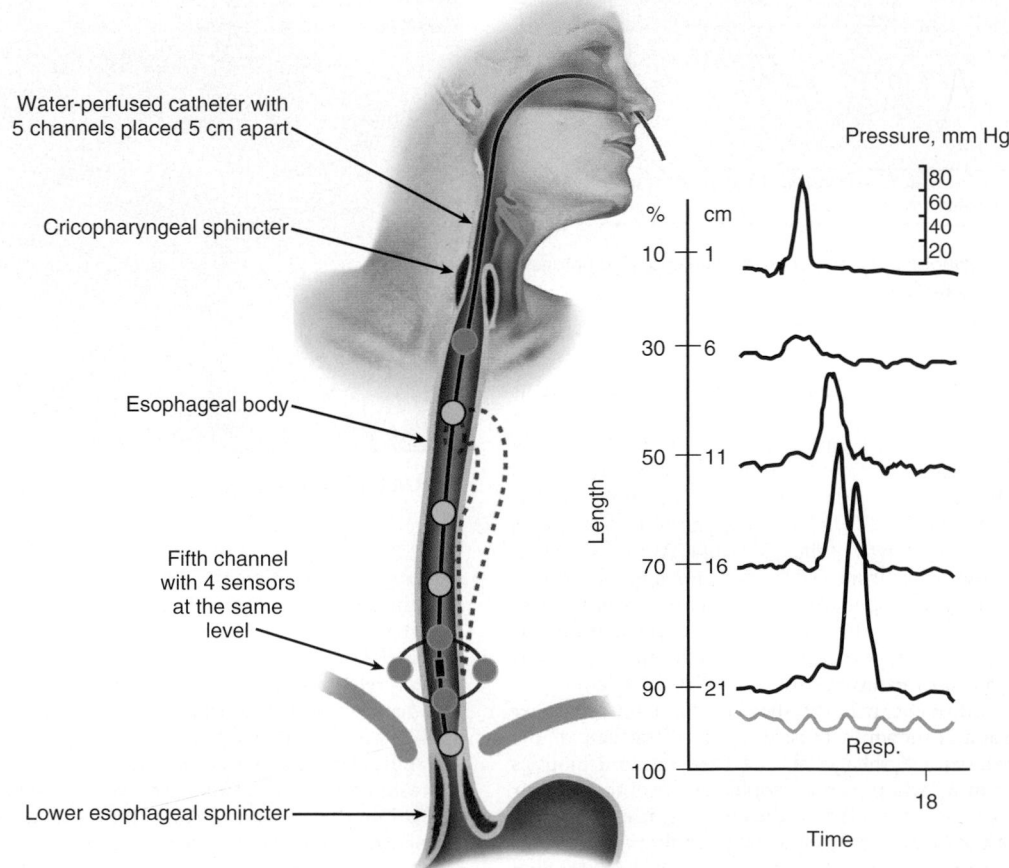

FIGURE 8 Esophageal manometry. A water-perfused or solid-state catheter is positioned in the esophagus. The sensors here are 5 cm apart, and the manometry shows normal wave propagation. Newer catheters that have sensors every 1 cm are termed *high-resolution manometry*.

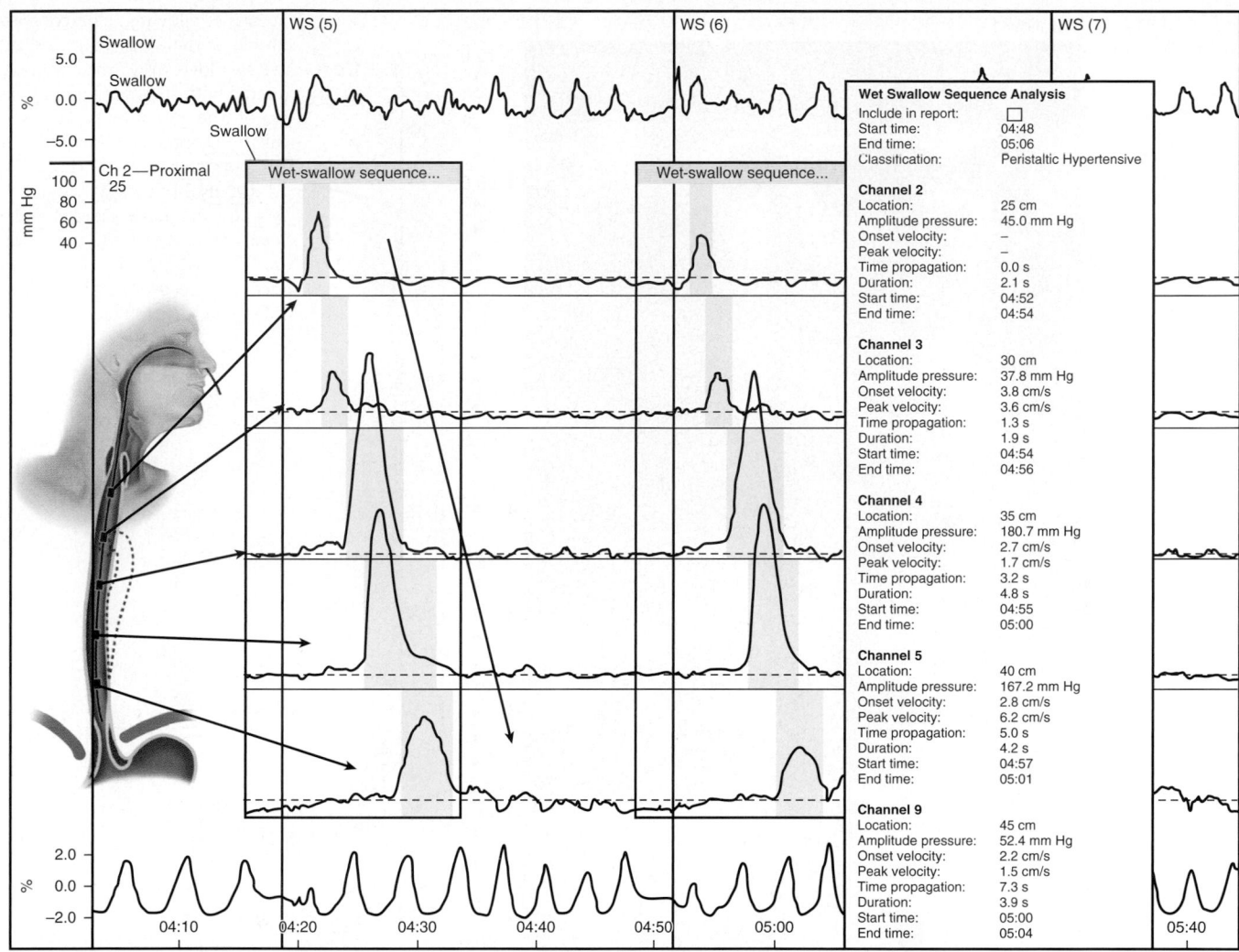

FIGURE 9 Normal esophageal body study. The channels are positioned at 5-cm intervals. The values shown are calculated for each wet swallow.

TABLE I: Normal LES Parameters in 50 Healthy Volunteers

LES Measurements	Mean	SD	Median	Maximum	Minimum	Percentile 2.5	5
Pressure (mm Hg)	14.87	5.14	13.8	25.6	5.2	6.1	8
Abdominal length (cm)	2.18	0.72	2.2	5	0.8	0.89	1.1
Overall length (cm)	3.65	0.68	3.5	5.5	2.4	2.4	2.6

Zaninotto G, DeMeester TR, Schwizer W, et al. The lower esophageal sphincter in health and disease. *Am J Surg.* 1988;155:104-111.

LES, Lower esophageal sphincter; *SD,* standard deviation.

However, these pressure measurements are displayed as a topographic pressure reading over time. A typical scan of a high-resolution swallow in achalasia is shown in Figure 10. This figure also shows impedance in magenta, as the catheter used included impedance monitoring. Figures 5 and 10 are also examples of high-resolution manometry.

Despite HRM providing more details of esophageal motility and ushering in the new era of the Chicago Classifications, it also has its limitations. (1) The Chicago classification is limited to those abnormalities or diagnoses detected by HRM with abnormalities of the UES, for example, not incorporated. (2) It is more expensive than traditional manometry in an era in which healthcare costs are an increasing concern. (3) HRM seems not to be applicable to nonobstructive dysphagia. (4) Although normative values do exist, there is still not a long enough experience to account for the myriad variables involved in diagnosing subtle differences between normal and abnormal in all patients.

Diagnostic Tests for Gastroesophageal Reflux

A surgeon performing a procedure for GERD should order four principal tests before performing a fundoplication or hiatal hernia

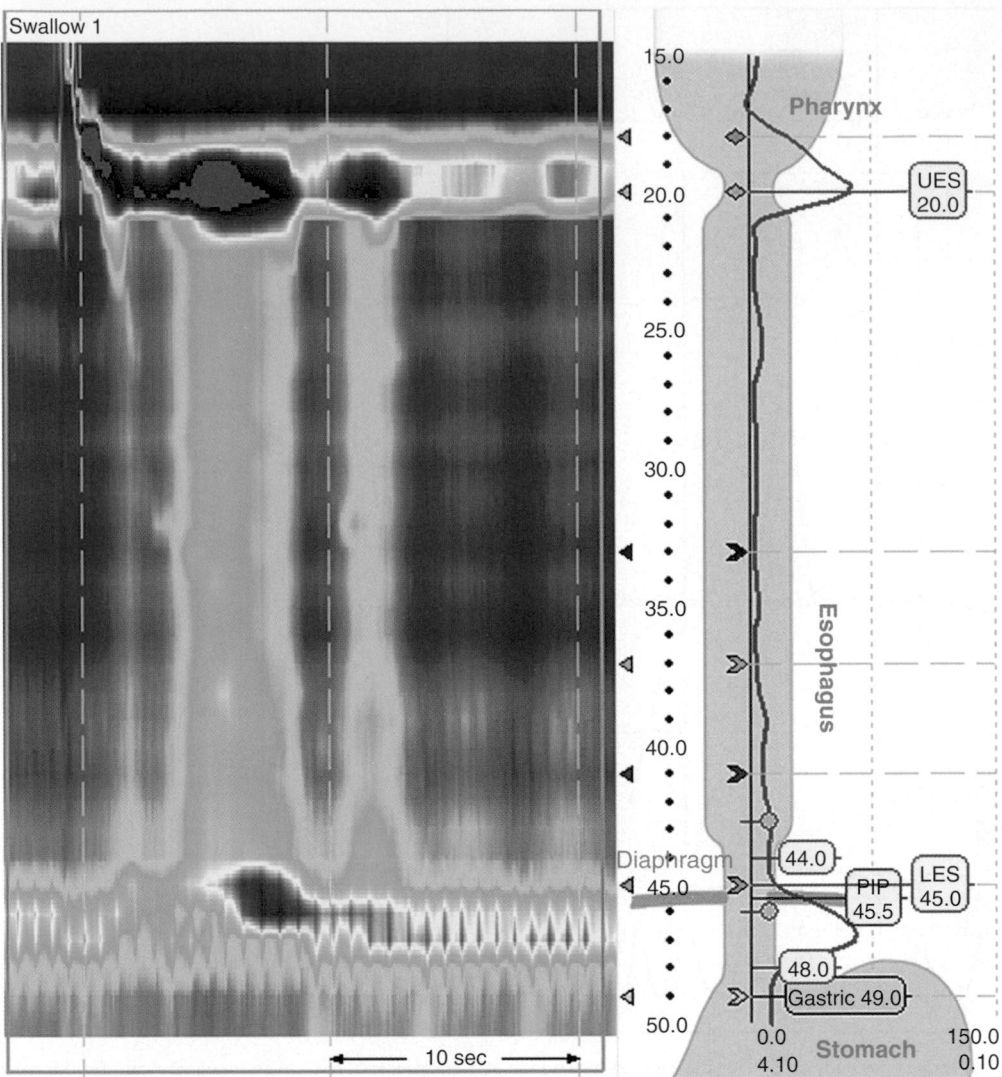

FIGURE 10 High-resolution manometry in a patient with achalasia. Note the simultaneous contractions and lack of swallow propagation. The lower esophageal sphincter is not hypertensive, but complete relaxation is not seen. *LES,* lower esophageal sphincter; *PIP,* pressure inversion point; *UES,* upper esophageal sphincter.

repair. First, an acid exposure test is used to document the presence of reflux because many patients with heartburn do not actually have GERD. Second, manometry is essential to ensure that esophageal dysmotility is not contributing to reflux as patients with dysmotility may not be able to clear physiologic reflux. Surgeons must be careful when operating on patients with documented GERD and impaired motility because postoperative dysphagia can be a significant problem. A partial fundoplication or a floppy complete fundoplication may prevent dysphagia in these patients. Third, a barium swallow helps with identification of the presence and size of a hiatal hernia and may alert the surgeon to the presence of a short esophagus. A tension-free intra-abdominal GEJ at the end of the procedure is imperative, and a variety of esophageal lengthening procedures can be used if necessary. Finally, an EGD should be performed to rule out malignant disease and to identify Barrett's esophagus in patients with severe GERD. We typically perform the EGD in the operating room at the same setting as the procedure.

Acid exposure in the esophagus is measured with an intraluminal pH probe with one of two methods: either an intraluminal tube with a nasopharyngeal catheter or a wireless Bravo pH probe (Medtronic, Minneapolis, MN). Both methods provide the physician with similar data, particularly relating to the amount of time the esophagus is

BOX 2: Measured Parameters During 24-Hour Esophageal pH Monitoring

1. Percent total time pH <4
2. Percent upright time pH <4
3. Percent supine time pH <4
4. Number of reflux episodes
5. Number of reflux episodes ≥5 minutes
6. Longest reflux episode (in minutes)

exposed to acid reflux. When the information is correlated with a symptom log, determination is possible of whether the patient's symptoms are related to acid exposure within the esophagus. This information is commonly expressed with use of six standard parameters (Box 2) to calculate a DeMeester score, or a composite pH score. A score of less than 14.72 (95th percentile of normal) is considered physiologic reflux, whereas a score greater than 14.72 is considered abnormal. Acid exposure in the esophagus may be physiologic, and it is recorded according to the position of the patient (supine or

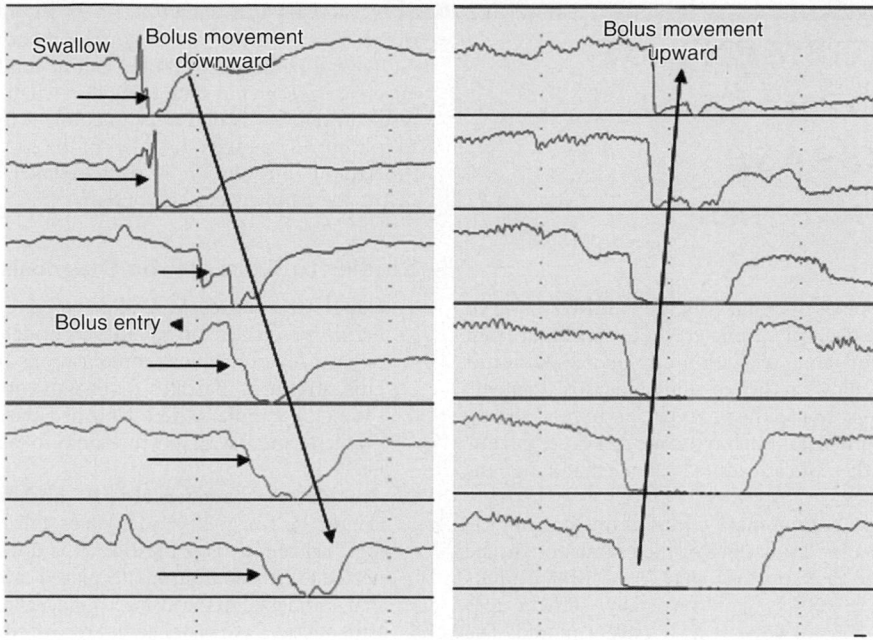

FIGURE 11 Impedance study showing antegrade and retrograde movements of a swallowed bolus.

upright) and the relation of acid exposure to meals. pH monitoring also may be used while the patient is on acid-suppressing therapy to determine whether there is adequate acid suppression with the current medication regimen. The data collected from each individual's tests are compared with normal values derived from data from healthy volunteers. The Bravo probe often is preferred by patients for pH monitoring because it is placed at the time of upper endoscopy and does not require an extended time with a nasopharyngeal catheter. The Bravo probe is placed 5 cm above the LES and wirelessly transmits data to a recorder worn by the patient. It measures ph for 48 hours while a wired probe is worn for 24 hours, which gives a larger sampling of pH changes in the esophagus and is more accurate.

Esophageal Impedance

Impedance monitoring measures bolus transport by measuring the resistance to electrical conductivity of the esophagus and its contents. Impedance testing is an important adjunct to traditional pH testing because it can be useful for patients taking PPIs and for evaluation of bile (nonacid) reflux. Impedance measurement works by using low AC voltage to apply an electrical potential between two electrodes on a catheter separated by an isolator. The circuit then is closed by the surrounding material spanning the electrodes. Because air, liquid, and esophageal mucosa have unique impedance characteristics, identification of the material that is bridging the electrodes is easy. Air is resistant to current flow and has a high impedance; liquid has a low impedance value. Esophageal tissue has an indeterminate range and is used as a baseline during monitoring. With multiple electrodes along a catheter system, identification of changes in impedance makes possible determination of the direction of bolus transport within the esophagus and identification of reflux of a bolus that has cleared the esophagus but comes back up from the stomach (Figure 11).

Multichannel intraluminal impedance (MII) is a new technology that incorporates impedance transducers for pressure measurement and a pH probe in one catheter. As a result, MII is used for the same indications as esophageal manometry and for detection and measurement of acid and nonacid reflux.

■ SUMMARY

The diagnosis of esophageal function disorders can be made from a careful history and the use of appropriate diagnostic testing. Several tests frequently are needed for the thorough evaluation of these disorders. Surgeons must understand the utility of these tests to evaluate whether a patient is a good surgical candidate for intervention and to determine the best treatment for a particular patient. A surgeon who is not familiar with these tests is not able to achieve optimal outcomes in the management of complex esophageal disorders. We also stress the importance of close collaboration between the radiologist, gastroenterologist, and surgeon in evaluating and treating this complicated group of patients.

■ ACKNOWLEDGMENTS

We recognize Philip W. Carrott, Jr., MD, James A. Mann, MD, and Benjamin D. Kozower, MD, MPH, Vinay Chandrasekhara, MD, and Sanjay Jagannath, MD, the authors of this chapter in the tenth and eleventh editions, as we have revised and updated their excellent work.

SUGGESTED READINGS

de Bortoli N, Martinucci I, Bertani L, et al. Esophageal testing: what we have so far. *World J Gastrointest Pathophysiol*. 2016;7:72-85.

Hamer PW, Holloway RH, Crosthwait G, et al. Update in achalasia: what the surgeon needs to know. *ANZ J Surg*. 2016 Mar 18.

Kahrilas PJ, Bredenoord AJ, Fox M, et al. The Chicago Classification of esophageal motility disorders, v3.0. *Neurogastroenterol Motil*. 2015;27:160.

Moore M, Afaneh C, Benhuri D, et al. Gastroesophageal reflux disease: A review of surgical decision making. *World J Gastrointest Surg*. 2016;8: 77-83.

Pandolfino JE, Gawron AJ. Achalasia: a systematic review. *J Am Med Assoc*. 2015;313:1841-1852.

THE MANAGEMENT OF GASTROESOPHAGEAL REFLUX DISEASE

Abbas El-Sayed Abbas, MD, MS, FACS

Patients with gastroesophageal reflux disease (GERD) have an incompetent lower esophageal sphincter (LES), resulting from transient relaxation, permanent relaxation, or increased intra-abdominal pressure. This allows reflux of duodenogastric contents into the esophagus and possibly also the pharynx, larynx, and airway. Whether acidic, alkaline, or neutral, such refluxate can cause inflammatory changes at each of these sites, leading to all the manifestations of GERD.

GERD is one of the most common afflictions of the human race. In Western countries it affects 10% to 20% of the population. In the United States, it is estimated that approximately 7% to 10% of adults experience gastroesophageal reflux symptoms daily, 10% to 20% at least once weekly, and 25% to 45% at least once a month. The economic impact of this disease is significant with direct costs of almost $10 billion and indirect costs related to lost productivity of $75 billion.

Its impact on quality of life is no less devastating when untreated, refractory, or complicated (e.g., erosive esophagitis, stricture, aspiration, asthma, Barrett's esophagus, adenocarcinoma).

■ CLINICAL MANIFESTATIONS OF GASTROESOPHAGEAL REFLUX DISEASE

GERD generally is defined as the occurrence of symptoms and/or mucosal damage produced by the abnormal reflux of gastric contents into the esophagus. It is often a chronic and relapsing condition.

Certain risk factors are associated with increased incidence of GERD, including obesity, hiatal hernia, pregnancy, delayed gastric emptying, and connective tissue disorders.

A degree of "physiologic" reflux is normal and is characteristically postprandial, asymptomatic, and not nocturnal. On the other hand, GERD typically is characterized by symptoms which are often nocturnal or while supine and may be associated with mucosal injury.

Symptoms of GERD can be classified as typical (esophageal), atypical (extraesophageal), and those of complications (alarms).

Typical esophageal symptoms include burning chest pain (pyrosis aka heartburn), regurgitation of sour or tasteless fluid into the mouth (water brash), sensation of a lump, or tightness in the throat (globus sensation), and pain on swallowing (odynophagia).

Atypical extraesophageal symptoms are due to irritation of structures other than the esophagus and include cough, wheezing, hoarseness, sore throat, postnasal drip, dental erosion, and ear pain. When these symptoms occur in the absence of typical ones, the condition is also called *silent reflux*. Patients with such manifestations should be evaluated by laryngoscopy and pH testing for possible laryngeal pharyngeal reflux.

Alarm symptoms can alert to the presence of complications and include dysphagia, early satiety, hematemesis, melena, vomiting, and weight loss. These may be sentinels of erosive esophagitis, strictures, or cancer and should be investigated aggressively.

■ DIAGNOSIS AND PREOPERATIVE EVALUATION

Symptom-based diagnosis of reflux disease has a sensitivity and specificity of only about 60% each. Despite this, if classic symptoms in the absence of the "alarm symptoms" exist, medical treatment for GERD can be initiated. Proton pump inhibitor (PPI) therapy is so effective in resolving symptoms that when such treatment does not result in relief, it is necessary to confirm the presence of reflux and to rule out any motility disorders of the esophagus or stomach. When procedural intervention is contemplated, it is also important to define the esophagogastric anatomy.

Studies to Confirm the Diagnosis

1. **Upper GI endoscopy:** Endoscopy is useful to identify a hiatal hernia, predict a short esophagus, or detect other esophagogastric disease. It can diagnose complications of GERD such as esophagitis, strictures, Barrett's esophagus, or cancer. The endoscopist should be familiar with established classifications for esophagitis (Table 1) and have a low threshold to take appropriate biopsies as needed.

2. **Ambulatory esophageal pH and impedance monitoring (Figure 1):** The gold standard in establishing a diagnosis of pathologic acid reflux is pH testing. It is done using a pH sensor connected to either a transnasally placed catheter or a wireless capsule that is attached to the distal esophageal mucosa during endoscopy. Patients eat a normal diet and record time of symptoms. A reflux episode is defined when the esophageal pH drops below 4. With PPI therapy, some patients actually may suffer from weak acid or non–acid reflux symptoms. This may not be apparent by pH testing and for this reason, multichannel intraluminal impedance (MII) is employed to allow the detection of any intraesophageal bolus reflux. After a period of at least 24 hours, the sensor is removed and the tracing is computer analyzed with the results expressed using standard parameters.

Studies to Rule Out Motility Disorders

1. **Esophageal manometry:** The presence or absence of esophageal dysmotility is of utmost importance in evaluating patients who are not improving on medical treatment or are being considered for surgery. The value of esophageal manometry is to rule out alternate diagnoses, which may mimic GERD in symptomatology such as achalasia. Another benefit is to accurately define the location of the LES while placing the pH probe. Finally, it is important when deciding on the type of fundoplication; total versus partial. Patients with esophageal dysmotility may be at more risk for dysphagia, regurgitation, and heartburn after a total fundoplication as opposed to a partial one.

2. **High-resolution esophageal manometry (HREM)** uses numerous longitudinally and radially distributed sensors on the catheter, which allow for simultaneous pressure readings of the entire esophagus and sphincters and the ability to create a three-dimensional plot of the esophageal pressures.

3. **Gastric scintigraphy:** A standardized meal tagged with ^{99m}Tc sulfur colloid is ingested and images are acquired to calculate the residual radiolabeled meal in the stomach at 2 hours (normal <60%) and at 4 hours (normal <10%). Delayed gastric emptying (gastroparesis) can cause or exacerbate symptoms of GERD. It is important to identify this *before* surgery because it is difficult to differentiate an iatrogenic vagal nerve injury from preexisting gastroparesis. Also, when diagnosed preoperatively, pyloric drainage such as pyloromyotomy or pyloroplasty can be added to the procedure, and the patient can be counseled regarding the higher likelihood of gas bloat syndrome after fundoplication.

Studies to Define the Anatomy

Once the decision is made to proceed with antireflux surgery (ARS), it is important to determine the anatomy of the esophagus and stomach. In addition to endoscopy, imaging studies allow the surgeon

TABLE 1: The Los Angeles Classification of Esophagitis

Grade A	One (or more) mucosal break no longer than 5 mm that does not extend between the tops of two mucosal folds
Grade B	One (or more) mucosal break more than 5 mm long that does not extend between the tops of two mucosal folds
Grade C	One (or more) mucosal break that is continuous between the tops of two or more mucosal folds but which involve less than 75% of the circumference
Grade D	One (or more) mucosal break which involves at least 75% of the esophageal circumference

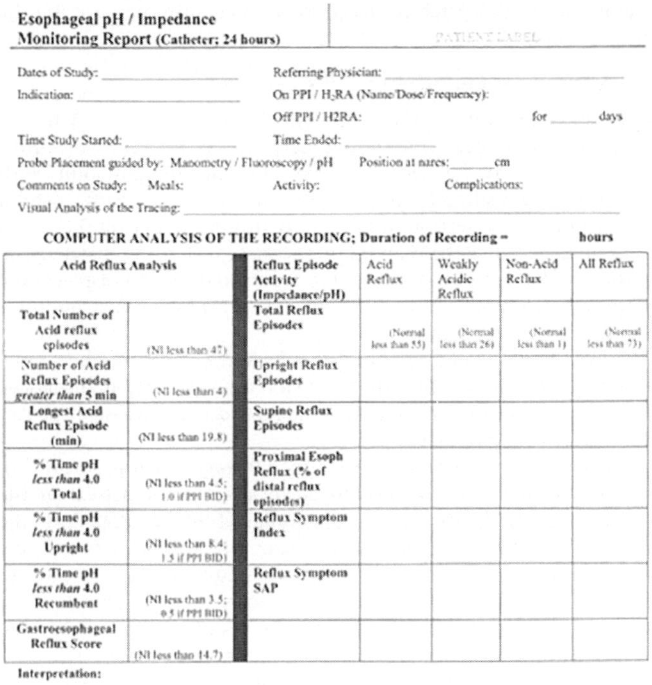
Esophageal pH / Impedance Monitoring Report (Catheter; 24 hours)

PATIENT LABEL

Dates of Study: ______ Referring Physician: ______

Indication: ______ On PPI / H_2RA (Name/Dose/Frequency):

Off PPI / H2RA: for ______ days

Time Study Started: ______ Time Ended: ______

Probe Placement guided by: Manometry / Fluoroscopy / pH Position at nares: ______ cm

Comments on Study: Meals: Activity: Complications:

Visual Analysis of the Tracing: ______

COMPUTER ANALYSIS OF THE RECORDING; Duration of Recording = hours

Acid Reflux Analysis		Reflux Episode Activity (Impedance/pH)	Acid Reflux	Weakly Acidic Reflux	Non-Acid Reflux	All Reflux
Total Number of Acid reflux episodes	(Nl less than 47)	Total Reflux Episodes	(Normal less than 55)	(Normal less than 26)	(Normal less than 1)	(Normal less than 73)
Number of Acid Reflux Episodes *greater than* 5 min	(Nl less than 4)	Upright Reflux Episodes				
Longest Acid Reflux Episode (min)	(Nl less than 19.8)	Supine Reflux Episodes				
% Time pH *less than* 4.0 Total	(Nl less than 4.5; 1.0 if PPI BID)	Proximal Esoph Reflux (% of distal reflux episodes)				
% Time pH *less than* 4.0 Upright	(Nl less than 8.4; 1.5 if PPI BID)	Reflux Symptom Index				
% Time pH *less than* 4.0 Recumbent	(Nl less than 3.5; 0.5 if PPI BID)	Reflux Symptom SAP				
Gastroesophageal Reflux Score	(Nl less than 14.7)					

Interpretation:

FIGURE 1 Chart with typical format for reporting a combined multichannel intraluminal pH/impedance study.

to plan the operation beforehand. An upper gastrointestinal series (UGIS) is a double-contrast barium esophagogastrogram followed by videofluoroscopic evaluation. It can assess the presence and size of a hiatal hernia, the presence of a short esophagus, esophagogastric dysmotility, and even the presence of reflux. It is important, however, to remember that this test is just a snapshot of the overall picture and cannot be used to establish or rule out the diagnosis of reflux or dysmotility.

MANAGEMENT

Management of patients with symptoms of GERD, as previously mentioned, usually is begun with an empirical medical therapeutic trial. This involves lifestyle modifications and once-daily PPI therapy. When this treatment is not effective, it is important to proceed with a diagnostic workup to establish the diagnosis and rule out complications. This entails endoscopy, pH/impedance ambulatory testing, and

BOX 1: Indications for Surgical Treatment

Failed medical management
Patient preference
GERD complications
Contraindication to PPI therapy, osteoporosis
Lung transplant patients or candidates with GER
Medical complications attributable to a large hiatal hernia
Atypical symptoms with reflux documented on 24-hour pH monitoring

GER, Gastroesophageal reflux; *GERD,* gastroesophageal reflux disease; *PPI,* proton pump inhibitor.

HREM. Once the diagnosis is confirmed, the PPI dosage can be increased and given twice daily in addition to adding nighttime HRA to the regimen.

Medical management is so effective in symptom control that it is rare for a patient who is fully complying with it to have a relapse unless there is an error in diagnosis or a complication such as stricture or cancer. However, there are many reasons why a patient may not be able to continue this therapy. It is extremely difficult to maintain the rigorous and demanding changes a "lifestyle modification" requires, such as abstaining from certain foods, losing weight, and avoiding stress. Numerous reports also have shown evidence of long-term adverse effects of PPI therapy on bone density, which is a concern for older patients who may have osteoporosis or younger ones who can expect a cumulative effect of lifelong therapy. Some may find the cost of medication prohibitive or may simply desire to be medication free. Finally, despite the high efficacy of maximal medical management, some patients with a clear diagnosis do fail.

When medical therapy cannot be continued, consideration is given for ARS. A complete workup (as outlined earlier) then is undertaken by a multidisciplinary team that should include an experienced foregut surgeon, an esophagogastrologist, an esophageal radiologist, otorhinolaryngologist, and pulmonologist. A final discussion among this team before surgery is important in reassuring the patient and referring physicians on the diagnosis and management plan.

Indications and Contraindications of Antireflux Surgery

Indications for antireflux surgery (ARS) are failure of therapy, the presence of complications despite therapy, the presence of silent GER (atypical symptoms), or the desire to discontinue therapy (Box 1). Evidence suggests that patients with typical symptoms that are worse when supine and who have had a good response to PPIs tend to have a better response to ARS.

In addition, certain patient populations with established GERD should be considered earlier for ARS, including those with a large hiatal hernia, those with risk of osteoporosis, children with GERD-associated complications, and lung transplant candidates. The presence of GER after lung transplant has been associated with an increased risk of acute and chronic rejection and diminished graft survival. Evidence suggests a benefit to ARS in this group of patients if done either before or within 6 months of lung transplant.

The one absolute contraindication is medical inoperability because of any number of causes. However, ignoring the "relative contraindications" sets the patient and surgeon up for failure. These include surgeon (and multidisciplinary team) inexperience, a hostile abdomen because of previous major surgeries, and morbid obesity. Of course, patients with established esophageal cancer or high-grade dysplasia would not and should not be offered ARS unless done in addition to a definitive plan to treat the malignancy. Numerous reports have shown no benefit of ARS in preventing progression of dysplasia in Barrett's esophagus. However, such patients who have had successful endoscopic ablation or resection of their disease are indeed candidates for ARS.

Patients with morbid obesity should be advised to consider Roux-en-Y gastric jejunal bypass but not sleeve gastrectomy, which may worsen preexisting GERD and make its management extremely difficult. For those who do not desire weight loss surgery, which certainly can be associated with its own risks, ARS can be offered with the understanding that surgery tends to have a higher recurrence rate and less symptom control.

Surgical Technique

Antireflux surgical procedures have been performed for more than 70 years with the first published report by Belsey in 1955. Soon after, Nissen described circumferential gastric fundoplication with anterior gastropexy. Later, Dor reported on transabdominal anterior fundoplication in 1962, Toupet on posterior fundoplication in 1963, and Hill on posterior gastropexy in 1967. Regardless of the name of the procedure, they all offer comparable and excellent relief and share the same basic principles:

1. Reduction of any hiatal hernia
2. Tension-free restoration of the intra-abdominal esophagus
3. Approximation of the diaphragmatic hiatal crura
4. Performance of a fundoplication (except the Hill repair, which does not include one)

Much debate has been made over several concepts of surgical management:

- Whether the fundoplication should be total or partial
- Whether the operation should be done through the chest or through the abdomen
- Whether the operation should be open or minimally invasive
- Whether the hiatus should be repaired primarily or with mesh
- Whether the esophagus needs a lengthening procedure

Each of these options may at times be necessary, and a foregut surgeon should be familiar and comfortable with all of them. It is important to select the correct and most appropriate approach after a thorough evaluation to ensure the most optimal outcome for the patient.

Deciding on the Type of Fundoplication

Several randomized trials of total versus partial fundoplication have shown that overall symptomatic relief, patient satisfaction, quality of life measures, and long-term outcomes are fairly equivalent between the two procedures, whereas side effects such as postoperative dysphagia and gas bloating are less common with partial fundoplication. My approach is to perform total fundoplication except in cases with significant esophageal dysmotility or weak peristalsis.

Deciding on the Approach

The advantages of the abdominal approach include the ability to explore for other causes of abdominal pain and to perform additional procedures such as pyloric drainage or vagotomy. They also include better general surgeon familiarity with the abdomen and less pain compared with a thoracotomy.

The advantages of the thoracic approach are several. In obese patients, because of the paucity of intrathoracic fat, the exposure of the hiatus is usually simple. In addition, creating a Collis gastroplasty for a "short esophagus" is much simpler in the chest. This is also true for very large hiatal hernias. Finally, a thoracotomy is an excellent option for a patient with a hostile abdomen resulting from multiple previous open abdominal surgeries. The most common approach is by left thoracotomy.

Despite the benefits of open surgery in regard to exposure, ability to palpate, and surgeon control, there is little doubt that laparoscopy is better tolerated than open surgery as evidenced by numerous randomized trials demonstrating less pain, shorter hospital stay, and faster recovery with equivalent antireflux efficacy.

For these reasons, laparoscopy has become the most common approach to ARS.

Deciding on Whether to Use Mesh

Repairing the widened hiatus by approximating the diaphragmatic crural pillars is the bulwark to prevent future rehernation and recurrence. This repair becomes subjected to intra-abdominal pressures and is thus at risk for future failure. It therefore has been proposed to place a prosthetic mesh to reinforce this repair. The concern with this is the possibility of erosion and infection with potentially catastrophic results. A modification of this approach is to use biologic mesh reinforcement. A recent randomized trial demonstrated a significant reduction in the incidence of hernia recurrence when using biologic porcine small intestine submucosa at 6 months; but long-term follow-up revealed loss of this benefit. Another approach advocated by some is to create "release incisions" in the lateral diaphragm to allow a tension-free repair followed by patch repair of those incisions, away from the esophagus.

I prefer to use prosthetic mesh only if there is evidence of diaphragmatic attenuation or tension on the crural repair. This tends to be more common in cases with very large hernias. A polytetrafluoroethylene (PTFE) patch is placed in an onlay fashion, covering the primary repair.

Deciding on a Lengthening Procedure

The presence of a true "short esophagus" has been debated. Often, it is merely a result of a large sliding hiatal hernia. However, occasionally it also may be secondary to chronic inflammation with subsequent transmural fibrotic strictures. Almost always, careful paraesophageal dissection in the mediastinum can deliver 3 to 4 cm of esophagus below the diaphragmatic hiatus without tension. Also, closure of the crura from a caudal to cephalad direction displaces the hiatus anteriorly and more cephalad, creating a longer intraabdominal esophageal segment.

When these maneuvers fail to create sufficient intra-abdominal esophageal length, which is the key to a tension-free repair, it may be necessary to perform a "lengthening procedure." Two such procedures have been popularized.

Collis gastroplasty was first described through a left thoracotomy. A linear stapler is introduced to create a 4- to 5-cm tube of the proximal stomach after passing a bougie (48F to 50F) into the stomach and holding it against the lesser curvature. A laparoscopic modification has been described using a circular stapler (35-mm) to create a "buttonhole" in the stomach adjacent to the bougie. A linear stapler then is passed into this buttonhole and fired parallel to the bougie toward the angle of His, creating a neoesophagus. The neofundus then is brought as either a total or partial fundoplication around this neoesophagus. Because the gastric tube still contains acid-secreting mucosa, there is concern for ongoing acid reflux, especially in patients with Barrett's esophagus. Also, when done for a failed Nissen fundoplication in which the short gastric vessels were previously divided, the proximal end of the Collis gastroplasty or fundus may become ischemic, predisposing to leak or stricture.

Another simpler approach is to create a transabdominal wedge gastrectomy, which consists of removing a triangular portion of the proximal gastric fundus. Once the short gastric vessels have been divided and the fundus is completely freed, a bougie is passed into the esophagus. A linear stapler then is fired across the fundus from the greater curve towards the lesser curve, just below the esophagogastric junction (EGJ) and just short of the bougie. A second firing of the stapler completes the wedge resection by firing adjacent and parallel to the bougie, creating a 4- to 5-cm neoesophagus. A fundoplication then is performed, using the remaining but smaller fundus, and care is taken to avoid making a wrap that is too tight.

Technique

Regardless of approach, the principles of ARP as outlined earlier must be followed. In general, the steps are the very similar and can be summarized as follows (Figures 2 through 7):

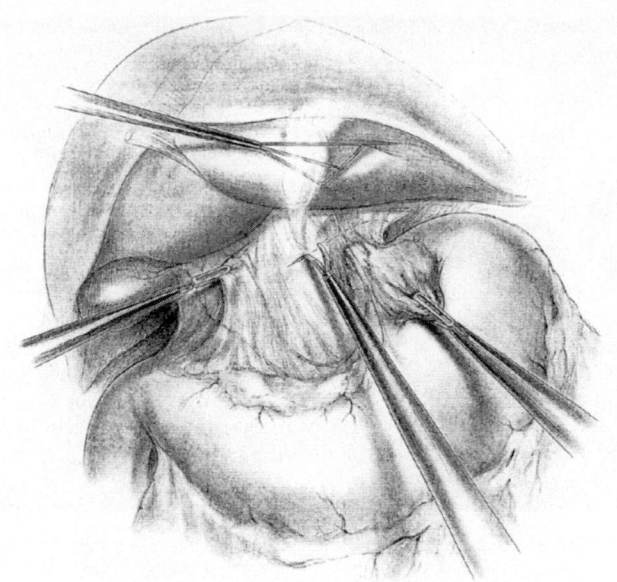

FIGURE 2 Division of gastrohepatic ligament. The dissection begins in the pars flaccida. *(From Soper NJ, Swanstrom LL, Eubanks WS, eds. Mastery of Endoscopic and Laparoscopic Surgery. 2nd ed. Philadelphia: Lippincott Williams & Wilkins; 2005:198.)*

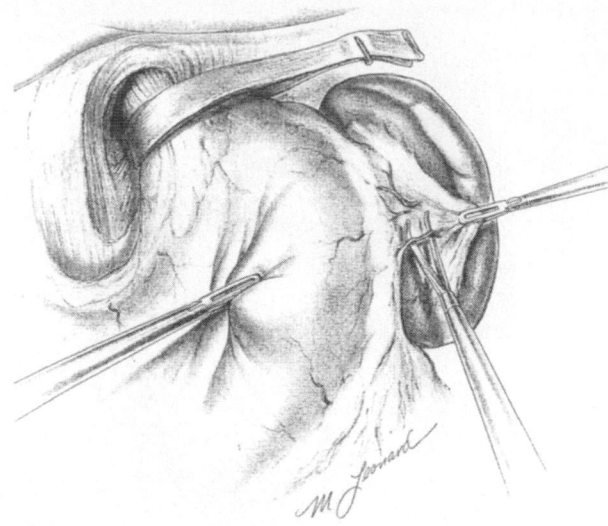

FIGURE 4 Division of gastrosplenic ligament. The division of the short gastric vessels allows for complete fundic mobilization. *(From Soper NJ, Swanstrom LL, Eubanks WS, eds. Mastery of Endoscopic and Laparoscopic Surgery. 2nd ed. Philadelphia: Lippincott Williams & Wilkins; 2005:199.)*

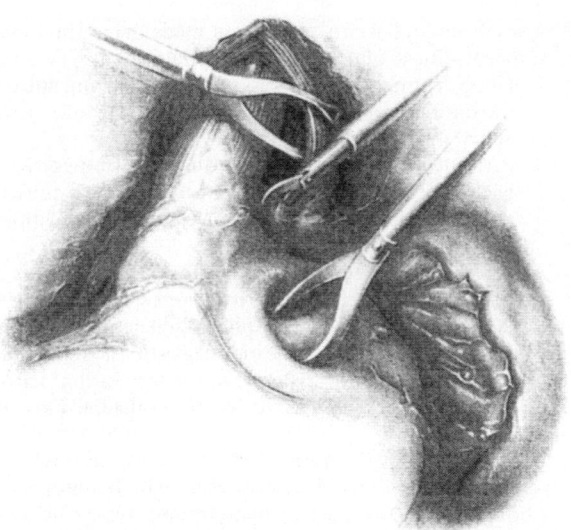

FIGURE 3 Dissection of left crus. The esophagus is gently retracted to the right using a blunt instrument.

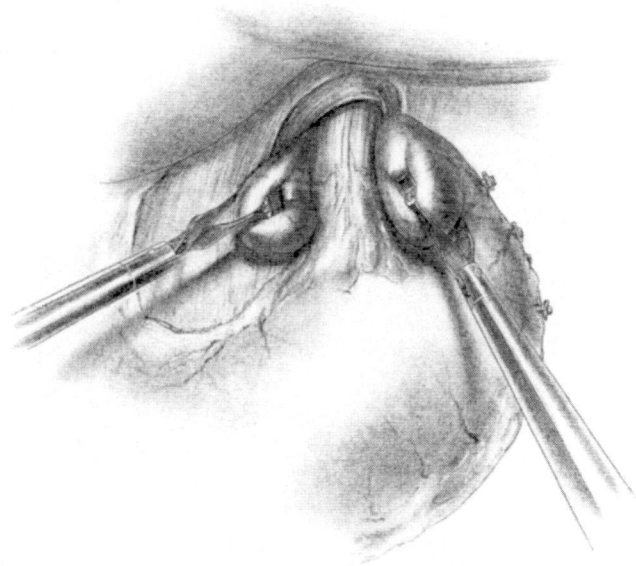

FIGURE 5 Performing the "shoeshine maneuver." This wrap is visualized before placement of sutures. *(From Soper NJ, Swanstrom LL, Eubanks WS, eds. Mastery of Endoscopic and Laparoscopic Surgery. 2nd ed. Philadelphia: Lippincott Williams & Wilkins; 2005: 200.)*

1. Mobilization of the EGJ and reduction of hiatal hernia:
   - The pars flaccida of the gastrohepatic ligament is divided. Care is taken to preserve any accessory (or rarely completely replaced) left hepatic artery, which may arise from the left gastric artery. However, if it impairs the positioning of the fundoplication, it may be divided and typically is of no consequence.
   - The right crus is identified and the phrenoesophageal ligament then is opened, mobilizing the anterior right crus away from the esophagus with careful blunt dissection. This dissection is carried anteriorly and circumferentially toward the left crus, ensuring that the anterior vagus nerve is identified and preserved. The hernia sac and EGJ fat pad are resected.
   - The greater omentum then is divided just below the spleen before dividing the short gastric vessels using an ultrasonic or bipolar electrosurgical instrument. The surgeon must stay about 1 cm off the greater curvature of the stomach to avoid thermal injury and delayed gastric necrosis.
   - The hiatus and both crura along with the posterior vagus nerve are identified posterior to the esophagus. Paraesophageal circumferential dissection is performed into the mediastinum until there is delivery of 3 to 4 cm into the abdomen without tension.
   - Approximation of the crura is then done using 3 to 4 nonabsorbable pledgeted sutures to recreate a hiatus that is nonobstructive (about 2 cm in diameter wider than the EGJ). Decision is made at this point regarding the use of onlay mesh.

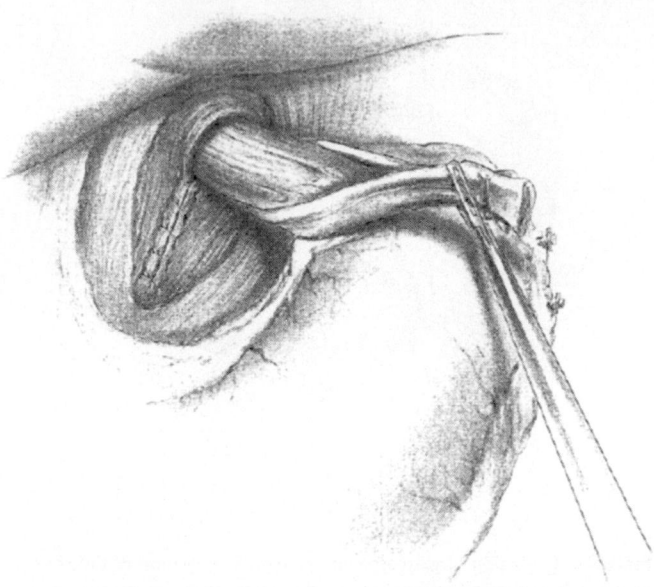

FIGURE 6 Closure of the crura. A posterior hiatal closure is performed with interrupted sutures. *(From Soper NJ, Swanstrom LL, Eubanks WS, eds. Mastery of Endoscopic and Laparoscopic Surgery. 2nd ed. Philadelphia: Lippincott Williams & Wilkins; 2005:200.)*

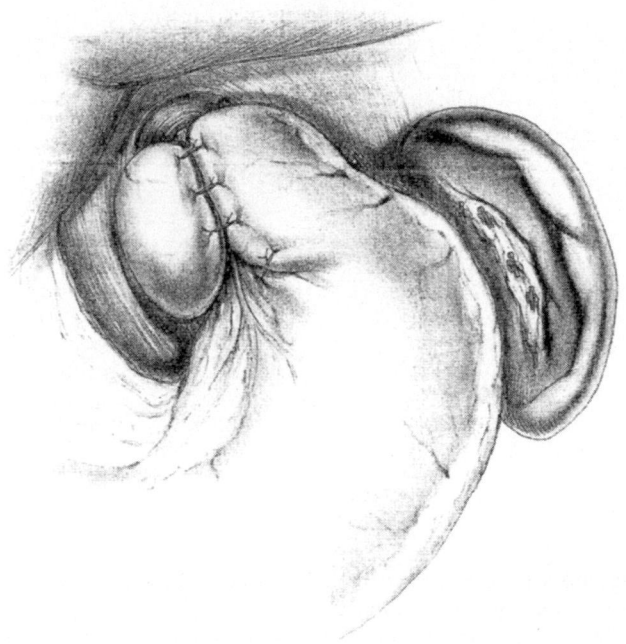

FIGURE 7 Completed fundoplication. The completed wrap lies to the right of the anterior midline. *(From Soper NJ, Swanstrom LL, Eubanks WS, eds. Mastery of Endoscopic and Laparoscopic Surgery. 2nd ed. Philadelphia: Lippincott Williams & Wilkins; 2005:201.)*

2. Creation of the fundoplication.
   ■ After ensuring sufficient fundic mobility, the surgeon then carefully grasps the gastric fundus and passes it behind and to the right of the esophagus, where it should remain in place after it is released. A fundus that retracts back when released is a sign that more dissection of the attachments to the spleen or diaphragm is still necessary.

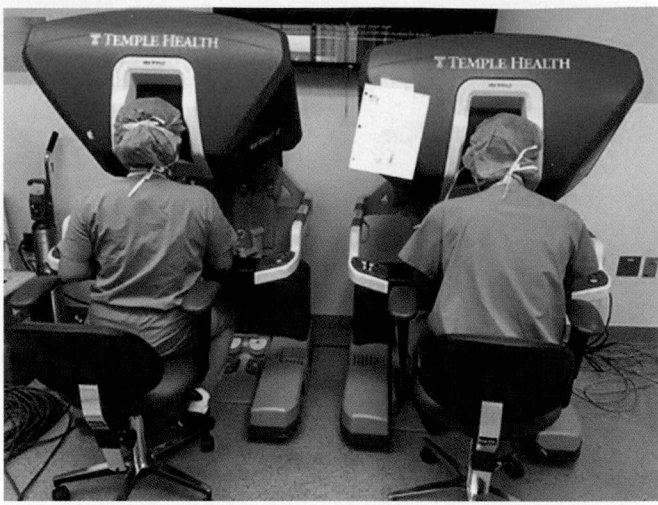

FIGURE 8 Completed Toupet fundoplication. *(Zucker KA. Surgical Laparoscopy. 2nd ed. Baltimore: Lippincott Williams & Wilkins; 2000:406.)*

■ A "shoeshine" maneuver then is performed by grasping both sides of the fundus, which then are pulled back and forth as if the back of the esophagus was the vamp of a shoe being shined. This helps to ensure proper orientation and tension.
■ A total fundoplication (Nissen) is made using three nonabsorbable sutures and fashioned as follows:
   1. Floppy enough to allow passage of an instrument between the fundus and the esophagus
   2. Short, only 2 to 3 cm in length
   3. Perfectly straddling the LES and not the stomach.
   4. Each stitch must incorporate the esophageal muscularis and the fundal seromuscular layer to prevent slipping of the wrap migration.
■ A posterior partial fundoplication (Toupet, Figure 8) is made by wrapping the fundus posteriorly and securing the fundus to the lateral wall of the esophagus bilaterally. Sutures are placed from the fundus to the esophagus on each side to create a 2- to 3-cm posterior 270-degree fundoplication. Each side of the fundus is also sutured to the ipsilateral crus of the diaphragm.
■ Some surgeons prefer to place a 50F to 56F bougie while fashioning the wrap to avoid making it too tight. In my experience, a bougie can distort the EGJ anatomy and create tension while manipulating the fundus. It also can cause an inadvertent esophagogastric perforation. I therefore prefer to perform the wrap in a floppy fashion without the use of a bougie.

Laparoscopy Technique

Laparoscopy has become the gold standard against which other procedures must be judged (Figures 9 through 12). Many surgeons prefer to stand between the abducted legs of the patient, who is placed in the lithotomy position, giving the surgeon a direct angle to the EGJ. Other surgeons stand on the patient's right side. The assistant stands at the patient's left, and two monitor screens are placed on both sides of the patient's head, eye level with both surgeon and assistant. The abdomen is insufflated to 15 mm Hg and a 10-mm, 30-degree endoscope is used. After port placement (Table 2), the patient is placed in reverse Trendelenburg position. The previous steps are then followed in the same order. When crural closure is performed, it is wise to decrease the pneumoperitoneum pressure to about 10 mm Hg to approximate the final anatomy after release of the pneumoperitoneum.

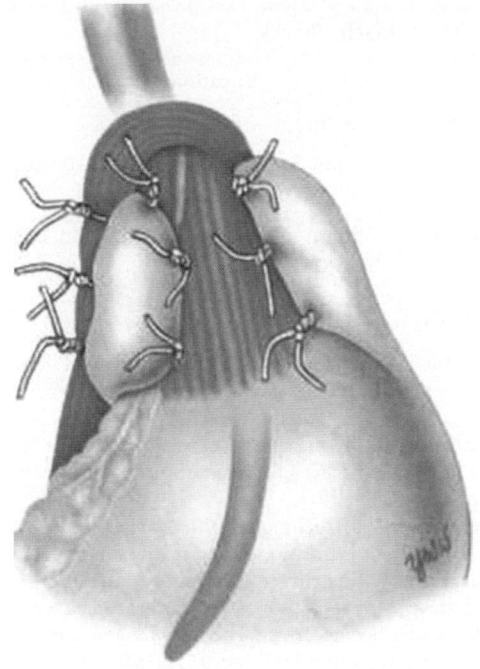

FIGURE 9 Partial wrap.

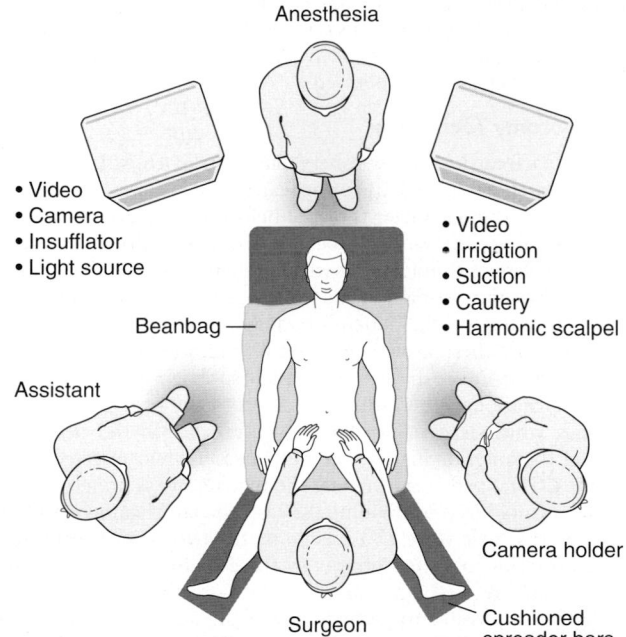

FIGURE 10 Layout of operating room. The surgeon is situated comfortably between the patient's legs. *(From Baker RJ, Fischer JE, eds. Mastery of Surgery. 4th ed. Philadelphia: Lippincott Williams & Wilkins; 2001:793.)*

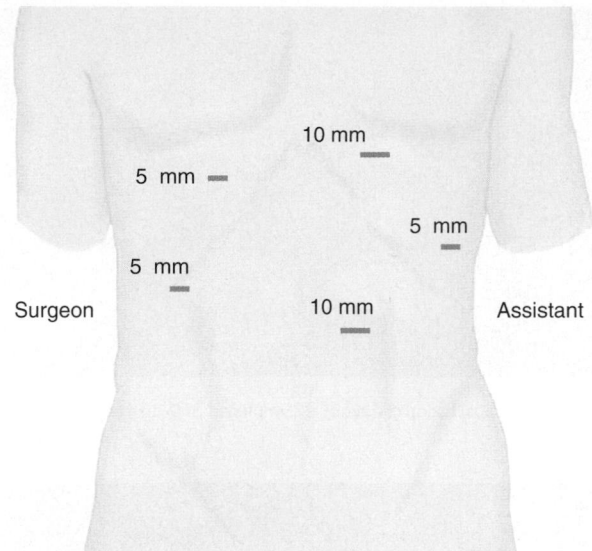

FIGURE 11 Port positioning for laparoscopic fundoplication.

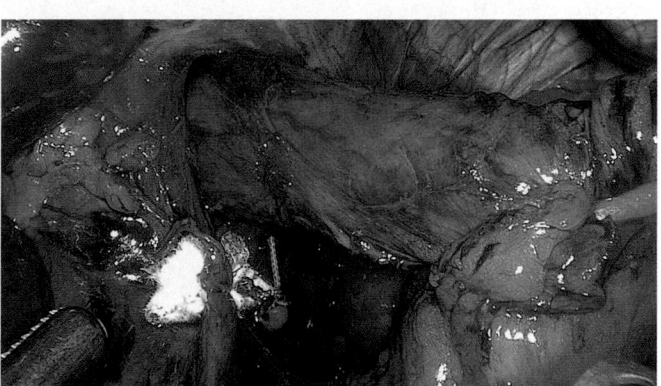

FIGURE 12 Laparoscopic closure of the diaphragmatic hiatus.

TABLE 2: Laparoscopy Ports

Function	Size	Location
Camera	10 mm	Midline supraumbilical
Surgeon's right hand	10 mm	Left subcostal, midclavicular line
Surgeon's left hand	5 mm	Right subcostal, midclavicular line
Assistant	5 mm	Left subcostal, anterior axillary line
Liver retractor	5 mm	Subxiphoid or right flank

Robotic-Assisted Laparoscopic Technique

The technical advantages of the da Vinci robotic system (Intuitive Surgical, Sunnyvale, CA) include the three-dimensional high-definition stereoscopic visualization with magnification and tremor eradication (Figures 13 through 15). They also include the wristed instruments, which facilitate the ability to perform complex dissection with precision and dexterity similar to that achieved with open surgery. The surgeon can direct the camera while simultaneously having two (or three) free hands to operate. With the use of a double console, it is also an excellent tool for teaching and training. During foregut procedures, this greatly facilitates access to the narrow mediastinum, delicate bimanual handling of the fundus, and precise placement of sutures for hiatal repair and fundoplication. It allows the ability to place square knots on the crura without needing

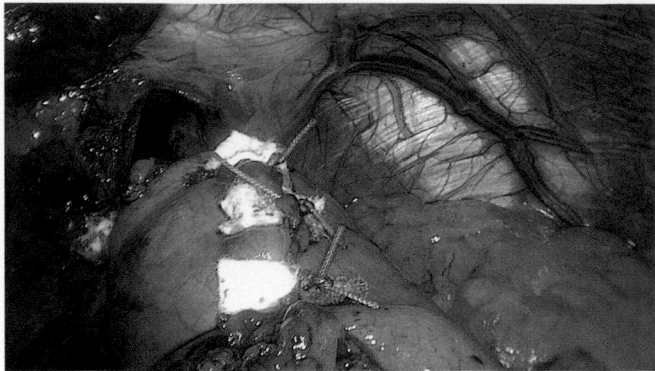

FIGURE 13 Laparoscopic view of a completed 360-degree fundoplication.

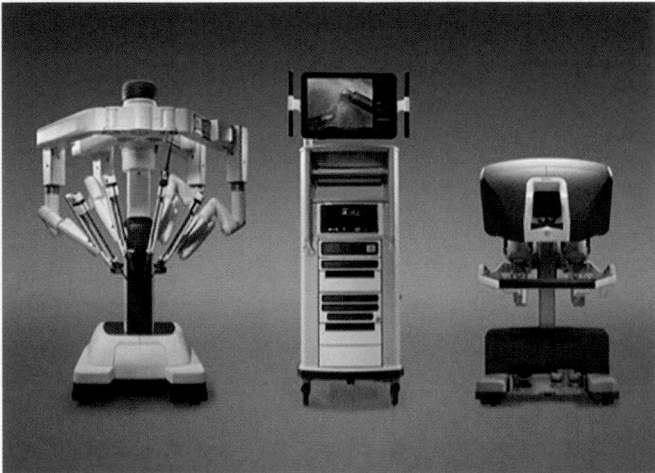

FIGURE 14 Port positioning for robotic-assisted fundoplication.

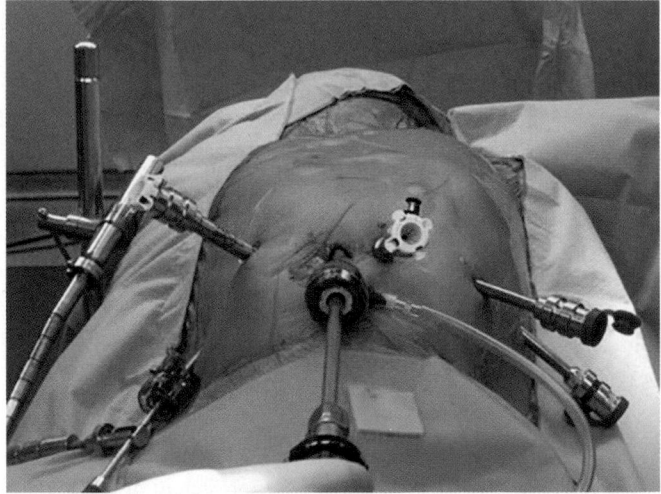

FIGURE 15 Port positioning for robotic-assisted fundoplication.

TABLE 3: Robotic Ports

Function	Size	Location
Assistant	10 mm	Above umbilicus
Camera	8 mm	Left paramedian, 10 cm from umbilicus.
Right Arm (#1)	8 mm	Right subcostal, midclavicular line
Left Arm (#2)	8 mm	Left subcostal, midclavicular line
Third arm (#3)	8 mm	Left flank, subcostal
Liver retractor	5 mm	Subxiphoid or right flank

robotically. In addition, with more experience by the surgeon and the team, operative times and costs approach those of standard laparoscopy.

We use a four-arm technique with ports placed 10 cm apart (Table 3). The patient is positioned supine in reverse Trendelenburg. Robotic articulating instruments are used, including a double-fenestrated grasper for retraction, a bipolar grasper, a wristed bipolar vessel sealer, and a needle driver. The bedside assistant suctions and delivers and removes suture and mesh. The same steps are followed as described earlier.

Laparotomy Technique

This usually is needed when laparoscopy is attempted but cannot be completed because of adhesions, technical difficulties, bleeding, or unexpected perforations. An upper midline laparotomy from the xiphoid process to the umbilicus is made. The left triangular ligament is divided, and the left lobe of the liver is retracted medially. The steps described earlier then are followed.

Thoracotomy Technique

This approach can be extremely helpful in cases of a hostile abdomen, a predicted short esophagus, or an extremely large diaphragmatic hernia. An epidural catheter is placed before general anesthesia, and a double-lumen endotracheal tube or left bronchial blocker is placed. A left dorsolateral thoracotomy with the patient in the right lateral decubitus position is made through the sixth or seventh intercostal space, depending on the patient's body habitus and position of the diaphragm on chest x-ray. The inferior pulmonary ligament and mediastinal pleura are divided. The distal esophagus is encircled with a Penrose drain and then dissected down to the phrenoesophageal ligament, which is divided allowing entrance into the peritoneal cavity at the anterior hiatus. The hernia sac is then resected along with the EGJ fat pad, ensuring that the vagus nerve is preserved. The stomach is mobilized by dividing the gastrohepatic ligament and the upper short gastric vessels. At this point, the two crura are approximated posterior to the esophagus by three or four interrupted silk sutures that are tied only after creation of the fundoplication. Although it is possible to perform any of the described fundoplications, the anterior 270-degee Belsey-Mark IV lends itself well to this approach, recreating the angle of His and reinforcing the LES. The proximal stomach is pulled up into the chest and three horizontal mattress sutures are placed 1 cm from the EGJ between stomach and esophagus to create the 270-degree wrap. A second row of sutures is then placed 1 cm proximal to the first row, including the diaphragm and tied down after reduction of the fundus into the abdomen. Finally, the sutures between the crura are tied, ensuring that the residual hiatus easily allows a finger to pass through.

■ POSTOPERATIVE CARE

After laparoscopic or robotic ARS, patients are admitted overnight. Intravenous ketorolac and acetaminophen are used in lieu of

extracorporeal knot-tying devices and greatly facilitates sewing of mesh to the overlying diaphragm with a running suture. These advantages are significant when performing reoperative ARS. No randomized studies have compared standard to robotic-assisted laparoscopy in ARS. Despite criticism of higher costs and operative times for the robotic procedure, it is my opinion that the technical benefits may increase the safety and accuracy of this operation when done narcotics. Nausea is treated with intravenous ondansetron. A naso-gastric tube is not used routinely unless indicated for severe nausea and vomiting. A barium esophagogastrogram is obtained the next morning to establish a baseline for any future comparison. Afterward, the patient begins consuming a soft diet and is discharged.

Patients stay on a soft diet for 6 weeks to allow for any surgery-related swelling to resolve. The medication list is reviewed carefully, PPIs are stopped, and all necessary pills are crushed if possible. They are advised to avoid undue straining such as heavy lifting, constipation, or coughing. Patients are followed closely to ensure compliance. Any onset of sudden chest pain or unexplained distress should be immediately evaluated with UGIS to rule out acute reherniation.

■ OUTCOME AND COMPLICATIONS

There is strong evidence of long-term success rate (both symptomatic and functional) of greater than 90% after first-time laparoscopic ARS. This is clearly superior to medical management. The rate of patients on PPI within 10 years of ARS is 5% to 25%, although only 20% to 30% of patients with "reflux-like" symptoms have positive pH studies.

In general, side effects are mild and transient, usually resolving within 4 to 6 weeks of surgery. During that time patients are advised to adhere to a soft and bland diet. However, persistent side effects may persist, including gas bloating, dysphagia, and GERD-like symptoms. Many of these complications of ARS, including postoperative dysphagia, gas-bloat syndrome, recurrence, and the need for reoperation, have been shown to be dependent on surgical experience.

■ **Dysphagia:** Patients commonly experience a mild but transient (<6 weeks) degree of dysphagia, but it may persist in 3% of patients. If dysphagia persists, further workup is warranted with UGIS and endoscopy. If it is secondary to an overtight wrap, not from slippage or reherniation, endoscopic dilation may resolve this problem and can be performed safely after 6 weeks from surgery.

■ **Gas bloat syndrome:** Fundoplication can impede the ability of the stomach to eliminate swallowed air by belching, leading to an accumulation of gas in the stomach and bowel. Symptoms include epigastric pain, inability to belch or vomit, early satiety, abdominal distension, and increased flatus. This is reported in up to 40% after total fundoplication but less after partial fundoplication. It is usually self-limiting within 6 weeks, and conservative treatment includes dietary restrictions and counseling to avoid aerophagia. If severe and persistent, endoscopic dilation should be attempted before consideration of surgical revision of fundoplication.

■ REOPERATIVE FUNDOPLICATION

Recurrence, persistence, or new development of symptoms after ARS is a challenging problem. This requires a thorough workup, including HREM, 24- to 48-hour pH/impedance testing, gastric emptying study, and UGIS to demonstrate reflux, identify any esophagogastric dysmotility, and rule out anatomic complications.

The causes for failure of surgery include the following:

1. **Recurrent GERD:** if documented in the absence of motility or anatomic complications may be treated medically or considered for revisional fundoplication
2. **Esophageal dysmotility:** either present before surgery or is a result of an obstructive wrap.
3. **Gastroparesis:** unless present before surgery, it may be a result of iatrogenic vagal injury. This may cause or exacerbate GER. Options include medical treatment (e.g., domperidone), pyloric Botox injection, gastric pacing, and pyloric drainage procedures.
4. **Anatomic failures** (Figure 16): The most common of these is a herniated wrap. Other complications include a slipped wrap, a disrupted wrap, paraesophageal hernia, a wrap that is too tight, and wrap that was erroneously placed on the stomach not the esophagus.

FIGURE 16 Pattern of failure of primary repair: four types of failure. **A,** Complete disruption; **B,** slipped Nissen; **C,** malpositioned wrap; **D,** transhiatal herniation. *(Reprinted from Hinder RA. Gastro-esophageal reflux disease. In: Bell RH Jr, Rikkers LF, Mulholland MW, eds. Digestive Tract Surgery: A Text and Atlas. Philadelphia: Lippincott-Raven Publishers, 1996:19, with permission.)*

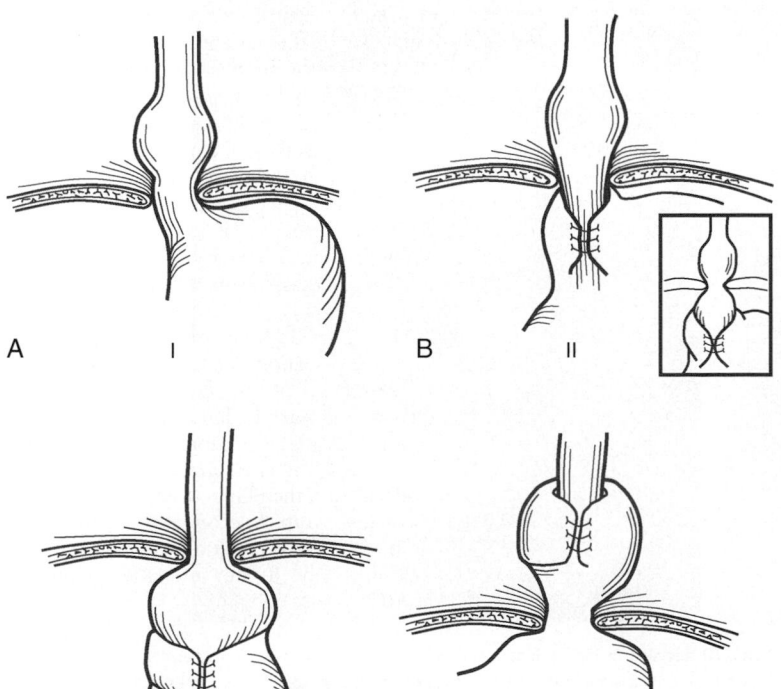

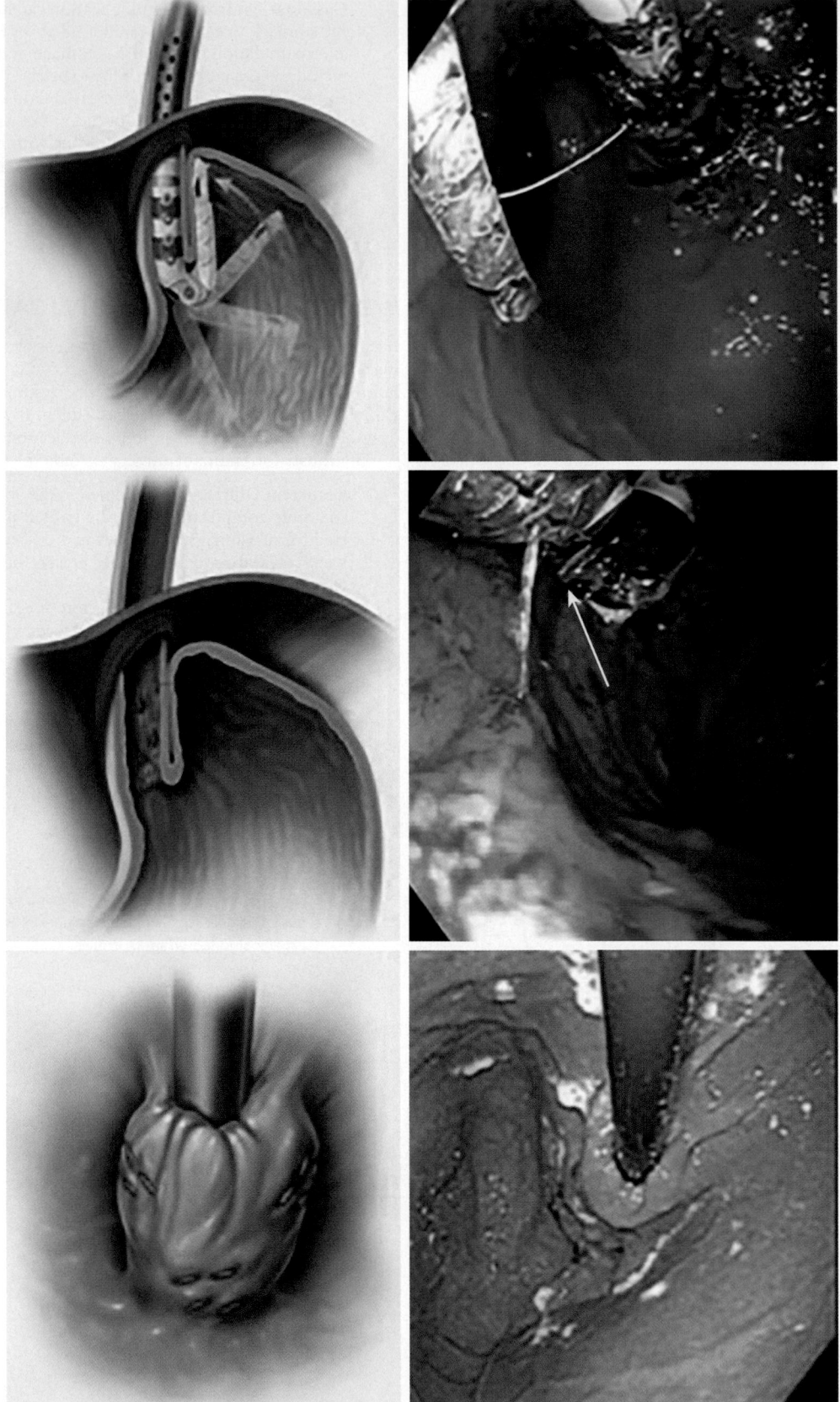

FIGURE 17 Transoral fundoplication creates a 3-cm flap valve, 180 to 270 degrees in circumference. *(Reprinted with permission from Hunter JG, et al. Efficacy of transoral fundoplication vs omeprazole for treatment of regurgitation in a randomized controlled trial. Gastroenterology. 2015;148:324-333.e5.)*

After LARS, the rate of revisional surgery is 3% to 7%. When the decision is made to consider this, several important points must be made:

1. Patients are counseled on both the risks and reduced expectations compared with initial ARS.
2. Not every patient with a failed fundoplication needs reoperation. Symptoms and complications must justify the risk.
3. Identification of the reason for failure. There is no role for "exploratory surgery" in this high stakes operation.
4. Consideration to refer the patient to a center with experience in reoperative foregut surgery.
5. Consideration for thoracotomy in cases of multiple prior laparotomies.
6. Consideration for pyloric drainage procedure in cases of associated gastroparesis.
7. A laparoscopic approach can be attempted with a low threshold to convert to laparotomy. Robotic-assisted laparoscopy offers a distinct advantage in reoperative ARS because it allows meticulous two-handed dissection with articulating instruments and superior visualization.

Technique

Dense adhesions frequently are found between the stomach and left lobe of the liver, which must be divided carefully to avoid gastrotomies, enterotomies, or esophagotomies. The previous fundoplication must be unwrapped completely. The hiatus is reinforced and mesh may be necessary especially in cases of rehernation. If 3 cm of esophagus cannot be reduced without tension into the abdomen, a lengthening procedure is done. Finally, a fundoplication is made.

■ EMERGING SURGICAL THERAPIES FOR GASTROESOPHAGEAL REFLUX DISEASE

Given the huge social and economic impact of a disease that affects a large portion of the population, emerging therapies remain an area of extensive research.

■ EsophyX (Endogastric Solutions, Redwood City, WA) creates an anterior partial fundoplication with endoscopically placed H-shaped fasteners made of polypropylene (Figure 17). Long-term functional data are not yet available.

■ Stretta (Mederi Therapeutics, Greenwich, CT) is an endoscopic device to induce heat-mediated remodeling of the lower esophageal sphincter by radiofrequency energy.
■ Linx (Torax Medical, Shoreview, MN) is a ring of magnetic beads, laparoscopically sized and placed around the EGJ to augment the LES. Although simpler than fundoplication, it is contraindicated in patients with a hiatal hernia greater than 3 cm, allergies to metals, or electrical implants and those who may require future MRIs.

More long-term data are needed before the efficacy of any of these devices can be compared with the current gold standard of laparoscopic fundoplication, a minimally invasive procedure that is extremely efficacious, extensively studied, and well tolerated.

SUGGESTED READINGS

Brown SR, Gyawali CP, Melman L, et al. Clinical outcomes of atypical extraesophageal reflux symptoms following laparoscopic antireflux surgery. *Surg Endosc.* 2011;25:3852-3858.

Katz PO, Gerson LB, Vela MF. Guidelines for the diagnosis and management of gastroesophageal reflux disease. *Am J Gastroenterol.* 2013;108:308-328, quiz 329.

Kilic A, Shah AS, Merlo CA, Gourin CG, Lidor AO. Early outcomes of antireflux surgery for United States lung transplant recipients. *Surg Endosc.* 2013;27:1754-1760.

Markar SR, Karthikesalingam AP, Hagen ME, Talamini M, Horgan S, Wagner OJ. Robotic vs. laparoscopic nissen fundoplication for gastro-oesophageal reflux disease: systematic review and meta-analysis. *Int J Med Robot.* 2010;6:125-131.

Oelschlager BK, Pellegrini CA, Hunter JG, et al. Biologic prosthesis to prevent recurrence after laparoscopic paraesophageal hernia repair: long-term follow-up from a multicenter, prospective, randomized trial. *J Am Coll Surg.* 2011;213:461-468.

Patcharatrakul T, Gonlachanvit S. Gastroesophageal reflux symptoms in typical and atypical GERD: roles of gastroesophageal acid refluxes and esophageal motility. *J Gastroenterol Hepatol.* 2014;29:284-290.

Peters MJ, Mukhtar A, Yunus RM, et al. Meta-analysis of randomized clinical trials comparing open and laparoscopic anti-reflux surgery. *Am J Gastroenterol.* 2009;104:1548-1561, quiz 1547, 1562. doi:10.1038/ajg.2009.176.

Skinner DB, Belsey RHR. Surgical management of esophageal reflux and hiatal hernia: long-term results with 1,030 cases. *J Thorac Cardiovasc Surg.* 1967;53:33-54.

Stefanidis D, Hope WW, Kohn GP, et al. Guidelines for surgical treatment of gastroesophageal reflux disease. *Surg Endosc.* 2010;24:2647-2669.

Yao G, Liu K, Fan Y. Robotic Nissen fundoplication for gastroesophageal reflux disease: a meta-analysis of prospective randomized controlled trials. *Surg Today.* 2014;44:1415-1423.

NEW APPROACHES TO GASTROESOPHAGEAL REFLUX DISEASE (LINX)

Tom R. DeMeester, MD

Between the early 1960s and early 1970s Drs. Rudolf Nissen, Ronald Belsey, and Lucius Hill introduced the golden era of antireflux surgery. These physicians designed procedures that took down a hiatal hernia, altered the anatomy of the gastroesophageal junction with a fundoplication of various degrees, and stopped reflux of gastric juice into the esophagus. In 1975 the first randomized controlled study confirmed the superiority of surgical over medical therapy with antacids. Surgery was off and running.

All came to a dramatic halt when the Nobel Prize was awarded to Sir James W. Black in 1988. He discovered an approach to drug development called *rational drug design structure.* Simply stated; if the pathophysiology of a disease is properly understood, a specific drug could be synthesized to interrupt key points in the pathogenesis and cure the disease. He used this concept to discover the beta and H2 receptor antagonists, propranolol and cimetidine. Cimetidine became the first drug ever to exceed $1 billion a year in sales. The methodology eventually led to the development of proton pump inhibitors (PPIs), which block the secretion of acid by the parietal cells. The aim of the drug was to increase the pH of the gastric juice, which along with the lower esophageal sphincter, were the two determinants of gastroesophageal reflux disease (GERD). By the 1980s the clinical benefits of PPIs were demonstrated dramatically by the abolishment of GERD symptoms and the virtual elimination of acid-induced reflux esophagitis, strictures, and giant Barrett's ulcers. Now medicine was off and running.

■ WHY A NEW SURGICAL ANTIREFLUX PROCEDURE?

After 35 years of experience with more than 20 million GERD patients on prescribed PPIs, physicians have developed some concerns. Despite the introduction and use of the new powerful acid-suppression drugs over this time period, the incidence of GERD continues to increase by 30% every 10 years, and 30% to 40% of patients on PPI therapy have only partial relief of their symptoms. Between 2% and 3.5% of the 20 million patients with GERD receiving PPI therapy develop Barrett's esophagus every year, of which 0.5% to 1% progress to esophageal adenocarcinoma. Despite this high percentage of patients with a partial response and disease progression on PPI therapy, less than 1% seek surgical therapy. These concerns have given rise to the thought that the time has come for a change in the treatment strategy of GERD. The current treatment strategy focuses only on one of the two determinants of the disease, the acid composition of the gastric juice, whereas the other determinant, failure of the lower esophageal sphincter (LES), is ignored. This focus on PPIs and disregard for the LES is likely the result of a historical misunderstanding that GERD is primarily an acid peptic disease. The primary abnormality in GERD is the loss of an effective LES to keep the gastric juice in the stomach. This was pointed out in 2003 in a unique publication by Dr. G. Wetscher and colleagues from Innsbruck, Austria. They showed that the recurrence of reflux symptoms and/or endoscopic esophagitis in patients on PPIs was related to the functional status of the LES and esophageal body. Patients with both a defective LES and esophageal contractions had an 80% recurrence rate compared with 39% in those patients with a defective LES and normal esophageal body contractions, or 8% in those with both a normal LES and normal esophageal contractions. They concluded that the status of the LES is a critical factor in the effectiveness of PPI therapy. The medication works well in patients with a normal LES and not so well in patients who have a defective LES. In the latter situation reflux episodes continue at the same frequency whether the patient is off or on the medication. The only difference is a change in the pH of the refluxed gastric juice. As a consequence, 85% of patients on PPIs still experience GERD-related symptoms, and in 35% the symptoms have reached the level to cause dissatisfaction with PPI therapy. In an effort to improve symptom control the prescriptions for double-dose PPIs has increased by 50% in the past 7 years, and 42% of patients supplement their prescription with other acid suppression medication in an effort to gain relief. Of greatest concern is that 10% to 15% of patients have progression of their disease while on PPI therapy, and the longer the disease persists the greater the number of patients who progress.

Over the past 35 years antireflux surgery has not fared much better. Even though the surgery can be performed through a laparoscope and achieve effective control of reflux symptoms and heal esophagitis, the outcomes vary in their effectiveness and durability, and the early surgical revision rate is too high. The procedures have significant side effects in that patients are unable to belch or vomit, risk having increased flatulence and postprandial bloating, and have a small possibility of bothersome dysphagia. When performed by the occasional surgeon, only 61% of patients are completely satisfied with their operation. These results discourage patients against antireflux surgery and at present less than 1% of GERD patients have surgical therapy. Unless there are some fundamental improvements in surgical therapy, it appears that the use of surgery for the treatment of GERD will reach a standstill.

■ NEW SURGICAL APPROACH TO GERD

The ideal surgical procedure to improve the function of the LES in a patient with GERD would be a minimally invasive, short, outpatient procedure that augments the LES function without causing anatomic alterations. Based on the effectiveness of the Nissen fundoplication it should have a greater than 80% probability of

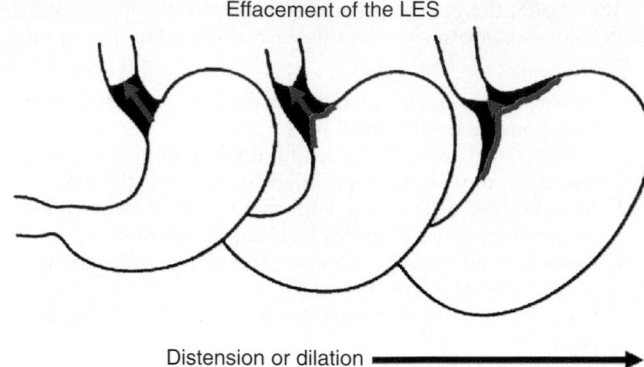

FIGURE 1 Effacement and shortening of the length of the lower esophageal sphincter (LES) that occurs with gastric distension or dilation after meals and, as a consequence, loss of its competency. The process exposes the effaced squamous mucosa of the distal esophagus *(red line)* and the underlying muscle of the LES *(black area below the red line)* to gastric juice.

normalizing esophageal acid exposure and a 90% probability of eliminating GERD-related symptoms. It should allow an unrestricted diet and cause no long-term side effects such as persistent dysphagia, symptomatic bloating, increased flatus, or the inability to belch or vomit. Further, it must be reversible without sequelae.

Over the past 10 years, studies on the pathophysiology of the LES have opened the door for technology to design a new device that meets the ideal requirement for a new surgical procedure for the treatment of GERD. These studies have shown that gastric distension or dilation after meals can cause effacement of the LES, resulting in progressive shortening of its length and, as a consequence, loss of its competency (Figure 1). This process exposes the effaced squamous mucosa of the distal esophagus and the underlying muscle of the LES to gastric juice. The inflammatory injury that occurs destroys the squamous mucosa, heals by the induction of metaplastic cardiac mucosa, and induces permanent damage to the muscle of the LES, resulting in a loss of its abdominal length, overall length, and pressure. The resulting structurally defective LES allows repetitive LES effacement to occur with ease, resulting in an escalation of the degrees of esophageal exposure to acidic bile containing gastric juice. Placing a loose ligature or ring around the inferior border of the LES can stop the effacement and has formed the basis for the design of new devices to augment LES function.

■ LINX ANTIREFLUX DEVICE

One of the new devices is the LINX Reflux Management System (Torax Medical, St. Paul, MN). It is a simple procedure, performed laparoscopically, that does not alter gastric or gastroesophageal junctional anatomy, augments the LES as a functional barrier to reflux, and can be reversed easily if necessary, thereby preserving the option for fundoplication or other therapies in the future. The LINX procedure is designed to limit technical variability, which will result in more standardization of antireflux surgery and more consistent clinical outcomes. The LINX device consists of a series of titanium beads with magnetic cores hermetically sealed inside (Figure 2). The beads are interlinked with independent titanium wires to form a dynamic ring designed to conform to the changing physiologic movements of the esophagus during swallowing. The device was designed to use the magnetic attraction between adjacent beads to prevent the opening of the LES by distal to proximal effacement and shortening of its length caused by episodes of gastric distension or postprandial gastric dilation secondary to adaptive relaxation. The device is sized to fit around the external circumference of the esophagus at the distal end of the LES without compressing the esophageal musculature.

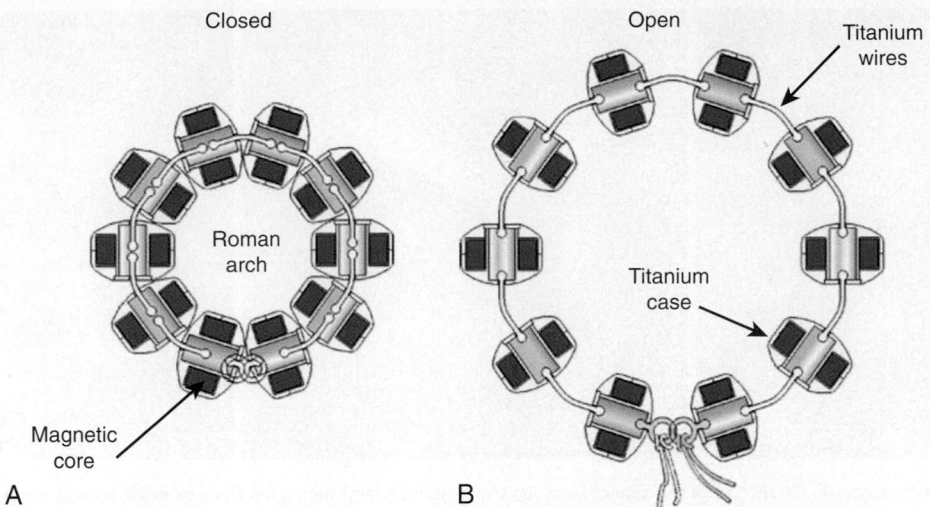

Closed

Open

Titanium
wires

Roman
arch

Titanium
case

Magnetic
core

A

B

FIGURE 2 An engineering schematic of the magnetic sphincter augmentation device. The device consists of an expansible bracelet of magnetic beads designed to be placed surgically around the exterior surface of the distal end of the lower esophageal sphincter (LES). Each bead is composed of a titanium case containing a magnetic core of small disk-shaped magnets. The beads are connected by titanium wires of specific lengths that limit the distance any two individual beads can move apart. When the device is closed (**A**), the magnetic force is sufficient to prevent effacement and opening of the LES yet is weak enough to allow the device to open (**B**) with the esophageal peristalsis. When the device is closed, the Roman arch construction prevents compression of the esophageal tissues.

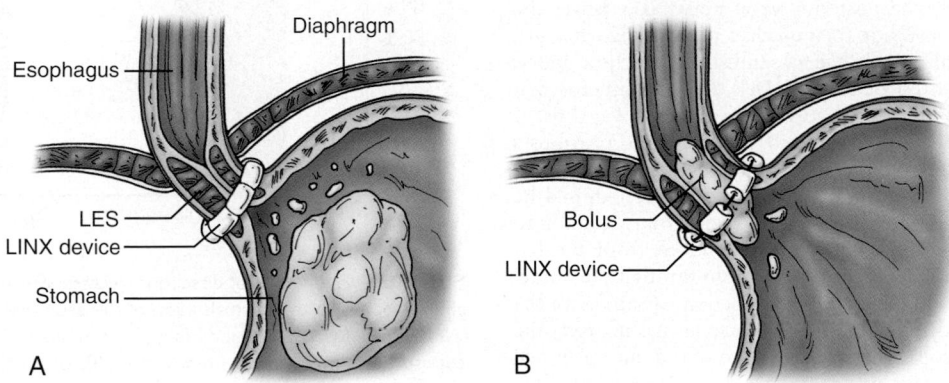

Diaphragm

Esophagus

LES
LINX device

Stomach

Bolus

LINX device

A

B

FIGURE 3 The LINX magnetic sphincter augmentation device is implanted around the inferior border of the lower esophageal sphincter (LES) as shown. **A** shows the magnetic device in the closed position, which prevents effacement and opening of the LES and subsequent reflux. Each magnetic bead rests on the adjacent beads to prevent compression of the esophageal tissues. **B** shows the device in the open position, which allows transport of food by esophageal peristalsis, belching of an overdistended stomach, and vomiting when necessary.

The beads separate to allow the transport of a food bolus into the stomach, to relieve gastric distension by belching or nausea by vomiting (Figure 3).

The LINX device was not designed to deter reflux episodes caused by pressure challenges that affect the whole abdominal environmental. To deter these challenges requires sufficient esophageal length in the abdominal domain to allow the LES to be compressed by changes in the abdominal environmental pressure that occur with daily living and working. For this reason, it is recommended that, if possible, the LINX device be implanted with minimal disruption of the phrenoesophageal ligament to preserve sufficient length of esophagus in the abdominal domain.

■ LINX IMPLANTATION PROCEDURE

The LINX device is implanted laparoscopically under general anesthesia. Surgical ports are placed similar to the pattern used for the laparoscopic Nissen fundoplication with one exception. The dissection port in the patient's right upper quadrant is placed far laterally to optimize the visualization and sizing of the esophagus at the gastroesophageal junction. A limited focus dissection is ideal for the implantation of the LINX device in a patient without a hiatal hernia. When performing a limited focus dissection, the surgeon must preserve and not dissect the phrenoesophageal ligament.

The surgical dissection begins by mobilizing the posterior gastric fundic wall off the lateral surface of the left crus to expose the caudal anterior edge of the left crus. In doing so, as few short gastric vessels as possible are divided. A 1-cm segment along the anterior margin of the left crus just above the crural decussation is identified. At this location a medial dissection is performed just beneath the esophagus to form a pocket target for the right-sided tunnel dissection. In performing this dissection care is taken not to enter the mediastinum. After the pocket target is made, the dissection is switched to the right side of the esophagus. The gastrohepatic ligament is opened by making two windows, a small one just superior to the hepatic branch of the anterior vagal nerve and a larger one

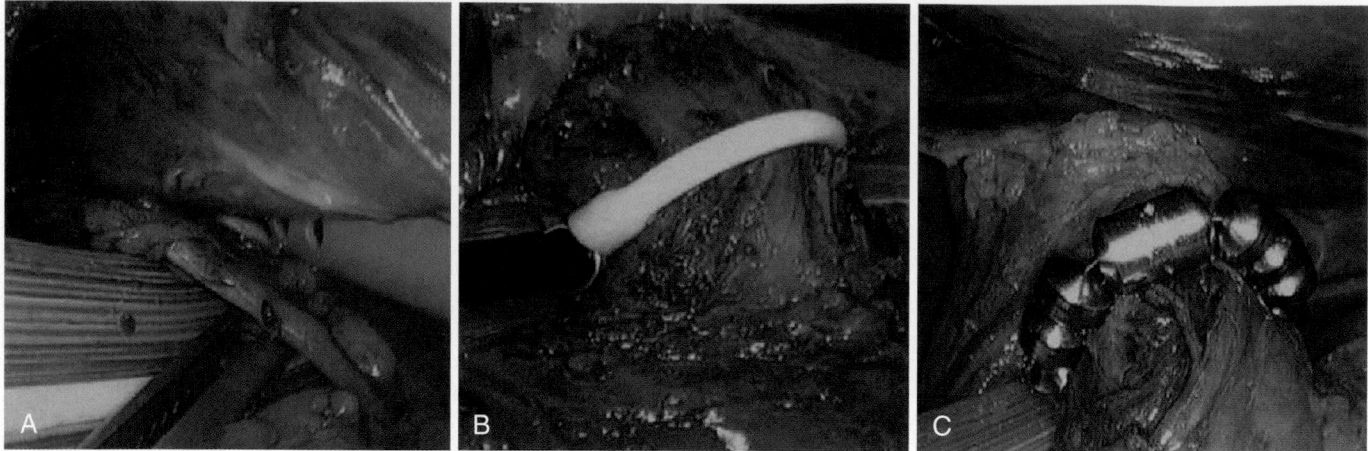

FIGURE 4 Intraoperative images. **A,** Dissection of the tunnel between the posterior vagal nerve and the posterior esophageal wall at the inferior border of the lower esophageal sphincter (LES). **B,** The position of the sizing tool to measure the circumference of the esophagus at the lower border of the LES. **C,** Completed implantation of the LINX device around the lower border of the LES with the clasps connected.

inferior to the hepatic branch. The inferior window allows access to construct a retroesophageal tunnel through a 1- to 2-cm incision in the peritoneum along the anterior edge of the right crus just above the crural decussation. Using a dissector placed through the far lateral right upper quadrant port and the inferior window in the gastrohepatic ligament, a gentle dissection is made towards the left crus just to identify the posterior vagal nerve as it leaves the esophagus and drops posterior to the celiac plexus (Figure 4, *A*). Bleeding from the small vessels can obscure the dissection and is controlled with judicial use of cautery. Delicately, a tunnel is dissected in a right-to-left direction, between the posterior vagal nerve and the posterior esophageal wall, to connect with the previously constructed pocket target on the anterior margin of the left crus. Entering the mediastinum during the tunnel dissection should be avoided. The dissector is passed through the pocket target and into the left upper quadrant. The dissector is removed from the left upper quadrant drawing a $\frac{1}{4}$-inch Penrose drain through the tunnel and securing its right and left ends for retraction. In line with the expected position of the device the fibroareolar tissue from the right and left lateral esophageal surfaces is removed, and a trench is constructed through existing fat on the anterior surface of the esophagus below the inferior leaf of the phrenoesophageal ligament. The circumference of the esophagus then is measured to choose the proper size of the LINX device to be implanted. The sizing tool is a laparoscopic instrument with a soft, circular curved tip that is actuated by coaxial tubes through a handset. The handset contains a numerical indicator that corresponds to the size range of the LINX device. The sizing tool is inserted through the far lateral placed right upper quadrant port, passed through the dissected tunnel between the posterior vagal nerve and esophageal wall and around the esophagus (Figure 4, *B*). Anterior retraction on the previously placed Penrose drain simplifies this maneuver. When making the measurement, the surgeon must not intubate the esophagus nor compress its muscular wall by the measuring device. Two measurements should be taken. If the measurement is between two sizes, the larger size is selected. The most common size is 14, and smaller sizes should be used sparingly and with caution. The appropriate size of device is selected and pulled through the tunnel in a left to right direction. Again, anterior retraction of the Penrose drain simplifies this maneuver. The ends of the device are brought anteriorly around the esophagus, the left end around the Angle of His and the right end over the gastrohepatic branch of the anterior vagal nerve. The clasps are connected together and the anterior portion of the device placed in the trench if present (Figure 4, *C*). If the right and left crura appear to diverge from one another above the crural decussation one or two figure-of-8 sutures can be placed to

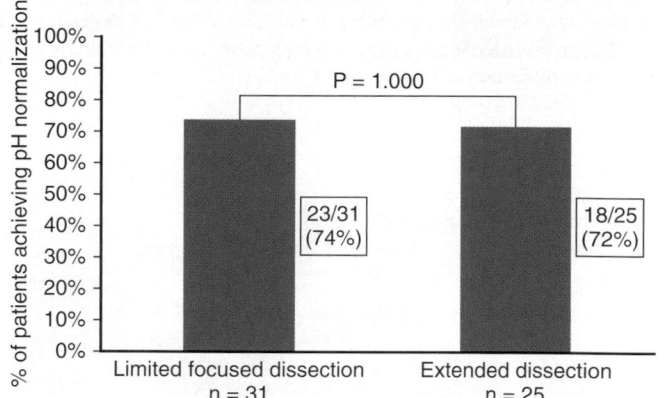

FIGURE 5 The degree of dissection necessary to implant the LINX anti-reflux device and normalization of the esophageal acid exposure. With either dissection (limited focus or extended) the esophageal acid exposure was normalized in more than 70% of patients. The durability of competency with a limited focus dissection is beyond 5 years. The durability of competency with an extended dissection is unknown.

approximate them, provided no further dissection is required. A small hiatal hernia less than 3 cm in size can be effectively repaired by this maneuver. The surgical time is usually under 1 hour. The patient is discharged the same day or, if an afternoon procedure, the next morning. The patient is to slowly return to a normal diet over the next week and discontinue the use of acid-suppression medication.

For patients with a hiatal hernia greater than 3 cm, a more extended and less focused dissection can be done to allow dissection and reduction of the hernia into the abdomen, approximation of the crura around a 2- to 3-cm length of abdominal esophagus, and implantation of the LINX device. An extended dissection also provides a fallback solution when greater exposure is necessary to implant the LINX device for reasons other than a hiatal hernia. Normalization of esophageal acid exposure is similar in patients after a limited focus or extended dissection (Figure 5). Again, when doing an extended dissection, it is important to approximate the crura around the esophagus in a manner that maintains 2 to 3 cm of esophagus in the abdominal environment. When this is not done, the ability to deter the reflux of gastric juice into the esophagus caused by episodes of increased abdominal environmental pressure is compromised.

■ LONG-TERM CLINICAL OUTCOMES OF THE LINX MAGNETIC SPHINCTER AUGMENTATION DEVICE

Long-term outcomes of patients who had the LINX magnetic sphincter augmentation implanted for GERD have been reported recently. The final 5-year results of the U.S. Food and Drug Administration's approved trial provides a careful analysis of the safety and effectiveness of the LINX device. The studied population consisted of 100 adults with gastroesophageal reflux disease for at least 6 months or more, who were partially responsive to daily PPIs and had abnormal esophageal acid exposure on 24-hour pH testing. The LINX device

was placed using standard laparoscopic techniques. Eighty-five subjects were followed for 5 years and evaluated for quality of life (GERD-HRQL score), reflux control (postoperative 24 hour pH testing at 1 year), use of PPIs, and side effects. Quality of life questionnaire was administered at baseline to patients on and off PPIs and after placement of the LINX device yearly for 5 years. Over the follow-up period, no device erosions, migrations, or malfunctions occurred. At baseline, the median GERD-HRQL scores were 27 when patients were not taking PPIs, 11 when on PPIs, and at 5 years after LINX placement the score decreased to 4 (Figure 6). All patients were taking daily PPIs at baseline, and this decreased to 15.3% at 5 years (Figures 7 and 8). Moderate to severe heartburn occurred in 89% of

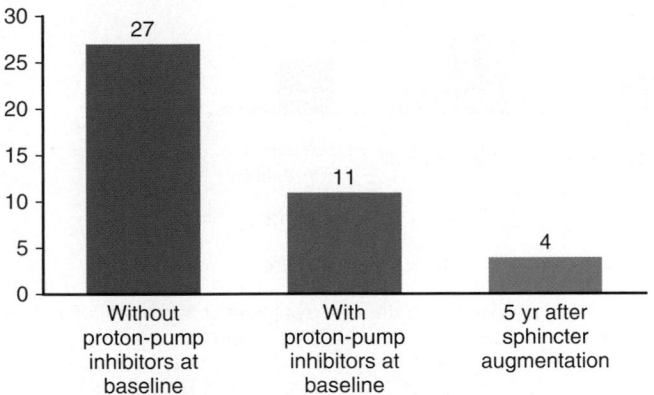

FIGURE 6 Median total GERD-HRQL scores measured at baseline without and with proton-pump inhibitors, as compared with 5 years after implantation of the LINX sphincter augmentation device. Higher scores indicate worse symptoms. (*P* < 0.001 for all comparisons with baseline.)

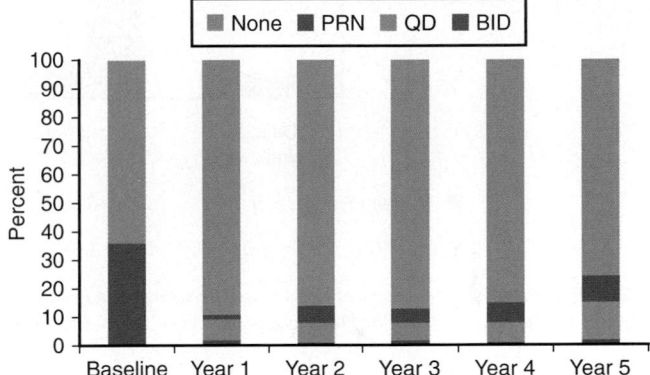

FIGURE 8 The use of PPIs at baseline and yearly throughout the 5 years. PPI use was categorized as none, as needed (PRN), once a day (QD), and twice a day (BID) at each yearly visit based on the prior 30 days. Patients who required BID PPIs decreased from 36% at baseline to 2.4% at 5 years.

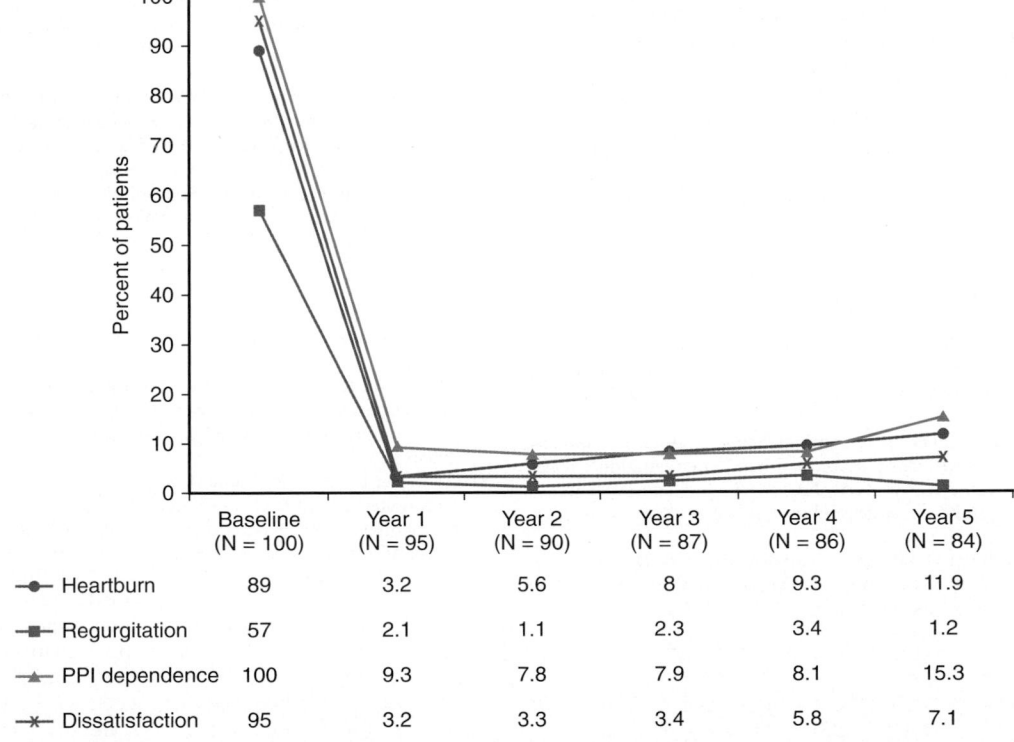

	Baseline (N = 100)	Year 1 (N = 95)	Year 2 (N = 90)	Year 3 (N = 87)	Year 4 (N = 86)	Year 5 (N = 84)
Heartburn	89	3.2	5.6	8	9.3	11.9
Regurgitation	57	2.1	1.1	2.3	3.4	1.2
PPI dependence	100	9.3	7.8	7.9	8.1	15.3
Dissatisfaction	95	3.2	3.3	3.4	5.8	7.1

P <.001 for comparision between baseline and all follow-ups

FIGURE 7 Reflux control of moderate-severe heartburn, moderate-severe regurgitation, PPI dependency and dissatisfaction with therapy. *P* < 0.001 between baseline and yearly follow-up evaluation out to 5 years for all comparisons. Of the six patients who were dissatisfied at 5 years, five reported daily use of PPIs.

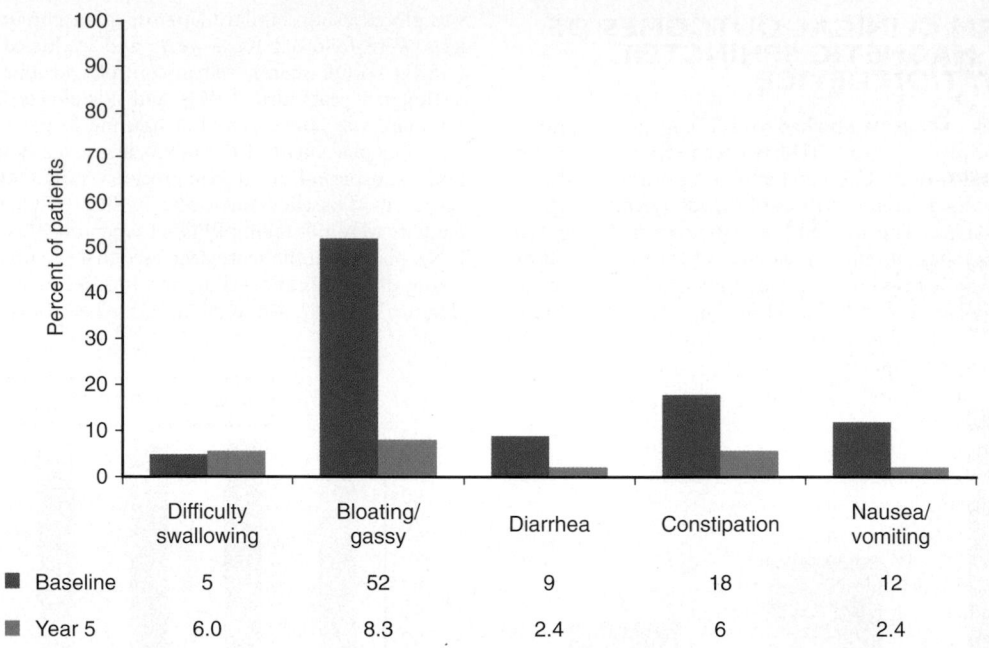

	Difficulty swallowing	Bloating/ gassy	Diarrhea	Constipation	Nausea/ vomiting
■ Baseline	5	52	9	18	12
■ Year 5	6.0	8.3	2.4	6	2.4

FIGURE 9 Potential side effects of LINX magnetic sphincter augmentation at 5 years when compared with the same symptoms at baseline. $P = 0.739$ for difficulty swallowing, $P < 0.001$ for bloating/gassy feeling, $P = 0.103$ for diarrhea, $P = 0.008$ for constipation, and $P = 0.003$ for nausea and vomiting.

patients at baseline but only 11.9% at 5 years (see Figure 7). Moderate to severe regurgitation occurred in 57% of patients at baseline, but only 1.2% at 5 years (see Figure 7). All patients reported the ability to belch and vomit if needed. Bothersome dysphagia was present in 5% at baseline and in 6% at 5 years (Figure 9). Bothersome gas bloat was present in 52% at baseline and decreased to 8.3% at 5 years (see Figure 9). No significant complication occurred. No new safety risks emerged over the 5 years of follow-up. On the basis of this and other reported studies, LINX is an effective fundic-sparing, antireflux procedure with minimal side effects. It is applicable to patients who have a partial response to PPIs, a desire to be off PPIs, or endoscopic/histologic signs of progression while on PPI therapy. A hiatal hernia is likely not a contraindication to the use of the LINX device, but long-term result regarding the recurrence rate of the hiatal hernia is needed.

SUGGESTED READINGS

Ayazi S, Tamhankar A, DeMeester SR, Zehetner J, Wu C, Lipham JC, Hagen JA, DeMeester TR. The impact of gastric distension on the lower esophageal sphincter and its exposure to acid gastric juice. *Ann Surg*. 2010;252: 57-62.

Bonavina L, DesMeester T, Fockens P, Dunn D, Saino G, Bona D, Lipham J, Bemelman W, Ganz RA. Laparoscopic sphincter augmentation device eliminates reflux symptoms and normalizes esophageal acid exposure—one and 2 year results of a feasibility trial. *Ann Surg*. 2010;252: 857-862.

Bonavina L, Saino GI, Bona D, Lipham J, Ganz RA, Dunn D, DeMeester T. Magnetic augmentation of the lower esophageal sphincter: results of a feasibility clinical trial. *J Gastrointest Surg*. 2008;12:2133-2140.

Bonavina L, Saino G, Lipham JC, DeMeester TR. LINX reflux management system in chronic gastroesophageal reflux: a novel effective technology for restoring the natural barrier to reflux. *Therap Adv Gastroenterol*. 2013;6: 261-268.

DeMeester TR, Peters JH, Bremner CG, Chandrasoma P. Biology of gastroesophageal reflux disease: pathophysiology relating to medical and surgical treatment. *Annu Rev Med*. 1999;50:469-506.

Ganz RA, Edmundowicz SA, Taiganides PA, Lipham JC, Smith CD, DeVault KR, Horgan S, Jacobsen G, Luketich JD, Smith CC, Schlack-Haerer SC, Kothari SN, Dunst CM, Watson TJ, Peters J, Oelschlager BK, Perry KA, Melvin S, Bemelman WA, Smout AJPM, Dunn D. Long-term outcomes of patients receiving a magnetic sphincter augmentation device for gastroesophageal reflux. *Clin Gastroenterol Hepatol*. 2016;14: 671-677.

Ganz RA, Gostout CJ, Grudem J, Swanson W, Berg T, DeMeester TR. Use of magnetic sphincter for the treatment of GERD: a feasibility study. *Gastrointest Endosc*. 2008;67:287-294.

Ganz R, Peters JH, Horgan S, Bemelman WA, Dunst CM, Edmundowicz SA, Lipham JC, Luketich JD, Melvin SW, Oelschlager BK, Schiack-Haerer SC, Smith DC, Smith CC, Dunn D, Taiganides PA. Esophageal sphincter device for gastroesophageal reflux disease. *NEJM*. 2013;368: 719-727.

Klaus A, Gadenstaetter M, Muhlmann G, Kirchmayr W, Profanter C, Achem SR, Wetscher GJ. Selection of patients with gastroesophageal reflux disease for antireflux surgery based on esophageal manometry. *Dig Dis Sci*. 2003;48:1719-1722.

Malfertheiner P, Nocon M, Vieth M, Stolte M, Jaspersen D, Koelz HR, Labenz J, Leodolter A, Lind T, Richter K, Willich N. Evolution of gastro-esophageal reflux disease over 5 years under routine medical care—the ProGERD study. *Aliment Pharmacol Ther*. 2012;35:154-164.

THE MANAGEMENT OF BARRETT'S ESOPHAGUS

Steven R. DeMeester, MD

■ DEFINITION OF BARRETT'S ESOPHAGUS AND TREATMENT OBJECTIVES

Barrett's esophagus (BE), defined by the presence of an endoscopically visible segment of columnar-lined esophagus with goblet cells on histology, develops as a consequence of gastroesophageal reflux disease (GERD). Consequently, any patient with BE has GERD because reflux is the only known cause for BE. In addition, BE is the precursor for esophageal adenocarcinoma, one of the world's fastest increasing and deadliest cancers. Consequently, in the management of a patient with BE there are two important issues: (1) therapy for the GERD that led to the BE and (2) prevention of progression or treatment of BE that has progressed toward adenocarcinoma.

■ GOALS AND OPTIONS FOR THERAPY IN BARRETT'S ESOPHAGUS

Accepted therapies for long-term management of GERD include medical therapy, typically with proton pump inhibitors (PPIs), or an antireflux procedure, typically a fundoplication, with the goal of relief of the reflux symptoms. In patients with BE there is controversy about the goal of reflux therapy. Many physicians suggest that the focus should be on relief of symptoms similar to any patient with reflux disease. This approach is based largely on the belief that no therapy can alter the natural history of BE and that progression, although rare, is inevitable in some patients. Although relief of symptoms is an important goal in the treatment of any patient with GERD, in a patient with BE at least some consideration should be given to the impact of therapy on Barrett's mucosa. Recent studies, although controversial, have suggested that treatment with PPIs may reduce the risk of progression in patients with BE. Likewise, there is evidence that, in patients with BE, antireflux surgery often leads to regression of dysplasia and may reduce the risk of progression toward adenocarcinoma. Unfortunately, there is also evidence that failed antireflux surgery is a significant risk factor for progression of disease in a patient with BE. Therefore the decision to recommend antireflux surgery in a patient with BE must not be taken lightly and should involve a careful analysis of the likelihood of long-term success of the procedure.

■ EVALUATION OF THE PATIENT WITH BARRETT'S ESOPHAGUS

Evaluation of a patient with BE begins with a careful endoscopy using white light and narrow band imaging or similar enhancement feature to facilitate identification of not only columnar replacement of the esophagus but also areas of irregularity within the columnar segment. It is recommended that the Prague classification system be used to record the circumferential and maximal length of the columnar segment. The presence and size of a hiatal hernia should be noted. Any lesion or nodule within the columnar lined mucosa must be evaluated carefully because this may represent an area of dysplasia or invasive adenocarcinoma. Four-quadrant biopsies should be obtained every 1 to 2 cm throughout the columnar segment.

In patients with BE a pH test to confirm the presence of increased esophageal exposure is, in general, not necessary, because the presence of BE is in itself verification of GERD. However, in patients with only an irregular squamocolumnar junction and no obvious columnar-lined segment of esophagus, a pH test is valuable. Before consideration of an antireflux procedure a motility test should be performed because esophageal body motility can be compromised by long-standing GERD. I also consider a videoesophagram invaluable to assess esophageal bolus transport with solids and liquids, to evaluate for a stricture, and to assess the size and reducibility of a hiatal hernia to assist in making the decision for surgery and in operative planning.

■ MANAGEMENT OF BARRETT'S ESOPHAGUS WITHOUT DYSPLASIA

A patient with nondysplastic BE should be managed like any other patient with GERD. The goal is symptom relief and quality of life, with the added twist that protection of the Barrett's mucosa from continued reflux-induced injury may lead to a reduced risk of progression to cancer. However, this concern in and of itself is insufficient to recommend surgery, and patients should be reassured rather than scared into surgery because of their BE. A patient found to have BE should rarely, if ever, die from esophageal cancer if appropriate surveillance endoscopy is performed (see the section on surveillance). Therefore the indication for surgery in patients with BE should be the presence of GERD symptoms inadequately controlled with acid suppression medication or impaired quality of life related to the dietary and lifestyle modifications required by their reflux disease.

Ideal candidates for antireflux surgery are patients with no or a small hiatal hernia, good esophageal body function, and classic heartburn and regurgitation symptoms that respond well to acid-suppression therapy. Some patients with BE fall into this group, whereas many more have sizeable hernias, impaired esophageal body function, or extraesophageal reflux symptoms related to nocturnal regurgitation and aspiration. A Nissen fundoplication has an excellent track record for control of GERD and usually is favored over a partial fundoplication in patients with BE, provided esophageal body motility is preserved. Patients with impaired motility may be best served with a partial fundoplication, although in the absence of achalasia the need for a tailored approach to the type of fundoplication is debated by some surgeons.

Whether antireflux surgery is performed or the patient is maintained on acid-suppression therapy, surveillance endoscopy is indicated to evaluate for progression of disease. The role or benefit of mucosal ablation with radiofrequency or other devices is unproven in patients with nondysplastic BE. In the setting of ultra-long segment (≥8 cm) BE ablation may reduce the tedious complexity of appropriate four-quadrant surveillance biopsies every 1 to 2 cm throughout the length of the columnar segment. Likely there is little role for ablation of short-segment, nondysplastic BE because surveillance endoscopy is still necessary given reports confirming recurrence of intestinal metaplasia over time after ablation.

■ MANAGEMENT OF BARRETT'S ESOPHAGUS WITH LOW-GRADE DYSPLASIA

Low-grade dysplasia (LGD) is associated with an increased risk for progression to adenocarcinoma compared with nondysplastic BE. However, pathologic determination of true dysplasia from inflammatory atypia can be difficult. If the endoscopy showing LGD did not include careful four-quadrant biopsies, the endoscopy should be repeated to confirm the absence of more advanced disease. These patients then typically start taking a PPI if not taking one already, and if they are, then the dose is increased or it is given twice a day. The endoscopy and biopsies should be repeated in 6 months to evaluate for a response. Alternatively, these patients can be offered antireflux surgery, given evidence that in most patients, LGD regresses after a fundoplication to nondysplastic BE. Persistent LGD after these measures is an indication for mucosal ablation.

MANAGEMENT OF BARRETT'S ESOPHAGUS WITH HIGH-GRADE DYSPLASIA

High-grade dysplasia (HGD) is an indication for intervention in most patients given the proven high risk for progression to adenocarcinoma. Often there is already a focus of invasive adenocarcinoma in these patients. Typically the first step in the management of these patients is a careful repeat endoscopy with a search for any nodules or lesions in the columnar mucosa; both white light and narrowband imaging or similar modality are used. Topical acetic acid spray also may help delineate areas of concern. Small lesions should undergo endoscopic resection (ER). ER is performed with a cap attached to the end of the endoscope within which the lesion is sucked up, snared, and removed. A good ER excises the full thickness of the mucosa and submucosa, leaving intact the muscularis propria. The ER specimen then is sent to the pathology laboratory for determination of whether cancer is present and, if so, the depth of invasion. Lesions larger than 1 to 2 cm should prompt an endoscopic ultrasound to evaluate depth of invasion and the presence of enlarged regional lymph nodes. If no lesion or only a very small lesion is present, the benefit of endoscopic ultrasound evaluation is unclear and likely not useful because the accuracy of T-staging is poor and these small lesions are unlikely to have associated malignant adenopathy. If an ER specimen of a nodule shows adenocarcinoma, the critical issue is whether the lesion is confined to the mucosa (T1a) or has invaded into the submucosa (T1b). The risk of lymph node metastases is 2% or less for T1a lesions but increases to approximately 25% with submucosal invasion. Other important features that can be determined from the ER specimen include the presence of lymphovascular invasion (LVI) and high grade (poor differentiation). Both of these features, if present, increase the likelihood of lymph node metastases. In most circumstances T1b lesions are best treated with an esophagectomy and lymph node dissection.

In patients with only HGD or pathologically confirmed T1a adenocarcinoma without LVI after ER of a lesion, the options are endoscopic therapy with the goal of esophageal preservation or an esophagectomy. Typically, endotherapy consists of ER for visible lesions and mucosal ablation for the residual flat columnar mucosa. Advantages of endoscopic therapy are very low morbidity and mortality with similar oncologic efficacy as an esophagectomy. However, multiple endotherapy sessions are usually necessary to eradicate all the intestinal metaplasia, long-term surveillance endoscopy is necessary to evaluate for recurrent mucosal disease, and recurrence or inadequately treated cancer is a risk. An alternative is an esophagectomy. Advantages of esophagectomy include immediate disease eradication with rare recurrence and no need for continued surveillance endoscopies. However, esophagectomy comes with a price related to significant short-term and long-term potential morbidity. Mortality should be uncommon (under 1%) in patients with early tumors treated at a high-volume center. Esophagectomy should be strongly considered for ultra-long segment BE, multifocal adenocarcinoma, poor esophageal body function with large hiatal hernia or dysphagia symptoms, and reflux disease poorly controlled on twice-daily PPI therapy. In these patients a vagal-sparing laparoscopic esophagectomy can eradicate the disease and minimize the long-term gastrointestinal morbidity associated with bilateral vagotomy.

OUTCOME OF ANTIREFLUX SURGERY IN BARRETT'S ESOPHAGUS

Numerous studies have shown that the 3- to 5-year failure rate of a fundoplication is increased in patients with BE up to 15% to 20% compared with 5% to 10% in patients without BE. Selection of appropriate patients for a fundoplication is critical to minimize this risk because a failed fundoplication is a risk factor for disease progression. A functioning fundoplication has been associated with frequent regression of LGD to nondysplastic BE and in patients with short-segment BE regression to no intestinal metaplasia. Furthermore, a functioning fundoplication likely reduces the risk of progression of BE to adenocarcinoma. Some patients with BE have end-stage GERD with dysphagia in the absence of a stricture, regurgitation and aspiration events, large nonreducing hiatal hernia, or very poor esophageal body function. In these patients antireflux surgery is complicated and at high risk for poor outcome, and an esophagectomy may be the best option even in the absence of dysplasia or cancer.

SURVEILLANCE ENDOSCOPY FOR BARRETT'S ESOPHAGUS

The role of surveillance endoscopy is to detect progression of BE before the development of invasive adenocarcinoma. The rate of progression appears variable in patients with BE, but the risk is higher in patients with longer segments of BE. General recommendations for surveillance in patients with nondysplastic BE are every 3 to 5 years and more frequently if LGD is present. Surveillance is seldom appropriate for HGD given the availability and efficacy of ablation techniques. Recent studies have raised questions about the efficacy of surveillance because earlier cancers were not detected and survival was not improved in those undergoing routine surveillance. The issue here is likely the surveillance interval. An interval of 3 to 5 years, although perhaps cost effective, is too long to reliably detect progression at an endoscopically treatable and curable stage. Annual surveillance endoscopy is my practice for nondysplastic BE, and with this approach disease progression beyond what can be treated endoscopically has not occurred. In patients with LGD or those undergoing endotherapy for HGD or T1a adenocarcinoma, even more frequent surveillance is appropriate.

CONCLUSION

BE often is associated with advanced reflux disease, and although antireflux surgery can be beneficial to eradicate GERD symptoms, improve quality of life, and perhaps induce regression of dysplasia or prevent progression to cancer, patients must be selected carefully to ensure good outcomes. Unfortunately, fundoplication failure and recurrent hiatal hernia occurs more often in patients with BE than in patients with GERD without BE, and a failed fundoplication is a risk factor for progression of BE to cancer. Endoscopic therapy has revolutionized the treatment for BE with HGD or intramucosal adenocarcinoma, but in some patients an esophagectomy is a better choice to address the mucosal disease and severity of GERD. Surgeons with a focused interest in esophageal disease should remain on the forefront of the evaluation and therapy of patients with BE to maximize long-term successful outcomes.

SUGGESTED READINGS

DeMeester SR. Barrett's oesophagus: treatment with surgery. *Best Pract Res Clin Gastroenterol.* 2015;29:211-217.

DeMeester SR. Reflux, Barrett's, and adenocarcinoma of the esophagus: can we disrupt the pathway? *J Gastrointest Surg.* 2010;14:941-945.

Grant KS, DeMeester SR, Kreger V, et al. Effect of Barrett's esophagus surveillance on esophageal preservation, tumor stage, and survival with esophageal adenocarcinoma. *J Thorac Cardiovasc Surg.* 2013;146:31-37.

Hofstetter WL, Peters JH, DeMeester TR, et al. Long-term outcome of antireflux surgery in patients with Barrett's esophagus. *Ann Surg.* 2001;234:532-538, discussion 538-539.

Oelschlager BK, Barreca M, Chang L, et al. Clinical and pathologic response of Barrett's esophagus to laparoscopic antireflux surgery. *Ann Surg.* 2003;238:458-464, discussion 464-456.

Zehetner J, DeMeester SR, Hagen JA, et al. Endoscopic resection and ablation versus esophagectomy for high-grade dysplasia and intramucosal adenocarcinoma. *J Thorac Cardiovasc Surg.* 2011;141:39-47.

THE ENDOSCOPIC TREATMENT OF BARRETT'S ESOPHAGUS

Lara Schaheen, MD, and James D. Luketich, MD

Barrett's esophagus (BE) is an acquired condition in which the normal stratified squamous epithelium of the esophagus is replaced with metaplastic, intestinal-type columnar epithelium containing goblet cells (Figure 1). Various prevalence rates can be found in the literature with several studies finding BE in 1% to 2% of all adults in North America. The relationship between BE and chronic gastroesophageal reflux has been well established. The metaplastic process is believed to be a protective response of the lower esophagus to gastric acid exposure and is detected in 15% of patients with chronic gastroesophageal reflux disease. Although there remains debate regarding the true incidence of BE, the management presents a growing concern because it is the most significant known risk factor and only known precursor to esophageal adenocarcinoma.

Patients with BE have a thirtyfold increased risk of developing adenocarcinoma of the esophagus. The risk of progression to esophageal adenocarcinoma arises in a stepwise fashion with nondysplastic Barrett's carrying an annual rate of cancer progression of 0.2% to 0.5%, BE with low-grade dysplasia of 0.7%, and BE with high-grade dysplasia of 7% per year. The AIM-Dysplasia trial, in which patients with dysplasia were randomized to continued surveillance or ablative therapy, reported a 19% annual rate of progression to cancer in the high-grade dysplasia (HGD) surveillance arm. The increasing incidence of esophageal adenocarcinoma over the past three decades has led to esophageal adenocarcinoma becoming one of the fastest rising solid cancers in the Western world. Despite advances in diagnosis and management, the overall 5-year survival remains only 17%.

■ SURVEILLANCE AND MANAGEMENT ALGORITHM FOR BARRETT'S ESOPHAGUS

Because the survival of patients with esophageal cancer is stage dependent and early spread before the onset of symptoms is characteristic of the disease, the best hope for improved survival lies in detection at an early and potentially curable stage. Screening and surveillance programs for BE have been shown to identify malignant progression at an earlier and less advanced stage, providing opportunities for curative interventions. A number of observational studies suggest that BE patients in whom esophageal adenocarcinoma (EAC) was diagnosed as part of a surveillance program have their cancers detected at an earlier stage and with markedly improved survival compared with patients not undergoing routine endoscopic surveillance. Other population-based retrospective cohort studies demonstrated improved survival among surveillance-detected EAC patients compared with those who underwent diagnostic examination because of the onset of symptoms. Furthermore, nodal involvement is far less likely in surveyed patients compared with nonsurveyed patients. Because esophageal cancer survival is stage dependent, these studies suggest that survival may be enhanced by appropriate endoscopic surveillance.

Current clinical guidelines from the American College of Gastroenterology recommend screening in men with chronic (>5 years) and/or frequent (weekly or more) symptoms of heartburn or acid regurgitation and two or more risk factors for BE or EAC. These risk factors include age over 50 years, Caucasian race, central obesity (waist circumference above 102 cm or waist–hip ratio above 0.9), current or past history of smoking, and a history of BE or EAC in a first-degree relative. Given the substantially lower risk of esophageal cancer in women with chronic reflux disease, screening for BE currently is not recommended.

If initial endoscopic evaluation is negative for BE, repeating endoscopic evaluation for the presence of BE is not recommended. If endoscopy reveals esophagitis, proton pump inhibitor (PPI) therapy should be initiated and repeat endoscopic assessment performed in 3 months to ensure healing of esophagitis and exclude the presence of underlying BE. Studies report a BE prevalence of 9% to 12% on repeat endoscopy after treatment of esophagitis with PPIs, making repeat endoscopy advisable.

Once a patient is diagnosed with BE, the screening algorithm is determined by the presence and grade of dysplasia because dysplasia remains the best clinically available marker of cancer risk in patients with BE. Patients with BE without dysplasia should undergo surveillance endoscopy at 3-year to 5-year intervals. In patients with BE and confirmed low-grade dysplasia (LGD) in which endoscopic therapy is not performed, annual surveillance is recommended until two consecutive examinations are negative for dysplasia, after which the patient can return to surveillance at 3- to 5-year intervals.

HGD is a high-risk lesion and, if detected, should be confirmed by a second pathologist because of the substantial interobserver variation in establishing the diagnosis. In patients with HGD, endoscopic therapy or esophagectomy is warranted because these patients are at high risk for development of esophageal adenocarcinoma. The presence of features such as ulceration, an endoscopically visible lesion, or multifocal HGD confers a higher risk of development of EAC and have been found to have an estimated risk of concurrent EAC of 60% to 78%.

Intensive endoscopic surveillance using the Seattle protocol, which includes four quadrant biopsies using jumbo forceps at 1 cm intervals every 3 months, is designed to identify patients that progress from HGD to adenocarcinoma. Proponents of intensive endoscopic surveillance argue that not all patients with HGD will go on to develop cancer. In a study of 30 patients with HGD who underwent esophagectomy, 43% were found to have occult adenocarcinoma on pathologic examination. When HGD is confirmed, patients have several treatment options, which include endoscopic eradication therapy via ablative or resection techniques and esophageal resection. Several studies have demonstrated that, in appropriately selected patients with HGD or T1a EAC endoscopic eradication, therapy can achieve good results. However, a careful examination of the patients excluded from these trials is warranted because the good outcomes seen with endoscopic therapy are not necessarily widely applicable to all patients. Criteria for determining which patients should be selected for endoscopic therapy versus esophagectomy remain unclear. Patients with multifocal and long segments of HGD, those at a higher risk of lymph node metastasis, a family history of esophageal cancer, and younger patients in whom a lifetime of surveillance may not be a good choice may be better served with an esophagectomy.

In patients with T1b EAC, consultation with a multidisciplinary surgical oncology team and surgical evaluation for esophagectomy by an experienced esophageal surgeon in a high-volume center should occur before any endoscopic therapy. Proponents of intensive endoscopic surveillance point to the potentially high morbidity and mortality of esophagectomy. However, high-volume surgical centers have mortality rates of less than 1%, with associated low morbidity rates. In our recent review of more than 1000 consecutive minimally invasive esophagectomies at the University of Pittsburgh Medical Center, the 30-day operative mortality was 0.9%. In carefully selected patients with high-grade dysplasia, esophagectomy can be performed with reasonably low morbidity and mortality rates. Esophagectomy should be considered in patients with T1b EAC, in whom the risk of nodal metastases can be as high as 27%, because endoscopic resection would leave nodal disease untreated. In a review of 1225 patients from 2004 to 2010, Dubecz and colleagues demonstrated a

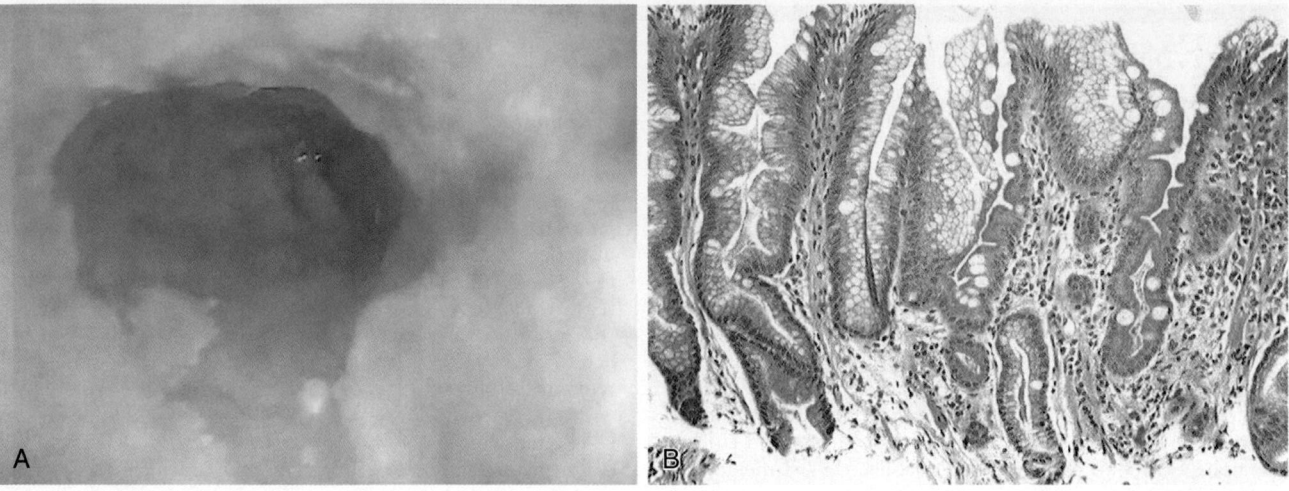

FIGURE 1 Barrett's esophagus. **A,** Salmon-colored Barrett's mucosa is seen extending above the proximal extent of the gastric folds. **B,** Microscopic features of Barrett's mucosa highlighting metaplastic columnar epithelium containing mucin-producing goblet cells. *(From Hornick JL et al.* Am J Surg Path. *2005;29:372-380.)*

TABLE 1: Modalities for Endoscopic Treatment of Barrett's Esophagus

Modality	HGD Resolved	BE Resolved	Recurrence Rate	Subsquamous BE Rate	Stricture Rate	Complication Rate	Advantages	Disadvantages
APC	67%-98.6%	38%-98%	33%-68% low power	25%-45% low power 0-30% high power	4%-10%	24% low power 40%-60% high power	Noncontact, technically simple	Requires several treatment sessions
MPEC	–	25%-88%	7%	7%	2%	41%-43%	Noncontact, technically simple, relatively inexpensive, readily available	Requires several treatment sessions
PDT	77%-88%	13%	5%-11%	2%-24%	4.8%-53%	4.8%-53%	Easy to perform; only FDA-approved ablation method for treatment of precancerous lesions in BE	Photosensitivity, relatively high stricture rate
EMR	59%-97%	53%	4%-30%	–	3%-30%	12%-60%	Histologic assessment; Complete removal of circumferential short-segment BE; 1-2 sessions	Difficulty treating long-segment BE

APC, Argon plasma coagulation; *BE,* Barrett's esophagus; *EMR,* endoscopic mucosal resection; *FDA,* U.S. Food and Drug Administration; *HGD,* high-grade dysplasia; *MPEC,* multipolar electrocoagulation; *PDT,* photodynamic therapy.

prevalence of lymph node metastasis in patients with esophageal adenocarcinoma and adenocarcinoma of the esophagogastric junction of 6.9% and 9.5% in patients with pT1a and 19.6% and 22.9% for pT1b tumors. Because the risk of lymph node metastasis is significant even in patients with early T1 esophageal cancers, endoscopic treatment should be considered only in a select group of patients.

■ PRINCIPLES OF ENDOSCOPIC THERAPIES

More recently, endoscopic ablative treatments have been developed to provide a less invasive approach to eradicating BE, HGD, and focal carcinoma in patients who are unable or unwilling to undergo intensive endoscopic surveillance or esophagectomy (Table 1). The observation that thermally damaged Barrett's mucosa can be replaced by normal squamous epithelium, particularly in an acid-free environment, spawned the development of multiple techniques designed to selectively eradicate Barrett's mucosa and minimize the risk of progression to cancer.

The goals of endoscopic therapies include removal of the abnormal Barrett's epithelium while preserving the overall integrity of the esophagus and accurately staging dysplasia or invasive disease.

Although ablation is effective in eliminating high-grade dysplasia in many patients, the importance of buried BE must be considered.

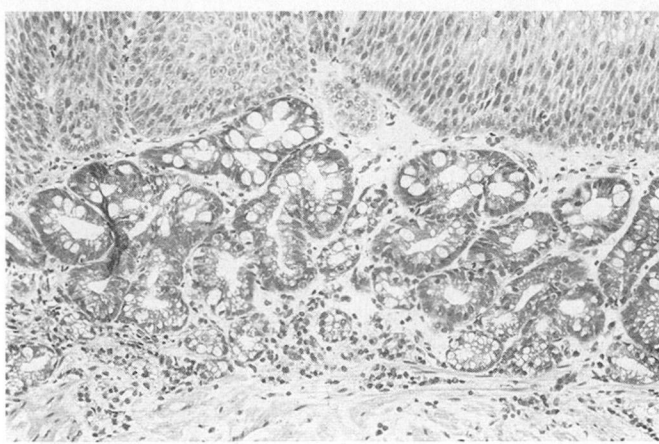

FIGURE 2 Subsquamous Barrett's epithelium. *(From Peters FP et al. Gastrointest Endosc. 2005;61:506-514.)*

Buried or subsquamous BE refers to the persistence of glandular epithelium beneath the new squamous epithelium, which is capable of undergoing dysplastic changes without detection. All described ablative techniques have revealed a cohort of patients that have residual subsquamous Barrett's epithelium (Figure 2). The presence of subsquamous Barrett's epithelium remains at risk for progression to adenocarcinoma and complicates surveillance endoscopy because the metaplastic mucosa is difficult to identify and biopsy. Currently published ablation techniques have rates of residual subsquamous Barrett's epithelium ranging from less than 2% to 69%. These rates loosely correlate with the depth of mucosal ablation, with more superficial penetration techniques often associated with a higher rate of subsquamous BE mucosa.

In patients being considered for ablation therapy, it is important to ensure the absence of nodular disease or invasive cancer in the ablative field because its presence can result in inaccurate staging and insufficient treatment. Endoscopic ultrasound with fine-needle aspiration of suspicious lymph nodes, and CT scan with contrast of the chest and abdomen should be performed to assess lymph node involvement or tumor extension beyond the submucosa before proceeding with endoscopic therapies. However, the risk of missing small nodal metastases in T1a and T1b by endoscopic ultrasound (EUS) has been demonstrated clearly. It is well known that the incidence of nodal metastasis can be as high as 27% in T1b; thus a negative EUS for nodes does not equate to a node-negative T1b patient.

Although endoscopic ablative therapies often are considered less invasive, there are certain limitations to this technique. Greatest success with endoscopic ablative therapy has been seen in patients with less than approximately 8 cm of metaplastic mucosa, frequently requires multiple treatments before eradication is achieved, and notably requires lifetime intensive post-treatment endoscopic surveillance. With these limitations in mind, medical professionals should identify reliable, motivated, and cooperative patients before offering endoscopic eradication therapy.

■ ENDOSCOPIC ABLATION TECHNIQUES

A number of different endoscopic modalities have been described to manage Barrett's epithelium. Available techniques include thermal ablation with argon plasma coagulation (APC), cryotherapy, chemical ablation (photodynamic therapy [PDT]), and radiofrequency ablation (RFA).

Argon Plasma Coagulation

APC induces coagulation of the tissue surface through the use of a high-frequency monopolar electrical current conducted via ionized argon gas. The depth of penetration usually ranges from 1 to 3 mm but may reach 6 mm by varying the power, distance, gas flow, and duration of treatment. At least 12 different centers have evaluated APC treatment on 444 patients with BE. Elimination of BE was reported in 38% to 88% of patients after follow-up ranging from 12 to 51 months. However, long-term relapse of intestinal metaplasia was as high as 68%. Complications of APC occur with an incidence as high as 24% and include chest pain, odynophagia, ulceration, stricture 4% to 10%, bleeding, perforation, pneumatosis, pneumoperitoneum, perforation, and even death. Subsquamous Barrett's epithelium was seen in 0 to 30% of these patients treated with high-power APC. More recent studies suggest that complete ablation of BE can be achieved in 38% to 98.6% of patients treated with APC with an associated recurrence rate of 33% to 68%.

Cryotherapy

Cryotherapy is a noncontact ablation technique that involves freezing of the surface epithelium through the use of liquid nitrogen or rapidly expanding carbon dioxide. Cell injury and death is secondary to the generation of free radicals in the frozen tissue during reperfusion. Johnston and colleagues published the first pilot study describing the use of cryotherapy in 11 patients with BE. They showed that 78% of patients had reversal of BE at 6-month follow-up without any major complications. Since then, other retrospective and smaller prospective studies have shown the efficacy of cryotherapy, with remission of HGD achieved in 94% to 97% of the patients and complete eradication of intestinal metaplasia in 53% to 81% patients. In the largest prospective, multicenter trial of cryotherapy for BE, eradication of BE with HGD was seen in 91% of patients, eradication of all dysplasia was seen in 81% of patients, and 65% of patients had eradication of all intestinal metaplasia after a mean follow-up of 21 months and an average of 3.5 spray cryotherapy sessions. Cryotherapy can be applied in the presence of bleeding and to nodular lesions. However, there is a relative lack of long-term data about the efficacy of cryotherapy compared with the most commonly used technique of RFA.

Photodynamic Therapy

PDT employs a photosensitizing drug that is absorbed and retained at higher concentrations in neoplastic tissue. Exposure of the esophagus to light of the proper wavelength at the time of endoscopy produces an oxidative photochemical reaction that elaborates singlet oxygen and reactive oxygen species resulting in mucosal destruction. Photofrin is a systemic photosensitizer, which, when injected at a dose of 2 mg/kg approximately 24 to 72 hours before endoscopic treatment, is activated by red light at 630 nm. Photofrin is retained selectively in the tumor cells at the submucosal or muscularis level, thus allowing for deeper penetration than RFA. An international multicenter randomized trial comparing PDT and omeprazole therapy to omeprazole therapy alone demonstrated that 77% of patients achieved complete ablation of high-grade dysplasia, compared with 39% in the omeprazole group. In addition, 52% of PDT/omeprazole patients achieved complete replacement of all Barrett's metaplasia/dysplasia compared with only 7% in the omeprazole group. Although improved cancer-free survival was seen in the PDT/omeprazole group, 13% of these patients advanced to adenocarcinoma during a mean follow-up of 24.2 months, and strictures occurred in 36% of patients.

Common complications after PDT include cutaneous photosensitivity, chest pain, nausea, pleural effusions, candida esophagitis, atrial fibrillation, and odynophagia. A common long-term side effect of PDT is the formation of esophageal strictures, which occurs in 4.8% to 53% of patients. Such strictures are usually responsive to endoscopic dilation. Esophageal perforation and tracheoesophageal fistulas are rare and seen in less than 1% in most large series. Virtually all studies using PDT report subsquamous intestinal metaplasia, with detailed pathologic studies reporting prevalence as high as 51.5%. A study performed by Badreddine and colleagues examined factors associated with recurrence of BE in patients who had received PDT. Among 261 patients included in the analysis, 86 patients had persistent nondysplastic Barrett's esophagus (NDBE) on postablation biopsies, 30 patients had LGD, 13 patients had HGD, and 2 had carcinoma. Multivariate analyses showed that advanced age, a history of tobacco use, and the inability to completely eradicate BE were all associated with an increased risk of recurrence. PDT is no longer used as a first-line treatment because of its complication profile of skin photosensitivity lasting for weeks to months, high rate of symptomatic strictures, high cost, and risk of buried BE in 58% of patients.

Radiofrequency Ablation

RFA has become the ablative treatment of choice in the management of dysplastic BE. RFA involves the delivery of high-frequency bipolar energy via direct contact with esophageal mucosa. Thermal injury to the superficial 0.5 mm of the esophageal mucosa results in tissue necrosis, allowing for the regrowth of normal squamous mucosa (Figures 1 and 2). Energy can be applied either circumferentially with a balloon sized to the patient's esophagus or focally with applicators available in different sizes. Initial RFA treatment should be delivered circumferentially using a sizing balloon catheter. Subsequent RFA treatments then can be delivered focally through a targeted ablation catheter mounted to the end of an endoscope.

Before RFA is delivered, the lesion should be examined to ensure that the mucosa is flat to allow for effective application, and any nodules should be resected to ensure that submucosal disease extension is not present, making the lesion unsuitable for endoscopic treatment.

Multiple prospective trials have shown that RFA is a safe, effective, and reliable treatment for BE. The Ablation of Intestinal Metaplasia containing dysplasia (AIM dysplasia) trial was a multicenter, randomized, sham-controlled trial that studied the outcomes of RFA in BE patients. In their initial study, 127 patients with dysplastic BE were randomized 2:1 to either RFA ablation or a sham procedure. The trial found that at 12 months follow-up, complete eradication of dysplasia was achieved in 81% of patients with RFA, compared with only 19% patients in the sham group. The rates of complete eradication of intestinal metaplasia and dysplasia approached 89% and 93%, respectively, at the 2-year follow-up in patients with HGD. A European study demonstrated a 90% remission at 5-year follow-up after RFA for BE with HGD. However, other studies have shown a significant rate of recurrence of BE after RFA ranging from 20% to 33% at long-term follow-up of 2 years. Although 78% to 86% of recurrent BE is nondysplastic and can be treated endoscopically, the importance of careful surveillance after RFA should not be overlooked. Characteristics such as older age, longer length of BE segments, and non-Caucasian race have been associated with higher rates of recurrence.

The low incidence of pain, bleeding, and stricture formation (4% to 12%) has led RFA to become the preferred ablative modality. Limitations of RFA therapy include high cost, requirement for multiple treatments, and increased likelihood of suboptimal ablation in patients with a tortuous esophagus, such as those with a hiatal hernia. Among the currently available ablative therapies, the long-term data regarding the safety and efficacy of RFA are most conclusive, making it the ablative modality of choice in the treatment of BE.

■ ENDOSCOPIC RESECTION TECHNIQUES

More recently, endoscopic resection techniques such as endoscopic mucosal resection and endoscopic submucosal dissection have emerged as techniques for the management of BE, high-grade dysplasia, and focal carcinoma in patients unable or unwilling to undergo intensive endoscopic surveillance or esophagectomy. Endoscopic resection allows for the removal of nodular tissue not suitable for

ablation, as well as pathologic analysis of suspicious lesions leading to more accurate staging. Most important, endoscopic resection of early esophageal cancers confined to the mucosa can offer an esophageal sparing, curative, oncologic tissue retrieval in appropriately selected cases.

Before proceeding with any endoscopic resection, patients with nodular disease or biopsy-proven invasive cancer should undergo computed tomography (CT) with contrast of the chest and abdomen and endoscopic ultrasound with fine-needle aspiration of suspicious lymph nodes to assess for lymph node involvement or tumor extension beyond the submucosa. Endoscopic resection techniques should not be used on lesions that are known to be deeper than the submucosa or do not lift on submucosal injection because the perforation risk is greatly elevated and the likelihood of achieving adequate resection is poor.

Endoscopic Mucosal Resection

Endoscopic mucosal resection (EMR) was introduced in 1984 and involves the removal of mucosal lesions through several steps: (1) raising the mucosal/submucosal target area by intramural saline injection or suction and (2) endoscopic snare resection (Figure 3). EMR provides a histologic specimen for pathologic evaluation and is thought to remove the genetic alterations associated with neoplasia, therefore reducing the risk of recurrence from metachronous lesions in the remaining segment. Lesions less than 2 cm can be removed en bloc, but larger lesions must be removed piecemeal. En bloc resection is preferred because it allows for more accurate assessment of the resection margins. Endoscopic mucosal resection can be performed in the endoscopy suite without the need for general anesthesia. Multiple techniques and devices exist for EMR. The most common techniques include submucosal saline injection to raise the lesion followed by snare polypectomy, suction of the lesion into a special endoscopic cap followed by snare polypectomy, or the application of bands around the base of the lesion to facilitate snare polypectomy.

Multiple studies have shown that EMR leads to better interobserver agreement on the degree of dysplasia and can lead to change in the final histologic stage when compared with biopsy specimens in up to 49% of the patients; therefore because of higher incidence of advanced histology and also better staging, EMR of all visible lesions is recommended.

The benefits associated with EMR include a shorter learning curve, shorter operative time, and lower perforation rate compared with ESD. However, several studies demonstrate a greater risk of local recurrence when lesions are not removed en bloc, and piecemeal resection of larger lesions make accurate pathologic assessment of margins inaccurate. Complete Barrett's eradication with EMR also has been described and achieves remission rates comparable with RFA in patients with high-grade dysplasia and nondysplastic BE. Although this technique may provide highly accurate staging of the entire Barrett's field, widespread adoption is limited because it often requires more than one session to achieve complete resection and is associated with a stricture rate of up to 44%.

Hybrid therapy that involves EMR of visible lesions, followed by endoscopic ablation of metaplastic epithelium (see Figure 2), has been shown to be an effective strategy for the management of BE. Harrero and colleagues studied EMR of visible lesions followed by RFA in 26 patients and showed that complete remission of neoplasia and intestinal metaplasia were achieved in 83% and 79% of patients, respectively, after a mean follow-up period of 29 months, without any severe complications. Despite the excellent outcomes of hybrid therapy, there has been some concern about a high incidence of synchronous and metachronous HGD, as well as recurrent high-grade lesions after focal EMR (14% to 24%). A recent systematic review showed that RFA and complete EMR were equally effective in the short-term treatment of BE but that complete EMR was associated with higher rates of complications; therefore complete EMR

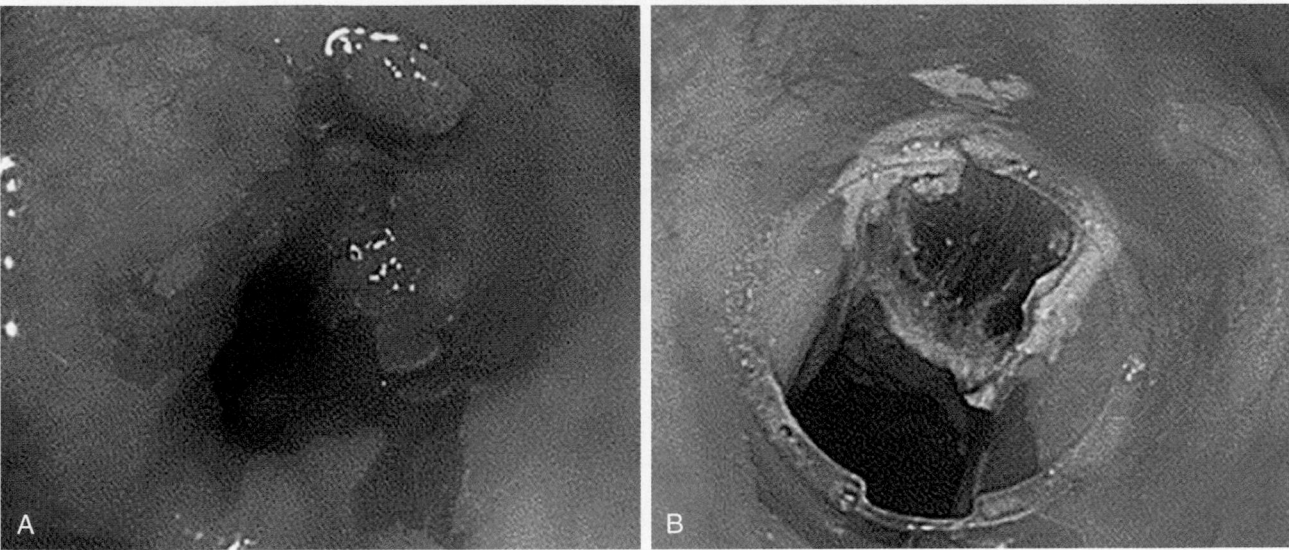

FIGURE 3 Endoscopic mucosal resection. **A,** Before. **B,** After.

should be considered only in patients with multifocal high-grade dysplasia or early esophageal adenocarcinoma.

In a pooled analysis of several EMR studies performed by Chadwick and colleagues, EMR was found to have a short-term adverse event rate of 12% with the most frequent complication being bleeding. Venous bleeding is not uncommon but usually can be managed endoscopically. The most common long-term adverse event associated with EMR is stricture formation, which is seen in 38% of patients. The risk of stenosis increases particularly after multiple or circumferential treatments. Stenosis can take months to develop and often can be managed with serial dilations.

Endoscopic Submucosal Dissection

With traditional EMR techniques lesions greater than 2 cm in size are unable to be resected en bloc and often are resected in a piecemeal fashion, leading to an increased risk of recurrence from residual dysplastic tissue. Endoscopic submucosal dissection (ESD) is an endoscopic resection technique developed in Japan that allows for the en bloc resection of flat, large (>2 cm), or ulcerated esophageal tumors and the surrounding mucosa. Endoscopic submucosal dissection is performed commonly under general anesthesia, requires specialized endoscopes and dissection tools, and is a time-consuming, technically challenging procedure with a steep learning curve. The procedure includes multiple steps, including marking the tumor circumferentially, lifting it off the submucosa by injection of glycerol, saline, and methylene blue dye, a circumferential mucosal incision, and dissection in the submucosal plane beneath the lesion, allowing for removal.

ESD has been used successfully for treatment of early esophageal squamous cell cancer, but the data regarding ESD in Barrett's neoplasia are limited. Studies from Asia and Europe have shown that ESD can achieve en bloc resection in 90% to 100% of patients with early EAC, with R0 resection achieved in 64% to 85% of patients. Similar to the complications seen with EMR, ESD carries a risk of bleeding, perforation as high as 10%, and stricture formation of 60%. The risk of stricture formation appears to be decreased if the resection area is limited to focal lesions and less than 50% of the esophageal circumference. ESD may offer several advantages over EMR in terms of higher rates of R0 resection, a more detailed histologic diagnosis, and lower recurrence rate. On the other hand, ESD is technically demanding and associated with more acute events than EMR; thus it has not gained wide acceptance in the management of early neoplastic lesions associated with BE.

■ CONCLUSION

Optimal management of dysplastic BE remains a subject of some debate. In recent years there has been a shift toward less invasive endoscopic therapies, including ablation and EMR. An understanding of the indications and limitations of these endoscopic treatments is necessary to appropriately apply these therapies in the treatment of this complex disease. When making decisions regarding choice of endoscopic treatment, one must consider the merits and limitations of each technique. Patients with BE and dysplasia should undergo careful endoscopic examination and targeted biopsies to rule out more advanced disease. Patients found to have nodular disease should undergo endoscopic resection with complete pathologic evaluation of tumor grade, depth, and margins. Complete EMR has the advantage of providing the entire BE segment for histologic evaluation, resulting in a change in staging in 30% of cases. This change in stage can affect treatment decisions and highlights the importance of resecting nodules before ablative therapy.

Patients with biopsy proven invasive carcinoma should undergo staging with EUS and CT scan in an effort to determine the extent of disease before proceeding with any endoscopic therapies. Only patients who receive complete endoscopic resection and are deemed to be low risk for lymph node involvement can be offered adjuvant ablative therapy and intensive post-treatment surveillance, whereas all others should be offered esophagectomy. Patients for whom there is concern of submucosal extension, inability to obtain complete endoscopic resection, or increased likelihood of lymph node involvement should be referred for surgical evaluation. For patients with T1b, we would recommend minimally invasive esophagectomy in our high-volume center rather than risk EMR in this population, where nodal metastasis ranges from 20% to as high as 27%. In our center, even patients with T1a invasive EAC are considered for minimally invasive esophagectomy (MIE) if they are of reasonable surgical risk, are younger patients, or where there is extensive long-segment BE in addition to a focal T1a lesion. Although recommendations regarding the management of patients with dysplastic BE and early invasive carcinoma exist, treatment plans should be individualized to each patient and created in collaboration with providers experienced in endoscopy and esophageal surgery. In all cases of HGD or early invasive EAC, an experienced surgical opinion should be obtained before committing to endoscopic therapy.

SUGGESTED READINGS

Abbas G, Pennathur A, Keeley SB, Landreneau RJ, Luketich JD. Laser ablation therapies for Barrett's esophagus. *Semin Thorac Cardiovasc Surg.* 2005;17: 313-318.

Conio M, Cameron AJ, Chak A, Blanchi S, et al. Endoscopic treatment of high-grade dysplasia and early cancer in Barrett's oesophagus. *Lancet Oncol.* 2005;6:311-321.

Luketich JD, Pennathur A, Awais O, et al. Outcomes after minimally invasive esophagectomy: review of over 1000 patients. *Ann Surg.* 2012;256:95-103.

Overholt BJ, Lightdale C, et al. Photodynamic therapy with porfimer sodium for ablation of high-grade dysplasia in Barrett's esophagus: international, partially blinded, randomized phase III trial. *Gastrointest Endosc.* 2005;62:488-498.

Shaheen NJ, Falk GW, Iyer PG, et al. ACG clinical guideline: diagnosis and management of Barrett's esophagus. *Am J Gastroenterol.* 2016;111:30-50.

THE MANAGEMENT OF PARAESOPHAGEAL HIATAL HERNIA

Avedis Meneshian, MD

Although the term often is used more generally, a true paraesophageal hernia (type II hiatal hernia) is characterized by an upward herniation of the gastric fundus/body into the chest, alongside a normally positioned, intra-abdominal esophagogastric (EG) junction, through an enlarged esophageal hiatus. More commonly, a mixed hernia defect exists (type III hiatal hernia), wherein the EG junction also has been displaced into the chest. The incidence of these hernias in the general population is unclear because many patients seeking evaluation are asymptomatic and have had the finding discovered incidentally in the context of chest and/or abdominal imaging for unrelated conditions.

■ SURGICAL INDICATIONS

There is general agreement that any *symptomatic* paraesophageal hernia (PEH) in a patient without prohibitive operative risk should be corrected surgically. Because the hernia is the underlying cause of symptoms and poses the potential risk of life-threatening complications, surgery is the only definitive therapy for this condition. Associated symptoms can include heartburn, frank regurgitation, postprandial epigastric fullness or pain, dysphagia, vomiting, weight loss, or dyspnea. Although currently conservative management in elderly asymptomatic patients is generally recommended, repair should be considered for asymptomatic patients in whom a paraesophageal hernia is documented incidentally and who are in otherwise excellent health; the small but real risk of catastrophic complication related to strangulation outweighs the minimal surgical and anesthetic risk in these otherwise healthy patients. Those who carry a more significant operative risk, whether symptomatic or asymptomatic, require the evaluation and judgment of an experienced surgeon, with particular attention given to perioperative pulmonary complication risk, especially in the context of a large hernia in which intra-abdominal domain and consequent difficulty with diaphragmatic excursion pose a significant recovery challenge.

■ PREOPERATIVE EVALUATION

Although there is no clear consensus regarding the necessity of preoperative studies, some anatomic documentation of the extent of disease (either contrast-enhanced upper gastrointestinal radiographic study or oral contrast-enhanced computed tomography [CT] scan of the chest and abdomen), as well as a functional assessment of esophageal motility (esophageal manometry or cine-esophagogram) should be considered. In our practice, contrary to conventional teaching, we consider a CT scan of the chest and abdomen the most useful study to ascertain the three-dimensional anatomy of the hernia and surrounding structures and to plan surgical repair (Figure 1). We use motility studies sparingly and reserve them for patients who present with dysphagia as a significant symptom component. In those patients, we typically begin with a cine-esophagogram and reserve manometry for patients found to have transit abnormalities on the cine study. We rarely, if ever, use 24-hour pH testing to assess reflux because all of our patients will have a loose Nissen-type fundoplication performed at the time of repair.

Perioperative cardiopulmonary risk assessment and related testing is performed on a case-by-case basis, particularly because these patients are often elderly. Patients who are obese are enrolled in a diet and exercise program with a goal of initiating healthy weight control before embarking on repair whenever feasible. An upper endoscopy to evaluate the distal esophagus and stomach and exclude concomitant peptic ulcer disease, Barrett's esophagus changes, stricture, neoplasm or other pathology is mandatory and, in our practice, is performed at the time of the planned surgical repair.

■ SURGICAL TECHNIQUE

The principal tenets of any paraesophageal hernia repair include the following:

1. Reduction of herniated abdominal contents into abdomen
2. Excision of hernia sac
3. Return of esophagogastric junction into abdomen
4. Mobilization of intrathoracic esophagus to ensure 2 to 3 cm of tension-free, intra-abdominal esophagus
5. Repair of diaphragmatic hernia defect (esophageal hiatus)

Laparoscopic Approach

The majority of our patients are managed with a laparoscopic, transabdominal approach. Preoperative deep venous thrombosis prophylaxis with subcutaneous heparin is used routinely in these patients. An upper endoscopy is performed to exclude any esophageal or gastric pathology that may have been undetected during prior imaging. Patients are maintained in the lithotomy position, with a contour-adjustable sand bag beneath them and their legs carefully padded and secured in stirrups. Both arms are abducted at 90 degrees on padded arm boards. The operating surgeon stands at the foot of the bed, between the patient's legs. The surgical table is placed into a steep reverse Trendelenburg position to allow the abdominal viscera to fall with gravity.

A small stab incision is made just above the umbilicus (Figure 2, point V), the abdominal wall pulled up firmly with two towel clamps, and the peritoneal cavity entered with a Veress needle after ensuring a normal saline drop test and low pressure on peritoneal manometry. Insufflation is maintained at 12 to 15 mm Hg until an adequate pneumoperitoneum has been achieved. Then the Veress needle is removed and a camera port incision placed (5 mm) in the midline (see Figure 2, point C), high enough above the umbilicus to allow the camera to travel well into the posterior mediastinum to allow an extended intrathoracic esophageal dissection. This location varies with patient anatomy, but we recommend erring high with this port placement. Once the 5-mm port is placed, a 5-mm, 30-degree

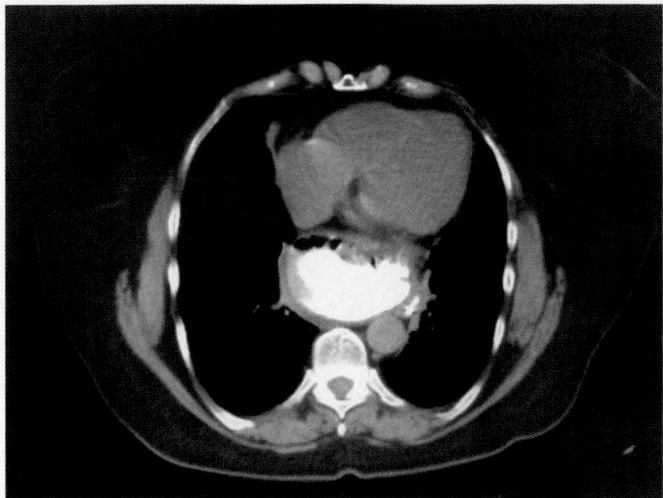

FIGURE 1 Single axial image from an oral contrast-enhanced computed tomography scan of the chest and abdomen documenting paraesophageal hernia.

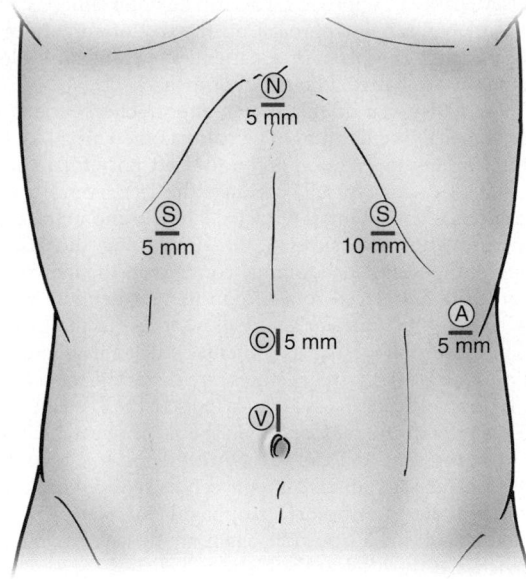

FIGURE 2 Illustration of laparoscopic abdominal port incision placement. *N*, Nathanson retractor; *S*, surgeon ports; *A*, assistant port; *C*, camera port; *V*, Veress needle insertion site.

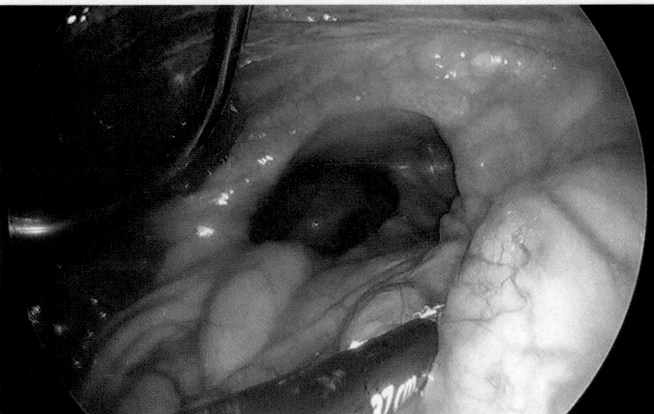

FIGURE 3 Intraoperative image of hiatal defect after loose abdominal contents have been reduced but before sac excision and reduction of herniated stomach and esophagogastric junction into the abdomen.

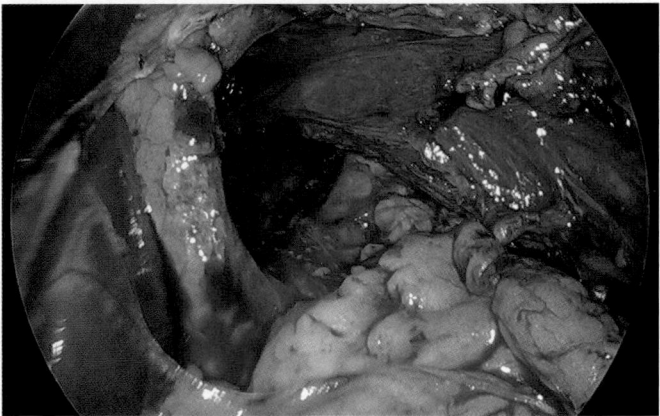

FIGURE 4 Intraoperative image of hiatal defect after sac excision, reduction of herniated stomach and esophagogastric junction into the abdomen, and extended proximal dissection of intrathoracic esophagus.

laparoscope is used and the abdomen explored. Next a Nathanson liver retractor is placed from a small stab incision just to the right of the xiphoid process (see Figure 2, point N), and with this the left lobe of the liver is elevated and retracted toward the right, thereby exposing the esophageal hiatus. Three additional port incisions then are made. A 5-mm port in the right upper quadrant and a 10-mm port in the left upper quadrant (see Figure 2, points S), triangulating with the xiphoid process, are used by the operating surgeon and are again placed high enough to allow ready access high into the posterior mediastinum. The fifth and final 5-mm port incision (see Figure 2, point A) is made laterally in the left upper quadrant to be used by the assistant, who also operates the camera (see Figure 2, point C).

First, all loose herniated contents are grasped and delivered back into the abdomen, leaving only fixed structures and the hernia sac in the chest (Figure 3). Irrespective of the size of the defect and the contents of the hernia, the majority of the abdominal contents generally can be reduced, commonly leaving only a portion of the stomach more firmly in the mediastinum. At this point, it is often helpful to enter the lesser sac along both the greater and lesser curvatures of the stomach and to pass a $\frac{1}{2}$-inch Penrose drain around the body of the stomach. The assistant surgeon then can grasp this loop and firmly retract toward the patient's feet. The hernia sac then is identified, retracted as completely into the abdomen as possible, then incised and dissection carried out to expose the right or left crus using a LigaSure (Medtronic, Dublin, Republic of Ireland). Once the crus on either side is identified, this plane is followed circumferentially and the sac is dissected free of the crura and excised until the entire hiatus is exposed. Next, taking care to preserve the vagus nerve, we dissected well into the posterior mediastinum, freeing the esophagus from the surrounding mediastinal pleura up at least to the level of the inferior pulmonary veins, and higher if feasible (Figure 4). This is arguably the most critical step in ensuring that a 2- to 3-cm, tension-free length of esophagus resides below the diaphragm and within the abdominal cavity after the hernia repair is complete. This limits the risk of recurrence and returns the EG junction to the most normal physiologic location possible. Using an extended intrathoracic esophageal dissection also obviates the need for any Collis-type esophageal lengthening procedure, which in our practice is rarely, if ever, used.

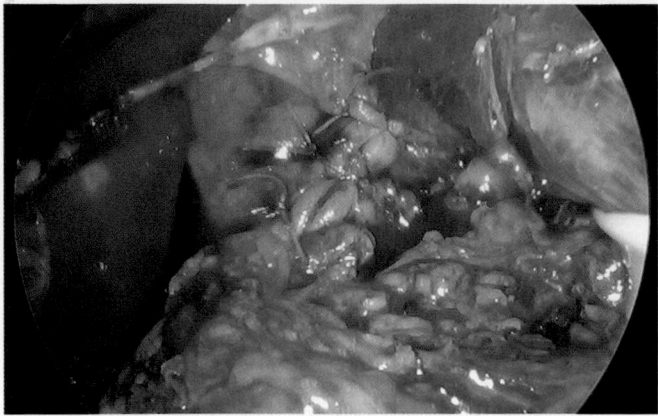

FIGURE 5 Completed primary cruroplasty around 56F bougie.

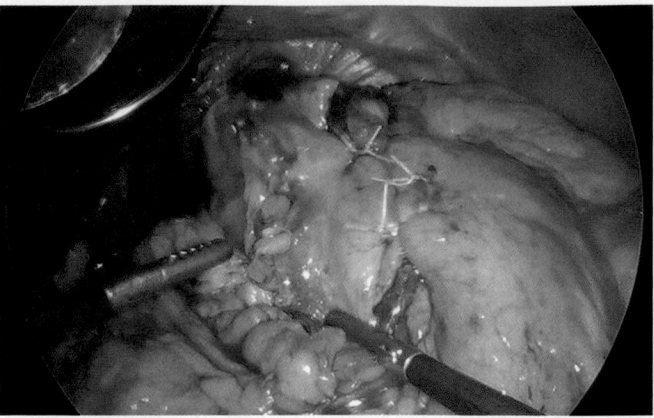

FIGURE 6 Completed Nissen fundoplication around 56F bougie.

Once the esophagus has been mobilized completely, attention is turned to dividing the short gastric vessels to sufficiently mobilize the fundus to allow for a loose Nissen fundoplication. With the exception of patients in whom there are known severe esophageal motility issues, we prefer using this approach in all patients to provide a degree of antireflux prophylaxis and to help anchor the repair below the diaphragm. Once the fundus is mobilized adequately and able to pass readily behind the EG junction, we carefully pass a 56F bougie dilator into the stomach, which we leave in place during the hiatal repair and subsequent fundoplication.

At this point, attention is turned to assessing the integrity of the diaphragmatic crura. Whenever possible, we prefer to repair the esophageal hiatus primarily and without the use of any form of mesh or pledgeted sutures. Ideally, we would have dissected the crura free without disruption of their investing fascia, thereby allowing us to reapproximate the hiatus primarily using 0-Surgidac endosutures. We do this by placing serial figure-of-8 sutures posteriorly in the crura and working forward until the repaired hiatus is opposing gently the esophagus with indwelling bougie (Figure 5). It is often helpful to begin with a simple retention suture placed slightly more anteriorly in the esophageal hiatus than the location of the planned final suture, on which the assistant surgeon can apply gently downward traction to relieve tension and facilitate suturing and tying the posterior crural repair stitches. This can be placed through a separate stab incision in the left upper quadrant, typically with a Carter-Thomason needle, and then is removed after the repair. We do not routinely employ pledgets for this repair. If the crura are thinned out or if we feel we cannot obtain a tension-free, durable repair with primary cruroplasty alone, then we consider the placement of a prosthetic reinforcement. We prefer a biologic prosthesis, which we can incorporate over time and is less apt to pose the risk of esophageal erosion. Once placed over the posterior repair, it is secured in position in four corners with interrupted 0-Surgidac endosutures.

Once the hiatus has been repaired adequately, we pass the mobilized gastric fundus behind the EG junction from left to right, ensure it has plenty of tension-free mobility, and then secure it to itself and the anterior wall of esophagus/EG junction anteriorly with additional interrupted 0-Surgidac endosutures in figure-of-8 fashion to complete the loose, 360-degree fundoplication (Figure 6). Next, we remove the bougie, release and remove the Nathanson retractor to allow the left lobe of the liver to fall back into its normal anatomic position, close the fascia of the single 10-mm port with 2-0 Vicryl suture using the Carter-Thomason closing device, then release the pneumoperitoneum, remove all trocars and the camera, and close the skin of all incisions with 4-0 Monocryl and Histoacryl glue. The patients then are awakened, extubated, and taken to the recovery room.

Left Thoracotomy Approach

In our experience, a challenging laparoscopic paraesophageal hernia repair is not made more feasible by converting to an open laparotomy. Therefore, if a laparoscopic approach fails to allow safe and complete reduction of herniated contents, we prefer a left thoracotomy (Belsey Mark IV) approach. This can be done either as a transition from a laparoscopic approach on the day of surgery or as an electively planned approach in a patient in whom multiple prior laparotomies have created a hostile abdomen.

For these patients, a double lumen endotracheal tube is placed and used to isolate the left lung. The patients then are placed in the right lateral decubitus position and a low left posterolateral thoracotomy is performed, typically through the left seventh or eighth interspace. The isolated lung is retracted laterally and in the cephalad direction, providing exposure to the descending thoracic aorta, esophagus, and herniated abdominal contents in the left chest. Stay sutures of 0-silk are placed routinely in the left hemidiaphragm to retract it laterally and inferiorly and allow access to the hiatus. The portions of the hernia sac and its contents, which are adherent to the mediastinum and left chest structures, are dissected free circumferentially. Typically, the hernia sac then is incised, the dissection carried down to the level of the crus, and then the sac is released circumferentially from the crus and excised. Once the sac has been released from the crus, the abdominal contents can be reduced back into the abdomen, and the intrathoracic esophagus completely mobilized, well up to beneath the aortic arch, again taking care to preserve the vagal branches at the level of the hiatus.

Next, from the chest, the proximal-most three or four short gastric vessels are divided to provide mobility to the gastric fundus. A 56F bougie then is inserted carefully into the stomach. Reflecting the esophagus and EG junction anteriorly, the posterior crural repair sutures then are placed (0-silk in figure-of-8 fashion) but not tied, until the repair gently opposes the esophagus and indwelling bougie. Pledgeted sutures are used only if the crura are attenuated. These sutures are not secured until after the fundoplication has been completed. Next, a 270-degree anterior Belsey Mark IV type fundoplication is performed using interrupted 2-0 silk sutures, taking horizontal mattress stitches from the esophagus to the stomach (2 cm below the EG junction), for a total of three such sutures placed 1 cm apart in circumference. Two such rows of sutures are fashioned, with the last one centrally incorporating the diaphragm. Next, the wrap and distal esophagus are returned without tension to beneath the diaphragm, the esophagus reflected anteriorly with a sponge-stick, and the posterior crural repair sutures secured. Once the hiatal repair has been completed, the bougie is removed, a 28F chest tube is placed into the left pleural space to minimize the accumulation of left pleural fluid overnight (removed the following morning), the lung is reinflated, and the thoracotomy is closed.

POSTOPERATIVE CONSIDERATIONS

Patients managed with laparoscopic paraesophageal hernia repair typically are admitted overnight to ensure adequate pain control. The morning after surgery, a contrast upper GI study is obtained to ensure adequate gastric emptying. Patients then are sent home on postoperative day 1 with a clear liquid diet for 72 hours, followed by soft food for 1 week. They are instructed to avoid eating large volumes early in the postoperative period in an effort to minimize gastric distension. Patients are reassessed symptomatically at 3 weeks and again at 6 months.

Outcomes

Failures reported in the literature are often broken down into symptomatic and radiographic recurrences. More than 90% of patients have durable, long-term symptom relief after laparoscopic paraesophageal hernia repair, whereas up to 40% of these same patients will have some degree of radiographic recurrence. The clinical significance of an asymptomatic radiographic recurrence remains unclear, and as such, we do not advocate any form of surveillance imaging modality in the long term. As in the preoperative setting, careful counseling regarding long-term dietary habits and weight control are paramount to successful, symptom-free, durable outcomes.

Controversies

Historically, there have been three principal controversies in the surgical management of paraesophageal hernias:

1. Should an open versus laparoscopic approach be used?
2. Should antireflux operations be performed at the time of PEH repair?
3. Should prosthetic hiatal reinforcement be used?

Although there are few randomized controlled trials that address each of these issues definitively, at least two of these issues should be laid to rest. There are abundant data that suggest that a laparoscopic approach is safe and effective in the majority of patients and should be considered the standard of care, even for massive and/or recurrent paraesophageal hernias. As long as a surgeon remains unbiased and considers open approaches whenever indicated, most PEH repairs can be initiated and completed laparoscopically. As noted, in our practice, a failure of the laparoscopic approach leads to a left thoracotomy approach to complete the procedure. This is based not upon any specific data but upon experience recognizing that a challenging laparoscopic PEH repair is an equally challenging open, transabdominal PEH repair. A left thoracotomy approach provides a unique vantage point from which to complete these challenging cases.

The use of an antireflux operation (most commonly a Nissen fundoplication) also should be used liberally, even in the absence of clear-cut reflux symptomatology preoperatively. If the wrap is performed over a tension-free intra-abdominal EG junction and over a reasonable size bougie (we use 56F), there is little added risk and/or operative time involved in this step, and little postoperative morbidity reported. Because a well-reconstructed EG junction and hiatal anatomy do not guarantee perfect LES function, the added value of limiting reflux and potentially anchoring the repair into the abdomen make this low-risk adjunct well worth using routinely.

Much more debate remains surrounding the need for buttressing the hiatal repair with a prosthetic. A recent randomized controlled trial of PEH repair and Nissen fundoplication with or without posterior onlay polytetrafluoroethylene (PTFE) mesh reinforcement documented a significant reduction in recurrence in the PTFE group. However, long-term complications (esophageal erosion/esophageal stenosis) were not assessed. Whenever possible, we prefer a primary repair of the hiatus because any prosthetic material poses the risk of esophageal erosion because the EG junction is a dynamic structure. When the crura are too attenuated for tension-free repair, we prefer reinforcement with a biologic material, ideally one that incorporates and/or reabsorbs over several months. Data suggest these biologic materials can minimize recurrence risk in the short term while limiting the risk of foreign body–related complications in the long term.

SUMMARY

Paraesophageal hernias should be repaired in all symptomatic and select asymptomatic patients who are reasonable surgical candidates. A laparoscopic approach should be used in most patients, with a left thoracotomy approach reserved for challenging cases. Extensive mobilization of the intrathoracic esophagus can ensure an adequate segment of tension-free esophagus below the diaphragm. Primary hiatal repair with a concomitant fundoplication should be used whenever possible, with onlay biologic prosthetic reinforcement used on a case-by-case basis.

SUGGESTED READINGS

Cooke DT. Belsey Mark IV repair. *Oper Techn Thorac Cardiovasc Surg*. 2013;215-229.
Frantzides CT, Madan AK, Carlson MA, et al. A prospective, randomized trial of laparoscopic polytetrafluoroethylene (PTFE) patch repair versus simple cruroplasty for large hiatal hernia. *Arch Surg*. 2002;137:649-652.
Furnee EJ, Draaisma WA, Gooszen HG, et al. Tailored or routine addition of an antireflux fundoplication in laparoscopic large hiatal hernia repair: a comparative cohort study. *World J Surg*. 2011;35:78-84.
Luketich JD, Nason KS, Christie NA, et al. Outcomes after a decade of laparoscopic giant paraesophageal hernia repair. *J Thorac Cardiovasc Surg*. 2010;139:395-404.
Stylopoulos N, Gazelle GS, Rattner DW. Paraesophageal hernias: operation or observation? *Ann Surg*. 2002;492-500.

THE MANAGEMENT OF ZENKER'S DIVERTICULUM

Jinny Ha, MD, and Richard Battafarano, MD, PhD

BACKGROUND

Zenker's diverticulum is a saclike outpouching of the pharyngoesophagus through Killian's triangle and is the most common type of esophageal diverticulum. Zenker's diverticulum is considered a false diverticulum because it does not involve all the layers of the esophagus; only the mucosa protrudes through the muscle layers. A pouch composed of the mucosa and submucosa of the pharyngoesophageal segment forms from pulsion forces in areas of relative hypopharyngeal wall weakness between the oblique fibers of the inferior pharyngeal constrictor and the horizontal fibers of the cricopharyngeus muscle. There is an incomplete understanding of the pathophysiology of the development of Zenker's diverticulum. However, it is presumed to be secondary to the development of high pulsion forces generated from the impaired relaxation of the upper esophageal sphincter.

CLINICAL FEATURES

Zenker's diverticulum typically affects elderly patients within the seventh and eighth decades of life. Zenker's diverticulum is found predominantly in males. The most common symptom is dysphagia, which may be caused by incomplete opening of the upper esophageal sphincter (UES) and/or extrinsic compression of the cervical esophagus by the diverticulum. As the diverticulum enlarges, patients can develop worsening dysphagia associated with weight loss and even malnutrition. Other typical symptoms include regurgitation of undigested food, choking, chronic cough, chronic aspiration, halitosis, and hoarseness. One of the few physical examination findings is Boyce's sign, which is defined as cervical borborygmus in the setting of a palpable neck mass and emaciation. Ulcers in the diverticulum occasionally can lead to significant bleeding, requiring intervention. Rarely, a Zenker's diverticulum may harbor a malignancy and patients may experience hematemesis, esophageal obstruction, or a sudden worsening of chronic symptoms.

DIAGNOSIS

A contrast esophagram with video fluoroscopy is the best imaging modality in the diagnosis and characterization of the diverticulum. The contrast esophagram typically demonstrates an esophageal pouch with retained contrast. The study provides information on the size and location and may identify abnormalities of the mucosal lining of the diverticulum. An upper gastrointestinal endoscopy is not performed routinely, unless the patient's symptoms or the contrast esophagram findings suggest a malignancy. Esophageal manometry is not required but can be helpful if the contrast study suggests an existing esophageal motility disorder such as esophageal spasm or achalasia. However, it is often difficult to perform these studies because the esophageal manometry catheters often coil within the diverticulum.

OPEN SURGICAL TREATMENT

There are two general surgical approaches for the management of Zenker's diverticula: open and transoral. The various surgical options are summarized in Table 1. With the development of new devices and techniques, less invasive approaches have gained popularity. Open surgical options are well established and include myotomy with diverticulectomy, diverticulopexy, or inversion. A few authors have described myotomy alone without specific management of the

TABLE 1: Summary of Operative Techniques for Management of Zenker's Diverticulum

Technique	Description
Endoscopic diverticulotomy	Transoral endoscopic division of cricopharyngeus muscle and the septum between the diverticulum and esophagus using electrocautery, laser, or stapler
Open diverticulectomy with myotomy	Excision of diverticulum with myotomy of the cricopharyngeus muscle
Open diverticulopexy with myotomy	Mobilization of the diverticulum with suture fixation above the neck of the diverticulum to the prevertebral fascia with myotomy of the cricopharyngeus muscle
Open myotomy alone	Myotomy of the cricopharyngeus muscle

diverticulum. However, persistent symptoms may occur in some patients using this approach.

The open surgical approach typically is performed under general anesthesia through a left cervical incision. Alternatively, this procedure can be performed under local anesthesia or selective C5-6 spinal anesthesia. The cervical esophagus is exposed after the division of the subcutaneous tissue and plastyma muscle. The sternocleidomastoid and carotid sheath are retracted laterally to reveal the underlying diverticulum. The diverticulum is dissected from the surrounding structures down to its base that is protruding through fibers of the upper esophageal sphincter. The myotomy then is performed by dividing the cricopharyngeus muscle fibers and extending the myotomy onto the cervical esophagus. If the surgeon chooses to perform a diverticulectomy, the neck of the sac can be divided using a stapling device. Alternatively, it can be divided with a scalpel and the defect closed with suture. It is best to first place a 52F Maloney dilator in the true lumen of the esophagus before excision of the diverticulum to decrease the risk of developing a mucosal stricture at the site of the diverticulectomy. Proponents of diverticulectomy state that it eliminates the potential for having retained food or liquid after eating and the very small risk of carcinoma that may develop in a residual diverticulum.

Diverticulopexy is performed by suturing the tip of the diverticulum to the prevertebral fascia in a nondependent position. Alternatively, the redundant mucosa of the diverticulum can be inverted or invaginated into the esophageal lumen and oversewn. The primary advantage of diverticulopexy and diverticular inversion is that the mucosa is not violated and left intact, resulting in a lower leak rate. These latter two techniques also allow for earlier resumption of oral intake and shorter hospital stays. Comparisons of these open techniques have not been performed in a randomized control study.

It is widely accepted that a complete cricopharyngeal myotomy must be performed no matter what technique is used to deal with the diverticulum because incomplete myotomy is associated with a high rate of recurrence. The division of the cricopharyngeal muscle reduces the UES resting pressure and normalizes the intrabolus pressure. During the myotomy, the cricopharyngeal muscle is divided completely. Because the upper esophageal muscular cuff also may be implicated in the pathogenesis of Zenker's diverticulum, many surgeons recommend extending the extramucosal myotomy 2 to 3 cm onto the esophagus. Potential complications with extension of the myotomy include perforation and associated neck and upper mediastinal infection. A myotomy alone may be sufficient for treatment of small diverticula (<2 cm).

RIGID ENDOSCOPIC TECHNIQUES

The first successful endoscopic treatment of Zenker's diverticulum was described in 1917 by Mosher and since has evolved with the improvements in visualization with newer endoscopes and novel devices such as lasers. The endoscopic approach can be performed using either rigid or flexible endoscopes. Because Zenker's diverticulum is a disease of the elderly, who often have comorbidities that make them high-risk surgical candidates, less invasive endoscopic techniques may offer potential advantages. These advantages include less postoperative pain, reduction in length of hospitalization, and quicker return to oral intake.

Endoscopic stapling diverticulotomy uses a bivalved Karl Storz Weerda diverticuloscope. This is performed under general anesthesia with endotracheal intubation with the neck fully extended. The bivalved diverticuloscope is introduced into the esophagus in the closed position. With the scope positioned in the esophageal inlet, the diverticuloscope is withdrawn to open the self-retaining valves to expose the septum. The anterior blade of the diverticuloscope is placed in the esophagus while the posterior blade is placed inside the diverticulum, straddling the septum. Care must be taken to prevent perforation of the diverticula with the lip of the diverticuloscope. Firing of the stapler simultaneously divides and seals the anterior wall of the diverticulum and the posterior wall of the esophagus. Diverticula smaller than 3 cm are not amenable to endoscopic stapling; these are too shallow to accommodate the anvil of the stapler and allow for complete transection of the septum and the performance of an adequate myotomy (recurrence rates as high as 35% have been reported for these smaller diverticula). The largest reported series using the endoscopic stapling approach (Bonavina et al) with 181 patients demonstrated a complication rate of 1.7% (two cases of dental injury and one case of mucosal tear). Eight of the cases were converted to open because of poor exposure or mucosal injury. The study reported that 92% of the patients were symptom free with a mean follow-up time of 27 months.

Dohlman's transoral technique divides the cricopharyngeus muscle using electrocautery or, more recently, CO_2 laser (introduced by van Overbeek in 1981). After the necessary exposure is achieved with the diverticuloscope, an operative microscope is used to focus the CO_2 laser and divide the esophageal mucosa and cricopharyngeus muscle while preserving the integrity of the extraluminal mucosa of the diverticulum. Using this technique, van Overbeek reported a 6% complication rate in his published series of 216 patients. Another series of 119 patients (Hoffman et al) reported a complication rate of 3.4%, which included mediastinitis, salivary fistulas, and dental injuries. The latter series included a follow-up period of 1 to 3 years, and 93% of the patients were symptom free.

A more recent technique uses the endoscopic harmonic scalpel to divide the partition between diverticulum and the esophagus. The harmonic scalpel simultaneously cuts and coagulates the tissue with minimal thermal spread. The smaller diameter of the harmonic scalpel allows it to be maneuvered into small diverticula, which is an advantage over the endoscopic stapler. Although this technique has been demonstrated effective for smaller diverticula, long-term outcomes have not been studied.

FLEXIBLE ENDOSCOPIC TECHNIQUES

Flexible endoscopic diverticulotomy can be performed under conscious sedation and without extension of the neck. In the literature, the flexible endoscope has been reserved for poor operative candidates with difficult head and neck anatomy for rigid esophagoscopy. The septum can be exposed using a variety of accessories (nasogastric tube, hood, endoscopic cap, and overtube). The diverticulotomy then can be made using the monopolar forceps, hook cautery, argon plasma coagulation, and needle knife. Multiple sessions may be required to avoid perforation and mediastinitis, ranging from one to three sessions in the literature. Repeat treatment can be performed the next day or the treatment completed over several weeks. Further studies are needed to understand the role of flexible endoscopy for the treatment of pharyngeal diverticulum. The optimal cutting technique is unknown and based largely on the endoscopist's preference.

CONCLUSION

Randomized control trials directly comparing open versus endoscopic techniques are lacking. In a single center study, Gutschow and colleagues compared open operative approaches versus endoscopic stapling and laser division and reported better symptom relief with open techniques (diverticulum size <3 cm, 85% vs 25%; ≥3 cm, 86% vs 50%). Salivary fistulas were the only type of complication associated with diverticulectomy with myotomy and pexy with myotomy group. The complications of the endoscopic CO_2 laser cohort included dental injury, upper mediastinitis, and carotid artery and jugular vein injury. The overall incidence of postoperative complications was low in the open and endoscopic group; however, the category of complications differed between the open versus endoscopic group. The combined complication rate for this series of patients was reported to be 5.3%. Rizzetto and colleagues demonstrated better long-term results with open surgical approaches compared with transoral techniques. Recurrent or persistent symptoms were reported in 21.5% of the patients in the endoscopic treatment group compared with 5.2% of the patients in the operative group (p < 0.05) with a median follow-up period of 40 months. There was no difference in the postoperative complication rates between the two approaches in this study. The outcomes for open surgical techniques were found superior to endoscopic approaches, particularly with smaller diverticula (<3 cm). In contrast, a review study by Chang and colleagues compared publications from 1990 to 2002. This study found that endoscopic stapling had a lower major complication rate and mortality rate compared with open surgery (2.6 vs 11.8% and 0.3% vs 1.6%, respectively). However, the included studies had complications rates that varied from 0 to 26%. The heterogeneity among the studies makes it difficult to soundly draw conclusions on whether the open or transoral technique is superior.

The treatment of pharyngeal diverticulum has evolved in recent years, and the role of endoscopic techniques is being investigated. Current available studies have shown both open and endoscopic techniques are safe and effective in the treatment of these Zenker's diverticulum in the short term, but long-term outcomes data for less invasive techniques are still pending.

The various surgical approaches have advantages and disadvantages. Open diverticulectomy with myotomy is safe, and the durable long-term outcomes have been well established in the literature. An open surgical approach may be contraindicated in severely debilitated patients who are poor operative candidates. The less invasive endoscopic techniques, especially flexible endoscopic techniques, may be advantageous in these cases. Endoscopic approaches have their limitations in cases of small and large diverticula, whereas open surgical diverticulectomy has no size limitations. As the surgical experience with minimally invasive techniques continues to increase, it may be important to consider the patient characteristics and understand the pros and cons of various techniques to individualize the best surgical approach for patients.

SUGGESTED READINGS

Bonavina L, Bona D, Abraham M, et al. Long-term results of endosurgical and open surgical approach for Zenker diverticulum. *World J Gastroenterol.* 2007;13:2586-2589.

Chang CY, Payyapilli RJ, Scher RL. Endoscopic staple diverticulostomy for Zenker's diverticulum: review of literature and experience in 159 consecutive cases. *Laryngoscope.* 2003;113:957-965.

Gutschow CA, Hamoir M, Rombaux P, et al. Management of pharyngoesophageal (Zenker's) diverticulum: which technique? *Ann Thorac Surg.* 2002;74:1677-1682.

Hoffmann M, Scheunemann D, Rudert HH, et al. Zenker's diverticulotomy with the carbon dioxide laser: perioperative management and long-term results. *Ann Otol Rhinol Laryngol.* 2003;112:202-205.

Mosher HP. Webs and pouches of the esophagus: their diagnosis and treatment. *Surg Gynecol Obstet.* 1917;25:175-187.

Rizzetto C, Zaninotto G, Costantini M, et al. Zenker's diverticula: feasibility of a tailored approach based on diverticulum size. *J Gastrointest Surg.* 2008;12:2057-2065.

Wouters B, van Overbeek JJ. Endoscopic treatment of the hypopharyngeal (Zenker's) diverticulum. *Hepatogastroenterology.* 1992;39:105-108.

THE MANAGEMENT OF ACHALASIA OF THE ESOPHAGUS

Rodney J. Landreneau, MD, Blair A. Jobe, MD, FACS, and Fahim Habib, MD, MPH, FACS

■ BACKGROUND

Although rare, achalasia is the most common of the primary esophageal motility disorders. Its incidence increases with age, from 0.25 per 100,000 in children to 35 per 100,000 in those over 85, with an average incidence of 1 per 100,000 per year. Because of its chronic nature prevalence is much higher at 10 per 100,000. Although the exact cause remains unknown, autoimmune, infectious, and neurodegenerative basis have all been proposed. Current thinking points towards an autoimmune response in a genetically susceptible individual triggered by an infection that results in destruction predominantly of the inhibitory postganglionic neurons of the distal esophagus and the lower esophageal sphincter (LES). The unopposed cholinergic action that results leads to a failure of the LES to relax in response to swallowing and a lack of coordinated peristalsis in the distal esophagus, the manometric demonstration of which defines the disease.

Dysphagia, the most common symptom, is progressive, occurring with both solids and liquids, and predates the development of other symptoms. Heartburn, regurgitation of undigested foods, chest pain, halitosis, and odynophagia are also common. Retention of food in the esophagus because of decreased clearance predisposes the patient to aspiration and respiratory symptoms, which are seen in up to 40% of patients, including cough, asthma, aspiration, hoarseness, and sore throat. Inability to maintain an adequate oral intake and sitophobia (the fear of eating) results in unintentional weight loss. Severity of achalasia, stage of disease, and response to treatment are assessed using the Eckardt score (Table 1).

■ DIAGNOSIS

The symptoms of achalasia overlap with those of a number of other disease processes, making diagnosis difficult. The differential diagnosis includes gastroesophageal reflux disease with peptic strictures, esophageal rings or webs, eosinophilic esophagitis, radiation or medication-induced strictures, nonachalasia motility disorders, previous fundoplication or bariatric surgery procedures, systemic disease including amyloidosis and sarcoidosis, malignancy, extrinsic compression of the esophagus, and paraneoplastic neuropathy-induced achalasia as seen with prostate or pancreatic cancer.

We begin with a *contrast esophagogram*, which demonstrates distal esophageal narrowing with a classic "bird's-beak" appearance (Figure 1). Other features include esophageal dilatation, a contrast-filled esophagus with slow or absent emptying, an air-fluid level, and a "corkscrew appearance" in the subset with vigorous distal esophageal contractions. In advanced cases the dilated tortuous esophagus may show substantial deviation from its normal straight axis, termed a *sigmoid esophagus*. The esophagogram provides a roadmap for the subsequent endoscopy. *Esophagogastroduodenoscopy* reveals a dilated or tortuous esophagus with retained food, esophagitis, and resistance to passage of the scope through the gastroesophageal junction. *Esophageal manometry* is the gold standard for establishing the diagnosis of achalasia. Demonstration of incomplete relaxation of the LES and absence of coordinated peristalsis in the distal esophagus is sine qua non. The presence of a hypertensive resting LES is not a criteria for diagnosis. Conventional manometry has been replaced largely by high-resolution manometry systems (HRM) that use a solid-state assembly with 36 circumferential sensors placed 1 cm apart that dynamically capture the pressure change along the entire length of the esophagus. Ten 5-mL water swallows are performed in the supine position and used to generate an esophageal pressure topography (Clouse) plot that allows classification of achalasia into clinically and prognostically relevant subtypes. This is termed the *Chicago Classification of motility disorders* and continues to undergo refinement.

The current version (Chicago Classification v3.0) divides achalasia into three distinct subtypes. Type I (55%) achalasia (classic achalasia) is associated with impaired LES relaxation, absence of peristalsis with complete loss of contractile activity in the body of the esophagus, and a dilated esophagus with a "bird's beak" on contrast esophagogram. In type II (40%) achalasia the impaired LES relaxation is associated with increased panesophageal pressures and absence of a peristaltic contraction. In type III (5%) achalasia in addition to impaired relaxation, premature simultaneous spastic contractions occur, which compartmentalize the bolus, giving rise to the characteristic corkscrew appearance. Esophagogastric outflow obstruction is another well-recognized manometric pattern in which impaired LES relaxation is associated with normal peristalsis and may represent early achalasia, where organized contractility of the body is as of yet preserved (Figure 2).

■ TREATMENT

Achalasia has no cure. The goal of therapy is to reduce the tone of the LES, allowing the esophagus to empty adequately. This may be achieved by medical, endoscopic, or surgical means.

Medical Therapy

Nitrates, calcium channel blockers, and more recently phosphodiesterase-5 inhibitors have been used to lower EGJ pressure. Nitrates increase nitric oxide concentration in the smooth muscle cells of the LES, increasing cyclic adenosine monophosphate levels, which promotes muscle relaxation. Isosorbide dinitrate, 5 to 10 mg, is given 15 minutes before meals. The oral calcium channel blocker nifedipine in doses of 10 to 30 mg given 30 to 45 minutes before meals acts by blocking entry of calcium into the smooth muscle cells of the LES reducing contractility. Sildenafil blocks phosphodiesterase-5 inhibiting the degradation of cyclic guanosine monophosphate induced by nitric oxide leading to impaired muscle contraction. The occurrence of significant side effects of the medications, development of tolerance, uncertain efficacy, and poor absorption because of the disease itself preclude routine use. Use of medical therapy is limited to patients who are not candidates for more invasive therapies.

Endoscopic Therapies
Botulinum Toxin

Botulinum, a neurotoxin derived for *Clostridium botulinum,* blocks the release of acetylcholine from nerve endings causing paralysis of the muscle. The effect is temporary and is reversed over the course of 3 to 4 months as a consequence of axonal regeneration. 100 U of Botox A (Allergen Inc, Irvine, California) are endoscopically injected in equal aliquots into the LES in four quadrants just above the Z-line using a sclerotherapy needle. Higher doses are not more effective. Although initially efficacious, the benefit fades over the ensuing year. Subsequent interventions are made more difficult by the use of Botox. Its use should therefore be limited to patients who are not candidates for either pneumatic dilatation (PD) or a laparoscopic Heller myotomy (LHM).

TABLE 1: Eckardt Score: Clinical Scoring System for the Grading and Staging of Achalasia

Score	Dysphagia	Regurgitation	Retrosternal Pain	Weight Loss (kg)
0	None	None	None	None
1	Occasional	Occasional	Occasional	<5
2	Daily	Daily	Daily	5-10
3	Each meal	Each meal	Each meal	>10

From Eckardt VF, Aignherr C, Bernhard G. Predictors of outcome in patients with achalasia treated with pneumatic dilatation. *Gastroenterology.* 1992;103:1732-1738.

Stage 0: score 0-1; Stage 1: score 2-3; Stage 2: score 4-6; Stage 3: score >6

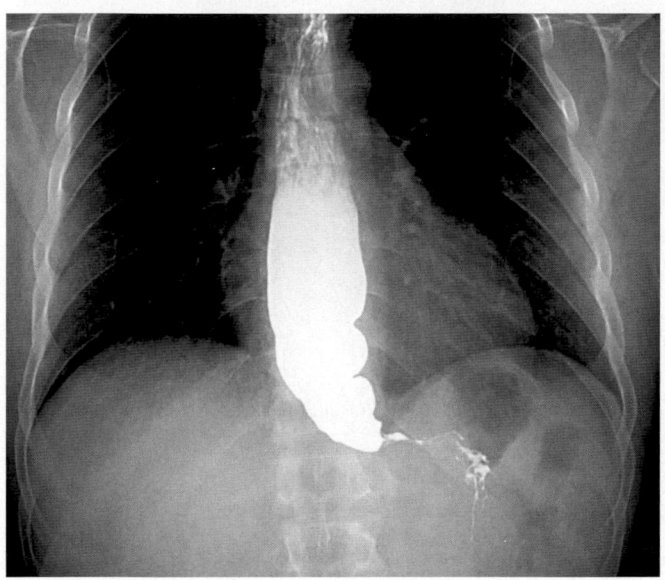

FIGURE 1 Bird's-beak appearance on barium swallow.

Pneumatic Dilatation

Under fluoroscopic guidance, a pneumatic balloon device (Micro-invasive Rigiflex balloon system, Boston Scientific Corp, Boston, MA) mounted on a flexible catheter and placed over an endoscopic guide wire is positioned across the LES. Using a handheld manometer, the selected balloon (30, 35, or 40 mm) is inflated to a pressure of 7 to 15 psi until the waist is fully flattened, and held for 15 to 60 seconds. This disrupts the circular fibers of the LES, providing relief. A graded dilatation protocol is followed starting with the 30-mm balloon, with additional dilatations using larger diameter balloons as needed based on response and symptoms. In patients with an uneventful dilatation a contrast esophagogram first with water-soluble contrast and if negative with barium is obtained to rule out occult perforation. If the patient develops pain and a perforation is clinically suspected, then a computed tomogram is obtained to assess for free air. If a leak is identified, a covered stent is used to seal it. The patient must remain cautious for severe chest pain or fever especially if postprocedure vomiting occurs because this may result in a delayed perforation with potentially devastating consequences. PD produces relief of symptoms in 60% to 90% of patients. Greater relief is seen with balloons of larger diameter; therefore a graded dilation approach is advocated. Within 5 years, more than a third of the patients will relapse and additional dilatations will be required. Outcome of PD is best in patients older than 45 years, females, a postdilatation LES pressure of less than 10 mm Hg, and a type II achalasia pattern on HRM. GERD can occur in 15% to 30% of patients after PD, necessitating acid-suppression therapy. In spite of a randomized trial performed as far back as the late 1980s demonstrating the superiority of LHM, PD continues to be performed frequently.

Per-Oral Endoscopic Myotomy

Per-oral endoscopic myotomy (POEM) is a novel endoscopic technique initially described for the treatment of achalasia that is now being applied across the spectrum of esophageal motility disorders. In 2010 Inoue and colleagues reported on 17 patients who underwent the procedure. Multiple subsequent reports have demonstrated POEM to be feasible and safe and with equivalent short-term outcomes compared with LHM with initial success rate of more than 90%. We started out with the adoption of POEM for type II achalasia and have now expanded its use to a broader spectrum of esophageal motility disorders.

Because of the high incidence of candidal esophagitis associated with retained food in the esophagus, nystatin swish and swallows are started 5 days before the intervention. The patient is placed on a clear liquid diet for 3 days before the procedure. The procedure is performed in the operating room, under general anesthesia, in the supine position. A single dose of perioperative antibiotics consisting of a first-generation cephalosporin and 200 mg of fluconazole are given before induction of anesthesia. Endoscopy is performed using CO_2 for insufflation and the location of the anatomic esophagogastric junction identified. Methylene blue admixed with saline is injected into the submucosal space 15 cm proximal to the EGJ. This creates a cushion and reduces the risk of inadvertent perforation of the esophagus. We avoid using epinephrine in the solution because of concern for mucosal sloughing as a consequence of its vasoconstrictor effect. A 1.5- to 2-cm longitudinal incision is made in the mucosa using a triangle-tip knife (TT knife, Olympus USA, Center Valley, PA) on the anterior wall of the esophagus at the 1 o'clock position. Once access to the submucosal space is gained, a gastroscope with a transparent plastic cap is introduced into the opening, and a submucous tunnel is created. Coagulation graspers are used to cauterize any large bridging vessels. The submucosal tunnel is carried onto the stomach for a distance of at least 3 cm. Myotomy is initiated 2 cm distal to the distal end of the mucosectomy and the plane between the circular and longitudinal muscles identified. A proximal to distal myotomy of the circular layer then is performed, extending it onto the gastric cardia for 2 to 3 cm. Identification of large submucosal gastric vessels is an indicator of an adequate distal myotomy. The gastroscope is now passed back through the esophageal lumen to assess the adequacy of the myotomy and the ease of passing the gastroscope through the EGJ. After confirming hemostasis, 80 mg of gentamicin in 20 mL of normal saline is instilled into the submucosal tunnel. The mucosal incision can be closed with over the scope clips (OSTC Clips, Ovesco, Tübingen, Germany) or sutured using an endoscopic suturing system (OverStitch endoscopic suturing System, Apollo Endosurgery, Austin TX) (Figure 3). As the POEM procedure theoretically does not involve division of the phrenoesophageal membrane or alteration of the angle of His, the intrinsic antireflux barrier may be preserved. However, it appears in practice that the

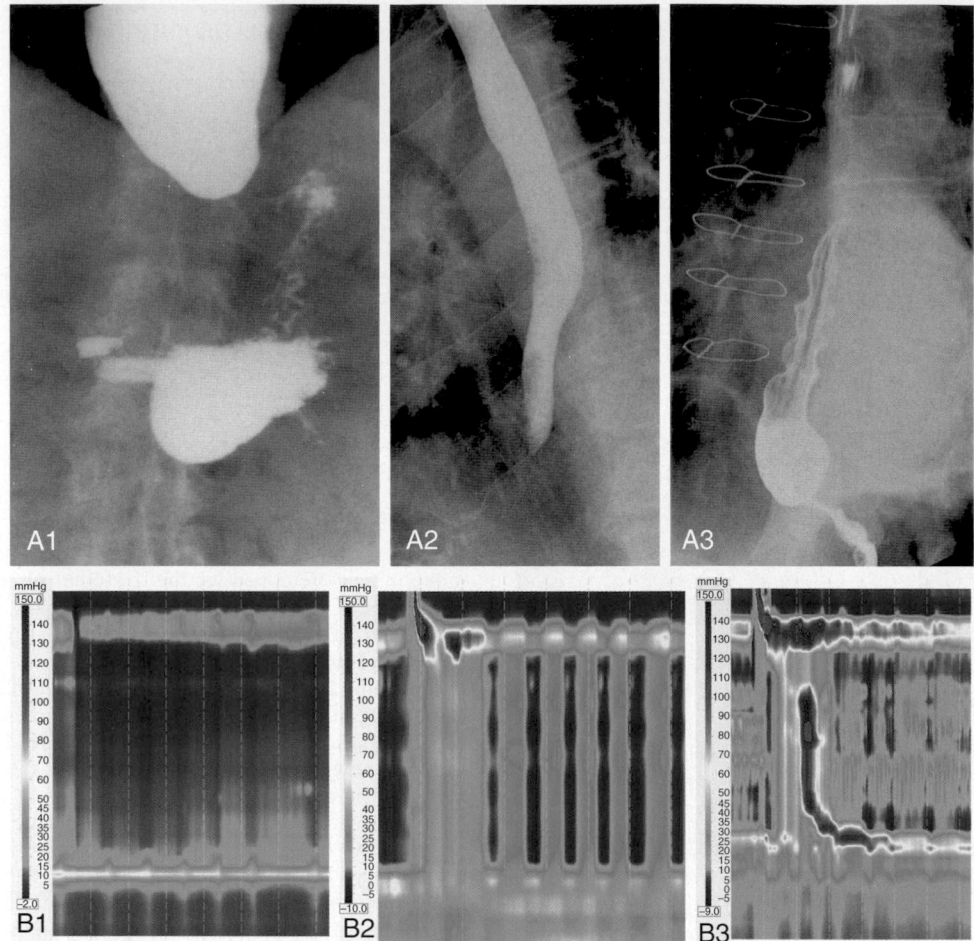

FIGURE 2 A1 and **B1,** Type I or Classic Achalasia: Impaired LES relaxation with absence of peristalsis. **A2** and **B2,** Type II: Impaired LES relaxation with panesophageal pressurizations and absent peristaltic contractions. **A3** and **B3,** Type III or Spastic Achalasia: Impaired relaxation of the LES with premature simultaneous spastic contractions.

postoperative reflux rate parallels that seen after forceful pneumatic dilation or surgical myotomy without partial fundoplication. An esophagogram is obtained the day after surgery. If no esophageal obstruction or leak is identified, a clear liquid diet is initiated. Low-dose proton pump inhibition is administered. Whenever possible, prolonged esophageal pH testing is performed 6 months after the procedure to assess pathologic reflux exposure. Although the initial results are promising (Figure 4), long-term efficacy in terms of durability of symptom control, development of reflux, and esophageal dilatation will become evident over time.

Surgical Treatment

Laparoscopic Heller Myotomy With Partial Fundoplication

Ernst Heller in 1913 described the performance of an anterior and posterior myotomy of the distal body of the esophagus for the treatment of achalasia. Zaaijer in 1923 modified the technique to a single anterior extramucosal myotomy with equivalent results. This modified Heller remained the standard until Pelligrini in 1992 described the thoracoscopic approach to myotomy. The explosion of minimally invasive techniques of laparoscopic surgery led to the development of the LHM, which in conjunction with a partial fundoplication provides excellent relief from dysphagia, less postoperative reflux, a shorter hospital stay, less postoperative pain, and earlier return to function. As a result, LHM with a partial fundoplication now is considered the gold standard for the treatment of achalasia in the United States (Figure 5).

Extreme caution must be exercised at time of induction of general anesthesia because of the potential risk of aspiration of retained esophageal contents. Thus a rapid sequence approach to endotracheal intubation and control of the airway is recommended. Once anesthetized, endoscopy is performed to evacuate any residual material, lavage the lumen with copious amounts of irrigation fluid. On occasion, the operative intervention actually may have to be delayed should significant esophageal debris be present that is difficult to clear for an initial endoscopic evaluation. We leave the endoscope in place to allow for intraoperative assessments as needed. The patient is then placed in a supine, split-legged position with footboards and adequate padding of the knees to prevent sliding during the steep reverse Trendelenburg position employed for the laparoscopic procedure. Pneumatic compression devices are applied to prevent deep vein thrombosis. The surgeon stands between the patient's legs and the assistant to the left side of the patient.

Access to the abdomen is gained by use of an 11-mm Visiport trocar system (Covidien, Mansfield, MA) inserted in the left paramedian location two thirds of the way between the xiphoid and umbilicus. This will be the site of the 10-mm 30-degree laparoscope for video optics. Alternatively, insertion of a Veress needle in the left upper quadrant close to the costal margin is used for CO_2 insufflation of the abdomen if previous abdominal surgery has been performed. The remaining trocars are placed under direct vision. A 10-mm port

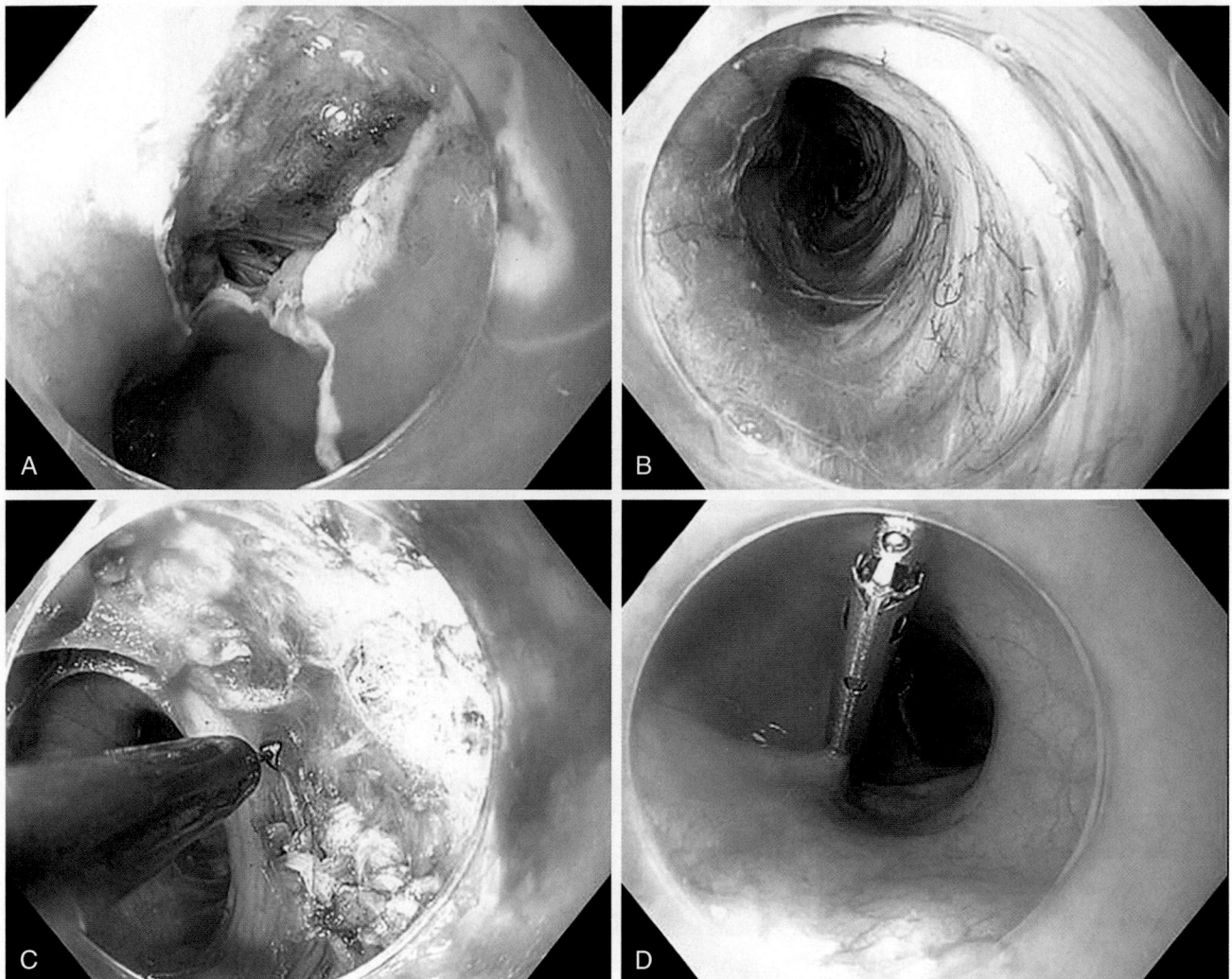

FIGURE 3 Endoscopic views of the POEM procedure: **A,** Mucosal entry site. **B,** The submucosal tunnel; the muscle layer is on the right and mucosa on the left. **C,** Myotomy to divide the circular layer of muscle. **D,** Closure of the mucosal defect using clips.

for the surgeon's right hand is placed in the left midclavicular line, 2-cm below the costal margin. A 5-mm trocar is placed in the anterior axillary line just under the costal margin for the assistant's right hand. A 5-mm trocar is placed in the epigastrium just to the right of the xiphoid and used to place a Nathanson liver retractor (Cook Medical, Bloomington, IN), which is connected to a table-mounted holder and is used to retract the left lateral segment away from the hiatus. A final 5-mm trocar is placed 2 to 3 cm below the costal margin just to the right of the falciform ligament and is used for the surgeon's left hand.

The gastric fat pad is grasped with a locking grasper and retracted inferiorly and laterally by the assistant. The gastrohepatic ligament is opened using harmonic shears (Harmonic Ace 7, Ethicon Endo-Surgery, Cincinnati, OH) and identification of the upper aspect of the right crural arch and the phrenoesophageal ligament is accomplished. The phrenoesophageal membrane is incised at approximately the 10 o'clock position along the crural arc and extended clockwise over the anterior aspect of the esophagus to the left side of the crural arch. The highest short gastric arterial arcades are divided to achieve adequate mobilization of the upper fundus and delineation of the gastroesophageal junction at the "angle of His" for future partial fundoplication (Dor fundoplication).

The hiatus is evaluated for a hiatal hernia, which is exceedingly uncommon. If none is present, no posterior dissection is attempted, and the attachments are left intact. If a hiatal hernia is present, or in the case of a sigmoid esophagus, circumferential dissection is performed and a posterior window is created between the posterior vagus and the wall of the esophagus. A Penrose drain is passed through this opening and used to provide traction for continued circumferential dissection of the esophagus into the lower mediastinum. The gastroesophageal fat pad is dissected off the anterior surface of the stomach in a left to right orientation, exposing the area where the myotomy is to be performed.

Intraoperative endoscopy is performed to locate the exact site of obstruction at the EGJ by using a combination of transillumination and slight esophageal insufflation.

We begin the myotomy by instilling saline with 0.5% epinephrine solution into the muscular wall of the distal esophagus, gastroesophageal junction, and cardia of the stomach in the area of the proposed esophagomyotomy. This maneuver assists in control of oozing during the dissection and also elevates the muscular wall of the esophagus from the esophageal submucosa, facilitating identification of the proper plane of dissection and myotomy.

The esophagomyotomy is then initiated 2 cm above the gastroesophageal junction using sharp dissection with endoscopic scissors and augmented with harmonic scalpel dissection. Once the circular muscle fibers are identified, they are elevated and divided until the submucosal plane is identified. In this plane, the myotomy is carried

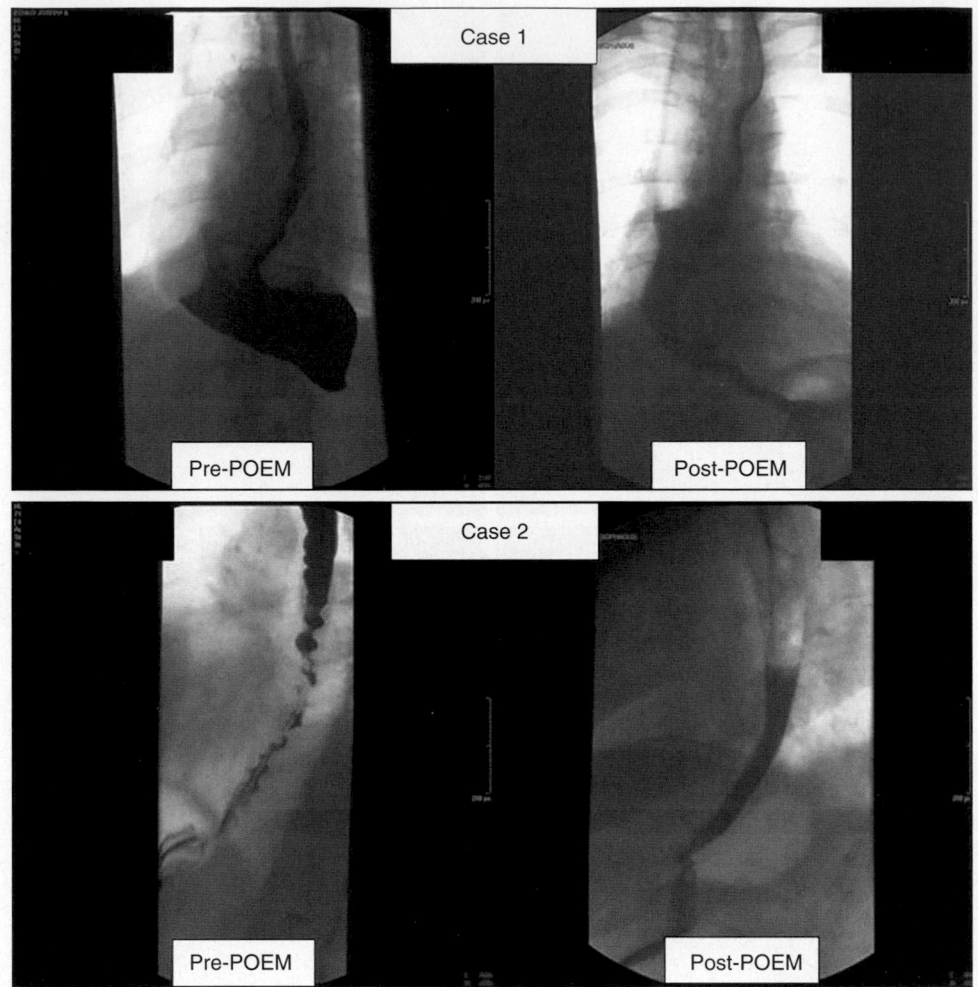

FIGURE 4 Barium swallow performed pre- and post-POEM: **A,** for a longstanding achalasia with a sigmoid esophagus and **B,** in distal esophageal spasm.

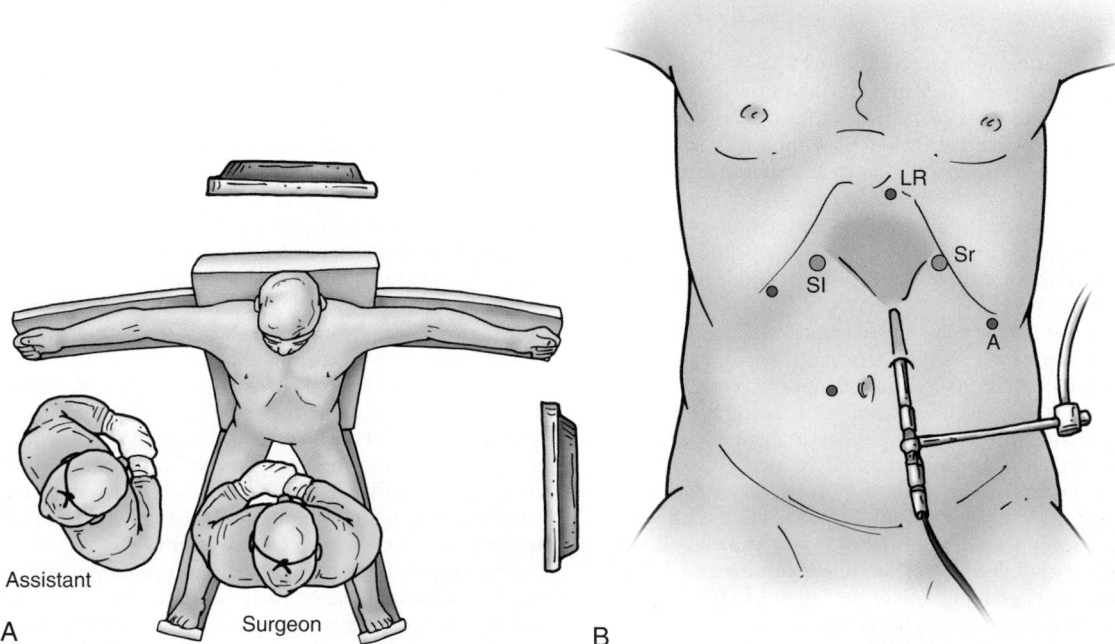

FIGURE 5 Technique of laparoscopic Heller myotomy and the Dor partial fundoplication for achalasia. **A,** Patient positioning: a split-leg table that allows for steep reverse Trendelenburg position is used. The surgeon stands between the legs of the patient with the assistant to the left. **B,** Shows our preferred sites for port placement. *C,* Camera, *Sl,* Surgeon's left hand, *Sr,* Surgeon's right hand, *A,* assistant's port. The unmarked trocar sites are additional 5-mm ports that may be required occasionally to provide adequate exposure or retraction.

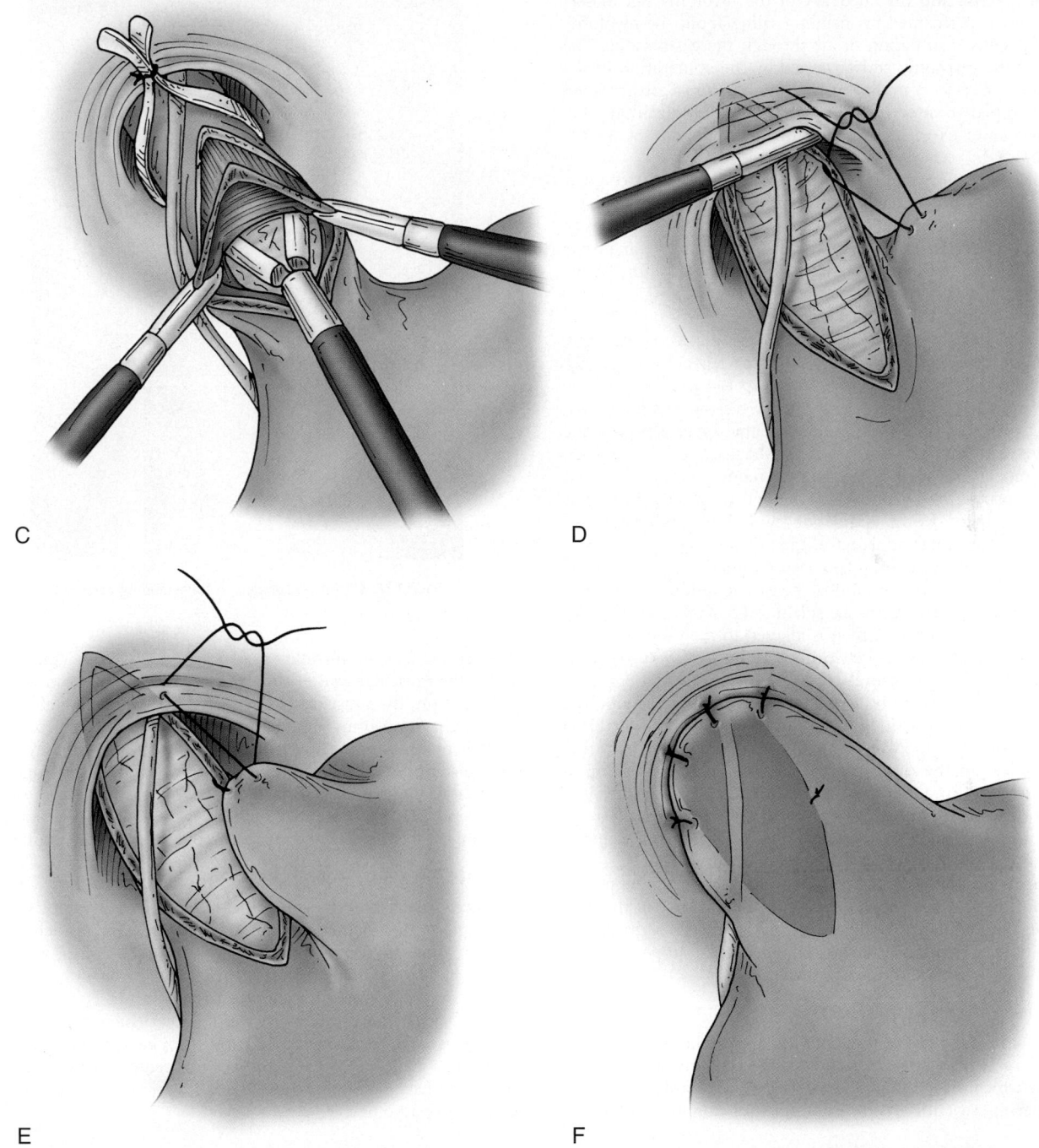

C

D

E

F

FIGURE 5, cont'd C, Division of the outer longitudinal muscle layer followed by that of the inner circular layer exposing the submucosal layer.
D, The first stitch of the Dor fundoplication anchors the greater curvature of the stomach about 2 cm from the angle of His to the right cut edge of the myotomy at the 4 o'clock position. Note the extensive myotomy that has been performed, which requires the anterior vagus nerve to be dissected off the anterior esophagus. **E,** The apical suture incorporated the diaphragm and the cut edge of the two layers of muscle. **F,** Application of sutures between the greater curvature, the edge of the hiatus, and the cut edge of the muscle allows the fundus of the stomach to roll over the defect in the muscle created by the myotomy.

upward for a distance of 5 cm from the EGJ and distally for a distance of 2.5 cm onto the gastric cardia until the large veins of the transverse submucosal venous plexus are identified. The muscle fibers are then separated from the underlying mucosa on both sides of the myotomy using endoscopic Kittner dissectors to ensure that at least 50% of the mucosal circumference is exposed.

It is important to emphasize that the critical aspect of the myotomy involves the transition from the distal esophagus toward gastroesophageal junction. It is often surprising how thin the muscular wall is as the myotomy transitions from the esophagus to the cardia of the stomach. Extreme caution is required at this point to avoid inadvertent perforation of the mucosa.

Endoscopy again is performed to confirm the integrity of the esophageal mucosa and the adequacy of the myotomy. An underwater seal test is performed by instilling saline about the myotomy and simultaneous insufflation of air through the gastroscope. The adequacy of the myotomy is determined by the obliteration of the rosette of mucosa seen preoperatively at the site of obstruction, and the unimpeded entry of the scope into the stomach. Transillumination allows us to identify and divide any bands of muscle that remain.

A partial fundoplication is performed to reduce the risk of postoperative reflux. If posterior dissection has not been performed, we prefer to create a Dor fundoplication. For this, the first suture is taken on the greater curvature of the stomach, 2 cm from the anatomic GEJ. This is sutured to the left crus at the 2 o'clock position, incorporating the cut edge of the myotomy, thus accentuating the angle of His. Subsequent sutures are taken along the greater curvature at 2 cm intervals and secured to the hiatus from the left to the right, thereby folding the anterior surface of the stomach over the myotomy. This aspect of the fundus then is sutured to the right side of the myotomy and the right crura arc at the 11 o'clock position. Final sutures between the mobilized fundus and the upper aspect of the arcuate ligament are performed. The esophagoscope is introduced into the stomach during this suturing to reduce the likelihood of esophageal obstruction by an overzealous suturing of the fundus to the arcuate ligament. Upon completion, mobilized fundus now lies in contact with the anterior aspect of the myotomized esophagus.

When a posterior dissection has been required, we prefer to use a modified "Toupet" fundoplication. The gastric fundus is passed in the retroesophageal space from the splenic side of the esophagus to the right. The fundoplication then is aligned to the esophagus and bilateral triangulation sutures between the mobilized fundus, myotomized esophagus, and the crural arc at the 11 o'clock and 2 o'clock positions, respectively. Finally, the fundus is grasped and mobilized from left to right and sutured to the right side of the crus at the 11:30 o'clock position to drape over the esophagomyotomy. As with the Dor fundoplication, the esophagoscope is maintained in the stomach to avoid excessive fundoplication and esophageal obstruction. It is important to avoid a total fundoplication (Nissen procedure) as significant obstruction to esophageal emptying is commonly a problem, thus defeating the very purpose of the esophagomyotomy.

An esophagoscopy is performed after completion of the procedure to confirm adequacy of the myotomy, the integrity of the fundoplication, and to again evaluate for any mucosal perforations. Postoperatively, a barium swallow is obtained on postoperative day 1. If negative, a clear liquid diet is initiated.

Transthoracic Myotomy

For the most part the use of transthoracic approaches to esophagomyotomy largely have been abandoned and used almost exclusively in cases in which an abdominal approach is not feasible. A lateral muscle sparing seventh interspace mini-thoracotomy commonly is used.

After careful intubation with a single-lumen endotracheal tube, esophagoscopy is performed to clear and clean the esophagus. A dual-lumen endotracheal tube, or bronchus blocker, then is placed to allow for single-lung ventilation of the right lung and ipsilateral atelectasis of the left lung to facilitate the esophageal dissection. The patient is placed in a right lateral decubitus position.

The muscle-sparing thoracotomy is performed, and the inferior pulmonary ligament is divided to approach the distal esophagus. The esophagoscope is left in place for periodic transillumination and insufflation. The esophagus is dissected from the level of the inferior pulmonary ligament to the anterior properitoneal membrane. The esophagus is encircled with a ½-inch Penrose drain with the esophagoscope in place within the esophagus. Care is taken to avoid injury to the vagal nerve trunks. The peritoneal reflection is incised. The crural opening is expanded, and the upper short gastric arcades are divided. The gastroesophageal junction and gastric cardia

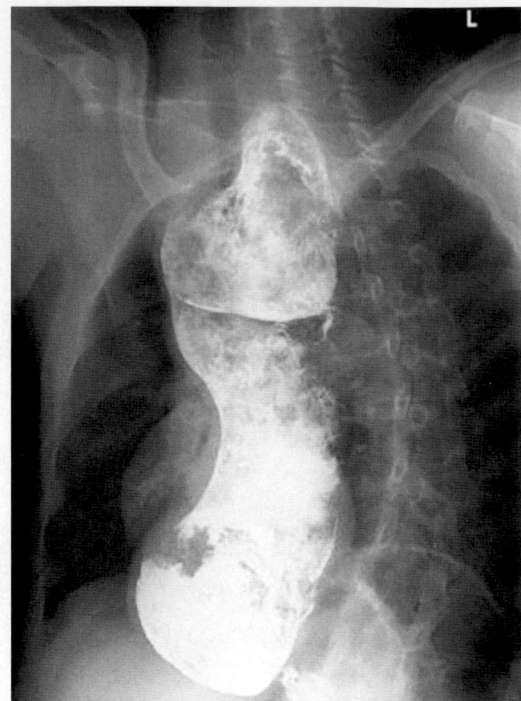

FIGURE 6 Megaesophagus in longstanding achalasia.

are identified. After instillation of saline with 0.5% epinephrine within the muscular wall of the distal esophagus and gastroesophageal junction, the muscular wall is separated from the submucosa. The esophagomyotomy is performed similarly to that performed in the laparoscopic approach. After esophagomyotomy, a Belsey partial fundoplication is performed. The chest is drained with a single, soft 24F Silastic chest tube placed to underwater seal drainage system. Postoperative barium esophagram and diet restoration is similar to the clinical pathway taken for laparoscopic esophagomyotomy.

Esophagectomy

Advanced achalasia with development of a dilated, tortuous sigmoid esophagus with a diameter of more than 6 cm was considered, until recently, an indication for esophagectomy (Figure 6). This was based on the perception that the peristaltic body would not be able to empty effectively even after an adequate myotomy. However, recent studies have demonstrated symptom improvement in more than 90% of patients treated with an LHM. Esophagectomy therefore is reserved as a measure of last resort in patients in whom all other modalities have failed or require resection because of concomitant esophageal pathology.

■ SUMMARY

Even though achalasia is a relatively rare disorder, its incidence and prevalence increase with age. Given the changing demographic in the United States, clinicians will likely encounter the disease more frequently. Surgical therapy with a laparoscopic Heller myotomy offers the best and most sustainable relief of dysphagia and the addition of a partial fundoplication protects against postoperative reflux. The type of fundoplication performed, Dor or Toupet, does not appear to matter. The endoscopic approach myotomy, POEM, has been shown to be feasible and safe. Its availability is limited, however, and long-term efficacy is yet to be determined. Pneumatic dilatation is not as effective as surgery and is ideal for patients who are poor surgical candidates. Medical therapy is reserved for patients who will not tolerate any intervention because of age or comorbid disease.

SUGGESTED READINGS

Bowers SP. Esophageal motility disorders. *Surg Clin North Am.* 2015;95: 467-482.

el-Sherif AE, Adusumilli PS, Pettiford BL, d'Amato TA, Schuchert MJ, Clark A, DiRenzo C, Landreneau JP, Luketich JD, Landreneau RJ. Laparoscopic clam shell partial fundoplication achieves effective reflux control with reduced postoperative dysphagia and gas bloating. *Ann Thorac Surg.* 2007;84:1704-1709.

Hoppo T, Thakkar SJ, Schumacher LY, Komatsu Y, Choe S, Shetty A, Bloomer S, Loyd EJ, Zaidi AH, VanDeusen MA, Landreneau RJ, Kulkarni A, Jobe BA. A utility of peroral endoscopic myotomy (POEM) across the spectrum of esophageal motility disorders. *Surg Endosc.* 2016;30:233-244. doi:10.1007/s00464-015-4193-y.

Inoue H, Sato H, Ikeda H, Onimaru M, Sato C, Minami H, Yokomichi H, Kobayashi Y, Grimes KL, Kudo SE. Per-oral endoscopic myotomy: a series of 500 patients. *J Am Coll Surg.* 2015;221:256-264.

Kilic A, Owens SR, Pennathur A, Luketich JD, Landreneau RJ, Schuchert MJ. An increased proportion of inflammatory cells express tumor necrosis factor alpha in idiopathic achalasia of the esophagus. *Dis Esophagus.* 2009;22:382-385.

Little AG, Soriano A, Ferguson MK, Winans CS, Skinner DB. Surgical treatment of achalasia: results with esophagomyotomy and Belsey repair. *Ann Thorac Surg.* 1988;45:489-494.

Novais PA, Lemme EM. 24-h pH monitoring patterns and clinical response after achalasia treatment with pneumatic dilatation or laparoscopic Heller myotomy. *Aliment Pharmacol Ther.* 2010;32:1257-1265.

Pellegrini C, Wetter LA, Patti M, Leichter R, Mussan G, Mori T, Bernstein G, Way L. Thoracoscopic esophagomyotomy. Initial experience with a new approach for the treatment of achalasia. *Ann Surg.* 1992;216:291-296.

Rawlings A, Soper NJ, Oeschlager B, Swanstorm L, Matthews BD, Pellegrini C, Pierce RA, Pryor A, Martin V, Frisella MM, Cassera M, Brunt LM. Laparoscopic Dor versus Toupet fundoplication following Heller myotomy for achalasia: results of a multicenter, prospective, randomized-controlled trial. *Surg Endosc.* 2012;26:18-26.

Rebecchi F, Giaccone C, Farinella E, Campaci R, Morino M. Randomized controlled trial of laparoscopic Heller myotomy plus Dor fundoplication for achalasia: long term results. *Ann Surg.* 2008;248(6):1023-1030.

Richards WO, Torquati A, Holzman MD, Khaitan L, Byrne D, Lufti R, Sharp KW. Heller myotomy versus Heller myotomy with Dor fundoplication for achalasia: a prospective randomized double-blind trial. *Ann Surg.* 2004;240:405-412.

Schuchert MJ, Luketich JD, Landreneau RJ, Kilic A, Gooding WE, Alvelo-Rivera M, Christine NA, Gilbert S, Pennathur A. Minimally-invasive esophagectomy in 200 consecutive patients: factors influencing postoperative outcomes. *Ann Thorac Surg.* 2008;85:1729-1734.

Schuchert MJ, Luketich JD, Landreneau RJ, Kilic A, Wang Y, Alvelo-Rivera M, Christine NA, Gilbert S, Pennathur A. Minimally invasive surgical treatment of sigmoid esophagus in achalasia. *J Gastrointest Surg.* 2009;13: 1029-1035.

Wiechmann RJ, Ferguson MK, Naunheim KS, Hazelrigg SR, Mack MJ, Aronoff RJ, Weyant RJ, Santucci T, Macherey R, Landreneau RJ. Video-assisted surgical management of achalasia of the esophagus. *J Thorac Cardiovasc Surg.* 1999;118:916-923.

THE MANAGEMENT OF DISORDERS OF ESOPHAGEAL MOTILITY

Lee L. Swanstrom, MD, and Kristin Wilson Beard, MD

Disorders of esophageal motility present a diagnostic and therapeutic challenge to gastroenterologists and surgeons. Achalasia, the most prevalent and best understood of these disorders, was addressed in the chapter "The Management of Achalasia of the Esophagus." Nonachalasia esophageal motility disorders are less prevalent than achalasia, incompletely understood, and often difficult to treat. The optimal classification scheme for this group of disorders is a work in progress. Management strategies are also controversial and there is no universally accepted standard of care. In this chapter, we attempt to guide the surgeon in a review of nonachalasia esophageal motility disorders and the application of their most current classification, with recommendations for management based on recent data.

■ PRESENTATION

Patients with disorders of esophageal motility may present with chest pain, dysphagia, regurgitation, heartburn, globus sensation, upper respiratory complaints, or some combination of these. Because these symptoms are nonspecific and esophageal motility disorders are rare, workup for other life-threatening conditions is necessary. Cardiovascular and pulmonary causes usually have been ruled out already in the patient with chest pain before referral to the surgeon. A negative cardiac workup is reassurance enough for some patients who may be able to conservatively manage mild symptoms. Anxiety, depression, somatoform disorder, and other psychiatric diagnoses are more common in the population of patients with esophageal motility disorders, so psychiatric history is an important part of the evaluation.

Gastroesophageal reflux disease (GERD) is another common cause of noncardiac chest pain. A trial of a proton pump inhibitor (PPI) is warranted, and if troublesome symptoms persist, further diagnostic testing should be carried out. Other alarm symptoms, especially dysphagia with weight loss, should heighten suspicion for a mechanical or malignant process and prompt expedient and careful evaluation.

■ DIAGNOSTIC TESTING

All patients evaluated for esophageal motility disorders must undergo a comprehensive diagnostic workup. This includes a contrast esophagram to help visualize anatomy, esophageal length, and the presence of a diaphragmatic hernia or esophageal diverticulum. A pH study with or without impedance is important to identify GERD, which may be a primary or contributing cause of symptoms, and can help guide therapeutic decisions of the surgeon or gastroenterologist. Endoscopic evaluation with biopsy is also mandatory to identify Barrett's esophagus, malignancy, peptic stricture, or esophagitis related to acid exposure, eosinophilia, or infection. In the absence of mechanical obstruction or mucosal abnormalities, esophageal motility is evaluated next by manometry.

High-resolution manometry (HRM) with esophageal pressure topography (EPT) is becoming the standard of care for evaluation of esophageal motility. HRM precisely defines esophageal contractile function, peristalsis, and bolus transit when impedance evaluation is included. Compared with conventional manometry, study acquisition is faster, more comfortable, and better tolerated by patients. For technicians and physicians, the topography contour plots increase diagnostic yield and provide an intuitive visual permutation of anatomic and physiologic characteristics.

■ CLASSIFICATION OF DISEASE

Classifying esophageal motility disorders is an evolving process. Definitions of disease phenotype have changed over time with improvements in diagnostic technology and better understanding of the clinical importance of various manometric patterns. In 2001 Richter systematically classified esophageal motility disorders using

THE CHICAGO CLASSIFICATION V3.0
Hierarchical analysis

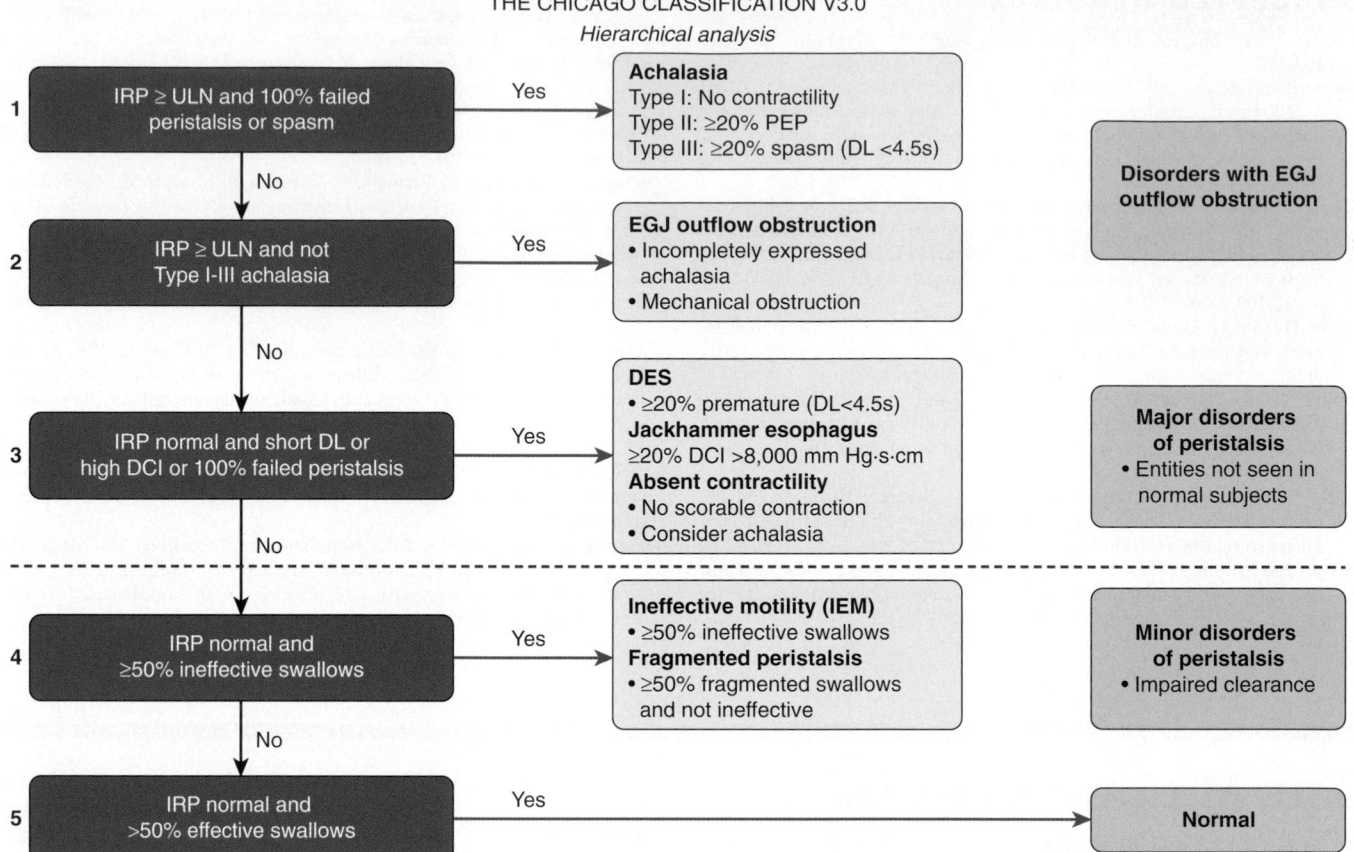

FIGURE 1 Chicago Classification v3.0. *DCI,* Distal contractile integral; *DES,* distal esophageal spasm; *DL,* distal latency; *EGJ,* esophagogastric junction; *IRP,* integrated relaxation pressure; *PEP,* pan-esophageal pressurization; *ULN,* upper limit normal. *(From Kahrilas PJ, Bredenoord AJ, Fox M, et al. The Chicago Classification of esophageal motility disorders, v3.0. Neurogastroenterol Motil. 2015;27:160-174.)*

conventional manometric criteria. Using high-resolution manometry, Kharilas and colleagues redefined this scheme in 2008 with the first edition of the Chicago Classification of esophageal motility disorders. The Chicago Classification is currently in its third edition (CC v3.0), which intended to simplify and clarify recognition of EPT patterns and physiologic metrics to better define clinically relevant phenotypes of esophageal dysmotility. CC v3.0 classifies the various manometric entities as *Esophagogastric outflow obstruction, Major disorders of peristalsis,* or *Minor disorders of peristalsis* (Figure 1). Manometric findings that do not meet criteria for these categories are considered normal. This chapter reviews nonachalasia disorders of esophageal motility according to the hierarchic analysis of the most current version of the Chicago Classification.

Esophagogastric Outflow Obstruction

Esophagogastric junction outflow obstruction (EGJOO) may be the result of intrinsic or extrinsic pathology, which highlights the importance of the comprehensive esophageal workup. Hiatal hernia, peptic stricture, stiff esophageal body resulting from scarring or radiation, prior surgical interventions, pseudoachalasia resulting from malignancy, or vascular obstruction from a diseased aortic arch are potential sources of mechanical outflow obstruction (Figure 2, *A*). Prominent vascular artifact on manometry or history suggestive of malignancy should prompt adjunct evaluation with endoscopic ultrasound (EUS) or CT scan. In a retrospective study, findings on selective EUS altered clinical management in as many as 15% of concerning cases. When other mechanical causes of esophagogastric outflow obstruction and achalasia have been ruled out, idiopathic cases remain. This is identified by incomplete relaxation of the EGJ, currently defined by HRM as elevated integrated relaxation pressure

(IRP) in the setting of preserved peristalsis (Figure 2, *B*), differentiating EGJOO from achalasia.

It is hypothesized that EGJOO may represent an incompletely expressed or precursor variant of achalasia, but this has not been verified in large numbers of patients. There are few data specific to this new entity since it has been redefined in CC v3.0. Cases previously classified as hypertensive lower esophageal sphincter (HTLES) by older versions of the Chicago Classification would now likely meet criteria for EGJOO. Interestingly, patients diagnosed with HTLES were found to have paradoxically elevated esophageal acid exposure about 25% of the time, despite relative EGJ obstruction. Therefore treatment of patients in this group should be tailored based on symptoms. PPIs should be considered if GERD is the major complaint. If dysphagia without abnormal esophageal acid exposure is identified, then medications directed to esophageal smooth muscle relaxation can be attempted. Endoscopic pneumatic dilation (PD) or botulinum toxin (Botox) injections are moderately effective options for relief of obstructive symptoms. Surgical therapy may be indicated in cases of severe or refractory symptoms. Esophageal myotomy, fundoplication, or a combination of the two may be tailored to the patient's symptoms and objective pathophysiology. Antireflux surgery without myotomy has been found to achieve good long-term results for patients with reflux and mild EGJOO caused by acid-induced spasm and inflammation, although preoperative dysphagia was found to predict a higher rate of failure. With dysphagia as the primary symptom, and either treated or normal esophageal acid exposure, laparoscopic Heller myotomy with partial fundoplication and per oral endoscopic myotomy (POEM) have been used successfully. In disorders such as EGJOO that do not affect the esophageal body, abdominal approaches for surgery are favored over thoracic because adequate proximal dissection is possible without accessing the

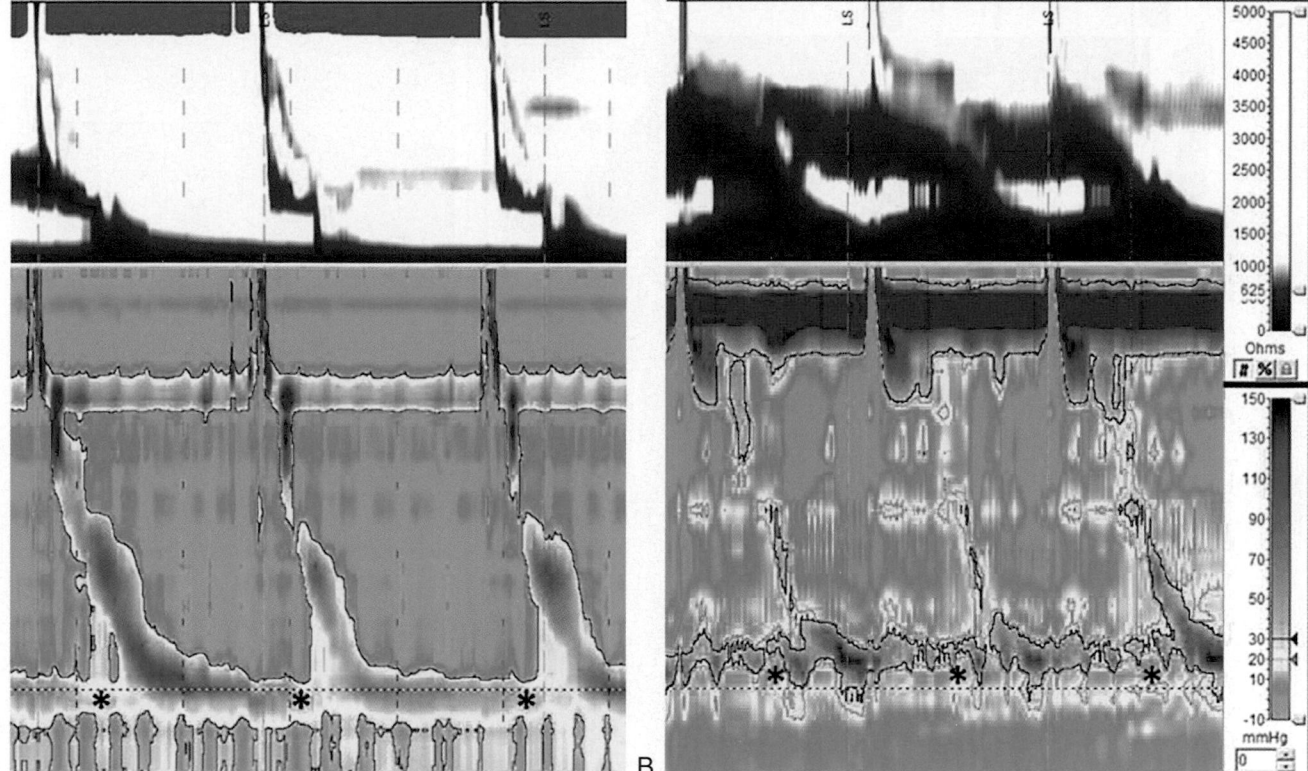

FIGURE 2 Esophagogastric junction (EGJ) outflow obstruction. Note the high-pressure, nonrelaxing EGJ *(asterisk)*. **A,** In this case caused by a hiatal hernia. **B,** Idiopathic, in the setting of ineffective motility and incomplete bolus clearance. *(Courtesy The Oregon Clinic.)*

thoracic cavity. Abdominal fundoplication options also offer greater symptom relief and generally are considered less technically challenging.

Major Esophageal Motility Disorders

This group of disorders is defined by manometric parameters that are *always* associated with symptoms. *Distal esophageal spasm (DES)*, also frequently referred to as *diffuse esophageal spasm,* is sometimes grouped with jackhammer esophagus or nutcracker esophagus, and achalasia type III as hypercontractile or "spastic" motility disorders. Patients with DES are symptomatic with chest pain, dysphagia, or regurgitation resulting from spastic contractions. The cause of DES is thought to be an impaired neurologic inhibitory pathway, allowing premature esophageal smooth muscle contractions. This disorder may overlap with or progress to achalasia. *Rapid* contractions previously categorized as DES by conventional manometry have been found to be nonspecific. With HRM these rapid contractions sometimes are identified in patients with EGJOO, GERD, and even in normal controls and therefore are no longer used to define DES. DES currently is defined by *premature* contractions in more than 20% of swallows. This is indicated manometrically as a low distal latency (DL); a truncated interval between initiation and deceleration of peristalsis (Figure 3, *A*). Barium esophagram classically shows a "corkscrew" pattern of simultaneous contractions, although this pattern is actually uncommon and not required for diagnosis (Figure 3, *B*). Treatment options for DES vary. Patients initially may benefit from reassurance with dietary and behavioral modifications or pharmacologic therapy. Persistent cases may require endoscopic intervention with PD or Botox, or surgical myotomy of variable length. Surgical approaches are discussed in more detail in the treatment section of the chapter.

Jackhammer esophagus was named to describe extreme hypercontractility and avoid confusion with DES. This disorder's cause is thought to be excessive cholinergic drive, causing asynchronous contractions of circular and longitudinal muscle. Jackhammer is defined manometrically by at least two swallows with significant hypercontractile vigor as measured by a distal contractile integral (DCI) exceeding 8000 mm Hg·s·cm (Figure 4, *A*). The hypercontractile segment may involve the esophageal body or may be limited to the esophagogastric junction, with EGJ relaxation pressure usually in the upper limit of normal.

Patients with jackhammer esophagus are *consistently* symptomatic with chest pain, dysphagia, and or regurgitation. This differentiates jackhammer by CC v3.0 criteria from *nutcracker esophagus,* defined as hypertensive peristalsis with DCI between 5000 to 8000 mm Hg·s·cm (Figure 4, *B*). Although some patients with DCI in this range are symptomatic, some asymptomatic control patients also fall into this range. For this reason the clinical relevance of nutcracker esophagus has been questioned. Some patients previously meeting criteria for nutcracker esophagus by manometry will now be classified as "normal" by CC v3.0, and the effect of that change has yet to be determined. Since CC v3. was redefined, few case reports have been made specifically for management of jackhammer esophagus, so further study of outcomes for this hypercontractile group will be required with time. Treatment is aimed at controlling spasm and can include dietary and behavioral modifications, pharmacologic therapy, or endoscopic or surgical treatments, which subsequently are discussed in greater detail.

Absent contractility is another new clinical entity under Chicago Classification v3.0. This disorder is defined by HRM with hypocontractility and failed peristalsis in 100% of swallows in the setting of an EGJ with normal relaxation pressure. Premature hypocontractile swallows with failed peristalsis are grouped here. In cases with borderline EGJ relaxation and evidence of esophageal pressurization, achalasia should be considered and the patient managed accordingly.

Systemic sclerosis (scleroderma) falls into the absent contractility category (Figure 5). This figure demonstrates complete hypocontraction of esophageal smooth muscle, with preserved skeletal muscle

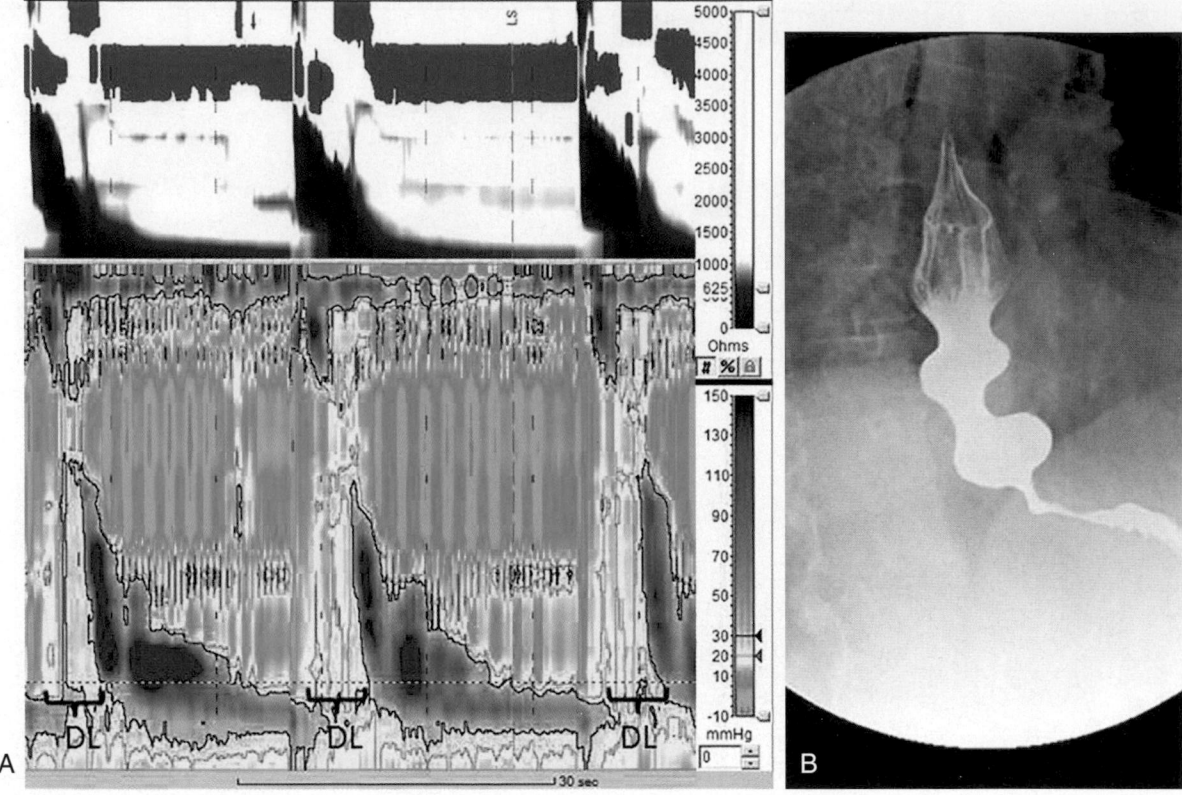

FIGURE 3 Distal esophageal spasm. **A,** Premature contractions with low distal latency (interval between initiation and deceleration of peristalsis). **B,** Esophagram with "corkscrew" pattern of simultaneous tertiary esophageal body contractions. *(Courtesy The Oregon Clinic.)*

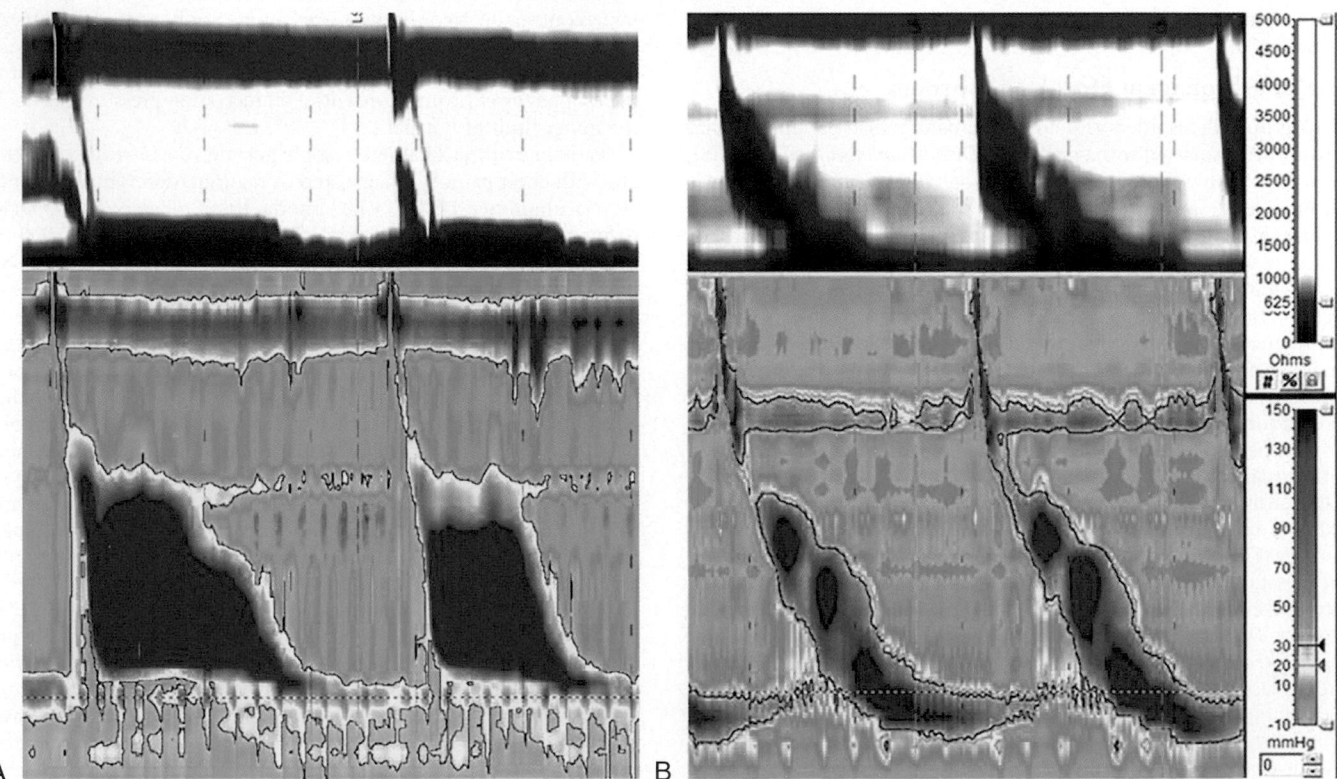

FIGURE 4 Hypercontractile disorders. **A,** Jackhammer esophagus. Extremely elevated contractile vigor (DCI in this case ranged from 12,000 to 50,000). **B,** Nutcracker esophagus. Peristaltic, vigorous contractions with DCI 5000 to 8000. *(Courtesy The Oregon Clinic.)*

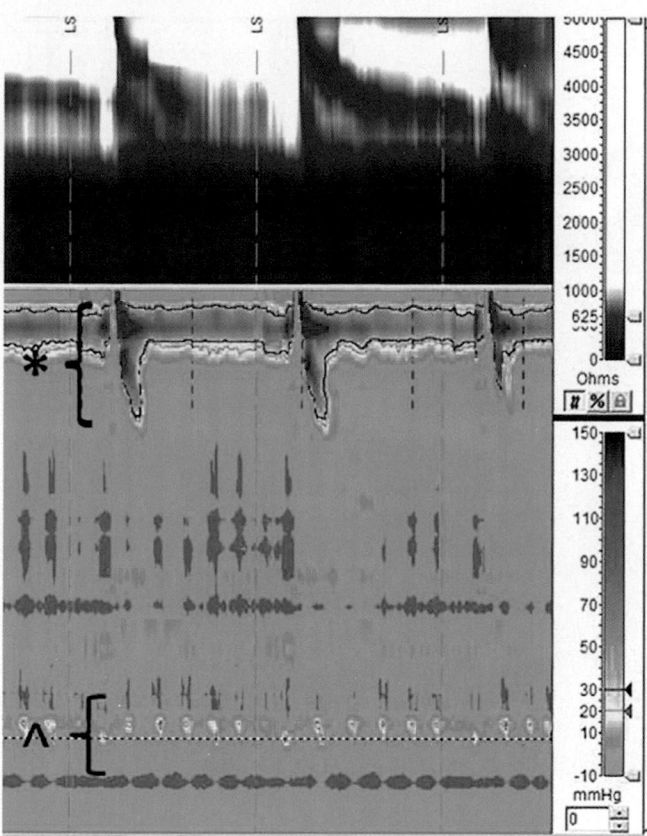

FIGURE 5 Absent contractility. This is a case of scleroderma with complete hypomotility of esophageal smooth muscle; note preserved function of skeletal muscle of the upper esophageal sphincter *(asterisk)* and diaphragm *(circumflex)*. *(Courtesy The Oregon Clinic.)*

contraction in the upper esophageal sphincter and diaphragm. Therapeutic options specific to diminished esophageal motility are limited, so treatment is directed primarily at the underlying systemic disorder, as well as relief of symptoms. Unfortunately no specific pharmacologic therapy improves contractility and function of esophageal smooth muscle. Prokinetic agents are fraught with side effects and now primarily are avoided. GERD has been identified frequently in these patients and should be treated aggressively with PPIs. Antireflux surgery can be considered carefully for refractory GERD cases in this setting but should be approached with caution at the risk of exacerbating dysphagia. Because connective tissue disorders such as scleroderma also can affect gastric motility, one should be aware that GERD symptoms may be a result of overflow reflux and should not be treated by fundoplication alone. A small retrospective review of scleroderma patients treated with fundoplication or Roux-en-Y gastric bypass (RYGBP) revealed improvement in control of reflux and dysphagia in the RYGBP group compared with fundoplication. In very carefully selected cases, RYGBP may be considered for primary management of refractory GERD in scleroderma. Less invasive endoscopic procedures such as suture plication or radiofrequency ablation may be more appealing for GERD in such fragile patients but are less effective at reducing reflux.

Minor Esophageal Motility Disorders

Patients with minor motility disorders often have minimal symptoms and require fewer interventions over time, and as such the prognosis of these patients is overall better than for those with major esophageal motility disorders. *Ineffective esophageal motility (IEM)* is a minor esophageal motility disorder defined by a significant number of weak or failed swallows. Presentation may include heartburn and

regurgitation with or without dysphagia, and symptoms tend to be mild. GERD often plays a significant role in the underlying cause of IEM because many of these patients are found to have underlying abnormal esophageal acid exposure. IEM is defined by HRM criteria as at least 50% of swallows with low or absent contractile vigor, indicated by DCI less than 450 mm Hg·s·cm (Figure 6, *A*). In the IEM patient, the manometry technician may elect to perform additional provocative testing with multiple repetitive swallow (MRS) assessment. Deglutitive inhibition of the esophageal body and EGJ occurs during MRS, usually followed by augmented esophageal contraction vigor and improved bolus transit. Augmented contraction with MRS may be reassuring to the physician who is considering an antireflux procedure to treat underlying GERD while avoiding iatrogenic postoperative dysphagia. When MRS does not augment subsequent contraction, it is predictive of late dysphagia after fundoplication. Although evidence would indicate that there is a relatively low risk of postoperative dysphagia with Nissen for patients with IEM, many surgeons choose to carefully tailor a partial fundoplication to avoid the risk of postoperative dysphagia. Clinical implications of MRS findings in this setting have yet to be defined clearly and require further study as these provocative maneuvers are used more frequently with HRM.

Therapeutic options are limited for IEM patients. Because many, if not most, IEM cases are related to chronic reflux disease, correction of GERD may result in correction of the motility disorder. Reassurance along with dietary and behavioral modifications may be helpful. As in other motility disorders, prokinetic drugs generally are not recommended. Low-dose antidepressants, especially tricyclic antidepressants or trazodone, may reduce functional chest discomfort, heartburn, and globus sensation but may not be effective for dysphagia.

Fragmented peristalsis is the final minor disorder of esophageal motility. It is defined manometrically by at least 50% of swallows with fragmented contractions, with a defect in peristaltic contraction of at least 5 cm, with preserved overall contraction vigor not meeting criteria for IEM (Figure 6, *B*). Outside of CC v3.0, no specific reports on this newly defined disorder have been made, and its clinical relevance is yet to be defined.

■ NONOPERATIVE MANAGEMENT

The main goals of any treatment for patients with esophageal motility disorders include reduction of chest pain and dysphagia. Treatment is focused on reducing spasm, GERD, and outflow obstruction to facilitate esophageal emptying. *Reassurance* alone can be beneficial. Reassurance not only helps to relieve anxiety but also has been shown to reduce severity of chest pain and frequency of health care utilization.

Dietary and Behavioral Modifications

Dietary and behavioral modifications can be very helpful for avoiding chest pain or dysphagia. These modifications include sitting upright and allowing plenty of time for meals, taking small bites, chewing thoroughly, and taking sips of liquid between bites. Foods such as bread, meat, and rice are notorious for worsening dysphagia and should be ingested with caution or avoided. Extremely hot or cold foods can exacerbate esophageal spasm. Choosing soft or liquefied foods can be helpful during symptom flares.

Pharmacologic Therapy

Before pharmacologic therapy is initiated, it is important to carefully review the patient's home medications and minimize those that affect esophageal motility. DES in particular is associated with chronic opioid use and has been shown to improve with opioid cessation. A few classes of drugs have been used with some success in providing symptomatic relief of esophageal spasm.

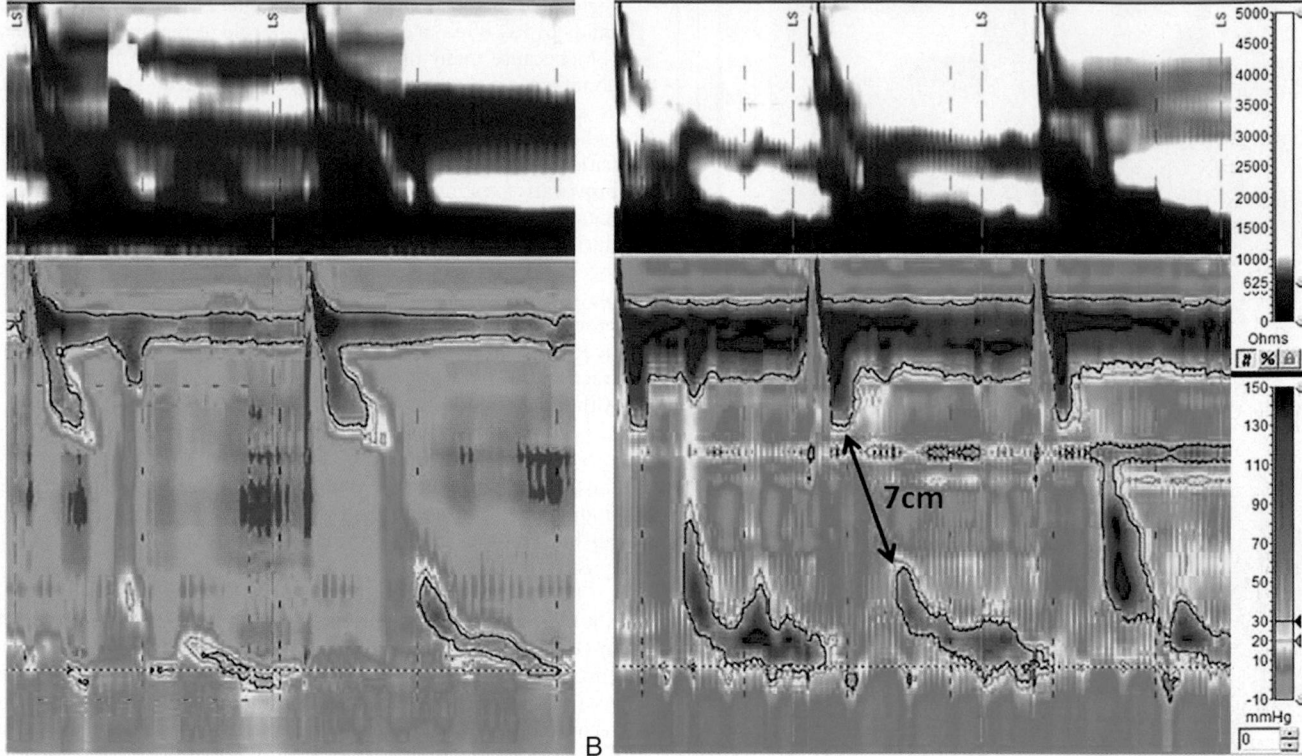

FIGURE 6 Minor disorders of peristalsis. **A,** IEM (ineffective esophageal motility), weak peristalsis (DCI <450). **B,** Fragmented peristalsis. Large breaks (>5 cm) with preserved contractile vigor (DCI >450). *(Courtesy The Oregon Clinic.)*

Smooth muscle–relaxing agents (nitrates or calcium channel blockers) may provide some symptomatic relief in spastic or hypercontractile disorders, including DES, some cases of EGJOO, and jackhammer esophagus. Phosphodiesterase-5 inhibitors such as Sildenafil, which acts by blocking degradation of nitric oxide, also can be effective. These drugs may be tolerated poorly because of lightheadedness, headache, or other side effects, and their efficacy may decline with time. Cost of Sildenafil may be prohibitive, and effects of daily long-term use of this agent in various populations of patients are unknown. Low-dose antidepressants, including tricyclic agents and trazodone, may provide pain modulation and anxiety relief for noncardiac chest pain. As previously discussed, GERD is frequently part of the clinical syndrome of esophageal dysmotility, although its role in pathogenesis is not understood completely. A trial of PPIs is warranted and may help reduce inflammation, pain, and spasm related to abnormal esophageal acid exposure.

Endoscopic Therapy

Pneumatic dilation (PD) has been used to treat spastic esophageal motility disorders affecting the EGJ, including EGJOO, DES, and nutcracker esophagus, with variable success. In small studies, 26% to 70% of DES and nutcracker patients had good response with PD, although there is concern that some of these cases may have been classified more accurately as achalasia. From the achalasia literature, there is a known risk of perforation with pneumatic dilation in the range of about 2% to 5% of cases performed by expert endoscopists. This rate of perforation is unacceptable to many endoscopists, who no longer use PD as first-line therapy.

Endoscopic injection of botulinum toxin (Botox) may be temporarily effective in relief of spasm in EGJOO, DES, or jackhammer disorders. The technique for administration of botulinum toxin has not been standardized; some report injection of the EGJ alone and others include the esophageal body. Botox to the esophageal body

may be helpful in cases such as DES or jackhammer, although it is uncertain exactly where and how much drug should be injected. Infection is an uncommon but serious risk of Botox injections. One mortality resulting from mediastinitis has been reported in a DES case treated with Botox, although other serious adverse events have been rare. Endoscopists may elect to use EUS to guide positioning and depth of injections into the thinner-walled esophageal body. In small studies of patients with EGJOO and DES, successful relief of symptoms with botulinum toxin injections was achieved in more than 50% of patients at 6 months, with further improvement from serial on-demand treatments thereafter. This was comparable to efficacy in achalasia. Fall off of symptom relief is present in each of these disorders with time, which may require repeat treatments or escalation to surgical intervention. Prominent symptoms and spastic features may predict early recurrence of symptoms. Botulinum toxin before surgical myotomy has been noted to increase difficulty in identifying and maintaining the proper dissection plane. Prior Botox is not a contraindication to surgery and is sometimes useful as a trial to determine if a patient may respond well to surgical myotomy.

■ SURGICAL MANAGEMENT

Surgical therapy is an option for nonachalasia esophageal motility disorders, but optimal timing and approach are controversial. Surgery generally has been reserved for medically refractory cases because outcomes are variable, somewhat unpredictable, and may be associated with surgical morbidity. As mentioned before, IEM patients with GERD, whether they also have dysphagia, tolerate antireflux surgery well, and treatment of the reflux often corrects the motility disorder as well. Classically, these patients have a partial fundoplication, most commonly a 270-degree posterior wrap (Figure 7). Nissen fundoplication also has been shown to be well tolerated in this setting; however, we reserve a full wrap for IEM patients with minimal symptoms of dysphagia preoperatively. Endoluminal antireflux procedures such as Stretta (radiofrequency) and transoral incisionless fundoplication (TIF), which provide less aggressive valve reconstructions, also may be good options for these patients.

Data on surgical outcomes for EGJOO, DES, and hypercontractile disorders are limited to a few series, mostly small and nonrandomized over the last 50 years. As diagnostic modalities have improved and disease classifications have evolved, these data become even more difficult to interpret. In general, outcomes for surgery are better for relief of chest pain and dysphagia compared with medical or endoscopic therapy. In DES, which is the most frequently studied esophageal motility disorder aside from achalasia, good symptomatic outcomes are reported in about 70% of cases treated with surgical myotomy via abdominal or thoracic approach at highly skilled centers. These outcomes are notably less successful than those for surgical myotomy for achalasia, so surgery often is reserved as a last resort for patients with nonachalasia motility disorders. Therefore many of these patients endure long courses of medical or endoscopic therapy because there is no clear definition of "medical failure."

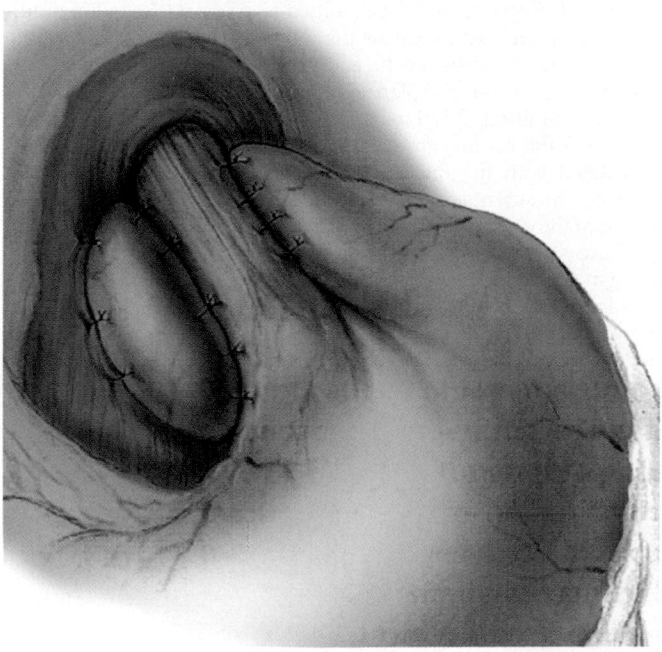

FIGURE 7 A completed laparoscopic 270-degree posterior Toupet fundoplication.

Surgical techniques for esophageal myotomy are varied. Traditional open surgery largely has been replaced by minimally invasive techniques, and new endoscopic options are available. Length of the esophageal body myotomy, inclusion of the EGJ in the myotomy, and addition of a concomitant antireflux procedure are variable from surgeon to surgeon. Previous authors in this text have recommended a long thoracic myotomy for the treatment of DES or other esophageal body motility disorders and have described the technique in detail (Figure 8). Thoracic access allows myotomy extension for the full length of the esophageal body, which is not possible with laparoscopic Heller myotomy. However, thoracic myotomy has the disadvantage of requiring single lung ventilation, chest tube placement, and typically a longer length of stay. The thoracic approach is complicated further if the surgeon desires a fundoplication or extended gastric myotomy.

We prefer a less invasive surgical technique for hypercontractile esophageal motility disorders: POEM. POEM offers several advantages for esophageal myotomy. This NOTES (natural orifice transluminal endoscopic surgery) procedure is completely endoscopic and incisionless. It provides the ability to tailor the length of myotomy with ease because the entire affected esophageal body and EGJ are accessible endoscopically. POEM allows the surgeon to produce a selective circular myotomy and avoids the risk of vagus nerve injury or disruption of the diaphragmatic crural component of the EGJ. Single lung ventilation, lateral or prone positioning, and chest tubes are not required, and postoperative pain is usually minimal.

POEM was first applied clinically for achalasia by Inoue in 2008, and since then more than 4000 cases have been performed worldwide with an excellent safety profile and good clinical results, mostly for patients with achalasia. Until recently, studies of POEM for nonachalasia esophageal motility disorders included only a few such cases and have not always been stratified by subtype. POEM is employed in our practice for cases of hypercontractile and spastic esophageal motility disorders, including DES, jackhammer esophagus, and EGJ outflow obstruction (including cases of nutcracker esophagus and HTLES as classified before CC v3.0) with good results. POEM has reported success rates of 70% to 80% for these disorders with relatively low morbidity at expert centers. Although these studies are small, they suggest comparable outcomes for extended POEM with low morbidity compared with traditional open or laparoscopic/thorascopic approaches for extended esophageal myotomy.

There is controversy as to whether myotomy for esophageal body motility disorders should be extended through the EGJ. Given the subsequent weakening of peristalsis after esophageal body myotomy, we favor extension of the myotomy through the EGJ onto the stomach to prevent relative outflow obstruction and postoperative dysphagia, even in the setting of a normally relaxing EGJ. At our center, POEM

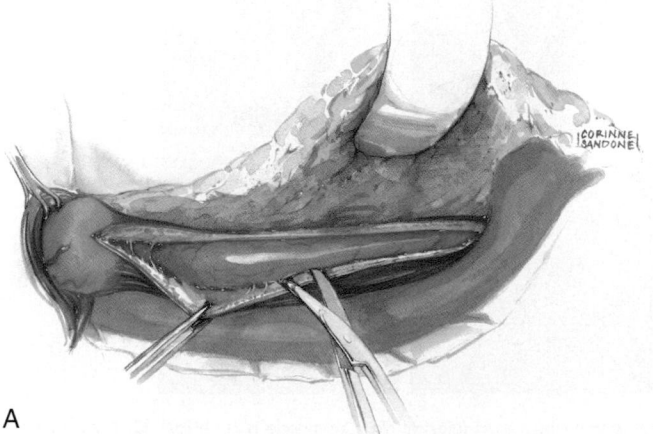

A

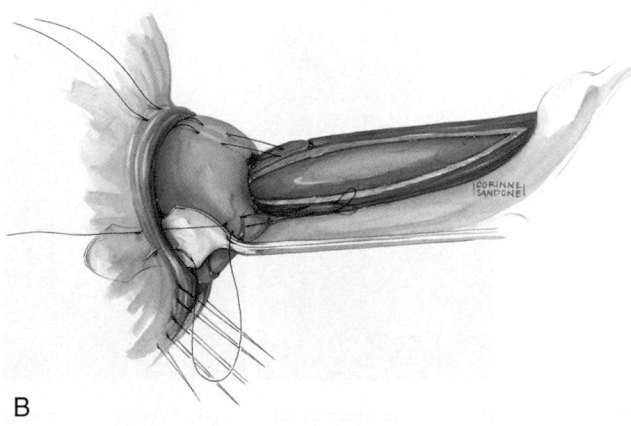

B

FIGURE 8 Thoracic myotomy and Belsey fundoplication.

myotomy length has been tailored based on HRM topography and endoscopic measurement of the high-pressure zone and has been extended proximally anywhere between 6 and 23 cm above the gastric cardia in such cases. In our recent experience, POEM with variable length of myotomy was comparable to other surgical techniques for relief of dysphagia and chest pain and had less morbidity.

A disadvantage of POEM is the requisite learning curve, which is about 20 cases for experienced endoscopists as demonstrated by Kurian and colleagues. GERD is also a long-term risk of POEM, currently with a 20% to 46% risk based on cumulative data. This sounds high but is in fact comparable to Heller with partial fundoplication, which has a postoperative rate of GERD between 21% and 42%, depending on fundoplication technique. Postoperative GERD is asymptomatic in half of patients, so routine follow-up pH testing or endoscopy is prudent. Patients identified with GERD have been treated successfully with PPIs with avoidance of long-term sequelae of reflux thus far. POEM results in a low rate of clinically significant leak or stricture and has been shown to be safe and effective in revision after Heller myotomy, Botox, and pneumatic dilation. POEM does not preclude subsequent endoscopic, laparoscopic, or thoracoscopic procedures should they be required. Because of these benefits, we feel that extended myotomy by POEM is the preferred approach for primary spastic motility disorders requiring surgery.

■ OPERATIVE TECHNIQUE

The POEM approach for extended myotomy for spastic esophageal motility disorders is reviewed here. Previous chapters in this and other texts have described esophageal myotomy with or without fundoplication via abdominal and thoracic approaches, so these are not repeated in detail here.

POEM is performed in the operating room under general anesthesia. The procedure requires a high-definition endoscope for optimal visualization and CO_2 insufflation because it has a better safety profile than room air. The patient is placed in supine position to allow access to the abdomen or chest. For a few days before the procedure, patients are given Nystatin rinse prophylactically to clear any *Candida* esophagitis related to esophageal stasis and allowed only

a liquid diet for 1 day to allow clearance of retained food. A preoperative antibiotic is administered as well as a single preoperative dose of intravenous steroid to prevent development of mucosal edema.

Upper endoscopy is performed to evaluate the anatomy, rule out *Candida* spp., and clear any fluid or food debris within the esophagus before proceeding. We use EndoFLIP (endoscopic functional lumen imaging probe) to measure baseline esophageal diameter, pressure, cross-sectional area, distensibility, and compliance. An overtube is used for distal myotomy to stabilize the scope from overtorquing. No overtube is used for extended myotomy. The gastric wall is tattooed with indigo carmine 2 cm distal to the EGJ in the anterior position along the lesser curvature, marking the target for the distal extent of the myotomy. The location and extent of the myotomy and mucosotomy are calculated based on careful evaluation of the preoperative manometry and intraoperative evaluation of the high pressure zone. An angled dissecting cap is attached to the high-definition (HD) endoscope to facilitate dissection and visualization. A mucosal lift is created with injectable saline with dilute indigo carmine in the anterior esophagus 2 to 4 cm proximal to the proximal extent of the planned myotomy (Figure 9).

An endoscopic cautery knife is used to create a 1.5-cm longitudinal mucosal incision to expose the submucosa. Using the dissecting cap, the surgeon advances the endoscope through the mucosotomy and into the submucosal plane. Once inside, spray cautery and serial injections of lifting solution are used to create a submucosal tunnel, separating the mucosa from the circular muscle. Visible vessels are coagulated with the dissecting knife or grasped with hot biopsy forceps. The submucosal tunnel is extended distally across the GEJ and onto the gastric wall until the distal darker blue tattoo is reached.

Once satisfied with the extent of the tunnel, the endoscope is brought back and the myotomy is created by selectively dividing the circular muscle layers. The thin longitudinal muscle layer is left intact whenever possible. Full-thickness breaches of the muscle are usually not critical as the mediastinal adventitial tissue is left intact. The myotomy is extended across the EGJ and onto the proximal gastric wall. During the procedure, exiting the tunnel to deflate insufflated gas from the stomach may be required to relieve gastric distension. Capnoperitoneum may develop in up to 30% of cases; it is often

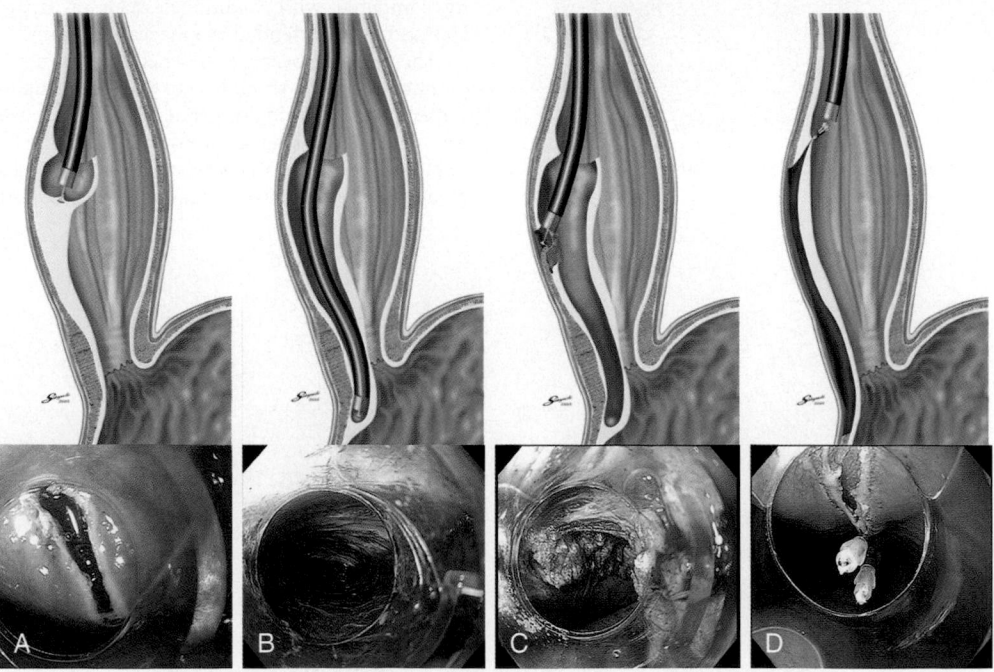

FIGURE 9 POEM. **A,** Entry into submucosal plane. **B,** Creation of submucosal tunnel (mucosa is inferior, circular muscle is superior). **C,** Myotomy of circular muscle. **D,** Closure of mucosal entry site with clips. *(From Inoue H, Sato H, Ikeda H, et al. Per-oral endoscopic myotomy: a series of 500 patients. J Am Coll Surg. 2015;221:256-264.)*

minor and self-limited but is evacuated easily with a Veress needle if abdominal overdistension or respiratory compromise develops.

After the myotomy is completed, the surgeon withdraws the endoscope, checking for hemostasis. Completion endoscopy identifies any inadvertent mucosal injuries, which are treated with endoscopic clips. The EndoFLIP catheter is replaced and measurements are compared with those obtained preoperatively to ensure adequacy of the myotomy before closure. Endoscopic clips then are used to close the proximal mucosotomy in a longitudinal fashion from distal to proximal.

Postoperative Care

The patient is kept NPO overnight, and a routine contrast esophagram is performed on the first postoperative day. If no leaks or obstruction are identified, the patient is allowed clear liquids and crushed medications. The patient may be discharged on postoperative day 1 if liquids are tolerated and should maintain a puree consistency diet for 1 week to avoid disruption of the mucosal closure clips. In most cases, postoperative pain is minimal and usually does not require narcotics.

Complications

Acute postoperative complications can include intratunnel bleeding, mucosal leak or dehiscence, or mediastinitis. The incidence of these complications is rare in reported series, and there have been no mortalities reported. Bleeding may require transfusion and repeat endoscopy to achieve hemostasis. Mucosal leaks or dehiscence may seal with conservative management but often require repeat endoscopy and repair with additional clips or suturing. Mediastinitis is treated with antibiotics and may require percutaneous or surgical drainage.

■ CONCLUSION

There is work to be done in the realm of nonachalasia esophageal motility disorders as HRM diagnostics and treatment options evolve.

To achieve the best possible outcome, therapeutic options should be considered carefully and individually tailored. Patients should be advised on expectations because treatment outcomes are somewhat unpredictable and may be disappointing in some cases. POEM is a promising, minimally invasive treatment option for hypercontractile and spastic disorders and perhaps will be considered as an early surgical intervention rather than salvage therapy given its relative success and safety profile. For hypomotility disorders associated with GERD, partial fundoplications remain the gold standard, although Nissen fundoplication also has been shown to be well tolerated in all but the most extreme cases. There also may be a role for newer endoscopic antireflux procedures, although there are insufficient data at this time to define their application for these relatively rare disorders.

SUGGESTED READINGS

Almansa C, Hinder RA, Smith CD, et al. A comprehensive appraisal of the surgical treatment of diffuse esophageal spasm. *J Gastrointest Surg.* 2008;12:1133-1145.

Inoue H, Sato H, Ikeda H, et al. Per-oral endoscopic myotomy: a series of 500 patients. *J Am Coll Surg.* 2015;221:256-264.

Irving JD, Owen WJ, Linsell J, et al. Management of diffuse esophageal spasm with balloon dilatation. *Gastrointest Radiol.* 1992;17:189-192.

Kahrilas PJ, Bredenoord AJ, Fox M, et al. The Chicago Classification of esophageal motility disorders, v3.0. *Neurogastroenterol Motil.* 2015;27:160-174.

Roman S, Kahrilas PJ. Distal esophageal spasm. *Curr Opin Gastroenterol.* 2015;31:328-333.

Sharata A, Dunst C, Pescarus R, et al. Peroral endoscopic myotomy (POEM) for esophageal primary motility disorders: analysis of 100 consecutive patients. *J Gastrointest Surg.* 2015;19:161-170.

Vanuytsel T, Bisschops R, Farré R, et al. Botulinum toxin reduces dysphagia in patients with nonachalasia primary esophageal motility disorders. *Clin Gastroenterol Hepatol.* 2013;11:1115-1121.e2.

Woltman TA, Oelschlager BK, Pellegrini CA. Surgical management of esophageal motility disorders. *J Surg Res.* 2004;117:34-43.

Zerbib F, Roman S. Current therapeutic options for esophageal motor disorders as defined by the Chicago Classification. *J Clin Gastroenterol.* 2015;49:451-460.

THE MANAGEMENT OF ESOPHAGEAL CANCER

Blair A. Jobe, MD, FACS, Rodney J. Landreneau, MD, and Fahim Habib, MD, MPH, FACS

■ EPIDEMIOLOGY

Worldwide, esophageal cancer (EC) is the eighth most common solid organ tumor and the sixth leading cause of cancer deaths. Of the two predominant histologic subtypes esophageal squamous cell carcinoma (ESCC) is the most common form globally. It is endemic in certain countries such as China, Central Asia, and India (the esophageal cancer belt) with a predilection for those of low socioeconomic status. Key etiologic factors (Box 1) contributing to its development include smoking, alcohol consumption, nutritional deficiencies, exposure to environmental carcinogens, longstanding achalasia, and caustic injury. Esophageal adenocarcinoma (EAC) in contrast occurs more commonly in North America and Western Europe. In the United States, EAC is the fastest increasing

solid organ malignancy and has shown a 600% increase in incidence since the 1970s. In 2015 alone, it is estimated that 16,980 people will be diagnosed with EC, and that 15,590 will die of their disease. The increased incidence is due largely to the epidemic of reflux disease with the development of intestinal metaplasia of the esophagus and its subsequent progression to high-grade dysplasia and invasive carcinoma. Risk factors include advancing age, male gender, Caucasian race, obesity, and certain genetic conditions such as tylosis.

■ CLINICAL PRESENTATION

EC may be diagnosed in the context of one of two clinical scenarios. First, the patient may be seen initially with symptoms, most commonly dysphagia. Because dysphagia does not develop until more than two thirds of the lumen is obstructed by tumor and patients initially adapt by adopting a diet of semisolid and liquid foods, the disease is often advanced at the time of presentation. Many of these patients have a history of long-standing reflux disease with or without a hiatal hernia, which has not been treated adequately or followed, and have associated regurgitation, odynophagia, and hematemesis. Hoarseness of voice resulting from involvement of the recurrent laryngeal nerve by the tumor or nodes containing

BOX 1: Causative Factors for Esophageal Carcinoma

Squamous Cell Carcinoma

Tobacco: increased with increasing use, associated with all forms of tobacco, including cigarettes, cigars, pipes, and chewing tobacco

Alcohol: increase proportional to amount consumed, usually more than 3 drinks/day. Effect synergistic with smoking

Nitrosamines: from a diet rich in nitrates and nitrites

Vitamin deficiency: retinol, riboflavin, ascorbic, and alpha-tocopherol

Trace element deficiency: selenium, zinc, molybdenum

Water impurities: petroleum

Caustic injury: alkalis more than acid

Chronic ingestion of hot liquids (>70° C)

Achalasia

History of ionizing radiation

Prior head and neck cancers

Chewing betel nut

Human papilloma virus infection

Plummer-Vinson syndrome

Celiac disease

Adenocarcinoma

Chronic gastroesophageal reflux disease

Obesity

Male gender

Caucasian race

Smoking

Dietary factors: increased consumption of red meats, increased iron intake, saturated fats

Adapted from Schuchert MJ, Luketich JD, Lanreneau RJ. Management of esophageal cancer. *Curr Probl Surg.* 2010;845-946.

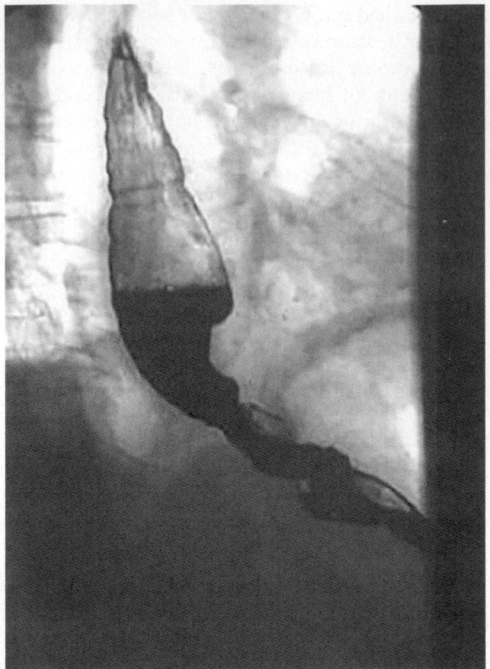

FIGURE 1 Barium Swallow Showing Obstruction.

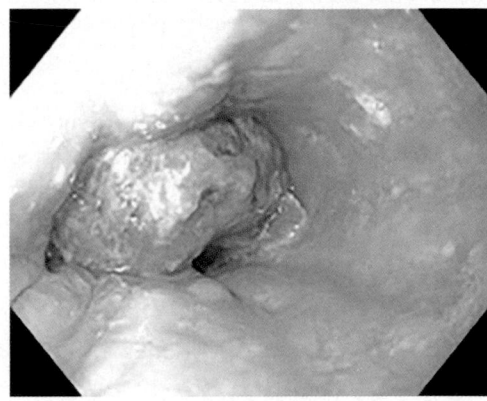

FIGURE 2 Endoscopic appearance of an esophageal cancer.

metastatic deposits, hiccups because of phrenic nerve involvement, and significant weight loss resulting from swallowing difficulties also indicate advanced disease. In the second instance, EC may be diagnosed on scheduled surveillance biopsy in patients with known reflux disease and Barrett's esophagus. EC here usually is diagnosed at an early stage, is often amenable to esophagus preserving treatment strategies, and carries a better prognosis.

■ DIAGNOSIS

We initiate workup by obtaining a barium swallow. Not only is it inexpensive and easy to perform but also it provides critical information regarding location and degree of esophageal obstruction and gives a roadmap for the esophagogastroduodenoscopy (EGD) to follow (Figure 1). EGD remains the gold standard for evaluation of symptoms suggestive of an EC. It not only accurately identifies the location of the tumor, its extent, topographic characteristics, and relation to the esophagogastric junction but also allows tissue to be obtained for histologic evaluation to confirm the diagnosis and determine grade (Figure 2). We use the Seattle protocol with four quadrant biopsies obtained along every centimeter of apparent disease using jumbo forceps. Additional biopsies are obtained of any suspicious lesions identified. In spite of such an aggressive biopsy protocol, only a small proportion of the mucosa at risk is obtained for evaluation, and the risk of sampling error is substantial especially in early disease. The use of advanced endoscopic techniques such as chromoendoscopy, narrow-band imaging, autofluorescence imaging, and confocal laser endomicroscopy increase the detail of mucosal and cellular architecture discerned,

allow biopsy of areas most likely to harbor pathology, and thereby reduce sampling error.

■ STAGING TECHNIQUES

Once diagnosis has been made, stage of the disease must be established (Figure 3). Accurate staging allows selection of an optimal management strategy for an individual patient, avoiding the burden of overtreatment or the risk of undertreatment. In addition, stage at presentation has prognostic significance and correlates well with survival. The 5-year survival is reported to be 90% for pTis, 75% for pT1, 45% for pT2, 30% for pT3, and 15% for pT4. Survival rates range from 30% to 60% for node-negative disease and drop significantly to 15% to 25% for node-positive disease. Finally, accurate staging is critical for comparing the outcomes of different treatment strategies.

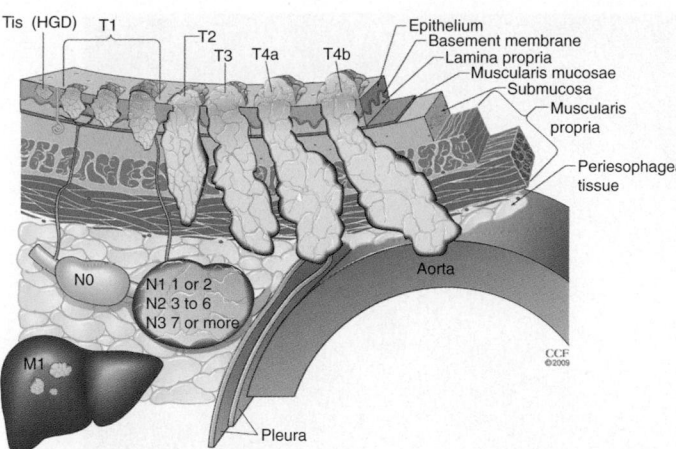

FIGURE 3 Staging of adenocarcinoma. *(From Rice TW, Blackstone EH. Esophageal cancer staging. Thorac Surg Clin. 2013;23:461-469.)*

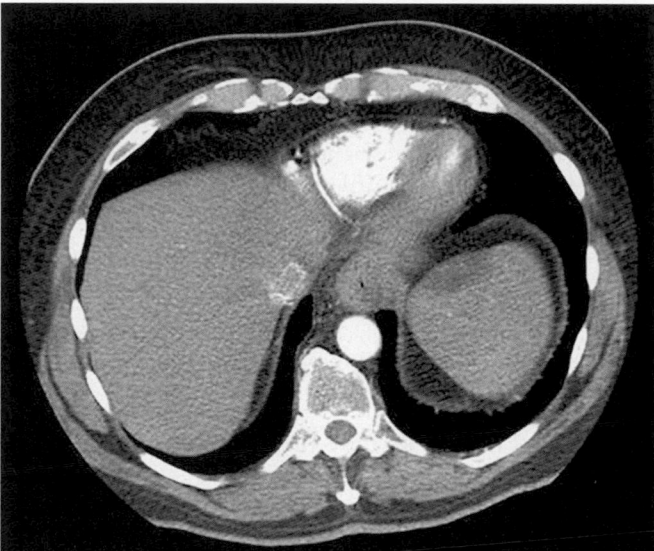

FIGURE 4 Computed tomography of the chest showing abnormal thickening of the esophagus suggestive of malignancy.

Staging should be carried out in an expeditious manner to avoid delay in therapy, potentially compromising outcome. The current staging system involves assessment of the depth or penetration of the tumor into the esophageal wall and surrounding structures, determination of lymph node involvement, the presence of distant disease and important nonanatomic characteristics, including histologic grade and location.

First, computed tomography (CT) of the chest and abdomen with oral and intravenous contrast is performed with the primary purpose to detect the presence of metastatic disease. Secondary purposes are to assess the locoregional extent of the disease and evaluation for indicators of unresectability. CT has poor sensitivity for early stage disease and is also limited in its ability to distinguish T3 from T4 lesions. However, esophageal thickening of more than 5 mm clearly is considered abnormal (Figure 4). Although CT is sensitive in detecting the presence of lymphadenopathy, it cannot clearly determine the cause of the lymph node enlargement especially in patients who may have an inflammatory basis for their lymphadenopathy because of local interventions or associated esophagitis. In general, lymph nodes

larger than 1 cm in the short axis are considered abnormal and must be further evaluated. CT signs of advanced disease that precludes resection includes contact of the tumor with the aorta for greater than 90 degrees of its circumference, bulging of the tumor into the posterior membranous portion of the airway, and loss of the retrocrural fat planes indicating invasion of the diaphragm, peritoneal studding, and omental caking.

Fluorodeoxyglucose positron emission tomography (FDG-PET) and CT-PET have a higher sensitivity for metastatic disease (Figure 5). In about 20% of patients, PET will identify distal metastasis that was not seen with conventional techniques, including CT and bone scans. Its key limitations lie in its failure to identify minimal disease, detect metastasis in lymph nodes that lie close to the primary tumor, and get masked by its signal, the so-called "halo-effect," and false positives that result from the inflammation associated with esophagitis or as a result of previous interventions. Because of this potential for false positives, PET-positive foci must be confirmed with biopsy and histologic evaluation.

Endoscopic ultrasound (EUS) is a useful staging modality with high sensitivity for detection of the depth of tumor invasion, the presence and characteristics of paraesophageal lymph nodes, and the presence of distant disease in the abdomen. Nodes are considered suspicious for harboring metastatic disease if they on EUS have distinct borders, a rounded appearance, hypoechogenic architecture, and a size exceeding 1 cm (Figure 6). EUS also can identify unresectability when the tumor extends into critical structures such as the aorta, left atrium, pulmonary artery, pulmonary vein, and the tracheobronchial tree. EUS cannot be performed in the face of advanced disease, in which luminal obstruction precludes passage of the probe; such obstruction is, however, invariably indicative of advanced disease representing a T3 or T4 tumor in more than 90% of cases. Its main limitations are its inability to detect superficial disease and to detect nodes more than 2 cm from the esophageal wall because of limited penetration of the high-frequency EUS employed. EUS-guided fine-needle aspiration of suspicious lymph can be performed to increase the accuracy of staging. EUS-FNA is not feasible if the path to the target lymph node passes through the tumor.

Endoscopic mucosal resection (EMR) is emerging as a valuable staging modality in patients with suspicious nodular lesions in the background of widespread mucosal changes such as Barrett's esophagus. EMR can be performed using a variety of techniques. It provides an adequate tissue sample that allows accurate determination of the depth of penetration of the tumor. In tumors smaller than 2 cm the EMR usually resects the entire lesion and therefore may be both diagnostic and therapeutic.

Laparoscopy improves the accuracy of staging in patients with tumors around the gastroesophageal junction. It is used to assess the peritoneal surface for occult deposits and evaluate the liver for small metastatic foci not visualized on imaging; it allows sampling of the celiac nodes. Accurate identification of nodal status can not only help appropriately stage the patient but also plan the extent of the radiation field. Improvements in noninvasive imaging and development of tissue sampling techniques such as endobronchial ultrasound with FNA, navigational bronchoscopy, and percutaneous image-guided biopsy largely have replaced thoracoscopy as a staging modality. Its use is restricted to cases in which suspicious findings are identified on noninvasive imaging and cannot be sampled adequately using the aforementioned techniques.

In spite of the advances made in staging patients with EC, the occurrence of nodal and distal recurrence after potentially curative therapy is not infrequent. Therefore there is great interest in evaluation of molecular markers in assessing the presence of micrometastasis in lymph nodes and identifying the presence of tumor DNA in circulating blood. Carcinoembryonic antigen mRNA expression using reverse transcription polymerase chain reaction improves ability to identify occult micrometastasis in nodal tissue.

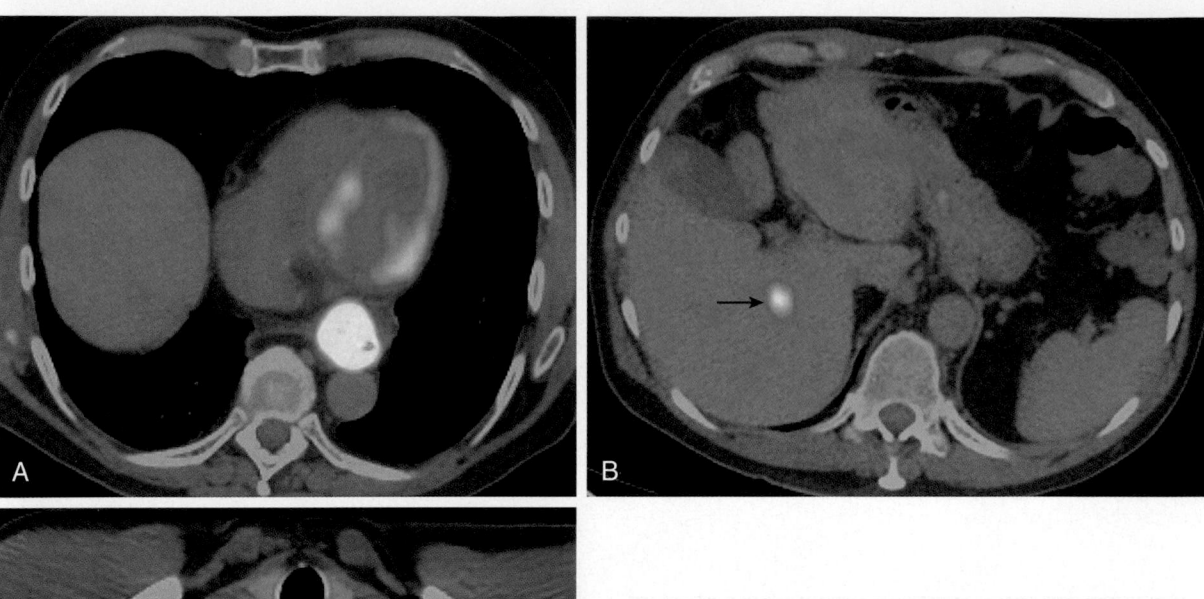

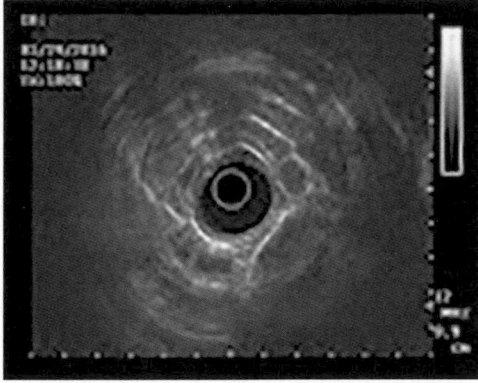

FIGURE 5 Positron-emission tomography-computed tomography demonstrating the primary tumor (**A**) and distant metastasis (arrows; **B** and **C**). *(From Erasmus JJ, Rohren EM, Hustnix R. PET and PET/CT in the diagnosis and staging of esophageal and gastric cancers. PET Clin. 3:135-145.)*

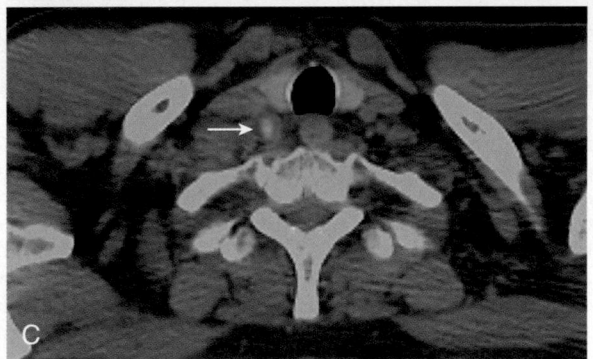

FIGURE 6 Endoscopic ultrasound of esophageal malignancy showing a lymph node highly suspicious for harboring metastatic disease.

■ STAGING

The current staging system employed for staging EC is the first evidence-based iteration that was constructed using de-identified data from more than 4000 patients and first was published in the seventh edition of the *Cancer Staging Manual* in 2010. It is based on the tumor-node-metastasis system that defines the anatomic extent of the cancer and takes into account nonanatomic characteristics of the tumor that have been recognized to be of importance, including the cell type, histologic grade, and location of its epicenter. Key changes in the new staging system are enumerated in Box 2. We individualize our treatment approach to individual patients primarily based on the stage of their disease; however, the patients' general health, functional status, and desires also must be taken into account.

■ STAGE-BASED TREATMENT STRATEGIES

Tis N0M0, T1a N0M0, Low-Risk T1b sm1 N0M0

In TisN0M0 disease or high-grade dysplasia (HGD), malignant change is confined to the mucosa and does not penetrate the basement membrane, therefore carries no risk for lymph node involvement. Options for the management of HGD include intensive surveillance endoscopy, endoscopic mucosal ablation, and esophagectomy. Proponents of surveillance argue that not all patients with HGD will go on to develop invasive cancer, and more aggressive therapies can be reserved for ones that do. Such an approach is prone to the risk of sampling error because foci of synchronous invasive carcinoma are present in 40% to 60% of patients identified with HGD. For this reason, esophagectomy until recently has been considered the standard of care in patients with HGD. Although curative, with 5-year survival rates in excess of 90%, esophagectomy has operative mortality rates of 3% to 12%, serious postoperative complication rates of 30% to 50% and the lifelong loss of esophageal function. Therefore esophagus-preserving therapies that eradicate the dysplastic mucosa while preserving function are emerging as the preferred approaches for the management of the patient with HGD. In T1aN0M0 disease, the tumor invades into the lamina propria or muscularis mucosae. Because of the general lack of lymphatics in these layers, the incidence of lymph node metastasis is reported to be less than 2% without potential for systemic spread. Esophageal-sparing local therapy that adequately eradicates the neoplastic tissue is gaining acceptance for the treatment of this stage of disease. T1bN0M0 tumors represent a watershed in the depth of tumor invasion, in which approach to management is less well defined. Because of the abundance of lymphatics in the submucosa and the resultant propensity for nodal involvement, esophagectomy has been the standard approach. More recently it has become recognized that not all

BOX 2: Changes in the Seventh Edition of the *AJCC Cancer Staging Manual*

Anatomic Characteristics

T Classification

T is redefined as high-grade dysplasia
T4 tumors subclassified
    T4a: invade adjacent structures that can be resected such as pleura, pericardium, and diaphragm
    T4b: invade adjacent structures that cannot be resected such as the aorta, airway, and vertebral bodies

N Classification

Regional lymph nodes reclassified as any periesophageal lymph nodes from the cervical region to the celiac plexus nodes
Nodal Status classified according to the number of positive nodes
    N0: No positive nodes
    N1: 1-2 positive nodes
    N2: 3-6 positive nodes
    N3: 7 or more positive nodes

M Classification

Redefined into two subtypes
    M0: No distant metastases
    M1: Distant metastases present
Nonanatomic Characteristics

Histologic Type

Adenocarcinoma
Squamous Cell Carcinoma

Histologic Grade

G1: Well differentiated
G2: Moderately differentiated
G3: Poorly differentiated
G4: Undifferentiated

Cancer Location

Upper thoracic: 20-25 cm from the incisors
Middle thoracic: 25-30 cm from the incisors
Lower thoracic: 30-40 cm from the incisors

Data from the *AJCC Cancer Staging Manual,* 7th ed. New York: Springer; 2010.

depths of ingression into the submucosa carry the same risk of nodal metastasis. T1b cancers are further classified as sm1, sm2, and sm3, by dividing the thickness of the submucosa into equal thirds. For low-risk T1b sm1 lesions, in which the tumor is smaller than 2 cm, is well or moderately well differentiated, and does not show lymphovascular invasion, incidence of lymph node metastasis is low (around 6%) with acceptable 5-year survival rates of 84% after esophageal-sparing treatment strategies. This subset of T1b patients therefore may be offered the option of esophageal preservation, which is particularly attractive in the frail patient with poor functional status and multiple comorbidities as is not infrequent in patients with esophageal cancer.

Current esophagus preserving strategies include radiofrequency ablation, photodynamic therapy, cryotherapy, and endoscopic mucosal resection. Radiofrequency ablation (RFA) uses a delivery system that transmits high energy (10 to 12 joules) directly to the mucosa that it is in contact with, generating heat, leading to coagulative necrosis and the destruction of 500 to 1000 µm of the most superficial tissue with which it is in contact. The HALO 360 (Covidien, Sunnyvale, CA) allows for the circumferential ablation of a 3-cm length of esophageal mucosa, and repositioning of the balloon allows ablation of additional segments. Residual islands, tongues of abnormal mucosa, and focal abnormalities can be treated using alternative delivery devices such as the HALO 90, HALO 60, and HALO Ultra. Performed under endoscopic guidance, multiple ablations can be performed at each endoscopic session and have to be repeated every 2 months until all the dysplastic epithelium has been eradicated. The annual rate of progression to EAC is 0.55% per patient per year. The most common complication is chest pain after the procedure and resolves over a week as the ablated mucosa heals. Gastrointestinal hemorrhage can result from mucosal erosions. A complication unique to RFA is the persistence of metaplastic epithelium under the normal squamous epithelium that cannot be detected on endoscopic evaluation and may serve as the focus for the development of EAC. Potential for recurrence of dysplastic epithelium mandates continued surveillance, every 3 months for the first year, every 6 months for the second year, and yearly thereafter. In addition, RFA does not provide tissue for pathologic evaluation.

Photodynamic therapy (PDT) is another ablative technique in which a photosensitizing agent (porfimer sodium) is administered 24 to 72 hours before treatment. The agent is accumulated and stored in higher concentrations in the neoplastic tissue as compared with normal tissue. Stimulation of the agent in vivo with a 630-nm laser light induces a photochemical reaction that results in the generation of reactive oxygen species and destruction of the tissue. PDT results in complete destruction of the dysplastic epithelium in 50% to 75% of cases. In more than half the ablated mucosa is resurfaced completely with normal squamous epithelium. As with RFA, subsquamous patches of intestinal metaplasia may persist and serve as the foci for the development of EAC. The most common complications of PDT are the development of strictures, cutaneous photosensitivity, candidal esophagitis, atrial fibrillation, and odynophagia.

Cryotherapy results in tissue destruction by inducing alternating cycles of rapid freezing and slow thawing using either liquid nitrogen or carbon dioxide directed toward the area to be treated through a catheter passed through the working channel of an endoscope. At each session, one third or one half of the circumference of the esophagus can be treated for a distance of about 3 cm. Multiple sessions therefore are required and are performed 6 to 8 weeks apart. Although the technique is highly efficacious in eradicating dysplastic epithelium, it is associated with a high potential for stricture formation that will require endoscopic dilatation. Like RFA, no tissue is available for histologic evaluation.

Endoscopic mucosal resection (EMR) is another option for these superficial early stage lesions. The lesion must be small enough to be removed completely by endoscopic means and hence is applicable to lesions smaller than 2 cm. First a thorough endoscopy is performed to identify the lesion of interest as well as to evaluate the remainder of the mucosa for additional areas of concern. If resources and expertise allow, advanced endoscopic techniques are used to increase yield. The target to be resected is marked using electrocautery. This overcomes the inability to identify the lesion accurately after the submucosal injection of saline, loss of orientation once a scope with a resection cap is introduced, and allows the specimen to be appropriately positioned on a corkboard for pathologic evaluation. We prefer the cap-and-snare technique in which a suction polyp is created to include all the mucosa within the marked area. A cauterizing snare then is used to resect the resultant polyp down to the submucosal level. Clear liquids are initiated on the first day and advanced as the symptoms of chest discomfort and odynophagia abate. Healing of the resultant ulcer can result in dysphagia, which usually resolves over the ensuing 6 to 8 weeks. The obtained specimen can be evaluated for the size of the tumor, its depth of invasion, the presence of lymphovascular invasion, and the degree of differentiation. After EMR of the lesion of interest, RFA can be performed to ablate the remainder of the abnormal mucosa. If the pathology reveals high-risk tumor characteristics, an esophagectomy can be performed. Potential complications include strictures, bleeding, and perforation. If HGD persists, a repeat of EMR and endoscopic ablation is performed until all diseased mucosa is eradicated. After repeated EMR, its subsequent performance may no longer be possible because of scarring. Here, cryotherapy is a potential option.

After esophageal preserving therapy, intense high-dose proton pump inhibitors, twice daily H2-blocker therapy, and sucralfate ("the kitchen-sink") are given to provide an acid-free environment that promotes healing. Surveillance endoscopy is performed every 3 months for 1 year with adequate four quadrant biopsies at every 1 cm of treated mucosa. Once two subsequent biopsies show no evidence of dysplasia, the surveillance interval may be increased. Once eradication of dysplastic epithelium is confirmed, antireflux surgery may be performed to eliminate further acid exposure. As alluded to earlier, contraindications to esophageal-preserving therapy include the presence of multifocal disease because of the high probability of sampling error, submucosal invasion beyond the outer third, squamous histology resulting from the higher propensity for lymph node involvement, lymphovascular invasion, poorly differentiated tumors, and nodules greater than 3 cm in diameter.

T1b sm2, sm3 N0M0

In contrast to T1b sm1 disease, tumors that invade into the middle and inner thirds of the submucosa have a significant propensity for spread to regional nodes. Hence esophagectomy with regional lymphadenectomy is the ideal approach in this subset of patients assuming that they are good surgical candidates able to withstand a major operative undertaking and its attendant morbidity.

T2-4a, Any N, M0

This represents locally advanced resectable esophageal cancer. The CROSS trial has added significant clarity to the approach to this stage of disease. The use of neoadjuvant chemoradiotherapy before surgical resection significantly increased to ability to achieve an R0 resection (no tumor within 1 cm of the resection margin), and a longer median survival of 49 months when compared with 24 months for surgery alone. A long-term follow-up (median follow-up 45 months, mean follow-up 84 months) has just been published and confirms the survival benefit of neoadjuvant therapy. The median survival of patients with SCC was 81.6 months with CRT, compared with 21.1 months with surgery alone. This raises the possibility of using CRT as definitive therapy for operable SCC. The proposed benefits of neoadjuvant therapy are that it increases the probability of achieving a R0 resection, sterilizes the regional lymph nodes reducing local recurrence, and treats micrometastatic disease, reducing the risk of systemic recurrence.

The particular surgical approach employed must be individualized for each patient taking into account tumor stage, type, location, extent of nodal dissection planned, patient comorbidities, body habitus, and surgeon experience and preference. The selected approach must allow for a R0 resection, performance of an adequate lymphadenectomy, reconstruction of the GI tract, and must be commensurate with the patients' ability to tolerate the operative insult. Surgical intervention may be undertaken using open, minimally invasive, and more recently robotically assisted techniques (Box 3).

The Ivor Lewis esophagectomy combines a laparotomy with a right thoracotomy. The laparotomy is performed via a midline incision, the abdomen is explored first to rule out undetected metastatic disease and to ascertain resectability. Use of a self-retaining upper abdominal retractor is critical for adequate exposure. Dividing the triangular ligament and retracting the lateral segment of the liver medially exposes the region of the hiatus. The gastrohepatic omentum then is taken down and dissection continued to the right crus taking down the phrenoesophageal ligament. The anterior surface of the esophagus then is dissected. The greater omentum then is dissected to gain access to the lesser sac.

We begin the dissection in the clear area of the pars flaccida and proceed cranially dividing the short gastrics between the stomach

---

BOX 3: Operative Options for Esophageal Carcinoma

Open, minimally invasive, or robotically assisted Ivor Lewis esophagectomy
  Ideal for adenocarcinoma of the lower and middle third of the esophagus
Open, minimally invasive, or robotically assisted McKeown esophagectomy
  Ideal for adenocarcinoma of the middle or upper third of the esophagus, and for squamous cell carcinoma of the esophagus
Open, minimally invasive, or robotically assisted transhiatal esophagectomy
  Ideal in patients who will not tolerate the pulmonary sequela of the thoracic component of an Ivor Lewis or McKeown esophagectomy
Left thoracoabdominal esophagectomy: ideal for bulky tumors in the region of the hiatus

---

and the spleen. Additional dissection of the attachments of the spleen to the diaphragm allows it to fall away from the operative field, exposing the right crus. The esophagus now is dissected circumferentially at the hiatus and a Penrose drain placed to provide traction for dissection into the mediastinum. The gastrocolic omentum now is divided caudally, taking care to stay wide of the right gastroepiploic vessels so as not to compromise the vascular supply of the conduit. The stomach now is reflected upward and medially and dissected free off its posterior attachments to the pancreas and retroperitoneum. The lymphatic tissue at the origin of the left gastric vessels is swept into the specimen, and the vessels are divided using a vascular stapler. Care is taken to preserve the right gastric artery. Additional mobilization can be achieved by performing a Kocher maneuver. Augmentation of gastric drainage can be achieved by a variety of methods. We prefer to inject 100 units of botulinum toxin onto the pylorus. Alternatively a pyloromyotomy or pyloroplasty can be performed. The gastric conduit then is prepared by several firings of the GIA stapler, ensuring that an adequate distal margin has been obtained and that the conduit will reach the site of anastomosis without tension. The hiatus is enlarged to allow the conduit to pass into the posterior mediastinum without compression and possible compromise of the vascular supply. A heavy nonabsorbable silk or polyester suture is used to attach the conduit to the esophagogastric specimen. A feeding jejunostomy tube is placed, following which the abdomen is closed.

The patient then is placed in the left lateral decubitus position to perform a right posterolateral thoracotomy through the fifth or sixth interspace. A dual lumen endotracheal tube is used to isolate the right lung. The esophagus along with all periesophageal tissue and associated lymphatic tissue is resected from the apex down to the hiatus, taking care not to injure the thoracic duct or its major branches. Division of the azygous vein greatly facilitates the dissection. The esophagogastric specimen and gastric conduit then are drawn into the chest. The proximal esophagus is divided well above the azygous vein. Either a stapled or hand-sewn anastomosis is performed after removing all redundancy in the conduit and passing a nasogastric tube past the anastomosis. The conduit is then tacked to the diaphragmatic hiatus to prevent visceral herniation. A drain is placed alongside the anastomosis, and apicoposterior and basilar chest tubes (#29 Blake) placed before closure of the chest. If the stomach cannot be used as a conduit because of either disease or previous surgery, the colon or jejunum can be used as a conduit. For use of the colon as a conduit, complete bowel prep is essential before surgery. The left colon is preferred because of its better size match and more reliable blood supply from the left colic artery.

The most commonly employed modification of the McKeown or three-hole esophagectomy begins with a right posterolateral thoracotomy completing the thoracic portion first to ensure resectability. In contrast to the Ivor Lewis esophagectomy, the dissection of the esophagus along with its associated lymphatic tissue is continued superiorly all the way to the thoracic inlet. The patient then is placed in the supine position and the abdominal portion of the procedure performed. After completion of the abdominal portion of the operation, an oblique left neck incision is made along the anterior border of the sternocleidomastoid muscle. After division of the platysma, the trachea is retracted medially and the carotid sheath laterally. Ligation of the middle thyroid vein and inferior thyroid artery is often necessary to gain adequate exposure. Dissection then is carried out lateral to the esophagus down to the prevertebral fascia, where blunt dissection is used to create a posterior plane. Finally the esophagus is separated from the trachea, taking care to remain close to its wall to avoid injury to the recurrent laryngeal nerve. A Penrose drain is placed around the esophagus and used to provide traction, facilitating continued dissection into the superior mediastinum. Application of gentle but firm pressure allows the esophagogastric specimen and gastric conduit to be drawn into the neck. The proximal esophagus is divided, and an anastomosis between the esophagus and gastric conduit performed. Either a side-to-side functional end-to-end stapled anastomosis or an end-to-end hand-sewn single layer anastomosis using absorbable suture is performed.

For a transhiatal esophagectomy the patient is positioned supine, with a shoulder roll to extend the neck, and the head is turned to the right. A midline abdominal incision is used and the initial portions of the operation are identical to the abdominal portion of an Ivor Lewis esophagectomy. Once the stomach has been mobilized fully, incising the diaphragm anteriorly from the apex of the crura enlarges the diaphragmatic hiatus. Using blunt finger dissection the esophagus is dissected off the aorta and spine posteriorly and the pericardium anteriorly. At this stage, an oblique left neck incision is made and the cervical esophagus circumferentially dissected free as previously described. A Penrose drain is placed around the esophagus and used to provide traction facilitating dissection into the superior mediastinum. The right hand is reintroduced through the hiatus and the esophagus bluntly dissected into the superior mediastinum. Simultaneously the left hand dissects into the mediastinum via the cervical incision until the fingers meet, indicating that circumferential mobilization of the esophagus in the mediastinum has been achieved. The esophagus is divided in the neck using a GIA stapler, with the superior end of a long 1-inch–wide Penrose drain incorporated into the staple line. The esophagus then is withdrawn into the abdomen, and the long Penrose drain trails along from the cervical incision into the abdomen through the posterior mediastinum. The stomach then is wrapped in a plastic bag to reduce friction during passage through the posterior mediastinum. The bag is attached to the abdominal end of the Penrose drain, which then is drawn into the neck by pulling on the end of the drain that remained in the cervical incision. Care is taken not to allow the conduit to twist during its passage through the posterior mediastinum. A hand-sewn or stapled anastomosis is performed. Any redundancy in the conduit is removed and the hiatus reduced in size to allow three finger-breadths to be accommodated with ease. A tight closure may result in bowstringing of the conduit, causing obstruction and may compromise blood flow. A drain is placed near the cervical anastomosis.

A left thoracoabdominal esophagectomy is ideal for large, bulky esophageal tumors around the hiatus because it affords excellent visualization of the anatomy. With the patient in the right lateral decubitus position, an oblique upper abdominal incision is made halfway between the xiphoid and the umbilicus in line with the sixth interspace. The abdomen first is entered and evaluated for presence of metastatic disease precluding resection. If none are identified, the chest is entered through the sixth interspace. Dividing the costal margin and taking down the diaphragm through a circumferential incision made about 2 cm from its attachment to the chest wall improve visualization. An extensive dissection of the thoracic esophagus along with the regional lymph nodes and adjacent pleura is performed. The esophagus is divided 8 to 10 cm above the upper extent of the tumor, after which attention is directed towards resection in the region of the hiatus. If needed, portions of the crura can be resected to achieve an R0 resection. Dissection now returns to the abdomen, where the distal esophagus along with an adequate margin of stomach is resected, the conduit prepared, a gastric emptying procedure performed, and a jejunal feeding tube placed. The conduit then is delivered into the chest through the hiatus and anastomosed to the native esophagus using a stapled or hand-sewn technique. After any redundant portion of the conduit is reduced back into the abdomen, the hiatus is reduced in size, and the conduit is secured to the crura. The diaphragm and costal margin are reapproximated before closing the chest over a 28F chest tube. The abdomen then is closed in standard fashion. A modification of this approach is to add a left neck dissection with dissection of the cervical and superior mediastinal esophagus with its associated lymphatic tissue and the performance of a cervical anastomosis.

The abdominal and/or thoracic portions of these operations can be performed using minimally invasive techniques with comparable oncologic outcomes and are significantly better tolerated by patients. Robotic assistance also has been added recently to the available armamentarium. These approaches are, however, complex and technically challenging and should be performed by surgeons with significant experience. Using a combination of laparoscopy and thoracoscopy, the McKeown and Ivor Lewis esophagectomy can be performed minimally invasively. For the thoracic portion of the McKeown esophagectomy, the patient is placed in the left lateral decubitus position and ventilated with a dual-lumen endotracheal tube to allow collapse of the right lung. We use a four-port technique. A 10-mm, 30-degree camera is introduced through an incision in the seventh intercostal space just anterior to the middle axillary line. Another 10-mm trocar is placed in the eighth space 2 cm posterior to the posterior axillary line. Two additional 5-mm trocars are placed, one below the tip of the scapula, and another in the fourth intercostal space anterior to the anterior axillary line. A polyester suture placed through the central tendon of the diaphragm and brought out using an Endo-Close needle through a 1-mm incision in the anterior inferior chest wall allows the diaphragm to be retracted improving visualization of the esophagus. Dissection is started by dividing the mediastinal pleura posterior to the esophagus beginning at a distance from the tumor. The esophagus is dissected circumferentially at this level, and the dissection in this plane is continued from the thoracic inlet to the diaphragm. Division of the azygous vein invariably is required. Care is taken to ligate the thoracic duct and its major branches using clips to avoid development of a chyle leak postoperatively. After placement of a 28F chest tube, the port sites are closed. The patient now is placed supine, and the abdominal portion of the procedure is performed using a 5-trocar approach similar to that for a Nissen fundoplication. Steps of the abdominal phase of the operation are identical to those of an open operation and include esophagogastric resection, preparation of the conduit, gastric drainage procedure, and placement of a jejunal feeding tube. The last step of the abdominal portion is to take down the phrenoesophageal ligaments and dissect the esophagus off the left and right crura. The crura may be divided to enlarge the hiatus to allow the conduit to pass through without compression. This step is left to the end to prevent decompression of the pneumoperitoneum into the chest. After this the cervical portion of the operation is performed, as previously described. After completion of the cervical anastomosis, the abdomen is reinsufflated and the redundant portion of the conduit drawn back into the abdomen and tacked to the hiatus using an endostitch device (Covidien, Mansfield, MA).

Minimally invasive Ivor Lewis esophagectomy is performed by first completing the abdominal portion of the operation laparoscopically with the patient in the supine position. The patient then is placed in the left lateral decubitus position, ports are inserted as for the thoracoscopic portion of a McKeown esophagectomy, and the esophagus along with lymphatic tissue is dissected circumferentially to above the level of the azygous vein, which must be transected to allow adequate exposure. The proximal esophagus then is transected, and the esophagogastric specimen along with the created conduit attached to it is drawn into the chest. The specimen is removed after placing it in a protective bag through the posterior port. The anastomosis is created using a 28-mm EEA stapler, the anvil of which may be introduced through the chest or orally (OrVil; Covidien, Mansfield, MA), with the handle of the stapler being passed through a gastrotomy that is subsequently closed using an Endo GIA stapler (Covidien, Mansfield, MA). A drain is placed alongside the anastomosis, and a 28F chest tube is placed posteriorly before closing the trocar sites.

Complications of Esophagectomy

Esophagectomy is a complex operative undertaking that is best performed in high-volume centers by experienced trained surgeons. This recommendation is supported by a recent meta-analysis, which demonstrated a threefold increase in mortality when performed in a low-volume center. Even in experienced hands, the overall complication rate is nearly 50%. Respiratory complications remain the most common, contributing to 50% to 65% of deaths after surgery. Preoperative optimization of pulmonary function, cessation of smoking, preemptive analgesia with epidural catheters, generous use of intercostal blocks, aggressive pulmonary toilet, and the use of minimally invasive techniques are integral to their prevention. Because of loss of protective sphincter mechanisms the patients are prone to reflux and aspiration, and pneumonia remains a major threat that must be recognized and prevented.

Development of a chyle leak is characterized by increased chest tube output, typically on reintroduction of enteral feeds. Output is generally 2 to 4 L a day, and the presence of chylomicrons and a triglyceride level of more than 100 mg/dL is diagnostic. Initial management is expectant with discontinuation of enteral feeds and provision of total parenteral nutrition. If high outputs persist, operative intervention by open or thoracoscopic means is indicated. Cream is administered before the operation to better identify the area of leak, which then can be oversewn. If no specific area of leak is identified, mass ligation of all the tissue between the azygous vein and aorta is performed, thus ligating the thoracic duct at the hiatus. Anastomotic leak is suspected clinically because of the change in character or output from the drain placed alongside at the end of surgery.

Any suspected leak is evaluated initially with an esophagogram using water-soluble contrast. If no leak is identified, the study is repeated with dilute barium. Additional evaluation can be performed with a contrast CT of the neck and chest. Endoscopy previously was considered contraindicated because of concerns that the necessary insufflation would result in either a disruption of the anastomosis or worsening of any present disruption. Recent experience, however, shows that when performed carefully, endoscopy can be performed safely and is useful not only to identify the presence of a leak and its extent but also to determine if there is conduit necrosis that is contributing to the leak. Limited leaks, which drain back into the conduit, or are completely evacuated by the indwelling drain, can be treated expectantly. Free leaks into the pleural cavity require operative intervention. Small leaks can be repaired, whereas larger leaks and those resulting from conduit necrosis require revision of the anastomosis. In both cases the repair must be buttressed with healthy vascularized tissue, such as the diaphragm, the pleura, or the pericardium. The use of esophageal stents is emerging as a valuable adjunct in the available armamentarium in the management of anastomotic leaks. When there is a delay in diagnosis and there is significant inflammatory response of the surrounding tissue, a repair is not possible because of the friable nature of the tissue. Here the affected portion

of the esophagus is resected, the proximal segment is exteriorized, and extensive drainage is provided with delayed reconstruction planned. Anastomotic stricture is accompanied by dysphagia and is usually the result of technical factors or ischemia of the conduit. It can be treated using dilatation or stents. Atrial fibrillation is common and usually is associated with the development of other complications, including anastomotic leaks and pulmonary complications. Its occurrence can be reduced by the prophylactic administration of amiodarone and the use of minimally invasive techniques. Recurrent laryngeal nerve injury is more common when a cervical anastomosis is performed as with a McKeown esophagectomy. In addition to the hoarseness of voice, the swallowing difficulties that result cause a significant increase in respiratory complications.

Adjuvant therapy is indicated in patients at high risk of local and/ or systemic recurrence. These include patients with T3 or T4 tumors, an R1 or R2 resection, or with multiple positive lymph nodes. A recent randomized controlled trial demonstrated significant improvement in the 3-year survival, increased duration of relapse-free survival, and reduced rate of local recurrence. Adjuvant CRT therefore should be offered to those able to tolerate it.

T4b Any N Any M or Any T, Any N, M1

T4b cancers invade structures that cannot be resected, such as the aorta, left atrium, and spine, whereas in M1 disease there is systemic spread of the malignancy. Patients with either are not candidates for curative therapy and should be offered the option of palliative care. Goals of palliative care include the treatment of specific symptoms, delaying death from metastatic disease with minimum morbidity, and improving the quality of remaining life. These goals are achieved best in the context of a multidisciplinary effort and should include a palliative care specialist. Providing continued psychologic support is paramount.

Oncologic palliation aims to achieve long-term control of the disease process potentially prolonging survival and can be achieved using CRT, chemotherapy, or radiation therapy. Chemoradiation achieves long-term disease control and prolongs survival. Its systemic consequences do, however, require the patient to have a good performance status and minimal comorbidities. It is also efficacious at resolving dysphagia, but it may take up to 6 weeks to achieve results. Chemotherapy alone is indicated when the predominance of symptoms is due to disseminated disease. Results are best when a combination of agents is used; this, however, results in greater toxicity of the agents made worse by the advanced age and comorbidities of the patient. Response should be assessed objectively halfway through the treatment. If no response is observed, the regimen should be changed. Radiation therapy is indicated for local symptoms including mediastinal pain, dysphagia, and local bleeding. It takes several weeks before improvement is seen. The two options for radiation therapy include external beam radiation and brachytherapy. External beam therapy is most effective for bulky tumors. However, it requires several visits, which may be difficult for patients living far away from the treatment facility. Brachytherapy involves the implantation of a radioactive source into the tumor endoscopically. It is suited best for exophytic lesions, in which it provides high-dose radiation to the tumor with minimum damage to the surrounding structures. Complications of brachytherapy include ulceration, bleeding, and stricture formation.

Endoscopic palliation is preferred when immediate results are desired. Endoscopic insertion of self-expanding stents provides effective and immediate palliation of dysphagia related to obstruction of tumor (Figures 7 and 8). Endoscopic dilatation is another effective technique and can be performed using either hollow-core polyvinyl dilators or through the scope balloon dilators. Although the effect is immediate, it is often short lived, and dilatation is required every 10 to 14 days. Alcohol sclerotherapy, argon plasma coagulation (APC), Nd:YAG laser therapy, and photodynamic therapy are other endoscopic techniques that result in tumor

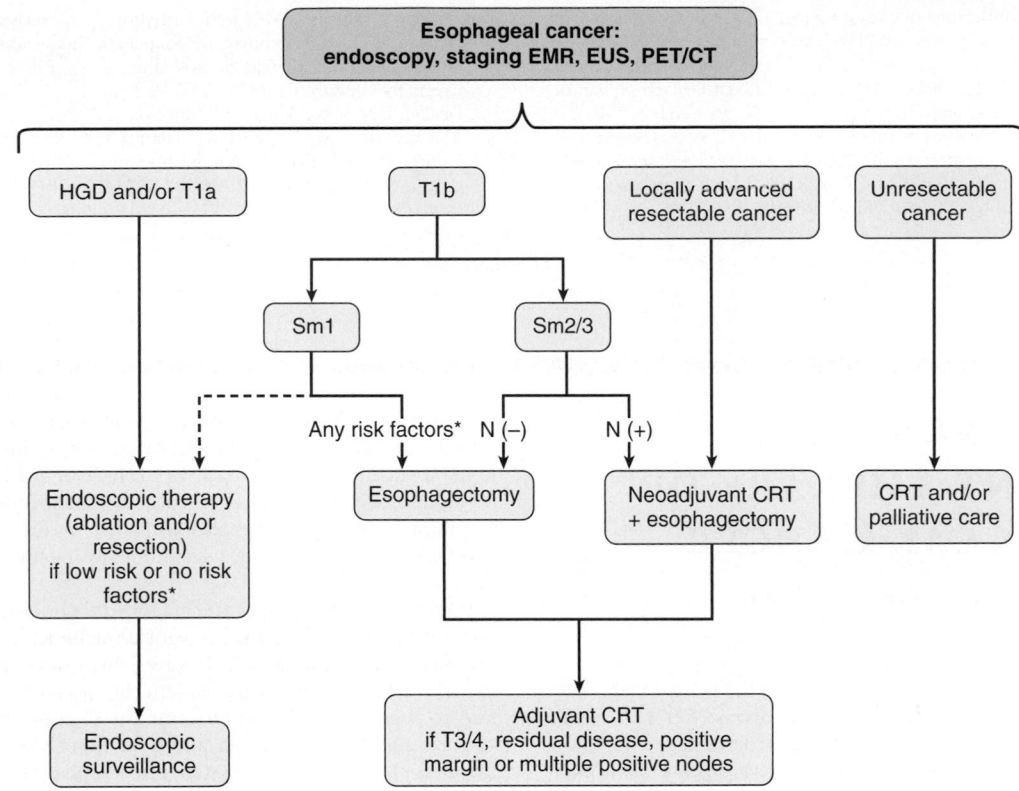

FIGURE 7 Treatment algorithm for esophageal carcinoma. *(From Hoppo T, Jobe B. Personalizing therapy for esophageal cancer patients. Thorac Surg Clin. 2013:473.)*

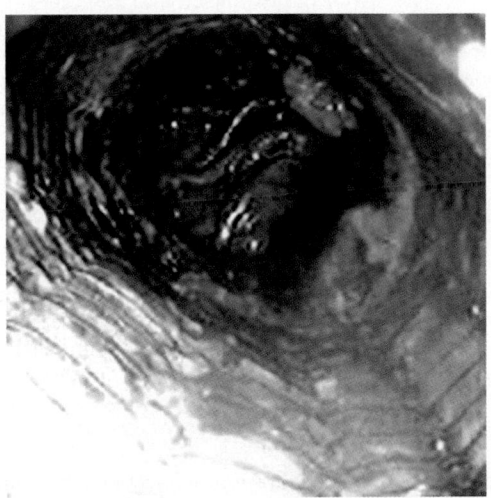

FIGURE 8 Palliative treatment of esophageal cancer using stents.

destruction, reestablishment of the esophageal lumen, and relief of dysphagia. APC and laser therapy are also highly effective in the management of bleeding from the surface of tumors.

■ SUMMARY

Esophageal cancer remains a highly lethal disease, the incidence of which is increasing at an alarming rate related largely to the epidemic of gastroesophageal reflux. High-quality endoscopy with adequate biopsies is critical to establishing a diagnosis. Once diagnosed, a comprehensive and expeditious staging workup must be performed with high-resolution contrast CT, PET imaging, EUS, EUS/FNA, bronchoscopy, and laparoscopy/thoracoscopy as necessary. Therapy must be individualized for patients based on the extent of disease, their age, performance status, comorbidities, and desires. Early stage disease with low likelihood of nodal involvement can be treated with esophagus-preserving treatments, including RFA, cryotherapy, and EMR. For resectable locally advanced disease, neoadjuvant chemoradiation followed by surgical resection remains the best option. For patients who are not surgical candidates, palliation using chemoradiation, chemotherapy, or radiation is employed to prolong survival. Endoscopic palliation of dysphagia is effective and improves quality of life. Research into molecular targets that govern or guide malignant transformation, proliferation, and spread of esophageal cancer may provide the next paradigm shift in the treatment of these patients.

SUGGESTED READINGS

Hoppo T, Jobe BA. Personalizing therapy for esophageal cancer patients. *Thorac Surg Clin.* 2013;23:471-478.

Luketich JD, Pennathur A, Franchetti Y, Catalano PJ, Swanson S, Sugarbaker DJ, De Hoyos A, Maddaus MA, Nguyen NT, Benson AB, Fernando HC. Minimally invasive esophagectomy: results of a prospective phase II multicenter trial—the Eastern Cooperative Oncology group (E2202) study. *Ann Surg.* 2015;261:702-707.

Nieponice A, Badaloni AE, Jobe BA, Hoppo T, Pellegrini C, Velanovich V, Falk GW, Reavis K, Swanstorm L, Sharma VK, Nachman F, Ciotola FF, Caro LE, Cerisoli C, Cavadas D, Figueroa LD, Pirchi D, Gibdosn M, Elizalde S, Cohen H. Management of early-stage esophageal neoplasia (MESEN) consensus. *World J Surg.* 2014;38:96-105.

Rice TW, Blackstone EH, Rusch VW. A cancer staging primer: esophagus and esophagogastric junction. *J Thorac Cardiovasc Surg.* 2010;139:527-529.

Schuchert MJ, Luketich JD, Lanreneau RJ. Management of esophageal cancer. *Curr Probl Surg.* 2010;47:845-946.

Shapiro J, van Lanschot JJ, Hulshof MC, van Hagen P, van Berge Henegouwen MI, Wijnhoven BP, van Laarhoven HW, Nieuwenhuijzen GA, Hospers GA, Bonenkamp JJ, Cuesta MA, Blaisse RJ, Busch OR, Ten Kate FJ, Creemers GJ, Punt CJ, Plukker JT, Verheul HM, Bilgen EJ, van Dekken H, van der Sangen MJ, Rozema T, Biermann K, Beukema JC, Piet AH, van Rij CM, Reinders JG, Tilanus HW, Steyerberg EW, van der Gaast A, CROSS study group. Neoadjuvant chemoradiotherapy plus surgery versus surgery alone for oesophageal or junctional cancer (CROSS): long-term results of a randomized control trial. *Lancet Oncol.* 2015;16:1090-1098.

van Hagen P, Hulshof MC, van Lanschot JJ, Steyerberg EW, van Berge Henegouwen MI, Wijnhoven BP, Richel DJ, Nieuwenhuijzen GA, Hospers GA, Bonenkamp JJ, Cuesta MA, Blaisse RJ, Busch OR, ten Kate FJ, Creemers GJ, Punt CJ, Plukker JT, Verheul HM, Spillenaar Bilgen EJ, van Dekken H, van der Sangen MJ, Rozema T, Biermann K, Beukema JC, Piet AH, van Rij CM, Reinders JG, Tilanus HW, van der Gaast A, CROSS Group. Preoperative chemoradiotherapy for esophageal or junctional cancer. *N Engl J Med.* 2012;366:2074-2084.

Neoadjuvant and Adjuvant Therapy of Esophageal Cancer

Ronan Kelly, MD, and Adrian Murphy, MD

The rates of esophageal cancer are rising in the United States with almost 20,000 people dying from this disease per year. Taken together upper GI tumors (esophageal, gastroesophageal junction, and gastric cancer) are second only to lung cancer in terms of incidence and mortality worldwide. The location of upper GI tumors in western countries has changed dramatically in recent years. Distal esophageal adenocarcinomas once represented only 0.8% to 3.7% of all esophageal neoplasms. This has changed dramatically with a sevenfold increase in the incidence of lower esophageal adenocarcinomas being recorded among U.S. white males over the past three decades. Lower esophageal adenocarcinoma now accounts for more than 80% of the cases of newly diagnosed esophageal cancer. This has been attributed in part to declining chronic infection rates by *Helicobacter pylori* and an increased incidence of gastroesophageal reflux disease and obesity.

The mainstay of curative treatment for nonmetastatic esophageal cancer involves surgical resection; however, most agree that a significant proportion of patients with resectable disease require multimodality interventions. The selection of patients who require preoperative or perioperative multimodality therapy has been assisted by improvements in staging investigations such as positron emission tomography (PET) and endoscopic ultrasound (EUS). In particular, EUS is the optimal modality to accurately stage locoregional disease in esophageal cancer.

In general, the consensus is that all nonsuperficial esophageal tumors (greater than stage 1) should be considered for multimodality therapy in addition to surgical resection.

In this chapter, the first part provides a summary of the indications and evidence for neoadjuvant (preoperative and perioperative) multimodality therapy. The second part discusses the indications and evidence for adjuvant (postoperative) multimodality therapy.

■ INDICATIONS AND RATIONALE FOR NEOADJUVANT THERAPY FOR LOCOREGIONAL ESOPHAGEAL CANCER

Patients with locoregional advanced esophageal cancer are candidates for multimodality therapy. This includes patients with T2-T4 tumors and those with nodal involvement that are nonmetastatic (M0) (Table 1). PET imaging is considered the gold standard for identification of patients with nonmetastatic disease because most esophageal tumors are (18)F-fluoro-2-deoxy-D-glucose (FDG) avid and EUS is optimal for determining the depth of tumor invasion. Although nodal disease can be visualized with CT, EUS, or PET, these imaging modalities are imperfect in accurately determining nodal status. Combining cytologic diagnosis with fine-needle aspiration (FNA) and EUS is the most specific way of diagnosing the presence of nodal disease.

Originally esophageal cancer staging did not differentiate between the two major histologic subcategories: adenocarcinoma and squamous cell carcinoma (SCC). However, the observation of differences in survival between esophageal adenocarcinoma compared with SCC lead to separate staging criteria for these subtypes, particularly in stages I and II (Table 2). In addition, the TNM (tumor-necrosis-metastasis) classification system in esophageal cancer includes the histologic grade (G) of the tumor. The anatomic location of SCC is also an important factor in differentiating T2-3 tumors (stages IB-IIB).

Clinical T1 Tumors

Based on the American Joint Committee on Cancer (AJCC) staging system for esophageal cancer, T1 tumors are subdivided into those that invade the lamina propria or muscularis mucosae (superficial, T1a) or T1b, which invades the submucosa (deep). Although it is accepted universally that those with T1a tumors should undergo definitive curative resection with endoscopic mucosal resection, the evidence for T1b tumors is less definitive. T1b tumors can be subdivided further based on their depth of submucosal invasion (deep: >50% invasion, superficial: <50% invasion) because this predicts the risk of nodal metastasis. EUS can often under-stage T1b tumors and so ideally should be combined with FNA to obtain further cytologic assessment of draining regional lymph nodes. If nodal metastasis is confirmed, then this upstages the tumor, and multimodality therapy should be considered.

Clinical T2 Tumors

In general, the poor outcome of surgical resection alone and the risk of locoregional recurrence form the rationale for including neoadjuvant chemoradiotherapy in patients with resectable esophageal cancer. T2 lesions are often overstaged with EUS, and the presence of dysphagia can assist with clarifying the distinction between T2 and T1b lesions because the latter rarely present with dysphagia. The difficulty regarding recommending neoadjuvant therapy for T2 lesions lies in the inherent inaccuracies in correctly identifying it. Although some centers advocate for esophagectomy as primary therapy for T2 tumors, this usually is recommended only for low-risk lesions (<2 cm, grade 1).

Clinical T3-T4 Tumors

Diagnosis of clinical T3 tumors is accomplished most reliably with EUS with a high level of confidence. T4 lesions usually are

TABLE 1: Definitions of Tumor-Necrosis-Metastasis Staging

PRIMARY TUMOR (T) STAGING

TX	Primary tumor cannot be assessed
T0	No evidence of primary tumor
Tis	High-grade dysplasia
T1	Tumor invades lamina propria, muscularis mucosae, or submucosa
T1a	Tumor invades lamina propria or muscularis mucosae
T1b	Tumor invades submucosa
T2	Tumor invades muscularis propria
T3	Tumor invades adventitia
T4	Tumor invades adjacent structures
T4a	Resectable tumor invading pleura, pericardium, or diaphragm
T4b	Unresectable tumor invading other adjacent structures, such as aorta, vertebral body, trachea

REGIONAL LYMPH NODES (N)

NX	Regional lymph nodes cannot be assessed
N0	No regional lymph node metastasis
N1	Metastases in 1-2 regional lymph nodes
N2	Metastases in 3-6 regional lymph nodes
N3	Metastasis in seven or more regional lymph nodes

DISTANT METASTASIS (M)

M0	No distant metastasis
M1	Distant metastasis

From Edge S, et al. *AJCC Cancer Staging Manual.* 7th ed. p. 109. New York: Springer; 2010.

TABLE 2: Anatomic Stage/Prognostic Groups

Stage	Tumor	Node	Metastasis	Grade	Location
SQUAMOUS CELL CARCINOMA					
0	In situ	0	0	1, X	Any
1A	1	0	0	1, X	Any
IB	1	0	0	2-3	Any
	2-3	0	0	1, X	Lower, X
IIA	2-3	0	0	1, X	Upper, middle
	2-3	0	0	2-3	Lower, X
IIB	2-3	0	0	2-3	Upper, middle
	1-2	1	0	Any	Any
IIIA	1-2	2	0	Any	Any
	3	1	0	Any	Any
	4a	0	0	Any	Any
IIIB	3	2	0	Any	Any
IIIC	4a	1-2	0	Any	Any
	4b	Any	0	Any	Any
	Any	3	0	Any	Any
IV	Any	Any	1	Any	Any
ADENOCARCINOMA					
0	In situ	0	0	1, X	
IA	1	0	0	1-2, X	
IB	1	0	0	3	
	2	0	0	1-2, X	
IIA	2	0	0	3	
IIB	3	0	0	Any	
	1-2	1	0	Any	
IIIA	1-2	2	0	Any	
	3	1	0	Any	
	4a	0	0	Any	
IIIB	3	2	0	Any	
IIIC	4a	1-2	0	Any	
	4b	Any	0	Any	
	Any	3	0	Any	
IV	Any	Any	1	Any	

From Edge S, et al. *AJCC Cancer Staging Manual.* 7th ed. p. 109. New York: Springer; 2010.

detected with CT/PET with the distinction of T4a lesions being considered resectable (pleural/pericardial/diaphragmatic invasion), whereas T4b lesions are considered unresectable (aortic/vertebral/tracheal involvement). Although T4b lesions still are treated with chemoradiotherapy, this is considered definitive therapy with alternative radiation doses/regimens from those used for neoadjuvant therapy.

Clinical Node Positive Tumors

Determining nodal status is particularly important in early T1-T2 lesions, where its detection would alter radically the treatment plan. This is best done with EUS-FNA because CT and PET are unreliable in detecting lymph node metastasis in superficial esophageal tumors. Accurate distinction between N1-N3 statuses cannot be reliably made preoperatively because this is a pathologic definition. However, the presence of extraregional lymph nodes such as those in the mesentery/para-aortic region is an indicator of unresectability. Celiac, mediastinal, and supraclavicular nodes are defined as regional lymph nodes in the seventh AJCC staging system; however, at a multidisciplinary clinic careful upfront consideration about radiation field size and resectability is important before therapy is initiated.

Restaging After Preoperative Therapy

After completion of preoperative therapy, restaging of patients before surgery usually incorporates a CT scan to evaluate the response to treatment and to ensure that the tumor is still resectable and a PET scan to exclude the interim development of metastatic disease. Some clinicians also advocate for repeat esophagoscopy to evaluate the endoluminal extent of disease, but repeat EUS has limited utility in this setting.

■ NEOADJUVANT THERAPY FOR LOCOREGIONAL ESOPHAGEAL CANCER

Although esophageal SCCs and adenocarcinomas differ in terms of their prognosis and now have separate AJCC staging systems,

TABLE 3: Prospective Randomized Trials Comparing Preoperative Chemoradiation to Surgery Alone

Trial	No. of Patients	Tumor Type	Clinical Stage	Staging Workup	Chemotherapy	Radiation	Median Survival Rate	Significance
Nygaard (1992)	53	Squamous cell	All stages	CT, EGD	Cis, bleomycin	35 Gy	17%, 3-y	NS
	50				None	None	9%, 3-y	
LePrise (1994)	41	Squamous cell	All stages	CXR, ultrasound	Cis, 5-FU	20 Gy*	19.2%, 3-y	NS
	45				None	None	13.8%, 3-y	
Bosset (1997)	143	Squamous cell	All stages	CT, EGD, bronchoscopy	Cis	37 Gy	18.6 mo	NS
	139				None	None	18.6 mo	
Walsh (1996)	58	Adenocarcinoma	All stages	CXR, EGD, ultrasound	Cis, 5-FU	40 Gy	16 mo	P = 0.01
	55				None	None	11 mo	
Urba (2001)	50	Adenocarcinoma (50%)	All stages	CT, bone scan, endoscopy	Cis, 5-FU, vinblastine	45 Gy	16.9 mo	NS
	50	Squamous cell (50%)			None	None	17.6 mo	
Burmeister (2005)	128	Adenocarcinoma (62.9%)	All stages	CT, EGD	Cis, 5-FU	35 Gy	22.2 mo	NS
	128	Squamous cell (37.1%)			None	None	19.3 mo	
Tepper (2008)	30	Adenocarcinoma (75.0%)	All stages	CT, EGD	Cis, 5-FU	50.4 Gy	53.8 mo	P = 0.002
	26	Squamous cell (25.0%)			None	None	21.5 mo	
CROSS (2012)	178	Adenocarcinoma (75.0%)	≥Stage II	CT, EUS, EGD	Carbo, paclitaxel	41.4 Gy	49.4 mo	P = 0.003
	188	Squamous cell (25.0%)			None	None	24.0 mo	

*Sequential.

Carbo, Carboplatin; Cis, cisplatin; CT, computed tomographic scan of chest and abdomen; CXR, chest x-ray; EGD, esophagoscopy; EUS, endoscopic ultrasound scan; 5-FU, 5-fluorouracil; NS, not significant.

there are few data to guide incorporating histologic subtype into treatment planning. SCCs tend to respond more favorably to chemoradiation and relapse locoregionally when compared with adenocarcinomas.

Historically, surgical resection for esophageal cancer alone resulted in 5-year survival rates of 10% to 20%. Adding preoperative radiotherapy alone did not improve outcomes likely because of the undertreatment of microscopic metastatic disease. However, the combination of chemotherapy and radiotherapy (chemoradiation, CRT) has been shown to reduce the rates of local and distant recurrences and as a result, improve overall survival rates. Many historical studies of preoperative CRT did not include modern staging techniques, thereby questioning the accuracy of the stages of the trial participants. Furthermore, these trials often treated an undefined number of patients with early stage disease, with the presence of any nonmetastatic disease as the sole trial cancer-related entry criterion (Tables 3 and 4).

Preoperative Radiotherapy

The role of radiotherapy (RT) alone to treat preoperative esophageal cancer has been supplanted by CRT as a result of improved clinical outcomes. A Chinese study compared surgery with RT alone in patients with esophageal SCC using modern RT techniques (3D-conformal and intensity-modulated RT) and found that overall survival rates did not differ significantly in those treated with surgery versus RT. In general, most preoperative RT regimens involve 1.8 to 2 Gy/fraction for a total of 45 to 50.4 Gy administered over 5 to 6 weeks. The RTOG 94-05 trial compared 50.4 Gy with 64.8 Gy as a definitive concurrent CRT dose. This trial determined that the higher dose was associated with higher complication rates, including fistulae and deaths, without any survival benefit. These data were then extrapolated for use as preoperative therapy in

deciding the optimal tolerable preoperative radiation dose. In reality, many of the complications seen in the higher radiation group in the RTOG trial occurred before even reaching the 50.4 Gy dose, so whether higher doses necessarily result in higher complications is unclear.

Preoperative Chemoradiation Therapy

Several studies have compared surgery with or without preoperative CRT and have shown a survival benefit using a concurrent rather than sequential approach. Not all studies consistently show the superiority of CRT versus surgery alone because some were underpowered statistically. Despite these limitations, there is a consensus that patients with greater than T2 resectable disease require neoadjuvant concurrent CRT. The Dutch CROSS study compared preoperative carboplatin/paclitaxel and RT with surgery alone in 363 patients with potentially resectable esophageal cancer. After a median follow-up of 7 years, CRT resulted in improved overall survival compared with surgery (48.6 vs 24 months, HR = 0.68, 95% CI 0.53-0.88, p = 0.003). Survival was dramatically better for patients with SCC compared with those with adenocarcinomas, although multivariate analysis showed that the overall survival benefit was not skewed entirely by patients with SCCs. Patients who received CRT also had improved complete resection (R0) and pathologic complete response (pCR) rates. The preoperative regimen was well tolerated, with 7% patients experiencing at least a grade 3 hematologic toxicity, but there were no differences in postoperative morbidity or mortality between the groups. The CALGB 9781 study was a small study that included 56 patients with stages I to III esophageal cancer comparing neoadjuvant CRT versus surgery alone. It showed a 40% pCR rate without any increase in morbidity or mortality with CRT. This study also demonstrated a trend towards improved survival with neoadjuvant CRT.

TABLE 4: Prospective Randomized Trials Comparing Preoperative Chemotherapy to Surgery Alone

Trial	No. of Patients	Tumor Type	Clinical Stage	Chemotherapy	5-Year Survival Rate	Significance
MRC (2002)	400	Adenocarcinoma (66%)	All stages	Cisplatin, 5-fluorouracil	25.0%	$P = 0.004$
	402	Squamous cell (31%)		None	15.0%	
RTOG 8911 (1998)	233	Adenocarcinoma (53%)	All stages	Cisplatin, 5-fluorouracil	18%	$P = 0.53$
	234	Squamous cell (47%)		None	20%	
MAGIC (2006)*	250	Adenocarcinoma	≥Stage II	Epirubicin, cisplatin, 5-fluorouracil	36.3%	$P = 0.008$
	253			None	23.0%	

*25% Gastroesophageal junction tumors.

MAGIC, Medical Research Council adjuvant gastric infusional chemotherapy trial; *MRC,* Medical Research Council; *RTOG,* Radiation Therapy Oncology Group.

Selective Chemoradiation Versus Chemotherapy in Adenocarcinoma

The data supporting the benefits of preoperative CRT are most convincing in SCC, whereas the data in adenocarcinoma are more tenuous. The Burmeister trial compared neoadjuvant 5FU/cisplatin/RT with surgery alone in 128 patients (~60% with adenocarcinoma) and did not demonstrate any improvements in progression-free or overall survival. This difference in the CROSS versus Burmeister trials raises the question whether adenocarcinoma is better treated with preoperative chemotherapy instead of CRT. Proponents of this selective preoperative approach based on histologic type also extrapolate the results from the Cunningham trial, which included primarily gastric cancer trials but also 25% of participants had esophageal and gastroesophageal junction (GEJ) adenocarcinomas. Proponents of the addition of radiation to the management of adenocarcinoma, however, point to the higher likelihood of achieving R0 resections with the addition of radiation, with several studies showing a correlation between R0 resection and survival. There is no strong evidence to compare these approaches.

The German POET trial randomized 126 patients with GEJ adenocarcinoma to induction chemotherapy (cisplatin/5FU/leucovorin) followed by preoperative cisplatin/etoposide/RT compared with preoperative CRT alone. The pCR rate was significantly higher in those who received induction chemotherapy (16% vs 2%) with a trend toward improved 3-year survival (47% vs 28%, P = 0.7), although it was underpowered to detect a survival advantage. Because of concerns over local recurrence and the absence of strong data to justify omitting preoperative RT, most clinicians favor CRT over chemotherapy alone.

Definitive Chemoradiation

SCCs tend to respond more favorably to CRT than adenocarcinomas. One obvious implication of this finding is whether surgery should be used only as salvage therapy in SCCs after definitive chemoradiotherapy.

Although the use of CRT followed by esophagectomy for locoregional advanced esophageal cancers has become accepted by most surgeons as the standard of care, this acceptance is not necessarily true of all physicians. Some clinicians feel that definitive CRT is the most appropriate treatment for all esophageal cancers and that surgery should be relegated to salvage recurrent disease. Although omitting surgery prevents the associated morbidity and mortality, there is likely to be reduced locoregional control with this approach.

The most important study that evaluated the marginal benefit of surgery after CRT (Stahl, et al) did not show a survival advantage with the addition of surgery. In this study, patients were randomized to either chemoradiation followed by surgery or to CRT alone.

Although this study raises important questions about the added benefit of surgery in this patient population, it is also important to note that all these patients had SCCs, the mortality rate of the operative arms was high (11.3%), and the local recurrence rate was higher in the nonsurgical arm. Given the fact that adenocarcinoma is far more common in the western world, it is not possible to extrapolate results from this study to all cases of locally advanced esophageal cancer.

Selective Definitive Chemoradiation

Selective definitive chemoradiation implies definitive treatment with CRT followed by a formal evaluation of clinical response during or at the completion of the therapy. Only those whose tumors have not responded to CRT are offered surgical resection. The Bedenne trial adopted this approach for 259 patients with SCCs who received CRT comprising 5FU/cisplatin/RT, and the researchers concluded that there was no benefit for the addition of surgery after CRT.

Subgroup analysis of trials shows that SCCs are most likely to respond to CRT, but the conflicting issue of salvage esophagectomy in patients whose cancer recurs after definitive CRT suggests that there may be increased risks of complications and death. There are considerably less data available for adenocarcinomas to rationalize the option of nonsurgical management. For patients who receive endoscopic complete response after CRT, there is the option of deferring surgical management after discussion of avoiding the risks of surgical complications versus potentially inferior locoregional disease control.

Timing of Surgery After Preoperative Chemoradiotherapy

A persistent concern about the use of preoperative CRT has been the potential of increased postoperative complications. Most of the data regarding the added risks of preoperative chemoradiation compared with surgery alone, as seen in the CROSS trial, do not support any added risks. The caveat in these data is that the average patient receiving preoperative therapy tends to be younger and healthier than the average esophageal cancer population. However, data support increased postoperative morbidity in older patients (>70 years) who received preoperative therapy.

Most clinicians aim to have a 5- to 7-week interval between the completion of preoperative CRT and surgical resection; however, the optimal interval has not been identified. This interval allows further tumor regression and the resolution of most acute inflammatory changes induced by RT while preventing fibrotic changes that render surgery more technically difficult. On the other hand, no data suggest that extending the interval allows further tumor regression and improves survival outcomes.

PET-Directed Therapy

PET scans performed after preoperative CRT can identify patients who have progressed and therefore avoid surgery. However, there is evidence that PET also can be prognostic in that those who achieve a metabolic response from neoadjuvant therapy have better long-term prognostic rates. Some advocate the idea that those who achieve a complete metabolic response on PET can avoid surgery altogether. The Municon II trial performed PET imaging in 56 patients with esophageal/EG tumors 14 days after initiation of neoadjuvant chemotherapy. Those without metabolic responses on PET were taken off chemotherapy and had earlier tumor resection. Those who responded continued to receive a full course of chemoradiotherapy followed by surgery. Survival rates at 1 year were equivalent in both groups (~80%), but there was a trend toward improved survival at 2 years in the responder group (71% vs 42%, p = 0.10). Early response to PET also is being used in patients participating in the CALGB 80803 trial with esophageal adenocarcinoma. This aims to determine the rate of pathological complete response in metabolic nonresponders who receive induction chemotherapy (FOLFOX-6 or carboplatin/paclitaxel) with radiotherapy. Patients may cross over to the alternative chemotherapy regimen if they do not respond by PET and will proceed to surgical resection. However, further prospective data are required to validate this approach.

Targeted Therapies in the Neoadjuvant Setting

Improvements in our knowledge of the molecular biology of esophageal cancer have identified differences between esophageal SCCs and adenocarcinomas, such as NOTCH1 mutations being specific to SCCs. Most trials involving targeted therapies focus on metastatic esophageal cancer. Attempts to improve clinical benefits in the neoadjuvant setting by adding cetuximab, a monoclonal antibody targeting EGFR, did not improve clinical response or overall survival in the RTOG 0436 study. There are ongoing studies looking at the role of anti-HER2 therapy in the neoadjuvant management of esophageal cancer (particularly GEJ tumors). The RTOG 1010 study aims primarily to determine if trastuzumab (anti-HER2 antibody) improves disease-free survival in combination with trimodality therapy (carboplatin/paclitaxel/RT/surgery) in patients with HER2-overexpressing esophageal adenocarcinoma. The NCT01212822 trial is a phase II trial currently examining the role of bevacizumab, a monoclonal antibody against VEGF, in combination with FOLFOX chemotherapy in patients with resectable esophageal cancer followed by surgical resection with additional adjuvant FOLFOX/bevacizumab.

■ INDICATIONS FOR ADJUVANT THERAPY

Very little data exist regarding the optimal management for patients initially managed surgically who subsequently are found to have a more advanced stage of disease for which multimodality therapy is appropriate. Options include observation, adjuvant chemotherapy, or adjuvant CRT. Another area without clear guidelines is the management of patients with involved radial margins, especially in patients who did not receive preoperative radiation. Although radiation is frequently added in this situation, no evidence is found to support any particular treatment approach.

Summary of Evidence for Adjuvant Therapy

There are no randomized trials to guide the management of patients in the postoperative setting. Retrospective data suggest that CRT can reduce the rates of local recurrence and improve overall survival for patients with T4 or node positive tumors who did not receive preoperative therapy. The benefit for adjuvant chemotherapy alone is less clear. The ECOG 8296 study was a phase II trial in which cisplatin/paclitaxel was given to patients with T2N+, T3-T4, N0/1 tumors. It showed a survival rate of 60% at 2 years (statistically improved to historical control). In general, postoperative therapy is considered more difficult to tolerate than preoperative therapy.

■ SUMMARY

Multimodality therapy has become the standard of care for the management of locoregional advanced esophageal cancer, with concurrent chemoradiation as the most universally accepted preoperative therapy approach. In the future, further attempts will be made to define which subset of patients are treated most appropriately with definitive chemoradiation, reserving surgery for palliation of either persistent or recurrent disease. In addition, the role of molecularly targeted therapies and immunotherapeutics, most notably antibodies inhibiting the PD-1/PD-L1 axis, must be investigated in the neoadjuvant/adjuvant setting to improve clinical outcomes.

SUGGESTED READINGS

Bedenne L, Michel P, Bouché O, et al. Chemoradiation followed by surgery compared with chemoradiation alone in squamous cancer of the esophagus: FFCD 9102. *J Clin Oncol.* 2007;25:1160.

Burmeister BH, Smithers BM, Gebski V, et al. Surgery alone versus chemoradiotherapy followed by surgery for resectable cancer of the oesophagus: a randomised controlled phase III trial. *Lancet Oncol.* 2005;6:659.

Cunningham D, Allum WH, Stenning SP, et al. Perioperative chemotherapy versus surgery alone for resectable gastroesophageal cancer. *N Engl J Med.* 2006;355:11.

Shapiro J, van Lanschot JB, Hulshof MCCM, et al. Neoadjuvant chemoradiotherapy plus surgery versus surgery alone for esophageal or junctional cancer (CROSS): long-term results of a randomized controlled trial. *Lancet Oncol.* 2015;16:1090-1098.

Stahl M, Walz MK, Stuschke M, et al. Phase III comparison of preoperative chemotherapy compared with chemoradiotherapy in patients with locally advanced adenocarcinoma of the esophagogastric junction. *J Clin Oncol.* 2009;27:851.

van Hagen P, Hulshof MC, van Lanschot JJ, et al. Preoperative chemoradiotherapy for esophageal or junctional cancer. *N Engl J Med.* 2012;366: 2074-2084.

THE USE OF ESOPHAGEAL STENTS

Todd C. Crawford, MD, Jinny Ha, MD,
and Daniela Molena, MD

■ BACKGROUND

Stenting for malignant esophageal strictures first was described in the surgical literature as early as the late nineteenth century, when Sir Charles James Symonds, a Canadian surgeon operating in London, placed a rigid tube across a malignant stricture in the esophagus. Maintenance of esophageal luminal patency remains the primary goal of stenting malignant esophageal strictures today. By providing alleviation of dysphagia, preservation of oral intake, and improvement of regurgitation and aspiration, stents have been shown to improve quality of life in patients with esophageal cancer. Over the last decade, improvements in stent design and durability have facilitated the expanding role of stent therapy from merely a palliative tool to a therapeutic remedy for a variety of esophageal conditions.

This chapter reviews modifications in stent design, indications for esophageal stenting, techniques for stent placement, challenges associated with stent deployment, positioning, and longevity, and finally, addresses future directions for this invaluable intervention.

■ STENT EVOLUTION

The first models of esophageal stents were rigid plastic conduits. Because these prostheses required significant esophageal dilatation before placement and malignant lesions were friable and often bulky, initial experiences with stenting resulted in a high incidence of perforation, aspiration, and stent migration. In a seminal paper published in 1993, Knyrim and colleagues were the first to demonstrate the safety and efficacy of self-expanding metal stents (SEMS). SEMS not only have revolutionized the palliation of malignant dysphagia but also have emerged as a nonoperative solution to many other benign or iatrogenic esophageal lesions, including tracheoesophageal fistulas, perforations, anastomotic leaks, and benign strictures.

In the 1990s SEMS quickly replaced rigid plastic prostheses because of the ease of deployment and reduction in periprocedural complications. Although the initial cost of SEMS far outweighed that of plastic conduits, the need for re-intervention and the frequency of complications seen with plastic stents rendered SEMS a more cost-effective option. Nitinol (an alloy of titanium and nickel) has been the primary component of most SEMS. Its elasticity allows for conformation to different anatomic angulations and degrees of stenosis and offers sufficient radial traction during stent expansion.

Initially, all SEMS were uncovered, indicating that the mesh interstices were exposed, thus permitting tissue or tumor ingrowth (Figure 1). This design facilitated satisfactory incorporation into the esophageal wall and therefore maximized fixation. However, its inherent vulnerability to epithelialization and tumor ingrowth led to a high rate of restenosis, recurrent dysphagia, and difficult stent removal. In response, partially covered stents were developed, using polyurethane, silicone, and other polymers to coat the mesh (Figure 2). Exposed wire struts remained at the proximal and distal aspects of these stents to facilitate incorporation into the esophageal wall. In a multi-center trial comparing partially covered to uncovered SEMS, the incidence of recurrent dysphagia trended higher in the uncovered stent group and the need for re-intervention was reduced significantly from 27% in those receiving uncovered stents to 0 in the group randomized to partially covered SEMS. More recently, fully covered stents have been developed to facilitate removal (see Figure

2), and some of them have an antireflux valve to reduce esophageal reflux when the stent crosses the esophagogastric junction.

Self-expandable plastic stents (SEPS) are composed of a polyester netting that is embedded within a silicone membrane, generating an outer polyester mesh with an inner silicone lining that spans the entire length of the stent (see Figure 2). At the proximal and distal ends, silicone coating is present to prevent impaction. By comparison to SEMS, SEPS exert more radial force on the esophageal wall. Since their introduction in 2011, SEPS have gained popularity as a result of their ease of removal at completion of therapy. This attribute is the result of a reduction in tissue reactivity seen after deployment. However, because of bulky stent delivery systems, deployment may be difficult in cases of severe stenosis. Increased radial force in combination with reduced incorporation into the esophageal wall predisposes these stents to migration. Proximal external flares have been fashioned to minimize the risk of migration. Although their efficacy remains uncertain, SEPS offer an attractive strategy in the management of benign lesions and are the only stents that have received FDA approval for such conditions. Multiple randomized trials comparing SEPS with partially covered SEMS in the management of malignant dysphagia have not demonstrated a significant difference in dysphagia relief or overall survival. However, complication rates were significantly higher in those receiving SEPS. Early data from van Boeckel and colleagues comparing fully covered SEMS to partially covered SEMS and SEPS in the management of benign esophageal lesions suggest that fully covered SEMS also may be safely used in the conservative treatment of benign esophageal ruptures and anastomotic leaks. Stent removal 5 to 6 weeks after the time of placement has been advocated for benign pathologies, although this has not been validated in prospective studies. Commonly used esophageal stents that are commercially available in the United States are listed in Table 1.

■ CLINICAL EVALUATION

A thorough understanding of patient symptomatology and medical history is imperative to determine a patient's candidacy for esophageal stenting. A standardized dysphagia scoring system developed by Ogilvie and colleagues is pictured in Table 2 and helps to better understand severity of disease at time of presentation and to evaluate response to treatment. Quality of life surveys also help to objectify results of stenting and often are used in comparative studies.

Radiographic evaluation of the esophagus provides an anatomic framework that will educate the endoscopist on the type and length of stent that will be most effective. This includes esophagram, endoscopy, and PET-CT in the case of malignancy. Barium esophagram may delineate the severity and length of stenosis. In cases of a known or suspected perforation, leak, or fistula, a water-soluble contrast study may inform the surgeon of the location, size, and severity of the esophageal defect. Endoscopy allows the provider to directly visualize the lesion or, alternatively, to determine whether the patient's symptoms are attributable to extrinsic compression. Intrinsic esophageal lesions can be sampled for histologic evaluation. PET-CT enables a better understanding of the anatomic relationship of the tumor to mediastinal structures, in particular the airway and the aorta, and also may demonstrate extension of disease in case of cancer. Bronchoscopy is necessary when aerodigestive fistulas are suspected, when the tumor is compressing the airway or extrinsic compression of the esophagus is caused by a tumor of pulmonary origin.

■ INDICATIONS

Current FDA indications for esophageal stenting include maintenance of esophageal luminal patency for intrinsic or extrinsic malignant tumors and occlusion of esophageal fistulas that may arise concurrently. In addition, SEPS have been approved for the treatment of benign esophageal lesions. Commercially available stents are now

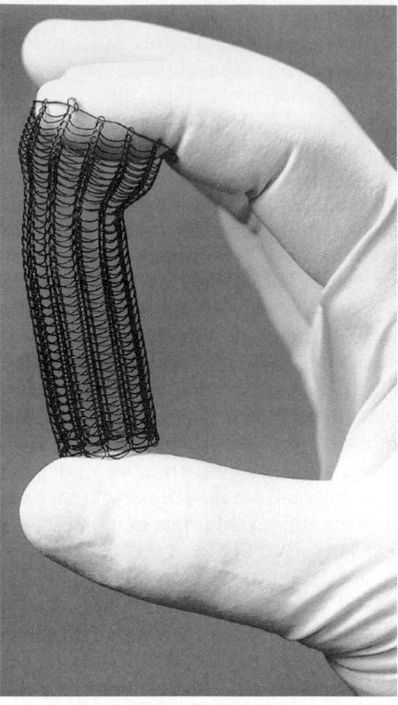

FIGURE 1 Self-expanding metallic stent (SEMS).

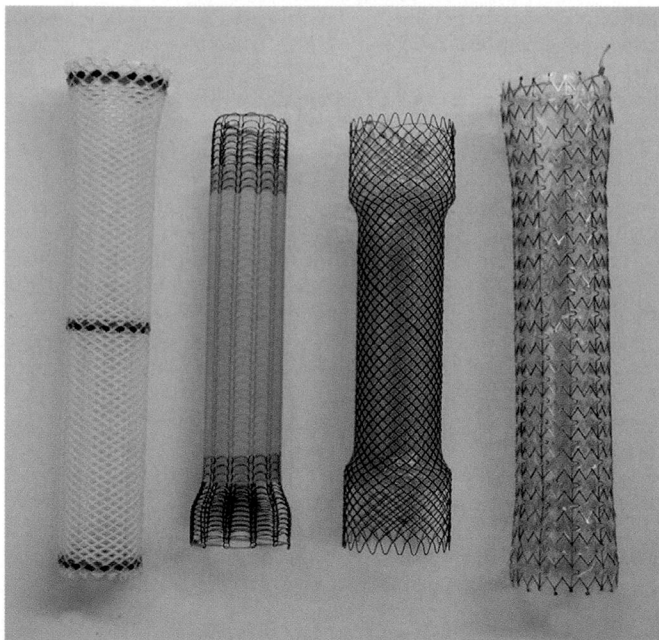

FIGURE 2 *From left to right:* Self-expandable plastic stent (SEPS), partially covered SEMS, double-layer fully covered SEMS, fully covered SEMS.

being used for off-label esophageal pathologies, including benign strictures, esophageal perforations, and anastomotic leaks related to surgery of the alimentary tract. More recently, esophageal stenting has demonstrated utility in the management of achalasia and even esophageal variceal bleeding. Although many stent devices have been subjected to observational studies only in a nonrandomized, uncontrolled setting, the scope of esophageal stenting continues to expand. The following paragraphs describe the current evidence for a variety of indications for esophageal stenting.

Malignant Esophageal Strictures

Despite improvements in detection, operative techniques, and neo-adjuvant multimodality therapy, the overall prognosis for esophageal cancer remains dismal, with a 5-year survival rate approaching 20%. As a result of their insidious growth, a large number of these tumors become clinically apparent late in their course and resultantly are unresectable. Progression of esophageal tumors of mucosal origin culminates in intraluminal obstruction and resultant dysphagia. Esophageal stenting represents a novel form of palliation in that its impact on dysphagia relief is immediate and does not subject the patient to the morbidity of an open operation.

Soon after Knyrim's landmark paper demonstrated a significant drop in complications and a decline in postprocedural mortality from 29% with rigid plastic conduits to 14% with SEMS, multiple additional studies have confirmed a reduction in complications with SEMS placement. Significant improvements in dysphagia score and quality of life after stenting also have been noted. However, a significant mortality benefit has not been observed with this intervention, which is likely a reflection of the aggressive and lethal nature of esophageal malignancies. Technical success rates of greater than 90% have been documented in most studies, suggesting that esophageal stenting is feasible even for locally advanced tumors. Recent work by Bassi and colleagues demonstrated effective palliation with fully covered SEMS, even for tumors within 4 cm of the upper esophageal sphincter (UES). Historically, a distance of 2 cm between UES and the upper aspect of the stent has been advocated. Unique risks related to proximal esophageal stenting include airway compromise and globus sensation.

Malignant Esophageal Fistulas

Aerodigestive fistulas result from esophageal tumor infiltration into the airway or conversely, from invasive malignancies originating in the respiratory tract and mediastinum and invading posteriorly. Multiple prospective studies have demonstrated efficacy of esophageal stents in sealing malignant fistulae with success rates approaching 70% to 100%. Tracheobronchial stenting may supplement esophageal stents in achieving closure of aerodigestive fistulae, and dual stenting recently was shown by Schweigert et al to improve oral intake and candidacy for adjuvant therapy (Figure 3). The juxtaposition of an airway stent and an esophageal stent should, however, be used with caution. The pressure of both stents on each other can lead to necrosis of the common tracheoesophageal wall with increase in size of the fistula often with disastrous consequences. Although covered stents have gained favor in the management of malignant fistulae, a superior design has not yet been elucidated. In a large study by Shin et al investigating the role of SEMS in the palliation of malignant aerodigestive fistulae in 61 patients, early clinical improvement, associated with fistula closure significantly improved mean survival from 6.2 to 15.1 weeks. Approximately one third of patients enrolled in this series experienced fistula recurrence; however, many were amenable to repeat endoscopic intervention.

Gastroesophageal Junction Tumors

Historically, tumors at the gastroesophageal (GE) junction with resultant dysphagia have been difficult to manage. Stenting across the GE junction remains controversial. Opponents express concern that stenting predisposes to gastroesophageal reflux. Although this may be true, the clinical repercussions of unabated reflux appears to be overestimated. Esophageal stents with anti-reflux mechanisms have been used in the management of GE junction strictures with mixed results. In these stent models, a one-way valve is attached to the distal end of the stent, inhibiting reflux of gastric contents into the esophageal lumen. Because of the size mismatch in luminal diameters of the esophagus and stomach, stents placed across GE junction tumors are prone to migration. Although early migration is uncommon with a

TABLE 1: Commercially Available Esophageal Stents in the United States

Stent Manufacturer and Stent Product Name	Material	Covered Design	Additional Features
BOSTON SCIENTIFIC			
Polyflex	Polyester netting lined with silicone	Covered (double layer)	
Ultraflex	Nitinol	Uncovered or covered	
WallFlex	Stainless steel	Partially or fully covered	
COOK MEDICAL			
Esophageal Z-Stent	Stainless steel (polyurethane coating)	Fully covered	Available Dua Anti-Reflux Valve
Evolution	Nitinol (internal and external silicone coating)	Partially or fully covered	Controlled-release system
ENDOCHOICE			
Bonastent	Nitinol (silicone coating)	Fully covered	Hook & Cross technology
MEDTRONIC			
Esophacoil	Nitinol	Uncovered	
MERIT MEDICAL ENDOTEK			
Alimaxx-ES	Nitinol (covered with polyurethane)	Fully covered	
TAEWOONG MEDICAL			
Niti-S Double Stent	Inner layer: covered with polyurethane; outer layer: uncovered nitinol wire	Fully covered (double layer)	
Niti-S	Nitinol (covered with polyurethane)	Fully covered	Available Polytetrafluoroethylene antireflux skirt

Adapted from Hindy P, Hong J, Lam-Tsai Y, Gress F. A comprehensive review of esophageal stents. *Gastroenterol Hepatol.* 2012;8:526-534.

TABLE 2: Dysphagia Scoring Scale

0	Able to consume normal diet
1	Dysphagia with certain solid foods
2	Able to swallow semi-solid soft foods
3	Able to swallow liquids only
4	Unable to swallow saliva (complete dysphagia)

Data from Ogilvie AL, Dronfield MW, Ferguson R, Atkinson M. Palliative intubation of oesophagogastric neoplasms at fibreoptic endoscopy. *Gut.* 1982;23(12):1060-1067.

tight stricture, late migration may denote an advantageous response to adjuvant therapy.

Bridge-to-Surgery

Patients with potentially resectable gastroesophageal malignancies may benefit from preoperative stent placement. Malnutrition represents an important barrier to successful completion of neoadjuvant therapy and predisposes to poor outcomes after surgical intervention. Enteral nutrition is favorable in comparison with alternative sources of caloric intake. Esophageal stents play an integral role in maintaining esophageal patency in the bridge-to-surgery model, especially in those requiring neoadjuvant therapy. In a recent

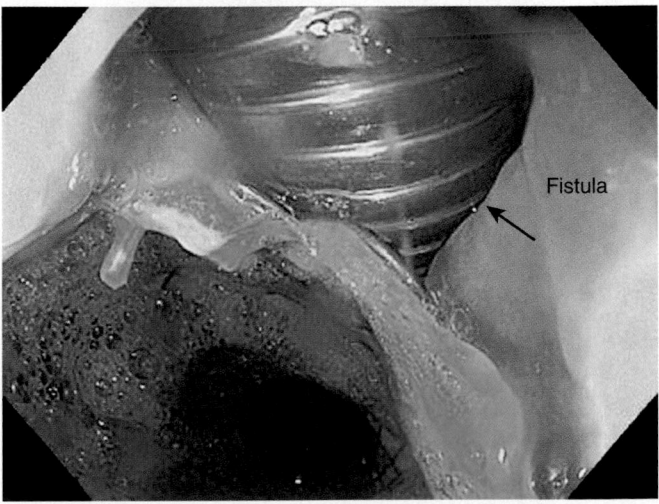

FIGURE 3 Endoscopic view of aerodigestive fistula managed with dual airway *(top of screen)* and esophageal *(bottom of screen)* stents.

publication by Martin and colleagues, SEPS placed in 52 patients before neoadjuvant chemotherapy and/or radiation were shown to improve enteral nutritional intake and quality of life. Historically, concerns related to preoperative stenting reflect the potential for stents, especially SEMS, to obscure tissue planes as a result of the

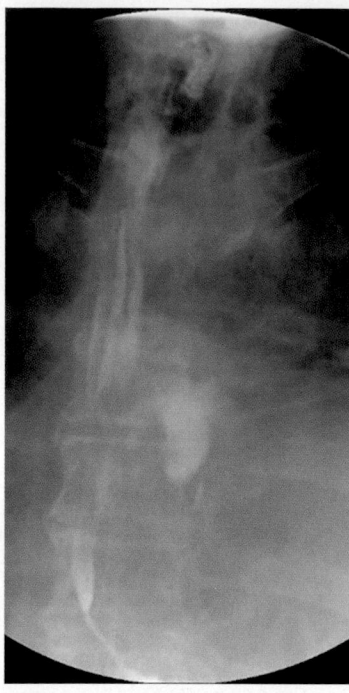

FIGURE 4 Upper GI series with water-soluble oral contrast demonstrating extraluminal extravasation of contrast from the left side of the esophagus approximately 2 cm below the level of the carina, consistent with esophageal perforation.

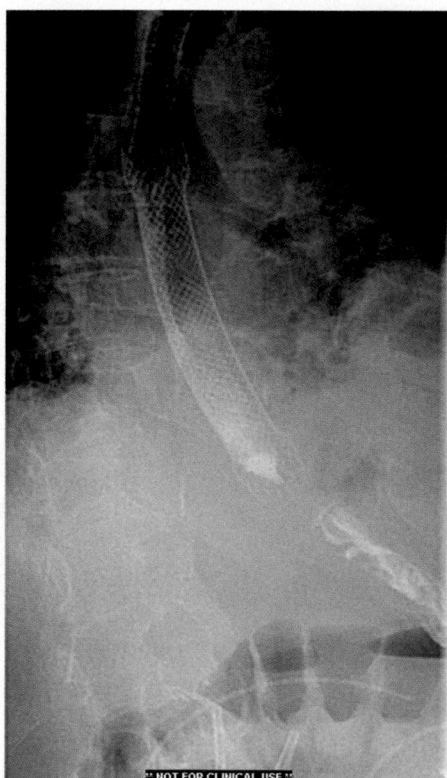

FIGURE 5 Repeat upper GI series with water-soluble oral contrast in the same patient as Figure 4 demonstrates a distal esophageal stent in good position. There is no evidence of contrast extravasation to suggest a persistent leak.

tissue injury they produce, cause microperforations leading to tumor dissemination, and exacerbate complications related to chemoradiotherapy. Despite reassuring findings from initial prospective studies, a recent large retrospective study by Mariette and colleagues, which included 38 patients that received SEMS before neoadjuvant therapy, documented significantly worse R0 resection rates (71.0% vs 85.5%, p = 0.041), median time to recurrence (6.5 vs 9.0 months, p = 0.040), and 3-year overall survival (25% vs 44%, p = 0.023). SEPS, however, have not been shown to increase postsurgical complications or anastomotic leak rates.

Benign Strictures

Benign esophageal strictures may result from caustic injury to esophageal mucosa, peptic ulcer disease, radiation, and the healing of an anastomotic leak. Although esophageal dilation has been the mainstay of therapy for over a century, patients with persistent or recurrent strictures often require more aggressive therapy. Conceptually, providing continuous esophageal dilation for a period of 6 weeks or greater should improve esophageal luminal patency. This can be accomplished with an endoprosthesis. Concerns related to stenting for benign lesions stem from the associated risks of hemorrhage, perforation, fistula formation, and traumatic stent removal. In addition, mechanical irritation from imbedded stents precipitates fibrosis and may lead to new stricture formation. Longer indwelling time appears to correlate with an increased risk of complication.

Stent selection for benign strictures requires a delicate balance between the risk of migration and the feasibility of removal. Although fully covered metal stents succumb to a greater rate of migration, they are easier and safer to remove.

SEPS also have been investigated in the management of benign strictures. Traditionally, SEPS have been designed with the intention of impeding epithelial ingrowth or overgrowth. Given their lack of incorporation into the esophageal wall, these stents rely heavily on radial force for stabilization within the esophageal lumen, resulting in a migration rate above 20% and in a prospective study by Dua et al, and a high incidence of complications, including bleeding, perforation, pain, fistula formation, and recurrence of dysphagia. Despite the risk of migration and the aforementioned complications, SEPS have been granted FDA approval in the treatment of benign esophageal strictures. Both SEMS and SEPS should be used with caution for selected patients with benign stricture.

Esophageal Perforations, Anastomotic Leaks, and Benign Fistulae

Esophageal perforations may be idiopathic, iatrogenic, or traumatic in origin (Figure 4). Postoperative enteric anastomotic leaks have become increasingly prevalent as the number of esophagectomies performed annually continues to rise. Benign airway-esophageal fistulae may arise from radiation, trauma, or pressure necrosis secondary to prolonged endotracheal intubation or nasogastric tube placement. Historically, surgical intervention was required for the aforementioned problems and carried significant morbidity and mortality. Although enteric spillage into the mediastinum or pleural spaces necessitates adequate drainage (often surgical), contained esophageal perforations and anastomotic leaks in otherwise stable patients no longer require immediate operation.

Despite limited prospective evidence, multiple retrospective case analyses have demonstrated excellent outcomes with esophageal stenting (Figure 5). In these studies, resolution of enteric leakage was observed in 85% of cases. No stent design was superior with regard to closure of the perforation or leak. Multiple case series have revealed successful implementation of SEPS in the management of anastomotic leaks with a resolution rate of 70% to 80%. Traumatic esophageal perforations also may benefit from stenting. One series by Siersema and colleagues revealed a greater than 80% rate of leak occlusion with SEMS placement. In a recent meta-analysis by van

Halsema and van Hooft, stenting for benign esophageal fistulae resulted in successful closure of the fistula tract in approximately 65% of patients.

COMPARISON OF ESOPHAGEAL STENTING TO OTHER TREATMENT MODALITIES

Laser therapy for malignant dysphagia has been compared retrospectively with esophageal stenting with no difference in rates of dysphagia relief or mean survival. Similarly, a large multi-center randomized trial again demonstrated comparable rates of dysphagia improvement and median survival among patients randomized to stenting or brachytherapy, although relief of dysphagia occurred more rapidly in the group that underwent stenting. Complication rates were significantly greater in the group that received stents compared with less invasive therapies. Despite these results, the increased need for rescue stenting in patients undergoing brachytherapy and the rapid relief of dysphagia achieved with esophageal stenting have curtailed the popularity and acceptance of laser therapy or brachytherapy as first-line treatment modalities.

TECHNICAL DETAILS

Esophageal stents may be placed under general anesthesia or conscious sedation. General anesthesia often is preferred to minimize the risk of aspiration and to facilitate ease of stent repositioning, when necessary. Typically, stents are placed under endoscopic or fluoroscopic guidance.

Initial endoscopy is undertaken to assess the location and length of the esophageal lesion and to gain a better understanding of the integrity of surrounding tissue. Occasionally, severely stenotic lesions require initial gentle dilation to facilitate safe passage of the endoscope. In these circumstances, the minimum dilation necessary to afford successful stent placement should be undertaken as excessive dilation can impair stent fixation and lead to early migration.

After thorough evaluation of the esophageal lesion, the appropriate stent should be selected and should have adequate length, enough to extend at least 2 cm beyond the lesion in each direction. The esophageal stent should have a slightly larger diameter than the esophageal lumen after expansion to exert sufficient radial force on the esophageal wall. Through the endoscope, a guidewire is inserted and advanced beyond the distal margin of the esophageal lesion to ensure adequate purchase. The endoscope is then withdrawn and the stent deployment device is advanced over the guidewire. Finally, the endoscope is reinserted to directly visualize stent deployment. The stent can be moved under direct visualization before complete deployment to ensure best coverage of the lesion.

Alternatively, fluoroscopy may be used to monitor stent expansion. A similar Seldinger technique is used involving initial insertion of a guidewire and then advancement of the stent deployment device over the wire under fluoroscopic surveillance. This modality requires radiopaque markers, extracorporeally and within the esophageal stent, to ensure appropriate stent position before deployment.

Stent delivery systems typically proceed with either proximal or distal release mechanisms. During or shortly after deployment, adjustments in stent position can be made with endoscopic graspers or toothed forceps. Oversizing of the stent can lead to perforation or incomplete stent expansion with resultant compromise of the esophageal lumen. In cases of incomplete expansion of an appropriately sized stent, balloon dilatation may be undertaken carefully. After successful deployment, repeat endoscopy is used to confirm proper stent positioning (Figure 6).

COMPLICATIONS

A review of frequently encountered complications should prepare the endoscopist for potential challenges related to stenting. Most esophageal stenting series document a complication rate of 30% to 35%. Recognizing the variability in physiologic reserve and tissue integrity among patients with malignant and benign esophageal pathologies will help the endoscopist to remain vigilant and anticipate potential consequences related to this procedure. Complications historically have been divided into immediate, early, and late. Thus strategies to minimize complications should be catered around technical considerations at time of placement and close surveillance postprocedurally.

Because rigid plastic conduits largely have been supplanted by SEMS and SEPS, concerns for immediate complications such as esophageal perforation at time of placement have been replaced with new complications related to severity of stenosis, anatomic relationship to the airway, and stent design. A thorough understanding of the cause of the esophageal lesion and its relationship to mediastinal structures will help to mitigate airway compromise after stent deployment. In patients with esophageal fluid columns related to severe stenosis, lateral decubitus positioning and continuous suctioning of the oropharynx may prevent aspiration. Finally, knowledge of previous esophageal interventions may inform the endoscopist of potential challenges related to stent positioning and deployment.

Immediate stent malpositioning or migration often denotes a technical failure. Knowledge of stricture length will inform the endoscopist of the proper stent size, which should be 3 to 4 cm longer than the stricture. A thorough understanding of the delivery system and directional sequence of stent deployment can prevent early mishaps. Intrinsic or external fluoroscopic markings ensure the stent is properly located. If malposition is detected soon after deployment,

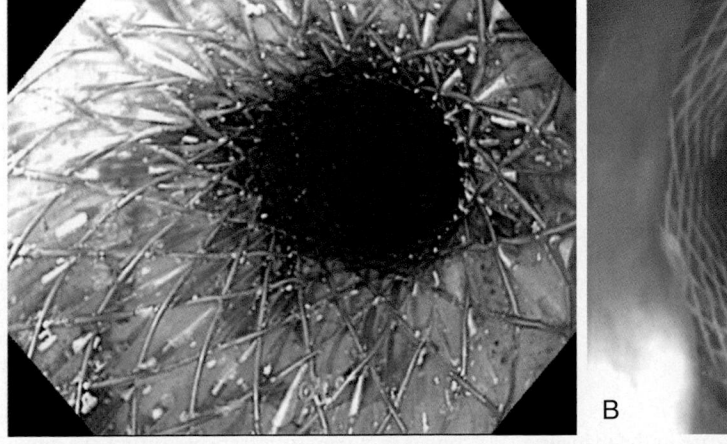
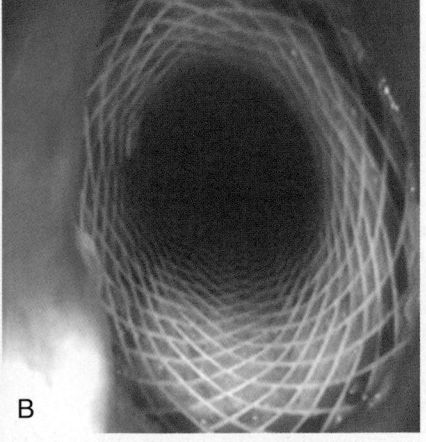

FIGURE 6 Endoscopic, intraluminal view of deployed and expanded SEMS (**A**) and SEPS (**B**).

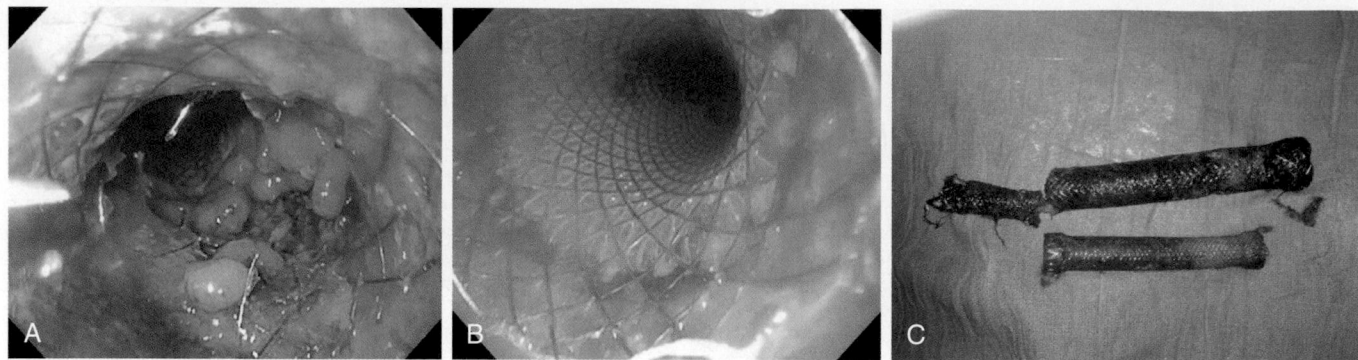

FIGURE 7 A, Endoscopic view of a fractured SEMS with associated ingrowth of esophageal mucosa. **B,** Interval placement of a SEMS within the lumen of the preexisting, fractured SEMS to facilitate removal. **C,** Successful extraction of both fractured SEMS *(top)* and intact SEMS *(bottom).*

distal stents may be amenable to proximal repositioning or placement of a more proximal overlapping stent. Stent dislodgement also may be iatrogenic and related to passing of the endoscope to assess stent position. This step is often avoidable by using fluoroscopic assessment or careful endoscopic examination. Fixation methods should be used if migration is anticipated. Finally, although rare, esophageal perforations may occur. In these cases, a covered stent may be used to seal the mucosal defect. Perforation often is related to trauma from the guidewire, and use of floppy-tipped guidewires may reduce the likelihood of this complication.

Early complications occur within 1 week of successful stent deployment. These include hemorrhage, pain, and nausea. Hemorrhage is often unavoidable and frequently reflects the friability of the esophageal lesion and the degree of luminal narrowing of the esophagus. Chest pain and nausea are underappreciated complications of stenting. These symptoms are often self-limited after stent placement but, when intractable, may indicate pathologic stent erosion into the mucosa.

Late complications occur after 1 week from successful stent placement. The myriad of late complications reflects variations in esophageal pathology and stent design. The most common late complications are stent migration and recurrent dysphagia. Migration is more common with the use of fully covered SEMS or SEPS and also may occur after stenting across the GE junction. Short strictures also predispose to distal migration. Stent removal after migration is controversial in asymptomatic patients, especially when the stent remains within the stomach; however, symptomatic patients merit intervention.

Recrudescence of dysphagia after stenting has multiple causes, including tumor ingrowth or overgrowth, epithelialization, and food impaction. Stent length is an important consideration in the case of a malignant stricture because shorter stents may be overtaken more rapidly by malignant tumors. Ingrowth is much less common in the era of covered stents; however, when partially covered stents are used, care should be taken to avoid deploying the uncovered portion of the stent in close proximity to tumor. Mechanical soft diets, sufficient chewing, and copious fluid intake may be effective in preventing food bolus impaction. Occasionally, repeat stenting is necessary to alleviate discomfort.

Finally, stent disruption can occur very rarely with tissue ingrowth between the broken mesh wires. Deployment of a covered stent within the disrupted stent will lead to tissue necrosis and sloughing of the ingrown tissue and will facilitate stent removal, preventing injury to the esophageal wall (Figure 7).

■ FUTURE DIRECTIONS

Although stenting has emerged as a standard of care in the management of malignant esophageal strictures, its acceptance as a first-line

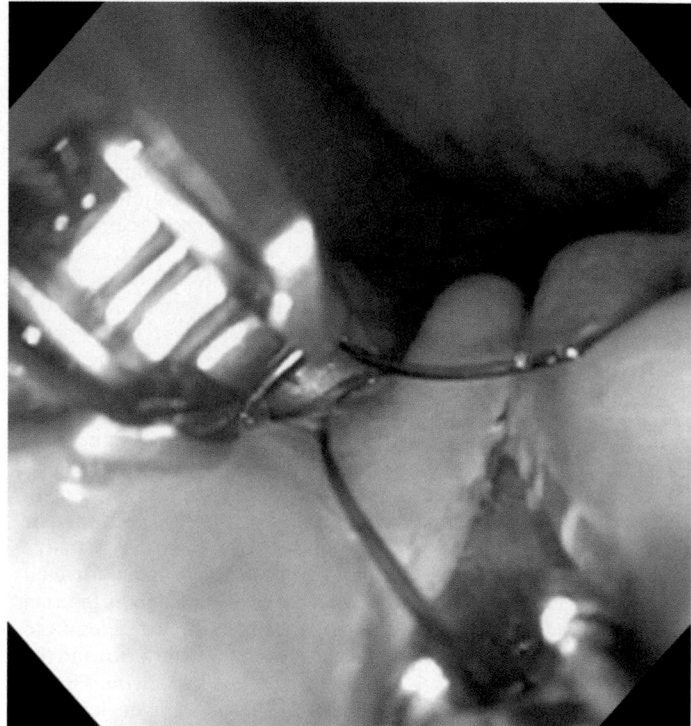

FIGURE 8 Endoscopic view of the Apollo Overstitch device, used for suture fixation of the proximal aspect of an esophageal stent to the esophageal mucosa.

therapy in benign pathologies has been hindered by challenges related to stent migration and ease of removal. Anti-migration technologies are now emerging to combat the high rates of stent migration observed with endoscopic stenting of benign lesions. Anchoring techniques are at the forefront of this frontier and include endoscopic suturing or clipping. Biodegradable stents recently have emerged as an attractive alternative to SEMS because they obviate the need for stent removal upon completion of therapy.

Recently, the Apollo Overstitch, an endoscopic suturing device, was approved for clinical use by the FDA. Now in its second generation, this product is indicated for prophylaxis against stent migration and in the correction of previously migrated stents. The unique design of the Overstitch facilitates suture reloading and deploying while maintaining visualization of the esophageal stent and enables a single provider to effectively suture the proximal aspect of the stent to the esophageal mucosa (Figure 8). Early data suggest the

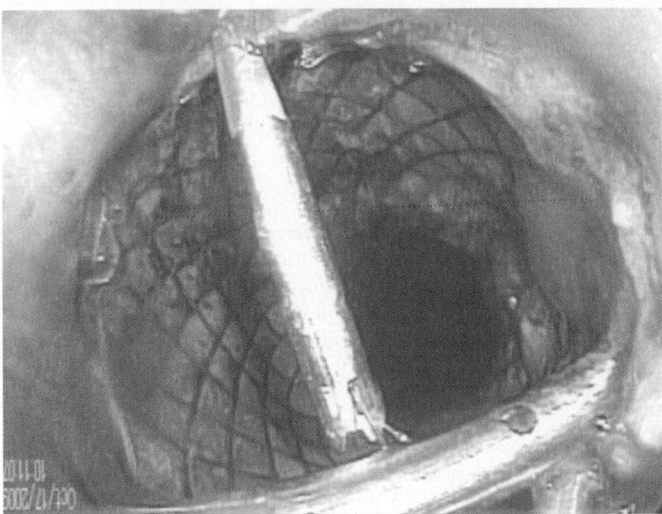

FIGURE 9 Endoscopic view of an esophageal clip, which stabilizes the proximal aspect of an esophageal stent.

Overstitch is safe, cost effective, and may decrease the need for re-intervention after stenting. Encouraging results also have been seen with endoscopic clipping, which fixes the proximal end of the stent to the esophageal mucosal layer. In addition, clipping has resulted in a significant reduction in stent migration in various trials (Figure 9).

Biodegradable stents confer several advantages in the management of benign strictures. First, the biocompatible composition induces minimal mechanical irritation and granulation tissue formation, leading to favorable remodeling of the esophageal wall. This may be helpful in preventing recurrent stricture. Biodegradation of stents alleviates the need for removal, which is often traumatic because of tissue embedding. Early studies have shown that biodegradable stent implantation is safe and technically feasible. In addition, no major complications were observed and the rate of stent migration was low. Dysphagia recurrence was similar to that observed in published studies using SEPS for the management of benign strictures. Future prospective studies are needed to better elucidate the effectiveness of biodegradable stents.

CONCLUSION

Esophageal stenting remains a first-line therapy in the palliation of unresectable, malignant esophageal strictures. As advances in stent design have made deployment safe and technically feasible for a variety of esophageal pathologies, indications for stenting continue to expand. Although the evidence for stenting malignant strictures is clear, insufficient evidence exists to uniformly advocate esophageal stenting for benign pathologies such as stricture, perforation, or anastomotic leak. Apprehensions related to stenting benign lesions stem from concerns for traumatic removal, high rates of stent migration, and dysphagia recurrence. Covered stents and plastic stents have emerged to combat challenges related to tissue ingrowth and recurrent strictures. Novel endoscopic procedural advancements, including endoscopic suturing or clipping, may help to reduce migration. The use of biodegradable stents may alleviate benign strictures without subjecting the patient to an increased risk of complications. Finally, individualized approaches to a variety of esophageal pathologies may pair esophageal stenting with adjunct therapies to optimize patient care and quality of life.

SUGGESTED READINGS

Conio M, Repici A, Battaglia G, et al. A randomized prospective comparison of self-expandable plastic stents and partially covered self-expandable metal stents in the palliation of malignant esophageal dysphagia. *Am J Gastroenterol.* 2007;102:2667-2677.

Kantsevoy SV, Bitner M. Esophageal stent fixation with endoscopic suturing device (with video). *Gastrointest Endosc.* 2012;76:1251-1255.

Knyrim K, Wagner HJ, Bethge N, et al. A controlled trial of an expansile metal stent for palliation of esophageal obstruction due to inoperable cancer. *N Engl J Med.* 1993;329:1302-1307.

Mariette C, Gronnier C, Duhamel A, et al. Self-expanding covered metallic stent as a bridge to surgery in esophageal cancer: impact on oncologic outcomes. *J Am Coll Surg.* 2015;220:287-296.

Repici A, Vleggaar FP, Hassan C, et al. Efficacy and safety of biodegradable stents for refractory benign esophageal strictures: the BEST (Biodegradable Esophageal Stent) study. *Gastrointest Endosc.* 2010;72:927-934.

Sharma P, Kozarek R. Role of esophageal stents in benign and malignant diseases. *Am J Gastroenterol.* 2010;105:258-273.

van Boeckel PG, Dua KS, Weusten BL, et al. Fully covered self-expandable metal stents (SEMS), partially covered SEMS and self-expandable plastic stents for the treatment of benign esophageal ruptures and anastomotic leaks. *BMC Gastroenterol.* 2012;12:19.

van Halsema EE, Wong Kee Song LM, Baron TH, et al. Safety of endoscopic removal of self-expandable stents after treatment of benign esophageal diseases. *Gastrointest Endosc.* 2013;77:18-28.

THE MANAGEMENT OF ESOPHAGEAL PERFORATION

Robert Maxwell, MD, FACS, and Jessica K. Reynolds, MD

Esophageal perforation is a life-threatening condition that requires a high index of suspicion and early diagnosis for optimal outcomes. Even with early diagnosis and appropriate management, mortality rates reported in the literature continue to range from 10% to 40%. Factors that influence mortality include the patient's clinical condition and comorbidities, the interval to diagnosis and treatment, and the cause and location of the perforation. Recent literature has focused on nonoperative management; however, we cannot overemphasize the importance of early aggressive surgical management when appropriate.

The most frequent cause of esophageal perforation is iatrogenic during upper endoscopy procedures and transesophageal echocardiography (60%) followed by spontaneous rupture, otherwise known as *Boerhaave's esophagus* (15% to 30%). Less frequently encountered causes include foreign body or caustic ingestion, malignancy, and trauma. Patients often present with a history of recent upper endoscopy procedures involving biopsy or dilation and may have underlying predisposing factors such as reflux esophagitis, hiatal hernia, stricture, or achalasia.

DIAGNOSIS

A detailed history and physical examination is of utmost importance in early diagnosis of esophageal perforation. Patients may have a recent history of esophageal instrumentation or retching. Often patients present with vague complaints. Some may experience pain localized to the chest, shoulder, or epigastrium, dyspnea, nausea, dysphagia, or fever. On physical examination, patients may remain hemodynamically stable or present with signs of septic shock or mediastinitis such as tachycardia or hypotension. Laboratory values generally reveal a leukocytosis. Although nonspecific for esophageal perforation, chest x-ray may reveal presence of pneumomediastinum, pleural effusion, pneumothorax, subcutaneous emphysema, or an abnormal cardiomediastinal contour. Further diagnostic imaging is necessary for better evaluation of the extent of injury, degree of contamination, and location.

Esophagography

Esophagography is a noninvasive diagnostic tool used to determine the level of perforation. Esophageal perforation may be represented by esophageal irregularity or extravasation of contrast. Gastrografin is preferred over barium because of the risk of mediastinitis; however, barium has been shown to have better resolution for contained injuries. It is our practice to first obtain a Gastrografin swallow followed by dilute barium if necessary for improved sensitivity and specificity. Real-time images under fluoroscopy also help better identify the location of the perforation. If Gastrografin demonstrates free perforation into the pleural space or abdominal cavity, the procedure is terminated. Barium can be given after Gastrografin for perforations contained within the mediastinum for better characterization. Barium leaking into the pleura or peritoneum causes extensive soiling and is difficult to remove. Figure 1 shows evidence of esophageal perforation on Gastrografin esophagography.

Computed Tomography

Computed tomography (CT) scans are readily available in the acute setting and are helpful in determination of the presence of contained or noncontained perforation. CT of the chest and upper abdomen with oral contrast allows for evaluation of the location of injury as

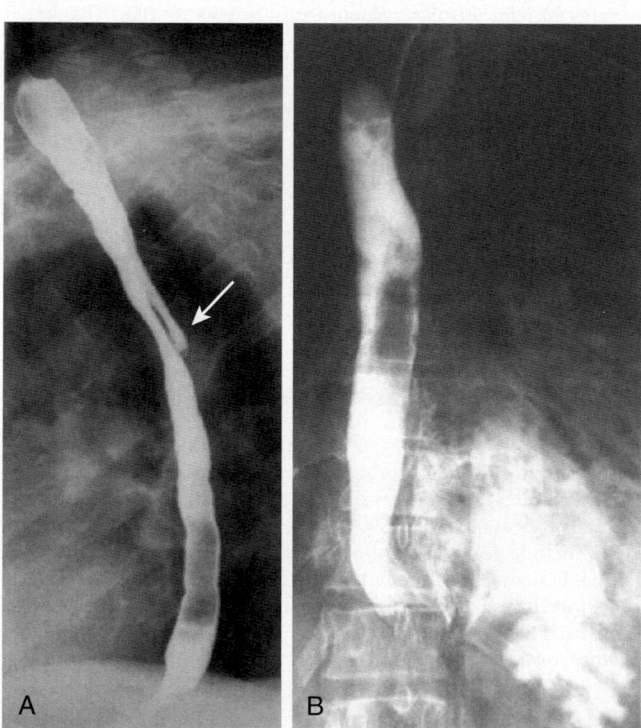

FIGURE 1 Esophageal perforation on Gastrografin esophagography. **A,** Perforation after endoscopic dilation of caustic stricture. Contained extravasation of contrast material *(arrow)*. **B,** Boerhaave syndrome. Massive left pleural extravasation of contrast material. *(Chirica M, Champault A, Dray X, et al. Esophageal perforations. J Visc Surg. 2010;147:e117-e128.)*

well as the severity of mediastinal or pleural space contamination. Imaging may reveal evidence of mediastinal fat stranding, pneumomediastinum, pleural effusion, empyema, pneumoperitoneum, or contrast extravasation. Figure 2 shows evidence of esophageal perforation on CT of the thorax.

Endoscopy

Flexible endoscopy should be considered in patients with high suspicion for perforation and nondiagnostic radiographic imaging. For diagnosis of esophageal perforation, endoscopy allows for careful inspection of mucosal integrity and viability. Direct visualization of the esophagus and stomach also allows the endoscopist to rule out underlying disease or malignancy. Because of the potential of insufflation of the thoracic cavity through a free perforation, the endoscopist must maintain a high index of suspicion for development of a tension pneumothorax. Endoscopic management of esophageal perforation requires a multidisciplinary approach with an experienced endoscopist. Figure 3 shows evidence of esophageal perforation on upper endoscopy managed with stent placement.

■ INITIAL MANAGEMENT

To determine which patients are candidates for nonoperative management, physiologic stability first must be assessed. The esophageal perforation also must be classified as free or contained. Nonoperative treatment of contained perforations has been demonstrated efficacious in selected patient populations. Patients who have contained leaks, heart rate below 100, normotension, white blood cell count (WBC) below 12,000 to 14,000 mm³ and no evidence of ongoing sepsis may be considered for nonoperative management. Individuals meeting these criteria are admitted to the ICU for 48 to 72 hours of observation. Patients should be maintained on NPO status with head of bed elevated, started on 72 hours of broad-spectrum antibiotics and a proton pump inhibitor (PPI), and dependent on premorbid nutritional status, considered for parenteral nutritional support. For distal perforations with potential for gastric reflux, antifungal coverage should be considered. Repeat imaging is obtained in 72 to 96 hours. If repeat imaging demonstrates no evidence of free perforation, a liquid diet with nutritional supplement may be started.

It is important to remember that these patients require close observation to ensure that they continue to meet nonoperative criteria. Should the patient's clinical condition deteriorate with fever, leukocytosis, tachypnea, tachycardia, or mental status changes, operative management is indicated. Patients who present with evidence of uncontained intrathoracic or intra-abdominal leak may progress quickly to septic shock secondary to mediastinitis, pleuritis, or peritonitis. These patients require emergent intervention for source control, aggressive IV fluid resuscitation for hemodynamic support, and close monitoring of urine output.

■ OPERATIVE MANAGEMENT

Decisions made in operative management of esophageal perforation are multifactorial and depend on the location and size of the injury, degree of contamination, and hemodynamic stability of the patient. For patients who require operative intervention, we recommend aggressive surgical management with primary repair, even in patients presenting more than 24 hours from the time of perforation. When feasible, two-layer closure is recommended, with the addition of a buttress procedure. In cases of delayed perforation, single-layer closure may be more practical. In rare circumstances, primary muscle flap closure may be considered.

Any underlying pathology may affect the ability to repair a perforation. If possible, inquire if the patient has a history of dysphagia or other functional disorder. In circumstances such as malignancy and stricture, necrosis or distal obstruction may prevent primary repair or re-establishment of continuity. Regardless of the

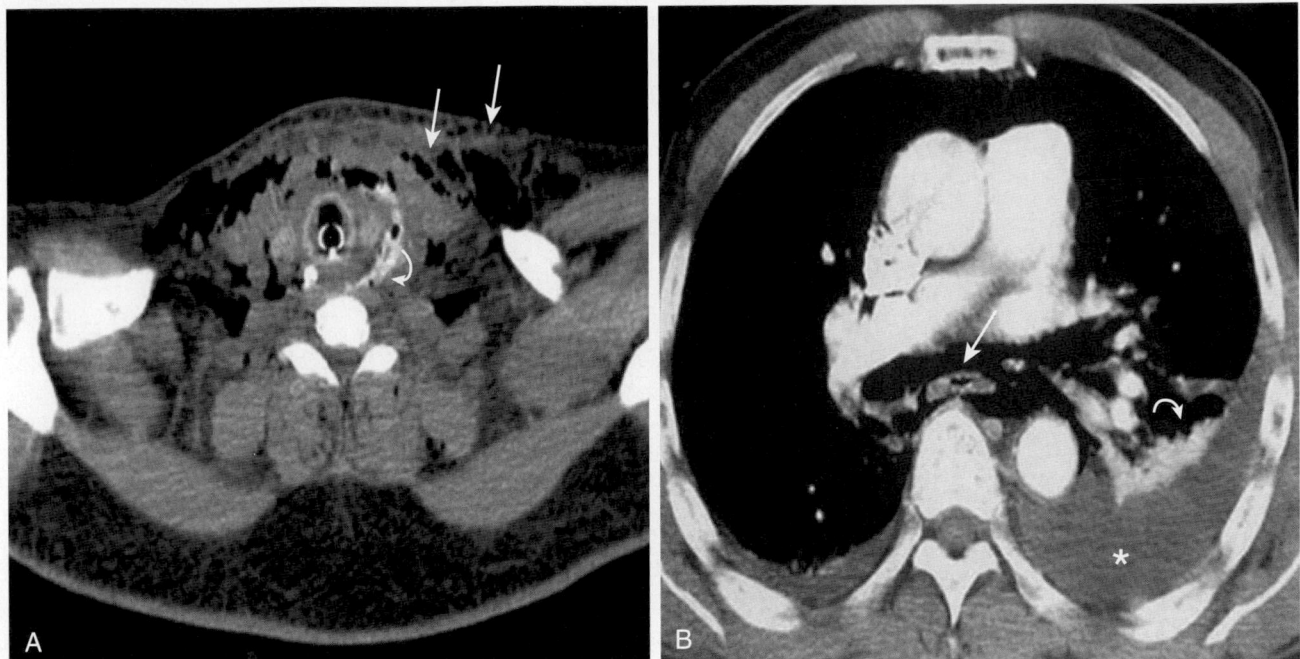

FIGURE 2 Esophageal perforation on CT of the thorax. **A,** Spontaneous perforation of cervical esophagus: ingested contrast-enhanced CT scan. Extravasation of contrast material *(curved arrow)* and subcutaneous emphysema *(full arrows)*. **B,** Boerhaave syndrome: atelectasis *(curved arrow)*, pneumomediastinum *(full arrow)*, pleural effusion *(asterisk)*. *(Chirica M, Champault A, Dray X, et al. Esophageal perforations. J Visc Surg. 2010;147:e117-e128.)*

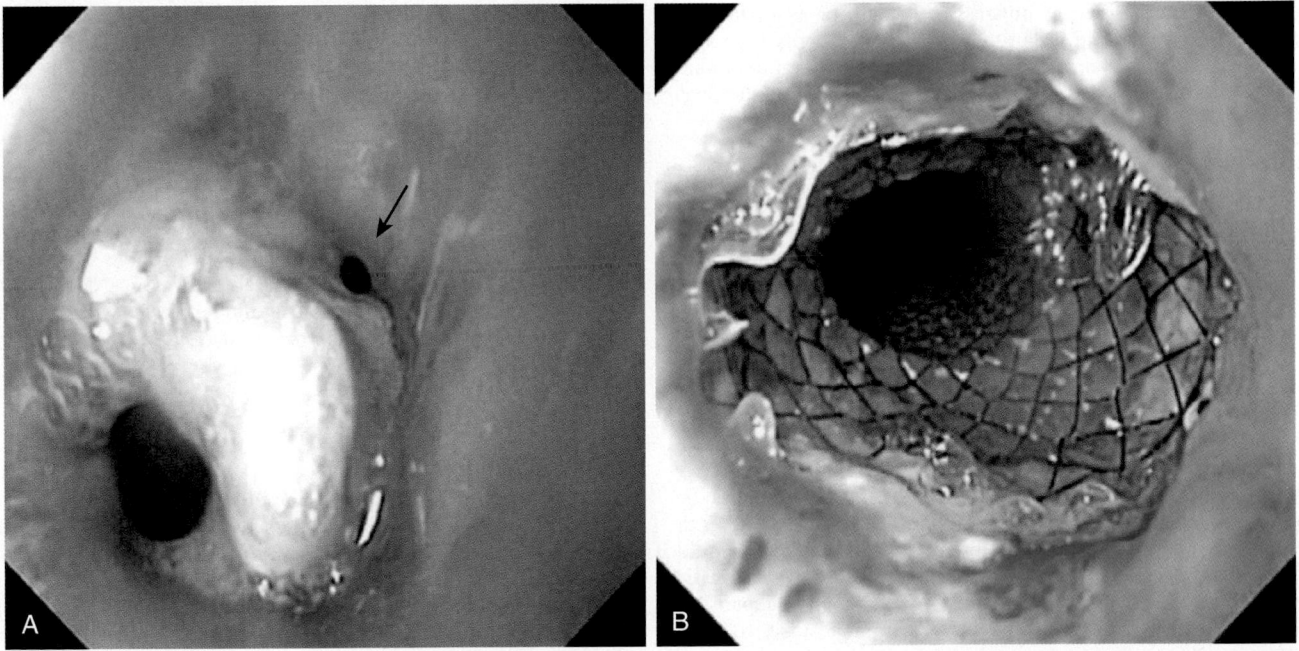

FIGURE 3 Endoscopic treatment of esophageal perforation. **A,** Endoscopic view: perforation middle third of esophagus *(arrow)*. **B,** Endoscopic view: stent in place. *(Chirica M, Champault A, Dray X, et al. Esophageal perforations. J Visc Surg. 2010;147:e117-e128.)*

circumstances, exposure, repair, drainage procedures, or diversion require meticulous technique for optimal outcomes.

Cervical Perforation

The preferred method of exposure for cervical esophageal perforation is a left-sided neck incision along the anterior border of the sternocleidomastoid muscle (SCM). It may be necessary to ligate the middle thyroid vein for improved exposure. The trachea and thyroid gland are retracted medially for exposure of the esophagus (Figure 4). The retroesophageal space is entered bluntly along the prevertebral fascia, with care taken to preserve the recurrent laryngeal nerve. Blunt dissection should be continued down to the posterior mediastinum to drain all fluid collections. If the perforation is identified, the defect is repaired primarily with absorbable suture. If the defect is not clearly identified, closed drainage is performed. The

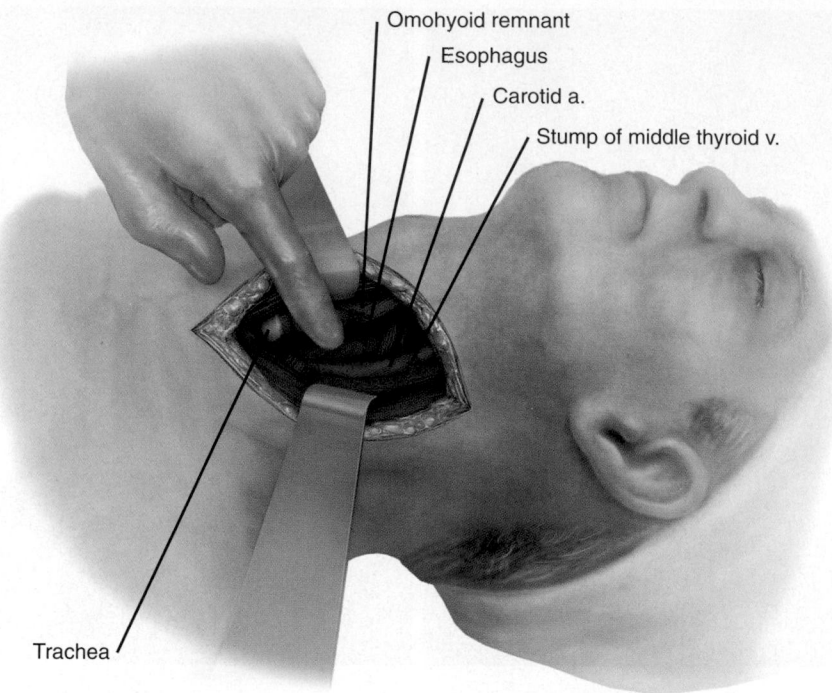

Omohyoid remnant
Esophagus
Carotid a.
Stump of middle thyroid v.
Trachea

FIGURE 4 Make an incision over the anterior border of the sternocleidomastoid muscle. If necessary, ligate the middle thyroid vein and inferior thyroid artery. Retract the trachea and thyroid gland medially to help expose the esophagus. *(From Cooke DT, Lau CL. Primary repair of esophageal perforation. Op Tech Thor Cardiovasc Surg. 13:126-137, 2008.)*

strap muscles can be used to buttress the repair, or as a patch for perforation not amenable to suture repair. For patients who have undergone primary repair or patch closure, a Gastrografin esophagogram is advisable on postoperative day 5 to demonstrate healing.

Thoracic Perforations

Perforations of the upper two thirds of the esophagus are best approached through a right posterolateral thoracotomy via the fifth interspace. The pleura is opened in the area of the perforation and the esophagus dissected for clear visualization of the perforation. The edges of the perforation should be débrided to determine the full extent of the injury. In fresh perforations, the mucosa may be closed with running absorbable suture and the muscularis closed with interrupted silk suture. The wound should be irrigated copiously. To buttress the repair, a vascularized intercostal muscle flap harvested from the fifth interspace is used. Drainage is provided with a 32F thoracostomy tube adjacent to the injury.

Perforations of the lower third of the esophagus should be approached through a left posterolateral thoracotomy in the seventh interspace. Again, primary repair is preferred and the repair should be buttressed with either an intercostal muscle flap or diaphragmatic flap (Figure 5). The majority of benign thoracic esophageal perforations will be amenable to primary repair. Again, repeat Gastrografin imaging is obtained on postoperative day 5.

Given the morbidity of esophageal exclusion, cervical esophagostomy and gastrostomy for delayed perforation is not recommended. This procedure should be reserved for unstable patients with severe ongoing sepsis and those with malignant perforations in which an esophageal stent is not applicable. Should this approach be necessary, the cervical esophagostomy is performed through a left-sided neck incision along the anterior border of the SCM. The esophagus should be dissected circumferentially with care taken to avoid injury to the recurrent laryngeal and vagus nerves. Once mobilized from the prevertebral fascia and posterior mediastinum, the esophagus is elevated to the skin level where either an end esophagostomy or loop esophagostomy is created. Loop esophagostomy is preferred for future reconstruction, and open jejunostomy for enteral feeding is

preferable after occluding the distal esophagus with a stapling device. A 45-mm thoracoabdominal stapler suffices for this purpose. A gastrostomy tube should be avoided if the stomach may be used later for reconstruction.

Abdominal Perforations

Perforations of the abdominal esophagus can be approached via an upper midline incision. One exception, although rare, is the patient who has an esophagus that is perforated into a large hiatal hernia. This exposure may require a left thoracotomy. Once debrided, the perforation should be closed primarily and buttressed with omentum, a rotational flap, or the fundus of the stomach via a Dor or Thal-type fundoplication.

Rotational Flaps

Diaphragmatic Flap

The technique of diaphragmatic flap buttress is illustrated in Figure 5. A posteriorly based full-thickness flap of adequate length and width is mobilized to reach the area of primary repair. The flap is secured to the esophagus with interrupted silk suture. The diaphragm then is closed primarily with nonabsorbable suture. For benign disease with a perforation not amenable to suture repair, primary diaphragmatic flap repair may be sutured to the débrided edges of the opening. Advantages of diaphragmatic flap use include the thickness, ease of mobility, and the extent of mobility because appropriately mobilized flaps are capable of reaching the level of the mid-esophagus.

Intercostal Muscle Flap

Pedicle muscle flaps are an effective technique for buttressing a primary repair or anatomic resection of the esophagus. Because the pleura is often too thin and the pericardial fat pad is frequently inconsistent with unreliable blood flow, the use of an intercostal muscle (ICM) flap is preferred. The ICM flap generally is harvested with the patient in the posterolateral thoracotomy position. The ICM overlying the sixth rib is mobilized using electrocautery. The cautery

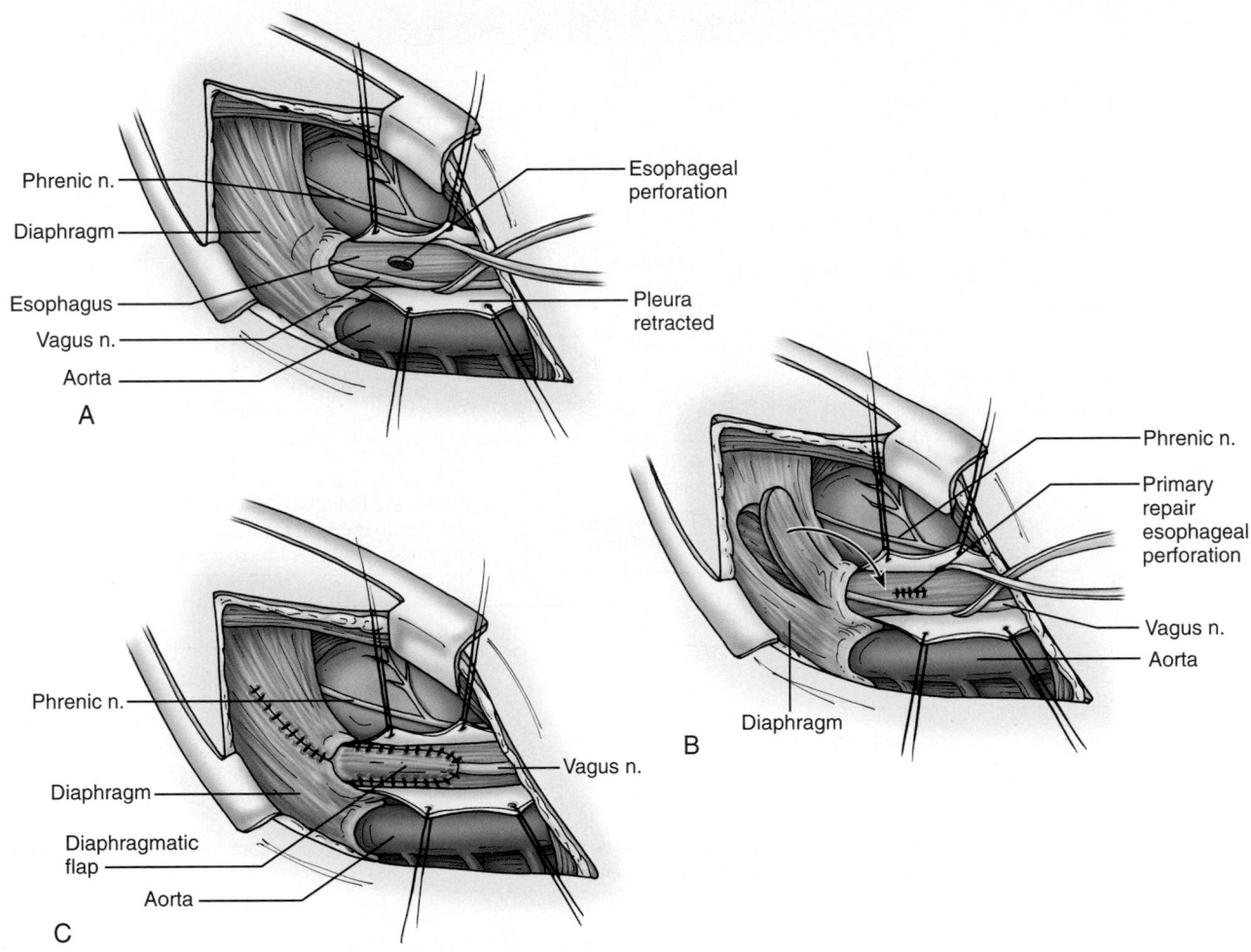

FIGURE 5 Diaphragmatic flap buttress technique for distal esophageal perforation. A posteriorly based full-thickness flap of diaphragm is mobilized to reach the area of primary repair. The flap is secured to the esophagus with interrupted silk suture. The diaphragm is then closed primarily with nonabsorbable suture. *(Illustration by Vicente A. Mejia, MD.)*

tip is positioned near parallel with the surface of the rib to avoid injury to the neurovascular bundle. The ICM is freed from the rib posteriorly to the level of the lumbar-dorsal fascia. Care must be taken to identify this landmark because further dissection risks injury to the intercostal vein. The ICM flap is transected anteriorly and reflected posteriorly to buttress the suture line. The buttress may be completed with interrupted silk suture.

Esophageal Stents

Esophageal stents were introduced first for palliation of malignant esophageal strictures in the early 1990s. Since that time, off-label esophageal stent use has resulted in multiple case series involving iatrogenic perforations, emetogenic rupture (Boerhaave's syndrome), and anastomotic leaks. The advantage of an esophageal stent is that the leak may be controlled with a minimally invasive technique in frail patients at high risk for general anesthesia or those with poor nutritional status. The role of stenting in the management of esophageal perforation is to limit sepsis from continued leak and to allow early resumption of enteral feeding. Most patients treated with an esophageal stent benefit from early video-assisted thoracoscopic surgery (VATS) 1 to 2 days after stent placement for débridement of the pleural space. Thoracostomy tube placement alone is often inadequate and may later necessitate thoracotomy.

Although minimally invasive, use of esophageal stents is not without complications. Patients may experience chest discomfort, fever, gastroesophageal reflux, or globus sensation. More serious complications such as bleeding, perforation, or stent migration also are seen. Later complications include tumor ingrowth, stent occlusion, fistula, and recurrent stricture. Stent migration rates can be as high as 30%, with stents crossing the gastroesophageal junction having a higher propensity for migration. Furthermore, placement of a stent in a nonstrictured lumen could be associated with significant rates of stent migration, resulting in technical and clinical failure. Considering use of an esophageal stent requires a multidisciplinary approach with local expertise in advanced endoscopy. Although technical success rates reported range from 90% to 100%, clinical success rates are approximately 80% with patients often requiring multiple procedures.

■ SPECIAL SITUATIONS

Malignancy

When esophageal perforation involves a malignancy, special consideration must be given to the treatment of both problems. If drainage is adequate, placement of an esophageal stent to control contamination is favored, reserving resection and anastomosis for a later time. If the patient is found to have massive contamination with hemodynamic instability not amenable to stent placement, cervical esophagostomy and gastrostomy should be considered. Stable patients with malignant perforation where stenting is not available are probably best served in a setting where esophageal resection is performed routinely. An algorithm is demonstrated in Figure 6 for summary of management pathways.

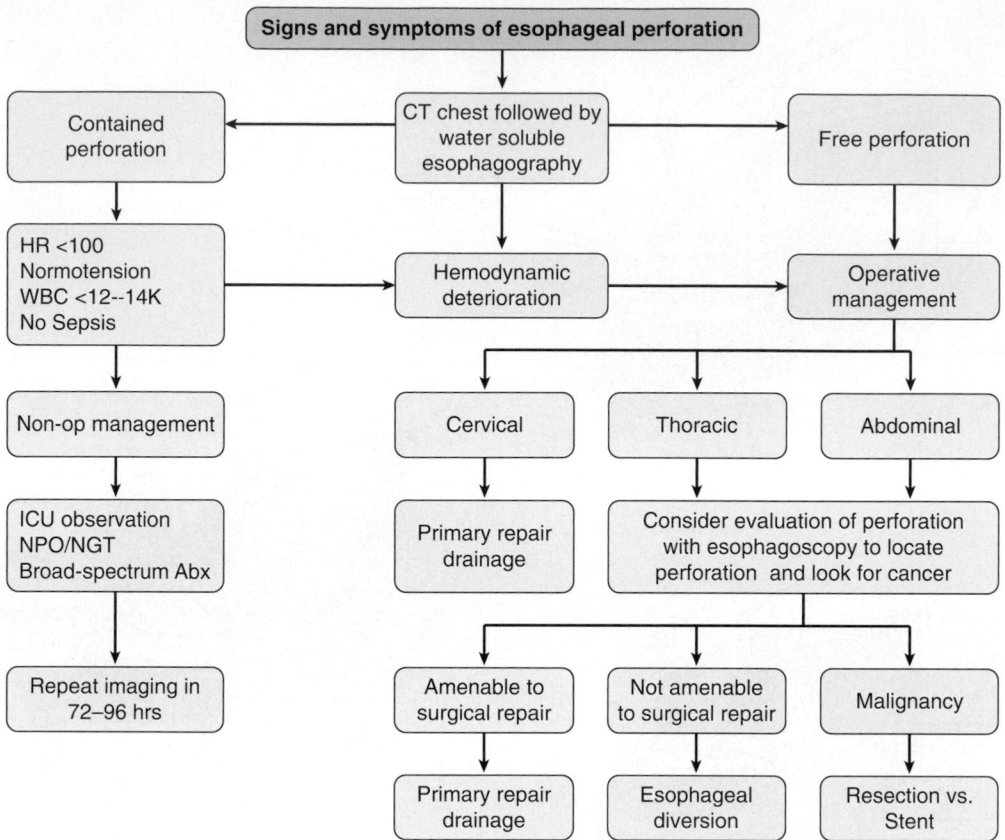

FIGURE 6 Algorithm for management of esophageal perforation. *Abx,* antibiotics; *CT,* computed tomography; *HR,* heart rate; *ICU,* intensive care unit; *NGT,* nasogastric tube; *NPO,* nothing by mouth *(nil per os)*; *WBC,* white blood cell count.

Achalasia

Patients with a known diagnosis of achalasia with perforation above the lower esophageal sphincter require special consideration. These patients may experience esophageal perforation during pneumatic dilatation, at the time of myotomy, or with other previously mentioned mechanisms. Because of the elevated intraluminal pressure proximal to the esophageal sphincter, healing of the repair often is precluded. Because the majority of these patients will experience distal esophageal perforation, exposure is performed best through a left anterolateral thoracotomy through the seventh interspace. The esophagus should be dissected circumferentially with care taken to avoid injury to the vagus nerves. As previously described, the perforation is closed in two layers with absorbable suture and buttressed with a rotational flap. These patients require myotomy for adequate healing. The myotomy should be performed on the opposite side of the esophagus from the perforation.

Nissen Fundoplication

Esophageal perforation after Nissen fundoplication is a known postoperative complication. One must have a high index of suspicion for perforation in patients who present with abdominal pain, fever, tachycardia, and leukocytosis postoperatively. Esophagography or CT imaging generally will reveal presence of a leak. These cases are best addressed with laparotomy, dismantling of the fundoplication, primary repair of the esophagus, and repeat Nissen fundoplication.

Esophagogastrostomy Leak After Esophagectomy

Anastomotic leak is a known and dreaded complication of Ivor Lewis esophagectomy. Management of the leak depends on the viability of the gastric conduit, the size of the leak, and the degree of contamination. Consideration must be given first to the viability of the gastric conduit, which may be evaluated by diagnostic thoracoscopy. If the gastric conduit is viable and contamination may be controlled with a drainage procedure, thoracoscopy or thoracotomy with chest tube placement should be performed to drain the pleural and mediastinal spaces with consideration given to endoscopic stent placement.

If the gastric conduit is found to be necrotic, the gangrenous stomach will have to be resected via a right thoracotomy and the gastric remnant reduced into the abdomen. Cervical esophagostomy and gastrostomy should be performed. Once the patient is no longer in critical condition, delayed reconstruction of the esophagus may be performed.

SUGGESTED READINGS

Dasari B, Neely D, Kennedy A, et al. The role of esophageal stents in the management of esophageal anastomotic leaks and benign esophageal perforations. *Ann Surg.* 2014;259:852-860.

Keeling WB, Miller DL, Lam GT, et al. Low mortality after treatment for esophageal perforation: a single-center experience. *Ann Thorac Surg.* 2010;90:1669-1673.

Neel D, Davis EG, Farmer R, et al. Aggressive operative treatment for emetogenic rupture yields superior results. *Am Surg.* 2010;76:865-868.

Richardson JD. Management of esophageal perforations: the value of aggressive surgical treatment. *Am J Surg.* 2005;190:161-165.

Schweigert M, Beattie R, Solymosi N, et al. Endoscopic stent insertion versus primary operative management for spontaneous rupture of the esophagus (Boerhaave syndrome): an international study comparing the outcome. *Am Surg.* 2013;79:634-640.

THE MANAGEMENT OF BENIGN GASTRIC ULCERS

Amy L. Lightner, MD, and F. Charles Brunicardi, MD

The management of benign gastric ulceration is becoming increasingly one of *Helicobacter pylori* treatment and antacid administration rather than surgical intervention. The majority of the 100,000 new cases of gastric ulcers diagnosed each year are related to *H. pylori* infection and nonsteroidal anti-inflammatory drug (NSAID) usage. Other causes worth noting include smoking, steroid usage, and Zollinger-Ellison syndrome. Thus the need for surgery is limited to cases of hemorrhage, perforation, obstruction, and refractory disease.

PRESENTATION AND DIAGNOSIS

The majority of patients experience epigastric pain that is relieved with food or antacids but recurs after a short interval. Initial evaluation of the patient should rule out pancreatitis, hepatobiliary disease, and aortic aneurysmal disease in the emergent setting using laboratory and imaging parameters. Often patients have had an upright abdominal x-ray or computed tomography (CT) scan to evaluate their epigastric discomfort, but definitive diagnosis relies on esophagogastroduodenoscopy (EGD). EGD can localize and characterize the lesion and provide tissue diagnosis for *H. pylori* and malignancy. In a nonoperative or operative setting, *H. pylori* should be treated and eradication confirmed 4 to 6 weeks later with a urease breath test. Treatment will decrease not only recurrence but also the risk of associated gastric cancer. Proton pump inhibitors (PPIs) often are administered in parallel with *H. pylori* treatment, and the patient is re-evaluated by endoscopy at 8 to 12 weeks. PPI therapy is discontinued only if and when ulcer healing is confirmed by upper endoscopy. Duration of surveillance for ulcer eradication is variable based on patient characteristics but can extend up to 12 weeks. After this, the ulcer will likely require surgical management based on "refractory" disease.

In the emergent setting of bleeding, perforation, or obstruction, the patient may have laboratory abnormalities, an upright abdominal x-ray demonstrating free air or a massive distended stomach, and a CT scan showing the same with nearby inflammation or extraluminal fluid. Depending on the severity of the situation, the patient may be treated with nonoperative conservative (e.g., medical management of ulcer) or endoscopic intervention (e.g., small bleed, small contained perforation, or obstruction amenable to dilation or stenting). If recurrent abdominal examinations or hemodynamic changes suggest lack of improvement or decompensation, the management plan should change accordingly, and the patient likely will need an operation. If, on initial presentation, there are signs of significant bleeding or uncontained perforation, the patient should be taken immediately to the operating room.

RISK OF CANCER

It is important to rule out gastric malignancy when diagnosing these patients. Biopsies should be taken at the time of EGD and/or operation and sent for frozen section. When in the operating room, frozen section positive for malignancy will change the extent of resection and add lymphadenectomy and omentectomy in the setting of a stable patient who can tolerate the additional operative time. One third of giant ulcers, ulcers larger than 2 cm in diameter, harbor malignant disease. Thus, if a giant ulcer is found on EGD, eight biopsies should be taken at the ulcer base and edge to rule out cancer, and earlier surgical intervention is warranted if the ulcer is suspicious or not rapidly healing. Ulcers that do not heal at 12 weeks despite maximal medical management also raise suspicion for malignancy. In addition, perforated ulcers, more than obstructing ulcers, may harbor a malignancy. Thus frozen sections should again be sent in the operating room to rule out a malignancy.

GASTRIC ULCER TYPES AND LOCATION

Johnson proposed a classification system that has been adopted universally for localizing and determining optimal treatment practices for gastric ulcers (Table 1). Type I ulcers, located along the lesser curvature, are the most common, making up 60% of benign gastric ulcers. Although the cause of these ulcers is not understood, they are not associated with acid hypersecretion, and *H. pylori* infection is found in the majority of patients. For the minority of patients who have refractory disease, antrectomy and vagotomy with Billroth I reconstruction is the procedure of choice (Figure 1). Type II and III gastric ulcers also are found along the lesser curvature near the incisura and prepyloric, respectively. Even though these ulcers are associated with acid hypersecretion, a vagotomy is recommended only in the setting of previously failed antacids or an unreliable patient because recurrence can be prevented with *H. pylori* eradication and antacids. Billroth I is the preferred surgical reconstruction, but the distal nature of type III ulcers may necessitate a Billroth II or Roux-en-Y creation (see Figure 1) if extensive kocherization of the duodenum has not created sufficient mobilization. Type IV ulcers, unrelated to acid hypersecretion, can present an anatomic challenge given their proximity to the gastroesophageal (GE) junction along the proximal lesser curve. When a surgeon is forced to operate in the setting of failed conservative management, a Pauchet's or Csendes' procedure (Figure 2) can be used to preserve as much stomach as possible. Type V is diffuse ulceration related to NSAID or steroid use. These are treated successfully with cessation of NSAIDs and an addition of a PPI or histamine blocker. If bleeding persists, the use of EGD with injection or cautery can be used. If this does not work, the patient may need to proceed to the operating room, where an anterior gastrostomy with inspection and oversewing any major sites of bleeding can be tried. Total gastrectomy should be used only in the setting of a life-threatening diffuse bleed.

For all the aforementioned locations, *H. pylori* and antacid therapy have significantly decreased the operative volume. In the

TABLE 1: Modified Johnson Classification

Type	Location	Acid Hypersecretion
I	Lesser curvature, incisura	No
II	Body of stomach, incisura, and duodenal ulcer (active or healed)	Yes
III	Prepyloric	Yes
IV	High on lesser curve, near gastroesophageal junction	No
V	Anywhere (medication induced)	No

setting of obstruction, conservative nasogastric tube (NGT) may be used in the setting of edema and inflammation, or dilation and stenting via EGD may be effective. In the setting of perforation, many ulcers can be wedged out with primary repair and/or a Graham patch rather than a formal gastric resection with an acid-reducing operation. However, if the patient has been on antacids and already had *H. pylori* eradication, then an operation involving removal of the acid-producing parietal cells of the stomach combined with an acid-reducing operation may be prudent.

■ SURGICAL TECHNIQUES

The goals of surgery in the setting of benign gastric ulcers are to (1) remove the ulcerogenic tissue and send it for pathologic examination

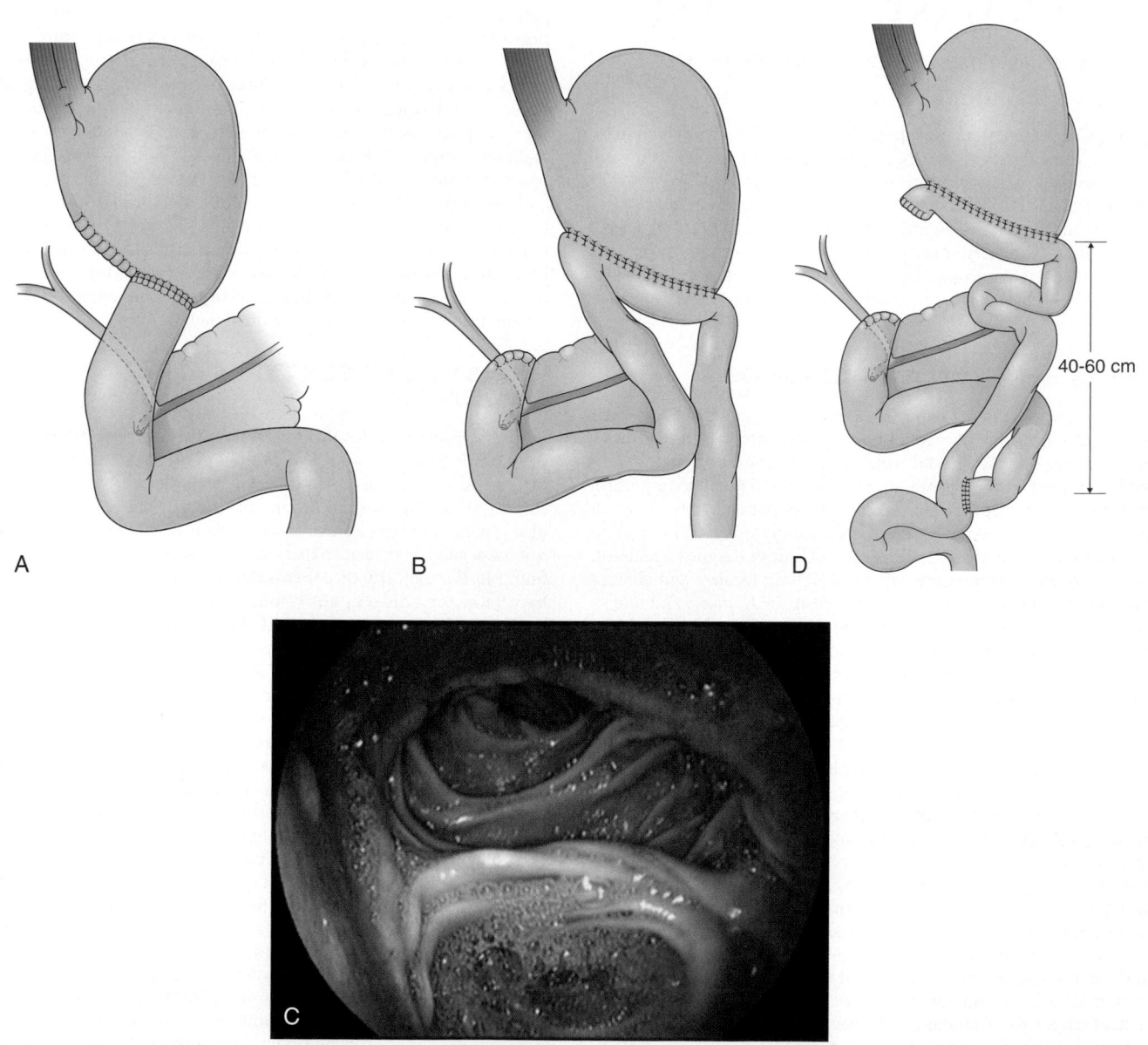

FIGURE 1 Three types of reconstruction after partial gastrectomy. **A,** Billroth I: A gastroduodenostomy is performed toward the greater curvature. **B,** Billroth II: A gastrojejunostomy is created to reestablish the alimentary transit. Several variations may be observed in this type of reconstruction. **C,** Frothy bile coming from the anastomotic opening linked to the lesser curvature indicates the afferent limb (anisoperistaltic anastomosis). **D,** Roux-en-Y: A gastrojejunostomy only is created with the efferent limb to prevent biliopancreatic reflux into the stomach. A 40-cm to 60-cm efferent limb leads to the jejunojejunostomy and afferent limb. *(From Ginsburg GG, Kochman ML, Norton ID, Gostout CJ. Clinical Gastrointestinal Endoscopy. 2nd ed. Philadelphia: Elsevier, 2011, Fig. 11.2, A through D.)*

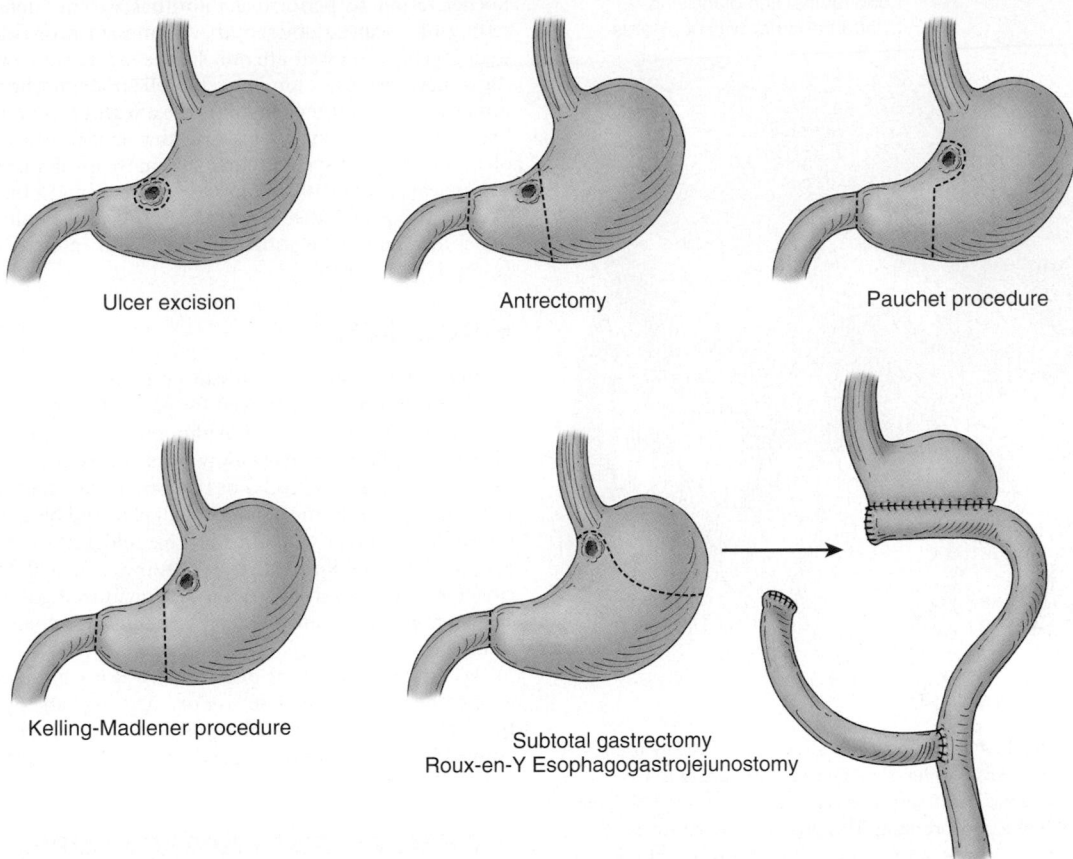

Ulcer excision

Antrectomy

Pauchet procedure

Kelling-Madlener procedure

Subtotal gastrectomy
Roux-en-Y Esophagogastrojejunostomy

FIGURE 2 Some useful operations for gastric ulcer include the Pauchet's operation (excision of a "tongue" of proximal lesser gastric curvature in continuity with distal gastrectomy), the Kelling-Madlener procedure (excision or biopsy of proximal ulcer and distal gastrectomy), and the Csendes' operation (subtotal gastrectomy to include part of the cardia with reconstruction with Roux esophagogastrojejunostomy). These procedures are particularly useful for gastric ulcer high on the lesser gastric curvature (type IV gastric ulcer). *(From Zuidema GD, Yeo CJ, editors.* Shackelford's Surgery of the Alimentary Tract. *5th ed. Saunders; 2002, pp. 74-85.)*

and, in the setting of medically refractory disease, (2) reduce gastric acid secretion. Reduction in acid secretion can be accomplished by removing vagal stimulation via vagotomy, gastrin-driven acid secretion by an antrectomy, or both. Vagotomy alone decreases peak acid output by 50%, whereas vagotomy plus antrectomy decreases peak acid output by 85%.

Vagotomy and Drainage

The purpose of any form of vagotomy is to eliminate the parasympathetic innervation of any remaining acid-producing stomach tissue. A truncal vagotomy involves dividing the right posterior and left anterior vagus nerves at the level of the distal esophagus, 4 cm proximal to the gastroesophageal (GE) junction. This requires mobilization of 5 to 6 cm of esophagus to carefully identify the common trunks before branching. When struggling to identify the posterior nerve, the surgeon can place the nerves on stretch by placing downward traction on the proximal stomach, keeping the GE junction in between the index and middle fingers, and pulling the esophageal muscles on stretch. The posterior vagus nerve then feels like an isolated cord. Once identified, clips are placed proximally and distally, and the trunks are transected and sent to the pathology laboratory to ensure removal of nerve tissue.

A selective vagotomy divides the left and right vagus nerves just below the posterior celiac branches that innervate the pancreas and small intestine and anterior hepatic branches that innervated the liver and gallbladder. These branches are typically just proximal to the GE

junction. Although the ulcer recurrence rate is the same, postoperative diarrhea and dumping may be lower with this technique.

A highly selective vagotomy, or parietal cell vagotomy, preserves Latarjet's nerves, which provide motor function to the pylorus. Thus this is the only technique that does not require a drainage procedure; both a truncal and selective vagotomy require a longitudinal pyloroplasty with a transverse closure, as described by Heineke-Mikulicz (Figure 3). The anterior and posterior branches of the vagus nerves are identified at the junction of the corpus and antrum of the stomach, usually 6 cm proximal to the pylorus. These branches have a characteristic "crow's foot" appearance and are divided, leaving the trunks intact.

Resection of Ulcer

If a formal acid-reducing operation is not performed, most ulcers can be managed by either (1) cleaning the edges for primary repair after biopsy or (2) wedging out with a stapler and sending tissue for frozen section. So long as there is no malignancy and the patient has not been on prior antacid treatment, the area of resection can be left alone, oversewn, or patched, and the patient can be put on antacids and *H. pylori* treatment.

In the setting of a formal resection (e.g., antrectomy), the ulcer location dictates the extent of dissection. When located on the distal aspect of the stomach, distal stomach with frozen sent to the pathology laboratory until antral glands containing G cells can to mark the proximal extent of dissection can be used. In the setting of a

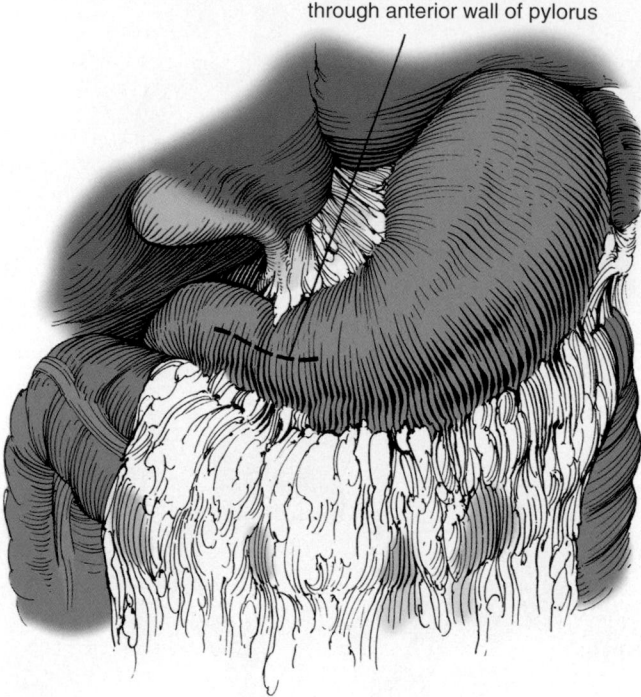

Longitudinal line of incision
through anterior wall of pylorus

FIGURE 3 The Heineke-Mikulicz procedure is the most widely used pyloroplasty. In a strict sense, a Heineke-Mikulicz pyloroplasty is a two-layer closure, whereas most surgeons actually perform the one-layer modification: the Weinberg pyloroplasty. This procedure is acceptable if there is minimal scarring at the pylorus and no foreshortening of the proximal end of the duodenum. After kocherization of the duodenum, a longitudinal incision is centered over the anterior pylorus and extends 2 to 3 cm proximally and distally. *(From Yeo CJ, et al: Shackelford's Surgery of the Alimentary Tract. 6th ed. Philadelphia: Elsevier, 2007, Fig. 57-22.)*

proximal lesser curve, the resection may be more difficult, requiring a Pauchet's procedure (see Figure 2) as previously discussed to preserve gastric tissue. The distal extent of dissection is nearly universally transection through healthy duodenal tissue just distal to the pylorus.

Options for Reconstruction

A Billroth I is the preferred form of reconstruction in benign gastric ulcer disease because it avoids the problem of retained antrum syndrome, duodenal stump leak, and afferent loop obstruction associated with a Billroth II reconstruction. A Billroth I is a gastroduodenostomy made via an anastomosis of the end of the duodenum to the distal greater curvature of the stomach. This can be performed in a hand-sewn fashion using permanent suture or stapled fashion with an end-to-end anastomosis (EEA) stapler through an anterior gastrotomy (see Figure 1). Postoperatively, a nasogastric tube is left in overnight to monitor for bleeding and removed on postoperative day 1, at which point the patient can be started on clear liquids and advanced quickly to a regular diet.

A Billroth II is a gastrojejunostomy, performed in the setting of inadequate reach and mobility of the duodenum after extensive

Kocherization to perform a Billroth I without tension, or in the setting of a scarred duodenum. An afferent limb, ideally no longer than 20 cm to prevent afferent limb syndrome, is brought through the transverse mesocolon in a retrocolic fashion. The retrocolic anastomosis minimizes the length of the afferent limb and decreases the likelihood of twisting or kinking that could lead to afferent loop obstruction, predisposing the patient to a devastating duodenal stump leak. A duodenal stump leak occurs in 1% to 3% of patients, usually at postoperative day 6 to 10. A drain should be left next to the stump and more widely drained with internal drainage if the stump is questionable.

■ ROUX-EN-Y

A Roux-en-Y reconstruction can be used in the same settings as a Billroth II but may be reserved for patients who have complications associated with a Billroth II. Although a Roux-en-Y reconstruction diverts the bilious drainage away from the gastric remnant resulting in less reflux than a Billroth I or II, a patient can develop gastric atony, resulting in a syndrome of abdominal pain and bloating, "Roux stasis syndrome." Patients who already have undergone a vagotomy are at increased risk of Roux stasis syndrome, and a Billroth II may be preferred in this setting. Without previous vagotomy, Roux-en-Y may be preferred because of decreased reflux esophagitis and remnant gastritis.

When the operation is performed, a Roux limb length of at least 40 cm helps prevent bile reflux. During an open procedure, both retrocolic and antecolic positions for the Roux limb appear equivalent in terms of outcomes, but a retrocolic approach provides greater length.

■ OPEN VERSUS LAPAROSCOPIC APPROACH

As the experience with laparoscopic surgery is increasing, more and more foregut procedures are being performed laparoscopically. First and foremost, the stability of the patient must be taken into account. If a large perforation with long duration of contamination is found, then a laparoscopic approach may not be warranted. Second, the experience of the operating surgeons and their comfort level for reconstruction must be evaluated. If the patient is stable and the operating surgeon facile with laparoscopic techniques, laparoscopic ulcer surgery is feasible, safe, and equally effective. It may even be particularly useful for vagotomy because of improved visualization of the nerve fibers or an isolated Graham patch for which a minimally invasive operation may allow for a faster recovery.

SUGGESTED READINGS

Bertleff MJ, Halm JA, Bemelman WA, et al. Randomized clinical trial of laparoscopic versus open repair of the perforated peptic ulcer: the LAMA Trial. *World J Surg.* 2009;33:1368-1373.

Howden CW, Hunt RH. The relationship between suppression of acidity and gastric ulcer healing rates. *Aliment Pharmacol Ther.* 1990;4:25-33.

Hsiao FY, Tsai YW, Wen YW, Kuo KN, Tsai CR, Huang WF. Effect of *Helicobacter pylori* eradication therapy on risk of hospitalization for a major ulcer event. *Pharmacotherapy.* 2011;31:239-247.

Siu WT, Leong HT, Law BK, et al. Laparoscopic repair for perforated peptic ulcer: a randomized controlled trial. *Ann Surg.* 2002;235:313-319.

Wu CY, Kuo KN, Wu MS, Chen YJ, Wang CB, Lin JT. Early *Helicobacter pylori* eradication decreases risk of gastric cancer in patients with peptic ulcer disease. *Gastroenterology.* 2009;137:1641-1648, e1641-1642.

THE MANAGEMENT OF DUODENAL ULCERS

Daniel T. Dempsey, MD, MBA

Duodenal ulcer is the result of localized acid/peptic injury to the duodenal mucosa caused by increased luminal acid and/or weakened mucosal defense. Common predisposing factors are *Helicobacter pylori* infection, nonsteroidal anti-inflammatory drugs (NSAIDs, including aspirin) use, and smoking. Other possible causes include gastrinoma (Zollinger-Ellison syndrome), stress, radiation, Crohn's disease, cocaine, and gastroduodenal dysmotility.

The most common symptoms of duodenal ulcer are abdominal pain, nausea, vomiting, and anemia. To current surgeons, the most common presentations are upper gastrointestinal (GI) bleeding, perforation, obstruction, and chronic abdominal pain. Peptic ulcer (duodenal, gastric, and marginal) is the most common cause of upper GI bleeding requiring hospitalization, but the majority of these patients (more than 90%) do not require an operation. Currently the most common indication for operation in duodenal ulcer patients is perforation. Operation for bleeding and obstruction are equally uncommon, and operation for intractable duodenal ulcer is very uncommon.

After operation for duodenal ulcer, recurrent ulcer can be minimized by chronic acid suppression, eradication of *Helicobacter* spp., diligent and permanent avoidance of NSAIDs and aspirin, and long-lasting abstention from smoking. Daily low-dose aspirin can be taken with impunity if medically indicated, provided a daily proton pump inhibitor (PPI) is taken too. If compliance with these management principles cannot be followed, ultimately ulcer recurrence is likely. Whether definitive ulcer operation in the current era is as effective in preventing recurrent ulcer as it once was is unclear. The acid suppressive effect of vagotomy may be no more profound than a daily PPI, but the former does not depend on patient compliance. However, the concept that bigger is better should be used sparingly today in ulcer surgery, particularly during emergency operation, which now is more common than elective operation for duodenal ulcer disease. Gastrectomy for ulcer should be avoided in thin patients.

Perforated Duodenal Ulcer

Clearly the most common indication for an operation today in duodenal ulcer patients is perforation. Duodenal ulcer perforation presents as an acute abdomen. The patient usually can pinpoint the onset of severe abdominal pain. There may or may not be a history suggestive of duodenal ulcer. Usually the patient appears very uncomfortable and is loathe to move. Tachycardia is frequently the only early vital sign abnormality. Fever and tachypnea then ensue, and hypotension is a late finding. On examination the abdomen is rigid and there is obvious peritonitis. Leukocytosis is common, and an upright chest x-ray usually shows pneumoperitoneum (absent in 10% to 15% of cases). Computed tomography (CT) scan is unnecessary, but when performed this nearly always shows extraluminal air in the upper abdomen, often with some free peritoneal fluid.

The mortality risk of perforated duodenal ulcer in the modern era is high, up to 25% in some series. Although this may be due in part to the frailty of the patient population affected, there is no doubt that delayed treatment increases mortality risk. Prompt fluid resuscitation and intravenous (IV) antibiotics are important, but so is prompt operation. Medical optimization, although necessary, should not be an excuse for prolonged delay in surgical treatment for patients with perforated duodenal ulcer. In addition to empiric broad-spectrum perioperative antibiotics, antifungal treatment should be considered particularly in the sicker patients. The very occasional stable patient without peritonitis and with a radiologically documented sealed perforation may be cautiously managed nonoperatively.

Laparotomy or laparoscopy with peritoneal washout (5 to 10 L) and omental patch closure of the perforation is the treatment of choice for most patients with perforated duodenal ulcer. We routinely send the peritoneal fluid for culture and sensitivity (including fungal studies). Routine biopsy is not necessary for perforated duodenal ulcer but should be performed if there is any suspicion of malignancy. We also leave a closed suction peritoneal drain for a few days, near but not on the closure site. Occasionally in the patient with documented chronic duodenal ulcer who has developed a perforation despite good medical management, a definitive ulcer operation may be considered if the patient has not been in shock and if the peritonitis is not severe or chronic.

Closure of the Perforation

In perforated duodenal ulcer, usually the hole is small (5 mm or less). Typically the actual perforation is not sutured closed because the sutures may pull through the friable tissue, making the hole bigger. Even if the sutures do not pull through, primary closure of the perforation may narrow further an already scarred gastric outlet. Therefore omental patch (Graham patch) is the preferred closure technique in most cases of perforated duodenal ulcer. An appropriate-size, tension-free, well-vascularized tongue of omentum is used to plug the hole. This omental patch is held in place by interrupted sutures placed through healthy duodenum on either side of the perforation. We usually place two or three interrupted bridging sutures, then lay the patch on, then tie the sutures gently but snugly over the patch. If necessary, additional sutures may be placed circumferentially between the healthy duodenum and the omental patch. Once the patch is secure, the adequacy of the seal can be tested by submerging the site under irrigation fluid while injecting air into the nasogastric (NG) tube. Methylene blue also may be used.

Rarely, the perforation is large (2 cm or 3 cm in diameter), and these holes can be difficult to close adequately with omental patch. In this situation, a tension-free two-layer anastomosis can be created between the débrided duodenal opening and a Roux limb. If the ampulla is deemed to be at risk, a biliary Fogarty can be advanced from above via the cystic duct or common bile duct. The duodenojejunal anastomosis can be checked with air insufflation and/or methylene blue instillation. In our opinion this is a more secure closure of a large duodenal perforation from peptic ulceration than a jejunal "serosal patch." Gastrostomy and jejunostomy tubes are placed. If desired, postoperative duodenal decompression can be accomplished with transpyloric NG tube (secured to nose with suture or bridle), lateral duodenostomy tube, or retrograde jejunostomy (our preferred approach). In giant perforated duodenal ulcer, definitive ulcer operation should be considered in the stable patient. Truncal vagotomy and either gastrojejunostomy or antrectomy would be the best definitive options in this situation. Depending on the quality of the duodenal repair, exclusion may be desirable and can be accomplished with pyloric occlusion and gastrojejunostomy, or antrectomy with Billroth II anastomosis. Care should be taken not to complicate the situation by creating a difficult duodenal stump however.

Definitive Ulcer Operation

As mentioned above, most patients with perforated duodenal ulcer should be washed out and patched and then medically managed (see later in this chapter). There are old data that suggest that a definitive ulcer procedure during an emergency operation for duodenal ulcer is safe and decreases ulcer recurrence. Such data are largely lacking

BOX I: Decreasing Recurrence After Emergency Duodenal Ulcer Operation

Rule out gastrinoma
Treat *Helicobacter* infection
Chronic acid suppression
No smoking
No NSAIDs/aspirin
Definitive ulcer operation

TABLE I: Emergency Operation for Duodenal Ulcer (NSQIP 2005-2010)

	Patch/ Oversew	Vagotomy/ Resection	Vagotomy/ Drainage	Total
Perforation	1149	70	23	1242
Bleeding	365	73	107	545
Total	1514	143	130	1787

in the modern era. Patients getting emergency duodenal ulcer operation today are sicker than ever, and definitive ulcer operation is only one of many steps to decrease ulcer recurrence (Box 1). Occasionally it may be appropriate to add a definitive ulcer operation to closure of perforated duodenal ulcer. When indicated, either truncal vagotomy and gastrojejunostomy, or proximal gastric vagotomy (parietal cell vagotomy) are reasonable considerations. In experienced hands, either operation can be performed open or laparoscopically. However, experience with these procedures is dwindling. The Taylor operation (posterior truncal vagotomy and anterior highly selective vagotomy) is a good alternative to parietal cell vagotomy. Table 1 shows the operations performed 2005 to 2010 for perforated and bleeding duodenal ulcer in the NSQIP database. Thirty-day operative mortality for emergency operation for bleeding peptic ulcer (gastric and duodenal) was 19%, and for perforation 12%.

Minimally Invasive Treatment

Laparoscopic operation for perforated duodenal ulcer is increasingly more common. It appears to be at least as safe and effective as open operation, and some studies suggest that the laparoscopic approach is preferred. We concur with this opinion. Laparoscopy confirms the diagnosis, and peritoneal irrigation can be readily accomplished laparoscopically. Laparoscopic patch closure of the perforation is usually straightforward. Even when conversion to open operation is necessary (uncommon), the laparotomy incision is smaller and optimally placed. Finally, it is likely that over the next decade, an increasing number of peptic ulcer perforations will be closed endoscopically with a NOTES (natural orifice transluminal endoscopic surgery) approach.

Postoperative and Long-Term Management

Modern surgical intensive care unit (ICU) care, with attention to optimization of critical organ function, fluid management, and treatment of sepsis is beneficial to most patients after closure of duodenal ulcer perforation. The decision to remove the NG tube and initiate oral liquids is made on clinical grounds. Postoperative contrast study usually is performed to rule out ongoing leak and to demonstrate gastric emptying. Antibiotics and antifungals are continued for 3 to 5 days, or until the patient is afebrile and without leukocytosis. The peritoneal drain is removed 24 hours after the initiation of oral

liquids if drainage is benign and the patient is doing well. Reoperation sometimes is required for persistent leakage from the perforation site, or abdominal wound dehiscence. We think emergency operation for duodenal ulcer is an indication for chronic PPI therapy and empiric treatment of *Helicobacter pylori* infection. Patients are advised strongly to avoid NSAIDs, aspirin, and smoking. Low-dose aspirin is permissible provided chronic PPI treatment is continued.

■ BLEEDING DUODENAL ULCER

The most common reason for hospitalization in the duodenal ulcer patient is bleeding. However, bleeding has become an infrequent indication for operation in duodenal ulcer largely because of the effectiveness of medical and endoscopic treatment. There also has been an increased appreciation of the risk of operation for bleeding duodenal ulcer, including rebleeding, postoperative complications, and mortality.

Three quarters of the patients with bleeding duodenal ulcer will stop bleeding with only IV fluid and PPI infusion. The other 25% will continue to bleed or rebleed, and essentially all the deaths related to bleeding duodenal ulcer occur in this group. Therefore it is important to identify patients who are in this group. Not surprising, these are the patients with the bigger bleeds. They are more likely to have hematemesis, hypotension, multiunit transfusion requirement, and/or endoscopic stigmata (visible vessel and/or active bleeding). The bleeding duodenal ulcer patient with any of these findings should be seen in consultation by a surgeon and watched carefully in hospital, perhaps initially in the ICU. Endoscopic findings and treatment plan should be understood by the surgeon if he or she is not the admitting physician. Deep posterior bleeding ulcers in the proximal duodenum are particularly worrisome because they may involve the gastroduodenal artery, which can cause exsanguinating hemorrhage.

Hemostasis usually can be achieved with PPI infusion and endoscopic treatment (bipolar cautery, epinephrine injection, clips). Rebleeding should prompt repeat endoscopic treatment and consideration of arteriography and possible angioembolization. An operation should be considered for persistent or recurrent bleeding in patients with hemodynamic instability or transfusion requirement in excess of 6 units of red cells. Although developed more than 20 years ago, the Rockall score (Table 2) is still useful to help stratify rebleeding risk and mortality risk in patients with upper GI bleeding, including bleeding duodenal ulcer. An 82-year-old patient with bleeding duodenal ulcer, hypotension, chronic obstructive pulmonary disease (COPD), and visible vessel on esophagogastroduodenoscopy (EGD) has a mortality risk of 40%.

Operation for Bleeding Duodenal Ulcer

Three options exist for surgical treatment: oversewing alone, oversewing with vagotomy and drainage, and vagotomy and antrectomy. Clinical trials from a previous era suggest that the ultimate result (i.e., survival) is similar to either of the two latter surgical options, but reoperation for rebleeding is less common after vagotomy and antrectomy. However, resection for bleeding duodenal ulcer rarely is done because most surgical patients are high risk. Furthermore, the duodenal stump can be difficult because the bleeding ulcer either must be resected, or, if not resected, it must be oversewn. Recent review of NSQIP data suggests that vagotomy and drainage for bleeding peptic ulcer has a significantly lower 30-day postoperative mortality rate (12%) than vagotomy and resection (23%) and oversewing alone (27%).

Oversewing of bleeding duodenal ulcer starts with exposure of the lesion, usually through a longitudinal duodenotomy or pyloroduodenotomy. Kocher maneuver is done first because this facilitates manual control of a bleeding gastroduodenal artery with the left hand of the surgeon standing on the patient's left side (long fingers behind the head of the pancreas, thumb in front). Deep posterior ulcers usually require placement of two or three heavy suture

TABLE 2: Rockall Score to Assess Rebleeding and Mortality Risk in Upper Gastrointestinal Bleeding

Points	0	1	2	3
VARIABLE				
Age	<60 yr	61-79 yr	>80	
Shock	None	P >100; BP >100 syst	BP <100 syst	
Comorbidity	None		CHF, ASCVD, COPD	Renal or liver failure; metastatic cancer
Diagnosis	Mallory-Weiss	All other	GI cancer	
Bleeding stigmata	None		Visible vessel, active bleeding	

ASCVD, Atherosclerotic cardiovascular disease; *BP,* blood pressure; *CHF,* congestive heart failure; *COPD,* chronic obstructive pulmonary disease; *GI,* gastrointestinal; *P,* pulse; *syst,* systolic.

ligatures placed in figure-of-8 or over and over fashion. The u-stitch has been well described. Once hemostasis is achieved, the ulcer bed should be abraded gently with the sucker tip to ensure rebleeding does not occur. The gut incision then can be closed either longitudinally or as a pyloroplasty. If the patient is stable and exposure straightforward, truncal vagotomy can be performed, along with pyloroplasty or gastrojejunostomy. Definitive operation is particularly appropriate for patients with bleeding duodenal ulcer larger than 2 cm. Postoperative management is similar to that after repair of perforated duodenal ulcer. High-dose PPIs in the early postoperative period may decrease rebleeding; avoidance of NSAIDs and smoking is imperative.

GASTRIC OUTLET OBSTRUCTION

Acute duodenal ulceration can result in reversible gastric outlet obstruction from edema and possibly dysmotility. Chronic duodenal ulcer can lead to obstruction from scar formation. History and endoscopic findings usually can differentiate between an acute potentially reversible obstruction and chronic obstruction.

Operation may be necessary for the patient with chronic gastric outlet obstruction from duodenal ulcer disease. These patients usually experience nausea, nonbilious vomiting, epigastric distension, and weight loss. The differential diagnosis obviously includes cancer because most patients experiencing these symptoms have malignant gastric outlet obstruction (pancreatic, duodenal, or gastric cancer). Evaluation includes EGD and biopsy, upper gastrointestinal fluoroscopy with oral barium and CT. Endoscopic dilation and medical ulcer treatment can delay operation for months or years in at least half the patients with benign gastric outlet obstruction from duodenal ulcer.

Surgical Treatment

The gold standard operation for obstructing duodenal ulcer is vagotomy and antrectomy (V/A), but vagotomy and gastrojejunostomy (V/GJ) is a very good alternative. The advantage of V/A is lower recurrence rate and reassurance that the cause of the obstruction is benign. The disadvantage is higher operative mortality risk. The advantage of V/GJ is a lower operative mortality and the potential for reversal of the GJ in the event that dumping becomes intolerable. Another advantage is that V/GJ can be done laparoscopically. A disadvantage of V/GJ is that obstructing cancer may be missed, and marginal ulcer may occur.

Vagotomy and antrectomy can be done through an upper midline or transverse incision. A mechanical retractor is helpful. Exploration of the gastroduodenal area for any evidence of malignancy is done. We prefer to do the truncal vagotomy first. The peritoneum over the abdominal esophagus is incised, and the gastrohepatic ligament is opened above the hepatic vagal branches. Pulling down on these branches makes the anterior vagal trunk stand out, and it is clipped and severed easily; a short segment is sent to pathology. The

phrenoesophageal ligament then is opened along the right crus and the retroesophageal space entered where the posterior vagus is reliably located, clipped, and severed and a biopsy is performed.

Unless it appears that duodenal stump closure would be difficult, we then proceed with antrectomy; otherwise loop gastrojejunostomy may be performed. The lesser curvature neurovascular bundle is divided at the angularis incisura, and the right gastroepiploic arcade is divided on the greater curvature at a point directly opposite. This is where the stomach is transected with a green or purple or black GIA cartridge (sometimes the chronically obstructed stomach is very thick walled). The gastrocolic ligament attached to the antrum (i.e., the specimen) is taken down usually outside the gastroepiploic arcade and the right gastroepiploic pedicle ligated and divided. The right gastric is ligated and divided. The postpyloric duodenum then is transected with a GIA or TA stapler. The duodenal staple line typically is not oversewn, but we cover it with well-vascularized omentum held in place by two or three strategically placed sutures. Antecolic isoperistaltic Billroth II gastrojejunostomy is performed (efferent limb on lesser curvature side). We eschew Roux reconstruction with a large gastric remnant because we are concerned about marginal ulceration and/or delayed gastric emptying. We continue to place a closed suction right upper quadrant (RUQ) drain, although routine peritoneal drainage after gastrectomy is not supported by clinical evidence.

Loop gastrojejunostomy is done to the dependent greater gastric curvature. We divide the little branches from the gastroepiploic to the stomach for a length of 6 to 8 cm, creating a target for the hand-sewn or stapled antecolic isoperistaltic gastrojejunostomy. Patients with obstructing chronic duodenal ulcer disease who are treated with vagotomy and gastrojejunostomy should be followed closely for 2 years to ensure that an obstructing cancer was not missed. We also continue some form of acid suppression despite the vagotomy to guard against marginal ulceration.

DIFFICULT DUODENAL STUMP

The routine closure of the proximal duodenum during distal gastrectomy is accomplished most easily with a GIA or TA type stapler (blue cartridge). A two-layer suture closure is also straightforward in the routine case. However, occasionally ulcer location or size or the extensiveness of the inflammation and/or scar may render secure duodenal closure very difficult. Although best avoided, this situation can test the mettle of the experienced surgeon, who knows that operative mortality skyrockets with postoperative duodenal leakage. If the ulcer has destroyed the posterior duodenal wall, the anterior edge of the open duodenum is sewn to the proximal or distal "lip" of the ulcer with interrupted suture. Secure hemostasis in the ulcer bed must be accomplished. The integrity of the closure is tested by placing the tip of the nasogastric tube at the ligament of Treitz (through the gastrojejunostomy) and distending the duodenum with air. Additional sutures may be necessary to render the duodenal closure air tight. Then healthy omentum is sewn over the closure.

Postoperative duodenal decompression may be accomplished via duodenostomy placed retrograde through the proximal jejunum (our preference) or placed in the lateral duodenum ("lateral duodenostomy"). Only as a last resort should the duodenal stump be closed around a tube ("end duodenostomy") because leakage is the rule. Jejunal serosal patch is typically not helpful in closing the difficult duodenum, but a Roux limb anastomosed to the end of the open duodenum occasionally can be useful. Gastrostomy and feeding jejunostomy should be considered in patients with difficult duodenal closure. Although the aforementioned NG tube, strategically positioned with the tip in the afferent limb near the distal duodenum, can be relied on for postoperative decompression of the *routine* duodenal closure, it should not be relied on as the sole means of duodenal decompression for the unusually difficult duodenal stump.

SUGGESTED READINGS

Bingener J, Ibrahim-zada I. Natural orifice transluminal endoscopic surgery for intra-abdominal emergency conditions. *Br J Surg.* 2014;101:e80-e89.

Buck DL, Vester-Andersen M, Moller MH. Surgical delay is a critical determinant of survival in perforated peptic ulcer. *Br J Surg.* 2013;100:1045-1049.

Cheng H-C, Wu C-T, Chang W-L, et al. Double oral esomeprazole after a 3 day intravenous esomeprazole infusion reduces recurrent peptic ulcer bleeding in high risk patients: a randomized controlled study. *Gut.* 2014;63:1864-1872.

Rockall TA, Logan RF, Devlin HB, et al. Risk assessment after acute upper gastrointestinal hemorrhage. *Gut.* 1996;38:316-321.

Schroder VT, Pappas TN, Vaslef SN, et al. Vagotomy/drainage is superior to local oversew in patients who require emergency surgery for bleeding peptic ulcers. *Ann Surg.* 2014;259:1111-1118.

Soreide K, Thorsen K, Soreide JA. Strategies to improve the outcome of emergency surgery for perforated peptic ulcer. *Br J Surg.* 2014;101: e51-e64.

Wang YR, Richter JE, Dempsey DT. Trends and outcomes of hospitalizations for peptic ulcer disease in the United States, 1993 to 2006. *Ann Surg.* 2010;251:51-58.

Wilhelmsen M, Moller MH, Rosenstock S. Surgical complications after open and laparoscopic surgery for perforated peptic ulcer. *Br J Surg.* 2015;102: 382-387.

THE MANAGEMENT OF THE ZOLLINGER-ELLISON SYNDROME

Jeffrey A. Norton, MD, Geoffrey W. Krampitz, MD, and Robert T. Jensen, MD

■ INDICATIONS

Zollinger-Ellison Syndrome (ZES) is a syndrome of severe peptic ulcer disease and diarrhea caused by gastrin hypersecretion. In 1955 Zollinger and Ellison reported cases of pancreatic neuroendocrine tumors and gastric acid hypersecretion in association with unusual jejunal peptic ulcer disease. These recurrent ulcers were refractory to conventional acid-reduction surgery and ultimately required total gastrectomy for symptomatic control. Zollinger and Ellison postulated that pancreatic tumors were the cause of the severe peptic ulcer disease in these patients. It is now known that these tumors were gastrinomas.

Gastrinoma is the second most common functional neuroendocrine tumor with an incidence of 1 to 3 cases per million. ZES has been proposed to be the underlying cause in approximately 0.1% to 1% of patients with peptic ulcer disease, but most studies show it is less frequent. Because of an increased awareness of Zollinger-Ellison syndrome and accurate immunoassays for gastrin, gastrinoma increasingly is diagnosed. However, mean time from symptoms to diagnosis is still 8 years, so improvements are needed.

ZES occurs in sporadic and familial forms. Approximately 20% of patients with ZES have the familial inherited form as part of multiple endocrine neoplasia type 1 (MEN1); 50% of patients with MEN1 have ZES, making gastrinoma the most common functional neuroendocrine tumor in MEN1. Thus, during the workup for ZES, MEN1 always must be excluded.

Most (80%) gastrinomas are found within the gastrinoma triangle, an imaginary triangle that includes the head of the pancreas and the duodenum. Furthermore, primary gastrinomas have been reported in ectopic, extra-pancreatic, extra-intestinal sites, including stomach, bile duct, ovary, lung, heart, and lymph nodes. Occult gastrinomas are found most commonly in the duodenum. In contrast to the original studies of ZES, most gastrinomas (70% to 95%) are now found in the duodenum, not the pancreas. Furthermore, most occur in the first portion of the duodenum, and they decrease in number as you progress distally. Duodenal gastrinomas are often smaller than pancreatic tumors. Duodenal gastrinomas more commonly spread to lymph nodes and pancreatic tumors more commonly to liver. In MEN1, both pancreatic (5% to 15%) and duodenal (85% to 95%) gastrinomas occur and are multiple. Primary gastrinomas have been described in lymph nodes. Whether these represent lymph node primary tumors or metastases from occult pancreatic or duodenal tumors is controversial. However, patients have been cured of ZES by removal of only lymph nodes, suggesting that true lymph node primary gastrinomas can occur. Characteristics of gastrinomas are summarized in Table 1.

Gastrinomas are characteristically slow growing and well differentiated and have low proliferative grade (Ki67 1% to 2% to more than 90%), but most (60% to 90%) are malignant, as defined by metastases. Most patients have lymph node, liver, or distant metastases at the time of diagnosis. Further, in a minority of patients (approximately 25%), the tumors pursue an aggressive course. Gastrinomas have lymph node metastases in 50% to 80% of patients, but unlike most cancers, lymph node metastases have minimal impact on survival. Liver metastases have the most detrimental prognosis. Pancreatic gastrinomas that are less frequent have a higher incidence of liver metastases than the more common duodenal gastrinomas (50% vs 10%), whereas duodenal gastrinomas have a higher incidence of lymph node metastases (40% to 70%). In addition, gastrinomas to the left of the superior mesenteric artery more commonly metastasize to the liver than tumors within the gastrinoma triangle. Pancreatic gastrinomas have a poorer prognosis than duodenal tumors because liver metastases have a direct negative impact on survival. Patients without any liver metastases had a 95% 20-year survival, whereas patients with diffuse bilobar liver metastases had a 10-year survival of only 15%. Patients who had a solitary liver metastasis or fewer than five discrete metastases in both liver lobes had an intermediate survival (60% at 15 years). The extent of liver involvement is therefore the most important predictor of survival (Figure 1).

Patients with ZES commonly also have peptic ulcer disease. Gastrinomas secrete unregulated amounts of gastrin that stimulate the parietal cells to produce acid, which results in peptic ulceration and epigastric abdominal pain. Excessive acid secretion also results in diarrhea and malabsorption, so patients lose weight. Reflux disease and esophagitis with or without stricture can occur. Approximately 20% of ZES patients have MEN1, and this syndrome always must be excluded. A family history of ulcers and peptic ulceration occurring

TABLE 1: Characteristics of Gastrinoma

Incidence (people/million/year)	1-3
Hormone	Gastrin
Signs or symptoms	Peptic ulcer
Location (%)	
Duodenum	60-95
Pancreas	20
Lymph node only	10
Malignant (%)	60-90
MEN1 (%)	20

MEN1, multiple endocrine neoplasia type 1.

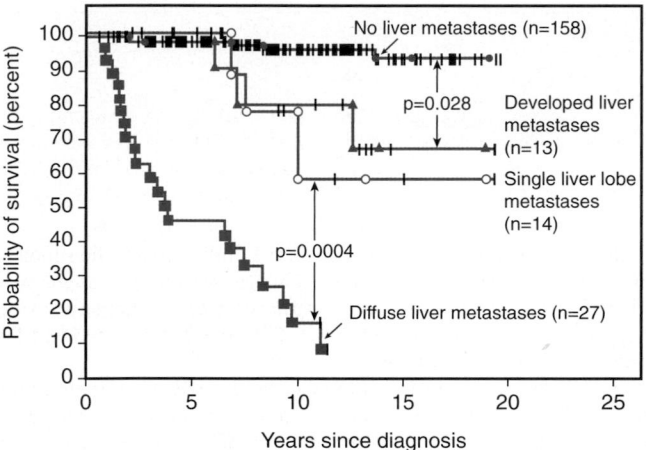

FIGURE 1 Survival of patients with liver metastases from gastrinoma.
(Modified from Norton JA, Jensen RT. Resolved and unresolved controversies in the surgical management of patients with Zollinger Ellison syndrome. Ann Surg. 2004;240:757-773.)

at a young age are clues to MEN1. Further, peptic ulcers in association with primary hyperparathyroidism and/or kidney stones, pituitary tumors, benign thyroid tumors, benign and malignant adrenocortical tumors, lipomas, and cutaneous angiofibromas are suggestive of MEN1 and should be excluded.

Patients with ZES usually have a solitary ulcer in the proximal duodenum similar to patients with non-ZES peptic ulcer disease. However, "atypical" presentations can occur with multiple ulcers or ulcers in unusual locations such as the jejunum. In addition, recurrent ulcers or persistent ulcers with appropriate treatment may occur in ZES. Any patient with unusual peptic ulcer disease should be screened for ZES. In addition, patients with peptic ulcer disease and diarrhea should be studied. However, some patients (20%) with ZES have only diarrhea and not peptic ulceration. Because ZES is rare and clinicians fail to consider its possibility, there is still a failure to diagnose it. The mean time from symptoms to diagnosis is 8 years in most studies.

◾ TECHNIQUES

The evaluation of a patient in whom ZES is suspected begins by obtaining a fasting serum concentration of gastrin. Hypergastrinemia occurs in almost all patients with ZES (if no recent resection,

chemotherapy) and is defined as a serum gastrin concentration greater than 100 pg/mL. Therefore a normal fasting serum gastrin concentration excludes ZES, but an elevated fasting gastrin alone does not establish ZES because numerous other more frequent conditions can cause this. Antacid medications such as histamine receptor antagonists or proton pump inhibitors must be discontinued and may cause a false-positive increase in serum gastrin concentration. Achlorhydria is a common false-positive cause of hypergastrinemia. Either gastric acid secretion or stomach pH level must be measured to exclude this condition. A normal adult basal acid output (BAO) is approximately 2 to 5 mEq/hr. A BAO greater than 15 mEq/hr (>5 mEq/hr in patients who have undergone previous acid-reducing operations) is diagnostic of ZES. Measurement of gastric pH at the time of endoscopy is a simpler, but less accurate, indicator of gastric acid hypersecretion. A gastric pH of more than 3 essentially excludes ZES, whereas a pH of 2 or less is consistent with ZES. All acid secretion–reducing medications (PPIs and H2 receptor antagonists) must be stopped before measuring acid output or stomach pH levels. The proper method for diagnosis of ZES is controversial. This occurred because abruptly stopping acid antisecretory drugs in a patient subsequently found to have ZES can lead to severe acid peptic side effects and is performed best by a group well versed in the diagnosis of ZES or with coverage with H2 blocker for a few days until the effect of the PPI wears off.

To exclude MEN1, patients should be screened for primary hyperparathyroidism by measuring a serum ionized calcium and parathyroid hormone level. MEN1 patients with ZES usually have primary hyperparathyroidism as the first manifestation of MEN1. It generally occurs before ZES, but infrequently some patients have ZES as the initial manifestation of MEN1. Hypercalcemia from hyperparathyroidism can exacerbate significantly the symptoms of ZES and further elevate serum gastrin levels a result of the underlying gastrinoma. As such, the diagnosis of hyperparathyroidism coexistent with ZES may alter the surgical management of the associated conditions.

An increased fasting serum gastrin concentration (>100 pg/mL) and abnormally elevated BAO (>15 mEq/L) are the strongest criteria to establish the diagnosis of ZES. However, gastric acid secretion rarely is measured in most centers. Furthermore, many patients (60% to 70%) with ZES have elevated fasting serum gastrin concentrations that overlap with a number of other conditions (elevated onefold to tenfold). Currently gastric pH in combination with fasting serum gastrin levels usually are used to establish the diagnosis. In a patient with a gastric pH of 2 or less and gastrin levels more than tenfold elevated, the diagnosis is secure. If the fasting gastrin is less than tenfold elevated with a gastric pH of 2 or less, it is recommend that a secretin test and gastric acid secretory test be performed if possible. After an overnight fast, secretin is administered intravenously (2 U/kg), and blood samples are collected immediately before and at 2, 5, 10, and 15 minutes after giving the secretin. An increase in serum gastrin concentration of 120 pg/mL above baseline after the administration of secretin is consistent with ZES. The test sensitivity is 94% and a specificity of 100%.

The diagnosis of ZES depends on the biochemical studies and secretin test as outlined. However, localization of the primary tumor and identifying metastases are critical to developing appropriate surgical strategies. Localization of gastrinomas should begin with noninvasive imaging to assess the true extent of tumor spread and exclude unresectable metastatic disease. Invasive modalities then may be used to localize the primary tumor prior to surgery. The sensitivities of various tumor localization modalities are summarized in Table 2.

Ultrasonography is often the initial imaging study obtained during the workup of abdominal symptoms. It is noninvasive, relatively inexpensive, and readily available. However, it seldom images the gastrinoma. On ultrasound, gastrinomas appear as well-defined, homogeneous sonolucent masses. However, transabdominal ultrasound has a low sensitivity (<30%).

TABLE 2: Sensitivities of Gastrinoma Localization Studies

Study	% of Tumors Localized			
	Overall	Pancreas	Duodenum	Liver Metastases
PREOPERATIVE				
Noninvasive				
Transabdominal ultrasonography	20-30			14
Abdominal computed tomography	50	80	35	50
Abdominal magnetic resonance imaging	25			83
Octreoscan	71-90		50	
DOTA scan	>90	>90	>60-90	>90
Invasive				
Endoscopic ultrasonography	85	75-100	28-57	
INTRAOPERATIVE				
Palpation	65	91	60	
Intraoperative ultrasonography	83	95	58	
Duodenotomy	–	–	100	

Endoscopic ultrasound (EUS) is an invasive procedure that combines endoscopy and ultrasound to produce high-quality, detailed, cost-effective images of gastrinomas within the pancreas and liver. It is less effective at imaging duodenal gastrinomas. EUS has a sensitivity of 85% (range 75% to 100%) for detecting pancreatic gastrinomas but only 43% (range 28% to 57%) for detecting duodenal gastrinomas. The differences in sensitivities are due to the fact that the gastrinomas are easier to detect as sonolucent masses against an echo-dense uniform background of the pancreas compared with the duodenum, which is composed of solid, air, and gas. Intraoperative ultrasound (IOUS) is another endoscopic study with similar limitations. It is very useful for localizing intrapancreatic gastrinomas and detecting liver metastases. IOUS can localize pancreatic and liver tumors as small as 5 mm and is therefore a powerful adjunct for detecting tumors not identified during preoperative imaging. However like EUS, IOUS is poor at detecting duodenal gastrinomas and thus is no substitute for duodenotomy with direct intraluminal palpation.

Duodenotomy at the time of surgery is a critical maneuver to detect small duodenal gastrinomas. These tumors usually cause dimpling of the mucosa and feel like a firm nodule between the thumb and forefinger. A prospective study of patients revealed a significantly higher cure rate after duodenotomy, both immediately and long term. Duodenotomy was particularly important in the detection of small duodenal tumors, allowing localization of 90% of tumors smaller than 1 cm versus only 50% discovered on preoperative imaging. Duodenal wall gastrinomas occur in greatest density more proximally in the duodenum but may still occur in the distal duodenum. Regional lymph nodes should be systematically sampled because lymph node metastases may be inapparent at exploration and will be found in 55% of patients with duodenal tumors. If a duodenotomy is performed, gastrinomas ultimately can be found in nearly all patients.

Because of increased vascularity, gastrinomas are imaged as a bright mass on the arterial phase of intravenous contrast-enhanced computed tomography (CT). Overall, abdominal CT detects approximately 50% of primary gastrinomas. However, the sensitivity of CT depends greatly on tumor size, tumor location, and the presence of metastases. CT reliably detects gastrinomas larger than 3 cm in diameter, whereas tumors smaller than 1 cm in diameter rarely are detected. Intermediate tumors between 1 and 3 cm are identified in 30% of cases. Primary gastrinomas that arise within the pancreas are identified much more reliably than those in extrapancreatic, extrahepatic locations (80% vs 35%). In addition, CT scanning identifies only 50% of liver metastases.

Gastrinomas are relatively hypervascular when compared with normal intra-abdominal tissues, and therefore gastrinomas have lower signal intensity on T1 imaging and higher signal intensity on T2 imaging compared with surrounding organs. Although abdominal MRI has a low sensitivity (25%) in localizing primary gastrinomas, it is particularly useful in detecting hepatic metastases (sensitivity of 83%). Gastrinoma metastases in the liver appear bright with distinct peripheral enhancement on dynamic T2-weighted images. In addition, MRI is especially useful to differentiate gastrinoma metastases within the liver from hemangiomas.

Somatostatin receptor scintigraphy (SRS), also called *octreoscan* or the *new DOTA scan,* is a nuclear medicine study for localizing primary and metastatic gastrinoma. SRS images gastrinoma based on the density of type 2 somatostatin receptors. Octreoscan has a sensitivity of 71%, specificity of 86%, positive predictive value of 85% and a negative predictive value of 52%. With a high pretest probability, as in the setting of ZES, octreoscan has an improved sensitivity of approximately 90%, specificity approaching 100%, and positive predictive value near 100%. The sensitivity of octreoscan for gastrinoma exceeds all other imaging modalities combined (angiography, MRI, CT, ultrasonography), except for the new and very promising DOTA scan.

Recent studies show that somatostatin receptor imaging with the DOTA scan using gallium (Ga)[68] DOTATOC PET/CT results in better imaging of the true extent of tumor in ZES patients. Because it is a whole body study, it is especially sensitive for metastases and will pick up primary tumors as well. It is more sensitive than octreoscan that uses ^{111}In-labeled pentetreotide with SPECT imaging. Ga[68] DOTATOC PET/CT was originally available only in Europe and now it is becoming increasingly available in the United States. True results are not yet known but, in our initial experience, are very positive. It images more than 90% of primary and metastatic gastrinomas (Figure 2). Currently it is the preoperative imaging study of choice for gastrinomas.

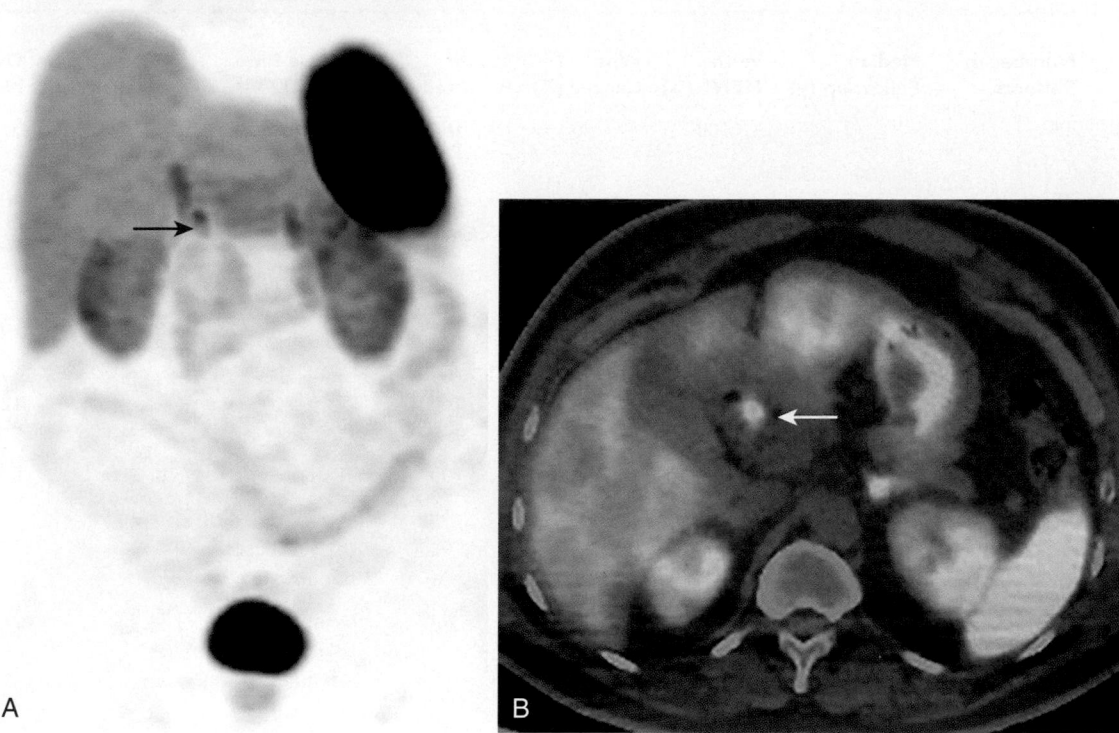

FIGURE 2 DOTA scan for imaging gastrinoma in a patient with Zollinger-Ellison syndrome (ZES). Patient with ZES and negative imaging, including a negative octreoscan. He decided not to have surgery until his tumor was imageable. DOTATOC PET scan was performed, and it identified the small gastrinoma in the first portion of the duodenum on the planar image (**A,** *arrow*) and the PET/CT scan (**B,** *arrow*). Subsequent surgery removed the tumor and adjacent lymph nodes.

■ RESULTS OF TREATMENT

Control of acid hypersecretion is the initial step in the treatment of patients with ZES. Proton pump inhibitors (PPIs) have made medical management of gastric acid hypersecretion possible in all patients with ZES. Oral omeprazole and intravenous pantoprazole must be dose adjusted in patients with ZES to normalize BAO levels to less than 15 mEq/hr (less than 5 mEq/hr in patients who have reflux esophagitis or who have had prior acid-reducing operations). Measuring BAO after initiating drug therapy is necessary because relief of symptoms alone is not a reliable indicator of effective acid control. The usual dose of omeprazole is 40 mg PO bid. Conversely, if acid hypersecretion is controlled, epigastric discomfort resolves, ulcers heal, and diarrhea ceases in virtually all ZES patients.

In MEN1, hypercalcemia resulting from primary hyperparathyroidism can exacerbate significantly the signs and symptoms of ZES. It further elevates serum gastrin levels resulting from the gastrinoma. Thus, in MEN1 ZES patients with coexistent primary hyperparathyroidism, neck exploration for 3 and ½ gland parathyroidectomy should be performed first before surgery aimed directly at gastrinoma removal. In these patients, subtotal parathyroidectomy (3 and ½ glands) can decrease significantly end-organ effects of hypergastrinemia, allowing for better medical control of ZES and its symptoms.

Gastrinomas associated with MEN1 are multiple, small, usually originate in the duodenum, and frequently develop lymph node metastases; however, these tumors may be more indolent than sporadic tumors and may have a more favorable long-term prognosis. In patients with MEN1 and ZES, surgical resection is seldom curative (0 to 10%) but may be effective to prevent or decrease the development of liver metastases. Increasing tumor size (>2 cm) correlates with progression to liver metastasis, which in turn is the strongest

predictor of survival (see Figure 1). Consequently, in patients who have MEN1, surgery is recommended only if there is an identifiable tumor greater than 2 cm. The operation should include resection of body and tail pancreatic NETs, enucleation of palpable pancreatic head tumors, duodenotomy with excision of duodenal tumors, and peri-pancreatic lymph node sampling. The goal of such an operation is to prevent liver metastases and thus decrease tumor-related mortality, not to cure ZES. However, some studies have documented cure of ZES in MEN1 patients by performing Whipple pancreaticoduodenectomy. We do not favor that approach because the long-term survival is excellent with the surgical approach described above and the morbidity is less (Table 3).

All patients with sporadic gastrinoma who do not have unresectable metastatic disease should undergo exploratory laparotomy for potential cure of ZES. A recent study demonstrated that routine surgical removal of gastrinoma increased survival by increasing disease-related survival and decreasing the development of distant metastases. A recent study shows if the diagnosis is made properly, even patients with negative preoperative imaging studies without MEN1 benefit from surgery. Surgical exploration and duodenotomy should be performed even in patients without an identifiable tumor on preoperative imaging, but with clear biochemical evidence of ZES because of the high probability of an occult duodenal gastrinoma. Gastrinomas localized to the duodenum may be locally resected with adequate margins. Resection should allow for nonconstricting closure of the remaining duodenum, and special attention is paid to avoid injury to the ampulla of Vater. Regional lymph nodes should be sampled and excised systematically, because lymph node metastases may be unapparent at exploration and are found in 55% of patients with duodenal tumors. Resection of a single duodenal gastrinoma and regional lymph node dissection resulted in a cure in 60% of patients with sporadic

TABLE 3: Outcomes of Surgery for Gastrinoma in Sporadic and MEN1 ZES

Author (year)	Number of Patients	Median Follow-up (y)	With MEN1 (%)	With Cancer (%)	Tumor Resected (%)	Disease-Free Survival (%)	Disease-Related Mortality (%)	Overall Mortality (%)
Norton et al (2001)	48	7	100	5	100	19 immediately, 0 at 5 y	2	3
Kisker et al (1998)	25	5	8	48	96	44	0 no liver mets 72 + liver mets	NR
McArthur et al (1996)	22	16	14	44	41	14	NR	19 at 10 y
Jaskowiak et al (1996)	17	2.3	13	94	100	35	6	12
MacFarlane et al (1995)	10	NR	100	60	70	NR	NR	0
Mortellaro et al (2009)	12	18	100	8	92	8 at 3 y, 0 at last follow-up	0	33
Norton et al (2006)	195 (160 surgery, 35 no surgery)	12	21 vs 26	54	94	51 immediately, 41 at last follow-up	1 vs 23	21 vs 54
Thompson (1998)	40 (40 surgery)	15	100	43	NR	68	0	97 at 5 y 94 at 10 y 94 at 15 y

MEN1, multiple endocrine neoplasia type 1; ZES, Zollinger-Ellison Syndrome.

gastrinoma. Multiple duodenal gastrinomas localized to either the upper or lower aspects of the duodenum may undergo partial resection of the duodenum. For patients with large tumors or ampullary involvement, a pylorus-preserving or standard pancreaticoduodenectomy may be indicated. Patients with pancreatic disease should undergo mobilization of the pancreas and palpation with intraoperative ultrasound. For disease in the body and tail of the pancreas, the patient should undergo a distal pancreatectomy with regional lymph node excision. Pancreatic head and neck tumors not involving major ductal or vascular structures are enucleated. For bulky large tumors localized to the pancreatic head, a pylorus-preserving pancreaticoduodenectomy may be necessary (results in Table 3).

Because 60% to 90% of gastrinomas are malignant, management of advanced disease is another significant problem. At the time of diagnosis of ZES, 25% to 33% of patients have liver metastases with 5% to 15% limited to one lobe of the liver. In these patients, cytoreductive surgery should be considered if all visible tumor can be removed safely. In contrast to patients with pancreatic adenocarcinoma, recent studies show many patients with possible vascular involvement on imaging studies by the gastrinoma will benefit from surgery because the tumor can be removed in most cases without vascular reconstruction. Other cytoreductive strategies, such as transarterial chemoembolization and radiofrequency ablation, may be performed preoperatively or in lieu of an operation in the case of liver metastases. Surgery remains the primary option for patients, because alternative therapies, including chemotherapy, radiofrequency ablation, transarterial chemoembolization, biotherapy, polypeptide radionuclide receptor therapy, anti-angiogenic therapy, and selective internal radiotherapy, have had some responses but have failed to demonstrate a long-term survival benefit.

■ SUMMARY AND RECOMMENDATIONS

In summary, ZES is a syndrome caused by gastrinoma usually located within the gastrinoma triangle and associated with symptoms of peptic ulcer disease and diarrhea. The diagnosis of ZES is achieved by measuring fasting levels of serum gastrin, gastric pH or basal acid output, and secretin testing. Because of the high association of ZES with MEN1, hyperparathyroidism must be excluded by obtaining a serum calcium and parathyroid hormone level. Treatment of ZES consists of medical control of symptoms with PPIs and evaluation for potentially curative surgical intervention. Noninvasive imaging studies including DOTA scan, SRS, CT, and MRI should be performed initially to evaluate for metastases and identify resectable disease. Invasive imaging modalities such as EUS may be performed to further evaluate primary tumors. IOUS, palpation, and duodenotomy are used for intraoperative localization of gastrinomas. In patients with MEN1, surgical resection should be pursued only if there is an identifiable tumor larger than 2 cm. All patients with resectable sporadic gastrinoma should undergo surgical exploration. In patients with liver metastases, surgery should be performed if all visible tumor can be removed safely.

SUGGESTED READINGS

Ito T, Igarashi H, Jensen RT. Zollinger-Ellison syndrome: recent advances and controversies. *Curr Opin Gastroenterol*. 2013;29:650-661.

Jensen RT, Cadiot G, Brandi ML, et al. ENETS Consensus guidelines for the management of patients with digestive neuroendocrine neoplasms: functional pancreatic endocrine tumor syndromes. *Neuroendocrinology*. 2012;95:98-119.

Norton JA, Alexander HR, Fraker DL, Venzon DJ, Gibril F, Jensen RT. Possible primary lymph node gastrinoma: occurrence, natural history, and predictive factors: a prospective study. *Ann Surg.* 2003;237:650-657, discussion 657-659.

Norton JA, Fraker DL, Alexander HR, Jensen RT. Value of surgery in patients with negative imaging and sporadic Zollinger Ellison syndrome. *Ann Surg.* 2012;256:509-517.

Norton JA, Fraker DL, Alexander HR, et al. Surgery to cure the Zollinger-Ellison syndrome. *N Engl J Med.* 1999;341:635-644.

Norton JA, Fraker DL, Alexander HR, et al. Surgery increases survival in patients with gastrinoma. *Ann Surg.* 2006;244:410-419.

Norton JA, Jensen RT. Resolved and unresolved controversies in the surgical management of patients with Zollinger-Ellison syndrome. *Ann Surg.* 2004;240:757-773.

Stabile BE, Passaro E Jr. Benign and malignant gastrinoma. *Am J Surg.* 1985;149:144-150.

Thompson NW, Vinik AI, Eckhauser FE. Microgastrinomas of the duodenum. A cause of failed operations for the Zollinger-Ellison syndrome. *Ann Surg.* 1989;209:396-404.

Wolfe MM, Alexander RW, McGuigan JE. Extrapancreatic, extraintestinal gastrinoma: effective treatment by surgery. *N Engl J Med.* 1982;306:1533-1536.

THE MANAGEMENT OF THE MALLORY-WEISS SYNDROME

Alan H. Tieu, MD, Vivek Kumbhari, MD, and Mouen A. Khashab, MD

■ DEFINITION, INCIDENCE, AND PATHOPHYSIOLOGY

The Mallory-Weiss syndrome (MWS) originally was described by Kenneth Mallory and Soma Weiss in 1929, who described patients with lacerations of the gastric cardia resulting from forceful retching and vomiting. It has been further defined as linear mucosal or submucosal lacerations of the gastroesophageal junction (GEJ) that may lead to upper gastrointestinal (UGI) bleeding. The syndrome should not be confused with Boerhaave's syndrome, which is defined as distal esophageal perforation as a result of vomiting.

Multiple studies have shown a 5% to 15% incidence rate of MWS in patients with acute UGI bleeding. Mallory-Weiss tears are the second most common cause of nonvariceal upper GI bleeding, superseded only by peptic ulcer disease. Hiatal hernia confers the greatest risk for developing Mallory-Weiss tear and can be found in 40% to 50% of cases. MWS usually occurs in the fifth and sixth decades of life.

The pathophysiology of Mallory-Weiss tears is thought to be the result of the rapid development of a large gradient between elevated intragastric pressure and negative intrathoracic pressure at the GEJ, which occurs in vomiting and retching. The forceful elevation of the GEJ above the diaphragm leads to the dilation and subsequent tearing of the gastroesophageal mucosa. Any bodily action that results in an abrupt increase in intra-abdominal pressure and gastric herniation may cause a Mallory-Weiss tear. These actions include forceful coughing, retching during endoscopy, and straining. Other mechanisms include direct trauma at the GEJ through the use of instruments such as a transesophageal echocardiography (TEE) probe. Alcohol and aspirin use may potentiate any tear and result in clinically significant bleeding.

■ CLINICAL MANIFESTATIONS AND DIAGNOSES

Patients generally present with hematemesis or coffee-ground emesis and typically have a history of recent nonbloody vomiting followed by hematemesis. However, as many as 50% of patients may not have a history of vomiting preceding hematemesis, and one fourth may have no identifiable risk factors. Mallory-Weiss tears do not often present with abdominal pain because the tears usually extend only to the submucosa. Although most patients present with hematemesis, 10% of patients may present with melena alone.

Flexible endoscopy is the current standard means for evaluation of patients with UGI bleeding. A standard view of the esophagus and a retroflexed view of the GEJ are needed to evaluate for tears. Notably, most tears occur below the GEJ, distally into a hiatal hernia sac, and along the lesser curve of the stomach. A retroflexed view in the stomach and GEJ may provide better visualization than the forward viewing position. Most tears occur within 2 cm of the GEJ; however, distal tear into the proximal portion of the stomach is common when a large hiatal hernia is present. Typically, a single tear is seen at endoscopy, most commonly along the lesser curve aspect of the cardia, although multiple tears may occur in up to 10% of patients. Most tears average 0.5 to 2.0 cm but may be up to 5 cm in length. Endoscopic visualization of Mallory-Weiss tears can include a clean base, oozing, or active spurting lesions (Figure 1).

■ PROGNOSIS AND TREATMENT

The prognosis of MWS is usually favorable; however, the reported mortality rates range from a low of 1.5% to as high as 10%. One prospective comparative study reported a 30-day mortality rate of 5.3% in MWS versus 4.6% for patients with peptic ulcer bleeding (p = 0.578), indicating similar mortality outcome. Identified risk factors for mortality include advanced age, low hemoglobin level, shock at presentation, and endoscopic finding of active bleeding.

In general, bleeding resulting from MWS is self-limited and can be treated with conservative medical management. Superficial mucosal Mallory-Weiss tears can start healing within hours and can heal completely within 48 hours. In general, medical treatment for patients with a Mallory-Weiss tear includes antiemetics if they have nausea or vomiting and a proton-pump inhibitor (PPI) to accelerate mucosal healing by raising intragastric pH to improve coagulation. Indications for endoscopic therapy include stigmata of active bleeding with either spurting or an oozing lesion.

Endoscopic therapy is the core treatment of MWS. In recent studies, surgical intervention is necessary in the less than 1% of patients given the excellent outcome by endoscopic techniques with reported 90% to 100% rate of successful hemostasis. Endoscopic hemostasis is accomplished with various techniques, including injection therapy, multipolar electrocoagulation, band ligation, hemoclipping, or combination treatment. Unfortunately, current data are insufficient to make a clear recommendation of one hemostasis modality over another.

Endoscopic injection therapy has been shown to significantly reduce further bleeding, transfusion requirements, and shorten the hospital stay as compared with medical management alone in MWS patients with high risk for persistent bleeding. In fact, randomized studies have shown that rebleeding occurred significantly more often in patients with a bleeding Mallory-Weiss tear who did not receive endoscopic hemostasis versus patients treated with epinephrine injection. Injection agents include vasoconstricting agents such as

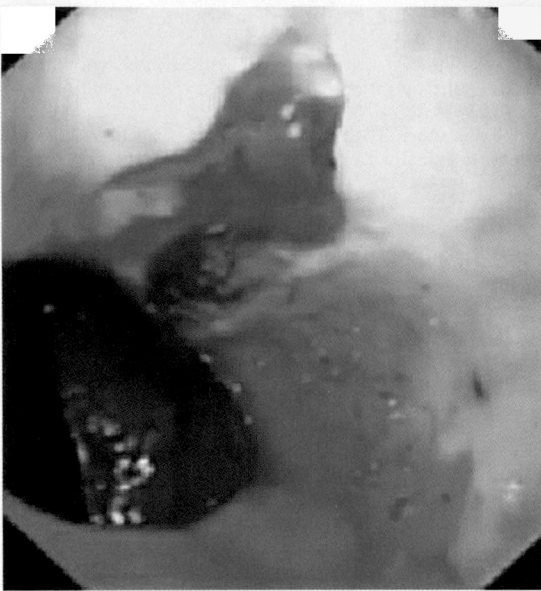

FIGURE 1 Endoscopic appearance of a Mallory-Weiss tear measured 2.5 cm in length with mild oozing. Note that the tear starts at the gastroesophageal junction and extends distally into the hiatal hernia.

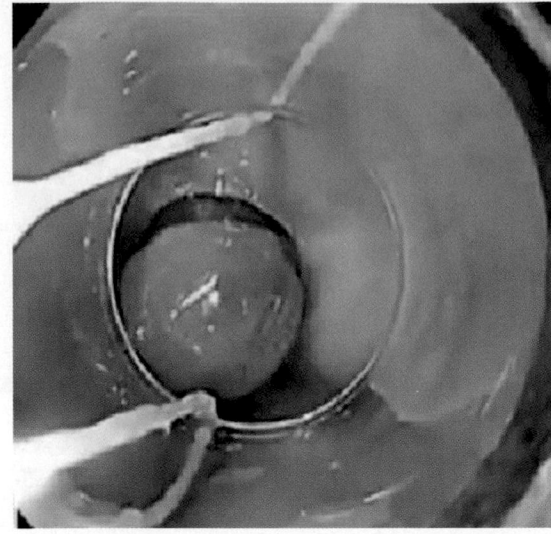

FIGURE 2 Endoscopic view through the endoscopic ligating device with deployed band encasing the tear.

epinephrine and sclerosing agents such as polidocanol or dehydrated ethanol. Epinephrine injection is used most commonly to treat Mallory-Weiss tears, although no optimal injection volume has been reported. In general, the endoscopic procedure of using epinephrine injection includes injection of 1 to 3 mL 1:10,000 epinephrine, prepared by mixing 1 mL 1:1000 epinephrine and 9 mL 0.9% saline solution, injecting into the area surrounding and close to the bleeding points with an injection needle. After therapy, the bleeding points are irrigated gently with sterile water to evaluate the hemostatic effect, and the process may be repeated as needed. The reported rates of primary hemostasis range from 93% to 100%, but rebleeding has been reported to occur in 5.8% to 44% of cases. Given the relatively high rebleeding rate, we recommend that epinephrine injection be combined with a second endoscopic therapy.

Electrocoagulation allows the simultaneous application of heat and pressure to the bleeding lesion and has been used as endoscopic therapy for MWS. However, the reported rate of initial hemostasis is 83.3% for patients with actively bleeding MWS, which is relatively lower than other therapeutic modalities. One explanation is that the application of the electrocoagulation in a wet field, as occurs when there is significant bleeding, decreases the effectiveness of coagulation because the liquid dissipates the heat quickly, thereby reducing the effect on the tissue. In addition, the correct positioning of the device has been relatively difficult for lesions located on the lesser curve of the cardia portion. Another consideration is that repeated coagulation has the risk of producing transmural injury and perforation because the esophagus lacks serosa and is very thin at the tear site.

Endoscopic band ligation (EBL), commonly used in variceal bleeding, also has been used to treat nonvariceal bleeding (Figure 2). For EBL, a single-band ligator often is used with or without an overtube. After endoscopic identification of the lesion, the endoscope then is reinserted with attachment of the band ligator. The hood of the ligator is placed over the bleeding site with suction applied and deployment of the elastic band. Typically, one or two elastic bands are used. One retrospective study comparing the efficacy of EBL versus hemoclips plus epinephrine in 56 MWS patients revealed that primary endoscopic hemostasis was achieved equivalently by both methods, but recurrent bleeding occurred in 18% in the hemoclips plus epinephrine group versus 0 in the EBL group (p = 0.02). The probable explanation for higher recurrent bleeding in hemoclips plus

epinephrine group was that treatment of Mallory-Weiss tears at the GEJ is probably more technically challenging when a hemoclip is used compared with band ligation. The authors suggested EBL as the treatment modality of choice for endoscopic treatment of bleeding MWS.

Endoscopic hemoclip placement has been studied as a therapeutic method for controlling bleeding from MWS. Clips include through-the-scope hemoclips (Figure 3) and the over-the-scope-clip (OTSC) (Ovesco Endoscopy, Tübingen, Germany). This "bear-claw" system is a new device developed for closure of luminal GI defects and hemostasis. However, there is no dedicated study investigating the efficacy and safety of OTSC in managing MWS patients. Hemoclip placement versus epinephrine injection has been compared in a randomized trial of 35 MWS patients and demonstrated similar primary hemostasis rates (bleeding, spurting, or oozing lesions), and the rebleeding rate was also similar. In a 2008 prospective, randomized trial comparing the efficacy and safety of endoscopic hemoclip placement and EBL in 41 MWS patients, it was concluded that both methods were equally effective and safe.

For patients with persistent bleeding refractory to endoscopic therapy, interventional embolotherapy may be considered as the next treatment option. Diagnostic angiography for UGI bleeding is centered on the anatomy of the celiac artery. Specifically for MWS, the left gastric artery (which arises from the celiac artery) is the primary target because it provides branches to the distal esophagus and fundus of the stomach. Small case series of embolotherapy for acute bleeding resulting from Mallory-Weiss tears reported technical success of 94% and clinical success of 88%. In comparison, the overall technical success rates and clinical success rates for embolization of nonvariceal UGI bleeding and of all causes are 92% to 100% and 51% to 94%, respectively. General complications of embolotherapy for MWS include access site hematoma, pseudoaneurysms, arterial dissection, contrast allergic reactions, and nephrotoxicity with the same frequency as with other endovascular procedures. Specifically for MWS, the risk of significant ischemia or stricture could be increased when potential collateral vessels are damaged from previous upper abdominal surgery, radiotherapy, or severe atherosclerosis.

■ SURGERY

Surgery for the treatment of MWS rarely is needed. It usually is reserved for patients who failed both endoscopic therapy and interventional angiotherapy (or when the latter is not available). Prior

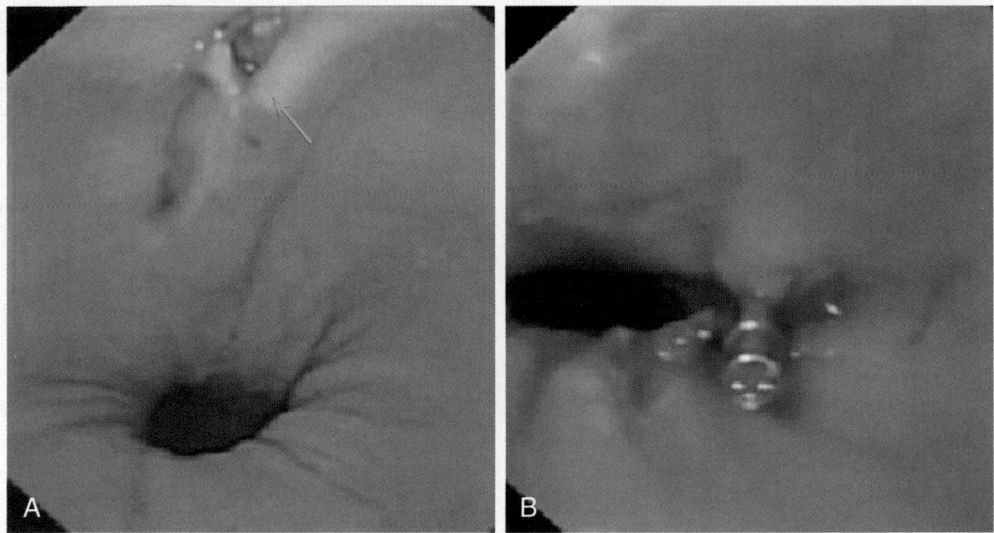

FIGURE 3 A, Endoscopic view of a Mallory-Weiss tear *(blue arrow)* at the gastroesophageal junction. **B,** After hemoclip deployed at the lesion with good hemostasis.

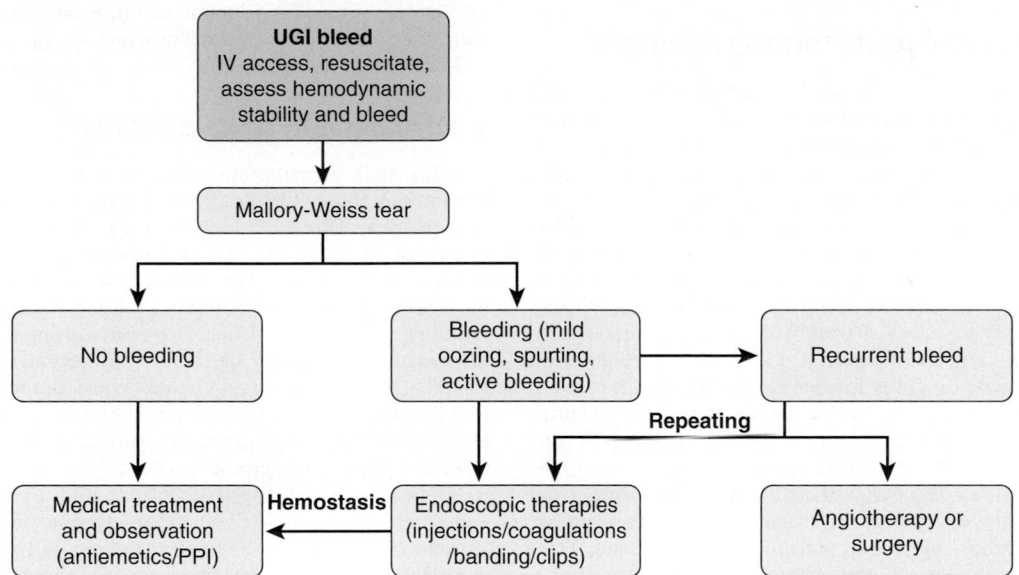

FIGURE 4 Treatment algorithm for Mallory-Weiss syndrome. *IV,* Intravenous; *PPI,* proton-pump inhibitor; *UGI,* upper gastrointestinal.

studies report a high rate of morbidity and mortality associated with the surgical treatment for acute UGI bleeding with 50% to 55% of patients suffering postoperative complications and 10% to 30% an in-hospital mortality.

Surgical approach to bleeding from Malloy-Weiss tears traditionally has been performed through open surgery with a high anterior longitudinal gastrotomy to gain access and visualization of the mucosa at the GEJ. Localization of the site of bleeding before laparotomy is imperative. Thus intraoperative endoscopy often is used in conjunction to identify the location and source of bleeding. Once the lesion is identified, simple oversewing technique of the tear with absorbable sutures is usually the technique of choice. Inspection for other sources of hemorrhage is advisable because Mallory-Weiss tears can coexist with other common causes of UGI bleeding. Recently, combined laparoscopic-endoscopic techniques for treating Mallory-Weiss tears have been reported. Laparoscopy is performed with port placement to access the abdominal cavity and GEJ. Endoscopy is used to localize the tear. Full-thickness absorbable sutures then are placed with endoscopic guidance over the bleeding mucosa.

Figure 4 describes our treatment algorithm for MWS. Initial management of acute UGI bleed includes early hemodynamic assessment and resuscitation. Once Mallory-Weiss tears are recognized endoscopically as the source of the UGI bleed, endoscopic therapy is the main treatment for bleeding tears. Recurrent bleeds may be managed by repeating endoscopic therapy before embolotherapy and/or surgery.

■ CONCLUSION

MWS is a relatively common cause of nonvariceal UGI bleeding, in which an abrupt rise in abdominal pressure caused by retching or vomiting induces linear tears near the GEJ. Because most patients stop bleeding spontaneously, mechanical treatment is reserved for those demonstrating active bleeding. When treatment is required, endoscopic therapy is the first-line therapy with excellent hemostasis rates. Embolotherapy is considered as the next line of treatment if endoscopic therapy fails. Surgery, which consists of simple oversewing of the bleeding mucosa, often is reserved as last resort.

SUGGESTED READINGS

Cho YS, Chai HS, Kim HK, et al. Endoscopic band ligation and endoscopic hemoclip placement for patients with Mallory-Weiss syndrome and active bleeding. *World J Gastroenterol.* 2008;14(3):2080-2084.

Clarke MG, Bunting D, Smart NJ, et al. The surgical management of acute upper gastrointestinal bleeding: a 12-year experience. *Int J Surg.* 2010;8:377-380.

Higuchi N, Akahoshi K, Sumida Y, et al. Endoscopic band ligation therapy for upper gastrointestinal bleeding related to Mallory-Weiss syndrome. *Surg Endosc.* 2006;20:1431-1434.

Lecleire S, Antonietti M, Iwanicki-Caron I, et al. Endoscopic band ligation could decrease recurrent bleeding in Mallory-Weiss syndrome as compared to haemostasis by hemoclips plus epinephrine. *Aliment Pharmacol Ther.* 2009;30:399-405.

Ljubicic N, Budimir I, Pavic T, et al. Mortality in high-risk patients with bleeding Mallory-Weiss syndrome is similar to that of peptic ulcer bleeding. Results of a prospective database study. *Scand J Gastroenterol.* 2014;49:458-464.

Shin JH. Recent update of embolization of upper gastrointestinal tract bleeding. *Korean J Radiol.* 2012;13(suppl 1):S31-S39.

Yin A, Li Y, Jiang Y, et al. Mallory-Weiss syndrome: clinical and endoscopic characteristics. *Eur J Intern Med.* 2012;23:e92-e96.

THE MANAGEMENT OF GASTRIC ADENOCARCINOMA

David W. McFadden, MD, and Bruce M. Brenner, MD

EPIDEMIOLOGY AND PATHOGENESIS

The incidence of gastric cancer in the United States has decreased considerably since the 1930s, when it was the leading cause of cancer mortality in the United States and Europe. In 2015, there will be an estimated 24,600 cases of and 10,700 deaths resulting from gastric cancer in the United States (Siegel et al, 2015). Worldwide, gastric cancer remains the fifth most common malignancy and third leading cause of cancer-related death (Siegel et al, 2015). Environmental and genetic factors play a role in gastric cancer development. There is considerable geographic variation in the incidence of gastric adenocarcinoma. Almost 50% of all cases worldwide occur in China. Japan, Korea, and areas of Central and South America also have high incidences, whereas gastric cancer is rare in North America, Australia, and portions of Northern Africa. In the United States the incidence is higher in men, as well as in certain ethnic groups, including African Americans, Hispanics, and Native Americans.

Overall, the incidence of gastric cancer has been decreasing. This is due predominantly to a decrease in distal gastric cancer, whereas the incidence of proximal, or gastric cardia tumors, is increasing. This suggests that the cause of gastric cancer may differ based on tumor location.

There are a number of known risk factors for gastric cancer. *Helicobacter pylori* infection increases the risk only of distal cancers. Other risk factors include gastric polyps, exposure to nitrosamines, tobacco use, previous gastric surgery, and pernicious anemia. Up to 15% of gastric cancers may occur in patients with a family history of gastric cancer, some of which are related to inherited syndromes. These include hereditary diffuse gastric cancer (E-cadherin/CDH1 mutation), familial adenomatous polyposis (FAP), and Lynch syndrome (hereditary nonpolyposis colorectal cancer). Appropriate genetic counseling and screening should be offered to patients and families affected by these syndromes. Prophylactic surgery may be discussed in CDH1 mutation carriers.

PATHOLOGY

More than 90% of malignant gastric tumors are classified as adenocarcinomas. There are two distinct histologic subtypes: intestinal (well differentiated) and diffuse (poorly differentiated). The former is seen more frequently in high-risk populations and older patients. It tends to form in glands, and the tumors appear as masses. There is a strong association with *H. pylori* infection. The diffuse type is more common in inherited syndromes and behaves more aggressively. It is associated with E-cadherin mutations and loss of cellular adhesion. These tumors infiltrate the gastric wall without forming glands. The finding of linitis plastica is associated with diffuse infiltration of the gastric wall by these tumors.

In recent years, proximally located and diffuse type tumors have been increasing in incidence in Western cultures, whereas there has been a substantial decrease in incidence of intestinal and more distal tumors. However, distal lesions continue to predominate in Japan and other parts of the world. The cause for this trend is unknown and likely multifactorial.

DIAGNOSIS AND STAGING

Unfortunately, the symptoms of gastric cancer are vague and in many cases mimic those of benign gastrointestinal disorders (i.e. epigastric pain, nausea). Screening for gastric carcinoma is performed commonly in the East but not recommended in Western countries because of the rarity of the disease. Thus the majority of tumors in the United States are diagnosed at advanced stages. Often physical examination is unremarkable. However, a palpable abdominal mass or one of the classically described findings, including Sister Mary Joseph's (periumbilical) and Virchow's (left supraclavicular) nodes as well as Blumer's shelf (prerectal metastases palpated during rectal examination because of tumor deposition in the rectovesical or rectouterine pouch) may be identified.

Endoscopy is the diagnostic examination of choice. Frequently, endoscopic ultrasound (EUS) is employed as an adjunctive test to determine the depth of the tumor (T stage) or lymph node involvement (N stage) with reported accuracies more than 75% and 60%, respectively. Traditionally, computerized tomography (CT) is used primarily for detection of metastatic disease; however, with newer technologies this modality may provide a level of accuracy for locoregional staging similar to that of EUS. Diagnostic laparoscopy can aid in the detection of unresectable disease because it identifies metastatic disease in up to 40% of patients with negative cross-sectional imaging. Peritoneal washings can be collected during these procedures and offer further prognostic information. This can be particularly relevant in patients who are scheduled to undergo neoadjuvant treatment. Positive peritoneal cytology is an independent predictor of poor survival. Because it carries a similar prognosis to other forms of stage IV gastric cancers, it has been classified as M1 disease in the seventh edition of the AJCC staging manual. The American Joint Committee on Cancer and International Union Against Cancer (AJCC/UICC) system remains the most commonly used pathologic staging criteria (Table 1). In the most recent update, tumors within 5 cm of and crossing the GE junction are staged using the esophageal cancer guidelines. The following guidelines apply to tumors more than 5 cm from and those that do not cross the GE junction: the depth of gastric wall invasion defines T stage. T1a lesions invade into the lamina propria or muscularis mucosa, whereas T1b lesions invade the submucosa. T2 tumors penetrate into the

TABLE I: **Seventh American Joint Committee on Cancer Staging System for Gastric Adenocarcinoma**

Primary Tumor	Tx	Primary tumor cannot be assessed.
	T0	No evidence of primary tumor.
	Tis	Carcinoma in situ: intraepithelial tumor without invasion of the lamina propria.
	T1	Tumor invades lamina propria, muscularis mucosae, or submucosa.
	T1a	Tumor invades lamina propria or muscularis mucosae.
	T1b	Tumor invades submucosa.
	T2	Tumor invades muscularis propria.
	T3	Tumor penetrates subserosal connective tissue without invasion of visceral peritoneum or adjacent structures. T3 tumors also include those extending into the gastrocolic or gastrohepatic ligaments or into the greater or lesser omentum, without perforation of the visceral peritoneum covering these structures.
	T4	Tumor invades serosa (visceral peritoneum) or adjacent structures.
	T4a	Tumor invades serosa (visceral peritoneum).
	T4b	Tumor invades adjacent structures, such as spleen, transverse colon, liver, diaphragm, pancreas, abdominal wall, adrenal gland, kidney, small intestine, and retroperitoneum.
Regional Nodes	Nx	Regional lymph node(s) cannot be assessed.
	N0	No regional lymph node metastasis.
	N1	Metastasis in 1 to 2 regional lymph nodes.
	N2	Metastasis in 3 to 6 regional lymph nodes.
	N3	Metastasis in 7 or more regional lymph nodes.
	N3a	Metastasis in 7 to 15 regional lymph nodes.
	N3b	Metastasis in 16 or more regional lymph nodes.
Metastases	Mx	Distant metastases cannot be assessed.
	M0	No distant metastases.
	M1	Distant metastases.

Stage Groupings	0	Tis N0 M0	IIIA	T2 N3 M0
	IA	T1 N0 M0		T3 N2 M0
	IB	T1 N1 M0		T4a N1 M0
		T2 N0 M0	IIIB	T3 N3 M0
	IIA	T1 N2 M0		T4a N2 M0
		T2 N1 M0		T4b N0 or N1 M0
		T3 N0 M0	IIIC	T4a N3 M0
	IIB	T1 N3 M0		T4b N2 or N3 M0
		T2 N2 M0	IV	Any T Any N M1
		T3 N1 M0		
		T4a N0 M0		

Adapted from American Joint Committee on Cancer. *AJCC Cancer Staging Manual,* 7th ed. New York:Springer; 2010. pp. 117-126.

muscularis propria. T3 lesions invade the subserosa but not the visceral peritoneum or adjacent structures. Finally, T4 lesions are characterized by invasion of the visceral peritoneum or adjacent organs. Nodal (N) status is determined by the number of lymph nodes involved. N1 involves metastases in up to two regional nodes, N2 from three to six, and N3 seven or more regional nodes. Regional nodes include the perigastric nodes, as well as the celiac, left gastric, splenic, and common hepatic artery nodes. To obtain accurate staging, the surgical specimen should contain a minimum of 15 lymph nodes for examination.

■ SURGERY

Primary Resection

Surgical excision remains the cornerstone of curative therapy for gastric cancer. The objective is to perform a complete resection with negative margins (R0 resection). This can be accomplished via subtotal or total gastrectomy because randomized controlled trials have shown no difference in survival in comparison of these operations. Because of the high propensity of gastric cancer to spread in the submucosa, gross margins of at least 5 cm are preferable. The management of microscopically positive margins (R1 resection) is a contentious issue. A number of studies have demonstrated a poor prognosis in patients with microscopically positive margins. More

recent studies have shown that this is predominantly true only in patients with T1 or T2 tumors and limited nodal involvement. Thus the decision to re-operate should be considered carefully based on the patient's overall condition and treatment goals, as well as on regional pathologic staging. NCCN guidelines currently do not recommend reoperation after R1 resection.

Lymphadenectomy

The extent of lymphadenectomy continues to be controversial. Historically, nodal resection has been defined by the proximity of the specimen to the stomach. A D0 dissection is when no effort is made to resect nodes, typically during palliative resection. D1 lymphadenectomy refers to excision of perigastric nodes, whereas D2 dissection includes nodes located along the main trunks of the celiac axis. The Japanese Society for Research in Gastric Cancer (JSRGC) standardized the extent of resection and lymphadenectomy in the early 1980s. Since that time, several retrospective studies from Japan have demonstrated significant survival advantage with extended D2 resection. However, several prospective randomized trials done in Western countries have not reproduced these findings. Notably, the Dutch Gastric Cancer Group trial comparing D1 and D2 lymphadenectomy, as defined by the JSRGC and performed under the tutelage of an experienced Japanese surgeon, did not show improvement

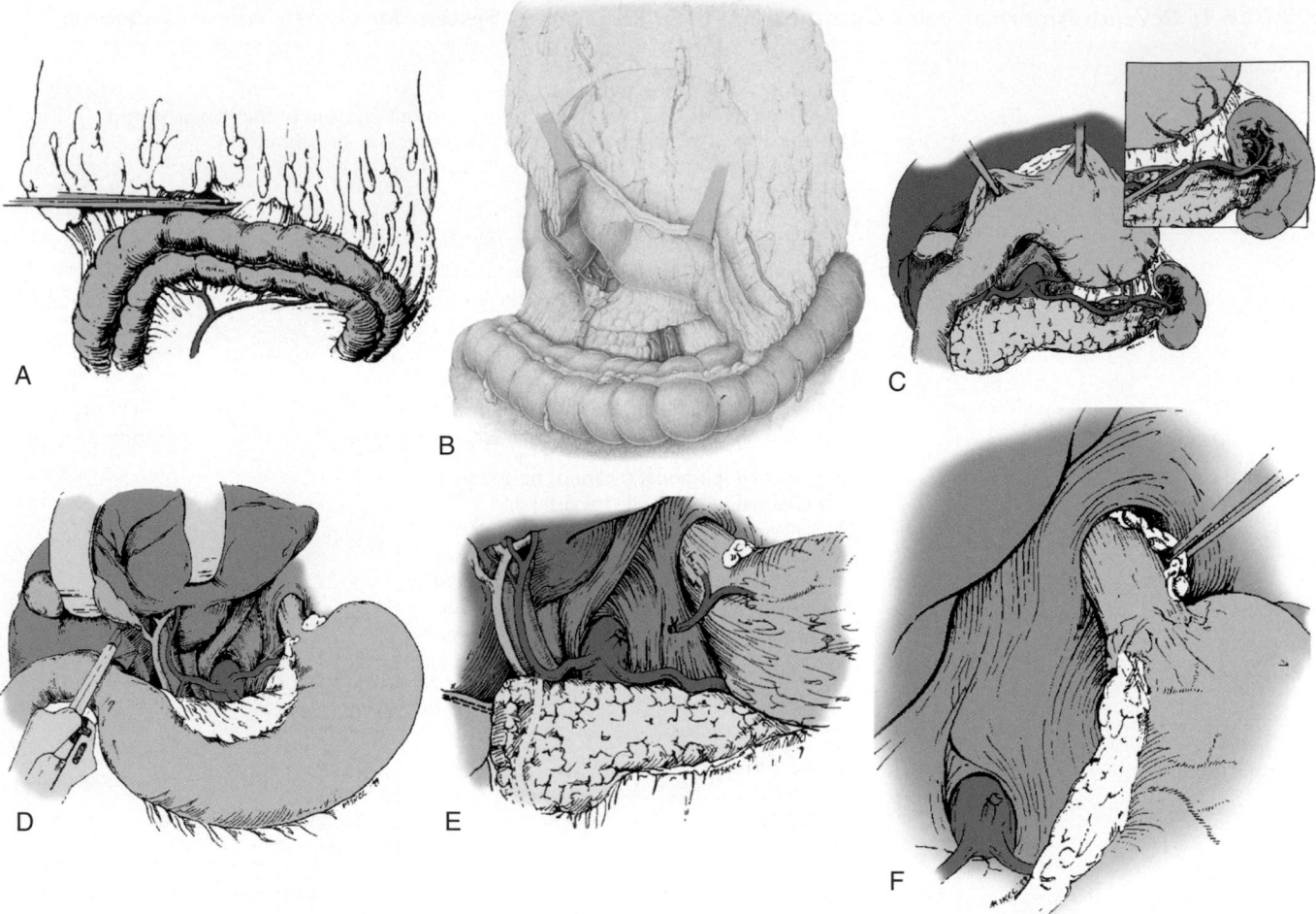

FIGURE I **A,** The avascular plane between the greater omentum and transverse mesocolon is incised. **B,** The greater omentum is dissected off of the colon along the avascular plane between the anterior and posterior sheaths of the transverse mesocolon. Dissection is carried down to the level of the pancreas. **C,** The lateral attachments of the stomach and short gastric vessels are divided. *Inset:* The splenic artery is dissected along the superior border of the pancreas. Nodal tissue is dissected down to the level of the splenic hilus. **D,** The duodenum is identified and divided with the GIA linear stapler. **E,** Nodal dissection proceeds from the porta hepatis toward the celiac axis along the superior border of the pancreas. The left gastric artery is divided at its origin. **F,** Nodal dissection continues along the right diaphragmatic crus and esophageal hiatus. The left paracardial nodes are taken during total gastrectomy.

in survival and was associated with higher postoperative morbidity. Similarly, the British Medical Research Council investigation of D1 and D2 lymphadenectomy showed a significant increase in postoperative morbidity without improvement in either overall or recurrence-free survival. In these trials, distal pancreatectomy and splenectomy were included in D2 resection, and subgroup analyses suggested that these procedures contributed to the morbidity of patients undergoing extended lymph node dissection. D1 and D2 resections without pancreatosplenectomy have been compared subsequently in nonrandomized, single-center trials that demonstrated comparable morbidity and improved survival after D2 resection. Aggressive lymphadenectomy is also beneficial because it allows for accurate staging. Several studies have indicated that survival is improved with an increased number of resected nodes. This observation is likely because of a reduction in understaging, or stage migration, when more lymph nodes are examined.

Operative Technique

Before resection and lymphadenectomy, the peritoneal cavity is examined for undiagnosed metastases. If not performed previously, diagnostic laparoscopy may be used based on the surgeon's preference to avoid unnecessary laparotomy. After this confirmation of resectability, the avascular plane between the transverse colon and greater omentum is divided sharply and the greater omentum dissected off the colon. The anterior sheath of the transverse mesocolon is separated along an avascular plane down to the pancreas. The pancreatic capsule should be taken selectively because there is limited evidence regarding the oncologic benefit. Next, the short gastric vessels and lateral omental attachments are taken down. The type of resection that is planned determines the extent of dissection along the greater curvature. The duodenum then is isolated and transected at least 1 cm distal to the pylorus, using a linear stapler, with close attention to avoid a retained antral remnant (Figure 1). Dissection continues along the porta hepatis toward the celiac vessels to include all nodal tissue anterior to the portal vein. Lymph nodes between the common hepatic artery and superior portion of the pancreas are reflected toward the celiac axis. The left gastric artery is identified and divided at its base and nodal tissue is swept off the right crus of the diaphragm and celiac trunk. The splenic artery is dissected along the superior portion of the pancreas and the lymph node dissection continues toward the splenic hilum. Here, the proximal portion of the specimen is divided either sharply for a total gastrectomy or with a linear stapler for a subtotal gastrectomy. Proximal margins are sent

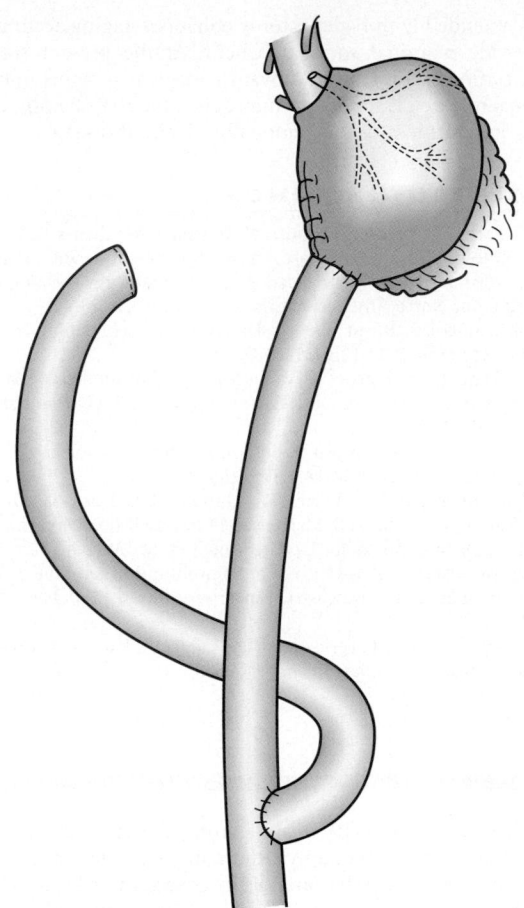

FIGURE 2 Roux-en-Y reconstruction.

routinely for frozen section to confirm microscopic tumor clearance. The gastrointestinal tract is reconstructed with Roux-en-Y esophago-jejunostomy after total gastrectomy or either Billroth II or Roux-en-Y gastrojejunostomy after subtotal gastrostomy. We prefer a 50- to 60-cm Roux-en-Y reconstruction to prevent the troublesome bile reflux gastritis experienced after a Billroth II (Figure 2).

The use of minimally invasive techniques in gastrectomy for gastric cancer remains controversial, but the frequency of its use is increasing. Laparoscopic resections once yielded a lower number of nodes because of technical issues with the procedure, but standardization of operative technique recently has shown comparable nodal harvests and overall survival. Nevertheless, there is a steep learning curve for this operation, and surgeons should seek adequate training at high volume centers before embarking on this route. Robotic procedures may alleviate this problem but are more expensive and take significantly longer to perform. Further studies are needed before these techniques can be implemented widely.

■ COMBINED MODALITY THERAPY

Adjuvant Therapy

Unfortunately even patients who undergo curative R0 resection have a high rate of recurrent disease after surgery. Locoregional and distant recurrences happen with comparable frequencies with most recurrences occurring within 2 years of surgery. Thus there has been significant interest in effective adjuvant therapies as an adjunct to resection of gastric cancer. In 2001 the Intergroup 0116 prospective randomized controlled trial comparing 5-fluorouracil and leucovorin plus external beam radiation to observation after curative resection of gastric cancer demonstrated improvement in overall and relapse-free survival in the treatment group. Based on this

investigation the inclusion of adjuvant therapy has become the standard of care for gastric cancer in the United States. However, this study has been criticized for poor standardization of surgical therapy. Complete resection with D2 lymphadenectomy was recommended in the study, but only 10% actually underwent this procedure. The majority of patients, 54%, underwent a D0 resection. Interestingly, this trial showed no difference in survival based on the extent of node dissection. More recent data have shown that the survival benefit of this therapy is maintained on long-term follow-up. A large study from Japan, the ACTS-GC trial, has investigated an alternative chemotherapeutic agent, S-1, but without the addition of radiotherapy. This drug is a combination of tegafur (prodrug of 5-fluorouracil), 5-chloro-2, 4-dihydropyridine (CDHP), and oxonic acid. This randomized phase III study demonstrated a significantly improved overall survival in patients with stage II or III disease who received this treatment after D2 resection. Importantly, these results assume that D2 resection is the standard resection and therefore may have limited application to treatment of Western patients. Ongoing studies also are evaluating currently the addition of targeted therapies such as trastuzumab, a targeted HER2 monoclonal antibody, to chemotherapy in the adjuvant setting.

Neoadjuvant Therapy

In addition to the criticisms of surgical therapy in the Intergroup 0116 trial, only 64% of patients were able to complete the regimen of postoperative chemoradiation. Likely benefits of preoperative administration include improved patient tolerance, ability to assess disease response in vivo, and tumor downstaging, which may improve R0 resection rate. Therefore significant interest exists in developing effective neoadjuvant or perioperative therapy regimens for gastric cancer. The British Medical Research Council's MAGIC trial comparing perioperative epirubicin, cisplatin, and 5-fluorouracil to surgery alone demonstrated improved overall and progression-free survival in addition to improved resectability. In addition, a significantly higher proportion of patients were able to tolerate the preoperative therapy. This study, however, has been criticized for the low rate of D2 dissection. More recent studies in the United States and Europe also have demonstrated improved survival and R0 resection rate with preoperative chemoradiotherapy. The RTOG 9904 trial, which was a phase II trial of neoadjuvant chemoradiotherapy, demonstrated a pathologic complete response in 26% of patients, with improved short-term survival in these patients. Presently, neoadjuvant therapy is recommended for patients with locoregionally advanced disease.

■ PROGNOSTICATION

Traditionally, outcomes have been predicted based on the AJCC staging system. However, there is significant variability within stage groups, making prognostication for individual patients difficult. The seventh edition of the AJCC staging system, as mentioned above, has separated cardia lesions and those that cross the gastroesophageal junction from more distal lesions and made several other changes that may improve the ability to accurately determine prognosis. Surgeons from Memorial Sloan-Kettering have developed a nomogram for predicting survival that was shown to be more accurate than older versions of the AJCC staging alone. This was accomplished by including age, sex, number of positive and negative lymph nodes, depth of invasion, and histotype. Subsequent analyses at large volume centers in the United States and Europe have validated this model. Using this model may allow for more careful stratification of treatment groups in future clinical trials. A similar nomogram developed in Korea compared favorably with the current AJCC staging system but may not be applicable to Western patients because of differences in extent of lymph node dissection. Discovery and implementation of additional prognostic markers, such as E-cadherin, HER2, and p53, could improve the accuracy of these nomograms.

◼ PALLIATION

Because of the grim prognosis of advanced gastric cancer and incapability to complete curative resection in about half of patients, understanding palliation is imperative when treating patients with gastric cancer. The utility of surgical therapy in palliation is controversial. Palliative gastrectomy is associated with significant morbidity (>50%) and mortality. Although this is presumably the result of the deconditioned state of patients with advanced gastric cancers, this procedure cannot be justified universally for prevention of symptoms. Follow-up studies of patients in whom elective gastrectomy was aborted because of detection of metastases at the time of operation found that only half required intervention for symptoms of advanced tumors and just more than 10% needed operative interventions. The development of newer chemotherapeutic regimens and the implementation of targeted therapies also may improve the ability to palliate patients with advanced gastric cancer.

◼ SUMMARY

Even though the incidence of gastric adenocarcinoma has declined significantly in the United States over the last century, there is a trend toward more proximal and biologically aggressive tumors. Surgical excision continues to be the foundation of curative therapy for patients with operable disease. R0 resection optimizes outcomes, whereas extended lymphadenectomy enhances staging accuracy and may provide marginal survival benefit. At the present time, the optimal timing and form of adjuvant treatment remains unknown. Additional research is needed to fully define the role chemoradiation will play in treatment of locoregionally advanced disease.

SUGGESTED READINGS

Knight G, Earle CC, Cosby R, Coburn N, Youssef Y, Malthaner R, Wong RK; Gastrointestinal Cancer Disease Site Group. Neoadjuvant or adjuvant therapy for resectable gastric cancer: a systematic review and practice guideline for North America. *Gastric Cancer.* 2013;16:28-40.

Lianos GD, Rausei S, Ruspi L, et al. Laparoscopic gastrectomy for gastric cancer. *Int J Surg.* 2014;12:1369-1373.

Newton A, Datta J, Karakousis GC, Roses RE. Neoadjuvant therapy for gastric cancer: current evidence and future directions. *J Gastrointest Oncol.* 2015;6:534-543.

Santoro R, Ettorre GM, Santoro E. Subtotal gastrectomy for gastric cancer. *World J Gastroenterol.* 2014;14:13667-13680.

Smalley SR, Benedetti JK, Haller DG, Hundahl SA, Estes NC, Ajani JA, Gunderson LL, Goldman B, Martenson JA, Jessup JM, Stemmermann GN, Blanke CD, Macdonald JS. Updated analysis of SWOG-directed intergroup study 0116: a phase III trial of adjuvant radiochemotherapy versus observation after curative gastric cancer resection. *J Clin Oncol.* 2012;30:2327-2333.

Torre LA, Bray F, Siegel RL, Ferlay J, Lortet-Tieulent J, Jemal A. Global cancer statistics, 2012. *CA Cancer J Clin.* 2015;65:87-108.

THE MANAGEMENT OF GASTROINTESTINAL STROMAL TUMORS

Michael J. Cavnar, MD, and Ronald P. DeMatteo MD, FACS

Gastrointestinal stromal tumor (GIST) is the most common sarcoma of the gastrointestinal (GI) tract and, in fact, represents the most common sarcoma subtype overall. Although it is relatively uncommon (1% of all GI neoplasms) compared with adenocarcinoma, dramatic improvement in treatment outcomes has resulted in an increasing cohort of surviving GIST patients, such that a practicing general surgeon should be familiar with the unique principles of management for this disease. In 1998 Hirota discovered a gain of function mutation in the proto-oncogene *KIT* in GIST. This quickly was translated to clinical medicine 3 years later, when Joensuu reported the first successful treatment of a patient with advanced GIST with imatinib mesylate (Gleevec, Novartis Pharmaceuticals), a tyrosine kinase inhibitor (TKI) of ABL, BCR-ABL, KIT, and platelet-derived growth factor receptor (PDGFR). Since these initial reports, understanding of the pathophysiology of this disease has advanced rapidly and currently is perhaps better than in any other GI malignancy. For example, current knowledge includes that the cell of origin is the interstitial cell of Cajal (ICC), and in most cases, development of GIST appears to require oncogenic activation of a tyrosine kinase in cooperation with the ICC lineage transcription factor ETV1. Approximately 75% of GISTs bear activating mutations in *KIT*, with *PDGFRα* mutated in another 10%. The remaining group of "wild type" GISTs has continued to shrink because alterations have been discovered in *BRAF, SDH,* and *NF1* in other patients.

Treatment of GIST with imatinib has been studied extensively. In patients with metastatic disease, imatinib prolongs median survival to more than 5 years from a historical median of 18 months. In the adjuvant setting after complete resection, imatinib prolongs recurrence-free survival (RFS), and chronic therapy may be required for high-risk patients. Neoadjuvant imatinib treatment may improve resectability for tumors that are locally advanced or located in anatomically difficult areas, and in some instances may allow organ-preserving resection. Imatinib therapy has expanded the role of resection of metastases. The ability to estimate the risk of recurrence in GIST patients increasingly is refined. In addition to traditional stratification using size, mitotic index, and site, specific mutations have a significant bearing on tumor behavior and sensitivity to TKIs. These remarkable advances in GIST have heralded a new era of targeted therapy in the treatment of cancer. Nevertheless, surgery remains the only potentially curative therapy for GIST. Consequently, an understanding of the surgical principles in GIST is critical.

◼ CLINICAL PRESENTATION

GIST is usually a disease of adults, with a median presenting age of approximately 60 years, with a slight male predominance. The incidence of GIST is estimated to be approximately 5000 new cases per year in the United States. The incidence of occult micro-GISTs smaller than 1 cm is actually much higher. In one study, one third of 98 consecutive autopsies were found to have small GISTs, usually in the proximal stomach. These micro-GISTs harbored *KIT* and *PDGFRα* mutations but had no mitotic activity.

Although GIST may arise anywhere from the esophagus to the rectum, the stomach is the most common site (40% to 60%), followed by small bowel (25% to 35%). The majority of small bowel tumors are found in the jejunum and ileum, with a minority (5%) arising in the duodenum. Rectal GISTs occur, although large bowel, esophageal, and extraintestinal GISTs are rare. The median size of GIST at presentation is 5 to 7 cm, although tumors may grow in excess of 30 cm. GISTs may be discovered by symptoms or incidentally by endoscopy or imaging during the workup for other conditions or at the time of unrelated surgery. Most symptoms are nonspecific, such as early satiety and bloating. Others experience abdominal pain or a noticeable mass. Although GIST is not a mucosa-based tumor like adenocarcinoma and instead grows from the muscle layer of the bowel wall, it still may be accompanied by bleeding in up to one quarter of patients because of erosion of the mucosa. Tumor bleeding also can occur from tumor rupture into the peritoneal cavity, which can lead to life-threatening hemorrhage. Bowel obstruction is infrequent because GIST tends to grow by displacing other structures rather than invading them. Metastasis typically involves the liver or peritoneal cavity. Lymph node involvement is rare in adult GIST, occurring less than 5% of the time.

Two rare subsets of GIST are worth noting. Pediatric GIST often is associated with succinate dehydrogenase (SDH) deficiency. Pediatric GIST exhibits a different biology that is overall indolent with female predominance, multifocal disease, frequent lymph node metastasis, and universal imatinib resistance. Familial GIST involving germline mutation of *KIT* or *PDGFRα* mutations is rare. Typically, the tumors are multifocal and indolent. GIST can occur rarely in association with the Carney-Stratakis syndrome (GIST and paraganglioma), Carney's triad (GIST, paraganglioma, and pulmonary chondroma), or neurofibromatosis type 1 (GIST, neurofibroma, glioma, and malignant peripheral nerve sheath tumor).

■ WORKUP

CT of the abdomen and pelvis with oral and intravenous contrast is the imaging test of choice for the initial evaluation of GIST. A typical GIST appears as an enhancing mass arising in the wall of the stomach or intestine (Figure 1). Large masses may exhibit heterogeneous enhancement resulting from necrosis. Small GISTs may not be visible

on CT, depending on the distention of the bowel and the amount of oral contrast. Alternatively, a large hypervascular GIST arising from the stomach may be misinterpreted as a primary liver tumor. Determining whether adjacent structures are involved by large tumors can be difficult based on CT alone. At exploration, such tumors often are found to be mobile and may not require multivisceral resection. For periampullary and rectal tumors, MRI can help further delineate anatomy. Although GISTs are typically glucose avid on [¹⁸F] fluoro-2-deoxy-D-glucose positron emission tomography (FDG-PET), this test is not necessary in the initial evaluation and should be reserved for assessment of metastatic disease when there is heterogeneity of response to TKIs.

Some GISTs are detected initially by endoscopic evaluation by the presence of a submucosal mass. A minority will show ulceration resulting from erosion of the mucosa, whereas others will not be visible because of primarily exophytic growth outside the bowel wall. Fine-needle aspiration (FNA) is 70% to 80% sensitive, usually revealing spindle cells that are CD117 (KIT) positive by immunohistochemistry. FNA may help differentiate GIST from other diagnoses such as leiomyoma, lymphoma, or adenocarcinoma, each of which requires different treatment. However, many times an FNA is inconclusive and a core biopsy is required. For lesions that would require potentially morbid operations (e.g., GE junction, periampullary, or in the rectum), it is reasonable to make several biopsy attempts if establishing the diagnosis would result in using neoadjuvant imatinib, which subsequently may reduce the magnitude of the

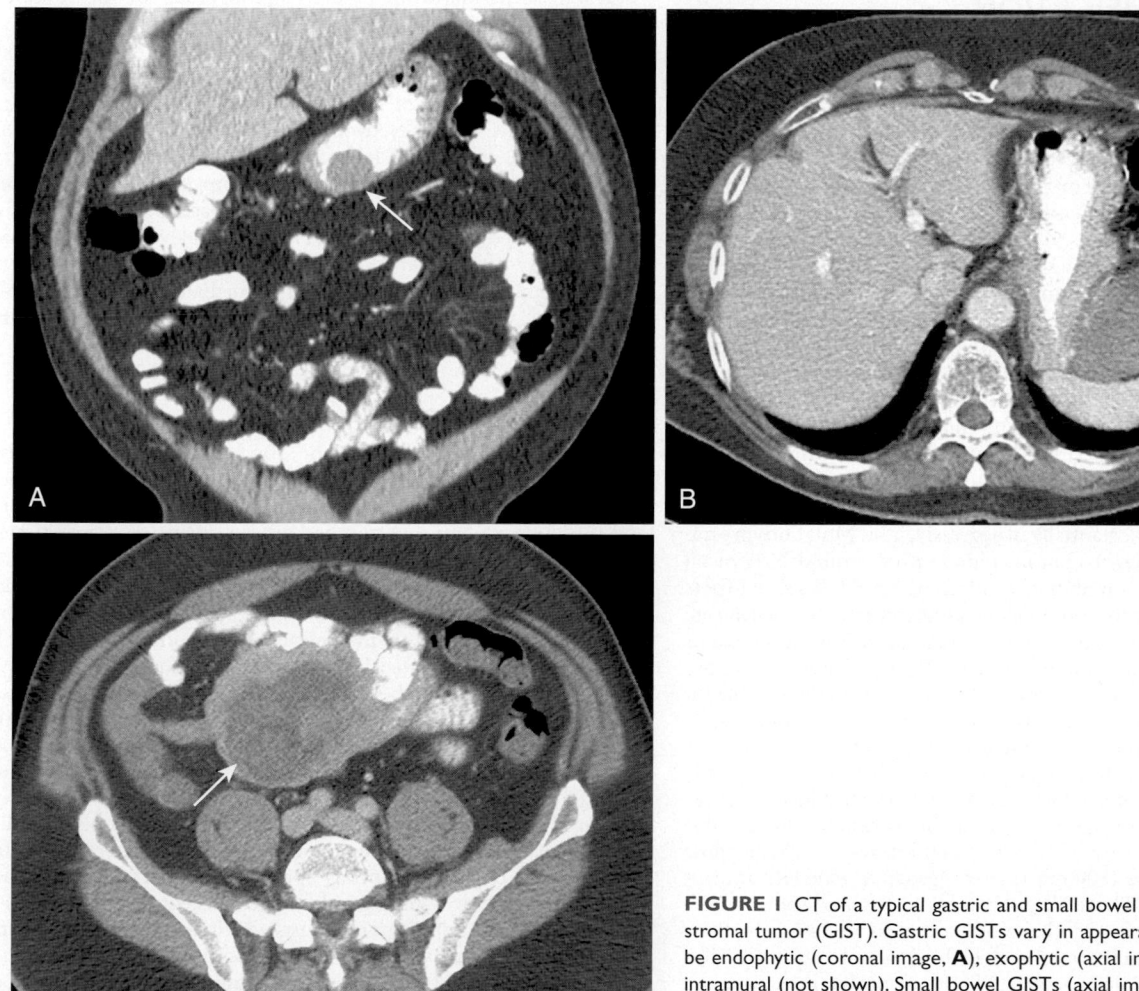

FIGURE 1 CT of a typical gastric and small bowel gastrointestinal stromal tumor (GIST). Gastric GISTs vary in appearance and can be endophytic (coronal image, **A**), exophytic (axial image, **B**), or intramural (not shown). Small bowel GISTs (axial image, **C**) typically do not cause obstruction. CT may not clearly delineate the origin from the bowel wall as in gastric GISTs. Arrows mark tumors.

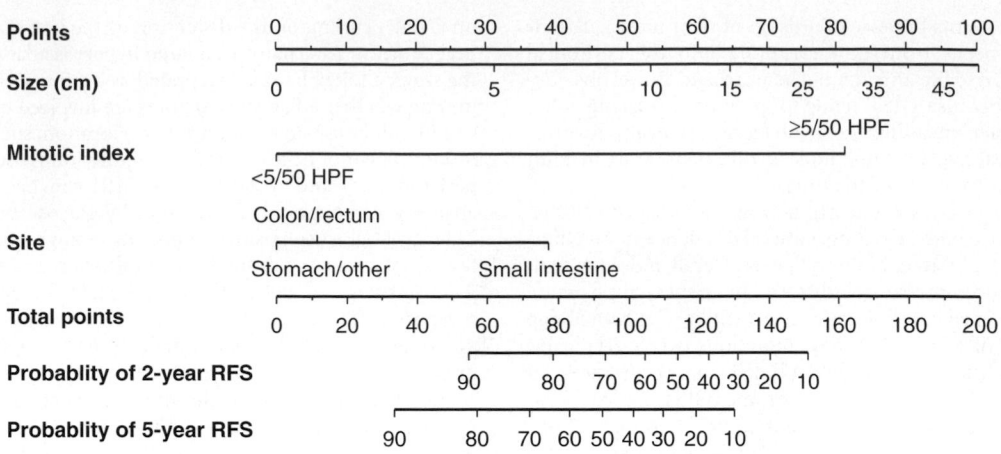

FIGURE 2 Nomogram for predicting 2- and 5-year recurrence-free survival (RFS) after resection of primary gastrointestinal stromal tumor. Points are assigned based on tumor size, mitotic index, and site by drawing a vertical line from each row to the "Points" row. The sum is then located in the "Total points" row, and a vertical line is drawn to "Probability" rows to estimate RFS. *(From Gold JS, Gönen M, Gutiérrez A, et al. Development and validation of a prognostic nomogram for recurrence-free survival after complete surgical resection of localised primary gastrointestinal stromal tumour: a retrospective analysis. Lancet Oncol. 2009;10:1045-1052.)*

operation. If the radiologic appearance is typical of GIST, biopsy is not necessarily required.

RISK STRATIFICATION

Three clinicopathologic parameters have been shown to independently predict risk of recurrence after complete resection of primary GIST: tumor size, mitotic rate, and tumor site. Size greater than 5 cm, mitoses larger than 5/50 high-powered fields, and nongastric site are poor prognostic variables. Several different risk stratification systems have been developed based on these variables. For example, the NIH-Fletcher criteria divide patients into very low, low, intermediate, and high risk of recurrence based on size and mitotic rate. We developed a nomogram that incorporates all three criteria (Figure 2) to provide a personalized estimate of 2- and 5-year RFS after complete resection of a primary GIST. The nomogram has been validated in three other datasets of patients and is available at *https://www.mskcc.org/nomograms/gastrointestinal/stromal-tumor*. The nomogram can be used to select patients for adjuvant imatinib.

Identification of the specific mutation in GIST, either after resection or preoperatively, provides useful additional information. Specific mutations are associated with disease biology and also response to imatinib. Three quarters of tumors harbor a *KIT* mutation; however, these vary substantially in aggressiveness. Mutations in exon 11 are by far the most common, representing around 65% of all GISTs. Among exon 11 mutations, codons 557 and 558 are hot spots for mutation, and tumors with deletions of this part of the gene are more likely to metastasize or recur as compared with point mutations or insertions in this area and others. Interestingly, patients with *KIT* exon 11 deletions in the ACOSOG Z9001 study were responsible for nearly all of the improvement in RFS achieved with 1 year of adjuvant imatinib, whereas other *KIT* mutations surprisingly showed little difference. *KIT* exon 9 mutations (about 10% of all GISTs) typically arise in nongastric tumors and have a worse natural history. Meta-analysis of two large trials of imatinib in metastatic unresectable GIST showed that patients with these mutations required higher dose imatinib for response (800 mg vs 400 mg daily). *PDGFRα*-mutant tumors (10% of GIST) are almost always gastric and show a more indolent biology. However, the most common mutation in these tumors, exon 18 D842V, is known to be imatinib resistant. Thus understanding the biology associated with a specific mutation, and its expected response to imatinib can help plan treatment and follow-up.

SURGERY FOR PRIMARY DISEASE

Indications

The long-term follow-up of the placebo group of the ACOSOG Z9001 study demonstrated that 70% of patients with tumors of 3 cm or larger were cured by surgery alone. In general, resection is indicated for GIST in patients who lack prohibitive comorbidities and have a life expectancy of more than a few years. NCCN (National Comprehensive Cancer Network) guidelines recommend that GISTs larger than 2 cm should be resected. It is reasonable to observe smaller tumors with serial endoscopy or imaging. In fact, a recent retrospective study of 989 subepithelial gastric tumors 3 cm or smaller showed that only 84 (8.5%) grew or developed concerning morphology during a median follow-up of 24 months. Of the 19 tumors removed, only seven were intermediate or high-risk GISTs, respectively, whereas the remainder were low or very low risk GIST, or not GIST at all.

General Technical Aspects

At the time of surgical exploration, the peritoneal surface and liver should be surveyed for metastatic disease. Identification of the primary tumor then is achieved with variable difficulty depending on the site. Exophytic anterior and greater curvature gastric tumors usually are immediately apparent. Posterior gastric tumors require extensive mobilization of the stomach, which is facilitated by retracting the left lobe of the liver to the right. Small, intramural, or intraluminal gastric tumors that are not easily identified externally or by palpation can be localized by intraoperative endoscopy or ultrasonography after filling the stomach with water. Duodenal tumors beyond the first portion require an extensive Kocher maneuver and possibly mobilization of the ligament of Treitz. Ileal and jejunal tumors are identified best by systematically running the small bowel from the ligament of Treitz to the terminal ileum.

Once the primary tumor is identified, all manipulation should be done with great care because these tumors are friable, especially after neoadjuvant treatment. During laparoscopic surgery, manipulation is achieved best by handling only tissue adjacent to the tumor (i.e., no-touch technique). Tumor rupture, whether spontaneous or iatrogenic, is associated with almost inevitable peritoneal recurrence. Likewise, GISTs recruit large arterial and venous collateral blood vessels, and careful dissection is required to prevent the potential for significant blood loss. During laparoscopic surgery, removal of the

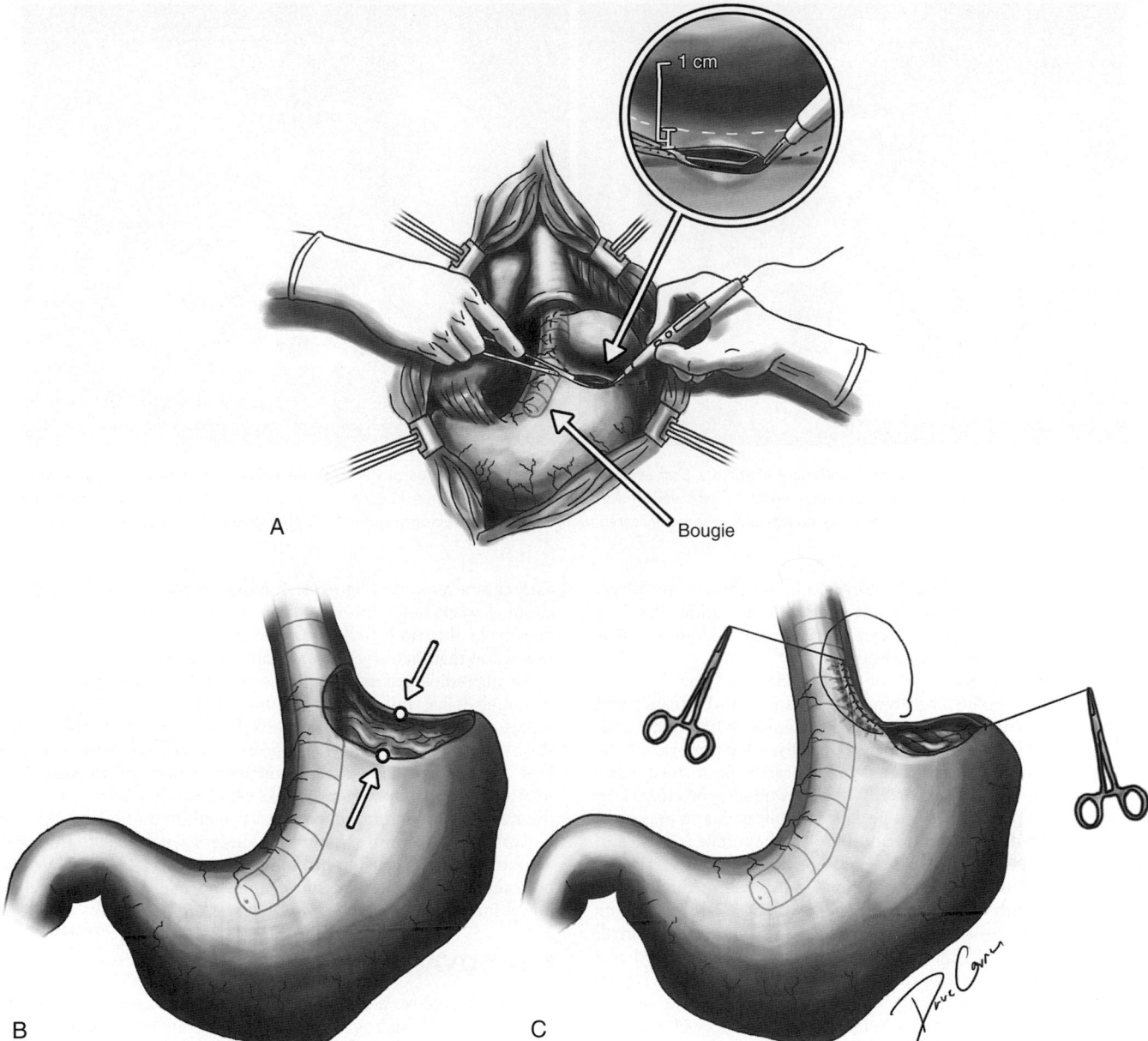

FIGURE 3 Illustration of resection of a large gastrointestinal stromal tumor at the gastroesophageal junction. After making a gastrotomy with cautery, the tumor is resected with a 1-cm margin (**A**). The defect (**B**) is then sewn closed (**C**) over a large bougie placed in the esophagus to prevent narrowing. *(Illustration by Dave Cavnar.)*

specimen should be done with a plastic specimen retrieval bag to prevent tumor seeding. Although GIST usually does not invade other organs and rather displaces them, any organ that is densely adherent should be at least partially resected en bloc.

Site-Specific Considerations

There are numerous site-specific considerations for the resection of GIST. Although adenocarcinoma requires formal anatomic gastrectomy with wide margins, resection of GIST does not require wide margins or lymphadenectomy. Although complete (R0) resection should be the goal, data from 819 primary GISTs 3 cm or larger resected in the ACOSOG Z9000 and Z9001 trials showed no difference in RFS in the 72 (8.8%) patients who had microscopically positive (R1) margins compared with those who underwent R0 resection, irrespective of imatinib treatment. This principle allows for one unique aspect of resection of gastric GIST, that is the technique of

gastrotomy and resection with a small negative margin (usually 1 cm) under direct visualization using cautery. Although many exophytic tumors with a narrow stalk or those on the greater curvature or fundus can be removed by wedge partial gastrectomy using surgical staplers without compromising the lumen, direct visualization facilitates safe resection while minimizing luminal narrowing in more difficult areas, such as the antrum, incisura, lesser curvature, or gastroesophageal junction (GEJ). For GEJ GISTs larger than a few centimeters, neoadjuvant imatinib usually is given (see below). Open surgery is preferred, particularly for tumors at the posterior aspect of the GEJ. After gastrotomy and removal of the tumor with a 1-cm margin, hand-sewn closure is done in the direction that provides the widest lumen (Figure 3). A bougie (usually 50F) should be placed in the esophagus during reconstruction to avoid narrowing. These techniques may obviate esophagogastrectomy, which carries substantially more morbidity than local resection of GIST from the GEJ. Although total gastrectomy is rarely necessary, it occasionally may be required

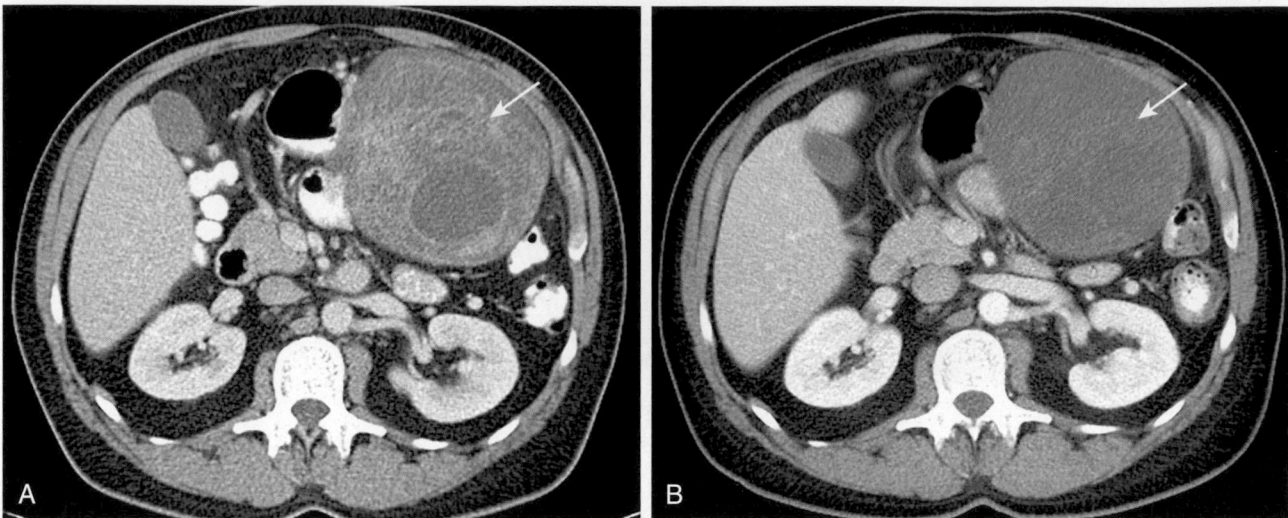

FIGURE 4 Initial tumor response to neoadjuvant imatinib is best assessed by changes in tumor density. A large gastric gastrointestinal stromal tumor (**A**) was treated with imatinib for 5 weeks, after which CT showed similar size (maximal dimension 12.6 cm pretreatment, 11.6 cm post-treatment) but decreased density (**B**). The patient eventually underwent an uncomplicated wedge partial gastrectomy, and pathology showed 98% treatment response.

for massive tumors. Such large tumors may be adherent to the spleen, distal pancreas, or colon, necessitating en bloc resection. If this is recognized preoperatively, we prefer to treat with neoadjuvant imatinib to accomplish organ preservation.

The next most common site of GIST is the small bowel. Jejunal and ileal tumors are the most frequent and are removed readily and reconstructed with a standard stapled side-to-side or functional end-to-end anastomosis. If done laparoscopically, after removal of the specimen in a retrieval bag, the anastomosis can be performed either intracorporeally or extracorporeally using a wound protector. Management of duodenal GISTs is especially complicated, and in general we prefer to use neoadjuvant imatinib unless the tumor is small and away from the pancreas. As discussed above, an extensive Kocher maneuver is required and may be extended to a full medial visceral rotation along with mobilization of the ligament of Treitz. Tumors near the ampulla usually require pancreaticoduodenectomy. Small tumors arising laterally in the second portion can be removed as a wedge resection and closed primarily if a tension-free closure is possible without compromising the lumen. Alternatively, reconstruction can be performed in Roux-en-Y fashion with a loop of jejunum anastomosed to the lateral duodenal defect. Tumors in the third or fourth portion of the duodenum can be reconstructed either with direct anastomosis to the jejunum, or by closure of the distal duodenum with a Roux-en-Y jejunal loop to the second portion.

Rectal GISTs are much more common than colonic GISTs. Neoadjuvant imatinib treatment of locally advanced rectal GIST may achieve sphincter preservation. Low rectal GISTs can be addressed transanally if small. Neoadjuvant imatinib also may downsize bulky distal rectal tumors to allow transanal excision.

■ NEOADJUVANT IMATINIB

As discussed above, for tumors that are locally advanced such that multivisceral resection would be required, or for tumors larger than a few centimeters located in difficult anatomic locations where tumor downsizing could allow less morbid surgery, we favor neoadjuvant imatinib treatment. Although change in metabolic activity is evident by FDG-PET within hours, actual decrease in tumor size can take many weeks or even several months on imatinib. In addition, responding tumors may even swell temporarily. As a result, traditional means of assessing tumor response to imatinib using RECIST criteria do not work well in GIST. Instead, the Choi criteria, which incorporate tumor density and size, are much more useful to evaluate

early tumor response (Figure 4). It is our practice to obtain a CT scan about 4 weeks after the initiation of therapy. Since a decrease in density in this time frame may be the only evident change, it is important that the surgeon personally review the images because the reporting radiologist may not be aware of this unique aspect of GIST. Although it has not been rigorously studied, it is our practice to repeat imaging at 3 and 6 months, beyond which further tumor shrinkage is unlikely. There have been no large prospective randomized clinical trials comparing immediate surgery with neoadjuvant imatinib followed by surgery. Unlike cytotoxic chemotherapy used in the neoadjuvant setting, neoadjuvant imatinib and other TKIs can be continued up until the time of surgery without compromising wound healing or causing immunosuppression. Likewise, they may be resumed when the patient is eating normally and has regained bowel function.

■ ADJUVANT IMATINIB

The initial large-scale studies of imatinib in metastatic unresectable GIST were highly successful, resulting in a dramatic improvement in survival from a historical median of 18 months to beyond 5 years. At the same time, imatinib was applied to the adjuvant setting. However, demonstrating similar improvement in survival has proven elusive, mostly because placebo-treated patients who develop recurrence or those who have recurrence after discontinuing imatinib are usually salvaged with imatinib and survive for extended periods of time. Also, since these patients are followed closely, recurrences often are found when they are small and amenable to re-resection. The ACOSOG Z9001 study was a phase III multicenter prospective randomized trial of imatinib compared with placebo for 1 year after resection of primary GISTs of at least 3 cm. The study was stopped early at interim analysis, when significantly improved RFS survival was noted in the imatinib group (98% vs 83% at a median follow-up of 19.7 months), and resulted in approval by U.S. and European regulatory agencies for imatinib treatment in GIST. We recently published the long-term follow-up of these patients. Interestingly, once the 1 year of prescribed imatinib was completed, the rate of recurrence increased (Figure 5). After 74 months of follow-up, the RFS curves of the placebo and imatinib arms have converged, indicating that imatinib was effective in controlling but not eradicating residual disease and is not curative. As discussed above, the majority of improvement in RFS was due primarily to the patients with exon 11 deletions, but not other mutations.

The SSG XVIII study was a phase III randomized study comparing 1 year to 3 years of adjuvant imatinib. This study showed improved 5-year RFS (66% vs 48%), with a slight improvement in overall survival (OS) (92% vs 82%), although the latter is of unclear significance because disease-specific survival was unchanged and there were few deaths in either group. Still, extended adjuvant imatinib seemed better. The PERSIST-5 trial is a phase II single-arm study of 5 years of imatinib in primary GISTs at high risk for recurrence (any site ≥2 cm with ≥5 mitoses/50HPF or any nongastric GIST ≥5 cm). Although the study is not complete, a planned interim 3-year analysis presented at the American Society of Clinical Oncology annual meeting in 2015 showed that of 91 eligible patients, only four

(4%) had developed recurrence, of which three had stopped the drug and the other was found to have the imatinib-resistant *PDGFRα* exon 18 D842V mutation. Our experience is similar, with very few recurrences occurring in high-risk patients continued on chronic imatinib after resection. It is thus our practice to prescribe chronic imatinib therapy in the adjuvant setting to high-risk patients whose goals of care are to remain recurrence free as long as possible, after explaining that it is unclear whether treatment will extend OS. Nevertheless, this decision must be weighed carefully with consideration that a 1-year supply of imatinib cost $92,000 in 2012.

■ RECURRENT, METASTATIC, AND RESISTANT DISEASE

In patients who develop recurrence after primary resection without adjuvant therapy, or for those who present with metastatic disease, imatinib is highly effective, with partial response or stable disease in the majority of patients. However, despite this initial efficacy, the median progression-free survival (PFS) with imatinib alone is 24 months, usually because of the development of secondary mutations in *KIT*. Clinically, during surveillance imaging on therapy, this may appear as viable tumor subclones that develop within a necrotic responding tumor (Figure 6), which should prompt concern for resistance. Sampling may reveal additional mutations, most commonly in exons 13, 14, or 17 of *KIT*. Additional mutations, although imatinib resistant, are often sensitive to second- and third-line TKIs. However, each further line of therapy provides sequentially diminishing returns. Second-line sunitinib improved PFS from 6 weeks to 27 weeks, whereas third-line regorafenib only improved PFS from 0.9 to 4.8 months.

Knowing the eventual outcome of TKI therapy alone for recurrent/metastatic patients, we have advocated surgical resection in well-selected patients with limited disease. In a study of 40 such patients from our institution treated with a median of 15 months of imatinib, 20 patients with responsive disease had better 2-year PFS and OS (61% and 100%) compared with 13 patients with focal resistance (one tumor growing; median PFS 12 months, 2-year OS 36%), and 7 patients with multifocal resistance (multiple tumors growing; median PFS 3 months, 1 year OS 36%). A study of 69 patients from Brigham and Women's Hospital/Dana Farber Cancer Institute showed similar results. Thus, in selected patients, it seems reasonable to resect metastatic disease that is responsive to therapy or is focally

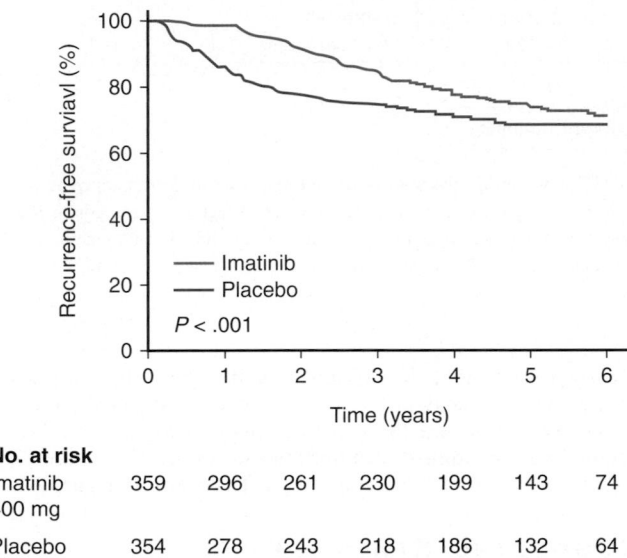

FIGURE 5 Recurrence-free survival in patients with primary gastrointestinal stromal tumor of 3 cm or greater after complete resection, randomized to 1 year of adjuvant imatinib versus placebo. *(From Corless CL, Ballman KV, Antonescu CR, et al. Pathologic and molecular features correlate with long-term outcome after adjuvant therapy of resected primary GI stromal tumor: the ACOSOG Z9001 trial. J Clin Oncol. 2014;32:1563-1570.)*

No. at risk							
Imatinib 400 mg	359	296	261	230	199	143	74
Placebo	354	278	243	218	186	132	64

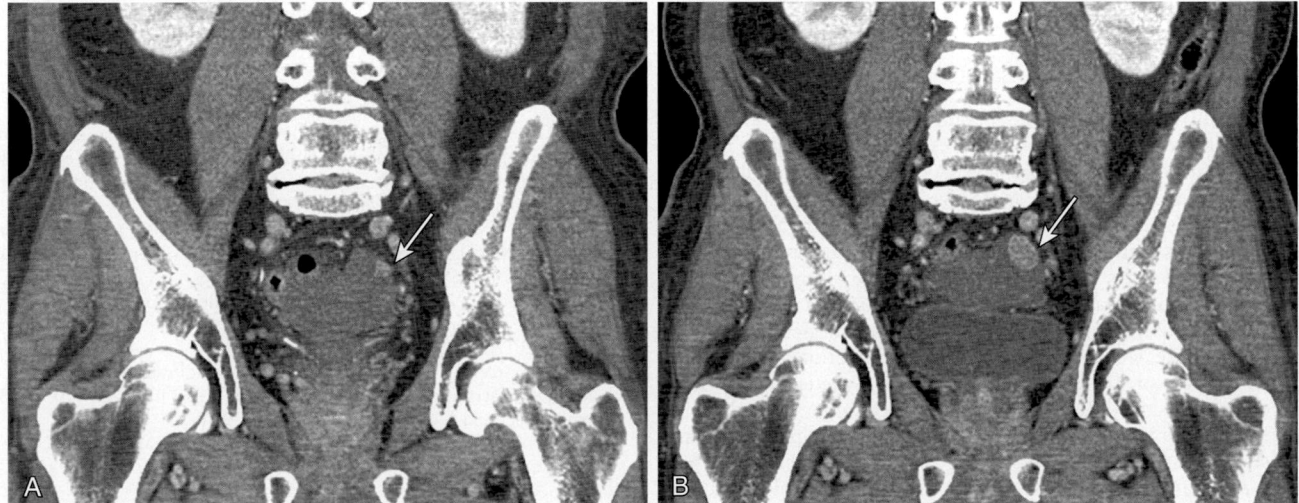

FIGURE 6 Development of a resistant tumor subclone within a tumor responding to imatinib. A patient with a pelvic recurrence of gastrointestinal stromal tumor was treated with chronic imatinib therapy. After 4 years of treatment, serial imaging (coronal CT images) separated by 4 months shows an enlarging enhancing nodule *(arrow)* within a necrotic tumor (**A,** first detection of a viable subclone; **B,** 4 months later). Pathology from resection showed 75% treatment response, but the viable nodule had a high mitotic rate and carried a new mutation in *KIT* exon 14 (original mutation was in exon *KIT* 11).

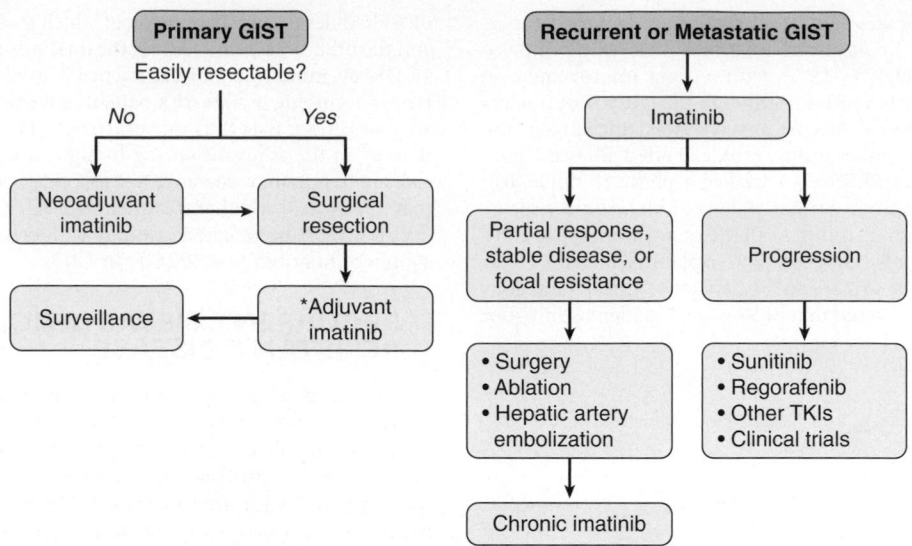

FIGURE 7 Schematic approach to patients with gastrointestinal stromal tumor (GIST). For locally advanced primary tumors treated with adjuvant imatinib, tumor density should be assessed by CT at 4 weeks to document response to therapy. If GIST nomogram predicts a high or intermediate risk of recurrence, adjuvant imatinib (*) should be continued for at least 3 years, possibly chronically. Surveillance after resection of GIST should include a CT of abdomen and pelvis every 3 to 6 months for 3 to 5 years and then annually. *(Adapted from Gold JS, DeMatteo RP. Combined surgical and molecular therapy: the gastrointestinal stromal tumor model. Ann Surg. 2006;244:176.)*

resistant. Those with multifocal resistance should be transitioned to second-line TKI therapy or referred for clinical trials. Still, this strategy has not been proven prospectively in a randomized trial of surgery plus TKI compared with TKI alone. Several attempts at such a trial have failed because of poor accrual. One such Chinese trial published its underpowered initial accrual, nevertheless showing a trend towards increased PFS in the surgery group. From a technical standpoint, resection of GIST liver metastases should be approached similarly to colorectal liver metastases, where resection is focused on clearing the liver of disease with attention to maintaining an appropriate future liver remnant. For multifocal disease, various ablative techniques can be used to supplement resection while preserving parenchyma. For resection of peritoneal metastases, resection may require en bloc removal of adjacent organs. After resection of liver or peritoneal metastases, adjuvant imatinib should be continued, likely indefinitely or until recurrence.

■ CONCLUSION

GIST is a relatively rare disease arising throughout the GI tract, most commonly in the stomach and small intestine, with activating mutations in *KIT* or *PDGFRα*. Disease biology varies from clinically irrelevant micro-GISTs to highly aggressive tumors presenting with widespread metastases to the liver and/or peritoneum. Surgery for GIST requires extreme care to avoid tumor rupture and bleeding from collateral vessels but is curative for 70% of patients with primary tumors of at least 3 cm. Diverse anatomic locations of GIST require numerous highly technical, site-specific surgical considerations, which are facilitated by neoadjuvant imatinib for locally advanced tumors or those larger than a few centimeters at the GEJ, duodenum, or rectum. Risk of recurrence after surgery is independently predicted by tumor size, mitotic rate, and site. Specific mutation also can help predict disease biology and responsiveness to TKI therapy. Adjuvant imatinib should be used in patients at high risk for

recurrence and should be continued for at least 3 years and possibly chronically. In patients with recurrent or metastatic GIST, resection should be considered for patients with limited disease who are responding to imatinib or demonstrate only focal resistance. An algorithm for multimodality therapy of GIST is shown in Figure 7.

SUGGESTED READINGS

Corless CL, Ballman KV, Antonescu CR, et al. Pathologic and molecular features correlate with long-term outcome after adjuvant therapy of resected primary GI stromal tumor: the ACOSOG Z9001 trial. *J Clin Oncol.* 2014;32:1563-1570.

DeMatteo RP, Lewis JJ, Leung D, et al. Two hundred gastrointestinal stromal tumors: recurrence patterns and prognostic factors for survival. *Ann Surg.* 2000;231:51-58.

Dematteo RP, Ballman KV, Antonescu CR, et al. Adjuvant imatinib mesylate after resection of localised, primary gastrointestinal stromal tumour: a randomised, double-blind, placebo-controlled trial. *Lancet.* 2009;373:1097-1104.

DeMatteo RP, Maki RG, Singer S, et al. Results of tyrosine kinase inhibitor therapy followed by surgical resection for metastatic gastrointestinal stromal tumor. *Ann Surg.* 2007;245:347-352.

Gold JS, Gönen M, Gutiérrez A, et al. Development and validation of a prognostic nomogram for recurrence-free survival after complete surgical resection of localised primary gastrointestinal stromal tumour: a retrospective analysis. *Lancet Oncol.* 2009;10:1045-1052.

Joensuu H, DeMatteo RP. The management of gastrointestinal stromal tumors: a model for targeted and multidisciplinary therapy of malignancy. *Annu Rev Med.* 2012;63:247-258.

Joensuu H, Eriksson M, Sundby Hall K, et al. One vs three years of adjuvant imatinib for operable gastrointestinal stromal tumor: a randomized trial. *JAMA.* 2012;307:1265-1272.

Rutkowski P, Gronchi A, Hohenberger P, et al. Neoadjuvant imatinib in locally advanced gastrointestinal stromal tumors (GIST): the EORTC STBSG experience. *Ann Surg Oncol.* 2013;20:2937-2943.

von Mehren M, Bejamin RS, Bui MM, et al. Soft tissue sarcoma, version 2.2012: featured updates to the NCCN guidelines. *J Natl Compr Canc Netw.* 2012;10:951-960.

THE MANAGEMENT OF MORBID OBESITY

Thomas Magnuson, MD,
and Michael A. Schweitzer, MD

The prevalence of morbid obesity has continued to increase in the United States and throughout the world. In the United States, nearly one third of adults are classified as obese with a body mass index (BMI) of greater than 30 kg/m^2, with more than 6% being severely obese (BMI > 40 kg/m^2). Medical therapies for weight reduction are, on the whole, unsuccessful at achieving and maintaining significant weight loss. Bariatric surgery continues to be the only durable method to obtain sustained weight loss and improvement of obesity-related medical disease for most patients.

Weight loss surgery first came into prominence in the 1970s, but early procedures were abandoned largely because of unacceptable complications (jejunal-ileal bypass) or poor long-term results (vertical banded gastroplasty). In the late 1990s weight loss surgery saw a resurgence, largely because of the development of improved bariatric procedures and application of minimally invasive surgical techniques. Currently, more than 150,000 bariatric procedures are performed in the United States annually. Over the last decade, numerous well-designed clinical trials have demonstrated the safety, efficacy, and durability of weight loss surgery. The four most common bariatric operations performed include Roux-en-Y gastric bypass, laparoscopic adjustable gastric band, duodenal switch with biliopancreatic diversion, and vertical sleeve gastrectomy. These operations achieve weight loss either by restriction of calorie intake (gastric band and sleeve gastrectomy), intestinal malabsorption of calories (duodenal switch), or a combination of restriction and malabsorption (gastric bypass). Weight loss surgery also has been demonstrated to have significant metabolic and neurohormonal effects (independent of restriction and malabsorption), which also may play an important role in the beneficial effects of these procedures.

■ PATIENT SELECTION

The National Institutes of Health issued a consensus statement in 1991 regarding the effectiveness of bariatric surgery and outlined patient selection criteria that are still in place today. Patients are considered candidates for bariatric surgery if they have a BMI of 40 kg/m^2 or greater or a BMI between 35 and 40 kg/m^2 if an obesity-related comorbidity such as diabetes or hypertension is present. In general, appropriate candidates for surgery should demonstrate prior unsuccessful attempts at nonsurgical weight loss options such as dietary intervention, pharmacologic therapy, or behavioral modification and have realistic expectations regarding the long-term outcomes achieved with surgery (Box 1). Relative contraindications include inability to comply with postoperative requirements, active alcohol or substance abuse, and uncontrolled psychiatric disease.

The evaluation of potential patients for bariatric surgery should involve a multidisciplinary team approach. This team should include a dietician and a mental health professional familiar with bariatric surgery. Their purpose is to obtain a complete past dietary and behavioral eating history, educate the patient on postoperative dietary expectations, examine social support structure, and ensure that any psychiatric or behavioral disorders are optimally controlled. At the Johns Hopkins Center for Bariatric Surgery, all patients are required to attend a multidisciplinary preoperative education seminar. Participation in postoperative support group meetings also is encouraged.

The age limits for surgery have expanded considerably over the last decade. Select centers now offer surgery to adolescent patients and to patients over the age of 70 years, with overall good results.

■ OPERATIVE PROCEDURES

Most bariatric surgical procedures are performed laparoscopically, with a hospital length of stay of 48 hours or less. Open surgery may be necessary and planned for patients who undergo revision surgery, those with prior extensive abdominal operations, or patients with a high BMI (more than 70).

On the morning of surgery, all patients should receive appropriate antibiotics as well as subcutaneous unfractionated or low-molecular-weight heparin to help minimize venous thromboembolic complications. Laparoscopic surgery involves the use of steep reverse Trendelenburg position, and the patient must be placed appropriately on the operating room table with use of a footboard and arms and legs secured. Initial laparoscopic entry in a morbidly obese patient can be difficult. We have found that the safest way to enter is in the left upper quadrant with direct vision, using a device that allows visualization of the abdominal wall layers during entry with a zero-degree laparoscope (12-mm Visiport; Covidien, Norwalk, CT). Once proper placement is confirmed, the abdomen then can be insufflated and the remaining laparoscopic trocars placed.

Laparoscopic Roux-en-Y Gastric Bypass

Gastric bypass (Figure 1) is the second most common bariatric procedure performed in the United States (30% to 40%). Numerous reports have shown that gastric bypass results in durable long-term weight loss and remission of metabolic disease with a reasonably low complication rate.

A 45-degree angled laparoscope is inserted, and the operation is performed using a total of 5 laparoscopic trocars (three 12-mm and two 5-mm). The omentum and transverse colon are retracted cephalad until the ligament of Treitz is visualized. The jejunum then is transected approximately 40 cm distal to the ligament of Treitz with a 60-mm white stapler cartridge (Endo-GIA Universal XL, Covidien, Norwalk, CT). The mesentery is divided with the gray stapler cartridge and the ultrasonic shears (AutoSonix XL, Covidien, Norwalk, CT). The proximal biliopancreatic limb of jejunum then is anastomosed to the distal segment of jejunum 75 to 100 cm distal to the point of division. We perform this anastomosis in a side-to-side fashion using a white Endo GIA stapler cartridge. The resulting mesenteric defect is closed with a running permanent suture to help minimize the risk of internal hernia.

Next the patient is placed in steep reverse Trendelenburg position, and the gastric pouch is created. The left lateral segment of the liver is retracted using a Nathanson retractor (Cook Medical, Bloomington, IN) through a subxiphoid 4-mm puncture and is held in position with a movable arm that attaches to the bed. We next dissect the peritoneal attachments at the angle of His to expose the left crus, follow the bare area of the gastrohepatic ligament, and enter the lesser sac. Division of the neurovascular bundle on the lesser-curve side of the stomach just distal to the left gastric artery and vein is accomplished using a gray vascular cartridge. Multiple 60-mm blue staple or black tri-staple cartridges then are used to transect the stomach up to the angle of His, creating a vertically oriented, 20-mL proximal gastric pouch. Any bleeding staple lines are controlled easily with clips or suture ligation.

We routinely bring the Roux limb up to the gastric pouch in an antecolic-antegastric orientation. This seems to reduce the incidence of internal hernias and is simpler to perform than a retrocolic-retrogastric approach. The side of the Roux limb is sutured to the gastric pouch staple line. A small enterotomy is made just proximal to the end of the Roux limb, and a similarly sized gastrotomy is made in the pouch for the placement of the Endo GIA. The stapler is loaded with a 45-mm blue cartridge to create the gastrojejunostomy, using only the first 30 mm of the staple cartridge. After the stapler is fired, a stay suture is placed on the lesser curve (right) side of the opening, and the suture then is used to retract the anastomosis to the left and

BOX 1: Indications for Bariatric Surgery for Morbid Obesity

1. BMI of 40 kg/m² or greater
2. BMI 35 to 39 kg/m² with significant obesity-related comorbidities (diabetes, hypertension)
3. Unsuccessful attempts at weight loss by nonoperative means
4. Clearance by dietician and mental health professional
5. No medical contraindications to surgery

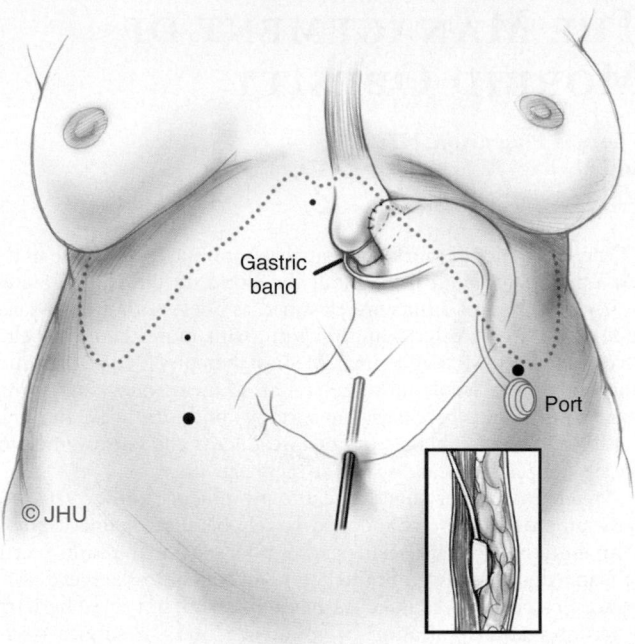

FIGURE 2 Laparoscopic adjustable gastric band. (Courtesy Corinne Sandone, Johns Hopkins University.)

Gastrografin swallow study can be performed on postoperative day 1 or 2 to check for leakage or obstruction.

Laparoscopic Adjustable Gastric Band

The laparoscopic adjustable gastric band (LAGB) received United States Food and Drug Administration approval in 2002 and has been in clinical use since that time. The band is adjustable via fluid injection into a subcutaneous port to allow for tightening or loosening of the band. Advantages of the band include reversibility, lack of intestinal stapling or manipulation, and ease of placement. The band requires an average of five to six adjustments in the first year after surgery, and its success depends in part on patient compliance and close follow-up. Relative contraindications for band placement include the super obese, large paraesophageal hernia, prior gastric resection or Nissen fundoplication, and chronic inflammatory changes at the gastroesophageal junction. Over the last several years, enthusiasm for the LAGB has diminished. This is related largely to studies suggesting inferior long-term weight loss compared with other operative options and a high rate of reoperation for band-related complications. The LAGB currently accounts for less than 10% of bariatric surgical procedures in the United States.

The LAGB procedure (Figure 2) is performed routinely via the pars flaccida technique, with two 12-mm trocars, one 5-mm trocar, and a 15-mm trocar for band insertion. The liver is retracted with a Nathanson retractor. Dissection is performed bluntly at the angle of His, freeing up attachments for later insertion of the band. The gastrohepatic ligament adjacent to the lesser curve of the stomach is then divided with electrocautery. The right crus is identified, and the anterior peritoneal tissue is divided. If a hiatal hernia is identified, reinforcement of the hiatus is important, either anteriorly or posteriorly, to discourage further herniation once the band has been placed. Two graspers are used to carefully dissect the plane of tissue posterior to the gastroesophageal junction to provide a tunnel for the LAGB.

An articulating dissector then is placed from the right crus toward the angle of His. The dissector arm then is flexed to create a right angle and locked into place. The adjustable band is placed into the

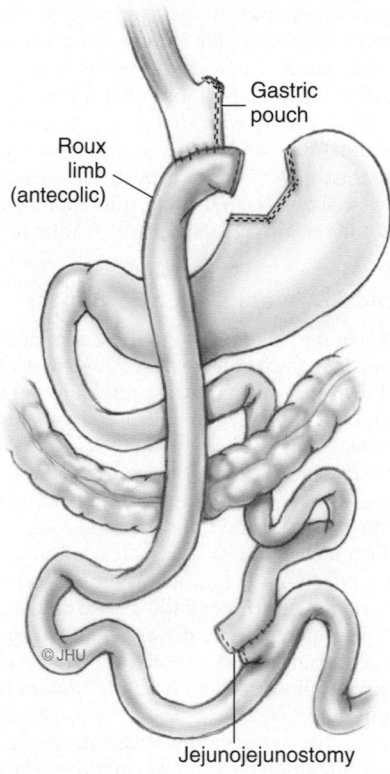

FIGURE 1 Antecolic-antegastric Roux-en-Y gastric bypass. (Courtesy Corinne Sandone, Johns Hopkins University.)

anterior, thereby exposing the posterior side. A running 2-0 suture is placed posterior on the left side and continuously run to the stay suture on the right side to which it is tied. A 32F, blunt, round-end bougie then is passed from the mouth through the gastrojejunal anastomosis and into the Roux limb. The bougie can be seen through the opening that was formed after the stapler was removed. A stay suture is placed at the halfway point of the opening between the end stay sutures. This stay suture and the stay suture on the left (angle of His side) are used to elevate the tissue so that the 60-mm length blue load cartridge can be used to close the openings. The stapler is brought down on top of the bougie while the tissue to be transected is retracted. This firing will close most of the opening, and the small remaining defect on the right side is closed readily with a 2-0 suture. The gastrojejunostomy is completed by running a 2-0 suture to cover the entire anterior portion in a second layer. The resultant anastomosis is approximately 12 mm in diameter. A leak test can be performed by clamping the Roux limb just distal to the anastomosis and insufflating air (via endoscope or orogastric tube), while the gastric pouch and anastomosis are submerged in saline.

The mesenteric defect then is closed between the Roux limb mesentery and the transverse mesocolon, up to the transverse colon. If desired, a drain can be placed adjacent to the gastric pouch, which usually is removed before hospital discharge. If clinically indicated, a abdomen through the 15-mm trocar in the left upper quadrant. The band is secured to the articulating dissector and brought around the stomach while the instrument is withdrawn. The band then is locked into place with approximately a 45-degree angle toward the patient's left shoulder. A minimum of two sutures then are placed from the fundus to the proximal gastric tissue around the band to secure the band into place. This reduces the possibility of band migration or herniation. It is important to ensure that the balloon portion of the band has not been compromised while either placing the band or suturing it into position.

The band tubing is brought out through the left upper quadrant port and secured externally to the subcutaneous injection port. When securing the port to the fascia, the surgeon must clear a sufficient space along the rectus sheath. After hemostasis has been achieved in the pocket, the port can be sutured or deployed into position while care is taken to leave the majority of the tubing in the abdomen. Finally, the port can be tested via Huber needle to ensure that the tube and band are functional and not kinked or malpositioned.

We do not perform a band fill before 6 weeks after surgery so that the site heals appropriately. If manual palpation of the subcutaneous port is difficult, fluoroscopy can be of assistance to fill the band. In patients with very thick subcutaneous tissue, placement of the band at the costal margin may be advantageous, for better palpation of the port during fills. Bands typically are filled approximately six times during the first year after placement. Each fill volume is 0.5 to 1 mL, depending on the amount of restriction desired. The patients must be able to swallow liquid without difficulty before leaving the clinic.

■ LAPAROSCOPIC VERTICAL SLEEVE GASTRECTOMY

Laparoscopic vertical sleeve gastrectomy (LVSG) is the most recent to be introduced of the bariatric surgery procedures (Figure 3) and is currently the most commonly performed weight loss operation in the United States (60% to 70%).

The LVSG is primarily restrictive, as the lateral aspect of the stomach is removed to create a sleeve-like tube or reservoir. The gastric resection also may assist with weight loss by causing hormonally assisted satiety. The fundus produces the proappetite hormone ghrelin, and because the fundus is removed, these hormone levels are reduced after LVSG. Although this bariatric procedure is not reversible, it can be converted into a Roux-en-Y gastric bypass or duodenal switch if greater weight loss is desired.

The LVSG typically is performed with one 5-mm, two 12-mm, and one 15-mm trocar. With the liver retracted with the Nathanson, the short gastric vessels are divided along the greater curve of the stomach. A LigaSure device (Covidien, Norwalk, CT) typically is used to accomplish this. A 40F blunt-tip bougie is placed in the stomach and directed along the lesser curve. The stomach is divided at the greater curvature, beginning 6 cm proximal to the pylorus. Green and blue staple loads (or black tri-stapler) are used adjacent to the 40F bougie and extending to the angle of His. The staple line is oversewn or an absorbable buttress material can be used with the staples to assist with hemostasis. To test the anastomosis, an endoscopic air test or liquid dye infused through an orogastric tube can be used.

The partial gastrectomy specimen is removed through the 15-mm trocar site. Care should be taken to repair the fascial opening of this enlarged trocar site to prevent postoperative herniation. We typically place a drain in the left upper quadrant that is removed before discharge. As with Roux-en-Y gastric bypass, a UGI study is performed only if clinically indicated.

Laparoscopic Duodenal Switch With Biliopancreatic Diversion

The laparoscopic duodenal switch with biliopancreatic diversion (DS-BPD) is primarily a malabsorptive operation that involves preservation of the pylorus and creation of a short, 100-cm ileal "common channel" (Figure 4). The DS-BPD is the least common bariatric

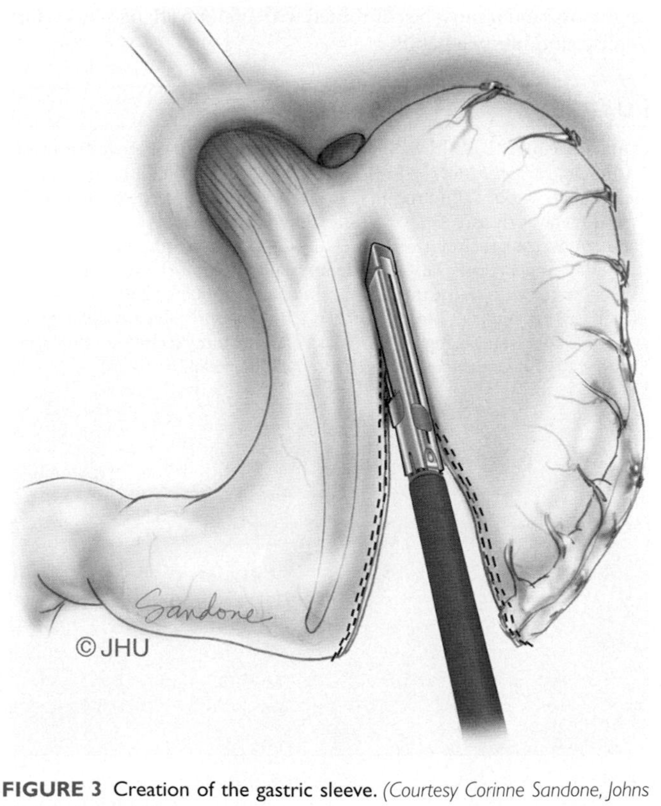

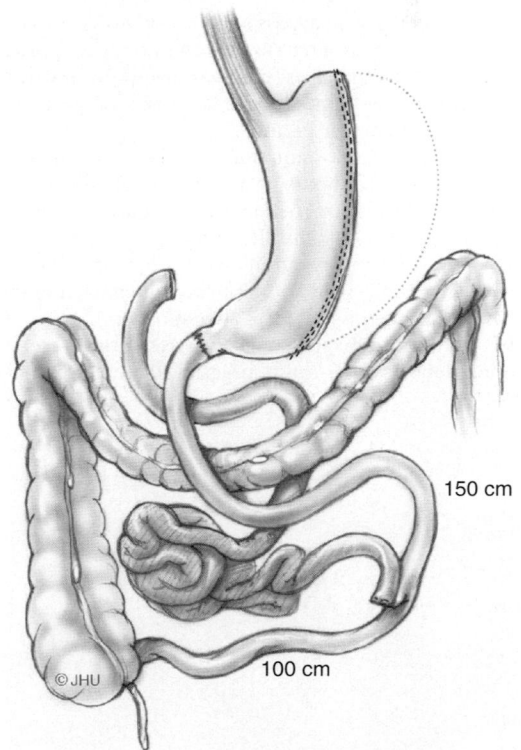

FIGURE 3 Creation of the gastric sleeve. (*Courtesy Corinne Sandone, Johns Hopkins University.*)

FIGURE 4 Antecolic duodenal switch with biliopancreatic diversion. (*Courtesy Corinne Sandone, Johns Hopkins University.*)

procedure performed because of its surgical complexity and potential for severe malabsorptive nutritional deficiencies.

This procedure can be performed in a single operation, or in two stages if the patient has a high BMI (>70). The first stage is similar to LVSG with the creation of a gastric sleeve. After approximately a 1-year period of weight loss, the patients can be converted to DS-BPD and malabsorptive second stage performed. This is performed by dividing the small bowel 250 cm from the ileocecal valve. The proximal end of bowel then is anastomosed to the distal ileum 100 cm from the cecum.

The patient then is placed in steep reverse Trendelenburg position, and the liver is retracted. If the sleeve gastrectomy portion has not been performed previously, then partial gastrectomy proceeds as previously described. The duodenum is then divided approximately 3 to 4 cm distal to the pylorus with a blue Endo GIA 60-mm stapler.

The Roux limb is directed in an antecolic fashion, and a side-to-side anastomosis is performed with the duodenum. An air leak or dye test can be performed to check for leaks at the stomach staple line and new duodenal-jejunal anastomosis. Finally, the mesenteric defect then is closed between the Roux limb mesentery and the transverse mesocolon.

■ OUTCOMES AND COMPLICATIONS

After any of the bariatric procedures, patients are seen in follow-up at 2 weeks to ensure that they are well hydrated, tolerating oral intake, and without wound complications. They are then seen at 3, 6, 12, 18, and 24 months and annually thereafter to follow weight loss and nutritional issues. Patients are encouraged to meet with dieticians and remain with their support groups indefinitely.

For 1 month after surgery, patients are all maintained on a high-protein puree consistency diet; after that they gradually are advanced to solid food. They also receive multivitamins, calcium, and vitamin B_{12} supplements. This is especially important for patients with gastric bypass and DS-BPD who are at higher risk for malabsorption and possible malnutrition. Supplemental iron always is considered for menstruating women.

Weight loss after gastric bypass and DS-BPD occurs primarily in the first 12 to 18 months after surgery and averages approximately 70% and 80% excess weight loss (EWL), respectively. Gastric banding and sleeve gastrectomy typically have less EWL, on average 40% to 50% over a 2-year to 3-year period.

One of the most important outcome measures after bariatric surgery is remission of obesity related metabolic diseases, such as type 2 diabetes. More than 70% to 80% of patients with diabetes experience complete remission after undergoing gastric bypass or DS-BPD. The restrictive operations have a 50% remission rate of diabetes. Hypertension, sleep apnea, hyperlipidemia, and fatty liver disease have similar remission rates after surgery.

Overall complication rates after bariatric surgery are less than 15% in most reports. Like most surgeries, there are early and late complications for bariatric surgery. Early or perioperative complications include bleeding, anastomotic leakage, and deep venous thrombosis. The mortality rate is less than 1% and is usually attributable to a pulmonary embolus or sepsis from anastomotic leak. Persistent unexplained tachycardia higher than 120 beats/min may be an early sign of sepsis, and an appropriate workup should be considered.

Vitamin B_{12}, calcium, iron, vitamin D, and protein deficiencies are long-term complications that can occur within the first year after surgery. Rigorous monitoring of nutrition status is necessary. Vitamin B_1 deficiency also can occur in patients with protracted vomiting after surgery, and they may experience extremity paresthesias and confusion. Lower extremity weakness and paresthesias also can be seen with vitamin B_{12} deficiency. Anastomotic stenosis and obstruction at the gastrojejunostomy in the first few months after surgery occur in less than 5% of patients after gastric bypass and usually can be managed with endoscopic dilation.

Internal hernias are also a possible complication and can occur at any time after surgery. The symptoms of internal hernia can be similar to an acute bowel obstruction or be chronic and described as postprandial cramping pain. If internal hernia is suspected, operative intervention may be required to avoid possible bowel ischemia.

In general, the results of weight-loss surgery are excellent, with most patients losing more than 50% of their excess weight with dramatic improvement or remission of metabolic disease. Approximately 10% to 15% of patients either do not achieve significant weight loss or partially regain their weight after 2 to 3 years. Ideally, these patients respond to dietary counseling, although some may need operative revision or conversion to a more malabsorptive procedure, such as the DS-BPD.

Unfortunately, no perfect method exists for choosing the best operation for each individual patient. Certainly, a multidisciplinary team approach is helpful in providing patient support throughout the preoperative and postoperative course. Reducing obesity-related diseases should be the major goal, not merely cosmetic improvement. Patients must understand that bariatric surgery is a tool to assist with weight loss, and it must be combined with lifelong changes in dietary, exercise, and lifestyle habits.

SUGGESTED READINGS

Adams TD, Gress RE, Smith SC, et al. Long-term mortality after gastric bypass surgery. *N Engl J Med*. 2007;357:753.

Buchwald H, Avidor Y, Braunwald E, et al. Bariatric surgery: a systemic review and meta-analysis. *J Am Med Assoc*. 2004;292:1724.

Melton G, Steele K, Schweitzer MA, et al. Suboptimal weight loss after gastric bypass surgery: correlation of demographics, comorbidities, and insurance status with outcomes. *J Gastrointest Surg*. 2008;12:250.

Schweitzer MA, Lidor A, Magnuson TH. 251 consecutive laparoscopic gastric bypass operations using a 2-layer gastrojejunostomy technique with a zero leak rate. *J Laparoendosc Adv Surg Tech*. 2006;16:83.

MANAGEMENT OF SMALL BOWEL OBSTRUCTION

Sandra R. DiBrito, MD and Mark Duncan, MD

Small bowel obstructions (SBOs) are responsible for one out of five surgical admissions for nontraumatic acute abdominal pain and are the most common surgical disorder of the small intestine. The majority of SBOs are attributed to postoperative adhesions. The prevalence of postoperative adhesive disease suggests that there are probably patients with subclinical SBOs that resolve spontaneously, not requiring hospitalization, with more frequency than we record. Despite the increasing utilization of laparoscopic surgery and presumed decrease in adhesive burden associated with laparoscopy, there has been no definitive evidence that the rate of SBO secondary to adhesions is decreasing concomitantly.

Management of SBOs varies widely based on clinical presentation and underlying cause, ranging from conservative care with fluids and nasogastric decompression to emergent operative intervention. Idiomatic surgical wisdom warns clinicians to "never let the sun rise or set on a bowel obstruction," encouraging expeditious and thorough investigation to prevent unnecessary morbidity and even mortality, recently estimated at 6% by a retrospective review. Management has not changed much since the time of Cope's discussion of the acute abdomen; however, studies suggest a high predictive value of innovative imaging techniques in guiding the surgeon toward or away from the operating room.

■ CLINICAL PRESENTATION

When patients are evaluated in the emergency department or even in clinic for colicky abdominal pain, bloating, nausea, and emesis, small bowel obstruction appears on the differential. These symptoms, in conjunction with a medical history of abdominal surgery, known herniae, prior small bowel obstruction, or malignancy should further raise clinical suspicion. It is imperative to assess the quality, frequency, and duration of symptoms, and ascertain other symptoms such as fever, chills, diarrhea, constipation, or obstipation. This historical evaluation can assist in differentiating between a patient who should be admitted to the floor (nausea, bloating, vague pain) and a patient who should proceed directly to the operating room (OR; fever, obstipation).

From a physiologic standpoint, direct manipulation or compression of the bowel does not result in the sensation of pain, and therefore the presence of adhesive disease at baseline does not cause chronic pain. Visceral pain is sensed by distension of the bowel wall, which occurs during small bowel obstruction of any cause, including adhesive disease. Following the Law of LaPlace, the larger the diameter of the bowel, the higher the pressure on the bowel wall. This results in the sensation of sharp, acute, variable pain usually described as colicky or cramping because peristalsis continues in the bowel despite obstruction. As the bowel becomes extremely dilated,

peristalsis ceases, and pain is perceived as constant and intense. The pressure within the lumen can overcome the capillary pressure in the bowel wall, resulting in bowel ischemia. Symptoms of chronic, vague abdominal pain could be suggestive of chronic, low-grade, partial obstruction, but this is not an indication for operative exploration.

When a patient with suspected bowel obstruction is examined, abdominal distension revealed by inspection is the hallmark of obstruction, particularly in the presence of visible surgical scars on the abdomen. Teachings traditionally suggest that auscultation should reveal "high-pitched tinkling" bowel sounds, but auscultation also may reveal a silent abdomen. This is not a sensitive or specific marker for obstruction, and although worth noting, it is unlikely to aid in clinical decision making. Percussion reveals tympany and may elicit pain as the examiner creates more pressure on an already distended bowel wall. Signs of focal or generalized peritonitis such as guarding and rebound pain merit exploration. A thorough examination for herniae, particularly for patients without a surgical history, is imperative, including point tenderness at common sites (umbilical, groin). A rare obturator hernia can be discovered with a rectal examination. Because a small bowel obstruction is a largely clinical diagnosis the examiner should be confident in the diagnosis after history and physical examination; however, the underlying cause may not be clear.

■ ETIOLOGY

Published studies suggest 4% to 10% of patients with a history of abdominal or pelvic operations are admitted for small bowel obstruction. Many terms have been used in an attempt to classify obstructions: partial vs complete, low grade vs high grade, open vs closed loop, but ultimately the clinician must assess patients on a case-by-case basis, analyzing individual factors to guide therapy.

The differential diagnosis for cause underlying small bowel obstruction is extremely broad, encompassing mechanical obstructions, malignancy, infection, trauma, and inflammatory conditions. Although by no means exhaustive, the most clinically relevant causes can be found in Box 1.

For patients without an operative history, hernia is the most common cause of small bowel obstruction. Presentation can range from complete obstruction to partial obstruction, but clinicians always should be wary of signs of strangulation or incarceration. Particularly, Richter's hernias, in which only a portion of the intestinal wall is within the hernia defect, must be considered, with bowel wall incarceration and ischemia and only partial obstruction. Any history of prior cancer should raise suspicion of metastasis. The likelihood of a new malignancy with the primary presenting symptom of obstruction is low, but in the population of patients with obstruction in the absence of prior surgery and with no demonstrable hernia, the chance of malignancy is high and should be investigated thoroughly with imaging and laboratory studies. Notably, adhesive disease can be secondary to peritonitis, diverticulitis, radiation enteritis, or even pelvic inflammatory disease, making adhesive disease a possible cause even in patients who have never undergone operations.

BOX 1: Causes of Small Bowel Obstruction

Adhesions

Hernia

- Incisional, port site*
- Umbilical
- Inguinal, femoral
- Internal*
- Parastomal*
- Abdominal wall, flank
- Obturator
- Paraesophageal

Inflammatory, Infectious

- Crohn's disease
- Stricture*
- Abscess
- Mesenteric adenitis
- Radiation enteritis
- Endometriosis

Malignancy

- Ileocecal, colon mass
- Lymphoma
- Metastases
  - Colon, ovarian, gastric, pancreatic, melanoma
- Primary small bowel tumor
  - Carcinoid, GIST, adenocarcinoma

Other

- Gallstone ileus
- Traumatic mural hematoma
- Foreign body
- Intussusception
- Congenital issues such as malrotation

*Included in the differential diagnosis of patients who have had previous operations.

Gallstone ileus, a commonly discussed but much less commonly encountered cause of small bowel obstruction, is a misnomer. It is not actually an ileus, but a true mechanical obstruction at or proximal to the ileocecal valve caused by erosion of a large gallstone into the small bowel via a biliary-enteric fistula. Presence of air in the biliary tree often is identified on imaging. Repair of the biliary fistula is indicated, preferably at the time of index surgery; however, based on the clinical status of the acutely obstructed patient, may not be appropriate on primary operation to relieve obstruction and could require a second operation after stabilizing the patient.

For patients in the immediate postoperative period, it is important to differentiate small bowel obstruction from adynamic ileus. The symptomatology of these two conditions is very similar: pain, nausea, emesis, distension, decreased passage of stool, and flatus. Plain radiographs demonstrate dilated loops of bowel with air fluid levels, which is neither sensitive nor specific for either condition. The underlying cause of ileus can be local inflammation or infection (as with perforated appendicitis), or simply postoperative, postanesthetic bowel akinesia. In either case, ileus can be treated with fluid resuscitation, nasogastric decompression, and the tincture of time. Ileus does not pose a threat of bowel ischemia, however, because the presentations are so similar, workup for small bowel obstruction should be considered whenever ileus is diagnosed. Although ileus is certainly more common in the immediate postoperative period, it is possible to have a small bowel obstruction caused by mechanical stricture, early adhesive band formation, laparoscopic port site, or other hernia, including internal hernia, or intraoperative error, which may necessitate prompt operative intervention.

DIAGNOSIS AND WORKUP

After a thorough history and physical examination, laboratory values can aid in identifying which patients require urgent operative management. Persistent leukocytosis after resuscitation is worrisome for strangulation, bowel compromise, or perforation. Prolonged emesis can cause hypokalemic, hypochloremic metabolic alkalosis, whereas bowel ischemia can cause a concomitant lactic acidosis. Urine electrolytes can be assessed for a paradoxic aciduria after the metabolic alkalosis if the clinical picture is still unclear; however, this is mostly of academic interest and not in our practice. Bowel could be compromised without an elevation of serum lactate if a closed loop obstruction is present, as the venous return from the compromised segment is cut off from circulation. Operative decompression of the loop allows for admixing of venous blood, resulting in a surge of lactate and cytokines, propagating a dramatic systemic inflammatory response. Trending electrolytes and white blood cell count helps to manage resuscitation and to inform operative decision making in patients who do not require urgent intervention but may still require a trip to the OR during their hospitalization.

In the case of a stable patient, plain films are an appropriate choice for a primary evaluation (Figure 1). When flat and upright views are obtained, films have 67% to 83% accuracy of diagnosing SBO. Signs include distension of small bowel more than 3 cm diameter, decompressed distal loops, paucity of air in the colon, and air fluid levels on upright films. Patients also may have gastric distension and a fluid level. A "gasless" abdomen suggests that all bowel loops are filled with fluid, consistent with either SBO or ileus. A chest x-ray or high KUB is indicated to look for free air pointing to a perforation. Imaging studies are not necessary if a patient has hemodynamic instability and physical findings of intra-abdominal catastrophe.

With ready access to CT scans, clinicians can obtain a much more valuable picture of the patient in the same amount of time it takes to perform a set of plain films. To evaluate the perfusion of the bowel wall, administration of IV contrast is recommended. Oral contrast can sometimes improve visualization of bowel loops; however, it usually is not well tolerated and can even obscure findings such as bowel wall ischemia that are best delineated with IV contrast only. It is imperative to search for and localize hernias, transition points, and general location of the obstructed segment, as well as to examine for any masses or intra-abdominal lymphadenopathy. The authors make a point to first identify the very reliably located descending colon on the CT scan, following it proximally to delineate colon and small bowel anatomy and ascertain the degree of distension or decompression in the colon (Figure 2).

Sensitivity and specificity of CT scans in identifying SBO are both more than 95%, with 90% specificity for identifying strangulated bowel. With a negative predictive value of nearly 100% for bowel ischemia, CT scan is a reliable test to rule out bowel compromise (Box 2). Although axial views are the historical standard for CT interpretation, we find coronal images superior in the evaluation of small bowel obstruction. The coronal plane allows appreciation of the overall gestalt of the abdomen in relationship to the stomach, colon, and small bowel simultaneously, often allowing for quick identification of transition points and decompressed distal bowel (Figure 3). More certain characterization of the transition point(s) can inform operative management. Limitations of CT scan include poor discernment of partial obstructions because bowel is less distended with more subtle transition points.

Any findings on CT that are suggestive of small bowel ischemia such as pneumatosis (Figure 4) should prompt urgent operative intervention. Free fluid is commonly present in small bowel obstructions, even if low grade or partial. However, a large volume of ascites is known anecdotally to portend poor spontaneous resolution and often is seen with bowel compromise.

Featured heavily in the recent Bologna Guidelines, fluoroscopy and contrast follow-through examinations are recommended in Europe as a measure for further evaluation of bowel obstructions.

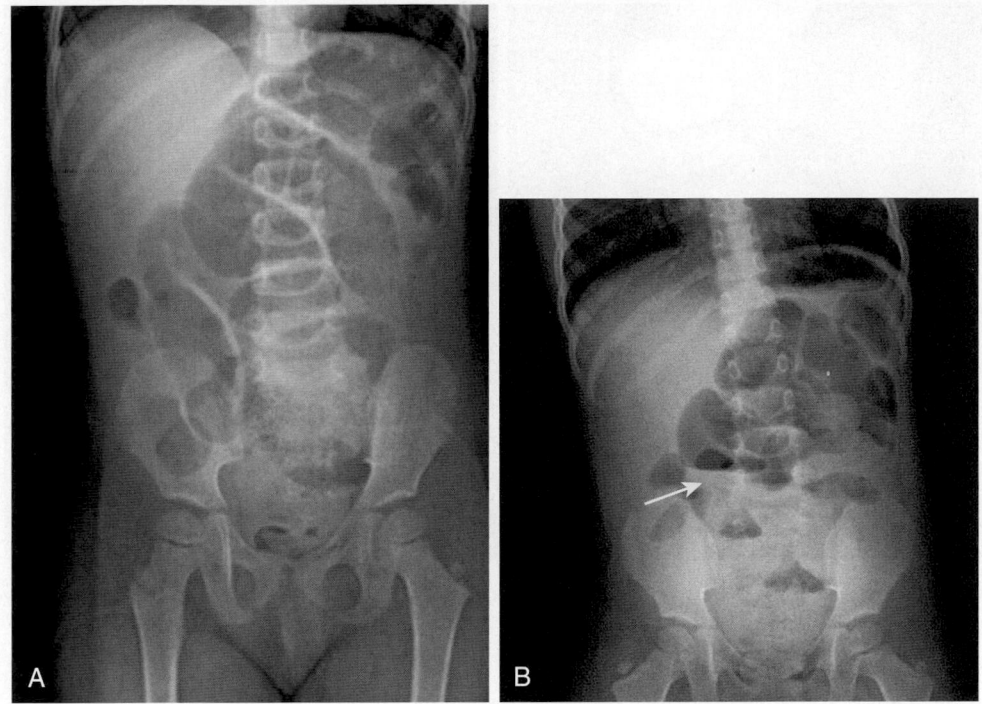

FIGURE 1 Flat (**A**) and upright (**B**) radiograph of small bowel obstruction in a pediatric patient; arrow identifies air-fluid level.

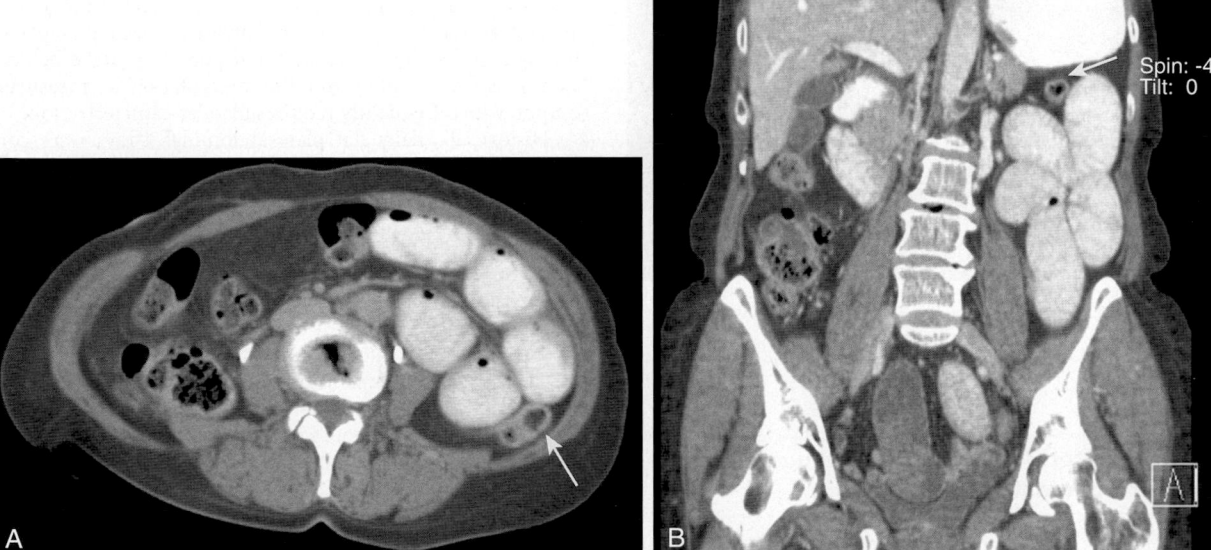

FIGURE 2 Axial (**A**) and coronal (**B**) CT views of abdomen with small bowel obstruction. Arrows indicate decompressed left colon.

Administration of water-soluble contrast medium allows for visualization of partial versus complete obstruction and further defines the transition point. This option is used less commonly in the United States because these examinations are poorly tolerated, contrast often dilutes in bowel contents, and they require several hours to complete, potentially delaying operative treatment decisions. Nevertheless, global reviews find that presence of contrast in the colon within 24 hours of administration portends resolution of obstruction without operative intervention, encouraging surgeons to continue conservative management. It also is suggested that in behaving as a hyperosmotic agent, contrast draws water and edema out of the bowel wall and into the lumen, theoretically aiding in the resolution of the obstruction.

■ NONOPERATIVE MANAGEMENT

Conservative management is preferred, when possible, to avoid the risks of operations. However, to safely manage a small bowel

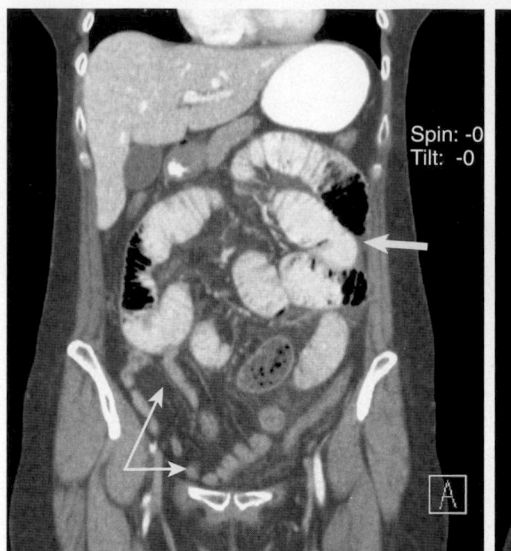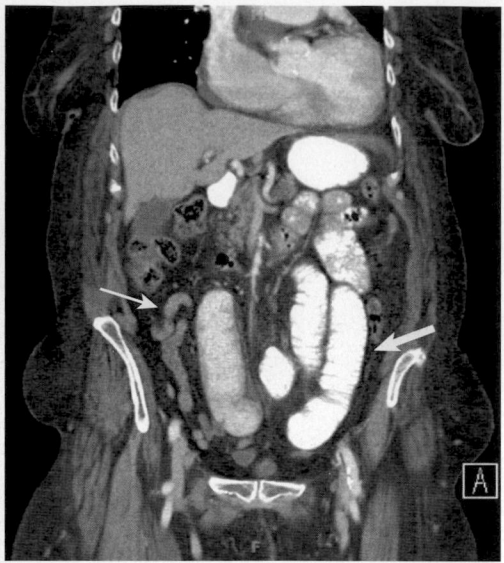

FIGURE 3 Coronal CT of two separate patients with small bowel obstructions. Thin arrows indicate decompressed distal small bowel; thick arrows indicate dilated proximal small bowel containing oral contrast.

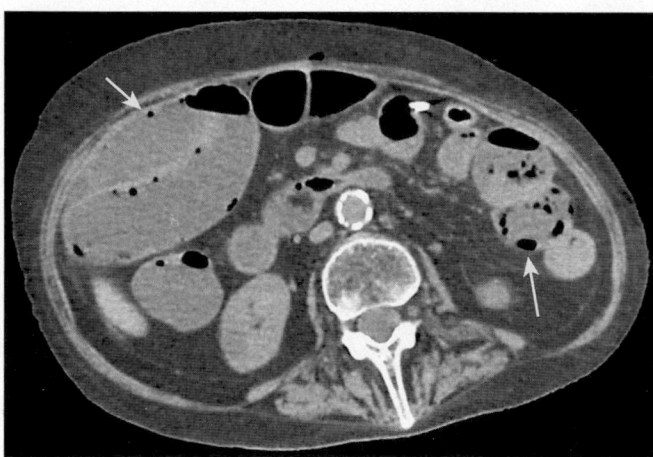

FIGURE 4 Axial CT demonstrating pneumatosis of small bowel wall, indicated by *arrows*.

BOX 2: Computed Tomography Findings Associated With Bowel Ischemia

Bowel Wall
- Decreased, delayed enhancement
- Mural thickening
- Pneumatosis

Mesentery
- Venous congestion, engorgement
- Mesenteric edema
- Mesenteric hemorrhage

Other
- Portal, mesenteric venous gas
- Free fluid, ascites

obstruction nonoperatively, the patient must be hemodynamically stable, must resolve acidosis and leukocytosis with initial resuscitation, and should not have signs of strangulation or perforation. Mainstays of therapy are nasogastric decompression and supportive care. Nasogastric decompression is accomplished best with a Salem sump tube that is flushed vigilantly with air and water to maintain optimal patency. Fluid resuscitation with Lactated Ringer's solution, as well as replacement of electrolytes as needed, replaces losses through gastric decompression and poor PO intake before admission. It is important to monitor resuscitation by measuring urine output, which frequently requires bladder catheterization.

Historically, daily flat plate abdominal x-rays were considered imperative to follow progress of evolving bowel obstruction. This is not necessary. Deciphering whether a patient is improving has more to do with the physical examination, decreasing NG tube output, decreasing pain, and passage of flatus, than findings on daily images, which do not inform treatment decisions reliably. That being said, if patients are not progressing after a 48- to 72-hour trial of conservative management, follow-up imaging is suggested.

A trial of conservative management is reasonable for patients who are early in their course of obstruction with low-grade nausea and manageable pain. Patients with suspicion of hernia or neoplasms as the obstructive point should not be treated conservatively. Clinicians also must consider the patient's individual risk factors for surgery and balance that against the risks of conservative management if the patient is truly a poor operative candidate.

If patients have not experienced resolution after 72 hours of decompression and supportive care, this predicts failure of conservative management in most cases. A recent meta-analysis suggests patients with more than 500 mL of nasogastric output on the third day of obstruction, or pain that is persistent for 4 days after hospitalization often are better served with an operation. Re-imaging patients at this stage with oral contrast allows for visualization of any progress, and if contrast still does not pass to colon 24 hours beyond the study, operative management is recommended. This does not apply for patients with history of frequent, recurrent small bowel obstructions. Patients with Crohn's disease may require 1 to 2 weeks of decompression, medical management of inflammation, and even a course of total parenteral nutrition to avoid reoperation. The rare patient with bowel obstruction secondary to mesenteric or mural hematoma associated with trauma can require 2 to 4 weeks to regain bowel function as the swelling of bowel and surrounding mesentery resolves.

■ OPERATIVE MANAGEMENT

As mentioned previously, patients with peritonitis, closed loop obstructions, or strangulation require emergent operative management. In addition, patients with irreducible hernias and those who are readmitted within 6 weeks of a recent operation are likely to require operative intervention. In these cases, the rate of bowel resection increases concomitantly with time-to-OR. A retrospective review demonstrated that for patients taken to OR within 24 hours, the rate of small bowel resection was 12%, whereas those delayed longer than 24 hours had a small bowel resection rate of 29%.

A midline approach is usually appropriate for entry into the abdomen, taking care to avoid damaging underlying bowel that may be adhesed to the abdominal wall from prior surgery. Lysis of adhesions is appropriate to allow for safe visualization of the bowel, but complete lysis of all adhesions is not necessary to achieve resolution of a bowel obstruction and can cause unnecessary damage to otherwise healthy bowel. Once the source of obstruction is located and rectified, it is imperative to run the bowel with particular attention to the distal aspect toward the ileocecal valve to ensure no downstream sites of obstruction are present. Herniae that are the source of obstruction should be repaired at the time of operation. Biologic mesh is preferred for hernia repair in cases that involve spillage of bowel contents; however, synthetic mesh is appropriate if no contamination has occurred and no bowel resection or repair is required. Bowel should be evaluated for any damage, including iatrogenic injury that may have occurred on entry into abdomen or with lysis of adhesions. If an injury is present, primary repair with silk suture using interrupted Lembert technique is indicated. Injury involving more than 50% of the circumference of the small bowel loop requires formal resection and reanastomosis.

When perforated or frankly ischemic bowel is encountered, it must, of course, be resected. When bowel is felt to be marginally viable, the surgeon may choose to leave the patient with an open abdomen for a short duration, to allow the bowel to reperfuse to its full capacity and to limit unnecessary resection. This may be particularly useful in situations that require large volume resuscitation or in which the bowel is extremely swollen. Historically, fluorescein dye (500 to 1000 mg intravenous administration in a 10% solution) has been used in conjunction with a Wood's lamp to identify areas of poor perfusion and may be helpful in identifying which sections of marginally viable bowel should be left versus resected. If a mass or neoplasm is encountered on exploration, this should be resected in an oncologic manner with 8- to 10-cm margins along the intestine as well as including the associated lymphatic tissue with the resected specimen. The liver and peritoneal cavity should be investigated for any evidence of metastases. On exit of the operating room, patients should be equipped with a functioning nasogastric tube whose position is confirmed intraoperatively. There are new (and old) strategies that have been developed in an effort to decrease adhesion formation, but the authors do not advocate for empiric use outside of controlled studies because there is no definitive research demonstrating benefit.

There is a limited role for laparoscopic evaluation of small bowel obstruction, particularly for patients in the early postoperative period after a recent laparoscopic surgery, cases that are thought to be related to a single band (having a short, very distinct transition point) and those in which the bowel is dilated but not to the degree that it would impair visualization. Laparoscopic management has resulted in 74% to 95% success for resolution of single-band adhesive

obstruction; however, the conversion rate for laparoscopic intervention in small bowel obstruction ranges from 30% to 50%. An open Hasson approach, away from prior surgical scars is recommended to decrease iatrogenic damage to the bowel. Those cases that are converted to an open approach typically are done so because visualization is inadequate (too many adhesions, bowel too dilated) or because of iatrogenic injury to the bowel, which occurs in up to 3% to 17% of laparoscopic operations for obstruction. The reported incidence of inadvertent enterotomy is nearly 20% in open cases as well. A recent survey of general surgeons revealed that surgeons who have been practicing less than 15 years and are located at academic/teaching centers are more likely to start a small bowel obstruction case laparoscopically than their counterparts further out from training. Surgeons perhaps are becoming more facile with laparoscopic techniques. It still is important to carry out a thorough evaluation of the bowel for more distal points of obstruction all the way to the ileocecal valve and to ensure that there has been no missed enterotomy. Although we recognize and appreciate the enthusiasm of the surgical community surrounding laparoscopy, this technique must be applied with caution, and the open approach remains safe and effective in most all circumstances.

■ PALLIATION OF MALIGNANT OBSTRUCTION

The surgical approach to small bowel obstruction in advanced malignancy requires special attention, addressing goals of care when choosing the appropriate operative management. Carcinomatosis, omental caking, and other end-stage malignancy can cause frequent, recurrent, and incapacitating small bowel obstruction. These patients benefit most from palliative management as opposed to aggressive adhesiolysis or bowel resection. Palliative insertion of a gastric tube with percutaneous, image-guided, or small open technique enables patients to achieve decompression in an outpatient setting. This allows them to enjoy more freedom and an increased quality of life despite chronic obstruction. Management of end-stage disease requires discussions with patients and their caretakers about appropriate goals as their underlying disease progresses. Patients who are well informed about symptoms they can expect often are more satisfied with their care, even though they may be deteriorating. During these discussions, it is imperative to discuss end-of-life care, including what the patient would want in the case of perforation in the setting of a chronic obstruction. Surgery has a definitive place in the palliation of malignant bowel obstruction and requires a plan for decompression, symptom management, and goals of end-of-life care.

SUGGESTED READINGS

Diaz JJ, Bokhari F, Mowery NT, et al. Guidelines for management of small bowel obstruction. *J Trauma.* 2008;64:1651-1664. <http://doi.org/10.1097/TA.0b013e31816f709e>.

Di Saverio S, Coccolini F, Galati M, et al. Bologna guidelines for diagnosis and management of adhesive small bowel obstruction (ASBO): 2013 update of the evidence-based guidelines from the world society of emergency surgery ASBO working group. *World J Emerg Surg.* 2013;8:42. doi:10.1186/1749-7922-8-42.

Leung AM, Vu H. Factors predicting need for and delay in surgery in small bowel obstruction. *Am Surg.* 2012;78:403-407.

Min-Zhe L, Lei L, Long-bin X, et al. Laparoscopic versus open adhesiolysis in patients with adhesive small bowel obstruction: a systematic review and meta-analysis. *Am J Surg.* 2012;204.

Mullan CP, Siewert B, Eisenberg RL. Small bowel obstruction. *AJR Am J Roentgenol.* 2012;198:W105-W117. <http://doi.org/10.2214/AJR.10.4998>.

THE MANAGEMENT OF CROHN'S DISEASE OF THE SMALL BOWEL

Mark A. Talamini, MD

Crohn's disease is a chronic inflammatory transmural disease of the gastrointestinal tract. It is remarkable for the spectrum of intensity, range of anatomic geography, and historically stubborn resistance to therapy other than surgery. As often is stated in medical student lectures, it can affect the gastrointestinal tract anywhere from the mouth to the anus. Most commonly, and often initially it occurs in the distal small bowel. Clinically it tends to be a cyclical disease in symptoms and pathophysiology, alternating inflammation and repair in synchrony with the physician's best efforts to manage it. Its exact "cause" continues to be an enigma, even in the early twenty-first century despite intense investigation. The body of research points to a complex interaction of genetics, environment, and the microbiome, with the host immune system at the center of it all. Its incidence continues to increase worldwide. The epidemiology, even from the disease's initial description is fascinating and continues to be so in our current era of "big data." Why, for instance, is it more common in those who have had tonsillectomy or appendectomy, and less common in those who had a childhood vegetable garden (Gearry et al, 2010)?

Contrary to early surgical dogma, Crohn's disease cannot be cured surgically. However, this fact does not diminish the critical role of surgery in the management of the disease for a large cohort of afflicted patients. Rather, surgical therapy is the ultimate tool for management of the complications of the disease for the roughly two thirds of all Crohn's patients who will undergo surgery. The fact that surgery is not curative makes the appropriate application of surgery that much more challenging. Overall, the goals of surgical treatment are alleviating symptoms and improving quality of life.

The clinical hallmark of Crohn's disease is abdominal pain and diarrhea. The broader spectrum of associated symptoms may include hematochezia, fever, anorexia and weight loss, fatigue, nausea and vomiting, malnutrition, vitamin deficiency, and growth failure in the young. In its early presentation it must be differentiated clinically from acute gastrointestinal (GI) conditions such as appendicitis or bowel obstruction. The diagnosis depends upon a detailed history, including family history and environmental and historical factors, and a complete physical examination. Imaging, both direct via endoscopy and indirect, are critical to understanding and tracking a given patient's disease. Barium contrast studies in current practice are rare, having been replaced by computed tomography (CT) or magnetic resonance imaging (MRI) investigations focused upon the bowel (CT or MRI enterography). The images from these studies performed with current generation machines are truly remarkable. Endoscopic examination of the affected GI tract provides direct observation and tissue diagnosis, as well as precise mapping of the disease, particularly in the colon and the upper tract. Capsule endoscopy allows for direct examination of the small bowel. At initial presentation, 40% of patients will have terminal ileal disease, 20% will have colonic disease, 10% will have more proximal small bowel disease, 10% will have perianal disease, and 20% will have disease in more than one anatomic location.

MEDICAL AND TEAM MANAGEMENT

The optimal surgical management of Crohn's disease occurs within a team environment anchored by the surgeon and gastroenterologist. Input from radiology, pathology, social work, and associated specialists as needed is important. The medical treatment of Crohn's disease has advanced exponentially in the last decade, following upon the introduction and application of anti-TNF (anti–tumor necrosis factor) biologic agents (Box 1). Much has been written on the medical management of Crohn's disease in previous editions of this text and in the literature. Recent important advances include the use of combination therapy with anti-TNF and azathioprine early in the disease leading to high mucosal healing rates and high steroid-free remission rates (Colombel et al, 2010). Newer agents, including anti-interleukin 12/23 antibody (ustekinumab) and anti–alpha-4 beta-7 integrin antibody (vedolizumab) for Crohn's disease, are showing great effect and broaden the biologic armamentarium (Sandborn et al, 2012; Sandborn et al, 2013).

INDICATIONS FOR SURGERY

Overall, the indications for surgery in the setting of small bowel Crohn's disease mirror the indications for bowel surgery in general (Box 2). Crohn's disease rarely perforates, but rather fistulizes. Bleeding is rarely an acute indication for surgery, but intermittent or chronic blood loss does occur. Obstruction is the most common indication for surgery in Crohn's disease. The natural history is that of gradual onset in the setting of this chronic relapsing disease. The cycling of inflammation and repair over time in a Crohn's-affected segment (usually the terminal ileum) eventually converts soft pliable bowel into constricted stovepipe. Clinically, as this process progresses, the symptomatology evolves from intermittent partial bowel obstruction experienced during episodes of transmural inflammation to chronic partial obstruction that exists between episodes of acute inflammation. The troika of the surgeon, gastroenterologist, and patient must determine when during this process surgical intervention is most appropriate to deal with "medically refractory" disease. Clearly the biologics have modified this process by reducing the inflammation and damage, but they have not prevented or reversed the process. Rather, they have probably drawn it out, allowing some patients to avoid surgery, while delaying surgery in others. Disease at multiple sites within the small bowel, or other sites along the GI tract (colon, duodenum) make these calculations more complex but do not alter the basic paradigm.

As a transmural inflammatory process, Crohn's disease also can create mischief that falls into the "fistulization" bucket. The common theme of this pathophysiology is the inflammatory process "burrowing" through the wall of the affected bowel into adjacent innocent structures, through the abdominal wall to the skin (enterocutaneous fistula), or into the peritoneal space (creating peritoneal collections). When the process creates a clean fistula into another portion of the GI tract without creating an abscess, the decision regarding surgery depends on the impact of the connection. If between two loops of small bowel, the short circuiting of succus entericus may have only minimal or no nutritional effect and therefore may not be a sole indication for surgery. However, even a clean fistula between the proximal jejunum and the transverse colon would have devastating nutritional and symptomatic effects and would have to be addressed with urgent surgery. Fistulas into other structures such as the bladder are usually not life threatening, but the recurrent infections and annoying symptoms of pneumaturia and fecaluria lead most patients to want an operation. Intraperitoneal collections occur when the pathophysiology of the "burrowing" does not successfully fistulize but instead creates an intraperitoneal collection. In Crohn's disease, this is rarely an isolated event. Rather, it is driven by a badly diseased segment of bowel. Generally, if a segment of diseased bowel has caused such a process that is sufficient indication for surgical resection.

Reduction or alteration of medication is also an important consideration in decision regarding surgery. A clear shift has occurred away from steroids as the mainstay of medical therapy for Crohn's, particularly with the effectiveness of the biologics. Many patients

BOX 1: Common Medications Used for Medical Therapy in Crohn's Disease of the Small Bowel

Mild Active Disease
5-ASA

Induction of Remission
Corticosteroids
Infliximab
Infliximab and azathioprine
New biologics

Maintenance of Remission
Azathioprine
6-mercaptopurine
Methotrexate
Infliximab
New biologics

BOX 2: Indications for Operation in Crohn's Disease

Failure of medical management
Intestinal obstruction
Fistula
Inflammatory mass/abscess
Hemorrhage
Perforation
Growth retardation
Reduction in medication burden

BOX 3: Guidelines for Operative Management

Determine length of healthy bowel.
Resect only the segment(s) causing complications.
Determine whether resection or stricturoplasty is more appropriate.
Resect to grossly negative margins.
Bypass only if the duodenum is involved, if resection is technically impossible, or in short bowel syndrome.
If there is a high risk for complications, protect the anastomosis with diversion.

■ TECHNICAL CONSIDERATIONS FOR SURGICAL INTERVENTION

Once a decision regarding elective surgery has been made, the patient's current disease state must be assessed to inform preoperative planning (Box 3). The patient's general medical condition must be assessed and maximized. If nutritional deficits exist, and time allows, nutritional improvement should be pursued. A standard bowel preparation should be performed preoperatively unless the patient has a long-term, high-grade obstruction. In these cases a prolonged period of clear liquid diet only, in combination with oral antibiotics just before surgery, will likely suffice. All patients are given prophylactic intravenous antibiotics just before surgery, and all patients perform preoperative showering and washing with a skin cleanser and antiseptic. Fluid and electrolyte imbalances and any existing anemia also should be corrected before surgery. If a diversion is possible, a stoma site should be marked preoperatively.

Perioperative management of steroids, antimetabolites, and biologic agents continues to be controversial in the setting of Crohn's surgery. To the extent possible, steroids should be reduced before surgery. The bigger recent question is whether to stop anti-TNF agents. The literature is mixed, with some studies showing no effect and others showing minimal effect (see selected literature). It is the current practice in most major IBD centers to not hold these agents for surgery, opting for control of disease over potential postoperative complications.

The exact state of disease should be known or fully pursued. Usually this involves a current axial imaging study focusing on the bowel (CT or MR enterography). If questions remain regarding the small bowel, capsule endoscopy or small bowel enteroscopy should be pursued. The colon should be examined via colonoscopy. The cecum and the terminal ileum in particular merit examination because the state of colonic disease is more difficult to assess laparoscopically in the operating room. If upper tract Crohn's exists or is suspected, upper endoscopy also should be performed. These imaging efforts share two goals: planning the extent of resection and seeking important disease in other areas of the GI tract.

In discussing the findings and the plan with the patient, important contingencies must be reviewed. The possible nutritional effects of surgery, as well as the possible role of a stoma should be discussed. The more information the patient and family understand regarding the plan, the better.

The mainstay of surgical therapy for Crohn's disease of the small bowel is resection. The most commonly faced initial operative scenario is a tight but reasonably short segment of chronically obstructed and scarred terminal ileum. The most common operation therefore is resection of this terminal ileum along with only the cecum if the right colon is otherwise uninvolved. Unless there are 6 inches or more of uninvolved terminal ileum distal to the segment that requires resection, the cecum should be resected. A remaining short segment directly adjacent to the cecum is highly likely to suffer recurrent Crohn's disease early. Thus this is an exception to the principle of attempting to preserve the ileocecal valve.

require multiple agents to control acute Crohn's flares, or for maintenance. Reducing or eliminating the burden of disease can provide patients with a "fresh start," off all agents except prophylactic postoperative medications. Eliminating steroids, given the long-term consequences of chronic steroids, can be in itself an indication for surgery. So too can reduction from multiple agents to a single maintenance or prophylactic nonsteroid agent with fewer side effects.

The timing of surgery for these and other complications of Crohn's disease is important in maximizing the clinical outcome. The patient's willingness or resistance to surgery affects decision making. However, the expert input of the surgeon and gastroenterologist regarding timing is paramount. Operating too soon, when the bowel is intensely inflamed is technically challenging and puts nondiseased bowel at risk. Allowing a flare time and space to settle down, if possible, can make a huge difference. Waiting too long in a patient unable to eat risks difficulties resulting from malnutrition. Any peritoneal collection should be drained percutaneously, and the local tissue given time to resolve the resulting inflammation before surgery, if possible.

Emergency indications for surgery in Crohn's disease rarely differ from indications in a non-Crohn's patient. Bleeding (Crohn's related or not), perforation, acute obstruction, and appendicitis can occur. The management largely is unaltered by the accompanying diagnosis of Crohn's disease. Patients with long-standing Crohn's of the small bowel are at increased risk of developing adenocarcinoma of the small bowel. The principles of surgical management of such a patient with adenocarcinoma arising in Crohn's diseased bowel are the same as a patient with de novo adenocarcinoma of the small bowel. Although unusual, a handful of rare diseases can masquerade as Crohn's disease of the small bowel. Two to bear in mind are tuberculosis of the small bowel, and Behçet's syndrome affecting the small bowel. Both have unique characteristics that would tip off the astute clinician. Both require therapy distinct from Crohn's disease. Both likely are associated with heritage or exposure outside of the United States.

In virtually all cases, an attempt is made at gaining laparoscopic access and at achieving a laparoscopic dissection and mobilization of the target diseased tissue. If the case will be shorter than 3 hours, we will have the patient void before arriving in the operating room and not use a urinary catheter. The laparoscope is placed in a periumbilical or umbilical position, with a 10-mm port. Once the laparoscope is in place, usually two additional 5-mm ports are placed. One is typically in the suprapubic region for cosmesis and to create a vector towards the expected site of dissection. The third trocar is placed after directly observing where the target tissue resides and selecting a location that will maximize the dissecting vector among the three trocars. During the case, visualization can be moved from port to port to gain additional exposure information. In general 30-degree scopes are used to maximize visual information from a variety of angles.

During the process of dissection and mobilization, the constant decision grid is whether the process can continue in a reasonably safe manner (there is no such thing as 100% safety), or whether the laparoscopic approach should be abandoned in favor of a larger incision (Schmidt et al, 2001). The initial dissection time rarely is wasted, as any dissection that can reduce the eventual length of total incision accrues to the patient's benefit in terms of recovery. The first step is full evaluation of the gastrointestinal tract laparoscopically, correlating the visual information with known preoperative evaluation. If a fistula exists, it must be identified. Once identified, can it be divided laparoscopically? If there was a previous collection with involved Crohn's bowel, can the bowel be mobilized?

The next step is to sufficiently mobilize tissue for resection or stricturoplasty. This almost always involves some mobilization of the cecum and right colon, as well as mobilization of terminal ileal mesentery from the retroperitoneum. Great care must be taken in this dissection to be in the proper dissection plane, thereby avoiding injury to vital retroperitoneal tissues. The ureter should be identified clearly. In rare cases of extreme mesenteric inflammation, the ureter may not be directly observable, but it should be pursued more distantly in the pelvis to understand its anatomic course. Straying into the retroperitoneal tissues or into the mesenteric vessels must be avoided, and if it cannot be avoided a larger incision should be made. A sufficient amount of the ascending colon toward the hepatic flexure also must be mobilized. In some patients this will require nearly full mobilization of the hepatic flexure. If the target diseased small bowel is more proximal, the cecum and ascending colon would not have to be mobilized.

The usual plan is for the diseased tissue to be extracted through the umbilicus because the origin of the mesenteric vessels is directly deep to the umbilicus. Extracting the tissue through a Pfannenstiel incision is more cosmetically acceptable but requires the mesentery to stretch further. The surgeon can assess whether the tissue is mobilized sufficiently by stretching the appendix and cecum towards the left upper quadrant. If these structures easily reach the left upper quadrant, they will exit through the umbilicus easily. Once adequate mobilization is ensured, a short 1- to 2-inch longitudinal incision is made in the skin about the umbilicus. The fascial incision can be 20% to 30% longer. The target tissue is grasped and gently delivered onto the abdominal wall. A wound protector always is used to enhance delivery and minimize surgical site infection.

The basic principle of small bowel resection for Crohn's disease is to remove all of the gross disease while preserving as much length as possible. This is best determined by both visual and tactile information. During resection of the bowel, division of the mesentery can be difficult. A vessel-sealing energy source normally is used, and it is nearly always sufficient and effective. However, 3-0 silk sutures and zero proline sutures always should be readily available to control any unexpected mesenteric bleeding. In controlling bleeding mesentery, finger pressure should be used while applying figure-of-8 sutures to crimp the bleeding vessels. Attempting to blindly clamp the thickened mesentery while bleeding can make things worse. The wise surgeon is wary of thickened and inflamed Crohn's mesentery, particularly if it extends all the way into the retroperitoneum. Bleeding in this situation can be treacherous and can put adjacent bowel at risk.

As old fashioned as it may seem, a two-layer, hand-sewn anastomosis is performed in an end-to-end manner with an outer layer of interrupted permanent suture and an inner layer of running absorbable suture. The greatest risk to the surgical Crohn's disease patient is leakage from the anastomosis. Although there are no level I data to prove that a stapled or hand-sewn anastomosis is superior, the confidence of controlling each suture is somehow reassuring. In addition, in Crohn's patients the blind end of a stapled side-to-side anastomosis has the theoretical potential of stasis of bowel contents, which may be a driver of recurrent disease. The mesenteric defect is always closed, if at all possible. If it cannot be closed, it is left fully open, to avoid internal herniation obstruction.

In the commonest Crohn's fistula scenario, diseased bowel fistulizes into normal "innocent" bowel. When this is the case, the fistula can be divided and the defect in the innocent bowel can be closed in a transverse manner, assuming the lumen of the bowel will not be compromised. The diseased bowel is then, of course, resected. If both sides of the fistula demonstrate gross Crohn's disease, then both segments must be addressed with resection, or possibly structuroplasty. If the innocent organ is the bladder, it can be closed in multiple layers and a catheter left in place.

A separate chapter in this text directly addresses the topic of stricturoplasty, a critical tool in the inflammatory bowel disease surgeon's armamentarium. Technically, a stricturoplasty can be accomplished laparoscopically without delivery of the tissue, if the surgeon's comfort level with laparoscopic suturing is sufficient.

The most challenging operative situation is diffuse jejunoileitis, requiring surgical therapy. In this situation, the surgeon is faced with many strictured sites separated by inches throughout the small bowel. Deciding what requires resection, what will resolve with stricturoplasty, and what can be left alone requires careful consideration and judgment. The most important principle in these cases is to not hurry and just accept a long day of suturing. The extent of the disease does not necessarily mandate an open procedure. The diseased segments can be eviscerated progressively segment by segment.

■ POSTOPERATIVE CARE

Postoperatively, patients are put on an enhanced recovery pathway, with maximal use of local blocks, minimal use of narcotics, no nasogastric tube, early mobilization, and early per-oral intake. Patients are discharged once there is clear evidence of sufficient bowel function to maintain hydration and nutrition independent of the hospital. Once home they are provided with information regarding warning signs of complications and given a quick and clear pathway back to the team should any concerns arise.

It is well known, and even assumed, that Crohn's disease will recur, and that at a microscopic level it will do so early at the anastomotic site. A recent and important advance in the team management of surgical Crohn's patients is early postoperative medical therapy, according to logical protocols. This is an active arena of investigation, worthy of monitoring (DeCruz et al, 2015). In those patients suffering from reduced bowel length affecting nutrition, the recent FDA approval of teduglutide (Gattex) for short bowel syndrome offers great promise (Jeppesen et al, 2011).

SUGGESTED READINGS

Bennett JL, Ha CY, Efron JE, et al. Optimizing perioperative Crohn's disease management: role of coordinated medical and surgical care. *World J Gastroenterol.* 2015;21:1182-1188. doi:10.3748/wjg.v21.i4.1182.

Colombel JF, Sandborn WJ, Reinisch W, et al. SONIC Study Group. Infliximab, azathioprine, or combination therapy for Crohn's disease. *N Engl J Med.* 2010;362:1383-1395.

De Cruz P, Kamm MA, Hamilton AL, et al. Crohn's disease management after intestinal resection: a randomised trial. *Lancet.* 2015;385:1406-1417.

El-Hussuna A, Krag A, Olaison G, et al. The effect of anti-tumor necrosis factor alpha agents on postoperative anastomotic complications in Crohn's disease: a systematic review. *Dis Colon Rectum.* 2013;56:1423-1433.

Gearry RB, Richardson AK, Frampton CM, et al. Population-based cases control study of inflammatory bowel disease risk factors. *J Gastroenterol Hepatol.* 2010;25:325-333.

Jeppesen PB, Gilroy R, Pertkiewicz M, et al. Randomised placebo-controlled trial of teduglutide in reducing parenteral nutrition and/or intravenous fluid requirements in patients with short bowel syndrome. *Gut.* 2011;60: 902-914.

Myrelid P, Marti-Gallostra M, Ashraf S, et al. Complications in surgery for Crohn's disease after preoperative antitumour necrosis factor therapy. *Br J Surg.* 2014;101:539-545.

Sandborn WJ, Feagan BG, Rutgeerts P, et al. GEMINI 2 Study Group. Vedolizumab as induction and maintenance therapy for Crohn's disease. *N Engl J Med.* 2013;369:711-721.

Sandborn WJ, Gasink C, Gao LL, et al. CERTIFI Study Group. Ustekinumab induction and maintenance therapy in refractory Crohn's disease. *N Engl J Med.* 2012;367:1519-1528.

Schmidt CM, Talamini MA, Kaufman HS, et al. Laparoscopic surgery for Crohn's disease: reasons for conversion. *Ann Surg.* 2001;233:733-739.

STRICTUREPLASTY IN CROHN'S DISEASE

Heather Yeo, MD, MHS, and Fabrizio Michelassi, MD

Crohn's disease (CD) is a chronic inflammatory bowel disease that can occur anywhere along the gastrointestinal tract, from mouth to anus. Characterized by transmural intestinal inflammation, it can lead to the development of strictures, septic complications such as abscesses and fistulas, hemorrhage, or malignant transformation. Despite improvements in medical therapy, the majority of patients require surgical treatment for such complications within 10 years of diagnosis.

Unfortunately, CD is a recurrent disease, and 20% to 60% of patients have postoperative clinical symptoms of recurrence; up to 50% need further surgical intervention after the index procedure. Because of the need for repeated intestinal resections, patients are at risk to develop intestinal insufficiency and short bowel syndrome, which can lead to the need for parenteral nutrition support. Surgical treatment of CD therefore should aim to address complications without jeopardizing bowel function.

Bowel-sparing surgical techniques, such as strictureplasty, have been proposed as an alternative to lengthy intestinal resections in the treatment of CD small bowel strictures. This chapter reviews indications, contraindications, technical aspects, and short- and long-term outcomes of various strictureplasty techniques.

■ OVERVIEW

Indications and Contraindications

Strictureplasty is the treatment of choice for patients with symptomatic non-phlegmonous jejunoileal CD fibrotic strictures, as highlighted in American and European guidelines for the management of CD. Symptoms may vary from postprandial crampy abdominal pain to complete bowel obstruction.

Several studies have also reported excellent results when strictureplasty techniques have been performed for strictures in other gastrointestinal locations, such as in the duodenum or at the site of a strictured ileocolonic anastomosis. In addition, strictureplasties have been reported in the treatment of isolated colonic strictures: however, the length and thickness of colonic strictures is usually not conducive to strictureplasty techniques.

Strictureplasties are contraindicated in the presence of local sepsis, such as phlegmon, abscess, generalized peritonitis, or for long strictures with thick, unyielding intestinal wall (Box 1). In these situations, strictureplasty may not be technically feasible or may be associated with a high risk of postoperative dehiscence. Suspicion of small bowel adenocarcinoma or dysplasia should lead to intraoperative biopsy and, if confirmed, resection of the bowel loop rather than a bowel-sparing procedure. Strictureplasty techniques are also contraindicated in the presence of constant low-grade hemorrhage associated with the diseased, strictured loop of intestine: if a strictureplasty is performed in these cases, the obstructive symptoms will be resolved, but usually the low-grade hemorrhage and the associated chronic anemia persist.

The presence of enteric fistulae was viewed previously as a contraindication for performing a strictureplasty, but more recent reports have suggested that strictureplasty may be performed in the presence of fistulae surrounded by chronic, rather than active, inflammation without increasing postoperative morbidity. The patient's nutritional status is a determinant in the consideration of performing a strictureplasty, and if profoundly impaired, it represents a contraindication to this technique. Finally, in the economy of a surgical procedure, if a stricture is located in close proximity of a diseased intestinal segment in need of resection, the resection usually is extended to include the stricture to minimize the length of the overall surgical procedure and the number of anastomoses.

Preoperative Preparation

As for all elective surgical procedures for CD, the extent of disease should be evaluated carefully radiographically and endoscopically before surgery. A complete assessment of disease extension should be performed using radiologic and endoscopic imaging. The use of magnetic resonance enterography (MRE) currently is preferred to study the small bowel based on increased sensitivity in distinguishing between inflammatory and fibrotic strictures, the former of which may be managed medically, whereas the latter are better managed surgically. A preoperative complete colonoscopy is the optimal imaging technique for the colon. It should be performed even in patients with CD apparently strictly limited to the small bowel as a downstream fistula, or the stricture may affect intraoperative management.

Preoperative identification of patients at risk of postoperative morbidity is important to risk stratify and help minimize postoperative complications. Several studies have focused on predictive risk factors of postoperative morbidity in CD surgery, showing that preoperative corticosteroid medication, poor nutritional status, and intra-abdominal phlegmon or fistula are independent predictors of poor outcome. Corticosteroid weaning is rarely feasible without worsening or reactivation of disease. Poor nutritional status can and should be addressed preoperatively by a short course of enteric or parenteral nutrition. Abdominal phlegmons and fistulae are frequently the reason for surgical intervention and must be dealt with surgically, but abscesses can be drained percutaneously, allowing time for inflammation to decrease.

Neither azathioprine nor infliximab have been demonstrated to have an impact on postoperative morbidity and can therefore be maintained in the perioperative course.

Intraoperative "Design of a Roadmap"

As with all CD cases, the operative approach should begin by a thorough examination of small bowel from the ligament of Treitz to the ileocecal valve with special care paid to recording all Crohn's-related findings. This can be performed either through a laparotomy or laparoscopically. The surgeon should be vigilant in identifying any strictures, phlegmonous masses, abscesses, or fistulae. This portion of the procedure helps to develop a "roadmap" and is crucial for planning the operation. A strategic approach to the patient's disease then is developed by studying the "roadmap" and includes the use of strictureplasties, intestinal resections, drainage of abscesses, repair of fistulous openings on target intestinal loops, or hollow viscera, or a combination of the above (Figure 1).

■ STRICTUREPLASTY TECHNIQUES

Strictureplasty techniques may be divided into three subgroups: short strictureplasties, including the well-known Heineke-Mikulicz technique; intermediate length procedures, including the Finney and

BOX 1: Contraindications for Strictureplasty in Crohn's Disease Surgical Management

Absolute Contraindications

Dysplasia or cancer at the stricture site
Hemorrhage
Locoregional sepsis
   Phlegmon
   Abscess
   Peritonitis

Relative Contraindications

Impaired nutritional status
Fistula
Stricture close to an area of resection
Long stricture with thick, unyielding intestinal wall

Jaboulay procedures; and long enteroenterostomies, such as the side-to-side isoperistaltic strictureplasty. The choice between these different techniques should be made according to the number of strictures and length of each one (Table 1).

Short Strictureplasties

The most common strictureplasty technique is the Heineke-Mikulicz technique. This strictureplasty was first introduced by Emmanuel Lee for the treatment of Crohn's disease in 1976 after he became aware of a similar technique on tubercular strictures of the terminal ileum described by Katarya. The technique is very similar to a Heineke-Mikulicz pyloroplasty from which it derives its name. The technique is optimal to address short strictures (≤7 cm) and is performed by making a longitudinal incision on the antimesenteric side of the bowel extending from 2 cm proximal to 2 cm distal to the stricture. The enterotomy then is closed in a transverse fashion in one or two layers. Our practice is to close this enterotomy in two layers using interrupted Lambert nonabsorbable 3-0 sutures for the outer layer and a running absorbable 3-0 suture for the inner layer (Figure 2).

TABLE 1: Choice of Strictureplasty Technique According to Disease Characteristics

Stricture Length	Technique
Short (≤7 cm)	Heineke-Mikulicz
Intermediate (>7 cm and ≤15 cm)	Finney/Jaboulay
Multiple short strictures clustered over a lengthy segment	Michelassi side-to-side isoperistaltic

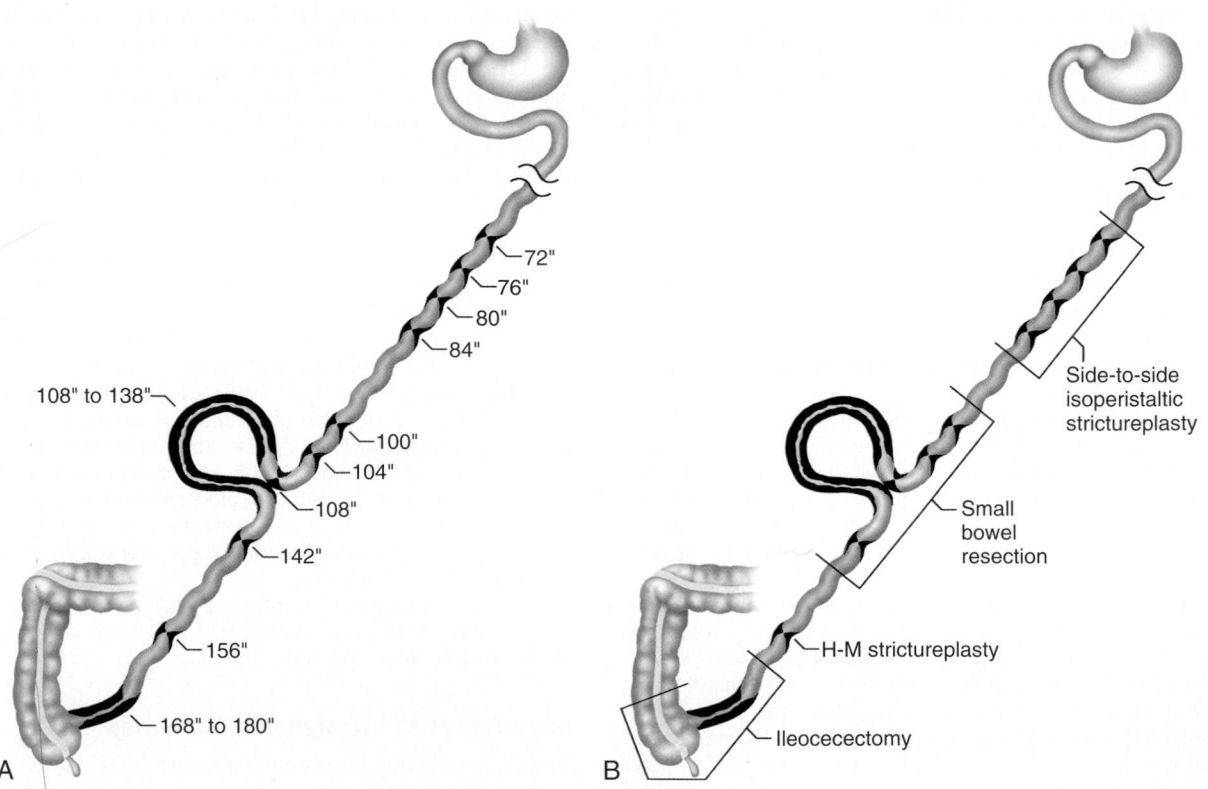

FIGURE 1 Design of a roadmap (**A**) and subsequent surgical plan (**B**) for extensive Crohn's disease.

The Judd strictureplasty is a variation of the Heineke-Mikulicz technique described for the surgical management of short strictures associated with a fistula opening. During this procedure, the longitudinal incision encompasses the fistula opening. After débridement of the fistulous opening to healthy tissue, the enterotomy then is closed as described in the Heineke-Mikulicz technique.

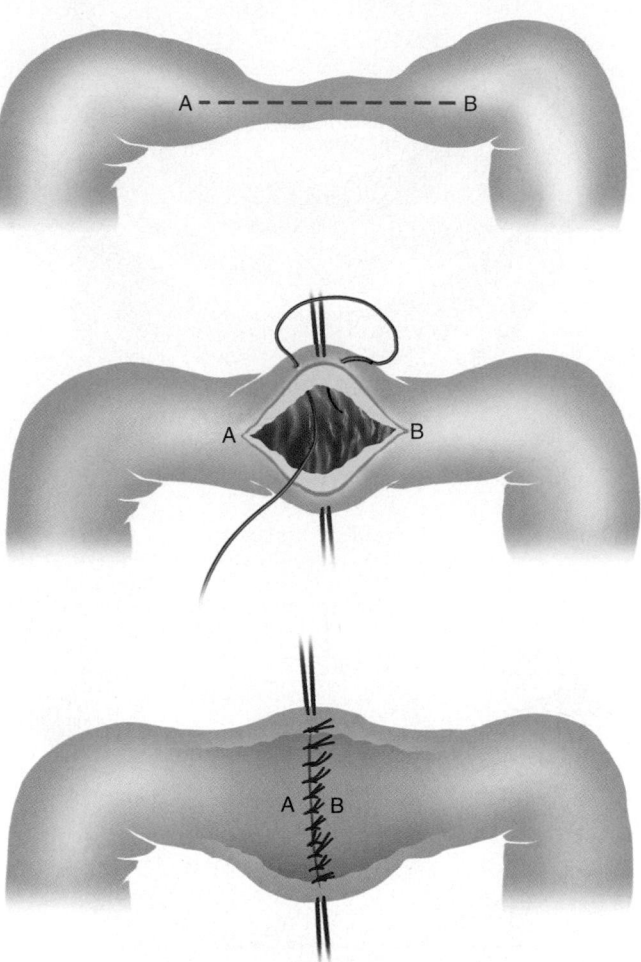

FIGURE 2 Heineke-Mikulicz strictureplasty on an isolated, short, small bowel stricture.

Intermediate Length Procedures

Additional procedures have been described to address longer strictures (>7 cm and ≤15 cm) than those manageable with the Heineke-Mikulicz technique or its variations. In this situation, the most commonly performed procedure is the Finney strictureplasty, named after the Finney pyloroplasty, firstly described in 1937. The strictured loop is folded over itself at its midpoint section, forming a U shape. A longitudinal enterotomy then is performed halfway between the mesenteric and the antimesenteric side on the folded loop. The opposed edges of the bowel are sutured together to create a short side-to-side isoperistaltic enteroenterostomy (Figure 3). Our preference is to use a two-layer closure similar to the one described for the Heineke-Mikulicz strictureplasty. Concerns about long-term complications, such as bacterial overgrowth in the bypassed segment, limit the length of the stricture to be addressed by this strictureplasty to less than 15 cm. The Jaboulay strictureplasty is used for strictures between 10 to 20 cm. The stricture is folded into a U shape, and the two enterotomies are created facing each other to allow for a side-to-side enteroenterostomy, which is not extended to the tip of folded loop as in a Finney. In this sense, the Jaboulay strictureplasty combines technical aspects of a bypass and a strictureplasty. The side-to-side enteroenterostomy is performed with a running continuous single layer or double layer as previously described for the Heineke-Mikulicz strictureplasty. Similar to the Finney strictureplasty, as the length of the side-to-side enteroenterostomy increases, so does the chance of developing a lateral diverticulum or blind loop, bacterial overgrowth, malabsorption, malnutrition, and persistent low-grade inflammation.

Long Enteroenterostomies

For longer intestinal segments affected by strictures, the Michelassi side-to-side isoperistaltic strictureplasty, first described in 1996 by the senior author, is the technique of choice to address multiple short strictures closely clustered over a lengthy small bowel segment (>15 cm).

In this technique, the small bowel loop affected by the stricture and its mesentery first is divided at its midpoint. The proximal intestinal loop then is moved over the distal one in a side-to-side fashion. Care is taken to ensure that stenotic areas of one loop are placed adjacent to the dilated areas of the other loop. The two loops are then approximated by a layer of interrupted seromuscular Lembert stitches, using nonabsorbable 3-0 sutures (Figure 4, *A*). A longitudinal enterotomy is performed on both loops, with the intestinal ends

FIGURE 3 Finney strictureplasty on an intermediate small bowel stricture.

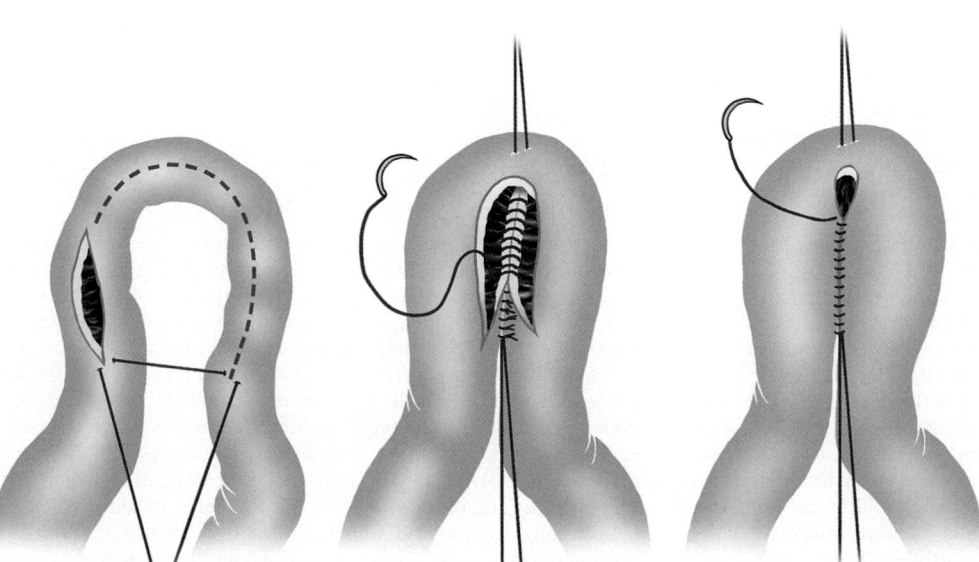

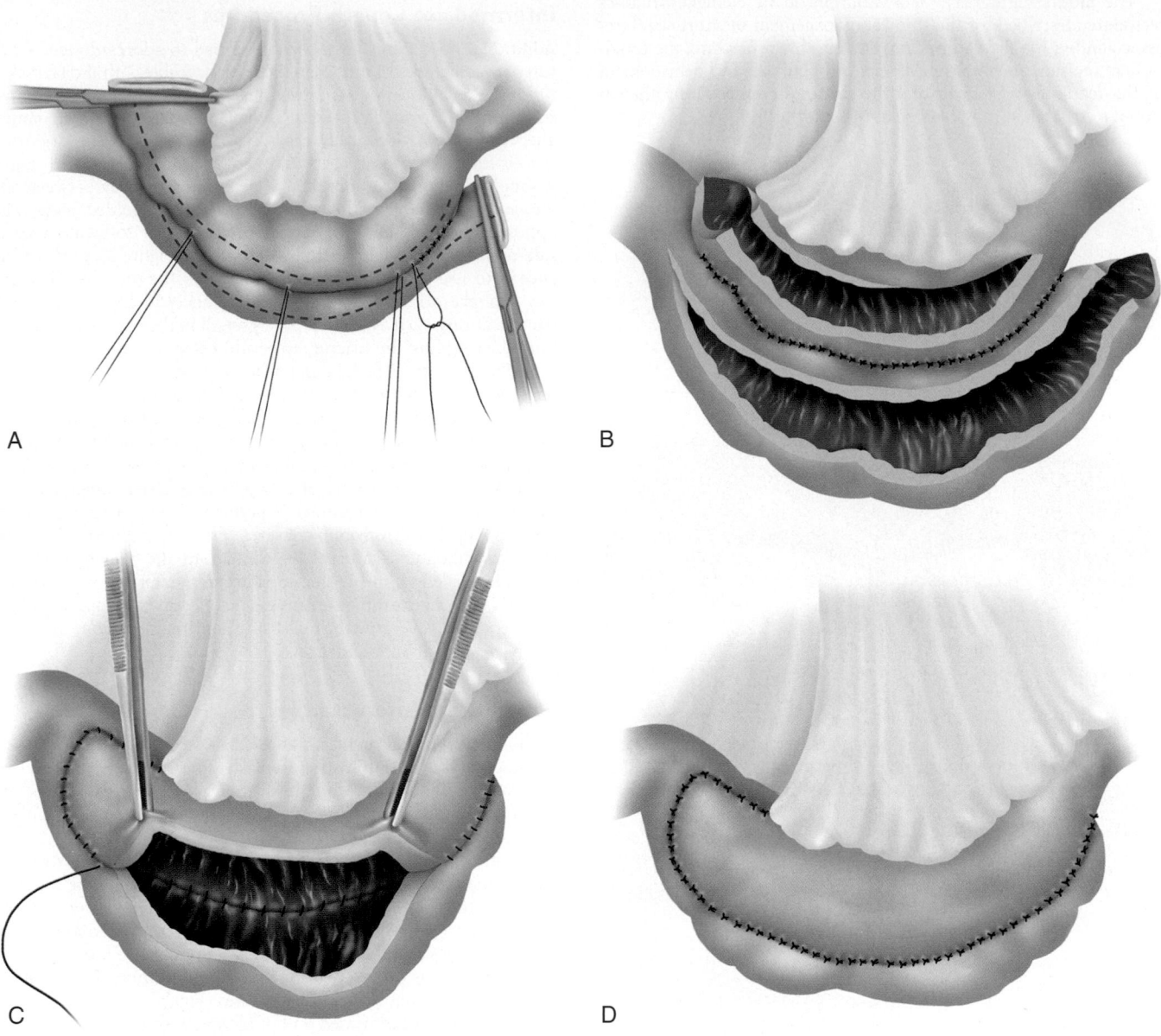

FIGURE 4 A to **D,** Side-to-side isoperistaltic strictureplasty.

tapered to avoid blind stumps (Figure 4, *B*). Frozen-section biopsies of suspicious areas of disease are obtained to exclude occult malignancy. Hemostasis is obtained with suture ligatures or electrocautery. The outer suture line is reinforced with an internal row of running, full-thickness 3-0 absorbable sutures, continued anteriorly as a running Connell suture (Figure 4, *C*); this layer is reinforced by an outer layer of interrupted seromuscular Lembert stitches using nonabsorbable 3-0 sutures (Figure 4, *D*).

Many variations of this side-to-side isoperistaltic strictureplasty technique have been described. These variations fall into five distinct categories: integration of other strictureplasty techniques (e.g., Heineke-Mikulicz or Finney techniques) with the side-to-side isoperistaltic strictureplasty technique usually at the inlet and/or the outlet of the strictureplasty; length of bowel selected for strictureplasty; use of diseased on diseased bowel vs. normal on diseased bowel; bowel location selected for procedure (jejunum, ileum, or terminal ileum, where the side-to-side isoperistaltic strictureplasty is performed between the ileum and the ascending colon); and condition for which this technique is applied (Crohn's, multiple NSAID-small bowel

strictures, and small bowel stricture arising from chronic ischemic enteritis).

■ RESULTS

Postoperative Short-Term Outcomes
A large number of publications have highlighted the safety of strictureplasties for CD. A meta-analysis by Campbell showed that the type of strictureplasty technique had no impact on short-term postoperative outcomes. Campbell analyzed 32 studies with 1616 patients who underwent 4538 strictureplasties. Short strictureplasties were the most commonly performed (81%), followed by intermediate procedures (10%), and long enteroenterostomies. Overall, 13% of patients developed postoperative complications, including 4% septic complications (anastomotic leak, fistula, and abscess) and 3% postoperative hemorrhages. The mortality rate was zero. In this study, there was no difference in short- and long-term morbidity between conventional techniques (Heineke-Mikulicz or Finney) and nonconventional techniques (Michelassi and its modifications).

Strictureplasty has been shown to have favorable outcomes when compared with small bowel resections for CD. The early postoperative complication rate of strictureplasty is lower than resection. In specific regard to functional outcomes, efficacy of strictureplasties has been largely demonstrated, with satisfactory relief of obstructive symptoms, improved food tolerance, and subsequent weight gain.

Long-Term Outcomes

Because CD is a chronic disease, patients often have recurrences regardless of mechanism of treatment. Endoscopic, radiologic, and histopathologic evaluations after strictureplasty have indeed highlighted complete CD regression at strictureplasty site in several reports. The mechanism associated with such inflammation regression remains unknown.

Several studies have shown that recurrence may be lower at strictureplasty sites than intestinal resection sites. In 2007 Yamamoto and colleagues performed a meta-analysis of the use and outcomes of strictureplasty that included more than 3250 strictureplasties in more than 1100 patients. In this study Yamamoto calculated that the strictureplasty recurrence rate was 3%.

Reports of development of small bowel adenocarcinoma arising at the site of strictureplasty have been documented. The incidence is fairly low and has been reported to be less than 0.4%. Given the rarity of this complication, most surgeons believe the risk of malignant transformation is not sufficient to dissuade performance of strictureplasty.

Long-term results associated with the side-to-side isoperistaltic strictureplasty technique have been reported by a multicenter study in 2007. This study demonstrated that only 14 of 184 total patients required surgery for recurrent disease at the side-to-side isoperistaltic strictureplasty site, after an average follow-up of 35 months. Recurrences occurred mostly at the inlet and at the outlet of the side-to-side strictureplasty, leading some authors to suggest the addition of a Heineke-Mikulicz strictureplasty at these sites during its original construction.

■ SUMMARY

Crohn's disease is a chronic and recurrent panintestinal inflammatory disorder. Surgical treatment is indicated to address complications of the disease or failure of medical treatment. Symptom alleviation expected from the procedure should be balanced with potential postoperative morbidity and long-term side effects. In this context, strictureplasty for CD-related small bowel stenosis has been demonstrated to be a safe and effective solution, relieving obstructive symptoms while preserving intestinal length for nutritional absorption.

Different strictureplasty procedures have been described to address different settings of CD. The choice of strictureplasty techniques should be made based on the length and the number of strictures and after complete evaluation of the gastrointestinal tract for evidence of gross Crohn's disease.

SUGGESTED READINGS

Ambe R, Campbell L, Cagir B. A comprehensive review of strictureplasty techniques in Crohn's disease: types, indications, comparisons, and safety. *J Gastrointest Surg.* 2012;16:209-217.

Campbell L, Ambe R, Weaver J, Marcus SM, Cagir B. Comparison of conventional and nonconventional strictureplasties in Crohn's disease: a systematic review and meta-analysis. *Dis Colon Rectum.* 2012;55:714-726.

Fearnhead NS, Chowdhury R, Box B, George BD, Jewell DP, Mortensen NJ. Long-term follow-up of strictureplasty for Crohn's disease. *Br J Surg.* 2006;93:475-482.

Fichera A, Lovadina S, Rubin M, Cimino F, Hurst RD, Michelassi F. Patterns and operative treatment of recurrent Crohn's disease: a prospective longitudinal study. *Surgery.* 2006;140:649-654.

Katariya RN, Sood S, Rao PG, Rao PLNG. Stricture-plasty for tubercular strictures of the gastro-intestinal tract. *Br J Surg.* 1977;64:496-498.

Lee EC, Papaioannou N. Minimal surgery for chronic obstruction in patients with extensive or universal Crohn's disease. *Ann R Coll Surg Engl.* 1982;64: 229.

Michelassi F, Hurst RD, Melis M, Rubin M, Cohen R, Gasparitis A, et al. Side-to-side isoperistaltic strictureplasty in extensive Crohn's disease: a prospective longitudinal study. *Ann Surg.* 2000;232:401-408.

Michelassi F, Taschieri A, Tonelli F, Sasaki I, Poggioli G, Fazio V, et al. An international, multicenter, prospective, observational study of the side-to-side isoperistaltic strictureplasty in Crohn's disease. *Dis Colon Rectum.* 2007;50:277-284.

Roy P, Kumar D. Strictureplasty. *Br J Surg.* 2004;91:1428-1437.

Yamamoto T, Fazio VW, Tekkis PP. Safety and efficacy of strictureplasty for Crohn's disease: a systematic review and meta-analysis. *Dis Colon Rectum.* 2007;50:1968-1986.

THE MANAGEMENT OF SMALL BOWEL TUMORS

Beth A. Helmink, MD, PhD, Christina E. Bailey, MD, MSCI, and John L. Tarpley, MD

Primary and metastatic tumors of the small bowel (SB) are exceedingly rare, constituting less than 3% of all tumors of the gastrointestinal (GI) tract. Approximately 9400 new cases of SB malignancy are diagnosed in the United States each year compared with 132,700 new cases of large bowel cancer. The mean age of diagnosis is 65.

Unfortunately, the diagnosis of SB malignancy often is delayed because of the lack of associated symptoms; when present, symptoms are vague and nonspecific in nature. Some studies report a delay in diagnosis of up to 30 weeks. Thus, despite their rare occurrence, SB tumors should always be included in the differential diagnosis in evaluation of patients with ongoing vague GI symptoms. SB tumors can present with obstruction, intussusception, and/or GI bleeding. In fact, it is estimated that up to 10% to 12% of all occult GI bleeds are due to SB tumors. Vague abdominal pain, nausea, vomiting, weight loss, and anemia are often late manifestations of locally advanced or metastatic disease. Location of the tumors can influence symptomatology. The presenting symptom of jejunal and ileal tumors often is obstruction, whereas that of duodenal tumors often is pain, biliary obstruction, gastric outlet obstruction, or occult bleeding. Unfortunately, many patients will be diagnosed retrospectively after exploratory laparotomy for an acute abdomen because of bowel perforation, intraperitoneal bleeding, complete obstruction, or intussusception caused by SB tumors.

It is curious that the SB composes more than 90% of the absorptive surface area of the GI tract but is relatively resistant to neoplastic transformation. Potential explanations include the rapid transit of mostly alkaline dilute liquid material, the robust immune system presence in the SB with numerous lymphoid follicles within the bowel wall and high IgA secretion, the rapid turnover of the epithelium, and the production of detoxifying enzymes, specifically benzpyrene hydroxylase within the SB epithelium. The relatively low bacterial load in the SB as compared with other regions of the GI tract is thought to play a part in preventing carcinogenesis by decreasing the conversion of bile acids into entities that are known to cause malignancy in the large bowel.

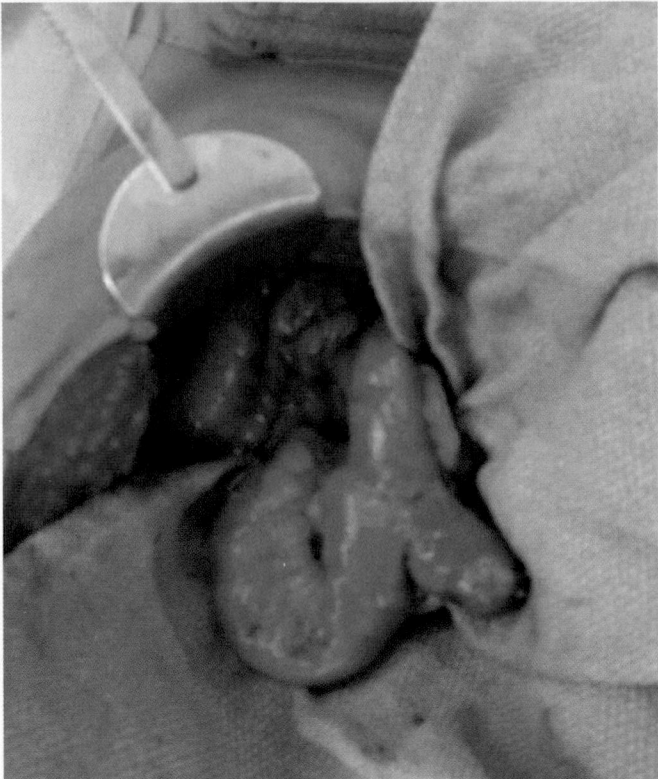

FIGURE I A small gastrointestinal stromal tumor in a Meckel's diverticulum.

Predisposing conditions for SB malignancy include genetic cancer syndromes such as familial adenomatous polyposis (FAP), hereditary nonpolyposis colon cancer (HNPCC), and Peutz-Jeghers syndrome (PJS). Chronic inflammation is cited as a risk factor as well, with increased frequency of malignancy in Crohn's and celiac diseases; the risk associated with these inflammatory conditions increases with severity and duration of disease. Structural abnormalities, including Meckel's diverticulum within the ileum, are also prone to the development of malignancy (Figure 1). Finally, dietary factors, including increased alcohol consumption as well as diets high in refined sugars and smoked or cured meats, predispose a person to SB malignancy.

■ IMPROVEMENTS IN SMALL BOWEL IMAGING

A combination of endoscopic techniques and cross-sectional scanning are requisite to detect intraluminal and extraluminal abnormalities suggestive of SB malignancy.

Endoscopy

Mucosal abnormalities are best detected by endoscopy. Until recently, the SB was a relatively unexplored territory endoscopically. Those with persistent GI symptoms, including recurrent obstruction or GI bleed of unknown origin after esophagogastroduodenoscopy (EGD) and colonoscopy, were left to diagnostic laparoscopy and/or exploratory laparotomy. Recent developments allow for the relatively noninvasive visualization of the entirety of the SB with diagnostic and often therapeutic potential.

EGD, push endoscopy, and double balloon endoscopy enable visualization of the stomach and proximal duodenum, early jejunum, and entire SB, respectively. An important feature is that these techniques allow for intervention, including biopsy, clipping, and tattooing. Push endoscopy and double balloon endoscopy, however, are time consuming and are limited to certain centers with facile technicians. In addition, all have risk of perforation and a slight risk of

pancreatitis. Video capsule endoscopy (VCE) was developed in the early 2000s and has low false-positive rate (2%) and relatively low false-negative rate (18%). The major limitation of VCE is the inability to intervene with biopsy. However, exciting advances in micromachine technology with the ability to "drive the capsule" may allow for this in the not-so-distant future. The use of VCE is contraindicated in the setting of motility disorders, obstruction, and stricture, specifically in the patient with Crohn's disease (CD), in whom capsule retention rates are prohibitively high. Retention rates of up to 8% are cited in patients with CD with known stricture. VCE use is also relatively contraindicated in the setting of conditions predisposing the patient to stricture, including NSAID use, prior abdominal operations, and history of radiation therapy.

Imaging Techniques

Imaging includes fluoroscopy and computed tomography (CT). Fluoroscopic imaging of the SB includes upper GI series with SB follow-through versus enteroclysis or SB enema, in which contrast agents are delivered in bolus to the SB via a nasojejunal tube. Both studies are simple, cheap, and widely available. SB enteroclysis is more invasive but provides more sensitivity because increased distention of the bowel reveals subtle luminal irregularities. The presence of SB tumor is suggested by the following findings: filling defects, stenosis, and irregular thickening of the folds of the bowel wall. Neither of these studies provides adequate evaluation of the bowel wall, mesentery, or adjacent lymph nodes. In this regard, CT imaging is superior and can demonstrate findings such as mesenteric foreshortening, fat stranding, lymphadenopathy, or distant metastatic disease that would indicate SB malignancy. CT enteroclysis or CT enterography combines the benefits of these two modalities to detect both intraluminal and extraluminal abnormalities. CT enterography is less invasive and often better tolerated by patients compared with CT enteroclysis because of less bowel distension.

■ BENIGN SMALL BOWEL TUMORS

Benign tumors of the SB include adenomas, leiomyomas, lipomas, hamartomas (and more rarely hemangiomas), lymphangiomas, fibromyxomas, and ganglioneuromas. Benign tumors are more likely to present with GI bleed and not abdominal pain. The decision to excise a benign small bowel tumor depends on the malignant potential of the tumor as well as symptomatology.

Hamartomas, often associated with PJS, and lipomas have very little malignant potential and should be resected only if causing significant symptoms. Leiomyomas can be large and should be resected because they are difficult to distinguish from the more sinister leiomyosarcoma or gastrointestinal stromal tumor (GIST) even with detailed histologic analysis. Adenomas vary in their malignant potential; tubular, tubulovillous, and villous adenomas have an increasing incidence of harboring adenocarcinoma, respectively. Tubular, tubulovillous, and some villous adenomas can be resected endoscopically. However, formal resection is recommended for villous adenomas containing even a small focus of invasive malignancy or carcinoma in situ no matter the location. Brunner's gland adenomas have a malignant potential similar to that of tubular adenomas and can be resected endoscopically. The duodenal adenomas seen in FAP have increased malignant potential, the extent of which varies with number, size, histology, and dysplasia of the polyps as assessed by the Spigelman classification. Prophylactic pancreaticoduodenectomy is recommended for Spigelman stage IV and above (Table 1). Prophylactic pancreaticoduodenectomy is recommended for duodenal adenomas with a Spigelman classification of stage IV or above.

■ MALIGNANT SMALL BOWEL TUMORS

In order of prevalence, malignant SB tumors include neuroendocrine tumor (NET), adenocarcinoma, lymphoma, and mesenchymal

TABLE 1: Spigelman Classification for Adenomas in the Setting of Familial Adenomatous Polyposis

	Number of Points		
	1P	2P	3P
Number of polyps	1-4	5-20	>20
Polyp size (mm)	1-4	5-10	>10
Histology	Tubulous	Tubulovillous	Villous
Dysplasia	Mild	Moderate	Severe
Stage	Spigelman score*		
0	0		
I	1-4		
III	5-6		
III	7-8		
IV	9-12		

*Addition of points.

Schulmann K, et al. Feasibility and diagnostic utility of video capsule endoscopy for the detection of small bowel polyps in patients with hereditary polyposis syndromes capsule endoscopy in hereditary intestinal polyposis. *Am J Gastroenterol.* 2005;100:27-37.

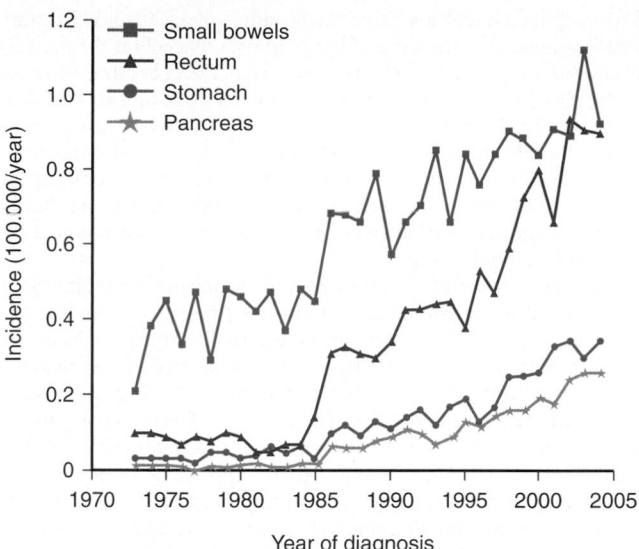

FIGURE 2 Graph depicting the marked increase in the incidence of neuroendocrine tumors.

tumors, including GIST. Few if any evidence-based guidelines exist for the diagnosis and treatment of SB tumors and relatively little information exists regarding prognosis given the low incidence and prevalence of these lesions.

Neuroendocrine Tumors

NETs are epithelial neoplasms that arise from enterochromaffin cells, also known as *Kulchitsky cells.* These tumors have the unique ability to synthesize and secrete bioactive substances. They are characterized by the expression of somatostatin receptors on their cell surface which has both diagnostic and therapeutic implications. NETs are rare, but their incidence is on the rise, having increased by more than 400% in the last 30 years (Figure 2). Given this increase as well as the relatively good prognosis for patients with these tumors, NET has surpassed adenocarcinoma as the most prevalent SB neoplasm.

There are certain familial predispositions to the development of NETs, including multiple endocrine neoplasia type I (MEN1) (gastrinoma) and neurofibromatosis (NF) (somatostatinoma). However, most familial syndromes are associated with foregut, not midgut carcinoids, sparing the majority of the SB. Other risk factors include the presence of breast and colorectal cancer. Smoking is a known environmental risk factor.

The presentation of NETs varies depending on the site of origin and the production of bioactive substances. Foregut NETs (i.e., duodenum) include gastrinomas (gastrin-producing) and somatostatinomas (somatostatin-producing). Gastrinomas are associated with Zollinger-Ellison syndrome and MEN1; patients present with heartburn, peptic ulcer disease, and chronic diarrhea. Patients with somatostatinomas classically present with diabetes mellitus or glucose intolerance, diarrhea, and cholelithiasis. Midgut (jejunal and ileal) NETs frequently are referred to as *carcinoid tumors,* a term coined by Oberndofer in the early 1900s to describe slow-growing tumors of the SB that unexpectedly had the ability to metastasize. These tumors are usually nonfunctional, and most patients present with vague abdominal symptoms related to mass effect. In addition, the strong desmoplastic reaction and dense fibrosis within the mesentery and its associated vessels can cause bowel obstruction and

ischemia secondary to venous congestion. Functional tumors can secrete serotonin, histamine, VIP, and prostaglandins, which can lead to intermittent flushing, bronchoconstriction, diarrhea, palpitations, and heart disease, specifically valvular fibrosis (i.e., carcinoid syndrome). Carcinoid syndrome is seen only when these tumors are bulky or metastatic (most commonly to the liver).

The diagnosis of NETs is made using a combination of tumor markers, endoscopy, and structural versus functional imaging. For those with functional tumors, selective biochemical evaluation should be performed; for example, a gastrin level and a secretin provocative test should be obtained for gastrinomas. For those with nonfunctional tumors, chromogranin-A, pancreatic polypeptide, neuron-specific enolase, and urinary 5-HIAA (a metabolite of serotonin) have been used as tumor markers. Structural imaging with contrast-enhanced CT has been used traditionally. Because of the expression of somatostatin receptors by the tumors, functional imaging also has a role in the diagnosis of NETs. 68-Ga-DOTATATE PET/CT is a relatively new modality that has proven superior to the traditional octreotide scan with regard to spatial resolution, the ability to detect small lesions, and the lower level of required radiation exposure.

Patients with NETs should be referred to high-volume centers for coordinated multidisciplinary treatment. In general, the degree and location of tumor involvement and tumor characteristics should dictate the aggressiveness of therapy. Surgical resection with curative intent is recommended for most patients with resectable disease. Unfortunately, only 20% of patients initially are seen with disease for which curative resection is a possibility; most have lymph node and/or liver metastases. However, even with metastatic disease, long-term survival is not uncommon with aggressive surgical intervention and medical therapy.

For resectable disease, exploratory laparotomy begins with a thorough exploration of the entirety of the SB because more than 30% of patients present with synchronous lesions. Segmental resection of the involved SB with lymphadenectomy should be performed. The exception to this is a small duodenal NET. Duodenal tumors less than 1 cm can be resected endoscopically; tumors between 1 and 2 cm can be enucleated via an open procedure; and all duodenal tumors greater than 2 cm require complete resection with lymphadenectomy, including pancreaticoduodenectomy if the position dictates as a result of the frequency of lymph node metastases with tumors of this size. Sporadic gastrinomas should be resected; those associated with MEN1 should not be resected given the multifocality of these tumors and frequent and early metastatic spread. Cholecystectomy is recommended at the time of laparotomy, especially if the need for octreotide therapy is anticipated because octreotide administration is associated with the development of biliary colic and cholecystitis. Nonresectable, symptomatic NETs can be palliated with subtotal resection of the lesion; whether this should be performed for patients with asymptomatic disease remains controversial. In addition, for patients with carcinoid syndrome, octreotide should be started before the induction of anesthesia and continued into the next day to avoid carcinoid crises.

Surgery also should be considered for recurrent locoregional and metastatic disease. For hepatic metastases, resection with curative intent is the goal if the criteria purported by the European Neuroendocrine Tumor Society (ENETS) consensus meeting is met: (1) resectable, well-differentiated tumor burden in the liver with acceptable morbidity and mortality; (2) absence of right heart insufficiency; and (3) absence of extra-abdominal or diffuse peritoneal disease. Metastatic liver disease can be approached with either a partial or formal hepatectomy. Ultrasound of the liver should be performed at the time of operation to detect any additional areas of metastatic disease. Radiofrequency ablation (RFA) commonly is used intraoperatively in combination with resection to address remaining lesions not amenable to resection. Embolization/chemoembolization and cryotherapy are also options for poor operative candidates or patients with multifocal disease not amenable to resection. Finally, in an otherwise young healthy patient, in the absence of extrahepatic disease or high risk of recurrence, liver transplantation has been performed but is not considered standard therapy. The role of resection of the primary lesion in the setting of unresectable metastatic disease is debated but is almost always completed.

According to the 2010 WHO consensus, NETs are separated based on their proliferative rate (i.e., Ki-67 index), into low-grade (G1, <2 mitoses/HPF, Ki-67 <3), intermediate-grade (G2, 2-10 mitoses/HPF, 3% < Ki-67 < 20%), and high-grade (G3, >10 mitoses/HPF, Ki-67 >20%) tumors. Low- and intermediate-grade tumors are grouped together and categorized as well differentiated, whereas high-grade tumors are categorized as poorly differentiated. Staging is by TNM staging by AJCC.

There are few effective cytotoxic agents available for the adjuvant treatment of NETs. For patients with metastatic disease, symptomatic management with somatostatin analogues including octreotide and/or lanreotide is common. Although the symptomatic control afforded by octreotide has long been known, only recently have studies shown antiproliferative effects of octreotide (PROMID and CLARINET studies) supporting their use in symptomatic and asymptomatic patients with low-grade and intermediate-grade tumors. These studies indicate that somatostatin analogues can increase progression-free survival (PFS) and possibly overall survival. Importantly, their use is not limited to those with positive octreotide scan. Traditional cytotoxic agents can be useful in the treatment of some poorly differentiated NETs. The role of radiation therapy is limited to radioisotope-targeted therapies.

Given the high recurrence rates, these patients require close follow-up every 3 to 6 months in the first 2 years and annually thereafter with measurement of CgA, 5-HIAA, and cross-sectional imaging. Five-year overall survival is approximately 60% to 90% for SB NETs, even with metastatic disease at presentation. Negative prognostic indicators include large tumor size, lymph node metastases, and distant metastatic disease, especially distant metastatic nodules larger than 1 cm.

Adenocarcinoma

Adenocarcinoma is the second most common tumor of the SB. Like colorectal adenocarcinoma, it is thought to arise from an adenomatous precursor. Also, similar to colorectal cancer, the size and character of the polyp determine malignant potential with large villous polyps being most likely to harbor malignancy. However, the cellular

pathways involved in carcinogenesis in the small bowel as compared with large bowel differ in intriguing ways. For example, although somatic mutations in APC are nearly omnipresent in colorectal cancer, they are rare in SB adenocarcinoma. The beta-catenin and Wnt signaling pathways, however, are still disrupted in SB tumors. SB adenocarcinoma is also more likely than colorectal cancer to have mutations in *SMAD4*; this suggests that mismatch repair pathways may be more important in carcinogenesis of the SB. SB adenocarcinoma is encountered more frequently in developed countries; risk factors include sedentary lifestyle and the consumption of a high-fat diet. However, it is interesting to note that the incidence of colorectal cancer is decreasing while that of SB adenocarcinoma is increasing within those affluent Western countries. Other risk factors for SB adenocarcinoma include smoking, alcohol use, and the presence of peptic ulcer disease. Diseases associated with SB adenocarcinoma include cystic fibrosis, celiac disease, and CD. Genetic cancer-predisposing conditions associated with SB adenocarcinoma include FAP, HNPCC, and PJS.

Symptoms, if present, include nonspecific GI complaints. Workup should entail CEA and CA 19-9 (CEA is elevated in a majority of SB adenocarcinomas), CT scan of the chest, abdomen, and pelvis as well as upper and lower endoscopy to evaluate for synchronous lesions. Of importance is that all patients presenting with adenocarcinoma of the SB should be evaluated for an occult underlying genetic condition.

SB adenocarcinoma is encountered most frequently in the setting of CD; patients with CD are more than 100 times more likely to develop SB adenocarcinoma typically within the area of bowel involved by CD. The distribution of tumors in the patient with CD reflects the differential involvement of the bowel, with the ileum being most likely involved. This feature complicates diagnosis. Most Crohn's flares exhibit signs and symptoms of obstruction; the same presentation is seen for SB adenocarcinoma. Those patients presenting with recurrent partial small bowel obstructions (SBOs) should heighten the suspicion for underlying malignancy. Imaging for SB tumors within areas of CD that are often strictured with thick, irregular walls is difficult. CT enterography versus enteroclysis can be helpful in these situations to delineate abnormalities within abnormalities. Finally, any area of bowel resected for active or uncontrolled CD, including fistulous tracts, should be evaluated closely for neoplasia.

Surgical resection with curative intent is recommended for most patients with SB adenocarcinoma and no evidence of distant metastasis; a recent review article cites 5-year survival rates of 54% and 0, respectively, for resected and nonresected disease. The goal of surgical resection is complete resection with negative margins and lymphadenectomy (at least 8 to 10 lymph nodes). For duodenal disease, this may require pancreaticoduodenectomy, depending on the location of the lesion. For distal ileal disease, right hemicolectomy may be required. The utility of adjuvant chemotherapy remains unknown because of the low incidence of SB adenocarcinoma, although, extrapolating from our experience with colorectal adenocarcinoma, it is likely beneficial. A global multicenter trial is ongoing to address this question.

Staging for small bowel adenocarcinoma is based on the TNM system (Table 2). Prognosis is fair with greater than 50% 5-year survival for stage I and IIa and 20% to 30% 5-year survival for stages IIa through IIIc. For metastatic or stage IV disease, 5-year survival is a dismal 5%. Factors predicting poor prognosis include incomplete or noncurative resection, lymph node involvement, and presence of distant metastases.

Lymphoma

Primary GI lymphomas constitute the largest subset of extranodal lymphomas and include disease originating in the stomach, SB, and colon. SB lymphomas arise from the lymphoid follicles of the intestinal submucosa; thus areas with the most lymphoid tissue (i.e., jejunum and distal ileum) have the highest rate of tumor formation.

TABLE 2: TNM Staging for Small Bowel Adenocarcinoma

Stage	Characteristics of Tumor-Node-Metastasis Classification System
T	**PRIMARY TUMOR**
TX	Primary tumor cannot be assessed
T0	No evidence of primary tumor present
Tis	Carcinoma in situ
T1a	Tumor invades the lamina propria
T1b	Tumor invades the submucosa
T2	Tumor invades the muscularis propria
T3	Tumor invades through the muscularis propria into subserosa or into nonperitonealized perimuscular tissue (mesentery or retroperitoneum), with extension of <2 cm
T4	Tumor penetrates the visceral peritoneum or directly invades other organs or structures
N	**REGIONAL LYMPH NODES**
NX	Regional lymph nodes cannot be assessed
N0	No regional lymph node metastasis
N1	Regional lymph node metastasis with one to three lymph nodes involved
N2	Regional lymph node metastasis with four or more lymph nodes involved
M	**DISTANT METASTASES**
MX	Presence of distant metastasis cannot be assessed
M0	No distant metastasis
M1	Distant metastasis
STAGE	**GROUPING**
0	Tis, N0, M0
I	T1-T2, N0, M0
IIA	T3, N0, M0
IIB	T4, N0, M0
IIIA	Any T, N1, M0
IIIB	Any T, N2, M0
IV	Any T, any N, M1

From Edge SB, Byrd DR, Compton CC, et al, eds. *AJCC Cancer Staging Manual.* 7th ed. New York: Springer; 2010:127-129.

TNM, tumor-node-metastasis.

SB lymphomas most often are accompanied by nonspecific abdominal pain, anorexia, and weight loss and, more rarely, diarrhea or a palpable abdominal mass. A significant fraction of patients present with perforation, and the diagnosis is made retrospectively. Lymphomas nearly always are associated with bulky lymphadenopathy, which is a distinguishing feature.

The most common histologic diagnosis is non-Hodgkin's lymphoma (NHL) of the B cell variety, but T-cell malignancies do exist and are often more sinister. Of the B-cell lymphomas, diffuse large B-cell lymphoma (DLBCL) and low-grade mucosa-associated lymphoid tissue (MALT) lymphoma are the most common. Other entities include Burkitt's lymphoma, mantle cell lymphoma, and follicular lymphoma. Burkitt's lymphoma can be endemic or sporadic; the more rare sporadic form typically involves the SB, whereas the endemic form associated with EBV infection primarily affects the face and orbit but also can involve the SB. Patients with HIV also are predisposed to Burkitt's lymphoma. Burkitt's has a characteristic cytogenetic abnormality with rearrangement of the *c-Myc* oncogene located on chromosome 8. SB Burkitt's lymphoma occurs near the ileocolic junction and often can cause intussusception. Burkitt's lymphoma of the SB is a very aggressive tumor. Mantle cell lymphoma of the SB is similarly aggressive. It typically involves both the spleen and small intestine and spreads early to mesenteric nodes and outside the abdomen to peripheral blood and nodes and bone marrow. It can present as a solitary lesion or with multiple lymphomatous polyposis. Follicular lymphoma, in contrast, is especially indolent.

Enteropathy-associated T-cell lymphoma (EATL) is a rare T-cell lymphoma representing 10% to 25% of all SB lymphomas and typically involves the jejunum. EATL may be either primary or secondary, the latter being associated with celiac disease; it is thought to be due to chronic stimulation of the intraepithelial lymphocytes. Although only 2% to 3% of all patients with celiac disease will develop EATL, 50% of those with disease refractory to a gluten-free diet will develop EATL. Greater than 75% of patients with EATL, especially the secondary form, have hypoalbuminemia and anemia on presentation, both of which are indicative of severe malnutrition and wasting. The lesions associated with EATL, unlike NHL, often are ulcerated with significant inflammatory changes. These patients frequently exhibit intestinal perforation, and, if left untreated, EATL almost invariably leads to death from abdominal sepsis.

Workup for suspected or confirmed SB lymphoma should include CT of the neck, chest, abdomen, and pelvis as well as PET scan in addition to endoscopic evaluation of the entire GI tract (Figure 3). Biochemical evaluation should include LDH and beta-2 microglobulin. Bone marrow biopsy is required. There are various staging systems for SB lymphoma; commonly used systems include the Lugano international staging, the Ann Arbor with Musshoff modification, and the Paris system (Table 3).

Historically, the surgeon was an important first player in both the diagnosis and treatment of SB lymphoma. However, with improved endoscopic and radiologic approaches to biopsy as well as the recognition of lymphoma as a systemic disease, the role of the surgeon in the treatment of SB lymphoma has waned. For most SB B-cell lymphomas with localized disease (Lugano stage I, II$_1$), surgical resection with adjuvant chemotherapy continues to be the treatment of choice. Surgical intervention requires a segmental resection with at least 12 mesenteric nodes. Adjuvant therapy includes the familiar CHOP or R-CHOP regimens. With the more indolent follicular lymphomas, a "watch and wait" strategy often is employed. Those with advanced disease (Lugano stage II$_2$ and greater) undergo chemotherapy only. Those with especially aggressive tumors are considered for high-dose chemotherapy and stem cell transplantation. For EATL, combined therapies are also more effective than resection alone; the additional benefit of consolidation therapy and autologous stem cell transplantation in these patients remains to be determined. Surgical intervention in patients with EATL is complicated by the malnourishment associated with celiac disease and chronic inflammation. The presence of CD30 on a majority of EATL tumors is being used to design targeted chemotherapies and is offering some hope to these patients. Unfortunately, the role of the surgeon in the treatment of patients with intestinal lymphoma often is for complications requiring urgent or emergent intervention (i.e., obstruction or perforation); this occurs in 11% to 64% of patients with SB lymphoma.

Gastrointestinal Stromal Tumor

GISTs represent one of the rare nonepithelial primary lesions of the GI tract; approximately 5000 new cases are diagnosed in the United

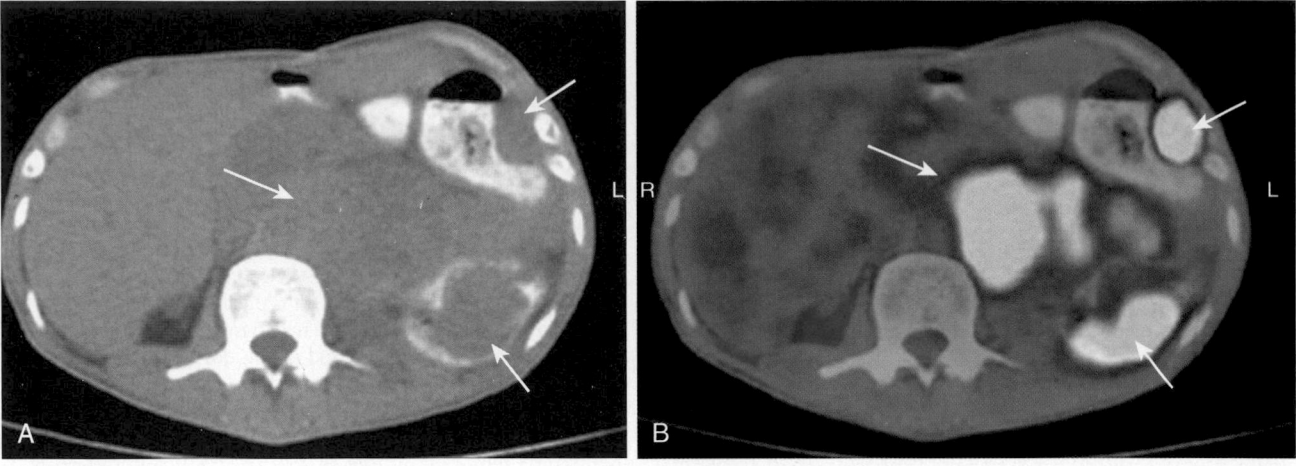

FIGURE 3 A and B, PET CT is useful in the detection of small bowel lymphomas (*arrows*).

TABLE 3: Lugano Staging System for Gastrointestinal Lymphomas

Stage	Extent of Lymphoma
I	Confined to GI tract (single primary, or multiple noncontiguous lesions)
II	Extending into abdomen from primary GI site II_1 = local nodal involvement II_2 = distant nodal involvement
IIE	Penetration of serosa to involve adjacent organ or tissues Specify site of involvement, e.g., IIE (pancreas) If both nodal involvement and involvement of adjacent organs, denote stage using both a subscript (1 or 2) and E, e.g., II_1E (pancreas)
IV	Disseminated extranodal involvement or concomitant supradiaphragmatic nodal involvement

Adapted from Rohatiner A, et al. Report on a workshop convened to discuss the pathological and staging classifications of gastrointestinal tract lymphoma. *Ann Oncol.* 1994;5:397-400.

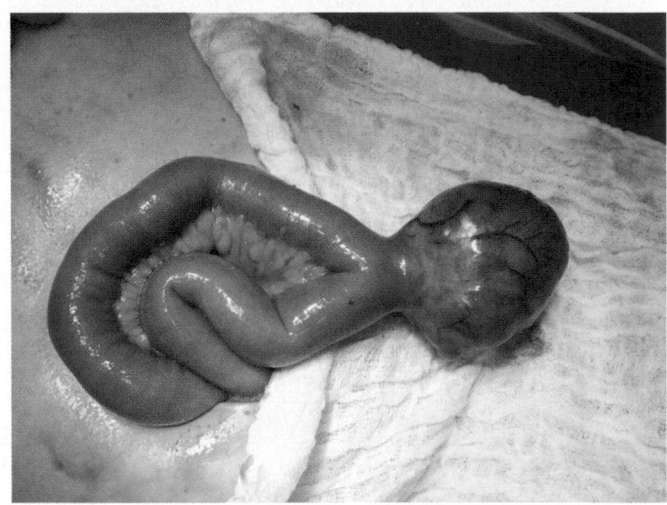

FIGURE 4 Small bowel gastrointestinal stromal tumor encountered during diagnostic laparoscopy for workup of gastrointestinal bleeding in elderly female after negative upper and lower endoscopy.

States each year. They are deceivingly benign in appearance: they can recur, metastasize, and ultimately prove fatal. They can occur anywhere in the GI tract, but most are found in the stomach (64%) and SB (35%) with the remainder found in the esophagus, colon, and rectum. In contrast to patients with other SB tumors, most patients with GIST are symptomatic. Symptoms include nausea/vomiting, early satiety, melena and anemia, abdominal pain, distension, fever, or leukocytosis (Figure 4). More than 50% of patients present with locally advanced or metastatic disease; 50% recur or metastasize despite initial optimal treatment of the primary lesion.

In the past, resection was the only possible intervention because GISTs are highly resistant to conventional chemotherapy. Fortunately, the approach to the treatment of GIST has changed radically in the last 15 years; this change was prompted by two related scientific discoveries made in the late 1990s. In 1998 there was a breakthrough discovery of a *c-KIT* mutation present in a majority of GISTs. c-KIT is a tyrosine kinase–linked cell surface receptor important for various cell signaling pathways involved in cell growth and differentiation. A *c-KIT* mutation leads to constitutive activation of the kinase; tumor growth and survival is absolutely dependent on that activity. The most common mutation in *c-KIT* is found in exon 11, followed by mutations in exons 9, 13, and 17. Since that time other less common

activating mutations have been discovered in various GISTs, including mutations in *PDGFRα, BRAF, N-ras, H-ras*, and succinate dehydrogenase. The second critical breakthrough came in the discovery of a novel small molecule inhibitor of the *BCR-abl* kinase for patients with CML. This kinase inhibitor called *STI 571, Gleevac,* or *imatinib* abruptly stops cellular division and induces apoptosis in nearly 100% of cells. Importantly, imatinib similarly inhibits the constitutively active *c-KIT* associated tyrosine kinase and various other kinases. Treating patients with nonresectable and widespread metastatic GISTs with imatinib had remarkable results with near elimination of tumor burden. Notably, the various *c-KIT* mutants have varying sensitivities to imatinib; specifically, those with exon 9 mutations are notoriously resistant to tyrosine kinase inhibitor (TKI) therapy. Thus knowing the sequence of the *c-KIT* mutant can help guide clinical decision making. Interestingly, imatinib is better than traditional chemotherapeutic agents even for those lacking *c-KIT* and/or *PDGFRα* mutation; this is an unexpected finding and suggests that this TKI may have other effects on tumor growth that are unknown at this time.

Surgical intervention depends on the overall health of the patient, presence or absence of metastatic disease, the size of the primary tumor, and the difficulty of the resection. In all cases, the goal should be negative margins with no rupture of the tumor capsule. No lymphadenectomy is necessary because GISTs infrequently metastasize to local nodes. Small tumors with low-risk features that are easily resectable can be excised with no adjuvant therapy. Resectable tumors with high-risk features should be excised followed by adjuvant TKI. High-risk features include tumor size greater than 2 cm, mitotic index greater than 5 mitoses per HPF, intraoperative tumor rupture, and inability to achieve an R0 resection. Adjuvant TKI therapy provides significant survival advantage as demonstrated by various phase III trials. For those presenting with nonresectable tumors resulting from involvement of critical structures/vasculature, TKI should be given preoperatively; significant tumor shrinkage is common and can allow subsequent resection. For those with mutations with poor response to TKI therapy (e.g., exon 9), a surgeon may be more inclined to perform a major operation first because it is unlikely that significant tumor shrinkage will occur with TKI administration. For those experiencing recurrent locoregional disease, re-resection is warranted and leads to increased survival. Finally, for those with widely metastatic disease responsive to TKI therapy, metastasectomy can lead to prolonged PFS and overall survival. However, operative intervention is not beneficial to patients with metastatic disease refractory to TKIs. It is important to note that nearly all patients who undergo metastasectomy ultimately will experience recurrence and then will need to be placed on continuous TKI therapy.

Prognosis for SB GIST is dependent on tumor size and location, mitotic activity, and adequacy of resection; long-term PFS ranges from more than 95% for small tumors with low mitotic rate to less than 10% for large tumors with high mitotic rate.

Metastatic Disease

Although primary SB tumors are rare, metastatic disease to the SB or its mesentery is not uncommon. The most common primary tumors that metastasize to small bowel include melanoma, colon, breast, kidney, and lung; melanoma represents approximately one third of all SB metastases (Figure 5). Patients most often present with vague abdominal pain, recurrent partial or complete obstruction, or occult GI blood loss. Up to 2% of patients with advanced malignancy eventually experience SB obstruction secondary to SB involvement.

SBO secondary to metastatic disease can be due to mechanical or nonmechanical problems. Pure mechanical problems include the presence of intraluminal tumors within the bowel wall, extrinsic compression from extraluminal tumors, and inflammation or infiltration of the bowel mesentery. There are often multiple areas of involvement. Nonmechanical GI paresis secondary to significant opioid use, immobility, poor oral intake, and paraneoplastic processes can complicate the diagnosis.

Operation can be considered in young patients or older patients with preserved functional status and a single area of involvement with otherwise reasonable prognosis. Surgical options include small bowel resection or palliative bypass. However, in most cases, SBOs secondary to metastatic disease, even when the result of purely mechanical cause, rarely lead to perforation and often resolve spontaneously. Obstruction in these patients is nearly always indicative of severe disease with an overwhelmingly poor prognosis. As such, in the case of SBO secondary to metastatic disease, surgical intervention rarely leads to increased survival. Exceptions include melanoma and renal cell carcinoma for which resection of metastatic lesions has

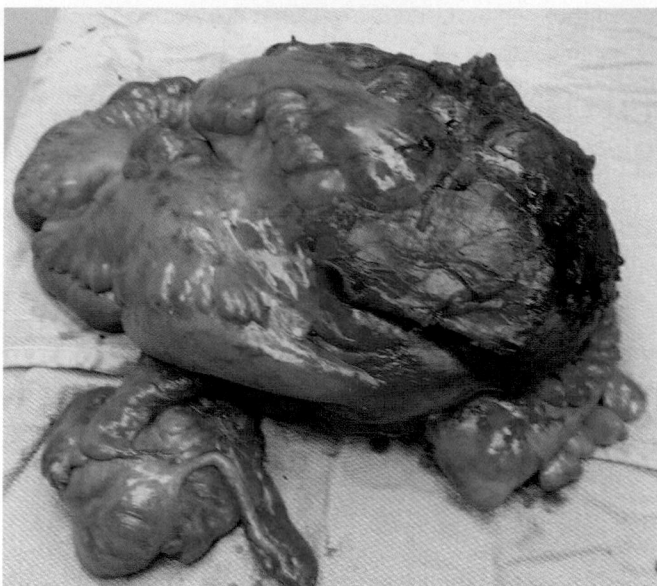

FIGURE 5 Large melanoma involving multiple loops of small bowel with bulky mesenteric lymphadenopathy resected en bloc.

been demonstrated to lead to increased survival. In a series studying the effect of surgical intervention for metastatic melanoma, a median survival of 48 months was observed in patients undergoing curative resection, whereas patients receiving optimal medical management survived only 5 to 6 months.

In lieu of operative therapy, interventions should include evacuation of the rectal vault, gastric decompression, and fluid resuscitation with correction of all biochemical imbalances, including hypercalcemia and hypokalemia. Adjunctive therapies should include antiemetics, analgesia, antisecretory agents, and steroids that have both antiemetic and anti-inflammatory effects. With regard to analgesia, fentanyl is thought to cause less gut immobility than other narcotic agents. Finally, given the poor prognosis, goals of care should be addressed as soon as possible. Involving the patient's oncologist and/or palliative care team is paramount.

■ ACKNOWLEDGMENT

The authors acknowledge the editorial and technical contributions of Margaret Tarpley, MLS, Senior Associate, Section of Surgical Sciences, Vanderbilt University School of Medicine.

SUGGESTED READINGS

Fernandes DD, et al. Cross-sectional imaging of small bowel malignancies. *Can Assoc Radiol J.* 2012;3:215-221.

Gold JS, DeMatteo RP. Combined surgical and molecular therapy: the gastrointestinal stromal tumor model. *Ann Surg.* 2006;244:176-184.

Grau AM, Broome J, Tarpley JL. Small bowel carcinoid/neuroendocrine tumors. In: Cameron JL, ed. *Current Surgical Therapy.* 10th ed. St Louis: Elsevier; 2011.

Raghav K, Overman MJ. Small bowel adenocarcinomas-existing evidence and evolving paradigms. *Nat Rev Clin Oncol.* 2013;10:534-544.

THE MANAGEMENT OF DIVERTICULOSIS OF THE SMALL BOWEL

Mark Hartney, MD, MS, Melissa Silva Zoumberos, MD, and Peter J. Fabri, MD, PhD, FACS

Although diverticulosis of the small bowel remains relatively uncommon, appropriate management is clinically important. The reported prevalence from multiple autopsy series ranges from 0.3% up to 5%. Diverticulosis of the small bowel has been observed in approximately 2% to 6% of small bowel contrast studies and in 7% of patients undergoing endoscopic retrograde cholangiopancreatography (ERCP). Most small bowel diverticula are asymptomatic, and it is estimated that less than 4% cause symptoms.

Small bowel diverticula can be congenital or acquired and can be classified as true diverticula (containing all layers of the intestinal wall) or false diverticula (containing only mucosa, submucosa, and serosa). They can occur in the duodenum, jejunum, and ileum but are most commonly found in the duodenum. Most asymptomatic small bowel diverticula are identified incidentally at celiotomy or on radiographic study and are usually managed nonoperatively. Advances in endoscopy have also increased the recognition and diagnosis. As jejunoileal diverticula are the most likely to become symptomatic or develop complications, resection of these diverticula has been recommended.

A fair amount of literature exists addressing the management of complications from diverticulosis of the small bowel. There have been hundreds of publications, most of which are case reports including reviews of the literature. Some larger series have attempted to extrapolate the findings to the general population; however, the utility remains limited.

■ DETECTION AND MANAGEMENT OF ASYMPTOMATIC (INCIDENTALLY DISCOVERED) SMALL BOWEL DIVERTICULOSIS

In the current era of radiologic imaging combined with advances in endoscopy, diverticulosis of the small bowel is being diagnosed more frequently. Despite the seeming increase in detection, there has not been a notable increase in symptomatic diverticula. Most truly are discovered incidentally and while still asymptomatic.

Duodenal and Intraluminal Diverticula

Duodenal diverticula are the most common diverticula of the small bowel, accounting for approximately 45% to 79%. They are usually solitary and asymptomatic. Although they are found in 1% to 6% of all upper gastrointestinal radiologic series, they are discovered even more commonly at autopsy. Fortunately, few (less than 1%) become symptomatic, as surgical intervention can carry significant morbidity and mortality.

Duodenal diverticula can develop congenitally or as an acquired entity. In addition to those classically described, pseudodiverticula or windsock diverticula also can occur congenitally in the duodenum as prolapses of mucosa or incompletely divided congenital septa. They typically arise from the second portion of the duodenum and can extend as far as the fourth portion. Frequently, pseudodiverticula are associated with other congenital anomalies: malrotation, omphalocele, annular pancreas, congenital biliary cysts, and various cardiac and urinary congenital abnormalities. Symptoms vary depending on the size and location, especially with regard to proximity to the ampulla of Vater.

Asymptomatic diverticula, by definition, are discovered incidentally upon radiographic or endoscopic examination and at celiotomy for another reason. Because most are asymptomatic and most remain asymptomatic, it has become the standard recommendation to not operate or resect any asymptomatic small bowel diverticula, especially because an asymptomatic patient cannot be made better.

There is statistical justification for operating only on symptomatic diverticula of the small bowel, which is infrequent because only 1% are symptomatic and less than that ever come to operation. Conversely, there is also statistical justification for not operating on asymptomatic diverticula. Zani and colleagues calculated that 758 patients with incidental Meckel's diverticulum would need to undergo intestinal resection to prevent 1 death.

Jejunoileal Diverticula

Diverticula arising in the jejunum and ileum account for 18% to 25% of all small bowel diverticulosis; however, about 10% of these are likely to become symptomatic. They are commonly multiple; 80% occur in the jejunum, 15% occur in the ileum, and 5% occur in both.

These jejunoileal (false) diverticula are thought to develop as a result of myoneural abnormalities, often dysmotility in the migrating motor complexes, leading to spastic contractions that result in prolonged, increased intraluminal pressures. Over the course of many years this is thought to lead to the formation of the false diverticula. Enteroclysis is the best radiographic study to evaluate jejunoileal diverticula, often to confirm the diagnosis. Computed tomography (CT)/magnetic resonance (MR) enterography likewise has been used increasingly in diagnosis. The use of capsule endoscopy also has a role in the diagnosis and evaluation of jejunoileal diverticula, especially symptomatic but not infected.

As with most other diverticula of the small bowel, surgical excision is not warranted in an asymptomatic patient with jejunoileal diverticula or those discovered incidentally; there has been no proven role for prophylactic resection.

Meckel's Diverticula

Meckel's diverticula are the most common congenital small bowel abnormality and account for the remaining 25% of small bowel diverticulosis. A Meckel's diverticulum is the remnant of a persistent portion (from failure of obliteration) of the proximal vitelline (omphalomesenteric) duct, which connects the embryonic midgut to the yolk sac. It only occurs on the antimesenteric border of the ileum as a true diverticulum, which contains all layers of the intestinal wall.

Meckel's diverticula are located approximately 2 feet from the ileocecal valve often containing one of two types of heterotopic tissue, most commonly gastric (75%) or pancreatic (15%) in one half of all Meckel's diverticula (50%) (Figure 1). The "rule of two" follows that Meckel's diverticula occur twice as commonly in males in 2% of the population and become symptomatic in 2% of cases usually within the first 2 years of life; they can extend over 2 inches in length and predominantly cause two types of symptoms: bleeding and obstruction.

The lifetime risk of an asymptomatic Meckel's diverticulum is very low. As well described, most Meckel's diverticula become symptomatic within the first 2 years of life and certainly by the age of 18. Based on 19 autopsy studies, in which 7 reported postnatal autopsies, Meckel's diverticulum has a prevalence of 1.23%. Mortality from Meckel's diverticulum is low (<0.001%) and is most common in the pediatric population. Incidentally discovered Meckel's diverticula should be left in situ, because the risk of postoperative complications from resection outweighs the risk of late complications.

A comprehensive systematic review done by Zani and colleagues concluded that there is no compelling evidence in the literature to

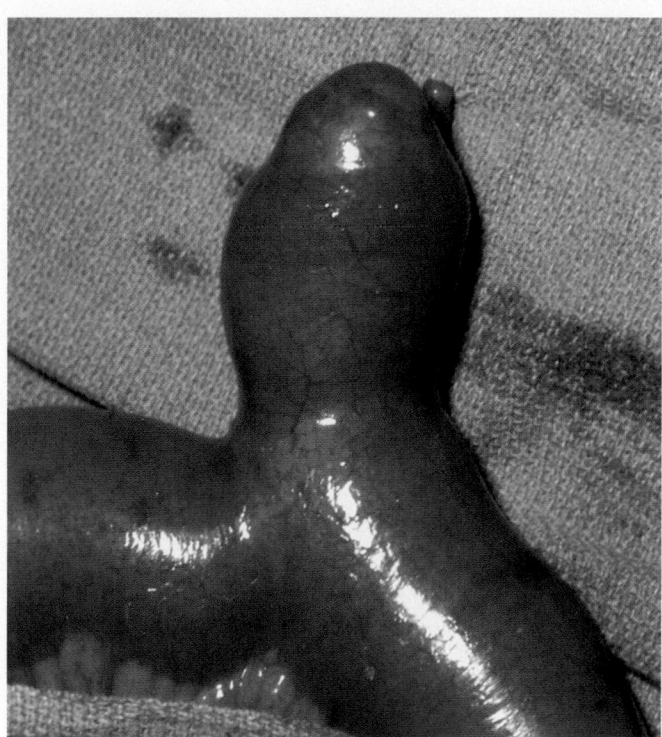

FIGURE 1 Common presentation of a Meckel's diverticulum projecting from the antimesenteric border of the ileum. *(From McKenzie S, Evers BM. Small intestine. In: Townsend CM Jr, ed: Sabiston Textbook of Surgery. 19th ed. Philadelphia: Elsevier Saunders; 2012.)*

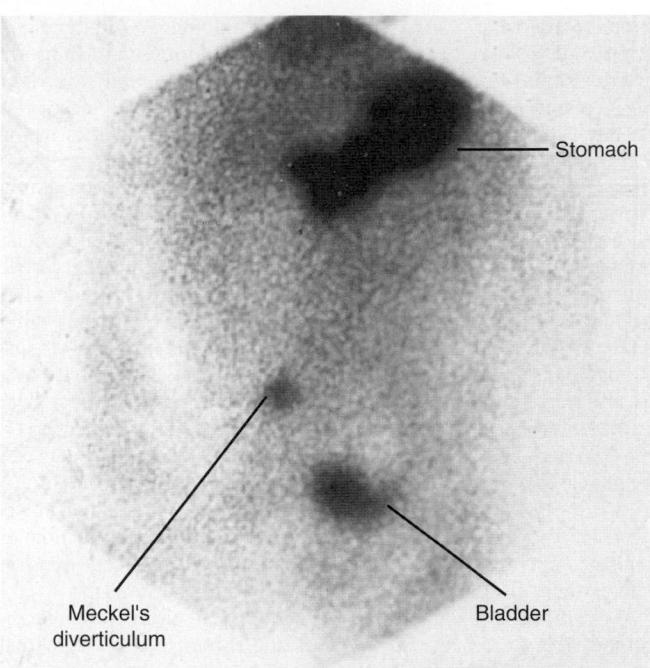

FIGURE 2 Technetium 99m-pertechnetate scintigram from a child with a Meckel's diverticulum clearly differentiated from the stomach and bladder. *(From McKenzie S, Evers BM. Small intestine. In: Townsend Jr CM, ed: Sabiston Textbook of Surgery. 19th ed. Philadelphia: Elsevier Saunders; 2012.)*

support prophylactic resection of an incidentally discovered Meckel's diverticulum at operation for an unrelated condition, even in young children. Nonetheless, palpable evidence of ectopic tissue intraoperatively; a prior history of diverticulitis, hemorrhage, or intussusception; or the presence of a mesodiverticular band serves as a relative indication. Most experts concur that a symptomatic or incidentally discovered Meckel's diverticulum in a young child should be resected.

■ MANAGEMENT OF SYMPTOMATIC SMALL BOWEL DIVERTICULA

Duodenal Diverticula

The investigational modalities of choice for duodenal diverticula include esophagogastroduodenoscopy (EGD) and endoscopic retrograde cholangiopancreatography (ERCP). These two modalities have become the cornerstone of visualizing duodenal diverticula, especially to clarify the relationship with and proximity to the ampulla of Vater and any contiguous biliary or pancreatic ductal structures. Increasingly, CT and MR enterography are being used for imaging, often ordered as a follow-up study to better characterize findings from standard contrast radiography.

Symptomatic duodenal diverticula are often the most difficult to manage because they usually include or are adjacent to the ampulla of Vater, specifically biliary and pancreatic ductal structures. Endoscopic therapy, including sphincterotomy as well as temporary stent placement, typically is attempted first. Operative management is reserved until after the inability to undergo endoscopic therapy or failure of endoscopic therapy.

Operative treatment of duodenal diverticula can be difficult and can be associated with significant morbidity and mortality, especially in inexperienced hands. Keys to the operative approach include a wide Kocher maneuver, clarification of the anatomic relationship of the diverticulum to biliary and pancreatic ductal structures, identification of ALL biliary and pancreatic ductal structures, liberal use of

intraoperative ductal stents, transverse or oblique closure of the duodenum, and sometimes a Thal patch, including cholecystectomy with any operation for duodenal diverticula. The diverticulum usually is resected, often with a stapler after extensive mobilization, or it can just be inverted.

Jejunoileal Diverticula

Symptomatic jejunoileal diverticulitis is diagnosed most often using CT/MR enterography. After enterography, uninfected, symptomatic jejunoileal diverticula also may be evaluated by push enteroscopy, double balloon endoscopy, and capsule endoscopy. Jejunoileal diverticula can present as diverticulitis, refractory inflammation, obstruction, perforation, and hemorrhage. Complicated jejunoileal diverticula often require surgical management, although jejunoileal diverticulitis usually can be managed nonoperatively, at least initially.

Most recommendations support segmental resection of jejunoileal diverticula, when necessary, especially to prevent narrowing of the small bowel. The real possibility of postoperative complications (reason to not operate when asymptomatic) is the usual reason offered for including incidental appendectomy at the time of operation.

Meckel's Diverticulum

Meckel's diverticula can become symptomatic in many ways. Most commonly, acid produced by ectopic gastric mucosa causes ulceration along the mesenteric border of the ileum; of those with hemorrhage, 95% contain gastric mucosa. Meckel's diverticulum can be a cause of chronic and acute GI hemorrhage in young patients. It is also an important cause of hemorrhage in the broader pediatric population but also occurs in adults.

Diagnostic modalities usually include a form of angiography or nuclear scintigraphy (Figure 2). Angiography can be useful during active hemorrhage, where it shows bleeding into the diverticulum or distal small bowel. Angiography is even more useful when it demonstrates a persistent right vitelline artery arising from the superior mesenteric artery or an enlarged, long, nonbranching, embryonic ileal artery leading to the diverticulum. The most useful arteriographic finding is a nonbranching end artery in the right lower abdomen containing a cluster of small, irregular arteries at its distal distribution. These often contain irregular arteries in the wall of the diverticulum and vitelline artery remnants as well as increased parenchymal blush from the ectopic gastric mucosa lining the diverticulum.

Meckel's scintigraphy uses technetium 99m pertechnetate, which is concentrated and then excreted by mucous-producing cells (gastric mucosa). It is important to remember that a Meckel's scan identifies ectopic gastric mucosa, not the hemorrhage. To obtain a quality study, it is often necessary to obtain oblique, lateral or postvoid films to distinguish a diverticulum from other activity. The activity in a Meckel's diverticulum should occur at about the same time as activity in the stomach. Depending on the center and radiologist, the sensitivity of a Meckel's scan is reportedly 75% to 85% and supposedly can be increased by pretreatment with pentagastrin or glucagon.

In adults, Meckel's diverticula commonly are seen as small bowel obstruction (45%). After adequate resuscitation, obstruction is managed operatively as quickly as possible, usually by wedge excision and primary closure or amputation with a surgical stapler.

Diverticulitis (25%) within a Meckel's diverticulum is often indistinguishable from acute appendicitis and is managed by segmental resection and primary ileoileostomy. Hemorrhage (20%) and ulcer also are managed by segmental resection and primary ileoileostomy. At operation for hemorrhage, segmental resection is recommended because the ulcer is typically on the mesenteric border of the ileum—opposite the antimesenteric border location of the Meckel's diverticulum and occasionally distal to it. Despite improved diagnostic modalities, most bleeding Meckel's diverticula are diagnosed at celiotomy.

Appendectomy should be considered at any operation for a symptomatic Meckel's diverticulum to prevent any future diagnostic dilemmas.

SUGGESTED READINGS

Akhrass R, Yaffe MB, Fischer C, Ponsky J, Shuck JM. Small-bowel diverticulosis: perceptions and reality. *J Am Coll Surg*. 1997;184:383-388.

Chiu EJ, Shyr YM, Su CH, Wu CW, Lui WY. Diverticular disease of the small bowel. *Hepatogastroenterology*. 2000;47:181-184.

Kouraklis G, Glinavou A, Mantas D, Kouskos E, Karatzas G. Clinical implications of small bowel diverticula. *Isr Med Assoc J*. 2002;4:431-433.

Thompson JN, Salem RR, Hemingway AP, Rees HC, Hodgson HJ, Wood CB, Allison DJ, Spencer J. Specialist investigation of obscure gastrointestinal bleeding. *Gut*. 1987;28:47-51.

Zani A, Eaton S, Rees CM, Pierro A. Incidentally detected Meckel's diverticulum: to resect or not to resect? *Ann Surg*. 2008;247:276-281.

THE MANAGEMENT OF MOTILITY DISORDERS OF THE STOMACH AND SMALL BOWEL

KMarie Reid Lombardo, MD, and Michael G. Sarr, MD

■ MOTILITY DISORDERS OF THE STOMACH

Dysmotility of the stomach more typically occurs as a result of damage of the vagus nerve that can result from chronic illness, such as poorly controlled diabetes. More often surgeons see gastric dysmotility after surgical interventions that disrupt the vagal nerve function, such as truncal vagotomy, gastrectomy, or disruption of the continuity of the jejunum with the duodenal pacemaker that occurs in the creation of the Roux-en-Y with the required transection of the proximal jejunum (Figure 1). Emptying can be either delayed (causing mild or severe gastroparesis) or increased (leading to dumping and/or diarrhea).

When functioning normally, the proximal stomach is responsible for relaxation (receptive relaxation) to accommodate the entry of solids and liquids by providing a reservoir necessary for temporary storage and the start of enzymatic breakdown of the ingested content. This relaxation is mediated by the vagus nerve. In addition, protein and fat digestion begins by way of pepsin and hydrochloric acid; the presence of amino acids will lead to hormonal signaling that causes a slow tonic contraction of the proximal stomach. This tonic contraction increases the intraluminal pressure in the proximal stomach, thereby leading to emptying of chyme into the duodenum. Gastric emptying mediated by the enteric nervous system can be disrupted by surgical procedures as previously listed. Little is known about specific cause(s) that lead to altered gastric emptying after gastroesophageal surgery, but it appears to be multifactorial. The surgical process itself in addition to patient-related factors, such as the presence of diabetes, hypothyroidism, chronic narcotic use, or cancer, can contribute to this process. As aging occurs, the rate of gastric emptying declines, so older patients are more susceptible to this syndrome. This section focuses on motility disorders after surgical interventions, postsurgical gastroparesis syndrome (PGS), and rapid gastric emptying.

Delayed Gastric Emptying

Although uncommon, delayed gastric emptying can occur after truncal vagotomy, Roux-en-Y gastrojejunostomy, gastric resections, or even after an antireflux fundoplication. The risk of delayed gastric emptying after truncal vagotomy increases twofold and continues to plague patients undergoing pancreatoduodenectomy with Roux-en-Y reconstruction with a rate of up to 30%. The exact cause is unknown, but certainly vagus nerve dysfunction is a key contributor. Disruption of the continuity of the proximal jejunum with the duodenal pacemaker after duodenal resection may lead to incomplete emptying or gastric stasis. Truncal vagotomy causing disruption of neural signaling also may lead to stasis or even gastric atony.

Clinical Presentation and Diagnosis

Patients often experience epigastric fullness or pain. They will complain of early satiety that may be accompanied with nausea or vomiting, usually of solids more than liquids. Delayed vomiting may be associated with undigested food, often the day after ingestion of the solid food; this type of vomiting is almost pathognomonic of gastroparesis provided there is no mechanical gastric outlet obstruction. Liquid intake may be better tolerated over solids, but anorexia or even inability to ingest enough calories because of symptoms can be severe enough that patients may experience dehydration, weight loss, or even malnutrition.

A detailed history is necessary to evaluate risk factors such as prior upper abdominal surgery (esophageal, gastric, duodenal, or pancreatic), metabolic disturbances such as diabetes or hypothyroidism, or structural conditions or structurally directed pathologies such as scleroderma. During the diagnostic phase, it is necessary to

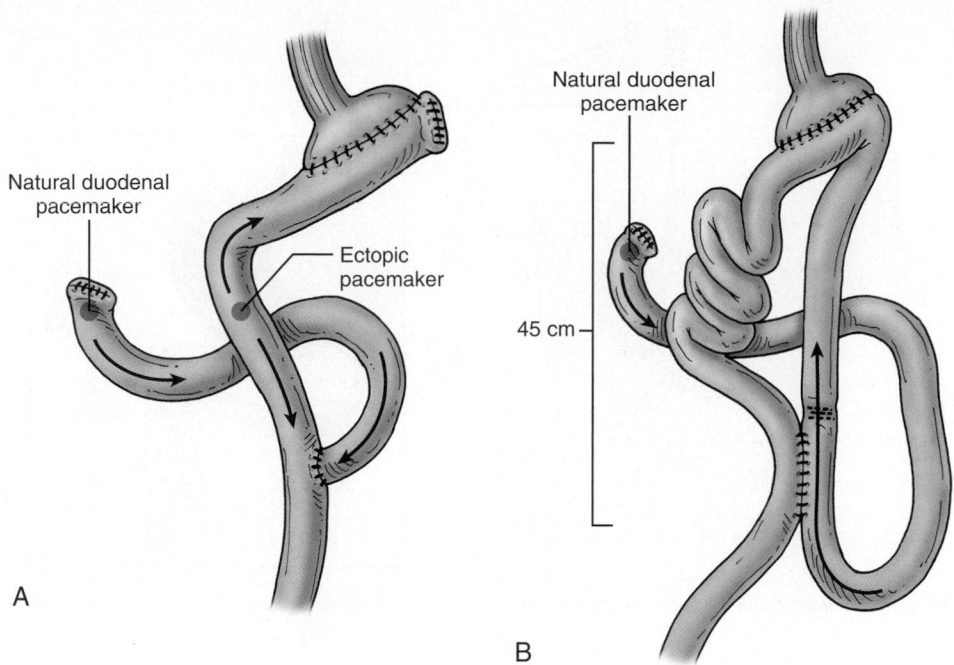

FIGURE 1 A, Ectopic duodenal pacemaker in a cut Roux limb after Roux-en Y gastrojejunostomy. **B,** In contrast, the normal pacemaker is maintained in an uncut Roux limb. *(Modified from image provided courtesy Mayo Clinic, Rochester, MN.)*

specifically exclude a mechanical obstruction presenting as efferent limb syndrome, anastomotic stricture, or rarely an intussusception after a gastroenterostomy. Once mechanical obstruction is excluded, clinicians must evaluate for metabolic derangements that can be observed from persistent vomiting or contributing causes such as diabetes and hypothyroidism. It is important to evaluate the nutritional state with an examination of serum levels of nutritional parameters such as serum albumin levels. Because albumin levels may be normal (they take a month or more to decrease substantially) ordering prealbumin, which has a shorter half-life, will help determine a more acute or subacute process. If patients do have a mechanical obstruction at the anastomosis that is identified as a stricture, ensure that they are not abusing nonsteroidal anti-inflammatory drugs (NSAIDs) and thereby contributing to anastomotic inflammation.

Imaging can begin with abdominal x-rays to rule out a mechanical obstruction. Gastric distention will likely be a finding. Upper endoscopy will allow visibility of undigested food in the stomach (always an abnormal sign), elimination of the possibility of anastomotic stricture, and the means by which to obtain biopsies. Postvagotomy gastroparesis is not associated with a dilated, distended stomach. Remember, gastric accommodation is prevented; if the gastric reservoir is very large, then think more of a mechanical obstruction. Gastric emptying studies can be performed using gastric scintigraphy, barium swallow, or gastric manometry when available, but with the presence of retained solid food in the gastric reservoir, these studies are usually not necessary.

Treatment

Treatment begins with the management of contributing factors, such as obtaining tighter glucose control or treatment of hypothyroidism. Modification of the diet is essential with a focus on liquids more than solids and adapting smaller and more frequent meals (ideally six while awake). The authors recommend a low-residue diet (i.e., lower fiber content) and softer foods. If dietary modification does not manage symptoms, a trial of a prokinetic drug such as metoclopramide, domperidone (if the patient still has an antrum, which is where domperidone takes effect), or low-dose erythromycin (125 mg,

not the usual doses of 250 or 500 mg) may help stimulate emptying. Total parental nutrition may be required in severe and life-threatening cases of malnutrition.

Operative intervention is limited to patients with medically refractory, severe symptoms affecting quality of life and challenging nutritional health. A jejunal feeding tube (percutaneous or open) (Figure 2) may be indicated but first with a trial of nasojejunal feeding to evaluate for tolerance of such feedings; such a trial is essential, because some patients have a poorly understood postvagotomy small bowel dysmotility. A venting gastrostomy tube may assist with the feeling of gastric fullness.

In a small subset of patients, near total (95%) or completion gastrectomy may play a role. A multidisciplinary discussion is mandatory before recommending this controversial strategy. An examination of 20 years of Mayo Clinic's experience of providing near total or completion gastrectomy in patients with severe PGS after a prior partial gastrectomy with truncal vagotomy showed that only about half the patients were able to maintain their nutrition orally. A similar trial of near total gastrectomy after a prior Nissen fundoplication in patients with PGS presumed to be related to vagal nerve injury found no benefit; the majority had persistent symptoms and required supplemental nutrition after the gastric resection. The authors do not recommend near or total gastrectomy as a routine strategy for PGS.

Alternative treatment options include implantation of an electrical gastric stimulator (Figure 3) into the stomach wall. This may be an option for patients with severe and refractory gastroparesis and who have diabetes or with predominant symptoms of nausea or vomiting. Although these nerve stimulators do appear to help with nausea and vomiting, they are controversial because they do not increase the effective gastric emptying. Acupuncture has been shown anecdotally to have some benefit in the management of selected patients with gastroparesis.

Rapid Gastric Emptying

Rapid emptying of gastric contents from the stomach into the duodenum, also known as *dumping*, can result from gastric operations that lead to "dumping" of a bolus of liquid or hyperosmolar chyme

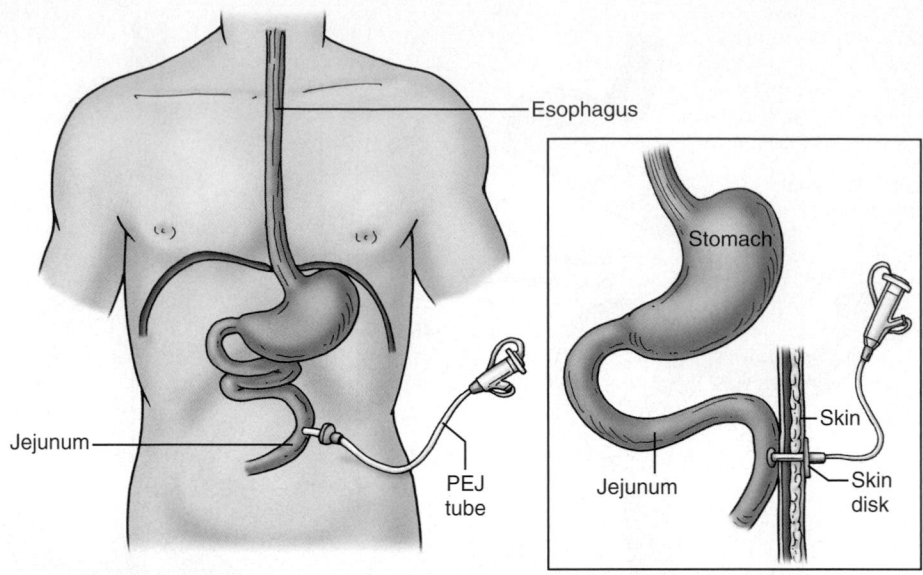

FIGURE 2 Percutaneous jejunostomy tube. *(Modified from image provided courtesy Mayo Clinic, Rochester, MN.)*

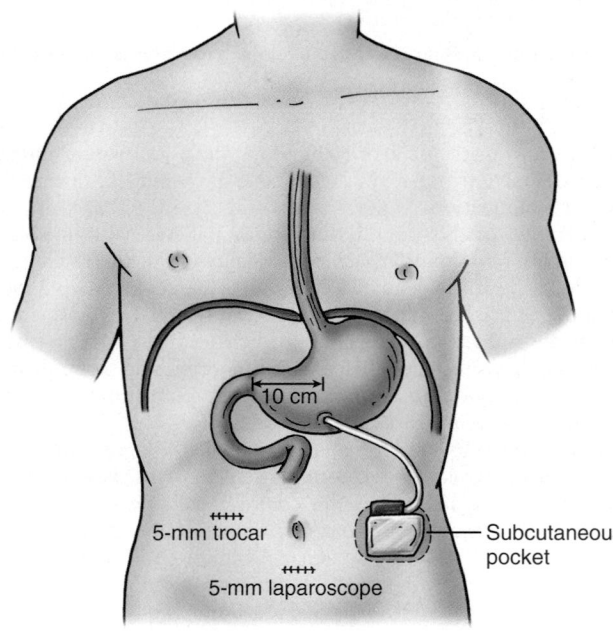

FIGURE 3 Laparoscopic approach for electrical gastric stimulator with gastric wall electrodes and subcutaneous battery. *(Modified from Ginsburg GG, et al. Clinical Gastrointestinal Endoscopy. 2nd ed. Philadelphia: WB Saunders; 2012.)*

into the duodenum. If the contents are only liquid, then the symptoms are minimal. Approximately 10% to 15% of patients experience dumping after gastric surgery. If the contents are of high osmolarity, such as a carbohydrate-rich bolus, then the resultant symptoms can be very unpleasant for the patient to experience. Because of increased tonicity, the rapid shift of fluid into the lumen of the small bowel can be unpleasant, but the majority of the symptoms arise from the release of vasoactive substances related to the high osmolality of the intraluminal content. The old theory of a "may result in relative hypovolemia" from the fluid shift has been disproved and is not the primary cause of the symptoms. Also, many relate dumping to diarrhea; this is neither appropriate nor accurate because many patients with dumping have no diarrhea.

Dumping can be seen after virtually any gastric operation, but the greatest frequency is after subtotal gastrectomy with vagotomy and the least frequency is after pyloroplasty alone. Patients who have undergone a truncal vagotomy and pyloroplasty will experience dumping at greater rates than those who had pyloroplasty alone. The symptoms occur early within 30 minutes of eating; there is also a form of dumping called "late dumping," in which the symptoms occur 2 to 3 hours after eating. There is really no difference in the patient symptoms except for timing. Symptoms are likely to be elicited after a large, rapidly ingested meal and are much worse with high osmolarity meals. In the past, dumping was a common feature after truncal vagotomy and pyloroplasty, but in the current era, dumping is observed primarily after Roux-en-Y gastric bypass surgery. Thankfully, dumping rarely is a permanent state especially after gastric bypass, in which the majority of patients will not have symptoms after 3 months. Predicting who will develop dumping is challenging.

Clinical Presentation and Diagnosis

The majority of patients, 75%, will present with early rather than late symptoms of dumping. The differential includes excluding the afferent loop syndrome, pancreatic insufficiency, bowel obstruction, and bile acid reflux after surgery. A detailed history will help to differentiate between dumping and these other important complications after gastric surgery. With *early dumping,* patients will complain of early satiety, abdominal pain, nausea, and evidence of autonomic dysfunction, such as a racing heartbeat, sweating, dizziness, and tremors. Unlike with early dumping, diarrhea is very common with late dumping. The symptoms may last for about an hour, because the high osmolarity causes release of vasoactive substances. Patients often are immobilized because of the severity of the ill feeling they experience. They will attempt to avoid a recurrence at all cost. *Late dumping* has similar symptoms but generally occurs approximately 2 to 3 hours or more after a meal. Additional features include fatigue, mental changes, or even fainting. Late dumping is associated with reactive hypoglycemia that occurs because of the rapid shifts in glucose levels after eating simple sugars and the subsequent over release of insulin. The high carbohydrate load in the small intestine leads to hyperinsulinemia resulting in rapid hypoglycemia. Recognition of this unfortunate sequela is important for patients to understand so that they can seek emergency care if needed.

Provocative testing to help to confirm the diagnosis of late dumping consists of using 50 g of orally administered glucose followed by serial measurements of glucose and plasma insulin levels as well as heart rate. Some suggest a concomitant, serum glucose and hydrogen breath test; an increase in the heart rate greater than 12 beats per minute and a rise in the hydrogen breath excretion allegedly has a sensitivity of 94% and a specificity of 92%. An upper GI series may help to define anatomy but is often not necessary.

Treatment

The primary treatment of dumping syndrome is dietary modification. Avoiding simple sugars (which includes alcohol and most dessert-type food items) and a high intake of carbohydrates helps to minimize symptoms. Simple measures such as avoiding drinking 30 minutes before or after a meal also may help. Adding fiber supplementation, complex carbohydrates, and drinking plenty of water during the day helps to slow transit and avoid dehydration as a result of dumping. Patients should avoid an upright posture while eating, because this may, in some patients, accelerate gastric emptying and instead recline if possible while eating. Although diarrhea is not the main presenting symptom, patients may have a late onset of diarrhea. As above, eating small frequent meals and having proteins and fats with meals help slow gastric emptying.

Dietary modifications alone may not help with dumping syndrome: 3% to 5% of patients will have refractory symptoms. In this population, a trial of octreotide may offer great relief of the dumping symptoms; if effective, as occurs in about 20% of patients, then a longer-acting formulation of octreotide should be used. In several randomized controlled trials, octreotide has been shown to improve symptoms in nearly all patients when compared with controls. Octreotide is given 30 minutes before or after a meal. The side effect of steatorrhea is treated typically with pancreatic enzyme replacement. Increasing the viscosity of the intraluminal contents by adding pectin and guar may slow the emptying process and alleviate symptoms.

The role of operative interventions to manage dumping is limited. The literature describes the use of a 10-cm reversed jejunal limb 100 cm from the ligament of Treitz as a measure to help patients who have severe diarrhea that may be associated with rapid gastric emptying. However, there are many complications with these reversed limbs, and the larger studies have not shown any substantial benefit to this now outdated procedure. For the late form of dumping associated with Roux-en-Y gastric bypass and its associated hypoglycemia (this syndrome has been called *noninsulinoma pancreatogenous hypoglycemia syndrome*), reversing the gastric bypass or redirecting the Roux limb into the duodenum may be the only option. The prior suggestion of subtotal pancreatectomy has proven to be ineffective in long-term outcomes.

■ MOTILITY DISORDERS OF THE SMALL INTESTINE

True motility disorders of the small intestine are actually unusual, and as a whole, represent a spectrum from reversible problems of motility, such as generalized adynamic ileus to the rare and progressive familial disorders of chronic idiopathic intestinal pseudo-obstruction and the acquired disorder of scleroderma. In addition, there are several unique clinical scenarios that involve motor abnormalities, such as the bypass enteropathy of the defunctionalized jejunoileum in patients after the original bariatric operation of the jejunoileal or "small bowel" bypass, small intestinal intussusception, and the dysmotility that can complicate small bowel function in patients who were born with intestinal atresia. This section will focus on adynamic ileus and the pseudo-obstructions of the small bowel.

Adynamic Ileus

A true small intestinal "ileus" after intra-abdominal operations actually is unusual. The "physiologic ileus" that occurs in the early postoperative period (first 1 to 4 days) after a laparotomy is often talked about. This ileus, or the inability to eat and have bowel movements,

is primarily a gastric and colonic phenomenon, not a small bowel "ileus" or dysmotility; indeed, the small intestinal contractile activity is present during the operation (in contrast to the stomach and colon, which have no contractile activity intraoperatively), also, intraintestinal feeding can be administered immediately postoperatively. In essence, the small intestine works relatively normally, whereas the motor activity leading to gastric emptying and colonic emptying is delayed for 3 to 4 days.

Adynamic ileus, however, is a generalized motor disorder of the entire gut, involving the small intestine as well. Adynamic (generalized) ileus involves a secondary blockade of effective contractile activity related most commonly to a systemic inflammatory disorder (such as sepsis) or after retroperitoneal operations (e.g., kidney transplantation) or with retroperitoneal conditions (e.g., trauma, hematoma) believed to interfere with the autonomic nervous innervation to the gut.

Clinical Presentation and Diagnosis

Diagnosis is based on the presence of vomiting, abdominal distention, obstipation of stool and gas, and the physical findings of tinkling bowel sounds and generalized bowel distention (small and large bowel) on diagnostic imaging, which occur in the appropriate clinical setting. With a heightened clinical suspicion, a simple abdominal radiograph will suffice. The differential diagnosis includes the exclusion of an obstructing rectal lesion, which may require proctoscopy or a transrectal contrast radiograph to exclude.

Treatment

Treatment should be directed at the cause of the ileus, most commonly sepsis. Specific pharmacologic or operative intervention is neither needed nor effective in an attempt to treat the ileus. Management is otherwise conservative, often including a nasogastric tube. Prokinetic agents are not effective. Adynamic ileus is transient and resolves when the systemic cause of the ileus has been controlled.

Chronic Idiopathic Intestinal Pseudo-Obstruction

This family of heritable disorders is uncommon, and the diagnosis, which mimics a mechanical small bowel obstruction, can be confusing and difficult if there is no obvious family history. There are three forms of chronic idiopathic pseudo-obstruction: a histopathologic myopathy of smooth muscle, a histopathologic neuropathy, and a less well-characterized form of neuromotor dysmotility that lacks any definitive histopathologic findings. All these disorders lead to disorganized motility with ineffective, uncoordinated contractile activity and markedly slowed propagation and transit of intestinal content.

Familial Visceral Myopathy

With this disorder of visceral smooth muscle, the amplitude of contractions is markedly abnormal, as is the coordination of propulsive contractile activity along the gut. This myopathy eventually affects the esophagus, stomach, small intestine, and colon, as well as the genitourinary system. The most common organs affected first by this myopathy can be the esophagus (megaesophagus), the duodenum (megaduodenum), the colon (megacolon), or the urinary system (megaureter). However, with time, all smooth muscle of the gut and genitourinary system becomes involved to some varied extent.

Familial Visceral Neuropathy

This disorder involves the autonomic nervous system of the gut, leading to discoordinated contractile activity with ineffective transit. Histologic findings are subtle and require a special expertise not only in the reading of the slides (which require a full thickness biopsy) but also in the staining of the tissue.

Neuromotor Dysmotility

This form of chronic idiopathic pseudo-obstruction mimics the primary visceral neuropathy form but lacks any discernible histopathologic findings. It is rare for a patient to develop a form of this dysmotility as a paraneoplastic phenomenon mediated by a humoral agent released by the neoplasm.

Clinical Presentation

Many times, the symptoms of dysmotility begin in one organ initially. A common presentation is severe constipation, which then progresses over a variable time (months to years) to also involve the small intestine. Some of these patients have been treated (inappropriately) by colectomy for a diagnosis of colonic inertia. Others present with megaesophagus, mimicking achalasia in some respects, but disease involvement of the distal gut develops eventually. In teenagers, one of the more common presentations is onset of megaduodenum often confused with the superior mesenteric artery syndrome (SMA syndrome); the latter itself is very rare and virtually always follows a marked weight loss rather than preceding or causing a weight loss as with pseudo-obstruction. Being a familial, heritable disorder, for patients other than the proband, there should be a family history of esophageal, colonic, or genitourinary problems.

The age of onset varies with the cause of intestinal pseudo-obstruction. Often the symptoms begin insidiously during late childhood/early teenage years with vague, chronic GI complaints. Other forms appear in the twenties and thirties in patients with a prior past history of such complaints as substantial constipation, dysphagia, gastroesophageal reflux, or intermittent abdominal distention/cramping. A clear implication of the clinical presentation/ diagnosis is that all too frequently, these patients have been operated on for a prior presumed mechanical "small bowel obstruction" secondary to a presentation of abdominal pain, distention, and markedly dilated small intestine, usually with no real objective or convincing site of mechanical obstruction found. The disease and symptoms often wax and wane, which raises the question if the current symptoms are secondary to adhesions rather than to a dysmotility.

Diagnosis

The diagnosis of chronic idiopathic intestinal pseudo-obstruction is most often one of exclusion (unless, of course, there is a strong family history). Because of its rarity, the diagnosis often is not considered, and patients are treated operatively as if they have a mechanical obstruction. Even when there is no definitive site of obstruction, the assumption is that the obstruction resolved. Thereafter, because the disease is intermittent at first, when the patient presents again with abdominal distention and a clinical picture of a mechanical small bowel obstruction, the concern of an adhesive obstruction is always present despite the concern of pseudo-obstruction from the prior operation. This makes the diagnosis and treatment very difficult.

Marked small intestinal distention (and often gastric as well) is the hallmark of diagnosis on radiographic imaging, and the distention goes all the way down to the cecum without a transition point. Early in the course of the disease, megaesophagus or megaduodenum may be the first sign, but later in the course, the entire small bowel is dilated, mimicking a very distal small bowel mechanical obstruction. The prior history of a negative exploration in the past or this presentation without any history of abdominal operation or hernia should raise the suspicion of the diagnosis, but obviously no one wants to mismanage or delay definitive treatment of a mechanical obstruction by delaying necessary definitive operative intervention.

There is no definitive or objective means of preoperative diagnosis other than a well-defined family history. A prior operation(s) without an obvious site of obstruction (and often it is necessary to read between the lines of the previous operative note by the surgeon who is trying to convince himself or herself that there was a site of obstruction) should raise suspicion of pseudo-obstruction, but nevertheless, there is always the worry of an adhesive cause being present.

Multiple attempts at diagnosis by characterizing the motor (contractile) pattern have been largely unsuccessful. Although the amplitude of contractions is decreased markedly in the visceral myopathic

form, measuring true amplitude in the presence of intestinal distension is not reliable whatever the cause. The most reliable method of diagnosis probably is best carried out by a "diagnostic" laparoscopic exploration. This approach offers objective visualization of the bowel with the least risk of subsequent adhesion formation. The finding of intestinal distention throughout the entire small intestine down to the cecum without any convincing site of concurrent or prior obstruction (adhesions, hernia, localized thickening of the bowel, or intraluminal mass that may have caused a transient intussusception) should raise suspicion of a motility disorder.

Treatment

Treatment of intestinal pseudo-obstruction is symptomatic and supportive only. Being a progressive disorder that involved the entire small intestine, any resections or internal bypasses should be avoided. Indeed, repeated laparotomies should be avoided if at all possible, because of the subsequent development of more adhesions, which only confuse the picture and complicate future decision making. When the diagnosis is suspected, laparoscopy rather than laparotomy should be used to confirm the diagnosis; whether a full-thickness biopsy is indicated or not is debatable, because there usually is no definite pathology evident, and most centers do not have the expertise to really look into the autonomic nervous system with the specialized staining needed. Similarly, for patients operated on previously, laparoscopy may allow the least invasive confirmatory approach as opposed to open laparotomy.

Because the symptoms and severity tend to wax and wane early in the course of the disease, any treatment should be conservative. As the disease progresses, chronic parenteral nutrition becomes the mainstay of treatment. In the latter stages of the disease, when the abdominal distention becomes chronic, a decompressive enterostomy may provide some benefit for the small intestinal distention. This should be considered in light of the known complications of any enterostomy tube, such as discomfort, fluid loss, or infection. Similarly, if vomiting is problematic, a tube gastrostomy also can be entertained, but again, all fluid loss from the tube must be replaced, making intravenous support more difficult.

Intestinal transplantation is a therapeutic possibility in selected individuals only. This approach brings its own problems, such as immunosuppression and infections. Whether intestinal transplantation is state-of-the-art currently is a quality judgment for each individual patient. With improvements in immunosuppression, transplantation represents the best alternative for this progressive and otherwise untreatable disease.

Postvagotomy Diarrhea

Postvagotomy diarrhea is a very rare form of dysmotility that is poorly understood and has no known effective treatment. Now that the era of vagotomy for duodenal ulcer disease is over, this very rare disorder should be even rarer.

Clinical Presentation

Although presenting as diarrhea, the underlying pathophysiology is believed to be a dysmotility, causing a rapid transit through the small intestine and not a malabsorption as such. The symptoms are diarrhea and cramping after eating but specifically without diarrhea or cramping in between meals. There is no real malabsorption as such in terms of fat (steatorrhea), protein (azotorrhea), or vitamins or minerals, but rather pain and fluid and electrolyte balance predominates. When analyzed, the diarrhea is a watery form, but the presence of undigested foodstuffs is evidence of rapid transit.

Diagnosis and Treatment

The diagnosis is often not thought of, is rare, and is one of exclusion. Endoscopies show normal mucosa confirmed on biopsy. Every form of diarrhea should be excluded before this diagnosis is made. This is important, because there is no effective treatment. Pharmacologic attempts at slowing transit with opiates or decreasing absorption, even with the use of octreotide have been uniformly unsuccessful. Prior attempts to slow transit by operative means such as reversed segments of small intestine are also not indicated because they just do not work. Once all other forms of diarrhea have been excluded, the treatment is supportive.

SUGGESTED READINGS

Clark CJ, Sarr MG, Arora AS, Nichols FC, Reid-Lombardo KM. Does gastric resection have a role in the management of severe post fundoplication gastric dysfunction? *World J Surg*. 2011;35:2045-2050. doi:10.1007/s00268-011-1173-9.

Forstner-Barthell AW, Murr MM, Nitecki S, Camilleri M, Prather CM, Kelly KA, Sarr MG. Near-total completion gastrectomy for severe postvagotomy gastric stasis: analysis of early- and long-term results in 62 patients. *J Gastrointest Surg*. 1999;3:15-23.

Mason RJ, Lipham J, Eckerling G, Schwartz A, DeMeester TR. Gastric electrical stimulation: an alternative surgical therapy for patients with gastroparesis. *Arch Surg*. 2005;140:841-848. doi:10.1001/archsurg.140.9.841.

National Institute of Diabetes and Digestive and Kidney Diseases. *Dumping syndrome*. <http://www.niddk.nih.gov/health-information/health-topics/digestive-diseases/dumping-syndrome/Pages/facts.aspx>. Accessed 15.11.01.

THE MANAGEMENT OF SHORT BOWEL SYNDROME

Jon S. Thompson, MD

Short bowel syndrome (SBS) is characterized by malabsorption and malnutrition, which generally occur when less than 180 cm of functional intestine remains in adults. The severity of the clinical features of SBS depends on several factors, including not only the extent of resection but also the site of resection, the underlying intestinal disease, the presence or absence of the terminal ileum and ileocecal valve, the functional status of the remaining digestive organs, and the adaptive capacity of the intestinal remnant. Three fourths of these instances result from massive intestinal resection and 25% from multiple sequential resections of the small intestine. Approximately two thirds of patients who develop SBS survive from that hospitalization, and a similar percentage are alive 1 year later. Patients' long-term outcome is determined primarily by their age and underlying disease. However, a number of deaths are caused by complications directly related to the management of SBS.

The pathophysiologic changes that occur in SBS relate to the loss of intestinal absorptive surface and more rapid intestinal transit. Malabsorption of nutrients results in malnutrition and weight loss, diarrhea and steatorrhea, vitamin deficiency, and electrolyte imbalance. Other specific complications include an increased incidence of nephrolithiasis from hyperoxaluria, cholelithiasis secondary to altered bile salt and bilirubin metabolism, and transient gastric hypersecretion. Bacterial overgrowth can also occur secondary to mechanical obstruction or primary motor abnormalities. In patients dependent primarily on parenteral nutrition (PN), liver disease remains an important factor in mortality. Functional and structural adaptation of the remaining intestine occurs after massive intestinal resection, resulting in improved absorption of nutrients and a decrease in diarrhea within the first few months after resection. The degree of adaptation that occurs depends on the extent and site of resection, the provision of enteral nutrients, and the response to gastrointestinal hormones and other regulatory polypeptides.

Early management of the patient with SBS is that of the critically ill surgical patient having recently undergone intestinal resection and other concomitant procedures. Thus controlling sepsis, maintaining fluid and electrolyte balance, and initiating nutritional support are important in the early management of these patients. Beyond this phase, the primary goals of management of SBS are to maintain adequate nutritional status, maximize the absorptive capacity of the remaining intestine, and prevent the development of complications related to the underlying pathophysiology and the nutritional therapy itself. Surgical approaches have become increasingly important and generally include preserving the intestinal remnant, maximizing or improving the function of the intestinal remnant, and augmenting intestinal length via transplantation.

■ THERAPEUTIC GOALS

Maintain Nutritional Status

The most important therapeutic objective in the management of SBS is to maintain the patient's nutritional status. By necessity this is achieved primarily by PN support in the early postoperative period. Enteral nutrition support can be started early after operation when the ileus has resolved. With time, an increasing amount of nutrients will be absorbed via the enteral route; this is important for maximizing intestinal adaptation and for preventing complications related to PN. As their conditions improve and intestinal adaptation occurs, many patients are able to absorb the necessary nutrients entirely via the enteral route. Intestinal remnant length has important prognostic implications in this regard. Patients with more than 180 cm small intestine remaining generally require no PN, those with more than 90 cm small intestine and particularly with colon will generally require PN for less than 1 year, and those with less than 60 cm small intestine will likely require permanent PN.

During the transition from parenteral to enteral nutrition support, the primary objectives are to maintain a stable body weight and prevent large fluctuations in fluid balance. Metabolic monitoring is necessary to detect and correct any metabolic abnormalities and micronutrient deficiency. A marked increase in gastrointestinal fluid loss is a sign that further increases in enteral feeding will not be tolerated. As parenteral requirements diminish, intermittent PN can be instituted, reducing hours of therapy during the day and eventually alternating days.

Maximize Enteral Nutrient Absorption

Dietary management for an individual patient with SBS is determined by a variety of factors, including intestinal remnant length and location, any underlying intestinal disease, and the status of the remaining digestive organs. The existence of a stoma is also an important consideration because diarrhea and perianal complications may markedly diminish oral intake. Thus patients with stomas may be more likely to take a greater percentage of their calories enterally. Patients with SBS, in fact, may develop hyperphagia to overcome their inefficient absorption. Continuous rather than intermittent enteral feeding may permit greater absorption of nutrients in patients with remnants less than 90 cm. Separating solid and liquid meals may aid absorption of solids.

The optimal diet for patients with SBS is determined primarily by whether the colon is in continuity. Initially a high-carbohydrate, high-protein diet is appropriate to maximize absorption. Fat absorption requires more digestion unless the fat is supplied in the form of medium-chain triglycerides. Stool fat increases markedly, however, with remnants less than 60 cm. The ability to absorb these nutrients does improve with time, thus the diet should be modified continually.

BOX 1: Medical Treatment of Short Bowel

Slow Transit

Loperamide, Lomotil, narcotics

Reduce GI Secretion

H_2 receptor antagonists
Proton pump inhibitors
Octreotide*
Clonidine*

Treat Bacterial Overgrowth

Antibiotics
Probiotics
Prokinetics

Treat Pharmacologically

Growth hormone
Teduglutide

*Off-label use.

BOX 2: Restoration of Intestinal Continuity

Advantages

Absorptive capacity increased
Energy from short-chain fatty acids
Intestinal stoma avoided
Infectious complications reduced
Transit time prolonged

Disadvantages

Bile acid diarrhea
Dietary restrictions
Perianal complications
Risk of nephrolithiasis

BOX 3: Complications in Short Bowel Syndrome

Therapy-Related

Metabolic
Nutritional
Infectious
Liver disease

Physiologic

Bacterial overgrowth
Cholelithiasis
Nephrolithiasis
Gastric hypersecretion

Other problems, such as lactase deficiency, also may be present. Patients with colon in continuity should have fat restricted to 20% to 30% of caloric intake and should have oxalate restricted to prevent nephrolithiasis. Because jejunal mucosa is relatively permeable, isotonic feedings are particularly important with jejunal remnants. Ingestion of a glucose-electrolyte oral rehydration solution with a sodium concentration of at least 90 mmol/L optimizes water and sodium absorption in the proximal jejunum and prevents secretion into the lumen. The role of specific nutrients (e.g., glutamine) remains controversial.

Another important aspect of the dietary management is to provide a diet that will maximize the intestinal adaptive response. Provision of fat, particularly long-chain triglycerides, and dietary fiber may be particularly important in this regard. Glutamine may be trophic to the gut. Although these nutrients may act directly to stimulate intestinal adaptation, the meal also may stimulate intestinal adaptation via endocrine or paracrine effects. Growth factors (e.g., growth hormone and GLP-2) also may stimulate intestinal adaptation and are currently available in the clinical setting.

Minimizing gastrointestinal secretion and controlling diarrhea are also important goals for maximizing absorption (Box 1). The addition of dietary fiber is useful in patients who are net fluid secretors. Several agents are useful for improving absorption via their antisecretory and antimotility effects, including narcotics such as codeine and diphenoxylate and atropine (Lomotil) and the peripherally acting narcotic loperamide. The long-acting somatostatin analogue octreotide improves diarrhea by increasing small intestinal transit time, reducing salt and water excretion, as well as gastric hypersecretion. However, it may not remain effective long term and has potentially deleterious effects, including steatorrhea, inhibition of intestinal adaptation, and increased incidence of cholelithiasis. Thus octreotide should not be used routinely for the management of chronic diarrhea. Both H_2 receptor antagonists and proton pump inhibitors have been shown to be effective in controlling gastric hypersecretion. Recent studies suggest that the alpha 2-adrenergic receptor against clonidine also may reduce fluid loss in those patients. Cholestyramine also may be beneficial when the diarrhea is related to the cathartic effect of unabsorbed bile salts in the colon and less than 100 cm of ileum has been resected.

Pharmacologic therapy for SBS is a rapidly expanding area of investigation. A variety of growth factors and hormones have been identified that promote intestinal growth or enhance absorptive function. Growth hormone has trophic and proabsorptive effects on the gut, as well as other metabolic effects. It is available for clinical use. However, growth hormone alone has not had a consistent

beneficial effect in clinical trials. Teduglutide, a GLP-2 analog, recently has been approved for use in SBS and promotes intestinal absorption and adaptation. Initial studies suggest therapy reduces need for supplemental fluids and nutrients.

An important clinical issue is whether to establish intestinal continuity in patients who have a colonic remnant. There are both advantages and disadvantages to restoring continuity (Box 2). The colon may in fact improve intestinal absorption by increasing the absorptive surface area, deriving energy from short-chain fatty acids and prolonging transit time. It also improves quality of life by avoiding the stoma. However, the response of the colon to luminal contents is somewhat unpredictable. Bile acids may in fact cause a secretory diarrhea. Perianal problems can be disabling and decrease the patient's oral intake. Oxalate is absorbed primarily in the colon, and patients are thus at increased risk for the formation of calcium oxalate stones. Historically, only one fourth of patients who initially had a stoma formed ultimately had continuity restored with a satisfactory outcome. However, medical professionals have become more aggressive about restoring continuity. This decision should be considered on an individual basis, depending on the length of the intestinal remnant and other anatomy, and the patient's overall condition. Generally, at least 60 cm of small intestine are required to prevent severe diarrhea and perianal complications.

Prevent Complications

Metabolic complications are common in SBS patients (Box 3). Patients are at risk for dehydration and renal dysfunction. Hypocalcemia is a common problem related to poor absorption and binding by intraluminal fat. Maintaining adequate levels of calcium, magnesium, and vitamin D supplementation are important to minimize bone disease. Hyperglycemia and hypoglycemia are frequent complications of patients receiving a large amount of their calories parenterally. Metabolic acidosis and alkalosis can occur. A specific problem is D-lactic acidosis, which results from bacterial fermentation of unabsorbed nutrients, particularly simple sugars.

Specific nutrient deficiencies must be prevented and monitored closely. These include iron and vitamin deficiencies as well as micronutrients such as selenium, zinc, and copper. Because fat is poorly absorbed, fatty acid deficiency also can occur. Serum free fatty acid levels and triene-to-tetraene ratios may have to be monitored periodically to determine the need for supplementation and response to treatment. In general, the enteral intake must greatly exceed the absorptive needs to ensure that these needs are being met.

Catheter-related sepsis is an important problem that often necessitates rehospitalization and replacement of catheters. Attention to technique and meticulous patient education are important to prevent this complication. Catheter thrombosis is another frequent problem. In patients who require total parenteral nutrition permanently, this may become an important factor in the patient's survival because vascular access may not be achievable indefinitely.

PN-induced liver disease is another potential long-term problem. This appears to be a multifactorial process that is often reversible but may lead to severe steatosis, cholestasis, and eventually cirrhosis. It occurs more frequently in children and accounts for one third of deaths of patients on long-term PN. It can be minimized by providing as large a portion of the calories as possible enterally, avoiding overfeeding, using mixed fuels (<30% fat), lipid minimization, and preventing specific nutrient deficiencies. Treating bacterial growth and preventing recurrent sepsis are also important.

Bacterial overgrowth may result from impaired motility or stasis caused by obstructive lesions. Depending on the bacterial species present, secretory diarrhea also may occur. Bacterial overgrowth requires a high degree of suspicion for diagnosis. This complication should be suspected when a patient's absorptive capacity and stool habits change acutely. This may result from a mechanical obstruction or a blind loop, which can be relieved by operation. However, it is often a primary motor abnormality, which requires intermittent therapy with antibiotics. Colonization of the lumen with probiotics is another potential therapy.

Cholelithiasis occurs in 30% to 40% of SBS patients. Long-term PN causes altered hepatic bile metabolism and gallbladder stasis. Biliary sludge forms within a few weeks of initiating PN if there is no enteral intake but rapidly disappears when enteral nutrition is resumed. Patients receiving PN are at risk for cholelithiasis and hepatocellular dysfunction and thus require careful clinical evaluation. Intestinal mucosal disease and resection, particularly of the ileum, cause bile acid malabsorption, leading to lithogenic bile and the formation of cholesterol stones. The risk for cholelithiasis is significantly increased if less than 120 cm of intestine remains after resection, the terminal ileum has been resected, and PN is required. The incidence of cholelithiasis can be minimized by providing nutrients enterally whenever possible and using therapies to intermittently stimulate gallbladder emptying. Cholelithiasis is more likely to be complicated in patients with SBS and requires more extensive surgical treatment. Prophylactic cholecystectomy should be considered when laparotomy is being undertaken for other reasons.

Nephrolithiasis, primarily calcium oxalate stones, also occurs with some frequency. Oxalate normally is bound to calcium in the intestinal lumen and is not absorbed. Decreased availability of calcium secondary to reduced intake or binding by intraluminal fat leaves free oxalate in the lumen. Thus the oxalate is absorbed in the colon and forms calcium oxalate in the urine. Nephrolithiasis is unusual in patients with intestinal resection and jejunostomy but occurs in one fourth of such patients with an intact colon within 2 years of resection. Nephrolithiasis can be prevented by maintaining a diet low in oxalate, minimizing intraluminal fat, supplementing calcium orally, and maintaining a high urinary volume. Cholestyramine, which binds oxalic acid in the colon, is another potential treatment.

Gastric hypersecretion is a potential problem in patients with SBS. Massive intestinal resection can cause gastric hypersecretion as a result of parietal cell hyperplasia and hypergastrinemia. This phenomenon is usually transient, lasting several months, and presumably involves loss of an inhibitor from the resected intestine. The associated hyperacidity exacerbates malabsorption and diarrhea. About one fourth of patients undergoing massive resection develop peptic ulcer disease. Treatment of gastric acid secretion may improve absorption and prevents peptic ulcer disease. Control of acid secretion by H_2 receptor antagonists or proton pump inhibitors should be initiated in the perioperative period after resection and maintained until the increased acid production resolves. A few patients eventually require surgical intervention, but gastric resection should be avoided when possible.

■ SURGICAL STRATEGIES

Preservation of Intestinal Remnant

Abdominal reoperation is required in approximately 50% of patients with SBS after their discharge from the hospital. Intestinal problems are the most frequent indication. An important goal in any reoperation in patients with SBS is to preserve the intestinal remnant length. Resection often can be avoided by using intestinal tapering to improve the function of dilated segments, employing strictureplasty for benign strictures, and using serosal patching for certain strictures and chronic perforations. Resection should be limited in extent when it cannot be avoided. Depending on the previous operations performed, patients occasionally have intestinal segments that can be recruited into continuity at the time of reoperation. It is always important to document the length of intestine remaining during any operation on a patient with SBS.

Surgical Therapy for the Short Bowel Syndrome

There are several goals of surgical therapy for the short bowel syndrome (Figure 1). One goal has been to slow intestinal transit by reversing intestinal segments, interposing colonic segments into the small intestine, and other innovative approaches. Another goal has been to improve the function of existing intestine. For example, stenotic segments cause partial obstruction, which could lead to malabsorption. This can be managed by relieving the obstruction, often with a simple approach such as a strictureplasty. Furthermore, dilatated dysfunctional segments aggravate malabsorption. These can be treated by tapering enteroplasty. For patients with particularly short remnants, increasing intestinal surface area is the best option for improving nutrient absorption. Intestinal lengthening procedures combine tapering with lengthening and are applicable in some patients. However, intestinal transplantation may be the final solution to this problem.

The surgical approach to the patient with SBS depends on several factors. The nature of nutritional support is obviously the primary determinant as to whether operation should be considered. In our experience, half of patients with SBS are able to sustain themselves on enteral nutrition alone. Operation should be considered cautiously and generally performed in these patients only if they demonstrate worsening malabsorption, are at risk for requiring PN, or have other symptoms related to malabsorption. Almost half of patients who are stable on long-term PN are candidates for operation, with the goal in this group being primarily to get the patient off PN. Patients who develop significant complication while dependent on PN have more compelling reasons to undergo operation. Most of these patients should undergo intestinal transplantation because many will die. Although liver disease is a frequent indication for transplantation, difficult vascular access and recurrent sepsis are also considerations. Patient age and underlying disease are also important factors. Children are much more likely to adapt to enteral nutrition but are also more likely to be candidates for operative treatment. In our experience, adult patients with mesenteric vascular disease and malignancy undergo operation less frequently.

The choice of operation for SBS is influenced by intestinal remnant length, intestinal function, and the caliber of the intestinal

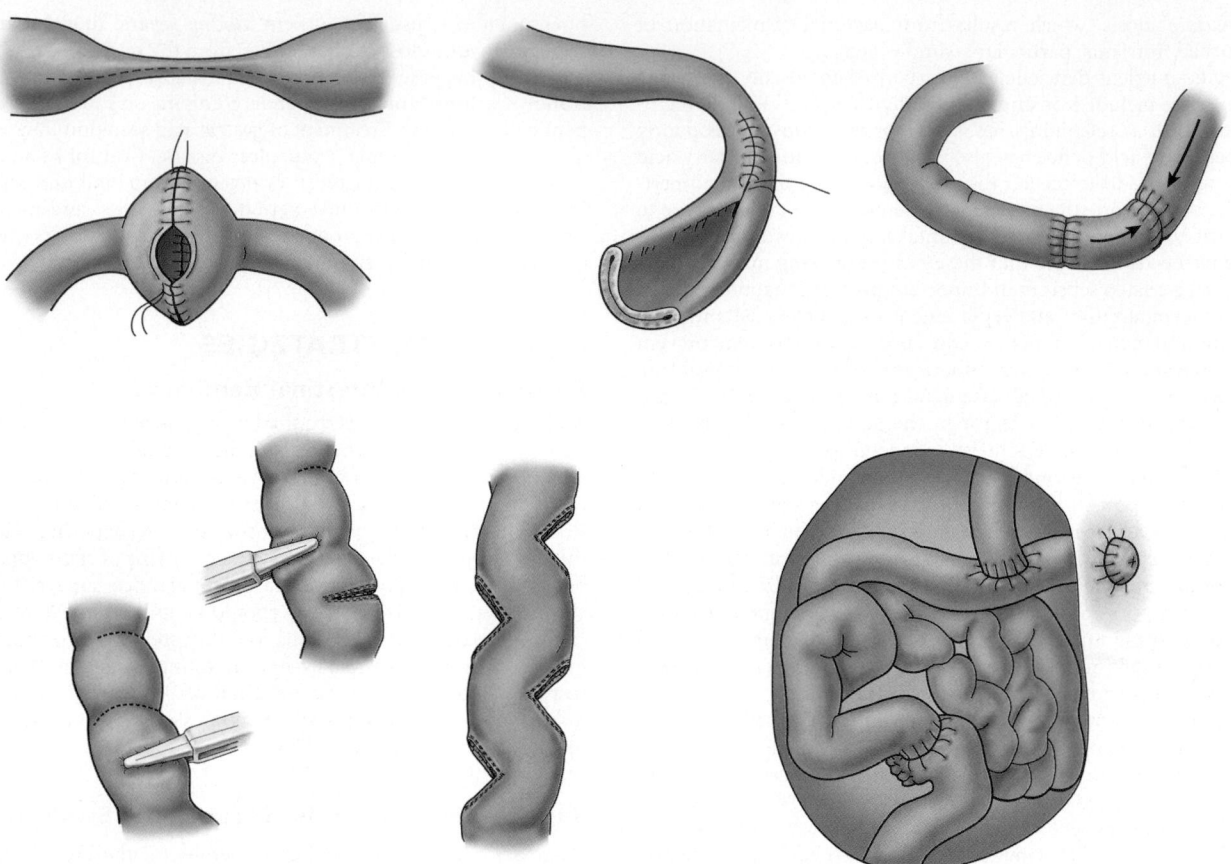

FIGURE 1 Surgical procedures for improvement of intestinal function in short bowel. *(Modified from Thompson JS, Langnas AN, Pinch LW, et al. Ann Surg. 1995;222:600; Kim HB, Fauza D, Garza J, et al. Serial transverse enteroplasty [STEP]: a novel bowel lengthening procedure. J Pediatr Surg. 2003;38:425-429, 2003.)*

remnant (Figure 2). These factors allow identification of several patient groups that might be treated by specific surgical procedures.

Adequate Remnant Length With Dilated Bowel

Adult patients with intestinal remnants greater than 120 cm are likely to be sustained on enteral nutrition alone, particularly if the ileocolonic junction is intact. However, these patients may develop dilated bowel secondary to obstruction, often at the site of a previous anastomosis. A useful approach to these patients is to relieve the intestinal obstruction, often with a strictureplasty, although other procedures may be necessary. Children with remnants greater than 60 cm usually are sustained on enteral nutrition alone. Dilatation of the intestinal remnant occurs more frequently in children and appears to have a different pathophysiologic basis. This may be a variant of intestinal pseudo-obstruction. Only one fourth of children with a significantly dilatated bowel have mechanical obstruction, but they routinely have bacterial overgrowth. Thus, for children, a tapering enteroplasty is often the appropriate therapy and also deals with any obstructive component present. This can be accomplished either by excising the redundant bowel along the antimesenteric border or simply imbricating it; the latter is our preferred approach. Motility is generally slow to return. Recurrent dilatation is a concern.

Moderate Remnant Length With Rapid Transit

A challenging group of patients are those who have shorter remnant (90 to 120 cm in adults) and signs of rapid transit. Slowing the rapid intestinal transit may permit these patients to be supported by enteral means alone. There are several possible approaches to this problem. Reversing 10- to 15-cm intestinal segments has been used most frequently in SBS. Longer reversed segments are more likely to be associated with chronic obstruction, whereas the shorter segments have less influence on intestinal transit and function. Almost 100 patients have

been reported in the literature, and although documentation is usually not extensive, clinical improvement has been reported in at least one half of patients. Some concerns have been raised about long-term function with the procedure. Both isoperistaltic and antiperistaltic colon interposition have been attempted. Although it appears that transit time may be prolonged because of the intrinsic differences in motility between the colon and small intestine, actual benefit has been difficult to show in a few anecdotal reports. Creation of various artificial valves to replace the ileocecal valve has been attempted. I have performed the valve procedure by creating a sphincter similar to that used in the continent ileostomy procedure but of shorter length (2 cm). I have had a favorable result in one adult and one child with this valve, but outcomes have not been as successful in the few other reports.

Patients With Short Remnant and Dilatated Bowel

Patients with short remnant length (<90 cm in adults and <30 cm in children) and dilatated intestinal segments represent a more difficult problem. Even though the dilatated segment could be tapered, this still does not result in enough functional bowel to avoid PN. In this situation, many surgeons have found intestinal lengthening to be the optimal treatment. The initial technique involved longitudinal intestinal tapering and lengthening, known as the *Bianchi procedure*. This involves dissection along the mesenteric edge of the bowel to allocate terminal blood vessels to either side of the bowel wall. Longitudinal transection of the bowel then is performed, usually with a stapling device that creates two parallel limbs of a smaller caliber. These then can be anastomosed to lengthen the intestinal remnant. More than 100 cases have been reported, mostly in children. Segments have been lengthened up to 55 cm, and overall improved nutrition resulted in approximately 90% of patients. This is a technically challenging procedure. Complications have been reported in 20% of procedures,

SURGICAL MANAGEMENT OF THE SHORT BOWEL SYNDROME

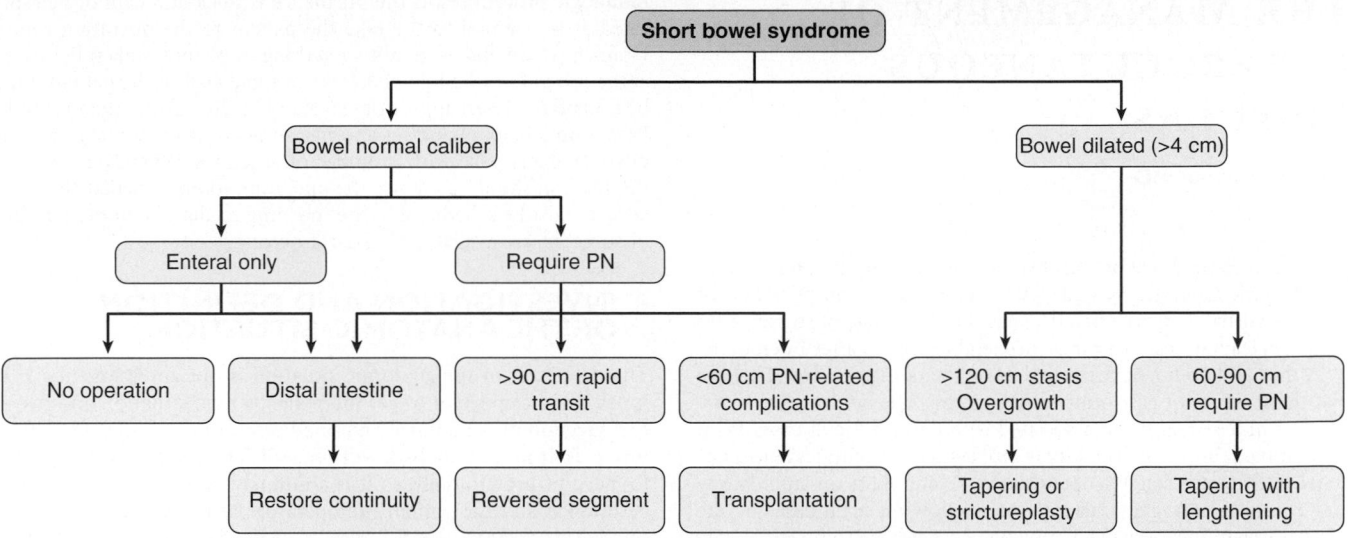

FIGURE 2 Surgical management of the short bowel. *PN,* Parenteral nutrition.

which not surprisingly include ischemia and anastomotic leaks. Recurrent dilatation has been a concern. However, follow-up for longer than 10 years suggests that this procedure has long-term benefit.

More recently, an alternative method of lengthening, termed *serial transverse enteroplasty procedure* (STEP), has been introduced (see Figure 1). This involves serial transverse applications of a linear stapler from opposite directions, dividing the bowel from either the mesenteric and antimesenteric sides or transversely. The length of the transverse division is determined by the intestinal diameter. This procedure avoids the difficult dissection along the mesenteric border of the Bianchi procedure and the end-to-end anastomosis. The bowel may have to be more dilatated to use this technique. It is more feasible in challenging areas such as near the ligament of Treitz. Complications are less with this technique. This procedure can be repeated if recurrent dilation occurs. Thus this technique has become the procedure of choice for intestinal lengthening.

One of the limitations of the intestinal lengthening procedures is that they can be applied only to a fairly select group of patients who have both a short intestinal remnant and an intestinal diameter greater than 3 to 4 cm. To improve the applicability of this technique, surgeons have used sequential operations employing first a procedure such as inserting an artificial valve to produce intestinal dilatation and then performing the lengthening at a later time.

Short Remnant Length and Parenteral Nutrition–Related Complications

Patients with short intestinal remnants (<60 cm in adults and <30 cm in children) who develop complications related to PN represent a challenging group. For these patients, intestinal transplantation is the ideal solution. Patients with liver failure and SBS have been candidates for combined liver and small intestine transplantation. The patients who have reversible liver dysfunction or who have adequate liver function but other complications such as difficult vascular access and recurrent infection are candidates for solitary intestinal transplantation. More recently, isolated liver transplantation has been advocated for patients with irreversible liver failure and SBS that can be rehabilitated. The significant mortality rate among patients developing PN-induced complications justifies what continues to be a formidable operative approach.

Almost 3000 intestinal transplantations have been performed worldwide. These have included primarily isolated small intestinal grafts (50%) with combined liver and small intestinal grafts (25%),

and multivisceral grafts (25%). The majority of the transplant recipients are children. Although the morbidity and mortality rates remain significant, 80% of patients who survive the procedure long term have been able to discontinue PN and return to more normal function. Long-term graft loss remains an important issue. Reported patient survival is 76% at 1 year, 56% at 5 years and 43% at 10 years.

It is hoped that with greater experience and improved results, this therapy can be extended to other patients with SBS. The more successful recent outcome has been related, in part, to the use of the new immunosuppressive agents and other innovative approaches to modifying the immune response. Of all of the surgical approaches, intestinal transplantation has the greatest potential for treating these patients, both in terms of the number of patients who would benefit and the functional improvement derived. Transplantation is clearly appropriate for individuals with anticipated survival of less than 12 months related to PN-induced complications. A more aggressive approach to the use of intestinal transplantation, particularly solitary transplantation, is justified in patients with signs of early liver dysfunction and other severe complications of nutritional therapy.

■ MULTIDISCIPLINARY APPROACH

Comprehensive care of intestinal failure patients requires a multidisciplinary approach. A physician leader with expertise in gastrointestinal disease should coordinate the efforts. Gastrointestinal surgical expertise in both adult and pediatric patients is required, and the presence of a transplant surgeon broadens the therapeutic options. Administrative support to coordinate the process and database is essential. A nurse coordinator is indispensable in day-to-day management. A nutritionist is essential. Psychologists and social workers are important for addressing psychosocial issues. This multidisciplinary effort should optimize patient outcome.

SUGGESTED READINGS

Abu-Elmagd K. The concept of gut rehabilitation and the future of visceral transplantation. *Nat Rev Gastroenterol Hepatol.* 2015;12:108-120.

Grant D, Abu-Elmagd K, Mazariegos G, et al. Intestinal Transplant Registry Report: global activity and trends. *Am J Transplant.* 2015;15:210-219.

Sudan D, Thompson JS, Botha J, et al. Comparison of intestinal lengthening procedures for patients with short bowel syndrome. *Ann Surg.* 2007;246:593-601.

Thompson JS, Rochling FA, Weseman RA, et al. Current management of short bowel syndrome. *Curr Probl Surg.* 2012;49:52-115.

THE MANAGEMENT OF ENTEROCUTANEOUS FISTULAS

Josef E. Fischer, MD

Gastrointestinal cutaneous fistulas are among the most catastrophic outcomes of gastrointestinal surgery. Complications of gastrointestinal surgery include anastomotic leaks, abscesses after drainage, leaving residual purulence, and abscesses after operation.

Although I do not have much data on the point to follow, I believe that the training of gastrointestinal surgeons has become less rigorous, less independent, and associated with fewer difficult cases. With the emphasis on work hours there are fewer cases with less independence and greater faculty supervision. The emphasis on laparoscopy may result in a greater leak rate than following open cases by the comparatively inexperienced surgeon. As new gastrointestinal surgeons sign contracts, they often have comparatively rigid and attractive work hours, which should not be denigrated because they allow the surgeons more time to spend with their families. There is more emphasis on oversight and having a senior surgeon in the operating room, especially in difficult cases.

In a complicated situation such as a patient with a gastrointestinal cutaneous fistula, it is probably easier to divide the history into various periods and the attempts to have the patient recover. The phases of treatment outlined in Box 1 are somewhat different and more detailed than the five steps that I have written about in the past (stabilization, investigation, decision, definitive therapy, and healing). To a certain extent, this updated schedule is the result of good and bad experience. What I have learned in the past is that there is little room for error. Meticulous care and meticulous operation will result in lower mortality. A review of the last 50 gastrointestinal cutaneous fistulas I have performed shows that there has been no patient mortality. I believe that this is largely the result of waiting 5 or 6 months after the discovery of the fistula for reoperation. At this point the adhesions have softened and are often filmy, resulting in fewer enterotomies and an easier operation.

STABILIZATION AND RECOGNITION

The most important aspect of initial treatment for the patient suspected of a gastrointestinal cutaneous fistula is the restoration of blood volume. In the past 20 years there has been some movement away from colloid and blood; however, in the case of the gastrointestinal cutaneous fistula, crystalloid alone is inadequate. Albumin, occasionally plasma, or occasionally fresh frozen plasma for clotting factors, and blood, especially fresh whole blood when the surgeon suspects that the patient has a clotting abnormality, are the best option. I am aware that the blood banks typically dispense the oldest blood to the patient. Although staff members of blood banks say that old blood is just as good to administer as fresh blood, there is evidence to the contrary, especially in patients who are critically ill. The surgeon in charge should insist on the freshest blood available and, when necessary, components such as platelets, fresh frozen plasma, and other components of blood, which will be essential.

DRAINAGE OF OBVIOUS ABSCESSES

Unfortunately patients discovered to have a gastrointestinal cutaneous fistula often have an accompanying abscess. This often is associated with a high fever. The fever is associated with catabolism and an increase in the loss of protein. If the abscess is recognized, it should be delineated as best as possible. This can be done with various radiologic procedures. If the purulence is thick and cannot be aspirated, it is essential to the take the patient to the operating room. Drainage of an abscess is not something to be undertaken lightly or at the end of the schedule. If one is in a small facility, the patient must be transferred to an appropriate tertiary facility. The surgeon should have ample help, including another surgeon of known skill and, if possible, experience with drainage of abscesses. Whenever possible, the surgeon should convince the operating room staff that this procedure must be scheduled in the morning so that an ample number of surgeons are available to assist if necessary.

■ INVESTIGATION AND DEFINITION OF THE ANATOMIC SITUATION

The definition of the anatomic situation is not an emergency. It is much more important to get the patient's fluid situation and his or her infection under control and stabilize nutrition so that anabolism proceeds. If not, catabolism will proceed. These patients can lose up to 500 g of protein daily, so it is absolutely essential that purulence be drained and the patient's temperature return to normal so that catabolism decreases. A CT scan may not be necessary, unless an abscess is suspected, and drainage is urgent. If there is an obvious abscess, this should be drained with a catheter if possible. If the surgeon cannot drain it, once the patient is stabilized, drainage should proceed in the operating room with adequate help, adequate colloid, crystalloid, and blood, and the sepsis is eradicated as best as possible.

■ NUTRITIONAL ASSESSMENT AND BEGINNING NUTRITIONAL SUPPLEMENTATION

Nutritional support cannot be delayed because patients may lose 500 g of protein daily. It is highly unlikely that the patient can begin enteral nutrition quickly when major nutritional support is required. Thus one starts the patient with total parenteral nutrition. An experienced surgeon should place a subclavian line under good conditions with adequate help and under strict asepsis. Nutritional support should begin immediately and the blood sugar should be checked so that fulminating hyperglycemia does not occur. After the anatomic situation is stabilized and abscesses are drained so that sepsis is eliminated, decision making can begin. Supplying the patient with enteral nutrition as meeting the entire needs of the patient may not be possible, but there is reasonable evidence that the combination of enteral and parenteral nutrition may result in better anabolism. In some patients, enteral nutrition may not be possible.

■ SPONTANEOUS CLOSURE

Spontaneous closure occurs in approximately 30% to 35% of patients. In a few patients with specific types of fistulas, the percentage may be higher. The anatomy will usually predict which fistulas will close. Sepsis prevents closure. The fistula may open and close depending on the anatomy, sepsis, and cleaning up the abdominal wall. A cleaner healthier abdominal wall around the fistula may aid spontaneous closure.

Aids to Closure

Keep the edges of the fistula clean, especially from gastrointestinal contents. Sumps (Figure 1) may help in using a soft latex tube, usually of urologic design and various sizes. An extra hole with a #14 whistle-tip catheter to gentle suction within a 22 or 24 yellow latex sump will help aspirate gastrointestinal contents from around the fistula. The protection may be with powders such as karaya powder or more recently with some of the better plastic material, which is adherent to the edge of the fistula and protects the skin (Figure 2).

BOX 1: Phases of Care of Patients With Gastrointestinal Fistulas

I. Recognition: first 24 hours
   A. Stabilization
      1. Restoration of blood volume
         a. Minimize crystalloid
         b. Albumin
            Plasma: especially fresh frozen, for clotting factors
         c. Fresh blood: avoid the "old blood"
            A practice of many blood banks
         d. Platelets when necessary
II. Recognition and drainage of obvious abscesses 24-48 hours
   A. High fever
   B. An accelerated rate of catabolisms: up to 500 g of protein daily
   C. Radiologic investigation
      1. The most experienced surgeon and collaborating radiologist
      2. Transfer when necessary to a tertiary facility
      3. Drainage in the operating room: cases should be done in the morning with adequate assistance
      4. When possible use a soft latex catheter (see Figure 1)
III. Nutritional assessment and beginning nutritional supplementation 24-48 hours
   A. Minimize delays
      1. Patients may lose 500 g of protein daily
      2. Enteral nutrition cannot make up all needs quickly
   B. Start parenteral nutrition
      1. A central line should be placed by an experienced surgeon
   C. Repeated measuring of blood sugar to avoid significant hyperglycemia
   D. After stabilization
      1. A combination of enteral and parenteral nutrition is probably best 48-72 hours
   E. How much nutrition
      1. 80-120 g of protein daily 48-96 hours
      2. Calories: 2200 calories to 3600 calories (depending on fever, sepsis)
      3. 20% fat
      4. Adequate
         a. Trace metals
         b. Vitamins
         c. Essential fatty acids

IV. Spontaneous closure up to 60 days
   A. Occurs in 30% to 35% of patients
      1. The anatomy usually predicts which fistulas will close
      2. Sepsis prevents closure
      3. Some fistulas may open and close
      4. Healthier nonseptic abdominal wall more likely to close
   B. Aids to closure
      1. Keep edges protected and clean
      2. Sumps with gentle suction
         a. Keep stool and pus away from edges
V. Operation
   A. If no closure has occurred in 60 days, operation
      1. 60 days for infected hernia
      2. 120-150 days for clean hernia
   B. The incision
      1. The incision must be closed; if not, fistula will reopen
      2. Go to areas that are easier
      3. The operation should begin early
      4. Keep skin edges clean with antibiotic-soaked blue towels or plastic drapes
VI. Lysis of adhesion
   A. Scissor dissection is safer
   B. Free everything up before attacking the fistula
   C. You will probably have to resect 18 inches of small bowel in resecting the fistula
VII. The anastomosis
   A. 2 layers of interrupted permanent suture
VIII. Postoperative care 150-170 days
   A. Do not be in a rush to feed the patient
   B. When feeding maintain calories and protein until bowel function is normal
   C. Make certain caloric and protein intake are adequate before stopping TPN
IX. Maintain nutrition and start rehabilitation 6 months
   A. Patients have lost protein, muscle, and neurologic function
   B. Patients may take up to $1\frac{1}{2}$ years before regaining total neural function
   C. Warn patients; tell them the length of time it will take
   D. Tell patients not to quit their jobs

Suction is broken by urologic type soft sumps, keeping the irritating material away from the edges of the sump (see Figure 2). Notice that the area is large and sumps themselves may be multiple, making certain that bowel or other noxious material does not irritate the skin and prevent healing.

■ OPERATION

Operation will be required in most patients, between 50% and 65%. This should only be attempted after an adequate trial of soft sumps, antibiotics, nutrition, and keeping the patient's abdomen clean. My rule is to allow the patient to be treated with sumps and wound protection that keep the wound clean for 60 days without sepsis. When the absence of sepsis, suction, and other protection of the wound have been successful for 60 days and show no sign of closing, the surgeon prepares for operating.

The incision is an extremely important part of the operative procedure (Figure 3). If you cannot close the incision after a resection, it is likely that an open-ended closure of the fistula will fail. The incision should be made in a clean area so that it is likely to allow the lysis of adhesions away from the fistula and, if possible, to avoid making further enterotomies. The surgeon should start in clean soft abdomen. My practice is to allow $5\frac{1}{2}$ to 6 months to elapse so that the adhesions within the abdomen become filmy, and entering the abdomen and freeing up the bowel avoids enterotomies. The surgeon must start far away from the fistula and must not force the lysis of adhesions. If you are not making progress in one area, put some soft laparotomy packs soaked in antibiotic solution (Kantrex is my favorite) and go elsewhere. Start early in the morning and do not put any other procedures on the operative schedule. The worst thing you can do is hurry the procedure because you undoubtedly will make unintended enterotomies. These procedures will take between 6 and 8 hours, so be prepared; you may want some nourishment and hydration in the middle of the case.

After you have made the incision and mobilized the skin and the fascia and have some freedom, my practice is to take blue towels, soaking the edges in Kantrex and sew them in place; that way you will not contaminate the edges with stool or septic material, and the case will remain clean until you get to the fistula (Figure 4).

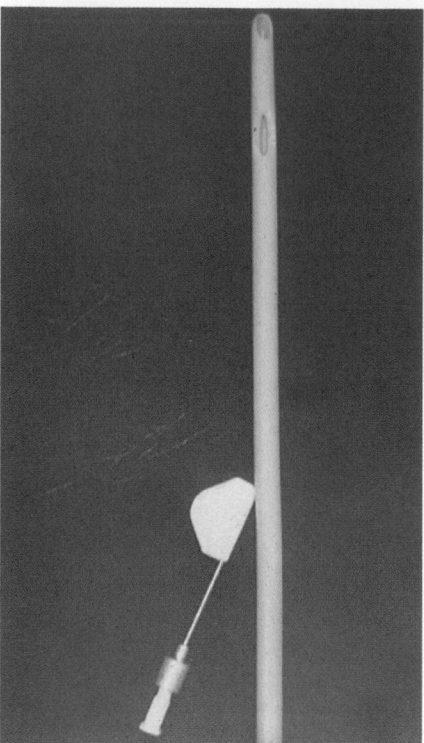

FIGURE 1 Sump system for management of fistulae. *(From Fischer JE, et al, eds. Fischer's Mastery of Surgery. 6th ed. Philadelphia: Lippincott, Williams, and Wilkins, 2012: Fig. 1, p. 1568.)*

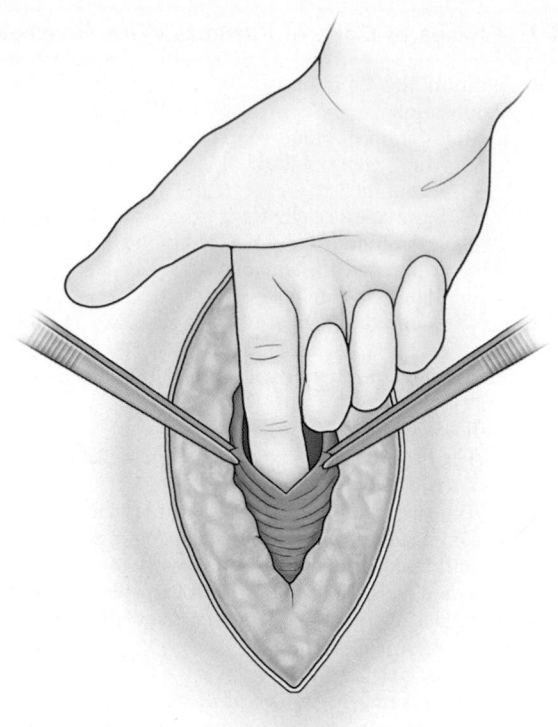

FIGURE 3 Once the surgeon has made the skin incision and clears the subcutaneous tissue from the fascia, the surgeon lifts the fascia with Kocher clamps so that one can see and then uses either index finger to separate the bowel from the underside of the fascia, without making an enterotomy. *(From Fischer JE, et al, eds. Fischer's Mastery of Surgery. 6th ed. Philadelphia: Lippincott, Williams, and Wilkins, 2012: Fig. 3, p. 1571.)*

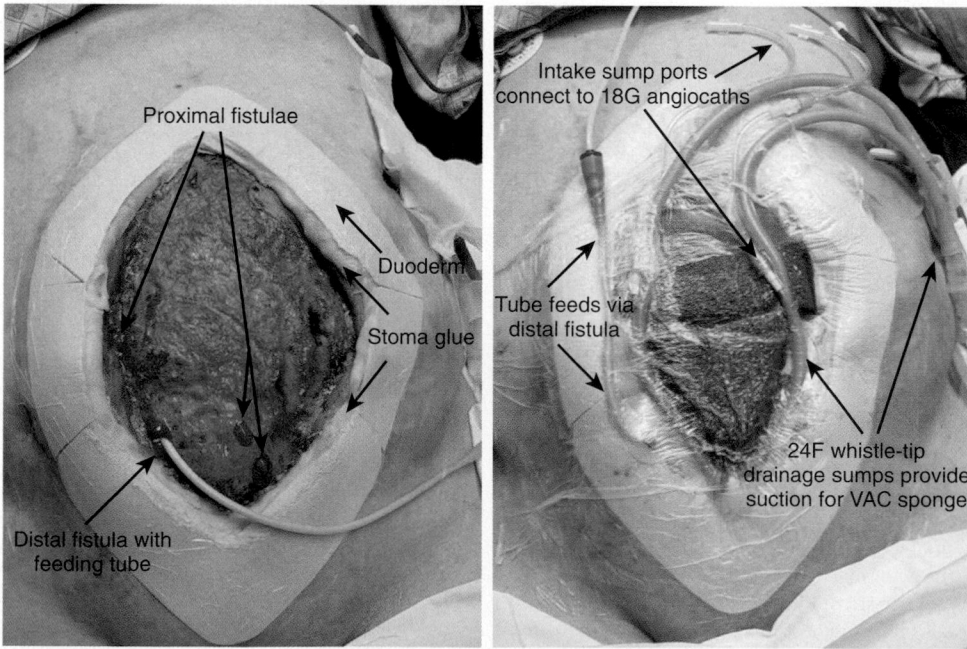

FIGURE 2 A and **B,** Vacuum-assisted closure dressing in situ. *(From Fischer JE, et al, eds. Fischer's Mastery of Surgery. 6th ed. Philadelphia: Lippincott, Williams, and Wilkins, 2012: Fig. 2, p. 1568.)*

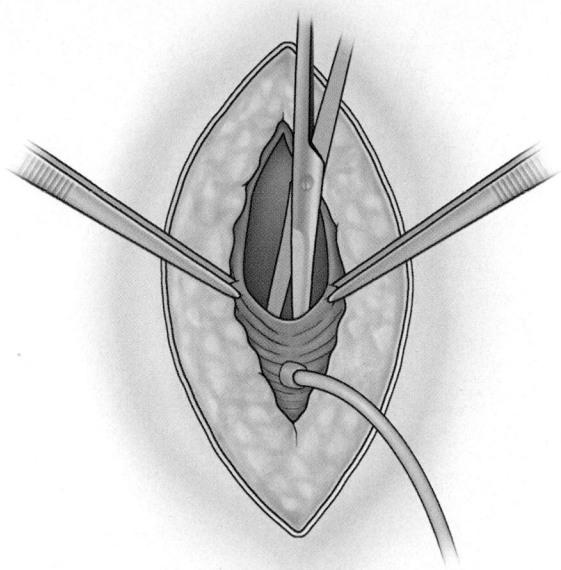

FIGURE 4 Both the skin incision and the fascia incision are lengthened carefully as the underside of the fascia is separated from the bowel and one can see clearly. The fascia may be divided with Metzenbaum scissors or a 15 blade scalpel. (*From Fischer JE, et al, eds. Fischer's Mastery of Surgery. 6th ed. Philadelphia: Lippincott, Williams, and Wilkins, 2012: Fig. 4, p. 1571.*)

■ LYSIS OF ADHESIONS

You should go from where the incision was made to freeing up everything else. Scissor dissection is safer. Once everything else if free, you must attack the fistula. It is usually not possible to free up the skin around the fistula and mobilize the fistula without enterotomies. As much as 18 inches of small bowel, which is dissected in and around the fistula, will likely be sacrificed. If you begin making enterotomies, take a break and sit down, you will have to resect shorter lengths of bowel with enterotomies and will have less chance of short bowel syndrome (Figures 5 and 6).

The anastomosis should be a two-layer interrupted anastomosis carried out with permanent suture. Do not use an absorbable suture. Do not test the anastomosis for a period of time by giving oral intake. If you give oral intake too early, the anastomosis may disrupt and there may be a leak.

■ POSTOPERATIVE CARE

The patient should be ambulated, and the wound should be reinforced with bulky dressings.

Do not be in a rush to feed the patient, especially solid food. You may continue with enteral nutritional support but certainly do not let total parenteral nutrition (TPN) decrease to a point at which the patient is not getting adequate protein and calories. Wait until the patient is having repeated bowel movements (preferably soft).

If the area in which you will be working and the anastomosis had infected contents, do not rush to stop the antibiotics.

If the area in which you were working had drainage, maintain the suction until the drainage dries for a period of time.

■ MAINTAIN NUTRITION AND START REHABILITATION

Remember that most of these patients have lost body mass. Allow nutrition to proceed before putting them through a vigorous aspect

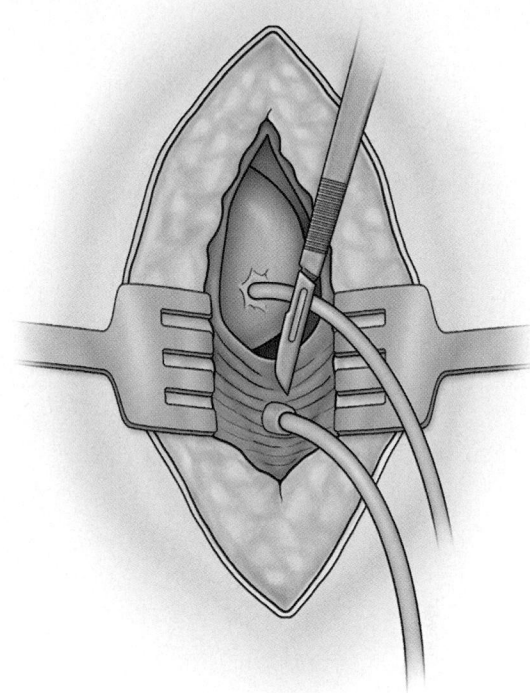

FIGURE 5 Further dissection of the abdomen: the bowel and fistula are clearly seen at the bottom of the wound. The fascia can be incised without fear of enterotomy. The goal is to reach the area where the fistulas are. The really adherent area is rarely longer than 12 inches of bowel. Enterotomies are unavoidable, but only 8 to 12 inches of bowel must be resected. (*From Fischer JE, et al, eds. Fischer's Mastery of Surgery. 6th ed. Philadelphia: Lippincott, Williams, and Wilkins, 2012: Fig. 5, p. 1572.*)

of rehabilitation. Make certain that bowel movements are regular and above all do not use a cathartic in the presence of a fresh anastomosis.

Allow 4 to 6 months of rehabilitation before the patients should think about returning to work. They have lost much protein, they will have also lost some of their neurologic function, and they will complain of the fact that they cannot think clearly. Resumption of function is important but if done too early, the patient will get depressed.

■ RESUMPTION OF FUNCTION

Most of these patients have lost body mass and neurologic function. If they return to work too early, particularly if they have a position of responsibility, they will find that they cannot think clearly and make mistakes. They will then retire prematurely. My experience is it will take up to 18 months for the nervous system to recover. I insist that patients wait 18 months before going back to work and make certain that they do not attempt to run their business early on but rely on a loyal work associate. Once they return slowly to the job, they will find that they can think as clearly as in the past. That will avoid depression that will occur by returning to work too early.

A fistula is a devastating event for a patient. Muscle protein and neurologic function are likely to deteriorate. Do not let patients return to work too soon. They should return slowly over months. That will keep them, their families, and their jobs intact.

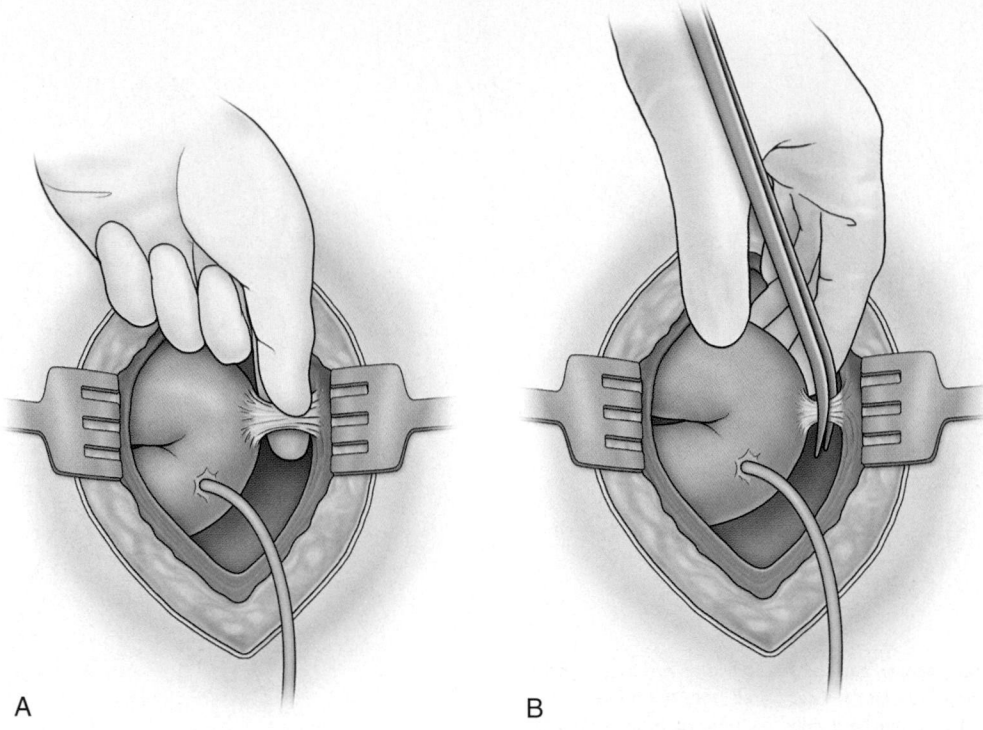

A   B

FIGURE 6 A and **B,** Adhesions can sometimes be dealt with by compressing the adhesions from a broad base to a narrow base. When the adhesion is narrowing and is easily visible, the narrowed adhesion can be sharply divided. *(From Fischer JE, et al, eds. Fischer's Mastery of Surgery. 6th ed. Philadelphia: Lippincott, Williams, and Wilkins, 2012: Fig. 6, p. 1572.)*

SUGGESTED READINGS

de Weerd L, Kjaeve J, Aghajani E, et al. The Sandwich Design: a new method to lose a high-output enterocutaneous fistula and an associated abdominal wall defect. *Ann Plast Surg.* 2007;58:580-583.

Edmunds LH, Williams GH, Welch CE. External fistulas arising from the gastrointestinal tract. *Ann Surg.* 1960;152:445. (classic).

Fischer JE. A Cautionary Note: use of VAC Systems may be associated with a higher mortality from fistula development in the treatment of gastrointestinal cutaneous fistulas. *Am J Surg.* 2008;196:1-3.

Fischer JE. On the importance of reconstruction of the abdominal wall following gastrointestinal fistula closure. *Am J Surg.* 2008;197:131-132.

Fischer JE. The importance of reconstruction of the abdominal wall after gastrointestinal fistula closure. *Am J Surg.* 2009;197:131.

Jamshidi R, Schechter WP. Biologic dressings for the management of enteric fistulas in the open abdomen: a preliminary report. *Arch Surg.* 2007;143:793-796.

Joyce MR, Dietz DW. Management of complex gastrointestinal fistula. *Curr Probl Surg.* 2009;46:384 (a nice monograph).

Kuvshinoff BW, Brodish RJ, McFadden DW, et al. Serum transferring as a prognostic indicator of spontaneous closure and mortality in gastrointestinal fistulas. *Ann Surg.* 1993;217:615.

Osborn C, Fischer JE. How I do it: gastrointestinal cutaneous fistulas. *J Gastrointest Surg.* 2009;13:2068.

Schechter WP, Asher H, Chang DS, et al. Enteric fistulas: principles of management. *J Am Coll Surg.* 2009;209:484. (a massive and classic review).

Soeters PB, Ebeid AM, Fischer JE. Review of 404 patients with gastrointestinal fistulas: impact of parenteral nutrition. *Ann Surg.* 1979;190:189.

Tawadros PS, Simpson J, Fischer JE. Abdominal abscess and enteric fistulae. In: Zinner MJ, ed. *Maingot's Abdominal Operations.* 12th ed. China: The McGraw-Hill Companies; 2013:197-216.

PREOPERATIVE BOWEL PREPARATION: IS IT NECESSARY?

Julia R. Berian, MD, and Neil H. Hyman, MD

The human intestine hosts most of the 100 trillion microbial cells in the body, and it is no wonder that infectious complications have plagued bowel surgery for centuries. Colorectal resection consistently carries high rates of surgical site infections and is associated with a formidable risk of anastomotic leak, intra-abdominal abscess, and sepsis. Before the routine use of prophylactic antibiotics, surgeons could expect postoperative wound infections in up to 40% of their patients. In modern series, rates of surgical site infection after colon or rectal resection are variable but still may reach as high as 25%.

Given the considerable morbidity and mortality associated with surgical site infections (SSI), colorectal SSI remains a high priority target for quality improvement efforts and risk reduction strategies in modern health care. The Centers for Medicare and Medicaid Services (CMS) have identified SSI (specifically for colon procedures and abdominal hysterectomies) as a hospital-acquired condition affecting hospital payments. Postoperative infectious complications are a salient endpoint for surgeons, health care payers, and patients. In this context, the question of bowel preparation and its role in reducing infectious complications remains controversial.

Myriad investigations, including many randomized controlled trials (RCTs), systematic reviews, meta-analyses, and large observational studies, have failed to produce a simple answer to the effectiveness and necessity of bowel preparation before surgery. This perhaps is due to strict assessments of mechanical and antibiotic bowel preparation in isolation. In contrast, several recent large observational database studies suggest that the true benefit may be derived from mechanical and oral antibiotic preparation in combination.

■ RATIONALE FOR PREPARATION

The biologic plausibility of bowel preparation seems undeniable. The goal of mechanical preparation is to decrease the fecal load in the colon to reduce the burden of bacteria, thereby reducing the risk of infectious complications. Studies in the 1930s and 1940s combined multiple strategies of mechanical and antibiotic preparation. By the 1970s, the Nichols/Condon neomycin-erythromycin-mechanical bowel preparation strategy was widely adopted. It was believed that mechanical cleansing facilitated the action of nonabsorbable oral antibiotics. However, as bowel preparation moved to the outpatient setting in recent decades, the oral antibiotic component was often omitted, considered unnecessary if intravenous antibiotics were administered at the time of incision. As it turns out, this may have been a significant error.

■ MECHANICAL BOWEL PREPARATION

Oral mechanical bowel preparation comes in several forms. Polyethylene glycol (PEG) solutions typically are given in large volume (4 L) or reduced volume (2 L) with the addition of bisacodyl. PEG solutions are osmotically balanced and provide colonic cleansing through washout, whereas the addition of bisacodyl stimulates colonic peristalsis. Hyperosmotic preparations with insoluble salts containing phosphate or magnesium achieve cleansing by drawing water into the bowel lumen. The risk of electrolyte imbalances is higher with hyperosmotic preparations. Multiday regimens using nasogastric tubes for whole-gut irrigation are historic artifacts and no longer widely practiced. See Table 1 for additional details on available mechanical preparations and their use.

■ DATA FOR MECHANICAL PREPARATION

Between the 1970s and 2015, many observational and randomized studies failed to show a difference in key outcomes between mechanical bowel preparation (MBP) and no preparation. Surgeons have been questioning the value of MBP almost since its inception. Indeed, there is substantial, level-one evidence from large randomized trials clearly indicating that mechanical bowel preparation offers no advantage, at least without oral antibiotics. The *Cochrane Database of Systematic Reviews* first addressed this topic in 2003 and has since published three updates (2005, 2009, and 2011). The most recent update (2011) includes data from 19 published RCTs and 1 unpublished RCT, encompassing 5805 patients. Examining a series of outcomes, including wound infection, anastomotic leak, peritonitis, reoperation and mortality, the authors conclude that mechanical bowel preparation (and rectal enema) may be omitted safely without any statistically significant difference in postoperative complications.

One often-cited weakness of prior studies (and their subsequent meta-analyses) is the heterogeneity of mechanical preps and, fundamentally, the inclusion of a range of different operations. In 2014 the Agency for Healthcare Research and Quality (AHRQ) conducted a clinical effectiveness review to expand upon the Cochrane reviews. The authors aimed to examine additional factors such as anatomic location of surgery, operative approach, and even a range of mechanical preparations used. Despite a broad array of sixty studies (including 44 RCTs, 10 nonrandomized comparative studies, and 6 single-group cohorts), the authors concluded that the evidence base is weak. They could not identify evidence of any benefit of mechanical bowel preparation; however, they could not exclude modest effects (30% to 50%) in either direction for overall mortality, anastomotic leak, wound infection, or peritonitis. In the end, it was concluded that the heterogeneity of study methods, small sample sizes, and inadequate reporting prohibited meaningful comparisons of MBP strategies. In examination of anatomic location of surgery, only one outcome, anastomotic leak, had sufficient data for analysis, and the results showed no difference between MBP and no MBP in either colon or rectal location.

TABLE 1: Mechanical Bowel Preparations

Preparation Type	Product Example	Volume	Administration	Notes on Use
PEG (Electrolyte lavage)	Colyte *Note: Flavored options are available* GoLYTELY *Note: Flavored options are available*	3785 mL 4000 mL	No solid food for at least 2 hours before ingestion of the solution; 240 mL (8 oz) every 10 minutes until rectal output is clear or 4 L are consumed.	Divided dose regimens (3 L the night before procedure, 1 L morning of procedure) may improve patient tolerance. PEG considered safer than osmotic laxatives/NaP for patients with electrolyte/fluid imbalances, renal or liver insufficiency, CHF or renal or liver failure
Sulfate-free PEG (improved smell/taste, more palatable for patients)	NuLYTELY *Note: Flavored options are available.* TriLyte *Note: Flavored options are available.*	4000 mL 4000 mL	No solid food for at least 2 hours before taking the solution; 240 mL (8 oz) every 10 min until rectal output is clear or 4 L are consumed	Similar efficacy to PEG
Low-volume PEG and bisacodyl tablets (decrease volume-related discomfort, e.g., bloating, cramping)	HalfLytely and bisacodyl tablet bowel prep MiraLAX	2000 mL 255 g in 2,000 mL	Only clear liquids on the day of the preparation. Dosage is four bisacodyl delayed-release tablets (5 mg) at noon. Wait for bowel movement or maximum of 6 hours; 240 mL (8 oz) low-volume PEG (i.e., HalfLytely) or 240 mL (8 oz) of clear liquid containing one capful of MiraLAX or other PEG-3350 regimen every 10 minutes until 2 L are consumed.	Equally effective as 4 L solutions, additional studies needed regarding safety
Aqueous NaP solutions	Fleet	90 mL with 48 oz additional liquid	Only clear liquids can be consumed on the day of preparation. Two doses of 30 to 45 mL (2-3 tbsp) of oral solution are given at least 10 to 12 hours apart. Each dose is taken with at least 8 oz of liquid followed by an additional minimum of at least 16 oz of liquid. The second dose must be taken at least 3 hours before the procedure.	May cause significant fluid shifts. Not for use in pediatric or elderly patients, bowel obstruction, gut dysmotility, other structural intestinal disorders, renal or liver or congestive heart failure. NaP may cause ulceration or mucosal abnormalities, do not use in patients with inflammatory bowel disease. Patients with compromised renal function or those taking ACE inhibitors or ARBs are at risk for phosphate nephropathy. In 2006 the FDA issued an alert regarding the risk for acute phosphate nephropathy, a type of acute renal failure, with the use of oral sodium phosphate solution or tablets.
Oral sodium phosphate (tablet)	Visicol (now discontinued)	32-40 tablets with 48 oz clear liquid	Dosage is 32 to 40 tablets: 20 tablets on the evening before the procedure and 12 to 20 tablets the day of the procedure (3-5 hours before). The 20 tablets are taken as 4 tablets every 15 minutes with 8 oz of clear liquid. Bisacodyl is prescribed by some physicians as an adjunct.	Early tablet composition included higher concentration of microcrystalline cellulose per tablet, which left residue obscuring mucosal surface. Later tablet composition decreased microcrystalline cellulose concentration. Overall, tablet NaP not associated with significantly improved patient tolerance when compared with aqueous NaP

TABLE 1: Mechanical Bowel Preparations—cont'd

Preparation Type	Product Example	Volume	Administration	Notes on Use
Adjuncts to mechanical preparation	Agent	Volume / Dose	Mechanism	Use
Enemas	Tap water Soap suds Fleet enema Fleet bisacodyl Enema Fleet mineral oil	500-1000 mL 500-1000 mL 135 mL 10 mg 1.25 oz 37.5 mL 480 mL	Distention and lavage of rectum and distal colon	Routine addition of enemas to oral preparation does not improve the quality of bowel cleansing, yet increases patient discomfort. Use enemas in patients presenting for endoscopy with poor distal colon preparation and in patients with defunctionalized distal colon (e.g., Hartmann's)
Bisacodyl	Bisacodyl	5 mg tablet	Poorly absorbed diphenylmethane that stimulates colonic peristalsis, used as adjunct for NaP or PEG preparations	Has been found to decrease the volume of PEG preparation required
Saline laxatives	Magnesium citrate (liquid) Picolax (sodium picosulfate/magnesium citrate)	250-300 mL	Hyperosmotic saline laxatives that increase motility by increased intraluminal volume	Addition of magnesium citrate to PEG allows for lower volume preparation. Use with extreme caution in patients with renal insufficiency or renal failure because of exclusive renal excretion of magnesium
Senna	Senna Senokot X-Prep Syrup (8 mg/5 mL)		Anthraquinone derivatives (glycosides and sennosides) are activated by colonic bacteria and directly increase the rate of colonic motility, with a subsequent increase in colonic transit and reduced water and electrolyte secretion	Senna with PEG may improve the quality of preparation and reduce volume required
Simethicone	Gas-X Mylicon Mylanta Generic formulations (80 mg)		Antiflatulent, often used to prevent foam formation after PEG preparation. Mechanism of action is unclear	May improve lumen visualization and patient toleration of bowel prep
Metoclopramide	Reglan Generic formulations also available	5 mg	Dopamine antagonist gastro-prokinetic, increasing the amplitude of gastric contraction, with increased peristalsis in duodenum and jejunum but without change in colonic motility	May reduce nausea, bloating. Does not improve colonic cleansing
Carbohydrate-electrolyte solutions	Gatorade E-Lyte Generic formulations	20 oz	Used with PEG and/or NaP solution to improve flavor and prevent NaP-related fluid and electrolyte shifts	Carbohydrate-based solutions more palatable for patients, however, associates with a theoretical risk of cautery-induced explosion if these carbohydrates are metabolized by colonic bacteria into explosive gases

Adapted from Wexner SD, Beck DE, Baron TH, Fanelli RD, Hyman N, Shen B, Wasco KE. A consensus document on bowel preparation before colonoscopy: prepared by a task force from the American Society of Colon and Rectal Surgeons (ASCRS), the American Society for Gastrointestinal Endoscopy (ASGE), and the Society of American Gastrointestinal and Endoscopic Surgeons (SAGES). *Dis Colon Rectum.* 2006;49:792-809.

ACE, angiotensin-converting enzyme; *ARB,* angiotensin receptor blocker; *CHF,* congestive heart failure; *FDA,* Food and Drug Administration; *NaP,* sodium phosphate; *PEG,* polyethylene glycol.

Because of little or no suggestion of benefit, patient complaints of prep-related discomfort, and physician concerns regarding electrolyte imbalances, dehydration, mucosal injury, and other adverse events, MBP has been abandoned in many areas of the world. Adverse events from bowel preparations are reported poorly in the literature, and the prep actually may increase the risk of contamination at surgery because liquid stool may be more likely to leak from the cut edge of the bowel than solid stool. Based on the available evidence, MBP alone generally is not recommended for routine colon operations.

■ DATA ON ORAL ANTIBIOTIC PREPARATION

A 2014 Cochrane review on antimicrobial prophylaxis for colorectal surgery showed that combined oral and intravenous prophylaxis reduced the risk of surgical site infection by 44% when compared with intravenous antibiotic administration alone (relative risk [RR] 0.56, 95% confidence interval [CI] 0.43 to 0.74). The data, derived from 14 studies including 2445 participants, was deemed high quality, such that further research is very unlikely to change the authors' confidence in the estimate of effect. Refer to Table 2 for examples of oral antibiotic prophylaxis.

Recent publications from statewide and nationwide data registries support this conclusion; combined preoperative oral antibiotic and mechanical bowel preparation is associated with reductions in surgical site infections, anastomotic leakage, ileus, and health services utilization outcomes such as length of stay and readmission. This includes several studies using data from the American College of Surgeons' National Surgical Quality Improvement Program (NSQIP), which have identified decreased infectious complications associated with combined oral antibiotic and mechanical bowel prep. Analyses using data from 2011 and 2012 consistently reveal lower rates of surgical site infection (rates reduced by 43% to 77%), as well as decreased anastomotic leak and procedure-related hospital readmission. An analysis of Veterans Affairs data came to similar conclusions, with lower readmission rates for infectious complications and shorter length of stay seen among the patients receiving oral antibiotic bowel preparation when compared with mechanical only or no preparation groups. Studies from the Michigan Surgical Quality Collaborative also have identified a decreased rate of abdominal abscess (1.6% vs 3.1%) or surgical site infection (5.0% vs 9.7%) between propensity matched pairs receiving mechanical bowel preparation and oral antibiotics compared with those with neither mechanical nor oral antibiotic preparation. The Michigan data also have been used to evaluate postoperative *C. difficile* colitis, revealing lower rates (0.5% vs 1.8%) among the oral antibiotic group.

■ CONCLUSIONS

Recent literature indicates that oral antibiotic preparation reduces complications for patients undergoing colorectal procedures. Although mechanical bowel preparation alone does not appear to provide a benefit, oral antibiotic without mechanical bowel preparation is rarely used. The effects of oral antibiotic prophylaxis without first cleansing the colon are not known and should be a focus for future research. Additional areas for further research include the use of bowel preparation in laparoscopic or minimally invasive approaches and in rectal surgery.

The current literature does not support routine use of purely mechanical bowel preparation. Mechanical bowel preparation may still be indicated for cases in which enhanced tactile feedback is required (such as for small lesions) or in cases that may require intraoperative colonoscopy. Bowel preparation in rectal surgery or laparoscopic approaches also may be warranted and deserves further study.

TABLE 2: Oral Antibiotic Regimens

Oral Antibiotic Prophylactic Regimen*	Use in Prior Literature (First Author, Year)
Neomycin + erythromycin	Nichols, 1973; Kaiser, 1983; Coppa, 1988; Lau, 1988; Khubchandani, 1989; Stellato, 1983
Metronidazole + neomycin	Hanel, 1980; Reynolds, 1989; Nohr, 1990 (included bacitracin); Lewis, 2002; Epsin-Basany, 2005
Metronidazole + kanamycin	Lazorthes, 1982; Monrozies, 1983; Takesue, 2000
Tinadazole + neomycin	Peruzzo, 1987
Kanamycin + erythromycin	Ishida, 2001; Kobayashi, 2007

Adapted from Bellows CF, Mills KT, Kelly TN, Gagliardi G. Combination of oral non-absorbable and intravenous antibiotics versus intravenous antibiotics alone in the prevention of surgical site infections after colorectal surgery: a meta-analysis of randomized controlled trials. *Tech Coloproctol.* 2011;15:385-395.

*Note that each of these oral antibiotics was combined with a range of intravenous antibiotics in the studies listed.

SUGGESTED READINGS

Dahabreh IJ, Steele DW, Shah N, Trikalinos TA. *Oral Mechanical Bowel Preparation for Colorectal Surgery.* Rockville, MD: Agency for Healthcare Research and Quality (US); 2014.

Güenaga KF, Matos D, Wille-Jørgensen P. Mechanical bowel preparation for elective colorectal surgery. *Cochrane Database Syst Rev.* 2011;CD001544.

Nelson RL, Gladman E, Barbateskovic M. Antimicrobial prophylaxis for colorectal surgery. *Cochrane Database Syst Rev.* 2014;5:CD001181.

Scarborough JE, Mantyh CR, Sun Z, Migaly J. Combined mechanical and oral antibiotic bowel preparation reduces incisional surgical site infection and anastomotic leak rates after elective colorectal resection: an analysis of colectomy-targeted ACS NSQIP. *Ann Surg.* 2015;262:331-337.

Toneva GD, Deierhoi RJ, Morris M, Richman J, Cannon JA, Altom LK, Hawn MT. Oral antibiotic bowel preparation reduces length of stay and readmissions after colorectal surgery. *J Am Coll Surg.* 2013;216:756-762, discussion 762-763.

THE MANAGEMENT OF DIVERTICULAR DISEASE OF THE COLON

Azah A. Althumairi, MD, and Susan L. Gearhart, MD

Diverticular disease is one of the most common gastrointestinal disorders in Western countries, and its incidence is thought to be increasing. Acute diverticulitis accounts for nearly 300,000 hospital admissions, and this is associated with a direct annual medical cost of $1.8 billion. The incidence increases proportionally with aging such that 60% of affected individuals are older than 80 years, whereas only 10% of affected individuals are younger than 40 years. The disease is rare in underdeveloped countries, suggesting a role of the environment in the pathogenesis. Furthermore, in U.S. and European populations, diverticulosis occurs more frequently in the sigmoid colon, whereas in Asian countries, more than 70% of diverticula are located in the right colon.

The most common type of diverticulum affecting the colon is a pseudodiverticulum. A pseudodiverticulum is a protrusion of only the mucosa through the muscularis propria of the colon usually at the point of penetration of the nutrient artery (vasa recti) that supplies the mucosa and submucosa. This is in contrast to a true diverticulum, which contains all layers of the bowel wall. The pathophysiology of diverticulitis is not fully understood. It has been thought to be an infectious process caused by bacterial overgrowth. Recently, this mechanism has been challenged by new reports suggesting that diverticulitis is primarily an inflammatory process of the colon similar to the autoimmune inflammatory bowel diseases. Evidence for this theory is seen in histopathologic sections of the diseased colon, where there appears to be an excess of mast cells in all layers of the bowel wall, and the process is thought to be initiated by the release of proinflammatory cytokines. Several studies also have examined the role of genetics in the development of diverticular disease. The relative risk for siblings of individuals with diverticular disease is nearly three times greater than the general population. The contribution of genetics to the development of diverticular disease also is noted in monozygotic twin studies as well and is estimated to contribute to 50% of the relative risk.

■ SYMPTOMATIC DIVERTICULITIS

Diverticular disease is usually an asymptomatic disorder. Contrary to old reports suggesting that up to 25% of individuals with diverticulosis will have symptoms, recent reports suggest that only 4% of patients with diverticulosis will have acute diverticulitis. Diverticulitis is the most common clinical presentation of diverticular disease. It is characterized by inflammation and/or infection of the diverticula. The theory is that the diverticulum becomes affected by fecaliths or inspissated waste leading to focal necrosis, bacterial overgrowth, and ultimately microperforation or macroperforation. The difference in the distribution of colonic diverticulosis leads to different clinical presentations. The most common cause for lower gastrointestinal bleeding is diverticular disease. Although often life threatening, the incidence of bleeding diverticular disease among patients with known diverticulosis is low (<20% of patients with known diverticulosis).

■ PRESENTATION

The classical symptoms of acute diverticulitis are left lower quadrant pain, fever, and obstipation. Confirmation of the presence of acute diverticulitis is made with blood tests demonstrating a leukocytosis and an abdominal computerized tomography (CT) demonstrating inflammation/stranding around the colon with or without free perforation. Approximately 15% of patients will have all the symptoms of diverticular disease; however, they will lack confirmatory imaging or blood tests demonstrating inflammation of their diverticulosis. Patients with these findings have been labeled as having *symptomatic uncomplicated diverticular disease (SUDD)*. Unlike acute uncomplicated diverticulitis, patients with SUDD tend to have cyclic episodes of left lower quadrant abdominal pain. Many of the symptoms of SUDD overlap with irritable bowel disease, a common disorder of the gastrointestinal tract associated with frequent cyclic generalized abdominal pain and bloating.

Complicated diverticular disease can be associated with symptoms of persistent abdominal pain and sepsis, despite treatment, suggestive of an intra-abdominal abscess or free perforation. In 1978 Hinchey published a grading system for diverticular disease with abscess formation or free perforation. This classification system was based on older methods of imaging and has been modified after the introduction of more sophisticated CT imaging. Nevertheless, European studies and studies from the United States often present data based on Hinchey class. Table 1 outlines the definition of each class, and Figure 1 provides a pictorial presentation of the classification system. Symptoms of fecaluria, pneumaturia, pyuria, or recurrent urinary tract infections are suggestive of the development of a colovesical fistula after an intra-abdominal–free perforation and abscess formation. Passage of stool through the vagina is suggestive of a colovaginal fistula complicating diverticular disease. This typically is seen only in women who have had a hysterectomy. Finally, worsening constipation in patients with long-standing diverticular disease may indicate the development of a colonic stricture.

On physical examination, patients often have tachycardia and fever. Abdominal findings often reveal guarding and signs of localized peritonitis that may be a result of microperforation and abscess formation. In cases of macroperforation and remote abscess, patients have generalized peritonitis. Free perforation and fecal peritonitis may be accompanied by life-threatening sepsis. In patients who have the passage of stool through the vagina, a gynecologic examination may reveal a fistulous connection at the vaginal apex. If a colonic stricture is present, abdominal distension often is noted.

■ EVALUATION

Initial evaluation should include laboratory investigations and urinalysis. In general, a leukocytosis will be present. CT imaging is the standard method to diagnose and stage acute diverticulitis. When performed with thin cuts after oral and intravenous contrast, CT has a sensitivity that approaches 98% and specificity of 99%. The key CT findings associated with acute diverticulitis include colonic wall thickening and pericolonic stranding around diverticula. On occasion there may be free extraluminal air present. Several studies have examined the role of CT colonography in the management of diverticular disease. The benefit of CT colonography is its ability to also demonstrate luminal narrowing and identify other luminal findings. However, CT colonography cannot be performed in the acute setting and is reserved for patients with long-standing recurrent disease. High-resolution ultrasound (US) and magnetic resonance imaging (MRI) are useful alternative modalities in patients with contraindications to CT scanning. US has a diagnosis accuracy of 97%; however, it is operator dependent and may be difficult to perform in patients with abdominal tenderness. MRI has a sensitivity of 94% and specificity of 92% and is not constrained by the limitations of US.

TABLE 1: Hinchey Classification and Modified Hinchey Classification

Hinchey Classification	Modified Hinchey Classification
I Pericolic abscess or phlegmon	0 Mild clinical diverticulitis
II Pelvic, intra-abdominal, or retroperitoneal abscess	Ia Confined pericolic inflammation, phlegmon Ib Confined pericolic abscess
III Generalized purulent peritonitis	II Pelvic, distant intra-abdominal, or retroperitoneal abscess
IV Generalized fecal peritonitis	III Generalized purulent peritonitis IV Generalized fecal peritonitis

■ MANAGEMENT

Management of diverticular disease depends on the patients' presentation. Asymptomatic diverticulosis discovered at the time of colonoscopy or abdominal imaging studies is managed with diet alterations. A recent study from the Los Angeles Veterans Association demonstrated that only 4% of patients noted to have diverticulosis on colonoscopy actually had diverticulitis. The mean time to disease was 7 years, and young patients were more likely to develop diverticulitis than older patients. Therefore patients (especially young ones) with asymptomatic diverticulosis should be instructed to increase the fiber (30 g per day) and water intake and to avoid foods high in fats. In the case of patients with SUDD, several medical therapies have been tried, including nonsteroidal anti-inflammatory drugs (NSAID), 5-ASA derivatives, probiotics, and rifaximin. Most studies evaluated mesalamine and rifaximin either as monotherapy or in combination and only demonstrated a modest benefit; however, further studies are needed. Treatment of acute diverticulitis is based on the severity of the disease and varies by whether it is complicated or uncomplicated acute diverticulitis.

Management of Uncomplicated Diverticulitis

Currently, the management of uncomplicated diverticular disease is being re-evaluated. Medical therapy can be successful in 75% to 91% of patients. However, many individuals seek surgical therapy because of the effect the disease has on their quality of life. In general, uncomplicated diverticular disease can be managed as an outpatient. The DIVER trial randomized patients with acute uncomplicated diverticulitis after receiving the first dose of antibiotic intravenously to outpatient management with oral antibiotics versus hospitalization with intravenous (IV) antibiotics. The outpatient management was more cost effective with no difference in the treatment failure rate or quality of life. However, diverticular disease often is associated with several comorbidities, such as immunosuppression, renal disease, and heart disease, and patients with significant comorbidities and acute diverticulitis may need to be hospitalized.

In otherwise healthy patients with absences of systemic signs of sepsis or severe abdominal pain, treatment initially involves bowel rest and antibiotics with aerobic and anaerobic coverage. A combination of ciprofloxacin and metronidazole for 7 to 10 days is usually effective. Recently, some studies have suggested that diverticulitis is an inflammatory process rather than infection caused by microperforation and questioned the need for antibiotics. The AVOD study is a multicenter randomized controlled trial (RCT) that treated 623

patients with uncomplicated diverticulitis with either IV fluids or IV fluids and IV antibiotics. They found that antibiotic treatment did not accelerate recovery nor prevent complications or recurrence. However, the recent practice parameters of the American Society of Colon and Rectal Surgeons (ASCRS) strongly recommend the use of antibiotics in the treatment of diverticulitis until better quality evidences are available to support the antibiotic-free treatment of diverticulitis. Clinical improvement is assessed with resolution of abdominal pain and fevers. With a good response to medical treatment, diet can progress gradually. In those individuals who fail to improve, a CT scan should be performed to rule out complicated disease.

Management of Complicated Diverticulitis

As mentioned previously, perforated diverticulitis can be staged on the basis of imaging studies with the Hinchey classification (see Table 1). This classification will assess the severity of disease, help plan the treatment, and correlate the risk of failure of nonoperative treatment and predict outcomes after surgical treatment of complicated diverticulitis. Complicated diverticulitis can be seen acutely with free perforation or as a late or chronic complication, including obstruction, stricture, and fistula.

Management of Diverticular Abscess (Hinchey I or II)

Small abscesses up to 3 to 4 cm usually resolve spontaneously. In the absence of clinical improvement or presence of a large abscess, percutaneous drainage under CT or US guidance should be performed and patients continued on IV antibiotics and bowel rest. With this approach, 52% to 74% of patients will avoid the need of urgent operation. The abscess drain is left in place till the clinical symptoms improve and output is minimal (<30 mL per day). The resolution of the abscess cavity also can be assessed with CT imaging before removal of the drain. Significant improvement in temperature, abdominal pain, and leukocytosis usually is seen within 48 hours after initiation of treatment. Surgical intervention may become necessary if the abscess is not accessible for drainage, or if symptoms either persist or worsen. Immunocompromised patients are at risk of delayed diagnosis as well as decreased ability to limit the spread of the infection. The mortality rate with medical treatment of diverticular disease in patients with significant comorbidities is high (up to 60% in some trials), and the threshold for surgical intervention should be low.

Management of Free Perforation (Hinchey III and Hinchey IV)

Patients with generalized purulent peritonitis (Hinchey III) or fecal peritonitis (Hinchey IV) are typically acutely ill with symptoms and signs of sepsis. Reported mortality rates are 6% for purulent and 35% for fecal peritonitis. Immediate aggressive fluid resuscitation and broad-spectrum IV antibiotics should be administered. Emergency surgical intervention is required to control the source of sepsis.

Historically, the standard of care for perforated diverticulitis was a two-stage approach with resection of sigmoid colon, including the perforation, closure of the rectal stump, and creation of proximal colostomy (Hartmann's procedure) at the acute phase. This is followed with colostomy takedown and anastomosis at 3 to 6 months after the initial surgery. This procedure is associated with mortality rates of 10% to 18%, with morbidity rate of 43%, and 10% stoma-related complications. It requires a second laparotomy for stoma closure and is associated with a prolonged hospitalization. Often restoration of bowel continuity is technically challenging, and nearly 30% to 45% of patients will end up with permanent colostomy.

Recognizing that urgent colectomy is associated with substantial morbidity, some authors have suggested a limited procedure with

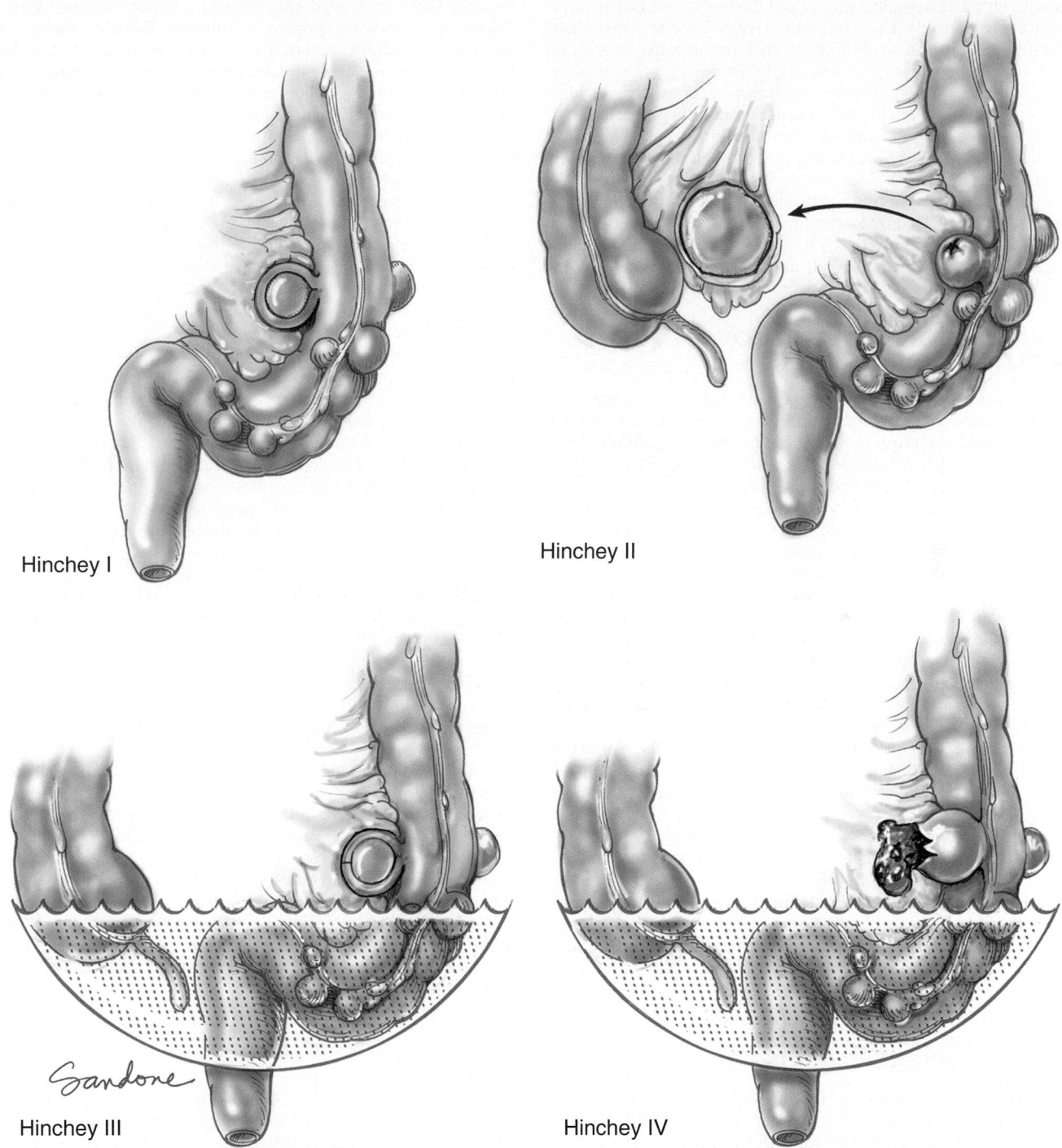

Hinchey I

Hinchey II

Hinchey III

Hinchey IV

FIGURE 1 Schematic of the Hinchey classification of complicated diverticular disease. *(Courtesy Corinne Sandone, University of Johns Hopkins School of Medicine.)*

laparoscopic peritoneal lavage to control the peritoneal sepsis and as a bridge to elective definitive surgery. The recent SCANDIV trial is a multicenter randomized trial that enrolled 199 patients to undergo either a Hartmann's procedure or laparoscopic peritoneal lavage for the surgical management of Hinchey III perforated diverticular disease. Although there was no difference in mortality between the two groups, patients undergoing laparoscopic peritoneal lavage had a significantly higher rate of reoperation for persistent abdominal sepsis (20% vs 5.7%, respectively). With these findings, currently

most guidelines do not support the use of laparoscopic peritoneal lavage unless the operative findings prohibit colon resection.

A primary anastomosis with or without colonic lavage and with or without diversion is another attractive alternative with acceptable morbidity and mortality in selected patients. This procedure negates the need for a second laparotomy for reversal of Hartmann's procedure and avoids stoma-related complications. The pooled morbidity rates are 31.7%, 23.7%, and 49.5%, and the pooled mortality rates are 3.8%, 7.2%, and 17.4% for resection and primary anastomosis, resection with primary anastomosis and diversion, and Hartmann's procedure, respectively. However, these results must be interpreted with caution because most of the literature is retrospective with some degree of selection bias. The only RCT comparing patients with Hinchey III and Hinchey IV who underwent Hartmann's procedure or primary anastomosis with diverting ileostomy with planned stoma reversal was stopped after interim safety analysis showed that Hartmann's reversal was associated with significantly more serious complications compared with ileostomy reversal (20% vs 0). Morbidity and mortality rates were not significantly different after the initial colon resection followed by Hartmann's reversal or primary anastomosis with diverting ileostomy (67% vs 75% and 13% vs 9%, respectively). However, stoma reversal rate after primary anastomosis with diverting ileostomy was higher (90% vs 57%, $P = 0.005$).

■ EVALUATION AFTER RECOVERY FROM ACUTE DIVERTICULITIS

After successful nonoperative management, current recommendations are to perform a colonoscopy after 6 to 8 weeks to evaluate for luminal disease. The purpose of this examination is to confirm the diagnosis of diverticular disease and exclude other diseases such as inflammatory bowel disease and colon cancer. About 3% to 5% of patients who have acute diverticulitis are found to harbor a colon cancer in subsequent colonoscopy examination. A recent retrospective analysis of 633 patients demonstrated an increased risk of colon cancer identified in complicated diverticular disease versus uncomplicated diverticular disease (10.8% vs 0.7%, respectively). The authors recommended that patients with complicated diverticular disease should undergo colonoscopic evaluation; however, routine colonoscopy for CT-proven uncomplicated diverticular disease may be unnecessary. CT colonography is an alternative to colonoscopy with equivalent results in identification of synchronous lesions in the setting of diverticular disease.

Patients can have late complications as a consequence of acute diverticulitis. Diverticular abscess or phlegmon may extend and rupture into an adjacent organ, resulting in formation of fistula in 12% of patients. The most common fistula to form is a colovesical fistula. Diagnosis is confirmed with a CT cystogram, and on occasion, the fistula can be seen on cystoscopy. Colovaginal fistula can be identified on gynecologic examination or by CT with rectal contrast. The inflammatory process associated with diverticulitis may cause progressive fibrosis resulting in colonic stricture formation. Biopsy to distinguish between diverticular stricture and cancer causing stenosis of the lumen in indicated.

■ ROLE OF ELECTIVE SURGERY AFTER RECOVERY FROM ACUTE DIVERTICULITIS

The traditional teaching was to recommend elective sigmoid colectomy for diverticular disease after recovery from a second episode of uncomplicated diverticulitis. The rationale behind this approach was based on a report by Parks in 1969, which found that the mortality rate increased from 4.7% in the first episode to 7.8% with each subsequent episode. Old data also suggested that after the second episode, there is a higher recurrence rate with more severe subsequent attacks and increased risk of perforation. Therefore elective sigmoid colectomy was intended to prevent subsequent complicated episodes that would necessitate stoma formation with an increased overall morbidity and mortality.

Recent data that examined the natural history of disease have challenged this approach, and suggested that, in most patients, complicated diverticulitis is the first manifestation of their disease. Moreover, the rate of recurrence in uncomplicated diverticulitis treated nonoperatively is 13% to 23%, with only 6% experiencing subsequent complicated recurrence requiring surgery. Additional studies have demonstrated the risk of free perforation to be 25% in the first

episode, 12.7% at second episode, and 5.9% at the third episode. Therefore the ASCRS practice parameters do not consider the number of episodes as an indication for elective surgery. The decision to perform elective sigmoid colectomy after recovery from uncomplicated diverticulitis should be performed on a case-by-case basis and individualized to each patient, considering his or her medical condition, operative risks, severity of the attacks, persistent symptoms, effect of recurrent attack on patient's personal and professional lifestyle, and inability to exclude carcinoma.

There are exceptions to these guidelines. Historically, diverticulitis in young patients (i.e., younger than 50 years) has been associated with a more virulent course and higher rate of recurrence. Recent data suggest that younger and older patients have similar severity of disease. Although younger patients have a higher cumulative risk of developing recurrent disease because they have much longer life span, the recurrence rate remains low, at 27% with 2.1% to 7.5% requiring subsequent emergency surgery. Therefore routine elective surgery in patients younger than 50 years is no longer recommended. Patients who are immunocompromised, with chronic renal failure or collagen-vascular disease, and transplant patients on chronic corticosteroid therapy are at greater risk of recurrent complicated diverticulitis and a higher risk of complications from perforation. In these groups of patients, operative intervention as a definitive treatment during the first hospitalization may be required.

Unlike uncomplicated diverticulitis, elective sigmoid colectomy should be performed after recovery from complicated diverticulitis as long-term resolution is unlikely. Mesocolic abscess of at least 5 cm or pelvic abscess treated medically with or without percutaneous drainage need definitive surgical resection because they have a recurrence rate up to 40%. In patients with late complications such as fistula or stricture, elective surgery is indicated for symptomatic relief or in cases with inability to rule out carcinoma.

■ SURGICAL CONSIDERATIONS

Surgical resection should include the entire sigmoid colon. The distal resection margin must extend to the proximal rectum with the creation of a colorectal anastomosis. A more extensive resection with lower rectal anastomosis may be required in patients with inflammation extending to the rectosigmoid. Proximal resection margin should be a healthy descending colon with absence of thickened and inflamed tissue. For this to be achieved, it is often necessary to mobilize the splenic flexure of the colon and divide the inferior mesenteric artery and vein (Figures 2 and 3). Routine use of ureteric stent generally is not indicated; however, it may facilitate the dissection in morbidly obese patients, patients undergoing reoperation, or if minimally invasive approaches are used in complicated diverticulitis.

Minimally invasive surgery is the preferred approach in elective settings (Figure 4). The Sigma trial randomized patients with complicated diverticulitis to either open or laparoscopic approach. The conversion rate was 19.2%. Although laparoscopic procedures were longer ($P = 0.001$), it was associated with less blood loss ($P = 0.033$). More major complications including anastomotic leak occurred with open procedures (9.6% vs 25.0%; $P = 0.038$). In addition, patients who underwent laparoscopic procedures had less pain ($P = 0.0003$), systemic analgesia requirement ($P = 0.029$), shorter hospital stay ($P = 0.046$), and a significantly better quality of life. Similar results in regard to operative time, postoperative pain, and analgesia requirement were reported from another RCT. This trial also demonstrated that laparoscopic sigmoid resection was associated with a 30% reduction in the duration of postoperative ileus and hospital stay.

The mortality rate after elective surgery for diverticulitis is 1.0% to 2.3%, and the morbidity rate is 25% to 55%. Recurrence rates range between 2.6% and 12.5%. The most important predictor of recurrence is incomplete resection of the sigmoid colon, in which the distal sigmoid colon is left in place. The reported incidence of recurrence is 12.5% after colocolonic anastomosis and 6.7% if colorectal anastomosis was performed.

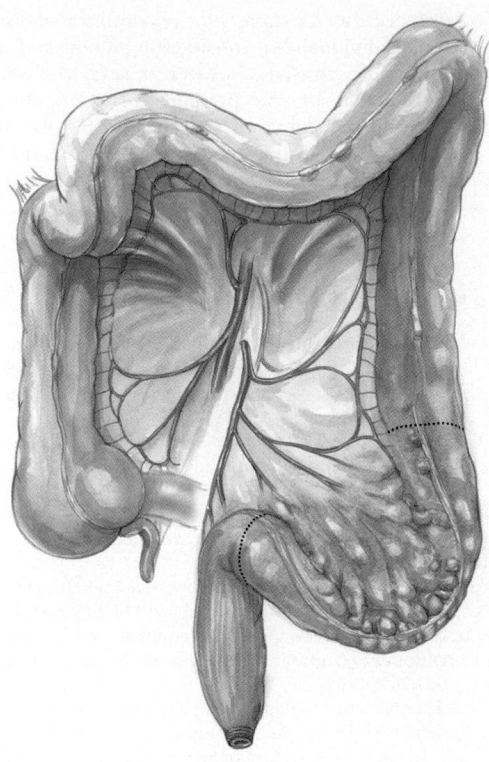

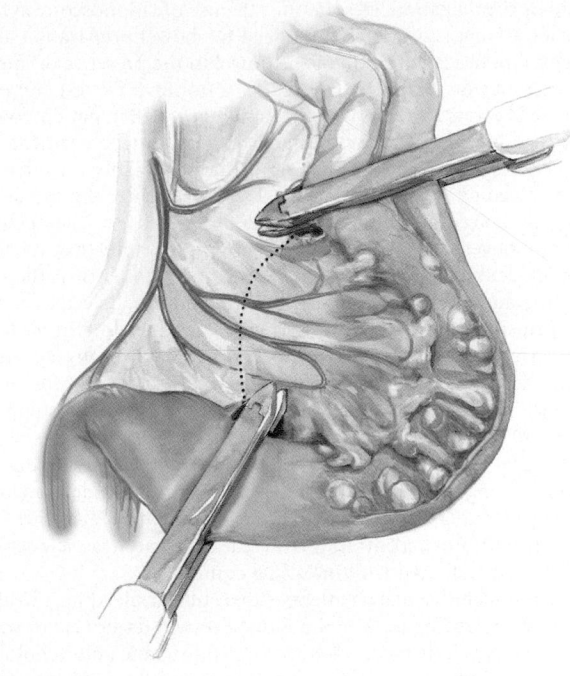

FIGURE 3 Sigmoid resection. *(From Cameron JL, Sandone C. Atlas of Gastrointestinal Surgery. 2nd ed. vol 2. Shelton, CT: People's Medical Publishing House; 2014.)*

FIGURE 2 Extent of sigmoid resection with division of inferior mesenteric artery and vein. *(From Cameron JL, Sandone C. Atlas of Gastrointestinal Surgery. 2nd ed. vol 2. Shelton, CT: People's Medical Publishing House; 2014.)*

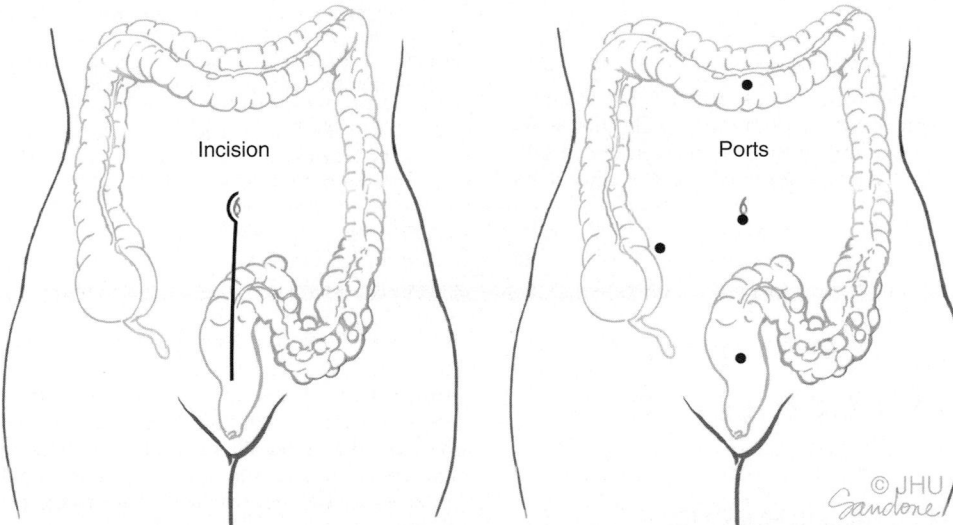

FIGURE 4 Open and minimally invasive sigmoid resection incisions. *(Copyright Corinne Sandone, Johns Hopkins University School of Medicine.)*

■ DIVERTICULAR BLEEDING

Risk factors for diverticular bleeding include history of hypertension, history of atherosclerosis, smoking, alcohol consumption, low-dose aspirin, non-aspirin antiplatelet medications, and regular use of NSAIDs. Patients typically experience abrupt onset of passage of red blood. Nonetheless, melena can happen with slowly bleeding right colon diverticula. Diverticular bleeding is usually self-limited and stops spontaneously with bowel rest in 70% to 80% of patients. Only 3% to 5% of patients experience severe bleeding. Immediate fluid and blood products resuscitation should be initiated as needed.

About 10% to 15% of patients with hematochezia have an upper gastrointestinal cause, which should be ruled out by performing upper gastrointestinal endoscopy.

Several diagnostic procedures are available to localize the bleeding site. These include colonoscopy, radionuclide scan, mesenteric angiography, and CT angiography. The choice of the diagnostic procedure is influenced by the patient's hemodynamic status, rate of bleeding, and the physician' experience to provide diagnostic and therapeutic procedures. For mild to moderate bleeding, colonoscopy can be both diagnostic and therapeutic. Hemostasis can be achieved with epinephrine injection or bipolar cautery and by placement of endoclip or band ligation. Despite this, the use of colonoscopy in the emergency setting is limited by the need for bowel preparation and by potential poor visualization of the bowel in the presence of intraluminal blood clots. Radionuclide scan is a noninvasive test and can detect bleeding rate as low as 0.1 mL/min. It is useful in patients with intermittent bleeding because red cell activity can be seen for 24 hours, allowing for repeated imaging. Although highly sensitive in detecting bleeding, radionuclide scan does not localize the source of bleeding or determine its cause and does not have a therapeutic potential. Conventional mesenteric angiography is an invasive test that can detect bleeding at a rate of 0.5 mL/min. It identifies the site of bleeding and allows for therapeutic intervention. Selective intra-arterial infusion of vasopressin can control the bleeding in 90% of patients. However, significant complications have been reported, including myocardial infarction and intestinal ischemia. Moreover, about 50% of patients will rebleed once the infusion is stopped. Another alternative is selective coil embolization. It is associated with less than 25% risk of rebleeding, and less than 10% risk of colonic ischemia. CT angiography is a noninvasive test and can detect active bleeding at a rate as low as 0.3 to 0.5 mL/min in 50% to 80% of patients. Intraluminal contrast extravasation is seen as a positive blush before it is diluted with intestinal content.

After nonoperative management of diverticular bleeding, the lifetime risk of rebleeding is 25%; therefore elective surgery is not warranted. Surgery is indicated if therapeutic endoscopic and radiologic options have failed. Indications of failure are the following: a requirement of more than 4 to 6 units of blood transfusion within 24 hours, continued bleeding after 72 hours, and rebleeding within 1 week of the initial episode. If the bleeding site is identified, segmental resection can be performed. Reported rebleeding rate is 6%. If the bleeding site could not be identified, subtotal colectomy is indicated. In the absence of significant comorbidities, primary anastomosis is a safe option; however, patients who received massive blood transfusion are at higher risk of anastomotic leak.

■ SUMMARY

Sigmoid diverticulitis can elicit mild symptoms amenable to outpatient management, or with colonic perforation and life-threatening sepsis requiring aggressive and urgent surgical intervention. Elective definitive surgery is indicated in complicated cases of diverticular disease. However, decision for surgery for uncomplicated diverticular disease should be individualized, considering patient and operative risk factors. Minimally invasive approach is safe with short-term benefits and preferable in the presence of surgical expertise. Diverticular bleeding is a common cause of lower gastrointestinal bleeding. It is usually self-limited and amenable to endoscopic or radiologic management. Urgent surgical interventions may be needed in severe cases.

SUGGESTED READINGS

Biondo S, Golda T, Kreisler E, Espin E, Vallribera F, Oteiza F, Codina-Cazador A, Pujadas M, Flor B. Outpatient versus hospitalization management for uncomplicated diverticulitis: a prospective, multicenter randomized clinical trial (DIVER Trial). *Ann Surg.* 2014;259:38-44.

Chabok A, Påhlman L, Hjern F, Haapaniemi S, Smedh K, AVOD Study Group. Randomized clinical trial of antibiotics in acute uncomplicated diverticulitis. *Br J Surg.* 2012;99:532-539.

Feingold D, Steele SR, Lee S, Kaiser A, Boushey R, Buie WD, Rafferty JF. Practice parameters for the treatment of sigmoid diverticulitis. *Dis Colon Rectum.* 2014;57:284-294.

Klarenbeek BR, Veenhof AA, Bergamaschi R, van der Peet DL, van den Broek WT, de Lange ES, Bemelman WA, Heres P, Lacy AM, Engel AF, Cuesta MA. Laparoscopic sigmoid resection for diverticulitis decreases major morbidity rates: a randomized control trial: short-term results of the Sigma Trial. *Ann Surg.* 2009;249:39-44.

Oberkofler CE, Rickenbacher A, Raptis DA, Lehmann K, Villiger P, Buchli C, Grieder F, Gelpke H, Decurtins M, Tempia-Caliera AA, Demartines N, Hahnloser D, Clavien PA, Breitenstein S. A multicenter randomized clinical trial of primary anastomosis or Hartmann's procedure for perforated left colonic diverticulitis with purulent or fecal peritonitis. *Ann Surg.* 2012;256:819-826, discussion 826-827.

Parks TG. Natural history of diverticular disease of the colon. A review of 521 cases. *Br Med J.* 1969;4:639-642.

Sallinen V, Mentula P, Leppaniemi A. Risk of colon cancer after computed tomography-diagnosed acute diverticulitis: is routine colonoscopy necessary? *Surg Endosc.* 2014;28:961-966.

Schultz J, Yaqub S, Wallon D, Bleic L, et al. Laparoscopic lavage vs. primary resection for acute perforated diverticulitis; the SCANDIV randomized clinical trial. *J Am Med Assoc.* 2015;314:1364-1375.

Shahedi K, Fuller G, Bolus R, et al. Long-term risk of acute diverticulitis among patients with incidental diverticulosis found during colonoscopy. *Clin Gastroenterol Hepatol.* 2013;11:1609-1613.

THE MANAGEMENT OF CHRONIC ULCERATIVE COLITIS

Chady I. Atallah, MD, Jonathan E. Efron, MD, and Sandy H. Fang, MD

Ulcerative colitis (UC) is a chronic and dynamic mucosal inflammatory bowel disorder (IBD), characterized by remissions and exacerbations. The disease starts with involvement of the rectum (proctitis) and may extend to include the sigmoid colon (proctosigmoiditis) or further contiguous involvement of the colon (proctocolitis). The more proximal gastrointestinal tract is not involved; however, diarrheal stool from severe inflammation in the cecum may cause an inflamed terminal ileum called "backwash ileitis" and must be differentiated from Crohn's ileitis.

IBD is multifactorial with genetic and environmental components. A family history of IBD is the most prominent risk factor. UC probands tend to have more relatives diagnosed with UC, and the same holds true for Crohn's disease. Seventy-five percent of patients with UC have perinuclear antineutrophil cytoplasmic antibodies. Environmental stimuli include increased sugar consumption, low-fiber diet, food allergies, food additives, infectious agents, and shortened breastfeeding time. Cigarette smoking is a protective influence in UC, whereas it is a risk factor for developing Crohn's disease.

Patients usually experience diarrhea and bleeding per rectum. Pain is an uncommon clinical feature except in severe active disease, when inflammation extends to the serosa. After long-term medical therapy, patients actually may experience constipation instead of diarrhea.

Diagnosis is made by endoscopy with multiple biopsies. Because inflammation starts in the rectum, proctoscopy or flexible sigmoidoscopy is usually all that is needed for confirmation of UC; however, complete colonoscopy with evaluation of the terminal ileum should be performed to define the extent of disease and to rule out other pathologic conditions, such as Crohn's disease or benign or malignant neoplasia. Surveillance endoscopy is recommended every 1 to 2 years, 8 years after diagnosis. Four-quadrant random biopsies are obtained at 10-cm intervals, for a total of at least 32 random biopsies, in addition to biopsies of suspicious lesions. A total colonoscopy is contraindicated in the face of an acute exacerbation, and in these cases, endoscopic evaluation is limited to the rectum and sigmoid colon. Other conditions that cause diarrhea and rectal bleeding must be ruled out, such as infectious etiology (*Clostridium difficile*, *Campylobacter* spp., *Salmonella enterocolitis*, *Escherichia coli* 0157:H7, amebiasis), collagenous colitis, and Crohn's colitis. Stool cultures for pathogenic bacteria, ova, and parasites should be sent for analysis.

■ INDICATIONS FOR SURGICAL THERAPY

Medically Refractory Disease

Medical therapy for UC refers to administration of a variety of immunosuppressive medications, which include 5-ASA compounds, steroids, antipyrine or pyrimidine compounds, and newer biologic therapy (tumor necrosis factor-α [TNF-α] antibodies). However, UC is chronic, often lasting for decades, and patients may progress to steroid dependence or a disease state that is medically refractory. Intractability to medical treatment defined by poorly controlled symptoms, poor quality of life, growth failure, or long-term effects of therapy (especially from steroids), remains the most common indication for surgical therapy in patients with UC (Figure 1). Between 15% and 30% of UC patients undergo elective or emergent surgery.

Fulminant Colitis and Toxic Megacolon

Severe colitis affects 5% to 15% of patients with UC and is characterized by bloody diarrhea, weight loss, volume depletion, fever, and severe anemia. Fulminant colitis refers to patients with severe colitis with progressive symptoms of toxicity. Attempts at conservative management with bowel rest, parenteral nutrition, parenteral steroids, and broad-spectrum antibiotics are required. If the disease progresses to fevers, leukocytosis, and distention despite maximal medical therapy, this indicates progression to toxic colitis. Toxic colitis refers to the triad of fever, tachycardia, and leukocytosis in patients with UC. When seen in patients who have distention of the transverse colon greater than 8 cm in diameter as seen on abdominal x-ray, this indicates toxic megacolon. Toxic colitis or toxic megacolon should be viewed as surgical emergencies because they indicate impending colonic perforation. Urgent or emergent resection is required. If a patient's condition with fulminant colitis does not improve or deteriorates within 48 to 96 hours of initiation of therapy, then second-line therapy or surgery should be considered. Ninety percent of patients with toxic colitis refractory to steroid therapy are able to avoid an emergent colectomy by the use of biologics, such as infliximab. Between 20% and 30% of patients with fulminant colitis require surgical intervention. If perforation ensues, the mortality rate after surgical intervention may be as high as 57%; therefore surgery is warranted.

Bleeding

The incidence of massive hemorrhage in UD is low, ranging from 0 to 4.5%. However, it accounts for 10% of all urgent colectomies performed for UC. Although colectomy for bleeding is rare, requirement of blood transfusions is common.

Cancer

Risk factors for malignancy in patients with UC include extensive involvement of the colon and long duration of disease. A historic meta-analysis demonstrates the cumulative risk of colorectal cancer as 2.1% at 10 years, 10% at 20 years, and after 30 and 40 years, the risk increases to 50% and 75%, respectively. However, recent population-based series show lower annual incidence rates of 0.06% to 0.2%. Endoscopic surveillance must begin 8 to 10 years after the onset of symptoms or sooner, depending on age of the patient, and be performed on an annual or biannual basis. If a patient also has primary sclerosing cholangitis or has a positive family history of colorectal cancer, surveillance intervals should shorten to annually. Ideally, colonoscopy should be performed while in remission to minimize confusion in the recognition of carcinoma because of inflammation. Because cancer may arise from flat mucosa, random serial four-quadrant biopsies should be obtained every 10 cm for a total of at least 32 biopsies as an adequate sampling for dysplasia or cancer.

If biopsy specimens are positive for high-grade dysplasia or cancer, a patient should undergo proctocolectomy. The risk of having an undetected cancer that is found after colectomy for high-grade dysplasia is 42%. In the setting of low-grade dysplasia, patients are encouraged to undergo elective prophylactic proctocolectomy. Unrecognized synchronous colorectal carcinoma is present in up to 20% of individuals who undergo surgery with the initial diagnosis

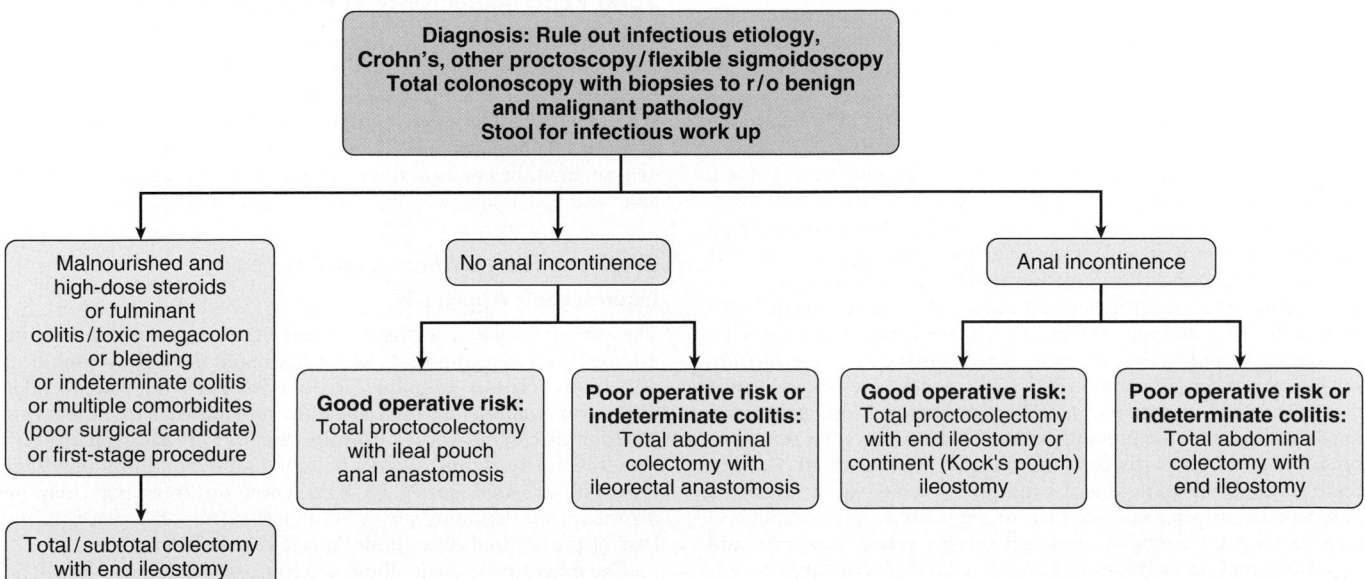

FIGURE 1 Surgical management of chronic ulcerative colitis.

of low-grade dysplasia. If the patient declines surgery, then close surveillance, every 3 to 6 months, is required. A biopsy of the polyps should be performed as per routine; however, the surrounding mucosa in four quadrants also should be sampled for dysplasia/carcinoma (DALM, non–adenoma-like dysplasia-associated lesion or mass). Resection of adenomatous tissue or a polyp is not an absolute indication for proctocolectomy, but when in conjunction with a DALM lesion is of greater concern. Typically patients with dysplastic changes have had their colitis for many years and no longer have inflammatory complaints. They are having normal bowel movements and therefore are often not as satisfied with their ileal pouch function. For this reason, patients are often reluctant to undergo surgery.

Stricture formation occurs in 5% to 12% of patients with 25% of the strictures being malignant. Thirty percent of cancers occurring in UC patients are diagnosed as a stricture. Malignant strictures appear late in the course of disease (61% after 20 years of disease), are usually located proximal to the splenic flexure (86%), and cause large bowel obstructions (100% vs 14% in benign strictures). Thus an oncologic resection of the colon and rectum is recommended for stricturing disease in patients with UC.

Extracolonic Manifestations

Hepatobiliary-associated disorders are the most likely to influence surgical management of the colon and rectum in UC patients. These patients may require orthotopic liver transplantation for primary sclerosing cholangitis. If a colectomy is required, permanent ileostomy creation is contraindicated because of the complications associated with peri-ileostomy varices from portal hypertension. Proctocolectomy for UC is beneficial for erythema nodosum (most responsive), arthritis, and eye diseases (episcleritis, uveitis, iritis, conjunctivitis) but does not affect outcomes for primary sclerosing cholangitis, ankylosing spondylitis, and sacroiliitis.

Growth Failure in Children

Surgery should be considered if children have growth retardation despite maximizing nutritional and medical therapy.

■ SURGICAL OPTIONS

Many surgical options exist for UC. Each surgical plan is tailored toward the individual patient according to his or her preoperative comorbidities, functional and continence status, and urgency of the operation. Patients should have extensive counseling regarding the potential for an ostomy. Several circumstances involve planning for future operations, in that patients may require multiple staged procedures, because of their disease status or whether they require an emergent operation.

Today, select patients are offered a minimally invasive approach. Advocates of the laparoscopic approach cite technical ease, improved patient comfort, better cosmesis, decreased lengths of hospital stay, and faster recovery as advantages over the open approach. Studies in minimally invasive IPAA creation have shown a decrease in adhesion formation and incisional hernias. There are many different approaches to minimally invasive proctocolectomy, including strict laparoscopy, laparoscopic-assisted, hand-assisted, or single-incision surgery. Specimen extraction of the ileal pouch may be performed through a lower midline incision, Pfannenstiel incision, right lower quadrant incision (the previously marked ileostomy site), or a periumbilical incision. If dissection is difficult because of anatomy or there are multiple adhesions, a hand port may be placed through a Pfannenstiel or lower midline incision. This hand port incision also may be used for an open approach for the pelvic dissection and pouch creation. Regardless of approach, all patients undergo a standard mechanical bowel preparation and receive perioperative intravenous antibiotics.

Subtotal Colectomy With End Ileostomy and Hartmann's Procedure

A subtotal colectomy with end ileostomy and Hartmann's procedure is the least morbid operation. It is the operation of choice in an emergent situation. It is indicated in moribund patients with fulminant colitis, toxic megacolon, perforation, and patients with numerous comorbidities. It also is used for those undergoing the first of a three-stage pouch procedure who are on high-dose steroids, multiple immunosuppression drugs, malnourished, or those patients who have indeterminate colitis. Indeterminate colitis patients whom the surgeons suspect may have Crohn's disease should undergo the three-stage procedure to allow for complete pathologic evaluation of the colon. For a planned first-stage procedure, it may be an option for those patients wanting to preserve fertility. In men, the risk of damaging the pelvic nerves is reduced by entering the pelvis with active rectal inflammation. Avoiding the proctectomy in women may prevent pelvic adhesions that may affect fertility.

In an emergency situation or when the colon wall is extremely fragile with a high risk of perforation, an open operation should be performed. The lower sigmoid colon is transected with a stapler just above the sacral promontory, leaving a rectal stump. The rectal stump then is imbricated with 2-0 Vicryl Lembert sutures. A rectal tube or Foley catheter is left in the rectum to decompress the rectal stump and avoids perforation of the stump. The Hartmann's pouch may be placed extrafascial, which lowers the risk of pelvic sepsis and subsequently facilitates future pelvic dissection. This often is done by bringing the divided colonic stump up through the most inferior aspect of the fascial incision and securing the colon in place.

The specimen is submitted for pathologic diagnosis. If the pathology test shows UC, a completion proctectomy and IPAA can be planned for a future definitive operation; however, if the pathology test shows Crohn's disease and the rectum is without disease, an ileorectal anastomosis is a future consideration.

A disadvantage of this procedure is that a diseased rectum remains. The fate of the retained rectum is not well known. There is believed to be a 10% risk of developing rectal cancer, so patients will require lifelong surveillance of the stump. Other issues include seepage and bleeding. Massive bleeding is rare. If the patient has massive hemorrhage from the rectum, an urgent proctectomy is completed with the rectum divided just above the levator muscle, leaving the opportunity for future creation of an ileoanal pouch.

Total Proctocolectomy and End Ileostomy

Total proctocolectomy (TPC) and end ileostomy is a procedure with a low morbidity rate and does not carry the functional problems associated with sphincter-preserving procedures. It remains an acceptable option for elective surgery in patients who have a high risk of pouch failure (impaired anal sphincter, previous anoperineal disease, multiple comorbidities). However, patients face the physiologic and psychologic sequelae associated with an ileostomy.

Total or Subtotal Abdominal Colectomy
Laparoscopic Approach

The patient is placed in the modified lithotomy position. For the minimally invasive approach, access is secured through an umbilical port by the Hassan technique. Right-sided ports are placed under direct visualization: four fingerbreadths superomedial to the anterior superior iliac spine with a 10-mm/12-mm port and four fingerbreadths superiorly and slightly oblique to the right lower quadrant port with a 5-mm port. The right lower quadrant port may be planned at the ileostomy site. A 5-mm left-sided port is placed at the level of the sigmoid colon under direct visualization.

The omentum is swept above the transverse colon and liver. The small bowel is tucked to the right side of the abdomen. The patient is positioned in steep Trendelenburg position with right side down.

The sigmoid colon is retracted anteriorly. The inferior mesenteric artery pedicle is identified and the peritoneum is incised parallel to the pedicle and inferiorly to the sacral promontory. A window is created to isolate the pedicle through medial to lateral dissection, taking the colon and its mesentery off the retroperitoneum, while making sure to protect the gonadal vessels and the left ureter, overlying the left iliac artery. The inferior mesenteric artery pedicle can be taken with an energy-based surgical device or endo stapler. The mesentery of the colon is dissected free from Gerota's fascia up to the splenic flexure. The lateral peritoneal attachments and the white line of Toldt are divided entering the previously dissected plane up to the splenic flexure. The splenic flexure is mobilized entering the lesser sac, by incising the gastrocolic ligament in reverse Trendelenburg position, joining the previous left colon mobilization. The sigmoid colon is retracted anteriorly, pulling the rectum out of the pelvis, and the proctectomy is performed (see Proctectomy). The rest of the colon is mobilized off the greater omentum and along the white line of Toldt, while the surgeon serially takes all major mesenteric vessels with an energy-based surgical device or vascular endo stapler. A second 5-mm port placed on the left may aid in the right colectomy. Placing the patient in slight Trendelenburg with the table tilted to the left allows the surgeon to perform the mobilization of the right colon. The ileocolic artery is isolated at its origin from the superior mesenteric artery, freeing it from the duodenum and retroperitoneum. The right colon mesentery is mobilized off of the retroperitoneum, and the surgeon identifies the right ureter. The lateral peritoneal attachments are divided entering the previously dissected plane and the mesentery based on the superior mesenteric artery is completely freed up to the duodenum. The hepatic flexure is mobilized by dividing the hepatocolic ligament and omentum with a vessel-sealing device. The remainder of the colonic mesentery is divided with the vessel-sealing device and the terminal ileum is divided with an endovascular stapler. If performing an ileal J pouch, the surgeon must completely mobilize the small intestine mesentery off of the duodenum to provide maximum reach to the pelvis.

Open Approach

The colon is mobilized along the white line of Toldt, as the surgeon is careful to identify and lateralize the left ureter and gonadal vessels. The splenic flexure is mobilized, with the surgeon entering the lesser sac and either dividing the omentum below the gastroepiploic artery thereby resecting the omentum, or mobilizing the omentum off of the transverse colon in the avascular plane that exists between the two structures.

The right colon is mobilized along the white line of Toldt, identifying the right ureter and gonadal vessels. The hepatic flexure is mobilized by dividing the colohepatic ligament. Complete mobilization of the superior mesenteric artery to its base is required, completely exposing the C loop of the duodenum. This is to facilitate reach of an ileal J pouch to the anus. The mesentery to the entire colon is divided down to the sacral promontory. The terminal ileum is divided with a stapler.

Proctectomy

Laparoscopic Approach

The patient is placed in steep Trendelenburg position and tilted to the right or left depending on the side of dissection. The rectosigmoid junction is retracted anteriorly and superiorly. The superior rectal vessels are taken at the sacral promontory. The peritoneum is incised over the sacral promontory, as the surgeon takes care to identify the right and left pudendal nerves and mobilize them off of the mesorectum. The presacral space is entered and dissection is continued inferiorly in this avascular plane. Rectal mobilization is facilitated by providing adequate traction and counter traction to help identify the correct plane of dissection. Posterior mobilization of the rectum is continued down through Waldeyer's fascia to the levator sling. The lateral avascular plane is identified inferiorly in the

previously dissected presacral space. Mobilization often is completed with electrocautery or a vessel-sealing device. Lateral to the rectum, the peritoneum and endopelvic fascia are incised. Retracting the rectum inferiorly and applying counter pressure with graspers on the uterus and vagina or seminal vesicles and prostate allows for the anterior dissection. Dissection is complete at the level of the anorectal ring. This is confirmed by digital examination with cross-clamping of the distal mobilized rectum.

At this point the rectum is divided with a stapler if a J pouch anastomosis is to be performed. This can be performed either by using Endo GIA staplers or by making a small incision above the pubis to facilitate placement of a TA stapler. Great care must be taken in women to ensure the vagina is kept free from the staple line and that there is approximately 1 cm of mobilized rectum distal to the staple line to allow a safe double-stapled ileal pouch anal anastomosis. The colon and rectum then are removed through either a periumbilical or suprapubic incision. If a mucosectomy is required or the patient is undergoing an intersphincteric dissection, the perineal dissection is initiated after completing the rectal mobilization. In this case the specimen often is removed via the anus.

Closed suction drains are placed into the presacral space before the perineal dissection because pneumoperitoneum will be lost after the specimen is removed. The terminal ileum is mobilized and the ileum is brought through the abdominal wall in the right lower quadrant for maturation after the perineal phase is complete. The rest of the anorectal dissection is performed through the perineal approach.

If the surgeon requires conversion to an open procedure, every effort is made to mobilize the entire colon (may convert to hand port) and take down the mesentery before starting the proctectomy portion of the procedure. Mobilization, especially at the hepatic and splenic flexures, often is better visualized with the laparoscope.

Open Approach

The sacral promontory is identified and entered taking care to mobilize the hypogastric nerves from the mesorectal fascia. To obtain ample visualization of the adherent fibers in an open approach, a St. Mark's retractor with a lip is placed behind the posterior rectum, while a malleable retractor is used for counter traction. Dissection is continued posteriorly in the avascular plane of the presacral space. Mobilization posteriorly should continue past Waldeyer's fascia to the levator ani muscles. Lateral rectal dissection is facilitated by lateral retraction of the pelvic sidewall with the St. Mark's retractor while the surgeon places medial traction on the rectum and mesorectal fascia. The anterior dissection is completed last with use of the St. Mark's retractor to retract the anterior structures superiorly while the surgeon applies posterior pressure on the rectum. The dissection is complete with the rectum fully mobilized to the levator ani muscles. The level of division is confirmed with digital palpation through the anus while clamping the distal rectum. The rectum should be divided at a level to allow room for stapling of the pouch to the anus, typically 1 to 2 cm above the dentate line. Great care is taken not to incorporate anterior or lateral structures into the staple line. Anterior retraction with the St. Mark's retractor helps facilitate rectal division. In women, before firing a TA stapler, the surgeon should perform digital examination of the vagina to ensure the vagina is not incorporated in to the TA staple line. If a mucosectomy is required or the patient is undergoing an intersphincteric dissection, the perineal dissection is initiated after completing the rectal mobilization. When the procedure is performed open, closed suction drain placement and ileostomy creation may be performed after the perineal phase.

Perineal Approaches to Remove the Distal Rectum

These dissections are enhanced by the use of a self-retaining retractor to efface the anus. For patients who are undergoing resection with permanent ileostomy, an intersphincteric dissection of the distal rectum and anus is favored. This allows the perineum to be closed with a complete muscular tube and significantly reduces the risk of perineal wound complications. An exception is when performing the operation in a patient with a low rectal cancer in whom an abdominoperineal resection is required.

Intersphincteric Proctectomy

A Lone Star retractor or other self-retaining retractor is sutured to the perineum, and the anus is effaced. A skin incision is created in the intersphincteric groove. The intersphincteric dissection is carried out in the avascular plane, preserving the external sphincter and the levator ani muscles. This avascular plane allows for easy dissection and is initiated in the posterior aspect of the anus extending laterally, reserving the anterior dissection last. The surgeon continues in this plane proximally until the abdominal-pelvic dissection is reached and the peritoneal cavity is entered. The entire specimen is removed through the perineum. An omental pedicle flap can be rotated into the pelvis to fill the dead space if it has not been resected with the specimen. Closed suction drains are positioned in the pelvis and the perineal wound is closed in layers with all muscular layers being closed with absorbable suture.

After both abdominal and perineal incisions are closed, a Brooke ileostomy is matured in the right lower quadrant at the previously marked ileostomy site.

Complications

Postoperative complications include intestinal obstruction, delayed healing of the perineal wound, sexual dysfunction (including postoperative infertility), and issues related to the ileostomy. Patients who have a chronically draining perineal wound should be investigated for retained mucosa, foreign bodies, and Crohn's disease. Sexual dysfunction after a low pelvic dissection in men consists of impotence and retrograde ejaculation; in women, 30% complain of dyspareunia. Obstacles of having an ileostomy—dehydration, skin irritation, stomal stenosis, prolapse, hernias—exist.

Total Proctocolectomy With Ileal Pouch-Anal Anastomosis

Total proctocolectomy with ileal pouch–anal anastomosis (TPC with IPAA) is the procedure of choice for many patients with UC undergoing elective surgery. It is associated with a 19% to 27% morbidity rate, low mortality rate (0.2% to 0.4%), and a good quality of life. It eliminates all active disease, in addition to being a sphincter-preserving procedure without the emotional concerns of having an ileostomy. Patients, on average, have 8 to 12 bowel movements per day. Because stool output from the pouch is more liquid, good anal sphincter control is a prerequisite for continence. Patients who have poor anal continence are not candidates for IPAA and require an end ileostomy. In light of concomitant carcinoma of the colon and rectum, IPAA is contraindicated in metastatic disease. Adjuvant radiation therapy should be performed before pouch creation because postoperative radiotherapy is associated with radiation enteritis, poor pouch function, and consequent failure. Finally, in UC patients with cecal cancer, a long segment of distal ileum with its associated mesenteric vessel may have to be resected, precluding the formation of a tension-free IPAA.

Typically, the ultimate goal of the TPC with IPAA is accomplished through staged procedures. In a select group of patients, a single-stage procedure may be performed by an experienced surgeon. These patients are usually younger, healthier, less obese, and not on immunosuppressive agents. Furthermore, the technical aspects of the operation must be straightforward, with minimal bleeding, good blood supply to the pouch, and no tension at the anastomosis. Most often, however, patients undergo a two-stage procedure: (1) TPC with IPAA and diverting loop ileostomy, (2) reversal of the ileostomy. Those who go through a three-stage procedure—(1) subtotal colectomy and end ileostomy, (2) restorative proctectomy with ileoanal pouch anastomosis and diverting loop ileostomy, (3) reversal of ileostomy—usually are malnourished patients receiving high-dose steroids and

are too sick to undergo a total proctocolectomy. Those with fulminant colitis or toxic megacolon have been shown to have a high risk of intra-abdominal sepsis, and thus simultaneous IPAA should not be performed at the initial operation because of the high risk of pouch failure.

A laparoscopic approach for the one-stage procedure has been shown to be associated with similar length of stay, morbidity, mortality, and readmission rates when compared with the open approach. Laparoscopy produces better cosmesis but longer operative time. For the two-stage procedure, laparoscopy is associated with a shorter time to ileostomy closure, and lower adhesion formation. Therefore a laparoscopic approach is recommended. The patient's positioning and mobilization of the colon and rectum are as described above. The terminal ileum is transected flush to the cecum, making sure to preserve the ileal branch of the ileocolic vessels. The rectum is transected just above the levator ani muscle. The root of the small bowel mesentery is mobilized to the level of the ligament of Treitz.

J Pouch Creation

In the laparoscopic technique, the terminal ileum may be exteriorized through the planned diverting loop ileostomy site or a small Pfannenstiel incision. Otherwise, the J pouch is formed through the hand port or an open midline incision. The limbs of the J pouch should be 15 to 18 cm in length, and the exact length is determined by identifying which point of the antimesenteric edge of ileum provides maximal reach to the pelvis. Adequate reach for the pouch is confirmed when the distal aspect of the pouch reaches 6 cm below the pubic symphysis, without tension. Sutures are placed to approximate the antimesenteric border of the planned J pouch. A 2-cm curvilinear incision is created at base of the J. Multiple (two or three) firings of the linear stapler are used to create the J pouch. The tip of the J pouch is oversewn to prevent a leak. The mucosal border of the staple line is inspected to ensure hemostasis and is oversewn if needed (Figure 2).

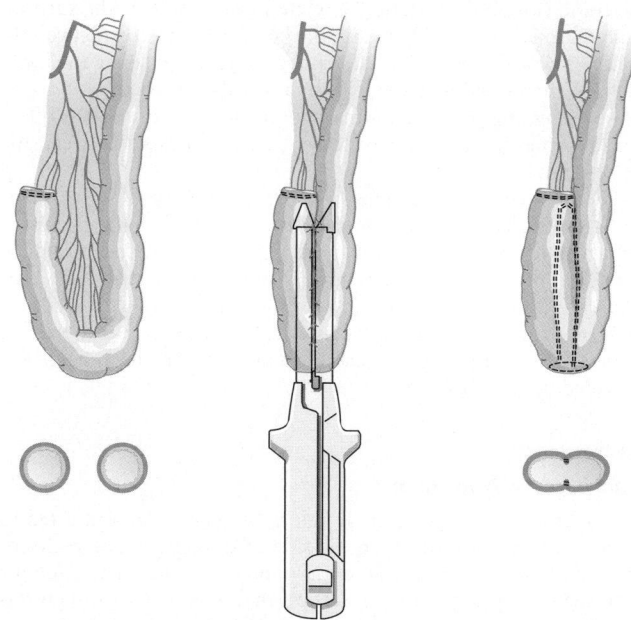

FIGURE 2 Creation of an ileal J pouch with a cutting linear stapler. For replacement of the rectum, a reservoir is created from the distal ileum. The stapler joins two limbs of intestine with staples while dividing the intervening wall. The diameter of the pouch created is twice as large as the original diameter of the ileum. (*From Townsend CM, Beauchamp RD, Evers BM, Mattox KL, editors. Sabiston Textbook of Surgery. 18th ed. Philadelphia: Elsevier Saunders; 2008, pp 1381, Fig 50-33.*)

Before creation of the anastomosis, the anorectal stump should be tested for a leak, either with an air leak test or with instillation of betadine.

Stapled Versus Handsewn Ileal Pouch Anal Anastomosis

A double-stapled pouch anal anastomosis is thought to provide better postoperative pouch function by maintaining the anal transition zone. It is our preferred method except in patients with rectal dysplasia or in patients with rectal carcinoma. In those cases mucosectomy with handsewn anastomosis is performed.

Double-Stapled Anastomosis

The curvilinear incision in which the stapler was inserted to create the J pouch is used for the ileal pouch anal anastomosis. For a double-stapled pouch anal anastomosis, the anvil is inserted into the base of the J pouch and secured with a double purse-string suture. The stapler is inserted transanally and the pin advanced posterior to the staple line of the anorectal stump to create the anastomosis (Figures 3 and 4). Great care must be taken to ensure the pouch is not twisted on its mesenteric pedicle and that the anterior structures, most commonly the vagina, are not incorporated into the anterior or lateral staple line. These are key points whether performing a laparoscopic or open procedure. A loop ileostomy then is formed 40 cm from the ileal pouch at a previously marked ileostomy site.

Mucosectomy and Handsewn Anastomosis

After the surgeon has completed the abdominal and pelvic dissection, attention is turned towards the anus. A self-retaining retractor, such as the Lone Star retractor, is secured to the perineum and the anus is effaced. The entire mucosa from the anal canal and distal rectum are removed transanally with the specimen. Normal saline or lidocaine with 1% epinephrine may be injected in the submucosal plane to aid in dissection. The mucosa is elevated with the electrocautery, generating a circular tube of tissue and initiating dissection at the dentate line. The peritoneal cavity is entered posteriorly, dividing the muscularis propria above the level of the puborectalis sling. The rectum is divided completely and the specimen is removed. The ileal pouch is grasped through the anus by using an empty sponge stick or Babcock clamp. Great care is made to keep the correct orientation of the pouch to avoid twisting the pouch on its vascular pedicle. The pouch is sutured to the anus by anastomosing to the denuded anorectal cuff with interrupted absorbable sutures. A closed suction

drain is placed in the presacral space behind the pouch and the pouch itself is drained. A loop ileostomy is formed 40 cm from the ileal pouch at the previously marked site in the right lower quadrant.

It has been suggested that the retraction and stretching of the anal canal used to perform an endoanal mucosectomy causes damage and issues with postoperative fecal incontinence. Hence, some surgeons prefer leaving the anal transitional zone epithelium without

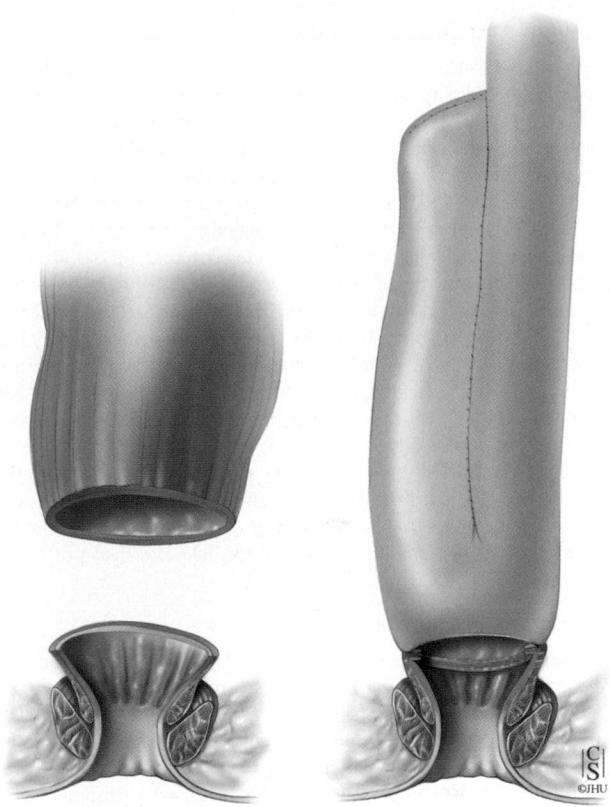

FIGURE 3 Creation of the J pouch. *(From Johns Hopkins Sidney Kimmel Comprehensive Cancer Center. <http://www.hopkinskimmelcancercenter.org/images/coloncancer/J-pouch2.jpg.> Accessed July 13, 2012.)*

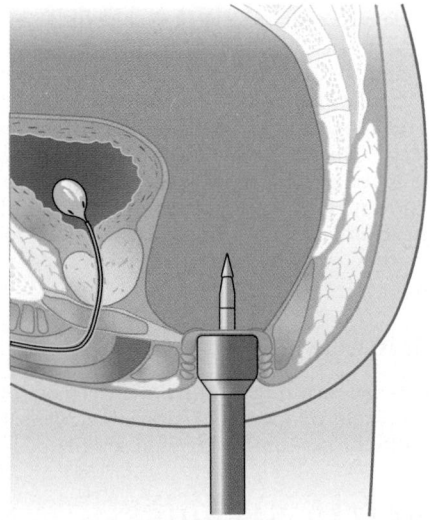
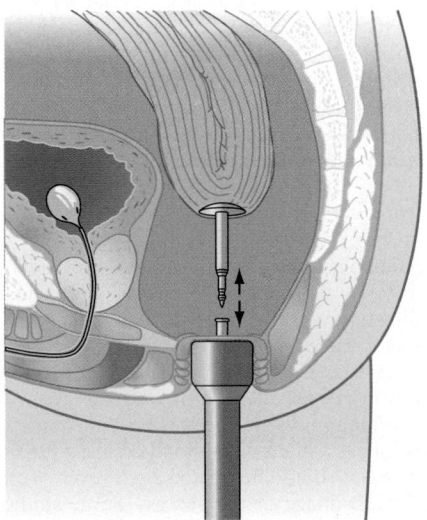

FIGURE 4 Fashioning of stapled ileal pouch–anal anastomosis. *(From Townsend CM, Beauchamp RD, Evers BM, et al, editors. Sabiston Textbook of Surgery. 18th ed. Philadelphia: Elsevier Saunders; 2008, pp 1382, Fig 50-34.)*

mucosectomy and using the double-stapled technique as described previously. The risk of the inflammation and dysplasia of the anal transitional zone left behind is low. Similarly in a mucosectomy procedure, there is a risk of inadvertently leaving small islands of mucosa. For these reasons, long-term annual examinations and biopsies are recommended for all IPAA patients, regardless of the anastomotic technique. These exams include pouchoscopy and are performed annually. Biopsies of any retained rectal cuff or suspicious areas in the ileal pouch are required.

Maneuvers to Ensure Reach of the J Pouch

The J pouch should reach comfortably, without tension to the anorectum. Maneuvers to achieve length of the ileum include complete mobilization of the superior mesenteric artery off the retroperitoneum (including mobilization off the anterior duodenum). The ileocolic artery may be divided to increase length, as the surgeon takes care to maintain collateral flow. The superior mesenteric venous pedicle may be divided with the knowledge that up to 20 cm of terminal ileum may be sacrificed because of loss of blood supply. Backlighting to outline mesenteric vessels is helpful in identifying mesenteric vessels, while the surgeon is working on the mesentery. Scoring the mesentery overlying the superior mesenteric artery helps increase the mesenteric length, as does opening mesenteric windows between collateral vessels near the border of the small intestine. After formation of the J pouch, the surgeon should wait 15 minutes to reassess viability of the J pouch.

If the J pouch still will not reach, the procedure is aborted by dropping the J pouch into the pelvis and creating a loop ileostomy. Often the pouch mesentery will stretch over time and in 6 months, the patient can be reoperated on to complete the ileal pouch anal anastomosis.

Other Types of Pouches

An S pouch has two 10- to 12-cm limbs and uses its efferent limb (end of the terminal ileum) as the anastomosis to the anus. Evacuation difficulties are high, so functional results are not as beneficial as with a J pouch. The S pouch does provide extra length and therefore is reserved for cases in which the J pouch cannot reach. A lateral isoperistaltic H pouch has a long outlet tract with similar sequelae of pouch distention, stasis, and pouchitis. A four-loop reservoir (W pouch) was developed to increase capacity; however, studies have shown there is no difference in reservoir function in terms of incontinence, urgency, and soiling, as compared to the J pouch.

Postoperative Course

Before closure of the ileostomy, the pouch should be studied to investigate for a leak, manifested by a fistula or abscess. Digital rectal examination is performed to assess sphincter tone and anastomotic stricture or defects. Endoscopy shows the course of healing of the suture lines. The pouch is studied with gastrografin to detect evidence of leak, abscess, fistulas, or sinus tracts. Only after confirmation that there is no abnormality with the pouch should the ileostomy be closed.

Complications

Small bowel obstruction occurs in 20% of patients who undergo ileal pouch operations. Patients also encounter similar issues with sexual dysfunction (including postoperative infertility) and ileostomy complications after a total proctocolectomy. Between 5% and 19% of patients have pelvic sepsis after an IPAA resulting from anastomotic dehiscence (with early or late manifestations as an abscess or fistula) or an infected pelvic hematoma. This rate may be higher and patients who have pelvic sepsis have a higher likelihood of subsequent pouch failure. Hence, pelvic sepsis should be treated aggressively with intravenous antibiotics and drainage of the abscess. Some studies have shown pouch failure rates for patients having a leak after a handsewn anastomosis to be higher than those who had a stapled anastomosis. The incidence of pouch-vaginal fistula ranges from 3% to 16%. It

requires surgical correction either through an abdominal or perineal approach. Ileoanal anastomotic stricture occurrences vary from 5% to 38%. Management includes finger dilation or repeated dilations under anesthesia and rarely a transanal approach with excision of the stricture and pouch advancement. The incidence of intraluminal or intra-abdominal hemorrhage varies from 1.5% to 3.5%, most of which occur within 7 days of surgery. The majority of cases are self-limited. If bleeding persists, irrigation of the pouch with adrenaline solution is recommended. Patients also may require endoscopy with inspection of the staple line with hemostasis maneuvers, such as cauterization, epinephrine injection, or clipping. Unstable patients must be taken to the operating room for endoscopy and possibly exploratory laparotomy.

The most frequent long-term complication is pouchitis or nonspecific inflammation of the ileal pouch. Medical management with oral metronidazole or ciprofloxacin, probiotics, and budesonide enemas are usually successful. For pouchitis that is refractory to the aforementioned medical therapy, immunosuppressive therapy is effective in 20% of cases. For those in whom all medical therapy has failed, a patient may require diversion or pouch excision.

Colectomy With Ileorectal Anastomosis

The colectomy with ileorectal anastomosis (IRA) rarely is performed for UC. A select group of patients are considered for this procedure—those who have indeterminate colitis and those who are young with good anal continence and good rectal compliance, with only mild inflammation of the rectum. It may be considered in young females who want to preserve fertility and avoid an ostomy, but it is rare to have patients with UC who require surgery but have minimal rectal inflammation. Moreover, the lack of a pelvic dissection negates the risk of sexual dysfunction. However, patients tend to have more bowel movements per day. In addition, disease and the potential for malignancy are left behind. The risk of malignancy of the rectum after IRA is approximately 10%. After IRA 25% of patients require a proctectomy resulting from severe proctitis. IRA is contraindicated in patients who have moderate to severe inflammation of the rectum, dysplasia or cancer of the rectum, perianal disease, and known anal incontinence.

Total Proctocolectomy With Continent Ileostomy (Kock's Pouch)

The continent ileostomy was introduced by Kock for patients who did not want to wear an ostomy appliance for a Brooke end ileostomy. A nipple valve is created by intussusception of a portion of ileum into the planned reservoir. The procedure has been abandoned in the management of UC because of the excellent outcomes with the ileal J pouch and the large complication rate associated with the Kock pouch. These complications include obstruction and incontinence, usually resulting from nipple valve slippage or dysfunction in 50% of patients. Patients have difficulty with catheterization of their pouch. Surgical reconstruction is the only option for repair. Approximately 25% of patients also suffer from pouchitis, 25% from intestinal obstruction, and 10% from pouch fistulas. Most patients with Kock pouches eventually require resection and formation of an end ileostomy.

■ CONCLUSION

Many options exist in the surgical management of chronic UC. An approach is tailored according to the individual patient's preferences as well as his or her comorbidity and severity of disease.

SUGGESTED READINGS

Biondi A, Zoccali M, Costa S, et al. Surgical treatment of ulcerative colitis in the biologic therapy era. *World J Gastroenterol.* 2012;18:1861-1870.

Cohen JL, Strong SA, Hyman NH, et al. Practice parameters for the surgical treatment of ulcerative colitis. *Dis Colon Rectum*. 2005;48:1997-2009.

Francone TD, Champagne B. Considerations and complications in patients undergoing ileal pouch anal anastomosis. *Surg Clin North Am*. 2013;93:107-143.

Holubar SD, Larson DW, Dozois EJ, Pattana-Arun J, Pemberton JH, Cima RR. Minimally invasive subtotal colectomy and ileal pouch-anal anastomosis for fulminant ulcerative colitis: a reasonable approach? *Dis Colon Rectum*. 2009;52:187-192.

Ross H, Steele SR, Varma M, Dykes S, Cima R, Buie WD, Rafferty J. Practice parameters for the surgical treatment of ulcerative colitis. *Dis Colon Rectum*. 2014;57:5-22.

Wick EC, Efron J. Minimally invasive rectal procedures for ulcerative colitis, rectal prolapse, and rectal cancer. *US Gastroenterol Hepatol Rev*. 2010;6:85-89.

The Management of Toxic Megacolon

Azah A. Althumairi, MD, and Jonathan E. Efron, MD

Toxic megacolon was first recognized and described as a clinical entity by Marschak in 1950. It is an infrequent, potentially life-threatening condition that results as a complication of ulcerative colitis (UC), Crohn's disease (CD), and some infectious colitides, commonly with *Clostridium difficile*–associated (pseudomembranous) disease (CDAD). Toxic megacolon results as a progression from fulminant colitis. Although fulminant colitis is not precisely defined, this term generally refers to severe inflammation of the colon with associated systemic toxicity with or without colonic dilatation. According to the diagnostic criteria of Truelove and Witts for the disease activity in UC, fulminant colitis is diagnosed by the presence of more than 10 times bloody diarrhea, heart rate higher than 90 beats/min, temperature above 37.5° C, requirement of blood transfusion, erythrocyte sedimentation rate (ESR) more than 30 mm/hr, with the presence of abdominal distension and tenderness on clinical examination, and dilated colon on x-ray. In the context of CDAD, according to the Dallal classification of CDAD severity, fulminant colitis is diagnosed by the presence of heart rate above 120 beats/min, leukocytosis with more than 30% bands, severe oliguria, and requirement of mechanical ventilator and vasopressors. Toxic megacolon is defined as segmental or total colonic distension of 6 cm in the presence of acute colitis and systemic toxicity. Radiologically, it typically exhibits dilatation of the proximal colon with thickened inflamed distal colon and associated pneumatosis. Unlike colonic obstruction, in which cecal dilation with perforation is a concern, the transverse colon is the area of greatest concern in toxic megacolon.

Given the other conditions that cause colonic destination, such as colonic pseudo-obstruction and Hirschsprung's disease, toxic megacolon is distinguished from these conditions by its systemic manifestations of toxicity. Early diagnosis and aggressive medical management are pivotal to prevent progression to the associated high morbidity and mortality. Moreover, prompt recognition of disease progression and severity and timely surgical intervention may be lifesaving.

■ CAUSE, INCIDENCE, AND PATHOGENESIS

Any inflammatory condition of the colon can result in toxic megacolon. These include inflammatory bowel disease (IBD), infectious causes including pseudomembranous colitis caused by *C. difficile* or other bacteria, such as *Salmonella, Shigella, Campylobacter,* or *Entamoeba,* and ischemic colitis (Box 1).

The incidence of toxic megacolon varies by the underlying cause. In patients with UC, it is estimated to be 5%, and the risk is higher early on in the disease. Historically, the reported incidence of CDAD ranged between 0.4% and 3%. However, with the changes

in the epidemiology of *C. difficile* infections and with emergence of new strains, there has been a 23% annual increase in the rate of hospitalizations resulting from CDAD in the United States.

The pathogenesis of the toxic dilatation of the colon is not understood fully. However, it is thought to be a result of severe inflammation of the colon that is associated with release of inflammatory mediators that induce colonic smooth muscle relaxation and inhibit colon motility. The acute severe mucosal inflammation becomes transmural and extends into the smooth muscle layer, resulting in loss of motor tone and paralysis. The severely inflamed smooth muscle produces nitric oxide, which is released into the colonic wall and further inhibits smooth muscle tone and causes dysmotility and atony. This generally causes dilatation of the colon proximal to the colonic segment that is severely inflamed. The toxic systemic response results from bacterial translocation and subsequent bacteremia.

Several other factors, such as hypokalemia, hypomagnesemia, opiates, anticholinergic or antimotility agents, antidepressants, barium enemas, and colonoscopy may affect adversely colonic motility and exacerbate colon dilatation.

■ DIAGNOSIS

The diagnosis of toxic megacolon is based on both clinical and radiologic findings. Therefore a thorough history and physical examination are crucial. The diagnosis must be suspected in patients who have diarrhea, abdominal distension, and signs of systemic toxicity.

The patient's history typically reveals symptoms of severe colitis that preceded the acute onset of colonic dilatation. These include severe diarrhea (usually bloody), abdominal pain, fever, chills, and tachycardia. Obtaining a history about a previous diagnosis of IBD with the extent of colonic involvement and medical therapy and recent use of antibiotic or other medications such as steroid, antimotility, and chemotherapeutic agents will help in determining the underlying cause.

Physical examination reveals significant localized or generalized abdominal tenderness and reduced bowel sounds accompanied with signs of systemic toxicity, such as fever, tachycardia, and hypotension. Presence of signs of peritonitis may indicate colonic perforation. However, it is not uncommon that the abdominal signs are masked by steroid treatment in patients being treated with high-dose steroids.

The best acceptable clinical criteria for the diagnosis of toxic megacolon were described by Jalan et al in 1969. The presence of three of the following criteria is required for the clinical diagnosis: fever higher than 101.5° F (38.6° C), heart rate higher than 120 beats/min, white blood cell count above 10.5 ($\times 10^9$/L), or anemia. In addition, patients should have one of the following criteria: dehydration, mental changes, electrolyte disturbances, or hypotension.

Plain abdominal x-ray is useful in making the diagnosis as well as following the disease course and the rate of colon expansion. It typically shows dilatation of the ascending and transverse colon that varies from 6 cm up to 15 cm. Once the transverse colon is dilated past 8 cm, there should be great concern for pending perforation. Other radiologic features include presence of air fluid levels and the

BOX 1: Causes of Toxic Megacolon

Most Common

Ulcerative colitis
Clostridium difficile–associated colitis

Less Common

Crohn's disease
Salmonella
Shigella
Campylobacter
Yersinia
Cytomegalovirus
Entamoeba histolytica
Cryptosporidium
Ischemia colitis
Chemotherapy
Colonoscopy
Barium enema
Drugs that slow colonic motility (narcotics, antidiarrheal drugs, anticholinergic drugs)

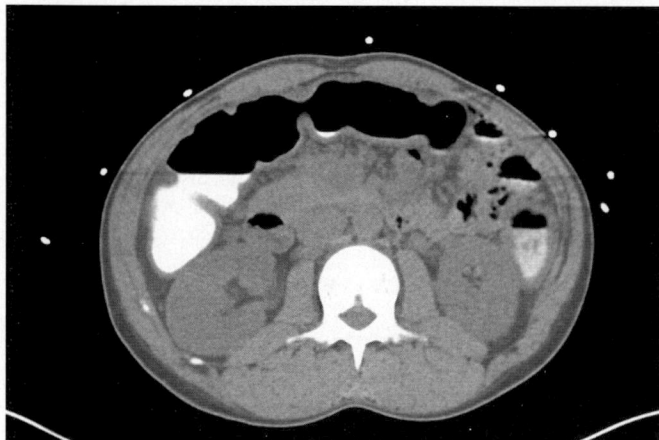

FIGURE 1 Computed tomography scan of the abdomen showing dilated and thickened wall of the colon.

TABLE 1: Laboratory Tests for the Diagnosis of *Clostridium difficile* Infection

Test	Sensitivity	Specificity
Cell cytotoxicity assays	60%-100%	96%-99%
Cell culture neutralization assay	67%-86%	97%-100%
Enzymatic detection of glutamate dehydrogenase	71%-91%	76%-98%
Enzyme immunoassay tests for toxins A and B	39%-76%	84%-100%
Nucleic acid amplification test for toxins A and B	84%-100%	94%-100%

loss of normal haustral pattern in the colon with thickening and edema of colonic wall. Small bowel and gastric distension may be seen as well, and they have been shown to be a significant predictor of toxic megacolon and progression to multisystem organ dysfunction in UC.

Computed tomography (CT) scan of the abdomen and pelvis is useful in confirming the diagnosis, excluding other causes of colonic dilatation, such as obstructing colonic cancer or diverticular stricture, and helping to exclude other abdominal complications, such as colonic perforation and ascending pyelophlebitis. Presence of colonic wall thickening, submucosal edema, pericolic stranding, and thickened haustra are indicative of severe colitis. In addition, the presence of dilatation of the transverse colon (greater than 6 to 8 cm) confirms the diagnosis of toxic megacolon (Figure 1).

Laboratory tests are not specific and show the findings of systemic inflammatory response with leukocytosis, anemia, elevated erythrocyte sedimentation rate or serum C-reactive protein, and electrolyte abnormalities with hypokalemia, hypomagnesemia, and hypoalbuminemia. These findings, if not corrected, may exacerbate the condition.

Stool sample for culture, sensitivity, and *C. difficile* toxin assay should be sent as well as blood culture because bacteremia occurs in up to 25% of patients with toxic megacolon. Several tests to detect

C. difficile are available. Sensitivity and specificity of each test vary; therefore it is recommended to perform a two-stage test approach to improve the diagnosis accuracy. Stool culture is highly sensitive; however, it does not differentiate between the presence of *Clostridium* bacteria and active infection. It generally is used in conjunction with other diagnostic tests. Other diagnostic tests with their sensitivity and specificity are listed in Table 1. The commonly used two-stage test approach includes initial screening with glutamate dehydrogenase assay followed by confirmation of a positive test with cell cytotoxicity assay. Some centers use toxin B gene PCR testing with nucleic acid amplification test as a single test to diagnose *C. difficile*.

Limited endoscopy may be considered to determine the cause of toxic megacolon in patients who are not known to have IBD. It can differentiate between the infectious causes of toxic megacolon because the finding of pseudomembranes is suggestive of CDAD, whereas the presence of inclusion bodies in the biopsies indicates cytomegalovirus (CMV) colitis as an underlying cause. It should be performed with extreme caution, without bowel preparation, and with minimal air insufflation; the endoscope should be advanced only as far as necessary to make a diagnosis. Complete colonoscopy should not be performed because of the high risk of perforation.

■ THERAPY

Management of toxic megacolon requires coordination between medical and surgical services with aggressive attempts of medical therapy and early surgical intervention in the absence of improvement, development of complications, or deterioration.

Medical Therapy

Regardless of the underlying cause of toxic megacolon, immediate aggressive supportive management in an intensive care unit must be initiated.

There is no evidence to support the use of nasogastric tube decompression because it does not decompress the colon. Frequent patient repositioning has been described as a method of colon decompression based on the observation that gas tends to accumulate in the transverse colon if the patient remains in the prone position and may be redistributed to the distal colon and rectum with frequent repositioning. There is no strong evidence to support use of this technique; however, it is simple and may be attempted.

Complete bowel rest with adequate intravenous fluid replacement is required. Electrolyte abnormalities, especially hypokalemia, dehydration, and anemia can exacerbate colonic dysmotility and must be corrected aggressively. Any medications that affect colonic motility, such as opiates, antimotility agents, and anticholinergics should be discontinued immediately. Prophylaxis for deep venous thrombosis and gastric ulcer should be administered. Broad-spectrum

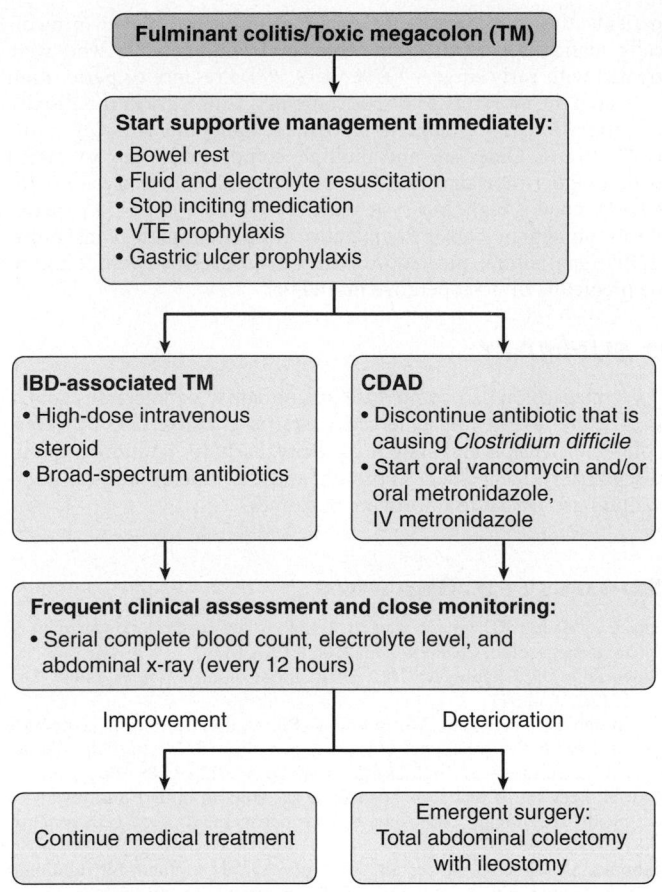

FIGURE 2 Management algorithm for toxic megacolon.

Intravenous metronidazole is also acceptable. If a patient cannot tolerate oral vancomycin because of severe ileus, it may be administered via an enema or nasogastric tube.

Surgical Therapy

Timing of surgical intervention is paramount in decreasing the morbidity and mortality of toxic megacolon and improving the patient's overall outcome. Medical management has been reported to be effective and successful in 50% to 70% of patients with toxic megacolon. However, delay in surgical intervention carries the risk of development of abdominal complications such as colonic perforation and abdominal compartment syndrome, which increases the mortality rate from 9% to 40%.

The possible need for surgical intervention and the nature of surgery must be discussed with patients and their families on admission. All patients must be evaluated and marked by a stoma therapist, who should mark the best site of an end ileostomy if needed.

Surgery is absolutely indicated in the presence of progressive colonic dilatation, uncontrolled hemorrhage, development of complications such as free perforation, and with general clinical deterioration. This includes progressive sepsis with continued tachycardia, hypotension, or the need for presser agents to maintain blood pressure. Lack of improvement within 48 hours is also a relative indication for surgical intervention. It is better to proceed to the operating room sooner as opposed to later, and any of the previously mentioned findings should push the surgeon to operate.

Mechanical bowel preparation is contraindicated, and the surgery typically is performed through an open approach for two reasons. The significant colon dilatation and friability of the colonic wall do not allow for a workable space or graspable tissue and therefore preclude a laparoscopic approach. The patient is often unstable and needs significant resuscitation from sepsis, requiring a quick efficient operation.

The current surgical standard of care for patients with toxic megacolon who require surgery is total colectomy with end ileostomy. This removes the diseased colon and allows restoration of intestinal continuity after patient recovery. The rectum should not be resected at the time of this emergent operation, despite how inflamed it may appear. The bowel is often fragile with a high likelihood of intraoperative perforation with manipulation resulting from the significant dilatation and inflammatory process, and thus it should be handled with extra care. During hepatic and splenic flexures mobilization, the colonic mesentery is divided close to the bowel wall to avoid damage to retroperitoneal structures.

The rectal stump may be severely inflamed and therefore difficult to manage. If the rectosigmoid junction appears too inflamed to hold staples or sutures, then the surgeon should leave a short segment of sigmoid colon to form a mucous fistula to decompress the remaining colon and rectum. In obese patients the rectal stump may be brought through the inferior aspect of the midline fascial incision and left buried in the subcutaneous space. This will be removed at time of stoma reversal, and if the stump blows out, it allows for decompression through the wound as opposed to in the peritoneal cavity. If a rectal stump is left in the peritoneal cavity, it should be decompressed in the operating room with a rectal tube that is left in place to allow for further postoperative decompression and possible vancomycin enemas. Drains should be left on top of the stump. A rectal stump leak typically occurs 5 to 10 days after surgery; therefore if a patient manifests signs of peritonitis 5 to 7 days after surgery after initially recovering well, the surgeon should have a high suspicion for rectal leak. Emergent return to the operating room with washout and drainage is necessary.

Postoperative care requires transferring the patient to an intensive care unit, where all supportive measures are continued as needed. Preoperative antibiotics are discontinued within 24 hours, and intravenous steroids are tapered to a maintenance dose (equivalent of 10 to 20 mg of prednisone per day). On restoration of gastrointestinal

antibiotics were found to reduce the mortality from septic complications that result from associated bacteremia or colonic perforation and should be initiated, while discontinuing any agent that may have led to *C. difficile* overgrowth. Frequent clinical assessment and close monitoring with physical examination, serial complete blood counts, electrolyte monitoring, and abdominal x-rays must be performed (Figure 2).

Management of Patients With Inflammatory Bowel Disease

High-dose intravenous steroid (hydrocortisone 100 mg every 6 hours) should be administered immediately to patients known to have IBD who have symptoms of fulminant colitis to prevent progression to toxic megacolon. There is no evidence that the steroid therapy increases the risk of perforation; however, it may mask the signs of colonic perforation, so again close surveillance is required.

Aminosalicylic acid products are used in mild to moderate cases of UC; however, there are no data to support their benefit in toxic megacolon. Similarly, cyclosporine and anti-tumor necrosis factor-alpha (TNF-α) are immunosuppressant medications used in severe cases of UC, but they have no role in the treatment of toxic megacolon.

Management of Patients With *Clostridium difficile*–Associated Disease

If toxic megacolon is thought to be caused by CDAD, the antibiotics thought to have initiated the *C. difficile* infection should be withdrawn immediately, and treatment with oral vancomycin (125 to 500 mg four times a day) and/or oral metronidazole (200 to 500 mg four times a day, or 500 to 750 mg three times a day) is initiated.

motility, enteral feeding is given. The rectal tube is removed on the fifth to seventh postoperative day.

An alternative, less invasive, colon-preserving surgical approach for the treatment of CDAD has been described recently. In a case-controlled study, Neal et al treated 42 patients with creation of loop ileostomy after visual assessment of colon viability. Intraoperatively, colonic lavage with 8 L of warmed polyethylene glycol 3350/electrolyte solution was performed via the ileostomy and drained via rectal tube. Postoperatively, patients received antegrade vancomycin enema (500 mg in 500 mL of Lactated Ringer's every 8 hours for 10 days) via the efferent limb of the ileostomy. All patients received intravenous metronidazole (500 mg every 8 hour for 10 days). These patients were compared with matching historical controls treated with total colectomy and end ileostomy. In the study cohort, 35 (83%) cases were performed laparoscopically. The colon was pre-served in 39 (93%) patients, and subsequent colectomy was required for continued sepsis in one patient and for abdominal compartment syndrome in two patients. When compared with a historical popula-tion, mortality was reduced from 50% to 19%.

Although this novel surgical approach may represent a less inva-sive surgical treatment with promising outcomes, the results of this study are limited by the retrospective nature and lack of randomiza-tion that introduce a selection bias. Furthermore, there are no clear criteria to suggest which patient may benefit from this approach. Finally, the results were never reproduced by other investigators. The 2015 practice parameters of the American Society of Colon and Rectal Surgeons for the management of *C. difficile* infection consid-ered that the evidence of this approach is weak and strongly recom-mend the standard of care surgical approach (subtotal colectomy with end ileostomy). This novel less invasive technique should not be considered in the severely septic patient requiring significant (presser or ventilatory) support.

■ OUTCOMES

The mortality rates from IBD-associated toxic megacolon have changed dramatically over the years. In an early review (1976) of 604 patients, the overall mortality was 19%, and it was higher in medi-cally managed patients when compared with patients who were treated with early surgery (27% vs 19.5%). Presence of perforation increased the mortality to 41.5% compared with 8.8% in the absence of perforation. In more recent reports, mortality rate after colectomy is 2% to 5%. Older age and multiple comorbidities are associated with a higher mortality rate. The mortality rate after colectomy for CDAD remains high. In a systematic review (2009) of 1433 patients, it was found to be 41.3%. Preoperative intubation, acute renal failure, multiorgan failure, and requirement of vasopressors were found to be predictors of postoperative mortality.

■ SUMMARY

Toxic megacolon can complicate inflammatory or infectious colitis. It is a life-threatening emergency that is characterized by severe colonic distension and systemic toxicity. Early recognition, a multi-disciplinary management approach, and the time of surgical inter-vention are crucial to improving outcomes.

SUGGESTED READINGS

Ausch C, Madoff RD, Gnant M, et al. Aetiology and surgical management of toxic megacolon. *Colorectal Dis.* 2006;8:195-201.
Autenrieth DM, Baumgart DC. Toxic megacolon. *Inflamm Bowel Dis.* 2012;18:584-591.
Carchman EH, Peitzman AB, Simmons RL, et al. The role of acute care surgery in the treatment of severe, complicated *Clostridium difficile*-associated disease. *J Trauma Acute Care Surg.* 2012;73:789-800.
Gan SI, Beck PL. A new look at toxic megacolon: an update and review of incidence, etiology, pathogenesis, and management. *Am J Gastroenterol.* 2003;98:2363-2371.
Klobuka AJ, Markelov A. Current status of surgical treatment for fulminant *Clostridium difficile* colitis. *World J Gastrointest Surg.* 2013;5:167-172.
Neal MD, Alverdy JC, Hall DE, et al. Diverting loop ileostomy and colonic lavage: an alternative to total abdominal colectomy for the treatment of severe, complicated Clostridium difficile associated disease. *Ann Surg.* 2011;254:423-427, discussion 427-429.

THE MANAGEMENT OF CROHN'S COLITIS

James W. Fleshman, MD, and Walter R. Peters, MD

Initially described as a transmural inflammatory process of the terminal ileum, Crohn's disease now is recognized to involve any part of the gastrointestinal (GI) tract. It is a chronic disease state that has no cure, and thus all treatment is directed at amelioration of symptoms and preservation of bowel function. The Montreal Classification of 2005 defines the distribution of Crohn's disease as ileal, colonic, ileocolic, or isolated upper intestinal. This chapter focuses on the surgical management of Crohn's disease involving the colon.

■ CLINICAL FEATURES

The cause of Crohn's disease is not yet completely understood, but it is increasingly clear that the disease results from the complex inter-action of genetic predisposition, environmental factors, the gut microflora, and intestinal immune function. From the physician's standpoint, Crohn's disease is fascinating because of the myriad clini-cal presentations and the variability in the distribution and behavior of the disease. From a patient's standpoint, it is an unremitting process that can affect quality of life greatly.

There is a bimodal distribution of age of onset with one peak in the 20s and 30s and a second peak around 60 years. The Montreal Classification characterizes the behavior of Crohn's disease as stric-turing, penetrating, or nonstricturing/nonpenetrating. It may be an obstructing process resulting from fibrosis with subsequent stricture formation; as a penetrating process with development of an abscess, fistula, or free perforation; or as an acute inflammatory process with pain, sepsis, and bleeding. Regardless of the distribution and behav-ior of the intestinal component of the process, many patients have anal manifestations of the disease, including fissures, ulcerations, strictures, abscesses, fistulae, and large skin tags. The incidence of perianal disease is higher in patients with colonic Crohn's disease than with more proximal disease. Perianal disease may represent the initial manifestation of Crohn's, and the presence of large, thick skin tags, fissures off of the midline, and complex fistulae should raise suspicion and prompt further evaluation.

In evaluation of a patient with Crohn's colitis, it is helpful to categorize the activity of the disease as acute/severe, acute fulminant, active/chronic, chronic, or dormant. This helps determine the urgency of care needed to appropriately respond to the patient's symptoms.

In addition to intestinal disease, Crohn's disease is associated with many extraintestinal manifestations, including pyoderma gangreno-sum, erythema nodosum, ankylosing spondylitis, and sclerosing cholangitis. The mechanism for these associations is not understood fully, but it has been observed that some of these conditions may improve with resection of the active intestinal disease, whereas others may not.

■ DIAGNOSIS

Crohn's disease remains a clinical diagnosis supported by other findings; no pathognomonic marker exists. Symptoms of Crohn's colitis include cramping abdominal pain associated with bloody diarrhea, fever, tenesmus, peritonitis, ileus, weight loss, anorexia, obstipation, and partial large or small bowel obstruction. Endoscopic findings may include either continuous or discontinuous pattern of inflammation (skip areas), rectal sparing, strictures, and longitudinal ulcers or fissuring. Histologic findings are often nonspecific, with crypt abscesses, destroyed mucosa, transmural inflammation, and ulceration and deep fissures to the serosa. Only a minority of biopsies demonstrate granulomas. Associated laboratory findings are nondiagnostic and include an elevated C-reactive protein or erythrocyte sedimentation rate, anemia, iron deficiency, and hypoalbuminemia.

In patients with evidence of small bowel or anal disease as well as colonic disease, differentiation from ulcerative colitis (UC) is simplified. For patients with isolated colonic disease, it is often impossible to be certain if the diagnosis is Crohn's disease or UC. The term *indeterminate colitis* has been used for these patients. Even when the entire colon is available for histologic evaluation, a definitive diagnosis sometimes cannot be made. The diagnosis is especially difficult to make when the disease is in a fulminant state, as defined by fever, abdominal pain, or local peritonitis, elevated white blood cell count (>16,000), and severe diarrhea tapering to obstipation as the situation worsens. Crohn's colitis can involve the entire colon and rectum, and the typical intermittent distribution with skip lesions may not be present when the disease is most severe. The presence of associated anal disease does not exist in UC and helps distinguish Crohn's from UC.

Commonly used serologic markers include antibodies against *Saccharomyces cerevisiae* (ASCA) and perinuclear antineutrophil cytoplasmic antibodies (p-ANCA). A pattern of ASCA positive and p-ANCA negative is suggestive of a diagnosis of Crohn's disease but is less than 100% specific, especially in the setting of indeterminate colitis. Therefore the surgeon often will be faced with a degree of uncertainty as to the precise diagnosis while planning intervention for what may be Crohn's colitis.

Few patients initially have fulminant colitis, but there is no set of predisposing factors for fulminant colitis. The old axiom of barium enema in a patient with active colitis causing severe fulminant colitis is historical. Antidiarrheal medications may contribute in the same way by slowing passage of stool.

■ MEDICAL MANAGEMENT

Medical management of Crohn's has changed dramatically over the past three decades with the emergence of new therapeutic agents. The use of 5-aminosalicylate medications, topical corticosteroids, and oral corticosteroids decreased with the advent of anti-TNF-α blockers and the increasing use of azathioprine. A nationwide cohort study in Denmark demonstrated a decreased risk for initial major abdominal or minor anorectal surgery that paralleled this shift in medical management (Rungoe et al, 2014). It is unclear whether the lifetime risk of surgery will decrease or whether surgery only will be postponed. Newer biologic agents targeting α-4 integrin such as natalizumab and vedolizumab may further contribute to improved medical outcomes and a decrease in the need for surgical intervention. It is possible that improved medical therapy may, in the future, change the relative frequency of the various complications of Crohn's disease that necessitate surgical intervention.

Interpretation of older literature regarding the behavior of Crohn's disease after surgical intervention also must take into consideration the potential impact of these newer agents on patients who have an indication for surgery. It is possible that improved medical therapy will significantly alter the likelihood of that patient requiring surgical treatment for recurrent disease in the future.

The new medications introduced into the armamentarium for Crohn's disease have not increased the difficulty or morbidity of surgical intervention. All of these biologic medications can be used without increasing the risk of poor wound healing or anastomotic leaks.

■ SURGICAL MANAGEMENT

Surgical resection of Crohn's disease never can be considered a curative therapy. It is important therefore for the surgeon to clearly identify the indication for surgery and to clarify the anticipated benefit to the patient. The type and extent of the operative procedure will be determined best by consideration of the physiologic condition of the patient, the goal of surgical intervention and the natural history of the disease, especially the potential need for future surgical intervention. Although intestinal preservation is emphasized in the treatment of small bowel Crohn's disease, only preservation of the rectum and anal sphincter is emphasized in the surgical management of Crohn's colitis. Salvage or sparing of the normal segments of the colon is not as important. Even so, the ability to preserve the right colon in a patient with short small intestine can make the difference between the requirement for intravenous supplementation of fluid and the ability to rely on oral intake to maintain homeostasis.

Indications for Surgery

Massive Lower Gastrointestinal Bleeding

It is rare for a patient with colonic Crohn's disease to have massive lower GI bleeding that would require urgent surgical intervention. Severe bleeding in a patient with Crohn's disease more commonly is due to an associated condition, such as gastritis or peptic ulcer disease. Anemia resulting from hematochezia and chronic disease is a more typical presentation. In the case of severe lower GI blood loss, initial intervention should focus on hemodynamic resuscitation and attempts to localize the source of the bleeding with nuclear medicine bleeding scans, angiography, or colonoscopy. As with other causes of lower GI bleeding, localization of the site of bleeding may allow a more limited surgical resection. Hemorrhage from small intestinal Crohn's disease is localized best with angiography and may be treated with highly selective embolization. In the case of Crohn's colitis complicated by severe hemorrhage, diagnosis is best made by careful colonoscopic evaluation. This may be of limited value, however, because it is most likely that a total abdominal colectomy will be necessary because the bleeding is likely to be diffuse. The decision to perform an anastomosis, an end ileostomy, or an anastomosis protected by an ileostomy will depend on many factors, including the hemodynamic stability of the patient, the extent of resection required, the nutritional status of the patient, and the use of chronic steroids or immunosuppression.

Severe Colitis, Fulminant Colitis, and Toxic Megacolon

Initial treatment of severe pancolitis should consist of hemodynamic resuscitation, broad-spectrum antibiotics, and bowel rest. The patient must be evaluated for the existence of an indication for urgent operation such as diffuse peritonitis, free intraperitoneal air, or unstable hemodynamics unresponsive to fluid resuscitation. Frequent reevaluations must be performed until the patient's condition clearly has improved or until there is evidence of deterioration, in which case urgent surgery is indicated. If urgent or emergent resection of fulminant colitis is required, a total abdominal colectomy with creation of end-ileostomy is the procedure of choice. In such an unstable patient, an anastomosis carries an unacceptable risk of leak.

Proctectomy is usually not necessary to control the acute colitis and would add significant time to the procedure and expose the patient to substantial additional morbidity. There is some debate as to the optimal management of the distal rectal segment. One option is to leave the stapled end of the distal segment in the subcutaneous tissue in an attempt to minimize the consequences of a leak from the rectal staple line. This approach, however, requires leaving a longer distal segment and may be technically difficult. A frequent result, in our experience, is a draining mucus fistula in the lower abdomen resulting from breakdown of the sigmoid closure. An alternative approach is to divide the upper rectum at the level of the sacral promontory and leave a rectal tube in place to decompress the shorter rectal stump.

Histologic evaluation of the entire resected colon may allow confirmation of the diagnosis. Further definitive surgery, either completion proctectomy or ileorectal anastomosis, then can be performed electively at a later date in a fully evaluated and optimally prepared patient.

In the absence of an indication for emergent surgery, the patient should be started on a course of intense medical management with IV fluids, bowel rest, and nutritional support. *C. difficile*, cytomegalovirus, and other infectious causes should be ruled out with stool testing. Extremely cautious sigmoidoscopy undertaken with minimal insufflation will assess the nature and severity of the colitis. Slowing agents and narcotics should be avoided to minimize the risk of toxic dilation of the colon. Treatment with IV corticosteroids or biologic agents should be initiated in an attempt to induce remission of the colitis. Broad-spectrum antibiotic coverage should be added if the patient exhibits fever, leukocytosis, or other signs of sepsis. The patient must be monitored closely for any signs of progressive deterioration, such as worsening pain or tenderness, progressive leukocytosis, fever, tachycardia, or hypotension. If no improvement in the clinical condition is noted over the first 3 to 5 days of intense medical therapy, or if there is any evidence of worsening, urgent surgery is indicated. It is important to intervene decisively before perforation of the colon. Morbidity and mortality are increased in patients who undergo surgery only after having a colonic perforation. As noted previously, total abdominal colectomy with ileostomy is the treatment of choice for severe, fulminant Crohn's colitis.

Stricture and Obstruction

Long-standing colonic Crohn's disease may produce significant fibrosis, leading to the development of strictures. These strictures may extend over varying lengths and may or may not produce symptoms of obstruction. These strictures typically do not respond well to attempts at colonoscopic dilatation, and aggressive attempts at balloon dilation may result in colonic perforation. Symptomatic strictures should be resected with the extent of resection (segmental or total colectomy) determined by the extent of Crohn's disease in the remaining portions of the colon and small intestine. It is important to recognize the increased risk of adenocarcinoma of the colon developing in chronically inflamed colonic mucosa. Approximately 7% of colonic strictures will harbor an occult adenocarcinoma. Even if asymptomatic, consideration should be given to resection of colonic strictures because of the difficulty in diagnosing these cancers. This is especially a concern with strictures that cannot be surveyed colonoscopically because of a more distal stricture. As in patients with UC, the risk of cancer is greatest in patients with long-standing extensive disease.

There are several reports of the use of self-expanding metallic stents in the treatment of strictures resulting from Crohn's disease. Most cases involve anastomotic strictures, in which the risk of malignancy is much less than in a colonic stricture because of long-standing fibrotic disease. Stenting has been reported to successfully treat anastomotic strictures but has a significant risk of stent migration. It is possible that the development of novel stents, either biodegradable or drug-eluting, may make this approach more attractive.

Perforation, Fistulae, and Abscess

Colonic perforation resulting from Crohn's disease may manifest as a free perforation, a pericolonic abscess or a fistula to the small bowel, duodenum, bladder, ureter, vagina, fallopian tube, or abdominal wall. Except for the rare situation of a free perforation with diffuse peritonitis, surgical intervention should be undertaken only in an optimally prepared patient by a surgeon prepared for a complex, multiorgan procedure. Attention should be given to optimizing the patient's nutritional status with oral supplements or total parenteral nutrition, if necessary. Active infection should be controlled by appropriate use of antibiotics and percutaneous drainage of abscesses. The patient should be offered preoperative education about the potential need for an ostomy, and all possible stoma sites should be marked before surgery. The extent of the Crohn's disease should be defined preoperatively with imaging and colonoscopy. The extent of the colonic resection will be determined by the extent and location of the inflammatory process. For patients with pelvic or retroperitoneal abscesses or those with fistulae involving pelvic organs, ureteral stents are helpful in the identification of ureteral injures.

In the case of fistulae between two segments of bowel, it is important to recognize whether there is active Crohn's disease present. If both segments of bowel have active disease, resection of both segments is indicated. Often, however, a segment of diseased bowel will perforate and create a fistula to an adjacent loop of otherwise normal bowel. This commonly is seen when diseased terminal ileum creates a fistula to an otherwise normal sigmoid colon. In this situation, resection of the ileum and repair of the secondarily involved sigmoid colon is an appropriate option.

In the uncommon situation of a free colonic perforation, emergent surgery must be undertaken with a primary goal of removing the source of sepsis, the perforated segment. The extent of resection will depend on the extent of disease activity in the rest of the large bowel but will most likely require a total abdominal colectomy. Anastomosis is unlikely to be appropriate in this setting, and the patient should be counseled to expect an ileostomy and be marked for such preoperatively.

Neoplasia

The incidence of colorectal cancer in patients with Crohn's disease is at least two to three times that of the general population. Current clinical practice guidelines published by the American Society of Colon and Rectal Surgeons call for routine colonoscopic surveillance in patients with Crohn's colitis, beginning no later than 8 years after diagnosis and continuing every 1 to 3 years. Patients with primary sclerosing cholangitis, a family history of colorectal cancer, inflammatory pseudopolyps, strictures, or ongoing inflammation may warrant more frequent evaluation. Sporadic adenomas may occur in patients with Crohn's disease and may be managed, as would an adenomatous polyp in any other patient. The finding of a nonadenomatous dysplasia-associated lesion or mass is an indication for resection of the colon because the risk of an associated cancer may be as high as 40%.

Extracolonic Manifestations of Crohn's Disease

There are a variety of extraintestinal manifestations of Crohn's disease. Some of these conditions, such as pyoderma gangrenosum and erythema nodosum, are likely to improve after resection of the active intestinal disease. Other manifestations, such as primary sclerosing cholangitis and ankylosing spondylitis, seem to progress independent of the status of the intestinal disease. For patients in whom the extraintestinal symptoms are sufficiently severe, resection of the active intestinal disease may be considered with the goal of controlling the extraintestinal manifestation.

Operations for Crohn's Colitis

Diversion

Internal bypass of symptomatic Crohn's disease is rarely an appropriate intervention. Only in the case of intense inflammation that would make resection hazardous, internal diversion with a bypass may be used as a temporizing procedure to allow for resolution of the inflammatory process before definitive resection. Permanent bypass leaves inflamed tissue at risk for malignant degeneration. Fecal diversion with an ileostomy or colostomy may be performed for temporary control of severe symptoms of colonic or anal Crohn's disease in selected patients who are unwilling to undergo definitive resection or who are in poor physiologic condition for major surgery. Fecal diversion occasionally results in clinical remission of the active inflammation, but only a minority of patients maintain that remission on restoration of intestinal continuity. Diversion should be used as a temporizing measure only in anticipation of definitive resection or local management of anorectal fistulae by means of flap advancement or transfer of muscle or skin into the diseased area.

Segmental Colectomy or Total Abdominal Colectomy With Anastomosis

Patients with rectal sparing may undergo a segmental colectomy, total abdominal colectomy, or total proctocolectomy. The risk of recurrent disease necessitating further surgery after a segmental or total colectomy must be weighed against the additional morbidity of a proctectomy and the impact of an ileostomy on quality of life. For patients with multiple segments of colonic disease, total proctocolectomy generally has been favored. For disease isolated to a single segment, segmental resection has been accepted as an appropriate alternative. In light of the introduction of newer biologic agents for the medical treatment of recurrent disease, it is possible that previous estimates of the likelihood of recurrence requiring surgery may be overstated, lending further support to the selective use of segmental resection.

For patients undergoing a total abdominal colectomy with ileorectal anastomosis, care must be taken to avoid kinking the small intestine, leading to early postoperative partial small bowel obstruction. Although the anastomosis can be performed with a circular stapler in an end-to-end or end-to-side manner, we prefer a functional end-to-end anastomosis created with a 75-mm linear cutter stapler because it results in an anastomosis with a larger cross-sectional area that may help prevent partial obstruction at the level of the anastomosis. We also have noted that it is not unusual for patients with an ileorectal anastomosis to develop a prolonged secondary ileus that has been termed the "ileorectal syndrome." The presence of an intact and functional anal sphincter just 12 to 15 cm distal to the ileum may increase the intraluminal pressure in the ileum, resulting in the physiologic changes found in an acute small bowel obstruction or an obstructed ileostomy. These changes include increased intraluminal fluid secretion and powerful muscular contractions in the bowel proximal to the anastomosis. The functional end-to-end anastomosis may allow greater rectal distension by splitting the circular muscle layer of the rectum over the length of the anastomosis, thus reducing the pressure within the distal ileum.

Total Proctocolectomy With End Ileostomy

Most patients with extensive colonic and rectal Crohn's disease will undergo total proctocolectomy with end ileostomy. The decision to perform the procedure in one or two stages will be based on the urgency of the procedure and the physiologic condition of the patient. Special care should be taken to avoid injury to the nerves of sexual function (the hypogastric nerves at the pelvic brim, the sympathetic nerves at the base of the inferior mesenteric artery (IMA), and the parasympathetic plexi deep in the pelvis). Ureteral stents may be helpful to identify and protect the ureters if there has been significant pelvic inflammation, hydronephrosis, or prior resections.

The importance of perioperative nursing care to the patient's recovery cannot be overstated. Preoperative education and site marking by a nurse trained in ostomy care will improve the patient's postoperative quality of life and rate of recovery. Studies have documented that up to a third of patients with a new ileostomy will require readmission to the hospital within 30 days of surgery. The most common complication leading to readmission is dehydration. Perioperative education and enhanced recovery care plans have been shown to be an effective means of decreasing the incidence of readmission.

Proctectomy

In patients who have undergone total abdominal colectomy with end ileostomy for Crohn's colitis, the clinical status of the retained rectum will determine the next step in their surgical care. For patients who are asymptomatic and satisfied with the quality of life offered by their ileostomy, there is no urgent need to resect the rectum. However, the retained rectal mucosa does have an increased risk for malignancy, and there are no published evidence-based guidelines for surveillance. The development of symptoms of bleeding, pain, or mucus discharge warrants evaluation with proctoscopy or flexible sigmoidoscopy for the presence of cancer, diversion proctitis, or active Crohn's disease.

The presence of rectal stricturing that precludes endoscopic evaluation is especially worrisome. In the absence of known or suspected malignancy, completion proctectomy with intersphincteric anal dissection is recommended. If a malignancy is identified, appropriate preoperative staging and therapy are performed as for any other rectal adenocarcinoma. Abdominoperineal resection with appropriate resection margins, including a negative circumferential margin and complete total mesorectal excision, should be performed.

Perineal wound healing is often problematic after proctectomy, especially in the face of long-standing anal fistulae. Wide excision, or at least fistulectomy, to remove all active Crohn's tissue should improve healing. In cases of extensive perineal disease, a vacuum-assisted wound device may speed healing and simplify wound care. An alternative for patients with severe perineal disease or nonhealing perineal wounds is the use of myocutaneous flaps to achieve healing.

Ileal Pouch-Anal Anastomosis

Creation of an ileal pouch-anal anastomosis in a patient with known Crohn's disease usually is not recommended because of the risk of the development of recurrent Crohn's in the ileal pouch as well as the frequent presence of anal disease in association with Crohn's colitis. Centers with a high volume of patients with inflammatory bowel disease will perform ileal pouch surgery for Crohn's colitis in carefully selected patients who are well counseled regarding the potential need for subsequent pouch removal. Selection criteria include the absence of small bowel or anal involvement, a normal anal sphincter, and a long interval after colectomy without evidence of recurrent disease. Given the complexity of the surgery and the potential for subsequent morbidity, this procedure is performed most appropriately in a specialized center with significant experience with this procedure.

The Role of Laparoscopic and Robotic Surgery for Crohn's Colitis

Laparoscopic resection has been demonstrated to be a safe and effective management option for the resection of Crohn's disease. Numerous studies have documented improved outcomes compared with open resection with regard to return of bowel function, length of stay, and postoperative complications. Long-term outcomes do not appear to be compromised by a laparoscopic approach. There is little evidence regarding the use of robotic-assisted surgery for Crohn's disease beyond small series and case reports, but robotic-assisted proctectomy for cancer has been shown to be safe and to result in a lower conversion rate than laparoscopic proctectomy. As with any colorectal resection, the choice of surgical technique must take into account the surgeon's experience and expertise with minimally invasive colectomy.

Technical Tips

1. Positioning the patient in a low lithotomy position allows the surgeon maximal flexibility should unexpected findings dictate a change in operative strategy. Given the unpredictable nature of Crohn's disease, this is a common occurrence, and the modified lithotomy position should be used for most procedures.

2. Exposure for the perineal dissection for a proctocolectomy or completion proctectomy can be maximized if the patient is placed in a prone jack-knife position. After completion of the abdominal portion of the procedure and creation of the ileostomy, the patient is moved onto a cart and then turned back onto the operating table face down. This allows the buttocks to be taped apart, the perineum to be well prepped, and the surgeon and assistant to have an optimal view of the surgical field. This is especially important with a small perineal incision and intersphincteric dissection.

3. Crohn's disease is unpredictable, and it is impossible to know which patients will undergo further surgery or require a stoma. Therefore care should be taken to avoid placing incisions in any area that may one day be required for a stoma. Transverse and paramedian incisions may sacrifice abdominal wall locations that may be required for a stoma in the future and should be avoided.

4. Mobilization of the inflamed colon is performed best using the natural embryologic retroperitoneal planes. On the left side, this plane is identified most easily and accurately at the level of the mid-descending colon, where the mesocolon overlies Gerota's fascia. The proper plane is much easier to identify at this level than at the sigmoid colon, where numerous false, secondary planes may exist. A second option is to enter the avascular presacral plane behind the superior hemorrhoidal vessels at the level of the sacral promontory and then dissect upwards to the mesosigmoid.

5. Blunt dissection with a finger-fracture technique often separates seemingly fused surfaces in the proper planes. This may be used to "pinch" inflamed bowel off of the abdominal wall, bladder, or adjacent bowel loops.

6. In patients with evidence of significant inflammation overlying the course of the ureters, or in patients with evidence of hydronephrosis, ureteral stents placed preoperatively may provide tactile feedback during dissection. In patients with severe inflammation or fibrosis, the stents may not be palpable but will increase the likelihood that a ureteral injury will be noted at the time of surgery when repair is accomplished most easily. It is important that the surgeon communicate with the urologist to request a large stent because a very small, pliable stent is more difficult to palpate.

7. The mesentery may be significantly thickened in patients with Crohn's disease. Energy devices applied to the full thickness of involved mesentery may have difficulty obtaining sufficient tissue compression to achieve hemostasis. One solution is to divide the mesentery in layers, taking initially a superficial layer of peritoneum and fat, which allows division of larger vessels individually as they appear.

8. It is often necessary to place suture ligatures on major vessels if the tissue is too thick for effective sealing. Cut mesenteric vessels tend to retract into the thickened mesentery, which quickly results in a visible enlarging hematoma. Suture ligatures placed after dividing the mesentery may not achieve hemostasis in the face of a large hematoma. Horizontal mattress sutures, placed before mesenteric division or behind clamps, approximately 1 cm from the cut edge of the mesentery are usually effective in preventing hematoma formation.

9. The splenic flexure is often difficult to mobilize in the setting of Crohn's colitis. Prior inflammation or subclinical perforations may cause dense adherence of the omentum to this portion of the colon. It is helpful to first mobilize the colon off of Gerota's fascia posteriorly. The lesser sac is entered medially between the greater curve of the stomach and the transverse colon to allow better visualization of the splenic flexure before attempting to free it from the omentum.

10. Chronic Crohn's disease may result in colonic shortening and a medially retracted, rounded splenic flexure. This actually facilitates flexure mobilization unless mesenteric inflammation adheres to the pancreas and perinephric fat. Beware of mobilizing the kidney along with the specimen in this circumstance.

11. If intense inflammatory changes in the terminal ileum and right colon preclude identification of the duodenum, iliac vessels, and right ureter, a safe but temporizing option is to perform a proximal diverting ileostomy or ileotransverse colon bypass, recognizing that resection of the diseased intestine will be necessary at a subsequent operation. Although not commonly necessary, this is a safe option that reduces the likelihood of a major life-threatening vascular, ureteral, or duodenal injury.

12. During reoperation for recurrent disease at an ileocolic anastomosis, an enteroduodenal fistula may be encountered. Complete mobilization of the proximal and distal bowel should be performed before any attempt to divide the fistula. This will allow accurate identification of the fistula site and may allow the duodenal end of the fistula to be resected transversely by applying a mechanical stapler to the side of the duodenal wall. The staple line should be inverted with seromuscular sutures, which will produce the final appearance of a horizontal stricturoplasty.

13. Chronic Crohn's colitis may result in significant fibrosis and thickening of the colonic wall. We have noted that fulminant colitis in this setting may result in perforation without antecedent dilation. In fact, the area most likely to perforate is not the dilated normal proximal colon but the atonic, thickened, transmurally inflamed diseased portion at the site of obstruction.

14. When an ileosigmoid anastomosis is performed, it is important to try to avoid creation of a large internal hernia. The small bowel may be rotated counterclockwise to allow the mesenteric defect to lie against the left retroperitoneum after completion of the functional end-to-end anastomosis. Alternatively, the sigmoid colon can be mobilized completely so that it can be flipped over to the right side of the abdomen, allowing the mesenteric defect to lie against the right retroperitoneum. In either case, the surgeon avoids draping the cut surface of the ileal mesentery across the entire small intestine, creating an internal hernia. It is sometimes helpful to suture the edges of the sigmoid and small bowel mesentery to prevent twisting of the bowel proximal to the anastomosis.

15. Resection margins are defined by grossly normal-appearing bowel. Frozen sections have no role in the surgical management of Crohn's disease because it is not necessary to obtain microscopically normal margins of resection. Inspection and palpation of the bowel and the junction of the bowel and mesentery best judge the extent of small bowel disease. The extent of colonic disease is more difficult to ascertain and is best judged by colonoscopic inspection of the mucosa.

16. Preservation of the ileocecal valve is not valuable as a means to reduce rapid transit of bowel contents. Saving the right colon absorptive capacity is worthwhile if a distal anastomosis is planned and the right colon is spared.

Operative Procedures

Intersphincteric Proctectomy

For patients requiring total proctocolectomy with ileostomy or a completion proctectomy who have no evidence or suspicion of distal rectal cancer, the perineal portion of the procedure can be performed in the intersphincteric plane. This offers the advantage of leaving intact external sphincter to reapproximate, resulting in superior wound healing.

- The patient is placed in the prone jack-knife position. The anus is sutured shut and the perineum then is prepped and draped in sterile fashion. A vaginal prep should be performed in women and a Foley catheter must be in place.
- An elliptic incision is made with cutting current at the anal verge. Extensions may be required to excise any fistula tracts that may be present.
- A self-retaining retractor, such as a Gelpi retractor or a disposable Lone Star retractor (Lone Star Medical Products, Stafford, TX) facilitates exposure.
- Dissection is carried cephalad circumferentially in the intersphincteric plane. Identification of the proper plane is aided by observation of contractions in the external sphincter in response to electrocautery while the internal sphincter is unresponsive. The terminal longitudinal fibers of the rectum are found in the intersphincteric plane and act as a guide to the dissection.
- Special care must be taken anteriorly, where the external sphincter may be very thin, to avoid injury to the posterior vaginal wall or urethra. Frequent palpation of the posterior vaginal wall or of the urethral catheter will assist in staying in the proper plane.
- At the top of the anal canal, the incision is carried into the perirectal fat either to meet the dissection performed from the abdominal approach or to completely release a short rectal remnant.
- The specimen is removed transanally, a suction drain is positioned in the pelvis and the wound reapproximated in multiple layers (puborectalis, external sphincter, subcutaneous fat, and skin) with absorbable suture. The defect is best closed linearly anterior to posterior by placing figure of 8 or horizontal mattress sutures to bring the lateral walls together in the midline.

Laparoscopic Total Abdominal Colectomy

Many patients with Crohn's colitis will require a total abdominal colectomy (TAC), either with ileorectal anastomosis or ileostomy. A laparoscopic TAC offers patients the benefit of minimally invasive surgery but is a technically demanding procedure that is not performed commonly by most surgeons. The following outlined approach is one way to perform a minimally invasive TAC. The steps may be performed in a different sequence or with a different operative approach, but the surgeon must be capable of mastering each of the steps to safely perform a laparoscopic TAC. A hand-assisted laparoscopic technique may be preferred and has been shown to offer equivalent outcomes to the laparoscopic approach but with shorter operative times. The difficulty and complexity of the procedure also demands that the surgeon be assisted by a surgical team well trained in advanced laparoscopic surgery, patient positioning, and the safe and efficacious use of advanced energy devices.

Initial Steps:
- The patient is placed in a modified lithotomy position in low stirrups. It is essential that the patient be secured adequately to the table with a beanbag or disposable foam pad because the bed may have to be moved into extreme degrees of tilt during the procedure. Both arms are tucked at the patient's side, and a soft strap is placed across the chest and fixed to the table. Sequential compression devices and a bladder catheter are placed.
- The initial trocar is placed at the umbilicus, and the abdomen is insufflated. One typical trocar placement is illustrated in Figure 1. The camera operator uses the umbilical port while the surgeon begins operating through the left abdominal and suprapubic ports. A flexible or 30-degree to 45-degree angled laparoscope is essential to provide adequate visualization.

- Atraumatic laparoscopic graspers should be used, but the surgeon should avoid grasping the bowel directly. A better technique is to sweep bowel gently or to grasp mesenteric, epiploic or omental fat to position the bowel.
- A variety of energy sources are available and appropriate for the procedure. Ultrasonic or advance bipolar devices have the ability to control larger vessels than monopolar cautery. The surgeon and the surgical team must be proficient in the proper use and understand the limitations of the device chosen.
- After an initial inspection of the abdomen, the patient is placed in the Trendelenburg position and tilted to the left. The omentum is flipped over the stomach in the left upper quadrant (LUQ), and the small bowel is retracted out of the pelvis into the LUQ.

Right Colon Mobilization:
- Mobilization of the colon begins at the cecum by lifting the cecum to the anterior abdominal wall and incising the peritoneum at the right pelvic brim, anterior to the iliac vessels, from the abdominal midline to the base of the terminal ileum and cecum. This incision allows access to the proper embryologic plane between the mesentery above and the ureter and gonadal vessels below. This plane can be developed in a cephalad and lateral direction with gentle blunt dissection and minimal use of energy. The duodenum will become visible and should be dissected posteriorly away from the overlying ileocolic mesentery.
- Dissection continues laterally and superiorly until the entire cecum, ascending colon, and hepatic flexure are lifted free of the retroperitoneum.
- The patient is then brought into a reverse Trendelenburg position, and the cecum is placed back into its anatomic position in the right lower quadrant. The hepatic flexure is released by dividing the peritoneum starting just lateral to the second portion of the duodenum and progressing laterally and inferiorly around the flexure, entering the previously dissected space behind the right colon. The omentum is freed from the proximal transverse colon to enter the lesser sac and free the transverse mesocolon from the pancreas and posterior gastric wall.
- The patient is returned to a slightly Trendelenburg position, and the medial surface of the mesentery of the cecum is grasped with anterior and caudal traction to put tension on the ileocolic vessels. This maneuver will expose the ileocolic vessels as a "bow-string" within the mesocolon.
- Avascular windows leading to the previously dissected space are found on both sides of the ileocolic vessels and are opened to isolate the vessels. The duodenum is found immediately posterior to the SMA and proximal ileocolic vessels and is at risk of injury from aggressive use of energy during this dissection. The ileocolic vessels are divided near their origin from the SMA with an appropriate energy device or clips. It is important to have a plan to regain control of the proximal ileocolic artery and vein should there be any bleeding. The proximal vessels can be controlled with clips, suture, or endoloops if necessary for secondary hemostasis.
- The right colon is finally released from its lateral peritoneal attachments and the mobilization is compete.

Left Colon Mobilization:
- The patient is now rolled right side down and placed in steep Trendelenburg position, and the surgeon moves to the patient's right.
- The small bowel is swept out of the pelvis to expose the sacral promontory and base of the sigmoid mesentery.
- The sigmoid mesentery is grasped and retracted anteriorly to expose the superior hemorrhoidal artery and the triangular space between the artery and promontory. The peritoneum is incised at the base of the triangle, and gentle blunt dissection is used to develop the plane between the mesosigmoid

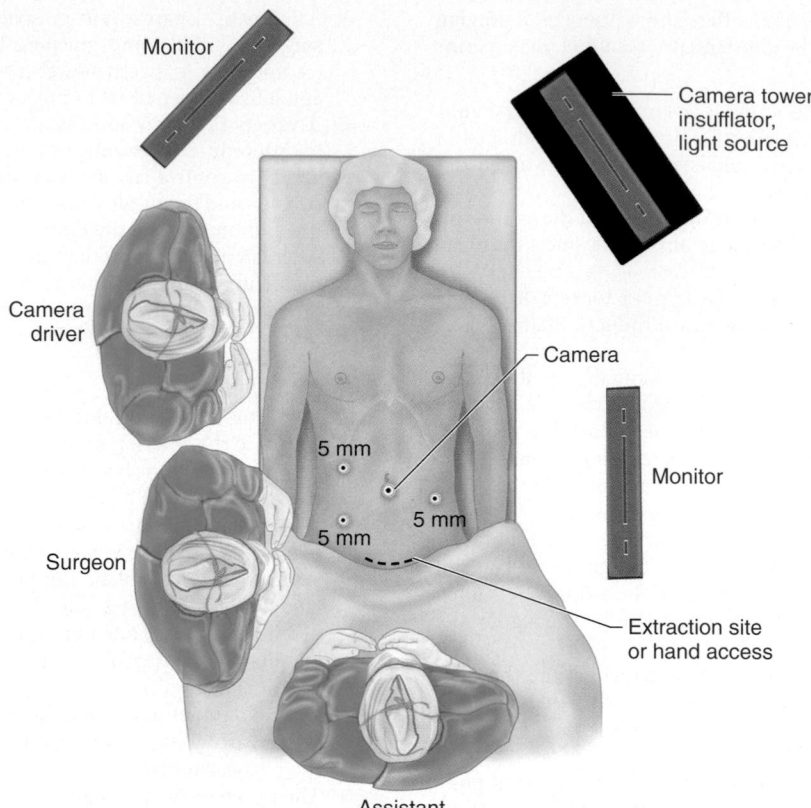

FIGURE 1 Trocar placement for laparoscopic total abdominal colectomy. *(Fleshman JW. Laparoscopic total abdominal colectomy and ileorectal anastomosis. In Fleshman JW, Birnbaum EH, Hunt SR, Mutch MG, Kodner IJ, Safar B.* Atlas of Surgical Techniques for the Colon, Rectum, and Anus. *Philadelphia: Saunders; 2013:102-125.)*

anteriorly and the ureter and gonadal vessels posteriorly. The plane is developed laterally beyond the left colon to the abdominal wall and superiorly to allow isolation of the IMA. The surgeon must remember that the dissection plane runs at an angle up and away from the midline to avoid injury to the iliac vessels.

■ Traction on the mesosigmoid in a caudal and anterior direction will expose a second window in the peritoneum just superior to the IMA between the aorta and inferior mesenteric vein (IMV). Incision of the peritoneum will complete the isolation of the IMA. The IMA may divided with the same considerations described for the ileocolic vessels.

■ The retrocolic plane is then developed with blunt dissection in a cephalad direction to the inferior border of the pancreas and laterally to the abdominal side wall.

■ The IMV is isolated and divided with clips or energy near its origin adjacent to the duodenum at the ligament of Treitz.

■ The left colon then is freed by dividing the lateral peritoneal attachments to the abdominal wall.

■ The patient is placed in a reverse Trendelenburg position to better expose the splenic flexure. The lateral dissection of the descending colon is continued cephalad and medially to release the splenic flexure from its attachments to Gerota's fascia, tail of pancreas, and spleen. With the omentum still flipped anterior to the stomach and spleen, the colon is freed from the undersurface of the omentum.

Transverse Colon:

■ The middle colic vessels are isolated by freeing the distal transverse mesocolon from the inferior edge of the pancreas from the splenic flexure to the IMV.

■ With a hand-assisted approach, the surgeon's hand can be used to encircle and lift the middle colic vessels under tension to

facilitate exposure and protect the superior mesenteric artery (SMA) and superior mesenteric vein (SMV) from injury. With a pure laparoscopic approach, care must be taken to retract the transverse mesocolon anteriorly to provide adequate visualization of the vessels. They may be divided individually with an energy device and/or clips, or they may be divided en masse with an endoscopic stapler. If the stapling option is chosen, it is extremely important to obtain adequate visualization of the entire staple line to be sure there is no injury to the SMA, SMV, or posterior gastric wall.

■ The suprapubic port site incision is extended and a wound protector is placed. The mesosigmoid at the level of the sacral promontory will be directly beneath incision. The mesentery and superior hemorrhoidal vessels are divided with energy or with traditional suture ligatures at the level of the promontory. The rectum is divided with a linear stapler, a linear cutter, or an endoscopic stapler, and the colon is retrieved through the opening. The terminal ileum then is delivered into the incision and divided with a linear cutter stapler.

Final Steps:

■ If the patient is to have an ileorectal anastomosis, the ileum is returned to the abdomen and allowed to curve down into the pelvis. A functional end-to-end anastomosis is fashioned with the linear cutter stapler and the resulting enterotomy closed with either a linear cutter or a linear stapler.

■ If the patient is to have an ileostomy, the skin is excised at the site marked preoperatively by the ostomy care nurse. The fat and anterior rectus sheath are incised in a longitudinal manner. The rectus muscle fibers are separated bluntly to allow incision of the posterior sheath and/or peritoneum. The end of the ileum is grasped with an Allis clamp passed through the ileostomy site and gently brought through the abdominal wall.

- The extraction site and larger trocar sites then are closed with absorbable suture and the ileostomy, if present, is matured.

SUGGESTED READINGS

Fleshman JW. Laparoscopic total abdominal colectomy and ileorectal anastomosis. In: Fleshman JW, Birnbaum EH, Hunt SR, Mutch MG, Kodner IJ, Safar B, eds. *Atlas of Surgical Techniques for the Colon, Rectum, and Anus.* Philadelphia: Saunders; 2013:102-125.

Rungoe C, Langholz E, Andersson M, Basit S, Nielsen NM, Wohlfahrt J, et al. Changes in medical treatment and surgery rates in inflammatory bowel disease: a nationwide cohort study 1979-2011. *Gut.* 2014;63:1607-1616.
Strong S, Steele S, Boutrous M, Bordineau L, Chun J, Stewart DB, et al. Clinical practice guidelines for the surgical management of Crohn's disease. *Dis Colon Rectum.* 2015;58:1021-1036.

THE MANAGEMENT OF ISCHEMIC COLITIS

Uri Netz, MD, and Susan Galandiuk, MD

Ischemic colitis (IC) is a condition that develops when the blood supply to the colon does not meet the cellular metabolic demands. It is the most common type of intestinal ischemia with an annual incidence of 15.6 to 17.7 per 100,000. IC presents with a wide spectrum of severity, ranging from a mild self-limiting form up to severe transmural colitis and gangrene. Considering the variable clinical findings, and in most cases relatively mild disease, the incidence is probably much higher than reported. This condition may be responsible for up to 1 in every 1000 hospital admissions. It is important to distinguish IC from acute mesenteric ischemia, a condition usually caused by an obstruction of the major vessels of the bowel that is accompanied by sudden, severe pain out of proportion to objective physical findings and necessitates immediate intervention (not dealt with in this chapter). IC is generally a disease of the small blood vessels, and in most cases, demonstrates a more subtle presentation. Approximately 20% of patients presenting to the hospital with IC will require surgery, stressing the importance of a high index of suspicion and a careful workup.

IC occurs in adults of all ages but is most prevalent in the elderly, in patients with multiple comorbid conditions, and in women. Several medical conditions have, in particular, been associated with IC (Box 1). Patients undergoing aortic or abdominal surgery in which the inferior mesenteric artery is ligated are especially predisposed to colonic ischemia. Another important at-risk population includes patients who have low flow states, such as those with septic shock or heart failure. A high index of suspicion is warranted after endovascular abdominal procedures. Evaluation for conditions predisposing to thrombosis should be considered in young patients with IC and patients with recurrent IC. Several drugs have been implicated in IC. A partial list is provided (Box 2). Constipation-inducing drugs also can cause IC, most likely as a result of reduced blood flow and increased intraluminal pressure. Immunomodulator drugs can affect thrombogenesis, and chemotherapeutic drugs can cause direct epithelial toxicity. Cocaine and methamphetamines cause ischemia by vasoconstriction.

ANATOMIC CONSIDERATIONS

The colon receives its arterial blood supply from the superior mesenteric artery (SMA) and the inferior mesenteric artery (IMA). The SMA gives the blood supply to the right colon via the ileocolic, right colic, and middle colic arteries. The ascending colon is supplied by the ileocolic and right colic arteries, and the transverse colon is supplied predominantly by the middle colic artery. The IMA gives rise to the left colic, sigmoid, and superior rectal arteries, which supply from the distal transverse colon to the proximal rectum. The SMA

and the IMA communicate through an extensive collateral circulation that limits the risk of ischemia to the colon (Figure 1). The arch of Riolan, also referred to as the *meandering mesenteric artery,* is a collateral vessel that is not often present, which connects the proximal SMA with the proximal IMA at the base of the mesentery. This collateral vessel is variable in caliber and may serve a vital role in delivering blood to the colon in cases of either SMA or IMA stenosis or occlusion. The marginal artery of Drummond forms a continuous arterial arcade that runs along the distal mesentery near the colonic wall and serves as a connection between the SMA and the IMA. Despite this collateral circulation, specific areas of the colon are more susceptible to ischemia. These "watershed" areas of the colon include the right colon, splenic flexure (Griffith's point), and the rectosigmoid junction (Sudeck's point). The right colon is vulnerable to ischemic insults arising from low flow states caused by hypotension resulting from hemorrhage, sepsis, or heart failure. The right colon is also at risk for ischemia from embolic events because the ileocolic artery is the terminal branch of the SMA and susceptible to embolic occlusion based on its straight take-off from the SMA. Another watershed area is the splenic flexure because of its location at the distal extent of the arterial supply of the left colic (IMA) and middle colic arteries (SMA). The collateral circulation of the splenic flexure is the most inconsistent and accounts for its predisposition for local ischemia. In some individuals, the marginal artery of Drummond is either diminutive or absent, limiting the collateral circulation and placing this segment of colon at greater risk for ischemia. The rectosigmoid junction also is considered a watershed area, because it receives its arterial supply from the distal branches of the sigmoid artery branches and from the superior hemorrhoidal artery, both terminal branches of the IMA. The increased incidence of significant atherosclerotic IMA stenosis with age and the need for IMA ligation during aortic surgery place the rectosigmoid region at greater risk for ischemia.

■ CLINICAL PRESENTATION

The signs and symptoms of IC are often nonspecific and require a high index of suspicion to make a prompt diagnosis. Patients presenting with IC frequently experience sudden abdominal cramping and/or mild to moderate left lower-abdominal pain that is not well localized, often with an urgent desire to defecate, and hematochezia or bloody diarrhea beginning within 24 hours of the onset of the abdominal pain. Associated bleeding is usually minor and rarely requires blood transfusion. The combination of these three symptoms (abdominal pain, tenesmus, hematochezia/bloody diarrhea) is present in about half of the patients; the pain usually precedes the bleeding. Abdominal tenderness is usually present over the involved area. Patients also may experience nausea, vomiting, and a low-grade fever. Medical history is important in establishing the diagnosis, with specific focus on cardiovascular risk factors, a history of hypercoagulability, prior surgery (especially aortic and abdominal surgery), recent invasive interventions, gastrointestinal symptoms, and low flow states. Also important are drugs such as opioids, immunomodulators, cocaine, contraceptives, and serotoninergics.

BOX 1: Medical and Surgical Conditions Associated With Ischemic Colitis

Cardiovascular/Pulmonary

Atherosclerosis*
Atrial fibrillation
Chronic obstructive pulmonary disease
Hypertension

Gastrointestinal

Constipation
Diarrhea
Irritable bowel syndrome

Low Flow State

Septic shock
Congestive heart failure
Hemorrhagic shock
Hypotension

Surgery

Abdominal surgery
Aortic surgery
Cardiovascular surgery

Invasive Interventions

Postendovascular abdominal manipulations (e.g., chemoembolization)
Postcolonoscopy

Metabolic/Rheumatoid

Diabetes mellitus
Dyslipidemia
Rheumatoid arthritis
Systemic lupus erythematosus

Miscellaneous

Hypercoagulable states[†]
Sickle cell disease
Long-distance running

---

*For example, ischemic heart disease, cerebrovascular disease, peripheral vascular disease.

[†]Antiphospholipid syndrome, factor V Leiden deficiency, protein C and S deficiency.

BOX 2: Drugs Associated With Ischemic Colitis

Constipation-inducing drugs (opioids and nonopioids)
Immunomodulator drugs (anti-TNFα, type 1 interferon-α, type 1 interferon-β)
Chemotherapeutic drugs (e.g., Taxanes)
Cocaine and methamphetamines
Female hormones
Oral contraceptive medications
Antibiotics
Pseudoephedrine
Serotoninergic (e.g., Alosetron, Sumatriptan)
Diuretics

IC tends to be segmental, based on the affected blood supply. The left colon (including the splenic flexure) is the most commonly affected segment, followed by the sigmoid colon (see Figure 1). About 25% of patients demonstrate isolated right-sided IC. Patients with right-sided IC are more likely to have atrial fibrillation, coronary heart disease, and chronic renal failure than patients with IC at other locations. They are also more likely to present with abdominal pain without rectal bleeding, have a higher chance of requiring surgery, and have a worse prognosis. Pancolonic IC is associated with a similarly poorer prognosis.

Most episodes of IC are mild and self-limiting. After resolution, about 10% of patients will have a recurrence, usually similar in intensity and location to the initial incident. A small proportion will continue to have chronic colitis lasting more than 3 months with continued symptoms such as pain; bleeding; bloody diarrhea; recurrent septic episodes suggested by signs such as fever; elevated leukocytes; tachycardia and tachypnea, with or without positive blood cultures; and a biopsy consistent with IC on colonoscopy. These patients have a higher rate of complications, including septic shock and multiorgan failure, stricture, and malnutrition from protein-losing enteropathy, and they eventually may require surgical resection of the involved segment.

■ DIAGNOSIS

After clinical suspicion, patients will generally undergo an extensive workup. Plain film radiographs of the abdomen may show rounded densities along the sides of a gas-filled colon (thumb printing), colonic dilation, or mural thickening. "Thumb printing," which is indicative of submucosal edema, is the most common radiographic finding in patients with ischemic colitis. It is, however, nonspecific and may be seen with other causes of colonic inflammation.

Computed tomographic (CT) scans of the abdomen have become the most common method for the initial diagnosis of colonic disease. For patients with suspected IC, CT scans of the abdomen and pelvis performed with both intravenous and oral contrast can reveal involved areas, demonstrate the severity of colitis, and exclude the presence of other diseases. Findings suggestive of IC include bowel thickening and pericolonic fat stranding of moderately long segmental distribution, thumb printing, and the presence of ascites. These findings are, however, relatively nonspecific. Pneumatosis (the presence of gas in the colonic wall), portal venous gas, and the presence of megacolon usually indicate severe disease favoring immediate surgical intervention. Multiphasic CT angiography should be performed to exclude acute mesenteric ischemia in cases of pain of sudden onset that is out of proportion to physical and laboratory findings. Multiphasic CT angiography also is recommended *after* an endoscopically or CT-diagnosed isolated right colon IC because this may be an indicator of SMA occlusive disease. However, in general, vascular imaging is not indicated in cases of ischemic colitis because this is usually a disease of small vessels. In the past, barium enema was used commonly to diagnose ischemic colitis; however, the utility of this technique is diminishing with the improved images obtained with CT scanning and because of the danger of barium peritonitis in the event of barium extravasation into the peritoneal cavity in the case of perforation or during surgery.

Ultrasound has been described mainly in combination with the Doppler flow evaluation of the colonic vasculature but, in general, is not used in the standard emergency evaluation of IC. Several studies have been published regarding the use of magnetic resonance imaging (MRI) in the diagnosis of ischemic colitis. MRI does not provide additional information as compared with CT scans but may play a role in patients with poor renal function or in cases in which repeat imaging is needed.

Flexible endoscopy is the gold standard for the diagnosis of IC. Colonoscopy or sigmoidoscopy can be used to visualize the colonic mucosa for signs of ulceration or ischemic changes. Early colonoscopy should be performed (within 48 hours), except in cases of acute peritonitis or if there are ominous signs suggestive of ischemia such as portal venous gas, intestinal pneumatosis, or pneumoperitoneum on imaging. Endoscopy usually is performed without mechanical bowel preparation, apart from a small volume saline enema to cleanse the distal bowel. In contrast to the expected increased risk of

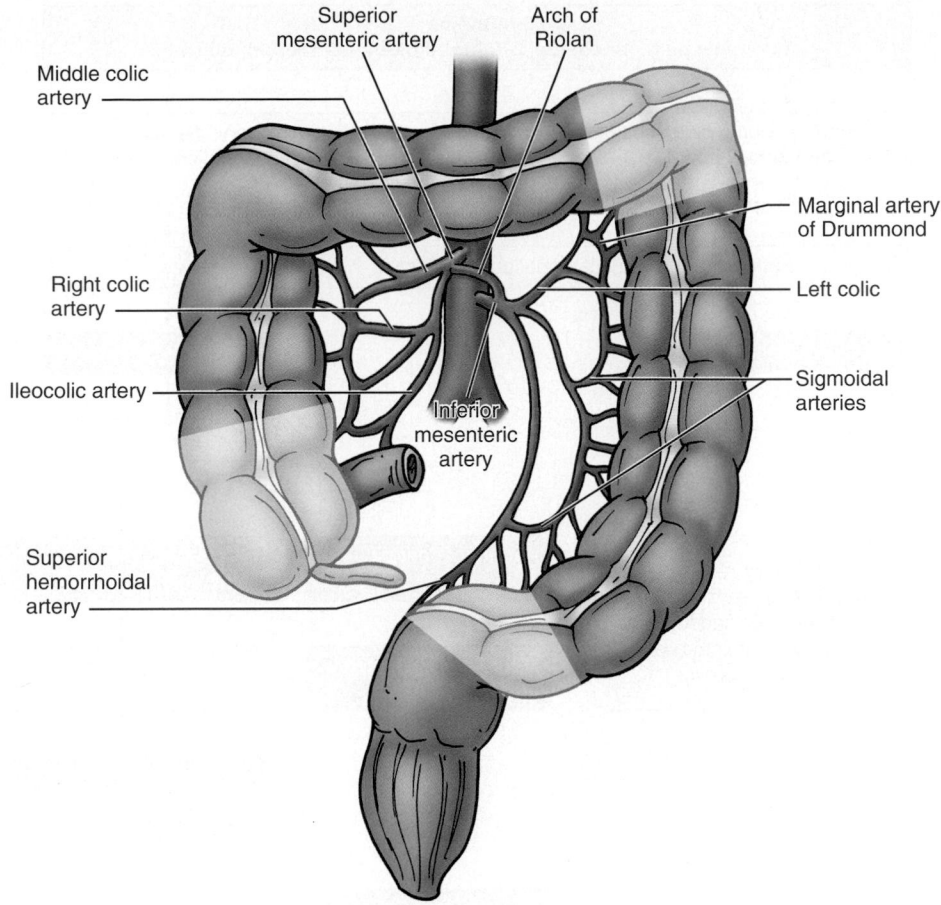

FIGURE 1 Arterial supply to the colon. Shaded areas depicting potential watershed regions.

perforation during endoscopy in the evaluation of IC, there does not seem to be a higher rate of perforation compared with other patients. Surgeons should, however, minimize insufflation and refrain from advancing beyond the most distal extent of the disease. Endoscopic findings characteristic of mild IC include mucosal edema, erythema, petechial hemorrhage, and mucosal ulceration. A single longitudinal ulcer called the "single-stripe" sign is seen uncommonly but believed to be specific for IC. More severe ischemia is characterized by a dusky appearance of the mucosa, submucosal hemorrhaging, and hemorrhagic ulcerations that can progress to frank necrosis. IC is usually segmental in distribution with an abrupt transition to normal mucosa in the nonaffected regions of the colon.

Biopsies should be taken from involved areas. Pathognomonic histologic changes include mucosal infarction and ghost cells; however, these cells are found in a minority of cases. Common histologic findings include an inflammatory cell infiltrate, mucosal edema and sloughing, altered crypt morphology, and hemorrhage within the lamina propria. In addition, macroscopically, the endoscopist can visualize the degree of bleeding from the biopsy site as an indicator of the degree of colonic perfusion.

Abnormalities in basic laboratory tests are nonspecific but can help predict disease severity. An elevated white blood cell count, blood urea nitrogen, and LDH, as well as a decreased hemoglobin and serum albumin have been shown to be associated with more severe IC. Arterial blood gases and serum lactate also can be helpful, with acidosis and decreased bicarbonate as well as increased serum lactate, all implying a greater risk of severe IC.

The differential diagnosis for patients believed to have IC includes *acute* mesenteric ischemia, infectious colitis, inflammatory bowel disease, diverticulitis, and colon cancer. It is important to differentiate IC from acute mesenteric ischemia, which affects primarily the

small intestine and requires urgent intervention. Patients with acute mesenteric ischemia generally experience severe *acute* onset abdominal pain, out of proportion to their physical examination results. In contrast to patients with IC, they generally do not have bloody diarrhea until late in their clinical course. Infectious colitis also should be considered in patients being evaluated for potential IC. Stool culture studies should be used to evaluate invasive bacteria, most commonly *E. coli* O157:H7, *Salmonella,* and *Shigella* spp. An important point is that, in many institutions, *E. coli* O157:H7 is not cultured routinely unless specifically requested. Patients with a recent hospitalization or recent antibiotic use should be evaluated for *C. difficile* colitis. This may be associated with the presence of pseudomembranes on endoscopic evaluation.

■ TREATMENT

The initial treatment of the patient with IC should focus on determining the severity of ischemia and whether surgery is required (Figure 2). Patients with suspected *acute* mesenteric ischemia should undergo immediate CT angiography or proceed immediately to surgery. Patients presenting with generalized peritonitis implying nonviable bowel or perforation also should undergo laparotomy immediately. Most patients with IC, however, present with mild to moderate disease that responds to supportive, nonsurgical management, and in whom an orderly diagnostic evaluation can proceed.

Nonsurgical Management

Nearly 80% of the patients with IC respond to conservative treatment, with resolution of their symptoms within a few days. Patients

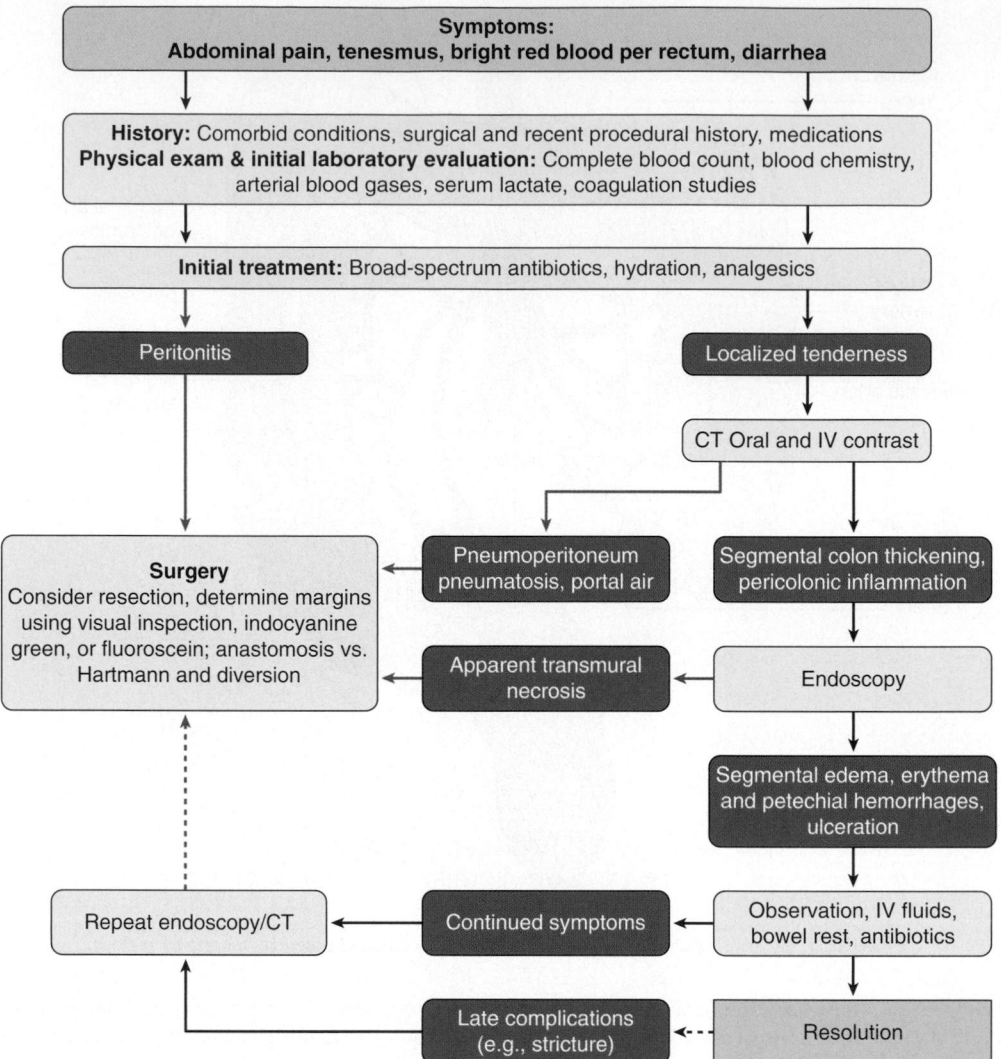

FIGURE 2 Treatment algorithm for ischemic colitis.

should be placed initially on bowel rest with aggressive fluid resuscitation, as needed, if hypovolemia is believed to be a factor in the development of the colonic ischemia. Bowel ischemia results in intestinal epithelial barrier failure. This, in turn, may lead to bacterial translocation, leading to fever, elevated leukocytes, tachycardia, and tachypnea, but it also may deteriorate to septic shock and multisystem organ failure. For this reason, empiric broad-spectrum antibiotics against both anaerobic and aerobic coliform bacteria are recommended to cover the normal colonic bacterial flora whenever IC is suspected, despite a lack of clinical trials supporting their efficacy. These antibiotics probably should be continued for at least a week. Nasogastric tube decompression is not needed routinely but should be considered in patients with nausea and vomiting. Cathartics should be avoided because they may lead to colon perforation. Glucocorticoids are not recommended, unless they are being used to treat a pre-existing condition such as lupus or rheumatoid arthritis. Serial abdominal radiographs may be useful to follow changes in colonic dilation. In critically ill patients in whom ischemic colitis develops as a complication of another illness, treatment should focus on limiting vasopressor use, if possible, to optimize mesenteric blood flow. Cardiac output also should be optimized with pulmonary artery catheterization or other noninvasive hemodynamic monitoring tools to guide fluid resuscitation strategies. Patients are at increased risk of IC after abdominal aortic aneurysm

(AAA) repair because of ligation of the IMA in open aortic surgery or coverage of the IMA takeoff during endovascular AAA repair. Patients in whom fever, leukocytosis, bloody diarrhea, abdominal pain, abdominal distention, or unexplained acidosis develops after AAA repair should be evaluated for potential colon ischemia. Supportive measures should be initiated as described previously, in addition to an urgent, flexible endoscopy to evaluate for colonic ischemia. In the absence of an indication for urgent exploration, the patient should receive supportive management with consideration for repeat endoscopy to re-evaluate for signs of worsening ischemia.

Surgical Management

The mortality rate approaches 50% in patients who require acute surgical intervention for IC. Indications for acute surgical exploration in patients with IC include peritonitis, pneumoperitoneum, massive hemorrhage, or signs of transmural necrosis on abdominal imaging, including pneumatosis or portal venous gas (Box 3). In addition, patients with ongoing or worsening abdominal pain, increasing leukocytosis, acidosis, oliguria, or signs of sepsis during treatment with supportive measures should be considered for abdominal exploration. Right-sided colonic ischemia tends to be more severe with an increased likelihood for the need of operative

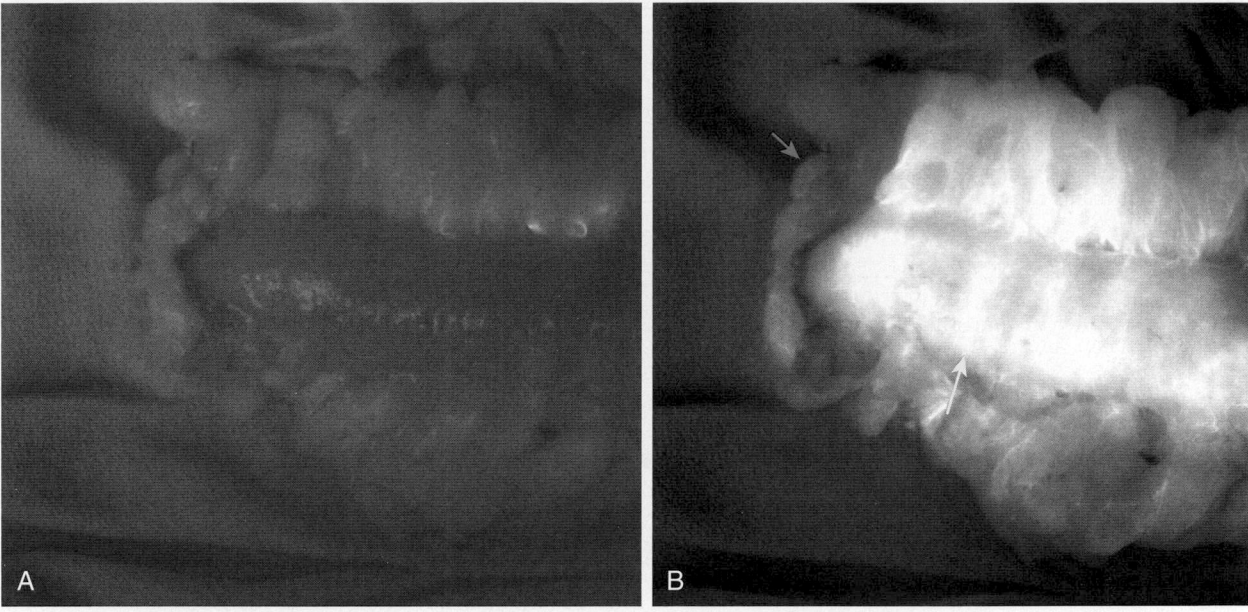

FIGURE 3 Indocyanine green–based infrared angiography. **A,** Colon before injection. **B,** Colon after injection: *(short blue arrow)* ischemia of resection margin; *(yellow arrow)* normal perfusion of colon.

BOX 3: Indications for Surgical Intervention in Patients With Ischemic Colitis

Acute

Peritonitis
Bowel perforation
Bowel necrosis
Fulminant colitis
Massive hemorrhage
Sepsis

Chronic

Intractable symptoms (abdominal pain, bloody diarrhea, etc.)
    lasting >2 weeks
Recurrent sepsis
Chronic colitis
Ischemic stricture
Malnutrition from protein-losing enteropathy

intervention and increased mortality compared with left-sided colon ischemia, as does pancolitis.

Surgical intervention for patients with IC should include a thorough exploration of the abdomen through a midline incision. The entire small and large intestine should be visualized and evaluated for signs of ischemia. Clearly necrotic or perforated bowel should be resected. In many cases, however, deciding whether a specific portion is likely to survive or how much to resect can be a challenge. Visual examination is the most common practice but tends to be imprecise, especially when the bowel has a dusky appearance. Intravenous injection of fluorescein followed by illumination with ultraviolet light (Wood's lamp) is a well-known technique used to help assess intestinal viability, but it has the distinct drawback of the inability to perform repeated assessments, as the dye remains in the tissue.

Intraoperative infrared angiography is a new method that has been gaining popularity in bowel surgery as an adjunct for decisions of whether to resect, in determining margins, and the integrity of intestinal anastomoses. It is based on the intravenous injection of indocyanine green (ICG), which is distributed throughout the circulation and which after laser excitation can demonstrate real-time tissue perfusion with a commercially available imaging system (Figure 3). In contrast to the ultraviolet-based system, it can be used repeatedly as the dye is cleared rapidly. Most cases of IC that require an urgent operation will require a colon resection. In general, a segmental colon resection of the involved segment should be performed with exteriorization of a diverting end ileostomy or colostomy in the urgent setting. Creation of an anastomosis is not advised in the acute setting because of the presence of potential tenuous blood flow to the newly created anastomosis and the presence of physiologic derangements that are likely to be present in a patient requiring emergent operation for colon ischemia. Because IC usually occurs in watershed areas, an anatomic colon resection should be performed so that the remaining colon is supplied by sufficient arterial inflow. In cases of extensive or patchy involvement of the large bowel, a temporary abdominal closure with planned second-look laparotomy after 24 hours may be advisable to determine the need for further resection. In rare cases of ischemia of the entire colon or massive hemorrhage that is not localized, a subtotal colectomy and end ileostomy may be required. In contrast to mesenteric ischemia of the small intestine, interventions that are aimed at revascularizing the large bowel in patients with IC are not indicated.

Patients initially treated nonoperatively, with ongoing colitis causing continued symptoms of abdominal pain, bloody diarrhea, or recurrent sepsis lasting more than 2 weeks from the initial diagnosis should be re-evaluated for colon resection. Colonic stricture and chronic colitis may develop as a chronic consequence of ischemic colitis. In cases of continued symptoms, patients should undergo repeat colonoscopy with biopsy and stool culture to exclude an infectious or malignant cause of colitis. Surgical resection rarely is indicated for chronic colitis caused by ischemia; however, malnutrition or intractable symptoms, recurrent bacteremia, or stricture may prompt the need for elective surgical resection of the affected colon.

■ SUMMARY

Ischemic colitis exists as a spectrum of disease that ranges from mild, transient self-limiting ischemia to severe, permanent disruption of blood flow and necrosis. Ischemic colitis is typically a disease of the elderly but should be considered in younger patients with symptoms of colonic ischemia. Although most patients have the mild form of ischemic colitis, nearly 20% need immediate or eventual operative intervention, which is associated with a significant increase in morbidity and mortality. Maintaining a high index of suspicion and promptly identifying patients with irreversible ischemic injury is paramount in achieving prompt surgical treatment to correct the physiologic derangements caused by large bowel ischemia.

SUGGESTED READINGS

Brandt LJ, Feuerstadt P, Longstreth GF, et al. ACG clinical guideline: epidemiology, risk factors, patterns of presentation, diagnosis, and management of colon ischemia (CI). *Am J Gastroenterol.* 2015;110:18-44.

Castleberry AW, Turley RS, Hanna JM, et al. A 10-year longitudinal analysis of surgical management for acute ischemic colitis. *J Gastrointest Surg.* 2013;17:784-792.

Foppa C, Denoya PI, Tarta C, et al. Indocyanine green fluorescent dye during bowel surgery: are the blood supply "guessing days" over? *Tech Coloproctol.* 2014;18:753-758.

O'Neill S, Yalamarthi S. Systematic review of the management of ischaemic colitis. *Colorectal Dis.* 2012;14:e751-e763.

Taourel P, Aufort S, Merigeaud S, et al. Imaging of ischemic colitis. *Radiol Clin North Am.* 2008;46:909-924, vi.

THE MANAGEMENT OF *CLOSTRIDIUM DIFFICILE* COLITIS

J. Daniel Stanley, MD, FACS, FASCRS, and Benjamin W. Dart IV, MD, FACS

*C*lostridium difficile is a gram-positive, spore-forming anaerobic bacillus that is the leading cause of nosocomial infectious colitis and a significant source of morbidity and mortality in the United States. The organism was first identified more than 100 years ago, and pseudomembranous colitis, which is most commonly caused by *C. difficile* infection (CDI), was first reported in 1893 during the preantibiotic era by the first president of The American College of Surgeons, John Finney. It was not identified as the causative agent for antibiotic-associated pseudomembranous colitis until 1978 by Dr. John Bartlett and others. The incidence of CDI has increased twofold to fourfold over the last two decades as a result of changing patterns of antibiotic use, an aging and more susceptible population, and the emergence of hypervirulent strains. Once recognized almost exclusively in hospital environments, community-acquired CDI, which is occurring in less vulnerable groups, is being reported increasingly. There are now approximately 3 million CDI cases in the United States each year with hospitalization costs nationwide estimated at $8.2 billion per year.

The presentation of CDI ranges from mild to severe, and the manifestations may be somewhat nonspecific, especially in the postoperative patient. A high degree of suspicion is important with stool studies confirming the clinical diagnosis. First-line medical treatment in most cases is with oral vancomycin or oral or IV metronidazole, depending on the severity or history of previous infection. Progressive or recurrent CDI may necessitate the use of fecal microbiota transplant (FMT), which recently has been established as a very effective treatment. Surgical intervention, most commonly a total colectomy with ileostomy, is required in some cases of moderate CDI and frequently in severe and fulminant cases. Because of the increasing frequency and the severity of CDI, it is important that the surgeon be familiar with the diagnosis and the medical and surgical management of these challenging patients.

■ PATHOGENESIS

Primary risk factors reflect the most commonly recognized elements of CDI pathogenesis: a source of colonization, a change in intestinal microflora and host debility or altered immunity (Box 1). A fourth important factor in the pathogenesis is the degree of toxin production related to the emergence of hypervirulent strains of *C. difficile.*

Asymptomatic carriers (3% of adults and 25% to 80% of infants) as well as patients with active disease serve as reservoirs for the spread of *C. difficile* by a fecal-oral route. Control of transmission is difficult in the institutional setting because *C. difficile* spores can survive in the dormant state for weeks to years on inanimate objects and may be carried from patient to patient by caregivers. Colonization rates of 20% to 50% may result after hospitalization of 1 and 4 weeks, respectively.

Progression to an active infection usually requires that the protective effects of an individual's normal intestinal flora be weakened as with antibiotic usage. Almost all antibiotics have the potential of causing CDI, and this risk increases with administration of multiple antibiotics or with prolonged treatment. The antibiotics most frequently associated with the development of CDI are fluoroquinolones and cephalosporins. Bowel preparation and chemotherapy also may alter the colonic microflora resulting in CDI.

One patient population that is particularly susceptible to CDI is the postsurgical patient. In addition to having multiple established risk factors for CDI (routine perioperative antibiotic exposure, aging population, and hospitalization), surgical patients are relatively immunosuppressed in the postoperative period.

The clinical manifestation of CDI is the result of toxin production. Toxinogenic strains of *C. difficile* typically produce both toxins A and B, although toxicity may occur when only one of these toxins is present. These toxins affect the enterocyte cytoskeleton, alter cell function, and disrupt tight junctions. This leads to edema and an inflammatory response, which may result in the characteristic pseudomembrane formation. The systemic alterations may be not only secondary to the inflammatory response but also a result of direct toxemic effects of the toxins because toxin B has been found to be a direct cardiotoxin. Hypervirulent strains of *C. difficile* are capable of producing toxins A and B in quantities sixteenfold to twentyfold higher than less virulent strains and are associated with increased mortality rates. The most frequently identified hypervirulent strain is known as *Bi, NAP-1/O27, toxigenotype III*, or *polymerase chain reaction (PCR) ribotype 027*. The NAP-1 strain has been shown to have a lower response rate to fidaxomicin and an increased resistance to fluoroquinolones. Cytolethal distending toxin (CDT), also known as *binary toxin*, is present in 6% to 12% of toxinogenic strains and is present in NAP-1/027 hypervirulent strains. Although it is cytotoxic in cell culture, its role in producing clinical symptoms is unclear regarding to what degree it may cause symptoms when not accompanied by toxin A or B. CDT may in part exert its effects by improved colonization rather than direct toxicity. There is a PCR test for this toxin, which can be used as a surrogate for identifying the hypervirulent NAP-1/027 strains.

CLINICAL MANIFESTATIONS

The clinical manifestations of CDI are of variable severity. The most common presentation is a mild antibiotic-associated diarrhea. This typically consists of less than 10 nonbloody stools per day with abdominal cramping and without systemic symptoms. CDI is the most common cause of antibiotic-associated colitis. Classically, the colitis resulting from CDI has been synonymous with pseudomembranous colitis, but this is somewhat of a misnomer because pseudomembranes are not always present.

Surgeons must be keenly aware of worsening symptoms because progression beyond mild disease significantly increases the likelihood of an eventual surgical intervention. Moderate to severe CDI consists of profuse diarrhea, fever, nausea, abdominal pain, leukocytosis, abdominal distention, and a varying degree of abdominal tenderness or peritoneal signs. Fulminant CDI (FCDI), which occurs in 1% to 8% of cases, is characterized by a severe systemic inflammatory response and is associated with mortality rates in the range of 30% to 90%. To further complicate the clinical presentation, as many as 37% of patients with FCDI may present without diarrhea because of an ileus.

BOX 1: Risk Factors for *Clostridium difficile* Infection

Primary Risk Factors

Age greater than 65 years
Antibiotic use within the previous 3 months
Hospitalization

Secondary Risk Factors

Female gender
Double-occupancy rooms
    ICU admission
    Admission to a long-term care facility within the last year
Postpyloric tube feedings
Chemotherapy
Acid-reducing therapy with proton pump inhibitors or histamine
    receptor blockers
Gastrointestinal procedures
Renal disorders
Organ transplantation
HIV
Autoimmune disease
Hypoalbuminemia
Inflammatory bowel disease

HIV, human immunodeficiency virus; *ICU,* intensive care unit.

DIAGNOSIS OF *C. DIFFICILE* INFECTION

The prompt and early diagnosis of CDI is important because there is evidence that the length of time from onset of symptoms to initiation of treatment directly correlates with mortality. Once a clinical suspicion of CDI is entertained, there are a number of options for establishing the diagnosis while assessing the severity of the disease. The most useful diagnostic tests are stool analysis, imaging studies, and occasionally, endoscopic evaluation.

Although several types of stool studies are available for establishing a definitive diagnosis of CDI, enzyme immunoassay for toxins A and B (ToxA/ToxB EIA) and PCR to identify DNA coding for the toxins are the two most commonly used (Table 1). Tox A/ToxB EIA is very specific for the presence of clinically relevant *C. difficile;* it lacks sensitivity. PCR, on the other hand, is very sensitive but detects clinically irrelevant carriers as well. Other laboratory studies that are useful in evaluating and stratifying patients with CDI include white blood cell count (WBC), serum lactate, and albumin. All three have been reported as important in identifying those patients with severe and fulminant CDI. The finding of a WBC in the range of 30,000 to 60,000 may be particularly useful when considering CDI because this degree of leukocytosis is much less common in other types of bacterial infection.

Plain abdominal x-rays may reveal a megacolon, ileus, and/or colonic wall edema.

Abdominal CT scan may be particularly sensitive in the patient with a severe or fulminant presentation; the most common findings are localized or diffuse colonic thickening and ascites. A thickened colon may result in an "accordion sign" configuration of either intraluminal contrast or air outlined by thickened mucosa.

Endoscopic evaluation may be useful in the presence of colonic pseudomembranes and in the correct clinical setting will render an almost certain diagnosis of *C. difficile.* Colonoscopy generally is preferred over sigmoidoscopy because colitis is limited to the right colon in approximately one third of cases. It also may be used for decompression and placement of a long colonic tube for vancomycin irrigation.

MEDICAL TREATMENT

Treatment recommendations for CDI depend on the severity of disease. Asymptomatic carriers do not require medical treatment, but some general principles should be applied to both carriers and symptomatic patients. Hospital infection control practices should be implemented in patients with *C. difficile* to limit spread within the institution (Box 2). General contact precautions and hand hygiene with soap and water must be observed. Routine hand cleaning with alcohol-based products is not adequate protection against CDI because spores can be resistant to alcohol.

TABLE 1: Diagnostic Tests for CDI

Test	Reported Sensitivity	Reported Specificity	Comments
Enzyme immunoassay for toxin A and B (Tox A/ToxB EIA)	48%-96%	94%-100%	Commonly used; commercially available; 30-minute turnaround
Polymerase chain reaction (PCR) for toxins A/B genes	87%-100%	90%-100%	Emerging as test of choice because of improved sensitivity, 45-minute turnaround
PCR for the binary, cytolethal distending toxin (CDT)	95%-100%	95%-100%	Indicates likely hypervirulent strain if toxin A/toxin B PCR also positive
Glutaraldehyde dehydrogenase (GDH or common antigen)	99%-100%	60%	Less commonly used as a cheap, sensitive, but nonspecific screening test

BOX 2: Infection Control Practices to Limit the Spread of *Clostridium difficile* Infection

Avoidance of Inoculation

Minimize ICU stay
Private room
Use of gloves
Hand washing with soap or chlorhexidine instead of alcohol-based solutions
Use patient-dedicated stethoscopes and instruments
Wash all nondedicated instruments between patient contacts
Follow isolation precautions

Interventions

Minimize antibiotics
    Follow guidelines for perioperative antibiotics
    Avoid broad-spectrum or multiple antibiotics
    Avoid prolonged courses of antibiotics
Avoid proton pump inhibitors and H2 blockers
Avoid unnecessary bowel preps
Avoid antidiarrheals
Minimize GI intubation for feeding or decompression

Institutional Measures

Consider antibiotic formulary changes in case of institutional epidemic

GI, gastrointestinal; *ICU,* intensive care unit.

BOX 3: Characteristics of Moderate, Severe, and Fulminant *Clostridium difficile* Infection

Moderate Colitis

Pulse >90, SBP >100, Temp 100° F-101.5° F, WBC 12,000-15,000
Pseudomembranes on colonoscopy
Colonic thickening on CT
Colon >6 cm
Oliguria responsive to volume
Normal lactate
Mild abdominal tenderness
Mild tachypnea

Severe Colitis

Moderate colitis and the following:
Pulse >120, SBP <100, WBC >15,000
Renal failure
Respiratory distress or intubation
Albumin <2.0
Lactate >2.0
Mental status changes
Moderate abdominal tenderness

Fulminant Colitis

Severe colitis and any of the following:
    Unimproved after 12-24 hours of treatment
    Need for vasopressors
    Ventilator dependence
    Abrupt rise in WBC

CT, computed tomography; *SBP,* systolic blood pressure; *WBC,* white blood cell count.

Medical management consists of stopping the offending antibiotic if possible and avoidance of antidiarrheals and narcotics, which may lead to toxic megacolon. European guidelines recommend no directed antibiotic therapy in mild cases because they generally resolve without further treatment. However, SHEA (Society for Healthcare Epidemiology of America) guidelines recommend metronidazole, 250 to 500 mg PO tid-qid for 10 to 14 days for mild to moderate cases and vancomycin 125 mg PO qid for 10 days. IV metronidazole is useful when the enteric route is unavailable because IV vancomycin does not result in adequate intraluminal levels. Vancomycin enemas or irrigations through a colonic tube may be of benefit in these patients. The typical dose is 500 mg in 100 mL of normal saline given as a retention enema or irrigation administered every 6 hours and may be given in addition to intravenous metronidazole. Fidaxomicin 200 mg PO bid for 10 days has been shown to be equivalent to vancomycin with a decreased recurrence. It is more effective than vancomycin in patients who must remain on other therapeutic antibiotics. Fidaxomicin is much more expensive than vancomycin and therefore is not a first-line treatment. Intravenous tigecycline is a useful antibiotic in patients who need a broad-spectrum antibiotic that is also active against *C. difficile.*

Fecal microbiota transplant (FMT) for recurrent CDI was reported in 1983. There have been multiple reports touting the safety and efficacy of FMT with a success rate of greater than 91%. FMT can be administered via NG, upper endoscopy, enema and colonoscopy. The FDA allows physicians to use FMT if standard therapies are not successful and if adequate informed written consent is given to include the disclosure that FMT for CDI is investigational. It is very important to follow donor selection guidelines and check for communicable diseases in the fecal donor. Indications for FMT currently include at least three episodes of CDI unresponsive to standard treatment, CDI not responding to therapy after a week, and recurrent or nonresponsive severe CDI.

■ SURGERY

It is important that the surgeon be involved early in the assessment and treatment of CDI. In addition to increased survival rates for patients on a surgical service, earlier surgical intervention also may improve survival in patients with severe and fulminant CDI. Surgical intervention is required in approximately 20% of patients who are critically ill with CDI. The classic indications for surgery include toxic megacolon or colonic perforation, and less clearly fulminant disease or failure of medical therapy within 48 to 72 hours for patients with continued signs of toxicity. Toxic megacolon in CDI has been defined as a cecal diameter of greater than 12 cm or a colonic diameter of greater than 6 cm on radiographic imaging. Not uncommonly, CDI patients with a toxic megacolon may have a conspicuous lack of diarrhea. This finding should not be misinterpreted as an improvement of the disease process. A very low threshold for operative intervention must remain when toxic megacolon exists. The presence of colonic perforation with CDI has an especially poor prognosis, and emergent surgical treatment is the only option for survival.

Classification of the disease process as fulminant is problematic because standardized definitions of disease severity are not well established. Likewise, failure of medical therapy in patients with severe colitis has remained a subjective indication of the need for surgery. A severity classification scheme or scoring system would be ideal to guide appropriate treatment algorithms that include early surgical intervention. Although several such systems have been proposed and appear promising, validated studies are needed before widespread adoption. However, several observations can be made from the collective experience regarding the characteristics of moderate, severe, and fulminant colitis (Box 3). Patients who meet these criteria need close clinical monitoring typically in an intensive care setting. On the basis of severity of illness and response to aggressive medical management, we recommend consideration for surgical intervention as described in Box 4. The presence or absence of a hypervirulent strain (based on serotyping or PCR for cytolethal distending toxin) also may affect decision making.

BOX 4: Guidelines for Surgery in *Clostridium difficile* Infection

Immediate surgical intervention:
    Peritonitis
    Perforation
    Fulminant colitis
    Recalcitrant severe colitis
Surgery if not improving within 12 hours of initial resuscitation:
    Severe colitis with megacolon
    Severe colitis and history of inflammatory bowel disease (IBD)
    Severe colitis and age >65 years
Surgery if not improving within 12 to 24 hours*:
    Severe colitis
Surgical consultation for consideration of surgery within 48 to 72
    hours if not improving on medical management*:
    Moderate colitis

*Consider early fecal microbiota transplant if immediately available and patient is stable.

Once the decision has been made to pursue surgical treatment, the operation must be performed in an expeditious and aggressive manner. Removal of the entire colon with preservation of the rectum and end ileostomy is necessary. A segmental colonic resection should not be performed for CDI regardless of the perceived extent of disease.

An anastomosis is not recommended. Because of the need to perform a rapid colectomy and the critical illness of the patient, a laparoscopic approach generally is not recommended but may be considered in a relatively stable subset of patients.

In preparation for surgical intervention, invasive cardiopulmonary monitoring with arterial line placement and central venous access is recommended. Aggressive fluid resuscitation is critical. Marking of a site for a planned ileostomy by an enterostomal specialist is ideal but not always immediately possible. The patient should be placed supine on the operating table. The abdomen is prepped and draped widely. A large midline laparotomy incision should be made. The length of the incision should allow for rapid mobilization of the colon. The gross appearance of the colon can vary from normal to markedly edematous, ischemic, or frankly necrotic. At this point, the surgeon must resist the temptation to perform a less aggressive operation based on the external appearance of the colon itself. If the diagnosis of CDI is secure and laparotomy is performed, the surgeon should proceed with a total colectomy and end ileostomy. The distal ileum and the rectum can be divided quickly with linear staplers, and the mesentery can be ligated with a clamp-and-tie technique. Alternatively, bipolar or ultrasonic tissue sealing and cutting devices can be helpful to quickly divide the mesentery and maintain adequate hemostasis. The omentum can be removed from the colon or divided and resected along with colon, whichever is most expeditious. Once the colon has been removed from the abdomen, the distal ileum is brought through an opening in the rectus muscle and fascia and the stoma matured after closure of the midline wound. Rarely, the patient may remain in extremis or the retroperitoneal and bowel edema may preclude closure. In this event, a damage control philosophy may be used. Delayed maturation of the stoma and/or use of an open abdomen strategy may be required to quickly conclude the operation.

Stoma reversal may be considered once the patient has recovered fully. Reversal rates are low, ranging from 20% to 35% with a median interval to closure of 234 days.

The mortality after colectomy for CDI has been reported to be 34% to 57%. Likely contributors to this finding include delays in the initial diagnosis or surgical consultation, poor patient selection, and difficulty predicting the disease course. Recognition of unacceptably high perioperative mortality has led many surgeons to reconsider whether total colectomy is the best surgical procedure for CDI.

An alternative surgical procedure for the treatment of CDI has been proposed recently. A loop ileostomy is constructed (often laparoscopically). The colon then is irrigated with warmed polyethylene glycol 3350/electrolyte solution via the ileostomy. Postoperative antegrade irrigation of vancomycin solution through the ileostomy is continued for 10 days. Early data demonstrate decreased mortality and high stoma closure rates. Although very intriguing, it is premature to recommend this procedure as standard first-line surgical treatment. After an operation for CDI, the patient should be taken to the intensive care unit. Although some patients demonstrate almost immediate improvement in their condition after removal of the diseased colon, ongoing critical care is necessary to limit morbidity and mortality. Hemodynamic support including vasopressors and large volume fluid resuscitation may be required. Likewise, aggressive treatment of multisystem organ failure may be necessary in the postoperative period.

■ RECURRENT INFECTION

Recurrence is a major challenge in the treatment of CDI with reports of rates between 6% and 47% within the first 2 weeks after completion of initial treatment. This risk is increased further with each subsequent recurrence. For patients with a first recurrence of CDI, it is reasonable to repeat standard dosing regimens of metronidazole or vancomycin. In severe cases of first recurrences, oral vancomycin alone or combination therapy to include intravenous metronidazole is recommended. Subsequent recurrences require consideration of additional treatment options such as tapering and pulsed antibiotic strategies, FMT, and combination or adjunctive drug regimens. Tapering is accomplished by decreasing the dosage of antibiotic over a 4- to 6-week time period. Because spores of *C. difficile* are resistant to antibiotics, pulsed dosing can be added to the end of a taper to allow for residual *C. difficile* spores to germinate. Although published dose tapering and pulsed strategies may differ slightly, it generally is believed that vancomycin should be the drug of choice in this setting because prolonged use of metronidazole can lead to peripheral neuropathy. Other options include fidaxomicin, rifaximin, tigecycline, rifampin, cholestyramine, and monoclonal antibodies. Treatment for recurrent CDI must be individualized based on the number of recurrences, the severity of disease, comorbidities, and available resources. The role of surgical therapy for recurrent CDI has not been established but is a consideration as a last resort.

■ *CLOSTRIDIUM DIFFICILE* INFECTION AND INFLAMMATORY BOWEL DISEASE

It is well established that CDI is increased in patients with inflammatory bowel disease (IBD), especially ulcerative colitis. These patients typically experience an increased hospital length of stay, an increased need for surgical intervention, and higher morbidity and mortality independent of the stress of surgical intervention. A diagnostic dilemma certainly can exist because many of the symptoms of IBD can mimic CDI. It is therefore important for the clinician to check for CDI in patients with worsening or relapsing IBD.

Treatment of CDI in patients with IBD differs little from that in the general population with few exceptions. Oral vancomycin is recommended as first-line therapy, which may be given in combination with IV metronidazole in more severe cases. It is important to minimize corticosteroids and other immunomodulators as well as broad-spectrum antibiotics. There should be a low threshold for total colectomy with ileostomy in patients with severe, fulminant and persistent CDI, which may serve as the first stage of restorative proctocolectomy.

■ *CLOSTRIDIUM DIFFICILE* ENTERITIS

CDI may manifest as an enteritis of variable severity. This may occur as pouchitis in a patient who has an ileal J pouch after a restorative proctocolectomy for familial polyposis or ulcerative colitis. Patients who have had a colectomy with ileostomy for fulminant CDI or some other diagnosis may develop life-threatening CDI of the small bowel. It is important to keep this in mind when caring for patients with high-output ileostomies or who develop an otherwise unexplained systemic inflammatory response so that stool studies may be sent for early diagnosis. Supportive care and treatment with oral vancomycin or metronidazole (PO or IV) should be initiated. FMT has been used successfully in treating CDI pouchitis.

■ CONCLUSION

With the increasing incidence and severity of CDI, surgeons will be called on more frequently to manage these often challenging patients. Mitigation of risk factors, early diagnosis, and aggressive treatment must be realized to improve outcomes. A high index of suspicion in those at risk will help the surgeon identify the patient with an early, atypical, or subtle presentation. CDI must be considered in any patient with a history of recent antibiotic use, unexplained abdominal pain, abdominal distention, fever, or leukocytosis, even in the absence of diarrhea.

It is important that the surgeon be familiar with the medical treatment of CDI as well as the role for FMT in recurrent and even moderate to severe cases. This often requires coordination of care with gastroenterologists and infectious disease specialists.

Unfortunately the mortality rate of those who require surgical intervention for CDI remains high. To improve mortality rates, the current consensus is that early and expeditious surgery is of likely benefit and that patients ideally will receive surgical intervention before reaching a fulminant state. It is clear that when the surgeon encounters a patient with CDI who has peritonitis, perforation, or fulminant colitis, the first consideration after resuscitation is to proceed to operative intervention. Patients with severe CDI who fail to promptly respond to nonsurgical therapy also should be considered strongly for surgical intervention even in the face of contributing comorbidities. Although total colectomy with ileostomy is the accepted procedure of choice, laparoscopic ileostomy with vancomycin lavage may emerge as a promising treatment option for severe and fulminant CDI.

SUGGESTED READINGS

Bartlett JG. *Clostridium difficile*: progress and challenges. *Ann N Y Acad Sci.* 2010;1213:62-69.

Efron PA, Mazuski JE. *Clostridium difficile* colitis. *Surg Clin North Am.* 2009;89:483-500.

Neal MD, Alverdy JC, Hall DE, et al. Diverting loop ileostomy and colonic lavage: an alternative to total abdominal colectomy for the treatment of severe, complicated *Clostridium difficile* associated disease. *Ann Surg.* 2011;254:423-427.

Stanley JD, Burns RP. Invited commentary: *Clostridium difficile* and the surgeon. *Am Surg.* 2010;76:235-244.

THE MANAGEMENT OF LARGE BOWEL OBSTRUCTION

Anne C. Fabrizio, MD, and Elizabeth C. Wick, MD

Obstruction of the large bowel is a serious and progressive disease process that traditionally has been managed with urgent surgery. Large bowel obstruction may result from of a variety of causes and occurs in all age groups. The management of large bowel obstruction varies by cause and thus rapid evaluation and diagnosis is essential in appropriately managing patients with obstructive symptoms.

■ CAUSE

The causes of large bowel obstructions can be categorized broadly as mechanical or functional (Box 1). Large bowel obstructions most often are due to neoplastic processes. Colorectal adenocarcinoma alone accounts for more than half of all large bowel obstructions (Figure 1). In fact, up to one third of patients with colorectal cancer have near or complete mechanical obstruction because of tumor burden. Malignant obstruction most commonly occurs in the descending colon and rectosigmoid.

Volvulus is the second most common cause of large bowel obstruction and results from an axial rotation of bowel around the mesentery (Figure 2). The sigmoid colon is the most common location for volvulus followed by the cecum and transverse colon.

Diverticular disease is the third most common cause of large bowel obstruction. Large bowel obstruction from diverticular disease may be chronic or acute. Diverticular stricture accounts for

approximately 10% of large bowel obstructions. Acutely, a diverticular large bowel obstruction can be caused by inflammation, stricture, or compression by an adjacent abscess.

Other mechanical causes of large bowel obstruction include cecal bascule, intussusception, inflammatory bowel disease, extrinsic tumors, fecal impaction, foreign body, infection, and adhesion-related obstruction.

Functional or adynamic causes of large bowel obstructions include colonic pseudo-obstruction, narcotic-associated adynamic ileus, and an adynamic state caused by systemic illness such as sepsis and toxic megacolon from *Clostridium difficile* infection or other severe causes of acute colitis. Treatment of the underlying cause in these patients often improves the manifestation of bowel obstruction.

■ CLINICAL PRESENTATION

Large bowel obstructions can present with a wide range of symptoms. The typical symptoms associated with large bowel obstruction are abdominal pain, distension, and obstipation. Emesis is usually a late presentation of large bowel obstruction, unless there is a concomitant small bowel obstruction. Often patients present with signs of hypovolemia and electrolyte imbalances, secondary to fluid loss into the dilated intestine.

Clinical signs and symptoms that suggest perforation, strangulation, or ischemia such as high fever, tachycardia, peritonitis, point tenderness, pain out of proportion to examination, or shock indicate a surgical emergency and the need for an urgent laparotomy.

■ DIAGNOSIS

History and Physical Examination

Rapid evaluation and diagnosis beginning with a focused history and physical examination should occur in patients presenting with signs and symptoms of a large bowel obstruction.

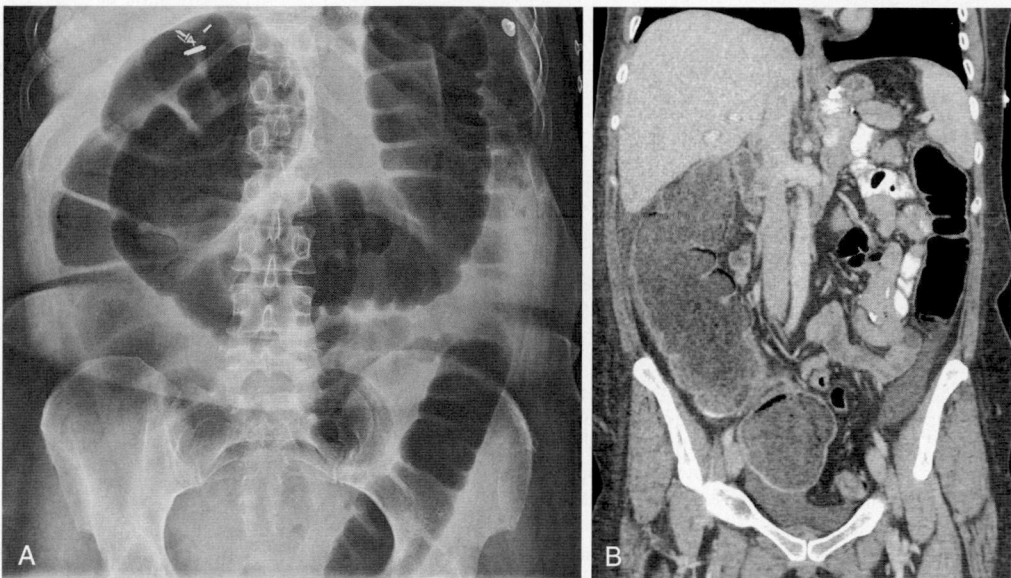

FIGURE 1 A and **B,** Obstructing sigmoid colon cancer. *(Courtesy Harisinghani Mukesh, MD, MGH Radiology.)*

BOX 1: Causes of Adult Large Bowel Obstruction

Mechanical

Neoplasm
Volvulus (sigmoid, cecal, transverse colon)
Diverticulitis
Cecal bascule
Intussusception
Inflammatory bowel disease
Incarcerated hernia
Infection (abscess, inflammation)
Fecal impaction
Adhesion-related obstruction
Foreign body

Functional

Acute toxic or chronic megacolon
Colonic pseudo-obstruction (Ogilvie's syndrome)

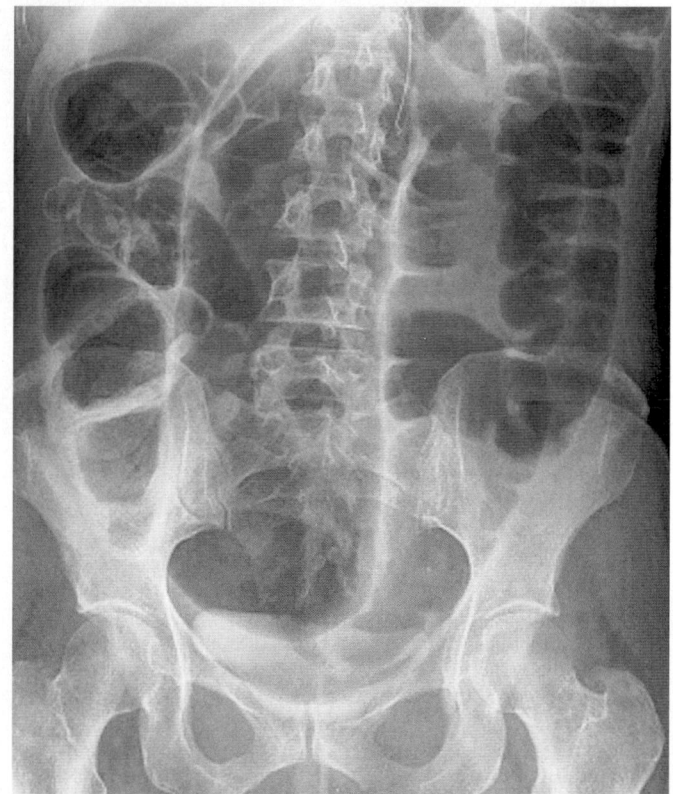

FIGURE 2 Sigmoid volvulus. *(Courtesy Harisinghani Mukesh, MD, MGH Radiology.)*

If the disease process is chronic or progressive in nature, such as malignancy, patients may report a preceding period of bloating or constipation with narrowing caliber of stools and gradually increasing cramping abdominal pain. In contrast, obstructive symptoms may progress on a much quicker time course in an acute disease process such as volvulus.

The review of systems should include changes in bowel function, changes in weight, or factors that incite pain. In terms of medical history it is important to elicit a history of chronic constipation or diarrhea, narcotic use, malignancy, and any prior surgery.

Physical examination findings consistent with a large bowel obstruction include abdominal distension and tympany. Other findings to note include palpable abdominal masses, point tenderness, or peritonitis. It is also essential to perform a nodal examination to evaluate for possible metastatic disease associated with a malignancy. A digital rectal examination also should be performed to assess for a possible rectal mass or blood. If possible, proctoscopy should be done to evaluate for a volvulus or sigmoid mass.

Labs

Basic labs should be obtained in any patient presenting with signs and symptoms of a large bowel obstruction, including a complete blood cell count (CBC) and complete chemistry. A CBC allows for assessment of anemia or elevated white blood cell count (WBC), and the complete chemistry evaluation is useful in the evaluation of electrolyte imbalances. A lactate also should be included in the workup if there is any suspicion of ischemia.

Imaging

Typical radiographic findings in large bowel obstruction include air/fluid levels within dilated loops of colon, failure of contrast to pass distally, and luminal caliber change.

The flat and upright abdominal x-ray is a quick and useful tool for diagnosing large bowel obstruction. Abdominal x-rays are 84% sensitive and 72% specific for identifying large bowel obstruction. Furthermore, with a good abdominal x-ray, it is possible to distinguish cecal or sigmoid causes of obstruction and rule out free air.

If patients are stable, additional imaging can be performed. The gold standard in diagnosing large bowel obstruction is a contrast enema examination, which has 96% sensitivity and 98% specificity and occasionally can be therapeutic. However, computed tomography (CT) of the abdomen and pelvis is overtaking rapidly the contrast enema examination as the preferred imaging for diagnosis of large bowel obstruction. With multiplanar reconstruction, CT scans provide an 83% sensitivity and 93% specificity for diagnosing large bowel obstruction. CT also can provide detailed information about the severity of obstruction resulting from a number of causes, such as diverticular disease, obstructive masses, or internal hernias.

A finding of large cecal diameter on imaging is important to note. Cecal dilation of 12 cm or greater is associated with an increased risk for ischemia and perforation. However, there is no direct correlation between cecal diameter and risk of perforation. Perforation can occur at smaller cecal diameters.

Endoscopy

For patients who are stable, endoscopy via flexible sigmoidoscopy or colonoscopy can be vital in the workup of patients with large bowel obstruction. Endoscopy allows diagnostic biopsy of masses in the case of malignancy and also can be therapeutic in reducing volvulus. Risk of perforation is low with rates of less than 1%. However, CO_2 insufflation should still be used to reduce the risk of perforation.

■ TREATMENT

Initial Management

An emergent laparotomy should be performed in any patient with signs of perforation, closed loop obstruction with ischemia, or peritonitis. In patients who are stable, preoperative preparation is essential to improving outcomes. Patients often present with intravascular depletion because of sequestration of fluids and should undergo aggressive fluid resuscitation and correction of electrolyte abnormalities. Close monitoring of urine production with a urinary catheter is important for evaluating adequate resuscitation. Decompression with a nasogastric tube should be performed early. Patients undergoing surgery should receive appropriate preoperative antibiotics and preoperative stoma marking because frequently an ostomy is required.

Surgical Techniques

Colostomy

A loop colostomy proximal to the obstruction is a good option in urgent operations for patients who are acutely ill, are septic, have signs of peritonitis, hemodynamic instability, have gross contamination because of perforation, or have other barriers to healing such as severe malnutrition or immunocompromised state as a means to decompress the colon. A loop colostomy usually is used because, in an end colostomy, a blind end of the distal bowel is left in the abdomen, with progressive obstruction this segment of colon can perforate. The colostomy relieves patients of obstructive symptoms with the benefit of limiting concerns subsequently for an anastomotic leak. However, colostomies can be associated with significant morbidity, including parastomal hernias, decreased quality of life, and low rates of closure.

Segmental Colectomy

In patients with right-sided obstruction, urgent right hemicolectomy with primary anastomosis should be considered and can be performed laparoscopically if the patient is stable and the proximal bowel is not overly dilated. This procedure is associated with low rates of anastomotic leak if the bowel appears viable and not excessively dilated and the patient is hemodynamically stable.

There is more debate regarding the preferred surgical procedure in left-sided obstruction. Traditionally, primary anastomosis during the initial procedure was avoided because of higher rates of anastomotic leak (near 20%).

In the unstable or high-risk patient, the Hartmann procedure often is selected as the surgery of choice for left-sided obstruction. Introduced in 1923 by Henri Hartmann specifically for the management of large bowel obstructions, the Hartmann procedure involves resection of the distal obstruction with an end colostomy. However, morbidity for the Hartmann procedure has been reported in up to 35% of patients undergoing the procedure. Furthermore, up to 45% of patients who undergo the surgery remain with a permanent colostomy.

Segmental colectomy with primary anastomosis is a good option for carefully selected patients if the proximal colon is not dilated severely. Retrospective reviews have shown similar rates of operative mortality and anastomotic leak in segmental colectomy for left-sided lesions as compared with right-sided segmental colectomies. Furthermore, the procedure also has been associated with improved quality of life. A good option in high-risk patients is a segmental colectomy with proximal diverting loop ileostomy. This still allows for the diversion of fecal stream and, in the event of anastomotic leak, intra-abdominal sepsis is contained and usually can be managed with percutaneous drainage of abscesses and antibiotics. Loop ileostomy reversal is a less invasive procedure and patients are more likely to undergo this procedure and have their intestinal continuity restored as compared with Hartmann's reversal. The disadvantage is that ileostomy management can be more challenging as compared with colostomy management with respect to intravascular volume and electrolyte shifts.

Subtotal Colectomy

Subtotal colectomy with removal of the compromised, dilated colon can be performed with either an ileosigmoid or ileorectal anastomosis or end ileostomy and Hartmann's pouch with plan for reversal at a later date. During this procedure, it is important to avoid size discrepancy in luminal diameter between two ends of bowel to be anastomosed. This is usually the operation of choice for patients with medically refractory functional large bowel obstructions. It is rarely used for mechanical large bowel obstructions unless there is concern about a synchronous lesion in the proximal colon.

Endoscopic Stenting

Endoscopic stenting for large bowel obstruction was first used in the 1990s. Stenting can be used for palliation or as a bridge to surgery.

Palliation with stenting is used in patients who are poor candidates for surgery, have complex disease, either locally advanced or metastatic cancer, and would benefit from neoadjuvant chemotherapy and/or radiation before surgery. Stenting provides alleviation of obstructive symptoms and has good success rates.

Technically and clinically successful stent deployment can be accomplished in approximately 90% of patients. However, the rates of complications associated with stenting may be significant, including stent migration, regrowth into the stent causing obstruction, and perforation.

Stenting is a viable option to use as a "bridge to surgery." Acute obstruction is relieved and patients are able to avoid emergency surgery. This allows patients to undergo treatment with neoadjuvant chemotherapy and/or radiation without a delay. In the case of rectal cancer, the use of neoadjuvant chemotherapy and radiation will improve the likelihood of a negative radial margin on the total mesorectal excision. In addition, stenting enables decompression of the proximal bowel over days to weeks and allows for other diagnostic investigations such as additional endoscopic evaluation for synchronous lesions. Once the acute obstruction is relieved by the stent, patients can be optimized nutritionally and medically for a semielective resection. Surgical mortality is reduced in elective surgery from around 20% to 5% as compared with emergency surgery. Studies also have shown higher primary anastomosis rates with preoperative stenting and lower stoma rates.

However, it is important to state that, in general, unless the oncologic operation can be optimized by additional treatment, surgery is still the preferred management if a patient can tolerate surgery. When compared with stenting, surgery has a higher clinical success with similar rates of morbidity and mortality.

■ SPECIAL CASES

Sigmoid Volvulus

If a patient is stable and is diagnosed with volvulus of the sigmoid colon, initial management should include a flexible sigmoidoscopy with an attempt at endoscopic detorsion. The classic finding on endoscopy is a "swirl sign." Decompression by sigmoidoscopy is successful in detorsing 85% to 95% of patients with sigmoid volvulus but is contraindicated in patients with an acute abdomen or if there are signs of ischemia. If detorsion is unsuccessful, urgent surgery is needed. There is a 60% rate of recurrence, so it is recommended that the patient undergo sigmoid resection during the original admission.

Cecal Volvulus or Bascule

In contrast to sigmoid volvulus, colonoscopic reduction of a cecal volvulus or bascule has a less than 30% success rate. The cecum also has higher rates of ischemia; up to 20% of patients have a gangrenous cecum. The primary treatment for this disease process is primary surgical resection with primary anastomosis if the patient is stable. Other procedures such as detorsion with cecopexy or cecostomy have a higher rate of complications and recurrence.

Pseudo-Obstruction

Pseudo-obstruction, or Ogilvie's syndrome, is associated with a number of underlying conditions such as postoperative conditions, cardiopulmonary disorders, other systemic disorders, and trauma and is more common in the elderly. It is difficult to distinguish from mechanical obstruction. CT imaging will reveal dilated colon without a transition point or a definitive area of caliber change.

Initial treatment of pseudo-obstruction involves conservative measures such as correcting electrolyte and fluid balance, discontinuation of opiates, and constipating or antimotility medications. If this is unsuccessful, medical therapy with neostigmine can be attempted. This should be done in a cardiac-monitored setting because neostigmine can cause severe bradycardia. Next, colonic decompression via endoscopy can be performed. This should be done by an experienced endoscopist because the goal is to remove air from the colon. If the pseudo-obstruction still fails to resolve, surgical intervention with a subtotal colectomy and end ileostomy can be performed.

■ SUMMARY

Large bowel obstruction is a serious disease process that often necessitates surgical resection. Rapid evaluation and diagnosis is essential to providing appropriate management. Emergent laparotomy should be performed in patients who present with peritonitis, signs or symptoms of ischemia, or shock. Preoperative optimization of patients with fluid resuscitation and correction of electrolyte imbalances should be performed whenever possible. Segmental resection with primary anastomosis can be considered in patients who are stable and have minimal barriers to healing. Endoscopic stenting can be considered for palliation or as a bridge to surgery in select patients.

SUGGESTED READINGS

Cirocchi R, Farinella E, Trastulli S, et al. Safety and efficacy of endoscopic colonic stenting as a bridge to surgery in the management of intestinal obstruction due to left colon and rectal cancer: a systematic review and meta-analysis. *Surg Oncol.* 2013;22:14-21.

Masoomi H, Stamos MJ, Carmichael JC, et al. Does primary anastomosis with diversion have any advantages over Hartmann's procedure in acute diverticulitis? *Dig Surg.* 2012;29:315-320.

Oren D, Atamanalp SS, Aydinli B, et al. An algorithm for the management of sigmoid colon volvulus and the safety of primary resection: experience with 827 cases. *Dis Colon Rectum.* 2007;50:489-497.

Ponec RJ, Saunders MD, Kimmey MB. Neostigmine for the treatment of acute colonic pseudo-obstruction. *N Engl J Med.* 1999;341:137-141.

Salem L, Anaya DA, Roberts KE, et al. Hartmann's colectomy and reversal in diverticulitis: a population-level assessment. *Dis Colon Rectum.* 2005;48:988-995.

ENTERAL STENTS IN THE TREATMENT OF COLONIC OBSTRUCTION

David F. Hutcheon, MD

Colonic obstruction may be benign or malignant in origin and traditionally is treated with emergency surgery. Between 10% and 30% of colon cancers cause complete or partial obstruction, as may a small number of pancreatic cancers, ovarian cancers, or lymphomas. The majority of obstructions are in the left colon, where the stool is more formed and the lumen narrower than in the right and transverse colon. Causes of colonic obstruction are listed in Table 1.

Emergency surgery is associated with mortality rates of 15% to 20% and morbidity rates of 40% to 50%. A recent study showed a mortality rate of 14.9% for emergency surgery versus 5.8% for elective surgery. Surgical mortality is increased in patients with older age, low socioeconomic status, high-grade obstruction, metastatic or locally advanced disease, and emergency surgery.

Patients may have associated medical problems that increase the risk of emergency surgery, including hypovolemia, sepsis, electrolyte disturbances, cardiac or renal compromise, and multiorgan failure. Stenting may allow time to stabilize the patient before surgery; however, the toxic patient with intestinal perforation, ischemia, peritonitis, or other surgical emergencies should be taken directly to the operating room.

Surgery ideally entails relief of the obstruction through resection of the tumor or other source of obstruction, and anastomosis of the bowel. In the setting of emergency surgery, the patient more frequently needs a multistage approach with a diverting colostomy or ileostomy for colonic decompression.

■ INDICATIONS

The major indications for colonic stent placement in patients with colon cancer are the following:

1. Palliation of advanced disease
2. Preoperative decompression as a bridge to surgery

Endoscopic decompression allows clinical stabilization of the patient before surgery. It also allows colonic cleansing before surgery, as well as preoperative colonoscopy to rule out synchronous colonic neoplasms. Finally, it usually avoids the need for a temporary or permanent colostomy and allows one-stage resection and anastomosis rather than initial colonic diversion. It also may allow preoperative chemotherapy and/or radiation in selected patients.

Treatment of benign lesions such as colonic fistulae and benign strictures is more controversial.

■ TECHNIQUES AND EQUIPMENT

Endoscopic metal stents may be uncovered or covered. The covered stents have a plastic coating over the metal mesh to prevent ingrowth of tumor. This advantage of diminished tumor ingrowth is balanced by an increased rate of stent migration. A Korean study compared covered (c) and uncovered (uc) stents for colonic obstruction. Results showed stent migration rates of 21.1% (c) versus 1.8% (uc) and stent occlusion rates of 3.8% (c) versus 14.5% (uc). The mean patency rate was greater than 6 months in both groups. Most colonic stents are uncovered and deployed through the endoscopic channel (TTS, through the scope). Available colonic stents are listed in Table 2.

The majority of stents deploy from the distal end proximally (Figures 1 and 2). The exception is the Ultraflex precision nitinol

stent by Boston Scientific (Marlborough, MA). A water-soluble contrast enema or computed tomography with water-soluble rectal contrast is usually helpful before endoscopy to delineate the lesion and the degree of obstruction. This allows planning of the endoscopic procedure, and the hypertonicity of the contrast usually provides cleansing of the distal colon. Care should be taken to perform a limited study to delineate the lesion and not place a large amount of hypertonic contrast proximal to the lesion.

Colon cleansing before endoscopy can be accomplished with cleansing enemas in distal complete colonic obstruction. Patients with nontotal obstruction can be prepped gently with an isotonic osmotic prep, such as polyethylene glycol. Prophylactic antibiotics should be administered to decrease the risk of procedure-associated bacteremia. Colonic overdistension proximal to the obstruction should be avoided by limiting air insufflation. Use of carbon dioxide rather than air insufflation is preferable to decrease the risk of proximal colon overdistension.

Endoscopy usually is performed with a therapeutic endoscope with a channel sufficient to allow passage of the stent. The scope is passed to the lesion and an attempt made to pass the lesion with gentle pressure only. A smaller scope also can be used to pass the lesion, although this is not essential. Dilation of the lesion is no longer performed because of the increased risk of perforation. A 0.035-inch, flexible-tip, long-length biliary guidewire is passed through a biliary catheter or sphincterotome and through the stricture under fluoroscopic guidance. Water-soluble contrast can be injected through the biliary catheter or sphincterotome to delineate the lesion. The guidewire is left in place and the biliary catheter or sphincterotome removed. The stent is then passed over the wire, through the therapeutic scope channel and into place, straddling the lesion. Deployment in 1- to 2-cm increments under intermittent fluoroscopic guidance should allow placement of the stent with at least 2 cm of stent both proximal and distal to the lesion. Ideally, a "waist" is seen fluoroscopically in the midportion of the stent with distal and proximal ends of the stent "flared" during and after full deployment. Many stents can be "resheathed" before being two thirds deployed, allowing repositioning. If stent placement is not satisfactory after deployment, a second stent can be placed, overlapping the first. If an endoscope with a channel diameter insufficient to allow passage of the stent is used initially, this can be removed, leaving the guidewire in place, and a large channel scope positioned by backloading the proximal end of the guidewire through the endoscopic metal stent preloaded through the scope. Stents also may be deployed without the endoscope, under fluoroscopic control, or alongside the endoscope, after placing the guidewire through the stricture.

After stent placement the patient should be maintained on a low-residue diet with laxatives sufficient to maintain a soft-to-loose stool consistency, which will not obstruct the stent. Vegetables, fruits, and whole grains should be avoided.

TABLE 1: Causes of Colonic Obstruction

Colorectal carcinoma	70%
Colonic volvulus	5%-15%
Strictures/adhesions	1.7%-10%
Hernia with colonic incarceration	2.5%

Crohn's disease, ischemic colitis, intussusception, and retroperitoneal fibrosis.

TABLE 2: Colonic Stents

	Diameter (mm)	Length	Through Scope
BOSTON SCIENTIFIC*			
Wallstent	20, 22	60, 90 mm	Yes
Wallflex nitinol	22, 25	60, 90, 120 mm	Yes
Ultraflex precision nitinol	25	5.7, 8.7, 11.7 cm	No
COOK MEDICAL†			
Z-Stent	25	40, 60, 100, 120 mm	Yes
Evolution Duodenal	22	60, 90, 120 mm	Yes

*Marlborough, MA.

†Bloomington, IN.

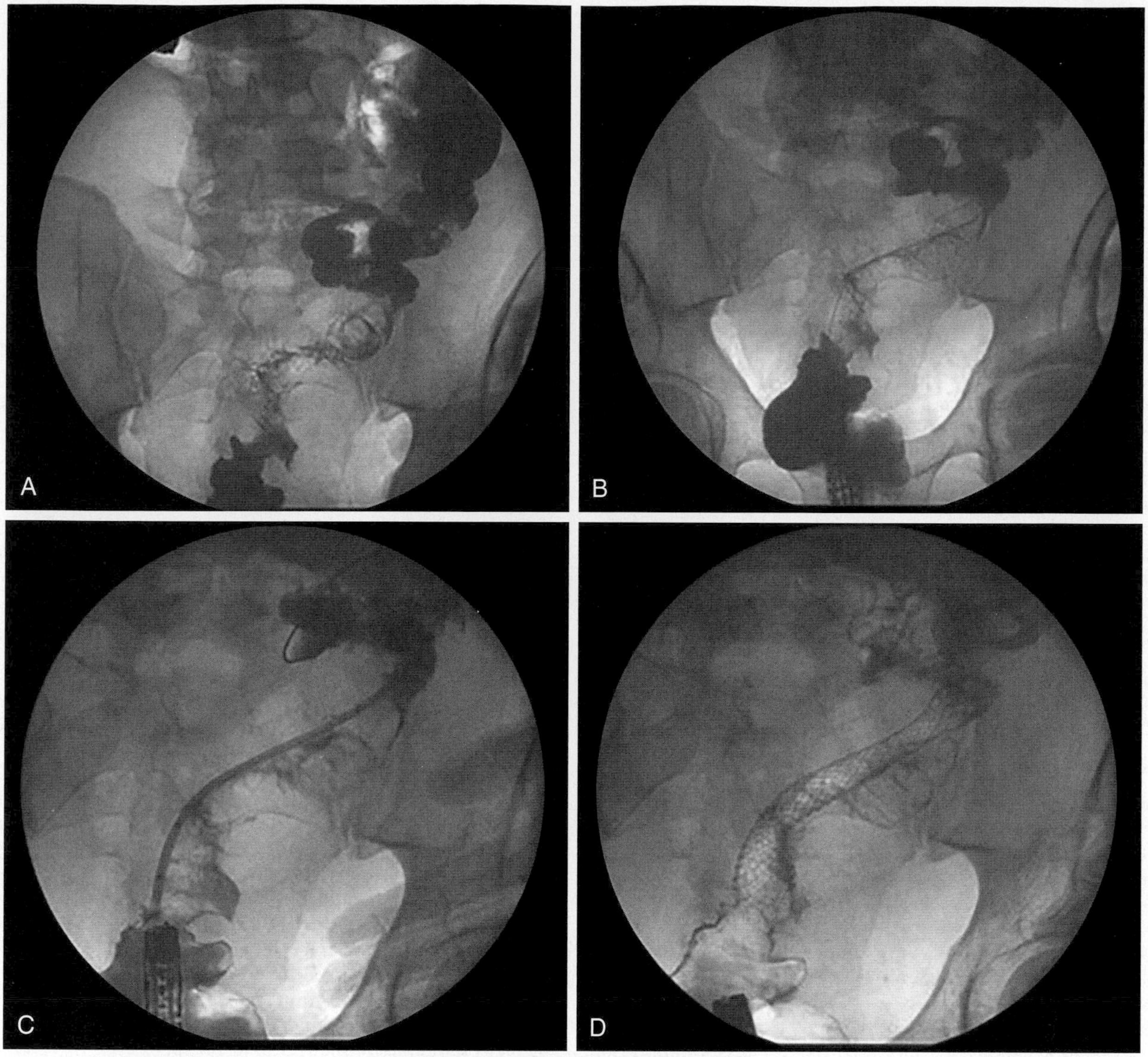

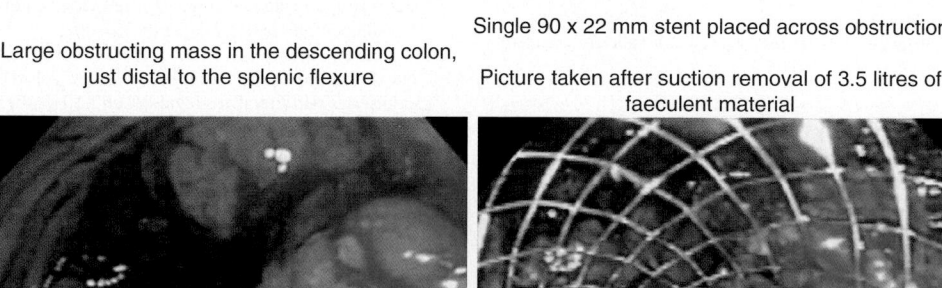

FIGURE 1 **A,** Contrast enema of sigmoid stricture. **B,** Guidewire passed through the stricture. **C,** "Through the stent" (TTS) stent passed through the stricture. **D,** Stent deployed through the stricture.

Large obstructing mass in the descending colon, just distal to the splenic flexure

Single 90 x 22 mm stent placed across obstruction

Picture taken after suction removal of 3.5 litres of faeculent material

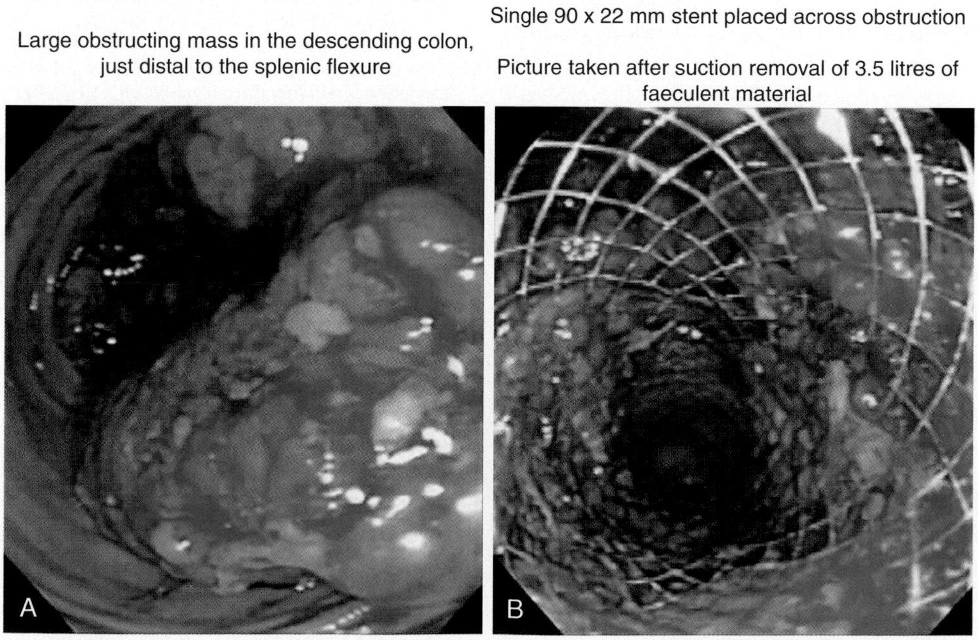

FIGURE 2 **A,** Malignant sigmoid stricture prestenting. **B,** Malignant sigmoid stricture poststenting.

Full expansion of the stent may take up to 72 hours. Abdominal x-rays can give information regarding stent expansion. After full stent expansion, the patient may be prepped for colonoscopic inspection of the entire colon.

■ EFFICACY

In a large meta-analysis of colonic stenting as a bridge to colonic resection, technical success defined as successful stent placement ranged from 46.7% to 100% with a weighted mean of 96.9%. Clinical success defined as adequate bowel decompression within 96 hours of stent insertion ranged from 40% to 100% with a weighted mean of 97.0%.

In a study of patients treated for palliation, stent patency at follow-up or death was 90.7%. Median stent patency was 106 days.

In patients treated for palliation, the median rate of reintervention, defined as unplanned surgical intervention, placement of a second or subsequent stent, or interventions to maintain stent patency such as laser ablation or colonic irrigation/enemas, was 20%. In patients with stents placed as a bridge to surgery the stents were in place for a shorter period, and median rate of reintervention was 7%.

■ COMPLICATIONS

The major complications of endoscopic metal stent placement are perforation and stent migration.

Perforation

Dilation of obstructing lesions has been associated with an increased risk of perforation. Because dilation now rarely is performed before stent placement, the risk of perforation has decreased to 5%, or less, in experienced hands. Perforation may be immediate, caused by the scope, stent, or guidewire, or delayed, usually because of erosion or pressure necrosis of bowel wall caused by the flared end of the stent abrading the colon. This occurs more frequently in colonic segments with sharp angulation, in which the stent ends abut and abrade the colonic wall.

Stented patients receiving chemotherapy with bevacizumab appear to be at a significantly increased risk for perforation. Prior therapy with bevacizumab does not appear to increase the risk of colonic perforation. Bevacizumab should be avoided in stented patients, and vice versa. The option of chemotherapy with bevacizumab should be considered before placement of endoscopic metal stents for palliation.

Anecdotal reports suggest a possible increased risk in patients treated with radiation.

Stent Migration

Migration of uncovered stents occurs in approximately 11% of patients. Migration happens more frequently in benign lesions, or lesions extrinsic to the colon. The stents appear to become less embedded in these lesions than in malignancies. Other causes of migrations are stents that are too short to adequately cover the structuring lesion, stents not wide enough to embed into the lesion, and shrinkage of tumors because of chemotherapy or radiation. About 25% of stent migrations occur within the first 3 days after placement. Not surprisingly, the longer the stents are in place, the higher the migration rate.

Abdominal Pain

Abdominal pain after stent placement is usually mild and resolves within hours to days, in the absence of perforation.

Rectal Bleeding

Minor bleeding may occur because of tumor friability. Significant bleeding is rare.

Recurrent or Persistent Obstruction

In a small percentage of patients, stenting will not relieve colonic obstruction. Initially this may be due to slow stent expansion, which may take up to 72 hours. Early stent migration or incomplete stenting of the entire tumor length can be rectified by stent replacement, or placement of an overlapping stent to totally bridge the tumor length. The stent also may become obstructed with fecal material. A second or extraneous lesion, such as synchronous lesion or extrinsic compression from carcinomatosis, also may lead to unsuccessful colonic decompression. Most of these issues can be diagnosed with a water-soluble retrograde contrast enema followed by repeat colonoscopy and placement of a second endoscopic stent.

Tumor ingrowth through the stent or at the ends of the stent also may be a cause of colonic obstruction, usually occurring weeks to months after stent placement. Tumor ingrowth can be treated by tumor ablation with argon photocoagulation or laser. A second stent also may be placed through the original stent. Tumor overgrowth at the ends of the stent is treated by overlapping a second stent with the first.

The rate of successful relief of colonic obstruction is lower in tumors greater than 10 cm. In one study of patients treated for palliation, stent obstruction was due to tumor ingrowth in 62%, stent migration in 13%, and fecal impaction in 25%.

■ CONCLUSIONS

Colonic stenting has a well-established role in the palliative care of patients with malignant obstruction that is not resectable or metastatic and in patients with multiple comorbid conditions. It also may be used as a bridge to surgery in patients with resectable malignant obstruction, allowing stabilization of the patient and a decrease in the rate of diverting colostomies. The planned use of bevacizumab and possibly radiation should temper the enthusiasm for stent placement, as should lesions longer than 10 cm.

SUGGESTED READINGS

De Ceglie A, Filiberti R, Baron TH, et al. A meta-analysis of endoscopic stenting as a bridge to surgery for left-sided colorectal cancer obstruction. *Crit Rev Oncol Hematol.* 2013;88:387-403.

Imbulgoda A, MacLean A, Heine J, et al. Colonic perforation with intraluminal stents and bevacizumab in advanced colorectal cancer: retrospective case series and literature review. *Can J Surg.* 2015;58:167-171.

Morris E, Taylor E, Thomas J, et al. Thirty day post operative mortality for colorectal surgery in England. *Gut.* 2011;60:806-813.

Vandiervliet G, Bichard P, Demarquay JF, et al. Fully covered self expanding metal stents for benign colonic strictures. *Endoscopy.* 2013;45:35-41.

Van Hooft J, Bemelman W, Oldenburg B, et al. Colonic stenting versus emergency surgery for acute left-sided malignant colonic obstruction: a multicentre controlled trial. *Lancet Oncol.* 2011;12:344-352.

Zahid A, Young CJ. How to decide on stent insertion or surgery in colorectal obstruction. *World J Gastrointest Surg.* 2016;8:84-89.

Zhao X, Liu B, Zhao E, et al. The Safety and efficiency of surgery with colonic stents in left sided colonic obstruction: a meta-analysis. *Gastroenterol Res Pract.* 2014;1-11.

The Management of Acute Colonic Pseudo-Obstruction (Ogilvie's Syndrome)

Nitin K. Ahuja, MD, and Marshall S. Bedine, MD

Acute colonic pseudo-obstruction is, as its name suggests, a condition of relatively sudden onset marked by the clinical and radiologic appearance of mechanical obstruction in the absence of a discrete obstructing lesion. The associated eponym, Ogilvie's syndrome, recognizes the surgeon who first reported the entity in 1948. Its exact pathophysiologic mechanism is unknown. Dominant thinking has dwelled for decades on putative autonomic dysregulation as triggered by various medical or traumatic processes.

Acute colonic pseudo-obstruction typically is noted in hospitalized patients with severe comorbid illness. The most frequently associated conditions include infection, cardiac disease, and operative and nonoperative trauma. Colonic pseudo-obstruction in a postsurgical context is most likely to follow abdominal and orthopedic procedures, with an average onset 4 days after surgery.

■ DIAGNOSIS

Signs and symptoms of colonic pseudo-obstruction include abdominal pain and distension, in the majority of cases, often associated with nausea and vomiting and an alteration in bowel habits. Constipation and diarrhea have been reported at a frequency of 40% to 50%. Physical examination reveals a protuberant abdomen that is tympanic to percussion, with bowel sounds usually present on auscultation. The primary differential diagnosis for acute colonic pseudo-obstruction includes acute mechanical obstruction, chronic intestinal pseudo-obstruction, and toxic megacolon.

Radiology often aids significantly in establishing the diagnosis of pseudo-obstruction. Computed tomography (CT) of the abdomen and pelvis typically demonstrates proximal colonic dilation with sparing of the descending colon (Figure 1). Dilation sometimes also extends to the rectum. CT is useful for excluding discrete obstructing lesions as well as neighboring structural abnormalities. Contrast enemas also may be helpful in delineating pseudo-obstruction but carry a risk of precipitating complications such as perforation via increased colonic pressure. Plain abdominal radiographs, although not specific enough for diagnosis of pseudo-obstruction, are often useful for monitoring interval changes in the degree of colonic dilation (Figure 2).

■ MANAGEMENT

Once acute uncomplicated pseudo-obstruction is recognized, management centers on the resolution of colonic dilation to prevent complications. Perforation risk increases markedly when cecal diameter exceeds 12 cm. Distension is possible above this threshold, however, as is perforation below it. A variety of therapeutic algorithms have been proposed, typically proceeding from conservative to progressively more invasive measures (Figure 3). Regular monitoring is advised throughout the timeline of care through serial physical examinations, laboratory testing, and plain radiographs every 12 to 24 hours. If and when a sustained response is achieved, administration of daily low-dose polyethylene glycol is advised to prevent recurrence.

Supportive Care

Initial management for uncomplicated pseudo-obstruction is primarily supportive. Bowel rest and intravenous fluids should be maintained while attempting to correct potential underlying causes. Efforts should be made to recognize and treat infections, cardiopulmonary instability, and electrolyte imbalances. In the latter circumstance, maintenance of serum potassium above 4 mg/dL and magnesium levels above 2 mg/dL is recommended. A review of medications should be performed to identify and discontinue, when possible, the use of gut-slowing agents such as opiates, antidiarrheals, anticholinergics, antipsychotics, and calcium-channel blockers.

Decompression via nasogastric tube typically is performed but with no clear data to support its effectiveness. Laxatives are discouraged given the risk of increased intraluminal pressure associated with their use. Mobilization should be encouraged, through ambulation if possible, or else through assisted transferring in and out of bed and alternating positions at least hourly among prone, supine, left and right lateral decubitus.

Neostigmine

For patients who fail to demonstrate improvement after 24 to 48 hours of conservative management, or in patients who initially have cecal dilation greater than 12 cm in diameter, a trial of neostigmine may be considered (Table 1). As a potent acetylcholinesterase inhibitor, neostigmine has demonstrated efficacy rates in the literature ranging from 60% to 100%. The drug typically is administered as a one-time intravenous dose of 2 mg, with effects demonstrated in 30 minutes or less. If signs and symptoms of pseudo-obstruction recur or persist, a second dose may be administered, commonly after an interval of 24 hours, although optimal timing has not been studied formally.

Neostigmine induces bradyarrhythmias at a frequency of 5% to 10%, in light of which the medication usually is administered with continuous cardiac monitoring in place and atropine readily available at the bedside. Other potential side effects include bronchoconstriction, hypotension, agitation, abdominal cramps, nausea/vomiting, salivation, and diaphoresis. Simultaneous administration of intravenous glycopyrrolate at a dose of 0.4 mg has been shown to attenuate some of these side effects.

Dose adjustments of neostigmine are required in patients with renal insufficiency. Doses typically are reduced by 50% for a creatinine clearance of 10 to 50 mL/min and by 75% for a creatinine clearance of less than 10%. Some practitioners view a serum creatinine greater than 3 mg/dL as a relative contraindication to this agent's use. Absolute contraindications include peritonitis and the presence of mechanical obstruction of either the intestinal or urinary tracts. Additional relative contraindications include a preintervention heart rate of less than 60 beats per minute, a systolic blood pressure less than 90 mm Hg, reactive airway disease, recent myocardial infarction, and concomitant beta-blocker use.

Neostigmine has not been well studied in the setting of pregnancy and therefore is listed as a Category C agent. Other medical therapies, including promotility agents such as metoclopramide, cisapride, and erythromycin, have been tried with anecdotal but inconsistent success.

Colonoscopic Decompression

Among patients who do not improve with conservative management and either cannot tolerate or fail therapy with neostigmine, endoscopic decompression should be considered (Table 2). The risks of colonoscopy in this setting are considerably increased, with a reported perforation rate of 2% to 3%; as such, the procedure should be performed only by an experienced endoscopist after risks and benefits

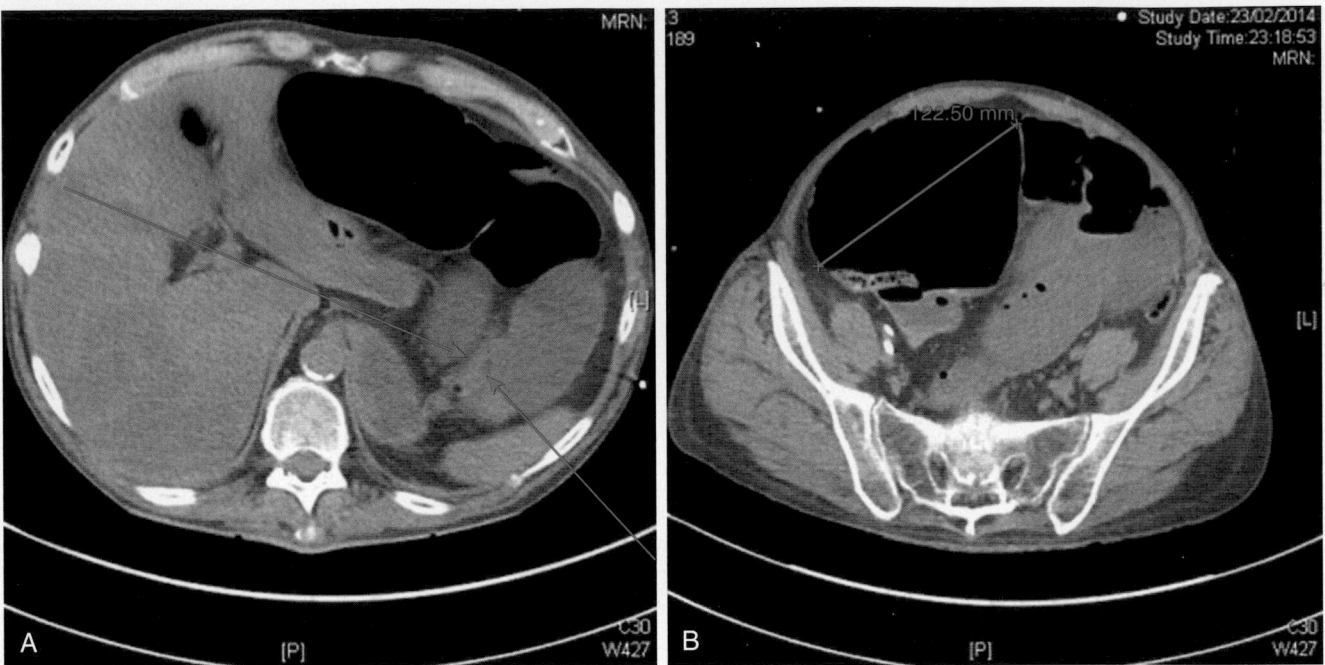

FIGURE 1 CT images of colonic dilation, with arrows denoting transition point in the absence of mechanical obstruction, consistent with Ogilvie's syndrome (**A**), and a ruler demonstrating cecal diameter at the typical threshold of concern for perforation (12 cm) (**B**). *(From Pereira et al. Ogilvie's syndrome—acute colonic pseudo-obstruction. J Visceral Surg. 2015;152:99-105.)*

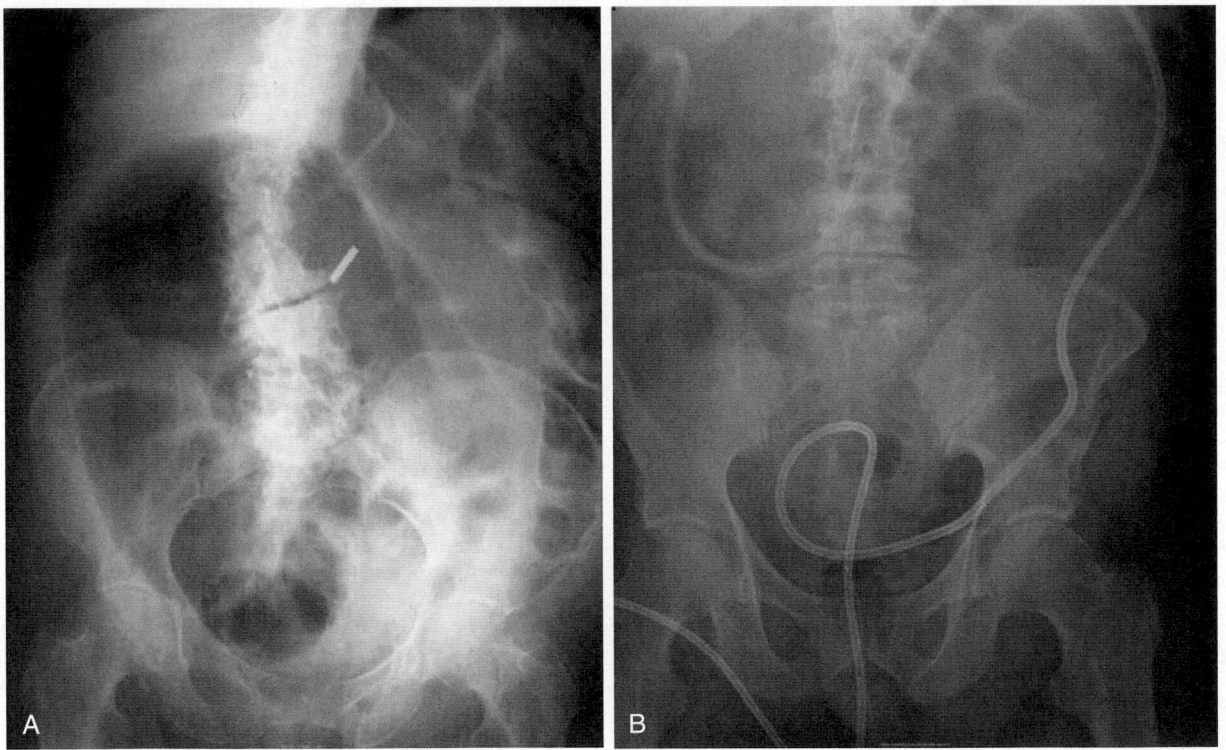

FIGURE 2 Upright abdominal plain films demonstrating acute colonic pseudo-obstruction before (**A**) and after (**B**) placement of a decompression tube. *(From Saunders MD. Acute colonic pseudo-obstruction. Best Pract Res Clin Gastroenterol. 2007;21:671-687.)*

have been weighed judiciously and communicated clearly to the consenting party.

Colonoscopic decompression typically is performed without any form of bowel preparation, given the risks of increased intraluminal pressure associated with enema instillation. A large-bore suction channel is preferred to remove gas and stool as rapidly and completely as possible. Air insufflation during the procedure should be minimized. Advancement to the cecum may be attempted, but if it cannot be safely reached, decompression up to the hepatic flexure is often sufficient for clinical benefit.

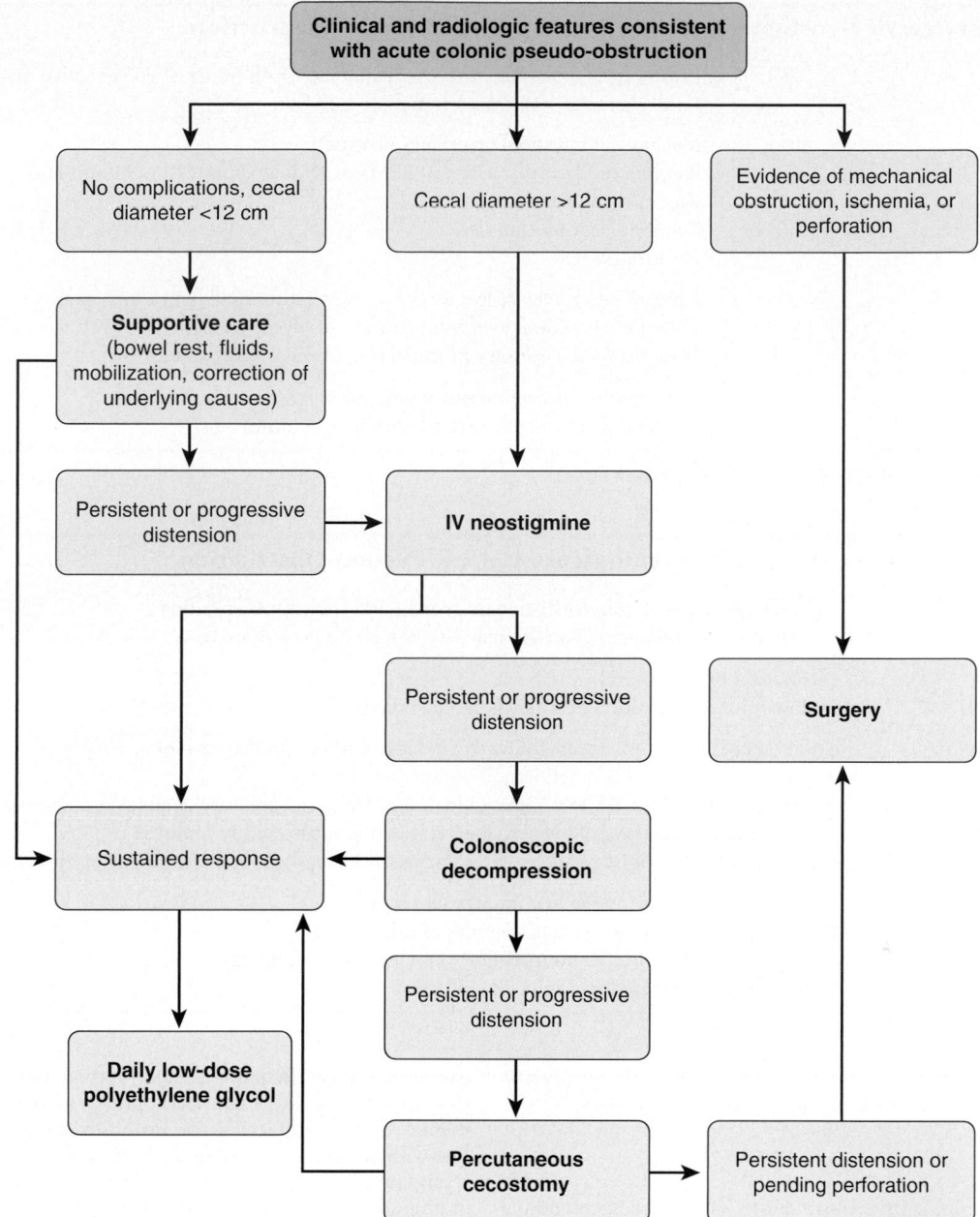

FIGURE 3 Algorithmic approach to stepwise therapy in acute colonic pseudo-obstruction.

Decompression alone has been definitively effective in approximately 50% of patients studied in case series. However, success rates may be augmented to 80% to 90% with placement of a decompression tube. Placement usually is performed over a guidewire, advanced either through the accessory channel as the colonoscope is withdrawn or under fluoroscopic guidance. Once placed, the decompression tube should be applied to low intermittent suction and flushed every 4 to 6 hours with a small volume of saline to prevent clogging. It is common for tubes to spontaneously dislodge with the restoration of peristalsis, although they should be manually removed if still in place after 72 hours.

A minority of patients may require repeat colonoscopic decompression to achieve a durable clinical response. Absolute contraindications to endoscopic intervention include perforation and peritonitis. Retrospective data suggest that gross evidence of colonic ischemia is present in about 10% of cases undergoing decompression. Per expert guidelines, ischemia remains a relative rather than absolute

contraindication to colonoscopy. If a frankly ischemic mucosal pattern endoscopically is visualized, however, immediate withdrawal is usually appropriate given the high risk of subsequent perforation.

Percutaneous Cecostomy

Among patients who fail conservative, pharmacologic, and endoscopic interventions, and among patients whose perioperative risk is high, percutaneous cecostomy may be considered for proximal colonic decompression. Percutaneous cecostomy tubes may be placed endoscopically or with radiologic guidance. Hybrid techniques also have been pursued to attempt percutaneous decompression in the ascending colon or more rarely in the descending colon.

Percutaneous cecostomy tends to be a highly specialized procedure for which robust safety and efficacy data are not available given the infrequency with which it is performed. However, reported complications are qualitatively similar to those of more conventional

TABLE 1: Overview of Neostigmine Use in Acute Colonic Pseudo-Obstruction

Indications	Failure to demonstrate improvement after 24-48 hours of conservative management
	Cecal diameter >12 cm on initial presentation
Contraindications	Mechanical intestinal or urinary obstruction
	Baseline bradycardia (HR <60 BPM) or hypotension (SBP <90 mm Hg)
	Recent myocardial infarction
	Ongoing beta-blocker use
	Peritonitis
Dosing	2 mg IV once; may repeat this dose after 24 hours if symptoms persist
	Consider simultaneous administration of glycopyrrolate 0.4 mg IV to attenuate side effects
	Dose decrease necessary in the setting of renal insufficiency
Monitoring	Continuous cardiac monitoring required before administration
	Effects typically demonstrated within 30 minutes

BPM, Beats per minute; *IV,* intravenous; *SBP,* systolic blood pressure.

TABLE 2: Use of Colonic Decompression in Acute Colonic Pseudo-Obstruction

Indications	Failure to respond to conservative management and trial of neostigmine
	Persistent pseudo-obstruction with inability to tolerate neostigmine
Contraindications	Perforation or peritonitis
	Endoscopic visualization of frankly ischemic mucosa
Placement	Colonoscope advanced at least to hepatic flexure (and cecum if possible)
	Air and stool removed through large-bore suction channel
	Guidewire placed under fluoroscopic guidance or through accessory channel as colonoscope is withdrawn
	Decompression tube placed over guidewire, which is subsequently removed
	Experienced endoscopist preferred given increased intraprocedural risk of perforation
Maintenance	Place decompression tube to low intermittent suction
	Flush every 4-6 hours with small volumes of saline
	Manually removed after 72 hours if not spontaneously dislodged
	Replacement considered in a minority of cases

percutaneous tube placements and include bleeding, cellulitis, peritonitis, perforation, and bumper-associated pressure necrosis.

Surgery

In the event that minimally invasive efforts fail to relieve pseudo-obstruction that has been present for longer than 6 days, surgical intervention may be considered. Practically speaking, this patient population is one in which perforation either is fast approaching or already has occurred. It should be emphasized that at this stage in the therapeutic algorithm, morbidity and mortality increase significantly. Rates of death range from 30% to 60% among patients with acute colonic pseudo-obstruction who undergo surgery of any kind. Less invasive surgical options include laparoscopic or open cecostomy or colostomy. In the event of structural complications, laparotomy with subtotal or total colectomy may be performed with either primary anastomosis or stoma formation, the latter typically preferred if a perforation has taken place.

■ SUMMARY

Acute colonic pseudo-obstruction is a motility disorder of the large intestine characterized by signs and symptoms of mechanical obstruction in the absence of discrete structural lesions. It most often is noted in hospitalized patients with comorbid medical illness and/or recent surgery or trauma. Cross-sectional imaging often helps to exclude alternative causes for colonic distension. Risks of complication with ischemia and perforation merit early recognition, close monitoring, and a stepwise approach to management. First-line therapy for uncomplicated pseudo-obstruction involves supportive care with bowel rest, intravenous fluids, and attempts to identify and resolve precipitating abnormalities. When colonic distension persists or progresses despite conservative management, intravenous neostigmine should be considered. If pharmacologic therapy fails or is contraindicated, colonoscopic decompression with or without guided intraluminal tube placement is the next most appropriate step, followed by percutaneous cecostomy if experienced practitioners are available. In cases of impending or known bowel perforation despite less invasive measures, operative intervention is imperative, recognizing the high mortality burden of any form of surgery in the treatment of Ogilvie's syndrome.

SUGGESTED READINGS

De Giorgio R, Knowles CH. Acute colonic pseudo-obstruction. *Br J Surg.* 2009;96:229-239.

Elsner JL, Smith JM, Ensor CR. Intravenous neostigmine for postoperative acute colonic pseudo-obstruction. *Ann Pharacother.* 2012;46:430-435.

Harrison ME, Anderson MA, Appalaneni V, et al. The role of endoscopy in the management of patients with known and suspected colonic obstruction and pseudo-obstruction. *Gastrointest Endosc.* 2010;71:669-679.

Ramage JI, Baron TH. Percutaneous endoscopic cecostomy: a case series. *Gastrointest Endosc.* 2003;57:752-755.

Vanek VW, Al-Salti M. Acute pseudo-obstruction of the colon (Ogilvie's syndrome): an analysis of 400 cases. *Dis Colon Rectum.* 1986;29:203-210.

THE MANAGEMENT OF COLONIC VOLVULUS

Alan Herline, MD, and Timothy M. Geiger, MD

Colonic volvulus refers to a twisting of the colon that causes obstruction. Unlike small bowel obstruction that normally occurs in the setting of prior operation(s) and adhesions; colonic volvulus occurs most commonly because of a twisting of the sigmoid colon or cecum that generally is believed to be from an acquired condition of the colon. Volvulus of other sections of the colon, including transverse and splenic flexure, are rare and account for less than 1% of all volvulus in the United States.

Current theory is that the mesenteric base becomes relatively narrow and the colon becomes elongated and without normal lateral attachments to the right- or left-side wall, a twisting of the colon occurs (Figure 1). Volvulus of the colon accounts for approximately 2% of all bowel obstructions (small and large bowel together) in the United States. It is estimated that volvulus causes 10% to 15% of large bowel obstructions. This differs from the higher rates of volvulus worldwide. Unlike many other conditions of the colon, the Western hemisphere actually has a lower incidence of colonic volvulus than other regions worldwide.

The differential diagnosis of volvulus includes all other causes of large bowel obstruction. This includes colonic and extrinsic neoplasms, inflammatory bowel disease, diverticulitis, Ogilvie's syndrome, adhesions, and constipation.

■ PRESENTATION

Volvulus usually is an urgent or emergent situation. It also can occur as a relapsing chronic form of recurrent obstructions based on the patient's history of intermittent episodes of pain and distension followed by sudden relief of the pain and the distension. The approach to these patients is similar. Sigmoid volvulus generally manifests as a large bowel obstruction, and cecal volvulus manifests as a small bowel obstruction. Patients generally have signs of distension and tachycardia and, in later presentation, may have decreased urine output, hypotension, and changes in mental status. The patient will have symptoms of cramping, abdominal pain, and constipation. If ischemia, perforation, or necrosis occurs, then there will be signs and symptoms consistent with sepsis.

■ DIAGNOSIS

If a patient presents with peritonitis and abdominal films demonstrating large or small bowel obstruction, the surgeon must proceed to the operating room once appropriate resuscitation has occurred. Sigmoid volvulus patients are more likely older, male, and institutionalized. If the patient's symptoms are less urgent, then tomographic imaging is accurate for sigmoid and cecal volvulus (70% to 90%). Classically abdominal films are described as a bent inner tube for sigmoid volvulus. In cecal bascule the abdominal films demonstrate findings of a kidney bean on the right side of the abdomen. In a cecal volvulus the distended colon projects into the left upper quadrant.

Another test commonly reported in the literature is a contrast enema (water-soluble contrast is preferred). Again, in a review of U.S. patients, 35% of cecal volvulus patients underwent a contrast enema with a correct diagnosis in 33% of patients. It was used in 46% of sigmoid cases and correctly diagnosed in 78% of patients. Historically, water-soluble enema was used for detorsion of the sigmoid colon, but this has been replaced with endoscopic decompression.

Neither of these treatments has a role in cecal volvulus if a diagnosis has been secured because of the risk of perforation.

■ TREATMENT OPTIONS

The surgical management of colonic volvulus depends on the location. In general the treatment algorithm for acute volvulus can involve endoscopic or operative detorsion for sigmoid volvulus followed by resection. Cecal volvulus treatment proceeds with surgery, detorsion, and either resection or colopexy. Detorsion (other than operative) methods are used rarely. All patients should be resuscitated appropriately and comorbid conditions maximized in an urgent manner if possible. Bowel preparation (for the small benefit it may offer) can be avoided, and second-generation perioperative antibiotics suffice. In the setting of sepsis and/or peritonitis then antibiotics covering a broader range of bacteria should be used. The Anesthesia team should be consulted immediately once the decision is made to proceed to the operating room. If available, consultation for ostomy marking is ideal in the event a stoma is needed, but this should not delay the time before proceeding to the operating room.

Cecal Volvulus

In the acute setting, surgical treatment and not endoscopic/ fluoroscopic treatment is used most commonly.

Surgery in the acute setting is divided into two categories, fixation and resection. There have been many reported techniques for fixation of the cecum, all with the goal of recreating the anatomic position of the cecum and keeping it from having the ability to rotate. The two most common fixation procedures are cecopexy and placement of a cecostomy tube. In large series pexy is shown to be performed 3% to 12% of the time and has at least a 26% recurrence and a mortality of 5% to 10% (similar to resection).

A cecopexy is performed by mobilizing the peritoneum off the right lateral and retroperitoneal surface. This can be performed laterally or medially. Attempting to start this plane laterally at the cecum may be difficult because the normal attachments of the cecum do not exist, and the surgeon may need to start at the hepatic flexure and proceed inferiorly. Pexy is made difficult because of the inherent thinness of the colon, and in the setting of distension this can be made more difficult. The colon then is sutured into position using the surgeon's suture of choice in either a running or interrupted fashion.

Cecostomy tube placement is infrequent (less than 2% of cases) and a description is given for completeness. Cecostomy has a mortality double that of resection. A cecostomy is created by placing a purse-string suture (usually two layers) on the anterior surface of the cecum, then creating an enterotomy in the middle and placing a drainage tube (typically a Malecot tube [28F to 32F]) into the lumen of the cecum. This is tied into position and the tube then is drained externally providing a fixation point and relieving distension.

Surgical resection involves removal of the cecum and portion of the ascending colon with (1) primary anastomosis; (2) resection and end ileostomy; or (3) primary anastomosis and proximal loop ileostomy. The amount of bowel resected is determined by areas of ischemia and or redundancy. The choice of anastomosis or ileostomy depends on patient factors and the condition of the abdominal cavity (perforation of gross contamination vs no perforation) and of the bowel. Typically this is accomplished via laparotomy, but laparoscopic approaches are reported. If there are concerns regarding whether to anastomose, assuming the bowel appears viable, an option is to perform a diverting loop ileostomy. Resection also can be performed with a long Hartmann's with rare need for a mucous fistula or resecting additional colon to avoid additional length of the defunctionalized colon. Surgical resection has far less than 1%

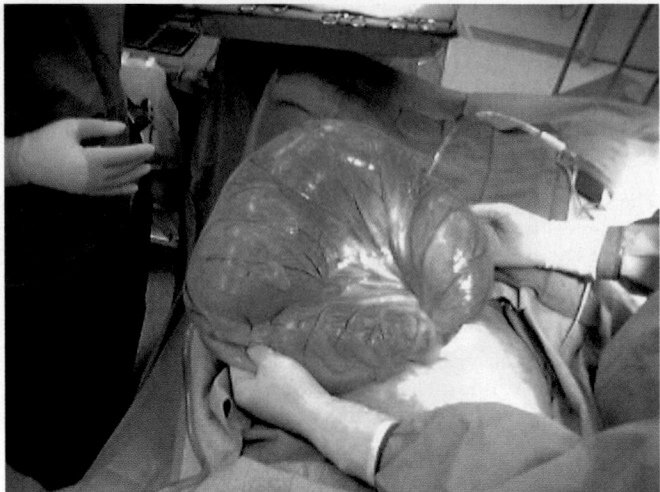

FIGURE 1 Twisting of the colon.

TABLE 1: Outcomes for Colonic Volvulus in the United States

n	Sigmoid Volvulus (n = 19,220)	Cecal Volvulus (n = 23,392)
Total charge ($)	80,352 (33,685-90,800)	68,935 (26,712-73,525)
Length of stay, d	15 (8-18)	11 (6-13)
Mortality		
Died	9.4	6.7
Missing	.28	.04
Postoperative complications		
Cerebrovascular accident	0.1	0.2
Cardiac complications	2.7	3.1
Respiratory failure	13.6	11.9
Pneumonia	10	7.5
Ileus/bowel obstruction	20.5	19.4
Anastomotic complications*	15.8	15.2
Acute renal failure	14.5	11.8
UTI	18.1	8.9
Urinary retention	3.2	2.3
Postoperative bleeding	2.6	3.0
Wound complications	6.3	6.6
DVT	1.0	0.6

From Halabi W, Jafari M, Kang C. Colonic volvulus in the United States. *Ann Surg.* 2014;259:293-301.

Continuous variables such as total charge and length of stay are reported as mean and interquartile range; categoric variables are reported as percent proportions.

*Including anastomotic leak, fistula, and intra-abdominal abscess.

DVT, Deep vein thrombosis; *UTI,* urinary tract infection.

recurrence and a mortality of 5% to 10%. Anastomotic complications (to include leak/abscess/fistula) are as high as 15%.

Sigmoid Volvulus

Sigmoid volvulus is amenable to endoscopic detorsion, operative detorsion, and pexy as well as resection. Patients present with distension and abdominal pain. Once a diagnosis is made using either plain films or tomographic imaging, proceed with endoscopic decompression. Endoscopic decompression alone has an extremely high recurrence (50% to 70%) and still carries a mortality of 6%. Decompression can be performed with a rigid or flexible endoscope.

If endoscopic decompression is completed and the patient is stable, then additional preoperative resuscitation can be completed. Ideally endoscopic decompression can be performed in the operating room before laparotomy, and this technically makes any operative procedure more feasible. Flexible endoscopy allows for visualization of the mucosa to rule out ischemia. If mucosa appears ischemic or necrotic, then the surgeon knows that resection will be necessary. If during endoscopic decompression perforation is suspected or decompression is unsuccessful, then the surgeon should proceed with laparotomy. Although sigmoid pexy is technically possible, Figure 1 demonstrates the potential difficulties with attempting to reduce and then suture the sigmoid to its anatomic lateral sidewall.

Just as in cecal volvulus, there are two general options for surgery: fixation versus resection. There have been many described procedures for fixation of the sigmoid colon. Including tube fixation (either by operative placement or even through the same technique used to place PEG tubes), fixation by pexy to the abdominal wall or transverse colon, and even mesenteric lengthening procedures to increase the length between the loops of the sigmoid colon to reduce the chance of recurrence. However, all of these fixation techniques carry a recurrence risk of 25% or greater. Because of this high risk, resection of the sigmoid colon generally is accepted as the best method to address acute and chronic sigmoid volvulus. Whether it is a resection with primary anastomosis or resection with end colostomy and Hartmann's closure of the rectum is dependent on patient factors. Laparoscopic approaches to the operation also are reported.

The patient is taken to the operating room once appropriately resuscitated, and flexible endoscopy is performed and the colon decompressed. Lower midline laparotomy is performed. This incision allows for adequate visualization, and incision length should not be a factor inhibiting performance of the operation. Many times the colon easily mobilizes out of the incision. Division of the distal rectosigmoid junction is performed initially. This allows for operative decompression to be performed on the table. There are multiple ways to perform operative decompression; all of which cause contamination of the operative field. Toweling off the field and opening the colon into a basin controls this with a modicum of success. Proximal division of the colon is based on the presence of ischemia. Colostomy is performed approximately 50% of the time, and the decision to anastomose is based on the condition of the patient and the bowel. Anastomotic complications occur approximately 15% of the time. A loop ileostomy can be performed to potentially reduce the effects of an anastomotic complication. Total colectomy is performed if the condition of the colon necessitates this or unusually if the surgeon finds synchronous cecal and sigmoid volvulus. Total colectomy carries the highest mortality.

Other Colonic Volvulus

Although transverse and splenic flexure volvulus is described, there is no consensus or large population of patients from which to draw conclusions. There have been reports of endoscopic decompression, but surgical intervention is recommended because of the belief of high recurrence rate with endoscopic treatment alone. However, the principles of surgical management remain to remove the area that has torsed, including any ischemic or compromised portions of colon, and then diversion or anastomosis is chosen based on the patient's systemic condition at the time of operation.

TABLE 2: Results of Colonic Volvulus Surgery by Patient Characteristics

Characteristic	Detorsion ± Colopexy (n = 209)	Right Colectomy (n = 728)	Left Colectomy (n = 781)	Total Colectomy (n = 56)	P
Age, mean ± SD, y	60.4 ± 21.1	64.7 ± 17.3	69.5 ± 16.9	67.6 ± 15.2	0.0001
Female, %	64.6 (57.9-70.8)	75 (71.7-78.0)	31.9 (28.7-35.2)	46.4 (34.0-59.3)	0.0001
Black, %	4.8 (2.6-8.6)	3.4 (2.3-5.0)	9.7 (7.8-12.0)	5.4 (1.8-14.6)	0.0001
Private payer, %	36.0 (29.7-42.6)	34.2 (30.9-37.7)	18.2 (15.6-21.0)	10.7 (5.0-21.5)	0.0001
Congestive heart failure, %	13.9 (9.8-19.2)	12.0 (9.8-14.5)	16.2 (13.8-19.0)	23.2 (14.1-35.8)	0.03
Comorbidity, mean ± SD	0.7 ± 1.3	0.8 ± 1.6	0.9 ± 1.6	0.9 ± 1.2	0.2

From Kasten K, Marcello P, Roberts P. What are the results of colonic volvulus surgery? *Dis Colon Rectum.* 2015;58:502-507.

Data are n (range) unless otherwise specified.

■ SUMMARY

Cecal or sigmoid volvulus is the cause of large bowel obstructions approximately 10% to 15% of the time. Other areas of colonic volvulus can occur and are rare. Tomographic imaging is the most accurate method to diagnosis, and many times abdominal films provide the diagnosis. Resection in either diagnosis offers the lowest recurrence and the lowest mortality. These patients are often older and ill, and mortality with the best of care occurs 6% to 20% of the time (Tables 1 and 2). Cecostomy or sigmoidostomy tubes carry a high morbidity and some mortality and are not usually performed.

Pexy does not decrease mortality and has a 26% recurrence. Endoscopic decompression only adds risk in the setting of cecal volvulus and is reserved for sigmoid volvulus as part of the intraoperative or preoperative preparation.

SUGGESTED READINGS

Halabi W, Jafari M, Kang C. Colonic volvulus in the United States. *Ann Surg.* 2014;259:293-301.

Kasten K, Marcello P, Roberts P. What are the results of colonic volvulus surgery? *Dis Colon Rectum.* 2015;58:502-507.

THE MANAGEMENT OF RECTAL PROLAPSE

Nicole M. Saur, MD, and Steven D. Wexner, MD, PhD(Hon)

Complete rectal prolapse is defined as a protrusion of all of the layers of the wall of the rectum outside of the anus. Partial mucosal prolapse involves only protrusion of the mucosa outside of the anus. Complete prolapse is identified on examination by circular mucosal folds and partial prolapse by radial folds. Internal rectal intussusception is defined as the rectum descending within itself but not protruding outside of the anus.

■ CAUSE

Although the cause of rectal prolapse remains partly elucidated, historically, two leading theories have emerged. Moschowitz described a sliding hernia through a defect in the pelvic fascia, whereas Broden and Snellman proposed that the mechanism involves the circumferential intussusception of the rectum. Regardless of the mechanism, risk factors have been identified for developing rectal prolapse that include (1) a deep pouch of Douglas, (2) laxity of the muscles of the pelvic floor and anal canal, (3) weakness of internal and external sphincter muscles, (4) pudendal neuropathy, and (5) lack of rectal fixation with mobile, redundant rectosigmoid and lax lateral ligaments.

■ PRESENTATION

Ninety percent of patients with rectal prolapse are females, often older than 50 years with a history of vaginal childbirth. Men with rectal prolapse typically are younger, 20 to 40 years. Unlike in women, the incidence rate in men decreases with advancing age. An increased incidence is found in nursing home–bound and psychiatric patients.

Symptoms typically associated with prolapse include a sensation of tissue outside of the anus after defecation or continuously, depending on the severity and chronicity of the prolapse. Rectal bleeding or mucous discharge after defecation may be noted in patients with chronically incarcerated prolapse. Fecal incontinence often is associated with prolapse secondary to the impairment of anorectal sensation and laxity of the sphincters and pelvic floor secondary to the chronically extruded mass. Other symptoms include a sensation of incomplete evacuation, tenesmus, constipation with straining, and urinary incontinence.

■ EVALUATION

The evaluation of a patient with rectal prolapse always should start with a history and physical examination. During examination, especially in the prone jack-knife position, the prolapse often is reduced. Patients frequently have a patulous anus and diminished resting tone and squeeze pressures during digital rectal examination. The best method to diagnose the type and degree of prolapse is with the patient sitting on a commode and bearing down to simulate a bowel movement. As previously noted, full-thickness prolapse is distinguished from mucosal prolapse by the appearance of circular folds; superficial mucosal ulcerations may be present, and examination also may reveal a concomitant cystocele and/or uterine prolapse.

Additional evaluation should include colonoscopy to exclude colonic or rectal disease, especially in patients who are older than 50 years. Manometry can assess and quantify sphincter damage that may result from chronic prolapse. Traditional contrast or newer MRI defecography can be used to assess occult prolapse or internal intussusception, which has been described in up to 33% of patients with disordered defecation. In addition, defecography can identify concomitant disease and determine the amount of redundant colon. Patients with a history of chronic constipation may benefit from colonic transit evaluation, which may affect the procedure chosen. If evidence of slow transit constipation or colonic inertia is identified, a subtotal colectomy may be the procedure of choice.

■ TREATMENT

Surgery is the only definitive form of treatment. In patients who are not surgical candidates, stool-bulking agents or stool softeners may provide symptomatic relief. Surgical goals include some combination of the following: narrowing of the anal orifice, obliteration of the pouch of Douglas, restoration of the pelvic floor, decreased rectosigmoid redundancy with bowel resection, and fixation of the rectum to the sacrum.

However, because the pathophysiology is imprecise and procedures imperfect there is no "perfect" procedure, and care must be individualized for each patient. The operation of choice for the given patient is based on consideration of the patient's age, gender, operative risk, presence of associated pelvic floor defects, degree of incontinence, presence of sphincter defect, history of constipation, and the surgeon's experience. Goals of surgery are to improve the anatomic abnormality, correct the functional disorders, limit morbidity, and minimize postoperative recurrence.

Surgery typically is classified into abdominal and perineal approaches. Traditionally, the perineal approaches have been reserved for older patients with more comorbidities who are not appropriate surgical candidates for a more invasive abdominal operation or general anesthesia. Abdominal surgeries are thought to be more effective, with lower rates of recurrence. Because full-thickness rectal prolapse is relatively rare and long-term follow-up studies are limited, there is no clear algorithm. The outcomes from the individual approaches are summarized in Table 1.

Preoperative Management

A full mechanical cathartic and oral antibiotic bowel preparation is performed before all procedures. Perioperative antibiotics and deep venous thrombosis prophylaxis are administered as per Surgical Care Improvement Project and institutional guidelines.

Perineal Procedures

Perineal procedures typically are reserved for elderly patients with significant comorbidities. Patients usually have minimal pain and earlier return of bowel function, tolerance of a regular diet, and ambulation than patients who undergo an abdominal operation. Current perineal approaches include mucosal sleeve resection, and perineal rectosigmoidectomy. Stapled transanal rectal resection (STARR) typically is used for internal intussusception and obstructed defecation but also can be used an as alternative to mucosal sleeve resection. Traditional anal encirclement operations have been abandoned because of poor success rates and high incidence of morbidity.

Mucosal Sleeve Resection (Delorme's Procedure)

Delorme's procedure was first described in 1900 and often is considered the treatment of choice for mucosal and short-segment full-thickness prolapse.

The procedure can be performed either in the prone jack-knife or the lithotomy position under general or regional anesthesia. A circumferential incision is made in the mucosa 1 cm proximal to the dentate line, and the submucosa and mucosal layers are dissected from the muscularis. Injection of local anesthesia with epinephrine or saline with epinephrine in the submucosa facilitates this dissection and aids in hemostasis. The stripped mucosa is excised, and a series

TABLE 1: Comparison of Operative Techniques for Rectal Prolapse

	Number Published Cases	Follow-Up in Months (Range, Mean)	Recurrence (%)	Constipation* (%)	Continence* (%)
PERINEAL PROCEDURES					
Delorme					
Total experience	609	11-43, 30	0-27	7-100+	25-85+
Last decade	158	12-43, 27.5	7-20		
Perineal Rectosigmoidectomy					
Total experience	799	12-228, 49.6	3-16	12-61+	6-80+/–
Last decade	168	13-44, 28.5	8.9-11.4		
ABDOMINAL PROCEDURES					
Ripstein's Procedure	595	12-83, 54.7	2-12	17-69+, 8-17-	18-78+, 8-10-
Abdominal Resection Rectopexy					
Open	516	17-98, 46	0-5	18-80+, 25-	11-78+
Laparoscopic	185	7-62, 24.7	0-12.5	64-69+	33-100+
Abdominal Suture Rectopexy					
Open	206	65-144, 76	3-9	27-83+/–	15-67+, 12-
Laparoscopic	191	6.9-48, 30.4	6-12.5	14-76 +, 11-	50-82+
Laparoscopic Ventral Rectopexy	675	28.8, 3-106	0-15	6-83+, 10-14-	14-67+

From Madiba TE, Baig MK, Wexner SD. Surgical management of rectal prolapse. *Arch Surg* 2005;140:63-73.

*When significant, + improvement, – worsening.

of four to eight parallel plicating stitches are placed by taking several sequential bites in the circular muscle. The mucosa with plicated muscle ultimately is anastomosed to the mucosa just proximal to the dentate line (Figure 1).

Morbidity and mortality rates have been reported as 4% to 33% and 0 to 2.5%, respectively. Complications include bleeding, anastomotic leak, stricture, and diarrhea. Recurrence rates have been reported to range from 6% to 26%. Up to 50% of patients reported an improvement in incontinence after the procedure without associated constipation.

Lieberth and colleagues performed the largest to date retrospective review of 76 patients of a median age of 74 years undergoing Delorme's procedure with a follow-up of an average of 36 months. The authors reported no mortality and 25% morbidity rates.

The most common postoperative complication was urinary retention (12%). They also reported anastomotic complications of bleeding (4%), leak (3%), and stricture (1%). The overall recurrence rate was 14.5%, with a mean time to recurrence of 31 months (1 to 60 months). The authors did not identify any predictors of recurrence in their cohort.

Stapled Transanal Rectal Resection

STARR is used primarily for internal intussusception or partial thickness prolapse but is preferred by some surgeons over the mucosal sleeve resection for full-thickness prolapse. In a similar procedure to stapled hemorrhoidopexy, a circular stapler is used and transanally placed to perform a double-stapled technique. One to three anterior purse-string sutures and one posterior purse-string suture are placed at least 5 cm proximal to the dentate line, and the stapler is secured. A defined amount of mucosa and full-thickness bowel wall thus is resected circumferentially, and the anorectal junction is reinforced with the staple line. The redundant tissue is removed and the anatomic abnormalities associated with obstructed defecation theoretically are corrected. Reported problems include high rates of recurrence, need for reoperation, and postoperative complications (severe pain, bleeding, pelvic sepsis, incontinence, stricture). In a large series (123 patients), Gagliardi and colleagues showed that after a median follow-up of 17 months, 29% of patients had recurrent rectocele and 28% had recurrent internal intussusception. Bleeding was the most frequent postoperative complication and occurred in 9.7% of patients. Nineteen percent of patients required reoperation. The most common postoperative complaints were perineal pain (53%), constipation with recurrence (50%), and incontinence (28%). Three patients developed rectovaginal fistulas, and one patient died secondary to a necrotizing pelvic soft tissue infection.

In response to these outcomes, the Transtar contour stapling device (Ethicon, Piscataway, NJ) and the transanal repair of rectocele and rectal mucosectomy (TRREMS) procedure have been proposed as alternatives to the original STARR operation. Rosen and colleagues evaluated the efficacy of the Transtar contour stapler in full-thickness prolapse. They reported a 20% (3 out of 15 patients) recurrence rate. Ribaric and colleagues evaluated the safety of a Transtar approach and reported an 11% complication rate secondary to bleeding (5%), staple line complications (3%), urinary retention (2%), and persistent pain (1%). Cruz and colleagues reported on a prospective multicenter trial including 75 patients who underwent TRREMS procedure. They showed that 13 patients required suture ligation of a staple line bleeding. Two patients had incomplete stapling. Three patients complained of persistent rectal pain, and seven developed a stricture. Eight patients had persistent grade I anorectoceles on postoperative defecography. Further studies are needed to determine the safety, efficacy, and long-term outcomes of the techniques.

Perineal Rectosigmoidectomy (Altemeier's Procedure)

The perineal rectosigmoidectomy first was performed by Mikulicz in 1889 but was later popularized by Altemeier in the 1970s.

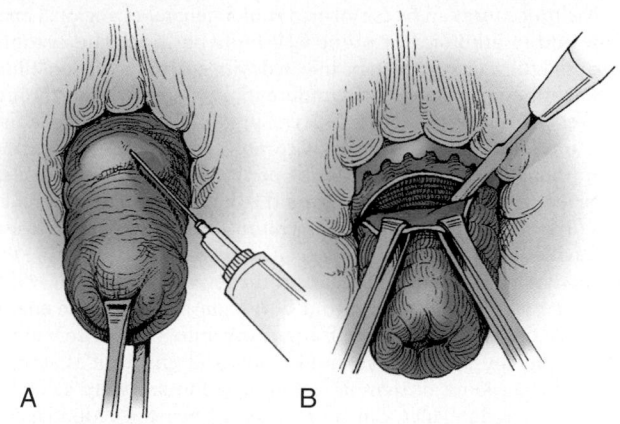

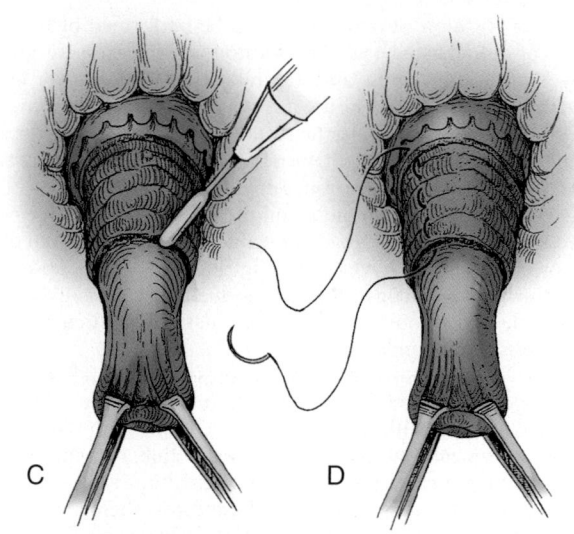

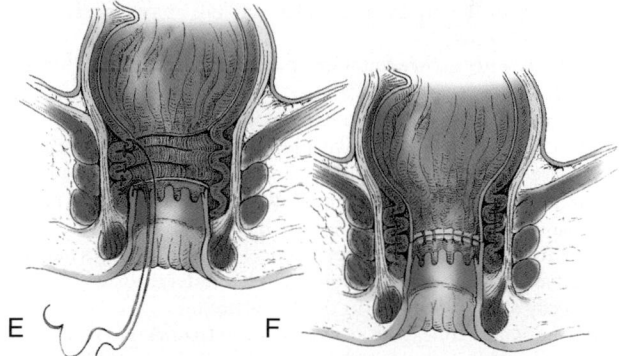

FIGURE 1 Delorme's procedure. **A,** Submucosal infiltration is carried out with saline or local anesthetic with epinephrine. **B,** Partial-thickness circumferential incision is made 1 to 2 cm proximal to the dentate line. **C,** The incision is carried through the mucosa, and the mucosa is dissected off the underlying muscle. **D** and **E,** Plication suture is placed. **F,** Mucosa is amputated and anastomosis is completed. *(From Garely AD, Krieger BR. Rectal prolapse. In Cameron JL, Cameron AM, eds. Current Surgical Therapy, 11th ed. Philadelphia: Elsevier; 2014.)*

The procedure can be performed under general or regional anesthesia and in lithotomy or prone jack-knife position. The rectum is prolapsed fully and then can be injected with epinephrine-containing local anesthesia or saline. A circumferential incision is made through all layers of the rectal wall 1 to 2 cm proximal to the dentate line. Once the full-thickness incision is complete, the redundant rectum is continually reduced. The anterior peritoneal reflection/hernia sac is opened and further rectum/sigmoid colon are reduced until there is no further redundancy. The mesorectum/mesocolon then is ligated and divided with an energy device. Great care is taken to ensure that the mesentery is not divided beyond the level of colon that will be used for the anastomosis to avoid devascularization of the anastomosis. A finger then is passed anteriorly into the peritoneum to palpate the course of the sigmoid colon and ensure it is straight. Often, further loops of sigmoid colon or redundancy are identified, and further redundancy can be reduced. When the redundancy is eliminated, the mesentery is divided to the level of the chosen point of bowel resection.

Levator plication (levatorplasty) can be performed before completion of the anastomosis. The levator ani muscles are grasped gently with Allis clamps, and several figure-of-8 sutures of 2-0 absorbable monofilament suture are placed with care taken to avoid incorporating the vagina into the sutures. Levatorplasty is associated with improved postoperative continence, decreased recurrence rates, and increased length of recurrence-free intervals.

The descending or sigmoid colon then is divided, and the end is anastomosed to the cut edge of the anus. We find it useful to divide the bowel sequentially while placing sutures of 2-0 absorbable braided suture in each quadrant and gradually completing the suturing in each of the four quadrants. Alternatively, a circular-stapled anastomosis can be undertaken.

Whenever sufficient redundancy is present, our preference is to perform a colonic J pouch with a pouch-anal anastomosis. An 8-cm J pouch is created with firing(s) of the GIA or endo-GIA stapler through an apical enterotomy. The staple line is reinforced for hemostasis where necessary, and the efferent limb is secured to the afferent limb. A handsewn coloanal anastomosis then is performed, initially taking sutures at 90-degree intervals, incorporating the anal mucosa, internal anal sphincter, and cut edge of the colonic pouch. As is mentioned earlier, a circular-stapled anastomosis can be performed (Figure 2).

Mortality rates associated with this procedure are low (0 to 6%), and most of the morbidity (5% to 24%) arises from the patient's underlying medical problems. However, the main surgery-related complications are postoperative bleeding and anastomotic dehiscence. Care must be taken to resect the appropriate amount of colon: resecting too much colon and mesentery can create an anastomosis that is under tension and prone to dehiscence, but not resecting all of the redundancy can lead to recurrence. Recurrence rates have been reported as 0 to 10% but are thought to be underreported secondary to relatively short follow-up in the literature.

Altomare and colleagues performed a retrospective review of 93 patients who had undergone Altemeier's procedure and had at least 1 year of follow-up to attempt to quantify long-term recurrence. Fifteen percent of the cohort were undergoing redo surgery after recurrence. After an average follow-up of 41 months, 18% had recurrence of full-thickness prolapse and 6% developed mucosal prolapse. The only predictor of recurrence identified was previous unsuccessful repair (odds ratio 3.8; $P = 0.042$).

Abdominal Procedures

Ripstein's Procedure

This technique was first described by Ripstein and Lanter in 1963. They believed that rectal prolapse was primarily the result of intussusception of the rectum secondary to the loss of rectal attachments. Therefore the surgical technique that developed affixes the rectum to the sacrum and thus prevents rectal prolapse.

Initially, the technique was described using fascia lata to create a sling used to fix the rectum to the sacrum, but subsequent modifications of the technique used prosthetic mesh. The procedure involves mobilization of the rectum down to the coccyx with dividing the lateral peritoneal attachments but preserving the lateral ligaments. While the rectum is pulled upward, a 5-cm piece of mesh is wrapped anteriorly around the rectum at the level of the peritoneal reflection and then sutured bilaterally to the presacral fascia approximately 5 cm below the sacral promontory. The sling should allow the passage of one to two fingers between the rectum and fascia to avoid too tight of a wrap, which can cause obstruction.

Studies have shown that this procedure is best suited for the patient without preexisting constipation. Up to 50% of patients had improvement of incontinence; persistence of constipation occurred in 57%, and new onset constipation developed in 10%. Recurrence and mortality rates after this procedure are relatively low, 0 to 8% and 0 to 1.6%, respectively.

Unfortunately, Ripstein's procedure does have a significant morbidity associated with it and therefore it is no longer performed frequently. Complication rates are reported from 17% to 33% and are largely related to the placement of the sling. The most common problem was constipation and fecal impaction, but presacral hemorrhage, stricture, small bowel obstruction, impotence, and fistula formation also were reported. Severe complications associated with placement of a mesh are the development of infection or erosion into the bladder, both of which require mesh removal. Modifications of the procedure to include a posterior wrap or substitution of polyvinyl alcohol sponge for the mesh have reduced the complication rates to 20%.

Abdominal Suture Rectopexy and Sigmoid Resection

This technique, originally described in 1955, remains one of the most commonly used and effective treatment options for full-thickness rectal prolapse. Frykman described four essential steps to this procedure: (1) complete mobilization of the rectum down to the levator complex, with the lateral ligaments left intact; (2) elevation of the rectum with suture fixation to the presacral fascia just below the sacral promontory; (3) obliteration of the cul-de-sac with suturing the endopelvic fascia anteriorly to the rectum; and (4) resection of the redundant sigmoid colon with an end-to-end anastomosis. The procedure remains essentially the same today, but many surgeons, including the authors, choose to omit the obliteration of the cul-de-sac. In addition, the authors modify the technique with placement of fixation sutures (0-polypropylene) into the sacral bone cortex rather than the presacral fascia. Adequate suture fixation through the cortex is ensured by performing this portion of the procedure via a Pfannenstiel access incision after laparoscopic mobilization to the level of the levators with care to preserve the lateral stalks.

A recent meta-analysis of 418 patients reported a recurrence rate of 0 to 9% and morbidity and mortality rates of 0 to 23% and 0 to 6.7%, respectively. Complications related to the procedure included colonic and small bowel obstructions, anastomotic leak, and presacral bleeding. Most patients reported an improvement in bowel habits after the procedure. Huber and colleagues found a reduction in constipation from 44% to 26% and in incontinence from 67% to 23%.

Abdominal Suture Rectopexy

Rectopexy without a sigmoid resection also can be used for the treatment of rectal prolapse. Fixation of the rectum to the sacrum can be accomplished with placement of interrupted nonabsorbable sutures to the lateral stalks or with use of a mesh (Ripstein's). Recurrence rates also range from 0 to 9%, but the functional outcomes are different as compared with a resection rectopexy. Frequently, constipation is worsened in these patients and incontinence improved.

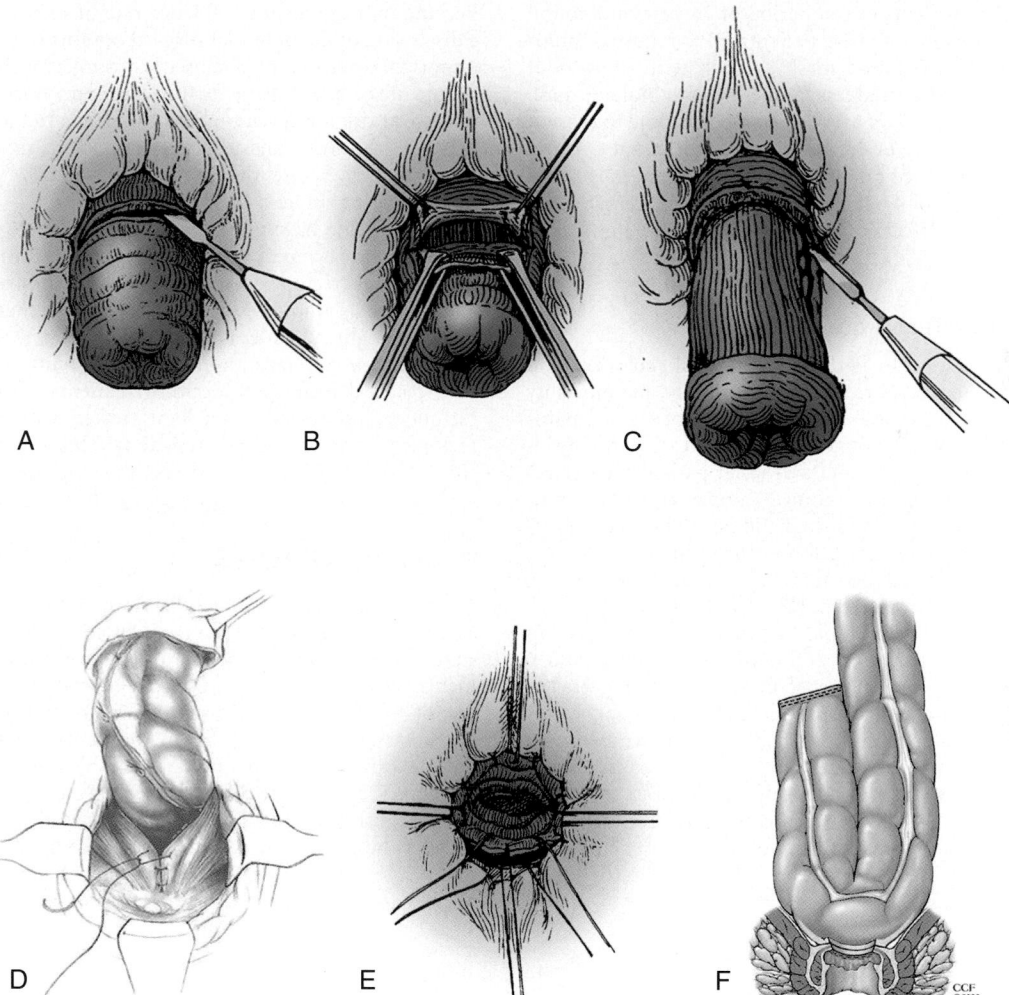

FIGURE 2 Perineal rectosigmoidectomy. **A** through **C,** Full-thickness excision of redundant bowel. **D,** Levatorplasty is performed with several figure-of-8 sutures, if possible. **E,** Incision of bowel at level of chosen anastomosis after all redundancy was removed. **F,** If adequate length is present, colonic J pouch is performed. *(A through E, Adapted from Gordon PH. Rectal procidentia. In: Gordon PH, Nivatvongs S, eds.* Principles and Practice for Surgery for the Colon, Rectum, and Anus. *3rd ed. New York: Informa Healthcare; 2007:415-450. F, Adapted from Wexner SD, Fleshman JW, eds.* Colon and Rectal Surgery: Abdominal Operations [Master Techniques in General Surgery]. *Philadelphia: Lippincott, Williams and Wilkins; 2012.)*

Ventral Rectopexy

Mesh can be used to facilitate rectopexy, and, as with the placement of mesh in other procedures, mesh infection and erosion are the most feared complications.

Ventral rectopexy has evolved from the approach described by Orr and Loygue and, most recently, is being performed laparoscopically with focus on anterior rectal dissection. Minimal posterior dissection is undertaken to expose the sacrum, and a mesh is secured on the anterior aspect of the distal rectum and the sacral promontory. Evans and colleagues performed a retrospective multicenter study to evaluate the frequency of mesh erosion and other sources of morbidity. They studied 2203 patients over a period of 14 years and found a 2% rate of mesh erosion. Of these patients, 51% required minor excision and 18 patients required mesh excision with or without bowel resection. Erosion occurred less frequently with biologic mesh than with synthetic mesh (0.7 vs 2.4%). The median time to erosion was 23 months. Consten et al. evaluated 919 consecutive patients and reported a 10-year recurrence rate of 8.2%. In addition, they noted a mesh complication rate of 4.6%, with a 1.3% rate of vaginal mesh erosion. Both obstructed defecation and incontinence were improved significantly.

Minimally Invasive Techniques

Laparoscopy has been used to perform abdominal rectopexy and resection rectopexy. The rates of recurrence, morbidity, and mortality have been shown to be comparable between the open and laparoscopic techniques. However, as with other procedures, laparoscopy is associated with shorter hospital stays and faster patient recovery. A meta-analysis of 467 patients undergoing 275 open and 192 laparoscopic procedures showed no significant difference between recurrence and improvements in constipation or incontinence.

Some enthusiasts have claimed that the robotic platform may confer an advantage in rectopexy because robotic suturing is purported to be easier than laparoscopic suturing. However, a recent systematic review of the literature evaluated 340 patients from 6 studies and did not show any difference in the rates of recurrence, conversion, or reoperation between robotic and laparoscopic rectopexy. Another study of 82 patients found higher recurrence rates with laparoscopy and robotics as compared with open procedures. Thus, despite marketing claims, scientific scrutiny has failed to reveal any statistically significant advantage to the robotic approach. In the meantime, we perform a hybrid approach of laparoscopic mobilization with a Pfannenstiel or lower midline access incision for suture placement and anastomosis.

Management of the Lateral Stalks

Tou and colleagues performed a Cochrane review meta-analysis and found three studies examining the effect of dividing versus preserving the lateral stalks during rectal mobilization in 64 patients undergoing open mesh rectopexy. They concluded that division of the ligaments was associated with a decreased recurrence rate (0 vs 19%) but increased rates of constipation (67% vs 43%).

■ RECURRENT PROLAPSE

Because of a significant incidence rate of recurrent rectal prolapse, a discussion of the potential surgical options is important. The most important determinant of subsequent surgery is the remaining blood supply of the bowel. Patients who have previously undergone resection are at risk for development of ischemia to the segment of bowel between the two anastomoses should a second resection be attempted. Therefore the surgeon must know the details of the patient's prior surgery.

Patients who have undergone a perineal rectosigmoidectomy are candidates for a repeat perineal resection, Delorme's procedure, or an abdominal rectopexy without resection. In this group of patients, addition of a sigmoid resection could cause ischemia in the remaining rectal segment. Patients who have undergone a previous abdominal rectopexy can have a redo rectopexy with or without resection or a perineal rectosigmoidectomy. Patients with prior abdominal rectopexy and resection are best treated with a redo abdominal rectopexy with or without resection. This treatment algorithm is summarized in Figure 3, and results are discussed in Table 2.

■ CONCLUSIONS

Rectal prolapse can be a difficult and frustrating condition to manage. The surgical technique of choice is based on the patient's functional status, bowel habits, and history of prior operations. The ideal treatment will minimize morbidity and mortality while decreasing the risk of recurrence for the given patient. In addition, surgical preferences vary between surgeons in the United States and Europe. A recent study by Formijne Jonkers et al. highlights some of these differences. Treatment of recurrent prolapse requires special attention to prior disruption of the blood supply to the remaining bowel to prevent the potentially catastrophic outcome of bowel perforation. Again, the treatment should be tailored to the individual patient because there is no panacea for primary or recurrent rectal prolapse.

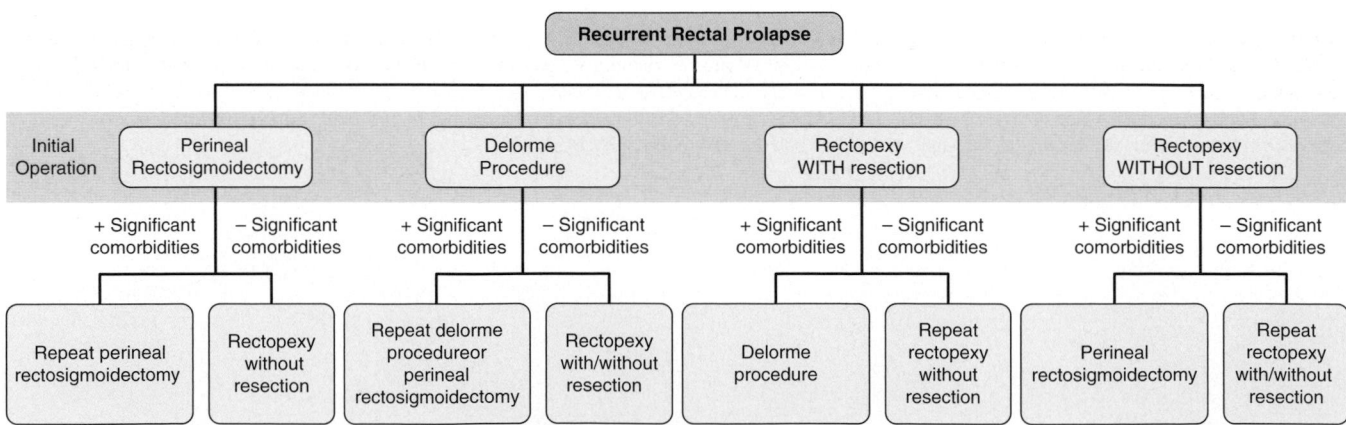

FIGURE 3 Algorithm for treatment of recurrent rectal prolapse. *(Adapted from Maron DJ, Nogueras JJ. Approaches to failed rectal prolapse surgery. In: Zbar AP, Madoff RD, Wexner SD, eds. Reconstructive Surgery of the Rectum, Anus and Perineum. 1st ed. Springer, London: 2013:551-558.)*

TABLE 2: Recurrent Rectal Prolapse: Summary of Studies

First Author	Year	Design	Procedure (Numbers: Total, Recurrence)	Previous Repair (n)	Complications (%)	Follow-Up (Months)	Recurrence Rates (%)	Functional Outcomes
La Greca	2014	Case report	Altemeier with laparoscopic control	Altemeier procedure	0	24	0	NR
Fazeli	2013	Prospective	Delorme (52, 6)	Abdominal repair (4), Delorme (2)	15.4	30	50	Constipation improved in 69.6%, incontinence improved in 71.4%
Ding	2012	Retrospective	Altemeier (113, 23)	Altemeier	17.4	37.5	39	NR
Boccasanta	2012	Prospective	Transobturator colonic suspension during Altemeier	Altemeier	0	30	0	Significant improvement in Wexner and quality of life scores
Steele	2006	Retrospective	Altemeier with levatorplasty (23) or without levatorplasty (25) Abdominal rectopexy (17) with resection (10) Delorme procedure (3)	Altemeier (53) Delorme (7) Theirsch (7) Rectopexy with resection (12) Rectopexy without resection (5)	Major: Abdominal: 15 Perineal: 10 Minor: Abdominal: 11 Perineal: 10	8.8	Abdominal: 15 Perineal: 37	NR
Tsugawa	2002	Case report	Laparoscopic rectopexy	Gant-Miwa operation (2)	0	24	0	Preoperative incontinence disappeared within 1 month.
Pikarsky	2000	Retrospective	Altemeier (14) resection rectopexy (8) rectopexy (2) pelvic floor repair (2) Delorme (1)	Rectopexy (7) Delorme (7) Altemeier (7) Anal encirclement (4) Resection rectopexy (2)	Anastomotic leak and wound infection after Altemeier	NR	14.8 (compared with primary group: 11)	NR
Watts	2000	Retrospective	Delorme (100, 20)	One previous Delorme (17) Two previous Delormes (3)	Mortality (n = 4)	16	50	Grade of incontinence was improved in 15/17 patients after 2nd Delorme despite recurrence
Araki	1999	Retrospective	Transsacral rectopexy with Dexon mesh	Perineal surgery (2) Anal encirclement (3)	0	12-36	0	Improvement in incontinence

Continued

TABLE 2: Recurrent Rectal Prolapse: Summary of Studies—cont'd

First Author	Year	Design	Procedure (Numbers: Total, Recurrence)	Previous Repair (n)	Complications (%)	Follow-Up (Months)	Recurrence Rates (%)	Functional Outcomes
Takesue	1999	Retrospective	Altemeier (10, 5)	Thiersch combined with Gant-Miwa (4) Unknown (1)	Anastomotic leak (n = 1)	42	0 or 24	7/10 preoperative incontinence, all continent postoperatively
Fengler	1997	Retrospective	Perineal proctectomy with levatorplasty (7) Rectopexy (3) Anterior resection with rectopexy (2) Delorme (1) Anal encirclement (1)	Perineal proctectomy and levatorplasty (10) Anal encirclement (2) Delorme (1) Anal encirclement (1)	NR	50	0	No improvement in fecal incontinence (n = 3)
Hool	1997	Retrospective	Ripstein (18) Anterior resection (3) Frykman-Goldberg (3) Rectal suspension (1) Altemeier (2) Anal encirclement (2)	Abdominal repair (15) Perineal repair (9)	Abdominal operations: 32 Perineal operations: 0	81	17	Constipation: 6/24 preoperative, 7/24 postoperative Incontinence: 10/24 preoperative 7/24 postoperative
Loygue	1984	Retrospective	Rectopexy (257, 61)	Thiersch (49) Simple colopexy (10) Rectopexy (5) Perineal resection (2)	Mortality n = 2 Morbidity: Reoperation for bleeding (n = 1), intervertebral disc infection (n = 3), pelvic sepsis (n = 1)	60-276	5.6	121/257 with preoperative incontinence, normal continence in 90% of patients postoperatively
Keighley	1983	Retrospective	Marlex mesh abdominal rectopexy (100, 26)	Theirsch (19) Rectopexy with polyvinyl alcohol sponge (Invalon; 5) Pelvic floor repair (2)	>24	0	0	67/100 with preoperative fecal incontinence; 24/67 with persistent incontinence

Adapted from Hotouras A, Ribas Y, Zakeri S, et al. A systematic review of the literature on the surgical management of recurrent rectal prolapse. *Colorectal Dis.* 2015;17:657-664.
NR, Not reported.

Suggested Readings

Altomare DF, Binda G, Ganio E, et al. Long-term outcome of Altemeier's procedure for rectal prolapse. *Dis Colon Rectum.* 2009;52:698-703.

Cadeddu F, Sileri P, Grande M, et al. Focus on abdominal rectopexy for full-thickness rectal prolapse: meta-analysis of literature. *Tech Coloproctol.* 2012;16:37-53.

Consten EC, van Iersel JJ, Verheijen PM, et al. Long-term outcome after laparoscopic ventral mesh rectopexy: an observational study of 919 consecutive patients. *Ann Surg.* 2015;262:742-747.

Formijne Jonkers HA, Maya A, Draaisma WA, et al. Laparoscopic resection rectopexy versus laparoscopic ventral rectopexy for complete rectal prolapse. *Tech Coloproctol.* 2014;18:641-646.

Hotouras A, Ribas Y, Zakeri S, et al. A systematic review of the literature on the surgical management of recurrent rectal prolapse. *Colorectal Dis.* 2015;17:657-664.

Lieberth M, Kondylis LA, Reilly JC, et al. The Delorme repair for full-thickness rectal prolapse: a retrospective review. *Am J Surg.* 2009;197:418-423.

Madiba TE, Baig MK, Wexner SD. Surgical management of rectal prolapse. *Arch Surg.* 2005;140:63-73.

Tou S, Brown SR, Malik AI, et al. Surgery for complete rectal prolapse in adults. *Cochrane Database Syst Rev.* 2008;CD001758.

Watkins BP, Landercasper J, Belzer GE, et al. Long-term follow-up of the modified Delorme procedure for rectal prolapse. *Arch Surg.* 2009;197:418-423.

Wexner SD. Reaching a consensus for the stapled transanal rectal resection procedure. *Dis Colon Rectum.* 2015;58:821.

The Management of Solitary Rectal Ulcer Syndrome

Anthony J. Senagore, MD, MS, MBA

The solitary rectal ulcer syndrome (SRUS) represents a spectrum of distal rectal mucosal/wall abnormalities, ranging from solitary ulceration to nodular lesions distributed along the anterior rectum. Cruvheiler initially described the solitary rectal ulcer in 1829. A subsequent larger case series including 68 patients with SRUS was published in 1969 by Madigan and Morison. In addition to the visualized rectal wall alterations, SRUS is associated almost exclusively with disorders of defecation and/or rectal prolapse.

■ PATHOGENESIS

The precise pathophysiology of SRUS remains unclear; however, it is associated with paradoxical puborectalis contraction and internal or external full-thickness rectal prolapse. This association strongly suggests a primary role for altered anorectal function leading to repetitive injury of the anterior rectal wall during defecation. Trauma resulting from chronic straining may lead to ischemic injury of the rectal mucosa and the range of response from erythema to ulceration. Ultimately, the repetitive injury and healing may produce nodular scarring within the rectal wall. The reported incidence of SRUS in patients with abnormal puborectalis contraction during straining is 50% to 77%. Other less common causative agents include ergotamine suppositories (a potent vasoconstrictor), radiotherapy, anal intercourse, or digitation. It is essential to exclude an underlying malignancy leading to the formation of an ulcer within the rectum, as demonstrated by a series from the Johns Hopkins Medical Institution, in which seven cases of SRUS ultimately were diagnosed as carcinoma.

■ PRESENTATION

Although SRUS is not particularly common, it occurs frequently enough to be considered when endoscopic abnormalities are seen in the distal anterior rectal wall. According to a study from Ireland, the incidence of SRUS was 1 in 100,000 per year. SRUS generally affects adults with a mean age at presentation of 49 years, and there appears to be a consistent female predominance. On average, patients will have had symptoms for 3.5 to 5.3 years, findings of internal or external rectal polyp prolapse, or anismus before definitive diagnosis.

The syndrome is characterized clinically by excess rectal mucus, bleeding, anismus, tenesmus, and difficult evacuation. The diagnosis of SRUS is based on the presence of the following criteria: (1) straining and a feeling of incomplete evacuation leaving the passage of blood and mucus through the rectum; (2) internal or external rectal prolapse; (3) solitary multiple erythematous ulcerated lesions or polypoid lesions on proctosigmoidoscopy; or (4) histologic evidence of distortion of the muscularis mucosa, fibrous obliteration of the lamina propria, and extension of the smooth muscle fibers into the lamina propria. The disorder can be misdiagnosed in more than 25% of cases. The differential diagnoses of the condition includes acute infectious or inflammatory proctitis, endometriosis, and neoplasia.

Evaluation

Endoscopy is the optimal way to confirm the diagnosis in symptomatic patients. Most patients present with endoscopic evidence of SRUS. Initial evaluation should include a complete GI and sexual social behavior history. A diary regarding bowel habits may be useful. Because the population presents with altered defecation, all patients need a colonoscopy or barium enema to exclude a colorectal malignancy or associated colitis. Symptoms or findings of pelvic organ prolapse should be evaluated thoroughly before embarking on surgical therapy. Patients with associated pelvic floor prolapse often complain of worsening anterior compartment syndromes, which may have to be addressed as part of the therapy.

Endoscopy reveals the typical ulcerative changes on the anterior rectal wall, which strongly support the diagnosis. Macroscopically, other findings of SRUS include erythematous, friable, thickened patches of rectal wall. Lesions may occur anywhere in the rectal wall but usually are located 5 to 12 cm from the verge. A generous biopsy of the lesion is essential to exclude other disorders, including malignancy. On microscopic examination, the mucosa and the muscular layer are thickened with fibrous extensions throughout. These findings also may be seen in patients with rectal prolapse, prolapsing hemorrhoids, and prolapsing stomas. Findings associated with SRUS included nodular induration of the circular muscle layer, grouping of the longitudinal muscle, and superficial ulceration. The superficial ulcerations seen on microscopic examination may have a transitional mucosa appearance because of regeneration of the epithelium. On occasion, the glandular epithelium may be trapped in the submucosa during repeated healing episodes, resulting in the entity known as *colitis cystica profunda*. Biopsy of this may be confused easily with a cancer.

Histologic findings consistent with SRUS are not mutually exclusive of carcinoma. A series of cases of rectal malignancy were reported from our institution in patients whose initial diagnosis was SRUS based on histologic evidence. It was the recommendation of the authors that large to jumbo biopsies be obtained to evaluate deeper within the rectal wall to exclude underlying malignancy. Discovery of atypical cells in the biopsy specimen may be highlighted by immunohistochemistry for cytokeratin. If the suspicion of malignancy remains high, further imaging such as computed tomography positron emission tomography scanning may be beneficial.

Radiographic evaluation may include defecating proctogram or dynamic pelvic magnetic resonance imaging to assess pelvic descent and/or internal rectal prolapse. Defecation will demonstrate a significant abnormality in more than 73% of patients with SRUS. The findings include abnormal puborectalis contraction during straining and internal or external rectal prolapse. Other findings in SRUS included poor rectal emptying and perineal descent. Unfortunately findings on preoperative imaging may not predict outcomes after surgery for SRUS. A careful evaluation for associated pelvic floor abnormalities, including urinary incontinence and uterine prolapse, should be performed.

Anal physiologic studies may assist in the diagnosis and determination of the cause of SRUS. The presence of abnormal or paradoxical puborectalis contraction with straining can be determined by the balloon expulsion test or surface electromyography (EMG) studies. Surface EMG studies record muscle activity during attempted defecation. During contraction of the sphincter muscles, findings on EMG would demonstrate an increase in activity. However with Valsalva or straining to defecate relaxation of the sphincter muscle should take place, resulting in a decrease in EMG activity. An increase in EMG activity during straining is pathognomonic for abnormal paradoxical puborectalis contraction. Other findings consistent with

the diagnosis of SRUS and commonly found in rectal prolapse include pudendal neuropathy and perineal descent. Pudendal neuropathy is demonstrated by prolonged pudendal nerve terminal motor latency (PNTML). PNTML is determined with a St. Mark's electrode inserted into the rectum attached to the gloved index finger with stimulation applied near Alcock's canal and recorded at the level of the anal sphincter.

More recently endoanal ultrasound has been used to evaluate patients who experience symptoms consistent with an SRUS. In full-thickness rectal prolapse the circular muscle within the rectum is thickened and condensed into bundles. Reports have indicated that more than 91% of patients with SRUS have a significant degree of internal rectal prolapse or intussusception as well as a thickened internal anal sphincter. The medium thickness was 3.9 mm (2.9 to 8.6 mm). This may be an indication of the potential progression of internal prolapse to full-thickness external prolapse.

Management of SRUS is primarily symptomatic. Although symptomatic improvement occurs more readily, complete endoscopic histologic resolution rarely is achieved. Initial management should include elimination of all potentially harmful suppositories and home remedies. The patient should consume a high-fiber diet (more than 15 g per day). This is very difficult to achieve with diet manipulation alone; therefore supplementation with an over-the-counter fiber supplement is recommended. Patients taking fiber supplements should be encouraged to drink at least six glasses of noncaffeinated fluids per day.

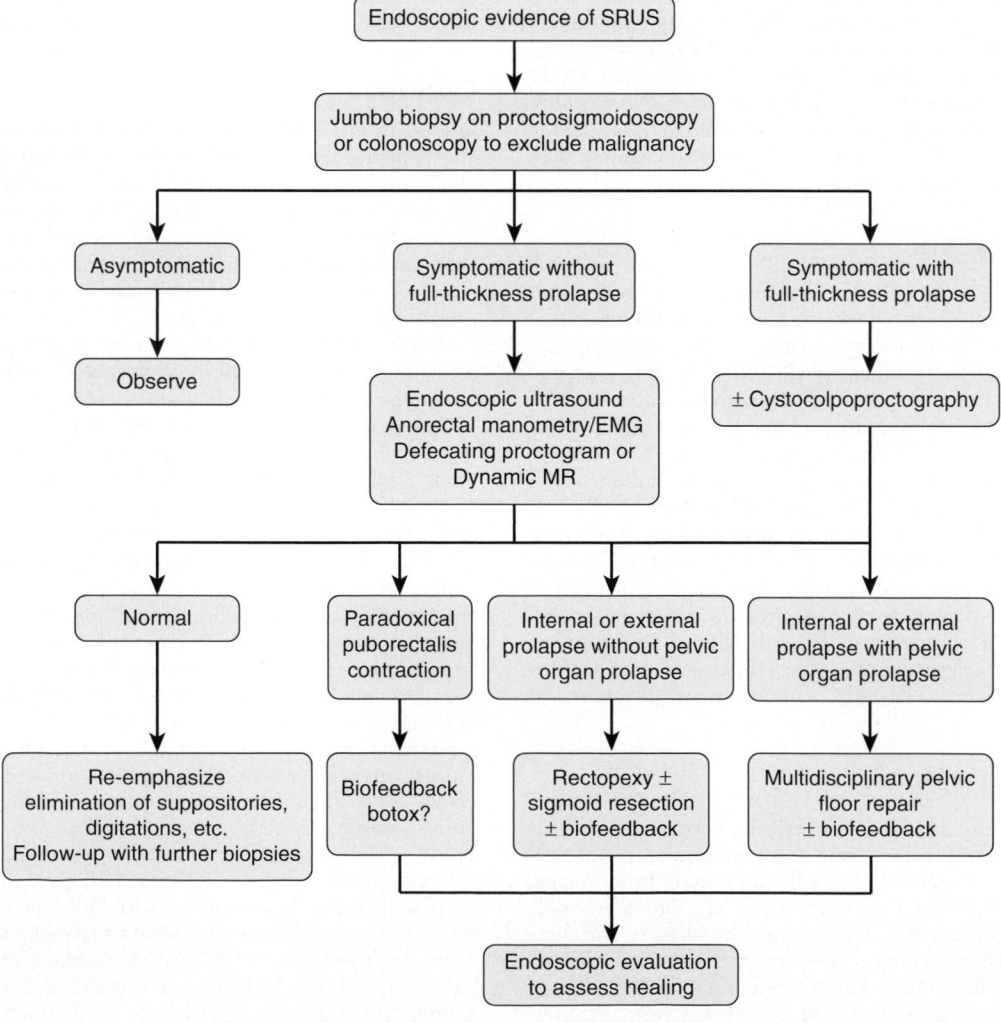

FIGURE 1 Schematic for the management of solitary rectal ulcer syndrome.

■ TREATMENT

Biofeedback is a form of behavior modification that is conducted in four to five sessions. Treatment of SRUS with biofeedback has been successful in patients in the short term; however, recidivism occurs in more than 50% of patients. Although conclusive evidence does not exist, those caring for patients with SRUS agree that biofeedback is more effective in patients with tenesmus. This would favor the use of biofeedback in patients with less structural injury to the rectum because retraining patients in active defecation may avoid disease progression. Recently, botulinum toxin type A Botox has been demonstrated to be a successful measure in more than 50% of patients with tenesmus, although data are limited.

Surgical treatment has been successful for SRUS associated with full-thickness rectal prolapse, in which an abdominal rectopexy with or without sigmoid resection is associated with symptomatic improvement in 55% to 66% of patients. Again, patients should be assessed for an anterior pelvic floor disorder that may dictate combined treatment with a urologist or urinary gynecologist. Patients with long-standing constipation and risk for intestinal motility disorder should undergo a Sitz marker study. A positive study demonstrating retention of more than 20% of markers in 5 days suggests slow transit constipation, which may require an abdominal colectomy at the time of rectopexy. However, it may be wise to just perform a sigmoid colectomy and assess function in this complex patient population. Laparoscopic rectopexy has become a frequent minimally invasive solution, whether by the posterior or ventral pexy technique.

Surgical resection of the rectal wall abnormality either by transanal excision or low anterior resection has not been associated with favorable outcomes and is best avoided. Ultimately, proctectomy with permanent stoma may be required in the most difficult cases of severely symptomatic patients. Perineal approaches to rectal prolapse may be successful; however, the failure rate is higher compared with abdominal approaches.

■ SUMMARY

A summary schematic representation of the management approach to SRUS is seen in Figure 1. SRUS is a relatively rare disorder associated with disorders of defecation. Symptoms include passage of blood and mucus of the rectum, tenesmus, straining, and incomplete evacuation. The best results achieved with biofeedback occur in patients with tenesmus in the absence of full-thickness rectal prolapse. Successful surgical management is achieved in patients with full-thickness external rectal prolapse with an abdominal antiprolapse procedure.

SUGGESTED READINGS
Choi HJ, Shin EJ, Hwang YH, Weiss EG, Nogueras JJ, Wexner SD. Clinical presentation and surgical outcome in patients with solitary rectal ulcer syndrome. *Surg Innov.* 2005;12:307-313.

Felt-Bersma RJ, Tiersma ES, Cuesta MA. Rectal prolapse, rectal intussusception, rectocele, solitary rectal ulcer syndrome, and enterocele. *Gastroenterol Clin North Am.* 2008;37:645-668, ix.

Jarrett ME, Emmanuel AV, Vaizey CJ, Kamm MA. Behavioural therapy (biofeedback) for solitary rectal ulcer syndrome improves symptoms and mucosal blood flow. *Gut.* 2004;53:368-370.

Kang YS, Kamm MA, Engel AF, Talbot IC. Pathology of the rectal wall in solitary rectal ulcer syndrome and complete rectal prolapse. *Gut.* 1996;38:587-590.

Mackle EJ, Parks TG. The pathogenesis and pathophysiology of rectal prolapse and solitary rectal ulcer syndrome. *Clin Gastroenterol.* 1986;15:985-1002.

Martin CJ, Parks TG, Biggart JD. Solitary rectal ulcer syndrome in Northern Ireland. 1971-1980. *Br J Surg.* 1981;68:744-747.

Sharara AI, Azar C, Amr SS, Haddad M, Eloubeidi MA. Solitary rectal ulcer syndrome: endoscopic spectrum and review of the literature. *Gastrointest Endosc.* 2005;62:755-762.

Tjandra JJ, Fazio VW, Petras RE, Lavery IC, Oakley JR, Milsom JW, Church JM. Clinical and pathologic factors associated with delayed diagnosis in solitary rectal ulcer syndrome. *Dis Colon Rectum.* 1993;36:146-153.

THE SURGICAL MANAGEMENT OF CONSTIPATION

Joshua H. Wolf, MD, and Eric G. Weiss, MD

Constipation is a common gastrointestinal complaint with a wide spectrum of causes. Its prevalence has been estimated to be as high as 28% in the general population. In the United States, it is responsible each year for 2.5 million office visits, 300,000 emergency room visits, and a cost of $1.6 billion to the healthcare system. Only a small percentage of patients have constipation that is due to a surgically correctable cause; however, for certain subsets of patients, surgery often is the most viable long-term option. Identification of these surgically correctable causes is possible only through careful evaluation and physiologic testing. In this chapter, we present the surgical approach to patients with constipation, including the use of anorectal physiologic testing in patient selection and operative strategies.

■ DEFINITION AND SCORING

Constipation often has subjective, self-reported symptoms that do not lend themselves well to precise definitions. It was recognized in the 1980s, however, that objective criteria were necessary to establish thresholds for treatment and to standardize research. The Rome diagnostic criteria for functional gastrointestinal disorders were introduced for this purpose in 1988 and were revised in 2006 as Rome III (Box 1). According to Rome III, a diagnosis of constipation requires two or more of the following criteria being present for at least 3 months: "(1) straining with at least 25% of defecations; (2) lumpy or hard stools in at least 25% of defecations; (3) sensation of incomplete evacuation for at least 25% of defecations; (4) sensation of anorectal obstruction/blockage for at least 25% of defecations; (5) manual maneuvers to facilitate at least 25% of defecations (digital evacuation, pelvic floor support); (6) fewer than three defecations per week." This definition excludes those patients who meet criteria for irritable bowel syndrome (IBS). To be diagnosed with IBS, a patient should exhibit recurrent abdominal pain or discomfort for at least 3 months, along with at least two of the following three features: pain/discomfort that is relieved with defecation, a change in stool frequency, or change in stool appearance.

A multitude of scoring systems have been devised for constipation that each use different parameters. The most commonly used scores are listed in Table 1 along with an associated description. For the Bristol stool scale (BSS), patients select one of seven pictures that best characterizes their bowel movements on the basis of stool consistency and appearance. Lower numbers indicate harder stool, with 1 and 2 representing severe and mild constipation, respectively. Advantages are its simplicity and ease of patient participation, but BSS is limited in scope because stool is the only variable. In contrast, most other scoring systems are based on patient or physician evaluation of functional symptoms. The Wexner constipation score (WCS) system is

BOX 1: Rome III Criteria (2006)

Present in at least 25% of defecations:
- Straining
- Lumpy or hard stools
- Sensation of incomplete evacuation
- Sensation of anorectal obstruction/blockage
- Manual maneuvers to facilitate evacuation

Fewer than 3 defecations per week

Does not meet IBS criteria

From Longstreth GR, et al. Functional bowel disorders. *Gastroenterology.* 2006;130:1480-1491.

IBS, Irritable bowel syndrome.

TABLE 1: Scoring Systems for Constipation

Name	Description
BSS	Pictures of stool ranging from loose (7) to severe constipation (1)
WCS	8 variables scored either 0-4 or 0-2 for a total of 30
SSS	9 variables scored 0-4 for a total of 36
PAC-SYM	12 variables scored 0-4 for a total of 48
PAC-QoL	28 variables with a range of scoring options and a possible total of 96
KESS	11 variables with a range of scoring options and possible total of 39

BSS, Bristol stool scale; *KESS,* The Knowles Eccersley Scott symptom score; *PAC-SYM,* patient assessment of constipation symptom score; *PAC-QoL,* patient assessment of constipation quality of life questionnaire; *SSS,* symptom severity score; *WCS,* Wexner constipation score.

based on a set of eight variables related to the action of defecation. These are displayed in Table 2 and include (1) frequency, (2) difficulty, (3) completeness, (4) presence of abdominal pain, (5) time in the lavatory, (6) need for laxatives or digital assistance, (7) failure, and (8) duration of symptoms. The first 7 are graded on a 5-point Likert scale (0 = none of the time; 4 = all of the time), and the last is graded on a scale of 0 to 2. The total possible score is 0 to 30, with 0 as normal and 30 as severe constipation. Any patient with a WCS score above 15 is considered constipated. Other systems include the symptom severity score (SSS), the patient assessment of constipation score (PAC-SYM), the patient assessment of constipation quality of life questionnaire (PAC-QoL), the Knowles Eccersley Scott symptom score (KESS), and the Longo scoring system for obstructed defecation syndrome (ODS).

■ CLASSIFICATION AND SURGICAL SELECTION

Because there are a myriad of presentations, constipation can be sorted and classified in several different ways. Some have advocated classification on the basis of general cause (colonic vs extracolonic; functional vs nonfunctional; primary vs secondary causes). Such schemes can be useful in selecting patients for initial medical treatments but are not adequate to identify patients who may benefit from surgical treatment.

For selection of patients for surgery, a more practical classification is based on the anatomy and physiology of the colon and the pelvic floor (i.e., whether colonic transit is normal or delayed, and whether the pelvic floor is functional or dysfunctional). Answers to these questions segregate patients into four different categories: (1)

TABLE 2: Wexner Constipation Scoring System

Frequency of bowel movements	Score
1-2 times per 1-2 days	0
2 times per week	1
Once per week	2
Less than once per week	3
Less than once per month	4

Difficulty: painful evacuation effort	
Never	0
Rarely	1
Sometimes	2
Usually	3
Always	4

Completeness: feeling incomplete evacuation	
Never	0
Rarely	1
Sometimes	2
Usually	3
Always	4

Pain: abdominal pain	
Never	0
Rarely	1
Sometimes	2
Usually	3
Always	4

Time: minutes in lavatory per attempt	
Less than 5	0
5 to 10	1
10 to 20	2
20 to 30	3
>30	4

Assistance: type of assistance	
Without assistance	0
Stimulative laxatives	1
Digital assistance or enema	2

Failure: unsuccessful attempts for evacuation per 24 hours	
Never	0
1 to 3	1
3 to 6	2
6 to 9	3
More than 9	4

History: duration of constipation (years)	
0	0
1 to 5	1
5 to 10	2
10 to 20	3
More than 20	4

From Agachan F, et al. A constipation scoring system to simplify evaluation and management of constipated patients. *Dis Colon Rectum.* 1996;39:681-685.

slow-transit constipation (STC), or colonic inertia; (2) pelvic floor dysfunction (PFD); (3) mixed disorder (STC + PFD); (4) normal-transit constipation (NTC) and IBS. Treatment for NTC/IBS is nonsurgical and therefore is not reviewed in this chapter. In Figure 1, we present an algorithm to help sort constipated patients (with nonacute presentations) into these categories. The first step, after reaching a diagnosis that is based on Rome III criteria, is to rule out a mechanical blockage with either a colonoscopy or a contrast enema and

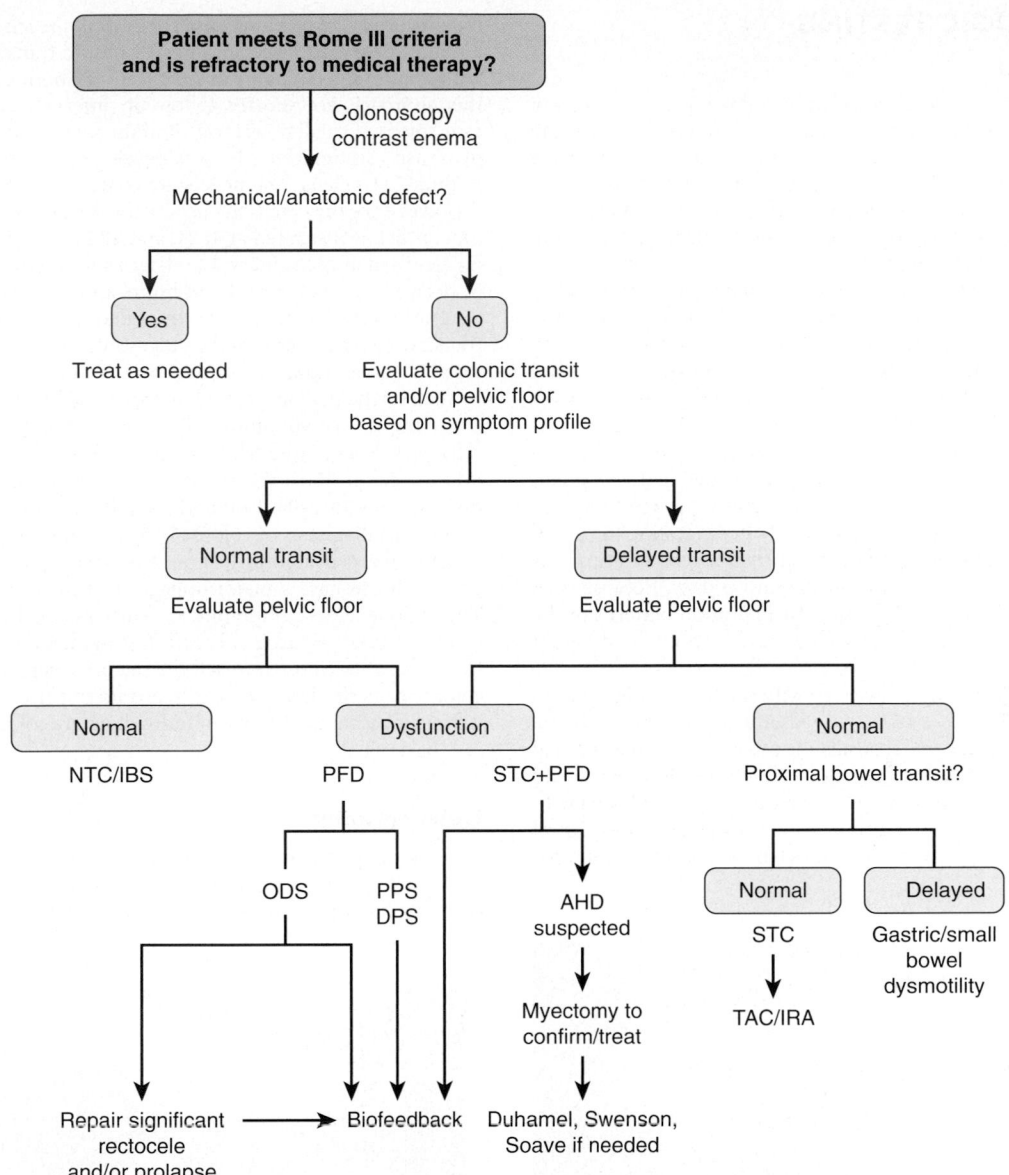

FIGURE 1 Algorithm for surgical management of chronic constipation. *AHD,* Adult Hirschsprung's disease; *DPS,* descending perineum syndrome; *IBS,* irritable bowel syndrome; *IRA,* ileorectal anastomosis; *NTC,* normal transit constipation; *ODS,* obstructed defecation syndrome; *PFD,* pelvic floor dysfunction; *PPS,* paradoxical puborectalis syndrome; *STC,* slow transit constipation; *TAC,* total abdominal colectomy.

flexible sigmoidoscopy or proctoscopy. It is important to perform a thorough history and physical examination directed at questions and examinations that will help in classifying patients. If no anatomic abnormalities are noted, the patient should undergo medical therapy. First-line medical treatment involves twice-daily fiber with soluble supplementation (psyllium, ispaghula), which has been shown to be more efficacious than insoluble fiber (wheat bran). Although often recommended, there is no evidence that addition of overall fluid intake improves symptoms in the absence of underlying dehydration. If symptoms persist after several weeks of fiber supplementation, an osmotic agent such as polyethylene glycol (PEG) or lactulose should be added, along with a stimulant such as glycerin or bisacodyl to be used intermittently as an adjunct. Newer drugs including "secreta-gogues" (lubiprostone and linaclotide) and serotonin 5HT agonists are significantly more expensive with no proven advantage over tra-ditional treatment and therefore generally are reserved as last-line medical agents.

If an at least 6-month trial of maximal medical treatment has failed, further evaluation with physiologic testing is warranted; this workup can be targeted on the basis of the patient's clinical presenta-tion. Symptomatic complaints suggestive of PFD should lead to an initial workup with anal manometry, which may include balloon expulsion, followed by defecography. Together these tests help confirm the diagnosis and to look for any surgically correctable fea-tures (rectocele, sigmoidocele, enterocele, intussusception). Accord-ing to guidelines from the American Gastroenterology Association, colonic transit testing should be deferred until the diagnosis of PFD has been ruled out or confirmed because if PFD is present, the addi-tional diagnosis of STC does not alter management significantly and may falsely prolong it. In cases in which transit studies confirm STC, gastric emptying and small bowel transit studies are performed as well to rule out a more proximal transit delay. If present, such a delay suggests a more global motility problem that would not be fully cor-rectable with surgery. Results from these tests will place the patient into one of the four categories listed previously, which in turn will determine the appropriate treatment. In the remainder of this chapter, we review the physiologic tests in more detail and then discuss the available surgical options for STC, PFD, and STC+PFD.

■ PHYSIOLOGIC TESTING

Transit Studies

Colonic transit is assessed radiologically by following the progression of ingested radio-opaque or radionuclear markers through the gastrointestinal tract (Figures 2 and 3). In the most widely used method, the patient ingests 24 radio-opaque markers within a single capsule. The capsule dissolves and the markers do not and therefore can be followed subsequently as they progress through the colon. Normal transit time through the colon on average is 31 hours in men and 39 hours in women. X-ray imaging is obtained at 3 and 5 days, and *slow* transit is defined by the retention of 20% or more of the markers (five markers) in the colon at 5 days. Marker location can help elucidate the type of dysfunction. If at 5 days the markers are scattered widely throughout the entire colon, this is suspicious for colonic inertia. If, however, all the markers at 5 days are aggregated in the sigmoid colon or proximal rectum, this is suspicious for pelvic outlet dysfunction. It is possible to obtain a more detailed assessment of colonic transit with segmental transit times. One method is to obtain daily serial imaging starting on day 3 after ingesting the initial 24 markers. In an alternative method, the patient ingests multiple sets of differently shaped markers for 3 consecutive days. Because each set has a different characteristic shape, the migration patterns of the different shapes are used to determine transit speed in different colonic segments.

Colonic transit also may be assessed with nuclear scintigraphy, in which the patient ingests a traceable radionucleotide rather than a set of radio-opaque markers. Typically the patient eats a dual-labeled meal, consisting of scrambled eggs with technetium-99 sulfur colloid and 300 cc of water with indium-111. The isotopes are followed with a gamma camera every 30 minutes in an upright position until gastric emptying, after which the patient is positioned supine for imaging every 30 minutes until the isotopes reach the colon (usually an additional 90 to 180 minutes). Colonic transit then is followed with scintigraphy imaging at 24, 48, and 72 hours. The advantages of this approach are shorter follow-up intervals and more accurate assessment of small bowel transit in the same study. Another method of transit scintigraphy that was developed at the Mayo Clinic uses indium-111 pellets. The pellets are coated in a pH-sensitive gel that dissolves once they cross the ileocecal valve and releases the radioisotope, which is measured at 4, 24, and 48 hours. The geometric mean is calculated at each interval to determine whether transit is normal or delayed (normal is <1.4 at 4 hours and 1.7 to 4.0 at 24 hours).

The SmartPill is another method that uses colonic pH to measure transit time. The SmartPill is an ingestible capsule that transmits data for pH, temperature, and luminal pressure to an external receiver that is worn by the patient. A sudden drop in pH by more than one unit, occurring at least 90 minutes after gastric emptying, is characteristically what is measured when the pill passes across the ileocecal valve into the colon. With the SmartPill, colonic transit is defined as the time between this pH drop and the pill's exit from the body.

When a diagnosis of colonic inertia is considered, more proximal or generalized dysmotility should be ruled out as well because, if present, it can have a major impact on success or failure of surgery. This is done with scintigraphy as mentioned earlier or with a hydrogen breath test. Hydrogen breath testing measures the time it takes for a dose of lactulose to reach the cecum, where it is metabolized by colonic bacteria that release a byproduct of hydrogen gas. This test is limited because only 75% of individuals are colonized by the necessary bacteria.

Defecography

Defecography is a dynamic evaluation of the pelvic floor during active defecation. It may be accomplished either fluoroscopically (cinedefecography) or with magnetic resonance imaging (MRI).

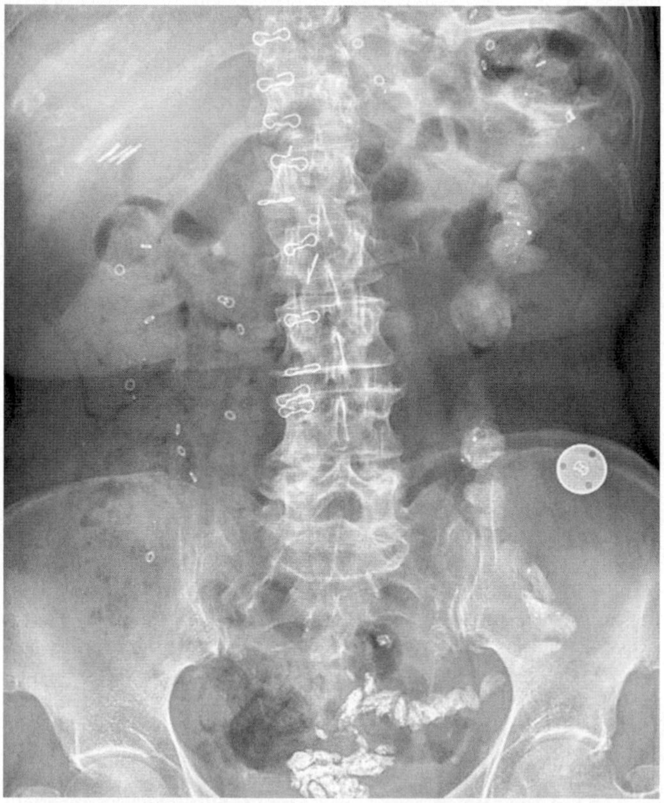

FIGURE 2 Colonic transit study on day 1. Abdominal radiograph demonstrating the presence of radio-opaque markers in right colon at the onset of the transit study.

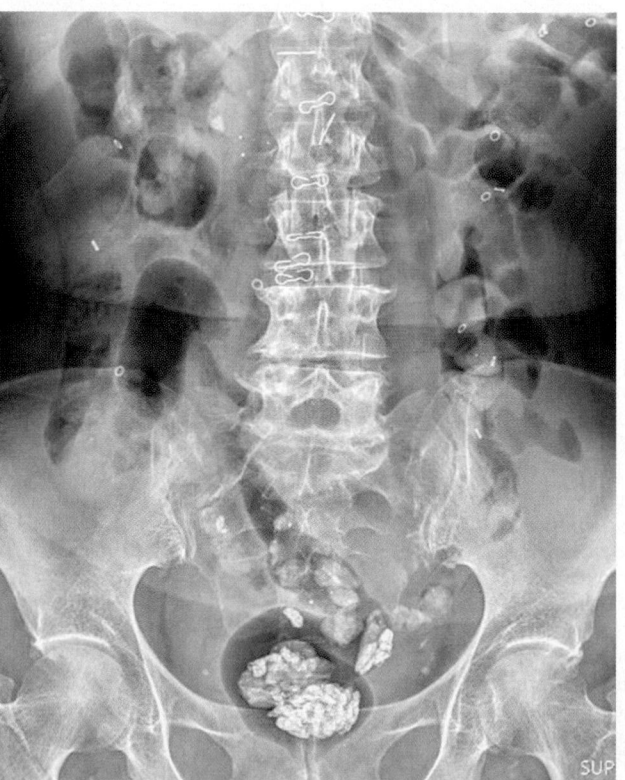

FIGURE 3 Colonic transit study on day 5. Follow-up radiograph showing retention of markers at 5 days, suggestive of slow-transit constipation.

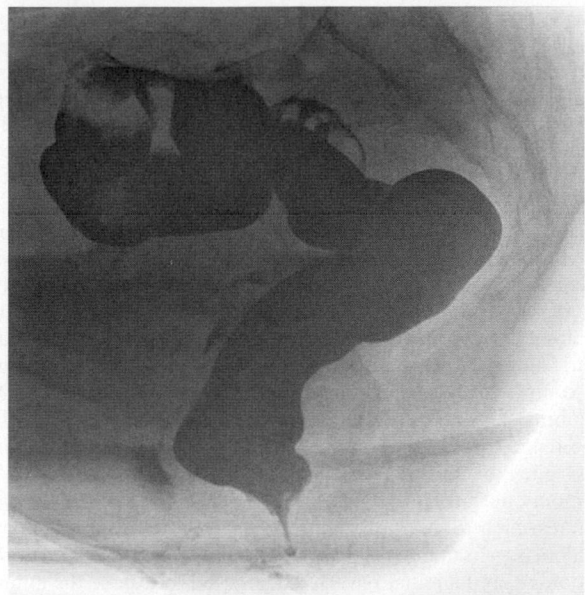

FIGURE 4 Cinedefecography. Sagittal pelvic view with moderate anterior rectocele.

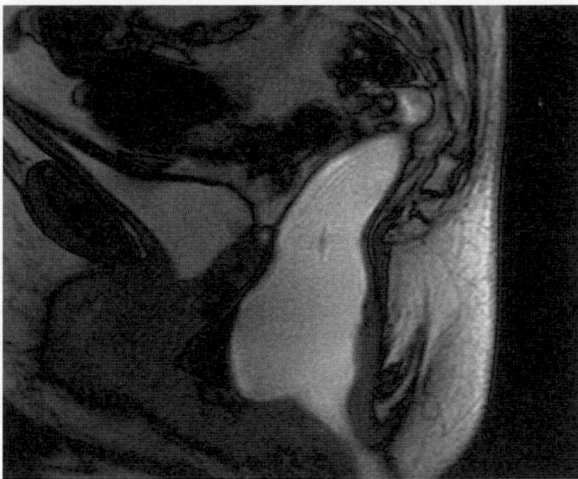

FIGURE 5 MRI-defecography. Diffusely abnormal descent of the pelvic floor with associated rectocele.

There are several different protocols for cinedefecography described in the literature, with a variety of methods used to opacify the rectum and in some institutions the vagina, bladder, and small bowel as well. Opacification of the latter three organs has been shown to improve diagnostic accuracy for lesions associated with PFD that are not opacified with rectal contrast alone and widen the rectovaginal septum (such as enterocele or sigmoidocele), or that lead to migration of the vagina during straining (such as a cystocele). Our practice is to use rectal contrast alone. Patients take an enema before the procedure. The patient then is placed in a left lateral decubitus position on the radiology table, and the rectum is infused with 50 cc of thin barium and air insufflation. After this, a caulking gun injector is used to inject 500 g of thick barium paste into the rectum. With the patient sitting on a radiolucent commode, static images are obtained during rest, squeeze and push, and dynamic fluoroscopic images are obtained while the patient defecates (Figure 4).

In MRI-defecography, patients are assessed in a similar manner (static and dynamic) with gel or air infused into the rectum and vagina (Figure 5). The examination can be done supine, or while sitting if an open-configuration magnet is available. Although more expensive, advantages of MRI over cinedefecography are the ability to evaluate all three pelvic compartments simultaneously and the lack of radiation exposure. Whether MRI-defecography has equal sensitivity or specificity for PFD compared with cinedefecography is the subject of ongoing controversy, particularly with regard to detection of intussusception and rectocele. Because the techniques are extremely operator dependent, test selection should, to a large extent, be based on the experience and familiarity of the radiology department performing the study.

Manometry

Anorectal manometry measures pressure, reflex, and sensation inside the anus and rectum under various conditions with a transanal probe. In conventional manometry, a 4- to 5-cm balloon is fixed to the shaft of the probe and three to six transducers are spaced out at regular intervals. Conventional probes are either "solid-state," in which the transducers are calibrated at atmospheric pressure before testing, or "water-perfusion," which generates a continuous pressure along the device. Pressure values are obtained during rest and

squeeze, and push. The rectoanal inhibitory reflex (RAIR) is tested by inflating a balloon at the distal tip of the probe, thereby distending the rectum. Intact RAIR causes relaxation of the internal anal sphincter (IAS) in response to increased rectal distension and is characterized by a drop in IAS pressure by 10 mm Hg for at least 5 seconds from the naturally tonic state. Absence of RAIR should raise suspicion for certain pathologic conditions, including Hirschsprung's disease, Chagas disease, dermatomyositis, and scleroderma; however, repeat testing should be performed to ensure the result is not related to technical problems with the study. Rectal sensation is measured by increasing the balloon volume inside the rectum until the patient is able to feel it is present. Balloon expulsion testing assesses the ability of the patient to expel a 50-cc balloon during defecation.

High-resolution anorectal manometry (HRAM) is a more recent technique that provides more detailed information. There are currently two types of HRAM probes available, a solid-state 4.2-mm diameter probe with 12 circumferential sensors and a "3D" 10.75-mm diameter probe with 256 sensors. In comparison with conventional manometry, HRAM is capable of measuring a "topographic" pressure map over the entire length and circumference of the anal canal. In a study comparing HRAM with conventional manometry, authors found that mean resting and squeeze pressures were higher when measured with HRAM.

■ SURGICAL OPTIONS AND TECHNIQUE

Slow-Transit Constipation

Slow-transit constipation (STC) is a failure of colonic propulsion, with abnormal prolongation time on colonic transit studies. If STC is present without co-existing PFD, and if further testing rules out proximal motility dysfunction, the patient may benefit from surgical resection. Total abdominal colectomy with ileorectal anastomosis (TAC/IRA) has been the most successful operation for STC, although several others have been reported, including subtotal colectomy with ileosigmoid (SC/ISA), subtotal with cecorectal anastomosis, segmental colonic resections, and diverting stomas. McCoy and Beck reviewed 22 studies through 2011 that reported TAC/IRA for STC and found "success" rates ranged from 50% to 100%, with only 4 under 80%, although the measure of success was not standardized across the different studies. In most, it was obtained subjectively through patient-reported quality of life assessments. Complications after TAC/IRA are reported in a highly variable manner. Small bowel obstruction has an incidence of 8% to 41%, requiring intervention in 44% to 100% of cases. Recurrent constipation occurs in anywhere from 0 to 33% of patients. Diarrhea and incontinence are 0 to 46% and 0 to 52%, respectively.

From a technical standpoint, TAC/IRA is the same for STC as in other benign contexts. The colon is fully mobilized from the terminal ileum to the rectosigmoid junction without high ligation of the vessels. Bowel continuity is restored with an IRA, which may be configured as an end-to-end or side-to-end anastomosis, both with similar functional outcomes. Some have argued that an antiperistaltic side-to-side IRA or ileal J pouch anastomosis to the rectum can reduce postoperative diarrhea, but conclusions from these studies are limited by small cohorts. Severe postoperative diarrhea is reported in a wide range, 0 to 46%. To date, most studies have reviewed open techniques, but recent data have shown equivalent outcomes in hand-assisted and laparoscopic approaches.

Alternatively, others have advocated for subtotal colectomy, including SC/ISA, subtotal colectomy with cecorectal anastomosis (SC/CCA), and segmental colectomy. Each has significant drawbacks that have limited its use over TAC/IRA. SC/ISA has a high rate of reoperation and conversion to completion colectomy/IRA because of persistent constipation. SC/CCA never gained traction in the United States because of early reports of cecal distension and conversion to TAC/IRA. However, despite this, the method has become increasingly popular in China and has been advocated strongly by the Roncoroni group in Italy. Supporters believe that preservation of the ileocecal valve maintains a colonic reservoir and a degree of colonic function that reduces postoperative diarrhea and electrolyte imbalances. Reports from European studies (Italy, France) have shown favorable outcomes, but those from China have reported mixed results. A third alternative to TAC/IRA is segmental colectomy. This theoretically would be an ideal option for patients with a purely segmental inertia; however, this is difficult to discern in a precise manner from radiologic transit studies. Segmental resection therefore has a high rate of failure and is not recommended for STC.

Pelvic Floor Dysfunction

PFD includes obstructed defecation syndrome (ODS), paradoxical puborectalis (PP), and descending perineum syndrome (DPS). PP and DPS are diagnosed definitively with defecography (Table 3), and because they do not have surgical solutions, treatment relies on bowel retraining programs and biofeedback. However, there are several structural abnormalities that are associated with ODS (rectocele, enterocele, sigmoidocele, intussusception, and prolapse) that may be addressed surgically. Often the prolapse and dysfunction in the posterior pelvic floor is associated with a more global pelvic floor prolapse, requiring a joint surgical approach with urogynecology. Repair of intussusception is similar to that of external rectal prolapse, and rectopexy alone, resection rectopexy, and Delorme procedure have been described.

Rectocele, Enterocele, and Sigmoidocele

A rectocele is a prolapse of the anterior rectal wall into the posterior wall of the vagina that is found incidentally in up to 80% of patients undergoing defecography. It is not known whether it is a cause or effect of ODS symptoms, and there is no general agreement regarding indications for operative repair, nor in the appropriate method of repair. Some have suggested surgery for size larger than 2 cm, significant contrast retention in defecography, and nonresolution of ODS symptoms. Surgical options include midline fascial plication with or without levatorplasty, or a site-specific repair, through transanal, transvaginal, or transperineal approaches. An alternative option less commonly performed in the United States is the stapled transanal rectal resection (STARR procedure).

In open transanal repair, the patient is placed in jack-knife prone positioning, and an anal retractor is inserted to expose the anterior wall of the rectum. A finger is placed in the vagina to define the size and borders of the rectocele. After submucosal injection of a mixture of lidocaine and epinephrine, a mucosal flap is raised to approximate the dimensions of the rectocele, and the underlying muscle is plicated with absorbable sutures. Excess tissue from the flap is excised and the mucosa is reapproximated with interrupted absorbable suture. Transvaginal repair typically consists of a posterior colporrhaphy. The patient is placed in lithotomy, and an incision is made along the midline of the posterior vaginal wall to expose the underlying tissue within the rectovaginal septum. The septum is then reapproximated with Vicryl suture (Ethicon, Somerville, NJ), and the vaginal wall is repaired. Some have advocated a "site-specific" repair of the rectovaginal fascia, as opposed to a complete midline plication. In the limited data comparing the two approaches, there was a higher rate of recurrence for the site-specific technique. In the transperineal approach, a transverse incision is made in the soft tissue above the anterior external anal sphincter, and dissection is carried out into the rectovaginal space. The fascia then is plicated with absorbable suture. If a traditional levatorplasty is performed, it involves suturing the perineal body and puborectalis in the midline and thereby bolstering the rectovaginal septum.

TABLE 3: Physiologic Testing in the Workup of Chronic Constipation

	Colonic Transit	Defecography	Manometry
NTC	Normal	Normal	Normal
STC	Delayed: 20% of radiologic markers remain in colon at 5 days	Normal	Normal
PFD	Normal	ODS: increased anorectal angle during defecation and inability to expel contrast* PPC: contraction of the puborectalis during defecation DPS: generalized descent of the perineum below the pubococcygeal line during defecation, with thinning of the pelvic musculature	Can be normal or abnormal; abnormal findings include increased resting anal pressure (>90 mm Hg), or low rectoanal gradient during evacuation

*Both rectocele and intussusception are reported with PFD but are not sufficient for the diagnosis.

DPS, Descending perineum syndrome; NTC, normal transit constipation; ODS, obstructive defecation syndrome; PFD, pelvic floor dysfunction; PPC, paradoxical puborectalis contraction; STC, slow transit constipation.

Transvaginal and transanal repairs have been compared in several prospective studies, which were then in turn evaluated through a Cochrane meta-analysis. Results of this analysis show that transvaginal approaches led to lower recurrence rates than transanal, measured with both subjective and objective (radiographic) output measures. Transvaginal approaches also were associated with shorter operative times, but length of overall hospitalization was greater. From the few prospective comparisons, use of mesh as an adjunct to repair has not improved outcomes.

STARR is another alternative to the previously mentioned approaches. This operation uses the same circular-stapler technique devised by Longo for treatment of internal hemorrhoids. Many variations have been proposed, but all use a circular stapler, either the PPH-01 or Contour stapler (Ethicon Endo-Surgery, Blue Ash, OH). The head of the circular stapler is inserted above the lesion, which is sutured with a purse-string stitch and gently retracted into the stapler, between the head and the shaft. After activation of the stapler it is removed and the staple line reinforced with absorbable suture.

Despite a consensus meeting being held in 2006 to discuss the STARR procedure, there are still ongoing debates regarding its long-term efficacy, as well as its true indications. There was general agreement that the procedure should be reserved for individuals who have failed medical management. Short-term results for STARR in ODS have overall been encouraging. Data from the largest report, the European STARR registry, evaluated 2171 patients with ODS who underwent STARR during a 3-year period (2006 to 2009). Follow-up at 12 months revealed significant improvement in multiple scoring systems aimed at assessing symptoms and quality of life. Complications included urgency (26.1%), acute urinary retention (9.6%), bleeding (3.6%), perianal sepsis (3.4%), and rectovaginal fistula (0.05%). There were no mortalities. Some reports with smaller cohorts have shown higher recurrence rates, and one group has noted that recurrence becomes more likely after 12 months. Long-term data for STARR are currently lacking.

Mixed Disorder: Slow-Transit Constipation and Pelvic Floor Dysfunction

Cases of PFD with coexisting STC are classified as combined disorders. As in cases of isolated PFD or STC, the first step is a prolonged trial of medical management, including biofeedback and bowel retraining. Should these measures fail, surgery has been used with only limited success. In most reported cases, the PFD was not known preoperatively and was diagnosed postoperatively in the setting of otherwise unexplained symptom recurrence. Because there has been some success in salvaging function in these cases with postoperative biofeedback, some authors have advocated a combined approach upfront for carefully selected patients: TAC or subtotal colectomy for the STC, with perioperative biofeedback for the PFD. Whether biofeedback is done preoperatively or postoperatively in this setting varies between surgeons.

Adult Hirschsprung's Disease

There has been more success in the surgical treatment of adult Hirschsprung's disease (AHD), which is a special case of combined constipation. AHD, like its pediatric counterpart, is caused by congenital absence of submucosal and myenteric ganglion cells in the internal anal sphincter. The length of proximal aganglionosis is variable, but more commonly in adults the length is a short segment, prone to more mild symptoms that can delay diagnosis until adulthood. Lack of these ganglion cells leads to an impaired rectoanal inhibitory reflex, which leads to stasis and distension in the more proximal bowel. In patients diagnosed as adults, there is often a history of lifelong constipation. Clinical suspicion can be investigated with anal manometry, but the patient must undergo a full-thickness rectal biopsy to confirm the diagnosis pathologically. Posterior anorectal strip myectomy is a technique that has been described for

diagnostic and therapeutic purposes. In this procedure, an incision is made in the rectal mucosa proximal to the dentate line to expose the underlying muscularis. A portion of internal sphincter muscle is excised and ideally contains ganglion cells at the proximal surgical margin. In short-segment disease, this procedure may be curative.

If myectomy is unsuccessful, AHD requires either bypass or resection of the dysfunctional rectum. In a meta-analysis and review of AHD from 2010, a total of 490 patients were identified in the literature. The most common surgical procedures performed in this cohort were Duhamel (47%), Swenson (10%), myectomy alone (9%), Soave (8%), and low anterior resection (5%). There are no recently published comparative data to evaluate the relative success of these techniques in adults.

The Duhamel procedure, first described in 1956, is a retrorectal transanal pull-through operation, in which the posterior wall of the rectum and anterior wall of the colon form a wide anastomosis. It has been adapted several times and has been simplified by the use of GIA staplers (Covidien, Mansfield, MA) (original procedure used a crushing clamp to be left in place for several days). The main advantage of this approach is the avoidance of rectal mobilization and associated morbidity. The disadvantage is the preservation of a blind rectal stump with the diseased segment left in situ. In contrast, the Swenson procedure involves sequential biopsies along the antimesenteric border of the colon and rectum, until the most proximal aganglionic segment is identified. This then is mobilized fully, intussuscepted through the anus, and resected. The colon is pulled through for a coloanal anastomosis. The Soave procedure involves a rectal mucosectomy up to the level of the peritoneal reflection and retraction of the colon through the remnant sleeve of rectal muscle. The colon is anastomosed to the anal canal after confirming the presence of ganglion cells on frozen biopsy.

Additional Surgical Options for Refractory Constipation in All Classes

Ostomy Formation

Diverting colostomies and ileostomies have been used for surgical management of refractory constipation, STC as well as other categories. Ileostomy generally is considered a last option, reserved for patients who have already failed another surgical method and have a dysfunctional colon, whereas patients with normal colonic transit and outlet constipation usually can be treated with a colostomy. Isolated cases of ileostomy formation have been noted in several series examining TAC/IRA, but the only series exclusively focused on ileostomy formation for STC was described in 2005 by Scarpa et al (N = 24). These authors found a reoperation rate of 30%, although all were stoma "refashionings" via parastomal incisions. Symptom recurrence was 4%.

Anterograde Continence Enema

Malone antegrade continence enema (MACE) is a treatment modality taken from pediatric surgery that has been used to treat adults with combined idiopathic constipation and incontinence. Malone's report in 1990 describes a nonrefluxing, continent stoma, formed from a reversed appendix. In this technique, the proximal right colon and appendix are mobilized through a right lower quadrant gridiron incision. The appendicocecal junction is transected with careful preservation of the appendiceal artery and the cecotomy is closed. The appendix is reversed and brought back into the cecum through a submucosal tunnel made underneath one of the tenia coli. It then is anastomosed to the cecal mucosa, and the seromuscular layers of cecum are closed over the submucosal portion, creating a valve. The original proximal end of the appendix is exteriorized through the abdominal wall and secured with a tubularized skin flap that effectively covers the stoma and minimizes spillage. In cases in which the appendix is absent, the ileum has been used instead with successful results. This technique is similar in principle to MACE but uses the ileocecal valve to prevent reflux up the stoma. Results from the largest reported series with a group of patients that included both methods (total N = 69) found that at a mean follow-up period of 75 months, 62% of patients were still using their enemas, and 12% did not require them any longer. The main technical complication reported in several series has been stenosis of the channel.

Sacral Nerve Stimulation

Sacral nerve stimulation (SNS) has been used to treat chronic constipation and has been the subject of several prospective studies. Kamm et al conducted a relatively large multicenter trial in Europe in 62 patients with chronic constipation. Temporary SNS stimulators were tested for a period of 21 days and transitioned to a permanent stimulator if the patient experienced benefit. For the 45 patients who proceeded to this second phase, bowel movement frequency improved from 2.3 to 6.6 per week. Despite these encouraging findings, a 2015 Cochrane review that evaluated the available published data as a whole for SNS in constipation did not find any clear benefit.

■ SUMMARY

Surgery rarely is indicated for chronic constipation. It has been estimated that only 3% to 5% of surgical referrals for constipation actually meet criteria for surgical intervention. Nonetheless, for properly selected patients it can improve symptoms substantially. The surgeon should proceed cautiously with careful examination and physiologic testing to identify patients with true indications for surgery who do not have occult conditions that will predispose them to postoperative recurrence.

SUGGESTED READINGS

Agachan F, et al. A constipation scoring system to simplify evaluation and management of constipated patients. *Dis Colon Rectum.* 1996;39: 681-685.
Bharucha AE, Pemberton JH, Locke GR 3rd. American Gastroenterological Association technical review on constipation. *Gastroenterology.* 2013; 144:218-238.
Denoya P, Sands DR. Anorectal physiologic evaluation of constipation. *Clin Colon Rectal Surg.* 2008;21:114-121.
Longstreth GF, et al. Functional bowel disorders. *Gastroenterology.* 2006;130:1480-1491.
McCoy JA, Beck DE. Surgical management of colonic inertia. *Clin Colon Rectal Surg.* 2012;25:20-23.
Muller-Lissner SA, et al. Myths and misconceptions about chronic constipation. *Am J Gastroenterol.* 2005;100:232-242.
Pemberton JH, Rath DM, Ilstrup DM. Evaluation and surgical treatment of severe chronic constipation. *Ann Surg.* 1991;214:403-411, discussion 411-413.
Thaha MA, et al. Sacral nerve stimulation for faecal incontinence and constipation in adults. *Cochrane Database Syst Rev.* 2015;(8):CD004464.

THE MANAGEMENT OF RADIATION INJURY TO THE SMALL AND LARGE BOWEL

Bradley J. Champagne, MD, FACS, FASCRS, and W. Conan Mustain, MD

Radiation therapy is an important component of the treatment of many forms of cancer. Ionizing radiation imparts damage to cancer cells through direct transfer of energy to macromolecules such as DNA, proteins, and membrane lipids, as well as through the generation of reactive oxygen species and inflammatory cytokines. As with any cancer therapy, limitations on the effectiveness of radiation are less related to its inability to kill cancer cells than the ability to do so without causing excessive harm to the patient. The therapeutic effects of radiation on a target organ must be balanced against the damaging effects on normal, adjacent tissues. Despite strategies to improve the differential response to radiation of tumor cells versus normal tissue, radiation-induced toxicity remains a significant cause of treatment-associated morbidity.

Radiation-induced injury to the intestinal tract is a common complication of radiation therapy for cancers of the abdomen, pelvis, and retroperitoneum. Effects on the bowel may be acute and self-limited, often beginning during therapy and resolving within months. Chronic radiation damage may manifest months to years after treatment with complications arising from disordered tissue remodeling and revascularization. Attempts have been made to improve delivery methods and modify host factors to minimize the damaging effects of radiation on normal bowel, but the long-term effects of these strategies remain to be seen. Despite their frequency, gastrointestinal (GI) symptoms in patients undergoing radiation therapy may be underreported by patients and underrecognized by providers. Studies have shown that in clinical trials, higher rates of toxicity symptoms were described in patient-reported studies in comparison with those of clinicians, underscoring the importance of addressing bowel function when caring for patients with a history of radiation exposure.

■ THERAPEUTIC AND TOXIC EFFECTS OF RADIATION

The cellular effect of radiation on tumors and normal tissue involves a complex interplay of direct cellular damage with secondary inflammatory and immune responses. In normal tissues reactive oxygen species are derived from multiple sources, including macrophages, leukocytes, and fibroblasts, and are a normal part of wound healing and the innate immune response. Cells contain numerous antioxidant systems that protect them from oxidative damage. Ionizing radiation interacts with intracellular water and target macromolecules to generate damaging free radicals, which overwhelm the cells' normal defense mechanisms, inducing cellular damage and apoptosis. Furthermore, reactive oxygen species stimulate production of numerous proinflammatory cytokines, including TGF-β, TNF-α, and IL-1, which enhance the cytotoxic effects of radiation on tumor cells but may lead to epithelial injury, inflammation, and fibrosis in normal tissues.

The injurious effects of radiation on normal tissue may be acute or chronic and vary by tissue type. Tissues with high cell turnover rates, such as skin and intestine, are especially sensitive to the acute cytotoxic effect of radiation on epithelial cells and the microvasculature. Other tissues, such as lung and brain, have acute toxicity primarily as a consequence of the inflammatory effects of radiation. Most acute tissue injury resulting from radiation is self-limited and requires only supportive care. Classically, the chronic effects of radiation on normal tissue have been attributed to depletion of vascular endothelial cells and tissue progenitor cells, leading to chronic ischemia, disordered revascularization, tissue loss, and fibrosis. Increasingly a more complex interaction of the vasculature, epithelium, and stroma, including infiltrating immune cells, is recognized as mediating ongoing tissue remodeling and injury. Late radiation injury may occur months to years after treatment and can lead to permanent,

TABLE 1: QUANTEC Appropriate Dose and Dose/Volume Parameters for Several Organs

Organ	Dose (Gy)*† Dose/volume parameters*
Heart	Mean dose <26 Gy (pericardium) V_{25} <10%
Lung	Mean dose <20 Gy V_{20} ≤30%
Kidney	Mean dose <15-18 Gy V_{20} <32%
Liver	Mean dose <30-32 Gy (<13 in 3 fractions, <18 in 6 fractions)
Esophagus	Mean dose <34 Gy
Stomach	Max point dose <30 Gy in 3 fractions V_{22} <4%
Small bowel	Max point dose <30 Gy in 3-5 fractions V_{15} < 120 cc for individual loops; V_{45} < 195 cc for entire peritoneum
Bladder	Max dose <65 Gy V_{65} ≤50%

Adapted from Marks et al. *Int J Radiat Oncol Biol Phys.* 2010;76:S10-S19.

*Dose or dose/volume parameters associated with <20% rate of serious organ-specific toxicity.

†Dose delivered at standard fractionation (1.8-2.0 Gy per daily fraction), unless otherwise noted.

QUANTEC, Quantitative Analysis of Normal Tissue Effects in the Clinic.

sometimes fatal, complications. The calculation of normal tissue complication probability has evolved since the seminal paper by Emami and colleagues in 1991. More recently, a collaborative effort of the American Society for Radiation Oncology and the American Association of Physicists in Medicine resulted in the publication of the *Quantitative Analysis of Normal Tissue Effects in the Clinic,* which provides updated dose/volume/outcome information for many organs and is used to guide treatment planning (Table 1).

The effectiveness of radiation on a particular tumor and its unintended effects on adjacent organs at risk are influenced by a number of factors beyond simply the characteristics of the tissue and the total dose received. Patient factors that affect tissue perfusion and immunity may influence the chronic response of normal tissue to radiation. Systemic diseases such as diabetes, atherosclerosis, or collagen vascular disease increase susceptibility to chronic radiation toxicity. Smoking and low body weight are additional risk factors for complications. Treatment characteristics such as the method of delivery and fractionation regimen affect the amount of normal tissue exposed and its ability to recover from the insult. A number of different methodologies are available for the delivery of therapeutic radiation that affect not only the effectiveness of cancer killing but also the side effect profile. New technologies and techniques for external beam therapy including 3D conformal radiotherapy, intensity-modulated radiotherapy (IMRT), stereotactic body radiotherapy (SBRT), volumetric modulated arc therapy, and other arc-related therapies such as CyberKnife (Accuray, Sunnyvale, CA) allow the accurate delivery of increasing doses to tumors while minimizing toxicity to nontarget organs. The need to treat areas of possible microscopic disease and the need for a treatment margin to account for target motion and setup error limit the ability to completely exclude normal tissue from the treatment field.

Brachytherapy involves the direct placement of radioactive material in proximity to a tumor for a short period to maximize tumor effects and minimize exposure to surrounding tissues. Radiation can be delivered by transient insertion of endocavitary or interstitial tubes, which house a removable radiation source or by the implantation of radioactive seeds with a predetermined half-life. Although the exposure of remote organs is limited by concentrating treatment in a focused area, tissue that is close to the source may incur toxicity. The type of radionucleotide and the placement have a significant influence on the amount and duration of radiation exposure to normal tissue. Studies in prostate and cervical cancer have shown favorable rectal toxicity profiles for patients treated by brachytherapy as opposed to external beam. Prostate cancer patients treated by brachytherapy showed significantly lower rates of acute and chronic rectal toxicity compared with patients treated by external beam radiation. Although rare, rectourethral fistula is a well-known and serious potential complication of prostate brachytherapy.

The effectiveness of radiation therapy and the extent of unintended side effects may be influenced by the presence of compounds that alter the susceptibility of tissues to radiation injury. These agents are referred to as *radiation modifiers.* The therapeutic index of radiation therapy may be enhanced by the administration of compounds that either limit toxicity in normal tissue or selectively enhance tumor sensitivity. Agents that selectively enhance radiation-induced killing of cancer cells while exhibiting no toxicity on normal tissue are referred to as *radiosensitizers.* The effects of radiosensitizers may be additive, if the agent imparts some direct tumoricidal effect that reduces the number of surviving cells, or synergistic, if the primary effect is to enhance the cytotoxicity of the radiation. Most agents used clinically as radiosensitizers are cytotoxic chemotherapies, which have additive and synergistic effects by inducing DNA damage and preventing DNA repair. Other strategies include the selective redistribution of tumor cells to cell cycle phases that are more sensitive to the effects of radiation, or blocking mutant pathways, which allow tumor cells to recover from the effects of radiation. It is important that any agent used as a radiosensitizer have selective uptake and activity in cancer cells versus normal tissue, or no therapeutic gain will be realized. The use of chemical radioprotectors to selectively impart protection to normal tissue is discussed in the section on prevention of radiation injury.

■ RADIATION INJURY TO THE BOWEL

The damaging effects of radiation on the intestine were recognized more than 100 years ago, shortly after the discovery of the x-ray. Any part of the GI tract may be at risk for injury during radiation for cancers in the chest, abdomen, pelvis, or retroperitoneum. The small bowel is particularly radiosensitive but is protected somewhat by its mobility within the abdomen. Fixed locations such as the terminal ileum, cecum, and rectum are the most common sites of injury. Previous surgery and the presence of adhesions may increase the risk of small bowel injury during pelvic radiation. The cellular effects of radiation on the bowel are biphasic. The acute phase of injury is mediated by activated oxygen radicals causing direct epithelial cell injury and mucosal inflammation through stimulation of proinflammatory cytokines. The result is a cascade of epithelial barrier disruption, mucosal atrophy, and inflammatory cell infiltration. Chronic injury is characterized by fibrosis as a consequence of progressive obliterative vasculitis and chronic ischemia, as well as mucosal atrophy due to the loss of crypt progenitor cells. Often viewed as two distinct entities, acute and late phase toxicity may progress on a continuum with the initial insult underlying the development of chronic symptoms. Studies have shown the development of acute symptoms to be a significant risk factor for chronic toxicity.

Clinically the symptoms of radiation toxicity are classified as early if they occur within 3 months of beginning therapy or late if they occur beyond 3 months. The Radiation Therapy Oncology Group and the European Organization for Research and Treatment of

TABLE 2: RTOG/EORTC Radiation Toxicity Grading

Grade	0	1	2	3	4	5
RTOG Acute radiation morbidity score*	None	Increased frequency or change in quality of bowel habits not requiring medication Rectal discomfort not requiring analgesics	Diarrhea requiring parasympatholytic drugs Mucous discharge not necessitating sanitary pads Rectal or abdominal pain requiring analgesics	Diarrhea requiring parenteral support Severe mucous or blood discharge necessitating sanitary pads Abdominal distension	Acute or subacute obstruction, fistula, or perforation GI bleeding requiring transfusion Abdominal pain or tenesmus requiring tube decompression or bowel diversion	n/a
RTOG/EORTC Late radiation morbidity score	None	Mild diarrhea and cramping Bowel movement ≤5 times daily Slight rectal discharge or bleeding	Moderate diarrhea and colic Bowel movement >5 times daily Excessive rectal mucus or intermittent bleeding	Obstruction or bleeding requiring surgery	Necrosis, perforation, or fistula	Death resulting from radiation late effects

*The acute morbidity criteria are used to score/grade toxicity from radiation therapy. The criteria are relevant from day 1 through day 90. Thereafter the EORTC/RTOG late radiation morbidity index is to be used.

RTOG/EORTC, Radiation Therapy Oncology Group/European Organization for Research and Treatment of Cancer.

Cancer (RTOG/EORTC) have published acute and late radiation morbidity scoring schema for a variety of organs. The various degrees of severity for GI toxicity are listed in Table 2. Other scoring systems include the Late Effects Normal Tissue/Subjective Objective Management Analytic (LENT/SOMA) and the National Cancer Institute Common Terminology Criteria for Adverse Events, version 4. Unfortunately neither the LENT/SOMA nor the RTOG/EORTC are well correlated with health care–related quality of life questionnaires and may underestimate the true incidence and severity of GI symptoms in patients undergoing radiation treatment.

Acute GI toxicity may manifest shortly after initiating therapy, typically peaking in the fourth or fifth week. Severity is variable, and common symptoms include diarrhea, cramping, and minor bleeding. Treatment is mostly supportive with antimotility agents and avoidance of dehydration. Symptoms are typically self-limited and resolve within weeks of completing treatment. Surgery rarely is required for acute GI toxicity, and only a minority of patients require modification or interruption of their planned therapy. Late complications arise months to years after completing therapy and are attributable to remodeling of the bowel wall with resultant mucosal atrophy, fibrosis, and vascular sclerosis. The consequences may be functional, resulting in malabsorption or disordered motility, or structural with stricture formation, fistulization, or refractory bleeding from telangiectasias. Chronic radiation damage to the intestine is a challenging clinical problem and can be associated with major morbidity. Colon and rectal radiation injury has a better prognosis and is less likely to require surgical intervention than small bowel complications.

The true incidence of GI toxicity during radiation therapy is difficult to define and is dependent on a number of factors, most importantly the dose of radiation and the amount of bowel exposed. Overall, symptoms of acute bowel toxicity occur in 60% to 90% of patients undergoing radiation for abdominal tumors. In patients treated with external beam radiation for retroperitoneal soft tissue sarcomas, acute grade 3 or 4 GI toxicity has been reported in 20% to 30% of patients. The rectum is especially vulnerable to radiation damage during treatment of prostate and cervical cancer. In prostate cancer, 40% to 60% of men undergoing external beam radiation therapy have symptoms of acute rectal toxicity. The estimated incidence of chronic rectal toxicity grade 2 or higher is less than 10%.

High-grade chronic rectal toxicity after treatment for cervical cancer has been reported in 10% to 15% of women at 20 years. Recent studies have shown that in all, more than 50% of patients receiving pelvic radiation report a permanent adverse effect of radiation-related GI symptoms on their quality of life.

Another late consequence of radiation injury to the bowel is the risk of malignancy. Increased rates of colorectal cancer have been reported in patients treated with pelvic radiation for cervical and prostate cancer. Two recent analyses of the Surveillance, Epidemiology, and End Results registry characterized the risk of rectal cancer in men treated with radiation for prostate cancer. Reviewing more than 85,000 men treated for prostate cancer between 1973 and 1994, Baxter and colleagues (2005) found an increased risk of rectal cancer in patients treated with radiation as opposed to surgery alone, with an adjusted hazard ratio of 1.7 (95% CI: 1.4 to 2.2). Colorectal cancers related to radiation exposure tend to be of a mucinous phenotype more frequently than sporadic tumors, suggesting a possible alternate carcinoma pathway in the radiated bowel.

■ PREVENTION

A number of strategies have been developed to reduce the risk of radiation injury to the bowel during therapy. During pretreatment simulation 3D imaging, patient immobilizers, and skin markings are used to carefully calibrate the planned course of therapy. Ensuring consistent positioning by daily imaging at each treatment session is practiced in some facilities. Prone positioning, treating with a full bladder, and elevating the hips with a belly board are strategies to reduce the risk of inadvertent small bowel exposure during pelvic radiation. Modern delivery systems such as SBRT and IMRT are able to deliver nonuniform doses over a carefully contoured treatment field, minimizing exposure to nontreatment organs.

A number of chemical agents have shown therapeutic promise in preventing or decreasing the severity of radiation-induced bowel injury, including angiotensin-converting enzyme inhibitors, statins, glutamine, arginine, and probiotics. Amifostine is the only FDA-approved radiation protector. It has selective uptake in normal tissue through differences in cellular pH and differential activity of alkaline phosphatase in tumor versus normal tissue. Intracellularly it is metabolized to a free radical scavenging thiol, which minimizes the damaging effects of reactive oxygen species. The effectiveness in preventing radiation-induced injury to the bowel is still unknown, but one study did show a positive effect on the rates of clinically significant rectal inflammation in a series of 20 patients undergoing pelvic radiation.

Perhaps one of the best prevention techniques is the use of preoperative rather than postoperative radiation. Especially with pelvic and retroperitoneal tumors, the risk of bowel entering the treatment field increases substantially after resection of the primary tumor. In the seminal German Rectal Cancer Trial, the use of preoperative chemoradiation was associated with significantly lower rates of acute and late toxicity than the postoperative approach, especially with regard to acute and chronic diarrhea and anastomotic stricture. In situations in which postoperative radiation is deemed necessary, a variety of surgical techniques may be used to exclude the small bowel from the predicted treatment field. The simplest of these is the use of omentum or a retroverted uterus to exclude small bowel from an empty pelvis after proctectomy. Closing the pelvic inlet with retroperitoneal tissue, taking care not to incorporate the ureters, is also possible. A variety of more elaborate techniques have been described, including creation of an omental envelope, placement of absorbable mesh slings, or implantation of prosthetic tissue expanders.

■ SPECIFIC INJURIES

Acute Radiation Enteritis

Acute radiation injury to the small bowel is a frequent side effect of abdominal and pelvic radiotherapy. The diagnosis usually is made by symptoms alone in patients who currently are undergoing treatment. Early symptoms include nausea and loss of appetite, with diarrhea and abdominal pain typically developing after a few weeks of treatment. The initial treatment of acute radiation enteritis is supportive. Diarrhea, the most commonly reported symptom, can be treated with antimotility or antisecretory agents such as loperamide, Lomotil (Pfizer, New York, NY), or octreotide. Octreotide was shown in one randomized controlled trial to be more effective than Lomotil in controlling symptoms of diarrhea resulting from acute radiation enteritis, with quicker resolution of symptoms and fewer patients requiring interruption of therapy. Adoption of a low-residue diet may benefit some GI symptoms, and patients should be encouraged to note and avoid foods that aggravate symptoms. Ensuring adequate fluid and caloric intake is crucial and requires a careful history and low threshold for checking lab work. Severe cases with persistent symptoms may require hospitalization with bowel rest, pain control, and parenteral nutrition. Severity is variable, but 15% to 20% of patients require some alteration of their intended therapy. Symptoms are typically self-limited and often resolve within 3 months. Surgery rarely is required for acute GI injury and generally should be avoided in patients receiving ongoing treatments.

Chronic Radiation Enteritis

The chronic effects of intestinal radiation may occur from 6 months to 30 years after treatment. Symptoms generally are related to alterations of structure and function, which impair normal absorption and transit. Malabsorption may manifest as chronic diarrhea, steatorrhea, weight loss, or nutritional deficiencies. Diarrhea is one of the most common symptoms, and its cause may be multifactorial. Patients with chronic damage to the terminal ileum may lose the ability to absorb bile salts, causing an osmotic diarrhea. With time this may result in depletion of the bile salt pool and subsequent fat malabsorption and steatorrhea. Stasis within a stenotic or bypassed segment of bowel may lead to bacterial overgrowth. Treatment should be aimed at controlling diarrhea, avoiding dehydration and electrolyte depletion, and ensuring adequate nutrition. Diarrhea may be treated with antimotility and antisecretory agents. Cholestyramine may be effective in reducing osmotic diarrhea from excess bile salts. Patients suspected of having bacterial overgrowth should be treated with oral antibiotics. Replacement of specific vitamin and electrolyte deficiencies should be addressed. In patients who are malnourished, it is important to determine if there is a problem with intake, which may suggest a mechanical cause of symptoms rather than simply malabsorption resulting from loss of functional bowel. Surgical removal of radiated bowel will restore function but is unlikely to alleviate symptoms of malabsorption.

Disordered intestinal transit may result from impaired motility in fibrotic segments or from true mechanical obstruction in areas of chronic stricture. Obstructive symptoms may be insidious, with intermittent colicky pain, intolerance of high-residue foods, or alternating constipation and diarrhea. Alternatively patients may present acutely with symptoms of obstruction or perforation. Oral contrast studies may help localize areas of stricture and determine extent of stenosis. Computed tomography (CT) and magnetic resonance (MR) enterography are especially useful to identify pathology not visible on conventional imaging (Figure 1). Pill enterography generally is not advised in the workup of radiation-induced injury because of the high risk of pill trapping. Endoscopic evaluation of the rectum and distal colon is indicated if a colonic anastomosis is considered a possibility.

Attempts to localize the site of disease should be coordinated with an aggressive search for recurrence of the original malignancy because complications from chronic radiation damage can be difficult to discern from recurrent tumor. Positron emission tomography (PET)-CT may provide additional information regarding the likelihood of recurrent cancer and should be interpreted along with measurements of appropriate tumor markers. In patients with recurrent or metastatic cancer a careful assessment of the patient's prognosis, well-being, and goals is essential to planning appropriate therapy. A significant number of patients undergoing surgery for radiation-associated complications will die from their original cancer within 2 years.

Indications for surgery in chronic radiation enteritis include obstruction, perforation, fistulization, or severe bleeding. Because patients frequently have had progressive disease for an extended period before presentation an assessment of their nutrition and functional status is indicated. Decompression by nasogastric tube, initiation of parenteral nutrition, control of sepsis with antibiotics, and drainage of intraabdominal collections should be accomplished first.

Radiation is associated with the formation of dense, obliterative adhesions, which require meticulous dissection and adhesiolysis. Extreme care should be taken to avoid enterotomies and the associated risk of leak and fistula formation. Liberal use of diverting stomas is recommended when colonic resection is required. Surgical options for the management of the injured bowel include resection with anastomosis or bypass of affected segments (Figure 2). Bypass has been advocated as a simpler and potentially safer option than dissecting out matted, fibrotic loops of bowel but obviously does not remove the diseased segments and may lead to ongoing symptoms from bacterial overgrowth, perforation, or abscess. Regimbeau and colleagues (2001) retrospectively analyzed outcomes of 109 patients treated surgically for chronic radiation enteritis and found lower rates of reoperation and better 5-year survival in patients treated by resection and anastomosis rather than bypass. In general, resection and anastomosis is preferable over bypass alone. An exception to this may be in the setting of a single loop fixed in the pelvis, where resection may risk severe bleeding or injury to vital pelvic structures. Strictureplasty may be used in select cases of chronic radiation injury with multiple, short-segment stenoses in a patient at high risk for short bowel syndrome. It is not indicated for perforation, bleeding, fistula, or in patients with limited disease and adequate intestinal reserve.

Radiation Proctitis

Acute rectal toxicity is a very common finding in patients undergoing pelvic radiation, typically occurring within the first few weeks of

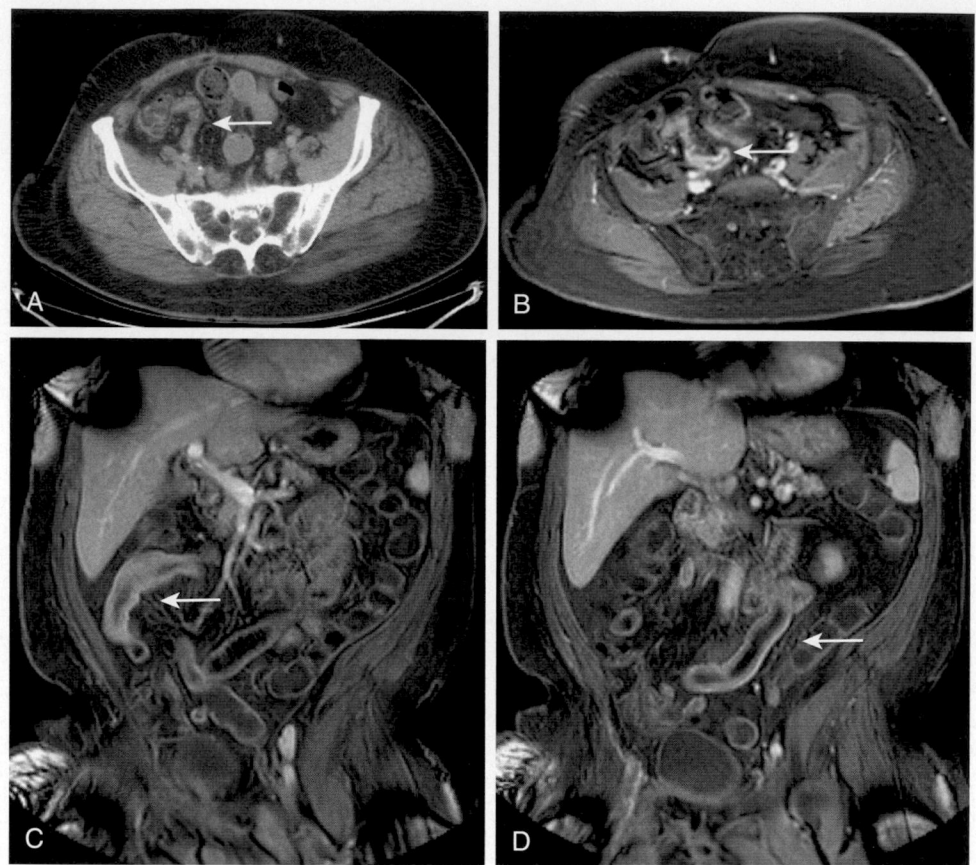

FIGURE 1 Chronic radiation injury to the small bowel. A 66-year-old male with prior abdominal radiation for testicular cancer with partial small bowel obstruction. **A,** Computed tomographic scan suggested an isolated stricture of the terminal ileum. Symptoms resolved with conservative management. **B,** Outpatient magnetic resonance enterography confirmed the ileal stricture but also showed multiple, long segments of radiation damage in a skip-lesion pattern involving more than 100 cm of small bowel (**C** and **D**).

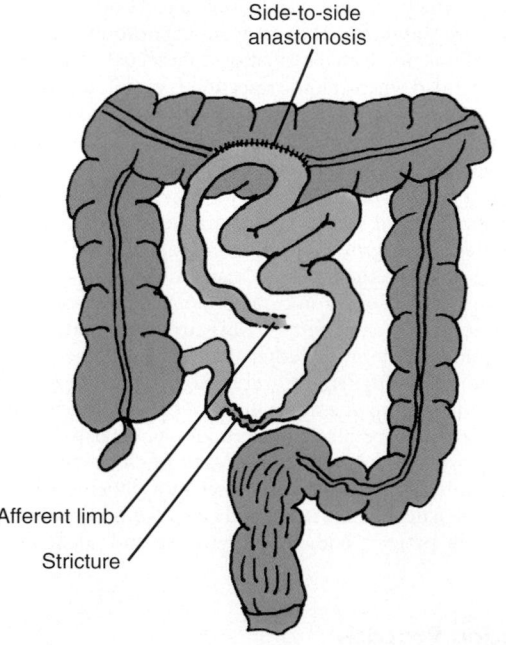

FIGURE 2 Side-to-side small bowel–transverse colon anastomosis bypassing a strictured segment of terminal ileum.

therapy and resolving shortly after cessation of therapy. The most frequent symptoms are diarrhea and tenesmus, although bleeding, mucous discharge, and fecal urgency may occur. Bleeding in the acute phase typically is related to mucosal sloughing, and massive hemorrhage is uncommon in this setting. Treatment is supportive and typically does not require interruption of therapy. Most patients recover spontaneously and remain asymptomatic with no further effects of radiation injury.

Chronic Radiation Proctitis

Symptoms of chronic radiation proctitis are related to the histologic changes of progressive fibrosis and disordered revascularization. Although fibrosis can lead to diarrhea, urgency, and incontinence, the development of mucosal telangiectasias can lead to significant bleeding. Chronic fibrosis leads to alterations of rectal sensation and compliance that have been well documented in patients with a history of previous pelvic radiation. Yeoh et al (2012) reported decreased basal pressure, squeeze pressure, volume at first perception, and rectal compliance in patients with prior external beam radiation for prostate cancer. The resultant fecal urgency can be a distressing problem and difficult to treat. Symptoms of chronic diarrhea and incontinence should be worked up thoroughly before settling on chronic rectal radiation toxicity and decreased compliance as the cause. A multitude of different entities can cause diarrhea in a patient with history of cancer and radiation treatment. These include but are not limited to infections, neutropenia, radiation damage to the small bowel, bacterial overgrowth, and dietary intolerances. Some of these conditions may be correctable, and others may be managed by simple measures such as antimotility agents.

The evaluation of a patient with a history of rectal radiation who experiences rectal bleeding should include a thorough history and physical examination followed by flexible sigmoidoscopy. In patients who are within 3 years of treatment, who had appropriate screening for colorectal cancer before treatment, the risk of malignancy as a cause of bleeding is low. Deep biopsies should be avoided to minimize risk of worsening bleeding, perforation, or fistula. The endoscopic appearance of the rectum does not directly correlate with symptoms because telangiectasias and mucosal congestion are seen in more than half of asymptomatic patients at 2 years after pelvic radiation for prostate cancer. Initial management includes optimizing bowel function through the medical treatment of constipation or diarrhea. Minimally symptomatic patients with mild bleeding may require no further treatment if bleeding is not affecting quality of life or causing significant anemia. Sucralfate enemas are an effective first-line treatment for radiation proctitis and may improve bleeding and tenesmus. Using 20-mL enemas of 20% rectal sucralfate suspension, most patients have significant improvement in symptoms within a few weeks. Short-chain fatty acid enemas have been studied with mixed results and may be used to treat acute radiation proctitis. 5-ASA derivatives have been shown to be of no benefit. Hyperbaric oxygen therapy is emerging as a potentially beneficial treatment for chronic radiation proctitis with a few prospective trials demonstrating mucosal healing and some benefit in bowel-related quality of life. High cost, need for repeated treatments, and limited availability are persistent barriers to hyperbaric oxygen therapy.

Patients with severe bleeding from radiation proctitis may require interventional therapies for hemorrhage control. The application of topical formalin is one of the oldest and most effective treatments for bleeding from chronic radiation proctitis. Spot treatment of bleeding sites with 10% formalin solution is performed via long cotton-tipped applicators through a rigid proctoscope. Alternatively, a more dilute solution of 4% formalin can be instilled directly into the rectum in 50-mL aliquots or on formalin-soaked gauze. The solution is kept in contact with the rectal wall for 2 to 3 minutes before removal followed by saline irrigation. Care must be taken to protect the surrounding perianal skin. Complications are rare, and repeat applications may be performed on a biweekly basis as necessary until symptoms resolve.

Endoscopic options for bleeding control include lasers, bipolar energy, or argon plasma coagulation (APC). Because of cost, safety, and the availability of other treatments the use of laser modalities has fallen out of favor. Bipolar or heater probes frequently are used for other types of upper and lower GI bleeds and may be used in select cases of chronic radiation proctitis when a visible vessel is identified. APC works by conduction of electrical current through a beam of inert argon gas, creating a superficial burn, which can be applied over a large area. Repeat treatments may be required, and treatment may be less effective in the setting of active bleeding. Studies have found topical formalin and APC to be equally efficacious in refractory bleeding from chronic radiation proctitis.

Surgery is needed infrequently for either acute or late rectal toxicity from radiation. The quality of long-term data is variable, but most studies report an incidence of surgical intervention for fistulae, bleeding, or intractable symptoms at less than 1%. In rare cases of severe, debilitating diarrhea and incontinence linked to chronic radiation change, diverting colostomy may be required to improve quality of life. In cases of severe uncontrollable hemorrhage, abdominoperineal resection or inter-sphincteric proctectomy is the procedure of choice.

Fistulae

Intestinal fistulae from radiation are a complex clinical problem and can occur in any location within the treatment field. In addition,

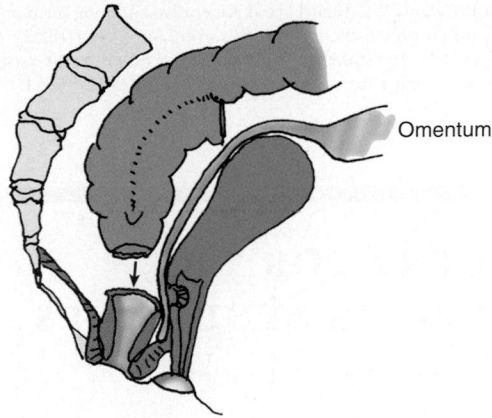

FIGURE 3 Abdominal approach to a midlevel rectovaginal fistula, demonstrating the use of a colon J pouch. The coloanal anastomosis is below the level of the posterior vaginal defect, which is left open to granulate closed. This also may be done with a straight anastomosis. The omental flap is an important additional buttress between the vagina and colon, separating the strictures and reducing the probability of recurrent fistulization.

fistulae may develop from a technical complication incidentally incurred in a radiated field. Management of fistulizing disease is dependent on the location of the fistula, the timing of presentation, the state of the surrounding tissues, and the overall condition of the patient. The principles of management for enterocutaneous and enteroenteric fistulae are much the same as they are in nonradiated patients, aside from the increased difficulty of dissection and the need to identify nonradiated bowel for anastomosis. Enteric fistulae to the bladder or vaginal cuff still can be managed by resection and anastomosis but, in cases where this cannot be accomplished safely, may be excluded and left attached to the affected organ as a well-vascularized patch, accepting the possibility of persistent mucous drainage.

Rectal fistulae from radiation are uniquely challenging, and several general management principles should be observed. Mid to upper rectal fistulae are treated appropriately by resection with anastomosis of healthy, nonradiated colon to the distal rectum or anal canal. The interposition of a well-vascularized tongue of omentum or a pedicled rectus muscle between the anastomosis and the affected organ may be considered (Figure 3). Temporary proximal diversion should be performed. Low rectal fistula to the vagina or the prostatic urethra can be treated by an abdominal, perineal, transsacral (Kraske), or trans-sphincteric (York-Mason) approach. Fecal and/or urinary diversion is indicated almost universally before reconstruction. Native tissue repairs have a high rate of failure, and the incorporation of healthy, well-vascularized tissue is advisable. A number of possible tissue grafts exist, including omentum, rectus muscle, gracilis muscle, buccal mucosa, or labial fat pad (Martius flap). In select patients diversion alone, with colostomy and suprapubic tube may be offered as definitive therapy. As always, recurrent malignancy should be excluded before undertaking repair.

SUGGESTED READINGS

Baxter NN, Tepper JE, Durham SB, et al. Increased risk of rectal cancer after prostate radiation: a population-based study. *Gastroenterology.* 2005;128: 819-824.

Hauer-Jensen M, Denham JW, Andreyev HJ. Radiation enteropathy—pathogenesis, treatment, and prevention. *Nat Rev Gastroenterol Hepatol.* 2014;11:470-479.

Kim JH, Jenrow KA, Brown SL. Mechanisms of radiation-induced normal tissue toxicity and implications for future clinical trials. *Radiat Oncol J.* 2014;32:103-115.

Regimbeau JM, Panis Y, Gouzi JL, et al. Operative and long term results after surgery for chronic radiation enteritis. *Am J Surg.* 2001;182:23-42.

Sauer R, Becker H, Hohenberger W, et al. Preoperative versus postoperative chemoradiotherapy for rectal cancer. *N Engl J Med.* 2004;351:1731-1740.

Yeoh EK, Holloway RH, Fraser RJ, et al. Pathophysiology and natural history of anorectal sequelae following radiation therapy for carcinoma of the prostate. *Int J Radiat Oncol Biol Phys.* 2012;84:e593-e599.

SURGERY FOR THE POLYPOSIS SYNDROMES

Scott R. Kelley, MD, FACS, FASCRS

Colorectal polyps can be classified as adenomatous, hamartomatous, hyperplastic, neoplastic, and inflammatory. The development of multiple polyps is considered a polyposis syndrome, and several have been described. Each syndrome has different characteristics, including presentation, genetic basis, extracolonic manifestations, and malignancy risk. Management options include strict surveillance for the early detection of cancer, chemopreventive medications, and surgery. A detailed family history and genetic evaluation are imperative, and siblings and offspring should be offered genetic counseling and testing. Multidisciplinary care (clinical services, support, counseling) and referral to a polyposis registry is recommended. This chapter focuses on the most common polyposis syndromes.

■ ADENOMATOUS POLYPOSIS SYNDROMES

Familial Adenomatous Polyposis

Familial adenomatous polyposis (FAP) is an autosomal dominant inherited disease resulting from a mutation in the adenomatous polyposis coli (APC) tumor suppressor gene located on chromosome 5q21. Most mutations are found between codons 168 and 1640, with two of the most significant being 1061 and 1309. FAP is defined as greater than 100 synchronous adenomas or less than 100 with a positive family history. Polyps, found predominantly in the rectum and left colon, develop in adolescence and are present in up to 15% of patients by 10 years of age and 75% by 20. If untreated, the risk of colorectal malignancy is nearly 100% by 35 to 40 years of age. Approximately 25% to 30% do not have a family history and will have FAP de novo. The most common presenting symptoms are bleeding, diarrhea, abdominal pain, and mucous discharge.

For those with a family history or identified APC mutation a screening colonoscopy should be performed at 10 to 12 years of age and continue annually. With the predilection for polyp development in the left colon and rectum, a yearly flexible proctosigmoidoscopy can be done instead of a formal colonoscopy. If adenomatous polyps are appreciated on sigmoidoscopy, a formal colonoscopy should ensue.

Extracolonic Intestinal Disease

Extracolonic intestinal disease is a common manifestation of FAP. More than 80% to 90% of patients will have gastric fundic gland hyperplastic polyps with very low malignant potential. Gastric adenomas are rare (10%), typically occur in the antrum, and are associated more commonly with Japanese and Korean heritage.

Duodenal adenomas, most commonly found around the ampulla of Vater and macroscopically different than colonic adenomas, are found in more than 95% of patients with FAP and develop approximately 15 years later than colonic polyps. Duodenal cancer, typically diagnosed around 50 years of age, occurs in 5% to 10% of patients and is the second leading cause of death associated with FAP. A screening esophagogastroduodenoscopy (EGD) typically is performed around 20 years of age, and the Spigelman severity score and staging system (Table 1) is used to determine surveillance intervals (Table 2). The risk of developing cancer after 10 years of follow-up for stage I is 0, stage II and III 2%, and 36% for stage IV. Small tubular adenomas, as well as those with low-grade dysplasia, can undergo biopsies and be observed. High-risk adenomas (villous, >1 cm), severe duodenal polyposis, high-grade dysplasia, or stage IV disease should be offered a pancreas-preserving duodenectomy, and those with cancer a pancreaticoduodenectomy. Chemoprevention with nonsteroidal anti-inflammatory agents (sulindac, celecoxib) can result in polyp regression in those with a lesser polyp burden, although overall the effect is minimal at best.

Extraintestinal Manifestations

Common extraintestinal manifestations of FAP include osteomas, congenital hypertrophy of the retinal pigment epithelium (CHRPE), epidermoid cyst, and dermoids. Benign osteomas of the mandible, skull, and tibia are the most common extraintestinal finding occurring in more than 80% of patients. Although CHRPE is not specific to FAP, having four or more areas of large, patchy fundic discoloration is pathognomonic and will be present in around 75% of individuals. Epidermoid cysts occur approximately 50% of the time.

Other extraintestinal manifestations, although rare, include supernumerary teeth, cerebellar medulloblastoma, and cancers of the liver, biliary tree, adrenal glands, and thyroid.

Desmoid Tumors

Desmoids develop in 15% to 30% of patients. These locally invasive abdominal wall and intraabdominal/retroperitoneal myofibroblastic tumors typically develop 2 to 3 years after surgery and occur around 30 years of age. They can develop spontaneously, are the third most common cause of death associated with FAP, and have been noted to be associated with trauma. Risk factors associated with the development of desmoids are mutations in the 3′ end of the APC gene, female gender, extraintestinal manifestations, and a family history of desmoid disease. Of desmoids, 10% grow rapidly, 10% resolve spontaneously, 30% vacillate between cycles of growth and regression, and 50% remain stable or grow very slowly.

Extra-abdominal desmoids are best treated with surgical extirpation with a 1-cm margin, although recurrence is high with documented rates of 20% to 50%. Early excision is recommended to decrease the size of the resultant abdominal wall defect.

Intraabdominal/retroperitoneal desmoids can invade the mesentery and surrounding structures resulting in obstruction, hemorrhage, fistulization, ischemia, and perforation. The primary treatment is medical and includes nonsteroidal anti-inflammatory agents (sulindac, celecoxib), estrogen antagonists (tamoxifen, toremifene, raloxifene), and chemotherapy (vinblastine, methotrexate, doxorubicin, dacarbazine). Radiotherapy can be used for palliative measures but is associated with small bowel necrosis and fistulas. Surgical removal is difficult and often impossible if the root of the mesentery is involved. Resection with completely uninvolved margins (R0) will result in recurrence 50% of the time. If possible, nonresective procedures such as diversion and bypass can be pursued for palliation. Ureteral obstruction is best treated with stenting.

There is not a defined screening regimen for desmoid tumors, although computed tomography (CT) and magnetic resonance

TABLE 1: Spigelman Staging System* for Upper Gastrointestinal Manifestations of Familial Adenomatous Polyposis

Points	1	2	3
Number of polyps	1-4	5-20	>20
Size of polyps (mm)	1-4	5-10	>10
Histology	Tubular	Tubulovillous	Villous
Dysplasia	Mild	Moderate	Severe

*Spigelman stage I, score 1-4; stage II, score 5-6; stage III, score 7-8; stage IV, score 9-12.

TABLE 2: Derivation of Spigelman Stage From Scores

Total Points	Spigelman Stage	Suggested Interval to Next Duodenoscopy (Years)
0	0	5
1-4	I	3-5
5-6	II	3
7-8	III	1
9-12	IV	Duodenectomy; if not, rescope in 6 months

imaging (MRI) can be used, especially for those with an increased risk of developing desmoids.

Attenuated Familial Adenomatous Polyposis

In contrast to classic FAP, attenuated FAP (aFAP) occurs at a later age (30s and 40s), with fewer than 100 polyps found predominantly in the right colon. If untreated, the risk of colorectal malignancy is nearly 100% by 59 years of age. Extracolonic and intestinal manifestations, including gastric adenomas, desmoids, and CHRPE, typically are not seen in aFAP.

For those with a family history or identified APC mutation suggestive of aFAP, screening colonoscopy should begin at 20 years of age and be repeated every 1 to 2 years. With the predilection for polyp development in the right colon a formal colonoscopy is recommended.

Mutation Y-Homolog–Associated Polyposis

Mutation Y-homolog (MYH)–associated polyposis (MAP) is an autosomal recessive inherited form of FAP resulting from a biallelic mutation in the MYH gene located on chromosome 1p34. The number of polyps associated with MAP is variable (tens to hundreds) with a median around 50. Polyps are found most commonly in the left colon and occur at a median age of 48. If untreated, the risk of colorectal malignancy is around 80% by 70 years of age. Extraintestinal manifestations are associated with MAP, although exceedingly rare.

Because of the phenotypic overlap with FAP, genetic testing for the MYH typically is performed when no APC mutation is detected, there are fewer than 100 adenomatous polyps, and the family history is irrelevant or does not reveal a dominant mode of inheritance.

Although there is no defined endoscopic screening criteria for MAP, an initial endoscopic (colonoscopy and EGD) evaluation should be performed starting around 25 to 30 years of age. If no polyps are appreciated, endoscopy should be repeated every 3 to 5 years and more frequently if present.

■ CHEMOPREVENTION

Although clinic trials have shown that nonsteroidal anti-inflammatory drugs (sulindac, exisulind, celecoxib) and aspirin can reduce the size and number of adenomas in the colon and rectum, there was not an appreciable reduction in cancer. Chemoprevention is not recommended as a primary therapy for polyposis syndromes and is not an appropriate alternative to prophylactic surgery. Situations in which chemoprevention can be entertained include treating ileal pouch anal anastomosis polyps, a high family risk of desmoid tumors, delayed surgery, and unwillingness or inability to tolerate polypectomy or completion proctectomy.

■ SURGERY

The primary goal of surgery is to prevent colorectal cancer. The timing and type of surgery offered depends on a multitude of factors, including clinical presentation, family history, and if known, the site of the chromosomal mutation. Severe polyposis (more than 1000 colonic or 20 rectal polyps) and APC mutations between codons 1250 and 1464 carry a higher risk of cancer and surgery should be offered as early as possible. Surgery also should be pursued early for symptomatic disease. For those with a high risk of desmoid disease (family history, mutation in the 3′ end of the APC gene, female gender, extracolonic manifestations), surgery should be delayed as long as possible to decrease the chance of desmoid tumors developing. Young patients should have surgery delayed, if possible, to allow for adequate physical, social, and intellectual maturity. For patients with classic FAP, surgery typically occurs around 16 to 20 years of age.

Surgical options include open or minimally invasive total proctocolectomy (TPC) with creation of an end or continent ileostomy, total abdominal colectomy (TAC) with creation of an ileorectal anastomosis (IRA), and a total proctocolectomy with creation of an ileal pouch anal anastomosis (IPAA).

Proctocolectomy With End Ileostomy

A proctocolectomy with end Brooke ileostomy has a low rate of complications but leaves the patient with an incontinent stoma. Indications for this approach are patient preference, low rectal cancer requiring an abdominoperineal resection, rectal cancer requiring postoperative pelvic radiation, inability to create an IPAA (inadequate mesenteric length), and poor sphincter function.

The procedure is carried out in an oncologic approach secondary to the risk of a preoperatively unrecognized cancer. A perineal intersphincteric dissection is carried out preserving the external sphincter and levator ani muscles. The perineum is closed in layers and the greater omentum, if present, is mobilized and placed in the pelvis to prevent future bowel obstructions. After closure of the abdomen the ileostomy is matured in a standard evaginated Brooke fashion, with an attempted ideal projection of 2.5 cm.

Proctocolectomy With Continent Ileostomy

Initially described by Nils Kock, the continent ileostomy still remains a viable alternative for motivated patients who are not candidates for an IPAA. Modifications and revisions to the original Kock continent ileostomy have been described (Barnett continent ileostomy reservoir and T pouch), although without evidence to suggest they are better than the Kock pouch. Contraindications to construction of a continent ileostomy include Crohn's disease, obesity, marginal small bowel length, and a psychologic or physical disability that would preclude understanding or being able to perform daily stomal intubation.

Total Abdominal Colectomy With Ileorectal Anastomosis

Colectomy with ileorectostomy should be considered only in cases of attenuated or mild polyposis (fewer than 20 rectal or 1000 colonic adenomas), rectal polyps smaller than 3 cm, no colorectal dysplasia or cancer, a distensible and compliant rectum, and in patients with an intact sphincter mechanism that are willing to adhere to strict follow-up. Ileoproctostomy is an appealing alternative in younger patients of reproductive age to decrease the risk of impotence and reduced fecundity. Strict rectal surveillance (every 6 to 12 months) must be adhered to because of the increased risk of future neoplastic changes. The risk of rectal carcinoma can reach up to 40% by 30 years, although this is based on literature from the pre-IPAA era. In patients who require a completion proctectomy, an end ileostomy, restorative IPAA, or continent ileostomy are all options.

Restorative Proctocolectomy and Ileal Pouch Anal Anastomosis

Initially described in 1978 by Parks and Nicholls, the restorative proctocolectomy has become the most common continence-preserving procedure performed in patients who are appropriate candidates. Indications include severe polyposis (more than 20 rectal, more than 1000 colonic adenomas), rectal polyps larger than 3 cm in size, colonic dysplasia or cancer, dysplastic rectal polyps, and in patients with an intact sphincter mechanism willing to adhere to strict follow-up. The restorative pouch can be fashioned in two limbs (J), three limbs (S), four limbs (W), or isoperistaltic (H) configurations. The J pouch, because of its ease of construction and excellent functional outcomes, has become the most common choice for surgeons.

A total colectomy is performed in an oncologic fashion, and the ileum is transected flush with the cecum (Figure 1). To provide adequate perfusion to the pouch it is imperative to preserve the ileal branches of the ileocolic and distal mesenteric arteries. Evaluation for adequacy of reach of the small bowel to the deep pelvis should be undertaken before creation of the pouch. If the proposed apex of the pouch-anal anastomosis can be advanced 3 to 4 cm below the inferior edge of the pubis, one can feel confident of successful reach for anastomosis. Strategies to decrease tension at the anastomosis include complete mobilization of the small bowel mesentery to the root of the superior mesenteric artery cephalad to the head of the pancreas (Figure 2), proximal division of the ileocolic artery

(Figure 3), and relaxing incisions of the mesentery over tension points along the superior mesenteric artery (Figure 4). Rectal dissection is completed in the TME plane, and transection of the rectum with a 30-mm transverse stapler should occur 2 to 3 cm above the dentate line in the anal transition zone (Figure 5). After reach has been verified, a J configuration is fashioned with each limb measuring between 12 and 15 cm in length. The limbs are paired in an antimesenteric fashion and are held in orientation with interrupted stay sutures. For those without evidence of adenomas in the anal transition zone, or dysplasia in the lower rectum, a double-stapled

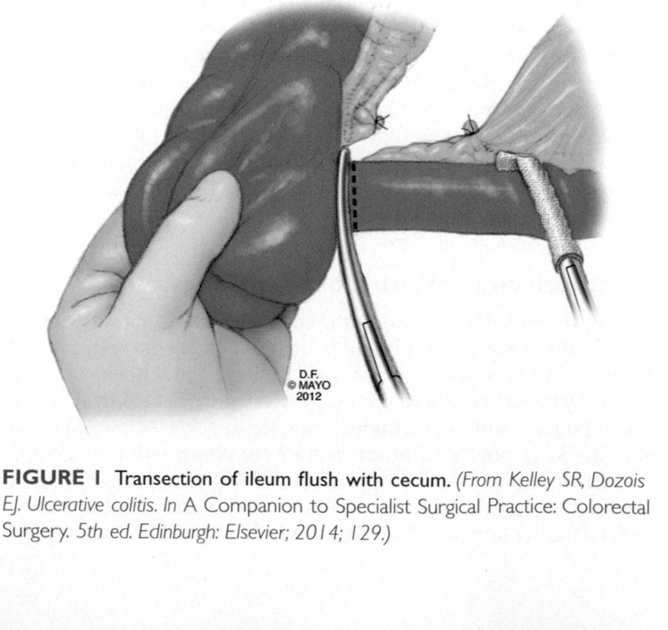

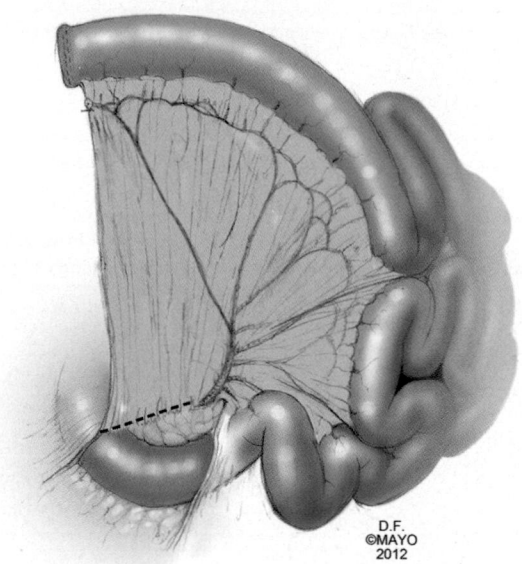

FIGURE 2 Mobilization of the small bowel mesentery to the root of the superior mesenteric artery. *(From Kelley SR, Dozois EJ. Ulcerative colitis. In A Companion to Specialist Surgical Practice: Colorectal Surgery. 5th ed. Edinburgh: Elsevier; 2014:131.)*

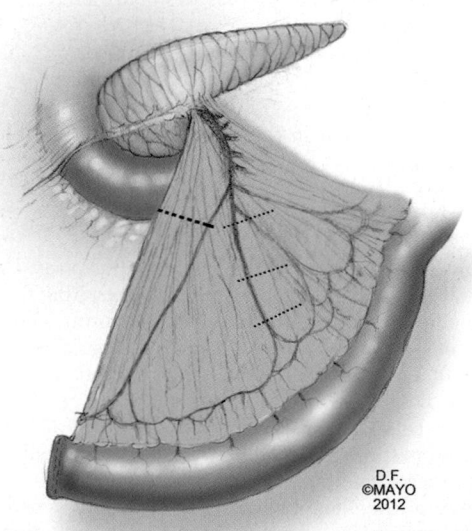

FIGURE 3 Division of the ileocolic artery. *(Used with permission of Mayo Foundation for Medical Education and Research, all rights reserved.)*

FIGURE 1 Transection of ileum flush with cecum. *(From Kelley SR, Dozois EJ. Ulcerative colitis. In A Companion to Specialist Surgical Practice: Colorectal Surgery. 5th ed. Edinburgh: Elsevier; 2014; 129.)*

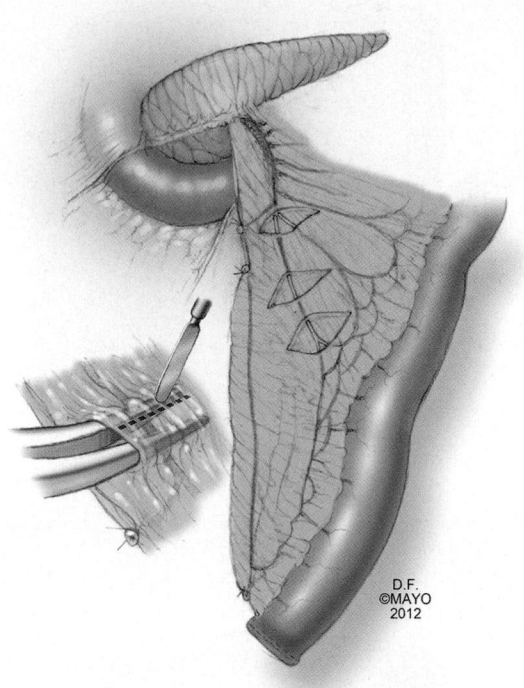

FIGURE 4 Mesenteric relaxing incisions. *(Used with permission of Mayo Foundation for Medical Education and Research, all rights reserved.)*

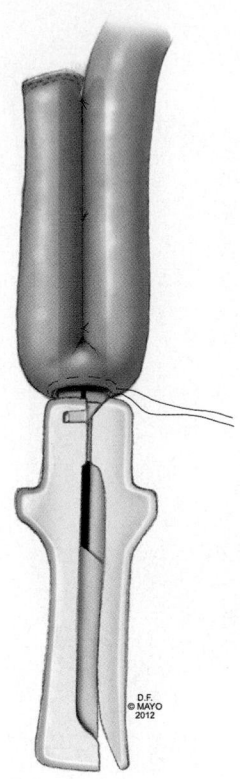

FIGURE 6 J pouch creation. *(Used with permission of Mayo Foundation for Medical Education and Research, all rights reserved.)*

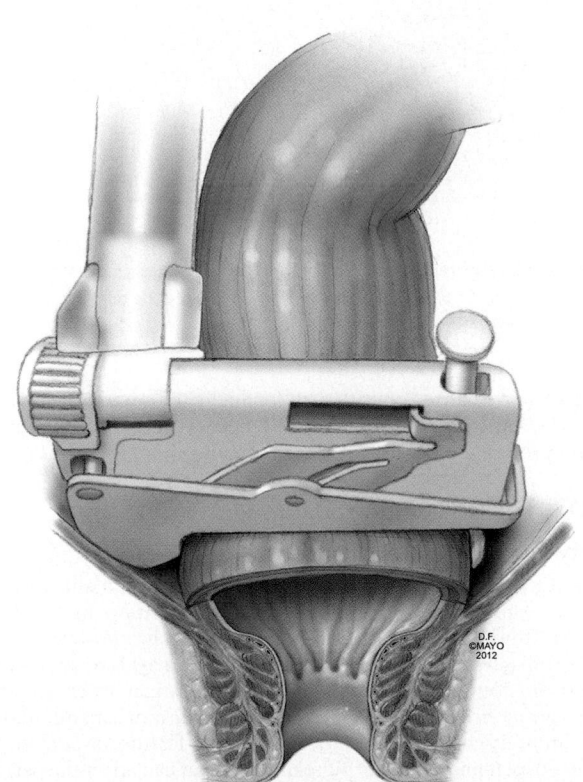

FIGURE 5 Rectal transection. *(From Kelley SR, Dozois EJ. Ulcerative Colitis. In A Companion to Specialist Surgical Practice: Colorectal Surgery. 5th ed. Edinburgh: Elsevier; 2014:132.)*

IPAA can be fashioned; otherwise an anal mucosectomy and hand sewn IPAA is recommended. After creation of the IPAA, an air insufflation leak test is performed and, if necessary, a protective loop ileostomy fashioned, which should be created as close to the pouch as possible to decrease issues with high output. In selected patients the operation can be completed with good results without the creation of a diverting loop ileostomy.

Double-Stapled Technique

An enterotomy is made in the antimesenteric apex of the pouch, and a linear cutting stapler is used to divide the walls of the two limbs, creating a common channel (Figure 6). A purse-string suture then is fashioned around the enterotomy, and the anvil from a circular stapler is placed inside the pouch where it is held in place by tightening the purse string (Figure 7). The circular stapler then is placed transanally. After appropriate orientation the circular stapler cartridge spike is advanced either above, or below, the transverse rectal staple line and attached to the anvil. The stapler then is closed, approximating the pouch and anus (Figure 8).

Hand-Sewn Technique

An anal canal mucosectomy is performed starting at the dentate line. Raising the mucosa with a submucosal injection (Figure 9) of dilute saline and epinephrine (1:200,000) facilitates dissection of the mucosa away from the internal sphincter muscle (Figure 10), which can be completed sharply or with electrocautery. After the mucosa and proximal rectum have been removed circumferentially, the pouch is brought down gently to the level of the dentate line. An enterotomy is made in the apex of the pouch, if not already created, and it is anchored in position by placing a suture in each of the four quadrants, incorporating a full-thickness bite of the pouch, internal sphincter muscle, and mucosa. Sutures are placed between the anchoring stitches to complete the anastomosis (Figure 11).

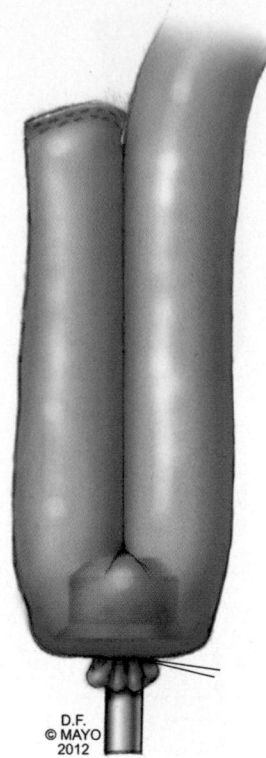

FIGURE 7 Anvil in J pouch. *(Used with permission of Mayo Foundation for Medical Education and Research, all rights reserved.)*

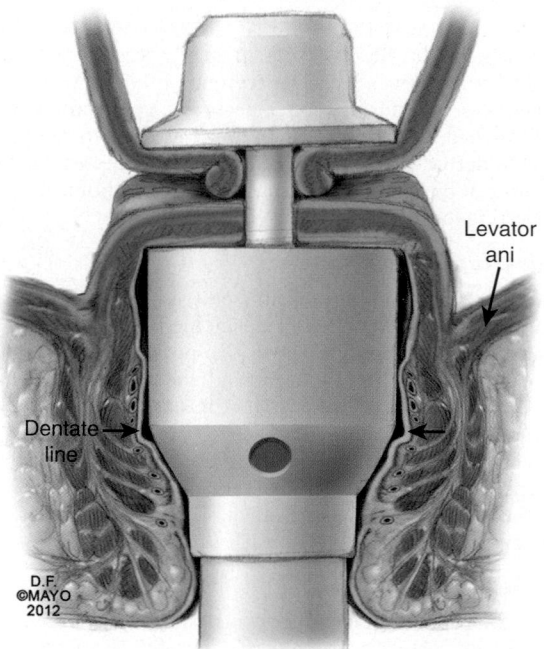

FIGURE 8 Stapled ileal pouch anal anastomosis. *(Used with permission of Mayo Foundation for Medical Education and Research, all rights reserved.)*

Postoperative Surveillance

After creation of an end ileostomy, IPAA, or IRA, annual endoscopic surveillance for adenomas, dysplasia, and carcinomas will continue for a patient's lifetime. Histologic evaluation of random biopsies and polyps should be performed to exclude dysplasia and cancer. More

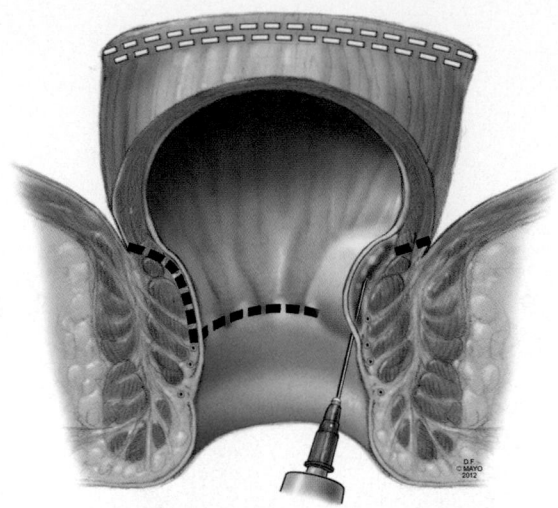

FIGURE 9 Submucosal injection. *(Used with permission of Mayo Foundation for Medical Education and Research, all rights reserved.)*

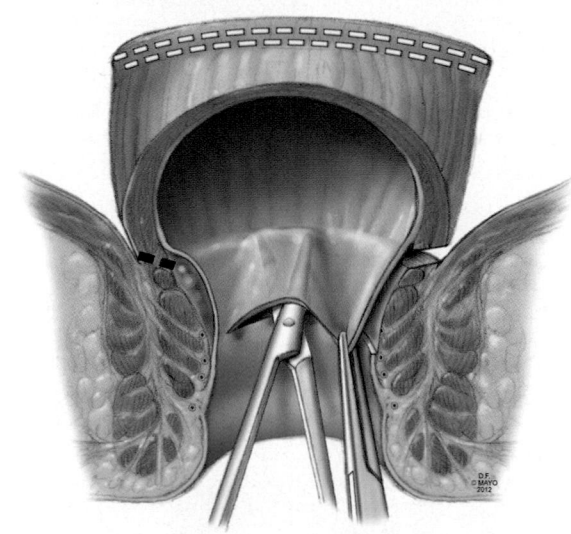

FIGURE 10 Anal mucosectomy. *(From Kelley SR, Dozois EJ. Ulcerative Colitis. In A Companion to Specialist Surgical Practice: Colorectal Surgery. 5th ed. Edinburgh: Elsevier; 2014:134.)*

frequent surveillance is performed for increased numbers or size of polyps. Severe dysplasia and villous adenomas more than 1 cm in size should prompt a completion proctectomy in those with an IRA.

■ OTHER POLYPOSIS SYNDROMES

Peutz-Jeghers Syndrome

Peutz-Jeghers Syndrome (PJS) is an autosomal dominant inherited disease resulting most commonly from a mutation in the *LKB1* (*STK11*) tumor suppressor gene located on chromosome 19p13. Approximately 30% to 40% will occur de novo. Hamartomatous polyps are found throughout the gastrointestinal tract, although most commonly the small intestine. Extraintestinal manifestations are common with the hallmark phenotypic feature in adolescence being mucocutaneous hyperpigmentation that can affect the perioral and buccal region, eyes, nostrils, perianal region, fingers and toes, and hands and feet. Hyperpigmentation dissipates as one ages. Hamartomatous polyps and mucocutaneous pigmentation confirms a diagnosis of PJS. Presenting symptoms can include abdominal pain,

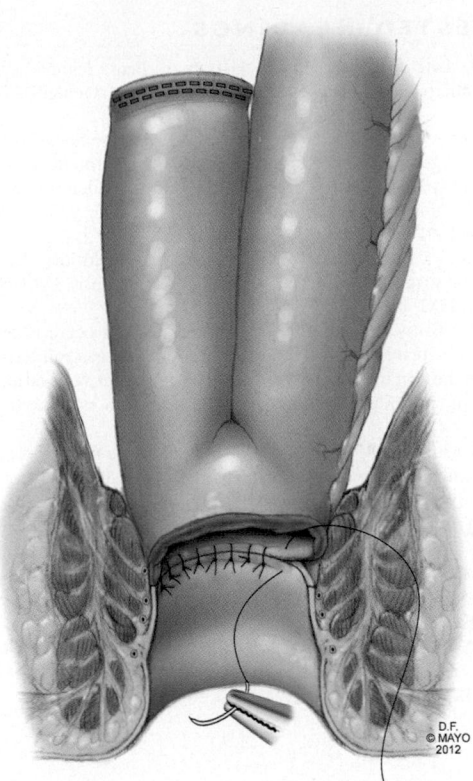

FIGURE 11 Hand-sewn ileal pouch anal anastomosis. *(Used with permission of Mayo Foundation for Medical Education and Research, all rights reserved.)*

are associated with some *SMAD4* mutations. Diagnosis of JPS is confirmed when five or more juvenile polyps are found in the colon or rectum, multiple polyps are appreciated in other regions of the gastrointestinal tract, or after identification of polyps with a positive family history. Presenting symptoms can include hematochezia and melanotic stools, anemia, intussusception, obstructing, and passage of autoamputated or prolapsed polyps. Colorectal cancer is the most common associated malignancy with lifetime rates as high as 39%. Other malignancies include gastric, duodenal, and pancreatic.

Asymptomatic patients should begin with screening colonoscopy by 15 years of age, and earlier for those with symptoms. If no polyps are detected evaluation can be repeated every 2 to 3 years, otherwise annually. EGD is recommended by age 25. Those with an *SMAD4* mutation should have periodic screening for AVMs.

Colorectal surgery is reserved for symptomatic disease, dysplasia, or cancer. For those with a relatively spared rectum, a TAC with IRA can be pursued; if the rectum is significantly involved, a TPC with IPAA is advisable. Surgeries in the remaining GI tract also may be warranted.

Cowden's Syndrome

Cowden's syndrome is an autosomal dominant disorder resulting from a mutation in the *PTEN* tumor suppressor gene located on chromosome 10q23. Polyps typically occur in the colon and stomach, and colonic polyps can include hamartomas, fibromas, adenomas, lipomas, and neurofibromas. Extraintestinal manifestations include pathognomic trichilemmomas, macrocephaly, and a wide variety of tumors and hamartomas of various organ systems (breast, thyroid, uterus).

The risk of developing colon and rectal cancer is thought to be no greater than the general population, although the risk for thyroid and breast cancer is noted to be around 10% and 50%, respectively. Screening recommendations are not standardized, but some recommend colonoscopy, mammography, and thyroid ultrasound beginning around 30 years of age. Treatment is based on symptoms.

Bannayan-Riley-Ruvalcaba Syndrome

Bannayan-Riley-Ruvalcaba syndrome (BRRS) is an autosomal dominant disorder resulting from a mutation in the *PTEN* tumor suppressor gene located on chromosome 10q23. Common findings associated with BRRS include pigmented penile macules, macrocephaly, hamartomas, hemangiomas, and mental retardation in more than 50%.

The risk of developing colon and rectal cancer is thought to be no greater than the general population. Treatment is based on symptoms.

Cronkite-Canada Syndrome

Cronkite-Canada Syndrome (CCS) is a noninherited disorder resulting from a mutation in the *PTEN* tumor suppressor gene located on chromosome 10q23. Hamartomatous gastrointestinal polyps in addition to alopecia, macrocephaly, onycholysis, and cutaneous pigmentation are common findings. Diffuse gastrointestinal inflammation resulting in malabsorption, diarrhea, and protein-losing enteropathy can occur.

The risk of developing colon and rectal cancer is thought to be no greater than the general population. Treatment is based on symptoms.

Hereditary Mixed Polyposis Syndrome

Hereditary mixed polyposis syndrome (HMPSS) is thought to be an autosomal dominant inherited syndrome, although a specific mutation has yet to be identified. HMPSS involves multiple different colon and rectal polyps (adenomatous, hamartomatous, and hyperplastic).

alteration in bowel habits, weight loss, bowel intussusception, anemia, hematochezia and melanotic stools, and small bowel obstruction. The risk of malignancy increases with age (thirteenfold higher than the general population); the most common cancers are colorectal, breast, pancreatic, and genitourinary.

Colonoscopy and EGD should be initiated around 10 years of age. If polyps are detected, endoscopic evaluation should continue every 2 to 3 years. If no polyps are found, repeat endoscopy and small bowel follow-through or capsule enteroscopy should be initiated by 20 years of age and repeated every 2 to 3 years. Other surveillance recommendations with low levels of evidence include an annual clinical examination, annual testicular examination starting at birth with ultrasound for abnormalities detected, monthly breast examination starting at 18, and annual breast MRI and cervical smear starting at 25.

Gastrointestinal surgery is reserved for symptomatic disease or cancer. Any polyp larger than 1.5 cm should be removed, if possible, at the time of surgery. Intraoperative on-table endoscopy can be used to evaluate the entire gastrointestinal tract.

Juvenile Polyposis Syndrome

Juvenile polyposis syndrome (JPS) is an autosomal dominant inherited disease resulting most commonly from mutations in the *SMAD4* and *BMPR1A* genes, which are located, respectively, on chromosomes 18q21 and 10q22. Polyps can be found throughout the gastrointestinal system; the colon is affected 100% of the time. Extraintestinal manifestations occur around 15% of the time and can include cleft lip and palate, polydactyly, genitourinary anomalies, intestinal malrotation, hydrocephalus, and congenital heart disease. Hereditary hemorrhagic telangiectasia and bleeding arteriovenous malformations (AVMs) in the GI, pulmonary tracts, brain, and mediastinum

The risk of developing colon and rectal cancer is thought to be greater than the general population, although this is unsubstantiated at this time. Treatment is based on symptoms.

Serrated Polyposis Syndrome

Serrated polyposis syndrome (SPS) is a disorder characterized by multiple polyps (hyperplastic or serrated) throughout the colon. A heritable pattern and genetic cause has not been identified. The World Health Organization has proposed three criteria for diagnosing SPS, of which diagnosis is made on fulfillment of any of the criteria. The criteria include (1) at least five serrated polyps proximal to the sigmoid colon, two of which are greater than 10 mm in diameter, (2) any number of serrated polyps occurring proximal to the sigmoid colon in an individual who has a first-degree relative with serrated polyposis, (3) more than 20 serrated polyps of any size distributed throughout the colon.

The risk of developing colon and rectal cancer is increased with rates of up to 30% to 50% documented in those with multiple polyps. The average age for developing colon and rectal cancer is 50 to 60 years. Treatment is based on polyp burden, dysplastic, or neoplastic changes.

Strict surveillance with colonoscopy every 1 to 2 years is advisable. First-degree relatives are at an increased risk of SPS and developing colon and rectal cancer (fivefold) and should be offered the same surveillance starting at 40 years of age or 10 years younger than the index case.

SUGGESTED READINGS

Beggs AD, Latchford AR, Vasen HF, et al. Peutz-Jeghers syndrome: a systematic review and recommendations for management. *Gut.* 2010;59: 975-986.

Church J, Simmang C, Standards Task Force, American Society of Colon and Rectal Surgeons. Practice parameters for the treatment of patients with dominantly inherited colorectal cancer (familial adenomatous polyposis and hereditary nonpolyposis colorectal cancer). *Dis Colon Rectum.* 2003;46:1001-1012.

da Luz Moreira A, Church JM, Burke CA. The evolution of prophylactic colorectal surgery for familial adenomatous polyposis. *Dis Colon Rectum.* 2009;52:1481-1486.

Dunlop MG, British Society for Gastroenterology, Association of Coloproctology for Great Britain and Ireland. Guidance on gastrointestinal surveillance for hereditary non-polyposis colorectal cancer, familial adenomatous polyposis, juvenile polyposis, and Peutz-Jeghers syndrome. *Gut.* 2002; 515:V21-V27.

Groves CJ, Saunders BP, Spigelman AD, et al. Duodenal cancer in patients with familial adenomatous polyposis (FAP): results of a 10 year prospective study. *Gut.* 2002;50:636-641.

Kalady MF, Jarrar A, Leach B, et al. Defining phenotypes and cancer risk in hyperplastic polyposis syndrome. *Dis Colon Rectum.* 2011;54:164-170.

Latchford AR, Neale K, Phillips RK, et al. Juvenile polyposis syndrome: a study of genotype, phenotype, and long-term outcome. *Dis Colon Rectum.* 2012;55:1038-1043.

Latchford AR, Sturt NJ, Neale K, et al. A 10-year review of surgery for desmoid disease associated with familial adenomatous polyposis. *Br J Surg.* 2006;93:1258-1264.

THE MANAGEMENT OF COLON CANCER

Joselin L. Anandam, MD, and Michael A. Choti, MD

Colorectal cancer affects more than 1 million people worldwide, and more than half will die from the disease. In the United States alone, this malignancy is the second leading cause of cancer deaths, affecting men and women equally. Large bowel cancer can be divided further by the anatomic location of the tumor into colon and rectal cancer. Colon cancers are those that arise within the portion of the large bowel that is within the peritoneal cavity, from the cecum to the peritoneal reflection, where the large bowel becomes the rectum. The distinction from rectal cancer, although seemingly somewhat arbitrary, is important to make for several reasons, including differences in clinical presentation, operative management, and type of adjuvant therapy offered. Of all large bowel cancer, the colonic site makes up approximately 70%. Like rectal cancer, colon cancer management requires a multidisciplinary team approach to optimize detection, treatment, and subsequent surveillance.

■ CLINICAL PRESENTATION: IMPORTANCE OF SCREENING AND EARLY DETECTION

Screening for colorectal cancer before it becomes clinically apparent has been shown to reduce cancer-related mortality. The success of screening programs is one of the reasons cited for the decline in mortality rates from colorectal cancers over the past 20 years. Screening generally is recommended to begin at age 50, unless risk factors including family history are present. On the basis of current guidelines, options for screening include annual fecal occult blood test, annual fecal immunochemical test, flexible sigmoidoscopy every 5 years, colonoscopy every 10 years, double-contrast barium enema every 5 years, or computed tomographic colonography (virtual colonoscopy) every 5 years. Stool DNA testing is also now an acceptable screening method for colorectal cancer; however, the interval between tests has not been determined. Unfortunately, even today, the majority of patients with colon cancer come to medical attention through symptomatic presentation rather than from screening.

The most common presenting symptoms are abdominal pain, blood per rectum, anemia, constipation, diarrhea, or change in stool character. In contrast to rectal cancer, colon cancer rarely presents with anal pain, tenesmus, or incontinence. The location of the tumor within the colon often dictates the type of symptoms experienced. Right-sided tumors tend to present with anemia or the constitutional symptoms produced by such. Obstruction from right-sided tumors is more commonly in the region of the ileocecal valve. Left-sided tumors are more likely to present with obstruction, largely because of the narrow bowel caliber, circumferential lesions, and firmer stool consistency. Evident blood in the stool and a change in stool caliber are also seen more commonly with distal colon cancer.

■ DIAGNOSIS AND EVALUATION

Patients with symptoms should undergo a diagnostic colonoscopy with histologic analysis of the colon lesion. Injection of an intramural permanent tattoo adjacent to the lesion circumferentially is recommended for surgical planning. There is a 6% to 8% chance of a synchronous lesion; therefore the entire colon should be examined. If this is technically not feasible because of a near-obstructing lesion, a colonoscopy should be performed 3 months after surgery.

A thorough history and physical examination and routine laboratory analysis, including carcinoembryonic antigen (CEA), should be part of the initial evaluation. An elevated preoperative CEA more likely is associated with advanced disease and is an independent predictor of poor outcome. Although a preoperative CEA level is advocated as a guide to postoperative management, it is important to realize that a normal preoperative CEA should not influence the utility of CEA for postoperative surveillance. Patients with normal levels at presentation, when the disease is localized clinically, often will develop CEA elevation with recurrence. Liver function tests also can be useful as a preoperative indicator of metastatic liver disease. Cross-sectional imaging should also be a routine part of the evaluation, most commonly computerized tomographic (CT) scan. This is important because approximately 20% of patients have metastatic disease at presentation. Positron emission tomography (PET) is not routinely recommended, particularly for patients without evidence of metastatic disease.

■ SURGICAL MANAGEMENT

The management of colon cancer depends on the stage at presentation. Patients can be divided into two categories: patients with a tumor amenable to resection with curative intent and patients in whom palliation is the goal. In patients with localized and potentially curable disease, surgical resection is generally the primary and initial therapy, followed by adjuvant chemotherapy in some cases. When patients present with advanced disease, chemotherapy is often the first line of therapy, and palliative resection is reserved for cases of locally symptomatic disease.

The goals of surgical therapy with curative intent are to achieve complete removal of the primary cancer with adequate tumor-free margins, an anatomically complete lymphadenectomy of the draining lymph nodes, en bloc resection of any involved adjacent organs, and avoidance of contamination of the surgical field with tumor cells. Between 80% and 90% of patients are appropriate candidates at presentation for an attempt at curative resection. The extent of colonic resection is determined by the vascular pedicles to achieve an adequate regional lymphadenectomy. Often this requires resection of a larger segment of bowel beyond that necessary simply to obtain negative margins.

The extent and type of bowel preparation before elective colon resection is controversial and often based on surgeon preference. On the basis of a recent Cochrane review, there is no evidence that mechanical bowel preparation improves the outcome for patients, including surgical site infections. However, mechanical preparation removes solid material, improving the ability to manipulate and remove the colon. When performed laparoscopically, this can be particularly advantageous. Evidence for the role of preoperative oral antibiotic administration has similarly been controversial. Recent evidence suggests that oral antibiotic administration after a mechanical bowel preparation has the lowest incidence of surgical site infection. However, use of the full mechanical/oral preparation has not been adopted widely by many surgeons. Prophylactic intravenous antibiotics should be administered within 60 minutes of incision. Prolonged antibiotic use after surgery has no benefit and therefore is not recommended beyond 24 hours after the surgery.

Colon Resection

The pericolic and surrounding draining lymph nodes are removed as part of a curative resection. Regional nodes are located along the course of the major vessels supplying the colon, along the vascular arcades of the marginal artery, and adjacent to the colon along the mesocolic border. Resection of these regional nodes requires ligation and division of the main vascular trunks to the affected colon segment. In tumors that are located between vascular pedicles (e.g., hepatic or splenic flexures), extended colectomy is performed to remove nodes along both associated vascular pedicles. More extensive colonic resections, including subtotal or total colectomy, typically are reserved for those patients with multiple tumors or in cases in which a prophylactic component is being performed for those at risk for metachronous disease.

All operations with curative intent must include a through exploration of the abdominal cavity for evidence of metastatic disease. Peritoneal surfaces, omentum, and paraaortic nodes should be assessed grossly. Particular attention should be paid to the liver, the most common site for metastatic disease. Visualization and careful manual palpation of all segments of the liver should be conducted when possible, including the periportal nodal region. Intraoperative ultrasound (IOUS) can be used in some cases to more carefully assess the liver. In cases in which liver metastases are known to be present on the basis of preoperative imaging, IOUS should be considered to assess potential resectability of the hepatic metastases.

Tumors of the cecum and ascending colon typically are managed with a *right hemicolectomy*. This involves resection of the terminal ileum, cecum, and ascending colon including the hepatic flexure. High ligation of the ileocolic and right colic vessels provides for an adequate lymphadenectomy. Tumors of the transverse colon often are managed with an extended left or right colectomy depending on the proximal or distal location of the tumor, including the middle colic and lymphatics. *Left hemicolectomy* is performed for tumors arising in the descending colon and includes ligation of the left colic artery. The splenic flexure is mobilized, and the transverse colon is anastomosed to the proximal rectum. For sigmoid cancers, either a left hemicolectomy or a sigmoid colectomy can be performed. When the bowel anastomosis is performed, various methods can be used, including hand-sewn or stapling techniques.

From several large studies, it has been proposed that a minimum of 12 lymph nodes be examined to accurately stage the cancer. High lymph node yield is correlated positively with survival. Inadequate nodes and therefore understaging may be due to the pathologist not identifying and examining all lymph nodes present in the specimen or the surgeon not removing enough lymph nodes.

Operative Approach: Open Versus Laparoscopic Versus Robotic Colectomy

Laparoscopic colectomy has gained complete acceptance in the surgical management of colon cancer. Large, multicenter randomized controlled trials have confirmed that colorectal cancer resection is comparable to open resection regarding oncologic efficacy, including nodal harvest, survival and locoregional recurrence (CLASICC, COST, COLOR, MRC trials). Moreover, this approach typically is associated with less postoperative pain, reduction in narcotic and oral analgesics requirements, and earlier resumption of diet. More recently, the use of robotic surgery has been advocated by some as an alternative minimally invasive approach. Early data show equivalent oncologic outcomes and lower conversion rate compared with standard laparoscopy, but longer operative times and added cost have limited the widespread use of this technique.

Surgeon and hospital volume play a role in colorectal cancer outcomes. Multiple studies have demonstrated that surgeon volume is a predictor of outcome following primary resection for colon cancer and that high-volume surgeons achieve a lower mortality rate. The probability of requiring a reoperation was found to be 30% less for patients treated by high-volume surgeons and 25% fewer complications. Providing patients with this information is important so that they can receive the best care.

Enhanced Recovery Pathways in Colorectal Cancer Management

Enhanced recovery pathways initially were designed to standardize medical care, improve outcomes, and lower health care costs for various surgical procedures, including colectomy. The key factors that delay recovery and discharge are the need for parenteral analgesia, intravenous fluids secondary to persistent gut dysfunction, and bed rest caused by lack of mobility. These pathways address each of these issues and involve all phases of the perioperative period: preoperative, intraoperative, and postoperative management. Specifically, the steps include preoperative patient information/psychologic preparation, maintenance of normothermia and oxygen delivery, nausea and ileus prevention, early feeding, opioid-sparing analgesia, and evidence-based postoperative care (e.g., early Foley catheter removal, VTE prophylaxis).

Management of Obstructing or Perforated Colon Cancer

The management of obstructing or perforated colon cancer presents unique considerations. When patients present with urgent evidence of obstruction without the opportunity to prepare the bowel, they must be expediently resuscitated and undergo immediate surgical exploration. If the obstruction is due to a proximal lesion near the ileocecal valve, a right hemicolectomy with primary anastomosis may be performed safely in most cases. More distal obstructions are problematic because the proximal colon is dilated and typically full of stool. Once the involved segment of colon is resected, on-table lavage can be performed. This involves mobilization of the colon, attachment of large bore sterile tubing to drain the effluent, and instillation of a large volume of warm saline through a catheter placed through an appendicostomy or the terminal ileum. The distal segment of bowel can be washed out from below. This technique can allow for a primary anastomosis in some cases, provided the bowel is relatively nondilated and healthy appearing.

Perforations at the tumor site can present either as locally contained abscesses or as free perforation with peritonitis. In addition, obstructing tumors can result in colonic perforation, typically proximal to the tumor or at the cecum. In the case of contained perforations, abscesses can be drained percutaneously with subsequent investigations and elective surgical management. Free perforation with peritonitis is a surgical emergency that necessitates rapid resuscitation and operation. In the setting of gross fecal contamination, resection of the tumor and perforation are performed when possible with a proximal colostomy or ileostomy (Hartmann's procedure). In some cases, a primary anastomosis can be performed with a protecting proximal ostomy. An unprotected anastomosis without diversion is ill advised in these unstable patients.

■ ADJUVANT TREATMENT

Patients with node-positive (stage III) colon cancer should be considered for postoperative adjuvant chemotherapy because multiple large randomized trials have demonstrated risk reduction of approximately one third. The most commonly used regimen is oxaliplatin combined with fluoropyrimidine (e.g., FOLFOX) for a 6-month duration. In those patients who may be more frail or have contraindications to oxaliplatin, fluoropyrimidine monotherapy can be considered. Several trials are currently underway comparing 3 months versus 6 months of therapy. These results are being eagerly awaited because it may significantly change the tolerability and cost of adjuvant therapy.

For patients with node-negative disease, the role of adjuvant chemotherapy is more controversial. In those patients with "high-risk" stage II colon cancer—poorly differentiated tumors, lymphovascular invasion, bowel perforation, inadequate tumor margins, T4 lesions,

or low nodal counts—adjuvant chemotherapy can be considered. Unlike with rectal cancer, adjuvant radiation therapy for colon cancer rarely is indicated.

■ SURVEILLANCE AND FOLLOW-UP

Following patients after treatment for colon cancer serves several functions. First, surveillance attempts to identify recurrent disease at a stage potentially resectable for cure. Second, following patients with colonoscopy can identify metachronous polyps or cancers at an early stage. Finally, surveillance reassures the patient. A balance must be struck between accomplishing these goals and providing care that has minimal morbidity and is cost effective.

On the basis of available data, guidelines for follow-up have been developed, including by the National Comprehensive Cancer Network (NCCN). Patients with T3 or greater tumors should be followed with history and physical examination and a CEA level every 3 months for the first 2 years after treatment and then every 6 months for the next 3 years. If rising CEA is identified, further testing should be performed, including imaging studies and colonoscopy. Annual radiologic surveillance is also recommended with cross-sectional imaging of the chest, abdomen, and pelvis, most commonly CT. In cases in which the primary tumor is of early stage (Tis, T1) or in which the patient may not be a candidate for aggressive treatment of recurrent disease, follow-up testing can be more limited.

Colonoscopy should be performed at 1 year postoperatively or within 6 months if a complete colonoscopy was not possible preoperatively because of obstruction or perforation. If the postoperative colonoscopy is free of polyps, repeat surveillance every 3 years generally is recommended. In patients in whom adenomas are found or if a hereditary syndrome is present, annual colonoscopy should be considered.

SUGGESTED READINGS

Adamina M, Kehlet H, Tomlinson GA, et al. Enhanced recovery pathways optimize health outcomes and resource utilization: a meta-analysis of randomized controlled trials in colorectal surgery. *Surgery.* 2011;149: 830-840.

Gustafsson UO, Scott MJ, Schwenk W, et al. Guidelines for Perioperative Care in Elective Colonic Surgery: Enhanced Recovery After Surgery (ERAS) Society Recommendations. *World J Surg.* 2013;37:259-284.

Levin B, Lieberman DA, McFarland B, et al. Screening and Surveillance for the Early Detection of Colorectal Cancer and Adenomatous Polyps, 2008: a Joint Guideline from the American Cancer Society, The US Multi-Society Task Force on Colorectal Cancer, and the American College of Radiology. *CA Cancer J Clin.* 2008;58:130-160.

National Comprehensive Cancer Network. *NCCN clinical practice guidelines in oncology: colon cancer, version 3.2015,* Fort Washington, PA, 2015.

Nelson H, Sargent D, Weiand HS, et al. COST Study Group: A comparison of laparoscopically assisted and open colectomy for colon cancer. *N Engl J Med.* 2004;350:2050-2059.

Zerey M, Hawyer LM, Awad Z, et al. SAGES evidence-based guidelines for the laparoscopic resection of curable colon and rectal cancer. *Surg Endosc.* 2013;27:1-10.

THE MANAGEMENT OF RECTAL CANCER

David A. Kleiman, MD, MSc,
and Jose G. Guillem, MD, MPH

According to the American Cancer Society, an estimated 134,490 new cases of colorectal cancer are expected to be diagnosed in

the United States in 2016, about one third of which will be found in the rectum. Colorectal cancer remains the second leading cause of cancer-related deaths in the United States with an estimated 49,190 deaths expected in 2016.

Anatomically, the rectum extends from the point at which the three taenia coli fuse into a single longitudinal smooth muscle layer (rectosigmoid junction) to the anal canal (Figure 1). However, from an oncologic standpoint, it is the distal 12 cm (withstanding individual variation) in the extraperitoneal pelvis that constitutes the rectum. Cancers that occur proximal to this level in the average body

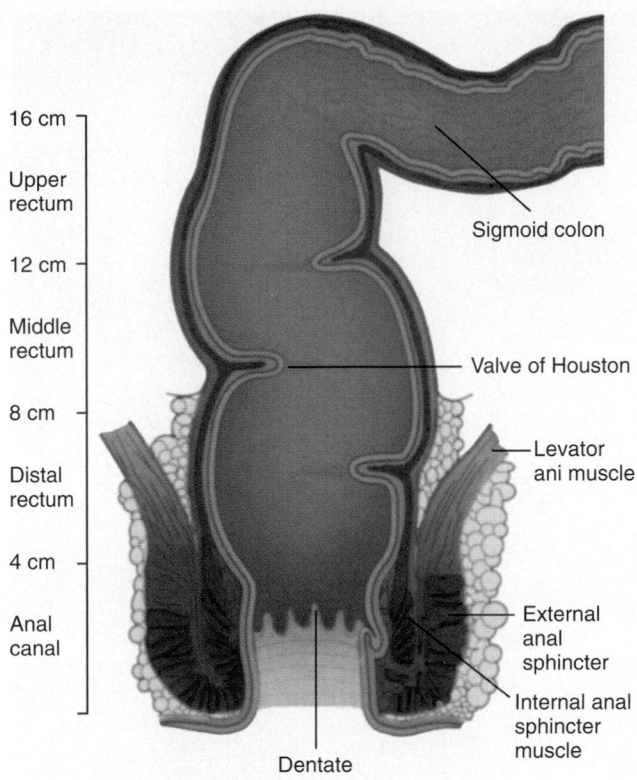

16 cm

Upper
rectum

12 cm

Middle
rectum

8 cm

Distal
rectum

4 cm

Anal
canal

Sigmoid colon

Valve of Houston

Levator
ani muscle

External
anal
sphincter

Internal anal
sphincter
muscle

Dentate

FIGURE I Anatomy of the rectum.

habitus behave more like colon cancers with regard to recurrence patterns, treatment, and prognosis.

This chapter reviews the preoperative evaluation and clinical staging of patients with rectal cancer and management options based on stage of disease, highlighting in particular a multidisciplinary approach, careful preoperative planning, and sequential multimodal therapy when indicated. These include surgery, short-course radiation therapy, induction or consolidation chemotherapy, and/or long-course chemoradiation therapy. Important practical considerations regarding surgery and other technical approaches for patients with rectal cancer also are discussed.

■ PREOPERATIVE EVALUATION

History, Physical Examination, and Laboratory Studies

A complete history and physical examination by the surgeon are essential components of the initial evaluation of rectal cancer patients. The history should elicit changes in bowel habits, presence of incontinence to either stool or flatus, previous colonoscopies, and a detailed family history to assess for the possibility of a hereditary or familial syndrome. In addition, when an ostomy is a consideration, preoperative counseling with an enterostomal therapist should be offered when available. A complete physical examination of patients with rectal cancer includes a digital rectal examination (DRE) and proctosigmoidoscopy. The DRE enables assessment of size, degree of fixation, and location of disease relative to the proximal extent of the anorectal ring. Proctosigmoidoscopy usually is performed in conjunction with the DRE. This allows delineation of tumor orientation (anterior, lateral, or posterior), circumferential involvement (evaluated as a percentage of the entire bowel wall circumference), and extent of proximal involvement. This information is useful in preoperative planning to help determine the need for neoadjuvant treatment and the likelihood of preserving anorectal function. A full colonoscopy also should be performed, if possible, because at least 5% of patients with rectal cancer have synchronous lesions that may

alter treatment plans. If a full colonoscopy is not possible, then a double-contrast barium enema or a computed tomography (CT) colonography may be used as an alternative. In addition to basic laboratory blood tests, a baseline carcinoembryonic antigen level also is recommended, mainly for postoperative surveillance purposes. Histologic confirmation of the diagnosis of an invasive adenocarcinoma should be obtained whenever possible, especially if neoadjuvant therapy is being considered.

Preoperative Imaging Studies

Accurate pretreatment imaging is needed to (1) delineate the depth of tumor penetration through the rectal wall, (2) assess whether locoregional lymph nodes (LN) are involved, and (3) determine the absence or presence of distant metastatic disease. The most common imaging studies currently used to acquire this information for rectal cancer are endorectal ultrasound (ERUS), magnetic resonance imaging (MRI), CT, and positron emission tomography (PET) scans.

ERUS and pelvic MRI can provide important preoperative locoregional staging information (Figure 2). Pelvic MRI with high-resolution T2-weighted images, including a narrow field of view of the rectum, provides the best evaluation of the rectal wall and perirectal fat and is considered the best modality for distinguishing T2 from T3 tumors. Postgadolinium 3D fast spoiled gradient echo sequences and diffusion-weighted images are useful adjuncts to the MRI study that can be useful for accentuating the primary tumor and locoregional lymph nodes. On T2-weighted images, there are three easily discernible layers of the rectal wall that have a characteristic alternating signal intensity pattern: an inner hyperintense layer represents the mucosa and submucosa, a hypointense middle layer represents the muscularis propria, and finally a hyperintense outer layer represents the perirectal fat. Distinguishing a T1 (invasion through the muscularis mucosa into the submucosa) from a T2 (through the submucosa into the muscularis propria) can be difficult on MRI because it is often difficult to discern the transition from the submucosa to the muscularis. However, distinguishing T3 (invasion into perirectal fat) from T4 (invasion into adjacent structures) tumors can be done with a high degree of accuracy. MRI also provides accurate information on the relationship of the tumor to the mesorectal fascia, which is crucial in predicting the likelihood of achieving a negative circumferential resection margin (CRM) and carries significant prognostic value. A meta-analysis of 21 studies evaluating the accuracy of preoperative MRI in rectal cancer reported a 77% sensitivity and 94% specificity in identifying invasion of the mesorectal fascia and a 77% sensitivity and 71% specificity of identifying lymph node involvement. MRI also provides useful information about overall pelvic anatomy and the relationship of the tumor to adjacent pelvic organs, which can assist with preoperative planning.

ERUS is an office-based procedure that can be used to clinically assess the depth of bowel wall penetration (T stage) and LN involvement (N stage) (Figure 2). Its overall accuracy in assessing T stage and N stage is comparable to MRI. The main advantage of ERUS over MRI is the ability to distinguish T0, T1, and T2 tumors, which may be particularly helpful when considering local versus radical resection. However, MRI is superior to ERUS at evaluating the mesorectal fascia and pelvic LN that are remote from the rectum.

CT of the abdomen and pelvis are used mainly in primary rectal cancer to assess for intra-abdominal metastasis and to evaluate other tumor-related complications such as perforation and obstruction. CT also may provide some information regarding adjacent organ involvement in advanced cases, but it is less accurate than MRI and ERUS for T- and N-staging purposes.

PET, or more commonly PET-CT, often is used as part of the initial staging of many cancers, but data are mixed regarding its utility in primary rectal cancer. PET has not been shown to offer an advantage over MRI or ERUS with regard to locoregional staging. However, PET and PET-CT may increase detection of distant

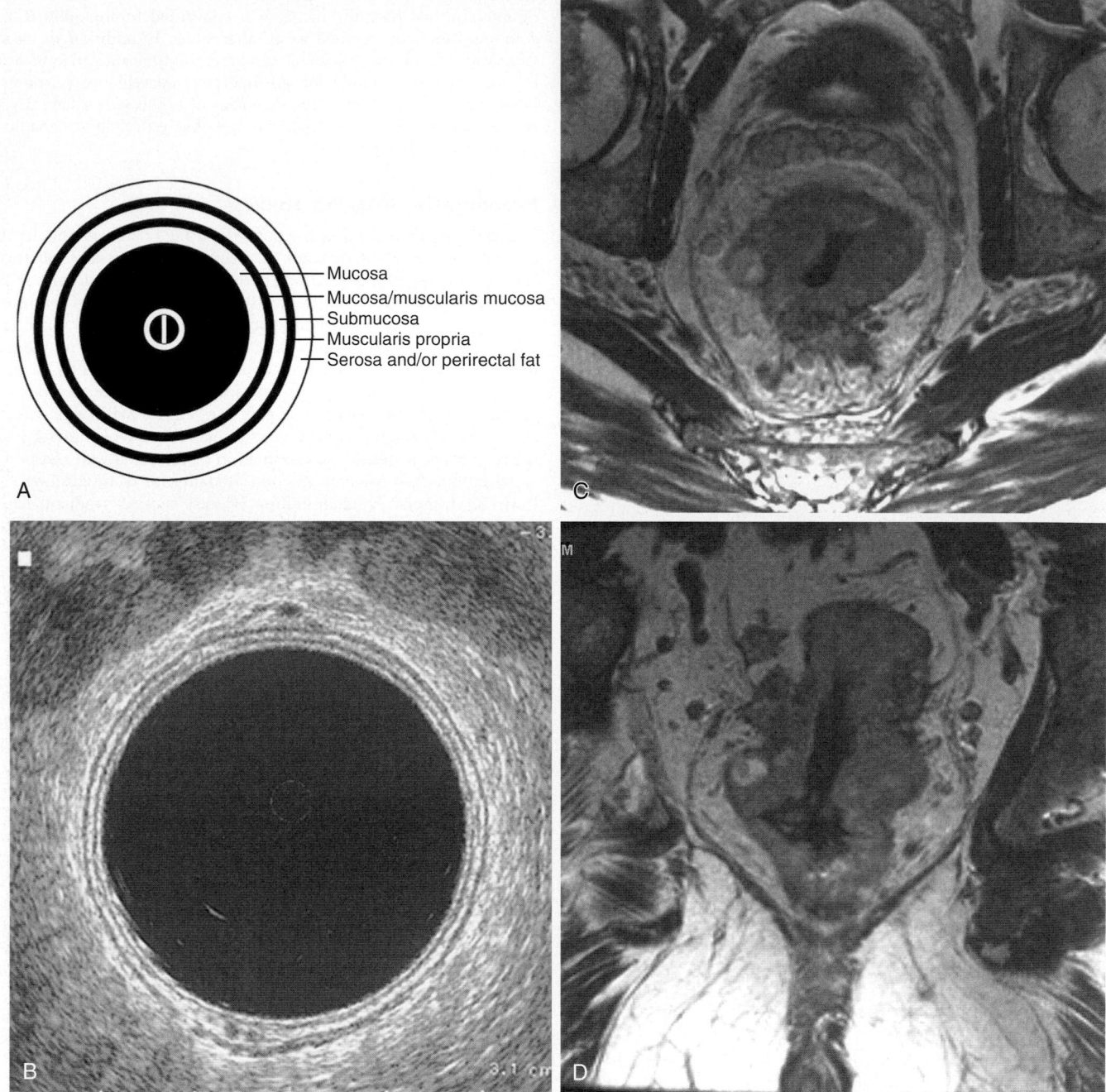

Mucosa
Mucosa/muscularis mucosa
Submucosa
Muscularis propria
Serosa and/or perirectal fat

FIGURE 2 Local staging of rectal cancer may be performed with endorectal ultrasound (ERUS) or magnetic resonance imaging (MRI). **A,** Schematic drawing of the layers of the rectal wall seen on ERUS. **B,** Example of an ERUS image of the normal layers of the rectal wall in a male patient. Cross-sectional (**C**) and coronal (**D**) T2-weighted MRI images of a T3N1 rectal cancer. In addition to assessing depth of invasion and nodal involvement, MRI provides additional information that is important for operative planning, such as involvement of adjacent organs, proximity to the sphincter muscles, and relationship to the peritoneal reflection. (**B** *from Kim HJ, Wong WD. Role of endorectal ultrasound in the conservative evaluation of rectal cancer.* Semin Surg Oncol. *2000;19:360;* **C** *and* **D**, *courtesy Dr. Marc Gollub, Department of Radiology, Memorial Sloan Kettering Cancer Center, New York, NY.)*

metastasis and may help to better characterize lesions that are suspicious for distant metastases found on CT or MRI. A study of 93 patients with locally advanced rectal cancer reported an overall accuracy, sensitivity, and specificity of PET in detecting distant disease of 94%, 78%, and 99%, respectively. However, some have argued that although additional or discordant findings identified on PET or PET-CT may affect medical management, they are unlikely to alter surgical management and have not been shown to improve outcomes. Therefore routine use of PET or PET-CT in the preoperative setting is not recommended universally.

The ultimate goal of the preoperative workup is to accurately stage the patient's disease in a timely and cost-effective manner. During the initial workup of primary disease, our practice is to perform locoregional staging and assess resectability with a rectal MRI, as well as obtaining an intravenous contrast-enhanced CT of the chest, abdomen, and pelvis to assess for intra-abdominal and lung metastasis. We selectively obtain PET-CT scans when it is necessary to further characterize indeterminate distant lesions found on CT, although modern high-quality CT scans that are read by a team of radiologists who are adept at performing oncologic assessments has enabled us to confidently characterize most lesions without needing a PET-CT.

Staging

After the diagnosis of rectal cancer, the patient is staged clinically by integrating the history, physical examination, proctosigmoidoscopy findings, and the results of preoperative imaging studies. The clinical stage then is used to select the most appropriate treatment strategy for each individual patient. Although the imaging studies described earlier form the current standard of care, there are clear limitations to these studies, and the implications of either clinically understaging or overstaging disease must be recognized.

Definite pathologic staging is carried out after surgical resection. Currently, the American Joint Committee on Cancer Tumor, Lymph Node, and Metastases (AJCC TNM) classification is the preferred system to stage rectal cancer. The most recent version of the AJCC TNM staging system (seventh edition, 2010) further subdivides stage II, III, and IV disease to better reflect prognosis within these groups (Table 1). One notable addition to this most recent version of the AJCC staging system is the recognition of satellite tumor deposits that lay within the subserosa, mesentery, or nonperitonealized pericolic or perirectal tissues but do not involve regional lymph nodes. This is now given the designation N1c, but its exact impact on prognosis remains unclear.

The AJCC recommends the histologic examination of a minimum of 12 lymph nodes to adequately assess nodal status and accurately stage patients. However, with increased used of neoadjuvant chemotherapy and/or chemoradiation, there is a growing awareness that neoadjuvant treatment may reduce the number of identifiable lymph nodes in the surgical specimen after total mesorectal excision (TME). Therefore less than 12 lymph nodes may still be considered adequate in this setting.

■ MANAGEMENT BASED ON CLINICAL STAGE

Deciding on the optimal treatment plan for patients with rectal cancer can be a complex and highly individualized process. Multimodal therapy that combines radiation therapy (RT), chemotherapy, and surgery is accepted as the standard of care for patients with rectal cancers, although the precise type and sequence of modalities depends on the stage at presentation. The complexity of the various multimodal treatment algorithms has evolved significantly in recent years, and it is now recommended that most rectal cancer cases should be reviewed by a multidisciplinary team after their initial presentation to formulate an individualized treatment plan. A proposed algorithm for the treatment of patients with rectal cancer is presented in Figure 3.

Even with the advances made in combined modality therapy, surgery remains the cornerstone of curative treatment for rectal cancer. Early rectal cancers (stage I) can be treated definitively by surgery alone; however, patients with more advanced (stage II and III) rectal cancers typically are treated with neoadjuvant therapy (chemotherapy and/or chemoradiation) before surgery to decrease the risk of recurrence and optimize oncologic outcomes.

The surgical options depend largely on the location and extent of disease, although patient factors, such as comorbid medical conditions and baseline anorectal function, also are considered. The main surgical approaches for rectal cancer include local excision procedures, such as transanal excision (TAE), transanal endoscopic microsurgery (TEM), or transanal minimally invasive surgery (TAMIS), and radical procedures that involve en bloc resection of the rectum along with the blood vessels and lymphatics that lay within the mesorectum. Radical resections can be subdivided further into sphincter-preserving procedures and those in which the sphincters cannot be salvaged without compromising a negative resection margin and therefore result in a permanent end colostomy. The goals of surgical

TABLE 1: AJCC TNM Definitions and Stage of Rectal Cancer (Seventh Edition)

PRIMARY TUMOR (T)

Tx	Primary tumor cannot be assessed
T0	No evidence of primary tumor
Tis	Carcinoma in situ: intraepithelial or invasion of lamina propria
T1	Tumor invades submucosa
T2	Tumor invades muscularis propria
T3	Tumor invades through the muscularis propria into pericolorectal tissue
T4a	Tumor penetrates to the surface of the visceral peritoneum
T4b	Tumor directly invades or is adherent to other organs or structures

REGIONAL LYMPH NODES (N)

Nx	Regional lymph nodes cannot be assessed
N0	No regional lymph node metastasis
N1	Metastasis in 1-3 regional lymph nodes
N1A	Metastasis in 1 regional lymph node
N1b	Metastasis in 2-3 regional lymph nodes
N1c	Tumor deposit(s) in the subserosa, mesentery, or nonperitonealized pericolic or perirectal tissues without regional nodal metastasis
N2	Metastasis in 4 or more regional lymph nodes
N2a	Metastasis in 4-6 regional lymph nodes
N2b	Metastasis ≥7 regional lymph nodes

DISTANT METASTASIS (M)

M0	No distant metastasis
M1	Distant metastasis
M1a	Metastasis confined to 1 organ or site
M1b	Metastases in >1 organ/site or the peritoneum

Stage	T	N	M
0	Tis	N0	M0
I	T1-T2	N0	M0
IIA	T3	N0	M0
IIB	T4a	N0	M0
IIC	T4b	N0	M0
IIIA	T1-T2	N1/N1c	M0
	T1	N2a	M0
IIIB	T3-T4a	N1/N1c	M0
	T2-T3	N2a	M0
	T1-T2	N2b	M0
IIIC	T4a	N2a	M0
	T3-T4a	N2b	M0
	T4b	N1-N2	M0
IVA	Any T	Any N	M1a
IVB	Any T	Any N	M1b

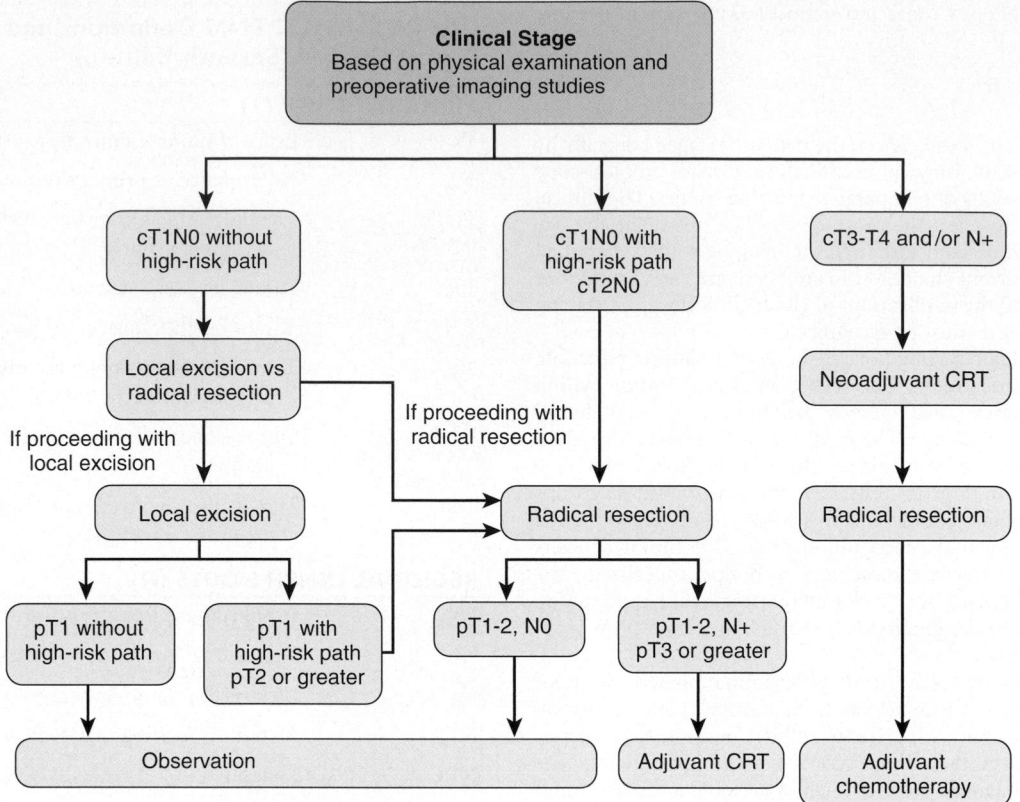

FIGURE 3 Treatment algorithm based on clinical stage of disease for patients with rectal cancer and no evidence of distant metastasis. *High-risk path* refers to (1) poor differentiation, (2) the presence of lymphovascular or perineural invasion, or (3) deep submucosal invasion (sm2 or sm3). *c,* Clinical stage; *CRT,* chemoradiation therapy; *p,* pathologic stage.

resection with curative intent are complete resection of the primary tumor with adequate margins, an anatomically complete lymphadenectomy of draining lymph nodes, and en bloc resection of contiguously involved structures.

Carcinoma in Situ and T1N0 Rectal Cancer

Local excision can be used to manage early stage rectal cancer (Tis-T1, N0). The goal of this procedure is to fully excise the lesion with negative margins without attempting to remove regional lymph nodes. These procedures are appealing because they are associated with lesser operative morbidity and better preservation of long-term anorectal function and may allow some patients to avoid a permanent colostomy compared with radical resections. However, the main limitation of local excision is that potentially involved regional lymph nodes are not removed, and therefore there is a risk of understaging and undertreating the patient. Therefore careful patient selection is essential to identify those patients who would most benefit from a localized rather than radical surgical approach.

Many authors have defined criteria that aid in selecting patients with low-risk T1 cancers who may be suitable for treatment by local excision as definitive therapy without compromising oncologic outcomes (Box 1). However, even when strict selection criteria for local excision are applied, local recurrence rates are in the range of 11% to 29% in most series with long-term follow-up. A retrospective review of nearly 300 patients who underwent surgery for T1 rectal cancers at Memorial Sloan Kettering Cancer Center (MSKCC) found that compared with patients who underwent radical resection, patients with similar rates of high-risk pathologic features, including lymphovascular invasion and poor differentiation, who underwent local excision had a significantly higher 5-year local recurrence rate (13% vs 3%) as well as decreased 5-year disease-specific survival

(87% vs 96%), which highlights the need for careful patient selection when considering a localized surgical approach.

There are two common circumstances in which patients who initially undergo local excision ultimately may require radical resection. The first is if the final pathology of the specimen reveals a more locally invasive tumor than was suggested on preoperative imaging and/or the lesion has other high-risk pathologic features. The second scenario is if the patient experiences a local recurrence and requires a salvage procedure. These patients tend to fair worse than comparably staged patients who underwent radical resection initially. This may be due in part to the fact that the local excision patients may have been understaged initially by not sampling regional lymph nodes. Subsequently, these patients do not receive the adjuvant therapy that they ordinarily would have received had the extent of their disease been appreciated fully at the time of initial surgery. In a review from the University of Texas MD Anderson Cancer Center of 46 patients with recurrent rectal cancer after local excision, 80% of patients achieved an R0 resection rate with reoperation, but 33% of patient required multivisceral resection, 5% required total pelvic exenteration, the sphincter preservation rate was only 33%, and the perioperative morbidity was 50%.

Therefore in general local excision should be offered only to patients who have low-risk disease and fully understand that local excision is associated with a significantly higher risk of recurrence. It also may be offered to patients who have a significant medical contraindication to major abdominal surgery, or those who are unwilling to accept the risk of having a temporary or permanent ostomy.

T2N0 Rectal Cancer

For tumors that appear to invade the muscularis propria without LN involvement (T2N0) on preoperative evaluation, the standard treatment is radical resection with total mesorectal excision in patients who are acceptable operative candidates. If lymph nodes are found to be involved on final pathologic examination, postoperative adjuvant chemoradiation (CRT) is recommended.

In very select clinical T2N0 rectal cancers, neoadjuvant chemoradiation can be considered when a bulky tumor in proximity to the upper part of the anorectal sphincter precludes sphincter preservation. A good response to RT may sufficiently reduce tumor bulk to allow the surgeon to preserve the sphincter and avoid a permanent colostomy, which may not have been possible otherwise. In the American College of Surgeons Oncology Group Z6041 prospective multicenter phase II clinical trial, patients with T2N0 rectal cancers were treated with long-course capecitabine and oxaliplatin during radiation followed 6 weeks later by local excision. Among 79 eligible patients, 44% achieved a complete pathologic response, and 64% of tumors were downstaged to either T0 or T1. However, after a median follow-up of 56 months, the 3-year disease-free survival (DFS) was lower than anticipated (88%) and a substantial amount of adverse gastrointestinal (29%), pain (15%), and hematologic (15%) events were observed during chemoradiation. Therefore it generally is advised that neoadjuvant chemoradiation followed by local excision be considered only for carefully selected patients with T2N0 tumors who refuse or are not candidates for radical resection.

Locally Advanced Rectal Cancer

In patients with transmural and/or node-positive (T3-T4/Nx or Tx/N1-N2) disease without evidence of distant metastases, multimodality therapy involving a combination of TME, chemoradiation therapy (CRT), and chemotherapy is indicated. The optimal sequence and timing of these modalities continues to evolve and may vary by institution. It is essential that these complex cases be discussed by a multidisciplinary disease management team at the outset of treatment. In general, a standard treatment regimen involves neoadjuvant CRT, then TME with either a low-anterior resection or abdominoperineal resection, followed by adjuvant chemotherapy. There is ample debate on the relative risks and benefits of alterations on this sequence, which are discussed in greater detail in Neoadjuvant and Adjuvant Therapy later in this chapter. In a report of 297 consecutive patients with T3-T4 and/or N1 rectal cancer who were treated at MSKCC with standardized neoadjuvant CRT regimens followed by TME, the recurrence rate was found to be 23% (2% local recurrence only, 19% distant recurrence, and 2% local and distant recurrence) after a median follow-up of 44 months, with an estimated 10-year recurrence-free survival of 62% and a 10-year overall survival (OS) of 58%.

Distant Metastatic (M1) Disease

Patients with distant metastasis represent a heterogeneous population for whom it is difficult to define an all-encompassing strategy. These complex and challenging cases should be discussed within the context of a multidisciplinary team. Treatment strategies are based mainly on factors related to (1) the primary lesion (related symptoms, resectability), (2) the extent of metastases (sites, resectability), and (3) the patient (age, comorbidities, ability to withstand major surgery, wishes regarding quality of life).

A strategy directed at curative intent can be adopted in patients with a resectable primary tumor and limited, resectable metastatic disease. In these cases, systemic chemotherapy is used commonly as the initial treatment modality. After restaging, resection of the primary and metastatic disease can be considered as either combined or staged operations. Alternatively, upfront surgical resection, as either combined or staged procedures, can be considered in patients with limited metastatic disease.

In selected patients with stage IV disease, systemic chemotherapy may provide effective palliation that obviates the need for surgery. However, some patients may experience symptoms such as pain, obstruction, or bleeding that do not respond to chemotherapy and require a palliative intervention such as a resection or diverting ostomy to alleviate symptoms. Although often used in obstructing descending and sigmoid colon cancers, endoscopic stents generally are avoided in rectal cancer because of the tendency for them to migrate and cause intolerable local symptoms such as pain and tenesmus.

Up to 60% of patients with colorectal cancer eventually develop liver metastases, and therefore the approach to the treatment of colorectal liver metastases (CRLM) deserves specific attention. With oligometastatic disease in an accessible location, complete resection when possible remains the best option, with 5-year survival rates of approximately 50% and a 20% chance of cure. More commonly, however, patients have borderline resectable or unresectable disease (80% to 90%). Traditional combination chemotherapy regimens may convert patients who were initially inoperable to potentially resectable, which results in similar 5-year survival as that of patients who were resectable initially.

More recently, hepatic artery infusion (HAI) chemotherapy has emerged as an attractive adjunct to systemic chemotherapy and may increase the conversion rate to resectable disease. In a phase II prospective trial conducted at MSKCC, 49 patients with initially unresectable CRLM were treated with best-available systemic chemotherapy (oxaliplatin/irinotecan/bevacizumab or irinotecan/5-FU/leucovorin/bevacizumab) along with HAI floxuridine.[10] Overall response rate was 76%, with four patients showing a complete response. Forty-seven percent of patients were converted to resection at a median of 6 months from treatment initiation, and patients who underwent resection had improved OS than those who did not undergo resection (3-year OS 80% vs 26%). Similarly, a recent meta-analysis of 1514 patients from 11 studies with initially unresectable CRLM treated with HAI with or without concurrent systemic chemotherapy found a 50% overall response and an 18% conversion to resectable disease. Those who underwent hepatectomy had a median overall and 5-year survival of 53 months and 49%, respectively, compared with 16 months and 3% for those who did not undergo surgery.

■ NEOADJUVANT AND ADJUVANT THERAPIES

The Swedish Rectal Cancer Trial was the first randomized trial to assess whether administering preoperative RT (5 Gy/day × 5 days) within 1 week of surgery improved outcomes. The preoperative RT group had decreased local recurrence at 5 years (11% vs 27%,

$P < 0.01$), increased 5-year OS (58% vs 48%, $P = 0.004$), and increased 9-year cancer-specific survival (74% v 65%, $P = 0.002$).

This was followed several years later by the Dutch Colorectal Cancer Group trial, which also assessed whether adding preoperative RT (5 × 5 Gy) to TME surgery improved oncologic outcomes in patients with locally advanced rectal cancers. On long-term follow-up, RT was found to improve 5-year local recurrence rates (5.6% for the RT plus TME group vs 10.9% for the TME-alone group), but no difference in OS was found. This study established a benefit with preoperative RT, even when optimal surgical resection with TME is performed.

The German Rectal Cancer Group compared preoperative with postoperative CRT (long-course RT with concurrent chemotherapy) for patients with stage II or III disease. Preoperative CRT was found to be associated with fewer acute and chronic toxicities and an improved 5-year local recurrence rate (6% vs 13% for the preoperative and postoperative groups, respectively). Long-term follow-up data show that at 10 years there was still a significant improvement in local control, but there was no effect on OS.

Locally advanced tumors are now treated with either short-course radiation therapy (5 Gy/day × 5 days) followed by surgery within 1 week, or long-course chemoradiation (1.8 to 2.0 Gy/day over 5 to 6 weeks to a total dose of 45 to 50 Gy along with 5-fluorouracil-based intravenous or oral capecitabine chemotherapy) followed by surgery 8 to 12 weeks later. Multiple studies comparing short-course and long-course regimens have shown that they both reduce local recurrence rates by more than half, but the benefits on OS are less clear. Short-course radiotherapy remains popular in many European centers, but long-course chemoradiation has become the preferred treatment regimen within the United States, largely because of increased local toxicity of the more concentrated doses of radiation that are administered with short-course therapy.

However, there is some debate as to whether all patients with locally advanced rectal cancer require neoadjuvant CRT. Several retrospective analyses suggest that a subset of patients with low-risk disease (T3N0M0 lesions with negative margins and favorable histologic features) may not derive a significant benefit from RT. Unfortunately limitations with current imaging modalities make it impossible to preoperatively select with certainty those patients with low-risk T3N0 disease. A large multi-institutional review found that 22% of patients who received preoperative CRT for clinically staged T3N0 rectal cancer by ERUS or MRI actually had node-positive disease on pathologic review of resected specimens. Because preoperative CRT may reduce the total number of LNs and also may sterilize mesorectal LNs, the true rate of patients clinically staged as having T3N0 who actually have node positive disease may be even higher. Although the risks of overstaging T3 rectal cancer have been recognized (18% of patients with clinically staged T3N0 disease actually had T2N0 disease, according to data from the German Rectal Cancer Group), it is possible that twice as many are understaged based on the earlier findings. These data would support preoperative CRT for patients with clinical T3N0 rectal cancers staged by ERUS or MRI because understaged patients would otherwise require postoperative CRT, which is associated with inferior local control, higher toxicity, and poor functional outcomes. Moreover, these data highlight some of the limitations of clinical staging by ERUS and MRI and clearly underscore the ongoing need to improve the pretherapy staging of rectal cancer.

Another ongoing question is whether neoadjuvant chemotherapy can be given alone without routine chemoradiation before TME. In the phase II/III PROSPECT (Chemotherapy Alone or Chemotherapy Plus Radiation Therapy in Treating Patients With Locally Advanced Rectal Cancer Undergoing Surgery) trial, patients with stage II or stage III rectal cancer are being randomized to receive either six cycles of neoadjuvant FOLFOX (fluorouracil, leucovorin, oxaliplatin) followed by immediate TME if the tumor has decreased in size by at least 20% (responders) or neoadjuvant CRT followed by TME if the tumor is stable or has progressed (nonresponders), or a control arm

of neoadjuvant CRT for 5½ weeks immediately followed by TME and eight cycles of adjuvant FOLFOX. This trial is still ongoing and final results are not yet available, but results from a pilot trial of 32 patients who were treated according to the experimental arm are encouraging. The authors found that only two patients (6.3%) did not respond to neoadjuvant chemotherapy alone, and the R0 resection rate was 100%. The pathologic complete response rate of chemotherapy alone was 25% and the 4-year DFS and OS were 84% and 91%, respectively.

After surgical resection, the current guidelines recommend further adjuvant chemotherapy for all patients with stage III disease as well as considering it for high-risk stage II disease. Recently, there has been increased awareness of the fact that many patients never begin or complete the prescribed course of adjuvant chemotherapy after radical surgery without significant delays resulting from postoperative complications, overall functional decline, or dehydration/malnutrition associated with delayed closure of a protective loop ileostomy. In fact, less than 50% of patients receive the complete course of chemotherapy without interruptions, and it is estimated that each 4-week delay in treatment may decrease OS by 14%. This has led some to advocate for delivering the chemotherapy before surgery as either induction chemotherapy (chemotherapy → CRT → TME) or consolidation chemotherapy (CRT → chemotherapy → TME). When compared with the traditional sequence of CRT followed by TME then adjuvant chemotherapy, the consolidation chemotherapy approach has been shown in a prospective clinical trial to be well tolerated and increase the pathologic response rate.

■ SURGICAL CONSIDERATIONS

Transanal Excision

Lesions considered amenable to a TAE must be accessible from the anal canal and located below the peritoneal reflection. The proximal limit of the resection is usually 6 to 8 cm from the anal verge. The goal of TAE is full-thickness excision of the rectal lesion with negative margins. The patient is placed in either the lithotomy or prone jack-knife position and the anus is effaced gently with a self-retaining retractor. We use electrocautery to mark a 1-cm margin circumferentially around the tumor, and then we incise the rectal wall full thickness down to the perirectal fat. The specimen is removed in one piece, pinned on a surface, oriented and delivered to the pathologist for examination. We prefer to close the defect in the rectum with absorbable suture, and we are careful to ensure that the rectal lumen is not significantly narrowed. Postoperative complications are usually minor and may include bleeding, local infection, and urinary retention.

Transanal Endoscopic Microsurgery and Transanal Minimally Invasive Surgery

TEM and TAMIS can be used to excise mid and upper rectal lesions that may otherwise be inaccessible with a standard transanal approach. TEM requires a specialized 40-mm diameter endoscope and long endoscopic operating equipment. Carbon dioxide insufflation facilitates exposure, while a binocular microscope on the TEM endoscope provides a constant, sixfold magnified 3D 220-degree view of the operative field. The technical principles that apply to transanal local excision, with respect to full-thickness excision and negative circumferential margins, also apply to TEM excision. Tumors as high as 10 cm anteriorly, 15 cm laterally, and 18 cm posteriorly can be excised with the TEM approach. However, the cost of the specialized resectoscope has limited the widespread use of TEM in the United States.

TAMIS is a newer technique that uses any of the commercially available single incision laparoscopic port systems and conventional laparoscopic equipment to reach lesions in the mid or upper rectum. The port is introduced into the rectum, CO_2 is used for insufflation, and a conventional laparoscopic camera (most commonly a 5-mm

30-degree or 45-degree scope) is used to visualize the lesion. A full-thickness resection with a 1-cm margin then is performed with laparoscopic graspers and thermal devices. The rectal defect is closed transversely with absorbable sutures.

A limitation of TEM and TAMIS is that very distal lesions (<5 cm from the anal verge) are often not amenable to either approach because of difficulty maintaining an adequate seal required for pneumorectum. For these distal lesions, a transanal excision is preferred. In addition, inadvertent entry into the abdominal cavity may occur during resection of lesions that are located above the peritoneal reflection, which may lead to peritonitis and sepsis if not identified and repaired promptly. This may be repaired transanally but sometimes may require conversion to laparotomy.

TEM and TAMIS have been shown to be more likely to result in a negative margin and have decreased local recurrence compared with TAE, likely because of improved visualization during the procedure. However, all three local excision techniques have a higher local recurrence rate for T1 and T2 adenocarcinomas compared with radical resection (10% to 30% vs 3% to 7%, respectively). This may be due to the fact that a number of preoperatively staged T1N0 and T2N0 lesions may have been understaged because current imaging modalities may have missed small, yet involved lymph nodes. Another possible explanation for the higher local recurrence rate noted with TAE, TEM, and TAMIS may be the inadvertent inoculation of the mesorectum with cancer cells that may occur during any local rectal cancer procedure.

Radical Resection

Radical resection for rectal cancer involves resection of the tumor and rectum en bloc with its blood and lymphatic supply and surrounding mesorectum. A sphincter-preserving low anterior resection (LAR) is the preferred approach to radical resection, as long as it is technically feasible and oncologically appropriate. With proper training and experience, it usually can be performed safely when cancers are located more than 1 cm from the upper portion of the anorectal ring, as long as the patient has a favorable body habitus and pelvic anatomy. Generally, slender patients with wide pelvises provide more favorable conditions for sphincter-preserving surgery, whereas obese patients and those with long, narrow pelvises pose a technical challenge that can preclude a restorative procedure.

Contraindications to LAR include tumor invasion into the anal sphincter or levator muscles. Significantly impaired preoperative anorectal function is a relative contraindication because it often leads to poor postoperative bowel function. An abdominoperineal resection is preferred in situations in which a margin-negative resection would result in loss of anal sphincter function leading to fecal incontinence.

During the planning and conduct of radical surgery for rectal cancer, the following must be considered: (1) TME, (2) autonomic nerve preservation, (3) negative circumferential and distal margins, and (4) sphincter preservation and restoration of bowel continuity and function, when possible. The following sections discuss each of these principles.

Total Mesorectal Excision

In 1979 Heald and colleagues popularized the TME technique for rectal cancer, which has since gained widespread acceptance. Even though it has never been assessed in a large, prospective, randomized trial, the TME technique has been associated consistently with significantly lower locoregional failure rates, ranging from 3% to 7%, compared with historic and contemporary controls. The markedly low local recurrence rates associated with TME have made it the standard of care in the surgical management of rectal cancer.

TME is defined as the complete excision of the visceral mesorectum with pelvic nerve preservation; the *mesorectum* refers to the fatty tissue that encompasses the rectum, contains the lymphatic drainage

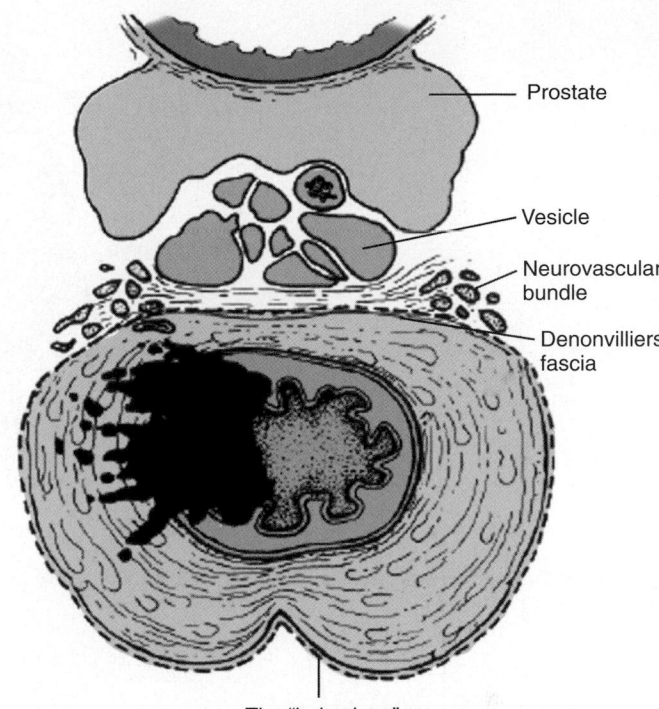

FIGURE 4 Schematic representation of the relationship of the mesorectum to the anterior anatomic structures in a male patient. The neurovascular bundle contains the nerves responsible for erection, ejaculation, and aspects of bladder function. *(From Heald RJ, Moran BJ. Embryology and anatomy of the rectum.* Semin Surg Oncol. *1998;15:70.)*

from the rectum, and is encased by visceral fascia. TME entails sharp dissection in the avascular areolar plane between the visceral fascia that envelops the rectum and mesorectum and the parietal fascia overlying the sacrum and pelvic sidewall structures (Figure 4). When properly performed, TME results in en bloc removal of the primary rectal cancer and mesorectum as an intact "package." The TME sharp dissection technique facilitates the identification and preservation of the pelvic autonomic nerves and also is associated with high negative CRM rates. For most middle and low rectal cancers, the entire mesorectum is mobilized and resected. Cancers in the upper rectum, usually located above 10 cm from the anal verge, can be treated with a tumor-specific excision, in which the mesorectum is divided at a right angle to the bowel 5 cm distal to the mucosal edge of the tumor.

Autonomic Nerve Preservation

Autonomic nerve preservation, as promoted by Enker and colleagues (1995), requires an understanding of the anatomy of the pelvic nerves (Figure 5). The sympathetic nerves of the pelvis originate from the T12 to L3 ventral nerve roots, which form the superior hypogastric plexus. Distal to the aortic bifurcation, the superior hypogastric plexus gives rise to the hypogastric nerves, and these may be associated intimately with the visceral fascia of the mesorectum.

The parasympathetic nerves of the pelvis, *nervi erigentes,* arise from the S2 to S4 ventral nerve roots. These join the sympathetic hypogastric nerves on the pelvic sidewall to form the inferior hypogastric plexus.

Injury to the pelvic autonomic nerves can be associated with significant genitourinary dysfunction and morbidity. Damage to the sympathetic hypogastric nerves can result in increased bladder tone and reduced bladder capacity, as well as with retrograde ejaculation in men. Damage to the parasympathetic system can result in voiding difficulties from increased tone in the bladder neck, as well as with erectile dysfunction in men and impaired vaginal lubrication in women.

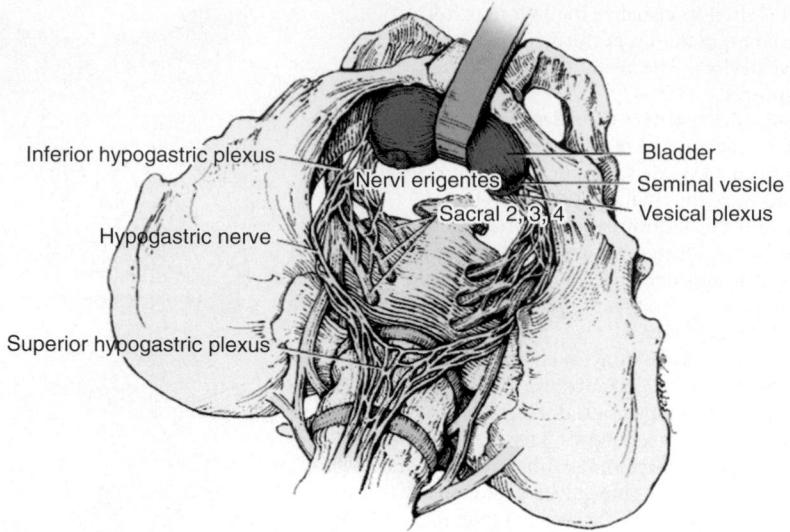

FIGURE 5 Diagram of pelvic nerve anatomy. *(From Guillem JG. Ultra-low anterior resection and coloanal pouch reconstruction for carcinoma of the distal rectum. World J Surg. 1997;21:722.)*

Circumferential Resection Margin

The CRM status refers to the adequacy of the surgical resection margin relative to the 360-degree radial extension of the primary tumor, which may include extension into the mesorectum and adjacent extrarectal soft tissue. The prognostic significance of a negative CRM in the presence of an intact mesorectum has been well established. A review of patients enrolled in the Dutch TME study found that CRMs smaller than 2 mm were associated with a local recurrence rate of 16% versus only 6% if the margin was 2 mm or larger. Moreover, CRMs 1 mm or less were associated with a significantly higher risk of distant metastasis (78% vs 13% for margins >1 mm) and shorter survival. In the preoperative setting, high-resolution rectal MRI with diffusion-weighted sequences can accurately predict involvement of the CRM.

Distal Resection Margin

Distal resection margins (DRMs) of 2 to 5 cm have been the traditional standard in rectal cancer surgery. However, multiple recent studies have narrowed these limits by showing that occult disease extending beneath the mucosal edge of the tumor is uncommon, especially after CRT. Recent whole-mount pathologic analyses on specimens from selected patients who underwent CRT followed by resection found intramural extension beyond the gross mucosal edge of residual tumor in only 2 (1.8%) of 109 patients. Moreover, when extension was present, it was limited to a distance of 0.95 mm or less in both cases. These results compare very favorably to data in the literature documenting distal spread beyond the mucosal edge of tumor in only 10% of patients, all of which occurred in poorly differentiated, node-positive lesions. Retrospective data suggest that margins as small as 1 cm may not compromise oncologic outcomes. A review from our institution found that local control and RFS with 3 years of follow-up after neoadjuvant CRT and TME-based resection were not significantly different when patients with DRMs less than or equal to 1 cm were compared with those with DRMs greater than 1 cm. We advocate striving for a DRM of at least 2 cm for most rectal cancers, even after preoperative CRT. However, a histologically negative DRM less than 1 cm is acceptable in carefully selected patients in the absence of adverse histologic features, particularly in situations in which an APR may be required for a wider margin. In cases in which the DRM status is uncertain, we suggest obtaining an intraoperative frozen section of the distal margin.

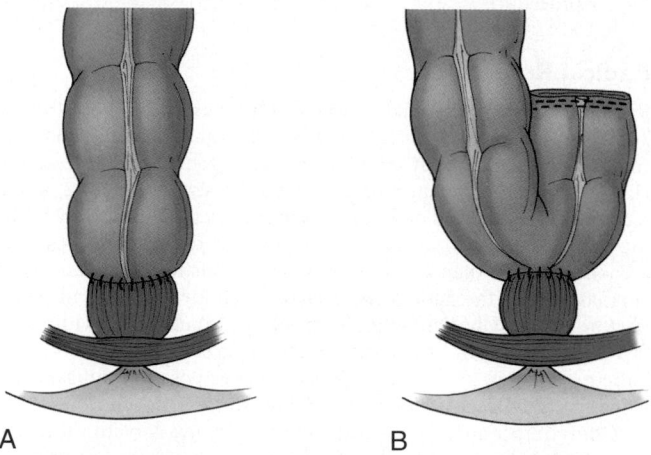

A   B

FIGURE 6 Illustrated comparison of a straight coloanal anastomosis *(left)* and a coloanal anastomosis with a colonic J pouch *(right)*. *(From Sailer M, Fuchs KH, Fein M, Thiede A. Randomized clinical trial comparing quality of life after straight and pouch coloanal reconstruction. Br J Surg. 2002;89: 1109.)*

Reconstruction Options After Low Anterior Resection

Reconstruction techniques after an LAR can be divided into straight coloanal anastomoses (SCA) in either an end-to-end or side-to-end fashion, or creation of a colonic reservoir with either a colonic J pouch (CJP) or a transverse coloplasty pouch (TCP) (Figure 6). The colonic reservoir techniques were developed in an attempt to improve functional outcomes over an SCA after a very low anterior resection, but they are technically challenging, and some fear that they have a higher leak rate. Multiple prospective randomized studies have compared these various options, and the majority of these show better short-term (within the first postoperative year) functional outcomes in terms of urgency and number of bowel movements per day with CJPs, but there do not seem to be any long-term (>1 year postoperatively) differences in terms of continence, leak rate, and overall quality of life. A recent meta-analysis of reconstruction techniques after LAR examined the results of 21 trials including 1636 patients and noticed that that CJP was associated with decreased frequency and antidiarrheal medication use for the first postoperative year compared with SCA. TCP and side-to-end coloanal anastomosis had similar functional outcomes to CJP, and all three techniques had similar leak rates.

Taken together, these data support an early functional benefit to reconstruction with a CJP over SCA, but the long-term benefits remain uncertain. In general, we consider a CJP after a very low anterior resection if the patient's pelvic anatomy is conducive to this procedure (narrowed colon lumen, limited colonic mesenteric fat, and a wide pelvis). However, when a CJP is not technically feasible, we favor performing an SCA.

Temporary Diversion After Low Anterior Resection

A large randomized trial from Sweden found that diverting stomas decreased the symptomatic anastomotic leak rate (10.3% in the diverted group compared with 28% in the nondiverted control group) after restorative LAR for rectal cancer. Their study also demonstrated the low likelihood of stoma reversal in patients who were not diverted initially but who later developed anastomotic leaks. A large population-based study suggested that factors associated with anastomotic leakage after low anterior resection included male gender, a low anastomosis (≤6 cm from the anal verge), preoperative RT, and the presence of adverse intraoperative events. Although exceptions do exist, we tend to perform a diverting loop ileostomy on most patients with a coloanal anastomosis and on those who have received preoperative external-beam RT. The ileostomy reversal is usually scheduled 3 months after surgery. However, when postoperative chemotherapy is required, reversal is postponed for several weeks beyond completion of chemotherapy. In all cases, an interim office visit with DRE and an enema study with water-soluble contrast are recommended to ensure that the anastomosis has remained patent and not narrowed and there is no evidence of leak before closure of the ileostomy.

Abdominoperineal Resection

The abdominoperineal resection (APR) refers to a combined abdominal and perineal approach to resecting the rectum, mesorectum, anus, surrounding perineal soft tissue, and pelvic floor musculature en bloc. The patient is placed in the lithotomy position and a TME is carried down to the level of the levators via the abdominal incision. The perineal dissection then begins by removing the anus and external anal sphincter muscles as widely as possible to their point of insertion and proceeding proximally until the TME dissection plane is reached. Great care must be exercised to avoid straying medially during both the perineal or abdominal-pelvic dissections. A permanent end colostomy then is created. An APR is indicated if the tumor directly involves the sphincter muscles, if adequate margins cannot be obtained during a restorative resection, or if the patient already has fecal incontinence preoperatively.

Beginning in 2007, several European centers began reporting on a more radical resection of the perineal component of the APR. With this approach, the patient is placed in the prone position for the perineal dissection, which is carried widely along the levator muscles to the point where they originate on the pelvic sidewall before traversing the levators and joining the mesorectal dissection. In so doing, the levators are left in their anatomic location attached to the rectal wall and a more cylindric surgical specimen is created.

Authors who endorse this cylindric or extralevatory abdominoperineal excision (ELAPE) technique contend that the more cylindric specimen decreases the rate of tumor perforation and positive CRM and improves outcomes. However, this procedure creates a larger perineal defect and typically requires tissue-flap reconstruction of the pelvic floor, which is associated with increased morbidity, especially in the setting of neoadjuvant therapy. Therefore one must consider all of these issues and chose the procedure that he or she is most comfortable performing.

Minimally Invasive Approaches to Radical Resection

The introduction of minimally invasive techniques to TME-based resection, including laparoscopy, robotic surgery, and most recently transanal TME, represents a significant advancement in the surgical management of rectal cancer. Several multi-institutional prospective randomized controlled trials have demonstrated that laparoscopic techniques can be performed safely for rectal cancer without compromising oncologic outcomes.

Four large multicenter prospective randomized trials have compared open and laparoscopic TME for rectal cancer. The Conventional versus Laparoscopic-Assisted Surgery in Colorectal Cancer (CLASICC) trial from the UK Medical Research Council randomized 794 patients with colorectal cancer, of whom 381 (48%) had rectal primaries, to laparoscopic assisted or open resection. In the subgroup of rectal cancer patients who underwent LAR, a trend was seen toward a higher rate of involved CRMs in the laparoscopic-assisted group compared with the open-resection group, but this did not translate into any significant differences between groups with regard to local control, 3-year DFS, or OS. There was, however, a trend toward worsened sexual function for men in the laparoscopic-assisted group. Results of the CLASICC trial must be interpreted with caution, however, because that trial was conducted in the very early days of laparoscopic surgery, and the surgeons who participated in that study had widely different levels of laparoscopic experience.

In the COLOR II (Laparoscopic Versus Open Rectal Cancer Removal) trial, 1044 patients from 30 international centers with solitary rectal cancers within 15 cm of the anal verge were randomized to either open or laparoscopic surgery. At 3 years, local recurrence (5% vs 5%), DFS (75% vs 71%), and OS (87% vs 83%) were nearly identical in the laparoscopic and open groups, respectively.

In the COREAN (comparison of open versus laparoscopic surgery for mid or low rectal cancer after neoadjuvant chemoradiotherapy) trial, 340 patients who had received neoadjuvant CRT were assigned randomly to either open or laparoscopic surgery. Three-year DFS and OS were also similar between the groups, although the study was powered only to detect a noninferiority margin of 15% for DFS.

A fourth prospective multicenter trial sponsored by the American College of Surgeons Oncology Group Z6051 randomized 486 patients with stage II or III rectal cancer within 12 cm of the anal verge to either laparoscopic or open resection after completion of neoadjuvant therapy. The primary outcome assessing efficacy was a CRM more than 1 mm, negative distal margin, and completeness of TME. Successful resection occurred in 82% of laparoscopic resections and 87% of open resections, which did not support noninferiority. Operative time was significantly longer for laparoscopic resections (266 minutes vs 220 minutes, $P < 0.001$), but there were no significant differences in length of stay, readmission, major complications, negative CRM, negative distal margin, or completeness of TME. The authors concluded that laparoscopic resection failed to meet criterion for noninferiority for pathologic outcomes and therefore should not be used in these patients.

Recently, there has been growing interest in adopting robotic surgical platforms for the surgical treatment of rectal cancer. Robotic surgery offers superior visualization and multidimensional range of motion, which can lead to improved ergonomics and precision during difficult pelvic dissections. However, critics point to the high cost of purchasing and maintaining the robotic platforms as well as the lack of haptic feedback that is inherent to robotic surgery as reasons why they hesitate to convert from conventional laparoscopy to robotic surgery. The existing literature to date comparing conventional laparoscopy with robotic surgery is limited to retrospective reviews and institutional case series, with most studies reporting that robotic surgery is associated with increased operative time, decreased blood loss, decreased conversion to open surgery, and similar oncologic outcomes. The Robotic Versus Laparoscopic Resection for Rectal Cancer trial is a multicenter, prospective randomized controlled trial that is still ongoing and is not scheduled to be complete until 2018.

SUGGESTED READINGS

Bonjer HJ, Deijen CL, Abis GA, Cuesta MA, van der Pas MH, de Lange-de Klerk ES, Lacy AM, Bemelman WA, Andersson J, Angenete E, Rosenberg J, Fuerst A, Haglind E. A randomized trial of laparoscopic versus open surgery for rectal cancer. *N Engl J Med.* 2015;372:1324-1332.

Fleshman J, Branda M, Sargent DJ, et al. Effect of laparoscopic-assisted resection vs open resection of stage ii or iii rectal cancer on pathologic outcomes (The ACOSOG Z6051 Randomized Clinical Trial). *J Am Med Assoc.* 2015;314:1346-1355.

Garcia-Aguilar J, Chow OS, Smith DD, Marcet JE, Cataldo PA, Varma MG, Kumar AS, Oommen S, Coutsoftides T, Hunt SR, Stamos MJ, Ternent CA, Herzig DO, Fichera A, Polite BN, Dietz DW, Patil S, Avila K. Effect of adding mFOLFOX6 after neoadjuvant chemoradiation in locally advanced rectal cancer: a multicentre, phase 2 trial. *Lancet Oncol.* 2015;16:957-966.

Garcia-Aguilar J, Shi Q, Thomas CR Jr, Chan E, Cataldo P, Marcet J, Medich D, Pigazzi A, Oommen S, Posner MC. A phase II trial of neoadjuvant chemoradiation and local excision for T2N0 rectal cancer: preliminary results of the ACOSOG Z6041 trial. *Ann Surg Oncol.* 2012;19:384-391.

Guillem JG, Chessin DB, Cohen AM, et al. Long-term oncologic outcome following preoperative combined modality therapy and total mesorectal excision of locally advanced rectal cancer. *Ann Surg.* 2005;241:829-836.

Jeong SY, Park JW, Nam BH, Kim S, Kang SB, Lim SB, Choi HS, Kim DW, Chang HJ, Kim DY, Jung KH, Kim TY, Kang GH, Chie EK, Kim SY, Sohn DK, Kim DH, Kim JS, Lee HS, Kim JH, Oh JH. Open versus laparoscopic surgery for mid-rectal or low-rectal cancer after neoadjuvant chemoradiotherapy (COREAN trial): survival outcomes of an open-label, non-inferiority, randomised controlled trial. *Lancet Oncol.* 2014;15:767-774.

Nash GM, Weiser MR, Guillem JG, et al. Long-term survival after transanal excision of T1 rectal cancer. *Dis Colon Rectum.* 2009;52:577-582.

Peeters KC, Marijnen CA, Nagtegaal ID, et al. The TME trial after a median follow-up of 6 years: increased local control but no survival benefit in irradiated patients with resectable rectal carcinoma. *Ann Surg.* 2007;246:693-701.

Sauer R, Becker H, Hohenberger W, et al. Preoperative versus postoperative chemoradiotherapy for rectal cancer. *N Engl J Med.* 2004;351:1731-1740.

Schrag D, Weiser MR, Goodman KA, Gonen M, Hollywood E, Cercek A, Reidy-Lagunes DL, Gollub MJ, Shia J, Guillem JG, Temple LK, Paty PB, Saltz LB. Neoadjuvant chemotherapy without routine use of radiation therapy for patients with locally advanced rectal cancer: a pilot trial. *J Clin Oncol.* 2014;32:513-518.

Skandarajah AR, Tjandra JJ. Preoperative loco-regional imaging in rectal cancer. *ANZ J Surg.* 2006;76:497-504.

THE MANAGEMENT OF TUMORS OF THE ANAL REGION

Megan Winner, MD, Joseph M. Herman, MD, and Nita Ahuja, MD, FACS

◼ ANATOMY AND OVERVIEW

As defined by the American Joint Commission on Cancer, the anatomic anal canal begins where the rectum passes the puborectalis portion of the levator ani muscle at the apex of the anal sphincter complex (palpable on digital rectal examination as the anorectal ring), approximately 1 to 2 cm above the dentate line. It extends distally to the junction of squamous mucosa and perianal skin, roughly at the point where the intersphincteric groove (the outermost boundary of the internal sphincter muscle) is palpable (Figure 1). Thus defined, the anal canal corresponds to the extent of the sphincter complex and is approximately 4 cm in length. At the midpoint is the dentate line, which is defined macroscopically by the anal valves and bases of the anal columns.

The arterial blood supply of the anal canal derives from the superior, middle, and inferior rectal arteries, the terminal branches of which reach the anal submucosa. Three main arterial trunks in the right anterior, right posterior, and left lateral positions can be isolated below the dentate line and originate primarily from the superior rectal artery. The upper anal canal is drained by the middle rectal veins and then into the systemic system via the internal iliac veins. The inferior anal canal is drained by the inferior rectal veins, which communicated first with the pudendal veins before draining into the internal iliac veins. Lymphatic drainage of the anal canal varies based on the level: below the dentate line drainage is to the inguinal lymph nodes; above, lymphatic drainage goes to the mesorectal, lateral pelvic, and inferior mesenteric nodes.

Microscopically, the anal canal is divided into three zones of mucosa of different histologic types (glandular, transitional, and nonkeratinizing squamous). The anal canal proximal to the dentate line is lined by colorectal type glandular mucosa. Immediately proximal to the dentate line lies a narrow zone (called the *anal transition zone,* or *ATZ*) of transitional mucosa, which is histologically similar to uroepithelium and is variably present. The ATZ epithelium may contain mucin-producing cells, endocrine cells, and melanocytes. Distally, the canal is lined with nonkeratinized squamous mucosa, which is absent of epidermal appendages, and which merges with the true epidermis of the perianal skin. The junction is called the anal *"verge,"* or *margin,* and is macroscopically indistinct (Figure 2). The various histologic elements of the anal canal explain the distinct categories of neoplasm that arise in the anal region. Tumors that develop from any of the three types of mucosa lining the anal canal are termed *anal canal cancers.* Although these anal canal tumors as a group account for only about 1.5% of all gastrointestinal neoplasms, their diagnosis and management can be challenging for pathologists and clinicians alike.

◼ SQUAMOUS NEOPLASMS

Human Papilloma Virus and Squamous Neoplasms

Human papilloma virus (HPV) is the most common sexually transmitted infection in the United States, affecting approximately 15% of the U.S. population. Although more than 100 different HPV types have been sequenced, one third of which can infect the anogenital epithelium, only a few have been associated with cancer, particularly serotypes 16 and 18. There is a strong association between oncogenic HPV strains and premalignant and malignant lesions of the genital tract, anus, rectum, and oral cavity/pharynx. In epidemiologic studies, up to 93% of anal squamous cell carcinomas (SCC) are associated with HPV infection, and HPV DNA has been isolated from 46% to 100% of in situ and invasive SCC of the anus. HPV infection explains, at least in part, the link between sexual activity and anal cancer, and between index and second cancers of the anogenital tracts and oral cavity/pharynx; the utility of vaccines against oncogenic HPV types in the prevention of anal neoplasia is currently under study. A minority of anal cancers are not associated with HPV infection. However, they do not appear to differ in terms of histology or natural history and frequently are grouped with HPV-associated anal cancers.

Condyloma Acuminatum (Anal Wart)

Condyloma acuminatum, or anal wart, is one manifestation of HPV infection. Between 500,000 and 1 million new cases of genital warts

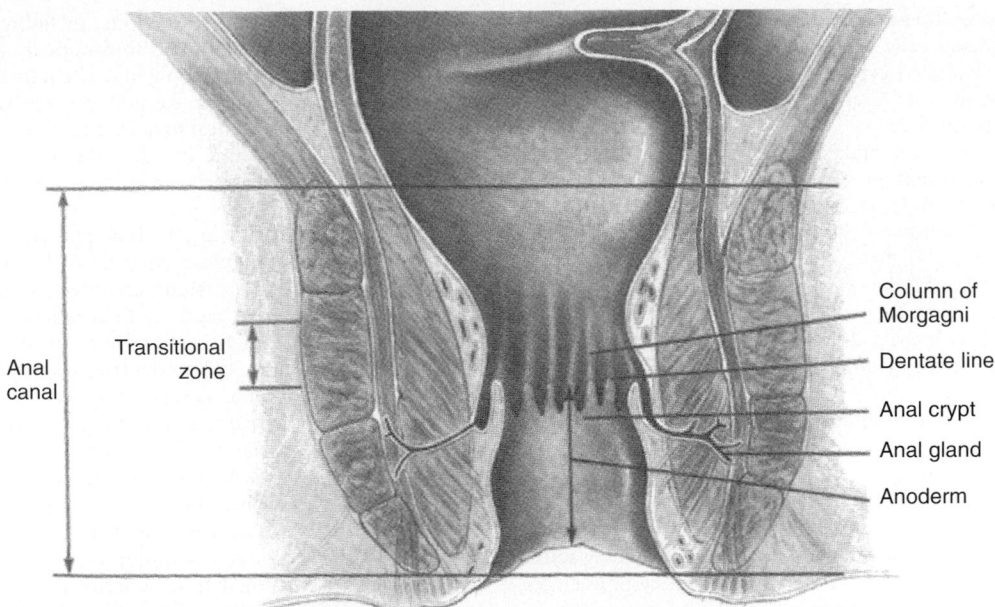

FIGURE I The anal canal. *(Adapted from Gordon PH, Nivatvongs S. Principles and Practice of Surgery for the Colon, Rectum, and Anus. 3rd ed. Informa Healthcare; 2007.)*

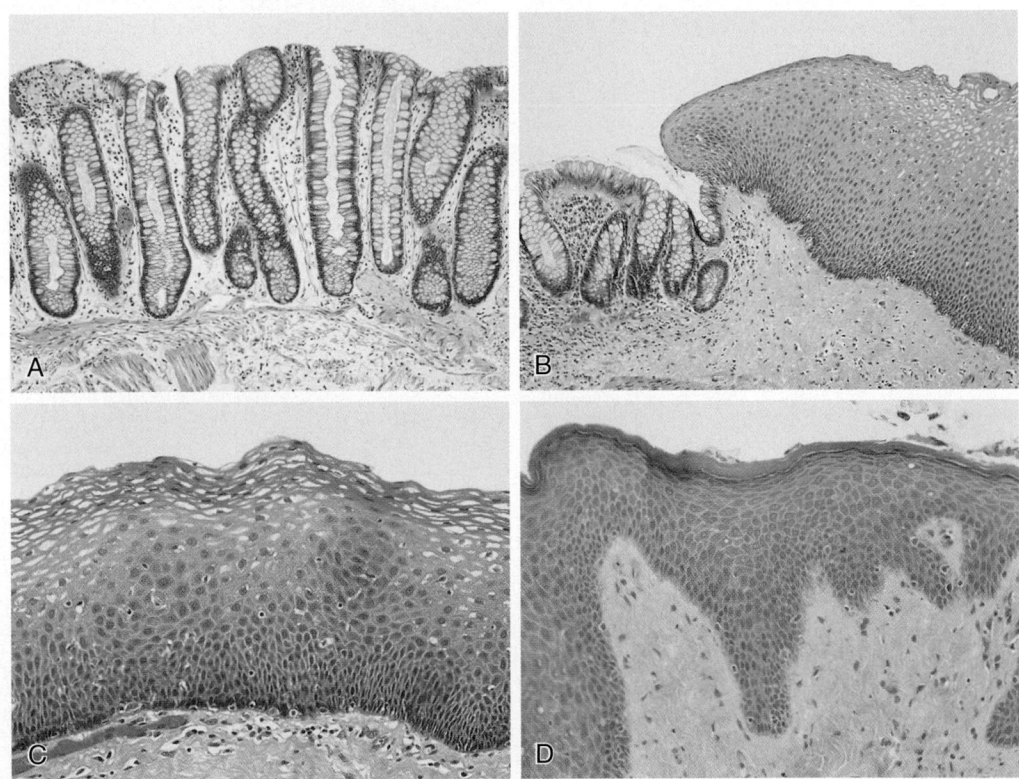

FIGURE 2 A, Normal columnar epithelium lining the upper zone of the anal canal. **B,** Normal mix zone transition from proximal to distal *(left to right)*. **C,** Normal, nonkeratinized **(C)** and keratinized **(D)** stratified squamous epithelium of the distal anal canal.

are believed to occur annually, resulting in 600,000 healthcare provider visits per year. Individuals with condyloma acuminatum are at increased risk for developing anogenital and head and neck cancers for 10 years or more after a diagnosis of anal warts, with large epidemiologic studies suggesting a standardized incidence ratio of these cancers between 1.5 and 20 times that of the unaffected population.

Although we are still learning about the natural history of condyloma acuminatum, anal warts generally are regarded as a premalignant lesion.

The key histologic features of condyloma acuminatum are a verrucous architecture composed of papillary excrescences and hyperkeratosis, and the presence of koilocytic changes within a maturing squamous epithelium (see Figure 3, *D*). The appearance of koilocytes—epithelial cells with changes characteristic of HPV infection such as vacuolated cytoplasm, wrinkled, hyperchromatic, and sometimes multiple nuclei, and perinuclear halos—can regress when viral infection subsides.

Several different medical and surgical approaches have been proposed for the treatment of anal condylomata, but there are limited clinical data to support one approach over another. The preferred approach depends on the number and extent of lesions, but patients with large (1 to 2 cm at the base or greater) or intra-anal lesions should be referred to a surgeon because treatment likely will require surgery at some point. Male and female patients also should undergo a thorough genital examination, and women diagnosed with condyloma should undergo a Papanicolaou (Pap) smear.

There are multiple topical therapies available for the treatment of anal warts, all of which work in different ways. They include podophyllotoxin (an antimitotic agent), imiquimod cream (an inducer of local cytokines), 5-fluorouracil (an antimetabolite), trichloroacetic acid (an inducer of protein coagulation), and sinecatechins (unclear mechanisms but has both antioxidant and immune-enhancing activity). Topical agents have moderate efficacy; in general, response rates in placebo-controlled trials of these agents are approximately 40% to 50%. Their use for large lesions is limited because all can be associated with significant side effects, including oncogenicity and teratogenicity (podophyllin and 5-fluorouracil) and significant local irritation or ulceration (podophyllin, trichloroacetic acid, imiquimod). Podophyllin (related to podophyllotoxin) rarely is used because of its significant local toxicity and need for provider administration. Local or systemic interferon-alpha has been used in an off-label setting for anal warts but is limited by systemic toxicity and recurrence.

Ablative or excisional surgical therapy may be considered when warts are amenable to surgical removal or when medical therapy has failed. Surgical therapies include cryotherapy, argon plasma beam treatment, and excision and/or fulguration. Cryotherapy often requires multiple treatment sessions but can be achieved in an office setting by the application of liquid nitrogen spray or swab, or a cooled nitrous oxide cryoprobe. Laser therapy with carbon dioxide or neodymium-doped yttrium aluminum garnet is expensive, requires anesthesia, and necessitates specialized protective equipment for the operator; however, it is highly effective in the initial clearance of warts. Anal warts also may be excised sharply or cauterized in the operating room. When large lesions are excised, skin bridges must be left intact between wounds to minimize scarring and to avoid anal stenosis (Figure 3). Whether an ablative or excisional approach is taken, multiple samples should be submitted for pathologic evaluation to identify the presence of dysplasia.

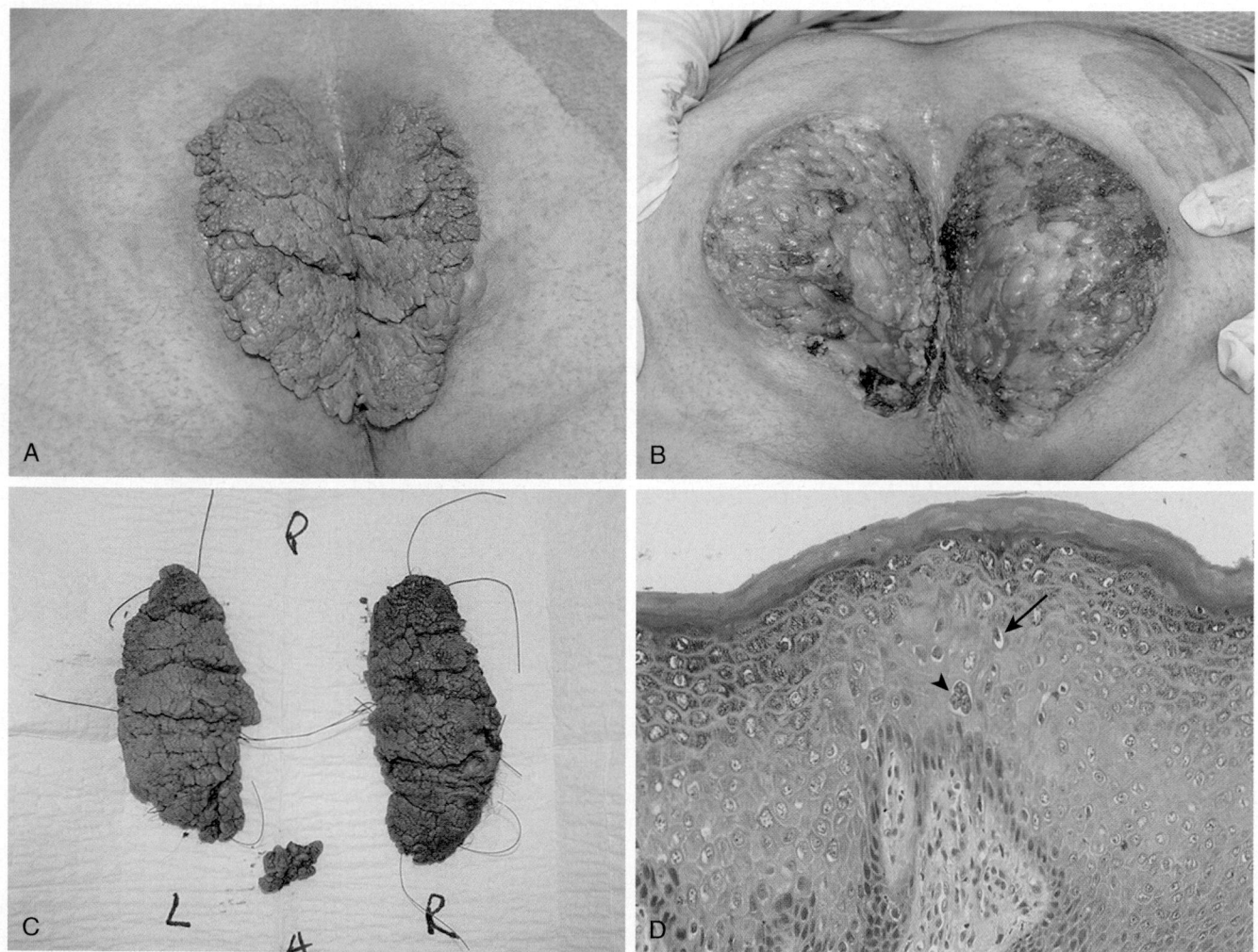

FIGURE 3 A, Condyloma acuminatum: large masses that involve the perianal area circumferentially. **B,** Surgical excision: intact skin bridges anteriorly and posteriorly to minimize the risk of stenosis. **C,** Surgical specimen. **D,** Papillae of squamous mucosa with features of human papillomavirus (HPV) infection: hyperkeratosis, koilocytic change *(arrow)* and trinucleation *(arrowhead)*.

Irrespective of treatment approach, between 20% and 50% of patients experience recurrence of anal condylomata, and it is unclear whether this is the result of inadequate treatment, recrudescence, reinfection, or other factors related to an individual's immune response. Genital HPV types can be identified in plucked pubic and perianal hair, suggesting that an endogenous reservoir for HPV may play a role in recurrence. Because both topical and surgical treatments are aimed at eradication of visible lesions only, available treatments likely do not fully address the underlying infection.

There is evidence that the immune system plays a major role in regression of genital HPV disease. There are significant differences in the epidermal and dermal concentration of CD4+-activated memory lymphocytes in patients with spontaneous regression of HPV infection compared with those without regression. Moreover, surgically treated anal condylomata in immunocompromised patients recur more often and more quickly than in immune-competent individuals. Thus in patients with human immunodeficiency virus (HIV)-seropositive conditions and anal condylomata, CD4 counts should be maximized to prevent or delay recurrence after treatment. Of the available pharmacologic treatments for anal warts, imiquimod and interferon are the only ones that have antiviral activity, and both drugs are associated with lower recurrence rates after surgical therapy compared with other topical agents. There is other evidence that, particularly in immunocompromised patients, immunostimulation may lead to a reduction in the size of lesions and in recurrence after surgery. Despite these data, the role of the immune system in modulating HPV infection is not understood fully. Although there is an association of serum antibodies to HPV proteins with HPV-related diseases, their role is uncertain because their presence does not correlate with wart regression. Although there is evidence that T cells in both male and the female genital epithelium secrete protective antibodies against HPV infections, the significance of this is as yet unclear.

The Buschke-Lowenstein tumor (named and described in 1925), verrucous carcinoma, or giant condyloma, is a rare, slow-growing neoplasm that is an intermediate form between condyloma acuminatum and squamous cell carcinoma. Like conventional condylomata, these lesions are likely to be associated with low-risk HPV, although they do not represent malignant transformation of a condyloma. The histologic appearance on a biopsy specimen may be identical to that seen in common condyloma acuminatum; however, excised specimens often demonstrate an endophytic component not present in ordinary condylomata. The biology of such lesions is typically that of local invasion without metastasis, and they have a tendency to form abscesses and fistulae and to recur after excision. Treatment consists of complete wide local excision that often requires flap closure; an abdominoperineal resection may be required in case of deep tissue involvement (Figure 4). The role of chemoradiotherapy is still unclear and seldom indicated.

Anal Intraepithelial Neoplasia

Epidemiology and Histologic Features

Anal intraepithelial neoplasia (AIN) is a necessary but not obligate precursor to invasive squamous anal carcinoma (SCC) and is stratified into three grades: AIN I, AIN II, and AIN III (indicating low-, moderate-, and high-grade dysplasia, respectively). AIN may involve the perianal skin and the anal canal, including the anal transition zone, but anal canal lesions without evidence of perianal involvement are very unusual. AIN is a multifocal disease process strongly associated with human papillomavirus (usually HPV types 6, 11, 16, and 18). There are strong etiologic and clinical similarities between AIN and cervical and vulvar intraepithelial neoplasia.

Histologically, AIN is characterized by cellular and nuclear abnormalities within squamous epithelial cells that are limited by the basement membrane. In AIN, nuclear pleomorphism, enlargement, hyperchromasia, and/or increased mitotic activity are observed above an expanded basal layer. The extent of basal layer expansion (or loss of maturing epithelium) is the basis for grading dysplasia in tissue biopsies of anal lesions. In AIN I, nuclear abnormalities are confined

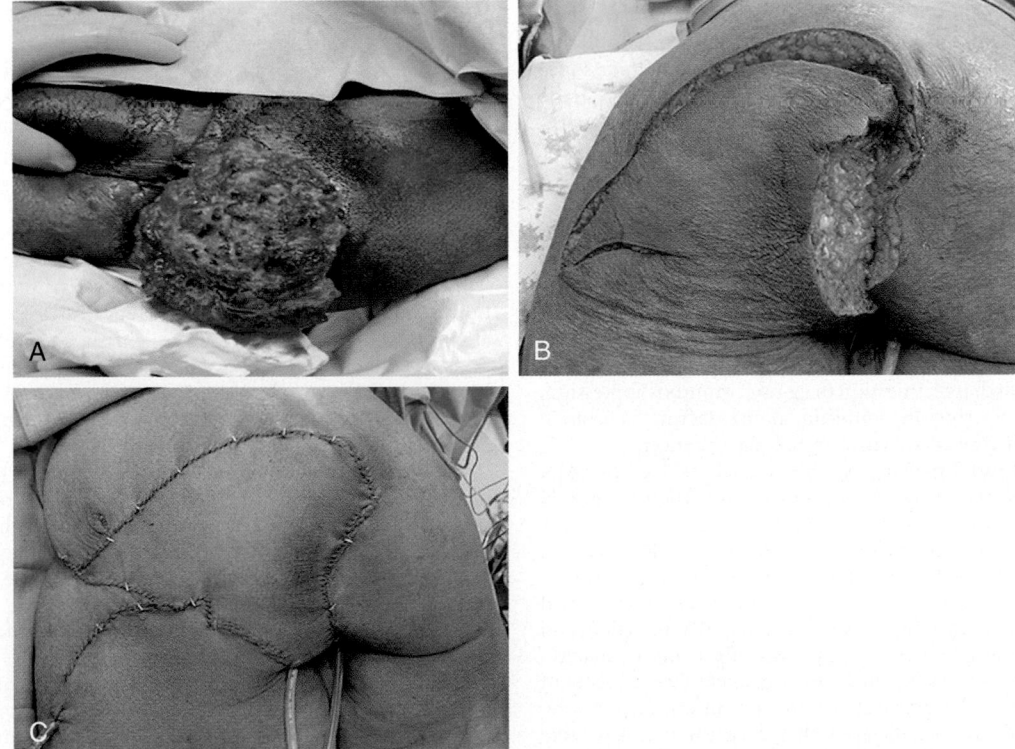

FIGURE 4 A, Verrucous carcinoma: clinical presentation. **B,** Wide local excision. **C,** Flap closure.

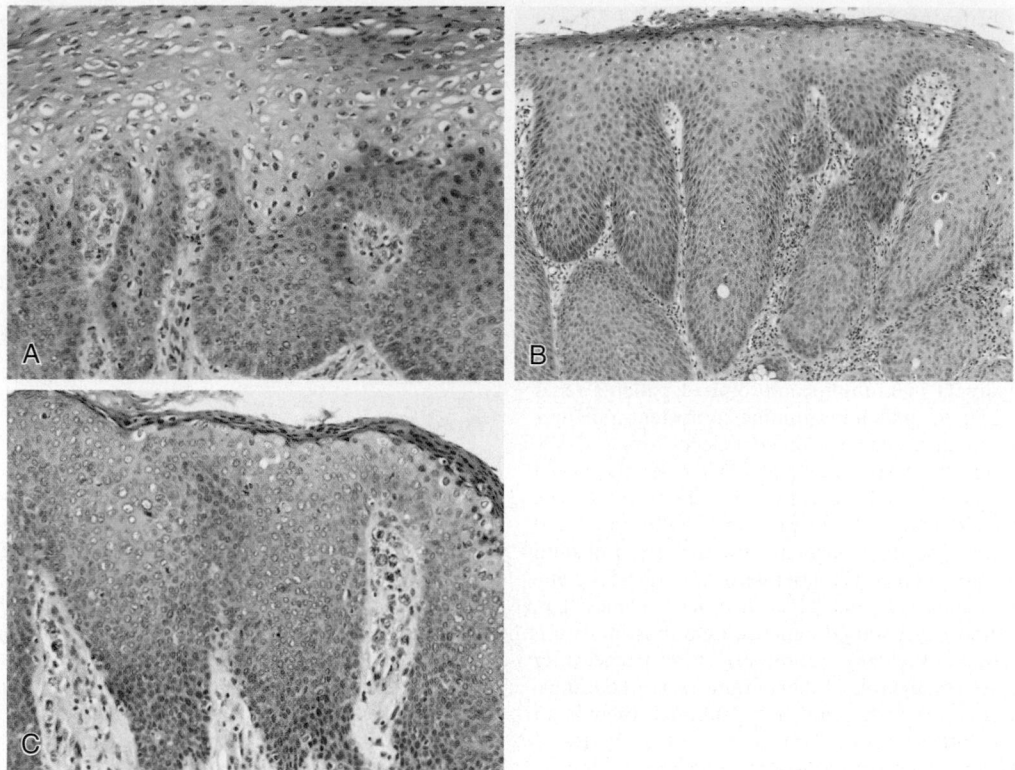

FIGURE 5 A, HPV infected epithelial cells can become dysplastic. The earliest form of dysplasia, anal intraepithelial neoplasia I (AIN I), is limited to the lower one third of the epithelium. **B,** In AIN II the grade of dysplasia increases as evidenced by expansion of cellular abnormalities and increased mitotic activity into the lower two thirds of the epithelium. **C,** Dysplastic cells take over the entire epithelium in AIN III, the highest grade of dysplasia. Note the complete loss of an identifiable basal layer with the top of the epithelium identical in appearance to the bottom. Further progression leads to invasive squamous cell carcinoma.

to the lower one third of the epithelium; AIN II is limited to the lower two thirds; and AIN III involves full thickness of the epithelium and is synonymous for carcinoma in situ (Figure 5). A different system is used to categorize cytologic specimens, for instance, those collected by anal Pap smear. In the Bethesda grading system, low-grade squamous intraepithelial lesions are equivalent to AIN I, and high-grade intraepithelial lesions to AIN II and III. Newer terminology is emerging for pathology specimens: low-grade intraepithelial neoplasia is synonymous with AIN I and high-grade intraepithelial neoplasia with AIN II/III.

Diagnosis

The exact prevalence rate of AIN in the general population is unknown, but it is thought to be less than 1%. Risk factors for AIN among men include HPV infection, anal warts, multiple sexual partners, anoreceptive intercourse among men who have sex with men, a history of rectal discharge, injection drug use, immunosuppression, and current cigarette smoking. Additional risk factors in women include a history of cervical or vulvar dysplasia or cancer.

Although AIN I and II may regress, this is much less likely for AIN III lesions. Although the frequency of progression of high-grade AIN to anal SCC is based on relatively small patient populations, data suggest that the risk of progression approximates 10% at 5 years in immunocompetent patients but can be as high as 50% in the immunosuppressed. Risk factors for AIN progression include HIV-related immunosuppression with a low CD4 count, anal HPV infection, and the presence of multiple HPV types. Cost-effectiveness analyses suggest that periodic screening with anal Pap smear (see subsequent discussion) of both HIV-uninfected and HIV-infected men who sleep with men may be beneficial, with the caveat that screening programs should be instituted only where there is local expertise in test interpretation and a referral structure for positive screens.

Prevention and Management

Vaccines directed against the HPV types associated with anal neoplasia (6, 11, 16, and 18) have demonstrated a decrease in AIN in men who sleep with men, as well as a decrease in persistent HPV infection.

There is no consensus as to the best management strategy once AIN develops, and no randomized trials have compared active treatment with observation. Proposed strategies range from watchful waiting to aggressive surgery, but the primary goal—whether AIN is treated immediately or observed—is to prevent the development of or identify early anal SCC because prognosis is associated strongly with disease stage at diagnosis. A conservative approach of observation is supported by the high recurrence rates seen after aggressive attempts at complete eradication. This is particularly true among patients with HIV and is likely the result of persistent HPV infection. Moreover, the rate of progression of high-grade AIN to invasive cancer is relatively low, with the possibility of detection of invasive disease at an early and still treatable stage.

Once the decision to ablate AIN has been made, treatment options include CO_2 laser ablation, cryotherapy, and electrocautery fulguration. All treatment strategies are burdened by high recurrence rates and significant morbidity, and lesions that make up more than 50% of the circumference of the anal canal may require staged treatment to avoid stenosis.

Excision of small lesions for histologic evaluation is preferred to purely ablative therapy because the latter precludes the possibility of a definitive diagnosis to guide further management. Anal mapping and anal Pap smear generally are used for definition of the extent of disease at the time of diagnosis, with excision and/or ablation of suspicious areas. This should be done with the assistance of high-resolution anoscopy (HRA), which, compared with conventional

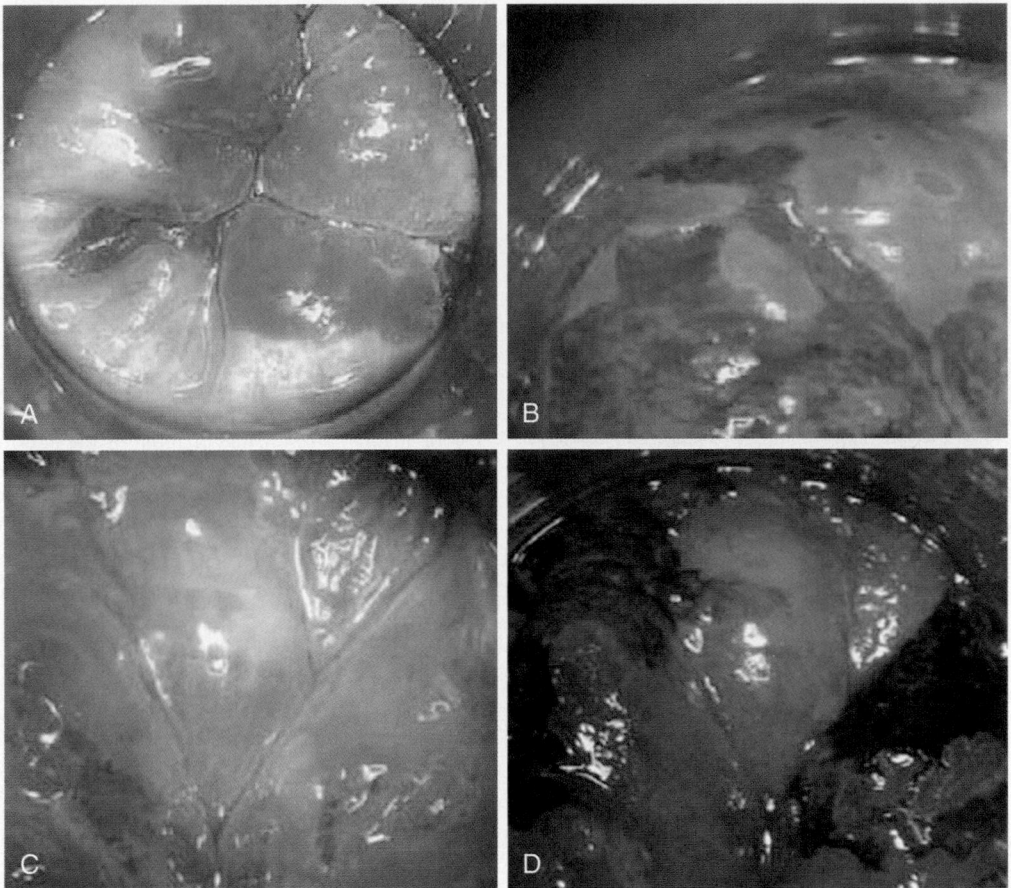

FIGURE 6 **A,** View of the normal squamocolumnar junction of the anal and rectal epithelia. **B,** Acetowhite gland openings and islands of columnar epithelia surrounded by the fully mature squamous epithelium, indicating an area that has undergone metaplasia. **C,** High-grade anal epithelial neoplasia with indistinct margins after application of acetic acid. **D,** The same lesion after application of Lugol's iodine. Note the more distinct and larger lesion margins than seen in **C**. *(Adapted from Apgar BS, Brotzman GL, Spitzer M, eds.* Colposcopy Principles and Practice. *2nd ed. Philadelphia: Saunders; 2008.)*

anoscopy, allows for more accurate identification of suspicious lesions and minimization of damage to healthy tissue. In HRA, dilute acetic acid is applied to the epithelium of the anal canal and perianal region, eliciting distinct changes and patterns in dysplastic anal mucosa: tissues that harbor AIN turn acetowhite (Figure 6). Aceto-whitening alone is nonspecific; rather, it provides a background on which clinicians can identify, with the assistance of magnification, the characteristic vascular changes of low-grade and high-grade dysplastic lesions. Lugol's solution may be applied in areas of diagnostic uncertainty. Failure of a region of tissue to stain with Lugol's solution is suspicious for dysplasia, and biopsy of these areas should be obtained. A high index of suspicion is required for diagnosis of AIN, and about 10% of AIN lesions are diagnosed as an incidental finding after excision of an "innocent" anal tag or condyloma-like lesion. The presence of ulceration in a (visible) lesion suggests invasion, as do symptoms of pain, bleeding, or tenesmus.

Once AIN is diagnosed and invasive cancer ruled out, patients should continue to be followed with anal Pap smear, excision of suspicious areas, and fulguration of less-concerning lesions. Other treatments, such as photodynamic therapy, topical immunomodulation therapies (such as imiquimod cream), and HPV immunotherapy, have been proposed; although promising, current data are too limited to draw any definitive conclusions regarding their long-term efficacy.

Bowen's Disease

Bowen's disease is a specific perianal manifestation of AIN III/SCC in situ. Patients with Bowen's disease typically have minor symptoms, such as burning or pruritus and up to a third will report a mass or bleeding. Clinically, Bowen's disease is characterized by erythematous, occasionally brown/red pigmented, scaly, or crusted plaques that sometimes have a moist or nodular surface (Figure 7). The differential diagnosis is extensive and includes benign dermatologic conditions such as psoriasis, eczema, and leukoplakia. The standard treatment is wide surgical excision. Before excision, to ensure clear resection margins and to identify multifocal disease, biopsies are taken from four quadrants at the dentate line, the anal verge, and the perianal skin and are submitted for frozen section (Figure 8). Despite wide excision, recurrence rates of up to 30% have been reported. The major disadvantage of wide local excision is difficulty with primary closure, which may require skin flaps.

Squamous Cell Carcinoma

Presentation

Most patients have a slow-growing intra-anal or perianal mass (Figure 9). Bleeding is common (45%), as is pain (30%); however, 20% may be asymptomatic. The diagnosis of SCC often is delayed because the nonspecific symptoms are attributed initially to other benign conditions such as hemorrhoids. Once the diagnosis of SCC is suspected, a disease-specific history should be performed, emphasizing symptoms, risk factors including sexual history, and signs of advanced disease (such as groin pain, indicating regional involvement of inguinal lymph nodes). A history of previous radiation or inadequately controlled HIV is important to establish because they may prove to be limiting or contraindications to chemoradiation therapy or radical surgery.

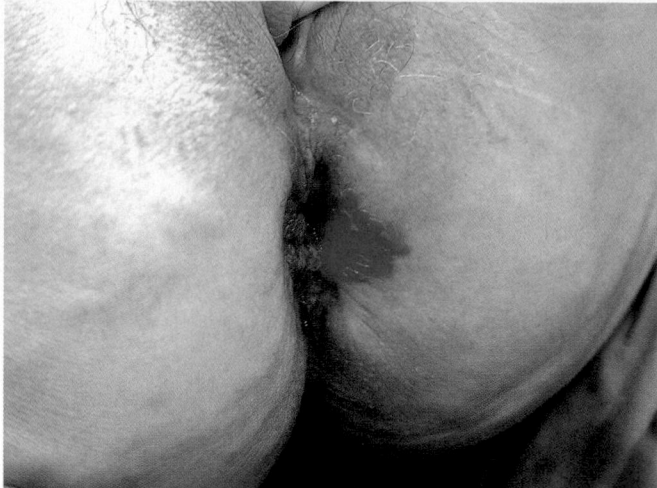

FIGURE 7 Bowen's disease: clinical presentation as brown-red pigmented, noninfiltrating, scaly plaques, with a moist surface and nodules.

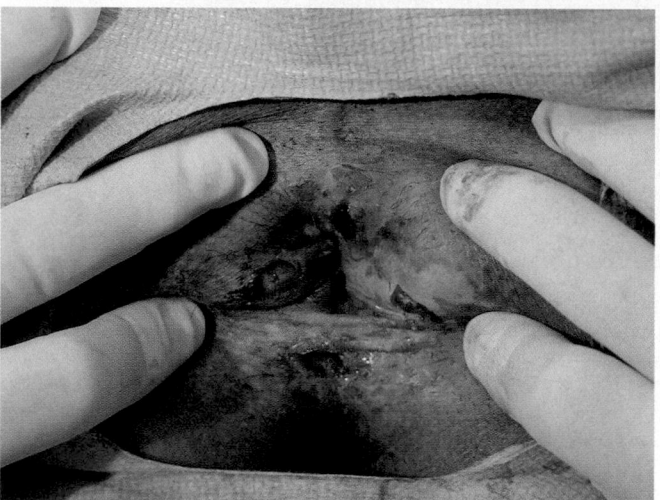

FIGURE 8 Anal mapping for Bowen's disease. Four-quadrant biopsies are obtained, starting at the dentate line, at the anal verge, and on the perianal skin. They are sent separately to the pathologist for permanent section.

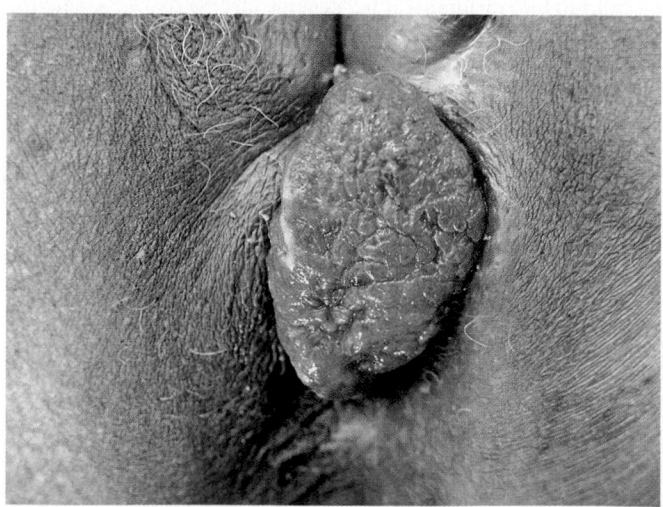

FIGURE 9 Anal squamous cell carcinoma: fungating mass at the anal verge.

Staging

Tumors are staged according to tumor size and invasion of surrounding tissues and nodal and distant metastases (TNM, Table 1). Historically, both staging and treatment of anal SCC were accomplished by radical and morbid surgery in the form of an abdominoperineal resection (APR) and inguinal lymph node dissection. Combined definitive chemoradiotherapy is now the preferred method of treatment, and staging occurs before treatment initiation. Physical examination by digital rectal examination and anoscopy, with biopsy of the primary tumor, helps to confirm the diagnosis and define the local extent of disease. Histologically, SCC is defined, and differentiated from AIN, by invasion of tumor cells beyond the basement membrane. Clinicians should palpate the inguinal area for signs of lymphatic spread, which can be confirmed by fine-needle aspiration cytology. Computed tomography (CT) of the chest, and CT or magnetic resonance imaging of the abdomen and pelvis are recommended by National Comprehensive Cancer Network guidelines to complete local and systemic staging. Positron emission tomography may be considered for T2-T4 tumors or any nodal disease. Primary rectal SCC are rare and are difficult to distinguish from anal cancers; they are treated with the same approach as that for anal SCC.

Treatment

Before 1974, the management of SCC of the anal canal consisted of primary surgical treatment in the form of an abdominoperineal resection, which left patients with a permanent colostomy, a difficult-to-heal perineal wound, and carried a 3% chance of perioperative mortality. The 5-year overall survival rate was between 40% and 70% in early series. Building on observations of the radiation-potentiating effect of fluoropyrimidines, investigators at Wayne State, led by Dr. Norman Nigro, constructed a protocol designed to decrease surgical failure rates. Dr. Nigro's original protocol consisted of continuous infusion 5-fluorouracil (5-FU) at 1000 mg/m^2 per day over treatment days 1 to 4 and 29 to 32, mitomycin (15 mg/m^2 mitomycin on day 1), and 3000-rad full-pelvis dose radiation calculated to the midplane of the pelvis, delivered in 15 treatments of 200 rad each over a 3-week period. Results from the first three patients who underwent what would later be termed the "Nigro" protocol demonstrated remarkable, complete pathologic responses and revolutionized the treatment of SCC of the anal canal, transforming it from a surgical disease into a "medical" one. Now, surgery is indicated only as salvage therapy for persistent or recurrent disease after chemoradiotherapy.

The combined modality therapy, which has undergone several revisions since the first regimen, is delivered to the primary tumor and the locoregional lymph nodes and can result in 5-year overall survival rates as high as 92%. Synchronous lymph node metastases reduce 5-year overall survival rates to 58%. Metachronous lymph node disease occurs in 10% to 25% of cases, and controversy persists about the optimal approach to treat the inguinal lymph node basins at the time of initial therapy. Some favor prophylactic inguinal irradiation, and others reserve inguinal irradiation for only those patients with histologically proven inguinal metastases. Arguments for delayed treatment include a high (48%) acute and late toxicity associated with inguinal irradiation. Moreover, in series of patients treated with the "Nigro" protocol, avoiding the inguinal fields, metachronous inguinal disease was observed in only 7% to 8% of patients, placing the hypothetical overtreatment associated with prophylactic inguinal radiation as high as 93%. However, modern radiation technologies such as intensity-modulated radiation therapy have lower treatment-related toxicities, and at our institution, patients with known or suspected inguinal node involvement will receive bilateral nodal irradiation at doses of 36 to 45 Gy or higher if bulky disease is present (>54 Gy). Irrespective of the approach to the inguinal nodal basins, surveillance of the inguinal regions is critically important to detection of early nodal metastases. Ten to fifteen percent of patients will eventually develop distant metastases, most commonly in the liver

TABLE 1: TNM Staging for Anal Squamous Cell Carcinoma

PRIMARY TUMOR (T)

TX	Primary tumor cannot be assessed
T0	No evidence of primary tumor
Tis	Carcinoma in situ (Bowen's disease), high-grade squamous intraepithelial lesion, anal intraepithelial neoplasia II–III (AIN II–III)
T1	Tumor 2 cm or less in greatest dimension
T2	Tumor more than 2 cm but not more than 5 cm in greatest dimension
T3	Tumor more than 5 cm in greatest dimension
T4	Tumor of any size that invades adjacent organ(s), e.g., vagina, urethra, bladder*

REGIONAL LYMPH NODES (N)

NX	Regional lymph nodes cannot be assessed
N0	No regional lymph node metastases
N1	Metastasis in perirectal lymph node(s)
N2	Metastasis in unilateral internal iliac and/or inguinal lymph node(s)
N3	Metastasis in perirectal and inguinal lymph nodes and/or bilateral internal iliac and/or inguinal lymph nodes

DISTANT METASTASIS (M)

MX	Distant metastasis cannot be assessed
M0	No distant metastasis
M1	Distant metastasis

AMERICAN JOINT COMMITTEE ON CANCER (AJCC) SUMMARY STAGE

Stage	T	N	M
0	Tis	N0	M0
I	T1	N0	M0
II	T2	N0	M0
	T3	N0	M0
IIIA	T1	N1	M0
	T2	N1	M0
	T3	N1	M0
	T4	N0	M0
IIIB	T4	N1	M0
	Any T	N2	M0
	Any T	N3	M0
4	Any T	Any N	M1

From Edge SB, et al. *AJCC Cancer Staging Manual.* 7th ed. New York: Springer; 2010:169-171.

*Note: Direct invasion of the rectal wall, perirectal skin, subcutaneous tissue, or the sphincter muscle(s) is not classified as T4.

and lungs. Treatment for metastatic disease is cisplatin and 5-FU; no other regimens have been shown to be effective.

Role of Surgery

Surgery generally is reserved for recurrent or persistent disease after chemoradiotherapy. For most persistent or recurrent disease, APR will be the only appropriate surgical therapy, although some small tumors may be appropriate for sphincter-preserving local resection (see The Management of Rectal Cancer chapter for APR technique). Given the limited evidence in support of good, nonsurgical salvage options, patients with persistent or recurrent disease who are appropriate surgical candidates with a reasonable life expectancy should be offered APR. Although long-term survival after APR is possible, prognosis among patients who do not completely respond to or relapse after chemoradiotherapy is poor compared with those who respond to medical therapy. Five-year overall survival after salvage surgery for persistent disease is about 30%, and for recurrent disease is closer to 50%. The status of the surgical margins, perineural and/or lymphatic invasion, and nodal involvement significantly influence prognosis.

When to declare a patient a nonresponder is a matter of debate. Results from the Cancer Research United Kingdom Anal Cancer Trial (ACT II), which compared mitomycin with cisplatin in treatment that included 5-FU and radiotherapy and added a randomized post-radiation chemotherapy, suggest that disease regression after radiation effects can continue for up to 6 months. A considered approach is to stage patients 8 to 12 weeks after treatment ends and, for those with persistent disease, wait an additional 4 weeks to see if there is further improvement. Those with suspicion or evidence of persistent disease at 26 weeks should undergo biopsy and salvage surgery, if appropriate.

Role of Inguinal Lymphadenectomy

Inguinal lymph node dissection carries an overall wound infection rate of 24% and a rate of moderate to severe infection of 16% and results in lower extremity edema in 40% of patients. As such, inguinal node dissection should not be performed prophylactically, or after a good response to initial chemoradiation in those patients with known, pretreatment inguinal metastases. Instead, it should be reserved for those who have either recurrent or persistent disease in the groin. In this setting, metastasectomy may improve long-term survival, although the rate of systemic disease in this population is high.

Inguinal lymph node dissection for persistent or recurrent disease starts with the superficial nodal basin. A diagonally oriented or S-shaped skin incision is made from a point medial to the anterior superior iliac spine caudally to the apex of the femoral triangle. Alternatively, two incisions can be made to access the superficial and deep inguinal nodal basins above (parallel to the inguinal ligament) and below (S-shaped) the inguinal ligament, thus avoiding an incision in the groin crease (Figure 10). The fat and lymph nodes are dissected from the femoral triangle, starting medially at the lateral edge of the adductor longus and proceeding laterally. The femoral vessels are preserved, and the saphenous vein is ligated and divided. Finally, the lymph nodes are dissected free from the femoral nerve. The deep nodal basin is accessed either by division of the inguinal ligament, which preserves the specimen in continuity, or by accessing the deep inguinal nodes through a counter incision on the abdominal wall parallel to the inguinal ligament, which preserves the ligament and avoids weakening the abdominal wall. The deep circumflex iliac vessels are ligated, and the peritoneum is separated from the preperitoneal fat and nodes by means of blunt dissection. The chain of lymph nodes along the external iliac vessels is dissected until the origin of the internal iliac vessels. The dissection incorporates the nodes overlying the obturator foramen. If the inguinal ligament is divided, the inguinal canal must be reconstructed to prevent hernias.

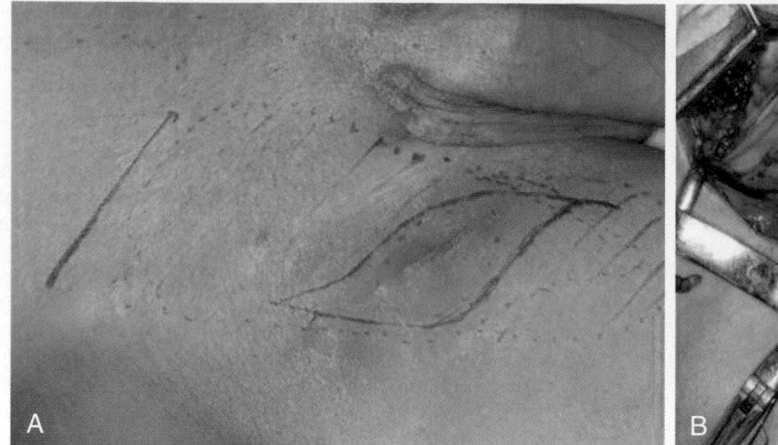
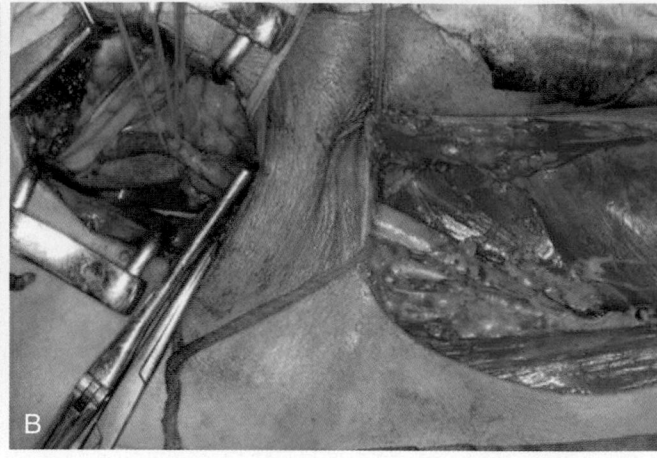

FIGURE 10 Ilioinguinal lymph node dissection with paired incisions. **A,** Incision lines. In this case, the incision below the inguinal crease is fusiform to include the skin overlying a metastatic node on which a biopsy was previously performed. **B,** Operating field after dissection. The abdominal wall was incised parallel to the inguinal ligament, which was preserved under the bipedicle flap. *(From Nakamura Y, Otsuka F (2013). Sentinel Lymph Node Biopsy for Melanoma and Surgical Approach to Lymph Node Metastasis, Melanoma—From Early Detection to Treatment., Dr. Ht Duc (Ed.), InTech,DOI: 10.5772/53625. Available from:http://www.intechopen.com/books/melanoma-from-early-detection-to-treatment/sentinel-lymph-node-biopsy-for-melanoma-and-surgical-approach-to-lymph -node-metastasis.)*

Post-Treatment Surveillance

For patients who demonstrate complete response after chemoradiotherapy, guidelines published by the National Comprehensive Cancer Network suggest digital rectal examination, anoscopy, and inguinal lymph node palpation every 3 to 6 months for 5 years, with the addition of annual imaging of the chest, abdomen, and pelvis for those with pretreatment T3-T4 or N1 disease or with initially persistent disease that later regressed or for those who undergo APR for persistent or recurrent disease.

Metastatic Disease

Options for patients with metastatic anal cancer are limited and primarily involve combination chemotherapy. A regimen consisting of 5-fluorouracil and cisplatin has been the most frequently studied and results in overall response rates of around 60%, most of which are partial responses. The median survival time is approximately 12 months. There are limited data on successful hepatic resection for limited metachronous lesions amenable to margin-negative resection; although recurrence after resection is the rule, some long-term survival is possible in highly selected patients.

Perianal Skin Cancers

Tumors arising in the hair-bearing skin at or distal to the squamous mucocutaneous junction have been referred to as *anal margin cancers;* however, the preferred term is *perianal skin cancers,* because, with the exception of anal melanoma, they behave biologically like cutaneous malignancies. They are classified and staged as skin cancers rather than anal canal cancers; however, the regional nodal drainage is specific to the anal canal. A standard treatment approach for these is electron beam radiation therapy. However, if the tumor extends into the anal canal, it should be treated with definitive chemoradiation or an APR.

■ ADENOCARCINOMA

Adenocarcinoma of the anal canal accounts for about 10% of all anal canal cancers. Most show a colorectal phenotype and originate from the columnar epithelium in the upper portion of the anal canal or from the glandular cells of the ATZ zone. Adenocarcinoma also can arise from anal glands and within established fistulas; the World Health Organization categorizes these entities as extramucosal (perianal) adenocarcinomas.

Although the distinction between these tumors and the true low-rectal adenocarcinomas that extend directly into the anal canal is often very difficult, the difference is purely semantic because the treatment algorithm is the same. For stage II and III lesions, treatment consists of neoadjuvant 5-fluorouracil–based combined modality therapy, then surgery, often as an APR, followed by 5-fluorouracil–based consolidation chemotherapy. For stage I disease surgery alone is sufficient. As in rectal cancer, the role of local excision is currently in dispute for small, superficial T1 lesions with favorable histologic features.

■ PAGET'S DISEASE

Perianal Paget's disease is a rare clinical entity with only a few hundred cases reported in the literature. In its early stages symptoms are limited, and the condition can be confused with eczema or dermatitis. As a result diagnosis and treatment usually are delayed; however, in many patients, the disease can be present for several years without progressing. Paget's disease may represent a true primary lesion arising from apocrine glands or may represent synchronous or metachronous lesions in patients with internal malignancies. The latter theory is supported by the fact that 33% to 86% of patients with Paget's disease have a history or concurrent lower gastrointestinal or genitourinary carcinoma.

The treatment for localized Paget's disease is surgical. However, because Paget's disease typically extends microscopically beyond the visible lesion, it is difficult to obtain a negative margin without sacrificing large skin areas. Recurrence rates between 30% and 70% after surgery have been reported; however, Mohs micrographic surgery, during which successive surgical resection margins are submitted for frozen section until negative, appears to result in lower recurrence rates (8% to 28%) and less morbidity. Surgery is not appropriate for medically unfit patients or those who wish to avoid radical surgery, or for those with multifocal, widespread disease that precludes complete resection. Radiotherapy can be used as a primary treatment in these cases and also can be used in the adjuvant setting. Recurrence rates after primary radiotherapy vary widely in the literature (0 to 60%). Systemic chemotherapy has been used in the adjuvant and neoadjuvant setting. Applied in combination with radiotherapy, it appears to improve overall response rates, but the use of systemic chemotherapy alone requires further investigation.

OTHER TUMORS

Melanoma

Anal melanomas account for about 4% of anal canal tumors and less than 1% of all melanomas. Anal melanoma is frequently not pigmented and does not have a macroscopically suspicious appearance. The prognosis of anal melanoma is poor; despite the fact that most patients have localized and apparently curable primary tumors, median survival after excision is only 2 years. Surgery is the treatment of choice because anal melanoma does not respond to chemoradiation. The extent of surgical resection (APR vs wide local excision) does not seem to significantly affect outcome because patients often die of distant metastases.

Neuroendocrine

Neuroendocrine neoplasms occasionally may occur in the anal canal. Most such tumors probably originate from neuroendocrine cells residing in colorectal type mucosa, although neuroendocrine cells are known to exist in ATZ mucosa as well. Because these lesions are often small, the treatment is typically a local excision. Definitive or neoadjuvant chemoradiation may be indicated for high-grade neuroendocrine neoplasms.

Mesenchymal Tumors

The most commonly diagnosed anorectal soft tissue tumor is the gastrointestinal stromal tumor (GIST), but anorectal leiomyosarcoma, rhabdomyosarcoma, angiosarcoma, malignant fibrous histiocytoma, dermatofibrosarcoma protuberans, schwannoma, and solitary fibrous tumor also have been reported in the literature. Anorectal mesenchymal tumors are heterogeneous with respect to behavior and prognosis and present particular challenges with respect to diagnosis and management in this complex anatomic area. Management preferably should be at centers with expertise in both sarcomas and colorectal surgery. The rarity of these tumors warrants full imaging, pathologic review, and discussion at a multidisciplinary tumor board. Some cases may require consideration of neoadjuvant chemotherapy or radiotherapy, although there is scant evidence to support specific treatment regimens. Postoperative radiation often is used in cases of close or positive margins but should not be used as a justification to perform less-than-adequate surgery. The curative-intent surgical approach is wide local excision, which may require APR to achieve negative margins. Recurrence and survival primarily depend on curative resection; Mohs surgery or endoscopic or transanal excision therefore should be reserved for small, low-grade tumors with a low risk of recurrence.

Malignant Lymphoma

Primary lymphoma of the anal canal is rare. However, cases of both Hodgkin's disease and non-Hodgkin's lymphomas have been reported. Immunocompromised patients are particularly at risk and in this population, the lymphomas are primarily of a high-grade, B-cell type. The treatment is chemoradiation.

SUGGESTED READINGS

Kanaan Z, Mulhall A, Mahid S, et al. A systematic review of prognosis and therapy of anal malignant melanoma: a plea for more precise reporting of location and thickness. Am Surg. 2012;78:28-35.

Kyriazanos ID, Stamos NP, Miliadis L, et al. Extra-mammary Paget's disease of the perianal region: a review of the literature emphasizing the operative management technique. Surg Oncol. 2011;20:e61-e71.

Nassif MO, Trabulsi NH, Bullard Dunn KM, et al. Soft tissue tumors of the anorectum: rare, complex and misunderstood. J Gastrointest Oncol. 2013;4:82-94.

Scholefield JH, Harris D, Radcliffe A. Guidelines from management of anal intraepithelial neoplasia. Colorectal Dis. 2011;13:S3-S10.

Simpson JAD, Scholefield JH. Diagnosis and management of anal intraepithelial neoplasia and anal cancer. BMJ. 2011;343:d6818.

Steele SR, Varma MG, Melton GB, Ross HM, Rafferty JF, Buie WD. Practice parameters for anal squamous neoplasms. Dis Colon Rectum. 2012;55:735-749.

THE USE OF PET SCANNING IN THE MANAGEMENT OF COLORECTAL CANCER

Linda Ferrari, MD, and Alessandro Fichera, MD, FACS, FASCRS

^{18}F-FDG is a glucose analogue that carries a positron-emitting isotope (^{18}F). Following the Warburg effect, ^{18}F-FDG is preferentially uptaken by metabolically active cells with upregulated cell surface glucose transporters and increased rate of glycolysis; unlike glucose, fluorodeoxyglucose (FDG) cannot be metabolized and accumulates inside cells. The emission of photons and the intensity of the positron emission tomography (PET) signal are proportional to the accumulation of FDG in the metabolically active cancer cells, resulting in different signal intensity between the tumor and adjacent normal tissue.

Cancer cells are not the only metabolically active cells with increased glucose uptake; rather every cell with increased activity acts in a similar fashion (i.e., inflammatory tissue or even benign lesions). This leads to low sensitivity and specificity, inadequate differentiation between cancer and inflammation, or between polyps and cancer. Furthermore FDG-PET has low signal in slow-growing tumors or tumors with low cellularity, such as mucinous carcinomas.

The positron-emitting radioisotopes used in PET imaging are short lived and thus minimize the radiation absorbed by the patient. Tissue activity is measured at a fixed point and normalized to body surface area; this technique is called *standardized uptake value (SUV)*.

The main limitation of PET imaging is the lack of anatomic correlation; for this reason it is often integrated with contrast-enhanced CT scan, to provide better anatomic information.

INCIDENTAL DETECTION OF COLORECTAL CANCER

Incidental focal ^{18}F-FDG uptake within the gastrointestinal tract frequently represents malignant or premalignant lesions. The rate of detected colorectal incidental foci ranges from 1% to 3% of FDG-PET/CT scans done for other reasons and subsequent colonoscopy detects cancer or polyps in more than 50% of these patients.

Recently Keyzer published a retrospective study of 9073 patients who underwent PET/CT over a 4-year period for a variety of reasons, including cancer (lung, melanoma, lymphoma, head and neck, breast, gastroesophageal) and nononcologic disorders (indeterminate pulmonary nodules, fever of unknown origin, sarcoidosis). A total of 82 patients without history of colonic disease had focal colonic FDG uptake and underwent colonoscopy. Overall 107 foci of colonic FDG uptake on PET/CT were noted, and in those patients 150 lesions were found at colonoscopy for a total of 60% of new lesions only detected on colonoscopy. The authors concluded that colonoscopy should not be restricted to the segment of FDG uptake but the entire colon should be investigated. The lesions visible only on colonoscopy were benign or smaller than 5 mm. Among the 107 foci of uptake 65 (61%) corresponded to a lesion on colposcopy (true positive), whereas 42 (39%) did not (false positive). The metabolic volume (MV) was lower in true-positive findings (4.0 ± 0.4 cm^3 vs 6.2 ± 0.7 cm^3, $P = 0.006$) than in false positive, whereas the SUV$_{max}$ did not differ significantly between groups (7.4 ± 0.5 vs 7.7 ± 0.5; $P = 0.649$). For premalignant lesions MV was lower ($P = 0.005$) and SUV$_{max}$ did not differ ($P = 0.103$) when compared with false-positive findings. In incidental findings SUV$_{max}$ values cannot be used to discriminate between true- and false-positive findings or between malignant and nonmalignant lesions. Incidental findings of FDG-uptake in the colon on PET/CT should be further investigated with full colonoscopy.

■ TUMOR STAGING

Initial staging of the primary tumor is paramount in colorectal cancer (CRC) to determine the best treatment strategy that may include early surgical intervention, neoadjuvant chemotherapy, or chemoradiation. After histologic diagnosis of CRC, computed tomography (CT) should be done in the initial staging imaging modality to rule out metastatic disease; in rectal cancer, magnetic resonance imaging (MRI) and/or transrectal ultrasound (TRUS) should be done for local staging. FDG-PET/CT does not play a significant role during the initial clinical assessment but can be added value in patients with advance disease (stages III and IV).

■ COLORECTAL CANCER

The role of FDG-PET/CT in primary CRC is considered limited (Table 1). In 2013 Cipe and colleagues prospectively evaluated 64 patients with CRC, mostly nonmetastatic at initial diagnosis. In this series FDG-PET/CT changed surgical management only in 2 (3.2%) patients (one liver metastasis and one supraclavicular lymph node). The authors concluded that FDG-PET/CT should not be recommended for initial staging in nonmetastatic patients.

In a retrospective analysis, Petersen and colleagues reviewed 67 patients with advanced CRC. They underwent FDG-PET/CT in addition to conventional imaging for initial staging. Among these patients, 20 (30%) had a change in patient management, in terms of curative intent (palliation vs cure) and treatment sequence and modalities. The differences in findings between the two studies should be attributed to the different patient populations.

Engelmann and colleagues prospectively studied 66 patients with FDG-PET/CT for staging of primary CRC. The diagnostic accuracies for tumor, nodal disease, and metastases by FDG-PET/CT were 82%, 66%, and 89%, respectively, versus 77%, 60%, and 69% for patients staged exclusively with conventional CT. FDG-PET/CT was particularly helpful in discriminating and characterizing "indeterminate lung lesions" found on CT. They concluded that PET/CT-based metastatic staging showed better specificity and higher accuracy than CT for unusual metastatic deposits.

Therefore FDG-PET/CT is not used routinely to stage primary early CRC, but it is useful in selected patients with advanced disease and/or suspected distal metastases, thus leading to a more effective and timely treatment planning.

■ RECTAL CANCER

Preoperative staging for rectal cancer dictates sequence of treatment modalities, and therefore staging accuracy is critical. The factors involved include depth of tumor penetration through the rectal wall, presence of lymph node metastases, adjacent organ involvement, and distant metastases. Traditional treatment options available based on staging include local excision, radical surgery, preoperative chemoradiation, adjuvant chemotherapy, or neoadjuvant chemotherapy in presence of metastatic disease.

Accurate primary staging includes MRI and TRUS to define T and N stage and contrast CT to evaluate potentially distant metastases and define M stage. Only a few studies have looked at the contribution of FDG-PET/CT to staging of primary rectal cancer (Figure 1).

In 2014 Ozis and colleagues evaluated 97 patients with primary diagnosis of rectal adenocarcinoma who underwent a conventional imaging and FDG-PET/CT. The majority of these patients were stage II or higher. FDG-PET/CT detected positive pelvic lymph nodes (Figure 2) in 15 patients and distant metastasis in 24 involving liver, lung, bone, distant lymph nodes, uterus, and sigmoid colon, resulting in a more advanced stage in 14 patients, a change in treatment strategy in 10 patients and change in the planned operation in 4. Median SUV$_{max}$ of metastatic and nonmetastatic lymph nodes was calculated as 2.23 ± 1.9 and 0.4 ± 1.0, respectively ($P > 0.05$).

The role of FDG-PET/CT for primary staging of rectal cancer remains to be fully elucidated. Currently it is reserved to cases in which CT scan and MRI are equivocal in patients with advanced disease.

■ LIVER METASTASES

Colorectal liver metastases (Figure 3) are present in 20% of patients at the time of initial diagnosis of CRC. An additional 70% of patients will develop metastases during follow-up. Liver is the most common

TABLE I: Change Management in Patients With Newly Diagnosed Colorectal Cancer

Author	Year	n	Study Design	Modality	Changes Resulting From PET Imaging
Park et al	2006	100	Prospective	FDG-PET/CT	Change in management in 24%
Davey et al	2008	83	Prospective	FDG-PET/CT	Change in management in 8% Change in overall management in 12%
Cipe et al	2013	64	Prospective	FDG-PET/CT	Change in management in 3.2% Restaging in 21%
Llamas-Elviras et al	2007	104	Prospective	FDG-PET	Change in therapy in 50% of nonresectable patients Restaging in 13% Modified scope of surgery in 12%
Heriot et al	2004	46	Prospective	FDG-PET	Change in management in 17% Change in disease stage in 39%
Petersen et al	2014	67	Retrospective	FDG-PET/CT	Change in management in 30%

CT, Computed tomography; *FDG-PET,* fluorodeoxyglucose–positron emission tomography.

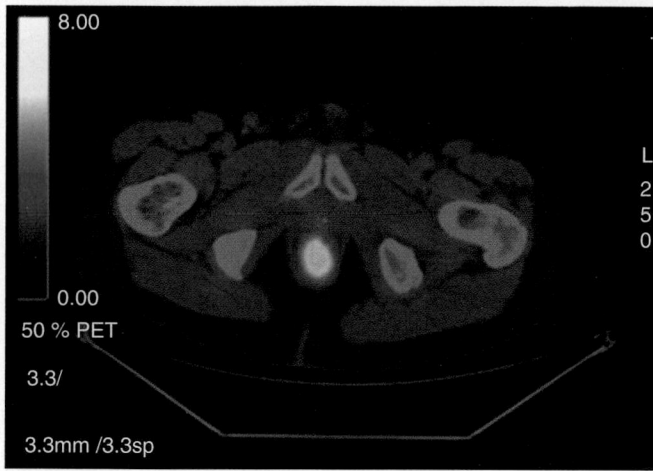

FIGURE 1 Patient with primary rectal cancer. Uptake at the primary site.

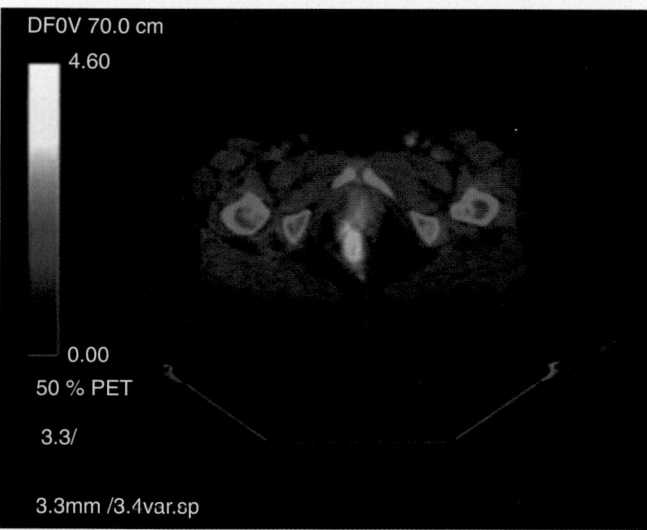

FIGURE 2 Detection of metastatic pelvic lymph nodes.

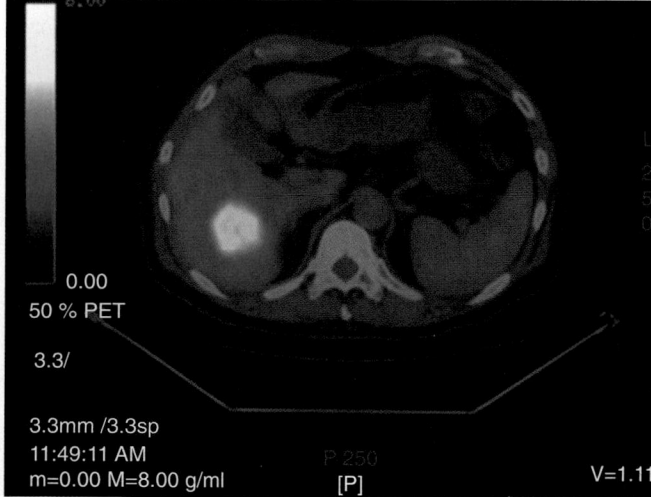

FIGURE 3 Single liver metastasis in a patient with rectal cancer.

site of hematogenous spread, and in 40% of cases this is the only organ involved. Resection of liver metastases in the only potentially curative therapy and can achieve a 5-year overall survival in 40% of patients; predictors for early recurrence and poor survival are presence of extrahepatic disease, carcinoembryonic antigen (CEA) of more than 200 ng/mL, more than one tumor, size of tumor exceeding 5 cm, and short disease-free interval.

Several anatomic factors should be considered before planning hepatic resection, especially the numbers of segments involved, proximity of lesions to arteries, veins, bile ducts, and predict the amount of remnant liver after resection. With the exception of planned two-stage hepatectomy, the goal of liver surgery for metastatic disease is removal of all metastatic lesions with negative margins while preserving sufficient amount of liver parenchyma. Often more than one modality is necessary to garner the preoperative information. Routine contrast-enhanced computed tomography (CECT) is used to evaluate the presence of metastases and is used for primary stage of all colorectal cancer; liver metastases are hypovascular during the portal venous phase, but suboptimal accuracy has been reported for lesions measuring less than 1 cm. MRI has a greater sensitivity, compared with CECT (95% vs 63%), especially for lesions smaller than 1 cm, and can detect low signal (hypointensity) compared with normal liver parenchyma on pre-contrast T1w images, hyperintensity on T2w, and hyperintensity on diffusion weighted imaging sequences. Currently MRI is considered the gold standard of imaging when liver metastases are detected by CECT.

FDG-PET and FDG-PET/CT in colorectal liver metastases is useful primarily to detect extrahepatic metastatic disease and to avoid unnecessary laparotomies or palliative liver resections.

Two randomized control trials analyzed the value added from FDG-PET and FDG-PET/CT in staging of colorectal liver metastases. Ruers and colleagues looked at 150 patients with CRC liver metastases found on CT scan and selected for surgical treatment. Patients were assigned to CT only (n = 75) or CT plus FDG-PET (n = 75). The primary outcomes were futile laparotomy, defined as a laparotomy that did not result in complete tumor clearance because of either intrahepatic or extrahepatic disease, disease-free survival (DFS), and overall survival (OS). None of these patients received preoperative chemotherapy, an important factor because chemotherapy significantly decreases FDG uptake in tumors, which results in less accurate detection of cancerous lesions. A significantly greater proportion of patients underwent futile laparotomy in the CT-only arm (45%) than in the FDG-PET (28%) (P = 0.042). In the latter group additional extrahepatic disease was noted in seven patients. Furthermore five patients were found to have focal liver lesions with low uptake and therefore classified as benign. Despite fewer laparotomies performed in the FDG-PET group 3-year OS and DFS were similar (61.3% and 35.5% vs 65.8% and 29%, respectively).

Moulton and colleagues randomized 404 patients with metastatic colorectal cancer; 270 were assigned to the FDG-PET/CT group, and 134 to the CT only as a control group. About 70% of the patients received chemotherapy within 12 weeks of surgery, which decreased FDG uptakes in tumors, resulting in more false-negative results. Surgical management was changed in 21 patients (8%) in the FDG-PET/CT group. However "curative" liver resection was performed in 91% of cases in the FDG-PET/CT group and 92% of the control group.

A prospective study by Georgakopoulos and colleagues has shown that FDG-PET/CT detected extrahepatic disease, missed by conventional imaging, in 9 out of 19 patients (47.3%) and these findings altered the management in 7 patients (36.8%). In addition in the group of patients scheduled for radiofrequency ablation FDG-PET/CT detected additional extrahepatic disease in 4 out of 16 patients (25%) and altered management in all of them. Overall, in 11 out of 35 patients (31.4%), FDG-PET detected extrahepatic metastatic disease.

In a retrospective study by Briggs and colleagues 94 patients with liver metastases were included and all underwent FDG-PET/CT, resulting in major treatment changes in 31 patients (30%);

TABLE 2: Management Changes by FDG-PET or FDG-PET/CT of Patients With Colorectal Liver Metastases

Study, Year	Number Patients	Design	Management Changes (%)	Investigators Conclusions
Ruers et al, 2002	51	Prospective	20%	FDG-PET/CT as a complementary staging method optimizes therapy of patients with CRC liver metastases, by detecting extrahepatic disease
Selzner et al, 2004	76	Prospective	21%	PET/CT provides important additional information in patients with presumed resectable CRC liver metastases, resulting in management changes
Briggs et al, 2011	94	Retrospective	30%	FDG-PET/CT improves staging accuracy, characterizes indeterminate lesions, and helps assign patients with metastatic CRC to the appropriate treatment
McLeish et al, 2012	54	Retrospective	67%	FDG-PET/CT can profoundly affect the management of patients with resectable CRC liver metastases
Georgakopoulos et al, 2013	19	Prospective	37%	FDG-PET/CT provides relevant additional information for patients with CRC liver metastases
Chua et al, 2007	75	Retrospective	25%	FDG-PET/CT performed better in detecting both colorectal and noncolorectal liver metastases and frequently altered patients management
Lake et al, 2014	133	—	20%	FDG-PET/CT may prevent futile operations, guide the resection of locoregional nodal disease, and downstage many patients thought to have extrahepatic disease on conventional imaging

CT, Computed tomography; *FDG-PET,* fluorodeoxyglucose–positron emission tomography.

extrahepatic disease was found in 9 patients, inoperable metastatic disease was found in 16, secondary primary tumor was identified in 3, and 3 were downstaged. Overall futile laparotomy was prevented in 16 patients (16%).

Several other studies found that FDG-PET or FDG-PET/CT offers additional benefit in selecting patients with CRC for hepatic resection by detecting extrahepatic disease (Table 2).

Yip and colleagues looked at the survival of patients with colorectal liver metastases. Their patients were divided in three groups: palliative group with occult extrahepatic disease found by FDG-PET/CT (n = 80); extensive multisite disease recognized on conventional imaging or disease progression during chemotherapy (n = 161); and finally patients with resected hepatic disease (n = 291). The 5-year overall survival was higher for the patients who underwent resection compared with the first and second groups (43%, 6.5%, and 6.1% respectively; $P < 0.001$). FDG-PET/CT seemed to be effective in selecting patients with occult extrahepatic disease, with poor survival, thus avoiding unnecessary surgery.

In conclusion FDG-PET or FDG-PET/CT can improve staging accuracy for colorectal liver metastases, especially when extrahepatic disease is suspected, leading to improved survival of selected patients.

■ LUNG NODULES

The lungs are the most common extra-abdominal site of metastases in CRC. Several studies have reported a 5-year overall survival between 24% and 67.8% after resection of pulmonary metastases, whereas still only 4.1% of patients with synchronous pulmonary metastases are treated with surgical curative intent. Indeterminate lung lesions (ILL) are found in 4% to 42% of the patients when staged with CECT.

FDG-PET and FDG-PET/CT are well-established imaging modalities to assess ILL greater than 1 cm in diameter with a sensitivity of 97% and specificity of 78%. A study of 186 pathologically proved ILL by Sim and colleagues proved that PET/CT had an

accuracy of 81% in diagnosing malignant lung nodules. In this study the likelihood of malignancy increased as SUV_{max} increased with SUV_{max} threshold of 2.5. Small lesions (<1 cm) are challenging because of limited spatial resolution of PET, which is approximately 7 mm for modern scanners. The partial volume effect leads to considerable underestimation of true intensity or activity within the lesion. In general, negative FDG-PET/CT results for nodules smaller than 1 cm, even more if smaller than 7 mm, do not confidently exclude malignancy. In fact a nodule smaller than 7 mm should be considered highly suspicious with an SUV_{max} threshold of 1.

Recently Jess and colleagues prospectively analyzed 238 patients operated for CRC followed for a median 24 months. In 20% of them an ILL was detected by preoperative CECT. Patients with ILL had a FDG-PET/CT scan performed at 3 months and low-dose chest CT performed 6, 12, 18, and 24 months postoperatively. Four of these patients (8.5%) had lung metastases detected at a median of 9 months postoperatively, whereas 2 (4.3%) had other lung malignancies. Instead in patients with normal staging CECT 10 of the 185 patients (5.4%) developed lung metastases detected median 16 months postoperatively ($P < 0.001$). The authors concluded that despite the relative low number of ILL that turned out to be malignant, it appears to be cost effective to use FDG-PET/CT in follow-up to detect lung metastases as early as possible to provide better resectability.

FDG-PET/CT can be used to characterize ILL during primary staging of CRC and follow-up of these lesions for early detection and surgical management.

■ ASSESSMENT OF TREATMENT RESPONSE

Patients with metastatic colorectal cancer usually are treated depending on the location and extent of disease with systemic chemotherapy and monitored by CECT. The rationale for the use of FDG-PET/CT in evaluating response to treatment is based on the amplified glucose metabolism of neoplastic cells. The increased glycolytic activity is typical of some neoplasms and is maintained in both hypoxic and normoxic conditions as a result of a multifactorial interaction between the neoplastic cells and the environment. On the basis of changes in neoplastic glucose metabolism, FDG-PET/CT is able to detect response to therapy and cell death during the early phases of treatment before morphologic changes become evident.

Colorectal Cancer

Treatment effect during chemotherapy is measured by the Response Evaluation Criteria in Solid Tumors (RECIST), which looks at changes in the size of the lesion. The limitation of RECIST is that decreasing in tumor size does not necessarily translate into an improvement in prognosis, and it may take several weeks before it becomes apparent. Patients often receive full course of therapy with the full range of toxicity before definite effects are detectable. Because FDG-PET/CT focuses on metabolic changes, it may be able to measure tumor response before anatomic changes occur, thus defining early response to treatment.

Hendlisz conducted a prospective trial looking at 40 patients who underwent FDG-PET/CT at baseline and at day 14 after one cycle of chemotherapy, to assess the predictive value of early FDG-PET changes on tumor response and treatment outcome. Twenty-three patients (58%) showed metabolic response 2 weeks after the first treatment. The patients showing a response had a significantly longer overall survival compared with patients showing no response at a follow-up of 28 months (hazard ratio 0.38 [95% CI 0.15 to 0.94]). The authors concluded that FDG-uptake changes in metastatic colorectal cancer patients can be used to predict treatment outcome and can be used to stop or change treatment in patients who do not show a response as early as the first cycle.

In another study Mertens prospectively studied 18 patients with resectable liver metastases, who underwent 5 cycles of neoadjuvant chemotherapy. Liver resection was performed after a median of 48 days after the last cycle of chemotherapy in 16 patients followed by additional 7 cycles of adjuvant chemotherapy. FDG-PET was performed before the start of neoadjuvant chemotherapy and 15 days after the last cycle of chemotherapy. Morphologic treatment response was evaluated by RECIST criteria: 8 patients showed a partial response, 9 stable disease, and 1 patient progressed. According to FDG-uptake imaging, SUV_{max}, standardized added metabolic activity (SAM) and ΔSAM (difference between baseline and follow-up SAM) were prognostic factors for progression-free survival and OS. Patients with SUV_{max} greater than 2.85 showed a median progression-free survival of 10.4 months, compared with 14.7 months in the group of patients with SUV_{max} less than 2.85 ($P = 0.01$). In addition patients with SUV_{max} greater than 2.85 showed a median overall survival of 32 months compared with a median overall survival that had not yet been reached in the group of patients with SUV_{max} less than 2.85 ($P = 0.003$). The patients with high follow-up SAM and low ΔSAM had a median progression-free survival and OS of 9.4 months and 32 months, respectively; instead patients with low follow-up SAM and low ΔSAM had a median progression-free survival and OS of 14.7 months ($P = 0.002$) and a median OS that had not yet been reached ($P = 0.002$). FDG-PET/CT then was thought to be a predictor of the clinical outcome in patients with metastatic colorectal cancer who undergo preoperative chemotherapy before liver resection.

Lau and colleagues reviewed 80 patients who underwent FDG-PET before liver resection. Fifty-one of them (63.8%) received preoperative chemotherapy; median follow-up time was 42.6 months. All metabolic parameters following preoperative chemotherapy were prognostic for 2-year OS. The absolute decrease in SUV_{max} was strongly discriminative for 2-year OS and recurrence-free survival (RFS); SUV_{max} was the most discriminative parameter with an Area Under Curve (AUC) of 0.84 for 2-year OS and AUC of 0.73 for 2-year RFS. Metabolic response once was again found to be a strong prognostic indicator that could offer an indirect appraisal of chemosensitivity of micrometastatic disease.

In conclusion, baseline parameters measured by FDG-PET/CT do not correlate with prognosis in patients with colorectal liver metastases; instead variations of these parameters before and after chemotherapy can measure metabolic response and can be used as prognostic indicators.

Rectal Cancer Response to Neoadjuvant Chemoradiation

Patients with locally advanced rectal cancer (LARC) are offered neoadjuvant chemoradiation as standard of care followed by surgery and adjuvant chemotherapy.

Accurate evaluation of preoperative treatment efficacy remains challenging by conventional body imaging. Post-treatment MRI, CT, or TRUS often cannot differentiate between fibrosis, necrosis, or inflammatory tissue and residual tumor foci. Studies have suggested that FDG-PET is more accurate in assessing treatment response than CT or MRI. The major limitation of these studies is the lack of standardization of timing of imaging evaluation.

Calvo prospectively studied 38 LARC (cT3-4, cN+) patients with FDG-PET/CT before and 5 weeks after completion of neoadjuvant therapy. They all underwent total mesorectal excision after approximately 6 weeks. The authors measured SUV_{maxPRE} at baseline, $SUV_{maxPOST}$ after neoadjuvant therapy, and tumor volume, and they correlated them with the final surgical specimen. On the basis of the tumor regression grade 19, patients showed a pathologic response, and 19 were classified as pathologic nonresponders. Significant differences between responders and nonresponders were seen in $SUV_{maxPOST}$ values (median 2.0 range 1.2 to 3.2 vs 4.8, 0-8.8; $P < 0.001$) and $\Delta SUV_{max\%}$ (median 72.2% range 38.0%-87.0%, vs 47.3%, range 0.9%-100%; $P < 0.0001$). OS and DFS at 5 years were 78.9% and 72.4% respectively; histopathology responders had significantly better DFS and OS compared with nonresponders ($P = 0.002$ and $P = 0.0018$, respectively). Metabolic nonresponders ($\Delta SUV<65\%$) showed a statistically significant worse 5-year DFS (54.1% vs 93.8%, $P = 0.007$) and OS (64.3% vs 94.1%, $P = 0.01$) than responders ($\Delta SUV>65\%$).

More recent studies have focused on detecting early response after 1 to 2 weeks of therapy to either modify therapy or to spare unnecessary morbidity of radiation therapy.

In a study by Cascini and colleagues, FDG-PET was performed at baseline, 12 days after the start of neoadjuvant chemoradiation (n = 33) and after completion (n = 17). As early as 12 days after the start of treatment they were able to correctly identify responders by decreases in SUV_{mean} (median value of SUV) (with decreases of >52%, the accuracy was 100%) and SUV_{max} (with decreases of >42%, the accuracy was 94%). Similarly Jansen and colleagues showed that a significant reduction in SUV_{max} was detectable after the first week of treatment ($P < 0.001$) in responders.

In a recent meta-analysis by Maffione and colleagues, 10 studies were included with a total of 302 patients to evaluate the value of FDG-PET/CT to detect early response of patients with LARC receiving neoadjuvant chemoradiation. FDG-PET/CT was found to have sensitivity and specificity of 79% and 78%, respectively. Interestingly another meta-analysis by Zhang and colleagues showed a higher sensitivity and specificity for FDG-PET/CT obtained during chemoradiation (sensitivity 86% and specificity 80%) than after completion of treatment (sensitivity 78% and specificity 62%).

Patients who achieve a pathologic complete response have a better OS and DFS compared with partial responders or nonresponders. On the basis of these preliminary results, nonoperative management of patients showing a clinical complete response has been proposed with a "watch and wait" approach with frequent clinical and radiologic follow-up. The suboptimal accuracy of conventional body imaging modality as stated makes such an approach less appealing to some investigators and clinicians.

Proponents of this approach have suggested the use of FDG-PET/CT for this treatment algorithm. Perez and his colleagues prospectively followed 99 patients who underwent FDG-PET/CT at baseline, after 6 weeks and 12 weeks after completion of neoadjuvant treatment before clinical assessment. Of these 99 patients 16 (16%) had a clinical complete response and were managed nonoperatively. These patients underwent FDG-PET/CT studies during the strict follow-up program. The authors showed that FDG-PET/CT at 6 weeks was able to accurately detect less than 50% of true complete responders; FDG-PET/CT performed closer to the time of surgery has a higher accuracy in detecting complete responders with lower false-positive findings because of radiation-induced inflammation and lower false-negative findings because of radiation-induced fibrosis, and they based the decision to pursue nonmanagement on the basis of the FDG-PET/CT findings at this time point.

Guillem and colleagues in New York reported somewhat conflicting results. They evaluated 121 patients, who underwent FDG-PET/CT scan before and 4 to 6 weeks after completion of neoadjuvant treatment. All the patients underwent surgical resection and 26 (21%) achieved pathologic complete response. FDG-PET/CT scan was not able to reliably distinguish pathologic complete from incomplete responders.

At this time there is no consensus regarding the use of FDG-PET or FDG-PET/CT to assess response after neoadjuvant therapy for LARC. Although this imaging modality seems to be useful to detect early responders, it falls short in detecting true complete responders who are potential candidates for nonoperative management.

■ DETECTION OF RECURRENCE

Local and systemic recurrence after colorectal cancer surgery occurs in up to 30% of patients during the first 2 years. Early detection allows for higher resectability and better survival with 5-year survival rates of 30% to 40% in selected patients with single organ metastatic disease. The most common sites for recurrence are liver, locally especially for rectal cancer (Figure 4) and lung, more common in low rectal cancer.

Postoperative surveillance protocols based on the site and stage of the original cancer include clinical visits with physical examination, CEA levels, endoscopy (sigmoidoscopy or colonoscopy) and CT scan for 5 years after surgical resection.

Several studies have shown that FDG-PET is sensitive and specific in detecting recurrence in patients with colorectal carcinoma, thus affecting patients' management, and this remains the main area of PET use to date. However the clinical value and overall efficacy of FDG PET/CT in surveillance are not yet fully established. Sobhani and colleagues evaluated 130 patients with colorectal cancer after curative surgical therapy randomly assigned to be followed with conventional imaging or with FDG-PET. The recurrence rates were similar in the two groups, but recurrences were detected sooner in the FDG-PET group with a higher rate of curative resections. Scott and colleagues conducted a multicenter prospective trial including 93 patients with recurrent CRC and demonstrated that FDG-PET/CT detected additional lesions in 45 patients (48.4%). FDG-PET/CT changed management plans in 61 patients (65.6%), resulting in 13 patients in whom a curative plan was changed to palliative and in 14 patients the plan was changed from palliative to curative.

Maas and colleagues, in their meta-analysis, looked at studies comparing body-imaging modalities in terms of accuracy in detecting local and distant CRC recurrence in patients with clinically or biochemically suspected treatment failures. They included 14 observational studies, comparing FDG-PET, FDG-PET/CT, CT, and/or MRI. They calculated the area under the receiver-operating characteristic curve (AUC) and established that FDG-PET and FDG-PET/CT were more accurate than CT with AUC of 0.94 (0.90 to 0.97) for FDG-PET, 0.94 (0.87 to 0.98) for FDG-PET/CT, and 0.83 (0.72 to 0.90) for CT. In patient-based analyses FDG-PET/CT had a higher diagnostic performance than FDG-PET with AUC of 0.95 (0.89 to 0.97) for FDG-PET/CT versus 0.92 (0.86 to 0.96) for FDG-PET. They concluded that FDG-PET and FDG-PET/CT were very accurate in

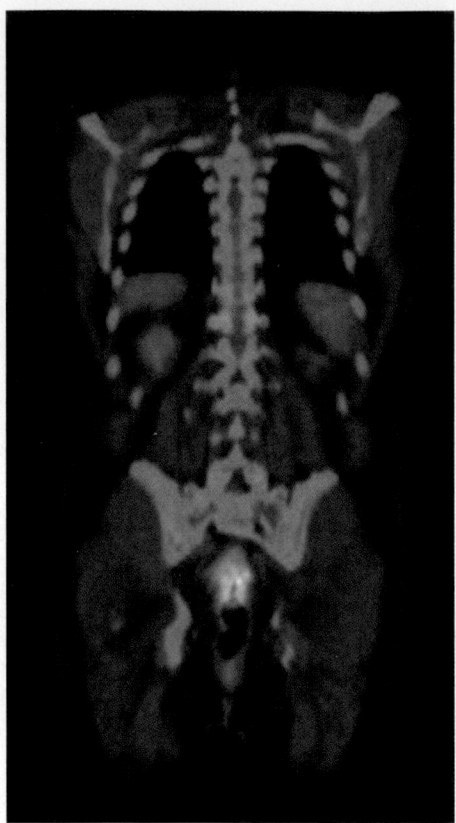

FIGURE 4 Local recurrence detected during follow-up after rectal cancer surgery.

detecting local and/or distant disease in CRC patients suspected to have recurrence; CT has the lowest diagnostic performance probably because of the lower accuracy of CT for detection of extrahepatic metastases (including local recurrence) and advocated for FDG-PET/CT to be considered the modality of choice for evaluation of patients with suspicion of recurrent disease.

Detection of Recurrence in Patients With Elevated Carcinoembryonic Antigen

Carcinoembryonic antigen is produced by the columnar and goblet cells of the colon, as well as colonic cancer cells, and has a half-life of 3 to 11 days.

Currently CEA monitoring is the most cost-effective modality for follow-up of patients with CRC, given the fact that serum CEA levels may increase 4.5 to 8 months before the development of symptoms. However, CEA levels often are increased in smokers, patients with inflammatory bowel disease, or other epithelial tumors. For these reasons CEA measurements have only 60% to 70% sensitivity and 80% of specificity in the diagnosis of colorectal cancer. In addition studies have demonstrated a median lead-time of up to 9 months between serum CEA elevation and detection of disease recurrence. Furthermore normal CEA levels do not exclude tumor recurrence, and an increased CEA level does not provide any information regarding the site of recurrence.

For all these reasons when serum CEA levels are elevated, imaging is necessary to confirm and localize the recurrence.

In 2013 Lu and colleagues conducted a systematic review and meta-analysis to assess the role of FDG-PET or FDG-PET/CT in patients with increased CEA levels and suspected recurrence. They included 11 studies (10 retrospective) and a total of 510 patients. These patients were included on the basis of high suspicion for recurrence, and both FDG-PET and PET/CT performed very well with high sensitivity (90.3% and 94.1%, respectively, for FDG-PET and FDG-PET/CT) and specificity (80.0% and 77.2%, respectively). FDG-PET and PET/CT showed excellent accuracy (89.03% and 92.38%, respectively). In addition FDG-PET or FDG-PET/CT detected 20% of patients with CEA elevation resulting from other causes. The pooled estimation of sensitivity and specificity for CT scan in the detection of tumor recurrence was 51.3% and 60.2% versus 94.1 and 77.2% for FDG-PET/CT.

Furthermore in a recent study by Giacomobono and colleagues quantitative measurement of SUV_{max} was used in patients with suspected recurrence with elevated CEA, as prognostic marker. In their retrospective study, they showed a worse OS in patients with SUV_{max} greater than 5.7 (median survival, 16 vs 31 months; $P = 0.002$).

When compared with standard CT imaging FDG-PET/CT appears to be superior in detecting recurrent disease in patients with elevated CEA. Ozkan and colleagues confirmed these results in a retrospective study that included 69 patients, showing a sensitivity of 97% and a specificity of 61% for FDG-PET/CT, versus 51% and 61% for CT scan.

Detection of Recurrence in Patients With Normal Carcinoembryonic Antigen

More recently studies have been demonstrated that FDG-PET/CT also could be useful in detecting recurrence in patients with normal CEA levels and suggested that this imaging modality should be included routinely in the follow-up of CRC patients.

Sanli and colleagues compared the diagnostic performance of FDG-PET/CT in patients with normal CEA levels (<5 ng/mL), or elevated CEA levels (>5 ng/mL), among 235 patients. Sensitivity and specificity for detecting recurrence were 100% and 84%, respectively, in the group with normal CEA, not significantly different from 97.1% and 84.6% in patients with elevated CEA. The authors concluded that FDG-PET-CT can detect accurately tumor recurrence, even in patients with normal CEA levels.

Peng and colleagues studied the ability of FDG-PET/CT in early detection of resectable recurrences of CRC. They conducted a retrospective study with 128 patients, 49 with elevated CEA levels and 79 with a clinical suspicion of recurrence but normal CEA levels. The overall sensitivity, specificity, and accuracy were 98.4%, 89.2%, and 93.8%, respectively, for the group with increased CEA levels and 100%, 88.9%, and 95.9% for the group with normal CEA levels. FDG-PET/CT changed clinical management in 63.6% of patients in the elevated CEA group and 39.2% in the normal CEA group.

Zhang and colleagues evaluated retrospectively the diagnostic performance of FDG-PET/CT in 106 patients. Patients were divided into four groups according to CEA levels: group 1 (CEA<3.4 ng/mL), group 2 (CEA 3.4 to 10 ng/mL), group 3 (CEA 10 to 30 ng/mL), and group 4 (CEA>30 ng/mL). The OS, specificity, and accuracy of FDG-PET/CT were 95.2%, 82.6% and 92.5%, and they did not differ statistically between groups based on CEA levels. When compared with standard CT (sensitivity, specificity, and accuracy of 80.7%, 73.9%, and 79.3%) sensitivity and accuracy were significantly higher for FDG-PET/CT compared with CT ($P = 0.004$ and $P = 0.013$). They concluded that regardless of CEA levels FDG-PET/CT can evaluate accurately metastases and recurrence during follow-up better than standard CT imaging.

■ CONCLUSIONS

PET imaging is an imaging modality in evolution. New tracers are under investigation to further its applications in the management of CRC. Currently the application of PET imaging in staging of early primary CRC is limited and not cost effective. Detection of metastatic disease and determination of resectability are areas in which PET imaging is used when CT, MRI, and ultrasound are inconclusive. The major area of investigation is the early assessment of response to therapy. Identifying responders could avoid unnecessary toxicity in patients that will not benefit from treatment or may allow for adjustment of therapy.

PET imaging provides useful information to help manage patients during CRC follow-up, in patients with elevated and normal CEA levels. Exact determination of the extent of disease may avoid unnecessary surgery and delay initiation of chemotherapy, which in the palliative setting may prolong survival.

SUGGESTED READINGS

Keyzer C, Dhaene B, Blocklet D, De Maertelaer V, Goldman S, Gevenois PA. Colonoscopic findings in patients with incidental colonic focal FDG uptake. *AJR Am J Roentgenol.* 2015;204:W586-W591.

Marcus C, Marashdeh W, Ahn SJ, Taghipour M, Subramaniam RM. FDG and colorectal cancer: value of fourth and subsequent post therapy follow-up scans for patients management. *J Nucl Med.* 2015;56:989-994.

Mertens J, De Bruyne S, Van Damme N, Smeets P, Ceelen W, Troisi R, Laurent S, Geboes K, Peeters M, Goethals I, Van de Wiele C. Standardized added metabolic activity (SAM) IN ^{18}F-FDG PET assessment of treatment response in colorectal liver metastases. *Eur J Nucl Med Mol Imaging.* 2013; 40:1214-1222.

Perez RO, Habr-Gama A, Gama-Rodrigues J, Proscurshim I, Julião GP, Lynn P, Ono CR, Campos FG, Silva e Sousa AH Jr, Imperiale AR, Nahas SC, Buchpiguel CA. Accuracy of positron emission tomography/computed tomography and clinical assessment in the detection of complete rectal tumor regression after neoadjuvant chemoradiation: long-term results of a prospective trial (National Clinical Trial 00254683). *Cancer.* 2012;118: 3501-3511.

NEOADJUVANT AND ADJUVANT THERAPY FOR COLORECTAL CANCER

Nilofer Azad, MD, and Melinda Cherie Myzak, MD, PhD

Colon and rectal cancer, or colorectal cancer (CRC), is a common disease in the United States with an estimated 132,700 new cases in 2015. The mortality and incidence rates have been declining over the last few decades, but 49,700 deaths a year in the United States are attributable to CRC. The decline in both incidence and mortality likely is due to several factors, including cancer prevention, improved screening, and potentially curative therapies.

For early stage CRC (stages I through III), surgical resection has been the main approach for curative treatment. Recurrence despite appropriate surgical resection is common and thought to be due to micrometastatic disease that is not readily detectable by current methods. The goal of neoadjuvant and adjuvant therapy is to eradicate these micrometastatic sites of disease to effect a total cure and prolong survival. Currently, our ability to determine which patients will benefit from additional therapy beyond surgical resection is somewhat limited. The decision to add neoadjuvant or adjuvant therapy still is based generally on anatomic tumor staging, although some clinicopathologic features and molecular profiling can add to

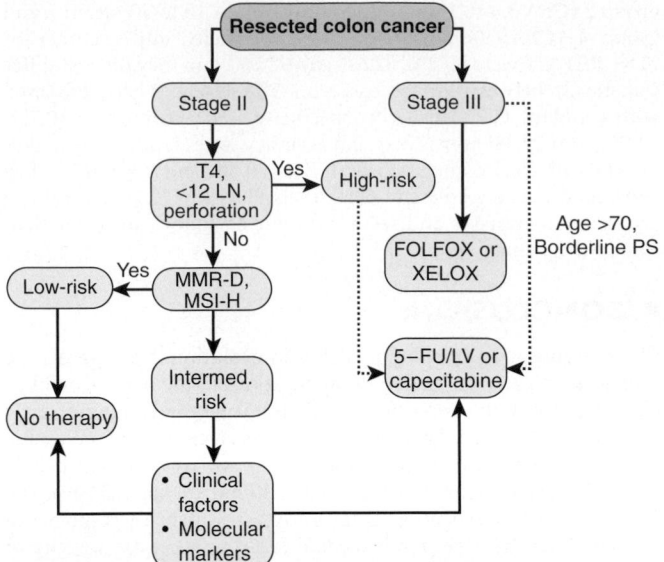

FIGURE I Algorithm for use of adjuvant treatment for colorectal cancer. *FOLFOX,* Folinic acid, 5-fluorouracil, oxaliplatin; *5-FU/LV,* 5-fluorouracil and leucovorin; *LN,* lymph nodes; *MMR-D,* defective mismatch repair; *MSI-H,* microsatellite instability; *PS,* performance status; *XELOX,* capecitabine and oxaliplatin.

risk stratification. Surgical, adjuvant, and neoadjuvant treatment approaches for CRC are different in colon versus rectal cancer and are discussed separately in this chapter (Figure 1).

■ STAGING

Formal CRC staging remains essential to establish the risk of recurrence after surgical resection for each individual patient to choose appropriate curative-intent treatment. Guidelines from the National Comprehensive Cancer Network (NCCN) for preoperative workup of newly diagnosed CRC should include the following: colonoscopy; complete blood counts; liver and kidney function tests; carcinoembryonic antigen (CEA) serum level; computed tomographic (CT) scan of chest, abdomen, and pelvis; and pathologic assessment of tumor tissue. Patients with rectal cancer also should undergo pelvic imaging with either magnetic resonance imaging (MRI) or endorectal ultrasonography to accurately define depth of tumor invasion and degree of lymph node involvement. The sensitivity and accuracy of endoscopic ultrasound is correlated with operator experience. Preoperative staging in rectal cancer is important because radiation therapy often is incorporated into neoadjuvant treatment, which may result in down-staging at the time of surgical excision. Positron emission tomography is not recommended routinely for staging of localized CRC but may be used to confirm metastatic disease if there are suspicious findings on CT scan to suggest distant metastatic disease (NCCN Guidelines, 2015).

CRC is staged based on the TNM staging system (T, primary tumor; N, regional lymph nodes; M, distant metastasis) adopted by the American Joint Committee on Cancer (AJCC; Table 1). In the most recent version of the *AJCC Cancer Staging Manual* (7th edition, 2010), several modifications were made, including the additional subdivision of stage II CRC into stage IIA, IIB, and IIC, as well as changes to how stage III disease is subclassified to reflect the prognostic impact of the number of involved regional lymph nodes. The importance of accurate staging is reflected in Table 2, which outlines the predicted 5-year survival rates. As is presented in the following sections, further prognostic features have been recommended to aid in discussions about the potential risk versus benefit of neoadjuvant and adjuvant therapies.

■ ADJUVANT THERAPY FOR COLON CANCER

Stage II Colon Cancer

Although adjuvant chemotherapy in stage III colon cancer has a significant survival benefit and is the standard of care, the consensus for use of adjuvant chemotherapy in stage II colon cancer is controversial. Trials for adjuvant chemotherapy in stage II disease have not shown a clear benefit, although some studies have shown a small effect in relative trend of disease-free survival (DFS) toward better outcomes, especially in patients with high-risk disease. According to the most recent survival data from AJCC (Table 2), most patients with fully resected stage II disease have an overall good predicted 5-year survival rate, thus adjuvant chemotherapy for stage II disease would have to show an excellent benefit to demonstrate improved overall outcomes. Original adjuvant chemotherapy trials enrolled stage II and stage III patients; because clinically and statistically significant benefits in those trials were seen only in stage III patients, large trials to specifically address the benefit of fluoropyrimidine-based chemotherapy regimens in predominantly stage II disease then were enrolled. In the QUASAR study, 3239 patients with stage II disease were randomized to receive adjuvant 5-fluorouracil (5-FU) plus leucovorin (LV) with or without levamisole (an immunomodulatory agent) after surgical resection. Adjuvant chemotherapy was associated with lower risk of disease recurrence and reduction in death, resulting in 3% to 4% absolute benefit in 5-year overall survival (OS), although the trend was not statistically significant in stage II disease (hazard ratio 0.86, 95% confidence interval 0.54 to 1.19).

The Intergroup Analysis, a meta-analysis to evaluate the benefit of adjuvant 5-FU-based chemotherapy regimens in patients with colorectal cancer, pooled individual data from 3302 patients with stage II or stage III colon cancer enrolled in seven randomized trials comparing LV- or levamisole-modulated 5-FU versus surgical resection alone. With multivariate analysis adjusted for T stage, histologic grade, and nodal status, there was a statistically significant improvement in 5-year DFS favoring chemotherapy (76% vs 72%), but the differences in OS were not statistically significant (81% vs 76%, an absolute benefit of 5%). The Multicenter International Study of Oxaliplatin/5-FU/LV in Adjuvant Treatment of Colon Cancer (MOSAIC) showed a small survival benefit for stage II patients with "high-risk" features (as defined by T4 lesions, perforation, obstruction, undifferentiated tumors) with the addition of oxaliplatin, but no overall improvement in outcome with FOLOX (5-FU/LV, oxaliplatin).

Although the majority of large studies have shown at best small improvements with adjuvant chemotherapy in stage II disease in unselected patients, these aforementioned trials have not defined high-risk individuals on the basis of consistent clinicopathologic features or molecular predictive factors. In a prospective analysis that stratified by risk factors (including T4 tumors, preoperative CEA serum level higher than 5, lymphovascular invasion, or perineural invasion), the DFS at up to 8 years after resection was 95%, 85%, and 57% for zero risk factors, one risk factor, or two or more risk factors, respectively. The NCCN, American Society of Clinical Oncology (ASCO), and the European Society for Medical Oncology define the following combination(s) of clinicopathologic features as high risk: T4 tumors; poorly differentiated histology (except with microsatellite instability-high [MSI-H] or mismatch-repair deficiency [dMMR]); lymphovascular invasion; perineural invasion; bowel obstruction; lesions with localized perforation or close, indeterminate, or positive margins; inadequately sampled lymph nodes (fewer than 12); or high preoperative CEA levels. Although these are recognized as prognostic factors for stage II colon cancer, there are no clear data to indicate that adjuvant chemotherapy in patients with high-risk prognostic factors will improve outcomes. A number of gene assays (Oncotype DX Colon; Coloprint) have been developed in attempt to predict recurrence and prognosis and thus assist in

TABLE 1: American Joint Committee on Cancer TNM Classification of Colon Cancer

PRIMARY TUMOR (T)

TX	Primary tumor cannot be assessed
T0	No evidence of primary tumor
Tis	Carcinoma in situ: intraepithelial or invasion of lamina propria*
T1	Tumor invades submucosa
T2	Tumor invades muscularis propria
T3	Tumor invades through the muscularis propria into pericolorectal tissues
T4a	Tumor penetrates to the surface of the visceral peritoneum[†]
T4b	Tumor directly invades or is adherent to other organs or structures[†,‡]

REGIONAL LYMPH NODES (N)

NX	Regional lymph nodes cannot be assessed
N0	No regional lymph node metastases
N1	Metastasis in one to three regional lymph nodes
N1a	Metastasis in one regional lymph node
N1b	Metastasis in two to three regional lymph nodes
N1c	Tumor deposit(s) in the subserosa, mesentery, or nonperitonealized pericolic or perirectal tissues without regional nodal metastasis
N2	Metastasis in four or more regional lymph nodes
N2a	Metastasis in four to six regional lymph nodes
N2b	Metastasis in seven or more regional lymph nodes

DISTANT METASTASIS (M)

M0	No distant metastasis
M1	Distant metastases
M1a	Metastasis confined to one organ or site (e.g., liver, lung, ovary, nonregional node)
M1b	Metastases in more than one organ/site or the peritoneum

From American Joint Committee on Cancer. *AJCC Cancer Staging Manual.* 7th ed. New York: Springer; 2010.

*Note: This includes cancer cells confined within the glandular basement membrane (intraepithelial) or mucosal lamina propria (intramucosal) with no extension through the muscularis mucosae in the submucosa.

[†]Note: Direct invasion in T4 includes invasion of other organs or other segments of the colorectum as a result of direct extension through the serosa, as confirmed on microscopic examination (e.g., invasion of the sigmoid colon by a carcinoma of the cecum) or, for cancers in a retroperitoneal or subperitoneal location, direct invasion of other organs or structures by virtue of extension beyond the muscularis propria (i.e., respectively, a tumor on the posterior wall of the descending colon invading the left kidney or lateral abdominal wall; or a mid or distal rectal cancer with invasion of prostate, seminal vesicles, cervix, or vagina).

[‡]Note: Tumor that is adherent to other organs or structures, grossly, is classified cT4b. However, if no tumor is present in the adhesion, microscopically, the classification should be pT1-4a, depending on the anatomic depth of wall invasion. The V and L classifications should be used to identify the presence or absence of vascular or lymphatic invasion, whereas the PN site-specific factor should be used for perineural invasion.

TNM, Tumor node metastasis.

determining which patients may benefit from adjuvant chemotherapy. These assays have been demonstrated to have prognostic value in terms of recurrence but have not been shown in prospective trials to help select which patients benefit from adjuvant chemotherapy.

Promising ongoing research has identified several tumor molecular factors that appear to have an impact on prognosis and potentially predict response to adjuvant chemotherapy. These include 18q deletion, thymidylate synthase overexpression, *K-ras, BRAF,* and *p53* mutations, microsatellite instability or deficient mismatch repair, hypermethylation, and presence of circulating tumor cells. Despite advances in improved risk stratification for stage II disease, no one

biomarker, or combination of biomarkers, has been proven to be useful in predicting response to adjuvant therapy, with the exception of MSI-H or dMMR. This subset of patients has a favorable prognosis but may have resistance to 5-fluorouracil (5-FU)–based chemotherapy. Interestingly, patients with MSI-H phenotype with previously treated metastatic disease respond extremely well to treatment with PD-1 immunotherapy, as demonstrated in a recent Phase II trial.

The actual benefit to adjuvant chemotherapy in patients with stage II disease remains controversial. Stage IIC patients have a poorer OS at 5 years compared with stage IIIA patients, which suggests that there may be a subset of patients who would derive improved long-term outcomes with adjuvant chemotherapy. Despite

TABLE 2: AJCC TNM Staging and Overall Survival for Colorectal Cancer

	Stage	5-Year Overall Survival (%)
T1-T2N0	I	74.0
T3N0	IIA	66.5
T4aN0	IIB	58.6
T4bN0	IIC	37.3
T1-T2N1, T1N2a	IIIA	73.1
T3-T4aN1, T2-T3N2a, T1-T2N2B	IIIB	46.3
T4aN2a, T3-T4aN2b, T4bN1-N2	IIIC	28.0

Data from American Joint Committee on Cancer. *AJCC Cancer Staging Manual.* 7th ed. New York: Springer; 2010.

the lack of randomized controlled trials, ASCO and NCCN do emphasize that adjuvant chemotherapy should be addressed in medically fit patients with resected stage II high-risk colon cancer on individual patient basis, including assessment of relapse risk, estimated benefit from adjuvant chemotherapy, and potential side effects, centering on patient choice. These conversations can be facilitated by online tools to provide visual representation of calculated benefit of therapy on the basis of several clinical and pathologic features (e.g., Adjuvant! Online and Numeracy). At this time, unselected patients with resected stage II colon cancer should not be offered routinely adjuvant chemotherapy because of minimal survival benefit in large studies. However, for low-risk or average-risk patients, NCCN recommends discussion of observation versus clinical trial versus 6 months of adjuvant 5-FU/LV or capecitabine. For high-risk patients, NCCN recommends discussion of clinical trial versus standard adjuvant regimens for stage III disease, including infusional 5-FU/LV and oxaliplatin (FOLFOX), capecitabine-oxaliplatin (CapeOx), infusional 5-FU/LV and oxaliplatin (FLOX), or 5-FU/LV versus capecitabine without oxaliplatin.

Stage III Colon Cancer

Adjuvant chemotherapy in stage III colon cancer has been accepted as standard-of-care since 1990, with several large randomized clinical trials showing OS and DFS benefit. As in stage II disease, the goal of adjuvant chemotherapy is to eradicate any micrometastatic disease to improve cure rate and reduce likelihood of disease recurrence. In stage III colon cancer, the addition of adjuvant chemotherapy to surgical resection results in an approximately 30% reduction in disease recurrence and 22% to 32% reduction in mortality. OS historically has been used to define benefit from adjuvant therapy; however, DFS has been accepted as a surrogate for 5-year OS for adjuvant studies in stage III colon cancer. The National Surgical Adjuvant Breast and Bowel Project (NASBP) C-01 was the first trial to demonstrate survival benefit for adjuvant therapy in colon cancer; 1106 patients were randomized, and the treatment arm, semustine, vincristine, 5-FU (MOF), was associated with a significant improvement in 5-year OS. The North Central Cancer Treatment Group (NCCTG) trial was the first to show benefit for adjuvant 5-FU plus levamisole; however, this regimen and the MOF regimen proved to have unacceptable side effects, and further studies (e.g., NASBP C-03) demonstrated inferiority of MOF to 5-FU/LV regimens. Additional studies examined the differences between bolus and short-term infusional 5-FU; a lack of superiority but more favorable side effect profile was demonstrated for continuous infusional 5-FU over bolus 5-FU in four trials. Later, an oral fluoropyrimidine, capecitabine, which is metabolized to fluorouracil, proved to be at least as effective

as 5-FU/LV. Six months of adjuvant 5-FU/LV was the standard until newer chemotherapeutic agents were introduced to trials in the adjuvant stage III setting on the basis of beneficial outcomes observed in metastatic colon cancer.

The pivotal MOSAIC trial (n = 2246) proved a benefit for addition of oxaliplatin, the only platinum-type agent shown to be active in CRC, to 5-FU/LV. The primary endpoint was 5-year DFS and was significantly higher with FOLFOX (73% vs 67%, hazard ratio [HR] 0.8). Forty percent of patients were stage II disease, and, as mentioned in the previous section, the OS rates were statistically significantly higher for patients with stage III disease treated with FOLFOX, but not stage II disease. With regard to side effects, peripheral neuropathy, febrile neutropenia, and grade 3 or 4 diarrhea were more common with FOLFOX. The NSABP C-07 trial also had improved outcomes with addition of oxaliplatin to 5-FU/LV regimens, although the regimen they used (weekly bolus 5-FU/LV plus oxaliplatin, or FLOX) proved to have an untoward toxicity profile, and, in the metastatic setting, FLOX has proven inferior to FOLFOX. Oral capecitabine has been proven to be at least equivalent to infusional 5-FU. The combination of capecitabine and oxaliplatin (XELOX or CapeOx) was compared directly with bolus 5-FU/LV; DFS was significantly superior with XELOX than with bolus 5-FU/LV (HR for DFS 0.80, 95% CI 0.69 to 0.93) after a median follow-up of 74 months.

Unlike oxaliplatin, which has been shown to improve outcomes in stage III adjuvant setting as well as metastatic disease, irinotecan has not proven to be beneficial in resected stage III disease. CALGB 89803 randomly assigned patients with resected stage III colon cancer to bolus 5-FU/LV with or without irinotecan; OS was not improved with addition of irinotecan, and there were significantly higher rates of treatment-related side effects. Similarly, the use of targeted agents such as bevacizumab and cetuximab in adjuvant resected stage III disease have shown no DFS or OS benefit despite improved outcomes when added to chemotherapy regimens in the metastatic setting. Postoperative adjuvant radiotherapy generally is not included in treatment of colon cancer that has been completely resected, in contrast to rectal cancer. However, local failure rates in high-risk disease can be up to 30%; a retrospective, single-institution series suggested that local failure rates were decreased in patients treated with radiotherapy. At this time, the role of adjuvant radiotherapy is not standard in resected colon cancer.

Currently, the recommendations for adjuvant therapy in resected stage III colon cancer include 4 to 6 months of an oxaliplatin-containing regimen such as FOLFOX or XELOX. For patients with significant comorbidities, underlying peripheral neuropathy, and elderly patients older than 70 years of age, 6 months of infusional 5-FU/LV or capecitabine can be considered. As new agents become available and additional biomarkers to predict prognosis and/or sensitivity to antineoplastic agents are discovered, these recommendations will likely be refined further.

■ NEOADJUVANT AND ADJUVANT THERAPY FOR RECTAL CANCER

Although surgical resection is the cornerstone of curative therapy for rectal cancer, neoadjuvant and adjuvant therapies play important roles in the treatment of these patients because the likelihood of local recurrence is high. Local failure after surgery alone is estimated to be less than 10% in patients with T1-T2 disease, 15% to 35% with T3N0 disease, and 45% to 65% in T3-T4, node-positive disease, although these rates are significantly lower when the surgical approach involves total mesorectal excision (TME). Rates of distal recurrence after TME are as high as 18% in stage II disease and 37% in stage III disease. Although the pathogenesis and molecular phenotypes of colon and rectal cancer are similar, it is thought that both tumor factors (e.g., anatomic location, difference in vasculature drainage patterns, lymph node invasion) and surgical factors (e.g., excision of mesorectum, extent of lymphadenectomy) may explain the difference in local recurrence rates. Given the considerable morbidity (pain, bleeding, obstruction, abscess, fistulas) of local disease recurrence, efforts have focused on abolishing local recurrence, as well as preventing recurrence in terms of distal metastases.

Adjuvant Therapy

Initial trials focused on adjuvant pelvic radiation therapy (RT) in an attempt to decrease local recurrence. A meta-analysis of eight randomized trials of surgery with or without adjuvant RT showed a significant reduction of 5-year local recurrence (17% versus 28%) when compared with surgical resection alone, although OS was similar in both groups. Subsequent trials examined postoperative combined modality therapy, with concurrent use of chemotherapy and pelvic RT. Although the chemotherapy regimens used in these early trials are no longer favored, they did determine a benefit for addition of fluoropyrimidine-based chemotherapy to adjuvant RT. For example, in the Gastrointestinal Tumor Study Group trial, 227 patients were randomized to observation, postoperative RT alone, chemotherapy alone, or postoperative RT with concurrent chemotherapy; recurrence rates were 55% with observation, 46% with chemotherapy, 48% with radiation therapy, and 33% with combined modality treatment. The combined modality chemoradiation arm also had a longer OS compared with observation alone, although not statistically significant.

In the United States, the favored approach is neoadjuvant therapy for rectal cancer, as will be discussed in the following section. Indications for upfront surgical resection include inability to distinguish between cT2 or T3 tumor in preoperative staging and proximal cT3N0 tumors for which RT may not be recommended after TME. Concurrent use of postoperative chemoradiation with 5-FU/LV or capecitabine and radiation with five daily fractions of 1.8 Gy per week to a total of 45 Gy. Chemotherapy regimens are similar to those used in adjuvant resected colon cancer (e.g., FOLFOX, 5-FU/LV, FLOX, capecitabine), although the optimal number of chemotherapy courses has not been established nor has the sequencing of adjuvant chemoradiotherapy and chemotherapy. Two regimens that are widely used include 2 months of chemotherapy, 6 weeks of concomitant chemoradiation, followed by 2 additional months of chemotherapy versus 4 months of chemotherapy followed by 6 weeks of concomitant chemoradiation. Adjuvant chemoradiation was standard of care in the United States until a seminal trial established the benefit and role of neoadjuvant chemoradiation in resectable rectal cancer, as will be discussed in the next section.

Neoadjuvant Therapy

The current approach to neoadjuvant therapy followed by the majority of United States centers involves a combined modality with radiosensitizing chemotherapy (5-FU/LV or capecitabine) and concurrent radiotherapy (50.4 Gy total radiation dose over the course of 5 to 6 weeks) with surgical resection 3 to 4 weeks after completion of chemoradiotherapy. This is based largely on a pivotal study, the German Rectal Cancer Trial, which randomized patients with T3-T4 or node-positive tumors to receive either preoperative or postoperative chemoradiation. All patients underwent TME followed by four additional cycles of 5-FU. Preoperative chemoradiation was associated with a significantly lower local recurrence (6% versus 13% with postoperative therapy). Although the benefit of addition of adjuvant chemotherapy after neoadjuvant chemoradiation followed by surgical resection remains controversial, the majority of patients do receive adjuvant chemotherapy similar to adjuvant therapy for resected colon cancer (such as 6 months postoperative FOLFOX, 5-FU/capecitabine, FLOX).

Neoadjuvant therapy is now the standard of care for resectable rectal cancer, with the exceptions as noted previously for indications of adjuvant therapy. A T3-T4 tumor is the only definitive indication for neoadjuvant therapy supported by multiple randomized clinical trials, demonstrating a more favorable long-term toxicity profile and

fewer local recurrences when compared with adjuvant therapy. Relative indications include clinically evident node-positive disease (positive findings on MRI or transrectal ultrasound), distal rectal tumors, and tumors that invade the mesorectal fascia on preoperative imaging. Combined modality chemoradiation is not without significant acute and long-term complications; preoperative RT versus postoperative RT have some overlapping side effects but also are unique to each situation. Both preoperative and postoperative chemoradiation have similar profiles in terms of acute grade 3 or 4 gastrointestinal toxicity (diarrhea). Sexual dysfunction is a risk for patients in both preoperative and postoperative settings, as is a long-term side effect of sacral insufficiency fracture. Benefits to preoperative chemoradiation include increased sphincter preservation, decreased local recurrence, and significantly lower rate of chronic anastomotic strictures. Another advantage to preoperative chemoradiation is the decrease in likelihood of chronic enteritis, which can cause significant morbidity in patients undergoing postoperative chemoradiation. Neoadjuvant chemoradiation does not affect perioperative morbidity or mortality. Other side effects of pelvic radiation in general include proctitis, cystitis, and, particularly in combination with chemotherapy, bone marrow suppression.

In light of the significant morbidity with treatment for resectable rectal cancer, both neoadjuvant therapy and the surgical resection itself, as well as the delay to systemic chemotherapy with neoadjuvant therapy, several small studies have been undertaken to determine if alternatives to the current standard of care may be feasible without compromising overall outcomes. A pilot trial of 32 patients addressed the use of preoperative chemotherapy (FOLFOX and bevacizumab) with selective use of chemoradiotherapy. After six cycles of chemotherapy, patients were assessed for clinical response; those with stable/progressive disease went on to receive chemoradiation, whereas responders immediately went on to TME. Thirty patients completed preoperative chemotherapy alone, with tumor regression and R0 resections, followed by 6 months of chemotherapy. Two patients did not tolerate the FOLFOX/bevacizumab chemotherapy and underwent standard chemoradiation followed by TME and 6 months of adjuvant chemotherapy. At 4 years, local recurrence rate was 0 and DFS was 84% (95% CI, 67% to 94%). This study suggests that selected patients with stage II or III rectal cancer may forgo neoadjuvant chemoradiation, eliminating the use of pelvic radiation, without compromising outcomes. A larger randomized phase III trial is currently open to further assess these findings.*

A prospective observational study focused on high-dose chemoradiotherapy followed by "watchful waiting." Patients with distal (lower 6 cm of rectum) resectable rectal cancer were given chemoradiation for 6 weeks with endoscopies and biopsies done throughout the course of treatment and 6 weeks after completion. Forty of fifty-one patients had complete clinical response (measured by complete tumor regression, negative tumor site biopsies, and no nodal or distant metastases by CT and MRI 6 weeks after treatment completion). These 40 patients were allocated to observation only. Local recurrence for the observation group at 1 year was 15.5% (95% CI, 3.3% to 26.3%). This study suggests that "watchful waiting" after high-dose chemoradiotherapy without TME may not compromise outcomes, at least in a selected group of patients. There also has been increasing interest and data to support the concept of endorectal brachytherapy for select patients with rectal cancers. Endorectal brachytherapy is administered via an endorectal probe over 4 consecutive days, with a higher dose of radiation given to the tumor and mesorectum than with standard pelvic radiation or intensity-modulated radiotherapy with less chronic toxicity. Good candidates for this emerging technique include patients with mid-distal rectal cancers not involving the anal sphincters and lymphadenopathy confined to the mesorectum. A randomized phase II trial of neoadjuvant endorectal brachytherapy versus standard radiation is presently underway.

As in colon cancer, there does appear to be a heterogeneity in patients with stage II and stage III rectal cancer in that some patients do not seem to require the same approach to effect a cure. Primary examples of this include the previously mentioned trials, in which some patients responded differently to the respective interventions. Similarly to colon cancer, studies are ongoing in an attempt to find molecular profiles and biomarkers that may predict which patients will benefit (or not benefit) from specific therapies.

■ SURVEILLANCE

Despite potentially curative surgical resection with adjuvant chemotherapy in CRC (and/or adjuvant or neoadjuvant chemoradiotherapy in rectal cancer), distant and local recurrence rates reach as high as 40%, underscoring the importance of surveillance after initial definitive treatment is complete. Although there is some variability in surveillance programs, most professional societies agree with an aggressive approach because early identification of recurrence or second primary tumors may allow for potentially curative therapy (surgical resection or systemic therapy), DFS, and improved overall outcomes.

The NCCN guidelines for surveillance after curative surgery are in line with most professional guidelines and reflect that recurrence is most common in the first 18 to 24 months after completion of adjuvant therapy. Per the NCCN guidelines, for patients with stage II and III colon cancer and stages I through III rectal cancer, recommended surveillance is as follows: history and physical examination with serum CEA (only if patient is candidate for further intervention) every 3 to 6 months for 2 years, then every 6 months for years 3 to 5; colonoscopy within 1 year of resection, unless not completed preoperatively, in which case it should occur within 3 to 6 months, and subsequent colonoscopies dependent on findings at most recent procedure; and chest, abdomen, and pelvis CT annually for 5 years after resection. In addition, proctoscopy can be considered every 6 months for 3 to 5 years for patients with rectal cancer after low anterior resection or transanal excision. For patients with stage I colon cancer, surveillance recommendations are colonoscopy 1 year after resection and subsequent colonoscopies dependent on findings (NCCN Guidelines, 2015).

SUGGESTED READINGS

Alberts SR, Sargent DJ, Nair S, et al. Effect of oxaliplatin, fluorouracil, and leucovorin with or without cetuximab on survival among patients with resected stage III colon cancer: a randomized trial. *JAMA.* 2012;307: 1383-1393.

André T, Boni C, Navarro M, et al. Improved overall survival with oxaliplatin, fluorouracil, and leucovorin as adjuvant treatment in stage II or III colon cancer in the MOSAIC trial. *J Clin Oncol.* 2009;27:3109-3116.

Appelt AR, Harling H, Jensen FS, et al. High-dose chemoradiotherapy and watchful waiting for distal rectal cancer: a prospective observational study. *Lancet Oncol.* 2015;16:919-927.

Benson AB 3rd, Schrag D, Somerfield MR, et al. American Society of Clinical Oncology recommendations on adjuvant chemotherapy for stage II colon cancer. *J Clin Oncol.* 2004;22:3408-3419.

Birgisson H, Påhlman L, Gunnarsson U, et al. Adverse effects of preoperative radiation therapy for rectal cancer: long-term follow-up of the Swedish Rectal Cancer Trial. *J Clin Oncol.* 2005;23:8697-8705.

Kapiteijn E, Marijnen CA, Nagtegaal ID, et al. Preoperative radiotherapy combined with total mesorectal excision for resectable rectal cancer. *N Engl J Med.* 2001;345:638-646.

Krishnamurthi SS, Seo Y, Kinsella TJ. Adjuvant therapy for rectal cancer. *Clin Colo Rectal Surg.* 2007;20:167-181.

Kuebler JP, Wieand HS, O'Connell MJ, et al. Oxaliplatin combined with weekly bolus fluorouracil and leucovorin as surgical adjuvant chemotherapy for stage II and III colon cancer: results from NSABP C-07. *J Clin Oncol.* 2007;25:2198-2204.

O'Connor ES, Greenblatt DY, LoConte NK, et al. Adjuvant chemotherapy for stage II colon cancer with poor prognostic features. *J Clin Oncol.* 2011;29: 3381-3388.

QUASAR Collaborative Group, Gray R, Barnwell J, et al. Adjuvant chemotherapy versus observation in patients with colorectal cancer: a randomised study. *Lancet.* 2007;370:2020-2029.

*Referenced with permission from the NCCN Clinical Practice Guidelines in Oncology (NCCN Guidelines) for Colon Cancer V.3.2015. Copyright National Comprehensive Cancer Network, Inc 2013. All rights reserved. Accessed September 25, 2015. To view the most recent and complete version of the guideline, go online to www.nccn.org. NATIONAL COMPREHENSIVE CANCER NETWORK, NCCN, NCCN GUIDELINES, and all other NCCN Content are trademarks owned by the National Comprehensive Cancer Network, Inc.

Sauer R, Becker H, Hohenberger W, et al. Preoperative versus postoperative chemoradiotherapy for rectal cancer. *N Engl J Med.* 2004;351:1731-1740.

Schrag D, Weiser MR, Goodman KA, et al. Neoadjuvant chemotherapy without routine use of radiation therapy for patients with locally advanced rectal cancer: a pilot trial. *J Clin Oncol.* 2014;32:513018.

Smith JA, Wild AT, Singhi A, et al. Clinicopathologic comparison of high-dose-rate endorectal brachytherapy versus conventional chemoradiotherapy in the neoadjuvant setting for resectable stages II and II low rectal cancer. *Int J Surg Oncol.* 2012.

Vuong T, Devic S, Podgorsak E. High dose rate endorectal brachytherapy as a neoadjuvant treatment for patients with resectable rectal cancer. *Clin Oncol (R Coll Radiol).* 2007;19:701-705.

THE MANAGEMENT OF COLONIC POLYPS

Amy L. Lightner, MD, and Kellie L. Mathis, MD, MSc

A colorectal polyp is a macroscopically visible protuberance into the colonic lumen resulting from overgrowth of the epithelial lining of the mucosa. Other lesions that are covered by histologically normal mucosa, such as carcinoids, lipomas, and leiomyomas, are not polyps by definition. Polyps are typically asymptomatic but rarely present with bleeding, tenesmus when in the rectum, obstruction, or intussusception. The majority of polyps require simple endoscopic removal, but a review of the histology is necessary to determine the polyp's malignant potential.

Polyps are categorized into non-neoplastic (hyperplastic, mucosal, inflammatory, and hamartomatous polyps) and neoplastic lesions (adenomas). Rarely polyps occur in the setting of hereditary syndromes, whereas the majority are sporadic. Thus flexible endoscopy with complete excision and histopathologic review determines the management of colonic polyps. This chapter focuses on the management of sporadic polyps, their risk factors for malignancy, and guidelines for future screening. Hereditary polyposis syndromes are discussed elsewhere.

■ NON-NEOPLASTIC POLYPS

Hyperplastic Polyps

Hyperplastic polyps are the most common non-neoplastic polyp, accounting for 50% of polyps 1 to 5 mm, 28% of polyps 6 to 9 mm, and 14% of polyps larger than 10 mm. They occur as a result of normal epithelial cells accumulating on the mucosal surface, creating a pale appearance, and they are typically sessile. These are the most frequently reported polyps on sigmoidoscopy and are found most often in the rectum. Previous literature focused on whether finding hyperplastic polyps in the distal colon was a risk for advanced neoplasia elsewhere, but the majority of studies do not find this relationship. The American Gastroenterological Association guidelines consider small hyperplastic lesions (smaller than 10 mm) limited to the sigmoid and rectum benign, and this finding should not shorten the standard recommended screening interval of 10 years.

Mucosal Polyps

Mucosal polyps are typically smaller than 5-mm lesions and are caused most often by prolapse of the mucosa. Histologically, these comprise normal mucosa, and they have no clinical significance.

Inflammatory Pseudopolyps

Inflammatory pseudopolyps are irregularly shaped islands of intact colonic mucosa neighboring areas of mucosal ulceration and regeneration in the setting of inflammatory bowel disease (IBD). These polyps are located typically in the colitic region of the colon. When found in clusters, they may be associated with surrounding dysplasia. Thus careful attention to biopsy of these areas should be used.

Hamartomatous Polyps

Hamartomatous polyps are polyps made up of normal tissue, which is growing in a disorganized mass. When sporadic, hamartomas are often referred to as *juvenile polyps* because they are commonly found in children. Nonsporadic hamartomas are associated with one of three autosomal dominant familial syndromes: juvenile polyposis, Peutz-Jeghers syndrome, and Cowden's syndrome. The hamartomas are not premalignant, but all of these syndromic patients are at higher-than-average risk of developing colorectal carcinoma (CRC).

Juvenile polyposis coli is defined as the presence of 10 or more juvenile polyps in the gastrointestinal tract. If similar lesions are found in at least one first-degree relative, the patients are considered to have familial juvenile polyposis, which is associated with a 50% rate of CRC. Screening colonoscopy should begin at the onset of symptoms or age 15 if asymptomatic and repeated every 3 years if no polyps are seen and every 1 year when polyps are seen.

Patients with Peutz-Jeghers syndrome have a characteristic phenotype with mucosal hyperpigmentation. These patients have multiple hamartomatous polyps throughout the small bowel and colon, which can lead to intussusception, bleeding, and/or obstruction at a young age. Colonoscopy is recommended every 3 years starting with the onset of symptoms or in the early teenage years in asymptomatic patients resulting from a 2% to 13% risk of gastrointestinal cancer.

Cowden's disease, characterized by hamartomatous neoplasms of the skin, mucosa, gastrointestinal tract, thyroid, endometrium and breast, has up to a 16% risk of CRC. Thus patients should undergo colonoscopy beginning at the age of 45 and continuing every 5 years.

■ NEOPLASTIC POLYPS

Adenomas

Adenomas differ from hyperplastic polyps in that they have cellular atypia and are recognized as precursors for invasive CRC. They are the most common neoplastic polyp found on colonoscopy, accounting for more than half of all colonic polyps. The histology is classified as tubular (65% to 85%), tubulovillous (10% to 25%), or villous (10%). Advanced adenomas are those that are larger than 1 cm or have villous architecture, severe dysplasia, or a focus of invasive carcinoma. Risk factors for adenomas include increasing age, increased body mass index (BMI), lack of physical activity, male sex, and African American ethnicity as well as smoking history. The prevalence of adenomas is approximately 25% at the age of 50 and reaches 50% by the age of 70, as compared with 1% to 4% among patients in their 20s. Similarly, the prevalence of advanced adenomas increases

with age, with 3.8% prevalence in patients younger than 65 and 8.2% in patients older than the age of 65 years.

More than 80% of CRC are known to develop from adenomas. The adenoma-carcinoma sequence, or loss of heterozygosity or chromosomal instability pathway, is a well-established cascade of genetic mutations that end in a CRC. One of the first mutations leading to the sporadic adenomatous polyp is loss of the tumor suppressor adenomatous polyposis coli gene, the same mutation found in familial adenomatous polyposis (FAP). The next gene thought to be affected is the oncogene *K-ras* followed by the loss of deleted in colon cancer (DCC), which likely plays a key role in transitioning from an adenoma to an advanced adenoma. The final step in development of a cancer from an adenoma is a mutation in the *p53* gene, a gene that regulates the cell cycle, allowing for time for either DNA repair or apoptosis. The average time for the development of adenoma to a cancer is thought to be 7 to 10 years, and shorter for advanced adenomas (Figure 1).

The adenoma-carcinoma sequence is supported clinically by the following: almost all colon cancers arise within an adenoma; the incidence of synchronous adenomas in a colon cancer resection specimen is 30%; the risk of colon cancer increases with larger and increasing numbers of adenomatous polyps; the incidence of CRC in patients with FAP is high; and the risk of cancer in unresected polyps is 4% at 5 years and 14% at 10 years. Thus the finding of adenomas on sigmoidoscopy should prompt a full colonoscopy, and the finding of an adenoma during colonoscopy should prompt complete polypectomy. Subsequent surveillance after polyp removal depends on the number, size, and histopathology of removed polyps and is discussed later.

Risk factors for focal cancer within an individual adenoma include villous histology, increasing polyp size (larger than 1 cm), and high-grade dysplasia. Risk factors for finding metachronous adenomas include histologically advanced adenomas and cancer. The risk for metachronous colon cancer (cancer diagnosed within 6 months of removal of index cancer or polyp) increases with the number of advanced adenomas present.

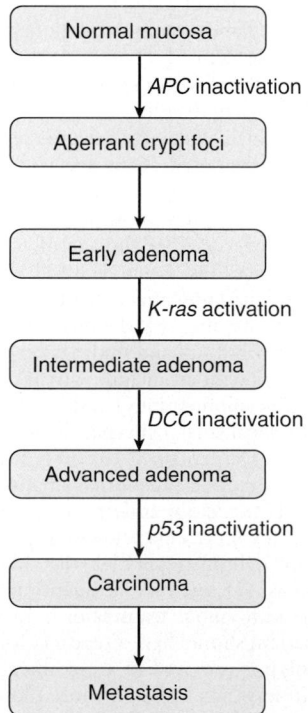

FIGURE I Adenoma to carcinoma sequence.

Sessile Serrated Adenomas

Sessile serrated adenomas (SSAs) were classified previously as hyperplastic polyps, but they are now known to be associated with an increased risk of colon cancer. SSAs are relatively uncommon, accounting for 0.5% to 4% of colorectal polyps. They are difficult to distinguish from normal mucosa, and their margins may be difficult to delineate endoscopically. They tend to be larger than 5 mm, are more often located in the right colon, and have an increased incidence in females. There appears to be a separate oncogenic or "serrated" pathway, which includes *BRAF* genetic mutation, high levels of CpG island methylation, and *MLH1* gene hypermethylation. The concern has been raised that the serrated polyp to adenocarcinoma progression may occur much more rapidly than the adenoma-carcinoma sequence for tubular adenomas.

■ GUIDELINES FOR COLONOSCOPY SCREENING AND SURVEILLANCE

Screening asymptomatic individuals for colorectal cancer has a known survival advantage, and in the United States, colonoscopy is the most commonly used screening modality. The National Polyp Study found that during long-term follow-up of more than 20 years, patients who had adenomas removed had an estimated 53% reduction in mortality from colon cancer compared with the expected number of deaths in the general population. Screening and surveillance intervals are based on prevention of interval cancers and, ultimately, improved survival as a result. The recommendations continue to evolve, and there is an increasing amount of evidence to suggest that up to 17% of lesions more than 1 cm are missed on initial colonoscopy, and 50% to 80% of interval cancers are attributed to these missed lesions. If the polypectomy is incomplete, residual neoplastic tissue can progress to malignancy. This is supported by the finding that nearly a quarter of interval cancers occur in the same site as a previous polypectomy. Current recommendations for colonoscopy surveillance are based on the premise that the baseline colonoscopy was performed with high quality (polyp and adenoma detection rates are considered the most important markers of quality) and adequate bowel preparation. If either of these are compromised, repeat colonoscopy should be performed at a shorter interval.

Screening and surveillance recommendations are made by several societies, including the United States Multi-society Task Force (MSTF). For average risk individuals, a 10-year interval is appropriate after negative findings on baseline colonoscopy, which should be done at age 50. Individuals with a first-degree relative with CRC or a high-risk adenoma diagnosed at an age younger than 60 years should start screening early and continue surveillance at a 5-year interval. The age at which to stop colonoscopy screening has been an area of ongoing controversy. After the age of 85 years, the United States Preventative Services Task Force (USPSTF) determined the risk of colonoscopy outweighed potential benefit and should be stopped. For patients ages 75 to 85, the USPSTF recommends individualization according to comorbidities and findings on prior colonoscopy.

Other screening modalities include virtual colonoscopy (i.e., computed tomography colonography) and stool DNA testing.

For patients with distal small hyperplastic polyps, the interval for surveillance endoscopy can remain at 10 years. If the baseline examination shows one to two tubular adenomas smaller than 10 mm with low-grade dysplasia, patients can undergo a repeat colonoscopy in 5 to 10 years because this represents a low-risk patient cohort. If the baseline examination demonstrates high-risk adenomas defined as (1) 3 to 10 adenomas, (2) one tubular adenoma 1 cm or larger in size, or (3) a polyp with villous features or high-grade dysplasia of any size, then the patient should have a repeat colonoscopy in 3 years. If a large sessile polyp is removed in a piecemeal fashion, consider repeat endoscopy in less than 1 year. If more than 10 adenomas are found, endoscopy should be repeated in less than 3 years, and genetic consultation should be advised. Finally, if a single SSA smaller than

TABLE 1: Current Guidelines for Colorectal Cancer Screening After Polypectomy

Risk Category	Recommended Colonoscopy Interval
1-2 small tubular adenomas	5-10 years
3-10 small adenomas *or* 1 adenoma >1 cm *or* A polyp with villous or high-grade dysplasia	3 years
>10 adenomas	<3 years
Sessile adenomas removed piecemeal	3-6 months

10 mm is found with no dysplasia, endoscopy should be repeated in 5 years, and if multiple SSAs, larger than 10 mm or dysplastic, are found, endoscopy should be repeated in 3 years (Table 1).

■ COLONOSCOPIC POLYPECTOMY

Advances in endoscopy have had a large impact on the management of colonic polyps. A variety of techniques are available to endoscopists for removal of polyps. These include hot and cold biopsy forceps, hot and cold snare excision, fulguration with argon plasma coagulation, piecemeal excision, endoscopic mucosal resection (EMR), and endoscopic submucosal dissection (ESD). Relative contraindications to colonoscopic polypectomy include anticoagulation therapy, bleeding diathesis, acute colitis, and evidence of invasive malignancy, such as central ulceration, a hard or fixed lesion, necrosis, or inability to raise the lesion with submucosal injection.

Biopsy Forceps Polypectomy

Cold forceps biopsy polypectomy is fast, easy, and inexpensive, but studies suggest that only diminutive polyps (smaller than 2 to 3 mm) are regularly completely excised with this technique. When larger polyps are removed in this fashion, there is a high rate of incomplete polypectomy. Jumbo forceps may be used as an alternative to the conventional forceps. Although the addition of electrocautery (hot biopsy technique) was once favored, it is associated with a higher complication rate and poor quality of the resected specimen, so it should not be used routinely.

Snare Polypectomy

Snare excision is preferred for polyps larger than 4 mm, achieving a higher complete polypectomy rate than biopsy forceps removal. The endoscopist advances a snare through a sheath, opens the snare (varying sizes available) to entrap the polyp, and slowly closes the snare around the base of the polyp, fracturing it from the surrounding tissue. The specimen then is suctioned through the scope channel or retrieved with a basket. It is generally accepted that cold snare is superior to the addition of electrocautery, but some pedunculated polyps are better treated with the hot technique. Lifting the lesion by injecting the submucosa is an effective technique to safely remove larger sessile lesions. Saline solution (with or without epinephrine or methylene blue) can be used to increase the distance between the mucosa and the muscularis propria.

Endoscopic Mucosal Resection and Endoscopic Submucosal Dissection Techniques

Large (more than 2 cm) and giant (more than 3 cm) polyps may require advanced techniques for removal. EMR and ESD techniques both involve a deeper plane of resection than a traditional polypectomy. EMR involves injecting the submucosal layer with saline or other suitable injectate under the lesion followed by snare excision in one or multiple pieces. The margins of seemingly incomplete polypectomy sites then can be treated with argon plasma coagulation. Predictors of recurrence after EMR are lesions larger than 4 cm, use of argon plasma coagulation, and piecemeal resection with more than six pieces. Most recurrences occur within the first few months of the procedure, so surveillance scoping should occur 3 to 6 months after the index procedure.

ESD offers benefits over EMR, primarily that the specimen is removed en bloc, allowing for optimal histologic evaluation. ESD involves injecting the submucosal layer at the edges of the lesion, incising the edge, and performing an exact dissection of the submucosal layer with endoscopic knives until the entire lesion is removed en bloc. Polypectomy with ESD is accomplished for 85% of lesions, and margins are negative 75% of the time. It is technically difficult and time intensive. Recurrence rates are lower with ESD, but EMR and ESD result in similar rates of colon preservation because most recurrences can be managed endoscopically.

It is important to tattoo the area adjacent to the polypectomy site with India ink anytime a large or suspicious polyp is removed because further endoscopic evaluation or surgical resection will be required.

Complications

Diagnostic colonoscopy is a safe procedure. Complications related to colonoscopic polypectomy are uncommon and typically minor. The risk of death is 1 in 14,000. Bleeding is the most frequent complication, occurring in 0.5% to 2.2% of patients. Bleeding may occur immediately or less likely in a delayed fashion. Immediate bleeding is treated with hemostatic clip placement or epinephrine injection. Most delayed postpolypectomy bleeds will stop spontaneously, but a few will require endoscopic injection or clipping. Colonic perforation occurs in 0.1% of patients and is related most often to use of electrocautery. Perforation rates are approximately 1% for EMR and 4% for ESD techniques. Conservative treatment is usually successful and includes inpatient observation, bowel rest, and intravenous antibiotics. If there are any signs of deterioration, the patient requires urgent laparoscopy or laparotomy. Perforations that are identified early with good tissue quality can be repaired primarily. Patients with significant peritoneal contamination will require a resection. Keep in mind that if a large polyp was removed and histopathology is pending, consideration for an oncologic resection should be entertained. Postpolypectomy syndrome occurs rarely in 0.3% of patients, most often when cautery has been used. Patients typically present 0 to 3 days after colonoscopy, with abdominal pain, tenderness, fever, and leukocytosis. On computerized tomographic scan, fat stranding typically is seen in the mesentery and the colonic wall is thickened at the polypectomy site, but there is no pneumoperitoneum. The symptoms are likely caused by a microperforation resulting in bacterial translocation. Patients should be treated with bowel rest, antibiotics, and close observation.

Large Polyps in the Rectum

Adenomatous polyps found in the distal rectum on endoscopy generally should prompt a surgical consultation. A transanal excision is preferred to polypectomy for very low lesions, and lesions more proximal can be resected with transanal endoscopic microsurgery or transanal minimally invasive surgery. These techniques offer a greater likelihood of removing the specimen in one piece, allowing the specimen to be fixed and sectioned to accurately determine depth of invasion, grade of differentiation, and margin status of a potential malignancy. This technique is also more likely to be definitive treatment for a high-risk adenoma or early stage malignancy.

Combined Endoscopic and Laparoscopic Surgery

A new series of techniques have been described and now used with increasing frequency for the removal of complex polyps that are not amenable to endoscopic resection. At least three variations are described in the literature, including laparoscopic-assisted EMR and ESD as well as laparoscopic full-thickness excision. In laparoscopic-assisted EMR and ESD, the endoscopist performs the polypectomy, while the surgeon watches with the laparoscope. The surgeon may invaginate the bowel to assist the endoscopist. The defect is examined closely by both proceduralists, and if there is a concern of perforation, the bowel is repaired via laparoscopy. In laparoscopic-assisted full-thickness resection, the endoscopist guides the surgeon to the location of the polyp, the surgeon performs a full-thickness excision of the lesion, and the surgeon closes the bowel wall defect with sutures or staples. A leak test can be performed with all of these techniques. Frozen section is used. Most patients are hospitalized until return of bowel function.

■ APPROACH TO THE MALIGNANT POLYP

Up to 5% of polyps contain a focus of invasive cancer, and the risk increases with increasing polyp size. A malignant polyp is defined as adenocarcinoma that invades into, but no deeper than, the submucosal layer of the bowel wall, representing a T1 CRC. This is an important distinction from carcinoma in situ or high-grade dysplasia, in which changes are confined to the mucosa and lamina propria, both of which are considered noninvasive but still require margins free of neoplastic tissue.

The depth of submucosal invasion found on polypectomy can be used to predict the risk of lymph node metastasis. Haggitt level also has been used but is less reliable. Submucosal invasion in a sessile polyp is classified as Sm1 (upper third), Sm2 (middle third), and Sm3 (lower third). Finding a sessile polyp with lower third (Sm3) invasion is an indication for a formal colonic resection. Other risk features associated with the presence of lymph node metastases include high tumor grade, extensive tumor budding, and lymphovascular invasion (Table 2). Without any of these features, the risk of lymph node metastasis is less than 1% but increases to 20% with a single feature and to 36% if two or more features are present.

Close surveillance after polypectomy can be used in the setting of all of the following features: a complete excision, a microscopic

TABLE 2: Pathologic Features of Malignant Polyps

Haggitt level	Submucosal invasion in polyp head (1), neck (2), stalk (3), and base (4) or submucosal invasion in a sessile polyp (4)
Submucosal invasion	Invasion in upper third of submucosa (Sm1), middle third (Sm2), or deep third (Sm3)
Tumor grade	Well, moderately, or poorly differentiated
Tumor budding	Absence or presence of clusters of malignant cells in the submucosa remote from the main site of submucosal invasion

Listed in order of escalating risk of lymph node metastasis.

margin greater than 2 mm, no lymphovascular or perineural invasion, moderately differentiated to well-differentiated histology, Haggitt level 1/2/3, and Sm1/2. Apart from this, a formal oncologic resection should be recommended in fit patients because of the high risk of lymph node metastasis.

SUGGESTED READINGS

Aarons CB, Shanmugan S, Bleier JI. Management of malignant colon polyps: current status and controversies. *World J Gastroenterol.* 2014;20:16178-16183.

Ahlquist DA. Multi-target stool DNA test: a new high bar for noninvasive screening. *Dig Dis Sci.* 2015;60:623-633.

Allen JI. Quality measures for colonoscopy: where should we be in 2015? *Curr Gastroenterol Rep.* 2015;17:10.

Bordacahar B, Barret M, Terris B, et al. Sessile serrated adenoma: from identification to resection. *Dig Liver Dis.* 2015;47:95-102.

Chandrasekhara V, Ginsberg GG. Endoscopic management of large sessile colonic polyps: getting the low down from down under. *Gastroenterology.* 2011;140:1867-1871.

Currie AC, Cahill R, Delaney CP, et al. International expert consensus on endpoints for full-thickness laparoendoscopic colonic excision. *Surg Endosc.* Jun 27, 2015.

Kahi CJ. How does the serrated polyp pathway alter CRC screening and surveillance? *Dig Dis Sci.* 2015;60:773-780.

Lieberman DA, Rex DK, Winawer SJ, et al. Guidelines for colonoscopy surveillance after screening and polypectomy: a consensus update by the US Multi-Society Task Force on Colorectal Cancer. *Gastroenterology.* 2012;143:844-857.

Nakajima K, Sharma SK, Lee SW, et al. Avoiding colorectal resection for polyps: is CELS the best method? *Surg Endosc.* Jun 20, 2015.

Rutter MD, Chattree A, Barbour JA, et al. British Society of Gastroenterology/Association of Coloproctologists of Great Britain and Ireland guidelines for the management of large non-pedunculated colorectal polyps. *Gut.* 2015;64:1847-1873.

Szylberg L, Janiczek M, Popiel A, et al. Serrated polyps and their alternative pathway to the colorectal cancer: a systematic review. *Gastroenterol Res Pract.* 2015;2015:573814.

MANAGEMENT OF PERITONEAL SURFACE MALIGNANCIES OF APPENDICEAL OR COLORECTAL ORIGIN

Jesus Esquivel, MD

Peritoneal surface malignancies encompass a series of gastrointestinal and gynecologic tumors that are characterized for their metastatic distribution throughout the abdomen and pelvis. This spread is not a random event but rather follows (1) the laws of intraperitoneal fluid flow, which is directed in a clockwise fashion toward the undersurfaces of the diaphragm; (2) the phagocytic activity of both the lesser and greater omentums as well as the appendix epiploicae of the sigmoid colon, and (3) gravity, with tumor deposits in the pelvis and pelvic organs. Therapeutic options for this particular group of patients have increased significantly over the last two decades, and patients that were considered candidates only for hospice care are now being evaluated by multidisciplinary teams with great success and long-term survival in selected cases. Cytoreductive surgery (CRS) that includes peritonectomy procedures to remove all visible disease coupled with hyperthermic intraperitoneal chemotherapy (HIPEC) to eradicate microscopic residual disease is playing an ever-increasing role with a significant impact on the quantity and quality of life on these patients. Systemic chemotherapy continues to have better response rates and also has increased the survival in those patients who have unresectable metastatic disease. However, selection criteria for treatment type and sequence of currently available therapies continue to represent an unmet need in oncology because there is no established nonsurgical stratifying parameter that helps to guide the order and duration of current therapies. In this chapter, I focus on peritoneal surface malignancies of colorectal cancer and appendiceal origin and review some proposed clinical pathways that will provide assistance in the management of these patients from the time of the diagnosis of their peritoneal metastases. In addition, I review what to do in the operating room when you encounter peritoneal metastases during an elective operation.

■ APPENDIX CANCER FOUND DURING A LAPAROSCOPIC APPENDECTOMY

Mucinous appendiceal neoplasms can manifest in a variety of ways. An ovarian mass is the most common presentation in female patients. In advanced cases with extensive pseudomyxoma peritonei (PMP), an increasing abdominal girth constitutes a frequent mode of presentation. Acute appendicitis also constitutes a frequent presentation in male and female patients. Routinely, these patients will go to the operating room for a laparoscopic appendectomy, and sometimes a noninfectious process will be identified (Figure 1). If the appendectomy can be performed laparoscopically and the appendiceal tumor does not involve the base of the cecum, then the surgeon should perform an appendectomy. In addition, it is extremely important for the surgeon to evaluate all abdominopelvic regions as described in Box 1 because frequently other sites of disease can be identified even if they were not seen in a preoperative computed tomography (CT) scan (Figure 2). A generous biopsy of one or two of the peritoneal implants should be performed as well. Both positive and negative findings should be included in the operative note. This will assist the peritoneal surface malignancy surgeon to determine the next step and to have a good estimate of the possibility of a complete cytoreduction without having to repeat the laparoscopic examination. Further management will depend on three important factors: (1) the nature of the primary tumor (low grade vs high grade), (2) whether

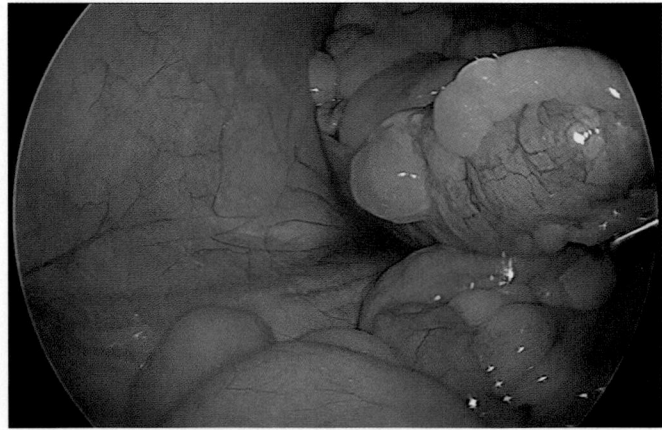

FIGURE 1 Ruptured mucinous appendiceal neoplasm identified during a laparoscopy for suspected acute appendicitis.

BOX 1: Abdominopelvic Regions That Must Be Evaluated and Reported When Peritoneal Metastases Are Discovered During an Elective Operation

1. Undersurface of the right and left hemidiaphragms
2. Lesser omentum and porta hepatis
3. Proximal small bowel
4. Distal small bowel
5. Pelvic peritoneum and pelvic organs

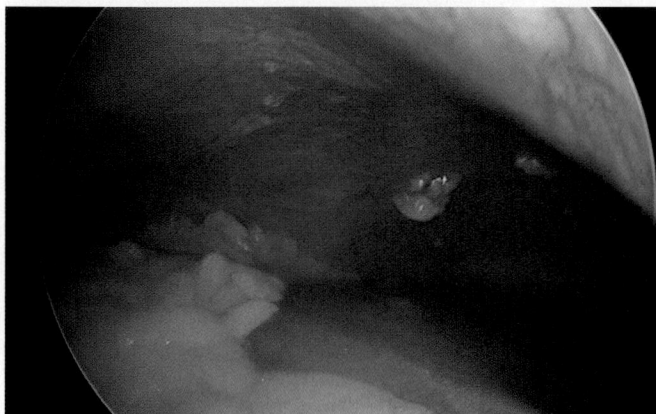

FIGURE 2 Mucinous deposits on the undersurface of the right hemidiaphragm.

the primary tumor is ruptured, and (3) the burden of disease. Mucinous appendiceal neoplasms, without invasion and nonruptured, would not require additional therapy after the appendectomy. High-grade tumors with significant involvement of the small bowel may benefit from systemic therapy first and then a repeat laparoscopy; low-grade tumors such as PMP with low burden of disease even can be treated with a laparoscopic CRS and HIPEC.

◼ PERITONEAL SURFACE DISEASE SEVERITY SCORE IN MUCINOUS APPENDICEAL NEOPLASMS

Recently, a new staging classification for mucinous appendiceal neoplasms with or without peritoneal dissemination and based on a pathologic evaluation of the primary tumor (G), histologic description of their peritoneal disease (P), and burden of disease (E), has been reported as the Peritoneal Surface Disease Severity Score (PSDSS) in 229 patients to assist with the management of these patients (Table 1).

Patients' characteristics included 135 (59%) females and 94 (41%) males. The median age was 52 years (range 21 to 79). One hundred and seventy-three patients underwent CRS and HIPEC (75.5%). Mean follow-up of all 229 patients was 34.6 months. There were 19 (8.3%), 67 (29.3%), 59 (25.8%), 43 (18.8%), and 41 (17.9%) patients with PSDSS 0, I, II, III, and IV, respectively.

Primary Appendiceal Neoplasm (G)

Five pathologic features were analyzed in each primary tumor with a slight modification of the original description by Pai and colleagues: (a) cytologic grade (low or high), (b) architecture (simple or complex), (c) periappendiceal mucin (present or absent), (d) extra-appendiceal epithelium (present or absent), (e) invasion (present or absent) (Box 2).

TABLE 1: PSDSS Stage of Mucinous Appendiceal Neoplasm

Stages		G	P	E
0		1-3	0	0
I	A	2-3	1-2	1-2
	B	4-5	0	0
II	A	4	1-2	1-2
	B	2-3	1-2	3
	C	4	3	1-2
III	A	5	Any	1
	B	4	Any	3
IV		5	Any	2-3

PSDSS, Peritoneal Surface Disease Severity Score.

Evaluation of the Peritoneal Dissemination (P)

This evaluation consists primarily of describing the histopathologic features of the peritoneal implants, regardless of the primary appendiceal neoplasm. Five groups were classified (Box 3).

Extent of Peritoneal Dissemination (E)

This is the volume of tumor burden assessed by the Peritoneal Cancer Index (PCI); the PCI could be the one at the time of surgery or by CT scan in those patients without surgery (Box 4).

◼ SURVIVAL IN 210 PATIENTS WITH MUCINOUS APPENDICEAL NEOPLASMS

There were no operative mortalities in the entire cohort of patients having surgery with or without HIPEC. Median overall survival (OS) of the 173 patients in the CRS and HIPEC group was 80.0 months (95% CI: 58.1-NR) and in 37 patients in the no-HIPEC group was 25.7 months (95% CI: 9.0-NR) ($P < 0.001$). The rate of 3-year and 5-year OS was 73% and 57% in the CRS and HIPEC group and 43% and 43% in the no-HIPEC group, respectively. The 19 patients with PSDSS 0 were excluded from the survival analysis of the no-HIPEC group because they were never considered candidates for CRS and HIPEC. At a mean follow-up of 18.1 months, all 19 patients were alive and free of disease. All 67 patients (55 in the CRS and HIPEC group and 12 in the no-HIPEC group) with PSDSS I are alive. Median survival for the 59 patients (56 in the CRS and HIPEC group and 3 in the no-HIPEC group) with a PSDSS II has not been reached (NR). Median survival of 39 patients with CRS and HIPEC and 4 patients in the no-HIPEC group with PSDSS III were 39.5 months (95% CI: 30.1-58.1) and not reached, respectively ($P = 0.008$). Median survival of 23 patients with CRS and HIPEC and 18 patients in the no-HIPEC group with PSDSS IV were 25.5 months (95% CI: 12.8-31.4) and 9.0 months (95% CI: 4.1-23.3), respectively ($P = 0.045$) (Table 2).

When the 173 patients undergoing CRS and HIPEC were stratified by the severity of their peritoneal disease (PSDSS), 5-year OS was 100%, 79.2%, 23.3%, and 6.9% in PSDSS I, II, III, and IV, respectively ($P < 0.001$) (Figure 3).

A univariate and multivariate analysis was performed on the survival of patients undergoing CRS and HIPEC. With the univariate analysis, significant difference in survival was associated with female sex versus male sex ($P < 0.001$); PSDSS Stage I, II, III, or IV $P < 0.001$; PSDSS groups I versus II $P = 0.015$, PSDSS groups III versus IV $P = 0.003$ and PSDSS groups I/II vs. III/IV $P < 0.001$; primary appendiceal neoplasm group (G) (G 2-3 vs G 4-5) $P < 0.001$; type of peritoneal dissemination (P) (P 1-2 vs P 3-4) $P < 0.001$ and tumor burden (E) 1, 2, or 3 $P < 0.001$. When these factors were re-examined in the

BOX 2: Primary Appendiceal Neoplasm (G)

Pathologic Criteria for Invasion

Unequivocal involvement of appendiceal wall, subserosal
  peritoneum, or omental fat
Destructive pattern of invasion with or without desmoplasia
Irregular/haphazard invasion of neoplastic glands
Complex glandular architecture
Cytologic atypia

   On the basis of evaluation of these features, five groups were
created to evaluate the primary tumor.

Group I Mucinous Appendiceal Neoplasm; Nonruptured

Cytologic grade: Low
Architecture: Simple
Periappendiceal mucin: Absent
Extra-appendiceal epithelium: Absent
Invasion: Absent

Group 2 Mucinous Appendiceal Neoplasm, Ruptured; LOW Risk of Recurrence

Cytologic grade: Low
Architecture: Simple
Periappendiceal mucin: Present or absent
Extra-appendiceal epithelium: Absent
Invasion: Absent

Group 3 Mucinous Appendiceal Neoplasm, HIGH Risk of Recurrence

Cytologic grade: Low
Architecture: Primarily simple/focally complex in the absence of
  invasion
Periappendiceal mucin: Present
Extra-appendiceal epithelium: Present
Invasion: Absent

Group 4 Low-Grade Mucinous Carcinoma

Cytologic grade: Low
Architecture: Simple, well to moderate differentiated, mucinous
  carcinoma (WHO Grades 1-2)
Periappendiceal mucin: Present or absent
Extra-appendiceal epithelium: Present or absent
Invasion: Present

Group 5 High-Grade Mucinous Carcinoma

Cytologic grade: High
Architecture: Complex, poorly differentiated/signet ring
  mucinous carcinoma (WHO Grades 3-4). Also includes goblet
  cell carcinoids
Periappendiceal mucin: Present or absent
Extra-appendiceal epithelium: Present or absent
Invasion: Present

WHO, World Health Organization.

BOX 3: Peritoneal Dissemination (P)

P 0: No peritoneal dissemination identified.
P 1: Only extracellular mucin; no tumor of any type identified.
P 2: In addition to extracellular mucin, there will be epithelial
  cells identified. These cells could consist of bland-looking
  epithelial cells, adenomatous epithelium with mild atypia, or
  even dysplastic adenomatous epithelium. However, there will
  be no signs of invasion.
P 3: Tumor identified, well or focally moderately differentiated
  adenocarcinoma, with invasion.
P 4: Tumor identified, poorly differentiated or signet ring cell
  adenocarcinoma, with invasion.

BOX 4: Peritoneal Dissemination (E)

E0: No peritoneal dissemination identified by imaging studies
  and/or during surgery
E1: Low volume. PCI of 10 or less
E2: Moderate volume. PCI more than 10 but less than 20
E3: High volume. PCI greater than 20

TABLE 2: Median Overall Survival in No-HIPEC and HIPEC Group

	N	Median Survival* (95% CI)	P Value†
PSDSS (I-IV)	210		<0.001
-HIPEC	173	80.0 (58.1-NR)	
-NO HIPEC	37	25.7 (9.0-NR)	
PSDSS I	67		
-HIPEC	55	NR	
-NO HIPEC	12	NR	
PSDSS II	59		0.005
-HIPEC	56	NR	
-NO HIPEC	3	NR	
PSDSS III	43		0.008
-HIPEC	39	39.5 (30.1-58.1)	
-NO HIPEC	4	NR (2.9-NR)	
PSDSS IV	41		0.045
-HIPEC	23	25.5 (12.8-31.4)	
-NO HIPEC	18	9.0 (4.1-23.3)	

*Months.

†*P*-value based on log-rank test.

CI, Confidence interval; *HIPEC,* Hyperthermic intraperitoneal
chemotherapy; *PSDSS,* Peritoneal Surface Disease Severity Score; *NR,* not
reported.

multivariate analysis sex (HR female vs male 0.44 (95% CI: 0.23-
0.82) and PSDSS stage (I, II, III, or IV) (HR I vs IV NR, HR II vs IV
0.20 (95% CI: 0.05-0.81), HR III versus IV 0.31 (95% CI: 0.15-0.65)
($P = 0.005$) were identified as independent predictors of survival
(Table 3).

■ PERITONEAL METASTASES FOUND DURING AN ELECTIVE LAPAROSCOPIC OR OPEN COLON RESECTION

About 8% of the near 150,000 new cases of colorectal cancer in the
United States will have peritoneal metastases at the time of
the original diagnosis. Many of them also will have other sites of
hematogenous dissemination and will be diagnosed with current
imaging modalities such as CT scan, magnetic resonance imaging,
and/or positron emission tomography scans. A few of these patients
will go to the operating room, and this will be the first evidence of
peritoneal metastases. What to do when this situation is encountered
represents a dilemma for many reasons, but the strategy can be
straightforward. Proceed with the intended colorectal resection *only*
if there is evidence of perforation, acute colonic obstruction, or
uncontrolled bleeding. These latter two situations are extremely rare.
Again, as in those patients with mucinous appendiceal metastases, it
is extremely important to perform a biopsy on specimens from a few
of them and describe the intraoperative findings as in Box 1.

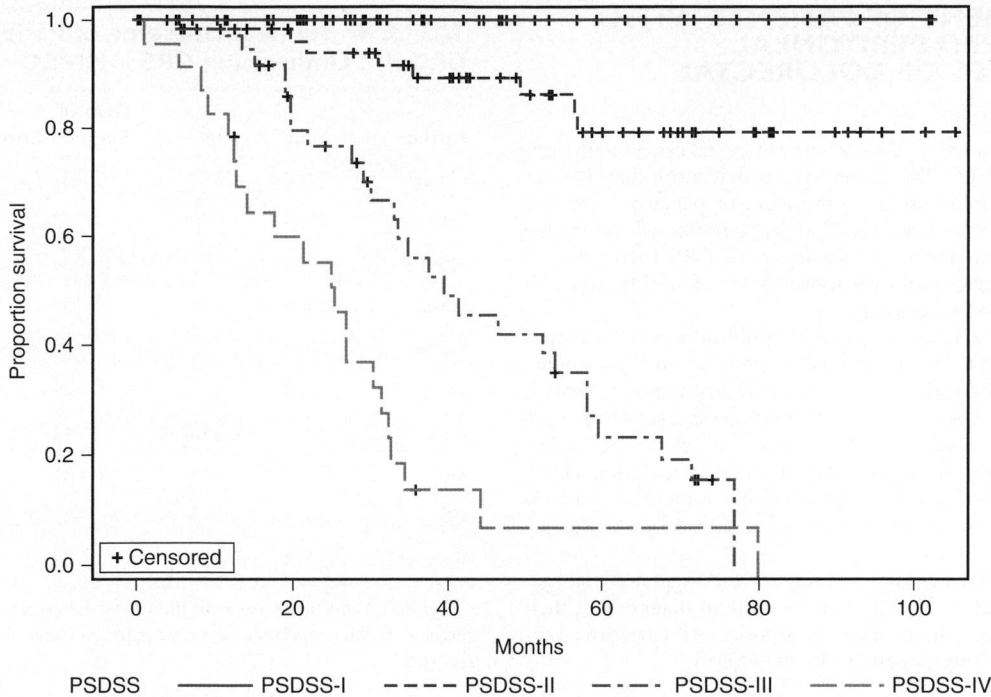

FIGURE 3 Survival analysis in patients with cytoreductive surgery and hyperthermic intraperitoneal chemotherapy classified by Peritoneal Surface Disease Severity Score.

TABLE 3: Univariate and Multivariate Analysis of Factors Associated With Survival in HIPEC Group

| Characteristic | N | Univariate | | Multivariate | |
		Median Survival* (95% CI)	P Value (1)	HR (95% CI)	P Value (2)
Age (years)			0.368		0.328
<50	72	67.8 (44.2-NR)			
50-70	90	NR (59.7-NR)			
>70	11	57.0 (27.6-NR)			
Sex			<0.001		0.010
F	100	NR (77.1-NR)		0.44 (0.23-0.82)	
M	73	49.5 (33.0-80.0)			
PSDSS			<0.001		0.005
Stage I	55	NR (NR-NR)		NR (NR-NR)	
Stage II	56	NR (NR-NR)		0.20 (0.05-0.81)	
Stage III	39	39.5 (30.1-58.1)		0.31 (0.15-0.65)	
Stage IV	23	25.5 (12.8-31.4)			
PSDSS			<0.001		
Stages I-II	111	NR (NR-NR)			
Stages III-IV	62	32.4 (26.9-37.6)			
Group (G)			<0.001		0.994
2-3	86	NR (NR-NR)			
4-6	87	39.5 (32.4-58.1)			
Peritoneal dissemination (P)			<0.001		0.993
1-2	94	NR (NR-NR)			
3-4	72	33.5 (29.1-41.4)			
Tumor burden (E)			<0.001		0.115
1	46	NR (77.1-NR)			
2	38	NR (56.4-NR)			
3	82	53.9 (34.9-71.5)			

*Months.

CI, Confidence interval; HIPEC, hyperthermic intraperitoneal chemotherapy; HR, hazard ratio; NR, not reported.

■ MANAGEMENT OF PATIENTS WITH ESTABLISHED PERITONEAL METASTASES OF COLORECTAL ORIGIN

An analysis of treatment of patients with colorectal cancer with peritoneal metastases (CRC-PM) demonstrates that more than 90% of patients will be treated with a combination of palliative cytotoxic chemotherapy and a biologic agent, and about 5% will be treated with a combined modality that incorporates CRS to remove all visible metastatic disease to the peritoneal cavity and HIPEC to eradicate microscopic residual disease.

Table 4 includes a summary of recent publications from centers around the world that include at least 50 patients on their studies, treated with CRS and HIPEC. Median survival of almost 3 years is very common with a few studies reporting median survivals of 40 plus months, with median 5-year survival of about 30%. The common denominator for a good long-term result includes achieving a complete cytoreduction and avoiding surgery in patients with large tumor burden and poorly differentiated/signet ring cell histologies.

Figure 4 represents a clinical pathway for the suggested management of patients with CRC-PM from the time of diagnosis of their peritoneal metastases. The pathway incorporates all currently available therapies and stratifies patients by the PSDSS.

TABLE 4: Survival Outcome of Patients With CRC-PM Undergoing CRS + HIPEC

Author	Year	N	Overall Survival (mo)	Five-Year Survival (%)
Glehen	2004	377	32	40
Da Silva	2006	70	33	32
Shen	2008	121	34	26
Chua	2009	54	33	NR
Franko	2010	67	34	26
Elias	2010	523	32	30
Quenet	2011	146	41	42
Ung	2013	211	47	42
Chua	2013	722	33	43
Esquivel	2014	705	41	NR

CRC-PM, Colorectal cancer with peritoneal metastases; *CRS*, cytoreductive surgery; *HIPEC*, hyperthermic intraperitoneal chemotherapy; *NR*, not reported.

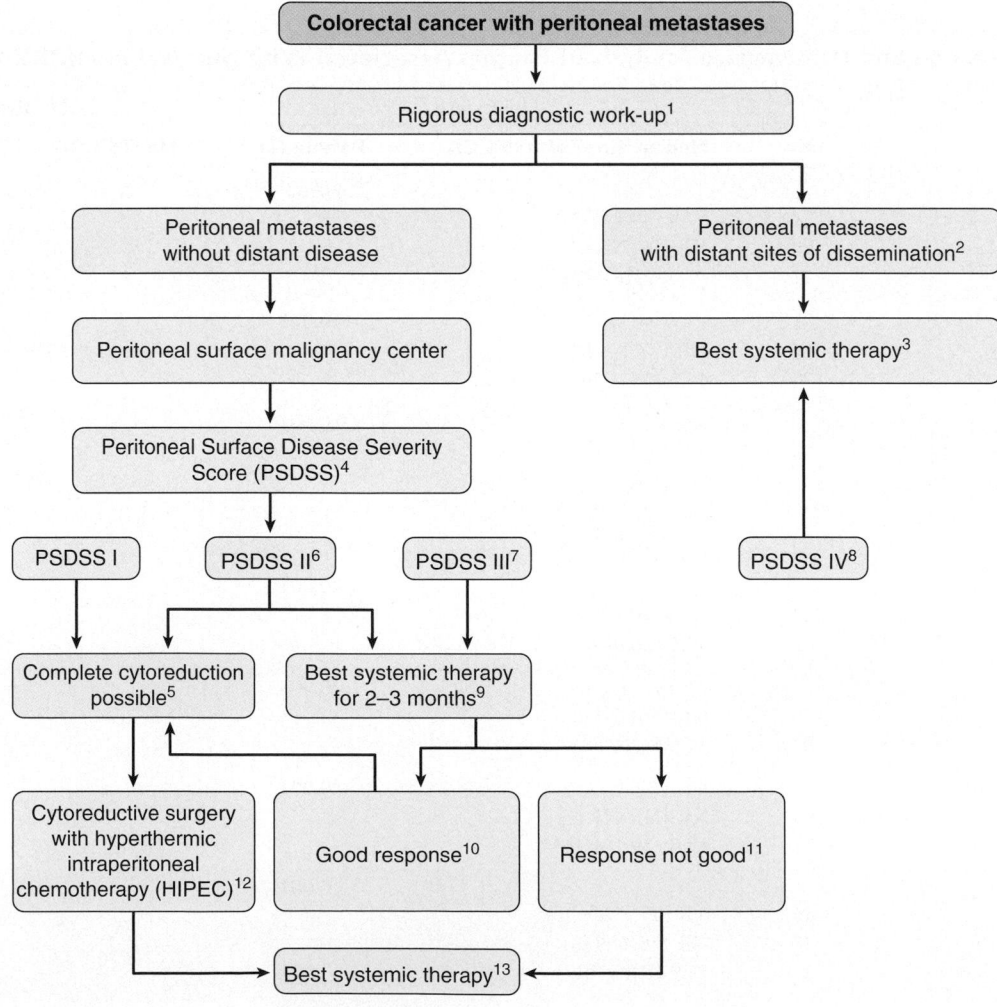

FIGURE 4 Clinical pathway for the management of peritoneal surface malignancies of colorectal origin.

1. This should include a recent colonoscopy. A CT scan of the chest, abdomen, and pelvis with maximum oral and intravenous contrast. A PET scan should be done in those patients in whom there is evidence or suggestion of hematogenous dissemination on the CT scan. K-ras status should be determined in all patients.

2. Patients with peritoneal metastases and liver or lung metastases should be referred to a medical oncologist for systemic therapy. Patients with three or fewer small, liver metastases can be considered for cytoreductive surgery and HIPEC if they had a good response to the first 3 months of systemic therapy.

3. Best systemic therapy includes a combination of cytotoxic chemotherapy and biological agents. Cetuximab or Panitumumab should be considered in those patients who could potentially become surgical candidates and are K-ras wild type.

4. The Peritoneal Surface Disease Severity Score (PSDSS) was introduced in an attempt to stratify patients with colorectal cancer with peritoneal metastases according to four tiers of estimated disease severity based on a 3-point scale that includes: (1) symptoms, (2) extent of peritoneal dissemination, and (3) primary tumor histology.

Peritoneal Surface Disease Severity Score (PSDSS) of Colorectal Cancer With Peritoneal Metastases

Clinical		CT- PCI		Histology	
No symptoms	0	PCI < 10 (Low)	1	G1 G2 N- L- V-	1
Mild symptoms	1	PCI 10-20 (Medium)	3	G2 N+ and/or L+ and/or V+	3
Severe symptoms	6	PCI > 20 (High)	7	G3 signet ring	9

Score	Stage
2-3	Stage I
4-7	Stage II
8-10	Stage III
>10	Stage IV

Clinical Symptoms:

Mild symptoms   = weight loss < 10% of body weight
                                Mild abdominal pain, some ascites

Severe symptoms = weight loss > 10% of body weight
                                unremitting pain, bowel obstruction, symptomatic ascites

Peritoneal Cancer Index (PCI)

By imaging (CT, PET, MRI) or exploration (laparoscopy or evaluation at time of first operation [in synchronous peritoneal carcinomatosis])

Histology

G 1: Well differentiated, G 2: Moderately differentiated, G 3: Poorly differentiated
N: Lymph nodes   L: Lymphovascular invasion   V: Vascular invasion

5. Variables associated with increased chances of having a complete cytoreduction:

Complete cytoreduction means that no macroscopic residual disease was left after the operative procedure. The following are clinical and radiographic variables that are usually associated with increase chances of achieving a complete removal of all tumor greater than 2.5 mm.

FIGURE 4, cont'd

ECOG Performance status 2 or less
No evidence of extra-abdominal disease
Up to three small, resectable parenchymal hepatic metastases
No evidence of biliary obstruction
No evidence of ureteral obstruction
No evidence of intestinal obstruction at more than one site
Small bowel involvement: No evidence of gross disease in the mesentery with several segmental sites of partial obstruction.
Small volume disease in the gastro hepatic ligament

6. PSDSS II patients that have a low CT-PCI (PCI < 10) and are good candidates for a complete cytoreduction can go directly to surgery and have systemic therapy after.

7. PSDSS III have a very low chance of having an upfront complete cytoreduction and therefore should have best systemic therapy first. Re-staging and re-evaluation should be done after 2 or 3 months of systemic therapy.

8. PSDSS IV patients do not have a good long-term outcome even when achieving a complete cytoreduction. These patients should have best systemic therapy first and should have cytoreductive surgery and HIPEC under a clinical protocol.

9. Best systemic therapy includes a combination of cytotoxic chemotherapy and biologic agents. Consider cetuximab or panitumumab in those patients who are K-ras wild type. If using bevacizumab, it appears to be prudent to hold the bevacizumab after Cycle #5 and use only the cytotoxic agents for Cycle #6.

10. The three parameters evaluated to judge the response to the "neo-adjuvant" systemic therapy include: (a) performance status, (b) CEA, and (c) imaging studies. Improvement of at least one of these parameters with the other two remaining unchanged should be the minimum requirement to consider a response as good. Patients with PSDSS II and III, who had a good response, should be evaluated for cytoreductive surgery and HIPEC.

11. Worsening of any of these three parameters while receiving systemic therapy should be considered as not having a good response. In this situation, systemic therapy should be continued, and changing the cytotoxic and/or biologic regimen should be considered.

12. American Society of Peritoneal Surface Malignancices Standardized HIPEC delivery in patients with colorectal cancer with peritoneal dissemination

1. HIPEC Method: Closed
2. Drug: Mitomycin C
3. Dosage: 40 mg
4. Timing of drug delivery: 30 mg at time Zero; 10 mg at 60 minutes
5. Volume of perfusate: 3 L
6. Inflow temperature: 42° Celsius
7. Duration of perfusion: 90 minutes

13. Patients with a PSDSS I that had cytoreductive surgery and HIPEC should receive standard best systemic therapy. Patients with a PSDSS of II or III that had a poor response to their first 3 months of systemic therapy and then have a good response after changing systemic agents should be considered for cytoreductive surgery and HIPEC.

FIGURE 4, cont'd

Prodige 7

Prodige 7 is a prospective randomized multicenter phase III trial by the French group, in which patients with colorectal cancer and limited peritoneal dissemination were taken to the operating room. The study was designed to evaluate what is the added benefit of HIPEC to a complete CRS. If a complete CRS was achieved, the patients were randomized in the operating room to either receive or not receive HIPEC. This study finished accrual at the end of 2013, and I am anxiously awaiting the results. In this study, HIPEC was delivered with oxaliplatin (460 mg/m²) in 2 L/m² of dextrose 5% over 30 minutes at a minimal temperature of 42° C. One hour before the HIPEC, 20 mg/m² of leucovorin and 400 mg/m² of 5-fluorouracil were given intravenously.

Outcomes After Complete Cytoreductive Surgery and Systemic Therapy Only

Recently, Desoineux and colleagues recognized that although the efficacy of surgery in patients with CRC-PM has been

demonstrated, the evidence to support the role of HIPEC is less certain. To address this issue, they reported the OS, progression-free survival (PFS), and morbidity on 50 consecutively included patients treated for CRC-PM with complete CRS and systemic chemotherapy only.

The median PCI was 8 (range 1 to 24); 23 three patients had liver or lung metastases (LLM); 22 patients had synchronous metastases. Median follow-up was 62.5 months (95% CI: 45.4-81.3) and median survival was 32.4 months (95% CI: 21.5-41.7). The 3-year and 5-year OS were 45.5% (95% CI: 0.31-0.59) and 29.64% (95% CI: 0.17-0.44), respectively. Presence of LLMs with peritoneal metastases was significantly associated with poorer prognosis, with survival at 5 years of 13.95% (95% CI: 2.9-33.6) versus 43.87% (95% CI: 22.2-63.7) when no liver or lung metastases were present ($P = 0.018$). Median PFS was 9.5 months (95% CI: 6.2-11.1).

They concluded that with an equivalent PCI range and despite one of the highest rates of LLM in the literature, their survival data of CRS + systemic chemotherapy only compare well with results reported after additional HIPEC. The therapy was well tolerated with acceptable morbidity without any mortality.

■ CONCLUSION

At the present time, much of our efforts regarding the treatment of patients with peritoneal surface malignancies must be directed at trying to establish precise pretreatment-stratifying parameters that will help in the evaluation of the role of all currently available therapies and will assist in identifying relative and absolute prognostic indicators that can be the basis of prospective trials.

Currently, genomic profile analysis only can help in the identification of patients with tumors that are "bad actors," but hopefully in the near future it will help in the treatment of patients with more targeted therapies. The future goal should be to increase the resectability of patients with peritoneal surface malignancies through the improvement of selection criteria and early referrals and through the use of systemic therapies in a neoadjuvant setting in those patients with more aggressive diseases. Better outcomes will be tied to therapies that help to maintain the complete surgical response and whether that includes HIPEC and/or more systemic therapies will have to be determined.

SUGGESTED READINGS

Desoineux G, Maziere C, Vara J, et al. Cytoreductive surgery of colorectal peritoneal metastases: outcomes after complete cytoreductive surgery and systemic chemotherapy only. *PLoS ONE*. 2015;10:1-12.

Esquivel J, Averbach A. Laparoscopic cytoreductive surgery and HIPEC in patients with limited pseudomyxoma peritonei of appendiceal origin. *Gastroenterol Res Pract*. 2012;98124.

Esquivel J, Garcia SS, Hicken W, et al. Evaluation of a new staging classification and a Peritoneal Surface Disease Severity Score (PSDSS) in 229 patients with mucinous appendiceal neoplasms with or without peritoneal dissemination. *J Surg Oncol*. 2014;110:656-660.

Esquivel J, Lowy A, Markman M, et al. The American Society of Peritoneal Surface Malignancies (ASPSM) Multiinstitution Evaluation of the Peritoneal Surface Disease Severity Score (PSDSS) in 1,013 Patients with Colorectal Cancer with Peritoneal Carcinomatosis. *Ann Surg Oncol*. 2014; 21:4195-4201.

Pelz O, Stojadinovic A, Nissan A, et al. Evaluation of a Peritoneal Surface Disease Severity Score in patients with colon cancer and peritoneal dissemination. *J Surg Oncol*. 2009;99:9-15.

THE MANAGEMENT OF ACUTE APPENDICITIS

Aqsa Shakoor, MD, and Walter Pegoli, Jr., MD

Appendicitis remains one of the most common disease conditions under the purview of the general surgeon. It has a lifetime risk of 7%, with the highest incidence in boys aged 10 to 14 years and girls aged 15 to 19 years. There are 250,000 appendectomies performed each year. Abraham Grooves performed the first elective appendectomy more than 130 years ago in 1883. This was followed by Reginald Fitz's seminal publication, *Perforating Inflammation of the Vermiform Appendix* in 1886, advocating for early appendectomy for appendicitis. Since the late 1800s the principles for diagnosing and treating appendicitis have been examined and refined. Despite improving diagnostic technology, there is still no single test or clinical finding that is 100% reliable. Given the consequences of missing true appendicitis, and the potential quality adjusted life years lost to a curable disease with highest incidence in teenagers, the surgical community has accepted a negative appendectomy rate of 5% to 15%. In this chapter, we elucidate the pathophysiology, diagnostic workup, and the evolving management paradigm of this disease process.

■ ANATOMY AND PATHOPHYSIOLOGY

The appendix, or vermiform (Latin for *worm shaped*) appendix, is an immunologic organ that plays an active role in the secretion of immunoglobulins, especially IgA. It develops as a protuberance off the terminal cecum, landmarked by the convergence of the three taenia coli. During antenatal and postnatal development, the appendix is pushed ahead of the cecum until the cecum becomes fixed to the right lower quadrant. During this process, the appendix adopts various positions, ostensibly at random, as noted in Figure 1. Although the base of the appendix is found reliably in the proximity of the ileocecal valve, the tip may be found in any number of recesses. The most common are retrocecal, retroileal, preileal, and pelvic.

The average length of the appendix is 9 cm in adults, but it may vary from 5 to 35 cm. The upper limit of normal for the transverse diameter is approximately 6 mm; however, it may be larger in the elderly population. The appendiceal artery, a branch of the ileocolic artery, provides the main blood supply to the organ.

A number of causes have been proposed for appendicitis. The most common is mechanical obstruction with a fecalith or an appendicolith. Lymphoid hyperplasia, parasitic infections, and neoplasm are less common causes. Given that the base of the appendix is relatively narrow compared with its luminal diameter and length, any proximal obstruction behaves like a closed loop obstruction. This is compounded by the fact that the luminal capacity of a normal appendix at atmospheric pressures is essentially zero. Increasing its volume to just 0.5 mL results in an increase in the intraluminal pressure by 60 cm of water.

Obstruction of the lumen results in a cycle of progressive inflammation and pressure by not only bacterial overgrowth but also ongoing mucosal secretions. This increased intraluminal pressure and subsequent distension of the appendix results in the stretch of visceral afferent nerve fibers resulting in vague epigastric or periumbilical pain experienced by the patient. As outflow obstruction worsens, it leads first to venous and lymphatic congestion followed by progressive obstruction of arterial inflow. This may be seen as infarcts along the antimesenteric border with resultant mucosal ischemia. Once the inflammation involves the appendiceal serosa, it then extends to the surrounding parietal peritoneum. By then, pain is localized to the right lower quadrant. Perforation usually occurs just beyond the point of obstruction, where the pressure is highest and the blood supply most limited.

The most commonly isolated bacteria associated in acute appendicitis are *E. coli*, *Bacteroides fragilis*, *Klebsiella pneumonia*, *Streptococcus*, *Enterococcus*, and *Pseudomonas aeruginosa*. *E. coli* and *Bacteroides* spp. are isolated from almost all perforated or gangrenous appendices. Appropriate antibiotic selection is essential for prophylaxis of surgical site infections or alternately for patients in whom nonoperative management is elected.

■ CLINICAL PRESENTATION AND DIAGNOSTIC MODALITIES

History and Physical Examination

In most cases, the diagnosis of acute appendicitis depends heavily on the clinical presentation. Patients typically complain of anorexia followed by epigastric or periumbilical abdominal pain. This may be followed by emesis; however, if emesis precedes abdominal pain, the diagnosis of appendicitis should be questioned. The pain typically reaches its peak at 4 hours and migrates from the periumbilical region to the right lower quadrant.

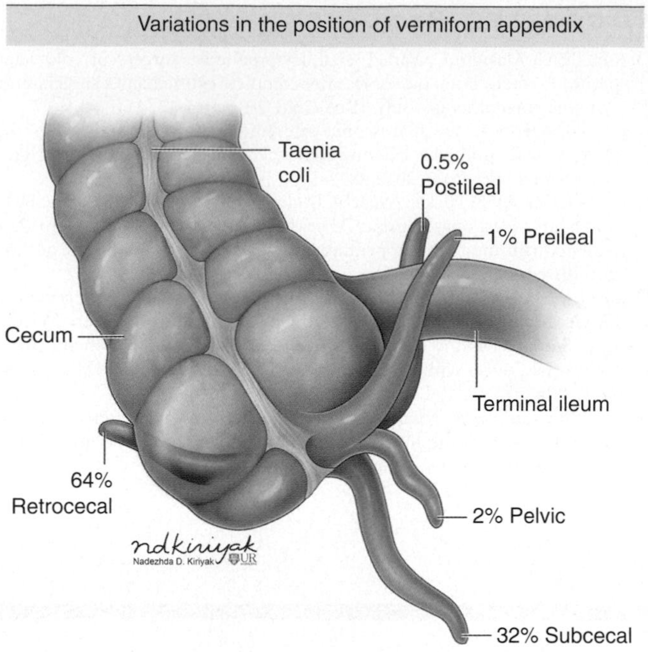

FIGURE I Variations in the position of the vermiform appendix.

The physical findings will be dictated by the location of the appendiceal tip and the degree of inflammation. The classic right lower quadrant pain, maximal at McBurney's point, correlates with an anterior appendix. Associated findings include guarding and rebound tenderness. The Rovsing's sign is indicative of localized peritoneal irritation and is elicited when palpation of the left lower quadrant results in pain in the right lower quadrant. A pelvic appendiceal tip is examined best by the obturator sign. This finding is elicited by positioning the patient supine and performing passive internal rotation of the flexed right thigh. A retrocecal appendix is associated with the psoas sign, which indicates a focus of inflammation in proximity to the muscle. The patient is positioned on the left side, and the right thigh is extended, stretching the iliopsoas muscle. The test is positive if this maneuver elicits pain.

Laboratory Examination

Common laboratory abnormalities include leukocytosis with or without a left shift and an elevated C-reactive protein (CRP) level. Although the diagnostic value of these inflammatory markers has been extensively studied, no consensus has been reached. One study has quoted a white blood cell count (WBC) cut-off of at least 9000 cells/mm^3 with a resultant reduction of negative appendectomy rates by 77%. However, many have approached heavy reliance on laboratory markers with skepticism. In general, a normal leukocyte count and CRP makes the diagnosis very unlikely, and a high WBC of more than 20,000 cells/mm^3 with an elevated CRP raises the index of suspicion.

Diagnostic Imaging

The age, body habitus, and gender of the patient guide the clinician on which imaging modality to use. Ultrasound (US) is considered the initial imaging study of choice in the pediatric population, females of childbearing age, and patients with a thin body habitus. It has been shown to have an overall sensitivity of 0.86 and specificity of 0.81. Pertinent findings for appendicitis include a distended, noncompressible appendix with an at least 6 mm diameter as noted in Figure 2. Color Doppler imaging can demonstrate hypervascularity in the wall of an inflamed appendix. The main limitations of this

modality are operator variability and limited visualization in obese patients and those with overlying bowel gas.

Compared with US imaging, computed tomography (CT) imaging has an overall sensitivity of 0.94 and specificity of 0.95. Given the higher sensitivity of CT scans, it is considered the favored imaging modality in cases of suspected perforated appendicitis or a retrocecal appendix or in obese patients or in those with severe abdominal pain with intolerance to graded compression. Pertinent findings on CT include a distended fluid-filled appendix, often with periappendiceal fat stranding as seen in Figure 3. Circumferential wall enhancement may be seen with contrast administration. The findings associated with complicated appendicitis are well visualized on CT.

Specific imaging considerations may be required in the evaluation of obese pediatric patients and pregnant patients. The combination of a rising rate of obesity in children and increasing frequency of appendicitis is a significant concern for surgeons. As noted earlier, obesity limits the utility of ultrasound. Given the risks of radiation exposure, arguments for foregoing a CT scan in patients with a high clinical suspicion, but a nondiagnostic US, have been proposed. When the diagnosis remains uncertain after an US, magnetic resonance imaging (MRI) has been shown to be equivalent to a CT scan as a diagnostic imaging modality and is a viable alternative.

In the pregnant patient, unruptured appendicitis is associated with 3% to 5% fetal loss as compared with 20% to 25% fetal loss with ruptured appendicitis. US with graded compression is the imaging study of choice in the first trimester. In later stages of pregnancy, the ability to visualize the appendix is severely limited. In one study, the ultrasound was unable to detect the appendix in 71% of patients with surgically proven appendicitis. Although CT is a quick and sensitive test to perform, it delivers between 29 and 43 mGy of radiation to the fetus, depending on the trimester of pregnancy. According to the International Commission on Radiological Protection, the best quantitative estimate of risk is about 1 cancer per 500 fetuses exposed to 30 mGy of radiation. The most vulnerable period for the fetus is from 8 to 15 weeks' gestation, during which radiation can result in intrauterine growth retardation and CNS defects. During this period, CT imaging should be obtained with extreme caution. MRI is a diagnostic modality with reported 89% to 100% sensitivity and 94% to 97% specificity. In one study, the routine use of MRI for suspected appendicitis in pregnant patients led to a significant decrease in the negative appendectomy rate, without a significant change in the perforation rate. Hence, at institutions where MRI is available, its use as a first-line imaging modality in pregnant patients with suspected appendicitis has been advocated.

■ MANAGEMENT OF ACUTE APPENDICITIS

Timing of Surgery

Traditionally, immediate appendectomy has been the standard of care for the treatment of acute appendicitis. However, this management paradigm is being challenged. Using ACS-NSQIP data on more than 32,000 appendectomies, Ingraham et al compared those performed within 6 hours of presentation with those performed after more than 12 hours. In contrast to previously held beliefs, a delayed appendectomy did not adversely affect 30-day outcomes. This finding has been confirmed in both the adult and pediatric populations. Adult patients with pathologically confirmed acute appendicitis who underwent appendectomy within 12 hours of diagnosis did not have statistically significant differences in the length of stay, operative time, or rates of complication from those whose operations were performed between 12 and 24 hours. For children, those who underwent appendectomy within 6 hours of diagnosis showed no difference with respect to operative time, perforation rate, or complications compared with those with operations after 6 hours. This undeniable shift in paradigm from an emergent to an urgent intervention allows for more efficient allocation of physician and hospital resources.

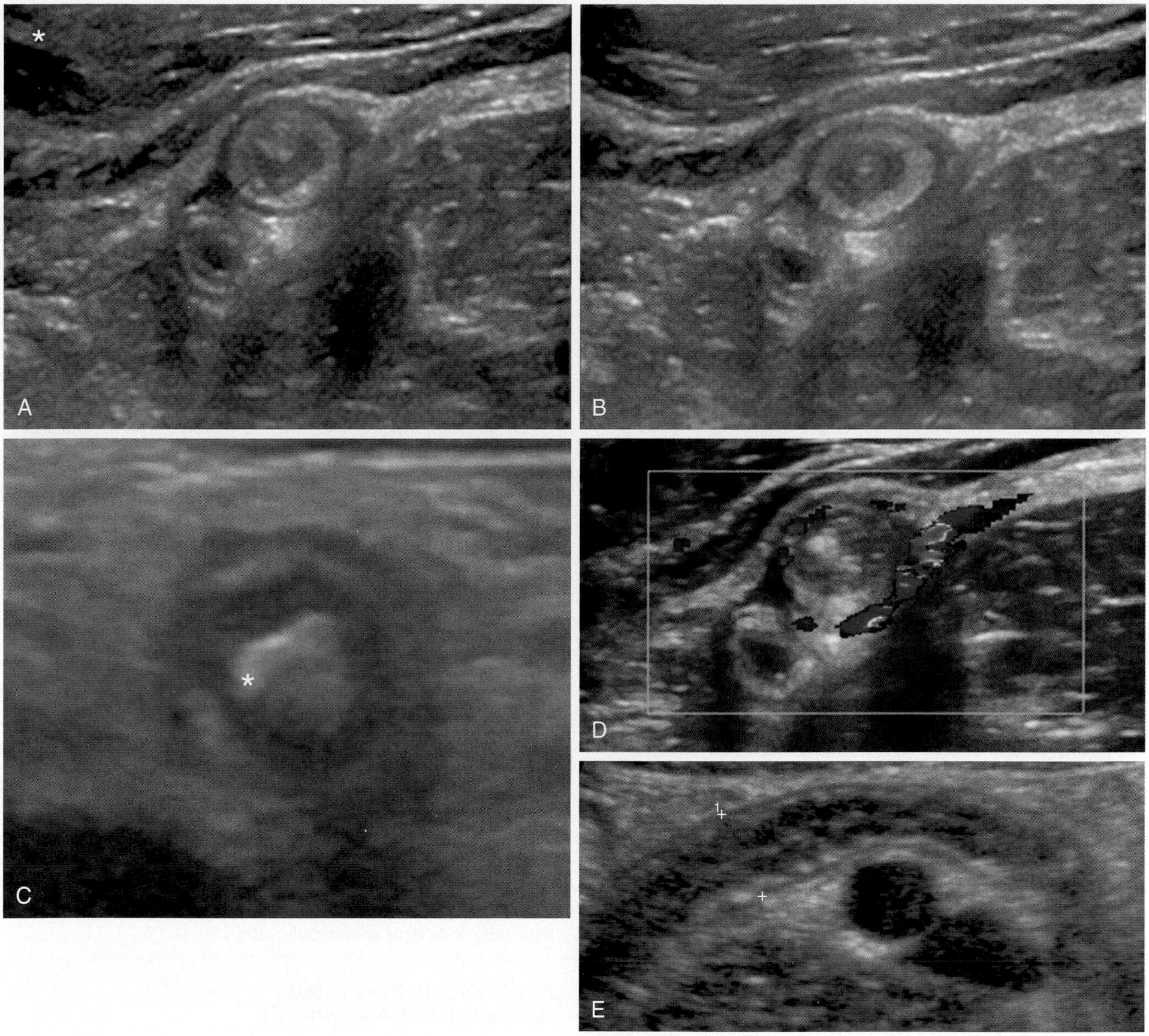

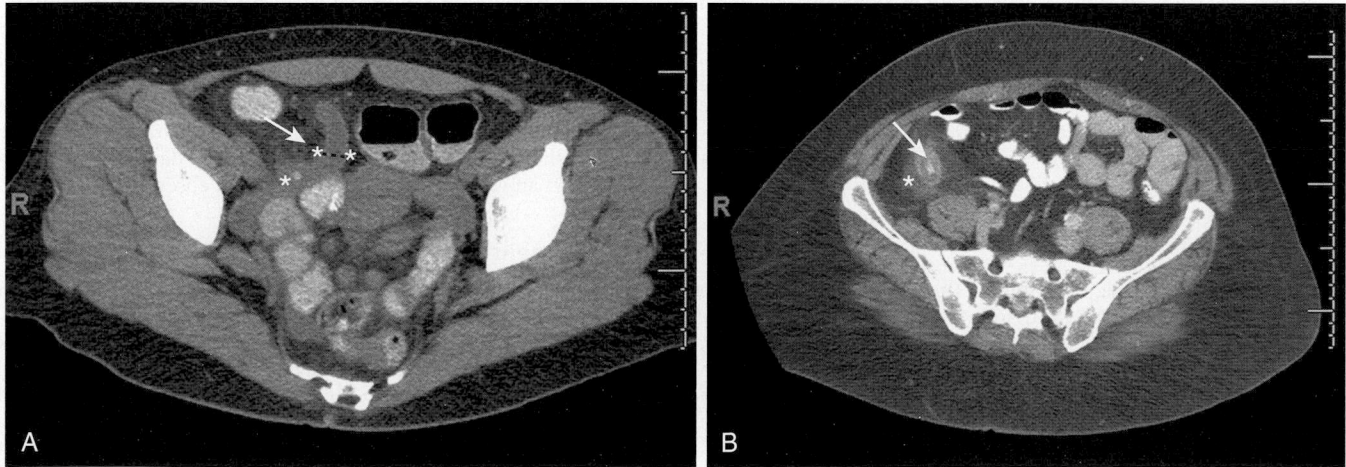

FIGURE 2 Ultrasound images of appendicitis. **A,** Noncompressed appendix with surrounding free fluid, marked by asterisk. **B,** Compressed appendix, with failure to change the luminal diameter compared with Figure 2A. **C,** Fecalith with a target appearance. **D,** Color Doppler can evaluate for presence or absence of blood flow within the wall of an inflamed appendix. **E,** Dilated appendix. *(Images courtesy Dr. Katherine Kaproth-Joslin.)*

FIGURE 3 CT images of appendicitis. **A,** Dilated appendix, marked by white arrow, in setting of an obstructing appendicolith, marked by white asterisk. **B,** Presence of periappendiceal fat stranding and inflammation noted by asterisk and appendicolith marked by arrow. *(Images courtesy Dr. Katherine Kaproth-Joslin.)*

Laparoscopic Surgery

The patient is positioned supine with both arms tucked and monitors placed at the foot of the bed. The sterile field is prepped from the xiphoid to the pubis. Access to the abdomen can be achieved through the umbilicus with the Veress needle or a Hassan trocar based on surgeon preference. To place a Veress needle, elevate the umbilicus with two towel clips and make a stab incision through the skin. Insert the Veress needle perpendicular to the skin, attentive of two audible clicks as the spring loaded needle retracts. The first point occurs as the needle meets and transverses the fascia and the second as it meets and transverses the peritoneum. A saline drop test is performed to confirm entry into the peritoneal cavity. The abdomen then can be insufflated before insertion of a 12-mm trocar.

The Hassan trocar is inserted by cutdown. An incision in the supraumbilical fold is made and carried through the subcutaneous tissue. Next, dissection is performed through the subcutaneous tissue with S-retractors, until the rectus fascia is visualized. Two retention sutures are placed into the fascia on either side of the midline incision. With the electrocautery, a vertical incision is made through the fascia that is elevated with the retention sutures. The peritoneal cavity is entered bluntly with a Kelly clamp. The Hasson cannula is placed into the peritoneal cavity under direct visualization and anchored with the previously placed sutures.

The abdomen is insufflated with carbon dioxide to a pressure of 12 to 15 mm Hg and is inspected to ascertain that no injuries occurred from initial trocar insertion and for other intra-abdominal diseases. There are a number of arrangements for the placement of the remainder of the trocars as seen in Figure 4. However, our preference is the use of an umbilical camera port and the working ports in the right upper quadrant and left lower quadrant to maximize triangulation (Figure 4, *A*).

A 5-mm trocar is inserted in the left lower quadrant lateral to the rectus with care taken to avoid injury to the inferior epigastric vessels and bladder. Another 5-mm trocar is placed in the right upper quadrant in between the umbilicus and the right costal margin. A four-quadrant exploration is performed quickly to rule out other intra-abdominal diseases. The patient is placed in reverse Trendelenburg position with right side up to gain exposure to the appendix.

With atraumatic graspers, the cecum is followed to the point where the taenia converge and lifted toward the left upper quadrant to help identify the appendix. The appendix is elevated and freed of any omental attachments. In the case of a retrocecal appendix, the lateral peritoneal attachments, the white line of Toldt, must be divided to mobilize the cecum and expose the appendix.

A window then is created in the mesoappendix between the base of the appendix and the cecum. A linear gastrointestinal endoscopic stapler with a blue load then is introduced through the umbilical port and base of the appendix is stapled and divided (Figure 5, *A*, and Figure 6). The stapler is then reloaded with a white, vascular, load, and the mesoappendix divided (Figure 5, *B*). The appendix is withdrawn from the umbilical port with a retrieval bag.

Once the appendix is extracted, the cecal staple line is inspected and hemostasis is achieved, if necessary. The working ports are removed under direct vision and bleeding controlled with electrocautery or sutures. Desufflation occurs through the umbilical port and all trocar sites greater than 5 mm are closed.

Open Appendectomy

Although the laparoscopic technique is the procedure of choice in most patients, open appendectomy remains an essential alternative. The patient is positioned and prepped in the manner noted earlier. A line is marked between the anterior superior iliac spine (ASIS) and umbilicus with McBurney's point noted at one third of the way from ASIS (Figure 4, *D*). A skin incision is made within a natural skin crease. The dissection is carried down until the aponeurosis of the external oblique is identified. The muscle is divided in the direction

of its fibers and spread bluntly to expose the underlying internal oblique muscle. It too is dissected similarly to expose the transversus abdominis. The transversalis is split to expose the peritoneum. The peritoneum is elevated and incised using Metzenbaum scissors with care taken to avoid injury to underlying bowel.

Once inside the abdomen, the cecum is identified and lifted through the incision to identify the attached appendix. A stapling device can be used to ligate the appendiceal base and mesoappendix. The "classic" technique, however, involves dividing the mesentery between two Kelly clamps with ligation of the free ends using 3-0 silk ties. The base of appendix is then identified and crushed with a Kelly clamp. The clamp is then moved 1 cm toward the tip. The appendix then is ligated with a 0 chromic suture and subsequently divided. The stump may then be cauterized, or a purse-string suture, or a Z-stitch may be placed in the cecum to invaginate the appendiceal stump.

The incision is closed in layers: first the peritoneum and transversalis fascia with a running absorbable suture. Next, the rectus sheath and the internal oblique are closed with interrupted suture, followed by the external oblique. Last, the skin is closed with a running subcuticular suture. In the case of perforation, however, the skin may be approximated loosely.

Postoperative antibiotics in cases of nonperforated appendicitis are not recommended. Studies have shown that postoperative antibiotics do not decrease the incidence of superficial surgical site infections (SSIs), deep SSIs, or organ space infections. However, they did result in a higher rate of *Clostridium difficile* infections, urinary tract infections, and longer length of stay.

Nonoperative Management of Nonperforated Appendicitis

Either laparoscopic or open appendectomy is the treatment of choice for uncomplicated appendicitis as recommended by the American College of Surgeons and the Society for Surgery of the Alimentary Tract. However, nonoperative management of acute appendicitis has been an evolving debate. Should medical management be chosen, the surgeon must remain extremely vigilant. Serial examinations and imaging are necessary to monitor for treatment failure. The rate of recurrence of appendicitis treated with antibiotics alone is up to 7% to 14% at 1 year from the index episode and frequently is associated with the presence of an appendicolith.

Antibiotics in Perforated (Complicated) Appendicitis

An appendiceal abscess or phlegmon is found in 3.8% of patients with appendicitis. The initial antibiotic regimen should have empiric coverage of gram-negative rods and anaerobic organisms. Coverage can be obtained with a beta-lactam (piperacillin-tazobactam) alone or a third-generation cephalosporin (ceftriaxone) and metronidazole. This can be narrowed further once cultures from a percutaneous drain or surgery are finalized. Patients usually can be converted to oral antibiotics once tolerating a diet. Initial intravenous (IV) antibiotics with IV ceftriaxone and metronidazole followed by conversion to oral amoxicillin/clavulanate (Augmentin) for a total 7-day course has been shown to be as efficacious as a total of 7 days of IV antibiotics without an increased risk of postoperative abscess formation.

Management of Perforated Appendicitis

Immediate surgical intervention can be associated with a more than threefold increase in morbidity compared with nonoperative management. Hence, the treatment algorithm for perforated appendicitis can be divided into two arms: patients with sepsis and generalized peritonitis and those with a contained abscess or phlegmon and localized peritonitis. The first require fluid resuscitation, antibiotics, and prompt surgical exploration. The management of patients with contained perforation is evolving. On the basis of retrospective

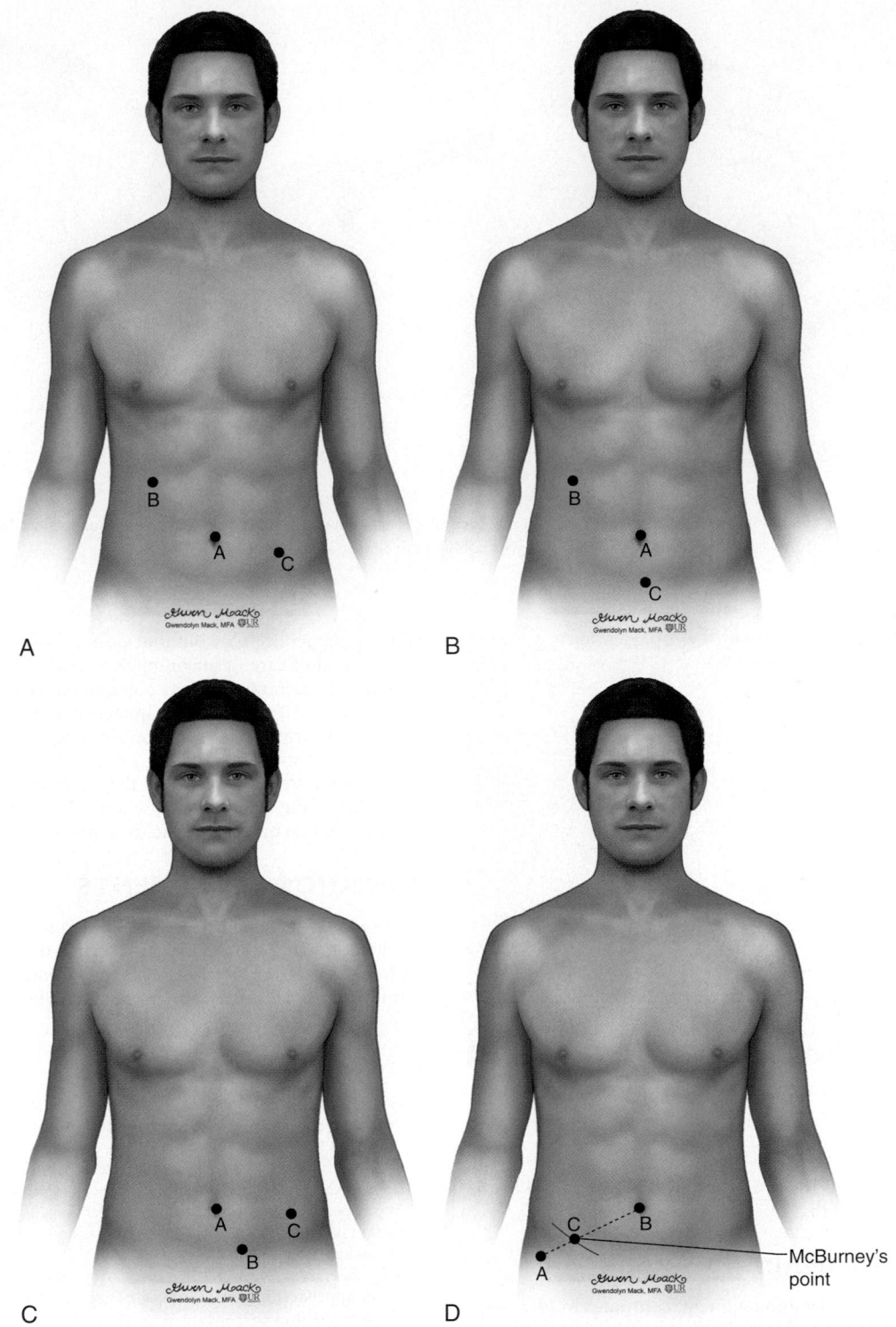

FIGURE 4 Laparoscopic and open incisions for appendectomy. **A,** Umbilical port, RUQ port, and LLQ port. **B,** Umbilical port, RUQ port, and suprapubic port. **C,** Umbilical port, LLQ port, and suprapubic port. **D,** McBurney's point one third the distance from the ASIS and umbilicus, with surgical incision made over the McBurney's point in a natural skin crease.

cohort studies, the current management paradigm for this subgroup of patients with complicated appendicitis is intravenous antibiotic therapy and placement of a percutaneous drain.

The practice of interval appendectomy is currently a topic of controversy. In adults, elective interval appendectomy remains fraught with significant morbidity with one study quoting a rate of 11%. Hence, after successful nonsurgical treatment, no interval appendectomy is indicated. This practice has been abandoned in the adult population. Although the risk of missing an underlying condition such as inflammatory bowel disease or a neoplasm is low, it cannot be eliminated. Hence, patients older than 40 years should undergo follow-up colonoscopy and/or CT or US imaging. Unlike adults, interval appendectomy is proposed in children with complicated appendicitis. The main reason for this is a higher risk of

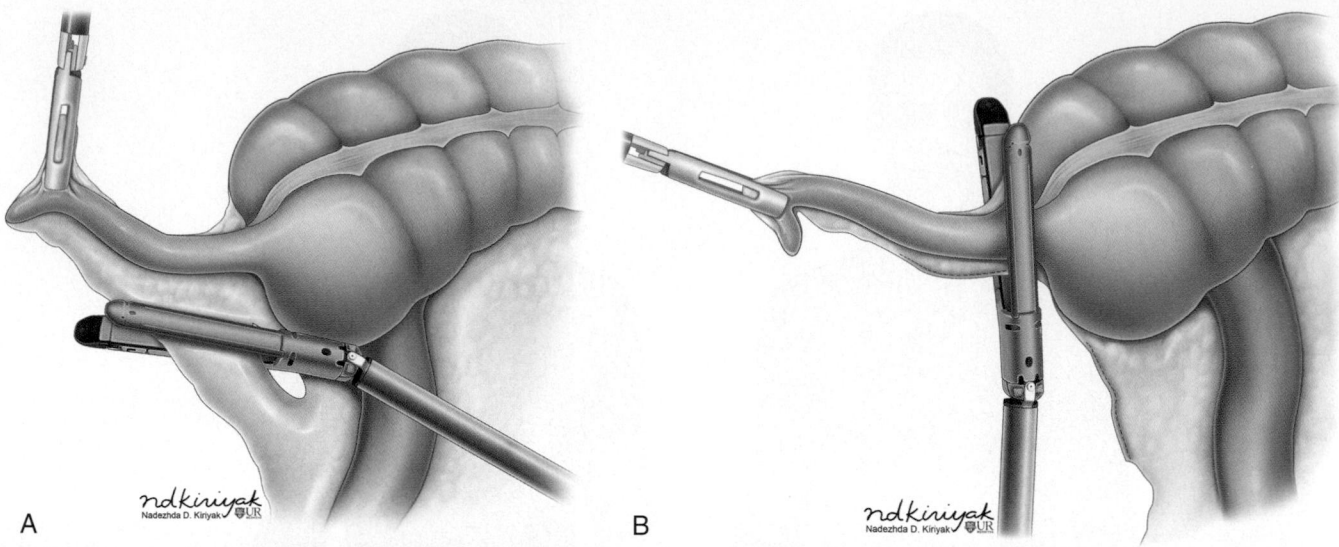

A B

FIGURE 5 A, A window is created in the mesoappendix between the base of the appendix and the cecum, and the mesoappendix is divided with a white, vascular, load. **B,** Base of the appendix is stapled and divided with a blue gastrointestinal staple load.

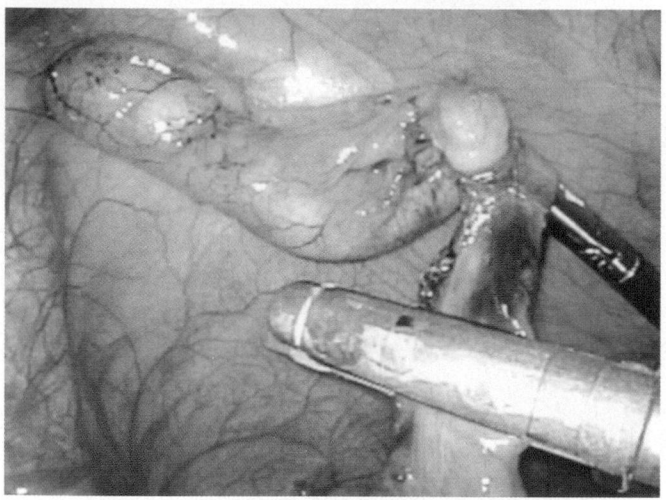

FIGURE 6 Base of the appendix is stapled and divided.

recurrent appendicitis, up to 72% in the presence and 26% in the absence of an appendicolith.

■ CLOSING SUMMARY

Appendicitis, although a common ailment, continues to be a diagnostic and management challenge. Its diagnosis is an exercise in clinical decision making. It presses surgeons to combine patient history, physical examination, laboratory values, and imaging studies to make the correct diagnosis. Some aspects of its management are evolving. Appendectomy without postoperative antibiotics remains the standard of care in uncomplicated cases. However, complicated appendicitis warrants antibiotics, drainage if possible, and nonoperative management without early appendectomy in adults. However, in children an early or interval appendectomy remains the practice in complicated appendicitis. In the future, these treatment algorithms will continue to be modified as they have over the past 130 years especially as the practice moves toward less invasive approaches. However, at this time, appendicitis remains a surgical disease.

■ ACKNOWLEDGEMENTS

We would like to acknowledge Dr. Katherine Kaproth-Joslin for her assistance in the diagnostic imaging section of this chapter, as well as Nadezhda D Kiriyak, Sarah Klingenberger, and Gwen Mack for their assistance in the illustrations and photographs.

SUGGESTED READINGS

Coakley BA, et al. Postoperative antibiotics correlate with worse outcomes after appendectomy for nonperforated appendicitis. *J Am Coll Surg.* 2011;213:778-783.

Fraser JD, et al. A complete course of intravenous antibiotics vs a combination of intravenous and oral antibiotics for perforated appendicitis in children: a prospective, randomized trial. *J Pediatr Surg.* 2010;45:1198-1202.

Ingraham AM, et al. Effect of delay to operation on outcomes in adults with acute appendicitis. *Arch Surg.* 2010;145:886-892.

Simillis C, et al. A meta-analysis comparing conservative treatment versus acute appendectomy for complicated appendicitis (abscess or phlegmon). *Surgery.* 2010;147:818-829.

St. Peter SD, Aguayo P, Fraser JS, et al. Initial laparoscopic appendectomy versus initial nonoperative management and interval appendectomy for perforated appendicitis with abscess: a prospective, randomized trial. *J Pediatr Surg.* 2010;45:236-240.

THE MANAGEMENT OF HEMORRHOIDS

Jennifer Blumetti, MD, and Jose R. Cintron, MD

Hemorrhoids are specialized vascular cushions that are located in the submucosal space in the anal canal. They are a normal part of human anatomy and contribute about 15% to 20% of anal resting pressure. Hemorrhoids help with closure of the anus and relay information regarding the composition of the rectal contents (i.e., solid, liquid, or gas). Hemorrhoids are described anatomically as three cushions located in the left lateral, right anterior, and right posterior positions. Internal hemorrhoids are located proximal to the dentate line and are covered in anoderm. External hemorrhoids are located distal to the dentate line and are covered with skin (Figure 1).

■ SYMPTOMS

Symptoms from hemorrhoids are very common and occur with increases in intra-abdominal pressure, such as with constipation or straining to defecate. The prevalence of hemorrhoids is approximately 4.4%, with more than 10 million people in the United States suffering from hemorrhoid symptoms. About half of these are older than 50 years. Common symptoms of hemorrhoids include bleeding, mucoid discharge, burning, itching, and prolapse. Pain typically is not associated with hemorrhoids, unless there is an acute thrombosis (Figure 2). Hemorrhoids are classified as internal or external and by degree of prolapse (Table 1).

Because patients typically believe that all anorectal symptoms can be attributed to hemorrhoids, it is important for the practitioner to differentiate hemorrhoid symptoms from other benign or malignant anorectal conditions. A thorough history and physical examination should be performed, with special attention to anorectal symptoms and bowel habits. Bleeding from hemorrhoids typically is described as bright red and occurring with bowel movements. Symptoms of constipation or straining should be elicited, including number of bowel movements and amount of time spent on the toilet. Amount of prolapse also should be documented and whether the patient has to assist with reduction. It is essential to differentiate prolapse resulting from hemorrhoidal disease compared with true rectal prolapse (Figure 3). A family history of colon cancer or polyps should be documented. A thorough examination of the anorectum, including anoscopy, should be performed. Patients with bleeding as one of their symptoms should be offered colonoscopy.

■ TREATMENT

Dietary and Lifestyle Modification

Once the patient has been diagnosed with symptomatic hemorrhoids, conservative treatment is first-line therapy for the vast majority of patients. Patients should be started on a fiber supplement such as psyllium, methylcellulose, or calcium polycarbophil and encouraged to drink eight glasses of water daily. Patients also should be counseled in reducing straining with defecation. Reading while sitting on the toilet should be discouraged. In many patients with grade I and II hemorrhoids, this conservative therapy is the only treatment necessary and has been shown to decrease symptomatic bleeding and prolapse in a large systematic review. Warm baths two to three times daily for 20 minutes (sitz baths) also may help with hygiene and provide some symptom relief. Topical over-the-counter therapies, which are used by many patients, may make the patient feel better, but these have not been shown to reduce hemorrhoid symptoms or address the underlying disease.

For patients who fail conservative therapy, there are several types of procedures that may be offered to patients. These include in-office procedures, such as rubber band ligation (RBL), sclerotherapy, infrared coagulation (IRC), and use of the HET bipolar system, and operative procedures (Table 2).

Rubber Band Ligation

RBL is the most commonly used office-based procedure for symptomatic internal hemorrhoids. It can be performed in grade I, II, or III hemorrhoids and does not require an anesthetic. The patient is placed in the left lateral decubitus or prone jack-knife position for office-based procedures. On anoscopy, the hemorrhoids are visualized, and the largest is addressed at the initial banding session. The rubber band is then placed 2 cm above the dentate line, which is above the level of somatic pain sensation (Figure 4). There are several types of rubber band ligators available; our preference is shown. Suction ligators are also available, which may be deployed without the need for an assistant. Benefits of RBL include removal of hemorrhoidal tissue with resultant fibrosis and scarring, which leads to decreases in bleeding and prolapse symptoms. It is successful in more than 90% of cases. It often does require multiple sessions to address all the hemorrhoidal disease. Some advocate banding only one hemorrhoid at a time; alternately, if the patient tolerates the first session well, two hemorrhoids can be banded at the subsequent session. Patients who are on anticoagulation cannot undergo RBL because the band will slough in approximately 1 week, causing bleeding. Blood thinners and aspirin typically are stopped for 1 week before and after each banding session. If the patient cannot be off anticoagulation, then an alternate treatment should be used, such as sclerotherapy.

Complications of RBL are typically minor and include pain, minor bleeding, vasovagal symptoms, and thrombosis of the adjacent external hemorrhoid. Severe pain immediately after placement indicates that the rubber band was placed too low near the dentate line. Immediate removal is required. Pelvic sepsis, with fever, severe pain, and urinary retention, is an extremely rare but serious complication that requires admission, intravenous antibiotics, and urgent examination under anesthesia, with wide drainage/débridement of necrotic tissue.

Sclerotherapy

Sclerotherapy is a less commonly used office procedure for grades I and II hemorrhoids. A sclerosant is injected into the hemorrhoids, resulting in fibrosis, scarring, and fixation. Sclerosing agents include 5% phenol (typically in almond oil), hypertonic salt solution, or ethanolamine. Using a 25-gauge needle, the surgeon injects sclerosant 1 cm above the dentate line into the submucosa of each hemorrhoid. The volume injected varies by the type of sclerosant used. For phenol, 2 to 3 mL are injected into each hemorrhoid, in a single treatment session. The benefit of sclerotherapy is that it can treat all three hemorrhoids in one setting, and patients can be anticoagulated fully during the treatment. Needle site bleeding is controlled easily with manual pressure. Long-term results of sclerotherapy are inferior to RBL. Sclerotherapy can be repeated at subsequent sessions for ongoing symptoms. Risks of sclerotherapy are rare and typically the result of incorrect injection of the sclerosing agent into the muscle or mucosa, leading to pain, ulceration, and sloughing of the mucosa. Repetitive sclerotherapy can result in scarring and/or stricture, but this is rare.

Other Office-Based Procedures

IRC also is used commonly for grade I or II hemorrhoids. It also has the advantage of being able to treat all three hemorrhoids in one

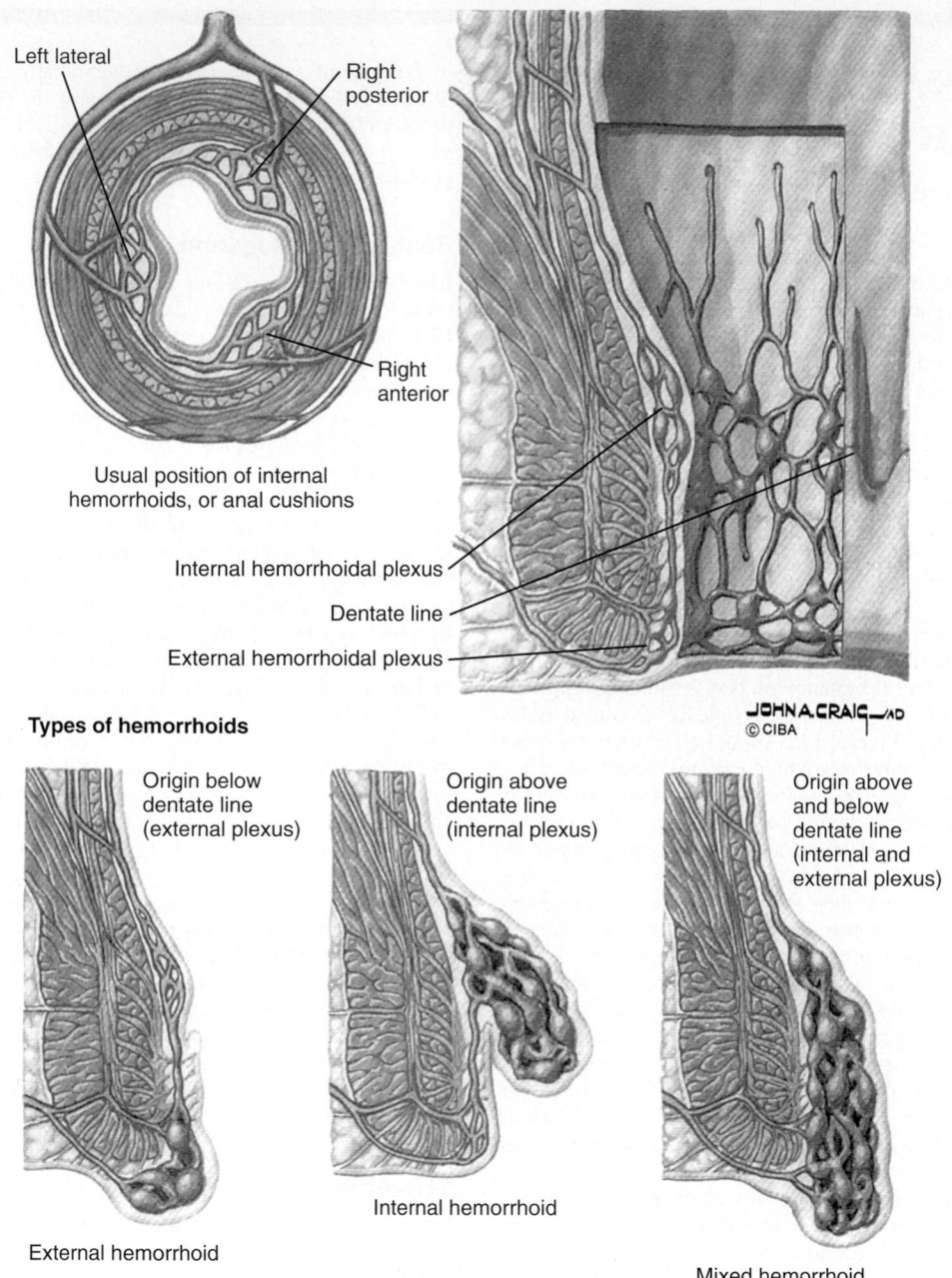

Left lateral

Right posterior

Right anterior

Usual position of internal hemorrhoids, or anal cushions

Internal hemorrhoidal plexus

Dentate line

External hemorrhoidal plexus

JOHN A. CRAIG—AD
©CIBA

Types of hemorrhoids

Origin below dentate line (external plexus)

Origin above dentate line (internal plexus)

Origin above and below dentate line (internal and external plexus)

External hemorrhoid

Internal hemorrhoid

Mixed hemorrhoid

FIGURE I Location and types of hemorrhoids.

setting. The tip of the infrared coagulator (IRC 2100, Redfield Corporation, Rochelle Park, NJ) is placed at the apex of the hemorrhoid, and a 1- to 1.5-second pulse is applied. This results in a 4-mm^2 focus of coagulation with 2.5-mm deep ulcer. Typically three to four applications are made for each hemorrhoid. The infrared energy results in thrombosis and tissue destruction, leading to scarring and fixation of the hemorrhoid. IRC is typically better tolerated and causes less pain than RBL. It is more expensive and is less effective in higher-grade hemorrhoids than RBL (Figure 5).

The HET system (HET bipolar system, Covidien, Boulder, CO) is a new modality used to treat internal hemorrhoids in the office. It is applied to the apex of the hemorrhoid, which is clamped between the specialized anoscope, and bipolar energy applied (Figure 6). All three hemorrhoid bundles can be treated in one setting. This technique may be beneficial for grades I and II hemorrhoid disease.

Operative Treatment

Operative treatment typically is reserved for patients with grades III or IV hemorrhoids and those who have persistent symptoms despite conservative and office-based procedures. It is estimated that only about 5% to 10% of patients with symptomatic hemorrhoids require surgical treatment of hemorrhoids. Surgery is typically superior to office-based procedures but does result in more complications such as pain, urinary retention (2% to 36%), bleeding (0.03% to 6%), anal stenosis (0 to 6%), infection (0.5% to 5.5%), and incontinence (2% to 12%).

Ferguson Hemorrhoidectomy

Ferguson, or "closed" hemorrhoidectomy, is the most common surgical hemorrhoid procedure. It involves removal of the hemorrhoid tissue with ligation of the pedicle, and closure of the defect. Our

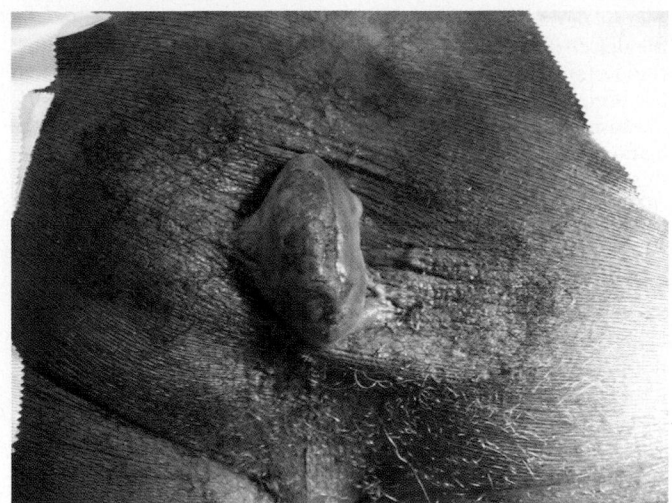

FIGURE 2 Acutely thrombosed external hemorrhoid.

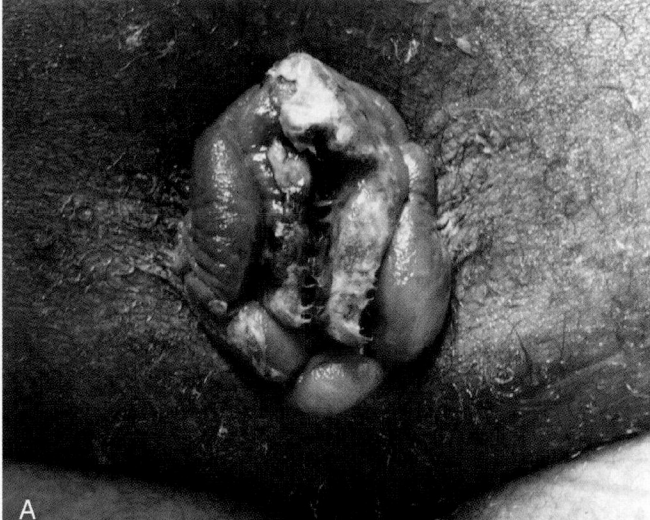

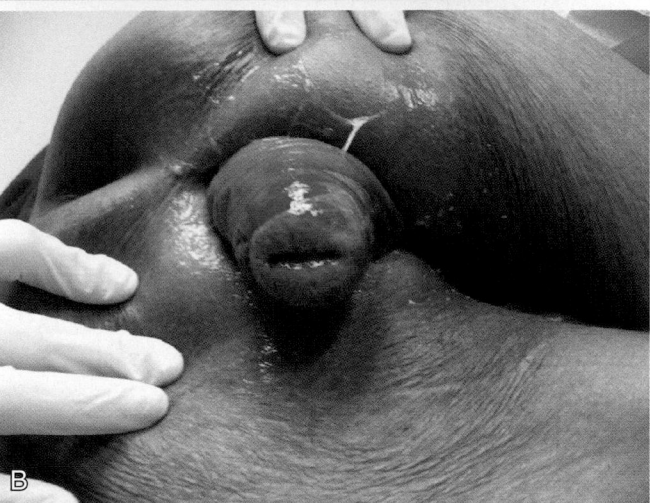

FIGURE 3 Differentiating hemorrhoidal prolapse from true rectal prolapse. **A,** Incarcerated, strangulated internal hemorrhoids with visible radial folds. **B,** True rectal prolapse with visible circular folds.

TABLE 1: Classification of Internal Hemorrhoids

Grade	Location	Symptoms
1	Bulge into anal canal	Painless bleeding
2	Prolapse, reduce spontaneously	Bleeding, burning, itching
3	Prolapse, must be manually reduced	Bleeding, itching, mucoid drainage
4	Prolapse and cannot be reduced	Pain, bleeding, mucoid drainage

preference is to perform this procedure under regional (spinal) anesthesia with the patient in the prone jack-knife position. Lidocaine with epinephrine is injected into the hemorrhoid. A V-shaped incision is then made on the perianal skin toward the anal canal, and the hemorrhoid is elevated initially off of the external sphincter and subsequently off of the internal sphincter muscle as the dissection proceeds into the anal canal. Once the sphincter muscles have been identified clearly, the skin incision is then continued onto the mucosa, thus ensuring that there is no damage to the sphincter muscle. The apex of hemorrhoid with the vascular pedicle is then clamped, and the hemorrhoid is excised. The pedicle is suture ligated, and the defect then is closed in a running locked fashion in the anal canal and continued in a simple running fashion on the perianal skin (Figure 7).

Milligan Morgan Hemorrhoidectomy

The Milligan-Morgan, or "open" hemorrhoidectomy, is performed more commonly in the United Kingdom. The technique begins similarly to the Ferguson hemorrhoidectomy, with dissection of the hemorrhoid off of the sphincter muscles in the perianal skin and in the anal canal. The hemorrhoid is excised and the apex is suture ligated, and then the wounds are left open to heal by secondary intention. Outcomes between the two techniques are similar, although wound healing is longer in the open technique.

Modifications of Excisional Technique

Energy devices may be used in the surgical treatment of hemorrhoids. The technique involves grasping the hemorrhoid, and the

TABLE 2: Treatment Options for Hemorrhoids

Treatments	1°	2°	3°	4°	Acute Prolapse
Dietary	x	x	x	x	x
Banding	x	x	x		
Sclerotherapy	x	x	x		
IRC	x	x	x		
Excision		x	x	x	x
Stapled		x	x	x	
THD/HAL		x	x		
HAL/RAR			x	x	

HAL, Hemorrhoidal artery ligation (A.M.I. Inc., Natick, MA); *IFC,* infrared coagulation; *RAR,* rectoanal repair or mucopexy; *THD,* transanal hemorrhoidal dearterialization (THD America, Ankeny, IA).

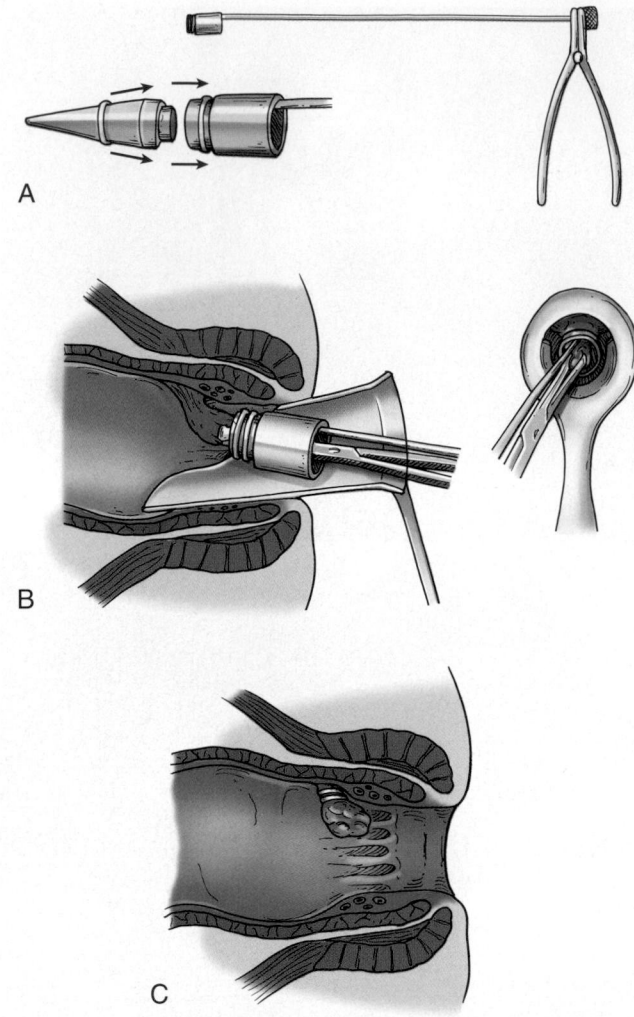

FIGURE 4 Rubber band ligation of internal hemorrhoids **A,** Rubber band placed onto banding gun. **B,** Hemorrhoid is grasped 2 cm above the dentate line and the band advanced over the hemorrhoid. **C,** Band in correct position after ligation.

energy device is then used to excise the hemorrhoid and seal the defect. This technique is faster than standard Ferguson hemorrhoidectomy and results in less pain at 1 day postoperatively, but pain has been shown to be equal at 2 weeks postoperatively. The cost is increased compared with Ferguson hemorrhoidectomy. Because the hemorrhoid is not dissected from the sphincters before excision in this technique, care must be taken to avoid damage to the underlying sphincter muscles, and avoidance of excessive removal of anoderm, which can result in anal stenosis.

Stapled Hemorrhoidopexy

Stapled hemorrhoidopexy typically is reserved for grades II through IV circumferential internal hemorrhoids. It was developed to reduce the pain associated with excisional hemorrhoidectomy. The technique uses a specialized circular stapler, which removes a circumferential area of mucosa and submucosa proximal to the hemorrhoids. This does not remove hemorrhoidal tissue but rather disrupts the vascular supply and puts the hemorrhoids back into their proper position. There are no external wounds, so pain is improved compared with excisional hemorrhoidectomy. Stapled hemorrhoidopexy does not address external hemorrhoid disease.

Stapled hemorrhoidopexy is performed with similar anesthesia and positioning to excisional hemorrhoidectomy. The hemorrhoidopexy "kit" contains a dilator, clear plastic anoscope, operating anoscope, and stapler (Figure 8, *A*). The dilator is placed into the anal canal, and the clear plastic anoscope then sutured to the perianal skin to evert the dentate line. The operating anoscope then is used as a guide to place a submucosal purse string 3 to 4 cm proximal to the dentate line (about 2 cm proximal to the hemorrhoid apex). Care must be taken to avoid full-thickness suture placement, especially in women as injury to the vagina can occur. Once the purse string has been placed, the purse string then is tied around the anvil of the stapler, and the stapler is then fired (Figure 8, *B*). The specimen appears as a "doughnut" of mucosa and submucosa.

Stapled hemorrhoidopexy has similar complication rates to excisional hemorrhoidectomy and has the benefits of faster operating time and less pain. Staple lines placed too close to the puborectalis can result in pelvic pain, so care must be taken to place the purse string appropriately. Staple line bleeding at the time of the initial operation is controlled easily with oversewing of the staple line. Rare complications such as rectovaginal fistula or rectal perforation have occurred. These are technical because of misplacement of the purse-string suture. Outcomes are similar to excisional

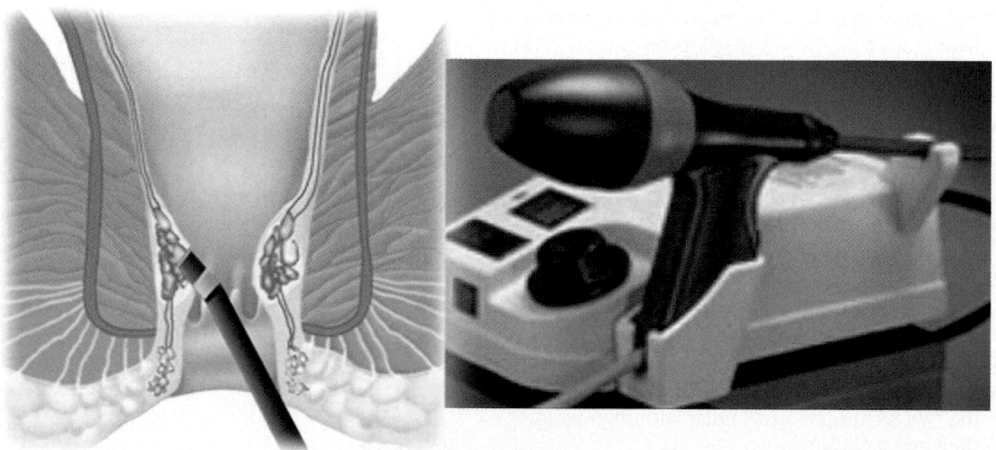

FIGURE 5 Infrared coagulation of internal hemorrhoids *Left,* applicator is applied to the apex of the hemorrhoid. *Right,* IRC device. (IRC 2100, Redfield Corporation, Rochelle Park, NJ.)

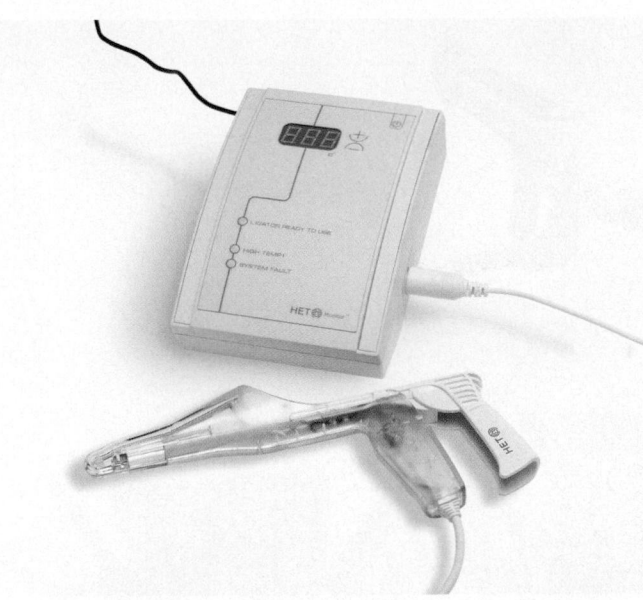

FIGURE 6 HET temperature monitor and HET bipolar forceps for treatment of internal hemorrhoids. *(All rights reserved. Used with permission of Covidien.)*

hemorrhoidectomy, although long-term recurrence is slightly higher in stapled hemorrhoidopexy.

Doppler-Guided Hemorrhoid Artery Ligation and Rectoanal Repair

A newer technique in the treatment of symptomatic hemorrhoids is Doppler-guided hemorrhoid artery ligation. This technique involves the use of one of two specialized patented anoscopes, the THD, transanal hemorrhoidal dearterialization (THD; America, Ankeny, IA), or the HAL, hemorrhoidal artery ligation (A.M.I. Inc, Natick, MA), both of which use Doppler guidance to isolate hemorrhoidal arteries for ligation. The technique is used typically for grade II to III hemorrhoids and allows for selective ligation of the hemorrhoidal arteries, which reduces arterial inflow to the hemorrhoids and restores normal physiologic conditions. In studies, up to 90% of patients had symptom improvement with this technique, with less postoperative pain than in other surgical techniques because all suturing is done proximal to the dentate line.

The ligation procedure is performed in the operating room. Positioning and anesthesia is similar to other hemorrhoid procedures. The specialized anoscope is placed into the anal canal to 6 to 7 cm from the anorectal junction. The vessels are localized with the attached Doppler, which is typically at about 2 cm above the anorectal junction (Figure 9). A Z-stitch or figure-of-8 stitch is placed at this location, with the slot in the anoscope, and a total of six sutures are typically placed at 1, 3, 5, 7, 9, and 11 o'clock positions in the anal canal.

For patients with larger (grade III or IV) hemorrhoids, the addition of a mucopexy, also called a *rectoanal repair,* has been advocated

Excision technique for mixed hemorrhoids

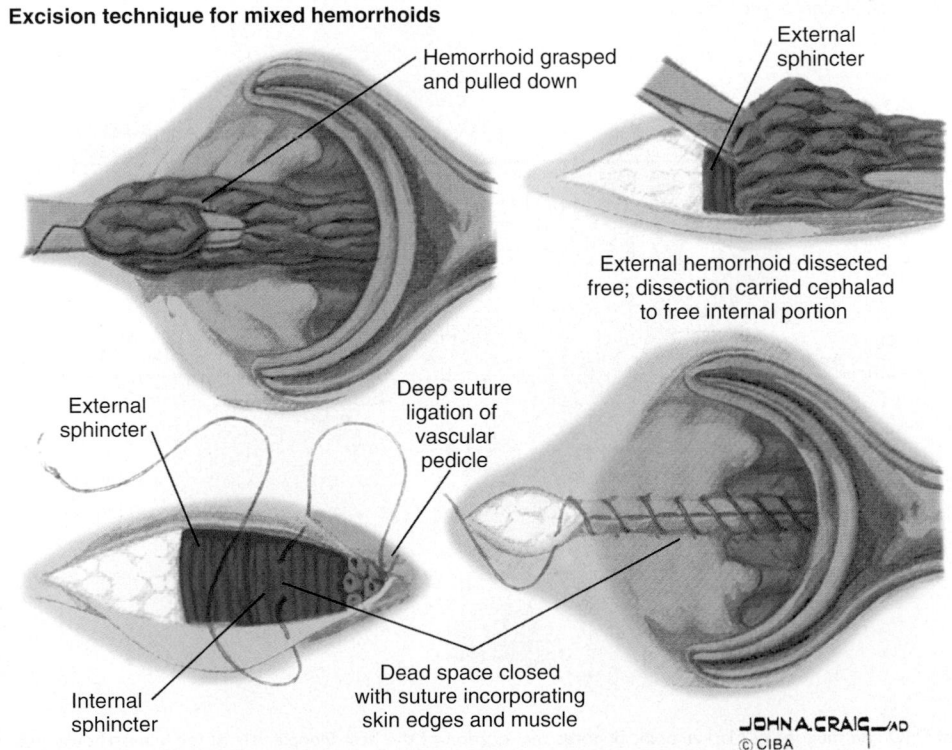

Hemorrhoid grasped and pulled down

External sphincter

External hemorrhoid dissected free; dissection carried cephalad to free internal portion

External sphincter

Deep suture ligation of vascular pedicle

Internal sphincter

Dead space closed with suture incorporating skin edges and muscle

JOHN A. CRAIG—AD
© CIBA

FIGURE 7 Ferguson hemorrhoidectomy.

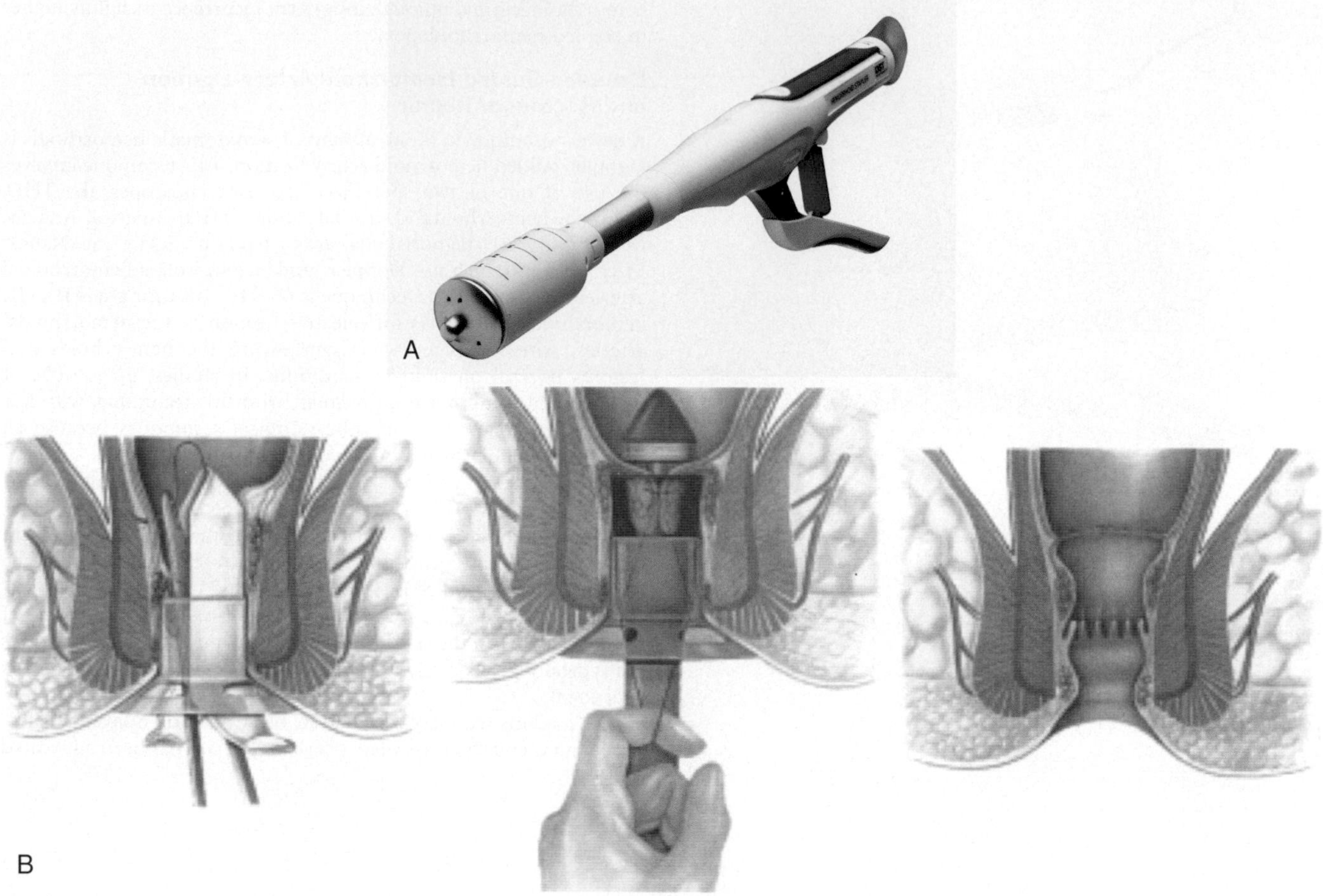

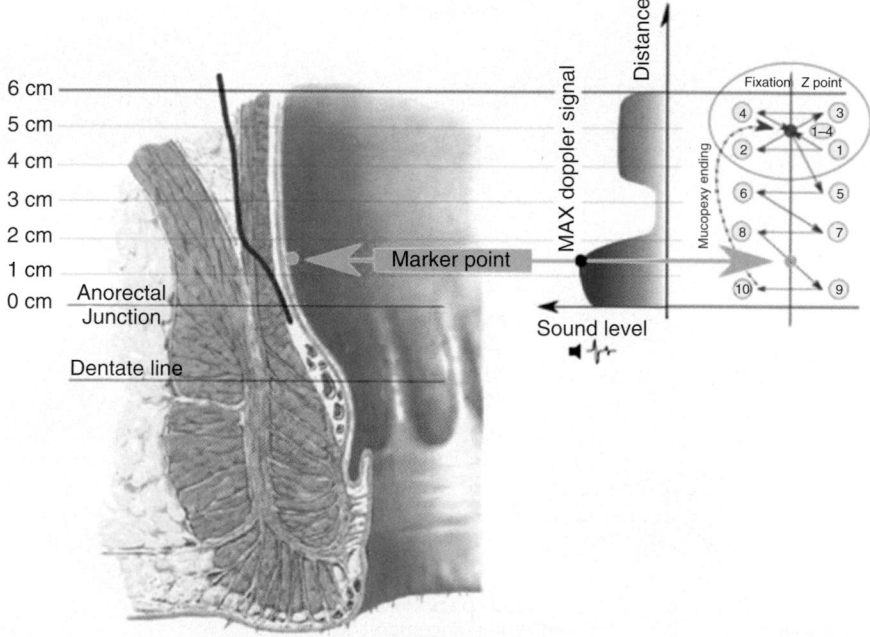

FIGURE 8 A, EEA hemorrhoid and prolapse stapler with DST Series technology. *(All rights reserved. Used with permission of Covidien.)* **B,** Stapled hemorrhoidopexy technique. *Left,* Purse-string suture applied 4 cm above the dentate line. *Center,* Stapler advanced into rectum, and traction held on the suture. *Right,* Staple line after completion of procedure.

FIGURE 9 Schematic of THD and mucopexy. Marker point denotes the location of the best Doppler signal for hemorrhoidal ligation. A Z-stitch is placed at this location for ligation alone. For higher grade hemorrhoids, mucopexy with running suture is performed starting proximally and encompassing the ligation point, pulling the redundant mucosa up into the rectum (right side of image). *(From Ratto C, de Parades V. Doppler guided ligation of hemorrhoidal arteries with mucopexy: a technique for the future. J Visc Surg. 2015;152:S15-S21.)*

to reduce symptoms. The technique begins similarly with Doppler-guided identification of the hemorrhoidal vessel (see Figure 9). A mark is made in this location with cautery. The anoscope once again is inserted proximally to 6 to 7 cm, and a Z-stitch placed at this point. This suture then is run distally, with bites placed 0.5 cm apart, ending at the apex of the hemorrhoid. This suture includes the hemorrhoidal artery to be ligated. The two ends of suture then are tied together to pull the redundant tissue back up into the distal rectum. The hemorrhoid itself is not sutured but instead pulled back into its anatomic position. This is done for each hemorrhoidal bundle. Pain is typically less than in excisional hemorrhoidectomy, and efficacy has been described in up to 90% of patients.

External Hemorrhoids

External hemorrhoids typically cause few symptoms, unless there is an acute thrombosis (see Figure 2). For patients with symptomatic internal hemorrhoids who also have large external hemorrhoids, excisional hemorrhoidectomy is preferred because this will address the internal and external disease. If the external hemorrhoids are soft and not fibrotic, then stapled hemorrhoidopexy may result in flattening of the external disease.

For patients with thrombosed hemorrhoids, treatment is based on relieving the patient's pain symptoms. Pain after thrombosis typically peaks in 48 to 72 hours, and patients who are seen during this window of time may benefit from excision of the thrombosed hemorrhoid. This can be performed with a local anesthetic, and an elliptical incision made over the hemorrhoid, and the thrombus excised. For patients seen 3 to 4 days after onset of symptoms, excision will not typically improve pain. Symptomatic treatment with analgesics, fiber supplementation, and sitz baths should be given, and the thrombus will resolve with time.

Acute Hemorrhoidal Disease or Strangulated Hemorrhoids

Patients who have acute prolapse that cannot be reduced are considered to have acute hemorrhoidal disease or strangulated hemorrhoids. There is significant edema, which does not allow for reduction (see Figure 3, *A*), and the hemorrhoids then can become ischemic, leading to ulceration and necrosis. Management of this is typically with urgent hemorrhoidectomy. With liberal use of an epinephrine-containing local anesthetic to reduce the edema, the hemorrhoids are reduced gently in the operating room, and standard Ferguson hemorrhoidectomy performed, taking care to leave normal anoderm between suture lines to avoid postoperative anal stenosis.

■ SUMMARY

Hemorrhoidal disease is a very common entity for which patients seek care. The vast majority of hemorrhoidal symptoms can be managed conservatively, with dietary modifications and sitz baths. Both office-based and operative procedures can be used in those patients refractory to conservative management.

SUGGESTED READINGS

Hall JF. Modern management of hemorrhoidal disease. *Gastroenterol Clin North Am*. 2013;42:759-772.

Kantsevoy SV, Bitner M. Nonsurgical treatment of actively bleeding internal hemorrhoids with a novel endoscopic device (with video). *Gastrointest Endosc*. 2013;78:649-653.

Ratto C, de Parades V. Doppler guided ligation of hemorrhoidal arteries with mucopexy: a technique for the future. *J Visc Surg*. 2015;152:S15-S21.

Rivadeneira DE, Steele SR, Ternant C, Chalasani S, et al. Practice parameters for the management of hemorrhoids. *Dis Colon Rectum*. 2011;54:1059-1064.

Singer M. Hemorrhoids. In: Beck DE, Roberts PL, Saclarides TJ, et al., eds. *ASCRS Textbook of Colon and Rectal Surgery*. New York: Springer; 2011.

THE MANAGEMENT OF ANAL FISSURES

Jonathan B. Mitchem, MD, and Todd D. Francone, MD, FACS, FASCRS

Anal fissure or fissure-in-ano is a common cause of anal pain. The true prevalence of the disease, however, is difficult to measure because patients are often reluctant to discuss perianal issues and may be misdiagnosed. Patients commonly have severe pain during or after defecation and/or bright red blood per rectum. Often patients describe a tearing sensation with bowel movements and blood on the toilet paper when wiping. The diagnosis of anal fissure is suggested by this history and confirmed by physical examination. For examination, the patient should be placed in the prone jack-knife or lateral decubitus position. Examining the external anus is generally all that is necessary to make the diagnosis. When the buttocks are gently separated, the fissure or a sentinel tag will be evident (Figure 1). Touching this with a cotton-tipped swab will reproduce the pain associated with defecation, and the diagnosis can be confirmed. If the diagnosis is not apparent during this examination, digital examination and office anoscopy should be performed to look for other diagnoses. If a diagnosis cannot be established, it is our practice to perform an examination under anesthesia for further evaluation. It is important to take the time to discuss findings and the diagnosis with patients because they often have heard different diagnoses and explanations from providers, leading to understandable frustration.

More than 75% of anal fissures are found in the posterior midline. The anterior midline position makes up the majority of the remainder. Anterior midline fissures are seen more commonly in women than men (up to 20% vs 5%) and are associated more commonly with an external sphincter defect. It is important to take this into consideration when evaluating a patient with an anterior midline fissure. Together, midline fissures make up more than 95% of fissures. This is related to the presumed pathophysiology of the disease. Manometric studies have demonstrated increased resting internal anal sphincter (IAS) tone in patients with an anal fissure. Increased IAS pressure results in diminished perfusion of the overlying anoderm. Given that the blood supply to the anoderm is most tenuous in the posterior and anterior midline, it logically follows that the majority of fissures occur in these locations. In younger women (younger than 40 years of age) with an anterior midline fissure it is important to consider a "low-pressure" fissure, commonly associated with obstetric trauma. Given the low sphincter pressure and external sphincter defect, alternative methods of surgical intervention such as anoplasty should be entertained in place of traditional sphincterotomy (Jenkins et al, 2008). Fissures not located in the midline should prompt a workup for other disease processes, including Crohn's disease, cancer, tuberculosis, and sexually transmitted diseases (human papilloma virus, human immunodeficiency virus, syphilis (Figure 2).

Patients with symptomatic fissure of less than 6 to 8 weeks in duration are considered to have an acute anal fissure (Figure 3). During this early time period, the fissure will likely consist of a tear or an ulcer in the skin of the anal canal beginning at the dentate line. After 6 to 8 weeks, fissures take on a chronic appearance characterized by fibrosis, a skin tag at the distal extent of the fissure, and/or a hypertrophied papilla at the proximal end (Figure 4). Often the internal sphincter muscle may be visible at the base of the fissure. The duration of symptoms is an important consideration when deciding on how to treat these patients.

■ TREATMENT

Acute Anal Fissure

For patients who have symptoms early in the course of their disease, approximately 50% will heal with stool softeners, fiber supplementation, and symptomatic control. We generally recommend 25 g of fiber per day, stool softeners for patients with constipation, and sitz

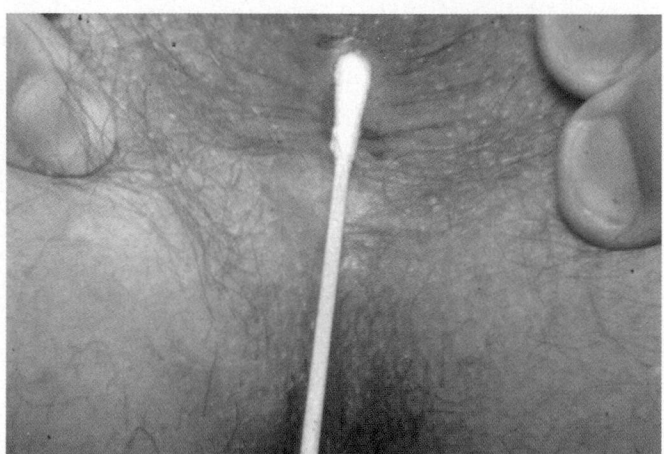

FIGURE I Examining the anus. Examining the external anus is generally all that is necessary to make the diagnosis.

baths or soaking in a tub after evacuation. Heat of any source (soaking, heating pad, hot water bottle) will help to alleviate the spasm of the anal musculature. Topical anti-inflammatory creams or suppositories also can be given to patients to help with symptom control. Patients are given a follow-up appointment to reassess in 6 to 8 weeks but are told that they may cancel this appointment if symptoms have resolved and follow up on an as needed basis. It is important to stress to patients that if the pain resolves but bleeding persists, they need to follow up for further evaluation.

Chronic Anal Fissure

Chronic fissures are those that have had prolonged symptoms before presentation or have failed 6 weeks of conservative management. There are a multitude of medical and surgical options for treating these patients. It is important to consider the likelihood of an alternative diagnosis in any patient with a prolonged nonhealing fissure. The gold standard of surgical therapy for chronic anal fissure is lateral internal sphincterotomy (LIS); however, there is some risk to continence with sphincterotomy, so it is important to reflect on this when undertaking the treatment of anal fissure. Conversely, the long-term risk of altered continence is unclear and different among studies. In one large long-term study, less than 10% of patients experienced difficulties with incontinence at more than 5 years of follow-up, and 3% experienced significant changes in lifestyle (Nyam and Pemberton, 1999). A second study detailed up to 15% to 30% of patients experiencing soilage or inability to control gas at an average of 36 months (Garcia-Aguilar et al, 1996). The latter study, however, had a lower rate of response (63% vs 87%) and was an "average" not a median follow-up, so these patients may have been experiencing early symptoms that resolved with time as suggested by Nyam and Pemberton. When embarking on treatment of anal fissures, a frank discussion with the patient regarding treatment modalities, time of healing, recurrence, and risk to future continence is critically important.

Medical Therapy

The mainstays of medical therapy for chronic anal fissure are fiber, pain control, and chemically induced relaxation of the IAS. Many different medications have been used in attempts to achieve relaxation of the IAS. The most commonly used topical therapies are either nitric oxide (NO) donors or calcium-channel blockers (CCB). Alpha-adrenergic antagonists also have been evaluated but have not demonstrated benefit. Glyceryl trinitrate (GTN) is the most widely used NO donor. After a 6- to 8-week course of topical 0.4% GTN

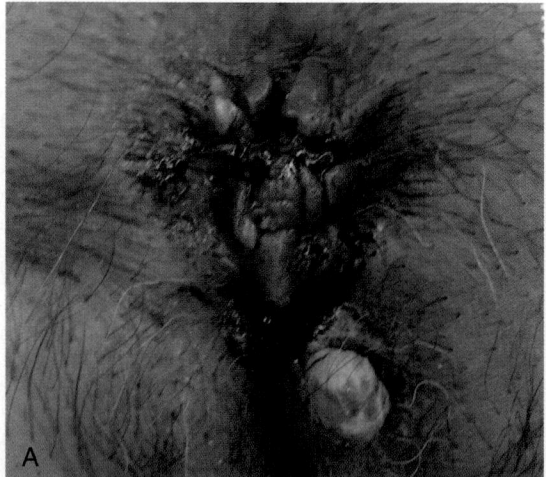

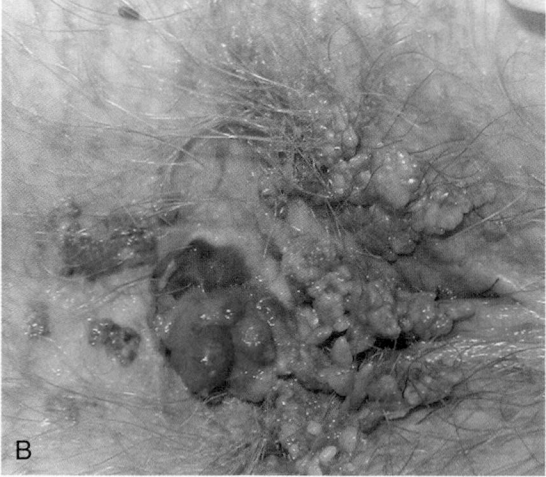

FIGURE 2 Fissures located in the lateral aspect of the anus should raise suspicion for other disease process such as anal carcinoma (**A**) and anal condyloma (**B**).

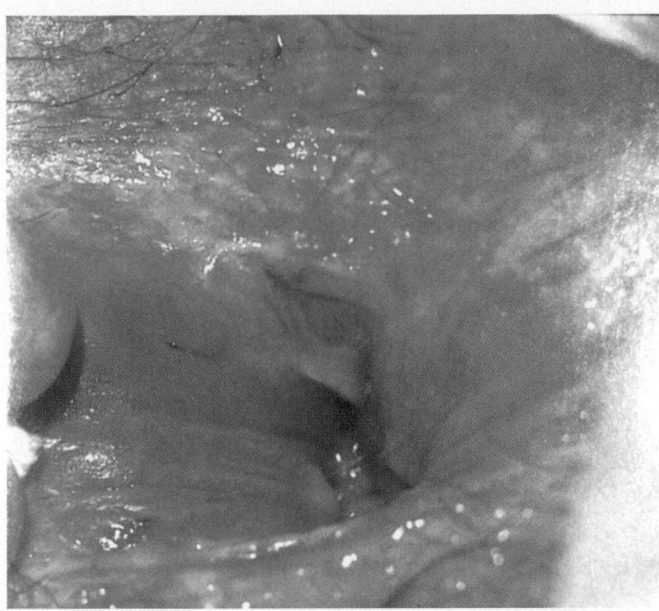

FIGURE 3 Fissures less than 8 weeks old typically are considered acute and are likely to respond to conservative treatment with fiber, stool softeners, and warm baths.

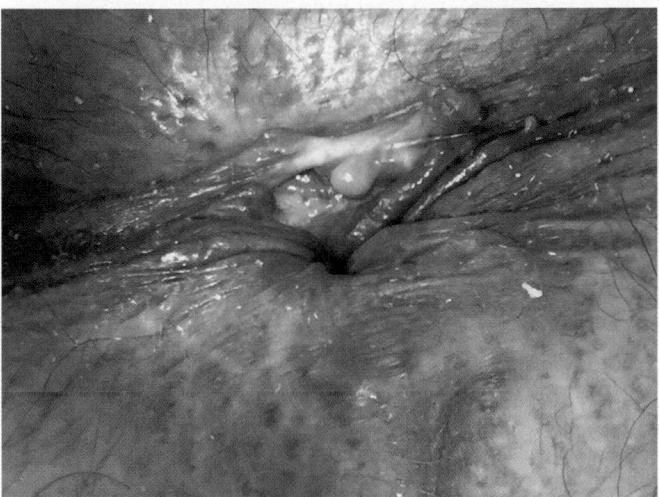

FIGURE 4 Chronic fissures are characterized by fibrosis, a skin tag at the distal extent of the fissure, and/or a hypertrophied papilla at the proximal end. The internal sphincter muscle may be visible at the base of the fissure.

ointment, GTN modestly improved healing rates when compared with placebo (48.9% vs 35.5%, Nelson et al, 2012); however, there was a high rate of recurrence at 1 year (50%), and a significant number of patients did not complete therapy secondary to headaches. Nifedipine and diltiazem have been used topically for the treatment of anal fissures with results similar to topical nitrates. Similarly, the most common side effect of CCB therapy was headache, although this was not as severe as GTN and rarely led to a disruption in therapy (<20% of patients). Both NO donor and CCB oral therapy have been used in trials with rates of dropout greater than 40% and headaches in excess of 30% leading to diminished efficacy (Nelson et al, 2012). In our current practice, we often use 2% diltiazem with 1% lidocaine.

Botulinum toxin (Botox) injection is another means of chemically induced sphincter relaxation. The effect of Botox is mediated by blocking acetylcholine release at the neuronal junction, therefore decreasing IAS tone. This effect begins within hours of injection and lasts 3 to 4 months. Fissure healing rates are comparable with GTN and CCB with fewer side effects, most notably some transient minor incontinence; however, recurrence rates were more than 50% after 1 year (Nelson et al, 2012). The injection may be performed in the office without sedation, although some patients may have severe discomfort with examination, and in this instance the operating room is the preferred location for treatment. A major issue with the use of Botox therapy is the wide variety of application dosages and methods. It is our practice to inject 20 u at 10 and 2 o'clock anteriorly in the intersphincteric groove (Figure 5), regardless of the area of the fissure, because data suggest this is the most effective method of application (Maria et al, 2000). If the fissure does not respond to medical therapy, an examination under anesthesia along with definitive surgical treatment is warranted to rule out other causes. The procedure should include endoscopic evaluation of the colon if not already performed. If the workup is negative, then definitive surgical management may be used in the same setting.

Surgical Therapy

The mainstay of surgical therapy and the current gold standard for the treatment of anal fissure is sphincterotomy. Complete long-term healing rates exceed 90%, and no current chemically induced IAS relaxation method has matched these results. Several different methods of sphincterotomy have been studied. Posterior midline sphincterotomy has rates of fissure healing that are similar to LIS but has been associated with keyhole sphincter deformity and poor wound healing, so this has been abandoned largely in favor of LIS. LIS can be performed via either "open" or "closed" technique with similar results (Nelson et al, 2011), although some have suggested there is a reduced risk of incontinence with closed LIS at the expense of slightly increased recurrence rates in long-term follow-up (Garcia-Aguilar et al, 1996). The "open" sphincterotomy is undertaken by making a small, radially oriented incision over the intersphincteric groove, dissecting out the internal sphincter muscle, and cutting approximately 60% defect in the muscle. The overlying incision is then closed with absorbable suture (Figure 6). A "closed" sphincterotomy is undertaken by placing the index finger of the surgeon in the anal canal, inserting an 11-blade scalpel in the intersphincteric groove and cutting the muscle toward the finger (Figure 7).

The main complication associated with LIS is incontinence. One of largest series reporting incontinence after LIS, more than 500 patients, reported that up to 50% of patients experienced transient degrees of incontinence, including inability to control gas, soiling or loss of stool, but at more than 5-year follow-up these rates were 6%, 8%, and 1%, respectively, and only 3% of patients reported this affecting their quality of life (Nyam and Pemberton, 1999). Tailoring the sphincterotomy to the length of the fissure rather than performing a complete sphincterotomy to the dentate line has helped to minimize this risk (Nelson et al, 2011). As mentioned earlier, closed LIS has been shown to have lower rates of incontinence symptoms when compared with open LIS (Garcia-Aguilar et al, 1996).

The surgeon may consider fissurectomy with or without advancement flap as an alternative to sphincterotomy. This procedure is used particularly when patients have a low baseline sphincter resting pressure. This is accomplished by curettage or excision of the fissure (Figure 8) and creating a cutaneous flap, which is then mobilized and advanced into the anal canal covering the area of the fissure (Figure 9). This can be accomplished with a variety of flap techniques, most commonly a V-Y or rectangular advancement flap, although some groups have reported using cutaneous island flaps, such as a "house" flap (Figure 10). In one study of 60 patients randomized to either LIS or fissurectomy with flap closure and median follow-up of >70 months all patients in both arms had healed fissures without recurrence with a significant decrease in "mild anal incontinence" in patients with fissurectomy (5.7% vs 47.1%) although this study had only 57% response rate in the fissurectomy group

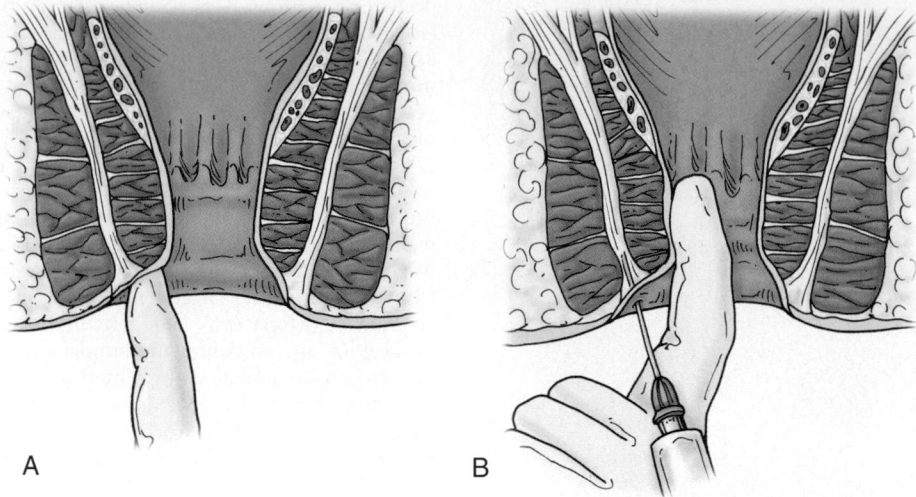

FIGURE 5 Botox injection is performed by injection of Botox at 10 and 2 o'clock anteriorly in the intersphincteric groove. First the index finger palpates the intersphincteric groove (**A**) and the needle is then placed within the groove (**B**) to inject the Botox. *(Reprinted with permission from In Braasch, Sedgwick, Veidenheimer, Ellis, eds. Atlas of Abdominal Surgery. Philadelphia: WB Saunders; 1991:199.)*

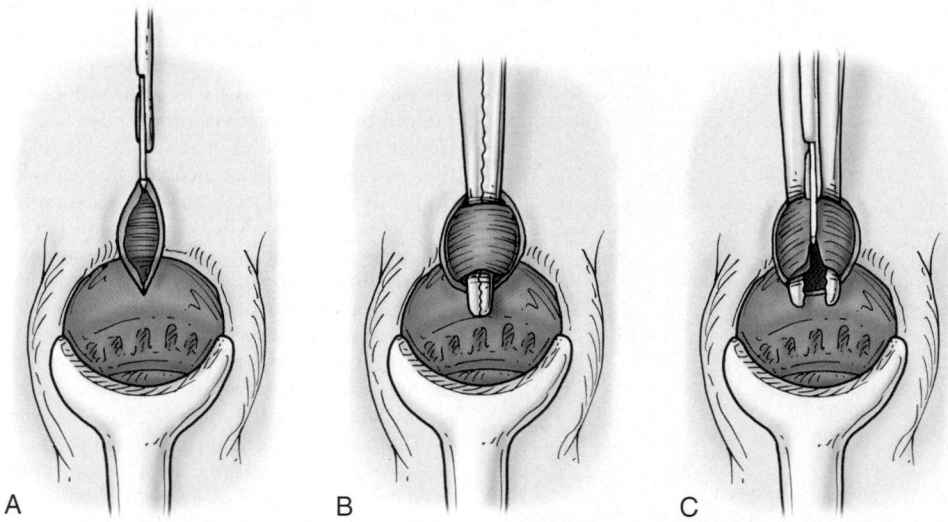

FIGURE 6 Open lateral internal sphincterotomy. **A,** First the overlying anoderm is incised. The internal sphincter muscle is then dissected free (**B**) and divided (**C**). *(Reprinted with permission from Wexner SW, Beck DE, eds. Fundamentals of Anorectal Surgery. 2nd ed. London: WB Saunders; 1998:214-215.)*

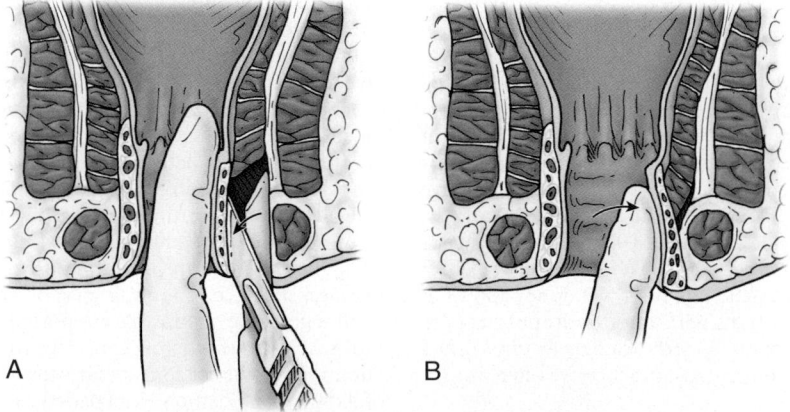

FIGURE 7 Closed lateral internal sphincterotomy. **A,** After anesthetizing the perianal area, the finger is inserted into the anal canal, an 11-blade scalpel is inserted in the intersphincteric groove and the muscle is cut toward the finger. **B,** After cutting the muscle, a wedge defect should be felt in the internal sphincter muscle. *(Reprinted with permission from Wexner SW, Beck DE, eds. Fundamentals of Anorectal Surgery. 2nd ed. London: WB Saunders; 1998:214-215.)*

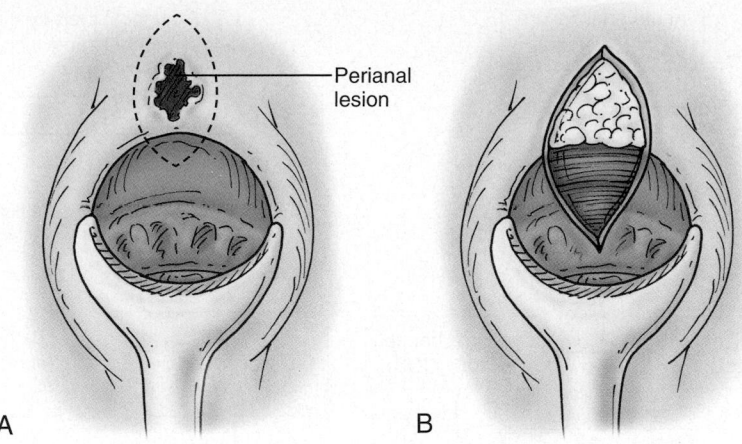

Perianal lesion

A   B

FIGURE 8 Fissurectomy may be used as an alternative approach to LIS. The fissure is either excised (**A**) such that the fissure base is visible (**B**) or curetted. At that time the wound maybe primarily closed or an anoplasty may be performed (see Figures 9 and 10). *(Reprinted with permission from Braasch, Sedgwick, Veidenheimer, Ellis, eds. Atlas of Abdominal Surgery. Philadelphia: WB Saunders; 1991:212.)*

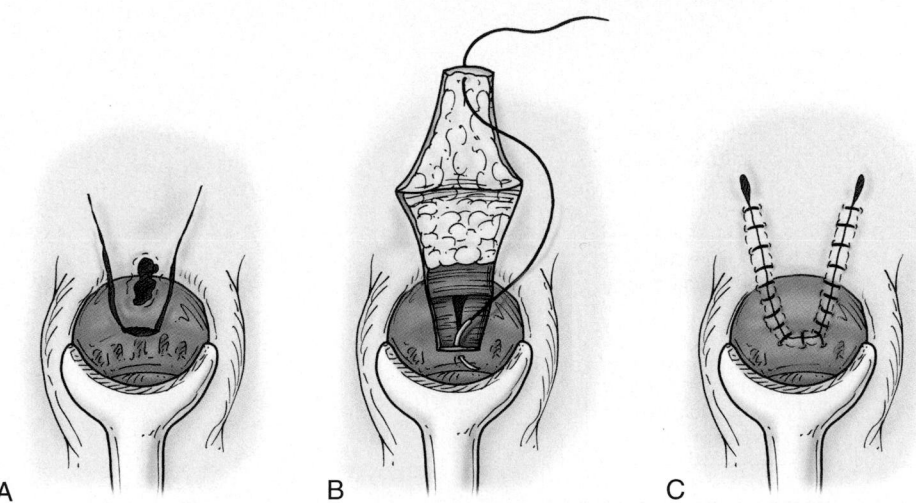

A   B   C

FIGURE 9 Anoplasty with a cutaneous anal flap may be used after fissurectomy to cover the remaining defect. *(Reprinted with permission from Braasch, Sedgwick, Veidenheimer, Ellis, eds. Atlas of Abdominal Surgery. Philadelphia: WB Saunders; 1991:212.)*

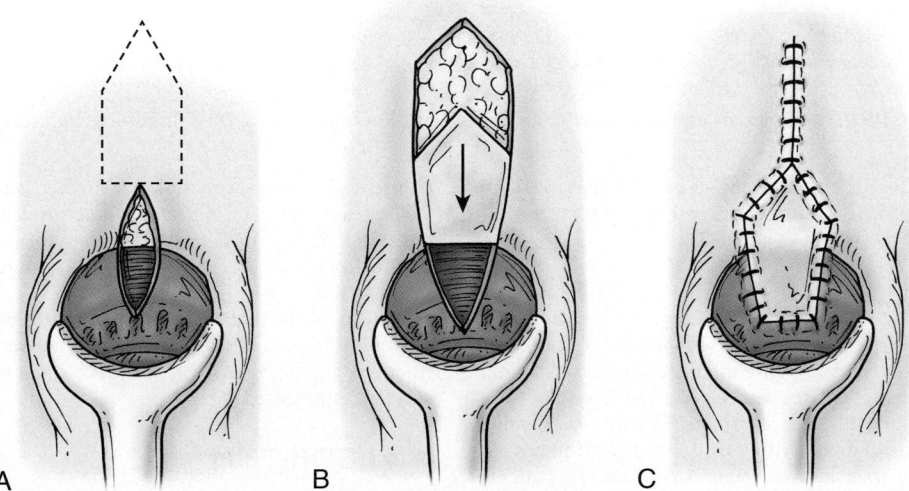

A   B   C

FIGURE 10 Cutaneous flap anoplasty for larger defects or fissures may best be accomplished with an island flap, such as a "House" advancement flap. *(Reprinted with permission from Liberman et al. Am J Surg. 2000;179:325-329.)*

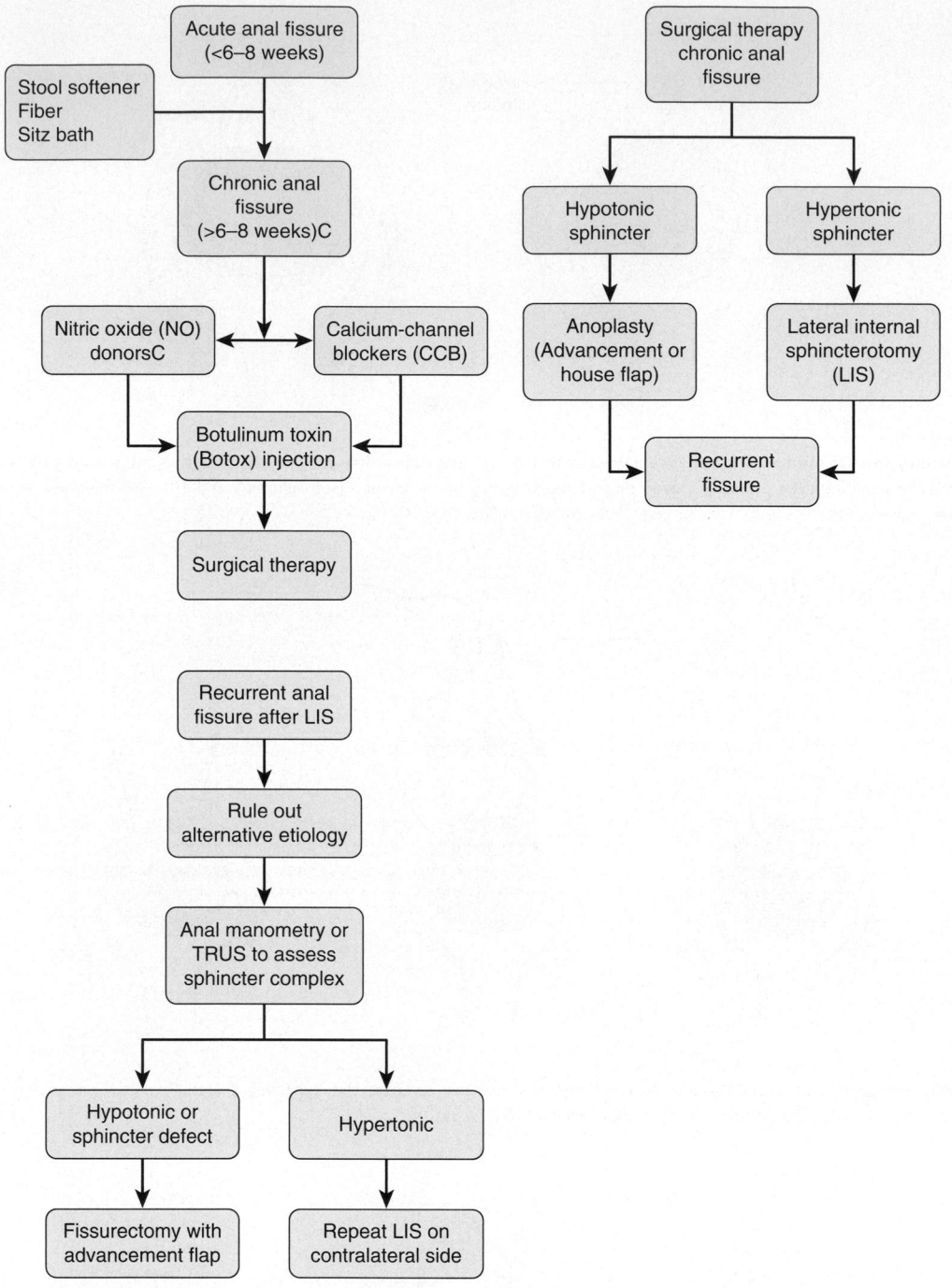

FIGURE 11 Algorithm: management of acute, chronic, and recurrent fissures. *TRUS,* Transrectal ultrasound.

(Hancke et al, 2010). This technique may be particularly useful in those patients with anterior midline fissures, which often are associated with sphincter defects (Nyam et al, 1995).

Recurrent Anal Fissures

Long-term recurrence in patients treated with medical therapy is common; however, long-term recurrence after LIS is rare and should prompt further investigation. The surgeon should consider why LIS has failed. Most commonly, the internal sphincter was divided incompletely, leaving the patient with persistent hypertonicity of the IAS; however, there may be an alternative cause. In patients with recurrent fissures, biopsy of the fissure edge should be considered to rule out other disease, and anal manometry should be considered before undertaking further surgical intervention. In well-chosen patients, repeat LIS has proven to be effective (Liang and Church, 2015). The procedure typically is performed on the contralateral side because there is likely residual scarring at the original site.

Alternatively, patients with hypotonic sphincters are unlikely to respond to repeat LIS, and this may increase the risk for fecal incontinence. For these patients, anoplasty with may be a more prudent surgical intervention.

■ ALGORITHM

The algorithm we typically use for the treatment of anal fissure is outlined in Figure 11.

Suggested Readings

Garcia-Aguilar J, et al. Open vs. closed sphincterotomy for chronic anal fissure: long-term results. *Dis Colon Rectum.* 1996;39:440-443.

Hancke E, et al. Dermal flap coverage for chronic anal fissure: lower incidence of anal incontinence compared to lateral internal sphincterotomy after long-term follow-up. *Dis Colon Rectum.* 2010;53:1563-1568.

Jenkins JT, Urie A, Molloy RG. Anterior anal fissures are associated with occult sphincter injury and abnormal sphincter function. *Colorectal Dis.* 2008;10:280-285.

Liang J, Church JM. Lateral internal sphincterotomy for surgically recurrent chronic anal fissure. *Am J Surg.* 2015;210:715-719.

Maria G, et al. Influence of botulinum toxin site of injections on healing rate in patients with chronic anal fissure. *Am J Surg.* 2000;179:46-50.

Nelson RL, et al. Non surgical therapy for anal fissure. *Cochrane Database Syst Rev.* 2012;(2):CD003431.

Nelson RL, et al. Operative procedures for fissure in ano. *Cochrane Database Syst Rev.* 2011;CD002199.

Nyam DC, et al. Island advancement flaps in the management of anal fissures. *Br J Surg.* 1995;82:326-328.

Nyam DC, Pemberton JH. Long-term results of lateral internal sphincterotomy for chronic anal fissure with particular reference to incidence of fecal incontinence. *Dis Colon Rectum.* 1999;42:1306-1310.

The Management of Anorectal Abscess and Fistula

Dara H. Christante, MD, and Amy J. Thorsen, MD

Approximately 100,000 patients in the United States seek care for anorectal sepsis each year. The mean age of presentation is at 40 years; males are twice as likely as females to have the condition. Fifty percent of patients treated for an acute anorectal abscess develop a fistula-in-ano requiring further surgical treatment. Principles of management have evolved to three basic tenets: control the septic process, define the involved anatomy, and attend to symptoms without compromising sphincter function. Although many presentations are straightforward, complex and recurrent disease challenge even the most experienced surgeon. It is crucial for the surgeon managing this disease to understand the regional anatomy, treat patients in the context of their comorbid conditions, and apply the proper surgical technique. Improper management can lead to potentially life-threatening sepsis or significantly affect a patient's quality of life by causing chronic discomfort and socially inhibiting problems with personal hygiene.

■ ANORECTAL ABSCESS

Cause and Classification

The anal glands empty into the rectum through 10 to 15 crypts of Morgagni located circumferentially at the dentate line. When this drainage is blocked, pressure builds as the septic source grows and propagates along paths of least resistance within or through the intersphincteric space. The potential pathways of suppurative extension delineate the anatomic spaces of anorectal sepsis: intersphincteric, submucosal, perianal, ischiorectal, postanal, and supralevator space (Figure 1).

The intersphincteric abscess, located at the site of the anal glands, tracks craniocaudally between the sphincter layers. A submucosal abscess represents the least extensive suppurative process, located just beneath the mucosa above the dentate line. Perianal abscesses descend through the intersphincteric space to the subcutaneous tissue around the anus and below the sphincter complex. The ischiorectal abscess has extended from the intersphincteric space through or above the external sphincter to the ischiorectal space. This space encircles the external sphincter caudal to the levators and medial to the ischial tuberosities. The postanal space is located posteriorly, between the levators (cranially) and the external sphincter (caudally); this space may be solely involved, or infection may extend laterally to the ischiorectal fossa, forming the so-called *horseshoe abscess*. Supralevator abscesses, located above the levators as the name implies, are caused by cranial extension of cryptoglandular sepsis or by caudal extension of an intra-abdominal process, such as diverticular disease, that perforates through the peritoneum.

Understanding the anatomic spaces of anorectal sepsis is imperative in deciphering the patient's presentation and planning the appropriate intervention that attains adequate drainage and reduces complications such as systemic sepsis, recurrence, fecal incontinence, and complex fistula formation. Although the cryptoglandular theory is believed to be responsible for the majority of anorectal abscesses, it is crucial to identify contributing conditions or alternate causes such as those displayed in Box 1. The impact of these factors and causes on the nature of the disease and treatment strategy is discussed later in the chapter.

Presentation and Diagnosis

Anal pain independent of defecation is the most common complaint. Swelling and fever are often present. Associated symptoms and medical history suggestive of or including inflammatory bowel disease or immunocompromise also should be gathered. On anorectal examination, an indurated bulge with fluctuance and cellulitis near the anal verge is indicative of perianal abscess. Intersphincteric abscesses are unique in their lack of external findings but cause exquisite tenderness on digital rectal examination. Ischiorectal abscesses typically have gluteal findings of induration, tenderness, and fluctuance without tenderness on digital rectal examination. Abscesses limited to the postanal space may have localized tenderness posterior to the anal verge, but without apparent induration or fluctuance. Supralevator abscesses may have no anorectal findings; further evaluation with pelvic imaging should be considered to exclude their presence. Bedside anoscopy can be performed but often is not tolerated and should not be pressed. Patients who cannot tolerate an examination should undergo an examination under anesthesia (EUA). Sigmoidoscopy is rarely helpful or indicated.

The majority of patients with a suggestive history and examination can be managed with bedside drainage or operative evaluation and treatment. Additional imaging, however, is useful in some acute situations. A CT scan is helpful in patients with associated abdominal symptoms or findings, or with clinical suspicion of a supralevator abscess. A CT scan should not be relied on to exclude drainable anorectal infection. Undrained anorectal infection can lead to severe systemic infection and destruction of the anal sphincter complex, resulting in functional morbidity. Transanal ultrasound and magnetic resonance imaging (MRI) are not generally available or tolerated in the acute setting of an anorectal abscess. Both are used as adjuncts in delineating fistula-in-ano.

Operative Evaluation and Drainage

Surgical drainage remains the definitive treatment of anorectal abscesses. Bedside drainage under local anesthesia using 1% lidocaine with dilute epinephrine often is well tolerated for perianal

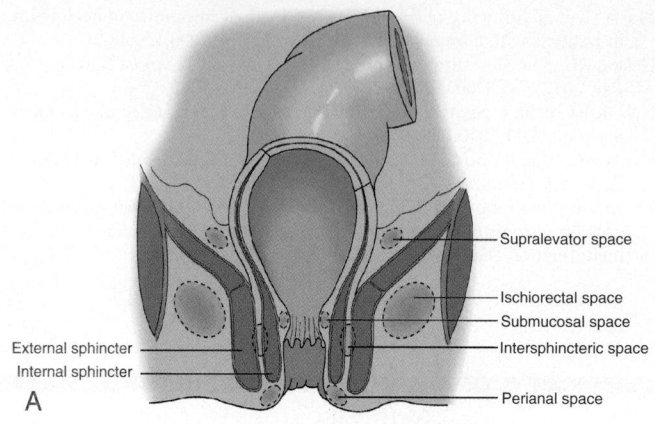

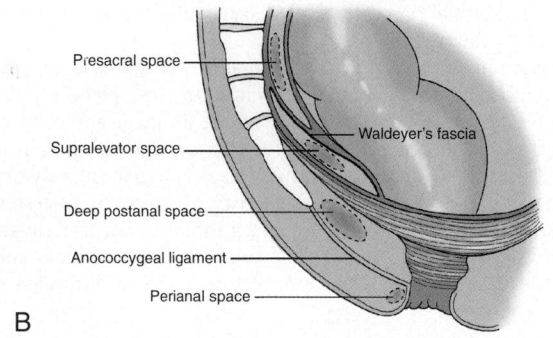

FIGURE 1 Anal sepsis and fistula. Classification of anorectal abscesses by location. **A,** Coronal view. **B,** Sagittal view. *(From Yeo CJ, et al. Shackelford's Surgery of the Alimentary Tract. ed 7. Philadelphia: Saunders; 2007.)*

BOX 1: Cause of Anorectal Abscess

Cryptoglandular
Iatrogenic (anorectal or genitourinary surgery)
Perineal trauma
Radiation injury
Inflammatory bowel disease
Acquired immunodeficiency syndrome
Invasive fungal infection
Hidradenitis suppurativa
Diverticulitis
Anal fissure
Osteomyelitis
Foreign body
Malignancy (carcinoma, adenocarcinoma, hematologic
    malignancy)

Adapted from Cameron Dietz chapter and Becks DE, et al, eds. *The ASCRS Textbook of Colon and Rectal Surgery.* 2nd ed. New York: Springer-Verlag; 2011.

abscesses and small ischiorectal abscesses. After infiltrating the area with local anesthetic, the surgeon makes a curved incision over the abscess. The incision should be oriented over the side of the abscess closest to the anal verge without transgression into the sphincter complex; this is done so that if a fistula forms, it is more likely to have a simple, short tract. A hemostat or finger is used to probe the wound, breaking down all loculations and defining the extent of disease. An ellipse of skin incorporating the initial incision is excised to prevent premature closure of the skin. The cavity is irrigated, and dry gauze is applied externally with the expectation of ongoing drainage.

Large abscesses and those that must be approached transanally are most appropriately done in the operating room under monitored anesthesia care or general anesthesia. A preoperative antibiotic with gram-negative coverage is administered. The anorectal region is best exposed with the patient in the prone jack-knife position and the buttocks taped widely apart, but high lithotomy is often adequate. A headlamp is recommended. Commonly used instruments are the Hill-Ferguson, Fansler, or Pratt bivalve retractors, fistula probes, and curettes. The perianal region is inspected, noting any induration, fluctuance, or dermatologic abnormalities. A digital rectal examination is performed followed by anoscopy, looking for mucosal bulging or other abnormality. Biopsies should be performed on ulcerations, suspicious nodules, or perianal lesions to exclude neoplasia. Biopsies should be performed on recurrent abscess or fistula tracts as well in an effort to diagnose underlying inflammatory bowel disease or the rare malignancy. If the site of purulence is not obvious, an 18-gauge needle can be used to aspirate in suspected areas. Culture data are rarely helpful but may be so in patients with recurrent infections, a history of methicillin-resistant *Staphylococcus aureus,* or patients with underlying HIV infection in whom atypical microbes may be present.

For large ischiorectal abscess, ipsilateral counter incisions can establish adequate drainage rather than a large incision that resects overlying healthy tissue and prolongs healing unnecessarily. Digital exploration of the abscess cavity is prudent to ensure that extension into the postanal space or the contralateral fossa is not present. Packing is usually not necessary and impractical for the patient to exchange. An alternate means of drainage uses a stab incision overlying the abscess, as close to the anal verge as possible, and the insertion of a 10F to 16F mushroom catheter into the cavity. The catheter is secured with an anchoring suture and left in place for a week. The catheter is removed once a tract is well established, although catheters can be left in for prolonged periods in cases of large or recurrent infections.

Drainage of a postanal space abscess deserves special note. A radial incision is made from the posterior anal verge toward the coccyx. Subcutaneous tissue is divided and the underlying fibers of the external sphincter are spread with a hemostat clamp. The anococcygeal ligament then is divided to access the postanal space. A digit is inserted to explore the extent of suppuration. If a horseshoe abscess is present, elliptical counter incisions over the involved ischiorectal fossa are created. Penrose drains can be looped between incisions to maintain patency. If an underlying fistula is noted, a noncutting seton is placed to prevent recurrent sepsis (Figure 2).

Intersphincteric abscesses are addressed transanally. Mucosa overlying the bulging anal canal is divided vertically with cautery. The underlying internal sphincter muscle, with circumferential transversely oriented muscle fibers, thus is exposed. A finely tipped hemostat is passed through the internal sphincter into the suppurative intersphincteric space and directed cephalad. The internal sphincter is divided over the hemostat with electrocautery. This generally does not compromise fecal continence, but patients should be informed of that small risk as part of informed consent. An alternate but less common method involves a stab incision at the anal verge in the intersphincteric groove and insertion of a small mushroom catheter into the affected intersphincteric space. The catheter is removed after sepsis has resolved.

The source of the supralevator abscess determines its treatment. Descending abdominal or pelvic sources typically are addressed with CT-guided percutaneous drainage; more complex or severe intra-abdominal disease may warrant transabdominal surgery or fecal diversion. Ascending cryptoglandular sepsis travels either through the intersphincteric space or through the levators from the ischiorectal fossa. The intersphincteric source is treated with transanal or transrectal drainage; incorrect surgical drainage through the ischiorectal fossa creates a suprasphincteric fistula. Conversely, the supralevator abscess with an ischiorectal source should be drained via skin incision to drain the ischiorectal fossa; transrectal

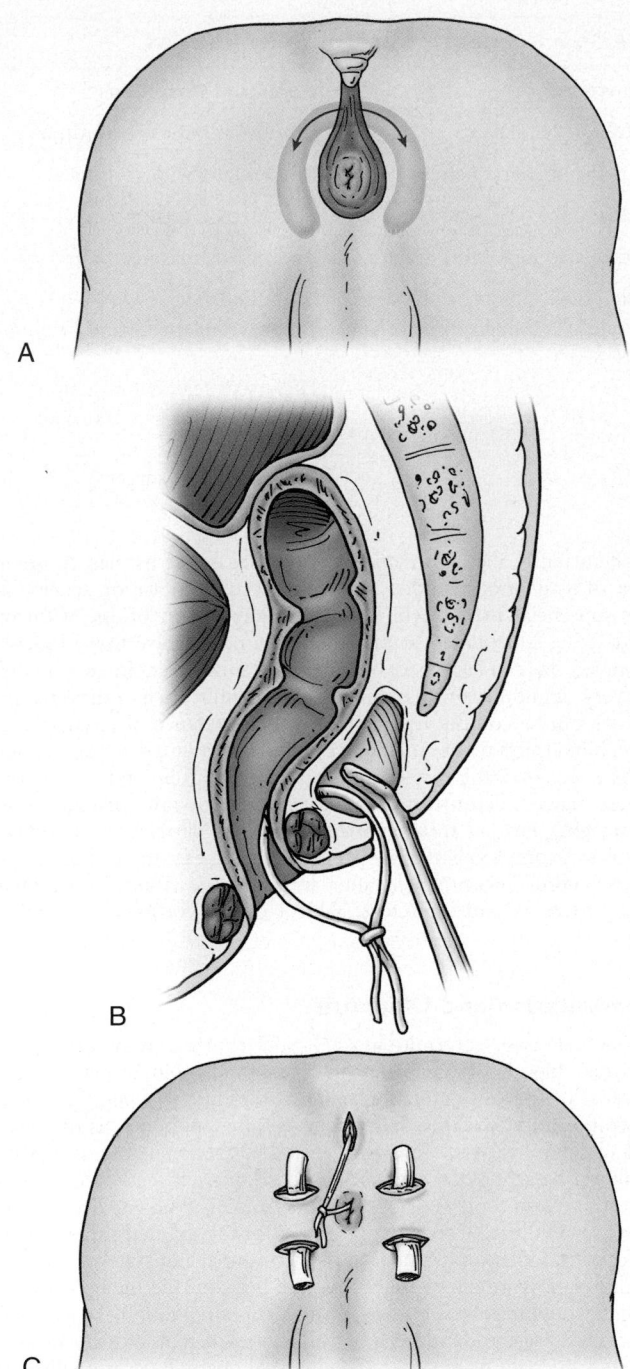

FIGURE 2 A, Horseshoe abscess with arrows shows that the deep postanal space is a window to the ischiorectal fossa bilaterally. **B,** The deep postanal space is drained through a radial incision in the posterior midline. A clamp is placed in the postanal space to ensure adequate drainage. If an internal opening is identified, a seton is placed through the fistula tract, encircling the posterior sphincter. **C,** Counter incisions drain the ischiorectal fossa. Placement of Penrose drains through the tracts ensures adequate drainage of the abscess cavities without significant soft tissue loss. *(Drawings courtesy Gaio Lakin, PhD.)*

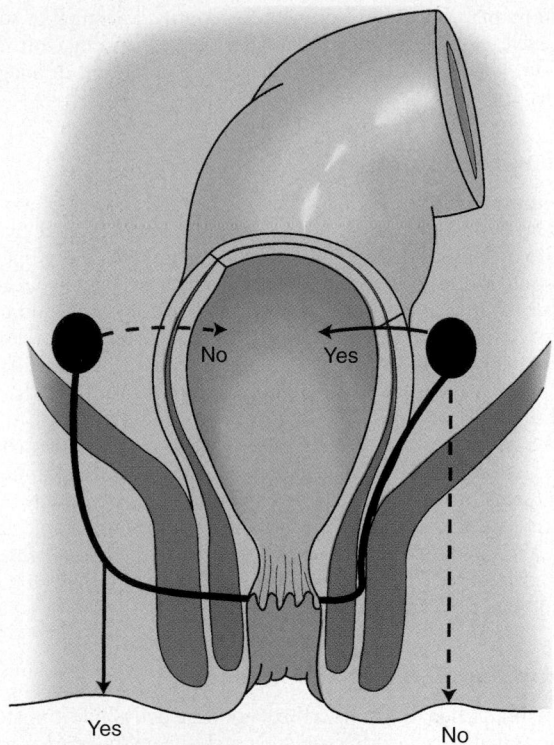

FIGURE 3 Drainage of a supralevator abscess. The supralevator abscess is denoted by the black oval. On the right, the supralevator abscess is associated with a transsphincteric fistula and passage through the ischiorectal fossa, often there are associated findings of an ischiorectal abscess. This abscess is drained via the skin and ischiorectal fossa; transrectal drainage would be inappropriate because it would result in an extrasphincteric fistula. On the left, the supralevator abscess is associated with an intersphincteric fistula and should be drained transrectally; drainage across the ischiorectal fossa would create a suprasphincteric fistula. Supralevator abscesses also may be addressed via CT-guided percutaneous drainage (alone or in combination with transrectal/transgluteal approaches), particularly when they are due to downward extension of an intra-abdominal process such as diverticulitis. *(From Yeo CJ, et al. Shackelford's Surgery of the Alimentary Tract. ed 7. Philadelphia: Saunders; 2007.)*

drainage would be inappropriate and create an extrasphincteric fistula (Figure 3).

Antibiotics and the Immunocompromised Patient

Most patients do not require antibiotic therapy after surgical drainage. In certain populations, however, antibiotics are warranted. Patients with large areas of cellulitis, signs of systemic sepsis or shock, prosthetic heart valves, or various conditions of immunocompromise warrant prolonged oral or parenteral antibiotics. Immunocompromised patient groups include those with diabetes mellitus, chronic corticosteroid use, acquired immunodeficiency syndrome, a history of bone marrow transplant, or active chemotherapy.

In contrast to all other patients with anorectal infection, profoundly neutropenic patients often are not addressed with surgery. The degree and duration of neutropenia is related directly to the incidence and prognosis of anorectal infections. In general, patients with absolute neutrophil counts (ANC) below 500 per cubic millimeter often do not mount sufficient immune response to develop suppuration. Therefore patients with low ANC and without fluctuance do not have a target for surgical drainage; prolonged, broad-spectrum antibiotics are recommended. This vulnerable patient population must be monitored closely, and imaging or EUA with aspiration may be useful adjuncts to identify a drainable source. Progressive sepsis, obvious fluctuance, or expanding soft tissue infection is an indication for surgical evaluation, drainage or débridement.

Primary Fistulotomy

Fistulotomy at the time of incision and drainage of the anorectal abscess was once a contentious issue. Proponents argued that the presence of sepsis aided in defining the fistula tract; laying open the tract would reduce recurrence. A general consensus has been reached, however, that primary or "prophylactic" fistulotomy submits a majority of patients who would never have recurred or developed a fistula to sphincterotomy and its attendant risks of fecal incontinence. Primary fistulotomy should be considered only in the most straightforward of superficial or low transsphincteric fistulas. Care must be taken to avoid creating false passages in the inflamed field while searching for the internal opening. Once the tract is cannulated with a fistula probe, the overlying tissue is divided and the wound is left open to drain. Primary fistulotomy is contraindicated in the elderly and in women with anterior fistulas, as well as in patients with compromised fecal continence, Crohn's disease, AIDS, and high transsphincteric fistulas.

Necrotizing Perianal Skin Infection

Necrotizing perianal skin infections are destructive, life-threatening infections that must be differentiated quickly from the more common anorectal abscess on the initial presentation because immediate surgical débridement offers the only chance at survival. Rapid development of severe anorectal pain that is out of proportion to findings on examination is the classic harbinger of a necrotizing infection. Risk factors include diabetes, chronic renal disease, obesity, smoking, and underlying neurologic disease (such as dementia or spinal cord injury) that prevents early detection or communication of symptoms and previous anorectal infections. Tender, irregular red, violaceous, or black macules and blisters in the perianal region are early signs of this dangerous entity; this may be associated with crepitus, induration, or gangrene. Septic shock and electrolyte disturbances may develop. Radical débridement of all nonviable tissue is necessary. Patients will require supportive management in the intensive care setting and empiric coverage with broad-spectrum antibiotics. Transfer to a tertiary center with hyperbaric oxygen capability should be considered. By limiting the growth of anaerobic and other forms of bacteria, and by boosting the effects of antibiotics and the immune system, hyperbaric oxygen is emerging as a powerful adjunct in treating this disease process and promoting healing. The need for fecal diversion is debated but should be considered only in the subacute setting after hemodynamic stability is well established.

■ FISTULA-IN-ANO

Cause and Classification

The cryptoglandular theory suggests that the acute suppurative process of anorectal sepsis originates at one of 8 to 10 anal glands located at the dentate line. These glands, whose ducts penetrate the internal sphincter and end in the intersphincteric space, allow bacteria to cause infection, which propagates along the path of least resistance until the growing pressure is released by surgical or spontaneous drainage. A fistula is the chronic sequelae of this process if the tract fails to heal and epithelializes. Although the cryptoglandular process is responsible for the vast majority of fistulas, Box 1 presents other causes that can instigate chronic inflammation and epithelialization along an abnormal communication between the skin and anorectum.

Fistulas are classified by their route between an internal opening in the anal canal and an external opening on the perianal skin. In 1976 Park and colleagues published the classification system that is

TABLE 1: Features of Complex Fistulas

Anatomy	Comorbid Conditions
Multiple fistulas	Compromised fecal continence
Suprasphincteric fistulas	Inflammatory bowel disease
Extrasphincteric fistulas	Refractory diarrhea
Associated high blind tract(s)	Anterior fistulas in women
High transsphincteric fistulas (>30% of anal sphincter length)	Immunodeficiency or compromised wound healing
	History of regional radiation
	History of obstetric trauma
	Elderly patients
	Prior anorectal surgery

used currently. Figure 4 depicts the four classes of fistulas. Another type of fistula not included in the anorectal classification scheme is the superficial fistula, which is essentially a skin bridge with an underlying subcutaneous tract that does not involve the sphincter complex; this can be a result of scarring after recurrent infections and surgery, or another process, such as hidradenitis. Each of these fistula classes can be complicated further by the presence of circular and high blind tracts that branch off the fistula tract into the intersphincteric space or ischiorectal fossa, but do not drain independently. These may be identified by careful exploration with a fistula probe or imaging. Fistulas are categorized further as "simple" or "complex" fistulas. A complex fistula has features that increase the risk of recurrence and/or incontinence after intervention, either by its own anatomy or by patient factors. Table 1 defines features of complex fistulas.

Presentation and Diagnosis

Patients describe intermittent anal pain; pruritus; drainage that is mucoid, bloody, or feculent; or occasionally blood per rectum because of friable granulation tissue at the internal opening. Cyclic discomfort and swelling that is relieved after spontaneous drainage is a common feature. A previous episode of perianal abscess may or may not be reported. Patients should be queried regarding gastrointestinal symptoms suggestive of inflammatory bowel disease and their current level of fecal continence. A history of anal surgery, anal infections, radiation, trauma, obstetric trauma, and systemic disease including inflammatory bowel disease, hematologic malignancy, or immunosuppression should be elicited. On examination, the external opening is easily identifiable; a palpable cord may be present and suggest the path of the tract. The internal opening occasionally can be palpated on digital rectal examination as a nodule or pit. Anoscopy, when tolerated, can assist in visualizing the internal opening as well as assess whether a distal proctitis is present. Further endoscopy can be considered in a patient with symptoms suggestive of inflammatory bowel disease.

Surgical Treatment

There are three tenets of fistula surgery: define the fistula anatomy, ensure resolution of sepsis, and preserve anal sphincter function. Maintaining these principles is critical at each step of treatment.

Define Fistula Anatomy

The anatomy of a fistula includes the internal external openings, the course of the intervening tract(s), and the presence of any blind tracts. Fistula anatomy is established most often by EUA. The patient is placed in prone jack-knife with the buttocks taped widely apart.

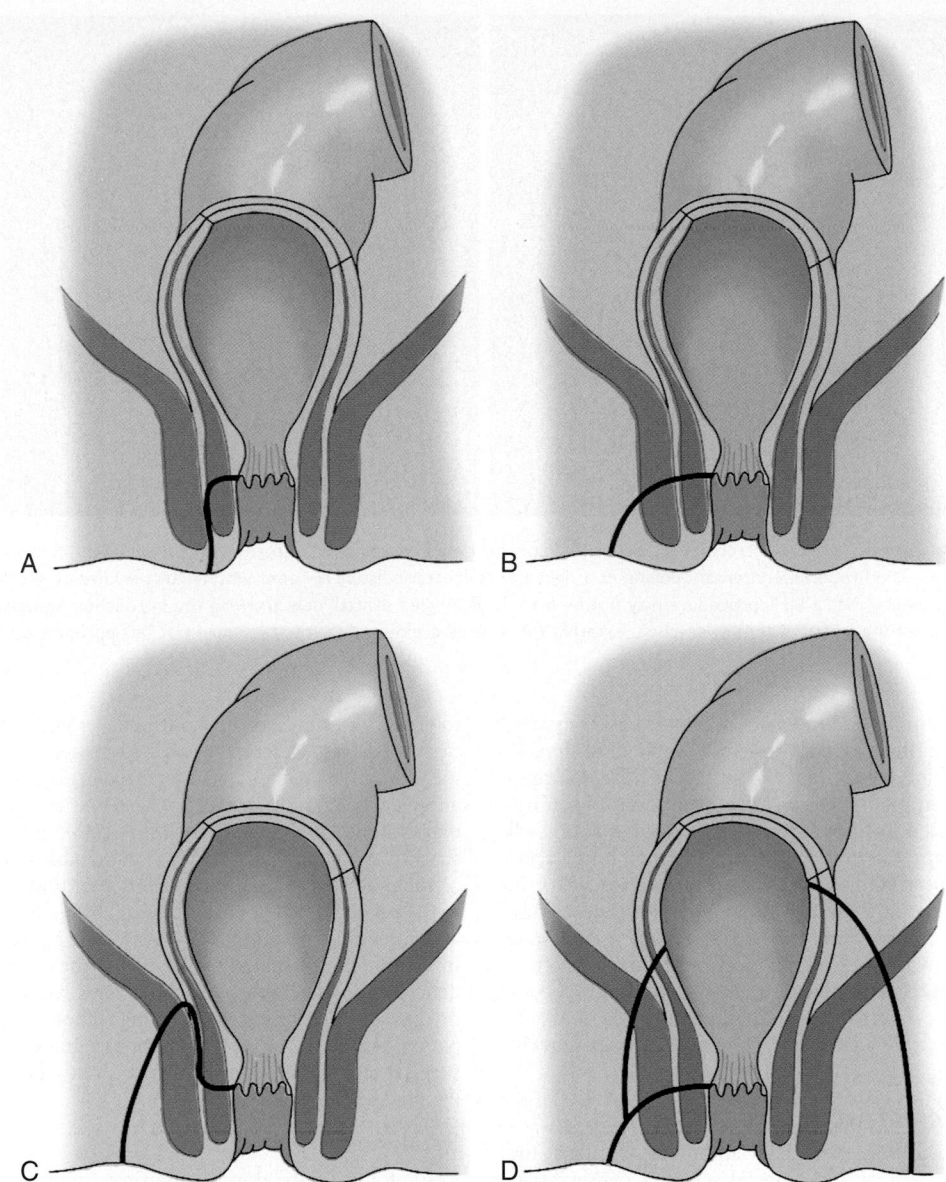

FIGURE 4 Classification of anal fistulas. **A,** Intersphincteric: The tract remains in the intersphincteric plane. 1, Simple. **B,** Transsphincteric: The fistula tract passes from the intersphincteric plane through the external sphincter muscle. 1, Uncomplicated. **C,** Suprasphincteric: There is an upward extension of the fistula tract in the intersphincteric plane. The tract then passes above the level of the puborectalis muscle and continues downward through the ischiorectal fossa to the perianal area. **D,** Extrasphincteric: There is a tract that passes from the skin of the perineum through the ischiorectal fossa and the levator muscles before entering the rectal wall. This fistula may be a consequence of an extension of a transsphincteric fistula or secondary to trauma, anorectal disease, or pelvic inflammation. *(Adapted from Yeo CJ, et al.* Shackelford's Surgery of the Alimentary Tract. *ed 7. Philadelphia: Saunders; 2007.)*

The perianal region is inspected, identifying evident external openings, suspicious lesions, or scars. Goodsall's rule predicts that an external opening posterior to a transverse line across the anus drains to a posterior midline internal opening; those that open anterior to the line have short, radial courses to the internal opening. Although Goodsall's rule is accurate for a majority of the posterior external openings, it has been shown to be less accurate in women with anterior openings.

Digital rectal examination is performed to assess for undrained sepsis and location of the internal opening. Anoscopy is used to identify the internal opening as well as note any signs of proctitis or malignancy. A fistula probe is inserted into the external opening and gently advanced toward the anticipated internal opening with subtle redirection as resistance dictates. The fistula tract easily should accept the probe without the sensation of tissue destruction; a false tract must not be created because it will only complicate the disease and neglect the primary tract. The internal opening also may be identified by injecting hydrogen peroxide into the external opening with an angiocatheter. Once cannulated, the type of fistula is established by determining its relationship to the internal and external sphincter complex, the levators, and presence of multiple fistulas or blind tracts. The percentage of sphincter complex caudal to the tract is determined; low transsphincteric fistulas are defined as those with less than 30% of the external sphincter involved. If the tract cannot be cannulated fully, the external opening is enlarged toward the anal verge, and a curette is used to débride the tract, and the operation is terminated. Adjunctive imaging is performed after 3 to 6 weeks to allow for inflammation related to surgery to subside.

When a fistula is recurrent, thought to be complex, or if anatomy cannot be identified by EUA, imaging can help identify sites

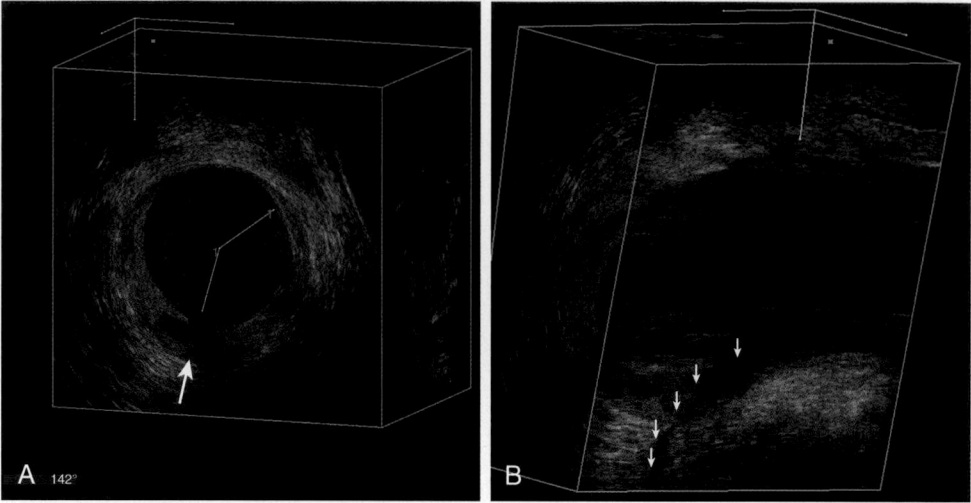

FIGURE 5 Ultrasound of right posterior transsphincteric fistula. **A,** Coronal view revealing a 142-degree internal sphincter defect on the left side from a previous hemorrhoidectomy. The hypoechoic internal opening of a right transsphincteric fistula is noted with an arrow. Given the edge of the internal sphincter defect abuts the fistula tract, a LIFT procedure may not be feasible. **B,** Angled sagittal view showing the hypoechoic transsphincteric fistula. Note the internal opening nears half the length of the hyperechoic external sphincter; therefore a fistulotomy would not be appropriate. *(Photo credit Amy Thorsen, MD.)*

of persistent infection and define the relevant anatomy. Transanal ultrasound and MRI are the principal modalities applied. Both have reliable accuracy with high concordance to surgical findings. Transanal endosonography can predict successfully the amount of sphincter that would be divided if primary fistulotomy is performed, as well as identify undrained sepsis, complex anatomy, and high blind tracts (Figure 5). MRI has been shown to alter surgical approach and decrease recurrence rates, and it appears to be superior at identifying suprasphincteric or extrasphincteric tracts. CT scan lacks adequate resolution to identify tracts and their relationship to the sphincters and levators with comparable accuracy. Fistulography, in which contrast is injected into the external opening and the fistula course is traced with fluoroscopy, rarely is undertaken in light of these technologic advancements.

Ensure the Resolution of Sepsis

For many patients with complex fistulas or an obvious fistula at the time of operative treatment of an anorectal sepsis, a conservative, staged approach with the initial placement of a seton is most appropriate. For a patient treated initially with a seton, a second stage procedure can be considered when the internal opening is less than 5 mm and the tract is simple, narrow, and without an associated cavity. Ongoing sepsis, as evidenced by pus, cellulitis, induration, or a persistent cavity, prevents healing and closure of the tract; any efforts to close the fistula definitively will likely fail. If persistent infection is present with a simple intersphincteric or low transsphincteric, a fistulotomy can be performed to simultaneously address the sepsis and the fistula. Complex fistulas with persistent sepsis should be treated with débridement of the tract around the seton, widening of the external opening, and a search for a high blind or circular tract. If additional treatable sources of the persistent sepsis cannot be identified or sepsis continues despite these approaches, imaging is pursued.

Assess and Preserve Anal Sphincter Function

Although a controlled anal fistula can cause significant discomfort and problems with personal hygiene, fecal incontinence is far more disruptive to a patient's quality of life. For that reason, preservation of continence is always a priority when choosing the proper management strategy. Division of the internal sphincter usually is well tolerated; division of distal third of the external sphincter is considered "safe" in healthy male individuals. The degree of sphincterotomy

tolerated without affecting continence is undoubtedly patient dependent, however. Careful analysis of patients' risk for incontinence includes an assessment of their current degree of continence, prior anorectal surgery or trauma, associated conditions that may cause diarrhea or inhibit healing, and likelihood of further anorectal surgery. Women in particular are vulnerable to incontinence because of their shorter sphincter complex, anatomic and neurologic injury to the pelvic floor sustained during childbirth, and to loss of elasticity and muscle attenuation associated with aging. Patients with active inflammatory bowel disease involving the anorectum and immunodeficiencies often heal poorly and have recurrent or metachronous fistula disease. Sphincter-preserving techniques are preferred in these patient populations. Table 2 provides a guide to choosing the proper surgical technique, although it does not take into account relevant patient factors.

Fistulotomy

Fistulotomy can be done at the time of abscess presentation, at the time of initial fistula presentation, or as a second stage procedure in appropriately selected patients. Regardless of timing, a fistulotomy is appropriate only in low-risk patients with a superficial, low intersphincteric or low transsphincteric fistula. Once the anatomy of the fistula is determined, the fistula is cannulated and the tissue overlying the probe is divided with electrocautery. The tract is débrided with a curette to remove debris and granulation tissue. For larger wounds, wound healing can be accelerated by marsupialization of the wound; the wound edges are sewn to the base of the wound with a continuous locking absorbable suture. Sphincter-sacrificing procedures have the highest success rates, generally more than 90%. This is at the untenable cost of compromised fecal continence; hence fistulotomy is not appropriate for high or complex fistulas.

Seton

A noncutting seton allows for ongoing drainage of sepsis and promotes fibrosis and maturation of the fistula tract, often in preparation for a second-stage procedure. After the fistula tract has been defined and débrided, the external opening is opened toward the anal verge. Circular, high blind tracts, and long subcutaneous tracts are appropriately laid open or drained and curetted. The seton, a thin Silastic band, vessel loop, or nonabsorbable suture, is threaded through the tract and secured in a loop or omega shape with several

TABLE 2: Management Strategy by Fistula Classification

Type of Fistula	Fistulotomy	Seton*	LIFT	Advancement Flap	Fibrin Glue	Collagen Plug	Address Intra-Abdominal or Pelvic Source
Superficial/ intersphincteric	•						
Low transsphincteric	•	•	•	•	•	•	
High transsphincteric		•	•	•	•	•	
Suprasphincteric		•		•		•	•
Extrasphincteric						•	•

*Seton placement can be a first stage or definitive treatment option.

LIFT, Ligation of intersphincteric fistula tract.

interrupted silk sutures. The seton should not be tight; a hemostat should fit easily between the skin and loop without tension. The second-stage procedure, either fistulotomy or a sphincter-preserving operation, usually is performed 6 to 10 weeks later. Setons used in this fashion for complex fistulas have success rates from 62% to 100%, depending on patient factors and the choice of the secondary procedure. For some Crohn's or other high-risk patients, seton placement can be the definitive operation; it is left in place for prolonged periods to prevent recurrent sepsis without the intention to perform a second stage procedure because of the likelihood of failure or iatrogenic incontinence.

Ligation of Intersphincteric Fistula Tract

Ligation of the *i*ntersphincteric *f*istula *t*ract procedure, or LIFT procedure is a relatively new sphincter-preserving technique first described in 2007. This is performed most often as a second-stage procedure for a transsphincteric fistula after a mature tract has developed.

With the patient in the prone jack-knife position with the buttocks taped widely apart, the fistula tract is cannulated with a probe. The external opening is widened to allow for drainage (Figure 6). A 1- to 2-cm curvilinear incision is made with electrocautery over the palpated intersphincteric groove above the fistula tract. A Lonestar retractor (Cooper Surgical, Trumbull, CT) deployed along the anoderm edges provides excellent exposure. The intersphincteric plane is developed bluntly with a fine-tipped hemostat. The fistula tract is isolated circumferentially with care to avoid disrupting it. The probe is removed and either end of the intersphincteric tract is suture-ligated with 3-0 absorbable suture. The tract is divided sharply with a scalpel. The external opening is injected with hydrogen peroxide; if there is a persistent leak, the intersphincteric opening of the external sphincter is oversewn until there is no longer a leak. Some authors test the internal opening with peroxide as well to ensure proper closure of the proximal portion of the tract. The anoderm is reapproximated with a running absorbable suture. Very high fistula tracts, or those that track long distances within the intersphincteric space may be difficult to properly isolate in the intersphincteric plane and are not good candidates for this approach.

Sirany and colleagues recently published a detailed literature review regarding the LIFT procedure and several technical variations. Primary healing rates varied between 47% and 95%. The impact on incontinence was not widely reported, but worsening of bowel continence was rare in studies that did report it. In general, the success rate is higher than that with bioprosthetics and comparable to endorectal advancement flap.

Endorectal Advancement Flap

The endorectal advancement flap is considered the "gold standard" sphincter-preserving operation. It is used as a second-stage

procedure for high fistula tracts, suprasphincteric tracts, and low tracts in high-risk patients with healthy rectal mucosa (see Table 1). For lesions below the dentate line, fistulotomy or a dermal advancement flap is preferred to prevent the creation of a mucosal ectropion that can form if the rectal mucosa is brought down to near the anal verge. Patients undergo a preoperative bowel preparation to forestall postoperative bowel movement. The prone jack-knife position is preferred for most fistulas, although lithotomy position often is used to address posterior midline anal fistulas. The seton is removed and the internal opening serves to mark the apex of the flap as depicted in Figure 7. Beginning at the internal opening, a flap is created by distal to proximal dissection with electrocautery, including mucosa, submucosa, and a few fibers of the internal sphincter (partial thickness). To ensure adequate perfusion, it is crucial that the base (proximal end) of the flap is wide, at least two to three times the width of the apex. The tongue-shaped flap is typically 2 to 4 cm long to allow for tension-free closure. The fistula tract is débrided with a curette, and the external opening is widened to allow for drainage. Absorbable suture is used to close the internal opening, and the integrity of the closure is tested with injection of hydrogen peroxide at the external opening. The tip of the flap with the internal opening is excised, and the flap gently is retracted distally over the internal opening to the dentate line, but not below it, to prevent ectropion formation. Wound edges are reapproximated with interrupted absorbable suture. Some surgeons place a small length of Penrose drain beneath the flap for drainage to decompress dead space and prevent seroma formation. Some authors describe maintaining the patient on antibiotics for 7 days postoperatively.

A recent systemic review of the procedure reported a success rate of 79.2% after an average of 28.9 months of follow-up; the success rate varied significantly, however, anywhere between 36.6% and 98.5%. Factors including obesity, history of radiation, prior attempts at repair, smoking, and inflammatory bowel disease have variably been found to predict failure. Although the sphincter muscle is not divided, worsening of bowel continence has been reported in 7% to 38% of patients treated with the procedure (ASCRS Practice Guidelines, 2011).

Fibrin Sealant and Collagen Plug

Synthetic and biologic materials have been new additions to the armamentarium of fistula treatment in the last 20 years. Their general principle is obliteration of the internal opening and fistula tract. Their primary benefit is a minimal risk profile because they pose no risk to continence, are easily repeated in the case of recurrence, and do not preclude subsequent surgical management. Fibrin sealant is a combination of fibrinogen and thrombin that is injected into the fistula tract (e.g., Tisseel). After sepsis has resolved, usually by means of a seton, the tract gently is débrided and irrigated. An angiocatheter is threaded from the external to the internal site, and the sealant is

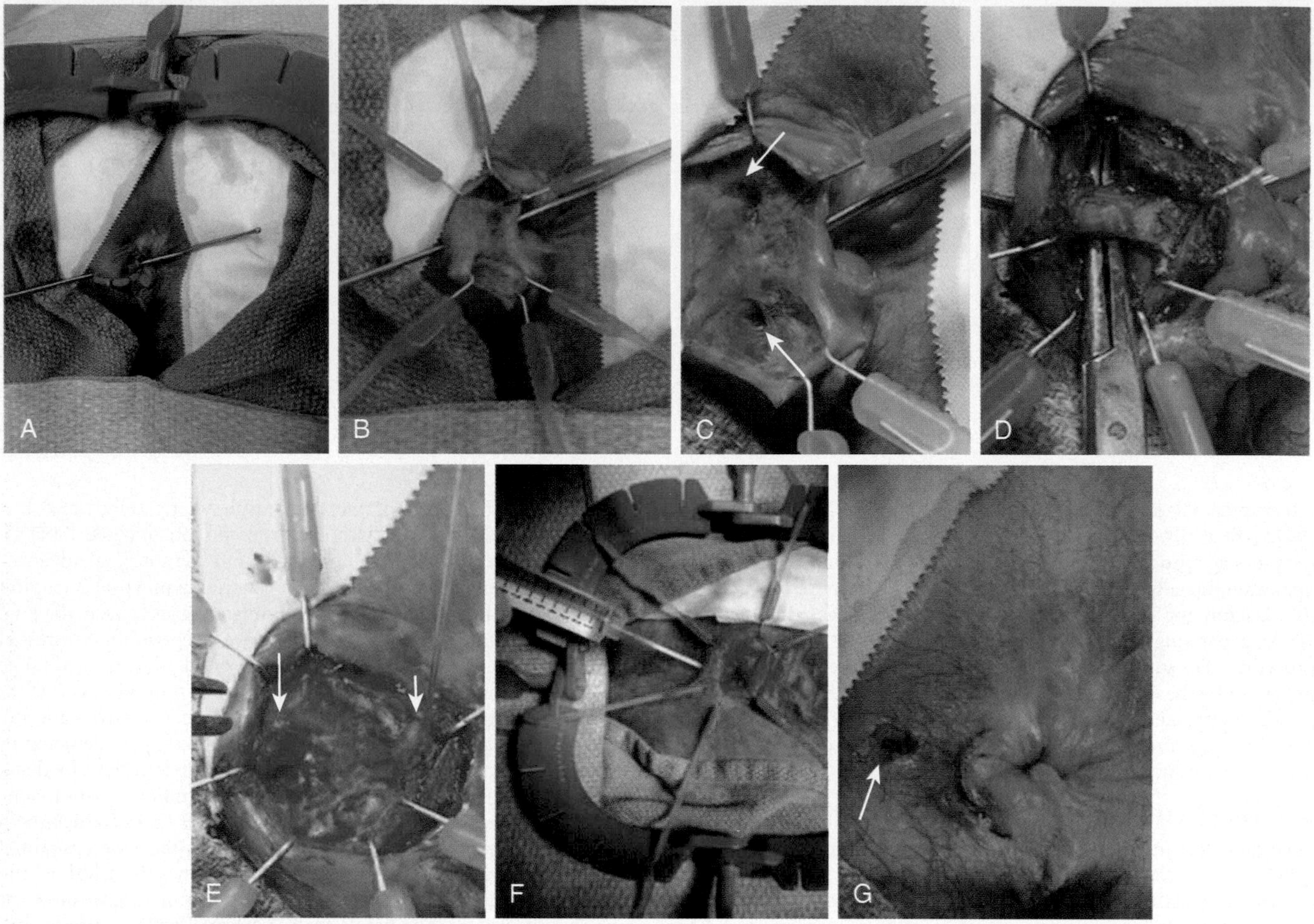

FIGURE 6 A, The fistula tract is cannulated. **B,** A curvilinear incision is made overlying, or slightly distal to, the intersphincteric groove. A Lonestar TM retractor is helpful for exposure. **C,** The intersphincteric plan is developed on either side of the tract *(arrows)*. **D,** Dissection continues around the tract until it is isolated. The probe is removed. **E,** Division and ligation of fistula tract. The tract is encircled with a Vicryl (Ethicon, Somerville, NJ) tie and the tract is ligated at the border of the internal anal sphincter *(small arrow)*. If a long tract is present, it can be excised and the tract near the external anal sphincter is either ligated or imbricated with Vicryl suture *(large arrow)*. **F,** The repair is tested by injecting hydrogen peroxide into the internal and external openings. The ligated ends can also be probed to ensure closure. If there is a leak, the fistula opening is further imbricated. **G,** The external opening *(arrow)* is slightly enlarged and the distal aspect of the tract is débrided with a curette. *(Photos provided by Jeffery J. Morken, MD.)*

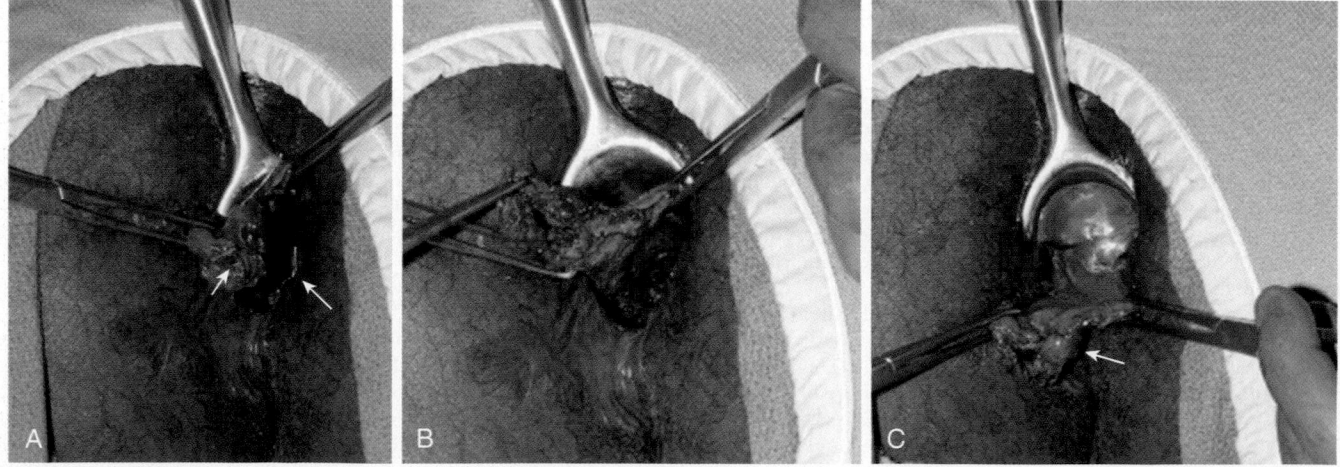

FIGURE 7 A, A wide-based flap is harvested. The arrow points to a fistula probe through the internal opening. The short arrow denotes the location of the internal opening at the edge of the flap. **B,** The flap should be full-thickness rectal wall and dissected as far proximally as possible to allow adequate advancement. Meticulous hemostasis must be achieved before advancing the flap. **C,** The arrow denotes the portion of the flap to be trimmed. The remainder of the flap is advanced and sutured with interrupted Vicryl stitches. *(Photo credit Amy Thorsen, MD.)*

injected such that a bead of sealant is formed at the internal opening. The angiocatheter is removed as the tract is filled with sealant. Another bead is developed at the external site to inhibit migration. The sealant material at the internal opening is sutured into place. Healing rates are low, ranging from 10% to 67%, but the low morbidity of the procedure allows for it to be considered a reasonable option.

Results and the risk profile are similarly low with bioprosthetic anal plugs applied in complex fistula, although some successes are durable. The fistula is cannulated, and a large silk suture is threaded through the tract. Curettage of the tract is not recommended. The suture is tied to the narrow end of the plug at the internal opening and then pulled through the tract until the plug exits the external opening. It is trimmed flush at both openings. The trimmed plug is sutured about the internal opening to secure it and close the internal opening.

Fistula-in-Ano and Crohn's Disease

The management of anal fistula in Crohn's disease is especially challenging. Fistulas develop according to the cryptoglandular theory as well as the underlying inflammatory condition of Crohn's disease. Fistulas in Crohn's patients often originate in the rectal mucosa creating high, complex fistula anatomy. They are often multiple and associated with high blind tracts. Treatment strategies are uniformly conservative because of poor wound healing, high recurrence rates, and vulnerability to incontinence related to frequent diarrhea, poor rectal compliance, and repeated insult to the sphincter complex with recurrent anal sepsis and need for intervention.

The initial surgical goal is to treat sepsis while maintaining sphincter integrity; this usually is addressed with a loose seton and widening of the external opening to allow for drainage. Consideration for medical management and an assessment of the extent of disease in conjunction with a gastroenterologist is recommended.

Improved healing rates with metronidazole, fluoroquinolones, and immunomodulators have been reported. The ACCENT II trial demonstrated patients who received infliximab compared with those in the placebo group experienced a significantly higher rate of anal fistula resolution (36% vs 19%). A common strategy is to initiate or escalate medical therapy with a seton in place and then remove the seton with the hope that it will heal in the quiescent disease state.

Asymptomatic fistulas do not require surgical management. Fistulotomy may be considered in patients with simple, low fistulas, but only in highly selected patients with careful consideration of the patient's individual risks of incontinence. Prolonged wound healing up to 3 to 6 months should be expected. Endorectal advancement flaps and LIFT procedures have been successful in patients without proctitis, but results are heavily dependent on patient selection. Long-term (indefinite) draining setons are a safe alternative to attempts at definitive management. If sepsis cannot be captured with local intervention and medical therapy, fecal diversion should be considered. Although diversion often leads to an improvement of symptoms and perianal sepsis, the perianal disease frequently recurs with reestablishment of intestinal continuity. Proctectomy is undertaken in refractory disease.

SUGGESTED READINGS

Becks DE, et al., eds. *The ASCRS Textbook of Colon and Rectal Surgery.* 2nd ed. New York: Springer-Verlag; 2011.

Sirany AM, Nygaard RM, Morken JJ. The ligation of the intersphincteric fistula tract procedure for anal fistula: a mixed bag of results. *Dis Colon Rectum.* 2015;58:604-612.

Soltani A, Kaiser AM. Endorectal advancement flap for cryptoglandular or Crohn's fistula-in-ano. *Dis Colon Rectum.* 2010;53:486-495.

Steele SR, Kumar R, Feingold DL, et al. Practice parameters for the management of perianal abscess and fistula-in-ano. *Dis Colon Rectum.* 2011;54: 1465-1474.

THE MANAGEMENT OF ANORECTAL STRICTURE

Jessica N. Cohan, MD, and Madhulika G. Varma, MD

Anal stricture is a rare but debilitating condition most often occurring after previous anorectal surgery. Mild to moderate strictures may be treated successfully with a bowel regimen and manual dilation. Severe or refractory strictures are managed using stricturoplasty or anoplasty with tissue flap coverage. Procedure type is selected based on the cause, location, and severity of the stricture. Principles include division or excision of the fibrotic, strictured tissue and reconstruction with a well-vascularized tissue flap, resulting in generally good outcomes.

■ CAUSE

Anorectal stricture describes the process of abnormal narrowing occurring anywhere along the anal canal from the anal verge to the levator ani complex because of fibrotic replacement of the normally pliable anoderm or distal rectal mucosa. It is distinct from anal stenosis, which describes a functional narrowing of the anal canal secondary to muscle hypertrophy or spasm.

The majority of anorectal strictures occur as a complication of previous anorectal surgery. The most common is hemorrhoidectomy, in which narrowing occurs secondary to excessive anoderm excision. There are a variety of other causes related to other colorectal surgical procedures, neoplasia, inflammation, and trauma, which are listed in Box 1.

■ EVALUATION

The most common symptom is pain with bowel movements. Patients also report difficulty with evacuation, bleeding, narrow caliber stools, fecal incontinence/seepage, tenesmus, and urgency. Patients may use laxatives frequently to avoid impaction or pain associated with bowel movements. A history should be obtained, specifically looking for previous anorectal surgery, Crohn's disease, or perianal trauma.

A diagnosis of anorectal stricture is made easily on physical examination. The physical examination further allows determination of the cause and the severity of the stricture, which are important for treatment planning. Visual inspection of the anal canal and perianal skin may reveal an active disease process, such as infection or tumor, or may show evidence of trauma. Digital rectal examination is used to determine the location and severity of the stricture. A mild stricture allows passage of the finger but will feel abnormally tight. In patients in whom the examination is limited by pain or the presence of a moderate to severe stricture, examination under anesthesia is used. This will facilitate examination in patients who have sphincter spasm, causing anal stenosis; however, it will have no effect on the fibrotic process underlying a true anorectal stricture. Anorectal strictures can be classified by severity and location, as shown in Table 1.

■ TREATMENT

Cause is an important consideration during treatment planning. For inflammatory lesions, treatment of the underlying condition may

BOX 1: Cause of Anorectal Stricture

Surgical Procedures

Hemorrhoidectomy
Low anterior resection
Ileal pouch-anal anastomosis
Anopexy
Excision of perianal skin lesions

Neoplastic

Bowen's disease
Paget's disease
Anal squamous cell carcinoma
Rectal adenocarcinoma
Condyloma acuminata

Inflammatory

Anal fistula
Crohn's disease
Tuberculosis
Actinomycosis
Lymphogranuloma venereum

Trauma

Radiation therapy
Perineal burns
Hot water enemas
Ibuprofen suppositories
Chronic laxative abuse

TABLE 1: Classification of Anorectal Stricture

Severity	Location
Mild: Stricture present, but allows passage of well-lubricated finger or medium Hill-Ferguson retractor	**Low:** At least 0.5 cm distal to the dentate line
Moderate: Passage of well-lubricated finger or medium Hill-Ferguson retractor only with forceful dilation	**Middle:** 0.5 cm on either side of the dentate line
Severe: No passage of well-lubricated finger or medium Hill-Ferguson retractor	**High:** At least 0.5 cm proximal to the dentate line

Adapted from Liberman H, Thorson AG. How I do it. Anal stenosis. *Am J Surg.* 2000;179:325-329.

treat the stricture and therefore should precede surgical therapy. Any underlying sepsis should be drained, and antibiotics initiated if indicated. Patients with underlying Crohn's disease should undergo biopsy to rule out cancer and be considered for a trial of biologic therapy. Patients seen within weeks of an anorectal surgical procedure may benefit from a period of observation for up to 2 months to allow wound healing and resolution of inflammation.

Conservative and Medical Management

Initial treatment includes hydration, fiber supplementation, and stool softeners. This prevents impaction, reduces pain associated with hard bowel movements, and causes gentle autodilation during bowel movements. This should be instituted in all patients, regardless of severity. It may be an effective treatment in patients with mild to moderate anorectal strictures and is a temporizing measure for patients who will ultimately require surgery.

Patients with mild to moderate anorectal strictures, or patients at high risk for failure of surgical management (e.g. history of Crohn's or radiation), should undergo a trial of manual dilation, which in combination with medical and dietary changes, often result in complete cure. Severe anorectal strictures are unlikely to benefit from manual dilation and are best managed operatively.

The initial dilation is performed as a clinic procedure, or in the operating room if needed because of patient discomfort. Well-lubricated Hegar dilators of increasing size are inserted gently, beginning with size 5, and in most patients, continuing to size 18. Subsequent dilations are done by the patient at home using a size 14 Hegar dilator. Patients lubricate the dilator, bear down on the toilet, and gently insert the dilator. Excessive force is avoided because any injury to the anoderm or sphincter complex could result in additional fibrosis, stricturing, and fecal incontinence.

Surgical Treatment

Patients with severe strictures or those not responsive to a trial of conservative management warrant surgical treatment. However, the risk of failure increases in immunocompromised patients, smokers, and people with diabetes. These patients should undergo a maximal trial of conservative management and be optimized as much as possible before intervention. Outcomes in patients with radiation injury and Crohn's disease are poor owing to underlying poor-quality tissue and compromised wound healing.

Strictures associated with malignancies require resection. Anastomotic strictures and those associated with Crohn's disease are best managed using incision with or without stricturoplasty. This procedure is performed with the patient in prone jack-knife position. The stricture is visualized with an anoscope or anorectal rectractor, depending on the location and severity, and divided longitudinally. This can be performed in all four quadrants if needed. The wounds can be left to heal by secondary intention or closed transversely (stricturoplasty) with 3-0 absorbable suture, if closure can be achieved without undue tension. Case reports in patients with anastomotic strictures have described the use of endoscopic techniques, staple cutters, and circular staplers, although none have yet become standard of care.

Anoplasty is the mainstay of surgical treatment for anorectal strictures. Although several variations of anoplasty have been described, the principle of anoplasty is release or excision of the fibrotic, strictured tissue and replacement with normal, pliable tissue with a tension-free, well-vascularized tissue flap. A variety of techniques are described later. Simple flap techniques, such as the lateral mucosal advancement flap, Y-V advancement flap, and rotational S-flaps, derive their blood supply from a skin bridge. Full-thickness flaps, such as the house and V-Y flaps, are supplied through the subcutaneous tissues. Procedure selection is guided by surgeon preference and individual patient factors, such as location and degree of the stricture. Bowel preparation and preoperative intravenous antibiotics are indicated. Patients are placed in the prone jack-knife position to facilitate visualization. The stricture is dilated serially with Hegar dilators. Any anoscope or anorectal retractor then can be used, although a nasal speculum may be necessary in patients with severe stenosis. Long-acting, local anesthetic generously is infiltrated into the area of the stricture, flap site, and pudendal nerve to provide postoperative analgesia and to facilitate flap dissection. The indications and important considerations for each procedure are described in Table 2.

Mucosal Advancement Flap

This flap is a variation of Martin's advancement flap. It is used for localized middle or high strictures and is the only flap discussed that involves moving healthy tissue distally in the anal canal. The strictured, fibrotic tissue is incised or excised, creating an oval defect. A

TABLE 2: Surgical Management of Anorectal Stenosis: Indications and Considerations

Category	Procedure	Indications	Considerations
Primary closure	Incision with or without stricturoplasty	Localized, low, very short length strictures	Safe in Crohn's disease. Can be done in four quadrants for anastomotic strictures
Simple flap	Mucosal advancement flap	Localized middle or high strictures	Allows lateral internal sphincterotomy, if required. Distal wound left to heal by secondary intention
Simple flap	Y-V advancement flap	Localized low strictures	Tapered proximal tip increases risk of ischemia and provides limited coverage
Simple flap	S-flap	Long, diffuse, or recurrent strictures associated with ectropion	Most complex technique, useful when treatment requires removal of substantial anoderm, and >50% of the anal canal needs coverage
Full-thickness advancement flap	House flap	Long, diffuse, or recurrent strictures associated with ectropion	Widely used technique, good for long or severe strictures, especially those that extend into the perianal skin. Up to four flaps can be performed in a single patient if needed
Full-thickness advancement flap	V-Y advancement flap	Localized middle or high stricture associated with ectropion	Tapered distal end limits utility in longer strictures

Adapted from Maria G, Brisinda G, Civello IM. Anoplasty for the treatment of anal stenosis. *Am J Surg.* 1998;175:158-160.

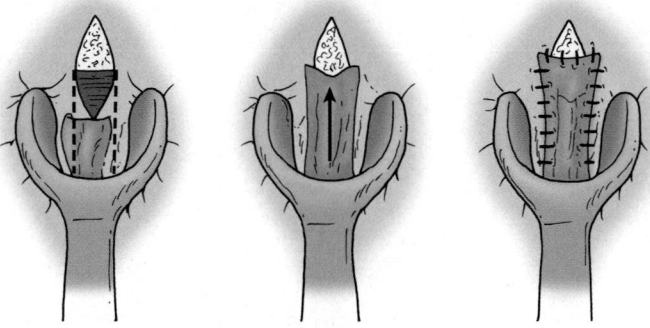

FIGURE 1 Mucosal advancement flap. *(Reproduced with permission from Liberman H, Thorson AG. How I do it. Anal stenosis. Am J Surg. 2000;179:325-329.)*

mucosal advancement flap is created by dissecting the mucosa off the internal sphincter in a rectangular area proximal to the oval defect (Figure 1). The flap is anchored to the distal internal sphincter with interrupted absorbable sutures, and the distal aspect of the oval defect is left open to heal by secondary intention. This allows drainage and minimizes the risk of ectropion formation.

Y-V Advancement Flap

The Y-V advancement flap begins with an incision or excision of a low, localized stricture, resulting in an oval defect. A V-shaped incision is made, with the apex at the distal tip of the wound, and the anoderm is advanced proximally to fill the defect (Figure 2). Because the tapered end of the V is used to fill the previously diseased area, this flap provides limited tissue coverage and therefore is used only in localized strictures that occupy less than 25% of the anal canal. The flap is secured with interrupted 3-0 absorbable suture, with great care taken at the tip, which is prone to ischemia.

S-Flap

This is a rotational flap technique that allows for complex reconstruction of the perianal area in patients with recurrent stenosis or those

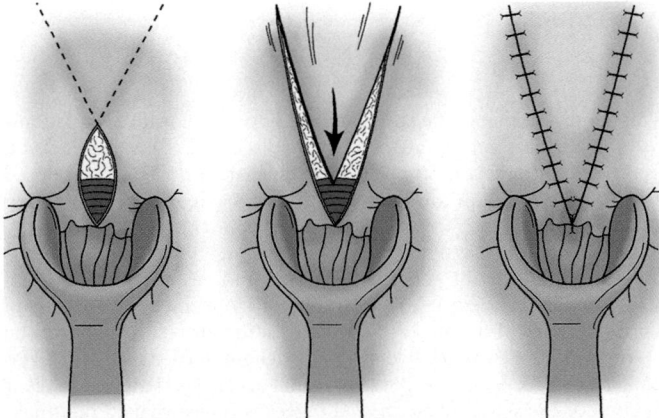

FIGURE 2 Y-V advancement flap. *(Reproduced with permission from Liberman H, Thorson AG. How I do it. Anal stenosis. Am J Surg. 2000;179:325-9.)*

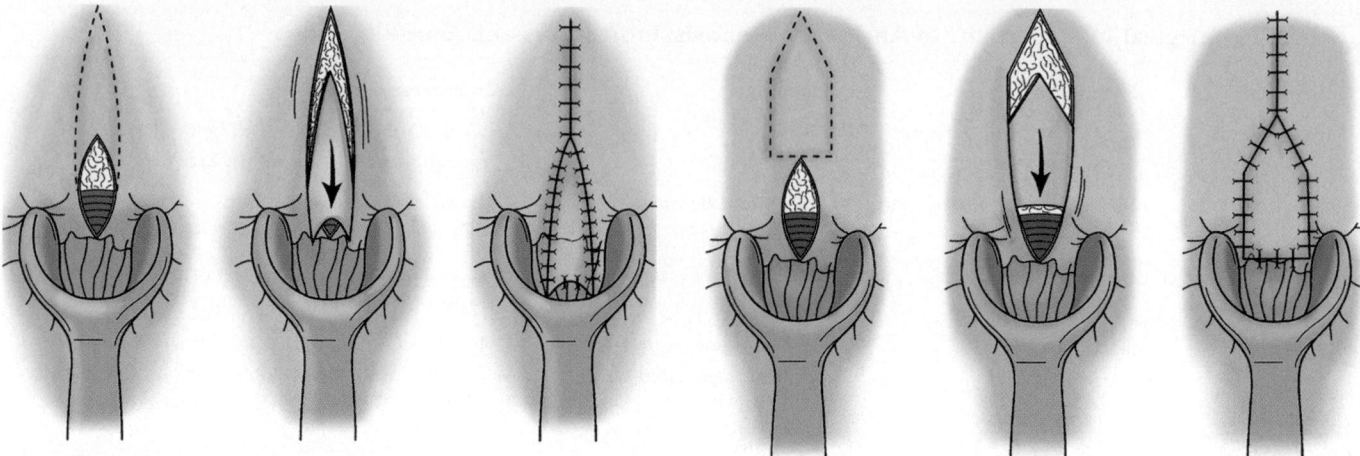

FIGURE 3 S-flap. *(Reproduced with permission from Liberman H, Thorson AG. How I do it. Anal stenosis. Am J Surg. 2000;179:325-9.)*

FIGURE 4 House flap. *(Reproduced with permission from Liberman H, Thorson AG. How I do it. Anal stenosis. Am J Surg. 2000;179:325-9.)*

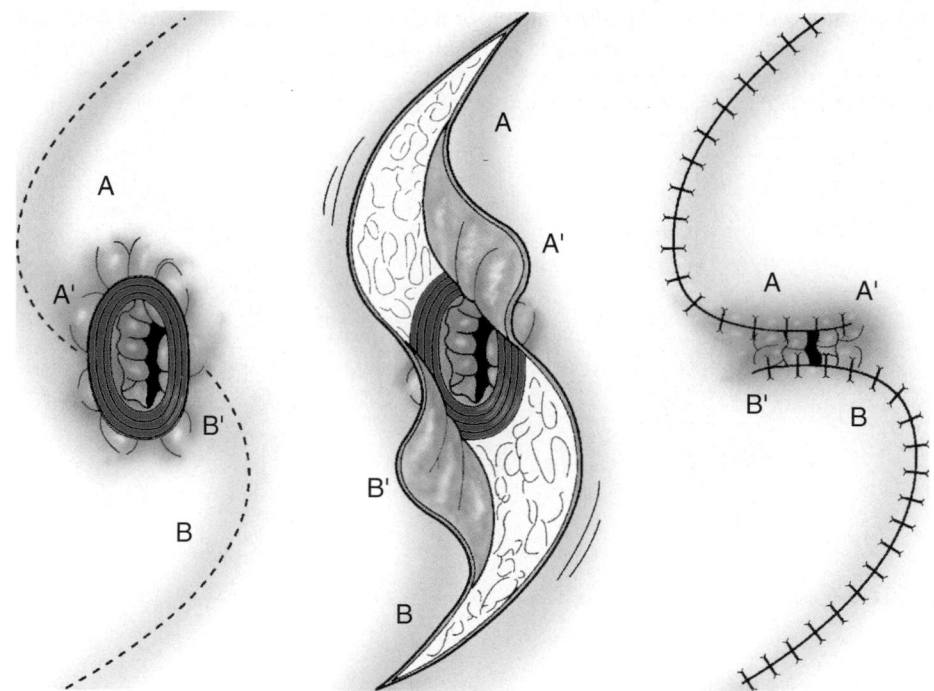

FIGURE 5 V-Y advancement flap. *(Reproduced with permission from Liberman H, Thorson AG. How I do it. Anal stenosis. Am J Surg. 2000;179:325-9.)*

who require excision of a large amount of perianal skin, as in patients with condyloma acuminata or Bowen's disease. An S-shaped incision is created, with the anus in the center. The flaps are rotated and closed without tension with interrupted 3-0 absorbable suture (Figure 3).

House Flap

The house flap is the most widely used and versatile technique. If necessary, the procedure can include up to four distinct flaps, one in each quadrant of the anal canal to treat severe or recurrent anorectal stenosis. This technique also offers the length needed to treat lesions that extend the length of the entire anal canal. The strictured area is incised or excised, leaving an oval defect. A house-shaped full thickness flap is then advanced proximally with its subcutaneous tissue. Care is taken to mobilize the flap circumferentially to ensure a tension-free closure (Figure 4). The base of the house is anchored to the internal sphincter proximally with 2-0 absorbable suture, whereas the walls, roof, and donor site are closed with 3-0 absorbable suture.

V-Y Advancement Flap

This is a modification of the Y-V advancement flap that protects the ischemia-prone tapered end by placing it distally in the repair, away from the anal canal. Because the base of the triangle is used to close the defect (Figure 5), this flap is more appropriate for strictures that involve more than a minimal area of anoderm. However, unlike the house flap, this technique results in a tapered distal end, which limits its use in long strictures. Similar to other flaps, the proximal end is anchored to the internal sphincter with 2-0 absorbable suture, whereas the donor site and lateral edges are closed with 3-0 absorbable suture. The distal end is closed loosely to allow drainage.

Postoperative Care

Patients undergoing examination under anesthesia, incision, and sphincteroplasty or simple flap techniques are discharged on the day of surgery and prescribed a bowel regimen of stool softeners, hydration, and fiber supplementation. Patients undergoing complex or multiple anoplasty techniques require admission for pain control, generally for 1 to 2 nights after surgery. Nonsteroidal anti-inflammatory agents, topical ointments, such as lidocaine with or without nifedipine, and sitz baths are the mainstays of pain management. A short course of oral narcotics is often necessary.

Patients are followed in the perioperative period for the development of surgical complications such as urinary tract infection, flap necrosis, suture line disruption, hematoma, infection, and abscess. Recurrence, chronic pain, and ectropion are possible long-term complications.

Outcomes

Anoplasty offers generally good results, although recurrence and flap failure are possible. Options include performing an additional anoplasty in another quadrant or performing a more extensive procedure, such as an S-flap. Patients at highest risk of treatment failure are those with Crohn's disease, severe stricture, immunosuppression, diabetes, radiation injury, or current smoking. The impact of surgery on pre-existing fecal incontinence is variable. In some patients, restoration of normal, pliable tissue in the anal canal and removal of the partial obstruction decreases soiling. In other patients, an underlying problem with anorectal sensation, rectal compliance, or anal sphincter tone requires further evaluation and management. In the rare patient who fails treatment with anoplasty, a permanent colostomy is considered.

■ ACKNOWLEDGEMENT

Jessica Cohan is supported by the Crohn's and Colitis Foundation of America (A123669) and the American Society of Colon and Rectal Surgeons (A124496). The funding sources had no involvement in study design, data collection, statistical analysis, manuscript preparation, or the decision to submit the article for publication.

SUGGESTED READINGS

Brisinda G, Vanella S, Cadeddu F, et al. Surgical treatment of anal stenosis. *World J Gastroenterol.* 2009;15:19211928.

Brochard C, Siproudhis L, Wallenhorst T, et al. Anorectal stricture in 102 patients with Crohn's disease: natural history in the era of biologics. *Aliment Pharmacol Ther.* 2014;40:796-803.

Liberman H, Thorson AG. How I do it. Anal stenosis. *Am J Surg.* 2000;179:325-329.

Maria G, Brisinda G, Civello IM. Anoplasty for the treatment of anal stenosis. *Am J Surg.* 1998;175:158-160.

THE MANAGEMENT OF PRURITUS ANI

Bradley Davis, MD

Pruritus ani, also known as *anusitis,* is a cutaneous sensation characterized by unpleasant itching and burning of the perianal skin. This condition affects up to 5% of the general population on a daily basis and exhibits a male predominance in a 4 : 1 ratio. Most patients who have pruritus ani are in the fifth to seventh decades. Pruritus ani may be localized or diffuse in the perianal region. The onset of symptoms is typically gradual and is often worse at night or in warm, moist climates. Pruritus ani can be subdivided further into idiopathic (primary) pruritus ani and secondary pruritus ani. Idiopathic pruritus ani is a diagnosis of exclusion, whereas secondary pruritus ani is attributed to a specific cause.

■ CAUSE

Idiopathic Pruritus Ani

Idiopathic pruritus ani accounts for anywhere from 20% to 75% of reported cases, and its diagnosis is predicated on a thorough patient evaluation and exclusion of secondary causes. The key inciting factor in idiopathic pruritus ani is fecal contamination leading to local irritation. Fecal matter contains allergens, bacteria, and bacterial enzymes capable of activating C-type nerve fibers within the dermis. The anoderm, in particular, has been shown to be more sensitive to fecal matter when compared with other areas of the body. Fecal contamination is often the result of poor anal hygiene, chronic diarrhea, fecal incontinence, or mucous leakage.

In a mechanism known as *pruritoceptive itching,* the repetitive trauma of scratching over time stimulates release of local proinflammatory cytokines, leading to chronic activation of C-type nerve fibers. This is also referred to as the *itch-scratch cycle* and is well described in dermatology literature.

In addition, dietary factors have been associated with the development of perianal pruritus. These so-called *pruritogenic foods* include coffee, colas, citrus fruits, chocolate, tea, energy drinks, and spicy foods. Proposed mechanisms by which pruritogenic foods trigger symptoms include local irritation, alteration of stool pH, histamine release, and inappropriate relaxation of the internal sphincter. The excessive consumption of liquids also can predispose to seepage and fecal contamination.

Poor anal hygiene is a common factor among patients with perianal pruritus, but overzealous hygiene also has been implicated in its pathogenesis. Elaborate cleansing routines, along with the use of irritating soaps and lotions, can destroy the natural skin barriers and further traumatize the anoderm.

Secondary Pruritus Ani

Sources for secondary pruritus ani generally fall into one of five categories: infectious, anorectal, dermatologic, malignant, and systemic disease. A list of common causes resulting in secondary pruritus is listed in Box 1.

Infectious agents resulting in perianal pruritus include bacteria, viruses, yeast, and parasites. Common bacterial offenders include *Staphylococcus aureus,* beta-hemolytic *Streptococcus pyogenes,* and *Corynebacterium minutissimum* (erythrasma). Sexually transmitted infections also have been implicated, including *Neisseria gonorrhoeae* (gonorrhea), *Chlamydia trachomatis,* and *Treponema pallidum* (syphilis); although these are rarely responsible for chronic symptoms. According to literature, *Candida* is responsible for up to 15% of secondary pruritus ani. Fungal infections with *Candida* species and other dermatophytes often proliferate in people with diabetes, or after treatment with antibiotics or immunosuppressant medications, such as steroids. Fungal lesions are characterized by a diffuse, erythematous, and often macerated plaques. In the setting of pruritus ani, the presence of any dermatophytes should be considered pathologic and treated with either topical or systemic antifungal medications. Viral agents include herpes simplex virus and human papillomavirus, the latter of which may manifest as condyloma acuminata in human immunodeficiency virus–positive patients. Herpes zoster, also referred to as *shingles,* also can affect the perineal region in a dermatomal pattern. Nocturnal symptoms in the pediatric population should alert suspicion towards a parasitic infection with *Enterobius vermicularis* (pinworms). Other parasites that induce pruritic

BOX 1: Selected Causes of Secondary Pruritus Ani

Infectious

Bacterial infection (*Staphylococcus, Streptococcus,* erythrasma)
Sexually transmitted infection (*Gonococcus, Chlamydia*)
Fungal infection (*Candida,* dermatophytes)
Parasites (pinworms, scabies)
Viral infection (herpes virus, condylomata, *Molluscum*)

Anorectal

Hemorrhoids (external, prolapsing internal)
Fistula-in-ano
Anal fissures
Hidradenitis suppurativa
Fecal incontinence
Perianal Crohn's disease
Skin tags
Chronic diarrhea
Pilonidal disease

Dermatologic

Contact dermatitis
Atopic dermatitis
Perianal psoriasis
Lichen sclerosus
Seborrheic dermatitis

Malignant

Anal canal cancer
Anal margin cancer
Rectal cancer
Bowen's disease
Extramammary Paget's disease

Systemic Disease

Diabetes mellitus
Leukemia
Lymphoma
Chronic renal failure
Iron-deficiency anemia
Hyperthyroidism
Hyperbilirubinemia

TABLE 1: Washington Hospital Staging Criteria

Stage 0	Normal-appearing perianal skin
Stage I	Erythematous and inflamed perianal skin
Stage II	White, lichenified perianal skin
Stage III	Lichenified skin with coarse ridges and ulceration

dermatitis, psoriasis, and lichen sclerosus. Contact dermatitis results from local irritants, commonly deodorants, perfumes, soaps, and certain foods. A detailed history focusing on postdefecation cleansing habits and anal hygiene can elucidate whether irritants may be involved. Allergic dermatitis often occurs in those who have other dysregulated allergic conditions, including asthma, atopic dermatitis (eczema), and hay fever. Lichen sclerosus is a poorly understood condition that commonly affects perimenopausal women. Most patients with lichen sclerosus have vulvovaginal pruritus, although perianal symptoms are also common. These patients respond well to topical steroids. Chronic nonresponders, however, carry a 5% risk of malignant degeneration into squamous cell carcinoma and should have biopsies performed should symptoms persist. Psoriasis frequently involves the scalp and flexor surfaces of the knees and elbows but less frequently can involve the perianal skin. Radiation dermatitis also can involve the perineum, although it is less commonly seen since the development of high- and medium-energy accelerators. The standard of care for radiation-induced dermatitis involves topical steroids and routine skin care with mild, unscented soap.

Neoplastic diseases should be considered in the differential diagnosis of any patient with perianal pruritus. These include anal cancer, anal margin cancer, rectal cancer, Bowen's disease (squamous cell carcinoma in situ), and extramammary Paget's disease (cutaneous adenocarcinoma in situ). In the setting of malignancy, pruritic symptoms often are more severe and persistent in comparison with idiopathic pruritus ani. If malignancy is suspected, biopsies and endoscopic evaluation is crucial to the workup.

Systemic diseases associated with perianal pruritus include diabetes mellitus, leukemia, lymphoma, chronic renal failure, iron-deficiency anemia, hyperthyroidism, and cholestatic disease. Uremic pruritus, or pruritus resulting from chronic renal failure, is a common symptom among dialysis patients. At present time, the only known cure is kidney transplantation. Cholestatic pruritus is a common symptom among patients with hepatic dysfunction, which may be alleviated with medications such as cholestyramine. In these cases, pruritus is rarely the sole symptom, and definitive treatment should be directed toward the underlying disease process.

■ PATIENT EVALUATION

A detailed history and physical examination are critical to the evaluation of any patient with perianal pruritus. The history should focus on the following points: onset and duration of pruritus; toileting behaviors and postdefecation cleansing habits; anal hygiene; mucous leakage or perianal moisture; travel history; dietary history specific to pruritogenic foods and beverages; and any accompanying symptoms. In addition, current medications and allergies should be reviewed.

The goal of the physical examination is to identify any secondary causes of pruritus. Physical examination should include close inspection of perianal skin and anoderm, genitalia, inguinal lymph nodes, and digital rectal examination. Anoscopy also should be performed to evaluate the anal canal for evidence of disease, and if malignancy is suspected, biopsies and further endoscopic evaluation should be pursued.

Developed at the Washington Hospital Center, the Washington criteria often are used to stage the appearance of perianal skin according to severity of disease (Table 1). Stage I disease consists of

symptoms include *Sarcoptes scabiei* (scabies) and *Pediculosis pubis* (crabs).

A variety of anorectal diseases are associated with pruritus ani, including external hemorrhoids, prolapsing internal hemorrhoids, fistula-in-ano, anal fissures, hidradenitis suppurativa, perianal Crohn's disease, skin tags, pilonidal disease, and chronic diarrhea. Anorectal conditions resulting in pruritus can be divided into two broad categories based on their pathophysiologic mechanism: fecal contamination and local inflammation.

Fecal contamination can result from seepage and suboptimal perianal hygiene, which in turn leads to irritation of the anoderm. The presence of hemorrhoidal disease and skin tags, for example, may impair perianal hygiene, leaving fecal matter within the perianal skinfolds. Fistula-in-ano results in chronic drainage of fecal matter onto the perianal skin. Other common factors resulting in fecal contamination include fecal incontinence because of impaired sphincter tone, decreased stool bulk, and chronic diarrhea. Hidradenitis and perianal Crohn's disease, on the other hand, are examples of pruritus mediated by inflammatory mechanisms. As is the case with idiopathic pruritus ani, secondary causes of perianal pruritus also are exacerbated by pruritoceptive itching.

The most common dermatologic conditions resulting in chronic pruritus ani include contact dermatitis, allergic dermatitis, atopic

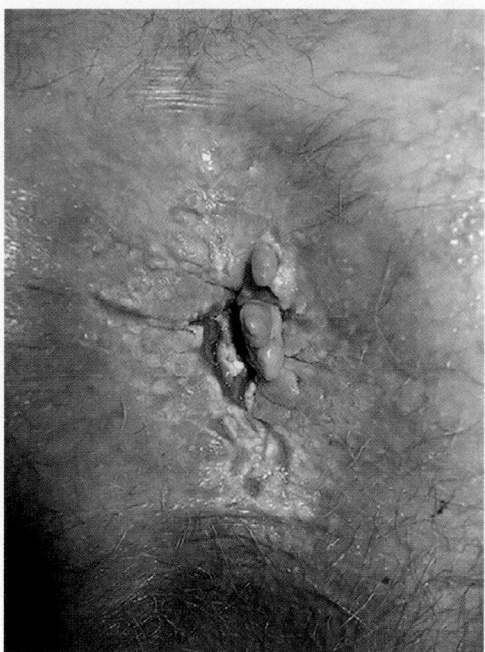

FIGURE 1 Clinical appearance of stage III pruritus ani.

erythematous and inflamed skin; stage II disease consists of licheni-fied changes in addition to perianal erythema; and stage III disease reveals coarse ridges and ulcerations (Figure 1). In a small minority of patients, perianal skin may appear normal (Washington stage 0). Biopsies should be performed on any suspicious lesions in the office with a simple (3- to 4-mm) punch biopsy, including normal-appearing perianal skin and the lesion in question. If Bowen's disease (carcinoma in situ) or condyloma acuminata are suspected, applica-tion of 3% to 5% acetic acid can help guide the biopsy. Infectious causes of pruritus can be evaluated with aerobic, anaerobic, and fungal swabs. If there has been any exposure to children harboring pinworm *(Enterobius vermicularis),* a transparent tape test can be performed easily, although this is done ideally in the early morning on consecutive days. All children who have pruritic symptoms should be evaluated with the transparent test.

■ TREATMENT

Once the diagnosis of idiopathic pruritus ani has been reached, patient education and treatment modalities should proceed simulta-neously. Successful treatment of pruritus ani begins with proper perianal hygiene, bowel augmentation, topical steroids, and the dis-continuation of any offending agents. Most patients achieve symp-tomatic relief and reversal of morphologic features with these conservative measures. Patients with idiopathic pruritus ani fre-quently have chronic symptoms and resultant social anxiety; thus patient reassurance and counseling are invaluable adjuncts to medical therapy.

The goal of perianal hygiene is to restore clean and dry perianal skin. Whenever possible, patients should bathe after each bowel movement. Otherwise, simple cleansing with disposable moist towels, such as baby wipes, is sufficient. Afterward, the skin should be patted dry with unscented toilet paper or a soft towel because vigorous wiping results in further trauma to the area. Clean and dry skin should be maintained throughout the day. Moist areas can be kept dry with cornstarch, talcum powder, or a simple cotton ball. If chronic diarrhea or mucous leakage impede proper perianal hygiene, bowel augmenting medications (e.g., fiber supplements) may be pre-scribed. These should be tailored to achieve soft, well-formed stools, while minimizing fecal soiling. Tap water enemas also may be a helpful adjunct if incomplete evacuation remains a problem.

Patients should be advised to avoid perfumed cleansers, lotions, and tight-fitting garments, which may abrade the already trauma-tized perianal skin. Other factors that contribute to the disease process are listed in Box 2 and also should be eliminated once identi-fied. These include specific medications, pruritogenic foods, topical agents, and lifestyle changes. Individual foods may be reintroduced gradually over the course of several weeks, one at a time, until the offending food and level of tolerance are identified. Nocturnal scratching also contributes to the itch-scratch cycle and can be avoided with trimmed nails and/or cotton gloves worn at night.

Topical steroids may serve as an effective adjunct to the afore-mentioned measures. Evidence for the use of topical steroids is conflicting, but in the setting of refractory disease, a short course of betamethasone or 1% hydrocortisone cream may alleviate pruritic symptoms. A small randomized controlled trial comparing 1% hydrocortisone cream versus placebo noted a 68% reduction in symptoms and 75% improvement in quality of life after a 2-week course. The use of topical steroids should be limited to several weeks because chronic use may result in atrophic changes to the perianal skin.

Treatment of secondary pruritus ani should be tailored to the specific underlying cause and is reviewed elsewhere.

■ RECENT ADVANCES

The majority of patients who have idiopathic pruritus ani respond favorably to conservative measures. There exist a subset of patients, however, who remain refractory to treatment despite strict adherence to hygienic and dietary modifications. After 4 weeks of conservative therapy, and secondary causes are again excluded, one of several second-line interventions may be pursued. These include topical cap-saicin, topical tacrolimus, and methylene blue injection. Several studies have been performed in recent years to support the use of these second-line agents.

Capsaicin is a product of *Capsicum* chili peppers and is postulated to increase the resting threshold for depolarization in local C-type nerve fibers. Topical capsaicin (0.006%) can be applied in a thin layer over the perianal skin, up to three times daily for 4 weeks. This is diluted from the usual concentration of capsaicin at 0.025%, which reduces the local burning sensation. Patients undergoing topical capsaicin therapy should be advised against specific side effects, including burning sensation and urticaria on application.

A randomized, placebo-controlled trial performed in 2003 com-paring active capsaicin versus menthol ointment noted symptomatic relief in 70% in the capsaicin arm. After a mean follow-up period of 10.9 months, 94% of original responders remained symptom free but continued to use topical capsaicin on a near-daily basis. The study also noted that capsaicin treatment was associated with higher burning sensation scores on application. A more recent systematic review published in 2010 analyzed six randomized controlled trials comparing topically applied capsaicin in treating pruritus in any medical condition, including the aforementioned study. After investigating the results, the authors concluded that there was no convincing evidence for the use of capsaicin in pruritus. Their criticism of the 2003 trial was that the study design did not report a statistically significant carryover effect between the two 4-week periods of intervention.

Tacrolimus, an immunosuppressive agent, is used commonly in the treatment of eczema. A dermatologic study performed on 2013 aimed to compare topical tacrolimus with Vaseline placebo, in patients with refractory pruritus ani. Notably, these patients also had atopic dermatitis. Topical tacrolimus ointment (0.03%), applied twice daily, resulted in a significant decrease in symptoms after a 4-week period. The study is not without its limitations, namely its small size and lack of long-term follow-up, so topical capsaicin may be preferable as the initial second-line agent.

Several studies have investigated intradermal methylene blue as a treatment modality for refractory pruritus ani. Methylene blue is believed to be directly toxic to the sensory nerves supplying the perianal skin. A 15-mL solution of 1% methylene blue can be injected with a 22-gauge needle and mixed with local anesthetics if desired. The injection should be localized to the affected perianal area, up to the level of the dentate line. A repeat injection may be performed at 4 weeks for partial response. A prospective study performed in 2004 noted complete relief of symptoms with methylene blue therapy in 24 of 30 patients after 1 month. After a 12-month follow-up 23 of 30 patients remained symptom free. A more recent prospective study in 2009 demonstrated similar results: symptomatic improvement in 96% and complete resolution in 57% of patients after a single treatment. Patients should be informed about the side effects of methylene blue before injection, including numbness and discoloration at the injection site. Skin necrosis and anaphylaxis are rare, but severe side effects of methylene blue injection may occur; neither of these were observed during the clinical trial.

■ SUMMARY

Pruritus ani is a common ailment, affecting up to 5% of the population on a daily basis. Diagnosis relies heavily on a focused history and physical examination. Any secondary causes of pruritus ani should be elucidated if present, and treatment guided towards the underlying condition. Simple procedures, such as punch biopsies or anal swabs, may be performed in the office setting to aid in unclear situations. The majority of cases can be managed with adequate perianal hygiene, topical agents, and the elimination of any offending agents. Patient education and reassurance are critical adjuncts to the healing process.

SUGGESTED READINGS

Al-Ghnaniem R, Short K, Pullen A, Fuller LC, Rennie JA, Leather AJ. 1% hydrocortisone ointment is an effective treatment of pruritus ani: a pilot randomized controlled crossover trial. *Int J Colorectal Dis.* 2007;22:1463-1467.

Garcia LS. Practical guide to diagnostic parasitology. *Am Soc Microbiol.* 2009;246-247. ISBN 1-55581-154-X.

Gooding SMD, Canter PH, Coelho HF, Boddy K, Ernst E. Systematic review of topical capsaicin in the treatment of pruritus. *Int J Dermatol.* 2010;49:858-865.

Lacy BE, Weiser K. Common anorectal disorders: diagnosis and treatment. *Curr Gastroenterol Rep.* 2009;11:413-419.

Lockhart-Mummery P. Discussion on pruritus ani. *Proc R Soc Med.* 1921;14:172-175.

Lysy J, Sistiery-Ittah M, Israelit Y, et al. Topical capsaicin—a novel and effective treatment for idiopathic intractable pruritus ani: a randomised, placebo controlled, crossover study. *Gut.* 2003;52:1323-1326.

Markell KW, Billingham RP. Pruritus ani: etiology and management. *Surg Clin North Am.* 2010;90:125-135.

Mentes BB, Akin M, Leventoglu S, Gultekin FA, Oguz M. Intradermal methylene blue injection for the treatment of intractable idiopathic pruritus ani: results of 30 cases. *Tech Coloproctol.* 2004;8:11-14.

Samalavicius NE, Poskus T, Gupta RK. Lunevicius R. Long-term results of single intradermal 1% methylene blue injection for intractable idiopathic pruritus ani: a prospective study. *Tech Coloproctol.* 2012;16:295-299.

Scarborough RA. Pruritus ani: its etiology and treatment. *Ann Surg.* 1933;98:1039-1045.

Siddiqi S, Vijay V, Ward M, et al. Pruritus ani. *Ann R Coll Surg Engl.* 2008;90:457-463.

Sutherland AD, Faragher IG, Frizelle FA. Intradermal injection of methylene blue for the treatment of refractory pruritus ani. *Colorectal Dis.* 2009;11:282-287.

Ucak H, Demir B, Cicek D, et al. Efficacy of topical tacrolimus for the treatment of persistent pruritus ani in patients with atopic dermatitis. *J Dermatolog Treat.* 2013;24:454-457.

SURGICAL MANAGEMENT OF FECAL INCONTINENCE

Muneera R. Kapadia, MD, and Irena Gribovskaja-Rupp, MD

■ PREVALENCE AND ETIOLOGY

Fecal incontinence may have a profound negative effect on quality of life. It affects 18 million adults in the United States, and the incidence increases with age. After age 50, up to 11% of men and 26% of women have fecal incontinence, although the true prevalence may be higher because social stigma likely limits reporting. Fecal incontinence is the second leading reason for admission to nursing homes and is recorded in up to 50% of institutionalized patients.

There are many causes that can contribute to fecal incontinence; the general categories include anal sphincter injury, anorectal diseases, neurologic etiologies, congenital malformation, and aging (Table 1). The most common cause of fecal incontinence in women is obstetric injury. Although women sustain these injuries at a younger age, they often do not experience fecal incontinence until after menopause, when supporting pelvic floor musculature weakens and compensatory mechanisms are lost. Obstetric injury can occur by causing anal sphincter disruption or injury to the pudendal nerves.

■ DIAGNOSTIC EVALUATION

Obtaining a complete history is important and should include stool consistency and frequency. In females, obstetric history may be revealing. Comorbidities and medications should be reviewed. Fecal incontinence scores and quality of life questionnaires can help quantify the severity of fecal incontinence. Physical examination should include external inspection, specifically looking for perineal body size and scars resulting from trauma or obstetric injury. Digital rectal examination is important to evaluate baseline tone, anal sphincter squeeze, and use of gluteal muscles. Other anatomic abnormalities that may contribute to fecal incontinence that should be identified on examination include rectocele, rectal prolapse, rectal mass, stricture, or fistula. Anoscopy and proctoscopy may help diagnose other

TABLE I: Causes of Fecal Incontinence

Anal sphincter injury	Obstetric injury
	Traumatic injury
	• Perineal impalement
	• Voluntary anoreceptive intercourse
	• Foreign bodies
	• Sexual abuse
	Iatrogenic
	• LIS, fistulotomy, hemorrhoidectomy
	• Anal and pelvic radiation
Anorectal disease not managed	Rectal prolapse
	Prolapsing internal hemorrhoids
	Inflammatory bowel disease
	Radiation proctitis
	Distal rectal cancer
Neurologic causes	Obstetric injury
	Multiple sclerosis
	CNS disease
	• Spinal cord injury
	• Tumor
	Diabetes mellitus
	Cerebrovascular accident
Congenital malformation	Spina bifida
	Imperforate anus
	Meningomyelocele
Aging	Diminished muscles bulk and strength
	Dementia

CNS, Central nervous system; *LIS*, lateral internal sphincterotomy.

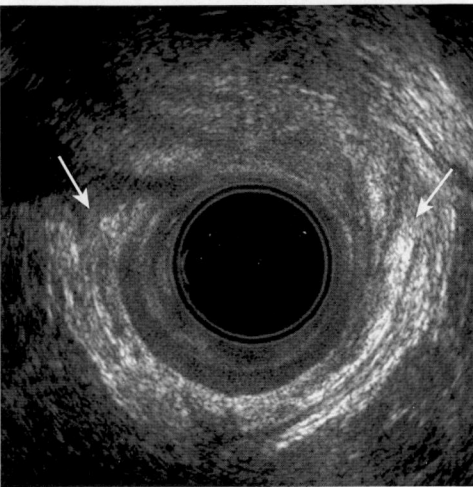

FIGURE I Anterior anal sphincter defect in a woman with incontinence. The distance between the two arrows represents an anterior defect in both the internal and external anal sphincters.

conditions, such as proctitis or rectal cancer, which may contribute to fecal incontinence.

Diagnostic testing for fecal incontinence may include endoanal ultrasound, anorectal physiology testing, pudendal nerve terminal motor latency, and defecography. In patients with suspected sphincter injury, endoanal ultrasound is helpful to confirm and characterize the degree of injury (Figure 1). Although ultrasound has excellent sensitivity and specificity in identifying sphincter defects, sphincter defect may not correlate with degree of incontinence. Anorectal physiology testing, including manometry (which determines resting and squeeze pressures) as well as anorectal sensation, volume tolerance, and compliance, may help to define the elements of dysfunction. Pudendal nerve terminal motor latency provides assessment of pudendal nerve function and measures the time to response at the external sphincter muscle. It has a limited impact in diagnosis and management of fecal incontinence and is not recommended routinely. Defecography is a contrast study that gives dynamic information regarding the pelvic floor. Contrast is instilled into the rectum, and the patient evacuates it into a commode while under fluoroscopic examination. It may demonstrate incomplete evacuation, overflow incontinence, intussusception, or rectal prolapse, which may contribute to fecal incontinence. Colonoscopy is appropriate in patients with new bleeding or change in bowel habits. Not all diagnostic testing modalities may be necessary for every patient, and testing should be tailored to the individual.

■ MEDICAL MANAGEMENT

The goal of medical management focuses on improving stool quality such that stools are more solid and evacuated completely. Medical management should be attempted before any more invasive therapies are implemented. Up to 20% to 50% of patients can improve after counseling regarding diet changes, fluid consumption, and medication management. Fiber can add bulk to stools, create more solid stools, and prevent seepage. Fiber supplements are available in several natural and synthetic preparations and can be ingested in pill form or mixed with liquids. Constipating agents such as loperamide, diphenoxylate/atropine, and codeine prolong whole gut transit time and firm stool consistency. In patients with a history of cholecystectomy or terminal ileal resection, the bile salt binding resin cholestyramine may be helpful. Amitriptyline, a tricyclic antidepressant with anticholinergic properties, and narcotics may be helpful in decreasing bowel motility. For the treatment of significant constipation with overflow incontinence, laxatives and stool softeners can be used. Finally, daily enemas may reduce incontinence episodes by decreasing the rectal stool load.

■ BIOFEEDBACK

Biofeedback is a therapy aimed at improving continence through sphincter exercises, rectal sensory retraining, and learning to coordinate voluntary external anal sphincter contraction with the onset of rectal distension. It is noninvasive and performed by a qualified nurse or physical therapist. The patient is monitored during the biofeedback sessions and counseled on appropriate muscle contraction, relaxation, abdominal pressure, and breathing techniques. Patients typically undergo four to six sessions. Biofeedback currently is recommended in patients with some degree of preserved voluntary sphincter contraction. Nonrandomized series report improvement in fecal incontinence between 64% and 89%. However, biofeedback is time intensive for the patient, and providers and may not have a sustained benefit. Overall, this therapy has no associated risks and offers potential benefits; if the patient is willing, biofeedback should be considered.

■ SURGICAL MANAGEMENT

There are several surgical options for the management of fecal incontinence for those patients who have had little to no improvement from medical management and/or biofeedback. The options for surgical management of fecal incontinence are listed in Box 1. Many of the available therapies are complex, have a high complication rate, or are not widely available in the United States. The more commonly offered procedures include injectable bulking agents, sacral nerve stimulation (SNS), sphincteroplasty, and stoma creation.

Injectable Bulking Agents

Several injectable bulking agents have been studied in clinical trials. These provide an enhanced mechanical barrier to fecal loss. There are three commercially available products; however, only NASHA Dx (stabilized hyaluronic acid dextranomer gel) is available in the United States. Injections typically are performed in the office setting with the patient positioned either prone jack-knife or left lateral decubitus. With anoscopy, the bulking agent is injected into the submucosa just above the dentate line, typically in four areas evenly spaced around the anal canal.

In a randomized controlled trial between NASHA Dx and sham injections, patients in the treatment arm experienced more benefit, which was defined as 50% or greater reduction in the number of incontinence episodes. At 6 months, 52% of patients who received NASHA Dx had benefit versus 31% of patients who had sham injections. At 3 years, this improvement was sustained, and quality of life scores were improved in the treatment group compared with baseline. Longer-term data are necessary to determine the durability of injectable bulking agents. This procedure is low risk and easy to perform; however, it is probably most appropriate for patients with only mild fecal incontinence.

Sacral Nerve Stimulation

Sacral nerve stimulation initially was developed as a treatment for urinary incontinence but subsequently was demonstrated to have benefits for fecal incontinence as well. The exact mechanism of action is unknown. It has been approved in Europe for the treatment of fecal incontinence for a number of years but only was approved in 2011 for use in the United States.

This therapy involves stimulating the S3 nerve root by delivering mild electrical pulses. Before the procedure, the patient should keep a fecal incontinence diary for 2 weeks. The procedure then is performed in two stages. The first stage is a testing phase in which a tined lead is placed under fluoroscopic guidance along the S3 nerve root. The patient is positioned prone with axillary rolls and a pelvic roll. The procedure may be conducted under either monitored anesthesia care or general anesthetic, but if the latter is chosen, it is important that only a short-acting paralytic agent be used during induction. The lower back and buttocks should be included in the prepped field. Access to the S3 foramen is obtained with a hollow needle under fluoroscopic guidance. Appropriate needle placement is confirmed by stimulating the needle with an electrical impulse and confirming the appropriate motor response, which should include pelvic bellows and ipsilateral big toe plantar flexion. If an alternate response is achieved, it indicates suboptimal needle placement. With Seldinger technique, a wire and subsequently a tined lead then is placed through the S3 foramen and along the S3 nerve root. Again, appropriate placement of the tined lead is confirmed with fluoroscopy and motor response corresponding to S3 nerve root stimulation. The tined lead

then is tunneled laterally to a subcutaneous pocket and coupled with an external wire. The external wire then is tunneled to the midline, where it is brought out of the skin and coupled with the external battery pack. The incisions should be closed in layers, and the patient should be maintained on oral antibiotics until the second procedure. The patient should be instructed against showering or bathing during the testing period. The patient again is instructed to keep a second fecal incontinence diary for 2 weeks.

The two diaries are compared to determine patient benefit. If there is a 50% or greater reduction in the number of incontinence episodes during the testing phase, the second stage involves implantation of the permanent device (Figure 2). The second procedure should be performed under monitored anesthesia care with the patient positioned prone, similar to the first stage. The lateral subcutaneus pocket should be opened and implantation of the permanent battery pack should proceed provided there is no evidence of infection. The external wire is uncoupled from the tined lead and removed. The permanent battery then is coupled to the tined lead and placed into the subcutaneous pocket. The skin is closed in layers. The battery typically lasts 3 to 5 years and will have to be replaced surgically after that time. If a 50% decrease in the number of incontinence episodes was not achieved during testing, at the second procedure, both the external wire and tined lead are removed.

The SNS study group reported results of a prospective multi-institutional trial conducted on 133 patients with fecal incontinence who underwent test stimulation, and 120 (90%) had a 50% or greater reduction in the number of incontinence episodes and therefore were implanted with a permanent battery. At 12 months, 83% of implanted patients achieved therapeutic success, and therefore of the initial patients, 75% achieved success. The mean number of incontinence episodes markedly decreased from 9.4 to 1.9 per week at 12 months. The risks associated with SNS are generally minor and include pain at the incision site and surgical site infection, both of which occur in less than 5% of patients. Infection often leads to the need for device explantation; however, implantation may be attempted again after the infection has cleared. The SNS study group also reported 5-year data, which demonstrated 89% of patients had sustained benefit, and 36% of patients reported perfect continence. However, 36% of patients required device revision or replacement. Overall, SNS represents an exciting therapy for the treatment of fecal incontinence.

Overlapping Anterior Sphincteroplasty

Sphincteroplasty is a direct repair of the anal sphincter and may be performed when there is an anterior anatomic defect. This occurs in women as a result of a vaginal childbirth injury, which is a leading cause of fecal incontinence. If obstetric sphincter injury is suspected, ultrasound imaging should be performed to confirm.

Patients typically undergo preoperative mechanical bowel preparation. The procedure should be performed under general anesthesia and patients may be positioned in either lithotomy or prone jack-knife. A curvilinear incision is made anterior to the anus, and the two sides of the sphincter are mobilized. The associated scar should be preserved because this is important for the repair and allowing the sutures to hold. Care is taken not to extend the dissection too far posteriorly so as not to injure the pudendal nerves. Once the dissection is completed, an anterior levatorplasty often is performed in conjunction with the sphincter repair to approximate the levator muscles. The two sides of the sphincter are reapproximated in an overlapping fashion with 2-0 monofilament mattress sutures. The skin is closed loosely with deep dermal sutures to allow for drainage (Figure 3).

Short-term results regarding continence after this procedure indicate that up to 80% of patients report good to excellent functional results. However, the benefit deteriorates over time such that with longer follow-up, few patients remain continent. This option remains most useful in the setting of an associated rectovaginal fistula or if

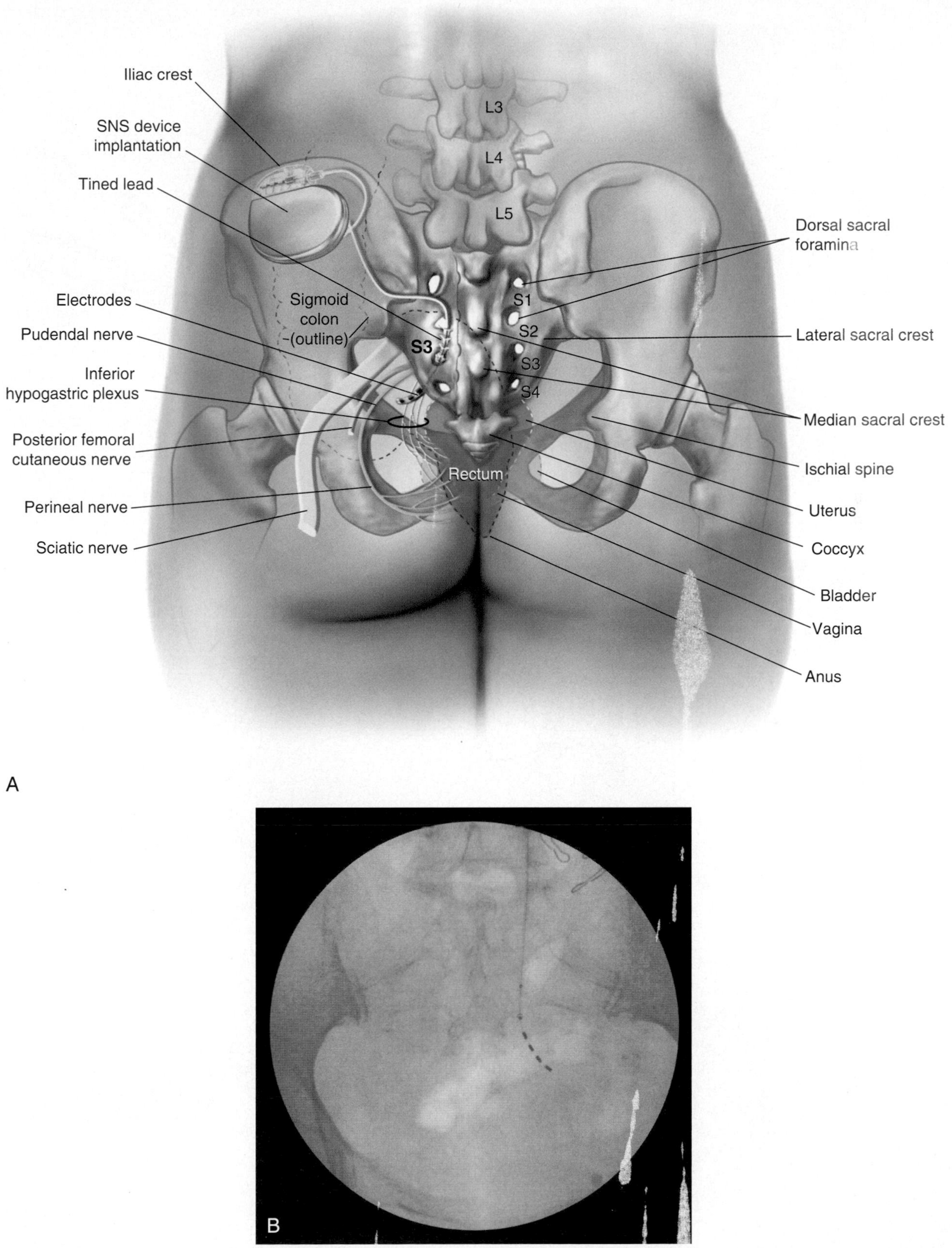

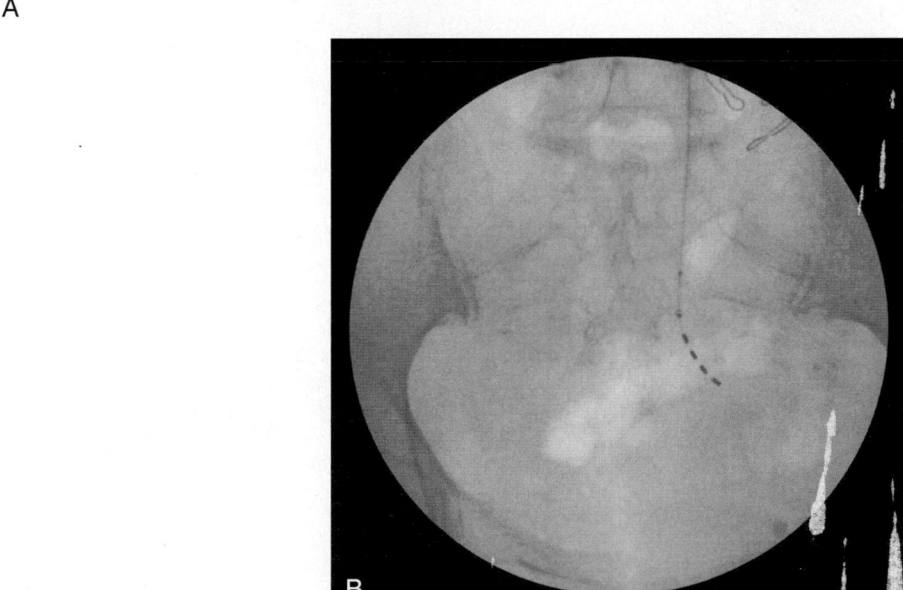

Iliac crest

SNS device implantation

Tined lead

Electrodes

Pudendal nerve

Inferior hypogastric plexus

Posterior femoral cutaneous nerve

Perineal nerve

Sciatic nerve

L3

L4

L5

Sigmoid colon –(outline)

S3

S1

S2

S3

S4

Rectum

Dorsal sacral foramina

Lateral sacral crest

Median sacral crest

Ischial spine

Uterus

Coccyx

Bladder

Vagina

Anus

A

B

FIGURE 2 Sacral nerve stimulation. **A,** Tined lead with implanted permanent battery. **B,** Anteroposterior abdominal x-ray image of the tined lead in the appropriate position. *(A, From Hull T. Posterior Pelvic Floor Abnormalities. Philadelphia: Elsevier; 2011.)*

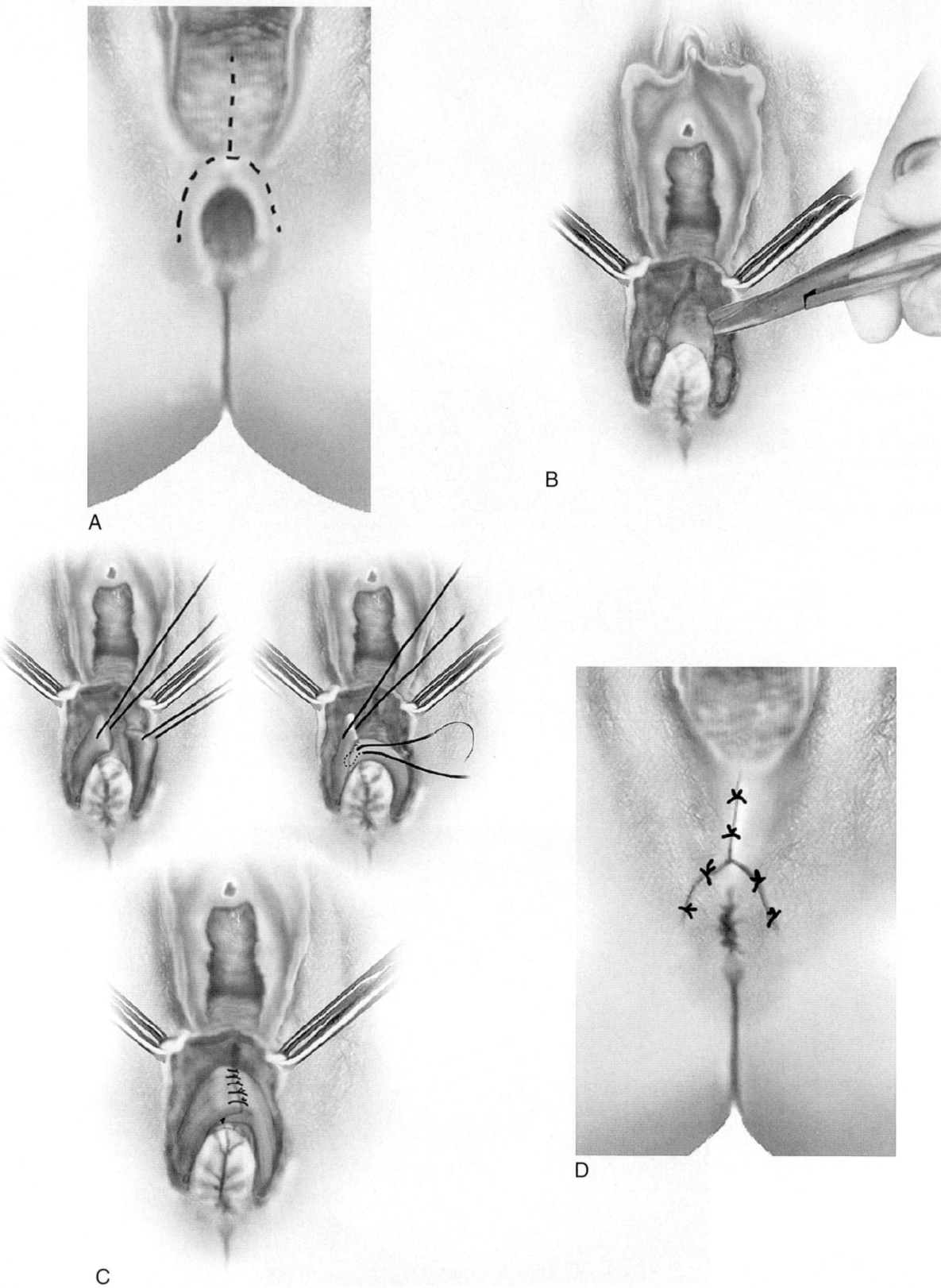

FIGURE 3 Overlapping anterior sphincteroplasty. **A,** A curvilinear incision is made anterior the anus. **B,** Both sides of the sphincter and associated scar are overlapped. **C,** The sphincter is secured in the overlapping position with mattress sutures. **D,** The skin is loosely approximated to facilitate drainage. *(From Baggish M. Atlas of Pelvic Anatomy and Gynecologic Surgery. Philadelphia: Elsevier; 2011.)*

there is significant fecal incontinence immediately after an obstetric injury, suggesting a severe injury. In these cases, operative intervention should not be undertaken for at least 3 to 6 months after delivery.

Stoma Creation

Stoma creation can offer an effective solution for fecal incontinence, albeit an invasive one. Indications for stoma creation include failure of medical therapy and other surgical therapies, or patient preference. In most patients with fecal incontinence, creation of a sigmoid colostomy is appropriate, although in patients with both fecal incontinence and slow transit constipation, an ileostomy may be beneficial. Stoma creation often can be created in a laparoscopic fashion. Regardless of approach, a stoma nurse should be involved both preoperatively and postoperatively. Survey data collected from patients with a stoma created for fecal incontinence demonstrated that 83% of patients reported improvement in quality of life, and 84% of patients would have chosen a stoma again.

■ CONCLUSIONS

Fecal incontinence is a prevalent and distressing problem. Stool bulking and constipating agents are appropriate initial treatments. There are several surgical treatments that are available, although SNS currently seems to be most efficacious for improving significant fecal incontinence. Other commonly offered options include injectable bulking agents and sphincteroplasty. Stoma creation usually is undertaken as a final option. Additional therapies for fecal incontinence are being developed and tested and may hold promise for future patients.

SUGGESTED READINGS

Bleier JI, Kann BR. Surgical management of fecal incontinence. *Gastroenterol Clin North Am.* 2013;42:815-836.

Graf W, Mellgren A, Matzel KE, Hull T, Johansson C, Bernstein M, Nasha Dx Study Group. Efficacy of dextranomer in stabilised hyaluronic acid for treatment of faecal incontinence: a randomised, sham-controlled trial. *Lancet.* 2011;377:997-1003.

Halverson AL, Hull TL. Long-term outcome of overlapping anal sphincter repair. *Dis Colon Rectum.* 2002;45:345-348.

Hull T, Giese C, Wexner SD, Mellgren AA, Devroede G, Madoff RD, Stromberg K, Coller JA, SNS Study Group. Long-term durability of sacral nerve stimulation therapy for chronic fecal incontinence. *Dis Colon Rectum.* 2013;234-245.

Malouf AJ, Norton CS, Engel AF, Nicholls RJ, Kamm MA. Long-term results of overlapping anterior anal-sphincter repair for obstetric trauma. *Lancet.* 2000;355:260-265.

Norton C, Burch J, Kamm MA. Patients' views of a colostomy for fecal incontinence. *Dis Colon Rectum.* 2005;48:1062-1069.

Tjandra JJ, Dykes SL, Kumar RR, Ellis CN, Gregorcyk SG, Hyman NH, Buie WD. Colon Standards Practice Task Force of The American Society of, and Surgeons Rectal, Practice Parameters for the Treatment of Fecal Incontinence. *Dis Colon Rectum.* 2007;50:1497-1507.

Wexner SD, et al. Sacral nerve stimulation for fecal incontinence: results of a 120-patient prospective multicenter study. *Ann Surg.* 2010;251:441-449.

THE MANAGEMENT OF RECTOVAGINAL FISTULA

Nicole M. Saur, MD, and Joshua I. Bleier, MD

Rectovaginal fistulas present challenges for the patient and the surgeon. Despite limited mortality, rectovaginal fistulas are associated with significant morbidity involving a significant negative impact in social, sexual, and overall quality of life. Because of the complexity of the disease and the surgical repair options, many patients fail multiple procedures before going to a tertiary care center.

The literature is made up of case series with small numbers of patients and the systematic reviews analyzing them. Therefore it is difficult to advocate for one repair technique or directly compare the results between techniques.

With these limitations in mind, in this chapter we discuss the surgical management of rectovaginal fistula and propose a broad treatment algorithm based on current reported literature.

■ CAUSE

Obstetric injury is the most common cause of rectovaginal fistula. Approximately 2% of all vaginal deliveries are associated with third- and fourth-degree perineal tears with 3% of these patients subsequently developing rectovaginal fistula; this accounts for 0.1% of all vaginal births. Fistulas arising from obstetric injury often are associated with anterior anal sphincter defects that lead to fecal incontinence of varying severity.

Crohn's disease is the second most common cause of rectovaginal fistulas; up to 10% of female Crohn's disease patients develop rectovaginal fistulas. Rectovaginal fistulas associated with Crohn's disease have a high recurrence rate and often require multiple procedures before lasting repair.

Iatrogenic injuries also make up a substantial number of rectovaginal fistulas. Up to 10% of female patients develop rectovaginal fistulas after low anterior resection. Neoplasia, infectious causes, anorectal or vaginal neoplasia, and radiation therapy make up the remainder of causes. A summary of causes of rectovaginal fistulas is included in Box 1.

■ CLINICAL MANIFESTATIONS

The most common presenting symptoms are passage of stool or gas via the vagina, which often can be misinterpreted as fecal incontinence. However, often the clinical picture is less clear: patients have symptoms of repeated urinary tract infections, dyspareunia, or vaginal discharge.

An indurated fistula tract often can be identified on digital examination in the office. Anoscopy or vaginal speculum examination often is used to visualize granulation tissue at the level of the tract. Gentle probing at that level often reveals the tract. Not all rectovaginal fistulas are identified on an initial clinical examination in the office. To further evaluate for the presence of a rectovaginal fistula in the office, a *tampon test* can be undertaken. A tampon is placed in the vagina, and an enema of diluted methylene blue dye is given as an enema. The patient is asked to ambulate, and later (i.e., after 20 to 30 minutes), the tampon is removed and inspected for evidence of blue dye. If dye is identified on the tampon, a fistula is highly suspected.

In a patient with inflammatory bowel disease, an examination under anesthesia (EUA) should be undertaken as the initial step after clinical examination as a means to identify the fistulous anatomy and evaluate for the degree of inflammation of the anus and rectum. Barring an obvious tract identified in the office, EUA is the best modality to define the fistula tract and plan surgical treatment. If the primary opening is identified, but with difficulty identifying the secondary opening, hydrogen peroxide or methylene blue can be used. A fistula probe can be placed into the fistula tract (Figure 1).

The goals of preoperative evaluation are to (1) identify the fistula, (2) determine the cause, (3) evaluate the extent of the disesae, and (4) identify surrounding injuries. Endoanal ultrasonography (EAUS) is the diagnostic test of choice to determine anal sphincter defects and to define occult collections and can be used with hydrogen peroxide to map complex fistulas. Pelvic magnetic resonance imaging (MRI) and endorectal coil MRI are also useful diagnostic modalities that can be used to identify sphincter defects and be used with hydrogen peroxide to identify fistulas. The use of ultrasound or MRI is operator and institution specific.

Pelvic floor physiologic testing is indicated when there is a history of anal sphincter injury or the presence of fecal incontinence because undiagnosed sphincter or pudendal nerve injuries can cause recurrent symptoms of incontinence after a successful fistula repair. Anorectal manometry is the test of choice to evaluate for sphincter dysfunction, and pudendal nerve terminal motor latency testing is the test of choice to detect nerve damage.

Especially in cases of malignancy and inflammatory bowel disease, a complete evaluation of the small bowel or colon and rectum may be necessary to determine the extent of involved organs. This workup may include small bowel series, enteroscopy, computed tomography/magnetic resonance (CT/MR) enterography, CT/MR colonography, colonoscopy, or contrast enema.

BOX 1: Cause of Rectovaginal Fistulas

Obstetric Injury

Episiotomy, third- and fourth-degree perineal lacerations

Inflammatory Bowel Disease

Crohn's disease

Iatrogenic

Anorectal surgery (fistulotomy)
Vaginal surgery (hysterectomy, rectocele repair)
Abdominal surgery (hysterectomy, low anterior resection, J pouch, procedure for prolapse and hemorrhoids)

Infectious

Cryptoglandular abscess, diverticulitis, tuberculosis

Neoplastic

Anal cancer, rectal cancer, vaginal cancer, cervical cancer

Radiation-Induced

External beam radiation, brachytherapy

■ CLASSIFICATION

Classification of rectovaginal fistulas not only is a descriptive exercise but also helps determine how they are managed. Rectovaginal fistulas may be classified according to their relation to the sphincter complex. *High fistulas* are defined as those above the sphincter complex and *low fistulas* are those at or below the level of the sphincters; these also are referred to as *anovaginal*. Trauma after vaginal delivery is almost always the cause of low fistulas, which often are associated with an associated sphincter injury.

Rectovaginal fistulas alternatively may be classified as *simple* or *complex*. *Simple* fistulas are located in the middle or lower portion of the rectovaginal septum, are less than 2.5 cm in diameter, and are

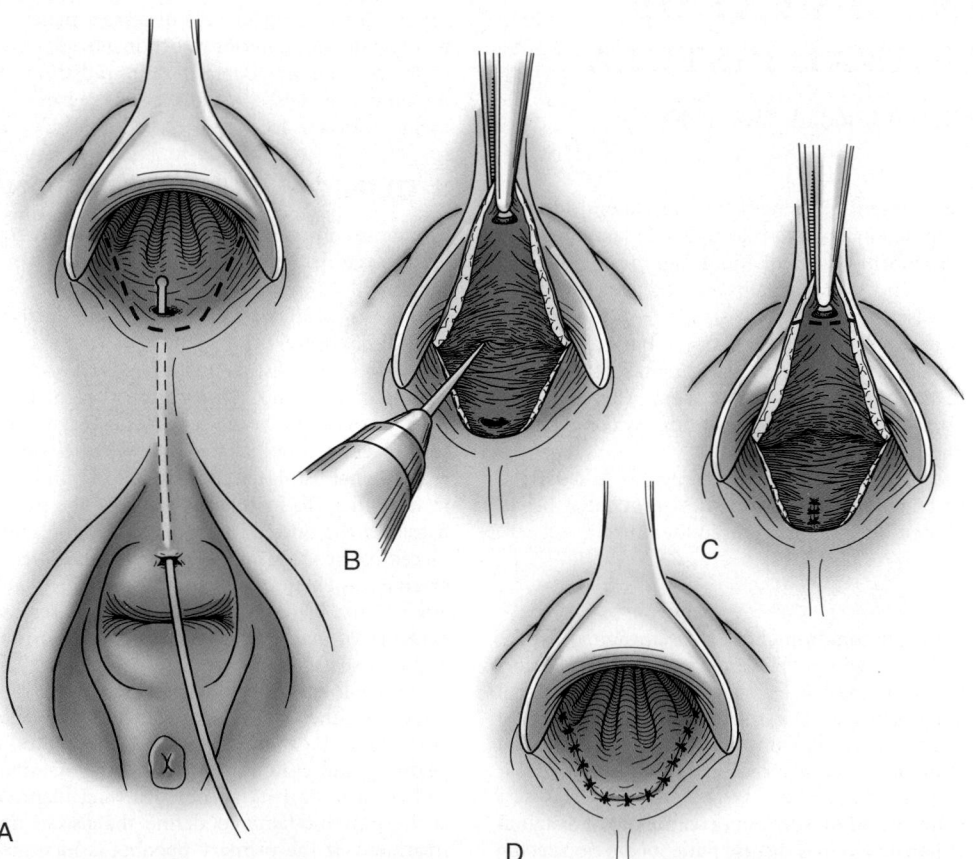

FIGURE 1 Endorectal advancement flap. **A,** Probe is placed through the fistula tract. **B,** The flap is started distal to the fistula tract. **C,** The flap is raised 4 to 6 cm, and the fistula tract is excised. The internal opening is suture ligated. **D,** The flap is sutured in place with interrupted sutures.

caused by local trauma or infection. In contrast, *complex* fistulas are usually greater than 2.5 cm, located in the upper portion of the rectovaginal septum, or are secondary to causes other than trauma and infection, such as neoplasia, diverticulitis, or inflammatory bowel disease.

■ PREOPERATIVE MANAGEMENT

The extent of preoperative preparation is largely subjective but usually varies with the type of procedure planned for the repair. For simple repairs and vaginal-based repairs, a phosphate enema on the morning of the procedure is adequate. For more extensive repairs, such as an overlapping sphincteroplasty or an interposition flap, and especially when fecal diversion is anticipated, a full mechanical and antibiotic bowel preparation is performed. Perioperative antibiotics and deep venous thrombosis prophylaxis are administered as per Surgical Care Improvement Project (SCIP) and institutional guidelines.

■ SURGICAL MANAGEMENT

Because of the complex nature of the disease and surgical techniques, optimum conditions must be present before undertaking any surgical repair. Goals of treatment are to preserve continence while achieving healing of the fistula.

The presence of active sepsis is an absolute contraindication to any attempt at surgical repair; drainage of any abscesses and resolution of sepsis is the first and most important step. A low threshold is maintained to place a draining seton until the infection is controlled and drainage stops, which can take 3 to 6 months or longer.

On the basis of a similar rationale, treatment of fistulas in the immediate postpartum period is delayed for a period of at least 3 to 6 months to allow acute inflammation to subside and fibrosis to develop. Symptomatic relief often is achieved with bulking agents and antidiarrheals. Before operative repair, an evaluation of the sphincter is undertaken with EAUS.

There are four general categories of surgical approaches to a rectovaginal fistula: *transanal, transvaginal, transperineal,* and *transabdominal.* Table 1 summarizes the indications and outcomes for the various treatment approaches currently in use. The first three categories of approach generally are reserved for low fistulas.

Transanal Approach

Fistulotomy

A fistulotomy, by definition, is the laying open of the fistula tract, which also may be excised. This often is performed as a two-stage procedure: first, a draining seton is placed and then removed after fistula tract maturation and fibrosis. The second stage involves cutting of the remaining tissue to lay open the tract.

Although a fistulotomy achieves the goal of almost 100% successful healing of the fistula, it involves division of varying thicknesses of the sphincter muscles and risks varying degrees of fecal incontinence. The incontinence is often permanent. Therefore, although lay-open fistulotomy theoretically is indicated for superficial fistulas, it very rarely is used today. Episioproctotomy, which involves fistulotomy followed by subsequent sphincter repair, is discussed later.

Endorectal Advancement Flap

Endorectal advancement flap (ERAF) is a mainstay of treatment for low rectovaginal fistulas, particularly in patients without concomitant sphincter defects. The procedure typically is performed in the prone jack-knife position, which offers excellent exposure of the anterior rectal wall. Both the anus and vagina are prepared, and a probe is inserted through the fistula from the vagina into the rectum. A gentle U-shaped flap then is outlined with the base cephalad and twice the width of the apex. The U shape and 2:1 dimensions ensure that there are no flap corners to become ischemic and the flap pedicle

is adequate to ensure blood supply to the anastomosis. The flap is started 1 cm distal to the fistula and consists of the rectal mucosa, submucosa, and a portion of the underlying internal sphincter, including the fistula opening at the apex; this is raised in cephalad manner with the use of needle-tip electrocautery. A sufficient length of flap should be mobilized 3 to 4 cm proximal to the fistula opening to ensure a tension-free closure after excision of the fistula. Injection of a dilute epinephrine solution facilitates dissection and minimizes blood loss (Figure 1).

After the flap is elevated, the fistula tract is curetted to remove all granulation tissue, and the defect in the remaining internal sphincter is closed with simple interrupted absorbable sutures. The apex of the flap then is excised to remove the fistula opening, and the flap is advanced caudad and ensured to be tension free. The flap is sutured in place with 2-0 interrupted absorbable sutures to close the wound by first placing sutures at either end of the wound and then continually bisecting the wound with sutures until closed. The vaginal opening is left open to facilitate drainage. Postoperative care includes a high-fiber diet, laxative to avoid fecal impaction, and sitz baths.

The ERAF offers the advantages of performing the repair from the high-pressure side of the fistula as well as sphincter preservation. Short-term success rates for rectal advancement flaps alone vary from 42% to 71% in the small series in the current literature with varying and often short follow-up. The primary downside of the ERAF is the need for dissection of otherwise healthy rectal wall and sphincter. Flap failure and ischemia may result in flap loss and a subsequent rectal defect that is much larger than the original opening. Rates of early (within 1 week) flap loss have been reported as high as 6% with late flap loss/failure rates ranging from 16% to 37%.

Fibrin Glue

At the time of examination under anesthesia, the rectal and vaginal fistula tract openings are identified. The fistula tract then is curetted and fibrin adhesive is injected into the fistula tract until it exits the secondary opening. The goal of fibrin glue placement is to plug the fistula with material that allows fibrous tissue ingrowth and results in autologous fistula healing with no disruption of the surrounding structures or sphincters. However, experience with fibrin glue in rectovaginal fistulas has been very limited and plagued by disappointing results predominantly secondary to glue extrusion because of short fistula length.

Bioprosthetics

Two bioprosthetics have been used for rectovaginal fistulas: the bioprosthetic mesh (Surgisis mesh; Cook Surgical, Bloomington, IN) and the rectovaginal fistula plug (Surgisis Biodesign Button; Cook Surgical, Bloomington, IN). Both products are made from lyophilized porcine intestinal submucosa, which provides a matrix for ingrowth of connective tissue.

The bioprosthetic mesh is used as an interposition graft. The rectovaginal septum is dissected through a perineal incision, and the fistula is excised. After closure of the rectal and vaginal openings, the rehydrated mesh is placed between the rectum and vagina with an adequate overlap over the rectal and vaginal closures; it is sutured in position with interrupted absorbable sutures, with the mesh kept as taut as possible. The bioprosthetic mesh is useful when tissue grafts are not suitable options.

The bioprosthetic rectovaginal fistula plug is tapered at one end to facilitate insertion. A fistula probe is introduced from the vaginal to the rectal opening, and the tapered end of the plug is tied to the probe with a suture. The probe is then withdrawn, the plug is pulled with it, and the button is lodged with the broader end at the rectal opening. The excess plug material at the rectal end is then excised, and the plug is sutured in position with absorbable sutures, which close the rectal mucosa over the plug. The vaginal side is left open, and the excess plug is trimmed at this level. The short length of the fistula tract poses the same problem with the plug as with fibrin glue,

TABLE 1: Types, Indications, and Outcomes of Surgical Options for Rectovaginal Fistulas

	Number of Published Cases	Closure Rate (%; Range, Mean)	Follow-Up (Months, When Recorded)	Complications	Fistula Type
TRANSANAL APPROACHES					
Endorectal advancement flaps	515	33.3-91, 68.8	7-40	Incontinence, Recurrence, Larger Fistula	Low, occasionally high
Fibrin glue	16	33-75, 56	3-26	Recurrence	Unclear
Bioprosthetic (Surgisis) plug	49	20-85.7, 45.9	3-22	Recurrence, Cost	Low, occasionally high
Bioprosthetic Mesh (Surgisis) repair	48	71-81.5, 76.3	12-22	Recurrence, Larger fistula, Cost	Low + high
TRANSVAGINAL APPROACHES					
Vaginal advancement flap	41	50-92.9, 55.3	30-55	Recurrence	Low
TRANSPERINEAL APPROACHES					
Transperineal ligation with sphincteroplasty for + sphincter defect	72	64.7-100*	3-120	Incontinence, Sexual dysfunction, Wound dehiscence	Low
Episioproctotomy	50	62.2	49.2	Incontinence, Sexual dysfunction	Low
Gracilis muscle flap	99	43-100	14-35	Sexual dysfunction, Cosmesis, Wound dehiscence	Low + high
Martius flap	104	65-100	23-120	Sexual dysfunction, Cosmesis	Low
TRANSABDOMINAL APPROACHES					
Transabdominal fistula ligation with omental flap	49	95-100	22-28	Bleeding, Intraperitoneal Rectal injuries	High
Rectal resection	20	92.3-100	25	Anastomotic leak, bleeding, intraperitoneal injuries	High

Adapted from Göttgens KW, Smeets RR, Stassen LP, et al. The disappointing quality of published studies on operative techniques for rectovaginal fistulas: a blueprint for a prospective multi-institutional study. *Dis Colon Rectum.* 2014;57:888-898.

*Several studies with unclear data, recurrent operations.

which makes the plug suitable only for rectovaginal fistulas that are more than 1 cm in length.

The experience with bioprosthetics as a whole in rectovaginal fistulas is very limited. Success rates of fistula closure by interposition techniques have been reported to be from 66% to 86% with short follow-up. Complications are rare and generally benign and include primarily infection and plug extrusion.

Transvaginal Approach

Vaginal Advancement Flap

In a technique similar to the rectal advancement flap, a flap of vaginal mucosa is raised, and the fistula tract is excised. The rectal mucosa is closed separately, over which the defect in the rectovaginal septum is approximated with interrupted absorbable sutures. The apex of the flap then is trimmed to excise the fistula opening and is sutured into position to close the wound.

The primary advantage of a vaginal flap is the use of healthy, pliable, and well-vascularized vaginal tissue, although the disadvantage remains that the repair is on the low-pressure side of the fistula. A vaginal flap is easier to mobilize than a rectal flap, especially in the presence of anorectal stenosis. A comparative analysis of 11 studies showed no statistically significant difference in the closure rates between a rectal and vaginal advancement flap closure in rectovaginal fistulas resulting from Crohn's disease. Therefore, especially when fibrostenotic disease is present in the anus or a transanal approach has failed, a transvaginal advancement flap is a viable option.

Transperineal Approach

Episioproctotomy and Layered Closure

This repair converts the fistula into a fourth-degree perineal tear by dividing all the tissue between the rectum and vagina through the perineal body. A layered closure then is performed to close the rectal mucosa, the rectal and vaginal muscular walls, and finally the vaginal mucosa. The greatest disadvantage of this procedure is the creation of a full-thickness defect in a previously uninjured part of the anal sphincter. Therefore a repair dehiscence risks significant incontinence, which may not have been the case preoperatively. This procedure should be attempted only by experienced surgeons and in patients with documented existing sphincter defects with fecal incontinence. In experienced hands, healing rates superior to ERAF closure (57.5% vs 42.5%) have been reported with improved sexual function ($P = 0.04$) and decreased rates of fecal incontinence (improved in episioproctotomy group, unchanged in ERAF group, $P < 0.001$) when compared with ERAF.

Transperineal Ligation With a LIFT procedure, Overlapping Sphincteroplasty

Simple transperineal ligation of the fistula tract can be undertaken with the ligation of the intersphincteric fistula tract (LIFT) procedure. A perineal incision is made over the intersphincteric groove and carried through the intersphincteric space, while a fistula probe is traversing the fistula tract. The fistula tract is ligated with absorbable sutures and divided. In a patient with a rectovaginal fistula and a concomitant sphincter defect, sphincteroplasty is an effective approach. If a sphincter defect is present, a sphincteroplasty is performed as described later. If there is no sphincter defect, the wound is irrigated and closed in layers.

If a sphincter defect is present, healthy ends of the external sphincter muscle are identified and skeletonized. The sphincter then is mobilized to the midline to ensure overlap without tension. Often the sphincter is so attenuated at the site of injury that the healthy ends of the sphincter can be overlapped and sutured into position without the need to divide or excise any tissue. The sphincter is overlapped and sutured in place with 2-0 absorbable interrupted mattress sutures. The wound is approximated loosely with the center of the skin incision left open for drainage. The technique should achieve similar results of episioproctotomy and, if it should fail, will not result in worse than preoperative incontinence. In addition, when a sphincter injury is present, the addition of an overlapping sphincteroplasty to an ERAF has been reported to increase both the rate of fistula closure (up to 100% in series of 20 patients) and restore continence (70% of patients).

Interposition Flaps

The interposition of healthy, vascularized tissue in the rectovaginal septum aims to increase the chance of successful closure of ischemic tissues caused by previous failed repair attempts. The potential for dyspareunia is a disadvantage of the technique. The gracilis and bulbocavernosus flaps are the two most described pedicled flaps for rectovaginal fistulas. Although not mandatory, fecal diversion typically is recommended and generally is undertaken before the flap procedure.

The approach is usually via a perineal incision, which is deepened to expose the rectovaginal septum and then is dissected at least 2 to 3 cm proximal to the level of the fistula. The fistula then is excised completely, or repaired via one of the previous techniques, and the rectal and vaginal defects are closed primarily.

The gracilis muscle has only vestigial function, and a reliable vascular pedicle enters the muscle at a constant location laterally in its upper third. The muscle of either leg can be used and is harvested through an incision in the medial aspect of the thigh. The harvested muscle then is tunneled through the subcutaneous tissue at the groin and maneuvered into the perineal incision. This then is parachuted between the rectum and vagina and held in position with interrupted absorbable sutures. The success rate of the gracilis muscle flap has been reported to be as high as 75% to 80%.

The Martius flap, which involves harvesting of the bulbocavernosus muscle with the overlying fat in the labia majora, is based on the perineal branch of the pudendal artery and is placed in the rectovaginal septum in similar fashion. As with all interposition flaps, this repair has the potential risk for increased postoperative dyspareunia, but labial function and cosmesis do not appear to be compromised. The success rate with this procedure has been reported to vary from 50% to 93.8%.

Transabdominal Approach

Rectal Resection/Advancement

Sleeve advancement is indicated in circumferential or structuring disease as is the case with Crohn's disease and for fistulas classified as high and complex. The procedure involves mobilization of the proximal rectum, resection of the diseased distal rectum, and restoration of continuity with an anorectal anastomosis.

Primary Repair With Omental Interposition

This transabdominal approach is best suited to repair high rectovaginal fistulas, which are usually a complication of surgical injuries or diverticulitis. The rectum is dissected down to the level of the fistula, which then is divided to expose the rectal and vaginal openings. If the rectal wall is healthy, the fistula tract can be débrided and closed primarily. The vaginal opening then is closed primarily, and a pedicled omental flap is placed between the two closures and held in position with interrupted sutures. However, if the surrounding rectum is indurated or diseased, sleeve advancement can be undertaken as described earlier.

Sometimes, a low rectovaginal fistula may require a transabdominal approach after multiple failed transanal, transvaginal, or transperineal approaches. A transabdominal approach in this setting has the advantages of resecting all ischemic tissue and bringing down well-vascularized tissues to the anal canal.

The procedure entails mobilization of the rectum and separation of the rectovaginal septum down to the pelvic floor. The fistula openings in the rectum and vagina then are débrided and closed primarily with interrupted absorbable sutures. A pedicled omental flap of sufficient length and based on either the left or right gastroepiploic artery, is prepared and placed in the pelvis. From the perineum, the lower rectovaginal septum is dissected free. The omental flap then is brought down into the rectovaginal septum and sutured to the subcutaneous tissue of the perineum. Additional sutures are placed to anchor the omentum to the levator ani along the lateral pelvic walls for tension-free interposition. Although this is a major surgical procedure, it brings vascularized omentum into the rectovaginal septum between the rectal and vaginal closures and may be the last, best option for successful closure in patients with multiple failed procedures.

Other Surgical Considerations

Fecal Diversion

There is no consensus on the indications of proximal fecal diversion in rectovaginal fistulas because it has been shown that a stoma does not necessarily ensure the success of a repair. However, after two failed attempts or the necessity of a pedicled flap closure, surgeons are more likely to proceed with diversion before or during the subsequent repair.

Choice of Repair

Considering the diverse causes, the large number of surgical options, and the lack of good-quality comparative studies, there is no clear guideline on the choice of procedures to undertake first for rectovaginal fistula repair. The choice of procedure is determined largely by the type of fistula (low or high, simple or complex), the cause, whether a sphincter defect exists, the number of prior failed attempts,

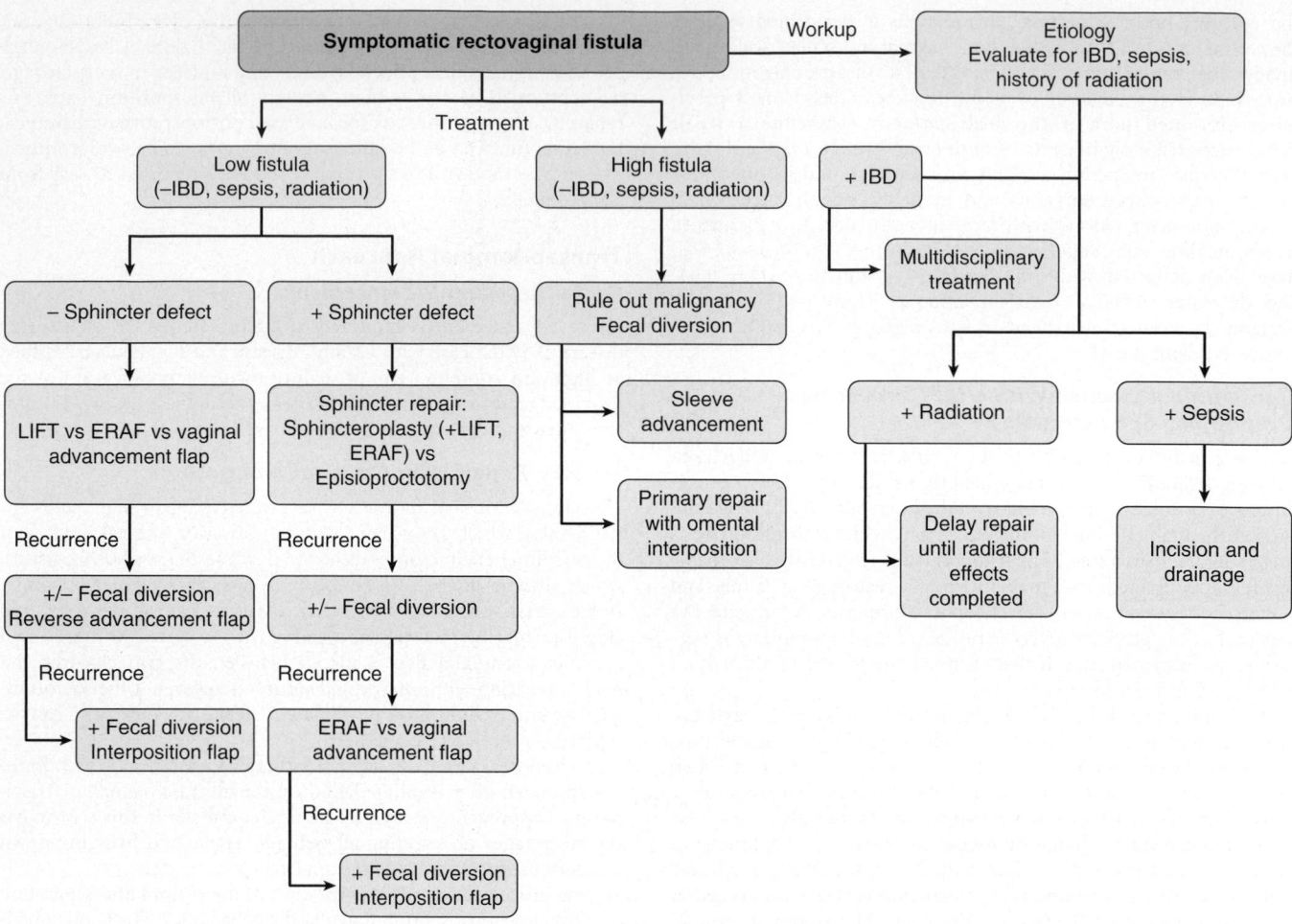

FIGURE 2 Proposed treatment algorithm for primary and recurrent rectovaginal fistula. *ERAF,* Endorectal advancement flap; *IBD,* inflammatory bowel disease; *LIFT,* ligation of the intersphincteric fistula tract.

and the functional status of the patient. A proposed algorithm for first-line treatment and subsequent repairs is explained later and listed in Figure 2.

Reported success rates vary greatly for each procedure. Experience likely plays a large role in this; however, even in experienced hands a certain failure rate is expected. Therefore all attempts should be made to avoid sphincter division and anal canal scarring in early repairs.

The first decision point in a proposed algorithm is whether a sphincter defect and associated incontinence are present. Overlapping sphincteroplasty will address the fistula and incontinence and is first-line treatment in this patient population, typically those with obstetric trauma. An ERAF can be added to increase the fistula healing rate.

In those patients without sphincter defect, either a rectal or vaginal advancement flap can be undertaken as first-line options. Although the results for both procedures are thought to be similar, a rectal advancement flap puts the repair on the high-pressure side of the fistula but requires healthy rectal mucosa, whereas the vaginal flap saves the rectal mucosa from scarring and internal sphincter from disruption but places the repair on the low-pressure side of the fistula.

If either the rectal or vaginal flap fails, the subsequent step is the opposite procedure. After failure of both a rectal and vaginal flap, the options are repeating a flap procedure or proceeding with an interposition pedicled flap, with the addition of fecal diversion. If the local tissues are still healthy with minimal scarring, a repeat flap can be attempted. However, with every subsequent failed procedure,

increased tissue ischemia is produced, and the chances of failure increase further. At this point, either gracilis or Martius interposition flaps should be considered with appropriate counseling in view of the reported dyspareunia with these repairs.

Because experience with bioprosthetics is limited, there is no formal recommendation for their use currently. However, because bioprosthetics rely on tissue ingrowth from surrounding tissue, a bioprosthetic-enhanced repair is not likely to succeed in an ischemic rectovaginal septum. In the presence of ischemia, a pedicled flap is a viable option. In addition, in the presence of a healthy proximal rectum, a distal proctectomy with a coloanal anastomosis will resect the diseased rectum and bring healthy proximal rectum to the anal canal, and a pedicled omental flap can be used as interposition.

■ SPECIAL CONSIDERATIONS

Radiation-Induced Fistulas

With the widespread use of radiation for locally advanced pelvic malignancies, the number of radiation-induced complications will continue to increase. The first step in management of radiation-induced rectovaginal fistulas is to rule out the presence of malignancy, either primary or recurrent. This requires detailed imaging and an examination with the patient under anesthesia with multiple biopsies of areas of irregularity or random biopsies if no irregularity exists. Once the presence of malignancy has been ruled out, the condition of the rectum, vagina, and surrounding perineal tissues must be evaluated.

No definitive repair should be undertaken for at least 6 months after the completion of radiation treatment to allow for the resolution of the acute inflammatory effects of radiation and for the recovery of the surrounding tissue. If the local tissues are viable, a rectal or vaginal advancement flap can be attempted. However, it should be noted that the repair is less likely to succeed because it is performed in radiated tissue. Therefore only one attempt at primary tissue repair should be undertaken. Enteric diversion and subsequent interposition flaps with gracilis muscle or sleeve advancement, if healthy proximal rectum is present, are the best available options in the setting of primary failure.

Crohn's Disease

Almost every patient with Crohn's proctitis and a rectovaginal fistula will require an examination under anesthesia and seton before definitive repair. Optimization of medical management is mandatory before surgical repair. Multidisciplinary management is critical: any repair is doomed to fail if all disease is not rendered quiescent. The ACCENT II study showed that patients who initially responded to infliximab (at least 50% reduction in fistula) had a 50% rate of full closure of the fistula. If medical management fails or is not an option, surgical treatment is undertaken. If the rectum is healthy, either rectal or vaginal advancement flaps can be undertaken first. However, if the rectum if inflamed or scarred, vaginal advancement flap is the preferred first choice. There should be a low threshold for diversion in these cases.

Crohn's disease–associated rectovaginal fistulas have an overall poor prognosis, with a recurrence rate that varies from 25% to 50%. It is therefore very important to appropriately counsel patients and set realistic treatment goals. In patients with poorly controlled proctitis, surgical options are very limited. Often patients are symptomatic from the abscesses associated with the repeated flare-ups of Crohn's proctitis and require optimization of medical management and prolonged seton drainage. With multiple failed procedures and recurrent fistulas, proctectomy with end colostomy is the definitive treatment of last resort.

Malignancy

The definitive treatment of malignant rectovaginal fistulas is an *en bloc* surgical resection of the malignancy, contiguous organs involved, and the fistula tract. This often requires a pelvic exenteration. A diverting stoma often is placed to control symptoms and decrease pelvic and perineal sepsis, while the patient receives neoadjuvant therapy. The patient is reevaluated after neoadjuvant treatment to determine the extent of treatment response and to suitability to undergo a major operation. In patients with good performance status and a satisfactory response to neoadjuvant therapy, a pelvic exenteration can be considered. However, in most patients who are not suitable candidates for exenteration, the treatment focus is palliation.

SUGGESTED READINGS

Ellis CN. Outcomes after repair of rectovaginal fistulas using bioprosthetics. *Dis Colon Rectum.* 2008;51:1084-1088.

Göttgens KW, Smeets RR, Stassen LP, et al. The disappointing quality of published studies on operative techniques for rectovaginal fistulas: a blueprint for a prospective multi-institutional study. *Dis Colon Rectum.* 2014;57:888-898.

Hull TL, El-Gazzaz G, Gurlund B. Surgeons should not hesitate to perform episioproctotomy for rectovaginal fistula secondary to cryptoglandular or obstetrical origin. *Dis Colon Rectum.* 2011;54:54-59.

Lefèvre JH, Bretagnol F, Maggiori L, et al. Operative results and quality of life after gracilis muscle transposition for recurrent rectovaginal fistula. *Dis Colon Rectum.* 2009;52:1290-1295.

Ruffolo C, Scarpa M, Bassi N, et al. A systemic review on advancement flaps for rectovaginal fistula in Crohn's disease: transrectal versus transvaginal approach. *Colorectal Dis.* 2010;12:1183-1191.

Schouten WR, Oom DM. Rectal sleeve advancement for the treatment of persistent rectovaginal fistulas. *Tech Coloproctol.* 2009;13:289-294.

THE MANAGEMENT OF ANAL CONDYLOMA

Laila Rashidi, MD, and Raman Menon, MD

Condyloma acuminata, commonly known as *anogenital warts,* is one of the most common sexually transmitted diseases in the United States. It is caused by the highly contagious human papilloma virus (HPV), which infects squamous epithelia. HPV is a small, non-enveloped, double-stranded DNA virus from the *Papovaviridae* family. The incubation period ranges from 3 weeks to 8 months. Most infections are transient and are cleared within 2 years.

There are more than 120 distinct HPV subtypes, of which approximately 35 types target the anogenital epithelium and have varying malignant potential. High-risk (oncogenic) types are 16, 18, 31, 33, 35, 39, 45, 51, 52, 56, 58, 59, 68, 69, and 82. Low-risk (nononcogenic) types are 6, 11, 40, 42, 43, 44, 54, 61, 72, and 81. Ninety percent of condyloma harbor HPV types 6 or 11. HPV types 16, 18, 31, 33, and 35 occasionally are identified in condyloma and are often a coinfection with subtypes 6 or 11. Growth patterns range from focally grouped diminutive warts to large and exophytic carpet-like lesions.

■ INCIDENCE

An accurate incidence of condyloma acuminata cannot be obtained because the size of the population at risk is unknown and because many cases are likely to be undiagnosed or subclinical. It is estimated that there are 500,000 to 1 million new cases of genital warts annually in the United States. Twenty-four million people in the United States currently are infected with HPV. Although condyloma affect both genders, recent data revealed that women accounted for 67% of the patient population.

■ RISK FACTORS

HPV is highly contagious and transmitted primarily through sexual activity. Unprotected vaginal, anal, and oral intercourse along with intercourse at a younger age are risk factors for transmission. Transmission from mother to child during delivery can also occur. Risk factors for development of condyloma include immunosuppression because of HIV or transplantation, use of injectable drugs, cigarette smoking, and diabetes.

■ PATHOGENESIS, PRESENTATION, DETECTION

HPV invades and infects the basal keratinocytes of the epidermis. The general appearance of condyloma ranges from small, solitary, flesh-colored plaques to distinct 1- to 2-mm flesh-colored papules, which may occur in large clusters (Figure 1).

The symptoms of infection may vary depending on the number of lesions and their location. The most common sites of occurrence are the perianal skin, anal canal, and genital region. Patients with a small number of warts may be asymptomatic. Other patients, especially those with larger disease burden, may have pruritus, bleeding, burning, tenderness, discharge, or pain. Larger exophytic masses can interfere with defecation, intercourse, or vaginal delivery. Lesions involving the proximal anal canal also may cause stricture.

The lesions often are visualized easily during physical examination of the external anal skin in the office. The extent of involvement should be documented by physical examination and anoscopy, sigmoidoscopy, colposcopy, and/or vaginal speculum examination, as indicated. Application of 5% acetic acid causes the lesions to turn white and can aid with identification. Other lesions also may resemble anal condyloma, and the differential diagnosis includes benign skin tags, hypertrophic anal papillae, molluscum contagiosum, seborrheic keratoses, hypertrophied sebaceous glands, condylomata lata

(secondary syphilis), dysplastic nevi, and anal cancer. A biopsy with histopathologic analysis will confirm the diagnosis.

■ MANAGEMENT OF ANAL CONDYLOMA

The management of anal condyloma is individualized to the patient and predicated on the size, number, anatomic distribution, and presentation of the lesions. Spontaneous resolution of condyloma has been reported, but most patients require an intervention. The goal of treatment is complete destruction of all condyloma, understanding that the underlying viral infection may persist. The choice of medical management, outpatient office treatment, or treatment in the OR, in our opinion, is based on whether it is the initial outbreak or recurrent disease, the number and distribution of the lesions, and presence or absence of intra-anal lesions (Figures 2 and 3). There is no evidence to suggest that one treatment is significantly superior to another, and patients should be counseled, in advance, that recurrence is common and generally occurs within the first few months after treatment. A summary of the common treatments is listed in Table 1.

We have found that managing the initial presentation in the OR under conscious sedation allows for excellent results. This allows for careful inspection of the perianal skin and anal canal and identification of all lesions with or without the use of counterstaining with acetic acid. In addition, excision of representative samples from all quadrants with submission for pathologic examination can confirm the putative diagnosis and identify potential patients who may have high-grade squamous intraepithelial lesion (see further discussion later). Fulguration of the remaining condyloma with electrocautery is the mainstay in addressing the small to moderate lesions. (Our practice eschews use of laser for fulguration because there can be viable virus in the smoke plumes with isolated case reports of transmission to healthcare providers.) Use of the needle-tip cautery is very useful because it can target more precisely the remaining small condyloma with decreased damage to the surrounding tissue. In this manner, the lesions are fulgurated, first turning white and then forming an eschar that can be removed with a curette. What may appear to be a large carpet of numerous condyloma can be treated in this fashion because the condyloma often have a narrow base and islands of normal perianal skin can be identified between them. This approach has been shown to be safe and without significant risk of anal stenosis even with confluent condyloma.

On rare occasions, one may encounter carpeting of condyloma with a wide base and minimal to no intervening normal perianal skin. In this circumstance, we recommend staging the treatment of the lesions to minimize anal scarring and stenosis. Such patients

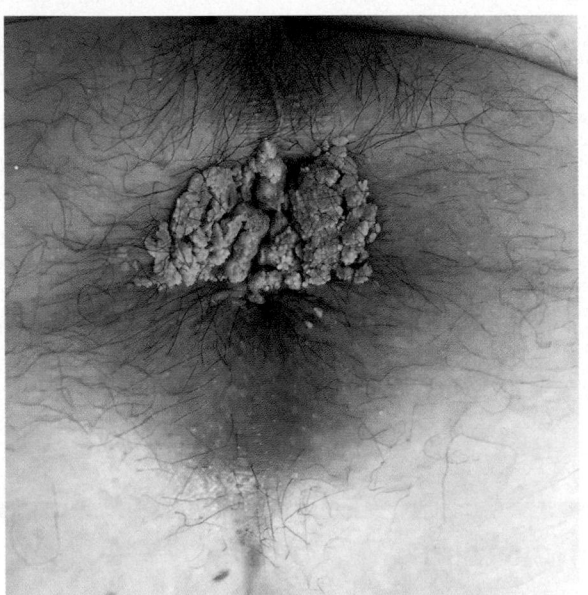

FIGURE 1 Anal condyloma.

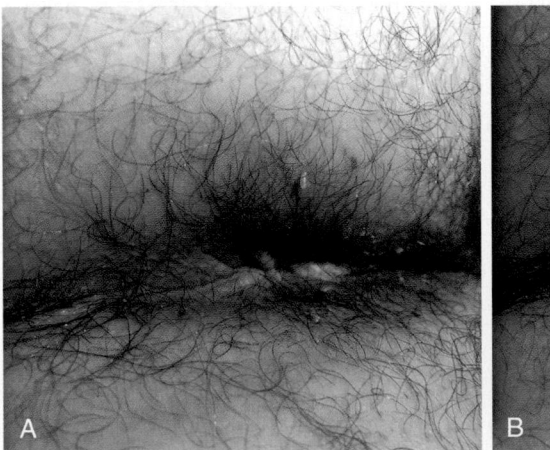 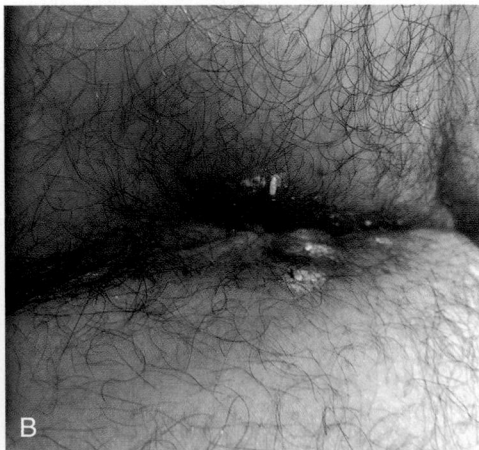

FIGURE 2 Treatment of anal condyloma before (**A**) and after (**B**) treatment in office with trichloroacetic acid.

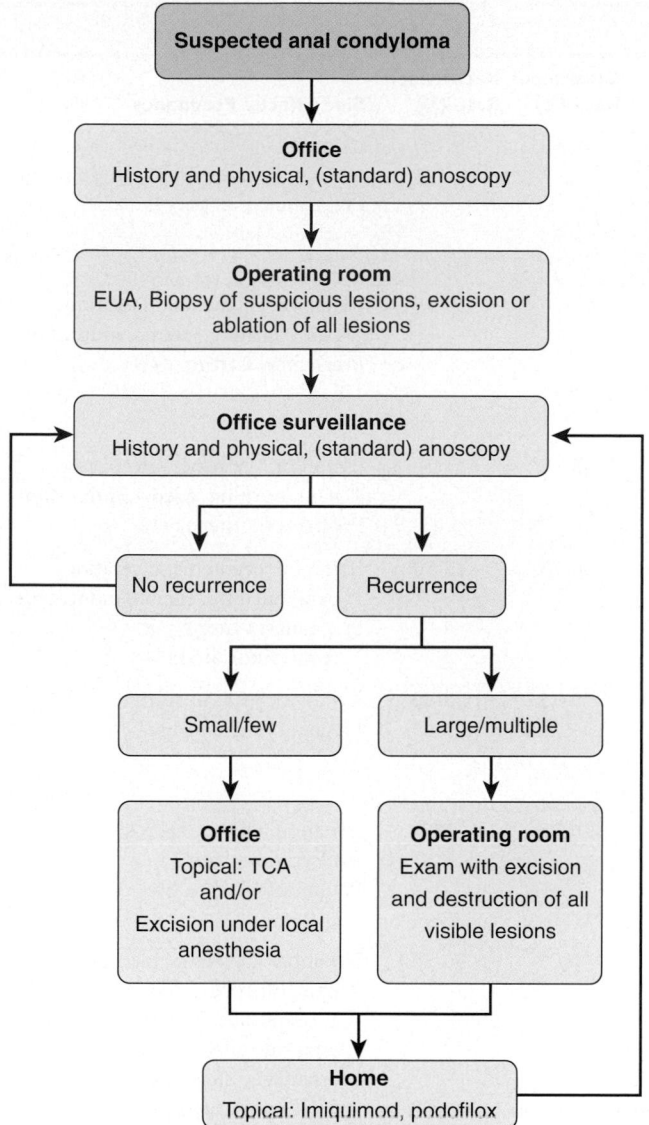

FIGURE 3 Treatment algorithm for anal condyloma.

however, it is now believed that up to 50% of GCA may contain foci of squamous-cell carcinoma. The disease is characterized by large, slowly progressive, exophytic, ulcerative, cauliflower-shaped tumors that infiltrate the adjacent tissue. It affects men more than women and is associated with immunodeficiency, smoking, and multiple sexual partners.

Clinical examination may reveal a palpable tumor mass with bleeding, pain, fistulas, and clinical pruritus. Most practitioners recommend operative management with a wide-local full thickness excision with 1 cm tumor-free margins. In lesions that involve the anal sphincter complex, abdominoperineal resection may be necessary. Adjuvant treatment with chemotherapy and radiation also may be considered in light of the high risk of recurrence.

Anal Squamous Intraepithelial Lesion

The incidence of squamous intraepithelial lesions is increasing. It has been recognized that these HPV-associated anal dysplastic lesions may be the precursor for anal squamous cell cancer, although the exact timing of transformation is unclear. Risk factors for progression include HIV infection, anoreceptive intercourse, transplantation, and a history of cervical or vulvar neoplasia.

In patients who are at higher risk for malignant transformation, anal cytology akin to the cervical Pap smear may be considered. The terminology used in describing cytologic findings is similar to that of the cervical Pap: atypical squamous cells of undetermined significance (ASC-US) and low-grade squamous intraepithelial lesion (LSIL) or high-grade squamous intraepithelial lesion (HSIL). The finding of HSIL or LSIL from either anal cytology or on biopsy of a condylomatous lesion, requires further investigation and workup.

There is controversy on the optimal management and surveillance strategy of patients with HSIL or LSIL. The two general approaches to managing these patients are high-resolution anoscopy or expectant management. High-resolution anoscopy (HRA) involves careful inspection of the anal canal with a high-resolution microscope after application of acetic acid (with Lugol's solution counterstaining) to identify other putative dysplastic regions for biopsy or ablation. Expectant management (EM) involves frequent office examinations with operative excision of any visible lesions. In a recently published, single-institution, retrospective, cohort series, Crawshaw et al analyzed the outcomes for 424 patients with biopsy-proven LSIL or HSIL, who underwent either HRA (220 patients) and EM (204 patients). Only three patients progressed to anal squamous cell cancer (one in the HRA group and two in the EM group), with all three patients noncompliant with either treatment or follow-up. Our practice has been to follow the EM pathway for these patients.

■ HUMAN PAPILLOMAVIRUS VACCINE

HPV vaccination is an effective method to prevent HPV infection. Three different vaccines are available in United States: a quadrivalent vaccine (HPV4- Gardasil) targeting HPV 6, 11, 16 and 18, a 9-valent vaccine (HPV9- Gardasil 9) targeting HPV 6, 11, 16, 18, 31, 33, 45, 52 and 58 and a bivalent vaccine (HPV2- Cervarix) targeting HPV 16 and 18.

For women, the United States Advisory Committee on Immunization Practices (ACIP) recommends administering the HPV vaccine series (HPV9, HPV4, or HPV2) routinely at age 11 to 12 years or up until age 26 years if not started previously. These vaccines can be administered to females as young as age 9. Catch-up vaccination also is recommended for females aged 13 to 26 years who have not been previously vaccinated or who have not completed their vaccine series. HPV vaccine is not recommended during pregnancy.

In males, the ACIP recommends administration of the HPV9 or HPV4 series at age 11 to 12 years, or up until age 21 years if not started previously, and vaccination for males aged 22 to 26 years on

benefit from treatment in the OR, in which only half the perianal skin is treated and allowed to heal before returning to the OR in 3 to 4 weeks to treat the other half.

After clearance of all lesions in the operating room, close office surveillance is critical. Typically, recurrence is limited to a few lesions, which are amenable to topical treatment by the physician in the office or by the patient at home. Trichloroacetic acid (TCA) is a keratolytic and acts to chemically cauterize the skin. It can be applied very precisely in the office with a small cotton-tipped swab with minimal damage to the surrounding normal skin (see Figure 2). The most commonly used self-administered topical treatments are imiquimod and podofilox. The best approach to recurrence may be a combination of ablative therapy and topical therapy, with reduced recurrence of condyloma when imiquimod was used as an adjunct to conventional ablation.

Giant Condyloma Acuminata

Giant condyloma acuminata (GCA) is a rare, poorly defined condyloma variant. No formal size criteria have been established, although reports in the literature vary from 1.5 to 30 cm in maximum diameter. It originally was described as lacking malignant potential;

TABLE 1: Common Treatments for Anal Condyloma

Forms of Treatment	Mechanism of Action	Treatment Instructions	Clearance Rate (%)	Recurrence Rate (%)	Side Effects/ Pregnancy
Imiquimod (Aldara) (patient-applied)	Induction of pro-inflammatory cytokines	5% cream, applied at bedtime and washed off in the morning 3 times per week (Mon., Wed., Fri.) for up to 16 weeks	40-80	10-20	Irritation, erythema, ulceration, pain, burning, edema, induration Pregnancy: Category C
Podofilox (Condylox) (patient-applied)	Interrupts mitosis	0.5% gel, applied twice daily for 3 consecutive days, followed by 4 days without treatment. Not to exceed 4 weeks	65-70	20-35	Irritation, erythema, ulceration, pain, burning, edema, induration Pregnancy: Category C
Sinecatechins (Veregen) (patient-applied)	Unknown	15% ointment, applied 3 times per day for up to 16 weeks	55-60	5-10	Irritation, erythema, ulceration, pain, burning, edema, induration Pregnancy: Category C
5-Fluorouracil (Efudex) (patient-applied)	Interrupts mitosis	5% cream applied daily for up to 10 weeks or 1% cream applied twice a day for 2-6 weeks	50-75	25-50	Irritation, erythema, ulceration, pain, burning, edema, induration Pregnancy: Category X (contraindicated)
Trichloroacetic acid (Tri-Chlor) (physician-applied)	Chemical cauterization	80-90% solution applied to lesions while avoiding uninvolved surrounding skin. May repeat monthly	70-75	20-40	Irritation, pain, burning Pregnancy: Safe to use
Liquid nitrogen (Physician-applied)	Cryoablation	Apply with applicator whitening the surrounding skin. May repeat monthly	70-75	30	Irritation, edema, necrosis, ulceration, pain Pregnancy: Safe to use
Podophyllin (Podocon-25) (physician-applied)	Interrupts mitosis	25% extract applied to lesions once per week to be washed off by patient 4 hours later for up to 6 treatments. Not to exceed 0.5 cc per application	40-70	30-55	Irritation, erythema, ulceration, pain, burning, edema, induration; Systemic absorption may cause fatal side effects Pregnancy: Category X (contraindicated)
Electrocautery (physician-applied)	Electrocauterization	Target lesions while minimizing damage to normal skin. Repeat as needed	60-90	35	Pain, scarring Smoke plumes may contain viable virus and may pose an infectious risk to healthcare provider Pregnancy: Safe to use
Laser (physician-applied)	Vaporization	Target lesions while minimizing damage to normal skin. Repeat as needed	80	30-50	Pain, scarring Smoke plumes have been shown to contain viable virus and pose an infectious risk to healthcare provider Pregnancy: Safe to use
Surgical excision (physician-applied)	Removal by tangential excision	Target lesions while minimizing damage to normal skin. Repeat as needed	60-90	40	Pain, bleeding, scarring Pregnancy: Safe to use

the basis of increased risk factors such as HIV or anal-receptive intercourse. This strategy for vaccination showed reduced rates of anal intraepithelial neoplasia in homosexual males aged 16 to 26 years as compared with placebo.

No data exist regarding the long-term efficacy of administration of the HPV vaccine in the setting of active or previous HPV infection. Some practitioners advocate vaccinating in this setting because it may confer protection against the other HPV strains to which the patient may not already have been exposed. Our practice has been to refer high-risk patients to an infectious disease specialist for further discussion.

SUGGESTED READINGS

Beck DE, Roberts PL, Saclarides TJ, et al., eds. *The ASCRS Textbook of Colon and Rectal Surgery*. 2nd ed. New York: Springer-Verlag; 2011.

Crawshaw BP, Russ AJ, Stein SL, et al. High-resolution anoscopy or expectant management for anal intraepithelial neoplasia for the prevention of anal cancer: is there really a difference? *Dis Colon Rectum*. 2015;58:53-59.

Klaristenfeld D, Israelit S, Beart RW, et al. Surgical excision of extensive anal condylomata not associated with risk of anal stenosis. *Int J Colorectal Dis*. 2008;23:853-856.

Palefsky JM, Giuliano AR, Goldstone S, et al. HPV vaccine against anal HPV infection and Anal intraepithelial neoplasia. *N Engl J Med*. 2011;365:1576-1585.

Trombetta LJ, Place RJ. Giant condyloma acuminatum of the anorectum: trends in epidemiology and management. *Dis Colon Rectum*. 2001;44:1878-1886.

Workowski KA, Bolan GA, Centers for Disease Control and Prevention. Sexually transmitted diseases treatment guidelines, 2015. *MMWR Recomm Rep*. 2015;64:1-37.

THE MANAGEMENT OF PILONIDAL DISEASE

Eric K. Johnson, MD, FACS, FASCRS, and Scott R. Steele, MD, FACS, FASCRS

Pilonidal disease (PD) represents a spectrum of disorders ranging from a simple asymptomatic sinus in the skin to a large, complex open wound with multiple draining sinuses and infection. It is for that reason that the old nomenclature of *pilonidal cyst* or *sinus* likely should be replaced by the more appropriate term *pilonidal disease*. Pilonidal is derived from the roots "pilus" (hair) and "nidus" (nest). This term was coined in 1880 and has been defying surgeons ever since. PD is believed to be an acquired disease related to trapping of hairs in the natal cleft, which leads to local trauma and inflammation. It is common, and although it can affect anyone, typically it is seen in hirsute individuals who have deep natal clefts. Elevated body mass index, poor hygiene, prolonged sitting, and excessive sweating may be additional risk factors.

The typical individual experiences drainage or pain in the area of the gluteal cleft. Patients often have acute abscesses that require immediate drainage. Definitive surgical management in the face of active infection is to be discouraged. Simple abscess drainage may be all that is required or may act as a bridge to definitive surgery. Management with oral antibiotics will fail in the setting of acute abscess but may be successful in the inflammatory phase before abscess formation. Diagnosis is rather simple and requires no laboratory or radiographic testing. The presence of midline pits in the sacrococcygeal region coupled with drainage, abscess formation, or an open wound suggest PD, whereas alternative diagnoses of hidradenitis suppurativa, anal fistula (Figure 1), and in rare cases neoplasm also should be considered.

■ TREATMENT

Treatment options range from simple shaving without surgery to wide local excision and complex flap reconstruction. There are many described methods of treatment, in fact far too many to adequately address in the text of this chapter. We believe that a surgeon should be familiar with three to four methods of surgical management that address the entire spectrum of disease severity, including managing those with recurrent disease and prior failures. The disease severity should drive the method selected for surgical treatment. Although

any method could be used in any situation, it would seem inappropriate to do a complex flap procedure such as a rhomboid flap in the setting of very minor disease (Figure 2). Less extensive methods will lead to optimal outcomes with lower risk in the setting of mild disease.

Principles of Treatment

There are several basic principles that should be considered when treating pilonidal disease so that optimal outcomes can be achieved:

1. **Control of sepsis:** Drain acute abscesses and avoid any attempt at definitive surgical management in the setting of active infection. All PD will be colonized with bacteria, but this is very different than active infection. Primary closure with or without flap reconstruction will fail in the setting of infection and will make future management more difficult.

2. **Disease severity and operative approach should match:** As stated previously, the anatomy or severity of disease should drive the selection of a treatment method. If the disease is minor, yet the patient requests surgery, a pit-picking procedure (description to follow) plus or minus a small amount of additional excision may be all that is needed. Complex and recurrent disease typically requires a wide excision and flap reconstruction.

3. **Avoid too much excision:** The old adage of excising all disease down to the postsacral fascia results in an extremely large and complex wound. This technique should be avoided if at all possible. Excision that is too deep or aggressive has been shown to correlate with disease recurrence/treatment failure.

4. **Unroof all disease, débride granulation tissue, remove hair:** This principle corresponds to principle 3. Removal or unroofing of skin overlying active disease may be essential, but do not be tempted to dissect any deeper. It is important, however, to account for all disease. Any hair or debris should be removed, and granulation tissue should be curetted or cauterized. It may be helpful to inject sinuses with methylene blue to ensure that no extensions are missed. Probes also may be used. If the wound is to be closed, adequate irrigation of the wound with saline is encouraged.

5. **Use an off-midline excision and closure when possible:** It is essential to attempt to perform an off-midline excision and closure. Wounds located in the midline of the gluteal cleft just do not seem to heal as well as those located elsewhere. Although it may be impossible to keep the entire wound out of the midline, there should be significant effort to minimize the amount of wound in the midline.

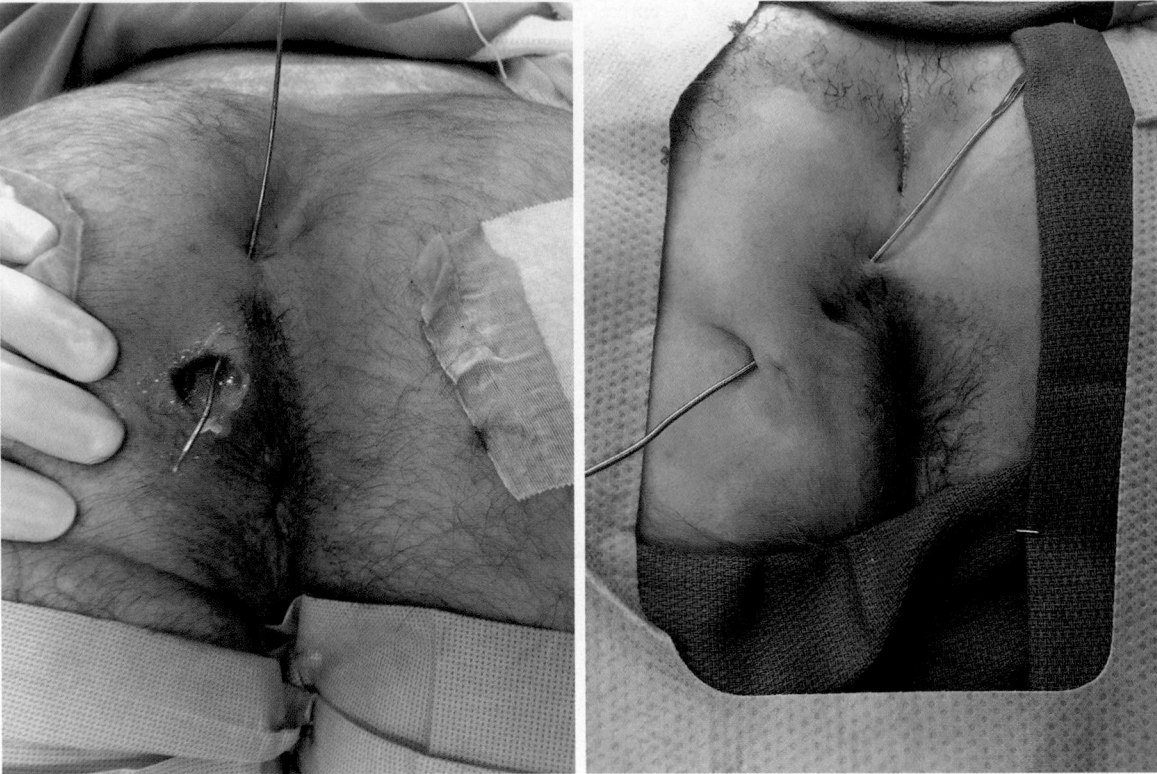

FIGURE 1 These images show two different patients who were suspected to have anal fistulas but were confirmed subsequently to have pilonidal disease. Disease in this location typically can be treated with a lay-open technique and will resolve rapidly.

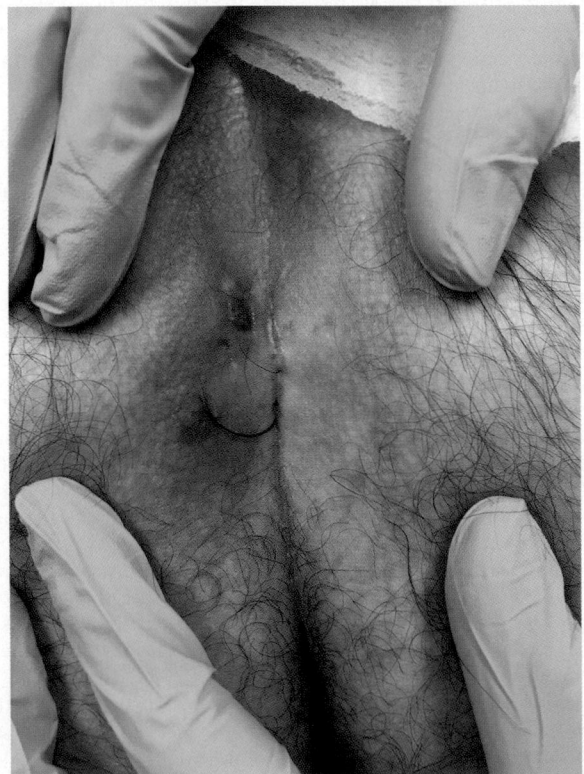

FIGURE 2 This image shows a patient with mild pilonidal disease that would not require treatment with a complex procedure such as a rhomboid flap.

6. **If the wound is closed, tension must be minimized:** Because of the inherent difficulty with wounds located in the region of the gluteal cleft, every effort should be taken to minimize wound morbidity. A "tension-appropriate" closure should be used. If this cannot be achieved initially, then tissue undermining or use of a flap should be considered. When flaps are used, it is important to ensure a lack of tension at both the excision and donor site. Tension seems to be better tolerated at the donor site, as is separation of the operative wound, especially because these sites are off the midline.

7. **Change the anatomy/flatten the natal cleft:** Because it is believed that deep natal cleft anatomy contributes to formation of pilonidal disease, it seems reasonable that any procedure designed to flatten cleft anatomy would lead to lower recurrence rates. Most flap procedures, and certainly the Bascom cleft lift procedure, are designed to do this. The cleft lift procedure, in particular, combines most, if not all, of the previously mentioned principles into one operation, which has likely contributed to its success. That stated, not all PD requires this action.

Nonoperative Treatment

In selected cases of minor disease, especially those with relatively asymptomatic or occasionally draining sinuses, nonoperative treatment consisting of shaving and hygiene measures can be successful. Older retrospective studies have shown that patients have better outcomes if shaving is used and surgery is avoided. These data are older and were compiled during the era when wide excision with healing by secondary intention was common. Although it is encouraged often, no study has ever shown benefit to laser hair removal. Despite this lack of data, it is not unreasonable to encourage the use of laser hair removal, or the use of depilatory agents, in the setting of minor disease as primary treatment. The risk is low but the cost to the

TABLE 1: Representative Studies From Modern Pilonidal Literature

Author	Year	Procedure	Number of Subjects	Mean Follow-Up	Rate of Healing
Lorant	2011	Sinus excision vs lay-open	39	12 mos	89%
			41	12 mos	97%
Colov	2011	Pit-picking	75	12 mos	80%
Bessa	2013	Karydakis flap vs rhomboid flap	120 total	20½ mos	98%
				20½ mos	97%
Gendy	2011	Local excision vs cleft lift	34	Not reported	74%
			39		97%
Altinoprak	2014	Rhomboid flap	345	33 mos	96%
Kaya	2012	Rhomboid flap	94	31 mos	96%
Arslan	2014	Rhomboid flap vs modified rhomboid flap vs Karydakis	96	33 mos	94%
			108		98%
			91		89%

patient may be high, and this should be considered. Shaving in the postoperative period has never been shown to be beneficial and in fact has been associated with higher recurrence rates by some investigators. Avoidance of prolonged sitting and weight loss also may help minimize symptomatic PD. We intentionally have omitted the discussion of fibrin glue injection or use of ablative agents such as phenol because we have little experience with these methods.

Operative Management

A description of every operative technique available to treat PD is beyond our scope, but we will focus on several procedures. These techniques can be grouped into basic or simple procedures, intermediate procedures, and complex flap procedures. The literature regarding the success of one procedure over another is mixed and consists mostly of small retrospective cases series with some randomized controlled trails comparing two or three methods (Table 1). It is possible to find data supporting the use of any procedure over another, and because of this, it is critical that a surgeon is familiar with personal outcomes as they relate to procedural approach. Aftercare by the patient and provider is likely as important as the procedural technique in success. It is imperative that patients keep the operative area clean, perform excellent wound care, and avoid strenuous activity until healing has taken place. Poor wound management and poor decision making will lead to failure.

Basic, Simple Procedures

Abscess Drainage

An individual with an acute pilonidal abscess requires only definitive incision and drainage. Typically, the abscess "points" to one side of the natal cleft, and this is visualized easily or is palpable. Our recommendation is to incise the abscess cavity just off midline under local anesthetic. Ensure that all loculations are broken up and that all purulence is drained. Initial packing often is employed for hemostasis, but we have not found continued packing to be necessary. Once- or twice-daily showering with soapy water aids in keeping the wound clean. These wounds typically close in 1 to 2 weeks, but in some cases the patient will be left with a chronic wound.

Pit-Picking and the Simple Bascom Procedure

In cases of mild chronic disease in which the primary complaint is related to the midline pits or in cases in which there is a small wound off-midline, this procedure may be considered ideal. It is simple and results in a healed wound rather quickly, usually in 1 to 3 weeks. In most cases, PD shows an affinity for one side of the natal cleft. In

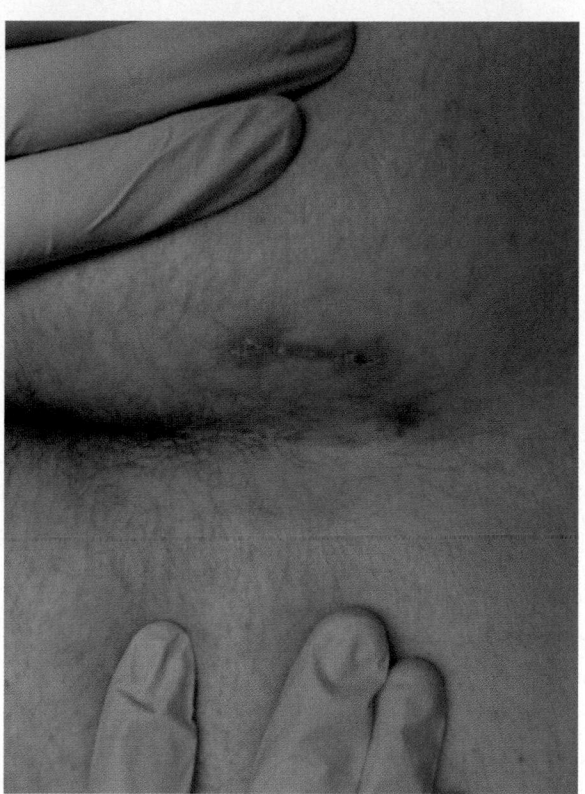

FIGURE 3 This image shows a patient seen 2 days after a simple Bascom procedure. The central pits and the off-midline incision have healed rapidly.

cases in which disease is localized purely to the midline in the form of pits, a pit-picking procedure alone is appropriate. In this technique the central pits are excised with a punch knife of appropriate size (just slightly larger than the pit itself). The knife is inserted to full depth, all pits are excised, hair and debris are removed, and the wounds are closed primarily with a variety of suture material. We prefer 3-0 Vicryl suture, but any absorbable or permanent suture may be used. It is not unusual to encounter a bit of bleeding after pit excision, and this can be controlled with needle-tip electrocautery.

In cases in which there is induration off the midline, a true simple Bascom procedure can be performed (Figure 3). Pits are excised

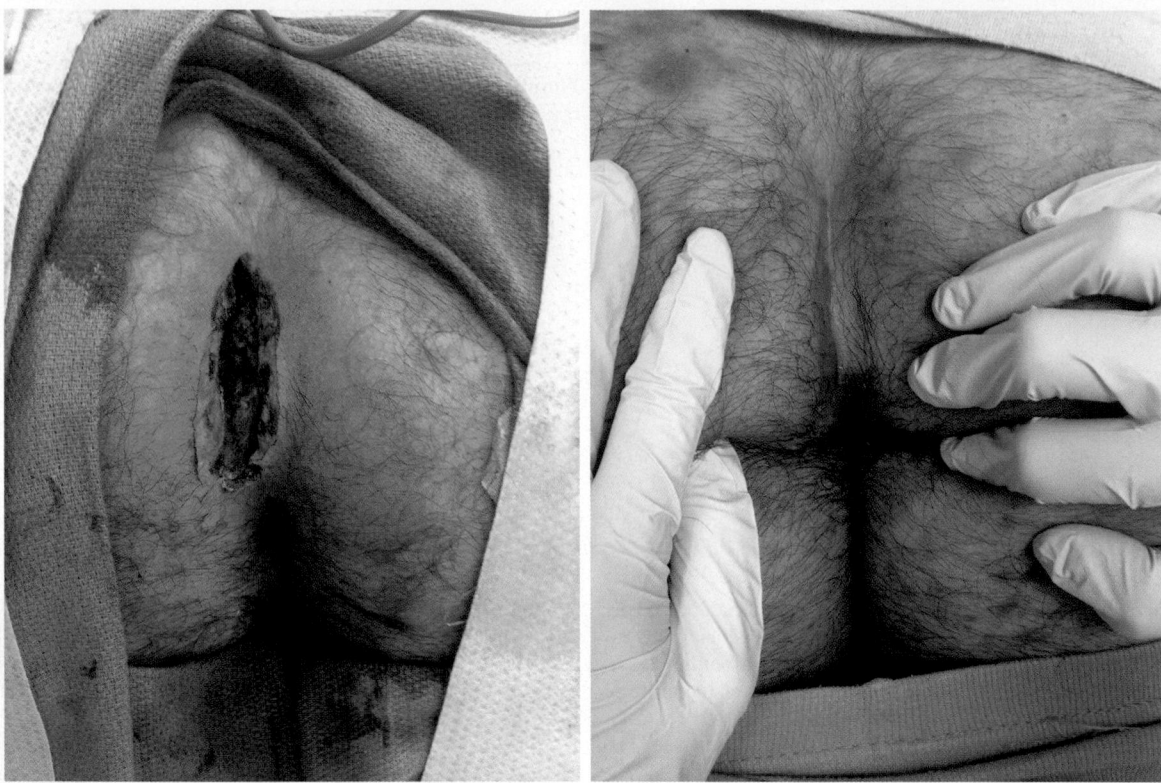

FIGURE 4 These images show a patient who was treated by unroofing the tissue over the sinus, and the wound was allowed to heal by secondary intention. Note that most of the wound is off the midline. He healed rapidly within 6 weeks.

similarly, and a 2- to 3-cm incision is created just lateral to the indurated area off the midline. A skin and subcutaneous flap is created by dissecting toward the midline pits, ultimately connecting the two areas of dissection. Indurated tissue is excised, and the wound is irrigated and then partially closed at the superior and inferior portions, leaving the central portion open. A small amount of packing is placed in the open portion of the wound and is removed the next day. Continued packing may be used or omitted per surgeon and patient preference.

Excision With or Without Primary Wound Closure

Many consider the gold-standard of surgical management to be simple excision with healing by secondary intention (Figure 4). It certainly still is performed commonly, although patients would tend to want to have primary closure. With use of the principles outlined earlier, the disease should be unroofed, ensuring that all hair, debris, and granulation tissue is removed, curetted, or cauterized. Every attempt should be made to minimize the tissue excised and to keep the majority of the wound off the midline. If possible, a simple primary closure can be performed, although our experience is that this often fails (Figure 5). The benefits to this approach include low risk of infection as well as the simplicity for the surgeon.

This procedure rarely results in a complex wound if patients are appropriately selected. If careful and meticulous wound care is employed postoperatively, the rate of success is reasonably high with this technique, again in appropriately selected individuals. Patients with extensive and destructive disease should not be managed this way because management results in a large and complex wound that rarely heals. Complete healing in the best of cases takes weeks to months. Some have reported the use of negative pressure dressings in this setting, but management of these devices in this location is often challenging. This option may be appropriate with larger wounds if resources are available.

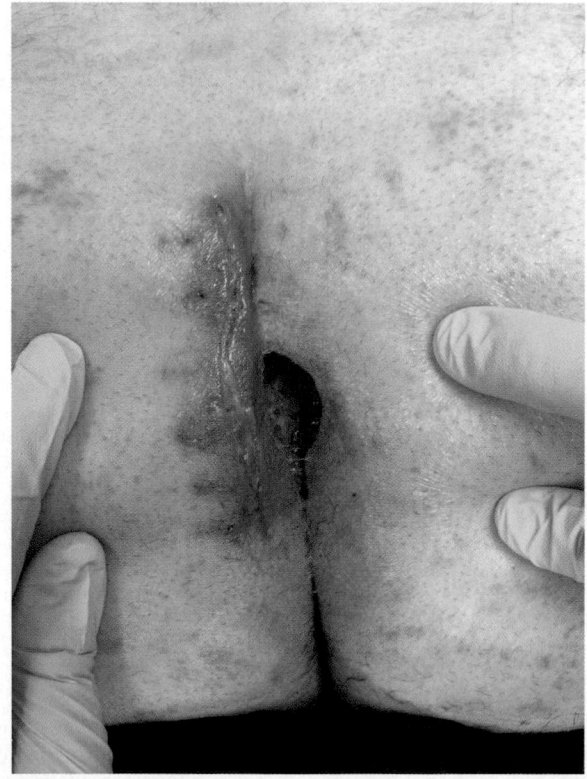

FIGURE 5 This image shows a patient who was managed with simple excision and primary closure. The wound dehisced within the first 2 weeks postoperatively, which led to a recurrence and the need for further surgery.

Intermediate Procedures

These procedures involve the excision of or unroofing of disease in the midline (or just off the midline) followed by subcutaneous flap mobilization and tension-appropriate closure, with or without the use of a closed-suction drain. They are designed to alter the cleft anatomy while minimizing the amount of excision. They also employ an off-midline closure. Patients with mild to moderate disease are ideal for these techniques (Figure 6). Those with extensive or destructive disease are not likely suitable for this type of management.

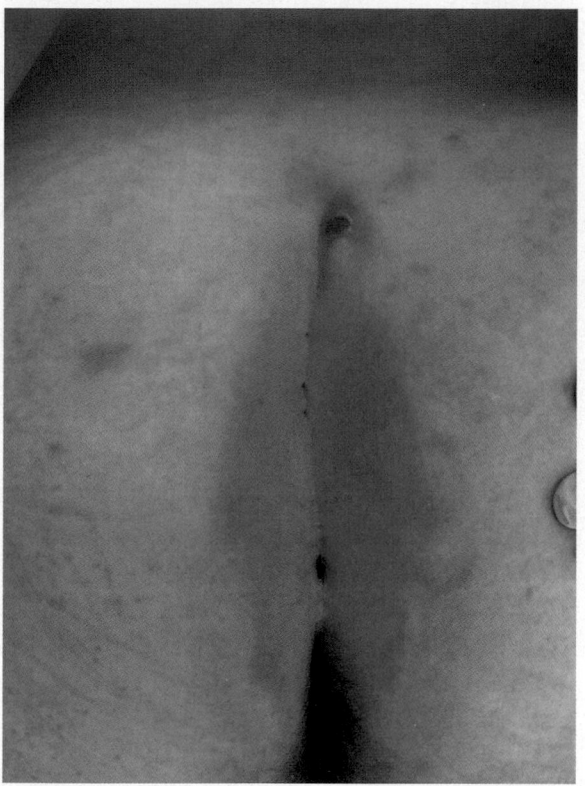

FIGURE 6 This image shows a patient with mild to moderate PD who would be a good candidate for a procedure such as the cleft lift.

Disease that is very close to or abuts the anal verge also may present a challenge if this type of management is considered.

Karydakis Flap

Initially, the affected tissue in the midline is excised, which results in an elliptical defect in the natal cleft. A skin flap with a beveled edge then is created and mobilized such that it will reach across midline to facilitate a tension appropriate primary closure. The wound is closed in layers to obliterate as much dead space as possible. Superficial wounds do not require drainage, but deeper wounds may require employment of a closed suction drain. Development of seroma places the repair at risk. If a drain is used, we leave it in place for a minimum of 3 days and require that the output be 20 mL or less per day for 2 consecutive days. This is a simple procedure to perform and results in some flattening of the natal cleft as well as a closure off the midline (Figure 7).

Cleft Lift Procedure (Video 1)

This is a simple yet creative procedure originally popularized by the late Dr. John Bascom. It uses all of the previously described principles and is suitable for most patients. Preoperative marking of the patient in the prone position in the operating room is essential to the correct performance of this procedure. This is our preferred procedure for patients with mild to moderate PD. Before a chlorhexidine prep, the "safe-zone" is marked with indelible marker by pressing the gluteal tissue together in the midline (Figure 8, A). The mark is drawn where the tissue from each side touches in the midline (Figure 8, B). The buttocks then are taped apart, revealing a "wish-bone"-shaped mark (Figure 8, C). This established a safe zone, beyond which dissection should not occur. This ensures a tension-appropriate closure. An additional elliptical/scimitar-shaped mark is placed over the area with more significant disease after skin preparation (Figure 8, D). This marks the skin that will be excised. The inferior portion of this mark is scimitar shaped to ensure appropriate closure near the anal verge. After instillation of epinephrine-containing local anesthetic, the skin outlined by the elliptical mark is excised (Figure 8, E). Not much, if any, subcutaneous fat should be excised. This invariably will expose some sinus tracts, hair, and granulation, which should all be removed, curetted, or cauterized. A skin/subcutaneous flap, about the thickness of a mastectomy flap, is created by dissecting toward the opposite side safe-zone boundary (Figure 8, F). Use of skin hooks facilitates this dissection. When the flap is raised inferiorly (near the scimitar), the dissection should be slightly deeper, providing additional thickness to this portion of the flap. Scar tissue in the midline

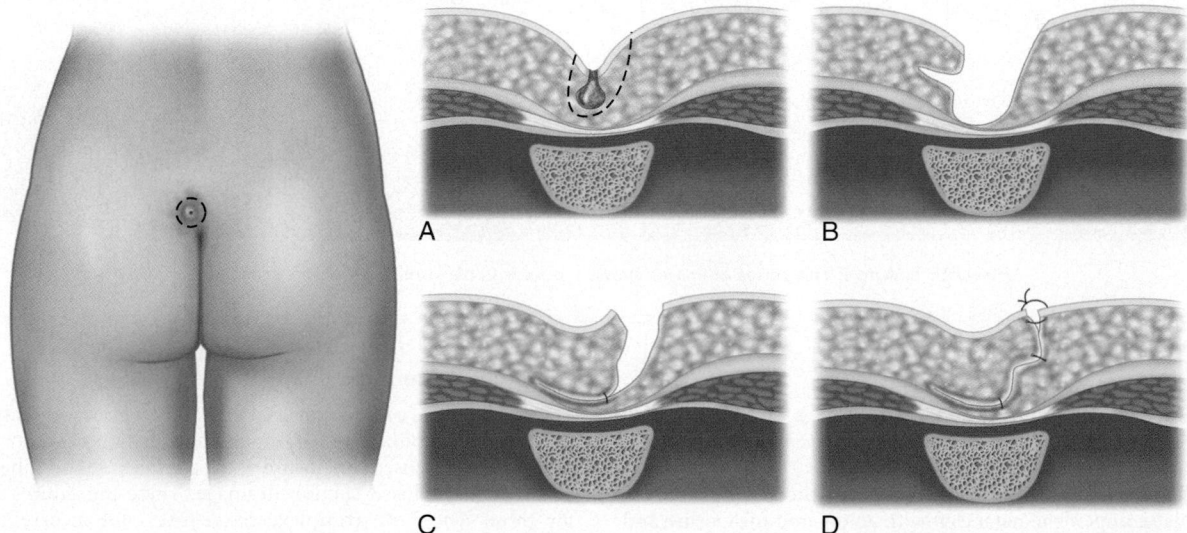

FIGURE 7 This series of images shows the steps in performing a Karydakis procedure.

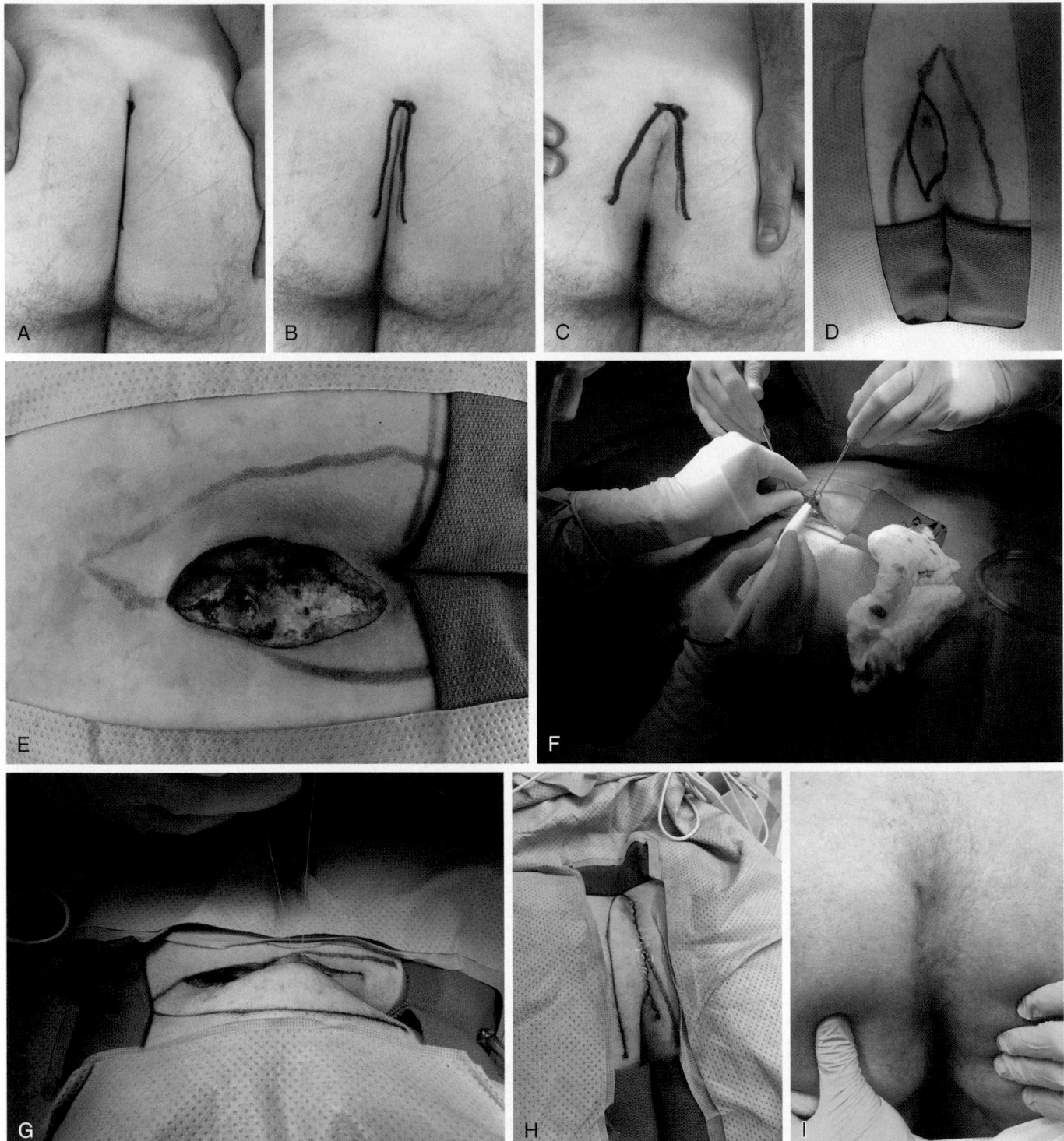

FIGURE 8 A to **I,** This series of images shows the steps in performing a cleft lift procedure.

then is released by dividing it into small cubes. The flap then is mobilized across the midline, and the wound is closed in layers, taking care to obliterate as much dead space as possible (Figure 8, *G*). In most cases, a closed suction drain will not be necessary, although when used it should be managed as described earlier. This procedure results in flattening of the natal cleft with an off-midline closure and is easy to perform (Figure 8, *H* and *I*).

Complex Procedures

These procedures consist of a wide excision of severely diseased tissue followed by mobilization of a lipocutaneous flap from an adjacent donor site that is used for closure of the complex wound. They almost always require closed-suction drainage. These procedures are ideal for those who have complex, destructive, and recurrent disease (Figure 9). The advantage of these techniques is that they bring thick

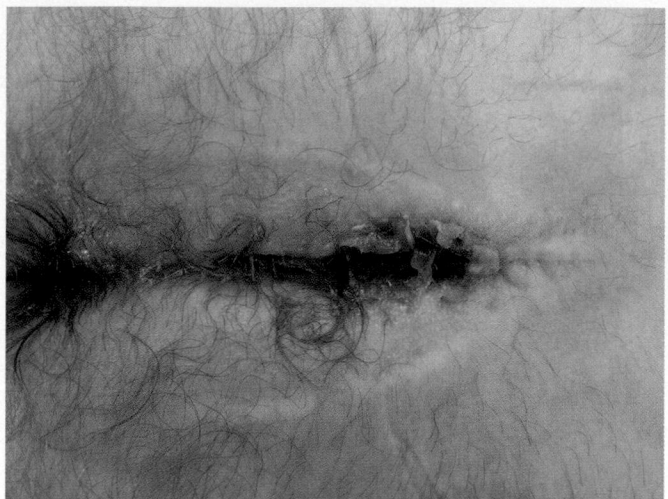

FIGURE 9 This image depicts an individual with locally destructive and recurrent disease that could be approached with a rhomboid flap technique.

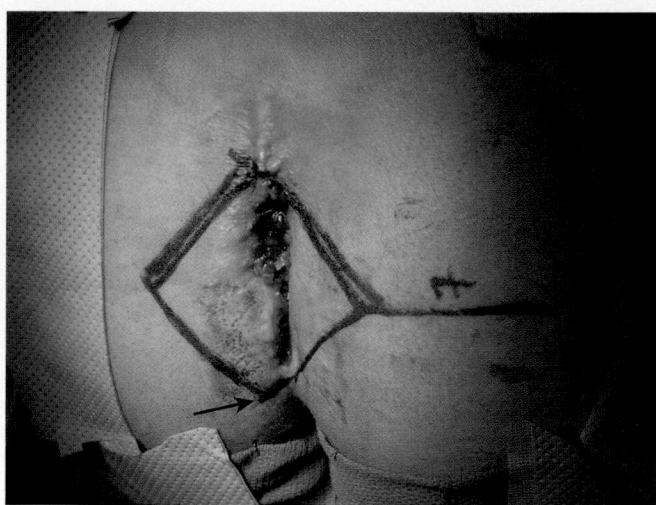

FIGURE 11 This particular image shows the preoperative marking of a patient undergoing a rhomboid flap procedure. Note the initial rhombus is oriented just off midline to ensure the tip is not immediately adjacent to the anal verge. The black arrow points this out.

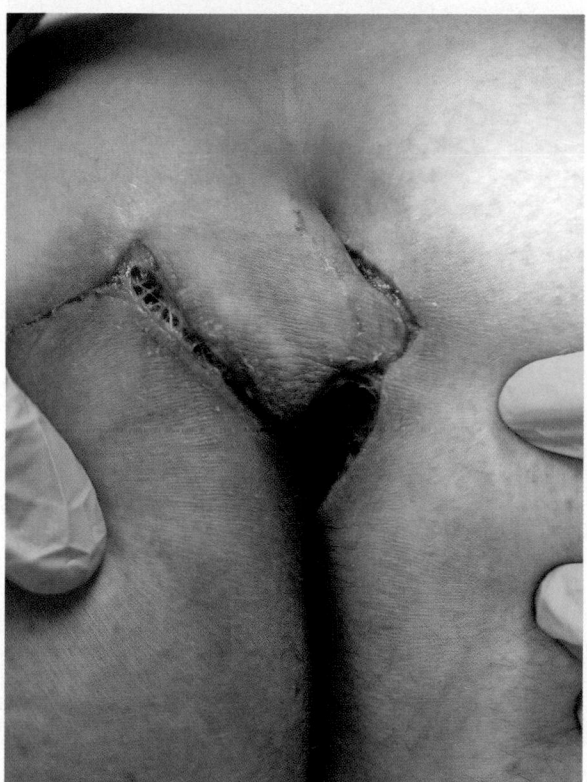

FIGURE 10 This image depicts a patient who underwent a rhomboid flap procedure, with the flap rotated inferiorly (instead of superiorly) from the left. He sustained a near complete dehiscence of the flap, but the flap remained viable and eventually healed with a relatively disfiguring scar.

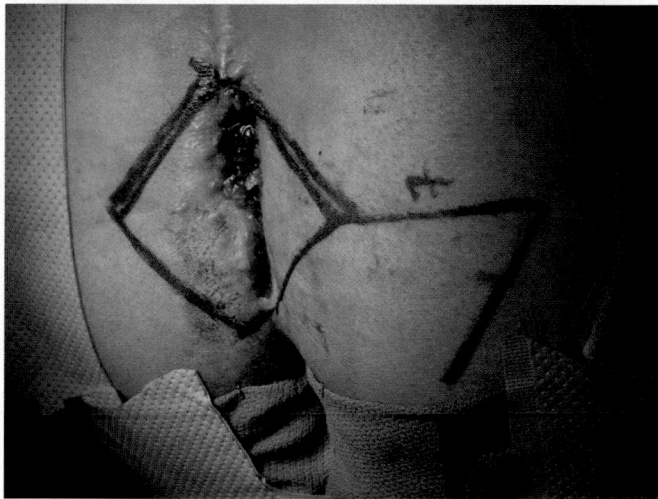

FIGURE 12 This image depicts all lines of incision for a rhomboid flap procedure.

and healthy tissue into the midline to fill and close large defects. They also flatten the natal cleft, potentially leading to lower recurrence rates. Disadvantages include the time and skill required to perform the procedures as well as the complexity of wounds that result from complete flap failure (Fig. 10). Fortunately, complete loss or dehis-cence of a flap is a relatively rare complication if patients are appropriately selected.

Rhomboid Flap (Video 2)

This is a more complex procedure that is useful in the setting of complicated PD. The patient again is positioned supine, and a chlorhexidine skin prep is performed. We administer intravenous antibiotics to cover skin flora. A diamond-shaped area of skin is excised, encompassing all disease. This typically is carried down to the postsacral fascia, although a more conservative excision may be performed on the basis of the amount of disease present. It is helpful to rotate the original diamond- or rhombus-shaped excision just slightly off midline (Figure 11). This ensures that the inferior tip of the rhombus is not located adjacent to the anus, the most likely area of postoperative wound separation. This technique is referred to as a *modified rhomboid* or *Limberg flap*. The flap then is mobilized from the donor site, typically the right buttock. The thickness of the flap

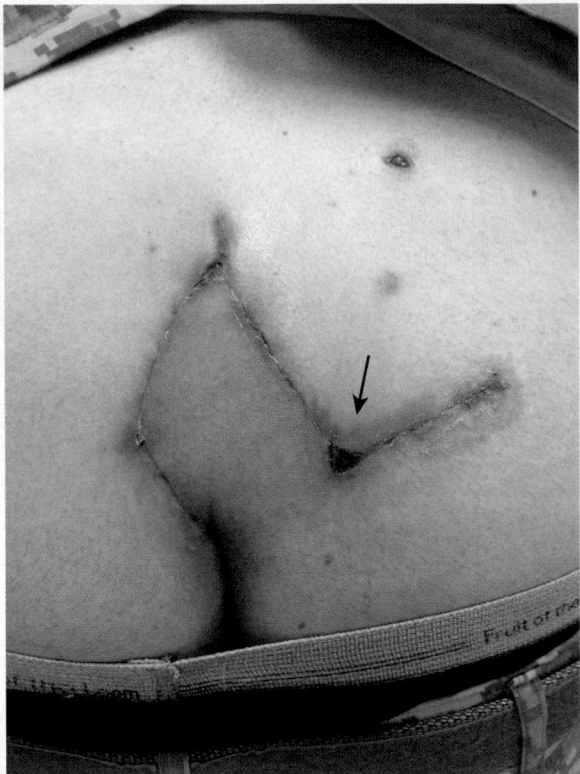

FIGURE 13 The black arrow in this image points out an area of the donor site, where there is always significant tension during closure. It is essential to undermine some in this area to facilitate minimal tension on this area of closure. This is a common site of minor incisional dehiscence.

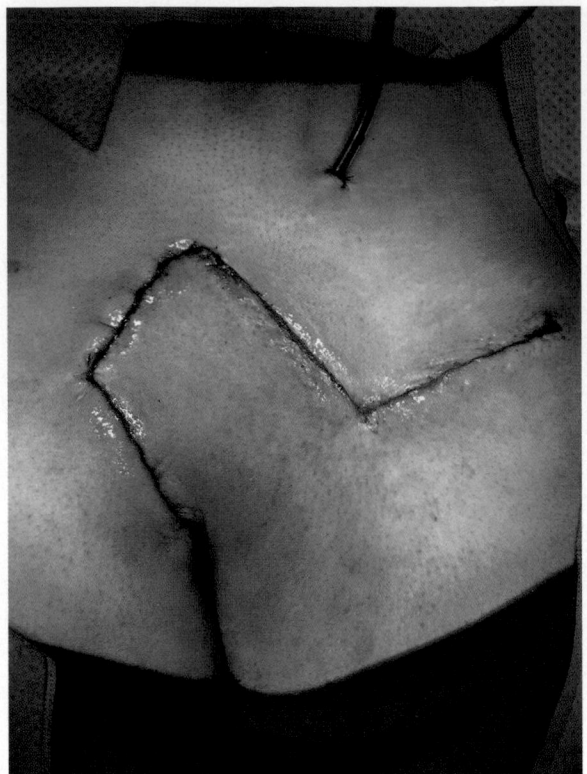

FIGURE 14 This image shows a closed suction drain exiting via a separate stab incision on the upper right buttock.

should be identical to the thickness of the tissue excised from the midline. The flap should be handled gently throughout the case. It is created by incising laterally from the right lateral tip of the rhombus onto the right buttock and then inferiorly (Figure 12). One must ensure preservation of a thick and wide pedicle to ensure adequate blood supply. It is also wise to mobilize some of the tissue above the flap on the right buttock to minimize tension at the donor site closure portion of the repair (Figure 13).

After adequate flap harvest, it is rotated in a counter-clockwise direction to cover the midline. We discourage harvesting the flap such that it requires downward rotation to close the defect. This results in a large portion of the incision residing near the anal verge, which we believe increases the likelihood of wound dehiscence (see Figure 10). The closed-suction drain should be placed, typically from the right side superiorly (Figure 14), and the flap then is secured to the mid-portion of the wound with a 2-0 absorbable suture. This often requires the help of an assistant. At this point, it is not unusual to feel just a bit unsure of one's ability to close this large wound. The surgeon should not worry, it will close. The wound then is closed in layers with absorbable suture. We prefer to close the skin with a 4-0 monofilament absorbable suture and then cover the wound with surgical skin glue. The drain is managed as referenced earlier. It is imperative to ensure that the patient does not engage in strenuous activity for 4 to 6 weeks after this procedure. This wound always is closed under some tension and is at risk for dehiscence during this period. It is not unusual to develop one or two small areas of wound separation that may drain in the first 1 to 2 weeks after surgery (Figure 15). This is not a serious complication but will require some minor wound care for 2 to 4 weeks. These areas almost always close. If they fail to close by 12 weeks postoperatively, we do not hesitate to return the patient to the operating room for minor débridement

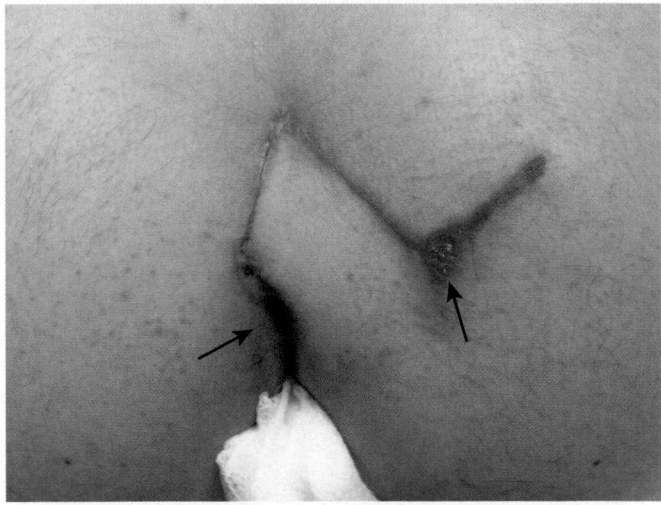

FIGURE 15 The black arrows point out the two most common areas of minor incisional dehiscence after a rhomboid flap procedure.

and primary closure of these areas, which has been uniformly successful.

Special Situations

In some patients, the extent of disease extends far enough up onto the lower back that it may be impossible to harvest a flap large enough to close the entire wound (Figure 16). We have encountered this several times and have a standard approach that we take in this setting. The key is to excise the portion of the wound involving the natal cleft and nothing more. The portion of the wound above the cleft can be débrided and treated like any open wound (Figure 17). It will heal because it is not in the low midline, as long as you have source control in the natal cleft. The rhomboid flap can be created in the standard fashion, rotated into place, and left with a free edge superiorly (Figure 18). A negative pressure wound dressing is an excellent adjunct in this setting and will assist with rapid healing.

Although we will not go into an extensive description, the V-Y flap technique is useful in the setting of failed flap repairs. It is a method that allows mobilization of a large amount of tissue into the midline to close large defects. This is the only setting in which we use this technique because the rhomboid flap is extremely effective as a primary complex technique. When these complex flap repairs are performed, patient selection is imperative. It is unwise to embark on an attempt in a patient who is a tobacco abuser or has uncontrolled diabetes. Those with collagen vascular disorders or documented problems with wound healing should be approached with caution. In terms of procedural timing, we will attempt definitive surgery after abscess drainage when there is no visual evidence of ongoing acute inflammation or infection. If a definitive procedure fails, we wait as long as possible before a salvage procedure, no sooner than 12 weeks (early and rare) and typically between 6 and 12 months. It is important to allow "failed" procedures time to heal because they often will.

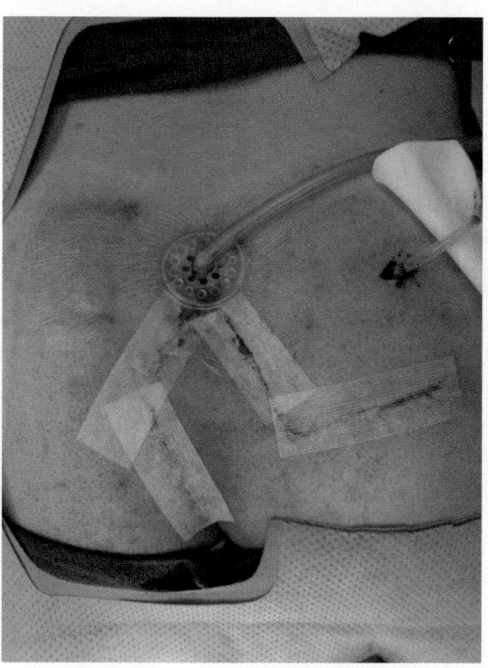

FIGURE 18 This is the patient from Figure 16 after undergoing a rhomboid flap procedure, leaving the upper portion of the wound open after débridement and placement of a negative pressure dressing. This wound healed without incident after 4 weeks.

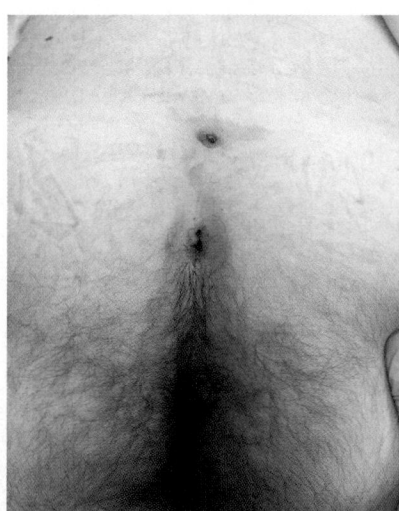

FIGURE 16 This patient had pilonidal disease that extended very far up onto the lower back. It would be difficult (but not impossible) to cover this entire area with a rhomboid flap. It is actually not necessary because the area higher up will heal after débridement because it is not in the natal cleft.

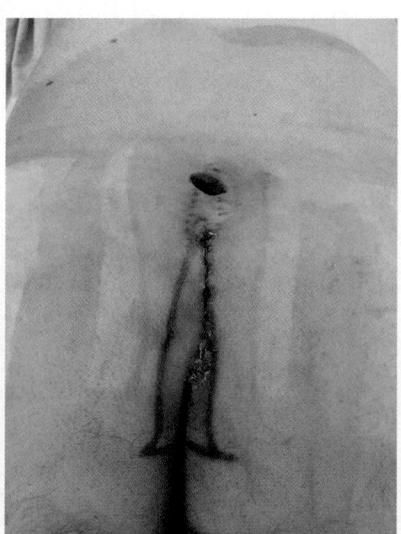
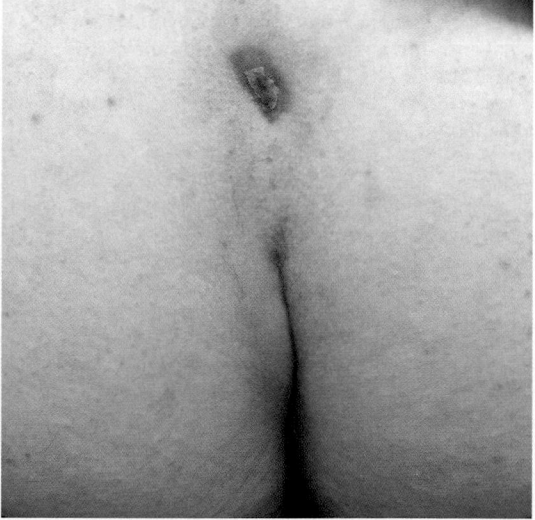

FIGURE 17 This series of images shows a situation similar to Figure 16. The pilonidal disease is treated with a cleft lift procedure, and the superior extension was simply débrided and allowed to heal by secondary intention, which it did after 3 weeks.

SUGGESTED READINGS

Can MF, Sevinc MM, Hancerliogullari O, et al. Multicenter prospective randomized trial comparing modified Limberg flap transposition and Karydakis flap reconstruction in patients with sacrococcygeal pilonidal disease. *Am J Surg.* 2010;200:318-327.

Guner A, Boz A, Ozkan OF, et al. Limberg flap versus Bascom cleft lift techniques for sacrococcygeal pilonidal sinus: prospective, randomized trial. *World J Surg.* 2013;37:2074-2080.

Lorant T, Ribbe I, Mahteme H, et al. Sinus excision and primary closure versus laying open in pilonidal disease: a prospective randomized trial. *Dis Colon Rectum.* 2011;54:300-305.

Rao MM, Zawislak W, Kennedy R, et al. A prospective randomized study comparing two treatment modalities for chronic pilonidal sinus with a 5-year follow-up. *Int J Colorectal Dis.* 2010;25:395-400.

Steele SR, Perry WB, Mills S, et al. Practice parameters for the management of pilonidal disease. *Dis Colon Rectum.* 2013;56:1021-1027.

THE MANAGEMENT OF LOWER GASTROINTESTINAL BLEEDING

Alison M. Wilson, MD, and Kevin Lynch, MS

Lower gastrointestinal bleeding (LGIB) is a complex problem becoming more prevalent as our population ages. Diagnostically, LGIB can be challenging because bleeds may arise from many different pathologic processes and originate at any point distal to the ligament of Treitz. Demographics help determine the likely cause of a patient's bleed; for example, most LGIB occurs in the elderly and results from diverticular or angioectasial bleeding. Children are affected more commonly by infectious gastroenteritis or anal fissures, whereas in the patient who is human immunodeficiency virus (HIV) positive, cytomegalovirus colitis or lymphoma are often to blame. Accurate diagnosis and localization of the bleed's origin is not trivial; preoperative localization decreases surgical morbidity and mortality and can lessen the scope of surgical resections. Accurate localization is one of the key concepts in the management and surgical approach to these patients. Fortunately, an arsenal of diagnostic techniques is available to aid today's surgeon.

■ EVALUATION AND LOCALIZATION

History, Clinical Examination, and Initial Evaluation

A thorough clinical examination and history may suggest an origin and cause of LGIB and are crucial to the selection of initial diagnostic tests. The clinician should inquire about past LGIB, prior abdominal or pelvic radiation, recent colonoscopy/polypectomy, use of nonsteroidal anti-inflammatory drugs, abdominal aortic graft surgery, liver disease or cirrhosis, HIV status, recent weight loss, and family history of colon cancer because each of these conditions yield important information.

Evaluation of the Large Intestine

Most commonly, LGIB is intermittent and of small volume, usually arising from a distal colonic or anorectal source. Flexible sigmoidoscopy and digital rectal examination (DRE) should be the initial tests in those younger than 40 years. Colonoscopy should be performed in patients older than age 50, particularly if they have any of the following: iron deficiency anemia, change in bowel habits, unexplained weight loss, or continued bleeding after a negative sigmoidoscopy. Controversy surrounds the optimal timing for colonoscopy in the evaluation of LGIB. Many suggest that with adequate bowel preparation, urgent colonoscopy, while the patient is actively bleeding, increases diagnostic yield relative to delaying to a later time in the hospital course. Significant hematochezia, particularly in conjunction with hemodynamic instability, should prompt additional evaluation for massive upper GI bleeding. Some "classic" presentations and sites of LGIB are reviewed in Table 1.

Nuclear scintigraphy (NSc) with technetium-99m–labeled RBCs can detect LGIB with relatively high sensitivity, although broad ranges have been reported. An important advantage of technetium-labeled RBC-Sc is its ability to detect bleeding occurring up to 24 hours after tracer injection, which grants NSc the ability to detect intermittent bleeds. NSc is considered more effective at detecting bleeding than at localizing it; false localization rates of 25% have been reported in pooled studies. Segmental resection guided by scintigraphy alone, led to unacceptably high rates of postoperative rebleeding. Therefore NSc is considered a screening test rather than a localization tool for resection.

Computed tomography angiography (CTA) is emerging as an important diagnostic tool for active LGIB. Extravasated contrast or hyperattenuation within the bowel lumen constitutes a positive finding. The sensitivity and specificity for acute GI bleeding ranges from approximately 85% to 90% and 85% to 92%, respectively. Although CTA can be sensitive, detecting bleeds of 0.3 mL/min, its efficacy depends on bleed severity. Localization accuracy has been reported to be up to 97% in patients with high transfusion requirements or hemodynamic instability. CTA also can be used to evaluate the small bowel, although capsule endoscopy and double balloon endoscopy are preferred. Disadvantages of CTA include the need for active bleeding at the time of the study, risk of contrast nephropathy, radiation exposure, and lack of direct therapeutic application.

When bleeding is too copious for colonoscopy to be efficacious, catheter angiography and embolization (CA) is a valuable tool both for localization and therapeutic management of LGIB. CA possesses a moderate to high sensitivity for LGIB, depending on how fast the patient is bleeding. CA is a better test in patients with active, overt bleeding than those with intermittent or low volume bleeding. In light of this, many screen for active bleeding with more sensitive tests, such as scintigraphy or CTA before angiogram. The likelihood of a positive angiography study may increase in patients with low hemoglobin, hemodynamic instability, or high transfusion requirements. Table 2 describes the strengths and weaknesses of each of the testing modalities commonly used in the workup for lower GI bleeding.

Evaluation of the Small Intestine

Although roughly 90% of LGIB is colonic, many obscure GI bleeds originate from the small bowel. Capsule endoscopy (CE) and double-balloon endoscopy (DBE) are the two diagnostic techniques of choice for evaluating SI bleeding. Widely considered the test of choice for small bowel evaluation, CE has high diagnostic yield and low complication rates and is noninvasive. In patients with obscure bleeding, sensitivity was approximately 90% and specificity was 95%. Diagnostic efficacy increases in patients with high transfusion requirements and acute and overt bleeding and in those taking warfarin. Lack of therapeutic capacity, inability to perform tissue biopsy, and premature battery failure are major disadvantages of CE. Complications of CE are rare but include capsule retention and rare instances of bowel perforation. DBE has diagnostic and therapeutic utility for small bowel bleeding. Diagnostic yield increases in patients who are actively bleeding or have positive esophagogastroduodenoscopy (EGD) or CE studies. Shortcomings of DBE include lengthy time requirement and a high rate of incomplete examinations. DBE typically requires at least 60 to 90 minutes and is labor intensive. Many consider CE and DBE complimentary studies for the evaluation of obscure LGIB. Because DBE can approach the small bowel from either oral or anal routes, some use CE findings to plan DBE approach.

TABLE 1: Classic Presentations of Lower Gastrointestinal Bleeding

Pathologic Condition	Classic Presentation	Origin
External hemorrhoid	Painful, sporadic low volume bleeds with red blood coating stool	Anal canal below pectinate line
Internal hemorrhoid	Painless, sporadic low-volume bleeds with red blood coating stool	Anal canal above pectinate line
Anal fissure	Tearing pain and bleeding with defecation	Anal canal
Diverticular bleeding	Painless or associated with mild cramping. Episodic bursts of arterial bleeding, high volume blood loss and passage of clots are possible. Increased prevalence in the elderly and with NSAID use	Right or left colon
Angiodysplasia	Painless or associated with mild cramping. Episodic venous bleeding, overt or occult bleeding are possible, often at low volume (but can be massive). Increased prevalence in the elderly	Often right colonic or cecal origin
Colon cancer	Cramping or painless hematochezia or melena with iron deficiency anemia. Increased risk with weight loss and positive family history	Left colon: hematochezia Right colon: occult bleeding, anemia

NSAID, Nonsteroidal anti-inflammatory drug.

■ THERAPY

Colonoscopy, angiography, and surgery are strategies used to treat LGIB. These modalities are all used for management of diverticular bleeding and angioectasia, the two most common causes of acute hematochezia. In general, surgery is reserved for hemodynamically unstable patients refractory to resuscitation, when other interventions have failed, or in good surgical candidates who have had recurrent bleeding.

Resuscitation

Resuscitation should begin as soon as it is recognized that the patient is bleeding. For patients with evidence of substantial bleeding, multiple comorbidities, or hemodynamic instability, a critical care environment is advised. Reversal of anticoagulants should be done early to assist technical efforts to control the bleeding. For patients therapeutic or supratherapeutic on Coumadin, a prothrombin concentrate complex (PCC) should be considered for reversal. Advantages of the PCC include rapid and effective reversal and avoidance of high volume often needed with the FFP. Therapeutic levels of antithrombin can be assessed with a variety of rapid assays. Although not widely available yet, new reversal agents for the direct Xa inhibitors are being developed. With rapid rates of blood loss, coagulopathy can develop and must be monitored closely and corrected.

Resuscitation and subsequent timing of therapeutic intervention are the keys to minimizing mortality and complications. The massive LGIB patient is very similar to a trauma patient. Activation of a Massive Transfusion Protocol is helpful in getting the correct blood and blood products. Early use of FFP and platelets is advised. Using trauma algorithms such as use of thromboelastography (TEG) or empiric blood to blood product ratios such as 1:1:1 to correct coagulopathy has been shown to be effective in massively bleeding patients. Active measures should be taken to avoid over-resuscitation or overuse of crystalloids. Crystalloids can contribute to bowel edema, abdominal compartment syndrome, and ARDS. Before surgical intervention, coagulopathy and metabolic acidosis should be corrected.

Nonsurgical Management and Therapeutic Options
Diverticular Bleeding

Diverticular bleeding is the most common cause of painless, acute hematochezia in the elderly. Given the high prevalence of diverticulosis, bleeding should be attributed only to diverticula with stigmata of recent hemorrhage (SRH), defined as visualized bleeding, exposed blood vessels, or adherent clots. Diverticular bleeding resolves spontaneously in 80% of patients overall and in 98.5% of those receiving fewer than four transfusion units per day; however, intervention

TABLE 2: Summary of Tests for Evaluation of the Large Intestine

Test	Therapeutic Utility	Active Bleeding During Test Required	Evaluates Small Intestine	Notes
Colonoscopy	+	–	–	Efficacy decreases if hemorrhage is massive or bowel prep inadequate
Angiography	+	+	+	Efficacy increases if hemorrhage is massive
Computed tomography angiography	–	+	+	Accurately localizes many bleeds and can be performed quickly
Scintigraphy	–	–	+	High sensitivity localization accuracy is suboptimal if scans are infrequent

often is considered necessary in patients requiring more than six units of blood transfusion per day. Unfortunately, up to a third of spontaneously remitting diverticular bleeds recur within 6 months to a year.

Colonoscopy has become the first-line treatment option for diverticular bleeding. Endoscopic hemostasis can be achieved with epinephrine injections, bipolar cautery, rubber band ligation, or endoclip placement. Endoscopic clipping achieved hemostasis in 75% to 100% of active diverticular bleeds, but efficacy may be location dependent; bleeding diverticula in the ascending colon may have increased risk of hemorrhage refractory to clipping. Although diverticula with SRH had similar rebleeding frequency as patients with presumptive diverticular bleeding, clipping diverticula with SRH increased time to rebleeding. Bipolar electrocoagulation and heater probe cautery are also effective; however, the minimal effective power should be used to lessen the risk of perforation, particularly in the ascending colon. Endoclips are recommended over heater probe cautery when SRH is localized to the diverticular dome because of perceived increased perforation risk. Rubber band ligation reduced early right colonic rebleeding relative to endoclips, but concerns about higher initial hemostatic failure rates and increased procedural time have been raised. Epinephrine injections often are used to diminish massive bleeds and facilitate bleed site identification, but their effects are somewhat temporary, and other hemostatic measures should follow. Tattooing of bleeding diverticula commonly

is recommended to facilitate rapid identification in the event of rebleeding.

Because of the diagnostic and therapeutic capacity, angiography and embolization has emerged as a favored option in patients with unstable vitals requiring more than five units of blood transfusion, particularly in the frail or those with severe comorbidities, in whom an emergent operation would carry a particularly high mortality. Clinically successful embolization rates have ranged from 63% to 90% and may decrease the need for emergency surgery. Super subselection with microcatheters and intra-arterial infusion vasoconstrictors, such as vasopressin, have been shown to be effective in stopping, or substantially decreasing, bleeding rates. This may convert an emergent operation to an urgent or elective one when the patient is better resuscitated. For embolization in the colon, microcoils are the preferred option. Unfortunately the rebleeding rate is not insignificant. Potential adverse effects include colonic ischemia (less common with microcoils), femoral hematoma, and contrast nephropathy.

Angioectasia

Angioectasia is the second most common cause of LGIB in the Western world. Like diverticular bleeding, angioectasial bleeding usually resolves spontaneously (up to 90%), but up to half recur within 1 year. Typically asymptomatic, angioectasia is the most common cause of obscure LGIB and is responsible for about 35% of

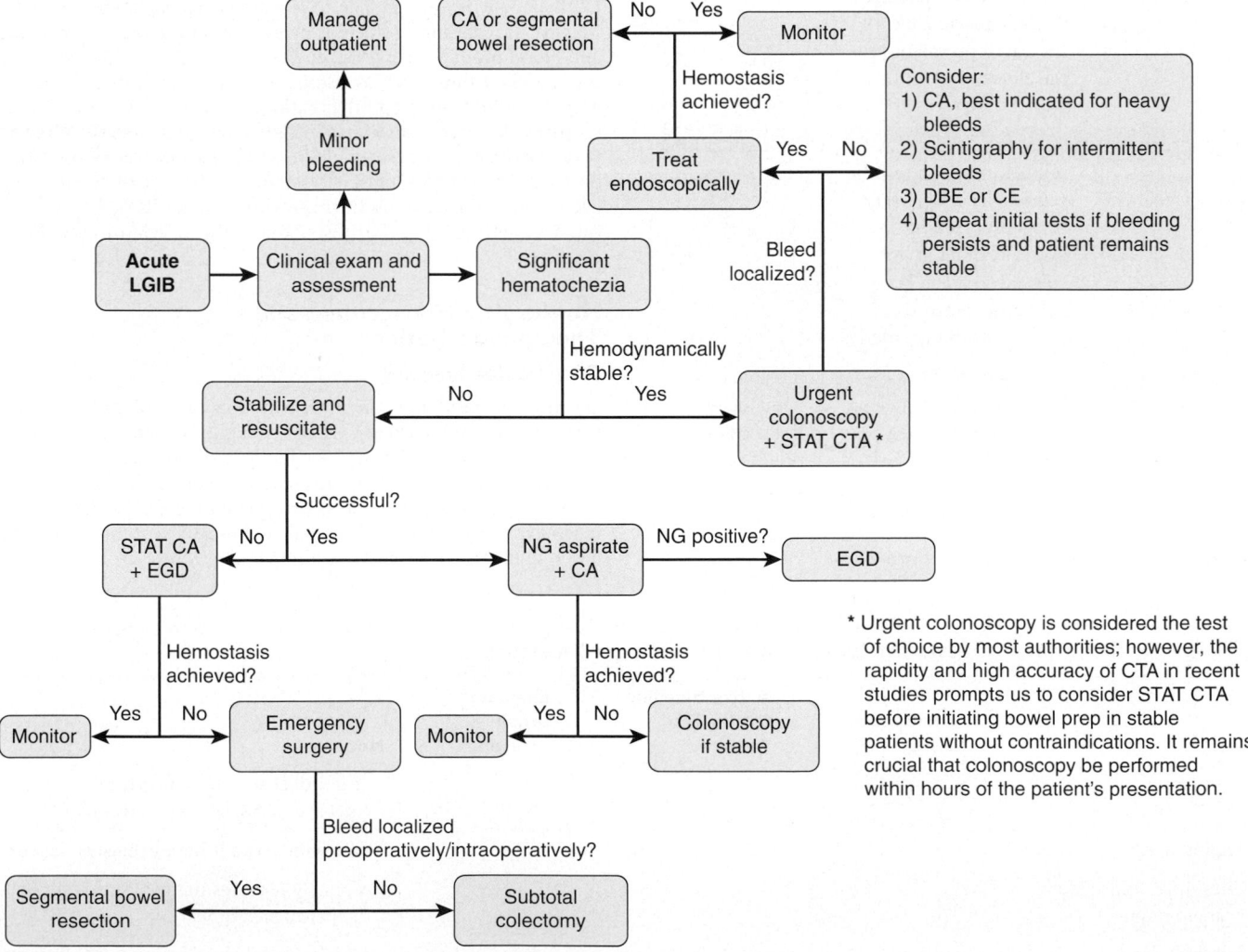

FIGURE 1 Algorithmic approach to acute lower gastrointestinal bleeding. *CA,* catheter angiography; *CE,* capsule endoscopy; *CTA,* computed tomography angiography; *DBE,* double-balloon endoscopy; *EGD,* esophagogastroduodenoscopy; *LGIB,* lower gastrointestinal bleeding; *NG,* nasogastric.

severe obscure LGIB. Colonic lesions are typically right sided in Westerners. Angioectasia has been associated with aortic stenosis, chronic heart failure, chronic renal failure, and von Willebrand's disease.

Argon plasma coagulation (APC), or APC followed by endoclips, is considered the endoscopic treatment of choice for bleeding angioectasia. APC has a high technical efficacy, and rebleeding rates were only 10% after 2 years for colonic bleeds but were 33% after 30 months for small intestinal bleeds. Recurrence of small bowel bleeding increased when more than two lesions were present. Although rare, APC has been associated with bowel perforation; this risk may be reduced by adequate bowel preparation, use of short bursts at low power, and submucosal saline injection before coagulation of large or right-sided lesions.

In addition to endoscopic management, other treatment modalities, including catheter embolization, surgery, and pharmacologic therapies, may be helpful. Angioectasial bleeding is often more challenging to treat through embolization than diverticular bleeding and has a higher recurrence rate. Thalidomide and octreotide have demonstrated efficacy in treating chronically bleeding angiodysplasia. Segmental resection of the bleeding bowel, although curative, is used only in patients with severe hemorrhages or those who have failed other treatment options.

Surgical Approaches

Given the advancements in technology, surgery often is not required to treat LGIB. When surgery is required it is often a salvage procedure after other methods have failed or it is due to recurrent bleeding. The surgical techniques are fairly straightforward; it is the timing and decision making that are the key to success. The diagnostic methods previously mentioned are paramount in localizing the bleed so that appropriate surgical intervention can be performed. Surgery is considered conventionally necessary for patients with hemodynamic instability refractory to resuscitation, ongoing hemorrhage requiring more than six units of transfusion despite negative colonoscopy and CTA, and for localized bleeds after failure of endoscopic or angiographic hemostasis. Emergency surgery for LGIB carries up to a 40% mortality risk and a substantial complication risk. If surgery is required, resuscitation to correct acidosis and coagulopathy should be done before general anesthesia. Ideally, the bleed is localized, allowing a segmental resection. If the bleed cannot be localized, then subtotal colectomy is the appropriate option. Blind segmental resection is not appropriate.

In cases in which the hemorrhage is massive and the patient cannot be resuscitated despite adequate blood and blood products, a damage control approach can be used. In this approach the goal is to stop the bleeding and perform a planned abbreviated laparotomy. If the bleed has been localized, a segmental resection should be done, if not a subtotal colectomy. In either case, the bowel is left in discontinuity and the patient returned to the ICU to continue resuscitation. With the bleeding source removed, the patient's physiology should improve within 12 to 24 hours if resuscitation is appropriate. At that time, a planned return to the OR can be done, and either an anastomosis or ostomy can be performed. These damage control approaches have been validated in the severely injured, and data continue to emerge regarding positive impact of these same techniques in emergency surgery as well.

■ CONCLUSION

LGIB is a growing problem in our aging population and represents a diagnostic challenge for clinicians. The surgeon should work with a team of endoscopic and imaging experts to ensure correct diagnosis and optimal therapy. General consensus has yet to be reached on an assessment algorithm; we prefer the algorithm depicted in Figure 1; however, the workup of LGIB should be tailored to each individual patient. Surgical resection of the bleeding bowel, although potentially curative, has become a salvage option.

SUGGESTED READINGS

Barnert J, Messmann H. Diagnosis and management of lower gastrointestinal bleeding. *Nat Rev Gastroenterol Hepatol.* 2009;6:637-646.
Duchesne J, Kimonis K, Marr A, et al. Damage control resuscitation in combination with damage control laparotomy: a survival advantage. *J Trauma.* 2010;69:46-52.
Ghassemi K, Jensen D. Lower GI bleeding: epidemiology and management. *Curr Gastroenterol Rep.* 2013;15.
Gunter O, Au B, Isbell J, et al. Optimizing outcomes in damage control resuscitation: identifying blood product ratios associated with improved survival. *J Trauma.* 2008;65:527-534.
Marion Y, Lebreton G, Pennec V, Hourna E, Viennot S, Alves A. The management of lower gastrointestinal bleeding. *J Visc Surg.* 2014;151:191-201.
Song L, Baron T. Endoscopic management of acute lower gastrointestinal bleeding. *Am J Gastroenterol.* 2008;103:1881-1887.
Strate L, Naumann C. The role of colonoscopy and radiological procedures in the management of acute lower intestinal bleeding. *Clin Gastroenterol Hepatol.* 2010;8:333-334.

ENHANCED RECOVERY AFTER SURGERY: COLON SURGERY

Liane S. Feldman, MD, FACS, FRCS

Great advances in surgical techniques have occurred in the last decades, particularly with the development of laparoscopic surgery. However, although outcomes have improved overall, 30% to 50% of patients experience a complication after colon surgery, and full functional recovery takes a month or longer. Significant variability is seen in outcomes but also in care processes. Overall median length of stay after uncomplicated colon surgery in National Surgical Quality Improvement Program (NSQIP) hospitals is 6 days, even though physiologic recovery can be achieved several days sooner in uncomplicated patients. There is significant variability between hospitals and clinicians for care processes and outcomes.

Perioperative care is a complex intervention, made up of many smaller interventions, involving multiple stakeholders (surgeons, anesthesiologists, nurses, and patients), each of which has the potential to accelerate or delay patient recovery. Most clinicians practice the way they were taught by their mentors. It takes clinicians a very long time to adopt new evidence into practice (estimated at 17 years) and perhaps even longer to stop doing things that provide no benefit or may even be harmful. Guidelines for best practices in perioperative care that accelerate patient recovery include up to 25 recommendations, many based on strong levels of evidence. In addition to laparoscopic surgery, these include pharmacologic (neural blockade, glucocorticoids, intravenous local anesthetics, nonsteroidal anti-inflammatory drugs [NSAIDs]), nutritional (limiting fasting, preoperative carbohydrate, immediate postoperative feeding), physical (maintaining normothermia, euvolemia, exercise), and hormonal (glycemic control) strategies that reduce the perioperative stress response (Figure 1).

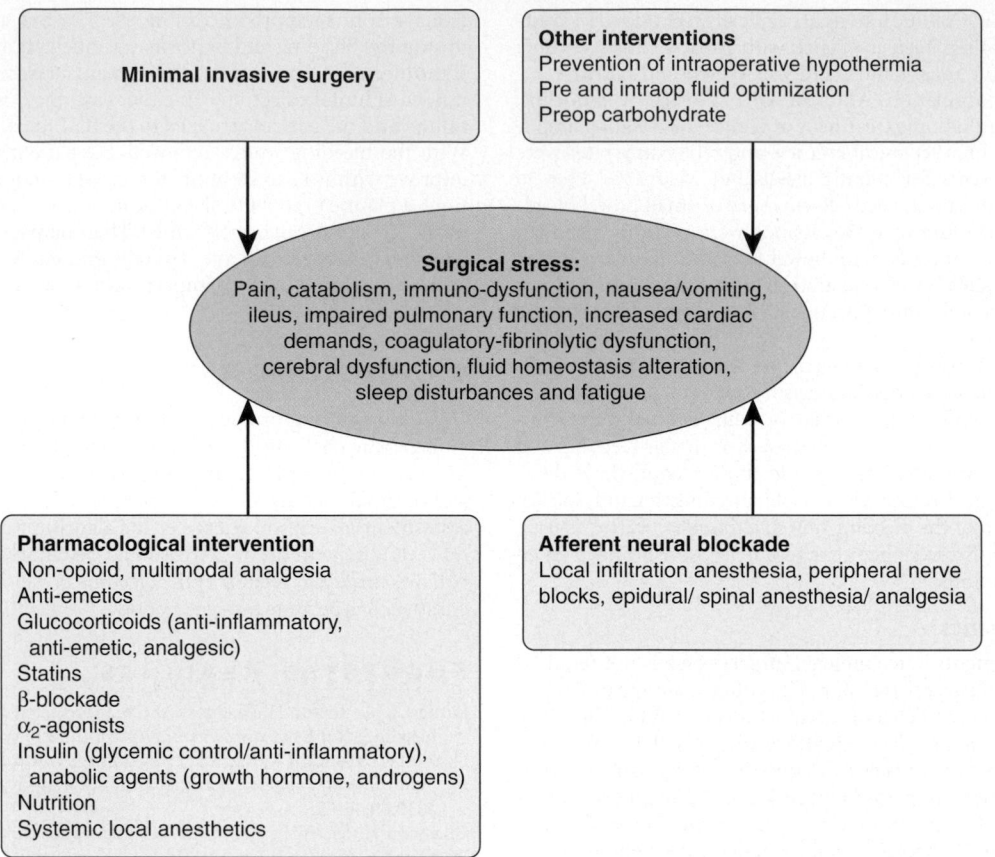

FIGURE 1 Approaches to reduce perioperative stress and improve recovery. Many listed interventions are outside the traditional purview of the surgeon, and optimization of perioperative care requires a multidisciplinary approach. *(From Kehlet H, Wimore DW. Evidence-based surgical care and the evolution of fast-track surgery. Ann Surg. 2008;248:189-198.)*

Surgeons are aware of new evidence in our field, but many of these potentially beneficial interventions are in the anesthesia, nursing, physiotherapy, or nutrition literature. For this evidence to be applied in clinical care, a multidisciplinary approach is required. Decisions made early in the perioperative process by one clinician will have an impact on what may be done downstream by another clinician. This requires a paradigm shift from traditional care, in which clinicians work in expertise-based silos and the patient moves from silo to silo, to an integrated, patient-centered model (Figure 2).

An Enhanced Recovery After Surgery (ERAS) pathway is an integrated, multidisciplinary, consensus-based approach to perioperative care. These plans combine evidence-based interventions from every phase of the perioperative trajectory into a single pathway aimed at attenuating the surgical stress response, reducing morbidity, and supporting early return of patient functioning. Earlier patient recovery and a standardized, consensus-based organized approach results in shorter hospital stay, lower costs, and less variability, without increasing complications or readmissions. The concept originated with Kehlet in the mid 1990s when he and his team reported hospital stays of 2 to 3 days after open colon surgery using a "fast track" pathway emphasizing thoracic epidural, early oral nutrition, and early mobilization. Since then, more than 15 randomized trials in colorectal surgery have investigated the effectiveness of what has since been named *ERAS* or *Enhanced Recovery Programs*. Meta-analyses of trials in colorectal surgery conclude that the ERAS approach is associated with a reduction in the risk of complications by about 30% and reduces hospital stay by an average of 2 days. Even though some resources are required to implement the program, ERAS pathways result in important institutional and societal cost savings because care is less expensive when length of stay and complications are reduced.

This chapter reviews the elements that can be included in an ERAS pathway for elective colon surgery, spanning the preoperative, intraoperative, and postoperative stages (Table 1). This includes prevention of surgical site infection and thromboprophylaxis that are addressed in other chapters. Implementation of an ERAS pathway begins with a multidisciplinary team with clinical champions from surgery, anesthesia, and nursing because the elements may require practice changes and gaining consensus form several clinical groups. The team should include representatives from all clinical areas that interact with surgical patients (Box 1). Ideally, if the program size allows, a coordinator is charged with managing the project and training personnel. A medical librarian is also a useful team member to provide help with summarizing evidence and best practices. Working from existing guidelines but modifying to fit the specific clinical context, the team will develop standard patient education materials, medical order sets, nursing standards, and an audit mechanism to monitor adherence and outcomes to promote implementation and make improvements. Although this chapter focuses on ERAS for colon surgery, the same principles can be applied to any procedure, although how each component is operationalized may differ. There is no clear evidence as to which elements are mandatory or how many must be used; it is not "one size fits all" or a magic recipe, but some of the most important elements include patient participation, laparoscopic surgery, early oral intake, early mobilization, fluid balance, and opiate-sparing analgesia.

■ PREOPERATIVE ELEMENTS

Patient Education

A successful ERAS program begins with an engaged, participating patient and requires a written or web-based educational resource that

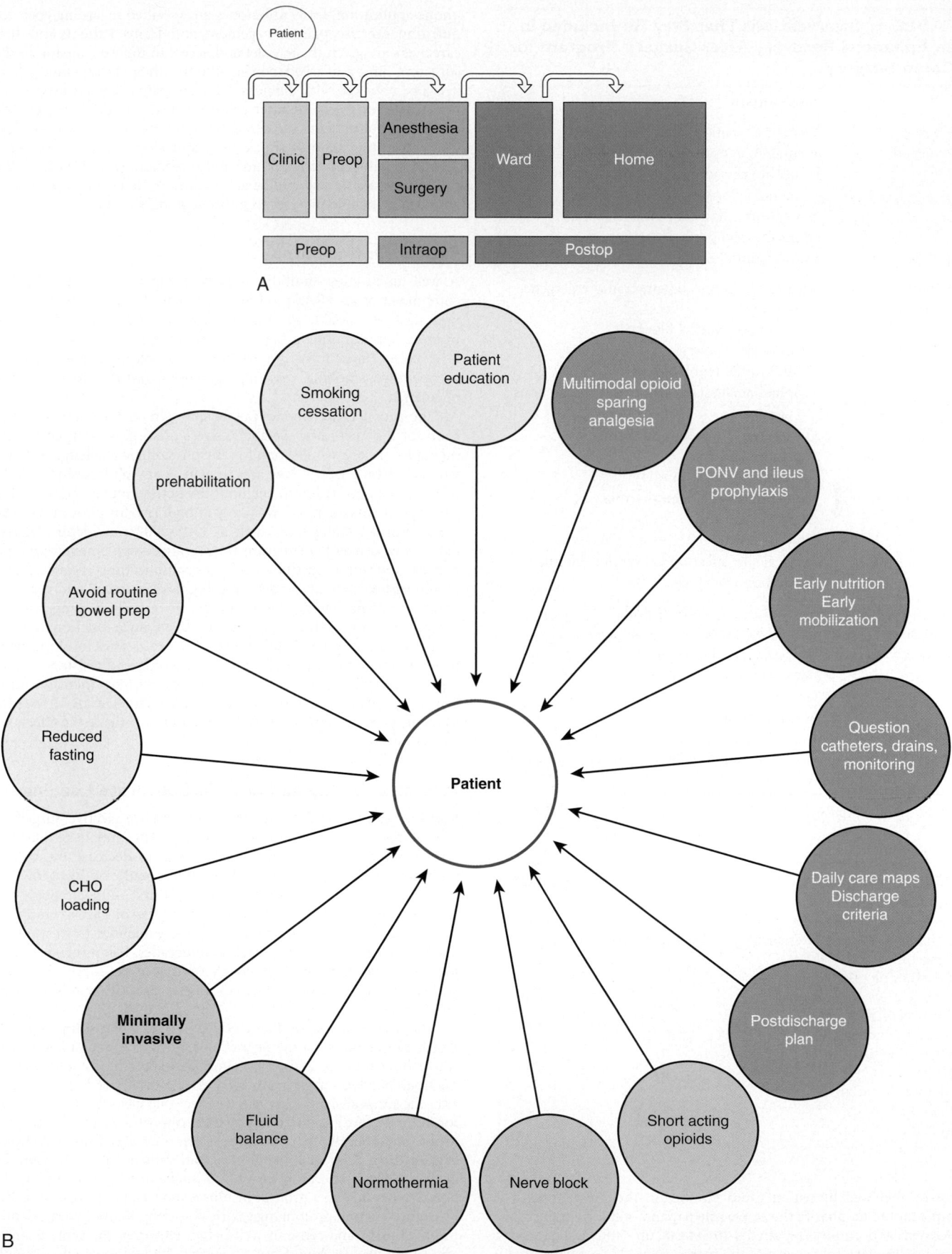

FIGURE 2 In the traditional approach to perioperative care (**A**), clinicians work in expertise silos, and the patient moves between these silos. In the ERAS approach (**B**), the entire perioperative trajectory is integrated into a standard, consensus-based pathway that organizes care around the patient and decreases variability in care processes and outcomes. *(From Feldman LS. Introduction to enhanced recovery programs: a paradigm shift in perioperative care. In Feldman LS et al, eds. The SAGES/ERAS Society Manual of Enhanced Recovery Programs for Gastrointestinal Surgery. New York: Springer; 2015.)*

TABLE 1: Interventions That May Be Included in an Enhanced Recovery After Surgery Program for Colon Surgery

	Intervention
Preoperative period	Written educational material Preoperative optimization (smoking and alcohol cessation, nutrition, correction of anemia, glucose control, exercise) Selective mechanical bowel preparation Minimize preoperative fasting Carbohydrate loading

Intraoperative period	Anesthetic agents allowing rapid emergence
	Open surgery
	  Thoracic epidural blockade
	Laparoscopic surgery
	  Abdominal trunk blocks
	  Spinal analgesia morphine or intravenous lidocaine
	Postoperative nausea and vomiting prophylaxis
	Minimally invasive surgery
	Maintenance of normothermia
	Glycemic control
	Fluid balance
	Surgical site infection prevention bundle
	Thromboprophylaxis

Postoperative period	No routine NG tube or drain Early removal of urinary catheter Immediate oral feeding Ileus prevention strategies Glycemic control Multimodal analgesia Immediate mobilization Criteria-based discharge
Throughout	Audit processes and outcomes

BOX 1: Members of the Enhanced Recovery After Surgery Team

Enhanced recovery after surgery (ERAS) nurse coordinator
Surgeons
Anesthesiologists
Preoperative clinic nurses
Surgical ward nurses
Nursing management
Physiotherapist
Nutritionist
Medical librarian
Pain service
Pharmacy

can be reviewed by patients and families in their own time. It is important to emphasize the active role patients will play in their own recovery and empower patients to "speak up" and ask questions. Essentially, a patient version of the pathway should be created that is aligned with the medical and nursing orders (Figure 3). This may be paper based or web based, or even may occur via a tablet or smart phone application. Daily milestones are specified regarding goals for nutrition, exercise, pain management, and drains. Patients and their caregivers are given the booklet and access to the web version in the surgeon's clinic and asked to bring it to the preoperative clinic, where it will be reviewed with the nurses. Postoperative day 3 is used as the target date for discharge after colon surgery. The discharge criteria are explicit for patients and caregivers (pain <4/10 with oral medications; tolerating solid diet; passing gas or stool; normal heart rate, blood pressure, and temperature; and agreement with discharge). All patient information should be at an appropriate health literacy level and ideally include pictures to improve understanding.

Patient Optimization

A well-functioning multidisciplinary preoperative clinic is a key component of an ERAS program. The goal of preoperative medical optimization should go beyond risk stratification and aim to improve surgical outcomes by increasing physiologic reserve, where it is compromised by pre-existing comorbidities. This includes preoperative smoking cessation, glucose control, and correction of anemia.

The preoperative period can be thought as an opportunity to train for the upcoming metabolic stress of surgery—physically and mentally—as one would train for any physiologic challenge. Patients who are already fit will have less to gain. A key philosophy in ERAS is to maintain nutrition throughout the perioperative period. Colon surgery patients are not particularly at high risk for poor nutritional status, but screening tools such as NRS-2002 can identify at-risk patients who may benefit from preoperative supplementation. Evidence that immunonutrition decreases complications is strongest for malnourished patients undergoing high-risk surgery and may not benefit patients having colon surgery in an ERAS program. An emerging concept is the use of exercise to enhance functional capacity before surgery (prehabilitation). A 3- to 4-week multipronged program including moderate-intensity exercise and resistance training, nutritional counseling, and psychologic support increases functional capacity before and after surgery, but larger trials are needed to identify who is most likely to benefit and investigate the effects on complications.

Minimize Fasting and Use Carbohydrate Loading

Keeping patients "NPO after midnight" before elective surgery is one of the best-known rules of surgery. The aim is to have an empty stomach at induction of anesthesia to decrease the risk of aspiration pneumonitis. This rule is simple and easy to follow but results in patient discomfort related to thirst, hunger, sleep disturbance, and anxiety. On the basis of studies of gastric emptying after intake of various foods and drinks, guidelines from multiple anesthesia societies in the past two decades recommend fasting for solids for 6 hours but conclude that clear fluids for most patients up to 2 hours before anesthesia are safe and should be encouraged.

The stress response is characterized by a state of insulin resistance that is proportional to the degree of surgical trauma and results in whole-body protein catabolism to mobilize substrate for glucose production. The loss of glycogen even after a brief fast is sufficient to alter the surgical stress response. The fact that clear fluids are safe up to 2 hours before anesthesia suggests the opportunity to enter surgery in the metabolically fed state rather than the starved state. Complex carbohydrate drinks act like a meal and shift metabolism from the fasting to fed state. Preoperative oral intake of 50 g of complex carbohydrate results in a prompt insulin response and decreases insulin resistance without prolonging gastric emptying. Carbohydrate drinks improve thirst and sense of well-being. However, the same benefits and safety profile should not necessarily be extrapolated to simple carbohydrate drinks such as Gatorade or juices that have not been studied formally.

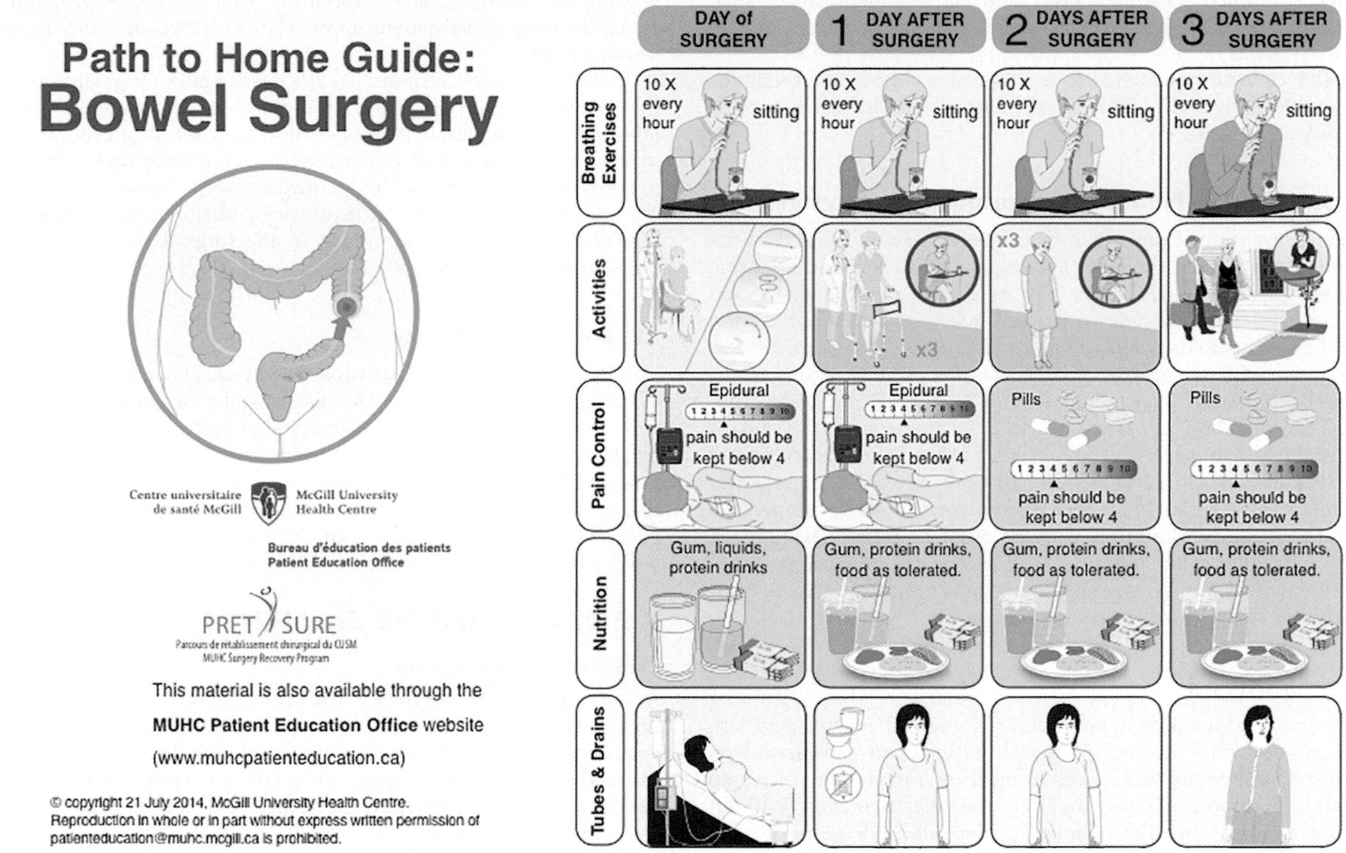

Path to Home Guide:
Bowel Surgery

Centre universitaire
de santé McGill   McGill University
Health Centre

**Bureau d'éducation des patients
Patient Education Office**

PRET / SURE
Parcours de rétablissement chirurgical du CUSM
MUHC Surgery Recovery Program

This material is also available through the

MUHC Patient Education Office website

(www.muhcpatienteducation.ca)

© copyright 21 July 2014, McGill University Health Centre.
Reproduction in whole or in part without express written permission of
patienteducation@muhc.mcgill.ca is prohibited.

FIGURE 3 Patient version of daily milestones to achieve in postoperative recovery in the ERAS pathway for bowel surgery at the McGill University Health Centre. The full patient information booklet is available at http://www.muhcpatienteducation.ca/DATA/GUIDE/170_en~v~bowel-surgery-montreal-general-hospital.pdf. *(Courtesy McGill University Health Centre Patient Education Office.)*

Bowel Preparation

Mechanical bowel preparation before colectomy is advocated to clean the bowel and prevent fecal spillage and infectious complications. However, bowel preparation is uncomfortable and results in fluid losses. A large body of randomized trials finds no clear benefit to bowel preparation for colon surgery with respect to infections, leak, and mortality. However, these trials did not adequately address the potential value of nonabsorbable oral antibiotics given in combination with bowel preparation. This field remains controversial: large population data sets suggest decreased superficial infections when the combination is used, without a benefit to mechanical preparation alone compared with no preparation (as was concluded from the randomized trials). Our current approach for colectomy is to combine mechanical bowel preparation with oral antibiotics for patients at higher risk of superficial surgical site infection in our institution, including open resection or high risk of conversion, when intraoperative colonoscopy is planned, or for rectal surgery with planned ileostomy. For laparoscopic right colectomy, bowel preparation is omitted; for laparoscopic sigmoid colectomy, two Fleet enemas are given the morning of surgery.

■ INTRAOPERATIVE ELEMENTS

Anesthesia and Analgesia Protocol

Close collaboration with anesthesiology is important for implementation of a well-functioning ERAS program. The anesthesiology team can play a large role in supporting early patient independent functioning or the opposite through modulation of the stress response,

fluid management, and analgesia. Long-acting anxiolytics are avoided, and short-acting anesthetic agents that facilitate early recovery are used. Deep muscle relaxation is necessary for laparoscopic cases to allow for lower pressure pneumoperitoneum that maintains hemodynamics and reduces postoperative pain.

The choice of analgesia in the operating room and postoperatively will have an impact on other elements of the ERAS program. An analgesic regimen that reduces metabolic stress and facilitates early nutrition and mobilization is the goal, so minimizing opiates and their side effects including ileus, nausea and vomiting, and respiratory depression is key. Multiple interventions are used. Because signals from the injury site carried by afferent nerves are important initiators of the stress response leading to activation of the immune-hypothalamic-pituitary-adrenal axis and sympathetic nervous system, it makes sense to block afferent and efferent nociceptive stimuli before tissue injury. This begins with infiltration of local anesthetics into the wounds before incision. Regional neural blockade with local anesthetics obtained by epidural and spinal decrease insulin resistance, provide excellent analgesia, and reduce opiate needs after open surgery. However, recent studies suggest that epidurals delay recovery after laparoscopic colectomy with an ERAS program. Intraoperative intravenous lidocaine infusion has anti-inflammatory and analgesic properties and is associated with lower opiate use, reduced nausea and vomiting, and reduced pain scores after laparoscopic surgery. Abdominal trunk blocks such as transversus abdominis plane (TAP) blocks can be placed by ultrasound for open surgery or under laparoscopic guidance. A minimal volume of 15 mL of long-acting local anesthetic is needed. After laparoscopic colectomy, they provide equivalent analgesia as epidural, especially when continued postoperatively. Adjuvant anesthetic drugs such as ketamine, dexmedetomidine, and dexamethasone have opiate-sparing effects.

Our current approach is to use thoracic epidural anesthesia for open colectomy and TAP blocks with intravenous lidocaine for most laparoscopic cases.

Postoperative Nausea and Vomiting Prophylaxis

Early resumption of oral nutrition is a key element of ERAS. Patients should be stratified for risk of postoperative nausea and vomiting (PONV) with available scores (e.g., Apfel) and prophylaxis tailored to risk level. Risks include female sex, history of PONV or motion sickness, nonsmoking, younger age, and laparoscopic surgery. Risk is increased with the use of volatile anesthetics and nitrous oxide, longer duration of surgery, and opioids. Patients receive dexamethasone at induction of anesthesia and ondansetron at the end of surgery. Fluid management should avoid excessive administration of crystalloids (which may contribute to ileus) as well as underhydration (which is a risk for PONV). Intraoperative and postoperative opiates should be minimized with the use of a multimodal approach with nerve blocks and adjuncts, including postoperative acetaminophen and NSAIDs. When prophylaxis fails, a different class of antiemetic should be used for rescue therapy.

Normothermia

Even mild perioperative hypothermia (34° to 36° C) is associated with adverse outcomes, including surgical site infection and blood loss. Shivering is very unpleasant and stressful and can result in increased heart rate, blood pressure, and cardiovascular demands. Without active interventions, the majority of patients undergoing general anesthesia will be hypothermic. Core temperature should be monitored. Forced air warmers are effective and safe and should be continued postoperatively until body temperature is more than 36°C. Fluid warmers should be used to prevent heat loss when more than 500 cc is given. The operating room should be kept warmer than 21° C at least until the patient is draped and active warming is started.

Fluid Balance

IV fluid should be thought of as a therapeutic intervention and used thoughtfully. Fluid overload of only 2.5 to 3 L, represented by weight gain exceeding 2.5 kg on postoperative day 1, is associated with worse outcomes, including ileus, impaired wound healing, altered coagulation, and pulmonary edema. Underhydration also increases morbidity, so fluid balance should be the goal. Fluid is managed at multiple points in the ERAS program. Preoperatively, patient education emphasizes taking preoperative clear fluids, and the active role of patients in early resumption of oral intake, allowing for early cessation of intravenous fluid. This cannot occur if patients experience nausea and vomiting, are oversedated, or are in pain. At induction of anesthesia, it is important to know whether the patient received a bowel preparation because the fluid losses will have to be replaced with an additional 1 L of fluid. Pumps should be used for fluid administration rather than just opening up IVs.

Insensible losses are lower than previously thought, especially with laparoscopic surgery, in the range of 3 to 5 cc/kg/hr, and are replaced with balanced crystalloid solution such as Lactated Ringer's. Intraoperative blood loss and fluid shifting resulting from increased endovascular permeability resulting from tissue injury lead to reduced intravascular volume that is replaced preferentially with colloids 1:1 and blood transfusion when necessary. However, intraoperative assessment of fluid status with heart rate, blood pressure, and urine output do not reflect early decreases in end-organ perfusion. Goal-directed therapy (GDT) technologies individualize fluid therapy by identifying patients who are fluid responsive (i.e., increase stroke volume in responsive to a fluid bolus). The value of GDT

to improve outcomes after colectomy with an ERAS program, especially when laparoscopic approaches are used, has not been demonstrated.

The surgical stress response results in salt and water retention in the early postoperative period, even in the absence of complications. Low urine output should be evaluated in the context of other signs of low perfusion such as hypotension before initiating large volumes of crystalloid resuscitation. Fluid homeostasis is facilitated by providing oral fluids immediately after surgery and stopping intravenous crystalloid infusions on admission to the surgical ward from the post-anesthesia care unit (PACU).

Laparoscopic Surgery

The laparoscopic approach is used when possible because it offers advantages independent of ERAS. Laparoscopy facilitates adherence with ERAS by decreasing pain, avoiding epidural, decreasing ileus, and facilitating early ambulation. The laparoscopic approach reduces inflammation and preserves immune function compared with open surgery within an ERAS program. Meta-analyses report shorter hospital stay and decreased total complications for laparoscopic compared with open surgery within an ERAS program.

■ POSTOPERATIVE ELEMENTS

Multimodal Analgesia

Acute surgical pain originates from nociceptive stimuli from the injured tissue, bowel manipulation, inflammation, sensitization of peripheral and central neurons, and inhibition of descending inhibitory pathways. Response to nociception contributes to activation and perpetuation of the stress response to surgery with its multiple negative consequences. Poorly controlled acute surgical pain is a risk factor for chronic pain. Because pain can be somatic, visceral, or neuropathic, a multimodal approach to pain is included throughout the ERAS program and involves the preoperative, intraoperative, and postoperative phases. A related goal is to avoid opioid side effects such as ileus, urinary retention, nausea and vomiting, sedation, and respiratory depression that will all delay recovery. Common components include local and regional blocks, intraoperative IV lidocaine, NSAIDs, and acetaminophen.

The role of preemptive analgesics, including acetaminophen, NMDA (N-methyl-D-aspartate) antagonists, COX-2 inhibitors, and gabapentinoids, remains unclear for colon surgery. Evidence is strongest for thoracic epidural as the best preemptive technique to reduce postoperative pain and analgesia use after open lower abdominal surgery but has rare but serious side effects, increases the risk of hypotension, leg weakness and pruritus, and becomes dislodged or fails to work in some patients. They are best used by specialized teams in which a postoperative pain service can troubleshoot and adjust. In our colon ERAS program, with a well-functioning pain service seeing patients every day, thoracic epidural is used mainly for open surgery.

When given routinely (not PRN), postoperative NSAIDs have important opioid-sparing effects, reduce opioid side effects, and improve postoperative analgesia. Some observational data raise concerns about increased risk of anastomotic leak when NSAIDs are used in the first 48 hours, but this is not consistent in the literature. They should be avoided in patients with renal failure. Acetaminophen improves analgesia and has an opioid-sparing effect. Use of acetaminophen in combination with NSAIDs is better than either used alone. The dose of acetaminophen should be reduced in patients with liver failure. Intravenous formulations of NSAIDs (ketorolac) and acetaminophen are available for patients with ileus but otherwise are given orally.

Immediate Oral Feeding

Oral intake is started as soon as the patient is awake as long as there is no nausea and vomiting. There no need to withhold intake until return of large bowel function as indicated by flatus or stool. In meta-analyses, early postoperative nutrition (within 24 hours) is associated with decreased total postoperative complications and does not increase the risk of leak, infection, or pneumonia. Early feeding decreases the time to solid diet but does not accelerate recovery of bowel function; it is simply that most patients tolerate feeding before full return of bowel function.

Patients are encouraged to resume oral intake when they arrive on the ward from the PACU. Patients are encouraged to drink more than 1 L fluid/day and the IV catheter is removed on postoperative day 1 if fluids are tolerated. Patients are encouraged to use nutritional supplements when oral intake may be decreased to preserve lean body mass. A structured plan for nutrition that is well understood by the patient, nurses, and residents is important. Simply starting clear fluids on postoperative day 1 does not prevent negative nitrogen balance.

Not all patients tolerate early feeding. In ERAS colon programs, about two thirds of patients will be eating a solid diet by postoperative day 2 with the remainder experiencing some symptoms of gastrointestinal dysfunction including nausea, vomiting, distension, and food intolerance along with no flatus or stool. Early feeding does not seem to increase the need for nasogastric tube insertion, but patients need to be closely monitored for symptoms of ileus and treated accordingly.

Promotion of Bowel Function

A multimodal approach to preserve or accelerate return of bowel function is critical to support early nutrition, early use of oral analgesics, and patient autonomy. This includes other ERAS interventions, such as avoiding fluid overload in the perioperative period, reducing opioids, laparoscopic surgery, and epidural analgesia for open surgery. Despite multiple interventions, in our experience, ileus remains a vexing problem for about 20% of patients.

Routine use of nasogastric tubes delays recovery of bowel function and should not be used. Chewing gum stimulates the cephalic-vagal response and is a sham feeding intervention. Although actual feeding does not seem to accelerate return of bowel function, meta-analyses of gum chewing trials suggest a modest benefit, and it is well tolerated and inexpensive. There is little evidence that laxatives such as bisacodyl or magnesium oxide accelerate return of bowel function after colon surgery, but use of a mild laxative often is included. Alvimopan is a peripheral mu receptor antagonist that accelerates GI recovery after open colorectal surgery when opioid analgesia is used. Its benefit after laparoscopic colectomy in ERAS requires further study. Although early mobilization often is encouraged by clinicians as a way to stimulate bowel function, there is little evidence to suggest this benefit.

Avoiding Drains

Drains and catheters cause pain and discomfort, impede independent mobilization, and pose a psychologic barrier to recovery. After colorectal surgery, routine nasogastric decompression should be abandoned with a meta-analysis 20 years ago demonstrating reduced atelectasis and pneumonia in patients without nasogastric (NG) tubes. If an NG tube is used in the operating room to evacuate air in the stomach as a consequence of ventilation before intubation, it should be removed in the operating room. As a consequence of ileus, about 10% of patients will require NG tube insertion, meaning 90% of patients will have avoided this uncomfortable intervention. After elective colon surgery, routine prophylactic closed-suction drainage of anastomoses provides no benefit concerning infections, leaks, or diagnosis of leak.

Urinary catheters are placed to drain the bladder during prolonged procedures, monitor urine output postoperatively, and prevent urinary retention, especially with an epidural catheter. However, urinary catheters may be uncomfortable and impede mobilization, and longer duration of use correlates with increased risk of

urinary tract infection. For patients at low risk of urinary retention (e.g., no benign prostatic hypertrophy, previous postoperative urinary retention, or other urinary tract abnormalities), without spinal or epidural undergoing uncomplicated right hemicolectomy, the catheter may be removed in the operating room. If the catheter is kept postoperatively and there was no extensive rectal dissection, it can be removed within 24 hours in low-risk patients, even when an epidural catheter is in place. A postoperative urinary retention protocol with bedside ultrasonography can be used to monitor bladder volumes and in-and-out catheterization performed if bladder volumes are more than 600 cc with the indwelling catheter replaced if more than two catheterizations are needed. This approach reduces the incidence of infection without increasing the need to replace the indwelling catheter compared with later removal.

Early Mobilization

The negative impact of bed rest on functional exercise capacity occurs after a relatively short time period and can be reversed or prevented by physical activity. Increased time out of bed aligns with the message of patient functional independence in ERAS. Increased ambulation is a predictor of early discharge in ERAS programs. It is unclear what "dose" of mobilization is required to achieve the benefits, but patients spend alarmingly little time ambulating in the absence of a structured program. Drains, pain, and ileus all impede mobilization. Different programs use different milestones, but having a structured program with daily goals reinforced through written material, ward posters, patient diaries, and use of a pedometer may increase adherence. Patients provided with a supervised preoperative "prehabilitation" program to increase physical activity remain more active postoperatively compared with those who begin a program after surgery.

Criteria-Based Discharge

Discharge criteria for colorectal surgery have been identified through international consensus work (Table 2). After uncomplicated colon surgery in an ERAS program, this is achieved on average by postoperative day 3, which is a reasonable target date for the program. There are some examples of ultrashort hospital stay (23 hours) after laparoscopic right hemicolectomy in selected patients in centers with well-experienced staff. Early discharge is facilitated by ongoing education of patients and families and a consistent message from clinicians emphasized in the daily care goals. The main advantage of ERAS on length of stay is for patients without complications who will be discharged on postoperative day 3 instead of day 5. Decreasing complications is the most important strategy to further decrease length of stay after that point.

Full recovery from surgery is, of course, incomplete at discharge; functional recovery requires weeks or months. Increasing functional capacity perioperatively with exercise and nutrition may also accelerate postdischarge recovery. Although the earlier discharge in ERAS programs does not increase readmissions or decrease patient satisfaction, it is important for patients and families to know where to go for help should complications arise.

Audit

It is critical to have information about adherence to the various components of the pathway to understand if the intended changes actually occurred and to relate changes in care processes with changes in outcomes. There is a strong association between adherence to the pathway and outcomes, including hospital stay and complications. It is best to start collecting these data even before the pathway is started to understand current practice and the gaps compared with guidelines, and follow changes as the ERAS program is adopted. Creating a process to record these measures in the medical record is an opportunity to discuss and troubleshoot ERAS implementation with the multiple team members involved in perioperative care. Audit can be a daunting task, so the minimum number of measures needed to get a sense of the program is a practical approach (Table 3). More complex audit tools are commercially available from the ERAS Society (ERAS Interactive Audit Tool) and colectomy-specific NSQIP now includes several Enhanced Recovery process measures and recovery outcomes. These data should be reviewed with the team on a routine basis to discuss areas for improvement and implement an action plan, then follow the results.

Making the Business Case

Some resources are required to begin an ERAS program, but there are clear institutional benefits to ERAS that must be communicated to have administrative support. Meta-analyses conclude that ERAS programs in colorectal surgery consistently decrease institutional costs through their impact on decreasing hospital stay and complications. In colorectal surgery, one can expect a decrease in hospital stay of between 1 and 4 days, depending on where it starts and whether laparoscopic surgery is used. Even when complications are not decreased with ERAS, length of stay should decrease simply by standardizing care between clinicians and by eliminating aspects of perioperative care that actually delay recovery and discharge (e.g., delaying feeding and using drains, opioid analgesia, and unnecessary blood tests). ERAS programs increase the value of laparoscopic surgery, with its increased equipment costs, by decreasing hospital stay and streamlining care.

American studies report savings of $1000 to $10,000 per patient with ERAS programs. However, many of these studies did not take implementation costs into account. Ideally, in a large program, there is a nurse coordinator responsible for keeping the project on track, managing meetings, coordinating the creation of the patient materials and order sets, training nurses and other personnel, and implementing the audit. A nurse with experience in the preoperative setting is an ideal person for this role. The cost of the program per patient decreases as more patients are cared for in the program. In a Canadian study in which implementation costs were taken into account, the ERAS approach remained dominant (i.e., less expensive and more effective), with the largest differences seen from the societal perspective. ERAS patients had lower productivity losses and required less care after hospital discharge.

TABLE 2: Criteria to Determine Readiness for Hospital Discharge After Colorectal Surgery

Criteria	Endpoint to Determine When Criteria Has Been Achieved
Tolerance of oral intake	Patients should be able to tolerate at least one solid meal without nausea, vomiting, bloating, or worsening abdominal pain. Patients should drink liquids actively (ideally >800-1000 mL/day) and not require intravenous infusion to maintain hydration
Recovery of lower gastrointestinal function	Patient should have passed flatus
Adequate pain control with oral analgesia	Patient should be able to rest and mobilize (sit up and walk, unless unable preoperatively) without significant pain (i.e., patient reports pain is uncontrolled or pain score ≤4 on a scale from 0 to 10) while taking oral analgesics
Ability to mobilize and self-care	Patient should be able to sit up, walk, and perform activities of daily living (e.g., go to the toilet, dress, shower, and climb stairs if needed at home) unless unable preoperatively

From Royse CF, Fiore JF Jr. Hospital recovery and full recovery. In Feldman LS, Delaney CP, Ljungqvist O, Carli F, eds. *The SAGES/ERAS Society Manual of Enhanced Recovery for Gastrointestinal Surgery.* New York: Springer; 2015.

■ ENHANCED RECOVERY AFTER SURGERY IMPLEMENTATION

At this point, a lot of information from other institutions with ERAS pathways is available; there is no need to start from scratch. An example of a multimodal perioperative care pathway for colon surgery is provided in Box 2. Standard order sets are created along with guidelines for intraoperative anesthesia protocols. There are several guidelines, textbooks, and websites dedicated to ERAS that

TABLE 3: A Clinical Dataset That Can Be Used to Audit Adherence With Enhanced Recovery After Surgery Measures and Outcomes

Preoperative	Intraoperative	Postoperative	Recovery Milestones
Written patient information	Preincision antibiotics	No NG or drain	Weight gain <2.5 kg POD 1
Clear fluids until 2-3 hr before anesthesia	Temperature ≥ 36°C when arrive in PACU	Urinary catheter <24 hr	Date first flatus/BM
Carbohydrate drink	Epidural for open cases	IV fluids <24 hr	Date tolerating solid food
	Trunk block/IV lidocaine for laparoscopic	Fluids POD 0	Date for pain control with oral analgesia
	Laparoscopic surgery	Solids POD 1	Hospital stay
	Balanced IV fluids	Out of bed POD 0 and POD 1	Readmissions
	PONV prophylaxis	Multimodal analgesia	

BM, Bowel movement; *IV,* intravenous; *NG,* nasogastric tube; *PACU,* post-anesthesia care unit; *POD,* postoperative day; *PONV,* postoperative nausea and vomiting.

BOX 2: Sample Enhanced Recovery After Surgery Pathway for Colon Surgery

Preoperative Assessment and Optimization

Evaluation of medication compliance and control of risk factors: hypertension, diabetes, COPD, smoking, alcohol, asthma, CAD, malnutrition, anemia

Psychologic preparation for surgery and postoperative recovery: provide written information and e-module link including daily milestones in perioperative pathway (diet, ambulation, presence of drains, pain management, and expected hospital stay [3-4 days])

Physical preparation with exercises at home: aerobic 30 minutes/day at moderate intensity (4-6 on Borg Scale) 3 days/week; resistance exercises; breathing exercises

Surgical considerations: operative approach (laparoscopic vs open)

Oral bowel preparation with antibiotics for rectal resections with planned ileostomy; fleet enemas for left sided resections

Stoma teaching as needed

Nutritional supplements if diminished oral intake, weight loss, low BMI

Day of surgery

Drink clear fluids with carbohydrates up to 2 hours before operation unless risk factors are present (e.g., gastroparesis, obstruction, dysphagia, previous difficult intubation, achalasia, pregnancy)

Preinduction

Short-acting sedative medication if needed for anxiety

Intraoperative Management

Anesthetic Management

Anesthesia protocol: Total intravenous anesthesia (TIVA)/desflurane/sevoflurane

Epidural catheter at appropriate level for postoperative analgesia for open surgery and infuse local anesthetics during surgery.

Bilateral transversus abdominis plane block for laparoscopic surgery

Intravenous lidocaine infusion 1.5 mg/kg bolus then 2 mg/kg/hr for duration of case if no epidural

Prevent PONV with dexamethasone and ondansetron plus others on the basis of baseline risk score

Avoid overhydration. IV Ringer's lactate maintenance at 3 mL/kg/hr for laparoscopic surgery, 5 mL/kg/hr open surgery. Additional 1 L of Ringer's lactate if bowel preparation used. Colloid 1:1 to replace blood loss.

Maintain normothermia (>36°C)

Maintain glucose <10 mmol/L

Antibiotic and DVT prophylaxis

Neuromuscular blockade to allow lower pressure pneumoperitoneum (12 mm Hg)

Titrate depth of anesthesia with bispectral index

Surgical Care

Minimize incision size. Laparoscopic surgery if feasible. Maximize use of small trocars.

Infiltrate incisions with long acting local anesthetic at beginning and end of procedure.

Anastomotic leak test and endoscopy

Remove NG tube before extubation

Remove urinary catheter after right hemicolectomy

Postoperative Care

Day of Surgery (Postoperative Day 0)

Gum chewing for 30 minutes TID (continue daily)

Full fluids with 1 can of nutritional supplement beverage if no PONV and no abdominal distension

Out of bed (sitting in chair) encouraged

Oral acetaminophen 650 mg every 4 hours and Celecoxib 200 mg BID for 72 hours routine

Glucose monitor and treatment if >10 mmol/L

Postoperative Day 1

Discontinue IV fluid infusion (heparin-locking catheter)

Discontinue urinary drainage catheter

Gum chewing for 30 minutes TID

Full oral diet as tolerated including nutritional supplementation beverage with each meal

Mobilize out of bed for 4 to 6 hours. Walk length of hallway with assistance TID

Glucose monitor and treatment if >10 mmol/L

Postoperative Day 2

Gum chewing for 30 minutes TID

Mobilize out of bed for 8 hours

Transition from epidural to oral medication (oxycodone + acetaminophen + NSAIDs) if stop test successful

Discharge criteria assessed: passing gas or stool, no fever, pain <4/10 with oral analgesia, walking unattended, eating

Postoperative Day 3

Discharge before lunch if discharge criteria met

Instructions for home including eating normal diet with supplements as needed, daily exercise, avoid opioids, accessing psychologic support

Schedule follow-up appointment in clinic 2 weeks after surgery

BID, Twice a day; *BMI,* body mass index; *CAD,* coronary artery disease; *COPD,* chronic obstructive pulmonary disease; *DVT,* deep vein thrombosis; *IV,* intravenous; *NSAIDs,* nonsteroidal anti-inflammatory drugs; *PONV,* postoperative nausea and vomiting; *TID,* three times a day.

will help teams create their own programs. Examples of patient education materials for a variety of ERAS pathways are available from the McGill University Health Centre patient education Office (http://www.muhcpatienteducation.ca). The Society of American Gastrointestinal and Endoscopic Surgeons has created the SMART Enhanced Recovery Program, which includes a recommended pathway, implementation timeline, and examples of order sets and educational materials from established programs (http://www.sages.org/smart-enhanced-recovery-program/). It may be daunting to consider changing so many things at once, and teams may decide to start with less complex programs, or parts of programs, or selected patients. Once experience is gained, more elements can be added. In addition, once the team gains experience with creating a pathway for colon surgery, many of these elements are applicable to other procedures and the benefits extended to more patients. The team that initiated the colon pathway will become the institutional ERAS steering committee and help other teams adopt pathways for their specific procedures.

Suggested Readings

Feldheiser A, Aziz O, Baldini G, et al. Enhanced Recovery After Surgery (ERAS) for gastrointestinal surgery, part 2: consensus statement for anesthesia practice. *Acta Anaesthesiol Scand*. 2016;60:289-334.

Feldman LS, Delaney CP, Ljungqvist O, Carli F. *The SAGES/ERAS Society Manual of Enhanced Recovery Programs for Gastrointestinal Surgery*. New York: Springer; 2015.

Gillis C, Li C, Lee L, et al. Prehabilitation vs rehabilitation: a randomized control trial in patients undergoing colorectal resection for cancer. *Anesthesiology*. 2014;121:937-947.

Gustafsson UO, Scott MJ, Schwenk W, et al. Guidelines for perioperative care in elective colonic surgery: Enhanced Recovery After Surgery (ERAS) Society recommendations. *World J Surg*. 2013;37:259-284.

Lee L, Mata J, Ghitulescu GA, Boutros M, Charlebois P, Stein B, Liberman AS, Fried GM, Morin N, Carli F, Latimer E, Feldman LS. Cost-effectiveness of Enhanced Recovery Versus Conventional Perioperative Management for Colorectal Surgery. *Ann Surg*. 2015;262:1026-1033.

Nicholson A, Lowe MC, Parker J, Lewis SR, Alderson P, Smith AF. Systematic review and meta-analysis of enhanced recovery programmes in surgical patients. *Br J Surg*. 2014;101:172-188.

Scott MJ, Baldini G, Fearon KC, et al. Enhanced Recovery After Surgery (ERAS) for gastrointestinal surgery part 1: Pathophysiologic considerations. *Acta Anaesthesiol Scand*. 2015;59:1212-1231.

THE MANAGEMENT OF CYSTIC DISEASE OF THE LIVER

Keri E. Lunsford, MD, PhD, and Fady M. Kaldas, MD, FACS

Cystic disease of the liver encompasses benign and neoplastic pathology. Benign liver cysts may be genetic, acquired, infectious, or parasitic. The majority of hepatic cysts are noninfectious and nonneoplastic. Neoplastic cysts are composed primarily of hepatic cystadenomas and cystadenocarcinomas. Although infectious and paracystic cysts are included in the classification of hepatic cysts, full discussion of these will be deferred until later in this book. The present chapter focuses primarily on the diagnosis, pathogenesis, and treatment of noninfectious cystic disease of the liver. A comparison of the features and treatment for the various types of hepatic cysts is shown in Table 1.

■ EVALUATION OF CYSTIC LIVER DISEASE

The majority of liver cysts are noted incidentally in asymptomatic patients on routine imaging, and the main rationale for further workup is to rule out malignancy. Routine liver function tests may be performed but are generally normal unless a cyst is very large and compressing major hepatic structures. Fever on presentation should raise concern for cyst infection or pyogenic liver abscess. In these cases, white blood cell count elevation and positive blood cultures may occur. Recent foreign travel, drinking of unfiltered water, or contact with livestock should prompt serologies for *Echinococcus* spp. or stool studies for *Entamoeba* spp. Cyst aspiration is rarely helpful in differentiating simple cysts from neoplastic cysts; no marker has been identified to distinguish malignant potential. Should *Echinococcus* spp. be suspected, aspiration should be avoided because of the risk for anaphylaxis. In addition, aspiration in suspected cystadenocarcinoma risks peritoneal spread of disease.

Radiologic imaging allows for the assessment of cyst size and characteristics, as well as the location within the liver. Simple cysts appear homogenous and anechoic with smooth borders on ultrasound. Neoplasia should be suspected with features of nodularity or thickening of cyst walls. Loculations, septations, or papillary projections also may be present. Debris within the cyst may represent malignancy or parasitic infection, although this more frequently represents layering from hemorrhage into a simple cyst. The presence of mural calcifications or "daughter" cysts should raise concern for echinococcal disease, and mural edema and enhancement often are seen with pyogenic liver abscesses.

Ultrasound is the most inexpensive available imaging modality, and it carries a sensitivity and specificity of more than 90% with an experienced operator. It is generally sufficient to evaluate the size and characteristics of a cyst. Either computed tomographic (CT) scan or magnetic resonance imaging (MRI) is more useful for evaluation of the location and surrounding structures of a cyst, and imaging is not operator dependent. It should be used in cases of any noted cyst atypia. Very small cysts may be indistinguishable from a hepatic mass on CT scan. Contrast imaging may be useful for determining the location of cysts with respect to vascular structures, especially for operative planning. Concern for communication with the biliary tree should prompt magnetic resonance cholangiopancreatography (MRCP) evaluation, endoscopic retrograde cholangiopancreatography (ERCP), or intraoperative cholangiogram (IOC).

■ MANAGEMENT OF BENIGN CYSTIC DISEASE OF THE LIVER

Simple Cysts

Simple cysts are the most common hepatic cyst and are noted on imaging in approximately 5% to 18% of the population. Cysts may be single or multiple but generally do not exhibit septations. The majority of cysts are less than 3 cm and asymptomatic. A single lining layer of cuboidal or columnar epithelium secretes serous fluid into the cyst cavity, and they generally do not communicate with the intrahepatic biliary tree.

Pathogenesis

Simple cysts of the liver are thought to arise congenitally from aberrant intrahepatic bile ducts that lose connection to the biliary tree. They are spheric or oval and range in size from a few millimeters to more than 20 cm. Very large cysts may cause atrophy of the surrounding hepatic parenchyma. Fluid contained within the cavity is generally serous but may appear brown if prior intracystic hemorrhage has occurred. The fluid results from retained secretory capacity of the epithelial lining of the cyst. In general, cysts will slowly expand over years as fluid accumulates with the largest cysts found in women older than the age of 50.

Indications for Intervention

In most cases, simple cysts are asymptomatic, have almost no malignant potential, and are rarely susceptible to rupture; thus intervention is not indicated unless symptomatic. Once the diagnosis of a simple cyst is established, further follow-up is not necessary unless symptoms develop. Gradual growth of cysts results in patients discounting symptoms for long periods. Symptoms are rare for cysts less than 5 cm but may occur with smaller, pedunculated cysts. Symptoms are most often a vague feeling of abdominal discomfort or fullness. Early satiety can occur when cysts compress the stomach. Abnormal liver function tests are rare unless bile duct compression occurs. An acute onset of abdominal pain may occur with hemorrhage into the cyst cavity.

Ultrasound most easily identifies simple cysts as round or oval anechoic, fluid-filled lesions with sharp borders. Septations are absent, but a false appearance of septations may occur with two adjacent cysts (Figure 1). With acute hemorrhage, imaging can

TABLE 1: Features and Management of Cystic Liver Lesions

Cystic Lesion	Clinical Findings	Radiographic Features	Management
BENIGN			
Simple cyst	Asymptomatic, may develop symptoms with pregnancy	Well-defined, unilocular round or oval cyst(s). Low fluid density	None unless symptomatic Alcohol sclerotherapy Laparoscopic fenestration
Ciliated foregut cyst	Pain at size <5 cm	Unilocular, subcapsular, single cyst near falciform ligament in segment IV. Four-layered wall on ultrasound.	Resection if >4 cm
Polycystic liver disease	Family history of PLD, history of PKD	Multiple cystic lesions on liver ± kidney. Gross hepatic enlargement	Open fenestration Liver resection Liver transplantation
Amebic abscess	Travel to endemic areas	Complex cyst with "double target" appearance	Metronidazole
Pyogenic liver Abscess	Clinical findings of infection	Complex cyst with rim enhancement	Percutaneous drainage and antibiotics Surgery if refractory
Hydatid cyst	Travel to endemic areas	Complex cyst with peripheral daughter cysts	Excision of cysts or pericystectomy
Traumatic cyst	History of trauma	Cystic liver lesions with variable density and intensity; density layering shifts with movement	None unless symptomatic or complications arise
NEOPLASTIC			
Cystadenoma	Absence of known infection, malignancy, or trauma, more common in females	Complex, multilocular cystic lesion with septations, microcalcification, and nodules. Contrast enhancement of septations	Enucleation Partial hepatectomy or lobectomy
Cystadenocarcinoma	Absence of known infection, malignancy, or trauma, more common in females	Complex, multilocular cystic lesion with septations, calcification, and nodules. Contrast enhancement of septations	Partial hepatectomy or lobectomy
IPMN-B	Absence of known infection, malignancy, or trauma, history of IPMN-P	Complex, multilocular cystic lesion with septations, calcification, and nodules. Biliary communication on ERCP or IOC. Bile duct dilation distal to tumor ± hepaticolithiasis	Partial hepatectomy or lobectomy with IOC ± extrahepatic biliary resection and portal lymphadenectomy
Embryonal sarcoma	Adolescent age	Large complex cystic lesion on CT or MRI. May appear solid on ultrasound.	Partial hepatectomy or lobectomy and chemotherapy
Cystic HCC	History of HBV, HCV, or cirrhosis	Complex hypervascular cystic lesion with portal venous washout	RFA TACE Partial hepatectomy or lobectomy Liver transplantation
Cystic metastasis	History of malignancy	Multiple complex cystic lesions with enhancement	Chemotherapy

CT, Computed tomography; *ERCP,* endoscopic retrograde cholangiopancreatography; *HBV,* hepatitis B virus; *HCC,* hepatocellular carcinoma; *HCV,* hepatitis C virus; *IOC,* intraoperative cholangiogram; *IPMN,* intraductal papillary mucinous neoplasm; *MRI,* magnetic resonance imaging; *RFA,* radiofrequency ablation; *TACE,* transarterial chemoembolization.

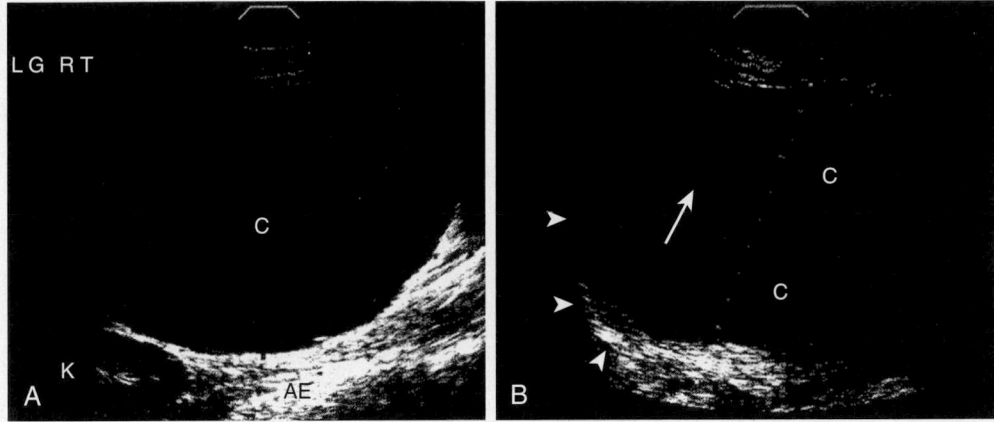

FIGURE 1 Ultrasound features of liver cysts. **A,** Simple cysts *(C)* have anechoic fluid, a thin imperceptible wall, and posterior acoustic enhancement *(AE)*. No internal features are present. *K,* Right kidney. **B,** Complex cysts have echogenic material within them, including internal septa *(white arrow)*, debris, and mural nodules or projections. These cysts *(C)* are multilocular. A thick, irregular wall *(white arrowheads)* is seen frequently in complex cysts.

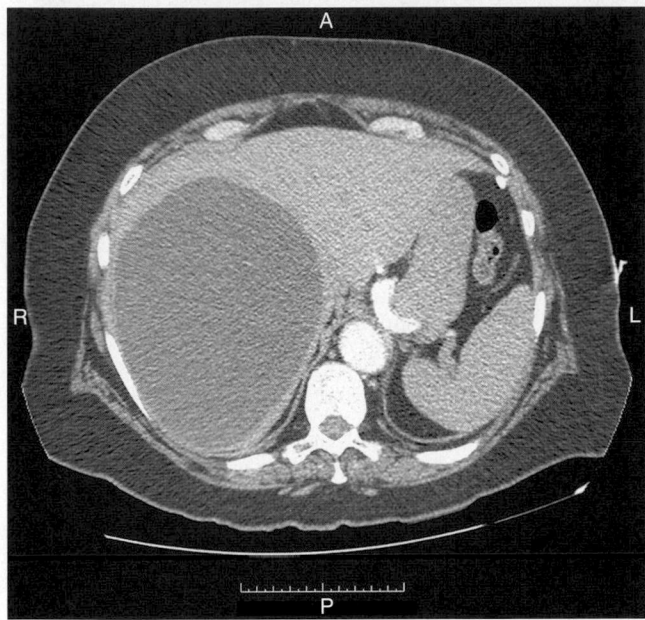

FIGURE 2 Computed tomography features of a simple liver cyst. CT scan of simple cysts will demonstrate a fluid density similar to water with no internal debris, projections, or nodules seen. The walls are thin and avascular, without contrast enhancement.

demonstrate increased fluid density and layering within the cyst cavity. The fluid density should move with patient rotation, unlike a cystic neoplasm. Other imaging modalities are generally not necessary but occasionally may be performed. CT scan will demonstrate avascular, water-dense, round lesions without septations (Figure 2). Very small cysts (<1 cm) can be difficult to distinguish from other liver lesions. On MRI, cysts are hypointense on T1-weighted imaging and hyperintense on T2-weighted imaging (Figure 3). Hemorrhagic cysts may become hyperintense on T1-weighted imaging. If concern for hydatid disease is present, MRI may be a useful tool for differentiation.

Techniques and Results of Therapy

Interventional Therapy

Ultrasound-guided cyst aspiration can be helpful to differentiate symptom causality. Temporary improvement of symptoms with aspiration should indicate that a patient's nonspecific symptoms are a result of the cyst. In this case, definitive therapy should be planned on the inevitable cyst reoccurrence. Sclerotherapy is the mainstay of interventional therapy for simple hepatic cysts. Ultrasound-guided puncture of the cyst followed by contrast instillation ensures the absence of biliary or peritoneal communications, which are contraindications to therapy. The aspirated cyst cavity is instilled with 95% ethanol or minocycline hydrochloride. For alcohol, the volume instilled should not exceed 120 mL to avoid severe ethanol intoxication. Alcohol is retained within the cyst for 2 to 4 hours, after which it is aspirated. Sedation often is required because of associated pain. The goal of therapy is ablation of the fluid-secreting epithelial lining of the cyst cavity. This process may be repeated if necessary. Therapy should be avoided in cases of biliary fistulization or recent intracystic hemorrhage. Severe hemorrhage may rarely occur, and inflammation induced by sclerotherapy can increase the difficulty of subsequent surgical therapy and imaging follow-up. Maximum efficacy may take up to 6 months for symptomatic relief. Ultimately, the cyst will often regress, with symptomatic reoccurrence in less than 5% of patients.

Surgical Therapy

The treatment of choice for a symptomatic, isolated, simple liver cyst is fenestration. Most commonly, this is performed laparoscopically; however, open fenestration may be considered. The cyst appears as a protuberant bulge on the liver surface. The cyst surface is punctured, and the anterior wall of the cyst is excised completely to open the cyst cavity (Figure 4). Produced fluid then may be absorbed by the peritoneum. Excision of the liver parenchyma should be avoided because this increases risk of postoperative bleeding or bile leaks. Large cysts can cause atrophy of surrounding hepatic parenchyma with relative sparing of vascular and biliary structures, which then may be in proximity to the cyst wall. The remaining cyst cavity epithelium may be fulgurated with an argon beam coagulator. It is important to send the cyst wall for pathologic evaluation to ensure that a cystadenoma or cystadenocarcinoma was not present. If identified, further resection of the cyst is indicated. Complications from fenestration are rare, but bleeding is the most common. Less than 5% of patients require open conversion. Bile leaks are the most concerning complication. If concern for biliary communication is present, an intraoperative cholangiogram should be performed. Most patients are discharged within 1 to 3 days; symptomatic improvements are experienced by 91% of patients. Symptomatic reoccurrence of the cyst is seen in less than 5% of patients.

Polycystic Liver Disease

Although simple cysts of the liver may be multiple, polycystic liver disease (PLD) is a distinct entity. A familial pattern of cystic liver disease suggests PLD. The degree of cystic liver involvement is highly

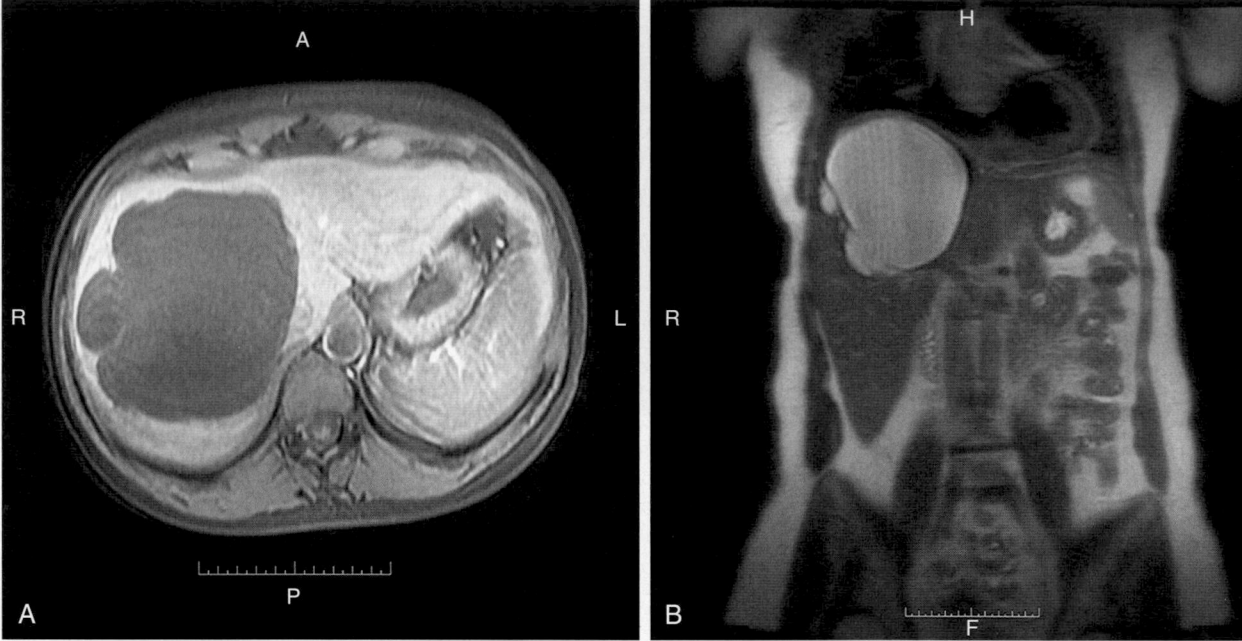

FIGURE 3 Magnetic resonance imaging of a simple liver cyst. **A,** Simple hepatic cysts appear hypointense on T1-weighted imaging. **B,** On T2-weighted imaging, cysts appear hyperintense. No internal debris or septations should be apparent.

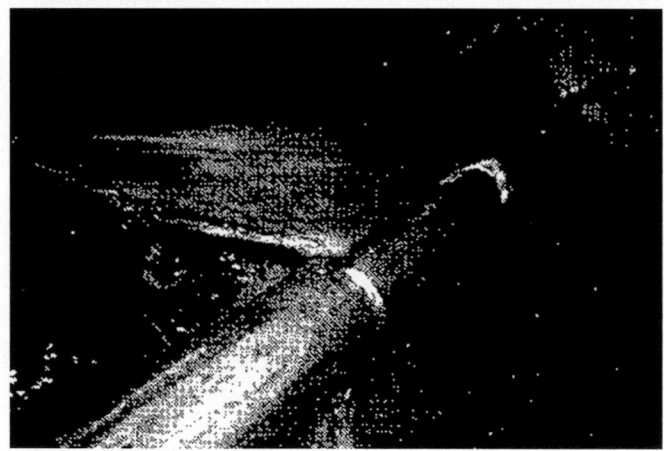

FIGURE 4 Laparoscopic cyst fenestration. The wall of the cyst should be excised completely with the transection plane at the interface between the cyst wall and the hepatic parenchyma. A coagulative heat source (not shown) or laparoscopic stapler may be used for excision.

TABLE 2: Gigot Classification of Polycystic Liver Disease

Category	Description
Type 1	Limited number (<10) of large cysts (>10 cm) with large areas of normal parenchyma
Type 2	Diffuse involvement of parenchyma by medium-sized cysts with large areas of uninvolved liver tissue
Type 3	Massive and diffuse involvement of the liver by small and medium-sized cysts with very little spared parenchyma

variable; thus distinction between these two entities may be difficult. PLD is staged on the basis of the Gigot classification (Table 2), which is defined by the number and size of hepatic cysts, as well as the remaining hepatic parenchyma. Determination of PLD classification is generally performed by CT or MRI imaging.

Pathogenesis

PLD may occur in isolation or, more commonly, in association with polycystic kidney disease (PKD). Both forms of the disease are associated with autosomal dominant transmission and a similar clinical course; however, responsible genetic mutations are distinct. Isolated PLD occurs more rarely, accounting for 10% to 20% of all PLD cases. Inherited genetic mutations of either the protein kinase C substrate 80K-H (*PRKCSH*) gene on chromosome 19 or the *SEC63* gene on chromosome 6 are responsible. Both responsible genes regulate early

secretory pathways of the cell. In approximately 90% of patients, PLD is associated with adult PKD. PKD is the most common genetically inherited renal disorder, resulting in progressive renal failure in 50% of affected individuals. PKD is caused by mutation of the *PKD1* or *PKD2* genes on chromosome 16, which encode polycystin-1 and polycystin-2, respectively. The familial pattern of inheritance results in early diagnosis; however, renal function generally is maintained until the fifth decade of life. Not all patients with PKD exhibit extrarenal cystic involvement. When present, liver cysts typically develop later than kidney cysts. Patients with symptomatic liver cysts are considered to have polycystic kidney and liver disease (PKLD). Other extrarenal manifestations, such as an increased incidence of cerebral aneurysms, require brain imaging as part of patient evaluation and especially before any planned operative intervention.

The liver cysts associated with PLD and PKLD are similar to simple cysts macroscopically and microscopically. They are lined with a single epithelial layer with phenotypic and functional characteristics of biliary epithelium. The genetic mutations associated with PLD result in abnormal intralobular bile ducts that fail to involute and/or connect with extralobular bile ducts, resulting in cyst formation. Growth results from proliferation of the epithelial cells in these complexes, and overgrown cells secrete fluid into the biliary microhamartomas.

Indications for Intervention

The majority of patients with PLD will not require surgical intervention. Therapeutic intervention should not be considered unless a patient becomes symptomatic. Even in the case of massive liver enlargement, patients may remain relatively asymptomatic. The most common clinical presentation is refractory pain resulting from increasing size of hepatic cysts and/or the liver as a whole. Additional symptoms may include early satiety, dyspnea, and lower extremity edema based on compression of the stomach, diaphragm, or inferior vena cava, respectively. Symptoms are thought only to occur once the cyst:parenchyma ratio is more than 1. Symptoms evolve over a prolonged period; thus patients often minimize their symptoms. Rapid progression or sudden onset of symptoms should raise concern for acute cystic complication, such as hemorrhage or infection. Biochemical hepatic deterioration is rare; however, hepatic failure may occur with massive PLD.

Symptomatic patients have a noted decrease in quality of life. Pain may become refractory, and patients may develop chronic wasting. Cyst fluid may become infected, cysts may rupture, or the patient may acutely hemorrhage into the cyst cavity. These complications are most common in hemodialysis patients. Additional serious complications such as hepatic venous outflow obstruction, biliary obstruction, and portal hypertension are indications for more urgent intervention (Table 3). Refractory ascites and/or pleural effusions may develop secondary to malnutrition or as a complication of fenestration. It remains controversial whether malignant transformation of cysts may occur. Cyst carcinoma and cholangiocarcinoma have been reported but are exceedingly rare.

Patients typically are referred for surgical evaluation after symptoms become incapacitating. Liver function tests should be evaluated, but the only laboratory abnormality that may be elevated is alkaline phosphatase or γ-glutamyl transpeptidase (GGT). Ultrasound imaging demonstrates multiple, fluid-filled, round cysts with sharp margins within the liver (and within the kidney in cases of PLKD). Coalescent cysts may give false impression of septations. Contrasted scans should be used judiciously given the commonality of concurrent PKD. On CT, cysts do not enhance and demonstrate a fluid attenuation of -5 to 20 Hounsfield units with distinct parenchymal margins. Vascular and biliary structures are often difficult to distinguish. On MRI, uncomplicated cysts are hyperdense on T2-weighted images and hypodense on T1-weighted images (Figure 5).

TABLE 3: Symptoms Associated With PLD

Symptom	Cause
Pain	Stretch of Gilson's capsule or irritation of parietal peritoneum
Early satiety	Gastric compression
Dyspnea	Diaphragmatic compression
Peripheral edema	IVC compression
Portal hypertension	Portal vein or hepatic venous outflow compression
Jaundice	Biliary compression
Ascites	Portal hypertension, malnutrition, or secondary to cyst fenestration
Esophageal varices	Portal hypertension

IVC, inferior vena cava.

Techniques and Results of Therapy
Medical Therapy

Medical therapies for PLD have been described with minimal efficacy. Because disease progresses with pregnancy, estrogen replacement should be avoided. Somatostatin analogues may decrease minimally liver volume in patients with massive PLD, but without symptomatic regression. The mTOR inhibitors have been associated anecdotally with liver and kidney cyst regression; however, the clinical impact of reduction is undetermined. Initial clinical trials of combined octreotide and everolimus therapy do not demonstrate significant regression over octreotide therapy alone.

Interventional Therapy

Transcatheter arterial embolization of liver cysts and kidney cysts also has been applied for treatment of PKLD, primarily in Japan. Hepatic arterial branches primarily supply hepatic cysts in PKLD patients, and branch embolization may increase parenchymal volume and reduce cyst volume. Patients did experience gradual symptomatic relief; however, the process is very labor intensive and time consuming. Cyst aspiration generally fails to alleviate in PLD given the large cyst burden. The best application for aspiration is the removal of infected fluid in cases of cyst infection. Percutaneous sclerotherapy similarly fails in most cases of PLD. Rigid parenchyma and surrounding cysts prevent collapse of treated cysts.

Surgical Therapy

In general, symptomatic patients should be referred for surgical evaluation. A small number of patients experience symptoms from a few very large cysts rather than the increased size of the entire liver. Open cyst fenestration alone may be helpful in these patients. The technique involves unroofing of superficial cysts to allow stepwise access to deeper cysts. Laparoscopic fenestration generally does not allow safe access to deeper cysts and at present should be considered only in patients with limited, large, superficial cysts.

In massive cystic disease, a combined resection and fenestration may be necessary. The aim of intervention is to decompress and debulk the liver and remove as many cysts as possible. Attention on imaging should be made to areas of the liver that are relatively spared from cystic involvement (often segments V or VI). Preservation of these areas allows for lobectomy or segmentectomy to debulk heavily involved segments combined with cyst fenestration of the remnant liver. Care must be taken intraoperatively to avoid damage to major vascular or biliary structures; cysts distort normal anatomic landmarks. Attention should be made on preoperative imaging to collateral circulation that may develop between the right and middle hepatic veins because of cystic compression of the right hepatic vein outflow. Fine-needle puncture of deeper septations before fenestration may be used to avoid unintentional resection of a compressed hepatic vein. Biliary injuries may result when cysts arise near the biliary confluence. As such, judicious use of IOC can ensure normal biliary drainage at case completion. Because of cystic compression of the hepatic or portal veins, approximately two thirds of patients with massive PLD may demonstrate fibrosis, centrilobular congestion, or nodular regenerative hyperplasia. This likelihood must be accounted for when planning resection to maintain sufficient liver volume.

The overall mortality is low from surgical debulking (<4%); however, morbidity ranges from an average of 30% for fenestration to 65% for resection. Most commonly, patients experience complications related to ascites and pleural effusion. Postoperative ascites results from continued secretion of fluid by cyst linings, liver outflow obstruction, and/or renal dysfunction. Ascites may delay wound healing or become secondarily infected. Reoperation for biliary leak or postoperative hemorrhage is required in approximately 10% of patients. Recurrent symptoms develop in approximately 35% of patients. Patients may experience a transient postoperative decline in renal function, and patients with preoperative renal dysfunction

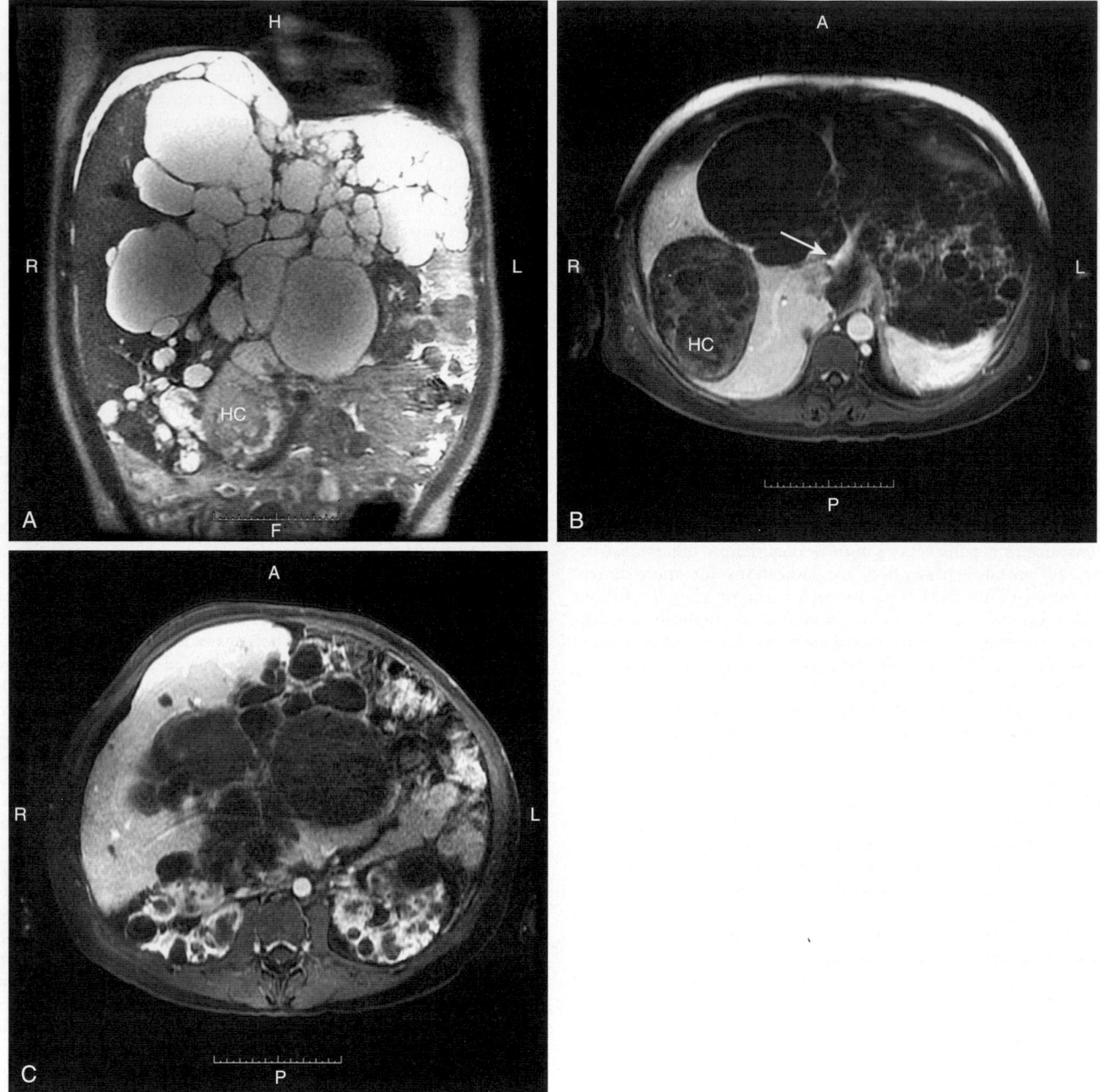

FIGURE 5 Magnetic resonance imaging of polycystic liver kidney disease. **A,** Multiple hepatic cysts are observed, nearly replacing the entire hepatic parenchyma. The liver is grossly enlarged, reaching nearly to the patient's pelvic brim. Uncomplicated cysts are hyperintense on T2-weighted imaging. The proximity of coalescing cysts gives the false impression of septations. Complicated cysts are observed (*HC*), indicating an evolving hemorrhagic cyst. **B,** On contrast-enhanced venous phase T1-weighted imaging, cysts appear hypointense. The vascular structures are difficult to identify, and the hepatic veins are compressed by surrounding cysts (*white arrow*). **C,** Concurrent polycystic kidney disease is commonly observed.

should be considered for simultaneous liver-kidney transplantation rather than surgery.

Transplantation

Liver transplantation is the single most definitive treatment for PLD. It offers a complete reversal of the symptoms and associated complications of the disease. Because of the high predilection for concurrent PKD, combined liver/kidney transplantation is required in approximately 40% of patients depending on the severity of kidney cysts and the degree of renal dysfunction. Thorough pretransplant evaluation of the patient's renal function is necessary to determine renal reserve.

Concurrent bilateral nephrectomy also should be considered for massively enlarged and symptomatic native kidneys.

Prioritization for liver transplantation is based on the severity of liver disease. The Model of End-Stage Liver Disease (MELD) scoring system determines the degree of biochemical liver dysfunction (measured by international normalized ratio and total bilirubin tests) and renal dysfunction (measured by serum creatinine level or need for dialysis). Because of the rare occurrence of biochemical liver disease, patients with PLD often cannot qualify for liver transplantation without additional MELD exception points. A particular patient's qualification for exception is granted subjectively by appeal to the

TABLE 4: Criteria for Obtaining MELD Exception in Listing Patients for Liver Transplantation With Polycystic Liver Disease

Criteria	Example
Massive PLD	Cyst:parenchyma ratio >1
Complications of PLD likely to resolve with transplantation	Biliary obstruction Venous outflow obstruction Portal hypertension Refractory ascites Recurrent cyst infections Refractory pain Chronic wasting
Not candidates for or have failed to respond to nontransplant interventions for symptom relief	Failed hepatic resection Malnutrition
Clinically significant manifestations of liver disease attributable to massive PLD	Cachexia Ascites Encephalopathy Portal hypertension Variceal bleeding Hepatic venous outflow obstruction Biliary obstruction Cholestasis Recurrent cyst infection
Severe malnutrition	Decreased lean body mass
Hypoalbuminemia	Serum albumin <2.2 mg/dL
Decreased lean body mass	Midarm circumference in nondominant arm between the acromion and olecranon process: <23.1 cm for females <23.8 cm for males

MELD, Model of End-Stage Liver Disease; *PLD,* polycystic liver disease.

regional review board, and the published exception point criteria are stringent (Table 4). In general, only patients with massive PLD, malnutrition, and significant complications are awarded qualifying points. Expected 5-year survival after liver transplant or simultaneous liver kidney transplant for PLD and PLKD is 80% to 85%.

Ciliated Hepatic Foregut Cysts

Ciliated foregut cysts may occur in any region of the embryonic foregut, including the liver and gallbladder. They are exceedingly rare and have a characteristic four-layered border with a ciliated columnar epithelial lining that may secrete fluid. Fluid may be watery, viscous, or mucous, leading to varied echogenicity on ultrasound. They generally demonstrate a subcapsular location, close to the insertion of the falciform ligament in segment IV. They are unilocular with a diameter of 2 to 6 cm. Most are discovered incidentally, but because of their subcapsular locations, even small cysts may cause pain. Because of their varied luminal contents, they occasionally may develop the appearance of an atypical solid tumor. Carbohydrate antigen (Ca) 19-9 may be elevated in cystic fluid and serum, making them difficult to distinguish from cystadenoma or

cystadenocarcinoma. Fine-needle aspiration may be helpful if it demonstrates ciliate, pseudostratified, columnar epithelium. Ciliated foregut cysts are generally benign, but malignant transformation has been described, especially with larger cysts. Resection is indicated for cysts that are larger than 4 cm, have wall abnormalities, cause pain, or enlarge rapidly.

Traumatic Cysts

Liver hematomas may occur as a result of traumatic, iatrogenic, or surgical damage to the liver. They may appear cystic but are not true cysts because they lack an epithelial lining. On occasion, they also may be associated with a ruptured liver lesion, such as a hepatic adenoma or hepatocellular carcinoma. Patients experience symptoms of severe acute pain, and generalized peritonitis or hemodynamic instability may occur with rupture of the liver capsule. Acutely, traumatic cysts appear echogenic on ultrasound. On CT scan, they demonstrate hyperdensity, and on MRI scan, they are hyperintense on T1-weighted imaging and hypointense on T2-weighted imaging. As the hematoma evolves, they take on a more cystic appearance as the clot liquefies. For unruptured cysts, management is conservative unless complications develop, such as bile leak, persistent pain, bleeding, or compression.

■ MANAGEMENT OF NEOPLASTIC CYSTIC LIVER DISEASE

Primary hepatic cystic neoplasms may be either benign (with malignant potential) or malignant. Rarely, other primary or secondary hepatic malignancies also may be cystic. This generally is due to tumor necrosis of portions of a solid hepatic malignancy. The overall incidence of all cystic liver tumors is low.

Hepatic Cystadenoma

There is some disagreement regarding the classification of hepatic cystadenomas. Approximately 85% of hepatic cystadenomas demonstrate ovarian-like stroma, and some exclude lesions without ovarian stroma from this category. Biliary cystic neoplasms have significant similarities to pancreatic mucinous cystic neoplasms and intraductal papillary mucinous neoplasms (IPMNs). A similar classification for hepatic cystadenomas has been proposed that is based on the cystic neoplasm's communication with the bile duct. For the purpose of this chapter, those with bile duct communication will be referred to as *intraductal papillary mucinous neoplasm of the bile duct* (IPMN-B).

Pathogenesis

Hepatic cystadenomas are the most common primary cystic tumor of the liver. Despite this, they likely account for less than 5% of all cystic hepatic lesions. They may arise from major biliary structures; however, most are intrahepatic. They carry a high risk of malignant transformation. Cystadenomas are solitary lesions ranging from 1 to 40 cm and may occur anywhere within the liver parenchyma. Grossly lobulated and multiloculated lesions are common; however, unilocular lesions do occur. Cyst contents are serous to mucinous in consistency. Hemorrhagic fluid is rare with adenomas and should alert to potential malignancy. Cyst walls demonstrate three distinct layers, inner epithelium, middle mesenchymal stroma, and an outer collagen connective tissue layer or pseudocapsule, which provides distinct separation from surrounding hepatic parenchyma. Epithelium may be cuboidal or columnar. Some areas may become denuded or demonstrate inflammation. Lumenal atypia, metaplasia, or dysplasia suggests high risk for malignant transformation. Eighty-five percent exhibit ovarian-like stroma and occur exclusively in women, whereas tumors without ovarian stroma occur in men and women and are more likely to have biliary communication.

Indications for Intervention

Hepatic cystadenomas with ovarian-like stroma occur almost exclusively in women with a peak incidence in the fourth or fifth decade of life. The symptoms may be similar to simple hepatic cysts. Because of the tremendous size potential of the lesion, increased abdominal girth and compressive symptoms are also common. The growth rate of these neoplasms is slow, leading to an insidious onset. With growth, adenomas may cause biliary compression and jaundice as well as acute pain. Rarely, rupture, hemorrhage, or superinfection may occur.

Diagnosis of hepatic cystadenomas relies primarily on imaging. Simple cysts, especially those with prior interventions or that have become atypical because of intracystic bleeding, may be difficult to distinguish. A mild elevation in serum alkaline phosphatase is sometimes seen. Ultrasound imaging demonstrates the presence of internal septations or papillary projections into the cystic space. On CT scan, adenomas appear as a hypodense, multiloculated mass with a well-defined border. Fluid attenuation is variable, and the septa may demonstrate fine calcifications and contrast enhancement (Figure 6). MRI is more reliable at demonstrating septations and loculations than CT scan. On MRI, cystadenomas are homogeneous and hyperintense on T2-weighted imaging and isointense or hypointense on T1-weighted imaging. Septations and loculations are seen, with septations demonstrating contrast enhancement. Cystadenomas are rarely multiple, and mild upstream dilation of bile ducts may be seen. Cytology is often nonspecific but may demonstrate chronic inflammatory exudate, bland cuboidal to columnar epithelial cells, or occasional papillary clusters. Analysis of cyst fluid may demonstrate increased Ca19-9 and carcinoembryonic antigen (CEA) levels; however, elevations are not diagnostic. Because of malignant potential all hepatic cystadenoma should be removed.

Techniques and Results of Therapy

Surgical therapy is the mainstay treatment for hepatic cystadenomas. There have been occasional reports of long-term success after fenestration with fulguration of the cyst lining; however, this is not recommended because of limited experience. Ablation may obscure follow-up imaging. When identified, cystadenomas may be removed either by partial hepatectomy or enucleation. The pseudocapsule surrounding the cyst generally makes separation from the surrounding parenchyma feasible. Care must be taken for lesions in segment 4 not to injure the biliary bifurcation. In these cases, an intraoperative

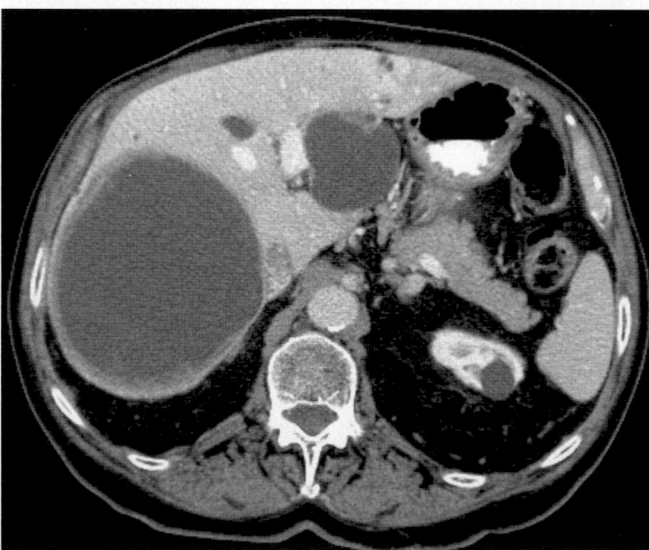

FIGURE 6 Contrast-enhanced computed tomography of hepatic cystadenoma. Two complex cystic lesions are observed with septations and contrast enhancement of the cyst wall, consistent with a diagnosis of cystadenoma.

cholangiogram is recommended to ensure the absence of biliary communication or tumor material within the bile duct. If bile is present within the cyst cavity or if biliary communication is identified, the diagnosis of IPMN-B should be excluded by frozen section analysis. Extrahepatic cystadenomas often require bile duct resection with bilioenteric reconstruction. Recurrence after either resection or enucleation is extremely rare.

Cystic Intraductal Papillary Mucinous Neoplasm of the Bile Duct

IPMN-Bs carry significant histologic and pathologic similarities to pancreatic IPMNs and hepatic cystadenomas. The main distinguishing factors from hepatic cystadenomas are a lack of ovarian-like stroma and communication with the bile ducts. Classification of these as a distinct pathologic category is relatively new.

Pathogenesis

IPMN-Bs are characterized pathologically by their ability to produce mucin and the presence of biliary intraluminal papillary proliferations. They are almost exclusively found in association with intrahepatic bile ducts. Two distinct variants exist: *cystic IPMN-B* and *duct ectatic IPMN-B*. Cystic IPMN-Bs generally occur as a large cystic mass of the liver. Similar to side-branch IPMNs of the pancreas, these entities are thought to arise from small peripheral bile ducts. They may resemble cystadenomas or cystadenocarcinomas because of the presence of cystic and solid mass components. Various degrees of atypia often are found within the biliary epithelium from low-grade dysplasia to invasive adenocarcinoma. Those with microinvasive or macroinvasive adenocarcinoma often are associated with large dilated ducts, mucobilia, and hepatolithiasis. They are often multilocular and occasionally hemorrhagic. They have an extremely high malignant potential, with in situ and invasive adenocarcinoma found in greater than 60% of cystic IPMN-Bs.

Indications for Intervention

Cystic IPMN-B typically occurs in the sixth decade of life. Most patients are asymptomatic, but jaundice, epigastric pain, and cholangitis may occur, especially in patients with concurrent hepaticolithiasis. On CT or MRI scan, cystic variants are difficult to distinguish from cystadenomas or cystadenocarcinomas. They occur as multilocular masses between 2 and 17 cm with septations and calcifications; however, they often contain large mural bile duct nodules with biliary ductal dilatation distal to the tumor. ERCP or IOC (but not MRCP) may demonstrate narrow biliary luminal communication. IPMN-B may occur concurrently with IPMN of the pancreas in some patients and should be excluded on preoperative imaging.

Techniques and Results of Therapy

Because of the high rate of malignancy seen in IPMN-Bs, intervention is indicated for all cystic IPMN-Bs. IOC should be performed to verify the presence of biliary communication. Retained mucin within the bile ducts must be excluded; it may result in postoperative biliary obstruction and cholangitis. The concern with IPMN-B in comparison with cystadenoma or cystadenocarcinoma is for superficial spread along the bile duct lumen; thus formal hepatectomy is the preferred operative approach. Enucleation is often insufficient to excise all involved biliary epithelium and may result in increased recurrence. Extrahepatic biliary resection and/or portal lymphadenectomy may be necessary in some cases. Overall, outcomes for hepatic resection with IPMN-B exceed that seen for cholangiocarcinoma, even in patients with malignant transformation, with 5-year patient survival ranging from 60% to 80%.

Hepatic Cystadenocarcinoma

Cystadenocarcinomas occur rarely, presumably arising from malignant transformation of a hepatic cystadenoma. Most are intrahepatic, and they tend to lack bile duct communication. Communication with the bile duct should raise suspicion of an alternative diagnosis, such as IPMN-B or a cystic variant of cholangiocarcinoma.

Pathogenesis

Similar to cystadenomas, cystadenocarcinomas may occur with or without ovarian-like stroma. Hepatic cystadenocarcinomas are generally solitary, which distinguishes them from hepatic metastases of pancreatic or ovarian cystadenocarcinomas. Their peak incidence occurs in the fifth and sixth decade. Patients often have a progressive abdominal mass, pain, or symptoms of obstructive jaundice (up to 20% of patients). Tumor rupture and acute intracystic hemorrhage may occur with some frequency, leading to a more acute presentation of abdominal pain. Evidence of intracystic hemorrhage or bilious content is common. As with other cystic hepatic masses, diagnosis may be delayed by the insidiously progressive nature of presenting symptoms.

Indications for Intervention

Hepatic cystadenocarcinomas range in size from 2 to 40 cm; thus size cannot be used as a discriminating factor to determine malignant potential. Tumor markers rarely are elevated; however, Ca19-9 occasionally may demonstrate a mild increase. Cyst fluid analysis is rarely helpful in differentiating diagnosis; atypical cells rarely are retrieved. Cyst fluid CEA and Ca19-9 are comparably elevated to cystadenomas and are not discriminatory. Caution should be used with even performing a cyst aspiration with suspected cystadenocarcinoma in the differential diagnosis because of a high risk of peritoneal seeding. On imaging, cystadenocarcinomas have similar appearance to cystadenomas and are generally difficult to distinguish. Intracystic hemorrhage or cyst wall nodularity is often present. Intracystic septae tend to be larger, and coarse calcifications are seen along cyst walls. Septa and nodules demonstrate enhancement with contrast administration.

Techniques and Results of Therapy

Surgical resection is the mainstay of treatment for hepatic cystadenocarcinomas. Intraoperative cholangiogram is recommended to exclude biliary communications and to distinguish them from IPMN-Bs. Microscopic tumor extension may exceed that demonstrated on preoperative or intraoperative imaging; thus formal hepatic resection or wedge resection with a wide margin is preferred over enucleation. Partial resection of the extrahepatic biliary tree with bilioenteric reconstruction may be necessary for tumors in proximity to the biliary confluence. Spillage of cyst contents should be avoided to prevent development of carcinomatosis. Given complete resection, patient survival and reoccurrence rates exceed that of hepatocellular carcinoma.

Embryonal Hepatic Sarcoma

Embryonal sarcomas are very rare tumors occurring in children 2 to 15 years of age; however, they occasionally may occur in early adulthood. They occur as very large, poorly differentiated tumors of the liver and may have both myxoid and necrotic contents. Because of tumor necrosis, they may become partially or, rarely, completely cystic; however, more commonly they appear cystic only on a CT or MRI scan because of high water content of the myxoid stroma. Ultrasound generally demonstrates solid tissues. Contrasted CT or MRI imaging may be helpful in distinguishing these from simple cysts or other cystic neoplasms because of the presence of late contrast enhancement.

Hepatocellular Carcinoma and Cholangiocarcinoma

Similar to embryonal sarcomas, hepatocellular carcinomas and cholangiocarcinomas may occasionally experience cystic degradation resulting from tumor necrosis. This may be either spontaneous or induced by therapy. Full discussion of the management of these tumors is presented elsewhere in this textbook (see Chapter 68).

Secondary Cystic Hepatic Neoplasms

Metastatic tumors to the liver rarely develop a complete or partial cystic component. This has been observed most frequently with neuroendocrine tumors, sarcoma, or melanoma. Metastatic carcinoma of the bronchus and breast, as well as ovarian or pancreatic cystadenocarcinoma also may develop cystic hepatic lesions. On CT or MRI scan, the presence of peripheral hypervascularity and multiplicity should raise suspicion of this diagnosis.

SUGGESTED READINGS

Arrazola L, Moonka D, Gish RG, et al. Model for end-stage liver disease (MELD) exception for polycystic liver disease. *Liver Transpl.* 2006;12(12 suppl 3):S110-S111.

Borhani AA, Wiant A, Heller MT. Cystic hepatic lesions: a review and an algorithmic approach. *AJR Am J Roentgenol.* 2014;203:1192-1204.

Farges O, Vilgrain V, Aussilhou B. Inflammatory, infective, and congenital: nonparasitic liver cysts. In: Jarnagin WR, Belghiti J, Buchler MW, et al., eds. *Blumgart's Surgery of the Liver, Biliary Tract, and Pancreas.* Philadelphia: Elsevier Saunders; 2012:992-1005.

Farges O, Vilgrain V. Cystic hepatobiliary neoplasia. In: Jarnagin WR, Belghiti J, Buchler MW, et al., eds. *Blumgart's Surgery of the Liver, Biliary Tract, and Pancreas.* Philadelphia: Elsevier Saunders; 2012:1268-1282.

Kelly K, Weber SM. Cystic diseases of the liver and bile ducts. *J Gastrointest Surg.* 2014;18:627-634.

THE MANAGEMENT OF ECHINOCOCCAL CYST DISEASE OF THE LIVER

Calvin Eriksen, MD, and Vatche G. Agopian, MD

■ BACKGROUND AND ETIOLOGY

Hepatic cystic echinococcosis, also termed *hydatid cyst disease,* is a zoonotic infection caused by the cestode of the genus *Echinococcus,* most commonly *Echinococcus granulosus* or *Echinococcus multilocularis.* Although archaeologic evidence of echinococcal infection dates as far back as 8000 years, it was not until Francesco Redi's observations in the seventeenth century that the disease was thought to be due to a parasitic infection. The life cycle of *E. granulosus* involves a canine primary host; sheep are the most common of large grass-eating mammals to act as the intermediate host. Infection in humans is incidental and is due to the fecal-oral transmission of the larval form of the tapeworm from the feces of intermediate hosts. *E. granulosus* is endemic in Africa, the Middle East, South America, Asia, and parts of Europe, with a reported incidence as high as 1% to 12% in pastoral communities. In comparison, *E. multilocularis* demonstrates a rodent-fox life cycle and has a much smaller endemic region limited to areas of Eastern Europe, Russia, and parts of China.

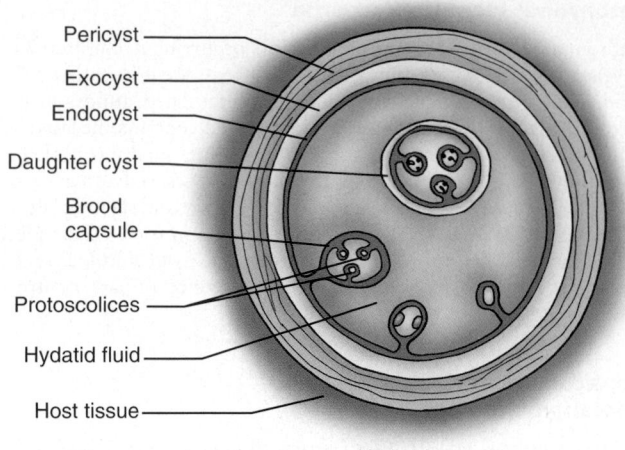

FIGURE 1 Schematic diagram of structure of echinococcal cyst showing pericyst, exocyst, endocyst, and protoscolices.

PATHOLOGIC SUBTYPES OF ECHINOCOCCAL INFECTION

Echinococcal infections are divided into two distinct types, cystic and alveolar. Cystic echinococcus (CE) is the predominant form and most commonly caused by *E. granulosus*, although two other species, *E. vogeli* and *E. oligarthrus*, also have been demonstrated to cause cystic disease. Although infection can occur in any organ, approximately 80% of infections involve a single organ; the liver (80%) and lung (20%) most commonly are affected. The cyst structure includes the pericyst, an outer adventitial layer of reactive host cells; the exocyst, a massive carbohydrate-rich acellular laminated layer; and the endocyst, an inner germinal layer that produces the brood capsules or "daughter" cysts containing the protoscolices (Figure 1). Daughter cysts can be present within the primary cyst or can extend beyond it. The cyst fluid is generally clear and may contain scolices or hooklets, with cloudy or discolored fluid suggesting communication with the biliary tree or secondary infection.

Alveolar echinococcal infections generally are caused by *E. multilocularis*, have a high affinity for the liver (only 1% of cases are primarily extrahepatic), and tend to behave more "tumor-like" with an invasive noncystic growth pattern. Parasitic vesicles can be seen on histopathologic assessment of a liver biopsy with period acid–Schiff staining. Polymerase chain reaction (PCR) can be used to detect *E. multilocularis*–specific nucleic acids on biopsy samples.

PRESENTATION AND DIAGNOSIS

The clinical presentation of hepatic cystic echinococcosis is highly variable. Nearly 50% of patients are asymptomatic at the time of diagnosis, with symptomatic patients demonstrating a wide range of clinical presentations from right upper quadrant pain to fevers, jaundice resulting from biliary obstruction, portal hypertension, Budd-Chiari syndrome resulting from venous outflow obstruction, and secondary cyst infection leading to liver abscess formation. Symptoms generally occur as the result of compression of adjacent structures; however, occasionally the cysts may rupture into the biliary tree or peritoneal cavity, potentially resulting in biliary obstruction or an acute abdomen with anaphylaxis, respectively. In cases of alveolar echinococcus resulting from *E. multilocularis*, similar compressive symptoms may occur, but cyst rupture and anaphylaxis are unlikely because alveolar echinococcus is not primarily a cystic disease.

The clinical diagnosis of echinococcal disease is based on patient history, laboratory evaluation, imaging studies, and histopathologic

findings in the aspirated cyst fluid or resected specimens. Laboratory evaluation usually includes a complete blood count (CBC) with differential looking for eosinophilia, liver function tests (LFTs), and most importantly serum antigen testing. Serum antigen testing largely has replaced the less specific complement fixation tests, such as the Casoni's skin test, which were previously the gold standard. The current enzyme-linked immunosorbent assay (ELISA) antigen testing has a sensitivity ranging between 85% to 89%, with some degree of cross-reactivity for other cestode or helminthic infections. When the diagnosis is in doubt, confirmatory testing for *E. granulosus* can be performed by either immunoblotting or ELISA techniques to assess for antigen 5 and antigen B. For patients with alveolar disease, the Em2 antigen has a 99% specificity for *E. multilocularis*.

Imaging

Cystic Echinococcus

Ultrasound is an excellent cost-effective modality for examining cystic lesions of the liver. In 1995 the World Health Organization Informal Working Groups on Echinococcus (WHO-IWGE) modified the previous echinococcal classification system of Gharbi with a subsequent modification in 2003 to the current classification system for CE based on ultrasonographic criteria (Table 1). CL lesions are cysts that are potentially parasitic, but confirmatory testing is required. CE 1 and CE 2 lesions are considered to be active echinococcal cysts, with either unilocular (CE 1) or multilocular (CE 2) ultrasonographic findings. CE 3 lesions are considered to be transitional and can be subdivided further into C3a, which have detached endocysts, or C3b, which are predominantly solid with daughter vesicles. CE 4 and CE 5 lesions are considered to be inactive cysts without viable, infectious protoscolices and often contain calcifications with a solid interior. Inactive cysts generally do not require treatment, whereas active and transitional cysts should be treated.

Computed tomography (CT) provides excellent characterization of cystic lesions and their relations to the hepatic vasculature and biliary anatomy and is useful for preoperative evaluation and planning (Figure 2). CT also can provide imaging of extrahepatic disease. Magnetic resonance imaging (MRI) is preferred to CT scanning whenever possible because it best discriminates echinococcal cysts from amebic cysts, congenital cysts, and cystadenomas; provides better visualization of cystic matrix; and along with magnetic resonance cholangiopancreatography (MRCP), can be used to evaluate for the presence of a cystobiliary communication (Figure 3).

Alveolar Echinococcus

In contrast to CE resulting from *E. granulosus*, ultrasound imaging of alveolar echinococcus (AE) resulting from *E. multilocularis* often reveals a pseudotumor, with nearly 70% of cases demonstrating areas of hypoechogenicity and hyperechogenicity with irregular borders, with occasional cystic components from central necrosis. In the remaining 30% of cases, alveolar lesions may have a hemangioma-like appearance, or the presence of small calcifications. CT imaging generally provides excellent anatomic depiction of the lesions and demonstrates calcifications easily (Figure 4). MRI with MRCP can be used to assess the relation of the lesion to the biliary tree. Positron emission tomography (PET) can be performed either with CT or MRI and is useful for detecting "metastatic" lesions as well as demonstrating active areas of infection within the liver. However, lack of uptake on PET imaging does not rule out the presence of infection but suggests that the inflammatory process is being suppressed.

Given the challenges in securing a definitive diagnosis of echinococcal cystic disease and distinguishing it from other cystic liver lesions, the World Health Organization (WHO) has defined categories of echinococcal disease based on clinical history (e.g., anaphylaxis secondary to cyst rupture), presence of serum antibodies, imaging findings consistent with hydatid disease, histopathologic findings in aspirated cyst fluid, and pathologic findings in resected specimens. Complicated echinococcal cystic disease is defined by

TABLE 1: Ultrasonographic Findings and Treatment Algorithm Adapted from WHO-IWGE

WHO-IWGE Classification	CL	CE 1	CE 2	CE 3	CE 4	CE 5
Representative ultrasonographic image						
Ultrasound Features	Unilocular, anechoic. Usually round. Cyst wall not visible	Unilocular, Anechoic Round or oval Cyst wall visible Hydatid sand *(snowflake)*	Multivesicular Septated Round or oval Cyst wall visible *Rosette, honeycomb-like*	Detached floating membrane Less round, complex *Water lily sign*	Heterogeneous, hypoechoic degenerating membrane No daughter cyst *Ball of wool*	Thick, calcified wall Arch-shaped *Cone-shaped shadow*
Medical treatment	Needs diagnosis from treatment	Yes	Yes	Yes	No†	No†
PAIR	—	Yes *	Yes*	Yes*	No†	No†
Surgery	—	No	Yes‡	Yes‡	No†	No†

Images taken from WHO-IWGE. *Acta Tropica*. 2003;85:253-261.

*For CE 1-CE 3 lesions <5 cm albendazole treatment is minimal requirement, PAIR alone also can be considered; however, optimal treatment should consist of albendazole + PAIR, when possible, especially for lesions >5 cm.

†For CE 4-CE 5 inactive lesions, a watch and wait approach is indicated.

‡Surgery is indicated for complicated cystic disease (i.e., intrabiliary cyst rupture with jaundice and cholangitis, intraperitoneal rupture, or aspiration of bilious or purulent fluid from within the cyst).

CE, Cystic echinococcus; *PAIR,* Puncture Aspiration Injection Reaspiration; *WHO-IWGE,* World Health Organization Informal Working Groups on Echinococcus.

intrabiliary cyst rupture with jaundice and cholangitis, intraperitoneal rupture, or aspiration of bilious or purulent fluid from within the cyst. A cystic lesion is a *possible case* of echinococcus when the clinical history and imaging *or* seropositivity is consistent with echinococcal infection, whereas a *probable case* has supportive clinical history, imaging, and two positive serologies. A *confirmed case* requires a clinical history, imaging studies, and serum testing consistent with echinococcal disease, *plus* (1) microscopic demonstration of protoscolices and/or hooklets *or* (2) changes in ultrasonographic imaging, showing a progression as defined by the WHO ultrasound classification (e.g., a CE 1 cyst progressing to a CE 3, either spontaneously or as the result of medical treatment). For cases of AE, confirmation is based on histopathology and detection of the *E. multilocularis* nucleic acid in a specimen by PCR.

■ TREATMENT

The goals of treatment for echinococcal liver disease are to mitigate symptoms, prevent progression of disease and the development of secondary complications, and eradicate the parasite with a combination of medical therapy and interventional strategies, including percutaneous and laparoscopic/open surgical procedures. The specific management varies by the type of infection, and treatment should be tailored to the particular presentation. Smaller, uncomplicated cysts may require minimal treatment with antiparasitic agents alone, whereas larger or complicated cystic disease usually requires surgical intervention to achieve cure. The WHO-IWGE recommendations generally are based on the imaging features; however, the availability

of local resources and surgical expertise are paramount when determining a treatment plan that will maximize the probability of cure while minimizing morbidity and mortality.

Medical Management

The mainstay of systemic treatment for echinococcal disease is with the benzimidazole class of antihelminthic drugs, the most effective of which is albendazole, given its excellent oral bioavailability and concentration in the cysts (10 to 15 mg/kg/day orally in two divided doses). However, mebendazole, praziquantel, and ivermectin also have protoscolicidal properties. Benzimidazoles are contraindicated in pregnancy because of teratogenic effects noted in animal studies and should be avoided in patients with chronic liver disease and bone marrow suppression because of their potential side effects, including hepatotoxicity, leukopenia, and thrombocytopenia. The combination of albendazole with 40 mg/kg/day of praziquantel once a week appears to be more effective in killing the protoscolices than albendazole alone. Patients with small (<5 cm), uncomplicated cysts (CE 1 and CE 3) respond well to medical treatment alone; however, for larger or more complicated cysts, the success rate of medical monotherapy is approximately 30%. In these circumstances, medical treatment should be used in combination with percutaneous or operative approaches to minimize recurrence and achieve cure. Medical treatment also is indicated for inoperable disease, multiorgan involvement, and in patients with peritoneal cysts. Monitoring of liver enzymes and blood counts is essential in patients on long-term treatment with benzimidazoles.

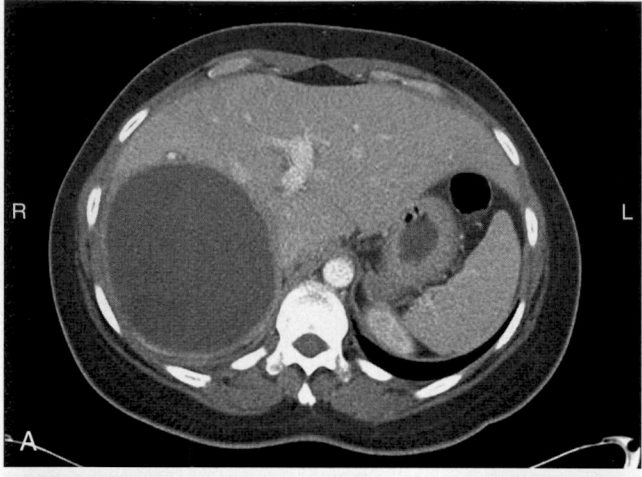

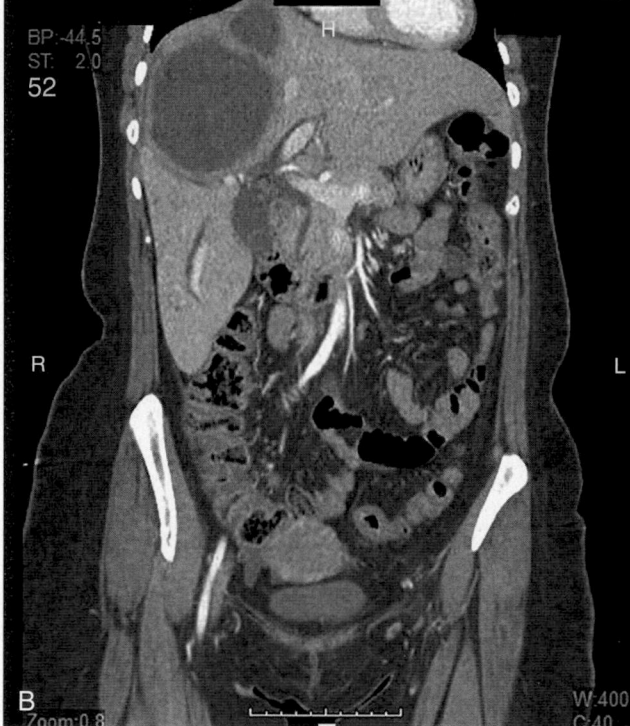

FIGURE 2 Computed tomography image showing a large echinococcal cyst in (**A**) axial and (**B**) coronal views. Note smaller daughter cyst superiorly in coronal view.

Percutaneous Approaches

Initially described in the early 1980s, percutaneous treatment of echinococcal cysts has had an increasing role in the management of select patients over the last several decades. Percutaneous therapy consists of simple catheter drainage aimed at evacuating the entire endocyst, or the PAIR treatment (*P*uncture, *A*spiration, *I*njection, and *R*easpiration) aimed at destroying the germinal cyst layer, reducing the size of the cyst, and eventually collapsing and solidifying the cyst. The PAIR technique uses ultrasound-guided percutaneous puncture of cyst via a transhepatic approach to avoid intraperitoneal spillage of cyst contents, followed by aspiration of the cyst fluid, injection of scolicidal agents (most commonly 20% hypertonic saline or 95% ethanol instilled for 10 to 15 minutes), and reaspiration of the fluid. PAIR generally is recommended for small (<5 cm), unilocular CE 1 and CE 3a lesions that are readily accessible percutaneously but can be considered in patients developing recurrence after operation,

inoperable cases, and pregnant patients or young children not fit for major surgery. Complicated cysts with infection, rupture, or evidence of biliary or pulmonary communication present an absolute contraindication to PAIR. The WHO recommends prophylaxis with a benzimidazole to start at least 4 hours before PAIR and to continue for 1 month after the procedure. Percutaneous catheter drainage usually is reserved for large (>10 cm), unilocular, uncomplicated disease; the catheter is left in place until the daily output is less than 10 mL/day.

The advantages of PAIR include its minimally invasive approach, lower cost compared with surgical therapy, and the ability to confirm diagnosis via testing of the cyst fluid. However, care must be taken to avoid spillage of daughter cysts, which may invoke anaphylaxis and seed the peritoneal cavity. Furthermore, recognition of the presence of cystobiliary communication is essential to avoid the risks for postprocedural biliary fistula, as well as the development of sclerosing cholangitis if the scolicidal agents enter the biliary tree. A large metaanalysis in 2003 compared PAIR plus benzimidazoles with surgical therapy and found that PAIR with medical therapy had superior cure rates with fewer recurrences and morbidity. However, the surgical comparison group was a historical control of mixed complexity cases; the majority did not receive concomitant drug therapy, making it difficult to draw any definitive conclusions. Although better data are necessary, PAIR appears to be an excellent choice in select patients with smaller, uncomplicated cysts when performed by experienced interventionalists.

Surgical Management

Before the introduction of percutaneous approaches, surgical management of echinococcal cystic disease of the liver was the primary therapeutic modality and continues to be the gold standard treatment for larger complex cysts. The WHO guidelines recommend surgical treatment for patients with large, complicated liver cysts, including cysts with infection, communication to the biliary tree, superficial cysts at risk of rupture, those with multiple daughter cysts, and cysts exerting pressure on adjacent vital organs. The diverse terminology used to describe operations performed for cystic echinococcus can be confusing and includes terms such as *capitonnage, fenestration, marsupialization, cystectomy,* and *pericystectomy.* To simplify our understanding, surgical treatment should be conceptualized broadly as "conservative" or "radical," depending on the extent of the operation.

The conservative approach essentially involves a partial or subtotal resection of the cyst, in which the endocyst is resected but the pericyst is left behind. As a result of leaving the pericyst, there is an obligatory residual cavity that must be managed appropriately to guarantee the success of the conservative approach. Although placement of an external drain has been used, this approach has now fallen out of favor, and evidence suggests that omentoplasty with securing of an omental pedicle into the cyst cavity reduces morbidity and recurrence compared with all other approaches. In contrast, the radical approach is aimed at removing the entire cyst, including the pericyst, and can be performed as a pericystectomy, a segmental or lobar liver resection, and in rare circumstances, liver transplantation. Although radical approaches tend to have decreased recurrence rates because the entire cyst is removed, there is an increased risk of perioperative morbidity because of the inherently more aggressive nature of the intervention.

Both conservative and radical operations can be performed either laparoscopically or with an open approach, with the overarching goals to safely evacuate the cyst contents, eradicate the parasite with a scolicidal agent, prevent spillage and subsequent recurrence, and minimize morbidity and mortality. The ultimate decision of the "best" surgical approach should be made based on surgeon experience as well as patient-specific factors, including location and size of the cyst and its proximity to and involvement of biliary or vascular structures. Regardless of the surgical approach, upfront treatment with a benzimidazole at least 1 day before surgery and up to 1 month

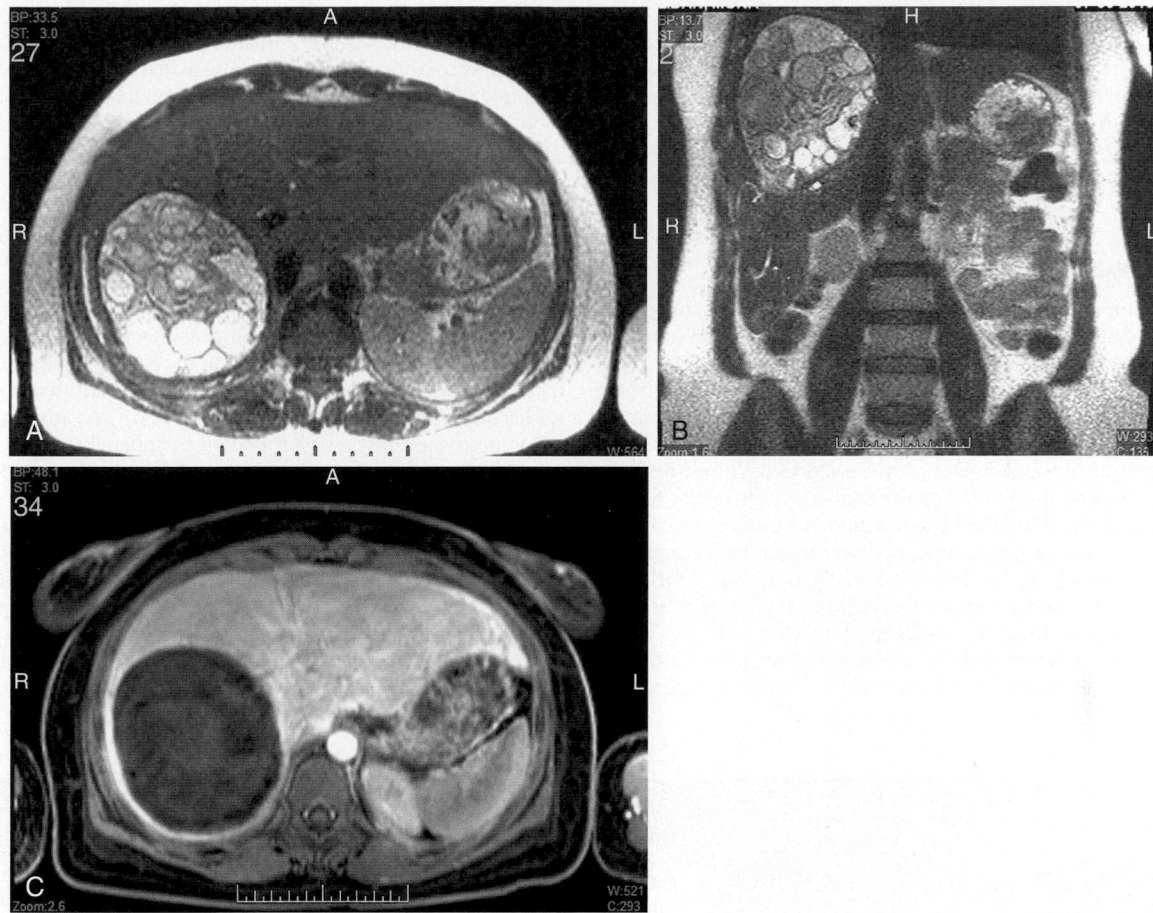

FIGURE 3 Magnetic resonance imaging of echinococcal cyst from a single patient in T2-weighted (**A**) axial and (**B**) coronal views and T1-weighted contrast enhanced image (**C**) demonstrating superior definition of septations and daughter cysts compared with the CT images of the same patient shown in Figure 2.

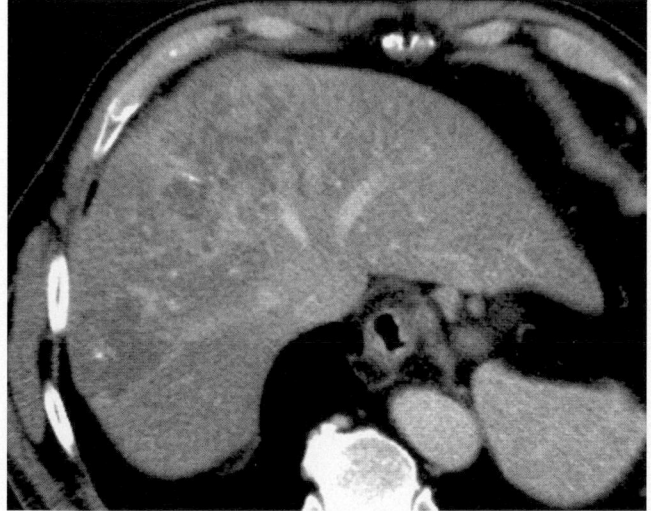

FIGURE 4 Computed tomography image showing the infiltrative pattern of alveolar echinococcus. *(From The Liver Imaging Atlas: www.liveratlas.org. Copyright © 2010 University of Washington. All rights reserved.)*

postoperatively is essential to decrease the risks of residual or recurrent disease.

Laparoscopic Drainage/Resection

Laparoscopy can be used for conservative and radical approaches, with multiple reports demonstrating safety and efficacy in well-selected patients. In general, we consider the laparoscopic approach for cysts that are located in easily accessible locations, such as the anterior/inferior liver segments 3, 4B, 5, and 6, which allows for minimization of the risk of spillage and adequate cyst content evacuation. Before entering the cyst cavity, scolicidal-soaked sponges should be placed through the trocars and surround the cyst to catch any spilled contents. The cyst then is punctured with a large-gauge needle and contents aspirated, allowing the endocyst to collapse. The trocars then can be upsized to allow for aspiration of the germinal membrane, with several recent reports describing large specialized trocars with attached suction ports that are effective in evacuating the cavity without spillage.

The advantages of the laparoscopic approach include more rapid recovery, shorter operative time and hospital stay, and decreased costs compared with conventional open surgery. However, disadvantages of laparoscopy include challenges in safely accessing posterior/superior segmental cysts and cysts located deep in the liver, as well as a limited ability to effectively drain all of the cyst contents with the standard laparoscopic suction equipment. In addition, laparoscopy has a slightly higher risk of cyst spillage into the peritoneal cavity, thought to be related to the increased abdominal pressures that occur with pneumoperitoneum. In a meta-analysis of outcomes for laparoscopic surgical approaches, including partial cystectomy, complete pericystectomy, and segmental resection, overall postoperative recurrence rates were remarkably low at 1%. We anticipate that this approach will gain popularity in well-selected patients as the collective experience with laparoscopy grows.

Open Operative Therapy

Open operation generally is recommend for large, multiloculated or complicated cysts and cysts in difficult to access posterior/superior segments of the liver and located deep within the hepatic tissue. The conservative open cyst evacuation should be performed with upfront systemic scolicidal therapy and with placement of hypertonic saline-soaked sponges and meticulous aspiration and drainage to avoid spillage. Removal of the daughter cysts, resection of the active germinal lining, and removal of debris is essential. A cyst-biliary fistula should be suspected if the fluid is bile stained or in large (>7.5 cm) cysts where the incidence is as high as 79%, prompting a search for the biliary communication and direct suture ligation with absorbable sutures followed by omentoplasty. Preoperative MRCP is very helpful in delineating the anatomy in these large cysts where a biliary communication can be anticipated and where use of intracyst scolicidal injection is contraindicated because of the risk of sclerosing

cholangitis. In these circumstances, placement of an external drain along the cyst cavity is recommended. Intraoperatively, we find that application of dilute hydrogen peroxide in the cyst cavity is extremely helpful in highlighting and identifying any small biliary communications. Rarely, a large biliary fistula requiring a bilioenteric anastomosis may be encountered. Despite operative measures to ensure identification and closure of a biliary fistula, occasionally a bile leak may persist postoperatively. In these circumstances, endoscopic retrograde cholangiopancreatography (ERCP) with sphincterotomy is usually therapeutic, with percutaneous transhepatic drainage a secondary option for recalcitrant leaks.

Ideally, given the morbidity that accompanies the abdominal incision when performing an open surgical intervention, we recommend a radical approach when feasible with the goal to perform a complete pericystectomy or a liver resection, excising the entire cyst with a rim of healthy liver tissue. Similar to the more conservative cyst evacuations, pericystectomy is best suited for peripherally located large cysts close to the surface of the liver. Although "closed" pericystectomy can be performed without draining the cyst contents, our preference during open pericystectomy of superficial cysts is to aspirate the cyst contents and ablate the cyst lining with injection of 20% hypertonic saline solution. We feel this approach best reduces the risk of accidental spillage during pericystectomy, in which the cyst may be entered inadvertently (Figure 5).

Liver resection is a more "radical" approach to echinococcal cyst disease of the liver and can range from nonanatomic wedge

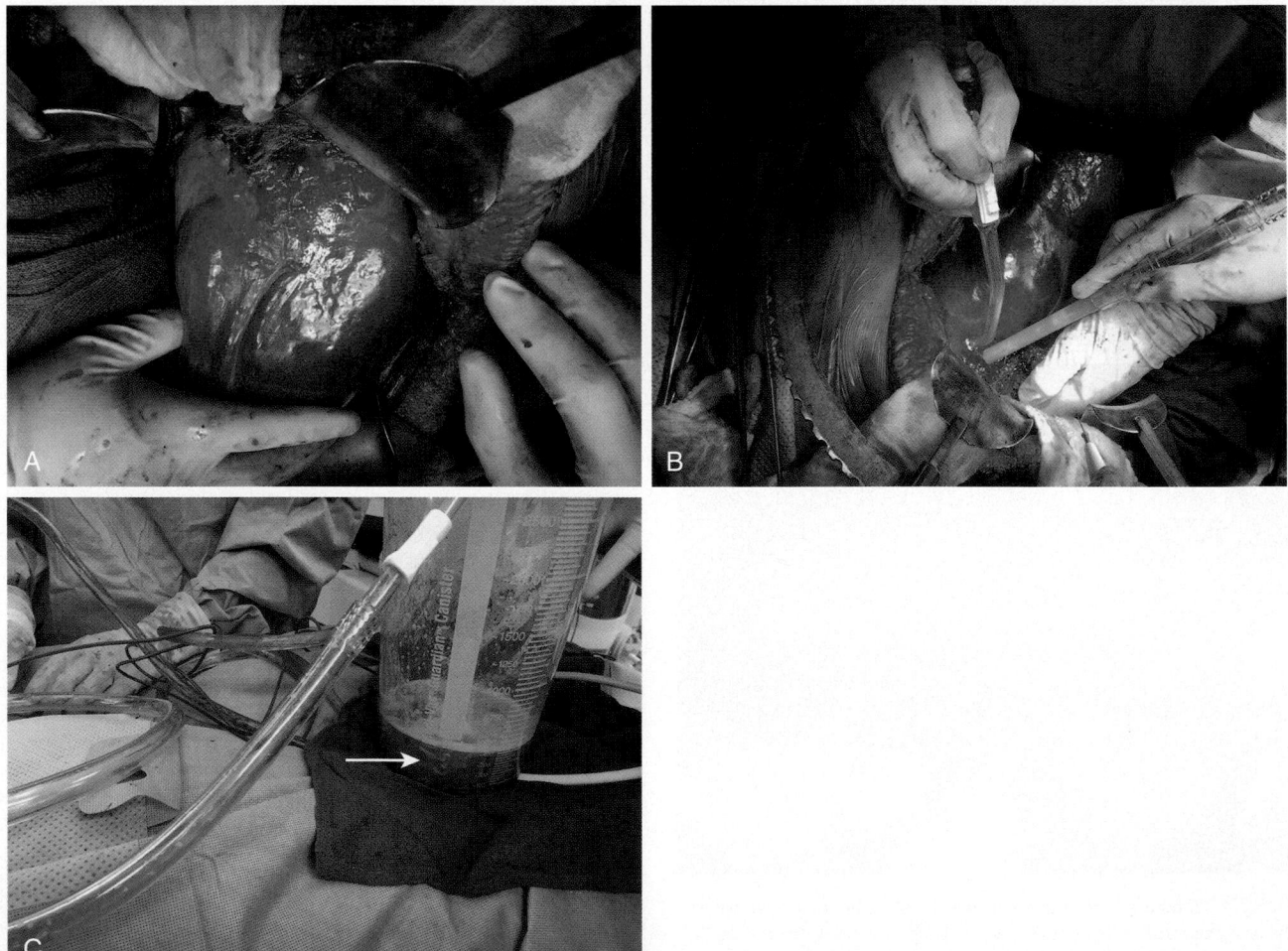

FIGURE 5 Intraoperative images of a large posterior dome hydatid cyst of the liver before (**A**) and during cyst evacuation (**B**) after placement of scolicidal soaked sponges and before definitive pericystectomy. **C,** Note the scolices and hooklets visible in the suctioned cyst fluid in image (*white arrow*).

resections to formal anatomic lobectomy. Liver resection should be considered for large complicated cysts deep within the hepatic parenchyma and those with cystobiliary fistulae and in smaller peripheral cysts where the cut surface of the liver is less with resection than with pericystectomy or cyst evacuation. Patients with failed prior percutaneous or conservative approaches also may benefit from a liver resection if complete excision of all the cysts is possible.

Transplantation, the most radical of all surgical management options, generally is not indicated for cystic echinococcal disease. It is reserved for cases with concomitant liver failure secondary to underlying liver disease and cirrhosis, or in exceptional cases in which there are severe consequences of the cyst compressing vital structures leading to problems with portal vein occlusion or Budd-Chiari syndrome, resulting in subsequent portal hypertension and/or liver failure.

Alveolar Echinococcus

The management of alveolar echinococcus, caused by *E. multilocularis,* deserves special comment. Unlike cystic echinococcus resulting from *E. granulosus,* alveolar echinococcus tends to be a much more aggressive disease with a more infiltrative component that may result in biliary obstruction, Budd-Chiari syndrome, and occasionally liver failure. As such, it has been classified by the WHO with a PNM staging system, with *P* indicating the extension of parasitic disease, *N* indicating the involvement of neighboring organs, and *M* indicating the presence of extrahepatic "metastasis" or involvement. Given the tumor-like nature of the disease, percutaneous management for alveolar echinococcus is not an option, and surgical treatment usually is mandated. The goals of surgery are to achieve an R0 surgical resection when possible, with no role for debulking or palliative procedures. Liver transplantation may be considered for unresectable patients without extrahepatic disease, or in patients developing liver failure resulting from secondary biliary cirrhosis and Budd-Chiari syndrome. Regardless of the surgical intervention, concurrent medical treatment with benzimidazoles is recommended for long-term management of the disease (at least 2 years) and may be required indefinitely for inoperable cases.

Long-Term Outcomes

Overall, the long-term cure rates for appropriately managed patients have improved tremendously worldwide and range from 90% to 95%. Percutaneous interventions with the PAIR technique have an acceptably low morbidity (8% to 13%) and negligible mortality (0.1%) compared with surgical therapy, where morbidity ranges from 25% to 33% with mortality rates of 0.7% to 4%. However, this must be interpreted with the understanding that patients requiring surgical therapy generally have more advanced disease that is not amenable to percutaneous therapy. Recurrence of disease tends to be lower with more radical surgical therapy (approximately 2%) and in general is less than 10% for uncomplicated disease managed either percutaneously or surgically. Given the endemic nature of the disease and risk for reinfection, WHO guidelines recommend follow-up visits with laboratory tests (CBC and LFTs) and ultrasound every 3 to 6 months to evaluate for potential recurrence. Patients with complicated disease and peritoneal or pleural rupture have a higher rate of recurrence approaching 25%. For alveolar disease, cross-sectional imaging with contrast-enhanced CT or MRI is recommended every 1 to 2 years for routine follow-up.

SUGGESTED READINGS

Brunetti E, Kern P, Vuitton DA. Expert consensus for the diagnosis and treatment of cystic and alveolar echinococcosis in humans. *Acta Trop.* 2010;114:1-6.

Buttenchoen K, Gruener B, Kern P, Beger HG, Henne-Bruns D, Reuter S. Long-term experience on surgical treatment of alveolar echinococcosis. *Langenbecks Arch Surg.* 2009;394:689-698.

Chautem R, Buhler LH, Gold B, et al. Surgical management and long-term outcomes of complicated liver hydatid cysts caused by *Echinococcus granulosus. Surgery.* 2005;137:312-316.

Jani K. Spillage-free laparoscopic management of hepatic hydatid disease using the hydatid trocar canula. *J Minim Access Surg.* 2014;10:113-118. doi:10.4103/0972-9941.134873.

WHO Informal Working Group. International classification of ultrasound images in cystic echinococcus for application in clinical and field epidemiological settings. *Acta Trop.* 2003;85:253-261.

THE MANAGEMENT OF LIVER HEMANGIOMA

Kevin C. Soares, MD, and Timothy M. Pawlik, MD, MPH, PhD

Liver hemangioma is the most common benign tumor of the liver and affects up to 20% of the population. Liver hemangiomas are four times more common in females and occur typically in the third to fifth decade of life. On presentation, roughly one half of patients have multifocal lesions. Although their cause remains unknown, the natural history of liver hemangiomas is benign. In turn, the management of liver hemangiomas is tailored to the probability of related complications, as well as the degree of symptoms.

Grossly most liver hemangiomas are well-defined, soft, dark lesions (Figure 1). Hemangiomas can range in size from less than 1 cm to extremely large. Hemangiomas greater than 5 cm are considered "giant"; however, size alone is not an indication for resection (Figure 2). Microscopically, hemangiomas have a single layer of endothelium lining with dilated, cavernous vascular channels surrounded by thin connective tissue containing occasional calcifications and fibrosis.

ETIOLOGY

The cause of hepatic hemangiomas is unclear. These lesions are either congenital lesions complicated by vascular ectasia or an acquired abnormality of normal hepatic vasculature with abnormal enlargement. The role of angiogenic factors in their pathogenesis remains debated; however, tumor regression after treatment with antivascular endothelial growth factor antibodies has been reported.

A hormonal association is suggested by the strong predisposition for female incidence. In addition, estrogen receptors are seen on surface of hemangiomas and increased rate of growth while on steroid therapy, oral contraceptives, or during pregnancy has been reported. There is no clear evidence, however, demonstrating a role of hormones in the cause of these tumors, and this association remains ambiguous.

CLINICAL PRESENTATION

The majority of hemangiomas (50% to 90%) are asymptomatic and most often identified as incidental findings at the time of cross-sectional imaging. Determining hemangioma-related symptoms is a critical component of the surgeon's evaluation because this is one of the few indications for surgical resection. Pain secondary to hemangiomas results from hemangioma thrombosis or stretching of Glisson's capsule, which leads to nonspecific visceral abdominal pain.

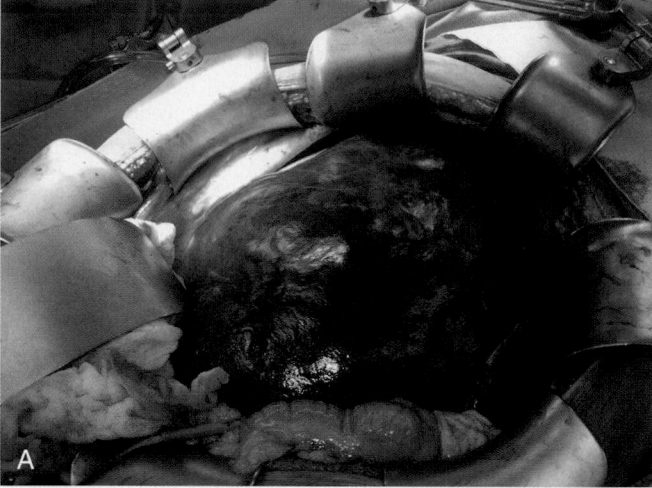

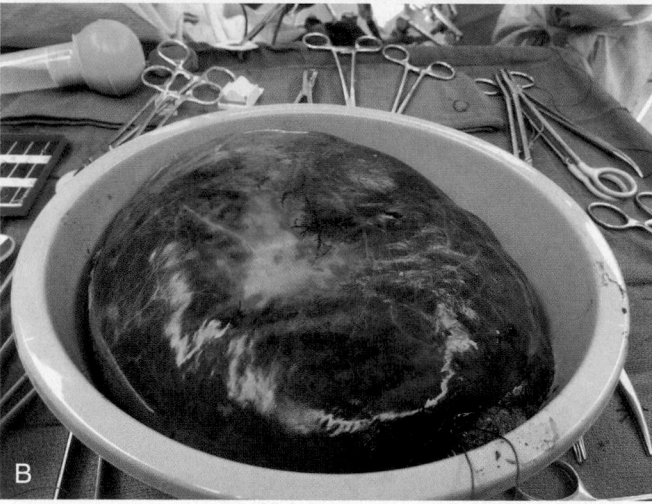

FIGURE 1 A, Intraoperative photograph of a giant hemangioma occupying the right hemiliver. **B,** Intraoperative view of giant cavernous hemangioma measuring 27.0 cm after extended right hepatectomy.

Accordingly, symptomatic hemangiomas generally are accompanied by nonspecific symptoms such as general abdominal pain, nausea, and early satiety. Hemangioma-related pain may present as right shoulder pain or abdominal pain with deep inspiration as a result of referred pain from diaphragmatic irritation. Mass effect of a large hemangioma on the stomach, duodenum, and biliary tree may result in early satiety, gastric outlet obstruction, and obstructive jaundice, respectively.

The likelihood of symptomatic lesions increases with larger hemangiomas. Large hemangiomas can lead to arteriovenous shunting and result in congestive heart failure. Life-threatening complications include rupture, hemorrhage, and Kasabach-Merritt syndrome. Although rupture is rare (occurring in less than 5% of cases), it is associated with significant morbidity, including disseminated intravascular coagulation and hypovolemic shock. One third of spontaneous hemangioma ruptures result in death. Kasabach-Merritt syndrome, or hemangioma thrombocytopenia syndrome, occurs when a large or rapidly growing hemangioma traps platelets, causing a consumptive thrombocytopenia, which progresses to a consumptive coagulopathy and eventually disseminated intravascular

coagulation. This often is triggered by a simple dental or surgical procedure and carries an estimated mortality of 30%.

DIAGNOSIS

The differential diagnosis of liver lesions is broad, and the management for each of these ranges from observation to therapeutic resection. Therefore it is imperative that the diagnosis of hemangioma be accurate to avoid unwarranted interventions. Diagnosis generally is accomplished radiographically. Ultrasound (US), contrast-enhanced computed tomographic (CT) scan, and magnetic resonance imaging (MRI) are the most common imaging modalities used.

The sonographic appearance of hemangiomas consists of a well-defined, hyperechoic homogeneous mass. This characteristic appearance can, however, vary as a result of central necrosis and fibrosis. CT is the most commonly used imaging modality in diagnosing hepatic hemangiomas. Unenhanced CT depicts hemangiomas as isodense liver lesions that often can be difficult to identify. However, a multiphase CT scan, including arterial, venous, and delayed phase imaging, has a sensitivity of nearly 90%. Classic findings include peripheral enhancement on arterial phase, centripetal filling on portal venous phase, and retention of contrast on delayed phase (Figure 3). A CT with these classic imaging characteristics is adequate for establishing the diagnosis, and further imaging modalities are not needed. However, these characteristics may not be seen in all cases. For example, peripheral enhancement on imaging may be missed on smaller lesions (less than 2 cm). In addition, larger lesions have a higher likelihood of fibrosis or thrombosis, thereby preventing complete centripetal filling. Regressed or thrombosed hemangiomas appear dense and fibrotic, therefore mimicking the appearance of malignancy. In cases in which the diagnosis remains ambiguous, further imaging modalities are indicated. This is particularly applicable to patients with potential neuroendocrine hepatic metastases, which have a similar CT appearance to hemangiomas.

Although more expensive, a dedicated hemangioma protocol MRI is the most sensitive (91%) and specific (95%) imaging modality. Low signal intensity on contrast-enhanced T1-weighted imaging and a bright signal on T2-weighted imaging with delayed relaxation times, also known as the "light bulb sign" (Figure 4), are characteristic and reliably differentiate hemangiomas from metastatic disease. Although MRI has improved sensitivity and specificity compared with CT in diagnosing hepatic hemangiomas, both are highly accurate, and a multiphase CT can be used to confirm the diagnosis. MRI is particularly helpful when the diagnosis is unclear and may be used for long-term surveillance to limit radiation exposure.

Percutaneous biopsy is contraindicated given the high likelihood of serious complications and low likelihood of a tissue sample supporting the diagnosis of hemangioma. Further imaging modalities seldom are needed. However, in cases in which the diagnosis is unclear, single photon emission CT with technetium-labeled red blood cells or angiography may be used. Of note, tagged red blood cell scans are limited for lesions located deep within the liver parenchyma. Technetium-99m sulfur colloid and hepatobiliary scintigraphy demonstrates a filling defect within the liver; however, this does not distinguish hemangiomas from other hepatic lesions and is therefore of limited value in the diagnosis of hepatic hemangioma.

Blood tests are generally normal except in cases of Kasabach-Merritt syndrome, where fibrinolysis within the tumor results in thrombocytopenia as a result of platelet sequestration and coagulation abnormalities. Obstructive jaundice from mass of the effect of the lesion on the biliary tree may result in elevated bilirubin and alkaline phosphatase levels. Tumor marker elevations including CA-19-9, carcinoembryonic antigen, and alpha-fetoprotein are unusual and warrant further evaluation.

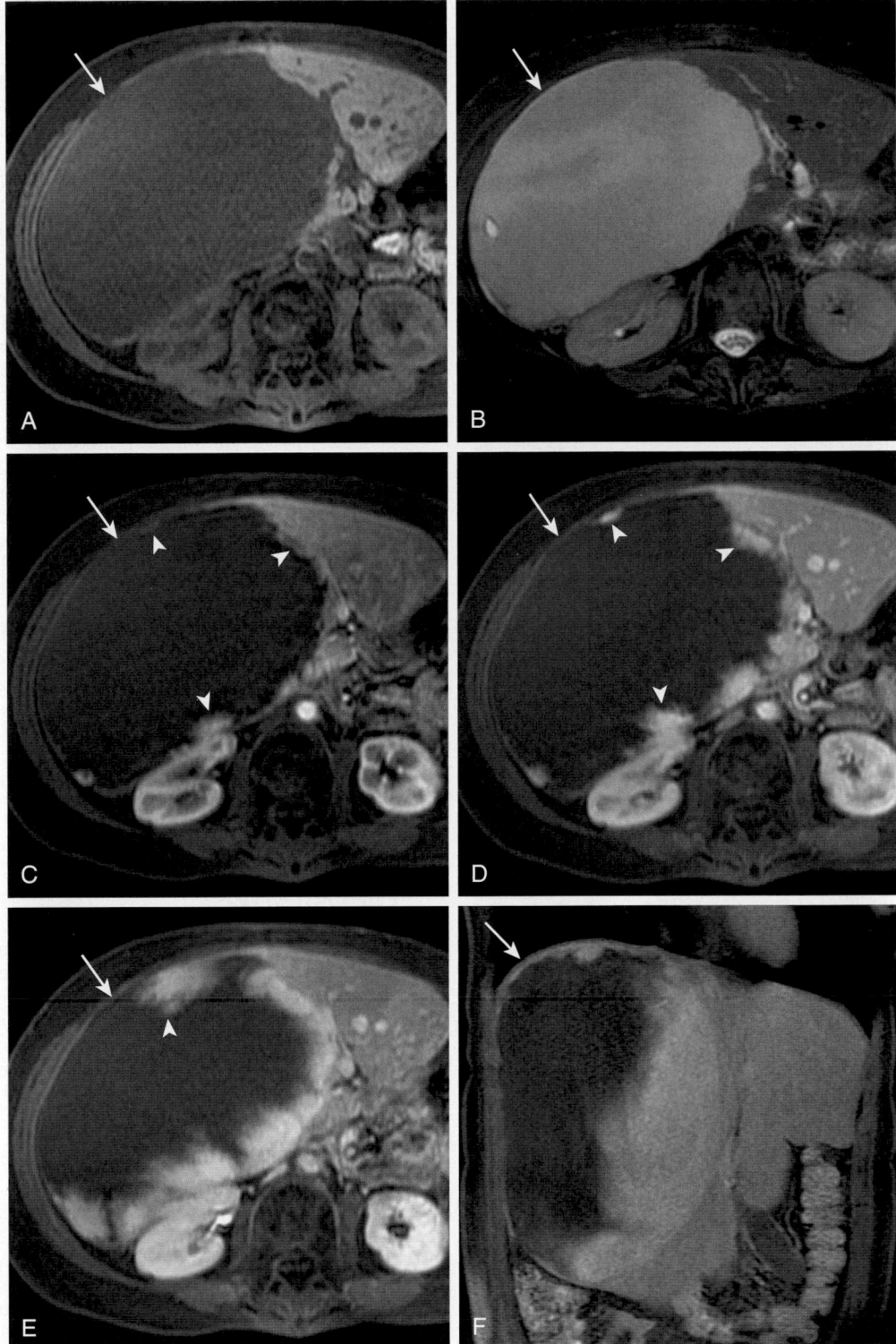

FIGURE 2 Giant hemangioma in a 41-year-old woman. Axial T1-weighted image of MRI shows a large mass in the right lobe of the liver that is hypointense to liver parenchyma (*arrow* in **A**). The mass is very hyperintense to liver on T2-weighted image (*arrow* in **B**). Axial T1-weighted images in the hepatic arterial phase (**C**), portal venous phase (**D**), and delayed phase (**E**) show progressive centripetal enhancement *(arrowheads)*. **F,** Coronal delayed phase image shows continued central enhancement of the mass *(arrow)*. These features are consistent with giant hemangioma. *(Courtesy Drs. I Kamel and M Ghasebeh, Department of Radiology, Johns Hopkins University School of Medicine.)*

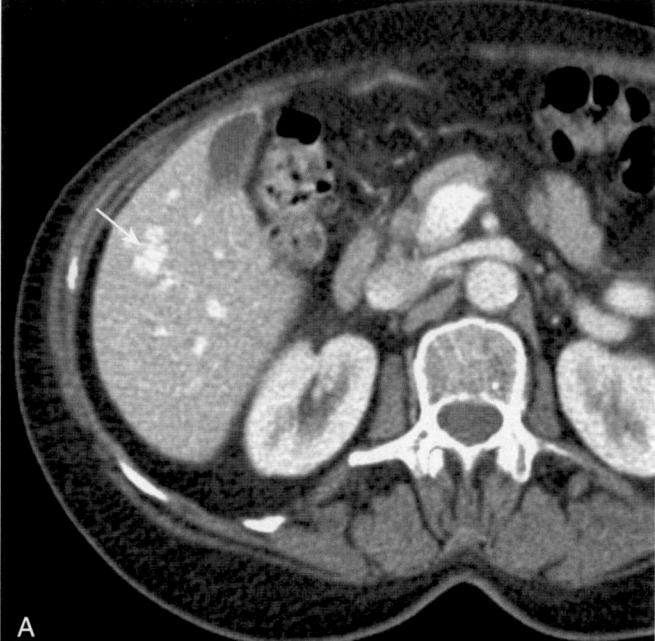

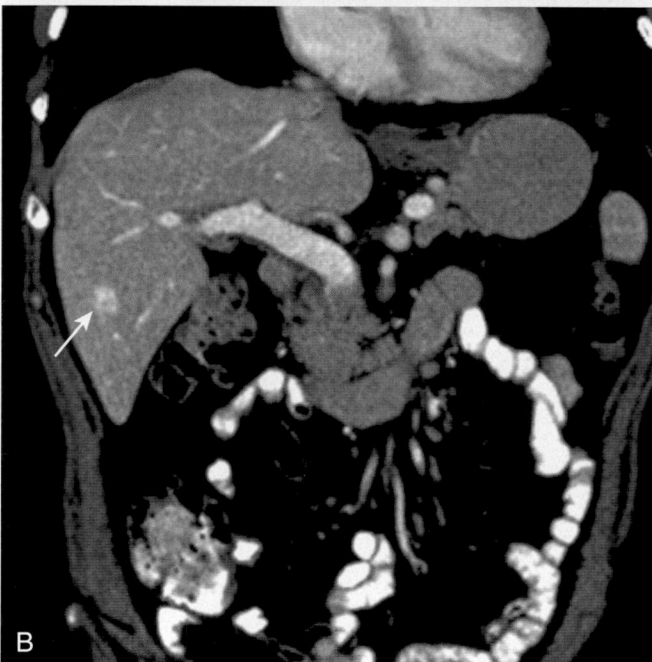

FIGURE 3 Computed topography appearance of a liver hemangioma. Axial (**A**) and coronal (**B**) CT in the portal venous phase show a hypervascular mass in the right lobe of the liver *(arrow)*. *(Courtesy Drs. I Kamel and M Ghasebeh, Department of Radiology, Johns Hopkins University School of Medicine.)*

■ MANAGEMENT

The natural history of hepatic hemangiomas is unremarkable; most lesions remain stable in size and 10% to 15% of lesions regress during follow-up. In a retrospective review of nearly 500 patients with hepatic hemangiomas and long term follow-up, observation versus operative intervention resulted in a similar incidence of hemangioma-related complications. Accordingly, the risk of rupture or size should not be used as a criterion for resection. Observation is indicated in asymptomatic patients even in pregnant patients and women taking oral contraceptive therapy.

The most common indication for surgical resection is severe hemangioma-related symptoms. Symptoms necessitating operative interventions include extreme pain or mass-effect related symptoms on adjacent gastrointestinal organs or the biliary tree. The decision to resect a symptomatic hemangioma must be weighed against the morbidity of the procedure. Specific factors to consider include location of the tumor, size of the tumor, and surgical risk factors of the patient. Moreover, other causes of abdominal discomfort or pain must be excluded before proceeding with resection.

Hemangioma-related complications, including intraperitoneal hemorrhage secondary to spontaneous or traumatic rupture, are an important indication for surgical resection. Resuscitation and embolization are first-line therapies in this situation followed by interval resection. In instances in which embolization is unsuccessful, emergent resection is indicated.

Kasabach-Merritt syndrome warrants emergent surgical resection despite concomitant coagulopathy, given that resection of the hemangioma will ablate the consumptive coagulopathy. Embolization is also appropriate, particularly when surgical resection is not feasible. Supportive care in an intensive care setting is often necessary to manage bleeding risks (i.e., intracranial hemorrhage) and prevent progression to disseminated intravascular coagulation and its associated complications.

Finally, diagnostic uncertainty and the inability to rule out malignancy is another indication for surgical resection. This typically is performed after all invasive and noninvasive diagnostic modalities have been exhausted. Rapid enlargement of a hemangioma is unusual and raises the possibility of malignancy. Both laparotomy and laparoscopy are appropriate followed by visual inspection of the lesion. Intraoperative biopsies may be warranted in select cases.

■ SURGICAL APPROACH AND TECHNIQUES

Hepatic hemangiomas may be resected by enucleation or via anatomic or nonanatomic liver resection. Enucleation is the most commonly used approach. When compared with anatomic or nonanatomic liver resection, enucleation is associated with decreased blood loss, decreased operative time, fewer operative complications, and increased preservation of hepatic parenchyma. In experienced hands, hemangioma liver resections are associated with low morbidity and mortality.

The blood supply of hepatic hemangioma is derived from the hepatic artery. Enucleation begins with control of the hepatic artery inflow. Larger lesions may even require ligation of the ipsilateral hepatic artery, whereas smaller hemangioma arterial inflow can be controlled by ligation of more distal branches. A Pringle maneuver is useful to help attenuate inflow in instances in which the hemangioma is inadvertently entered. This maneuver also may be used as a preemptive technique to decompress the tumor and ease dissection, especially in very large lesions that may be difficult to handle. Inflow occlusion of less than 30 minutes is generally well tolerated without ischemia reperfusion injury. In situations in which enucleation will require more than 30 minutes, intermittent unclamping for 5 minutes may be used. Gentle pressure on the hemangioma during the 5-minute reperfusion limits re-expansion of the decompressed hemangioma.

The presence of a pseudocapsule that is relatively avascular and does not contain bile ducts makes hemangiomas particularly amenable to enucleation. Dissection begins by incising through Glisson's capsule to identify the plane of the pseudocapsule. Initially, it may be necessary to divide normal parenchyma to identify the pseudocapsule. Intraoperative US may be used to identify deep lesions within

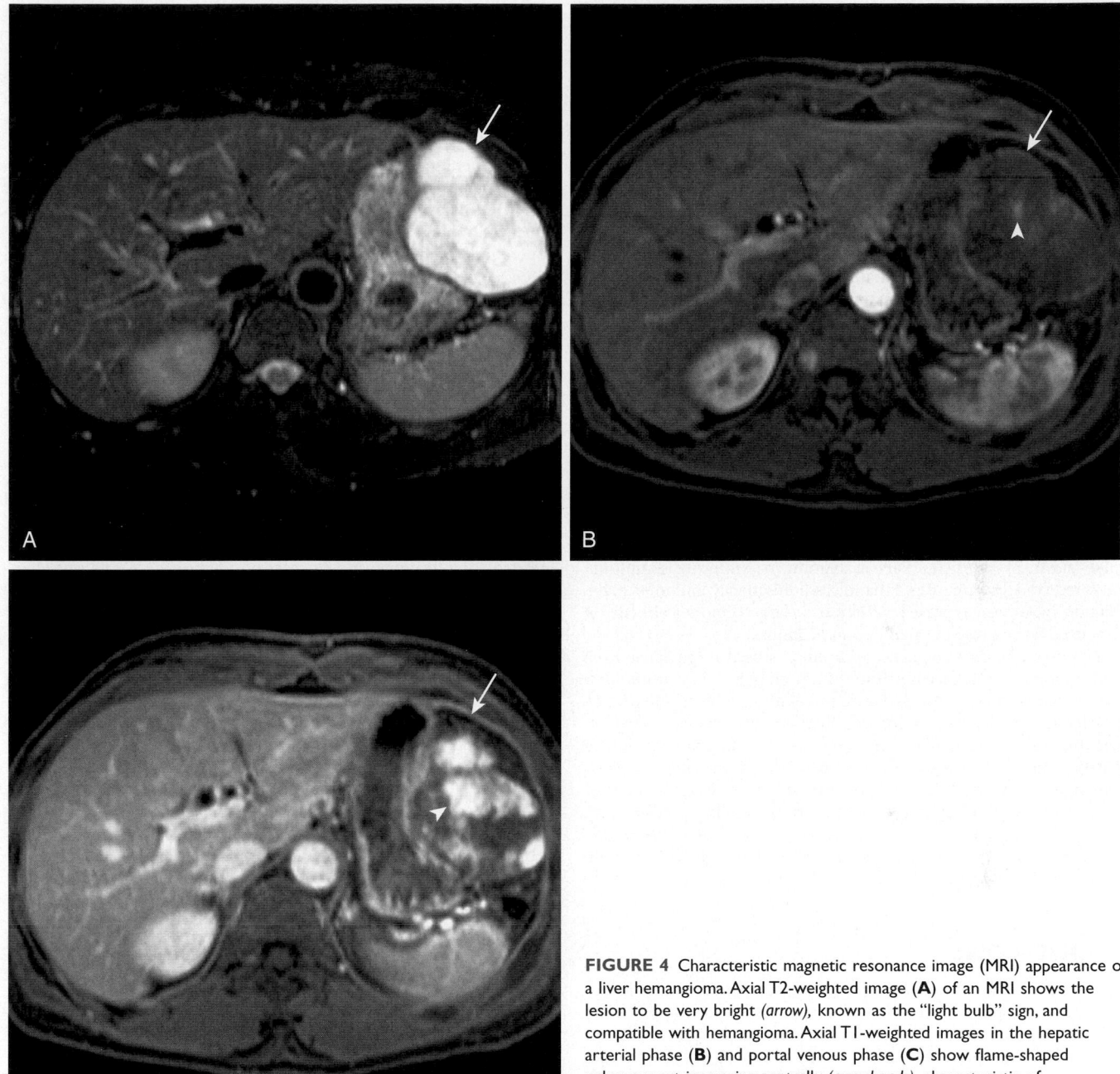

FIGURE 4 Characteristic magnetic resonance image (MRI) appearance of a liver hemangioma. Axial T2-weighted image (**A**) of an MRI shows the lesion to be very bright *(arrow)*, known as the "light bulb" sign, and compatible with hemangioma. Axial T1-weighted images in the hepatic arterial phase (**B**) and portal venous phase (**C**) show flame-shaped enhancement increasing centrally *(arrowheads)*, characteristic of hemangioma. *(Courtesy Drs. I Kamel and M Ghasebeh, Department of Radiology, Johns Hopkins University School of Medicine.)*

the liver parenchyma. Dissection along the plane of the pseudocapsule lowers the risk of entering the lesion and causing significant blood loss. In addition, it limits the potential for parenchymal injury and bile leaks. Ultrasonic dissection, blunt techniques, energy-based devices, and staplers are all appropriate techniques to separate the hemangioma from the surrounding liver parenchyma. Of note, certain hemangiomas have a poorly defined hemangioma to normal liver parenchyma interface, thus lacking an obvious fibrous pseudocapsule and complicating attempts at enucleation.

Anatomic versus nonanatomic resection of liver hemangiomas typically is used in cases of diagnostic uncertainty where the lesion is highly suspicious for malignancy. Tumor location, expectant morbidity, and surgeon comfort are important preoperative factors to consider when deciding on an optimal approach. Nonanatomic approaches are ideal for small, peripheral locations; particularly those located in Couinaud segments II and III. For deeper lesions, operative approach is dictated by surgeon comfort and diagnostic suspicion. Standard liver resection techniques and principles apply. Inflow occlusion often is used to decompress the tumor and facilitate resection.

Minimally invasive enucleation or resection has been described in the literature with acceptable outcomes. Small, peripheral, or superficial lesions are particularly amenable to this approach. Tumors in the right side of the liver are juxtaposed more commonly to major intrahepatic vessels, thus complicating a laparoscopic approach. Orthotopic liver transplantation has been reported in the literature for unresectable lesions and in patients with Kasabach-Merritt syndrome, but this is exceptionally rare.

NONOPERATIVE THERAPIES

Nonoperative treatment of hepatic hemangiomas generally is reserved for patients with spontaneous or traumatic hemangioma rupture. In addition, symptomatic patients who refuse surgery or have prohibitive surgical risk factors are also eligible for nonoperative therapy. Options include transarterial embolization, percutaneous radiofrequency ablation, percutaneous ethanol ablation, and hepatic radiation therapy. Transarterial embolization is used as a bridge to surgery in cases of intraperitoneal hemorrhage. Outcomes with these techniques are not well documented, and data describing their effectiveness are lacking. Elective embolization for symptomatic patients has been associated with transient pain relief, although long-term outcomes are unknown. In most cases, tumor size is unchanged, and recurrence or recurrent symptoms are common after embolization.

Thermal ablation also has been shown to reduce symptoms, although complete ablation is rarely possible given the nearby vascular and biliary pedicles. Partial ablation may improve symptoms but is reserved for rare cases. Ethanol, radiofrequency, and microwave ablation have been reported. Ablation of large tumors (>10 cm) is associated with a higher rate of complications.

Nonoperative management commonly is used in pediatric liver hemangiomas, which account for 10% of all pediatric liver tumors. Liver hemangiomas in the pediatric population are typically part of a systemic process and multifocal. Symptomatic pediatric hepatic hemangiomas carry a high mortality rate (70%). Embolization is first-line therapy along with cytotoxic drugs in children with hemangioma-associated congestive heart failure. Systemic corticosteroids are first-line agents. Corticosteroid-resistant proliferating tumors also can be treated with intravenous vincristine or interferon-alpha. Surgical resection in children may be indicated with severely symptomatic or ruptured tumors.

PROGNOSIS

Follow-up imaging of newly diagnosed hepatic hemangiomas is recommended despite the scarcity of data regarding the appropriate follow-up algorithm in asymptomatic patients. Despite increased costs, MRI is the preferred modality to reduce radiation exposure. An accepted algorithm consists of an MRI 3 months after diagnosis with a repeat MRI in 3 to 6 months if the lesion is atypical or if there is a low suspicion for malignancy. If the lesion is stable on repeat imaging, annual imaging is recommended with more infrequent follow-up for unchanging lesions.

The natural history of hepatic hemangioma is benign; most lesions remain stable. When indicated, resection generally is well tolerated and recurrence is rare. It is performed with extremely low morbidity and mortality in experienced hands. Females with large hemangiomas historically have been advised to avoid pregnancy for fear of rupture; however, this risk is small and evasion of pregnancy is not indicated. However, pregnant patients and those exposed to exogenous estrogens may have a higher likelihood to have their hemangiomas increase in size and therefore warrant careful observation.

In general, surgery for benign liver lesions such as a hemangioma is associated with high patient satisfaction and improved quality of life (QOL). Overall, most patients report satisfaction with their treatment, as well as a "better" or "much better" QOL. Presence of preoperative "moderate-to-extreme" pain predicts overall improved QOL after surgery. Given that patients with significant preoperative symptoms derive the most benefit from surgery, operative intervention for hepatic hemangioma is best reserved for this population of patients.

SUMMARY

The increased use of cross-sectional imaging has increased the detection of hepatic hemangiomas. The natural history is benign with few complications. Small asymptomatic lesions may be observed and initially followed with serial imaging to document tumor stability. Resection is indicated for severely symptomatic tumors, hemangioma-related complications, and in cases of diagnostic uncertainty. Hemangioma rupture is rare and embolization is appropriate in these instances followed by surgical resection. Enucleation is the most commonly preferred approach; however, both resection and enucleation are safe and associated with extremely low morbidity and mortality in experienced hands. Prognosis and long-term outcomes are excellent and recurrence is rare.

SUGGESTED READINGS

Colli A, Fraquelli M, Massironi S, et al. Elective surgery for benign liver tumours. *Cochrane Database Syst Rev.* 2007;(24):CD005164.

Donati M, Stavrou GA, Donati A, Oldhafer KJ. The risk of spontaneous rupture of liver hemangiomas: a critical review of the literature. *J Hepatobiliary Pancreat Sci.* 2011;18:797-805. doi:10.1007/s00534-011-0420-7.

Herman P, Costa ML, Machado MA, et al. Management of hepatic hemangiomas: a 14-year experience. *J Gastrointest Surg.* 2005;9:853-859.

Kneuertz PJ, Marsh JW, de Jong MC, Covert K, Hyder O, Hirose K, Schulick RD, Choti MA, Geller DA, Pawlik TM. Improvements in quality of life following surgery for benign hepatic tumors: results from a dual center analysis. *Surgery.* 2012;152:193-201.

Margonis GA, Ejaz A, Spolverato G, Rastegar N, Anders R, Kamel IR, Pawlik TM. Benign solid tumors of the liver: management in the modern era. *J Gastrointest Surg.* 2015;19:1157-1168.

Mezhir JJ, Fourman LT, Do RK, et al. Changes in the management of benign liver tumours: an analysis of 285 patients. *HPB (Oxford).* 2013;15:156-163.

Schnelldorfer T, Ware AL, Smoot R, et al. Management of giant hemangioma of the liver: resection versus observation. *J Am Coll Surg.* 2010;211:724-730.

Yoon SS, Charny CK, Fong Y, et al. Diagnosis, management, and outcomes of 115 patients with hepatic hemangioma. *J Am Coll Surg.* 2003;197:392-402.

THE MANAGEMENT OF BENIGN LIVER LESIONS

Katherine E. Poruk, MD, and Matthew J. Weiss, MD

Improvements in abdominal imaging have not only enhanced our ability to accurately diagnose disease but also have increased the identification of benign, often asymptomatic, lesions in the liver. The incidence of benign liver lesions is believed to be between 7% and 20% of the population. Although the management of benign liver lesions relies primarily on routine surveillance and a nonoperative approach, surgery may be necessary if the mass is symptomatic, has a risk of malignant transformation, or has a possibility of hemorrhage or rupture. Surgeons must be familiar with the clinical workup, accurate radiographic identification, and subsequent management of the most common benign liver lesions, including hepatic cysts, hemangiomas, adenomas, and focal nodular hyperplasia (FNH). A complete understanding of the natural history of benign liver lesions is mandatory to properly manage these neoplasms and avoid unnecessary interventions.

RADIOLOGIC WORKUP OF BENIGN LIVER LESIONS

A rise in the frequency of abdominal imaging for unrelated indications has resulted in an increase in the identification of asymptomatic, benign liver lesions. Fortunately, simultaneous improvements in imaging quality have resulted in more accurate diagnostic capability as well. Most asymptomatic lesions found incidentally in the liver are benign, especially in younger patients without a history of cancer or underlying liver disease such as cirrhosis. The vast majority of these liver lesions can be diagnosed accurately by imaging alone without the need for further invasive testing and managed without the need for surgery. However, given their incidence in the population, discovery on routine imaging studies can still lead to unnecessary surgery when incorrectly mistaken for an underlying primary hepatic malignancy. In addition, patients undergoing staging workup for extrahepatic malignancies who are found to have a liver lesion can be diagnosed erroneously as having a metastatic lesion, which leads to incorrect cancer staging and treatment. A complete understanding of benign hepatic lesions is therefore mandatory for surgeons to prevent unnecessary interventions.

Certain complementary findings on ultrasound, computed tomography (CT) scan, and/or magnetic resonance imaging (MRI) should lead a surgeon to suspect a hepatic simple cyst, hemangioma, adenoma, or focal nodular hyperplasia (Table 1). All three imaging modalities are complementary for the workup of a benign liver lesion, and usually more than one will be used to establish an accurate diagnosis. In the majority of patients, a benign liver lesion first is diagnosed incidentally on abdominal CT scan because these scans are widely available in most hospitals, have a high diagnostic sensitivity and specificity, and are relatively quick to obtain compared with other imaging modalities. Limitations to the use of CT scan often involve the need for intravenous iodinated contrast material to accurately diagnose a lesion, which may not be possible in patients with a contrast allergy or poor renal function. MRI provides additional characterization of a liver lesion because it is more accurate and sensitive in denoting subtle differences in liver parenchyma without the need for ionizing radiation. However, it is limited in some situations by the time required to complete each study and its relative contraindications, including patients with a pacemaker or implanted device. Ultrasound is a relatively accurate yet noninvasive imaging modality without the added risk of radiation and may be used first

in patients with nonspecific abdominal complaints. Given that the majority of benign liver lesions can be identified successfully by imaging with one or more of these modalities, fine-needle aspiration or percutaneous core liver biopsy rarely is required for diagnostic purposes, especially when there is little concern for underlying malignancy.

BENIGN LIVER CYSTS

Pathogenesis

Simple liver cysts occur in approximately 5% of the adult population, are frequently asymptomatic, and are almost always benign. These cysts are predominantly congenital in nature, arising from aberrant bile ducts, which have lost communication with the biliary tree. As a result, the buildup of serous, nonbilious fluid creates a spheric, nonseptated cyst lined with a single layer of biliary cuboidal epithelial cells and a rim of fibrous stroma. Congenital cysts are most often small and solitary and can be found anywhere in the liver, with a higher predilection for the right hepatic lobe. Simple cysts tend to remain stable in size over time, although some may increase gradually in size over time because of a continued production of serous fluid by the epithelial cells lining the cyst. Rarely, hepatic cysts larger than 20 cm have been reported, although the majority are only a few centimeters in diameter.

Presentation

Simple hepatic cysts can be diagnosed at any age, although they are seen more commonly in adults. These cysts often are diagnosed incidentally after a patient undergoes abdominal imaging for an unrelated cause, and a prevalence of between 2.5% and 5% has been reported in the adult population. There is a slight predominance in females, especially with increasing age, in whom large, symptomatic cysts are almost always diagnosed. The majority of patients with simple cysts are asymptomatic, but nonspecific symptoms can occur as a result of enlargement, hemorrhage, infection, or rupture of the cyst. Symptoms are much more common with cysts larger than 4 cm in diameter and those in the right hepatic lobe, which can cause pressure on the stomach or diaphragm, leading to abdominal pain, shortness of breath, early satiety, nausea, and vomiting. In rare cases, hepatomegaly or a mass may be palpated on abdominal examination. Other symptoms can be related to compression of nearby biliary, pulmonary, digestive, and vascular structures. In addition, larger cysts have a greater likelihood of spontaneous rupture or hemorrhage, leading to pain, fever, shock and, rarely, death.

Imaging

Abdominal ultrasound provides the most accurate imaging for the diagnosis of simple hepatic cysts in addition to its advantage as a noninvasive modality. On ultrasound, simple cysts appear as a round or oval anechoic lesion with few to no septations. Noninfectious hepatic cysts have a smooth, well-defined, imperceptible wall, posterior acoustic enhancement suggesting a well-defined border between tissue and serous fluid, and an absence of internal vascularity. Ultrasound also may be able to demonstrate an absence of communication with the intrahepatic bile ducts. Heterogeneity, layering of fluid, and internal echoes mimicking septations are often indicative of hemorrhage within the cyst, whereas intracystic debris on ultrasound may be seen with infection. The majority of simple cysts can be diagnosed by ultrasound alone, but CT or MRI may be necessary in difficult cases in which uncertainty remains. Abdominal CT scan will demonstrate a homogeneous, hypoattenuating, well-circumscribed lesion without enhancement of the cyst with the administration of intravenous contrast (Figure 1, *A*). Simple cysts appear as a hypointense lesion on T1-weighted MRI with T2-weighted

TABLE 1: Comparison of Ultrasound, CT, and MRI Findings for the Four Most Commonly Encountered Benign Liver Lesions

Type of Lesion	Ultrasound	CT Scan	MRI Scan
Simple hepatic cyst	Round anechoic lesion without septations Heterogeneity may be seen with hemorrhage	Homogeneous hypoattenuating, well-circumscribed lesion without contrast enhancement	T1: Hypointense, homogeneous lesion T2: Homogeneous, hyperintense lesion without contrast enhancement
Hepatic hemangioma	Well-demarcated hyperechoic lesion; blood flow rarely seen	Asymmetric peripheral enhancement with gradual central enhancement on delayed films	T1: Hypointense lesion T2: Hyperintense lesion; may have peripheral enhancement with gadolinium
Hepatic adenoma	Well-demarcated, heterogeneous hypoechoic or hyperechoic mass	Well-encapsulated lesion, isointense to hypointense on noncontrast CT. Heterogeneity possible because of areas of hemorrhage or necrosis, with a hyperintense signal seen with active bleeding	T1, T2: Isointense to hyperintense lesion; heterogeneity seen with recent hemorrhage or necrosis
Focal nodular hyperplasia	Variable; may be hyperechoic, isoechoic, or hypoechoic. Central scar is seen only in a minority of patients	Well-circumscribed lesion, hyperintense on arterial phase and isointense on venous phase. Central scar may remain hyperintense on venous phase	T1: Isointense to hypointense lesion without attenuation of central scar T2: Isointense to hyperintense lesion with hyperintense central scar

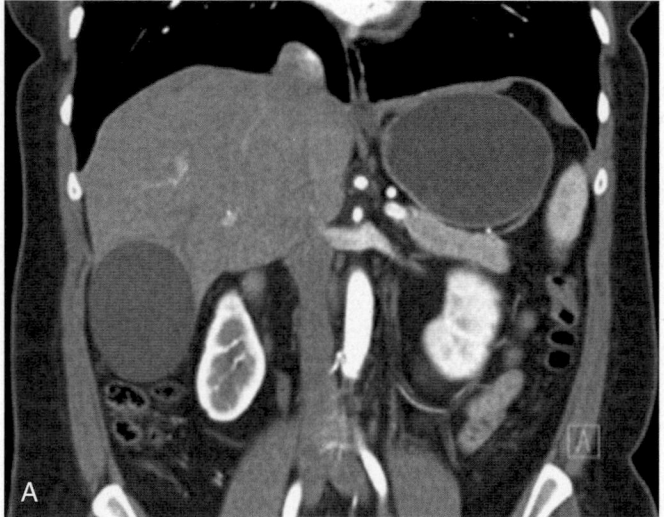
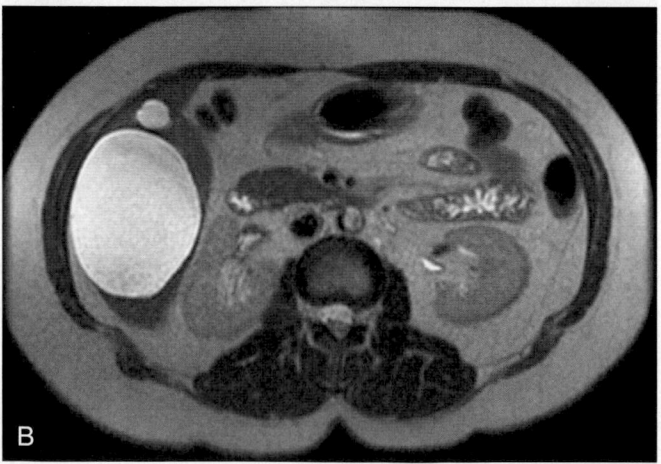

FIGURE 1 A, Coronal CT demonstrating a simple liver cyst in the right lobe of the liver in a 46-year-old woman, also viewed on T2-weighted MRI (**B**) as a hyperintense, spheric lesion.

imaging demonstrating a homogeneous, hyperintense lesion without enhancement after contrast injection (Figure 1, *B*). Aspiration of cyst fluid rarely is needed for diagnosis but may be performed before surgery to rule out an infectious cause and will demonstrate sterile fluid.

Management

The majority of simple liver cysts can be managed nonoperatively. Asymptomatic cysts smaller than 4 cm should be followed with routine imaging by ultrasound every 6 to 12 months to ensure stability, and any rapid increase in size should prompt further workup to rule out associated malignancy. If the cyst does not change after 2 to 3 years, further surveillance is usually unnecessary. Patients with rapidly enlarging cysts or with symptoms require treatment either with surgical resection or, in selected cases, sclerotherapy. Aspiration alone is not recommended because cyst fluid typically will reaccumulate, leading to recurrence, and there is no rationale for the placement of a percutaneous drain into the cyst.

Historically, simple cysts were treated by wide resection of the portion of the liver containing the lesion. However, in the majority of patients this has been replaced with surgical fenestration, or "unroofing," of the cyst, involving the removal of the roof or upper portion of the cyst close to its margin with the liver parenchyma to allow for free drainage into the abdomen. Fenestration can be undertaken by an open or minimally invasive (laparoscopic or robotic) approach, although posteriorly located cysts in segments VII and VIII are often inaccessible by laparoscopy. The goal of cyst fenestration is to resect the cyst wall along its margin with the liver, and care should be taken to avoid extending the incision into the parenchyma given a risk of damage to nearby biliary or vascular structures leading to a bile leak or uncontrolled bleeding. A flap fashioned from the greater omentum often is placed in the former cyst cavity to prevent recurrence. After removal, the resected cyst wall is sent for pathologic examination to rule out associated malignancy. Complete excision of the cyst is rarely necessary. However, wedge or anatomic resection is favored when there is concern for associated malignancy or in patients with multiple cysts when complete resection would be more effective. Large trials have demonstrated a recurrence rate of less than

10% to 15% for either approach, often related to incomplete unroofing of the cyst, especially when unfamiliar with the laparoscopic approach. Morbidity and mortality rates are low (morbidity 0 to 15%, mortality <5%), specifically depending on the operative method, and include bile leaks, hematomas, and surgical site infections.

In symptomatic patients with prohibitively numerous comorbidities, who are not surgical candidates, sclerotherapy has become an alternative method for treatment of benign liver cysts. Sclerotherapy involves the destruction of the epithelial lining of the cyst to prevent the secretion and accumulation of intraluminal fluid. A drainage catheter is placed percutaneously into the cyst so that fluid can be aspirated before injection of a sclerosing agent, such as ethanol, minocycline hydrochloride, or ethanolamine oleate. The sclerosing agent is allowed to instill before removal. As a result, patients with a communication between the cyst and the biliary tree or with a history of intracystic bleeding are not candidates for sclerotherapy. Although safe with relatively low postprocedure morbidity and mortality, sclerotherapy is associated with a high rate of recurrence when compared with surgical management.

■ HEPATIC HEMANGIOMA

Pathogenesis

Hepatic hemangiomas, also known as *cavernous venous malformations,* are the most common benign lesions of the liver. Hemangiomas are congenital abnormalities characterized by large cavernous spaces within the liver lined by endothelial cells and filled with blood, with vascular compartments separated by fibrous tissue. In rare cases, thrombi may be present. Grossly, these lesions are round and well encapsulated and may show evidence of hemorrhage or calcification. Liver hemangiomas have no metastatic potential and, unlike hepatic adenomas, have a very low risk of spontaneous rupture or hemorrhage. The majority of patients have a single lesion, although a significant minority have multiple lesions throughout the liver. Although hemangiomas can occur anywhere in the liver, they tend to be peripherally located, and there is a slight predominance for the right lobe. Most hemangiomas are small but can range anywhere from a few millimeters to upwards of 20 cm in diameter. Giant hemangiomas are defined by a size greater than 10 cm and in children may be associated with Kasabach-Merritt syndrome. In addition, patients with this syndrome have severe thrombocytopenia, coagulopathy, hypofibrinogenemia, and elevated fibrin degradation products.

Presentation

Hepatic hemangiomas are more common in females, especially between the ages of 20 and 50 years. The majority of patients with hemangiomas are asymptomatic. However, symptoms such as abdominal pain, early satiety, and nausea are possible, especially with lesions greater than 5 cm in size. However, some studies have suggested that many patients with hemangiomas who experience pain are discovered to have a different source of their abdominal discomfort on workup. Spontaneous rupture is rare, even in patients with hemangiomas greater than 10 cm. For the vast majority of patients, hepatic hemangiomas will be found incidentally on abdominal imaging at the time of workup for an unrelated complaint.

Imaging

Ultrasound typically shows a well-demarcated hyperechoic lesion, and blood flow is seen in only a minority of patients. CT scan with intravenous contrast demonstrates asymmetric peripheral enhancement of the lesion followed by gradual central enhancement with washout on delayed films related to the flow of blood, which is pathognomonic for hemangiomas (Figure 2, *A*). Hepatic hemangiomas on MRI are defined by a hypointense signal on T1-weighted

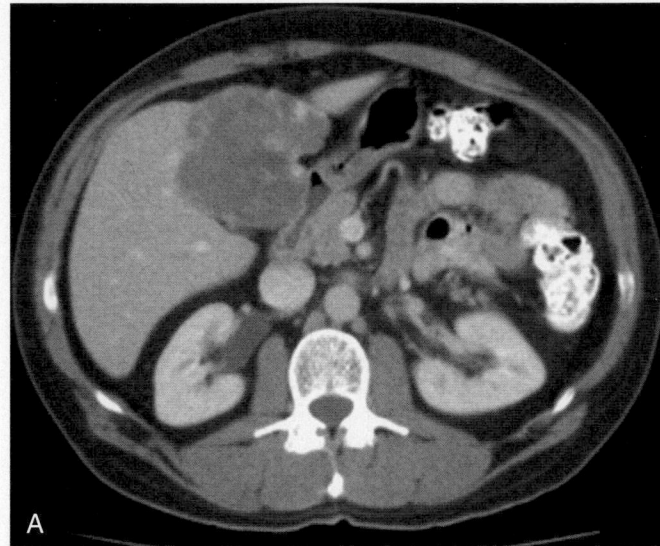

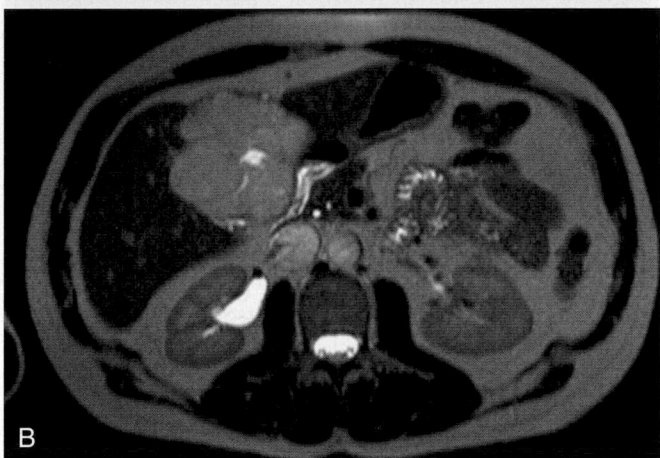

FIGURE 2 A, CT scan demonstrating peripheral enhancement of a hepatic hemangioma in a 52-year-old man. **B,** T2-weighted MRI demonstrating hyperintense staining of the same hemangioma in the left hepatic lobe.

imaging and hyperintensity of the lesion on T2-weighted imaging (Figure 2, *B*). Gadolinium administration on MRI often demonstrates peripheral enhancement similar to that seen on CT scan.

Management

Surgical resection rarely is indicated for hemangiomas. Resection may be indicated for symptomatic patients, patients with growth of their hemangioma, or in patients with the rare complication of rupture. Resection can be achieved either by wedge resection of the lesion or formal segmental resection, and the decision often is made based on the location and proximity of the hemangioma to biliary and vascular structures. Many lesions leave a pseudocapsule and actually can be shelled out. Some advocate the use of hepatic arterial embolization to shrink the size of the hemangioma or control potential bleeding before resection, but this is often not necessary. In addition, orthotopic liver transplant has been used in selected cases to treat patients with large, symptomatic, unresectable hemangiomas or individuals with Kasabach-Merritt syndrome with good long-term results. Most patients who are asymptomatic or have small lesions can be successfully managed conservatively with routine imaging to rule out any enlargement.

■ HEPATIC ADENOMA

Pathogenesis

Hepatic adenomas (HAs) are rare, benign tumors of the liver. Grossly, adenomas appear as well-circumscribed, soft tan lesions with or without a defined capsule. Histopathologic examination demonstrates sheets of hepatocytes containing glycogen and lipid deposits with an absence of Kupffer and bile ductules in the background of normal liver. These sheets of adenoma hepatocytes are separated by dilated sinusoids, perfused only by large peripheral arteries on their surface. As a result, hemorrhage is common and may spread to the surrounding liver if no capsule is present, whereas necrosis may be seen if the adenoma outgrows its blood supply. The majority of patients only have a single adenoma, although it is not uncommon to find multiple adenomas. HAs can be found anywhere in the liver, although they are more common in the right lobe. Size may vary from several millimeters to more than 30 cm, although most are only a few centimeters in diameter. The main concern with hepatic adenomas is a small portion of patients may transition from a benign adenoma to hepatocellular carcinoma (HCC). A large systematic review suggests the rate of malignant transformation of an HA is about 4.2%, with the majority occurring in adenomas greater than 5 cm. Laboratory tests such as alpha-fetoprotein (AFP) before surgical resection may help to delineate patients with associated malignancy.

Research has suggested the hepatic adenomas can be divided into four subtypes based on their genetic and pathologic features. Hepatocyte nuclear factor (HNF) 1α–inactivated HAs are the most common and are characterized by steatosis without inflammatory infiltrates or cytologic abnormalities. β-catenin-activated HAs are characterized by pseudoglandular formation with frequent cytologic abnormalities. These mutations are seen more frequently in male patients when compared with the other subtypes. Hepatic adenomas without either mutation include those with or without inflammatory features. HAs with focal or diffuse inflammatory infiltrates are more likely to have numerous dystrophic vessels, cytologic abnormalities, and ductal reaction. Comparatively, HAs without either mutation or inflammatory features have no specific clinical or morphologic features compared with the other three groups. However, these HAs had the highest risk of bleeding. Interestingly, there is an increased association between patients with beta-catenin mutations and HCC associated with adenomas or borderline lesions.

Presentation

HAs are diagnosed most commonly in young women of childbearing age, specifically between 20 and 40 years of age, although rarely they can be found in males. HAs were seldom seen until the 1970s, corresponding with the development and use of oral contraceptives in the prior decade. The main risk factor for their development is oral contraceptives (OCP) use, and this risk increases with longer durations of therapy and higher hormonal dosages. However, a small percentage of patients can develop adenomas even after only 6 months of OCP use. Early epidemiologic studies estimated the occurrence of adenomas to be 3 to 4 per 100,000 users of OCPs, compared with only 0.13 per 100,000 in nonusers, and numerous studies confirmed these results by showing a significantly higher incidence of adenomas in patients on contraceptives. Sporadic cases have been associated with anabolic androgenic steroid use by bodybuilders and patients requiring long-term steroid therapy. In addition, HAs are seen frequently in patients with glycogen storage diseases (GSD) types I and III. Studies have demonstrated that more than 50% of patients with GSD type I and 25% with GSD type III will develop adenomas. GSD-associated adenomas are found predominantly in young, male patients, usually younger than 20 years of age. Most patients with hepatic adenomas are asymptomatic and are only found incidentally while undergoing abdominal imaging. However, as these tumors grow in size, some patients experience sudden right upper quadrant or epigastric pain, usually related to

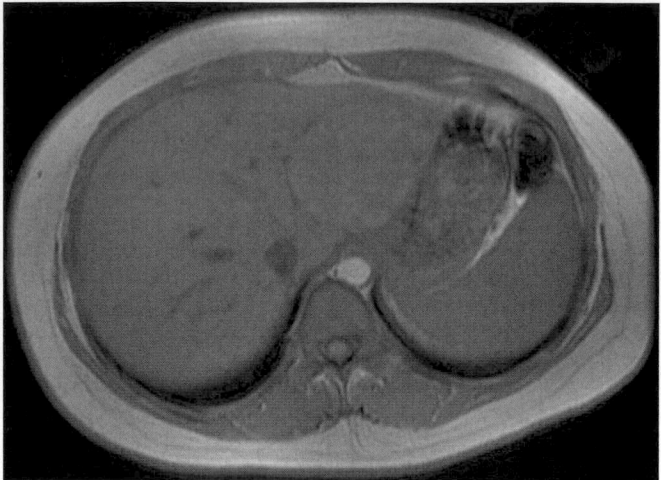

FIGURE 3 MRI demonstrating an isointense, homogeneous hepatic adenoma in the left hepatic lobe without evidence of hemorrhage in a 20-year-old woman.

spontaneous rupture and hemorrhage. In rare cases, rapid bleeding into the abdominal cavity can lead to hypovolemic shock and death.

Imaging

Imaging is often the first indication that a patient has an adenoma, especially in asymptomatic individuals. Ultrasound shows a well-demarcated, heterogeneous hypoechoic or hyperechoic mass, which in some cases can be confused for malignancy or metastases. CT demonstrates a round, well-encapsulated lesion that is isointense to hypointense on noncontrast CT or during the venous phase CT. Some adenomas may be heterogeneous in appearance because of areas of hemorrhage or necrosis, and hyperintensity will be seen on arterial phase CT when there is active or recent hemorrhage. On MRI, hepatic adenomas are isointense to hyperintense on both T1- and T2-weighted images, especially when hemorrhage is present, and further early enhancement is seen with gadolinium administration (Figure 3).

Management

Initial management for asymptomatic patients with adenomas smaller than 5 cm involves cessation of oral contraceptives or anabolic steroids. In some cases, this may lead to regression of the adenoma, although complete disappearance has been documented only in a minority of cases. In addition, there also have been reports of growth, rupture leading to hemorrhage, and malignant transformation after the cessation of OCP, making it a controversial management option. For patients who have growth of their adenoma off OCPs, have adenomas greater than 5 cm or are symptomatic, surgical resection is recommended to reduce the risk of hemorrhage and malignant transformation. The surgical approach should be that of resecting a malignant tumor to achieve negative margins, despite the fact that the vast majority will be benign. The choice of formal anatomic resections versus parenchymal sparing approaches should be guided by the underlying suspicion of malignancy, technical factors, and should follow the same oncologic principles as resecting HCCs. Intraoperative ultrasonography is useful to help identify adenomas that cannot be palpated or easily visualized in the operating room. A minimally invasive approach by laparoscopic or robotic means may be possible in patients with accessible adenomas without active hemorrhage. Radiofrequency ablation (RFA) has been suggested as a potential treatment for patients with small or multiple adenomas not amenable to surgical treatment. Although RFA appears safe, long-term data are lacking on future hemorrhagic risks.

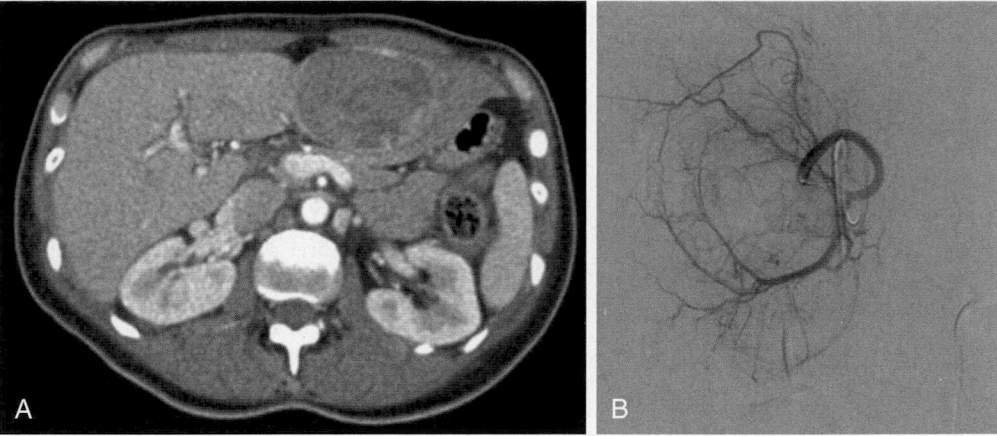

FIGURE 4 A, CT scan demonstrating a heterogenous mass in the left lobe of the liver, consistent with hemorrhage into a hepatic adenoma. **B,** Hepatic angiography demonstrating abnormal parenchymal blush and vasculature related to the hemangioma without active extravasation.

The management of patients with active or life-threatening hemorrhage from their adenomas will depend on the overall stability of the individual at presentation. If possible, embolization by interventional radiology is preferred in patients with evidence of active bleeding but stable vital signs, with elective resection of the adenoma during the same hospitalization (Figure 4, *A* and 4, *B*). In the minority of patients in whom embolization is not possible or who are hemodynamically unstable, emergent laparotomy may be necessary to gain control of bleeding. If an emergent operation is needed, a minimally invasive approach is not recommended. Mortality from intra-abdominal hemorrhage is high but is reported to decrease to between 5% and 10% after emergency resection or embolization. Pringle maneuver (inflow occlusion), packing of the liver, and hemostatic agents may be necessary to help control bleeding. Formal anatomic resection is not necessary unless it will help to quickly control hemorrhage. Selective arterial embolization is also a useful adjunct to treatment when bleeding cannot be controlled operatively, followed by elective resection at a later date.

■ FOCAL NODULAR HYPERPLASIA

Pathogenesis

FNH is the second most common benign hepatic lesion after hemangioma. These lesions have no identified malignant potential, and there is no risk of rupture or hemorrhage. Histopathology will demonstrate polyclonal proliferation of normal liver parenchyma, formed as a hyperplastic response to a fibrous scar of vessels found in the center of these lesions. However, approximately 20% of patients have an "atypical" lesion, defined by the absence of a central scar. The overwhelming majority of patients with FNH will have only one lesion; most are smaller than 5 cm. However, although rare, lesions greater than 10 cm have been reported.

Presentation

Similar to other benign liver diseases, FNH is diagnosed most commonly in females of reproductive age between 20 and 50 years, although no link with OCPs has been identified. However, it is suggested that FNH may be responsive to estrogen, and women taking OCPs have been noted to have larger, more symptomatic, and more vascular lesions. In rare situations, FNH is seen in children. FNH is identified in the majority of patients as an incidental finding on abdominal imaging. However, some individuals will be diagnosed after presenting with vague symptoms such as abdominal pain, discomfort, or a palpable liver mass. Liver function tests will be normal in the vast majority of patients, although an elevated alkaline phosphatase or bilirubin may be seen in patients with large lesions compressing the intrahepatic bile ducts.

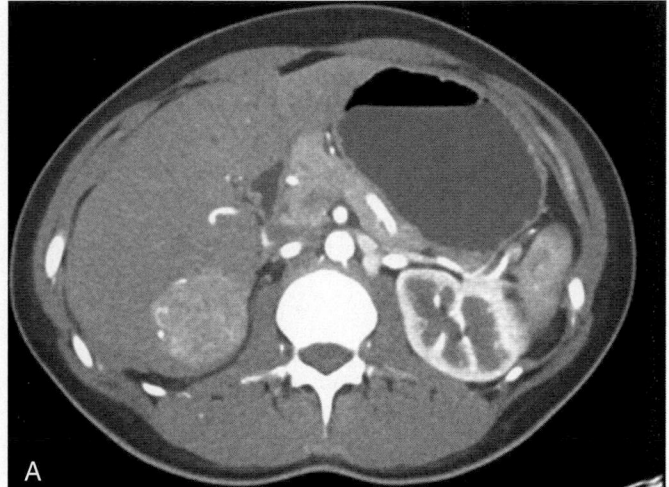

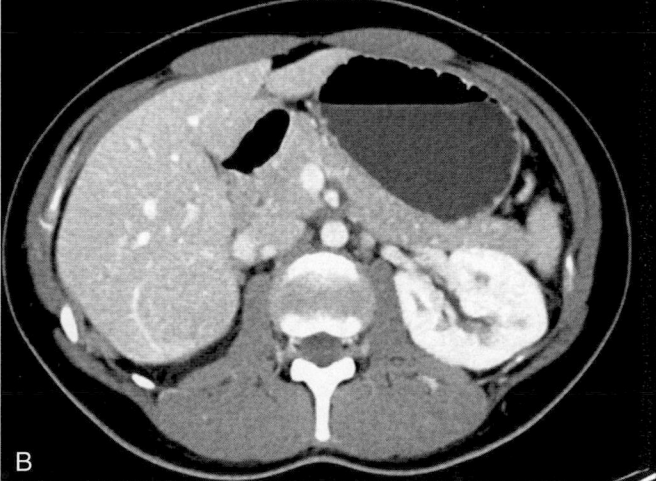

FIGURE 5 Arterial-phase (**A**) and venous-phase (**B**) CT scan demonstrating focal nodular hyperplasia in a 26-year-old woman.

Imaging

CT scan will demonstrate a well-circumscribed lesion that is hyperintense on the arterial phase scan (Figure 5, *A*) and isointense on venous phase (Figure 5, *B*), with a central scar that may remain hyperintense on venous phase because of the diffusion of contrast. If a noncontrast CT scan is obtained, the lesion will be isointense or hypointense, with a hypoattentuating central scar seen only in a minority of cases. On MRI, an isointense to hypointense lesion will be seen on T1-weighted images without attenuation of the central scar. T2-weighted imaging will show a hyperintense lesion with hyperintense central scar, with early enhancement if gadolinium is administered. Ultrasound is rarely useful for diagnosis because a central scar will be seen for only a minority of patients. Percutaneous biopsy for indeterminate lesions is generally not advisable, given a risk of tumor seeding if underlying malignancy is present as well as a low sensitivity and specificity for diagnosis.

Management

The majority of patients with FNH can be managed conservatively, and surgery is almost never necessary when the diagnosis is reached conclusively. In asymptomatic patients with typical imaging findings for FNH, resection is unnecessary and individuals may be followed with routine surveillance, although even this is not necessary long-term. It is also suggested that female patients with a newly diagnosed FNH discontinue OCPs, although this recommendation is controversial. A complete personal and family history in addition to laboratory values should be obtained to rule out the possibility of malignancy. Indications for hepatic resection are limited to only patients with symptoms, such as pain or weight loss, or the inability to conclusively rule out malignancy, often in those with atypical FNH and the absence of a central scar. FNH has no risk of malignant potential or bleeding, and surgery rarely is indicated. When necessary, hepatic resection can be performed by either an open or minimally invasive approach and should involve complete resection of the lesion with a rim of normal liver parenchyma. However, formal anatomic resection may be necessary based on the size and location of the lesion.

■ SUMMARY

Advances in imaging over the past several decades have not only improved our ability to accurately diagnose diseases but also have increased the frequency of incidentally discovered lesions, including those in the liver. An adequate workup is necessary to rule out malignancy for all incidentalomas. Fortunately, the most commonly found incidental liver lesions are benign and include simple cysts, hepatic hemangiomas, hepatic adenomas, and focal nodular hyperplasias. Most patients with asymptomatic, benign liver lesions can be monitored successfully with routine imaging and do not need surgical management. Hepatic resection is recommended for adenomas that are symptomatic, greater than 5 cm, or are growing because of the risks of hemorrhagic rupture or underlying malignancy. Hepatic cyst fenestration is recommended for symptomatic patients, or cysts with rapid growth during surveillance. Anatomic resection of cysts is necessary only when underlying malignancy (cystadenocarcinoma) is suspected or cannot be excluded. Hemangiomas of the liver should be resected only for truly symptomatic lesions or in rare cases of rupture. FNH is primarily managed conservatively, with operative management necessary only for symptomatic patients or when the possibility of underlying malignancy cannot be eliminated. The ability of a surgeon to understand the diagnostic characteristics and operative management of these four lesions is paramount to their proper treatment and prevention of unnecessary interventions.

SUGGESTED READINGS

Chun YS, House MG, Kaur H, et al. SSAT/AHPBA Joint Symposium on Evaluation and Treatment of Benign Liver Lesions. *J Gastrointest Surg.* 2013;17:636-644.

Gore RM, Newmark GM, Thakrar KH, et al. Hepatic incidentalomas. *Radiol Clin North Am.* 2011;49:291-322.

Kneuertz PJ, Marsh JW, de Jong MC, et al. Improvements in quality of life after surgery for benign hepatic tumors: results from a dual center analysis. *Surgery.* 2012;152:193-201.

Mezhir JJ, Fourman LT, Do RK, et al. Changes in the management of benign liver tumours: an analysis of 285 patients. *HBP (Oxford).* 2013;15:156-163.

Navarro AP, Gomez D, Lamb CM, et al. Focal nodular hyperplasia: a review of current indications for and outcomes of hepatic resection. *HPB (Oxford).* 2014;16:503-511.

Stoot J, Coelen RJS, de Jong MC, et al. Malignancy transformation of hepatocellular adenomas into hepatocellular carcinomas: a systematic review including more than 1600 adenoma cases. *HPB (Oxford).* 2010;12:509-522.

Yoon SS, Charny CK, Fong Y, Jarnagin WR, et al. Diagnosis, management, and outcomes of 115 patients with hepatic hemangioma. *J Am Coll Surg.* 2003;197:392-402.

Zucman-Rossi J, Jeannot E, Nhieu JT, et al. Genotype-phenotype correlation in hepatocellular adenoma: new classification and relationship with HCC. *Hepatology.* 2006;43:515-524.

THE MANAGEMENT OF MALIGNANT LIVER TUMORS

Richard D. Schulick, MD, and Ana L. Gleisner, MD

The most common malignant liver tumors are hepatocellular carcinoma (HCC), intrahepatic cholangiocarcinoma (ICC), and metastatic colorectal cancer (mCRC). In the Western world, metastatic liver tumors are more common than primary liver tumors.

Surgical resection is the mainstay of treatment for hepatic malignancies. Appropriate selection of patients for resection requires evaluation of the overall health status, oncologic appropriateness and, finally, resectability of the disease. A lesion is considered resectable if negative margins can be obtained while leaving an adequate amount of functional liver parenchyma with intact hepatic arterial and portal venous inflow, venous outflow, and biliary drainage. If this cannot be accomplished, other liver-directed therapies may be considered, such as tumor ablation, tumor embolization, and external radiation.

Tumor ablation can be performed with various techniques such as alcohol injection and thermal ablation with heat—microwave or radiofrequency ablation (RFA)—or cold (cryoablation); microwave and RFA are the most successful in hepatic malignancies. A newer technology called *irreversible electroporation* is emerging as an attractive alternative to thermal ablation for tumors near vascular structures. Irreversible electroporation uses short-duration, high-voltage pulses to create defects in the lipid bilayer that ultimately result in cell necrosis without the heat-sink effect that is associated with thermal ablation when used near vascular structures. Tumor embolization includes transarterial bland embolization (TAE), transarterial chemoembolization (TACE), or radioembolization. Finally, external-beam radiation therapy—either conformal or stereotactic—is emerging as yet another alternative for the treatment of malignant liver tumors not amenable to resection.

HEPATOCELLULAR CARCINOMA

HCC is the most common primary malignant liver tumor worldwide. Although the incidence is highest in Asia and sub-Saharan Africa, the incidence in the United States has been increasing in recent years. Risk factors include cirrhosis of any cause, including hepatitis B and C. In the absence of cirrhosis, HCC usually is associated with hepatitis B, although a variant type, fibrolamellar HCC, occurs in patients with no underlying liver disease. HCCs are characterized by homogeneous enhancement in the arterial phase and washout of the contrast material in the portal venous phase on computed tomography (CT) scan and magnetic resonance imaging (MRI).

For patients with cirrhosis, liver transplantation will address both the HCC and the underlying liver disease. However, because of limited organ availability and transplant-associated risks, such as organ rejection and immunosuppression-related complications, other treatment modalities often must be considered. The most widely used treatment modalities for HCC include TACE, ablation, and resection. Resection versus transplantation will be addressed in a separate chapter.

Surgical resection of HCC is a good option when feasible. The presence and degree of fibrosis/cirrhosis correlates with the incidence of postoperative liver failure, as well as with long-term survival. Therefore major liver resection generally is limited to patients with no cirrhosis or cirrhosis classified as Child's A with no evidence of portal hypertension. In these patients, mortality rates are lower than 5%. Although 5-year survival rates range from 30% to 60%, recurrence rates are considerable among patients with cirrhosis, with recurrence noted in about one third of patients within 5 years. Other factors negatively associated with long-term survival include invasion of major vessels, microvascular invasion, and both the number of tumors and tumor size. However, when adjusted for the presence of other prognostic features, tumor size is not a predictor of survival in patients with solitary lesions. Resection of tumors in patients with multifocal HCC and major vascular invasion are associated with poor prognosis and high recurrence rates (>95%) and should be considered only in highly selected cases.

In the appropriately selected patient, resection should be attempted only if negative margins can be obtained. Moreover, a recent randomized trial showed improved survival in patients after resection of HCC with 2-cm margins compared with resection with 1-cm margins. Ideally, anatomic resections of portal territories, including sectionectomies, segmentectomy, and subsegmentectomy, should be performed, because HCC tends to spread via portal venous tributaries. Anatomic resections have been associated with improved survival in patients with HCC in observational studies. However, thermal ablation of small (<3 cm) HCC has been shown to have long-term outcomes that are equivalent to surgical resection in recent randomized trials, with less morbidity and mortality. These data should be interpreted cautiously, however, because these studies had small sample sizes and were not designed as noninferiority trials. There are prospective studies that suggest inferior long-term outcomes for ablation compared with surgical resection, with local recurrence rates close to 10%. Ablation can be accomplished percutaneously or through an open or laparoscopic operation. Finally, ablation of tumors greater than 4 cm or close to major vascular structures should be avoided, because this approach is associated with high rates of incomplete tumor destruction and recurrence, with local recurrence rates as high as 40%.

Embolization (bland, chemoembolization, or radioembolization) is used typically for patients who are not candidates for curative treatment by resection, transplantation, or ablation. Embolization also may be used as a bridge to liver transplantation or before ablation for tumors between 3 and 5 cm. In the latter group, the combination of TACE and RFA has been shown to improve survival when compared with either modality alone. Response rates with TACE are as high as 80%, but the treatment usually must be repeated every 3 to 6 months. A total bilirubin greater than 3 mg/dL is a contraindication for these treatments. Portal vein thrombosis is a relative contraindication for TAE and TACE. These patients can be treated with radioembolization or external-beam radiation. In the right setting, superselective embolization can be considered even if the ipsilateral portal vein is thrombosed. External-beam radiation is an alternative for HCC with local control rates around 90%, although long-term data are limited.

Although surgical resection and transplantation are contraindicated in the presence of extrahepatic disease, liver-directed therapies may be used in the presence of limited extrahepatic disease, if the liver disease is thought to be rate limiting.

INTRAHEPATIC CHOLANGIOCARCINOMA

ICC is the second most common primary malignant liver tumor, accounting for 10% to 20% of such cases. Its incidence has increased markedly over recent decades for unclear reasons. Risk factors for the development of cholangiocarcinoma include sclerosing cholangitis (8% to 20% lifetime risk), choledochal cysts (3% to 28% lifetime risk), and cirrhosis. Of the three gross subtypes of ICC—mass forming, periductal infiltrating, and intraductal—the periductal infiltrating type is associated with the worst prognosis and unfortunately is the most common. ICCs are typically low in attenuation on CT scan, with minor peripheral enhancement and upstream biliary dilation. Capsular retraction also may be noted. The diagnosis often is made when a liver lesion is found to be adenocarcinoma from biopsy and a workup for the primary is undertaken with upper and lower endoscopy and sometimes PET scan without a source.

Surgical resection with the goal of obtaining negative margins is the only curative option. The hilar nodes should be dissected formally because they are positive in about one third of this patient population. Survival rates for resected patients range between 40% and 60% in 5 years. Positive margins and positive nodes are associated with worse prognosis, and adjuvant chemotherapy and radiation may be beneficial in these cases, although unproven by randomized controlled trials. ICC is associated with a significant risk of peritoneal carcinomatosis, and diagnostic laparoscopy sometimes is considered in these patients. Presence of extrahepatic disease including lymph nodes beyond the porta hepatis is a contraindication for resection. Multiple liver lesions, which represent intrahepatic metastases, are associated with a poor prognosis, and resection should be considered only in highly selected patients. The presence of gross lymph node metastases in the hilum also is associated with worse prognosis, but some of these patients may benefit from resection and adjuvant therapy. For locally advanced tumors, TAE, TACE, or radioembolization can be used. Radiographic response can be seen in 25% of the patients. Whether regional therapy is better than chemotherapy in locally advance tumors still remains to be determined.

METASTATIC COLORECTAL CANCER

Colorectal cancer is the third most frequent malignancy with approximately 130,000 new cases diagnosed every year in the United States. Synchronous or metachronous metastatic involvement of the liver will be diagnosed in about 50% of the patients with colorectal cancer. Consequently, mCRCs are far more common than primary liver tumors. These lesions are typically hypovascular and appear hypodense during the portal venous phases on CT scan. In this chapter, we focus on the resection of mCRC. Other liver-directed therapies for mCRC are addressed in other chapters.

Surgical resection is the best curative option in patients with colorectal liver metastasis. The goal of the procedure should be to remove all the metastases with microscopically negative margins. The width of the negative surgical margins has not been shown to be associated with increased risk of local recurrence in patients with mCRC. Parenchymal-sparing hepatectomies are preferred to major hepatectomies when applicable because these procedures are associated with decreased morbidity and increased rates of salvage ability in cases of recurrence, with no increase in recurrence rate or decrease in overall survival. For bilateral colorectal metastases, major resection can be combined with wedge resection or ablation of the lesions on the contralateral side. These procedures may be performed at the same time or with staged operations, as dictated by the anticipated volume of the liver remnant. In patients with colorectal cancer and synchronous hepatic metastasis, the primary tumor and the liver disease can be resected at the same time or separately. Concomitant liver and colorectal resection should be considered when only a minor liver resection is required or when the colon surgery is straightforward. Major liver resections should, however, be avoided when complex colorectal procedures are performed, such as those requiring extensive pelvic dissection or a low rectal anastomosis. In these situations, the hepatic metastases can be addressed first or after resection of the primary. Because the liver is usually the determining factor for complete disease resection, the "liver first" approach is an attractive option, especially for patients with extensive liver disease that may progress to unresectability and patients with rectal cancer that will require time between radiation and resection of the primary tumor. Occasionally, however, the primary tumor is symptomatic and must be addressed first. In contrast to patients with primary liver tumors, hepatic resection often is considered for patients with extrahepatic disease, so long as the extrahepatic disease is limited and resectable. This is a reflection of the very high response rates to the various systemic chemotherapy options currently available.

Preoperative chemotherapy typically is administered to assess tumor response, and in theory to address micrometastatic disease that is not seen on imaging, although it has not been shown to improve survival in candidates for hepatic resection of mCRC. However, prolonged modern chemotherapy for colorectal cancer may be associated with significant injury to the liver, with increased risk of postoperative complications after liver resection. Specifically, irinotecan-based treatment is associated with steatohepatitis, whereas oxaliplatin-based chemotherapy is associated with sinusoidal congestion. Moreover, small (<2 cm) lesions may disappear with chemotherapy. If not surgically resected, these lesions will recur in up to 80% of the patients. The surgeon and the medical oncologist must work closely to determine optimal duration of preoperative chemotherapy and timing for the surgical procedures. In general if preoperative chemotherapy is used, the duration should be limited to several months before bringing the patient to the operating room.

Prognostic factors for patients who have undergone curative resection of mCRC to the liver include the disease-free interval between the diagnosis of the primary tumor and the metastatic disease, size of the largest hepatic tumor, presence of extrahepatic disease, and nodal status of the primary tumor. Overall and disease-free survival range from 30% to 60% and 20% to 40% in 5 years, respectively.

PREOPERATIVE ASSESSMENT

Patients should undergo preoperative optimization and risk stratification according to the presence of medical comorbidities. Liver function is assessed with evaluation of total bilirubin, prothrombin time, albumin, presence of ascites, and history of encephalopathy. The Child-Turcotte-Pugh (CTP) scoring system (Table 1) is associated with perioperative mortality rates of 5%, 30%, and 80% in patients with classes A, B, and C, respectively. Thrombocytopenia (platelets <100,000/mm³), splenomegaly, and esophageal varices are indicatives of portal hypertension, which is associated with prohibitive rates of perioperative mortality after major liver resections.

The location of the hepatic lesions and their relationship to the main hepatic vessels and the biliary tree are determined with high-quality contrast-enhanced CT scan or MRI. The volume of the future liver remnant (FLR) then is estimated to minimize risk of postoperative hepatic failure. The minimal recommended volume of the FLR varies according to the quality of the liver remnant. For patients with

TABLE 1: Child-Turcotte-Pugh score*

Measure	1 Point	2 Points	3 Points
Total bilirubin (mg/dL)	<2	2-3	>3
Serum albumin (g/L)	>35	28-35	<28
PT/INR	<1.7	1.71-2.30	>2.30
Ascites	None	Mild	Moderate to severe
Hepatic encephalopathy	None	Grades I-II (suppressed with medication)	Grades III-IV (refractory)

*The score uses five clinical measures: class A, 5-6 points; class B, 7-9 points; class C, 10-15 points.

PT/INR, Prothrombin time/international normalized ratio.

a healthy liver, the FLR should be at least 20% of the total liver volume. Patients with some degree of liver dysfunction, such as those with chemotherapy-induced liver injury, should have a FLR of at least 30%, whereas those with evidence of cirrhosis should have a FLR of 40% or more depending on degree of dysfunction. Volumetry is calculated with three-dimensional CT scan or MRI. The volume of nonfunctional liver (parenchyma that is either nonperfused or replaced by tumor) is subtracted from the total liver volume, which is especially important for patients with large lesions. Alternatively, the estimated total liver volume can be calculated with the patient's body weight or body surface area (i.e., total liver volume in cm³ = $-794.41 + 1267.28 \times$ body surface area in m²). Patients with insufficient FLR volumes should undergo portal vein embolization (PVE) of the branches of the segments planned for resection to induce growth to the contralateral side. Volumetry is repeated about 4 weeks after PVE and in a few more weeks if the minimal recommended FLR has not been achieved. The degree of hypertrophy (hyperplasia) of the remnant (at least a 5% increase in the volume of the FLR or an increase of 2% per week or more) has been associated with decreased rates of postoperative liver insufficiency.

OPERATIVE APPROACH TO RESECTION

Liver resections can be categorized into anatomic and nonanatomic. Anatomic resections include segmentectomies, sectionectomies, hemihepatectomies, and extended hepatectomies. Although small peripheral lesions are usually amenable to nonanatomic resections, lesions that are either large or centrally located often require anatomic resections. These procedures can be performed either through an open technique or laparoscopically. Laparoscopic liver resections are addressed in a separate chapter.

Positioning, Incision, and Exposure

Patients are placed supine in 15 degrees Trendelenburg position to decrease the risk of air embolism with both arms extended at 90 degrees. Intravenous fluids should be restricted until transection of the parenchyma is completed to decrease bleeding from hepatic veins. Central venous cannulation is often unnecessary but should be considered in patients with extensive comorbidities. If used, a central venous pressure less than 5 cm H₂O should be maintained. Once the parenchymal transection has been completed, intravascular volume should be restored to achieve isovolemia.

In the open technique, a right subcostal incision with an upper midline extension provides adequate exposure for most tumors. The xyphoid should be removed to facilitate visualization of the suprahepatic inferior vena cava (IVC). An upper midline incision is usually adequate for resections of the left liver and may suffice for resection of the right liver in a thin patient. Lesions in the right liver near the dome may require a thoracoabdominal incision for better exposure of the suprahepatic vena cava. The abdominal cavity is explored for the presence of extrahepatic disease. The round ligament is ligated, and the falciform ligament is dissected up to the anterior surface of the hepatic veins. The gastrohepatic ligament is opened to expose the caudate lobe with care not to injure an accessory or replaced left hepatic artery. Intraoperative ultrasound is performed to identify all known lesions—as well as any new lesions—and their relationship with vascular and biliary structures, as well as the position of the main hepatic vessels relative to the transection plane.

Inflow and Outflow Control

For major hepatic resections, artery and portal vein inflow vessels can be dissected and controlled in the hilum of the liver, intraparenchymally, or through small hepatotomies (see Figure 1). The latter approach should be avoided if the tumors are close to the hilum (<2 cm). Selective inflow control before the transection will result in a vascular demarcation line that will guide the correct transection plane. After inflow has been controlled, control of the hepatic venous outflow is performed. This also can be done outside the liver or within the parenchyma, during the transection.

Occlusion of the portal triad (Pringle maneuver) can be performed in major and minor liver resections during the transection of the parenchyma to decrease blood loss. The liver can tolerate up to 1 hour of ischemia, but intermittent vascular occlusion with cycles of 15 to 20 minutes on and 5 minutes off will decrease the ischemia/reperfusion injury, which is especially important in cirrhotic livers. Total ischemic time always should be limited as much as possible. If proper transection planes are selected, often a Pringle maneuver is not necessary, especially if inflow vascular control to the portion of the liver to be removed has been performed.

Parenchymal Transection

Transection of the liver parenchyma can be performed with multiple techniques—most often a combination of techniques—according to the surgeon's experience and preference. Finger fracture (digitoclasy), clamp crushing, water jet devices, and ultrasound energy devices (i.e., CUSA or Cavitron Ultrasonic Surgical Aspirator) gently fracture the parenchyma while preserving vessels and bile ducts crossing the transection plane (Figure 2). These structures then are controlled with ties, clips, energy devices, or staplers for larger structures. Bipolar (i.e., LigaSure, Covidien, Mansfield, MA) and ultrasonic (Harmonic Scalpel, Ethicon Endo-Surgery, Cincinnati, OH) vessel-sealing devices can be used for control of vessels up to 7 to 8 mm—decreasing the need for ties and clips and thereby resulting in faster transection. Hemostatic devices such as the argon beam coagulator and the radio-frequency sealer devices (i.e., TissueLink and Aquamantys, Medtronic, Minneapolis, MN) are very useful to control bleeding from the cut edge of the liver. Finally, staple devices can be used for the division of large vessels.

Right Hepatectomy

If a right hepatectomy is to be performed, further dissection of the anterior surface of the hepatic veins is carried out to expose the right hepatic vein. The right coronary and triangular ligaments then are divided, exposing the bare area of the liver as the right liver is mobilized and rotated to the left and the short hepatic veins draining directly to the IVC are ligated. The retrocaval ligament (Makuuchi's ligament) is identified and transected with a vascular stapler (Figure 3). Further dissection between the liver and the IVC will expose the right hepatic vein, which is encircled. Attention is turned to the hilum, where the right hepatic artery and right portal vein are dissected and ligated. Alternatively, the right pedicle is controlled intrahepatically as a large curved clamp is passed through an incision made at the left base of the gallbladder fossa, exiting through an incision at the junction of segment VII and the caudate process (see Figure 1). A clear line of vascular demarcation then can be identified, and the right hepatic vein is ligated subsequently with a stapler (Figure 4). The right hepatic duct will be identified as the transection of the parenchyma approaches the left base of the gallbladder fossa. The transection plane follows the area of vascular demarcation.

For large tumors in the right hemiliver that are adhered to the diaphragm and the retroperitoneum, the parenchyma can be divided before the mobilization of the right liver. Inflow control initially is

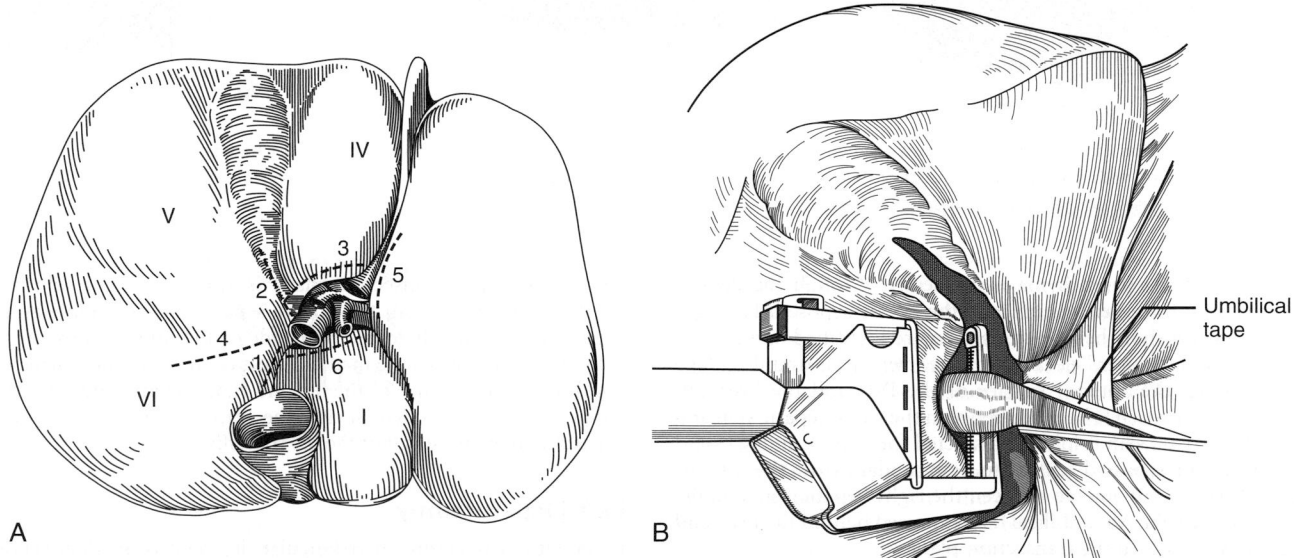

FIGURE 1 For the right portal pedicle to be accessed (**A**), hepatotomies are made in the gallbladder fossa (2) and in the caudate process (1). The pedicle is encircled with a renal pedicle clamp, and a vessel loop is passed around it. The vessel loop is used to retract the main portal vein/left portal vein to the left as a TA stapler is passed and fired to divide the right portal pedicle (**B**). *(From Fong Y, Blumgart LH. Useful stapling techniques in liver surgery. J Am Coll Surg. 1997;185:93.)*

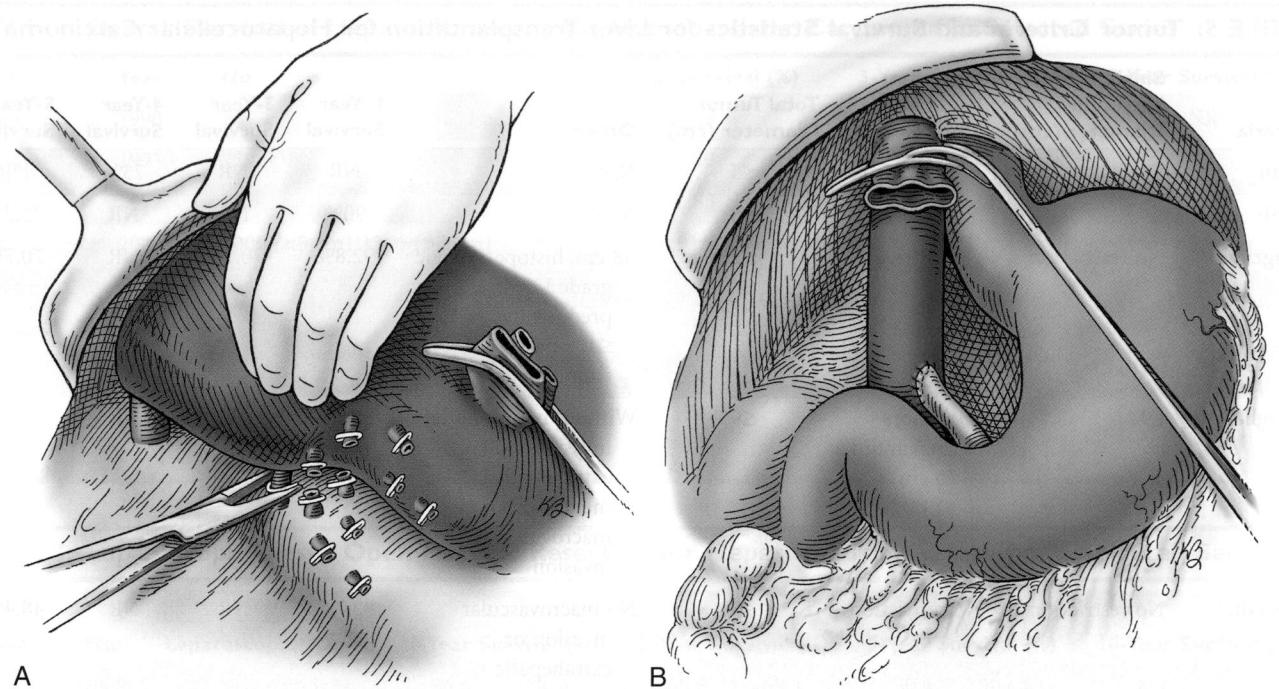

FIGURE 2 Piggyback explant technique. **A,** The division of short hepatic branches of the liver and separation of the liver off the inferior vena cava. **B,** Depiction of the explanted liver with native inferior vena cava intact. *(From Busuttil R, Klintmalm G, eds. Transplantation of the Liver. 3rd ed. Philadelphia: Elsevier; 2015, Figs. 45-16 and 45-17.)*

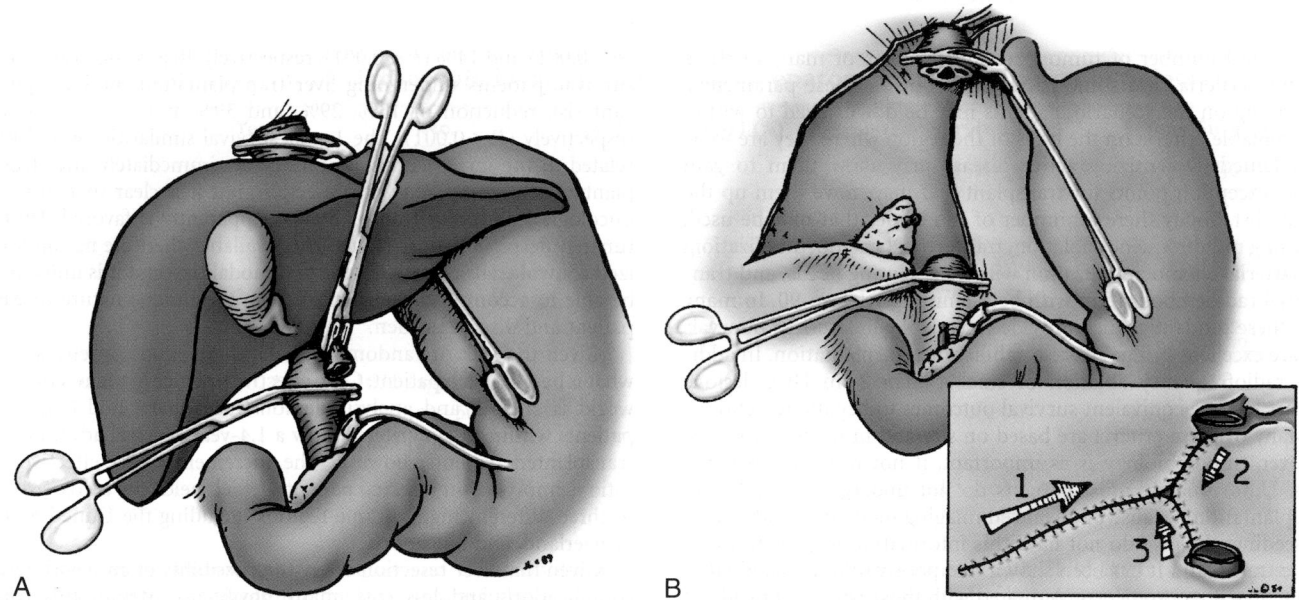

FIGURE 3 Classic bicaval explant technique. **A,** Clamps are placed on both the suprahepatic and infrahepatic inferior vena cava. **B,** Explanted liver showing orifices of all three hepatic veins. *(From Busuttil R, Klintmalm G, eds. Transplantation of the Liver. 3rd ed. Philadelphia: Elsevier; 2015, Figs. 45-9 and 45-10.)*

In addition, different techniques may be used in transplantation for HCC (Figures 2 and 3). There was initial concern regarding the use of the piggyback technique in HCC patients, which leaves the native inferior vena cava intact, because this theoretically may allow for a positive caval margin behind. Despite these concerns, in some hands the recurrence-free and overall survival is similar or even greater with the piggyback compared with conventional caval replacement. This is important given the use of living donor liver transplantation, which uses a piggyback technique.

Cholangiocarcinoma

Cholangiocarcinoma may be subdivided into perihilar and intrahepatic cholangiocarcinoma. The treatment options for intrahepatic cholangiocarcinoma are surgical resection, locoregional therapy, chemotherapy, and radiation, or a combination of these. The use of liver transplantation in these patients is not accepted widely, and patients are not granted exception points as in either HCC or perihilar cholangiocarcinoma.

Patients with perihilar cholangiocarcinoma may be resected, and concomitant liver resection can decrease recurrence rate and improve disease-specific survival. Unfortunately not all patients are amenable to resection; however, they may undergo transplantation and are granted MELD exception points if they meet certain criteria that vary from region to region. Transplant also may be used in the setting of severe liver disease and primary sclerosing cholangitis with cholangiocarcinoma. The most standardized therapy and protocol includes neoadjuvant chemoradiation followed by liver transplantation, and this has afforded a survival at 1, 3, and 5 years of 90%, 80%, and 71%, respectively.

SUGGESTED READINGS

Belghiti J, Fuks D. Liver resection and transplantation in hepatocellular carcinoma. *Liver Cancer.* 2012;1:71-82.

Bodzin AS, Busuttil RW. Hepatocellular carcinoma: advances in diagnosis, management, and long term outcome. *World J Hepatol.* 2015;7:1157-1167.

Ferreira MV, Chaib E, Nascimento MU, Nersessian RS, Setuguti DT, D'Albuquerque LA. Liver transplantation and expanded Milan criteria: does it really work? *Arq Gastroenterol.* 2012;49:189-194.

Goh BK, Chow PK, Teo JY, et al. Number of nodules, Child-Pugh status, margin positivity, and microvascular invasion, but not tumor size, are prognostic factors after liver resection for multifocal hepatocellular carcinoma. *J Gastrointest Surg.* 2014;18:1477-1485.

Llovet JM, Fuster J, Bruix J, Barcelona-Clinic Liver Cancer G. The Barcelona approach: diagnosis, staging, and treatment of hepatocellular carcinoma. *Liver Transpl.* 2004;10(2 suppl 1):S115-S120.

Sapisochín G, de Sevilla EF, Echeverri J, Charco R. Liver transplantation for cholangiocarcinoma: Current status and new insights. *World J Hepatol.* 2015;7:2396-2403.

Schroeder RA, Marroquin CE, Bute BP, Khuri S, Henderson WG, Kuo PC. Predictive indices of morbidity and mortality after liver resection. *Ann Surg.* 2006;243:373-379.

Simonetti RG, Camma C, Fiorello F, Politi F, D'Amico G, Pagliaro L. Hepatocellular carcinoma. A worldwide problem and the major risk factors. *Dig Dis Sci.* 1991;36:962-972.

Tranchart H, Di Giuro G, Lainas P, et al. Laparoscopic resection for hepatocellular carcinoma: a matched-pair comparative study. *Surg Endosc.* 2010;24:1170-1176.

Zheng Z, Liang W, Milgrom DP, et al. Liver transplantation versus liver resection in the treatment of hepatocellular carcinoma: a meta-analysis of observational studies. *Transplantation.* 2014;97:227-234.

ABLATION OF COLORECTAL CARCINOMA LIVER METASTASES

Zhi Ven Fong, MD, and Kenneth K. Tanabe, MD

Colorectal carcinoma is the third leading cause of new cancer incidence and cancer deaths in the United States, accounting for an estimated 49,700 cancer-specific deaths in 2015. Because of its portal venous drainage system, the liver is the most frequent site of colorectal carcinoma metastases. A third of patients with colorectal carcinoma have liver metastases, and up to a half of patients develop liver metastases throughout the course of their disease. Although surgical resection remains the mainstay therapy for isolated colorectal carcinoma liver metastases, many patients are not candidates for resection because of comorbidity or inability to spare sufficient liver.

Liver-directed locoregional ablative therapy represents a viable treatment option for some of these patients with unresectable colorectal liver metastases. Several liver ablation techniques use thermal energy to affect a zone of coagulative necrosis and irreversible damage to proteins and DNA, causing cell death. With an ablation electrode placed into the tumor, energy absorption by the cells produces heat and thermal coagulation of tumor cells and adjacent parenchyma. Since its introduction in the 1980s, ablation techniques have gone through significant evolution, with emerging technologies enabling quicker, more effective tumor ablation. In this chapter, we summarize the current ablative techniques (cryoablation, radiofrequency ablation [RFA], microwave ablation [MWA], and irreversible electroporation [IRE]) and review patient selection, outcomes, and follow-up after ablation.

CRYOTHERAPY

Cryotherapy first was described in 1951. It initially was used as a treatment for hepatocellular carcinoma, but its indication was extended to colorectal carcinoma liver metastases in the 1980s. Historically, liquid nitrogen was used to effect hypothermic cellular death by direct contact with the tumor surface. In more contemporary settings, cryoablation uses the Joule-Thomson effect with argon gas rather than liquid nitrogen to create repeated freeze-thaw cycles via insulated probes to cause tumor cell death. However, cryotherapy instrumentation is more cumbersome and more expensive and has been replaced by RFA in the majority of hospitals.

RADIOFREQUENCY ABLATION

RFA is the most widely used ablation technique. Metal electrodes (probes) are placed into the tumor and dispersive grounding pads placed on the patient. A generator creates high-frequency alternating currents of 350 to 500 kHz, which creates friction from ionic agitation within the current, primarily adjacent to the probe. The ion agitation generates extreme heat surrounding the probe, and further passive conduction into adjacent tissue. RFA electrodes are commercially available in different designs with the purpose of maximizing the size of ablation zones. Boston Scientific and Rita Medical use multitined, clustered electrodes to increase electrode surface area and create a larger ablation zone (Figure 1). Conversely, Valleylab and Celon use electrodes that are cooled internally via saline circulation, which minimizes desiccation and charring at the electrode-tissue interface. Charring is undesirable because it creates high electrical impedance and impedes current flow. This is critical because incomplete tumor ablation is the primary cause of local tumor recurrence. However, with all types of RFA probes, passive thermal conduction is necessary, and RFA efficacy decreases as tumor size increases. Studies have demonstrated significantly higher local recurrence rates when RFA is performed on tumors at least 3.5 cm in size. In addition, RFA is less effective when a tumor is very close to a large blood vessel because the continuous blood flow in the vessels keeps the tumor cells on the vessel wall very close to physiologic temperatures. This phenomenon is known as the "heat-sink" effect, the dissipation of thermal energy by blood flow.

There has been no randomized controlled trial evaluating the efficacy of RFA against other treatments for colorectal carcinoma liver metastases. In addition, it is difficult to analyze the comparative effectiveness of RFA from retrospective studies. Most studies comparing RFA with surgical resection for colorectal carcinoma liver metastases fail to overcome selection bias because the main indication for RFA is unresectability and patients who are unable to tolerate surgical resection. In addition, heterogeneity in the definition of unresectability by centers and disease (e.g., lesion size, number,

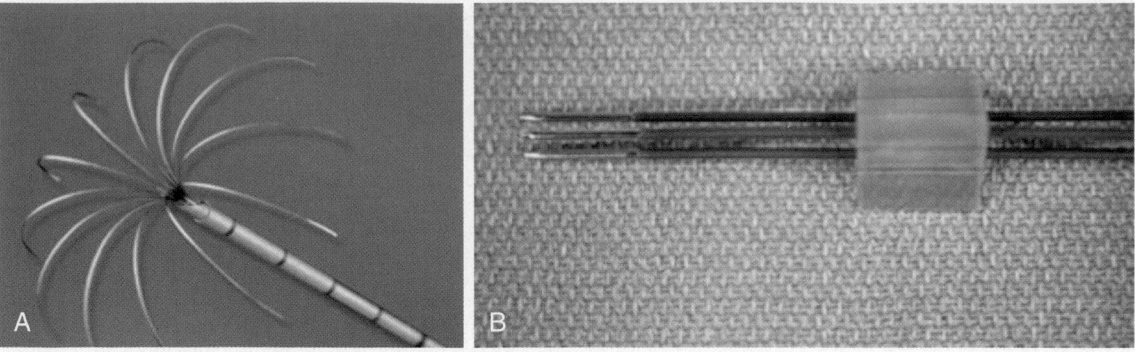

FIGURE 1 Radiofrequency electrode designs. **A,** Expandable multitined probe with its array deployed. **B,** Three clustered, straight electrodes spaced optimally to maximize ablation zones.

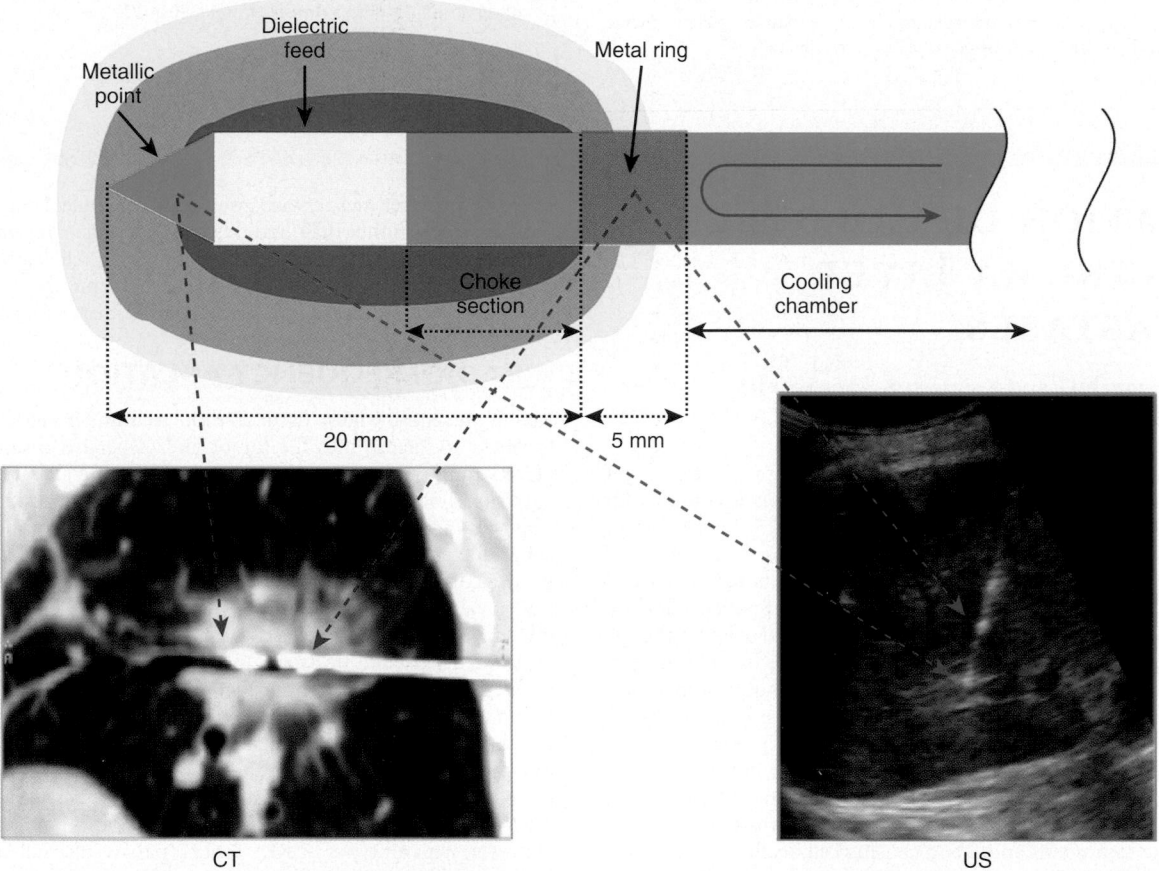

FIGURE 2 Microwave ablation electrode, with intraprocedural imaging of a computed tomography *(CT)*–guided ablation of a lung tumor *(left)* and ultrasound *(US)*-guided ablation of a liver tumor *(right)*. *(Images courtesy H.S. Hospital Services S.p.A, Rome, Italy.)*

location) further confounds the analysis, with multivariate regression often inadequate in controlling these important covariates. Such limitations notwithstanding, the liver-only and ablation site recurrence rates have been reported to be 44% and 9%, respectively. The 5-year survival rates reported by high-volume centers have been estimated to be 18% to 22%. In general, these outcomes are best when ablation is limited to solitary liver lesions that are smaller than 3 cm. Because of these data, resection is the preferred treatment whenever feasible. Prospective clinical trials with well-defined patient selection criteria and assessment of completeness of tumor ablation are needed to better delineate the true efficacy of RFA.

■ MICROWAVE ABLATION

MWA uses dielectric hysteresis to generate microwaves with frequencies ranging from 900 to 2500 mHz to cause coagulative necrosis. In contrast to RFA, microwave antennas are used as probes, which cause active heating of all tissues within their broadcasting range, thereby inducing a more homogenous zone of thermal destruction (Figure 2). In contrast to RFA, MWA does not require power control via temperature or impedance monitoring. When compared with RFA, experimental studies in mouse models have demonstrated that MWA is associated with a more rapid rise in temperature and larger ablation zone. In addition to producing less charring, MWA is better able to penetrate through biologic materials with low conductivity (i.e., charred tissue) and is nearly 25% less susceptible to the "heat-sink" effect because it does not rely as much on heating by thermal conduction. In one published report on MWA of hepatic tumors (50% colorectal liver metastases), successful ablation (defined radiographically) was observed in 100% of patients with an ablation site recurrence of less than 3% and overall hepatic recurrence of 37%. The overall survival was 38 months.

■ IRREVERSIBLE ELECTROPORATION

IRE represents the latest ablative technology and uses repeated electrical pulses to irreversibly increase the permeability of cells' lipid bilayer in targeted cell membranes and spares adjacent structures. Although cells themselves undergo apoptosis, the structural integrity of adjacent vital structures such as blood vessels and bile ducts is preserved. Accordingly, IRE is well suited to applications in which tumors are directly adjacent to critical vascular or biliary structures. Patients undergoing IRE require deep muscle paralysis because IRE generally triggers muscle contraction with each pulse of delivered energy. IRE should not be performed in proximity to the heart because of potential cardiac arrhythmias secondary to alterations in the ion transport initiated by the electrical current. Although the safety and efficacy of this modality requires further investigation, IRE represents a very promising modality with ongoing clinical trials enrolling patients prospectively.

■ PATIENT SELECTION

Surgical resection, whenever feasible, remains the mainstay of treatment of isolated colorectal carcinoma liver metastases. When patients are not candidates for resection, systemic chemotherapy and local ablative strategies should be considered. Despite advances in systemic chemotherapies that have led to response rates as high as 70%, durable complete clinical responses are still rare with systemic chemotherapy alone. It has been postulated that aggressive cytoreduction with ablation combined with chemotherapy may be more effective than chemotherapy alone. This concept was examined in the CLOCC trial, a study in which patients with colorectal carcinoma liver metastases were randomized to treatment with chemotherapy alone, versus chemotherapy plus RFA. Patients had up to nine colorectal carcinoma liver metastases lesions smaller than or equal to 4 cm and were considered unresectable. No difference in 30-month overall survival rate was observed between the two groups (61.7% for combined treatment vs 57.6% for chemotherapy only group, $P = 0.22$). However, the 3-year disease-free survival rate for the combined treatment group was higher than that of the chemotherapy-only group (27.6% vs 10.6%, $P = 0.025$). These results dispel the notion that chemotherapy combined with ablation is a superior approach to chemotherapy alone. However, use of ablation instead of chemotherapy or to allow for a chemotherapy holiday has merit in selected patients.

Some studies show better outcomes when ablation is performed on patients who have had an objective response to systemic therapy, which is not a surprising finding given that this is a biologically favorable cohort. Consideration of the ablative approach to patients who are candidates for combined therapy must involve integration of specific tumor-specific variables into treatment planning. As previously mentioned, RFA is the most commonly used ablation modality, but MWA should be considered when the tumor is at least 3 cm or is in proximity to a large vessel because it provides a more consistent radial heating distribution and is less susceptible to "heat-sink" effects. Larger tumors (>5 cm) are associated with an unacceptably high risk of recurrence when treated with ablation, most likely secondary to incomplete ablation. In selected patients with larger tumors, surgical resection can be combined with ablation to offer patients the best chance at long-term disease-free survival. For example, a patient with a large metastasis in the left lobe and two smaller metastases located deep in the right lobe may benefit from left hepatectomy combined with ablation of the two right lobe lesions. For lesions adjacent to major vessels or central bile ducts, IRE should be considered to minimize adjacent vessel or ductal injuries that may lead to strictures.

■ EVALUATION

It is important to emphasize that, as with all cancer care, patients with colorectal carcinoma liver metastases should be evaluated by a multidisciplinary team, including medical oncologists, surgical oncologists, and diagnostic and interventional radiologists. Although liver ablation is a treatment option for unresectable colorectal carcinoma liver metastases, not all lesions are amendable to ablation. For patients who are candidates for ablation, specific clinical features should be taken into consideration to appropriately plan which modality to use, appropriate timing, and specific approach to probe placements to ensure a complete and successful ablation.

Extrahepatic Metastases

In accordance to guidelines issued by the National Comprehensive Cancer Network (NCCN) and the American Society of Clinical Oncology, patients with metastatic colorectal carcinoma should undergo a computed tomography (CT) scan and positron emission tomography (PET) scan to evaluate for extrahepatic metastatic disease. Liver magnetic resonance imaging (MRI) with a hepatobiliary contrast agent is the most sensitive technique for detection of liver metastases. Patients whose colorectal carcinoma metastases are restricted to the liver are the best candidates for ablative therapy (in lieu of resection). Patients with lung metastases should be evaluated by a thoracic surgeon; ablation of liver metastases should be considered only in circumstances in which the lung metastases also will be extirpated, ablated, or radiated definitively. Patients with peritoneal metastases or distant nodal metastases (i.e., paracaval nodes) should not be considered for liver tumor ablation.

Baseline Hepatic Function

Candidates for hepatic ablation also should undergo evaluation of liver function. This includes assessment of biochemical liver function tests to assess for cholestasis or liver inflammation, inspection of scans in search of clues suggesting hepatic steatosis, and a search for any evidence of portal hypertension. Thrombocytopenia from splenomegaly combined with portal hypertension increases the risks of liver tumor ablation. A vast majority of patients have liver function sufficient to support liver tumor ablation. Chemotherapy-induced hepatotoxicity in the form of steatosis, steatohepatitis, and sinusoidal distension increases the risks of liver resection. However, these conditions appear to have little impact on risks associated with ablation.

Tumor-Specific Parameters

On the basis of the CT or PET scan, the surgeon should consider the size, number, and location of each lesion. Lesions larger than 3.5 cm likely will require multiple probe placements for complete ablation, and the need for overlapping ablation zones to eradicate a tumor significantly increases the risk of incomplete ablation and local recurrence. The lesion's proximity to major vessels (portal and hepatic vein) should be evaluated, and MWA can be considered versus RFA to mitigate any anticipated potential "heat-sink" effect. Lesions close to the central bile ducts should not be thermally ablated because of potential injury to bile ducts. For ablations performed percutaneously, proximity of the tumors to gallbladder, stomach, colon, and diaphragm should be taken into consideration to prevent burn injuries. This is not an issue for thermal ablations performed via laparoscopic or open surgery because tumors may be dissected away from these structures before ablation. For metastases in proximity to the heart, percutaneous positioning of electrodes is risky, and ablation of these tumors is best accomplished by operative approach. IRE should not be used for metastases in proximity to the heart for fear of induction of arrhythmia.

■ TREATMENT APPROACH

Percutaneous Versus Operative Approach

Ablation can be performed with a percutaneous or operative approach (open or laparoscopic) (Figure 3), each having its own benefits and tradeoffs. Percutaneous ablation is less invasive and is associated with lower morbidity rates and cost than operative ablation. This approach is ideal for patients not able to tolerate general anesthesia and whose tumors are not adjacent to visceral organs. It is also ideal for patients with lesions requiring repeat applications. For patients with liver lesions close to visceral organs, percutaneous infusion of dextrose fluid into the space can be used to create a separation between the lesion and adjacent structure (i.e., diaphragm) and is effective in mitigating adjacent thermal injury.

For patients requiring laparoscopy or laparotomy for other reasons such as combined hepatectomy with ablation, or colectomy for extirpation of the primary colorectal carcinoma, a surgical approach for ablation (open or laparoscopic) should be considered. Although open or laparoscopic ablation is associated with higher morbidity than percutaneous ablation, it offers the opportunity for surgical exploration of the abdomen, which improves staging. During

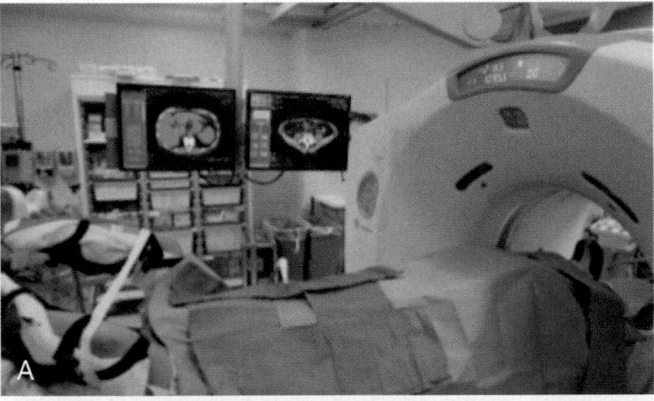
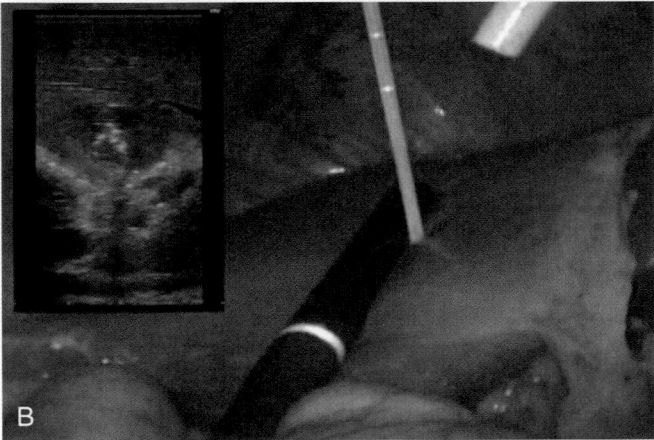

FIGURE 3 A, Patient set up for a computed tomography–guided percutaneous microwave ablation (MWA) of a hepatocellular carcinoma in an interventional radiology suite. **B,** Laparoscopic MWA of a hepatic tumor under the guidance of intraoperative ultrasound. *(Photo courtesy Dr. R. Santambrogio, HPB and Digestive Surgery, San Paolo Hospital, University of Milan, Italy.)*

laparotomy or laparoscopy, up to 10% to 20% of patients are found to have radiographically occult extrahepatic metastases, which are a relative contraindication to ablation. In addition, intraoperative ultrasound allows for accurate evaluation of tumor location and more precise electrode placements. Temporary hepatic blood flow occlusion maneuvers, such as the Pringle maneuver or hepatic artery occlusion, also minimize "heat-sink" effects during ablation. As a result of more complete tumor destruction, ablation via the operative approach has been reported to have an estimated ablation site recurrence of 3%, lower than that of the percutaneous approach (8%). Finally, the operative approach allows for ablation to be used adjunctively with surgical resection.

Technical Considerations for Operative Approach

Ablation via the laparoscopic approach often can be achieved with two ports: an umbilical port (for the laparoscope) and a second port for the laparoscopic ultrasound probe. The ablation probe can be placed percutaneously and does not require an additional port. The first step in performing operative ablation of colorectal carcinoma liver metastases is a thorough evaluation of the abdominal cavity to exclude extrahepatic metastases (e.g., peritoneal surfaces, diaphragm). Intraoperative liver ultrasound then should be performed to evaluate the location of the tumor(s), identify any additional tumors not seen on preoperative imaging, and assess the relationship of tumors to major vascular and biliary structures. The position of the probe placement must be planned carefully to achieve the most effective ablation zone. Gas produced during ablation creates ultrasonographic echogenicity, which obscures view of deeper areas. Therefore the ultrasonographically deepest portions of a tumor typically are ablated first. Once the tumor location is mapped out, visceral organs in proximity to the planned ablation zone should be dissected or retracted out of harm's way. If the tumor is in proximity to the gallbladder, a cholecystectomy may be necessary. Under intraoperative ultrasound guidance, the ablation electrode then is placed into the target lesion, and the array deployed within. A tourniquet may be placed around the porta hepatis for inflow occlusion.

Thermal ablation then is initiated, and specifically for RFA, monitoring is performed to maintain a maximum parenchymal temperature of about 100° C to 110° C to minimize charring. The monitoring is performed via different approaches depending on the manufacturer. Rita Medical uses temperature control via sensor electrodes embedded in the tips of the tines, whereas Boston Scientific uses impedance control, in which the ablation power is slowly ramped up until the tissue impedance reaches a preset threshold. Once the temperature or impedance level is reached, the energy source is turned off to allow tissue vaporization to settle and reapplied at a lower level or terminated completely.

■ COMPLICATIONS AND FOLLOW-UP

For all ablation techniques, the potential complications range from minor, such as skin burn under the grounding pads, to more serious, such as bile leak, bleeding, and liver abscesses. Cryoablation historically was associated with complication rates of 10% to 20%, which ultimately saw the technique being replaced with RFA and MWA. These more contemporary techniques have been demonstrated to be safer, with morbidity rates ranging from 2% to 5%. Reported determinants of complication rates, in addition to tumor size and location, include physician and institution experience, as well as ablation approaches (percutaneous vs operative).

Post-treatment imaging is performed to evaluate the efficacy of ablation. In contrast to hepatocellular carcinoma, colorectal liver metastases are often hypovascular, which makes it difficult to differentiate residual tumor from areas of necrosis. In general, it is most helpful to compare preprocedural and postprocedural images with regard to the size, shape, and location of the necrosis zone. Ideally, a 5- to 10-mm margin of ablation should be achieved

Successful tumor ablation

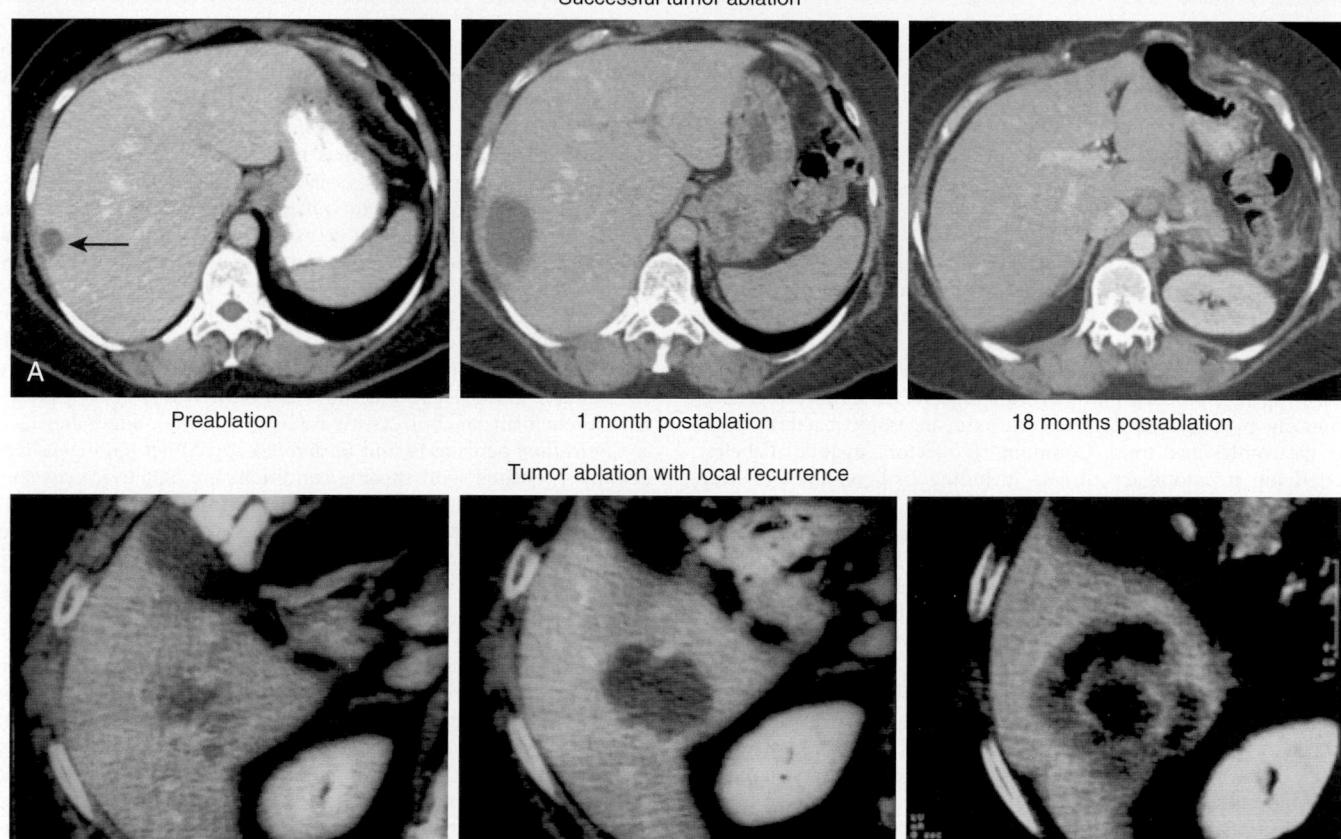

Preablation   1 month postablation   18 months postablation

Tumor ablation with local recurrence

Preablation   Incomplete tumor ablation   Tumor recurrence

FIGURE 4 A, Successful radiofrequency ablation of colorectal carcinoma liver metastases, with computed tomography (CT) imaging demonstrating the lesion in segment VI preablation (*arrow*), necrosis zone from ablation at 1 month, followed by radiographic resolution at 18 months postablation. **B,** Incomplete ablation of colorectal carcinoma liver metastases, with CT imaging showing the lesion preablation, postablation imaging demonstrating the irregularity in the contour of ablation affected by adjacent vessels, and postoperative CT revealing local ablation-site recurrence resulting from incomplete ablation.

circumferentially. The International Working Group on Image-Guided Tumor Ablation recommends a baseline study (CT or MRI) to be performed within 1 week and no more than 4 weeks post-ablation. This also ensures that residual disease as a result of incomplete ablation is picked up expediently and treated by repeat ablation. Subsequent follow-up imaging then can be spaced out to every 3 to 4 months. PET scans have been demonstrated to be sensitive for detection of recurrence in patients who are at least 3 months postablation when the inflammation has subsided. NCCN guidelines are similar and recommend imaging every 3 to 6 months for the first 2 years after ablation, which then can be spread out to annually thereafter (Figure 4).

SUMMARY

Surgical resection should be the mainstay therapy for patients with colorectal carcinoma liver metastases. However, for the majority of patients who are not candidates for resection, liver ablation represents a treatment modality that offers these patients a chance at disease-free survival. In addition, liver ablation plays a role as an adjunct to liver resection for local disease control. Clinical trials with clearly defined patient selection and outcomes measures are needed to better delineate the true utility of liver ablation in the primary or adjunctive treatment of colorectal carcinoma liver metastases. As newer ablation techniques with larger ablation zones and shorter

ablation times emerge, the selection criteria for ablation will continue to extend and outcomes improve.

SUGGESTED READINGS

Abdalla EK, Vauthey JN, Ellis LM, Ellis V, Pollock R, Broglio KR, Hess K, Curley SA. Recurrence and outcomes following hepatic resection, radio-frequency ablation, and combined resection/ablation for colorectal liver metastases. *Ann Surg.* 2004;239:818-825.

Adam R, Delvart V, Pascal G, Valeanu A, Castaing D, Azoulay D, Giacchetti S, Paule B, Kunstlinger F, Ghémard O, Levi F, Bismuth H. Rescue surgery for unresectable colorectal liver metastases downstaged by chemotherapy: a model to predict long-term survival. *Ann Surg.* 2004;240:644-657.

Martin RC, Scoggins CR, McMasters KM. Safety and efficacy of microwave ablation of hepatic tumors: a prospective review of a 5-year experience. *Ann Surg Oncol.* 2010;17:171-178.

Oshowo A, Gillams A, Harrison E, Lees WR, Taylor I. Comparison of resection and radiofrequency ablation for treatment of solitary colorectal liver metastases. *Br J Surg.* 2003;90:1240-1243.

Siperstein AE, Berber E, Ballem N, Parikh RT. Survival after radiofrequency ablation of colorectal liver metastases: 10-year experience. *Ann Surg.* 2007;246:559-565.

Wong SL, Mangu PB, Choti MA, Crocenzi TS, Dodd GD 3rd, Dorfman GS, Eng C, Fong Y, Giusti AF, Lu D, Marsland TA, Michelson R, Poston GJ, Schrag D, Seidenfeld J, Benson AB 3rd. American Society of Clinical Oncology 2009 clinical evidence review on radiofrequency ablation of hepatic metastases from colorectal cancer. *J Clin Oncol.* 2010;28:493-508.

THE MANAGEMENT OF HEPATIC ABSCESS

Christine M. Durand, MD

Hepatic abscesses are the most common type of visceral abscess. In the United States the incidence rate is around 3 per 100,000 and is higher in men than women. Without prompt recognition and treatment, liver abscesses are uniformly fatal.

Hepatic abscesses can be divided into three major categories: pyogenic, amebic, and fungal. Pyogenic abscesses are caused primarily by polymicrobial aerobic and anaerobic bacteria from the gastrointestinal tract. Common risk factors include diabetes, underlying hepatobiliary disease including malignancy, and liver transplantation.

Amebic abscesses are the result of *Entamoeba histolytica*, which has a high endemic prevalence in Mexico, the Indian subcontinent, Indonesia, and Africa. Most patients with amebic liver abscesses in the United States have a history of recent travel to an endemic area.

Fungal abscesses are increasing in frequency, particularly in immunocompromised patients with a cancer or history of solid organ or bone marrow transplant. They typically are caused by *Candida* species.

The treatment of liver abscesses has evolved. Many nonoperative treatment strategies are available, and a multidisciplinary management approach from interventional radiologists, biliary endoscopists, and infectious diseases specialists can be successful in most cases. However, surgery remains the definitive treatment for large, complicated abscesses or when less invasive approaches fail.

■ PYOGENIC LIVER ABSCESS

Pyogenic abscesses are a rare but highly morbid disease. Over time there have been shifts in cause. Early in the twentieth century, pylephlebitis, from appendicitis, was the most common cause, with an overall mortality rate that approached 75% to 80%. During the 1950s to 1970s, biliary obstruction from benign and malignant diseases accounted for most of the cases. Recently, the landscape has shifted again with the emergence of liver transplantation as treatment for end-stage liver disease and hepatic malignancy.

Pathophysiology

Pyogenic abscesses can arise from multiple sources: (1) the biliary ductal system from ascending cholangitis, (2) the portal blood flow, from pylephlebitis originating from appendicitis or diverticulitis, (3) direct extension from adjacent disease, such as cholecystitis, (4) injury from trauma or liver-directed therapy, (5) the hepatic artery, from septicemia originating from a distant source, and (6) a cryptogenic process. In one of the largest Western series at the Johns Hopkins Hospital, 40% of pyogenic liver abscesses were biliary in origin, and an underlying malignant disease was the cause in the majority of these patients in the nontransplant setting.

In liver transplant recipients, additional risk factors for pyogenic abscess include: (1) hepatic infarction from vascular thrombosis or anastomotic stenosis, (2) ischemic cholangiopathy (nonanastomotic biliary stricture) as a consequence of hepatic arterial compromise or the use of deceased-donor liver organs procured after cardiac death (donation after circulatory death; Figures 1 and 2), and (3) biliary anastomotic stricture. The use of partial liver grafts (from live and deceased donors) carries an increased risk of biliary leak from the cut surface of the liver that may result in perihepatic pyogenic abscess.

Although the infectious organisms and initial diagnostic and treatment algorithms are similar to non–transplant-related causes, the definitive treatment is based on patency of the hepatic vessels, viability of the bile ducts, and function of the hepatic allograft. In severe cases, retransplantation of the liver is the only option.

The microbiology is highly variable and depends on the underlying process (Table 1). *Escherichia coli*, *Klebsiella* spp., and *Enterococcus* spp. commonly are isolated in cases related to choledocholithiasis, whereas *Pseudomonas* spp., other multiple resistant gram-negative aerobes, vancomycin-resistant *Enterococcus* (VRE) spp., and yeast are the more likely pathogens in patients with biliary obstruction from malignancy who received multiple courses of antibiotics. Although cases with liver abscesses from diverticulitis and appendicitis are attributed to gram-negative aerobes and *Bacteroides fragilis,* patients with severe forms of cholecystitis are likely to harbor anaerobes such as *Clostridium perfringens* and *Bacteroides* spp. Other pathogens frequently associated with specific conditions are *Staphylococcus* spp. and methicillin-resistant *Staphylococcus aureus* (MRSA) from subcutaneous abscess, enterococcal and staphylococcal pathogens from endocarditis, and anaerobes in cryptogenic abscesses.

Diagnosis

The classic initial symptom of a pyogenic hepatic abscess is fever, which occurs in more than 90% of patients. Approximately one half of those with an abscess have abdominal or right upper quadrant pain. Other frequent symptoms include malaise, anorexia, and nausea. Occasionally, the diaphragm is involved, resulting in pleuritic chest pain, cough, or dyspnea. The mode of presentation also may include severe sepsis in patients with an underlying biliary malignancy and after liver-directed therapy or liver transplantation. On physical examination, the liver may be tender and enlarged, or the patient may appear jaundiced. Pyogenic liver abscesses rarely rupture, and frank peritonitis is unusual.

Over the past 40 years, advances in imaging have dramatically improved the diagnosis of pyogenic hepatic abscesses. Plain films may show an elevated right hemidiaphragm, right pleural effusion, right lower lobe atelectasis, abnormal extraluminal gas in the right upper quadrant, or portal venous gas if pylephlebitis is the source. Ultrasound (US) is a useful initial screening study for hepatic abscess because it has a sensitivity of 80% to 95% and is excellent in evaluation of the gallbladder and intrahepatic bile ducts. Computed tomography (CT) is more sensitive (95% to 100%) in the detection of abscesses, and the presence of gas and rim enhancement with intravenous contrast is suggestive of a hepatic abscess. CT also allows for a more thorough evaluation of the abdomen for detection of the underlying cause. Magnetic resonance imaging (MRI) of the liver is an equally sensitive technique in detection of liver abscesses and, in combination with magnetic resonance cholangiopancreatography, provides detailed information with regard to the relationship of the hepatic abscess to the biliary system.

Blood cultures should be drawn because they are positive in up to 50% of cases. Cultures obtained directly from an aspirate are critical, and both aerobic and anaerobic cultures should be requested. Cultures from existing drains are not appropriate because they typically are contaminated with skin flora and environmental organisms and will lead to misguided therapy.

Treatment

Pyogenic hepatic abscesses are associated with a significant mortality rate, and prompt diagnosis and treatment of hepatic abscesses are crucial for good outcomes. Management must include treatment of the liver abscess and the underlying source. Most pyogenic hepatic abscesses are managed with antibiotic administration and drainage.

Antibiotics

When a pyogenic hepatic abscess is suspected, first blood cultures should be drawn and then empiric intravenous antimicrobial therapy initiated. The antibiotic coverage subsequently is modified on the basis of results of blood cultures and a fluid sample from the abscess. As outlined previously, the bacteria found usually correspond to the source (see Table 1). As such, the choice of the initial antibiotic agents should be based on the presumed source of the hepatic abscess. For a presumed colonic source, the combination of fluoroquinolone or a third-generation cephalosporin with metronidazole provides appropriate coverage. For a presumed biliary source, a broad-spectrum penicillin such as piperacillin-tazobactam is a good choice and as empiric treatment for most gram-negative aerobes, anaerobes including *Clostridia* spp., and susceptible enterococcal species. If the patient is severely ill and has had recurrent cholangitis, meropenem to treat drug-resistant gram-negative bacteria and linezolid to treat VRE are reasonable choices. In liver transplant recipients, coverage for *Candida* spp. with fluconazole or an echinocandin should be considered. If a subcutaneous abscess or endocarditis is the presumed source, inclusion of vancomycin for MRSA coverage is appropriate.

If specific bacteria are isolated and sensitivities are determined, the antibiotic regimen should be targeted. Classically, antibiotic treatment has been recommended for 4 to 6 weeks; however, shorter antibiotic duration may be appropriate if adequate drainage has been achieved. Even when prolonged antibiotics are indicated for multiple small abscesses with no abdominal source, oral antibiotics with good bioavailability may be substituted for home intravenous antibiotics.

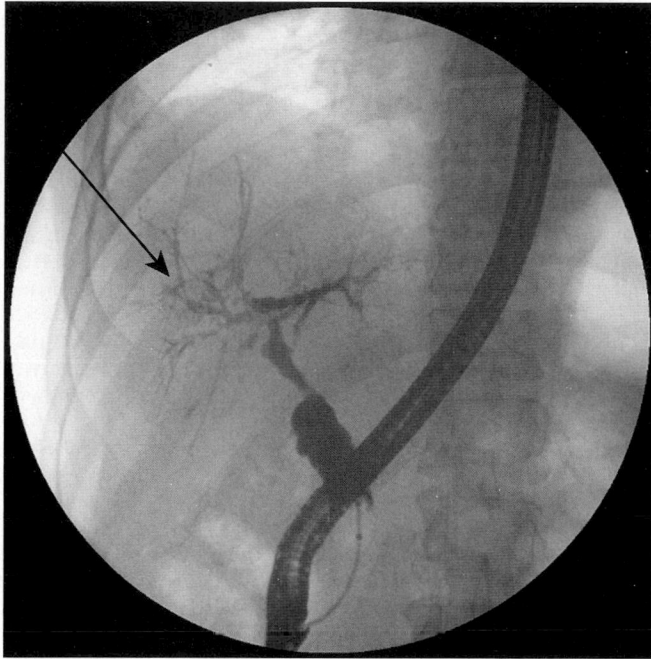

FIGURE 1 An endoscopic retrograde cholangiopancreaticography showing intrahepatic ischemic cholangiopathy after orthotropic liver transplantation with a graft procured after circulatory death.

TABLE 1: Underlying Processes and Typical Pathogens

Underlying Process	Typical Pathogens
Biliary, benign	• *Escherichia coli* • Anaerobes • *Klebsiella* spp. • *Enterococcus* spp.
Biliary, malignant	• *Pseudomonas* spp. • Multidrug-resistant GN aerobes • VRE • Yeast
Diverticulitis/appendicitis	• GN aerobes • *Bacteroides fragilis*
Severe cholecystitis	• See Biliary, benign • *Clostridium perfringens* • *Bacteroides* spp.
Subcutaneous abscess	• *Staphylococcus* spp. • MRSA
Endocarditis	• *Enterococcus* spp. • *Staphylococcus* spp.
Cryptogenic anaerobes	• Anaerobes

GN, Gram-negative; *MRSA,* methicillin-resistant *Staphylococcus aureus*; *VRE,* vancomycin-resistant *Enterococcus*.

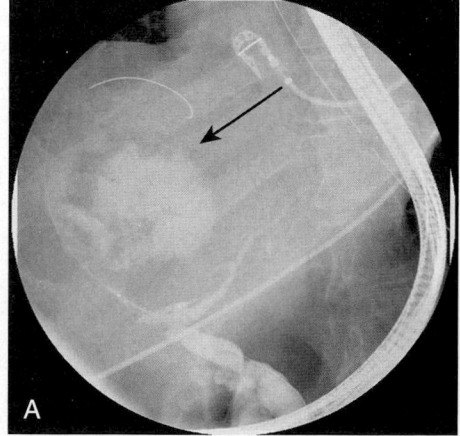
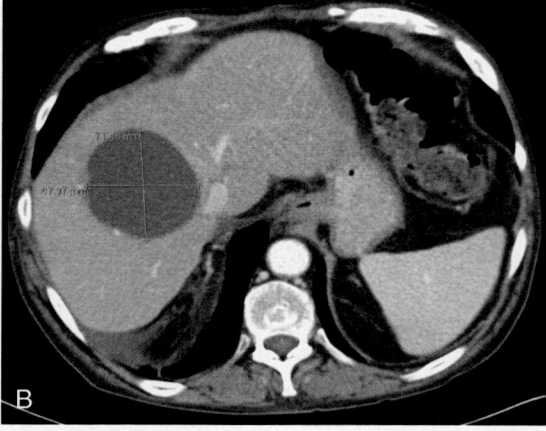

FIGURE 2 A, Endoscopic retrograde cholangiopancreaticography. **B,** Computed tomographic scan showing intrahepatic ischemic cholangiopathy progression to biloma and abscess formation.

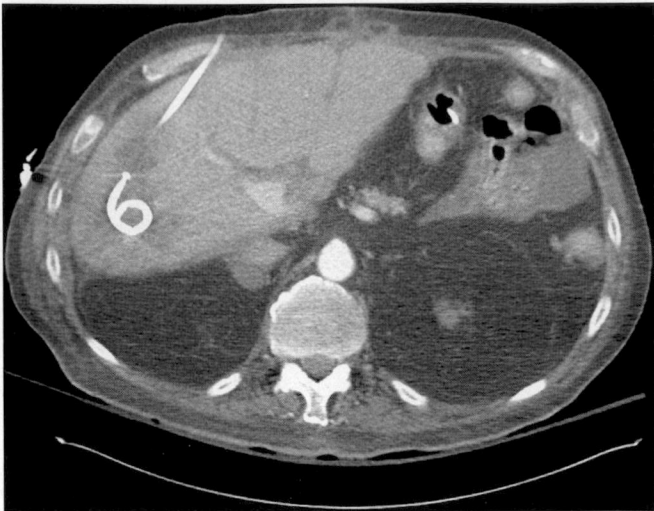

FIGURE 3 Radiograph showing percutaneous drainage of pyogenic abscess.

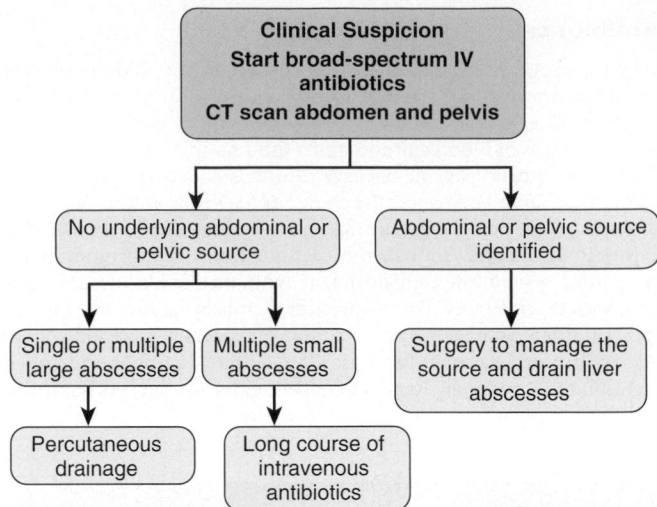

FIGURE 4 Algorithm for management of pyogenic hepatic abscesses. *CT*, Computed tomographic scan; *IV*, intravenous.

Drainage

Intravenous antibiotics have decreased the mortality rate of patients with pyogenic hepatic abscesses; however, most patients also need abscess drainage, either with percutaneous catheter placement, closed aspiration, or surgery. The surgical therapy of liver abscess has evolved to a multispecialty approach with advances in minimally invasive surgery, ablative therapies, and image-guided interventions.

Once the pyogenic abscess has been confirmed with imaging and no intra-abdominal source necessitates operative intervention, the initial management should include antibiotics and percutaneous drainage. At the Johns Hopkins Hospital from 1973 to 1993, 45% of patients were treated with a percutaneous drain; many of these cases, especially later in the series, involved multiloculated abscesses. Rajak and colleagues (1998) compared catheter placement with percutaneous aspiration and found that the success rate was superior with catheter placement (60% vs 100%). Percutaneous catheter placement involves the insertion of an 8F to 14F pigtail catheter over a guidewire with imaging guidance. The abscess cavity then is studied with the injection of contrast through the catheter. Finally, the catheter is left to gravity or suction, until complete resolution of the drainage and collapse of the abscess cavity have occurred (Figure 3). Percutaneous drainage is not appropriate for patients with multiple large abscesses, a known intra-abdominal source that requires surgery, ascites, or in whom transpleural drainage is required.

Percutaneous needle aspiration involves imaging-guided drainage of the abscess without placement of the catheter. The benefits of needle aspiration are decreased cost, traumatic complications, and avoidance of drain discomfort. Yu and colleagues (2004) compared outcomes after aspiration and drainage of liver abscesses and showed equivalent results between the two treatment modalities. Although aspiration resulted in less liver trauma, patient discomfort, and cost, this approach was associated with a higher recurrence rate requiring repeated aspiration procedures compared with catheter drainage.

Although patients with small hepatic abscesses and no biliary obstruction respond to prolonged intravenous antibiotics without drainage, a select group of patients requires surgical intervention.

When an intra-abdominal source for the infection requires an operation, the liver abscess can be drained surgically in concert with management of the primary problem (Figure 4). Surgical treatment also is required in cases of failed nonoperative therapies and remains the salvage procedure.

Before the availability of systemic antibiotics, an extraperitoneal approach for surgical drainage was performed to avoid contamination of the peritoneum. The availability of modern antibiotics and the current technique of a transperitoneal approach via a midline or right subcostal incision provide direct access to the liver abscess, abdomen, and pelvis. After the underlying disease in the abdomen is addressed, the liver is evaluated, and the hepatic abscess is located with palpation and intraoperative US. The area to be drained then is isolated from the rest of the abdomen with towels, and aspiration of the abscess is performed to obtain fluid for culture (Figure 5). A tract then is created through the hepatic parenchyma toward the cavity, ideally to drain the abscess in a dependent fashion. Next, the cavity is irrigated and suctioned to remove purulence and minimize contamination. The tract then should be enlarged and the abscess débrided to break up any loculated pockets of purulence. A large-caliber drain is placed in the abscess cavity, and the perihepatic area around the abscess also may be drained; however, these drains are brought out through separate incisions. All hepatic abscesses should be cultured to direct antibiotic therapy. Pathologic examination also is recommended to evaluate for malignancy and to look for trophozoites of *E. histolytica*.

Although drainage of a liver abscess in combination with systemic antibiotic is successful in most cases, hepatic resection is necessary in unusual circumstances. In patients in whom an inflammatory mass develops as a result of multiple percutaneous drainage procedures or chronic biliary obstruction from multiple biliary drainage procedures that involve one hemiliver, a hemihepatectomy is necessary to remove the diseased portion of the liver. However, these patients are prone to profound sepsis with liver manipulation; therefore partial hepatectomy should be undertaken cautiously (Box 1).

■ AMEBIC HEPATIC ABSCESS

Amebiasis is a relatively common global parasitic infection caused by the protozoan *E. histolytica*, with the highest incidence in tropical and subtropical climates. Amebiasis typically affects men between the ages of 20 and 40 years. Although uncommon in the United States, amebic abscesses should be included in the differential diagnosis in patients with a history of travel to or immigration from endemic areas of the world and in the presence of human immunodeficiency virus.

The liver is the most common extraintestinal location of amebiasis, and amebic liver abscesses occur in 1% of patients with amebiasis. Human infestation occurs with the ingestion of a mature cyst in fecal contaminated food, water, or hands. Excystation occurs in the small intestine, and trophozoites are released and migrate to the large intestine. The trophozoites produce cysts, which are passed in the feces.

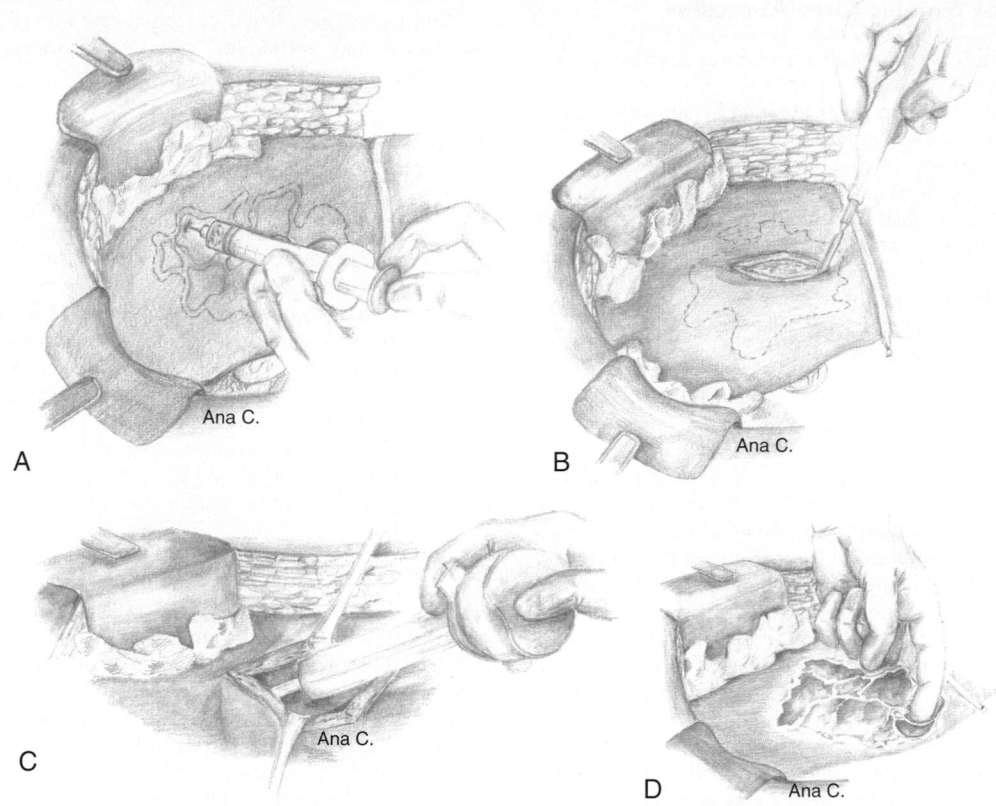

FIGURE 5 A, Abscess aspiration for aerobic and anaerobic culture. **B,** Incision of the liver capsule to drain the abscess. **C,** Irrigation of abscess cavity. **D,** Manual disruption of loculations. *(Illustrations by Ana Costache.)*

BOX 1: Pearls for Pyogenic Hepatic Abscesses

- The most common pathogens isolated from pyogenic liver abscess are gram-negative aerobes and anaerobic bacteria.
- With use of indwelling biliary stents, increasing antibiotic resistance, and growing numbers of immunocompromised patients, infection with fungal species, drug-resistant gram-negative organisms and gram-positive organisms, such as *Enterococcus,* also should be considered.
- Aspiration of liver abscess should be undertaken in most patients because it provides rapid relief of symptoms, microbiologic evaluation, and targeted antibiotic therapy.
- Percutaneous drainage usually is required, and open surgery should be reserved for selected patients.

In many cases, the trophozoites remain confined to the intestinal lumen of individuals who are asymptomatic carriers, passing cysts in their stool. In some patients, the trophozoites invade through the intestinal mucosa (intestinal disease), through the bloodstream, or via extraintestinal sites such as the liver, brain, and lungs (extraintestinal disease), where it forms into an abscess. The most common complication of amebic abscesses is rupture into the surrounding organs, such as direct extension into the pleuropulmonary space or rupture into the pericardium or peritoneum. The diagnosis and management of pyogenic and amebic abscesses differs, and these differences are reviewed.

Diagnosis

The presentation of amebic abscesses may be acute with fever and right upper quadrant pain or less specific with weight loss, fever, and abdominal pain. An amebic liver abscess usually does not present at the same time as colitis but within a year after the initial infection. Unlike a pyogenic abscess, the patient is not jaundiced and does not have underlying biliary disease. Also, most patients are younger than 50 years and have a history of travel to an endemic location. The definitive diagnosis of an amebic liver abscess is by identification of *E. histolytica* trophozoites in the pus or serum antibodies to the ameba. The majority of amebic liver abscesses (75% to 80%) show up as a single focus in the right lobe.

Treatment

With the introduction of metronidazole decades ago, drainage procedures (surgical or percutaneous) are only necessary in circumstances in which there are abscess complications, suspicion of bacterial coinfection, or diagnostic uncertainty.

Antibiotics

Treatment is based on amebicidal drugs to eliminate liver organisms and a luminal agent to eliminate intraluminal cysts even if not seen in the stool given the low sensitivity of microscopy to identify organisms. Preferred tissue agents include metronidazole 500 to 750 mg three times a day for 7 to 10 days. Tinidazole 2 g orally for 5 days is an alternative that may be better tolerated. To eradicate intraluminal cysts, the following regimens can be used: paromomycin (25 to 30 mg/kg per day orally three times a day for 7 days), diiodohydroxyquin (650 mg orally three times a day for 20 days), or diloxanide furoate (500 mg orally three times daily for 10 days for adults). Metronidazole treats intestinal and extraintestinal sites. Failure to use a luminal agent after metronidazole in cases of amebic abscess results in a 10% relapse rate.

BOX 2: Pearls for Amebic Liver Abscesses

- Only 10% to 20% of patients with amebic liver abscess have a history of diarrhea.
- Treatment should include an agent to target hepatic infection (e.g., metronidazole) as well as an intraluminal infection (e.g., paromomycin) to prevent relapse of amebic liver abscess.
- Failure to show response to antiamebic medication requires evaluation for polymicrobial infection with bacteria.
- Amebic abscess usually responds rapidly to antimicrobial therapy in 3 to 7 days, although follow-up imaging should be obtained and make take months to show resolution.
- Percutaneous drainage rarely is required.

Drainage

Blessmann and colleagues (2003) performed a prospective randomized trial to determine whether any significant benefit was obtained by adding aspiration to antibiotics for the treatment of amebic abscesses. In this study, aspiration did not improve the outcomes; therefore image-guided percutaneous treatment is used only in the following circumstances: (1) if no clinical response is seen after 5 to 7 days of antibiotics, and (2) if an abscess, especially a large one, is at high risk for rupture. If the complication of rupture or extension does occur, percutaneous drainage is useful in treating pulmonary, peritoneal, and cardiac complications. Although surgical drainage rarely is required for this disease, surgical intervention is required in unusual situations such as hemorrhage, erosion into surrounding organs, or sepsis from a secondarily infected amebic abscess that has failed percutaneous treatment.

Outcomes

The vast majority of patients with amebic abscesses respond after 3 days of therapy. However, if not treated in a timely fashion, this condition can be fatal, with mortality rates ranging as high as 15% to 20%. Several patient factors that are independent predictors of mortality include (1) a bilirubin value greater than 3.5 mg/dL, (2) encephalopathy, (3) an abscess volume greater than 500 mL, (4) an albumin value less than 2 g/dL, and (5) multiple abscesses. In addition, patients with complications of the abscess, rupture, or direct extension have worse outcomes. In conclusion, amebic abscesses respond well with medical management, and drainage procedures are reserved for rare circumstances. Clinical improvement precedes radiologic resolution, which may take up to 9 months. Follow-up imaging is advised (Box 2).

◼ FUNGAL HEPATIC ABSCESS

The incidence of fungal liver abscesses has been increasing because of the increasing numbers of immunocompromised patients and increasing exposure to broad-spectrum antibiotics. Increased risk occurs with liver transplantation and bone marrow transplantation in particular as well as with hepatobiliary tumors. Mixed bacterial and fungal abscesses often occur in patients with biliary malignancies who have had indwelling stents and frequent exposure to antibiotic.

Treatment

Treatment of fungal abscesses follows the same principles as treatment for pyogenic hepatic abscesses, focusing on antimicrobial agents and drainage. Drainage is, again, with simple aspiration, percutaneous drainage, or surgical drainage. About 80% of fungal abscesses contain *Candida* spp.; the next most common fungal organisms are *Aspergillus* and *Cryptococcus*. Historically, amphotericin B was the first-line therapy, but micafungin and caspofungin are currently the agents of choice. An adequate course must be used; an earlier analysis suggested that inadequate treatment with amphotericin B was associated with a high mortality rate. Oral fluconazole may be used after initial intravenous therapy if *Candida albicans* is the cause. Patients with mixed fungal and bacterial abscesses also should receive appropriate antibiotics for the isolated bacteria.

Outcomes

Fungal abscesses of the liver are a significant source of mortality. The series from Johns Hopkins that analyzed fungal infections from 1973 to 1993 reported that all four patients with monomicrobial fungal abscesses with fungemia died. However, those patients who received a complete course of amphotericin B and did not have fungemia survived. In mixed fungal and bacterial abscesses, the overall mortality rate was 50%; however, adequate amphotericin B treatment resulted in a lower mortality rate (20% vs 62%). In conclusion, although fungal hepatic abscesses carry a high mortality rate, early administration of modern antifungal agents for the prevention of fungemia should improve survival.

SUGGESTED READINGS

Blessmann J, Binh HD, Hung DM, et al. Treatment of amebic liver abscess with metronidazole alone or in combination with ultrasound-guided needle aspiration: a comparative, prospective and randomized study. *Trop Med Int Health.* 2003;8:1030.

Hong JC, Yersiz H, Petrowsky H, et al. Liver transplantation using organ donation after cardiac death: a clinical predictive index for graft failure free survival. *Arch Surg.* 2011;146:1017-1023.

Huang CJ, Pitt HA, Lipsett PA, et al. Pyogenic liver abscess: changing trends over 42 years. *Ann Surg.* 1996;223:600.

Jay CL, Lyuksemburg V, Ladner DP, et al. Ischemic cholangiopathy after controlled donation after cardiac death liver transplantation: a meta-analysis. *Ann Surg.* 2011;253:259-264.

Lipsett PA, Huang CJ, Lillemoe KD, et al. Fungal hepatic abscess: characterization and management. *J Gastrointest Surg.* 1997;1:78-84.

Rajak C, Gupta S, Jain S, et al. Percutaneous treatment of liver abscess: needle aspiration versus catheter drainage. *AJR Am J Roentgenol.* 1998;170:1035-1039.

Yu SC, Ho SS, Law WY, et al. Treatment of pyogenic liver abscess: prospective randomized comparison of catheter drainage and needle operation. *Hepatology.* 2004;39:932-938.

TRANSARTERIAL CHEMOEMBOLIZATION FOR LIVER METASTASES

Todd Schlachter, MD, and Jean-Francois H. Geschwind, MD

Image-guided therapies play an important role in the treatment of patients with primary and secondary hepatic malignancies. A variety of therapeutic modalities are available including intra-arterial approaches such as transarterial chemoembolization (TACE) and selective internal radioembolization therapy (SIRT). These therapies offer reduced systemic toxicity and effective local tumor control. As a result, some procedures have been included in the National Comprehensive Cancer Network treatment guidelines. In this chapter, we describe how intra-arterial therapies may be incorporated into a multidisciplinary approach with the goal to treat liver cancer.

■ HISTORY

The concept of liver-directed therapy was introduced originally in 1977 by Yamada and colleagues as a palliative therapy with the goal of treating patients having unresectable hepatocellular carcinoma (HCC). The scientific rationale for all intra-arterial therapies lies in the fact that in contradistinction to healthy liver tissue, which is supplied by the portal vein, most liver malignancies draw their blood supply from the hepatic artery. This characteristic allows for a high intratumoral concentration of chemotherapeutic agents, and the tumoricidal effects of vessel embolization.

The original therapies focused on embolizing the tumor-feeding hepatic arteries; since that time chemotherapeutic agents and radioactive spheres have been developed to improve on this basic concept. Transarterial embolization (TAE) of the tumor vessel is considered a bland embolic technique. TAE with the addition of one or multiple intra-arterially injected chemotherapeutic agents is referred to as *TACE*. In general, TACE may be performed with an oil emulsion, beads, or microspheres. The oil emulsion is referred to as *conventional TACE* or *cTACE*. When the beads elute a chemotherapeutic agent, this is referred to as *drug-eluting beads transarterial chemoembolization*, or *DEB-TACE*. The application of radioactive spheres, usually deploying a beta-emitting yttrium-90 (Y90) isotope, is referred to as *SIRT*.

■ TECHNIQUE

A thorough preprocedure workup is necessary before chemoembolization. The indication and contraindications to this form of therapy require clinical, laboratory, and imaging evaluation, and often the patient is reviewed in a multidisciplinary conference setting. Intra-arterial therapies can be used for the palliative treatment of patients with unresectable liver tumors, as an adjunctive option before tumor resection or as a bridge to orthotopic liver transplantation. In general, TACE can be indicated in patients with liver-dominant, unresectable hepatic malignancies. Thus several groups of patients with secondary liver malignancies can benefit from this therapy.

Before the start of the procedure, intravenous fluids, steroids, and an antiemetic often are administered. Locoregional intra-arterial liver-directed procedures share a common approach. Initially, arterial access is gained with the Seldinger technique, and multiple diagnostic angiograms are performed. This defines the hepatic arterial anatomy, assesses the blood supply of the tumor, determines portal venous patency, and establishes the ideal location for embolization. This is particularly important for transarterial chemoembolization, in which, as opposed to radioembolization, a super-selective placement of the catheter is crucial for optimal results.

On occasion, fluoroscopy is not sufficient to delineate the proper location of the microcatheter for embolization; in these cases, a computed tomography scan can be obtained immediately after injection to verify optimal positioning (XperCT, Philips, Netherlands; DynaCT, Siemens Medical, Germany) (Figure 1).

Postembolization care is centered on the arterial access site as well as pain control, nausea, and monitoring for injury to liver and kidney. Patients frequently are observed for an extended recovery before they are discharged to home. After discharge, patients are followed in clinic with new cross-sectional liver imaging and laboratory evaluations.

Conventional Transarterial Chemoembolization

In cTACE, the chemotherapeutic cocktail is emulsified with Lipiodol, an oily contrast medium. Lipiodol (Guerbet, Villepinte, France), an iodine ester derived from poppy seed oil, has unique properties as a drug carrier and embolizing agent. Because of the hypervascularized character of most liver tumors and the absence of Kupffer cells, Lipiodol persists within tumor nodules for several weeks.

Although no data show increased efficacy of one chemotherapeutic agent over another, the most common cocktail used in the procedure is cisplatin, adriamycin/doxorubicin, and mitomycin. These agents all have been shown to have good liver extraction and low systemic drug concentrations when administered into the hepatic artery. In addition, the intratumoral concentration of chemotherapeutic drug is reported to be 10 times higher than if it were delivered through the hepatic artery as compared with the portal vein.

The subsequent administration of embolic material (such as Gelfoam, polyvinyl alcohol particles, or trisacryl gelatin microspheres) causes stasis in subsegmental arterial branches. The primary reasons for the additional embolic agents is to help retain the chemotherapeutic agents within the tumor and to induce ischemic necrosis. Some data have suggested that postchemotherapy embolic agents help improve long-term arterial patency. Long-term arterial patency is necessary for repeated chemoembolization because its efficacy is related to the number of times it can be repeated.

Drug-Eluting Beads

The use of drug-eluting beads (DEB-TACE) or microspheres signaled a new frontier in interventional oncology. This agent, which incorporates the chemotherapeutic agent on a microsphere, has a dual function: the capability to slowly release chemotherapy in a controlled fashion over time and embolization of the treated artery.

In DEB-TACE, the drug-eluting beads are prepared hours before the embolization procedure in a complex mixture containing a single chemotherapeutic drug. The two types of drug-eluting microspheres are DC bead microspheres (Biocompatibles, Farnham, Surrey, UK) and QuadraSphere microspheres (Biosphere Medical Inc., Rockland, MA). The DC beads are loaded most commonly with doxorubicin and are used typically for the treatment of HCC, cholangiocarcinoma, and neuroendocrine metastases. The beads also can be loaded with irinotecan; this agent is used for treatment of colorectal metastases to the liver.

The pharmacokinetics of the profile of DEB-TACE is significantly different as compared with that of conventional TACE. The peak drug concentration occurs in both treatments within 5 minutes after injection, but it is significantly lower in the DEB-TACE group (78.97 ± 38.4 ng/mL vs 895.66 ± 653.1 ng/mL; $P = 0.001$). In addition, the variability of the maximal concentration of doxorubicin is considerably higher in the conventional TACE group as compared with the DEB-TACE group. In addition, the total systemic dose of doxorubicin of cTACE is also significantly higher as compared with DEB-TACE.

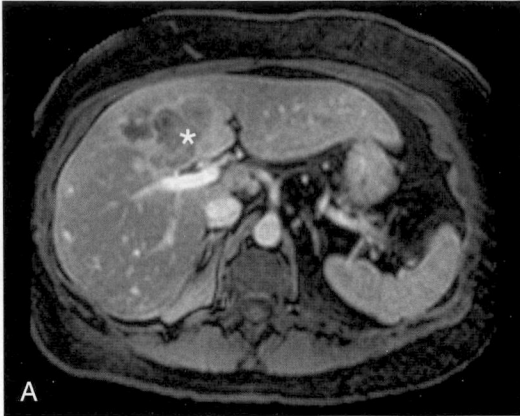

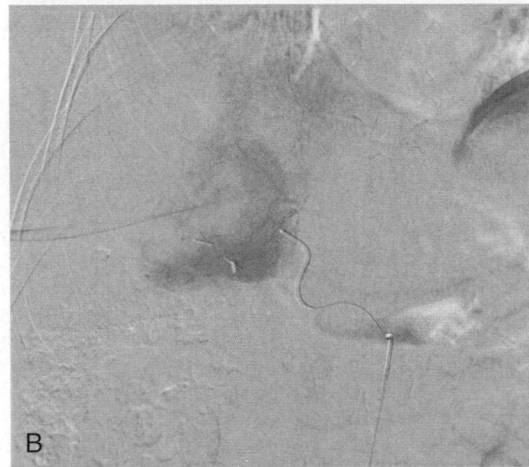

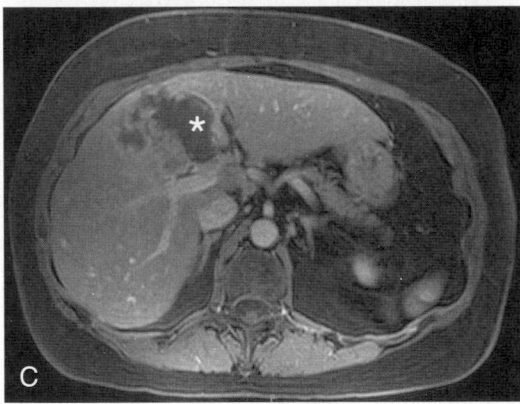

FIGURE 1 A, Magnetic resonance imaging (MRI) after contrast of 62-year-old woman showing segment IV cholangiocarcinoma with significant contrast enhancement (*star*). **B,** Angiogram before chemoembolization showing hypervascularity of lesion shown in **A**. **C,** MRI after contrast showing central necrosis in same lesion after chemoembolization (*star*).

This improved pharmacokinetic profile of DEB-TACE allows more selective dose delivery to the tumor and a reduction of systemic toxicity.

Selective Internal Radiation Therapy

SIRT is performed with the injection of microspheres carrying a dose of Y90. Y90 is a pure beta-emitter with a half-life of 64.1 hours and a mean soft tissue penetration of 2.5 mm. It deposits more than 90% of its energy in the first 5 mm of tissue and in the first 11 days. Two embolization agents are approved by the U.S. Food and Drug

---

BOX 1: Contraindication to Intra-arterial Local Regional Therapy

Absolute Contraindications

Curative surgical resection of tumor
Ongoing systemic infection
Uncorrectable coagulopathy
Leukopenia
Cardiac or renal failure
Hepatic encephalopathy
ECOG performance status >2

Relative Contraindications

Central biliary obstruction
Worrisome/worsening liver function tests
Tumor burden involving more than 50% of the liver
Significant tumor burden outside the liver
Ascites
Recent variceal bleeding
Intractable hepatic AV fistula
Surgical hepatojejunostomy anastomosis

AV, Arteriovenous; *ECOG,* Eastern Cooperative Oncology Group.

Administration for clinical use: the resin-based SIR-Spheres (Sirtex Medical Ltd., Australia) and the glass-based TheraSpheres (BTG, England).

With the catheter positioned properly in the hepatic artery, the microspheres will flow predominantly into the tumor vessels, releasing their payloads in tumor vessels. Both types of microspheres deliver high cumulative doses of radiation to the tumor, which can vary from 100 Gy to more than 3000 Gy. Because of the extremely small size of the microspheres, their highly aggressive payload, and locations of injection, radioembolization bears the risk of systemic distribution of radioactive isotopes via hepatopulmonary shunts or nontarget delivery into the gastrointestinal tract. For these reasons, a pretreatment angiogram and injection of ^{99m}Tc-labeled macroaggregated albumin must be performed to evaluate arterial anatomy and liver shunting fraction before approving the treatment with Y90 (Box 1).

■ TREATMENT OF HEPATOCELLULAR CARCINOMA

TACE has been included officially in treatment guidelines and according to the Barcelona Clinic Liver Cancer (BCLC) staging and treatment strategy; it can be applied as a palliative therapy in patients with intermediate-stage HCC. The level I evidence for survival benefits of patients treated with TACE was provided by two separate prospective phase 3 trials in 2002: Llovet in Barcelona compared either TAE or TACE to conservative therapy, and Lo in Hong Kong compared TACE with conservative measures. In 2003 Llovet's meta-analysis of 7 RCTs showed a 2-year survival of 41% treated with intra-arterial therapy and 27% receiving conservative care. A meta-analysis in 2004 by Marelli similarly showed a significant decrease in mortality with TACE over conservative care.

Lewandowski and colleges in 2010 published a retrospective, single-center study designed to assess treatment response and long-term survival outcomes in a large group of patients with unresectable HCC and included 172 mainly cirrhotic individuals (91%). According to the European Association for the Study of the Liver criteria (EASL), 64% of the treated tumors showed response with 23% showing complete response. The median OS (OS) for patients with early stage disease (BCLC A) was reported as 40.0 months. In patients with intermediate and advanced stage disease, OS was 17.4 months (for BCLC B) and 6.3 months (BCLC C).

The Precision V trial is the only prospective randomized trial comparing the DEB-TACE and conventional TACE. In this study, there were 212 total patients, 102 in the DEB-TACE group and 110 in the cTACE group. The authors concluded that DEB-TACE is a safe procedure, with a better side effect profile compared with conventional TACE, and is beneficial to patients with more advanced disease.

In a prospective randomized trial comparing DEB-TACE with bland embolization, 41 patients with HCC were assigned to the DEB-TACE group, and 43 patients were assigned to the bland embolization group. Tumor response was evaluated with the EASL criteria and alpha-fetoprotein levels. The results showed that the recurrence rate was higher at 9 months with the bland embolization group as compared with the DEB-TACE group. There was also a longer time to progression (TTP) for the DEB-TACE group (42.4 ± 9.5 vs 36.2 ± 9.0 weeks; $P = 0.008$).

The data on radioembolization for HCC are not as mature and complete as for TACE, but available studies have demonstrated good results with radioembolization. One of the very few existing long-term outcome studies of radioembolization to present prospectively collected data treated a total of 291 patients with Y90 in 526 sessions over the course of 5 years. There was an almost even split between Child-Pugh A (45%) and Child-Pugh B (52%) patients, with 52% of the patients classified as BCLC stage C (BCLC A 17%, BCLC B 28%). When patients were assessed with EASL criteria, the overall response rate was 57% (CR 23%, PR 34%), while stratified response rates were significantly better for Child-Pugh A patients with 66% responders (compared with 51% in Child-Pugh B patients). The time to progression for the entire cohort was 7.9 months. The data on median OS reported 17.2 months for Child-Pugh A patients and 7.7 months for Child-Pugh B patients, thus reinforcing the potential of radioembolization to treat unresectable HCC patients.

■ PALLIATION FOR OTHER LIVER TUMORS

TACE is used not only in the setting of HCC but also for palliation of cholangiocarcinoma. In addition, TACE also has been used for the palliation of numerous metastatic lesions to the liver, including ocular melanoma, neuroendocrine, colorectal carcinoma, renal cell carcinoma, some sarcomas, and breast cancer.

Cholangiocarcinoma

Intrahepatic cholangiocarcinoma (IHC) is a rare hepatic malignancy with a typically poor prognosis. The only curative option for cholangiocarcinoma is surgical resection (Figure 1). The prognosis is especially poor in those patients with unresectable disease (survival, 5 to 8 months), which usually makes up more than 70% of patients. Valle in the 2010 ABC-02 trial showed median OS increased from 8.1 months (gemcitabine only) to 11.7 months (gemcitabine and cisplatin). Just like HCC, most of the blood supply to IHC is derived from the hepatic artery, making intra-arterial therapy attractive. In the study by Burger and colleagues, 17 consecutive patients were treated with conventional TACE (multiagent). These patients were relatively healthy (15 of 17 patients had Child-Pugh A; 14 of 17 had ECOG [Eastern Cooperative Oncology Group] 1-2). The median survival time in this group was 23 months. Two patients with unresectable disease went on to resection after TACE. In another retrospectively analyzed study of 15 patients treated with cTACE (single agent), Herber and associates found that the median survival time was 16.3 months and that 1-year, 2-year, and 3-year survival rates were 51%, 27%, and 27%, respectively. In this study, the patients were generally healthy with good liver function (14 of 15 had Child-Pugh A). Both of these studies have shown improved survival in those patients undergoing TACE therapy.

In 2013 two studies, one by Mouli and another by Rafi, showed SIRT in the treatment of IHC to be safe and effective. For example, Mouli and colleagues showed that survival varied on the basis of presence of the following; multifocal (5.7 mo vs 14.6 mo), infiltrative (6.1 mo vs 15.6 mo), and bilobar disease (10.9 mo vs 11.7 mo). Most interesting is that large isolated disease could be converted to resectable status in five patients who successfully underwent curative (i.e., R0) resection.

Ocular Melanoma

Ocular melanoma is the most common intraocular malignant tumor in adults. Up to 50% of those patients diagnosed with ocular melanoma have subsequent development of systemic metastases within 2 to 5 years. The metastatic disease tends to involve the liver; greater than 70% of cases of metastatic ocular melanoma involve the liver, and the liver is generally the first site of metastases. Once the melanoma metastasizes to the liver, the prognosis worsens, and survival is typically between 2 and 9 months. In a study by Sharma and colleagues in 2008, 20 patients with ocular melanoma were treated with cTACE: 13 of 20 patients had stable disease, with an OS time of 9 months. In another study by Vogl in 2007, 12 patients were treated with cTACE. Three of 12 had a partial response, and 5 of 12 had stable disease. The OS time in these patients was 21 months.

Immunoembolization (not previously discussed) is the infusion of an immunologic stimulant into the hepatic artery followed by embolization. This therapy has shown promising but mixed success in patients with ocular melanoma to the liver; further research is ongoing.

In 2011 Eschelman and colleagues described 32 patients undergoing SIRT. Patients with less than 25% tumor burden had longer OS period of 10.5 months versus 3.9 months when tumor burden was more than 25%. SIRT for ocular melanoma to the liver may be of benefit in patients with low total tumor burden (<25%).

Colorectal Cancer

Colorectal cancer most commonly metastasizes to the liver and is the leading cause of death in these patients. At the time of initial diagnosis, 20% to 50% of patients already have liver metastases. Patients who only receive supportive therapy with colorectal metastases to the liver typically have a 7-month to 8-month survival time. The only curative option for these patients is surgical resection; surgical resection has a median survival time of 28 to 46 months, with 5-year survival rates from 24% to 40%.

In a study by Vogl and associates in 2009, 463 patients with unresectable colorectal hepatic metastases that were refractory to systemic chemotherapy were treated with TACE. By imaging characteristics, 68 patients (14.7%) had partial response, 223 patients (48.2%) had stable disease, and 172 patients (37.1%) had progressive disease. The 1-year and 2-year survival rates after chemoembolization were 62% and 28%, respectively. Median survival times from date of diagnosis of liver metastases and date of first chemoembolization were 38 months and 14 months, respectively.

DEB as a new platform for intra-arterial drug delivery to secondary liver tumors has been demonstrated in a retrospective analysis of 28 patients with metastatic colorectal cancer. Irinotecan-loaded drug-eluting beads (DEBIRI) were used and tumor response was assessed with mRECIST criteria in all patients. After an overall 47 procedures, 15% of the treated patients were classified as complete responders and 30% showed partial response, whereas 20% showed stable disease and 35%, progressive disease. Most importantly, a median OS of 13.3 months was achieved with this treatment, yet again proving the potential of DEB-TACE.

In one study, 55 patients underwent 99 treatments with irinotecan DEB. The median disease-free and OS time from the time of first treatment was 247 days and 343 days, respectively. A small trial with 11 patients performed by Aliberti and associates described preliminary results from treatment of intrahepatic cholangiocarcinoma with DEB-TACE. They reported a median survival of 13 months and

100% response evaluation criteria in solid tumors response from DC bead treatment.

Cosimelli in 2010 reported a multicenter phase II trial with 50 consecutive patients with unresectable and chemorefractory metastatic colorectal carcinoma for treatment with SIRT/Y90. As a result, median OS was 12.6 months, and the 2-year survival rate of 19.6% was achieved, thus proving the potential of radioembolization to stabilize end-stage liver metastases.

More recently, in the SIRFLOX study by Gibbs and associates in 2015, 530 patients with unresectable colorectal hepatic metastases of which 90% were synchronous, primary tumor not resected, were prospectively randomized to receive mFOLFOX6 or mFOLFOX6 and SIRT (Y90) as first-line therapy. This study showed statistically significant progression-free liver disease with a 31% reduction in disease progression in the liver. Kim and associates showed patients with KRAS wild type (wt) mutation receiving SIRT showed improved median OS of about 4 months over those patients without wt KRAS.

Metastatic Neuroendocrine Tumors

Metastatic neuroendocrine tumors represent approximately 10% of metastatic disease of the liver. Carcinoid and pancreatic islet cell have a predilection to metastasize to the liver, and those patients with liver metastases have a poorer prognosis and quality of life. Surgical resection is curative but is possible only in less than 10% of patients. TACE can be used in patients with unresectable, hormonally active neuroendocrine tumors and strongly contribute to the elimination of hormonal symptoms.

In a study performed by Gupta and colleagues in 2005, 69 patients with carcinoid metastases to the liver and 54 patients with pancreatic islet cell metastases to the liver underwent treatments with either hepatic arterial embolization or TACE. They found that carcinoid tumors had better outcomes than those with islet cell carcinomas in terms of response rate (66.7% vs 35.2%; $P = 0.001$), progression-free survival time (22.7 months vs 16.1 months; $P = 0.046$), and OS time (33.8 months vs 23.2 months; $P = 0.012$). Patients treated with TACE had a trend toward higher OS and improved response in islet cell tumors but not carcinoid tumors, but this difference was not statistically significant.

Touzios and colleagues performed TACE with cisplatin, doxorubicin, and mitomycin C. The median survival time and 5-year survival rate were 50 months and 50%, respectively. Ruutiainen and associates performed TACE with cisplatin, doxorubicin, mitomycin, iodized oil, and PVA. The 1-year, 3-year, and 5-year survival rates were 86%, 67%, and 50%, respectively. Most recently, Vogl and associates (n = 15) compared two separate chemoembolization protocols, one with mitomycin C alone and the other with mitomycin C and gemcitabine. Their results showed that the combined mitomycin C and gemcitabine had significantly better 5-year and OS rates as compared with the mitomycin C alone (5-year survival rate, 46.67% vs 11.11%; OS time, 57.1 months vs 38.67 months).

Renal Cell Carcinoma

Renal cell carcinoma rarely is metastatic to the liver. However, its metastases are extremely vascular, making it an ideal candidate for intra-arterial locoregional therapy. In a study performed by Nabil and colleagues in 2008, 22 patients were treated with TACE (either mitomycin C alone or mitomycin C with gemcitabine). Imaging showed a partial response in 13.7%, stable disease in 59%, and progression in 27.3%. Median survival times from diagnosis and from TACE were 68.6 months and 8.2 months, respectively. The 1-year and 2-year survival rates were 31% and 6%, respectively. Although these survival results are less than those achieved with surgery, those patients treated in this study had significantly more advanced disease as compared with those with surgical resection.

Breast Carcinoma

Distant metastases occur in approximately 6% to 7% of all patients with breast carcinoma. The 5-year survival rate in these patients with stage IV disease is 10% to 18%. Of these patients (stage IV), 3% to 12% have metastases limited to the liver. In a study performed by Giroux and colleagues, eight patients with metastatic breast cancer were treated with TACE. On imaging, five patients had a partial response, one had stable disease, and two had disease progression. All patients died within 13 months after receiving the treatment, with a mean of 49 months from primary diagnosis.

In 2014 Lewandowski and colleagues showed treatment with SIRT in chemotherapy-resistant breast cancer liver metastases was safe and provided disease stabilization in 98.5% of the treated liver tumors, and 24 patients had 30% reduction in tumor size. Median survival for patients with less than 25% versus 25% tumor burden or more was 9.2 months and 3.9 months. Unilobar versus bilobar disease conferred a median survival of 30.9 versus 6.5 months.

Abdominal Sarcomas

Approximately 64% to 70% of abdominal sarcomas metastasize to the liver. Once the sarcoma metastasizes to the liver, there is a median survival time of 14 months in those patients who receive supportive care only. In a study published by Rajan and associates, 16 patients with a variety of gastrointestinal sarcomas were treated. Postprocedure imaging showed 2 patients had a partial response, 11 patients had stable disease, and 3 had progression. Survival rate from diagnosis was 81% at 1 year, 54% at 2 years, and 40% at 3 years. Median survival time was 20 months.

In 2015 Chapiro and colleagues showed that enhancement-based volumetric assessment before and after treatment can best predict patient outcomes that help determine if additional therapy is beneficial.

■ CONTRAINDICATIONS TO TRANSARTERIAL CHEMOEMBOLIZATION

Although there are no absolute contraindications to the TACE procedure, relative contraindications can be identified according to the exclusion criteria in most clinical trials: advanced liver disease (Child-Pugh classification C or above), active gastrointestinal bleeding, biliary obstruction, encephalopathy, refractory ascites, vascular invasion or portal vein invasion from tumor, extrahepatic metastases, portosystemic shunts, contraindication to arterial intervention (INR >1.8, platelets <50,000, creatinine >1.5), and poor performance status (ECOG >2).

In the case of biliary obstruction, care must be taken to avoid biliary necrosis of the obstructed segments, which could result in abscess formation. In a study by Kim and colleagues, the authors recommend a reduction in the amounts of oil/gelatin sponge particles to reduce the amounts of biliary complications after TACE (bilomas and focal biliary strictures; Figure 2). If a reversible cause is found for the biliary obstruction, a percutaneous biliary tube should be inserted before TACE. In addition, prior biliary reconstructive surgery has been identified as an independent risk factor for the formation of abscesses after TACE.

Regarding portal vein thrombosis, numerous studies have shown that TACE is safe in these patients. In a study by Pentecost and associates, nine patients with portal vein thrombosis underwent transarterial chemoembolization. In these patients, eight patients responded to treatment. No patient had development of hepatic infarction or insufficiency as a consequence of the procedure. A larger study was performed by Georgiades and colleagues in which 32 consecutive patients with portal vein thrombosis were treated with TACE. In these patients, the median OS time was 9.5 months. The 30-day

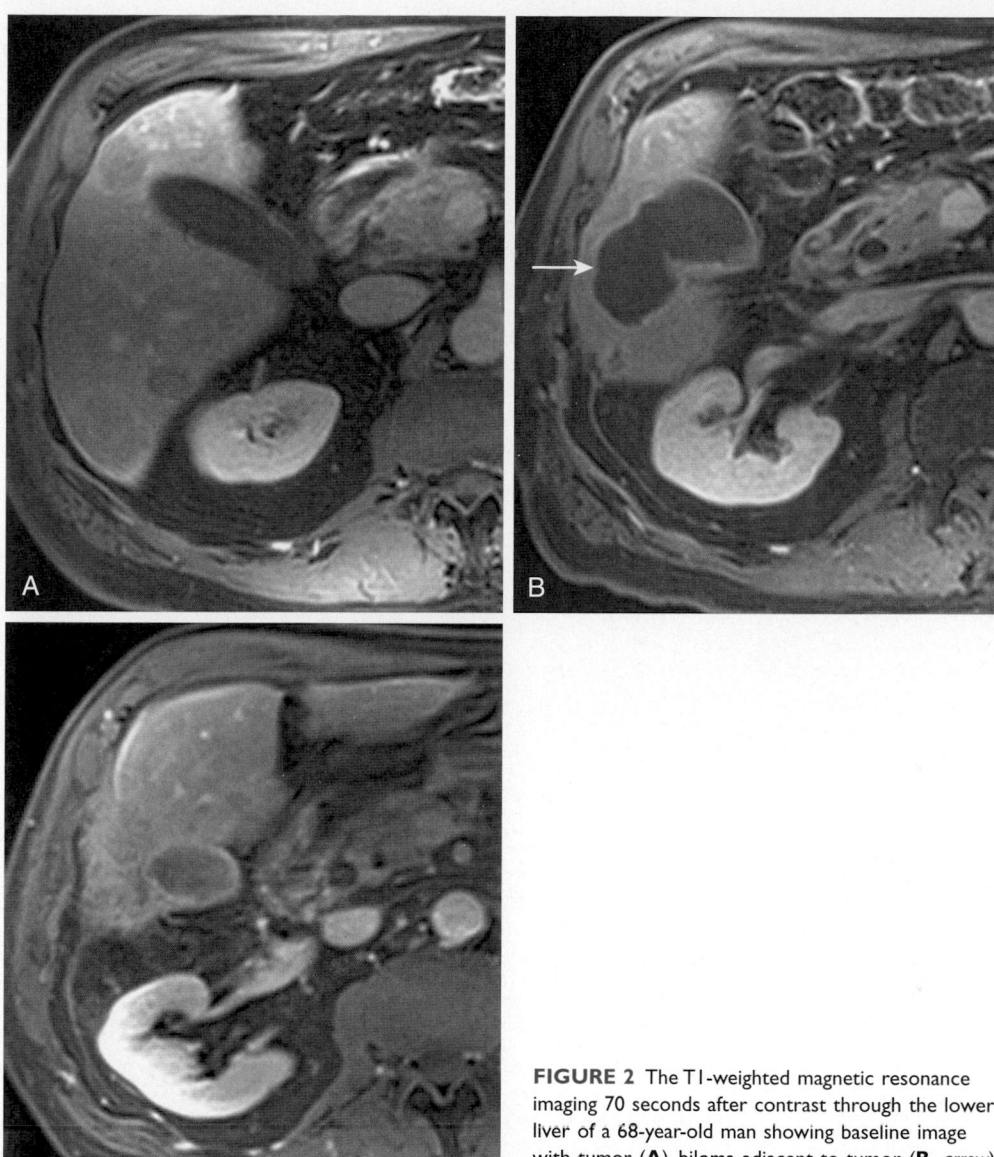

FIGURE 2 The T1-weighted magnetic resonance imaging 70 seconds after contrast through the lower liver of a 68-year-old man showing baseline image with tumor (**A**), biloma adjacent to tumor (**B,** *arrow*), and resolved biloma after drainage, now with mostly necrotic tumor (**C**).

mortality rate was 0, and there was no TACE-related hepatic infarction or acute liver failure. The 6-month, 9-month, 12-month, and 18-month survival rates were 60%, 47%, 25%, and 12.5%, respectively. The authors concluded that portal venous thrombosis should not be considered a contraindication to TACE.

Kothary and associates performed a study in which 52 patients underwent high-risk procedures. All patients had elevated serum bilirubin values, 76.9% of patients had serum albumin levels less than 3.5 mg/dL, and 25% of the patients had portal vein invasion. Greater than 50% had a Child-Pugh score of 9 or greater. Although patients with multifocal disease and lobar invasion had significantly higher mortality rates, the 1-year and 2-year survival rates were 67.9% and 37.7%, respectively. The authors concluded that patients at high risk did not have a higher rate of mortality as a consequence of the procedure.

■ COMPLICATIONS

The most common complication after TACE is the postembolization syndrome (PES). It happens in approximately 2% to 7% of patients after the procedure. Symptoms of PES include abdominal pain, nausea, vomiting, and mild fever. In a study performed by Leung and associates, the two factors associated with an increased risk of PES were gallbladder embolization and total chemoembolization dose administered. They also found that previous embolization was associated with a decreased risk of PES. Patel and colleagues performed a study in which they showed that no patient factors (age, laboratory values) or bland versus chemoembolization were associated with a higher risk of PES. The treatment of PES is supportive care only.

The most important and serious consequence of TACE is hepatic insufficiency or failure. Chan and associates found that acute hepatic decompensation occurred in 20% of all patients treated with TACE, with 3% of cases irreversible. Patient factors associated with a higher rate of hepatic decompensation included dose of cisplatin used, baseline bilirubin level, baseline prothrombin time, baseline aminotransferase level, and stage of cirrhosis.

Less common, but equally as serious, complications of TACE include cerebral lipiodol embolism and pulmonary embolism or infarction. The former is caused by an arteriovenous shunt in the liver with either an intracardiac shunt or pulmonary shunt. Five total cases of cerebral lipiodol embolism have been reported in the literature. Pulmonary embolisms or infarctions can occur from an arteriovenous shunt occurring in the liver. A study by Chung and colleagues showed that the incidence of pulmonary complications increases as the dose of lipiodol increases.

SUGGESTED READINGS

Bhagat N, Reyes DK, Lin M, et al. Phase II study of chemoembolization with drug-eluting beads in patients with hepatic neuroendocrine metastases: high incidence of biliary injury. *Cardiovasc Intervent Radiol*. 2013;36:449-459.

Chapiro J, Duran R, Lin M, et al. Transarterial chemoembolization in soft-tissue sarcoma metastases to the liver–the use of imaging biomarkers as predictors of patient survival. *Eur J Radiol*. 2015;84:424-430.

Duran R, Chapiro J, Frangakis C, et al. Uveal melanoma metastatic to the liver: the role of quantitative volumetric contrast-enhanced MR imaging in the assessment of early tumor response after transarterial chemoembolization. *Transl Oncol*. 2014;7:447-455.

Llovet JM, Real MI, Montana X, et al. Arterial embolisation or chemoembolisation versus symptomatic treatment in patients with unresectable hepatocellular carcinoma: a randomised controlled trial. *Lancet*. 2002;359:1734-1739.

Llovet JM, Ricci S, Mazzaferro V, et al. Sorafenib in advanced hepatocellular carcinoma. *NEJM*. 2008;359:378-390.

Sato T. Locoregional management of hepatic metastasis from primary uveal melanoma. *Semin Oncol*. 2010;37:127-138.

PORTAL HYPERTENSION AND THE ROLE OF SHUNTING PROCEDURES

Christine E. Haugen, MD, and Andrew M. Cameron, MD, PhD, FACS

Portal hypertension is defined as portal venous pressure greater than 5 to 7 mm Hg. The cause most commonly is due to increased portal venous resistance that can be classified anatomically as prehepatic, intrahepatic, or posthepatic. The most frequent causes of portal hypertension in the United States are cirrhosis resulting from alcoholic liver disease or hepatitis C virus infection.

One consequence of portal hypertension is the development of collateral vessels between the portal and systemic venous systems known as *varices*. The most clinically relevant variceal network is between the coronary and short gastric veins to the azygos vein forming esophageal varices; other sites include retroperitoneal, hemorrhoidal, and caput medusa. Larger size of varices and worsening hepatic function (Child's B or C) are risk factors for hemorrhage.

Fifty percent of patients with cirrhosis have esophageal varices, and up to one third will develop variceal hemorrhage. The staggering 15% to 20% mortality rate of each variceal hemorrhage event emphasizes the need for a structured management plan.

◼ MANAGEMENT

The treatment algorithm for portal hypertensive varices has evolved over time and involves an array of modalities. Medical therapy makes up the majority of management regarding esophageal varices, given that up to two thirds of patients will never experience a bleed. Use of nonselective beta-blockers and avoidance of hepatotoxins are the mainstays of medical management in patients with gastroesophageal varices. Nonselective beta-blockers decrease cardiac output as well as cause splanchnic vasoconstriction to reduce portal venous pressure.

In the one third of patients that will have a variceal bleed, acute hemorrhage should be managed in the intensive care unit setting and includes initial resuscitation followed by definitive management. The algorithm is seen in Figure 1. Airway protection with possible endotracheal intubation, large-bore IV access, and volume resuscitation are critical first steps in aggressive management to prevent death. Blood products should be transfused to maintain a goal hemoglobin of 7 to 8 g/dL. Over-resuscitation worsens portal hypertension and can increase variceal bleeding.

Prophylactic antibiotics should be started in cirrhotic patients at the time of an acute variceal bleed. Simultaneous infection and variceal bleeding is shown to be a risk factor for failure to control bleeding, early rebleeding, increased days of hospitalization, and death. Ceftriaxone or IV ciprofloxacin can be used for prophylaxis.

Vasoactive medications, such as vasopressin, can be used to decrease splanchnic blood flow. The unfavorable side effect profile of vasopressin may necessitate simultaneous administration of nitroglycerin to avoid extreme hypertension, myocardial ischemia, and arrhythmias.

Octreotide, a long-acting somatostatin analogue, is a splanchnic vasoconstrictor. A continuous octreotide infusion along with endoscopic management is used to control acute variceal bleeds. A proton pump inhibitor should be initiated at the time of acute variceal bleeding and continued for a short course after definitive therapy.

Luminal Tamponade

Tamponade with a Sengstaken-Blakemore tube or a self-expanding metal stent has been shown to control variceal hemorrhage in 90% of cases. The disadvantage to the technique is the 50% recurrent hemorrhage rate once tamponade is released. Complications with Sengstaken-Blakemore tube include esophageal rupture, esophageal necrosis, and aspiration in up to 30% of patients. It also must be removed within 24 to 36 hours of placement. Metal stents carry the risk of esophageal perforation, bronchial compression, and stent migration but can remain in place for up to 2 weeks. Given the high recurrent hemorrhage rate, tamponade is a temporary measure until a definitive plan to control variceal bleeding can be made.

Endoscopic Diagnosis and Therapy

Esophagogastroduodenoscopy (EGD) is the primary diagnostic and therapeutic modality used during acute esophageal variceal bleeding in conjunction with aggressive resuscitation measures. EGD should be performed on an emergent basis. Variceal banding and sclerotherapy are the primary interventions performed with successful hemorrhage control in 90% of patients.

Sclerotherapy involves injecting a sclerosing agent directly into the varix or surrounding tissue. Complications include esophageal ulceration, perforation, stricture, and fibrosis along with renal and pulmonary complications. Banding involves placing a tight band around the varix that stops bleeding and causes thrombosis of the vessel. It has a more favorable safety profile and has become the preferred standard for endoscopic intervention over sclerotherapy for acute variceal bleeding.

Transjugular Intrahepatic Portosystemic Shunt

Transjugular intrahepatic portosystemic shunt (TIPS) may be considered as rescue therapy for initial uncontrolled variceal bleeding after failed endoscopic management (10% to 20% of patients) or rebleeding. TIPS is a more definitive management option because it corrects the underlying problem of portal hypertension, at least temporarily. With the reduction in portal pressure, patients may experience improvement in portal gastropathy, ascites, and hydrothoraces.

TIPS involves the percutaneous guidance of a wire from usually the right internal jugular vein, into the right hepatic vein, then through hepatic parenchyma into a portal branch. The guidewire is

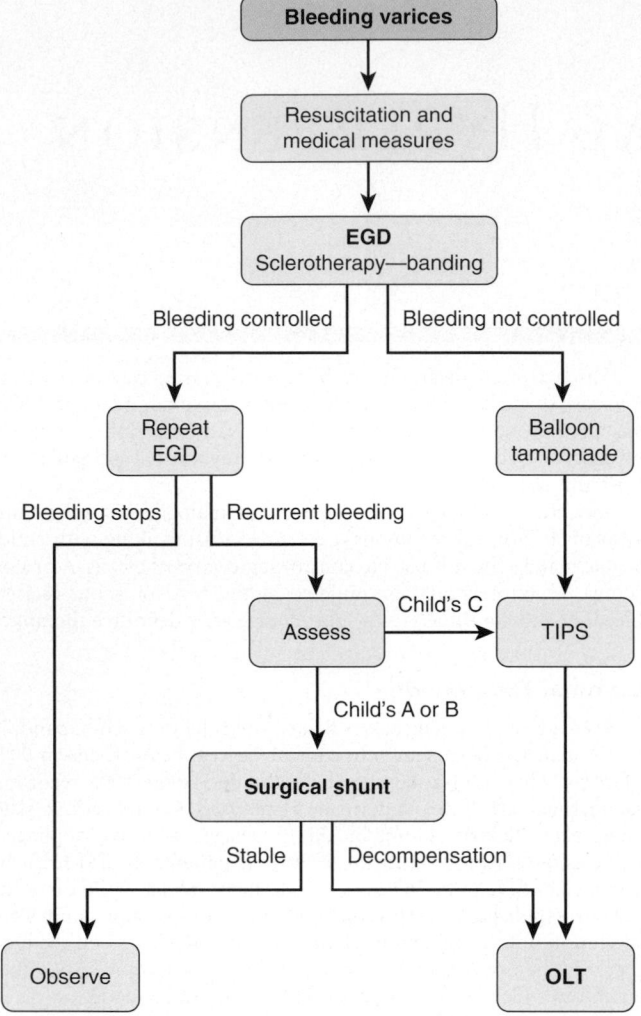

FIGURE 1 Management of acutely bleeding gastroesophageal varices. *EGD*, Esophagogastroduodenoscopy; *OLT*, orthotopic liver transplant; *TIPS*, transjugular intrahepatic portosystemic shunt.

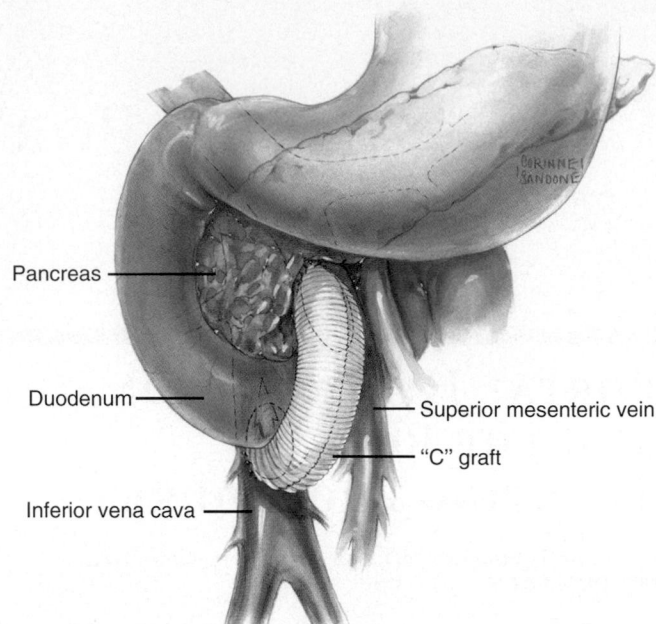

FIGURE 2 Interposition mesocaval shunt. *(From Cameron JL, Sandone C. Atlas of Gastrointestinal Surgery, 1st ed, vol 1. 1993.)*

passed most frequently into the right portal vein, the parenchymal tract is balloon dilated, and then after portography an expandable covered stent is inserted.

The most frequent complications of this procedure are inherent to stent placement and include stenosis or thrombosis. Other complications include encephalopathy, bleeding, sepsis, liver infarction, and liver failure. The mortality ranges from 5% to 40%, with higher mortality seen in poorly compensated cirrhotics and shunts placed on an emergent basis.

Surgical Shunts

With the success of endoscopic therapy and TIPS for acute variceal bleeding, surgical shunts typically are reserved for chronic or recurrent variceal hemorrhage in patients in whom TIPS have thrombosed repeatedly, but also rarely can be a salvage procedure in the acute setting. Surgical portosystemic shunts are classified, by varying degrees of portal venous shunting, as selective or nonselective. Selective shunts provide selective decompression of the portal-azygous system while preserving portal inflow into the liver, whereas nonselective shunts divert all portal flow away from the liver. All portosystemic shunts decrease gastroesophageal varices and reduce the risk of hemorrhage.

Nonselective portosystemic shunts divert large quantities of portal venous flow from the liver to the caval system. These include end-to-side portacaval shunts, side-to-side portacaval shunts, interposition shunts, or conventional splenorenal shunts. The end-to-side portacaval shunt completely diverts portal flow to the liver and is effective in preventing gastroesophageal variceal hemorrhage but is associated with unacceptably high rates of hepatic encephalopathy and is therefore of historic interest only (Figure 2). The side-to-side portosystemic shunts completely decompress the portal venous system and the intrahepatic sinusoidal system. The complete diversion of portal flow increases the risk of liver failure and hepatic encephalopathy. The dissection of the porta hepatis needed to construct portacaval shunting is discouraged if the patient is a potential liver transplant candidate. For reasons listed earlier, mesocaval shunts, also known as *H-grafts*, serve as a surgical shunt bridge to liver transplantation. These shunts avoid dissection in the porta hepatis and can be ligated at the time of liver transplantation.

Selective portosystemic shunts preserve portal flow to the liver and decompress gastroesophageal varices. The distal splenorenal shunt, introduced by Warren, involves the anastomosis of the distal splenic vein end to the left renal vein along with the ligation of collaterals, coronary vein, and gastroepiploic veins (Figure 3). This shunt continues to perfuse the liver through the superior mesenteric venous system. The distal splenorenal shunt should not be performed in patients with intractable ascites because maintained sinusoidal and mesenteric portal hypertension can worsen ascites. These shunts often are limited by technical difficulty and the development of pancreatic collaterals. Multiple studies have compared selective and nonselective shunts and demonstrated the rates of survival and recurrent bleeding are similar, but the incidence of postoperative hepatic encephalopathy is lower with selective shunts.

■ SUMMARY

Acute variceal hemorrhage in patients with portal hypertension carries a high morbidity and mortality. A multidisciplinary and structured approach is necessary to manage these patients. Medical therapy, endoscopic therapy, and TIPS are the primary treatment modalities of variceal hemorrhage. The role of surgical shunting is

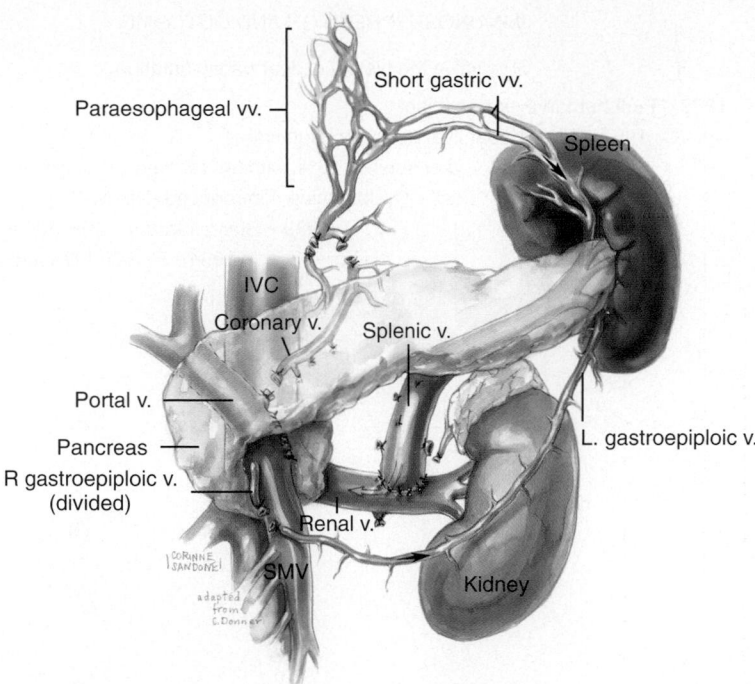

FIGURE 3 Distal splenorenal shunt. *(From Cameron JL, Sandone C. Atlas of Gastrointestinal Surgery, 1st ed, vol.1. 1993.)*

diminishing but still represents an effective and relatively safe means to control variceal hemorrhage in patients with recurrent bleeds.

SUGGESTED READINGS

Garcia-Tsao G, Sanyal AJ, Grace ND, Carey W. Prevention and management of gastroesophageal varices and variceal hemorrhage in cirrhosis. *Hepatology*. 2007;46:922-938.

Orloff MJ. Fifty-three years' experience with randomized clinical trials of emergency portacaval shunt for bleeding esophageal varices in cirrhosis: 1958-2011. *JAMA Surg.* 2014;149:155-169.

Zeppa R, Warren WD. The distal splenorenal shunt. *Am J Surg.* 1971;122: 300-303.

LIVER TRANSPLANTATION

Benjamin Philosophe, MD, PhD

The evolution of liver transplantation has been relatively rapid. The first human liver transplant was performed by Thomas Starzl in 1963. Between March 1 and October 4, 1963, Starzl performed 5 human liver transplants, with the longest survival at 23 days. The patients died with functioning grafts that had little evidence of rejection at autopsy. There was also a single failed attempt in Boston in 1963 and in Paris in 1964 before the operations came to a halt, perceived at that time to be too difficult. It was not until 1967 that the first liver transplant recipient survived for 1 year. Immunosuppression consisted of azathioprine, prednisone, and antilymphocyte globulin. It was not until cyclosporine was introduced in 1980 that 1-year survival was being achieved consistently (Figure 1).

As a result of these successes, the surgeon general initiated a consensus conference in 1983. It was then concluded that liver transplantation had become a "clinical service" and was no longer considered an experimental procedure. This led to a rapid expansion in the number of centers performing liver transplantation. As the waiting list for liver transplantation grew exponentially, surgical fellows flocked to train under Starzl, who had moved to the University of Pittsburgh. The resulting growth of qualified surgeons eventually caught up with the national and international need for liver transplants. The introduction of tacrolimus in 1989 pushed the 1-year survival rates even higher, exceeding 80%, leading to the approval of the drug by the U.S. Food and Drug Administration (FDA) in 1994. As a result of surgical techniques progressing, current 1-year patient survival for deceased donor transplantation is 86% (http://optn.transplant.hrsa.gov).

■ INDICATIONS FOR LIVER TRANSPLANTATION

Acute Liver Failure

Acute liver failure (ALF) is a rare but potentially fatal syndrome characterized by sudden loss of hepatic function in a person without pre-existing liver disease. ALF also can occur in patients with known diseases, such as Wilson's disease, autoimmune hepatitis, or hepatitis B. ALF affects approximately 2000 to 3000 Americans each year (Hoofnagle et al., 1995). It commonly is classified as fulminant or subfulminant. Fulminant liver failure is defined as the development of encephalopathy within 8 weeks of the development of symptoms such as jaundice (Bernal et al., 2013). Subfulminant hepatic failure is reserved for patients who have had liver disease for up to 26 weeks before the development of hepatic encephalopathy.

IMMUNOSUPPRESSION AND OUTCOME

Survival in the history of liver transplantation

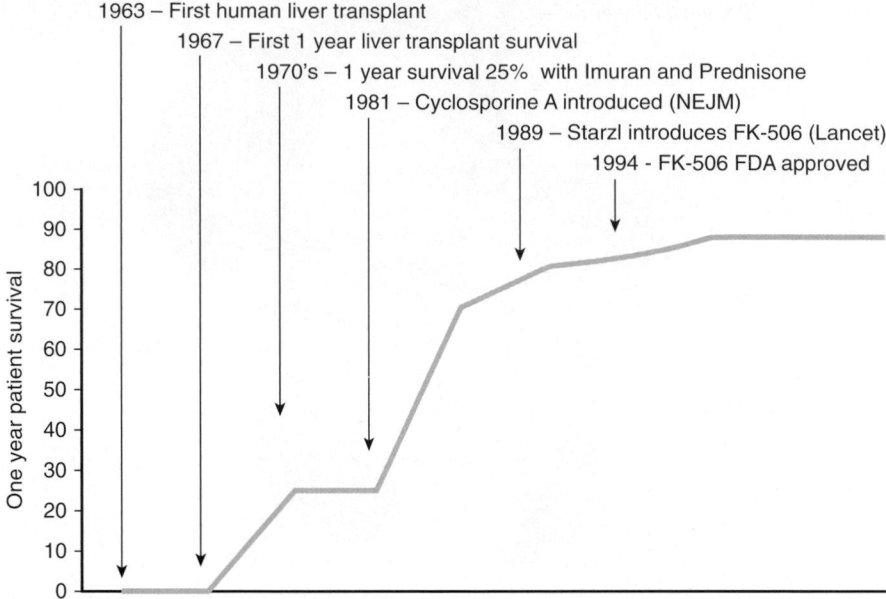

FIGURE 1 Immunosuppression and outcome: survival in the history of liver transplantation. *FDA*, U.S. Food and Drug Administration; *NEJM*, The New England Journal of Medicine.

Whether fulminant or subfulminant, encephalopathy is an essential component in the definition of ALF. The most common cause of ALF in the United States and Western Europe is drug-induced liver injury, which accounts for 50% of the cases. Acetaminophen is the leading cause of ALF. Patients who are at increased risk for acetaminophen-induced ALF include those with concomitant alcohol use, malnutrition, or use of medications known to induce cytochrome P450 (CYP450) enzymes (e.g., phenytoin, carbamazepine, rifampin). In 308 consecutive patients from 17 tertiary care centers participating in the U.S. Acute Liver Failure Study Group, acetaminophen was identified as the cause of ALF in 40% of patients. The other causes identified, in ascending order of prevalence, were malignancy (1%), Budd-Chiari syndrome (2%), pregnancy (2%), Wilson's disease (3%), hepatitis A virus infection (4%), autoimmune hepatitis (4%), ischemic hepatitis (6%), hepatitis B virus infection (6%), and idiosyncratic drug-induced liver injury (13%); 17% of cases were found to be indeterminate.

Patients suspected of having ALF should be transferred to a liver transplant center immediately because this can progress very rapidly to fulminant liver failure and then death. The development of complications, including cerebral edema, hemodynamic abnormalities, coagulopathy, renal failure, infection and sepsis, acid-base disturbances, and pulmonary dysfunction, requires immediate attention.

The common cause of death in patients with fulminant hepatic failure (FHF) is cerebral edema. Hyperammonemia is considered a critical factor in the development of cerebral edema and herniation. The grades of encephalopathy correlate with the degree of herniation. Cerebral edema develops in about 80% of patients who develop grade 4 hepatic encephalopathy. The resultant increased intracranial pressure (ICP) results in decreased cerebral perfusion pressure, in turn leading to ischemic brain damage and herniation. This accounts for more than half of ALF-associated mortality.

However, ALF-induced encephalopathy is different from that of cirrhosis despite the fact that ammonia levels are elevated in both. Cerebral edema does not develop in the setting of chronic liver disease. As such, lactulose, a nonabsorbable disaccharide used to decrease ammonia levels in patients with cirrhosis, has never been shown to improve survival in the setting of ALF. Rather, therapeutic measures focus on decreasing ICP, including elevation of the head of the bed and minimizing patient stimulation through sedation or paralysis.

The development of increased ICP is an ominous sign. Clinical changes on examination occur only after significant cerebral edema has developed and as such are not helpful. Head computed tomography (CT) is equally insensitive in the early stages of edema but helpful with more advanced encephalopathy to rule out other pathologic conditions such as intracranial hemorrhage. If cerebral edema is evident on CT, the likelihood of irreversible brain injury or uncal herniation is high, and transplantation is contraindicated at this point. ICP monitoring can help to diagnose intracranial hypertension and optimize management. There are various types of ICP monitors, but all carry a significant risk of intracranial hemorrhage after their placement. Whether the added benefit of ICP monitors is worth the risks remains controversial. Some transplant centers routinely use ICP monitors, whereas others do not and rely on clinical signs.

Without a doubt, predicting which patients with FHF will require a time-sensitive, lifesaving transplant or will recover with medical management alone can be very difficult. Many studies have attempted to identify prognostic indicators to guide this clinical decision. The most widely applied is from King's College Hospital in London. The King's College criteria are outlined in Box 1. The positive predictive value of the King's College criteria is 80% to 100% according to most studies, higher than many other criteria proposed.

In patients who meet the King's College criteria, liver transplantation is the only definitive treatment option for patients with fulminant liver failure. Farmer and colleagues performed a single-center retrospective analysis of 204 patients who underwent liver transplantation in an 18-year span. They showed a 73% 1-year patient survival and a 67% 5-year patient survival. Graft survival was 63% at 1 year and 57% at 5 years. More recent registry data showed significant improvement. One- and five-year graft survival was 80% and 73%, respectively (Scientific Registry of Transplant Recipients annual report, 2015).

Chronic Liver Disease

Causes of chronic liver disease are depicted in Figure 2. The indications for transplantation have changed over time. Figure 2 shows the diagnosis at the time of transplantation over the past 25 years.

Alcoholic hepatitis has always been a major cause of chronic liver disease and remains so today. Although alcohol is listed as a primary

---

BOX 1: King's College Criteria for Liver Transplantation

Acetaminophen Induced

pH <7.3 *or*
INR >6.5 and serum Cr >3.4 mg/dL

Nonacetaminophen Induced

INR >6.5 *or*
Any 3 of variables below
    INR >3.5
    Bilirubin >17.6 mg/dL
    Age ≤10 or >40 years
    Cause: drug toxicity
    Time from onset of jaundice to encephalopathy >7 days

Cr, Creatinine; *INR,* international normalized ratio.

---

diagnosis around 15% of the time, it is often a secondary diagnosis with an overall incidence of 40% to 50%. Hepatitis C has risen to become the primary cause of chronic liver disease in the past 10 years. For some transplant centers, hepatitis C is the cause in up to 60% of patients. However, with the advent of effective treatment and cure, the incidence is expected to decrease in the next 10 years.

Nonalcoholic steatohepatitis (NASH) is rapidly becoming a major cause of cirrhosis. NASH, often a "silent" liver disease, histologically resembles alcoholic liver disease but occurs in people who drink little or no alcohol. Steatosis with inflammation and cellular damage including ballooning of hepatocytes is the hallmark of NASH. People with NASH feel well and are not symptomatic until the cirrhosis is more advanced. NASH affects 2% to 5% of Americans. An additional 10% to 20% of Americans have fatty liver but no inflammation or liver damage, a condition called nonalcoholic fatty liver disease (NAFLD). It is unclear why some develop NASH and others do not. Both NASH and NAFLD are becoming more common, possibly because of the greater number of Americans with obesity. In the past 10 years, the rate of obesity has doubled in adults and tripled in children. It is predicted that NASH will become the leading indication for liver transplantation in the United States by 2020.

Another epidemic in the making is hepatocellular carcinoma (HCC). HCC is the third leading cause of cancer-related death worldwide and one of the leading causes of death in patients with cirrhosis (El Serag, 2011). Its incidence has more than doubled in the past 2 decades and will continue to increase over the next 20 years. As seen in Figure 2, HCC had become the most common indication for liver

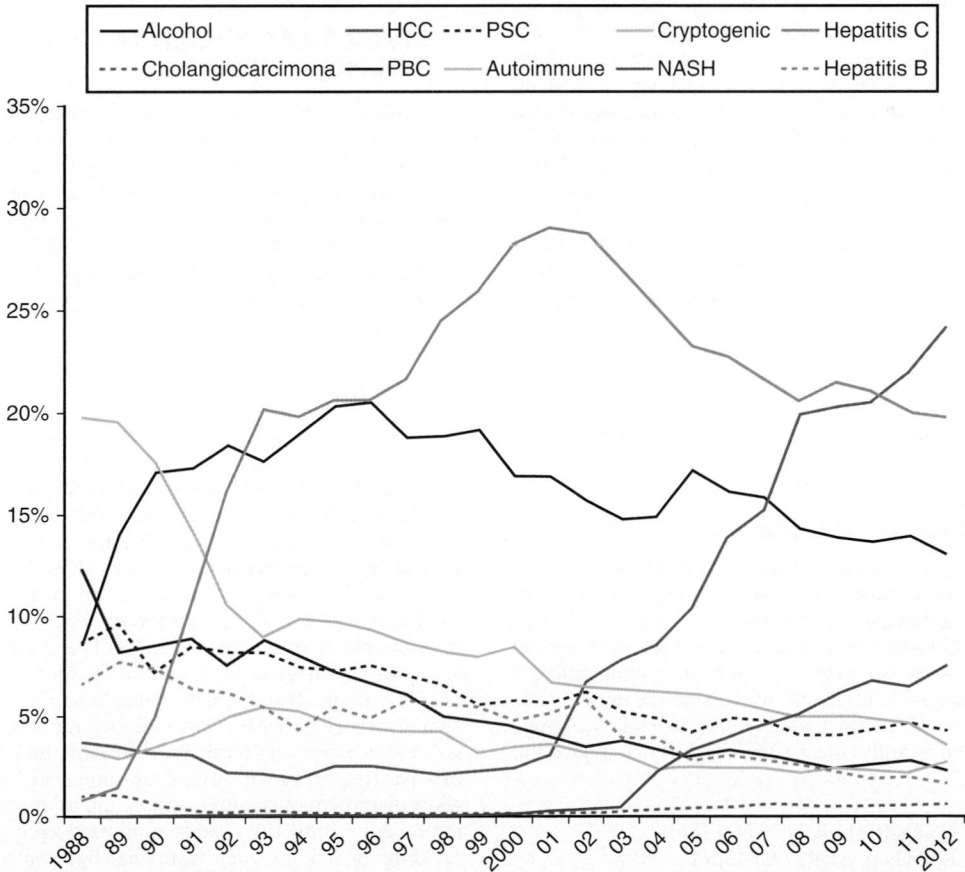

FIGURE 2 Diagnosis of liver disease at the time of transplantation. *HCC,* Hepatocellular carcinoma; *NASH,* nonalcoholic steatohepatitis; *PBC,* primary biliary cirrhosis; *PSC,* primary sclerosing cholangitis.

transplantation in 2012. This is partly related to the changes in allocation that have favored transplanting patients with HCC. In the United States, HCC is associated with cirrhosis in nearly 90% of the cases, and in some cases liver transplantation is the best chance for cure. A landmark article in 1996 by Mazzaferro and colleagues showed that for small HCCs, the outcomes after transplantation are excellent if they fall within certain criteria. Because the publication came from a group in Milan, these have become known as the Milan criteria. Milan criteria include HCC candidates with lesions that are stage T1 (one lesion <2 cm) or stage T2 (one lesion ≥2 cm but <5 cm, or as many as three lesions <3 cm each without any vascular invasion). Transplantation indeed is the treatment of choice for patients with HCC within the Milan criteria who also have cirrhosis. Five-year disease-free survival is vastly better after transplantation (82%) compared with resection (40%, P <0.001; Bellavance et al., 2008).

In 2002 the United Network of Organ Sharing (UNOS) changed the allocation of livers from a Child-Pugh categorized system to a Model for End-Stage Liver Disease (MELD)–based system that focuses on severity of disease and de-emphasizes waiting time. With the new policy, candidates with stage T1 or stage T2 HCC have priority beyond the degree of hepatic decompensation. The priority MELD score for stage T1 and stage T2 HCC ultimately was reduced first from 29 to 24 and then to 22 for stage T2 HCC only.

Cholangiocarcinoma, long considered a contraindication to transplantation, is re-emerging as an indication, especially in patients with primary sclerosing cholangitis (PSC). Early publications in the 1990s showed a 20% to 25% 5-year survival, with no improvement of neoadjuvant or adjuvant therapy. A sentinel paper from the Mayo Clinic appeared in 2005 and showed an 82% 5-year survival for patients who underwent a neoadjuvant chemoradiotherapy protocol. The protocol was very selective, including only patients with small hilar tumors and excluding those with previously attempted resections or those with extrahepatic disease on a protocol exploratory laparotomy (Rea et al., 2005). The study was criticized because of the loose diagnostic criteria that may have included PSC patients without cancer. Sixteen of the 38 (42%) patients transplanted showed no evidence of cancer on the explant. However, skepticism was abated when a multicenter trial with 12 participating centers showed similar results (Darwish Murad et al., 2012). This trial included a larger number of non-PSC (71) and PSC patients (143) who underwent liver transplantation for perihilar cholangiocarcinoma. The 10-year recurrence-free survival was 51% and 62%, respectively ($P = 0.06$). Although not as impressive as the initial Mayo Clinic report, these outcomes are significantly better than most of the surgical reports that exist. The 5-year survival for the cohort is even better (72%) if UNOS criteria are met (initial hilar mass <3 cm, no evidence of extrahepatic or lymph node disease on protocol exploration). On the basis of these two studies, UNOS now assigns 22 MELD points to patients with hilar cholangiocarcinoma who meet the criteria discussed earlier.

Model for End-Stage Liver Disease

MELD was first developed to predict survival in patients with complications of portal hypertension who are undergoing elective placement of transjugular intrahepatic portosystemic shunts (Malinchoc et al., 2000). The MELD score uses objective variables and has been shown to be an accurate predictor of survival among different populations of patients with advanced liver disease (Kamath et al., 2001). The formula used to calculate MELD is based on three variables found to significantly affect survival and their regression coefficients:

$$[0.957 \times \text{Log}_e(\text{Cr}) + 0.378 \times \text{Log}_e(\text{bili}) + 1.120 \times \text{Log}_e(\text{INR}) + 0.643] \times 10$$

where Cr is creatinine, *bili* is bilirubin, and *INR* is international normalized ratio.

TABLE 1: Model for End-Stage Liver Disease (MELD) Mortality Equivalents

MELD Score	3-Month Mortality
7	1%
20	8%
24	10%
26	15%
29	20%
31	30%
33	40%
35	50%
37	60%
38	70%
40	90%

Because MELD accurately predicts survival in patients with cirrhosis who have infections, variceal bleeding, cholestatic diseases, acute liver failure, and alcoholic hepatitis, it has been modified by UNOS and used to prioritize patients for liver transplantation. The modifications for transplantation maximize the score at 40 and assign a creatinine of 4 mg/dL for patients on renal replacement therapy. The 3-month predicted mortalities associated with MELD scores are outlined in Table 1.

■ LIVER TRANSPLANTATION TECHNIQUES

The techniques of hepatectomy and implantation have changed over time. The first attempts at liver transplantation used venovenous bypass (VVB) technique, which in itself has evolved to include a centrifugal pump and heparin-coated cannulas, thereby eliminating some of the fatal pulmonary embolisms initially encountered. In 1998 Chari and colleagues reported that 95% of centers were using VVB at least during the anhepatic phase. However, VVB is fading away as more and more centers successfully adopt caval preservation and partial clamping techniques.

Bicaval Anastomosis

With this conventional technique, the native liver is resected together with the retrohepatic inferior vena cava (IVC) and orthotopically replaced by a donor liver that includes the IVC (Figure 3). The native hepatectomy begins with dissection of the hepatic hilum. The dissection isolates the left and right hepatic arteries, which are divided separately. The proper hepatic artery (HA) is dissected beyond the gastroduodenal artery (GDA) to the common hepatic artery because a patch of the GDA and the common hepatic artery is often used for the subsequent arterial anastomosis. The cystic duct is divided, followed by the division of the common duct closer to the hilum to obtain maximal length on the duct. What is left at this point is the portal vein (PV) with surrounding lymphatic tissue. The vein is skeletonized from its bifurcation toward the pancreas, often to the first pancreatic branch. Several centimeters of vein are necessary to allow placement of clamps or for cannulation with VVB. PV division is not done until the liver is mobilized completely. This includes dividing the left and right triangular ligaments, mobilization of the right lobe off the diaphragm, and dissection of the retrohepatic IVC to completely mobilize it posteriorly. The adrenal vein is often divided to obtain adequate mobility of the IVC for clamping.

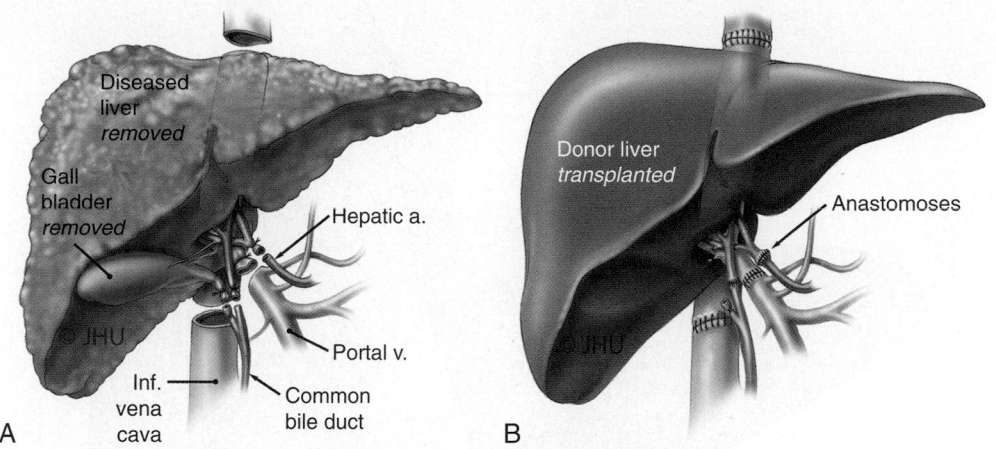

FIGURE 3 Classic bicaval anastomosis. The native liver is resected together with the retrohepatic inferior vena cava (IVC) (**A**) and orthotopically replaced by a donor liver that includes the IVC (**B**). *(Illustration Copyright © 1998-2003 by The Johns Hopkins Health System Corporation and The Johns Hopkins University; used with permission from the Johns Hopkins Division of Gastroenterology and Hepatology (www.hopkinsmedicine.org/gi). Illustration created by Mike Linkinhoker.)*

Complete venous clamping with or without VVB is necessary. Complete IVC and PV clamping can result in important hemodynamic consequences with decreased venous return, congestion in the caval and splanchnic bed, and a reduction of renal function. This should be done when the hepatectomy is nearly complete because the congestion leads to increased bleeding during hepatectomy. For this reason VVB was introduced in the mid-1980s. However, as anesthetic conditioning has improved, VVB can be avoided, especially when the vascular anastomoses are done expediently. Two IVC anastomoses are required, one suprahepatic and one infrahepatic end to end.

Piggyback Technique

In 1989 Tzakis and colleagues popularized the technique of orthotopic liver transplantation (OLT) with preservation of the IVC, called the "piggyback" technique. This technique involves complete mobilization of the liver off the IVC, including the hepatic veins that are individually oversewn. In the Tzakis report the transplant was still performed with the use of a VVB. Venous outflow reconstruction was performed between the suprahepatic donor IVC and a common orifice created by opening the native right, middle, and left hepatic veins or only the middle and left veins (Figure 4). Several studies, including a randomized trial, favored the piggyback technique over the traditional bicaval technique, with a shorter anhepatic phase, reduction of blood loss, and reduction of the cost of the procedure in favor of the piggyback technique.

Modifications of the Piggyback Technique

Several reports describing a venous outflow complication rate of up to 5% appeared. These complications included graft congestion and stenosis of the caval anastomosis. For this reason, modifications of the piggyback technique became more popular. In 1992 a side-to-side anastomosis between donor and recipient IVC without the routine use of VVB was described. In this modification both suprahepatic and infrahepatic ends of the donor IVC are closed, and the anastomosis is created between two new incisions, one made on the recipient IVC and another on the donor IVC (Figure 5). Cherqui introduced another venous outflow reconstruction. He enlarged the common orifice of three hepatic veins by a caudal incision on the anterior wall of the recipient IVC and anastomosed it with the suprahepatic end of the donor IVC (end-to-side anastomosis) (Tayar et al., 2011). This technique was further modified by closing all

hepatic veins and creating an anastomosis between a new incision on the anterior wall of the recipient IVC and a V-shaped incision on the donor IVC to avoid stricturing of the outflow anastomosis (Polak et al., 2006). In certain situations where the suprahepatic IVC cuff is very short, such as in domino liver transplantation, or in case of outflow complications after piggyback implantation, some authors advocate the use of the infrahepatic cavocaval anastomosis (Nishida et al., 2001).

Although there are studies comparing the different piggyback techniques, the essential message is to extend the cavostomy on the recipient to create a wide caval anastomosis and avoid some of the venous stricturing complications that ultimately lead to Budd-Chiari syndrome. One thing is clear, however: avoiding VVB with caval-preserving techniques is becoming the norm in many liver transplant centers.

Vascular Reconstruction

The PV reconstruction is usually performed end to end with fine polypropylene suture. There are several important technical considerations to uphold to avoid either stenosis or kinking that can ultimately lead to PV thrombosis. A technique that Starzl initially described is allowing for a "growth factor" when tying after circumferentially running the suture. This allows expansion of the anastomosis to accommodate the distension that occurs when flow is re-established. Failure to incorporate the growth factor will result in an "hourglass" anastomosis that may be prone to stenosis and thrombosis. The second concept is related to the length of donor PV. Typically during a liver transplant, the operative field is expanded with the use of surgical retractors. This has to be taken into account in assessing the length of the donor PV. It is not uncommon to find the PV kinking once the retractors are removed because it was sewn with too much donor length. To avoid this problem many surgeons will minimize the retraction inferiorly and place laparotomy pads above the liver to bring the liver down before the PV anastomosis. If this problem does occur, it is important to redo the anastomosis after cutting an adequate amount of donor PV. This can be performed with minimal hepatic sequelae if done expediently in the presence of arterial perfusion.

Portal Vein Reconstruction in the Presence of Native Portal Vein Thrombosis

PV thrombosis increasingly is being recognized in patients with advanced cirrhosis and in those undergoing liver transplantation.

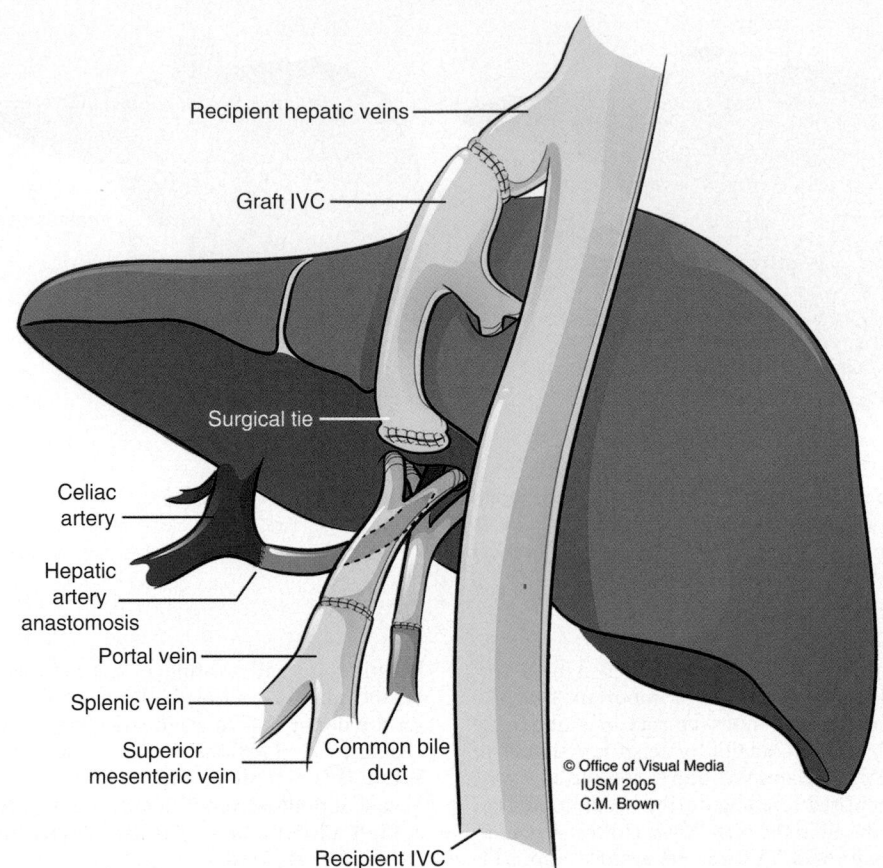

FIGURE 4 Piggyback technique. Venous outflow reconstruction is performed between the suprahepatic donor inferior vena cava (IVC) and a common orifice created by opening the native right, middle, and left hepatic veins or only the middle and left veins. (© *Office of Visual Media, Indiana University School of Medicine.*)

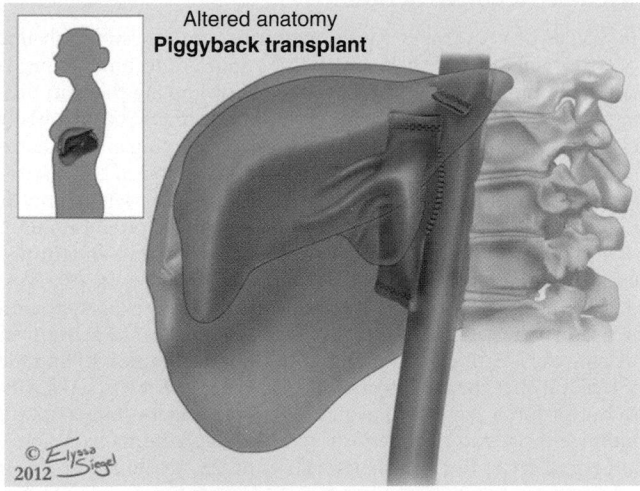

FIGURE 5 Modified piggyback technique. In this modification both supra- and infrahepatic end of the donor IVC is closed and the anastomosis is created between two new incisions, one made on the recipient IVC and another on the donor IVC. In this modification all hepatic veins are sewn over and a new incision on the anterior wall of recipient IVC is made. (*Used with permission from Elyssa Siegel, Art as Applied to Medicine, Johns Hopkins University.*)

Reduced portal flow and hypercoagulability that occurs with advanced liver disease is probably responsible for clotting in the porto-spleno-mesenteric venous system. The prevalence of PV thrombosis in patients without HCC has been reported to be as high as 25% in ultrasound-based studies, with the overall incidence increasing to nearly 40% with time (Maruyama et al., 2013). PV thrombosis was long considered a contraindication to liver transplantation, but as reports with good outcomes appeared, this is no longer the case. Techniques of native PV thrombectomy have been well described, with success rates exceeding 95%. The thrombus often extends to the confluence of the splenic and mesenteric veins, often sparing at least the superior mesenteric vein (SMV). For this reason thrombectomy is more successful when the dissection during the hepatectomy is carried out beyond the confluence to reach the tail of the thrombus. Although some authors advocate the use of Fogarty balloons, the clot is often organized and adherent to the vein wall. The extent of the clot can be examined manually and visually. If the thrombus completely occludes portal flow, the PV can be divided at the right and left confluence with the edges held apart with tonsil clamps. This allows the surgeon to separate the clot and the attached intimal layer from the media of the vein circumferentially using a dura elevator. This maneuver is extended as far as necessary, frequently entering the splenic and superior mesenteric veins. The free edge of the clot then is clamped with a tonsil or ring clamp and gently rotated and pulled out (Molmenti et al., 2002). Because hypercoagulability is considered a risk factor for PV thrombosis, often the recipients are placed on a full dose daily aspirin before discharge. With this technique, a bypass graft from the SMV that uses donor iliac vein to re-establish PV inflow is rarely necessary.

In cases of massive portal system thrombosis that involves the SMV and splenic vein, salvage revascularization techniques have been described. Cavoportal hemitransposition has been described by Tzakis and colleagues (1998) when no portal inflow can be achieved. This technique involves ligating (either completely or partially) the infrahepatic recipient IVC. The PV anastomosis is either done end to end inferior to the point of ligation or end to side with partial ligation. Overall survival was poor, so this technique should be reserved only as a salvage procedure intraoperatively.

Arterial Reconstruction

The arterial reconstruction is usually a direct anastomosis between the donor and recipient HA in an end to end fashion. The anastomosis should involve Carrel patches on the donor and recipient ends to decrease the incidence of hepatic artery thrombosis (HAT) (Merion et al., 1989). The donor artery typically involves the entire celiac trunk with a patch of aorta. This is sewn to a Carrel patch created by the recipient gastroduodenal artery and the proper HA coming off the common hepatic artery. In cases where donor arteriopathy exists, it is important to shorten the artery to a segment free of disease. A donor patch also can be made with the splenic artery takeoff if the remainder of the artery is disease free.

In other cases, the recipient HA is unsuitable for use because of poor inflow from more proximal stenosis, atherosclerosis, or intimal dissection. Options include dissecting more proximally on the recipient artery beyond the takeoff of the splenic artery. If the inflow is adequate at that point, an end-to-side anastomosis to both the celiac and the splenic artery confluence can be achieved while preserving flow to the spleen. Alternatively, an end-to-end anastomosis to the celiac artery can be performed while sacrificing the splenic artery (El-Hinnawi et al., 2013). Although this is an appropriate alternative, especially in retransplants, splenic infarcts and abscesses can result. The most common method used to deal with poor arterial inflow is an arterial conduit directly from the aorta with donor iliac artery graft. For this reason donor iliac graft is always procured with the liver. The anastomosis can be done to either the supraceliac or infrarenal aorta. The infrarenal aorta is used more commonly because it is safer and access is easier. The graft commonly is tunneled antepancreatic and retrogastric/retrocolic. However, the infrarenal aorta is more prone to calcification and atherosclerotic disease, especially in older patients. The supraceliac aorta is easy to access after the hepatectomy, so it may be used in cases where arterial reconstruction is planned (e.g., retransplantation with HAT). However, the supraceliac aorta does not hold sutures as well as the infrarenal aorta, and any complications with this segment can result in disastrous consequences. The use of arterial conduits is associated with excellent long-term outcomes and low HAT rates (Zamboni et al., 2002).

Aberrant donor arterial anatomy is present in up to 25% of cases and has to be recognized during the procurement. An accessory or replaced right HA arising from the superior mesenteric artery (SMA) often is preserved by procuring the SMA trunk with the celiac artery. The artery then can be reconstructed on the back table before implantation. A left accessory or replaced HA arising from the left gastric artery also should be preserved, although no reconstruction is necessary because it arises from the celiac trunk. Back table preparation of the accessory left HA requires careful dissection of the left gastric artery with ligation of all of its branches.

Biliary Anastomosis

The two main techniques of biliary tract reconstruction are direct duct-to-duct and Roux-en-Y hepaticojejunostomy or choledochojejunostomy. If the recipient duct is normal, a duct-to-duct anastomosis is preferable. This preserves the native physiology and anatomy and allows future biliary access via endoscopic retrograde cholangiopancreatography (ERCP). The end-to-end anastomosis commonly is performed with either running or interrupted dissolvable sutures. When a significant size discrepancy exists, a side-to-side anastomosis can be used. Both techniques are acceptable and yield equivalent results (Davidson et al., 1999).

Roux-en-Y reconstruction is often needed in retransplantation or for patients with PSC. However, the routine use of Roux-en-Y anastomosis for PSC has become a topic of controversy, as many are now advocating direct duct-to-duct anastomosis in PSC patients with normal appearing ducts (Sutton et al., 2014; Damrah et al., 2012).

The routine use of T-tubes during biliary anastomosis has been challenged for more than a decade and has lost favor in the majority of transplant centers. Several pivotal trials have shown that the incidence of biliary complications is actually lower when T-tubes are not used (Scatton et al., 2001; Weiss et al., 2009). Duct-to-duct biliary anastomosis, whether end to end or side to side, should be done without any biliary tubes.

■ OUTCOMES

Despite a progressive increase in the severity of liver disease in transplant recipients, graft survival continues to improve. The national 1-year graft and patient survival in 2014 was 86% and 90%, respectively. The incidence of acute rejection continued to decline, likely related to increasing induction immunosuppression and novel agents.

For patients who underwent liver transplantation in 2009, the 5-year overall graft survival rate was 70.2%. Survival was poorest for recipients aged 65 years or older, those with hepatitis C infection or malignancy, and those who underwent retransplantation. It is likely that the new direct-acting antiviral agents (DAAs) for hepatitis C will improve graft survival in this population.

■ COMPLICATIONS FOLLOWING LIVER TRANSPLANTATION

Vascular Complications
Arterial

The interruption or the reduction of arterial flow during liver transplantation frequently is associated with biliary ischemia and complications that include bile duct necrosis, liver abscesses, and graft dysfunction. This occurs because of the absence of collaterals in liver transplant recipients. In the native liver, HAT or ligation is usually well tolerated because of the abundant arterial collateral sources that avoid ischemia of the liver parenchyma. In contrast, disruption of these collaterals inevitably occurs when performing total hepatectomy for transplant. In cases of HAT, the allograft often survives because of portal flow and portal oxygen. The biliary tree, however, is dependent primarily on arterial flow and is therefore especially sensitive to interruption of arterial blood. Recognition and prompt management of HAT is of great importance for graft and patient survival. The incidence of HAT is 2% to 5%, about half of these cases occurring early within the perioperative period and half occurring late. Early HAT inevitably leads to graft loss and a high mortality rate. For this reason, diagnosed patients often have to be retransplanted. Rarely, HAT can be caught shortly after it occurs and graft failure can be thwarted with thrombectomy and revision or reconstruction of the artery.

Measurement of hepatic arterial flow can be accomplished easily with flow probes (e.g., Transonic). The flow probes are placed on the reconstructed artery to gently surround the vessel, excluding extraneous tissue. By immersing the flow probe in saline, a good acoustic contact occurs and the readings stabilize rapidly with little fluctuation. Hepatic arterial flow is dependent on both cardiac output and portal venous flow. However, it has been shown that arterial flow of less than 200 cc/min is associated with a sixfold increase in HAT, and that flow of less than 100 cc/min is associated with a significant increase in the incidence of primary nonfunction (Lin et al., 2002; Pratschke et al., 2011). Information on volumetric flow at the time of operation either can be reassuring or may indicate an unexpected problem that can be fixed at this time.

Hepatic artery stenosis (HAS) occurs in 2% to 10% of cases. Chen and colleagues (2009) reported an overall HAS incidence of 2.8%, with early (<30 days) HAS incidence accounting for 40% and late HAS incidence accounting for 60%. The mean time that elapsed between transplantation and diagnosis of HAS was 91 days. HAS can lead to an insidious form of graft disorder, in both the early and the later postoperative stages. Many patients with HAS are asymptomatic and most commonly have only mildly elevated liver function tests. Because of the insidious nature of HAS, some centers perform routine screening ultrasounds at regular time intervals.

The therapeutic management of HAS includes either surgical revision or percutaneous endovascular interventions, such as percutaneous transluminal angioplasty (PTA) with or without stent placement. In one study treating 42 cases of HAS, 81% were treated successfully by PTA, with an incidence of immediate complication, including dissection and arterial rupture, of 7% (Saad et al., 2005). These results compare favorably with surgical approaches, so PTA has become first-line therapy for HAS.

Venous

Venous complications are less frequent than arterial complications but also can result in graft failure, especially if they occur in the early postoperative period. Endovascular management has become the treatment of choice for the majority of venous complications.

Portal Vein

The incidence of PV complications is low, estimated around 1%. They are more common in pediatric and living donor transplants. The most common complications are PV thrombosis (PVT) and PV stenosis (PVS).

The risk factors for PVT include technical issues (kinking of the PV because of excess length), preoperative PVT in the recipient requiring intraoperative thrombectomy, hypercoagulability, small PV diameter, and reconstruction with a vein conduit. Early PVT can be devastating, leading to early graft dysfunction and loss, and generally is less well tolerated than early HAT. Excess length of the PV after anastomosis can occur easily because of the presence of retraction during the anastomosis. Once the retractors are released, the operative field collapses and kinking of the PV can occur. To account for this, laparotomy pads typically are placed behind the dome of the liver, essentially bringing the liver down and facilitating an anastomosis that will not have redundancy. In addition, a "growth factor" is included when tying the final knot to prevent wasting of the anastomosis when flow is reintroduced and the PV expands.

If flow is compromised for any of the reasons discussed earlier, the risk of PVT is increased. It is therefore important to ensure that once the retractors are removed the PV is not kinked or redundant. In addition, measurement of portal venous flow can be accomplished easily with flow probes. Portal venous flow is dependent on cardiac output and graft size. The range is wide, but in general PV flow should exceed 1 L/min to minimize the risks of PVT (Pratschke et al., 2011). PV hyperperfusion can affect arterial flow (Henderson et al., 1992) but is usually problematic only with small grafts and living donor liver transplantation.

PVS is a rare complication of liver transplantation, primarily because the majority of patients with PVS are asymptomatic. PVS is a bigger problem in pediatric and living donor transplants because size mismatch is more likely to lead to technical issues that result in PVS. When PVS does occur, the management is dependent on the timing. Early PVS within the perioperative period should be approached surgically. Late PVS is more amenable to percutaneous approaches, either transhepatic or transjugular. Percutaneous balloon dilatation has been reported with good success and has become the treatment of choice (Shibata et al., 2005). Asymptomatic PVS noted on ultrasound without any graft dysfunction should be observed without any intervention necessary.

Biliary Complications

The most common type of biliary reconstruction is a choledocho-choledochostomy (duct-to-duct anastomosis). Choledochojejunostomy is sometimes necessary in cases where the native bile duct is diseased or unusable, such as in patients with PSC or redo liver transplants. Duct-to-duct anastomosis has several advantages. The sphincter of Oddi function is preserved, which plays a role in decreasing the risk of ascending cholangitis, and this reconstruction also allows easy endoscopic access to the biliary tree for diagnostic and therapeutic purposes.

Bile Leak

Bile leaks occur early in up to 20% of cases after liver transplantation. Most are self-limited and seal within a few days without any further intervention as long as the leaks are well drained. If the leaks are not well drained, patients could be seen with abdominal pain, fever, or any sign of peritonitis. Ultrasound or CT scan often can identify a biloma or fluid collection near the porta hepatic, which should raise the suspicion greatly. Once bile leak is suspected, ERCP with sphincterotomy and stent placement becomes the diagnostic and therapeutic procedure of choice, assuming that there are no intraoperatively placed biliary tubes at the time of anastomosis. The success rate often exceeds 85%, and no further treatment is necessary. In the event that a bile leak is more extensive or involves necrosis of the distal donor duct, surgical reconstruction is necessary to avoid biliary strictures that will become problematic in the future.

Bile Duct Strictures

Biliary strictures are also a common biliary complication, occurring in up to 15% of cases with deceased donor transplants (Sharma et al., 2008). Strictures are classified as anastomotic and nonanastomotic. The approach to each type is markedly different, so it is important to distinguish the two. Anastomotic strictures early in the postoperative period often are related to technical issues, including surgical techniques, small caliber ducts, or burn injury from electrocautery. Later onset anastomotic strictures most likely are related to ischemia at the end of the donor duct leading to fibrotic healing. Nonanastomotic strictures likely result from ischemia secondary to preservation injury, donation after cardiac death, prolonged use of vasopressors, rejection, hepatic artery insufficiency, or recurrent disease.

Although magnetic resonance cholangiopancreatography (MRCP) has high sensitivity and specificity, the diagnostic procedure of choice is ERCP because therapeutic options often are required. For anastomotic strictures, balloon dilation with stent placement is more successful than dilation without stent placement. The stents generally are replaced by larger stents every 3 months to prevent clogging, cholangitis, or stone formation. Serial dilation with dual or multiple stents will prove successful in the vast majority of patients. Surgical intervention is rarely necessary.

Management of patients with nonanastomotic strictures is more difficult, as these strictures are prone to developing sludge, casts, and stones, rendering plastic stents less effective. The recent use of metallic wall stents may improve the success of endoscopic management of these strictures. If the disease is limited to the extrahepatic ducts, surgical revision is necessary and requires conversion to a Roux-en-Y hepaticojejunostomy. If the intrahepatic ducts also are involved, retransplantation may be necessary.

■ LIVING DONOR LIVER TRANSPLANTATION

Living donor liver transplantation (LDLT) for pediatric recipients was introduced in 1989 to overcome the severe shortage of deceased donor organs across the world (Strong et al., 1990). In 1993 Tanaka and colleagues reported the first adult-to-adult right liver LDLT using a right lobe, making liver transplantation feasible for adults in areas of the world where deceased donors are very limited (Tanaka et al., 1993). Since then, living donor grafts for adults have expanded to include right lobes with the middle hepatic vein and left lobes. Centers embarking on LDLT often face ethical issues regarding donor safety when a healthy adult must undergo a complicated major surgery without receiving any health benefit. The complication rate after LDLT ranges widely in the literature between 10% and 50%, depending on the severity. Unfortunately there have been a number of deaths after living donation. The risk for death is estimated to be 0.2% to 0.5% with left lobe donation and 0.3% to 1% with right lobe donation. Because of this, as well as a highly publicized death of a living donor in New York City, enthusiasm for LDLT has waned in the United States since 2001, despite a flat number of deceased donor liver transplants since 2006 (Figure 6). Five-year survival for living donor liver transplants is around 80%, equal to deceased donor transplants.

Graft function after LDLT is highly dependent on graft volume. Although left lobe donation is associated with a lower mortality rate, left lobe volumes are typically smaller and small-for-size syndrome is more prevalent, especially in the face of significant portal hypertension. As a result, right lobe grafts have been used more commonly in adults. The literature has suggested that a graft weight–recipient weight ratio of 0.8% or greater and a graft weight–standard liver volume ratio of 40% are the same limits for donor graft size to avoid small-for-size syndrome. Small-for-size syndrome is defined as prolonged cholestasis with ascites void of technical issues. Imaging techniques to predict vascular anatomy and graft weight include magnetic resonance imaging (MRI) with intravenous (IV) contrast and fine-cut CT scans with IV contrast. There are multiple software companies that reconstruct the CT or MRI images in three dimensions (3D) to allow the surgeon to more precisely assess graft volume, including segmental drainage of the liver (Figure 7). These 3D analyses enable the surgical team to better plan resection lines and the need for venous reconstruction. Parenchymal transection for right lobe grafts typically is performed immediately to the right of the middle hepatic vein (Figure 8). Large branches from segment 5 or 8 draining to the middle hepatic vein may need to be reconstructed to avoid hepatic congestion (Figure 9).

Biliary complications have been the Achilles heel of LDLTs. Biliary anatomy is highly variable, and the need to anastomose two bile ducts is not uncommon. As a result, the leak and stricture rate can be as high as 30%, higher than for deceased donor transplants.

Despite the technical challenges and higher rate of graft complications, LDLT remains a lifesaving procedure for patients with end-stage liver disease.

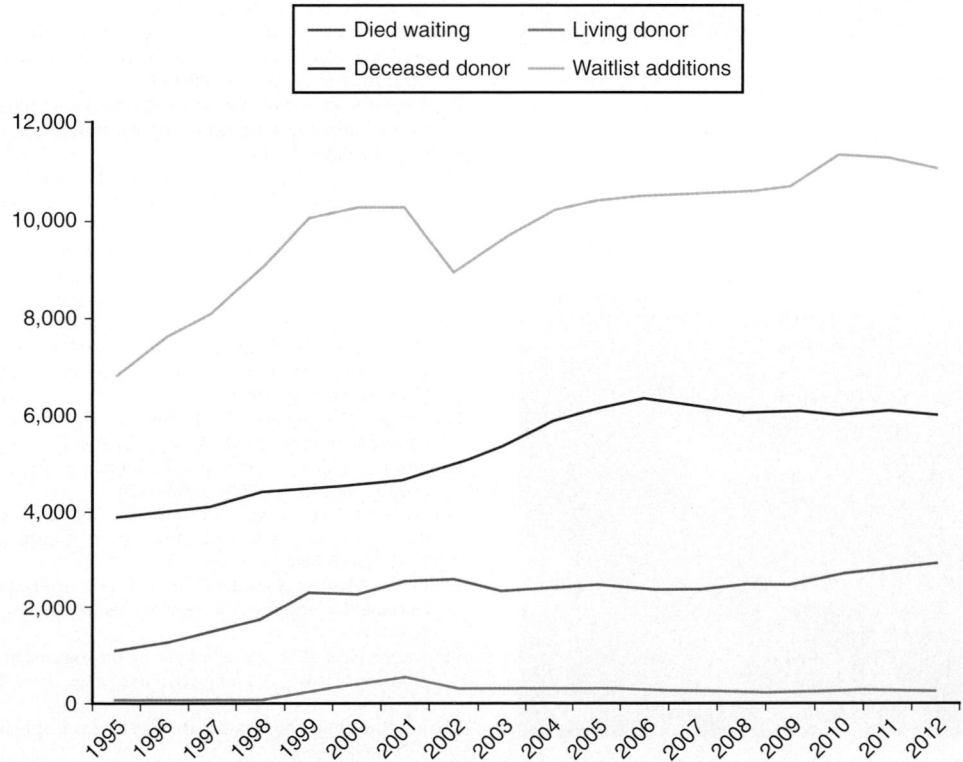

FIGURE 6 Waiting list additions, deaths, and liver transplantations over time. *(Data from United States Organ Procurement and Transplantation Network [OPTN].)*

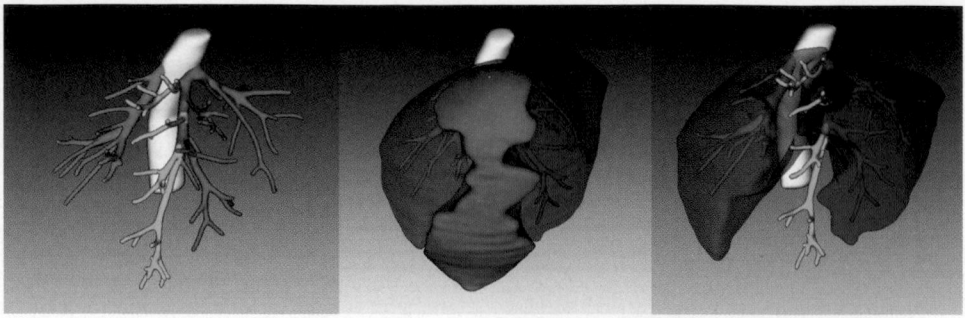

Geometry analysis of
hepatic vein

RT lobe Vol. (cm³)	505.52 (31%)
LT lobe Vol. (cm³)	658.77 (40%)
RT Middle HV Branches Vol. (cm³)	480.99 (29%)

FIGURE 7 Three-dimensional reconstruction to assess live donor liver graft. *HV*, Hepatic vein; *LT*, left; *RT*, right.

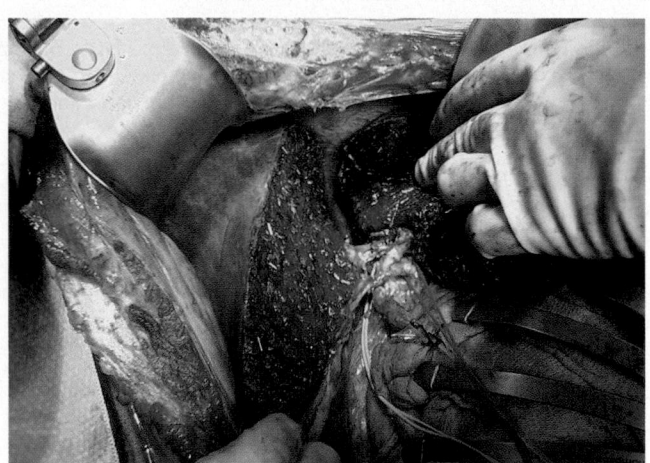

FIGURE 8 Parenchymal transection to the right of the middle hepatic vein.

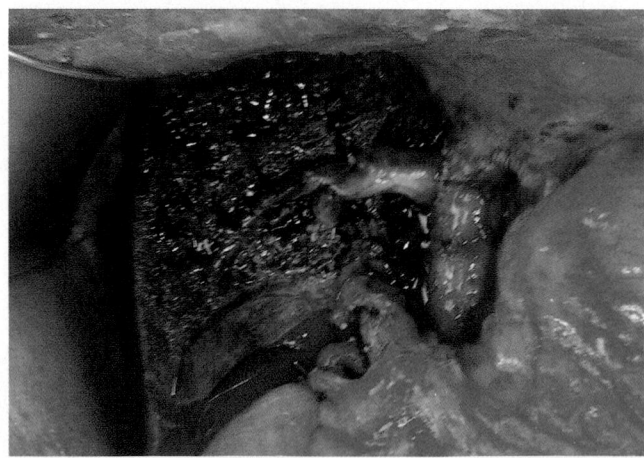

FIGURE 9 Right lobe graft after reperfusion with reconstruction of segment 5 vein.

SUGGESTED READINGS

Bellavance EC, et al. Surgical management of early-stage hepatocellular carcinoma: resection or transplantation. *J Gastrointest Surg.* 2008;12: 1699-1708.

Bernal W, Wendon J. Acute liver failure. *N Engl J Med.* 2013;369:2525-2534.

Chari RS, et al. Venovenous bypass in adult orthotopic liver transplantation: routine or selective use? *J Am Coll Surg.* 1998;186:683-690.

Chen GH, Wang GY, Yang Y, Li H, Lu MQ, Cai CJ, Wang GS, Xu C, Yi SH, Zhang JF. Single-center experience of therapeutic management of hepatic artery stenosis after orthotopic liver transplantation: report of 20 cases. *Eur Surg Res.* 2009;42:21-27.

Clemmenen JO, Larsen FS, Kondrup J, et al. Cerebral herniation in patients with acute liver failure is correlated with arterial ammonia concentration. *Hepatology.* 1999;29:648-653.

Damrah O, et al. Duct-to-duct biliary reconstruction in orthotopic liver transplantation for primary sclerosing cholangitis: a viable and safe alternative. *Transpl Int.* 2012;25:64-68.

Darwish Murad S, et al. Efficacy of neoadjuvant chemoradiation, followed by liver transplantation, for perihilar cholangiocarcinoma at 12 US centers. *Gastroenterology.* 2012;143:88-98.

Davidson BR, et al. Prospective randomized trial of end-to-end versus side-to-side biliary reconstruction after orthotopic liver transplantation. *Br J Surg.* 1999;86:447-452.

El-Hinnawi A, et al. Use of the recipient celiac trunk for hepatic artery reconstruction in orthotopic liver transplantation. *Transplant Proc.* 2013;45: 1928-1930.

El Serag HB. Hepatocellular carcinoma. *N Engl J Med.* 2011;365:1118-1127.

Farmer DG, et al. Liver transplantation for fulminant hepatic failure: experience with more than 200 patients over a 17-year period. *Ann Surg.* 2003;237:666-676.

Henderson JM, et al. Hemodynamics during liver transplantation: the interactions between cardiac output and portal venous and hepatic arterial flows. *Hepatology.* 1992;16:715-718.

Hoofnagle JH, Carithers RL Jr, Shapiro C, Ascher N. Fulminant hepatic failure: summary of a workshop. *Hepatology.* 1995;21:240-252.

Kamath PS, et al. A model to predict survival in patients with end-stage liver disease. *Hepatology.* 2001;33:464-470.

Lin M, et al. Hepatic artery thrombosis and intraoperative hepatic artery flow rates in adult orthotopic liver transplantation. *ANZ J Surg.* 2002;72:798-800.

Malinchoc M, et al. A model to predict poor survival in patients undergoing transjugular intrahepatic portosystemic shunts. *Hepatology.* 2000;31: 864-871.

Maruyama H, et al. De novo portal vein thrombosis in virus-related cirrhosis: predictive factors and long-term outcomes. *Am J Gastroenterol.* 2013;108: 568-574.

Merion RM, et al. The hepatic artery in liver transplantation. *Transplantation.* 1989;48:438-443.

Molmenti EP, et al. Thrombendvenectomy for organized portal vein thrombosis at the time of liver transplantation. *Ann Surg.* 2002;235:292-296.

Nishida S, et al. Domino liver transplantation with end-to-side infrahepatic vena cavocavostomy. *J Am Coll Surg*. 2001;192:237-240.

Ostapowicz G, Fontana RJ, Schiodt FV, et al. Results of a prospective study of acute liver failure at 17 tertiary care centers in the United States. *Ann Intern Med*. 2002;137:947-954.

Polak WG, et al. End-to-side caval anastomosis in adult piggyback liver transplantation. *Clin Transplant*. 2006;20:609-616.

Pratschke S, et al. Arterial blood flow predicts graft survival in liver transplant patients. *Liver Transpl*. 2011;17:436-445.

Rea DJ, et al. Liver transplantation with neoadjuvant chemoradiation is more effective than resection for hilar cholangiocarcinoma. *Ann Surg*. 2005;242: 451-458.

Saad WE, Davies MG, Sahler L, Lee DE, Patel NC, Kitanosono T, Sasson T, Waldman DL. Hepatic artery stenosis in liver transplant recipients: primary treatment with percutaneous transluminal angioplasty. *J Vasc Interv Radiol*. 2005;16:795-805.

Scatton O, et al. Randomized trial of choledochocholedochostomy with or without a T tube in orthotopic liver transplantation. *Ann Surg*. 2001;233: 432-437.

Sharma S, Gurakar A, Jabbour N. Biliary strictures following liver transplantation: past, present and preventive strategies. *Liver Transpl*. 2008;14: 759-769.

Shibata T, Itoh K, Kubo T, Maetani Y, Shibata T, Togashi K, Tanaka K. Percutaneous transhepatic balloon dilation of portal venous stenosis in patients with living donor liver transplantation. *Radiology*. 2005;235: 1078-1083.

Starzl TE, Marchioro TL, Von Kaulla KN, Hermann G, Brittain RS, Waddell WR. Homotransplantation of the liver in humans. *Surg Gynecol Obstet*. 1963;117:659-676.

Starzl TE, Todo S, Fung J, Demetris AJ, Venkataramanan R, Jain A. FK 506 for human liver, kidney and pancreas transplantation. *Lancet*. 1989;2: 1000-1004.

Strong RW, Lynch SV, Ong TH, Matsunami H, Koido Y, Balderson GA. Successful liver transplantation from a living donor to her son. *N Engl J Med*. 1990;322:1505-1507.

Sutton ME, et al. Duct-to-duct reconstruction in liver transplantation for primary sclerosing cholangitis is associated with fewer biliary complications in comparison with hepaticojejunostomy. *Liver Transpl*. 2014;20: 457-463.

Tanaka K, Uemoto S, Tokunaga Y, et al. Surgical techniques and innovations in living related liver transplantation. *Ann Surg*. 1993;217:82-91.

Tayar C, et al. Optimizing outflow in piggyback liver transplantation without caval occlusion: the three-vein technique. *Liver Transpl*. 2011;17:88-92.

Tzakis G, et al. Liver transplantation with cavoportal hemitransposition in the presence of diffuse portal vein thrombosis. *Transplantation*. 1998;65: 619-624.

Weiss S, et al. Biliary reconstruction using a side-to-side choledochostomy with or without T-tube in deceased donor liver transplantation: a prospective randomized trial. *Ann Surg*. 2009;250:766-771.

Zamboni F, et al. Use of arterial conduit as an alternative technique in arterial revascularization during orthotopic liver transplantation. *Dig Liver Dis*. 2002;34:122-126.

ENDOSCOPIC THERAPY FOR ESOPHAGEAL VARICEAL HEMORRHAGE

Patrick I. Okolo III, MD, MPH, FASGE, and Yen-I Chen, MD

Esophageal varices are venous collaterals that form as a consequence of portal hypertension. Every year 5% to 10% of patients with cirrhosis will develop esophageal varices. This is more likely to occur in patients with progressive cirrhosis and may be present in up to 60% of patients with decompensated cirrhosis. Hemorrhage from esophageal varices occurs in about 10% of cirrhotic patients annually and accounts for up to 70% of gastrointestinal bleeding in this population. Bleeding from gastric varices is less common, although it is often more profound and more difficult to manage.

■ CLINICAL PRESENTATION

Patients with variceal bleeding often have signs and symptoms of upper gastrointestinal bleeding, including melena and hematemesis. In many cases of acute bleeding, the patient may be seen in extremis characterized by physiologic decompensation. In this latter case, as with all cases of suspected gastrointestinal bleeding, a focused history and physical examination accompanied by supporting laboratory investigations and a high index of suspicion enable prompt diagnosis of variceal bleeding.

■ OVERVIEW OF THE ACUTE MANAGEMENT OF ESOPHAGEAL VARICEAL BLEEDING

The initial step in the management of patients with all manner of gastrointestinal bleeding is an assessment of severity. Assessment of severity and correction of physiologic derangements is essential to the proper management of patients with variceal hemorrhage. Any patient with upper gastrointestinal bleeding who has signs and symptoms or laboratory findings suggestive of portal hypertension should be suspected of having variceal hemorrhage until proven otherwise. These patients often require significant resources for their proper management, and transfer to an area capable of providing care across the continuum of acuity (such as an intensive care unit) is often necessary.

Meticulous resuscitation to a hemoglobin level of 7 to 8 g/dL and a systemic blood pressure of 100 mm Hg is essential. However, fluid overload should be avoided because animal models have shown risk for increase in portal pressure and bleeding exacerbation, whereas a randomized controlled trial demonstrated a mortality benefit with a restrictive strategy for blood transfusion with a 7 g/dL threshold versus a 9 g/dL target. The patient's airway should be controlled to avoid aspiration, and intravenous (IV) broad-spectrum antibiotics should be administered. Antibiotics in this setting have been shown to reduce mortality and mitigate bacterial sepsis, renal failure, and the likelihood of rebleeding. An IV octreotide infusion at 50 μg/hr should be started after an initial IV bolus of 50 μg. After initiation of octreotide in the appropriate setting, the infusion is continued for 2 to 5 days. A vasoconstrictor and a vasodilator can be synergistic in reducing portal pressure and can be used in combination in the initial management of variceal bleeding. Endoscopic options, including endoscopic variceal ligation (EVL) and sclerotherapy, are the mainstay of acute management of variceal hemorrhage. Esophageal stenting is emerging as a possible rescue modality for variceal bleeding refractory to EVL. Reduction of portal pressure by placement of a radiologically guided shunt (transjugular intrahepatic portosystemic shunt [TIPS]) and less frequently surgical portosystemic bypass remain options for management of variceal bleeding. TIPS is performed by interventional radiology and involves placing a covered metal stent between the portal vein and the hepatic vein, thus creating a shunt and lowering the portal pressure. Bypass frequently is associated with portosystemic encephalopathy, so patients should be selected carefully for treatment with this technique. TIPS placement is often considered in bleeding from gastric varices, as endoscopic banding has a very limited role in their management. In these patients, acute hemorrhage and its immediate aftermath can be managed endoscopically by the direct injection of cyanoacrylate. 2-Octyl cyanoacrylate is available in the United States and is used in an off-label manner to treat gastric varices after acute bleeding.

Endoscopic ultrasound (EUS) with or without fine-needle injection of coils may improve the precision of this technique. Balloon tamponade should be used as a temporary measure in patients with refractory bleeding. This enables cessation of bleeding before implementation of a more durable hemostatic strategy.

ENDOSCOPY AND ACUTE VARICEAL BLEEDING

Endoscopy remains the gold standard for the diagnosis and treatment of esophageal varices. Endoscopy permits direct visualization and characterization of varices, enabling the determination of the distribution of the varices and whether or not there is evidence of recent bleeding. Endoscopy allows comparative evaluation of varices and thus enables prognostication even when a patient has not experienced any prior gastrointestinal bleeding. Endoscopy has proven efficacy when used appropriately in the prevention of variceal bleeding before or after an index bleeding episode. This chapter, however, focuses on the role of endoscopy in the treatment of acute variceal bleeding.

Pre-endoscopy considerations are of significant importance and may influence the clinical outcome of any episode of variceal bleeding. The patient should be moved to an intensive care unit whenever appropriate. Resuscitation to a hemoglobin of 7 to 8 g/dL and systolic blood pressure of 100 mm Hg using blood and crystalloid should be achieved whenever possible. The patient ideally should be intubated to prevent aspiration before, during, and after the endoscopic procedure. Although systemic evidence for this is scant, anecdotal evidence suggests that it is indeed prudent. The timing of endoscopy is pivotal in patients with severe hemorrhage. A retrospective study demonstrated that delayed endoscopy was a risk factor for additional mortality. This lies in contrast to patients who have no evidence of hemodynamic compromise. There appears to be no significant differences in outcomes in endoscopies performed anytime within the continuum of the first 24 hours after presentation. The recent UK consensus guideline recommends immediate endoscopy after resuscitation in patients who are unstable and endoscopy within a period of 24 hours for all other bleeding. The decision regarding timing should be based on the severity of the hemorrhage, the patient's physiologic capacity, and the presence of comorbidities and nuanced by the availability of institutional resources and expertise.

Endoscopy is the mainstay of diagnosis and provides visual evidence of bleeding from esophageal or gastric varices. Attributable bleeding is denoted by the presence of active bleeding or stigmata of recent or remote bleeding (red wale markings, nipple sign, cherry red spots). An overlying clot and the presence of fresh blood without other identifiable causes also are considered highly suggestive of variceal bleeding. Strategies to improve endoscopic visualization, including enhanced suctioning and positional changes, may facilitate endoscopy and permit improved diagnosis and therapy.

Endoscopic Band Ligation

Endoscopic band ligation is the foundation of endoluminal treatment in esophageal variceal bleeding. In this technique the endoscope is coupled to a distal attachment that houses a multiband ligator. This distal attachment allows visualization and serves as the space to sequester portions of the varix and subsequently ligate them using an elastic band. The endoscope with the attached band applicator is advanced under direct vision to the distal-most portion of the offending varix or varices. Just above the gastroesophageal junction, the mucosa is thinnest, predisposing to bleeding but also permitting purchase of the varix by suction into the distal cap. While maintaining suction until the varix is captured completely within the cap, a band ligator is deployed by the endoscopist. Then this is repeated starting from the most distal esophagus and moving cephalad in a clockwise fashion until all high-risk varices have been eradicated. Immediate and sustained hemostasis is the main goal of endoscopy

in this setting. There are many band ligation devices available, and the endoscopist and his or her team should be familiar with setup and troubleshooting of all aspects of the locally available banding device.

The most logical approach to the management of acute variceal bleeding is to combine pharmacologic therapy with endoscopic therapy, as pooled analyses of available data demonstrate improved outcomes and lowered mortality with combination therapy versus endoscopic banding alone. Endoscopic banding is as effective as traditional sclerotherapy in achieving hemostasis in at least 95% of patients. However, it is more efficient, requiring 12% fewer sessions to achieve eradication, and is associated with fewer complications. Banding is the gold standard of endoscopic treatment, and other techniques largely are reserved for gastric varices or refractory cases of esophageal varices.

Endoscopic Sclerotherapy

Endoscopic injection techniques include traditional sclerotherapy and endoscopic venous obliteration using cyanoacrylate polymer. Endoscopic injection of sclerosing agents into or around a varix was the mainstay of endoscopic therapy but has been supplanted by variceal banding for the aforementioned reasons. Endoscopic venous obliteration and endoscopic injection of fibrin tissue sealants remain viable options in the management of gastric varices. Injection sclerotherapy should not be used routinely in the management of esophageal varices if endoscopic band ligation is available. Injection sclerotherapy should be used in cases where bleeding is refractory to endoscopic band ligation. Injection sclerotherapy usually is performed using a 23- or 25-gauge endoscopic needle. None of the various sclerosants in clinical use (including morrhuate sodium and ethanolamine) has demonstrated superior efficacy. Injection can be made into the varix (intravariceal) or between varices (paravariceal) without altering efficacy. Chest pain is seen in about 10% of patients after injection sclerotherapy and is not always caused by post-treatment ulceration. Esophageal strictures and other local extraesophageal serosities occur less frequently.

Self-Expanding Metal Stent Placement

The placement of a self-expanding metal stent as rescue therapy for refractory bleeding from esophageal varices has been emerging slowly since the development of fully covered removable esophageal stents. Ideally the stent placed under this circumstance should be removable and can be placed at the bedside without an absolute need for fluoroscopy. Placement of a stent in this situation potentially allows for hemostasis and optimization of a patient before other definitive therapies such as TIPS. Evidence from the use of these stents is mostly anecdotal from case series and expert opinion. The SX-ELLA Danis stent (Ella CS, Hradec Kralove, Czech Republic) is a removable, covered, self-expanding metal stent (SEMS) that has a bespoke design for treating esophageal varices; measuring 25 mm wide and 13.5 cm long, it very easily tamponades bleeding varices in the distal esophagus. This stent is not available in the United States, but at our institution we have placed similar sized stents endoscopically with good anecdotal results. The use of these stents continues to evolve, and they may emerge as an established modality for the treatment of endoscopically refractory acute bleeding from esophageal varices.

Gastric Varices

Gastric varices are discussed in this chapter to highlight how their treatment is similar to and different from the treatment of esophageal varices. Gastric varices are more challenging to treat because their clinical consequences can be more dramatic than those associated with esophageal varices. The optimal approach to gastric varices also depends on their anatomic classification and cause. Isolated gastric varices from splenic vein thrombosis should not be treated endoscopically. Gastroesophageal varices occurring in both the esophagus and the lesser curvature of the stomach, so-called GOV1, should be treated in the same manner as esophageal varices

Cyanoacrylate is a liquid agent that polymerizes rapidly on contact with blood. It has been utilized in the treatment of gastric varices. In the United States, cyanoacrylate is available as 2-octyl cyanoacrylate (Dermabond; Ethicon, Somerville, NJ) or *n*-butyl-2-cyanoacrylate (Histoacryl; Braun Medical, Bethlehem, PA). The technique is similar to injection sclerotherapy, but there are a few caveats. Fundal varices are best seen endoscopically in retroflexion, and the procedure often is performed using this approach. Precision in the "choreography" of injecting gastric varices is prudent to minimize complications and optimize outcomes. The patient should be well sedated to prevent movement around the time of injection. Typically 1 to 2 cc of cyanoacrylate is injected directly into the varix and then is followed by a 1-cc flush of sterile water. The needle is withdrawn from the varix in the same plane of entry. At our institution, care is taken not to withdraw the injection catheter back into the endoscope. A 1- to 1.5-cm length of catheter can be safely left outside the scope (needle retracted), thus minimizing the risk of glue damage to the endoscope. Repeat injections may be necessary in some cases, but the risk for embolization rises with increasing volumes of injection.

EUS-guided injection using a forward viewing or standard view linear scope also has been described. Anterograde injection in a transmural fashion is feasible when EUS guidance is used. Pre-injection of coils may confer the advantage of a platform for the cyanoacrylate to polymerize, thus reducing the risk of embolization.

Successful obliteration of the varix is confirmed by endoscopic assessment of the consistency of the varix or by endoscopic Doppler assessment.

Transient fevers, presumably secondary to bacteremia or pyrogens, can occur after endoscopic treatment of gastric varices. Other minor complications include self-limited chest and epigastric abdominal pain. Recurrent, usually delayed-onset bleeding may occur in a number of patients after ulceration at the injection site. Worsened hemorrhage during treatment can occur very rarely because of laceration or injury to a gastric varix in the setting of a poorly sedated patient. Embolization has been described in less than 1% of patients and is the most dreaded complication of cyanoacrylate injection. Endoscopy teams also are tasked with developing protocols and practices to avoid cyanoacrylate damage to endoscopes.

The use of detachable snares has been evaluated and is reportedly more effective than banding in the treatment of gastric varices but may confer no advantage over banding in the treatment of esophageal varices. Endoscopic topical treatment with the TC-325 nanopowder and a Turkish plant extract, Ankaferd BloodStopper, has been described. These agents have demonstrated early efficacy in the acute treatment of gastric variceal bleeding, and concerns about possible embolization in the setting of venous-based bleeding have not been observed; however, there are questions regarding its ability to achieve sustained hemostasis given its temporary luminal residency time of less than 24 hours. Therefore its use as a monotherapy in variceal upper gastrointestinal bleeding cannot be advocated at this time. Novel endoscopic Doppler probes have been developed and allow for objective auditory assessment of flow without the use of endoscopic ultrasound. Adequate hemostasis is denoted by the absence of flow through a treated vessel. Their use has not been evaluated systematically at present, so the incremental value in the routine treatment of gastrointestinal bleeding has not yet been clarified.

■ SUMMARY

Endoscopy is the cornerstone of managing bleeding from esophageal varices. It allows for diagnostic visualization, classification, treatment, and prognostication. Optimal outcomes result from coupling endoscopy with pharmacologic therapy in the treatment of variceal bleeding. Endoscopists and their teams must exhibit best practices in the management of esophageal varices. This requires proper training and communication among team members. Patient outcomes are optimized significantly by careful preprocedure and postprocedure management.

SUGGESTED READINGS

Bernard B, Grange JD, Khac EN, et al. Antibiotic prophylaxis for the prevention of bacterial infections in cirrhotic patients with gastrointestinal bleeding: a meta-analysis. *Hepatology*. 1999;29:1655-1661.

Bhat YM, Weilert F, Fredrick RT, et al. EUS-guided treatment of gastric fundal varices with combined injection of coils and cyanoacrylate glue: a large U.S. experience over 6 years (with video). *Gastrointest Endosc*. 2016;83:1164-1172.

Bhatia V. Endoscopic ultrasound (EUS) for esophageal and gastric varices: how can it improve the outcomes and reduce complications of glue injection. *J Clin Exp Hepatol*. 2012;2:70-74.

Castaneda B, Morales J, Lionetti R, et al. Effects of blood volume restitution following a portal hypertensive-related bleeding in anesthetized cirrhotic rats. *Hepatology*. 2001;33:821-825.

Chen PH, Hou MC, Lin HC, et al. Cyanoacrylate embolism from gastric varices may lead to esophageal variceal rupture. *Endoscopy*. 2011;43(suppl 2 UCTN):E149-E150.

Chen VK, Wong RC. Endoscopic Doppler ultrasound versus endoscopic stigmata-directed management of acute peptic ulcer hemorrhage: a multimodel cost analysis. *Dig Dis Sci*. 2007;52:149-160.

Chen YI, Barkun A, Nolan S. Hemostatic powder TC-325 in the management of upper and lower gastrointestinal bleeding: a two-year experience at a single institution. *Endoscopy*. 2015;47:167-171.

Cheung J, Soo I, Bastiampillai R, et al. Urgent vs. non-urgent endoscopy in stable acute variceal bleeding. *Am J Gastroenterol*. 2009;104:1125-1129.

Heresbach D, Jacquelinet C, Nouel O, et al. Sclerotherapy versus ligation in hemorrhage caused by rupture of esophageal varices: direct meta-analysis of randomized trials. *Gastroenterol Clin Biol*. 1995;19:914-920.

Hou MC, Lin HC, Liu TT, et al. Antibiotic prophylaxis after endoscopic therapy prevents rebleeding in acute variceal hemorrhage: a randomized trial. *Hepatology*. 2004;39:746-753.

Kuramochi A, Imazu H, Kakutani H, et al. Color Doppler endoscopic ultrasonography in identifying groups at a high-risk of recurrence of esophageal varices after endoscopic treatment. *J Gastroenterol*. 2007;42:219-224.

Martins Santos MM, Correia LP, Rodrigues RA, et al. Splenic artery embolization and infarction after cyanoacrylate injection for esophageal varices. *Gastrointest Endosc*. 2007;65:1088-1090.

Myers RP, Kaplan GG, Shaheen AM. The effect of weekend versus weekday admission on outcomes of esophageal variceal hemorrhage. *Can J Gastroenterol*. 2009;23:495-501.

Shim CS, Cho JY, Park YJ, et al. Mini-detachable snare ligation for the treatment of esophageal varices. *Gastrointest Endosc*. 1999;50:673-676.

Tripathi D, Stanley AJ, Hayes PC, et al. U.K. guidelines on the management of variceal haemorrhage in cirrhotic patients. *Gut*. 2015;64:1680-1704.

Villanueva C, Colomo A, Bosch A, et al. Transfusion strategies for acute upper gastrointestinal bleeding. *N Engl J Med*. 2013;368:11-21.

Zehetner J, Shamiyeh A, Wayand W, et al. Results of a new method to stop acute bleeding from esophageal varices: implantation of a self-expanding stent. *Surg Endosc*. 2008;22:2149-2152.

TRANSJUGULAR INTRAHEPATIC PORTOSYSTEMIC SHUNT

Arun Chockalingam, BS, Brian P. Holly, MD, and Kelvin Hong, MD

The creation of a transjugular intrahepatic portosystemic shunt (TIPS) was put forth as a possible treatment for the symptoms of portal hypertension in the early 1970s. Over the ensuing 2 decades, the work of many pioneers—including Rosch, Uchida, Colapinto, Palmaz, and others, many of whom lent their names to relevant apparatus—culminated in the introduction of TIPS to mainstream clinical practice.

TIPS can be a lifesaving procedure as well as one that alleviates severe symptoms related to portal hypertension. TIPS is also a durable solution with a long-term efficacy of 90%. It is, however, a double-edged sword, demanding meticulous technique and stringent patient selection to keep what was once a high morbidity and mortality at a minimum.

■ INDICATIONS

The list for causes of portal hypertension is long and is summarized in Box 1. Whatever the causative pathophysiology, TIPS can reduce or normalize the portal pressure and ameliorate the associated symptoms. As the technique for placing a TIPS became more refined and safer and the technology became more adapted to the specific physiology and anatomy of a portosystemic shunt, the indications for TIPS have expanded gradually. Box 2 outlines the indications and contraindications for TIPS.

Variceal Bleeding

Portal hypertension can cause varices along the entire gastrointestinal (GI) tract, including the small bowel and colon (hemorrhoids). Varices are more apt to bleed through the mucosa of the gastroesophageal junction, where the coronary vein is particularly disposed to dilatation. Varices are present in 30% of compensated cirrhotic patients and 60% of decompensated cirrhotic patients.

The primary treatment of bleeding gastroesophageal varices is medical management or endoscopic management. Even though endoscopic management is often successful, because of the progressive nature of chronic liver disease, recurrent bleeding should be expected in more than 50% of patients. Unlike medical or endoscopic management, shunting procedures such as TIPS address the underlying cause of variceal bleeding (portal hypertension). Portosystemic shunting is therefore the only definitive treatment for portal variceal bleeding. Meta-analysis of the literature has shown that TIPS has a lower rate of both variceal rebleeding and death due to rebleeding, with a strong trend toward increased survival (at the expense of increased hepatic encephalopathy). Most of the studies included in these meta-analyses predate the era of polytetrafluoroethylene (PTFE) covered TIPS stent-grafts, which have improved long-term patency over bare metal stents with a trend toward better overall survival. Head-to-head comparisons of TIPS created with stent-grafts and endoscopic and medical management is lacking.

Currently the primary indication for TIPS is to control portal variceal bleeding refractory to medical and endoscopic management. However, there is evidence from one randomized controlled study supporting the early use of TIPS in selected patients with advanced cirrhosis (Childs-Pugh classes B and C) and acute esophageal variceal bleeding. Additional studies are needed to confirm this finding before TIPS can be accepted as a first-line therapy for bleeding esophageal varices in patients with advanced liver disease.

Ascites

Ascites is the most common complication of cirrhosis. In addition to the severe limitations in lifestyle it creates, it poses a risk for bacterial peritonitis and other infections, renal failure, and increased mortality. No single cause for cirrhosis-related ascites has been identified. However, it is likely that a combination of causes, including decreased plasma albumin levels, increased bowel permeability, and cirrhosis-related hemodynamic changes (e.g., increased cardiac output, vasodilatation, increased plasma volume) factor together in the formation of ascites.

Initial management consists of sodium restriction and administration of loop diuretics and aldosterone antagonists. In advanced stages, ascites becomes refractory to medical management, and TIPS may be indicated. TIPS is very effective in eliminating ascites. Because the root causes are hemodynamic or hormone related, response to TIPS is not immediate. It may take 2 to 4 weeks after TIPS for ascites to resolve, during which time additional paracenteses may be necessary. Randomized controlled trials, meta-analyses, and systematic reviews of the literature have demonstrated that TIPS significantly improves transplant-free survival compared with repeated paracentesis.

Hepatic Hydrothorax

Hepatic hydrothorax is defined as the accumulation of at least 500 mL of pleural fluid in a patient with cirrhosis without cardiopulmonary disease. Even though this definition is not 100% specific to hepatic hydrothorax, additional signs, such as isolated right-sided hydrothorax and concurrent ascites, help to confirm the diagnosis. It occurs in less than 10% of patients with cirrhosis, as peritoneal fluid permeates via small diaphragmatic communications. Again, initial management is sodium restriction and diuretics. In nonresponsive patients, TIPS will eliminate hydrothorax in most and decrease the frequency of thoracentesis in the rest.

Hepatorenal Syndrome

Hepatorenal syndrome (HRS) portends a poor prognosis for the cirrhotic patient, as it occurs during the late stages of the hemodynamic changes related to cirrhosis. Alterations in vasoactive hormones responding to these hemodynamic changes result in splanchnic vasodilation, renal arterial vasoconstriction, and the opening of small intrarenal arteriovenous communications. The end result is renal hypoperfusion and ensuing renal failure.

Two distinct forms of HRS have been identified: *type 1 HRS,* which progresses rapidly, and *type 2 HRS,* which evolves slowly. Type 1 HRS is precipitated by an event that incites acute-on-chronic liver failure, an exaggerated systemic inflammatory response, and kidney dysfunction as part of broader multiorgan failure. Targeting the precipitating event is the hallmark of treatment for type 1 HRS. Type 2 HRS results in large part from a reduction in effective arterial blood volume created by a shift of fluid from the intravascular compartment to the extravascular compartment (i.e., ascites). Noncontrolled studies suggest that using TIPS to reduce the production of ascites may improve renal function in type 2 HRS. However, the use of TIPS in HRS should be undertaken after serious consideration because of the contrast load and acute hemodynamic changes it involves.

Hepatopulmonary Syndrome

Hepatopulmonary syndrome is the presence of intrapulmonary vasodilatation and multiple small, right-to-left shunts that result in

BOX 1: Causes of Portal Hypertension

Presinusoidal

Portal, splenic, or superior mesenteric vein thrombosis
Idiopathic portal hypertension
Mass effect (i.e., tumor)
Schistosomiasis
Precirrhotic stage, primary biliary cirrhosis
Alcoholic central sclerosis
Endothelitis (liver rejection, radiation injury)
Arterioportovenous fistula (traumatic or Osler-Weber-Rendu)
Hyperdynamic splenomegaly (infectious or myelodysplastic)
Nodular regenerative hyperplasia
Congenital extrahepatic portal vein occlusion

Perisinusoidal

Cirrhosis
Congenital hepatic fibrosis
Cystic liver disease
Sarcoidosis

Postsinusoidal

Budd-Chiari syndrome
Veno-occlusive disease (sinusoidal obstruction syndrome)
Chronic passive congestion (nutmeg liver)
Mass effect (i.e., tumor)

BOX 2: Indications and Contraindications for Transjugular Intrahepatic Portosystemic Shunt

Indications

Standard of Care

Portal variceal hemorrhage refractory to medical or endoscopic management
Ascites refractory to medical management
Budd-Chiari syndrome not responsive to anticoagulation
Hepatic hydrothorax refractory to diuretics and salt restriction

Emerging Indications

SUPPORTED BY CONTROLLED STUDIES
"Cirrhotic" portal vein thrombosis caused by slow blood flow in the portal vein
Childs-Pugh classes B and C with acute esophageal variceal bleeding (simultaneously treated with medical or endoscopic interventions)

SUPPORTED BY NONCONTROLLED STUDIES AND CASE SERIES
Hepatorenal syndrome (more so type 1 than type 2)
Hepatopulmonary syndrome
Portal gastropathy refractory to beta-blockers
Hepatic veno-occlusive disease

Contraindications

Absolute

Severely elevated right heart pressure
Severe tricuspid regurgitation
Severe pulmonary hypertension
Severe congestive heart failure
Severe encephalopathy
Uncorrectable bleeding diathesis
Active systemic or hepatic bacterial infection
Unrelieved biliary obstruction

Relative

Hepatic vein thrombosis
"Noncirrhotic" portal vein thrombosis caused by hypercoagulability or tumor thrombus
Poor liver function reserve
Polycystic liver disease
Central liver mass
Gastric antral variceal ectasia

impaired gas exchange. Because of the lack of data, TIPS cannot be recommended as a standard treatment for hepatopulmonary syndrome. In selected cases, however, especially in severely compromised patients who are on the liver transplant list, TIPS may prove to be a lifesaving bridge to surgery.

Budd-Chiari Syndrome

Budd-Chiari syndrome is caused by mechanical obstruction of the hepatic venous outflow and gradually results in cirrhosis and portal hypertension. Excluding the hepatic venous web, which can be treated successfully with simple balloon angioplasty, treatment for the fulminant form of Budd-Chiari syndrome is liver transplantation, although anticoagulation may help to stave off disease progression. TIPS has proven to be a valuable tool to bridge such patients to transplantation.

In the nonfulminant form of Budd-Chiari syndrome, anticoagulation is first-line therapy. When anticoagulation fails, TIPS is a reasonable and accepted next step, as is direct intrahepatic portosystemic shunt (DIPS) if access to the hepatic veins is occluded completely (Figure 1). The use of TIPS in this patient population was examined in a large retrospective study that showed 1-year and 10-year transplant-free survival much greater than expected. The American Association for the Study of Liver Diseases (AASLD) now recommends creation of a TIPS in patients with Budd-Chiari syndrome who fail to improve with anticoagulation.

Portal Hypertensive Gastropathy

Portal hypertensive gastropathy (to be distinguished from vascular ectasia) is the diffuse dilatation of gastric veins that, along with the inflamed and fragile mucosa of the stomach, predispose the patient to bleeding. TIPS, which normalizes the portal pressure, and mucosal protection (i.e., avoiding nonsteroidal anti-inflammatory drugs and alcohol) combine to minimize this risk. These types of lesions rarely induce bleeding, but TIPS has been shown to control bleeding in patients with portal hypertensive gastropathy.

▪ TECHNIQUE

Patient Preparation

Many of the complications related to the placement of TIPS can be avoided by proper patient workup. Review of pertinent cross-sectional imaging confirms a patent (nonthrombosed) portal vein and reveals the relative orientation of the hepatic and portal veins. This minimizes the number of attempts to engage the portal vein and therefore minimizes the associated risk for bleeding. Good hydration minimizes the risk of acute renal failure, and initiation of metronidazole (Flagyl) or lactulose mitigates the risk of encephalopathy. Type and crossmatching of blood may prove lifesaving if a bleeding complication is encountered. Finally, all involved should be cognizant of related risks, especially the 30-day mortality, which ranges from less than 5% for elective procedures in well-compensated patients to 50% for emergent procedures in unstable patients with advanced liver disease.

Access

Access through the right internal jugular vein is preferred, although the left internal jugular vein also can be used. Access is maintained

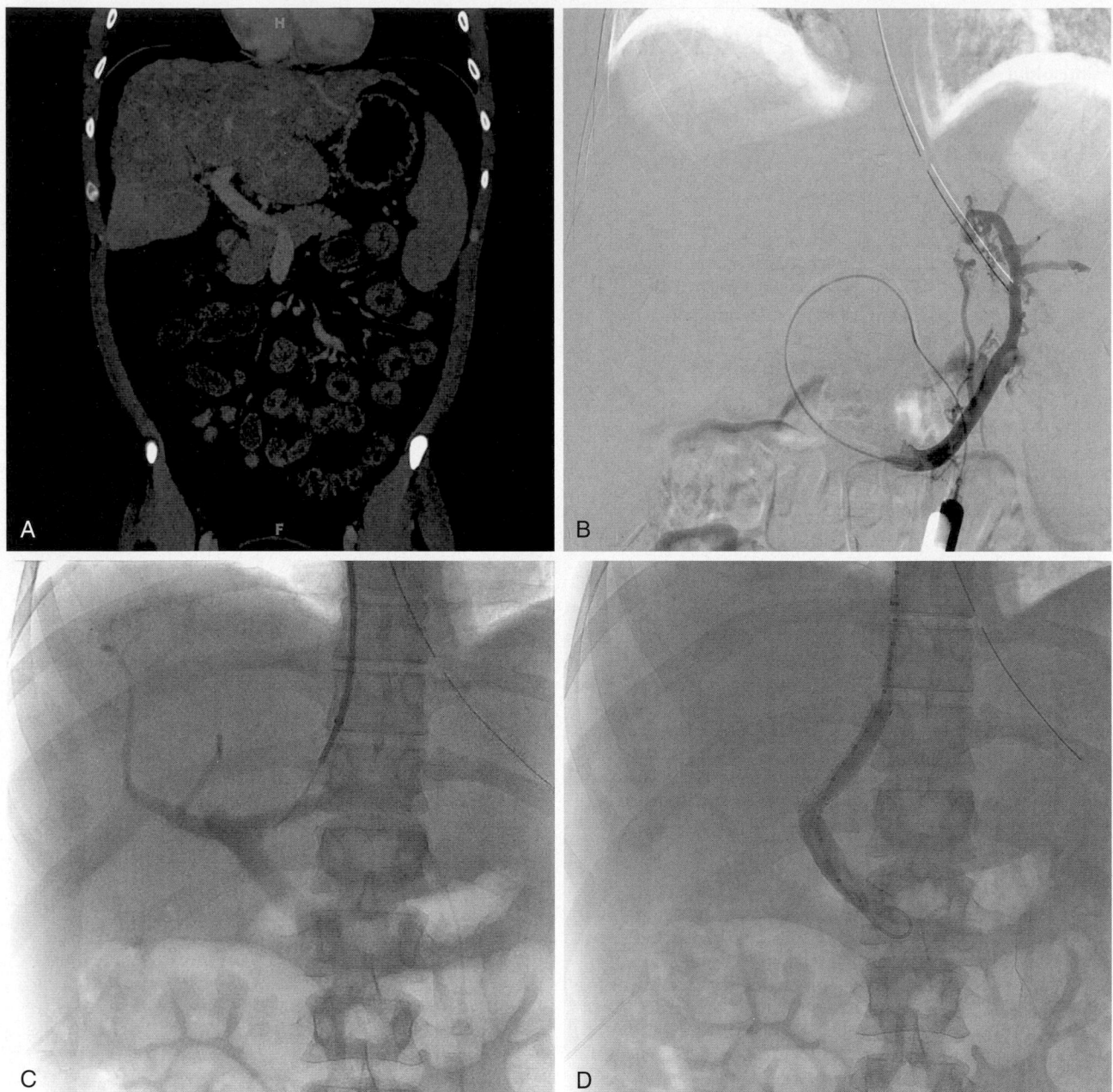

FIGURE 1 Direct intrahepatic portosystemic shunt (DIPS). **A,** Coronal reformatted computed tomographic scan pre-DIPS of Budd-Chiari syndrome. **B,** Direct transhepatic left hepatic venogram showing Budd-Chiari syndrome. **C,** Direct transhepatic left portal vein access with hepatofugal flow and portal hypertension and gastric varices. **D,** Direct DIPS needle throw from intrahepatic inferior vena cava and portal venogram.

with a long, large vascular sheath parked in the intrahepatic inferior vena cava to allow multiple catheter-wire exchanges without recrossing the right atrium (Figure 2).

Diagnostic Assessment

Optimizing the TIPS outcomes requires not only anatomic assessment but also functional assessment of the patient's hemodynamic status. One of the contraindications to TIPS is elevated right heart pressure. Ensuring that the right atrial pressure is not elevated severely is mandatory before shunting the portal venous blood to an already overburdened right heart. Right atrial pressures below 15 mm Hg are generally safe, whereas pressures above 20 mm Hg predispose the patient to acute right heart failure. There are no

specific guidelines, and sound clinical judgment is important. For example, a right atrial pressure of 16 mm Hg should not preclude creation of a TIPS in an unstable patient with ongoing variceal bleeding.

After selecting the right hepatic vein, free and wedged hepatic venous pressures are measured and usually confirm portal hypertension. Normal corrected pressures should not necessarily terminate the procedure, as these are not accurate in general and are wholly inaccurate in cases of presinusoidal portal hypertension.

Delineation of the portal venous system is accomplished by injection of carbon dioxide (CO_2) via a catheter wedged into the hepatic vein. CO_2 is not nephrotoxic and can be given in virtually unlimited quantity. Frontal and lateral views show the anatomic relationships, so that the right portal vein can be targeted for access (Figure 3).

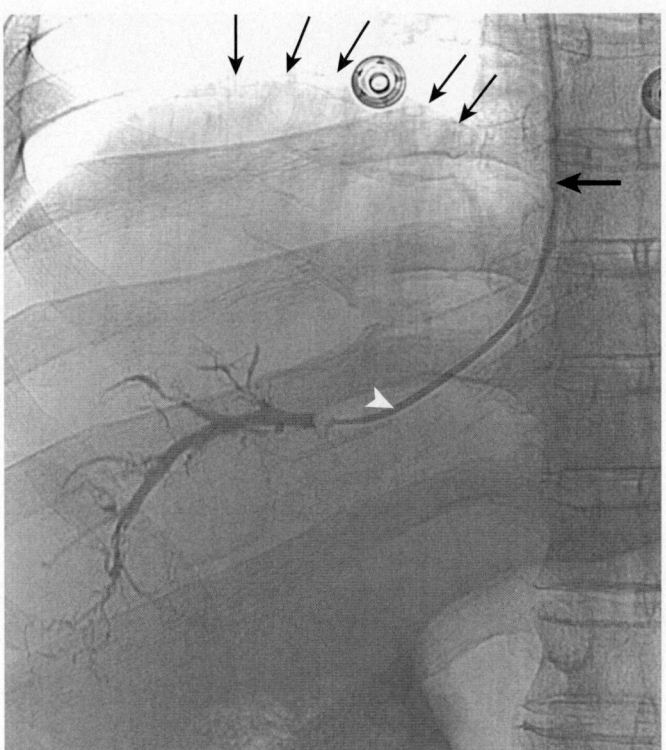

FIGURE 2 Right hepatic venogram performed via a selective catheter (*arrowhead*). The tip of the internal jugular sheath (*heavy black arrow*) is below the diaphragm (*black arrows*) to avoid catheter-wire manipulations in the right atrium. The steps of transjugular intrahepatic portosystemic shunt insertion shown in Figures 2 to 10 are all from the same patient.

In the vast majority of patients, the TIPS is placed from the right hepatic vein into the right portal vein because this is the shortest and most direct path for shunt creation. However, a recent randomized controlled trial found that using the left portal vein resulted in a significant reduction in the incidence of encephalopathy and rehospitalization during 2 years of follow-up after TIPS creation. These data must be confirmed in additional studies before the standard approach of targeting the right portal vein is abandoned.

Shunt Placement

The next step is the cannulation of the right portal vein from the right hepatic vein. To accomplish this, a curved metallic sheath is advanced via the existing right internal jugular sheath in the right hepatic vein. The new catheter is rotated based on the anatomy revealed during CO_2 portography, so that it targets the right portal vein. When the operator judges the curved sheath to be directed toward the right portal vein, a long needle is advanced toward it. Aspiration of blood suggests intravascular location, and contrast injection confirms that the tip is in the portal vein (Figure 4).

Once it is confirmed that the tip of the needle is in the right portal vein, a wire is passed distally through the main portal vein into the superior mesenteric vein or splenic vein for security (Figure 5). The traversed liver parenchyma is fibrotic and difficult to cross unless predilated. A small caliber (4- to 6-mm diameter) balloon is used to predilate the liver parenchyma between the right hepatic and right portal vein now crossed by the wire (Figure 6). A marking catheter then is passed over the wire into the portal venous system. This allows for direct portal pressure measurement and a portal venogram. The venogram will be used to select the appropriate length stent to be placed (Figure 7).

If the direct portal pressure is within normal limits, TIPS creation is abandoned irrespective of the clinical picture. If a TIPS is not

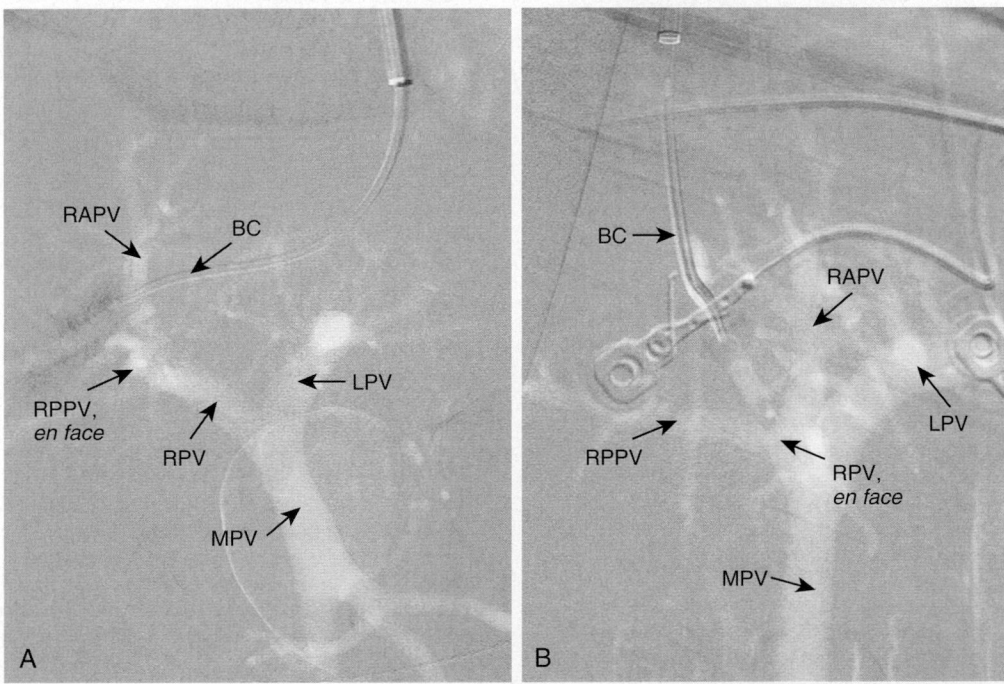

FIGURE 3 Frontal (**A**) and lateral (**B**) digital subtraction views of a carbon dioxide (CO_2) hepatic venogram. CO_2 is injected via a balloon occlusion catheter to force the CO_2 retrogradely into the portal system. The right portal vein and its first-order branches, the left portal vein, and the main portal vein are visualized easily. In the lateral view, the right portal vein is seen nearly en face. The operator usually targets the right portal vein from the right hepatic vein with a long needle introduced via the right internal jugular sheath. *BC*, Balloon occlusion catheter; *LPV*, left portal vein; *MPV*, main portal vein; *RAPV*, right anterior portal vein; *RPPV*, right posterior portal vein; *RPV*, right portal vein.

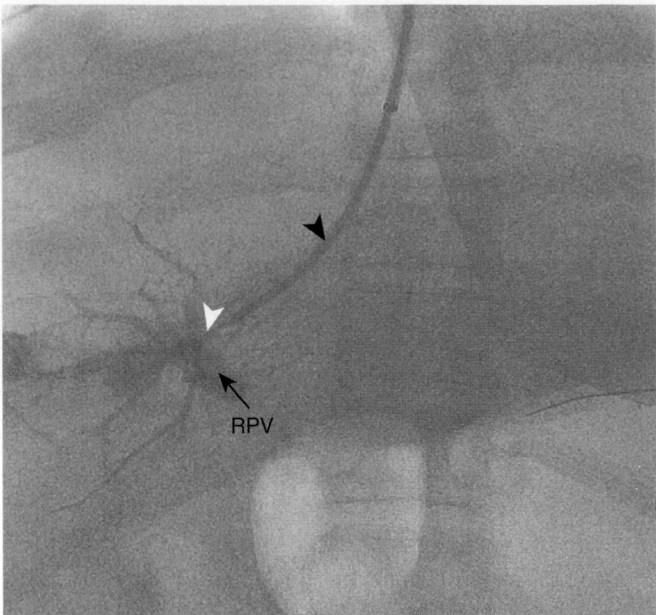

FIGURE 4 Frontal unsubtracted venogram via a needle (*white arrowhead*) after it was advanced from the right hepatic vein through a catheter (*black arrowhead*) toward the right portal vein (RPV). Contrast fills the branches of the right portal vein with hepatopetal blood flow.

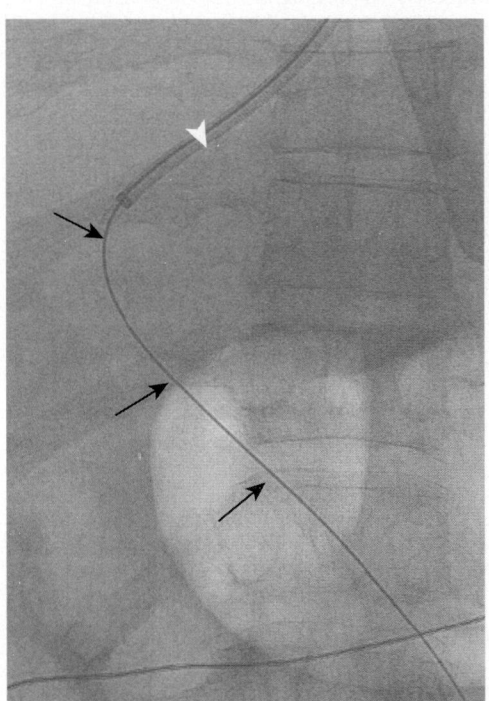

FIGURE 5 After the needle is confirmed to be in the targeted portal vein branch, a wire is advanced through it into the portal vein (*black arrows*). Note the location of the right internal jugular sheath (*arrowhead*). The wire now crosses from the right hepatic vein through a short segment of liver parenchyma and into the right portal vein.

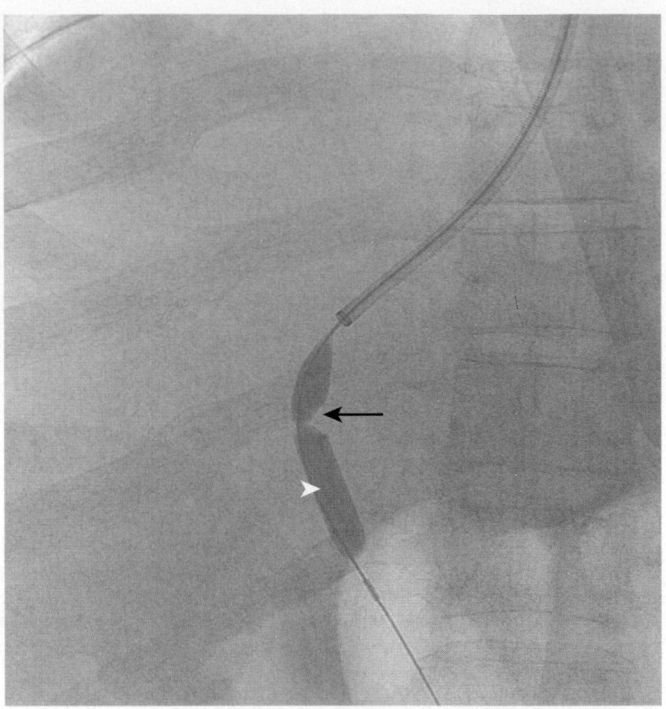

FIGURE 6 Because cirrhotic liver is difficult to cross, it is predilated with a small balloon (*arrowhead*) to facilitate the necessary sheath exchanges. The "waist" (*arrow*) in the middle of the balloon reveals just how hard the liver parenchyma can be.

possible or is contraindicated, the gastroesophageal varices can be embolized via a catheter to stop the hemorrhage without placing a TIPS. Although this is very effective, it is temporary; the ongoing portal hypertension likely will cause new varices to form.

The stent is advanced through the larger sheath, which keeps it constrained and in position. The sheath is pulled back into the right atrium, uncovering the stent. The distal 2 cm of the stent are uncovered and flare out on withdrawal of the sheath. The rest of the stent is "ripcorded" open once it is in the appropriate position (Figure 8).

Shunt Evaluation

Usually a 10-mm diameter stent is used, and initially it is balloon-dilated up to 8 mm in diameter. The direct portal pressure is measured again; if it is not satisfactory, a 10-mm balloon is used to open the stent to capacity (Figure 9). The smaller the stent diameter, the less chance of encephalopathy postprocedure. A final portal venogram is performed to document flow and lack of variceal filling (Figure 10).

■ SPECIAL CASES

Budd-Chiari Syndrome

The creation of a TIPS in a patient with Budd-Chiari syndrome is especially challenging because the hepatic veins are thrombosed. This appears as the classic spider vein appearance on a hepatic venogram (Figure 11). Although it is best if the TIPS is placed from hepatic vein to portal vein, the lack of patent hepatic veins may necessitate an inferior vena cava to portal vein TIPS through the caudate lobe, a so-called DIPS (see Figure 1).

Parallel Transjugular Intrahepatic Portosystemic Shunt

Rarely, despite a previous TIPS, the patient's symptoms may not be alleviated completely. If portal hypertension and variceal bleeding are

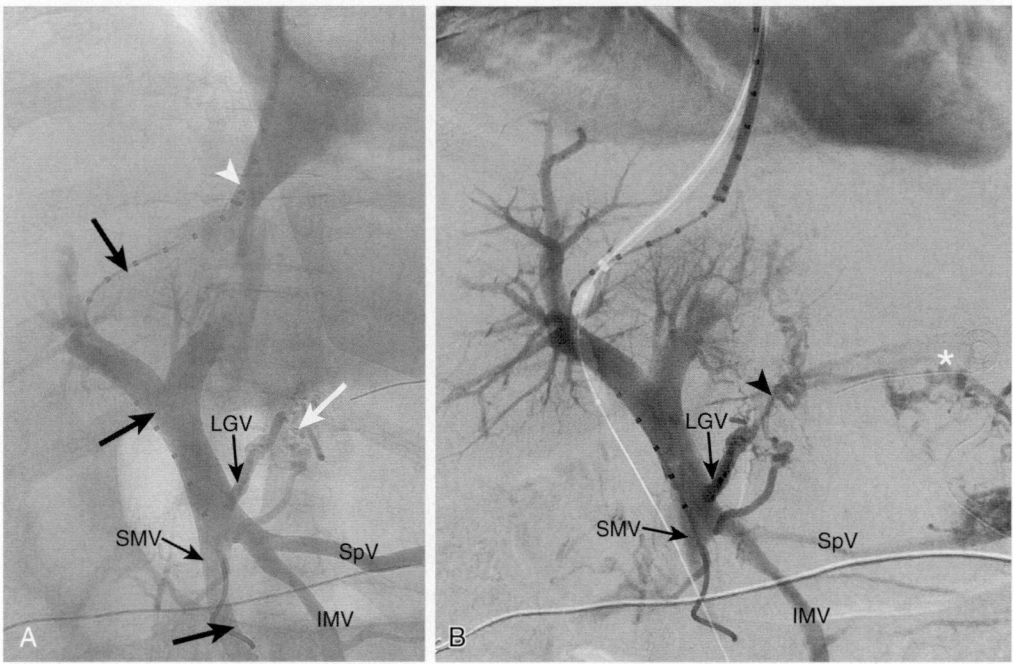

FIGURE 7 Frontal unsubtracted (**A**) and subtracted (**B**) venograms. **A,** Simultaneous contrast injection via the right internal jugular sheath (*arrowhead*) and marker catheter (*black arrows*) in the portal vein allows for calculation of the required length of the stent. Note the esophageal varices (*white arrow*) arising from the left gastric vein. **B,** A wider field of view with digital subtraction shows to greater effect the ominous esophageal (*arrowhead*) and gastric (*asterisk*) varices. *IMV,* Inferior mesenteric vein; *LGV,* left gastric vein; *SMV,* superior mesenteric vein; *SpV,* splenic vein.

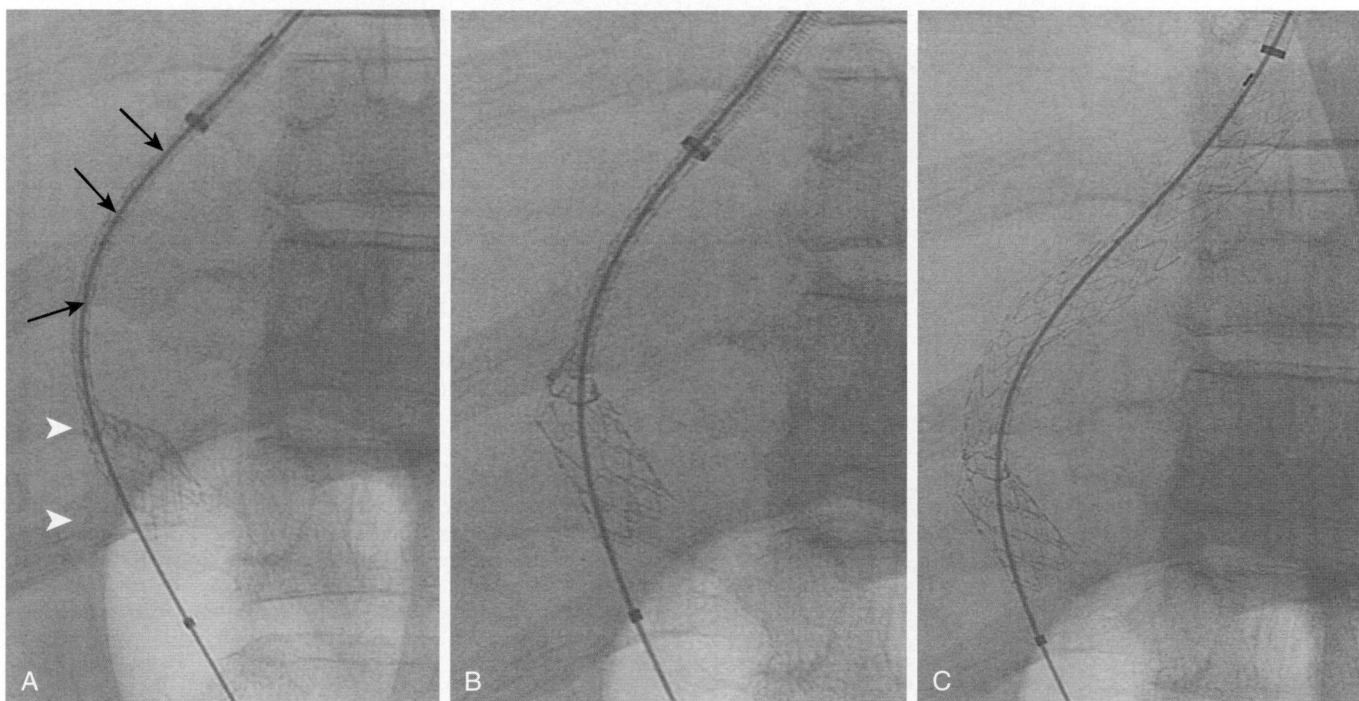

FIGURE 8 Frontal views of the deployment sequence of a transjugular intrahepatic portosystemic shunt stent. First, the stent is advanced via a sheath through the right hepatic vein, across the liver parenchyma, and into the portal vein. **A,** The stent's distal 2 cm (*arrowheads*) are constrained only by the sheath, and once the sheath is pulled back it springs open. The remainder of the stent (*arrows*) remains undeployed. **B,** The entire system then is withdrawn gently until the proximal end of the distal 2 cm hits the parenchymal tract. **C,** Once the operator judges the stent to be in proper position, the remainder of the stent is opened by pulling on the ripcord.

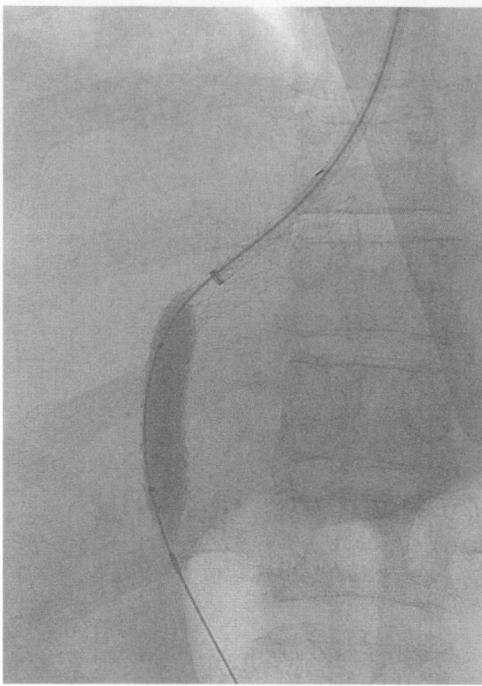

FIGURE 9 After transjugular intrahepatic portosystemic shunt placement a balloon is used to open the stent to the desired diameter. The objective is to open the stent to the minimum diameter required to reduce the portal pressure to the desired level.

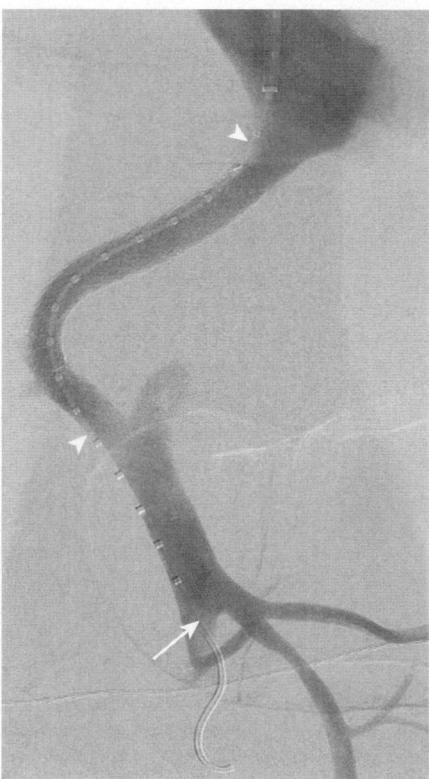

FIGURE 10 Frontal view of a portal venogram via a catheter (*arrow*) after transjugular intrahepatic portosystemic shunt placement (*arrowheads*). Note the antegrade flow of contrast into the right atrium and no contrast filling the varices. Compare with Figure 7.

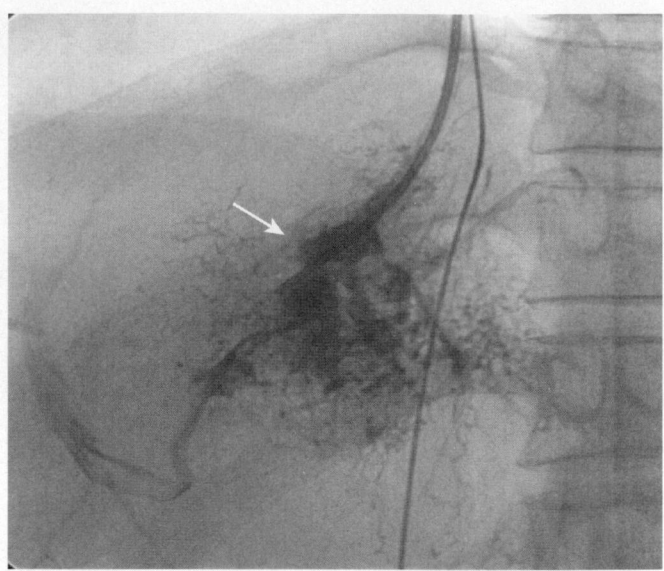

FIGURE 11 Frontal subtracted hepatic venogram in a patient with Budd-Chiari syndrome. Hepatic venogram shows the "spiderlike" appearance (*arrow*) of multiple small collateral draining veins.

a persistent problem despite a TIPS or if the first TIPS thromboses, a second TIPS may be placed utilizing the other hepatic and portal veins (Figure 12).

Transumbilical or Direct Portal Access

When access into the portal vein is challenging because of anatomy, the operator has two other options. First, access into the umbilical vein, which usually is dilated, provides a conduit into the left portal vein. A catheter there allows opacification of the portal venous system, which provides a better target for TIPS (Figure 13). Second, access through a naturally occurring portosystemic shunt, such as a splenorenal shunt, sometimes can be used to gain access to the portal circulation. When the umbilical vein is not accessible and a natural portosystemic shunt does not exist, direct percutaneous access into the right or left portal vein can allow for contrast opacification and targeting (Figure 14).

Reversal or Revision of Transjugular Intrahepatic Portosystemic Shunt

Occasionally a TIPS reversal or revision is necessary. Limited liver reserve or overzealous shunting may result in liver failure or intractable encephalopathy. In such cases the interventionalist has the option to decrease the shunting or shut down the TIPS altogether. Several maneuvers exist to reduce shunting, including placing a stent within the TIPS, two stents side by side, or even a "waisted" (hourglass-like) stent. If these interventions are not possible or are inadequate, the entire TIPS can be shut down. TIPS shutdown is a rarely performed and advanced procedure.

Direct Intrahepatic Portosystemic Shunt

DIPS is a recently developed modification to the TIPS procedure. Using intravascular ultrasound guidance, DIPS has been shown to decrease radiation dose and procedural time compared with TIPS. DIPS uses the caudate lobe as a parenchymal tract to create a side-to-side portocaval shunt, which removes the possibility of hepatic vein stenosis. Portal access is accomplished by advancing a 21-gauge trocar needle through the caudate lobe into the main portal vein. After the inner trocar is removed, a guidewire (0.018 in) can be

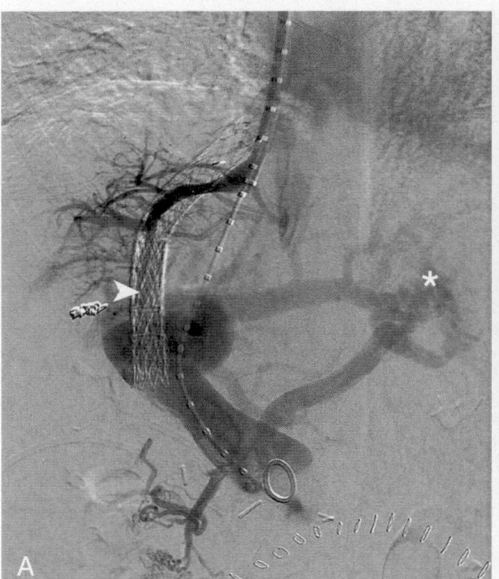
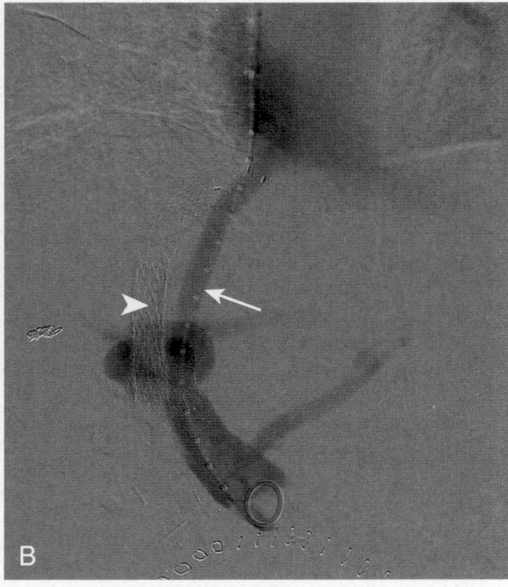

FIGURE 12 A, Frontal subtracted portal venogram via a catheter placed through the middle hepatic vein shows that the previously placed right hepatic to right portal vein transjugular intrahepatic portosystemic shunt (TIPS) (*arrowhead*) is occluded. Because of this, the patient had recurrent bleeding from gastric varices (*asterisk*). **B,** Repeat portal venogram after placement of a parallel TIPS (*arrow*) shows antegrade flow into the right atrium and decompression of the varices.

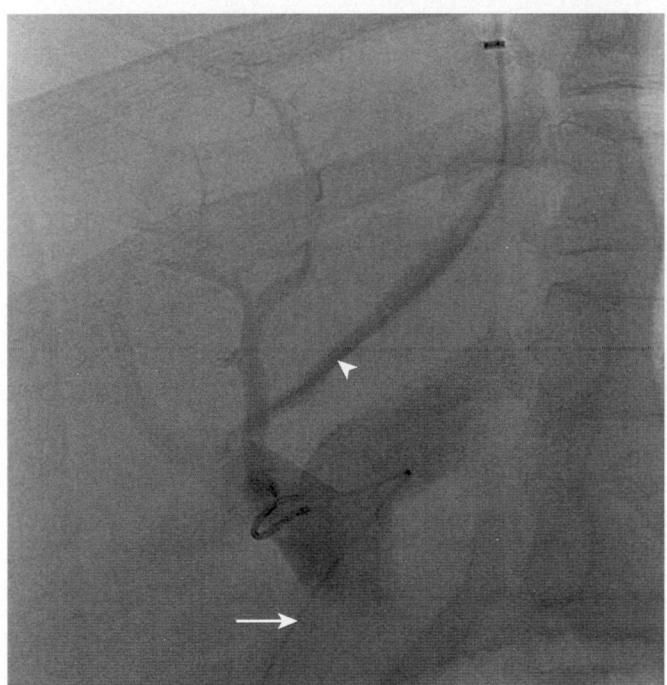

FIGURE 13 Superficially accessible portosystemic collateral vessels can be used to access and opacify the portal venous system for targeting before needle advancement. Here, a percutaneously placed transumbilical vein (*arrow*) opacifies the portal branches. A catheter (*arrowhead*) is seen traversing the parenchymal tract between the right hepatic vein and right portal vein.

advanced, followed by a 5F (5F Rösch Uchida) catheter. The needle and guidewire then can be removed, after which a 0.035-in guidewire (e.g., Amplatz) can be advanced into the portal vein. After portal vein access, a shunt can be created using a PTFE covered stent-graft. During the first ever DIPS procedure, the stent used was homemade, as there were no devices available to deploy. Over the last few years, the DIPS technique has been improved with creation of stent-graft devices (e.g., Viatorr; W.L. Gore & Associates, Flagstaff, AZ). Reported total procedure time for DIPS is less than 1 hour. In recent studies DIPS creation usually was successful in entire patient cohorts and has produced higher patency and real-time imaging compared with TIPS. In some interventional radiology practices, DIPS has replaced TIPS as a default procedure, especially in patients with occluded TIPS, challenging anatomy, calcification of the portal vein, or portal vein thrombosis due to hepatocellular carcinoma.

Transjugular Intrahepatic Portosystemic Shunt in Transplanted Livers

TIPS has been used to bridge liver transplants in patients in end-stage liver disease (ESLD). Before transplantation, TIPS is used to manage complications for portal hypertension and ensure that patients can remain transplant candidates. After transplantation, TIPS has a similar utility, in that post-transplant complications can cause recurrent disease. For this reason, indications for TIPS in transplanted livers are the same as those for patients pretransplantation. Studies have shown TIPS to be effective in addressing early complications such as portal vein thrombosis and delayed graft function. At first TIPS was more complex in patients with liver transplants because of the altered anatomy of hepatic vessels. The piggyback technique to TIPS has been effective in addressing this challenge. In this technique TIPS placement is done in the left internal jugular vein rather than in the right.

Fewer shunt stenoses and procedural complications have been recorded in post-transplant patients compared with pretransplant patients. Approximately 10% to 20% of stents in patients with transplants require revision, whereas up to 70% do in patients without transplants. However, patients with transplants who undergo TIPS have higher risks of infection, renal failure, and neurologic complications than patients without transplants. For example, 20% to 50% of cases result in death by sepsis, the most common post-transplant TIPS complication. Clinical success rate of TIPS in patients without transplants is much higher than in patients with transplants (93% vs 77%).

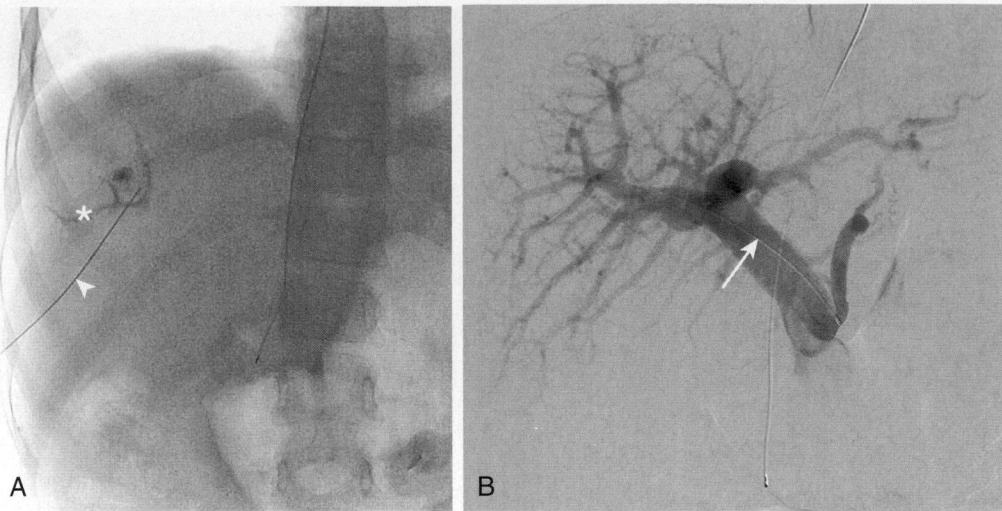

FIGURE 14 A, In cases where no other option is available, direct percutaneous portal vein access can be useful. A needle (*arrowhead*) is placed under ultrasound guidance into the portal venous system, which is then opacified with contrast (*asterisk*). **B,** A catheter (*arrow*) is advanced into the main portal vein where a portal venogram is performed and targeted for transjugular intrahepatic portosystemic shunt from the right hepatic vein.

TABLE I: Complications Related to Transjugular Intrahepatic Portosystemic Shunt (TIPS)

Complication	Frequency	Predisposing Factors	Mitigating Factors
TIPS dysfunction	Occlusion or stenosis: 18%-78% Thrombosis: 10%-15%	Uncovered stents Smaller diameter stents Stent migration or suboptimal placement	Choice of stent Precise deployment Venoplasty or restenting
Encephalopathy	In compensated liver disease: up to 12% In uncompensated liver disease: up to 50% Requiring TIPS reversal: 4%	History of encephalopathy High ammonia levels Limited reserve Increased age	Reduce or close the TIPS Metronidazole or lactulose
Bleeding	Hemobilia: <5% Intraperitoneal bleeding: 1%-2%	Difficult anatomy Abnormal coagulation profile	Correct coagulation profile
Sepsis	2%-10%	Active infection	Treat infection before TIPS
Renal failure	Highly variable	Elevated creatinine Dehydration Diabetes High contrast load	Hydrate Use carbon dioxide contrast
Liver failure or hepatic infarction	2%-4%	Limited reserve High bilirubin Overshunting	Reduce or close the TIPS

■ CLINICAL OUTCOMES

Clinical Response to Transjugular Intrahepatic Portosystemic Shunt

TIPS is the most effective option for treating gastroesophageal variceal bleeding. The rebleeding rate after TIPS placement is 4% per year, the lowest among all treatment options, including endoscopic management. TIPS is reserved for use after failure of endoscopic management only because of the greater risks associated with it, particularly encephalopathy. Cessation of bleeding is evident almost immediately after TIPS creation.

TIPS also has been shown to be very effective in treating ascites, and it reduces the risk of ascites by 50% to 80% over the life of the patient. In addition, TIPS has been shown to improve survival and transplant-free survival compared with other treatment options. Resolution of ascites may take up to 4 weeks after TIPS placement.

In patients with hepatorenal syndrome, TIPS improves renal function in 62% of patients. However, it is occasionally difficult to distinguish noncirrhotic-related chronic renal insufficiency from hepatorenal syndrome.

Complications and Management

The complications related to TIPS are shown in Table 1. The most feared complication is liver failure, which usually results from excessive portohepatic venous shunting in a liver with limited baseline reserve. If patients with no liver reserve are excluded appropriately, the risk of liver failure is 2% to 4%.

Encephalopathy can be seen in up to 12% of patients with compensated liver disease and in up to 50% of patients with noncompensated liver disease. Flagyl and lactulose provide significant relief for such patients, but a small percentage (~4%) will not respond and may require TIPS reversal.

Death from sepsis is rare (~4%). Bacteremia results in TIPS stent seeding ("endotipsitis"), which can be very challenging or impossible to treat. Broad-spectrum antibiotics may clear the bacteremia, but in some cases it recurs after cessation of treatment, as the seeded stent elutes more bacteria. Active infection is an absolute contraindication to TIPS, and any infection must be cleared before intervention.

The overall post-TIPS 30-day mortality ranges from less than 10% to 40%. Higher mortality rates are seen in patients with poorly compensated liver disease who are having a TIPS created on an emergent basis, usually for life-threatening variceal bleeding. For patients with compensated liver disease who are having a TIPS created on an elective basis, mortality is less than 5%. It is therefore important to carefully select patients and refer for TIPS placement before it manifests into an emergency. Vasoactive drug therapy has been shown to reduce the risk for mortality at 7 days, in addition to improving hemostasis and shortening length of stay.

The MELD (Model for End-Stage Liver Disease) score, routinely used to predict survival in patients with ESLD and allocate liver transplants, initially was developed to predict poor survival in patients after creation of a TIPS. The cut-off score for high-risk short-term mortality (expected survival less than 3 months after TIPS creation) in the initial MELD study was 18. The MELDNa score, which incorporates serum sodium (Na) with the serum international normalized ratio (INR), bilirubin, and creatinine of MELD, has been shown to be a more accurate predictor or risk post-TIPS (MELDNa ≥15). Both versions of the MELD score are more accurate predictors of risk after TIPS than the Child-Pugh score.

Follow-up

TIPS follow-up is based mostly on clinical signs and symptoms. Ultrasound surveillance can be useful. However, false-positive reports (of occluded stent) can result if ultrasound is performed too soon after TIPS creation. The newly placed TIPS has air trapped within it, which limits ultrasound penetration and can simulate the sonographic appearance of an occluded TIPS. Waiting at least 2 weeks after TIPS for the air to be absorbed is generally adequate to avoid this problem. Recurrent variceal bleeding or ascites is a very specific indicator of TIPS restenosis or occlusion and should prompt a diagnostic venogram or intervention. There is a 10% rate of reintervention for stenosed or occluded TIPS. The 1-year primary unassisted patency rate for expanded polytetrafluoroethylene (ePTFE) covered stents is 80% to 85%. There is no role for the use of uncovered bare metal stents, as their restenosis rate after TIPS creation is unjustifiably high.

■ SUMMARY

The most important determinant of clinical outcomes after TIPS placement is proper patient selection and preparation. Cirrhotic patients with portal hypertension should be under surveillance and should be referred for TIPS after conservative management fails but before the complications of portal hypertension manifest into an emergency. This, along with optimal patient preparation, can help to reduce the morbidity and mortality related to TIPS to the lowest possible levels. In addition, the introduction of ePTFE stents has improved the efficacy and patency rate of TIPS, and many patients survive for many years with a TIPS. The benefits of a TIPS include reduced drop-off risk from the transplant list, improved lifestyle quality (i.e., resolution of ascites), and reduction of the many portal hypertension–related complications. Most important, TIPS often is a lifesaving procedure for those with variceal hemorrhage.

SUGGESTED READINGS

Abraldes JG, Tandon P. Therapies: drugs, scopes and transjugular intrahepatic portosystemic shunt—when and how? *Dig Dis.* 2015;33:524-533.

Bai M, Qi X, Yang Z, et al. Predictors of hepatic encephalopathy after transjugular intrahepatic portosystemic shunt in cirrhotic patients: a systematic review. *J Gastroenterol Hepatol.* 2011;26:943-951.

Bonnel AR, Bunchorntavakul C, Reddy KR. Transjugular intrahepatic portosystemic shunts in liver transplant recipients. *Liver Transpl.* 2013;20:130-139.

Charon JP, Alaeddin FH, Pimpalwar SA, et al. Results of a retrospective multicenter trial of the Viatorr expanded polytetrafluoroethylene-covered stent-graft for transjugular intrahepatic portosystemic shunt creation. *J Vasc Interv Radiol.* 2004;15:1219-1230.

Chen L, Xiao T, Chen W, et al. Outcomes of transjugular intrahepatic portosystemic shunt through the left branch vs. the right branch of the portal vein in advanced cirrhosis: a randomized trial. *Liver Int.* 2009;29:1101-1109.

Eesa M, Clark T. Transjugular intrahepatic portosystemic shunt: state of the art. *Semin Roentgenol.* 2011;46:125-132.

García-Pagán JC, Caca K, Bureau C, Laleman W, et al. Early use of TIPS in patients with cirrhosis and variceal bleeding. *N Engl J Med.* 2010;362:2370-2379.

Guy J, Somsouk M, Shiboski S, et al. New model for end stage liver disease improves prognostic capability after transjugular intrahepatic portosystemic shunt. *Clin Gastroenterol Hepatol.* 2009;7:1236-1240.

Hausegger KA, Karnel F, Georgieva B, et al. Transjugular intrahepatic portosystemic shunt creation with the Viatorr expanded polytetrafluoroethylene-covered stent-graft. *J Vasc Interv Radiol.* 2004;15:239-248.

Hoppe H, Wang SL, Petersen BD. Intravascular US-guided direct intrahepatic portocaval shunt with an expanded polytetrafluoroethylene-covered stent-graft 1. *Radiology.* 2008;246:306-314.

Kirby JM, Cho KJ, Midia M. Image-guided intervention in management of complications of portal hypertension: more than TIPS for Success. *Radiographics.* 2013;33:1473-1496.

Lo GH, Liang HL, Chen WC, et al. A prospective, randomized controlled trial of transjugular intrahepatic portosystemic shunt versus cyanoacrylate injection in the prevention of gastric variceal rebleeding. *Endoscopy.* 2007;39:679-685.

Loffroy R, Favelier S, Pottecher P, et al. Transjugular intrahepatic portosystemic shunt for acute variceal gastrointestinal bleeding: indications, techniques and outcomes. *Diagn Interv Imaging.* 2015;96:745-755.

Malinchoc M, Kamath PS, Gordon FD, et al. A model to predict poor survival in patients undergoing transjugular intrahepatic portosystemic shunts. *Hepatology.* 2000;31:864-871.

Narahara Y, Kanazawa H, Fukuda T, et al. Transjugular intrahepatic portosystemic shunt versus paracentesis plus albumin in patients with refractory ascites who have good hepatic and renal function: a prospective randomized trial. *J Gastroenterol.* 2011;46:78-85.

Park JK, Saab S, Kee ST, et al. Balloon-occluded retrograde transvenous obliteration (BRTO) for treatment of gastric varices: review and meta-analysis. *Dig Dis Sci.* 2014;60:1543-1553.

Petersen BD, Clark TW. Direct intrahepatic portocaval shunt. *Tech Vasc Interv Radiol.* 2008;11:230-234.

Rössle M, Gerbes AL. TIPS for the treatment of refractory ascites, hepatorenal syndrome and hepatic hydrothorax: a critical update. *Gut.* 2010;59:988-1000.

Saad W. Balloon-occluded retrograde transvenous obliteration of gastric varices: concept, basic techniques, and outcomes. *Semin Intervent Radiol.* 2012;29:118-128.

Saad W. Transjugular intrahepatic portosystemic shunt before and after liver transplantation. *Semin Intervent Radiol.* 2014;31:243-247.

Salerno F, Cammà C, Enea M, et al. Transjugular intrahepatic portosystemic shunt for refractory ascites: a meta-analysis of individual patient data. *Gastroenterology.* 2007;133:825-834.

Senzolo M, M Sartori T, Rossetto V, et al. Prospective evaluation of anticoagulation and transjugular intrahepatic portosystemic shunt for the management of portal vein thrombosis in cirrhosis. *Liver Int.* 2012;32:919-927.

Silva RF, Arroyo PC Jr, Duca WJ, et al. Complications following transjugular intrahepatic portosystemic shunt: a retrospective analysis. *Transplant Proc.* 2004;36:926-928.

Wong F. Recent advances in our understanding of hepatorenal syndrome. *Nat Rev Gastroenterol Hepatol.* 2012;9:382-391.

Yang Z, Han G, Wu Q, et al. Patency and clinical outcomes of transjugular intrahepatic portosystemic shunt with polytetrafluoroethylene-covered stents versus bare stents: a meta-analysis. *J Gastroenterol Hepatol.* 2010;25:1718-1725.

Zheng M, Chen Y, Bai J, et al. Transjugular intrahepatic portosystemic shunt versus endoscopic therapy in the secondary prophylaxis of variceal rebleeding in cirrhotic patients: meta-analysis update. *J Clin Gastroenterol.* 2008;42:507-516.

THE MANAGEMENT OF REFRACTORY ASCITES

Rushabh Modi, MD, MPH, and Francisco A. Durazo, MD

Ascites is defined as an abnormal accumulation of fluid in the peritoneal cavity resulting from portal hypertension, renal function, plasma hydrostatic-oncotic pressure imbalance, and endogenous vasoactive substances. Although cirrhosis of the liver is the primary cause for more than 80% of patients with ascites, a small portion of ascites can be caused by other conditions such as malignancies (e.g., peritoneal carcinomatosis), infectious causes (e.g., abdominal tuberculosis), congestive heart failure, nephrotic syndrome, hepatic vein obstruction, pancreatic diseases, severe alcoholic hepatitis, and miscellaneous disorders of the peritoneum. It is vital to diagnose the cause of ascites initially because the management can differ greatly depending on the cause. Refractory ascites exists on a clinical spectrum of fluid overload from pre-ascites, characterized by subtle sodium retention, to diuretic responsive ascites and then to severe complications of refractory ascites, including hepatorenal syndrome (HRS) and hyponatremia. For a practicing surgeon, the presence of ascites is particularly important for preoperative risk assessment because most patients with ascites develop severe hepatic dysfunction, poor nutritional status, and electrolyte imbalances, which increase overall perioperative risks.

This chapter provides various pharmacologic and surgical treatment options and the rationale for them in the management of refractory ascites. The pathophysiology of ascites and diagnostic modalities are discussed briefly to provide a better understanding of the different therapeutic approaches.

■ PATHOPHYSIOLOGY

The first hypothesis of ascites formation was the "backward theory" in the early 1960s, in which portal hypertension and hypoalbuminemia led to excessive splanchnic lymph formation, which causes the thoracic duct to flow backward from the heart and then extravasate into the peritoneal space. This extravasation of accumulating ascites triggers a vicious cycle of intravascular depletion and subsequent renally induced sodium retention. However, in this theory, it would be expected that cardiac index and plasma volume would be diminished in the presence of portal hypertension. The backward flow theory was discredited later, though, when it was found that systemic vasodilatation in cirrhosis, characterized by decreased systemic vascular resistance, actually prompted increased plasma volume and cardiac output. The "overflow theory" then was dismissed later when studies showed that angiotensin II blockade induced a significant reduction of the wedged hepatic venous pressure without any change in the hepatic blood flow. This finding suggests that arterial vasodilation is not systemic but rather confined to the regional splanchnic circulation.

The currently accepted hypothesis for the mechanism of ascites in cirrhosis is the "peripheral arterial vasodilation" theory. The primary causative effect is sinusoidal portal hypertension secondary to progressive hepatic fibrosis. Portal hypertension induces the release of nitric oxide and vasodilator peptides, which causes the splanchnic arterial vasodilation. The arterial vasodilation in the splanchnic circuit leads to reduced effective arterial blood volume, which activates vasoconstrictors and sodium-retaining systems, resulting in renal sodium retention. Therefore high sodium concentration increases splanchnic capillary permeability and causes ascites formation.

■ REFRACTORY ASCITES

Refractory ascites is divided into resistant ascites and intractable ascites. Resistant ascites is defined as being unresponsive to diuretics (spironolactone 400 mg and furosemide 160 mg a day), and intractable ascites occurs when patients cannot tolerate diuretics because of side effects (i.e., azotemia, hyponatremia, or encephalopathy). True resistant ascites is associated with advanced cirrhosis, hepatorenal syndrome, and a poor prognosis. The responsiveness to therapy is determined by weight loss, urine output, and the negative balance of sodium. Practically, note that these metrics can be difficult to measure accurately, especially on the medical-surgical floor or in patients without Foley catheters. Ascites in patients who develop complications such as hepatic encephalopathy, renal insufficiency, and hyponatremia after diuretics therapy also are considered refractory. Refractory ascites represent less than 10% of all ascites.

Diagnosis of Ascites

All patients with new onset ascites or all patients with known ascites on admission should get diagnostic paracentesis because 10% to 25% of these patients can have spontaneous bacterial peritonitis (SBP) without overt clinical signs and symptoms.

Analysis of ascitic fluid can help to determine the etiology of the underlying conditions and detect causative micro-organisms in infectious processes. Cell counts, Gram stains, cultures, albumin, total protein, glucose, and lactate dehydrogenase (LDH) from ascitic fluid should be sent to the laboratory for analysis. Triglyceride levels should be added in suspected cases of chylous ascites. Cytology tests should be done in suspected malignancies. Serum albumin, total protein, and LDH should be sent at the same time to compare serum-ascitic gradients. Adenosine deaminase can be considered for tuberculous peritonitis. Testing serum for cancer antigen 125 (CA-125) is not necessary to make a diagnosis of ascites, as it is nonspecifically elevated in ascites and not indicative of reproductive malignancy. Its use is not recommended in patients with ascites of any type.

To determine the cause of ascites, the current recommendation is to calculate the serum-ascites albumin gradient (SAAG) rather than differentiate transudates from exudates. SAAG is based on the plasma oncotic-hydrostatic pressure balance and is directly related to portal pressure.

$$SAAG = Serum\ albumin - Ascitic\ albumin$$

The causes of ascites, according to SAAG, are shown in Table 1.

Paracentesis

Although most cirrhotic patients have prolonged prothrombin time and thrombocytopenia, there is no evidence supporting significant bleeding from paracentesis in this population. International normalized ratio (INR) is not an accurate reflection of coagulopathy in liver disease, as both procoagulant and anticoagulant production is diminished in chronic liver disease. In addition, studies have suggested 10 times greater von Willebrand factor activity leading to hyperfunctional platelets. Thus routine transfusion of platelets or fresh frozen plasma is not recommended to perform paracentesis. The major contraindication for paracentesis is disseminated intravascular coagulopathy (DIC).

The preferred site for needle entry is 3 cm medial and 3 cm superior to the anterior superior iliac spine on the left lower quadrant of the abdomen. The midline approach is not preferable because many patients are obese. The right lower quadrant also is not desirable because the cecum can become distended in patients who take lactulose. The distended cecum has a higher risk of perforation. The needle should not be inserted in areas with cutaneous infection, abdominal wall hematoma, scars, or visibly engorged subcutaneous veins. Bedside ultrasound, if available, is useful, especially in ascites accumulated in compartments.

The paracentesis needle can be inserted with either the angular technique or the Z-track technique. In the angular technique, the

TABLE 1: Causes of Ascites With or Without Portal Hypertension

SAAG ≥1.1 g/dL: Portal Hypertension	SAAG <1.1 g/dL: No Portal Hypertension
• Cirrhosis	• Peritoneal carcinomatosis
• Alcoholic hepatitis	• Nephrotic syndrome
• Vascular obstructions (Budd-Chiari syndrome or portal vein thrombosis)	• Pancreatitis
	• Peritoneal tuberculosis
• Congestive heart failure	• Serositis
• Metastasis to liver	
• Fatty liver disease of pregnancy	
• Myxedema	

SAAG, Serum-ascites albumin gradient.

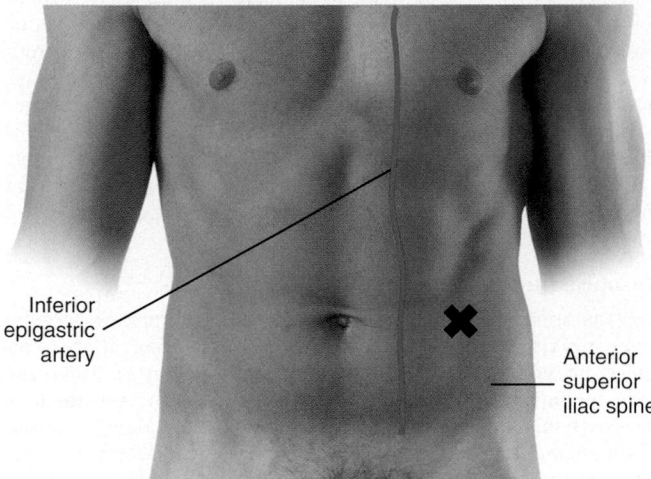

Inferior epigastric artery

Anterior superior iliac spine

FIGURE 1 Preferred needle entry site for paracentesis. *(From Drake R, Vogel AW. Gray's Atlas of Anatomy. Philadelphia: Churchill Livingstone; 2007.)*

needle is inserted obliquely from the cutaneous site into the peritoneum. In the Z-track technique, cutaneous tissues are pulled down, and the needle is inserted straight into the peritoneum. The purpose of these techniques is to ensure that cutaneous and peritoneal sites do not directly overlap each other, thereby minimizing ascitic fluid leakage (Figure 1).

Treatment of Ascites

Ascites formation from cirrhosis results from renal retention of sodium and water. Therefore the goal of the treatment is to mobilize the ascitic fluid by creating a net negative balance of sodium. Net negative sodium balance can be achieved with decreasing sodium intake and increasing sodium secretion. Urinary sodium (Ur Na^{++}) excretion in cirrhosis plays a role as a prognostic factor. Although a spot Ur Na^{++} less than 10 mg/dL correlates with only a 20% 2-year survival, that number increases to 60% in 2-year survival among cirrhotic patients when Ur Na^{++} is greater than 10 mg/dL. The treatment of low-SAAG ascites should concentrate on underlying causes.

Nonpharmacologic Therapies
Dietary Sodium Restriction

Restriction of dietary sodium intake is one of the most important nonpharmacologic treatments of ascites because renal sodium

retention is the key contributing factor to ascites formation. When sodium intake surpasses urinary and insensible losses of sodium, net positive sodium balance retains extra fluid, causing ascites and peripheral edema. The goal is to create a negative net balance of sodium, thereby contracting extracellular fluid volume. Fluid restriction is not necessary in patients with cirrhosis who are on diuretic therapy and sodium restriction.

A typical American diet usually contains 4 to 6 g of sodium per day. About one third of this sodium comes from salt, another one third comes from processed foods, and the rest is from water and other foods (e.g., meat, vegetables). Daily sodium restriction of 1.5 to 2 g is recommended. One teaspoon of table salt contains 2300 mg of sodium, which is more than the recommended daily sodium intake. It is very important for patients not to add any salt to their food at all. Staying away from all processed foods is also essential because processed foods contain a substantial amount of sodium for preservation. Patients should be instructed to replace processed meats and vegetables with fresh or frozen and also to avoid eating at fast-food restaurants because processed food is their main ingredient.

Patients should keep a record of what they eat, including portion size and sodium content. Patients should weigh themselves and record their weight every day as well. Compliance is the most important part of this treatment because most patients fail to stick to a low-sodium diet. The progress of treatment can be monitored simply with daily weight, but there are objective measures to prove noncompliance in patients. Although the most accurate measurement is 24-hour urinary sodium, this is not practical to obtain, especially in outpatient settings. On the other hand, a spot urinary sample can be collected easily. Spot Ur Na^{++} by itself does not provide a complete account of sodium excreted over a 24-hour period because of notable diurnal variations in renal sodium excretion. However, it has been shown that a spot urinary sodium-potassium (Na$^+$/K$^+$) ratio greater than 1 represents 24-hour sodium intake of more than 2 g, indicating noncompliance. In such patients, nutrition counseling with a registered dietician referral may be helpful.

In cirrhosis, only 15% to 20% of patients can achieve negative sodium balance by restricting dietary sodium intake only, without diuretics. Therefore diuretic therapy should be started in patients with cirrhosis along with sodium restriction from the beginning of treatment.

Fluid Restriction

Restriction of daily fluid intake to 1 to 1.5 L per day usually is not necessary in patients with ascites because an adequate negative sodium balance can help to eliminate excess free water. The only benefit of fluid restriction can be observed in patients with profound hyponatremia—that is, serum sodium less than 125 mg/dL. Fluid restriction with a serum sodium above this level risks prerenal azotemia because of exacerbation of relative underfilling of arterial circulation.

Pharmacologic Therapies
Diuretics

Most patients with cirrhosis need to take diuretic agents to control their ascites in addition to restricting dietary sodium. Diuretics increase renal sodium excretion, thereby achieving net negative sodium balance and eliminating excess fluid accumulated in extracellular spaces. The most commonly used diuretics are potassium-sparing aldosterone antagonists (e.g., spironolactone, amiloride) and loop diuretics (e.g., furosemide).

There are two strategies for treating ascites with diuretic agents. The first regimen begins with an aldosterone antagonist alone. The dose of spironolactone is increased every week to its maximal dose until the clinical response is achieved. If there is no response after maximal dose of spironolactone, furosemide should be added, and its dose should be increased every week. In the second approach, both spironolactone and furosemide are started as a combination from the beginning of treatment, and the doses are increased weekly based on clinical response and measurement of urinary sodium excretion. Studies have shown that there is no significant difference in terms of efficacy and incidence of complications between these two regimens.

The starting doses of diuretics for ascites are generally higher than the doses for hypertension or heart failure. The starting doses of spironolactone and furosemide are 100 mg and 40 mg per day, respectively, and the maximal doses are 400 mg and 160 mg per day, respectively. The therapeutic response can be monitored simply with daily weight. The goal of effective diuresis is losing 2 pounds per day in patients with peripheral edema and 1 pound per day in those without edema because the highest absorptive capacity of the peritoneal cavity is approximately 0.5 L per day. Overdiuresis can induce severe electrolyte imbalances and renal failure. A spot urinary Na^+/K^+ ratio greater than 1 has a 90% sensitivity in predicting a negative sodium balance (>78 mmol/day sodium excretion).

The advantages of using aldosterone antagonists and loop diuretics together are counter-regulatory effect on potassium reabsorption, greater natriuretic potency, and earlier onset of diuresis. Thiazide diuretics are not recommended, in general, despite their synergistic effect in blocking sodium reabsorption in distal tubules when used together with loop diuretics. Thiazides plus loop diuretics can cause significant hypokalemia and hyperammonemia via various mechanisms. In cirrhosis, hyperammonemia can result in hepatic encephalopathy. In individuals who develop gynecomastia because of spironolactone use, amiloride can be substituted. Other loop diuretic agents, such as torsemide and bumetanide, also can be used safely and effectively in cirrhotic patients with ascites. Some concern exists that intravenous loop diuretics, often used in hospitalized patients, may induce disproportionately severe prerenal azotemia. However, some data suggest that a single intravenous dose of furosemide may differentiate patients with diuretic-responsive versus diuretic-resistant ascites. Diuretic agents should be discontinued when there are diuretic-induced complications, such as severe hyponatremia (serum Na^+ <120 mg/dL), renal failure, or hepatic encephalopathy. A newer aldosterone antagonist, eplerenone, has been used with success in congestive heart failure but has not been studied rigorously in portal hypertension–induced ascites.

Albumin

Hypoalbuminemia is a common complication of liver failure in cirrhosis because albumin is synthesized mainly in the liver. Albumin is a plasma volume expander, and it plays a crucial role in maintaining plasma oncotic pressure. On the other hand, as mentioned previously, the pathogenesis of ascites is related to increased splanchnic arterial vasodilation, causing decreased effective plasma volume. In addition, intravenous albumin has a short half-life and is not cost effective. Therefore albumin should not be used routinely in the management of ascites. On the other hand, albumin infusions are very effective in preventing renal dysfunction associated with spontaneous bacterial peritonitis. Recently, concomitant use of albumin and vasoconstrictors has been shown to improve circulatory hemodynamics, renal function, and control of ascites.

Vasoconstrictors

Vasoconstrictors have been used in the management of hepatorenal syndrome and the prevention of hemodynamic instability after large volume paracentesis (LVP), along with albumin. Recent studies have shown that the use of vasoconstrictors in cirrhotic patients with preserved renal function improves sodium excretion, circulatory function, and ascites control. Various vasopressors have been studied for this purpose. Octreotide, a somatostatin analogue, can cause splanchnic vasoconstriction and improve renal perfusion. Midodrine, an alpha-1 receptor agonist, also can be used along with octreotide and albumin. A randomized pilot study showed that midodrine plus standard medical therapy (sodium restriction, diuretics, and LVP) is superior to standard medical therapy alone for the control of ascites without any renal or hepatic dysfunction. Terlipressin, a vasopressin derivative, also induces splanchnic vasoconstriction and can be used to control ascites. Although terlipressin is not available in the United States, it has been used widely for hepatorenal syndrome in Europe and other parts of the world. A recent study showed that terlipressin plus diuretics and albumin may improve the outcomes of refractory ascites by increasing urinary sodium excretion and decreasing the need for LVP (Table 2).

Vasopressin Receptor Antagonists

Vaptans are a class of medications that are vasopressin receptor antagonists that competitively block the V2 receptor at the renal collecting tubules, thereby preventing reabsorption of water and inducing aquaresis. They initially were used for the treatment of hyponatremia in patients with cirrhosis and ascites. However, initial studies demonstrated that electrolyte improvements stopped on cessation of the drug. Given the side effects of the medication as well as lack of long-term improvements in mortality and their expense, vaptans are not recommended, although they are used occasionally in Europe.

Drugs to Avoid

Nonsteroidal anti-inflammatory drugs (NSAIDs) are prostaglandin inhibitors. Their use can increase urinary sodium excretion and precipitate acute kidney injury in addition to risks for NSAID-induced

TABLE 2: Summary of Medical Therapy for Refractory Ascites

Category and Action	Drug	Dose	Remarks
DIURETICS			
Aldosterone antagonist	Spironolactone	100 mg to 400 mg PO daily	Monotherapy or combination with furosemide
Epithelial sodium-channel blocker	Amiloride	10 mg to 40 mg PO daily	Substitute for spironolactone in cases with gynecomastia
Loop diuretics (torsemide and bumetanide can be used)	Furosemide	40 mg to 160 mg PO daily	Combination with spironolactone
VASOCONSTRICTORS			
Somatostatin analogue	Octreotide	300 μg twice daily SQ	Can be used in combination with midodrine
alpha-1 receptor agonist	Midodrine	7.5 mg three times daily PO	Can be used in combination with octreotide and albumin infusion

PO, By mouth; *SQ,* subcutaneous.

nephropathy and peptic ulcer disease, both of which those with cirrhosis are at higher risk for. Nonselective beta-blockade traditionally has been recommended for variceal bleeding prophylaxis. Their use in patients with concurrent ascites is controversial. Some studies suggest that propranolol can make patients more diuretic resistant and worsen overall survival. More important, patients with cirrhosis have lower circulatory blood pressure because of arterial vasodilation. Use of nonselective beta-blockers can prompt hypotension. Lastly, antihypertensive medications such as angiotensin-converting enzyme (ACE) inhibitors and angiotensin receptor blockers should be used with caution. They minimize the effects of vasoconstricting hormones designed to counteract arterial vasodilation due to nitric oxide in patients with cirrhosis. Their use also can prompt hypotension and acute kidney injury.

Interventional Therapies

Patients with ascites, who are refractory to nonpharmacologic treatment options, often require additional interventional approaches to control their ascites. Interventional therapies include serial LVP, a transjugular intrahepatic portosystemic shunt (TIPS), a peritoneovenous shunt (PVS), and ultimately liver transplantation.

Large Volume Paracentesis

LVP, or therapeutic paracentesis, has been used in the management of cirrhotic patients with ascites for centuries, long before the discovery of diuretic agents. In LVP, 4 to 5 L of ascitic fluid are removed. Randomized controlled trials have demonstrated that LVP can be performed safely and effectively every 2 weeks, even in patients with minimal urine sodium excretion. It can be performed either in an outpatient clinic or in a hospital setting. One controversy that has erupted over LVP is postparacentesis albumin infusion. Many studies have failed to reveal that albumin infusion after LVP has mortality or morbidity benefits, but significant improvements have been observed in electrolyte imbalances, plasma renin, and creatinine levels. Because albumin is very expensive, it is not cost effective to use routinely after LVP of 4 to 5 L. In cases of larger amounts of ascitic fluid removal (i.e., 6 to 8 L), however, albumin infusion should be considered to maintain homeostatic fluid balance.

Indwelling Catheters

Permanent abdominal or pleural indwelling catheters, such as PleurX, that allow patients to self-perform paracentesis or thoracentesis are not recommended. Such catheters represent a notable infection risk. Moreover, they worsen the underlying problem. Protein leaking from excessive fluid removal drops oncotic pressure, which worsens ascitic fluid accumulation, thereby creating a vicious cycle.

Transjugular Intrahepatic Portosystemic Shunts

Although TIPS was pioneered by Dr. Josef Rösch in 1969, it was not used in clinical practice until the late 1990s because of technical difficulties. Later, TIPS was used to decrease portal hypertension in the management of refractory variceal hemorrhage. However, it was found that TIPS might be of benefit in eliminating refractory ascites by means of increasing natriuretic effects. The TIPS procedure essentially is performed by interventional radiologists in the United States, whereas some hepatologists perform TIPS in Europe. During the TIPS procedure, a shunt is created between the hepatic vein and the portal vein from a percutaneous jugular venous approach. A stent then is deployed across the shunt to maintain its patency. The major indications for TIPS placement are refractory ascites requiring LVP more frequently than every month, refractory variceal bleeding, and as a bridge to liver transplantation. The absolute contraindication for TIPS placement is worsening hepatic encephalopathy (Figure 2). A relative contraindication for TIPS is the presence of congestive heart failure, which can be worsened by increased systemic fluid after TIPS. Note that the Model for End-Stage Liver Disease (MELD) score originally was designed to provide prognostication of post-TIPS

mortality. A score above 15 should generate a discussion of relative risks and benefits.

Recently, new synthetic fluoropolymer-covered stents have been used in TIPS procedures. A randomized trial showed that polytetrafluoroethylene (PTFE)-coated stents yielded more than twice the duration of patency of metal stents in 1 year. Meta-analyses have established that TIPS can provide better control of ascites and possible improvement in survival, although there are higher rates of hepatic encephalopathy. Reinitiating and titrating up the doses of diuretic agents in post-TIPS patients are reasonable because better natriuresis can be achieved after portal hypertension has been reduced.

Because favorable outcomes have been shown in recent studies, it is recommended that TIPS be performed earlier as a first-line treatment for acute and recurrent variceal bleeding in patients who have hepatic venous pressure gradients higher than 20 mm Hg. Additional benefits of TIPS are potential improvements in nutrition, body mass index, and quality of life in severely malnourished patients with end-stage liver disease.

Peritoneovenous Shunts

A PVS is a shunt that drains ascitic fluid from the peritoneal cavity to the systemic veins, such as the internal jugular vein or the superior vena cava. It lies underneath the skin and runs from the abdomen to the upper part of the body. PVSs (also known as LeVeen shunts and Denver shunts) were introduced in the 1970s and widely used until the late 1980s. Currently PVSs are not used in clinical practice because of higher rates of complications and the development of newer and safer techniques such as TIPS. The complications associated with a PVS are obstructions (40% of shunt failure in first year) due to kinking or clogging of the shunts and thrombosis, serious infections such as peritonitis and bacteremia, postshunt coagulopathy leading to DIC, pulmonary edema, and increased risk for variceal bleeding secondary to increased venous return and hepatic encephalopathy.

■ SPONTANEOUS BACTERIAL PERITONITIS

SBP is an infection of the peritoneum that occurs spontaneously without any overt source that can be remedied surgically. It is a common complication in patients with portal hypertension and ascites. Approximately 30% of cirrhotic patients with ascites develop SBP, and it is associated with a 20% mortality rate. All hospitalized patients with ascites must have paracentesis for ascitic fluid analysis because clinical signs and symptoms are not sufficient to diagnose SBP. Patients with a previous normal ascitic fluid analysis who later develop abdominal pain, fever, encephalopathy, leukocytosis, or renal failure should have repeat paracentesis. Treating SBP only with empiric antibiotics, without a definitive bacterial culture, is not recommended because it can lead to inadequate therapeutic response and increased resistance of micro-organisms.

Treatment of Spontaneous Bacterial Peritonitis

Ascitic fluid with absolute neutrophil counts of more than 250 cells/mm^3 is diagnostic for SBP. Empiric antibiotics need to be initiated as soon as possible, before the result of bacterial culture is available. Most ascitic fluid culture will grow specific micro-organisms, and the antibacterial therapy should be narrowed down accordingly. Patients who have negative culture results but suspicious clinical symptoms of SBP also should be treated empirically with antibiotics. The recommended antibiotic therapies are summarized in Table 3.

Studies have shown that a decrease in mortality was observed in some patients with SBP who received intravenous albumin infusion along with empiric antibiotics. Current guidelines support giving 1.5 g/kg of albumin infusion within 6 hours of SBP diagnosis and

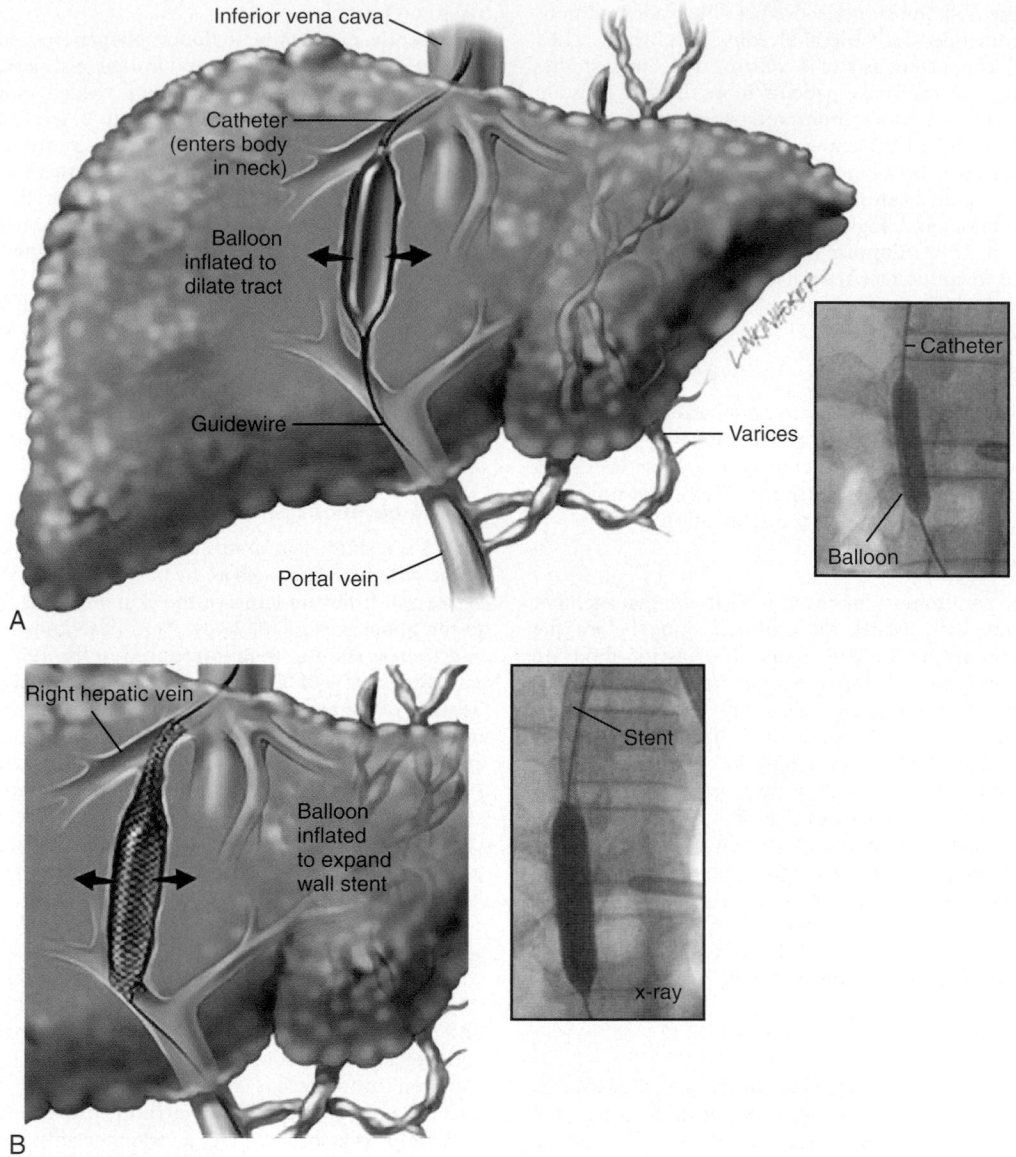

FIGURE 2 **A** and **B,** Transjugular intrahepatic portosystemic shunt placement. *(From Johns Hopkins Medical Institutions. Used with permission.)*

1.0 g/kg of albumin infusion on day 3 in patients with SBP who also have blood urea nitrogen less than 30 mg/dL, serum creatinine more than 1 mg/dL, or total bilirubin less than 4 mg/dL.

Patients with ascites also may develop secondary peritonitis involving bowel perforation or intra-abdominal abscess. Clinical signs and symptoms are not helpful in distinguishing secondary peritonitis from SBP, although SBP infection sometimes can be seen with mild symptoms. It is recommended to perform ascitic fluid analysis for total protein, LDH, and glucose to assist in the determination of secondary peritonitis. Elevated ascitic fluid absolute neutrophil counts (in thousands), multiple organisms on Gram stains and cultures (including fungi and enterococcus), ascitic fluid total protein more than 1 g/dL, ascitic fluid LDH more than half of the upper limit of the serum, and ascitic fluid glucose less than 50 mg/dL are suggestive of secondary peritonitis, with 100% sensitivity and 43% specificity. These patients should be evaluated immediately with emergent abdominal x-rays and computed tomographic (CT) scanning to look for signs of intra-abdominal perforations or abscesses.

Spontaneous Bacterial Peritonitis Prophylaxis

Secondary prophylaxis can be achieved with oral ciprofloxacin 750 mg once a week. Norfloxacin was discontinued in 2014 for unclear reasons by Merck, the sole manufacturer in the United States. Trimethoprim-sulfamethoxazole also is recommended in patients with ascites after the first episode of SBP. Primary prophylaxis for SBP in patients with cirrhosis and ascites is still controversial. Current guidelines support giving primary prophylaxis with oral ciprofloxacin to patients with ascitic fluid protein less than 1.5 g/dL and at least one of the following: serum creatinine more than 1.2 mg/dL, blood urea nitrogen more than 25 mg/dL, serum sodium less than 130 mEq/L, or Child-Pugh score greater than 9 with serum total bilirubin more than 3 mg/dL. Note that overzealous use of antibiotic prophylaxis when not indicated risks bacterial resistance. Data-supported indications should guide therapy selection. In patients with prior SBP who develop acute upper gastrointestinal bleeding, intravenous ceftriaxone therapy for 7 days is recommended. The antibiotic therapy for SBP prophylaxis is summarized in Table 3. A growing body of research suggests that proton pump inhibitors may

TABLE 3: Summary of Treatment and Prophylaxis in Spontaneous Bacterial Peritonitis

Antibiotics	Route and Dosages
EMPIRIC ANTIBIOTICS	
FIRST-LINE THERAPIES	
Cefotaxime	2 g IV every 8 hours (or)
Ofloxacin (patients with mild infection with no shock, vomiting)	400 mg PO every 12 hours
SECOND-LINE THERAPIES	
Ceftriaxone	1 g IV every 12 hours (or)
Ciprofloxacin	400 mg IV every 12 hours (or)
Piperacillin-tazobactam	3.375 g IV every 6 hours (or)
Ertapenem	1 g IV every day for resistant pathogens (or)
Cefepime	1-2 g IV every 8 hours for resistant pathogens
PROPHYLACTIC ANTIBIOTICS	
FIRST-LINE THERAPY FOR PATIENTS WITH GASTROINTESTINAL BLEEDING	
Ceftriaxone	1 g IV every day for 7 days
DAILY PRIMARY PROPHYLAXIS	
Trimethoprim-sulfamethoxazole	1 double-strength tablet PO every day
WEEKLY PROPHYLAXIS	
Ciprofloxacin	750 mg PO weekly

IV, Intravenous; *PO*, by mouth.

increase the risk of SBP. Removing this medication, if no strong indication exists, may help to prevent the development of SBP.

■ HEPATIC HYDROTHORAX

Hepatic hydrothorax is a development of pleural effusion in a cirrhotic patient with portal hypertension, without any underlying cardiopulmonary diseases. It commonly is seen on the right side, but left-sided and bilateral involvements also can be seen. The likely mechanisms for pathogenesis of hepatic hydrothorax are hypoalbuminemia, which reduces plasma osmotic pressure, azygos vein hypertension, transdiaphragmatic migration of ascitic fluid via lymphatic systems, and ascitic fluid leakage via diaphragmatic defects. Hepatic hydrothorax may occur in the absence of ascites. As in ascites, all patients who have hepatic hydrothorax or pleural effusion with unclear etiology should have a diagnostic thoracentesis. Hepatic hydrothorax can be seen with transudative pleural effusions but not always. Definitive diagnosis can be made with a technetium sulfur colloid study. Detection of passage of radiotracer into the chest cavity confirms diagnosis. Accuracy can be increased by performing this study after recent paracentesis.

However, as in ascites and SBP, hepatic hydrothorax can become infected spontaneously, called spontaneous bacterial empyema (SBEM). In this case, the pleural fluid analysis becomes exudative. The diagnostic criteria for SBEM are serum-pleural albumin gradient more than 1.1 g/dL, pleural fluid neutrophil counts more than 500/mm^3, and the absence of pneumonia or contiguous infectious process on chest radiography. SBEM occurs as a result of a direct microbial spread from the pleural cavity in the presence of portal hypertension. Rarely, SBEM can develop without clinically significant ascites. All patients with hepatic hydrothorax who develop fever, chest pain, dyspnea, and encephalopathy should have repeat thoracentesis to evaluate pleural fluid analysis.

The management of hepatic hydrothorax is basically the same as with refractory ascites. Conservative management includes sodium restriction and diuretic therapy. In refractory cases, therapeutic thoracentesis, TIPS, and peritoneovenous shunting can be performed. Tube thoracostomy with injection of a sclerosing agent can be a method of long-term management, but the evidence for its efficacy is not validated. In patients with documented SBEM, third-generation cephalosporins such as ceftriaxone (1 g intravenously daily for 10 days) can be given empirically. An antibacterial regimen should be narrowed down as soon as the results of bacterial cultures are obtained.

Hepatic hydrothorax is a late and serious complication of cirrhosis. Patients with hepatic hydrothorax generally have end-stage liver disease, and these individuals should be evaluated for liver transplantation.

SUGGESTED READINGS

Salerno F, Guevara M, Bernardi M, Moreau R, Wong F, Angeli P, Garcia-Tsao G, et al. Refractory ascites: pathogenesis, definition and therapy of a severe complication in patients with cirrhosis. *Liver Int.* 2010;30:937-947.

Wong F. Management of ascites in cirrhosis. *J Gastroenterol Hepatol.* 2012;27:11-20.

THE MANAGEMENT OF HEPATIC ENCEPHALOPATHY

Neha Jakhete, MD, and Amy K. Kim, MD

Hepatic encephalopathy (HE) is a complex, potentially reversible, neuropsychiatric syndrome seen in patients with cirrhosis or acute liver failure. A 2010 study of patients in the United States reported 22,931 hospitalizations because of HE in 2009, with an average length of stay of 8.5 days at a cost of $63,108 per case and with a mortality rate of 15% (Stepanova, et al., 2012).

■ CLINICAL PRESENTATION AND DIAGNOSIS

HE is a clinical diagnosis, with a presentation of a wide spectrum of psychiatric and neurologic symptoms. Symptoms are nonspecific and can be seen in many other medical conditions, including hypoglycemia, intoxication, or infection. Other causes of altered mental status must be excluded before making the diagnosis of HE (Box 1). Asterixis, a flapping tremor of the outstretched hands, is a common feature of HE but also can be seen in other metabolic encephalopathies.

Patients with HE may have symptoms ranging from subtle abnormalities, detectable only through specialized psychological testing, to frank coma. Focal neurologic deficits such as hemiplegia or

BOX I: Differential Diagnosis of Hepatic Encephalopathy (HE)

Overt HE or Acute Confusional State

Diabetic complications (hypoglycemia, ketoacidosis, hyperosmolar, lactate acidosis)
Alcohol (intoxication, withdrawal, Wernicke)
Drugs (benzodiazepines, neuroleptics, opioids)
Infections
Electrolyte disorders (hyponatremia and hypercalcemia)
Nonconvulsive epilepsy
Psychiatric disorders
Intracranial bleeding and stroke
Severe medical stress (organ failure and inflammation)

Other Presentations

Dementia (primary and secondary)
Brain lesions (traumatic, neoplasms, normal pressure hydrocephalus)
Obstructive sleep apnea
Hyponatremia and sepsis can both produce encephalopathy and precipitate HE by interactions with the pathophysiological mechanisms. In end-stage liver disease uremic encephalopathy and HE may overlap.

From *Hepatic Encephalopathy in Chronic Liver Disease, 2014 Practice Guideline by AASLD and EASL.* © American Association for the Study of Liver Diseases.

BOX 2: West Haven Criteria for Semiquantitative Grading of Mental State

Grade I

Trivial lack of awareness
Euphoria or anxiety
Shortened attention span
Impaired performance of addition

Grade 2

Lethargy or apathy
Minimal disorientation for time or place
Subtle personality change
Inappropriate behavior
Impaired performance of subtraction

Grade 3

Somnolence to semistupor, but responsive to verbal stimuli
Confusion
Gross disorientation

Grade 4

Coma (unresponsive to verbal or noxious stimuli

From Ferenci P, Lockwood A, Mullen K, Tarter R, Weissenborn K, Blei AT. Hepatic encephalopathy—definition, nomenclature, diagnosis, and quantification: final report of the Working Party at the 11th World Congresses of Gastroenterology, Vienna, 1998. *Hepatology.* 2002;35:716-721. doi:10.1053/jhep.2002.31250

hemiparesis are observed in less than 20% of patients, and seizures are rarely seen. Any focal neurologic deficiency should prompt imaging to exclude any structural lesions.

Diagnosis is made after excluding other causes of brain dysfunction and in patients with advanced liver disease or portosystemic shunt. Ammonia levels commonly are elevated in HE, but the level can vary, does not always correlate with severity of encephalopathy, and does not add any diagnostic or prognostic value in management of HE. Therefore it is not recommended to routinely check ammonia levels in patients with cirrhosis. Electroencephalography testing is always abnormal in overt HE, but observed changes, such as triphasic waves, are not specific.

In general, accepted stages for the broad spectrum of clinical manifestations of encephalopathy are based on level of consciousness, cognitive function, behavioral disturbances, and neuromuscular features (Box 2). In milder cases, patients with encephalopathy may be unaware of any deficits, and symptoms such as sleep pattern reversal, mild confusion, irritability, or personality changes may be apparent only to close contacts. Therefore it is important that family members or caregivers are available to corroborate history provided by the patient.

■ PATHOPHYSIOLOGY OF HEPATIC ENCEPHALOPATHY

The pathogenesis of HE is multifactorial, and despite a large body of research in both humans and animals it remains unclear. Most theories hypothesize that the brain is exposed to toxic substances produced in the gut by the actions of bacteria on nitrogenous compounds, which are cleared incompletely from the blood by the damaged liver. Ammonia was the first substance discovered and has been the most extensively studied; it is thought to be an important pathogenic factor in HE. Most patients with overt HE have elevated plasma levels of ammonia, and children with urea cycle enzyme deficits and otherwise normally functioning livers develop profound hyperammonemia and symptoms indistinguishable from HE.

Ammonia can affect central nervous system (CNS) function through several mechanisms (Figure 1). After crossing the blood-brain barrier, ammonia enters CNS astrocytes and combines with

the neurotransmitter glutamate to form glutamine through the action of glutamine synthetase. Astrocytic glutamine enters mitochondria, in which it is converted back to ammonia and glutamate. Mitochondrial ammonia contributes to the production of reactive oxygen species and upregulates aquaporin 4. This results in astrocytic swelling that causes histologic changes known as *Alzheimer type II astrocytosis.* Adverse effects of ammonia on cerebral perfusion and glucose metabolism also contribute to CNS impairment. There is evidence that y-aminobutyric acid (GABA), the primary inhibitory neurotransmitter in the CNS, may play an important role in the pathogenesis of HE. Increased GABA levels have been associated with liver injury and hyperammonemia. Increased production of endogenous benzodiazepine ligands by gut bacteria can result in increased GABAergic transmission and altered CNS function. This explains why some patients with HE respond to the benzodiazepine antagonist flumazenil even in the absence of exposure to exogenous benzodiazepines.

Other substances, such as mercaptans and neurosteroids, and manganese toxicity also may contribute to neuronal and astrocytic injury in HE. In all likelihood these factors have varying influences in individual patients, depending on the cause, acuity, and severity of the liver disease and hence the variable manifestations of HE.

■ CLASSIFICATION AND MANAGEMENT OF HEPATIC ENCEPHALOPATHY

There are four grades of HE (see Box 2). Grade 1 HE is mild and typically can be treated on an outpatient basis. Depending on the degree of confusion and the involvement of caregivers, grade 2 HE can be treated on an outpatient or inpatient basis. Grades 3 and 4 HE are much more severe and require hospitalization for close monitoring and treatment.

Minimal Hepatic Encephalopathy

Minimal HE (MHE) is a milder form of HE in which impairment in cognitive function is detectable only through neuropsychological testing. The number connection test and block design test have

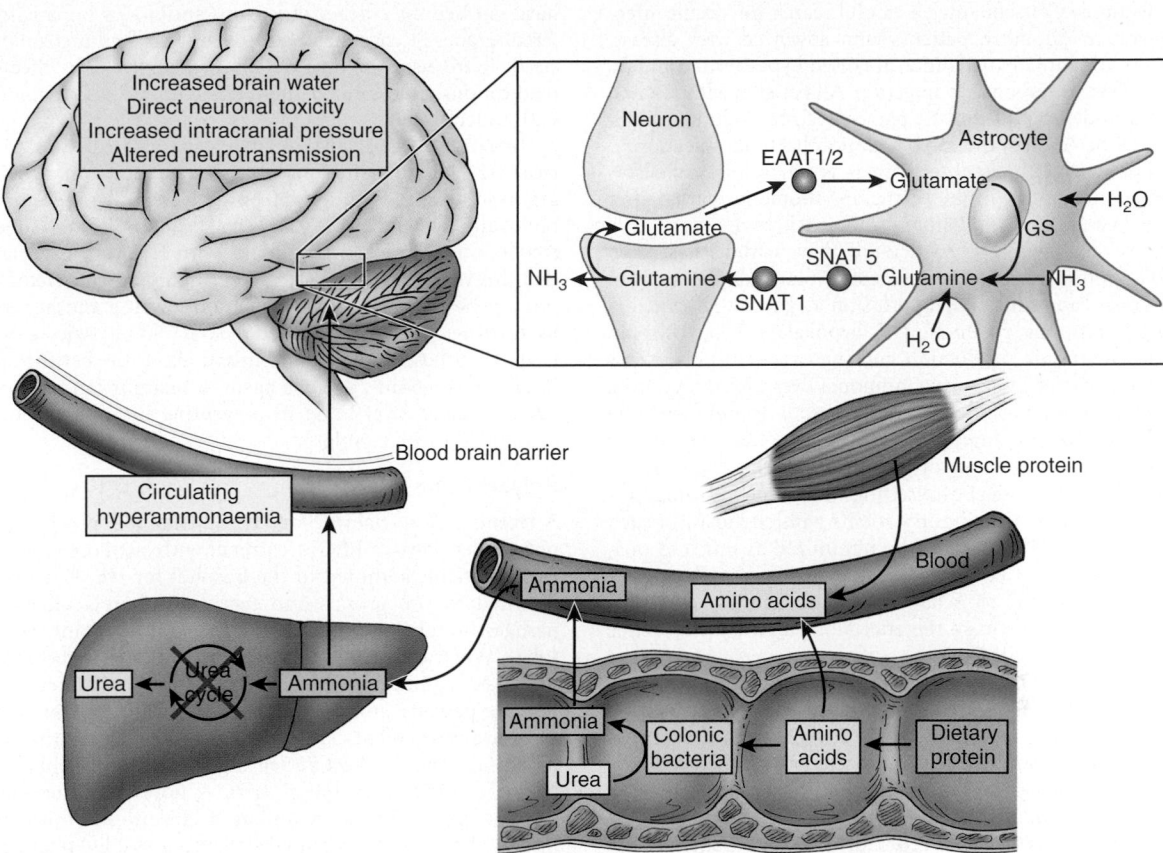

FIGURE 1 Pathophysiologic mechanisms of hepatic encephalopathy (HE) and the role of ammonia in the development of HE. Decreased hepatic urea cycle metabolism in the context of liver cirrhosis or portosystemic shunting leads to accumulation of ammonia (NH_3), a product of protein catabolism, in the systemic circulation. Ammonia readily crosses the blood-brain barrier and is metabolized in a cerebral detoxification pathway by glutamine synthetase (GS), with the formation of glutamine occurring exclusively in cerebral astrocytes. Accumulation of glutamine exerts an osmotic effect, with the influx of water (H_2O) leading to astrocytic swelling. Glutamine is shuttled via transporters (SNAT 5/SNAT 1) to presynaptic neurons, converted to γ-aminobutyric acid (GABA) or glutamate before release into the inhibitory or excitatory synaptic cleft, respectively, and subsequently scavenged by astrocytic reuptake transporters (EAAT1/2). *(From Tranah TH, Paolino A, Shawcross DL. Pathophysiological mechanisms of hepatic encephalopathy. Clin Liver Dis. 2015;5:59-63. doi:10.1002/cld.445.)*

reasonable specificities for MHE and are easy to administer. The deficits in MHE are related primarily to visuospatial orientation, attention problems, and impaired short-term memory. Oral and written skills show little impairment.

Neuroimaging studies have shown a correlation between MHE and changes in cerebral blood flow and abnormalities on neuropsychological testing. Although patients with MHE have no overt symptoms of encephalopathy, they may have diminished capacity to work or drive. Several recent controlled trials have suggested that both lactulose and rifaximin improve neuropsychological testing and quality of life in patients with MHE.

Overt Hepatic Encephalopathy in Patients With Cirrhosis

HE is a common complication of cirrhosis and remains one of the major burdens of disease in this population, in terms of quality of life and functional status. It can be episodic, developing over a short period with fluctuations in severity. It also may be persistent, with continuous overt neurologic or behavioral abnormalities. In most patients with episodic encephalopathy, a precipitating factor other than liver disease can be identified (Box 3), and correction of the precipitating factor can treat encephalopathy in most patients.

Gastrointestinal (GI) bleeding is the most common precipitant. This occurs through a combination of decreasing hepatic and renal perfusion and a large protein load to the gut, which results in

BOX 3: Precipitating Factors in Hepatic Encephalopathy

Gastrointestinal bleeding
Sedatives or analgesics
Dehydration
Renal failure
Hypokalemia
Metabolic alkalosis
Infection (spontaneous bacterial peritonitis, pneumonia, urinary tract infection)
Excessive dietary protein
Constipation

increased production of nitrogenous byproducts. Evaluation of GI blood loss and control of active bleeding must be performed in all patients with episodic HE.

A high prevalence of infection is found in patients with HE, suggesting a potential pathogenic link between the systemic inflammatory response and HE. Cytokines can exacerbate astrocytic swelling, and certain bacteria cell wall compounds can augment the effects of ammonia on compromising cerebral blood flow. It is important to note that cirrhotic patients frequently have baseline neutropenia from hypersplenism and may not exhibit leukocytosis in response to bacterial infections. Consequently, a careful search for occult infection is imperative. Similarly, patients with advanced liver disease, particularly fulminant hepatic failure, are often hypothermic and do not mount a fever in response to infection. All patients with HE and ascites should undergo a diagnostic paracentesis to exclude spontaneous bacterial peritonitis, the most common bacterial infection in hospitalized patients with cirrhosis. If there is a high index of suspicion for infection, empiric antibiotic therapy should be started after cultures have been drawn and before results are known.

Cirrhotic patients with HE, particularly those with ascites, often are exposed to potent diuretics. Intravascular volume depletion from vigorous diuresis can reduce renal perfusion and result in azotemia and increased ammonia production. A hypokalemic alkalosis can enhance renal ammonia production and increase transport across the blood-brain barrier by favoring ammonia over ammonium ion. In these patients, re-establishing intravascular volume and correcting electrolyte imbalances, including hyponatremia, often can reverse hepatic encephalopathy without any other specific therapy.

In postoperative or critical care settings, HE often is blamed for the prolonged effects of sedation in patients with cirrhosis. In such patients the use of sedatives should be minimized as much as possible, and clinicians must be aware that these drugs may have prolonged effects. Exposure to sedatives and analgesics, especially benzodiazepines, can potentiate the effects of putative neurotoxins in HE and should be avoided.

In patients with persistent encephalopathy or in those with episodic encephalopathy whose symptoms persist after precipitating factors have been treated, specific therapy directed toward encephalopathy is indicated. Modulating the gut bacteria with medication is the mainstay of treatment. The medications used reduce the gut production of ammonia through a variety of mechanisms. Despite maximal medical therapy, HE is refractory in some patients. The medications used for treatment of overt HE are used for all types of HE but are best understood in the context of overt HE.

Medications

As already mentioned, correction of the potential precipitating factor is the first step to treating patients with HE. The following medications are recommended after the initial management of the precipitating factor or in the absence of a clear trigger for HE. Medical management also is recommended to prevent recurrent encephalopathy.

Oral Disaccharides

For many years the nonabsorbable disaccharides lactulose and lactitol have been the mainstay of therapy for HE. Theoretically, lactulose increases ammonia clearance through its cathartic action and decreases ammonia absorption by increasing the stool pH. Many patients show improvement in symptoms of HE within hours of lactulose administration. These agents improve symptoms of encephalopathy, but it is important to note that they do not reduce the mortality rate.

Lactulose also is given to most patients with persistent HE at a dose sufficient to produce two to three soft bowel movements per day. For most patients, 30 mL given every few hours until the goal number of bowel movements is achieved is adequate. Excessive dosing may cause bloating and excessive diarrhea that may compromise patient compliance. Overuse of lactulose also can lead to complications, including dehydration, hypernatremia, and even worsening of HE. Despite these side effects, lactulose remains the most commonly used agent for the treatment of HE. For patients who are unable to take lactulose orally, it can be administered per rectum as a retention enema (300 mL lactulose with 700 mL water).

Low Absorbable Antibiotics

Suppression of toxin production by gut bacteria provides the basis for the use of poorly absorbed antibiotics. Numerous clinical trials have assessed the efficacy of various antibiotics in patients with different grades of encephalopathy. Neomycin and metronidazole classically were used to treat HE; however, the side effects of these medications have limited their use. Limited effectiveness is noted with vancomycin.

Rifaximin, a derivative of rifamycin, originally was developed to treat traveler's diarrhea and has broad-spectrum activity against gram-negative rods and gram-positive cocci. A randomized, double blind, multicenter trial (Bass, et al., 2010) showed superiority of rifaximin over placebo in patients with HE. It is important to note that this was done in the setting of ongoing use of lactulose. Rifaximin can be given safely for long periods of time, another great benefit to the drug. The recommended dose is 550 mg twice a day, in addition to lactulose. The data are mixed about the benefit of rifaximin in HE when used as a single agent. Rifaximin can be used for both overt episodes of HE and in preventing future episodes of HE in conjunction with lactulose.

Polyethylene Glycol

A recent clinical trial in 2014 (HELP trial; Rahimi, 2014) compared polyethylene glycol (PEG) treatment with lactulose treatment in cirrhotic patients admitted to the hospital for HE. Patients were randomized to two groups and received either lactulose (orally, by nasogastric tube, or rectally) or PEG (4 L by mouth or nasogastric tube). When compared with lactulose, patients who received PEG improved significantly faster (1 vs 2 days). It is interesting to note that the patients' ammonia levels did not necessarily correlate with clinical improvement. The theory behind PEG treatment for HE is its strong cathartic effect in clearing out the colon. Although this was only a single-center clinical trial, it poses the question of using cathartic agents for the treatment of HE instead of just lactulose, as discussed previously. Potential side effects of PEG treatment include dehydration and electrolyte imbalances.

Dietary Protein Management

The potential association between dietary protein intake and encephalopathy was first described decades ago. In theory, reducing dietary protein intake should reduce nitrogenous toxin production. Although improvement may be seen in individual encephalopathic patients with dietary protein restriction, this benefit has been difficult to demonstrate in controlled trials. In fact, in several studies of severe acute alcoholic hepatitis, the administration of high-protein, high-calorie diets improved rather than exacerbated encephalopathy. In addition, protein restriction to less than 40 g/day can accelerate catabolism and contribute to malnutrition. During episodes of severe encephalopathy, dietary protein intake is negligible during the first few days in the hospital. Continuing 1.2 to 1.5 g/kg/day protein is important given the high catabolic state of the body during illness.

Other Therapies

Many other therapies for HE have been studied throughout the years but have not become mainstays of treatment because of mixed results in research trials. Branched-chain amino acids in several different formulations improve symptoms but not length of survival, and they are relatively expensive. Probiotics, or isolated cultures of live organisms, are thought to help by reducing substrates available to other gut bacteria, but the evidence remains limited in terms of effectiveness. L-ornithine-L-aspartate (LOLA) lowers plasma ammonia concentrations by enhancing the metabolism of ammonia to glutamine and is used in the treatment of HE outside the United States (Khungar, 2012). Flumazenil, a benzodiazepine antagonist, showed improvement in HE but is not approved by the U.S. Food and Drug Administration (FDA) for the treatment of HE. It is thought to bind endogenous benzodiazepines that are created in the gut, thereby preventing systemic effects. Zinc lowers plasma ammonia by increasing ornithine transcarbamylase activity, but its benefits in HE have been inconsistent.

Hepatic Encephalopathy Associated With Acute Liver Failure

HE is a prominent component of acute liver failure, but it differs from that seen in cirrhosis. Although marked hyperammonemia can be seen in both disorders, cerebral edema with intracranial hypertension is common in acute liver failure but is rarely seen in chronic liver disease. The risk for cerebral edema is correlated to encephalopathic grade. The risk is very low in grades 1 and 2 HE but progresses to 35% in grade 3 and to 75% in grade 4. Some have proposed that markers of systemic inflammation commonly seen in acute liver failure may be a contributing factor. Excess free water with hyponatremia may exacerbate ammonia-induced cerebral edema.

Accurately assessing intracranial pressure (ICP) on clinical grounds is difficult. Physical findings such as papillary changes, abnormalities in oculovestibular reflex, and decerebrate posturing are indicators of intracranial hypertension but often are apparent at an irreversible stage. Consequently, some medical centers advocate the use of invasive monitoring devices, which accurately measure ICP. However, one retrospective report from the U.S. Acute Liver Failure Study reported a 10% complication rate associated with invasive monitoring, of which 5% could have contributed to death. There was also no significant improvement in outcomes in patients subjected to invasive monitoring. In the absence of ICP monitoring, frequent (hourly) neurologic assessment is recommended to identify intracranial hypertension early.

Patients with acute liver failure who develop grade 2 HE should be admitted to an intensive care unit with integrated monitoring and multiorgan support. Patients with grade 3 HE should be ventilated for airway protection, and the head should be elevated to 30 degrees. Intravenous hypotonic solutions should be avoided because of the risk of hyponatremia-induced cerebral edema. Bolus infusions of mannitol (0.5 to 1 g/kg) or hypertonic saline should be given to those patients with objective evidence of increased ICP. Hypothermia to a core body temperature of 34°C to 35°C can be considered as a bridge to liver transplantation. If the patient has acute renal failure and needs renal replacement therapy, continuous mode rather than intermittent dialysis is recommended for stability in cardiovascular and intracranial parameters. More detailed instructions for the management of patients with acute liver failure can be found in the recommendations published by the U.S. Acute Liver Failure Study Group and in the American Association for the Study of Liver Diseases practice guidelines.

SUGGESTED READINGS

Bass N, et al. Rifaximin treatment in hepatic encephalopathy. *N Engl J Med.* 2010;362:1071-1081.

Gentile S, Guarino G, Romano M, et al. A randomized controlled trial of acarbose in hepatic encephalopathy. *Clin Gastroenterol Hepatol.* 2005;3:184-191.

Khungar V, Poordad F. Hepatic encephalopathy. *Clin Liver Dis.* 2012;16: 301-320.

Rahimi RS, Singal AG, Cuthbert JA, Rockey DC. Lactulose vs polyethylene glycol 3350—electrolyte solution for treatment of overt hepatic encephalopathy: the HELP randomized clinical trial. *JAMA Intern Med.* 2014;174: 1727-1733.

Stauch S, et al. Oral L-ornithine-L-aspartate therapy of chronic hepatic encephalopathy: results of a placebo-controlled double-blind study. *J Hepatol.* 1998;28:856-864.

Stepanova M, Mishra A, Venkatesan C, et al. In-hospital mortality and economic burden associated with hepatic encephalopathy in the United States from 2005 to 2009. *Clin Gastroenterol Hepatol.* 2012;10:1034-1041, e1.

Tranah TH, Paolino A, Shawcross D. Pathophysiological mechanisms of hepatic encephalopathy. *Clin Liver Dis.* 2015;5:59-63.

Vilstrup H, Amodio P, Bajaj J, et al. Hepatic encephalopathy in chronic liver disease: 2014 practice guideline by the American Association for the Study of Liver Diseases and the European Association for the Study of the Liver. *Hepatology.* 2014;60:715-735.

THE MANAGEMENT OF BUDD-CHIARI SYNDROME

James P. Hamilton, MD

Budd-Chiari syndrome (BCS) refers to any pathophysiologic process resulting in hepatic venous outflow tract obstruction but most commonly refers to thrombosis of the hepatic veins or the intrahepatic or suprahepatic inferior vena cava (IVC). The vast majority of patients with BCS have an underlying risk factor for thrombosis, although usually this is unrecognized at the time of presentation. Myeloproliferative disorders are the most common underlying thrombotic risk factor for BCS. Others include factor V Leiden mutation; prothrombin G20210A mutation; antiphospholipid syndrome; deficiencies of protein C, protein S, or antithrombin; paroxysmal nocturnal hemoglobinuria; Behçet's disease; hyperhomocysteinemia; MTHFR mutation; ulcerative colitis; hypereosinophilic syndrome; granulomatous venulitis; recent pregnancy; and recent oral contraceptive use. For decades the optimal treatment of BCS involved the creation of a surgical shunt or liver transplantation to relieve the portal hypertension. However, improvements in outcomes with less invasive procedures (i.e., transjugular intrahepatic portosystemic shunt [TIPS]) have changed the management of this life-threatening condition.

■ PRESENTATION AND DIAGNOSIS

The presentation of BCS ranges from asymptomatic in 20% of cases to acute liver failure. Rapid recognition and diagnosis of BCS is critical for initiation of organ and lifesaving medical and interventional treatment strategies. Patients afflicted with this potentially devastating disorder are typically young (ages 20 to 40 years) and most often female. The female predominance (3:1) is thought to be related to the concomitant use of prothrombotic, estrogen-containing oral contraceptives in the setting of previously undiagnosed hypercoagulable state. The classic clinical presentation includes hepatomegaly, right upper quadrant pain, and ascites, followed by jaundice. These clinical findings are the direct consequence of the underlying pathophysiology: hepatic outflow obstruction. Lower extremity edema, portal hypertension–related gastrointestinal bleeding, and hepatic encephalopathy may occur. In acute and subacute presentations of BCS, ascitic fluid analysis typically reveals a serum-ascites albumin gradient of 1.1 g/dL or more, with a total protein greater than 3.0 g/dL. This pattern of laboratory values is indicative of hepatic congestion; therefore diagnostic transthoracic echocardiogram is required to help distinguish between BCS and right-sided heart failure. Ascitic fluid analysis in chronic BCS also reveals a serum-ascites albumin gradient greater than 1.1 g/dL, but the total protein is usually lower than 2.5 g/dL. Serum laboratory abnormalities are often nonspecific. In acute presentations, serum transaminases may be elevated up to 100 times the upper limit of normal. Alkaline phosphatase and bilirubin also may be elevated and gradually worsen with disease

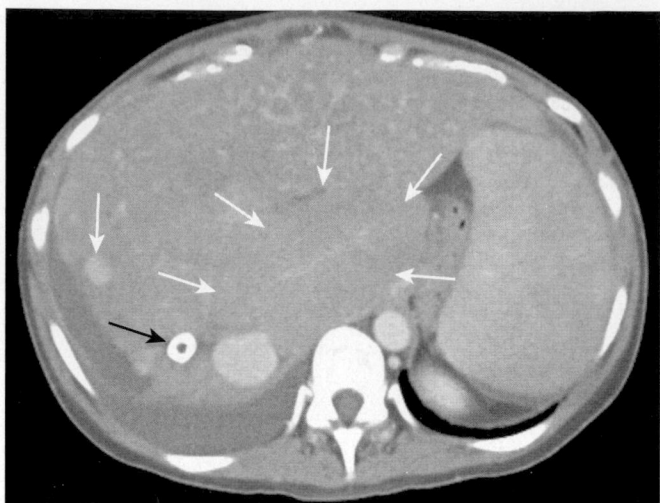

FIGURE 1 Typical computed tomographic scan of a patient with chronic Budd-Chiari syndrome. Note the heterogeneous appearance of the liver parenchyma, regenerative nodules (*small white arrow*), and caudate lobe hypertrophy (*white arrows*). The black arrow points to an occluded transjugular intrahepatic portosystemic shunt.

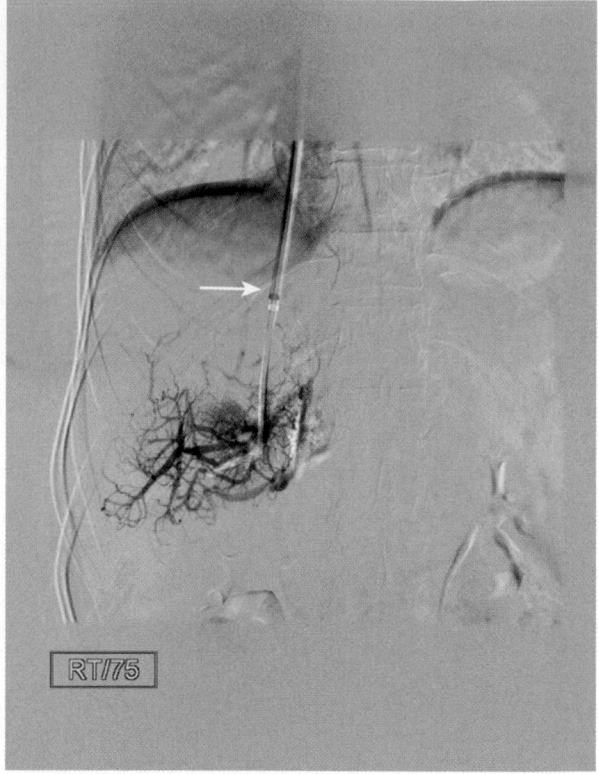

FIGURE 2 "Spiderweb" morphology of small portal venules in Budd-Chiari syndrome as seen on venography. A catheter is seen transcending the liver (*arrow*).

progression. Coagulation studies may be abnormal, with prolonged prothrombin time indicating hepatic synthetic dysfunction, and elevated activated partial thromboplastin time (aPTT) signifying an underlying disorder of coagulation. Interpretation of the complete blood cell count often requires recognition of the overall disease process. In cases where the hepatic vein thrombosis is caused by a myeloproliferative syndrome (i.e., essential thrombocytosis or polycythemia vera), the portal hypertension and associated splenomegaly or splenic sequestration may cause blood counts to fall into the normal range. Finally, a battery of laboratory tests is typically done in order to diagnose a hypercoagulable state, with results specifying a diagnosis in approximately 50% of cases.

In many centers, Doppler ultrasonography is the initial study of choice to evaluate hepatic venous patency. Findings are correlated highly with venography, and Doppler ultrasonography is relatively inexpensive and readily available. Other noninvasive imaging modalities for BCS include computed tomographic (CT) scan or magnetic resonance imaging (MRI), which in addition to characterizing hepatic outflow also may demonstrate parenchymal abnormalities, the degree of ascites, and the presence of caudate lobe hypertrophy. High-quality imaging can be both diagnostic and used to help plan therapeutic intervention. To best visualize the hepatic vessels, it is critical that these cross-sectional imaging modalities are performed with intravenous contrast and dedicated arterial, venous, and washout phases. A classic feature is caudate hypertrophy because the caudate lobe drains into the IVC and is spared from the outflow obstruction in BCS (Figure 1). Typical parenchymal perfusion patterns seen on CT scan or MRI in BCS are early central contrast enhancement with delayed patchy peripheral enhancement and prolonged peripheral retention of contrast. Ascites and splenomegaly may be seen; in addition, concomitant, extrahepatic portal vein thrombosis is present in approximately 15% of patients with BCS.

Hepatic venography remains the gold standard for diagnosing BCS. In addition to diagnosing difficult cases, venography can characterize the obstructive lesion and provides the opportunity to measure portocaval pressures and perform a liver biopsy. Characteristic features of venography in BCS are occlusion of the hepatic veins and a "spiderweb" morphology of the small intrahepatic venules, which are thought to represent collateralization (Figure 2). Histologic findings typical of BCS are centrilobular (zone 3) congestion, necrosis, fibrosis, and in some cases cirrhosis. Intrahepatic portal vein thrombosis can occur and lead to portovenous and portoportal

bridging fibrosis. Regenerative nodules are commonly seen in chronic BCS and may resemble focal nodular hyperplasia on histology and imaging. Hepatocellular carcinoma can develop in the setting of long-standing BCS and, because of alterations in the vascular supply of the liver, may be difficult to distinguish from regenerative nodules on imaging. In this case, targeted biopsies may be necessary to distinguish benign from malignant lesions.

■ TREATMENT

The goals of treatment for BCS are to prevent clot propagation, restore vascular patency, decompress hepatic congestion, and treat complications of portal hypertension. The choice of therapy depends on a variety of factors, including the experience of the center, the availability of interventional radiology, and the patient's clinical presentation (Figure 3). The patency of the portal vein is often a critical factor, as it may render TIPS or portacaval shunt technically impossible.

Medical Therapy

Immediately after diagnostic imaging is performed, anticoagulation with fractionated heparin should begin. The underlying cause of BCS should be investigated thoroughly and treated. The V617F point mutation in the Janus kinase 2 (*JAK2*) gene in myeloid cells is highly specific for myeloproliferative disorders and should be tested in all patients with BCS. Most patients with a predisposing thrombotic disorder will require indefinite anticoagulation, although hydroxyurea and aspirin may be as effective as anticoagulation at preventing thrombosis in some patients with myeloproliferative disorders. Medical treatment for portal hypertension, including sodium restriction and diuretic therapy, also should be initiated. Renal function should be monitored carefully, as the acute portal hypertension

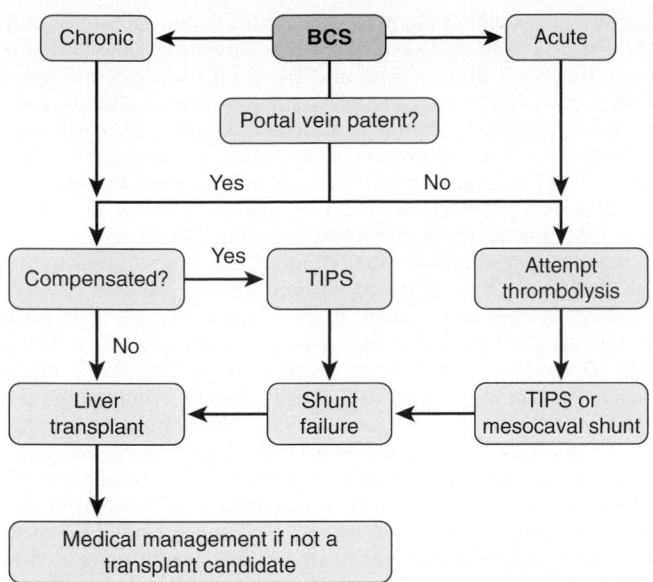

FIGURE 3 Treatment algorithm for patients with Budd-Chiari syndrome (BCS). *TIPS,* Transjugular intrahepatic portosystemic shunt.

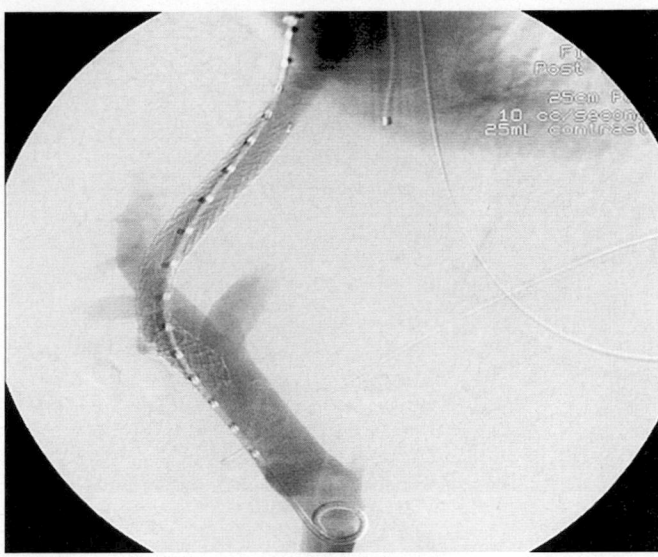

FIGURE 4 Transjugular intrahepatic portosystemic shunt extending from the right portal vein into the right atrium.

caused by BCS may precipitate hepatorenal syndrome. A subset of patients may demonstrate steady clinical improvement and may avoid invasive treatment. However, anticoagulation alone is unlikely to result in adequate venous recanalization, and patients receiving medical therapy only must be monitored closely for disease progression.

Systemic and in situ thrombolytic agents have been used to treat BCS, although this has been poorly studied in controlled trials. There is some evidence that directed thrombolysis is effective, and it can be considered in acute forms of BCS for patients without contraindications. In acute presentation, tissue plasminogen antagonist (TPA) may be delivered directly into the hepatic vascular system through cannulation of the portal vein. This strategy often is used over a period of 12 to 24 hours, with careful monitoring for hemorrhagic complications in an intensive care unit. Thrombolytic agents should not be used in chronic BCS given the low chance of venous recanalization and increased risk for bleeding complications in the setting of portal hypertension.

Interventional Radiology

Most patients with BCS will not improve with medical treatment alone. The role of interventional radiology in managing these patients has become increasingly important. Balloon angioplasty can be used in cases of focal occlusions, such as IVC webs, or short-length hepatic vein stenoses. Vascular reocclusion occurs commonly, and therefore stent placement is recommended if feasible. However, careful consideration must be made before stent placement, as it may interfere with vascular anastomosis if the patient eventually requires orthotopic liver transplantation (OLT). Successful stent placement leads to hepatic decompression, and clinical improvement can be sustained even despite reobstruction. Complications appear to be lower with the transluminal approach compared with the transhepatic approach.

TIPS placement is now the standard of care for the treatment of BCS that has not responded to medical therapy. The rationale for TIPS is to create an intrahepatic shunt from the portal venous system to the proximal hepatic vein or IVC to bypass the obstructed hepatic veins (Figure 4). Historically, TIPS was not considered a durable therapy for BCS because of very high rates of stent occlusion (up to 75% at 1 year). At that time TIPS was considered a bridge to definitive surgical therapies such as liver transplantation or creation of a surgical shunt. However, TIPS has been shown to be very effective even in

patients with severe BCS who have failed medical management. In 2008 Garcia-Pagan and colleagues demonstrated an overall 84% 5-year survival after TIPS for BCS. This same series demonstrated 88% 1-year and 78% 5-year liver transplantation–free survival. TIPS stents are now covered with polytetrafluoroethylene (PTFE). TIPS dysfunction due to stent occlusion is less than 25% annually with these stents. TIPS also can be performed in the setting of BCS and portal vein thrombosis, although the success rate is lower and the procedure may require an attempt of thrombolysis to the portal vein beforehand. TIPS remains a sophisticated procedure and is best performed by skilled interventional radiologists with much experience. Proper patient selection helps to increase the likelihood of success after TIPS. A right-sided echocardiogram should be performed, and TIPS should be avoided in patients with right heart failure. Patients with decompensated liver disease (e.g., Model for End-Stage Liver Disease [MELD] score >17) often do very poorly after TIPS, and these patients should be considered for liver transplantation. The major complication after TIPS is the development of hepatic encephalopathy. This can be managed with nonabsorbable antibiotics and synthetic sugars to induce catharsis. Hepatic encephalopathy is typically not a problem in cases of acute BCS.

Surgical Therapy
Portosystemic Shunting

Blakemore first described the portacaval shunt in the late 1940s (Figure 5). Since then multiple surgical variants have been developed, including splenorenal, mesocaval, and mesoatrial shunts. The choice of technique depends on individual patient factors such as patency of the IVC and extent of caudate lobe enlargement. Several studies show excellent short-term outcomes. However, among four multicenter retrospective analyses of patients with BCS who underwent portosystemic shunt, only one demonstrated a survival advantage with portosystemic shunting after adjusting for Child-Pugh score. In 2012 Orloff and colleagues published results of their prospective cohort of 77 BCS patients treated with surgical portosystemic shunt. Long-term survival was 95% among patients with isolated hepatic vein occlusion treated by side-to-side portacaval shunt after a mean follow-up of 15 years. Mesoatrial shunt for IVC occlusion was associated with a high failure rate and thus discontinued in the authors' series after 1990, but combined side-to-side portacaval shunt with cavoatrial shunt in this population yielded a 100% survival at a mean follow-up of 12 years.

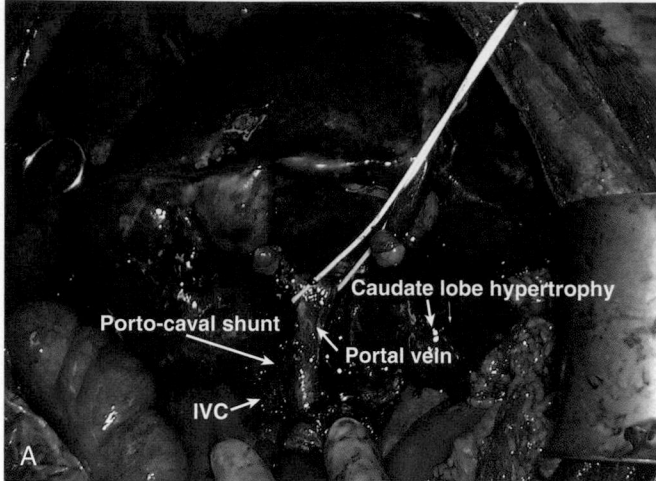

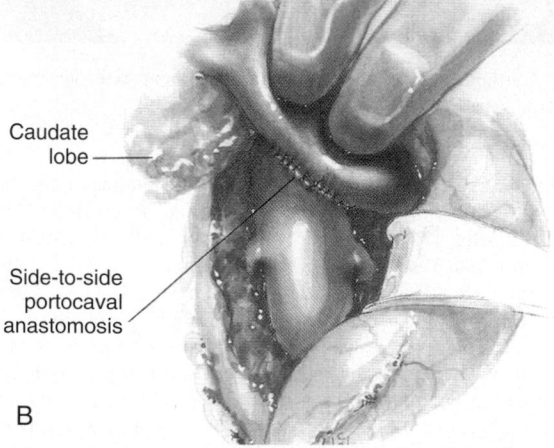

FIGURE 5 Budd-Chiari syndrome with previous portosystemic shunt procedure at the time of orthotropic liver transplantation. **A,** Caudate lobe hypertrophy. **B,** Side-to-side portal-caval shunt. *IVC,* Inferior vena cava.

Not surprisingly, shunt patency is essential to long-term success with portosystemic shunting. This was demonstrated by Bachet and colleagues, who followed 39 patients for a median of 100 months. Shunt dysfunction occurred in 20 patients and was associated with a significantly higher mortality (55% vs 16%). Shunt revision was successful for 7 of the 20 patients with shunt dysfunction, and none of these patients developed refractory ascites or died during follow-up. Because of the increasing availability and success of TIPS for BCS, surgical portosystemic shunting has become less commonly performed at some centers. Nevertheless, surgical portosystemic shunting can be associated with excellent long-term outcomes if performed early in the course of the disease before the development of irreversible liver damage. Referral to an experienced surgeon is essential, and a liver transplantation team should be consulted before performing a surgical shunt.

Liver Transplantation

In patients with decompensated cirrhosis due to BCS, OLT is the only curative option. In 1976 Putnam and Starzl reported the first case of OLT in a 22-year-old female with acute hepatic venous occlusion, noting excellent results at 16-month follow-up. Since then, experience with OLT in the setting of BCS has undergone a dramatic evolution. Early experience with OLT for BCS yielded inferior outcomes, with 3-year survival as low as 45%. In general, two factors have modified the approach and positively influenced outcomes: (1) aggressive initiation of medical and interventional therapy, and (2) anticoagulation. In the modern

era of transplantation for BCS, survival has improved significantly. Mentha and colleagues evaluated 248 patients in the European Liver Transplant Registry who underwent OLT for BCS and found 76% 1-year, 71% 5-year, and 68% 10-year survival. Twenty-seven patients developed venous thrombosis despite anticoagulation, including six with recurrent venous outflow obstruction. Segev and colleagues examined 510 patients transplanted for BCS and found 81% graft survival and 85% patient survival at 3 years post-OLT among those transplanted in the MELD era.

Liver transplantation in the setting of BCS poses several technical challenges. With acute or chronic disease, the liver may be markedly swollen and difficult to manipulate. As well, hyperplasia of the caudate lobe makes access to and dissection of the IVC a difficult endeavor. Concomitant stenosis of the IVC makes suprahepatic and infrahepatic control equally difficult. Although a prior TIPS procedure does not preclude OLT, distal migration of the stent may complicate the portal vein anastomosis. Substantial migration may require transection of the stent with the anastomosis performed directly to the portal vein remnant of the stent in situ. Noted by many institutional experiences, isolation of the hepatic veins for a piggyback anastomosis can be difficult with active outflow occlusion.

Portal vein thrombosis can be a difficult problem, and it requires a strategic plan before transplantation. The portal vein can be thrombectomized routinely, and reasonable flow established, if the superior mesenteric vein (SMV) is patent. If this is not possible, a vein graft with donor iliac vein can be constructed between the donor portal vein and the SMV.

In the setting of complete mesenteric occlusion, two possibilities exist. First, many times these recipients have an extremely large and patent coronary vein because of severe portal hypertension; this vein can be used for portal inflow. Second, anastomosis of the donor portal vein to the recipient's IVC (caval hemitransposition) is an option. Unfortunately, this approach can have extremely high morbidity and mortality.

Because of the aforementioned caudate lobe hyperplasia or caval stenosis, the recipient IVC may not be usable for living donor liver transplantation (LDLT). In 2006 Yan and colleagues reported the first case of an adult-to-adult LDLT for BCS using a cryopreserved iliac vein graft. The authors highlight several important technical issues. In this case it was necessary to incise the diaphragm and expose the pericardium to the level of the right atrium secondary to hepatic venous outflow occlusion. The iliac graft then was sewn to the suprahepatic and infrahepatic venae cavae. The right hepatic vein of the right hepatic lobe allograft then was sewn to the iliac graft in end-to-side fashion.

Alternatively, a large series from Japan reported the long-term outcome in eight patients with BCS who underwent LDLT. Of these patients, five underwent cavoplasty with a replacement vein graft after extensive resection of the thrombosed anterior IVC wall. Although the combined experience with LDLT for BCS is small, the current data suggest living donation as an emerging treatment option for this patient population.

Recurrence of hepatic venous outflow obstruction has been observed in up to 10% of patients, ranging from months to years post-transplant. Consequently, lifelong anticoagulation is currently recommended. Early experience with recurrent BCS post-OLT was associated with an extremely high mortality rate. However, interventional techniques have provided some alternatives to retransplantation or death. Recurrent BCS can be approached in two ways. Retransplantation is an option in patients with mild to moderate thrombus burden in the hepatic veins and IVC refractory to an interventional approach. However, the anatomic features of the recurrent thrombus must be delineated carefully; recipients with a completely occluded IVC and portal vein are unlikely to be candidates for retransplantation. In severe cases, TIPS can be used to re-establish flow in one or more hepatic veins in the setting of preserved liver function.

Finally, there is no evidence to suggest that OLT increases the risk of malignant transformation of underlying myeloproliferative disease in patients with BCS.

■ SUMMARY

Budd-Chiari syndrome is a life-threatening condition that can be treated successfully when a timely diagnosis is made and the proper therapy is applied. Initial treatment with anticoagulation followed by placement of a TIPS is the standard of care for patients with well-compensated liver function. Long-term follow-up of patients who undergo TIPS has demonstrated excellent transplant-free survival, and stent failure is now uncommon. Although select centers have a robust experience with surgical portosystemic shunt procedures, most institutions initially use interventional radiologic procedures for those with acute or subacute onset of disease.

Although long considered the most viable long-term treatment option for patients with all forms of BCS, liver transplantation typically is reserved for patients with decompensated liver disease or recurrent stent or shunt failure.

SELECTED READINGS

Cameron JL, Maddrey WC. Mesoatrial shunt a new treatment for Budd-Chiari syndrome. *Ann Surg.* 1978;187:402-406.

Darwish MS, Plessier A, Hernandez-Guerra M, Fabris F, Eapen CE, Bahr MJ, Trebicka J, Morard I, Lasser L, Heller J, Hadengue A, Langlet P, Miranda H, Primignani M, Elias E, Leebeek FW, Rosendaal FR, Garcia-Pagan JC, Valla DC, Janssen HL. EN-Vie (European Network for Vascular Disorders of the Liver). Etiology, management, and outcome of the Budd-Chiari syndrome. *Ann Intern Med.* 2009;151:167-175.

Menon KV, Shah V, Kamath PS. The Budd-Chiari syndrome. *N Engl J Med.* 2004;350:578-585.

Molmenti EP, Segev DL, Arepally A, Hong J, Thuluvath PJ, Rai R, Klein AS. The utility of TIPS in the management of Budd-Chiari syndrome. *Ann Surg.* 2005;241:978-983.

Srinivasan P, Rela M, Pracgalias A, et al. Liver transplantation for Budd-Chiari syndrome. *Transplantation.* 2002;73:973-977.

Zimmerman MA, Cameron AM, Ghobrial RM. Budd-Chiari syndrome. *Clin Liver Dis.* 2006;10:259-273.

recommended to patients with gallbladder polyps and concurrent gallstones. However, with regard to prevention of biliary complications from gallstone disease, prophylactic cholecystectomy for patients with both polyps and gallstones could be considered.

Gallbladder Wall Calcifications

There are two pathologic variations of calcification in the gallbladder. Selective mucosal calcification represents focal calcium deposits in the mucosa of the gallbladder wall. Diffuse intramural calcification (commonly called *porcelain gallbladder*) involves a diffuse band of calcium infiltrating the muscular layer of the gallbladder wall.

Older reports indicated a gallbladder malignancy incidence as high as 60% with a porcelain gallbladder, and historically, porcelain gallbladder has been an absolute indication for prophylactic cholecystectomy because of this association. In recent years, this axiom has been called into question. Chen and colleagues reviewed 192 patients with porcelain gallbladder between 2008 and 2013, of which 102 underwent cholecystectomy and 90 were observed. None of the cholecystectomy patients demonstrated malignancy on pathology review, and none in the observation group developed gallbladder malignancy during mean follow-up of $3\frac{1}{2}$ years. The cholecystectomy group did, however, have a higher risk of postoperative complications, some requiring additional endoscopic and percutaneous interventions leading to increased morbidity and costs associated with the procedure.

Stephen and colleagues reported a higher incidence of gallbladder malignancy among patients with selective mucosal calcifications compared with patients with diffuse intramural calcifications. A meta-analysis by Schnelldorfer demonstrated an overall 6% malignancy incidence among patients with gallbladder wall calcifications, compared with 1% of matched patients without calcifications. Furthermore, patients with focal gallbladder calcifications had a significantly higher rate of malignancy than those with diffuse calcification (35% vs 16%). These data suggest that the pattern of calcification dictates the risk of developing cancer because patients with complete calcification have no mucosa left to create an adenocarcinoma.

The decision to proceed with prophylactic cholecystectomy in an asymptomatic patient with gallbladder wall calcification should be individualized to the patient, given a potentially preventative or curative outcome of surgery, weighed against the perioperative morbidity and mortality.

Gastric Cancer

Cholelithiasis is seen more frequently in patients who have undergone surgery for gastric cancer. Several theories for this association exist. Denervation of the parasympathetic and sympathetic branches is a likely factor and is associated with the extent of lymphadenectomy and resection. Patients have a higher risk of developing gallstones after total gastrectomy, and D3 or D2 lymphadenectomy when compared with distal gastrectomy or D1 lymphadenectomy, respectively. Duodenal exclusion as part of reconstruction also is known to result in an increased rate of cholelithiasis, attributed to decreased secretion of cholecystokinin. Other proposed factors include the rapid weight loss that accompanies total gastrectomy, and biliary stasis resulting from edema and inflammation around the bile ducts.

Proponents of prophylactic cholecystectomy at the time of gastric surgery cite benefits that include avoiding reoperation in cases of acute acalculous cholecystitis, and avoidance of complex ERCP or common bile duct exploration in the presence of Roux-en-Y anatomy for postoperative choledocholithiasis or cholangitis.

Small Bowel Resection

Two groups of patients undergoing small bowel resection merit consideration for prophylactic cholecystectomy. Patients with short gut syndrome or those who will be left with short gut after surgery are at increased risk of developing symptomatic cholelithiasis. The pathophysiology is multifactorial but includes altered enterohepatic circulation of bile salts from ileal resection and prolonged parenteral nutrition requirements. The ongoing risk of acalculous cholecystitis should also factor into decision making in patients with severe illness. Although prophylactic cholecystectomy concomitant with extended small bowel resection may not extend life, it can prevent further complications in an otherwise palliative situation. Furthermore, prophylactic cholecystectomy in these patients can prevent the need for reoperation in an otherwise hostile abdomen, decreasing the risk of injury to small bowel and adjacent structures during future cholecystectomy.

The second group in which to consider prophylactic cholecystectomy are those patients with intestinal carcinoid syndrome who will require long-term somatostatin analog therapy. Somatostatin inhibits cholecystokinin resulting in decreased gallbladder motility and promotes lithogenesis. One study found new gallstones developed in 63% of patients treated with somatostatin analogues for intestinal carcinoid, with 17% requiring cholecystectomy within 5 years of initiating treatment. Prophylactic cholecystectomy therefore should be considered at the time of small bowel resection for carcinoid tumor if somatostatin therapy is to be used.

Hemoglobinopathy

Patients with sickle cell disease (SCD) are at a greater risk of gallstone disease and biliary complications compared with the general population. Cholelithiasis is observed in 70% of adults with SCD over the age of 30. The incidence of cholelithiasis in children nears 40% as they approach adulthood. Patients with SCD have a higher rate of biliary complications; 50% develop complications within 5 years of gallstone detection. Furthermore, it may be hard to distinguish an episode of vaso-occlusive crisis from biliary complications because both may be accompanied by fever, abdominal pain, leukocytosis, and jaundice.

Muroni and colleagues compared a cohort of SCD patients undergoing prophylactic cholecystectomy for asymptomatic cholelithiasis with those undergoing cholecystectomy for symptomatic cholelithiasis. The symptomatic group had a significantly higher rate of choledocholithiasis discovered during intraoperative cholangiography. There was no significant difference in postoperative morbidity or mortality between the two groups, although the study size may have been too small to appreciate a difference. Prophylactic cholecystectomy for adults with sickle cell disease with asymptomatic cholelithiasis is safe and should be considered strongly given the high rate of progression to symptomatic disease.

Similarly, patients with hereditary spherocytosis (HS) are at an increased risk of cholelithiasis. Long-term data have shown that patients without gallstones who undergo splenectomy are at minimal risk of developing gallstone disease in the future. Patients with symptomatic disease benefit most from combined splenectomy and cholecystectomy. Patients under the age of 50 with asymptomatic gallstones also will benefit from combined splenectomy and cholecystectomy, although this decision may have to be individualized. Given the fact that splenectomy abates the lithogenic process in patients with HS, there is no role for prophylactic cholecystectomy in these patients.

Not unsurprisingly, laparoscopic cholecystectomy can be performed safely in isolation or concomitantly with splenectomy for symptomatic cholelithiasis in patients with beta-thalassemia. There are limited data to evaluate the role of prophylactic cholecystectomy in thalassemia patients with asymptomatic cholelithiasis.

Transplant

The management of asymptomatic cholelithiasis deserves special consideration in the solid organ transplant population. In general, there is an increased prevalence of gallstones in transplant recipients, increased morbidity from infectious biliary complications, and increased mortality from emergent cholecystectomy post-transplantation.

Kao and colleagues demonstrated that kidney and pancreas transplant candidates and recipients benefit more from expectant management of asymptomatic cholelithiasis. On the other hand, cardiac transplant patients represent a different demographic. Kilic and colleagues used the Nationwide Inpatient Sample database to review heart transplant recipients who underwent cholecystectomy between 1998 and 2008. Heart transplant recipients who underwent urgent surgery, open cholecystectomy, or who had complicated gallstone disease were found to have high rates of inpatient mortality. These data suggest a role for prophylactic cholecystectomy in heart transplant recipients with asymptomatic or uncomplicated gallstone disease.

Spinal Cord Injury

Spinal cord injury patients are at increased risk of gallstone disease, with multiple studies demonstrating an incidence of 30% or more. That said, the incidence of biliary complications, 2.2%, is similar to the general population. The level of spinal cord injury and the mechanism (traumatic vs degenerative) have no proven correlation with presence of gallstone disease. Expectant management should be the rule for patients with asymptomatic cholelithiasis. Cholecystectomy is indicated for patients with symptomatic gallstone disease, although it is a difficult diagnosis to make in those with high spinal cord injuries.

Bariatric Surgery

Obesity has long been known to increase the risk of gallstone disease. Surgery for obesity, including Roux-en-Y gastric bypass, increases the risk of developing symptomatic gallstones, attributed to the rapid weight loss that follows. The incidence of symptomatic gallstones requiring cholecystectomy after bariatric surgery varies widely but is reported to be as high as 30%. The use of prophylactic cholecystectomy in patients undergoing laparoscopic Roux-en-Y gastric bypass surgery has not been answered definitively; however, three standard approaches to these patients have been applied widely: (1) prophylactic cholecystectomy for all patients undergoing gastric bypass surgery, (2) selective cholecystectomy in patients with gallstones or biliary symptoms, or (3) a watch-and-wait approach with or without prophylactic ursodeoxycholic acid.

Proponents of the first approach cite the possibility of late, severe biliary complications, such as choledocholithiasis or biliary pancreatitis, which can be difficult to treat in the setting of altered foregut anatomy. However, severe biliary complications have been shown to be rare, occurring in less than 1% of gastric bypass patients. Furthermore, most episodes of severe biliary complications are preceded by at least one episode of biliary colic, which can signal the need for early elective rather than urgent or emergent intervention. Data on the safety of concomitant prophylactic cholecystectomy vary. Some studies show no increase in perioperative morbidity, minimal additional operative time, and an unchanged length of stay. However, a nationwide study by Worni and colleagues noted a higher perioperative complication and mortality rate among patients who had concomitant cholecystectomy at the time of gastric bypass. Opponents to the routine cholecystectomy approach cite increased operative time and the technical difficulty of performing cholecystectomy in a patient with obese body habitus, compared with the postbypass patient with significant weight loss.

There are limited data on the management of patients with asymptomatic cholelithiasis who then undergo gastric bypass surgery.

Given the lack of evidence in this arena, some surgeons have adopted a more selective approach to gallstones, performing cholecystectomy at the time of gastric bypass only when gallstone pathology (cholelithiasis, sludge, polyps) or a history of biliary symptoms has been identified preoperatively.

Ursodeoxycholic acid has been used as prophylaxis against gallstone formation in the first 6 months after gastric bypass surgery. One meta-analysis of five randomized controlled trials revealed an 8.8% rate of gallstone formation in the ursodeoxycholic acid group compared with 27.7% in the placebo group. Cost and medication side effects limit patient compliance and therefore its general application.

Management of gallstones in patients undergoing bariatric surgery remains controversial. Concurrent cholecystectomy for patients with biliary symptoms identified preoperatively is supported by the data. Expectant management for patients with preoperative ultrasound demonstrating either a normal gallbladder or cholelithiasis without biliary symptoms is also acceptable. Subsequent laparoscopic cholecystectomy for patients who develop symptoms can be performed safely.

SUGGESTED READINGS

Cabarrou P, Portier G, Chalret Du Rieu M. Prophylactic cholecystectomy during abdominal surgery. *J Visc Surg.* 2013;150:229-235.

Chen GL, Akmal Y, DiFronzo AL, Vuong B, O'Connor V. Porcelain gallbladder: no longer an indication for prophylactic cholecystectomy. *Am Surg.* 2015;81:936-940.

Choi SY, Kim TS, Kim HJ, Park JH, Park DI, Cho YK, Sohn CI, Jeon WK, Kim BI. Is it necessary to perform prophylactic cholecystectomy for asymptomatic subjects with gallbladder polyps and gallstones? *J Gastroenterol Hepatol.* 2010;25:1099-1104.

Gracie WA, Ransohoff DF. The natural history of silent gallstones: the innocent gallstone is not a myth. *N Engl J Med.* 1982;307:798-800.

Gurusamy KS, Davidson BR. Surgical treatment of gallstones. *Gastroenterol Clin North Am.* 2010;39:229-244.

Kao LS, Flowers C, Flum DR. Prophylactic cholecystectomy in transplant patients: a decision analysis. *J Gastrointest Surg.* 2005;9:965-972.

Kilic A, Sheer A, Shah AS, et al. Outcomes of cholecystectomy in US heart transplant recipients. *Ann Surg.* 2013;258:312-317.

Marchetti M, Quaglini S, Barosi G. Prophylactic splenectomy and cholecystectomy in mild hereditary spherocytosis: analyzing the decision in different clinical scenarios. *J Intern Med.* 1998;244:217-226.

Moonka R, Stiens SA, Resnick WJ, McDonald JM, Eubank WB, Dominitz JA, Stelzner MG. The prevalence and natural history of gallstones in spinal cord injured patients. *J Am Coll Surg.* 1999;189:274-281.

Muroni M, Loi V, Lionnet F, Girot R, Houry S. Prophylactic laparoscopic cholecystectomy in adult sickle cell disease patients with cholelithiasis: a prospective cohort study. *Int J Surg.* 2015;22:62-66.

Norlen O, Hessman O, Stalberg P, Akerstrom G, Hellman P. Prophylactic cholecystectomy in midgut carcinoid patients. *World J Surg.* 2010;34:1361-1367.

Schnelldorfer T. Porcelain gallbladder: a benign process or concern for malignancy? *J Gastrointest Surg.* 2013;17:1161-1168.

Silen W. *Cope's Early Diagnosis of The Acute Abdomen.* New York: Oxford; 2010.

Stephen AE, Berger DL. Carcinoma in the porcelain gallbladder: a relationship revisited. *Surgery.* 2001;129:699-703.

Stinton LM, Myers RP, Shaffer EA. Epidemiology of gallstones. *Gastroenterol Clin North Am.* 2010;39:157-169.

Uy MC, Talingdan-Te MC, Espinosa WZ, Daez ML, Ong JP. Ursodeoxycholic acid in the prevention of gallstone formation after bariatric surgery: a meta-analysis. *Obes Surg.* 2008;18:1532-1538.

Worni M, Guller U, Shah A, Gandhi M, Shah J, Rajgor D, Pietrobon R, Jacobs DO, Ostbye T. Cholecystectomy concomitant with laparoscopic gastric bypass: a trend analysis of the nationwide inpatient sample from 2001 to 2008. *Obes Surg.* 2012;22:220-229.

THE MANAGEMENT OF ACUTE CHOLECYSTITIS

Peter J. Fagenholz, MD, and George Velmahos, MD, PhD, MSEd

Acute cholecystitis (AC) is acute inflammation of the gallbladder usually resulting from obstruction of the cystic duct with gallstones. Diagnosis is based on a combination of clinical signs and physical examination findings (most important, right upper quadrant abdominal pain and tenderness) and imaging showing cholelithiasis and/or gallbladder inflammation. Standard treatment is prompt laparoscopic cholecystectomy, although selected patients may be managed medically or with percutaneous cholecystostomy tube placement. Surgeons should be prepared to convert planned laparoscopic cholecystectomy to open cholecystectomy and be familiar with bailout options for the sometimes difficult cholecystectomies encountered in patients with AC.

■ CLINICAL PRESENTATION, EVALUATION, AND DIAGNOSIS

Patients with AC typically experience upper abdominal pain that localizes to the right upper quadrant and lasts for more than 6 hours. A history of prior similar episodes that were shorter in duration or less severe often can be elicited. Patients may have a known history of gallstones either identified during evaluation for prior episodes of abdominal pain or identified incidentally on imaging studies performed for other reasons. Nausea and vomiting are frequently present, fever less so. The most common physical examination finding is right upper quadrant abdominal tenderness. Murphy's sign, inspiratory arrest with palpation over the gallbladder, is the classic physical examination finding. All of these signs and symptoms may be muted or absent in patients who are obese, have diabetes, are on steroids or otherwise immunosuppressed, or have impaired sensorium.

The most important differential diagnosis is between AC and other biliary tract disease, such as biliary colic or choledocholithiasis. A number of other intra-abdominal diseases, such as pancreatitis, peptic ulcer disease, mesenteric ischemia, hepatitis, and colitis, and extraabdominal disease such as myocardial ischemia and pneumonia occasionally may resemble AC. History taking and physical examination should focus on narrowing this list to appropriately direct further laboratory and imaging tests.

There are no diagnostic laboratory studies. A mild leukocytosis is common. Liver function tests are typically normal or only mildly elevated and are helpful primarily in differentiating AC from other forms of complicated gallstone disease, such as choledocholithiasis and cholangitis, or medical liver disease such as acute hepatitis. Marked abnormalities in serum bilirubin, alkaline phosphatase, or transaminases should prompt consideration of an alternative diagnosis. Serum amylase and lipase should be sent to evaluate for acute pancreatitis.

The optimal choice of imaging test depends primarily on the pretest probability for AC relative to other forms of intra-abdominal pathology. Ultrasonography, computed tomography (CT), cholescintigraphy (HIDA scan), and magnetic resonance imaging (MRI) are capable of identifying AC with variable sensitivity and specificity and have different levels of cost and availability. Using them correctly depends on the clinical scenario. For patients with a typical presentation and a high clinical suspicion for AC, transabdominal ultrasound is the current diagnostic test of choice. It is inexpensive, requires no ionizing radiation, is widely available, and is more than 90% sensitive for detection of cholelithiasis. Signs of AC on ultrasound include pericholecystic fluid, gallbladder wall thickness greater than 4 mm, gallbladder distension, a gallstone lodged in the neck of the gallbladder, and a sonographic Murphy's sign. However, ultrasound, although very sensitive for the detection of gallstones, is only about 60% to 70% sensitive for detecting these "objective" signs of AC. Thus the scenario in which a patient has a convincing clinical presentation for AC, followed by an ultrasound showing gallstones, but no objective ultrasonographic signs of cholecystitis is a common one. In this scenario, for surgically low-risk patients, we recommend proceeding to cholecystectomy, confident that the patient either has AC (as diagnosed clinically) or at least significantly symptomatic gallstone disease that merits cholecystectomy.

Scenarios frequently arise in which the orderly progression from history, to physical examination, to laboratory evaluation, to ultrasonography, to a diagnosis of AC does not occur. It is very common for surgeons to be consulted in patients who come to the emergency department with abdominal pain and after initial evaluation undergo CT scanning as the first radiologic test. When the CT scan shows evidence of AC, is a subsequent ultrasound necessary? We would argue rarely or never. Although not the first-line test for AC and poorly sensitive for cholelithiasis, CT is actually more sensitive than ultrasound for detecting objective signs of AC such as pericholecystic fluid or inflammation and gallbladder wall thickening (Figure 1). It is also the most versatile test for evaluating the other entities usually considered in the differential diagnosis of AC. If a CT scan shows AC and no other diagnosis is suggested strongly by the clinical presentation or CT scan, there is little to no utility to performing ultrasonography just to demonstrate stones in the gallbladder.

Another common scenario is the patient with an atypical clinical presentation for AC, in whom ultrasonography demonstrates stones but no clear evidence of AC. Are these incidentally found stones in a patient with some other pathology, or are they the true source of the problem? After reviewing the patient and clinical data, the surgeon must decide whether there is a significant risk of intra-abdominal pathology not related to the biliary tract. If there is significant concern for other intra-abdominal pathology as the source of the patient's symptoms, we usually perform abdominal CT scanning with intravenous contrast. It is the test most likely to either confirm the diagnosis of AC and rule out an alternative diagnosis or to provide an alternative explanation for the patient's symptoms. The other commonly used test to evaluate for acute cholecystitis when the diagnosis is unclear after clinical evaluation and ultrasonography is HIDA. Although HIDA is highly sensitive and specific for cholecystitis, it is not as widely available as CT and if negative for acute cholecystitis, it provides no useful information regarding other possible diagnoses. Thus we use it very selectively.

■ MANAGEMENT

Cholecystectomy is the standard treatment for AC and has the advantage of not only treating the current episode but also removing the risk of subsequent bouts of AC and other biliary tract complications related to gallstones. All patients diagnosed with AC should receive appropriate antibiotics. The decision regarding which of the following treatment options to use depends on the overall medical condition of the patient and the severity and duration of symptoms. Patients with minimal medical comorbidities presenting early in their disease generally should be managed surgically, those with significant comorbidities but mild AC may merit a trial of medical therapy, and those who are critically ill or have severe medical comorbidities and severe AC are managed best with percutaneous cholecystostomy.

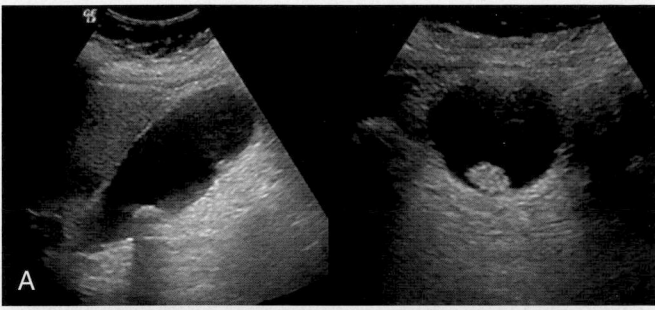

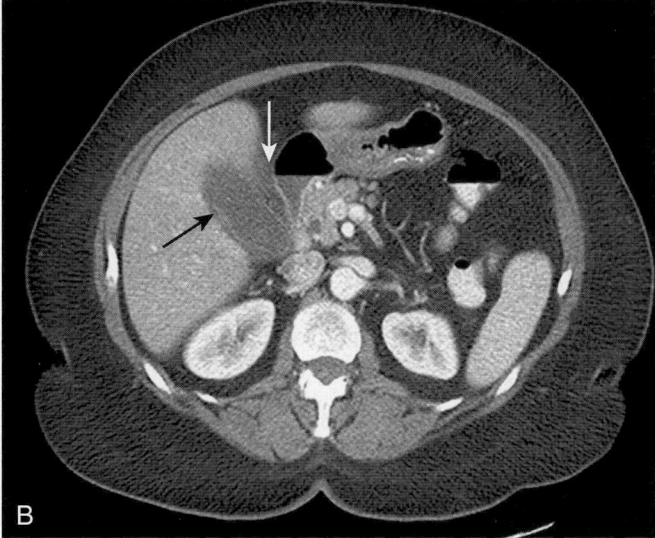

FIGURE 1 Computed tomographic and ultrasound images of a patient with acute cholecystitis. **A,** Ultrasound shows cholelithiasis without any objective evidence for acute cholecystitis. **B,** Computed tomography (B) shows pericholecystic fluid *(black arrow)* and stranding *(white arrow)*. Surgery revealed an inflamed gallbladder and pathology showed acute and chronic cholecystitis. *(From Fagenholz PJ, Fuentes E, Kaafarani H, et al. Computed tomography is more sensitive than ultrasound for the diagnosis of acute cholecystitis. Surg Infect [Larchmt]. 2015;16:509-512.)*

Cholecystectomy

Cholecystectomy is standard treatment for patients with AC and should be performed within 72 hours of onset of symptoms, the sooner the better. Alternatives to cholecystectomy and when to apply them are discussed later. Once the decision is made to operate, there is nothing to be gained by waiting, and prompt surgery provides quicker relief to the patient, limits overall hospital stay, and avoids progressive inflammation that can worsen as days pass and make dissection more difficult. Laparoscopic cholecystectomy is the procedure of choice, but surgeons must be familiar with both laparoscopic and open techniques because the conversion rate in AC is 10% to 20%.

Laparoscopic Cholecystectomy

Laparoscopic cholecystectomy is the approach of choice in AC because multiple studies have demonstrated less morbidity, shorter hospital stays, less time until return to normal function, and lower costs with the laparoscopic approach. The technique of laparoscopic cholecystectomy for AC is fundamentally the same as for elective cholecystectomy; for other indications, the procedures are just harder. The basic steps of patient positioning, equipment, abdominal access, exposure of the gallbladder and cystic structures, dissection of the cystic structures until a critical view of safety is obtained, and judicious use of cholangiography when needed to define the anatomy

are the same and are described in detail elsewhere in this book. We discuss a few factors specific to cholecystectomy for acute cholecystitis.

Simply grasping an inflamed gallbladder may be problematic, and this often can be aided by decompression. Occasionally decompression can be accomplished with a purpose made laparoscopic needle-aspirator, but this is often too small to achieve effective decompression in acute cholecystitis. A 14-gauge angiocatheter needle placed through a tiny stab incision has a better chance of success. If this does not achieve adequate decompression a 5-mm laparoscopic trocar can be driven directly into the fundus of the gallbladder and a suction aspirator used to evacuate the gallbladder. If this technique is used, an endoloop can be used to close the cholecystotomy to prevent stone spillage. Standard laparoscopic graspers may not be able to effectively grasp the thickened and edematous gallbladder wall in acute cholecystitis. This is not a mere nuisance, it is an actual danger because ineffective gallbladder retraction, especially laterally, is a risk factor for bile duct injury. Tripod graspers or large claw graspers may be able to effectively grasp an inflamed gallbladder when standard 5-mm toothed graspers cannot. It is worth identifying a piece of equipment at your home institution that is effective for this purpose.

Once the gallbladder is rendered graspable, the dissection begins. Adjacent structures, usually omentum, duodenum, and sometimes transverse colon or mesocolon must be peeled off the gallbladder. This is best done by identifying the plane where the structure meets the gallbladder and peeling bluntly downward parallel to the gallbladder wall rather than pulling outward. Adhesions to the adjacent liver capsule may be tougher than the capsule itself and so should be divided with scissors or electrocautery before this blunt dissection to avoid bleeding from a capsular tear. Once the gallbladder is exposed, the cystic dissection begins. As with any laparoscopic cholecystectomy the peritoneum and fatty tissue surrounding the cystic structures must be cleared. Inflammation may pull the gallbladder in close to the porta hepatis, and so we often begin in cases of acute cholecystitis by rotating the gallbladder medially and bluntly stripping the peritoneum and tissue lateral to the cystic structures. This is a relatively safe area to work in initially because it is away from the portal structures, and releasing this lateral peritoneum often improves the amount of lateral retraction that is possible when dissecting in Calot's triangle. Because of edema, electrocautery may be less effective in some cases of AC than in most elective cholecystectomies, and thus blunt dissection may be more useful. The suction irrigator or a laparoscopic peanut dissector can be used for this. Some small capillary oozing may be seen in cases of AC, and this usually can be swept away bluntly as the dissection continues. It is critical to maintain the same standards of visualization as during an elective cholecystectomy. Although it may be harder to obtain the critical view of safety, the same standards of anatomic definition must be applied in cases of AC. Some authors have advocated a "top-down" laparoscopic dissection, beginning at the gallbladder fundus, when inflammation impairs the initial cystic dissection. We are not advocates of this technique unless it is used regularly in elective cases because it leaves the surgeon using an unfamiliar technique in only the hardest cases.

Occasionally the cystic duct may be foreshortened and/or thickened because of acute and chronic inflammation. If it is too wide to safely close with standard clips, an endoloop or laparoscopic stapler may be used. In either case when a duct appears too large to clip, the surgeon must be absolutely sure, either by dissection or cholangiography, that it is in fact the cystic duct. Once that is clear, the endoloop or stapler should be applied so as not to narrow the common bile duct. If stapling, we usually use a 30-mm long linear cutting stapler with 2.5-mm staples. Once the cystic structures are divided safely, the gallbladder must be removed from the liver bed. This is a curiously underdiscussed portion of the operation that can still result in problems if not done correctly. A significant portion of bile leaks after laparoscopic cholecystectomy are related to subvesical ducts, most of which course through the liver parenchyma just deep to the gallbladder fossa. Maintaining adequate tension with the retracting instruments and staying in the correct areolar plane of dissection minimizes this complication as well as bleeding from the liver parenchyma.

Finally, although we have attempted to provide a few tips relevant to accomplishing laparoscopic cholecystectomy in cases of acute cholecystitis, when the anatomy cannot be defined clearly because of inflammation or other factors, there should be no hesitation to convert to an open procedure (described later). Although morbidity is increased somewhat by an open approach, this small increase is nothing compared with the morbidity of a major bile duct or vascular injury, which may occur when persisting laparoscopically with inadequate exposure or dissection. It is very hard to find a surgeon who regrets converting a laparoscopic cholecystectomy to open, but there is no shortage of surgeons who regret persisting laparoscopically in cases of unclear anatomy with sometimes disastrous results.

Open Cholecystectomy

Because laparoscopic cholecystectomy is the standard procedure in cases of acute cholecystitis, most open cholecystectomies in this setting occur as a conversion from a laparoscopic procedure. There are very few conditions that mandate open cholecystectomy with no attempt at laparoscopy, but there are a number of risk factors for conversion to open cholecystectomy, including obesity, long duration of symptoms, cirrhosis, and male sex. Keeping in mind these risk factors, there are some theoretical advantages to performing planned open cholecystectomy rather than converting from a laparoscopic approach. Operating time and equipment costs can be reduced and planning for postoperative analgesia, including regional anesthesia, can be performed prospectively. In some series the highest complication rates are in cholecystectomies converted to laparoscopic to open, often after laparoscopic misadventure. It is possible that correctly identifying these difficult cases and starting with an open approach could limit some of these complications.

Both upper midline and right subcostal incisions provide excellent exposure for open cholecystectomy. We prefer a fundus-down technique, in which the fundus is grasped and separated from the liver edge with electrocautery. The medial and lateral peritoneal leaves overlying the gallbladder are incised with cautery, and the hepatic attachments are dissected either with cautery or bluntly with fingers or a suction catheter. When the infundibulum is reached, lateral retraction helps expose the cystic duct and artery, which are ligated.

Bailout Options

Even experienced surgeons will encounter gallbladders that cannot be removed safely. Options depend on when this is recognized. Ideally it will be recognized preoperatively, and patients will be treated nonoperatively as described later. If difficulties are recognized while the gallbladder is relatively intact or if the patient has medical instability early in the procedure, cholecystostomy tube is an excellent option. If the problem is that the gallbladder is fused to the liver and efforts to separate it result in repeated injury to the hepatic parenchyma with bleeding and associated risk of bile leak, then the back wall of the gallbladder abutting the liver can be wholly or partially left in place and the mucosa cauterized to reduce the risk of mucocele. If the cystic structures cannot be dissected safely out from a hostile porta hepatis, then subtotal cholecystectomy is acceptable and far preferable to risking significant injury to adjacent structures. If subtotal cholecystectomy is performed, we remove all stones from the gallbladder and then either oversew a small remaining cuff of infundibulum attached to the cystic duct, or if that is not possible because of poor tissue

quality, we attempt to identify the cystic duct orifice from within the lumen of the gallbladder and oversew it from within. After performing any of these bailout maneuvers, we leave a closed suction drain.

Complications and Postoperative Care

Major bile duct injury is the most discussed, feared, and morbid complication of cholecystectomy and is discussed at length in different sections of this book. We only can reiterate that the key to prevention is complete dissection of the cystic structures with judicious use of cholangiography as needed to help define the anatomy. If injury does occur, the key is to recognize it. Partially visualized clipping to control bleeding should be avoided and, if performed, should be followed by a careful postclipping analysis of the anatomy. The source of any bile leakage in the field should be identified clearly. If it is rundown from a small grasper-related tear in the gallbladder fundus, there is no cause for worry, but that should be ascertained clearly rather than assumed. After completion of the cholecystectomy, the area should be surveyed actively for any bile leakage and the source identified. Techniques for repair of bile duct injury are discussed elsewhere, but even if the operating surgeon is not comfortable performing these, early identification, drainage, and transfer to a center of expertise for definitive management can limit morbidity.

Most bile leaks after cholecystectomy are not related to undiagnosed major bile duct injuries but to leakage from the cystic duct stump or small subvesical ducts. When the surgeon perceives a higher-than-average risk of this, closed suction drainage should be left. This can include cases in which the gallbladder was exceptionally adherent to the liver parenchyma so that subvesical ducts may be at risk, cases with poor cystic duct tissue quality, or cases in which bailout maneuvers described earlier were used. Leaks in these scenarios may not be immediately apparent in the operating room. Because most patients undergoing such difficult cholecystectomies for AC will at least spend the night in the hospital, we remove these drains immediately before discharge if there is no evidence for bile leak. If a small leak is present, it usually will heal with drainage alone. If patients have biloma because of an unanticipated leak in an undrained case, percutaneous radiologically guided drainage should be used. Once a bile leak is drained, the next decision is usually whether to perform endoscopic retrograde cholangiopancreatography (ERCP) with sphincterotomy and/or common bile duct stent placement to decompress the biliary tree. The advantages of ERCP in this setting are that it can identify the source of the leak, reduce the volume of bile leakage, and reduce the time to healing and drain removal. The disadvantage is that it is yet another procedure with its own risks of complications. In general, we tend to avoid immediate ERCP if we have an anticipated low-volume bile leak that is adequately drained, such as may occur after one of the bailout maneuvers described earlier. If we have an unanticipated or high-volume bile leak, then we tend to use ERCP to define the anatomy as well as decompress the biliary system.

Bile and gallstone spillage is common during cholecystectomy for AC. Bile should be irrigated and aspirated, and an effort should be made to retrieve any dropped gallstones. Sludge and small stones may be difficult to retrieve but also pose the lowest risk of postoperative complication. Larger stones can result in abscess formation and a more extensive effort to retrieve them should be made. Postoperative drainage should be used infrequently, generally in cases in which there is significant concern for postoperative bile leak. Postoperative antibiotics should similarly be used very rarely, typically only in cases with ongoing SIRS or sepsis. Pulmonary complications including pneumonia and reintubation are not uncommon after open cholecystectomy. Strong consideration should be given to regional anesthesia with transversus abdominis plane block, paravertebral block, or epidural anesthesia both for patient comfort and to limit the risk of serious pulmonary complications.

Medical Management

As discussed earlier, medical therapy generally should be used for patients with moderate to severe medical comorbidities and mild AC. Antibiotics are the cornerstone of medical management for AC. Although only about half of patients with AC will have positive bile cultures, there is no reliable method for identifying who these patients are, and there is no other medical therapy specific for the disease. The most common organisms are enteric gram negatives (*Escherichia coli, Klebsiella* spp., *Enterobacter* spp.), anaerobes (bacteroides, clostridium), enterococci, and streptococci; antibiotic therapy should cover these all empirically. A number of antibiotic regimens can provide needed coverage. A typical duration of coverage is 7 to 14 days, although there are very few data regarding the optimal duration of treatment. As noted earlier in patients undergoing surgery, antibiotics generally should be discontinued postoperatively. Analgesia with acetaminophen, nonsteroidal anti-inflammatories, and opiates should be used until pain resolves and supportive intravenous fluids until adequate oral intake is tolerated. If patients do not improve clinically within 72 hours, strong consideration should be given to using percutaneous or surgical treatment. Studies report a greater than 85% response rate for medical therapy with most patients untroubled by recurrent biliary events over short-term follow-up (1 to 3 years).

Percutaneous Drainage

Percutaneous cholecystostomy (PC) should be used in patients who fail medical therapy, have contraindications or are high risk for general anesthesia, have severe AC particularly with local complications such as adjacent liver abscess, or have a prolonged duration of symptoms (more than 3 to 4 days), which may increase the risk of cholecystectomy and the possibility of open conversion. PC is approximately 90% effective in relieving symptoms. It usually is performed under local anesthesia or light sedation with ultrasound guidance. Minor complications, such as catheter dislodgement or blockage, occur in about 15% of cases; more serious complications such as bleeding or bile leakage occur in less than 1% of cases.

We usually perform contrast injection of the tube in 4 to 6 weeks. If the cystic duct is patent, then the tube can be removed. The risk of recurrent AC or other biliary complications after PC is poorly defined, and reports range from 10% to 50%. Thus the decision about whether to perform interval cholecystectomy can be individualized on the basis of patient age and surgical risk. If the cystic duct remains occluded, we leave the tube in place until the time of cholecystectomy.

Endoscopic Therapy

Endoscopic therapy for AC can consist of transpapillary stenting or transmural drainage. Transpapillary stenting uses ERCP to place a stent into the gallbladder via the cystic duct. This is usually left to internally drain into the duodenum and eventually is removed endoscopically. Transpapillary stenting is technically successful in 80% to 90% of cases and is as effective (about 90%) as PC in resolving symptoms. The technique requires sphincterotomy and so incurs small risks of post-sphincterotomy bleeding, perforation, and pancreatitis. Transmural drainage involves puncturing the gallbladder under endoscopic ultrasound guidance, dilation of the tract, and placement of a stent. Newer lumen-apposing covered stents may provide long-term internal drainage.

Special Situations

Pregnancy

The differential diagnosis of AC in pregnant patients includes all of the entities mentioned earlier as well as several pregnancy-specific entities, such as HELLP syndrome and acute fatty liver of pregnancy. The traditional teaching that cholecystectomy should be avoided in the first and third trimesters of pregnancy is challenged by actual evidence suggesting that laparoscopic cholecystectomy is at least as safe as nonoperative management in all trimesters. Nonetheless, data less specific to cholecystectomy suggest that fetal organogenesis may be affected by laparoscopic surgery in the first trimester and that surgery during the third trimester may precipitate preterm labor. We typically pursue same admission cholecystectomy during the second trimester in low-risk patients (short duration of symptoms, medically low risk). In the first and third trimesters we usually attempt medical management followed by PC if needed as a bridge to cholecystectomy in the second trimester or postpartum period, respectively.

Acalculous Cholecystitis

Acalculous cholecystitis is an inflammatory condition of the gallbladder not resulting from gallstones. It results from gallbladder stasis and ischemia, often leading to secondary infection and typically occurs in critically ill patients. Treatment options are the same as for calculous AC. Because of the usually poor medical condition of patients with acalculous cholecystitis and the fact that they are not at risk for recurrent complications of gallstones, PC is a much better option as "destination therapy" in acalculous than in calculous disease. We usually reserve cholecystectomy for patients who have evidence for perforation or who fail to improve after PC, which may be due to gallbladder necrosis.

SUGGESTED READINGS

Baron TH, Grimm IS, Swanstrom LL. Interventional approaches to gallbladder disease. *N Engl J Med.* 2015;23:357-365.

Fagenholz PJ, de Moya MA. Acute inflammatory surgical disease. *Surg Clin North Am.* 2014;94:1-30.

Fagenholz PJ, Fuentes E, Kaafarani H, et al. Computed tomography is more sensitive than ultrasound for the diagnosis of acute cholecystitis. *Surg Infect (Larchmt).* 2015;16:509-512.

Yeh DD, Cropano C, Fagenholz P, et al. Gangrenous cholecystitis: deceiving ultrasounds, significant delay in surgical consult, and increased postoperative morbidity. *J Trauma Acute Care Surg.* 2015;79:812-816.

MANAGEMENT OF COMMON BILE DUCT STONES: LAPAROSCOPIC COMMON BILE DUCT EXPLORATION

Byron F. Santos, MD, and Steven M. Strasberg, MD

Choledocholithiasis is present in approximately 5% of patients who require surgery for symptomatic cholelithiasis. Common duct exploration and endoscopic retrograde cholangiopancreatography (ERCP) are two techniques available for stone removal. The classical surgical approach was open common duct exploration, which is rarely done today. Instead bile duct exploration may be performed laparoscopically in most cases via the cystic duct or through a choledochotomy. Although laparoscopic common bile duct exploration (LCBDE) techniques are highly successful, only about 7% of common duct stones are managed by LCBDE, with the vast majority being treated by ERCP. This chapter describes the two laparoscopic techniques for duct exploration. A short summary of the now uncommon technique of open exploration is also given at the end of the chapter.

A single-stage laparoscopic procedure is the preferred treatment for choledocholithiasis in the presence of symptomatic cholelithiasis in many centers. Several randomized trials have shown that LCBDE, which is done with laparoscopic cholecystectomy (i.e., a single-stage approach), is equivalent in terms of ductal clearance and morbidity to laparoscopic cholecystectomy plus preoperative or postoperative ERCP, but leads to shorter lengths of stay and lower costs. Postoperative ERCP also may have a failure rate of 4% to 10%, resulting in a risk of requiring a return to the operating room for open common bile duct exploration.

Although outcomes data support the use of LCBDE, a survey of practicing general surgeons has found that few actually perform this procedure. Reasons given for not performing laparoscopic exploration were time constraints, lack of equipment, inadequate endoscopic backup, and insufficient laparoscopic technical capabilities. There is a striking difference between the rapid and widespread adoption of laparoscopic cholecystectomy and the slow and localized use of laparoscopic bile duct exploration. Adoption of LCBDE should be encouraged and LCBDE should be used by surgeons able to perform this advanced laparoscopic technique in the management algorithm for choledocholithiasis.

■ PATIENT SELECTION

Patients in whom cholecystectomy is indicated for gallstones, regardless of the degree of suspicion for choledocholithiasis, may be advised to pursue a surgery-first approach consisting of laparoscopic cholecystectomy with intraoperative cholangiography (IOC) and LCBDE if necessary. Contraindications to a surgery-first approach include patients with hemodynamic instability from ascending cholangitis (better served with ERCP), patients in whom a malignant process is suspected (require appropriate workup to evaluate for malignancy), and patients with general contraindications to laparoscopic cholecystectomy (e.g., coagulopathy, hemodynamic instability).

Clinical characteristics that should alert the surgeon to an increased risk of choledocholithiasis include older age, jaundice, dark-colored urine, acholic stools, gallstone pancreatitis, cholangitis, elevated liver function tests, and a dilated common bile duct or cystic duct and choledocholithiasis on preoperative imaging. Although the overall incidence of choledocholithiasis in the United States likely has fallen, there may be populations in whom choledocholithiasis is still prevalent, including patients without access to regular health care, older patients, and veterans. In these patients, the incidence of choledocholithiasis during laparoscopic cholecystectomy may be up to 15% to 20%. Surgeons should be aware that choledocholithiasis may persist despite ERCP and that stones may enter the duct after ERCP and before surgery. Therefore intraoperative cholangiography should still be used liberally when ERCP has preceded cholecystectomy. Patients should be counseled preoperatively on the possibility of finding choledocholithiasis and the therapeutic options (LCBDE, open common bile duct exploration [OCBDE], or postoperative ERCP). Patients should be prepared for the possibility of additional procedures postoperatively (ERCP or reoperation) should LCBDE fail, as well as for the possibility of drain placement if necessary.

■ SURGICAL PLANNING FOR LCBDE

The ideal situation is when the surgeon has confirmation of choledocholithiasis preoperatively (positive imaging finding or preoperative ERCP with residual stones). The surgeon can then prepare the needed equipment and staff for the procedure ahead of time. More commonly, the diagnosis of choledocholithiasis is made intraoperatively. Having the necessary equipment (Table 1) readily available, preferably in a kit or cart, makes for an expedient procedure.

Routine considerations that are recommended for all laparoscopic cholecystectomy cases but are essential to LCBDE include having a C-arm compatible operating table and room. The C-arm should be positioned to enter the field from the left side of the patient, as the surgeon will utilize the right midclavicular trocar for cholangiography and LCBDE access. Trocar placement for LCBDE is similar to a standard four-port laparoscopic cholecystectomy except that the midclavicular trocar can be placed more cephalad and lateral than usual to facilitate transcystic manipulations. Additional 5-mm trocars may be placed for this purpose or to facilitate suturing during choledochotomy if necessary.

■ INTRAOPERATIVE IMAGING

Use of routine biliary imaging (cholangiography or ultrasound) not only is associated with a decreased risk and severity of bile duct injuries during laparoscopic cholecystectomy, but also allows the surgeon to evaluate the patient for the presence of choledocholithiasis with a sensitivity and specificity approaching 99%. Routine cholangiography, in particular, facilitates the performance of LCBDE, as the surgeon and operating team already will have performed the first key steps of LCBDE.

Technical aspects of cholangiography that facilitate LCBDE include the use of an Olsen clamp along with a 5F open tip catheter (Figure 1, A) through the midclavicular port. This allows for a precise and controlled cannulation and fixation onto the cystic duct. Routine use of a 5F catheter allows the surgeon to use a 0.035-inch hydrophilic wire for difficult cannulations or to gain wire access for transcystic LCBDE. Once the catheter is secured to the cystic duct, the instrument retracting the gallbladder fundus should be clamped to the drape or to the patient with a penetrating towel clip to maintain exposure while freeing up the assistant for other tasks.

■ DECISION MAKING

The cholangiogram should be evaluated to define the anatomy of the cystic duct and its junction with the biliary tree; the presence of filling defects, including their number, size, and location (proximal or distal to the cystic duct–common bile duct junction); and the diameter of the common bile duct. The 5-mm diameter of the cholangiogram clamp can be used as a reference measurement. Small distal stones

TABLE 1: Equipment List for Laparoscopic Common Bile Duct Exploration (LCBDE)*

Instrument	Manufacturer	Product No.
DISPOSABLE		
Cholangiogram catheter, 5F	Cook	G29145
Common bile duct exploration set:	Cook	G26908
0.035-inch hydrophilic guidewire	Cook	G09607
8-mm × 4-cm wire-guided dilation balloon	Cook	G36347
12F access sheath	Cook	G08297
High-pressure inflation device	Cook	G31027
Nitinol wire basket	Cook	G36251
Laparoscopic endobiliary stent, 7F	Cook	G13699
1 L normal saline irrigation bag with pressure cuff		
Tubing for continuous irrigation with connector to choledochoscope		
Laparoscopic ligating loop (absorbable)		
REUSABLE		
Olsen cholangiogram clamp	Karl Storz	28378CH
Flexible 8.5F choledochoscope	Karl Storz	11292AD1
Laparoscopic padded grasper (for grasping the choledochoscope)	Karl Storz	33551PG
Separate laparoscopy tower with camera, light source, and monitor		

*Note: Manufacturers and product numbers listed are examples. Other suppliers may be available for certain products.

(3 mm or less) sometimes can be successfully flushed past the ampulla with saline while administering intravenous glucagon (should be avoided in patients taking beta-blockers) or nitroglycerin to induce relaxation of the sphincter of Oddi.

A transcystic approach is possible when a limited number of small distal stones are encountered in a patient with favorable cystic duct anatomy. The advantage of a transcystic approach is that an incision in the common bile duct can be avoided. The disadvantages of a transcystic approach are that proximal stones may be impossible to reach and large stones may require fragmentation or choledochotomy to remove. The ideal situation is when the cystic duct is generous in size (at least 5 mm) and has a lateral insertion on the common bile duct. Transcystic LCBDE should not be performed when the common duct diameter is very small (i.e., 3 mm or less) because the possibility of bile duct injury is too great and the stones are so small that they likely will pass spontaneously or are actually air bubbles.

In contrast to transcystic LCBDE, transcholedochal LCBDE is performed through an incision in the common bile duct, just distal to the cystic duct–common hepatic duct junction. This approach requires the ability to suture the common bile duct once

stone extraction is completed but is favored by some surgeons, as it provides complete access to the upper and lower biliary tree and is more versatile when the surgeon encounters stones that are large in size or number. This approach carries a risk of bile leaks and common bile duct strictures, however. To minimize the risk of strictures, transcholedochal LCBDE should be avoided in patients with bile ducts smaller than 7 mm and should be performed only by surgeons who are facile with advanced laparoscopy and suturing.

■ TRANSCYSTIC LCBDE

Cystic Ductotomy

If the cystic duct is large and minimally tortuous, the ductotomy already made for the cholangiogram near the gallbladder neck can be used. Otherwise, an incision closer to the common bile duct may enable an easier cannulation into a larger and less tortuous segment of the cystic duct. Additional dissection closer to the cystic duct–common bile duct junction may be necessary in some cases and should be done with care.

Wire Access

With the cholangiogram catheter in place, a 0.035-inch hydrophilic guidewire can be passed through the catheter under fluoroscopy until it coils in the duodenum. The Olsen clamp is then withdrawn over the wire. The assistant can help by pinning the wire just above the level of the cystic duct with a grasper to maintain wire access during instrument exchanges. An access sheath is passed over the wire through the port to reduce internal bowing of the catheter-directed instruments and to create a better seal for pneumoperitoneum.

Balloon Dilation

Routine balloon dilation of the cystic duct is recommended, as it not only makes it easier to traverse the valves of Heister in the cystic duct with instruments, but also creates a larger channel for stone removal through the cystic duct. A balloon dilator (Figure 1, B) is advanced over the guidewire and positioned in the cystic duct with fluoroscopic guidance. Ideally this balloon should cross the cystic duct–common bile duct junction and the location of the ductotomy so that the entire cystic duct is dilated uniformly. If necessary, the cystic duct can be dilated sequentially if the balloon is not long enough. The cystic duct should not be dilated beyond the diameter of the common bile duct so as to avoid injuring the cystic duct–common bile duct junction. Dilation should be done under fluoroscopy and with a high-pressure balloon inflation device (Figure 1, C) filled with dilute contrast. Balloon inflation should be held for about 3 minutes to allow the duct to gently dilate.

Stone Clearance

Several methods of transcystic stone clearance have been described. Wire baskets (Figure 1, D) may be passed through the cystic duct into the common bile duct (preferably through a cholangiogram catheter to reduce trauma to the bile duct or the creation of false passages) to trawl for stones with or without fluoroscopic guidance. Fogarty biliary balloons also may be used to dislodge stones or pull them out retrograde through the cystic duct, but this method sometimes may cause proximal stone migration into the hepatic ducts.

The use of a flexible choledochoscope to directly visualize and capture stones with a wire basket is the most direct way to ensure clearance of the biliary tree during LCBDE. Traditional fiber optic choledochoscopes require a separate camera, light source, and monitor, but new video choledochoscopes have a distal video chip, integrated light source, picture-in-picture capability, and improved resolution. The choledochoscope is connected to a pressurized saline irrigation bag to distend the bile ducts and clear debris during choledochoscopy (Figure 2).

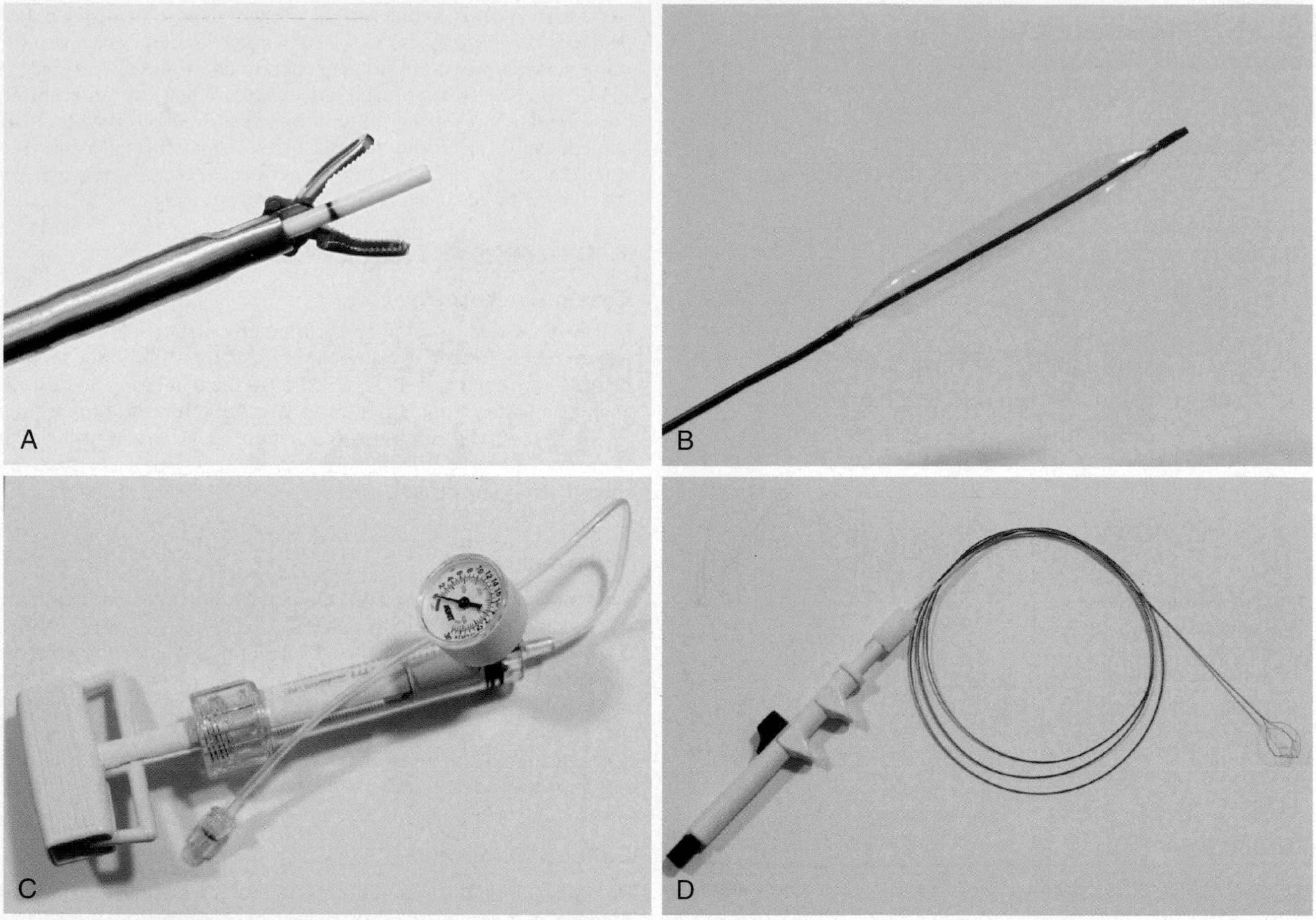

FIGURE 1 Instruments used during laparoscopic common bile duct exploration (LCBDE). **A,** Olsen cholangiogram clamp with 5F cholangiocatheter. **B,** Wire-guided balloon dilator. **C,** High-pressure balloon inflation device. **D,** Wire basket for use through a choledochoscope working channel.

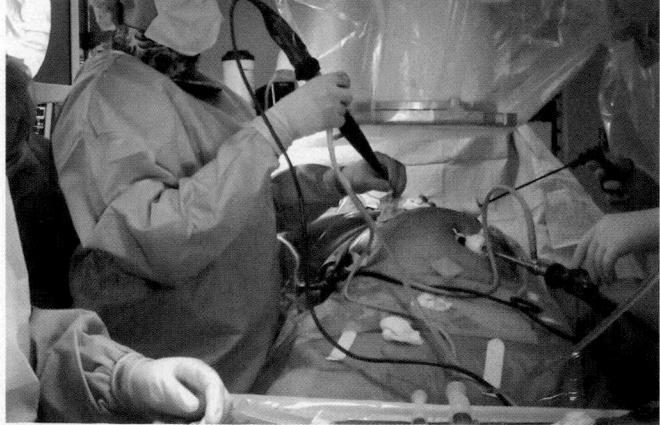

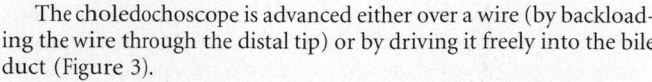

FIGURE 2 External view of room setup for laparoscopic common bile duct exploration (LCBDE). The surgeon uses the midclavicular trocar to pass the flexible choledochoscope. An assistant maintains the laparoscopic view and uses a grasper for assistance. A C-arm is in position for maneuvers performed under fluoroscopy (wire access and balloon dilation).

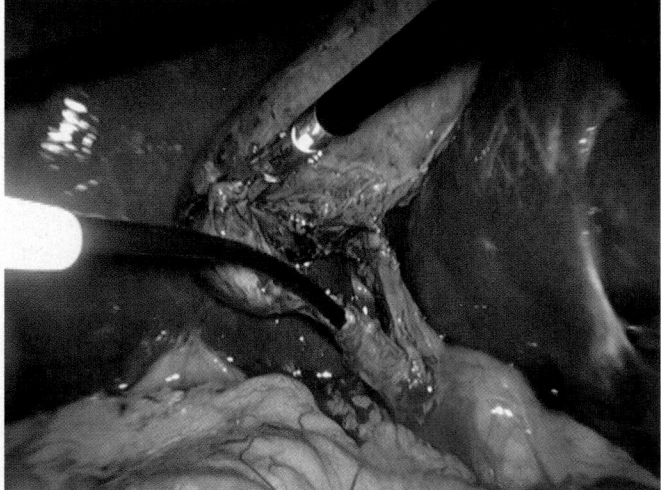

FIGURE 3 Transcystic laparoscopic common bile duct exploration (LCBDE). The flexible choledochoscope is advanced into the common bile duct through a cystic ductotomy.

The choledochoscope is advanced either over a wire (by backloading the wire through the distal tip) or by driving it freely into the bile duct (Figure 3).

The choledochoscope occasionally may be directed proximally toward the hepatic ducts but generally is limited to visualization of the distal common bile duct. Stones are visualized (Figure 4, *A*) and wire baskets are passed through the working channel of the scope in a closed configuration. Once the wire basket is advanced beyond the stone, the basket is opened and pulled back until it engages the stone (Figure 4, *B*). The scope and basket containing the stone are held

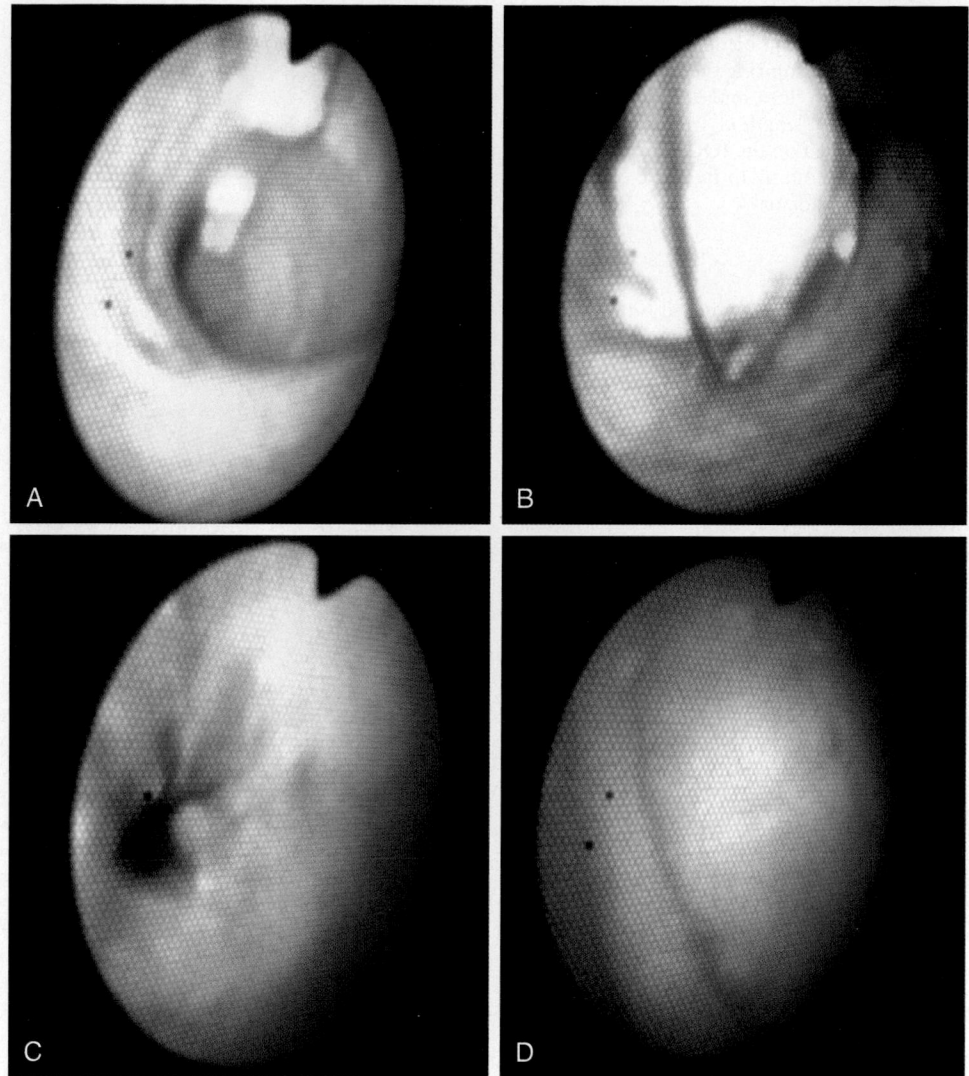

FIGURE 4 Flexible choledochoscope images seen during laparoscopic common bile duct exploration (LCBDE). **A,** Small common bile duct stones. **B,** Stone captured by a wire basket. **C,** Patent ampulla as seen from within the bile duct. **D,** Duodenal lumen with characteristic folds visible.

tightly together and pulled out through the cystic duct. After clearance of all visible stones, the choledochoscope usually can be advanced gently past the ampulla (Figure 4, *C*) until the folds of the duodenal mucosa are visualized (Figure 4, *D*). If the stones are too large for transcystic removal, laser lithotripsy can be used through the choledochoscope to fragment the stones for easier removal. Shock wave lithotripsy also may be used but may be more traumatic to the wall of the common bile duct. Small stones sometimes may be pushed or flushed past the ampulla with the choledochoscope. Dilation of the ampulla also may be done under fluoroscopy but should be done with caution, as this may cause pancreatitis or bile duct injury (if the balloon diameter is larger than the diameter of the common bile duct).

Duct Closure

A closing cholangiogram should be performed to check for residual stones and to rule out bile duct injury resulting from the procedure. It is preferable to use a ligating loop on the cystic duct stump for added security rather than clips, given that the cystic duct has been manipulated and may not hold clips well. Clips should be placed to mark the cystic duct stump radiographically. Drain placement is not routinely necessary.

■ TRANSCHOLEDOCHAL LCBDE

Transcholedochal LCBDE may be performed in patients unfit for a transcystic approach or in those where a transcystic approach has failed, although some surgeons use a transcholedochal approach exclusively. Alternatives to transcholedochal exploration in the case of a failed transcystic exploration include postoperative ERCP or conversion to OCBDE. Transcholedochal LCBDE should be reserved for patients with a common bile duct diameter of at least 7 mm to reduce the risk of long-term stricture. It should not be performed in the setting of severe inflammation of the porta hepatis. The final decision on management strategy should depend on the stone burden, surgeon skill and experience, and available local resources (e.g., ready access to a skilled endoscopist to perform ERCP).

Exposure and Ductotomy

The first step is to expose the anterior supraduodenal common bile duct. If there is doubt as to the location of the choledochus, a fine-needle aspiration may be used to aspirate bile to confirm its location. Lateral and upward traction on the cystic duct will help expose the anterior common bile duct. A longitudinal opening is made sharply on the anterior aspect of the bile duct. The ductotomy may be created with a specialized laparoscopic knife (Berci Micro Knife, Karl Storz, Tuttlingen, Germany), fine shears, or a #11 blade held with a locking grasper. Care should be taken to avoid injuring the arteries supplying the choledochus, typically at the 3 o'clock and 9 o'clock positions. The opening should be extended to a length of 1 to 2 cm or slightly larger than the largest stone identified on the IOC. Stay sutures may be placed on either side of the ductotomy to facilitate elevation of the bile duct but this step is not mandatory.

Stone Clearance

Once the ductotomy is made, stones may be flushed out of the bile duct or captured with the choledochoscope as previously described for transcystic LCBDE. The choledochoscope should be directed both proximally and distally in the biliary tree to ensure complete stone clearance.

Duct Closure

The traditional way to close the choledochotomy is with fine 4-0 absorbable sutures over a T-tube. T-tubes have been used with the goal of decompressing the biliary tree to protect the closure, holding the duct open to reduce stricture formation as it heals, and facilitating percutaneous access to the bile duct in the case of retained stones. Typically a 14F or larger T-tube is used and prepared by the surgeon by trimming and beveling the ends of the tube and removing a portion of the back wall of the intraductal portion of the tube to facilitate removal. The tube may be used to perform a postoperative cholangiogram before removal in the office, usually 3 weeks postoperatively.

The use of T-tubes for transcholedochal LCBDE is controversial, however, as T-tubes are known to be associated with problems such as discomfort and inconvenience for the patient, bile leaks or prolonged fistulas after removal, and early dislodgement. Also, they can make the closure of the ductotomy more technically challenging. Primary closure for laparoscopic choledochotomy appears to be a safe and acceptable option based on current literature. Closure is performed in a longitudinal, running, or interrupted fashion with fine 4-0 absorbable sutures. Adjuncts to primary closure also have been proposed, including ampullary stenting to decompress the biliary tree or external biliary drainage (through the cystic duct stump). After closure of the choledochotomy, a closing cholangiogram should be performed either through the T-tube or through the cystic duct stump to confirm a watertight closure. Closed suction drainage is recommended to monitor the closure for a postoperative bile leak.

Antegrade Biliary Stenting

The use of plastic stents placed in an antegrade fashion across the ampulla from a laparoscopic approach has expanded the armamentarium of the laparoscopic surgeon. Ampullary stents can be used when stone clearance is incomplete, when there is ampullary edema, when protecting a primary closure, or as an alternative to LCBDE (combined with postoperative ERCP). Compared with T-tubes, stents offer a way to decompress the biliary tree without the need for external biliary drains. Plastic stents may be passed through the cystic duct or through the choledochotomy used for LCBDE and positioned across the ampulla with conventional endoscopic delivery systems or with a 7F stent delivery system designed for laparoscopic placement (Figure 5). Transcystic placement of the stent typically requires the same initial procedures as transcystic LCBDE. A cholangiogram is performed and the position of the ampulla is marked on the screen for reference. Wire access across the ampulla is achieved and a balloon dilator is used to dilate the cystic duct to allow passage of the delivery system. Next, the stent delivery system is advanced over the wire and the stent is positioned across the ampulla and deployed under fluoroscopy. A closing cholangiogram confirms the

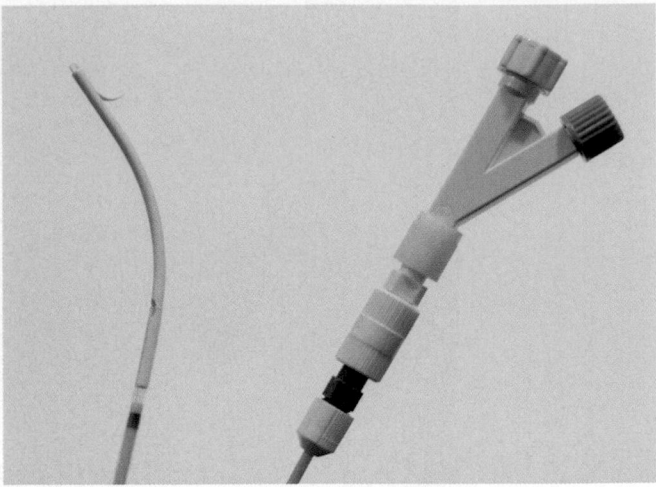

FIGURE 5 Ampullary stent deployment system. A 7F plastic stent is visible on the left of the image, with a wire-guided deployment mechanism on the right.

position of the stent and should demonstrate brisk emptying of contrast from the bile duct. When used in cases of retained stones or as an alternative to LCBDE, stent placement converts an urgent ERCP into an elective outpatient procedure that can be scheduled after the patient has recovered from the cholecystectomy. In addition, the presence of an ampullary stent facilitates cannulation of the bile duct, which may improve the success rate of postoperative ERCP, especially for less skilled endoscopists. Although useful as adjuncts in certain situations, biliary stents are not without risks, with reports of complications such as stent migration, occlusion, cholangitis, acute pancreatitis, stent erosion of the bile duct and duodenum, and early dislodgement. The ultimate role of biliary stents in the laparoscopic management of choledocholithiasis remains to be defined.

Results of LCBDE

The success rate of LCBDE in terms of stone clearance depends on whether a transcystic or transcholedochal approach is used. A transcystic approach may be successful in up to 70% of patients when using choledochoscopy and basket extraction through the cystic duct. A transcholedochal approach improves the success rate to around 95% to 98%, making it the preferred approach for some surgeons.

Complications specific to transcystic exploration may include bile leak, pancreatitis, retained stones, and bile duct injury from excessive traction or manipulation of instruments (wire baskets, balloons, etc.). Transcholedochal exploration has a similar complication profile but carries a higher risk of bile leak (around 5% to 15%) because of the need for choledochotomy closure.

To date, there have been several randomized trials that have compared single-stage management with two-stage management (preoperative ERCP plus laparoscopic cholecystectomy) for patients with suspected choledocholithiasis. These trials have demonstrated similar stone clearance rates and morbidity for each approach, with shorter hospital stays and lower costs for the single-stage approach.

The management of choledocholithiasis discovered intraoperatively has been studied in two randomized trials that demonstrated similar stone clearance rates and morbidity, but with potentially shorter hospital stays for the patients undergoing single-stage management.

The efficacy of LCBDE compared with the gold standard of OCBDE was also evaluated in a prospective randomized trial in 2012. This trial included 256 patients and showed that LCBDE could achieve a stone clearance rate of 71% with an initial transcystic approach. Subsequent laparoscopic choledochotomy increased the clearance rate to 94%, versus 97% for OCBDE through a choledochotomy. Complications were similar but LCBDE resulted in a lower wound infection rate and a shorter hospital stay.

Training Surgeons in LCBDE

The traditional surgical teaching paradigm of "see one, do one, teach one" has failed to educate a generation of surgeons in the techniques of CBDE, which were considered in the mainstream of general surgical practice during the "open" era. Except for residents who train at centers where LCBDE is the primary approach to choledocholithiasis, the majority of graduating chief residents in the United States perform on average less than one LCBDE during their entire residency, according to a study by Bell examining Accreditation Council for Graduate Medical Education (ACGME) case logs for graduating residents from 2005. This minimal experience is inadequate for competency in this procedure. Yet, despite this situation, there are factors that have the potential to increase the use of LCBDE in the future. Today's residents are trained in an environment where laparoscopy has become the standard of care for many operations and perform greater numbers of advanced laparoscopic cases during their training than did their predecessors. In addition, they are required to perform more flexible endoscopic procedures than in the past and they have greater exposure to wire-guided and catheter-based techniques as a result of the endovascular revolution. The skill set of advanced laparoscopy, flexible endoscopy, and catheter-based interventions makes today's residents uniquely suited to learn LCBDE. Economic pressures also may encourage the adoption of LCBDE, as it is more cost effective than two-stage management. The proliferation of bariatric surgery also has led to a large population of gastric bypass patients with high rates of symptomatic gallstones and anatomy that makes LCBDE more feasible than ERCP. On a national level, there is also a movement to change the culture of laparoscopic cholecystectomy. A group of Society of American Gastrointestinal and Endoscopic Surgeons (SAGES) leaders, in an editorial in *Surgical Endoscopy* in 2013, has called on surgeons to "first, do no harm; [and] second, take care of bile duct stones."

The training of surgeons in the techniques of LCBDE should start with the adoption of routine imaging as an essential component of laparoscopic cholecystectomy. In addition, simulation-based curriculums have been developed that have been shown to improve residents' performance in the techniques of LCBDE. Such initiatives have translated to increased clinical use of the procedure at tertiary care centers such as Northwestern University in Chicago. Although it may be unrealistic to train most surgeons to become competent in transcholedochal LCBDE, the techniques of transcystic LCBDE should be within the reach of most surgeons who perform laparoscopic cholecystectomy and may allow surgeons to once again provide comprehensive, single-stage management of patients with choledocholithiasis.

■ OPEN COMMON BILE DUCT EXPLORATION

OCBDE for extraction of gallstones is performed rarely today. Its chief indication is failure of other techniques.

Major principles of OCBDE are:

■ A bile duct of 5 mm or less is a relative contraindication and a bile duct of 3 mm or less is an absolute contraindication to OCBDE. Stones smaller than 3 mm in diameter usually pass spontaneously and pose little risk to a patient unless the patient previously has had acute pancreatitis. In cases of gallstone pancreatitis, stones identified by cholangiography should be removed endoscopically when the duct is very small. This is a rare event.

■ Avoid forceful manipulation of instruments in the bile duct, as this may result in false passages into the bowel or retroperitoneum

with consequent fistula or abscess and later stricture of the bile duct.

■ An operative cholangiogram should be performed before ductal exploration to delineate the position and number of stones and as a roadmap to ductal anatomy. Common duct exploration always should be completed by examination of the duct with choledochoscopy or cholangiography (or preferably both).

The procedure is performed through a right subcostal or upper midline incision. An extensive Kocher's maneuver is performed so that the retroduodenal and intrapancreatic bile duct can be palpated for stones. Exploration of the bile duct is often easier from the left side of the table. The common bile duct is identified by incising the overlying peritoneum and by following the cystic duct to its union with the common duct. Normally the structure is a green color and small blood vessels are visible on its surface. The size of the common duct and the midplane of the duct are noted. After placing two stay sutures in the common duct, the duct is incised with a #15 blade longitudinally at the level of the cystic duct entry. The incision initially should be made slightly to the left of the longitudinal midplane of what appears to be the common bile duct. This avoids opening into the septum of a fused cystic/common hepatic duct in the case of parallel insertion of the cystic duct that is present in about 20% of patients. Once the duct is opened the side walls should be palpated with an instrument such as a Potts scissors placed into the duct in order to identify the center line (midplane) of the duct. The duct is then opened for approximately 1.5 cm. Obvious stones are extracted. Stones palpated in the duct may be milked up (or down) until they appear in the choledochotomy and can be extracted. Next, the duct is explored with Randall stone forceps. The path of the duct is learned by allowing the closed forceps to find their way up and down the duct. The forceps are then reinserted in an open position and closed to grasp stones. One should be aware that when exploring upward the confluence of ducts can be grasped and mistakenly thought to be a stone. Once a stone is grasped it should be removed gently. Excessive force should not be used. Flexible spoons or scoops are also useful devices for removing stones. The bile duct should be irrigated with a catheter or directly with a bulb syringe whose tip has been wedged into the duct (Figure 6). Flushing the duct in this manner expands the duct around the stones and is particularly useful for intrahepatic stones. The choledochoscope may be used at open surgery to remove stones, as described in the laparoscopic section of this chapter. The biliary Fogarty catheter also may be used.

Ampullary patency can be proven by different means. One common technique is to use a metal sound such as a Bakes dilator. A small-diameter sound should be used and the ampulla should not be dilated with graduated sounds. Holding the sound between the thumb and index finger only avoids use of force. The presence of the sound in the duodenum is detected by the "steel sign" (i.e., seeing the tip of the sound through the duodenal wall). Use of a biliary Fogarty catheter is probably a superior way to prove patency. It is very flexible and tends to pass into the duodenum easily when there is no obstruction. When there is free passage of the catheter for 20 cm into the bile duct without resistance, the balloon may be inflated and pulled back to identify the position of the sphincter of Oddi. When there is doubt one should palpate the catheter in the duodenum before inflation.

Choledochoscopy is always performed with a flexible or rigid scope. At open surgery common bile duct (CBD) stay sutures are crossed to retain saline, which is flushed into the duct under pressure.

When stones are identified they may be removed with the techniques described earlier or with baskets passed via the scope as previously described.

Impacted stones represent a special case. Severely impacted stones remain one of the uncommon indications for open exploration after other approaches fail. The safest and most effective way of dealing with these stones is by electrohydraulic lithotripsy via the

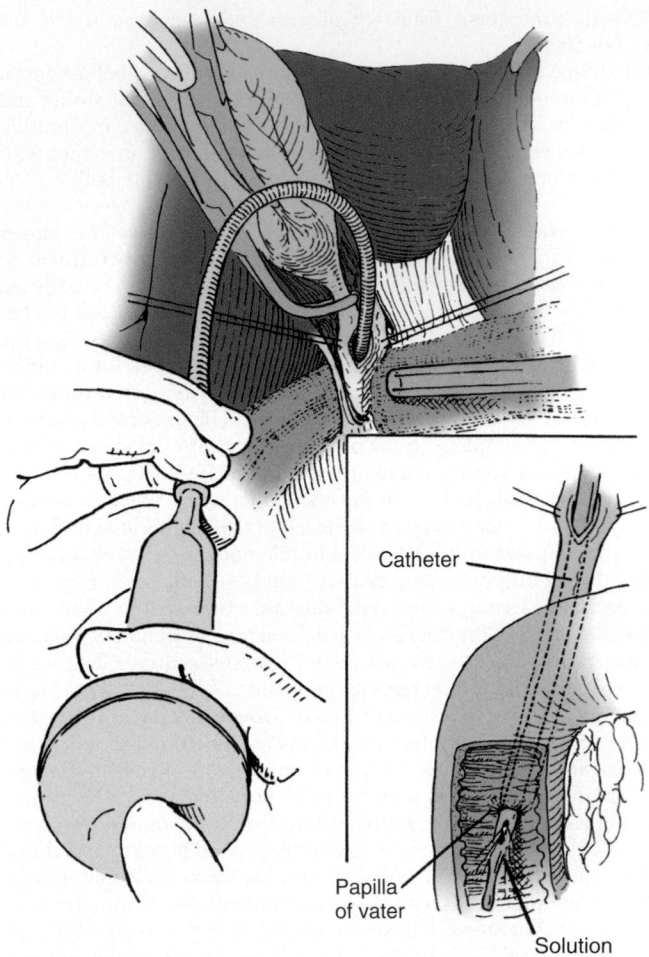

FIGURE 6 Technique of open common bile duct exploration (OCBDE). After placement of stay sutures, the common bile duct is incised longitudinally and cleared of stones with flushing, Randall stone forceps, or choledochoscopy. *(From Zollinger RM Jr, Zollinger RM. Atlas of Surgical Operations. 7th ed. New York: McGraw-Hill; 1993.)*

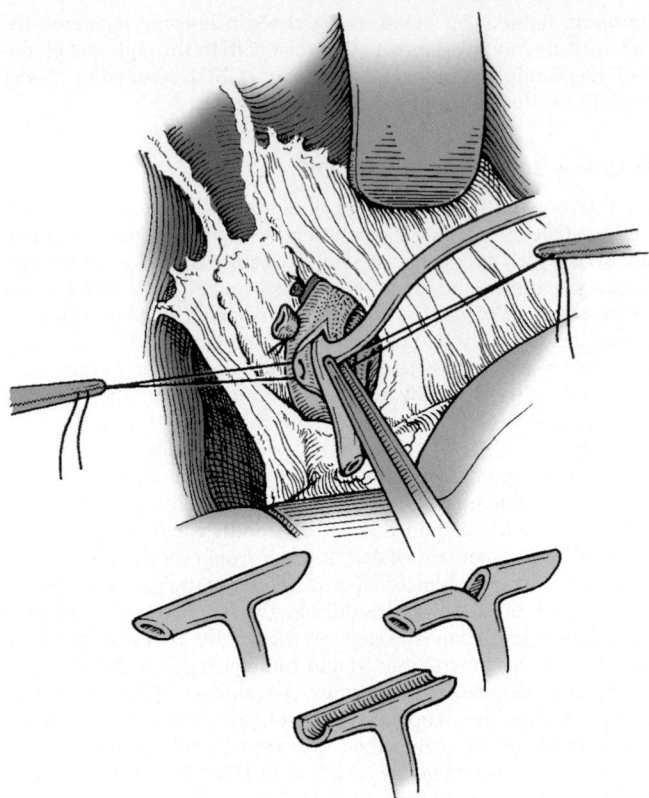

FIGURE 7 Closure of the common bile duct with a T-tube. A 14F or larger T-tube is prepared in one of the ways shown and inserted into the bile duct. The duct is then closed around the tube with fine absorbable sutures to create a watertight closure. *(From Zollinger RM Jr, Zollinger RM. Atlas of Surgical Operations. 7th ed. New York: McGraw-Hill; 1993.)*

choledochoscope. This technique breaks the stones into small pieces, which then can be extracted. Laser energy has been used to do the same but is more expensive. Electrohydraulic lithotripsy always must be done under direct vision and the active tip should be immediately adjacent to the stone and away from the walls of the CBD. In the past, impacted stones at the lower end of the bile duct have been extracted by duodenotomy and sphincteroplasty. This is almost never required and should be done only by surgeons who have experience in the technique. If an impacted stone cannot be removed and experience in lithotripsy or sphincterotomy is lacking, a T-tube should be placed and the operation terminated so that the patient may be referred for treatment of the stone. Removal can almost always be achieved by endoscopic or percutaneous means in specialized centers. This is preferable to duodenotomy and sphincteroplasty in our opinion because currently few surgeons have experience in this procedure.

After choledochoscopy is completed a T-tube is sewn into place (Figure 7). A 14F (4.7-mm) or larger tube should be used. Stones may be extracted through tube tracks of this size in the postoperative period, if they are discovered on postoperative T-tube cholangiography. The tube should fit loosely in the duct; if it is snug, it should be replaced with a smaller size tube. The tube should be moved down the duct so that the choledochotomy is sutured from above downward. This prevents the tube pulling on the suture line when it is extracted. The duct is closed with fine absorbable sutures (e.g., 3-0

chromic) taking bites of 1 to 2 mm in depth and about 2 mm apart with running or interrupted technique. The last bites are made alongside the exiting long limb of the T-tube to obtain a watertight seal. The T-tube is flushed with saline. The authors do this by inserting a 5F infant feeding tube down the T-tube, as this seems to best rid the tube and duct of air bubbles. A cholangiogram is obtained. Often dye will not enter the duodenum once the sphincter of Oddi has been instrumented. This should not be considered a reason for re-exploration if the choledochoscopy has been adequate.

SUGGESTED READINGS

Bansal VK, Misra MC, Rajan K, Kilambi R, Kumar S, Krishna A, Kumar A, Pandav CS, Subramaniam R, Arora MK, Garg PK. Single-stage laparoscopic common bile duct exploration and cholecystectomy versus two-stage endoscopic stone extraction followed by laparoscopic cholecystectomy for patients with concomitant gallbladder stones and common bile duct stones: a randomized controlled trial. *Surg Endosc.* 2014;28:875-885.

Berci G, Hunter J, Morgenstern L, Arregui M, Brunt M, Carroll B, Edye M, Fermelia D, Ferzli G, Greene F, Petelin J, Phillips E, Ponsky J, Sax H, Schwaitzberg S, Soper N, Swanstrom L, Traverso W. Laparoscopic cholecystectomy: first, do no harm; second, take care of bile duct stones. *Surg Endosc.* 2013;27:1051-1054.

Cuschieri A, Lezoche E, Morino M, Croce E, Lacy A, Toouli J, Faggioni A, Ribeiro VM, Jakimowicz J, Visa J, Hanna GB. E.A.E.S. multicenter prospective randomized trial comparing two-stage vs single-stage management of patients with gallstone disease and ductal calculi. *Surg Endosc.* 1999;13:952-957.

Grubnik VV, Tkachenko AI, Ilyashenko VV, Vorotyntseva KO. Laparoscopic common bile duct exploration versus open surgery: comparative prospective randomized trial. *Surg Endosc.* 2012;26:2165-2171.

Nathanson LK, O'Rourke NA, Martin IJ, Fielding GA, Cowen AE, Roberts RK, Kendall BJ, Kerlin P, Devereux BM. Postoperative ERCP versus laparoscopic choledochotomy for clearance of selected bile duct calculi: a randomized trial. *Ann Surg.* 2005;242:188-192.

Rhodes M, Sussman L, Cohen L, Lewis MP. Randomised trial of laparoscopic exploration of common bile duct versus postoperative endoscopic retrograde cholangiography for common bile duct stones. *Lancet.* 1998;351:159-161.

Rogers SJ, Cello JP, Horn JK, Siperstein AE, Schecter WP, Campbell AR, Mackersie RC, Rodas A, Kreuwel HT, Harris HW. Prospective randomized

trial of LC+LCBDE vs ERCP/S+LC for common bile duct stone disease. *Arch Surg.* 2010;145:28-33.

Spirou Y, Petrou A, Christoforides C, Felekouras E. History of biliary surgery. *World J Surg.* 2013;37:1006-1012.

Teitelbaum EN, Soper NJ, Santos BF, Rooney DM, Patel P, Nagle AP, Hungness ES. A simulator-based resident curriculum for laparoscopic common bile duct exploration. *Surgery.* 2014;156:880-887.

THE MANAGEMENT OF ACUTE CHOLANGITIS

Theodore N. Pappas, MD, and Morgan L. Cox, MD

Acute cholangitis is characterized by infection and inflammation of the biliary tract resulting from biliary obstruction. The spectrum of clinical severity can range from mild to potentially life-threatening disease accompanied by septic shock and multiorgan dysfunction. It is a morbid condition with a natural history of rapid deterioration, which makes expeditious diagnosis critical.

■ EPIDEMIOLOGY

Cholangitis occurs at median age of 50 to 60 years. Risk factors include smoking, increasing age, and biliary instrumentation. The risk factors for cholelithiasis apply to cholangitis, given gallstones are the most common cause. It affects males and females equally.

Acute cholangitis occurs in the setting of biliary obstruction, which leads to the stasis of bile. Up to 70% of cases are due to secondary choledocholithiasis (stones originating in the gallbladder). Other sources of obstruction include malignant and benign strictures, primary sclerosing cholangitis (PSC), and primary choledocholithiasis known as *recurrent pyogenic cholangitis*. Obstruction also can stem from iatrogenic manipulation, including anastomotic or ischemic strictures and obstructed biliary stents. Acute cholangitis is a common complication of previously placed internalized biliary drains. These drains can become kinked or clogged, leading to obstruction and subsequent infection. A complete list of acute cholangitis causes is listed in Box 1.

Given the incidence of secondary choledocholithiasis, the most common location of obstruction is "low" or distal in the common bile duct (CBD). Proximal obstruction most likely is due to malignancy or recurrent pyogenic cholangitis. The location of the obstruction is critical in determining the most appropriate therapy.

■ PATHOGENESIS

The body's mechanism for preventing biliary infection includes the continuous flow of bile, bile salts that are inherently bacteriostatic, and IgA. Bile is sterile at baseline. Bacteria can enter the biliary system via duodenal ascent typically prevented by the sphincter of Oddi. Hematogenous spread from the portal vein rarely occurs. Iatrogenic manipulation has the potential to introduce bacteria into the biliary tree, and stents are foreign bodies allowing bacterial colonization. Endoscopic retrograde cholangiopancreatography (ERCP) has been implicated in 0.5% to 1.7% of cases of cholangitis.

Once bacteria has entered the biliary system, it has the ability to proliferate, causing increased intrabiliary pressure. This in turn increases the permeability of the epithelium, allowing translocation of bacteria from bile to systemic circulation through lymphatic and venous channels, leading to sepsis.

Acute cholangitis is typically polymicrobial with the most common isolates being bowel flora, gram-negative in particular. The most frequently identified gram-negative bacteria are *Escherichia coli* (25% to 50% of cases), *Klebsiella* species (15% to 20% of cases), *Enterobacter* species (5% to 10% of cases), and *Pseudomonas* species. The most commonly isolated gram-positive bacteria are *Enterococcus* species (10% to 20% of cases). The contribution of anaerobes, such as *Bacteroides* and *Clostridium* species, to the pathogenesis of acute cholangitis is controversial. However, anaerobes are not uncommonly cultured in specimens obtained from elderly patients and those who have undergone biliary instrumentation.

Other rare pathogens include helminths, fungi, and viruses, including CMV and EBV. These atypical pathogens should be considered in endemic areas for parasitic infection and the immunocompromised.

■ PRESENTATION

In 1877 a French neurologist and professor in anatomic pathology, Jean-Martin Charcot, described the Charcot's triad of symptoms consisting of fever, right upper quadrant abdominal pain, and jaundice found in acute cholangitis. The triad is reported in up to 75% of cases but likely present in only 15% to 20%. The most common component is fever occurring in more than 80% of cases. The presentation was extended by B.M. Reynolds and E.L. Dargan in 1959 to include hypotension and altered mental status known as *Reynolds' pentad,* which is found in less than 5% of cases. The pentad suggests systemic disease and sepsis.

When a patient experiences the set of symptoms previously mentioned, an adequate differential diagnosis includes cholecystitis, Mirizzi's syndrome, liver abscess, infected choledochal cysts, and right lower lobe pneumonia or empyema. Remember to consider cholangitis in elderly and immunocompromised patients because they may not have these common symptoms. This can lead to a delay in diagnosis and poor outcome.

■ DECISION-MAKING ALGORITHM

In 2013 the Tokyo guidelines were updated to outline the management of acute cholangitis and cholecystitis, which has brought an evidence-based approach to the definition, diagnosis, and management of these conditions. The guidelines include clinical, laboratory, and imaging criteria. Criteria for suspected and definite diagnosis are seen in Box 2.

The workup of acute cholangitis begins with laboratory testing. Complete blood count (CBC) exhibits leukocytosis, neutrophilia, and likely a left shift. Elevated alkaline phosphatase, transaminitis, and conjugated hyperbilirubinemia will be revealed on comprehensive metabolic panel. Elevated amylase and lipase is a rare finding with cholangitis, unless the obstructing stone is located at the ampulla or has passed causing a gallstone pancreatitis. Along with basic labs,

BOX 1: Causes of Acute Cholangitis

Noniatrogenic

Benign Conditions

Choledocholithiasis
    Primary
    Secondary
Pancreatitis (chronic/acute), including pancreatic pseudocyst
Papillary stenosis
Mirizzi's syndrome
Choledochal cysts and Caroli's disease
Biliary strictures
    Ischemia
    Primary sclerosing cholangitis
    Recurrent choledocholithiasis
    Recurrent cholangitis
    Other inflammatory conditions

Malignancies

Pancreatic cancer
Cholangiocarcinoma
Duodenal/ampullary cancer
Primary tumor or metastasis to liver, gallbladder, or porta hepatis

Iatrogenic

Obstructed biliary endoprosthesis
Iatrogenic biliary stricture
    Direct surgical trauma
    Ischemia-induced stricture
    Anastomotic stricture (bilibiliary/bilioenteric anastomosis)

BOX 2: Diagnostic Criteria for Acute Cholangitis: Tokyo Guidelines

A. Clinical context and clinical manifestations
    1. History of biliary disease
    2. Fever or chills
    3. Jaundice
    4. Abdominal pain (right upper quadrant or upper abdominal)
B. Laboratory data
    1. Evidence of inflammatory response*
    2. Abnormal liver function tests†
C. Imaging findings
    1. Biliary dilation or evidence of an etiology (stricture, stone, stent, etc.)
D. Suspected diagnosis
    1. Two or more items in A
E. Definite diagnosis
    1. Charcot's triad (2 + 3 + 4)
    2. Two or more items in A + both items in B + item C

From Hirota M, Tadahiro T, Kawarada Y, et al: Tokyo guidelines for the management of acute cholangitis and cholecystitis. *J Hepatobiliary Pancreat Surg.* 2007;14:1-126, 2007.

*Abnormal white blood cell count, increased serum C-reactive protein level, and other changes indicating inflammation.

†Increased serum alkaline phosphatase, γ-glutamyl transpeptidase, aspartate aminotransferase, and alanine aminotransferase levels.

cultures should be sent from blood, bile, and removed biliary stents to allow for subsequent tapering of antibiotics.

After labs and cultures are sent, imaging studies are necessary to confirm dilated bile ducts, reveal the specific cause for obstruction, exclude differential diagnoses, and guide therapeutic interventions. A transabdominal ultrasound should be ordered as the first study in most cases with suspected biliary tree pathology, including acute cholangitis. An ultrasound is readily available, noninvasive, rapidly performed, and cost effective. Performing an ultrasound is feasible even in severe cases. It has low sensitivity for choledocholithiasis but a very high sensitivity for CBD dilation. It is possible ductal dilation will not be apparent in an early presentation.

There are several other primary imaging studies available to evaluate the biliary tree, but they do not have a role in the diagnosis of cholangitis. This includes HIDA scan, which is indicated only to identify cystic duct obstruction. Also infection in cholangitis reduces the secretion of the radiotracer used for HIDA. Endoscopic ultrasonography (EUS) has excellent sensitivity for choledocholithiasis but should not be used in the acute setting. It is helpful for further characterization of a mass as the cause of initial obstruction, but this would be performed after recovery from infection.

Computerized tomography (CT) and magnetic resonance cholangiopancreatography (MRCP) have the ability to diagnose a dilated biliary tract. CT can identify the site of obstruction but not necessarily the cause. It provides a global evaluation of abdominal anatomy and pathology. It has a poor sensitivity for intraductal stones. MRCP has greater sensitivity for choledocholithiasis, and it is the ideal test to characterize biliary strictures. However, both of these are unnecessary tests in the initial workup of acute cholangitis because transabdominal ultrasound and clinical presentation are sufficient for diagnosis before intervention. MRCP can be a valuable modality to confirm a stone has passed when the clinical picture is not clear.

After appropriate noninvasive imaging with transabdominal ultrasound, further indicated imaging consists of modalities that are also therapeutic, including ERCP or percutaneous transhepatic cholangiography (PTC) with percutaneous biliary drain (PBD). Both modalities allow for identification of obstruction location, drainage, culture, and biopsy or brushings.

■ PRINCIPLES OF MANAGEMENT

Patients with cholangitis require treatment on an inpatient basis. Therapy consists of three main components, including resuscitation, antibiotics, and biliary drainage outlined in the management algorithm (Figure 1). Treatment for severe cases should be implemented in the intensive care unit (ICU). Resuscitation begins with fluid, correction of electrolyte abnormalities and coagulopathies, and externalization of pre-existing biliary drains. Antibiotics should be given immediately. Ideally, cultures are drawn before antibiotics are started, but cultures should not cause a significant delay in treatment.

Antibiotic coverage should start broad covering gram-negative and gram-positive bacteria as well as anaerobes. Antibiotics can be tapered on the basis of final culture results. The length of treatment is based on clinical response and typically concludes after 7 to 14 days.

Several appropriate antibiotic choices exist for empiric therapy. Options include fluoroquinolones (ciprofloxacin, levofloxacin) alone or with metronidazole, carbapenems (imipenem or meropenem), extended-spectrum penicillins (piperacillin), penicillin/beta-lactamase inhibitor combinations (piperacillin and tazobactam, ampicillin and sulbactam, ticarcillin and clavulanate), and ampicillin with gentamicin. Gentamicin-based regimens are avoided because of the substantial risk of aminoglycoside-induced nephrotoxicity. Second-generation and third-generation cephalosporins have excellent activity against gram-negative bacteria, although poor coverage against *Enterococcus* species, and are not recommended. Zosyn is a great choice given its broad gram-negative, gram-positive, and anaerobic coverage; penetration into bile; and ease of administration.

All patients with signs or symptoms consistent with cholangitis, no matter the severity, should be started on broad-spectrum antibiotics and undergo transabdominal ultrasound. Once the patient is stabilized, biliary drainage should be considered based on severity. Remember some patients will not stabilize until the duct is cleared of obstruction. The severity assessment described in the Tokyo

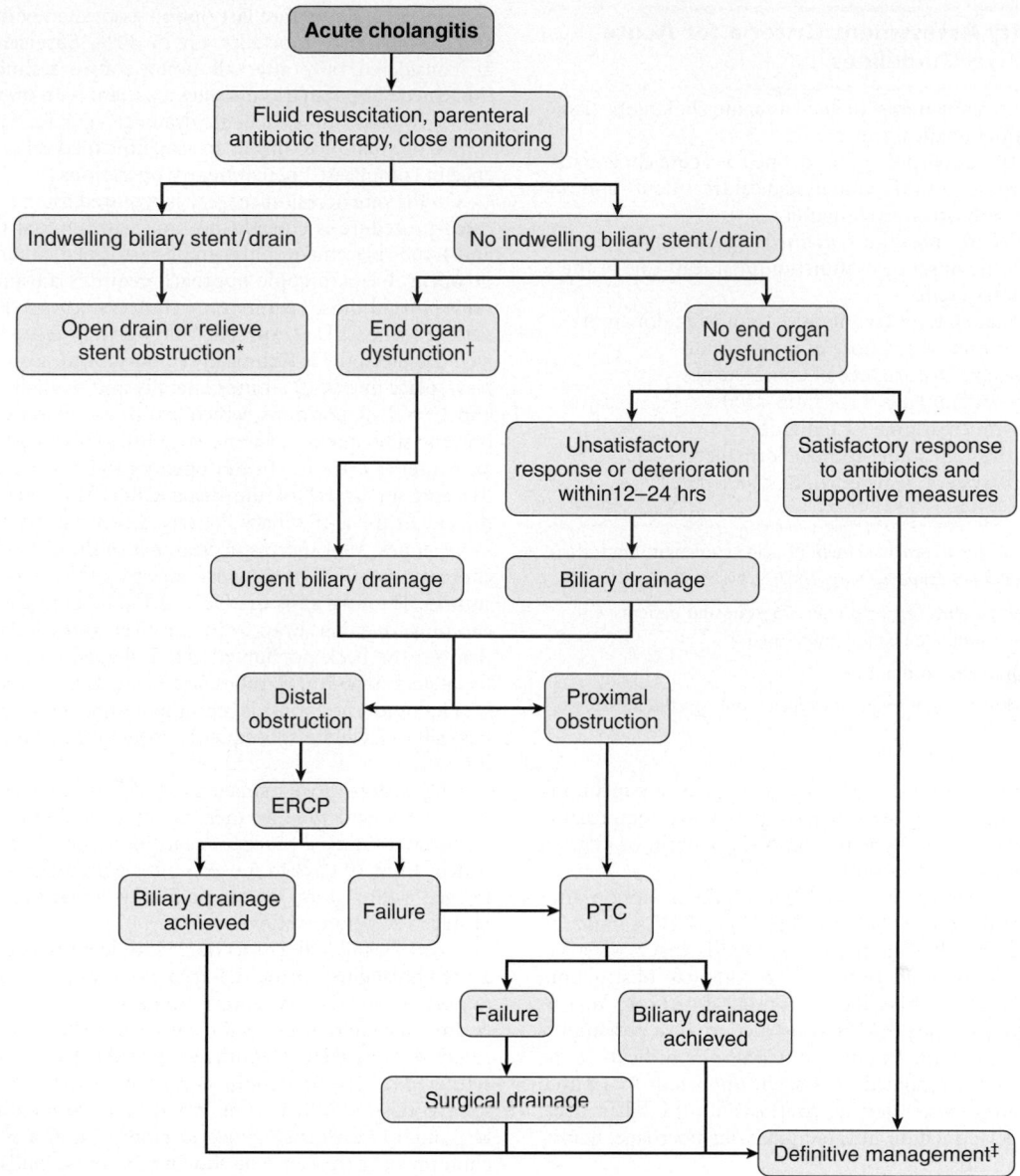

FIGURE 1 Clinical algorithm for management of acute cholangitis. *ERCP,* Endoscopic retrograde cholangiopancreatography; *PTC,* percutaneous transhepatic cholangiography.
*For changing internal stents, urgency is determined by presence or absence of end-organ dysfunction.
†For example, altered mental status or hemodynamic lability.
‡Timing of definitive management is determined by the severity of the episode of cholangitis and the comorbidities of the patient.

guidelines is shown in Box 3. Mild cases do not require drainage unless the patient has ongoing evidence of obstruction or relapse of infectious symptoms after medical therapy. Moderate and severe disease both are treated with biliary drainage but in different time frames. A moderate severity case requires early biliary drainage within 24 hours. Severe disease consistent with Reynolds' pentad or any end organ dysfunction should be drained emergently within hours.

Patients with pre-existing external biliary drains should be placed to gravity drainage as soon as the diagnosis of acute cholangitis is considered. Biliary drainage is not required if there is clear evidence the stone has passed. This includes obvious improvement in liver function. Typically, alkaline phosphatase and total bilirubin counts will lag behind improvement in transaminitis. If the patient is improving clinically, but lab results do not suggest the duct has cleared, an MRCP is the best study to determine duct patency and need for biliary drainage.

The optimal drainage technique depends on the site of obstruction, previous drainage attempts, available equipment, and physician expertise. The gold standard is ERCP, which is 90% to 98% effective in draining the biliary tract given the majority of obstructions are in the distal CBD. ERCP is a therapeutic and diagnostic intervention. It allows for clearing the CBD of obstruction, sphincterotomy, replacement of biliary stents, and/or dilation and stenting of strictures. Diagnostic options include biopsy and brushings. PSC is the only diagnosis in which instrumentation should be avoided if possible. Again, if the patient fails to improve, biliary drainage ultimately is indicated.

Overall, ERCP has a complication rate of 7% to 15%. Theoretically after gaining access to the biliary tree, bile should be aspirated before injecting contrast to prevent increasing already elevated biliary pressures. However even with aspiration, ERCP alone will still increase biliary pressures leading to transient bacteremia. Other complications include postprocedural pancreatitis and duodenal injury.

BOX 3: Severity Assessment Criteria for Acute Cholangitis: Tokyo Guidelines

Mild (grade I) acute cholangitis, defined as acute cholangitis that responds to initial medical treatment*

Moderate (grade II) acute cholangitis, defined as acute cholangitis that does not respond to the initial medical treatment* and is not associated with organ dysfunction

Severe (grade III) acute cholangitis, defined as acute cholangitis associated with the onset of dysfunction in at least one of the following organs/systems:

1. Cardiovascular system: Hypotension requiring dopamine >5 μg/kg per min or any dose of dobutamine
2. Nervous system: Disturbance of consciousness
3. Respiratory system: PaO_2/FiO_2 ratio <300
4. Kidney: Serum creatinine >2.0 mg/dL
5. Liver: Prothrombin International Normalized Ratio >1.5
6. Hematologic system: Platelet count <100,000/μL

From Tokyo Guidelines for the management of acute cholangitis and cholecystitis. *J Hepatobiliary Pancreat Surg.* 2007;14:1-126, 2007.

NOTE: Compromised patients (e.g., patients >75 years and patients with medical comorbidities) should be closely monitored.

*General supportive care and antibiotics.

FiO₂, Fractional concentration of inspired oxygen; *PaO₂*, partial pressure of arterial oxygen.

In some instances, it is unsafe to perform a sphincterotomy, including when the patient has an uncorrected coagulopathy. Temporizing biliary drainage can be achieved with a nasobiliary drain or internal biliary stent without a sphincterotomy.

PTC with PBD placement is a secondary drainage option after ERCP. It is successful about 90% of the time. PTC should be attempted only before ERCP if the biliary tree is inaccessible via endoscopic access. This could be due to a complete obstruction, inadvertent division of the bile duct as complication from laparoscopic cholecystectomy, Roux-en-Y reconstruction, or a periampullary duodenal diverticulum. Percutaneous access is difficult if the intrahepatic ducts are not dilated. It is again important to aspirate and obtain a culture before injecting contrast into the biliary tree. Complications of PTC include intraperitoneal hemorrhage, hemobilia, and bile peritonitis.

PTC should be considered for intrahepatic biliary dilatation without extrahepatic dilatation suggestive of proximal or hilar pathology. It allows for precise drainage of sectoral ducts if necessary. Keep in mind that cholangitis rarely develops behind tumors or strictures without previous instrumentation. Therefore only areas of the liver that were instrumented previously should be drained as treatment for cholangitis.

A percutaneous cholecystostomy tube can be unpredictable and not provide adequate drainage of the entire biliary system in the setting of acute cholangitis. However, a definitive diagnosis of cholangitis is not always obtained before intervention. Cholecystostomy tube placement is appropriate if there is concern for cholecystitis as the cause of symptoms. This requires a patent, nontortuous cystic duct to drain the CBD. The location of obstruction has to be distal to the junction of the cystic duct and common hepatic duct if any drainage is to be achieved. If a cholecystostomy tube is placed and clinical improvement does not occur, ERCP or PTC still is indicated for proper drainage of the biliary tree as treatment for cholangitis.

It is common for a patient to have a transient bacteremia after percutaneous intervention. Instrumentation of the infected biliary tract causes postprocedure SIRS that requires ICU support. Although this can produce hemodynamic instability, supportive care in the ICU is typically sufficient without further intervention unless the biliary tract is not drained adequately.

Surgery is a very rare last option associated with high morbidity and perioperative mortality up to 40%. Surgical options should be considered only after all nonoperative techniques have been exhausted. One scenario includes a patient with previous Roux-en-Y gastric bypass with inadequate drainage via PTC. Surgical treatment should be attempted only at an academic medical center with experience in complicated hepatobiliary operations.

On the rare occasion surgery is required for cholangitis, the indicated procedure is choledochotomy with limited CBD exploration and T-tube placement. This can be performed either laparoscopically or open. A laparoscopic approach requires advanced laparoscopic skills beyond those required for cholecystectomy. First, the anterior surface of the CBD is exposed. Although not necessary for treatment, a cholecystectomy is technically important for exposure to the CBD. Next, place fine (4-0) sutures laterally and medially on the CBD at 2 and 10 o'clock positions, which avoids the blood supply laterally to prevent subsequent ischemic stricture. This provides traction and exposure for a 15- to 20-mm opening to be made longitudinally on the anterior aspect of the distal CBD. Then place an endoscope directly or use a 4F biliary Fogarty catheter to try to remove one or more stones. After successful clearance of the duct, close the choledochotomy over a T-tube with interrupted 3-0 or 4-0 absorbable sutures. The tube exits the CBD at the inferior end of the choledochotomy, opening away from the liver and caudal to the sutures. Remove the back portion of the T-shaped end or cut a notch to facilitate extraction. T-tubes are customized from a 16F tube or smaller tube. The T-tube is brought out linearly through the abdominal wall to facilitate subsequent access for imaging or manipulation if needed.

The postoperative management of T-tubes depends on the clinical scenario and whether there is any suspicion of persistent stones in the duct. Clinical practice regarding removal of the T-tube varies widely, from 10 days to 6 weeks after placement. T-tubes should be imaged with T-tube cholangiography to ensure patency without obstruction before removal.

All of the following procedures should be avoided in patients with acute cholangitis: formal CBD exploration, transduodenal sphincteroplasty, and biliary enteric bypass. Interval definitive surgical treatment should be delayed until the initial episode of infection has resolved completely. Definitive treatment has no role in the acute setting of cholangitis. Cholecystectomy can be performed during the same admission if there is no end-organ dysfunction and the patient responds to treatment. Cholecystectomy is indicated during choledochotomy or if the cause of cholangitis was secondary choledocholithiasis or Mirizzi's syndrome.

More complex definitive surgery should be performed at a later date after infection has resolved. Further imaging, including CT, MRI, and EUS, can be beneficial in characterizing causative pathology other than secondary choledocholithiasis. This includes cases requiring biliary reconstruction because of benign biliary strictures or periampullary tumors.

■ PROGNOSIS

Most cases, up to 85%, are mild and respond to conservative management without biliary drainage. Overall mortality is 2.7% to 10%, with the poorest prognosis associated with end organ damage. Mortality rates of acute cholangitis have improved from greater than 50% in 1980 likely because of better drainage techniques.

SUGGESTED READINGS

Hirota M, Tadahiro T, Kawarada Y, et al. Tokyo guidelines for the management of acute cholangitis and cholecystitis. *J Hepatobiliary Pancreat Surg.* 2007;14:1-126.

Sabiston DC, Townsend CM. Biliary system. In: *Sabiston Textbook of Surgery: the Biological Basis of Modern Surgical Practice.* 19th ed. Philadelphia: Elsevier Saunders; 2012:1476-1514.

THE MANAGEMENT OF BENIGN BILIARY STRICTURES

Chad G. Ball, MD, and Keith D. Lillemoe, MD

Benign strictures of the biliary system are among the most challenging clinical problems faced by general surgeons. Mismanagement is frequent; however, short- and long-term complications such as sepsis, cholangitis, secondary biliary cirrhosis, portal hypertension, and complete biliary obstruction may be avoided by rapid and sage referral to centers with high-volume experiences in hepatobiliary surgery. Finally, biliary injuries and strictures remain extremely costly to patients in a medical and financial context, as well as to their overall quality of life.

This chapter briefly reviews the cause and classification of biliary injuries and strictures as well as the necessary steps to achieve diagnosis and effective treatment in the setting of iatrogenic bile duct injuries, chronic pancreatitis, autoimmune pancreatitis, sclerosing cholangitis, and pyogenic cholangitis.

■ IATROGENIC BILE DUCT INJURY AND STRICTURE

Benign biliary strictures are the end result of either traumatic injury or inflammatory processes, such as pancreatitis, biliary calculi, infection, and autoimmune disorders. However, by far the most common cause of a bile duct stricture is iatrogenic injury during an operation in the right upper quadrant, usually cholecystectomy. The incidence of biliary injury was stable and low (0.2%) in the last several decades of traditional open cholecystectomy. Subsequent to the rapid proliferation of laparoscopic cholecystectomy in the early 1990s, the incidence rose dramatically with numerous database/registry studies demonstrating the modern incidence of biliary injury to have stabilized at 0.4%. Although a recent report from New York State has suggested the true "modern" incidence may have returned to "pre-lap chole" levels, further studies are necessary. Regardless of the low incidence of injury, the large absolute number of laparoscopic cholecystectomies performed results in nearly 3000 iatrogenic biliary injuries per year in the United States alone.

Furthermore, there are estimates that one in three general surgeons will create a bile duct injury during their career. Of further concern is that, given the significant decrease in open biliary experience among surgical trainees in the modern era, conversion to open procedures may no longer represent the safest option in cases of a "difficult" cholecystectomy. Some experts now argue that attempts to complete a cholecystectomy after conversion from the laparoscopic approach to an open procedure are at high risk for an even more complex injury, including portal vascular strictures. Thus completing a partial cholecystectomy (with stone evacuation) or simply inserting closed suction drainage with subsequent transfer to a more experienced biliary surgeon is a safer and more reasonable option.

The impact of biliary injuries is substantial. The financial costs, disability, morbidity, and mortality are even more significant, considering the original intent was in many cases as an outpatient laparoscopic procedure with little to no disability. Bile duct injuries lead directly to multiple invasive procedures, reoperations, and readmissions to hospital. The estimated medical costs of managing these patients approximate $50,000 per event. Long-term follow-up of Medicare patients suffering bile duct injury also has shown a substantial (ninefold) increase in mortality compared with controls. Finally, bile duct injuries clearly affect the quality of life of patients.

Therefore bile duct injuries are a leading cause of medical malpractice claims filed against general surgeons.

Mechanisms of Bile Duct Injury

Iatrogenic injury during laparoscopic cholecystectomy is typically the result of a perceptual error in identifying biliary anatomy. Our visual system constructs an incredibly complex model that coalesces information based on multiple sensory inputs (texture, shadow, optic flow, binocular disparity). It also relies on our previous experience and learned anatomy. In addition, the most common laparoscopic injury occurs with either excessive cephalad retraction of the gallbladder fundus or insufficient lateral retraction on the infundibulum, resulting in an alignment of the cystic and common bile ducts. Therefore the classic misperception of the common bile duct is the cystic duct, resulting in subsequent clipping and complete ductal transection (Figure 1).

Additional issues that contribute to the occurrence of bile duct injuries include excessive thermal cautery medial to the gallbladder, aberrant biliary anatomy (most commonly a right posterior sectoral bile duct that drains directly into the common bile duct or gallbladder), and extensive inflammation (acute) and/or gallbladder retraction (chronic) within Calot's triangle, creating the perception of a "short cystic duct." The issue of visual alignment and laparoscope perspective has become even more topical with the proliferation of single-incision laparoscopic cholecystectomy. Single-incision techniques are known to be associated with a higher rate of common bile duct injury than the traditional four-incision laparoscopic methodology with an angled scope.

Preventing Iatrogenic Bile Duct Injury

Injury avoidance is clearly the stated goal of every general surgeon embarking on either an elective or urgent cholecystectomy. Although much has been written about preventing bile duct injuries, there are a number of core tenets. The first and most commonly stressed in obtaining the "critical view of safety" was described by Soper and Strasberg in the 1990s. This concept mandates that the fundus of the gallbladder is retracted superiorly while the infundibulum is retracted laterally. This exposure generally allows the surgeon to carefully dissect out Calot's triangle, leaving only two structures connected to the lower end of the gallbladder: the cystic artery and cystic duct. The critical view of safety also has been enhanced to describe both anterior and posterior views (Figure 2). Although this maneuver is the single most effective means of preventing a bile duct injury, the reality is substantially more complex. In scenarios of a short or nonexistent cystic duct, or a small common bile duct, these structures can be confused with each other. As mentioned earlier, inappropriate or overzealous traction then makes these associations even more challenging. Similarly, inflammation closes the space between the gallbladder and the bile duct. In extreme cases, they even may be fused and move as a single unit. This not uncommon reality makes identification of associated regional anatomy even more important for the surgeon in an attempt to orient the critical structures of interest and proceed with a safe procedure. These spacial-regional issues can be challenged further by a loss of perspective, given the tendency of many camera operators to move ever closer to the operative dissection.

The role of intraoperative cholangiography in preventing bile duct injuries is controversial. Similar to many smaller, individual series that have failed to demonstrate that either routine or opportunistic intraoperative cholangiography prevents biliary injuries, a recent Medicare-based study of 92,000 patients identified no statistically significant association between intraoperative cholangiography and common bile duct injury. The authors concluded that intraoperative cholangiography is "not effective as a preventive strategy

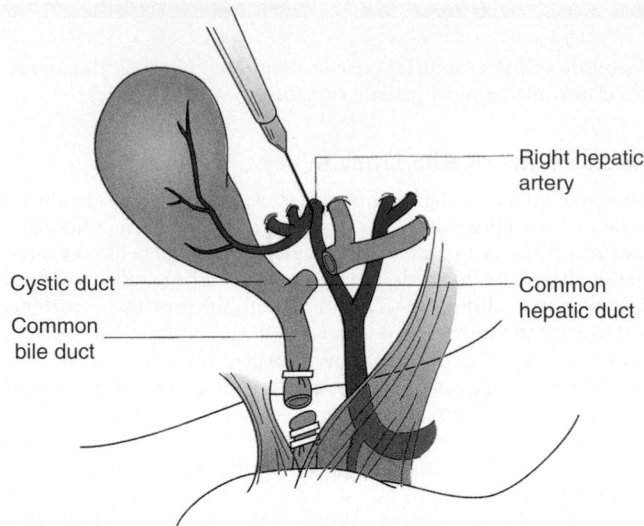

FIGURE 1 Classic laparoscopic bile duct injury. The common bile duct is mistaken for the cystic duct and transected. A variable extent of the extrahepatic biliary tree is resected with the gallbladder. The right hepatic artery, in background, also is often injured. *(Adapted from Branum G, Schmidt C, Baillie J, et al. Management of major biliary complications after laparoscopic cholecystectomy. Ann Surg. 1993;217:532.)*

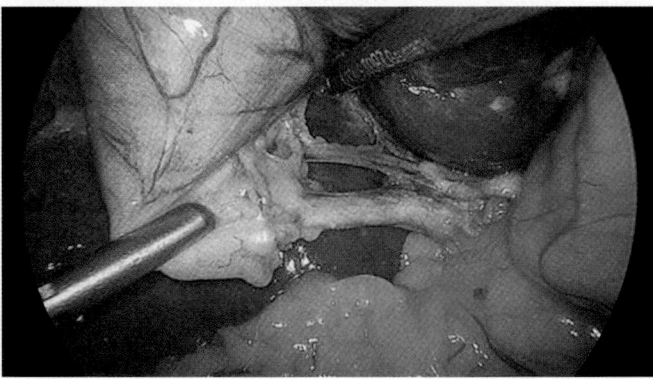

FIGURE 2 The critical view of safety is demonstrated showing only two distinct structures—the cystic duct and cystic artery—after developing a several centimeter plane between the neck of the gallbladder and the liver edge.

against common bile duct injury during laparoscopic cholecystectomy." Intraoperative cholangiography also is known to potentially underestimate the extent of the injury, as well as lead to misinterpretation of the images themselves by general surgeons in more than half of instances.

An additional confounding factor in preventing iatrogenic injuries surrounds the optimal timing of performing a laparoscopic cholecystectomy in the setting of acute inflammation of the gallbladder. Although 30-day postoperative morbidity and mortality may remain independent of timing, it is clear that patients who undergo laparoscopic cholecystectomy beyond 24 hours of presentation to a hospital are more likely to necessitate an open procedure, sustain a bile duct injury, require significantly longer postoperative and overall lengths of hospital admission, and increase total costs.

Classification of Injury

Numerous classification schemes are available to describe benign biliary strictures (Bismuth, Strasberg, Amsterdam, Neuhaus,

Stewart-Way, Hannover, Lau classifications). The most widely used system was developed in the prelaparoscopic era by Bismuth and defined the type of stricture based on the anatomic location with respect to the hepatic bifurcation (i.e., the level at which healthy tissue is available for surgical reconstruction). With advent of the laparoscopic technique, injuries became more complex, proximal, and common and also included biliary leakage. This reality mandated an update that was provided by Strasberg and colleagues (Figure 3).

The scenario of concurrent vascular trauma at the time of biliary injury is worthy of special note. Trauma to the hepatic artery at the time of a bile duct injury during laparoscopic cholecystectomy has been recognized at an increasingly higher incidence (as high as 50%, when investigated at the time of presentation). The true impact of an arterial injury, however, remains debated because often arterial injury does not appear to affect either early or late outcomes. The most common site of vasculobiliary injury is the right hepatic artery. Damage to this vessel can lead to a higher injury level on the bile duct than the gross observed mechanical trauma. Vasculobiliary injuries also can have specific effects on the arteries (pseudoaneurysm with delayed hemorrhage), bile ducts (necrosis, stenosis, cholangitis), and/or liver (necrosis, atrophy) over variable lengths of time. Concurrent hepatic artery and portal vein injuries can have catastrophic effects on the liver, including rapid necrosis. Finally, a more clinically important cause of ischemia can be unnecessary dissection around the bile duct during cholecystectomy or bile duct anastomosis, which can divide or injure the major arteries of the bile duct that travel in the 3 o'clock and 9 o'clock positions. This local ischemia clearly can influence the development of late strictures of both a native bile duct or an anastomosis.

Clinical Presentation

It is clear based on multiple large series that less than 40% of iatrogenic bile duct injuries are recognized during the index cholecystectomy. This reality mandates continued awareness and vigilance for any component of the procedure that is "off normal." Such findings include, but are not limited to, (1) evidence that a standard 9- to 10-mm clip is insufficient to completely occlude the ductal structure, (2) persistent leakage of bile from the liver, (3) identification of a "second" ductal structure, (4) "extra" soft tissue adjacent to the porta hepatis, (5) the presence of a large artery coursing behind the presumed cystic duct, (6) sustained bleeding from the area medial to the gallbladder, (7) an excessive number of required clips, and (8) the inability to adequately identify regional anatomic structures.

Because most biliary injuries are unrecognized at the original operation, the most common time for presentation is in the early postoperative period. Either the surgeon admits the patient immediately after a difficult procedure, or the patient returns to the hospital after an initial discharge home. In either scenario, abdominal discomfort, nausea, anorexia, vomiting, and general malaise are common. This clinical presentation is typically a direct result of incomplete clipping of a transected hepatic duct with sustained bile leakage into the peritoneal cavity as a biloma or bile ascites or through operatively placed drains. If the duct is ligated completely via clips, then the presentation is most commonly abdominal pain in the context of acute onset of jaundice, and less commonly signs of cholangitis. Any of these symptoms must be investigated thoroughly with a detailed examination, laboratory evaluations, and either ultrasonography or cross-sectional imaging to rule out a peritoneal fluid collection or biliary dilation.

Repair of the Immediately Recognized Injury

In the minority of cases in which the injury is recognized intraoperatively, the surgeon should engage in two crucial steps: (1) consult a second surgeon with significant hepatobiliary experience and (2) further characterize the bile duct injury via intraoperative cholangiography, or less commonly intraoperative ultrasound or direct

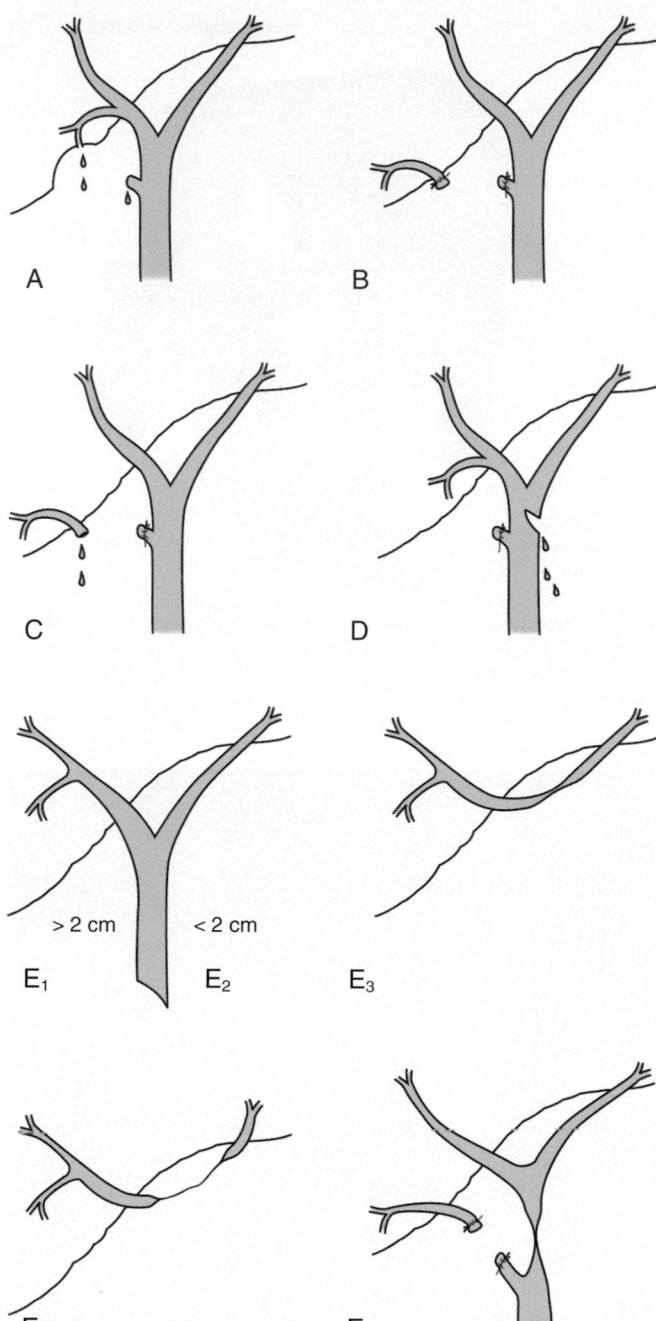

FIGURE 3 Classification scheme for benign biliary strictures. *Type A,* Cystic duct leaks or leaks from small ducts in the liver bed. *Type B,* Occlusion of part of the biliary tree, typically clipped and divided right hepatic ducts. *Type C,* Transection (but not ligation) of the aberrant right hepatic ducts. *Type D,* Lateral injuries to major bile ducts. *Type E₁,* Common hepatic duct division, more than 2 cm from bifurcation. *Type E₂,* Common hepatic duct division, less than 2 cm from bifurcation. *Type E₃,* Common bile duct division at bifurcation. *Type E₄,* Hilar stricture, involvement of confluence and loss of communication between right and left hepatic duct. *Type E₅,* Involvement of aberrant right hepatic duct alone or with concomitant stricture of the common hepatic duct.

evaluation after conversion to an open procedure. Regarding step 1, repair of a major common bile duct injury requires both the technical skills and unencumbered judgment of an experienced hepatobiliary surgeon. If such an experienced surgeon is not available, a telephone conversation and possible transfer to a tertiary institution should be

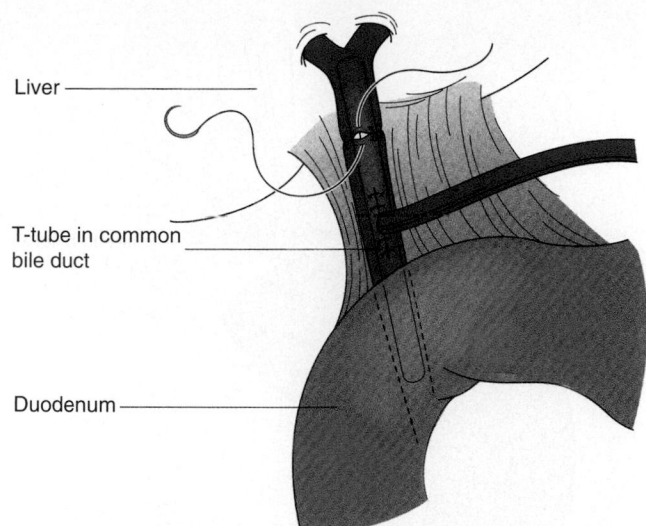

FIGURE 4 If the injured segment of the bile duct is short (<1 cm) and the two ends can be opposed without tension, an end-to-end anastomosis can be performed with placement of a T-tube through a separate choledochotomy either above or below the anastomosis. The T-tube should not be brought out directly through the anastomosis.

given strong consideration. Attempts to remove the gallbladder, if not already done, or ligate the proximal bile duct to allow dilatation should be avoided to prevent further damage. In most cases, simply drainage of the gallbladder bed and if possible, placing a catheter in the proximal transected duct is advisable to control the bile leak.

If a satisfactory repair by an experienced surgeon is possible, it is ideal to perform repair at the time of original operation. The identification of the proximal level of the injury is paramount in selecting the most durable and successful reconstruction technique. If a segmental or accessory duct smaller than 3 mm has been injured and cholangiography demonstrates segmental or subsegmental drainage of the injured ductal system, simple ligation of the injured duct is adequate. If the injured duct is 4 mm or larger, however, it is likely to drain multiple hepatic segments or the entire right or left lobe and thus requires operative repair. If the injury involves the common hepatic duct or the common bile duct below the bifurcation, it is reasonable to carry out the repair at the time of injury. The aims of any repair should be to maintain ductal length and not to sacrifice tissue, as well as to create a repair that will not result in postoperative bile leakage. As a result, all repairs at the time of initial operation should be drained externally.

If the injured segment of the bile duct is short (less than 1 cm) and the two ends can be opposed without tension, an end-to-end anastomosis can be performed with potential placement of a T-tube through a separate choledochotomy either above or below the anastomosis (Figure 4). Generous mobilization of the duodenum out of the retroperitoneum (Kocher's maneuver) will help approximate the injured ends of the bile duct. Although primary end-to-end repair carries a high rate of anastomotic stricture, such strictures are often amenable to endoscopic balloon dilatation and stenting with excellent long-term outcomes. An end-to-end repair, however, should be avoided if the ductal injury is near the hepatic duct bifurcation or if there has been excessive loss of bile duct tissue.

For proximal injuries or if the injured segment of the bile duct is greater than 1 cm in length, an end-to-end bile duct anastomosis should be avoided because of the excessive tension that usually exists in these situations. In these circumstances, the distal bile duct should be oversewn, and the proximal bile duct should be débrided of injured tissue and anastomosed in an end-to-side fashion to a Roux-en-Y jejunal limb (Figure 5). The use of a Roux-en-Y jejunal limb is

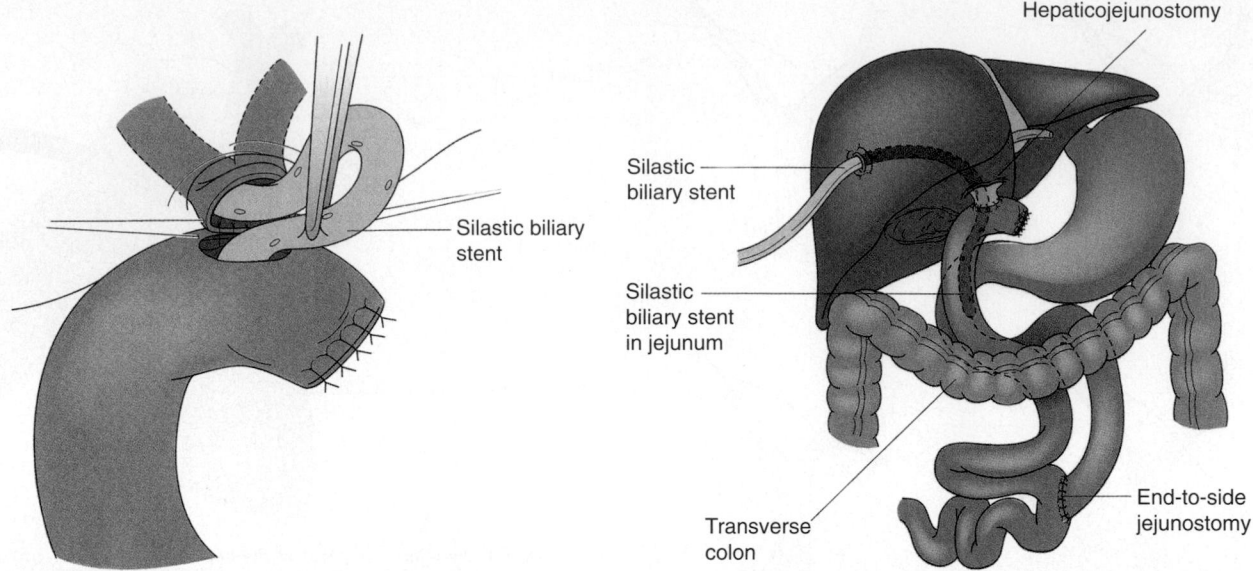

FIGURE 5 The Silastic stent is placed through the anastomosis. A completed Roux-en-Y hepaticojejunostomy with transanastomotic stent. *(Adapted from Cameron JL. Resection of benign bile duct stricture with reconstruction utilizing Silastic transhepatic biliary stents and hepaticojejunostomy. In: Atlas of Surgery. vol 1. Ontario: BC Decker; 1990:45, 55, 57.)*

preferable to anastomosis to the duodenum because, in the latter case, an anastomotic leak results in a duodenal fistula.

Unfortunately, most bile duct injuries during laparoscopic cholecystectomy occur during procedures by surgeons who are not experienced in performing complex biliary reconstruction (repairs by the primary surgeon are successful in less than 20%). This reality is highlighted by the average surgical trainee volume of 112 laparoscopic cholecystectomies during residency compared with 0.9 bile duct explorations and 1.6 choledochoenteric anastomoses. In these settings, the surgeon should consider *not* repairing the injury and therefore avoiding the risk of further worsening the situation. The biliary tree should be drained via a retrograde catheter to facilitate cholangiography, but the bile duct should not be ligated because ligation of the proximal bile duct stump most often leads to necrosis, subsequent bile leakage, and a more challenging reconstruction resulting from proximal migration of the injury. The subhepatic space should be well drained to control the biliary leak. Prompt transfer to a tertiary hepatobiliary center should then be made. Full disclosure to patients and their families is also paramount.

Initial Management After Delayed Recognition in the Postoperative Period

The initial management of a patient who seeks medical treatment in a typically delayed manner after an iatrogenic bile duct injury depends on the precise timing, mode, and anatomy of the injury. In the early setting (less than 72 hours), the patient most commonly has a bile leak, biloma, or bile ascites/peritonitis. In the context of an intraperitoneal bile leak, the associated inflammation within the field almost always demands a delay before reconstruction. The patient benefits from immediate control of the leak, evacuation of all fluid collection, control of sepsis, and sufficient time to allow resolution of the associated intra-abdominal inflammation. Parenteral antimicrobial therapy should be tailored to the biliary cultures and continued until the sepsis is resolved. Operative intervention, particularly by an inexperienced hepatobiliary surgeon, in this setting makes the identification of anatomy difficult and increases the risk of worsening the injury. To this end, biliary reconstruction under these circumstances frequently leads to long-term failure in the form of recurrent leak or biliary stricture.

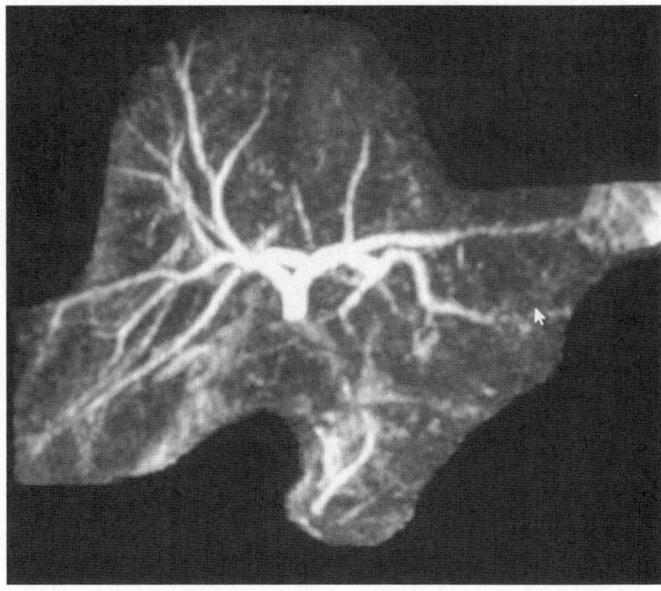

FIGURE 6 MRCP of patient with complete transection (with ligation by clips) of the common hepatic duct.

It is also imperative that before any attempt to repair a bile duct injury presenting in the postoperative period is made, *complete* cholangiography via percutaneous transhepatic cholangiography (PTC), magnetic resonance cholangiopancreatography (MRCP), and/or endoscopic retrograde cholangiography (ERCP) is essential. MRCP is worth considering early to noninvasively define the anatomy and nature of the injury and therefore the subsequent role of invasive procedures, including placement of transhepatic stents to control the bile leak (Figure 6).

Finally, complete arteriography (computed tomography angiography [CTA] or magnetic resonance angiography [MRA]) should be performed to rule out a concurrent right hepatic arterial injury, which occurs in 10% to 30% of cases and can lead to complications of false aneurysm formation, bleeding, or hepatic parenchymal or duct ischemia, all of which can prompt postoperative complications or poor long-term outcomes.

There remains some debate over the role and utility of preoperatively placed transhepatic stents. In our opinion, such stents are imperative in the setting of an uncontrolled bile leak, despite the recognized challenge of access of a nondilated intrahepatic ductal system. Even if the complete anatomy can be defined by MRCP, we feel that the presence of a biliary catheter, particularly if extending *below* the level of the injury/transection, can be extremely helpful in facilitating intraoperative identification and dissection of the hepatic ducts in the context of a very proximal/hilar injury. For injuries above the hepatic duct bifurcation, both the right and left main hepatic ducts should be stented individually. Finally, postoperative stenting can prevent a postoperative bile leak after a challenging biliary-enteric anastomosis and reduce the risk of an anastomotic stricture. To maintain percutaneous control of the biliary-enteric anastomosis in the postoperative setting, preoperative stents can be replaced at the time of the surgical repair with larger, soft Silastic stents ranging from 12F to 22F (Figure 7).

Definitive Management of Bile Duct Stricture

Given the significant maturation of endoscopic and percutaneous techniques in the management of biliary strictures, there is now frequently more than one acceptable methodology in treating a biliary stricture in the modern era. The management of benign bile duct strictures with the percutaneous transhepatic route traditionally has been indicated in patients with a failed prior biliary-enteric anastomosis to a jejunal limb. Access to the proximal biliary tree is gained and the stricture is traversed with a guide wire under fluoroscopic guidance and subsequently dilated with angioplasty-type balloon catheters. After the procedure, a transhepatic stent is left in place across the stricture to allow subsequent access to the biliary tree for repeat cholangiography, dilation, and maintenance of a lumen during the healing process. Signs of cholangitis are common in most patients after percutaneous instrumentation and must be treated expeditiously.

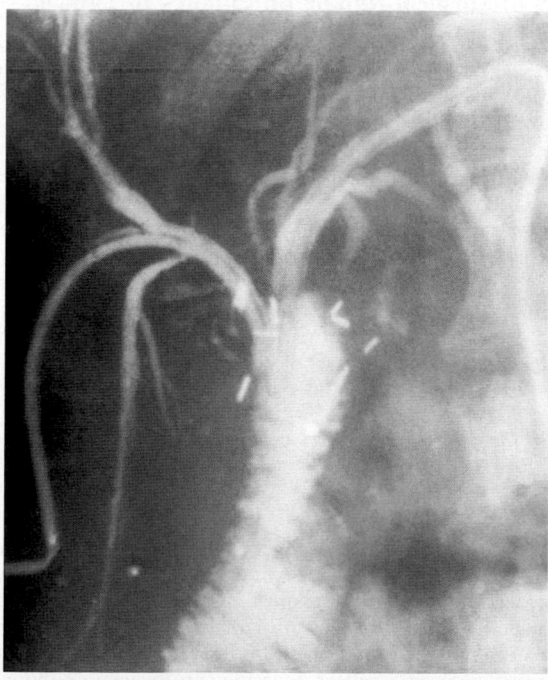

FIGURE 7 Postoperative cholangiogram demonstrating completed hepaticojejunostomy to the individual right and left hepatic ducts. Soft Silastic stents are placed across the anastomosis.

Endoscopic balloon dilation is another reasonable option but traditionally has been considered technically possible only in patients with primary bile duct strictures or with stenoses at a prior primary end-to-end repair or choledochoduodenal anastomosis. With the advent of double balloon enteroscopy, however, patients with a history of a prior hepaticojejunostomy may undergo ERCP. This technique begins with cholangiography and endoscopic sphincterotomy followed by traversing the stricture with an atraumatic guide wire, and sequential balloon dilation. One or usually multiple stents then are placed. Reevaluation with cholangiography is performed every 3 to 6 months. Although debates exist regarding which nonsurgical technique is superior, it is ideal when a given institution can offer multiple options. A recent study showed that patients with bile duct injuries were treated most commonly by endoscopists (40%), followed by surgeons (36%) and interventional radiologists (24%). However, success rates were higher for surgery (88%) compared with either endoscopy (76%) or interventional radiology (50%). Outcomes have improved dramatically over time among all approaches.

A number of alternative strategies are available with the specific type of treatment indicated varying depending on the site and extent of the biliary stricture. More specifically, Strasberg type A injuries are best treated with ERCP and biliary stent placement. Type B and C injuries (occluded or leaking posterior sectoral duct respectively) often do not require operative intervention, but if the patient experiences recurrent sepsis/cholangitis in the undrained sector, a right posterior hepatic sectionectomy is typically the best option given the high failure rate associated with an always technically demanding nondilated isolated posterior sectoral duct-enteric anastomosis. Management of type D injuries (less than 50% of the common bile or hepatic duct circumference) can be managed variably, depending on whether the injury was caused by diathermy energy–based devices. Endoscopic or IR dilatation and stenting may be successful for short segment strictures. If an operative approach is indicated, a primary end-to-end repair will lead to long-term failure in up to two thirds of cases, given the predictable fibrosis, retraction, and subsequent stricturing that accompanies thermal ductal injuries. Thus because the majority of iatrogenic ductal injuries are caused by a thermal source during a laparoscopic cholecystectomy, excising a portion of the duct back to healthy tissue and performing a Roux-en-Y hepaticojejunostomy reconstruction is preferred.

Invariably there is a loss of bile duct length; most bile duct injuries are a result of fibrosis associated with the injury. Thus simple excision of a bile duct stricture with end-to-end ductal anastomosis or repair is rarely technically feasible.

The goal of operative management of a bile duct stricture is the establishment of bile flow into the proximal gastrointestinal tract in a manner that prevents sludge, stone formation, cholangitis, restricture, and cirrhosis. Typically some version of a biliary-enteric anastomosis is required. Several principles guide successful biliary-enteric reconstruction: (1) exposure of healthy proximal bile duct that provides drainage of the entire liver, (2) preparation of a suitable section of intestine that can be brought to the area of the stricture without tension, and (3) creation of a biliary-enteric anastomosis that approximates biliary to enteric mucosa. In almost all cases, these principles mandate construction of a hepaticojejunostomy via a Roux-en-Y limb of jejunum. There are multiple options for hepaticojejunostomy, depending on the nature of the injury. If a segment of hepatic duct is intact and not ischemic, a simple end-to-end hepaticojejunostomy is adequate.

Strasberg type E injuries always require a biliary-enteric reconstruction in injuries that involve the hepatic duct bifurcation but still possess communication between the right and left hepatic ducts (intact hilar plate), it may be necessary to lower the hilar plate and/or extend the choledochotomy along the left hepatic duct to ensure a large common orifice (Figure 8). Strictures that completely separate the right and left systems require either creating a common "back" wall by sewing separate, but in close proximity, right and left ducts together, or alternatively creating distinct right and left biliary-enteric

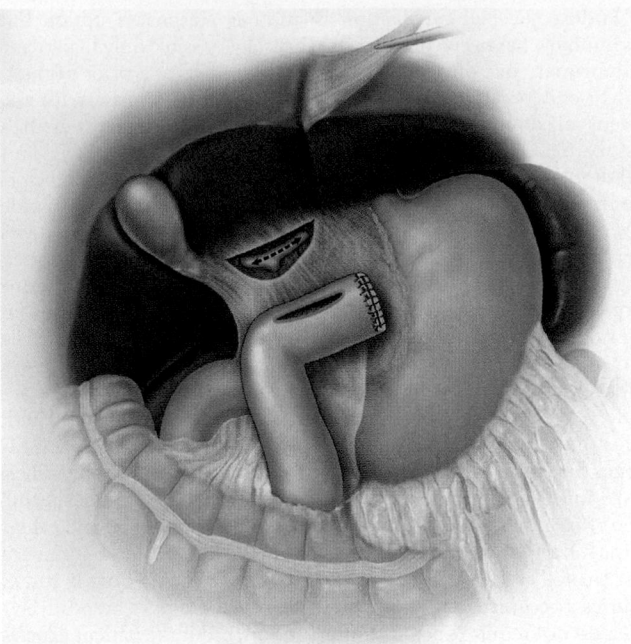

FIGURE 8 After the hilar plate is lowered, the left hepatic duct is exposed below at the base of segment IV. Careful dissection to the patient's left allows full exposure of the duct to its entry into the umbilical fissure, whereas dissection toward the patient's right provides access to the biliary confluence and the right hepatic duct.

anastomoses. The importance of the hilar arterial plexus (epicholedochal plexus) in such cases of proximal bile duct injuries is also worth mentioning because there is significant utility in performing a "high" hepaticojejunostomy reconstruction to an intact proximal hilar bridge between the right and left ducts (i.e., uses the crossing arterial anatomy to minimize the risk of subsequent biliary stenosis).

On occasion, suitable duct length outside of the hepatic parenchyma is unavailable, and the surgeon must solicit direct access to the intrahepatic biliary system. The segment II duct can be located and isolated as it courses superficially on the inferior posterior surface. The parenchyma is incised over the duct, and the duct is opened along its length for 2 cm in preparation for a biliary-enteric anastomosis. Similarly, the segment III duct can be isolated on the medial anterior surface of segment III just lateral to the insertion of the ligamentum teres. This duct is located more deeply within the liver parenchyma but is an excellent site of access for biliary drainage.

Technical considerations for performing a Hepp-Couinaud hepaticojejunostomy include the dominant goal of ensuring a gastrointestinal linkage (70 cm retrocolic Roux limb of jejunum) to a wide, long anastomosis with well-vascularized ductal tissue in a tension-free manner. Excessive dissection greater than 5 mm in the cephalad direction should be avoided, with the caveat of lowering the hilar plate at the base of segment 4b. The anastomosis itself usually is achieved with interrupted 5-0 absorbable sutures.

We support the routine use of transanastomotic stents, which should be placed through the anastomotic orifice after construction of the posterior wall, but before the anterior wall. Closed suction drainage adjacent to the anastomosis is also common. The length of time that the stents are left in place is variable and subject to debate. We usually remove the stents after 2 to 3 months in a healthy patient with a well-healed anastomosis as confirmed by both complete mechanical internalization and cholangiographic evidence of the absence of leakage or stricture.

Finally, in rare cases with failure of all standard surgical techniques of reconstruction with resultant end-stage liver disease, liver transplantation may offer an opportunity for survival. However, most liver transplants are indicated urgently after extreme vasculobiliary injuries caused during open cholecystectomy.

Long-Term Results of Surgical Reconstruction

The perioperative outcomes of surgical repair for biliary injuries after laparoscopic cholecystectomy have been reported in detail throughout the literature. Historically, excellent long-term results were achieved in 70% to 90% of patients who underwent repair of bile duct strictures. The definition of satisfactory results in most series required that patients have not required intervention for symptoms such as jaundice or cholangitis. The length of follow-up is particularly important in analyzing final results because recurrent strictures can occur up to 20 years after the initial procedure (although two thirds of restrictures are evident within 2 years, and 90% are observed within 7 years). The percentage of patients with good results is related inversely to the number of previous repairs. Other factors that favor a good outcome include young age at the time of stricture repair, use of a Roux-en-Y biliary-enteric anastomosis, absence of infection and hepatic fibrosis, and the use of transhepatic stents.

Stewart and Way have attempted to better delineate variables associated with successful reconstruction after biliary injuries from laparoscopic cholecystectomy. In their publication, four factors were found to predict the outcome of the repair: (1) the performance of complete preoperative cholangiography, (2) the choice of repair, (3) the details of the operative repair, and (4) the experience of the surgeon performing the repair. Ninety-six percent of the procedures in which cholangiograms were not obtained before surgery were unsuccessful. Sixty-nine percent of the procedures for which cholangiogram data were incomplete were unsuccessful. In contrast, 84% of repairs were successful when the cholangiographic data were complete. Further in support of the preceding literature, Roux-en-Y hepaticojejunostomies outperformed end-to-end anastomoses (63% vs 0 successful, respectively), and experienced biliary surgeons outperformed the index laparoscopic surgeons (84% vs 17% successful, respectively).

Effect of Surgical Repair on Quality of Life

Several studies have examined the impact of iatrogenic bile duct injuries on quality of life after surgical repair. Most demonstrate that the patients have either comparable or mildly diminished quality of life compared with matched controls. In one study, patients who reported pursuing a lawsuit after their injury had significantly worse quality-of-life scores in all domains when compared with those who did not entertain legal action. The most recent study, which spanned a 23-year period (169-month median follow-up), evaluated 62 patients who had generally undergone a Roux-en-Y hepaticojejunostomy reconstruction and confirmed that mental health concerns were more common than physical or general health issues after bile duct injuries. Although most patients displayed an eventual return to their physical baseline, psychologic quality of life was much more difficult to correct over time.

■ NONIATROGENIC BILIARY STRICTURES

Chronic Pancreatitis

Chronic pancreatitis is a cause of clinically relevant biliary strictures. In these cases, pancreatic fibrosis results in distal biliary strictures that involve the entire intrapancreatic portion of the bile duct and lead to dilation of the complete proximal duct. Although the clinical presentation of patients is variable, it often includes alcoholism with concurrent endocrine and/or exocrine insufficiency. Although the precise incidence of biliary stricture in patients with chronic pancreatitis is unknown, serum alkaline phosphatase appears to be the most sensitive marker of obstruction (chemical cholestasis). A confirmed diagnosis requires either ERCP or MRCP (identifying a long, smooth, gradual tapering of the distal bile duct on the cholangiographic component). These investigations also have the advantage of providing an update on the mechanical status of the pancreatic duct. As long as a periampullary tumor has been ruled out, therapeutic options are numerous but most commonly use a biliary bypass (either choledochoduodenostomy or choledochojejunostomy). The former procedure also has the advantage of leaving the duodenum intact for subsequent endoscopic procedures. In patients in whom malignancy cannot be excluded, or who have concurrent chronic pain and/or duodenal obstruction, pancreaticoduodenectomy is preferred to treat each of these complications in a single procedure. Two randomized trials have demonstrated the superiority of surgical versus endoscopic therapy for obstructive pathology with regard to the primary intervention success rate, pain relief, and quality of life. As a result, it generally is recommended that if an endoscopic approach has not resolved these complications effectively within 12 months, patients should be offered surgical therapy/bypass.

Autoimmune Pancreatitis

Autoimmune pancreatitis is a rare inflammatory disease that is almost uniformly responsive to steroid therapy. These patients can have obstructive jaundice and often have an associated pancreatic mass. This form of pancreatitis is subdivided into two distinct subgroups: type I (IgG4 [immunoglobulin 4]–related, relapsing) and type II (limited to the pancreas, rarely relapsing). Biliary obstruction can be associated with either pathology. A lack of prompt response to steroid therapy should trigger an immediate search for a different underlying cause, such as a periampullary cancer.

Primary Sclerosing Cholangitis

Primary sclerosing cholangitis is a chronic, progressive, and destructive cholangiopathy that is related to inflammatory bowel disease and results in an identifiable pattern of biliary strictures and dilations. The typical manifestation of these patients involves recurrent episodes of cholangitis leading to secondary biliary cirrhosis and not uncommonly biliary malignancy. Unfortunately, there is no simple definitive treatment beyond hepatic transplantation. More specifically, although ursodeoxycholic acid is known to reduce the time to transplantation, current guidelines do not recommend its usage. In

the setting of a dominant stricture, placement of a biliary stent via ERCP or on occasion, PTC, can be helpful. The presence of a concurrent malignancy as the cause of the stricture must be ruled out first, however (SpyGlass ERCP or MRCP; Boston Scientific, Natick, MA).

Recurrent Pyogenic Cholangitis

Recurrent pyogenic cholangitis is an inflammatory condition located within the liver and biliary tree that manifests as biliary structuring, dilatation, and stone formation secondary to recurrent cholangitis. Although described by many names, this cause of biliary strictures occurs most commonly in Asian patients with a history of discrete episodes of cholangitis-related symptoms. Diagnostic modalities include, but are not limited to, ultrasonography, cross-sectional imaging (CT or MRCP), and/or ERCP. Surgical therapies encompass the entirety of biliary surgery: (1) hepatic resection (disease [atrophy and stones] is located within an isolated section of the liver), (2) combined liver resection with biliary-enteric bypass, (3) choledochotomy and T-tube placement, (4) biliary access limbs (Hudson loop), and (5) hepatic transplantation. Selection of one surgical therapy over another depends on the distribution of the disease and the underlying health of the liver and patient. More commonly, however, this challenging disease requires multidisciplinary management from an experienced team of surgeons, endoscopists, and interventional radiologists.

SUGGESTED READINGS

Ejaz A, Spolverato G, Kim Y, et al. Long-term health-related quality of life after iatrogenic bile duct injury repair. *J Am Coll Surg*. 2014;219:923.

Melton GB, Lillemoe KD, Cameron JL, et al. Major bile duct injuries associated with laparoscopic cholecystectomy: effect on quality of life. *Ann Surg*. 2002;235:888.

Pitt HA, Sherman S, Johnson MS, et al. Improved outcomes of bile duct injuries in the 21st century. *Ann Surg*. 2013;258:490.

Sheffield KM, Riall TS, Kuo YF, et al. Association between cholecystectomy with vs without intraoperative cholangiography and risk of common duct injury. *JAMA*. 2013;310:812.

Stewart L, Way LW. Bile duct injuries during laparoscopic cholecystectomy. *Arch Surg*. 1995;130:1223.

Strasberg SM, Helton WS. An analytical review of vasculobiliary injury in laparoscopic and open cholecystectomy. *HPB (Oxford)*. 2011;13:1.

Strasberg SM, Hertl M, Soper NJ. An analysis of the problem of biliary injury during laparoscopic cholecystectomy. *J Am Coll Surg*. 1995;180:101.

The Management of Cystic Disorders of the Bile Ducts

Steven A. Ahrendt, MD

Choledochal cyst is a rare congenital dilation of the extrahepatic and/or intrahepatic biliary tract. Although choledochal cysts usually develop in infancy and childhood, the disease is commonly diagnosed in adults. The incidence of choledochal cyst is only between 1 in 100,000 and 1 in 150,000 people in Western countries but is much higher in East Asian populations. Choledochal cysts are four times more common in women than men. Choledochal cysts are associated with an increased risk of cholangitis and pancreatitis as well as a high risk of malignant degeneration.

■ ETIOLOGY AND CLASSIFICATION

The frequent presentation of choledochal cysts in infancy supports a congenital origin. An anomalous pancreatobiliary duct junction (APBDJ) has also been documented in between 80% and 90% of pediatric patients with choledochal cysts. In APBDJ, the pancreatic duct joins the common bile duct more than 15 mm proximal to the ampulla, resulting in a long common channel and free reflux of pancreatic secretions into the biliary tract. This reflux of pancreatic juice into the biliary tract results in increased biliary pressures and inflammatory changes in the biliary epithelium and may be related to the formation of choledochal cysts.

The current classification of choledochal cysts was initially proposed by Alonso-Lej and subsequently modified by Todani (Figure 1). Type I cysts (dilations of the extrahepatic biliary tract) are the most common and comprise 80% to 90% of choledochal cysts. Type I cysts further subdivide into cystic (IA), focal (IB), and fusiform (IC). Type IV cysts (cystic dilation of both the intrahepatic and the extrahepatic biliary tract) also occur frequently (15% to 20% of

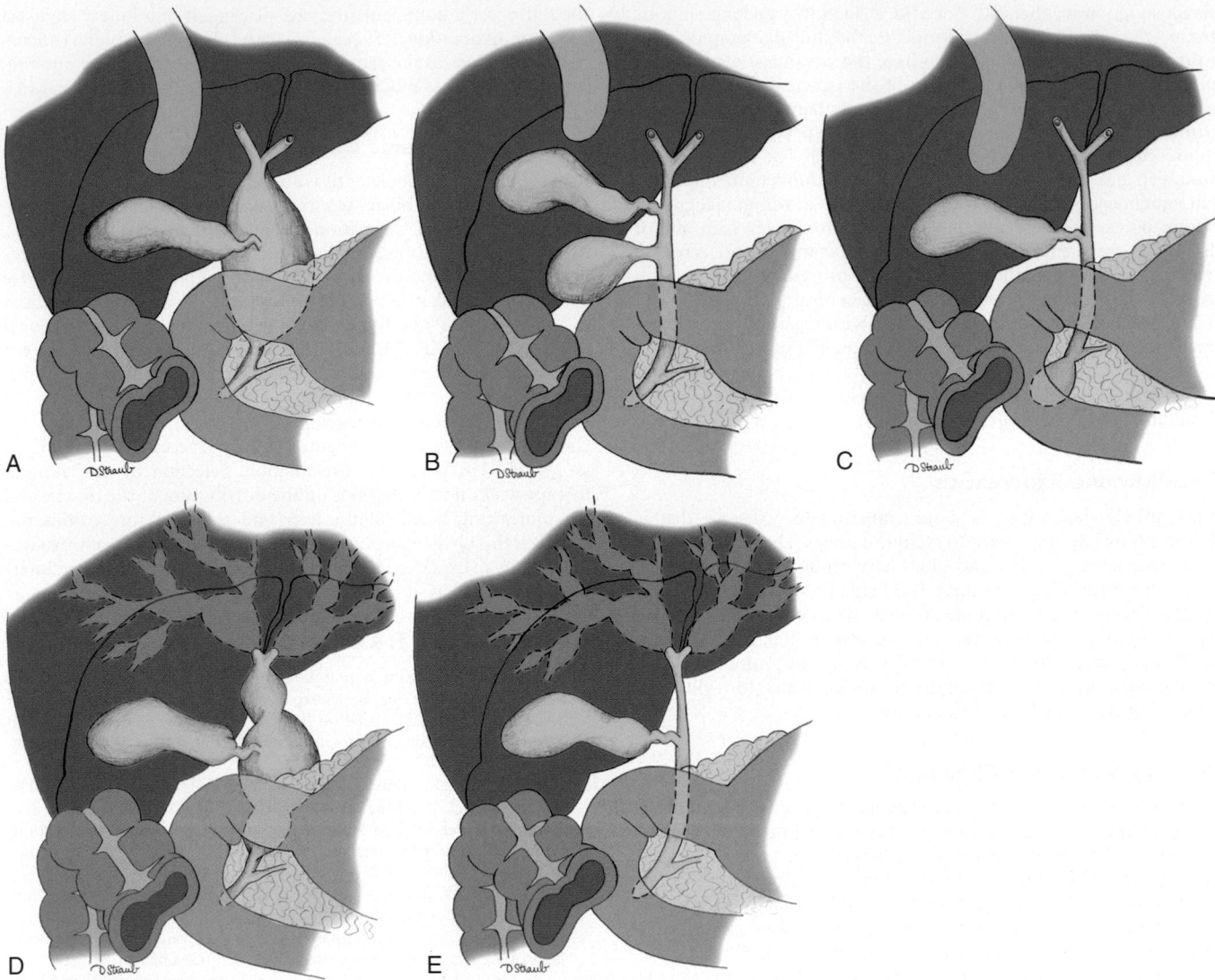

FIGURE 1 Classification of biliary cysts. **A,** Type I. **B,** Type II. **C,** Type III. **D,** Type IVA. **E,** Type V. *(From Lipsett PA, Pitt HA, Columbani PM, et al. Choledochal disease: a changing pattern of presentation. Ann Surg. 1994;220:644.)*

patients). Type II (saccular diverticulum of extrahepatic bile duct), Type III (bile duct dilation within the duodenal wall [choledochocele]), and Type V cysts (intrahepatic cysts [Caroli's disease]) are much less common, with each type being diagnosed in fewer than 10% of patients with choledochal cysts.

■ CLINICAL PRESENTATION

The classic clinical triad associated with choledochal cysts includes right upper quadrant pain, jaundice, and an abdominal mass; however, this presentation occurs in fewer than 10% of patients. The clinical presentation differs among children and adults. Children often have an abdominal mass and jaundice. In adults, biliary and pancreatic symptoms, including abdominal pain (87%) and jaundice (42%), are frequently present. Less common clinical findings include nausea (29%), cholangitis (26%), pancreatitis (23%), and an abdominal mass (13%). Symptomatic gallstones and acute cholecystitis occur commonly and adult patients diagnosed with choledochal cysts have frequently undergone prior cholecystectomy. The increased use of cross-sectional imaging has also led to the diagnosis of choledochal cyst in asymptomatic patients.

■ DIAGNOSIS

Laboratory evaluation may demonstrate mild liver function abnormalities in 60% of adult patients with choledochal cysts, and these findings are not specific. The diagnosis can be established with ultrasound or computed tomographic (CT) scanning but may be overlooked if the diagnosis is not considered. A common bile duct diameter exceeding 1 cm in an adult suggests a distal obstruction from a stone or neoplasm or the presence of cystic dilation of the biliary tract. In addition, the presence of a right upper quadrant cyst distinct from the gallbladder is suggestive of a choledochal cyst.

Cholangiography (endoscopic, transhepatic, or magnetic resonance) is required to determine the type of choledochal cyst and plan the extent of operative treatment. Magnetic resonance cholangiopancreatography (MRCP) is highly sensitive and specific in the diagnosis and classification of choledochal cysts and avoids the risks inherent in endoscopic and percutaneous techniques. MRCP is also accurate in defining the presence of an APBDJ and is useful in identifying the presence of biliary stones and cholangiocarcinoma.

■ MANAGEMENT

Traditionally, choledochal cysts were managed with internal drainage procedures (cystenterostomy) and cholecystectomy. This approach led to persistent biliary stasis and a high rate of cholangitis, pancreatitis, recurrent strictures, and liver fibrosis. More significantly, the risk of cholangiocarcinoma in the remaining biliary cyst was unacceptably high. The current approach includes cholecystectomy, complete resection of the choledochal cyst whenever possible to minimize the risk of malignant transformation, and a biliary enteric anastomosis to prevent further reflux of pancreatic juice into the biliary tract. Patients initially managed with cystenterostomy should undergo resection as outlined in the following sections because of the continued high risk of malignancy.

Type I: Extrahepatic Bile Duct Cyst

After cholecystectomy a Kocher's maneuver is performed. The anterior wall of the choledochal cyst is dissected distally until it narrows at the inferior portion of the cyst. The distal common bile duct is ligated at this level and divided, taking care not to injure the pancreatic duct. The cyst is then reflected anteriorly off of the portal vein. The cyst is mobilized to the level of the hepatic duct bifurcation. The common hepatic duct is divided just distal to the hepatic duct bifurcation. Frozen section of the proximal and distal bile duct margins is obtained to exclude the presence of cholangiocarcinoma. Biliary-enteric continuity is restored with an end-to-side Roux-en-Y hepaticojejunostomy. Roux-en-Y hepaticojejunostomy is preferred to hepaticoduodenostomy, which has a higher risk of postoperative bile reflux, gastritis, and gastric cancer.

Type II: Extrahepatic Biliary Diverticulum

Type II cysts usually can be managed by simple diverticulectomy with closure of the common bile duct at the cyst neck. These cysts are typically not associated with an APBDJ and do not have a high risk of malignant transformation.

Type III: Choledochocele

The majority of choledochoceles is small and can be managed with endoscopic sphincterotomy. These cysts also do not carry an elevated risk of cholangiocarcinoma. Larger cysts have been managed successfully with transduodenal excision.

Type IV: Intrahepatic and Extrahepatic Bile Duct Cyst

Management of type IV choledochal cysts is challenging. Diffuse involvement of the intrahepatic bile ducts can make complete excision impossible. The extrahepatic component is treated with cyst excision and reconstruction similar to type I choledochal cysts. Partial hepatectomy is recommended for any intrahepatic component likely to result in future complications such as intrahepatic stones or cholangitis.

Type V: Caroli's Disease

Initial treatment of Caroli's disease includes treatment of any symptoms, including cholangitis with antibiotics, biliary drainage procedures, and stone extraction. All patients should undergo surveillance for cholangiocarcinoma with serial imaging and serum cancer antigen 19-9 (CA19-9). Patients developing symptoms from localized intrahepatic cysts or cysts confined to one lobe of the liver are best approached with hepatic resection. Patients with complicated bilobar disease and recurrent cholangitis despite maximal medical therapy, portal hypertension, or suspicion of early cholangiocarcinoma are candidates for orthotopic liver transplantation.

■ PROGNOSIS

Perioperative morbidity and mortality in patients undergoing choledochal cyst resection are comparable to other major hepatobiliary procedures. Common complications include wound infection, anastomotic leak, and hemorrhage. Long-term complications are common (up to 40%) and include anastomotic stricture, cholangitis, and cholangiocarcinoma. Late complications are more common in patients with type IV and V biliary cysts. Five-year survival in patients with choledochal cysts managed with resection and biliary reconstruction exceeds 90%. Unfortunately, the risk of cholangiocarcinoma remains elevated after resection and thus patients should undergo long-term surveillance.

SUGGESTED READINGS

Edil BH, Cameron JL, Reddy S, et al. Choledochal cyst disease in children and adults: a 30-year single-institution experience. *J Am Coll Surg*. 2008;206: 1000-1008.

Lee SE, Jang JY, Lee YJ, et al. Choledochal cyst and associated malignant tumors in adults: a multicenter survey in South Korea. *Arch Surg*. 2011;146:1178-1184.

Soares KC, Arnaotakis DJ, Kamel I, et al. Choledochal cysts: presentation, clinical differentiation, and management. *J Am Coll Surg*. 2014;219: 1167-1180.

THE MANAGEMENT OF PRIMARY SCLEROSING CHOLANGITIS

Nicholas J. Zyromski, MD, and Henry A. Pitt, MD

Primary sclerosing cholangitis (PSC) is a chronic inflammatory disease characterized by strictures of the intrahepatic and extrahepatic biliary tree and a variable, but generally progressive, clinical course, ultimately leading to cholestasis and hepatic cirrhosis. Several systemic autoimmune diseases are associated with PSC, most commonly inflammatory bowel disease (IBD). Biliary malignancy is very common, developing in approximately 15% of patients with PSC, but cholangiocarcinoma (CCA) may be extremely difficult to diagnose in these patients with existing biliary strictures. No medical therapy effectively has delayed progression of disease. A wide variety of percutaneous, endoscopic, and surgical approaches are used to treat patients according to the pattern of stricture disease. No one interventional modality is clearly superior because the principal goals of treatment are to delay progression of disease (liver fibrosis/cirrhosis) and prevent malignant degeneration. Liver transplantation is clearly the treatment of choice once hepatic cirrhosis develops, but surgical resection of a dominant stricture may be effective in selected noncirrhotic patients.

NATURAL HISTORY

The incidence and prevalence of PSC in the United States and Europe range from 0.5 to 1.3 and 3.9 to 16.2 per 100,000, respectively. Current evidence suggests that the incidence may be increasing. Approximately two thirds of patients with PSC are male, with an average age in the 40s at the time of diagnosis. Large population series have shown that the median survival from time of diagnosis to death or liver transplantation ranges from 12 to 18 years. About 75% of PSC patients have involvement of both intrahepatic and extrahepatic bile ducts; 15% have only intrahepatic, and 10% have only extrahepatic bile duct involvement. The hepatic duct bifurcation nearly always is involved in patients with extrahepatic ductal disease.

The cause of PSC is poorly understood. The fact that most PSC patients have IBD has led many to consider autoimmunity as a cause. Evidence supporting this theory includes the common finding of autoantibodies (including atypical antineutrophil antibody, p-ANCA, which is found in 88% of PSC patients). The coexistence of PSC and IBD also supports the hypothesis of a bacterial cause. Bacterial translocation permitted by increased intestinal epithelial permeability may lead to Kupffer's cell activation, tumor necrosis factor-α (TNF-α) production, and subsequent biliary inflammation/fibrosis. Contemporary interest in the gut microflora has suggested a putative link between the microbiota, enteroportal circulation, and PSC development, particularly in the setting of IBD. Finally, a hereditary component to PSC almost surely exists; first-degree relatives of PSC patients have nearly a fourfold increased incidence of PSC diagnosis compared with the general population. The genetic pattern in PSC is complex and polymorphic, although many of the identified aberrant loci are related to the human leukocyte antigen complex.

ASSOCIATED DISEASES

Between 70% and 80% of PSC patients also have IBD, most commonly ulcerative colitis but also Crohn's disease. In contrast, only 10% of IBD patients will be diagnosed with PSC. Colon cancer is significantly more common in IBD patients with PSC; the risk of colon cancer in this population may increase after liver transplant. Colonoscopy therefore should be performed in all PSC patients with a more rigorous surveillance schedule than that recommended for the general public. Other autoimmune diseases associated less commonly with PSC include type 1 diabetes mellitus, thyroiditis, ankylosing spondylitis, autoimmune hepatitis, and celiac disease. PSC has been associated with a moderately increased risk for pancreatitis, pancreatic adenocarcinoma, and colorectal carcinoma.

Gallbladder disease is very common in PSC patients. Gallstones develop in more than 25% of PSC patients. Gallbladder polyps are diagnosed in about 5% of PSC patients; this incidence is substantially higher than that seen in the general population. In addition, adenocarcinoma is detected in nearly half of these polyps. Therefore cholecystectomy should be performed in any PSC patient diagnosed with gallbladder polyps, and some authorities recommend annual screening with gallbladder ultrasound. Hepatocellular carcinoma (HCC) also is common in PSC patients with end-stage liver disease. HCC is detected in 2% to 4% of explanted livers from PSC patients undergoing liver transplant. CCA develops in as many as 15% of PSC patients. Screening for and diagnosis of CCA are discussed in more detail later. Box 1 summarizes diseases associated with PSC.

CLINICAL PRESENTATION AND DIAGNOSIS

The widely variable presentation of PSC patients highlights disease heterogeneity. Patients may be completely asymptomatic and come to PSC diagnosis from the finding of abnormal liver function tests. The IBD patient screened for liver disease falls into this category. On

---

BOX 1: Diseases Associated With Primary Sclerosing Cholangitis

Ulcerative colitis
Crohn's disease
Type 1 diabetes mellitus
Thyroiditis
Autoimmune hepatitis
Ankylosing spondylitis
Celiac disease
Acute pancreatitis
Pancreatic adenocarcinoma
Gallstones
Gallbladder polyps
Colorectal adenocarcinoma
Cholangiocarcinoma
Hepatocellular carcinoma

---

the other hand, many PSC patients experience the typical biliary symptom of right upper quadrant pain, or with pruritus and fatigue. Patients with intrahepatic bile duct involvement also may have first end-stage liver disease and hepatic failure, whereas those with isolated extrahepatic biliary strictures may have jaundice as the first clinical sign.

Magnetic resonance cholangiography (MRC) has become the gold standard for diagnosis of PSC. MRC affords visualization of intrahepatic bile ducts proximal to high-grade strictures and provides information about liver morphology in addition to imaging other abdominal structures. MRC is a purely diagnostic test (Figure 1). Endoscopic retrograde cholangiography (ERC) accurately demonstrates the intrahepatic and extrahepatic biliary tree more than 95% of the time and also permits intervention such as stenting, brushing, and biopsy. ERC has a small, but real, potential for complications, including cholangitis, visceral perforation, pancreatitis, and hemorrhage. Percutaneous transhepatic cholangiography (PTC) is used less frequently in current practice. PTC is technically challenging even for an experienced interventional radiologist; however, this test is clearly useful in select cases. Like endoscopy, percutaneous access to the biliary system also permits biopsy and stenting.

Liver biopsy should be performed in all PSC patients to document the degree of hepatic fibrosis. The possibility of lobar atrophy/hypertrophy should be considered when performing a liver biopsy. As discussed earlier, colonoscopy is indicated in PSC patients on a more aggressive schedule not only to diagnose colonic neoplasia but also to secure or exclude the diagnosis of inflammatory bowel disease.

BILIARY MALIGNANCY IN PRIMARY SCLEROSING CHOLANGITIS

The specter of CCA looms large in the setting of PSC; CCA is diagnosed in 1% to 2% of PSC patients annually, with a lifetime risk of 15%. This CCA incidence represents an increased risk of up to 160 times that of the general population. Unsuspected ("incidental") CCA is found in 3% to 9% of explanted livers at the time of transplantation for PSC despite aggressive preoperative screening protocols. CCA is observed more frequently in the setting of IBD and in women. No correlation exists between CCA diagnosis and development of hepatic cirrhosis or duration of PSC. About half of patients who develop CCA will be diagnosed within 1 year of presentation with PSC; many of these patients are diagnosed concurrently. Unfortunately, no high-risk group within the PSC population has been identified to target with more intensive screening protocols.

The diagnosis of CCA is challenging in the setting of multiple intrahepatic and extrahepatic bile duct strictures, and outcomes after CCA diagnosis are uniformly poor. A rational screening program involves serial cross-sectional imaging (MRI/MRCP) and measurement of serum tumor marker carbohydrate antigen (CA) 19-9

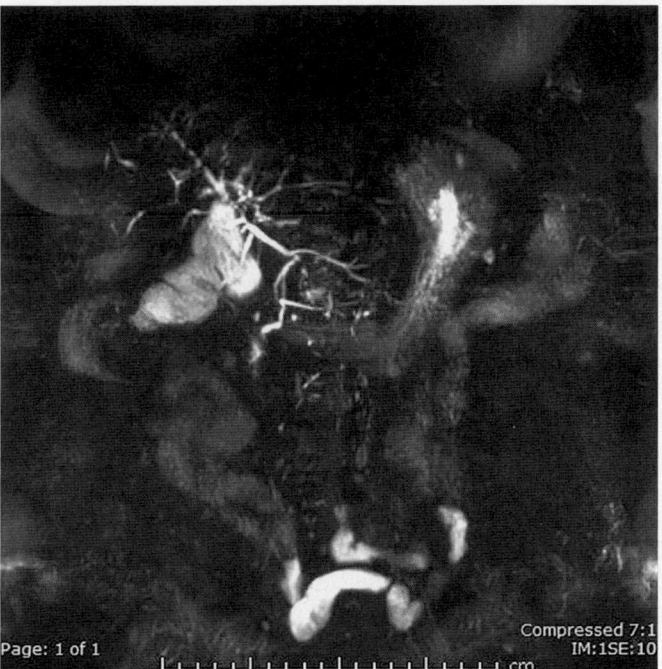

FIGURE I Magnetic resonance cholangiography demonstrating multiple intrahepatic bile duct strictures characteristic of primary sclerosing cholangitis. This patient has progressive disease; she underwent resection of extrahepatic biliary tree with cholangiojejunostomies for a dominant hilar stricture 9 years before this image was taken.

TABLE I: Select Medications Studied in Treatment of Primary Sclerosing Cholangitis and Their Category or Mechanism of Action

Agent	Category/Mechanism
UDCA	Hydrophilic bile acid
Prednisone	Corticosteroid
Budesonide	Corticosteroid
Colchicine	Mitotic inhibitor
Tacrolimus (FK 506)	Immunosuppressant
Methotrexate	Immunosuppressant
Mycophenolate mofetil	Immunosuppressant
Pirfenidone	Antifibrotic
Metronidazole	Antibiotic
Minocycline	Antibiotic
Etanercept	TNF-α inhibitor
Pentoxifylline	TNF-α inhibitor
Docosahexaenoic acid	Improves CFTR function

CFTR, Cystic fibrosis transmembrane conductance receptor; *TNF-α,* tumor necrosis factor-α; *UDCA,* ursodeoxycholic acid.

concentration. Although CA 19-9 is relatively specific, it suffers from poor sensitivity and may be spuriously elevated (giving a false positive) in the setting of jaundice. Serum concentration greater than 130 U/mL in the absence of jaundice or cholangitis should raise suspicion for CCA development. Endoscopic (ERC) evaluation is applied selectively to patients with increasing CA 19-9 or those in whom dominant strictures develop or progress.

Tissue histology is the gold standard for making the diagnosis of CCA; however, the sensitivity of biliary brushings and biopsy obtained at the time of ERC is less than 40%, although specificity is almost 100%. Currently, fluorescence in situ hybridization (FISH) has been applied more liberally. This test takes advantage of the fact that chromosomal abnormalities are present in approximately 80% of biliary malignancies. Indeed, patients with a dominant biliary stricture and polysomy were found to have an 88% incidence of CCA. Cholangioscopy, endoscopic and intraductal ultrasound, and confocal laser endomicroscopy are promising evolving technologies with which to interrogate the biliary tree. Proteomic analysis of serum, bile, and urine may aid CCA diagnosis in the future. The role of positron emission tomography (PET) in diagnosis of biliary malignancy has been evaluated recently; unfortunately, sensitivity and specificity of this test are poor. Complete surgical resection offers the best prognosis for those patients developing CCA in the face of PSC. Patients with recurrent dominant strictures or those with cellular atypia or dysplasia on cytologic brushing or biopsy therefore should undergo operative exploration rather than repeated attempts at endoscopic diagnosis.

PSC patients also have a significantly increased risk of having gallbladder neoplasia, although the precise incidence of this problem is difficult to quantitate. Some authorities recommend annual gallbladder ultrasound as part of a screening protocol, with cholecystectomy indicated for *any* size lesion identified because gallbladder cancer has been reported to arise even in small (less than 1 cm) polyps in PSC patients. Cholecystectomy obviously must be weighed against the generally increased perioperative risks attendant to end-stage liver disease.

MEDICAL THERAPY

Numerous agents aimed to abrogate the pathologic course of PSC have been tested in controlled clinical trials. Unfortunately, no medical therapy has slowed effectively disease progression, prolonged survival, or improved outcomes in patients with PSC (Table 1). The hydrophilic bile acid ursodeoxycholic acid (UDCA) is one of the most widely studied agents. Data from a large prospective, randomized trial of low-dose (12 to 15 mg/kg daily) UDCA demonstrated improvements in serum liver chemistry values but failed to show improvement in liver histology or transplant-free survival. Subsequent prospective studies with increased doses of UDCA have been analyzed by meta-analysis; similarly, this collective analysis failed to show a beneficial effect on symptoms, serum liver chemistry values, quality of life, or transplant-free survival.

Immunosuppressive agents are not beneficial in PSC. Administration of both topical and systemic glucocorticoids has been studied prospectively; no improvement in any objective outcome measure has been seen in PSC patients. In addition, glucocorticoid administration actually may be dangerous because it carries an increased risk of infection and may mask symptoms of biliary infection. Targeted therapy with antifibrotic agents, TNF-α inhibitors, T-cell modulators, and inhibitors of "toxic bile" formation (Farnesoid X agonists) all are in conceptual or early investigative phases.

ENDOSCOPIC AND INTERVENTIONAL RADIOLOGIC THERAPY

Since the late 1980s, percutaneous transhepatic stenting and endoscopic dilatation with or without stenting have been used to treat dominant strictures in PSC. A dominant stricture has been defined as narrowing 1.5 mm or less in the common bile duct or 1 mm or less in the common hepatic duct. With improvements in endoscopic techniques and technology, the majority of tertiary centers treating PSC patients currently favor the endoscopic over the percutaneous approach. Clinical response can be demonstrated in up to 80% of patients after endoscopic balloon dilatation. Placement of endobiliary stents has become limited generally to patients in whom balloon dilation fails to maintain luminal patency. Stenting duration of 6 to 8 weeks is probably optimal to avoid cholangitis, although some patients require extended periods of stenting (up to 12 months) before stricture resolution has been achieved. Complications of endoscopic therapy arise in approximately 10% of patients and include bleeding, perforation, pancreatitis, and cholangitis. The majority of these complications resolve with medical management. Advanced endoscopic techniques such as cholangioscopy and intraductal ultrasound are practiced more routinely at high-volume biliary centers and may be helpful particularly in diagnosing CCA.

Percutaneous approaches to the biliary tree are used less frequently in the current era. However, percutaneous stents remain important in select patient groups, including those who have had previous biliary bypass or a surgical bariatric procedure (Roux-en-Y gastric bypass or duodenal switch).

■ SURGICAL RESECTION

Highly selected patients with dominant extrahepatic strictures and no hepatic cirrhosis may benefit from resection of the extrahepatic biliary tree and reconstruction with a Roux-en-Y limb of jejunum. Surgical resection provides durable relief of jaundice, definitively confirms or excludes the diagnosis of CCA, and delays the progression of hepatic cirrhosis and the need for liver transplantation.

In what is now a classic study, Ahrendt and colleagues evaluated 146 PSC patients managed by surgical resection, percutaneous or endoscopic treatment, medical therapy alone, and transplantation. In noncirrhotic patients, the overall 5-year survival (85% vs 59%) and transplant-free survival (82% vs 46%) were significantly longer in the resection group compared with those managed endoscopically (Figure 2). With a greater than 5-year follow-up, no

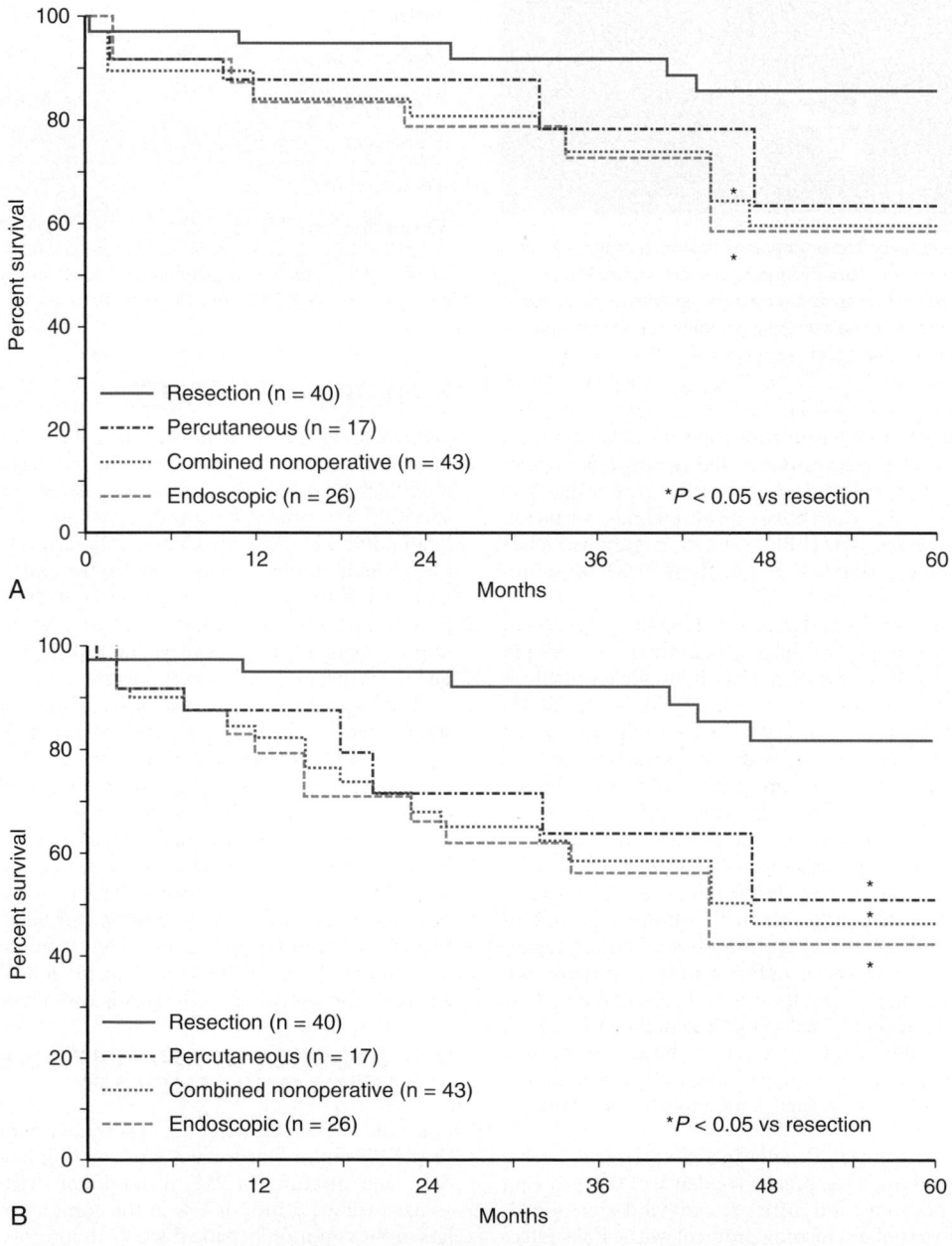

FIGURE 2 Overall (**A**) and transplant-free (**B**) survival curves for noncirrhotic patients undergoing resection, percutaneous, and endoscopic treatment of dominant extrahepatic biliary strictures in primary sclerosing cholangitis. *(From Ahrendt SA, Pitt HA, Kalloo AN, et al. Primary Sclerosing Cholangitis: Resect, Dilate, or Transplant? Ann Surg. 1998;227:412-423.)*

surgical patient had CCA. Patients with hepatic cirrhosis had longer survival after transplantation than after resection or endoscopic management.

High-quality cross-sectional imaging (computed tomography or magnetic resonance imaging) with intravascular contrast is important to assess hepatic vascular anatomy as well as the presence of liver atrophy/hypertrophy. The hepatic duct bifurcation is involved in most (80%) patients with dominant strictures; therefore percutaneous stents are placed preoperatively into the right and left hepatic ducts. This maneuver greatly facilitates dissection of the hepatic bifurcation and provides stenting for the reconstructive hepaticojejunostomy. Perioperative antibiotics are tailored to cover specific bacteria cultured from the bile and continued postoperatively for a few days to treat the mild cholangitis that occurs with intraoperative stent manipulation and cholangiography. Antibiotics may be discontinued when the patient has been afebrile for 24 hours.

The operative approach to resection of the extrahepatic biliary tree with Roux-en Y cholangiojejunostomy over transhepatic stents is illustrated in Figure 3. An upper midline incision provides excellent exposure of the hepatic bifurcation and allows optimal positioning of the transhepatic stents on the abdominal wall. Careful abdominal exploration is undertaken, and suspicious lymph nodes are biopsied for frozen section analysis. Intraoperative ultrasonography is applied routinely; suspicious intrahepatic nodules likewise are biopsied. The hepatic flexure of the colon is mobilized, and a wide Kocher's maneuver performed. Cholecystectomy is undertaken if the gallbladder is in situ, and the common bile duct is divided close to the pancreas to remove as much biliary epithelium as possible. The distal common bile duct at the edge of the pancreas is oversewn, and dissection continues, proximally lifting the bile duct off of the portal vein. The right hepatic artery should be anticipated at this point of the dissection because its usual course is posterior to the common hepatic duct. The right and left main hepatic ducts are divided proximal to the bifurcation, and frozen section analysis of the proximal and distal bile duct margins is performed to rule out malignant transformation.

The preoperatively placed transhepatic stents are exchanged retrograde for large Silastic catheters. A Roux limb of jejunum is brought through the transverse mesocolon to the right of the middle colic vessels, and cholangiojejunostomies are created over the Silastic catheters. Chromic sutures placed at the stent exit site from the liver minimize bile leakage. Completion cholangiography is performed in the operating room to ensure optimal stent positioning and exclude anastomotic leak. The Silastic stents are brought through the abdominal wall in a subcostal position away from the midline incision. Incorporation of a gentle curve as the stents pass through the abdominal wall is important to avoid kinking of the stent and to facilitate subsequent radiologic stent changes. Closed suction drains are placed behind the cholangiojejunostomies and at the sites of stent exit from the liver.

Overall morbidity after extrahepatic biliary resection with Roux-en-Y cholangiojejunostomy is approximately 30% to 40%, and perioperative mortality is less than 3%. Specific postoperative complications include cholangitis, bile leak, and hemobilia; these complications are generally amenable to nonoperative management. In addition, long-term follow-up suggests that less than 10% of these patients will never require a liver transplantation.

■ LIVER TRANSPLANTATION

The Mayo Model is a mathematic construct incorporating serum bilirubin, degree of hepatic fibrosis, presence of splenomegaly, and age. This model is used widely to predict survival and the optimal timing of liver transplantation. Approximately 5% of all liver transplants in the United States are performed for end-stage liver disease secondary to PSC. The perioperative mortality of liver transplantation is more than 5%, but survival of patients after liver transplant for PSC is good; 90% and 70% 1- and 5-year survival rates are common (Figure 4). Patients transplanted for PSC have a somewhat higher retransplant rate at 2 years versus those transplanted for other indications: 10% versus 5%. The major cause for retransplant is hepatic artery thrombosis. Relative to other indications, liver transplant for PSC is accompanied by somewhat higher rates of acute cellular and chronic ductopenic rejection as well as the development of biliary strictures. Recurrent PSC occurs in 20% to 25% of patients undergoing liver transplant. Patients with IBD and an intact colon

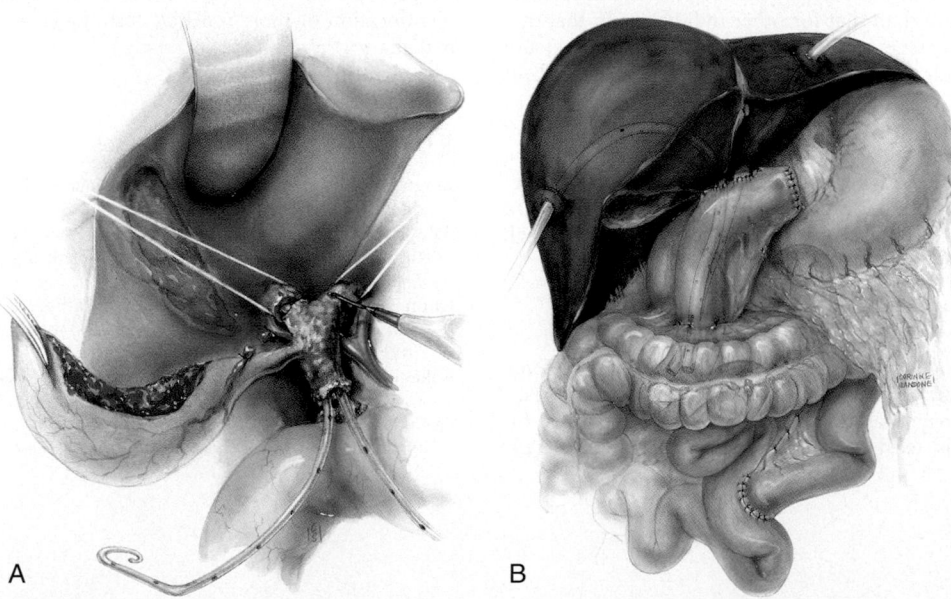

A　　　　　　　　　B

FIGURE 3 Technical steps involved in resection of the extrahepatic biliary tree (**A**) with reconstruction by Roux-en-Y hepaticojejunostomy over transhepatic biliary stents (**B**). *(From Cameron JL and Sandone C: Atlas of Gastrointestinal Surgery, vol 1. 2nd ed. B.C. Decker, Inc., Toronto; 2007.)*

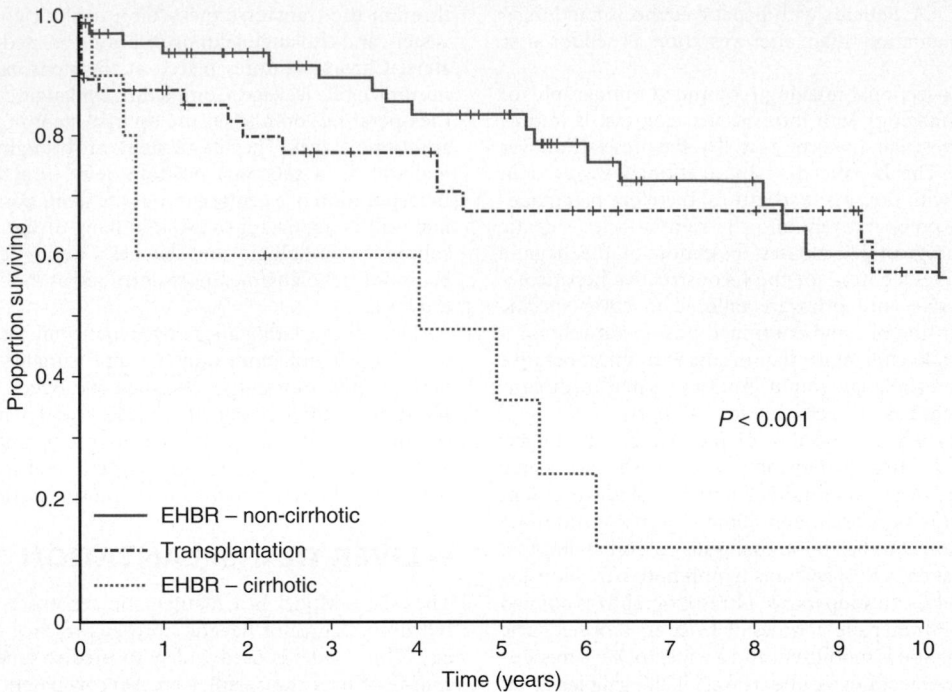

FIGURE 4 Survival rates for noncirrhotic primary sclerosing cholangitis patients treated with extrahepatic biliary resection (EHBR) were similar to those managed by transplantation. In comparison, cirrhotic patients treated with EHBR fared poorly ($P < 0.001$ vs others). *(From Pawlik TM, Olbrecht VA, Pitt HA, et al. Primary sclerosing cholangitis: role of extrahepatic biliary resection. J Am Coll Surg. 2008;206:822-832.)*

may be at increased risk for recurrent PSC after liver transplant. No specific medical therapy has been shown to decrease the incidence or PSC recurrence.

Unsuspected CCA is found in 3% to 9% of explanted livers of patients undergoing transplantation for PSC. However, small (less than 1 cm) unsuspected CCA does not appear to affect the long-term survival of these patients. In fact, these findings have stimulated the investigational protocol (with rigorous neoadjuvant chemoradiotherapy) for liver transplantation as a specific treatment for CCA in highly selected patients. The technical conduct of liver transplantation for PSC is different than that for other indications in that that the extrahepatic biliary tree is resected down to the pancreas, and the donor graft bile duct is anastomosed to a Roux-en-Y limb of jejunum.

Aggressive screening colonoscopy is warranted for post-liver transplant PSC patients with IBD because the risk of developing colonic malignancy in this population appears to be higher after liver transplant. Ursodeoxycholic acid is administered commonly to decrease the risk of colon cancer in PSC patients with IBD, although little evidence supports this practice.

■ SUMMARY

The cause and pathogenesis of PSC remain poorly understood, and no medical therapy affects the disease course. Magnetic resonance cholangiopancreatography has become the gold standard for diagnosis and also is used widely for surveillance. Endoscopic

intervention is reserved for therapy of dominant strictures or evaluation/biopsy of lesions suspicious for CCA. CCA develops in approximately 15% of patients with PSC, but the diagnosis of malignancy is notoriously difficult to differentiate from that of benign stricture. For select patients with a dominant extrahepatic stricture (10%) or concern for malignancy (10%), resection of the extrahepatic biliary tree provides durable therapy. In patients with established cirrhosis, liver transplantation is clearly the optimal therapy. Current research efforts are focused on elucidating the etiopathogenesis of PSC, development of medical therapy, and identification of more sensitive techniques with which to diagnose malignancy.

SUGGESTED READINGS

Ahrendt SA, Pitt HA, Kalloo AN, et al. Primary sclerosing cholangitis: resect, dilate, or transplant? *Ann Surg.* 1998;227:412-423.

Baluyut AR, Sherman S, Lehman GA, et al. Impact of endoscopic therapy on the survival of patients with primary sclerosing cholangitis. *Gastrointest Endosc.* 2001;53:308-312.

Eaton JE, Talwalkar JA, Lazaridis KN, et al. Pathogenesis of primary sclerosing cholangitis and advances in diagnosis and management. *Gastroenterology.* 2013;145:521-536.

Nakanishi Y, Saxena R. Pathophysiology and diseases of the proximal pathways of the biliary system. *Arch Pathol Lab Med.* 2015;139:858-866.

Pawlik TM, Olbrecht VA, Pitt HA, et al. Primary sclerosing cholangitis: role of extrahepatic biliary resection. *J Am Coll Surg.* 2008;206:822-832.

THE MANAGEMENT OF BILE DUCT CANCER

Naeem Goussous, MD, Shirali T. Patel, MD, and Steven C. Cunningham, MD, FACS

Bile duct cancer, also known as cholangiocarcinoma, accounts for approximately 3% of all gastrointestinal malignancies. There is high variability in the estimated incidence of bile duct cancer worldwide, with the highest incidence occurring in the northeast provinces of Thailand (113 per 100,000 person-years), as compared with the low incidence seen in the Western Hemisphere (0.5 to 1.5 per 100,000 person-years). Because cholangiocarcinoma is relatively resistant to chemotherapy and radiotherapy, surgical resection is the only realistic hope for a cure. Unfortunately, however, these patients usually have advanced tumors not amenable to resection, in which case survival is typically less than 1 year. Even after resection, prognosis is poor, with 5-year survival ranging from 10% to 48% depending on the series and the location of the tumor.

Among all bile duct cancers, 5% to 10% are intrahepatic, 60% to 70% are hilar (also known as Klatskin's tumors), and 20% to 30% are distal cholangiocarcinomas. Recent epidemiologic studies have shown a slight rise in the incidence of intrahepatic cholangiocarcinomas and a stable-to-declining incidence of extrahepatic tumors.

There are three different histologic subtypes: sclerosing, nodular, and papillary. Sclerosing tumors are the most common and tend to arise in the hilar area. Their infiltrative and fibrotic nature makes both diagnosis and surgical resection challenging because they tend to track along ducts and nerves. The nodular subtype is characterized by the formation of firm, irregular nodules that project into the lumen of the bile duct, and may coexist with the sclerosing subtype. Papillary tumors, by contrast, have a higher resectability rate and a better prognosis.

Bile duct cancer usually is seen in the sixth and seventh decade of life with a slight male predominance. Risk factors are uncommon but include primary sclerosing cholangitis, choledochal cyst disease, biliary parasites (*Clonorchis sinensis* and *Opisthorchis viverrini*), and bacterial infections of the biliary tree (*Salmonella*). Hepatitis C and B, alcohol abuse, and obesity have also been linked to increased incidence of bile duct cancer.

■ INTRAHEPATIC BILE DUCT CANCER

Presentation and Preoperative Evaluation

Intrahepatic tumors are often found incidentally during abdominal imaging for unrelated reasons. If symptomatic, these tumors usually are seen with nonspecific symptoms like abdominal pain, fatigue, weight loss, and decreased appetite. Physical examination is usually unremarkable, and jaundice is seen only if the stages are advanced or if the biliary tree is occluded near the hilum of the liver.

The diagnostic workup of intrahepatic cancers of the bile ducts follows the guidelines of other intrahepatic masses. Once identified, the hepatic mass requires further characterization with a dedicated multiphase, contrast-enhanced, liver-protocol magnetic resonance imaging (LPMRI). Several common lesions, such as hepatocellular cancer, focal nodular hyperplasia, and liver hemangioma, are readily diagnosed with a proper LPMRI alone, precluding the need for a biopsy. However, given that metastasis is the most common solid liver mass, a search for a primary lesion is often necessary and should include upper and lower endoscopy along with chest computed tomography (CT) and mammogram.

Laboratory evaluation includes a liver chemistry panel, which is often mildly abnormal; viral serologic tests for hepatitis; and tumor markers alpha-fetoprotein (AFP), carcinoembryonic antigen (CEA), cancer antigen 19-9 (CA19-9), and chromogranin-A (CGA), which

are neither specific nor diagnostic but can be useful for surveillance if elevated preoperatively.

Preoperative evaluation should include a careful and systematic review of functional status both of the patient in general and of the liver in particular. Given the potentially high risks of the operations typically done for bile duct cancers and given that many of these patients are older and have comorbidities, we routinely perform a formal preoperative functional assessment. Although there are many such oncogeriatric assessments, we use the following five common tools, all of which can be completed either in the waiting room or in just 2 to 3 minutes in the examining room:

- The Eastern Cooperative Oncology Group performance status (ECOG FS, ranging 0 to 5; *Am J Clin Oncol.* 1982;5:649).
- Vulnerable Elders Survey (VES-13, ranging 1 to 10, a score of 3+ vs 0 to 2 identifying 32% of individuals as vulnerable, with four times the risk of death or functional decline when compared with older persons scoring 3 or less; *J Am Ger Soc.* 2001;49:1691).
- The G-8 geriatric screening tool (ranging 0 to 17, a score of 14 or less identifying at-risk individuals; *Ann Oncol.* 2012;23:2166).
- Fried's Frailty (ranging 2 to 6, a score of 4 to 6 indicating a positive screen for exhaustion; *J Gerontol A Biol Sci Med Sci.* 2001;56:M146).
- American College of Surgeons Surgical Risk Calculator (http://riskcalculator.facs.org/).

Liver-specific evaluation includes consideration for biopsy and an assessment of resectability, which entails assessment of liver volumes and function. Biopsy of the mass is recommended principally for patients for whom surgical resection is not an option and tissue diagnosis is needed to guide chemotherapy. The volume of the future liver remnant (FLR) should be at least estimated if not measured with CT volumetrics before proceeding with any major resection. An FLR of at least 25% of normal hepatic parenchyma should be maintained postresection, with an intact arterial and portal inflow, hepatic venous outflow, and biliary enteric drainage. For patients with cirrhosis, the FLR should be 40% to 50% or more before attempting resection. Preoperative assessment of liver function is done with an indocyanine green elimination test in much of the world, but this is rarely used in the United States. The Child-Turcotte-Pugh (CTP) score and the Model for End-Stage Liver Disease (MELD) score are commonly used in the United States to assess liver function.

Criteria for unresectability include locally advanced tumor involving either inflow or outflow bilaterally, multiple bilateral intrahepatic tumors, and distant metastatic disease. Small localized satellite lesions, perihepatic lymphadenopathy, and portal hypertension are very poor prognostic factors and shift the risk/benefit balance toward nonoperative management.

Staging

Intrahepatic bile duct cancers are staged according to the seventh edition of American Joint Committee on Cancer (AJCC) tumor-node-metastasis (TNM) staging system (Table 1). The eighth edition is due to be released imminently.

Management
Resection

Resection ranges from nonanatomic wedge resection for small tumors to formal anatomic resections, such as extended hepatectomy, for larger lesions. If the FLR is too small, preoperative portal vein embolization on the side with the tumor can result in contralateral hyperplasia of the FLR, lowering the risk of postoperative liver failure. Even major liver resection combined with portal and/or caval resection and reconstruction has been performed safely in patients who are otherwise excellent candidates, but such resections should be performed only in high-volume centers, ideally liver-transplant centers.

TABLE 1: Tumor-Node-Metastasis (TNM) Staging System for Intrahepatic Cholangiocarcinoma

PRIMARY TUMOR (T)

TX	Primary tumor cannot be assessed
T0	No evidence of primary tumor
Tis	Carcinoma in situ (intraductal tumor)
T1	Solitary tumor without vascular invasion
T2a	Solitary tumor with vascular invasion
T2b	Multiple tumors, with or without vascular invasion
T3	Tumor perforating the visceral peritoneum or involving the local extrahepatic structures by direct invasion
T4	Tumor with periductal invasion

REGIONAL LYMPH NODES (N)

NX	Regional lymph nodes cannot be assessed
N0	No regional lymph node metastasis
N1	Regional lymph node metastasis present

DISTANT METASTASIS (M)

M0	No distant metastasis
M1	Distant metastasis present

ANATOMIC STAGE/PROGNOSTIC GROUPS

Stage 0	Tis	N0	M0
Stage I	T1	N0	M0
Stage II	T2	N0	M0
Stage III	T3	N0	M0
Stage IVA	T4	N0	M0
OR	Any T	N1	M0
Stage IVB	Any T	Any N	M1

From Edge SB, et al. *AJCC Cancer Staging Manual.* 7th ed. New York: Springer Inc; 2010:252-253.

Regarding open operative approach, a right subcostal incision, which depending on the lesion and its location may be limited or extended bilaterally to a chevron incision with or without a vertical midline extension, provides excellent exposure and is adequate for essentially every situation, although some have used a thoracoabdominal extension for extreme cases. A midline incision may be used for easily resectable left lesions, or when a liver resection is combined with a nonliver procedure requiring a midline incision. Depending on the results of the preoperative imaging, diagnostic laparoscopy may precede open operation to assess for carcinomatosis. Increasingly complex hepatectomies are carried out for malignant disease laparoscopically and robotically, and this decision regarding type of approach is surgeon dependent. At our institution, most difficult resection or major right resections are performed open, whereas most straightforward or left resections are performed minimally invasive.

The first step, whether open or minimally invasive, is confirming the absence of gross metastatic disease. For hemihepatectomy or extended hepatectomy, the liver is mobilized by dividing the triangular ligaments and widely mobilizing the liver. The gallbladder, if present, is removed. Intraoperative ultrasound (US) is used to assess intrahepatic anatomy, to identify the known lesion(s), to search for unrecognized lesions, and to further plan the resection. Inflow is controlled in the hilum of the liver. Hepatic venous outflow is controlled by dividing the appropriate hepatic vein(s), generally extrahepatically, before parenchymal transection. A Rumel clamp is always placed in preparation for a Pringle's maneuver but is uncommonly needed. When used, Pringle inflow occlusion is maintained for periods of 15 minutes, followed by 5-minute periods of perfusion. The parenchyma is then transected with a combination of energy devices, fracture techniques, and staplers. The use of drainage catheters after major liver resection is surgeon dependent, and we generally do not use them.

Other Treatments

Adjuvant therapy in the form of fluoropyrimidine-based or gemcitabine-based chemotherapy can be considered in high-risk patients after R0 resection. For patients with a positive microscopic disease or positive lymph nodes, for example, chemotherapy or chemoradiotherapy may be considered. Macroscopic residual disease should be managed as an unresectable disease.

Unfortunately, most patients with cancers of the intrahepatic bile ducts may not be candidates for curative-intent resection and these patients will be managed with palliative intent. Patients with unresectable tumors, either because of poor functional status of the patient or the liver or because of advanced disease, may still be candidates for external beam radiotherapy, transarterial chemoembolization, transarterial radioembolization, or ablation. Ablative techniques for cholangiocarcinoma include not only radiofrequency and microwave ablation, but also photodynamic therapy (PDT), which is increasingly used at select centers. Several small and generally low-quality studies have shown safety and efficacy in patients with unresectable disease undergoing these additional treatments, but there is no convincing evidence to support any one of these therapies over another.

■ HILAR CHOLANGIOCARCINOMA

Presentation and Preoperative Evaluation

Obstructive jaundice, usually painless, is the predominant presentation for patients with hilar cholangiocarcinomas. Other constitutional symptoms, such as nonspecific abdominal pain, anorexia, and weight loss, often accompany jaundice. Often the presence of hilar tumor is brought to attention by the finding of isolated intrahepatic biliary dilatation in the absence of dilatation of the common bile duct, seen on abdominal US imaging performed for a possibly unrelated complaint.

Cross-sectional imaging with either high-quality, multiphase, pancreas-protocol CT (PPCT) or LPMRI may confirm the presence of biliary dilatation upstream of a stricture. The finding of a hilar biliary stricture in the absence of a previous biliary intervention is highly suspicious for the presence of a malignancy. PPCT or LPMRI, ideally before stent placement (to avoid stent-related artifacts), also may be used to evaluate the status of the portal lymph nodes, the presence of metastatic disease, the extent of any liver atrophy, and the presence of vascular involvement. Right arterial invasion is more common than left arterial invasion because the right hepatic artery courses much closer to the confluence.

Endoscopic retrograde cholangiopancreatography (ERCP) or percutaneous transhepatic cholangiography (PTC) may add meaningfully to defining the anatomy of the biliary tree and provides the ability to drain an obstructed biliary system and to obtain brush or choledochoscopic forceps biopsy. Performing a biopsy of these cancers is difficult, however, and it is acceptable to proceed with resection in appropriate cases despite the absence of a tissue diagnosis. Preoperative drainage is associated with a slight increase in postresection infectious complications but is necessary in cases of severe jaundice because cholestasis impairs liver regeneration after major hepatectomy, which is often required in these cases to obtain tumor clearance and to achieve optimal survival and recurrence rates. An appropriate goal before resection is normalization of serum bilirubin, but depending on underlying liver function a goal of less than 6 to 7 mg/dL is also frequently used.

The preoperative evaluation of patients with hilar bile duct cancer, similar to that of intrahepatic cancer, should include a careful and systematic review of the functional status both of the patient in general, as described earlier, and of the liver in particular, especially because many hilar resections include liver resections. Because an extended right hepatectomy is commonly required and this resection in particular carries a high risk of leaving a small FLR causing postoperative liver failure, special attention should be paid during operative planning to the size and function of the FLR, as described for intrahepatic cancers.

Staging

- Bismuth-Corlette: This classification system is one of the oldest and most widely used systems. It classifies tumors into four categories based on the longitudinal spread of the tumor along the biliary tree (Figure 1). This system, although initially conceived to guide operative decision making, no longer does so, primarily because it lacks information about the radial extension of the tumor, vascular involvement, nodal disease, and distant metastases.
- Blumgart: This classification system was created in the Memorial Sloan Kettering Cancer Center. Integrating both the longitudinal and the radial growth of the tumor along with vascular involvement and the resultant presence of liver atrophy, it is composed of three stages of primary tumor growth (Table 2). This increasingly used preoperative staging system has been shown, principally at its parent institution, to predict tumor resectability (Table 2 and Box 1).
- TNM: Based on the seventh edition of the AJCC (Table 3), this is a pathologic staging system, and as such it has minimal contribution to preoperative planning but is useful for postoperative risk stratification and decision making.
- International Cholangiocarcinoma Group: This relatively new multicenter staging system is still under evaluation but has the potential advantage of including the best of each of the previously mentioned systems, or at least the advantage of combining important components from each of these systems. It includes information from the previously mentioned staging systems, such as the extent of the primary biliary tumor (B), tumor size (T), tumor form (F), involvement of the portal vein (PV), involvement of the hepatic artery (HA), liver volume remnant (V), presence of underlying liver disease (D), status of lymph nodes (N), and presence of metastatic disease (M) (Table 4).

Management

Resection

Because initial exploration may detect metastatic disease, this is sometimes performed laparoscopically. Although in select centers the definitive resection may also proceed laparoscopically or robotically,

TABLE 2: Blumgart Clinical Tumor Staging for Hilar Cholangiocarcinoma

T1	Tumor involving biliary confluence +/− unilateral extension to second-order biliary radicles
T2	Tumor involving biliary confluence +/− unilateral extension to second-order biliary radicles and ipsilateral portal vein involvement +/− ipsilateral hepatic lobar atrophy
T3	Tumor involving biliary confluence þ bilateral extension to second-order biliary radicles; or unilateral extension to second-order biliary radicles with contralateral portal vine involvement; or unilateral extension to second-order biliary radicles with contralateral hepatic lobar atrophy; or main or bilateral portal venous involvement

Data from AJCC Staging, Edge SB, et al. *AJCC Cancer Staging Manual*, 7th ed. New York: Springer Inc; 2010:252-253, and from Jarnigan WR, Fong Y, DeMatteo RP, et al. Staging, resectability, and outcome in 225 patients with hilar cholangiocarcinoma. *Ann Surg.* 2001;234:507.

BOX 1: Local Tumor-Related Criteria for Unresectability

1. Hepatic duct involvement up to secondary biliary radicals bilaterally
2. Encasement or occlusion of the main portal vein proximal to its bifurcation*
3. Atrophy of one hepatic lobe with contralateral encasement of portal vein branch
4. Atrophy of one hepatic lobe with contralateral involvement of secondary biliary radicals
5. Unilateral tumor extension to secondary biliary radicles with contralateral vein branch encasement or occlusion

Modified from Jarnigan WR, Fong Y, DeMatteo RP, et al. Staging, resectability, and outcome in 225 patients with hilar cholangiocarcinoma. *Ann Surg.* 2001;234:507.

*Relative criterion. Portal vein resection and reconstruction may be possible.

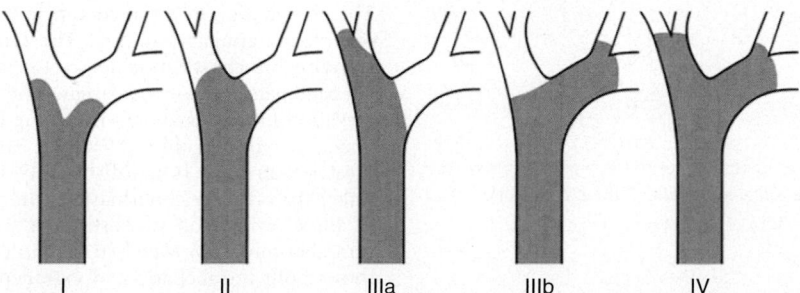

FIGURE 1 Bismuth-Corlette classification of hilar bile duct cancers. *Type I*, Tumors located distal to the hepatic confluence. *Type II*, Tumors involving the confluence. *Type IIIa*, Tumors involving the confluence and the right hepatic duct. *Type IIIb*, Tumors involving the confluence and the left hepatic duct. *Type IV*, Tumors involving both right and left hepatic ducts. *(From DeOliveira ML, Schulick RD, Nimura Y., et al. New staging system and a registry for perihilar cholangiocarcinoma. Hepatology. 2011;53:1363-1371.)*

TABLE 3: Tumor-Node-Metastasis (TNM) Staging System for Hilar Cholangiocarcinoma

PRIMARY TUMOR (T)

TX	Primary tumor cannot be assessed
T0	No evidence of primary tumor
Tis	Carcinoma in situ
T1	Tumor confined to the bile duct, with extension up to the muscle layer or fibrous tissue
T2a	Tumor invades beyond the wall of the bile duct to surrounding adipose tissue
T2b	Tumor invades adjacent hepatic parenchyma
T3	Tumor invades unilateral branches of the portal vein or hepatic artery
T4	Tumor invades main portal vein or its branches bilaterally; or the common hepatic artery; or the second-order biliary radicals bilaterally; or unilateral second-order biliary radicals with contralateral portal vein or hepatic artery involvement

REGIONAL LYMPH NODES (N)

NX	Regional lymph nodes cannot be assessed
N0	No regional lymph node metastasis
N1	Regional lymph node metastasis (including nodes along the cystic duct, common bile duct, hepatic artery, and portal vein)
N2	Metastasis to periaortic, pericaval, superior mesenteric artery, or celiac artery lymph nodes

DISTANT METASTASIS (M)

M0	No distant metastasis
M1	Distant metastasis

ANATOMIC STAGE/PROGNOSTIC GROUPS

Stage 0	Tis	N0	M0
Stage I	T1	N0	M0
Stage II	T2A-B	N0	M0
Stage IIIA	T3	N0	M0
Stage IIIB	T1-3	N1	M0
Stage IVA	T4	N0-1	M0
Stage IVB	Any T	N2	M0
OR	Any T	Any N	M1

From Edge SB, et al. *AJCC Cancer Staging Manual.* 7th ed. New York: Springer Inc; 2010.

this decision is surgeon dependent. A right subcostal incision is commonly used, and may be extended bilaterally and/or vertically. The round ligament is divided and may be left long for subsequent anastomotic wrapping and for cephalad and anterior retraction of the liver to help expose the hilum. The hepatoduodenal ligament is dissected, and its three main tubular structures are skeletonized. To assist with exposure of the portal vessels and to complete a portal lymphadenectomy, we transect the common bile duct early, as distal as possible above the pancreas. A frozen section biopsy is performed to confirm a negative margin without which a pancreaticoduodenectomy would be required to achieve a margin-negative resection. The bile duct is reflected upward with all lymph nodes, clearing the vessels. The gallbladder is dissected from the cystic plate and removed or maintained in situ as another handle attached to the biliary tree.

To facilitate the approach to the confluence of the hepatic ducts and to explore the vessels, the hilar plate is lowered according to the technique of Blumgart. This procedure nicely exposes the left hepatic duct, which is then divided and sent for frozen section biopsy. If the result is negative, this biopsy allows proceeding with an extended right hepatectomy with curative intent. If positive, an attempt should be made to divide the right hepatic duct with a negative margin, which would allow a curative-intent extended left hepatectomy. Because the left hepatic duct is longer than the right hepatic duct, it is generally more likely that a negative biopsy will be obtained on the left than on the right. A formal caudate resection is also sometimes required if there are any caudate branches close to the tumor. Some advocate for aggressive portal venous resection but this practice is controversial.

Reconstruction is performed via a Roux-en-Y hepaticojejunostomy. On either side the surgeon may encounter two or more radicles requiring anastomosis. This is more likely on the right after a left resection, given the shorter right hepatic duct that receives the right posterior and right anterior ducts. This situation may also occur at the confluence of the right and left hepatic ducts after resection of the extrahepatic biliary tree, including the hepatic duct confluence, as might be done for Bismuth-Corlette type I and II tumors. In such cases of multiple duct orifices, it is sometimes helpful to join two adjacent lumens with sutures to make a common wall, before single enteric anastomosis (Figure 2).

Other Treatments

Although these tumors are generally chemoresistant, adjuvant chemoradiotherapy is sometimes used in cases of positive margins or positive lymph nodes. Patients with unresectable disease should undergo biliary stenting (ideally internal and metal), with consideration for chemotherapy and radiotherapy. If the disease is found to be unresectable at laparotomy, operative bypass with segment III or IV hepaticojejunostomy is appropriate. The gallbladder, if present, should be removed at the same time. PDT is increasingly used and is associated with improved survival and quality of life, but this evidence is of low quality. Liver transplantation is offered at select centers for highly selected patients after neoadjuvant chemoradiation.

■ DISTAL BILE DUCT CANCER

Presentation and Preoperative Evaluation

The presentation of distal cholangiocarcinomas is similar to that of other periampullary tumors. The typical presentation is painless jaundice, but constitutional symptoms such as nonspecific abdominal pain, nausea, anorexia, fatigue, and weight loss are also common. Elevation in liver enzymes, including transaminases, alkaline phosphatase, and bilirubin, is almost universal. Hyperbilirubinemia greater than 8 to 10 mg/dL usually suggests a malignant process rather than choledocholithiasis or other benign biliary obstruction.

Initial evaluation of obstructive jaundice usually starts with a transabdominal US, which, unlike in cases of hilar bile duct cancer, shows both intrahepatic and extrahepatic biliary dilatation. High-quality, dedicated PPCT is very useful to identify and characterize even small cancers of the distal bile duct, arterial anatomy and anomalies, regional lymphatic and distant or hepatic metastases, and the relationship of the tumor to nearby vascular structures. Depending on where in the distal bile duct the cancer arises, there may or may

TABLE 4: International Cholangiocarcinoma Group Staging System for Hilar Cholangiocarcinoma

BILE DUCT (B)		LABEL SIDE/LOCATION* DESCRIPTION	
B1	Common bile duct	**Involvement (>180 degrees) of the Hepatic Artery (HA)**	
B2	Hepatic duct confluence	HA0	No arterial involvement
B3 R	Right hepatic duct	HA1	Proper hepatic artery
B3 L	Left hepatic duct	HA2	Hepatic artery bifurcation
B4	Right and left hepatic duct	HA3 R	Right hepatic artery
TUMOR SIZE (T)		HA3 L	Left hepatic artery
T1	<1 cm	HA4	Right and left hepatic artery
T2	1-3 cm	**Liver Remnant Volume (V)**	
T3	≥3 cm	V0	No information on the volume needed (liver resection not foreseen)
TUMOR FORM (F)		V%	Percentage of the total volume of a putative remnant liver after resection
Sclerosing	Sclerosing (or periductal)	**Underlying Liver Disease (D)**	
Mass	Mass-forming (or nodular)	Fibrosis	
Mixed	Sclerosing and mass-forming	Nonalcoholic steatohepatitis	
Polypoid	Polypoid (or intraductal)	Primary sclerosing cholangitis	
INVOLVEMENT (>180 DEGREES) OF THE PORTAL VEIN (PV)		**Lymph Nodes (N)**	
PV0	No portal involvement	N0	No lymph node involvement
PV1	Main portal vein	N1	Hilar or hepatic artery lymph node involvement
PV2	Portal vein bifurcation	N2	Periaortic lymph node involvement
PV3 R	Right portal vein	**Metastases (M)**	
PV3 L	Left portal vein	M0	No distant metastases
PV4	Right and left portal veins	M1	Distant metastases (including liver and peritoneal metastases)

From DeOliveira ML, Schulick RD, Nimura Y, et al. New staging system and a registry for perihilar cholangiocarcinoma. *Hepatology.* 2011;53:1363-1371.

*L, left; R, Right.

not be secondary pancreatic signs of a periampullary malignancy, such as atrophy and ductal dilatation. It is not uncommon to have all of the these clinical, laboratory, and secondary radiographic signs of a distal bile duct cancer, with no mass seen, because unlike pancreatic cancer, primary cancers of the distal bile duct typically occlude the lumen even when very small.

ERCP can be used as a diagnostic imaging modality characterizing a distal biliary stricture and has the advantage of obtaining tissue diagnosis and providing drainage of the biliary tree in cases of cholangitis. However, routine ERCP with stenting is not recommended because it colonizes the biliary tree with enteric organisms and increases the incidence of postoperative infectious complications after pancreaticoduodenectomy. Unlike intrahepatic and hilar cases, distal bile duct cancer essentially never requires a major hepatectomy, so the aforementioned need to allow jaundice to resolve preoperatively does not apply. Endoscopic US has the advantage of providing detailed images of the tumor, biliary tree, and vessels, and of obtaining a biopsy (fine or core needle) without colonizing the biliary tree.

The preoperative risk assessment for patients with distal bile duct cancer is similar to that of intrahepatic and hilar cancers and should

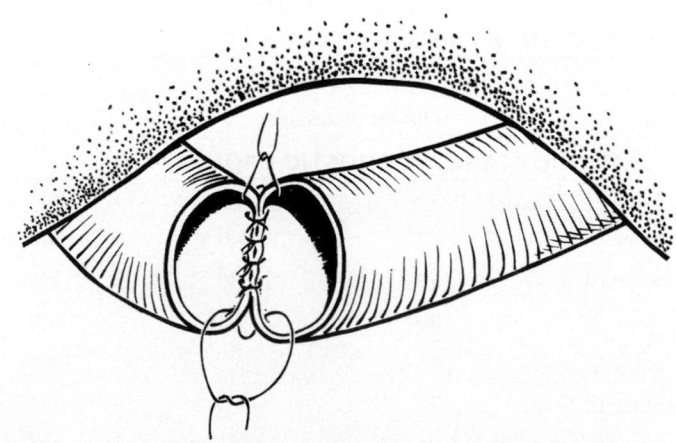

FIGURE 2 Joint anastomosis of adjacent ductal orifices. *(From Jarnagin WR. Blumgart's Surgery of the Liver, Pancreas, and Biliary Tract. 5th ed. Philadelphia: Saunders; 2012:Figure 29-10.)*

include a careful and systematic review of the patient's functional status, as described earlier.

Staging

Distal cholangiocarcinoma is staged on the basis of TNM staging system in the seventh edition of the AJCC (Table 5).

Management

Resection

Resection of distal cholangiocarcinomas requires a pancreaticoduodenectomy. Criteria for resectability include the absence of both metastatic and locally advanced disease. The approach is typically open but increasingly done laparoscopically or robotically at some centers. If open, an upper midline incision provides excellent exposure. An evaluation for metastatic disease is the first objective. Although this can be done with a laparoscopy, laparotomy is also an

TABLE 5: Tumor-Node-Metastasis (TNM) Staging System for Distal Cholangiocarcinoma

PRIMARY TUMOR (T)

TX	Primary tumor cannot be assessed
T0	No evidence of primary tumor
Tis	Carcinoma in situ
T1	Tumor confined to the bile duct histologically
T2	Tumor invades beyond the wall of the bile duct
T3	Tumor invades the gallbladder, pancreas, duodenum, or other adjacent organs without involvement of the celiac axis or the superior mesenteric artery
T4	Tumor involves the celiac axis or the superior mesenteric artery

REGIONAL LYMPH NODES (N)

NX	Regional lymph nodes cannot be assessed
N0	No regional lymph node metastasis
N1	Regional lymph node metastasis

DISTANT METASTASIS (M)

M0	No distant metastasis
M1	Distant metastasis

ANATOMIC STAGE/PROGNOSTIC GROUPS

Stage 0	Tis	N0	M0
Stage IA	T1	N0	M0
Stage IB	T2	N0	M0
Stage IIA	T3	N0	M0
Stage IIB	T1-3	N1	M0
Stage III	T4	Any N	M0
Stage IV	Any T	Any N	M1

From Edge SB, et al. *AJCC Cancer Staging Manual.* 7th ed. New York: Springer Inc; 2010.

appropriate first step in these cases, given that imaging is currently of very high quality, which results in very few missed liver metastases, and given that patients typically are seen earlier with distal cholangiocarcinoma than with other periampullary cancers because of the small size at which these cancers block the small bile duct. There are many appropriate ways to perform the pancreaticoduodenectomy, some highlights of which are presented here.

The right colon and hepatic flexure are mobilized and an extensive Kocher's maneuver is performed. A tunnel must be created cephalad along the anterior surface of the superior mesenteric vein (SMV) under the neck of the pancreas. The SMV can be encountered by continuing the Kocher's maneuver along the third portion of the duodenum to the SMV with mesenteric venous tributaries to assist in its location. A full right medial visceral rotation can be helpful at this point and provides excellent exposure to the SMV, the superior mesenteric artery (SMA), and the uncinate process of the pancreas.

Once the SMV tunnel is begun, attention is turned to the hepatoduodenal ligament. The gallbladder, if present, is removed and the major tubular structures of the hepatoduodenal ligament are skeletonized. The gastroduodenal artery is identified, test-clamped, and divided. This reveals the anterior surface of the portal vein, along which a tunnel is made caudad under the neck of the pancreas. When these two tunnels meet, a Penrose drain is passed through the tunnel. The common hepatic duct is divided (if the biliary tree is colonized, bile should be cultured to guide later therapy in case infection develops), the distal stomach or proximal duodenum is divided, and the neck of the pancreas is divided on the Penrose or a large clamp to protect the vein below. Frozen section biopsy of the bile duct and pancreas should be obtained to confirm a negative margin. Dividing the proximal jejunum a little more distal than is traditionally taught may provide a less edematous jejunal limb for the anastomosis. The uncinate process, the duodenal mesentery, and the jejunal mesentery are contiguous, and their division is the final step. If a wide right medial visceral rotation has been performed, inferior traction on the divided proximal jejunum provides excellent exposure to the uncinate process and the SMA for this final step, once the divided proximal jejunum has been brought under the SMA and SMV, from the left lower abdomen to the right upper abdomen.

Many options are available for reconstruction. If a medial visceral rotation has been performed all the way to the duodenum, the defect of the ligament of Treitz (DLoT) no longer exists, and the distal jejunum may be brought under the SMV and SMA. Otherwise, this DLoT should be closed and the jejunum brought through the bare area of the transverse mesocolon just to the right of the middle colic vessels in preparation for the pancreaticojejunostomy. The plethora of descriptions of the pancreaticojejunostomy is a testament to the lack of evidence supporting any single best technique. Whichever technique the surgeon is most comfortable with is likely the best one for that surgeon and that patient. A technique with excellent early results, the "Colonial Wig" pancreaticojejunostomy, combines invagination using full-thickness U-sutures, with wrapping the jejunum around the anastomotic corners, and an outer layer of interrupted sutures. An end-to-side hepaticojejunostomy then is created two inches downstream, followed by an antecolic duodenojejunostomy or gastrojejunostomy. In cases at especially high risk for pancreatic fistula (e.g., soft gland), the risk may be mitigated in at least three ways: by adding decompression of the pancreaticobiliary limb (e.g., with a Braun enteroenterostomy between the afferent and efferent limbs of the duodenojejunostomy or gastrojejunostomy), by wrapping the anastomosis in an omental flap, and by administering octreotide. Closed drains are placed near, but not on, the anastomosis.

Other Treatments

As with intrahepatic and hilar bile duct cancers, distal cholangiocarcinoma is not particularly chemosensitive, but adjuvant chemoradiotherapy may be used in cases of positive margins or lymph nodes. Unresectable disease warrants either durable stenting or biliary bypass and consideration for chemotherapy and radiotherapy. PDT is also used but the evidence supporting its use is generally of low quality.

■ OUTCOMES

As shown in Table 6, 5-year survival rates for bile duct cancer range from 10% to 48% depending on the study and the cancer site. Survival, not surprisingly, depends greatly on the status of resection margins, lymph node status, and differentiation. Tumor recurrence

occurs usually at the bile ducts, nodes, and liver. Given the extensive nature of these resections, the morbidity (27% to 76%) and mortality (0% to 15%) rates shown in Table 6 are acceptable.

■ SUMMARY

Bile duct cancers are a diverse group of diseases requiring vastly different resections, depending on the location within the biliary tree. All of these resections, however, are similar in requiring a careful

TABLE 6: Institutional Series of Resection for Bile Duct Cancer From the Last 10 Years

Author, Location, Year	N	Liver Rx (%)	5-Y-S, R0 (%)	5-Y-S, R1/2(%)	5-Y-S, All (%)	Morbidity* (%)	Mortality* (%)
			Intrahepatic				
DeOliveira, Baltimore, 2007	34	100	63	NR	40	NR	2
Endo, New York, 2008	77	100	NR	NR	NR	38	1
Paik, Korea, 2008	97	100	31	NR	31	NR	NR
Guglielmi, Italy, 2009	52	100	23	0	20	32	4
Ercolani, Italy, 2010	72	100	48	0	48	28	NR
Ali, Rochester, 2013	121	100	NR	NR	23-44‡	43	1
Li, China, 2013	124	100	NR	NR	15-17‡	NR	NR
Uenishi, Japan, 2008	113	100	34	0	29	NR	NR
Tamandl, Austria, 2008	74	100	NR	NR	28	27	10
Konstanoulakis, Greece, 2008	54	100	39	0	25	NR	7
Jonas, Germany, 2009	195	100	30	0	22	42†	7†
			Hilar				
DeOliveira, Baltimore, 2007	173	20	30	NR	10	NR	5
Miyazaki, Japan, 2007	161	88	36	0	NR	39	7
Chen, China, 2009	138	100	NR	NR	30	30	0
Hirano, Japan, 2010	146	94	NR	NR	35	45	3
Lee, Korea, 2010	302	89	47	8	33	43	2
Shimizu, Japan, 2010	224	100	37-42‡	0	NR	45	6
Unno, Japan, 2010	125	100	46	19	35	49	8
Li, China, 2011	215	95	41	0	30	41	4
Saxsena, Australia, 2011	42	100	NR	NR	24	45	2
van Gulik, Netherlands, 2011	99	38	NR	NR	20-33‡	68	10
Young, United Kingdom, 2011	83	93	33	8	20	64	7
Cannon, New Orleans, 2012	59	83	NR	NR	34	39	5
Nuzzo, Multicenter, 2012	440	86	32	6	26	47	9
Cheng, China, 2012	171	100	17	3	13	26	3
Cho, Korea, 2012	105	75	NR	NR	34	NR	14
De Jong, Multicenter, 2012	305	73	NR	NR	20	NR	12
Dumitrascu, Romania, 2013	106	73	NR	NR	27	52	7
Matsuo, New York, 2012	157	82	NR	NR	32	59	8
Song, Korea, 2012	230	77	NR	NR	33	NR	4

Continued

TABLE 6: Institutional Series of Resection for Bile Duct Cancer From the Last 10 Years—cont'd

Author, Location, Year	N	Liver Rx (%)	5-Y-S, R0 (%)	5-Y-S, R1/2(%)	5-Y-S, All (%)	Morbidity* (%)	Mortality* (%)
Hilar							
Wahab, Egypt, 2012	159	100	NR	NR	18	52	6
Nagino, Japan, 2013	574	97	76	24	32	57	5
Ebata, Multicenter, 2014	1352	97	47	22	40	NR	3
Furusawa, Japan, 2014	144	99	41	15	33	73	1
Nari, Argentina, 2014	45	78	32	0	21	73	15
Tamoto, Japan, 2014	49	100	NR	NR	51-59‡	31	2
Distal							
DeOliveira, Baltimore, 2007	229	0	27	NR	23	NR	3
Murakami, Japan, 2007	43	0	60	8	44	44	0
Tan, China, 2013	84	0	NR	NR	37	NR	2
Andrianello, Italy, 2015	46	0	NR	NR	18	76.1	0

Modified from DeOliveira ML, Cunningham SC, Cameron JL, et al. Cholangiocarcinoma: thirty-one-year experience with 564 patients at a single institution. *Ann Surg.* 2007;245:745.

*30-day.

†90-day.

‡For two different periods/groups.

5-Y-S, 5-year-survival; *NR,* not reported; *R0,* negative microscopic margins; *R1/2,* positive microscopic/macroscopic margins.

preoperative risk and functional assessment and in being challenging technically. Although surgical resection is the only therapy that is potentially curative, most patients have advanced, unresectable disease. Many other treatment strategies exist for these patients, albeit with generally low-quality data supporting their use. Given all of this, a multidisciplinary team approach should be the norm when bile duct cancer is evaluated and treated.

SUGGESTED READINGS

DeOliveira ML, Cunningham SC, Cameron JL, et al. Cholangiocarcinoma: 31-year experience with 564 patients at a single institution. *Ann Surg.* 2007;245:755.

DeOliveira ML, Schulick RD, Nimura Y, et al. New staging system and a registry for perihilar cholangiocarcinoma. *Hepatology.* 2011;53:1363-1371.

Lazaridis KN, Gores GJ. Cholangiocarcinoma. *Gastroenterology.* 2005;128:1655.

Matsuo K, Rocha FG, Ito K, et al. The Blumgart preoperative staging system for hilar cholangiocarcinoma: analysis of resectability and outcomes in 380 patients. *J Am Coll Surg.* 2012;215:343-355.

Shaib Y, El-Serag HB. The epidemiology of cholangiocarcinoma. *Semin Liver Dis.* 2004;24:115.

Singhal D, van Gulik TM, Gouma DJL. Palliative management of hilar cholangiocarcinoma. *Surg Oncol.* 2005;13:59.

Yang X, Aghajafari P, Patel ST, Cunningham SC. The "Colonial Wig" Pancreaticojejunostomy: Zero Leaks with A Novel Technique for Reconstruction After Pancreaticoduodenectomy. Oral presentation to New England Surgical Society 2016 Annual Meeting. Abstract book in press.

THE MANAGEMENT OF GALLBLADDER CANCER

Rebecca A. Marmor, MD, and Jason K. Sicklick, MD, FACS

Despite the fact that surgical resection is the only curative therapy for gallbladder cancer, many surgeons have approached this disease with fatalism. However, with improved surgical technique, a better understanding of the disease biology, and an increased willingness to intervene even in locally advanced cases, patient survival has improved over time. This chapter reviews data addressing the management of gallbladder cancer, beginning with a brief overview focusing on the epidemiology and natural history of disease, followed by a discussion of surgical and medical approaches. We also highlight emerging data on the genomics of gallbladder cancer and how this may guide medical therapy in the future. We conclude by providing an evidence-based algorithmic approach to treating patients with gallbladder carcinoma.

■ EPIDEMIOLOGY

There is geographic variation in the incidence of gallbladder cancer. High annual incidence countries (i.e., those with a rate >10 per 100,000 persons) include Bolivia, Chile, India, Pakistan, and Poland. Gallbladder cancer is considered a rare disease in the United States, with an annual incidence rate of 1.13 per 100,000 persons according to data from the Surveillance, Epidemiology, and End Results (SEER) Program of the National Cancer Institute. Overall, there are approximately 5000 new diagnoses in the United States each year, with a disease-specific mortality leading to approximately 2800 deaths. We now know that the annual incidence in the United States is affected by several factors, including sex and race. The annual incidence in females is 1.4 per 100,000 persons, whereas in males it is 0.8 per 100,000 persons. Consistent with these data, from 2003 to 2013 about two thirds of cases in the United States occurred in females. Besides differences in sex, the incidence in the United States is also variable according to race; the American Indian/Alaskan Native populations have the highest incidence rates at 3.2 cases per 100,000 persons. In light of the epidemiology of this cancer, we now know that incidence correlates with the prevalence of cholelithiasis in a given population.

■ RISK FACTORS

Gallstones are present in 70% to 90% of patients with gallbladder cancer; in fact, a history of gallstones appears to be one of the strongest risk factors for the development of this malignancy. The risk of carcinoma rises with increased stone size; one study demonstrated that stones larger than 3 cm had a tenfold increased risk of gallbladder cancer as compared with stones less than 1 cm. Other common risk factors include female sex; older age; obesity; history of chronic cholecystitis; occupational carcinogen exposure; poor diet; and American Indian, Alaskan Native, or black races. Because many of these risk factors (e.g., female sex, older age, obesity) are associated with development of cholelithiasis for which patients undergo cholecystectomy, gallbladder tumors are found in approximately 1% of all cholecystectomy specimens. Porcelain gallbladder (the intramural calcification of the gallbladder wall) is also associated with gallstone disease in more than 95% of cases. In turn, the rate of cancer associated with porcelain gallbladder is approximately 2% to 3%. Other less common risk factors include chronic *Salmonella* infections, biliary cysts, aberrant pancreaticobiliary duct junction (leading to a long common channel), and medications (e.g., methyldopa, isoniazid). Surgeons evaluating patients for cholecystectomy with any of the aforementioned risk factors must have an elevated index of suspicion for the possibility of gallbladder cancer during all phases of care.

■ PRESENTATION

Gallbladder cancer may be diagnosed in one of several ways: (1) preoperatively on workup for symptoms; (2) preoperatively as an incidental finding on imaging; (3) intraoperatively at the time of planned cholecystectomy for suspected benign gallbladder diseases; or (4) postoperatively on pathologic analysis after routine cholecystectomy (note that at early stages, gallbladder carcinomas may be difficult to grossly differentiate from chronic cholecystitis).

The point at which the disease is diagnosed informs the subsequent workup and management. Despite improved imaging techniques, only about 50% of gallbladder cancers are diagnosed preoperatively. This is likely related to the fact that the clinical presentation of gallbladder cancer is often identical to the clinical presentations of biliary colic or chronic cholecystitis. Thus the diagnosis requires a high index of suspicion on the part of the clinician. For patients with advanced disease, the presentation may be just as vague, with only complaints of constitutional symptoms such as weight loss and malaise. These patients also may have jaundice, which can result from the tumor obstruction of the extrahepatic biliary tree. Unfortunately, most gallbladder cancer is diagnosed at an advanced stage. One study from Memorial Sloan Kettering Cancer Center (MSKCC) found that 37% of patients initially were diagnosed with stage IV disease. This is consistent with national data demonstrating that about one third of gallbladder cancers have metastatic disease. Therefore diagnostic evaluation is imperative for guiding appropriate treatment planning.

■ DIAGNOSTIC EVALUATION

History and physical examination are inadequate to diagnose and stage gallbladder cancer. Laboratory tests, including a liver panel and tumor markers (e.g., carcinoembryonic antigen [CEA] and cancer antigen 19-9 [CA19-9]), also are not diagnostic for this disease. Moreover, the latter are not ordered routinely in patients suspected of having benign gallstone disease. Furthermore, a CEA level greater than 4 ng/mL is 93% specific for the diagnosis of gallbladder cancer but is only 50% sensitive. Likewise, a serum CA19-9 level greater than 20 units/mL is 79.4% sensitive and 79.2% specific. Although these tumor markers may be helpful for identifying disease in high prevalence areas, they are not considered useful as screening tools in lower prevalence areas, such as the United States. Because laboratory values are not used routinely in making the diagnosis, vigilance in examining preoperative imaging studies (e.g., ultrasound [US], computed tomography [CT], magnetic resonance images [MRI]) for tumors is essential. Any gallbladder mass, any gallbladder polyp larger than 1 cm, or the presence of a porcelain gallbladder should raise the suspicion of gallbladder cancer. However, other diagnoses should be considered. The differential diagnosis of gallbladder masses also includes many benign conditions, such as cholesterolosis, cholesterol polyps, adenomyomatosis, and intracholecystic papillary-tubular neoplasms (ICPN; formerly known as inflammatory polyps and adenomas); however, gallbladder cancer must be worked up in the presence of the aforementioned concerning findings.

For those patients who have jaundice with or without pruritus, as well as constitutional symptoms, a careful review of imaging is especially important. The diagnosis of gallbladder cancer may be overlooked and the signs and symptoms attributed to benign diseases, such as choledocholithiasis (with or without cholangitis) or Mirizzi's syndrome. However, the aforementioned diagnoses often will be associated with symptoms of acute pain, fevers, and leukocytosis. On the other hand, a tumor-associated obstruction of the extrahepatic biliary tree may be painless, and insidious without leukocytosis. A cancer should not be ruled out merely based on the aforementioned differences in presentation. Thus any mid–common bile duct obstruction should be considered a gallbladder cancer until proven otherwise, because tumors that arise in the gallbladder neck or within Hartmann's pouch also may infiltrate the common hepatic duct, making them clinically and radiologically indistinguishable from hilar cholangiocarcinomas.

■ ANATOMY AND PATHOPHYSIOLOGY

Approximately 60% of gallbladder tumors originate within the fundus, 30% within the body, and 10% within the neck. These tumors may grow in a diffuse or nodular pattern. Most commonly, tumors grow in a diffusely infiltrative pattern and tend to involve the entire gallbladder by spreading within the subserosal plane. This is the same plane that is dissected during routine cholecystectomy for benign diseases. As a result, if the tumor is not recognized at the time of operation, it is unlikely that a simple cholecystectomy will excise the disease completely. On the other hand, the nodular type of gallbladder cancer tends to have earlier invasion through the gallbladder wall and into the liver and/or adjacent structures. This type is often easier to treat surgically because the margins are better defined. In contrast to the nodular growth pattern, the diffuse growth pattern portends a better prognosis because even large tumors often have only minimal gallbladder wall invasion.

Because the gallbladder lies on segments IVb and V of the liver, tumors of the fundus or body often involve these segments. Direct extension into the porta hepatis structures (i.e., portal vein, hepatic artery, and bile duct) commonly occurs and is a frequent cause of signs and symptoms. Moreover, lymphatic invasion is also common and most frequently involves cystic and pericholedochal nodes (Figure 1). Tumor cells may then metastasize to lymph nodes posterior to the pancreas, portal vein, and common hepatic artery. Advanced disease ultimately may reach the celiac axis, superior mesenteric artery, and aortocaval lymph nodes. In addition, gallbladder cancers have an incredible propensity to seed and grow in other locations, including the peritoneum. This explains this tumor's ability to

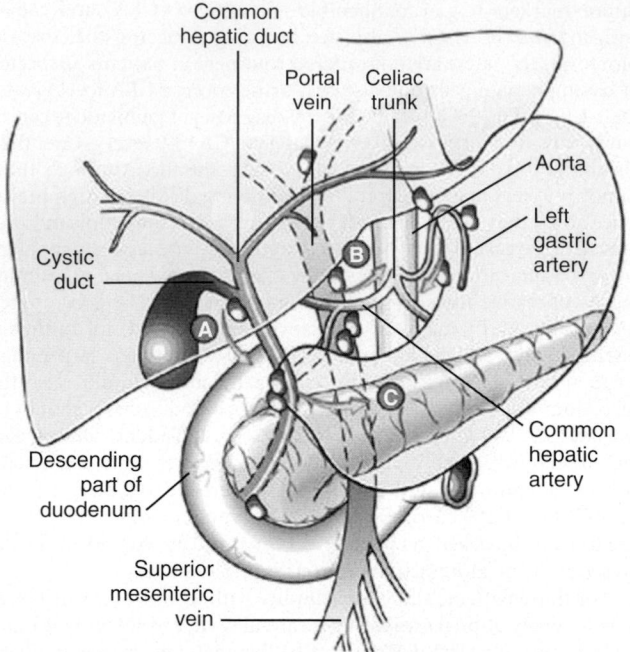

FIGURE I Patterns of lymphatic drainage from the gallbladder. **A,** The main pathway of lymphatic drainage, and thus lymph node metastasis from gallbladder cancer, is to the cholecystoretropancreatic nodes. This pathway drains from the gallbladder to nodes along the cystic duct and common bile duct and then to nodes posterior to the duodenum and pancreatic head. **B,** The cholecysto-celiac pathway courses from the gallbladder through the gastrohepatic ligament to celiac nodes. **C,** The third lymphatic drainage route is the cholecystomesenteric pathway, coursing from the gallbladder posterior to the pancreas to aortocaval lymph nodes. *(From Keefe DMK, Frei E, Holland JF, et al. Holland-Frei Cancer Medicine. 6th ed. Hamilton, ON: BC Decker Inc.; 2003. Figure 102–1.)*

cause carcinomatosis, as well as to grow along needle biopsy tracts and laparoscopic port sites. Growth in these sites may be exacerbated further by bile spillage during laparoscopic cholecystectomy. Hematogenous spread is less common but will be seen most often with noncontiguous liver metastases (91%) and more rarely as lung (32%) or brain (5%) metastases. In rare instances, distant subcutaneous metastases have been reported in the breasts, chest wall, axillae, and buttocks.

■ RADIOLOGIC WORKUP

Preoperative imaging can be essential to making a diagnosis, if clinicians have the proper degree of suspicion before surgery. However, radiologic workup can be equally important for those patients whose cancer is diagnosed intraoperatively or postoperatively. Careful review of any study (e.g., US, CT, MRI) is essential and may provide information concerning liver involvement, biliary extension, vascular involvement, presence of ascites, and/or metastatic disease, which can guide further management. Additional cross-sectional imaging studies are indicated for appropriate staging of disease if the patient has only undergone US for suspected benign gallbladder disease. Thus all patients suspected of having a gallbladder cancer preoperatively warrant CT of the chest, abdomen, and pelvis before surgery; all patients found to have tumors more advanced than T1a intraoperatively or postoperatively should undergo these studies after surgery.

Together, CT and US comprise the most frequently used combination for initial assessment; however, magnetic resonance cholangiopancreatography (MRCP) is becoming increasingly important for

the evaluation of suspected gallbladder tumors, as it is better for allowing an experienced radiologist to differentiate benign from malignant gallbladder lesions. MRCP may also be useful for visualizing invasion into the hepatoduodenal ligament structures and lymph node involvement.

Cholangiography, either endoscopic retrograde cholangiopancreatography (ERCP) or percutaneous transhepatic cholangiography (PTC), has low yield for diagnosing patients with suspected gallbladder cancer because the gallbladder is infrequently observed with this technique. However, it may be useful for patients who have jaundice in order to evaluate and treat (e.g., stent) suspected extrahepatic biliary tree involvement.

The role of fluorodeoxyglucose positron emission tomography (FDG-PET) in the management of patients with suspected or known gallbladder disease is not well elucidated. Although most (86%) gallbladder cancers are FDG-avid, prior studies reveal a low sensitivity for extrahepatic metastases or peritoneal carcinomatosis. However, it can be a useful adjunct when deciding whether to operate on a patient. A recent case series found that out of 100 patients who underwent preoperative PET scans, the management of only 5 patients was altered. However, the utility of PET was increased among patients without a prior cholecystectomy and in patients with suspicious nodal disease on CT. PET also can be a useful adjunct to detect radiographically occult advanced disease in patients being considered for surgical management. However, the clinician must be aware of the limitations of the study.

■ STAGING AND NATURAL HISTORY OF DISEASE

A multitude of systems have been used for staging gallbladder cancer. The most common system for evaluation worldwide has been the American Joint Committee on Cancer (AJCC) tumor node metastasis (TNM) staging system (Table 1), which was revised in 2010 (seventh edition) to better reflect resectability and patient prognosis.

According to the seventh edition AJCC staging system, tumors without perimuscular invasion are considered stage I disease, with 5-year survival rates from 39% to 43%. Tumors with invasion into the perimuscular connective tissue but without extension beyond the serosa or into the liver are considered stage II disease, with 5-year survival rates of approximately 12% to 14%. In the absence of regional lymph node metastases, tumors that perforate the gallbladder serosa and/or directly invade the liver and/or adjacent structures (e.g., stomach, duodenum, colon, pancreas, omentum, extrahepatic biliary tree) are stage IIIA disease. Tumors that also have local nodal metastases (e.g., nodes along the cystic duct, common bile duct, hepatic artery, and/or portal vein) without vascular invasion are stage IIIB disease. Combining these two groups, the 5-year survival rates for stage III disease are 2% to 5%. Finally, stage IVA disease includes those patients with vascular invasion and stage IVB disease includes those patients with distant metastases or with vascular invasion and distant nodal metastases (e.g., periaortic, pericaval, superior mesenteric artery, and/or celiac artery nodes). The 5-year survival rate for stage IV disease is 1% to 2%.

■ SURGICAL MANAGEMENT

A breadth of operations has been advocated for managing gallbladder cancer. These operations range from simple cholecystectomy to combined extended hepatectomy, common bile duct resection, and pancreaticoduodenectomy. Unfortunately, debate still exists regarding the appropriate extent of resection. The most practical way to approach gallbladder cancer is to base therapy on the clinical TNM stage of disease because there is a close correlation between stage and prognosis (Table 2). Knowing the likelihood of local, nodal, peritoneal, or distant disease allows for a rational therapeutic approach.

TABLE 1: AJCC Staging System for Gallbladder Cancer (7th Edition)

PRIMARY TUMOR (T)

Tis	Carcinoma in situ
T1	Tumor invades lamina propria (T1a) or muscular layer (T1b)
T2	Tumor invades perimuscular connective tissue
T3	Tumor perforates serosa and/or invades the liver and/or one adjacent structure
T4*	Tumor invades main portal vein or hepatic artery or invades two or more extrahepatic structures

REGIONAL LYMPH NODES (N)

N0	No regional lymph node metastasis
N1	Metastases to nodes along the cystic duct, common bile duct, hepatic artery, and/or portal vein
N2†	Metastases to periaortic, pericaval, superior mesenteric artery, and/or celiac artery lymph nodes

DISTANT METASTASIS (M)

M0	No distant metastasis
M1	Distant metastasis

STAGING GROUPS (TMN)

Stage 0	Tis	N0	M0
Stage I	T1	N0	M0
Stage II	T2	N0	M0
Stage IIIA	T3	N0	M0
Stage IIIB	T1-T3	N1	M0
Stage IVA	T4	N0-N1	M0
Stage IVB	Any T	N2	M0
	Any T	Any N	M1

From Edge SB, Byrd DR, Compton CC, et al., eds. *AJCC Cancer Staging Manual.* 7th ed. New York: Springer; 2010:211-217.

*T4 denotes locally advanced, unresectable tumors.

†N2 nodes are considered distant metastatic disease.

For patients with the earliest stages of the disease (i.e., incidental Tis or T1a gallbladder cancer discovered in specimens after laparoscopic cholecystectomy), there is no need for further surgical management if the disease is limited to the muscularis propria layer. In fact, current National Comprehensive Cancer Network (NCCN) guidelines do not recommend staging workup. Multiple studies have revealed that these patients have a 5-year survival rate exceeding 90%.

However, for patients with T1b or more advanced disease, an extended cholecystectomy may be considered. Although historically some surgeons argued that T2 tumors with negative margins required treatment with only a simple cholecystectomy, recent studies have demonstrated improved survival with a more aggressive surgical approach. A study by Abramson and colleagues found a median

survival advantage of more than 3 years with extended cholecystectomy as compared with simple cholecystectomy (9.9 years vs 6.4 years) in patients with T1b tumors. Data from MSKCC suggest that an improvement in survival can be achieved with extended or radical resection as compared with simple cholecystectomy alone. Another multi-institutional retrospective review from Japan, which included 1686 resections for gallbladder cancer, demonstrated significantly improved survival rates for patients undergoing radical resection versus simple cholecystectomy (5-year survival rates of 51% versus 6%, respectively). Even for patients with locally advanced (i.e., T3, T4, or TxN1) disease, extensive resection has been associated with improved overall survival. In fact, several studies document 5-year survival rates from 28% to 60% after radical resection for patients with TxN1 disease. It is clear from pathologic data that T2, T3, or T4 tumors are associated with more than a 50% chance of metastases to regional lymph nodes. As liver resections have become safer, increasing numbers of surgical centers are performing radical resections for this disease and data are consequently accumulating to justify such an aggressive approach.

Currently, the only absolute contraindications to surgery for gallbladder cancer are medical comorbidities, M1 disease (i.e., distant metastases including liver, peritoneum, etc.), involvement of N2 lymph nodes (i.e., celiac, peripancreatic, periduodenal, or superior mesenteric), malignant ascites, significant involvement of the hepatoduodenal ligament, or encasement of major vasculature. In the absence of these findings, surgical exploration should be attempted, as surgery is the only potentially curative therapy for gallbladder cancer. In the following sections, we further review the data supporting radical resection for gallbladder cancer at the various stages of disease.

Tumor Confined to the Lamina Propria (T1a)

There is now an abundance of data that indicate that early stage gallbladder cancers without perimuscular invasion (i.e., T1a) are adequately treated by simple cholecystectomy. In a large meta-analysis only 1.8% of 706 patients with T1a tumors developed lymph node metastasis and only 1.1% of patients died from disease. In patients who have a pathologic diagnosis of T1a gallbladder cancer after laparoscopic cholecystectomy for suspected benign biliary tract disease, a careful review of the pathologic features is imperative. Care must be taken to verify negative margins, including the cystic duct. Areas of deeper invasion should be ruled out by an experienced pathologist. If the gallbladder wall margin is found to be involved by tumor, a liver resection is warranted in the absence of advanced disease on cross-sectional imaging. If the cystic duct stump is involved, an excision of the common hepatic duct and common bile duct (including the confluence with the cystic duct stump) followed by Roux-en-Y hepaticojejunostomy is indicated. No nodal dissection is warranted in the latter case and no further staging workup is recommended according to current NCCN guidelines.

Tumor With Perimuscular Invasion (T1b)

Traditionally, T1b tumors were treated with simple cholecystectomy alone. However, recent data suggest that these tumors may be better managed with more aggressive resections. These data have revealed that T1b tumors have a higher rate of lymph node metastases as compared with T1a tumors. The meta-analysis mentioned in the previous section demonstrated a lymph node metastasis rate of 10.9% among 560 T1b tumors, with 52 patients dying of disease. In addition to a higher propensity for lymph node metastases as compared with T1a tumors, T1b tumors also have high rates (up to 13%) of residual disease found at the time of re-resection. It is therefore reasonable to offer re-excision with radical (or extended) cholecystectomy (i.e., segment IVb/V hepatic resection) and portal lymph node dissection to patients with T1b tumors who do not have medical contraindications to surgery or evidence of metastatic disease on

TABLE 2: Recommended Management by Stage

Stage	Surgical Management	Postoperative Management
T1a	Simple cholecystectomy	Review pathology report to confirm negative cystic duct margins No routine follow-up advised
T1b	Radical cholecystectomy (i.e., segment IVb/V resection [preferred], hepatic wedge resection, right hepatic lobectomy, or trisectionectomy with R0 resection) and portal lymphadenectomy	Staging workup with CT chest/abdomen/pelvis (or CT chest and MRI abdomen/pelvis) Adjuvant fluoropyrimidine chemoradiation versus gemcitabine-based or fluoropyrimidine-based chemotherapy Surveillance imaging
II	See above for T1b tumors	See above for T1b tumors
III	Consider diagnostic staging laparoscopy followed by operation for T1b tumors if no metastatic disease is identified	See above for T1b tumors
IVA	Stage IVA (T4 N0-1 M0) disease may be amenable to resection (see stage III).	Adjuvant fluoropyrimidine chemoradiation versus gemcitabine-based or fluoropyrimidine-based chemotherapy
IVB	N2 and M1 disease is a contraindication to attempts at curative resection. Patients may require palliative operation for relief of biliary obstruction but attempts at endoscopic/ percutaneous drainage should be considered first-line treatment.	Unresectable disease: combined gemcitabine/cisplatin therapy, fluoropyrimidine-based or gemcitabine-based chemotherapy regimens

CT, Computed tomography; *MRI,* magnetic resonance imaging.

staging workup. Along these lines, for incidentally discovered T1b tumors, review of the operative report or consultation with the original surgeon is of the utmost importance, to identify signs of disseminated disease at the time of simple cholecystectomy. Given the high rate of margin positivity, careful review of the pathology report is critical to identify whether margins were microscopically negative (i.e., R0) or positive (i.e., R1). Finally, current NCCN guidelines recommend a complete staging workup for patients with T1b tumors, including CT chest and cross-sectional abdominopelvic imaging.

Liver Resection

Over time, recommendations for liver resection for gallbladder cancer have ranged from a limited wedge resection around the gallbladder bed to routine extended right hepatectomy. In general, an anatomic segment IVb/V resection is now preferred when possible because this operation allows for the greatest chance of R0 resection while maximizing hepatic parenchymal preservation. For patients who have a T2 gallbladder tumor discovered at laparoscopic cholecystectomy, re-exploration and radical resection may be confounded by inflammation from the previous operation, which may make it difficult to determine the extent of disease. Frozen section biopsies are often helpful in assessing the extent and spread of disease. Depending on the extent of disease, a right hepatectomy or right trisectionectomy may be necessary to resect all disease.

Portal Lymphadenectomy

In the past, recommendations for lymph node dissection have ranged from excision of the cystic duct node alone (i.e., Calot's node) to en bloc portal lymphadenectomy with pancreaticoduodenectomy. However, combined liver and pancreatic resections have high operative mortalities approaching 20% and are not justified by long-term survival data. On the other hand, portal lymphadenectomy for T2 to T4 tumors is supported by the finding of positive nodes in more than 50% of patients. Currently, most surgeons resect cystic, periportal, and hepatic artery lymph nodes (Figure 2). Another prospective cohort study from MSKCC provides convincing evidence that for a

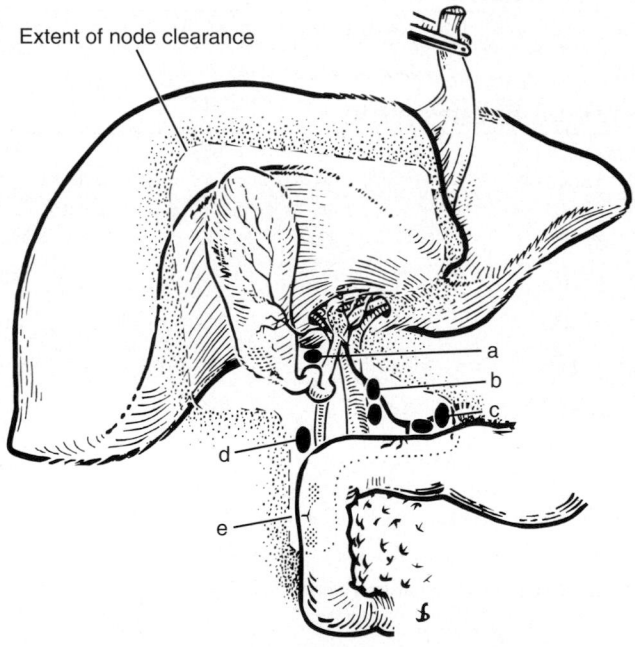

FIGURE 2 Diagrammatic representation of the extent of lymph node dissection in an extended or radical cholecystectomy. *a,* Cystic duct node(s); *b,* portal nodes; *c,* hepatic artery nodes; *d,* common bile duct nodes; *e,* retroduodenal nodes. *(From Blumgart LH, Fong Y. Surgery of the Liver and Biliary Tract. 3rd ed. Philadelphia: WB Saunders; 2000. Figure 53.8.)*

gallbladder cancer to be considered node negative, a minimum of six lymph nodes must be removed. In the past, resection of the common bile duct also was advocated during portal lymphadenectomy but current NCCN guidelines do not recommend this practice, as it is associated with increased morbidity and does not clearly extend survival.

Extrahepatic Bile Duct Resection

Resection of the common hepatic duct and common bile duct may be warranted in the case of tumor extension into the biliary tree, a positive cystic duct margin, or extensive skeletonization of the porta hepatis during lymphadenectomy, which results in concern for biliary ischemia. After resection, a Roux-en-Y hepaticojejunostomy should be performed to re-establish biliary-enteric continuity.

Excision of Laparoscopic Port Sites

Current NCCN guidelines do not recommend port site resection because a tumor identified at the port site is a marker for disseminated peritoneal disease and resection has not been shown to improve patient outcomes. In a study of 113 patients by Maker and colleagues, port site resection was not associated with improved overall or disease-free survival.

Reoperation for Incidentally Discovered Gallbladder Cancer

Historically, it was thought that patients who underwent two operations had worse prognoses than those who were treated with a single operation. In one early study, there was a median survival of 42 months for patients undergoing a curative resection at the first operation versus 12.5 months for those undergoing a curative resection at a second operation. More recent data suggest that there is no difference in outcomes in patients who have a radical resection after a previous laparoscopic cholecystectomy for incidental gallbladder cancer as compared with patients who undergo one operation. Moreover, there appears to be no difference in survival or recurrence in patients who have a second operation after an initial open or laparoscopic cholecystectomy. However, achieving an R0 resection is critical to improving survival in patients undergoing re-resection. A study from Johns Hopkins Hospital showed that there was no difference in survival between patients who underwent immediate conversion to an open resection for intraoperatively discovered gallbladder carcinoma (N = 6) and those patients who underwent laparoscopic cholecystectomy followed by later re-exploration for a tumor identified at histopathologic review (N = 33). Taken together, tumors incidentally discovered during laparoscopic cholecystectomy do not require conversion to an immediate open resection. Instead, patients should be referred to a tertiary care center for further evaluation and subsequent exploration. Moreover, to minimize the chance at peritoneal dissemination, biopsy is not recommended. On the other hand, when there is concern for an early gallbladder cancer, a hepatobiliary surgeon may (1) perform a simple laparoscopic cholecystectomy; (2) review the pathologic features intraoperatively on frozen section biopsy; and (3) proceed to perform a radical resection and lymphadenectomy if there is evidence of T1b or more advanced disease.

Tumor Invading Into the Subserosal Layer (T2)

By definition, T2 tumors invade the muscular coat of the gallbladder but do not penetrate the serosal plane. The recommended management for T2 disease, without evidence of metastases, is a radical cholecystectomy and portal lymphadenectomy with negative margins. The latter includes removal of periportal, peripancreatic, and hepatic artery lymph nodes. These recommendations are based on the pattern of disease spread and the high probability of lymph node metastases with T2 tumors. In diffuse gallbladder cancer, which is the most common type of disease, the cancer grows in a subserosal plane, which contains the lymphatic channels. When performing a simple cholecystectomy for benign gallbladder disease, the gallbladder is usually incompletely removed. The cystic plate (i.e., the gallbladder serosa on the liver side) is usually left behind because most of the dissection occurs within the subserosal plane, which is the least

bloody plane for dissection. For this reason, there is an increased likelihood of positive margins after simple cholecystectomy alone.

In a multicenter retrospective cohort study of patients undergoing re-resection for gallbladder cancer, 10.4% of patients with T2 tumors were found to have disease within the liver and 31.3% of patients had N1 lymph node involvement. Other studies have reported lymph node metastasis rates as high as 62% in patients with T2 tumors. Moreover, in 40% to 76% of cases, residual disease is found at re-exploration. Therefore it is perhaps this group of patients with T2Nx-1 lesions that may have the best chances of improved survival from definitive extended re-resection. In fact, extended cholecystectomy has been shown to increase the 5-year survival rates in patients with T2 tumors from 20% to 40% with simple cholecystectomy and to upward of 80% with extended cholecystectomy and portal lymphadenectomy.

Advanced Tumors (T3 and T4)

Patients with T3 or T4 gallbladder cancers have more advanced tumors. After laparoscopic cholecystectomy, not only will there be a microscopically positive margin on pathologic testing, but there likely will be a grossly positive margin (i.e., R2 resection) at cholecystectomy and there also will be a hepatic mass on cross-sectional imaging. Historically, there was debate over the justification for more radical forms of resection in patients with such advanced disease. However, as radical resections have become increasingly safe, reports of long-term survivors after aggressive surgical management are now more abundant in the literature. Dixon and colleagues showed that R0 resection led to significantly improved survival in patients with stage III disease. In this series of 99 patients who were stratified into 6-year treatment period cohorts, it was shown that as surgeons were increasingly willing to perform more aggressive resection for advanced disease, patient survival improved. These data would indicate that radical resection for advanced gallbladder cancer may be potentially curative in a subset of patients. Like patients with T1b or T2 tumors, patients who have T3 or T4 disease also should undergo a staging workup, including cross-sectional imaging studies of the chest, abdomen, and pelvis, to rule out signs of more advanced/metastatic disease, including noncontiguous metastases or signs of carcinomatosis.

Although current NCCN guidelines do not routinely mandate staging laparoscopy before an attempt at definitive resection, several studies have demonstrated the procedure's importance in identifying disseminated disease. A prospective series of 409 patients by Agarwal and colleagues diagnosed 23% of patients with disseminated disease based on laparoscopy alone. The yield of the technique was higher in locally advanced tumors and may be considered for T3 tumors before definitive resection. However, it is noteworthy that the NCCN guidelines do not recommend routine laparoscopy before resection but they do recommend the procedure for patients with an imaging finding that is concerning for gallbladder cancer. Finally, barring any contraindications to an operation (i.e., medical contraindications to major abdominal surgery, cirrhosis, or insufficient remnant liver volume to maintain adequate hepatic function), patients should be explored (or re-explored after laparoscopic cholecystectomy) for radical resection of the tumor.

■ OPERATIVE MORBIDITY AND MORTALITY

The operations described in the previous sections are extensive procedures with substantial risks. In particular, most patients undergoing treatment for gallbladder cancer are in their seventh or eighth decades of life and may be at increased risk for complications as a consequence of concomitant medical comorbidities. A review of National Surgical Quality Improvement Program (NSQIP) data of 613 patients undergoing surgery for gallbladder cancer between 2005 and 2009 demonstrated morbidity rates from 21% to 28% depending on the extent of resection. Mortality rates for patients undergoing extended hepatectomy were 16%, compared with those for patients undergoing cholecystectomy (7%) or partial hepatectomy (2%).

The most common complications are bile leak, liver failure, intra-abdominal abscess, and respiratory failure and wound infection. Therefore the risks of surgical resection need to be weighed against the benefits depending on the stage of disease.

■ ADJUVANT THERAPY

Because of the insidious nature of the disease, more than 50% of gallbladder cancers will be unresectable at the time of diagnosis, with approximately one third of patients having metastatic disease. Thus chemotherapy remains a mainstay of treatment for gallbladder cancer. Because of the rarity of gallbladder cancer and the infrequency of completely resected disease, there is only one prospective, randomized trial studying the utility of adjuvant therapy for gallbladder cancer. This study from Japan evaluated the 5-year overall survival rate in 140 patients who received adjuvant chemotherapy using mitomycin C and 5-fluorouracil (5-FU) after noncurative resection. Survival was improved with adjuvant therapy (26% vs 14%, P = 0.03). In a more recent but nonrandomized trial, the Southwest Oncology Group (SWOG) S0809 study reported that capecitabine and gemcitabine followed by capecitabine-based chemoradiation resulted in a 2-year survival rate of 65% in patients with pT2-4 Nx, pTx N1, or R1 disease. Thus current evidence suggests that there is a role for adjuvant chemoradiation and chemotherapy. At present, NCCN guidelines support the use of gemcitabine/cisplatin combination therapy or fluoropyrimidine-based or gemcitabine-based chemotherapy in the adjuvant setting for patients with pT1b-4 Nx or pTx N1 disease. Like other biliary tract tumors (i.e., intrahepatic and extrahepatic cholangiocarcinoma), gemcitabine combined with cisplatin is most often used as first-line chemotherapy based on the randomized controlled Phase III ABC-02 trial, which showed improved median overall survival with combination therapy versus gemcitabine alone (11.7 months vs 9 months).

Data regarding radiation therapy are more robust but not conclusive. One group evaluated intraoperative radiation therapy after complete resection T4N0-1 gallbladder (stage IV) cancer and reported a 3-year survival rate of 10.1% for patients receiving radiation therapy versus 0% for those having surgery alone. In addition, a study from the Mayo Clinic evaluated 21 patients with all stages of disease who received adjuvant external beam radiation therapy and 5-FU after curative resection. They had a 5-year survival rate of 64% versus a historical surgical cohort with a 5-year survival rate of 33% after R0 resection alone. Finally, in a large population-based analysis using the SEER database (1995-2005), patients with T2 to T4 or N1 disease derived the most improvement in survival from chemoradiation therapy. On the basis of these data and guidelines, adjuvant single agent chemotherapy with either (1) fluoropyrimidine or gemcitabine, or (2) fluoropyrimidine-based chemoradiation may be considered in patients with pT1b-4, pTxN1, or R1 disease.

■ MANAGEMENT OF UNRESECTABLE OR METASTATIC DISEASE

As previously mentioned, chemotherapy remains a mainstay of treatment for advanced gallbladder cancer. On the basis of several trials, active chemotherapy regimens include (1) gemcitabine with oxaliplatin or capecitabine; (2) capecitabine with cisplatin or oxaliplatin; (3) fluorouracil with cisplatin or oxaliplatin; (4) single agent fluorouracil; (5) single agent capecitabine; or (6) single agent gemcitabine. However, systemic chemotherapy has objective response rates of only 10% to 30%. Thus patients with unresectable disease and good functional status also may be directed to clinical trials to determine whether any novel therapies may be effective.

Palliative therapy also may be appropriate in the context of a median survival of approximately 6 months in patients who have unresectable or metastatic disease. The goal of palliation should be relief of pain, jaundice/pruritus, or bowel obstruction. Biliary bypass for obstruction can be difficult because of advanced disease in the porta hepatis. A segment III bypass is usually necessary if surgical bypass is chosen to relieve jaundice. However, such bypasses have a 30-day mortality rate of 12%. Therefore, in the jaundiced patient with advanced, unresectable gallbladder cancer, a radiologic (i.e., PTC) or endoscopic (i.e., ERCP) approach to biliary drainage is preferred. As there are higher rates of bile leaks and bleeding with the percutaneous approach and the percutaneous stent is most often externalized at least initially, a trial of endoscopic stenting usually is undertaken first.

■ DISEASE BIOLOGY AND FUTURE DIRECTIONS

Past research has identified two distinct pathways for the development of gallbladder cancer. In the first pathway, cholelithiasis resulting in chronic cholecystitis causes irritation of the gallbladder mucosa; this irritation may predispose the mucosa to malignant transformation. Historically, tumors thought to arise from chronic cholecystitis were characterized by early TP53 mutations with rare KRAS mutations. The second pathway is associated with an aberrant pancreaticobiliary duct junction, which may allow for pancreatic juice reflux into the biliary tree because the duct junction lies outside of the sphincter of Oddi. In contrast to those tumors associated with cholelithiasis, tumors associated with abnormal pancreaticobiliary duct junction were characterized by early KRAS mutations, with late onset of TP53 mutations.

More recent advances in next-generation sequencing of genes have allowed researchers to better characterize gallbladder cancer and identify possible targets for therapeutic intervention. It is now recognized that the most common genomic alterations in gallbladder cancer include PBRM1 underexpression (53%); TP53 mutations (4% to 41%); CDKN2A/B loss (19%); ERBB2 amplification/overexpression (15% to 16%); PIK3CA mutations (12% to 14%); ARID1A mutations (13%); KRAS mutations (4% to 11%); NRAS mutations (4%); APC mutations (4%); CTNNB1 mutations (4%); FGFR1-3 fusions/amplifications (3%); IDH1 mutations (1.5%); and BRAF mutations (1%). More broadly, the most commonly affected pathways include MAPK signaling; PI3K/AKT/mTOR pathway; TP53/MDM2/MDMX axis; and the Wnt/β-catenin pathway. To a lesser extent, affected pathways include apoptosis; cell cycle regulation; chromatin remodeling; double-stranded breaks of DNA; cytoplasmic NADPH production; FGF signaling; TGF-β signaling; JAK/STAT pathway; JNK signaling; PKC pathway; and the phospholipase Cγ pathway. Several of these genomic alterations may confer susceptibility to targeted therapies approved by the U.S. Food and Drug Administration (FDA), including inhibitors of the cell cycle (e.g., palbociclib), ERBB2 (e.g., afatinib, lapatinib, trastuzumab, pertuzumab, trastuzumab emtansine), PI3KCA/mTOR (e.g., everolimus, temsirolimus), MEK (e.g., trametinib), FGFR (e.g., pazopanib, regorafenib, ponatinib, lenvatinib), and BRAF (e.g., vemurafenib, dabrafenib). Although gallbladder cancer was historically treated like other biliary tract cancers, it is now clear that these tumors have distinct genomic alterations. Therefore by selecting agents that directly target the genomic alterations found in gallbladder cancers, outcomes in these patients may be improved. At present, several targeted agents are under investigation in gallbladder cancer. Overall, further clinical studies are needed to define the role of these agents in selected patients possessing tumors with the aforementioned alterations.

■ SUMMARY

Gallbladder cancer is an aggressive disease with a poor but slowly improving prognosis. Appropriate staging workup, radical resection, and adjuvant chemotherapy/chemoradiation can improve survival and may lead to cure in some patients. Given the similar underlying risk factors for gallstones and gallbladder cancer, malignancies are encountered in approximately 1 in 100 cholecystectomy specimens that are removed for presumed benign gallstone disease. Because these tumors can have an insidious course, any long obstruction of the mid–common bile duct or gallbladder mass detected on imaging should be considered gallbladder cancer until proven otherwise.

Gallbladder carcinoma commonly disseminates via four mechanisms: (1) direct extension and invasion into the liver and adjacent organs; (2) lymphatic spread; (3) shedding and peritoneal dissemination; and (4) hematogenous spread to distant sites. In order to investigate the extent of disease, workup may include US, MRCP, CT, PET-CT, and/or staging laparoscopy. Operative candidates may be selected based on evaluation of the patient's general medical condition and functional status, as well as a rigorous staging workup to rule out locally advanced disease with significant vascular involvement or disseminated disease. Evidence of nonregional nodal metastases (i.e., N2 disease) or distant metastases (i.e., M1 disease) on preoperative workup precludes a curative resection because no long-term survivors have been reported with N2 or M1 disease.

An evidence-based algorithm has been developed for the surgical management of gallbladder carcinomas. For T1a tumors, simple cholecystectomy is sufficient if the cystic duct margin is negative. For T1b to T4 tumors, a radical cholecystectomy (segment IVb and V resection) with portal lymphadenectomy should be performed, with microscopically negative margins (R0 resection). An extended hepatic resection (i.e., right hepatectomy or right trisectionectomy) may be necessary to achieve an R0 resection depending on the location and extent of the tumor. Lymphadenectomy should include resection of lymph nodes of the porta hepatis and along the hepatoduodenal ligament. In turn, if the extrahepatic biliary tree is involved with a tumor or rendered ischemic by an extensive resection/lymphadenectomy, it should be resected followed by Roux-en-Y hepaticojejunostomy reconstruction. On the basis of emerging data, port site resection is no longer indicated for gallbladder cancers identified after laparoscopic cholecystectomy for benign disease. Recent data suggest that there is a role for adjuvant chemotherapy/chemoradiation in patients with resected disease. For patients with evidence of widespread dissemination, there are no curative surgical options. These patients should be treated with systemic chemotherapy or palliative therapies for symptoms. In summary, gallbladder cancer is a complex disease process best managed by an interdisciplinary group, which includes surgical oncologists, medical oncologists, radiation oncologists, radiologists, interventional radiologists, gastroenterologists, pathologists, and palliative medicine specialists, in order to optimize patient care.

SUGGESTED READINGS

Abramson MA, Pandharipande P, Ruan D, Gold JS, Whang EE. Radical resection for T1b gallbladder cancer: a decision analysis. *HPB (Oxford)*. 2009;11:656-663.

Agarwal AK, Kalayarasan R, Javed A, Gupta N, Nag HH. The role of staging laparoscopy in primary gall bladder cancer—an analysis of 409 patients: a prospective study to evaluate the role of staging laparoscopy in the management of gallbladder cancer. *Ann Surg*. 2013;258:318-323.

D'Angelica M, Dalal KM, DeMatteo RP, Fong Y, Blumgart LH, Jarnagin WR. Analysis of the extent of resection for adenocarcinoma of the gallbladder. *Ann Surg Oncol*. 2009;16:806-816.

Dixon E, Vollmer CM Jr, Sahajpal A, Cattral M, Grant D, Doig C, et al. An aggressive surgical approach leads to improved survival in patients with gallbladder cancer: a 12-year study at a North American center. *Ann Surg*. 2005;241:385-394.

Henley SJ, Weir HK, Jim MA, Watson M, Richardson LC. Gallbladder cancer incidence and mortality, United States 1999–2011. *Cancer Epidemiol Biomarkers Prev*. 2015;24:1319-1326.

Kapoor VK, Pradeep R, Haribhakti SP, Sikora SS, Kaushik SP. Early carcinoma of the gallbladder: an elusive disease. *J Surg Oncol*. 1996;62:284-287.

Maker AV, Butte JM, Oxenberg J, Kuk D, Gonen M, Fong Y, et al. Is port site resection necessary in the surgical management of gallbladder cancer? *Ann Surg Oncol*. 2012;19:409-417.

Sicklick JK, Fanta PT, Shimabukuro K, Kurzrock R. Genomics of gallbladder cancer: the case for biomarker-driven clinical trial design. *Cancer Metastasis Rev*. 2016;35:263-275.

THE MANAGEMENT OF GALLSTONE ILEUS

Steven B. Goldin, MD, and John Mullinax, MD

Bowel obstruction secondary to a gallstone in the small bowel was first described by Bartholin in 1654 and again by Courvoisier in 1890. Gallstone ileus is a rare complication of cholelithiasis. Approximately 30% of the adult population have cholelithiasis but only 0.3% to 0.5% of patients with cholelithiasis will develop gallstone ileus. Gallstone ileus results from inflammation surrounding the gallbladder that results in a bilioenteric fistula. Similar complications include Mirizzi's syndrome, in which a large gallstone in the infundibulum erodes through the gallbladder wall into the common bile duct. Another such complication is Bouveret's syndrome, in which a gallstone erodes through the gallbladder wall into the stomach and impacts at the pylorus, resulting in gastric outlet obstruction. The most frequent location of a cholecystoenteric fistula is between the gallbladder and duodenum (Figure 1) followed by a fistula to the mid/distal small bowel. Cholecystocolic fistulae are much less common but have been described mainly to the hepatic flexure.

The pathophysiology for all of the cholecystoenteric fistulae is similar. Chronic luminal pressure from a large gallstone results in localized necrosis and perforation into the wall of adjacent bowel. The fistulous tract becomes an epithelialized conduit that allows transit of gallstones between the gallbladder and bowel. Small stones (typically smaller than 2 cm) often pass through the ileocecal valve and are evacuated. Larger stones (generally more than 3 cm in diameter) may result in a bowel obstruction. This unique cause of bowel obstruction is rare and responsible for only 3.7% of all cases of bowel obstructions. It is a significantly more common (22.5% to 25%) cause of bowel obstruction in elderly females without prior abdominal operations.

■ DIAGNOSIS

Clinical

The presentation of patients with gallstone ileus is much the same as for any other patient with small bowel obstruction. Typical symptoms include nausea, vomiting, and colicky abdominal pain. Classically, biliary colic followed 1 to 2 days later by signs of bowel obstruction. A clinical presentation unique to this entity is the "tumbling stone" phenomenon. This phenomenon involves a varied pain location throughout the abdomen during the several days preceding evaluation. The varied location and duration of pain are thought to be due to intermittent obstructions that occur at various locations as the stone moves though the small bowel.

Radiographic

Regardless of the symptoms reported by the patient, Rigler's triad describes the radiographic findings most classically associated with gallstone ileus. Rigler's triad first was described in 1941 when plain radiographs were the only available imaging modality (Figure 2) and consists of small bowel obstruction, pneumobilia, and an aberrant stone in the GI tract seen on radiographic imaging. Although

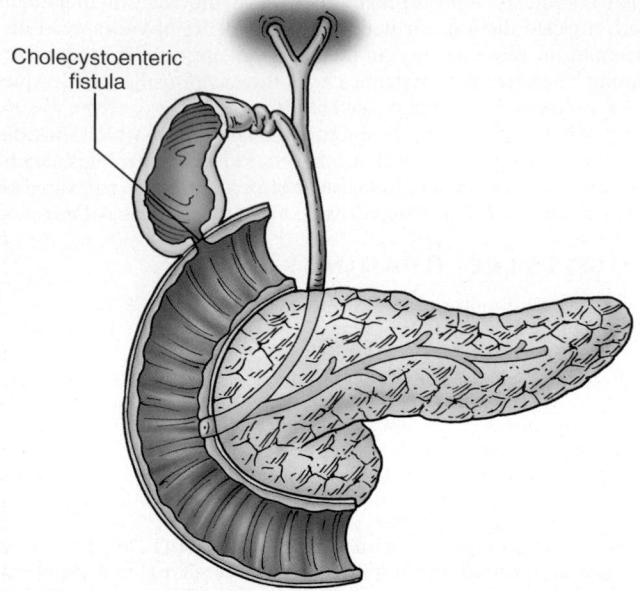

FIGURE 1 Cholecystoenteric fistula. The fistula responsible for gallstone ileus is most commonly between the fundus or infundibulum of the gallbladder and the second portion of the duodenum. *(Modified from Smith JA. Abdominal Ultrasound. 3rd ed. Philadelphia: Churchill Livingstone; 2011.)*

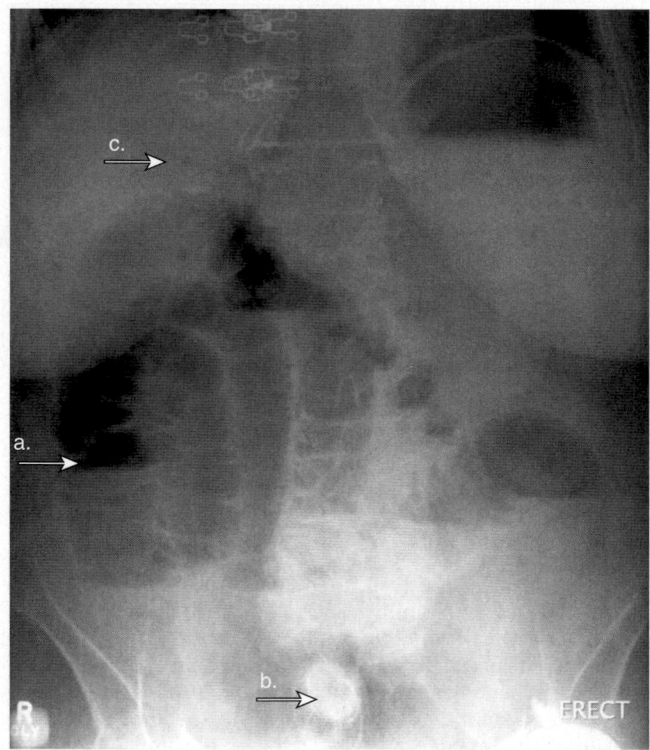

FIGURE 2 Abdominal radiograph demonstrating Rigler's triad. Dilated small bowel (*a*) proximal to enterolith (*b*). Pneumobilia (*c*) is also present, which completes the triad. *(Case courtesy Dr. Frank Gaillard, Radiopaedia.org, rID: 6906.)*

Rigler's triad is the most specific constellation of symptoms relating to the diagnosis, it is not the most common manner of presentation and is seen in only 20% to 50% of patients. In contemporary reports, computed tomography (CT) is the preferred imaging modality because it is 93% sensitive for the diagnosis (Figure 3). More

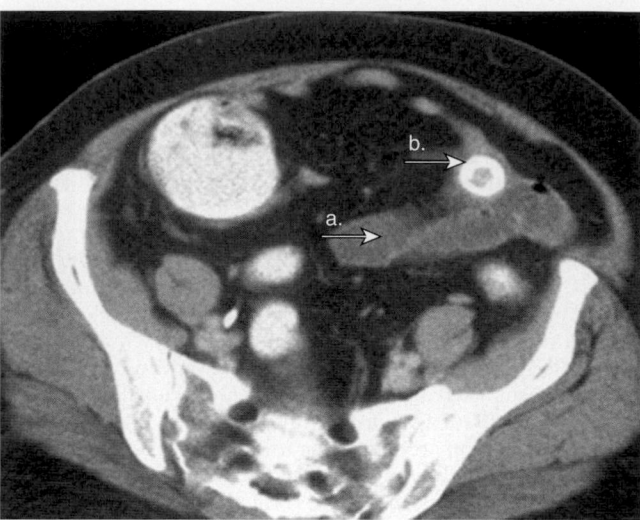

FIGURE 3 Computed tomography of abdomen/pelvis with (*a*) dilated bowel proximal to (*b*) enterolith. *(From Zaliekas J, Munson JL. Complications of gallstones: the Mirizzi syndrome, gallstone ileus, gallstone pancreatitis, complications of "lost" gallstones. Surg Clin North Am. 88:1345-1368; 2008.)*

important than the sensitivity of this diagnostic tool is the ability to recognize other calculi within the gastrointestinal (GI) tract, which occur in up to 12.5% of patients. Identification of additional stones within the GI tract preoperatively improves operative planning, but the small bowel and stomach always should be searched for additional stones during surgery to prevent an early recurrent postoperative bowel obstruction.

■ MANAGEMENT

Operative intervention is required in the management of patients with gallstone ileus. As with any other acute surgical conditions, attention should focus first on the general condition of the patient. Early intravenous resuscitation with isotonic crystalloid is important. Nasogastric tube decompression is important as in any type of bowel obstruction to decrease the risk of aspiration and decompress the bowel. Adjuncts such as an indwelling urinary catheter can be helpful to follow the response to resuscitation. The acuity of the patient dictates the timing of the operation, but prompt exploration is indicated once a definitive diagnosis is made. This occurs generally later than most other acute surgical conditions; the final diagnosis is made roughly 3 to 8 days after the onset of symptoms.

The primary objective during surgery is to remove the offending gallstone and relieve the bowel obstruction. The small bowel should be palpated manually from the ligament of Treitz distally to the point of obstruction, which is most often in the terminal ileum or at the ileocecal valve. Careful palpation along the entire length of the bowel is important to ensure that multiple stones are not overlooked. Once the stone is identified, an enterotomy is made in healthier bowel approximately 30 cm proximal to the bowel obstruction site in a longitudinal fashion on the antimesenteric side of the bowel. The stone is milked out of the bowel, and the enterotomy is closed in a transverse fashion with careful attention to not narrow the lumen of the bowel.

This enterolithotomy approach is the fundamental objective of surgical intervention. Whether to address the cholecystoenteric fistula at the time of the operation is controversial and is the source of much debate. Proponents argue that a single-stage operation resolves all disease and abrogates the risk of future similar events. The risk of recurrence, however, is low and is reported to be in the range of 5% to 9%; of patients with recurrent symptoms, only 10% require reoperation. This means that only 1% of patients who have not had the cholecystoenteric fistula addressed at the index operation will require reoperation. The low recurrence rate and infrequent need for repeat surgical intervention leads many to avoid the biliary pathology at the time of the initial operation.

A single-stage approach to encompass enterolithotomy, cholecystectomy, and closure of the cholecystoenteric fistula also conveys higher perioperative morbidity and mortality rates according to two large series. Doko and colleagues reported a perioperative morbidity rate of 27.3% for enterolithotomy alone compared with 61.1% for a single-stage approach ($P = 0.043$). In a large meta-analysis by Reisner and colleagues, the mortality rate for a single-stage approach was reported to be 16.9% compared with 11.7% for patients who underwent only enterolithotomy. Finally, another large series of patients treated with single-stage approach reported a perioperative mortality of 22.7%. Given these differences in morbidity and mortality, a single-stage approach should be undertaken infrequently and with great attention to patient selection.

Controversy also surrounds the need for delayed closure of cholecystoenteric fistula after enterolithotomy alone. Exploration of asymptomatic patients cannot, by definition, improve their quality of life, and the cholecystectomy is much more complicated because of the severe inflammation and need to repair the fistula. Furthermore, as mentioned earlier, the recurrence rate reported in multiple studies is very low, and of these patients, only 10% require intervention. Elective cholecystectomy to avoid recurrence of gallstone ileus in 1% of patients therefore does not seem warranted. If interval cholecystectomy is undertaken, it is important to also ensure that the common bile duct is not obstructed by a second gallstone.

Minimally invasive techniques have been used to treat gallstone ileus, but at this time, laparoscopic techniques should be avoided for several reasons. First, dilated small bowel increases the risk of inadvertent enterotomy. Second, many patients are hypovolemic at the time of operation and pneumoperitoneum may affect cardiac return negatively. Finally, the ability to thoroughly evaluate the small bowel for secondary stones is extremely limited. Although the short-term gain of less postoperative pain may be beneficial, the long-term sequelae of the laparoscopic approach may not be worth the additional risks.

■ DISCUSSION

Gallstone ileus is fortunately an infrequent complication of cholelithiasis. Patients have bowel obstruction, and the specific underlying cause can be difficult to ascertain preoperatively. Identification of Rigler's triad or "tumbling" pain is helpful but present only in a minority of patients with the condition. Imaging in the form of CT is the most helpful preoperative evaluation, and adequate resuscitation is paramount before exploration. The recommended approach for acute surgical intervention is enterolithotomy alone rather than enterolithotomy, cholecystoenteric fistula repair, and cholecystectomy at the index operation. This is due to the increased morbidity and mortality rates of the latter approach. Patients who undergo only enterolithotomy infrequently develop recurrence of symptoms when the gallbladder is not removed, and only a very small minority of those with recurrent symptoms require repeat exploration.

SUGGESTED READINGS

Ayantunde AA, Agrawal A. Gallstone ileus: diagnosis and management. *World J Surg.* 2007;31:1292-1297.

Doko M, Zovak M, Kopljar M, et al. Comparison of surgical treatments of gallstone ileus: preliminary report. *World J Surg.* 2003;27:400-404.

Lassandro F, Romano S, Ragozzino A, et al. Role of helical CT in diagnosis of gallstone ileus and related conditions. *AJR Am J Roentgenol.* 2005;185:1159-1165.

Luu MB, Deziel DJ. Unusual complications of gallstones. *Surg Clin North Am.* 2014;94:377-394.

Pavlidis TE, Atmatzidis KS, Papaziogas BT, et al. Management of gallstone ileus. *J Hepatobiliary Pancreat Surg.* 2003;10:299-302.

Reisner R, Cohen J. Gallstone ileus: a review of 1001 reported cases. *Am Surg.* 1994;60:441-446.

Warshaw AL, Bartlett M. Choice of operation for gallstone intestinal obstruction. *Ann Surg.* 1966;164:1051-1055.

TRANSHEPATIC INTERVENTIONS FOR OBSTRUCTIVE JAUNDICE

Arun Chockalingam, BS, Christos Georgiades, MD, PhD, FSIR, FCIRSE, and Kelvin Hong, MD

The patient with obstructive jaundice is managed with a multidisciplinary team approach. This may involve the combined expertise of multiple healthcare providers and specialists to include primary care physicians, gastroenterologists, surgeons, and interventional radiologists. Although there are many causes of obstructive jaundice (Box 1), percutaneous transhepatic techniques used for such patients are the focus of this chapter.

The interventional radiologist is involved through use of advanced diagnostic imaging techniques, providing percutaneous image-guided access into the bile ducts and offering endoluminal therapies. Since the introduction of percutaneous transhepatic dilation in 1978, percutaneous techniques have become alternatives to surgical and endoscopic treatments. Long-term data on percutaneous treatments are limited, but studies have reported 3-year success rates between 56% and 74%. Imaging modalities include fluoroscopy and ultrasound guidance and, less commonly, computed tomography (CT),

endoluminal cholangioscopy, and magnetic resonance imaging (MRI). Such therapies may include percutaneous management of benign biliary strictures, biliary ductal injuries and leaks, biliary decompression of cholangitis, biliary duct biopsy, stone removal (with fluoroscopy or cholangioscopy), palliation of malignant biliary obstruction with endoprostheses, and occasional endoluminal therapies such as radiation, photodynamic therapy, and drug infusion (Figures 1 through 5). Therapy also may include application of physiologic parameters, such as a biliary manometric perfusion test, to help decide when a biliary drainage catheter may be removed. A dialogue among gastrointestinal (GI) endoscopists, interventional radiologists, internal medicine specialists, oncologists, primary care physicians, nurses, and other team members is required to manage such patients effectively.

■ NONINVASIVE IMAGING

Biliary anatomy in the patient with obstructive jaundice is defined initially with noninvasive imaging techniques. Many centers use cross-sectional imaging techniques, and many have multidetector CT scanners that allow for rapid patient evaluation and reformatting of images in multiple anatomic projections. Ultrasound (US) is an inexpensive and generally available imaging modality that provides confirmation of dilated intrahepatic and extrahepatic ducts. It is operator dependent, but in skilled hands, it provides important information regarding the possible cause. For example, it is useful in confirming the presence or absence of dilated biliary ducts and detecting stone

BOX 1: Causes of Obstructive Jaundice

A. Benign
1. Choledocholithiasis
2. Papillary stenosis
3. Choledochal cystic disease
4. Postsurgical stricture
5. Mirizzi's syndrome
6. Pancreatic pseudocyst
7. Sclerosing cholangitis
8. Parasitic disease
B. Malignant
1. Pancreatic adenocarcinoma
2. Cholangiocarcinoma
3. Gallbladder carcinoma
4. Ampullary/gastroduodenal carcinoma
5. Periampullary/periportal lymphoma
6. Metastatic disease
7. Neuroendocrine tumors

From Mellinger J, MacFadyen B. Obstructive jaundice: endoscopic management. In Cameron J, ed. *Current Surgical Therapy.* ed 8. St Louis: Elsevier; 2004.

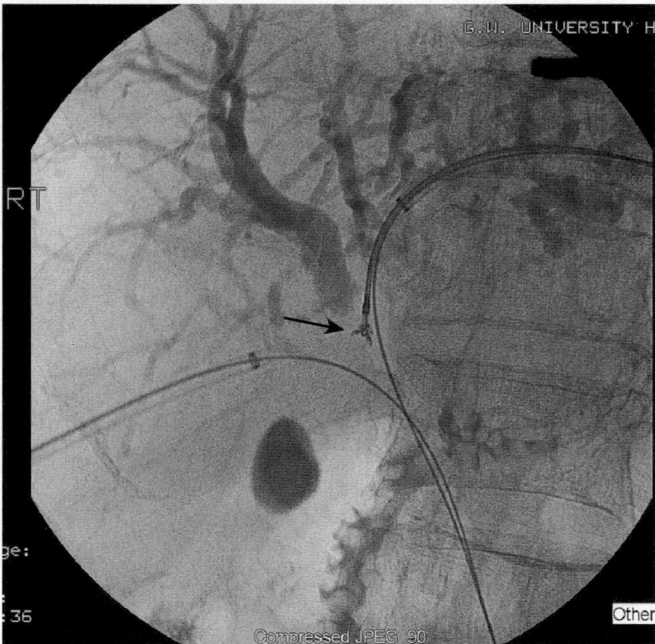

FIGURE 1 Digital spot fluoroscopic image in left anterior oblique projection showing "clam shell" biopsy *(black arrow)* being performed for a hilar mass lesion with the left-sided access. This patient presented with signs and symptoms of obstructive jaundice. Note the lack of contrast in the common bile duct. *(Adapted from Cameron JL. Current Surgical Therapy. 9th ed. Philadelphia: Mosby; 2008.)*

disease (e.g., cholelithiasis, choledocholithiasis) It is also advantageous in children because it uses no ionizing radiation. It also may be used at bedside in the critically ill patient to drain the gallbladder (percutaneous cholecystostomy).

When US is used to evaluate the liver, the addition of color-flow Doppler easily differentiates visualized tubular structures (dilated biliary ducts) from vessels (hepatic artery, hepatic vein, portal vein). Extrahepatic anatomy may not be visualized adequately in patients with extensive bowel gas (ileus or bowel obstruction), or it may not be technically feasible because of a limited "sonic window" for

imaging, such as in a patient with multiple drains, wound dressings that cannot be removed, and open abdominal incisions with a silo barrier.

As mentioned earlier, thin-section helical CT images, especially those taken with newer multidetector scanners, allow rapid evaluation of abdominal anatomy. Studies are reproducible, and axial images may be reformatted to provide anatomic detail of liver, biliary anatomy, and other adjacent organs, such as the pancreas and duodenum. CT is more expensive than US, and it uses ionizing radiation and generally requires administration of oral and intravenous contrast; however, initial images without contrast may be useful in detecting bile duct stones. Because of CT's greater sensitivity to density differences, poorly calcified or noncalcified stones on plain films may be detected readily on CT. On the downside, CT is not portable; therefore ill patients must be transported to and from the scanner.

MRI is useful, especially given the ability to reformat axial images and produce a magnetic resonance (MR) cholangiogram. The technique requires a significant amount of time, but when performed well, it can result in a detailed representation of bile duct anatomy. In some centers, magnetic resonance cholangiopancreatography has replaced routine endoscopic retrograde cholangiopancreatography (ERCP) for defining bile duct anatomy. Because it uses no ionizing radiation, MRI is useful in children. However, in such instances, sedation or anesthesia support may be required to complete the MR examination.

◼ ENDOSCOPIC AND PERCUTANEOUS EVALUATION

After clinical evaluation, laboratory blood work, and cross-sectional imaging, the patient must be evaluated endoscopically. ERCP is often the first invasive procedure performed in patients requiring biliary surgery and/or intervention. ERCP is especially useful in patients with coagulopathies, marked ascites, or in whom intrahepatic lesions, such as multiple hepatic cysts, preclude a safe transhepatic approach. Limitations of ERCP in patients with obstructive jaundice include the inability to cannulate the biliary system because of surgically altered anatomy (biliary–enteric anastomosis) and technical limitations in treating intrahepatic or hilar lesions from an endoscopic retrograde approach.

For the patient to be considered an operative candidate for biliary reconstruction, such as with choledochoenterostomy, precise anatomic definition of the intrahepatic and extrahepatic bile ducts is essential in planning the surgical reconstruction. When ERCP is unable to completely opacify the biliary system, percutaneous transhepatic cholangiography (PTC) is the preferred procedure. PTC accurately depicts the intrahepatic biliary tree, lesion length, and lesion numbers, and it defines whether the biliary disease involves the bifurcation. Should a bifurcation lesion be found, bilateral (right and left) PTC and biliary drainage procedures may be performed. At our institution, the placement of one or more transhepatic biliary drainage catheters facilitates biliary reconstruction, assisting the surgeon in creating one or more biliary-enteric anastomoses.

In a clinical situation in which the extrahepatic biliary system has been injured, such as with inadvertent complete clipping of the common hepatic or common bile duct, PTC alone may not fully define the distal extrahepatic bile duct anatomy. ERCP may be required to define distal anatomy up to the clip, and PTC and external percutaneous biliary drainage (PBD) may be used to define anatomy superior to the clipped duct. In this latter case, precise anatomic detail is delineated for eventual biliary reconstructive surgery. At times, combined ERCP and percutaneous transhepatic procedures are required to bridge and reconstruct biliary disruptions (rendezvous procedure) when either access point is insufficient to clearly define the entire biliary tree.

PTC is the first step to PBD. The only absolute contraindication to PTC/PBD performed as a means of access into the biliary system

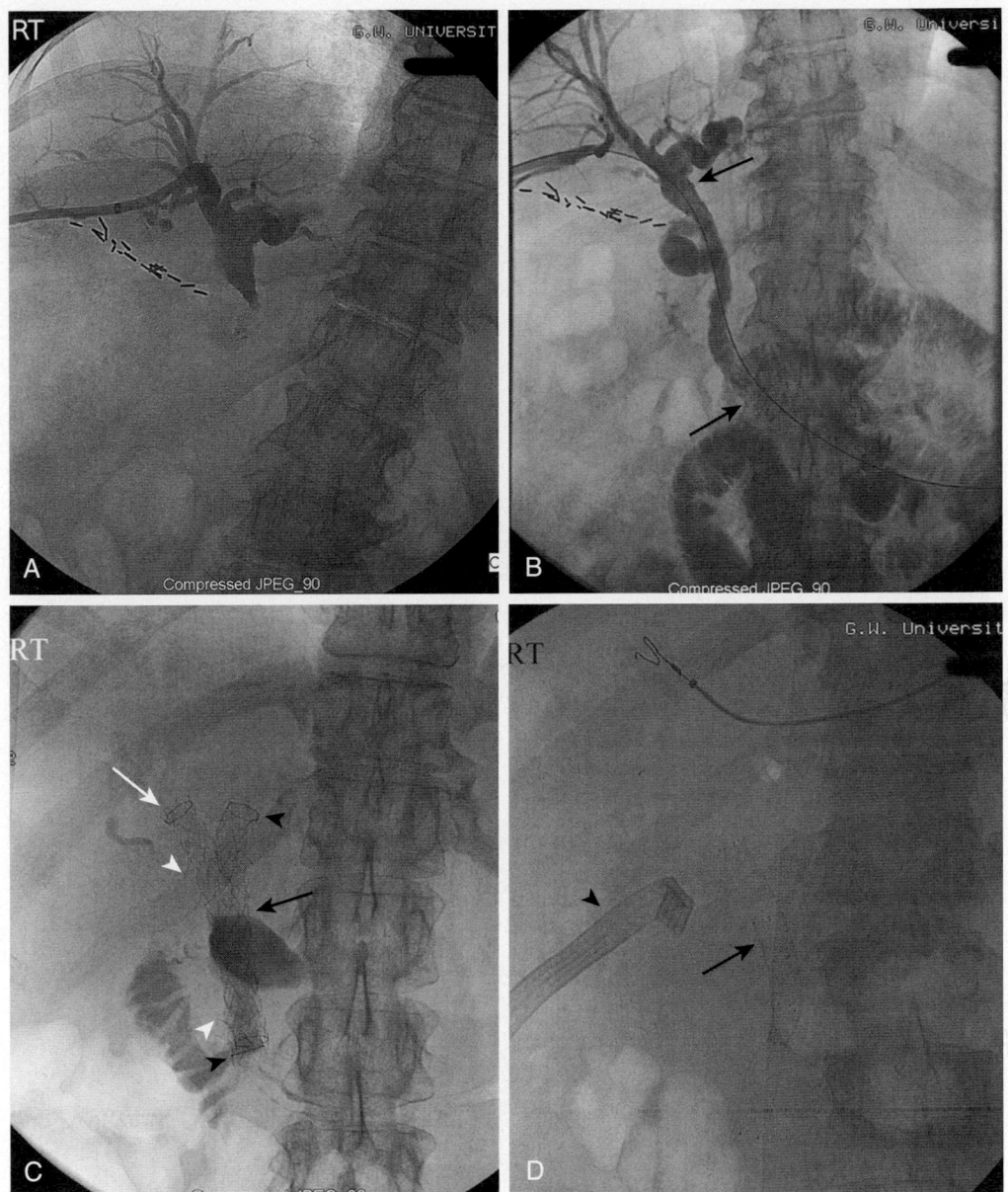

FIGURE 2 A, Digital spot fluoroscopic image of the right upper quadrant in right anterior oblique projection showing abrupt cutoff of contrast in the common hepatic duct. There is no opacification of the duodenum. Note the contrast injection via a preexisting right-sided external biliary drainage. **B,** Digital spot fluoroscopic image of the right upper quadrant in the same patient. Cholangiogram performed after placement of an expanded polytetrafluoroethylene (ePTFE) endoprosthesis (W.L. Gore & Associates, Flagstaff, AZ) shows rapid flow of contrast through the endoprostheses into the duodenum; *arrows* mark the extent of endoprosthesis. Because the pancreatic head mass was unresectable, an ePTFE endoprosthesis was placed. **C,** Another patient with cholangiocarcinoma who underwent bilateral ePTFE endoprostheses placement. Note the metallic stent "skeleton" *(black arrow)* and radiopaque rings indicating the edges of the ePTFE covering *(arrowheads)*. Also seen are uncovered metallic ends adjacent to the radiopaque rings *(white arrow)* and anchoring. **D,** Another patient with a pancreatic head mass who underwent internal bare-metal stent placement for common bile duct obstruction. Note the three overlapping bare metal stents *(arrow)* outlining the common bile duct. Also seen is a Jackson-Pratt drain in the gallbladder fossa *(arrowhead)*. *(Adapted from Cameron JL. Current Surgical Therapy. 9th ed. Philadelphia: Mosby; 2008.)*

for the treatment of patients with obstructive jaundice is a significant coagulopathy that cannot be corrected. PBD also should be avoided in patients with diffuse polycystic liver disease or in patients with hepatic cysts resulting from parasitic infections (e.g., *Echinococcus*). Occasionally, cross-sectional imaging and PBD under CT or US imaging guidance may be useful to find an appropriate safe "window" for access into the biliary system in patients with multiple intrahepatic lesions.

Ideally, the patient with obstructive jaundice undergoing PTC/PBD should not have a coagulopathy. At our institution, PBD

generally is not performed if the platelet count is below 50,000 or if the international normalized ratio (INR) is greater than 1.7. Should the platelet count or INR parameters be altered significantly, blood products—such as platelets, fresh frozen plasma, and vitamin K—may be administered to the patient for the biliary drainage procedure.

The presence of ascites presents a challenge for percutaneous transhepatic drainage. Should biliary drainage be required in a patient with ascites, ERCP with stent placement is the preferred means of drainage (i.e., "internal drainage"). The patient with

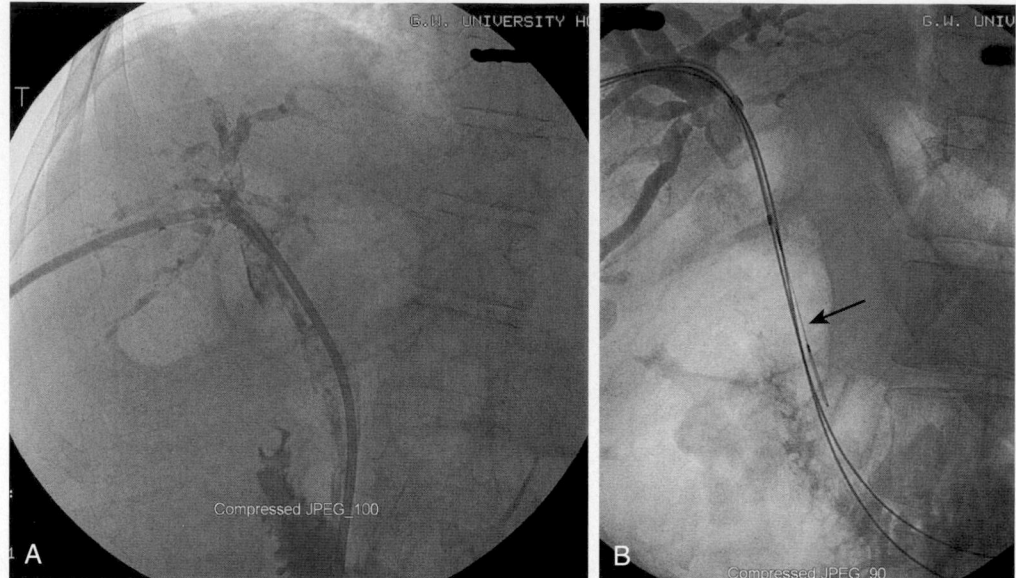

FIGURE 3 A, Digital spot fluoroscopic image of an adult patient who presented with obstructive jaundice. PTC/PBD revealed numerous intraluminal filling defects in both intrahepatic and extrahepatic bile ducts. **B,** Endoluminal brush biopsy *(arrow)* performed to confirm the diagnosis through a preexisting right-sided access. Pathologic analysis of the specimen later confirmed this to be metastatic colon adenocarcinoma. *(Adapted from Cameron JL. Current Surgical Therapy. 9th ed. Philadelphia: Mosby; 2008.)*

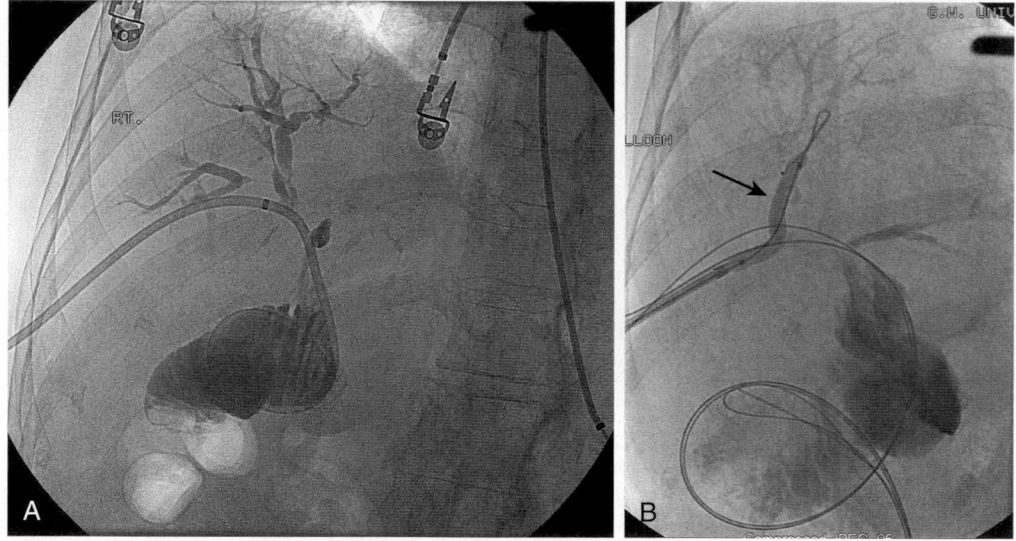

FIGURE 4 A, Digital spot fluoroscopic image of right upper quadrant in right anterior oblique (RAO) projection showing multiple intrahepatic biliary strictures in an adult patient who had undergone previous choledochojejunostomy. This patient has primary sclerosing cholangitis. **B,** Digital spot fluoroscopic image of right upper quadrant in RAO projection in the same patient. Patient underwent balloon cholangioplasty *(arrow)* for treatment of intrahepatic biliary strictures. *(Adapted from Cameron JL. Current Surgical Therapy. 9th ed. Philadelphia: Mosby; 2008.)*

significant ascites requiring a percutaneous transhepatic drainage catheter often is plagued with leakage of ascitic fluid around the tube, which soaks dressings, causes skin irritation and inflammation, and theoretically places the patient at risk of bile leakage into the peritoneum (bile peritonitis). Technically, the presence of ascites also can make percutaneous biliary drain placement difficult. Because the liver floats in fluid, it is moved easily during needle placement. This can make it difficult to accurately cross the liver capsule with the needle.

■ **PERCUTANEOUS TRANSHEPATIC CHOLANGIOGRAPHY AND PERCUTANEOUS BILIARY DRAINAGE TECHNIQUE SUMMARY**

The technique of PTC/PBD is well described and outlined later; it is an invasive procedure. Intravenous antibiotics are given immediately on admission if a patient is seen with clinical signs and symptoms of biliary sepsis or cholangitis. In patients who are not septic,

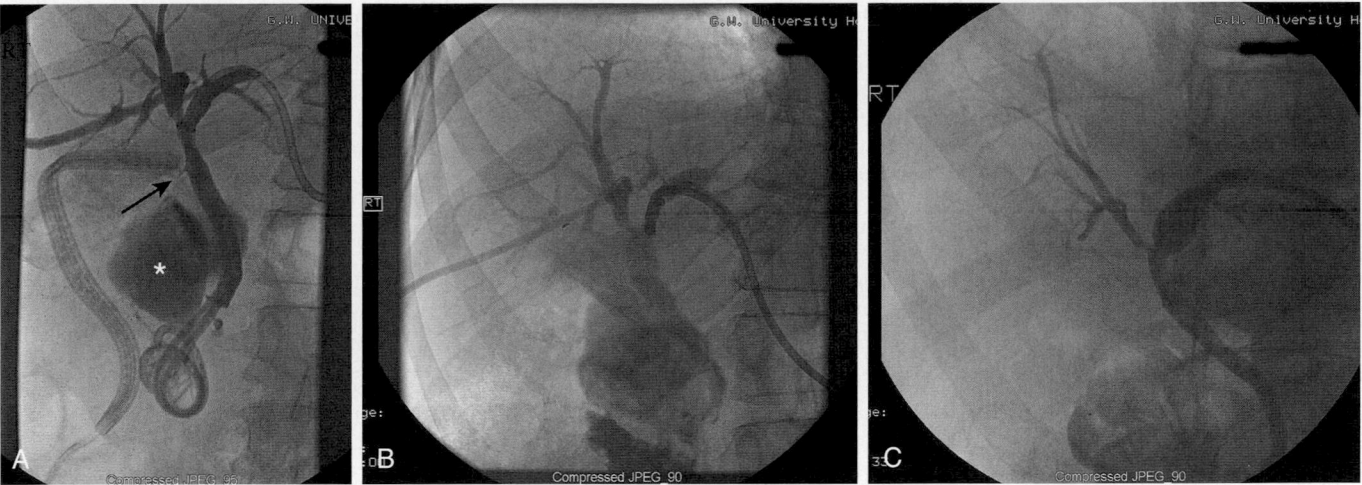

FIGURE 5 A, Digital spot fluoroscopic image of right upper quadrant in a patient who had undergone cholecystectomy. A postoperative cystic duct stump leak (*arrow*) was managed by bilateral percutaneous transhepatic internal/external drainage catheter placement to divert bile. The internal/external biliary drainage catheters were left in place for 6 weeks. Note contrast within the duodenal bulb (*asterisk*). **B,** Digital spot fluoroscopic image of right upper quadrant in right anterior oblique projection in the same patient. A trial was performed by keeping the catheter distal ends proximal to the confluence of right and left main ducts, allowing for internal drainage without assistance of drainage catheters across the site of postoperative bile leak. **C,** Digital spot fluoroscopic image of right upper quadrant in left anterior oblique projection showing adequate flow of contrast into the right main duct and common bile duct from a left-sided injection. External biliary drainage catheters were removed after 2 weeks. The patient remained asymptomatic at 6-month follow-up. (*Adapted from Cameron JL. Current Surgical Therapy. 9th ed. Philadelphia: Mosby; 2008.*)

intravenous antibiotics are administered on the day of the procedure and generally are continued for 24 hours afterward. As mentioned earlier, the complete blood count, coagulation studies, and liver function tests are done as part of our routine preprocedure laboratory analysis.

After counseling regarding the risks of the procedure, informed consent is obtained. The patient is placed in the supine position. Intravenous sedation and analgesia are administered under an institutional conscious sedation protocol, and physiologic monitoring of blood pressure, pulse, and oxygen saturation is recorded frequently. In patients with hypotension and biliary sepsis, the help of an anesthesiologist can be invaluable: they can secure the airway and actively manage blood pressure and pain control, allowing safe reliable procedure. Although some interventional radiologists prefer initial biliary access from the left subxiphoid approach, at our institution, a right midaxillary approach generally is used.

The first step is to anesthetize the skin and subcutaneous tissues inferior to the level of the costophrenic angle and above the level of the colon hepatic flexure. A thin needle (22G Chiba; Cook Medical, Inc., Bloomington, IN) is advanced under fluoroscopic guidance into the liver, entering at the midaxillary line parallel to the tabletop. The needle is directed medially and superiorly. After the stylet is removed, the hub of the needle is connected through tubing to a syringe containing diluted contrast (1:1 dilution of saline to contrast). As the needle is withdrawn, contrast is injected slowly under fluoroscopic guidance. If the tip of the needle is in a bile duct, contrast is seen to flow away from it. On opacification of the biliary anatomy, multiple images are obtained to accurately define anatomy.

Should PBD be considered, and if a peripheral duct has not been entered or the point of duct entry is unfavorable for advancement of a guidewire, a second thin needle (we use a 21G trocar needle) may be used to select a more peripheral right duct. Once the needle is placed in a more peripheral location, a coaxial system consisting of a small-caliber, platinum-tipped, steerable guidewire and dilator/stiffening cannula is advanced and used to secure biliary access. With use of this system, the initial small-caliber guidewire is exchanged for a larger, stiffer guidewire, and a biliary drainage catheter may then be advanced to achieve drainage across a specific bile duct lesion.

In those patients with a high-grade biliary stricture at the bifurcation isolating the right and the left ductal systems, a left PTC/PBD may be required. Anatomic depiction of the left biliary system requires access from a subxiphoid approach. As part of planning the left PTC/PBD approach, it is important that cross-sectional imaging studies be reviewed to determine whether major organs, such as the transverse colon, are interposed between the subxiphoid skin-entry site and the left lobe of the liver. Imaging also should be reviewed to determine if the left lobe is atrophic because of chronic left-sided biliary obstruction. If the left lobe is atrophic and requires drainage, an approach that is more medial than the standard left-sided subxiphoid percutaneous approach may be required.

Once percutaneous transhepatic access is achieved in the patient with obstructive jaundice, biliary catheter maintenance is required. Initially, the catheter is placed to external (bag) drainage. This is especially true for the patient with sepsis resulting from infected bile.

If the patient is critically ill and hemodynamically unstable, placement of an external drainage catheter alone will achieve biliary decompression (placement of a simple, locking perforated drainage catheter as an external drain). Once hemodynamically stable, the patient may return for conversion either to an external/internal biliary drainage catheter (biliary stent) or an internal drainage catheter made of plastic or metal (internal biliary stent, or *biliary endoprosthesis*). The latter generally is reserved for patients with surgically unresectable disease and limited life expectancy who are receiving palliative care. Specifics on the use of endoprostheses are covered later in this chapter.

Transhepatic external/internal biliary drainage catheter placement in the patient with obstructive jaundice requires crossing the obstructing lesion(s). The ultimate goal is to eventually reestablish the biliary-enteric "circulation." If left to external drainage alone (i.e., given the inability to advance the multiple-sidehole drainage catheter into the small bowel) the loss of bile may result in significant morbidity to the patient, including dehydration and electrolyte disturbances. In such a patient, replacement is with intravenous electrolyte-rich fluid (e.g., Lactated Ringer's solution) or orally with an electrolyte-rich sports drink if the patient is able to tolerate oral fluids.

Biliary drainage catheters generally are flushed once or twice a day, especially in patients with viscous or infected bile. The patient and healthcare providers must be instructed about the technique. In the patient with an external/internal biliary drainage catheter, the importance of flushing *into* the tube, "forward flushing," taking care not to aspirate fluid *back* into the syringe, must be emphasized. Forceful aspiration with a syringe may bring bacteria rapidly from the GI tract into the biliary system (i.e., under pressure), and sepsis may result.

If left in place on a chronic basis, external/internal biliary drainage catheters require a periodic exchange. In general, catheters are exchanged over a guidewire on an outpatient basis approximately every 2 to 3 months. For this procedure, the patient receives a single dose of intravenous antibiotics before the cholangiogram and biliary catheter exchange. If conscious sedation is required, the patient returns from the interventional suite to the recovery room (usually for 1 hour). During this time, the newly exchanged biliary drainage catheter is connected to an external drainage bag. If the patient is afebrile, he is discharged home with instructions to "cap" the biliary tube after 24 hours (i.e., the bag is removed). Should the patient become febrile after tube exchange, a decision is made regarding a subsequent course of therapy. The patient may be observed and later discharged on oral antibiotics with the biliary catheter left to external drainage until the patient is afebrile. The patient is told to return if symptoms worsen. Should an outpatient become septic, the patient should be admitted to the hospital and continued on intravenous antibiotics with the biliary drainage catheter left to external (bag) drainage. The clinical presentation of sepsis is fortunately infrequent after routine outpatient catheter exchanges.

Internal Drainage (Biliary Endoprostheses)

The patient who has undergone transhepatic biliary drainage for obstructive jaundice because of surgically unresectable malignant disease may receive a palliative biliary endoprosthesis (internal biliary stent). If clinically stable at the time of initial biliary drainage, the patient may have placement of the biliary endoprosthesis in a single step. This allows rapid treatment and reduces cost compared with placement of an external/internal drainage with later conversion to a completely internalized catheter system (i.e., a multistep procedure).

The endoprosthesis used is either polymer (plastic) or metallic (bare metal open mesh or a covered stent). The plastic endoprostheses are larger in caliber and require transhepatic tract dilation to 10F or 12F. This can cause considerable pain to the patient, and there is a theoretical risk of increased bleeding. Although inexpensive compared with metallic endoprostheses, there are few manufacturers of plastic endoprostheses for transhepatic deployment. The majority of plastic endoprostheses are placed endoscopically.

In contrast, metallic endoprostheses are smaller in caliber at deployment but have significantly larger luminal diameters. For example, self-expanding bare metal stents used as biliary endoprostheses may be deployed through a 6F or 7F sheath system and expand to 1 cm in diameter. These types of stents provide longer patency times and greater cost effectiveness compared with plastic stents. Thus for palliation, a patient could undergo PTC/PBD followed by placement of a metallic endoprosthesis in a single step.

For malignant biliary obstruction, placement of these self-expanding bare metal stents must be considered because the location of the stent can be a significant predictor of pancreatitis. To reduce chances of pancreatitis, literature suggests suprapapillary rather than transpapillary placement.

After endoprosthesis placement, the patient's transhepatic access may be removed if there is no significant bleeding. Should bleeding occur, such as with a friable tumor, a temporary external drainage catheter should be initiated for the patient's transhepatic access tract. This maintains access in the event that the endoprosthesis becomes acutely occluded with thrombus. Once thrombus has cleared, generally in 1 to 2 days, the catheter may be removed after a final cholangiogram confirms patency of the metallic endoprosthesis.

PBD followed by metallic biliary stent placement is extremely important in managing hilar biliary obstruction, but deciding whether to decompress the obstructed ducts in one or both hepatic lobes still must be considered. Very few data on unilobar versus bilobar drainage exist in literature. However, one study showed no difference in survival or stent patency between the two procedures.

Biliary endoprostheses used for palliation are considered permanent implants, hence their use in patients with limited life expectancy. The patency is generally 6 to 12 months. Patients should be warned of this and told that should the endoprosthesis occlude, repeat endoscopic or transhepatic access may be required to relieve the obstruction.

Covered biliary endoprostheses have been developed that have improved the long-term patency for palliation of malignant biliary obstruction. Percutaneous transhepatic placement of expanded polytetrafluoroethylene (ePTFE) covered stent-grafts has been approved (Viabil biliary endoprosthesis; W.L. Gore & Associates, Flagstaff, AZ). These stent-grafts have been modified to include perforations or fenestrations in the ePTFE covering so as not to occlude biliary branches that may otherwise be obstructed by a continuous covering. Such stent-grafts also have anchor "barbs" that prevent migration.

A recent meta-analysis has shown that covered self-expandable biliary endoprostheses have longer duration of patency compared with uncovered self-expandable stents (mean of 61 days). Greater long-term patency of stent-grafts provides an additional therapeutic option to enhance the quality of life in patients with unresectable malignant biliary disease. Although covered and uncovered biliary endoprostheses show similar rates of stent dysfunction, the mechanisms of stent dysfunction differ. Covered stent dysfunction usually involves tumor overgrowth around the stent edges, sludge formation, or stent migration. Uncovered stent dysfunction is more commonly the result of tumor ingrowth through the interstices of the stent. Available data show no statistically significant increase in episodes of cholecystitis or pancreatitis with covered biliary endoprostheses.

The relationship between stent outcomes and stent coating material remains undetermined. However, when plastic stents are used, stent diameter relates to stent patency such that 10F stents show longer stent patency duration as compared with 8F stents; smaller diameter predisposes to occlusion by biliary sludge.

Patients with benign disease and covered stent-grafts, regardless of material used (e.g., expanded polytetrafluoroethylene [ePTFE]), may be considered for endoscopic removal. This is not the preferred treatment for benign disease, but it may be used as an alternative in patients who could otherwise not undergo biliary reconstructive surgery or percutaneous transhepatic catheters. One study suggests a protocol of staged upsizing of internal/external biliary catheters, balloon dilation (8 mm), and prolonged stent treatment at maximum catheter size (18F) for benign biliary strictures. Results from this study showed stricture patency probabilities of 84%, 78%, and 74% at 1 year, 2 years, and 5 years, respectively.

■ COMPLICATIONS OF PERCUTANEOUS TRANSHEPATIC CHOLANGIOGRAPHY AND PERCUTANEOUS BILIARY DRAINAGE

Technical success rates of PTC/PBD are high, and major complication rates are generally low (5% to 8%). Some reported major complications include hemobilia or hemorrhage, sepsis, biloma, peritonitis, pancreatitis, pleural effusions, and, rarely, death. Another complication is cholangitis, which is found in up to 20% of patients. Fortunately, these episodes of cholangitis are usually brief and not associated with hypotension.

Hemobilia and Hemorrhage

Hemobilia occurs when blood enters the bile duct during catheter exchange. This complication has been reported in 2% to 8% of patients undergoing PTC/PBD. It is usually a result of injury to one of the major vessels, either a hepatic artery or vein or portal vein. These patients generally are seen with bleeding from the biliary drainage catheter with right upper quadrant pain. The patient also may have melena or hematochezia.

Hemobilia can occur from either the venous or arterial system. If it occurs from the hepatic or portal vein, it is generally nonpulsatile and dark in color; this generally is managed by either repositioning or upsizing the biliary drainage catheter.

If the bleeding occurs as a result of injury of an arterial branch, emergency consent should be obtained for hepatic arteriography. The bleeding is generally bright red and pulsatile and may be due to a hepatic artery–bile duct fistula or a pseudoaneurysm of the hepatic artery with communication to the biliary system. The treatment requires transcatheter arterial embolization, generally with embolic coils. Occlusion of the injured vessel is accomplished by advancing a catheter distal to the injury site and coiling across it. After hepatic artery branch embolization, the transhepatic access does not have to be abandoned.

Sepsis

If the patient develops a fever, rigors, and hypotension, sepsis should be suspected. Sepsis can arise even with prophylactic antibiotic treatment, and it can be treated with intravenous antibiotics, expansion of intravascular volume, and pressor support. Identification of the causative agent by bacterial culture is imperative to "tailor" the antibiotic use.

Pericatheter Leakage

Transhepatic access may result in leakage of bile around the catheter. This often is due to occlusion of the catheter lumen, and the problem may be addressed by catheter exchange. Occasionally, ascites also may leak around the catheter and may resemble bile leakage. The optimal way to drain the biliary system of a patient with ascites may be with an internal stent (endoprosthesis). If an endoprosthesis is not possible, the catheter may be upsized in an attempt to temporarily tamponade the site, allowing time for tract maturation. A purse-string suture on the skin placed around the catheter also may be used to reduce leakage of ascitic fluid.

■ BILIARY CATHETER REMOVAL

In addition to the routine biliary exchange every 8 to 12 weeks, the decision as to when to remove the biliary drainage catheter in a patient who has undergone treatment of benign biliary strictures is based on clinical and laboratory parameters and on biliary flow dynamics. As mentioned, the duration of stenting is controversial. Most interventionalists will leave a stent in place for at least 3 months before determining if it can be removed. At our institution, we often leave biliary stents in place for 6 to 12 months. Before removing a biliary tube, an "over-the-wire" cholangiogram is performed by pulling the biliary drainage catheter back over a guidewire. If the site of stented stricture looks patent based on an injection of contrast through the tube, a decision may be made to initiate a clinical trial. For this, a shortened biliary drainage catheter is reintroduced over the guidewire, but the tip is placed above the biliary stricture. This maintains percutaneous access and allows bile to flow across the nonstented, previously dilated stricture. The tube is capped for 1 or 2 weeks, and any signs or symptoms of cholangitis, right upper quadrant pain, fever, jaundice, or leakage around the biliary drainage catheter indicate a probable failure of the trial. Because percutaneous access has been maintained, the stricture can be redilated and re-stented easily; alternatively, the patient may require surgery.

If the patient remains asymptomatic during the clinical trial, and there is documented evidence of flow across the stricture on follow-up cholangiography, a biliary manometric perfusion test may be performed. Dilute iodinated contrast is infused in a stepwise manner via the shortened PBD. Biliary pressures less than 20 cm of H_2O are considered normal. In patients with an asymptomatic "clinical trail," and normal pressures during the biliary manometric perfusion test, the positive predicted value for biliary duct patency at 1 year approaches 90%. Patients are monitored carefully with follow-up liver function tests obtained at periodic intervals after tube removal.

In the medical literature, published data for results of percutaneous dilation and stenting indicate long-term patency of 55% to 76% with follow-up periods of 5 and 3 years, respectively. However, most of the data are retrospective in nature. Long-term patency rates for surgical repair of similar lesions are 89% at 72 months follow-up. Initial reports of percutaneous balloon dilation showed significant complications that included hemobilia, mainly resulting from cholangitis or transhepatic access. More recently, cutting balloon dilation has been shown to be safe for treating biliary-enteric anastomotic strictures that are resistant to conventional balloon techniques.

In patients with malignant biliary obstruction, the biliary drainage catheter may be removed after placement of an internal stent (endoprosthesis), either plastic or metallic. Patients with sclerosing cholangitis require a combined approached that may involve operative resection of the dominant strictures, PTC followed by drainage, and balloon dilation of intrahepatic strictures and periodic biliary catheter exchanges. A recent study has shown that percutaneous transhepatic biliary drainage and subsequent metallic stent placement are viable palliative treatment options in patients with metastatic gastric cancer; subsets of patients with differentiated histology of primary gastric cancer and serum bilirubin levels greater than 2 mg/dL after biliary drainage may benefit from combinatory therapy of metallic stent placement and chemotherapy.

■ OTHER INTERVENTIONS

Irreversible Electroporation

Irreversible electroporation (IRE) is a nonthermal ablation technique that induces cell death via pulsed direct current. Thermal ablation techniques have increased 5-year survival of hepatocellular carcinoma from under 1% to 33% to 54%. However, most patients are considered ineligible for these procedures because of having tumors in proximity to main biliary tracts. IRE induces cell death via formation of nanopores in the cellular membrane, but while leaving extracellular matrix intact so that bile ducts can retain function. One study has shown IRE to be effective in treating centrally located liver tumors adjacent to bile ducts, but more studies must be done to assess safety.

Cholangioscopy

As previously mentioned, the use of cholangioscopy is not as common in biliary interventions but is starting to become so in assessment of biliary disease. Peroral cholangioscopy (POC) was first described in the 1970s but was used rarely because of high costs. Now with recent developments, POC is becoming feasible.

There are two types of POC: indirect and direct. Indirect POC uses a catheter with an optical probe inside that is inserted within the duodenoscope. Direct POC is used more frequently and uses a very thin upper endoscope. Diagnostic uses of POC include visualizing indeterminate biliary structures, verifying bile duct stone clearance, and staging cholangiocarcinoma. For simple diagnostic POC, we allow the tract to mature for 2 weeks after placement of an 8F to 10F biliary drain. Cholangioscopy (Figure 6) then is performed with either a 9F access sheath or a bare tract technique without sheath. This method works for diagnostic visual inspection with or without use of 3F clamshell biopsy forceps.

Studies have shown POC to have higher sensitivity and positive/negative predictive value than ERCP. POC has been considered a safe procedure, with few incidences of complication (in less than 8% of patients). The most common complication reported was cholangitis (14% of cases in one study), with an overall complication rate of

FIGURE 6 Cholangioscope. **A,** The latest generation of flexible fiberoptic choledochoscopes (Model: CHF-CB30 L/S, Boston Scientific, Marlborough, MA) have an outer diameter of 8.4F and working length of 45 cm (S type) or 70 cm (L type, pictured here). This endoscope provides 120 degrees angulation in the up or down direction, and depth of view ranging between 2.5 and 50 mm. **B,** Two access ports on the cholangioscope feed into a single channel. Our irrigation system is attached to the anterior port *(straight arrow)*, whereas the posterior port *(curved arrow)* is used for passage of wires and instruments.

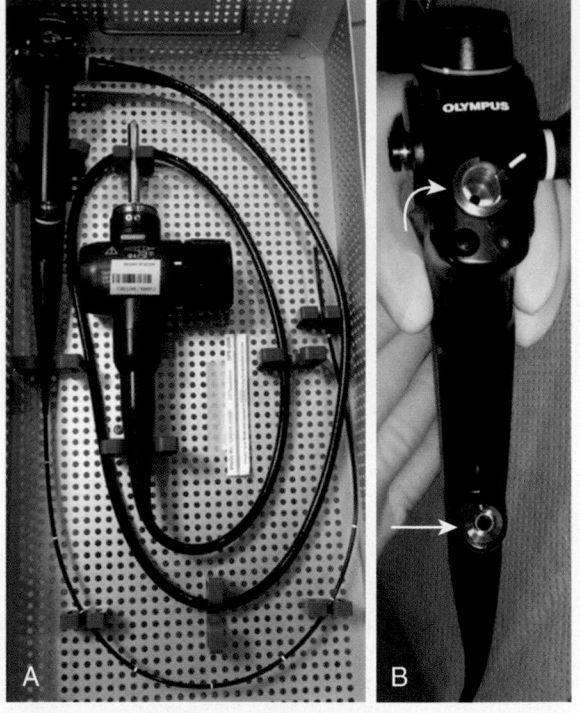

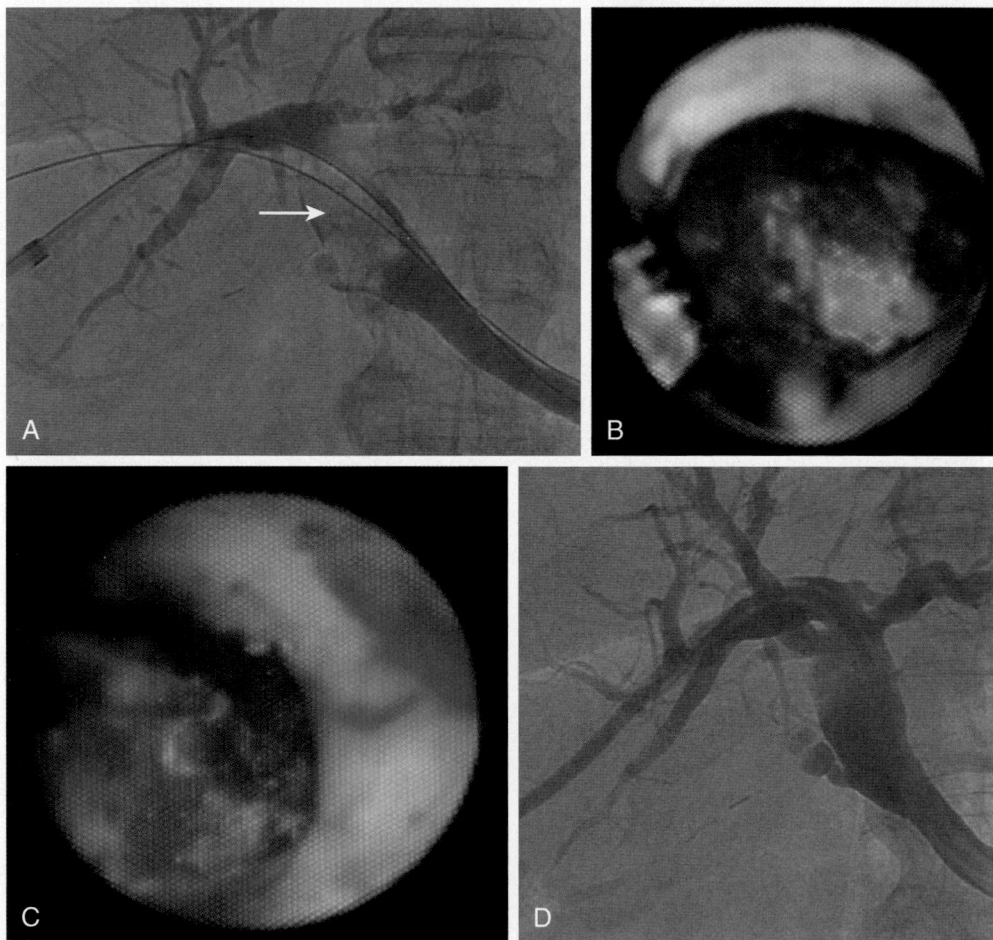

FIGURE 7 Laser lithotripsy. **A,** Diagnostic cholangiogram demonstrates a large filling defect *(arrow)* near the hepatic hilum. **B,** A large stone is visualized on cholangioscopy, partially covered with golden mucus. **C,** The laser fiber is positioned just proximal to the stone, which allows the laser light to reflect off the stone surface. Laser lithotripsy is performed with care to avoid nontargeted firing. Stone fragments are either removed with a basket or flushed down the biliary tract to allow passage through the ampulla. **D,** Post-treatment cholangiogram demonstrates complete removal of the large stone with restoration of bile flow.

7.5% (in an international multicenter study). Direct POC also has been shown to be effective in providing guidance for reinterventions involving occluded metal stents. Cholangioscopy can be used to treat obstructive stones in the biliary system as well (Figure 7). POC-guided removal of biliary stones is highly successful, with complete stone removal from bile ducts having a success rate of 90%.

Intraductal Radiofrequency Ablation

Intraductal radiofrequency (RF) ablation has been used to treat malignant tumors involving the bile duct with endoscopy. More recently, there have been a few studies investigating this type of ablation being used with PTC. One study showed that PTC and intraductal RF ablation followed by biliary stent placement was safe and effective in the short term. At 6 months postoperation, 2 out of 11 patients in an experimental group (PTC/RF) developed recurrent jaundice and received repeat procedures. In the same study, recurrent jaundice was observed in 3 months in the control group (without RF ablation).

■ SUMMARY

Transhepatic access for obstructive jaundice provides several therapeutic options for patients with both benign and malignant obstructions. A range of therapeutic options is available, including emergent drainage, endoluminal biopsy, biliary stricture dilation, long-term stenting, and endoprosthesis for palliation. In addition, direct visualization with endoscopic techniques (cholangioscopy) may assist in treatment of retained intrahepatic stones and may allow a significant reduction in radiation exposure to the patient, interventional radiologist, and personnel in the room.

Improvements in techniques of percutaneous transhepatic cholangiography, biliary drainage, and adjunctive biliary interventions provides the interventionalist with ready access to the biliary system to assist in multidisciplinary management of patients with complex biliary disease. The team *approach* is warranted because such patients often require management by surgeons, interventional radiologists, gastroenterologists, and primary care physicians.

The nonsurgical treatment of patients with transhepatic interventions for obstructive jaundice continues to expand. It is hoped that the previously mentioned information assists the reader in understanding some of the options available to these patients.

SUGGESTED READINGS

Abdel SA, Theilmann L. Fully covered self-expandable metal stents for treatment of both benign and malignant biliary disorders. *Diagn Ther Endosc.* 2012;article ID 498617.

Braasch WJ, Warren KW, Blevens PK. Progress in biliary strictures repair. *Am J Surg.* 1975;129:34-37.

Burhenne HJ. Nonoperative retained biliary tract stone extraction: a new roentgenologic technique. *Am J Roentgenol Radium Ther Nucl Med.* 1973;117:388-399.

Burhenne HJ. The technique of biliary duct stone extraction. *Radiology.* 1974;113:567-572.

Depietro DM, Shlansky-Goldberg RD, Soulen MC, et al. Long-term outcomes of a benign biliary stricture protocol. *J Vasc Interv Radiol.* 2015;26:1032-1039.

Dumonceau JM, Tringali A, Blero D, Devière J, Laugiers R, Heresbach D, Costamagna G. Biliary stenting: indications, choice of stents and results: European Society of Gastrointestinal Endoscopy (ESGE) clinical guideline. *Endoscopy.* 2012;44:277-298.

Ghersi S, Fuccio L, Bassi M, Fabbri C, Cennamo V. Current status of peroral cholangioscopy in biliary tract diseases. *World J Gastrointest Endosc.* 2015;7:510-517.

Gillman R, Alexander MS, Zucker KA, Bailey RW. The use of radionuclide imaging in the evaluation of suspected biliary damage during laparoscopic cholecystectomy. *Gastrointest Radiol.* 1991;16:201-204.

Gwon DI, Ko GY, Sung KB, Yoon HK, Kim KA, Kim YJ, Kim TH, Lee WH. Clinical outcomes after percutaneous biliary interventions in patients with malignant biliary obstruction caused by metastatic gastric cancer. *Acta Radiol.* 2012;53:422-429.

Huang X, Shen L, Jin Y, et al. Comparison of uncovered stent placement across versus above the main duodenal papilla for malignant biliary obstruction. *J Vasc Interv Radiol.* 2015;2:432-437.

Ikeura T, Shimatani M, Takaoka M, Masuda M, Hayashi K, Okazaki K. Reintervention for an occluded metal stent under the guidance of peroral direct cholangioscopy by using an ultra-slim enteroscope. *Gastrointest Endosc.* 2015;81:226-227.

Jo JH, Park BH. Suprapapillary versus transpapillary stent placement for malignant biliary obstruction: which is better? *J Vasc Interv Radiol.* 2015;26:573-582.

Krokidis M, Fanelli F, Orgera G, et al. Percutaneous treatment of malignant jaundice due to extrahepatic cholangiocarcinoma: covered Viabil stent versus uncovered wallstents. *Cardiovasc Intervent Radiol.* 2009;33:97-106.

Lammer J, Deu E. Percutaneous management of benign biliary strictures. In: Kadir S, ed. *Current Practice of Interventional Radiology.* Philadelphia: Decker; 1991:550-553.

Li TF, Huang GH, Li Z, et al. Percutaneous transhepatic cholangiography and intraductal radiofrequency ablation combined with biliary stent placement for malignant biliary obstruction. *J Vasc Interv Radiol.* 2015;26:715-721.

Liapi E, Georigiades C, Geschwind JF. Transhepatic interventions for obstructive jaundice. In: Cameron J, ed. *Current Surgical Therapy.* 9th ed. St Louis: Elsevier; 2008:456-467.

Lillemoe KD, Pitt HA, Cameron JL. Postoperative bile duct strictures. *Surg Clin North Am.* 1990;70:1355-1380.

Lillemoe KD, Pitt HA, Cameron JL. Current management of benign bile duct strictures. *Adv Surg.* 1992;25:119-174.

Mellinger J, MacFadyen B. Obstructive jaundice: endoscopic management. In: Cameron J, ed. *Current Surgical Therapy.* 8th ed. St Louis: Elsevier; 2004.

Mukund A, Rajesh S, Agrawal N, Arora A, Arora A. Percutaneous management of resistant biliary-enteric anastomotic strictures with the use of a combined cutting and conventional balloon cholangioplasty protocol: a single-center experience. *J Vasc Interv Radiol.* 2015;26:560-565.

Osterman FA Jr, Venbrux AC. Obstructive jaundice: percutaneous transhepatic interventions. In: Cameron JL, ed. *Current Surgical Therapy.* 5th ed. St Louis: Mosby-Year Book; 1995:394-399.

Picus D, Wyman PJ, Marx MV. Role of percutaneous intracorporeal electrohydraulic lithotripsy in the treatment of biliary tract calculi. *Radiology.* 1989;170:989-993.

Saleem A, Leggett CL, Murad MH, Baron TH. Meta-analysis of randomized trials comparing the patency of covered and uncovered self-expandable metal stents for palliation of distal malignant bile duct obstruction. *Gastrointest Endosc.* 2011;74:321-327, e1-3.

Savader SJ, Cameron JL, Pitt HA, et al. Biliary manometry versus clinical trial: value as predictors of success after treatment of biliary tract strictures. *J Vasc Interv Radiol.* 1994;5:757-763.

Silk MT, Wimmer T, Lee KS, et al. Percutaneous ablation of peribiliary tumors with irreversible electroporation. *J Vasc Interv Radiol.* 2014;25:112-118.

Thompson CM, Saad NE, Quazi RR, Darcy MD, Picus DD, Menias CO. Management of iatrogenic bile duct injuries: role of the interventional radiologist. *Radiographics.* 2013;33:117-134.

Trerotola SO, Savader SJ, Lund GB, et al. Biliary tract complications following laparoscopic cholecystectomy: imaging and intervention. *Radiology.* 1992;184:195-200.

van Sonnenberg E, Casola G, Wittich GR, et al. The role of interventional radiology for complications of cholecystectomy. *Surgery.* 1990;107:632-638.

Veal DR, Lee AY, Kerlan RK, Gordon RL, Fidelman N. Outcomes of metallic biliary stent insertion in patients with malignant bilobar obstruction. *J Vasc Interv Radiol.* 2013;24:1003-1010.

Venbrux AC, Ignacio EA, Soltes AP, Chun AK. Imaging and intervention in the biliary system. In: Klein AS, Pemberto JH, eds. *Shackelford's Surgery of the Alimentary Tract.* Vol. 2nd. 6th ed. Philadelphia: Saunders Elsevier; 2007.

Venbrux AC, Ignacio EA, Soltes AP, Washington SB. Malignant obstruction of the hepatobiliary system. In: Baum S, Pentecost MJ, eds. *Abrams Angiography and Interventional Radiology.* New York: Lippincott Williams & Wilkins; 2006.

Venbrux AC, Osterman FA Jr. Percutaneous biliary endoscopy. In: LaBerge JM, Venbrux AC, eds. *Biliary Interventions: Society of Cardiovascular and Interventional Radiology Syllabus.* Reston, VA: SCVIR; 1995:246-258.

Venbrux AC, Robbins KV, Savader SJ, et al. Endoscopy as an adjuvant to biliary radiology intervention. *Radiology.* 1991;180:355-361.

OBSTRUCTIVE JAUNDICE: ENDOSCOPIC THERAPY

Yamile Haito Chavez, MD, and Anthony N. Kalloo, MD

Obstructive jaundice is one of the most frequent and serious forms of hepatobiliary disease. It is caused by a mechanical interruption of bile flow through the biliary system. The etiology of biliary obstruction can be divided into benign and malignant causes (Box 1). Cholelithiasis and pancreatic cancer are the most common benign and neoplastic causes of jaundice, respectively, and comprise 40% of total cases. Evaluation of the biochemical tests of liver function reveals a cholestatic pattern. There is an elevation in the direct bilirubin with disproportionate elevation in the alkaline phosphatase compared with the serum aminotransferases. An accurate assessment of the cause and anatomic location of the obstruction is critical to gauge success in the management. Advances in biliary radiology with transabdominal ultrasound scan (US), computed tomographic (CT) scan, magnetic resonance imaging (MRI), and magnetic resonance cholangiopancreatography (MRCP) in recent years have allowed accurate, noninvasive imaging of the biliary tree and pancreas. Sensitivity and specificity of each test are described in Table 1. US is the study of choice for the initial evaluation of jaundice or symptoms of biliary disease (Figure 1). CT scan and MRCP play important roles in evaluating suspected malignancy before attempting treatment. Although MRCP has been widely adopted because of its availability, high sensitivity, and specificity, it has limitations, particularly in the setting of imaging for small gallstones. Endoscopic retrograde cholangiopancreatography (ERCP) and endoscopic ultrasound scan (EUS) are the endoscopic modalities used in the evaluation of patients with biliary obstruction. ERCP had been regarded as the gold standard for evaluation of the common bile duct and the biliary tree. However, because of the risks of post-ERCP pancreatitis, EUS has gained increasing favor as an auxiliary diagnostic study. Other emerging technologies that have been used in determining the cause of biliary strictures include intraductal ultrasound (IDUS), florescent in situ hybridization (FISH), and confocal laser endomicroscopy (CLE). In the past, obstructive jaundice was treated mainly with surgical interventions or percutaneous transhepatic cholangiography (PTC) drainage. However, endoscopic therapies have become the primary approach for management of obstructive jaundice. In many cases, they have become first-line therapy. This chapter focuses on the current standard of endoscopic therapy of obstructive jaundice.

■ ENDOSCOPIC THERAPIES FOR OBSTRUCTIVE JAUNDICE

Endoscopic Retrograde Cholangiopancreatography

Since its advent in 1968, ERCP has become the gold standard for diagnosis and treatment in the setting of biliary obstruction. ERCP is the most widely used diagnostic procedure in patients with biliary obstruction. Besides identifying the obstruction and determining its location and extent, it can provide tissue samples for cytologic evaluation. Once the biliary system is accessed, guidewire choice, the need for dilation, and stent choice are the three main technical decisions to consider. Cytologic testing should be done to exclude malignancy. A biliary sphincterotomy is recommended to ensure biliary access on subsequent ERCPs and facilitate stent placement. A guidewire should traverse the obstruction to secure access, directing the catheter into the correct segment, and can aid in minimizing contrast contamination of the biliary tree. Strictures can be dilated with either a balloon or a bougie system. There are no head-to-head comparisons between the two techniques. The degree of dilatation is guided by the size of

the bile duct distal to the stricture. Balloon dilation of focal strictures has the advantage of showing a waist fluoroscopically, the persistence of which indicates a need for further dilatation. Most strictures should be stented after dilatation because recurrence rates of nearly 50% have been described with dilatation alone, although this is not an absolute rule and does depend on the underlying cause. Plastic and metal stents are used for endoscopic drainage of the biliary tree. The advantage of a plastic biliary stent is the low cost and the large variety of sizes available. However, plastic stents can be used only in the short term because they can occlude within 2 to 3 months. Metal stents have the advantages of a large-diameter (8 mm to 11 mm) lumen, longer patency, and an easier deployment option, and do not require aggressive dilation before stent placement, but they are more expensive. Metal stents come in three different types: fully covered, uncovered, and partially covered. Uncovered stents have a median patency of approximately 20 months and reinterventions are frequently required to manage stent occlusion from high rates of reactive tissue hyperplasia. In addition, stent embedment into the bile duct wall makes them nonremovable. Partially covered stents, which leave proximal and distal ends bare, are consequently less prone to becoming embedded in tissue and thus have improved ease of retrieval. Uncovered and partially covered stents are used mostly in malignant conditions when the life expectancy is greater than 6 months. The advent of fully covered metal stents has changed the paradigm for management of biliary stricture because they can be removed. However, they have migration rates between 20% and 40%. The fully covered metal stents are now widely used in the setting of benign strictures.

The overall complication rate of ERCP ranges from 4% to 15%. The most common complication is post-ERCP pancreatitis (PEP), which is generally reported at between 5% and 10%; however, in high-risk situations such as clinically suspected sphincter of Oddi dysfunction and normal serum bilirubin in female patient, young age, difficult cannulation, pancreatic duct injection, or precut sphincterotomy, higher incidence of PEP has been reported. Pancreatitis can be prevented by inserting a prophylactic pancreatic stent and giving rectal indomethacin after the procedure, as shown in a recent randomized trial, especially for individuals at high risk. Other complications include bleeding and perforation, especially after sphincterotomy, at a rate of 1% to 2%. Most ERCP complications can be managed conservatively. Rarely do patients need surgical intervention.

Cholangioscopy

Peroral cholangioscopes are divided into two main systems: dual-operator mother-daughter systems and single-operator catheter-based slim or ultraslim standard endoscopes. The mother-daughter systems include a choledochoscope that is introduced through the therapeutic channel of the duodenoscope. Indications for cholangioscopy are divided into therapeutic and diagnostic (Box 2). By far, the two most common indications for cholangioscopy are management of difficult stones and assessment of indeterminate strictures. Direct visualization of the stone allows for reduced bile duct injury during lithotripsy and for differentiation among stone fragments, blood clots, air bubbles, and so forth. Intraductal lithotripsy is performed with either electrohydraulic lithotripsy (EHL) or pulsed laser. Cholangioscopy with EHL is associated with a high rate of success for removal of extrahepatic biliary stones that have failed extraction with conventional ERCP techniques. Clearance rates of 83% to 100% have been reported. Cholangioscopy provides valuable data used to evaluate indeterminate biliary strictures by providing direct assessment of the involved epithelium and the adjacent epithelium and by providing direct visualization for biopsies. Cholangioscopy in addition to cholangiographic images obtained during ERCP increased the diagnostic yield from 78%-85% to 93%-99% and the overall sensitivity from 58% to 100%. In addition, cholangioscopy can assess the extent of the disease and identify synchronous lesions not seen during cholangiography. Complications associated with peroral cholangioscopy often are associated with specific maneuvers performed during ERCP (e.g., sphincterotomy). Complications specific to the performance of cholangiopancreatoscopy include cholangitis, which is related to intraductal fluid irrigation and, uncommonly, hemobilia and bile leaks attributable to intraductal lithotripsy.

Endoscopic Ultrasound

EUS complements ERCP through its sonographic and tissue sampling capabilities. The role of EUS in management of obstructive jaundice has evolved from staging and sampling tumors to accessing bile ducts. ERCP biliary cannulation fails in 3% to 12% of cases, with failure being due to previous surgery, periampullary tumor infiltration, duodenum stenosis, complex hilar cholangiocarcinomas, or periampullary diverticulum. In these cases, alternative classical approaches included surgical interventions or PTC and drainage, with significant associated morbidity. PTC can be difficult to perform

or even be contraindicated in patients with obesity, ascites, or intervening structures, such as vasculature or lungs. Complication rates of PTC range from 10% to 20% and common complications include cholangitis, bile leak, bleeding, fistula formation, peritonitis, empyema, pneumothorax, and stent occlusion. The mortality rate associated with PTC has been reported to be as high as 6%. Surgical drainage is associated with 2% to 5% mortality and 17% to 37% morbidity. Moreover, surgery requires a longer recovery time.

Over the past two decades, the development of the linear array echoendoscope has led to various EUS-related therapeutic techniques for failed papillary cannulation (Figure 2). EUS-guided biliary drainage (EGBD) can be performed using one of three methods. First, direct transluminal stenting that uses a transgastric or

---

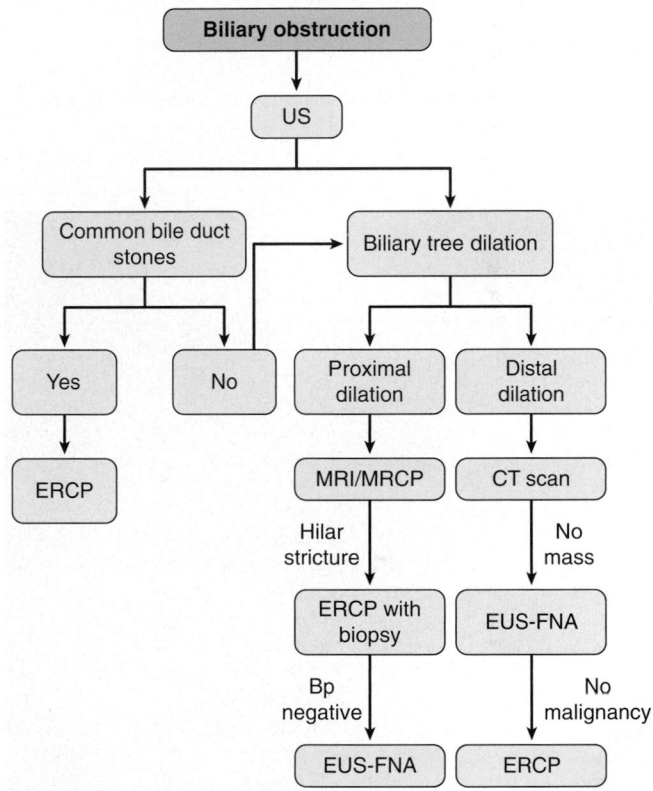

FIGURE 1 Algorithm of obstructive jaundice diagnosis. *CT scan*, Computed tomographic scan; *ERCP*, endoscopic retrograde cholangiopancreatography; *EUS*, endoscopic ultrasound scan; *FNA*, fine-needle aspiration; *MRCP*, magnetic resonance cholangiopancreatography; *MRI*, magnetic resonance imaging; *US*, ultrasound scan. *(From Singh A, et al. Biliary strictures: diagnostic considerations and approach.* Gastroenterol Rep (Oxf). *2015;3:22-31.)*

TABLE 1: The Sensitivities for Different Imaging Modalities for Common Bile Duct Stones and Malignancy

	US		CT		MRCP		EUS	
	Sensitivity	Specificity	Sensitivity	Specificity	Sensitivity	Specificity	Sensitivity	Specificity
Common bile duct stones	22%-33%	100%	65%-88%	73%-97%	85%-92%36 and 37<50% for stones <3 mm	93%-97%	81%-94%	94%-95%
Malignancy	71%	Unknown	40%-94%	97%	84%	76%-88%	78%	84%

From Hou LA, Van Dam J. Pre-ERCP imaging of the bile duct and gallbladder. *Gastrointest Endoscopy Clin N Am.* 2013;23:185–197.

CT, Computed tomography; *EUS*, endoscopic ultrasound scan; *MRCP*, magnetic resonance cholangiopancreatography; *US*, transabdominal ultrasound scan.

BOX 2: Indications for Cholangioscopy

Therapeutic

Lithotripsy
Tumor ablation
Control of bleeding
Guidewire advancement
Reopening occluded metal stents

Diagnostic

Biliary strictures
Staging
Filling defects
Ductal abnormalities
Choledochal cysts
Tissue acquisition
Confocal microscopy

From Raijman I. Choledochoscopy/cholangioscopy. *Gastrointest Endos Clin N Am.* 2013;23:237-249.

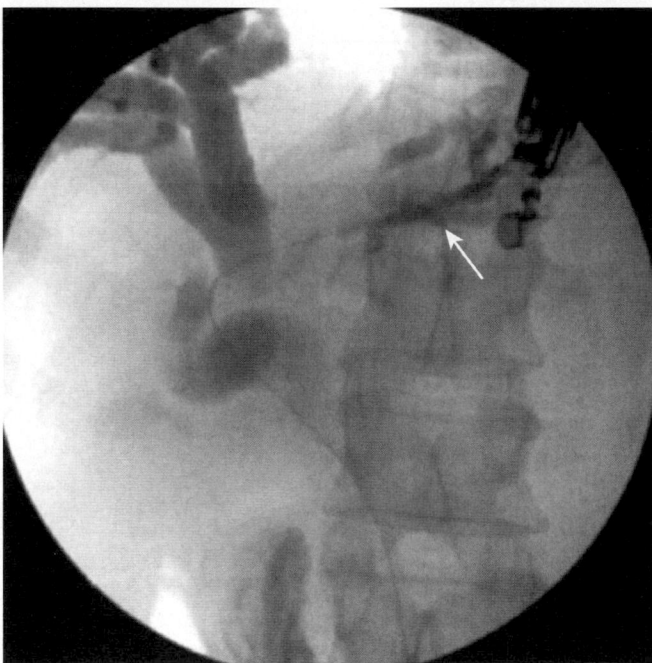

FIGURE 2 Fluoroscopic image during hepaticogastrostomy dilation (*arrow*). Transgastric endoscopic ultrasound scan (EUS) guided access of the left intrahepatic duct. A 0.025-inch hydrophilic guidewire was advanced into the distal common biliary duct. The hepaticogastrostomy was then dilated to facilitate the access of a metal stent for anterograde EUS-guided biliary drainage.

transduodenal approach may be performed without accessing the papilla. Second, a rendezvous technique may be considered, whereby a wire is placed into an intrahepatic or extrahepatic bile duct, passed through the papilla, and retrieved by a duodenoscope for biliary interventions. A third approach is EUS-guided antegrade transpapillary biliary stent placement. Among these, EUS-guided rendezvous therapy seems to be the safest approach. However, a major limitation of the rendezvous approach is that it can be attempted only with patients in whom the papilla is accessible by endoscopy. EGBD can be performed with high therapeutic success (87%) but is associated with 10% to 20% morbidity and rare serious adverse events.

BOX 3: Predictors of Failed Mechanical Lithotripsy

Size of the stone (>30 mm)
Ratio of stone to bile duct diameter >1
Impaction of the stone in the bile duct
Barrel-shaped and piston-shaped stones
Stones arising from the cystic duct takeoff
Periampullary diverticulum
Inverted papilla orientation (altered anatomy)
Bile duct anomalies (distal tapering or sigmoid shape)

■ BENIGN BILIARY OBSTRUCTION

Choledocholithiasis

Choledocholithiasis is a common condition that occurs in 10% to 20% of patients with cholelithiasis, 7% to 14% of patients who have undergone cholecystectomy, and 18% to 33% of patients with acute biliary pancreatitis. Choledocholithiasis can result in serious complications such as cholangitis and gallstone pancreatitis. Management of patients with suspected choledocholithiasis requires confirmation of stones in the common bile duct. Choledocholithiasis can be diagnosed in several ways. Even though ERCP has a high sensitivity to diagnose choledocholithiasis, it is associated with complications in 4% to 15% of patients. Thus it is critical that ERCP be used only for therapy and not for diagnosis. US has a high specificity (100% in multiple studies) but it is insensitive (22% to 33%) for detecting common bile duct stones. MRCP has a sensitivity of 90%, similar to ERCP. MRCP has largely replaced ERCP as the method of choice for diagnosing choledocholithiaisis. EUS is much more sensitive than any other modalities for stones that are smaller than 5 mm (see Table 1).

ERCP is indicated if choledocholithiasis is found on imaging, ERCP with sphincterotomy has achieved primacy in the management of bile duct stones. If used appropriately, the biliary endoscopist may remove 80% to 90% of stones and may expect complications in fewer than 10% of cases. During ERCP, biliary stones are removed with extractor balloon and basket after biliary sphincterotomy. Baskets, especially lithotripsy baskets, are preferred for large stones (>1 cm). Sphincteroplasty (balloon dilation of the sphincter) can be done to remove large stones but only after a biliary sphincterotomy has been performed because alone it increases the rate of PEP. Mechanical, electrohydraulic, or laser lithotripsies are used to fragment large stones. The success rate of mechanical lithotripsy is 70% to 80% and the factors associated with failure are the size of the stones (>30 mm), impaction of the stone at the bile duct, a ratio of stone to bile duct diameter greater than 1, and the type of lithotripter used (Box 3). EHL, laser-induced shock wave lithotripsy, and extracorporeal shock wave lithotripsy can be used for pulverizing stones. Cholangioscopy has increased the success of EHL and laser-induced shock wave lithotripsy. EHL can be used only with direct visualization with cholangioscopy to avoid ductal injury. In several retrospective series, clearance of difficult stones that have failed conventional ERCP treatments occurred in 90% to 100% of patients after one or two EHL sessions. The main risk of EHL is perforation, which has an overall risk of less than 1%. This occurs because of extreme elevation of the surface temperature of the stones and surrounding ductal tissues, which is usually caused by prolonged application of EHL. Bleeding can also occur. An alternative treatment is pulsed laser lithotripsy, which has success rates of 83% to 100% in removal of stones and clearing of bile ducts. A plastic stent is often left in situ if the duct is not clear of stones or until interval cholecystectomy is performed.

Postsurgical Complications

Biliary tract complications are an important cause of morbidity and mortality after liver transplants (LTs) and laparoscopic

BOX 4: Risk Factors for Postsurgical Strictures

Postcholecystectomy Strictures

Confusion of the cystic duct with the common bile duct (CBD)
Excessive traction on the gallbladder neck during resection
Biliary ischemia
Unintentional electrocautery injury
Extension of thermal injury applied to a correctly
  recognized CBD

Posttransplant Strictures

Risk Factors Related to the Recipient or Donor

Mismatched size between donor and recipient bile ducts
ABO incompatibility
Use of donor after cardiac death

Risk Factors Related to Surgical Technique

Type of biliary anastomosis
Use of a T-tube
Tension of the duct anastomosis

Other Risk Factors

Hepatic artery thrombosis
Prolonged warm and cold ischemia

cholecystectomy. The two main complications are biliary strictures and bile leaks. The incidence rate of these complications is very low (<2%) after laparoscopic cholecystectomy. Multiple factors contribute to stricture formation after laparoscopic or open cholecystectomy, with confusion of the cystic duct with the common bile duct as the most common cause of intraoperative injury. Other risk factors are listed in Box 4. The rate of post-LT complications is between 10% and 25%. Risk factors conditioning post-LT complications are multifactorial and could be grouped as related to the recipient or donor or related to surgical technique (see Box 4). The initial evaluation should begin with Doppler ultrasound scan, followed by MRCP, which has a sensitivity of 96% and specificity of 94% for diagnosis of postsurgical biliary complication.

Postsurgical Strictures

Benign Biliary Strictures After Cholecystectomy

Cholecystectomy remains a common cause of benign biliary strictures with an incidence of 0.2% to 0.7% among patients undergoing laparoscopic cholecystectomy. Postcholecystectomy stenosis develops as a consequence of bile duct injury that may occur intraoperatively (dissection, electrocautery, clip or suture placement, ligation) or postoperatively (adhesion formation). Endoscopic therapy has been associated with variable success, with reported response rates between 40% and 90%. The diverse response rates likely are related to different intervals of patient follow-up after stent removal because stricture recurrence can occur many months to years later. Long-term data of postsurgical strictures treated with multiple plastic stents and intermittent stent exchange (approximately every 3 months) over the course of a year have demonstrated promising success rates ranging from 80% to 100%, with a recurrence rate of 20% to 30% within 2 years of stent removal. This approach therefore has become the current standard of care when treating postsurgical strictures. It should be noted, however, that postoperative strictures located at the hepatic ductal confluence may be less responsive to endoscopic stenting than strictures located more distally (25% vs 80% resolution rate). There are limited data regarding the use of fully covered and partially covered self-expandable metallic stents (SEMSs) in the treatment of postcholecystectomy strictures.

Benign Biliary Strictures After Liver Transplant

Among patients who have undergone LT, biliary strictures are among the most common postoperative complications, with their incidence ranging from 5% to 15% after deceased donor LT and 28% to 32% after living donor LT, and even higher rates seen in cardiac death donor LT. Post-LT biliary strictures can manifest early (<30 to 90 days) or late (>90 days) in the post-LT course and may occur at the anastomosis (anastomotic biliary stricture, or ABS) or elsewhere in the biliary tree (nonanastomotic biliary stricture, or NABS). Patients usually have symptomatic or asymptomatic increase in liver function tests but, unlike other causes of biliary obstruction, dilatation of the donor bile ducts is an unreliable indictor of biliary obstruction. Endoscopic therapy is the first-line management approach for ABSs and for select NABSs, with percutaneous intervention and surgical revision or retransplantation being reserved for endoscopic treatment failures. ABSs are a consequence of local trauma at the surgical juncture between the recipient's and the donor's extrahepatic ducts (most commonly common bile duct–common bile duct choledochocholedochostomy) and account for 80% of post-LT biliary strictures. They appear as a short, single stricture localized to the anastomosis. Most ABSs arise within 12 months after transplantation. Earlier presentations (<30 to 90 days), usually caused by edema and inflammation, have a good response to therapy and are less likely to recur, with resolution of strictures over an average of 3 to 6 months. Delayed-onset ABSs, a consequence of fibrotic scarring, might require up to 1 to 2 years of stenting to avoid stricture recurrence based on the few available published series. Balloon dilation to a maximal diameter of the duct up to 10 mm, followed by insertion of multiple plastic stents, decreases stricture recurrence by 62% to 31% compared with balloon dilatation alone. ABSs also may be treated with metal stents but this has been less studied. Nonanastomotic stenosis accounts for 10% to 25% of post-LT biliary strictures and tends to occur earlier than ABSs. These are typically a sequela of donor-recipient ABO incompatibility, prolonged graft ischemic time peri-LT, or post-LT hepatic artery thrombosis. NABSs may be either unifocal or distributed diffusely throughout the extrahepatic or intrahepatic biliary tree, are more technically challenging to access and treat, and have lower long-term endoscopic treatment success rates (50% to 75%). Nevertheless, maximal stenting, as with ABSs, may result in graft preservation and overall favorable outcomes in a considerable proportion of patients with NABSs, although some ultimately will require retransplantation. Up to 30% to 50% of patients require retransplantation despite endoscopic therapy. The poor response is likely related to the presence of multifocal strictures, associated sludge and casts, and recurrence of an underlying disorder.

Primary Sclerosing Cholangitis

Primary sclerosing cholangitis (PSC) is a chronic cholestatic liver and biliary tract disease that has a highly variable natural history. The pathogenesis of the disorder remains elusive, although the complications of the disease are a direct result of fibrosis and strictures involving intrahepatic and extrahepatic bile ducts. PSC may be asymptomatic for long periods but also may have an aggressive course, leading to recurrent biliary tract obstruction and recurrent episodes of cholangitis, and may progress to end-stage liver disease. Up to 50% of patients with PSC will develop "dominant" strictures, which are loosely defined as a common biliary duct stenosis up to 1.5 mm in diameter or hepatic duct stenosis up to 1 mm in diameter, during their course. A major challenge in the setting of a PSC-associated dominant stricture is excluding underlying malignancy, which develops in up to 20% of patients with PSC. The diagnosis is now most frequently established using MRCP, although direct cholangiography may be more sensitive. The typical cholangiographic findings include focal structuring and saccular dilatation of the bile ducts, which may lead to a "beaded" appearance.

The endoscopic management focuses on the treatment of dominant strictures. The goals of endoscopic intervention are to dilate the strictures to 6-mm to 8-mm diameter and to reduce the serum alkaline phosphatase level to 1.5 times the upper limit of normal. The management of PSC with a dominant stricture is challenging on multiple fronts: the difficulty in distinguishing malignant from benign strictures, the difficulty in managing proximal and multiple strictures, the high rate of secondary bacterial cholangitis, and the lack of definitive therapeutic strategies aside from LT. Techniques used for endoscopic treatment of dominant strictures in PSC are not well standardized. Case series support the benefit of dilation, stent placement, and combinations of these methods for treatment of dominant strictures. A review of multiple case series showed that stent placement can lead to more frequent complications of cholangitis than dilation alone but that stenting for short duration will reduce the risk of stent occlusion and may allow stenting without increased risk of cholangitis. Bile duct stones frequently develop in PSC because of impaired bile outflow and bacterial overgrowth from biliary strictures. When intraductal stones are recognized, endoscopic dilation of obstructing strictures and stone extraction will reduce bile outflow obstruction. Cholangioscopy is used primarily to interrogate indeterminate strictures in an effort to enhance detection of cholangiocarcinoma but has the additional benefit of detection of unrecognized bile duct stones.

■ MALIGNANT OBSTRUCTION

Many disease processes arising from primary or metastatic disease can lead to malignant biliary strictures. Until the 1980s biliary-enteric surgical bypass was the treatment of choice for people with malignant pancreaticobiliary disease. However, in the last 20 years endoscopic decompression, primarily through stent placement, has emerged as a therapeutic option offering lower overall cost, shorter hospitalization, and lower morbidity when compared with surgical intervention. The endoscopic goal is for adequate biliary drainage to palliate obstructive symptoms but also to limit the number of interventions in the patients' remaining life. Preoperative biliary decompression may improve symptoms; prevent complications of cholestasis, especially if there is a delay in surgical resection; and allow time for neoadjuvant chemotherapy in patients with locally advanced malignancy.

Plastic stents and SEMSs are used to drain the biliary tree. Plastic stent diameters range from 7F to 12F. Plastic stents with a diameter larger than 10F increase the technical difficulty of placement without improving stent patency. Therefore a diameter of 10F is thought to be the best combination of patency and technical ease of placement. Plastic stents of 10F have patency rates of approximately 3 months, are very effective, and are inexpensive; however, the short duration of stent patency remains a disadvantage. Metal stents have a lumen diameter three to four times that of plastic stents and have significantly longer patency. Therefore placement of SEMSs for palliation

of malignant biliary strictures should be considered, especially for patients with a predicted life expectancy of more than 3 to 4 months. Uncovered, partially covered, and fully covered SEMSs are used for palliation of patients with malignant strictures. SEMS failure is usually related to tissue ingrowth with the uncovered type, whereas migration is usually the cause of stent failure with the covered type.

Malignant strictures are classified as intrahepatic or proximal, extrahepatic or distal, and hilar strictures. The most common malignant stricture is related to pancreatic cancer. For obstruction of the extrahepatic bile duct, a SEMS is the stent of choice. The role of endoscopic drainage in cases of intrahepatic strictures is limited. In hilar obstructions, when both hepatic ducts are occluded, the goal of endoscopic therapy is to place bilateral stents into the left and right common hepatic ducts. If bilateral stenting cannot be achieved, unilateral stenting of the most dilated duct is performed. In patients in whom access to the papilla is not possible, direct access to the bile duct via EUS-guided puncture can be performed. A metallic or plastic stent is inserted to form either a hepatogastrostomy or a choledochoduodenostomy, depending on the site of puncture. These procedures have an overall success rate of 92% but are limited by complications that include biliary leak, pneumoperitoneum, and infection. Many studies have shown no difference in mortality between palliative surgery and endoscopic drainage groups.

Endoscopic tumor ablations, such as photodynamic therapy (PDT) or radiofrequency ablation, are also options for management of malignant biliary obstruction. PDT is a palliative treatment that is considered promising for the local control of cholangiocarcinoma. It induces tissue necrosis by the application of a laser beam with a specialized wavelength through a translucent endoscopic catheter combined with a photosensitizer, which accumulates in the tumor. The main purpose of PDT is to achieve easy deployment of a stent across the tumor in the bile duct. Although endoscopic biliary drainage is a well-established method, it is not always possible to perform this procedure for all patients who have obstructive jaundice.

SUGGESTED READINGS

Baillie J. Endoscopic approach to the patient with bile duct injury. *Gastrointest Endos Clin N Am*. 2013;23:461-472.

Buxbaum J, et al. Modern management of common bile duct stones. *Gastrointest Endos Clin N Am*. 2013;23:251-275.

Divyesh S. Advancements in biliary stenting. *J Clin Gastroenterol*. 2012;46:191-196.

Lindor K, Kowdley K, et al. ACG clinical guideline: primary sclerosing cholangitis. *Am J Gastroenterol*. 2015;110:646-659.

Mangiavillano B, Pagno N, et al. Outcome of stenting in biliary and pancreatic benign and malignant diseases: a comprehensive review. *World J Gastroenterol*. 2015;21:30.

Webb K, Saunders M. Endoscopic management of malignant bile duct strictures. *Gastrointest Endos Clin N Am*. 2013;23:313-331.

THE MANAGEMENT OF ACUTE PANCREATITIS

Angela LaFace, MD, Donald Davis, MD,
and Vic Velanovich, MD

Acute pancreatitis is a pathologic condition with far-reaching consequences and is the leading cause of gastrointestinal-related hospitalizations in the United States. The annual incidence of acute pancreatitis ranges from 13 to 45 per 100,000 persons and appears to be on the rise. Common causes include gallstone disease, alcohol use, and hypertriglyceridemia, all of which are conditions concordant with the U.S. obesity epidemic. When a cause cannot be determined, the disease is considered idiopathic, which is not uncommon in acute pancreatitis. Acute pancreatitis affects men and women equally. Increasing age confers higher risk and a twofold to threefold increased risk is seen in African Americans as compared with Caucasians. Symptomatology ranges from a mild, self-limited course to severe, complicated disease that may lead to infected pancreatic necrosis, organ failure, and death. Although a low mortality rate of 1% is seen in acute pancreatitis overall, advanced age, comorbidities, and severe disease are associated with increased risk of mortality. There is a continuum of disease progression in which acute pancreatitis may become recurrent in 20% to 30% and chronic in 10% of patients.

■ DIAGNOSIS AND EVALUATION

The diagnosis of pancreatitis requires two of the three following criteria: clinical (upper abdominal pain), laboratory (serum amylase >3 times normal), and imaging (computed tomography [CT], magnetic resonance imaging [MRI], ultrasonography). A detailed medical history, including family history of pancreatic disease, should be taken on presentation. Important considerations include previous diagnoses of pancreatitis, gallstone disease, alcohol use, hypertriglyceridemia, trauma, medications, and recent biliary or pancreatic instrumentation including endoscopic retrograde cholangiopancreatography (ERCP). Careful physical examination is performed along with laboratory testing to detect hematologic, metabolic, or electrolyte disturbance. Measurement of transaminases and a right upper quadrant ultrasound may aid in diagnosing a biliary cause.

Radiologic evaluation with CT scan is not required for diagnosis of acute pancreatitis in most patients, although it may be necessary in cases of diagnostic uncertainty. Consequently, routine early CT scanning is not indicated and should be avoided. There is no evidence to support improved outcomes, clinical management is rarely influenced, and increased duration of hospitalization has been reported with this practice. However, early CT evaluation is indicated in patients who have acute pancreatitis as well as severe abdominal pain where bowel ischemia or hollow viscus perforation is suspected. The extent of pancreatic and peripancreatic necrosis typically becomes apparent 72 hours after symptom onset; therefore optimal initial CT assessment is performed after 72 to 96 hours. Several earlier guidelines advocated routine serial CT scans obtained weekly throughout the course of acute pancreatitis; however, current guidelines have abolished this practice, as there is no evidence to support its benefit. Follow-up imaging with CT or MRI is indicated in cases of treatment failure or clinical deterioration or before any invasive intervention. Both CT and MRI are excellent radiographic modalities to assess pancreatic tissue viability; however, MRI may be preferred to discriminate necrotic collections from pseudocysts and in patients where ionizing radiation is contraindicated.

■ ASSESSMENT OF SEVERITY

Numerous scoring systems historically have been used to predict disease severity and outcomes in acute pancreatitis. The oldest and best known, Ranson's criteria, published in 1974, uses several laboratory parameters gathered at presentation and at 48 hours to identify patients who are likely to have severe disease. One point is given for each criterion met and a score of 3 or greater supports a diagnosis of severe acute pancreatitis. The Atlanta classification, revised in 2012, is a comprehensive tool that combines early clinical assessment of severity with radiologic evaluation of late sequelae of acute pancreatitis. Four distinct pancreatic morphologies are described by this image-based classification system: (1) interstitial edematous pancreatitis, (2) necrotizing pancreatitis, (3) acute peripancreatic fluid collection, and (4) pancreatic pseudocyst. These data may be used to guide treatment in later disease stages. It appears, however, that the presence of systemic inflammatory response syndrome (SIRS) is the most predictive of severe acute pancreatitis. Presence of two or more of the following criteria defines SIRS: (1) temperature less than 36°C or greater than 38°C, (2) heart rate greater than 90/min, (3) respiratory rate greater than 20/min, (4) white blood cell count less than 4000 cells/mm^3 or greater than 12,000 cells/mm^3 or greater than 10% bands. Multisystem organ failure is associated with the persistence of SIRS physiology past 48 hours and, in turn, persistent multisystem organ failure (>48 hours) is the leading predictor of mortality in acute pancreatitis. A 25% mortality is associated with persistent SIRS, with a high sensitivity and specificity of 77% to 89% and 79% to 86%, respectively. Ultimately, a holistic approach that accounts for host risk factors, clinical risk stratification, and response to therapy is most appropriate and accurate for prognostication in acute pancreatitis.

■ INITIAL MANAGEMENT

Resuscitation

The presentation of patients with acute pancreatitis varies from mild abdominal pain to systemic shock. Many patients with acute pancreatitis need significant resuscitation at presentation. Initial aggressive fluid replacement is required as these patients are hypovolemic for multiple reasons, including vomiting, poor oral intake, increased respiratory losses, diaphoresis, and edema. Patients with signs of shock need aggressive fluid boluses and often vasopressive medications to restore end organ perfusion. Pancreatitis causes pancreatic edema and microangiopathic effects that decrease blood flow to pancreatic cells resulting in cellular death and unregulated release of pancreatic enzymes. This in turn leads to increased inflammation, vascular permeability, and edema with subsequent worsened perfusion of the pancreas. Restoration of the intravascular volume and perfusion is imperative to help prevent propagation of this cycle.

Classically, resuscitation of patients with acute pancreatitis has included continued isotonic solution infusion at up to 20 mL/kg/h after initial stabilization. However, recent evidence suggests that more judicious regimens for continued resuscitation significantly decrease morbidity and possibly mortality. Avoiding fluid overload is especially important in patients who have concurrent heart and renal disease. Avoiding overresuscitation reduces complications such as pulmonary edema, acute respiratory distress syndrome (ARDS), and abdominal compartment syndrome.

Initial resuscitation should aim at restoring normal hemodynamics and end organ perfusion. Lactated Ringer's solution is the fluid of choice for fluid resuscitation, as well-designed prospective studies have demonstrated its superiority over normal saline. Boluses should be given as quickly as possible in 500- to 1000-mL increments. Improvement or maintenance of normal values of surrogate markers, such as hematocrit, blood urea nitrogen (BUN), and creatinine, can be reassuring. Once initial resuscitation is completed and euvolemia is restored, appropriate vasopressive support should be provided if hemodynamic instability and shock persist. Determination of euvolemia or adequate resuscitation will vary by institution and critical care group.

As mentioned earlier, previous guidelines recommended continuous infusion with lactated Ringer's solution at a rate of 10 to 20 mL/kg/h for the first 24 to 48 hours. In recent years, many other groups, including the Surviving Sepsis Campaign, have advocated goal-directed guidelines for resuscitation. Both of these approaches may be appropriate at many institutions, especially those without the ability to provide continuous monitoring of patients by a multidisciplinary critical care team. Parameters for goal-directed therapy may include central venous pressure (CVP), pulmonary arterial wedge pressure (PAWP), mixed venous saturation (SvO₂), lactate level, and hourly urine output. However, multiple large, multicenter, randomized control trials in numerous countries have now demonstrated that early goal-directed therapy is not superior to careful resuscitation performed by experience critical care teams.

Indeed, many of these patients also have multisystem dysfunction, making their hourly urine output, lactate, and renal function inaccurate markers for resuscitation. Our experience has found that using these parameters in isolation or continuously infusing Lactated Ringer's solution at the recommended rates often results in fluid overload with increasing complications. Our institution's preference is to rely heavily on the SvO₂ measured by a pulmonary arterial catheter when euvolemia is in question. Numerous studies have challenged the reliability of both CVP and PAWP in measuring volume status. Similar to the Surviving Sepsis Campaign, we have found that an SvO₂ above 65% correlates with adequate tissue perfusion in most patients. It should be stressed that most patients can be resuscitated without a pulmonary artery catheter but we have found that it is an invaluable tool in patients with persistent hypotension and oliguria despite initial aggressive fluid resuscitation.

The method of resuscitation varies between groups and institutions. Resuscitation performed with goal-directed therapy or continuous infusion of resuscitative fluid may be appropriate, especially if intensive, continuous monitoring by a critical care team is not feasible. Hypervolemia may result but this is preferable to hypoperfusion. Otherwise, patients with signs of shock should be resuscitated in a thoughtful, diligent, and continuous manner by a critical care team in an intensive care unit (ICU) until SIRS physiology has resolved.

Antibiotics

Antibiotics should be given to patients with acute pancreatitis and an active infection. This may include cholangitis, urinary tract infection, pneumonia, catheter-related infections, bacteremia, and, indeed, infected pancreatic necrosis.

Acute pancreatitis itself may cause fever, tachypnea, tachycardia, hypotension, oliguria, and other symptoms that may be clinically indistinguishable from sepsis and septic shock resulting from a profound systemic inflammatory response. If an infection is suspected, broad-spectrum antibiotics should be initiated with antifungal coverage in select cases. Cultures should be obtained and antibiotic therapy tailored based on organism sensitivities; immediate cessation is warranted if culture results do not support concomitant infection.

Patients with infected pancreatic necrosis have a significantly higher mortality rate when compared with patients with sterile pancreatic necrosis. Historically, prophylactic antibiotics were given to patients with pancreatic necrosis to prevent conversion of sterile pancreatic necrosis to infected pancreatic necrosis, as previous studies suggested that prophylactic antibiotics may be able to prevent this transition. However, a meta-analysis of more recent, well-designed, randomized controlled trials demonstrated no significant benefit from prophylactic antibiotics in this setting. Currently, antibiotics do not appear to be beneficial in a prophylactic role in acute pancreatitis.

Nutrition

Long-held dogma in acute pancreatitis is that patients should be kept without enteral nutrition, allowing the pancreas to "rest" based on the belief that enteral feeding exacerbates pancreatic inflammation. To that end, many patients with acute pancreatitis have been maintained on total parenteral nutrition (TPN) to avoid additional enteral simulation. In recent years, multiple studies based on both clinical and laboratory observations demonstrate that such an approach is harmful to patients with acute pancreatitis, and the evidence does not support the claim that enteral feeding exacerbates pancreatic inflammation.

In mild pancreatitis (patients without SIRS or need for ICU admission), immediate enteral feeding should be initiated. Multiple studies have demonstrated that patients can be started safely on a low-fat solid diet and that restricting the diet to clear liquids is without benefit. Initiating a solid diet early increases caloric intake and shortens hospital stays.

The timing of initiation of enteral nutrition in severe pancreatitis is controversial but should be attempted before TPN is considered. Multiple randomized controlled trials and meta-analyses have shown that infectious complications, organ failure, and mortality were increased with the use of TPN in patients with severe pancreatitis. Enteral feeding prevents atrophy and breakdown of the gastrointestinal tract mucosal barrier and may prevent bacterial translocation. Some studies also demonstrate a decreased incidence of infected pancreatic necrosis.

In patients who are unable to maintain their nutritional requirement with oral intake alone, nutritional supplementation should be provided in the form of tube feedings. Nasojejunal positioning of the feeding tube was long considered optimal to avoid pancreatic stimulation but numerous studies have now demonstrated that nasogastric tubes are safe and effective for most patients with acute pancreatitis. Given the theoretical risk of aspiration with the use of this feeding modality and potential associated complications, an aspiration precaution protocol is advised. Placement of a nasojejunal feeding tube is often more difficult than a nasogastric tube and may require some form of radiographic assistance, but should be attempted if nasogastric feeding is not tolerated and before considering TPN.

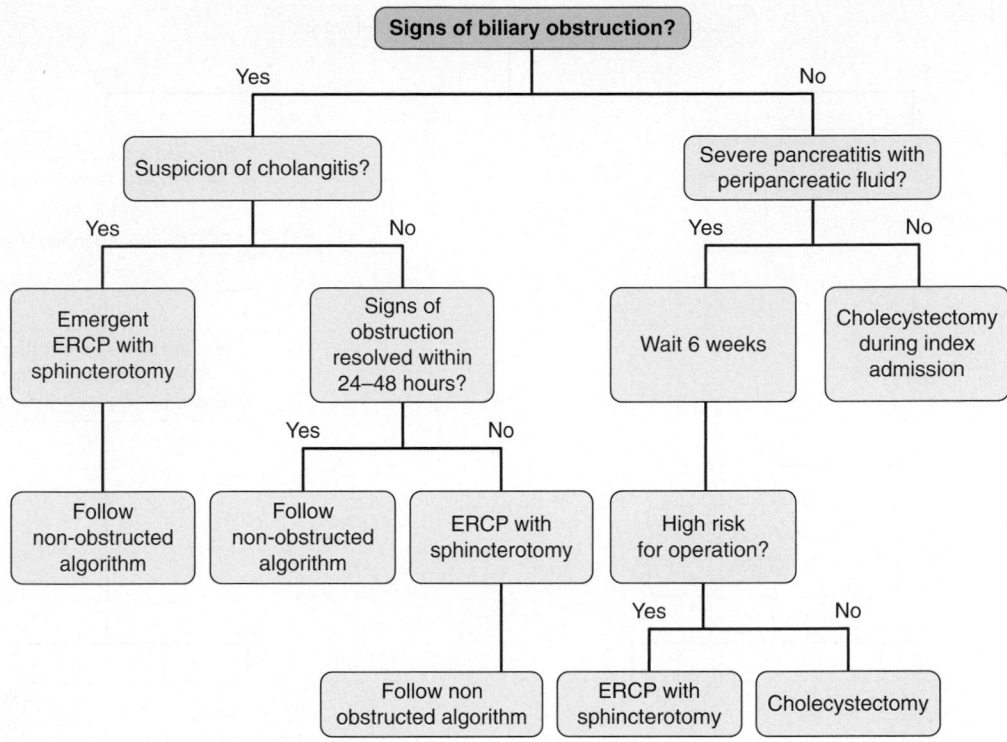

FIGURE 1 Management algorithm for acute pancreatitis resulting from gallstones with and without common bile duct obstruction. *ERCP*, Endoscopic retrograde cholangiopancreatography.

Endoscopic Retrograde Cholangiopancreatography and Cholecystectomy

The preferred treatment of biliary pancreatitis has changed and many previous questions about the role of ERCP and cholecystectomy have been clarified. Large randomized controlled trials and meta-analyses have failed to demonstrate benefit of routine ERCP and it should be avoided unless there is evidence of biliary obstruction. If cholangitis is suspected, urgent ERCP should be performed as soon as feasible, ideally within 24 hours of admission. Delay up to 48 hours is reasonable in patients who have biliary obstruction in the absence of cholangitis, as spontaneous stone passage may result in resolution of the obstruction without intervention (Figure 1).

Cholecystectomy is recommended for patients with biliary pancreatitis but optimal timing depends on disease severity. In mild cases of acute pancreatitis, surgery should be performed during the index admission. A 6-week interval before cholecystectomy should be granted for patients with severe disease and peripancreatic fluid collections. Allowing such fluid collections to resolve or mature decreases the incidence of infectious complications (Figure 2).

ERCP with sphincterotomy effectively prevents recurrent biliary pancreatitis and can be used alone in patients with life-threatening comorbidities and prohibitive surgical risk. Cholecystectomy should be performed after sphincterotomy in those who are deemed acceptable surgical candidates, as these patients remain at risk for gallstone-related disease complications.

■ SURGICAL MANAGEMENT

Historically, the treatment for necrotizing pancreatitis was pancreatic necrosectomy. This approach was abandoned because of the high morbidity and mortality of the procedure and the observation that many of these patients recovered without operation. Surgery was then reserved for infected pancreatic necrosis or other complications such as gastric outlet obstruction or bile duct obstruction. However, recent evidence suggests that necrosectomy often may

be unnecessary, even in infected cases. If infected pancreatitis is suspected or proven, either by imaging or culture obtained by image-guided fine-needle aspiration (FNA), empiric antibiotics with adequate pancreatic tissue penetration (i.e., carbapenems) should be initiated. If FNA is performed and is negative for infection, empiric antibiotic therapy should cease. FNA should not be performed routinely and should be avoided if clinical suspicion for infection is low or the patient is clinically improving.

In cases of antibiotic therapy failure in infected pancreatic necrosis, all attempts at stabilization should be made for at least 4 weeks before performing invasive procedures. Allowing time for sequestration of necrotic pancreatic tissue has been shown to decrease the morbidity of these procedures. The first invasive intervention that should be attempted is percutaneous drainage or endoscopic transluminal drainage. If a percutaneous approach is taken, this tract subsequently can be dilated for further débridement. Laparoscopic or open necrosectomy is indicated in cases of treatment failure with these modalities. This "step-up" approach should be utilized when feasible and has been shown to reduce major complication and multisystem organ failure.

An intra-abdominal catastrophe or persistent clinical instability necessitates the appropriate immediate intervention that may reach across multiple specialties. Indicated interventions may include angioembolization, endoscopic intervention, laparotomy with perforation repair, diverting ileostomy or colostomy, or even open necrosectomy with blunt removal of all pancreatic tissue and two large-bore drains for postoperative lavage. These interventions should be dictated by the individual patient's immediate, life-threatening needs.

■ SUMMARY

The management of acute pancreatitis continues to evolve. Everything from the diagnosis to the treatment of this disease has changed significantly over the last 20 years. Radiographic imaging, specifically CT scans, is no longer considered required for diagnosis and subsequent CT scans are no longer used to monitor the progression of the

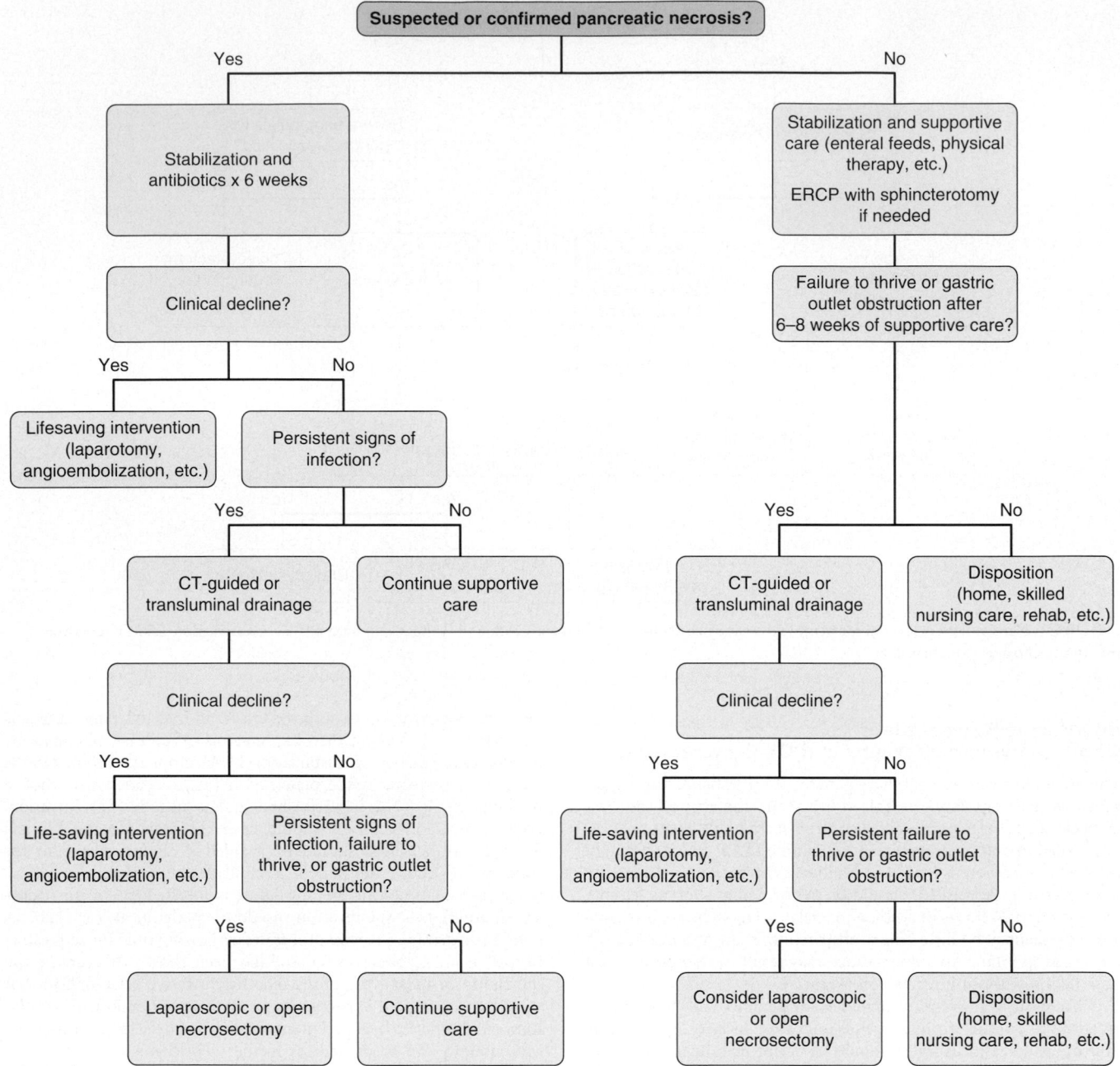

FIGURE 2 Management algorithm for acute pancreatitis associated with pancreatic necrosis. *CT*, Computed tomography; *ERCP*, Endoscopic retrograde cholangiopancreatography.

disease process. In fact, radiographic imaging is now considered useful only if the diagnosis of pancreatitis or infected pancreatic necrosis is in doubt.

Routine ERCP appears to be unnecessary but should be done as soon as feasible if cholangitis is present, if signs of biliary obstruction do not resolve, or if the patient with biliary pancreatitis is not a suitable candidate for cholecystectomy. Cholecystectomy should be done at the index admission if the pancreatitis is not severe and is of biliary origin.

Resuscitation is still of primary importance in patients with severe pancreatitis but there is increasing recognition that this must be done with substantial thought, care, and diligence to avoid fluid overload and once common complications such as ARDS and abdominal compartment syndrome.

Nutrition should be provided as soon as possible and in enteral form. If the patient is not able to eat adequate calories by mouth,

nasogastric or nasojejunal feedings should be initiated. There is no need to "cool down" the pancreas and TPN should be used only if enteral nutrition is not feasible.

The role of antibiotics has been clarified. Antibiotics should not be used for prophylaxis against infected pancreatic necrosis but have become the first-line treatment for this disease process. Only once antibiotics have failed should more invasive forms of treatment be pursued. Image-guided or transluminal drainage should be attempted before surgical intervention.

Surgical intervention was once the mainstay treatment for severe acute pancreatitis. This is no longer the case. Aggressive, surgical management has largely been replaced by more conservative, non-operative, supportive care. This has significantly reduced wasted resources while decreasing morbidity and mortality. Surgery is still an important part of the treatment of severe acute pancreatitis but only when all other measures have failed.

SUGGESTED READINGS

DeCosta DW, Boerma D, van Santvort HC, et al. Stages multidisciplinary step-up management for necrotizing pancreatitis. *Br J Surg.* 2014;101: e65-e79.

Dellinger RP, Levy MM, Rhodes A, et al. Surviving sepsis campaign: international guidelines for management of severe sepsis and septic shock, 2012. *Crit Care Med.* 2013;41:580-637.

Poropat G, Giljaca V, Hauser G, Stimac D. Enteral nutrition formulations for acute pancreatitis. *Cochrane Database Syst Rev.* 2015;(3):CD010605.

Tse F, Yuan F. Early routine endoscopic retrograde cholangiopancreatography strategy versus early conservative management strategy in acute gallstone pancreatitis. *Cochrane Database Syst Rev.* 2012;(5):CD009779.

Villatoro E, Mulla M, Larvin M. Antibiotic therapy for prophylaxis against infection of pancreatic necrosis in acute pancreatitis. *Cochrane Database Syst Rev.* 2010;(12):CD002941.

THE MANAGEMENT OF GALLSTONE PANCREATITIS, PART A

Kevin E. Behrns, MD, and Steven J. Hughes, MD

Acute pancreatitis is the most frequent gastrointestinal diagnosis for hospital admission in the United States with approximately 275,000 admissions in 2009. Gallstones are the most frequent cause of acute pancreatitis with about 15 cases per 100,000 persons per year resulting in an annual aggregate cost of $2.9 billion. The incidence of acute pancreatitis is increasing and likely related to the rising incidence and prevalence of obesity. Other risk factors include African American heritage, type 2 diabetes, hypertriglyceridemia, and alcohol abuse. Acute pancreatitis may be overdiagnosed because of the near-universal availability of laboratory tests that measure pancreatic enzyme serum concentrations that should be used to confirm, but not diagnose, clinically suspected acute pancreatitis.

■ CLINICAL PRESENTATION AND EVALUATION

Clinical Presentation

Patients with gallstone pancreatitis are seen emergently with the acute onset of midepigastric pain that radiates to the back. The pain is unrelenting and accompanied typically by severe nausea and occasional vomiting. Fever, jaundice, acholic stools, and dark urine are not frequent accompaniments to the pain, but, if present, should raise the suspicion of choledocholithiasis and/or acute cholangitis. The most common differential diagnoses include acute cholecystitis, choledocholithiasis, and peptic ulcer disease. The clinical diagnosis of gallstone pancreatitis may be confirmed by serum amylase or lipase concentrations that are increased threefold over the upper limit of normal values. The serum concentrations of pancreatic enzymes, however, do not predict disease severity. Patients with persistent (more than 72 hours), severe abdominal pain should have a contrast medium–enhanced computed tomography (CECT) scan to identify and define potential complications, but patients with mild to moderate disease should not be exposed to cross-sectional imaging on presentation.

Patients with severe pancreatitis occasionally may have hypotension, tachycardia, and tachypnea, mandating admission to the intensive care unit with multimodal management from surgeons, critical care specialists, and gastroenterologists. Clinical deterioration, however, more typically ensues in the hours after the initial assessment, mandating careful review of objective predictors of a severe clinical course (Table 1). Patients with at least three Ranson's criteria or an Acute Physiology and Chronic Health Evaluation (APACHE) score of more than 7 should be admitted preemptively to an intensive care unit.

Disease Severity

In general, patients with gallstone pancreatitis can be classified into one of three categories (mild acute pancreatitis, moderately severe acute pancreatitis, and severe acute pancreatitis) according to pancreatic morphology, the presence of organ failure, and local or systemic complications (Table 2). Morphologically as assessed by CECT, acute pancreatitis is defined as interstitial pancreatitis, which is characterized by edematous changes in the pancreatic parenchyma with or without accompanying acute peripancreatic fluid collections (APFC; Figure 1, *A*), or necrotizing pancreatitis with the presence of nonviable pancreatic parenchyma and, most typically, a surrounding acute necrotic collection (ANC; Figure 1, *B*) in the peripancreatic tissues. Organ failure in patients with gallstone pancreatitis may be transient (less than 48 hours) or persistent (more than 48 hours) and usually initially is accompanied by respiratory failure followed by renal failure and, in severe cases, cardiovascular failure. The 2012 revised Atlanta classification of acute pancreatitis uses the Modified Marshall scoring system to grade organ dysfunction, but for the purposes of categorizing patients with gallstone pancreatitis, the presence of transient or persistent single or multiorgan failure is adequate for management. Local complications of pancreatitis are defined as an APFC, ANC, pancreatic pseudocyst (PP), or walled-off pancreatic necrosis (WOPN). Briefly, an APFC is peripancreatic fluid in the presence of interstitial edematous pancreatitis without necrosis, and it often resolves spontaneously within weeks. An ANC is a collection of fluid and necrosis associated with necrotizing pancreatitis, and it may involve the parenchyma, the peripancreatic tissues alone, or both the pancreas and the retroperitoneal tissues. A pancreatic pseudocyst is an encapsulated, homogenous, enzyme-rich fluid collection with a well-defined wall that matures over 4 weeks. Finally, WOPN is a mature encapsulated collection of necrosis that develops over 4 weeks. Systemic complications of pancreatitis represent exacerbations of pre-existing comorbidities, such as coronary artery disease or chronic obstructive pulmonary disease.

Mild Acute Gallstone Pancreatitis

Patients with mild acute gallstone disease have abdominal pain, nausea, or vomiting, have an increased serum amylase or lipase concentration, and transient increases in serum bilirubin, alkaline phosphatase, or alanine aminotransferase concentrations. These symptoms and abnormal laboratory findings abate within 24 to 48 hours, and CECT is not indicated because an APFC is not present or is not significant clinically. These findings are consistent with a gallstone or sludge that has caused transient obstruction of the pancreatic duct. Abdominal ultrasonography, however, is indicated to confirm the presence of gallstones.

Moderately Severe Gallstone Pancreatitis

The clinical presentation of a patient with moderately severe gallstone pancreatitis is complicated by persistent typical abdominal symptoms that may be accompanied by the presence of a fever, leukocytosis, or persistently increased pancreatic- and/or liver-associated enzymes. These symptoms do not regress over the usual 48 hours and

TABLE 1: Severity Scoring Systems for Acute Pancreatitis

	Ranson's Criteria		Glasgow Criteria	APACHE (0-4 Points Each)
On admission	Within 48 hrs		Age > 55 yr	Temperature
Age >55	Hemoglobin ↓ below 10 mg/dL		WBC > 15 × 10⁹/L	Mean arterial pressure
WBC < 16 × 10⁴/L	Blood urea nitrogen ↑ > 5 mg/dL		PaO_2 < 60 mm Hg (8 kPa)	Heart rate
LDH > 350 U/L	Ca↓ < 8 mg/dL		LDH > 600 U/L	Respiratory rate
AST > 250 U/L	PaO_2 < 60 mmHg (8 kPa)		AST > 200 U/L	Oxygenation
Glucose > 200 mg/dL	Base deficit > 4 mEq/L		Albumin < 32 g/L	Arterial pH
	Fluid sequestration > 6 L		Ca < 2 mmol/L	HCO_3^-
			Glucose > 10 mmol/L	Na^+
			Urea > 16 mmol/L	K^+
				Creatinine
				Hematocrit
				WBC
				Glasgow coma scale

AST, aspartate aminotransferase; *Ca*, calcium; *HCO₃⁻*, bicarbonate; *K*, potassium; *LDH*, lactate dehydrogenase; *Na*, sodium; *WBC*, white blood cell count.

TABLE 2: Characteristics of the Various Forms of Gallstone Pancreatitis

	Mild Acute Pancreatitis	Moderately Severe Pancreatitis	Severe Acute Pancreatitis
Morphology	Interstitial/edematous	Necrotizing	Necrotizing
SIRS response	Absent	Transient	Persistent for 1-2 weeks
Organ failure	Absent	<48 hours	>48 hours
Local complications			
APFC	Occasional	Often	Present initially
ANC	Absent	Occasional	Present
PP	Absent	Rare	Occasionally
WON	Absent	Rare	Often
Risk of infection	Nil	Low	Moderate

ANC, Acute necrotic collection; *APFC*, acute peripancreatic fluid collection; *PP*, pancreatic pseudocyst; *SIRS*, systemic inflammatory response syndrome; *WON*, walled-off necrosis.

may be accompanied by transient organ failure manifest by increasing oxygen requirements and an abnormally elevated creatinine or blood urine nitrogen (BUN). Persistent symptoms for more than 3 days are an indication for CECT that may reveal interstitial, edematous pancreatitis with an APFC or sterile pancreatic necrosis without persistent organ failure. Patients with continually increased liver-associated enzymes (bilirubin > 4) may have biliary obstruction from gallstones, and magnetic resonance cholangiopancreatography (MRCP) is indicated to confirm or exclude the presence of an obstructing stone.

Severe Acute Gallstone Pancreatitis

Patients with severe acute gallstone pancreatitis have abdominal symptoms and develop single or multiple organ failure that is persistent. These patients exhibit signs of the systemic inflammatory response syndrome (SIRS) with tachycardia, hypothermia or hyperthermia, leukocytosis, and tachypnea. They require admission to the intensive care unit and often have progressive organ failure requiring intubation and mechanical ventilation, renal replacement therapy, and/or inotropic support. After resuscitation and stabilization, CECT may demonstrate pancreatic necrosis with local complications;

however, necrotizing pancreatitis evolves over days and weeks, and early CECT may not demonstrate significant pancreatic or peripancreatic findings. MRCP may be indicated in those patients with a high suspicion of acute cholangitis, and perhaps, in these critically ill patients, endoscopic retrograde cholangiopancreatography (ERCP) is the most efficient procedure for the relief of biliary obstruction.

■ DISEASE MANAGEMENT

The management of patients with gallstone pancreatitis ranges from relatively straightforward medical and surgical care to the most complex care, requiring state-of-the art facilities and highly trained medical and surgical specialists. The recommendations for management outlined later, therefore, are highly dependent on the resources available in local care settings. Herein, the management of gallstone pancreatitis will be described in the context of the severity of pancreatitis.

Mild Acute Gallstone Pancreatitis

The management of patients with mild gallstone pancreatitis may be accomplished at nearly all medical centers because the diagnosis is ascertained by history, physical examination, and routine laboratory tests. In addition, imaging requires only an abdominal ultrasound to confirm the presence of gallstones and/or sludge and exclude biliary dilation suggestive of choledocholithiasis (common bile duct diameter >11 mm). Patients' symptoms resolve over 1 to 3 days, at which time the patient should undergo laparoscopic cholecystectomy with intraoperative cholangiography. Cholecystectomy should be performed during the index hospitalization as confirmed by the PONCHO trial, which demonstrated that recurrent gallstone-related complications occur in 5% of patients with same-admission cholecystectomy compared with a 17% rate of recurrent gallstone-related complications in patients undergoing interval cholecystectomy. The

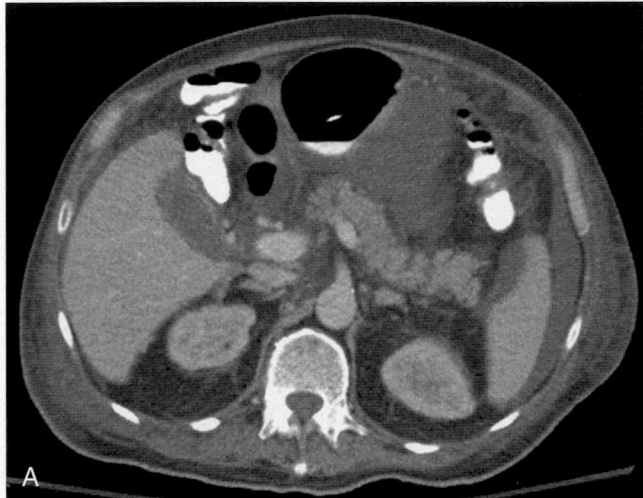

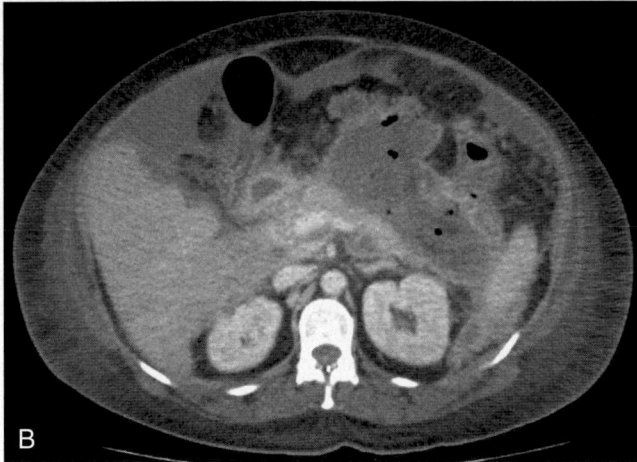

FIGURE I **A,** An acute peripancreatic fluid collection accompanying interstitial edematous pancreatitis. **B,** Walled-off necrosis with gas bubbles indicative of infected pancreatic and peripancreatic necrosis.

rate of complications from cholecystectomy was low (less than 1%) in both groups.

Intraoperative cholangiography should be performed routinely in these patients because there is no indication for preoperative ERCP or MRCP. Choledocholithiasis is identified infrequently because most gallstones have passed into the intestine. Patients with choledocholithiasis identified on intraoperative cholangiography may be managed by watchful waiting for symptoms, laparoscopic common bile duct exploration, or postoperative ERCP, all of which are options for management depending on patient health, number of stones in the bile duct, and size of the bile duct.

The outcomes of patients with mild acute gallstone pancreatitis are excellent without anticipated mortality, complications in less than 5% of patients, and a hospital duration of stay of approximately 3 days.

Moderately Severe Acute Gallstone Pancreatitis

Patients with moderately severe gallstone pancreatitis have evidence of local complications from pancreatic injury and transient organ failure, and thus should be managed in a monitored setting. Initial management of these patients should be directed toward prompt resuscitation with Ringer's lactate solution and the provision of supplemental oxygen. The goals of fluid therapy should be to ameliorate tachycardia and maintain a urine output of 0.5 to 1.0 mL/kg/hr. BUN can be trended for improvement in the patient's fluid status. Because organ failure is transient with this condition, rapid improvement is anticipated, and a prolonged intensive care unit stay should be unnecessary. However, the duration of hospitalization may be dependent on the local complications related to pancreatic injury. Edematous pancreatitis with an APFC should resolve relatively quickly, whereas sterile necrosis may cause persistent symptoms and limit per oral intake, necessitating institution of enteral nutrition in the infrequent patient. Occasionally, patients with moderately severe pancreatitis will have biliary obstruction manifest by persistently elevated liver associated enzymes, and these patients may require a MRCP or ERCP with sphincterotomy for relief of biliary obstruction. Nonetheless, the overall course of recovery should be progressive improvement without a need for intervention related to the pancreatic injury, and cholecystectomy with intraoperative cholangiography should be performed before hospital discharge for the usual patient. For patients who have sterile necrosis, follow-up CECT is recommended to ensure resolution of the pancreatic injury without complicating features such as the development of a pancreatic pseudocyst.

Patients with moderately severe gallstone pancreatitis should recover completely with no expected mortality and few complications (Table 3). The duration of hospital stay is dependent on resolution of symptoms and dietary intake, but overall duration should be 7 to 10 days.

Severe Acute Gallstone Pancreatitis

Patients with severe acute gallstone pancreatitis represent a management challenge for even the most experienced and skilled medical

TABLE 3: Outcomes of Interventional Approaches to Moderately Severe and Severe Pancreatitis

	Percutaneous Catheter Drainage	Endoscopic Therapy	Minimally Invasive Surgery	Open Surgery
Mortality (%)	0-34	0-15	0-40	4-47
Morbidity (%)	4-60	0-46	0-92	33-89
Reintervention (%)	0-79	0-31	8-40	
Anticipated length of stay	Days to weeks	Days to weeks	Weeks	Weeks to months

and surgical pancreatologists. These patients are managed best at quaternary institutions with well-equipped intensive care units, endoscopy and radiology suites, and operating rooms, all of which are staffed by critical care experts, surgeons, interventional radiologists, and gastroenterologists. Because these patients develop a profound SIRS response and often have rapid deterioration in their condition, they should be managed in an intensive care unit where their airway can be managed promptly and resuscitation commenced immediately. Airway intubation and mechanical ventilation requiring advanced techniques to maintain oxygenation are not uncommon, and the development of an abdominal compartment syndrome may affect ventilation and require a decompressive laparotomy. Likewise, renal failure requiring replacement therapies such as continuous venovenous hemofiltration may be present. This period of critical illness is driven by cytokine elaboration that persists for 1 to 2 weeks before waning. The goals of therapy during this period of critical illness include maintenance of oxygen delivery to the central nervous system and viscera by mechanical ventilation, adequate resuscitation with Lactated Ringer's solution, inotropic administration as needed to support blood pressure and decrease heart rate, maintenance of renal function with or without renal replacement therapy, and nutritional support. Nutrition should be delivered enterally either via a nasogastric tube or nasojejunal tube with a polymeric formula because elemental or immune-enhancing formulations offer no advantage.

During the initial evaluation, the gallbladder and biliary tree should be evaluated by ultrasonography and serum liver–associated enzymes. The presence of gallstones, elevated liver associated enzymes, and a dilated biliary tree are indications for an MRCP or ERCP. Evidence of acute cholangitis or biliary obstruction in these critically ill patients merits an emergent ERCP with endoscopic sphincterotomy (ES) for duct drainage. The routine use of ERCP with ES in patients with severe necrotizing gallstone pancreatitis, however, is not indicated.

As the systemic inflammatory response wanes over 1 to 2 weeks, these patients will develop local complications of necrotizing pancreatitis, including an ANC, PP, or WON. By 4 to 6 weeks, these processes should be mature, and management of these complications guided by symptoms. Interventions, unless required by a change in the patient's status, should not be undertaken until at least 4 weeks have passed since the onset of pancreatitis. The most ominous local complication is infection. The percentage of nonviable pancreas and the extent of peripancreatic necrosis may predict the likelihood of infected pancreatic necrosis, which increases the mortality rate significantly compared with sterile pancreatic necrosis (5% vs 20%). Despite the dire outcome with infected necrosis, the administration of prophylactic antibiotics to patients with necrotizing pancreatitis has not been shown to decrease the rate of development of infected necrosis or systemic infections, and thus prophylactic antibiotics are not warranted.

The management of the local complications of necrotizing pancreatitis is highly dependent on the nature of the local complication. An ANC accompanying pancreatic necrosis may be sterile or infected. Sterile necrosis often requires no intervention, and patients recover over time except for the infrequent patient who develops failure-to-thrive as a result of sterile necrosis. Patients with failure-to-thrive syndrome may require percutaneous drainage or endoscopic or operative débridement for full recovery. In contrast, patients with infected necrosis generally require drainage or débridement of the pancreas and peripancreatic tissues along with the administration of culture-directed antibiotic therapy. The mode by which infected pancreatic necrosis is drained or débrided is variable and dependent on institutional expertise. Percutaneous drainage with vigorous flushing and scrupulous attention to catheter patency may adequately address small-to-moderate sized collections. Alternatively, infected ANCs or WON may be managed by endoscopic débridement when the collection is in proximity to the stomach and may be approached transgastrically for drainage and manipulation. In addition, moderate-sized

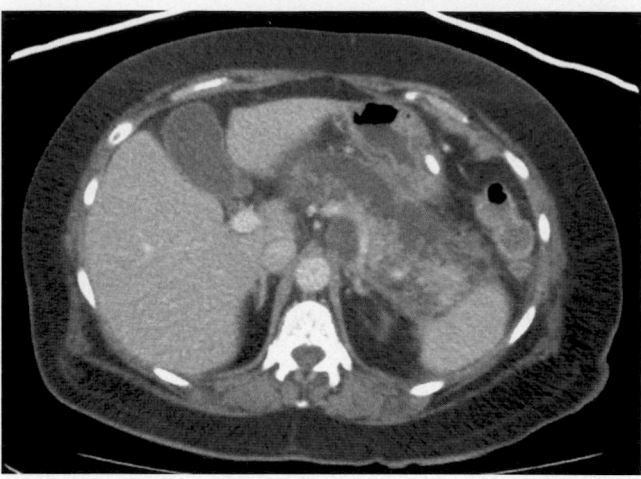

FIGURE 2 Contrast-enhanced computed tomography demonstrating necrotic pancreas in the region of the anatomic pancreatic neck, resulting in a disconnected pancreatic duct.

collections may be addressed laparoscopically via a transgastric approach or pure laparoscopic débridement. Large-volume débridements and extrapancreatic complications such as colonic ischemia may be handled best by open operative débridement or resection. More recently, combined approaches such as the step-up approach have been used to permit percutaneous drainage followed by laparoscopic retroperitoneal débridement as necessary. This approach, compared with open necrosectomy, decreased the incidence of new-onset organ failure (12% vs 40%) and new-onset diabetes mellitus (16% vs 38%).

Importantly, before débridement, a CECT should be obtained to ascertain the presence of the disconnected pancreatic duct syndrome (Figure 2). A viable pancreatic remnant in the tail separated by a substantial area of pancreatic necrosis in the neck of the gland should lead to the suspicion of a disconnected pancreas. Alternatively, a MRCP may show discontinuity of the pancreatic duct. Regardless, operative approaches for the disconnected pancreatic duct in the setting of severe pancreatitis include distal pancreatectomy and splenectomy accompanied by pancreatic débridement as necessary.

Finally, concomitant with or following pancreatic drainage or débridement, the patient must have a cholecystectomy to prevent further episodes of gallstone-induced pancreatitis.

The outcomes of patients with severe acute gallstone pancreatitis are variable depending on the patient's overall condition, the extent of the disease, the type of procedure performed, the expertise of the providers, and the institutional experience with such patients (Table 3). As noted previously, patients with sterile pancreatic necrosis require interventions infrequently, and therefore medical management results in a mortality rate of 5% or less with few complications. Patients with infected necrosis, however, often require drainage or débridement, which may be accomplished through percutaneous drainage (PCD) alone, PCD with video-assisted retroperitoneal débridement via a step-up approach, endoscopic methods, laparoscopic transperitoneal approach, or open necrosectomy. PCD alone has a mortality rate as low as 5% but up to 34% of patients in one series. Reported morbidity ranges from 4% to 60% with 5% to 79% of patients requiring a subsequent operation with duration of catheter drainage from 16 to 152 days. Laparoscopic approaches may be transperitoneal or retroperitoneal and are associated with mortality rates ranging from 0 to 40% with morbidity from 21% to 92% (Figure 3). Overall success rates for these approaches vary from 60% to 92%. The results with endoscopic therapy, either alone or with adjuvant techniques, demonstrated mortality rates from 0 to 15%, whereas morbidity ranged from 11% to 46%. Most patients require

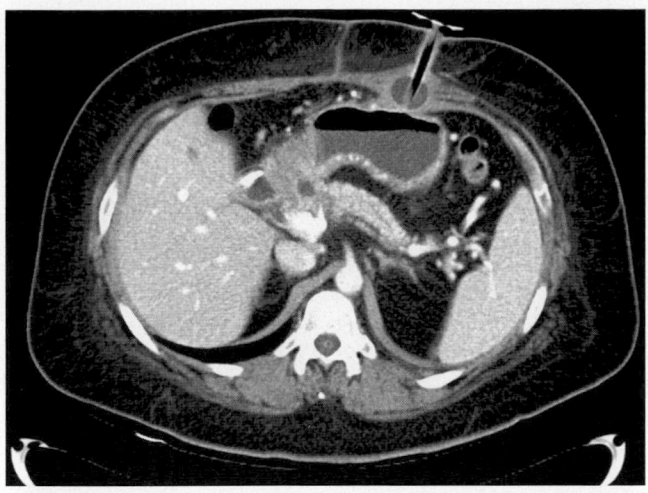

FIGURE 3 Contrast-enhanced computed tomography demonstrates viable pancreas draining into the stomach after laparoscopic transgastric necrosectomy.

necrotizing pancreatitis, which requires months to treat. Regardless, the disease is managed best by a multidisciplinary, evidence-based approach that uses multimodal interventions in patients with necrotizing pancreatitis complicated by failure-to-thrive or infection. Ultimately all patients should have a timely cholecystectomy, or an endoscopic sphincterotomy in infirm patients, to treat the origin of the disease.

three endoscopic sessions to adequately address the necrosis. The open surgical approaches are heterogenous, and some of these approaches are no longer used in contemporary management. Operative techniques such as open packing, planned relaparotomy, closed packing, and continuous lavage often are not required. When open surgery is necessary, a single operation timed 4 to 6 weeks after the onset of necrotizing pancreatitis should accomplish drainage, débridement, or resection of the pancreas as necessary. Mortality with open surgery ranges from 5% to 47%, and morbidity rates are often greater than 50%.

■ CONCLUSION

Acute gallstone pancreatitis presents a wide spectrum of disease that ranges from mild pancreatitis that resolves quickly to severe

SUGGESTED READINGS

Banks PA, Bollen TL, Dervenis C, et al. Classification of acute pancreatitis-2012: revision of the Atlanta classification and definitions by international consensus. *Gut.* 2013;62:102-111.

Da Costa DW, Bouwense SA, Schepers NJ, et al. Same-admission versus interval cholecystectomy for mild gallstone pancreatitis (PONCHO): a multicenter randomized controlled trial. *Lancet.* 2015;386:1261-1268.

Fischer TD, Gutman DS, Hughes SJ, et al. Disconnected pancreatic duct syndrome: disease classification and management strategies. *J Am Coll Surg.* 2014;219:704-712.

Freeman ML, Werner J, van Santvoort HC, et al. Interventions for necrotizing pancreatitis: summary of a multidisciplinary consensus conference. *Pancreas.* 2012;41:1176-1194.

Petrov MS, Loveday BP, Pylypchuck RD, et al. Systematic review and meta-analysis of enteral nutrition formulations in acute pancreatitis. *Br J Surg.* 2009;96:1243-1252.

Van Santvoort HC, Besselink MG, Bakker OJ, et al. A step-up approach or open necrosectomy for necrotizing pancreatitis. *N Engl J Med.* 2010;362: 1491-1502.

Villatoro E, Mulla M, Larvin M. Antibiotic therapy for prophylaxis against infection of pancreatic necrosis in acute pancreatitis. *Cochrane Database Syst Rev.* 2010;(5):CD002941.

Working Group IAP/APA Acute Pancreatitis Guidelines. IAP/APA evidence-based guidelines for the management of acute pancreatitis. *Pancreatology.* 2013;13:e1-e15.

Wu BU, Banks PA. Clinical management of patients with acute pancreatitis. *Gastroenterology.* 2013;144:1272-1281.

Yadav D, Lowenfels AB. The epidemiology of pancreatitis and pancreatic cancer. *Gastroenterology.* 2013;144:1252-1261.

THE MANAGEMENT OF GALLSTONE PANCREATITIS, PART B

Peter Dixon, MD, Madhumithaa Parthasarathy, MBBS, Gopal C. Kowdley, MD, PhD, FACS, and Steven C. Cunningham, MD, FACS

In the United States, acute pancreatitis continues to be a common gastrointestinal cause of hospital admissions and is associated with significant morbidity and healthcare expenditure. More than 300,000 hospitalizations and 20,000 related deaths cost more than $2 billion annually. Of the two most common causes of pancreatitis—alcohol and gallstones, which together account for more than 80% of the disease burden—gallstones are the most common, accounting for 40% to 60% of all cases. Most of these cases follow a mild course and are self-limited with supportive care, but approximately 20% progress to severe disease, requiring a prolonged hospital stay and intensive care, and are associated with a mortality rate approaching 30%. Three key areas in the management of patients with gallstone pancreatitis (GSP) are diagnosis, risk stratification with predictors of severity, and the type and timing of definitive intervention.

■ DIAGNOSIS

A definitive diagnosis of acute pancreatitis is not generally difficult to make. Two of the following three criteria are sufficient: (1) abdominal pain that is constant, severe, epigastric, often radiating to the back, accompanied by nausea, vomiting, and anorexia, and exacerbated by oral intake; (2) serum lipase (or amylase) level at least three times the upper limit of normal; and (3) characteristic imaging findings, ideally with a contrast-enhanced computed tomography (CT). In patients with typical abdominal pain and elevated lipase or amylase, it is often advisable to delay CT for 72 hours, and at that time to perform a dedicated pancreas-protocol CT (PPCT) with an early arterial phase and a delayed portal venous phase, ideally calibrated to cardiac output. Important advantages of this 72-hour delay in the PPCT include avoiding excessive radiation and contrast exposure associated with repeat CT imaging, allowing free fluid to begin to coalesce, and increasing the ability to distinguish pancreatic necrosis from transiently ischemic areas. In some cases of obviously mild pancreatitis, or frequently recurrent alcoholic pancreatitis, CT may be omitted.

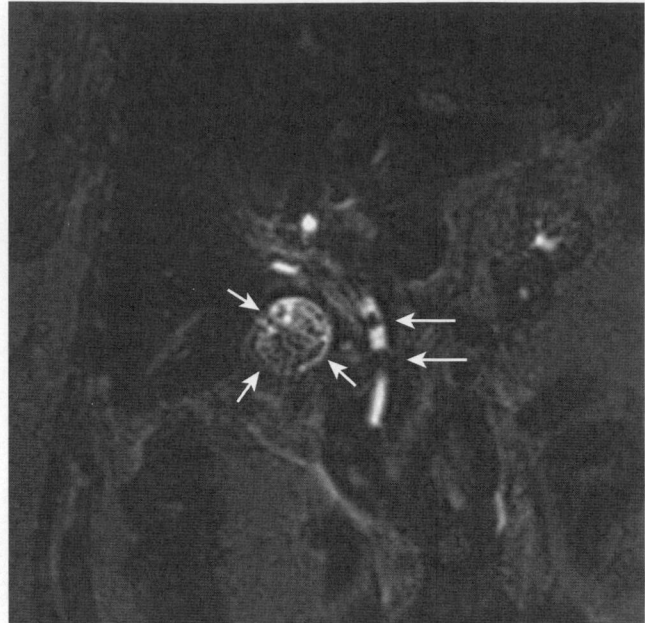

FIGURE 1 Magnetic resonance cholangiopancreatography (MRCP) in a patient with cholelithiasis (*3 short arrows*) and choledocholithiasis (*2 long arrows*).

TABLE 1: Severity of Acute Pancreatitis According to the 2012 Revision of the Atlanta Classification

Severity	Characteristics
Mild	No organ failure No local or systemic complications
Moderate	Organ failure that resolves within 48 h (transient organ failure) or Local or systemic complications without persistent organ failure
Severe	Persistent organ failure (>48 h) • Single organ failure • Multiple organ failure

Modified from Banks PA, Bollen TL, Dervenis C, Gooszen HG, Johnson CD, Sarr MG, Tsiotos GG, Vege SS, Acute Pancreatitis Classification Working Group. Classification of acute pancreatitis—2012: revision of the Atlanta classification and definitions by international consensus. *Gut.* 2013;62:102-111.

The diagnosis of gallstones as the cause of the pancreatitis is largely a diagnosis of exclusion. In brief, the presence of gallstones or sludge and the absence of other known causes are generally sufficient for the diagnosis of GSP. However, because both gallstone and nongallstone pancreatitis are very common, careful consideration of the many other causes is warranted. Alcohol and medications are probably the two most common nongallstone causes, but other possible causes include hypertriglyceridemia, autoimmunity, ductal obstruction by tumors or anomalies, nerve stimulators, and numerous dietary exposures. Careful history-taking is essential for patients who have acute pancreatitis to help rule out nongallstone causes.

In addition to ruling out other causes of pancreatitis, careful review of laboratory and imaging data can shore up the diagnosis of GSP per se. Several different laboratory values, such as elevated aminotransferases, bilirubin, and alkaline phosphatase, are useful in identifying a biliary origin of pancreatitis. Initial imaging is essential and satisfies three major needs in the management of GSP: confirmation of cause, identification of complications, and, as discussed later, assessment of severity. The most common initial modality is ultrasound (US), which is used to confirm the presence of gallstones or sludge and to measure the diameter of the common bile duct. Ultrasound is the least invasive and most widely available imaging modality and therefore generally precedes CT, magnetic resonance imaging (MRI), endoscopic ultrasound scan (EUS), endoscopic retrograde cholangiopancreatography (ERCP), and magnetic resonance cholangiopancreatography (MRCP). Although US is optimally 95% sensitive in detecting cholelithiasis, in GSP the sensitivity may decrease to 60% to 80% because of increased bowel gas caused by concomitant ileus. CT may detect both choledocholithiasis and cholelithiasis but may overestimate duct diameter compared with US, and is not nearly as highly sensitive as MRCP for choledocholithiasis (Figure 1).

STRATIFICATION AND SCORING

Acute GSP, like other causes of acute pancreatitis, can evolve rapidly. It is important to continually attempt to distinguish those patients in whom the disease may be severe and protracted from those who will go on to a rapid and full recovery. Risk stratification has major implications for patients because it not only predicts morbidity and mortality but also largely determines treatment. There are many scoring and classification systems and none is perfectly accurate in stratifying patients by severity.

According to the 2012 revision of the Atlanta Classification, acute pancreatitis is divided into three main categories: mild, moderate, and severe (Table 1), based predominantly on the presence and extent of organ failure and complications. This schema has been validated in several studies and has been shown to prognosticate morbidity and mortality. One of the greatest advances in recent years, largely thanks to the work of the Acute Pancreatitis Classification Working Group, is the standardization of the nomenclature used to describe the severity levels and the complications and to define organ failure (Tables 2 and 3).

The PPCT scan, ideally done 48 to 72 hours after diagnosis, is one of the most important tests performed to guide stratification and subsequent treatment of patients with GSP, both those with mild acute pancreatitis (MAP) and those with severe acute pancreatitis (SAP). When performed too early, however, it may be of limited utility and may not accurately reveal the still-evolving pancreatitis or local complications. For instance, what looks like necrotizing pancreatitis (NP) may be an area of transient ischemia, and what is initially free fluid, termed an acute peripancreatic fluid collection (APFC), may yet reabsorb and disappear or may coalesce into a pancreatic pseudocyst (PP). The CT Severity Index or Balthazar Score (Table 4) incorporates the grade of pancreatitis, including pancreatic and peripancreatic fluid collections, and the proportion of NP. Depending on the value of this score, the associated morbidity and mortality attributable to the pancreatitis ranges from 0% and 0% for the mildest MAP to 17% and 92%, respectively, for the worst SAP (see Table 4).

TREATMENT

For All Patients

Regardless of disease severity, in acute GSP intravenous fluid resuscitation is a mainstay of treatment. As this treatment begins, triage and patient stratification are ongoing, as discussed earlier. All patients require frequent serial re-evaluations because even patients with apparently mild GSP may go on to rapidly develop SAP and require intensive care, which may include mechanical ventilation and cardiovascular support.

For Patients With Mild Disease

Initial infusion should be in the form of boluses followed by an infusion rate targeted to urine output, heart rate, blood pressure, and

TABLE 2: Nomenclature of Pancreatitis

Term	Definition
Mild acute pancreatitis (MAP)	Pancreatitis without evidence of organ failure or local complications
Moderately severe acute pancreatitis (MSAP)	Pancreatitis with a local complication such as APFC, PP, ANC, or WON (all defined below) or with organ failure (defined below) lasting less than 48 hours
Severe acute pancreatitis (SAP)	Pancreatitis with a local complication such as APFC, PP, ANC, or WON (all defined below) or with organ failure (defined below) lasting more than 48 hours
Interstitial edematous pancreatitis (IEP)	Pancreatitis that lacks pancreatic or peripancreatic necrosis on imaging
Necrotizing pancreatitis (NP)	Pancreatitis with parenchymal, peripancreatic, or combined necrosis, identified by contrast-enhanced imaging
Acute peripancreatic fluid collection (APFC)	Peripancreatic fluid collection that occurs within the first 4 weeks of pancreatitis in the setting of IEP, without a well-defined wall
Pancreatic pseudocyst (PP)	APFC that has persisted more than 4 weeks and now has evidence of a well-defined wall
Acute necrotic collection (ANC)	Collection of both fluid and necrotic solid material, in NP, within the first 4 weeks, without a well-defined wall
Walled-off necrosis (WON)	ANC that has persisted more than 4 weeks and has developed a well-defined wall
Organ failure	A score of 2 or more for any organ system in the Marshall scoring system (see Table 3)

Modified from Sabo S, Goussous N, Sardana S, Patel ST, Cunningham SC. Necrotizing pancreatitis: a review of multidisciplinary management. *J Pancreas*. 2015;16:1. See text for further explanation.

TABLE 3: Modified Marshall Scoring System

Organ System	Score				
	0	1	2	3	4
PaO₂/FiO₂	>400	301-400	201-300	101-200	≤101
Serum creatinine (mg/dL)	<1.4	1.4-1.8	1.9-3.6	3.6-4.9	>4.9
Systolic blood pressure (mm Hg)	>90	<90, Fluid responsive	<90, Not fluid responsive	<90, pH <7.3	<90, pH <7.2

Modified from Thandassery RB, Yadav TD, Dutta U, Appasani S, Singh K, Kochhar R. Dynamic nature of organ failure in severe acute pancreatitis: the impact of persistent and deteriorating organ failure. *HPB (Oxford)*. 2013;15:523-528; and Sabo S, Goussous N, Sardana S, Patel ST, Cunningham SC. Necrotizing pancreatitis: a review of multidisciplinary management. *J Pancreas*. 2015;16:1.

Note: Organ failure is defined by a score of 2 or greater in any category. Assumes no pre-existing renal disease with creatinine >1.4 and no use of inotropic agents.

correction of any acidemia. Restriction of oral intake for patients with pancreatitis has been a traditional mainstay of treatment, and although it is still advised on presentation, subsequent enteral nutrition should be begun soon thereafter, as tolerated, typically within 24 hours. In mild GSP this is generally accomplished with an oral diet. If nausea and vomiting persist, however, nasogastric tube decompression can protect against vomiting and aspiration. Given that the primary complaint of patients with pancreatitis is pain, this complaint deserves serious attention. Intravenous opiates often form the cornerstone of pain treatment, with the understanding that all opioids cause spasm of the sphincter of Oddi and therefore theoretically will decrease the chance that small stones will pass the sphincter into the duodenum in patients with GSP. Antibiotics should not be administered routinely to patients with GSP unless an infection has been identified. For those patients with cholangitis and those who go on to develop extensive NP (see the following section), antibiotics may be warranted.

Patients with GSP who have significant cholangitis in addition to GSP should undergo urgent ERCP. Although some have advocated for early routine ERCP in cases of GSP, a 2013 Cochrane review of studies comparing this strategy with conservative, selective use of ERCP found no evidence that early routine ERCP significantly affected mortality or morbidity. This is especially relevant for patients with mild GSP: in a 2015 meta-analysis comparing early ERCP and sphincterotomy with conservative management, a decrease in complication rates was noted among patients with severe disease but not in those with mild disease.

Laparoscopic cholecystectomy should be offered to patients with mild GSP during the index hospitalization, generally as soon as the patient is stable with significant resolution of acute symptoms (Figure 2). In a recent Cochrane review, early cholecystectomy was associated with zero adverse events and with a shorter hospital stay and shorter operating times when compared with a group who underwent delayed cholecystectomy.

TABLE 4: Computed Tomography (CT) Severity Index

CT Grade		Necrosis			Outcome	
Grade	Points	Percentage	Additional Points	Severity Index	Mortality (%)	Morbidity (%)
A	0	0	0	0	0	0
B	1	0	0	1		
				2	0	4
C	2	<30	2	4	6	35
				6		
D	3	30-50	4	7	17	92
E	4	>50	6	10		

Modified from Balthazar EJ, Freeny PC, vanSonnenberg E. Imaging and intervention in acute pancreatitis. *Radiology* 1994;193:297-306, and from Sabo S, Goussous N, Sardana S, Patel ST, Cunningham SC. Necrotizing pancreatitis: a review of multidisciplinary management. *J Pancreas* 2015;16(2):1. See text for details.

Grade A, Normal pancreas; *Grade B*, pancreatic enlargement; *Grade C*, pancreatic inflammation or peripancreatic fat; *Grade D*, single peripancreatic fluid collection; *Grade E*, two or more fluid collections or retroperitoneal air.

For Patients With Severe Disease

As with mild GSP, early and aggressive fluid resuscitation is the cornerstone of initial therapy in SAP caused by gallstones, and improvements in systemic inflammatory response and urine output should be the clinical endpoints, ideally in an intensive care setting. Regarding nutrition, the enteral route is preferred in severe disease as in mild disease, but is less often possible. Still, every effort should be made to achieve enteral nutrition because it is associated with a lower incidence of infected pancreatic necrosis. Postpyloric feeds are not likely better than gastric feeds. Antibiotics are often used in severe acute GSP to prevent conversion of sterile necrosis to infected necrosis but the benefit is only marginal if the extent of necrosis is <30% and antiobiotic use is controversial even with more extensive necrosis. Use of octreotide is similarly controversial. After initial stabilization, transfer to a high-volume pancreatic surgery center should be considered, depending on local resources and expertise.

As discussed earlier, a recent GSP meta-analysis comparing early ERCP plus sphincterotomy with conservative management found a decrease in complication rates among patients with SAP. Once a generous sphincterotomy has been performed, the patient is generally protected from further choledocholithiasis for several weeks to several months.

Unlike in MAP, in which early (same-admission) cholecystectomy is recommended to prevent future episodes of GSP, in SAP early operation should be avoided, whether for cholecystectomy or pancreatic débridement. There are, however, a few notable exceptions, such as abdominal compartment syndrome, refractory hemorrhage, and colonic necrosis or perforation, in which case immediate operation is warranted (Figure 2). In most all other cases, operation should be delayed for as long as possible but ideally for at least 4 to 6 weeks. One benefit of this delay is that the NP becomes more clearly demarcated on CT and operatively, making débridement much safer. In addition, regarding the cholecystectomy, the aforementioned protection from future episodes of GSP that is afforded by the sphincterotomy makes the deferral of cholecystectomy safe. Up to two thirds of patients with NP are successfully managed without débridement. When an acute necrotic collection (ANC) has become infected, however, antibiotics and débridement or drainage are indicated. If débridement is required after 4 to 6 weeks, at which time the ANC is termed walled-off necrosis (WON), the gallbladder may be removed at the same time as débridement of the WON (Figure 2). If delayed pancreatic débridement or drainage is never required,

cholecystectomy may proceed electively, with a significantly lower complication rate compared with same-admission cholecystectomy. A complete review of the management of SAP is provided in Figure 2, illustrating that a range of interventions, from supportive care alone to open necrosectomy, may be required, including intermediate procedures such as combined percutaneous and endoscopic drainage (dual-modality drainage), endoscopic necrosectomy, and minimally invasive surgical necrosectomy.

Gallstone Pancreatitis in Pregnant Patients

Physiologic changes associated with pregnancy increase the risk of forming gallstones. The diagnostic criteria for GSP in patients who are pregnant are similar to those for nonpregnant patients. Abdominal US is the optimal initial test to confirm the presence of gallstone disease in pregnant patients but is limited in its ability to assess the pancreas. MRI, however, as shown in Figure 1, not only can provide the diagnosis of stones—both cholelithiasis and choledocholithiasis—but also can assess for the degree of pancreatitis, without the ionizing radiation that accompanies standard ERCP and CT.

Pancreatitis may lead to multiple prenatal complications, including preterm labor, prematurity, and in utero fetal death. Patients with GSP in the first trimester have the highest rates of fetal loss and a very low rate of term pregnancies, as well as a high rate of recurrence of stone-related symptoms. Because of this high likelihood of and risks associated with recurrent GSP, laparoscopic cholecystectomy and ERCP have a favorable risk/benefit ratio in these patients. Cholecystectomy is possible in all trimesters but safest in the second trimester. ERCP is also possible during pregnancy, the largest risk being from the radiation exposure during the procedure. Techniques that eliminate or minimize the use of radiation during ERCP, such as choledochoscopy, and careful attention to shielding effectively remove or mitigate radiation exposure.

A reasonable approach to GSP depending on trimester is the following: (1) first trimester—conservative treatment and laparoscopic cholecystectomy +/− ERCP; (2) second trimester—laparoscopic cholecystectomy +/− ERCP; (3) third trimester—conservative treatment +/− ERCP and a laparoscopic cholecystectomy in the early postpartum period. Intraoperative maneuvers that can minimize risks during cholecystectomy in pregnant patients include left lateral positioning and using lower insufflation pressures.

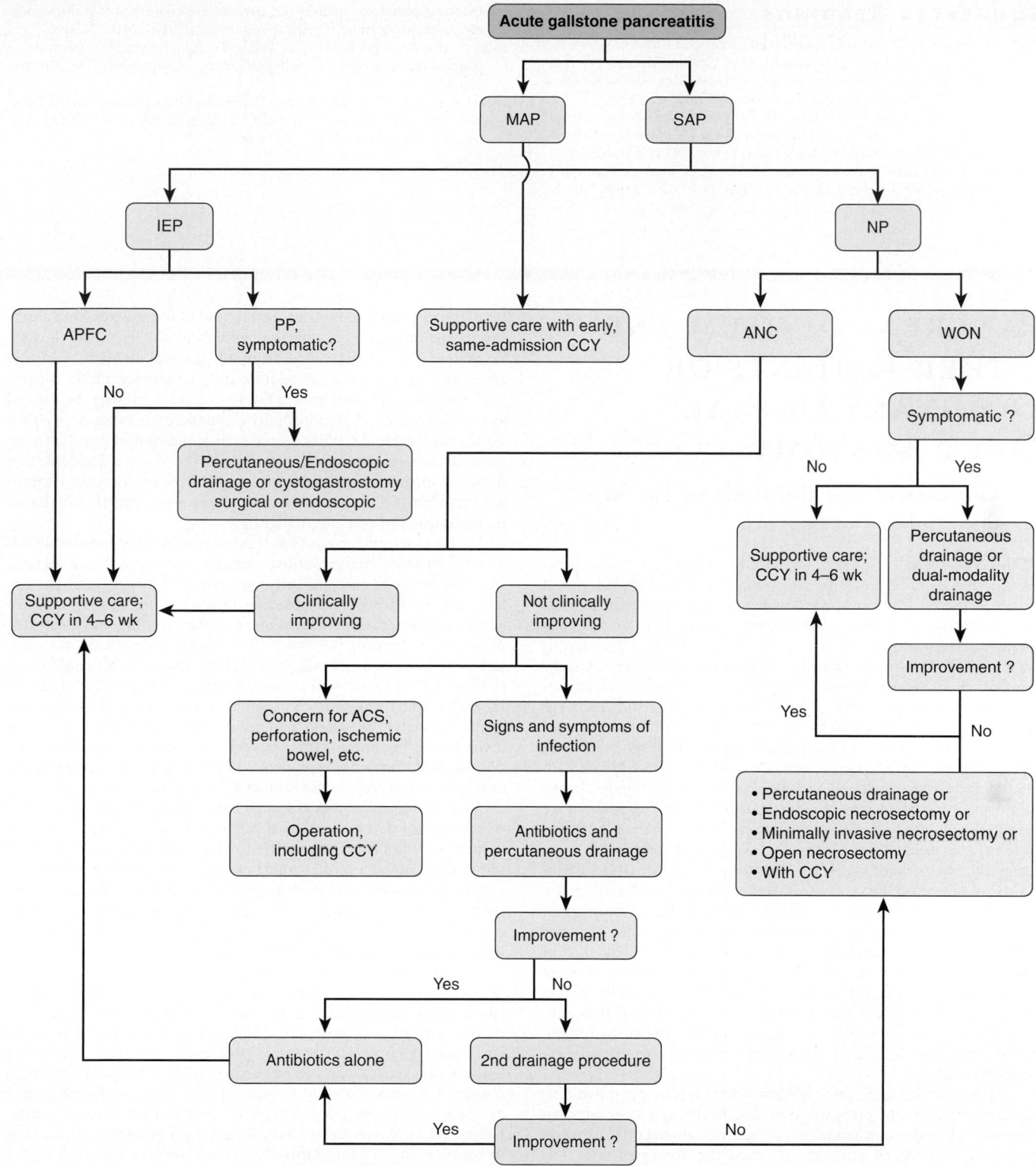

FIGURE 2 Algorithm for the management of gallstone pancreatitis (GSP). *ACS,* Abdominal compartment syndrome; *ANC,* acute necrotic collection; *APFC,* acute peripancreatic fluid collection; *CCY,* cholecystectomy; *IEP,* interstitial edematous pancreatitis; *MAP,* mild acute pancreatitis; *NP,* necrotizing pancreatitis; *PP,* pancreatic pseudocyst; *SAP,* severe acute pancreatitis; *WON,* walled-off necrosis. (*Modified from Sabo S, Goussous N, Sardana S, Patel ST, Cunningham SC. Necrotizing pancreatitis: a review of multidisciplinary management. JOP. 2015;16:125-135.*)

SUGGESTED READINGS

Banks PA, Bollen TL, Dervenis C, Gooszen HG, Johnson CD, Sarr MG, Tsiotos GG, Vege SS, Acute Pancreatitis Classification Working Group. Classification of acute pancreatitis—2012: revision of the Atlanta classification and definitions by international consensus. *Gut.* 2013;62:102-111.

Gurusamy KS, Nagendran M, Davidson BR. Early versus delayed laparoscopic cholecystectomy for acute gallstone pancreatitis. *Cochrane Database Syst Rev.* 2013;(9):CD010326, doi:10.1002/14651858.CD010326.pub2.

Maqsood H, Goussous N, Parthasarathy M, Horne C, Kaur G, Setiawan L, Sautter A, James S, Ferdosi H, Sill AM, Kowdley GC, Cunningham SC

Does computed tomography (CT) overestimate common-bile-duct diameter in the evaluation of gallstone pancreatitis? *JOP.* 2016;17:216.

Sabo S, Goussous N, Sardana S, Patel ST, Cunningham SC. Necrotizing pancreatitis: a review of multidisciplinary management. *JOP.* 2015;16:125-135.

Shmelev A, Abdo A, Sachdev S, Shah U, Kowdley GC, Cunningham SC. Energetic etiologies of acute pancreatitis: a report of five cases. *World J Gastrointest Pathophysiol.* 2015;6:243-248.

PANCREAS DIVISUM AND OTHER VARIANTS OF DOMINANT DORSAL DUCT ANATOMY

David B. Adams, MD, and Gregory A. Coté, MD, MS

Three strategies are used in the surgical management of inflammatory disorders of the pancreas: improve drainage, resect damaged tissue, or combine the first two with a simultaneous resection and drainage procedure. These principles apply to the management of recurrent acute pancreatitis and chronic pancreatitis associated with dominant dorsal duct anatomy, which is more commonly called pancreas divisum. The prudent surgeon always remembers that pancreas divisum is as common as left-handedness: 10 percent of the population has pancreas divisum. The anatomic variant known as pancreas divisum develops in the busy 6-week-old embryo (Figure 1). Migration, rotation, and vacuolization are happening everywhere in the 6- to 8-week embryonic foregut. During this developmental period the dorsal and ventral pancreatic buds fuse and realign their ductal systems. In the usual fusion of the ductal systems, the ventral duct or duct of Wirsung becomes the main pancreatic duct (Figure 2, *A, B*). The dorsal duct, the duct of Santorini, is the minor duct (Figure 2, *A*). When dorsal and ventral ductal fusion is incomplete, the duct of Santorini drains the majority of the pancreas through an orifice that is notably smaller than the orifice of a normal sphincter of Oddi (Figure 2, *C, D*). The duct of Santorini may have a narrow filamentous pathway to the duct of Wirsung or may drain a portion of the head independently (Figure 2, *E*). Hence the concept was promulgated in the 1970s that in pancreas divisum there is an anatomic impediment to the normal drainage of pancreatic exocrine secretions, which results in an obstructive pancreatopathy.

In pancreas divisum, which is the main pancreatic duct? Avoiding the descriptor "main" prevents confusion in discussion of pancreas divisum. When divisum anatomy is present, the dorsal duct, formerly known as the duct of Santorini, is called the dominant duct. The terms *complete fusion* and *incomplete fusion* have been used to describe variants of pancreatic ductal anatomy associated with dominant dorsal duct anatomy. Complete divisum typically denotes a dominant dorsal duct with no vestigial communication to the ventral system (duct of Wirsung). Incomplete divisum denotes a dominant dorsal duct with a residual, albeit miniscule communication between the dorsal duct and the ventral duct. Variations of the dominant dorsal duct are many and infrequent enough that radiologic and endoscopic delineation may be confusing. The classic radiographic image has the dominant pancreatic duct crossing the terminal bile duct and entering the descending duodenum (Figure 3). Usually a

small ductal system drains the ventral head of the pancreas and enters the duodenum through the major papilla with the terminal bile duct. Be aware of the entity called acquired pancreas divisum, which is associated with chronic pancreatitis and malignancy. Either process may result in total occlusion of the ventral duct, causing the duct of Santorini to assume responsibility for pancreatic exocrine outflow via the minor papilla. Whenever there is a question of acquired pancreas divisum (also called "pseudodivisum") without a demonstrated mass on magnetic resonance imaging (MRI) or computed tomographic scan (CT scan), endoscopic ultrasound scan (EUS) should be undertaken to rule out malignancy.

In the nineteenth century foregut surgeons were commonly talented anatomists. In the twentieth century physiology was of increasing importance to the innovative surgeon. The twenty-first century has seen the addition of molecular biology to the management of surgical disorders. The history of the understanding and treatment of pancreas divisum has followed a similar pathway. In the past, pancreas divisum was labeled a congenital anomaly that could cause obstructive pain and pancreatitis. With the development of diagnostic endoscopic retrograde cholangiopancreatography (ERCP) in the 1970s, idiopathic recurrent pancreatitis was attributed to pancreas divisum and became a target for surgical management with duodenotomy and minor duct sphincteroplasty. As therapeutic endoscopy developed, endoscopic minor duct sphincterotomy or papillotomy supplanted the open surgical approach. Although sphincteroplasty was successful in the majority of patients in early studies, long-term failures were not uncommon. Improving patient selection based on physiologic and anatomic parameters with measurement of pancreatic ductal response and exocrine output to hormonal stimulation of the exocrine pancreas was used. However, early optimism of improving patient selection via physiologic assessment did not meaningfully improve long-term outcomes (Figure 1).

Chronic pancreatitis and acute recurrent pancreatitis are disorders that lack strong evidence on which surgical practice can be based. Many other similar "gray zone" disorders are multifactorial in origin. Scurvy is a disease with a single and simple cause that can be cured with vitamin C. If chronic pancreatitis were like scurvy and had a single cause, it would be easily curable. Chronic pancreatitis has many known risk factors, many of which are overlapping, such as alcohol and smoking. Anatomic, environmental, and genetic factors are likely to interact with the divisum phenotype in causing or contributing to pancreatitis. Pancreas divisum is clearly associated with a higher prevalence of genetic mutations that predispose to pancreatitis; this has led to the current concept that pancreas divisum is not a cause of pancreatitis by itself but acts as a partner with genetic mutations. In patients with idiopathic pancreatitis, pancreas divisum is not an independent risk factor when compared with controls without pancreas divisum. However, pancreas divisum frequency is higher in patients with genetic mutations and pancreatitis, especially those with *CFTR* mutations or polymorphisms, suggesting a cumulative effect of these two cofactors. *SPINK1* and *PRSS1* functional genetic anomalies are also associated with pancreas divisum and acute recurrent and chronic pancreatitis.

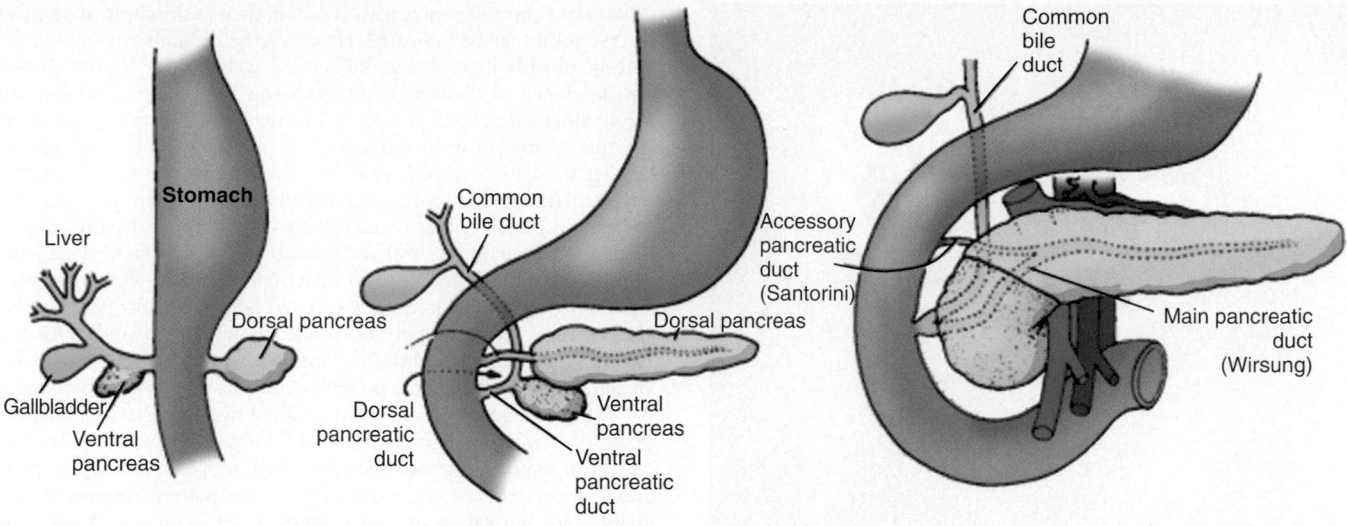

FIGURE 1 Embryologic development of the pancreas.

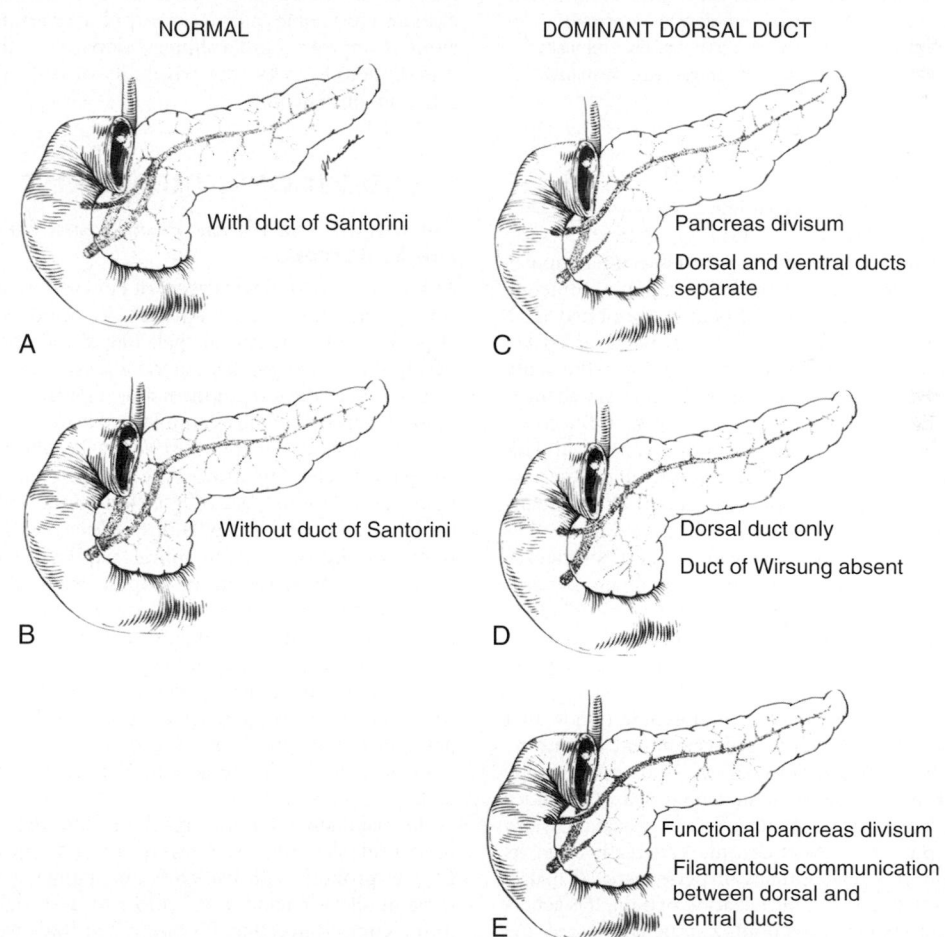

NORMAL

DOMINANT DORSAL DUCT

A   With duct of Santorini

B   Without duct of Santorini

C   Pancreas divisum
Dorsal and ventral ducts
separate

D   Dorsal duct only
Duct of Wirsung absent

E   Functional pancreas divisum
Filamentous communication
between dorsal and
ventral ducts

FIGURE 2 Line drawings of most common pancreatic ductal anatomy (**A, B**) and pancreas divisum and its variants (**C** to **E**).

■ DIAGNOSIS

The clinical presentation of pancreatitis associated with dominant dorsal duct anatomy has two variations: acute recurrent pancreatitis and chronic pancreatitis. Current concepts suggest that the former leads to the latter. Rarely does chronic pancreatitis associated with

pancreas divisum result in severe fibrosing pancreatitis associated with biliary, duodenal, or splanchnic venous obstruction. Pain intractable to medical management is the main reason patients with pancreas divisum seek the help of surgeons and gastroenterologists. Patients with acute pancreatitis associated with pancreas divisum present the same way other patients with pancreatitis do. Pain that

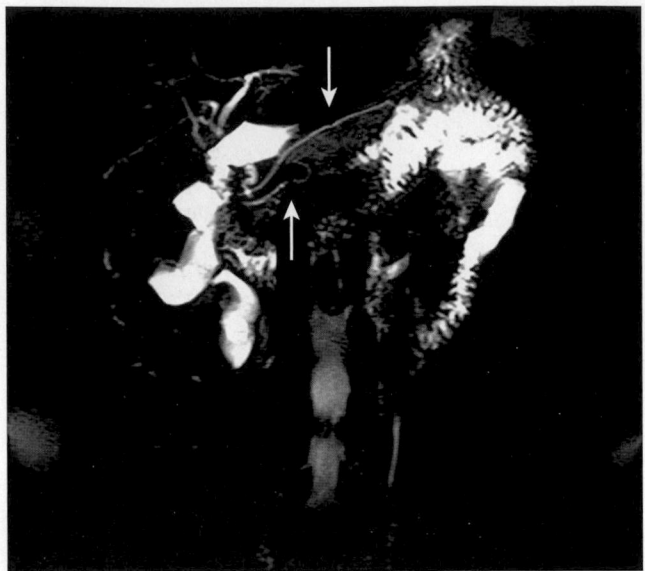

FIGURE 3 Pancreas divisum magnetic resonance cholangiopancreatography (MRCP) with the dorsal duct (Santorini labeled with downward arrow) crossing the terminal bile duct, which unites with the ventral duct remnant (Wirsung labeled with upward arrow). Dorsal and ventral ducts terminate respectively at major and minor papilla.

triggers nausea and vomiting is the predominant symptom. The pain is notable for its intensity, character, and location. Patients localize the pain to the epigastrium with radiation into the interscapular region. Pain is commonly characterized by the sensation of someone twisting a knife in the upper abdomen. The pain is often rated as 11 on a scale of 1 to 10. Serum lipase is elevated, as may be the leukocyte count and other inflammatory serologic markers. When the acute illness is severe, pancreatic and peripancreatic inflammatory changes will be seen on CT scan and MRI studies. If pancreatic necrosis develops in the presence of pancreas divisum, other pancreatitis risk factors should be considered. It is uncommon for acute pancreatitis associated with pancreas divisum to lead to pancreatic and peripancreatic necrosis. The usual course is that of a self-limited illness that resolves with expectant, nonoperative management and hospitalization of less than 1 week. With resolution of the acute illness, patients return to normal function and activities and pancreas morphology presumably returns to normal. If recurrent bouts of acute pancreatitis continue, changes of chronic pancreatitis may become evident on cross-sectional imaging.

A hopeful hypothesis recommends that endoscopic minor duct sphincterotomy be undertaken before the development of chronic inflammatory and fibrotic changes. The goals of endoscopic therapy are to (1) eliminate future episodes of acute pancreatitis; (2) reduce the frequency or severity of recurrent bouts of acute pancreatitis; and (3) prevent the development of overt chronic pancreatitis and its complications, primarily the development of peripancreatic neural inflammatory pathways that lead to centralization of pain. It is generally assumed that if acute pancreatitis bouts can be eliminated, the third objective would follow suit. On the other hand, the chief indication for surgical therapy of pancreas divisum is pain; endocrine and exocrine insufficiency is rare, as are biliary, duodenal, and splanchnic venous occlusion.

The more difficult patient is one who has had one bout of acute pancreatitis or no documented evidence of pancreatitis but who has pancreas divisum and chronic pain that is characteristic of pancreatitis. When patient quality of life is diminished by frequent emergency department visits, work absences, and loss of social contacts, evaluation with MRI and EUS is indicated. If objective evidence of

obstructive chronic pancreatitis is noted, then endoscopic or surgical intervention may be indicated. However, the difficulty in waiting for chronic morphologic changes to develop is that once chronic fibrosis has developed in the head of the pancreas, endoscopic and surgical minor duct sphincterotomy have a limited success rate. Division of the sparse smooth muscle fibers of the minor sphincter is unlikely to alter the hardened fibrosis of the surrounding pancreatic parenchyma. The prudent surgeon remembers that when you cut scar tissue, you get more scar tissue. When you operate for pain, you get pain. The splanchnic neural architecture is vast and lacks specificity. Biliary, gastric, esophageal, and intestinal disorders all may appear similar to pain and nausea associated with chronic pancreatitis. Nevertheless, surgeons and gastroenterologists who undertake the care of patients with chronic pancreatitis and pancreas divisum engage in changing what is possible and offer the hope of helping a patient whose quality of life is diminished by unpredictable hospital visits and isolation from work and family. This care requires the collaboration of pancreatic surgeons, endoscopic specialists in pancreatic disease, behavioral psychologists, and pain management specialists. In general, endoscopic therapy for pancreas divisum is typically recommended for pancreatic-type pain in association with obstructive morphology (e.g., a dilated pancreatic duct or santorinicele) or documented recurrent acute pancreatitis without another clear and reversible cause. Minor sphincterotomy for abdominal pain alone is unproven and a slippery slope; once the orifice is compromised, there is always the possibility of orifice restenosis and bona fide duct obstruction.

■ ENDOSCOPIC TREATMENT

Identifying the Minor Papilla and Positioning the Endoscope

Although the pathologic nature of pancreas divisum remains controversial, the endoscopic approach to minor papillotomy is more elegant. The first technical challenge to therapy is successfully identifying the minor papilla. Duodenoscopes are designed for optimal orientation at the level of the major papilla, so positioning the endoscope for minor papilla cannulation usually requires a "semi-long" position. This is illustrated in Figure 4, where the scope is resting along the greater curvature of the stomach. This position is less stable than the traditional "short" position of the duodenoscope used for the majority of major papilla cases. Nevertheless, the semi-long position typically orients the minor papilla directly in front of the working channel; the minor papilla is usually located 2 to 5 cm superior to the major papilla, along the medial wall but slightly lateral to the major papilla. In some cases, the minor papilla may be located underneath an overlying duodenal fold that requires retraction with a catheter or other device before cannulation ensues. Because this procedure requires a long scope position that is uncomfortable for patients who are prone on a fluoroscopy table, it is almost universally performed with anesthesia-administered sedation with or without endotracheal intubation.

Occasionally the minor papilla is patulous and the actual orifice unidentifiable after minutes of careful endoscopic observation. Blindly probing with catheters and guidewires rapidly may cause periampullary edema and transform a straightforward procedure into a complicated one. Probing often leads to false tracks adjacent to the true lumen, rarely causing perforation but often making cannulation impossible. Therefore if a minor papillary orifice is unidentifiable, the minor papilla can be sprayed with a dilute dye such as methylene blue or India ink. After this maneuver, pancreatic juice outflow should lead to clearing of the dye at the minor orifice (Figure 5). Alternatively, or in conjunction with this approach, secretin may be administered (0.2 μg/kg) intravenously over 1 minute to stimulate pancreatic juice flow. This often unveils the minor papillary orifice within minutes of administration and continued careful endoscopic observation.

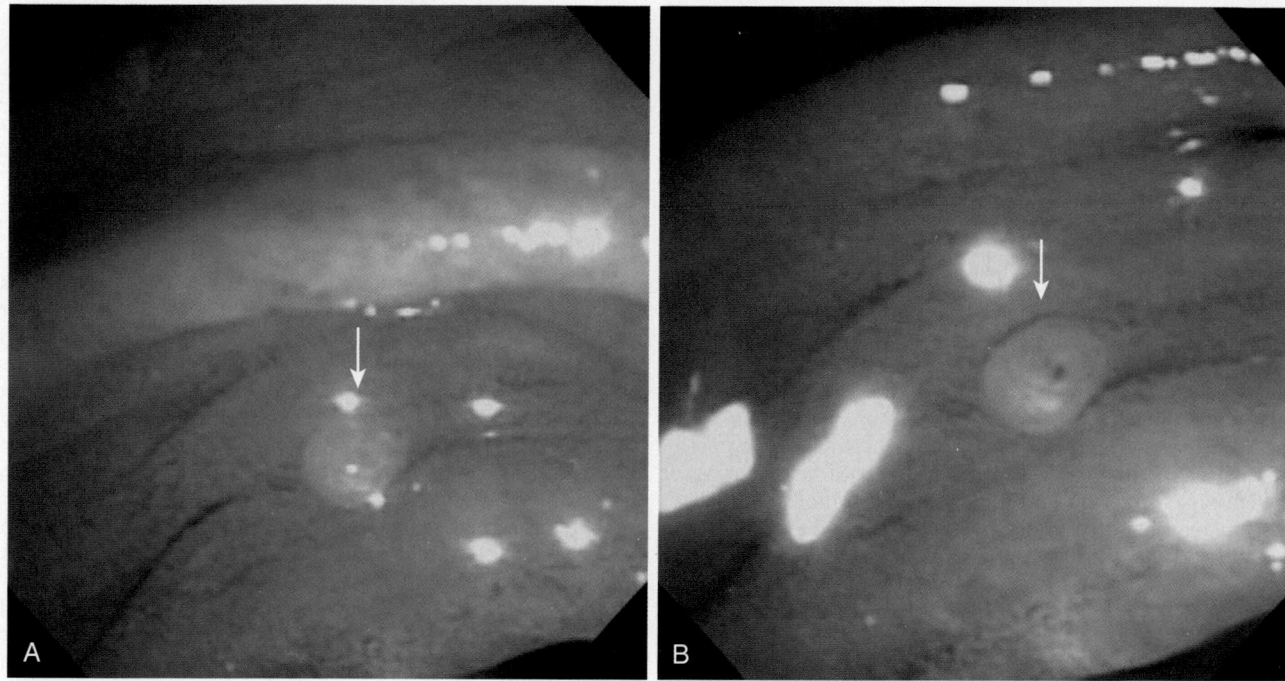

FIGURE 4 Endoscopic image of the minor papilla (*arrow*) with (**A**) a "closed" orifice and (**B**) an "open" orifice.

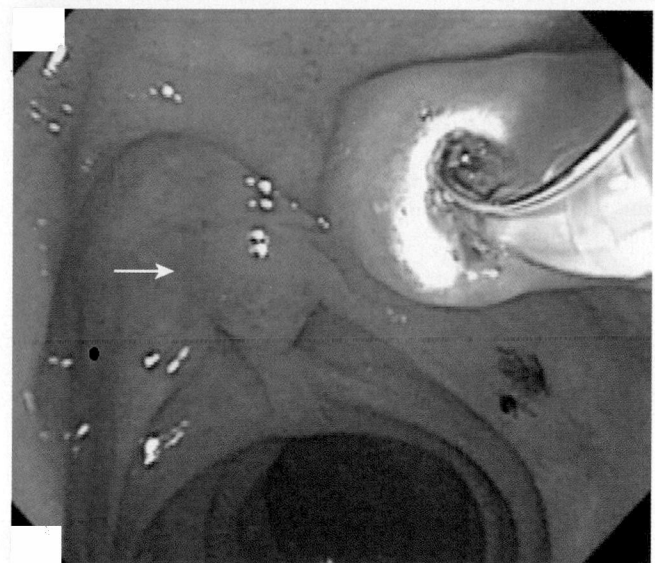

FIGURE 5 Endoscopic image of minor papillotomy "in progress," which also shows (beside the arrow) the major papilla downstream for reference.

An absolute last resort involves the use of a needle-tipped catheter that is gently pressed into the minor papilla, followed by light injection of radio contrast dye to delineate the configuration of the Santorini duct. If the needle is inserted into the submucosal layer of the minor papilla or duodenum, such an injection may result in a submucosal bleb and obliterate the papillary anatomy for a short period, often making minor papillary cannulation impossible during that procedure.

Cannulation

Once the minor papillary orifice is clearly delineated, most endoscopists prefer to gain access using a tapered cannula or sphincterotome

(3F or 4F tip) with a hydrophilic, straight guidewire. Most experts prefer a smaller caliber (0.018-, 0.021-, or 0.025-inch) guidewire because the orifice is considerably smaller than the major papilla. The leading 3 to 4 mm of guidewire protruding from the catheter tip is used to grip the minor orifice; at this point, the endoscopist or assistant may probe gently with the guidewire under fluoroscopic guidance; if the guidewire advances with minimal resistance, then 2 to 5 cm of guidewire may be advanced into the duct before contrast injection. Guidewires should not be advanced deeply to the body or tail of the pancreas without antecedent injection of a small amount of contrast to delineate the course of the duct and avoid side branch puncture. Alternatively, the cannula or sphincterotome may be inserted gently into the minor orifice first, followed by probing with the guidewire. This is suboptimal in many cases because the orifice is usually less than 1 mm (3F) and the smallest cannulating devices are 3F at the tip.

Once the guidewire is clearly seated in the main pancreatic duct, it should be advanced carefully along the main duct to the distal body or pancreatic tail. This provides adequate rail support over which the cannula or sphincterotome can be advanced deeply into the duct for further opacification and positioning for sphincterotomy.

Minor Endoscopic Sphincterotomy

There are two approaches to minor endoscopic sphincterotomy, each of which has advantages and disadvantages. There are no data to support one approach over the other. The first approach is a pull-type minor sphincterotomy that mimics the standard technique for biliary and pancreatic sphincterotomy at the major papilla. With a sphincterotome, the device is bowed within the minor orifice, and electrocautery is applied to cut the superior aspect of the "muscle." This word is in quotations because many minor papillae have no or miniscule smooth muscle, leaving the characterization as a "sphincter muscle" very much in doubt. Electrocautery is typically a blend of alternating/mixed cut and coagulation currents, to minimize char while permitting an adequate incision to enlarge the orifice. Some experts advocate using a pure cut current for minor sphincterotomy, to minimize the risk of orifice restenosis; this comes with a slightly higher risk of bleeding and has not been shown to affect long-term outcomes. The advantage of the pull-type technique is that it is most likely to minimize the risk of an incomplete incision; however, if an excessive amount of cut wire is left inside the pancreatic duct during the sphincterotomy, this is likely to induce post-ERCP pancreatitis and delayed high-grade strictures at the orifice.

An alternative and widely accepted approach is to perform a needle-knife sphincterotomy over a pancreatic stent. In this case, a small caliber (3F to 5F) pancreatic stent is deployed over the guidewire. With a needle-knife sphincterotome, the minor sphincterotomy is performed by cutting on the superior aspect of the stent until the stent is exposed within the duct itself. This technique is believed to have a lower risk of postsphincterotomy perforation but may be associated with a higher rate of incompletely dividing the minor orifice. In cases of failed minor cannulation, a precut or free hand (without the guidance of a pancreatic stent) needle-knife sphincterotomy may be attempted to expose the minor orifice for deeper access. Given the higher rates of post-ERCP pancreatitis and unproven technical benefits, this maneuver should be used very sparingly. Unlike the biliary sphincter complex, the duct of Santorini rarely has a long intraduodenal segment to guide the depth and orientation of the incision.

Pancreatitis Prevention

For the past two decades, the mainstay for preventing post-ERCP pancreatitis has been the use of small caliber pancreatic stents (3F to 5F). These have been shown to reduce the risk of post-ERCP pancreatitis in multiple randomized clinical trials, presumably by reducing intraductal pressure in the critical hours or days after ERCP and its associated papillary trauma. The efficacy of prophylactic stents after minor papilla endotherapy mirrors that for patients with standard pancreatic duct anatomy. Importantly, patients with pancreas divisum who undergo ERCP solely for major papilla therapy have a lower baseline risk of post-ERCP pancreatitis; once minor papilla cannulation is attempted, however, the risk approaches that of the highest-risk populations. Therefore most experts are uncomfortable performing an endoscopic minor sphincterotomy without placement of a small caliber pancreatic duct stent immediately before or after the incision. The stents pass out of the minor orifice spontaneously in more than 90% of cases; the minority require a second endoscopy to pull the stent if it is retained after 10 to 14 days on a follow-up x-ray.

Postprocedure, rectal indomethacin (100 mg) is the first widely accepted pharmacologic intervention to minimize the risk of post-ERCP pancreatitis. The medication is administered anytime immediately before, during, or at the completion of the ERCP, and presumably reduces the risk of post-ERCP pancreatitis by interrupting the earliest inflammatory cascades triggered by papillary trauma and intraductal hypertension. Its efficacy as a freestanding preventive modality—without pancreatic stents—remains unproven for patients with pancreas divisum undergoing minor endoscopic sphincterotomy. However, the medication is inexpensive and low risk, so has become widely popular as an adjunct for high-risk patients.

Postprocedure Management

The majority of patients undergoing ERCP may be discharged 1 to 2 hours after the procedure. Preprocedure and early postprocedure pain or nausea are important predictors of unplanned admission after ERCP. Intravenous fluids, preferably Lactated Ringer's solution, should be administered during ERCP and in the recovery room in case pancreatitis ensues. If there are no symptoms concerning for post-ERCP pancreatitis and the procedure was otherwise uneventful, patients may be discharged home after a short period of observation.

Approximately 10% to 15% of patients will require overnight observation after ERCP; admission rates after endoscopic minor sphincterotomy are unknown but the post-ERCP pancreatitis rate is also 10% to 15%. The majority of these patients will improve within 72 hours of the procedure but a small minority (1% to 2% of all patients with post-ERCP pancreatitis) may develop severe acute pancreatitis and local complications such as pseudocysts or necrosis. The possibility of post-ERCP pancreatitis—mild or severe—must be considered when weighing the risks and benefits of endoscopic therapy.

■ SURGICAL TREATMENT

Minor Duct Sphincteroplasty

Operative sphincteroplasty of the sphincter of Henle was the mainstay of therapy before the development of endoscopic sphincterotomy. It is hard to imagine how an operative sphincteroplasty can be better than an endoscopic sphincterotomy, given the sparseness of smooth muscle fibers that surround the pancreatic duct as it courses into the duodenum. Occasional patients with bypassed foregut anatomy may elect open surgical sphincterotomy and forgo a retrograde endoscopic approach or a hybrid laparoscopic and endoscopic prograde approach. Surgical outcomes with open sphincteroplasty are best when endoscopic sphincterotomy has not been done before. The first cut is the best one. It is tempting to undertake open sphincteroplasty in patients with altered foregut anatomy, such as gastric bypass patients. These patients may be well served by a hybrid procedure with concomitant laparoscopic gastrostomy of the bypassed stomach and endoscopic prograde sphincterotomy. A gastrostomy tube is left in place to secure access for removal of the anastomotic stent later. Patients with prior Billroth II gastrectomy are not candidates for endotherapy. A retrograde approach to the minor papilla does not provide angulation that allows for endoscopic sphincterotomy. Patients who previously have undergone successful endoscopic sphincterotomy with recurrent fibrosis may be candidates for operative sphincteroplasty. The concept is that open minor duct sphincteroplasty with loop magnification and fine absorbable suturing of the duct will have better outcomes than endoscopic sphincterotomy. The difficulty in undertaking this course of action is that patients with chronic fibrosis of the head of the pancreas do poorly with sphincteroplasty and preoperative identification of pancreatic fibrosis is imperfect.

Technique

The most recent ERCP and magnetic resonance cholangiopancreatography (MRCP) are displayed on the operating theater monitors closest to the surgeon, who has on a headlamp and magnifying loops. The abdomen is entered through an upper midline incision. The falciform ligament is divided when it limits placement of a wound protector or retraction of the liver. A self-retaining retractor is placed to retract the abdominal wall in order to divide the lateral duodenal attachments and the ligamentous attachments of the transverse colon to the duodenal pancreatic union. After the wide kocherization of the duodenum and mobilization of the hepatic flexure of the colon inferiorly and laterally, the duodenum is mobilized medially to the midline. Exposure is maintained with the self-retaining retractors placed around the wound circumference, retracting liver, stomach, and transverse colon out of sight. A laparotomy pad is placed behind the duodenum to elevate it toward the midline. A longitudinal duodenotomy is made in the descending duodenum, angled slightly from medial to lateral as the electrocautery knife goes from proximal to distal duodenum. Intraluminal exposure is maintained by grasping the medial and superior duodenal wall with a Babcock clamp or with stay sutures of 3-0 silk. The major papilla is identified with palpation and visualization of bile expressed with manual compression of the gallbladder and common bile duct. Centimeters proximal to the major papilla, the minor papilla can be palpated on the medial wall of the duodenum. Care is taken not to distort duodenal mucosa by direct suction and grasping with a forceps, as minor mucosal trauma can obscure visualization of the minor papilla. The minor papilla is palpated and cannulated with a lacrimal duct probe (Figure 6). When the papilla cannot be found, secretin stimulation can be used, but this increases the risk of postoperative pancreatitis, particularly if operative drainage has limited success. Sphincterotomy is accomplished by dividing the sphincter muscle with needle-knife low-energy cautery over the lacrimal duct probe. Care is taken to cut only red muscle fibers. When yellow pancreatic tissue is encountered, the sphincterotomy is complete. Two or three interrupted sutures of 5-0 monofilament absorbable sutures are placed to reapproximate duodenal and ductal mucosa (Figure 7). Minor duct sphincteroplasty is distinctly different from that of a biliary sphincteroplasty where the common bile duct lies parallel and juxtaposed to the duodenum, which allows for a lengthy sphincterotomy. The minor duct enters the duodenum at right angles from the pancreas. There is not a lot of room to cut this sphincter. A 3F or 5F double pigtail stent is placed across the anastomosis. It is removed endoscopically 6 weeks later. The duodenotomy is closed with a running suture of 3-0 absorbable monofilament suture, reinforced as needed with interrupted sutures of 3-0 silk. The fascia is reapproximated with interrupted zero absorbable sutures. The skin is closed with a 4-0 running subcuticular suture. Closed suction drainage of the retroduodenal space is not used routinely. Because stenosis of the major papilla is associated with pancreas divisum, some would advocate performing biliary sphincteroplasty and pancreatic ductal septoplasty whenever minor duct sphincteroplasty is undertaken. This indication is exceptional but not irrational.

Postoperative Management

Patients are managed on a fast track much as one would manage a patient after an open cholecystectomy. Nasogastric and urinary bladder intubation are avoided. Diet is advanced early as tolerated. Complications particular to this operation are pancreatitis and duodenotomy dehiscence (Table 1). Postoperative pancreatitis is uncommon and presents in typical fashion with pain, tachycardia, and serum lipase and leukocyte elevation. Duodenal dehiscence presents in a subtle fashion, similar to a duodenal stump leak after Billroth II gastrectomy. Vague upper abdominal pain and nausea precede by days the appearance of systemic toxicity with fever, tachycardia, tachypnea, and leukocytosis. Alert vigilance for this complication is needed because it is uncommon, subtle in presentation, and devastating if unrecognized early.

Lateral Pancreaticojejunostomy

Dominant ductal dilation is an indication for lateral pancreaticojejunostomy (LPJ) in chronic pancreatitis associated with pancreas

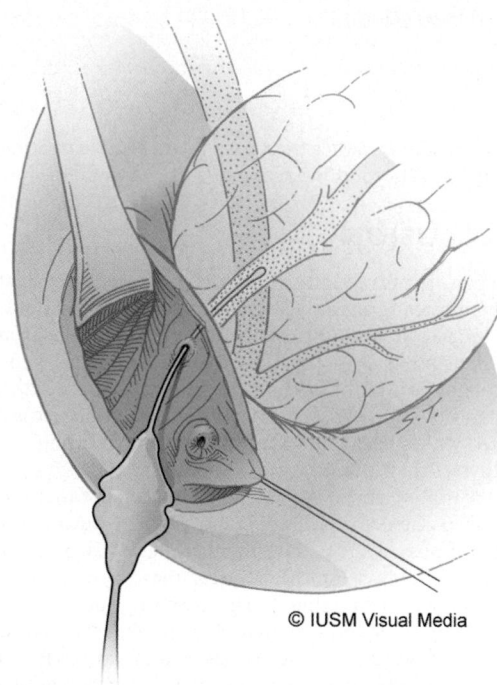

FIGURE 6 Through a longitudinal duodenotomy the minor papilla is identified and cannulated with a lacrimal duct probe.

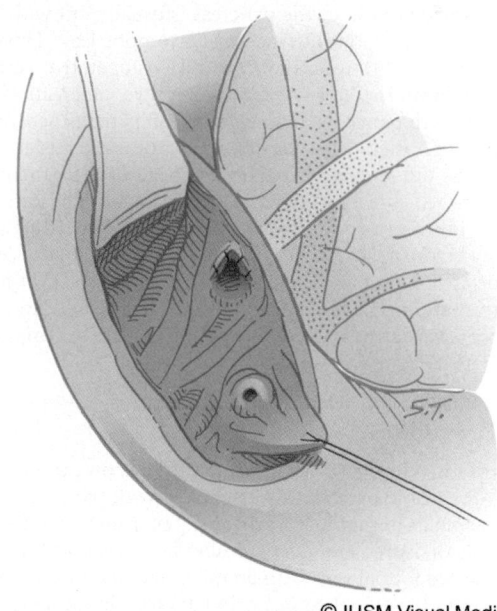

FIGURE 7 After division of the muscular fibers of the sphincter of Henle with needle-knife electrocautery, the termination of the dorsal pancreatic duct is anastomosed to the duodenal mucosa with interrupted sutures.

TABLE 1: Surgical Outcome After Minor Duct Sphincteroplasty in Patients With Pancreas Divisum

Author, Year	N	Morbidity	Mortality	Good Response	Mean Follow-Up, Months
Warshaw, 1990	88	NR	0	71%	53
Bradley, 1996	37	NR	0	54%	60
Madura, 2005	74	25%	0	64%	NR
Morgan, 2008	17	10%	0	54%	43

NR, Not reported.

divisum. Outcomes after LPJ are similar to those reported with chronic pancreatitis not associated with pancreas divisum. In particular, the patient with the borderline dilated pancreatic duct not greater than 7 mm in diameter may benefit from LPJ when diffuse fibrosis of the pancreas is present with a fibrotic encapsulation of the pancreas. LPJ has the theoretic advantage of releasing the pancreas from its so-called pancreatic compartment syndrome. Part of the discussion of LPJ in the management of chronic pancreatitis of all causes is that if LPJ fails and the patient progresses to consideration of total pancreatectomy with islet autotransplantation (TPIAT), islet yields are diminished in patients who have had LPJ, related to either the underlying disease state or technical challenges presented by islet isolation in patients who have a longitudinal disruption of the pancreatic duct. The technique of LPJ in pancreas divisum does not differ from that discussed elsewhere in this book. Because the pancreas ductotomy is extended medially adjacent to the duodenum, the gastroduodenal artery should be ligated before its division.

Whipple Procedure

Pancreatoduodenectomy may be indicated in patients with pancreas divisum who have failed minor duct sphincteroplasty when changes of chronic pancreatitis develop in the head of the pancreas. The operative technique is not different from that described elsewhere in this book. When a resection of the head is indicated in pancreas divisum, the divided neck of the pancreas is usually soft with a nondilated pancreatic duct, one at risk for anastomotic leak. Thus internal and external anastomotic stenting and postoperative octreotide infusion may diminish the risk of postoperative pancreatic fistulas. If head resection in pancreas divisum fails and patients become candidates for TPIAT, islet yields may be uncompromised. Islet volume is greater in the tail and body than in the head of the pancreas and islet loss is limited in a head resection for pancreas divisum. When anastomotic obstruction occurs after a Whipple procedure, acinar cells atrophy before destruction of the islets. The resultant islet-rich, acinar-poor atrophied pancreas may be favorable isolation for islet autotransplantation. The issue of whether pancreas divisum patients with chronic pancreatitis should undergo a speculative Whipple procedure or a TPIAT is unanswered.

Hybrid Procedures

Variations of the Whipple procedure and the Puestow procedure have been used in chronic pancreatitis associated with pancreas divisum in a fashion similar to their use in chronic pancreatitis not associated with pancreas divisum. Though typically the Beger and Frey procedures are selected for patients with an inflammatory mass in the head of the pancreas, they have been used in pancreas divisum not associated with enlargement of the head of the pancreas. The Frey procedure was developed because of the ascribed failure of the LPJ to drain the head and uncinate process of the pancreas. In pancreas divisum the head should be drained effectively with a longitudinal ductotomy. The use of multiple resection and drainage techniques is an indication of the difficulty in patient selection and management in chronic pancreatitis associated with pancreas divisum.

Total Pancreatectomy With Islet Autotransplantation

TPIAT is indicated in patients with chronic pancreatitis with intractable pain who have failed medical, endoscopic, and surgical management. Pancreas divisum is a risk factor for chronic pancreatitis in about 15% of the cohort in the reports of TPIAT in the management of chronic pancreatitis. Typical pancreas divisum patients who are selected to TPIAT have undergone endoscopic sphincterotomy, operative sphincteroplasty, and pancreatic head resection in succession over many years. The unanswered question is whether TPIAT should

TABLE 2: Management Strategies for Pancreas Divisum in the Setting of Chronic Pancreatitis Intractable to Medical Management or With Recurrent Acute Pancreatitis

Nonfamilial, dilated duct >7 mm	Lateral pancreaticojejunostomy
Familial	Total pancreatectomy with islet autotransplantation (TPIAT)
Nondilated duct with recurrent acute pancreatitis	Endoscopic minor papillotomy
Nondilated duct endotherapy failure	Operative sphincteroplasty
Nondilated duct endotherapy failure with moderate to severe chronic pancreatitis in the head	Pancreatoduodenectomy
Operative sphincteroplasty failure	Pancreatoduodenectomy
Pancreatoduodenectomy failure	TPIAT

be undertaken sooner rather than later if endoscopic treatment fails. That discussion is beyond the scope of this chapter.

■ CONCLUSION

Given the paucity of comparative effectiveness studies evaluating the impact of endoscopic or surgical minor papillotomy on nonobstructive recurrent acute and chronic pancreatitis, the management of pancreas divisum is primarily based on experience. Though the divisum anatomic variant is common, its association with chronic pancreatitis is by no means a *sine qua non*. When pancreas divisum is associated with intractable pain associated with chronic pancreatitis or with recurrent pancreatitis, alcohol and tobacco cessation is necessary. A trial of pancreatic enzyme replacement therapy should be undertaken. Genetic mutations and polymorphisms should be investigated if possible. A management strategy based on a regional experience extending with the surgical management of pancreas divisum is suggested in Table 2. The pathway outlined in Table 2 differs from much of the experience in the current literature and underscores the influence of regional population differences and their attendant practices. As the pathogenesis of pancreatitis is better understood, treatment strategies will become less intuitive and experience based and more effective.

To seek and to find evidence on which to base the management of pancreas divisum is to repeat Samuel Johnson's experience described in the preface to his 1755 *A Dictionary of the English Language*: "I saw that one inquiry only gave occasion to another, that book referred to book, that to search was not always to find, and to find was not always to be informed; and that thus to pursue perfection, was, like the first inhabitants of Arcadia, to chase the sun, which, when they had reached the hill where he seemed to rest, was still beheld at the same distance from them."

SUGGESTED READINGS

Bertin C, Pelletier AL, Vullierme MP, et al. Pancreas divisum is not a cause of pancreatitis by itself but acts as a partner of genetic mutations. *Am J Gastroenterol.* 2012;107:311-317.

Borak GD, Romagnuolo J, Alsolaiman M, et al. Long-term clinical outcomes after endoscopic minor papilla therapy in symptomatic patients with pancreas divisum. *Pancreas.* 2009;38:903-906.

Chacko LN, Chen YK, Shah RJ. Clinical outcomes and nonendoscopic interventions after minor papilla endotherapy in patients with symptomatic pancreas divisum. *Gastrointest Endosc.* 2008;68:667-673.

Cotton PB. Congenital anomaly of pancreas divisum as cause of obstructive pain and pancreatitis. *Gut.* 1980;21:105-114.

Lans JI, Geenen JE, Johanson JF, et al. Endoscopic therapy in patients with pancreas divisum and acute pancreatitis: a prospective, randomized, controlled clinical trial. *Gastrointest Endosc.* 1992;38:430-434.

Morgan KA, Romagnuolo J, Adams DB. Transduodenal sphincteroplasty in the management of sphincter of Oddi dysfunction and pancreas divisum in the modern era. *J Am Coll Surg.* 2008;206:908-914.

Pappas SG, Pilgrim CHC, Kelm R, et al. The Frey procedure for chronic pancreatitis secondary to pancreas divisum. *JAMA Surg.* 2013;148:1057-1062.

Schlosser W, Rau BM, Poch B, et al. Surgical treatment of pancreas divisum causing chronic pancreatitis: the outcome benefits of duodenum-preserving pancreatic head resection. *J Gastrointest Surg.* 2005;9:710-715.

Schnelldorfer T, Adams DB. Outcome after lateral pancreaticojejunostomy in patients with chronic pancreatitis associated with pancreas divisum. *Am Surg.* 2003;69:1041-1044.

Warshaw AL, Simeone JF, Schapiro RH, et al. Evaluation and treatment of the dominant dorsal duct syndrome (pancreas divisum redefined). *Am J Surg.* 1990;159:59-64.

THE MANAGEMENT OF PANCREATIC NECROSIS

Monika A. Krezalek, MD, and John C. Alverdy, MD, FACS

The majority of patients with acute pancreatitis experience a mild form of the disease limited to interstitial pancreatic edema without local and systemic complications. Such patients often experience a benign and self-limited course of the disease, which usually resolves within the first week of symptom onset. However, approximately 20% of patients with acute pancreatitis suffer significant complications, many of which can be catastrophic. Between 5% and 10% of patients can develop pancreatic parenchymal and/or peripancreatic tissue necrosis, which is the most feared complication of pancreatitis, carrying an approximate 15% risk of mortality. About one third of patients with necrotizing pancreatitis will develop infected necrosis, a feared and difficult-to-treat complication that carries an associated mortality up to 30%. Traditionally, infected pancreatic necrosis has been considered an absolute indication for urgent operative intervention. However, in the last decade there has been a major shift both in the way severe acute pancreatitis (SAP) and its complications are defined and classified and in the approach and timing of operative intervention. The traditional early open surgical débridement approach largely has been abandoned and replaced by minimally invasive approaches to evacuation and drainage of pancreatic and peripancreatic necrosis. Open operative intervention usually is delayed and mostly avoided because of its high incidence of morbidity and mortality. In this chapter, we describe the current indications and techniques for conservative and operative management of sterile and infected pancreatic necrosis.

■ DEFINITIONS AND DIAGNOSIS

A multidisciplinary consensus conference in Atlanta in 1992 provided a framework for a universally applicable classification system of complications of severe acute pancreatitis. However, improved understanding of the pathophysiology of acute pancreatitis and its complications, specifically organ failure and pancreatic necrosis, along with advances in diagnostic imaging modalities, have uncovered deficiencies in this system and identified the need for its revision. The "Acute Pancreatitis Classification Working Group" published the 2012 international expert consensus report that more precisely defined the various clinical manifestations of severity of acute pancreatitis (Tables 1 and 2).

Complications of acute pancreatitis should be suspected in a patient who displays a protracted course with persistent or worsening abdominal pain, fever, worsening organ failure, and sepsis.

Necrotizing pancreatitis most commonly involves necrosis of both the pancreatic parenchyma and peripancreatic tissues, less commonly necrosis of peripancreatic tissue alone, and rarely necrosis of pancreatic parenchyma alone. Clinically, isolated peripancreatic necrosis may be associated with improved outcomes when compared with the other two entities. However, the severity of organ failure that can accompany SAP does not necessarily correlate to the degree of pancreatic necrosis and vice versa.

Contrast medium–enhanced computed tomography (CECT) is particularly useful in establishing presence and extent of necrosis (Figure 1) as well as diagnosis of local complications of acute pancreatitis (such as venous thrombosis and pseudoaneurysms) (Figure 2). It remains the standard imaging modality for diagnosis of necrotizing pancreatitis. Administration of intravenous contrast is generally necessary, and images ideally should be taken during the pancreatic and portal venous phases. However, the development and demarcation of necrosis evolves over several days, and early CECT may underestimate or fail to detect the extent of necrosis. Therefore optimal timing of initial imaging should occur at least 72 to 96 hours after the onset of symptoms. In addition, there is no evidence that earlier detection of necrosis improves outcomes or necessarily influences treatment. Magnetic resonance imaging (MRI) and transabdominal or endoscopic ultrasound (EUS) also may be used and may be necessary to discriminate the degree of solid debris in the necrotic collections, which are not easily visualized with CECT (Figure 3). The combination of T1- and T2-weighted MRI sequences along with magnetic resonance cholangiopancreatography can be especially useful in defining the extent of necrosis and amount of solid debris, in defining the anatomy of and presence of stones in the biliary tree, and in determining the presence of a disconnected pancreatic duct. In patients with renal impairment, the fat-suppressed T1-weighted images of MRI can detect necrosis even without gadolinium infusion, thus minimizing any further harm to often already compromised renal function.

Local complications, by definition, typically occur in patients with moderately severe and severe pancreatitis and tend to clinically manifest late along the continuum of the inflammatory process. Anatomically there are typically two distinct collection entities that develop within the setting of necrotizing pancreatitis (see Table 2). The first is an acute necrotic collection, which usually is discovered within the first 4 weeks of disease onset. It contains variable amounts of fluid and necrotic material and lacks a well-defined capsule. Walled-off necrosis, in contrast, typically is diagnosed 4 weeks after disease onset and is characterized by a well-defined inflammatory capsule. Both types of collections may be loculated, multiple, distant from the pancreas, and associated with disruption of the main pancreatic duct. Pancreatic and peripancreatic necrosis can remain sterile or become infected. The majority of infections develop during the late phase of necrotizing pancreatitis and do not seem to correlate with the extent of necrosis. Infected necrosis often is suspected on the basis of clinical

TABLE 1: Definition of Severity of Acute Pancreatitis (2012 Revised Atlanta Classification)

	Organ Failure	Local or Systemic Complications
Mild	Absent organ failure	Absent local or systemic complications
Moderately Severe	Transient organ failure (<48 hr)	Local or systemic complications in the absence of persistent organ failure
Severe	Persistent organ failure (>48 hr)	One or more local complications

Table adapted and revised by the authors from Banks PA. Classification of acute pancreatitis–2012: revision of Atlanta classification and definitions by international consensus. *Gut.* 2013;62:102-111.

findings of persistent fever, tachycardia, adynamic ileus, worsening organ dysfunction, and sepsis. Approximately 40% of patients with acute pancreatitis and failure to thrive have infected pancreatic necrosis. Secondary infection of pancreatic necrosis can be confirmed on the CECT by the presence of gas or gas-fluid levels in the collection (Figure 4). Although percutaneous image-guided sampling for bacterial and fungal culture can be occasionally useful to distinguish infected from sterile necrosis, this practice has fallen into disfavor because of the high false-negative rate of the test. In addition, there is now more emphasis on supportive care and delayed procedural intervention regardless of suspected infection status. In general clinical signs and imaging dictate whether infected necrosis is present and tend to drive the decisions regarding procedural intervention. It is important to mention that the term *pancreatic abscess,* which was used historically to describe a localized collection of purulent material without significant necrotic component, is no longer included in the current classification because it is an extremely rare finding and a confusing term that overlaps with other definitions. Other local complications of acute pancreatitis can include gastric outlet

TABLE 2: Local Complications of Moderately Severe or Severe Acute Pancreatitis (2012 Revised Atlanta Classification)

Acute Pancreatitis Entity Local Complications	Definition	Contrast Medium–Enhanced Computed Tomography Findings*	Timing of Diagnosis Relative to Onset of Acute Pancreatitis (AP)
Interstitial edematous pancreatitis	Acute inflammation of the pancreatic parenchyma and peripancreatic tissues without recognizable tissue necrosis	Diffuse pancreatic parenchyma enhancement by IV contrast	
Acute peripancreatic fluid collection (APFC)	Peripancreatic fluid with no associated necrosis and no features of a pseudocyst	Homogenous collection with fluid density confined by normal peripancreatic fascial planes, without intraparenchymal extension, and without definable wall encapsulating the collection	<4 weeks after AP onset
Pancreatic pseudocyst	An encapsulated collection of fluid with a well-defined inflammatory wall usually outside pancreatic parenchyma	Homogenous, well-circumscribed fluid density completely encapsulated by a well-defined wall and no solid components	>4 weeks after AP onset
Necrotizing pancreatitis	Inflammation associated with pancreatic parenchymal and/or peripancreatic necrosis	Lack of pancreatic parenchymal enhancement by IV contrast and/or presence of peripancreatic necrosis	
Acute necrotic collection (ANC)	A collection containing variable amounts of both fluid and necrotic tissue associated with pancreatic parenchymal and/or peripancreatic necrosis; may be sterile or infected	Heterogeneous collection of liquid and nonliquid density of varying degrees without a definable wall encapsulating the collection in the setting of necrotizing pancreatitis; presence of gas indicates infection	<4 weeks after AP onset
Walled-off necrosis (WON)	A mature encapsulated collection of pancreatic and/or peripancreatic necrosis with a well-defined inflammatory wall; may be sterile or infected	Heterogeneous collection of liquid and nonliquid density and various degrees of loculations, completely encapsulated by a well-defined wall in the setting of necrotizing pancreatitis; presence of gas indicates infection	>4 weeks after AP onset

Adapted from Banks PA. Classification of acute pancreatitis–2012: revision of Atlanta classification and definitions by international consensus. *Gut.* 2013;62:102-111.

*Magnetic resonance imaging or endoscopic ultrasound may be necessary to confirm presence/absence of solid collection components.

IV, Intravenous.

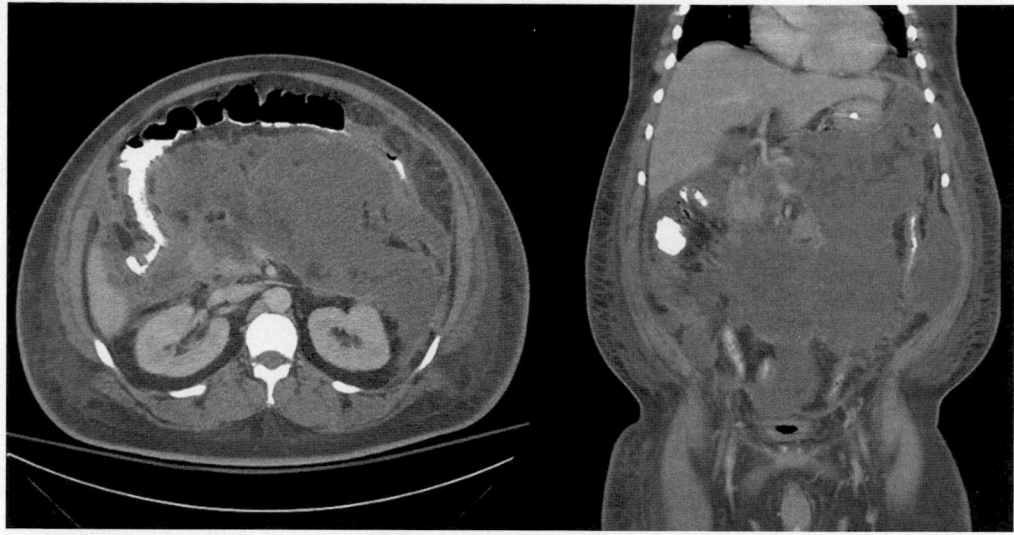

FIGURE 1 Computed tomographic scan with intravenous contrast showing extensive pancreatic and peripancreatic necrosis with virtually no remaining enhancing pancreatic substance. Partial encapsulation of the fluid-filled collection can be appreciated as well as significant infiltrative changes in the peripancreatic fat and ascending colon inflammatory wall thickening. *(Images courtesy Abraham Dachman, MD, Department of Radiology, The University of Chicago Hospitals.)*

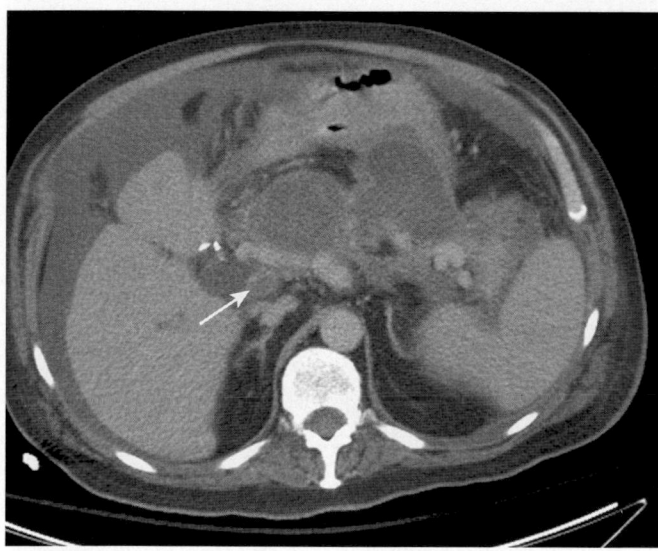

FIGURE 2 Computed tomographic scan with intravenous contrast showing portal venous thrombosis, a complication of necrotizing pancreatitis. Most of the pancreas does not enhance, although there is some residual enhancing parenchyma present in the body and tail. There is extensive thrombus formation within the main portal vein *(arrow)*. *(Image courtesy Abraham Dachman, MD, Department of Radiology, The University of Chicago Hospitals.)*

obstruction, splenic and portal vein thrombosis, pseudoaneurysms, and colonic infarction.

■ INITIAL TREATMENT AND ROLE OF PROPHYLACTIC ANTIBIOTICS

Necrotizing pancreatitis carries especially high mortality rates when associated with organ failure and infection. Therefore much attention has been focused on minimizing the risk of both complications. Evidence shows that decreased rates of persistent systemic inflammatory response syndrome (SIRS) and organ failure can be achieved with early goal directed fluid resuscitation within the first 24 hours of acute pancreatitis diagnosis. Recent evidence also suggests that early enteral nutrition given to patients with predicted severe acute pancreatitis decreases infectious complications, severity of organ failure, need for surgical interventions, and mortality compared with parenteral nutrition. On the basis of results of a recent randomized controlled trial, it is now recommended to provide enteral nutrition within 48 hours of diagnosis whenever possible because of improved outcomes. IAP/APA 2012 guidelines recommend that to improve outcomes of severe acute pancreatitis, it is necessary to manage these patients in an intensive care unit setting within a high-volume specialist center with unrestricted availability of interventional radiologists, endoscopists, and surgeons.

Multiple strategies have been proposed to prevent secondary infection of what is thought to be initially sterile necrosis. Approaches such as parenteral antibiotics, selective gut decontamination, and use of probiotics have been studied and routinely implemented. None of these approaches, however, has proven to be independently associated with improved outcomes. Routine use of prophylactic antibiotics in patients with severe acute pancreatitis and sterile necrosis is not recommended currently given conflicting evidence and concerns regarding the possible selection of resistant strains of bacteria and fungi. Selective gut decontamination has shown reduced rates of infectious complications of acute pancreatitis in animal models; however, these results have not been reproduced clearly in humans and are confounded by concurrent use of systemic antibiotics. Administration of probiotics also has been suggested to replenish health-promoting gut microflora. However, recent evidence has shown that there is no effect on infectious complications and, in one study, an increased mortality rate was observed in patients undergoing probiotic therapy. Therefore both selective gut decontamination and probiotic therapy are not recommended currently.

■ THERAPEUTIC INTERVENTION: INDICATIONS AND TIMING

Historically, severe acute necrotizing pancreatitis, particularly when accompanied by secondary infection, was considered to be an absolute indication for an early surgical intervention. However, recently numerous studies have provided compelling evidence that early intervention within the first 2 weeks of symptom onset is associated with unacceptable high mortality rates. In a retrospective series from

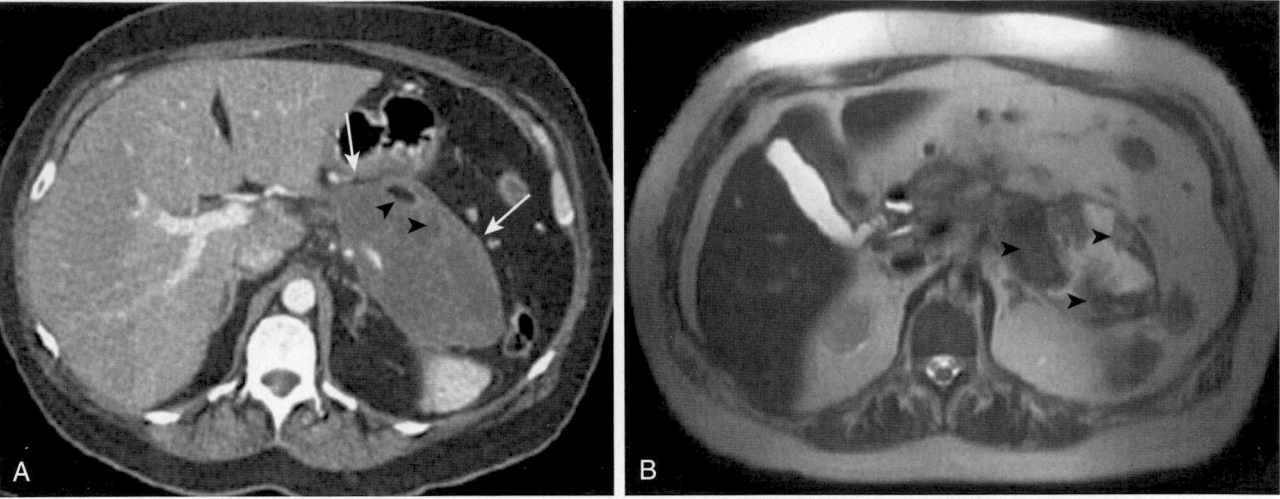

FIGURE 3 Comparison of sensitivity of computed tomography (**A**) and T2-weighted magnetic resonance imaging (**B**) in detecting solid components of pancreatic necrosis. Black arrowheads denote areas of solid necrotic debris, which are better visualized on MRI. White arrows indicate the extent of collection. *(Image adapted from Banks PA, Bollen TL, Dervenis C, et al [Acute Pancreatitis Classification Working Group]. Classification of acute pancreatitis—2012: revision of the Atlanta classification and definitions by international consensus. Gut. 2013;62:102-111.)*

the Netherlands, open necrosectomy was associated with up to 75% mortality when performed within the first 2 weeks of symptom onset, compared with 45% mortality with delay of operative intervention at 14 to 29 days, and striking reduction in mortality to 8% when surgery was delayed past 30 days. In addition, early surgery has been shown to be an independent predictor of poor outcome in acute necrotizing pancreatitis. A randomized controlled trial comparing early versus late necrosectomy demonstrated an unacceptably high mortality rate in the early intervention arm, and therefore the trial was closed before completion of the study. There are now several studies that provide strong evidence that mortality can be decreased significantly with delay of operative intervention beyond 4 weeks of symptom onset. This time frame is not chosen at random; the process of maturation of pancreatic and peripancreatic necrosis requires about 4 weeks and occurs via parenchymal demarcation, the development of a discrete inflammatory rind, and at least partial liquefaction of the contents of the collection. Débridement attempts of very friable and inflamed pancreas before this level of mature formation of a walled-off necrosis increase the risk of inciting an overwhelming inflammatory response, hemorrhage, and fistula development. Also débridement attempts before complete demarcation of necrosis risk removal of viable pancreatic tissue and place the patient at an unnecessary risk for pancreatic exocrine and endocrine insufficiency. Therefore, all invasive interventions should ideally be delayed past 4 to 6 weeks from symptom onset. However, in patients with infected necrotizing pancreatitis and clinical deterioration, the need for immediate source control can become evident and force procedural intervention. In such cases, the availability of less invasive techniques such as percutaneous or peroral transluminal drainage allows for deferment of surgical intervention and in some cases completely avoids the need for surgery.

Indications for either radiologic, endoscopic, or surgical intervention per the 2012 IAP/APA guidelines include suspected or documented infected necrotizing pancreatitis in the setting of clinical deterioration or unresolving organ failure preferably more than 4 weeks after symptom onset. Asymptomatic walled-off necrosis does not mandate surgical intervention. Even in select patients with proven or suspected infected pancreatic necrosis who are clinically stable and minimally symptomatic, expectant management with antibiotics is recommended. These patients must be monitored closely, and intervention is warranted with signs of clinical

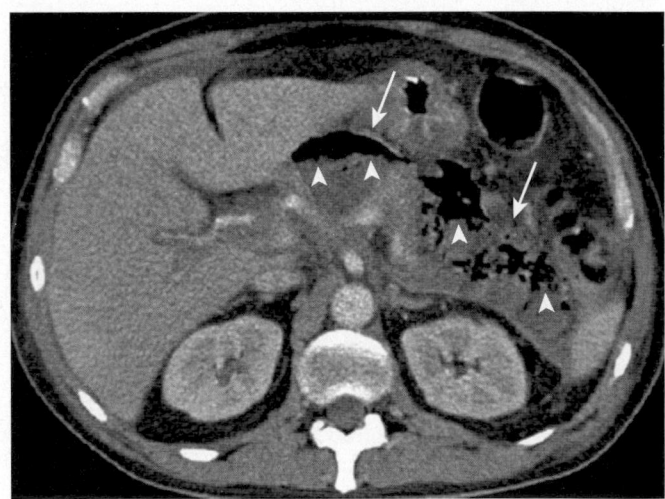

FIGURE 4 Computed tomographic scan with intravenous contrast showing necrotizing pancreatitis complicated by infected pancreatic necrosis. Acute necrotic collection of the pancreatic and peripancreatic area *(white arrows)* with associated gas *(white arrowheads)* indicating infection. *(Image adapted from Banks PA, Bollen TL, Dervenis C, et al [Acute Pancreatitis Classification Working Group]. Classification of acute pancreatitis—2012: revision of the Atlanta classification and definitions by international consensus. Gut. 2013;62:102-111.)*

deterioration. Collateral damage from SAP may develop, however, and result in the need for emergency surgical intervention, such as when there is intestinal ischemia, perforated viscous, acute bleeding, or abdominal compartment syndrome. In such cases, surgical débridement of sterile necrosis is to be avoided. Although rare, there are also situations in which intervention is warranted in the setting of sterile necrosis; these include intractable gastric outlet obstruction, intestinal or biliary obstruction from mass effect, persistent abdominal pain or "unwellness," and disconnected duct syndrome with persistent symptomatic collections. However, these interventions ideally should be delayed past 8 weeks after symptom onset.

■ CHOICE OF THERAPEUTIC INTERVENTION IN NECROTIZING PANCREATITIS

The optimal strategy and current standard for managing patients with suspected or confirmed infected necrotizing pancreatitis and clinical deterioration involves a multidisciplinary step-up approach. Recommendations call for initial image-guided percutaneous catheter drainage or endoscopic transluminal drainage with the use of endoscopic ultrasound, followed by endoscopic or surgical débridement, when necessary. The goal of this approach is to allow for deferment of formal débridement until safe, or avoidance of more invasive treatment strategies altogether.

Percutaneous Drainage

Image-guided percutaneous drainage of infected pancreatic necrosis performed by an interventional radiologist has been used traditionally as an adjunctive approach for drainage of residual collections after open necrosectomy. However, because of innovations in the field of interventional radiology and a growing understanding of the disease process, it has become the initial intervention of choice in patients requiring source control (Figure 5). This treatment strategy is especially useful when the collection is composed primarily of liquefied necrotic material. The goal is to temporize the patient in the early phase of infected necrosis, until a more definitive approach, such as endoscopic or surgical necrosectomy, becomes safer as the patient clinically stabilizes. In some cases, source control through percutaneous drainage in combination with prolonged antibiotic therapy is sufficient to achieve complete resolution and avoids the prospect of a more invasive surgical débridement. Percutaneous drainage is feasible in more than 95% of patients with infected pancreatic necrosis and prevents 23% to 50% of the need for a surgical necrosectomy. Moreover, data suggest that a decrease in the collection size of 75% or more 2 weeks after drainage predicts success of this technique without the need for further interventions. Preferably, the collection should be accessed through the retroperitoneal route to more easily allow, if needed, minimally invasive surgical approach (retroperitoneoscopy). Upsizing to large-bore catheters can be carried out to optimize the removal of solid debris. If percutaneous catheter drainage fails, endoscopic transluminal and minimally invasive approaches can be considered, although the optimal method of necrosectomy has not yet been defined. Close communication

between the radiologist, endoscopist, and surgeon is necessary to consider which approach is anatomically most feasible and safest for the patient. The decision to proceed in one direction versus the other depends on the degree of expertise and willingness of all team members to participate. Of course, open surgery is always an option; however, it should be reserved for cases that fail source control by other methods.

Endoscopic Drainage and Débridement

Endoscopic techniques used to treat necrotizing pancreatitis have their origins in peroral endoscopic drainage of pancreatic pseudocysts. Endoscopic transmural drainage may be considered safely as an alternative first step in treatment of suspected or confirmed infected necrotizing pancreatitis in centers with expertise in this technique. However, the collection must be located within 2 cm of the stomach or duodenum. The collection is accessed with electrocautery through the posterior wall of the stomach or medial wall of the duodenum. The site of transluminal entry into the collection may be identified by simply observing the bulging impression that the collection exerts onto the posterior wall of the stomach or duodenum. However, this potentially risks injury to vascular and other surrounding structures. Therefore concurrent use of endoscopic ultrasound (EUS) is recommended because it allows for better visualization of fluid collection and its solid necrotic component. EUS with duplex capability allows for avoidance of nearby vasculature. Once access to the collection is obtained, the tract is dilated with large-diameter balloon, and drainage is facilitated by placement of large-bore removable pigtail or self-expanding metallic stents. Nasocystic catheters may be left in place for irrigation. This technique is particularly useful in cases of necrotizing pancreatitis complicated by disconnected pancreatic duct syndrome, which requires stents to be left in place indefinitely to prevent fluid reaccumulation. Transluminal direct endoscopic necrosectomy (DEN) is a form of natural orifice transluminal endoscopic surgery introduced in 2000, and its efficacy has been established widely. Access is obtained in a similar manner as for simple endoscopic drainage. The flexible endoscope is passed through the transmural opening into the collection, and its placement is confirmed through fluoroscopy (Figure 6). Mechanical débridement is performed with irrigation and endoscopic instruments, such as forceps, baskets, and nets. Usually repeat débridements are necessary. In a pilot randomized controlled trial (PENGUIN) of 20 patients, transluminal endoscopic necrosectomy

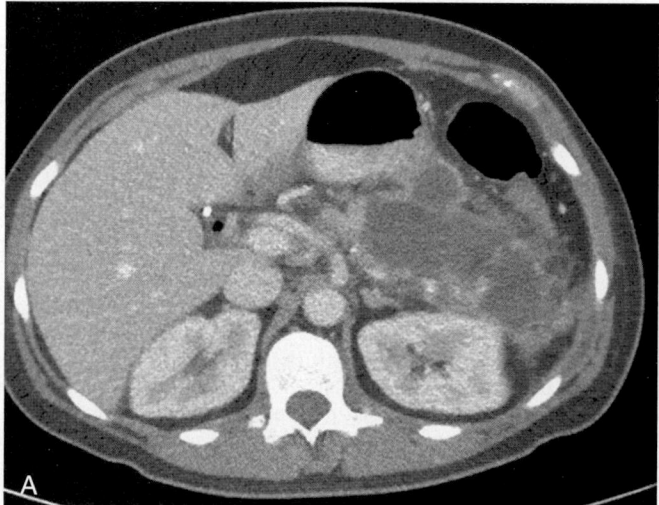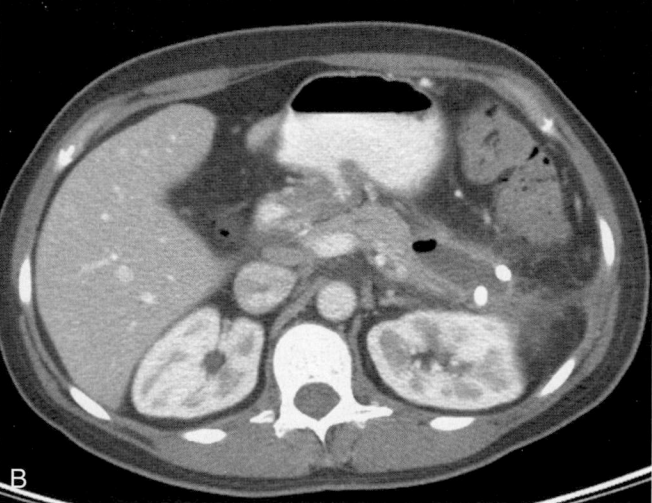

FIGURE 5 Computer tomographic scan with intravenous contrast showing walled of necrotic collections **(A)** and reduction in the volume of collections after percutaneous drain placement **(B)**. *(Images courtesy Abraham Dachman, MD, Department of Radiology, The University of Chicago Hospitals.)*

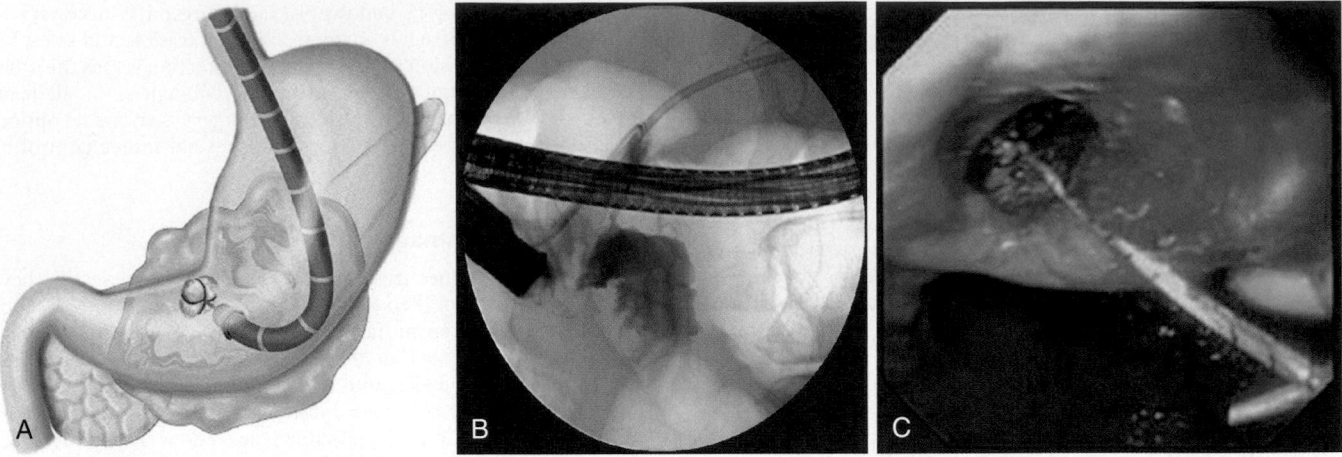

FIGURE 6 Endoscopic necrosectomy. **A,** Necrotic collection is endoscopically débrided by creating an opening in the posterior gastric wall via electrocautery. **B,** Position of the endoscope within the necrotic cavity is confirmed with fluoroscopy before débridement. **C,** Intraoperative image showing removal of necrotic material. *(Images courtesy Irving Waxman, MD, Department of Gastroenterology, The University of Chicago Hospitals.* **A,** *From Seewald S, et al. Aggressive endoscopic therapy for pancreatic necrosis and pancreatic abscess: a new safe and effective treatment algorithm [videos]. Gastrointest Endosc. 2005;62:92-100.)*

was shown to be associated with lower risk of organ failure, pancreatic fistulae, and overall complications compared with surgical necrosectomy. However, this approach may not be feasible for peripancreatic necrosis with wide retroperitoneal extension. The combination of transmural endoscopic and percutaneous approaches is also a feasible débridement approach, in which irrigation is performed through the percutaneous drains with intraluminal egress of fluid. The combined approach has been shown to minimize the development of pancreaticocutaneous fistulae, decrease the number of necessary débridement procedures, and decrease the need for subsequent surgical intervention.

Laparoscopic Transperitoneal and Video-Assisted Retroperitoneal Débridement

Gagner first described minimally invasive surgical treatment of necrotizing pancreatitis in 1996. Since then, this approach has been favored over the historical gold standard of open necrosectomy. The advantages of minimally invasive approach over open necrosectomy include reduction in systemic complications and organ failure. In a retrospective analysis of a prospective database comprising 189 patients, minimally invasive retroperitoneal necrosectomy was shown to significantly decrease the risk of complications and death when compared with open necrosectomy. However, mortality rates have not been reported consistently and compared across studies. Two approaches to minimally invasive necrosectomy exist: laparoscopic transperitoneal débridement and video-assisted retroperitoneal débridement (VARD). Laparoscopic transperitoneal débridement allows visualization of and access to all the compartments of the abdominal cavity, with the possibility of using a hand-assist port. Laparoscopic enteric drainage is also possible with this approach and entails creation of an anastomosis between the stomach or small bowel and an adjacent mature necrotic collection to allow continued internal drainage. However, laparoscopic transperitoneal approaches risk contamination of otherwise sterile spaces such as the peritoneal cavity. Reoperation rates after this approach reach 20%. VARD is currently the preferred method for minimally invasive access (Figure 7). Image-guided drains initially are placed through the retroperitoneal route. When surgery is deemed necessary, these tracts are subsequently upsized, allowing for visualization with the laparoscope, rigid nephroscope, or endoscope. With this approach morbidity is decreased to 10% to 30%, and mortality rates vary between 0 and 20%.

Step-Up Approach

Because of the frequent need for more definitive débridement after interventional drainage procedures along with high morbidity and mortality of early surgical intervention, the combination of these modalities (i.e., step-up approach), has gained popularity in recent years. It allows for source control in critically ill patients and has the advantage of temporizing while conservative and supportive management continues. The first step is percutaneous or endoscopic transgastric approach to drainage, followed by VARD if no improvement is noted. This approach has been studied widely in the clinical setting and is supported currently by feasibility, safety, and efficacy data. Step-up approach with percutaneous retroperitoneal catheter drainage followed, when necessary, by minimally invasive necrosectomy recently was compared with primary open necrosectomy in a landmark multicenter randomized controlled trial (PANTER). The results reveal reduction in major complications (such as multiorgan failure), new-onset diabetes, incisional hernias, as well as costs.

Open Pancreatic Necrosectomy

Open pancreatic necrosectomy is the traditional surgical approach with goals of complete drainage and removal of all necrotic tissue. Over the past decade, the shift away from open surgical interventions in favor of less invasive alternatives has been driven mainly by the high morbidity (34% to 95%) and mortality rates (6% to 25%) of open procedures, depending on the timing of surgery and patient selection. Nevertheless, open surgery for necrotizing pancreatitis remains a viable option in a select group of patients when the intervention is appropriately delayed and performed in centers with expertise. Access may be gained through a standard laparotomy incision or a retroperitoneal flank incision. The necrotic tissue is débrided manually with blunt and careful dissection with the goal of leaving as much vital pancreatic tissue as possible. There are three traditional ways in which to manage the patient after open necrosectomy: open packing, closed packing, and postoperative continuous lavage. Open packing entails packing of the marsupialized lesser sac, whereas the abdomen is left open for reassessments of débridement success (every 24 to 48 hours). Once no necrotic tissue remains, the abdomen often is allowed to heal entirely through secondary intention or rarely may be closed primarily. Closed packing technique uses the principle of planned staged relaparotomies (every

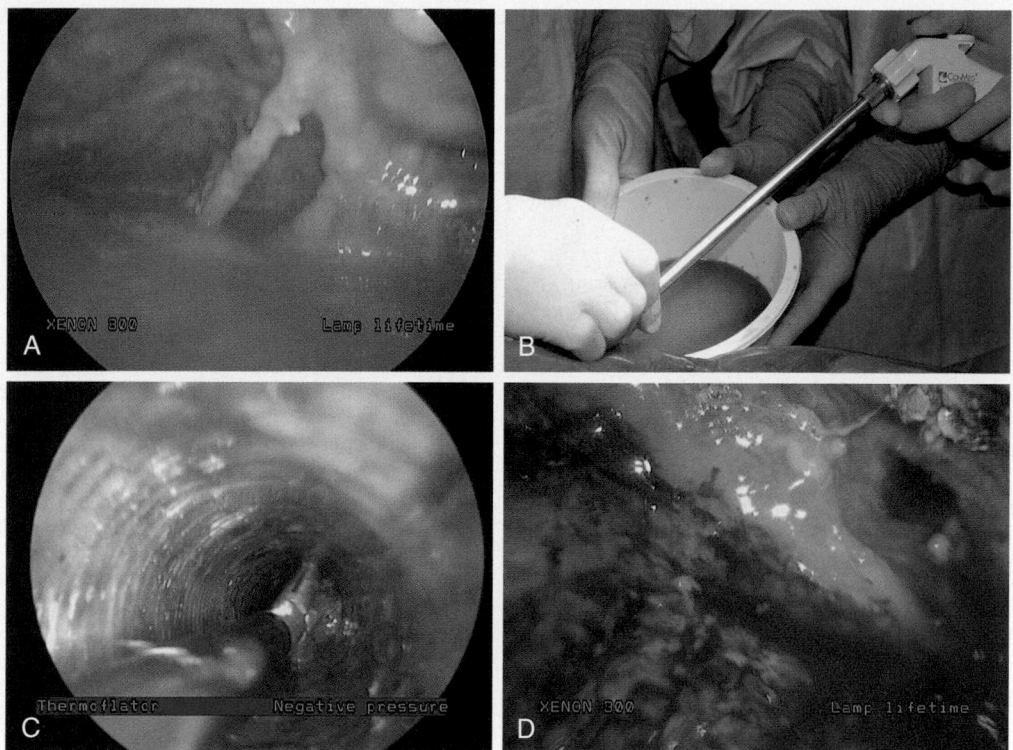

FIGURE 7 Technique for video-assisted retroperitoneal débridement. **A,** Necrotic cavity is accessed by following the tract of previously placed drains. **B,** Murky fluid is encountered and drained with laparoscopic suction device. **C,** Solid necrotic material is removed with laparoscopic graspers. **D,** Wall of cavity is free of necrotic material at conclusion of débridement.

48 hours) with closure of the abdomen, possibly over drains, in the interim. Closed continuous lavage technique uses large double-lumen drains that are left in place after débridement to continue large volume continuous irrigation after abdominal closure. This allows continued clearance of infected necrotic material, assessment of the effluent, and avoidance of the stress of relaparotomy. Postoperative continuous irrigation has been shown to be superior to open packing and planned relaparotomies in terms of reducing morbidity.

■ SUMMARY

Pancreatic necrosis is one of the most feared complications of acute pancreatitis and carries a high rate of morbidity and mortality. Recommendations regarding optimal treatment strategies recently have changed because of a clearer understanding of the disease process, advances in imaging and minimally invasive approaches. Early fluid resuscitation and enteric nutritional support remain the mainstays of initial supportive care. Antibiotic prophylaxis is no longer recommended in cases of sterile pancreatic necrosis. However, in patients with suspected or confirmed secondary infection, empiric antibiotic therapy should be initiated. An infused computed tomography scan or MRI is recommended for evaluation of the extent of necrosis and potential local complications. Patients requiring early source control because of suspected or confirmed secondary infection and clinical deterioration should be temporized with percutaneous drain placement or transluminal endoscopic drainage if the anatomy is amenable. In cases in which additional débridement is necessary, the choice of VARD, laparoscopic transperitoneal débridement, or DEN is appropriate, depending on patient anatomy, characteristics, and institutional expertise. Open necrosectomy remains

a valid approach in select cases in which the step-up approach is not feasible. The goals of débridement are common to all surgical interventions: to clear necrotic material leaving behind healthy pancreatic tissue and to allow continued drainage and irrigation of the cavity.

SUGGESTED READINGS

Bakker OJ, van Santvoort HC, van Brunschot S, et al (Dutch Pancreatitis Study Group). Endoscopic transgastric vs surgical necrosectomy for infected necrotizing pancreatitis: a randomized trial. *JAMA.* 2012;307: 1053-1061.

Banks PA, Bollen TL, Dervenis C, et al (Acute Pancreatitis Classification Working Group). Classification of acute pancreatitis—2012: revision of the Atlanta classification and definitions by international consensus. *Gut.* 2013;62:102-111.

Bello B, Matthews JB. Minimally invasive treatment of pancreatic necrosis. *World J Gastroenterol.* 2012;18:6829-6835.

Besselink MG, Verwer TJ, Schoenmaeckers EJ, et al. Timing of surgical intervention in necrotizing pancreatitis. *Arch Surg.* 2007;142:1194-1201.

Freeman ML, Werner J, van Santvoort HC, et al (International Multidisciplinary Panel of Speakers and Moderators). Interventions for necrotizing pancreatitis: summary of a multidisciplinary consensus conference. *Pancreas.* 2012;41:1176-1194.

Horvath K, Freeny P, Escallon J, et al. Safety and efficacy of video-assisted retroperitoneal débridement for infected pancreatic collections: a multicenter, prospective, single-arm phase 2 study. *Arch Surg.* 2010;145: 817-825.

Van Santvoort HC, Besselink MG, Bakker OJ, et al (Dutch Pancreatitis Study Group). A step-up approach or open necrosectomy for necrotizing pancreatitis. *N Engl J Med.* 2010;362:1491-1502.

Working Group IAP/APA Acute Pancreatitis Guidelines. IAP/APA evidence-based guidelines for the management of acute pancreatitis. *Pancreatology.* 2013;13(4 suppl 2):e1-e15.

THE MANAGEMENT OF PANCREATIC PSEUDOCYST

William Hawe Nealon, MD

The hallmark of significant episodes of acute pancreatitis (AP) is fluid collections and/or necrosis. In the majority of cases of AP there are generally only minimal physiologic consequences, and fluid collections are less common. Patients with mild "interstitial" AP, 75% to 80% of cases, recover without incident. Even in patients with moderate and in many episodes of more severe disease, fluid collections and pseudocysts (PSs) will resolve spontaneously without any need for intervention. Thus key to the understanding of PSs is the element of time. The amount of time transpired after the "index episode" is pivotal in considering intervention.

Historically in the pancreatic literature fluid collections qualify as PS only after persisting for more than 4 weeks. This definition is not followed commonly, particularly in nonsurgical reports and in day-to-day readings by radiologists in a clinical setting. This strict definition was established first by the Atlanta Symposium of 1992 and the subsequently published classification system. These terms have been updated. In the current nomenclature fluid collections that are seen in the first 4 weeks after the index episode are termed *acute peripancreatic fluid collections*. Once these fluid collections persist beyond 4 weeks, they are categorized as PS.

Further complicating this classification system is the fact that patients who experience an episode of severe necrotizing pancreatitis (NP) are given entirely different nomenclature. This is based on the presence of areas of necrotic pancreas and of necrotic peripancreatic soft tissue. Once again there is a distinction made between conditions present up to 4 weeks after the index episode. The imaging findings at this stage are termed *postnecrotic peripancreatic fluid collections* (PNFC). After 4 weeks the fluid-filled structures become consolidated with thick fibrous walls. These more mature structures are termed *walled-off pancreatic necrosis* (WOPN). Unfortunately, the confusion previously mentioned in regard to inconsistent use of the terms related to PS in daily clinical practice is also apparent to an even greater degree when discussing WOPN. It is extremely common, if not uniform, practice that formal readings on cross-sectional imaging of patients with WOPN are described as PSs by the radiologist. The hallmark of these images is the presence of necrotic debris within the cavity. These structures typically are composed of very thick walls with an irregular cavity, which will characteristically approximate the shape of the lesser sac and completely fill that space. Thus the collection is commonly somewhat sausage shaped. The mix of fluid and debris in these entities is striking.

This awkward mix of names does not represent confusion only with definitions. There are clear practical implications. In consideration of the fact that as many as 80% of acute peripancreatic fluid collections resolve spontaneously, failure to wait 4 weeks before intervention muddies the waters regarding outcomes. Can we be surprised with clinical successes for certain interventions performed in the first weeks of the disease course when most would have resolved spontaneously without any intervention at all? This practice carries the potential for reflecting unrealistically positive results for these interventions. As we evaluate the current literature on PSs, it is imperative to view the reports through the prism of this known course of disease. Many reports involving nonoperative interventions for PSs either do not report the time elapsed since the index episode of AP or they document performing interventions well before the 4-week limit. I cannot overstate the importance of delaying interventions, performing simple observation, and reimaging in fluid collections/PSs identified early in the course of an episode of AP.

The process of simple observation generally will yield the following progression seen by sequential imaging. At the outset there is typically generalized intra-abdominal fluid with some element of distorted pancreatic anatomy. There may be a delay of 24 to 72 hours before the first fluid collection appears. Many believe this is influenced by the timing and magnitude of fluid/crystalloid resuscitation. Follow-up imaging may be obtained after 2 to 3 weeks, at which time a more organized peripancreatic fluid collection is seen and later an actual PS, which either regresses or slowly develops a more thickened or "mature" wall. If you are considering operative drainage of PSs, the surgeon must make the determination that the wall has matured sufficiently to hold a suture.

The procedure called either *necrosectomy* or *débridement of pancreatic necrosis* has been applied liberally according to recent reports in patients many months past their index episode. Historically, débridement of pancreatic necrosis has been associated with high rate of morbidity, a need for multiple operations, and a not insignificant rate of mortality. Because operations are delayed later in the course of disease (a practice that I strongly endorse) much more favorable outcomes and survival after débridement may be expected.

I believe there is a place for segregating these two entities. The use of the term *débridement of pancreatic necrosis* should be limited to the urgent/emergent procedure performed within the first 4 weeks after the index episode of NP. This procedure is performed intentionally less frequently today as recognition of the poor outcomes experienced in patients managed with early débridement. In place of immediate surgery in patients whose clinical condition dictates some form of intervention successes have been reported repeatedly for percutaneous drainage. These reports demonstrate that in a high percentage of cases this intervention can serve as a bridge to definitive surgery later in the course of the disease, and in between 20% and 30% of patients drainage alone is sufficient. If, as I suggest, we segregate those patients who undergo débridement in the first 4 weeks after the index attack, those patients undergoing "true débridement" will experience consistently poor outcomes.

My colleagues and I have been interested in establishing a correlation between persistence of PS or of WOPN and injuries to the pancreatic duct. I have established a system by which to categorize the ductal distortions seen after an episode of pancreatitis. Very simply a type 1 duct has no injury, type 2 has sustained a ductal stricture, and type 3 is a complete disruption with complete and permanent disconnection between the duct in the head and distal body of the pancreas from the duct in the tail of the pancreas, the so-called "disconnected duct syndrome." Our data have confirmed a direct correlation between type 2 or type 3 changes and persistence of PS or WOPN and a correlation between these ductal injuries and the presence of infected necrosis. We have advocated for a practice guideline in which the condition of the pancreatic duct dictates the mode of intervention chosen. Either percutaneous or endoscopic drainage, perhaps even aspiration without drain placement, is appropriate for type 1 ducts. Transpapillary drainage (i.e., endoscopic placement of a pancreatic duct stent across the stricture) or surgery is best applied to type 2 ductal anatomy. We believe that type 3 ducts are managed best by surgery as the durability of either a percutaneous or endoscopic transmurally placed drain is not seen, likely because the isolated remnant of pancreatic parenchyma will continue to secrete. The remnant of pancreas is termed the *isolated pancreatic segment*. All pancreatic enzymes and bicarbonate-rich secretions from the left of the disconnection will continue to flow with no possible re-entry into the duct in the head of the pancreas or into the intestine without surgical intervention.

Finally, it is important for the reader to exercise some care when approaching pancreatic fluid collections to make certain that there is not a cystic neoplasm masquerading as a PS. The diagnosis of intraductal papillary mucinous neoplasm (IPMN) involves a cystic lesion that may be indistinguishable by imaging from a PS. Adding to the confusion is that a sizable percentage of patients with these lesions first come to the hospital with an episode of AP. As many as 40% are seen first in this manner. Clues to this diagnosis may be the imaging documentation of what appears to be a mature cyst essentially on admission to the emergency department. Recall that true PSs require weeks to mature. Suspicions also may be raised by the fact that in some of these patients the severity of the episode of pancreatitis is inconsistent with acute PS formation. Unfortunately, the existence of this lesion is not widely known outside of those physicians whose practice focuses on pancreatic diseases.

■ PATHOPHYSIOLOGY

Much of our knowledge of the pathophysiology of PS comes from assumptions. We know that the fluid in a PS and in a WOPN is essentially pure pancreatic juice, combined with cellular debris and products of inflammation, particularly in the acute setting. Cytokines and fibroblasts are present. Thus we can say with certainty that all PSs (and WOPN) have a communication with the pancreatic ductal system based on the fact that the contents include pure pancreatic juice, which could be present only if there is a communication. This observation collides with the often-referenced presence or absence of communication with the pancreatic duct, which is described in imaging reports. I use the term *radiographically demonstrable communication* to describe a PS in which clear communication can be demonstrated by endoscopic retrograde cholangiopancreatography (ERCP), by magnetic resonance cholangiopancreatography (MRCP), or during injection of contrast into a percutaneously placed drain. PSs can be seen in patients after an episode of acute pancreatitis and in the presence of chronic pancreatitis. With acute pancreatitis it is known that enzymes within the acinar cells of the pancreas are activated from their typically dormant, inactive state seen in physiologic circumstances. It is known that an element of autodigestion of the pancreas occurs, and that this may result in pancreatic duct disruption and leakage of pancreatic juice. The duct may be altered temporarily or permanently with either a stricture or complete disruption of the duct. As already stated, we have established a correlation between duct disruption and persistence of a PS.

If we ask for a plausible mechanism for the formation of the "mature" wall in the PS we go back to assumptions. Inert pancreatic juice does not induce a significant inflammatory response. This can be confirmed by the fact that "pancreatic ascites," which typically develops after rupture of a PS, has no suggestion of acute inflammation in the clinical setting. Perhaps the presence of the other components of inflammation, particularly fibroblasts and platelets, may contribute to the evolution of the fibrotic wall of a PS. We know that in nearly all areas of the body where fibrosis occurs, there will be a nearly identical histologic character with a fibroblast-mediated extracellular matrix formation. With necrosis it is conceivable that the necrotic debris induces classic wound-healing process of scar formation or fibrosis. It is known that a component of severe necrotizing pancreatitis is ischemia to parts or all of the gland. The segment of pancreas just overlying the spine has the classic vascular features of a "watershed" area and clinically this is precisely where the majority of ductal disruptions can be found.

Before the evolution of reliable imaging in the last quarter of the twentieth century the timing of intervention on a PS was dictated by the element of time. It was said that 6 weeks were required after the index episode before a "mature" wall would form. This was based on a questionably valid model in which a plastic bag was placed in the peritoneal cavity of dogs, and only after 6 weeks did a suitable scar form around it. Later Bradley evaluated serial ultrasound examinations of PS (the current state of the art imaging modality in the years before his 1979 publication) and with very poor follow-up again found 6 weeks as a meaningful interval, after which spontaneous resolution was unlikely and major complications were more likely to occur. The 6-week precept is not always followed now, but certainly the fact that many PSs will resolve spontaneously must be recognized.

The mechanism by which chronic pancreatitis (CP) progresses to PS is even more murky. The majority of patients with CP have not had a significant antecedent history of AP. No correlation has ever been made to show that the patients with CP who do develop PSs are part of the estimated 15% of CP patients with prior moderate to severe acute pancreatitis. Prolonged pancreatic duct stricture or occlusion after an episode of moderate to severe AP has a high rate of conversion to CP, for example, if no intervention is made to ameliorate the damage. We are actually even more challenged for scientific evidence to support any proposed mechanism for PS development in CP. We do know that as with the texture of the pancreas gland itself in CP, the PSs tend to have a rigid wall and often have calcifications in the wall. I have reported data to confirm that when operating on patients for the coexistent diagnosis of CP and PS, duct drainage with a Frey or Puestow procedure is sufficient. The concept that the behavior of a PS is determined entirely by PD dynamics is upheld in this observation. Unfortunately, transpapillary PD stent placement may have success in managing the PS, but it plays little role in managing CP. Since the 1980s it has been recognized that symptoms are unlikely to resolve unless both the PS and the underlying CP are addressed at the time of intervention.

The mechanism for WOPN formation may be easier to define because the residual necrotic debris may be expected to finally be replaced by scar or fibrosis. The wall in a WOPN is predictably much thicker, and its evolution as followed by serial imaging demonstrates that the WOPN grows out of the initial necrotic material in the lesser sac. The thickness of the walls of a WOPN and their consequent rigidity carries significant implications for management. Although the majority of PSs will collapse upon drainage, WOPN cavities will persist predictably after evacuation using any of the available modalities. This residual cavity affects time to complete resolution of symptoms after intervention.

PSs have been described in a wide variety of anatomic locations. I have seen three cases of mediastinal PS. They can be seen in the abdominal cavity somewhat remote from the pancreas. They have been described in the pleural space, overlying the kidney, in the subhepatic space, in the spleen, and other places.

■ PRESENTATION

The most common presentation of a PS is after an episode of AP or of pancreatic trauma. It is important to note that PSs have been seen after no identifiable recent episode of pancreatitis. The mechanism for this presentation is challenging, but it is key to understand that PS may arise after a relatively mild episode of pancreatitis. I prefer to immediately use the term *index episode* of pancreatitis in approaching this entity because some patients have repeated acute events. Recall that the time elapsed since a PS has been identified is a meaningful measure to inform the decisions for intervention.

More commonly a discrete episode of moderate to severe AP can be identified. With necrosis the likelihood of sustaining an injury to the pancreatic duct rises. A common mechanism for post-traumatic PS is a seatbelt injury after a car crash. As the pancreas crosses over the spine, the midbody of the pancreas is crushed between the seatbelt and the spine. The trauma can lead to disruption of the duct and result in a pancreatic ductal disconnection. This location of ductal disruption is nearly identical to the most common site for disconnection after an episode of severe necrotizing pancreatitis, in the area described as a "watershed" area of the pancreas. The classic presenting symptoms are upper abdominal pain, radiating to the upper back, associated with nausea, some with vomiting, loss of appetite, and weight loss since the episode. Although some patients, based upon severity of the initial attack, will have been recognized early in the course of the episode to be worthy of monitoring for the development of a PS, there are many cases in which the patient is sent home and then returns in 10 to 30 days after the index episode with the symptoms just mentioned.

BOX 1: Complications Associated With Pseudocysts

- Obstruction (intestinal, vascular, biliary)
- Infection
- Rupture (pancreatic ascites)
- Hemorrhage
- Fistula formation with the intestine (duodenum, colon, small bowel, pleura)

There is a risk for an error commonly encountered in my practice that merits emphasizing. If you review the symptoms just described and you factor in the observed frequency of about 50% of hyperamylasemia in serum of patients with a PS, then you may not be surprised to learn that these patients, upon transfer to my care, have carried a diagnosis of recurrent AP through their course. At the transferring hospital this routinely results in the decision to restrict oral (PO) intake without providing any form of nutrition. The actual diagnosis is symptomatic PS and its associated hyperamylasemia and not AP. In the absence of mechanical compression of the stomach or duodenum PO feeding is routinely tolerated in patients with PSs.

Signs of gastric or intestinal compression can lead to an inability to tolerate PO intake, and some form of alternative nutrition should be initiated. If the PS compresses the bile duct, jaundice may be visible. The classic list of potential complications seen in patients with PSs is in Box 1.

Pancreatic ascites is a key diagnosis to consider in a patient with a history of ethyl alcohol (ETOH) abuse. Often these patients are given the mistaken diagnosis of cirrhosis-related ascites and are assumed to be preterminal with hepatic failure. Pancreatic ascites is almost uniformly the result of a ruptured PS, and interventions aimed at the underlying pathology will forever rid the patient of ascites. Pancreatic enzymes that are not activated cause no acute intra-abdominal symptoms such as peritoneal irritation. A high index of suspicion may be necessary in this circumstance.

Infected PS is now termed *pancreatic abscess.* In the original taxonomy *pancreatic abscess* was the term used for infection in what was once called *pancreatic phlegmon.* These prior pancreatic abscesses carried a high rate of morbidity and mortality. That same entity is now under the category of infected pancreatic necrosis, which still carries a significantly higher mortality and morbidity when compared with infected PS, the entity currently described as *pancreatic abscess.* These can occur acutely and require urgent intervention. Similarly, hemorrhage will occur acutely, and urgent intervention is required. Surgical intervention in the setting of hemorrhage is fraught with hazards. Interventions via transcatheter angiographic methods are mandated. This can be through embolization or by placing coated vascular stents across the bleeding. The splenic artery is the most common source of the bleeding, but as mentioned, PS can be located in a variety of sites.

Regarding fistulas, I have observed a phenomenon countless times in the management of PS. As percutaneous drainages became more common through my career, I saw an increasingly frequent imaging diagnosis of spontaneous fistula formation between the PS and the intestinal tract. The historical surgical literature on the subject quoted the frequency of spontaneous fistula formation to the intestinal tract as less than 3%. The interventional radiology (IR) literature quotes the rate at 67%. I have performed upper and lower endoscopies on countless patients to confirm that the catheter traverses the lumen. We gain immense quality from our IR colleagues. The fact that the catheters traverse the intestine almost never results in a worse course for the patient.

There is literature on the management of asymptomatic PS. Studies suggest that no intervention is necessary in this setting, but the available literature has identified that past a diameter of 5 to 6 cm the likelihood of serious complications rises, even in the absence of symptoms. Furthermore, as mentioned previously, one must adopt a practice of surveillance for the possibility of a cystic neoplasm masquerading as a PS.

DIAGNOSTIC EVALUATION

The diagnostic workup for PS first requires a level of suspicion. In the simplest scenario one naturally considers a PS after an episode of AP. The trigger for exploring for this diagnosis is simply the persistence of symptoms after the characteristic 3 to 5 days typically required for resolution. Because computed tomography (CT) scans are difficult to avoid in emergency departments (EDs) suspicion may increase if large amounts of intra-abdominal fluid were identified in the initial CT scan. As stated, a patient may be discharged too promptly home after the acute episode and may have smoldering persistent symptoms. In spite of repeated visits to EDs it may take months or more before any effort is made to obtain cross-sectional imaging. In the physical exam one can palpate a large PS in the upper abdomen, but depending on body habitus and PS size this is not routinely possible. Serum amylase will be elevated in at least 50%. Symptoms suspicious for gastric or intestinal obstruction or of jaundice may signal the presence of a PS. As stated, the presence of a cystic neoplasm must be excluded. Because an episode of AP may be triggered by an IPMN there is added concern for confusion. If a patient admitted acutely with a diagnosis of AP has on imaging what appears to be a fully mature cyst, one should consider that this likely represents IPMN and not PS.

Cross-sectional imaging is the standard for the first step in imaging. Important elements in the visual evaluation are the thickness ("maturity") of the capsule or wall of the PS. The PS is typically round. Internal debris is rare, although with a history of blood loss anemia hyperdense material is visible in the PS. Using Hounsfield units this can be characterized as blood. Finding a WOPN is associated with a known history of necrotizing pancreatitis. In one study my colleagues and I performed every WOPN identified by imaging was given the term PS in the official reading. Hopefully the terminology will migrate to the radiology literature and be disseminated. Clues that this structure is a WOPN include the fact that the wall is typically very thick, the interior of the chamber is nearly always filled with necrotic debris, and the structure is very rarely circular, all in contradistinction to PS. The shape often approximates the lesser sac, although they may form in a variety of locations (Figures 1 and 2). Imaging allows assessment of the degree of compression of surrounding structures and the relation of the PS to these structures. It is often surprising that a patient can tolerate PO intake in spite of considerable compression of the stomach by the PS. If a patient is experiencing pain after meals and there is no gastric, duodenal, or intestinal compression, this should create suspicion that a degree of pancreatic ductal disruption has taken place. The presence of gland calcification and/or a dilated main pancreatic duct (MPD) can alert you to a diagnosis of CP. Associated pancreatic functional impairments can further establish this diagnosis. Finally, the most common cause of splenic vein thrombosis is pancreatitis. This can be assessed by contrast-enhanced CT scan (CE-CT). This commonly results in considerable formation of engorged collateral veins, which can raise the risks of injury and hemorrhage of these fragile veins during open, percutaneous, or endoscopic transluminal therapies. Less commonly combined splenic vein and portal vein/superior mesenteric vein thrombosis may be seen.

After the diagnosis of PS is made, there is no need to repeat imaging sooner than 4 weeks after the index episode. With worsening symptoms, particularly in the case of WOPN, imaging should be repeated sooner, primarily to exclude infection or of massive increase in size of the PS. With infection air may be seen within the cavity. In rare occasions this represents communication between the PS and the intestinal tract. In the past, this finding or the finding of deteriorating clinical status drove the decision to obtain CT-guided aspiration of the necrosis and sampling for culture. This practice has nearly vanished. In the past, the finding of infected contents, particularly

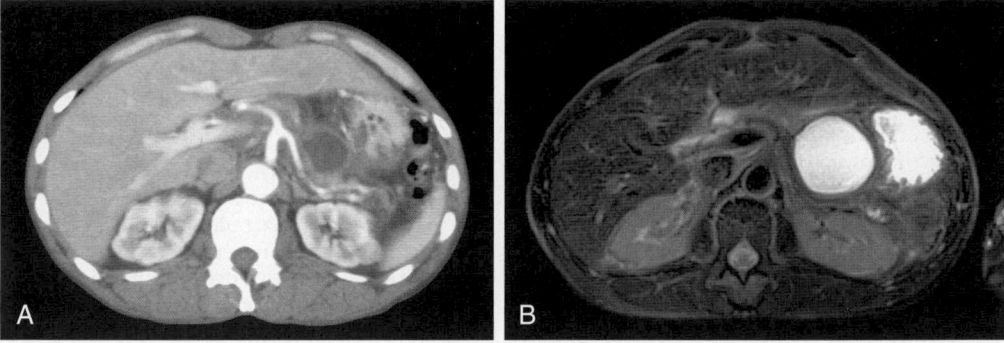

FIGURE 1 A pancreatic pseudocyst is well visualized with contrast-enhanced computed tomographic scan (**A**) as a simple fluid-filled structure with a hyperdense fibrous capsule in the body of the pancreas and with magnetic resonance (**B**) on T2-weighted imaging as a round, homogeneously enhancing lesion.

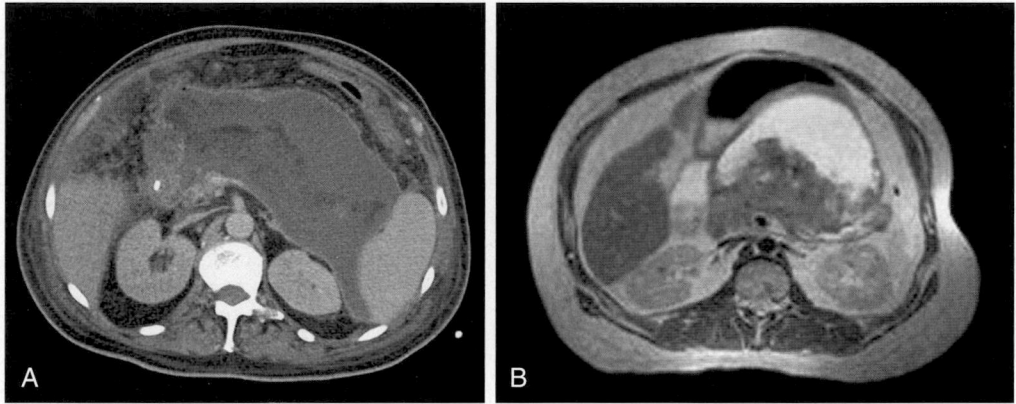

FIGURE 2 Walled-off pancreatic necrosis is shown on contrast-enhanced computed tomographic scan (**A**) as a peripancreatic fluid collection containing heterogeneous material representing solid necrotic debris and with magnetic resonance (**B**) on T2-weighted imaging as a rounded enhancing fluid-filled collection containing nonenhancing solid necrosis.

infected necrosis, mandated immediate surgical intervention. Given recent reports, particularly the prospective analysis performed and reported by the Dutch Pancreatitis Consortium in the *New England Journal of Medicine*, surgeons almost always should start with percutaneous drain placement. Thus a key element in the evaluation of the CT scan or other imaging modalities is the establishment of safe paths to follow for placement of percutaneous drains. These may be either transabdominal or retroperitoneal. The goal is to avoid penetrating bowel, the pleural space, major vascular structures, and the various solid organs in the path of the drain (kidneys, spleen, liver). Please note that there is literally no value in a noncontrast CT scan. In all circumstances a contrast-enhanced computed tomography (CE-CT) should be sought. If concerns for renal impairment exist, then either magnetic resonance imaging/magnetic resonance cholangiopancreatography (MRI/MRCP) or endoscopic ultrasound (EUS) should be considered.

My colleagues and I advocate for exploring and defining the anatomy of the pancreatic ductal system in the determination of the likelihood of spontaneous resolution of a PS over time as well as to direct therapy as discussed later in the chapter. In the past and in my personal experience ERCP had a value, particularly in defining MPD injuries. I advocated this practice with the admonition that some intervention be performed within 24 hours of the procedure if communication with the duct is demonstrated radiographically. Combined ERCP and MPD stent placement (transpapillary stents) may serve as a therapeutic measure for definitive management of PS. It is key to recognize that this intervention carries the risk of contaminating a previously sterile collection.

EUS can be used to assess ductal anatomy, the size of the PS, and many of the measures obtained in the other forms of imaging. This modality can be used to sample the fluid in an effort to distinguish cystic neoplasms from PSs. It can define mural nodules, which imply possible malignant progression in IPMN. The fluid can be sent for evaluation. In PS the fluid contains debris, macrophages, and no mucosal cells. In IPMN the carcinoembryonic antigen (CEA) level is elevated, and mucicarmine stains are positive. Cytology is of little value in this analysis. In addition, the historic use of endoscopic transluminal drainage of PS and of transgastric débridement of pancreatic necrosis in WOPN, EUS guidance has improved accuracy greatly and prevented or reduced the frequency of complications such as injury to major vascular structures.

Regarding MPD assessment, one can obtain clarity from all modalities mentioned. I prefer contrast-enhanced MRI/MRCP (Figure 1, *B*). MRCP can be enhanced by a simultaneous infusion of Secretin, which will stimulate secretion of high-volume bicarbonate and water from ductal cells. The resulting dilatation of the MPD may aid in delineation. I rarely use this added feature because the added detail does not merit the considerable added cost. Ductal disruption (the so-called *disconnected duct syndrome*), ductal stenosis, gland atrophy, and fine details of the chamber, including mural nodules and presence of necrosis, may be seen. Because the state of the MPD should drive decisions regarding modalities for intervention, this particular analysis of the pancreatic anatomy is key.

■ MANAGEMENT

As stated previously, the majority of PSs resolve spontaneously. Only in the rarest circumstances should interventions be considered until 4 to 6 weeks after the index episode. I have worried about the validity of reports, particularly in the nonsurgical literature, in which early

BOX 2: System for Categorizing Ductal Anatomy Seen After Pancreatitis

Type 1: Normal Duct
Type 2: Stricture in the Main Pancreatic Duct
Type 3: Complete Obstruction of the Main Pancreatic Duct
Type 4: Chronic Pancreatitis

interventions are performed, given the fact that the majority of these patients would have experienced complete resolution without intervention. All of my studies evaluating the management of peripancreatic fluid collections have had the specific aim of better assigning the appropriate modality to manage PSs and WOPN. The hypothesis has been that in patients with undisturbed MPD anatomy, either percutaneous or endoscopic transluminal (gastric or duodenum) drainage is preferred. There has arisen the use of the term *cyst-gastrostomy* or *cyst-duodenostomy* for what is no more than placement of one or several transluminal stents into the collection. I find that terminology misleading and a bit grandiose. I prefer using the term *transluminal endoscopic drainage.*

As mentioned, I have validated a categorization system for ductal injuries after pancreatitis (Box 2). In type 1 the MPD has no signs of injury. Type 2 ductal injury denotes a pancreatic ductal stricture. Type 3 represents a complete ductal disruption (disconnected duct syndrome), and type 4 ducts are those seen in patients with a diagnosis of CP. There is a failure rate of nonsurgical management of approximately 25% in patients with type 2 changes. From my experience type 3 changes only can be managed operatively.

In a paper presented at the recent meeting of the American Pancreas Club 2016 endoscopic transpapillary management of type 3 ducts was evaluated. In this procedure the distal stricture must be pierced blindly, hoping to find the opposite end of the MPD in the body and tail of the pancreas. Documented outcomes included a high rate of failure, a high frequency of repeated procedures, and a high rate of urgent hospitalizations in the postprocedure period. It seems unlikely that most gastrointestinal (GI) endoscopists would accept the risk of this procedure; few data support this modality.

Another creative measure has been reported in the endoscopic literature in which EUS guidance is used to identify the MPD to the left of the disconnection. With use of this imaging guidance a stent can be placed through the wall of the stomach into the MPD, thus achieving ductal drainage. Considering the fact that the viable pancreatic parenchyma in the tail of the pancreas will continue secreting through a lifetime, the durability of this intervention must be considered.

Thus my colleagues and I advocate nonsurgical interventions for all type 1 ducts. When managing PS associated with type 2 ducts, we advocate for nonsurgical interventions followed by definitive surgical drainage for treatment failures. Often missing from this algorithm is what number of failed nonsurgical interventions should, in good conscience, be performed before recognizing that this modality has failed. We see patients at times subjected to dozens of failed procedures before finally finding a pancreatic surgeon for definitive operative intervention. Too frequently, it is the patient who finally stops the experimental procedures. (The surgical management of type 3 and type 4 ducts with associated PS is discussed later in this chapter.)

In review, symptomatic cysts and cysts measuring less than 5 cm are not typically in need of intervention. Cysts that are symptomatic (i.e., causing pain, preventing PO intake, associated with obstruction of the stomach, duodenum, or small bowel, causing obstruction of the bile duct, rupture, hemorrhage, or associated with fistulae) require intervention. One caution to consider in managing a patient with biliary obstruction associated with a PS is whether the cyst alone is causing the obstruction or has the bile duct developed a primary stricture as a result of the acute inflammation in AP. In this case I

advocate a trial of nonsurgical modalities, even if anatomy such as type 3 ductal changes have been documented. In this case the advantage of performing a decompression of the PS is to see if this measure results in resolution of the bile duct obstruction or does not. If it does not, then at definitive operation for the pancreas one can add an operative drainage of the bile duct using either a choledochojejunostomy or choledochoduodenostomy. Finally I use nonsurgical techniques to decompress the PS even with a known type 3 duct if the patient is so metabolically, physiologically, and nutritionally debilitated that open operation represents excessive risk. This measure can serve as a bridge to definitive operation. Typically in this setting one sees either PS recurrence after endoscopic drainage or persistent drainage of pancreatic juice after percutaneous drainage. I favor percutaneous drainage in this bridging setting because injection of contrast into the drain can provide documentation of the ductal anatomy. Furthermore, this procedure routinely provides a view of the isolated duct in the left side of the obstructed MPD, details that are not visible by ERCP, although certainly available in a quality MRCP.

I rarely employ cyst-gastrostomy. The rate of the postoperative complication of hemorrhage after operative cyst-gastrostomy is unusually high compared with cyst-jejunostomy, in my experience. This has caused me to suspect that the stomach, not the PS, is responsible for this complication. There also are convincing data to demonstrate that operative cyst-gastrostomy in a cyst larger than 8 cm or in cysts located entirely inferior to the stomach have an increased rate of sepsis. This observation is even more dramatic in patients with WOPN. Surgical management of WOPN involves a less prompt recovery compared with that of PS. The rigid capsule in a WOPN, mentioned repeatedly in this chapter, results in persistence of the cavity after drainage, whereas PSs routinely collapse in the operating room once they are drained. In the WOPN and in the excessively large or inferior PS the assumed mechanism is the accumulation of food and debris in the cavity. With regard to WOPN complete recovery from interventions will be delayed until the cavity regresses. In particularly large and rigid WOPN I will place a closed suction drain in the cavity as well as creating a Roux-en-Y jejunostomy.

For operative cyst gastrostomy or cyst-duodenostomy either an open or a laparoscopic approach is appropriate. Palpation or laparoscopic ultrasound may be used to pinpoint the location of the cyst. Stay sutures should be placed to the left and right of the anticipated gastrotomy incision on the anterior surface of the stomach. Electrocautery can be used to create the gastrotomy. A length of approximately 10 cm should be sufficient in an open procedure. A smaller incision may be possible for the laparoscopic approach. Be aware that the stomach will collapse immediately. Use the stay sutures to assist in visualizing the posterior wall of the stomach, and be prepared to struggle with the great redundancy of the gastric mucosa. Once the location has been confirmed, use an 18-gauge angiocath to confirm that the PS is accessible. Make an incision in the posterior stomach wall and either place a running stitch circumferentially around the posterior gastrotomy using monofilament suture on a large needle such as a CT-1 to avoid struggling to rescue the needle from within the cavity. It is much simpler to use a circular end-to-end stapling device. As with other uses of the EEA-type device, a purse-string suture must be placed unless the gastrotomy is very snug around the shaft of the instrument without it. A biopsy of the wall of the PS is required. I recommend frozen section exam in the event that the eventual diagnosis would mandate reoperation. Any debris within the cyst should be evacuated. Neither cyst-gastrostomy nor cyst-jejunostomy should be undertaken without confirming a tight adherence between the PS and these structures.

For Roux-en-Y cyst-jejunostomy I create the Roux limb in the usual manner. In almost all cases I seek an access point through the transverse mesocolon to the left of the spine in body-tail PS and to the right of the spine or midline for PSs located toward the head of the pancreas. If this access point is not established easily, then other convenient areas should be sought. If possible a dependent site should be used for improved drainage. It should not be a challenge to extend the mesenteric dissection of the Roux limb to permit access to further remote targets.

I perform anastomoses by hand. It may be helpful to use a technique I first learned from Leslie Blumgart. I use monofilament, absorbable suture. I place the sutures for the anterior row into the anterior aspect of the incision in the PS, using an out-to-in direction for the sutures. Leave the needles on the sutures and be careful to avoid tangles. Next the posterior row of interrupted sutures can be placed and tied. This is done before opening the jejunum. Be careful not to create too large a jejunostomy. The previously placed anterior sutures are now very easy to place in the jejunum. Without this technique, placing the anterior sutures after the jejunum has been placed deep within the abdomen can be technically challenging. The management of WOPN and the management of the isolated pancreatic segment, the pancreatic tissue located to the left of the ductal disconnection in type 3 ducts, is discussed later in this chapter.

Walled-Off Pancreatic Necrosis

In the case of WOPN, as previously stated, I prefer to avoid drainage to the stomach. Considerable success has been reported by Baron and colleagues with very aggressive endoscopic entry into the necrosis in the lesser sac through a transgastric approach. Again leaving this rigid cavity vulnerable to permitting food and other nonsterile debris into the cavity should be avoided. Barron has shifted primarily to a retroperitoneal approach, possibly for that reason. Only a small subset of GI endoscopists are likely to be this aggressive. Débridement of pancreatic necrosis, or "necrosectomy," may be performed using several techniques, including open operative débridement, endoscopic transgastric retroperitoneal débridement, and retroperitoneal or transabdominal laparoscopic débridement. I have used flexible endoscopes for essentially the same procedure as others use laparoscopic equipment. I will restate that the literature on this subject may be misleading. In the historical literature, débridement of pancreatic necrosis was performed early in the course of acute necrotizing pancreatitis. Precise indications for intervention were not yet established. It was the norm to require multiple returns to the operating room (OR) for re-débridement, creating a mindset that the amount of débridement may be limited at the first or even subsequent operations because the surgeon anticipated a return to the OR. Unfortunately, this mindset has not vanished entirely even today.

Open abdomen was another practice in this prior era of early necrosectomy. Unfortunately, the open abdomen, a practice abandoned by pancreatic surgeons decades ago, has resurfaced in the wake of the valid data produced in trauma patients who have been victims of extreme crystalloid indiscretion. The data supporting the open abdomen in this setting are irrefutable. There is no such validation for the now-commonplace practice of open abdomen for the patient with infected pancreatic necrosis nor for any other intra-abdominal entity characterized by sepsis and a contaminated abdomen. In this historic era outcomes were poor and mortality high. As the data have evolved, every effort is now made to delay operative intervention until at least 4 weeks after the index episode. This can be achieved partly by simply recognizing the value in waiting. Where previously the surgeon may have believed the hazards of delaying intervention outweighed the value in permitting the process to evolve, the data now clearly dictate a delay unless clinical imperatives arise. If the patient's clinical status deteriorates or if infected necrosis is confirmed sooner than 4 weeks after the index episode, then some intervention must be considered. Starting with Patrick Feeney at Virginia Mason in Seattle in the 1990s and reproduced in many centers thereafter, it was discovered that percutaneous drainage could be used to offer a bridge until 4 to 6 weeks had elapsed. In the original report, it was discovered that 24% of patients with WOPN and infected necrosis could be managed definitively with percutaneous drainage alone. Other reports have recorded successes as high as 47%. The

Dutch group has similarly advocated for this management principle. Thus the early data looking at débridement of pancreatic necrosis focused on the older version, performed in the acute setting. Delaying the "débridement" for 4 to 6 weeks after the index episodes should be considered as an entirely unique entity. In this setting the patient typically has recovered from the extremes seen in the early weeks after the attack. Some patients will be nutritionally unsound, but the organ failure should have largely resolved. Operative outcomes and patient survival data should be equally superior.

For operative intervention in this setting it is important to determine the anatomy of the MPD using ERCP or MRCP. My colleagues and I have reported data that suggest that patients with WOPN who require débridement are highly likely to have underlying ductal pathology. For open débridement a midline incision is best. The lesser sac can be entered by carefully dividing the gastrocolic omentum, preserving the epiploic vessels, and avoiding injury to the mesocolon. At times it may be best to access the lesser sac through the remains of the mesentery by using the area to the left of the spine where colonic vessels are less likely to be encountered. The solid necrotic debris typically is separated easily from the underlying viable tissue as a result of the delay. The necrotic debris is much more likely to be densely adherent to the underlying pancreatic parenchyma when operation is performed early. It is mandatory to remove all necrotic material down to viable pancreas. Because of unfamiliarity with the anatomy, many fail to perform complete débridement, and multiple reoperations are required. In 2016 reoperation for débridement of pancreatic necrosis should be necessary in fewer than 10% of patients. Be aware that in cases of extreme necrosis of the pancreas, typically seen in the midbody of the pancreas, there may be no pancreatic tissue separating the floor of the retroperitoneum in the lesser sac and the splenic vein and artery. Care must be taken to avoid inadvertently entering these vascular structures. The lesser sac should be drained with large-bore drains.

All of the minimally invasive techniques, excluding the endoscopic transgastric approach, start with percutaneously placed drains. Although most of the literature has assessed the use of retroperitoneal drains using the left flank approach, sometimes you may be told that no safe access point can be seen from that approach. I have thus employed both left- and right-sided flank approaches to the lesser sac as well as a transabdominal approach through the epigastrium. An evolving technology can assist in maneuvering catheters through the turns and twists required to avoid injury. Much also depends upon just how intrepid the interventionalist proves to be. Although the literature is clear that because of the semisolid nature of the necrotic debris, it is safe and more effective to use large-bore drains (20F to 24F), resistance to using these large drains from the interventional radiologist is likely. However, the "step-up" approach advocated by the Dutch group used 7F catheters with success.

The tract should be permitted to mature for up to 7 days before operation. In the OR a guidewire is passed through the catheter and it is removed. With use of a balloon catheter with a channel for passing a wire, the tract can be balloon dilated to accommodate the instrument. Laparoscopic instruments have been used with success in techniques such as the videoscope-assisted retroperitoneal débridement, coined by the Seattle group. In this practice the access point can be enlarged to accommodate multiple ports. For my flexible endoscopic approach, I use an upper GI scope with multiple ports. I prefer the flexible endoscope for its ability to accommodate curves and angles because the cavities bear some resemblance to a cave with many different interconnected chambers. I have strived to establish access points for the left and the right flank in the same patient. In this manner I can use one port for vision and another port for débridement. After a tract is dilated further, it can be effective to use instruments typically used in open surgery, such as the ringed forceps, often called "the spongestick without the sponge." The rounded tip prevents perforation of structures, and the wide mouth permits grasping the necrotic debris without fragmenting it. Through the endoscopic channel it is possible to use a snare to grasp the necrosis.

There is a longer-mouthed endoscopic grasping instrument called an "alligator" forceps for the same purpose. Assuming the technology aimed at broadening the use of NOTES (natural orifice transluminal endoscopic surgery) continues to grow, we may see the development of more complex and more effective instrumentation that can pass through endoscopic channels. As with open débridement, the goal is to completely evacuate all necrotic material. Surgeons can irrigate aggressively and then place large-bore drains. If using this endoscopic approach, be certain that CO_2 insufflation is available. There is a well-reported fear of air embolus and potential death if air insufflation is used. Recovery from these minimally invasive methods is prompt.

Pseudocysts Associated With Disconnected Duct (Type 3 Ducts) and Management of the Isolated Pancreatic Segment

As previously described, one potential result of an episode of severe necrotizing pancreatitis is permanent destruction to the main pancreatic duct. The most common site is in the midbody of the pancreas. The tissue to the left of the ductal disruption is essentially viable parenchyma, which continues to secrete bicarbonate-rich water and inactive pancreatic enzymes (Figure 3). As outcomes for survival in patients with severe necrotizing pancreatitis have improved dramatically over the past two decades, the likelihood of a patient with this phenomenon has risen. Unfortunately, these patients frequently are dismissed as simply being fortunate to be alive. There is great resistance to consider intervention, particularly if prior débridement has been performed. Thus frequent in my practice are patients who have suffered through months to years of misery and who have bounced from doctor to doctor, including surgeons, only to be told there was no intervention capable of relieving the problem. Typically there is a PS at the site of the disruption. At times, if a percutaneous drainage was used, the disconnection is manifested as a persistent fistula from the drain. In this case, injecting contrast through the catheter will delineate the duct in the isolated pancreatic segment.

There are three potential operative strategies. As stated earlier, in my opinion, the endoscopic options hold minimal promise. The choices include Roux-Y cyst-enterostomy, Roux-Y lateral pancreatojejunostomy to the duct in the remnant, or distal pancreatectomy-splenectomy. In our reports on this subject, my colleagues and I found that distal pancreatectomy-splenectomy had several negative consequences. Because the density of beta cells are greatest in the tail of the pancreas, the risk of converting the patient to insulin dependence was greater than 50%. In addition, operative times were longer than in the other two procedures, hospital length of stay was longest, and the need for blood transfusion was highest of all three choices. This procedure may be associated with extensive scarring and adhesions in the left upper quadrant of the abdomen. Often the spleen is densely adherent to the lateral and anterior peritoneal surfaces and to the left hemidiaphragm, and its dissection can be a difficult and bloody affair.

Having said that, our follow-up data demonstrated that subsequent recurrent episodes of AP or pain occurred at a disturbing frequency in patients who had been managed by a cyst-jejunostomy. I no longer recommend this option. I thus advocate for open Roux-en-Y pancreatojejunostomy to the duct in the isolated segment. Access to the tail of the pancreas may require entering the PS. Familiarity with pancreatic surgery and of retroperitoneal anatomy is mandatory. Once the segment is found, it is possible to palpate the pancreatic duct, which often is dilated. Intraoperative ultrasonography may be used to locate the MPD. An 18-gauge angiocath should be placed into the duct, and crystal clear pancreatic juice must be confirmed. Once the duct has been accessed, electrocautery then can be used to extend the incision along the duct in both directions. This procedure may well be termed a *Puestow procedure* in the tail of the pancreas. We perform the procedure with interrupted absorbable monofilament suture. The posterior row is placed and tied before the jejunum is opened. Care must be taken to avoid creation of an excessively wide enterotomy. The size must approximate the size of the pancreatic duct incision. After the enterotomy has been created, the anterior row of sutures are placed with a sequence starting with both corners followed by the very middle of the anastomosis. Thereafter the gaps are divided by half with each suture. This ensures a well-matched attachment. Another helpful maneuver is that, if you are unable to locate the MPD, it is effective to carefully create a vertical incision in the midbody of the pancreas. In this manner you eventually will access the duct, at which time you convert to a horizontal incision in the duct. At times, when adhesions in the remainder of the abdominal cavity have been excessive, I have used a pancreaticogastrostomy to the posterior wall of the stomach, which is located just anterior to the pancreas.

Pseudocysts Associated With Chronic Pancreatitis

Freeark and Prinz made important contributions in the late 1980s to this field. They found that patients with the combined diagnosis of chronic pancreatitis (CP) and PSs who had undergone operation for PS returned with persistent symptoms because of a failure to address

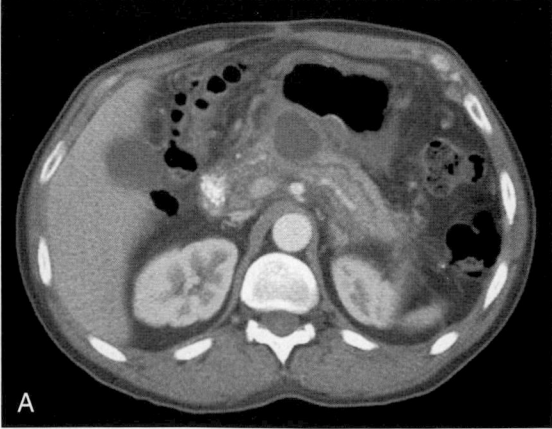 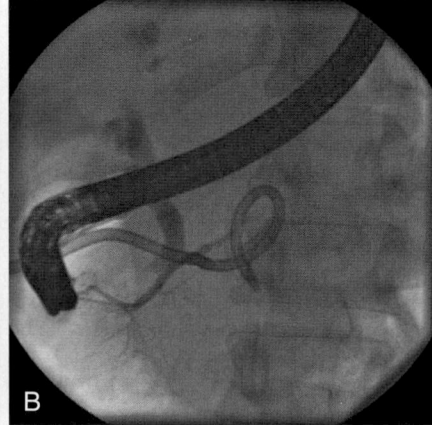 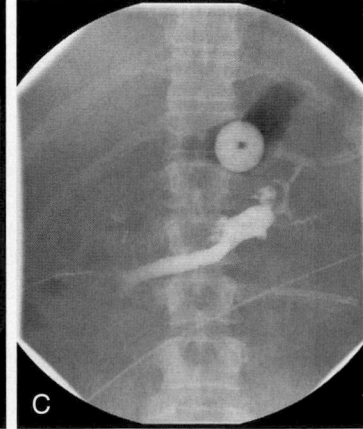

FIGURE 3 A disconnected left pancreatic remnant occurs after necrosis in the neck of the pancreas with resultant obliteration of the main pancreatic duct. The disrupted pancreatic duct from the viable left pancreas, now not in continuity, leaks and results in a midbody pseudocyst. This condition is visualized on contrast-enhanced computed tomographic scan (**A**). It is shown by an abrupt cut-off of the pancreatic duct at the neck on endoscopic retrograde pancreatography (**B**) and by a drain track fistulagram filling only a small tail remnant (**C**).

the underlying CP. They reported on combined cyst-jejunostomy drainage and Puestow procedure in one operation. As I have followed this subset of patients and as I developed my recognition of the dominant role played by the MPD in the course and in the persistence of PS, I performed a study in which I examined the theory that duct drainage alone is sufficient in the management of patients with PSs associated with CP. In this study I began by placing closed-suction drains in the PS after performing a definitive operation for CP (Puestow or Frey procedure). After the first five cases in which no pancreatic juice emerged from the drains, I no longer included the drains in the study. Outcomes were definitive that with duct drainage the PS can be ignored. This principle is also seen in the management of the isolated pancreatic segment. The associated PS can be ignored if adequate duct drainage is achieved. The data are convincing that endoscopic transpapillary stent placement holds little promise in this setting.

■ CONCLUSION

Thus several precepts must be remembered. The vast majority of PSs require no intervention. This is because the majority will resolve spontaneously without intervention and because small (<4 cm) asymptomatic PSs require none. One must exercise surveillance and recognize the distinctions between PSs, WOPN, and cystic neoplasms, particularly IPMN. Early intervention is never indicated for PS and is to be avoided in necrosis and for WOPN. The condition of the main pancreatic duct must be considered in the management of persistent PS and in WOPN. Ductal injury or disruption is common in persistent PS and WOPN. Our system of categorizing ductal injuries after

pancreatitis should be used to drive the choice of modality to treat PSs. Type 1 (normal ducts) can be treated successfully with nonsurgical interventions. Type 2 (duct stricture) should be given a trial of nonsurgical treatments, but a failure rate of at least 25% should be anticipated. At that point surgical interventions should be employed. Excessively repeating the failed nonsurgical intervention should be discontinued. Type 3 (ductal disruption) is essentially treatable only with operation and ideally with a lateral pancreaticojejunostomy. If this is not feasible, then distal pancreatectomy/splenectomy should be employed. Type 4 (PS associated with chronic pancreatitis) should address the CP, and the drainage of the duct will render any procedure aimed at the PS to be unnecessary.

Because some of the more difficult cases are recognized, referral to a specialized pancreatic center is optimal if not mandatory.

SUGGESTED READINGS

Beck WC, Bhutani MS, Raju GS, Nealon W. Surgical management of late sequelae in survivors of an episode of acute necrotizing pancreatitis. *J Am Coll Surg*. 2012;214:682-688, discussion 688-690.

Nealon WH, Bhutani M, Riall TS, Raju G, Ozkan O, Neilan R. A unifying concept: pancreatic ductal anatomy both predicts and determines the major complications resulting from pancreatitis. *J Am Coll Surg*. 2009;208:790-801.

Nealon WH, Walser E. Duct drainage alone is sufficient in the operative management of pancreatic pseudocyst in patients with chronic pancreatitis. *Ann Surg*. 2003;237:614-622.

Working Group IAP/APA Acute Pancreatitis Guidelines. IAP/APA evidence-based guidelines for the management of acute pancreatitis. *Pancreatology*. 2013;13:e1-e15.

PANCREATIC DUCTAL DISRUPTIONS LEADING TO PANCREATIC FISTULA, PANCREATIC ASCITES, OR PANCREATIC PLEURAL EFFUSION

Motokazu Sugimoto, MD, David Sonntag, MD, Richard A. Kozarek, MD, and L. William Traverso, MD

■ DEFINITIONS

The following is a list of terms that are commonly associated with pancreatic ductal disruption:

Pancreatic ductal disruption: A loss of ductal integrity anywhere in the pancreatic ductal system (i.e., a main pancreatic duct or tertiary ductules) demonstrated by computed tomography (CT), sinogram through a percutaneous drain that reveals a pancreatic duct, endoscopic retrograde cholangiopancreatography (ERCP), or magnetic resonance cholangiopancreatography (MRCP). Disruption also is suggested by a persistent finding of amylase-rich drain fluid.

Pancreatic fistula: Passage of pancreatic juice through a pancreatic ductal disruption that exits the pancreatic parenchyma. This fistula can reside totally within the capsule of the pancreas and

therefore can be minimal and self-healing. Alternatively, the fistula can breach the capsule of the pancreas, resulting in pancreatic juice entering the retroperitoneal or peritoneal cavities. A controlled pancreatocutaneous fistula is a condition in which an ongoing pancreatic fistula is well drained by a percutaneous catheter, preventing pancreatic juice from extending elsewhere.

Acute peripancreatic fluid collection: This term was defined according to the revised Atlanta classification of acute pancreatitis. It is an accumulation of pancreatic juice (enzyme-rich fluid) in the peripancreatic area to include the adjacent retroperitoneal or peritoneal cavities (Figure 1, *A*), and it appears within 4 weeks after onset of acute pancreatitis.

Pancreatic pseudocyst: This term was also redefined in the revised Atlanta classification. It is an intrapancreatic or peripancreatic fluid collection that develops a well-circumscribed wall, usually determined by imaging studies (Figure 1, *B*) and, in general, it appears more than 4 weeks after the onset of acute pancreatitis.

Pancreatic necrosis: Implies a *permanent* condition that occurs when a portion of the pancreas loses its blood supply because of severe inflammation. Contrast-enhanced CT shows lack of enhancement of the pancreatic parenchyma (Figure 1, *C*). Pancreatic parenchymal necrosis can be associated with a distinct nonparenchymal necrosis called *peripancreatic necrosis*. Multiple serial CTs during the entire clinical course should be interpreted carefully not to misread necrosis when the lack of enhancement may be due to inflammation or overlying fluid collections. According to the revised Atlanta classification, "acute necrotic collection" is a pancreatic or peripancreatic collection containing variable amounts of fluid and necrosis associated with necrotizing pancreatitis, whereas "walled-off necrosis" is a pancreatic or peripancreatic collection that has matured into an encapsulated collection with a well-defined inflammatory wall. Walled-off necrosis usually occurs more than 4 to 8 weeks after onset of necrotizing pancreatitis.

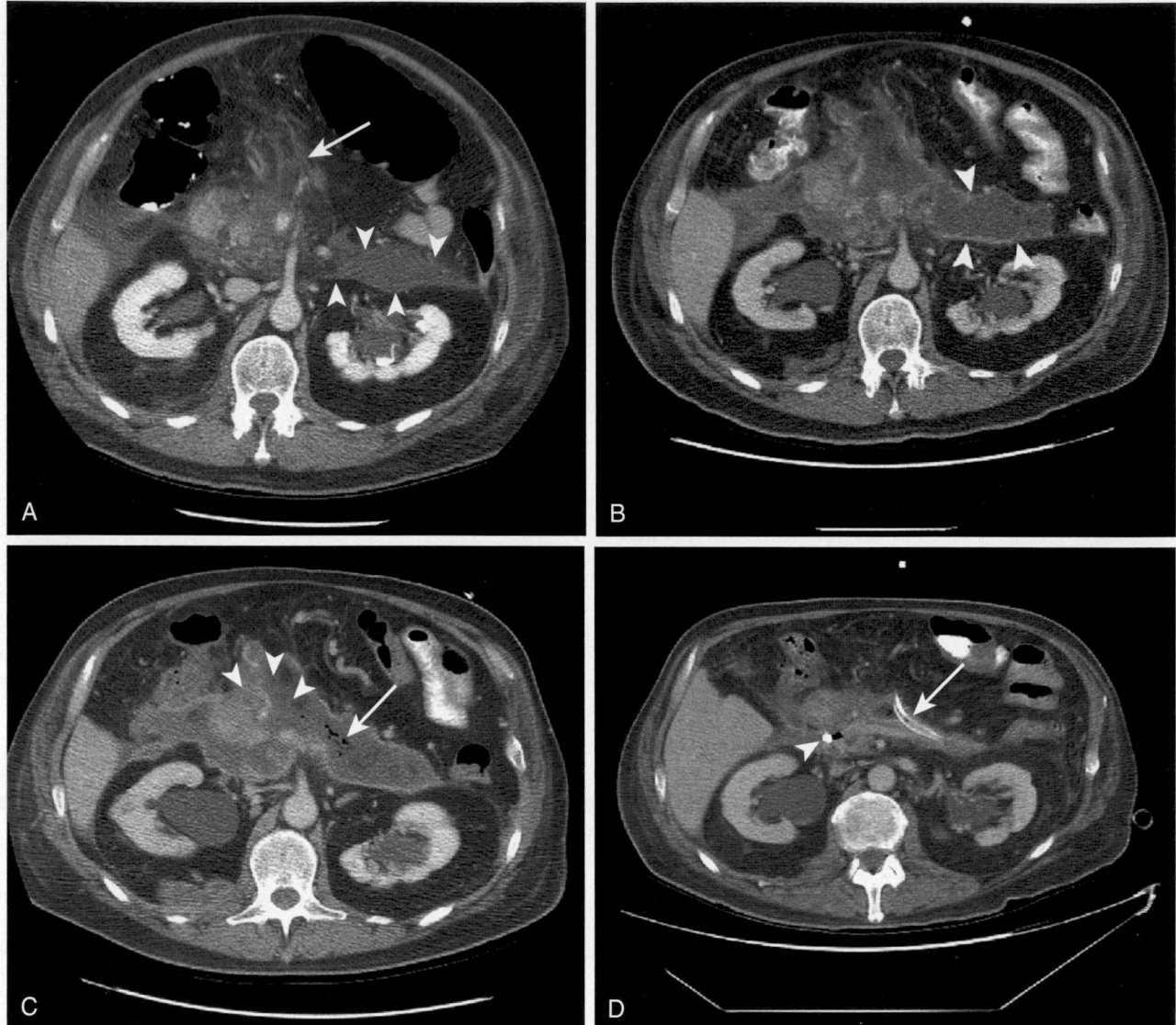

FIGURE I A 64-year-old male patient with acute pancreatitis with nausea and abdominal pain. **A,** The computed tomography (CT) image shows peripancreatic fluid *(arrowheads),* later proved to be amylase rich. There are extensive inflammatory changes at the root of the mesentery *(arrow).* **B,** Follow-up CT 20 days later reveals evolution of the peripancreatic fluid with development of an enhancing wall *(white arrowheads),* suggesting maturation of the collection. **C,** Fourteen days later, another CT shows small pockets of gas within the collection *(arrow)* and development of surrounding infected peripancreatic nonenhancement, suggesting necrosis *(arrowheads).* **D,** After aggressive drainage of abdominal fluid collections with catheters *(white arrow),* follow-up CT reveals near-complete resolution of the collection. Note the bile duct has a stent in place *(arrowhead).*

Pancreatic ascites: A collection of pancreatic juice from a pancreatic ductal disruption that communicates into the peritoneal cavity, usually from the lesser sac (Figure 2). This uncommon type of pancreatic fluid collection is not walled off to form a peripancreatic fluid collection or a pseudocyst and is usually well tolerated by the patient, unless the proenzymes in the ascites become activated as would occur if the ascites became contaminated with microorganisms. Approximately half the cases have a concomitant pseudocyst present, suggesting that the cause of the ascites may have been leakage from the pseudocyst.

Pancreatic pleural effusion: A collection of enzyme-rich pancreatic juice in the pleural cavity on either side of the chest (Figure 3). This collection originates from a pancreatic ductal disruption "fistulizing" into the retroperitoneum. The collection is not walled off in the extracapsular peripancreatic space but rather communicates through pleuroperitoneal foramina into the right or left pleural cavity. The location of the ductal disruption in the pancreatic ductal system determines whether the right or left

pleural cavity is the site of collection (i.e., a ductal disruption dorsally over the portal vein may accumulate in the right chest, whereas a disruption dorsally from the pancreatic tail may accumulate in the left chest). The presence of a right or left pleural effusion is a clue to the site of the ductal disruption within the pancreas.

Disconnected pancreatic duct syndrome: A condition in which proximal and distal sides of the pancreas are separated permanently by pancreatic ductal disruption. Flow from the upstream disconnected side of the pancreas is no longer possible to go through the downstream native pancreatic duct. Persistent secretion of the disconnected segment cannot enter the enteral stream, resulting in formation of peripancreatic fluid collection, peripancreatic necrosis, or pseudocyst. The disconnection in majority of patients occurs after pancreatic necrosis of the head or neck/body of the gland. A common site of disruption is at the pancreatic neck probably because of the watershed blood supply to the neck being from the pancreaticoduodenal artery and splenic artery

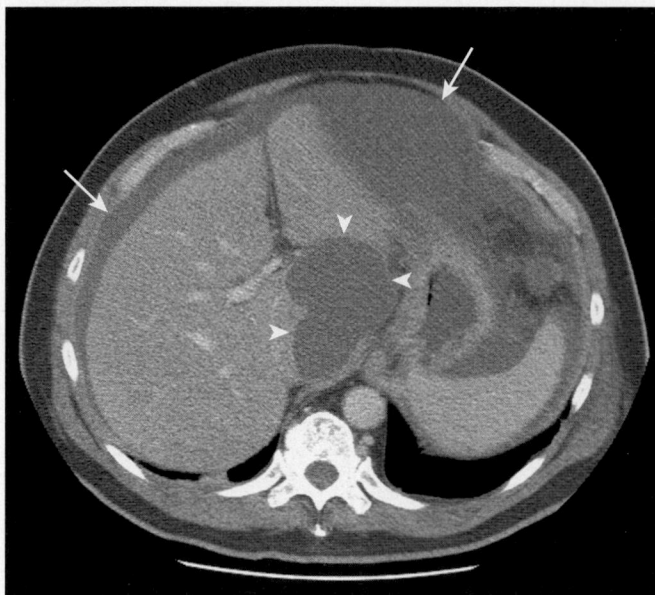

FIGURE 2 An abdominal computed tomography reveals pancreatic ascites around liver *(arrows)* and spleen. The patient was shown to have a downstream-duct disruption and disconnected gland in the area of the body of the pancreas. Pancreatic fluid leaked into the lesser sac *(arrowheads)* and then freely into the peritoneal cavity *(arrows)*.

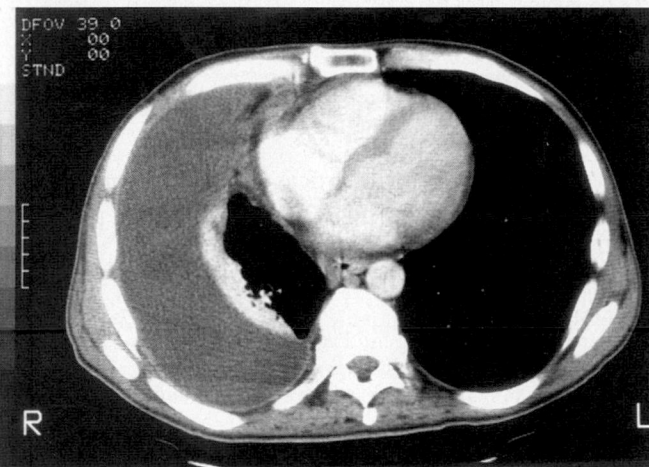

FIGURE 3 A right-sided amylase-rich pleural effusion is shown by computed tomography in a man with a dorsal-duct disruption at the genu of the pancreatic duct over the portal vein. The route to the right pleural cavity was through the retroperitoneum over the portal vein by way of the hepatoduodenal ligament through the pleuroperitoneal foramina of the diaphragm.

arcades (Figure 4, *A* and *B*). When the gland can be seen to be disconnected on CT, this represents the most extreme finding of the disconnected pancreatic duct syndrome and is a consequence of complete necrosis of a central portion of the pancreas (Figure 5).

■ CLINICAL PRESENTATION AND DIAGNOSIS

Identification of Pancreatic Ductal Disruption

Approximately 90% of patients developing acute pancreatitis experience a self-limiting course of abdominal pain and hyperamylasemia that resolves within 1 week. However, when clinical symptoms persist

longer than a week, then most likely a pancreatic ductal disruption is developing. Over decades of observing the pattern of anatomic findings during the sequence of CT scans, in each case of severe pancreatitis it has become prudent to focus on the status of pancreatic ductal anatomy. The first clue is if any patient develops acute peripancreatic fluid collection, pancreatic pseudocyst, or pancreatic necrosis.

Pancreatic ductal anatomy has been categorized successfully in association with pseudocyst regardless of the presence of pancreatic necrosis, in studies by Nealon and colleagues (Figure 6). According to the types of pancreatic ductal injury after acute pancreatitis, consequences were predicted and therapies were directed. A type III injury results in disconnected pancreatic duct syndrome and was associated with a more refractory clinical course: no spontaneous resolution, higher incidences of pancreatic fistula and recurrent pancreatitis, longer drainage time, and necessity of more aggressive treatment such as surgical débridement.

Diagnostic Approach

If patients with acute pancreatitis are not improving by 1 week of conservative treatment after the onset of symptoms, then an assessment to define possible ductal disruption must begin. Why? The key to success is controlling the leak at its source and not allowing the retroperitoneum to be continuously bathed with pancreatic juice. While the patient is managed by volume resuscitation, electrolyte replacement, pain control, and nutritional support in the acute phase, a contrast-enhanced CT is used to identify presence, location, and size of peripancreatic fluid collection or pancreatic necrosis. The CT findings as listed in the rest of this discussion may suggest the site of pancreatic ductal disruption; however, other subsequent imaging modalities will more precisely locate the site of leakage from a pancreatic ductal disruption. These more precise imaging techniques are fluoroscopic drain studies after percutaneous drainage, ERCP, or MRCP with or without secretin administration. Fluoroscopic drain studies or an ERCP may miss the leak site as sufficient volume of contrast must be injected to clearly delineate the ductal anatomy.

If the leak is ventral in the pancreas, then the pancreatic juice will accumulate inside the lesser sac. Peripancreatic fluid collections also can accumulate in the retroperitoneum by dorsal rupture through the pancreatic capsule from the tail to collect over the left renal space or from the dorsal head in the pancreaticoduodenal groove to collect over the right pararenal space. Pancreatic juice collections in these areas have difficulty traveling elsewhere, and they will form the classic pseudocyst. The inflammatory process ultimately results in a thickened wall. More commonly, lesser sac fluid collections will form a pseudocyst rather than leak out into the peritoneal cavity to result in pancreatic ascites.

Pleural effusions also are detected easily by CT. They are related to pancreatic juice leaking from a ductal disruption and then penetrating the pancreatic capsule into the retroperitoneal space. When undrained, the dissecting fluid can enter the left pleural cavity from a disruption in the pancreatic tail or body and communicate into the left chest through pleuroperitoneal foramina. The juice can enter the right pleural cavity from a ductal disruption of the pancreatic neck, dorsally over the pancreatic head but ventral to the portal vein. This space is a channel to the thorax because pancreatic juice can pass behind the hepatoduodenal ligament, through the pleuroperitoneal foramina, and into the right chest. On its way to either pleural cavity a fluid collection made up of pancreatic juice can approach the esophageal hiatus, resulting in a periesophageal fluid collection that can dissect into the mediastinum.

Indication and Rationale for Treatment

If a patient shows anatomic signs of persistent pancreatic juice leakage, such as persistent or enlarging peripancreatic collections, *and* that patient shows clinical deterioration such as by the signs,

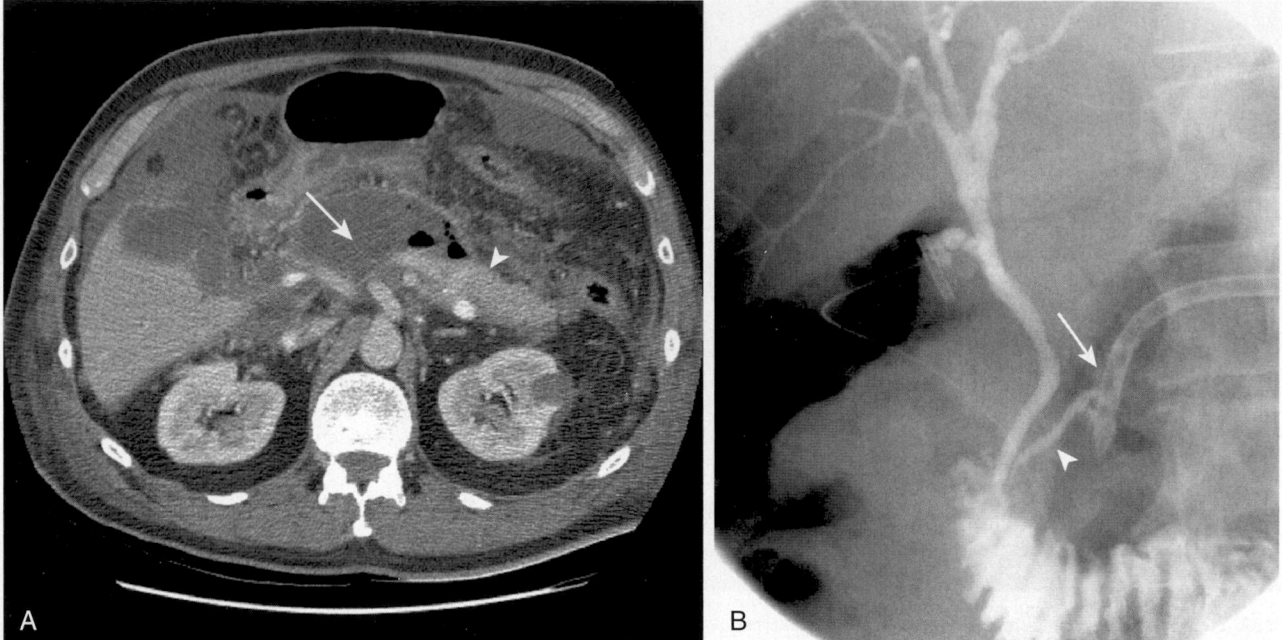

FIGURE 4 **A,** Necrosis in the region of the pancreatic neck *(arrow)* resulted in disconnection of the head from the body of the pancreas shown in this computed tomography. Note the enhancing body and tail of the pancreas *(arrowhead)*. **B,** An intraoperative cholangiogram through the cystic duct during necrosectomy showed free reflux of contrast up into the main pancreatic duct *(arrowhead)* and then into the cavity of necrosis where the pancreatic neck had been *(arrow)*. Overlying the latter is a percutaneous drain from the left anterior renal route that had been used in the preoperative period to allow for nonemergent necrosectomy after the inflammatory process had improved. Note the contrast filling the drain.

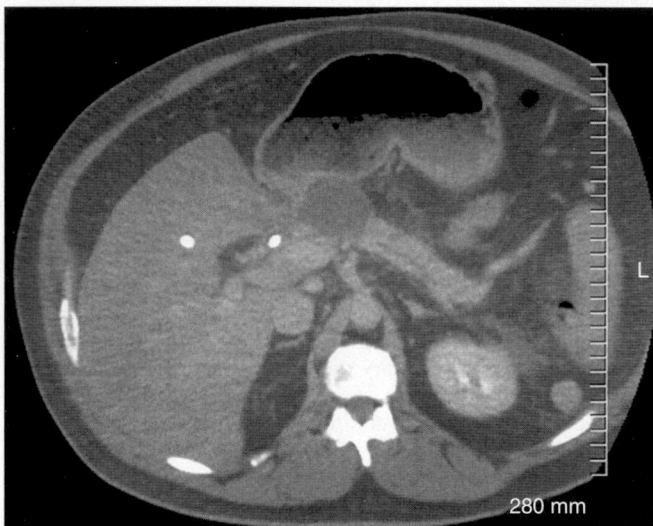

FIGURE 5 Proximal and distal sides of the pancreas are completely separated shown on computed tomography (CT). Pancreatic juice leakage secreted from the distal side of the pancreas must be controlled by external or internal drainage system.

BOX 1: Indications for Percutaneous Catheter Drainage

Presence of peripancreatic collections by computed tomography (CT) plus:
Symptoms
  Refractory abdominal pain despite use of narcotics
  Inability to begin oral intake
Clinical signs
  Persistent or enlarging fluid collection by CT
  Persistent abdominal distension/ileus
  Systemic inflammatory response syndrome and/or organ
    failure
  Persistent or increasing inflammatory data
  (C-reactive protein and/or white blood cell count)
  Persistent increase in serum amylase or lipase activity
    suggesting persistent pancreatic juice leakage

symptoms, and/or laboratory findings as listed in Box 1, then pancreatic collections (fluid or necrosis) should be drained. If pancreatic juice leakage is uncontrolled, the following patterns have been observed: (1) peripancreatic necrosis with or without infection, (2) formation of pseudoaneurysm (Figure 7, *A* and *B*), erosion into a blood vessel without pseudoaneurysm, or erosion into a hollow viscus, or (3) communication with the free peritoneal cavity, mediastinum, or pleural cavities. We have found that the likelihood of infection increases the longer the pancreatic juice is uncontrolled, which results in progressive peripancreatic damage. Peripancreatic

infection causes organ failure in the late phase and results in higher mortality rate, approximating 20% to 40%. Our premise is not to wait for infection but to halt the process.

A mature pseudocyst is more common in referred patients with a prolonged course but is uncommon in our own primary cases because of the proactive approach to fluid collections. This observation results from our bias: all fluid collections that are *symptomatic* should be drained proactively with minimally invasive methods before a thickened wall develops.

■ MANAGEMENT AND TREATMENT

Percutaneous Catheter Drainage

After initial resuscitation for acute pancreatitis, a contrast-enhanced abdominal CT will indicate most accurately the presence of

Categories of Ductal Anatomy

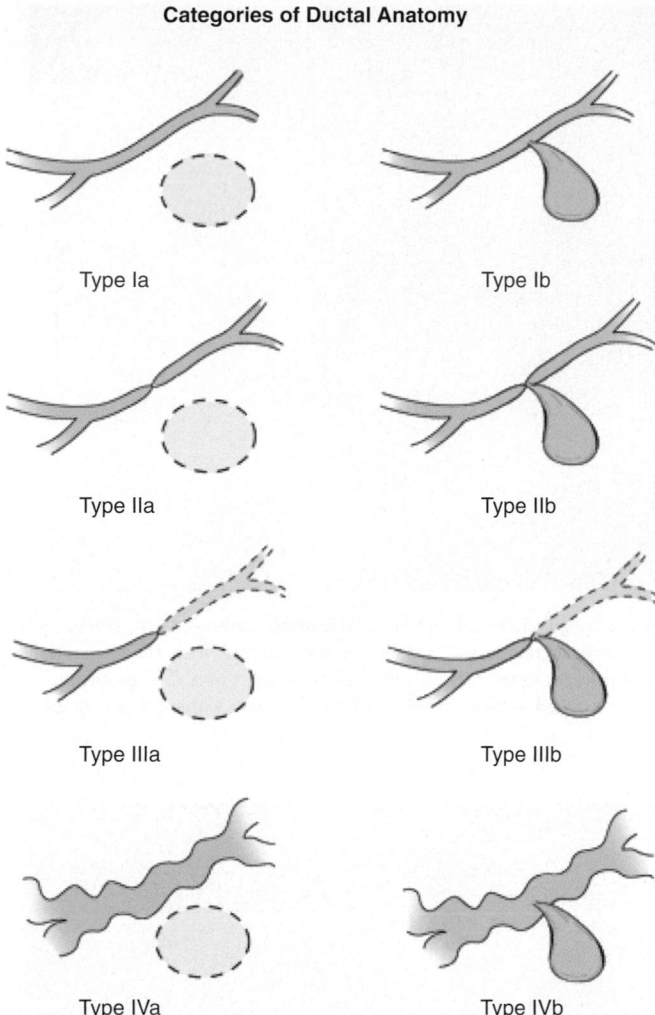

FIGURE 6 System to characterize pancreatic ductal anatomy after acute pancreatitis. Type I: normal duct. Type II: pancreatic duct stricture. Type III: pancreatic duct occlusion (disconnected pancreatic duct syndrome), Type IV: chronic pancreatitis. Type Ia represents no communication between the pancreatic duct and the pseudocyst. Type Ib represents communication between the pancreatic duct and the pseudocyst, and so on. *(From Nealon WH, Bhutani M, Riall TS, et al. A unifying concept: pancreatic ductal anatomy both predicts and determines the major complications resulting from pancreatitis. J Am Coll Surg. 2009;208:793.)*

collection. To minimize the radiation dose, CT technique is limited to the upper abdomen and to a single venous phase. Each CT is followed by a fluoroscopic drain study, allowing cavity lavage and drain reposition, exchange, or upsize (up to 18F). Frequent imaging allows detection and treatment of new peripancreatic collections that can be drained using additional PCD sites. The frequency of CT/drain studies is decreased to *once a week* as the patient becomes clinically stable and the cavities decrease in size. Drainage fluid can be monitored for appearance and volume throughout the clinical course. Samples of the fluid are assessed for amylase activity, Gram stain, and microbiologic culture at the time of PCD and anytime during the course for the presence of pancreatic juice and emerging microorganisms in the cavity. Drainage catheters are removed when the cavities are determined to be collapsed by CT and output is minimal.

The goal of PCD is to achieve "effective drainage." Effective drainage consists of two key elements to control pancreatic juice leakage: drain location and patency. Even though the drain may have been placed in the center of a fluid collection, subsequent CTs and serial fluoroscopic drain studies provide information regarding the presence and site of pancreatic ductal disruption; that is, communication of contrast between main pancreatic duct and peripancreatic space. Then, the drain can be maneuvered to the *site of leakage* from the pancreas (not necessarily the center of the original collection). This maneuver avoids long sinus tracts and extension of more fluid collections elsewhere (Figure 8). Drain patency can be maintained by frequent fluoroscopic drain studies, such as exchanging, upsizing, and lavage.

Once again, our PCD protocol provides continuous control of extravasated pancreatic juice by maintaining patent drains that are placed or ultimately maneuvered to the *site of leakage*. Once achieved, further progression of peripancreatic necrosis should be halted. Once imaging shows no progression of necrosis, we have observed the necrosum to eventually become liquefied. Necrosis cavities will collapse over time if associated with effective drainage, appropriate antibiotics, and adequate nutrition. There may be symptomatic ascites or pleural effusion during the clinical course, which can be managed by ultrasound-guided aspiration or PCD; however, the interventional challenge is not to focus on the peripheral collections but to control pancreatic juice leakage at the *site of leakage*. PCD is an attractive approach because it is less invasive to patients and can be used in a proactive manner earlier before severe sepsis requires traditional surgical necrosectomy. PCD and post-PCD fluoroscopic procedures should be diligently pursued to achieve "effective drainage" using repetitive procedures. Surgical débridement always is reserved as the last resort if conservative treatment fails. By making use of PCD, our series of 39 patients with pancreatic necrosis avoided surgical necrosectomy, and the patients had no pancreatitis-related mortality.

Percutaneous Transgastric Catheter Drainage

Percutaneous transgastric catheter drainage provides another option of drainage route when a better drainage window on CT other than the transgastric route is not available (Figure 9, *A* and *B*). This option enhances minimally invasive drainage techniques and avoids the default to surgical necrosectomy. Moreover, especially in the later clinical course, percutaneous transgastric catheter drainage facilitates internalization of external drains for those cases developing disconnected pancreatic duct syndrome and prevent development of a pancreatocutaneous fistula. Although we must acknowledge the possibility of introducing gastroenteric organisms into the peripancreatic space via the percutaneous transgastric catheter into the retroperitoneum, the drainage fluid can still be used to monitor appearance and volume and sample for amylase activity and microbiologic culture through the externalized catheter. Serial drain studies via this catheter provide important information regarding the site and presence of a pancreatic ductal disruption. In the later clinical course, a percutaneous transgastric drainage catheter can be internalized by two 10F × 10-cm pigtail catheters (Cook Inc., Bloomington,

pancreatic fluid collections, as well as their size and location, as mentioned above. At this point, persistent or enlarging peripancreatic collections plus clinical judgment and/or laboratory findings suggesting uncontrolled pancreatic juice leakage (see Box 1) prompt us to drain collections. Percutaneous catheter drainage (PCD) is a minimally invasive drainage method, allowing interventional radiologists to place a catheter with the shortest and safest route into the collections under CT-guide, with relatively less risk of introducing infection in the cavity compared with endoscopic transmural drainage. Safe access routes are considered to be those remote from intestines, large vessels, or pleural space.

The CT-guided PCD began, in general, with placement of a 12F pigtail drainage catheter (Cook Inc., Bloomington, IN), which is attached to a low-pressure, closed suction drainage system (TRU-CLOSE, UreSil, Skokie, IL). The catheters are flushed with 10 to 20 mL of sterile saline three times daily. Contrast-enhanced CTs are obtained *every 3 days* after PCD to observe the status of the

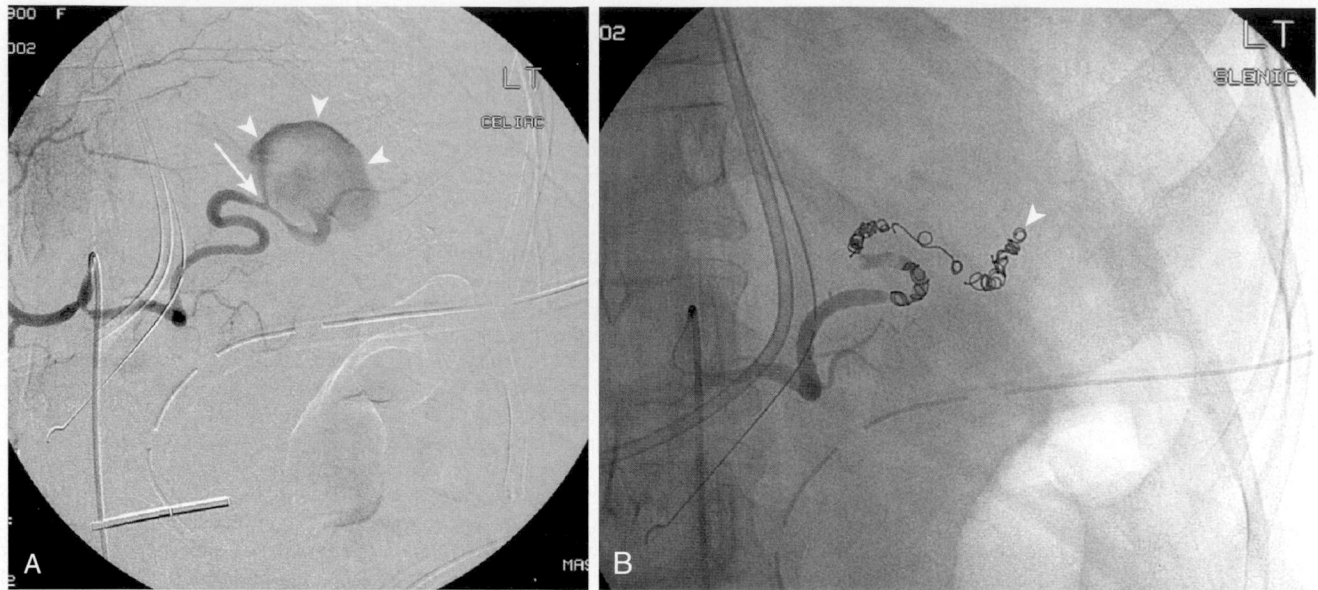

FIGURE 7 Digital subtraction arteriogram in a 46-year-old female patient with necrotizing pancreatitis and multiple drainage catheters with severe bleeding through drainage catheters with cardiopulmonary arrest. **A,** Emergent celiac arteriogram reveals extravasation of contrast from the midportion of the splenic artery into one of the drained cavities *(arrowheads)* through a pseudoaneurysm *(arrow)*. **B,** Selective splenic arteriogram after successful occlusion of the artery with Gelfoam (Pfizer, New York, NY) and multiple coils (one is marked with an *arrowhead*) shows no flow within the artery and no extravasation.

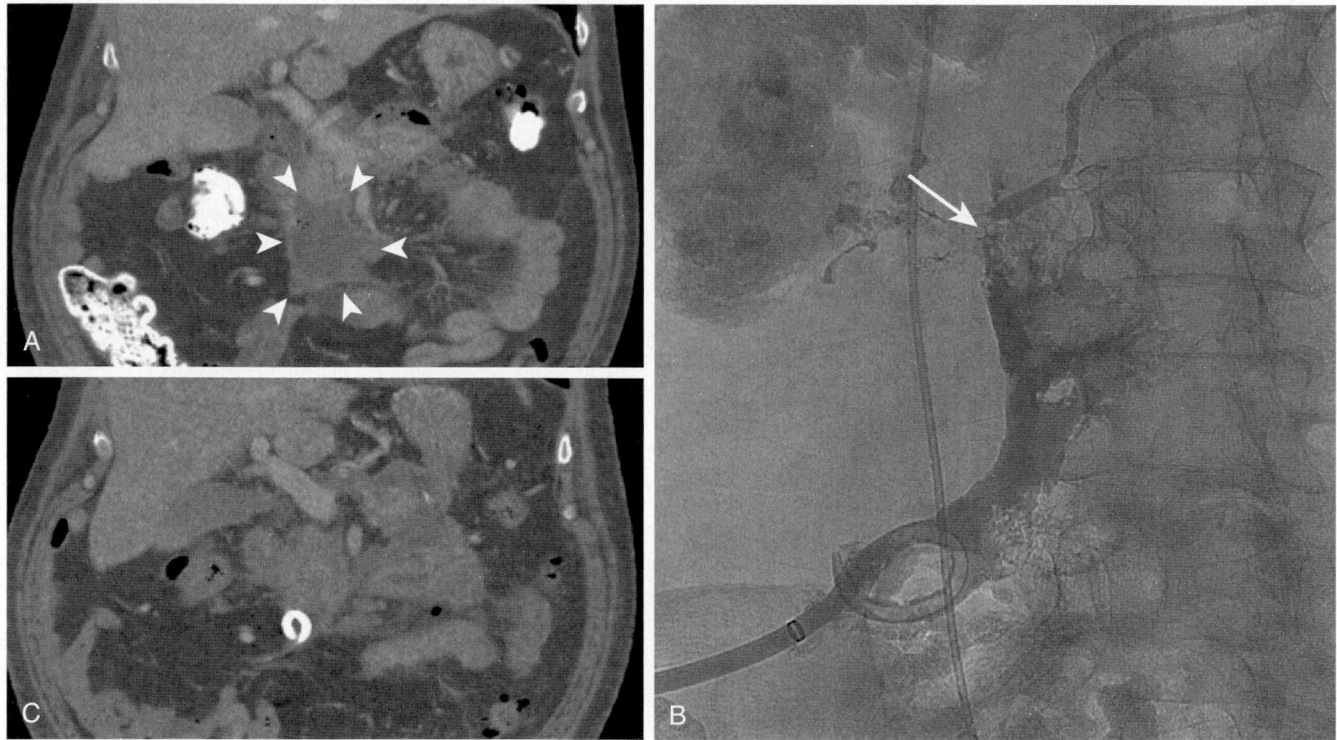

FIGURE 8 66-year-old male with severe acute necrotizing pancreatitis. **A,** An abdominal computed tomography shows peripancreatic fluid collection localized inferiorly to pancreatic head. **B,** A fistulogram drain study showed communication of contrast from peripancreatic fluid collection through main pancreatic duct *(arrow)*. **C,** Tip of the drain was placed at the site of pancreatic duct disruption.

IN) under fluoroscopy, providing internal transgastric drainage to treat a persistent pancreatic fistula (Figure 9, *C*). The percutaneous site does not have to be abandoned but can be used as a gastrostomy site for decompressing the stomach or placing a gastrojejunostomy tube for jejunal feedings.

Endoscopic Treatment

In contrast to PCD, a transpapillary stent placed by ERCP can relieve downstream obstruction and decompress the pancreatic ductal system. In patients with a disconnected pancreatic duct syndrome, it is desirable to place a transpapillary stent bridging from proximal

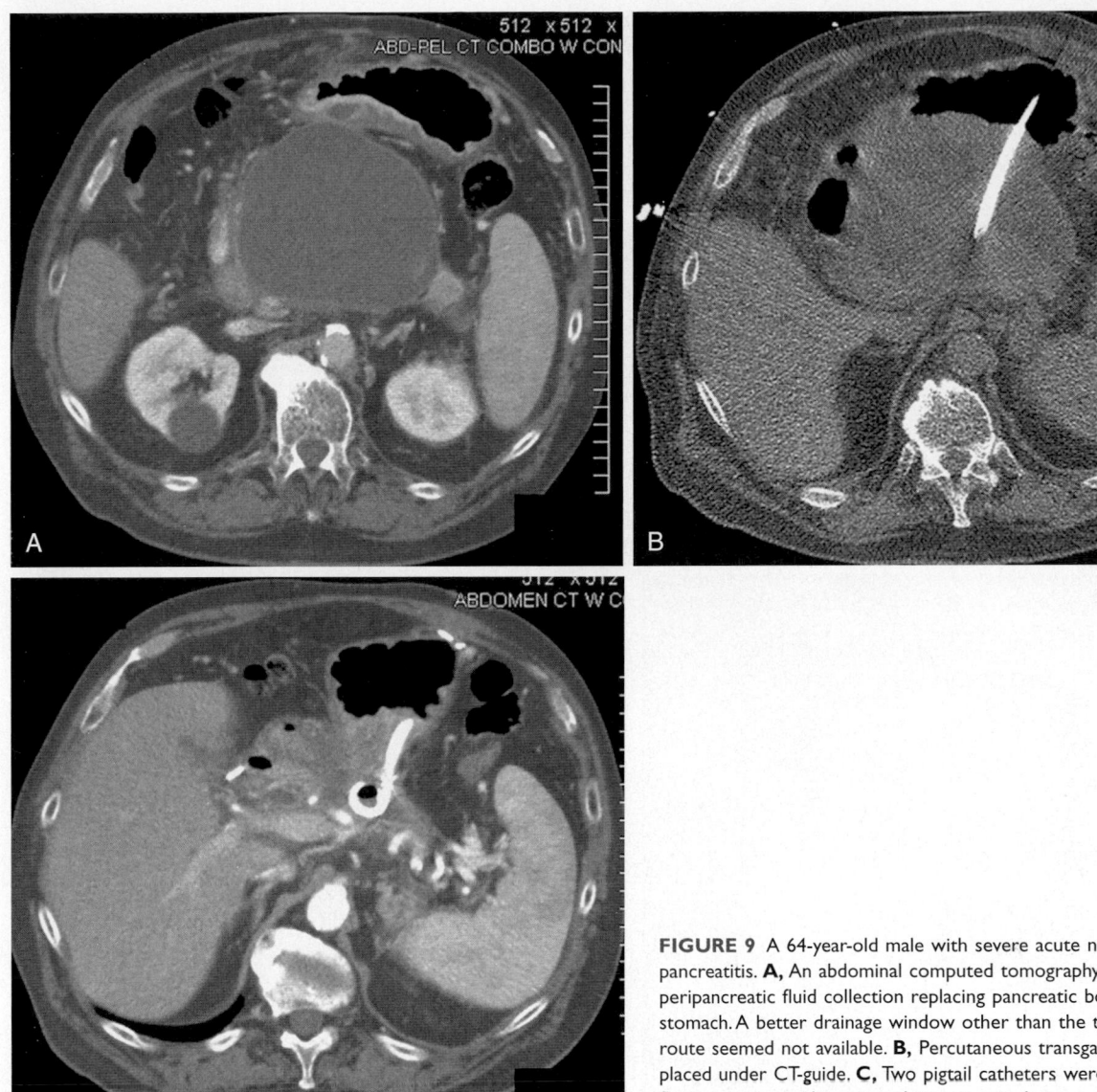

FIGURE 9 A 64-year-old male with severe acute necrotizing pancreatitis. **A,** An abdominal computed tomography (CT) shows peripancreatic fluid collection replacing pancreatic body behind stomach. A better drainage window other than the transgastric route seemed not available. **B,** Percutaneous transgastric drain was placed under CT-guide. **C,** Two pigtail catheters were placed under fluoroscopy, providing internal transgastric drainage to treat persistent pancreatic fistula.

(downstream) side of the pancreas to distal (upstream) side beyond the site of disruption. However, if not feasible, pancreatic juice leakage from the distal side of the pancreatic ductal disruption requires percutaneous or endoscopic drainage. Endoscopists also should be cognizant of the risk of ERCP pancreatitis that may exacerbate the underlying inflammatory process.

It is also possible to direct treatment simultaneously with other endoscopic techniques because ERCP defines the pancreatic ductal anatomy well. Endoscopic ultrasound (EUS)-guided transmural stenting (cyst-gastrostomy or cyst-duodenostomy) for treatment of walled-off pancreatic necrosis can be performed as an alternative to PCD. Endoscopic necrosectomy can be performed as an alternative to surgical necrosectomy. Endoscopic drainage procedures allow patients to avoid external catheter placement and to establish internal drainage of leaked pancreatic juice to the gastrointestinal tract, especially for patients with a disconnected pancreatic duct syndrome. However, pseudocysts or walled-off necrosis must be located adjacent to the gastric wall or duodenum to be eligible for the endoscopic drainage procedure, and there is no role for endoscopic transmural drainage for acute peripancreatic fluid collections. Moreover, the endoscopic procedure may introduce infection into the peripancreatic space, and one cannot repetitively assess the appearance, volume,

amylase activity, or microbiologic culture of the drainage fluid. Particularly for direct endoscopic necrosectomy, the incidence of procedure-related adverse events is an issue to be overcome to include the potential for bleeding, perforation, or air embolism. However, relatively mild cases with pancreatic ductal disruption often can be managed by endoscopic techniques alone.

Our group has advocated efficacy of a combined percutaneous and endoscopic approach (dual-modality drainage) for symptomatic walled-off pancreatic necrosis (Figures 10 and 11). After PCD, the patient is taken immediately to the endoscopy suite, and general anesthesia is administered. The necrosum is accessed either endoscopically (if a visible bulge was present intraluminally) with a needle-knife sphincterotome (Cook Endoscopy, Winston-Salem, NC) or under EUS control by using a 19-gauge needle or EUS-directed transenteric drainage system (Navix; Xlumena, Mountain View, CA). After wire-guide access is achieved, the tract is dilated by using either a 4F or 6F dilating catheter (Cook), needle-knife sphincterotome (Cook), or Navix device, subsequent to which further dilation is performed by using a 6- to 8-mm CRE balloon dilator (Boston Scientific, Natick, Mass) (or 8-mm balloon on the Navix catheter). Two 7F (varying lengths) double-pigtail stents (Cook) are placed across the gastric or duodenal wall to maintain the tract. In the case

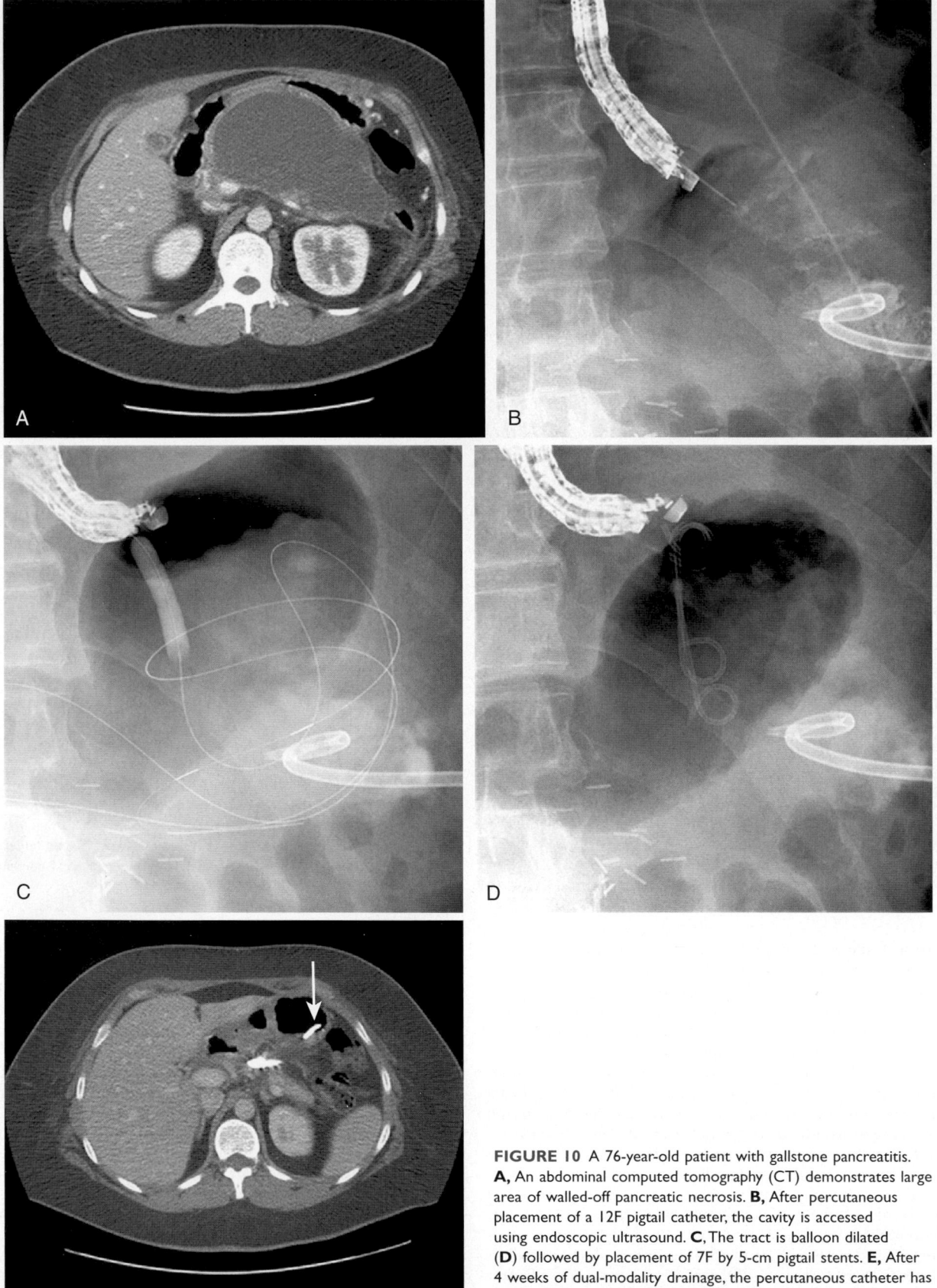

FIGURE 10 A 76-year-old patient with gallstone pancreatitis. **A,** An abdominal computed tomography (CT) demonstrates large area of walled-off pancreatic necrosis. **B,** After percutaneous placement of a 12F pigtail catheter, the cavity is accessed using endoscopic ultrasound. **C,** The tract is balloon dilated (**D**) followed by placement of 7F by 5-cm pigtail stents. **E,** After 4 weeks of dual-modality drainage, the percutaneous catheter has been removed leaving 2 transgastric pigtail stents *(arrow)* in this patient who was left with a disconnected duct syndrome.

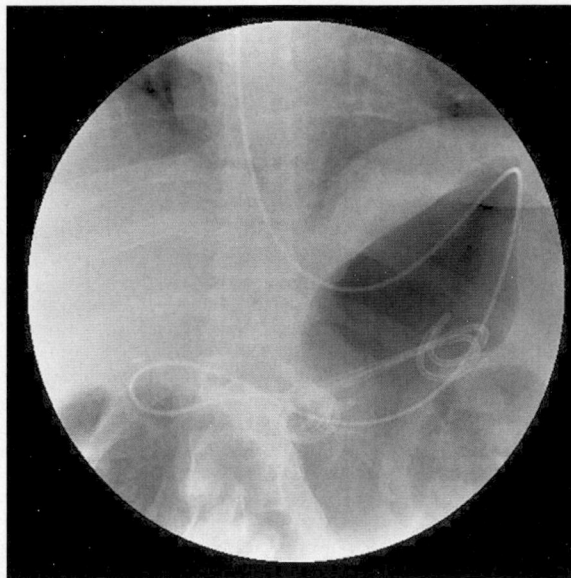

FIGURE 11 As originally described, following transgastric stent placement into walled-off pancreatic necrosis, a naso-lesser sac drain was placed alongside pigtail stents to allow saline irrigation.

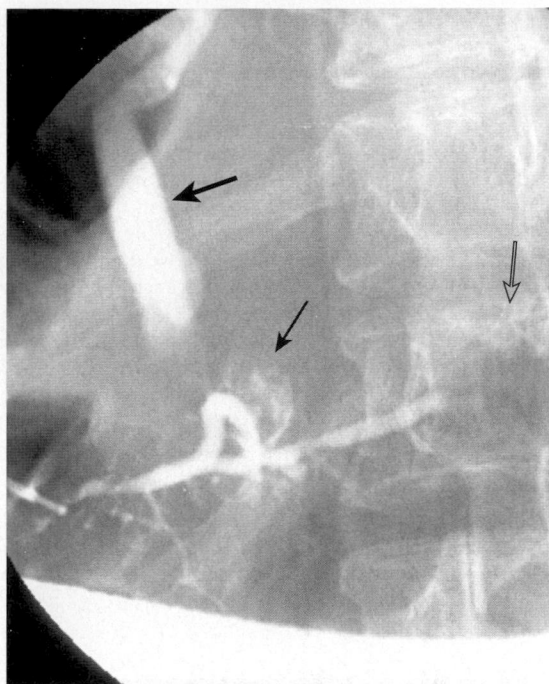

FIGURE 12 In a patient with pancreatic ascites and pancreas divisum, the dorsal pancreatic duct in the pancreatic head is leaking in two locations. The first is shown as contrast leaked through a disruption into the lesser sac *(thin closed arrow)*. The second is from the upstream pancreatic duct that is obstructed over the vertebral bodies. A faint collection of contrast in the lesser sac is marked with an open arrow. These disruptions accounted for the pancreatic ascites. Just before the pancreatic duct injection through the minor ampulla, the common bile duct *(large closed arrow)* had been filled from the major ampulla. After trans-minor-papilla stenting, the ascites resolved, but pain continued, and the downstream disruption did not seal. An uncomplicated pancreatoduodenectomy resolved these problems when the inflammation was at a minimum.

of multiple areas of walled-off necrosis, multiple percutaneous drainage catheters are placed; however, transenteric stents are placed into the necrosum, which is closest in proximity to the gastrointestinal tract. Once placed, transenteric stents are not manipulated intentionally throughout the course of treatment. With use of dual-modality drainage, our series with 117 patients with symptomatic walled-off necrosis demonstrated no need for surgical necrosectomy and no procedure-related mortality.

Surgical Management

Traditionally, sick patients with infected pancreatic necrosis underwent open necrosectomy, and high mortality of 20% to 40% was observed. In 2010 a Dutch multicenter randomized controlled study (the PANTER trial), comparing outcomes of primary open necrosectomy versus a minimally invasive "step-up" approach starting with PCD followed by a surgical procedure such as video-assisted retroperitoneal débridement (VARD) or open necrosectomy as needed, showed significant benefit of minimally invasive approach: 35% of the patients treated with a minimally invasive drainage procedure avoided any surgical procedure, while experiencing similar mortality (19%) to the patients with primary open necrosectomy (16%). Since then, PCD has been used more frequently, and open necrosectomy has decreased its role and is the last resort when other treatment modalities fail. Instead, VARD has been shown safe and effective. VARD can be used to avert more invasive procedures or as a bridging therapy between PCD and open necrosectomy. However, use of PCD earlier, before development of infection in peripancreatic space, severe sepsis, or organ failure, may preclude the need for these more invasive procedures. This hypothesis warrants a well-designed, prospective, randomized controlled trial to test the benefit of early minimally invasive intervention.

In symptomatic patients with a disconnected pancreatic duct syndrome, especially for those in whom pancreatic juice leakage from the distal side of the pancreatic gland is not efficiently drained, distal pancreatectomy to remove the focus of symptoms is indicated. Pancreatic head resection may be required for downstream obstruction in the pancreatic head and upstream duct disruption that is also in the head of the gland (Figure 12). Fortunately, the application of transmural internalized drainage by percutaneous or endoscopic technique may reduce the necessity of these more invasive and complex procedures. Exploring the peripancreatic space is a morbid procedure because of the dense scarring and left-sided portal hypertension resulting from splenic vein occlusion and the severe inflammation. We have observed a considerable number of patients in whom distal pancreas became more atrophic and reduced its secretion over time just with internalized drainage. Although longstanding placement of internalized drainage tubes is needed for these patients, they could avoid open surgical procedures and preserve pancreatic endocrine/exocrine function even with the atrophic small piece of the distal pancreas, which otherwise may be reduced peremptorily by the resection.

Multidisciplinary Team Approach

Patients with pancreatic ductal disruption should be managed during their entire clinical course in multidisciplinary fashion, involving a team of interventional radiologists, hospitalists, nurses, dieticians, pharmacists, infectious disease specialists, intensive-care specialists, gastroenterologists, and pancreatobiliary surgeons. In the treatment modalities and strategies we mentioned above, we cannot always say which treatment is superior to others, because of the paucity of sufficient evidence and the variability in the patients' presentation. Two important prerequisites are necessary for a tailored approach for each patient. First is the assembly of a team, which requires years of recruitment using influence and leadership at centers of expertise in the treatment of these patients. Second, and possibly just as difficult as team assembly, is the design and use of a common algorithm that allows the reporting of data supported with the "power of n."

■ SUMMARY

Pancreatic ductal disruptions are refractory complications after acute pancreatitis. Patients with suggestive findings of uncontrolled pancreatic juice leakage should be drained early in the clinical course before severe sepsis develops. PCD is more feasible and a less invasive technique than surgical necrosectomy. Effective drainage is achieved by patent drain(s) located at the site of pancreatic juice leakage. Dual-modality drainage with combined PCD and endoscopic transenteric drainage is useful for patients with symptomatic walled-off pancreatic necrosis. A multidisciplinary team approach is mandatory to successfully manage patients who manifest with a variety of presentations.

SUGGESTED READINGS

Banks PA, Bollen TL, Dervenis C, et al. Acute Pancreatitis Classification Working Group. Classification of acute pancreatitis—2012: revision of the Atlanta classification and definitions by international consensus. *Gut.* 2013;62:102-111.

Horvath K, Freeny P, Escallon J, et al. Safety and efficacy of video-assisted retroperitoneal debridement for infected pancreatic collections: a multicenter, prospective, single-arm phase 2 study. *Arch Surg.* 2010;145:817-825.

Nealon WH, Bhutani M, Riall TS, et al. A unifying concept: pancreatic ductal anatomy both predicts and determines the major complications resulting from pancreatitis. *J Am Coll Surg.* 2009;208:790-799.

Ross A, Gluck M, Irani S, et al. Combined endoscopic and percutaneous drainage of organized pancreatic necrosis. *Gastrointest Endosc.* 2010;71:79-84.

Ross AS, Irani S, Gan SI, et al. Dual-modality drainage of infected and symptomatic walled-off pancreatic necrosis: long-term clinical outcomes. *Gastrointest Endosc.* 2014;79:929-935.

Sugimoto M, Sonntag DP, Flint GS, et al. A percutaneous drainage protocol for severe and moderately severe acute pancreatitis. *Surg Endosc.* 2015;29:3282-3291.

Sugimoto M, Sonntag DP, Flint GS, et al. Better outcomes if percutaneous drainage is used early and proactively in the course of necrotizing pancreatitis. *J Vasc Interv Radiol.* 2016;27:418-425.

van Santvoort HC, Besselink MG, Bakker OJ, et al. Dutch Pancreatitis Study Group. A step-up approach or open necrosectomy for necrotizing pancreatitis. *N Engl J Med.* 2010;362:1491-1502.

THE MANAGEMENT OF CHRONIC PANCREATITIS

Alessandro Paniccia, MD, and Barish H. Edil, MD

Chronic pancreatitis (CP) is a progressive disease that culminates in the destruction of the normal pancreas with loss of its exocrine (acinar cells) and endocrine (islet cells) functions. The annual incidence of CP is estimated to range between 5 and 14/100,000; the prevalence of CP is approximately 50 per 100,000 persons with an annual treatment cost of approximately $17,000 per person. A diagnosis of CP is associated with a 10- to 20-year reduction in life expectancy and a 3.6-fold increase in mortality risk compared with the general population.

Histologically, CP is characterized by a sustained inflammatory process that leads to irreversible pancreatic fibrosis, resulting in deformation of pancreatic ducts and changes in the composition and arrangement of pancreatic islets.

The most common clinical manifestation of CP is abdominal pain (i.e., epigastric pain commonly radiating to the back), with a reported prevalence of 50% to 85%. Pancreatic exocrine insufficiency (PEI) is present in 40% to 50% of patients with CP; it usually manifests with steatorrhea characterized by loose, fatty, and malodorous stool. The occurrence of symptomatic PEI often indicates that more than 90% of pancreatic exocrine function is lost and is therefore a sign of advanced disease. Diabetes mellitus type 3c is a form of secondary diabetes that develops in more than half of patients suffering from CP. This form of diabetes arises from the complete loss of islet mass, which is typical of CP, and is characterized not only by the inability to release insulin but also by the loss of counter-regulatory hormones (i.e., glucagon, pancreatic polypeptide), subjecting these patients to episodes of severe hypoglycemia.

■ ETIOLOGY AND CLASSIFICATION

Chronic pancreatitis is a multifactorial disease with a strong genetic predisposition. Several risk factors known to contribute to the development of CP are summarized conveniently by the TIGAR-O classification system in six etiologic groups, including (1) toxic-metabolic, (2) idiopathic, (3) genetic, (4) autoimmune, (5) recurrent and severe acute pancreatitis, or (6) obstructive (Table 1). Alcohol remains the most common risk factor for the development of CP in Western countries. However, data obtained from the North American Pancreatitis Study (NAPS) suggest that alcohol is responsible for only 44.5% of CP patients, with the remaining cases attributed to nonalcoholic causes. Mutations in several genes, including cationic trypsin *(PRSS1)*, pancreatic secretory trypsin inhibitor *(SPINK1)*, and cystic fibrosis transmembrane conductance regulator *(CFTR)* contribute to the development and irreversible progression of CP. Although rarely sufficient alone, genetic variants of the above-mentioned genes can exacerbate the effect of environmental stressors such as alcohol. Worth mentioning is hereditary pancreatitis. This disease is responsible for 2% to 3% of CP in the United States and is caused by a germline mutation resulting in gain of function of the *PRSS1* gene. Affected patients experience early onset CP, developing symptoms before the age of 20 and often before the age of 5.

Autoimmune pancreatitis represents a particularly rare cause of chronic pancreatitis that is recognized in less than 5% of patients undergoing evaluation. It is characterized by distinct clinical and histologic features and by a propensity to respond well to corticosteroid therapy.

■ DIAGNOSIS

Early diagnosis of CP remains one of the most challenging aspects of this disease. The diagnostic approach relies on historical clinical information and is supported by the results of radiographic studies and laboratory tests of pancreatic function.

Abdominal pain is one of most common symptoms and often the main reason prompting patients to seek medical attention. Pain characteristics can vary, ranging from episodic postprandial epigastric pain, in the early phases of the disease, to a continuous pattern in more advanced disease stages. Although pain is a typical symptom, it is not necessary for the diagnosis because 20% to 45% of patients have no pain symptomatology despite radiographic and laboratory evidence of CP.

Imaging studies have a paramount role in the diagnosis of CP. The most common imaging findings in the setting of CP were described recently in the NAPS2 study and include pancreatic duct dilation (68%), atrophy (57%), calcifications (55%), pancreatic duct irregularity (51%), and pancreatic pseudocysts (32%).

TABLE 1: TIGAR-O Classification System of Causes of Chronic Pancreatitis

Toxic-metabolic	Alcohol
	Tobacco
	Hypercalcemia
	Chronic renal failure
	Toxins
Idiopathic	Early onset
	Late onset
	Tropical
Genetic	Hereditary pancreatitis (cationic trypsinogen mutation)
	CFTR mutations
	SPINK1 mutations
	Alpha-1 antitrypsin deficiency
Autoimmune	Isolated autoimmune CP
	Syndromic autoimmune CP (e.g., PSC, Sjögren's-associated.)
Recurrent and severe AP	Postnecrotic
	Recurrent acute pancreatitis
	Ischemic/vascular
Obstructive	Pancreas divisum
	Intrapapillary mucinous tumor
	Ductal adenocarcinoma

Adapted from Etemad B, Whitcomb DC. Chronic pancreatitis: diagnosis, classification and new genetic developments. *Gastroenterology.* 2001;120:682-707.

AP, Acute pancreatitis; *CP,* chronic pancreatitis; *PSC,* primary sclerosing cholangitis; *TIGAR-O,* Toxic Idiopathic Genetic Autoimmune Recurrent Obstructive.

TABLE 2: Cambridge Classification of Chronic Pancreatitis by Endoscopic Retrograde Pancreatography

Grade	Main Pancreatic Duct	Side Branches
Normal (grade 0)	Normal	Normal
Equivocal (grade 1)	Normal	<3 Abnormal
Mild (grade 2)	Normal	>3 Abnormal
Moderate (grade 3)	Abnormal	>3 Abnormal
Severe (grade 4)	Abnormal*	>3 Abnormal

Adapted from Muniraj T, et al. Chronic pancreatitis, a comprehensive review and update. Part II: diagnosis, complications, and management. *Dis Mon.* 2015;61:5-37.

*Large cavity >10 mm, duct obstruction, intraductal filling defect, severe dilation or irregularity.

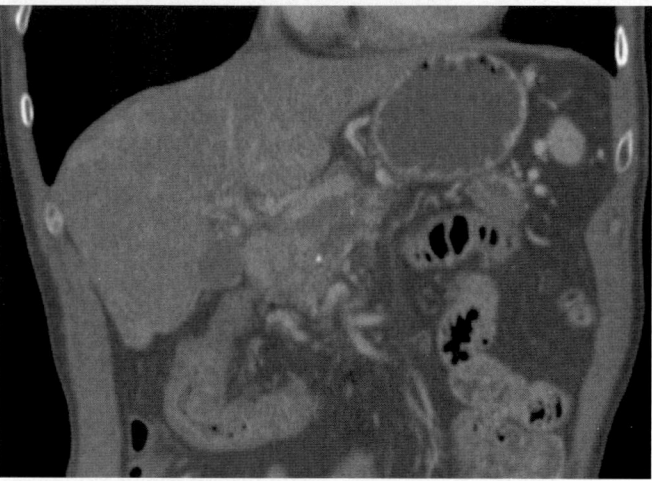

FIGURE 1 Computed tomography image of patient with evidence of changes of chronic pancreatitis with pancreatic duct dilation distal to pancreatic head stone.

Historically, plain abdominal x-ray was considered the gold standard imaging modality. This diagnostic approach relies mainly on the presence of diffuse calcification throughout the pancreatic parenchyma typical of alcohol-induced pancreatitis. However, plain abdominal x-ray has a poor sensitivity ranging from 30% to 40%.

Currently, computed tomography (CT) is often the primary imaging modality, having a sensitivity ranging from 47% to 80% and a specificity of 90% (Figure 1). Caution should be used in interpreting pancreatic calcification findings seen on CT. A study conducted by Ciampisi and colleagues found that CP was present in only 68% of patients with pancreatic calcifications seen on CT, whereas the remaining 38% had other disease, including neuroendocrine tumor (13.6%), intraductal papillary mucinous neoplasm (IPMN) (4.8%), malignant IPMN (5.8%), serous cystadenoma (3.9%), and pancreatic adenocarcinoma (3.9%). CT is also useful for the identification of the complications associated with chronic pancreatitis, such as pancreatic pseudocysts, infection, hemorrhage, pseudoaneurysm formation, pancreatic fistula, and biliary or gastrointestinal obstruction.

Magnetic resonance cholangiopancreatography produces detailed images of the hepatobiliary and pancreatic systems; in the setting of advanced disease it has a sensitivity of 75%, but it is of low yield in the early stages of disease, in which its sensitivity is only 25%.

Endoscopic retrograde cholangiopancreatography (ERCP) is arguably the most sensitive and specific test (ranging from 70% to 100%) for the diagnosis of CP (Figure 2). Abnormalities seen in the main pancreatic duct and its side branches can be used to grade the severity of CP according to the Cambridge classification (Table 2). However, because of its invasive nature and risk of complications, its use rarely is employed solely for diagnostic purposes, and it is reserved mainly to carry out therapeutic interventions and as a reference test to compare other diagnostic modalities during investigational studies.

Endoscopic ultrasound (EUS) can be a valuable aid in the diagnosis of CP in its early stages even before the development of the anatomic anomalies (e.g., calcifications, large duct obstruction, atrophy) that usually are recognized by other imaging modalities. Diagnosis is based on a series of ductal and parenchymal characteristics that are summarized in the endoscopic ultrasound–Rosemont criteria in Table 3.

■ MANAGEMENT

Therapeutic management of CP must be individualized to the specific patient. The choice of the appropriate treatment depends on a thorough understanding of the cause of the disease (see TIGAR-O classification), on the presence of obstruction of the pancreatic or biliary tract, on the existence of dilation of the pancreatic duct, and on the presence of CP-related complications.

Medical Management

Medical management strives to alleviate pain symptomatology, to replace pancreatic enzymes, and to achieve glucose homeostasis.

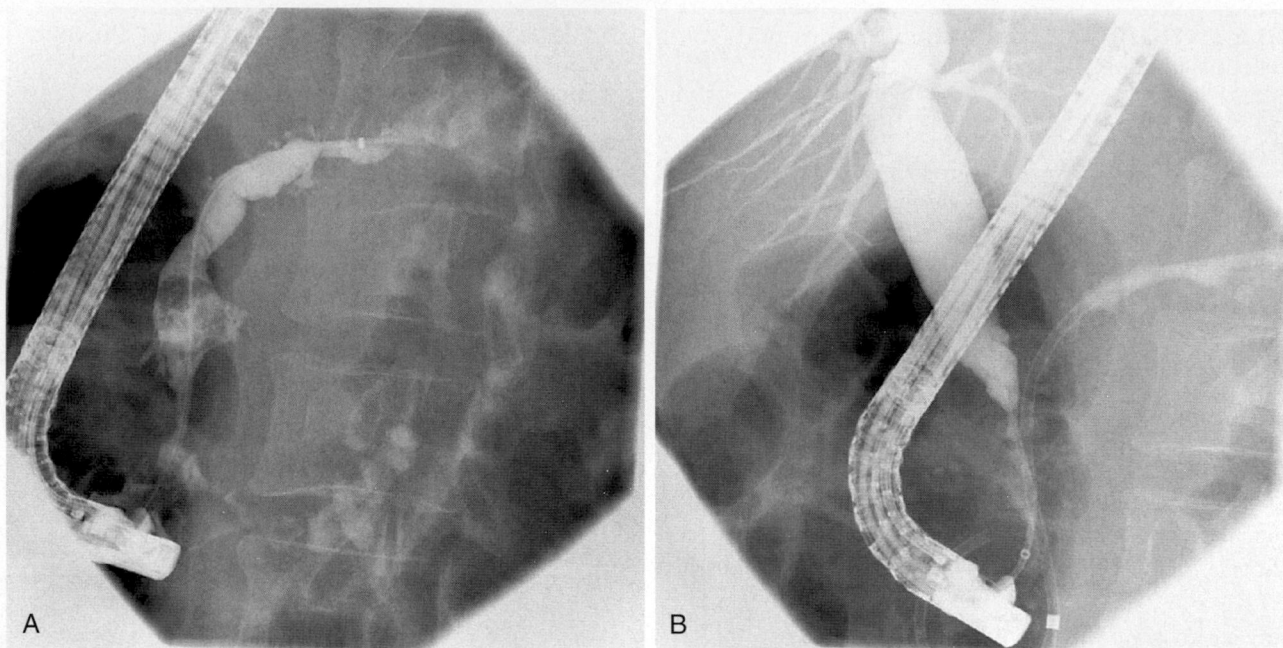

FIGURE 2 Endoscopic retrograded cholangiopancreatography images of patient with chronic pancreatitis and obstruction of pancreatic duct and distal bile duct. **A,** Evidence of focal localized benign-appearing stricture within the head of the pancreas. There is diffuse moderate upstream pancreatic duct dilatation with multiple enlarged side branches consistent with chronic pancreatitis. In addition there are several intraluminal stones within the downstream pancreatic duct. **B,** Injection of the biliary duct demonstrates marked common bile duct dilation with downstream irregular intrapancreatic bile stricture caused by an inflammatory mass in the head of the pancreas. A pancreatic duct stent is present and terminates in the upstream body of the pancreas.

TABLE 3: Endoscopic Ultrasound–Rosemont Criteria for Chronic Pancreatitis*

PARENCHYMAL FEATURES

Major A: • Hyperechoic foci with shadowing (B and T) **Major B:** • Lobularity with honeycombing (B and T)	**Minor:** • Lobularity and no honeycombing (i.e., noncontiguous) • Hyperechoic foci and no shadowing • Cysts • Stranding

DUCTAL FEATURES

Major A: • MPD calculi in H/B/T	**Minor:** • Irregular MPD contour • Dilated side branches • MPD dilation >3.5 mm in B and >1.5 mm in T • Hyperechoic duct margin

Adapted from Muniraj T, et al. 2015. Chronic pancreatitis, a comprehensive review and update. Part II: Diagnosis, complications, and management. *Dis Mon.* 2015;61:5-37.

*Most centers require at least 5 Rosemont criteria to diagnose chronic pancreatitis.

B, Body; *H,* head; *MPD,* main pancreatic duct; *T,* tail.

Opioids are the mainstay of pain management, demonstrating moderate success. Encouraging results are associated with the use of pregabalin (up to 300 mg twice a day), a centrally acting analgesic that, in addition to its "pain relief" effect, leads to a reduction of opioid use. Pancreatic enzymes replacement therapy should be offered to all patients with steatorrhea or excessive weight loss. Nonenteric coated formulations of pancreatic enzyme preparation (given concomitantly with a proton-pump inhibitor), containing a minimum dose of 40,000 to 50,000 U of lipase should be administered during each meal and titrated according to the clinical response (decrease in diarrhea, increase in body weight, and increase in serum levels of fat-soluble vitamins) up to 90,000 U per meal.

Endoscopic Therapy

Endoscopic therapies commonly are employed as first-line interventions in the setting of obstructive chronic pancreatitis. The goal of these therapies is to relieve pressure in the pancreatic duct and to facilitate drainage of pancreatic juices into the intestines. Endoscopic retrograde cholangiopancreatography (ERCP) is the mainstay of these treatment modalities because it allows dilation of pancreatic strictures, papillotomy of the papilla of Vater, placement of stents in the pancreatic duct, and in some cases removal of stones (with or without shock wave lithotripsy). ERCP-based therapies are most effective in the setting of main pancreatic duct obstruction caused either by strictures (preferably a single stricture in the head of the pancreas) or stones.

Pancreatic strictures can be dilated endoscopically and often require stent placement followed by serial stent exchanges or upsizes, usually every 3 months for a period of 2 years. Pancreatic stent removal is associated with a 30% to 40% risk of restenosis of the main pancreatic duct. Papillotomy of the papilla of Vater is performed commonly during ERCP in the setting of CP because it facilitates pancreatic duct decompression, stent placement, and stone extraction. Restenosis after papillotomy is seen in 14% of cases. Pancreatic duct stones can be removed endoscopically; however, stones greater than 5 mm in diameter often require mechanical or extracorporeal shock wave lithotripsy before ERCP extraction. Complications associated with ERCP treatment include bleeding, perforation, and post-ERCP pancreatitis.

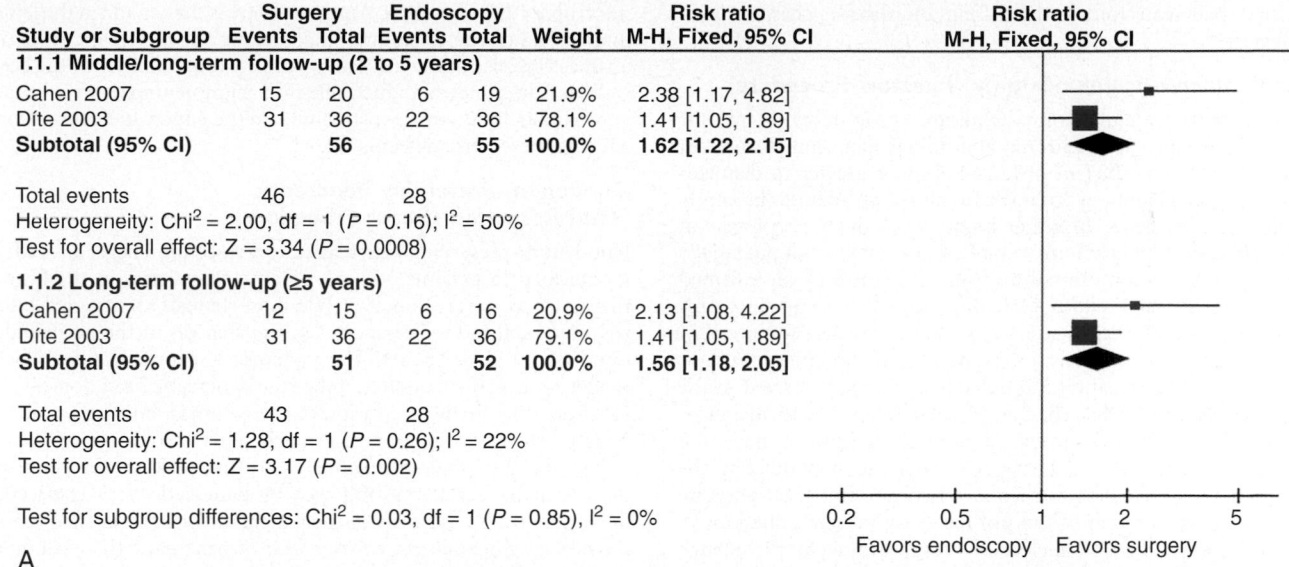

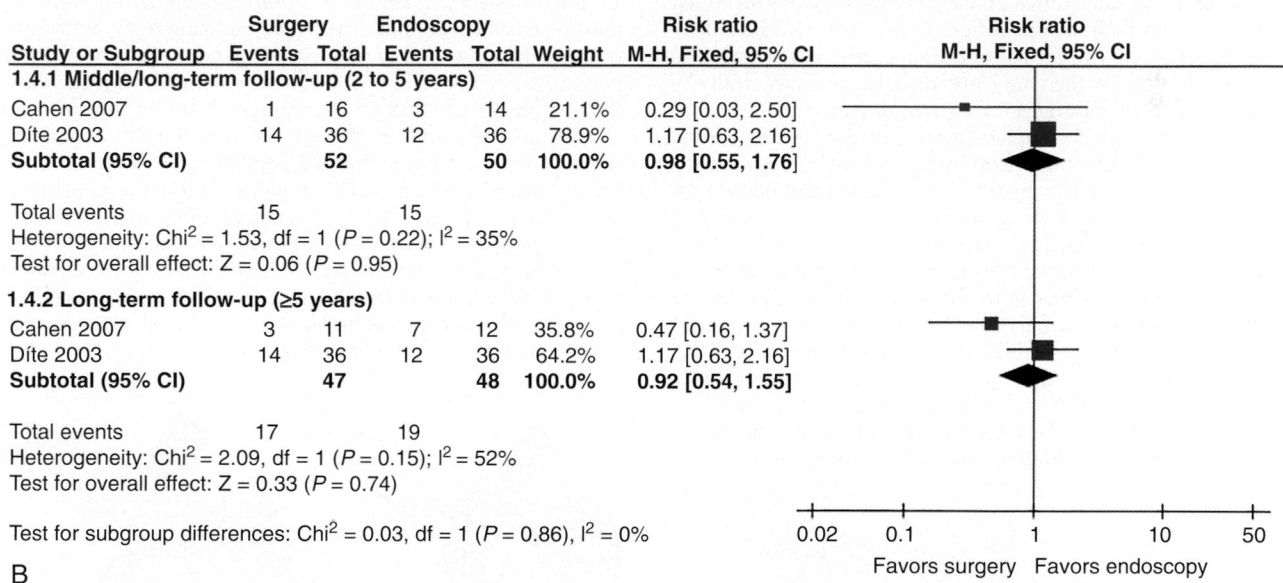

FIGURE 3 Meta-analysis comparing endoscopic versus surgical treatment for chronic pancreatitis. **A,** Pain relief; **B,** new-onset endocrine insufficiency. *(Data from Ahmed Ali U, et al. Endoscopic or surgical intervention for painful obstructive chronic pancreatitis. Cochrane Database Syst Rev. 2015;3:CD007884. Cahen DL, et al. Endoscopic versus surgical drainage of the pancreatic duct in chronic pancreatitis. New Engl J Med. 2007;356:676-684. Díte P, et al. A prospective, randomized trial comparing endoscopic and surgical therapy for chronic pancreatitis. Endoscopy. 2003;35:553-558.)*

Although multiple endoscopic treatments are often necessary, partial or complete pain relief can be achieved in approximately 74% of cases with about 50% remaining pain free at 5 years.

A meta-analysis conducted by the Cochrane group suggests that surgical drainage may be more effective than endoscopic therapy in achieving long-term pain control in the setting of obstructive chronic pancreatitis. Data derived from two randomized controlled trials enrolling 111 patients randomized to surgical treatments versus endoscopic therapy showed more than a twofold increased incidence of complete pain relief (risk ratio 2.45 [95% CI 1.18-5.09]) in the surgical group (Figure 3, *A*) and no significant differences in new-onset endocrine pancreatic insufficiency (Figure 3, *B*).

Surgical Management

Surgical therapies often are reserved for cases with disabling chronic pain after failure of medical and endoscopic therapies.

Approximately 40% to 75% of patients with chronic pancreatitis eventually require surgery. It is paramount that patients undergo a thorough preoperative imaging evaluation aimed at assessing the extent of pancreatic duct dilation, the presence and location of pancreatic strictures, and the existence of any malignant mass. The presence of correctable anatomic abnormalities, such as biliary obstruction, duodenal obstruction, large symptomatic pseudocyst, and lesions suspicious for neoplasia, is among the main indications for surgical intervention. The primary aims of surgical therapies include decompression of obstructed ducts, pain relief, and preservation of pancreatic tissue whenever possible. Therefore surgical intervention can focus primarily on pancreatic decompression (lateral pancreaticojejunostomy), be a hybrid procedure in which partial pancreatic resection and ductal decompression are performed at the same time (duodenum-preserving pancreatic head resection with or without lateral pancreaticojejunostomy), or be solely a resective procedure (pancreaticoduodenectomy, distal pancreatectomy, and total pancreatectomy), depending on disease characteristics and severity.

Lateral Pancreaticojejunostomy (Puestow Procedure)

Lateral pancreaticojejunostomy (Puestow procedure) is recommended in patients with chronic abdominal pain and dilation of the main pancreatic duct of at least 7 mm or greater in diameter (Figure 4). When planning this operation it is important to promptly identify the coexistence of either biliary duct dilation (present in 30% to 50%) or duodenal narrowing (less than 5%), both potentially caused by compression exerted on these structures by an inflamed pancreatic head that would not be addressed solely by a lateral pancreaticojejunostomy. Such a scenario would necessitate some sort of pancreatic parenchymal resection, especially if the anteroposterior diameter of the pancreatic head exceeds 4 cm, as illustrated in the following sections of this chapter. The lateral pancreaticojejunostomy can be performed through a midline incision. Initially, the pancreas is visualized by entering the lesser sac after dividing the attachments between the gastrocolic omentum and the transverse colon. The posterior wall of the stomach may present adhesions to the anterior aspect of the pancreas as a result of the chronic inflammatory process, requiring a careful lysis of adhesions to separate these structures. The dilated main pancreatic duct often is identified at the level of the body of the pancreas; this can be achieved by fingertip palpation or with the aid of intraoperative ultrasound. The correct identification of the pancreatic duct is confirmed with the use of a 20-gauge angiocatheter by aspirating pancreatic juice and eventually by threading the angiocatheter into the pancreatic duct to serve as a guide for the subsequent incision of the pancreatic duct. It is paramount that the pancreatic duct is incised and opened for its entire length, starting 1 or 2 cm from the duodenal wall and extending for at least 7 cm. The duct should be examined carefully, and all identified stones should be removed. Once the pancreatic duct is open, attention is turned to the identification of an area of jejunum approximately 15 cm past the ligament of Treitz. After transection, the jejunal limb is mobilized and passed through a defect created in the transverse mesocolon and laid along the pancreatic body with the transected end terminating over the pancreatic tail. The pancreaticojejunostomy can be performed by first securing the distal end of the jejunal limb to the tail of the pancreas using interrupted 2-0 silk suture. An enterotomy is then made in the jejunal limb to match the ductotomy made along the pancreatic duct, and an anastomosis completed with sutures taking full bites of the bowel wall and the pancreatic duct. Finally a jejunojejunostomy is created approximately 50-cm downstream from the pancreaticojejunostomy, and the mesenteric defect is closed.

Duodenum-Preserving Pancreatic Head Resection (Beger Procedure)

Duodenum-preserving pancreatic head resection (Beger procedure) is indicated in patients with an inflammatory mass in the head of the pancreas, severe common bile duct stenosis (that failed biliary stenting), and in the presence of severe stenosis of the peripapillary duodenum (Figure 5, A). The pancreas is exposed and a Kocher maneuver is performed to mobilize the pancreatic head dorsally; this is followed by the identification of the common bile duct, common hepatic artery, and superior mesenteric vein at a location just inferior to the uncinate process. A tunnel is created between the pancreatic neck and the portal vein followed by pancreatic neck transection. Subsequently, the majority of the pancreatic head is resected (cored-out), leaving behind just a 5-mm cuff of pancreatic tissue along the duodenal wall represented by a shell-like pancreatic remnant with an anteroposterior extension of approximately 20 to 30 mm. Care must be taken to avoid injuries to the intrapancreatic portion of the common bile duct and to preserve the pancreaticoduodenal arcades posteriorly. A Roux limb of jejunum is mobilized in a retrocolic fashion, and reconstruction is obtained via an end-to-side pancreaticojejunostomy between the left pancreas and the jejunal loop. A second anastomosis is performed approximately 8-cm distal of the left pancreatic anastomosis, in an end-to-side fashion, between the jejunal loop and the pancreatic remnant along the duodenal wall. In cases presenting with severe prepapillary common bile duct stenosis, which is not relieved by subtotal resection of the pancreatic head, an elliptical excision of the common bile duct wall may be necessary. This bile duct segment will be included in the jejunopancreatic anastomosis and does not require a separate anastomosis.

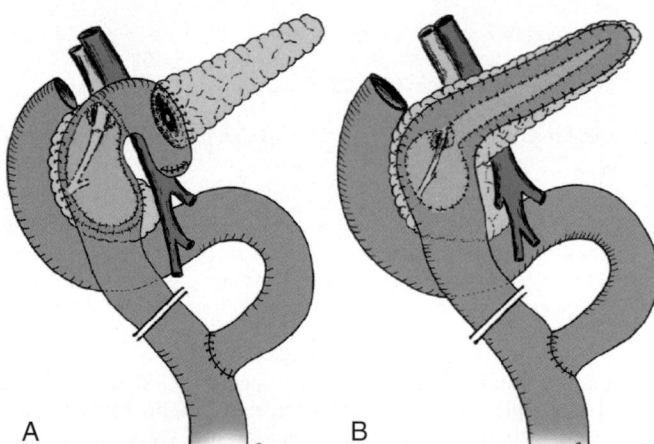

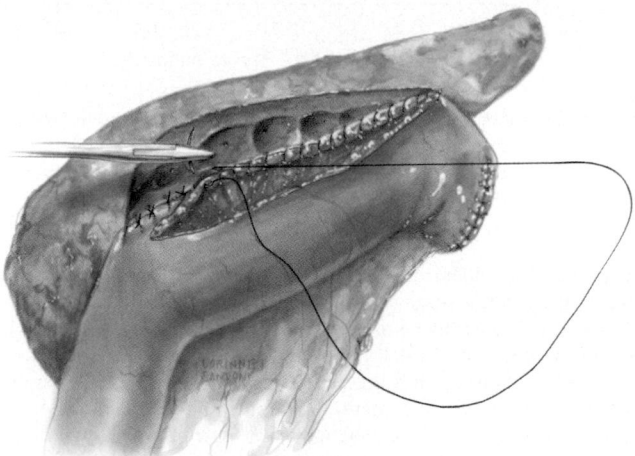

FIGURE 4 Lateral pancreaticojejunostomy (Puestow procedure). The original operation described by Puestow and Gillesby in 1958 included resection of the pancreatic tail and splenectomy. Currently, the Partington-Rochelle modification of the original Puestow procedure often is used; this consists of a spleen-preserving longitudinal side-to-side Roux-en-Y pancreaticojejunostomy, without pancreatic tail resection. *(From Cameron JL, Sandone C. Atlas of Gastrointestinal Surgery. vol 2. 2nd ed. 2014; Shelton, CT: PMPH-USA.)*

FIGURE 5 A, Duodenum-preserving pancreatic head resection (Beger procedure). The Beger procedure is associated with two major risks, including duodenal ischemia resulting from damage and inadequate flow via the posterior branch of the gastroduodenal artery and increased pancreatic leak rate in light of two separate pancreaticojejunostomy anastomosis. **B,** Local resection of the head of the pancreas with lateral pancreaticojejunostomy (Frey procedure). The coring of the pancreatic head is more limited in the Frey procedure compared with the Beger procedure and is created in continuity with a longitudinal ductotomy of the main duct in the body and tail of pancreas. *(Reprinted from Köninger J, et al. Duodenum-preserving pancreatic head resection—a randomized controlled trial comparing the original Beger procedure with the Berne modification (ISRCTN No. 50638764). Surgery. 2008;143:490-498.)*

Local Resection of the Head of the Pancreas With Lateral Pancreaticojejunostomy (Frey Procedure)

In 1986 Charles Frey described a modification of the duodenum-preserving pancreatic head resection that requires partial coring of the ventral part of the pancreatic head, in addition to a side-to-side pancreaticojejunostomy anastomosis (5B). This technique allows for simultaneous decompression of the intrapancreatic segment of the common bile duct in addition to drainage of the main pancreatic duct. The Frey procedure is best suited for patients with a dilation of the main pancreatic duct associated with a minor inflammatory mass in the head of the pancreas. As the pancreatic neck is not transected during the Frey procedure, a more limited dissection is necessary when compared with the Beger procedure; this can be advantageous especially in the setting of severe inflammation when the separation of the pancreatic neck from the portal vein and the superior mesenteric vein can be challenging.

Bachmann and colleagues recently reported data on long-term outcomes following the Beger and the Frey procedure showing equivalent efficacy with regard to pain and quality of life at a median follow-up of 16 years. In addition, the rate of endocrine insufficiency was similar, specifically 77% vs 83% ($P = 0.655$) after the Beger and the Frey procedure, respectively. The choice between the two procedures often rests with the surgeon's preference and expertise.

Resection-Only Procedures

Pancreaticoduodenectomy and Distal Pancreatectomy

Resection-only procedures include pancreaticoduodenectomy (PD), with or without pylorus sparing technique, distal pancreatectomy (DP), and total pancreatectomy (TP) with or without islet cell autotransplantation (IAT).

Pancreaticoduodenectomy remains the procedure of choice when a pancreatic malignancy is suspected. However, it can be argued that in the setting of CP, performing a PD presents a few disadvantages because it requires partial removal of pancreatic parenchyma in addition to removal of surrounding organs and interruption of intestinal continuity. A recent meta-analysis conducted by Sukharamwala and colleagues, including seven randomized controlled trials and three prospective nonrandomized controlled trials for a total of 569 patients, suggests that duodenum-preserving pancreatic head resection (DPPHR) procedures are superior to PPPD in achieving long-term results, such as quality of life, professional rehabilitation, and exocrine insufficiency; in addition no significant differences exist in postoperative pain relief, endocrine insufficiency, and perioperative morbidity (Table 4). Results from a multicenter randomized trial (European ChroPac trial [ISRCTN38973832]) designed to evaluate

DPPHR versus PD procedure propose to provide high-quality data to guide surgeons' choice between these two procedures.

Currently, distal pancreatectomy rarely is performed for CP because it is associated with only short-term pain relief. It is relegated primarily to the rare cases of isolated pancreatic tail strictures or complications such as pseudoaneurysm.

Total Pancreatectomy With Islet Cell Autotransplantation

Surgical removal of the entire pancreas is indicated for the most extreme cases of CP when medical, endoscopic, and prior surgical treatments have failed. However, severe endocrine pancreatic insufficiency, with new onset of brittle-diabetes (characterized by exaggerated variation in blood glucose level and ketoacidosis), historically has discouraged the use of this procedure. Furthermore, pain relief is not guaranteed, and as many as 30% to 50% of patients will continue to experience pain and require chronic opiate medications. Advancements in the field of pancreatic islet cell autotransplantation (IAT) propose to render total pancreatectomy (TP) a more appealing therapeutic option for severe CP with some authors advocating its use even in the setting of minimal change pancreatitis in light of a theoretical cost effectiveness. Isolation of pancreatic beta cells is technically demanding and is performed by only a few specialized centers in the United States. Isolated beta cells usually are infused via catheter into the portal vein or mesenteric venous tributaries for final engraftment into the liver (Figure 6). Caution should be used in selecting candidates for total pancreatectomy with IAT. A thorough metabolic examination aimed at the evaluation of pancreatic beta cell mass and C-peptide levels must be obtained, in addition verification of patency of the portal vein must be ensured. It is paramount to verify the absence of concomitant pancreatic malignant or premalignant lesions, substance abuse dependency (alcohol or illicit drugs), and poorly controlled psychiatric illness that could compromise the patient's ability to comply with the medical management of endocrine and exocrine pancreatic insufficiency. A successful IAT mostly eliminates the risk of brittle-diabetes; however, lifelong pancreatic enzyme replacement therapy is necessary, and up to 75% of patients still will require insulin.

■ SUMMARY

Chronic pancreatitis is a progressive disease that culminates in the destruction of the normal pancreas with loss of its exocrine (acinar cells) and endocrine (islet cells) function. Pain in CP patients is difficult to manage and often requires a multidisciplinary and multimodality approach. Medical management strives to alleviate pain symptomatology, to replace pancreatic enzymes, and to achieve

TABLE 4: Outcome of DPPHR Versus PPPD for Chronic Pancreatitis

Outcomes	Number of Studies	Participants	Odds Ratio (M-H, fixed, 95% CI)	Statistical Significance
Pain relief	6	311	0.73 (0.43, 1.24)	$P = 0.24$
Quality of life	6	354	−12.86 (−16.19, −9.54)	$P < 0.00001$
Professional rehabilitation	5	254	0.47 (0.28, 0.79)	$P = 0.004$
Exocrine insufficiency	5	236	2.16 (1.27, 3.69)	$P = 0.005$
Endocrine insufficiency	4	211	1.49 (8.86, 2.57)	$P = 0.15$
Length of stay	6	352	4.25 (3.10, 5.40)	$P = 0.00001$
Perioperative morbidity	6	403	1.52 (0.88, 2.63)	$P = 0.13$

Adapted from Sukharamwala PB, et al. Long-term outcomes favor duodenum-preserving pancreatic head resection over pylorus-preserving pancreaticoduodenectomy for chronic pancreatitis: a meta-analysis and systematic review. *Am Surg.* 2015;81:909-914.

CI, Confidence interval; *DPPHR,* duodenum-preserving pancreatic head resection; *M-H,* Mantel-Haenszel; *PPPD,* pylorus-preserving pancreaticoduodenectomy.

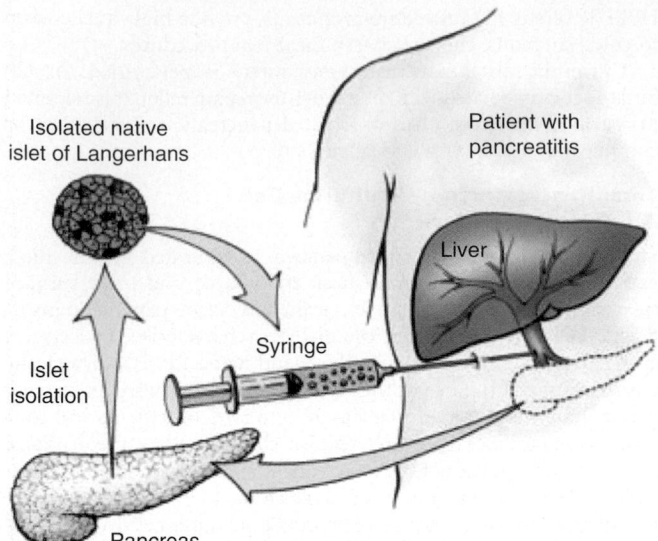

FIGURE 6 Pancreatic islet cell transplantation. When total pancreatectomy for islet cell isolation is performed, care must be taken to preserve the gastroduodenal artery and the splenic artery and vein until just before resection to minimize ischemia to the islet tissue. Pure islet cells are isolated via mechanical dispersion (semiautomated Ricordi method) and enzymatic digestion of the pancreatic specimen. Isolated and purified islet cells can be infused into the portal system via direct puncture of the portal vein or alternatively using a stump of the splenic vein or by cannulation of the umbilical vein. (Adapted from Witkowski P, Savari O, Matthews JB. Islet autotransplantation and total pancreatectomy. Adv Surg. 2014;48:223-233.)

glucose homeostasis. Endoscopic treatments, often used in addition to medical treatments, are employed commonly as first-line interventions in the setting of obstructive chronic pancreatitis. Surgical therapies often are reserved for cases with disabling chronic pain after failure of medical and endoscopic therapies. Approximately 40% to 75% of patients with chronic pancreatitis eventually will require surgery. The primary aims of surgical therapies include decompression of obstructed ducts, pain relief, and preservation of pancreatic tissue whenever possible. The optimal timing of surgical intervention remains a matter of much debate; however, mounting evidence suggests that earlier surgical intervention may be cost effective and associated with improved overall outcomes.

SUGGESTED READINGS

Ahmed Ali U, et al. Endoscopic or surgical intervention for painful obstructive chronic pancreatitis. *Cochrane Database Syst Rev.* 2015;(3):CD007884.

Bachmann K, et al. Surgical treatment in chronic pancreatitis timing and type of procedure. *Best Pract Res Clin Gastroenterol.* 2010;24:299-310.

Campisi A, et al. Are pancreatic calcifications specific for the diagnosis of chronic pancreatitis? A multidetector-row CT analysis. *Clin Radiol.* 2009;64:903-911.

Kesseli SJ, Smith KA, Gardner TB. Total pancreatectomy with islet autologous transplantation: the cure for chronic pancreatitis? *Clin Translat Gastroenterol.* 2015;6:e73-e78.

Muniraj T, et al. Chronic pancreatitis, a comprehensive review and update. Part I: epidemiology, etiology, risk factors, genetics, pathophysiology, and clinical features. *Dis Mon.* 2014;60:530-550, 2014.

Muniraj T, et al. Chronic pancreatitis, a comprehensive review and update. Part II_ Diagnosis, complications, and management. *Dis Mon.* 2015;61:5-37.

Sukharamwala PB, et al. Long-term outcomes favor duodenum-preserving pancreatic head resection over pylorus-preserving pancreaticoduodenectomy for chronic pancreatitis: a meta-analysis and systematic review. *Am Surg.* 2015;81:909-914.

THE MANAGEMENT OF PERIAMPULLARY CANCER

James F. Griffin, MD, Katherine E. Poruk, MD, and Christopher L. Wolfgang, MD

Periampullary cancer is a general term encompassing the four most common malignant neoplasms arising in the region of the ampulla of Vater. At this site the epithelium of the distal common bile duct (CBD), main pancreatic duct (MPD), and duodenum converge to form the ampulla of Vater, and each may serve as a primary site of malignancy. Despite their heterogeneous origins, these cancers often are discussed together because of similarities in their clinical presentation, preoperative assessment, and surgical management.

Pancreatic ductal adenocarcinoma (PDAC) accounts for the overwhelming majority of periampullary malignancies (75% to 85%), followed by distal cholangiocarcinoma, ampullary adenocarcinoma, and duodenal adenocarcinoma. A variety of additional cancers are encountered in the periampullary region, but they are much less common. These include neuroendocrine neoplasms, pancreatic cystic neoplasms, acinar and squamous cell carcinomas, gastrointestinal (GI) stromal tumors, sarcomas, lymphomas, and metastases from other cancers. Altogether, periampullary malignancies have a yearly incidence of approximately 50,000 cases and account for more than 30,000 deaths per year in the United States.

William S. Halsted performed the first successful operation for a periampullary cancer at the Johns Hopkins Hospital in 1898. He excised a segment of the second portion of the duodenum, including

the ampulla, followed by an end-to-end anastomosis of the duodenum with reimplantation of the pancreatic and common bile ducts. The patient lived for an additional 7 months but ultimately died from complications related to local tumor recurrence. Just 5 days before Halsted's procedure, the Italian surgeon Alessandro Codivilla attempted the first en bloc resection of the head of the pancreas and part of the duodenum, but the patient died from complications of a pancreatic fistula in the early postoperative period. Walther Kausch is credited with the first successful regional pancreaticoduodenectomy (PD) in 1909, but it was Allen O. Whipple's refinements to the procedure, presented before the American Surgical Association in 1935, that finally generated mainstream interest in PD as a legitimate surgical option for periampullary cancers. The technique continued to evolve in the years that followed, but outcomes remained poor, with perioperative mortality ranging from 20% to 40%, morbidity between 40% and 60%, and 5-year survival for PDAC of less than 5%. The turning point came in the 1980s with the centralization of care at high-volume centers where surgeon specialization, multidisciplinary approaches, and standardization of preoperative and postoperative care lowered perioperative mortality to less than 5%. Today, PD is the standard of care for all resectable periampullary cancers and is performed at high-volume centers with a mortality rate of less than 2%.

■ PERIAMPULLARY CANCER TYPES

Pancreatic Ductal Adenocarcinoma

In the United States PDAC is the tenth most common cancer overall and the fourth leading cause of cancer-related deaths, with 2015 projections estimating 49,000 new cases, 41,000 new deaths, and a 5-year relative survival rate of only 7%. Despite continued medical advances and decades of effort, long-term survival has not improved significantly. Compared with the other nonpancreatic periampullary cancers, PDAC is the most aggressive and tends to be seen with advanced disease so that only 15% to 20% of patients qualify as surgical candidates at the time of diagnosis. Among those who do undergo resection, median postoperative survival is still approximately 20 months, with a 5-year survival of only 20%.

PDAC generally is diagnosed in the sixth and seventh decades of life, with males and females affected equally. Smoking, obesity, and long-standing type 2 diabetes mellitus are all recognized risk factors. In addition, there are also inherited factors, evident in the 1.9-fold to thirteenfold increased risk of PDAC observed among patients with a family history of the disease (depending on the number and relatedness of those affected). Patients who have at least two affected first-degree relatives are defined as having familial pancreatic cancer (FPC), which accounts for an estimated 5% to 10% of cases.

Distal Cholangiocarcinoma

Cholangiocarcinoma accounts for only 3% of all GI malignancies but is the most common primary cancer of the biliary tract and second most common of the periampullary region (9% to 14%). It arises from the epithelial lining of the biliary tract and is divided into three types based on the anatomic location of disease: intrahepatic, hilar (Klatskin's tumor), and distal. The distal type arises in the CBD between the junction of the cystic duct and the ampulla of Vater and accounts for 20% to 40% of cholangiocarcinomas. It most commonly affects patients in the seventh decade of life and has a slight male preponderance. Five-year survival for patients with regional or localized disease ranges between 24% and 39% compared with only 2% for patients with distant metastases at the time of diagnosis.

There are several well-established risk factors for cholangiocarcinoma marked by a shared tendency for causing chronic biliary inflammation and stasis. Among these is primary sclerosing cholangitis (PSC), an autoimmune disorder characterized by progressive inflammation, fibrosis, and stricture of the bile ducts. The parasitic flatworms *Clonorchis sinensis*, *Opisthorchis viverrini*, and *Opisthorchis felineus* (liver flukes) also are known to increase the risk of cholangiocarcinoma, particularly in Southeast Asia, through chronic infection of the bile ducts. Other risk factors include chronic pancreatitis, hepatitis B and C infection, hepatolithiasis, and choledochal cysts.

Ampullary Adenocarcinoma

Ampullary adenocarcinoma is a rare cancer arising from the ampulla of Vater. It accounts for only 0.2% to 0.5% of GI malignancies and is third in incidence among periampullary cancers (6% to 8%), but its incidence has continued to rise steadily over the past 3 decades. It is diagnosed most frequently in the sixth and seventh decades of life and shows a slight male preponderance. Given the ampulla's function as the site of biliopancreatic outflow, patients with ampullary adenocarcinoma generally develop obstructive symptoms early in disease progression. Consequently they tend to be seen at an earlier stage with resectable disease in up to 80% of cases. A higher resectability rate and intrinsically lower biologic aggressiveness give ampullary adenocarcinoma a much better prognosis compared with PDAC and distal cholangiocarcinoma, with 5-year survival rates ranging from 34% to 68%.

Despite the overall survival statistics, ampullary cancer is well known for its inconsistent clinical behavior. Often this is attributed to the heterogeneous tissue composition of the ampulla, which contributes to misdiagnoses and likely influences the aggressiveness of disease. There is even speculation that ampullary adenocarcinoma is not one unique entity but a collection of cancers arising from the different epithelia of the ampullary complex. Pathologic evaluation lends support to this theory by demonstrating two primary subtypes, intestinal and pancreaticobiliary, that exhibit patterns of histologic tumor differentiation and immunohistochemical markers resembling cancers of their respective namesakes. Moreover, evaluating prognosis according to subtype reveals that pancreaticobiliary-type cancers have much poorer survival similar to PDAC and cholangiocarcinoma, whereas survival for intestinal-type cancers is comparable to duodenal adenocarcinoma.

Duodenal Adenocarcinoma

Duodenal adenocarcinoma is the least common of the major periampullary cancers, accounting for only 4% to 7% of disease at this location and 0.4% of GI malignancies overall. Despite its rarity, it is the most common site for small bowel adenocarcinoma, comprising 56% of all cases. It affects both sexes equally, and diagnosis usually is made in the sixth and seventh decades of life. Cancer is believed to arise within duodenal polyps through an adenoma-carcinoma progression pathway similar to that described in colorectal cancer. Although the majority of disease develops sporadically, patients with familial adenomatous polyposis (FAP) carry a 100% to 200% increased risk for cancer because of their tendency to form duodenal adenomas. Consequently these patients require strict, long-term endoscopic surveillance.

At presentation, duodenal cancers are often larger than the other periampullary cancers because of significant intraluminal growth before mass effect results in symptoms. However, more favorable tumor biology compared with PDAC and cholangiocarcinoma gives duodenal adenocarcinoma the best prognosis among all periampullary cancers, with 5-year survival rates reported between 45% and 71%.

■ CLINICAL PRESENTATION

The most common presenting symptom among patients with periampullary cancer is progressive jaundice resulting from malignant biliary outflow obstruction. This usually is accompanied by varying degrees of pruritus, dark urine, light-colored stools, and scleral icterus and may be associated with constitutional symptoms such as weight loss, anorexia, and fatigue. Despite the classical teaching of painless jaundice, it is not uncommon for patients to report vague abdominal discomfort or a dull ache in the midepigastric region that radiates to the back. However, severe abdominal pain is not common, and its presence may be indicative of advanced disease and tumor invasion into the retroperitoneal (celiac) nerve plexus. Patients also may experience cholangitis, symptoms of pancreatic exocrine or endocrine insufficiency, and GI bleeding with melanotic stools and anemia.

The initial encounter with a patient suspected of periampullary malignancy should include a thorough history to elicit any relevant risk factors such as a family history of malignancy or a personal history of predisposing conditions and habits. Physical examination is often nonspecific but may demonstrate signs of jaundice or vague abdominal tenderness, hepatomegaly, or a palpable nontender gallbladder (Courvoisier's sign) consistent with distal bile duct obstruction. Palpation of an enlarged periumbilical node (Sister Mary Joseph's nodule) or left supraclavicular node (Virchow's node) is an ominous sign indicative of advanced disease.

Basic laboratory testing should be performed, including a complete blood cell count (CBC), electrolytes, liver enzymes, coagulation studies, and tumor markers. The results often demonstrate a direct hyperbilirubinemia and elevated alkaline phosphatase levels consistent with biliary obstruction. In the setting of prolonged biliary obstruction, patients also may demonstrate a coagulopathy because of malabsorption of the fat-soluble vitamin K. This is evident on coagulation studies as a prolongation of the prothrombin time (PT) and an elevated international normalized ratio (INR). Malnutrition and weight loss may be reflected by hypoalbuminemia, and the CBC often shows anemia that can result from a combination of factors, including malnutrition, chronic disease, and GI bleeding. Finally, serum carbohydrate antigen 19-9 (CA 19-9) levels should be obtained as a means of evaluating the extent of potential subclinical tumor dissemination, response to therapy, and monitoring for recurrence. Unfortunately its utility as a diagnostic tool is limited for several reasons, the most important of which for periampullary cancers is that it becomes increasingly unreliable in the setting of biliary obstruction.

■ DIAGNOSIS AND STAGING

Imaging Evaluation

Diagnosis and staging of periampullary cancer relies primarily on high-resolution cross-sectional imaging using computed tomography (CT) and magnetic resonance imaging (MRI) in combination with endoscopic procedures. Multidetector computed tomography (MDCT) is the imaging study of choice for preoperative assessment of periampullary malignancies because it offers simultaneous evaluation of local-regional and metastatic tumor spread and three-dimensional (3D) multiplanar reconstructions detailing the tumor's relationship to adjacent vascular structures (Figure 1). A pancreas-specific CT protocol should be used to image the abdomen, which typically calls for orally administered water, intravenous contrast, and triphasic acquisition of fine cuts through the pancreas and liver. When performed correctly, CT imaging has a sensitivity of 91% and a specificity of 85% for detecting PDAC. For resectability, CT imaging is highly predictive of unresectable disease (89% to 100%) but has a lower predictive value for resectable disease (45% to 79%) because of difficulty detecting small liver metastases and peritoneal implants.

PDAC is identified best during the portal venous phase as an ill-defined hypodensity surrounded by normally enhancing pancreatic parenchyma. Ampullary adenocarcinoma appears as a nodular mass, bulging ampulla, or irregular periampullary thickening that enhances during the pancreatic and portal venous phases. Duodenal carcinoma may be seen as a masslike thickening of the duodenal wall or a discrete polypoid mass with heterogeneous attenuation and modest enhancement after contrast administration. It generally involves a short segment with or without luminal narrowing and may show internal necrosis, calcification, or ulceration. Finally, distal cholangiocarcinoma may show no obvious mass lesion at all. Instead, it often is seen as a short segment of asymmetric CBD wall thickening

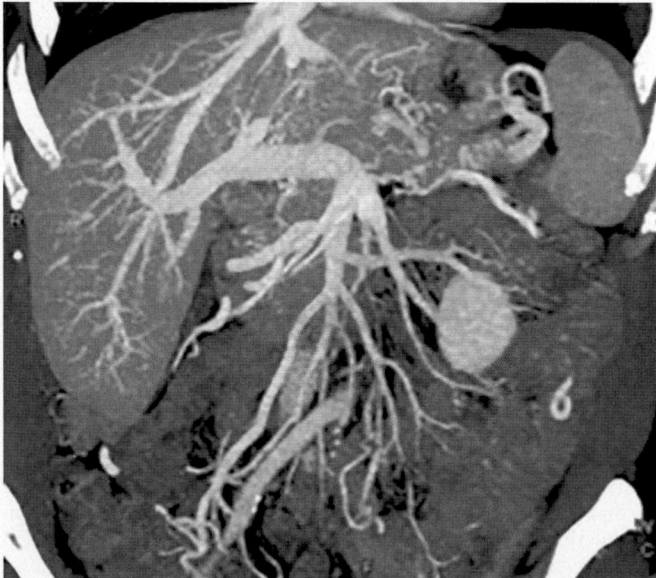

FIGURE 1 Three-dimensional computed tomographic reconstruction (coronal view) of the mesenteric vasculature in a patient with pancreatic adenocarcinoma.

or abrupt luminal obliteration with abnormal enhancement during the portal venous phase.

All periampullary tumor types may demonstrate varying degrees of pancreatic or biliary ductal dilatation on imaging as indirect evidence of tumor presence because of their shared proximity to the ampulla. It is not uncommon to observe both types of dilatation simultaneously, the so-called "double-duct" sign, although this most commonly is associated with PDAC. In some cases a distinct mass cannot be identified on imaging for distal cholangiocarcinomas, ampullary cancers, and duodenal cancers. In such cases an additional endoscopic evaluation such as esophagogastroduodenoscopy (EGD), endoscopic ultrasound (EUS), or endoscopic retrograde cholangio-pancreatography (ERCP) may be necessary to make the diagnosis.

Staging and Resectability

Periampullary adenocarcinomas are staged according to the American Joint Committee on Cancer (AJCC) tumor-node-metastasis (TNM) staging system. These criteria incorporate the size and extent of the primary tumor (T stage), lymph node involvement (N stage), and presence of distant metastases (M stage) into stratified groups designed to guide prognosis and treatment. A major aspect of staging is the assessment of tumor resectability, which depends on the T stage as it relates to important vascular structures, including the celiac axis, superior mesenteric artery (SMA), hepatic artery, superior mesenteric vein (SMV), and portal vein (PV). Although several groups have established specific criteria defining resectability in the setting of PDAC, no specific criteria currently exist for the remaining nonpancreatic primary cancers. As a result, questions of resectability in these tumors usually default to the PDAC criteria.

AJCC stages I and II represent conventionally resectable disease defined as localized, nonmetastatic tumors without extension into the major visceral vasculature. Stage III is composed of nonmetastatic tumors that exhibit some degree of major vascular involvement (T4). This appears on imaging as the loss of fat separation between tumor and vessel, which is referred to as "abutment" when involvement is less than 180 degrees of the vessel's circumference (Figure 2) and "encasement" when involvement is more than 180 degrees (Figure 3). Finally, stage IV is the most advanced form of disease and is marked by distant metastases that render it unresectable regardless of vascular involvement.

Borderline Resectable and Locally Advanced Unresectable Pancreatic Ductal Adenocarcinoma

PDAC is by far the most common form of periampullary cancer and the most frequent subject of studies evaluating tumor resectability in this region. Between 80% and 85% of newly diagnosed patients are seen with conventionally unresectable disease, the majority of which is attributable to distant metastases. However, up to 30% are seen with stage III disease characterized by some degree of major vessel involvement. For a subset of these patients who demonstrate more limited vascular involvement, margin-negative resection and long-term survival still may be possible. This has led to the division of stage III PDAC into two categories based on the degree of local involvement: borderline resectable pancreatic cancer (BRPC) and locally advanced unresectable pancreatic cancer (LAPC). In general BRPC refers to technically reconstructable involvement of the portovenous axis or abutment of a major artery, whereas LAPC refers to unreconstructable involvement of the portovenous axis or encasement of a main artery. In an effort to standardize this distinction, the Americas Hepato-Pancreato-Biliary Association (AHPBA), Society for Surgery of the Alimentary Tract (SSAT), Society of Surgical Oncology (SSO), and National Comprehensive Cancer Network (NCCN) have agreed on a definition of BRPC, which is presented in detail in Box 1. For additional details on borderline resectability, the reader is referred to the consensus statement recently published by the International Study Group for Pancreatic Surgery (ISGPS).

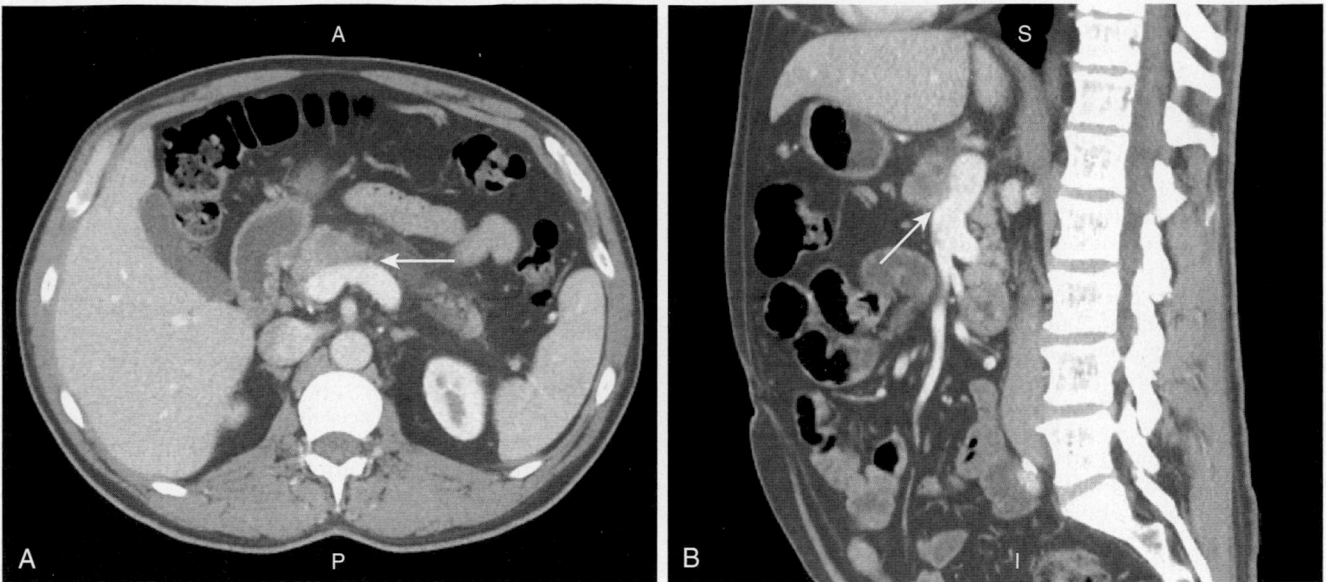

FIGURE 2 Venous phase computed tomographic imaging with (**A**) axial and (**B**) sagittal views demonstrating a pancreatic adenocarcinoma in the neck of the pancreas with abutment (less than 180 degree vessel involvement) at the portal vein–superior mesenteric vein (PV-SMV) confluence. The arrows point to the interface of the PV-SMV and tumor where loss of fat separation can be appreciated.

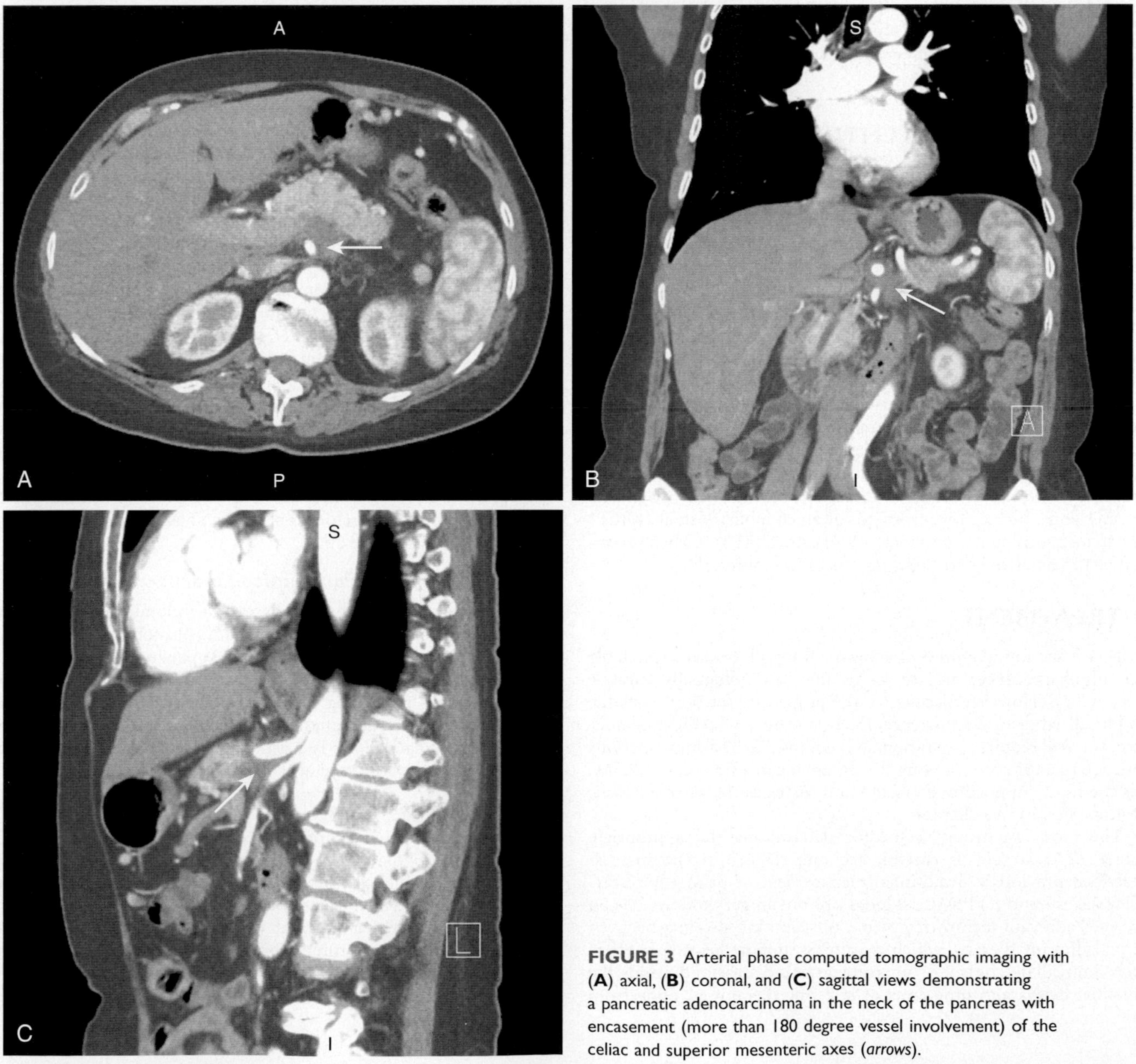

FIGURE 3 Arterial phase computed tomographic imaging with (**A**) axial, (**B**) coronal, and (**C**) sagittal views demonstrating a pancreatic adenocarcinoma in the neck of the pancreas with encasement (more than 180 degree vessel involvement) of the celiac and superior mesenteric axes (*arrows*).

BOX 1: AHPBA/SSAT/SSO/NCCN Criteria for Borderline Resectability in PDAC

1. No distant metastases
2. Venous involvement of the PV/SMV demonstrating tumor abutment with or without impingement and narrowing of the lumen, encasement of the PV/SMV but without encasement of the nearby arteries, or short segment venous occlusion resulting from either tumor thrombus or encasement but with suitable vessel proximal and distal to the area of vessel involvement, allowing for safe resection and reconstruction.
3. GDA encasement up to the hepatic artery with either short segment encasement or direct abutment of the hepatic artery, without extension to the celiac axis.
4. Tumor abutment of the SMA not to exceed >180 degrees of the circumference of the vessel wall.

Modified from Callery MP, Chang KJ, Fishman EK, Talamonti MS, William Traverso L, Linehan DC. Pretreatment assessment of resectable and borderline resectable pancreatic cancer: expert consensus statement. *Ann Surg Oncol.* 2009;16:1727-1733.

AHPBA/SSAT/SSO/NCCN, Americas Hepato-Pancreato-Biliary Association/ Society for Surgery of the Alimentary Tract/Society of Surgical Oncology/ National Comprehensive Cancer Network; *GDA,* gastroduodenal artery; *PDAC,* pancreatic ductal adenocarcinoma; *PV/SMV,* portal vein/superior mesenteric vein; *SMA,* superior mesenteric artery.

■ PROPERATIVE STENTING AND BIOPSY

Certain circumstances call for additional invasive workup, including the need for tissue diagnosis to guide neoadjuvant therapy or non-surgical treatment of unresectable disease. EUS has emerged as the most useful invasive imaging modality because it can detect small adenocarcinomas not visible on cross-sectional imaging and provide additional information regarding tumor relationship to the mesenteric vessels. When combined with fine-needle aspiration (FNA), it is the safest, most accurate means of tissue diagnosis and preoperative nodal staging. Unfortunately, EUS-FNA is not always readily available, and results are operator dependent.

ERCP and percutaneous transhepatic cholangiography (PTC) are additional means of imaging, sampling, and intervening in patients with obstructive jaundice, but they are utilized less frequently because of their invasiveness and potential for complications. Today these procedures are more useful as therapeutic rather than diagnostic interventions, such as for placement of an endobiliary stent (ERCP) or percutaneous biliary drainage (PBD) catheter (PTC) when preoperative or palliative biliary decompression is required.

■ TREATMENT

Surgery is the foundation of management for all forms of resectable periampullary cancer and serves as the only potentially curative intervention. However, because of the propensity for both systemic and localized disease recurrence, the best chance of achieving long-term survival requires multimodality therapy. The recommendations for such therapies vary among the different cancer types, but PDAC has the most supporting literature and serves as the primary focus of discussion in this chapter.

The most important factor for determining the appropriate course of treatment is careful, accurate staging in the manner described previously. Traditional management of primarily resectable (stages I and II) PDAC includes upfront surgery followed by an accepted adjuvant therapy regimen. Consideration also may be given to neoadjuvant therapy, which is gaining support because it offers more immediate control of micrometastatic disease and avoids the potential delays and omissions of systemic therapy resulting from

postoperative complications. In addition, it selects for more favorable tumor biology because disease progression during therapy is indicative of more aggressive disease unlikely to benefit from surgical resection. Patients with metastatic (stage IV) disease do not derive any survival benefit from surgical resection and instead should be offered systemic therapy or supportive care, depending on their overall health status.

Stage III PDAC in the form of BRPC has been targeted only recently for curative intervention. Once a diagnosis of BRPC is made, there are no set algorithms defining standard treatment pathways, and current management strategies vary depending on institutional experience and available resources. Our philosophy is that all patients with BRPC should undergo neoadjuvant chemotherapy or chemoradiotherapy before resection because this has been shown to "sterilize" surgical margins and better control micrometastatic disease. As noted previously, neoadjuvant therapy has the additional advantage of selecting for good tumor biology and may spare some patients an unnecessary operation. In the case of LAPC, most patients will not become candidates for a potentially curative resection; however, a small percentage may exhibit "downstaging" after induction chemotherapy or chemoradiotherapy. On completion of induction therapy these patients should undergo repeat cross-sectional imaging to evaluate their treatment response.

■ SURGICAL MANAGEMENT

Pancreaticoduodenectomy

PD is the method for oncologic resection of periampullary cancers. The two most common variations of PD are the standard PD, which involves an en bloc distal gastrectomy, and the pylorus-preserving PD (PPPD), which leaves the pyloric sphincter complex intact. Despite extensive research, the benefits of one approach over the other are not clear, and both techniques are commonly used.

Until relatively recently, open PD was the only accepted approach to the surgical management of periampullary cancers. Although the vast majority of PDs are still performed via the open approach, recent years have seen the evolution and expansion of minimally invasive surgical (MIS) techniques. Included among these are laparoscopic PD (LPD) and robotic PD (RPD), which have been shown to be as safe and effective as the open procedure when performed in select patient populations at high-volume centers. Minimally invasive resection techniques have shown a great deal of promise in delivering at least equivalent oncologic resections with the potential for faster recoveries and fewer wound-related complications. This has direct implications for ongoing management and long-term survival because wound-related complications and prolonged, complicated recoveries are major factors that delay or altogether prohibit the delivery of adjuvant therapy.

Surgical Technique: Pancreaticoduodenectomy

PD is divided into three broad phases: (1) abdominal exploration to confirm absence of extraregional spread; (2) mobilization of structures and formal tumor resection; and (3) pancreaticobiliary and GI reconstruction (Figure 4). There are many approaches to performing PD, and details pertaining to the specific order of operative steps, manner of exposure, and anastomotic techniques often vary between institutions. What follows is a generalized technique based on that most commonly performed at the Johns Hopkins Hospital.

Abdominal Exploration

The abdomen is entered through a vertical midline incision extending from the xiphoid process to just below the umbilicus or alternatively through a bilateral subcostal incision. In both cases exposure is greatly improved by the placement of a self-retaining retractor. The procedure begins with a thorough inspection of the peritoneal cavity to assess for evidence of tumor spread beyond the zone of resection, including all visceral and parietal surfaces of the peritoneum, the omentum, and all bowel from the ligament of Treitz to rectum. After

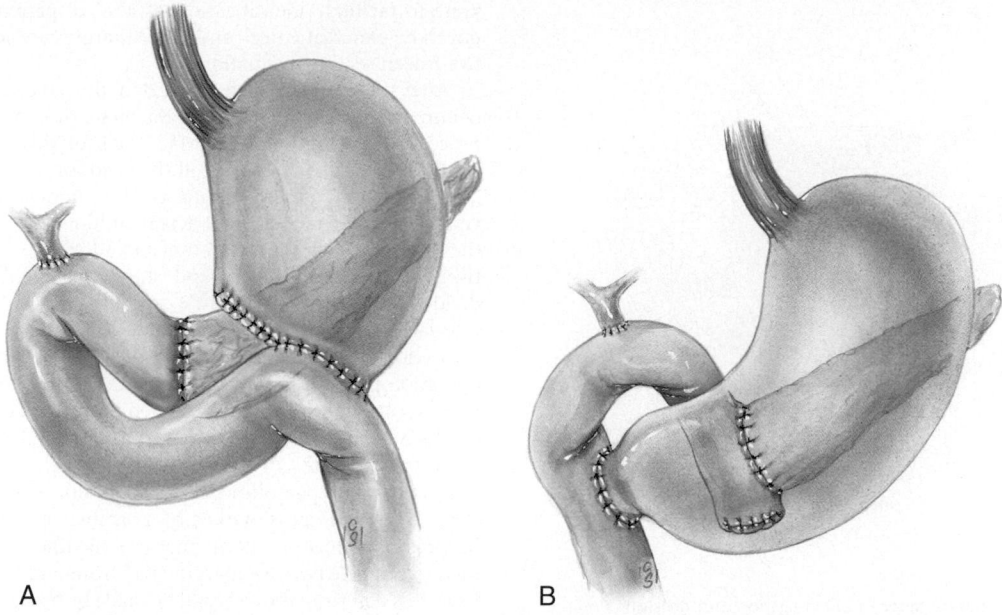

A   B

FIGURE 4 Standard pancreaticoduodenectomy with hemigastrectomy and gastrojejunostomy (**A**) versus pylorus-preserving pancreaticoduodenectomy with duodenojejunostomy (**B**). Illustrations by Corinne Sandone. *(From Wolfgang CL, Herman JM, Laheru DA, Klein AP, Erdek MA, Fishman EK, et al. Recent progress in pancreatic cancer. CA Cancer J Clin. 2013;63:318-348.)*

inspecting the liver surface during the initial exploration, its parenchyma also must be palpated to assess for deeper lesions or evaluated with intraoperative ultrasound if there is heightened clinical suspicion or questionable findings on preoperative imaging. If the patient is believed to be at high risk for occult tumor spread before surgery, initial abdominal exploration should be performed as a diagnostic staging laparoscopy to avoid the potentially unnecessary morbidity of a large abdominal incision.

Tumor Resection

Once extraregional dissemination has been ruled out, exposure of the pancreatic head is initiated by mobilizing the right colon and hepatic flexure from their retroperitoneal attachments. This may be extended into a complete right medial visceral rotation (Cattell-Braasch maneuver) to better expose the third and fourth portions of the duodenum, but it is not necessary in most cases. With continued medial dissection, electrocautery is used to free the transverse mesocolon from its loose alveolar attachments along the duodenum and pancreatic head. The lesser sac then is entered by dividing the gastrocolic ligament between the antrum and proximal transverse colon. Within the transverse mesocolon, the middle colic vein is identified and traced along its course to the anterior surface of the SMV. There it joins either directly or as a common tributary with the right gastroepiploic vein called the gastrocolic trunk of Henle. Depending on the anatomy, the middle colic vein or gastrocolic trunk is ligated and divided to avoid traction injury to the SMV. The right colon now may be reflected medially to maximize exposure of the duodenum and infrapancreatic SMV as it enters beneath the inferior border of the neck of the pancreas.

Next an extensive Kocher's maneuver is performed by dividing the lateral retroperitoneal attachments of the duodenum. The retroperitoneal dissection is carried medially to the left lateral border of the aorta, with care taken to include all fibroadipose and lymphatic tissues with the duodenum and pancreatic head as they are elevated out of the retroperitoneum. This results in a clean exposure of the inferior vena cava (IVC), bilateral renal and gonadal veins, right ureter, and medial edge of the left kidney. Anterior exposure of the SMV now may be completed by clearing any remaining peritoneal attachments and dissecting caudally to the level of the junction of

the first jejunal venous tributary. With the duodenum fully Kocherized, the tumor may be palpated to assess its relationship to the superior mesenteric vessels; however, the most accurate assessment is still provided by recent pancreas protocol CT imaging.

The dissection then moves to the hepatoduodenal ligament, where the overlying peritoneal membrane is divided to permit dissection of the portal structures within. At this point it is important to assess for any anomalous hepatic arterial vasculature because variant anatomy is common (in up to 50% of patients) and inadvertent ligation of a major artery can result in hepatic ischemia or breakdown of the bilioenteric anastomosis. The most common vascular anomaly encountered during PD is a replaced right hepatic artery (RHA), which may be present in up to 15% of patients and usually arises as the first branch off of the SMA. A replaced RHA typically runs posterolateral to the PV in the hepatoduodenal ligament and courses behind the head of the pancreas and CBD en route to the liver. Intraoperative clues that should raise suspicion for anomalous hepatic vasculature include a pulsation felt posterior to the PV or CBD, a diminutive hepatic artery, and any deviation from the expected vascular configuration.

Within the hepatoduodenal ligament, the bile duct and hepatic artery are both located anterior to the PV with the hepatic artery medial to the biliary structures. Dissection begins with removal of the common hepatic artery lymph node, which generally exposes the common hepatic artery (CHA) and its branch, the gastroduodenal artery (GDA). The CHA is dissected circumferentially proximal and distal to the takeoff of the GDA to clearly visualize its course. The GDA also is dissected circumferentially for a length of 1 to 2 cm in preparation for division, which must be performed in order to completely mobilize the neck of the pancreas. Before division the GDA is occluded with an atraumatic clamp, followed by confirmation of flow in the proper hepatic artery, either by direct palpation or with Doppler ultrasound. In patients with celiac stenosis, liver perfusion is dependent on retrograde flow through the GDA from the SMA. This step is crucial because dividing the GDA in the setting of critical celiac artery stenosis can result in fatal hepatic ischemia or breakdown of the bilioenteric anastomosis. Once adequate flow has been confirmed in the proper hepatic artery, the GDA is doubly ligated or suture ligated and then divided (Figure 5).

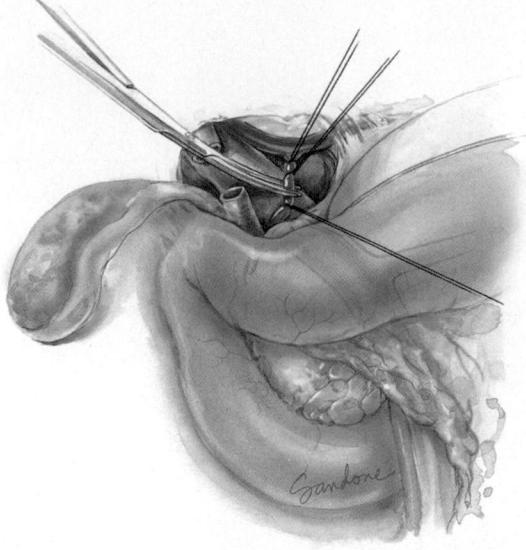

FIGURE 5 Gastroduodenal artery (GDA) ligation and division. After test clamping the GDA to ensure adequate perfusion through the celiac axis, the artery is doubly ligated and divided. Note that the common hepatic duct has been divided already, which may be performed before division of the GDA by some surgeons. *(From Cameron J, Sandone C. Pancreaticoduodenectomy (pylorus-preserving Whipple procedure). Atlas of Gastrointestinal Surgery, Volume 1. 2nd ed. Hamilton, Ontario: BC Decker Inc; 2007:284-305.)*

The hepatoduodenal ligament lymph node bundle lateral to the PV and CBD is identified, divided near the level of the cystic duct, and swept inferiorly for removal en bloc with the specimen. Before division, care should be taken to verify that there are no pulsations present in this tissue mass because, as mentioned previously, this lies within the usual course of a replaced RHA. The gallbladder, if present, is mobilized out of the gallbladder fossa, followed by cystic artery ligation and dissection of the cystic duct through its junction with the CBD. At this point the gallbladder may be removed by ligating and dividing the cystic duct or left in situ for removal with the main specimen. Taking care to avoid injury to the underlying PV, the common hepatic duct (CHD) and CBD are cleared circumferentially of any remaining peritoneal or fibroadipose attachments. The CHD then is divided near its junction with the cystic duct, after which the specimen side is retracted caudally to expose the dissection plane on the underlying anterior wall of the PV. For distal bile duct cancers or larger periampullary tumors of any kind, a more proximal resection on the hepatic duct may be required to obtain an adequate margin.

For PPPD, the first portion of the duodenum is transected at least 1.5 cm distal to the pylorus using a linear GIA stapler. For standard PD, the stomach is divided proximal to the antrum with multiple firings of the linear GIA stapler. In either case, the next step is division of the jejunum at a convenient point 30 to 40 cm distal to the ligament of Treitz. The stapled end is oversewn with nonabsorbable Lembert's sutures, and the intervening mesentery is divided between ties until the jejunum and third and fourth portions of the duodenum can be passed beneath the superior mesenteric vessels into the right upper quadrant. At this point the tunnel is developed under the neck of the pancreas using blunt but precise dissection from above and below the neck. Once completed, a soft Penrose drain is looped through the tunnel to elevate the neck of the pancreas and protect the underlying PV and SMV during transection. Figure-of-8 stitches are placed superiorly and inferiorly on either side of the intended transection site to control bleeding from the superior and inferior pancreaticoduodenal arteries. Then the neck is divided down to the Penrose drain using electrocautery for improved hemostasis or a

knife to facilitate identification of a small pancreatic duct. At this point the pancreatic neck and CHD margins are sent for intraoperative frozen section evaluation.

After the neck has been transected, the pancreatic head and duodenum are retracted laterally to facilitate dissection of the uncinate process off of the PV and SMV. Much of this is performed using gentle, blunt dissection without the need for ligation and division of any substantial venous tributaries. Two notable exceptions are the vein of Belcher (superior pancreaticoduodenal vein) draining into the PV and the first jejunal branch of the SMV. These are both relatively constant landmarks and should be identified, ligated, and divided. Next the PV and SMV are retracted medially to expose the interface of the uncinate process and the lateral wall of the SMA. Dissection of the uncinate off of the SMA is a critical step in the operation because failure to perform this properly can result in an unnecessarily positive margin. When performed correctly, dissection results in a completely skeletonized right lateral SMA border.

At this point the PD specimen may be delivered from the operative field and prepared for pathologic evaluation by properly orienting it with all margins marked by a distinctive suture or ink. Because histologic evaluation alone may be insufficient to distinguish a microscopically positive margin (R1) from a grossly positive margin (R2), this determination should be made by operative assessment and documented in the operative note.

Reconstruction

Re-establishment of pancreatic, biliary, and enteric continuity requires the construction of three anastomoses: pancreaticojejunostomy (PJ), hepaticojejunostomy (HJ), and gastrojejunostomy (GJ) for a standard PD or duodenojejunostomy (DJ) for PPPD. The reconstruction begins by passing the proximal jejunum retrocolic to the right of the middle colic vessels for the PJ and HJ anastomoses. Next, the GJ or DJ may be fashioned in a retrocolic fashion or as an antecolic Hofmeister anastomosis (for GJ).

Of the three anastomoses, the PJ is the most problematic because of its tendency to leak. To address this problem, a number of variations in PJ construction have been developed, most of which fall into the two broad categories of invagination versus duct-to-mucosa techniques. At our institution the most common technique is an end-to-side, duct-to-mucosa anastomosis performed in two layers (Figure 6). The back row of the outer layer is placed first using nonabsorbable silk sutures to imbricate the jejunal serosa onto the posterior surface of the pancreas. A jejunotomy of the same size and directly adjacent to the pancreatic duct is created, and the two are approximated using an inner layer of interrupted absorbable sutures. The anastomosis is completed by finishing the outer layer of imbricating Lembert's sutures anteriorly.

The HJ is constructed approximately 5 to 10 cm downstream from the PJ at a site that avoids tension or torque on either anastomosis. After creating an appropriately sized jejunotomy, the anastomosis is constructed in an end-to-side fashion using a single layer of interrupted absorbable sutures.

Finally the DJ or GJ is constructed downstream from the HJ using either a retrocolic or an antecolic anastomosis. In both cases the anastomosis itself is performed in an end-to-side fashion with an inner layer of running absorbable sutures reinforced by an outer layer of nonabsorbable inverting Lembert's sutures. Before closure, soft closed suction drains are placed in the vicinity of the PJ and HJ to identify and control leakage from these anastomoses during the postoperative period.

Major Vascular Resections

Portomesenteric Venous Resection and Reconstruction

Venous resection is performed at the PV-SMV confluence when the pancreas cannot be dissected free without leaving behind gross tumor or risking injury to the underlying PV and SMV (Figure 7). Once the decision is made to proceed with venous resection, the PV

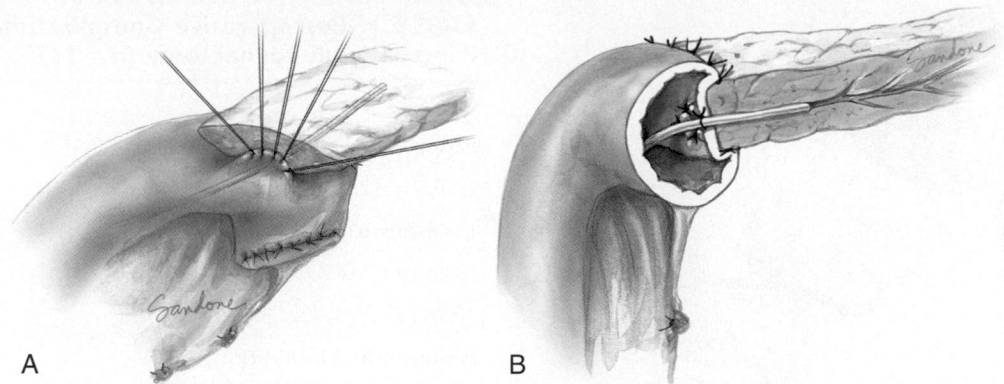

A   B

FIGURE 6 Duct-to-mucosa pancreaticojejunostomy construction in two layers. **A,** The inner layer is constructed by making a small jejunotomy for anastomosis to the pancreatic duct using absorbable sutures. **B,** The outer layer imbricates the jejunal serosa onto the pancreatic surface using nonabsorbable sutures. Some surgeons place a temporary pancreatic stent through the anastomosis at the time of its construction, as pictured here. *(From Cameron J, Sandone C. Pancreaticoduodenectomy (pylorus-preserving Whipple procedure). Atlas of Gastrointestinal Surgery, Volume 1. 2nd ed. Hamilton, Ontario: BC Decker Inc; 2007:284-305.)*

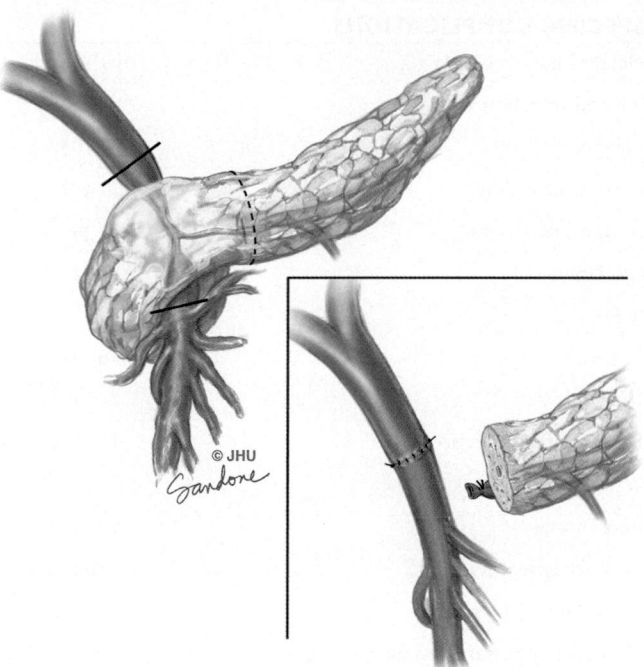

FIGURE 7 Resectable tumor involvement at the portal vein–superior mesenteric vein (PV-SMV) confluence. This is considered resectable because invasion is limited to a single target vessel above and below the necessary region of resection (*dark lines*) and does not extend too high on the PV. The vein segment and mass are resected en bloc, followed by a primary end-to-end reconstruction (*inset*). Ligation and division of the splenic vein, even absent direct involvement, is often necessary to mobilize the PV and SMV sufficiently for primary anastomosis. Illustrations by **Corinne Sandone.** *(From Wolfgang CL, Herman JM, Laheru DA, Klein AP, Erdek MA, Fishman EK, et al. Recent progress in pancreatic cancer. CA Cancer J Clin. 2013;63:318-348.)*

and SMV are cleared for 2 to 3 cm proximal and distal to the PV-SMV confluence, and vascular clamps are placed to isolate the involved segment.

The type of resection and reconstruction required varies depending on the location and degree of tumor involvement. When limited to a small aspect of the lateral or posterior wall (<⅓ vessel circumference), a tangential resection reconstructed with a patch such as greater saphenous vein or bovine pericardium is sufficient. More extensive tumor involvement generally requires full segmental resection with a primary venous anastomosis or interposition graft. The standard approach to segmental resection at the PV-SMV confluence involves ligation and division of the splenic vein (SV). This provides additional length to the SMV and PV for primary end-to-end anastomosis and allows medial access to the SMA to complete the dissection before segmental resection. When the SV is divided, resection defects up to 3 cm generally can be reapproximated for primary anastomosis. If the ends cannot be reapproximated without tension, an autologous vein graft of sufficient size (e.g., left renal vein or internal jugular vein) should be used for reconstruction. Synthetic grafts (e.g., ringed Gore-Tex prosthesis) also may be used but only in the absence of a suitable autologous source given the risk for postoperative infection and thrombosis.

Arterial Resection

Major arterial resections for PDAC are more controversial than venous resections because there are currently limited data evaluating morbidity and survival in this group. As such, encasement of the major visceral arteries remains a contraindication to resection in all but a few isolated cases. One such case occurs when a short segment of CHA is involved in the region of the GDA, where the tumor and associated arterial segment may be amenable to en bloc resection (Figure 8). Reconstruction by primary end-to-end anastomosis of the common and proper hepatic arteries is preferable, but a large defect may require interposition with an autologous vein graft (greater saphenous vein). Alternatively, arterial transposition or interposition using either the splenic artery or the left gastric artery may be performed, especially in situations where a larger segment of CHA must be resected.

■ POSTOPERATIVE CARE

Postoperative care after PD has become more standardized in recent years, resulting in decreased postoperative mortality, reduced length of hospital stay, and improved surgical outcomes. In the immediate 24-hour period after surgery, patients usually are admitted to a monitored unit for close care and volume resuscitation. Blood glucose is managed with an insulin drip, and nasogastric decompression is maintained through an intraoperatively placed nasogastric (NG) tube. On postoperative day 1, the NG tube and Foley catheter are removed, blood glucose management is transitioned to a subcutaneous insulin sliding scale, and the patient is transferred to a dedicated surgical nursing unit. Even before transfer out of the monitored unit, early ambulation and incentive spirometry are begun and continued

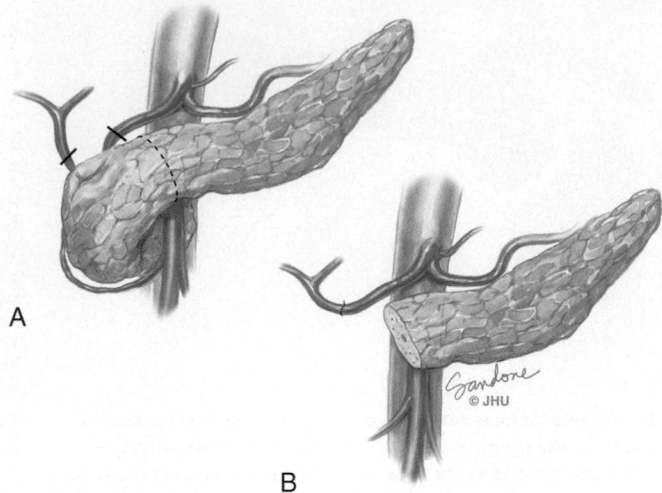

FIGURE 8 Short segment encasement of the common hepatic artery (CHA). Arterial encasement is generally indicative of locally advanced, unresectable disease, but short segment encasement of the CHA (**A**) is often amenable to en bloc resection (**B**) followed by primary anastomosis. Illustrations by Corinne Sandone. *(From Wolfgang CL, Herman JM, Laheru DA, Klein AP, Erdek MA, Fishman EK, et al. Recent progress in pancreatic cancer. CA Cancer J Clin. 2013;63:318-348.)*

throughout the admission. Dietary advancement begins with limited ice chips on postoperative day 1 followed by progression through clear liquids, soft diet, and the eventual postsurgical goal diet (usually a carbohydrate-controlled diet) over successive days, depending on whether the patient is passing flatus and without nausea or vomiting. The use of prokinetic agents such as erythromycin or metoclopramide is advocated by some surgeons to increase gastric emptying but is not routine.

Drains are often left in place until the patient is tolerating a regular diet (usually postoperative day 4 or 5), when drain amylase levels can be used to evaluate for the presence of a pancreatic fistula. If output volume has decreased sufficiently and amylase levels are low, drains are removed sequentially on successive days. More recently there has been a movement toward early drain removal by postoperative day 3, which has shown decreased fistula rates, length of hospital stay, and costs compared with the usual management approach based on drain amylase levels.

■ POSTOPERATIVE COMPLICATIONS

Although the perioperative mortality associated with PD has decreased steadily over the past 2 decades, the morbidity rate has remained largely unchanged, with major complications reported in 35% to 45% of cases. This point is illustrated clearly in the postoperative outcomes of 1175 consecutive PDs performed for periampullary cancers at Johns Hopkins Hospital over 4 decades (Table 1). The most common complications are delayed gastric emptying (DGE), postoperative pancreatic fistula (POPF), and wound infection. Delayed postpancreatectomy hemorrhage (PPH) (>5 days postoperative) occurs less commonly but carries potentially catastrophic consequences and is associated with a relatively high risk of mortality. In an effort to standardize the reporting of these complications and guide their clinical management, the ISGPS has proposed several validated consensus definitions.

Delayed Gastric Emptying

DGE is a functional gastroparesis occurring in 14% to 45% of patients after PD and is diagnosed once mechanical obstruction has been ruled out by upper GI contrast series or endoscopic evaluation.

TABLE 1: Postoperative Complications After Pancreaticoduodenectomy (n = 1175)

Category	n (%)
Perioperative Mortality	**26 (2)**
1970s (n = 23)	7 (30)*
1980s (n = 65)	3 (5)*
1990s (n = 514)	10 (2)
2000s (n = 573)	6 (1)
Perioperative Morbidity	**415 (38)**
1970s (n = 23)	No data
1980s (n = 65)	7 (30)
1990s (n = 514)	158 (31)*
2000s (n = 573)	250 (45)
Reoperation Rate (during index admission)	**35 (3)**
SPECIFIC COMPLICATIONS	
Delayed gastric emptying	161 (15)
Wound infection	91 (8)
Pancreatic fistula	52 (5)
Cardiac morbidity	27 (4)
Abdominal abscess	38 (4)
Cholangitis	26 (2)
Sepsis	19 (2)
Bile leak	16 (2)
Lymph leak	11 (1)
Urinary tract infection	11 (1)
Peptic ulcer	10 (1)
Pneumonia	10 (1)
Acute pancreatitis	5 (1)
Small bowel obstruction	3 (0.3)
Median Length of Stay, days (range)	**9 (4-375)**
1980s	16 (10-51)*
1990s	11 (7-373)*
2000s	8 (4-375)

Modified from Winter JM, et al. 1423 pancreaticoduodenectomies for pancreatic cancer: a single-institution experience. *J Gastrointest Surg.* 2006;10:1199-1210, discussion 1210-1211.

*P <0.05 compared with the present decade.

The ISGPS definition divides DGE into grades A, B, and C according to increasing clinical impact as determined by NG tube requirement, ability to tolerate oral intake, and need for prokinetic therapy (Table 2). Its cause remains unclear, but it is likely multifactorial and often associated with concurrent intra-abdominal abscess or POPF.

Management of DGE is predominantly supportive and includes discontinuation of oral intake, resumed nasogastric decompression, and initiation of prokinetic agents to improve symptoms and recovery time. Prolonged cases of DGE require some form of nutritional

TABLE 2: ISGPS Consensus Definition and Grading of Delayed Gastric Emptying After Pancreatic Surgery

Definition: Functional gastroparesis after surgery without mechanical obstruction as determined by upper gastrointestinal contrast series or endoscopic evaluation.

Grade	NGT Requirement	Days of PO Intolerance (POD)	Vomiting and Gastric Distension	Use of Prokinetics
A	4-7 days or reinsertion >POD 3	7	±	±
B	8-14 days or reinsertion >POD 7	14	+	+
C	>14 days or reinsertion >POD 14	21	+	+

Modified from Wente MN, et al. Delayed gastric emptying (DGE) after pancreatic surgery: a suggested definition by the International Study Group of Pancreatic Surgery (ISGPS). *Surgery.* 2007;142:761-768.

ISGPS, International Study Group of Pancreatic Surgery; *PO,* oral; *POD,* postoperative day; *NGT,* nasogastric tube.

TABLE 3: ISGPS Consensus Definition and Grading of Postoperative Pancreatic Fistula After Pancreatic Surgery

Definition: Drain output of any measurable volume of fluid on or after postoperative day 3 with amylase content >3 times normal serum activity. Once this criterion has been met, the grading system is applied.

Clinical Variable	Grade A	Grade B	Grade C
Clinical condition	Well	Often well	Ill-appearing or poor
Imaging results (if obtained)	Negative	Negative or positive	Positive
Supportive treatments (nutritional support, antibiotics, somatostatin analogue)	No	Yes or no	Yes
Persistent drainage ≥3 weeks (± drain)	No	Usually yes	Yes
Clinical signs of infection	No	Yes	Yes
Sepsis	No	No	Yes
Reoperation	No	No	Yes
Death related to fistula	No	No	Possibly yes
Readmission	No	Yes or no	Yes or no

Modified from Bassi C, et al. Postoperative pancreatic fistula: an international study group (ISGPF) definition. *Surgery.* 2005;138:8-13.

ISGPS, International Study Group of Pancreatic Surgery.

support and cross-sectional imaging to evaluate for secondary causes such as an intra-abdominal abscess. If the patient cannot resume oral feeding within 7 to 10 days, nutritional support in the form of enteral nutrition (EN) or parenteral nutrition (PN) should be initiated. EN is preferred if a feeding jejunostomy was placed at the time of surgery; otherwise total parenteral nutrition (TPN) should be used.

Postoperative Pancreatic Fistula

POPF is a common and costly complication after PD with a wide range of presentations that include transient anastomotic leak, intra-abdominal abscess, and frank fistula formation. Risk factors for development of POPF include a small pancreatic duct, a soft gland, and patients with nonpancreatic periampullary cancers because these usually have a normal parenchyma. Initial signs and symptoms are often nonspecific but may include vague abdominal discomfort, nausea, tachycardia, leukocytosis, and fever. According to the ISGPS consensus definition, POPF is defined as a drain amylase level more than three times the normal serum level on or after postoperative day 3, regardless of the output volume. This is then divided into grades A, B, and C based on increasing severity (Table 3) to help guide management.

Grade A POPFs have little to no clinical impact and require no specific interventions. Once detected, the surgeon may elect to remove the drain incrementally over successive days to ensure fistula closure, but this is not required. These patients may continue to eat normally, and hospital discharge generally is not delayed. By definition, only grades B and C are of any clinical significance requiring specific intervention. These fistulas usually result in increased cost from prolonged hospital stays, longer intensive care unit (ICU) admissions, additional procedures, and readmissions. Uncomplicated low-output fistulas can be managed conservatively with percutaneous drainage of intra-abdominal collections, restriction of oral intake, and nutritional support via TPN or EN using a distally positioned nasointestinal tube or feeding jejunostomy. Long-acting somatostatin analogues such as octreotide are used often as well because they function by reducing GI secretions; however, their efficacy is still under debate because current evidence remains inconclusive. Empiric antibiotics also may be started if there is concern for infection, and all drains should be maintained with outputs measured regularly. Conservative management results in spontaneous fistula closure in up to 90% of cases, usually within 4 weeks. On rare occasions, patients with severe clinical instability or signs of sepsis and organ dysfunction may require surgical re-exploration and repair or revision of the PJ anastomosis.

TABLE 4: ISGPS Consensus Definitions of Postpancreatectomy Hemorrhage

A. DEFINITIONS

TIME OF ONSET

- Early hemorrhage (≤24 hr after the end of the index operation)
- Late hemorrhage (>24 hr after the end of the index operation)

LOCATION

- Intraluminal (anastomotic suture lines, cut surface of the pancreas, stress ulceration, pseudoaneurysm)
- Extraluminal (arterial or venous vessels, diffuse bleeding from resection area, anastomosis suture lines, pseudoaneurysm)

SEVERITY OF HEMORRHAGE

Mild

- Decrease in hemoglobin concentration <3 g/dL
- No significant clinical impairment
- Transfusion of no more than 2-3 units packed cells within 24 hr of surgery or 1-3 units beyond 24 hr
- No requirement for reoperation or interventional angiographic embolization

Severe

- Decrease in hemoglobin concentration ≥3 g/dL
- Clinically significant impairment (tachycardia, hypotension, oliguria, hypovolemic shock)
- Transfusion requirement >3 units packed cells
- Need for invasive treatment (interventional angiographic embolization or relaparotomy)

B. GRADING SCALE

Grade	Onset, Severity, and Location	Clinical Condition
A	Early, mild, intraluminal or extraluminal bleeding	Good
B	Early, severe, intraluminal or extraluminal bleeding Late, mild, intraluminal or extraluminal bleeding	Good to moderately impaired
C	Late, severe, intraluminal or extraluminal bleeding	Severely impaired, life-threatening

Modified from Wente MN, Veit JA, Bassi C, Dervenis C, Fingerhut A, Gouma DJ, et al. Postpancreatectomy hemorrhage (PPH): an International Study Group of Pancreatic Surgery (ISGPS) definition. *Surgery.* 2007;142:20-25.

ISGPS, International Study Group of Pancreatic Surgery.

Postpancreatectomy Hemorrhage

Major postoperative bleeding is a less common but potentially lethal complication after PD. The matter is complicated by the fact that it may originate from a number of potential sites and have variable timing and severity. The most important clinical factor is time of onset because this tends to correlate with the mechanism and source of bleeding, which in turn determines the best course of intervention. According to the ISGPS consensus definition, presented in detail in Table 4, early PPH occurs within 24 hours of surgery and late PPH occurs anytime thereafter. Despite such efforts to standardize the definition, the precise distinction between early and late PPH remains controversial, and many institutions continue to use different time points. At our institution, early PPH encompasses all bleeding events occurring up to and including postoperative day 5.

Early PPH usually results from a failure to achieve adequate hemostasis that, if significant, is seen as surgical bleeding best managed by a return to the operating room. Late PPH is usually the result of an inflammatory process (i.e., pancreatic leak) that causes vascular erosion and formation of arterial pseudoaneurysms prone to bleeding. The most common site for pseudoaneurysm formation is the GDA stump, followed by the hepatic artery, SMA, and splenic artery. This form of bleeding is best managed endovascularly by selective coil embolization of the pseudoaneurysm, which has a success rate of approximately 85%. Alternatively, a covered stent can be deployed to exclude the pseudoaneurysm, particularly in the case of a GDA stump blowout where the target may be insufficient for coil embolization.

■ CONCLUSION

Periampullary cancer is composed of a heterogeneous group of malignancies all affecting the same region near the ampulla of Vater. Although these malignancies often are seen with similar symptoms and are all managed surgically with PD, prognosis varies greatly according to the specific type of cancer. PDAC not only carries the worst prognosis of the group, but also accounts for the majority of cases. Currently the management of PDAC and other nonpancreatic periampullary cancers is evolving by embracing new technologies for minimally invasive resections and applying neoadjuvant therapies to increase the number of surgical candidates and improve the rate of R0 resections.

SELECTED READINGS

Bassi C, Dervenis C, Butturini G, Fingerhut A, Yeo C, Izbicki J, et al. Postoperative pancreatic fistula: an international study group (ISGPF) definition. *Surgery.* 2005;138:8-13.

Bockhorn M, Uzunoglu FG, Adham M, Imrie C, Milicevic M, Sandberg AA, et al. Borderline resectable pancreatic cancer: a consensus statement by the International Study Group of Pancreatic Surgery (ISGPS). *Surgery.* 2014;155:977-988.

Boone BA, Zenati M, Hogg ME, Steve J, Moser AJ, Bartlett DL, et al. Assessment of quality outcomes for robotic pancreaticoduodenectomy: identification of the learning curve. *JAMA Surg.* 2015;150:416-422.

Callery MP, Chang KJ, Fishman EK, Talamonti MS, William Traverso L, Linehan DC. Pretreatment assessment of resectable and borderline resectable pancreatic cancer: expert consensus statement. *Ann Surg Oncol.* 2009;16:1727-1733.

Cameron J, Sandone C. Pancreaticoduodenectomy (*Pylorus-Preserving Whipple procedure*). *Atlas of Gastrointestinal Surgery.* Vol 1. 2nd ed. Hamilton, ON: BC Decker Inc; 2007:284-305.

Croome KP, Farnell MB, Que FG, Reid-Lombardo KM, Truty MJ, Nagorney DM, et al. Total laparoscopic pancreaticoduodenectomy for pancreatic ductal adenocarcinoma: oncologic advantages over open approaches? *Ann Surg.* 2014;260:633-640.

Griffin JF, Poruk KE, Wolfgang CL. Pancreatic cancer surgery: past, present, and future. *Chin J Cancer Res.* 2015;27:332-348.

He J, Ahuja N, Makary MA, Cameron JL, Eckhauser FE, Choti MA, et al. 2564 resected periampullary adenocarcinomas at a single institution: trends over three decades. *HPB (Oxford).* 2014;16:83-90.

Wente MN, Bassi C, Dervenis C, Fingerhut A, Gouma DJ, Izbicki JR, et al. Delayed gastric emptying (DGE) after pancreatic surgery: a suggested definition by the International Study Group of Pancreatic Surgery (ISGPS). *Surgery.* 2007;142:761-768.

Wente MN, Veit JA, Bassi C, Dervenis C, Fingerhut A, Gouma DJ, et al. Postpancreatectomy hemorrhage (PPH): an International Study Group of Pancreatic Surgery (ISGPS) definition. *Surgery.* 2007;142:20-25.

Winter JM, Cameron JL, Campbell KA, Arnold MA, Chang DC, Coleman J, et al. 1423 pancreaticoduodenectomies for pancreatic cancer: a single-institution experience. *J Gastrointest Surg.* 2006;10:1199-1210, discussion 1210-1211.

VASCULAR RECONSTRUCTION DURING THE WHIPPLE PROCEDURE

Warren R. Maley, MD, and Charles J. Yeo, MD

Despite recent advances in the chemotherapeutic treatment of pancreatic ductal adenocarcinoma (PDAC), margin-negative surgical resection (R0) remains the only potentially curative treatment for the disease. Pancreatic multiphase computed tomography (CT) or magnetic resonance imaging (MRI), including arterial, pancreatic parenchymal, and portal venous phases of contrast enhancement with thin cuts through the abdomen and three-dimensional (3D) reconstruction, allows for determination of the relationship of the primary tumor to the mesenteric vasculature and detection of metastatic disease to the liver or peritoneum. Clearly resectable lesions are defined as those without demonstrable metastatic disease where the primary tumor does not involve the celiac axis, the hepatic artery or superior mesenteric artery (SMA), the superior mesenteric vein (SMV), or the portal vein. Mesenteric venous resection has played an increasingly important role in achieving an R0 resection in "borderline" resectable or "locally advanced" lesions involving the SMV or portal vein. The development of active chemotherapeutic regimens against PDAC means that this technique may play an expanding role in the care of patients with "borderline" or "locally advanced" disease who are undergoing neoadjuvant therapy before attempted resection. A recent International Study Group of Pancreatic Surgery (ISGPS) consensus statement discussed borderline resectable PDAC and proposed a classification of venous resections.

■ DEFINING RESECTABILITY

The capacities of CT and MRI to predict vessel or nodal involvement are roughly equivalent. We tend to prefer a multidetector CT scan using oral water and intravenous (IV) contrast, with workstation reconstructions. MRI may be superior to CT in detecting liver or peritoneal metastases. PDAC is considered localized and resectable provided that (1) imaging does not demonstrate any distant metastases; (2) there is a lack of SMV or portal vein abutment, distortion, or encasement; and (3) there are clear fat planes around the celiac axis, hepatic artery, and SMA.

Tumors considered "borderline" resectable include those without metastases but with SMV or portal vein abutment, with or without narrowing of the lumen or encasement. Short segment venous occlusion still may be resectable provided that there are segments of the vein proximal and distal to the obstruction that allow for safe resection and reconstruction. Tumor involving either the gastroduodenal artery (GDA) or a short segment of the hepatic artery not involving the celiac axis and tumor abutting less than 180 degrees of the circumference of the SMA are also considered "borderline" for resection.

Primary lesions that demonstrate abutment of the celiac axis, more than 180 degrees of SMA encasement, or long segments of venous occlusion without optimal venous reconstruction are considered "locally advanced" and generally are not deemed candidates for resection without neoadjuvant therapy.

Evaluation for normal variants of hepatic arterial anatomy always should be performed. In particular, if the right hepatic artery or the entire common hepatic artery originates off of the SMA, these arteries may be involved by the primary lesion, which changes the assessment of resectability. Sagittal arterial views of the aorta should be reviewed before a Whipple procedure in order to rule out stenosis of the celiac axis origin. Enlargement of the GDA due to collateral flow from the SMA may suggest the presence of celiac stenosis (from either intrinsic aortic-celiac orifice plaque or median arcuate ligament compromise).

■ PREOPERATIVE PLANNING AND PREPARATION FOR SURGERY

We typically obtain operative consent well before the operation. This is done as part of a multidisciplinary team approach, with the patient being educated regarding the pancreaticoduodenectomy, vascular reconstruction, and perioperative expectations to include duration of surgery, length of hospitalization, and recovery. Patients typically are given a copy of the publication titled *Understanding Pancreatic Cancer*, Second Edition, which is published by the Lustgarten Foundation. They also are referred to websites for additional information.

In addition to signing previously prepared and detailed operative consent forms, patients are asked to consider participating in various clinical studies. This includes a discussion of consent for tumor harvest, which allows us to place individual patient's resected tumors into a biobank. In addition, the tumors typically are accessed using a pan-cancer mutation panel, not only for genomic analysis but also for proteomic and phosphoprotein analysis. As well, patients at Thomas Jefferson University Hospital often participate in prospective randomized trials that are investigator initiated, such as our recent HYSLAR trial.

■ SURGICAL TECHNIQUE: THE EXTIRPATIVE PHASE WHEN VASCULAR RESECTION IS CONTEMPLATED

On the day of surgery, patients receive preoperative intravenous antibiotic as well as subcutaneous heparin at a dose of 5000 units. TED stockings are applied before patients enter the operating room. After the successful induction of general endotracheal anesthesia, appropriate monitoring lines are placed, sequential compression devices are placed on the legs, and a Foley catheter is inserted in sterile fashion into the bladder. The abdomen, left neck, and both groins then are prepared and draped in routine fashion using chlorhexidine. Patients are identified and a preoperative timeout and preoperative briefing are performed, per the Thomas Jefferson surgical checklist.

We perform our pancreatic resections almost exclusively using a vertical midline incision. The incision is taken from the xiphoid to a little below the umbilicus using a skin knife, and the abdomen is entered cautiously using the electrocautery. A thorough exploration of the abdominal cavity is performed. Particular attention is paid to the peritoneal surfaces, stomach, small bowel, mesenteric root, liver, and colon. We examine for the presence of malignant ascites, carcinomatosis, or omental implants.

We then protect the skin edges and place our abdominal wall retractors. We typically commence the operation by taking the gallbladder down from the gallbladder fossa using the electrocautery and the fundus-down technique. The cystic artery is identified, tied with 2-0 or 3-0 silk, and divided. The cystic duct is dissected out right down to the common hepatic duct–common bile duct junction. We next work in the hepatoduodenal ligament, dissecting out the extrahepatic biliary tree. The common hepatic duct just proximal to the insertion of the cystic duct is identified, elevated off of the portal vein, and encircled with a vessel loop. We then divide the common hepatic duct with the electrocautery or knife and control the proximal hepatic duct with the silver bulldog, thereby preventing intraperitoneal contamination from ongoing bile drainage.

We typically then grasp the distal common hepatic duct and cystic duct junction with an Allis forceps, elevate them ventrally, and then work on the anterior aspect of the portal vein, dissecting this behind

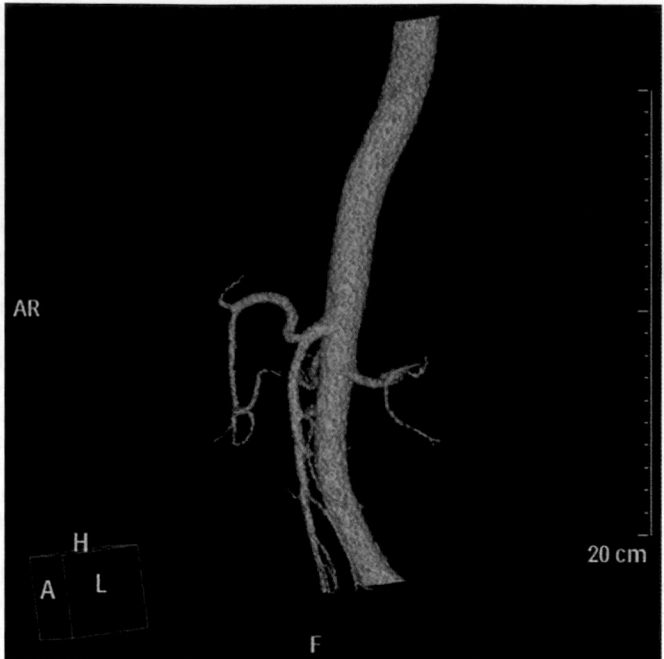

FIGURE 3 Common hepatic artery originating from the superior mesenteric artery—fully "replaced" arterial system to the liver.

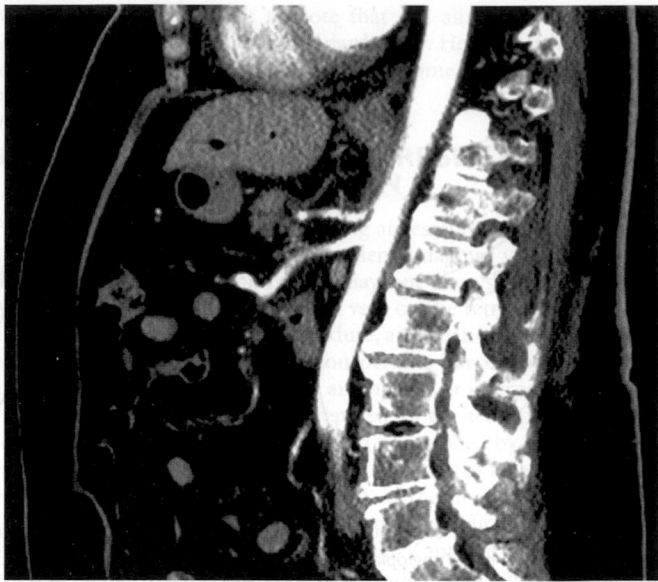

FIGURE 4 Sagittal view of the aorta demonstrating celiac stenosis at the orifice. Hepatic arterial flow was served by the gastroduodenal artery (GDA). The markedly dilated right gastroepiploic artery can be seen originating from the superior mesenteric artery, providing flow to the GDA retrograde.

reach the right lobe of the liver via passage in the porta hepatis just posterior to the common bile duct. Segments of these replaced or accessory right hepatic arteries can be resected if they appear to be involved by tumor. Accessory hepatic vessels with pulsatile back-bleeding from the liver typically can be ligated. However, totally replaced right hepatic arteries should be maintained by re-anastomosis to the GDA stump. Ligation of the replaced right hepatic artery frequently will result in lobar necrosis of the liver parenchyma previously injured by bile duct obstruction secondary to the pancreatic mass. Very rarely, the entire hepatic artery may be replaced off of the SMA, and this must be separated carefully from the head of the pancreas and preserved (Figure 3).

The presence of celiac artery stenosis should be determined preoperatively by viewing the arterial sagittal images (Figure 4). Celiac artery stenosis also can be recognized intraoperatively if the GDA is two to three times the normal diameter and the proper hepatic artery pulsation is lost when the GDA is test occluded. In the majority of cases this can be resolved by lysing the median arcuate ligament. All of the arcuate ligament fibers should be divided down to the anterior wall of the aorta superior to the takeoff of the celiac artery. After lysis of the arcuate ligament, the test occlusion of the GDA should be repeated to determine whether hepatic arterial flow has been improved by this maneuver. If this fails to augment hepatic arterial flow, reimplantation of the celiac artery (difficult to accomplish) or interposition saphenous vein graft from the aorta to the celiac artery may need to be considered.

If the hepatic artery proves to be encased over a short segment, this encased portion can be resected and either a primary reanastomosis may be performed or an interposition saphenous vein graft can be utilized if primary re-anastomosis would result in excessive tension. In general, arterial reconstructions are to be avoided unless absolutely necessary. They are a dramatic Achilles heel if they accompany a Whipple procedure and are prone to pseudoaneursym formation if a fistula ensues or infection occurs in the operative bed.

■ SURGICAL RECONSTRUCTION

After the extirpative phase of the Whipple procedure, we commence the reconstructive phase, which requires the performance of three anastomoses: the pancreaticojejunostomy (PJ), the hepaticojejunostomy (HJ), and the duodenojejunostomy (DJ). The rent at the level of the ligament of Treitz is closed with interrupted 3-0 silk pop-off sutures. The retained jejunum typically is brought up through a small rent in the right side of the transverse mesocolon. We mobilize the pancreatic remnant for a distance of approximately 2 cm and then commence our reconstruction with the PJ. In most cases this is performed as an end-to-side PJ to the uppermost portion of the available jejunum. We typically mention the texture of the gland and the size of the pancreatic duct in the operative notes, and we prefer to use a 5F or 8F pediatric feeding tube as a temporary internal stent. The pediatric feeding tube is removed during the performance of the HJ, when the jejunum is open. We prefer to perform an invagination PJ, with the inner layer being done with 3-0 Vicryl continuous suture and the outer layer being done with 3-0 silk interrupted suture.

Approximately 10 cm downstream from the PJ we typically perform a standard biliary reconstruction as an end-to-side HJ. This anastomosis is done using single-layer 5-0 PDS sutures, placing our posterior sutures first and then using a 10F to 14F T-tube (cut to be an I-tube) to temporarily stent the internal aspect of the anastomosis. Then the anterior sutures are placed and tied. The anastomosis then is checked for leaks and to ensure that it is without undue tension.

In cases with a firm pancreas, with a low chance of PJ leak, we typically go on to perform the DJ about 30 cm downstream from the HJ, above the transverse mesocolon. During the time that the jejunum is open, we retrieve the T-tube from the lumen of the jejunum. The DJ anastomosis is done using an outer layer of interrupted 3-0 silk sutures and an inner layer of running 3-0 Vicryl sutures. After completion of the DJ, we tack the efferent limb of the DJ to the right-sided transverse mesocolon, several centimeters downstream from the DJ.

In cases where the PJ appears to be at high risk of a leak, most notably when the gland is soft and friable and does not hold sutures well, we depart from the DJ reconstruction described and instead perform a "downstream" DJ either through a separate central rent in the mesocolon or in antecolic fashion. We do this at least 35 cm downstream from the HJ, so as to avoid reflux of ingested food and gastric juices back toward the HJ and the PJ. Again, during the time that the jejunum is open, we retrieve the I-tube from the lumen of the jejunum. This downstream DJ anastomosis also is done using an outer layer of interrupted 3-0 silk sutures and an inner layer of running 3-0 Vicryl sutures. After completion of the downstream DJ, we typically pull the DJ anastomosis down through the mesocolon, and we tack the stomach to the mesocolon about 4 cm cephalad to the DJ. In this scenario, we also tack the efferent limb of the HJ to the right side of the transverse mesocolon.

It is at this point that we check for hemostasis thoroughly throughout all of our operative sites. We carefully look at the gallbladder fossa and hepatoduodenal ligament and in the retroperitoneum surrounding the SMV, portal vein, and SMA. We also assess for hemostasis at the level at the ligament of Treitz. We then typically place two or more $\frac{3}{16}$-inch round drains through separate stab incisions, one or more in the right flank and one or more in the left flank. We go sufficiently lateral to avoid injury to the rectus muscles and to the inferior epigastric artery and vein. All drains are sewn in place with 2-0 steel wires. The superiormost right drain is cut to the proper length and brought into the right subhepatic space near but not touching the HJ, and it also resides posterior to the neoduodenum. The left-sided superior drain is brought through the gastrocolic ligament and placed near but not touching the PJ in the left subhepatic space. Additional drains (placed after venous reconstruction) are directed into the pelvis, particularly if the SMV clamp time has been long and if the small bowel shows evidence of petechiae or edema. These pelvic drains are placed to avoid abdominal compartment syndrome, should the patient have considerable acute, short-term fluid losses into the peritoneal cavity.

We then check the placement of the nasogastric tube, ensuring that it resides in proper position in the stomach. The abdomen then is irrigated copiously with warm, sterile antibiotic solution. We often place retention sutures using horizontal mattress #2 nylon sutures, particularly if the patient has received preoperative neoadjuvant chemotherapy or if we anticipate considerable abdominal distension. The abdominal fascia then is routinely closed using running #2 nylon sutures, taking 1-cm bites of the fascia with each stitch approximately 1 cm apart. The subcutaneous tissue and skin then are closed using running absorbable suture. The abdomen then is scanned with a radiofrequency chip wand to assess for retained sponges, and all counts are checked. A postoperative debriefing is always performed, and the patient is transferred from the operating room to a monitored bed.

■ POSTOPERATIVE MANAGEMENT

We have embraced the use of a postpancreaticoduodenectomy critical pathway for our patients, targeting hospital discharge on postoperative day 6 or 7. Approximately 80% of our patients are managed per this pathway and achieve timely discharge. Details of the pathway have been published by Kennedy and colleagues.

■ SUMMARY

Preoperative CT or MRI is essential for determining the presence of venous or arterial involvement by the pancreatic cancer. Awareness of hepatic arterial variants or celiac artery stenosis is vital to avoid liver ischemia potentially precipitated by the Whipple procedure. Anticipation of the need for vascular resection or reconstruction allows for the proactive procurement of autologous venous patch or conduit materials. Attending to all other aspects of the resection before dealing with the venous involvement permits rapid elimination of the specimen from the field, facilitating the reconstruction. Partnering with a liver transplant surgeon may be of assistance if these vascular resection techniques are outside the general scope of your practice.

SUGGESTED READINGS

Bockhorn M, Uzunoglu FG, Adham M, et al. Borderline resectable pancreatic cancer: a consensus statement by the International Study Group of Pancreatic Surgery (ISGPS). *Surgery.* 2014;155:977-988.

Katz MH, Fleming JB, Pisters PW, et al. Anatomy of the superior mesenteric vein with special reference to the surgical management of first-order branch involvement at pancreaticoduodenectomy. *Ann Surg.* 2008;248: 1098-1102.

Kennedy EP, Brumbaugh JP, Yeo CJ. Reconstruction following the pylorus preserving Whipple resection: PJ, HJ and DJ. *J Gastrointest Surg.* 2010;14: 408-415.

Kennedy EP, Rosato EL, Sauter PK, et al. Initiation of a critical pathway for pancreaticoduodenectomy at an academic institution: the first step in multi-disciplinary team building. *J Am Coll Surg.* 2007;204:917-924.

Lavu H, Sell NM, Carter TI, et al. The HYSLAR trial: a prospective randomized controlled trial on the use of a restrictive fluid regimen with 3% hypertonic saline (HYS) versus lactated ringers (LAR) in patients undergoing pancreaticoduodenectomy. *Ann Surg.* 2014;260:445-455.

Lustgarten Foundation for Pancreatic Cancer Research. *Understanding Pancreatic Cancer: A Guide for Patients and Caregivers.* 2nd ed. Bethpage, NY: Author; 2012.

Pessaux P, Varma D, Arnaud JP. Pancreaticoduodenectomy: superior mesenteric artery first approach. *J Gastrointest Surg.* 2006;10:607-611.

PALLIATIVE THERAPY FOR PANCREATIC CANCER

Brian Kadera, MD, and O. Joe Hines, MD

Over the past decade, our understanding of pancreatic ductal adenocarcinoma biology has improved substantially but little has changed in the outcomes for this disease. The 5-year survival rate remains at 6%. Of the 49,000 patients who will be diagnosed this year, most will be stage III or IV and considered unresectable. In order to serve this population it is important for surgeons to understand the treatment options that can help to maintain quality of life for these patients.

Multidrug therapy, most notably FOLFIRINOX (5-fluorouracil, leucovorin, irinotecan, and oxaliplatin), has a proven survival benefit in advanced stage disease. In our practice, those patients with stage IIb or stage III who respond to chemotherapy as evidenced by decrease in cancer antigen 19-9 (CA19-9) or decrease in the degree of vessel involvement are offered exploration and possible pancreaticoduodenectomy. A proportion of these patients are found to be unresectable because of metastatic disease or arterial invasion. Palliation of symptoms associated with locoregional tumor growth and invasion then becomes the focus of therapy.

Pancreatic cancer commonly occurs in the pancreatic head, which results in three main sequelae: biliary obstruction, duodenal obstruction, and tumor-related pain. Although traditionally managed by open operative approaches, less invasive endoscopic, laparoscopic, and radiologic methods are now accepted as preferred interventions.

BOX 1: Potential Advantages and Disadvantages of Neoadjuvant Therapy

Benefits of Neoadjuvant Therapy

The ability to deliver systemic therapy to all patients

Identification of patients with aggressive tumor biology (manifested as disease progression) at the time of post-treatment and preoperative restaging who thereby avoid the toxicity of surgery

Increased efficacy of radiation therapy; free radical production in a well-oxygenated environment

Decreased radiation-induced toxicity to adjacent normal tissue, as the radiated field is resected at the time of pancreatectomy

Decreased rate of positive resection margins; superior mesenteric artery margin in particular

Decreased rate of pancreatic fistula formation

Potential for the tumor size to decrease, especially in borderline resectable tumors, which may facilitate surgical resection

Disadvantages of Neoadjuvant Therapy

Potential for complications from pretreatment endoscopic procedures (endoscopic ultrasound scan and fine-needle aspiration, and endoscopic retrograde cholangiopancreatography)

Biliary stent–related morbidity; stent occlusion during neoadjuvant therapy

Disease progression obviating resectability; loss of a "window" of resectability may occur (rarely) in the borderline resectable patient

Coordination of multiple physicians during the preoperative phase; discrete handoff from surgeon to medical oncologist to radiation oncologist (as occurs with adjuvant therapy) is not possible in the neoadjuvant setting

---

of radiation and decreases the toxicity to adjacent normal tissue. The addition of radiation has important pathologic implications, with several series reporting decreased rates of positive margins (R1 or R2) and node-positive disease.

When neoadjuvant therapy was introduced as an alternative to a surgery-first approach, several concerns were raised regarding its safety and feasibility. Foremost was the concern that patients with localized PC may develop local disease progression that would prevent potentially curative surgical resection; in other words, the "window of opportunity" for surgery could be lost. As the experience with neoadjuvant therapy has matured, concerns regarding local disease progression have not been realized. In the largest combined experience with neoadjuvant therapy for patients with resectable PC (a broad definition of resectable was used in these studies), fewer than 2% of eligible patients were found to have isolated local disease progression at the time of restaging after neoadjuvant therapy (before planned surgery). Disease progression during or after neoadjuvant therapy, if it occurs, usually is seen at distant sites such as the liver, peritoneum, and lung. In addition, theoretical concerns over the toxicity of neoadjuvant therapy and the impact of treatment-related side effects on operative morbidity and mortality also were not observed. In fact, the incidence of pancreatic fistula, the most frequent serious complication associated with pancreatectomy, has been demonstrated to be reduced after neoadjuvant therapy, as the treated pancreas becomes more firm with a decrease in enzyme production. With regard to overall complications, a recent analysis of the National Surgical Quality Improvement Project (NSQIP) database demonstrated no differences in 30-day mortality and postoperative morbidity rates among patients treated with neoadjuvant therapy as compared with patients who received surgery first. However, neoadjuvant treatment sequencing does require successful tumor biopsy (endoscopic ultrasound–guided fine-needle aspiration) and, if the patient has biliary obstruction, the placement of a metal stent for biliary decompression.

■ STAGE-SPECIFIC TREATMENT PLANS

Stage-specific treatment plans as recommended by the NCCN and our recommended treatment sequencing are outlined in Table 3. It is important to note that consensus guidelines support the early administration of systemic therapy in three of the four stages of PC (borderline resectable, locally advanced, and metastatic). The use of neoadjuvant therapy for patients with resectable PC remains highly controversial. However, considering that surgery has a modest impact on the natural history of PC in most patients, a neoadjuvant approach to treatment sequencing is gaining support and will be the focus of critical analysis in the near future.

Resectable PC

Outside of a clinical trial, neoadjuvant treatment of resectable PC may consist of chemotherapy alone or chemoradiotherapy. If chemoradiotherapy is used, systemic gemcitabine combined with external beam radiation therapy is favored (Figure 2, *A*). This regimen is a slight modification of the neoadjuvant treatment schema reported by Evans and colleagues and includes a standard fractionation course of radiation therapy (1.8 Gy/day, M-F, 28 fractions) to a total dose of 50.4 Gy, with concurrent weekly gemcitabine given on day 1 (day –2 to +1) at a dose of 400 mg/m^2 at fixed dose rate over 40 minutes. This program resulted in a median survival of almost 3 years in those patients who completed all intended therapy to include surgery. Restaging with pancreatic protocol CT imaging is completed 4 weeks after the last radiation treatment and, in the absence of disease progression, patients are then brought to surgery. The recent reports of efficacious multidrug regimens, such as FOLFIRINOX (5-fluorouracil, leucovorin, irinotecan, and oxaliplatin) and gemcitabine/nab-paclitaxel, in patients with advanced disease has generated enthusiasm for their use in the neoadjuvant setting in patients with borderline resectable disease. Acknowledging that the use of chemoradiotherapy remains controversial, neoadjuvant FOLFIRINOX or gemcitabine/nab-paclitaxel delivered over approximately 2 months also represents a logical treatment alternative for patients with resectable disease.

Borderline Resectable PC

Patients with borderline resectable PC are fundamentally different from those with resectable disease in that they (1) are at higher risk for harboring radiographically occult distant metastatic disease, (2) are at the highest possible risk for a positive margin of resection due to tumor-artery abutment, (3) require a more complex operation usually involving vascular resection and reconstruction, and therefore (4) there is a greater possibility that, despite the best efforts of the physician team, a surgical procedure may yield no oncologic benefit for the patient. For these reasons, investigators have applied a more robust level of selection consisting of a longer period of induction therapy, often including chemotherapy followed by chemoradiotherapy, before considering surgery. The chemoradiotherapy portion of induction therapy has been thought to be particularly important for those patients with arterial abutment in the hope of sterilizing at least the periphery of the tumor and thereby preventing a positive margin of resection in the autonomic neural tissue that envelopes the visceral arteries.

Treatment sequencing in patients with borderline resectable PC aims to both treat presumed (radiographically occult) systemic disease without the delay imposed by a surgery-first treatment approach and avoid local disease progression that may sacrifice a window of opportunity for surgical resection of the primary tumor. Therefore our preferred off-protocol neoadjuvant treatment schema for patients with borderline resectable PC consists of an initial 2 months of systemic therapy followed by chemoradiotherapy

TABLE 3: Comparison of Treatment Sequencing Strategies for Patients With Pancreatic Cancer (outside of a clinical trial)

Stage	NCCN	MCW
Resectable	• Surgery • Restaging • Adjuvant therapy (+/– chemoradiotherapy; 6 months)	• Neoadjuvant chemoradiotherapy (5.5 wk)* • Restaging • Surgery • Restaging • Adjuvant therapy (4 months)
Borderline resectable	• Neoadjuvant therapy (regimen not specified) • Restaging • Surgery • Restaging • Consider adjuvant therapy	• Neoadjuvant chemotherapy (2 mo) • Restaging • Neoadjuvant chemoradiotherapy (5.5 wk) • Restaging • Surgery • Restaging • Adjuvant therapy (4 months)
Locally advanced	• Chemotherapy • Restaging • Chemoradiotherapy in selected patients	• Chemotherapy (minimum 4 months) • Restaging • Chemoradiotherapy • Restaging • Surgery in highly selected patients
Metastatic	• Systemic therapy (FOLFIRINOX or gem-nab) • Clinical trial	• Systemic therapy • Clinical trial

Note: Clinical trials are preferred in all patients with pancreatic cancer (regardless of stage of disease) who have a performance status acceptable for treatment.

*Systemic therapy alone (FOLFIRINOX, gem-nab) is being considered by many clinicians because of the efficacy of these regimens in advanced disease and the challenges of delivering FOLFIRINOX in the adjuvant setting after such a large operation.

FOLFIRINOX, 5-fluorouracil, leucovorin, irinotecan, and oxaliplatin; *gem-nab*, gemcitabine/nab-paclitaxel; *MCW*, Medical College of Wisconsin; *NCCN*, National Comprehensive Cancer Network.

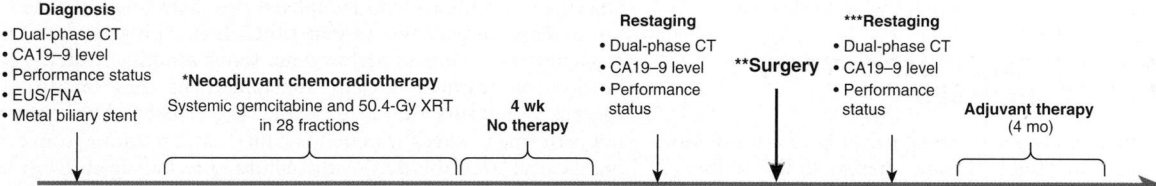

*Systemic therapy alone (FOLFIRINOX, gem-nab) is being considered by many clinicians because of the efficacy of these regimens in advanced disease and the challenges of delivering FOLFIRINOX in the adjuvant setting after such a large operation.
**Surgery is typically performed in the fifth week after the completion of XRT.
***Patients are restaged during postop week six if their recovery has been uncomplicated; however, there is no need to restage if recovery is complicated and the patient is not a suitable candidate to receive further systemic therapy.

A

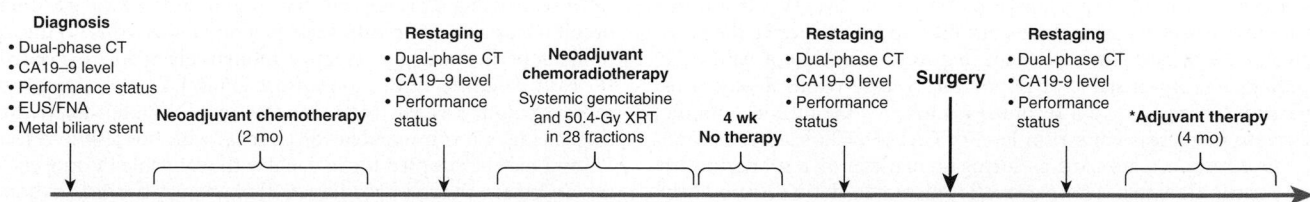

*The benefit of further postoperative/adjuvant systemic therapy after a more prolonged induction phase is being questioned, especially in those patients of advanced age or when postoperative recovery is slow.

B

FIGURE 2 Schematic representation of treatment sequencing in (**A**) resectable and (**B**) borderline resectable pancreatic cancer (PC). *CA19-9*, cancer antigen 19-9; *CT*, computed tomography; *EUS*, endoscopic ultrasound scan; *FNA*, fine-needle aspiration; *FOLFIRINOX*, 5-fluorouracil, leucovorin, irinotecan, and oxaliplatin; *gem-nab*, gemcitabine/nab-paclitaxel; *XRT*, external radiotherapy.

(Figure 2, *B*). The choice of systemic agents for initial treatment has evolved from single-agent gemcitabine to combination therapies, such as FOLFIRINOX or gemcitabine/nab-paclitaxel. After the delivery of systemic therapy, patients are restaged with particular attention to treatment response indicators (clinical, radiographic, biochemical). Patients who have stable disease after 2 months of chemotherapy (no change on CT imaging and a modest decline [or no decline] in cancer antigen 19-9 [CA19-9]) should transition to chemoradiotherapy. The importance of local disease control, especially in patients with potentially operable disease, cannot be overstated; in the absence of a dramatic response to the first 2 months of systemic therapy, patients with borderline resectable PC should be transitioned to chemoradiotherapy to avoid clinically significant local-regional disease progression that negatively may affect operability. More prolonged course neoadjuvant systemic therapy is the subject of current clinical trial development; such trials should all include detailed assessment of treatment response to minimize the risk of local tumor progression.

Locally Advanced PC

The majority of patients with locally advanced PC have unresectable disease. However, in a small proportion of patients, current systemic therapies (FOLFIRINOX, gemcitabine/nab-paclitaxel, GTX [gemcitabine, docetaxel, and capecitabine]) have been associated with significant radiographic response, which has enabled select patients to undergo surgical resection for what was previously thought to be unresectable disease. Such patients often have received a lengthy course (4 to 6 months) of systemic therapy, often followed by chemoradiotherapy, and are then found to have a good performance status with a low or normalized serum level of CA19-9. After such extended therapy, patients without disease progression have three options: a treatment break (rarely preferred by the asymptomatic patient with a normalized CA19-9), maintenance chemotherapy (however defined), or consideration of surgery. Surgery is often considered because there are few other attractive options and surgical resection of the primary tumor is thought to be the only option for possible cure or long-term survival, as complete histologic responses are rare with systemic therapy and chemoradiotherapy (the primary tumor is likely to harbor viable cancer cells). However, it is important to remember that such responding patients likely will realize a significant survival benefit even without surgery, as they have been preselected based on response to induction therapy. It is therefore critically important that surgery be applied only to carefully selected patients using objective criteria—and not because other therapies have been exhausted and the medical team is unsure of what to do next.

■ DEFINING CLINICALLY IMPORTANT TREATMENT RESPONSES

Stage-specific treatment strategies are designed to both treat radiographically occult micrometastatic disease (present in the majority of patients) and maximize local disease control. The assessment of treatment response is critically important and should be performed after the completion of any treatment modality. In patients with localized PC, defining response to therapy can be particularly challenging, as the majority of patients with localized PC are likely to have minimal to modest changes in tumor size on cross-sectional imaging. At the Medical College of Wisconsin (MCW), treatment response is assessed using three critically important criteria: the presence or absence of clinical benefit (e.g., the resolution of pain), CT findings to suggest stable or responding disease versus disease progression (change in cross-sectional diameter of the tumor), and the decrease or increase in serum level of CA19-9. Clinical benefit and CA19-9 response are used as surrogate markers of response under the assumption that extrapancreatic micrometastatic disease likely has responded to therapy if the condition of the patient improves and the level of CA19-9 declines. In general, neoadjuvant therapy should not be expected to "downstage" a tumor. Although tumors may demonstrate a decrease in overall size, the relationship of the tumor to adjacent vessels generally does not change. A change in clinical stage, reflecting a change in local tumor-vessel anatomy, in response to neoadjuvant therapy has been reported to occur in less than 1% of cases. Therefore the use of restaging imaging should be performed primarily to (1) identify local or distant disease progression, and (2) facilitate operative planning. Careful attention to radiographic findings allows for a detailed preoperative plan, especially when vascular reconstruction is anticipated. It is especially important

that vascular resections occur as planned events rather than as an emergent response to vascular injury, as unexpected vascular injuries ultimately can compromise the completeness of the resection, resulting in a positive margin.

CA19-9 has been demonstrated to be a useful prognostic marker in patients with PC. Among patients with localized PC, a decrease in CA19-9 in response to neoadjuvant therapy has been reported to correlate with overall survival. A greater than 50% reduction in CA19-9 levels in response to neoadjuvant therapy has been associated with an improved overall survival. Recent data from our institution have demonstrated that among patients who undergo neoadjuvant therapy and pancreatic resection, the normalization of CA19-9 in response to induction therapy (preoperative value) has been a highly favorable prognostic factor and has been associated with a median survival of 46 months. Equally important is the recognition that an increase in CA19-9 level after induction therapy correlates with disease progression. Although the majority of patients will experience a decline in CA19-9 in response to neoadjuvant therapy, approximately 20% of patients will have an increase in CA19-9; among these patients, metastatic disease will be detected (at restaging or laparoscopy) in 50%. Therefore clinicians should have a low threshold for expanding the diagnostic workup (MRI of liver or PET) before surgery in patients who have a rising CA19-9 level after neoadjuvant therapy.

After the completion of neoadjuvant therapy, at the time of restaging before surgery, it is important that a careful assessment of the patient's performance status and medical comorbidities be re-evaluated. Several studies have demonstrated that patients with poor performance status or uncontrolled comorbidities are likely to experience postoperative morbidity and mortality. The physiologic stress associated with preoperative therapy has the potential to identify or expose patients with poor physiologic reserve who may not tolerate a large operation. Neoadjuvant therapy has the potential to uncover otherwise subclinical comorbidities that may not have been readily appreciated at the time of diagnosis. In our recent experience, among older patients who completed neoadjuvant therapy but did not undergo surgery (because of either disease progression seen on restaging or a decline in performance status resulting from the combination of treatment toxicity and underlying comorbidities), the median overall survival was the same regardless of why surgery was not performed. A decline in performance status resulting from evolving medical comorbidities or the failure to recover from treatment-related toxicity was just as powerful a predictor of poor outcome as was the development of metastatic disease.

■ FUTURE DIRECTIONS

Increasingly, PC is acknowledged to be a systemic disease and treatment sequencing strategies are evolving to improve the treatment of occult metastases. Currently, there is tremendous focus on the development of increasingly sensitive biomarkers that are needed for the early diagnosis of PC, to improve clinical disease staging, and to more accurately assess treatment response. Neoadjuvant treatment sequencing is recommended for patients with borderline resectable PC and may be adopted for patients with resectable PC as well. With increasing acceptance, neoadjuvant therapy may be the backbone for most future studies of multimodality therapy in localized PC that will increasingly incorporate novel investigational drug therapies and evolving techniques and fractionation schemes for the delivery of radiation therapy.

SUGGESTED READINGS

Aldakkak M, Christians KK, Krepline AN, George B, Ritch PS, Erickson BA, et al. Pre-treatment carbohydrate antigen 19-9 does not predict the response to neoadjuvant therapy in patients with localized pancreatic cancer. *HPB.* 2015;17:942-952.

Appel BL, Tolat P, Evans DB, Tsai S. Current staging systems for pancreatic cancer. *Cancer J.* 2012;18:539-549.

Evans DB, Farnell MB, Lillemoe KD, Vollmer C Jr, Strasberg SM, Schulick RD. Surgical treatment of resectable and borderline resectable pancreas cancer: expert consensus statement. *Ann Surg Oncol.* 2009;16:1736-1744.

Evans DB, George B, Tsai S. Non-metastatic pancreatic cancer: resectable, borderline resectable, and locally advanced—definitions of increasing importance for the optimal delivery of multimodality therapy. *Ann Surg Oncol.* 2015;22:3409-3413.

Evans DB, Varadhachary GR, Crane CH, Sun CC, Lee JE, Pisters PW, et al. Preoperative gemcitabine-based chemoradiation for patients with resectable adenocarcinoma of the pancreatic head. *J Clin Oncol.* 2008;26:3496-3502.

Oettle H, Neuhaus P, Hochhaus A, Hartmann JT, Gellert K, Ridwelski K, et al. Adjuvant chemotherapy with gemcitabine and long-term outcomes among patients with resected pancreatic cancer: the CONKO-001 randomized trial. *JAMA.* 2013;310:1473-1481.

Sohal DP, Walsh RM, Ramanathan RK, Khorana AA. Pancreatic adenocarcinoma: treating a systemic disease with systemic therapy. *J Natl Cancer Inst.* 2014;106:dju011.

Winter JM, Brennan MF, Tang LH, D'Angelica MI, Dematteo RP, Fong Y, et al. Survival after resection of pancreatic adenocarcinoma: results from a single institution over three decades. *Ann Surg Oncol.* 2012;19:169-175.

Winter JM, Cameron JL, Campbell KA, Arnold MA, Chang DC, Coleman J, et al. 1423 pancreaticoduodenectomies for pancreatic cancer: a single-institution experience. *J Gastrointest Surg.* 2006;10:1199-1210.

UNUSUAL PANCREATIC TUMORS

Jashodeep Datta, MD, and Charles M. Vollmer, Jr., MD

Historically, the vast majority of pancreatic resections have been performed for either malignant pancreatic ductal adenocarcinoma (PDAC) or benign recalcitrant chronic pancreatitis. In a contemporary specialty pancreatic surgical practice, however, other less prevalent lesions may comprise a substantial proportion of resections performed. The inclusion of these lesions as valid surgical indications is justified by two phenomena. First, in the modern era of pancreatic surgery (i.e., the last 30 to 40 years) considerable experience has been accrued to indicate which diseases benefit from resection and which do not. This knowledge was garnered in an era when preoperative diagnostics were not as sophisticated as contemporary techniques; consequently, many "masses" were resected without knowledge of the actual diagnosis. As a result, the natural history of these lesions was deciphered via trial and error. Next, the advent and refinement of high-fidelity axial imaging and endoscopic diagnostics has ushered in the era of the *asymptomatic pancreatic lesion*, otherwise known as the pancreatic incidentaloma. Through these technological advances, numerous lesions are being identified whose natural history is less well defined—particularly cystic lesions—and whose evaluation and treatment remains to be refined. Although diagnostics have come a long way, obtaining an accurate and final diagnosis still frequently requires surgical resection in many circumstances. This chapter introduces some of these less appreciated lesions and their optimal diagnostic and therapeutic approaches.

■ PANCREATIC CYSTS

In the last decade, pancreatic cystic lesions have come to the forefront in pancreatic surgery and account for a significant number of referrals and, ultimately, resections. Cysts cause consternation for surgeons because of inaccurate diagnostics, ill-defined natural histories, and significant consequences from inappropriately performed operations. Evaluation of these cystic lesions should be approached systematically. Inflammatory pseudocysts are the most common cysts of the pancreas and their management is outlined elsewhere in this book. However, one should consider the category of pancreatic cystic neoplasms (PCNs), which now is recognized to account for up to 50% of pancreatic cysts.

In general, three categories of PCNs exist: mucinous cysts, serous cysts, and others. PCNs can be classified further into dysplastic (premalignant) and frankly malignant variants. Mucinous cysts can be broken down into intraductal papillary mucinous neoplasms (IPMNs), mucinous cystic neoplasms (MCNs), and nondysplastic mucinous cysts (NDMCs). Serous lesions are dominated by serous cystadenomas (SCAs) and also include the exceedingly uncommon serous cystadenocarcinomas. Most cysts in the "other" category are actually malignancies that uncharacteristically demonstrate cystic morphology. Many of the more commonly encountered cystic entities are delineated later in the chapter, with the exception of IPMN, which is discussed elsewhere in this book.

Serous Cystadenoma

Despite being the best-characterized PCN and readily identified by current axial imaging techniques, SCAs continue to vex surgeons, as they are all too frequently misdiagnosed and unnecessarily resected. They account for only 1% of *all* pancreatic neoplasms but a far larger proportion (i.e., nearly one third) of *cystic* neoplasms. They are ubiquitous throughout the entire gland and can have variable sizes and morphologies. Most are completely innocuous and asymptomatic but larger lesions have the capability of obstructing the bile duct (causing jaundice), the pancreatic duct (causing pancreatitis), or the outflow tract of the stomach (gastric outlet obstruction). This occurs not by invasion but rather by space-filling, compressive impingement or an associated local inflammatory effect. With larger lesions, epigastric abdominal pain can be a prelude to these more overt symptoms. Like many pancreatic cystic pathologies, SCAs are found more frequently in females but usually at a later age than others (i.e., sixth decade onward).

SCAs are benign lesions with a true epithelium lined with glycogen-rich, clear, cuboidal cells that stain positive for periodic acid-Schiff (PAS). They do not communicate with the pancreatic ductal system. Imaging displays a characteristic thin-walled capsule with a microcystic pattern with thin-walled septae. Most SCAs are readily identified by one of two characteristic imaging findings (Figure 1, *A–C*): a "starburst" pattern of a central (often calcified) scar or, more commonly, a "ground-glass," "cluster-of-grapes," or "honeycomb" appearance. Fine-needle aspiration (FNA) analysis of the cyst fluid yields a clear, serous fluid low in carcinoembryonic antigen (CEA) and mucin content. However, cytology obtained from these lesions sometimes shows "atypia" leading to diagnostic uncertainty and operative intervention, which proves to be inappropriate in most circumstances.

A variant of the overwhelmingly benign SCA is serous cystadenocarcinoma, which is felt to represent a malignant degeneration of SCA. In the handful of such cases (i.e., less than 50) described in the literature, this entity has been defined by metastatic carcinoma in the presence of a primary lesion that otherwise appears identical to SCA. In that SCA is a benign neoplasm with a fleetingly low risk of malignant degeneration—and consequent associated mortality—observation is the rule for asymptomatic lesions. Natural history studies indicate that some will increase in size with time after initial identification (approximately 0.5 cm/yr) but larger cysts (i.e., more than 4 cm in diameter) may progress at a greater rate (approximately

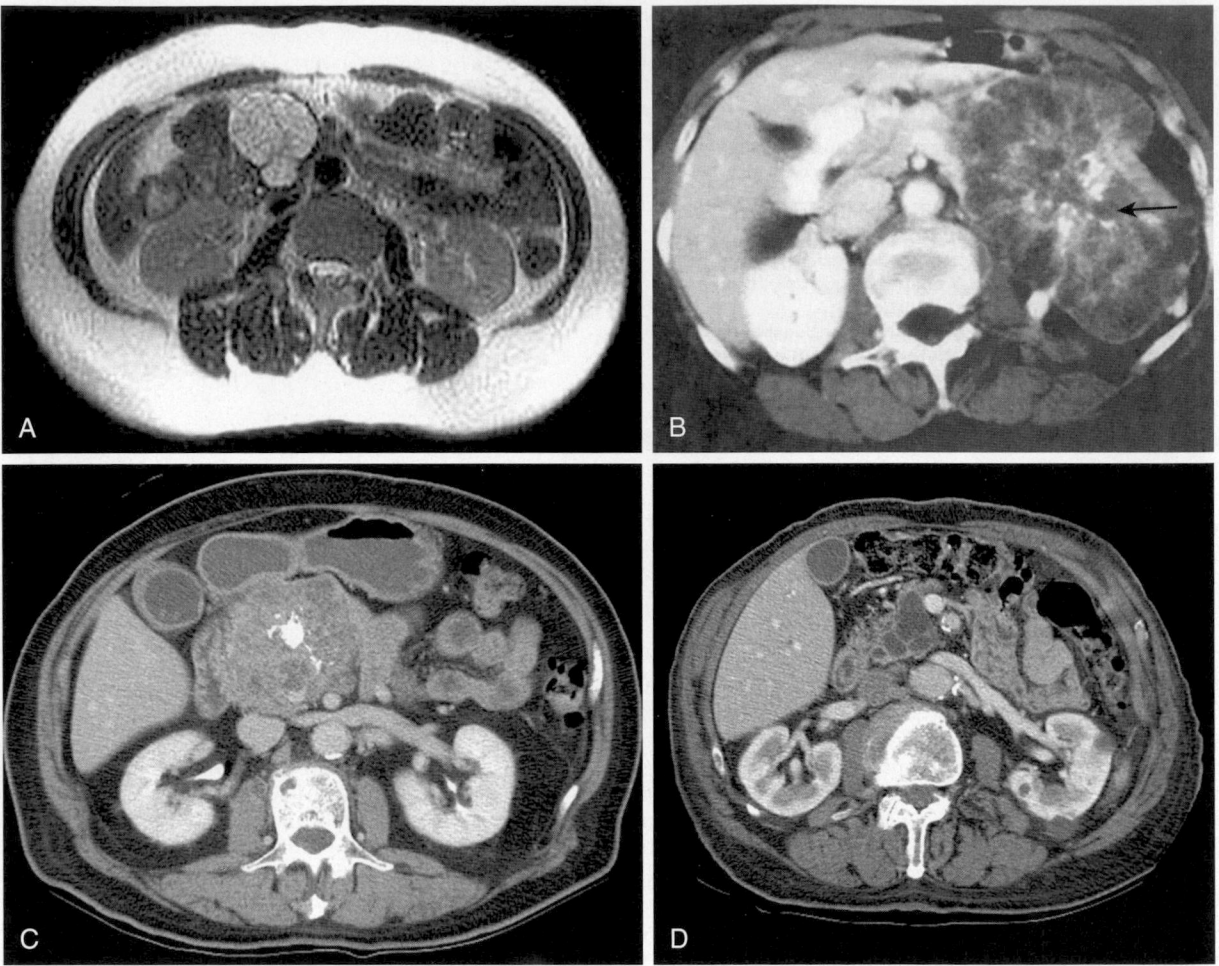

FIGURE 1 The variable appearances of serous cystadenomas (SCAs). **A,** T2-weighted magnetic resonance imaging shows the most common "honeycomb" appearance from numerous microcysts. **B,** A classic "stellate scar" in a large lesion in the tail of the pancreas. **C,** Internal calcification. **D,** The less common but clinically challenging macrocystic morphology, which is commonly confused for a mucinous neoplasm.

2 cm/yr) and are more likely to ultimately cause symptoms. In such cases, growth indicates progressive fluid accretion in the cyst, not accumulating dysplastic (i.e., solid) components as observed in other PCNs.

Although most SCAs are observed, surgical intervention is indicated for clearly symptomatic lesions and perhaps for larger cysts given their propensity for rapid growth (on an individualized case-by-case basis). As mentioned, far too often these lesions are diagnosed *after* resection for what was presumed to be a more aggressive entity such as MCN (see following section) or side-branch IPMN (discussed elsewhere). This is because a second, less distinct morphology exists for SCAs—the macrocystic form (Figure 1, *D*). Although they preserve the same histologic epithelial features of conventional SCAs, these lesions lack the classic features described earlier and have larger, more discrete cystic cavities separated by obvious septae. Often these are smaller (1- to 4-cm) lesions that are seen at a younger age (40s), more frequently in the head of the pancreas, and more often in males. These nontraditional features result in diagnostic ambiguity; as such, these lesions are confused with their more threatening cystic counterparts (i.e., MCNs and IPMNs). With the current epidemic of incidentally identified pancreatic cystic lesions, distinguishing these lesions from SCAs represents a key management dilemma. Often the distinction can be made by the identification of mucin and/or elevated CEA levels by FNA, along with scrutiny of clinical and radiographic features described earlier.

Mucinous Cystic Neoplasms

MCNs are dysplastic neoplasms with clear-cut malignant potential that represent 2% of all pancreatic neoplasms but up to a quarter of cystic neoplasms. Classically, they are singular, large, thick-walled cysts, lined with mucin-secreting columnar epithelium, and almost never communicate with the pancreatic ductal system (distinguishing them from IPMNs; Figure 2, *A*). Distinct "ovarian-type" stroma within the cyst capsule is a defining pathologic feature of MCNs; this is typically determined histologically after resection (Figure 2, *B*). There is a strong female predilection (9:1) and MCNs are most commonly situated in the body and tail of the organ. The classic clinical scenario is of a younger woman (40s to 50s but often as young as teens to 20s) who has vague abdominal pain; however, with more frequent use of cross-sectional imaging, these lesions are being identified incidentally. A mucinous cystic lesion situated in the head of the pancreas is more likely to be an IPMN.

Diagnosis is commonly made by pancreas protocol axial imaging—computed tomographic scan (CT scan) or magnetic resonance imaging (MRI)—which reveals either a single, unilocular lesion (more frequently) or a smaller macrocystic multilocular lesion with septations. Sometimes the wall contains calcium, a finding that adds to diagnostic confusion with chronic pseudocysts, which also can be calcified. In general, MCNs are most often misdiagnosed as pseudocysts and it is not uncommon to see cases where internal drainage operations were used initially, only to have persistent

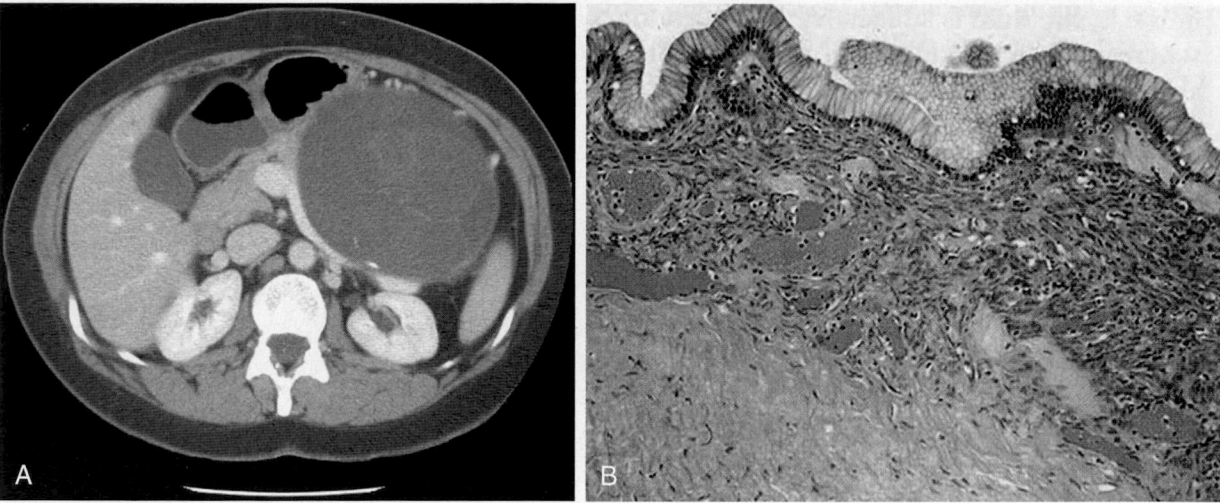

FIGURE 2 A, This large mucinous cystic neoplasm (MCN) situated in the tail of the pancreas presented as a palpable mass in an otherwise healthy, asymptomatic 22-year-old woman. Notice the macrocystic appearance with internal septations. **B,** The classic histologic appearance of a MCN demonstrating mucinous columnar epithelium with dysplastic features, associated with characteristic "ovarian-type" stroma.

symptoms and cyst recurrence because of neoplastic progression. To avoid this dilemma, after careful consideration of the clinical history endoscopic ultrasound scan (EUS) with cyst aspirate (FNA) is helpful, as it can demonstrate a viscous, "string-like" nature to the mucin-rich fluid. Furthermore, a CEA level greater than 200 from the cyst aspirate is strongly indicative of mucinous etiology (but not necessarily malignant transformation) of the cyst; conversely, pseudocyst fluid is generally high in amylase activity. Finally, cyst aspirate cytology can be obtained to determine whether invasive malignancy is present. Findings "consistent with malignant cells" are reliable when present, whereas "atypical" or "nondiagnostic" descriptors are not as trustworthy.

As is the case for their mucinous cystic counterpart IPMN, MCNs are dysplastic and felt to follow an "adenoma-to-carcinoma" sequence of degeneration to invasive malignancy. Older series of MCN resections demonstrate that nearly 30% to 50% of these lesions harbor either high-grade dysplasia or frankly invasive carcinoma; however, newer literature, utilizing more stringent pathologic criteria (e.g., ovarian-like stroma, mural nodules), estimate the malignancy risk somewhere between 5% and 15%. Identification of mural nodules, calcifications, positive aspirate cytology, or distant metastatic spread should alert to this possibility. For this reason, consensus guidelines from the International Association of Pancreatology (via Sendai Consensus Conference Guidelines and the subsequent Fukuoka modification) recommend that *all* suspected MCNs be surgically resected in suitable operative candidates. It should be emphasized, however, that the natural history of these lesions remains poorly defined, particularly in MCNs less than 3 cm and without mural nodules. Moreover, given this ambiguity in determining the true cancer risk of these lesions, a conservative approach may be considered in medically unfit patients in whom the risk of perioperative mortality and morbidity exceeds the cumulative risk of malignancy.

MCNs are amenable to definitive surgical resection, usually accomplished by a distal pancreatectomy (now more commonly achieved laparoscopically in select cases), given their most common position in the pancreas. However, caution must be exercised in adopting a minimally invasive approach for large lesions or those with imaging characteristics suspicious for malignancy because of the importance of maintaining capsule integrity and complete removal during operative dissection. Smaller lesions may be amenable for "targeted" parenchyma-sparing pancreatectomy (or even enucleation in very select circumstances). If margins are completely clear, recurrence after resection of a noninvasive MCN is rare, as is the threat of a metachronous MCN developing in the remnant

pancreas—these are generally singular lesions. However, *malignant* MCNs follow an oncologic trajectory similar to invasive PDAC and should be considered for adjuvant therapy and close surveillance after resection.

■ NONDYSPLASTIC MUCINOUS CYSTS

Common dogma that *every* mucinous cyst of the pancreas is dysplastic (and therefore has a certain malignant potential) has led to a general policy of resection for all such lesions. However, we have recently encountered a number of NDMCs of the pancreas. Over a 4-year period, 104 resections were performed for suspected cystic neoplasms, with IPMNs, SCAs, and MCNs predominating. Of these, 7 cases of mucinous cysts, devoid of dysplastic features, were identified, representing 6.7% of all resected cysts and 10.3% of the 68 cysts of mucinous etiology. Although FNA cytology was *atypical* in all cysts that were analyzed in this fashion, histologically these demonstrated a simple columnar mucinous epithelium with a pancreatobiliary phenotype without evidence of cytologic atypia, papillary growth, or ovarian-type stroma in any of the cases. *MUC1, MUC2,* and *MUC5AC* were expressed in 83%, 0%, and 100%, respectively. Unfortunately, these lesions masquerade as true MCNs of the pancreas clinically, radiographically, and biochemically, leading to surgical resection, perhaps unnecessarily. It is uncertain whether these cysts are entirely benign or represent the earliest stage of the tumorigenesis spectrum of MCNs; reassuringly, there has been no recurrence with a mean follow-up of 44 months in this reported series.

Solid Pseudopapillary Neoplasm

Solid pseudopapillary neoplasm (SPN), a moniker defined by the Word Health Organization (WHO) in 1996, is a unique entity also referred to by many other names in the literature, including Frantz's tumor, Hamoudi tumor, or papillary and cystic tumor. SPN is a solid tumor with a marked tendency for cystic degeneration and appears frequently as a primary cystic neoplasm. The third most prevalent cystic neoplasm of the pancreas (10%), it is yet another rare pancreatic neoplasm overall (1% to 2%), with fewer than 1000 cases reported in the literature. Although usually benign, it can be aggressive with invasion of local structures and has certain malignant and even metastatic potential (10% to 15% of patients). Distant spread occurs most commonly to the liver and peritoneal cavity and lymphatic spread also has been recognized but is inconsistent. This diagnosis should be considered for young patients (age 40 and below;

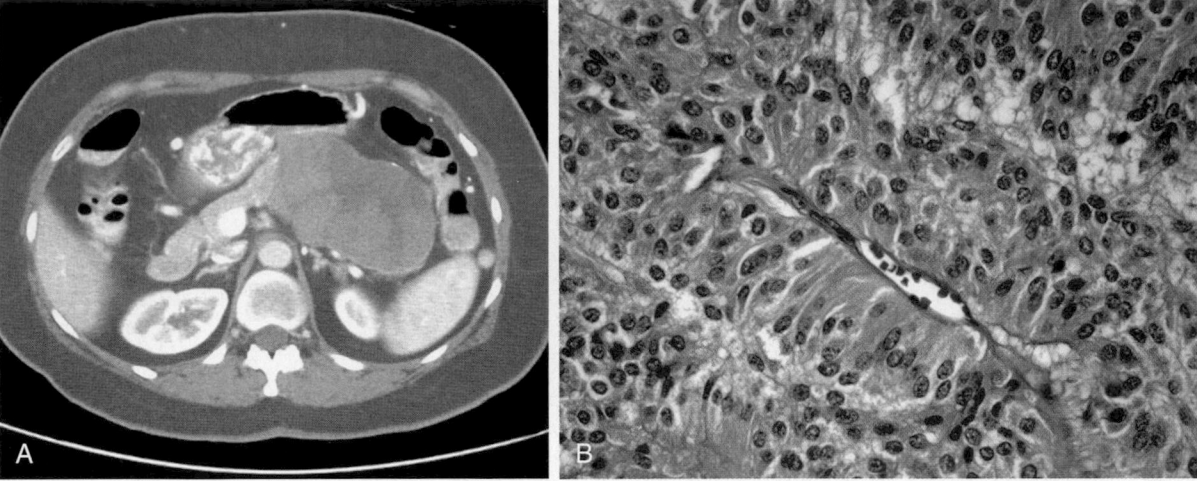

FIGURE 3 A, Solid pseudopapillary neoplasm of the distal pancreas in a 41-year-old woman. Note the typical large size and heterogeneous appearance indicative of internal cystic degeneration from necrosis and sloughing of the pseudopapillae. **B,** Histologic appearance of a "pseudopapilla" showing crowded sheets of cells arranged around vascular stalks. As the tumor enlarges, these cells slough from their vascular supply and cause necrosis, which simulates cystic qualities on axial imaging.

mean age 27) who have a large pancreatic mass (usually focused in the body or tail; mean size 11 cm); there is a marked female predilection (9:1). These tumors are generally asymptomatic but can cause abdominal pain, nausea, vomiting, or palpable masses when they become excessively large. Given their rarity, prognostic factors for malignancy and survival are lacking; however, perineural and lymphovascular invasion appear to augur a poor prognosis.

CT scan usually depicts well-circumscribed lesions with a heterogeneous appearance owing to mixed solid architecture, cystic components, and hemorrhagic degeneration. MRI reveals heterogeneous signal intensity reflecting the complexity of its components; moreover, areas of increased signal intensity on T1-weighted images can signify blood products. Because of this amorphous appearance (Figure 3, A), they are often categorized as cystic in etiology. As mentioned, however, the cystic appearance reflects necrotic degeneration of the primary cytoarchitecture, solid papillary vascular stalks, which slough and hemorrhage as the tumor progresses in size. Diagnosis by imaging is aided by attention to the four Cs: a **c**ircumscribed, **c**ystic-appearing lesion with a **c**apsule and, often, internal **c**alcification. There are no distinct tumor markers and the tumor does not typically produce a paraneoplastic syndrome. Because of its largely necrotic composition, FNA biopsies are usually unrewarding. Histologic analysis reveals sheets of polygonal epithelial cells with prominent stalks and an incohesive appearance (Figure 3, B). Foamy histiocytes and cholesterol crystals are common. Mitotic figures are rare and nuclear pleomorphism is unusual. The histologic progenitor cell is undefined and there are lines of evidence to support genesis from each of the endothelial, epithelial, or mesenchymal lineages. However, a consistent immunophenotype is observed, with vimentin, neuron-specific enolase, and α1-antitrypsin expression being near universal. Recently, nuclear expression of beta-catenin is regarded as a unique immunohistochemical feature of SPN, as it underlies the genetic mutation of catenin found in more than 90% of tumors; therefore abnormal nuclear labeling of beta-catenin strongly supports its diagnosis.

Given their unpredictable but real metastatic potential, all SPNs should be resected operatively. Although tumors may be extremely large and generally impinge on vital structures, they are usually completely resectable. Obviously, negative margins are desired and typically attainable. Excellent 5-year survival rates (i.e., >90%) can be achieved after total resection with uninvolved margins. This reflects the fact that many of these lesions are in fact noninvasive. However,

it is probably prudent to surveil patients with axial imaging after resection given the potential for distant spread. An aggressive approach to both synchronous and metachronous metastatic disease to the liver and elsewhere is justified, especially because most patients are generally young and healthy. Adjuvant therapies (including gemcitabine, 5-fluorouracil [5-FU]/cisplatin, streptozocin, or radiotherapy) for advanced disease not amenable to surgical clearance have been applied in selected circumstances.

Lymphoepithelial Cysts

Lymphoepithelial cysts (LECs) are exceedingly rare, entirely benign lesions that, like other unusual pancreatic tumors, cause diagnostic and therapeutic ambiguity. Despite their relatively large size (usually >5 cm), they are generally asymptomatic and are discovered incidentally distributed throughout the gland but most commonly in the body or tail. Unlike other cystic lesions, there is a fourfold male predominance. Imaging features include encapsulated, uniloculated or more commonly multiloculated cysts in and/or around the gland with an enhancing fibrous rim. Similar to MCNs, these cystic cavities are not in communication with the ductal system. The cyst contents are complex, containing keratin, cholesterol, and other debris that is sloughed from the epithelial lining. MRI can be useful in distinguishing these from other cystic lesions, by identifying bright, high-signal keratin on T1-weighted images. This is the opposite scenario in most cysts, where static fluid exhibits a bright signal during the T2 phase. Furthermore, the lipid content of the cholesterol can be discerned by MRI.

Histology of these lesions is unique. As its name implies, there is a combination of lymphoid stromal tissue surrounding a stratified squamous epithelial lining. The cyst cavity is cluttered with keratinized debris with or without lymphocytes, and cholesterol crystals. EUS analysis of the cyst fluid often will demonstrate high levels of tumor markers (CEA, cancer antigen 19-9 [CA19-9]) and sometimes amylase. However, as opposed to mucinous lesions (with dysplasia or malignant potential), analysis of the fluid aspirate from an LEC will not display mucin but rather demonstrate the histologic hallmarks of this lesion (squamous cells, lymphocytes, cholesterol). If diligent analysis yields any of this evidence in an asymptomatic scenario, then observation is appropriate management. However, for LECs that cause pain or obstructive features, surgical options exist. Complete resection through partial pancreatectomy may be necessary based on individualized factors; yet given the benign nature and natural history of these particular cysts, internal drainage procedures and operations are a reasonable alternative but only if the correct diagnosis is secured.

■ AUTOIMMUNE PANCREATITIS

Autoimmune pancreatitis (AIP) is a particularly important unusual condition of the pancreas in that, when properly recognized, it is treated medically (i.e., corticosteroid therapy) and not surgically. The primary dilemma is that it appears as a mass effect in the pancreas, which mimics PDAC both radiographically and clinically. At the advent of this disease, this fact led to most cases being diagnosed only through pathologic analysis of resected specimens after major pancreatectomy. More recently, other criteria, relying heavily on characteristic clinical, radiologic, and biochemical findings, have allowed for less invasive diagnosis and management. Two forms of AIP are recognized: (1) type 1 or lymphoplasmacytic sclerosing pancreatitis (LPSP) or AIP without granulocyte epithelial lesions (GELs) reflects a pancreatic manifestation of a specific subtype of serum immunoglobulin (IgG4)-related systemic disease, characterized by elevated serum IgG4 levels and extrapancreatic lesions such as primary sclerosing cholangitis, inflammatory bowel disease, Sjögren's syndrome, psoriasis, retroperitoneal fibrosis, sarcoid, and others. This entity represents an autoimmune destruction of the pancreatic parenchyma that is likely mediated by both humoral and cellular components; and (2) type 2 or idiopathic duct-centric pancreatitis (IDCP), which differs from LPSP predominantly by the presence of GELs and the relative paucity of IgG4-positive plasma cells.

The clinical picture of AIP is variable; although most patients have overt symptoms like jaundice, pancreatitis, progressive pain, and endocrine or exocrine insufficiency, which suggests malignancy, a minority may have more subtle findings such as weight loss, anorexia, fatigue, and lethargy. These symptoms may take months to manifest, distinguishing AIP from the more sudden presentations that occur with pancreatic malignancy. The clinical picture is distinctly different from generic acute pancreatitis from other causes; in fact, serum elevation of pancreatic enzymes, although possible, is not typical.

On imaging, AIP often appears as if the whole pancreas is "full" with a hypoenhancing mass effect that resembles a sausage with a characteristic enhancing rim (indicative of local edema). However, there also clearly can be focal hypoenhancing CT appearances, which more often resemble pancreatic adenocarcinoma. Sometimes evidence of autoimmune disease in other abdominal or thoracic organs is recognized (Figure 4). Endoscopic retrograde cholangiopancreatography (ERCP) or magnetic resonance cholangiopancreatography (MRCP) will show stricturing of the intrapancreatic (and sometimes extrapancreatic) common bile duct, as well as focal, segmental, or diffuse strictures of the pancreatic duct. Notably, the pancreatic duct usually seems diminutive and beaded and is rarely dilated (as observed in chronic non-autoimmune pancreatitis). Interestingly, concomitant recognition of pancreatic cysts in conjunction with AIP can perplex clinicians; recent evidence suggests that unilocular cysts associated with AIP are more likely to resolve with corticosteroid therapy than are multilocular cysts, which are more likely to harbor occult malignancy.

Diagnostic suspicion by imaging studies should then be confirmed by either serologic or histologic means. IgG4 is often but not always elevated (70% of cases). Other biomarkers such as anticarbonic anhydrase or anti-lactoferrin antibodies and specific serum microRNAs are emerging as useful. Histologic confirmation is more troublesome, as EUS-based FNA sampling is notoriously inaccurate. In some cases we have performed laparoscopic ultrasound-guided core biopsies to obtain certainty in a minimally invasive fashion. The last resort, of course, is open biopsy or, ultimately, pancreatic resection. Plasma cell infiltration of the pancreas (frequently IgG4

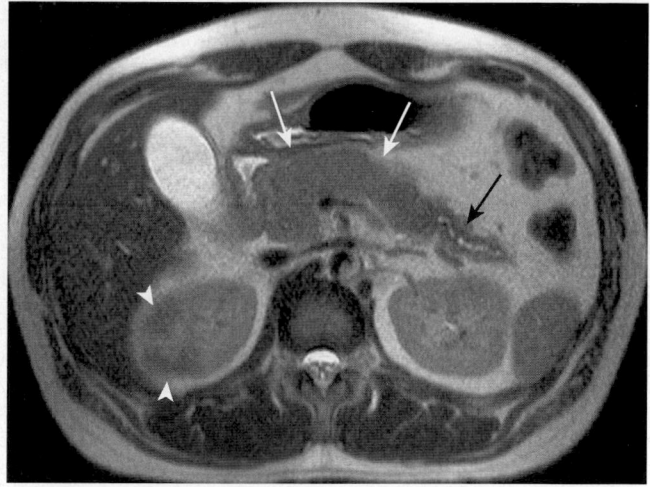

FIGURE 4 Axial T2-weighted image of the abdomen shows diffuse enlargement and loss of the normal acinar pattern in the head, neck, and body of the pancreas (*white arrows*). There is upstream dilation of the pancreatic duct and atrophy of the gland in the tail (*black arrow*). Note hypointense ill-defined lesions in the kidneys (*white arrowheads*) consistent with lymphoplasmacytic infiltrates. Both the pancreatic findings and the renal infiltrative lesions improved with therapy.

BOX 1: Mayo Clinic Extended Diagnostic Criteria for Autoimmune Pancreatitis

Imaging

Pancreas mass or enlargement, focal pancreatic duct stricture, pancreatic atrophy, pancreatic calcification, or pancreatitis

Serology

Elevated serum IgG4 level

Histology

At least one of the following: (1) periductal lymphoplasmacytic infiltrate with obliterative phlebitis and storiform fibrosis; or (2) lymphoplasmacytic infiltrate with storiform fibrosis *and* abundant IgG4 positive cells (>10 cells/high-power field)

Other Organ Involvement

Hilar or intrahepatic biliary strictures, persistent distal biliary stricture, parotid or lacrimal gland involvement, mediastinal lymphadenopathy, retroperitoneal fibrosis

Response to Steroid Therapy

Resolution or marked improvement of pancreatic or extrapancreatic manifestation with steroid therapy

positive) with ductocentric inflammatory destruction may be seen on pathologic analysis.

Optimal diagnosis of this heterogeneous disease is in constant flux. The Mayo Clinic has proposed advanced diagnostic guidelines that incorporate not only the original classification system of the Japanese Pancreas Society (imaging, serology, and histology) but also other organ involvement and/or response to steroid therapy (Box 1). From this, three categories of patients seem to segregate: (1) those with characteristic histology, (2) those who satisfy classic imaging features along with elevated IgG4 titers, and (3) those whose disease process responds to therapy in the setting of elevated IgG4 levels or unexplained pancreatic disease. The International Association of Pancreatology more recently has issued international consensus diagnostic criteria for AIP to facilitate categorization of AIP into type 1 and type 2 subtypes.

Treatment for both subtypes consists of high-dose systemic corticosteroids (0.6 to 1 mg/kg) with reassessment of imaging and CA19-9 after 2 weeks of treatment. If successful, repeat imaging at 4 to 6 weeks will demonstrate dramatic changes for the better. The natural history of AIP over the long term is poorly defined so far. Most patients can be weaned off their steroids entirely but clinical resistance can occur in about 25%. In that case, another cycle of treatment may be necessary and some patients even require lifelong therapy or conversion to another immunosuppressant like azathioprine (Imuran). In cases of jaundice, biliary strictures are treated first with temporary endobiliary stents and often will resolve completely within a few months of initiating steroid therapy. If no change is observed in radiographic appearance, serum IgG4 levels, or stricture morphology, and/or if rising CA19-9 levels are observed, then a misdiagnosis of AIP should be entertained and malignancy should be considered strongly instead. In certain cases of diagnostic uncertainty, inability to obtain an accurate histologic diagnosis, or failed medical treatment, surgical resection may be required.

ACINAR CELL CARCINOMA

Acinar cell carcinoma (ACC) has very unique characteristics that distinguish it from other pancreatic tumors, both unusual and common. As more experience accrues with this rare (less than 2%) pancreatic neoplasm, it appears that ACC biology is more favorable than PDAC. It is diagnosed earlier (mid-50s), more frequently in males, and tumors appear to be larger at diagnosis (around 5 cm), leading to nonspecific symptoms like weight loss, pain, and bloating. Jaundice is not as ubiquitous. On CT evaluation, ACCs mimic hypodense PDACs but the tumor borders are often less discrete, sometimes showing hyperenhancement. On gross inspection they are fleshy, rather than infiltrative, and histologic review often resembles neuroendocrine tumors with clusters of cells, hemorrhagic and necrotic areas. Immunohistochemistry analysis can distinguish between the two entities (pancytokeratin stains strongly for both but ACCs do not express chromogranin A or synaptophysin).

What distinguishes these unusual tumors is the regular generation and release of lipase, which account for paraneoplastic symptoms like polyarthralgia, eosinophilia, and subcutaneous fat necrosis and rashes (i.e., erythema nodosum)—known as Schmid's triad. This lipase expression can act as a tumor marker, as it regresses with surgical resection of the primary tumor; however, similar to other pancreas-related tumor markers (e.g., CA19-9), it has no role in predicting ultimate survival. Alpha-fetoprotein is similarly expressed by some of these tumors and serves a similar role in postresection surveillance.

Upfront surgery is typically used for suspected ACC that is considered resectable radiographically. The definitive diagnosis of ACC is generally made postoperatively after thorough histologic review. Evidence continues to accrue indicating a more favorable prognosis when compared with PDAC. One multi-institutional series of 17 patients showed 1- and 5-year survival rates of 92% and 53%, respectively, with a median survival of 61 months in resected cases. In another population-based review of 672 patients with ACC, 16% had localized disease, 26% had regional disease, and 58% had distant metastases; patients with local-regional disease were more likely to be resectable when compared with PDAC. In this broader patient sample, the reported 5-year survival for ACC was as high as 72%, markedly better than that observed with PDAC (approximately 20%); even 22% of unresectable ACC cases lived 5 years. Given that there is a clear propensity for metastasis, adjuvant chemoradiotherapy might contribute to improved survival; there are even reports of "neoadjuvant" conversion from an initially unresectable to a downstaged resectable tumor. Patients with metastatic disease might benefit from aggressive multimodality therapeutic approaches. However, no uniform multimodality regimen has emerged because of the rarity of this malignancy. Recent evidence indicates that ACC is moderately chemoresponsive to agents that have activity in PDAC and colorectal carcinoma; moreover, genetic analysis indicates that ACC is genomically distinct from other pancreatic cancers and has identified novel potential therapeutic targets that warrant further investigation.

PRIMARY PANCREATIC LYMPHOMA

Although the actual occurrence of primary pancreatic lymphoma (PPL) may be a once-in-a-career event for most surgeons, it is necessary to consider in any workup for an unusual pancreatic mass, given its unique treatment requirements. Non-Hodgkin's lymphoma can certainly manifest in any non-nodal tissue throughout the body but it is highly uncommon in the pancreas.

The clinical picture is vague, featuring weight loss, nausea or vomiting, pain, and sometimes B symptoms. Jaundice and back pain are surprisingly absent despite the size of the observed mass. Laboratory values, including the white blood cell count, are generally normal but an elevated lactate dehydrogenase may provide a clue. Usually the patient proceeds to axial imaging for workup of these nonspecific findings and the appearance is of a bulky lesion with considerable local lymphadenopathy—findings that exceed those expected for pancreatic adenocarcinoma (Figure 5). Because a definitive diagnosis of PPL is impossible from imaging alone, such an atypical lesion will usually proceed to EUS evaluation and a fine-needle tumor aspirate is frequently reliable in obtaining enough tissue to secure the diagnosis under skilled cytopathology review. If EUS-guided tissue yield is inadequate, CT-guided or operative (e.g., laparoscopic or open) techniques are utilized to obtain tissue.

The management and prognosis of PPL depend on the stage and grade of the tumor. The first-line therapy for PPL is systemic chemotherapy and not surgical resection. The prevalent regimen is CHOP (cyclophosphamide, hydroxydoxorubicin, oncovin, and prednisone); in cases of CD20-positive diffuse large B-cell lymphoma, rituximab is added to CHOP regimens and an improvement in the rate of remission is typically observed. Complete remissions occur in around three quarters of patients with early-stage, contained disease. Improved outcomes are now evident with the addition of targeted biologic therapies in addition to the CHOP approach, especially for more diffuse, advanced disease.

Surgeons generally will rue the decision to operate on bulky pancreatic lymphoma, as resection is both technically challenging

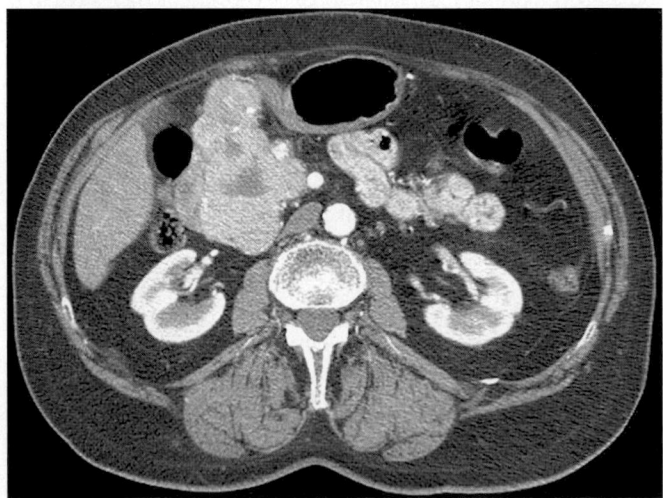

FIGURE 5 The typical appearance of a bulky, lobular primary lymphoma situated in the pancreatic head.

and fraught with potential complications that will impair the patient's recovery. However, a report from the Johns Hopkins University describes a few cases of early, smaller lymphomas that were resected under the assumption that they were actually pancreatic adenocarcinomas. Interestingly, these have resulted in complete 5-year remissions.

■ METASTATIC LESIONS

Very few cancers metastasize to the pancreatic parenchyma and this scenario represents well fewer than 1% of all pancreatic resections performed. The best characterized of these is renal cell carcinoma (RCC) but melanoma, breast, lung, colon, and gynecologic malignancies also have been reported. For the most part, metastatic tumors to the pancreas are indicative of advanced stage disease of the primary and associated with a dismal overall prognosis. Therefore complete and thorough staging, appropriate for the specific primary tumor in question, should be undertaken to determine if the pancreatic metastasis is indeed isolated. Most of these metastases characteristically appear as *hypervascular* tumors, rather than the more common hypoenhancing appearance of pancreatic adenocarcinoma. Accordingly, these can be confused with other rare conditions in the pancreas, including ectopic splenules or primary neuroendocrine tumors. Definitive tumor diagnosis may be obtained via EUS-guided FNA if there is doubt but generally is not required if there is an established cancer diagnosis of RCC, melanoma, or breast cancer.

RCC is the most common and best understood of these tumors. Interestingly, the pancreas appears to be a selective site for metastasis from RCC; this peculiarity has been reported by several studies. Most metastases are metachronous, with a relatively long disease-free interval (>10 years in many cases) from primary nephrectomy to discovery of metastasis. What makes it more unique, and validates aggressive surgical resection, is the fact that many patients achieve long-term survival postpancreatectomy (5-year survival rates exceeding 80%). RCCs appear as hypervascular masses (Figure 6) that may be distributed anywhere in the pancreatic substance and even may be multiple. In suitable operative candidates, it is reasonable to proceed with targeted pancreatectomy, based on extent and position of the lesion(s). Total pancreatectomy for isolated pancreatic metastasis with diffuse involvement of the gland also has been reported.

As a general rule for all metastatic lesions to the pancreas, like with RCC, surgical interventions are appropriate for instances where the disease is confined to the pancreas and there is no systemic burden otherwise in good candidates. More frequently, however, concurrent metastatic disease is found elsewhere; aggressive surgical resection therefore has little positive impact and more likely has negative consequences in light of a limited life span. However, resection (or palliative bypass) in select cases should be considered on an individual basis because these lesions may appear in a symptomatic fashion (such as transfusion-dependent upper gastrointestinal bleeding, frank hemorrhage, or obstructive jaundice) requiring intervention. Furthermore, with the advent of new biologic adjuvant therapies for RCC and melanoma, strategies relying on surgical debulking of dominant large tumor burden are gaining favor.

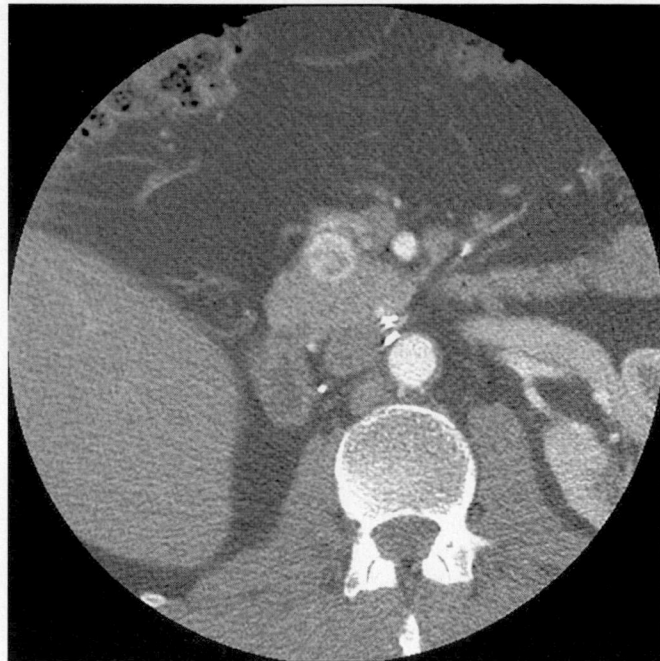

FIGURE 6 A solitary, well-circumscribed renal cell carcinoma metastatic to the pancreatic head demonstrates characteristic hypervascularity. This asymptomatic lesion presented 8 years after the index nephrectomy through active cancer surveillance.

SUGGESTED READINGS

Demirjian AN, Vollmer CM, McDermott DF, et al. Refining indications for contemporary surgical treatment of renal cell carcinoma metastatic to the pancreas. *HPB (Oxford)*. 2009;11:150-153.

Nadig SN, Pedrosa I, Goldsmith JD, et al. Clinical implications of mucinous nonneoplastic cysts of the pancreas. *Pancreas*. 2012;41:441-446.

Reddy S, Edil BH, Cameron JL, et al. Pancreatic resection of isolated metastases from nonpancreatic primary cancers. *Ann Surg Oncol*. 2008;15:3199-3206.

Sachs T, Pratt WB, Callery MP, Vollmer CM. The incidental asymptomatic pancreatic lesion: nuisance or threat? *J Gastrointest Surg*. 2009;13:405-415.

Tanaka M, Fernandez-del Castillo C, Adsay V, et al. International consensus guidelines 2012 for the management of IPMN and MCN of the pancreas. *Pancreatology*. 2012;12:183-197.

Tseng JF, Warshaw AL, Sahani DV, et al. Serous cystadenoma of the pancreas: tumor growth rates and recommendations for treatment. *Ann Surg*. 2005;242:413-419.

Vollmer CM, Dixon E, Grant DR. Management of a solid-pseudopapillary tumor of the pancreas with liver metastases. *HPB (Oxford)*. 2003;5:264-267.

Wisnoski NC, Townsend CM Jr, Nealon WH, et al. 672 patients with acinar cell carcinoma of the pancreas: a population-based comparison to pancreatic adenocarcinoma. *Surgery*. 2008;144:141-148.

INTRADUCTAL PAPILLARY MUCINOUS NEOPLASMS OF THE PANCREAS

Francesca M. Dimou, MD, Jennifer A. Perone, MD, and Taylor S. Riall, MD, PhD

Initially described by Ohashi and colleagues in 1982, intraductal papillary mucinous neoplasms (IPMNs) were not recognized formally as distinct lesions from mucinous cystic neoplasms (MCNs) until 1999. Over the past few decades the incidence of IPMNs has increased, likely secondary to both increased frequency of abdominal imaging and clearly defined diagnostic criteria. IPMNs are a group of intraductal pancreatic epithelial neoplasms characterized by (1) mucin production, and (2) diffuse or segmental involvement of the main pancreatic duct or major side branches. IPMNs lack the ovarian stroma characteristic of MCNs, differentiating them pathologically from these entities.

IPMNs represent a spectrum of epithelial changes, similar to the evolution of pancreatic intraepithelial neoplasias (PanINs) to invasive pancreatic adenocarcinoma. However, unlike PanINs, these lesions can be identified grossly and radiographically before the development of invasive cancer, providing an opportunity for early intervention analogous to the removal of colonic adenomatous polyps. The management of IPMNs is complicated by the fact that recurrences have been documented in the remnant pancreas after removal of both benign and malignant lesions. This biologic behavior suggests a field defect, with increased risk of neoplastic transformation in all pancreatic ductal epithelium. Further complicating factors include uncertainty surrounding the time for progression to malignancy, the differing malignant potential based on the anatomic and histologic characteristics of the IPMN, and the significant morbidity and mortality associated with pancreatic resections. The greatest controversy involves the appropriate timing and indications for resection and the criteria for safe observation of IPMNs with lower malignant potential. When resection is indicated, controversy remains regarding the extent of resection in the setting of residual IPMN at the pancreatic margin and surveillance of the pancreatic remnant.

■ CLASSIFICATION

Anatomic Classification

IPMNs are classified as main duct (MD-IPMN), branch duct (BD-IPMN), or mixed type IPMNs with both main and branch duct components. MD-IPMNs are characterized by diffuse or segmental involvement of the main pancreatic duct, with radiographic findings of main pancreatic duct dilation greater than 5 mm without any other causes of obstruction (Figure 1, A). Previously, criteria for MD-IPMN had a cutoff of main duct dilation greater than 10 mm. However, in developing the most current International Consensus Guidelines (2012) for the management of IPMN and MCN of the pancreas, expert review of available data concluded that using greater than 5 mm as the diagnostic criteria increased the sensitivity for radiologic diagnosis without losing specificity. The greatest concern with MD-IPMN is risk of high-grade dysplasia (carcinoma in situ) or invasive carcinoma; in retrospective case series of resected IPMNs, the rate of high-grade dysplasia or invasive cancer ranged between 35% and 100%, regardless of symptomatology (Table 1).

BD-IPMNs (Figure 1, B) involve the pancreatic duct side branches but not the main pancreatic duct, and typically occur in younger patients. They are more common than MD-IPMNs, at a rate of 10:1. BD-IPMNs can occur anywhere within the pancreas and 40% to 60%

are multifocal. Despite the high incidence of multifocal disease, there is no evidence that an increased number of lesions amplifies the risk of invasive disease. BD-IPMNs are thought to have a lower risk of malignant transformation. Because of this lower risk of malignancy, BD-IPMNs are more commonly observed, but in resected series the rate of malignancy ranged from 6% to 56%. The overall rate of malignancy in BD-IPMNs is likely much lower, as those with concerning features are more likely to be removed.

Mixed type IPMNs are characterized by the involvement of both the main and branch pancreatic ducts and behave clinically and pathologically like MD-IPMNs (Figure 1, C).

Histologic Classification

IPMNs are composed of mucin-producing columnar cells, which show papillary proliferation, cyst formation, and varying degrees of cellular atypia. Tumors are graded according to the most atypical area in the lesion, following an orderly progression from low-grade dysplasia to moderate dysplasia to high-grade dysplasia and finally to invasive carcinoma. The 2012 International Consensus Guidelines now favor using the terms *low-grade*, *moderate*, and *high-grade dysplasia* in lieu of the previously used terms *IPMN adenoma*, *borderline IPMN*, and *carcinoma in situ*.

Four histologic subtypes of IPMNs have been identified: gastric, intestinal, pancreatobiliary, and oncocytic (Table 2; Figure 2). All can have increasing degrees of dysplasia. Within the four subtypes there is increasing understanding of the proclivity of each subtype to develop into invasive disease, the type of invasive malignancy that develops, and the varying disease prognosis.

The gastric subtype occurs primarily in BD-IPMN and is the most common subtype overall (in keeping with the greater incidence of BD-IPMN than MD-IPMN). These neoplasms are found in the periphery of the pancreatic parenchyma and in the uncinate process. Histologically, they resemble gastric foveolar cells and form pyloric gland-like structures at the base of the papillae (see Figure 2, A). Based on immunohistochemistry, the gastric subtype expresses mucin 5AC (MUC5AC) and mucin 6 (MUC6) proteins, with scattered expression of mucin 2 (MUC2) and no expression of mucin 1 (MUC1). When compared with oncocytic and pancreatobiliary subtypes, the gastric subtype was found to have a superior 5-year survival rate and a lower likelihood of recurrent disease. They are typically low grade, with only 10% to 30% developing into invasive disease. However, once invasive disease develops, the overall prognosis is poor.

The intestinal subtype is the second most common type of IPMN and the most common type of MD-IPMN. As is characteristic of MD-IPMNs, these neoplasms are typically found in the pancreatic head but can involve the entire duct. They have a characteristic villous growth pattern and express MUC2, MUC5AC, and caudal-type homeobox 2 (CDX2). Thirty to fifty percent of patients with the intestinal subtype will develop invasive malignancy, which is a mucinous (colloid) carcinoma that behaves in a relatively indolent fashion when compared with tubular carcinoma.

The pancreatobiliary subtype also typically involves the main duct and is found in the pancreatic head. It is regarded by some as a high-grade version of the gastric type of IPMN, histologically characterized by complex papillae and cells that resemble pancreatic and biliary duct cells. This subtype expresses MUC1 and MUC5AC. Among all of the histologic subtypes, it is associated with the greatest likelihood of malignancy, with more than 50% of patients developing invasive disease. The invasive form of this subtype is histologically indistinguishable from a conventional ductal (tubular) adenocarcinoma and is differentiated by the presence of noninvasive IPMN in the specimen. The pancreaticobiliary type is associated with a high recurrence rate and an overall poor prognosis.

The oncocytic subtype, commonly misdiagnosed as cystadenocarcinoma, is a rare subtype found in the main pancreatic duct. This

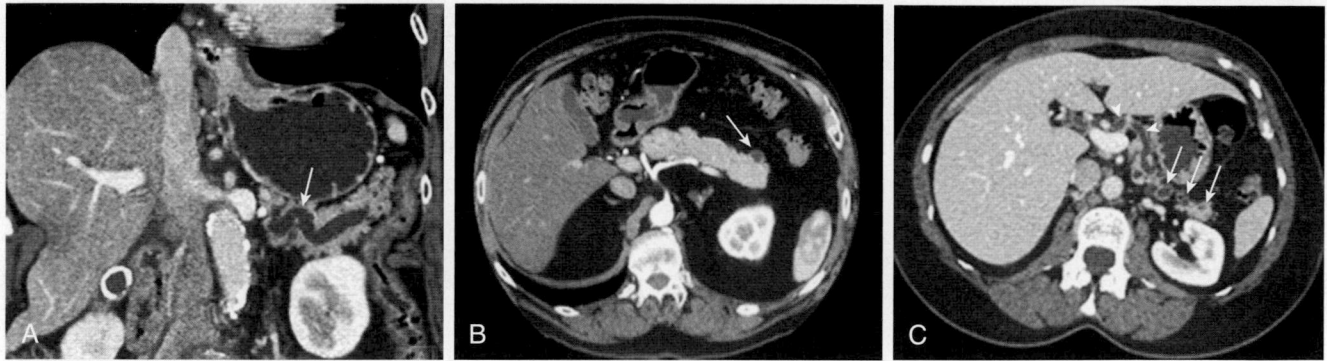

FIGURE 1 A, Sagittal multidetector computed tomographic (MDCT) image showing main duct intraductal papillary mucinous neoplasm (MD-IPMN) with notable dilatation (*arrow*) of the main pancreatic duct. **B,** Axial MDCT image showing a small cystic lesion in the pancreatic tail (*arrow*) consistent with branch duct IPMN (BD-IPMN). No dilation is observed in the main pancreatic duct. **C,** Mixed-type IPMN on CT scan. There is notable diffuse dilatation of the pancreatic duct in the head and body of the gland (*arrowheads*) and multiple small branch duct lesions throughout the body and tail (*arrows*).

TABLE 1: **Studies Investigating Malignancy in Main Duct and Branch Duct Intraductal Papillary Mucinous Neoplasms (IPMNs) Before and After Establishment of the Sendai Criteria**

First Author	Year	Total	Main Duct		Branch Duct		Additional Findings
			N	Malignant* N (%)	N	Malignant* N (%)	
Sugiyama	2003	62	30	21 (70.0)	32	13 (40.6)	Mural nodules and MPD ≥7 mm associated with malignancy
Salvia	2004	140	140	83 (59.3)			Jaundice and diabetes significantly associated with malignancy
Sohn	2004	136	36	18 (50.0)	60	18 (30.0)	Lymph node status predictive of survival for invasive disease in univariate analysis
Suzuki	2004	1024	201	120 (59.7)	509	150 (29.4)	Malignant disease more common in older patients, main duct disease, enlarged papilla orifice, and symptomatic older patients who were symptomatic, had main duct disease, or have an enlarged papilla orifice
Lee	2005	67	27	12 (44.4)	35	10 (28.6)	
Serikawa	2006	103	47	30 (63.8)	56	11 (19.6)	
Schmidt	2007	156	53	30 (56.6)	103	20 (19.4)	Mural nodularity and atypical cytopathologic features predictive of malignancy and/or invasive disease
Rodriguez	2007	145			145	32 (22.1)	Findings associated with malignancy included presence of mural nodules, cyst size ≥30 mm, and presence of a thick wall
Schnelldorfer	2008	208	76	49 (64.4)	84	15 (17.8)	In patients with invasive disease, 58% had recurrent disease compared with 10% in those without invasive disease
Kim	2008	118	70	25 (35.7)	48	3 (6.3)	Relative risk of malignancy was greatest when duct was ≥13 mm, tumor was ≥35 mm, and main duct disease was involved
Nagai	2008	72	15	15 (100)	49	25 (51.0)	In univariate analysis, CA19-9, MPD diameter, tumor size, and presence of mural nodules were significantly associated with malignancy in BD-IPMN and mixed type IPMN. Symptoms of abdominal pain and weight loss were also significant factors
Jang	2008	138			138	26 (18.8)	Cyst size >20 mm was a significant prognostic factor in MV analysis
Ohno	2009	87	14	11 (78.5)	48	20 (41.7)	Type III and IV mural nodules and symptoms significantly associated with malignancy in MV analysis

Continued

TABLE 1: Studies Investigating Malignancy in Main Duct and Branch Duct Intraductal Papillary Mucinous Neoplasms (IPMNs) Before and After Establishment of the Sendai Criteria

First Author	Year	Total	Main Duct		Branch Duct		Additional Findings
			N	Malignant* N (%)	N	Malignant* N (%)	
Nara	2009	123	26	26 (100)	59	26 (44.1)	Cyst size >40 mm, MD-IPMN or mixed type IPMN, and presence of mural nodules or a thick septum were prognostic factors associated with malignancy
Bournet	2009	47			47	10 (21.3)	
Hwang	2010	187	28	20 (71.4)	118	19 (16.1)	Main duct disease predictive of malignancy. In those with BD-IPMN, mural nodularity was a prognostic factor
Mimura	2010	82	39	34 (87.2)	43	20 (46.5)	Main duct disease and diabetes were prognostic factors of malignancy in MV analysis
Crippa	2010	389	81	55 (67.9)	159	34 (21.4)	
Sadakari	2010	73			73	79 (9.6)	MPD ≥5 mm and atypical cytologic features significantly associated with malignancy
Kanno	2010	159			159	59 (37.1)	Mural nodules ≥6.5 mm and CEA >5 ng/mL were significantly associated with invasive IPMN in MV analysis
Hodul	2012	105			105	62 (56.9)	Cyst size ≥20 mm more likely to harbor invasive cancer
Fritz	2012	287			287	69 (24.0)	24.6% were considered Sendai negative and harbored malignant features
Sahora	2013	226			226	52 (23.0)	MPD dilation and cyst size ≥30 mm significantly associated with malignancy
Shimizu	2013	310			310	160 (51.6)	Cyst size, mural nodule size, and MPD dilation significantly associated with malignancy
Abdeljawad	2014	52	52	40 (76.9)			MPD ≥8 mm significantly associated with malignancy
Kawada	2014	202			202	24 (11.9)	Mural nodule size ≥10 mm and positive cytology significantly associated with malignancy
Lee	2014	84			84	16 (19.0)	EUS scoring system including dilation of ducts, size of cyst, size of mural nodule, septal thickening, and patulous orifice
Marchegiani	2015	173	173	125 (72.3)			
Dortch	2015	66			66	12 (18.2)	
Kim	2015	177			177	39 (22.0)	Cyst size ≥30 mm and mural nodules significantly associated with malignancy

*Includes high-grade dysplasia and invasive cancer.

BD-IPMN, Branch duct IPMN; *CA19-9*, cancer antigen 19-9; *CEA*, carcinoembryonic antigen; *EUS*, endoscopic ultrasound scan; *MD-IPMN*, main duct IPMN; *MPD*, main pancreatic duct; *MV*, multivariate.

subtype is characterized by complex arborizing papillae, oncocytic cells, and intraepithelial lumina formation. It expresses MUC1, MUC2, MUC5AC, and MUC6 and tends to form large tissue nodules with limited mucous production.

■ CLINICAL PRESENTATION

IPMNs are thought to account for 1% to 3% of all exocrine pancreatic neoplasms and 20% to 50% of all cystic pancreatic neoplasms. They are most commonly diagnosed in the sixth to seventh decade of life and affect males and females equally. With the increase in abdominal imaging over the last few decades, most IPMNs are identified incidentally on imaging done for another purpose, presenting a

management dilemma. When patients do have symptoms, they are typically nonspecific, such as nausea, vomiting, abdominal pain, back pain, weight loss, or anorexia. When obstructive jaundice is present, the concern for malignancy is high. In addition, patients (primarily those with MD-IPMN) can develop pancreatitis-like symptoms due to blockage of the pancreatic duct with mucin; others may develop symptoms of exocrine and endocrine pancreatic insufficiency but this is usually a sign of advanced disease.

■ EVOLVING MANAGEMENT

Given the concern for malignant potential, when IPMNs were first characterized in the late 1990s many surgeons advocated for

TABLE 2: Histologic Classification of Intraductal Papillary Mucinous Neoplasms (IPMNs) and General Characteristics Commonly Found Within Each Subtype

	Gastric	Intestinal	Pancreatobiliary	Oncocytic
Main duct vs branch duct	BD-IPMN	MD-IPMN	Typically MD-IPMN	MD-IPMN
Incidence	Most common subtype overall (49%-63% of all IPMNs)	Most common subtype of MD-IPMN (18%-36% of all IPMNs)	Less common (7%-18% of all IPMNs)	Least common (1%-8% of all IPMNs)
Location	Uncinate process and pancreatic periphery	Pancreatic head, may involve entire duct	Pancreatic head	
Histologic features	Resemble gastric foveolar cells, form pyloric gland-like structures at the base of the papillae	Villous growth pattern	Complex papillae, cells resemble pancreatic and biliary duct cells	Complex papillae but with eosinophilic cytoplasm, and oncocytic cells
Immunohistochemical profile	• Scattered expression of MUC2 • MUC5AC • MUC6 • No expression of MUC1	• MUC2 • MUC5AC • CDX2	• MUC1 • MUC5AC	• MUC1 • MUC2 • MUC5AC • MUC6
Progression to invasive disease	10%-30%	30%-50%	>50%	Limited, but can be up to 30%
Invasive form	Conventional ductal (tubular) adenocarcinoma	Mucinous (colloid) carcinoma	Conventional ductal (tubular) adenocarcinoma	

BD-IPMN, Branch duct IPMN; *CDX2,* caudal-type homeobox 2; *MD-IPMN,* main duct IPMN; *MUC,* mucin.

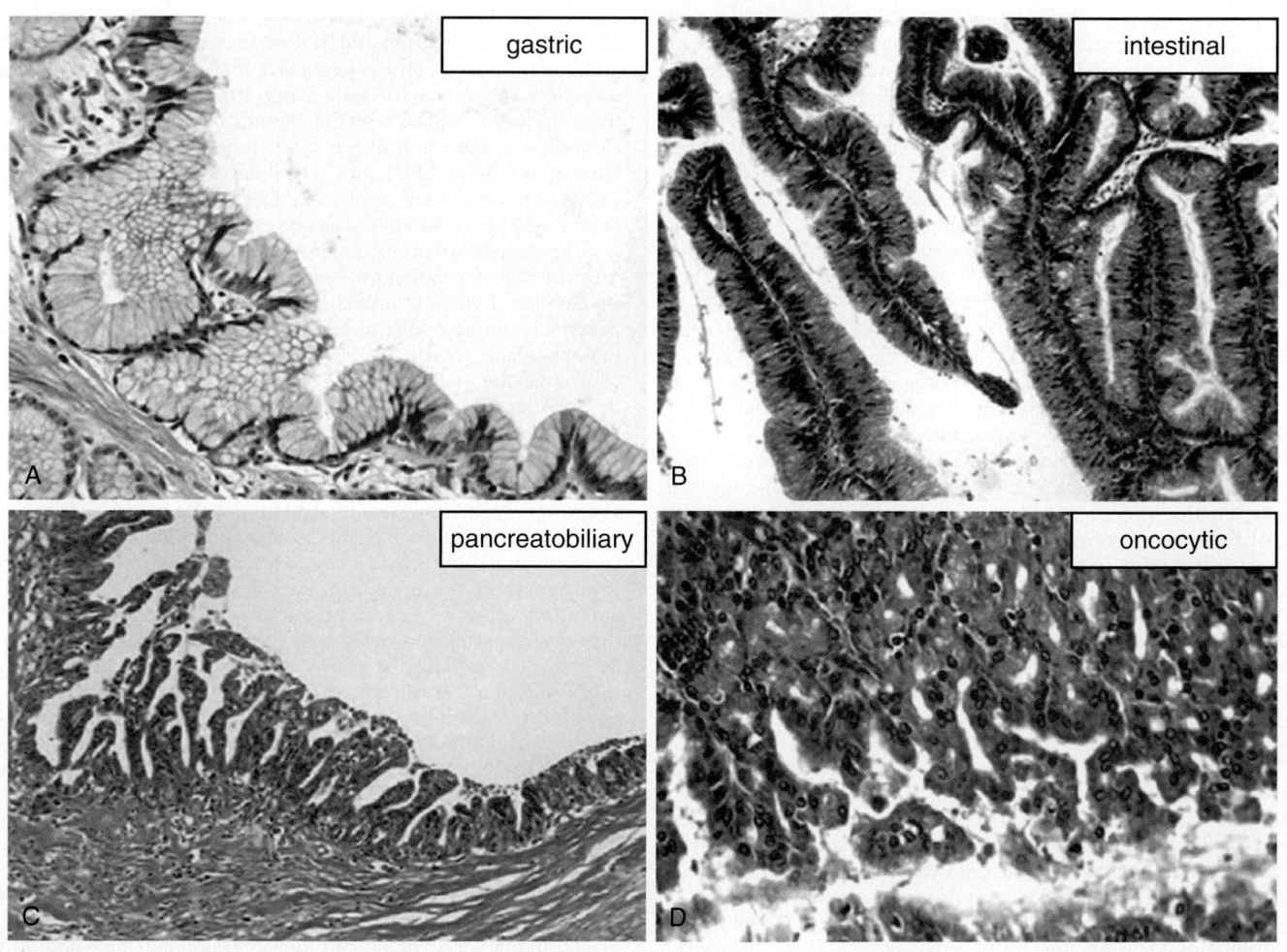

FIGURE 2 The four histologic classifications of IPMN are (**A**) gastric, (**B**) intestinal, (**C**) pancreatobiliary, and (**D**) oncocytic. *(From Tanaka M, Fernandez-del Castillo C, Adsay V, et al. International consensus guidelines 2012 for the management of IPMN and MCN of the pancreas. Pancreatology. 2012;12:183-187.)*

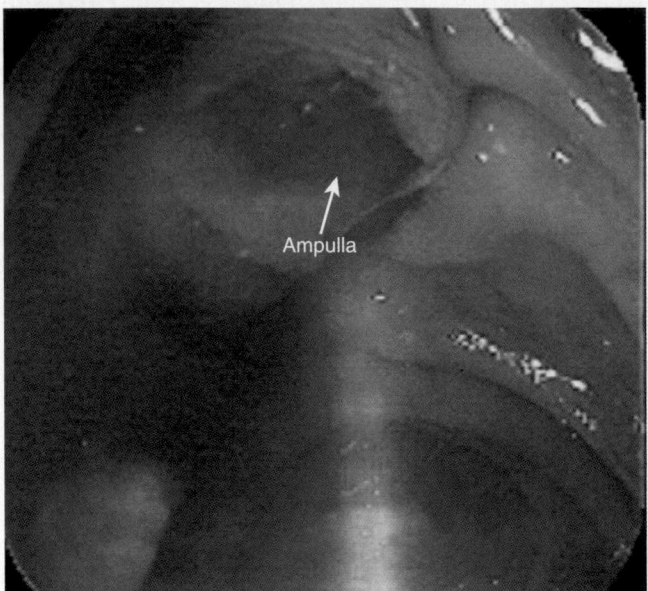

FIGURE 3 Upper endoscopy demonstrating dilated ampulla with secretion of mucin and "fish-mouth sign," which is pathognomonic for intraductal papillary mucinous neoplasm.

aggressive resection to prevent malignant transformation. However, as we learned more about the anatomic and histologic subtypes, it has become widely accepted that not all IPMNs need to be resected. Many incidentally found IPMNs may not pose a threat when considering a patient's life expectancy, associated comorbidities, and risk of postoperative complications. In addition, pancreatic resection is a high-risk operation with postoperative morbidity as high as 30% to 60%, making risk stratification of the likelihood of malignancy, as well as operative risk, essential to decision making.

When determining whether a patient should undergo resection or observation, it is important to use risk stratification to assess the lesion with regard to the likelihood of existing malignancy and overall malignant potential. In 2012 the International Consensus Guidelines (Sendai criteria) were updated and reported on features considered to be "high risk" and "worrisome" (Box 1). These criteria helped to establish a detailed algorithm for deciding whether a patient should undergo resection or surveillance. These guidelines provide an excellent roadmap for decision making; however, clinical circumstances (family history of pancreatic cancer, elevated cancer antigen 19-9 [CA19-9], inability to tolerate surgery, etc.) and patient preference offer the opportunity for shared decision making in this complex disease.

Diagnosis and Management

Diagnosis of IPMN should be made using a combination of thorough history and physical examination, noninvasive imaging, and endoscopy. It is extremely important to accurately differentiate IPMN from other pancreatic cystic lesions and correctly characterize it as main duct or branch duct, as this will determine optimal management.

At the time of presentation to a surgeon, most patients already will have had cross-sectional imaging with computed tomographic scan (CT scan) or magnetic resonance imaging (MRI). If this imaging is not adequate for evaluating pancreatic duct size and the presence of mural nodules, additional imaging should be performed. An upper endoscopy that demonstrates an enlarged ampulla or "fish-mouth sign" is pathognomonic for an IPMN (Figure 3). Once IPMN is in the differential diagnosis stage, clinicians can refer to the 2012 International Consensus Guidelines (Figure 4).

First, patients should be evaluated for the presence of high-risk stigmata (see Box 1), defined as (1) obstructive jaundice with presence of a cystic lesion in the head of the pancreas, (2) enhancing solid component with a cyst, and/or (3) main pancreatic duct 10 mm or greater in size. If a patient has any of these characteristics, surgery is recommended if the patient is an appropriate surgical candidate.

If there is no evidence of high-risk stigmata, the next step should be evaluation for worrisome features (see Box 1). These include (1)

cyst 3 cm or greater in size, (2) thickened, enhancing cyst walls, (3) main duct 5 to 9 mm in size, (4) nonenhancing mural nodule, and/or (5) abrupt change in caliber of pancreatic duct with distal pancreatic atrophy. If a patient meets any of these criteria, an endoscopic ultrasound scan (EUS) should be done to evaluate for definite mural nodules, main duct features suspicious for involvement, or cytology suspicious or positive for malignancy. If EUS demonstrates any of these findings, surgical resection should be considered strongly if clinically appropriate. If EUS is inconclusive, close surveillance with alternating MRI and EUS should be done every 3 to 6 months. If no worrisome features are identified on EUS, ongoing management is determined by the size of the largest cyst.

The surveillance protocol differs based on imaging modality and time interval, depending on the size of the largest lesion. In lesions smaller than 2 cm, multidetector 3D-CT with pancreatic protocol or pancreatic-protocol MRI should be the primary imaging modality. Lesions smaller than 1 cm should be imaged every 2 to 3 years and lesions that are 1 to 2 cm should be imaged yearly for the first 2 years; if the lesion remains stable, the surveillance interval may be lengthened. Both CT and MRI are equivalent with regards to the information they provide on tumor type, location, development of additional lesions, lymph node and organ metastasis, and invasion into adjacent structures. MRI, however, is able to provide better information regarding the presence of possible septae and mural nodules (or solid components) and provides more accurate information on the involvement of the main pancreatic duct, including detection of communications between side branch cysts and the main pancreatic duct that can be missed on CT scan. Ductal communication also may be evaluated via EUS (Figure 5).

Lesions that measure 2 to 3 cm should undergo EUS 3 to 6 months after diagnosis and then the surveillance interval may be lengthened, alternating between EUS and MRI, if there is no interval growth, development of worrisome or high-risk stigmata, or change in symptoms. If a patient is young and fit and may require prolonged surveillance, surgery should be considered. In lesions larger than 3 cm, MRI with EUS should be done every 3 to 6 months, and resection should be considered in young, fit patients.

Patients with two or more affected first-degree relatives should have more aggressive surveillance, as the risk for malignancy is far greater in this subset of patients. Imaging should include both MRI/

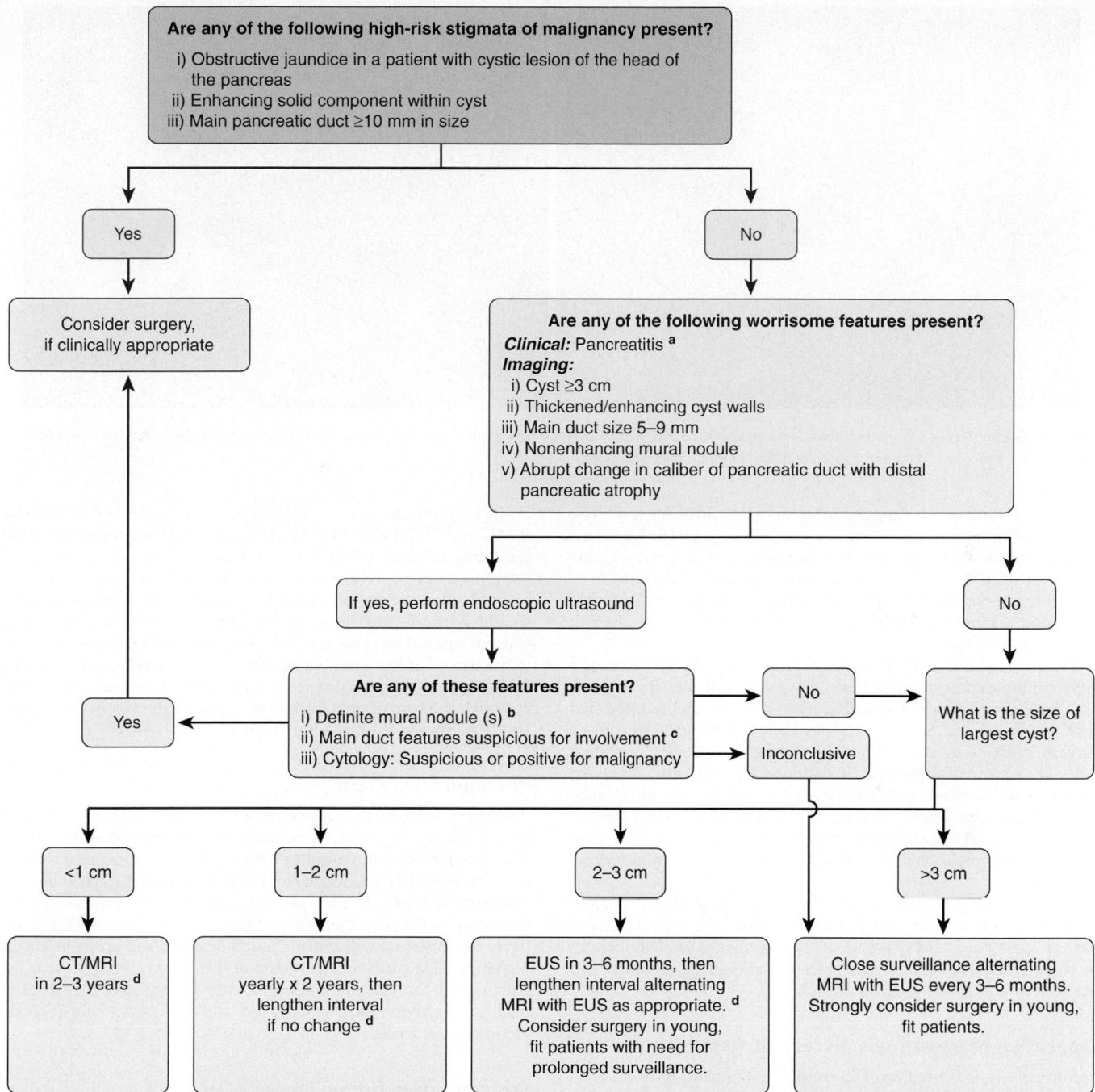

Are any of the following high-risk stigmata of malignancy present?

i) Obstructive jaundice in a patient with cystic lesion of the head of the pancreas
ii) Enhancing solid component within cyst
iii) Main pancreatic duct ≥10 mm in size

Yes → Consider surgery, if clinically appropriate

No →

Are any of the following worrisome features present?

Clinical: Pancreatitis [a]
Imaging:
i) Cyst ≥3 cm
ii) Thickened/enhancing cyst walls
iii) Main duct size 5–9 mm
iv) Nonenhancing mural nodule
v) Abrupt change in caliber of pancreatic duct with distal pancreatic atrophy

If yes, perform endoscopic ultrasound

No

Are any of these features present?

i) Definite mural nodule (s) [b]
ii) Main duct features suspicious for involvement [c]
iii) Cytology: Suspicious or positive for malignancy

Yes

No

Inconclusive

What is the size of largest cyst?

<1 cm → CT/MRI in 2–3 years [d]

1–2 cm → CT/MRI yearly x 2 years, then lengthen interval if no change [d]

2–3 cm → EUS in 3–6 months, then lengthen interval alternating MRI with EUS as appropriate. [d] Consider surgery in young, fit patients with need for prolonged surveillance.

>3 cm → Close surveillance alternating MRI with EUS every 3–6 months. Strongly consider surgery in young, fit patients.

a. Pancreatitis may be an indication for surgery for relief of symptoms.
b. Differential diagnosis includes mucin. Mucin can move with change in patient position, may be dislodged on cyst lavage, and does not have Doppler flow. Features of true tumor nodule include lack of mobility, presence of Doppler flow, and fine-needle aspiration of nodule showing tumor tissue.
c. Presence of any one of thickened walls, intraductal mucin, or mural nodules is suggestive of main duct involvement. In their absence main duct involvement is inconclusive.
d. Studies from Japan suggest that on follow-up of subjects with suspected BD-IPMN there is increased incidence of pancreatic ductal adenocarcinoma unrelated to malignant transformation of the BD-IPMN(s) being followed. However, it is unclear if imaging surveillance can detect early ductal adenocarcinoma, and, if so, at what interval surveillance imaging should be performed.

FIGURE 4 International Consensus Guidelines for surveillance and surgical resection of intraductal papillary mucinous neoplasm (IPMN) depending on high-risk stigmata, worrisome features, and size. *BD-IPMN,* branch duct IPMN; *CT,* computed tomography; *EUS,* endoscopic ultrasound scan; *MRI,* magnetic resonance imaging. *(Modified from Tanaka M, Fernandez-del Castillo C, Adsay V, et al. International consensus guidelines 2012 for the management of IPMN and MCN of the pancreas. Pancreatology. 2012;12:183-187.)*

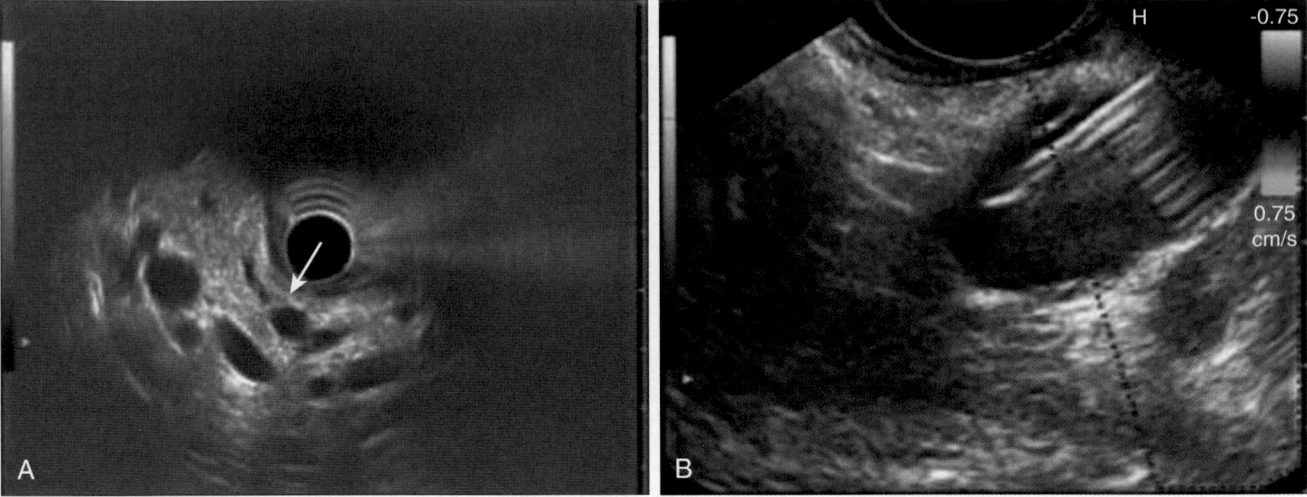

FIGURE 5 Endoscopic ultrasound done for intraductal papillary mucinous neoplasm demonstrating ductal communication between (**A**) the lesion and (**B**) the main pancreatic duct and subsequent fine-needle aspiration biopsy.

magnetic resonance cholangiopancreatography (MRCP) and EUS. Worrisome features in the setting of a family history certainly warrant strong consideration for resection. In higher-risk surgical patients where the decision to operate is more difficult, MRI/MRCP at 3-month intervals and annual EUS should be done for the first 2 years after diagnosis until the risk of malignancy outweighs the risk of surgical resection.

Certain patients may be deemed unfit for pancreatic resection given multiple comorbidities, frailty associated with advanced age, or even patient preference. Given that the risk of morbidity associated with pancreatic resection is as high as 30%, the risks and benefits of surgery must be discussed with the patient in order to provide a tailored treatment approach. In patients who are truly unfit for surgery, surveillance is not indicated, as it will not change ultimate management. In higher-risk patients, the number of worrisome or high-risk stigmata may shift the risk-benefit assessment of surgical resection; imaging is therefore indicated and shared decision making is essential.

Finally, some patients may prefer surgical resection to the concern associated with ongoing surveillance, whereas other patients may have circumstances that make adequate surveillance unlikely. In both of these circumstances, surgical resection should be considered in patients who are good surgical candidates.

Operative Management: Extent of Resection

Preoperatively, it is important to counsel patients on both the risks and the benefits of pancreatic resection and observation. This includes discussion of cancer risk, treatment risk, and the need for long-term surveillance in both settings. Especially in the setting of multifocal disease, the possibility of total pancreatectomy and its associated risks should be discussed. Possible postoperative complications and the risk of endocrine and/or exocrine insufficiency associated with even partial pancreatic resection also should be discussed with patients.

Options for resection include pancreaticoduodenectomy, distal pancreatectomy, enucleation, and total pancreatectomy. The choice of procedure depends on the location of the IPMN and pathologic features. Preoperative planning is essential and largely dependent on preoperative imaging, as well as intraoperative ultrasound. The entire gland should be evaluated intraoperatively given the high frequency of multifocal IPMN. Limited resections include enucleation, which also may be considered in the setting of benign BD-IPMN; however, nonanatomic resections may be associated with higher pancreatic fistula rates or, rarely, leakage of mucin.

In all cases, the goal of the surgery is resection of all invasive IPMN and IPMN with high-grade dysplasia. At the time of surgical resection, an intraoperative frozen section of the pancreatic neck margin should be performed. If the neck margin is positive for high-grade dysplasia or invasive cancer, re-resection to negative margins should be performed even if this requires total pancreatectomy. Current surgical thinking does not recommend total pancreatectomy in the setting of low-grade or moderate-grade dysplasia at the surgical margin, as the physiologic implications of total pancreatectomy outweigh the risks of ongoing surveillance and the risk of developing another lesion in the remnant pancreas.

Postoperative Care

Perioperative morbidity and mortality is similar to that for any other patient undergoing a pancreatic resection or major abdominal operation. Pancreas-specific complications of which the surgeon should be aware include delayed gastric emptying, pancreatic fistula, and other anastomotic leaks. Unlike patients with chronic pancreatitis or aggressive pancreatic adenocarcinoma, most patients with IPMNs have soft pancreata with normal-size bile ducts and are therefore at higher risk for pancreatic fistulas and bile leaks. Depending on the patient and the extent of resection, the patient also may require pancreatic enzyme supplementation and insulin to help regulate blood glucose levels.

Postoperative Surveillance

Surveillance protocols can be classified based on whether the patient underwent resection for BD-IPMN or MD-IPMN. In patients who undergo resection, surveillance depends on margin status and pathologic grade (Figure 6). In patients with a diagnosis of invasive IPMN, surveillance should mirror that of pancreatic adenocarcinoma, with CT scans every 3 months for the first year and every 6 months thereafter. In patients who undergo resection for high-grade dysplasia, MRCP or CT scans should be obtained every 3 to 6 months. For low-grade and intermediate-grade dysplasia, surveillance depends on surgical margin status. If margins are negative, surveillance with CT scans or MRCP at 2 and 5 years is appropriate. However, in those with low-grade or moderate-grade dysplasia at the resection margin, MRCP surveillance with history and physical examination should be done twice a year.

When performing surveillance after resection, it is important to identify whether a patient has a family history of pancreatic adenocarcinoma, positive surgical margins, development of new

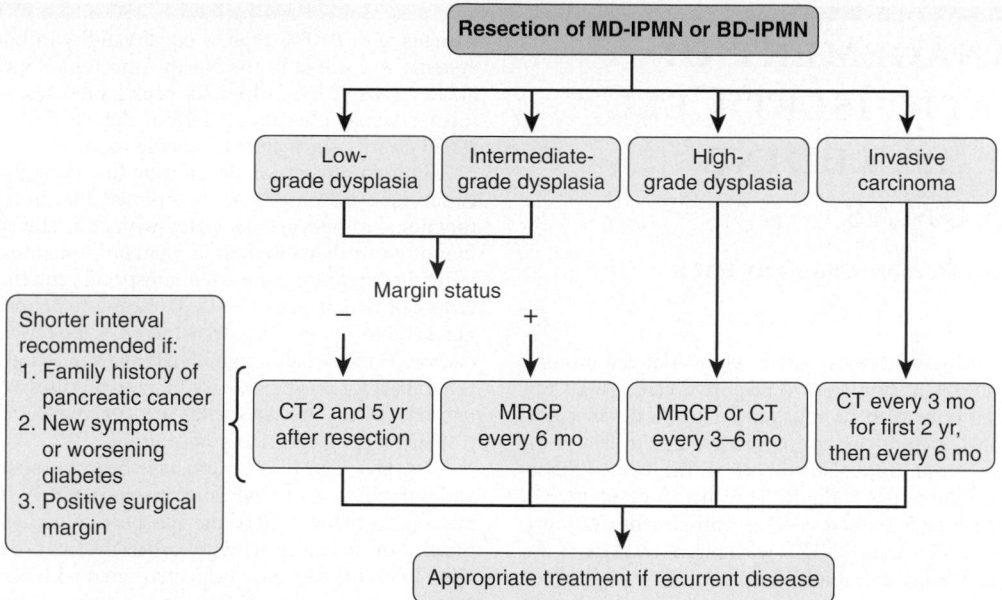

FIGURE 6 Proposed algorithm for management of main duct intraductal papillary mucinous neoplasm (MD-IPMN) and branch duct intraductal papillary mucinous neoplasm (BD-IPMN) after surgical resection. *CT*, Computed tomography; *MRCP*, magnetic resonance cholangiopancreatography.

symptoms, or worsening of diabetes. Such clinical factors may be worrisome for progression of the disease and these patients should undergo shorter-interval surveillance. In the case of both MD-IPMN and BD-IPMN, if additional lesions are identified on surveillance, management should be based again on the International Consensus Guidelines (see Figure 4).

Extrapancreatic Malignancy

Extrapancreatic malignancy has been reported in cases of both MD-IPMNs and BD-IPMNs; the incidence ranges from 10% to 45%. Frequent sites include breast, colon, and prostate. There are no current recommendations for screening extrapancreatic malignancies, but initial evaluation with up-to-date screening colonoscopy and mammogram should be done in addition to continuing recommended screening for these malignancies. Extra attention should be paid to this both preoperatively and postoperatively.

■ PROGNOSIS

The overall survival rate for patients with IPMN has been reported to range between 36% and 77%, with the presence of malignancy being the strongest predictor of survival. Once invasive disease develops, the behavior of IPMNs is very similar to that of tubular pancreatic ductal carcinoma. For noninvasive neoplasms, the 5-year survival rate after surgical resection is 70% to 100%; however, for those patients with invasive disease, the 5-year survival rate ranges from 30% to 60% based on the histologic subtype of invasive malignancy. Invasive tubular carcinomas occur in the setting of gastric and pancreaticobiliary histologic subtypes and can be found in both MD-IPMNs and BD-IPMNs. This type is morphologically indistinguishable from pancreatic ductal adenocarcinoma and, as such, has a greater likelihood of nodal metastasis as well as a higher incidence of perineural and vascular invasion. Therefore those with invasive disease are similarly treated with adjunct treatment, including chemotherapy and/or radiation similar to that used for pancreatic adenocarcinoma.

The 5-year survival rate for resected tubular type malignancy is 37% to 55%. In contrast, colloid carcinoma (i.e., mucinous carcinoma) has morphologic characteristics similar to other exocrine malignancies such as breast and skin. It is associated with the intestinal subtype, and overall has a better prognosis than the tubular carcinoma, with an estimated 5-year survival rate of 61% to 87% after surgical resection.

Other poor prognostic indicators related to survival include invasive disease at the surgical margin and presence of jaundice. Recurrence in all patients who undergo resection ranges from 7% to 43% in the remaining gland. However, good results have been reported in patients who underwent repeat resection for recurrence in the remaining gland.

■ CONCLUSIONS

IPMNs are an important clinical entity that surgeons should be aware of given the complex management and surveillance associated with these lesions. Multiple factors must be considered when diagnosing, treating, and surveilling these patients. Although the Sendai criteria serve as guidelines in the management of IPMNs, the overall patient and clinical characteristics of the lesion should be factored in when deciding on the optimal management plan given that the evolving management of IPMNs is not a simple one-size-fits-all approach. The decision to operate versus to surveil these patients is a complex one and involves frank discussion with the patient regarding operative risks, benefits, and the risk of malignant progression. The treatment option that is most appropriate should be tailored to the patient's needs and specific disease pathology.

SUGGESTED READINGS

Koh YX, Zheng HL, Chok AY, et al. Systematic review and meta-analysis of the spectrum and outcomes of different histologic subtypes of noninvasive and invasive intraductal papillary mucinous neoplasms. *Surgery.* 2015;57:496-509.

Machado NO, Hani Q, Wahibi K. Intraductal papillary mucinous neoplasm of pancreas. *N Am J Med Sci.* 2015;7:160-175.

Ohtsuka T, Tanaka M. Postoperative surveillance of branch duct. In: Tanaka M, ed. *Intraductal Papillary Mucinous Neoplasm of the Pancreas.* Japan: Springer; 2014:189-199.

Ohtsuka T, Tanaka M. Postoperative surveillance of main duct. In: Tanaka M, ed. *Intraductal Papillary Mucinous Neoplasm of the Pancreas.* Fukuoka, Japan: Springer; 2014:181-188.

Tanaka M, Fernandez-del Castillo C, Adsay V, et al. International consensus guidelines 2012 for the management of IPMN and MCN of the pancreas. *Pancreatology.* 2012;12:183-187.

THE MANAGEMENT OF PANCREATIC ISLET CELL TUMORS EXCLUDING GASTRINOMAS

Irene Lou, MD, and Herbert Chen, MD, FACS

Pancreatic neuroendocrine tumors (PNETs), or islet cell tumors, are rare malignancies arising from pluripotent cells within the pancreas. These tumors tend to be more indolent than pancreatic adenocarcinoma. PNETs comprise approximately 2% to 3% of all pancreatic tumors, with an annual incidence in the United States ranging from 4 to 5 cases per million. The incidence of PNETs increases with age, peaking in the sixth and seventh decades. Autopsy series report higher incidences of PNETs, with recent analysis of the Surveillance, Epidemiology, and End Results (SEER) registry of cancer patients confirming an increase in diagnosis over the last 30 years. PNETs are generally classified as functional or nonfunctional (Table 1). Tumors with hormonal overproduction resulting in clinical syndromes are considered functional whereas tumors that do not cause any symptoms and are often metastatic at presentation are considered nonfunctional.

PNETs are usually sporadic, but are also associated with autosomal dominant hereditary conditions such as multiple endocrine neoplasia type 1 (MEN 1) and even more rarely with other syndromes such as von Hippel-Lindau syndrome and neurofibromatosis 1. Genetic analysis has compared PNETs with pancreatic adenocarcinomas, with PNETs exhibiting 60% fewer genes mutated per tumor. The genes most often affected by pancreatic adenocarcinoma, such as TGF-β, K-ras, and TP53, are rarely altered in PNETs. Genes frequently altered in PNETs, such as MEN1 (mammalian target of rapamycin [mTOR]), DAXX (death-domain associated protein), and ATRX (α-thalassemia/mental retardation syndrome X-linked), similarly are not seen in pancreatic adenocarcinoma. On a molecular level, PNETs exhibit more C-to-G transversions compared with the C-to-T transitions found in adenocarcinomas. This difference may be attributed to exposure to different environmental carcinogens or different DNA repair pathways.

■ DIAGNOSIS AND PROGNOSIS

Because of diverse tumor biology, there is no uniform classification system for PNETs. The most commonly used are the World Health Organization (WHO) classification and the tumor node metastasis (TNM) staging systems suggested by the European Neuroendocrine Tumor Society (ENETS) and the American Joint Committee on Cancer (AJCC). The WHO classification, last updated in 2010, defines and classifies neuroendocrine tumor phenotypes based on degree of differentiation and primary tumor site. Important factors in classification include angioinvasion, mitoses, and proliferation index by Ki-67 level (Table 2). PNETs are also divided according to a grading scheme based on Ki-67 index and mitotic count, with higher Ki-67 and mitotic counts associated with a higher-grade tumor. Ki-67 has been found to be a major predictor of tumor progression, with every unit increase in Ki-67 corresponding to a 2% increased risk of progression.

The ENETS uses TNM staging, and its prognostic value has been validated as a good system for high-grade tumors. The AJCC proposed TNM staging based on that used for exocrine pancreas neoplasms. Multiple classification systems may lead to confusion, especially when the two systems have discordant findings. However, a recent study at the Mayo Clinic on the largest surgical cohort of patients with PNETs reports equal validity in both of these staging systems. According to the North American Neuroendocrine Tumor Society (NANETS) 2010 consensus guidelines, staging can be performed using either the ENETS or the AJCC system, as long as it is stated clearly which system is being used.

Clinical presentation depends on functionality, leading to distinct endocrine syndromes that are outlined later in this chapter. Because functional tumors are associated with clinically apparent symptoms, they often are diagnosed earlier than nonfunctional tumors. However, individual symptoms are often nonspecific and the complex of symptoms can remain unrecognized, leading to an average delay in diagnosis of 5 to 7 years. This delay increases the probability of metastatic disease. Therefore although PNETs are rare, a high index of suspicion is required for diagnosis. According to all cases available in the SEER registry, distant metastasis was present in 64% of patients with gastropancreatic neuroendocrine tumors.

Several serum biomarkers have been proposed in the diagnosis and surveillance of PNETs. Chromogranin-A (CGA) is often co-released in many PNETs and has been advocated to be a potential marker of secretory activity, especially in nonfunctional tumors. High levels of CGA have been associated with poorer prognosis, and an early decrease in CGA level on treatment has been reported to have more favorable outcomes. However, patients on proton pump inhibitors and with renal insufficiency may have falsely elevated CGA levels. 5-Hydroxyindoleacetic acid (5-HIAA) is not as useful in pancreatic neuroendocrine tumors, which do not secrete serotonin, but may be used if a nonfunctional PNET is suspected.

Advanced imaging has become a cornerstone in the diagnosis of PNETs. The most commonly used modalities of computed tomography (CT) and magnetic resonance imaging (MRI) can detect 22% to 45% of these tumors, with somatostatin-receptor CT scans able to detect noninsulinoma lesions in 57% to 77%. Endoscopic ultrasound (EUS) has greatly increased localization of PNETs and is able to detect these lesions with an overall sensitivity and accuracy upward of 90% (Figure 1). In addition, a fine-needle biopsy can be obtained using EUS. 18-fluorodeoxyglucose (^{18}FDG) positron emission tomography (PET) scanning has not proven useful for PNETs, except with exceptionally aggressive tumors. More recently, dynamic ultrasound and MRI with contrast, which allows temporal enhancement in arterial, venous, and delayed phases, have shown promise in detecting lesions as small as 3 mm. All of these available imaging techniques fail to provide prognostic information, however. Pathologic grading of tumors helps to guide treatment options, as higher-grade tumors are aggressive and treated like small cell lung cancers with chemotherapy.

■ FUNCTIONAL TUMORS

Functional tumors result in clinical manifestations resulting from hypersecretion of hormones. Therefore these PNETs are named according to the hormone that is being overproduced.

Insulinoma

Insulinomas are the most common of the functional PNETs. These tumors are typically small and benign, and more than 99% are located in the pancreas. Fewer than 10% are malignant, or multiple, and there is a slightly higher incidence in women.

Presentation

Patients typically are diagnosed between the ages of 40 and 45, with symptoms caused by hypoglycemia as a result of fasting. Typically, symptoms are caused by hypoglycemia of the central nervous system, resulting in headaches, confusion, and visual disturbances, or by an excess of catecholamines secondary to hypoglycemia, resulting in symptoms such as palpitations, sweating, and tremors. The original description of Whipple's triad suspecting insulinoma consists of

TABLE 1: Summary of Pancreatic Islet Cell Tumors

Tumor	Annual Incidence (per million)	Most Common Symptom(s)	Location	Malignant (%)	Association With MEN 1 (%)
Insulinoma	1-3	Hypoglycemia	Entire pancreas	<10	4-5
Glucagonoma	0.01-0.1	Necrolytic migratory erythema Glucose intolerance Deep vein thrombosis Diarrhea	Entire pancreas	50-80	3
VIPoma	0.1	Watery diarrhea Hypokalemia	Body and tail of pancreas	40-70	3
Somatostatinoma	Rare	Diabetes Diarrhea	Pancreas (55%) Duodenum/jejunum (44%)	>70	<1
Nonfunctional	2.2	Asymptomatic Abdominal pain	Entire pancreas	50	<1

MEN 1, Multiple endocrine neoplasia type 1; *VIPoma,* vasoactive intestinal polypeptide-secreting tumor.

TABLE 2: World Health Organization Classification System of Pancreatic Neuroendocrine Tumors

Grade	Ki-67	Mitotic Rate (per 10 hpf)
Low grade	≤2%	<2
Intermediate grade	3-20%	2-20
High grade	>20%	>20

hpf, High power field.

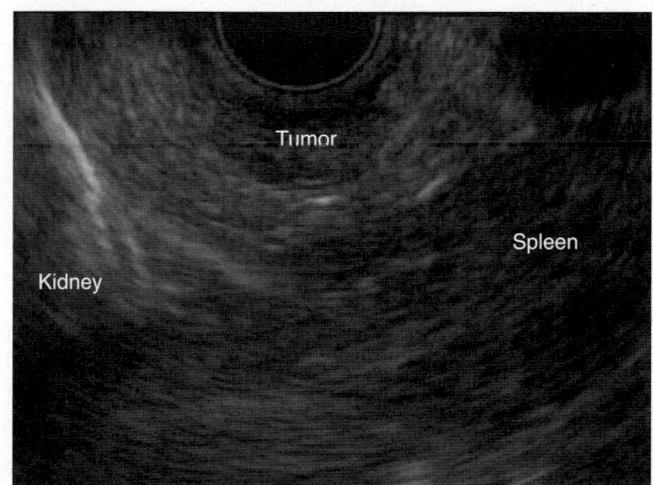

FIGURE 1 Endoscopic ultrasound image revealing a neuroendocrine tumor in the tail of the pancreas. The spleen and left kidney are also in view.

having symptoms of hypoglycemia, a plasma glucose less than 40 mg/dL, and relief of symptoms with the administration of glucose.

Diagnosis

Clinically, patients must demonstrate an elevated insulin to glucose ratio during fasting, with associated elevated levels of C-peptide. If factitious hypoglycemia is suspected, levels of urine or plasma sulfonylurea metabolites also can be measured. The gold standard for diagnosis is a 72-hour fast during which plasma C-peptide, proinsulin, insulin, and glucose levels are drawn every 6 hours until symptoms emerge. Failure of insulin suppression in the setting of hypoglycemia supports the diagnosis of an insulinoma. Symptoms appear in 75% of patients within the first 24 hours of fasting and in 95% of patients after 48 hours of fasting if an insulinoma is present.

Insulinomas usually occur within the pancreas, but because of their small size, with more than 80% of tumors smaller than 2 cm, they can be difficult to localize. Thin-section CT and MRI are easily available and the initial imaging modalities of choice but are positive in only 10% to 40% of cases. Somatostatin receptor scans can sometimes be useful but localize insulinomas in only 25% of cases because of either the low density or the lack of somatostatin receptors compared with other PNETs. EUS has been shown to be positive in 70% to 95% of cases and is the procedure of choice if other noninvasive studies are negative. EUS is particularly helpful in identifying small pancreatic lesions. Selective angiography also can be performed and when combined with hepatic venous sampling for insulin after calcium stimulation has reported high rates of successful localization.

Treatment

Insulinomas differ from other PNETs in that they have low potential for malignancy. Fewer than 10% are malignant; therefore more than 90% of patients can achieve cure with removal of the tumor. Insulinomas are located uniformly throughout the pancreas, with one third in the head, one third in the body, and one third in the tail. The majority of patients found to have an insulinoma undergo pancreatic enucleation, or less commonly pancreatic resection, with cure rates of 85% to 95%. Enucleation, increasingly being performed laparoscopically, can be done safely if the tumor is farther than 2 to 3 mm from the pancreatic duct. Otherwise a partial pancreatic resection is warranted. In most cases lymphadenectomy is not required, except in the rare exception when a malignant insulinoma is suspected.

If the patient is localized preoperatively, enucleation or pancreatic resection may be performed in a minimally invasive way (Figure 2). In a nonlocalized patient with sporadic insulinoma, surgical exploration is indicated. Because the majority of these tumors are intrapancreatic, intraoperative ultrasound (IOUS) is recommended in conjunction with manual palpation of the pancreas to locate the lesion, and this combination is successful in finding 92% of tumors. In addition to IOUS, frozen sections and intraoperative insulin sampling also may be used. When the insulinoma cannot be localized preoperatively or intraoperatively, blind distal resection is not recommended.

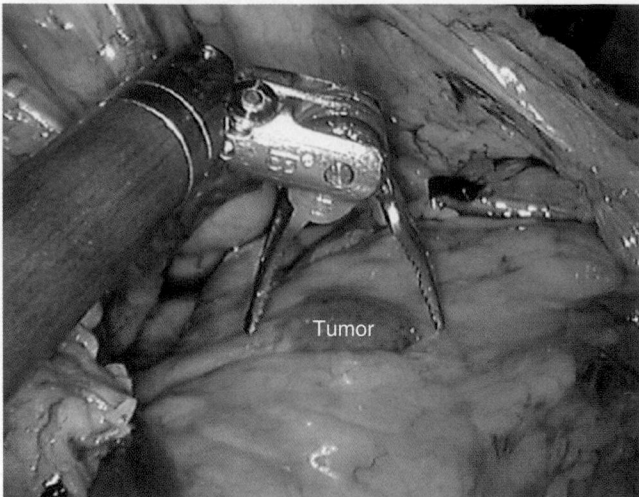

FIGURE 2 Minimally invasive resection of an insulinoma located in the tail of the pancreas.

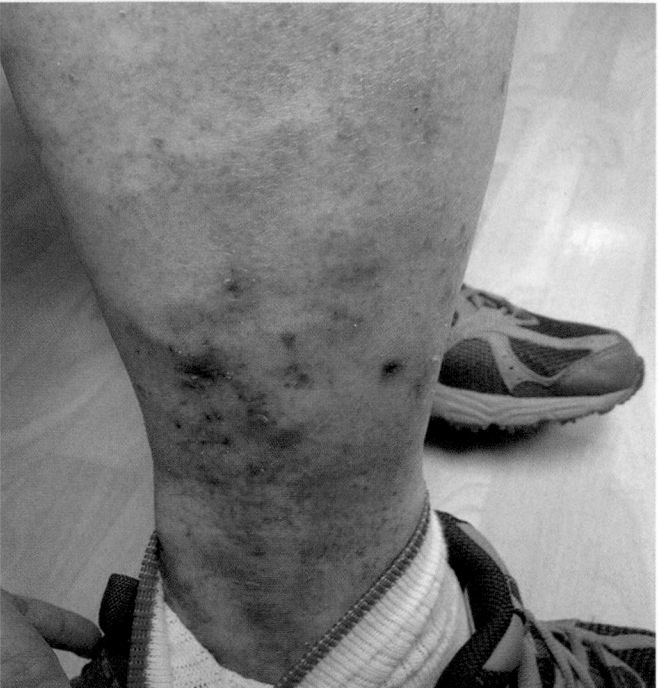

FIGURE 3 Necrolytic migratory erythema in the pretibial region of this patient is a characteristic rash associated with a glucagonoma. The lesion is intensely red and scaly and commonly also occurs in intertriginous areas.

Medical treatment for metastatic insulinomas requires small, frequent meals and control of hypoglycemia with medications such as diazoxide, somatostatin analogues, and glucocorticoids in refractory cases.

The overall 5-year survival after diagnosis of an insulinoma is excellent at 97%, with 100% disease-specific survival and 90% disease-free survival. A 25-year experience reported from the Massachusetts General Hospital revealed only lymphovascular invasion on multivariate analysis to be predictive of disease recurrence, with recurrences occurring within the first 5 years.

Glucagonoma

Glucagonomas are found almost exclusively in the pancreas and are malignant 50% to 80% of the time.

Presentation

Approximately 70% of patients with glucagonoma will have necrolytic migratory erythema, intense red lesions that primarily affect intertriginous sites like the perineum, as well as areas prone to minor trauma such as the trunk and legs (Figure 3). This dermatitis in addition to diabetes, diarrhea, and deep vein thrombosis (DVT) constitute the "4D syndrome" associated with glucagonomas.

Diagnosis

Hormonal analysis will reveal elevated plasma levels of glucagon, and often other pancreatic hormones such as pancreatic polypeptide, in the presence of appropriate symptoms. Biopsy of skin lesions also can be performed and characteristically reveals vacuolated keratinocytes in the upper epidermis. CT or MRI is useful in identifying and localizing the tumor.

Treatment

Surgical resection should be performed when possible. Normalization of serum glucagon either by surgery or by somatostatin analogues usually results in the rapid disappearance of the necrolytic migratory erythema. Sporadic cases usually are diagnosed late in the course of disease, resulting in at least 50% of patients having metastatic disease. Somatostatin analogues or interferon-α is effective in palliating symptoms, and dietary supplementation of zinc, amino acids, and essential fatty acids also has been reported to help. Chemotherapy regimens have not proven effective against metastatic glucagonomas; however, these tumors are slow growing and patients with metastatic disease often die of causes unrelated to the tumor.

Vasoactive Intestinal Polypeptide-Secreting Tumor (VIPoma)

VIPomas are located selectively in the body and tail of the pancreas, with more than 70% being malignant.

Presentation

The symptoms associated with VIPoma, also referred to as Verner-Morrison syndrome, include watery diarrhea, hypokalemia, and achlorhydria (WDHA). The chronic secretory diarrhea persists despite fasting and is the predominant presenting symptom. Excess vasoactive intestinal polypeptide (VIP) inhibits gastric acid secretion, bone resorption, and glycogenolysis and causes vasodilation, resulting in symptoms of hypochlorhydria, hypercalcemia, hyperglycemia, and flushing, respectively.

Diagnosis

Serum levels of VIP usually exceed 200 pg/mL but have been reported as high as several thousand in the setting of appropriate clinical symptoms. The majority of VIPomas are malignant, with 70% of patients having metastatic disease at the time of diagnosis. Most primary VIPomas in adults are located in the pancreas and often present at a size easily detectable by either CT or MRI. Up to 90% of VIPomas express somatostatin receptors; therefore somatostatin receptor scans also can be useful in localization.

Treatment

Before starting any treatment, potentially life-threatening issues of electrolyte imbalance and volume status need to be addressed and corrected. More than 80% of pancreatic VIPomas can undergo resection. Somatostatin analogues also result in excellent symptomatic control with or without surgery.

Somatostatinoma

The majority of somatostatinomas are solitary and generally quite large at the time of detection, with a slightly higher incidence in the pancreas over the proximal small bowel.

Presentation

The syndrome associated with pancreatic somatostatinomas classically involves diabetes, diarrhea or steatorrhea, and weight loss as a result of the great inhibitory effect of somatostatin.

Diagnosis

Diagnosis can be confirmed by a fasting plasma somatostatin level that is greater than three times the normal range with the appropriate symptoms. If the index of suspicion is high and plasma levels of somatostatin return within the normal range, a stimulatory or inhibitory test also can be performed to measure plasma values. Somatostatinomas are malignant in 60% to 70% of cases, with tumor size greater than 2 cm as a predictive factor of metastatic spread.

Treatment

As with other rare PNETs, 70% of pancreatic somatostatinomas have metastasized to regional lymph nodes or the liver at the time of diagnosis. Treatment depends on size, location, and the extent of disease at presentation. Complete surgical resection is ideal but often not possible; therefore tumor debulking, chemoembolization of the primary tumor as well as metastatic lesions, and chemotherapy have all been used to temper clinical symptoms.

Other Functional Tumors

Rare tumors can result in paraneoplastic syndromes such as those that produce ectopic adrenocorticotropic hormone (ACTH) or parathyroid hormone–related peptide. Diagnosis is made by the presence of a PNET on imaging with an appropriately elevated serum hormone level. These tumors may be difficult to diagnose because of the intermittent nature of hormone release resulting in fluctuating plasma levels and have a corresponding unusual clinical presentation of symptoms. Therefore these tumors are typically quite large at discovery. Curative surgery is always recommended when possible and requires pancreatic resection with lymphadenectomy because of the high rate of lymph node metastasis with these tumors. Somatostatin analogues also may be used to improve clinical symptoms.

■ NONFUNCTIONAL TUMORS

Up to 40% of PNETs do not have clinical symptoms of hormonal hypersecretion; however, this does not mean they do not produce any hormones. These tumors may produce but not secrete hormones, produce clinically inert hormones such as pancreatic polypeptide (PP), or secrete hormones in too low a concentration to induce symptoms. Because of their silent growth, they often appear as an asymptomatic abdominal mass or, if the tumor has grown large enough, with symptoms of compression or invasion of adjacent organs. Most commonly, patients will have abdominal pain, anorexia, jaundice, or weight loss. Improvements in cross-sectional imaging have decreased the mean tumor diameter over the last several decades, with more tumors being found incidentally. Nevertheless, the incidence of liver metastasis at initial diagnosis still ranges from 60% to 85%. Diagnosis of nonfunctional PNET can be made by the presence of a pancreatic mass in patients without hormonal symptoms, with an elevated CGA or PP level or a positive somatostatin receptor scan. CGA, when elevated in nonfunctional tumors, can be helpful in determining response to therapy and in surveillance of patients with liver metastasis.

The median overall survival of patients with nonfunctional PNETs is 38 months, with a 5-year survival rate of 43%. The most powerful predictors of poor prognosis are degree of tumor differentiation and presence of distant metastasis.

■ MANAGEMENT

In those with limited disease, resection remains the primary method of achieving cure. Those with advanced disease and a large tumor burden also may undergo cytoreductive surgery for palliation purposes. Surgical resection of regional and distant metastatic disease with or without cytoreductive intent also has been shown to provide symptom control and extend survival, although there are currently no prospective data to support this in PNETs.

■ TREATMENTS

Surgical Approaches

The primary method of cure in PNETs is surgery. However, because a large percentage of patients have either lymph node or liver metastasis, this presents a major limitation for surgical resection. Nevertheless, Hill and colleagues performed a national study of PNETs that revealed surgical resection was associated with improved survival across all stages of disease.

Localized

Surgery is the cornerstone of treatment for small, localized, malignant tumors with the goal of approximately 2-cm margins to achieve an R0 (negative margins) resection. Regional lymphadenectomy is also recommended, especially for nonfunctional PNETs. Most PNETs that are smaller than 2 cm can be treated by enucleation or local resection, with more advanced pancreatic surgery reserved for carefully selected patients (Figure 4). Except for sporadic insulinomas, which are rarely malignant, the majority of these operations are approached by laparotomy to appropriately explore the abdomen and regional lymph nodes.

Metastatic

The prognosis of metastatic PNETs depends on histologic grade. When possible, the primary tumor and corresponding lymph nodes are surgically removed. There are some single-center data to support the use of cytoreductive surgery when the metastasis is localized or if more than 90% of the tumor load is resectable, to both improve hormonal control and increase survival in metastatic PNETs. However, this type of resection is possible in only about 10% of patients, with a high tumor recurrence rate up to 76%. Resection of the primary pancreatic tumor despite metastatic spread also may be warranted in nonfunctional tumors to prevent life-threatening acute pancreatitis and obstructive complications.

More than 50% of PNETs have hepatic metastasis at the time of diagnosis. Many patients with PNETs undergoing treatment for liver metastasis will be given somatostatin analogues. If an abdominal exploration is planned, cholecystectomy also should be performed, as cholelithiasis is a common side effect of somatostatin therapy.

Local-regional methods such as hepatic arterial embolization and chemoembolization have been used as palliative measures in patients with liver metastasis who are not candidates for resection. Radiofrequency ablation (RFA) also can be used, either in conjunction with cytoreductive surgery or alone. RFA is limited to patients with unresectable metastatic disease 5 to 7 cm in diameter. Laparoscopic RFA can be used when there are fewer than 10 liver lesions and the largest tumor is ideally smaller than 3 cm, although the procedure can be used with tumors up to 5 cm in diameter. This results in symptom control in more than 90% of patients with malignant PNETs. Radioembolization with yttrium-90 microspheres is another approach to hepatic metastasis and shows promise, but definitive data are currently lacking.

Because most PNETs overexpress somatostatin, peptide receptor radionuclide therapy (PRRT) using labeled octreotide also has been investigated widely. The best objective partial response reported has ranged from 9% to 29%, with complete response in 2% to 6% of patients. Although currently approved in some European countries, this treatment is still under investigation in the United States.

There also has been discussion regarding the consideration of liver transplantation in patients with metastatic PNETs. Patients must be without extrahepatic metastasis, ideally have a tumor with a low proliferation rate, and have failed all other therapeutic options. Most transplanted patients will recur, however, either from

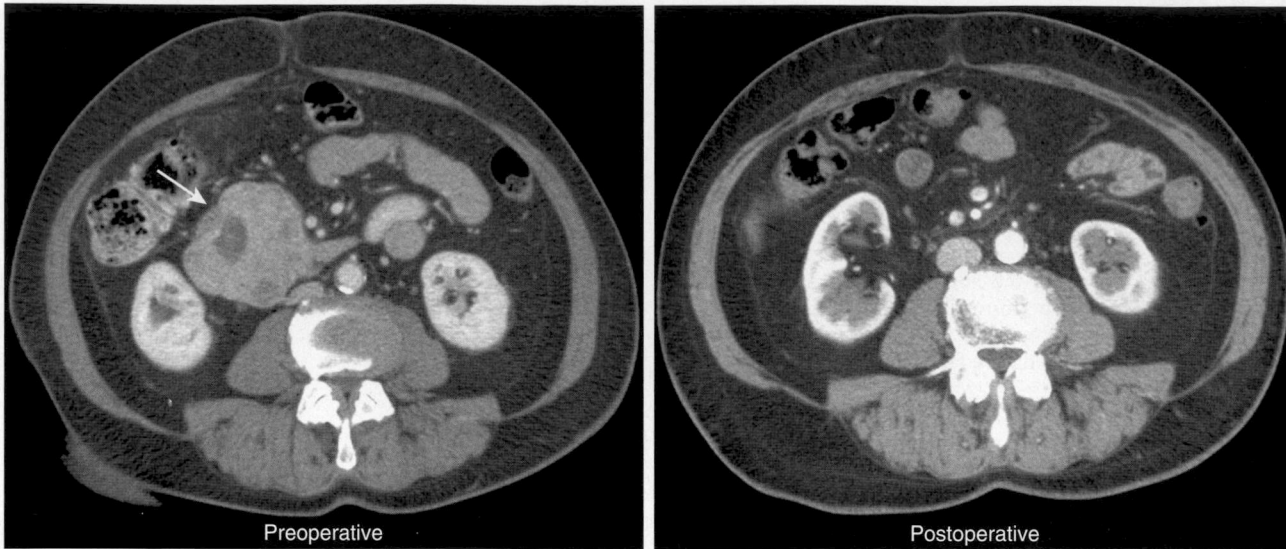

FIGURE 4 Axial computed tomography images of a well-differentiated neuroendocrine tumor (*arrow*) located in the head of the pancreas. The patient underwent successful pancreaticoduodenectomy. *(Courtesy Dr. Clifford Cho.)*

postoperative immunosuppression or from undiagnosed extrahepatic disease that existed before transplantation.

Nonoperative Approach

Small nonfunctional PNETs increasingly are being found incidentally with improvements in cross-sectional imaging, A retrospective analysis by Lee and colleagues examined patients with nonfunctional PNETs smaller than 2 cm without suspicious features who did not undergo surgery. The study reported minimal or no growth over an average follow-up period of 3 to 4 years. When weighed against the potential complications of pancreatic surgery, nonoperative management may be beneficial for this cohort. Tumor size, however, has not been a consistent independent prognostic indicator in PNETs, and large, prospective data with adequate long-term follow-up are still needed to validate this approach.

Systemic Treatments

Currently available treatments can prolong survival but do not cure metastatic disease. The goals of medical treatment for PNETs are to palliate symptoms and suppress tumor growth and spread.

Symptomatic Treatments

Somatostatin analogues, most commonly octreotide, remain the primary agent of choice to treat the symptoms of functional PNETs. Analogues have longer half-lives, without the rebound hypersecretion of hormones that occurs after native somatostatin injection, and come in both short-acting and long-acting formulations. Common side effects of somatostatin analogues include nausea, abdominal cramping, diarrhea, and injection site pain. These agents are overall well tolerated and safe and result in relief of symptoms in about 75% of patients. Because of their potent ability to control clinical symptoms, somatostatin analogues may continue to be given despite tumor progression. The duration of somatostatin analogue treatment continues indefinitely until there is a total loss of symptom control or the development of intolerable side effects. They previously have demonstrated a limited antitumor effect, with approximately 30% of patients showing disease stability and fewer than 5% of patients showing radiologic tumor regression. Recently, the CLARINET trial treated patients with well-differentiated or moderately differentiated, nonfunctional, somatostatin receptor–positive neuroendocrine tumors with somatostatin analogue lanreotide versus

placebo. The study recruited patients with 3 to 6 months of stable disease before enrollment, and reported prolonged progression-free survival at 24 months of 65% in the lanreotide group versus 33% with placebo.

Interferon-α also has been used to manage symptoms of neuroendocrine tumors, though it has been less well studied than somatostatin analogues for PNETs. However, interferon has significant adverse side effects that many patients find intolerable.

Antiproliferative Treatments

Chemotherapy is recommended for advanced PNETs, as they have been shown to be more sensitive to chemotherapy than other types of neuroendocrine cancers. Streptozocin-based chemotherapy regimens have been used since the 1980s. In combination with 5-fluorouracil (5-FU) and/or doxorubicin, the regimen has an objective response rate of 35% to 40% with median response duration of 9 months. Alkylating agents, such as dacarbazine, also have been used but are limited by high toxicity rates. Recently, temozolomide, an oral alkylator, in addition to capecitabine, an oral prodrug for 5-FU, have shown synergistic apoptotic effects in vitro. Strosberg and colleagues treated 30 chemotherapy-naive patients with well-differentiated or moderately differentiated metastatic PNETs with a combination of capecitabine and temozolomide and analyzed response rate, survival, and toxicity. Using capecitabine and temozolomide as first-line therapy, the study reported a 70% objective radiographic response with a median progression-free survival of 18 months. In addition to superior response and survival rates, the study also reported decreased toxicity compared with streptozocin-based regimens. Prospective randomized data regarding the use of temozolomide for PNETs are currently in progress.

Two agents for targeted therapy have emerged recently as treatment options for advanced or nonresectable progressive PNETs. Everolimus, an oral mTOR inhibitor, was approved for the treatment of locally advanced or metastatic PNET in 2011 as a result of the RADIANT-3 study. The randomized phase III trial demonstrated progression-free survival of 11.0 months on everolimus compared with 4.6 months on placebo, with a 73% crossover from the placebo to the everolimus group. However, the overall tumor response rate to everolimus was only 4%. Another randomized phase III clinical trial used sunitinib, an oral tyrosine kinase inhibitor, versus placebo. This trial was terminated early favoring sunitinib because of a clear progression-free survival benefit in the treatment group. This led the U.S. Food and Drug Administration (FDA), citing progression-free survival of 10.2 months in the treatment group versus 5.4 months in the placebo group, to approve sunitinib for use in progressive, well-differentiated neuroendocrine tumors in May 2011. Sunitinib had an overall objective response of 9%.

Because of the low response rates from monotherapy, a recently completed phase I/II study treated patients with temozolomide and everolimus. The results showed an acceptable safety profile as well as encouraging progression-free survival data. With improved understanding of the molecular pathways that result in PNETs, discovery of novel molecular targets and new combinations of therapy are paving the way for improved treatment options for this rare malignancy.

SUGGESTED READINGS

Caplin ME, Pavel M, Ruszniewski P. Lanreotide in metastatic enteropancreatic neuroendocrine tumors. *N Engl J Med.* 2014;371:1556-1557.

Carter Y, Jaskula-Sztul R, Chen H, et al. Signaling pathways as specific pharmacologic targets for neuroendocrine tumor therapy: RET, PI3K, MEK, growth factors, and Notch. *Neuroendocrinology.* 2013;97:57-66.

Hill JS, McPhee JT, McDade TP, et al. Pancreatic neuroendocrine tumors: the impact of surgical resection on survival. *Cancer.* 2009;115:741-751.

Kunz PL, Reidy-Lagunes D, Anthony LB, et al. Consensus guidelines for the management and treatment of neuroendocrine tumors. *Pancreas.* 2013;42(4):557-577.

Raymond E, Dahan L, Raoul JL, et al. Sunitinib malate for the treatment of pancreatic neuroendocrine tumors. *N Engl J Med.* 2011;364:501-513.

Strosberg JR, Fine RL, Choi J, et al. First-line chemotherapy with capecitabine and temozolomide in patients with metastatic pancreatic endocrine carcinomas. *Cancer.* 2011;117:268-275.

Yao JC, Shah MH, Ito T, et al. Everolimus for advanced pancreatic neuroendocrine tumors. *N Engl J Med.* 2011;364:514-523.

TRANSPLANTATION OF THE PANCREAS

Joseph K. Melancon, MD, and Jay A. Graham, MD

■ HISTORY

The origin of the pancreas transplant, like all solid organ transplantation, may be traced to the celebrated experimental surgeon Alexis Carrel, who was the first surgeon to properly execute the fine suturing techniques required for small vessel anastomosis. Carrel's genius centered on lack of vascular endothelial injury by avoiding the manual manipulation of blood vessels and instead tethering these vessels at triangulated anchors with fine ligatures before creating carefully sutured anastomosis. Legions of vascular surgeons have used this tried and true method of vascular anastomosis, and organ transplantation would have been impossible without the technique. In his small surgical laboratory in Lyon, France, at the turn of the twentieth century, Alexis Carrel transplanted any sort of canine organ from which he believed he could isolate reliably a dominant artery and vein; this included kidneys, spleens, ovaries, uteri, pancreata, and testes. Carrel even theorized correctly that his transplanted tissues failed only after achieving adequate blood supply because of a humoral process that was wholly separate from the technical feat of surgical organ transplantation.

Clinical pancreas transplantation began at the University of Minnesota in 1966 when Kelly and Lillihei performed a simultaneous kidney and pancreas transplantation in a young lady with type 1 diabetes and end-stage renal disease. The success of that operation ultimately compelled many other intrepid surgeons to offer pancreas transplants to their patients with diabetes. Although early attempts at pancreas transplantation often encountered many technical difficulties, chief among the clinical conundrums was how to adequately deal with the copious exocrine secretions that flowed through a graft duodenum that often had compromised blood supply. The other main technical problem was sluggish blood flow into and out of an organ that seemed especially prone to graft thrombosis. The pancreaticoduodenal graft also proved much more immunogenic than all other solid organ transplants, and therefore graft loss secondary to acute rejection was much more common. Throughout the 1980s and 1990s David Sutherland and his team at the University of Minnesota showed dogged determination in quelling the leviathan that seemed to work against making pancreas transplantation a successful clinical

exercise. Incremental technical improvements all built upon Carrel's simple caveat of minimal manipulation of vascular grafts, and avoidance of enteric activation of pancreatic enzymes by adopting Sollinger's technique of bladder drainage of exocrine effluent. Improved immunosuppressive therapies such as cyclosporine and then tacrolimus, as well as antiviral therapies that tamed the deadly cytomegaloviral infections, were also key advances to make pancreas transplantation successful.

■ PATIENT SELECTION

Pancreas transplantation is indicated for patients with diabetes who have had progressive signs of tissue injury under appropriate medical management. Patients with brittle diabetes who develop retinopathy, neuropathy, and/or gastroparesis/enteroparesis are candidates for pancreas transplantation. Progressive autonomic dysfunction is a hallmark of rampageous diabetic small vessel disease that manifests most dangerously in patients who exhibit hypoglycemic unawareness, a telltale sign that alone qualifies a patient for pancreas transplantation because of its high mortality and recalcitrance to exogenous insulin therapy. The main indication for pancreas transplantation is diabetic nephropathy, and therefore the most common type of pancreas transplant is a simultaneous kidney and pancreas transplantation; performed in patients with diabetes and end-stage renal disease. Although most patients with diabetes who require pancreas transplants are type 1, either type 1 or type 2 patients can qualify for pancreas transplantation, as long as the patients are not obese and are younger than age 55.

■ TYPES OF PANCREAS TRANSPLANTATION

Beta cell replacement therapy can proceed via five different surgical therapies:

1. Simultaneous kidney and pancreas transplant
2. Pancreas after kidney transplant
3. Pancreas alone transplant
4. Alloislet transplant
5. Autoislet transplant

The most successful type of beta cell replacement therapy is via a solid-organ pancreas transplant, typically with a kidney transplant. Pancreas after kidney transplantation and pancreas-alone transplants are performed more rarely but also can be performed with great success. Alloislet transplantation in the United States currently is performed only under experimental protocols at only a few licensed centers. The results of alloislet transplantation are not nearly as good as solid organ transplantation. Autoislet transplants are really an adjunct treatment for chronic pancreatitis, in which a patient's own islet cells are isolated from the surgically removed pancreatic gland and then inserted via the portal vein into the patient's liver. Autoislet transplants are much more successful than alloislet transplants because no immune response is elicited by the autologous tissue.

■ PANCREAS PROCUREMENT

A careful extrication of the pancreas during procurement must occur to ensure success of pancreas transplantation. In the initial dissection, which occurs during the warm phase, the pancreas gland is surveyed and palpated after opening the lesser sac to determine the suppleness of the gland and to make sure no signs of pancreatitis are present. Only young (younger than 50 years) and relatively thin (body mass index, BMI < 30) organ donors are considered ideal pancreas donors, and a pancreas from an ideal donor should be pink and soft throughout the gland with no firm nodules. During the initial dissection the splenic and superior mesenteric arteries are dissected circumferentially about and doubly looped with vessel ties that can be tightened later so that the infusion of preservation fluid in the cold phase can be minimized (<3 L) to prevent gland edema. When the cold phase begins after aortic cross-clamp and reverse perfusion of iced preservation fluid ensues, it is imperative to place copious amounts of ice directly upon the pancreas (anterior and posterior) to prevent any undue warming of the ischemic gland, which can lead to pancreatitis after transplantation. The duodenum is stapled proximally just distal to the pylorus and distally at the ligament of Treitz. The small bowel mesentery is stapled across with a large vascular TA stapling device. The splenic artery is cut and tagged at its origin on the common hepatic artery, and the superior mesenteric artery is cut at the aorta. The portal vein is cut halfway between the liver and the pancreas, and the gastroduodenal artery is simply ligated at its source. The gland is removed quickly with the spleen attached and placed directly into iced preservation fluid.

■ PANCREAS TRANSPLANTATION BACK TABLE

The hallmark of an uneventful pancreas transplant begins with the back table of the allograft. This is an operation that usually takes about 1½ to 2 hours to complete. Speed is not rewarded during this part of the procedure; rather a meticulous adherence to surgical technique is required. Moreover, because the back table of the organ takes place in 4° C University of Wisconsin (UW) solution, speed is relevant.

The stepwise back table of the pancreas organ includes the following:

- Arterial reconstruction
- Venous outflow management
- Duodenal C loop calibration
- Splenectomy
- Ligation of peripancreatic vascular branches

Arterial Reconstruction

Arterial reconstruction is paramount to successful graft inflow and viability. Moreover, complex revascularization is required because of the requisite technique of pancreas procurement. Given that liver is procured almost universally at the same time, standard procedure accepts that the celiac artery and distribution are kept in continuity for the hepatic allograft.

As such, the splenic artery and gastroduodenal artery (GDA) are divided to free the pancreas from the liver. Notably, the head of the pancreas and C loop of the duodenum are fed by a collateral network of superior and inferior pancreaticoduodenal arteries. Expectantly, the superior pancreaticoduodenal arteries (anterior and posterior)

descend from the GDA and the inferior pancreaticoduodenal arteries (anterior and posterior) *ascend* from the superior mesenteric artery (SMA). This dual organ blood supply from the foregut and midgut is unique to the pancreas and requires a creative approach to ensure adequate inline arterial flow.

The *Y-graft* is the solution to account for the dual blood supply. Y-grafts generally refer to the common iliac artery with bifurcation into the external and internal iliac artery. These arteries are removed delicately at the time of procurement. The brachiocephalic trunk and right subclavian and right common carotid artery also can be used as a Y-graft when confronted with hostile or diminutive iliac vasculature.

The Y-graft facilitates anastomosis to the splenic artery and SMA, thereby ensuring adequate perfusion to the entire organ. It is crucial to minimize any opportunity of anastomotic stricture in both limbs. In general, the iliac Y-graft matches the caliber of the splenic artery and SMA, but the brachiocephalic trunk is the alternative option available. Most problems in pancreas transplantation arise in the tail as manifested with thrombosis. Therefore, after seating a limb of the Y-graft on the splenic artery, it is recommended to perform the anastomosis using 7-0 Prolene sutures in an interrupted fashion.

Although running versus interrupted suture has never been studied with regard to the Y-graft in pancreas transplantation, anecdotally interrupted sutures may prevent stenosis. Moreover, because much of the morbidity comes from splenic vein thrombosis, it is imperative to abrogate any barriers to unimpeded flow through the Y-graft/splenic artery anastomosis. Regarding the donor SMA, the caliber is usually larger than the splenic artery, and therefore running or interrupted sutures may be used. Commonly, a 6-0 Prolene running suture can be used to anastomose the other limb of the Y-graft to the SMA.

There can be many pitfalls in arterial reconstruction, none more damaging than creating tortuosity with generous redundancy in the two arms of the Y-graft. It is recommended to cut the two arms of the Y-graft close to the bifurcation, mindful not to create anastomotic tension, but also close enough to prevent possible twisting or kinking. The common iliac artery or brachiocephalic trunk of the Y-graft also should be kept short during implantation to prevent the aforementioned problems.

Venous Outflow Management

The venous outflow of the pancreas allograft is through the portal vein after the splenic vein and foreshortened superior mesenteric vein (SMV) meet at the confluence. During implantation, the portal vein is seated on the inferior vena cava (IVC) if the pancreas is to be placed on the right. Extension grafts usually are not required with right-sided positioning of the pancreas because of the anterior nature of the IVC. Moreover, extension grafts may promote twisting with outflow impedence, all but ensuring graft loss. Infrequently, the pancreas allograft may have to be positioned on the left side because of a prior kidney transplant on the right. Here, a venous conduit may be necessary because the left external iliac vein is the target for outflow anastomosis and this vein is posterior.

The major feeding vessel to the portal vein is the splenic vein, and it generally provides the most consternation in the postoperative period because of a heightened propensity toward thrombotic events. This is a low-flow channel because ligation of the short gastric arteries during procurement of the allograft relegates the splenic artery to the sole source of blood entering the tail of the pancreas. As such, any chance of vessel wall incursion should be minimized to prevent endothelial injury and platelet aggregation.

Duodenal C Loop Calibration

The duodenal C loop represents segments 1, 2, and 3, whereas segment 4 generally is removed before implantation. More important, attempts are made to trim segments 1 and 3. Division of the bowel distal to the pylorus and proximal to the SMA yields an appropriate-size duodenum for exocrine drainage. As such, excessive duodenum should be minimized to abrogate the risk of ischemic ulceration and blind loop bacterial overgrowth. By contrast, while the surgeon is attempting to shorten the C loop, care should be taken to not stray too far into the second portion of the duodenum, where injury to the ampulla of Vater can occur.

As the C loop usually is shortened with ligation of the small feeding vessels juxtaposed to the pancreas and a gastrointestinal stapling device, it is prudent to oversew the staple line. Remember, the entire duodenal remnant relies on blood supply from inferior pancreaticoduodenal arteries arising from the SMA as the GDA is ligated. It therefore is recommended to reinforce the staple line because of potential ischemic challenges to the cut portions of the duodenum. Lambert sutures over the staple line provide an excellent bolster because these submucosal bites may give an added layer of tissue apposition.

Splenectomy

Although reperfusion with splenectomy has been described, numerous reports have discouraged this approach because of a potential for an augmented direct immune response with the exposure of a rich donor lymphocyte source. Given this inference, splenectomy usually occurs during the back table portion of the operation. Again a vascular device is employed to ligate and divide the splenic vasculature emanating from the tail of the pancreas. Care must be taken not to include and crush the tail of the pancreas with a stapling device, because this could lead to distal tip necrosis, pancreatitis, or even postoperative pancreatic fistula. It is also prudent to oversew the staple line given the potential of bleeding.

Ligation of Peripancreatic Vascular Branches

Bleeding after reperfusion from the peripancreatic vascular branches can cause significant morbidity. Inadequate attention to ligation of the periallograft branches may result in hemorrhage that can be considerable and difficult to control. To this end, it is important to account for the GDA before implantation. An unrecognized, improperly ligated GDA can lead to significant bleeding on the undersurface of the implanted pancreas. Nevertheless aside from the usually apparent GDA, identification of potential sites of bleeding can be challenging along the pancreatic allograft because of the diminutive size of the feeding vessels.

One technique to find these small vessels is to place the pancreas allograft in ice-cold normal saline. Flushing the pancreas in normal saline with UW solution through the Y-graft with intermittent clamping of allograft portal vein may reveal sites of potential bleeding. Practically, the Y-graft is cannulated and connected to a bag of cold UW solution and placed to gravity with the portal vein clamped with a small bulldog. Given the hyperviscosity and increased density of UW solution as it relates to normal saline, one can see more easily areas of inappropriate effluent from the graft. The venous pressure should be relieved occasionally with opening of the portal vein clamp. Using this novel technique, one mimics blood flow through the pancreas and reproduces sites of possible bleeding.

■ RECIPIENT OPERATION

Bowel or Bladder Drainage

Implantation techniques of the pancreas allograft have evolved since Kelly and Lillehei performed the first pancreas transplantation in 1966. Most notably, an improved surgical approach has yielded 1-year graft survival approximating 90%. Management of the exocrine drainage of the pancreas and the challenges afforded have dictated the lessening morbidity associated with this operation.

Initial attempts at ligation or scleroses of the pancreatic duct were met with dismal results. In 1985, Dr. Sollinger introduced bladder

drainage of the exocrine secretions to offset the morbidity of the aforementioned procedures. Although this novel technique did improve upon the past experience, bladder drainage was not without its own complications. Anastomosis of the duodenal C loop of the pancreas to the bladder can cause serious morbidity and requires conversion to enteric drainage about 15% of the time. Complications of bladder drainage that require conversions are hematuria, dehydration cystitis, and metabolic derangements through severe bicarbonate loss.

One of the arguments in favor of bladder drainage centers on the greater ability to account for rejection in the pancreas allograft through surveillance of amylase in the urine. However, with better induction therapy and immunosuppression regimens, rates of rejection are extremely low and probably do not necessitate the bladder drainage technique.

Given this propensity for problems arising from directing the exocrine function of the pancreas allograft into the bladder, most centers have moved to enteric drainage. Generally, the tail of the pancreas is directed down to facilitate bowel anastomosis to the duodenal C loop as opposed to bladder drainage that orients the tail up. Although the description of a Roux limb enteric has been described, a more simplistic approach is to anastomose in a side-to-side fashion jejunum approximately 30 to 50 cm distal from the ligament of Treitz. More importantly, enteric drainage is more physiologic because the bowel is teleologically designed to manage the enzymatic and bicarbonate load of the pancreas.

Venous Drainage

Venous drainage of the pancreas can either be systemic or portal. Portal venous drainage has been championed as a strategy to minimize extreme glycemic fluctuations. Anastomosing the donor portal vein to the SMV allows the insulin to be partially metabolized by the liver. In theory, this "first pass" of insulin can reduce the hypoglycemic episodes witnessed in the perioperative period. Given that much of this hypoglycemia is dictated by the ischemia reperfusion injury and early graft recovery, these extreme variations usually resolve in the weeks after transplantation.

Support of portal venous drainage also has arisen because of the belief that there may be decreased antigen presentation as the liver downregulates the allogeneic expression on donor lymphocytes. Importantly, outcomes and rejection rates are the same between portal and systemic venous drainage pancreas transplants. As such, most centers favor systemic venous drainage as this is a technically easier approach with portal vein anastomosis to the IVC or iliac veins.

Implantation

Techniques of implantation are predicated upon facilitating the simplest surgical approach. A midline incision from the pubis extending just above the umbilicus is preferred because this provides bilateral access to the inflow and outflow vasculature. The right colon and small bowel mesentery are mobilized to visualize the IVC and iliac vessels.

Favoring enteric systemic drainage, the pancreas allograft usually is implanted on the right because of ease of venous anastomosis as the IVC is in an anterior position. The arterial anastomosis is made between the Y-graft and common iliac artery. Notably, the Y-graft common channel should be kept as short as possible to prevent twisting and is cut approximately 1 cm from the bifurcation before implantation. The tail of the pancreas is directed down to aid in bowel anastomosis of the duodenal C loop and loop of jejunum. In simultaneous pancreas kidney (SPK) the kidney is placed commonly on the left side.

In pancreas after kidney (PAK) transplant, the pancreas can be placed on the left or right. In left-sided placement it is advisable to place a venous extension graft to the donor portal vein using procured donor iliac vein. The posterior location of the left external iliac vein usually demands this necessary length on the venous outflow.

Reperfusion of the pancreas allograft should be uneventful secondary to the care taken with the back table. Nevertheless, minute branches that are bleeding may be controlled with suture ligation. After reperfusion the exocrine function resumes immediately as manifested by an expanding duodenum. Careful observation of the ballotable character of the duodenum with increased pressure as the exocrine drainage pours into this viscus may require expeditious relief. A large-bore Angiocath can be introduced in the middle of duodenal C loop (the area of the ultimate bowel anastomosis) and suction applied to relieve the pressure until ultimate preparations are made to open the duodenum.

■ FINAL CONSIDERATIONS

Transplantation of the pancreas is one of the most challenging of solid organ transplants because the gland itself can be pugnacious and intemperate. The choice of pancreas donor and recipient are the two most important decisions that must be made correctly for the transplant to be successful. It is imperative that pancreas donor and pancreas recipients are relatively thin because ample research has shown increased complications when BMI of donors and/or recipients increases over 30. The transplant procedure must be accomplished in a way that minimizes tension at the vascular anastomosis and maximizes exposure at the insertion site of the graft because torsion or twisting of the gland markedly increases thrombosis risk. Pancreas recipients usually require more immunosuppression than other solid organ transplants, including a full dose of induction immunosuppression with T-cell–depleting antibodies such as thymoglobulin (4.5 to 6 mg/kg). Perioperative anticoagulation also is required often because of the more thrombophilic nature of the pancreas graft.

SUGGESTED READINGS

Demartines N, Schiesser M, Clauien PA. An evidence-based analysis of simultaneous pancreas—kidney and pancreas transplant alone. *Am J Transplant.* 2005;5:2688-2697.

Gruessner AC, Sutherland DE. Pancreas transplant outcomes for United States (US) and non-US cases as reported to the United Network for Organ Sharing (UNOS) and the International Pancreas Transplant Registry (IPTR) as of June 2004. *Clin Transplant.* 2005;19:433-455.

McCullough KP, Keith DS, Meyer KH, Stock PG, Brayman KL, Leichtman AB. Kidney and pancreas transplantation in the United States, 1998-2007: access for patients with diabetes and end-stage renal disease. *Am J Transplant.* 2009;9:894-906.

ISLET ALLOTRANSPLANTATION FOR DIABETES

A. M. James Shapiro, MD, PhD, FRSC

The concept of islet transplantation is simple. Diabetes results from a relative or absolute lack of the hormone insulin after autoimmune beta cell destruction (type 1), defects in receptor or postreceptor signaling (type 2), or from myriad other causes, including surgically induced total pancreatectomy. Subcutaneous insulin injection as first developed by Banting and Best in 1923 is lifesaving. However, exogenous insulin fails to prevent inexorable microangiopathic end-organ complications triggered by advanced glycation end products, leading to blindness, renal failure, limb amputation, cerebrovascular accident, myocardial infarction, and shortened lifespan. Intensive insulin therapy (four to five daily injections) or insulin pump therapy improves glycemic control and markedly reduces risk of secondary complications but substantially increases risk of iatrogenic hypoglycemia. Recurrent neuroglycopenia results in hypoglycemic unawareness or "brittle" diabetes that may become disabling in up to one fifth of type 1 diabetes (T1DM) patients over time. Progress with innovative technologies, including continuous glucose sensors, low-glucose suspend insulin pumps, and a "bionic pancreas" that infuses insulin and the counter-regulatory hormone, glucagon, may reduce hypoglycemia. However, these are cumbersome and expensive, require complex adjustment, and are not universally available. All still fall short of the physiologic, moment-to-moment precise glycemic control afforded by islets in the normal pancreas. Pancreas transplantation, first established in 1966 by William Kelly and Richard Lillehei in Minnesota, has advanced substantially; portal or systemic venous drainage together with enteric exocrine drainage effectively restores near-perfect glycemic control, stabilizes and even reverses some secondary diabetic complications, but requires major surgery and lifelong immunosuppression and is associated with morbidity and occasional mortality. The tantalizing concept of transplanting only the islets of Langerhans, eliminating all risk associated with the exocrine pancreas, first was established by Walter Ballinger and Paul Lacy in St. Louis MO in 1972, when rats with chemical diabetes were cured by islet transplantation. In the following year, they showed that intrahepatic islet delivery via the portal vein was the most efficient site for diabetes reversal in rodents. Remarkably, just 1 year later in 1974, David Sutherland and John Najarian carried out the first human intraportal islet allotransplants in Minnesota under steroid and azathioprine immunosuppression.

Today, the portal venous islet implant site remains the most effective site to routinely result in prolonged insulin independence in patients with T1DM. Highly purified islets are infused under therapeutic heparinization with continuous portal pressure monitoring, essentially eliminating risk of portal venous thrombosis. Access to the portal vein is acquired safely through percutaneous transhepatic approach in interventional radiology, and ablation of the liver parenchymal access track with thrombostatic paste has eliminated risk of postprocedural bleeding in major centers. Camillo Ricordi developed the "Ricordi chamber" in 1988 to facilitate enzymatic and mechanical dissociation of the human pancreas. This technique, coupled with rapid methods to bulk-purify pancreatic digest on continuous osmotic gradients, all performed in ultra-clean room clinical good manufacturing practice (cGMP) facilities, led to reliable isolation of high-quality human islets suitable for transplantation. In 2000 the Edmonton group was the first to consistently achieve high rates of insulin independence in T1DM after islet transplantation through the combined use of potent, corticosteroid-free immunosuppression and transplantation of sufficient islet mass usually prepared from two or more human organ donors. Lifelong immunosuppression is required to prevent allograft rejection and control risk of recurrent autoimmunity.

Once just an experimental curiosity, islet transplantation has become a routine clinical procedure for patients with unstable T1DM. Currently, more than 2000 intraportal islet transplants have been carried out internationally. The University of Minnesota recently celebrated their 600th islet autotransplant procedure, and the University of Alberta in Edmonton celebrated their 500th islet allotransplant. In Canada, the United Kingdom, and several European and Australian centers, islet transplantation has become fully integrated and government funded as part of standard care. In the United States, islet allotransplantation currently is designated as experimental, but recent completion of two major trials (CIT-07 and CIT-06) by the National Institutes of Health (NIH) will likely lead to approval with biologic licensure in 2016-2017. This will have major bearing on funding and activity of islet transplantation in US sites.

■ INDICATIONS

The indications for islet allotransplantation in T1DM are summarized in Box 1. Two groups are considered: Islet Transplant Alone (ITA), in which refractory hypoglycemia and glycemic lability are the major indications, and Islet After Kidney, in which the decision process is more straightforward as patients are already fully immunosuppressed to maintain a successfully transplanted kidney. In ITA, risks of lifelong immunosuppression must be offset by individualized risk of diabetes, and patients are selected only after all reasonable attempts have been made to stabilize refractory glycemic control by optimized insulin therapy, insulin pumps, and/or frequent glycemic monitoring under supervision of an expert independent diabetologist. Objective scores (Clark, Ryan hypo score) have been established to facilitate stringent review.

A limited islet supply and need for intensive, lifelong immunosuppression are the two perceived drawbacks that presently restrict broader application of islet transplantation. The dual risks of poorly controlled diabetes and immunosuppression may be defined clearly. Those unfamiliar with transplantation often overestimate the procedural and immunosuppressive risks. Indeed, we have yet to encounter a patient death directly resultant from the procedure or from exposure to immunosuppression in 227 patients receiving 516 intraportal infusions to date in Edmonton (0 risk). Perhaps as islet transplantation becomes more routine, and immunosuppressive management more streamlined, indications will broaden to include children and also those with more stable glycemic control; the earlier successful islet transplantation is applied in the course of diabetes, the greater the potential protective impact in preventing secondary complications. Only carefully controlled trials that randomize patients with T1DM to insulin or transplantation and provide lifelong follow-up

on an intent-to-treat basis in both arms will define if and when such a balance has been met. However, funding for such trials may be unattainable.

■ TECHNICAL CONSIDERATIONS

Donor Selection and Surgical Pancreas Procurement

Selection of organ donors for islet isolation is summarized in Table 1. Donation after neurologic brain death typically is chosen for islet isolation in circumstances in which the pancreas is unsuitable for whole pancreas transplantation. More recent limited experience with the processing of pancreata for islets from deceased cardiac death donors suggests that the obligate period of additional warm ischemia sustained during withdrawal of care and cardiac arrest is not detrimental to islet isolation and clinical outcome after transplantation. Exactly how much injury can be tolerated by the human pancreas in this setting remains unknown, but we generally accept organs for processing with up to 45 minutes of warm ischemia.

The best islet yields are obtained from donors on minimal inotropic support, and the ideal islet donor overlaps with the ideal donor used for whole pancreas transplantation. Donors with higher body mass index and more fatty pancreas tend to digest easier. However, donors with underlying type 2 diabetes have defects in insulin secretion that preclude suitability for processing, thus donors with hemoglobin A1C (HbA$_{1c}$) of at least 6.5% are excluded. Until recently, islet yields from younger donors (age 18 to 30) tended to be suboptimal, reflecting increased collagen and the more fibrous nature of the younger gland. However, refinements in enzymatic choice and delivery techniques have led to marked improvement in islet yield in several of the Clinical Islet Transplant Consortium (CIT, NIH)

BOX 1: Indications for Islet Transplantation

A. Islet Transplant Alone (ITA)

Type 1 diabetes, duration > 5 years
Age > 18 years, weight < 90 kg, insulin requirement < 1.0 U/kg/day
Absence of malignancy or untreated infection
Ability to comply with immunosuppression and close follow-up
Refractory hypoglycemia or lability despite:
  a. Optimal intensive insulin or insulin pump with appropriate monitoring
  b. Supervision of a diabetologist or endocrinologist
  c. Evidence of increased risk of hypoglycemia, using objective scores:
    i. Clark Score ≥ 4
    ii. HYPO Score ≥ 1000
    iii. Lability Index (LI) ≥ 400
    iv. Combined HYPO ≥ 400 and LI ≥ 300

B. Islet After Kidney (IAK)

Type 1 diabetes, successful prior renal allograft
Ability to tolerate immunosuppression, with prednisone dose ≤ 5 mg/day
Absence of BK virus, or other active opportunistic infection
Nonsensitized (PRA < 20%)

TABLE 1: Pancreas Donor Selection Criteria

Inclusion Criteria	Exclusion Criteria
DBD	Type 1 or 2 diabetes (HbA$_{1c}$ >6.5%)
Multiorgan donor	Malignancy other than primary brain tumor
Male or female	Untreated sepsis
Age 15-75	Hepatitis B and hepatitis B core positive
Warm ischemic time < 10 min	
Cold ischemic time < 12 hours	Hepatitis C
DCD	HIV or AIDS
Controlled setting	Syphilis
Warm ischemia < 45 minutes	Viral encephalitis
Warm ischemia < 45 minutes	Creutzfeldt-Jacob disease
	Rabies
	Tuberculosis
	Sustained periods of hypotension
	Elevated serum creatinine (>3× normal)
	Abnormal liver function (>3× normal)
	Elevated serum amylase or lipase
	High-risk sexual behavior (unless NAT testing available and negative)
	History of recent IV drug use

DBD, Deceased brain death donor; *DCD,* deceased cardiac death; *NAT,* nucleic acid testing for HIV.

BOX 2: Pancreas Procurement for Islet Isolation

1. Hemodynamic stability with minimal inotropic support
2. Absence of type 1 or 2 diabetes (HbA$_{1C}$ < 6.5%)
3. Minimal pancreas handling ("use spleen as a handle")
4. Maximize arterialized blood flow before cross-clamp, keep SMA, GDA, and splenic arteries patent
5. Avoid venous congestion during cold perfusion (avoid mesenteric venous cannula)
6. Minimize warm ischemia immediately after cross-clamp: open lesser sac, pack with ice-saline slush, then submerse explanted pancreas in chilled UW or KTK solution
7. Consider direct cannulation of pancreatic duct with low volume ductal injection with 30 cc of UW or HTK solution
8. Expedite transport to minimize cold ischemia where possible (<6 hours ideally)
9. Use the experienced procurement team from the receiving islet center when possible

HbA$_{1C}$, Hemoglobin A1C; *GDA,* gastroduodenal artery; *HTK,* histidine-tryptophan-ketoglutarate solution (Custodiol Inc., Brantford Ontario); *SMA,* superior mesenteric artery; *UW,* University of Wisconsin solution (Viaspan, Bristol-Myers-Squibb NY USA).

centers. This, combined with good clinical outcomes, may have important bearing on future allocation of pancreas organs for whole organ versus islet.

Surgical removal of the human pancreas from an organ donor for islet isolation requires similar meticulous care as that used for whole pancreas transplantation (Box 2). The pancreatic capsule must be maintained intact, and the duodenum and spleen are resected en bloc, to facilitate pancreatic cannulation and enzymatic distension when the pancreas arrives in the cGMP islet isolation laboratory. The cost of pancreatic acquisition in the United States varies up to $44,000, and the additional costs of islet processing are estimated at a further $25,000. The consequences of a failed islet isolation are therefore substantial, and much of this is within direct control of the surgical procurement team. Pancreas preservation in "intracellular" University of Wisconsin (UW) or "extracellular" histidine ketogluta-rate (HTK) solution appears to provide equivalent islet isolation outcomes. A switch in Canada from UW to HTK led to an increase in isolation success from 40% to 70%, at least suggesting that HTK is not detrimental and may indeed be beneficial.

Minimal pancreatic handling and use of the spleen as a "handle" is the optimal surgical approach. The lesser sac is opened, the anterior pancreatic capsule inspected for signs of trauma, pancreatitis, or tumor, and the duodenum is Kocherized, then staple-transected beyond the pylorus and again beyond the second part. The splenic artery is controlled with a vessel loop. A replaced right hepatic artery should not be a contraindication to pancreas procurement, and a superior mesenteric artery (SMA) vascular pedicle is not required for islet isolation. The gastroduodenal artery (GDA) is left patent until after cross-clamp then ligated and divided. Systemic heparinization is initiated with 500 units per kg donor weight, and after 3 minutes of circulation, and once teams are ready, the distal aorta is cannulated, proximally cross-clamped, and the abdominal organs are flushed with 4 to 6 L of chilled UW or HTK solution. Immediately after aortic cannulation and cross-clamp, iced slush-saline is packed behind and in front of the pancreas to facilitate rapid cooling. Once the distal common bile duct and distal portal vein are divided, the SMA and splenic arteries are transected, the pancreas may be removed first from the field and placed in chilled preservation solution on the back table in preparation for packaging and transport. This actually facilitates the completion of the dissection of the hepatic vasculature and optimizes visualization and protection of a replaced right hepatic artery.

Human islet cell isolation

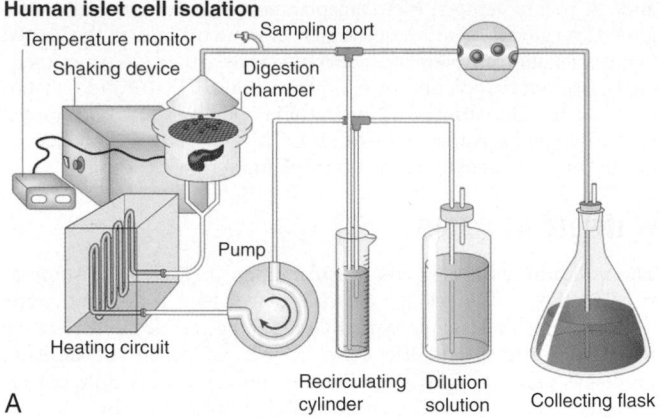

Purification of islets by density-gradient separation

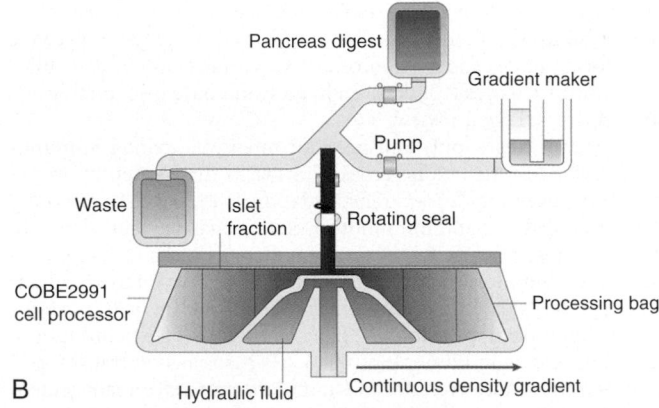

FIGURE 1 Schematic of Ricordi digestion chamber circuit for processing of the human pancreas for islet isolation in the cGMP isolation laboratory. **A,** Human islet cell isolation. **B,** Purification of islets by continuous density gradient centrifugation on a COBE 2991 cell apheresis system (adapted from Ricordi with permission). *(From Ricordi C, Strom TB. Clinical islet transplantation: advances and immunological challenges. Nat Rev Immunol. 2004;4:259-268.)*

Islet Isolation, Purification, and Culture

Once the pancreas is received in the cGMP isolation facility, it is surface-decontaminated, the duodenum and spleen removed, and the pancreatic duct is cannulated in antegrade and retrograde fashion at the level of the pancreatic body, then perfused for 10 minutes with recirculating cold collagenase enzyme (4°C to 10°C), then warmed for 4 minutes to 37°C (islet isolation schematic Figure 1). The pancreas is then transected into nine pieces and transferred to the Ricordi chamber (Figure 2). Here, enzymatic collagenase solution is circulated for approximately 10 to 15 minutes at 37°C with the pancreatic fragments gently shaken against a 500-μm mesh screen, facilitated by the presence of hollow steel marbles. Traditionally glass toy marbles were used, but theoretical risk of glass splinter led to their replacement. Samples of the circulating pancreatic digest are taken at frequent intervals, stained with dithizone dye to stain the intraislet zinc a deep red-orange, and once islets are liberated, the circuit is cooled rapidly, quenched with albumin solution to bind collagenase, and diluted to halt the digestion process. Expert judgment is required to determine when to halt digestion because both premature or late dilution results in inadequate fragment digestion or intact islet disintegration, resulting in isolation failure.

An inability to extract large numbers of high-quality human islets represented a formidable challenge in the 1970s and 1980s and precluded success in early clinical transplant attempts. The "automated method" was developed initially by Camillo Ricordi working in Paul

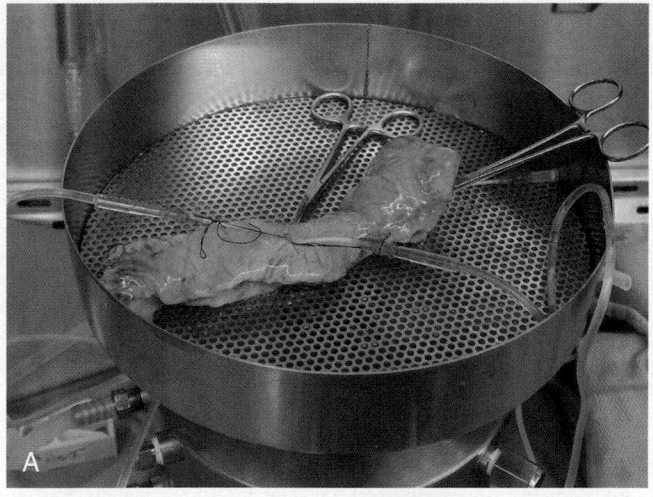

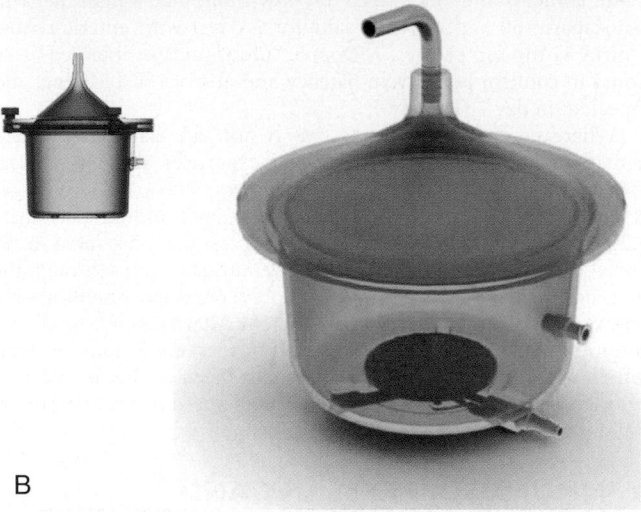

B

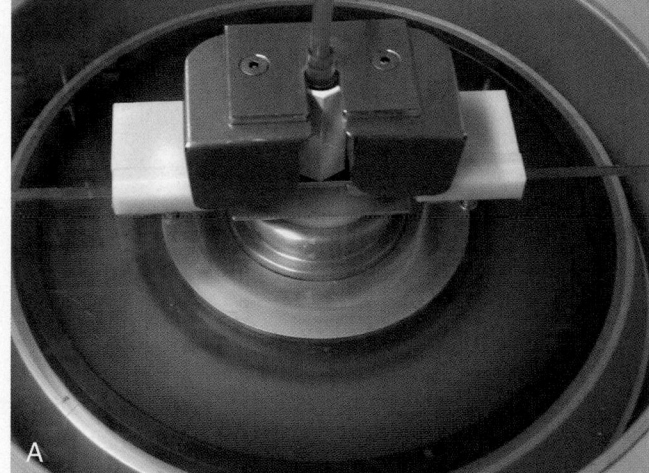

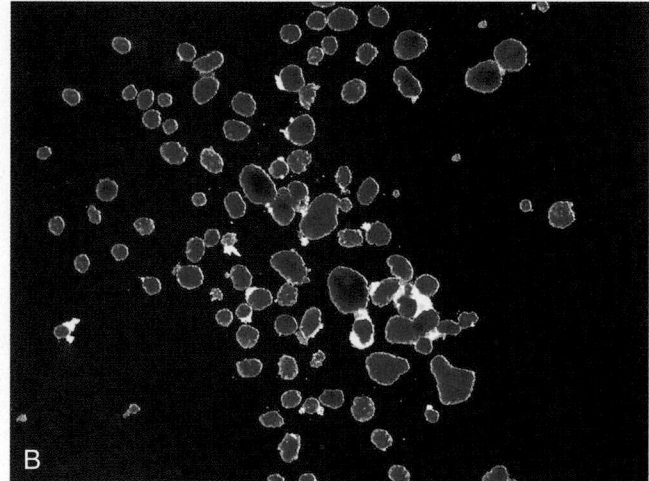

B

FIGURE 2 A, Perfusion of the human pancreas after dissection of the duodenum and spleen, and retrograde and antegrade cannulation of the pancreatic duct in the midpancreatic body. **B,** Schematic and photograph if a disposable Ricordi chamber used routinely for the digestion phase in human islet isolation (adapted from Ricordi with permission). *(A, Photo credit Doug O'Gorman and Dr. Tatsuya Kin, Clinical Islet Isolation Laboratory, University of Alberta—with permission. B, From Ricordi C, Strom TB. Clinical islet transplantation: advances and immunological challenges. Nat Rev Immunol. 2004;4:259-268.)*

FIGURE 3 A, COBE 2991 cell apheresis system loaded with pancreatic digest using continuous gradient separation in iodixanol. *(Photo credit Doug O'Gorman and Dr. Tatsuya Kin, Clinical Islet Isolation Laboratory, University of Alberta, with permission.)* **B,** Final islet product (postpurification and culture) stained with dithizone. Typical islets vary in size between 50 and 500 μm.

Lacy's laboratory in St. Louis in 1986, has proven over time to be the best method for mass islet isolation from the human pancreas, and was the cornerstone of Ricordi's success in early pilot clinical trials in Pittsburgh. The process has evolved over time and has been adopted universally by all clinical islet isolation laboratories. More recent refinements include optimized collagenase enzyme blends and delivery, better purification gradients, and stringent control and record of the entire cGMP process in manufacturing facilities.

Multiple wash steps ensue, followed by purification of the digest on continuous iodixanol (Optiprep, Axis-Shield, Oslo) gradients using a specially modified COBE2991 cell apheresis system. Islets are less dense than the exocrine debris, and a 10-minute centrifugal spin on these gradients allows islet fractions to be separated (Figure 3, *A*). This process reduces a 70 to 100 g human pancreas down to 3 to 5 cc of purified islets.

After further wash steps, purified islets are cultured usually at 22° C (or in some centers at 37° C) for up to 72 hours before they are released for clinical transplantation (Figure 3, *B*). This culture period results in a 10% to 20% loss of islet mass but

further increases purification and allows islets to be transplanted in a less inflammatory state. The islets lost during culture may be compromised already and may not have survived the early post-transplant period, but this is not known with certainty. The culture period clearly facilitates patient care by allowing time for recipient travel, immunologic screening including prospective cross-match if indicated, and an opportunity to condition the recipient with anti-inflammatory and induction T-cell–depletional therapies without exposing transplanted islets to injurious circulating cytokine products. The addition of insulin, transferrin, zinc, selenium, and pyruvate to CMRL-based culture (Miami media) with addition of nicotinamide appears to further optimize islet survival in culture. Islet culture also permits islet preparations to be shipped between cGMP isolation and clinical transplant centers, concentrating skill and expertise locally and minimizing costs associated with islet isolation.

Before islets are released for intraportal infusion, the final product release criteria must be met, as detailed in Box 3. These criteria ensure safety, sterility, ABO blood type, and immunologic compatibility, minimize infectious transmission, and ensure that an adequate mass of viable islets is provided. An islet mass of at least 5000 islet equivalents (IEQ) per kilogram based on the recipient's weight generally is required for transplantation to proceed. A single donor transplant is

BOX 3: Standard Islet Product Release Criteria

Sterility

Gram stain: no bacteria
Endotoxin content: <5 EU/kg based on recipient weight
Culture: no bacteria or fungal elements (available *post hoc* after
14 days culture)

Potency

Static insulin release: stimulation index > 1.0

Volume

Packed tissue volume ≤ 5.0 cc or settled tissue volume ≤ 7.5 cc

Purity

≥30% (based on dithizone staining)

Viability

≥70% (based on membrane integrity staining with FDA/PI or
Syto green)

Minimal Islet Mass (Protocol Dependent)

≥6000 IEQ/kg for single donor protocols
≥5000 IEQ/kg for routine initial transplants
≥4000 IEQ/kg for retransplant in multiple infusion protocols

Compatibility

ABO Blood group compatibility
Negative cytotoxic crossmatch (required if PRA > 10%, or
depending on protocol)

FDA/PI, Fluorescein diacetate/propidium iodide.

much more likely to lead to insulin independence if the islet transplant mass exceeds 6000 to 7000 IEQ/kg.

The final product release criteria are a conservative, minimal threshold. A reliable, predictive potency assay is much needed to correlate more closely with clinical islet efficacy. A predictive assay has been a challenge to identify. Standard tests of dye-exclusion viability are imprecise. Insulin release during static or dynamic glucose challenge fails to predict functionality reliably in vivo. Several approaches are being developed, including a high-throughput automated perfusion system and kinetic flux imaging system for beta cell potency, oxygen consumption rate analyses, and "sentinel" transplantation of a small proportion of the human islet product in diabetic immunodeficient mice.

Intraportal Islet Transplantation in the Recipient

The portal vein is accessed most readily through the percutaneous transhepatic approach under local anesthesia in interventional radiology, which has proven to be a safe and reliable approach in experienced, high-volume centers. A combination of ultrasound and fluoroscopic guidance through right-sided access can be accomplished within approximately 20 minutes. Initial access is attained with 22-gauge Chiba needle with Seldinger guidewire upsize technique to allow an 18-gauge guidewire to be positioned in the main portal vein (Figure 4). A single-lumen 4F or 5F angiocatheter (NEFF, Cook Canada, Stouffville, Ontario) or equivalent then is positioned to lie just above the portomesenteric confluence. A portal venogram is reviewed, and baseline portal pressure documented. A "time-out" briefing is completed, confirming that all product release criteria have been met and that the correct islet preparation has been assigned to the recipient.

The final islet preparation is suspended in transplant media in a closed, sterile gravity infusion bag, and therapeutic heparin is initiated intraportally by mixing heparin 70 units per kg recipient weight in the infusion bag. Islets are infused under gravity while the portal pressure is measured intermittently throughout. An intravenous infusion of heparin at 3 units per kg per hour then is maintained and adjusted to a PTT of 60 to 80 seconds. If the baseline portal pressure exceeds 20 mm Hg, or if the portal pressure rises above 22 mm Hg during infusion, no further islets are given until the pressure normalizes. Upon completion, the portal catheter is withdrawn slowly through the hepatic parenchyma, while infusing thrombostatic paste. We prefer Avitene paste for this purpose (1 g Avitene microfibrillary collagen powder [Medchem Products, Woburn, MA]) mixed with 3 cc radio-opaque contrast + 3 cc saline). The contrast allows clear delineation of deployment as the portal catheter is withdrawn (Figure 5). The previous alternative techniques of Gelfoam plugs (Pfizer, New York, NY) or metal coils are far less reliable in our experience.

Provided there is no evidence of post-transplant bleeding, the heparin infusion is continued for 48 hours, to minimize the Instant Blood Mediated Inflammatory Reaction and improve islet engraftment. Patients are discharged on low-molecular-weight heparin (enoxaparin 30 mg SC twice daily for 7 days) with enteric-coated aspirin 81 mg for 14 days. A Doppler ultrasound is obtained at 24 hours to confirm portal vein patency and absence of bleeding, and repeated on day 7 (Figure 6).

Where percutaneous liver access is not safe (large right-sided hemangioma or lack of local radiologic expertise), an open surgical approach may be considered for portal access (<1% of cases in larger centers). This requires general anesthesia, may induce peritoneal adhesions, and potentially may make re-access for subsequent intraportal transplantation more challenging. Surgical access through the umbilicus with recanalization of the obliterated left umbilical vein may provide access to the left portal system. Alternatively, a minilaparotomy and cannulation of an omental or mesenteric allows a dual-lumen 9F Broviac-type catheter to be advanced to the main portal vein. The second channel permits continual portal pressure monitoring during islet infusion.

■ IMMUNOSUPPRESSANT AND ANTI-INFLAMMATORY MANAGEMENT

Selection of the optimum antirejection therapy is especially challenging in islet transplantation. Although an islet transplant represents a relatively miniscule allogenic cell mass, these cells are at least, if not more, susceptible to immunologic rejection compared with any solid organ graft. Solid organs become less prone to allorejection over time through immunologic "accommodation," allowing for stepwise reduction in immunosuppressant dosing after 3 to 6 months. The added immunologic threat of recurrent islet autoimmunity in T1DM implies that stepwise reduction may cross the immunologic threshold for control of autoimmunity, leading to islet destruction. Without precision tools to guide personalized medicine-type dosing, immunosuppressive targets remain a challenge for islet transplantation. The final paradox is that the very immunosuppressants most effective in preventing rejection (calcineurin inhibitors tacrolimus, cyclosporine, and corticosteroids) are each uniquely toxic to beta cells, and the least "islet-friendly" from a metabolic and islet survival perspective.

Induction Therapy

Depletional T-cell induction antibodies are favored in islet transplantation as a strong adjunctive strategy in autoimmune regulation and tolerance to autoimmunity and alloimmunity, as supported by a wealth of preclinical studies. Thymoglobulin (rabbit antithymocyte globulin, Genzyme US, Cambridge, MA) was used effectively by Bernhard Hering and the Minnesota group to facilitate single-donor islet engraftment and has been adopted as the cornerstone for the CIT consortium registration trials in islet-alone and islet-after-kidney transplantation (CIT-07 and CIT-06 trials). Thymoglobulin

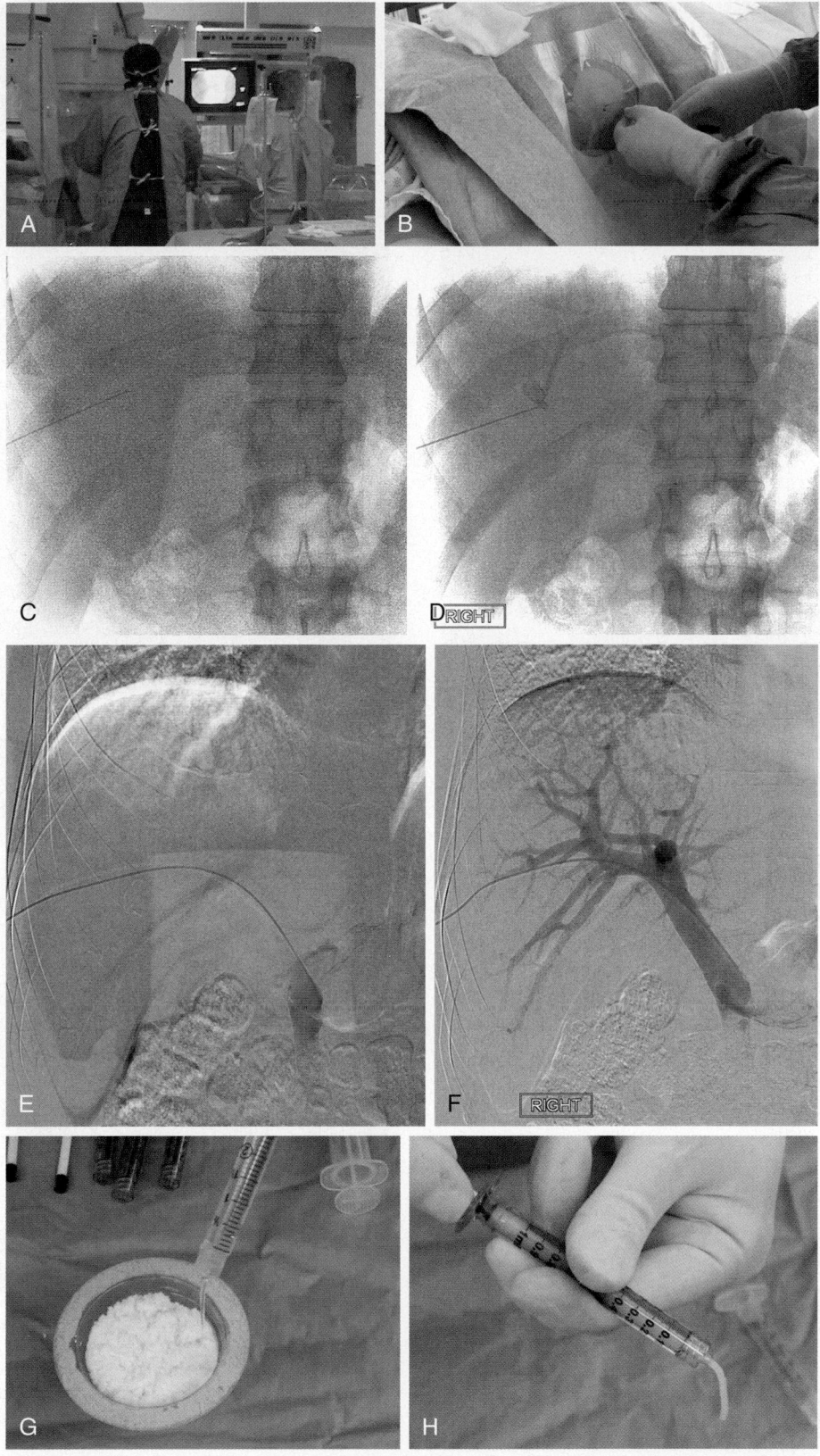

FIGURE 4 Steps involved in percutaneous portal venous access and subsequent track ablation after intraportal human islet transplantation. **A,** Modern interventional radiology suite. **B,** Local anesthesia for right sided transhepatic portal access, initially directed by Doppler ultrasound. **C,** Advancing 22G Chiba needle under fluoroscopic guidance. **D,** Access to a segment 7 portal radicle visualized by fluoroscopy. **E,** Exchange for an 18G guidewire and subsequent 4F catheter positioned at the portosplenic confluence. **F,** Portal angiogram confirming normal right and left portal tree branching pattern and satisfactory catheter position. Islets are delivered under gravity infusion with intermittent portal pressure monitoring, after therapeutic heparinization. **G,** Mixing of 1 g Avitene powder in 3 cc contrast and 3 cc saline to make a radio-opaque thrombostatic paste (**H**).

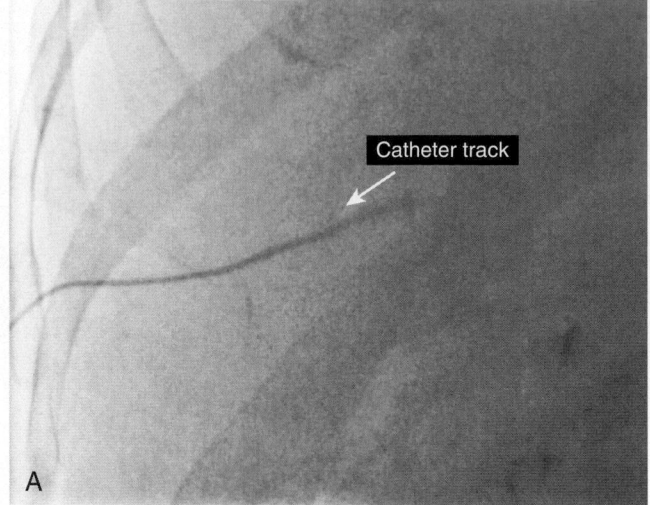

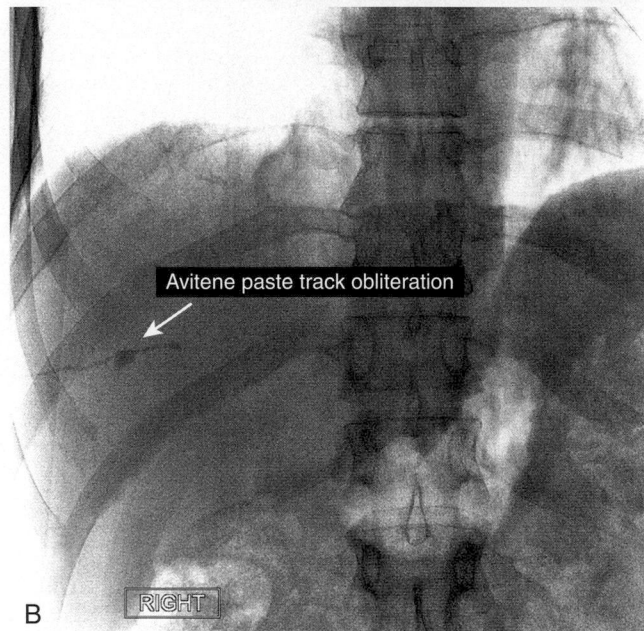

FIGURE 5 A, Contrast outline of the transhepatic parenchymal track with the catheter still in position. **B,** Deployment of Avitene paste and completion x-ray confirming effective track ablation outlined by the contrast contained in the paste.

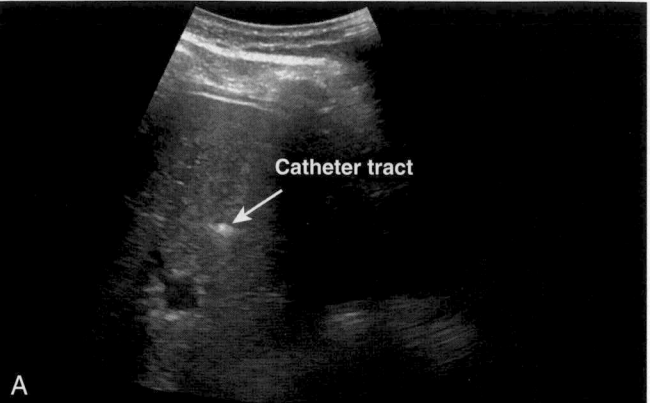

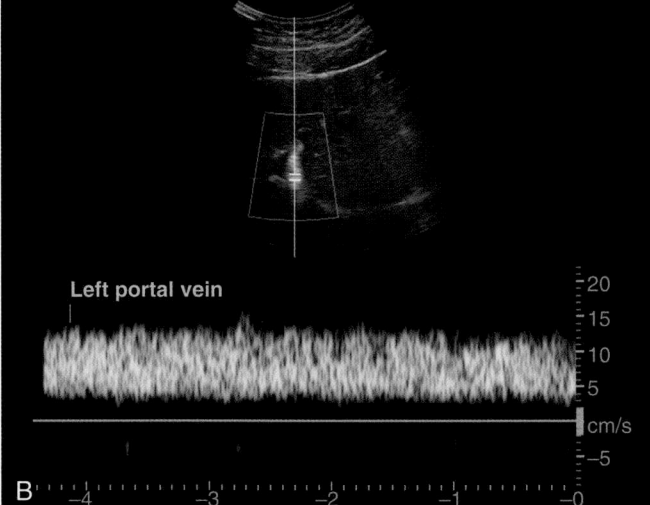

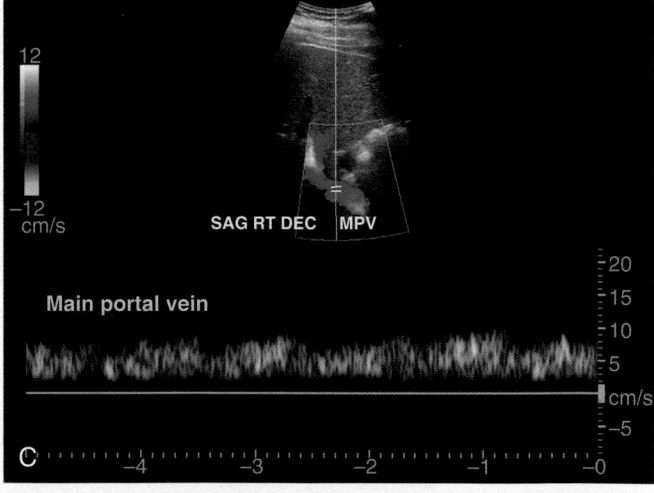

FIGURE 6 Doppler ultrasound of the liver and portal vein at 24 hours post-transplant. **A,** The catheter track and site of Avitene deployment can be visualized on ultrasound *(arrow)*. There is no free fluid and no sign of bleeding. **B,** Doppler ultrasound demonstrating normal flow within the left portal vein. **C,** Doppler ultrasound demonstrating normal flow in the right and main portal vein.

is administered by peripheral intravenous infusion in a cumulative dose of 6 mg/kg over 2 to 3 days, with the goal being to infuse at least 2 mg/kg before islet infusion while islets are maintained in culture.

Since 2002, we have favored alemtuzumab induction (Campath-1H, anti-CD52 monoclonal antibody that rapidly depletes all T cells) in Edmonton because it is cheaper than thymoglobulin, is administered over 3 hours after predosing with acetaminophen 650 mg, diphenhydramine 50 mg, and solumedrol 250 mg IV, and tends to have a more prolonged immunodepletive effect. Alemtuzumab recently has been rebranded for treatment of multiple sclerosis, which has severely limited access in some countries. We first used alemtuzumab in combination with the mTOR inhibitor sirolimus but found high rates of monocyte-mediated rejection similar to the initial experience in kidney transplantation. This issue was eliminated by switching from sirolimus to tacrolimus. Recently, detailed immune monitoring of alloimmunity with Bart Roep (Leiden) demonstrated marked IL-10 deviation, with marked suppression of CD8 autoimmunity,

suggesting that alemtuzumab provided highly synergistic protection in islet transplantation. We have found this approach to be safe and associated with low rates of opportunistic infection and malignancy.

Anti-IL2 receptor monoclonal antibodies were used in the original Edmonton Protocol patients. Although well tolerated without side effects, these agents add only marginal potency to immunosuppressive regimens and have minimal impact on T1DM autoimmunity. Basiliximab (Novartis, Hanover, NJ) is given at fixed dose of 20 mg IV on day 0 and 4. We tend to reserve basiliximab induction now for patients receiving second islet transplants under circumstances in which sustained T-cell depletion persists (absolute lymphocyte count <5% of baseline) after previous alemtuzumab.

Maintenance Therapy

The combination of high-dose sirolimus with low-dose tacrolimus was selected in the early Edmonton Protocol series to minimize exposure to calcineurin inhibitors while providing effective background immunosuppression. All of our first seven subjects were rendered insulin independent with that approach, and this garnered intense interest. We found by 3 to 5 years, however, that most patients needed to return to small amounts of insulin, and others experienced persistent side effects from sirolimus (mouth ulcers, ovarian cysts, peripheral edema, proteinuria). More recently we have stopped using sirolimus and now recommend tacrolimus (target level 10 ng/mL) and mycophenolate mofetil (1 g twice daily or less as tolerated) in combination with alemtuzumab induction. This improved our 5-year insulin independence rate to more than 50%, a level that matches outcomes to whole pancreas-alone transplantation. Furthermore, it considerably enhanced the side effect profile and improved compliance. Despite theoretical concerns regarding islet toxicity, in practice this combination has provided effective prophylaxis from rejection and recurrent autoimmunity.

The University of California San Francisco group used the combination of thymoglobulin either with maintenance costimulation blockade with belatacept (Bristol Myers Squibb, Hannover, NJ) or an antileukocyte functional antigen-1 (anti-LFA-1) antibody efalizumab to provide a unique but potent calcineurin-inhibitor free regimen with sirolimus or mycophenolate. This was well tolerated and led to high rates of single-donor islet engraftment. However, efalizumab has been withdrawn because of very low risk of progressive multifocal leukoencephalopathy in psoriasis subjects, and the ability to combine belatacept with other T-depleting therapies is being restricted by the manufacturer. Therefore an ideal calcineurin inhibitor (CNi)–free approach remains lacking for more widespread testing at present in clinical islet transplantation.

Anti-inflammatory Therapies

Bernhard Hering promoted the use of TNF-alpha blockade with etanercept (50 mg IV before transplant, then 25 mg SC on days 3, 7, and 10) in their single-donor series, and their local findings were supported additionally by analysis of Collaborative Islet Transplant Registry (CITR) data, demonstrating a profound positive impact of early TNF-alpha blockade upon late 5-year insulin independence. We further found that the combination of anti-IL1 beta receptor antibody with etanercept markedly improved human islet engraftment in mice, and we have extended that approach routinely in patients (anakinra 100 mg SC daily for 7 days).

Other Prophylactic Medications

Broad-spectrum antibiotics are given for prophylaxis before intraportal islet infusion. Valganciclovir (450 mg for 14 days, then increased to 900 mg daily for 12 weeks) is given for cytomegalovirus prophylaxis, especially when T-depletional induction is used. Sulphamethoxazole 400 mg–trimethoprim 80 mg is given daily for 6 months for *Pneumocystis jiroveci* prophylaxis. Glucagon-like peptide–1 (GLP-1) analogues have been used to improve islet function and improve single-donor success but are not well tolerated and discontinued in a third of subjects because of persistent nausea.

■ COMPLICATIONS

Procedural Risks and Consequences of Intraportal Transplantation

Compared with other solid organ transplants of heart, lung, liver, kidney, and pancreas, islet transplantation may be considered one of the safest transplant procedures, at least in expert hands. Islet transplantation involves percutaneous or occasionally open surgical access to the portal tributaries. Procedural risks include intraperitoneal bleeding and portal venous thrombosis, both of which are now avoidable if the islet preparation is purified (<5 cc packed cell volume), and therapeutic heparinization is maintained throughout and after intraportal delivery, and the catheter tract is ablated effectively (see above). The most common complication is mild pain or discomfort at the catheter insertion site, or referred to the right shoulder tip. This is generally transient, occurs in up to half of subjects, and generally resolves promptly.

With this approach, risk of portal thrombosis is exceedingly rare, and indeed we have yet to encounter complete thrombosis of the portal vein in more than 500 islet allograft infusions in Edmonton. Complete thrombosis of the entire portal system was originally one of the most feared complications of intraportal islet transplantation (first described by John Cameron in 1980), but in the current era of low-endotoxin collagenase, continuous gradient purification, routine islet culture, and protocol-driven portal pressure monitoring, this should be entirely avoidable. We occasionally have encountered small peripheral branch vein portal thrombosis on screening Doppler ultrasound in 3.7% of cases, but these are self-limiting and inconsequential. Patients with underlying thrombophilia (protein C, S, antithrombin 3 deficiency, Factor V Leiden mutation) may be at increased risk, and screening of those with a prior thrombotic history may lower risk. In long-term follow-up of more than 250 patients, some out beyond 16 years post-transplant, we have never encountered signs of portal hypertension.

Despite liberal use of therapeutic anticoagulation, bleeding from the liver puncture site is now rare (<1% at the University of Alberta). In our early experience, before track obliteration with Avitene, we found that laparoscopic evacuation of clot with direct cautery to the liver surface was a safe and effective method to manage this rare complication. Although laparoscopic control for liver bleeding usually would not be applied in the setting of liver trauma, prior knowledge of the localized site of capsular puncture mitigated need for more invasive surgical repair. Use of a small 4F to 5F catheter leaves a narrow parenchymal tract, and complete tract obliteration with Avitene thrombostatic paste for a length of at least 4 cm effectively prevents intraperitoneal bleeding. Using this technique, no subject has required blood transfusion or surgical intervention for bleeding on the most recent 250 cases in Edmonton.

Hepatic steatosis has been observed in long-term follow-up of intraportal islet autograft and allograft recipients on screening ultrasound or MRI in one fifth of cases. When identified on liver biopsy, the fat deposits are typically macrovesicular, focal, and reflect local high insulin release from functioning islets and are reversible when islets are rejected. These changes have not been associated with nonalcoholic steatohepatitis (NASH) in islet recipients and are not seen as a worrisome finding.

Concern has been raised regarding risk of hepatocellular carcinoma (HCC) in rats receiving intraportal islets after streptozotocin-induced chemical diabetes. There has yet to be a single case report of HCC or other malignant transformation in more than 2000 clinical intraportal islet infusions to date, thus this risk appears to be negligible.

Small arteriovenous fistulae may rarely be observed after percutaneous transhepatic access (risk <1%) and can be ablated safely by percutaneous hepatic arterial embolization.

■ OUTCOMES

Outcomes of islet transplantation in more than 864 islet recipients from the CITR registry and from a series of recent presentations from the leading islet transplant centers indicate substantial improvement in 5-year insulin independence. Furthermore, islet trials have demonstrated consistent and remarkable stabilization of glycemic control with sustained elimination of hypoglycemia irrespective of insulin-independent status. Four of the initial Edmonton Protocol patients currently remain insulin free, two with their original transplants, the longest free for almost 17 years currently. Six independent islet centers report 50% to 70% insulin independence rates at 5 years post-transplant (Figure 7). Implications of equivalent outcome between islet and pancreas transplantation will take time to resound among patients and the transplant community. The attraction of a simple, percutaneous cellular implant and avoidance of major surgery still must be offset by a need for more than one islet donor, a 50% failure rate during islet processing, and important, islet transplantation is not universally available. The expertise is restricted to centers with cGMP infrastructure, funding, and good outcomes (Figure 8).

■ FUTURE STEM CELL THERAPIES AND REGENERATIVE MEDICINE

Islet transplantation is currently a highly effective therapy for a limited subset of patients with T1DM complicated by severe refractory hypoglycemia. Outcomes continue to improve at an impressive pace. Immunosuppression may not be needed if scientific progress in immune tolerance induction continues in ongoing trials with tolerogenic graft facilitating cells, hematopoietic stem cells, and regulatory T-cell infusions. The acute organ donor shortage then will become the rate-limiting step in preventing further expansion of islet transplantation to patients with more stable forms of diabetes. Remarkable progress has occurred in the use of derived, expandable beta cells from potentially limitless sources. The company ViaCyte in San Diego has developed a human embryonic stem cell–derived pancreatic progenitor cell population that can be expanded routinely in vitro and further differentiated in vivo to cure diabetes in mice. Transplantation of these Cyt49 (PEC-01) cells within a macroencapsulating, immune-shielding device (Encaptra) may allow subcutaneous transplantation to proceed without need for lifelong immunosuppression. Clinical trials have been initiated to test the safety and preliminary efficacy of such an approach. Meanwhile groups in Boston (Doug Melton) and Vancouver (Tim Kieffer) are developing similar but more differentiated embryonic stem cell–derived islet-like products that shortly will also enter the clinical arena. The Nobel laureate Shinya Yamanaka and his group in Kyoto, Japan, are working on

inducible pluripotent stem cells (iPSC) derived from the patient's own skin and other expandable transdifferentiated cells. If successful, perhaps cell transplantation will be accomplished without need for immunosuppression. If such transplants are to succeed in T1DM, autoimmunity still will have to be effectively reversed by novel "immunologic reset" protocols. As these endeavors proceed, in parallel several clinical trials are moving forward to foster repair and regeneration in the injured native pancreas, which, if successful, could obviate a need for cellular transplantation entirely. What is abundantly clear is that future generations of surgeon-scientists are needed to play an ongoing pivotal role in transforming current cell transplant treatments to durable regenerative medicine cures of the future.

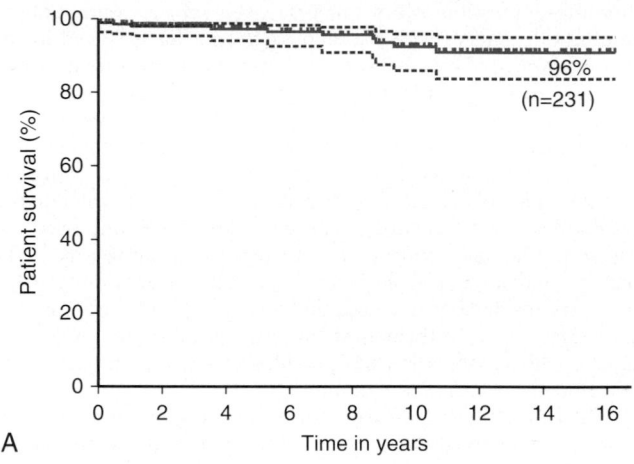

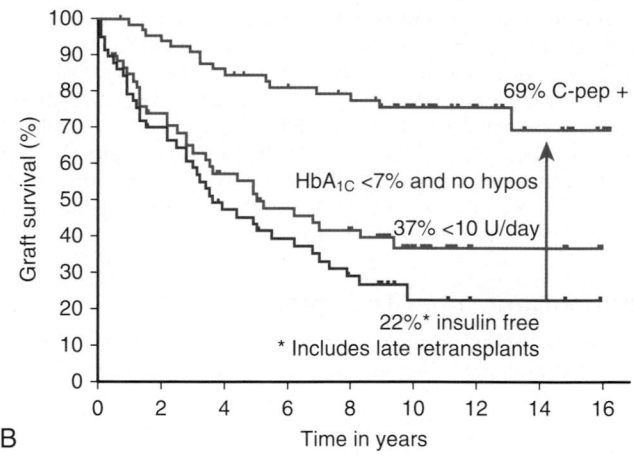

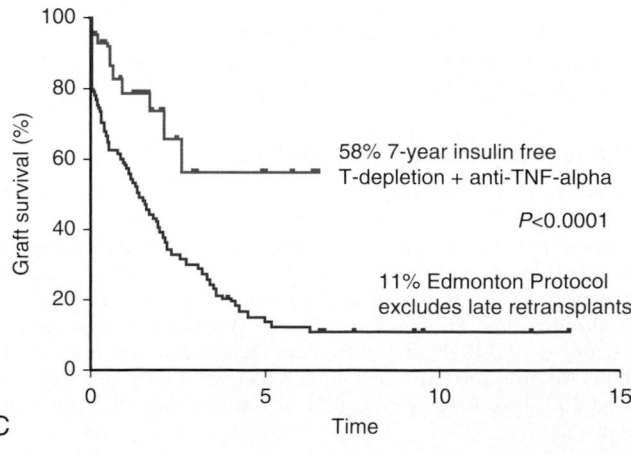

FIGURE 7 A, Sixteen-year follow-up with 96% patient survival (Kaplan-Meier) in 231 patients receiving islet allotransplants at the University of Alberta. No deaths were related to the islet implant procedure or to complications of immunosuppression. Occasional late deaths were mainly myocardial infarct related in those with longstanding diabetes (dotted red lines refer to 95% confidence interval). **B,** Islet transplant graft survival (insulin independence and C-peptide secretion by Kaplan-Meier) in the Edmonton Protocol expanded series. Twenty-two percent (lower red curve) remained insulin free beyond 16 years (including some that received late retransplants). Sixty-nine percent (upper blue curve) demonstrated persistent C-peptide secretion with either partial or full islet transplant function, sufficient to lower HbA1c below 7% and protect patients from hypoglycemia. Thirty-seven percent (middle green line) required less than 10 U insulin per day by 16 years of follow-up. **C,** Comparison of current state-of-the-art T-depletional and anti-inflammatory induction protocols where 58% remained insulin-free by 7 years post-transplant (upper blue curve), significantly better than the original Edmonton Protocol subjects excluding late retransplants (11% lower red curve, P < 0.0001).

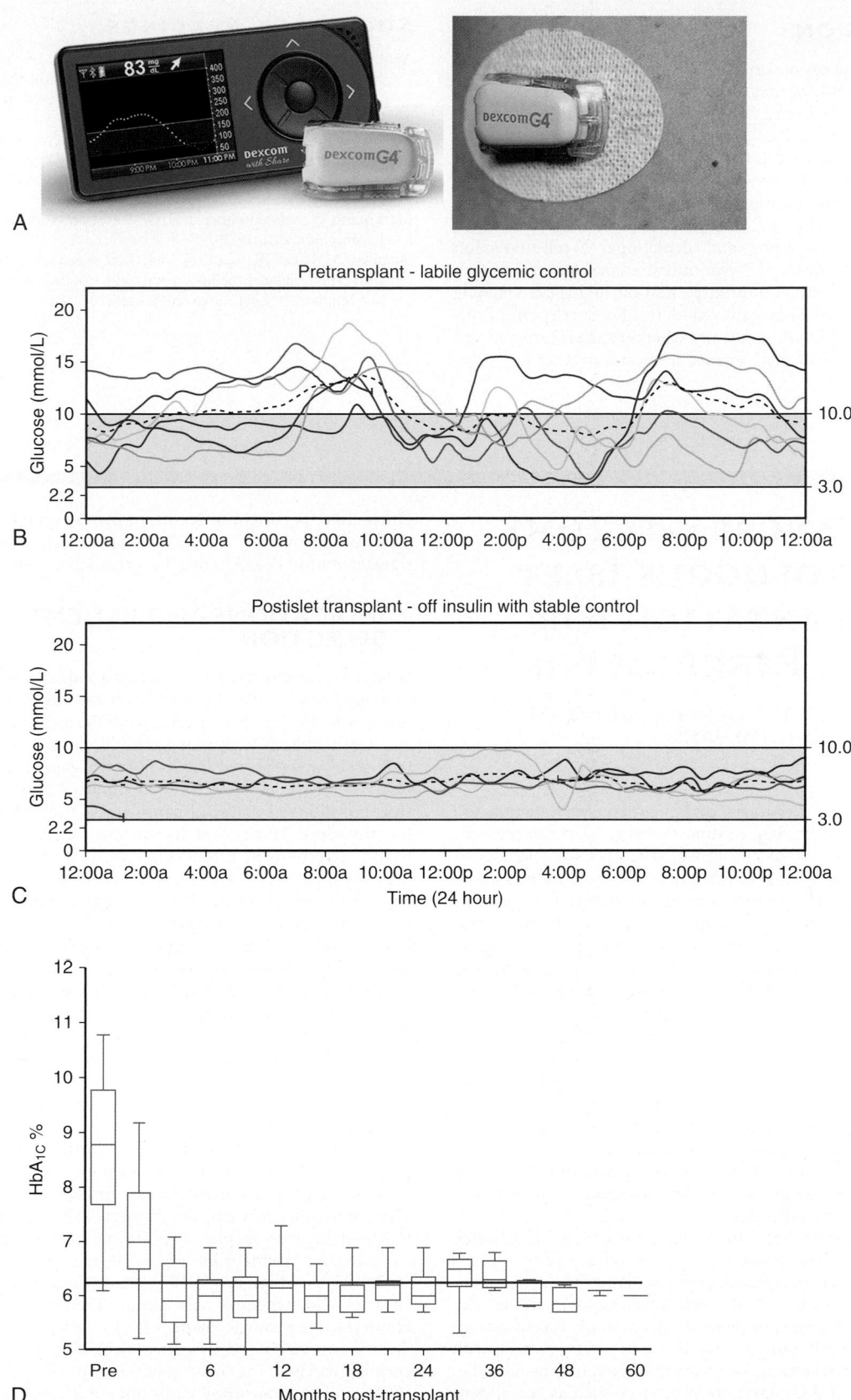

FIGURE 8 A, A continuous glucose meter (CGM) records 24-hour glycemic control protocols for hypoglycemia and hyperglycemia. **B,** CGM profiles in a typical subject selected for islet transplantation BEFORE transplant demonstrating wide fluctuations in glycemic control despite optimized insulin, with frequent hypoglycemia and hyperglycemia. **C,** CGM glucose profile in a patient AFTER islet transplantation, completely free of insulin, with normal glycemic control and full protection from hypoglycemia. **D,** Hemoglobin A1C (HbA$_{1c}$) profile before and for 5 years postislet allotransplantation in patients treated with T-depletional and anti-inflammatory induction therapy. The transverse line represents normal glycemic control (HbA$_{1c}$ <6.1%).

■ CONCLUSIONS

Remarkable progress has occurred in outcomes of clinical islet transplantation since Paul Lacy first established the concept 43 years ago. Reliable methods have been established for high-yield, high-quality purified islet isolation, and safe techniques for intraportal cell delivery developed. The Edmonton Protocol galvanized the field 16 years ago with unprecedented rates of early insulin independence using novel steroid-free immunosuppression and double transplants to provide sufficient endocrine reserve. Recent advances in anti-inflammatory anti-TNF-alpha and depletional T-cell induction therapy have further advanced 5-year outcomes in selected centers to match those of pancreas-alone transplantation in T1DM. Ongoing trials will determine whether stem cell–derived beta cells can substitute fully for human islets of today, and whether such transplants will succeed in the absence of maintenance immunosuppression.

SUGGESTED READINGS

Agulnick AD, Ambruzs DM, Moorman MA, et al. Insulin-producing endocrine cells differentiated in vitro from human embryonic stem cells function in macroencapsulation devices in vivo. *Stem Cells Transl Med.* 2015;4:1214-1222.

Barton FB, Rickels MR, Alejandro R, et al. Improvement in outcomes of clinical islet transplantation: 1999-2010. *Diabetes Care.* 2012;35:1436-1445.

Hering BJ, Bellin MD. Transplantation: sustained benefits of islet transplants for T1DM. *Nat Rev Endocrinol.* 2015;11:572-574.

Markmann JF. Isolated pancreatic islet transplantation: a coming of age. *Am J Transplant.* 2016;16:381-382.

Shapiro AM, Lakey JR, Ryan EA, et al. Islet transplantation in seven patients with type 1 diabetes mellitus using a glucocorticoid-free immunosuppressive regimen. *N Engl J Med.* 2000;343:230-238.

TOTAL PANCREATECTOMY AND AUTOLOGOUS ISLET TRANSPLANTATION FOR CHRONIC PANCREATITIS

Andrew J. Lee, MD, PhD, Piotr Witkowski, MD, PhD, and Jeffrey B. Matthews, MD, FACS

Chronic pancreatitis is characterized by progressive inflammation and parenchymal fibrosis, leading to irreversible morphologic changes, including ductal calcifications, strictures, and pseudocyst formation, as well as permanent loss of exocrine and, eventually, endocrine function. The most common associated risk factor is alcohol consumption, although the importance of genetic and hereditary factors increasingly has been recognized. Exocrine dysfunction (which is experienced by patients as steatorrhea, malabsorption, and malnutrition) can be managed by pancreatic enzyme replacement therapy. Clinically relevant endocrine dysfunction is usually not apparent until the later stages of disease and is managed by exogenous insulin. Clinically, the most troubling symptom is pain, which may be severe and unrelenting or only episodic. It is the symptom of pain that most negatively affects quality of life and leads to significant disability, including loss of employment, substance dependence, and social stigmatization. The management of pain remains challenging. Its severity does not always correlate with the extent of morphologic changes identified on imaging studies. Many patients become dependent on narcotic pain medications.

Surgical intervention for chronic pancreatitis may be indicated for patients with incapacitating pain that is refractory to medical management. A variety of operations are available for the treatment of chronic pancreatitis, and these are detailed elsewhere in this text. The choice of operation largely depends on anatomic considerations and the presumed mechanism of pain. For example, for patients with large duct disease in whom the mechanism of pain may be related to ductal obstruction, a decompressive procedure such as lateral pancreaticojejunostomy may be indicated. On the other hand, a partial pancreatic resection may be indicated for patients with a dominant inflammatory mass.

However, some patients with chronic pancreatitis or recurrent acute pancreatitis have no conventional surgical option because there is no suitable anatomic target (i.e., small duct disease, diffuse disease). Others have persistent or recurrent pain despite operative intervention. For this subset of patients, total pancreatectomy with islet autotransplantation (TPIAT) may be a reasonable option (Figure 1).

■ INDICATIONS AND PATIENT SELECTION

Total pancreatectomy (TP) for malignant disease of the pancreas was described first in 1943 by Rockey. In the 1960s a small number of series of TP for patients suffering from the intractable pain of chronic pancreatitis began to appear in the literature. Although significant pain relief was reported in a majority of patients, TP generally was reserved for the most exceptional clinical circumstances in the late stages of disease because of considerable morbidity associated with the procedure. TP removes diseased pancreatic parenchyma but also leads to the complete loss of islet cells. This results in brittle insulin-dependent pancreatogenic diabetes (type 3c). Glycemic control after TP is challenging because of the loss of glucagon-dependent counter-regulation, leading to frequent episodes of hypoglycemia and/or ketoacidosis. In addition, complete exocrine insufficiency after TP requires high-dose pancreatic enzyme supplementation.

To preserve islet cell function, Sutherland and colleagues at the University of Minnesota performed the first islet autotransplantation (IAT) in 1977. Since then, with advances in surgical techniques and improvements in islet cell preparation, a number of specialized centers have developed programs to treat patients with chronic pancreatitis by combining total, completion, or near-total pancreatectomy with IAT.

An expert panel at PancreasFest held in Pittsburgh in 2012 concluded that TPIAT is an effective treatment option for highly selected patients with severe painful chronic or recurrent acute pancreatitis. There was consensus that the primary indication for the procedure is intractable pain despite other treatment modalities and not amenable to conventional alternatives. Detailed patient selection criteria for TPIAT have been proposed by the University of Minnesota group (Box 1) and generally have been adopted by most institutions. However, morphologic changes in the pancreas such as atrophy or fibrosis can be caused by aging, alcohol intake, or diabetes. Also, chronic narcotic use may result in opioid-induced hyperalgesia (OIH) and narcotic bowel syndrome, which makes it difficult to differentiate pancreatitis from other sources of abdominal pain. Therefore patient selection for TPIAT remains challenging. TPIAT should be performed only after extensive discussion between the patient and the providers in a multidisciplinary setting.

The patients who suffer from certain forms of genetically linked chronic pancreatitis deserve special consideration for TPIAT. Gene

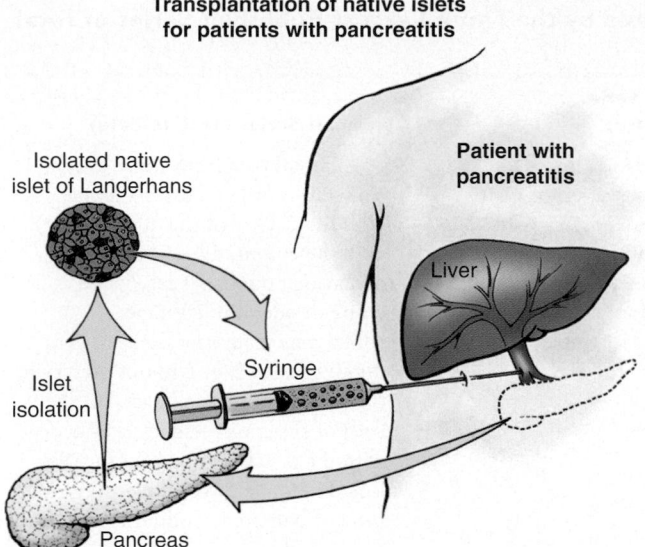

**Transplantation of native islets
for patients with pancreatitis**

Isolated native
islet of Langerhans

Islet
isolation

Pancreas

Syringe

**Patient with
pancreatitis**

Liver

FIGURE I Transplantation of islets in patients with chronic pancreatitis. *(From Witkowski P, Savari O, Matthews JB. Islet autotransplantation and total pancreatectomy. Adv Surg. 2014;48:223-233.)*

BOX 1: University of Minnesota Criteria for TPIAT*

Patient Must Fulfill Criteria Numbers 1–5:

1. Diagnosis of chronic pancreatitis, based on chronic abdominal pain of >6 mo duration and at least 1 of the following:
    - Pancreatic calcifications on computerized tomography scan
    - At least 2 of the following: ≥4/9 criteria on EUS, compatible ductal or parenchymal abnormalities on secretin MRCP; abnormal endoscopic pancreatic function tests (peak HCO_2 ≤80 mmol/L)
    - Histopathology confirmed diagnosis of chronic pancreatitis
    - Compatible clinical history and documented hereditary pancreatitis (*PRSS1* gene mutation)
    - History of recurrent acute pancreatitis (more than 1 episode of characteristic pain associated with imaging diagnostic of acute pancreatitis and/or elevated serum amylase or lipase >3 times upper limit of normal)
2. At least 1 of the following:
    - Daily narcotic dependence
    - Pain resulting in impaired quality of life, which may include: inability to attend school, recurrent hospitalizations, or inability to participate in usual, age-appropriate activities
3. Complete evaluation with no reversible cause of pancreatitis present or untreated
4. Failure to respond to maximal medical and endoscopic therapy
5. Adequate islet cell function (nondiabetic or C-peptide positive)[†]

From Bellin MD, Freeman ML, Schwarzenberg SJ, et al. Quality of life improves for pediatric patients after total pancreatectomy and islet autotransplant for chronic pancreatitis. *Clin Gastroenterol Hepatol.* 2011;9:793-799. Table 1.

EUS, Endoscopic ultrasound; *MCRP*, magnetic resonance cholangiopancreatogram.

*Criteria were implemented formally in 2008.

[†]Patients with C-peptide negative diabetes meeting criteria 1 through 4 are candidates for total pancreatectomy alone.

mutations in the cationic trypsinogen (*PRSS1*) gene, the cystic fibrosis transmembrane conductance regulator (*CFTR*), and serine protease inhibitor Kazal type 1 (*SPINK1*) all predispose carriers to recurrent acute and chronic pancreatitis. In particular, for patients with hereditary pancreatitis associated with *PRSS1* gene mutation, the lifetime risk of pancreatic cancer is approximately 40%, which represents a twenty-fivefold increased risk compared with smoking. Therefore a lower threshold for TPIAT may be reasonable in this patient population. It is important to note that TPIAT has not been studied formally as a method to reduce cancer risk. However, no pancreatic cancer has been reported in the post-TPIAT setting since the procedure's introduction nearly 40 years ago.

There are several contraindications for TPIAT. TPIAT should not be performed in patients with active alcoholism, active illicit drug use, or uncontrolled psychiatric illness that could impair compliance with complex medical management. In addition, TPIAT should not be performed in patients with C-peptide negative diabetes, type 1 diabetes, portal vein thrombosis, portal hypertension, end-stage liver disease, or high-risk cardiopulmonary disease. There are case reports, including our own report, of TPIAT being utilized in the setting of malignancy. However, because of risk of contamination of the islet prep with tumor cells and possible dissemination of malignancy, this approach is controversial and not currently recommended.

■ SURGICAL TECHNIQUE

Total Pancreatectomy

The surgical approach to total pancreatectomy varies among high-volume TPIAT centers, as summarized in Table 1. One common feature, however, is the effort to preserve the blood supply of the pancreas for as long as possible, to minimize the warm ischemia time for the islet cells. To achieve this, the gastroduodenal artery and the splenic artery and vein are preserved until just before resection. This is a crucial element of TPIAT because islet yield directly correlates with graft success rate in multiple studies.

In some centers, pancreatectomy is performed without transection of the pancreas to keep the pancreatic capsule intact and facilitate collagenase digestion of the parenchyma. However, others, including our group, feel that this prolongs the procedure and potentially increases the ischemia time. Therefore we usually divide the parenchyma at the neck of the pancreas and send the distal (left) pancreas for islet processing while we continue to complete removal of the head of the pancreas.

In initial reports, TP was performed with preservation of the duodenum in the setting of a benign disease. However, this approach was associated with increased complications, including stricture related to duodenal ischemia from disruption of the pancreaticoduodenal arcade. Today, partial duodenectomy is much more commonly performed in the setting of TP.

The spleen has important (though incompletely understood) immunologic functions, and some centers routinely strive to preserve the spleen during TPIAT. Splenic vessels are ligated near the spleen's hilum, and blood supply is preserved via the short gastric vessels. Occasionally, anatomy is favorable to enable pancreatectomy without sacrificing the splenic artery and vein. However, with splenic preservation there is a small risk of variceal transformation in the short gastric veins, which may lead to gastric bleeding. In addition, incomplete perfusion may cause painful splenomegaly in the postoperative period. For this reason, we and other groups usually prefer to perform splenectomy during TP, especially in adult patients. Greater effort to preserve the spleen in children may be warranted.

TP is most often performed by an open laparotomy, although a minimally invasive procedure using a laparoscopic and/or robotic approach recently has been described.

After removal of the pancreas, gastrointestinal continuity is restored by choledochojejunostomy and either duodenogastrostomy or gastrojejunostomy, depending on whether a pyloric preservation approach was used. The proximal jejunum usually is advanced in

TABLE 1: Comparison of the Surgical Approaches Adopted by the Three Largest Published Series of Total Pancreatectomy With Islet Autotransplantation

	Leicester Series (55 to date)	Minnesota Series (>200 to date)	Cincinnati Series (>130 to date)
Pancreatic resection and duodenectomy	Total with partial duodenectomy Pylorus preserving and preserving 4th part of duodenum Pancreas resected as a whole	Earlier series were near total with preservation of entire duodenum Past 15 years, partial duodenectomy, preserving pylorus and 4th part of duodenum Pancreas resected as a whole	For near-total pancreatectomy, a small rim (<5%) of pancreas left along with the C loop of the duodenum, with the common bile duct and pancreaticoduodenal artery and entire duodenum left intact For total pancreatectomy, partial duodenum with or without preserving the pylorus Pancreas divided at the level of superior mesenteric artery with the distal portion sent for islet isolation while dissection around the head of pancreas continues
Spleen	Spleen preserving, supplied by the short gastric vessels	Splenectomy performed unless it retains an absolutely normal appearance after hilar ligation	Routine splenectomy
Reconstruction	End-to-end duodenoduodenostomy or end-to-side duodenojejunostomy Choledochoduodenostomy	End-to-end duodenoduodenostomy or end-to-side duodenojejunostomy Choledochoduodenostomy	Not required in near-total pancreatectomy Side-to-side gastrojejunostomy or end-to-side duodenojejunostomy End-to-side hepaticojejunostomy

From Ong SL, Gravante G, Pollard CA, et al. Total pancreatectomy with islet autotransplantation: an overview. *HPB.* 2009;11:613-621. Table 2.

retrocolic fashion through the transverse mesocolon, and a biliary-enteric anastomosis is performed in an end-to-side configuration using a single layer of interrupted or continuous fine absorbable suture, depending on the diameter of the duct. An antecolic two-layered end-to-side duodenojejunostomy or Hofmeister-style gastro-jejunostomy is preferred. The abdomen is then irrigated, the viscera are covered with a single moist laparotomy pad, and the abdominal wall is covered temporarily with an occlusive iodine-impregnated transparent adhesive drape while the islet preparation proceeds. Attention is given to maintenance of core body temperature and systemic fluid balance, and a low-dose insulin infusion is initiated to keep serum glucose in the 120 to 140 mg/dL range.

Pancreas Processing

Immediately after resection of the pancreas (or, sequentially, the pancreatic body/tail portion followed by the head/uncinate portion), it is promptly removed and placed into cold preservation solution. Blood is then flushed with preservation solution via the splenic artery after opening a splenic vein. The pancreatic duct is then cannulated, allowing injection of digestion enzyme into the pancreas later on in the processing facility. The backbench preparation is complete when the duodenum and the spleen have been disconnected, and the pancreas is then packed in cold preservation solution and transported to the islet isolation laboratory. In the United States, islet isolation must be performed in a laboratory that meets all Food and Drug Administration (FDA) criteria (good manufacturing practice, or GMP) for processing human tissue.

The main goal of the islet isolation process is to disrupt the exocrine pancreas and release relatively pure islet cells into a small tissue volume that can be infused safely. Briefly, the digestion solution containing collagenase is injected into the pancreatic duct using a perfusion machine to distend the organ (Figure 2). Next, the pancreas is divided into smaller pieces and gentle mechanical dispersion is performed using the modified Ricordi method, freeing islets from the exocrine tissue. Upon completion of the digestion process, the cell

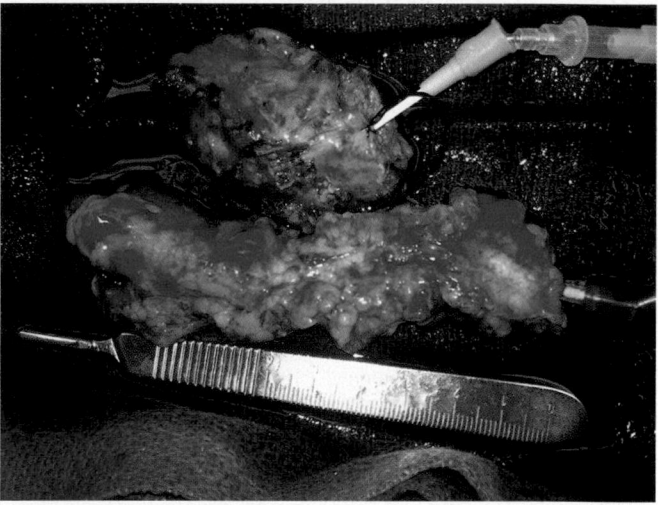

FIGURE 2 Total pancreatectomy specimen (a head and a body with tail) from a patient with chronic pancreatitis. The pancreatic duct is cannulated with an angiocatheter, allowing for subsequent perfusion with collagenase and organ digestion. *(From Witkowski P, Savari O, Matthews JB. Islet autotransplantation and total pancreatectomy. Adv Surg. 2014;48:223-233.)*

pellet is collected, islet cells are assessed for viability and counted under a microscope, and islet mass is expressed as islet equivalents (IEQs) (Figure 3). The cell pellet is also tested for endotoxin content, and Gram stain is performed to determine sterility. In the setting of islet autotransplantation, it is not unusual for there to be microscopic and culture evidence of bacterial contamination, given that the patient often has undergone multiple medical, endoscopic, and/or surgical interventions, such as gastric antisecretory therapy, sphincterotomy, or anastomosis. It is our practice to avoid extended

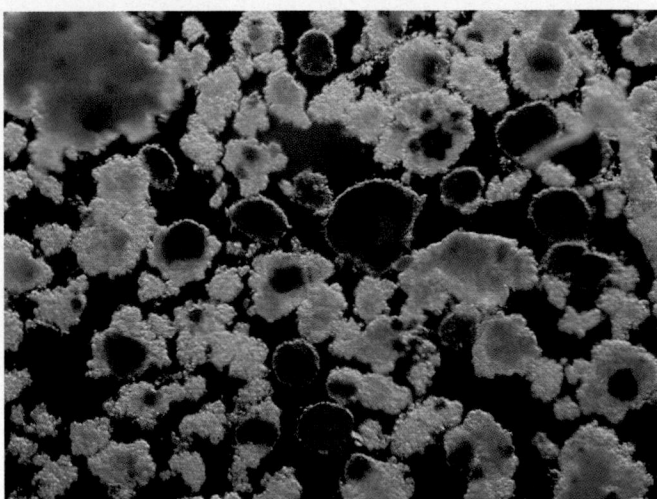

FIGURE 3 Pancreatic tissue after digestion seen under light microscopy (magnification 30×). Islets stained with dithizone are red, and acinar tissue remains unstained in yellow-brown. *(From Witkowski P, Savari O, Matthews JB. Islet autotransplantation and total pancreatectomy. Adv Surg. 2014;48:223-233.)*

prophylactic antibiotic therapy despite positive Gram stain or culture, but we use the information for culture-directed antibiotic therapy if the patient shows early signs of postoperative infection.

Direct infusion of a large tissue volume into the portal vein may lead to varying degrees of intrahepatic microembolization, inflammation, and portal hypertension. To reduce the risk of these complications, some TPIAT centers further purify islet cells from acinar tissue when the pellet volume exceeds 0.25 mL/kg body weight or 20 mL of tissue. It is important to remember that, inevitably, some islet mass will be lost during the purification process. Therefore the benefit of decreasing the risk of large volume infusion must be weighed against the risk of lower islet mass leading to decreased graft function. However, in the setting of chronic pancreatitis, the pancreas is usually so fibrotic and atrophic that the tissue volume of the preparation is small enough that purification is usually unnecessary.

Islet Infusion

During the islet isolation process, the patient remains in the operating room with the laparotomy incision temporarily covered after the reconstruction is completed. After islet processing is completed, the islet preparation is suspended in a balanced solution containing human albumin, placed into the infusion bag, and then transported from the islet laboratory back to the operating room. Surgical exposure of the portal vein is then obtained. Islets are then infused into the portal system under direct vision via the stump of the splenic vein, the umbilical vein, or direct puncture of the portal vein (Figure 4). Some groups prefer to close the patient's abdomen immediately after the reconstruction, leaving the islets to be cultured overnight and then infused postoperatively by a percutaneous approach under radiologic guidance.

Just before islet infusion, the baseline portal pressure is measured, and it is then monitored intermittently throughout the infusion period. In general, portal pressure should not exceed 20 to 25 mm Hg. When a large tissue volume is infused, portal pressure inevitably will rise, potentially leading to reduction in blood flow and portal vein thrombosis. Anticoagulation with heparin typically is used to prevent this complication. In our experience, when an islet volume less than 20 mL is infused into normal liver, portal pressure usually does not increase substantially. If portal pressure does rise above 25 mm Hg during islet infusion, the infusion should be discontinued. The remaining islets are then either dispersed instead into the peritoneal cavity or, preferably, injected into the leaves of the mesentery,

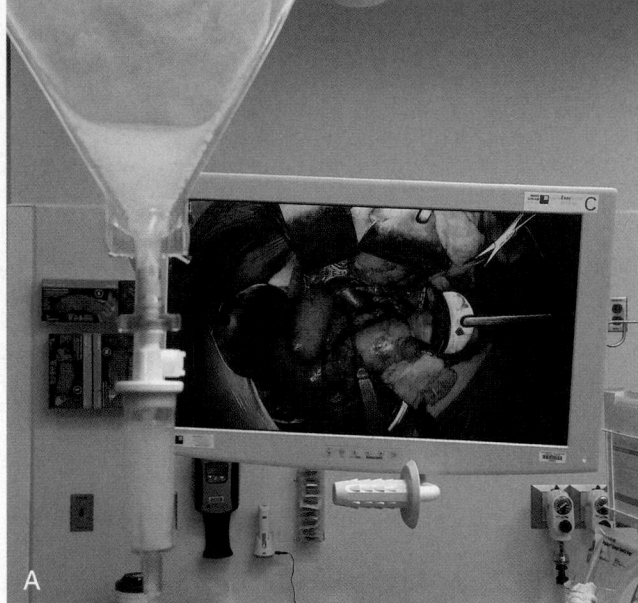

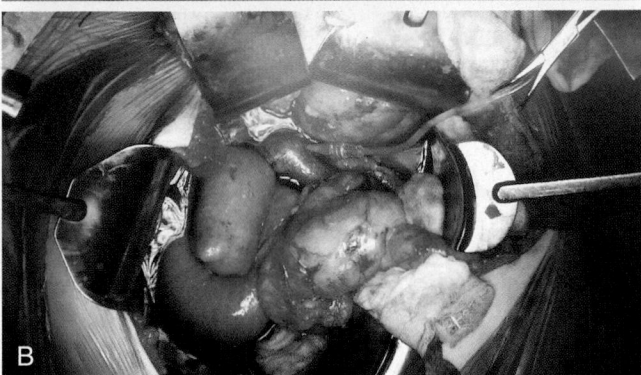

FIGURE 4 A, Islet preparation in the infusion bag is seen in the foreground. The operative field is visible on the operating room monitor. **B,** Close-up view of the operative field. The portal vein was cannulated under direct vision with an angiocatheter for islet infusion.

gastric submucosa, or intramuscular space, where at least some degree of islet engraftment might occur (this is unproven). Although islets transplanted into these alternative sites have been shown to survive in animal models, the efficacy of this approach in the clinical setting is unproven.

■ POSTOPERATIVE MANAGEMENT

Most elements of postoperative management after TPIAT are similar to those for any patient who undergoes major pancreatic resection. However, a number of important features of postoperative management deserve specific comment. Because of the importance of tight postoperative glycemic control, patients routinely are admitted to the intensive care unit so that continuous insulin infusion may be administered safely. During the isolation process, islet vasculature is disrupted, and the islet cells are exposed to mechanical, osmotic, and hypoxic stress, leading to upregulation of proapoptotic pathways. Also, in the immediate post-transplant period, the islet cells depend on diffusion of nutrients and oxygen until neovascularization occurs. Therefore newly transplanted islet cells do not function fully for the first few weeks and require time for recovery and engraftment. Tight glycemic control is necessary to protect islets from toxic hyperglycemia during this period. Therefore intensive insulin therapy with continuous insulin infusion begins immediately, with the goal that serum glucose is maintained at a target of 120 mg/dL. In the first few hours, a low continuous rate of 5% dextrose infusion may be necessary to avoid hypoglycemia. Typically, insulin infusion rates of between 0.5 and 2 U/hr are used. After 48 hours, transition to subcutaneous injection begins, initially with a long-acting formulation, supplemented by sliding-scale and postprandial regular insulin. Patients are weaned from insulin therapy gradually over the course of 3 to 6 months, if possible, as the autotransplanted islets achieve maximal function.

Extended prophylactic heparin or enoxaparin therapy is used for 30 days. Postoperative pain management can be difficult in some patients and is best managed with a team of expert acute pain specialists. Epidural, patient-controlled analgesia, local blocks, and ketamine infusion are particularly useful. Narcotic weaning must be managed carefully. After institution of an oral diet, all patients require pancreatic enzyme replacement therapy, usually with coated enzyme preparations to achieve 72,000 to 96,000 IU lipase with meals, and a lower dose for snacks. Attention should be paid to the potential for fat-soluble vitamin deficiency, with routine multivitamin supplementation and periodic nutritional assessment.

■ RESULTS OF TPIAT

The largest case series reporting TPIAT outcomes have come from the University of Minnesota, the University of Cincinnati, and the University of Leicester. The main endpoints of TPIAT to consider include relief of pain, overall improvement in quality of life, as well as endocrine function and insulin independence.

Pain Relief and Quality of Life

The primary goal of TPIAT is the relief of severe, unrelenting pain associated with chronic pancreatitis. Many patients become dependent on narcotics preoperatively, and the use of multiple high-dose formulations, including continuous infusion, is often encountered. It is not surprising, then, that the preoperative health-related quality of life (QOL) is significantly worse in patients with chronic pancreatitis compared with those in the matched general population. Significant or complete pain relief after total pancreatectomy usually can be achieved in well-selected patients, with approximately two thirds of patients achieving narcotic independence. Using a standard assessment tool (SF-36), the Cincinnati group has shown that QOL also improved significantly after TPIAT at mean follow-up of 19 months and remains improved over at least 5 to 10 years.

However, a significant minority of patients (approximately 10% to 20%) will continue to have persistent, minimally improved, or recurrent symptoms. The basis for failure is incompletely understood but includes continued substance dependence, central pain sensitization, and, on occasion, the possibility that the preoperative symptoms did not derive solely from the pancreas. Patients who continue to require narcotics postoperatively tend to have had higher narcotic requirements preoperatively as expressed in morphine equivalents (MEs). For patients with OIH, narcotic independence may not be feasible. More studies are needed to identify patients at risk for OIH and to develop effective methods for narcotic cessation.

Endocrine Function

Overall, reported postoperative insulin independence ranges from 10% to 40%, depending on the duration of follow-up. For example, after 3-year follow-up, a third of patients in the Minnesota series achieved insulin independence, and another third of patients had partial graft function defined by positive blood C-peptide. Even though patients with partial graft function require insulin supplementation, overall glycemic control was improved, as glycated hemoglobin (HgA1c) tended to be below 7% in the vast majority of cases. In addition, the primary goal of IAT is to prevent brittle diabetes and its attendant hypoglycemic and hyperglycemic episodes, not necessarily to achieve insulin independence. Cincinnati, Leicester, and other centers have published similar results, with insulin independence achieved in 22% to 40% of patients. Although there is some attrition of islet function over time, long-term survival of islet autograft has been documented.

Although considerable variability exists among all report series, islet yield tends to correlate with insulin independence. For example, in the Cincinnati series, the patients who achieved insulin independence received a mean of 6,635 IEQ/kg of body weight, whereas the patients who remained insulin dependent received a mean of 3,799 IEQ/kg of body weight. In turn, islet yield and quality depend on the quality of the pancreas. Advanced parenchymal damage caused by chronic inflammation and fibrosis lowers islet yield. In addition, prior pancreatic resection and pancreatic duct decompression (e.g., after Puestow's procedure) can decrease islet yield by up to 50%.

Therefore overall endocrine function after TPIAT depends on many factors, including patient selection, duration of disease, any prior surgical procedure, quality islet processing, and factors related to successful engraftment. This suggests that using TPIAT earlier in the disease process actually may improve the endocrine functional outcome. However, the ability to achieve improved islet yield should not in itself be the major determinant of the timing or selection of TPIAT.

■ SUMMARY

In appropriately selected patients, TPIAT achieves relief of pain and improves QOL while avoiding the risks of difficult-to-manage hyperglycemic and hypoglycemic episodes and, in a minority of patients, offering the possibility of insulin independence. Candidates for TPIAT should be counseled thoroughly regarding potential benefit (i.e., pain relief) and potential risk (i.e., lifelong exocrine insufficiency and likely type 3c diabetes). Setting realistic expectations should be a priority in preoperative discussions. Although long considered to be an experimental treatment, the reported outcomes over the last 40 years have established TPIAT as an effective treatment tool for chronic pancreatitis. TPIAT is now covered by most third-party payers in the United States and, for some patients, is clearly now the standard of care. Many patients who suffer from chronic pancreatitis may benefit from earlier consultation for the possibility of TPIAT.

SUGGESTED READINGS

Bellin MD, Freeman ML, Gelrud A, et al. Total pancreatectomy and islet autotransplantation in chronic pancreatitis: recommendations from PancreasFest. *Pancreatology*. 2014;4:27-35.

Bramis K, Gordon-Weeks AN, Friend PJ, et al. Systematic review of total pancreatectomy and islet autotransplantation for chronic pancreatitis. *Br J Surg*. 2012;99:761-766.

Chinnakotla S, Beilman GJ, Dunn TB, et al. Factors predicting outcomes after a total pancreatectomy and islet autotransplantation lessons learned from over 500 cases. *Ann Surg*. 2015;262:610-622.

Ong SL, Gravante G, Pollard CA, et al. Total pancreatectomy with islet autotransplantation: an overview. *HPB (Oxford)*. 2009;11:613-621.

Wilson GC, Sutton JM, Abbott DE, et al. Long-term outcomes after total pancreatectomy and islet cell autotransplantation: is it a durable operation? *Ann Surg*. 2014;260:659-665.

Witkowski P, Savari O, Matthews JB. Islet autotransplantation and total pancreatectomy. *Adv Surg*. 2014;48:223-233.

SPLENECTOMY FOR HEMATOLOGIC DISORDERS

John-Paul Bellistri, MD, and Peter Muscarella II, MD

■ INDICATIONS FOR SPLENECTOMY

Splenectomy continues to play an important role in the management of a number of hematologic disorders. Indications for splenectomy in patients in this population include symptoms related to splenomegaly and decreased blood counts related to sequestration or autoimmune destruction. Symptoms associated with splenomegaly include abdominal pain, early satiety, weight loss, and abdominal distension. Cytopenia is defined as a decrease in the circulating cell count of one or more blood components (anemia, leukopenia, thrombocytopenia). Hypersplenism is a common complication of hematologic disorders, whereby the spleen sequesters one or more blood cell lines. Hypersplenism is defined as cytopenia with a normal compensatory hematopoietic response by the bone marrow, splenomegaly, and correction of cytopenia with splenectomy. In addition, splenectomy should be considered for patients with unexplained splenomegaly. Splenectomy for hematologic conditions rarely leads to cure of the underlying hematologic disorder but may be beneficial for resolution of hematologic abnormalities and ameliorating symptoms of splenomegaly, thus leading to an overall reduction in the morbidity associated with these disorders. These may be classified broadly as autoimmune/acquired disorders, congenital disorders, neoplasms, and myeloproliferative disorders (Box 1).

Autoimmune and Idiopathic Disorders

Immune Thrombocytopenia

Immune thrombocytopenia (ITP; formerly idiopathic/immune thrombocytopenic purpura) is a condition characterized by platelet destruction secondary to platelet autoantibodies. This leads to thrombocytopenia (<100,000/L) with a relative underproduction of platelets by the bone marrow. Production of immunoglobulin G (IgG) directed towards platelet glycoproteins (GPIIb/IIIa, GPIb/IX) increases platelet destruction by the reticuloendothelial system of the spleen. In addition to humoral immune mediated factors, there is a component of cellular immunity involved in platelet and megakaryocyte destruction. ITP is a diagnosis of exclusion, and other illnesses that can cause secondary ITP, such as human immunodeficiency virus infection, systemic lupus erythematosus, antiphospholipid antibody syndrome, hepatitis C virus, and lymphoproliferative disorders, must be considered. Certain drugs also may elicit similar immune-mediated platelet destruction. A medication history of cocaine, gold, certain antibiotics, antihypertensives, anti-inflammatories, heparin, quinidine, and abciximab may result in this immune phenomenon.

The prevalence of ITP in adults is about 5 per 100,000 people, occurring nearly twice as frequently in women as in men. There is an approximately fourfold increase in prevalence in older adults (>55 years of age). Most patients with ITP have asymptomatic thrombocytopenia. Symptoms of bleeding usually do not occur unless platelet counts are less than 30,000/mm³. "Platelet-type bleeding" includes bruising, purpura, petechiae, bleeding from the oral mucosa, epistaxis, menorrhagia, and gastrointestinal bleeding. The most severe complication is intracerebral hemorrhage, and this occurs in approximately 1% of patients. The prevalence of ITP in children is approximately 12 and 9 per 100,000 in girls and boys, respectively. Children at a young age (approximately 5 years) may have a sudden onset of petechiae or purpura, usually days to weeks after an infectious illness. ITP is commonly self-limited in children, with more than 70% of patients achieving remission within 6 months of presentation. The risk of intracerebral hemorrhage in children is less than 0.2%.

Observation is a viable initial treatment option for selected patients, and this is most successful in the pediatric population when the platelet count is greater than 20,000/mm³. A trial of observation is reasonable in adults with platelet counts above 30,000/mm³, although this is rarely successful. Patients who exhibit persistent thrombocytopenia despite observation, or who exhibit platelet counts less than 30,000/mm³ (20,000/mm³ in children), should begin corticosteroid therapy. The standard initial dose is 1 to 2 mg/kg/day of prednisone for 2 to 4 weeks followed by a steroid taper. If platelet counts remain low after 6 to 8 weeks of steroid therapy, or if thrombocytopenia recurs after steroid taper, splenectomy should be considered. Intravenous immunoglobulin (IVIG; 1 mg/kg/day for 1 or 2 days) can be considered for patients who would benefit from a rapid increase in platelet count (e.g., in the setting of bleeding or in preparation for an invasive procedure) or for those who are unable to tolerate steroids. Careful coordination of IVIG administration with the referring hematologist is important before surgery because this usually can be performed as an outpatient.

Splenectomy is indicated for refractory thrombocytopenia, relapses requiring multiple rounds of therapy, or in patients who have suffered unwanted side effects. Splenectomy results in a 75% to 85% permanent response with no need for further therapy, and platelet counts will usually start to increase shortly after surgery. If perioperative platelet transfusion is required for persistently low platelet counts or bleeding, transfusion should be withheld until the splenic artery has been ligated. It has been our experience that splenectomy can be performed safely with minimal bleeding risk, even in patients with platelet counts below 10,000/mm³.

Thrombotic Thrombocytopenic Purpura

Thrombotic thrombocytopenic purpura (TTP) is a disorder in which a deficiency of the ADAMS13 protein leads to increased platelet aggregation and subsequent microvascular thrombosis. The interaction between von Willebrand Factor (vWF) and platelets usually is controlled by the ADAMS13 protein, which cleaves vWF and prevents platelet aggregation. TTP may occur spontaneously but often is precipitated by factors such as chemotherapy agents (gemcitabine, mitomycin C, or calcineurin inhibitors), quinine, cyclosporine, clopidogrel, ticlopidine, hematopoietic stem cell transplantation, or pregnancy.

The annual incidence of TTP is 4 to 10 cases per million. TTP is characterized clinically by a microangiopathic hemolytic anemia (MAHA), severe thrombocytopenia, fever, neurologic complications, and renal failure. Patients often have petechiae (most commonly on the lower extremities), fever, myalgia, and fatigue. Neurologic symptoms include headache, mental status changes, seizures, and even coma. Patients can develop congestive heart failure or cardiac arrhythmias. TTP usually is suspected with MAHA and thrombocytopenia in the setting of elevated lactate dehydrogenase (LDH), elevated bilirubin, a negative Coombs test, and a peripheral blood smear demonstrating schistocytes, nucleated red blood cells, and basophilic stippling.

Initial therapy consists of daily plasma exchange. Plasmapheresis is carried out with a goal of exchanging about 1 to 1.5 plasma volumes. Approximately 70% of patients will respond to this therapy. Platelet transfusions generally are not recommended for use in TTP because of the risk of severe clinical deterioration that has been reported after their administration. Rituximab (anti-CD20 antibody) and glucocorticoids are second-line therapies. Until the 1970s, splenectomy was the only modality available for the treatment of TTP. Currently, splenectomy generally is reserved for refractory thrombocytopenia or frequent relapses. When combined with high-dose steroid therapy, splenectomy has been shown to improve disease-free interval. The response rate for splenectomy for TTP is 40%, considerably lower than that seen for ITP.

Autoimmune Hemolytic Anemia

Autoimmune hemolytic anemia (AIHA) is a disorder in which autoantibodies are formed and directed against red blood cell antigens. AIHA should be suspected in patients with anemia, reticulocytosis, elevated LDH, low haptoglobin, and indirect hyperbilirubinemia. AIHA is classified as warm autoimmune hemolytic anemia (WAIHA) or cold autoimmune hemolytic anemia (CAIHA), based on the results of a direct agglutinin test (DAT). If the DAT is positive for IgG alone, or IgG and complement 3d (C3d), then the diagnosis is most probably WAIHA. Conversely, if the DAT is positive for C3d alone, then CAIHA is the most probable diagnosis.

In WAIHA, polyclonal IgG (sometimes IgA) autoantibodies, usually directed towards Rh antigens, form a light coat over red blood cells that then are removed by the spleen. The peak incidence of WAIHA occurs between the ages of 40 and 70 years, but it can occur at any age. In children, the disease is often self-limited, occurring after a viral infection and resolving over 2 to 3 months. Initial treatment with corticosteroid therapy (prednisone; 1 mg/kg/day) usually results in improved hemoglobin levels within several days, and remission occurs in 80% of patients. Children generally respond better to steroid therapy than adults. The steroid dose is tapered gradually to the lowest dose needed to control hemolysis. Splenectomy is indicated for patients who fail to achieve remission by 3 weeks, or for those in whom hemoglobin levels cannot be maintained with low-dose steroids. Response rates of 60% to 80% usually are seen within the first 2 weeks after surgery. Approximately 50% of patients will continue to require low-dose steroids (15 mg/day) to maintain hemoglobin concentrations after splenectomy.

In CAIHA, monoclonal IgM autoantibodies target red blood cells at low temperatures and cause hemolysis. Red blood cell destruction is complement mediated, and red blood cells are removed by the liver, rather than the spleen, as seen in WAIHA. CAIHA makes up 15% to 25% of AIHA. This disorder usually is caused by an infectious process such as Epstein-Barr virus (EBV) infection or by lymphoproliferative disorders. Signs and symptoms are usually more progressive. Patients also may complain of Raynaud's phenomenon. Treatment consists of avoiding cold temperatures by staying indoors and wearing appropriate clothing, which can prevent an acute hemolytic crisis. Alkylating agents such as chlorambucil and cyclophosphamide have been used successfully for treatment along with plasmapheresis. Steroids are usually not an effective treatment. Splenectomy is not indicated for the treatment of this disorder because the liver is the site of red blood cell destruction and not the spleen. If patients require transfusions for supportive care, a blood warmer is essential. Cross-matching blood products for transfusion can be challenging for these patients.

Congenital Diseases of the Blood

Hereditary Spherocytosis

Hereditary spherocytosis (HS) is characterized by the presence of spherocytes on peripheral blood smear, hemolytic anemia, and increased red blood cell clearance by the spleen. HS is the most common congenital anemia, prompting splenectomy with a prevalence of 1 in 5000 people in Europe and North America. The disorder is also common in Japanese and African populations. HS represents a heterogeneous group of membrane protein deficiencies with a common pathophysiology. Most protein defects exhibit autosomal dominant inheritance (spectrin, ankyrin, band 3 protein). However, some less common variants are inherited through an autosomal recessive pattern (protein 4.2). Membrane protein mutations lead to destabilization of the lipid bilayer with subsequent release of lipids from the membrane surface. The consequent decrease in cell membrane surface area results in sphering of the red blood cell with decreased deformability, impaired passage of the red blood cell through the splenic pulp, and increased osmotic fragility. The spherocytes then are destroyed prematurely within the spleen.

HS may manifest as mild or severe forms. In mild forms, patients may be asymptomatic or suffer only mild jaundice. Patients with more severe forms may have anemia, jaundice, splenomegaly, and cholelithiasis with pigmented (bilirubin) gallstones. Peripheral blood smear demonstrates spherocytes and reticulocytes. Treatment by splenectomy is curative for almost all patients with dominant forms of spherocytosis and is indicated in the presence of growth retardation, skeletal changes, symptomatic hemolytic disease, anemia-induced organ dysfunction, leg ulcers, or development of extramedullary hematopoietic tumors. There is some controversy over whether patients with mild or moderate forms of HS who do not exhibit these sequelae should undergo splenectomy. Preoperative abdominal ultrasonography should be performed for patients undergoing surgery for HS, and cholecystectomy should be performed at the time of splenectomy for patients with gallstones. Splenectomy usually is delayed until after age 5 to decrease the risk of overwhelming post-splenectomy infection (OPSI). There may be a role for partial splenectomy in children younger than 5 years because some studies have shown an improvement in anemia with potential maintenance of splenic immune function in this group.

Hereditary Elliptocytosis

Hereditary elliptocytosis (HE) is a rare disorder that results from mutation of the red blood cell membrane skeleton proteins spectrin, protein 4.1R, and glycophorin C. HE has a prevalence of approximately 3 to 5 per 10,000 in the United States. Inheritance usually follows an autosomal dominant pattern, and the disorder is more common in people of African and Mediterranean descent. The true incidence is unknown because of the wide variety of clinical presentations. Most patients with the dominant inheritance are asymptomatic with a mild compensated anemia or no anemia at all. Affected cells are morphologically characterized by biconcave elliptocytes, or rod-shaped, cells. These cells are much more deformable than spherocytes, and patients have a less severe clinical course. In contrast, the rare autosomal recessive form can lead to severe hemolysis. Patients with mild HE, who are asymptomatic and without evidence of hemolysis, do not require treatment. Patients with chronic hemolysis may require blood transfusions and daily folic acid. Splenectomy is indicated for patients with symptomatic anemia and is curative.

Hereditary Pyropoikilocytosis

Hereditary pyropoikilocytosis (HPP) is an autosomal recessive, severe hereditary hemolytic anemia in which red blood cells demonstrate striking micropoikilocytosis and thermal instability. HPP represents a subtype of HE, arising from the same molecular defects. Patients with HPP usually have a common hereditary elliptocytosis mutation from one parent and a milder subclinical defect in spectrin synthesis from the other parent. The disease usually is seen as anemia and jaundice in newborns and infants. Splenectomy is curative for patients with severe anemia.

Hereditary Stomatocytosis (Hydrocytosis) and Xerocytosis (Desiccytosis)

Hereditary stomatocytosis and xerocytosis are rare autosomal dominant hemolytic anemias characterized by a variable clinical course from asymptomatic to mild hemolytic anemia. In stomatocytosis, the underlying defect leads to increased erythrocyte cation permeability and an increased erythrocyte volume. In xerocytosis, there is a decrease in intracellular cation content and cell volume. Stomatocytes have a mouth-shaped area of central pallor, whereas target cells and spiculated cells are identified on peripheral blood smear in patients with xerocytosis. For cases of severe hemolysis, splenectomy may improve the anemia but does not fully correct the hemolysis. In patients with these conditions, the role for splenectomy should be considered carefully. Patients with stomatocytosis and xerocytosis can develop severe complications after splenectomy, such as hypercoagulability leading to catastrophic thrombotic episodes and chronic pulmonary hypertension. Fortunately, most patients with these rare forms of hemolytic anemia have a mild clinical course and do not require splenectomy.

Thalassemia

The thalassemias are a group of autosomally dominant inherited hematologic disorders caused by a defect in the synthesis of one or more of the hemoglobin chains. As a group, the thalassemias represent the most common genetic disorder known worldwide. The clinical manifestations associated with thalassemia arise from quantitatively imbalanced accumulation of globin subunits and inadequate hemoglobin production. Each subtype is characterized by the affected globin chain (alpha, beta, gamma, or delta). The beta subtype is the most common form of thalassemia in the United States and occurs mainly in patients of Italian and Greek descent.

Patients that have the heterozygous (thalassemia minor) form of beta-thalassemia are usually asymptomatic with a microcytosis and mild anemia. The homozygous form (thalassemia major or Cooley's anemia) is much more severe. Patients are usually asymptomatic until 6 months of age because of the presence of fetal hemoglobin (HgF). Patients then have severe hemolytic anemia, abdominal swelling, growth retardation, irritability, jaundice, pallor, splenomegaly, pigmented gallstones, and skeletal abnormalities. Laboratory values show a severe microcytic anemia with nucleated red blood cells, anisocytosis, and poikilocytosis. Patients also may have mild neutropenia and thrombocytopenia.

Treatment consists of periodic, lifelong blood transfusion and iron chelation therapy. Splenectomy is reserved for patients with increased blood transfusion requirements arising in the setting of hypersplenism. Massive splenomegaly is usually rare in appropriately transfused patients, and by itself, is not an indication for splenectomy. A transfusion requirement of more than 180 to 200 mL/kg/year of packed red blood cells usually represents excessive red blood cell requirements and warrants splenectomy. A 25% to 60% reduction in transfusion requirements can be expected after splenectomy. Splenectomy usually is delayed until the age 4 or 5 to decrease the risk of infectious complications (OPSI).

Sickle Cell Anemia

Sickle cell anemia is an autosomal recessive hemoglobinopathy characterized by an amino acid substitution on the beta chain of the hemoglobin molecule. The abnormal hemoglobin S (HgS) molecule confers red blood cells with the propensity to deform and take on a sickle shape when exposed to low oxygen tension. Sickle cells cause stasis and vasoocclusion in the microvasculature of the body, leading to tissue ischemia, severe pain, and chronic organ tissue damage. Exacerbations of symptoms are referred to as *sickle cell crises.* Patients who are homozygous for the disorder have sickle cell disease, and many undergo autosplenectomy by an early age as a result of multiple infarcts. Treatment is by avoidance of situations that can precipitate a sickle cell crisis, hydration, and transfusions.

Splenectomy rarely is indicated for sickle cell disease because of autoinfarction of the spleen but can be indicated for splenic abscesses and splenic sequestration. Splenic abscess can be a complication of splenic infarction and is an indication for splenectomy. Acute splenic sequestration has a high mortality (up to 15%). It is characterized by massive splenomegaly, acute exacerbation of anemia, and hypovolemia. This initially is treated with restoration of blood volume and red blood cell mass, but recurrence is common. Splenectomy should be considered to prevent further episodes of sequestration. It is important to maintain euvolemia and normothermia to prevent complications of an acute sickle cell crisis in the perioperative period.

Pyruvate Kinase Deficiency

Pyruvate kinase deficiency (PKD) is the most common genetic defect causing congenital nonspherocytic hemolytic anemia. PKD is an autosomal recessive disease that occurs when a defect in the glycolytic pathway results in a deficiency of adenosine triphosphate. Red blood cells are less deformable and often are destroyed in the spleen, leading to splenomegaly. Hemolysis can be exacerbated by acute infections and pregnancy. Patients with PKD have mild to severe anemia accompanied by splenomegaly. Clinically, the effects of hemolysis are often milder than in other hemolytic anemias because of elevated levels of 2,3-DPG in pyruvate kinase deficient red cells. These red blood cells permit more efficient delivery of oxygen to the tissues given the same concentration of hemoglobin in the blood. Splenectomy is indicated for patients with the severe hemolytic variants of PKD, or patients that require significant numbers of transfusions. As in the previous sections, splenectomy commonly is delayed until after the age of 5.

G6PD Deficiency

Glucose 6 phosphate dehydrogenase (G6PD) deficiency is the most common enzyme deficiency in the world. The disease is an X-linked disorder of the enzyme G6PD in the glutathione pathway that leads to damage of red cell macromolecules by toxic oxygen products. Hemolysis can be precipitated by acute infections, oxidant drugs (sulfas and antimalarials), and fava beans. Treatment is directed at inciting agent. Severe anemia is treated with transfusion. Splenectomy is rarely, if ever, indicated for the anemia associated with G6PD deficiency.

Neoplasms and Myeloproliferative Disorders
Hodgkin's Lymphoma

Hodgkin's lymphoma is a malignant neoplasm of lymphoreticular cell origin that usually affects young adults in their second and third decades. Primary treatment may consist of chemotherapy and/or radiation. Historically, splenectomy was performed as part of a staging laparotomy that included lymph node sampling and liver biopsy. Staging laparotomy is used rarely today and largely has been replaced by imaging modalities such as computerized tomography (CT) scanning and positron emission tomography scanning. Splenectomy rarely is indicated but may be beneficial for patients who develop thrombocytopenia or symptoms related to splenomegaly.

Non-Hodgkin's Lymphoma

Non-Hodgkin's lymphoma (NHL) is the most common type of lymphoma and comprises a diverse group of lymphomas varying in prognosis based on histologic subtype and clinical features. NHL represents the most common primary splenic neoplasm with splenic involvement occurring in 65% to 80% of cases. Splenectomy is indicated for symptoms related to massive splenomegaly and cytopenias resulting from splenic sequestration. It is not uncommon for hematologists to request splenectomy to assist with diagnosis to determine appropriate therapy. This may occur in situations in which patients have failed to respond to therapy or when inadequate tissue is available for proper histologic or cytometric analysis.

There are some subtypes of NHL that involve the spleen more than others. Splenic marginal zone lymphoma (SMZL) is an indolent B-cell lymphoma causing microvascular invasion of the spleen with marginal zone differentiation that occurs in older patients. Splenectomy is both diagnostic and therapeutic in SMZL. Splenectomy is an appropriate initial treatment and has been shown to lead to partial or complete remission in many patients because the spleen is the site of lymphoma origin. Chemotherapy may be recommended for some patients as the initial therapy at the discretion of the referring oncologist, and data suggest that this is appropriate.

Hairy Cell Leukemia

Hairy cell leukemia (HCL) is a rare leukemia, representing 2% of leukemias. Patients have fatigue, left upper quadrant abdominal pain, fever, infection, and/or coagulopathy. The disease is characterized by B-lymphocytes that possess cytoplasmic projections from the cell membrane ("hairy cells"). This is an indolent disease that commonly occurs in the fifth decade with splenomegaly (80% to 90% of patients), pancytopenia, neoplastic peripheral mononuclear cells, and bone marrow infiltration. Pancytopenia is caused by hypersplenism and replacement of bone marrow by leukemic cells.

In the past, splenectomy was an essential component of standard of treatment. Splenectomy results in symptomatic improvement from massive splenomegaly and a 40% to 70% improvement in the hematologic cell lines for up to 10 years irrespective of splenic size. Treatment with the purine analogues pentostatin and cladribine has supplanted the use of interferon-alpha2, other chemotherapeutic agents, and splenectomy as primary therapy. These agents have proven response rates of 92%, with complete remission rates of 80% and 10-year survival rates greater than 90%. Splenectomy rarely is indicated for the treatment of HCL and is reserved for cases of incomplete response to first-line therapy, persistent splenomegaly in the absence of bone marrow involvement, atraumatic splenic rupture, and severe bleeding from thrombocytopenia.

Chronic Lymphocytic Leukemia

Chronic lymphocytic leukemia (CLL) represents a B-cell leukemia in which there is progressive accumulation of functionally incompetent lymphocytes. CLL arises usually after the fifth decade of life and is more common in men than in women. Splenic infiltration is common in advanced stages and can lead to severe splenomegaly and substantial cytopenias because of hypersplenism. Splenectomy is indicated to relieve symptoms associated with massive splenomegaly, such as abdominal pain, distension, and early satiety. Splenectomy for the treatment of severe thrombocytopenia and anemia, in the setting of secondary ITP or AIHA, has a 60% to 70% hematologic response rate and has been shown to lead to improved overall survival.

Chronic Myelogenous Leukemia

Chronic myelogenous leukemia (CML) is a disorder of abnormal proliferation and accumulation of granulocytes. Ninety-five percent of CML patients will have the characteristic Philadelphia chromosome with a reciprocal translocation between chromosomes 9 and 22 [t(9;22)] leading to fusion of the breakpoint cluster region and Abelson leukemia virus gene. CML may occur in childhood but is found mainly in adults with a mean age of 65 at diagnosis. Diagnosis commonly is made during the chronic phase, which is commonly asymptomatic. Splenomegaly occurs in 40% of patients in the chronic phase. The disease can progress to an accelerated phase with the development of fever, night sweats, weight loss, bone pain, increased white blood cell count, and increasing splenomegaly despite medical therapy. An acute blastic crisis can develop, resulting in severe splenomegaly and hypersplenism, leading to severe anemia, bleeding complications, and infection. Current first-line therapy is with imatinib, a tyrosine kinase inhibitor. Bone marrow transplantation or interferon-alpha can be used in cases of poor response or relapse. Splenectomy has not shown any survival benefit in the early chronic phase or before bone marrow transplantation but may offer palliation in patients with severe symptoms of splenomegaly or hematologic disorders from hypersplenism.

Primary Myelofibrosis (Myelofibrosis With Myeloid Metaplasia)

Primary myelofibrosis (PMF) is a chronic malignant hematologic disorder that results in hyperplasia of abnormal myeloid precursor cells leading to marrow fibrosis and extramedullary hematopoiesis in the liver and spleen. This can lead to significant splenomegaly, cytopenias from splenic sequestration, and portal hypertension from venous thrombosis. PMF is prevalent in patients with history of radiation or toxic industrial agent exposure. It is more common in men than women with the average age of diagnosis being 65 years.

Splenectomy is indicated for patients who develop hemolysis requiring significant transfusions, thrombocytopenia, symptomatic splenomegaly, recurrent splenic infarctions, hypercatabolic symptoms (anorexia, fatigue, fever, night sweats, weight loss) and portal hypertension with refractory ascites and variceal hemorrhage. Splenectomy in PML has a substantial risk of morbidity (15% to 30%) and mortality (10%) and only should be performed in a select group of patients. Splenectomy in patients with PML has been associated with hemorrhage, infection, leukocytosis, severe thrombocytosis (18% to 50%), progressive hepatomegaly (12% to 29%), fatal hepatic failure (7%), and leukemic transformation (11% to 20%). Some studies have reported an increase in the complication rate with a laparoscopic approach versus open in PMF. The appropriate use of palliative splenectomy in PMF can result in improved quality of life for patients that are unresponsive to less invasive approaches. Postoperative use of platelet-lowering agents such as hydroxyurea, interferon-alpha, aspirin, and anagrelide has been shown to aid in reduction of thrombotic complications. Surgical technique involving ligation of the splenic vein flush at its confluence with the superior mesenteric vein has been described to improve laminar flow and decrease portal vein thrombosis. Compensatory massive hepatic enlargement can be treated with low-level radiation and chemotherapy.

Miscellaneous Disorders

Amyloidosis

Amyloidosis is a common disorder that results in extracellular deposition of insoluble fibrillar proteins in tissues and organs. Hepatosplenomegaly may occur in 25% of patients, and severe splenomegaly is seen in approximately 10% of individuals. These patients may develop functional splenic insufficiency. Splenectomy is indicated for signs and symptoms associated with a massively enlarged spleen. This does not, however, alter the ultimate course of the disease. In addition, patients with severe hepatic dysfunction from amyloid deposition may develop coagulopathy associated with factor X deficiency. In these patients, splenectomy may improve factor X levels. Perioperative administration of factor VIIa is important to control bleeding in patients undergoing splenectomy.

Gaucher's Disease

Gaucher's disease is a glycolipid storage disease in which a deficiency in beta-glucosidase (glucocerebrosidase) leads to deposition of glucocerebroside in the reticuloendothelial system. This deposition leads to severe organomegaly, pulmonary infiltrates, and bone marrow infiltration. Patients can have anemia, thrombocytopenia, osteopenia, bone pain, osteonecrosis, and massive hepatosplenomegaly. Splenectomy is indicated for severe and symptomatic splenomegaly and refractory cytopenia. Partial splenectomy has been advocated in some children with Gaucher's disease to preserve some splenic function. Splenectomy does not alter disease progression but can improve thrombocytopenia and reduce the risk of splenic rupture. Because the spleen is a reservoir for storage material, splenectomy for Gaucher's disease can result in redistribution and deposition in other organs resulting in severe bone disease (tenfold increased risk of osteonecrosis) and worsening lung or kidney function. Therefore careful patient selection is recommended before splenectomy in this patient population.

Felty's Syndrome

Felty's syndrome comprises rheumatoid arthritis, otherwise unexplained neutropenia, and splenomegaly. The size of the spleen may be variable, and splenomegaly is not essential for the diagnosis. The HLA DR4 antigen will be present in 85% of cases. Patients have severe or chronic infections as a result of the neutropenia, especially with neutrophil counts below $0.5 \times 10^9/mm^3$. Patients may have spontaneous remissions of their neutropenia. First-line treatment consists of low-dose methotrexate or disease-modifying antirheumatic drugs. Granulocyte colony-stimulating factor may be used for treatment failures, in cases of increased infection risk, or before planned joint surgery. Splenectomy is indicated when medical treatment has failed as manifested by recurrent infections or severe neutropenia. Splenectomy results in an 80% hematologic response rate. Unfortunately, infectious complications associated with Felty's syndrome may still ensue, and these do not always correlate with improvements in granulocyte counts.

Sarcoidosis

Sarcoidosis is a noncaseating granulomatous disease. Although 90% of patients have primary lung involvement, the disease can affect every organ in the body. Primary splenic sarcoid is very rare, and splenic involvement is often found as part of a multiorgan sarcoidosis. Up to 40% of patients with sarcoidosis have splenomegaly and 3% have massive splenomegaly. Splenic involvement occurs in 10% to 15% of patients with sarcoidosis. Treatment is primarily medical and generally includes corticosteroids or methotrexate. Indications for splenectomy include symptoms related to symptoms of splenomegaly, intractable pain, exclusion of a neoplastic process, and hypersplenism. Splenectomy does not alter the course of sarcoidosis but has been shown to aid in the treatment of refractory hypercalcemia in some case reports.

Idiopathic Splenomegaly

In the setting of splenomegaly without a clear cause, splenectomy has a diagnostic and therapeutic role. Historical series have revealed a 40% to 70% occurrence of lymphoma in this patient population. Most of these patients do not exhibit any clinical signs of lymphadenopathy to otherwise indicate malignancy. Tissue obtained through splenectomy may be the only means of performing the appropriate histopathologic or cytologic analyses to make a diagnosis. When hypersplenism is present, splenectomy can alleviate symptoms of splenomegaly and correct cytopenias. Early diagnosis of lymphoma can improve survival in this patient population because it provides the opportunity for early diagnosis and treatment.

■ PREOPERATIVE CONSIDERATIONS

Preoperative imaging is important for operative planning. Both CT and ultrasound are options for assessing splenic size. CT provides the advantage of providing information regarding anatomic relationships, vascular anatomy, presence of accessory spleens (Figure 1), perisplenic lymphadenopathy, and inflammation. Splenic artery embolization may be advantageous to prevent excessive blood loss in the setting of severe thrombocytopenia, or in patients who do not wish to receive blood transfusions for religious reasons. In addition, embolization may help to reduce the size of the spleen in cases of massive splenomegaly (Figure 2) to allow for laparoscopic resection. Patient selection is important in these cases because embolization may cause severe pain and ischemic complications.

Appropriate perioperative antibiotics are given within 60 minutes before making skin incision and should cover skin flora. Low-molecular-weight heparin should be administered subcutaneously

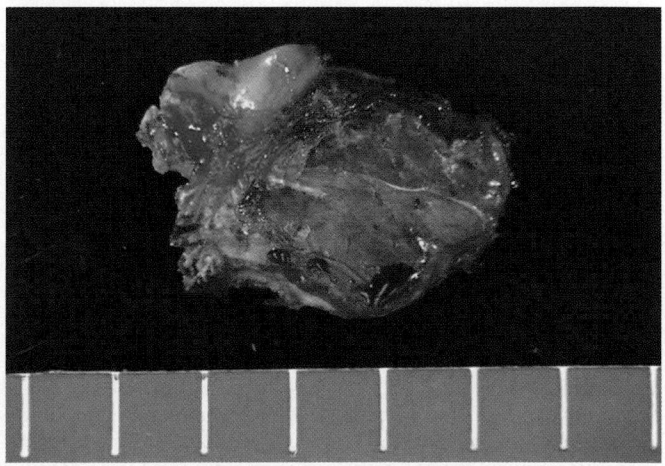

FIGURE 1 Accessory spleen.

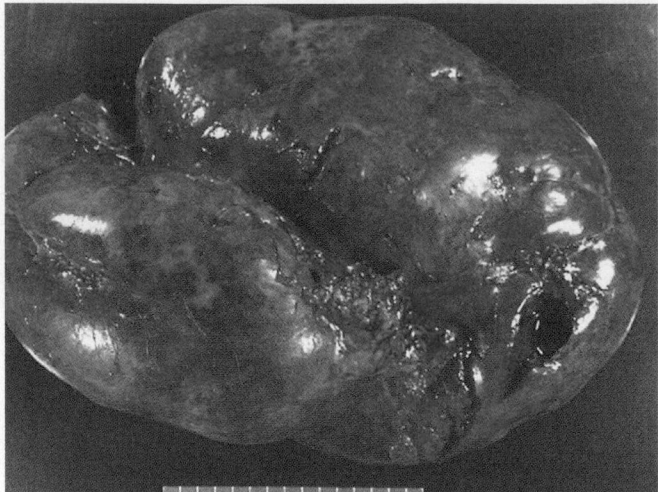

FIGURE 2 Massive splenomegaly in a patient who underwent splenectomy for complications of a lymphoproliferative disorder.

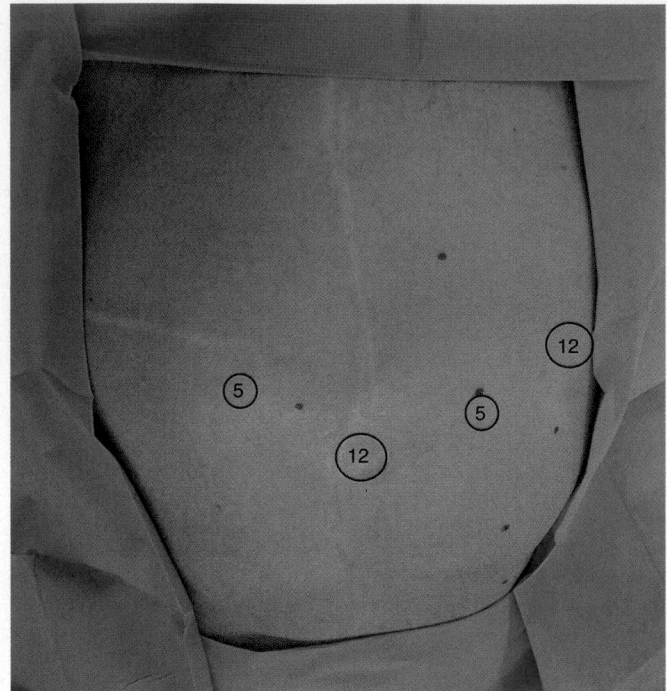

FIGURE 3 Port placement.

before induction of anesthesia and should be continued postoperatively for up to 1 month as prophylaxis for splanchnic thrombosis. The use of an orogastric or nasogastric tube can reduce gastric distension and can improve visualization and dissection of the short gastric vessels along the greater curvature of the stomach. Blood products should be available intraoperatively, especially in patients with severe thrombocytopenia. Platelets are transfused only as needed after ligation of the splenic artery. If patients have been treated with chronic corticosteroids, stress dose steroids should be administered with a rapid taper postoperatively. In elective cases, it is recommended to vaccinate patients against encapsulated organisms (*Haemophilus influenzae* B, polyvalent *Pneumococcus,* and *Meningococcus* vaccines) 2 weeks before splenectomy. If splenectomy is emergent, the patient should be vaccinated postoperatively.

■ SURGICAL PROCEDURE

Laparoscopic splenectomy has become the standard approach for performing splenectomy in patients with hematologic disorders. Laparoscopic splenectomy provides the advantages of shorter length of stay, decreased postoperative pain, and decreased morbidity. Recent studies have shown a trend toward shorter operative times that are comparable to open splenectomy in cases of normal or moderately enlarged spleens. Most data show comparable detection of accessory spleens that can result in disease recurrence in cases of autoimmune hematologic disorders. Much of the controversy surrounding laparoscopic splenectomy involves the size of the spleen. The normal adult spleen measures up to 11 cm in length and weighs approximately 80 to 300 g. Moderate splenomegaly generally is defined as a spleen that is 11 to 20 cm in greatest dimension, and massive splenomegaly represents a spleen that is more than 20 cm in greatest dimension. Laparoscopic splenectomy can be performed safely in patients with splenomegaly, even in cases in which the spleen is more than 20 cm in length. It has been our experience that the ability to perform laparoscopic splenectomy in cases of massive splenomegaly often is limited only by the size of the retrieval device. Regardless, the surgeon should exercise good judgment in patient selection for laparoscopic splenectomy. Factors to be considered should include medical comorbidities, splenic size, indication for surgery, blood counts, coexisting coagulopathy, and history of previous splenic irradiation. The hand-assisted laparoscopic approach may be useful for selected patients with splenomegaly and allows for rapid control of hilar blood flow and assistance with retraction. Nevertheless, open surgery should never be considered to be a failure and actually may be the safest approach for some patients.

For laparoscopic splenectomy, the patient may be placed in a lateral decubitus position or supine with a bump under the left side. A bean bag can be used to facilitate positioning for surgeons who prefer the left lateral decubitus position. A split-leg bed can be helpful when the patient is supine and allows the primary operating surgeon to stand between the legs during the dissection. Port placement generally includes a 12-mm periumbilical camera port, a 5-mm right upper quadrant port, a 5-mm left upper quadrant port, and a 12-mm left sided port placed more inferiorly and laterally to allow for passage of the endoscopic stapling device (Figure 3). Access to the abdomen can be gained using a Veress needle, an optical trocar, or an open approach depending on the preference of the surgeon. The patient generally is repositioned in reverse Trendelenburg position with the left side up, after port placement and camera insertion, to facilitate exposure of the spleen. For patients with a generous liver or splenomegaly, the use of a self-retaining liver retractor, such as the Nathanson device with a Fast-clamp, can facilitate visualization. This generally is placed through a 5-mm incision created at the groove between the xiphoid process and the left costal margin. The abdomen is explored, paying careful attention to identify any accessory spleens that may be present. The liver also should be inspected for signs of cirrhosis. The splenocolic ligament is mobilized and divided with an energy device. This allows for further mobilization and inferior retraction of the splenic flexure of the colon. The gastrosplenic ligament and the short gastric vessels then are divided using an ultrasonic vibrational energy device, endoscopic metallic clips, or bipolar energy device. This dissection should be carried up the level of the left crus, and the stomach can be retracted to the right. The splenorenal ligament then is dissected to identify the splenic artery and splenic vein within the splenic hilum (Figure 4). These structures then are divided using a vascular load on an endoscopic linear stapling device. The splenophrenic ligament is divided last because this structure maintains cephalad/lateral retraction of spleen during division of the hilar vessels.

The spleen then is placed into an endoscopic bag. The edges of the bag then are brought through the lateral trocar site. The spleen is morcellated using ringed forceps and extracted in a piecemeal fashion. After extraction, the splenic bed, hilum, and greater

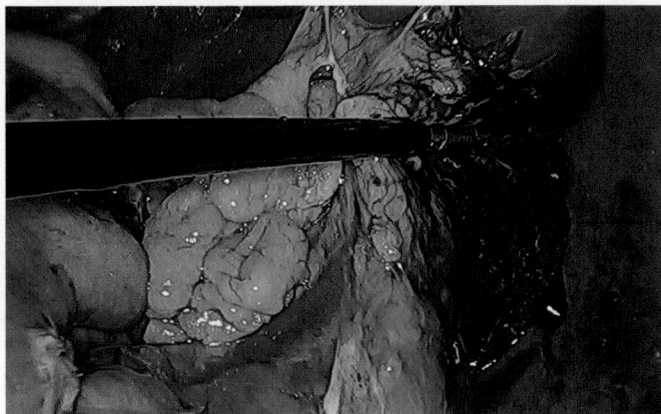

FIGURE 4 Laparoscopic view of splenic hilar vessels.

curvature of the stomach should be inspected thoroughly to ensure hemostasis. At this point the abdomen should be examined again for splenunculi or accessory spleens. The most common locations for splenunculi are the gastrosplenic ligament and greater omentum. For open splenectomy, a midline or left subcostal incision may be used. The midline incision may be preferable in patients with massive splenomegaly or a narrow costal margin.

■ POSTOPERATIVE MANAGEMENT AND COMPLICATIONS

Patients should be monitored for hemorrhage, atelectasis, and infection in the early postoperative period. The most common site of hemorrhage at re-exploration is from the undersurface of the diaphragm. Infectious complications include subphrenic abscess and OPSI. If patients were unable to receive preoperative vaccinations, they should be administered 2 weeks after surgery. If compliance is a concern, they may be administered before discharge from the hospital. Vaccinations should be held for 3 months after surgery in patients who have been treated with immunosuppressive agents. Patients should receive booster vaccinations every 5 years for pneumococcus and meningococcus. Prophylactic antibiotics have been recommended for at least 2 years in children but generally are not used in adults. Penicillin is the agent of choice (Box 2). In patients with penicillin allergies, trimethoprim-sulfamethoxazole or erythromycin may be used.

The risk for OPSI is highest in children under the age of 5 and within the first 2 years after surgery but does carry a lifelong risk. Risk factors for OPSI include age (14% in children younger than 5 years of age vs 0.5% in children older than 5 years of age), splenectomy for a hematologic disorder, and history of immunosuppressant therapy. OPSI has a reported fatality rate of 50%. *Streptococcus pneumoniae, Neisseria meningitides, Haemophilus influenza* type B, and group A *Streptococcus* account for most of the severe infections. *Escherichia coli, Capnocytophaga* species, and intraerythrocytic parasites also pose a risk. Patients typically have an upper respiratory infection that rapidly proceeds to sepsis and multisystem organ failure. A high index of suspicion is required, and early and aggressive treatment with broad-spectrum antibiotics and supportive measures can be lifesaving.

Other postoperative complications include a thrombocytosis, leukocytosis, pneumonia, pleural effusion, pancreatitis, pancreatic fistula, venous thrombosis, injury to adjacent organs, and hypersplenism resulting from the presence of a missed accessory spleen. Risk factors for postoperative complications include massive splenomegaly and myeloproliferative disorders (mainly PMF). Thrombocytosis can occur immediately postoperatively and peaks at 3 weeks. Antiplatelet therapy is indicated with thrombotic complications or

prophylactically when platelet levels reach 1 million. Patients with an accessory spleen will have an absence of Howell-Jolly, Heinz bodies, and target cells and may require re-exploration for accessory spleens or selective embolization.

Portal vein or mesenteric vein thrombosis can be a serious complication of splenectomy. Post-splenectomy splanchnic venous thrombosis has been reported in 20% to 50% of patients undergoing splenectomy, with higher rate for laparoscopic splenectomy. For this reason, patients can be maintained on prophylactic doses of low-molecular-weight heparin for 4 weeks postoperatively. Risk factors for thrombosis include myeloproliferative disorders, hemolytic anemias, a long splenic vein stump, postoperative thrombocytosis, hypercoagulable state, and splenomegaly. Patients have vague abdominal pain, distension, ileus, fever, and nausea and can develop intestinal infarction and portal hypertension. In the setting of splanchnic venous thrombosis, systemic anticoagulation is required with recannulation rates of more than 90% when treated promptly.

■ CONCLUSION

Splenectomy remains an important tool for the treatment of a wide range of acquired, congenital, and neoplastic hematologic disorders. Splenectomy also can serve as a diagnostic tool in the setting of idiopathic splenomegaly. Management of patients undergoing splenectomy requires careful preoperative preparation and postoperative management to ensure a safe perioperative course.

SUGGESTED READINGS

Carr JA, Shurafa M, Velanovich V. Surgical indications in idiopathic splenomegaly. *Arch Surg.* 2002;137:64-68.
Crary SE, Buchanon GR. Vascular complications after splenectomy for hematologic disorders. *Blood.* 2009;114:2861-2868.
Feldman LS, Demyttenaere SV, Polyhhronopoulos GN, et al. Refining the selection criteria for laparoscopic versus open splenectomy for splenomegaly. *J Laparoendosc Adv Surg Tech A.* 2008;18:13-19.

Habermalz B, Sauerland S, Neugebauer E, et al. Laparoscopic splenectomy: the clinical practice guidelines of the European Association for Endoscopic Surgery (EAES). *Surg Endosc.* 2008;22:821-848.

Ikeda M, Sekimoto M, Takiguchi S, et al. High incidence of thrombosis of portal venous system after laparoscopic splenectomy. *Ann Surg.* 2005;241: 208-216.

Mourtzoukou EG, Pappas G, Peppas G, Falagas ME. Vaccination of asplenic or hyposplenic adults. *Br J Surg.* 2008;95:273-280.

Price VE, Blanchette VS, Ford-Jones EL. The prevention and management of infections of children with asplenia or hyposplenia. *Infect Dis Clin North Am.* 2007;21:697-710.

Somasundaram SK, Massey L, Gooch D, et al. Laparoscopic splenectomy is emerging 'gold standard' treatment even for massive spleens. *Ann R Coll Surg Engl.* 2015;97:345-348.

THE MANAGEMENT OF CYSTS, TUMORS, AND ABSCESSES OF THE SPLEEN

Ory Wiesel, MD, and P. Marco Fisichella, MD

Splenic cysts and tumors are rare and most often discovered incidentally in the asymptomatic patient. Sometimes they can become symptomatic and be life threatening, mandating immediate surgery. Abscesses of the spleen are now seen less often after administration of antibiotics but when present can pose significant morbidity and mortality in the affected individuals. In this chapter we describe splenic cysts, tumors, and abscesses along with their presentation and specific treatments. We concentrate on laparoscopic splenectomy (LS) as the gold standard of splenectomy.

■ SURGICAL ANATOMY OF THE SPLEEN

In-depth knowledge of spleen anatomy is imperative for the operating surgeon. The spleen is located in the left upper abdominal quadrant and is protected by ribs 9 to 12. It is 10 to 12 cm long and weighs around 100 g in the healthy, normal individual. The anatomy of the splenic vasculature varies from patient to patient. In the majority of cases, the splenic artery arises from the celiac axis; however, in rare instances it may originate from the aorta, the superior mesenteric artery, the middle colic artery, the left gastric artery, the left hepatic artery, or the accessory right hepatic artery. The branching pattern of the splenic artery also can be variable and classically has been categorized into two types: distributed and magistral (Figure 1). In the distributed type, which accounts for the majority of cases, the splenic trunk is short and up to a dozen long but small branches fan out and insert over most of the medial surface of the spleen. The less common magistral type instead consists of a long splenic trunk, which divides closer to the hilum into three or four larger branches that enter the hilum in a more compact bundle and which may make the dissection of the individual vessels more challenging. The splenic trunk also gives rise to the left gastroepiploic artery, which courses along the greater curvature of the stomach and should be preserved during the operation. However, the inferior polar arteries, which arise from the left gastroepiploic artery, are ligated in the first stages of a splenectomy. The short gastric vessels originate from the fundus of the stomach and anastomose with the superior polar artery of the spleen. These vessels are taken during the operation to expose the splenic hilum. In addition to the variability of its vascularity, numerous ligaments that suspend the spleen contribute to its complex anatomy. A thorough understanding of these ligaments facilitates the execution of the operation laparoscopically, and their anatomy is routinely reviewed with the house staff before each operation (Figure 2). Anteriorly, the gastrosplenic ligament contains the short gastric and the gastroepiploic vessels. Posteriorly, the splenic vessels and the tail of the pancreas can be found within the splenorenal ligament. Laterally, the spleen is attached superiorly to the diaphragm by the phrenicosplenic ligament, part of the phrenicocolic ligament, and inferiorly to the splenic flexure of the colon by the splenocolic ligament. The phrenicocolic and splenocolic ligaments are usually avascular structures that can be divided safely during surgery.

■ SPLENIC CYSTS

Splenic cysts are rare; however, because of the current use of abdominal imaging, the incidence of splenic cysts is thought to be up to 1%. Several classification systems exist for splenic cysts (Figure 3). Martin classified splenic cysts into type 1 (or true cysts), which are cysts with an epithelial lining, and type 2 cysts (or false cysts), which are cysts that lack an epithelial lining. Pseudocysts are usually post-traumatic and originate in an organized subcapsular hematoma that failed to reabsorb. Rarely, splenic pseudocysts are secondary to prolonged splenic abscess or an infarct. Other classification systems are based on pathogenesis or the etiology of splenic lesions.

Fowler classified splenic cysts as parasitic cysts and nonparasitic cysts. Parasitic cysts are caused mainly by *Echinococcus granulosus* and usually are seen in endemic areas. Radiologic diagnosis can be made by identifying calcification in the cyst wall or daughter cysts. Serologic testing can assist in diagnosis. It is imperative to diagnose hydatid cysts before biopsy or surgery. As with hydatid cysts in the liver, extreme caution should be taken while manipulating the cysts to prevent rupture or spillage of the cyst contents into the abdominal cavity. Anaphylactic shock and death have been described after spillage and dissemination of the cyst contents. Injection of alcohol, 3% sodium chloride, or 0.5% silver nitrate can prevent this catastrophic event. Splenectomy or unroofing of the cyst with marsupialization is described. Primary true cysts of the spleen account for 10% of all nonparasitic cysts; they are lined with squamous epithelium and thought to be congenital. They are found incidentally in children and adolescents and are usually asymptomatic. They tend to have elevated cancer antigen 19-9 (CA19-9) and carcinoembryonic antigen (CEA) and are benign in nature. Most other nonparasitic cysts are pseudocysts and are secondary to trauma. Other rare primary nonparasitic cysts are of mesothelial and dermoid origin and are extremely rare.

The clinical significance of splenic cysts is attributed mainly to the mass effect (i.e., affecting nearby organs) and to their potential to rupture and bleed profusely.

■ PELIOSIS OF THE SPLEEN

Peliosis of the spleen is a rare condition characterized by multiple cystlike blood field cavities within the splenic parenchyma. It is thought to originate from sinusoidal dilatation and is usually an incidental finding in an asymptomatic individual. This rare condition harbors the dangerous potential of splenic rupture. On computed tomographic scan (CT scan), it appears as multiple cystlike, hypodense lesions, well defined. They may or may not enhance after contrast administration. The main differential from splenic lymphoma or metastasis is the fact that splenic peliosis involves nonsolid cystic lesions whereas the former involve cysts that are solid in nature.

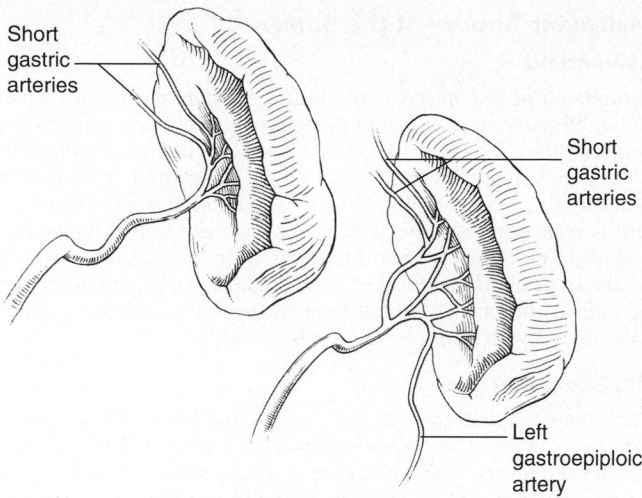

FIGURE I The most common variants of the vascular anatomy of the spleen: (*left*) distributed and (*right*) magistral). *(From Fisichella PM, Wong YM, Pappas SG, et al. Laparoscopic splenectomy: perioperative management, surgical technique, and results. J Gastrointest Surg. 2014;18:404-410.)*

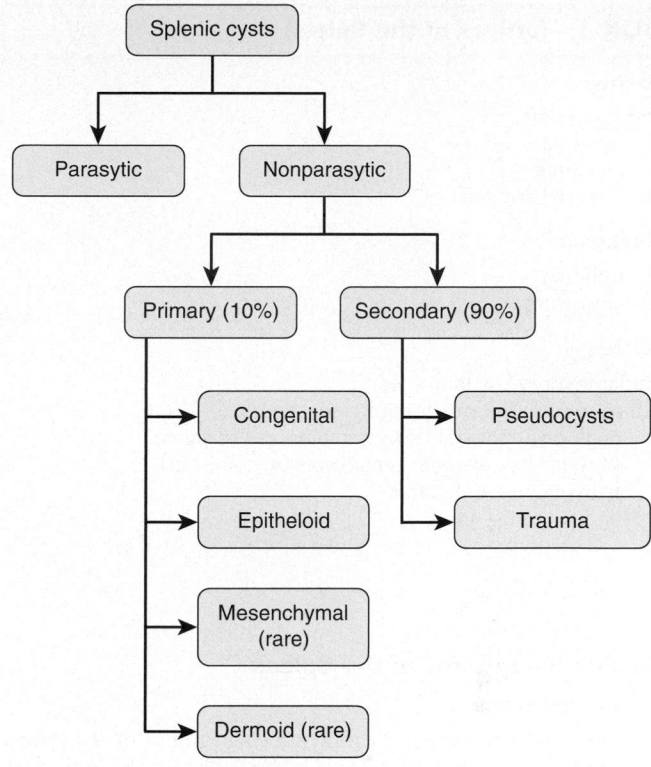

FIGURE 3 Cysts of the spleen.

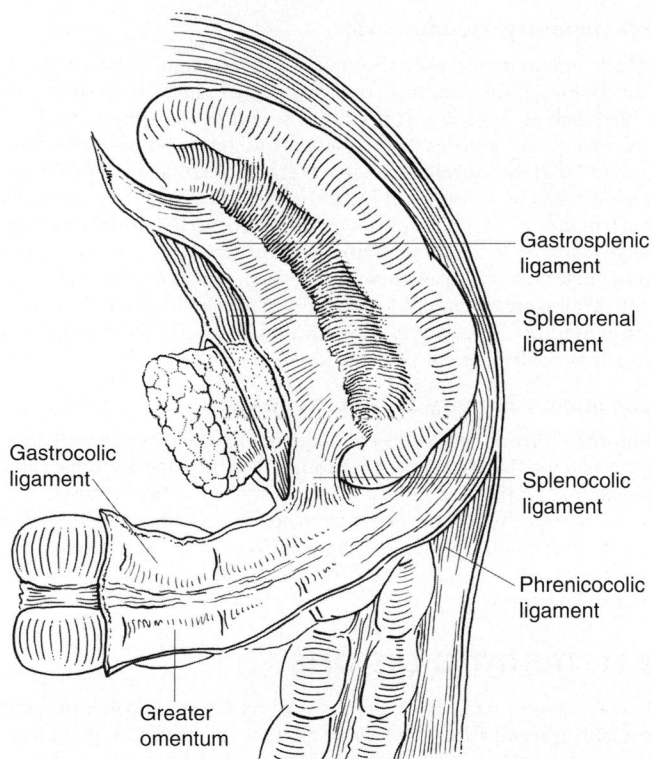

FIGURE 2 Ligaments of the spleen. *(From Fisichella PM, Wong YM, Pappas SG, et al. Laparoscopic splenectomy: perioperative management, surgical technique, and results. J Gastrointest Surg. 2014;18:404-410.)*

abscess or as part of systemic multiple abscesses in immunocompromised patients. Most splenic abscesses originate from hematogenic spread, and some originate from spread of infection from a nearby infected organ (pancreas: infected peripancreatic collection or abscess; colon: diverticulitis; kidney: pyelonephritis or renal abscess) or space (subdiaphragmatic, perinephric abscess). A few predisposing conditions, such as human immunodeficiency virus (HIV) infection, malignancies, septicemia, endocarditis, hemoglobinopathies, intravenous (IV) drug use, prior splenic trauma or infected pseudocyst/hematoma, and polycythemia vera, are key factors in the pathogenesis of splenic abscesses. Gram-positive cocci (*Staphylococcus, Streptococcus,* or *Enterococcus* spp) and gram-negative enteric organisms (*Salmonella* spp) typically are involved. *Mycobacterium* spp, *Actinomyces* spp, and fungal abscess (*Candida, Aspergillus* spp) also can occur, especially in the immunocompromised individual. Splenic abscess can be unilocular or multilocular. Unilocular abscess can be drained and treated with antibiotics, with a success rate of 75% to 90% in selected series, whereas multilocular abscess usually is treated with splenectomy.

■ SPLENIC TUMORS

Splenic neoplasms can be classified as primary or secondary. Primary splenic tumors can be benign or malignant and can be categorized further into vascular neoplasms (originating from the red pulp) and lymphoid neoplasms (originating from the white pulp). Secondary neoplasms of the spleen include metastases from nearby or distant tumors and non-neoplastic splenic lesions mimicking splenic neoplasms (such as granulomatous disease and sarcoidosis).

Primary Neoplasms of the Spleen

Most common primary neoplasms of the spleen are benign and originate from the vascular endothelium (Box 1).

■ SPLENIC ABSCESS

Splenic abscess is rare but has the potential to evolve into life-threatening disease with mortality ranging from 15% to 20% in the healthy patient and up to 70% to 80% in the immunocompromised patient. Pyogenic splenic abscess can be seen as an isolated splenic

BOX 1: Tumors of the Spleen

Benign

Hemangioma
Lymphoma
Hamartoma
Littoral cell angioma

Malignant

Lymphoma
Angiosarcoma

Other

Inflammatory pseudotumor
Uncommon: fibroma, fibrosarcoma, lipoma,
  angiomyolipoma, leiomyosarcoma and malignant
  fibrous histiocytoma, hemangiopericytoma, and
  hemangioendothelioma
Metastases to the spleen

Benign Neoplasms of the Spleen

Hemangioma

Hemangiomas are the most common benign tumor of the spleen. They usually are found incidentally in the asymptomatic individual. They usually are solitary and rarely are multiple or diffuse as seen in hemangiomatosis or associated with generalized angiomatosis syndrome. Most of them are smaller than 2 cm in diameter. Larger hemangiomas are associated with rupture and bleeding risk. Two principal patterns exist: cavernous hemangioma (most common) and capillary hemangioma.

Lymphangioma

Lymphangiomas are rare, benign, slow-growing lesions seen mainly in childhood. These lesions tend to be multiloculated and can be seen as an isolated splenic nodule or as part of systemic lymphangiomatosis. Large splenic lymphangiomas may be seen as a large abdominal mass in childhood, but in adults they usually are found incidentally in imaging.

They have three histologic types: simple (capillary), cavernous, and cystic.

Hamartoma

Hamartoma is a rare benign tumor of the spleen. Incidentally found at autopsy in 0.13% of individuals, these lesions are composed of malformed splenic red pulp elements without organized lymphoid follicles. They are usually smaller than 3 cm in diameter but can reach up to 18 cm in diameter. Spontaneous rupture of splenic hamartomas has been described, but most lesions are found incidentally in asymptomatic individuals. Although imaging findings may suggest the possibility of splenic hamartoma, a definite diagnosis based on needle biopsy or imaging may not be possible, and frequently splenectomy is needed.

Littoral Cell Angioma

Littoral cell angioma (LCA), first described in 1991, is a relatively new clinicopathologic entity arising from littoral cells lining the red pulp sinuses. These tumors involve the spleen diffusely, with multiple nodular masses leading to splenomegaly and hypersplenism. These usually are seen as multiple masses of varying sizes involving the entire spleen that are isodense on noncontrast CT scan, hypodense on the early portal phase after contrast administration, and isodense on the delayed phase.

Malignant Tumors of the Spleen

Lymphoma

Lymphoma of the spleen is the most common splenic malignant tumor. Primary involvement of the spleen by lymphoma is much less common than secondary involvement, accounting for less than 1% of all lymphomas. These are usually non-Hodgkin's lymphomas of B-cell origin. Secondary involvement of the spleen is more common and is seen in association with generalized abdominal lymphadenopathy. The most common finding is splenomegaly, but this may be absent in up to one third of cases. Radiologically lymphoma can be diffuse/infiltrative or small/focal with miliary nodules or bulky solid masses with multiple large nodular lesions.

Angiosarcoma

Hemangiosarcomas are rare and account for 1% to 2% of all soft tissue sarcomas. Hemangiosarcoma is the most common primary nonhematopoietic malignant tumor of the spleen. It is a highly aggressive tumor with poor prognosis. Splenomegaly is common and spontaneous rupture has been reported in up to 25% of cases. Liver metastases are commonly found at presentation. Special care should be taken before performing percutaneous needle biopsy because of the high risk of massive bleeding.

Other Nonvascular, Nonhematopoietic Neoplasms of the Spleen

Inflammatory Pseudotumor

Splenic inflammatory pseudotumor is a rare benign lesion of uncertain etiology, likely resulting from an unusual reparative response to injury such as infection. It usually is found in the spleen and liver and mainly is found as an incidental finding in an asymptomatic individual. Histologically, it is characterized by spindle cell proliferation admixed with abundant inflammatory cells, mainly plasma cells and lymphocytes. Clinical presentation is nonspecific, and the tumors range from 3.5 to 22 cm in diameter. Most reported cases are 10 cm in diameter. On CT scan these lesions appear as a hypodense mass with delayed enhancement, with a central scar without enhancement corresponding to collagen fibers around vessels. Final diagnosis usually is made after splenectomy.

Uncommon Primary Splenic Neoplasms

Fibroma, fibrosarcoma, lipoma, angiomyolipoma, leiomyosarcoma, and malignant fibrous histiocytoma, hemangiopericytoma, and hemangioendothelioma all have been described in the literature and are extremely rare. They have a nonspecific appearance (except for lipomatous lesions, which are characterized by the presence of fat) and nonspecific clinical symptoms. Final diagnosis usually is made after splenectomy.

■ METASTATIC LESIONS

Splenic involvement by metastasis is relatively uncommon and thought to result from the lack of afferent lymphatics, high antitumor activity of splenic lymphoid tissue, and sharp angle of splenic vessels.

Splenic metastases are found in metastatic melanoma, lung, breast, and ovarian carcinomas as well as, rarely, in pancreatic, colon, and stomach carcinomas. Most metastases to the spleen are seen as solitary or multiple masses; diffuse infiltration is a rare phenomenon. Radiologic appearance is variable and often found as cystic and necrotic lesions. Calcification in splenic metastatic disease is rare unless the primary tumor is a mucinous adenocarcinoma.

Implants on the serosal surface of the spleen are seen in patients with peritoneal carcinomatosis, commonly an ovarian or gastrointestinal (GI) primary lesion. Pseudomyxoma peritonei also often involves the spleen.

Direct tumor invasion of the spleen is uncommon but may be seen in tumors originating in nearby structures, such as the kidney, retroperitoneum, colon, stomach, and distal pancreas.

■ SYMPTOMS, SIGNS, AND DIAGNOSIS

Symptoms and signs of splenic cysts and tumors can be specific (i.e., as a result of hypersplenism or splenomegaly) but mostly are nonspecific. Patients with an enlarged spleen frequently have left upper quadrant (LUQ) discomfort and pain. Left shoulder pain (Kehr's sign) or left-sided pleuritic chest pain can occur as a result of diaphragmatic compression or subdiaphragmatic fluid collection or abscess. Acute splenic rupture or bleeding can occur indolently and quickly can evolve into hemorrhagic diathesis and shock. Splenic abscess involves symptoms of abdominal pain, fever, and malaise. Physical examination is nonspecific. LUQ tenderness or peritonitis, splenomegaly, and frequently petechiae or purpura (as a result of thrombocytopenia) can be splenic specific. Most of the splenic abnormalities have unique imaging patterns, and biopsy or an invasive procedure rarely is needed before treatment decision. Abdominal ultrasound (US), CT scan, or magnetic resonance imaging (MRI) is the gold standard for diagnosis, and contrast administration is recommended for differential diagnosis of bleeding or parenchymal abnormalities. In case of an occult infection or splenic abscess, positron emission tomography (PET) scan or pulled white blood cell (WBC) scintigraphy can be helpful to demonstrate splenic infections. When embolic splenic infarct or infection is suspected, aortic arch vascular imaging (computed tomographic angiography, or CTA) and echocardiogram are recommended to rule out the source of the embolic lesion. Hydatid cysts are uncommon in North America but rather more common in other parts of the world. Rupture of the cyst and expulsion of its content into the abdomen may be accompanied by anaphylaxis and peritoneal dissemination. Serologic testing is recommended when a hydatid cyst is suspected after imaging. Biopsies or punctures of the hydatid cyst should be avoided in order to prevent dissemination or rupture.

■ SURGERY

Preoperative planning is the key for every surgical procedure. Given the potential of bleeding during splenectomy, proper preoperative evaluation and planning should be performed in every patient.

Laparoscopic splenectomy is the standard surgical procedure performed in most centers worldwide. Open splenectomy is still indicated in abdominal trauma and in cases where the spleen size does not permit safe laparoscopic resection.

Although several methods of spleen-preserving surgery have evolved (e.g., unroofing of cysts, partial splenectomy), we describe LS, as it is the most common surgery performed today for splenic lesions.

Preoperative Evaluation and Planning

Our preoperative evaluation includes a detailed history and physical examination with focus on abdominal symptoms, a complete blood count, and a CT scan of the abdomen.

Although abdominal ultrasonography is useful to determine the size of the spleen and detect the presence of accessory spleens, which should be removed during surgery, we believe that a CT scan of the abdomen and pelvis with contrast provides superior information. In fact, the CT scan helps in determining the overall intra-abdominal geography, including the size, shape (not all spleens are shaped the same, especially when they are larger than normal), and relationship of the spleen to the tail of the pancreas; determining the presence of accessory spleens; and obtaining a clear interpretation of the vascular anatomy. The preoperative visualization of the hilar vasculature helps

tremendously during the procedure, and its variations are described in more depth later. This information is essential, as it helps in planning the operative approach, which becomes more difficult with larger spleens, and provides the surgeon with a roadmap to review before the operation. We consider a spleen with an interpole length of 25 cm or one that crosses the midline or enters the pelvis unfeasible for a laparoscopic approach.

Operative planning includes correction of any coagulopathy to the degree possible. Steroids and IV immunoglobulin are used to increase platelet counts preoperatively for patients with idiopathic thrombocytopenic purpura (ITP). In the operating room, packed red blood cells and platelets routinely are made available. However, platelet transfusions are seldom required. The transfused platelets are sequestered into the spleen, and we believe that this may make the spleen boggier and more prone to rupture when handled during the operation. Nevertheless, LS can be performed safely and effectively in patients with ITP who have platelet counts as low as 20,000/μL. In fact, recent studies support the notion that LS is feasible with platelet counts below 20,000/μL without transfusion. Nevertheless, when platelet transfusion is necessary during surgery, we prefer to administer it after controlling the splenic artery inflow at the hilum to prevent sequestration. Furthermore, we have never resorted to preoperative splenic artery embolization, even though some have used it in an attempt to reduce blood loss and the size of large spleens. This adjunct has shown equivocal results, and the ischemia caused by the embolization causes significant and very uncomfortable abdominal pain for patients. Nevertheless, in cases being considered for a laparoscopic approach where staplers may be applied, absorbable gelatin powder (e.g., Gelfoam), not coils, should be used for embolization.

Finally, patients are counseled about the lifelong potential of increased susceptibility to bacterial infections and the risk of overwhelming post-splenectomy sepsis. For these reasons, we routinely vaccinate patients against *Neisseria meningitidis, Haemophilus influenzae type b,* and *Streptococcus pneumoniae* at least 15 days before the operation or within 30 days after an emergent splenectomy in order to decrease this risk.

Laparoscopic Splenectomy

Although anterior, lateral, and posterior approaches to LS have been proposed, we focus on a semilateral approach, as we feel that this allows the surgeon more versatility and better adaptation to spleens of different sizes and shapes. A very brief description of the posterior approach is provided to illustrate the sporadic situations in which it may be adopted.

Laparoscopic Access and Initial Port Placement

After induction of anesthesia and general endotracheal intubation, an orogastric tube is inserted to decompress the stomach. This procedure is performed before the patient is positioned because insertion of an orogastric tube while the patient is in the lateral decubitus position is challenging and often unsuccessful. In most patients, invasive monitoring with a central line or an arterial line is preferred but not required. A Foley catheter is always inserted. If the patient has been treated chronically with large doses of steroids, we discuss with the anesthesiologist the plan for supplemental perioperative hydrocortisone dosing.

Positioning of the Patient

The patient is placed on the operating room table on a beanbag in the right semilateral decubitus position (at a 45-degree angle to the operating table).

Positioning the patient in this manner, with the stabilization offered by the beanbag, allows for proper adjustment during the course of the surgery so that a fully supine position (anterior approach) or fully lateral position (lateral or posterior approach) can

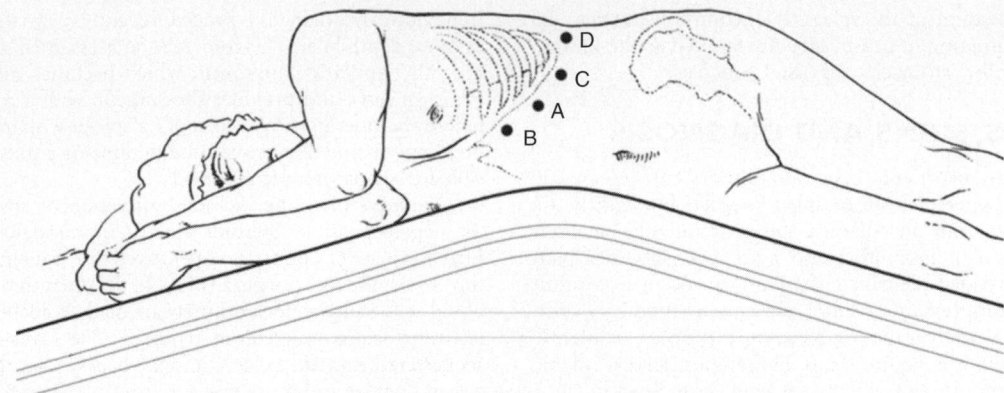

FIGURE 4 Patient positioning and port placement. The patient is placed in right semilateral decubitus position with the costal margin at the level of the operating table break. The first trocar (A) is placed 3 cm below the midline of the left costal margin, additional 5-mm trocars (B and C) are placed along the lower costal margin, and an 11-mm trocar (D) placed in the left flank will accommodate the endoscopic stapler. *(From Fisichella PM, Wong YM, Pappas SG, et al. Laparoscopic splenectomy: perioperative management, surgical technique, and results. J Gastrointest Surg. 2014;18:404-410.)*

be achieved at the discretion of the surgeon. In general, a more anterior approach is used for spleens that are longer than larger and in which the splenocolic ligament is positioned more inferiorly (toward the pelvis). Moreover, it is important to position the patient with his or her costal margin barely hanging from the break of the operative table, to effectively increase the distance between the left costal margin and the anterior superior iliac spine of the pelvis. This allows for greater freedom of movement for the most lateral port, placed into the patient's left flank. Liberal padding is then used on all pressure points.

Port Placement

After complete neuromuscular paralysis, a 5-mm incision is made 3 cm below the middle of the left costal margin. The Veress needle is inserted, a water drop test is performed, and the abdomen is insufflated to 14 mm Hg of carbon dioxide (CO_2). The Veress needle is then removed, and a 5-mm port followed by a 5-mm, 0-degree laparoscope is inserted into the abdominal cavity under direct visualization. The laparoscope is then exchanged for a 5-mm, 30-degree laparoscope, and the other trocars are placed under direct visualization in the order illustrated in Figure 4. In general, three 5-mm trocars, spaced 10 cm from each other, are placed anteriorly along the costal margin, and one 11-mm trocar that accommodates the endoscopic stapler is placed in the left flank, usually after the splenic flexure of the colon has been mobilized properly, as happens with longer spleens.

Mobilization of Splenic Ligaments

For mobilization of the splenic ligaments, we prefer to use the laparoscopic LigaSure vessel sealing system (Covidien, Mansfield, MA), which in our experience protects against injuries to the diaphragm and the spleen when the dissection is carried very close to these structures. The operation is started by taking down the splenocolic ligament, which contains the inferior polar vessels of the spleen. Once the inferior pole of the spleen has been mobilized completely, mobilization of the ligaments proceeds to the left by dividing the most lateral portion of the gastrocolic ligament in order to access the gastrosplenic ligament medially. The dissection continues medially and superiorly, so that the short gastric vessels are divided. This dissection continues upward toward the left pillar of the crus, with gentle medial retraction of the fundus of the stomach as progress is made toward the apex of the spleen. The entire stomach is then folded medially to fully expose the splenic hilum. This maneuver is facilitated greatly by emptying the stomach with the orogastric tube placed preoperatively and left on low, continuous suction. At this time, the superior pole of the spleen is mobilized completely by

taking down the uppermost portion of the splenorenal ligament. The complete mobilization of the superior pole of the spleen subsequently will facilitate the vascular control of the splenic hilum. After these steps, a thorough search is then performed for accessory spleens, which are excised and placed between the folded stomach and the left lobe of the liver for later retrieval with the principal specimen.

At this point, with proper operating table positioning and the meaningful use of gravity as a tool for retraction and exposure and with the spleen being suspended primarily by the splenorenal and phrenocolic ligaments, a clear view of the splenic hilum, upper pole, and lower pole is finally achieved so that the surgeon is left with the best strategy for addressing the hilar structures.

Management of Splenic Hilum

First, the tail of the pancreas is identified in relation to the splenic hilar structures. When the tail of the pancreas extends closer to the hilum of the spleen, the zone for transection of the splenic vessels is short. In this case or when a distributed anatomy is present, small (0.5-cm) hilar vessels may be sealed with the LigaSure system. In all other cases (e.g., difficult cases with a large amount of visceral fat and larger hilar vessels), we prefer applying careful serial firings of an endoscopic stapler loaded with vascular cartridges. Conversely, when a magistral anatomy is present, the hilum is taken with one firing of an endoscopic stapler loaded with a 60-mm vascular cartridge, provided that the tail of the pancreas is protected and that all hilar structures can be included between the jaws of the cartridge. To allow this maneuver, the superior and inferior poles of the spleen must be mobilized adequately, so that a posterior window can be developed behind the hilum to accommodate the stapler. These steps can be achieved by proceeding with the mobilization anteriorly or posteriorly to the spleen by adequate tilting of the operating table to the left or the right using the stabilization offered by the beanbag. In this way, the surgeon can tailor the best approach to the splenic hilum according to the spleen's size, shape, vascular anatomy, and relationship with the tail of the pancreas. Finally, in some cases, when a main splenic artery and vein can be easily dissected individually, we prefer to staple the splenic artery first and then staple the vein. In all cases, the remaining dissection of the splenorenal ligament and its vascular structures is completed with the LigaSure system away from all staple lines.

Extraction of the Spleen

The insertion of the spleen into the extraction bag often can be very frustrating after a well-executed LS. However, an effective manipulation of both the spleen and the bag can make this step a very rewarding conclusion to the operation. First, we transect the spleen from all of its attachments and carefully position it away from the left diaphragmatic dome using operating table positioning when appropriate. Then, we insert a reinforced, oversized plastic bag (Cook Medical, Bloomington, IN) through the most lateral, 11-mm port site. The bag is unfolded and positioned to form a "scorpion tail," with the open end of the bag grasped superiorly by the assistant and inferiorly in the surgeon's left hand while the tail of the bag is rolled up slightly and nestled in the LUQ. The spleen then slips inside the bag, guided by a grasper (which holds the cut ligaments of the spleen and not its parenchyma) held in the surgeon's right hand and by positioning the patient in the Trendelenburg position. In this scenario, the spleen is directed into the open bag, whose "tail" unfolds itself on the entry of the spleen. Once the spleen has been placed successfully into the bag, the strings of the bag are grasped with an instrument inserted through the 11-mm port. The port is then removed so that the bag can be opened to allow for the insertion of ring forceps for morcellization and extraction. In known cases of ITP, we always prefer to morcellate the spleen. In other cases, when an intact spleen should be sent to the pathology department, we resort to one of two options. In a male patient, we prefer to enlarge downward the most medial trocar incision, always placed at the midline in the epigastrium, to perform a laparotomy small enough to retrieve the specimen. In a female patient, we give her the option preoperatively to perform a Pfannenstiel's incision for cosmetic reasons. After the specimen is removed, the abdomen is reinsufflated and the dissection area reinspected to methodically check the staple lines, ensure hemostasis, and exclude injuries to the stomach, pancreas, diaphragm, and colon. Once bleeding from the port sites is adequately controlled, all trocars are removed. The 11-mm port site is always closed with a figure-of-eight 2-0 absorbable suture and infiltrated with local anesthetic. Drains are not placed routinely unless the pancreas was inadvertently injured or transected.

Posterior Approach

The truly posterior approach, with the patient in a fully lateral position, has been popularized in Europe but is rarely used in North America. However, one should be aware of the method, as it could be used for spleens that are more prominent anteriorly, obscuring the view to the hilum, and in which a magistral branching pattern of the splenic artery is present. This approach entails transecting the lateral ligaments of the spleen (phrenicocolic and splenocolic) to allow the spleen to fall and rotate medially, thus exposing directly the hilar vessels from behind. This maneuver is thought to allow for a safer and less challenging dissection of the individual vessels in selected cases.

Postoperative Care

Postoperatively, the orogastric tube and Foley catheter are removed at the completion of the case. Pain is controlled with intermittent parenteral narcotics, and the patient subsequently is transitioned to oral pain medication. All patients are encouraged to ambulate and are allowed unrestricted diet as early as possible. Most are discharged on postoperative day 1 and are advised to cater their activities according to their comfort level.

Patients are commonly seen in the clinic 2 weeks postoperatively, when a complete blood count is drawn. Administration of preventive immunization against overwhelming post-splenectomy infection (OPSI) and sepsis is warranted if the patient did not receive it before surgery.

Robotic Splenectomy

Robotic splenectomy is an evolving new technique and data are still accumulating. In the few studies conducted to date, the use of robotic surgery for splenic resection seems safe and feasible. Both straightforward splenectomies and complicated splenectomies in patients with cirrhosis or patients with splenomegaly have been described, and the high resolution of the robotic system allows safe and precise dissection of the splenic hilar vessels. A concern was raised about the ability to control significant bleeding using the current limitation of three arms, with the need to convert emergently to open surgery in cases of major bleeding. A recent paper demonstrated the superiority of robotic splenectomy in partial splenic resection where accurate vascular dissection is needed.

Outcome and Complications

Post-splenectomy complications usually are divided into early and late complications based on the proximity to the surgery. Early complications are surgery related (intraoperative and postoperative hemorrhage; left lower lobe atelectasis and pneumonia; left pleural effusion; subphrenic collection; iatrogenic pancreatic, gastric, and colonic injury) and non–surgery related.

Reactive thrombocytosis is observed frequently after splenectomy. Although post-splenectomy deep vein thrombosis, pulmonary embolism, and acute myocardial infarction have been described, the significance of post-splenectomy thrombocytosis and its contribution to the pathogenesis of these events is not clearly defined and subject to debate. Prophylactic antiplatelet therapy is not advocated. Mesenteric vein thrombosis is a well-described phenomenon after splenic vein ligation and can be seen in up to 30% of surgeries in selected series. OPSI is the most common fatal late complication of splenectomy. It can occur at any time after splenectomy. Most of the reported infections occur more than 2 years after surgery. The most frequently involved organisms are *S. pneumoniae, H. influenzae, N. meningitidis,* and *Salmonella* spp. The standard of care today for post-splenectomy prophylaxis includes administration of pneumococcal vaccine polyvalent (Pneumovax 23), *H. influenzae type b* conjugate, and meningococcal polysaccharide vaccine within 2 weeks of splenectomy or before surgery.

SUGGESTED READINGS

Avital S, Kashtan H. A large epithelial splenic cyst. *N Engl J Med.* 2003;349:2173-2174.

Fisichella PM, Wong YM, Pappas SG, et al. Laparoscopic splenectomy: perioperative management, surgical technique, and results. *J Gastrointest Surg.* 2014;18:404-410.

Giovagnoni A, Giorgi C, Goteri G, et al. Tumors of the spleen. *Cancer Imaging.* 2005;5:73-77.

Giza DE, Tudor S, Purnichescu-Purtan RR, Vasilescu C. Robotic splenectomy: what is the real benefit? *World J Surg.* 2014;38:3067-3073.

Ingle SB, Hinge Ingle CR, Patrike S. Epithelial cysts of the spleen: a minireview. *World J Gastroenterol.* 2014;20:13899-13903.

Kaza RK, Azar S, Al-Hawary MM, et al. Primary and secondary neoplasms of the spleen. *Cancer Imaging.* 2010;10:173-182.

SPLENIC SALVAGE PROCEDURES

Isaac W. Howley, MD, and Kent A. Stevens, MD

The management of splenic injuries has changed considerably over the past several decades, with a large increase in the use of nonoperative management (NOM). Most splenic injuries are now managed nonoperatively in most trauma centers because of an increase in the diagnosis of clinically inconsequential injuries and more restrictive indications for splenectomy. Angioembolization has an important role in nonoperative management. In addition, several operative techniques may be used to repair splenic injuries and control hemorrhage while leaving the spleen in situ. This chapter describes operative and interventional radiography splenic salvage procedures that may help avoid splenectomy and its consequent risks.

Although these procedures will obviate the need for resection in most cases, splenectomy remains the definitive procedure to control splenic hemorrhage. Especially in the severely injured patient being managed within the modern damage control paradigm, splenectomy should be viewed as a lifesaving operation.

■ BENEFITS OF SPLENIC SALVAGE

The spleen has a variety of hematologic and immunologic functions, including the removal of senescent and defective red blood cells, white blood cells, and platelets. Splenic tissue contains large concentrations of macrophages, lymphocytes, and antigen-producing cells and produces a variety of opsonins that play an important role in complement activation. Splenectomy puts patients at risk for overwhelming post-splenectomy infection (OPSI); this was reported first in 1952 in a series of five infants who had undergone splenectomy for hereditary spherocytosis. All were less than 6 months of age, and two of them died. Subsequent reports, before the widespread use of vaccinations against encapsulated organisms, have shown a 60- to 100-fold risk of severe infections among children younger than 5. The risk is significantly lower but still present among adult splenectomy patients. Estimates of lifetime risk range between 0.1% and 9%, with a fatality rate of 35% to 80%. Encapsulated bacteria, especially pneumococci, cause the bulk of OPSI. Vaccination against pneumococcus, *Haemophilus influenzae*, and meningococcus should be performed before hospital discharge for all splenectomy patients.

In addition to the immunologic consequences of splenectomy, the surgery itself has several potential complications. The gastric fundus and the tail of the pancreas lie in close proximity to the splenic hilum. Iatrogenic pancreatic injuries have been reported to occur in as many as 15% of patients receiving splenectomy. Deep venous thrombosis (DVTs), including portal vein thrombosis, may occur in 2% to 3% of splenic surgery patients, and these patients are at risk for surgical site infections as well. Of course, patients who receive laparotomies are at risk for incisional hernias and small bowel obstructions, although the incidence of small bowel obstruction after trauma laparotomy is less than 1%. NOM, in the appropriate patient population, allows most of these risks to be avoided.

■ NONOPERATIVE MANAGEMENT

Blunt splenic injuries once were viewed as an indication for splenectomy. Impetus for avoiding splenectomy grew in the 1960s as the spleen's immunologic functions became better appreciated. Selective NOM of blunt splenic injury was described first in the pediatric trauma population in 1968 and gradually gained acceptance in adult trauma management. This coincided with increasing availability and accuracy of computed tomography (CT) scans for diagnosis in hemodynamically stable blunt abdominal trauma patients. With this increase in the number of trauma patients undergoing CT imaging, more low-grade splenic injuries were detected. With better imaging, splenic injury could be graded without operation, and the American Association for the Surgery of Trauma developed an Organ Injury Scale (OIS) to aid in research and in clinical decision making (Table 1).

As NOM gained acceptance, it was attempted in a wider variety of patients, and over time its application has become broader. NOM has been attempted and often succeeds in a variety of clinical scenarios that were once seen as contraindications, including fluid-responsive hypotension, immunologic disease, and advanced age. The Eastern Association for the Surgery of Trauma (EAST) developed guidelines for NOM of blunt injuries to the spleen in 2003, which were last revised in 2012 (Box 1). Although significant practice variations exist between trauma centers, the majority of splenic injuries now are managed nonoperatively.

To consider NOM for a patient with a splenic injury, several criteria should be met. The patient should be kept in a monitored setting, in a facility with 24-hour operating room and surgeon availability in case the patient requires an emergency splenectomy. Patients should receive an arterial line to allow for continuous blood pressure monitoring and should have frequent abdominal examinations and repeated hemoglobin checks for the first 24 hours of admission. The EAST Guidelines list four criteria for considering NOM for blunt splenic injury (see Box 1). Patients who are hemodynamically unstable, require transfusion of more than two units of red blood cells, have peritonitis, have a neurologic injury and would be at risk for secondary injury in the setting of global hypotension, or have other injuries requiring operative intervention should be taken emergently to the operating room. If the patient requires laparotomy for other injuries and the spleen has a low-grade injury, a variety of splenorrhaphy procedures may be considered. Splenectomy, although not free of potential complications, remains the safest option in patients with a neurologic injury, coagulopathy, or a high physiologic burden from their injuries.

Role of Angioembolization

In the appropriate patient population, splenic artery angioembolization (SAE) may be a useful adjunct to NOM. The 2012 EAST guidelines for management of blunt splenic injury recommend SAE in hemodynamically stable patients with CT findings of active extravasation (Figure 1), pseudoaneurysm, or arteriovenous fistula; moderate pneumoperitoneum; persistent bleeding; or for grade IV and grade V injuries. Several studies with a variety of methodologies, including retrospective reviews of the National Trauma Data Bank, ecologic studies comparing trauma centers by rates of SAE, and prospective multicenter observational studies consistently have shown a correlation between SAE and avoidance of splenectomy in patients initially managed by NOM.

In the absence of CT evidence of active extravasation, selective angioembolization of splenic artery branches is not possible. However, there is still a role for empirical nonselective splenic artery embolization. This reduces blood pressure and flow to distal vascular and parenchymal injuries, allowing for clot formation and potentially obviating the need for splenectomy. An observational study from Florida has demonstrated the efficacy of SAE for preventing NOM failure in patients with blunt grade IV or V injury without a contrast blush on admission CT scan; a separate study from Norway demonstrated via historical controls that there is no benefit to empirical SAE in patients with blunt grade III injuries without active extravasation. Accordingly, in the absence of contrast blush or pseudoaneurysm on CT, we recommend angioembolization for grade IV and V, but not grade III, splenic injuries.

TABLE 1: Organ Injury Scale for the Spleen by the American Association for the Surgery of Trauma

Grade	Injury Type	Description of Injury
I	Hematoma	Subcapsular, nonexpanding, <10% surface area
	Laceration	Capsular tear, nonbleeding, <1 cm parenchymal depth
II	Hematoma	Subcapsular, nonexpanding, 10%-50% surface area; intraparenchymal, <5 cm in depth
	Laceration	Capsular tear, active bleeding, 1-3 cm parenchymal depth that does not involve a trabecular vessel
III	Hematoma	Subcapsular, >50% surface area or expanding; ruptured subcapsular or parenchymal hematoma with active bleeding; intraparenchymal hematoma ≥5 cm or expanding
	Laceration	>3 cm parenchymal depth or involving trabecular vessels
IV	Laceration	Laceration involving segmental or hilar vessels producing major devascularization (>25% of spleen)
V	Laceration	Completely shattered spleen
	Vascular	Hilar vascular injury with devascularized spleen

Progression of Care

Most NOM failures occur within 24 hours of injury, although delayed hemorrhage has been reported even several weeks after injury. NOM patients typically are managed with at least 24 hours of bed rest and NPO status. There are no high-quality studies or guidelines regarding the optimum duration of bed rest, invasive monitoring, hospitalization, and time to initiate deep venous thrombosis prophylaxis and resumption of activities. Given the paucity of evidence, a Delphi study published in 2013 found general consensus among trauma surgeons and interventional radiologists that patients should stay in a monitored setting for 1 to 3 days with serial hemoglobin checks and that routine follow-up imaging is not necessary.

An algorithm for the operative and nonoperative management of splenic injuries is shown in Figure 2.

Results of Nonoperative Management

Judiciously applied NOM should have a very high success rate, as defined by avoidance of delayed splenectomy or sequelae of hemorrhage. A multicenter study sponsored by EAST showed an 89% success rate for NOM without the use of SAE. Reports in the peer-reviewed literature on the benefit of SAE are difficult to assess because of differences in indications and definitions

BOX 1: Criteria for Nonoperative Management of Blunt Splenic Injury

1. Hemodynamic stability
2. Documented computed tomographic classification of injury
3. Absence of additional injuries requiring operative intervention
4. Transfusion of fewer than two units of packed red blood cells

From East Associated for the Surgery of Trauma (EAST) AdHoc Committee on Practice Management Guideline Development. Non-operative management of blunt injury to the liver and spleen 2003. <http://east.org.tpg.>

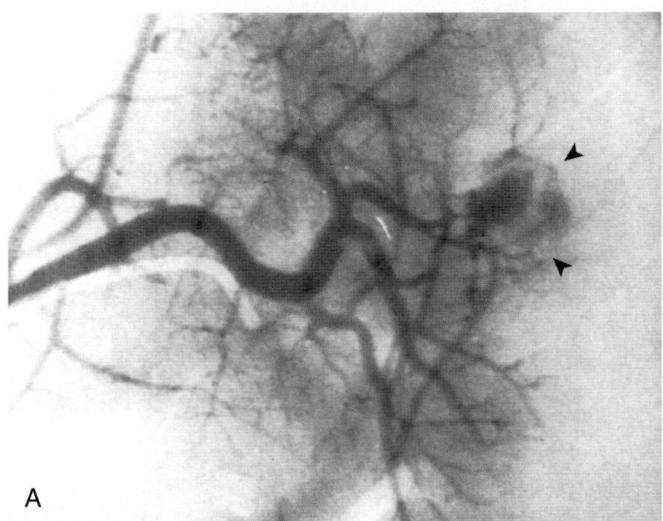
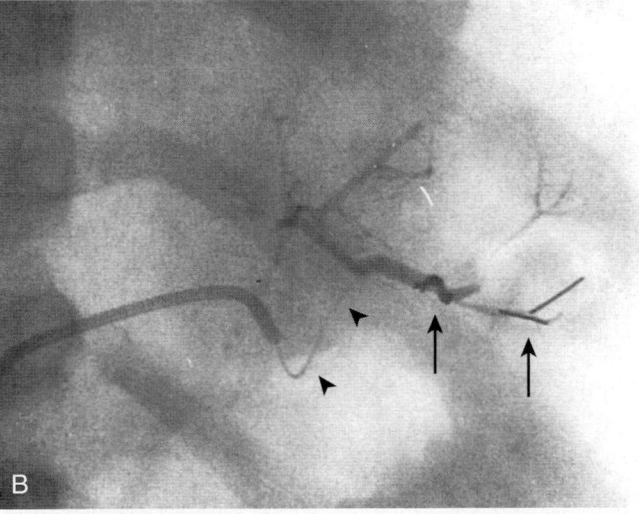

FIGURE 1 A, Splenic pseudoaneurysm (*arrowheads* indicate contrast within the pseudoaneurysm) after nonoperative treatment of blunt splenic injury. **B,** Successful angiographic embolization (*arrows* show occlusion of ruptured vessels). *(From Coran AG, et al. Pediatric Surgery. 7th ed. Philadelphia: Elsevier; 2012. Fig. 20-3.)*

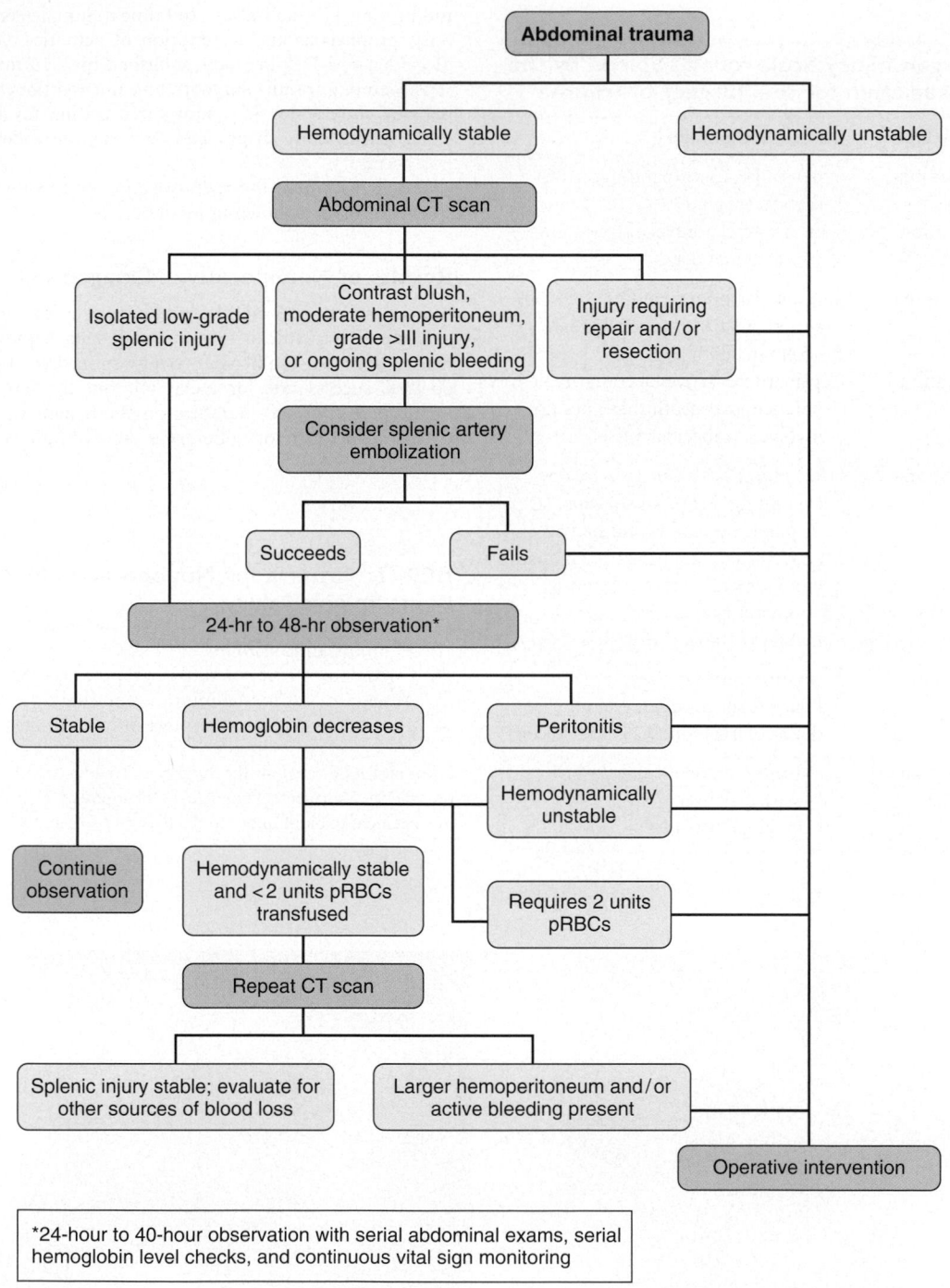

FIGURE 2 Algorithmic approach to the management of traumatic splenic injury. *CT,* Computed tomographic; *pRBCs,* packed red blood cells.

between studies; other series of patients in which SAE was used have described NOM success rates as high as 97%. Complications of NOM include delayed hemorrhage, splenic infarcts and abscesses, splenic artery pseudoaneurysms, and immunosuppression from SAE. Delayed hemorrhage may occur days to weeks after injury and should be treated by emergent laparotomy with splenectomy.

Immunosuppression does not seem to occur after SAE. There are no published long-term cohort studies of patients who have undergone SAE that would allow direct calculation of OPSI rates. However, several studies have looked at specific immunologic markers that require a competent spleen among these patients and have found function similar to that of healthy controls, much higher than for splenectomy patients. Vaccination against encapsulated organisms is not performed routinely in patients after SAE, unlike for patients after splenectomy.

PENETRATING SPLENIC TRAUMA

Most publications regarding the management of splenic injuries have focused on blunt trauma victims; the EAST guidelines apply specifically to this population. Penetrating abdominal trauma patients are also at risk for splenic injury. These injuries often happen in conjunction with injuries to nearby organs. The spleen is located superior and posterior to the splenic flexure of the colon and inferior to the left hemidiaphragm. Colonic injury mandates laparotomy for control of contamination and possibly hemorrhage, and left thoracoabdominal injuries should be evaluated with diagnostic laparoscopy or thoracoscopy to rule out left hemidiaphragmatic injury. Therefore the majority of patients with penetrating splenic injury need operative exploration to evaluate or manage associated injuries. Some of these patients will have high-grade splenic injuries with active hemorrhage mandating splenectomy. Other patients have multiple severe injuries, warranting an abbreviated damage control laparotomy. In this setting, even relatively minor splenic injuries should be treated by splenectomy to eliminate the risk of splenic hemorrhage should coagulopathy develop or bleeding restart once normotension is achieved and arterial vasospasm passes. As in blunt trauma, the combination of penetrating splenic and neurologic injuries should be treated by splenectomy to avoid the risk of splenic hemorrhage, hypotension, and possible secondary neurologic injury.

Although most patients with penetrating injuries to the spleen will need splenectomy, some patients will be better managed by less invasive means. NOM is appropriate for a subset of patients with isolated splenic injuries who fulfill the same criteria as for blunt splenic injuries. The failure rate for NOM may be significantly lower for penetrating injuries; in a series of 225 patients with penetrating injuries to the spleen at Los Angeles County–University of Southern California Medical Center (LAC+USC) over 11 years, 83% of patients underwent emergency surgery. Of the 38 patients in whom NOM was attempted initially, the failure rate was 37%, although a substantial portion of these patients had associated hollow viscus or diaphragmatic injuries that were diagnosed in a delayed fashion. There is a subset of hemodynamically stable patients with minor to moderate penetrating splenic injuries who are suitable candidates for operative splenic salvage. In the LAC+USC series, splenorrhaphy was performed in 19% of patients undergoing emergency surgery and 42% of patients receiving operations after an initial trial of NOM. In patients undergoing exploration for other injuries with minor splenic injuries that are not actively bleeding, strong consideration of splenorrhaphy should be made because the tamponade provided by a closed abdomen has been lost, and there are few additional operative risks once a laparotomy has been performed.

OPERATIVE SPLENIC SALVAGE

A variety of splenic salvage techniques exist that may control hemorrhage while avoiding the immunologic consequences of the lifelong asplenic state. These techniques should be approached with caution because they are more prone to failure and delayed bleed than is splenectomy. They are performed infrequently because most injuries can be managed nonoperatively, and the most severely injured patients usually require splenectomy.

As with any open abdominal exploration for trauma, a generous midline laparotomy should be performed, and the entire abdomen examined for injuries. After ruling out or addressing more pressing injuries, attention may be turned to the spleen. The omentum should be taken down from the splenic hilum and the short gastric vessels divided using either 2-0 silk ligatures or bipolar electrocautery, permitting full visualization of the splenic hilum. Dividing the lienophrenic, lienorenal, and lienocolic ligaments will mobilize the spleen, allowing it to be elevated toward midline on its vascular pedicle of the splenic artery and vein and the short gastric arteries. The tail of the pancreas will be close to the splenic artery, and care should be taken to avoid iatrogenic pancreatic injury. At this point, a decision must be made to attempt splenorrhaphy, partial splenectomy, or complete splenectomy.

Splenorrhaphy

Minor injuries may be managed by any of a variety of topical hemostatic devices and agents. Small capsular and parenchymal injuries can be cauterized using electrocautery or argon photocoagulation. Topical agents such as microfibrillar collagen (Avitene [Davol, Cranston, RI]), absorbable gelatin sponge (Gelfoam [Pfizer, New York, NY]), or methylcellulose (Surgicel [Johnson & Johnson, New Brunswick, NJ]) can be left in place over the cauterized surface of the spleen to provide a matrix for clot formation. Deeper lacerations can be repaired with large hemostatic mattress sutures using 2-0 polypropylene or 0 chromic catgut. Dacron strips or pledgets (Ethicon [Piscataway, NJ]) can be used to buttress the sutures (Figure 3), although the use of nonresorbable pledgets may increase the risk of SSI if the abdomen has been contaminated by a hollow viscus injury. A tongue of omentum may be incorporated into the mattress sutures for additional tamponade and hemostasis.

Splenic lacerations that cannot be easily repaired topically or with suture splenorrhaphy may be amenable to mesh wrap repair. In this technique, the mobilized spleen is wrapped completely with a sheet of synthetic absorbable polyglycolate mesh. The mesh is gathered around the splenic hilum and approximated with a purse-string suture. Care should be taken not to compromise the arterial perfusion or venous drainage of the spleen.

Partial Splenectomy

Hemorrhage from deeper lacerations involving the larger vessels near the splenic hilum may not be controlled with splenorrhaphy alone. In this situation, partial splenectomy can be used to resect the nonsalvageable portion of the spleen, leaving a functional remnant in which hemostasis can be achieved. This is an appropriate maneuver if ligating a splenic artery branch results in a major reduction in the rate of hemorrhage, and at least half of the splenic parenchyma from an identifiable vessel is viable.

Manual compression of the spleen with a laparotomy sponge, and/or temporary occlusion of the vascular pedicle with a DeBakey bulldog clamp may be required for control of bleeding. The splenic artery branch that feeds the lacerated splenic pole then is ligated and divided (Figure 4), as is the corresponding venous branch. The residual splenic parenchyma then is divided using a linear stapler device or electrocautery. The resected margin is oversewn with mattress sutures, with or without the use of pledgets or an omental buttress.

FIGURE 3 Horizontal mattress sutures with Dacron strips approximate the laceration. *(From Cameron JL, Sandone C. Atlas of Gastrointestinal Surgery. 2nd ed. Shelton, CT: People's Medical Publishing House-USA; 2013; used with permission from PMPH-USA, Shelton, Conn.)*

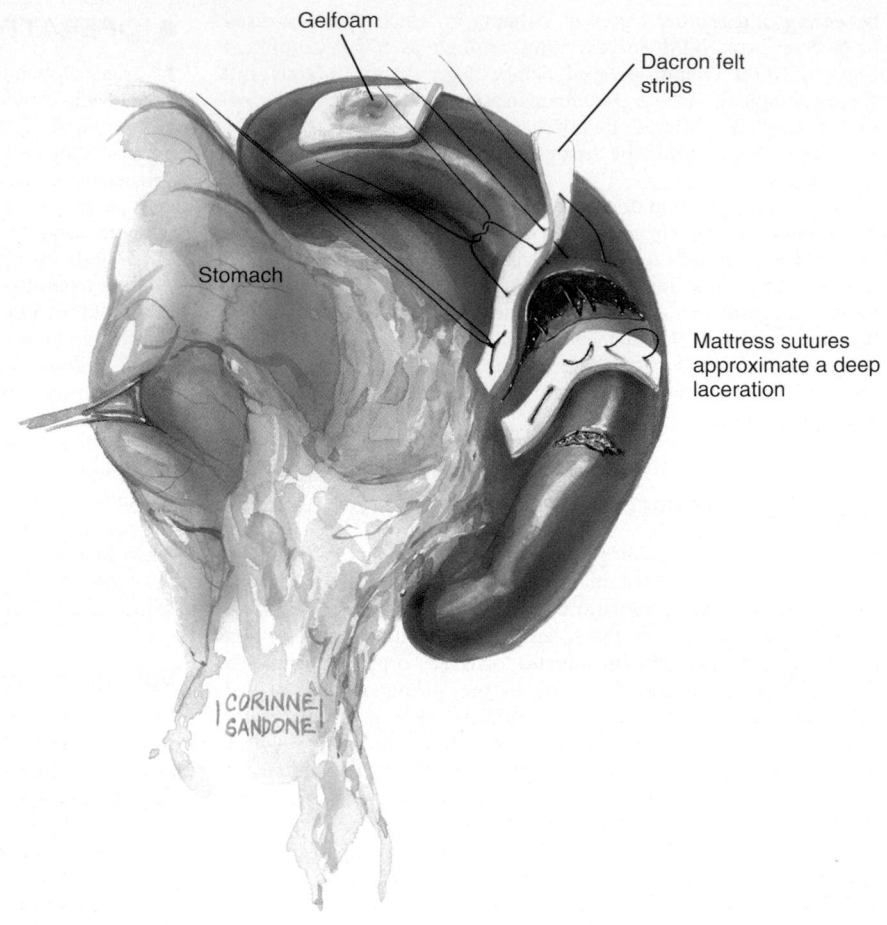

FIGURE 4 Partial splenectomy involves ligating and dividing the branches of the splenic artery and vein while applying manual compression as necessary. *(From Cameron JL, Sandone C. Atlas of Gastrointestinal Surgery. 2nd ed. Shelton, CT: People's Medical Publishing House-USA; 2013; used with permission from PMPH-USA, Shelton, Conn.)*

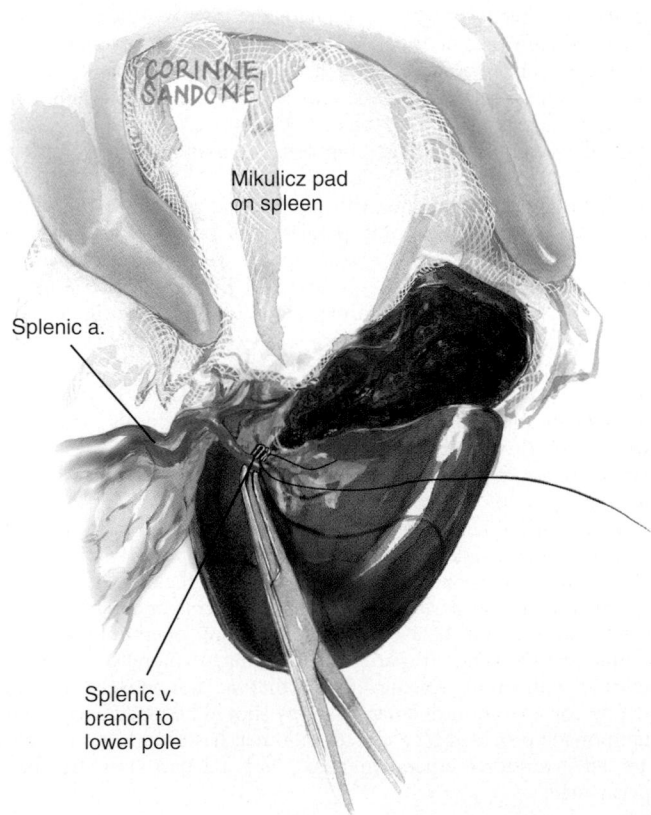

■ SUMMARY

The majority of splenic injuries may be treated without splenectomy. Intravenous contrast CT scans, serial physical and laboratory examination, and clinical decision making are crucial for successful NOM. In a subset of patients, SAE is a useful adjunct to NOM. A variety of operative maneuvers may be used to control splenic hemorrhage without splenectomy and the resulting loss of immune function. Although these splenic salvage maneuvers may reduce preventable morbidity in the appropriate patient, splenectomy is still the safest and most appropriate management for some patients, including those with hemodynamic instability, neurologic injury, or continuing hemorrhage.

SUGGESTED READINGS

Berg RJ, Inaba K, Okoye O, et al. The contemporary management of penetrating splenic injury. *Injury*. 2014;45:1394-1400.

Olthof DC, van der Vlies CH, Joosse P, et al. Consensus strategies for the nonoperative management of patients with blunt splenic injury: a Delphi study. *J Trauma*. 2013;74:1567-1574.

Stassen NA, Bhullar I, Cheng JD, et al. Selective nonoperative management of blunt splenic injury: an Eastern Association for the Surgery of Trauma practice management guideline. *J Trauma*. 2012;73:S294-S300.

Zarzaur BL, Kozar R, Myers JG, et al. The splenic injury outcomes trial: an American Association for the Surgery of Trauma multi-institutional study. *J Trauma*. 2015;79:335-342.

THE MANAGEMENT OF INGUINAL HERNIA

Timothy Kuwada, MD, and Dimitrios Stefanidis, MD, PhD, FACS, FASMBS

Inguinal hernia repair is one of the most common general surgical procedures, with more than 700,000 repairs performed in the United States every year. The procedure has a long history with many techniques described as it has evolved over the years. The contoured, three-dimensional anatomy of the groin is relatively complex, and there are a variety of different hernias that a surgeon may encounter within the groin. Although minimizing recurrence has been a long-standing premise of hernia repair, there are growing concerns about the risk of chronic groin pain. Regardless of the chosen approach (open vs laparoscopic), reducing morbidity and recurrence is dependent on meticulous technique and a thorough understanding of the groin anatomy. In this chapter we review the anatomy, presentation, diagnosis, and therapeutic options for groin hernias.

ANATOMIC CONSIDERATIONS

There are three weak points in the groin that account for almost all groin hernias: the internal ring (indirect hernia), the posterior "floor" of the inguinal canal medial to the epigastric vessels (direct hernia), and the femoral space (femoral hernia), which is medial to the femoral vessels and nerve and posterior to the inguinal ligament. The area encompassing these potential defects is called the *myopectineal orifice* (Figure 1). Most groin hernias are either direct or indirect inguinal hernias, both of which herniate into the inguinal canal. The inguinal canal is bounded by the inguinal ligament inferiorly, the transversus abdominis and internal oblique (the "conjoined tendon") superiorly, the transversalis fascia (the "floor") posteriorly, and the external oblique anteriorly. The cord structures (vas deferens, nerves, and testicular vessels) enter the inguinal canal through the internal ring and track inferior and medial to exit the canal at the external ring (Figure 2). When the peritoneum (sac) herniates through the internal ring, it resides anterior to the cord structures. Smaller hernias remain in the canal, whereas larger hernias breach the external ring and can extend well into the scrotum (inguinal-scrotal hernia).

There are three main sensory nerves that track through the inguinal canal: the iliohypogastric, the ilioinguinal, and the genital branch of the genitofemoral nerve. The ilioinguinal and iliohypogastric nerves enter the inguinal canal on the superior border exiting between the transversus abdominis and the internal oblique; they do not traverse the internal ring. These nerves provide sensation to the base of penis and scrotum in men and the mons and labia majora in women. During open inguinal hernia repair, these two nerves are at high risk for injury. There is debate as to whether they should be divided intentionally, creating a sensory deficit in favor of possible chronic pain from nerve injury. The genitofemoral nerve originates at the L1-2 plexus and courses inferiorly along the anterior psoas muscle, where it divides into a femoral and genital branch. The genital branch enters the inguinal canal via the internal ring, whereas the femoral branch parallels the iliac vessels, exiting the femoral canal and providing sensation to the inner thigh. The lateral femoral cutaneous nerve provides sensation to the upper lateral thigh. It initially tracks parallel to the ilioinguinal and iliohypogastric nerve but in a more inferior position. After crossing the psoas, it courses inferior, and anterolateral along the iliacus muscle, exiting the groin posterior to the inguinal ligament. During a laparoscopic preperitoneal dissection, dissecting into the side wall (iliacus muscle) can jeopardize this nerve (Figure 3).

PRESENTATION AND DIAGNOSIS

Groin hernias can occur at any age; however, they are more common in the middle to later years of life. Inguinal hernias are more common in men than women. However, femoral hernias, which make up less than 10% of groin hernias, are more common in women and more likely to have incarceration. Groin hernias are categorized as congenital (incomplete closure of the processus vaginalis) or acquired (because of weakening of the body wall tissues). Risk factors for hernia development include advanced age, male gender, Caucasian race, smoking, increased abdominal pressure, COPD, collagen disorders, and a personal or family history of hernia. There are conflicting data as to whether heavy lifting increases the risk of developing a hernia.

The most common presenting symptom of an inguinal hernia is a groin mass that is accentuated with coughing, straining (urination, defecation, or lifting), or prolonged periods of standing. The mass may disappear after lying down or with manual pressure. Many patients with a groin mass have few to no symptoms or pain. Alternatively, patients with groin pain and no definitive groin mass often are referred for surgical evaluation with the presumptive diagnosis of an inguinal hernia. Urinary or gastrointestinal symptoms, in the presence of an inguinal hernia, should raise suspicion for intermittent incarceration and lower the threshold for repair.

Most inguinal hernias can be diagnosed on physical exam and are classified as reducible, incarcerated, or strangulated. With the patient in the standing position, the examiner commences with a visual inspection of the groin. Any visual asymmetry of the groin is highly suggestive of a hernia. The groin then is palpated by invaginating the upper scrotum with the tip of the index finger and probing parallel to the spermatic cord to the level of the external ring. The patient then should cough or perform the Valsalva maneuver to accentuate any herniating contents. If a mass is present, it should be characterized further by size, degree of extension into the scrotum, ability to reduce the mass, and location relative to the inguinal ligament. If the mass is incarcerated, positioning the patient in the supine position may help with reduction of the hernia. Femoral hernias are more difficult to appreciate on exam and tend to elicit more pain and tenderness inferior to the inguinal canal in the region of the proximal inner thigh. The contralateral groin and umbilicus also should be examined carefully for the presence of an occult hernia. If repair is anticipated, the surgeon should discuss management of any

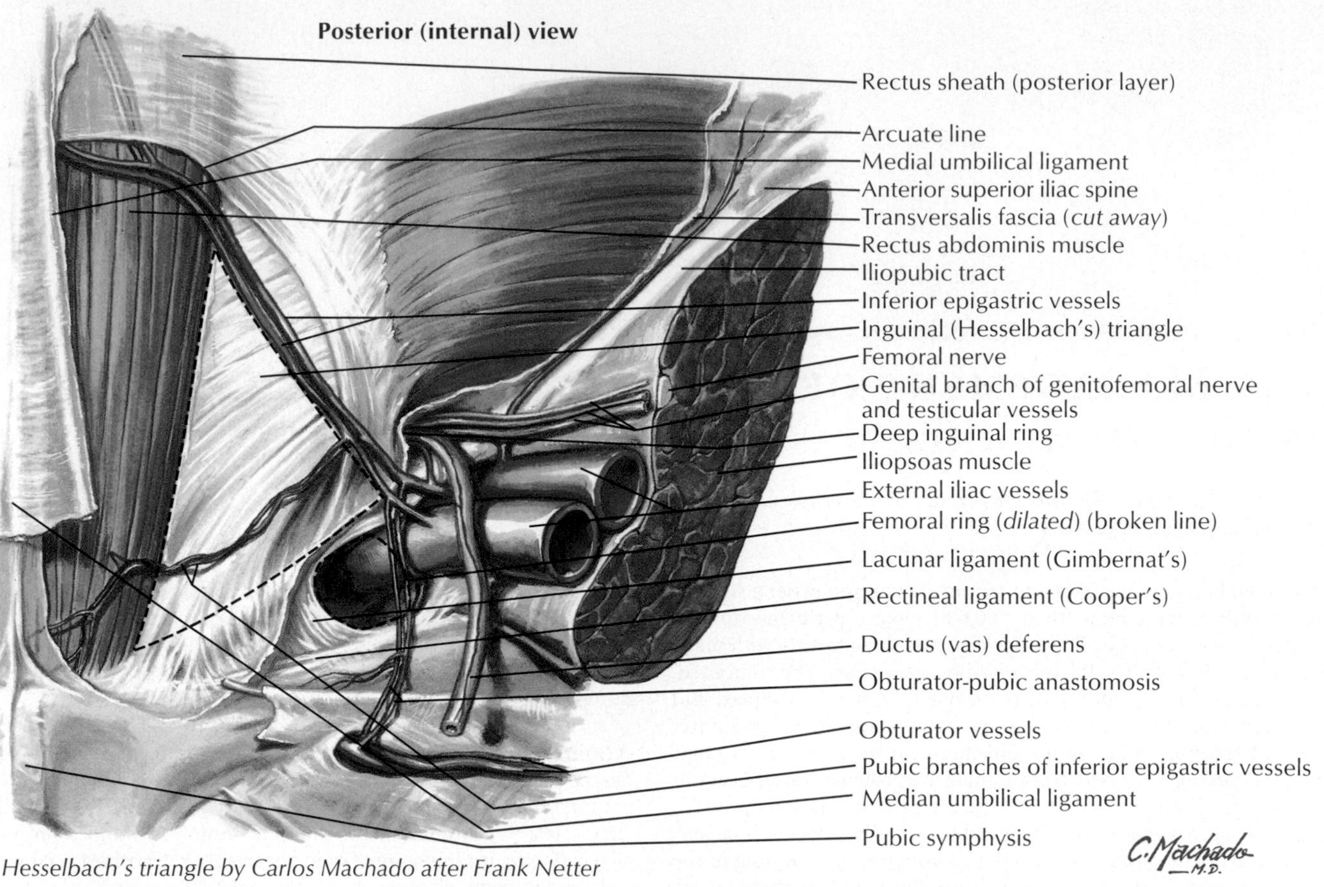

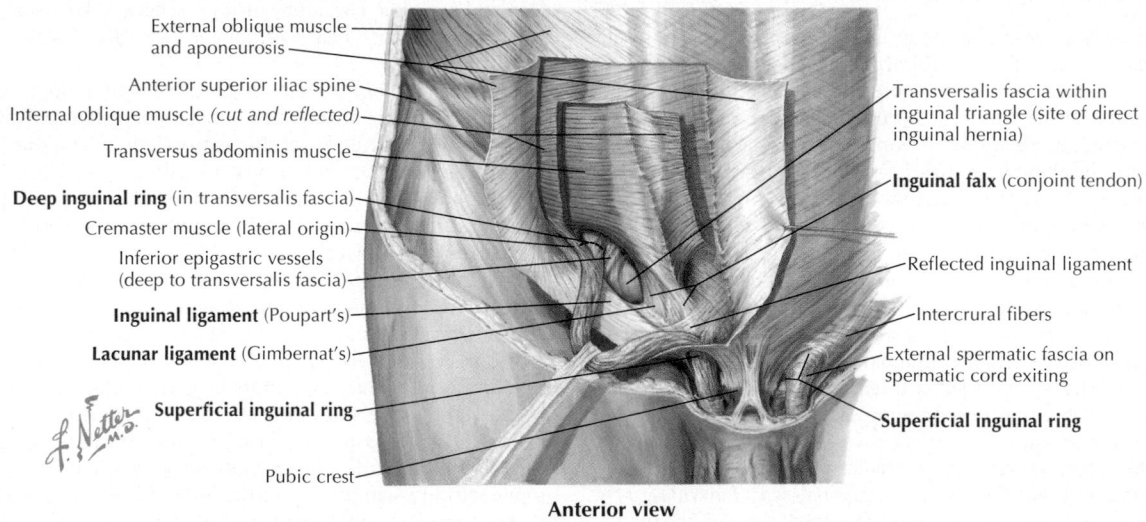

Posterior (internal) view

Rectus sheath (posterior layer)
Arcuate line
Medial umbilical ligament
Anterior superior iliac spine
Transversalis fascia (*cut away*)
Rectus abdominis muscle
Iliopubic tract
Inferior epigastric vessels
Inguinal (Hesselbach's) triangle
Femoral nerve
Genital branch of genitofemoral nerve and testicular vessels
Deep inguinal ring
Iliopsoas muscle
External iliac vessels
Femoral ring (*dilated*) (broken line)
Lacunar ligament (Gimbernat's)
Rectineal ligament (Cooper's)
Ductus (vas) deferens
Obturator-pubic anastomosis
Obturator vessels
Pubic branches of inferior epigastric vessels
Median umbilical ligament
Pubic symphysis

Hesselbach's triangle by Carlos Machado after Frank Netter

FIGURE 1 Anatomy of the groin from an intra-abdominal perspective. *(Copyright Elsevier, Inc., all rights reserved. www.netterimages.com.)*

External oblique muscle and aponeurosis
Anterior superior iliac spine
Internal oblique muscle *(cut and reflected)*
Transversus abdominis muscle
Deep inguinal ring (in transversalis fascia)
Cremaster muscle (lateral origin)
Inferior epigastric vessels (deep to transversalis fascia)
Inguinal ligament (Poupart's)
Lacunar ligament (Gimbernat's)
Superficial inguinal ring
Pubic crest

Transversalis fascia within inguinal triangle (site of direct inguinal hernia)
Inguinal falx (conjoint tendon)
Reflected inguinal ligament
Intercrural fibers
External spermatic fascia on spermatic cord exiting
Superficial inguinal ring

Anterior view

FIGURE 2 Inguinal anatomy. *(Copyright Elsevier, Inc., all rights reserved. www.netterimages.com.)*

co-existing hernias. In addition to a hernia, the differential diagnosis of a groin mass includes adenopathy, soft tissue neoplasm, and a venous varicosity. Any scars in the vicinity of the lower abdomen also raise the possibility of an incisional hernia. Finally, the position of the testicle should be documented because a high-riding or partially undescended testicle can mimic a hernia.

As opposed to a ventral hernia, it is very difficult to directly palpate a defect in the internal ring, inguinal floor, and femoral ring;

instead the diagnosis of a groin hernia is dependent on palpation of herniating contents. Lipomas of the spermatic cord ("cord lipoma") complicate the diagnosis because they can mimic an inguinal hernia. Thus it is possible for a patient to have a groin hernia in the presence of a normal exam (inability to reproduce herniating contents) or in the case of a cord lipoma to have no true defect in the presence of a groin mass. Finally, the specter of "sports hernia" has complicated further the diagnostic and therapeutic algorithm of groin pathology.

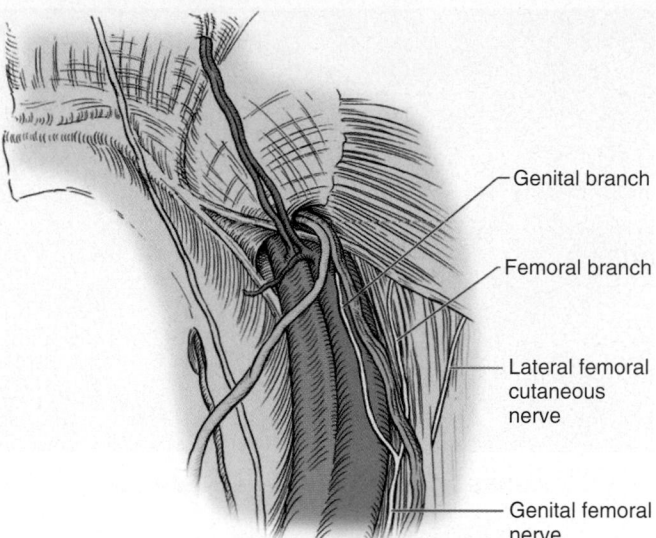

- Genital branch

- Femoral branch

- Lateral femoral cutaneous nerve

- Genital femoral nerve

FIGURE 3 Nerves at risk for injury during laparoscopic inguinal hernia repair. *(From Evans S. Surgical Pitfalls: Prevention and Management. Philadelphia: Saunders; 2009.)*

Sports hernia is a misnomer, and *athletic pubalgia* is a more appropriate term because there is no true tissue defect but rather pathology of the aponeurosis of the groin; typically this is associated with a sports-related activity. In carefully selected patients with specific radiographic and clinical findings, surgical repair (similar to inguinal herniorrhaphy) may be a viable treatment option. Athletic pubalgia is addressed in more detail in another chapter of this book.

As mentioned above, the majority of inguinal hernias can be diagnosed with a history and physical exam. However, for patients with groin pain and a normal or equivocal groin exam, imaging can assist in the diagnosis of a suspected occult groin hernia. Ultrasound is the most cost-effective modality, but it is user dependent, and it is difficult for the surgeon to interpret the images after the fact. In our opinion, computed tomography (CT) provides a more consistent, detailed view of the groin and pelvic anatomy and can be particularly useful in diagnosing occult groin hernias. If athletic pubalgia is suspected, pelvic magnetic resonance imaging is the optimal imaging modality.

■ TREATMENT

The decision to surgically repair or observe a groin hernia is based primarily on the type of hernia, the degree of symptoms, and the patient's ability to tolerate surgery. It is important to distinguish femoral and inguinal hernias because femoral hernias have a higher risk of strangulation and generally should be repaired expeditiously. Patients who have a strangulated or obstructing groin hernia require emergent operative intervention, and the likelihood of a bowel resection mandates that the surgeon carefully plan the incision and alternatives for repairing the hernia in a contaminated field. Nevertheless, the majority of patients with inguinal hernias have reducible hernias, many of which are minimally symptomatic.

The traditional recommendation has been to repair all hernias to prevent potential strangulation. However, a large randomized controlled trial by Fitzgibbons and colleagues comparing watchful waiting to surgery for asymptomatic inguinal hernias in men has cast doubt on this established dogma. Over a 4-year period, none of the 364 patients assigned to watchful waiting progressed to strangulation, and only two patients required emergent surgery for incarcerated obstructing groin hernias (risk of incarceration of 1.8/1000 patient years). Furthermore, watchful waiting did not increase the risks of future hernia repair. Although watchful waiting appears to be safe,

recently published long-term data from this study (>10 years) indicated that more than two thirds of the patients in the watchful waiting group ultimately underwent inguinal hernia repair. The authors concluded that men with minimally symptomatic inguinal hernias should be counseled that, although watchful waiting is a reasonable and safe strategy, symptoms will likely progress and an operation will be needed eventually. It is important to realize that the results of these studies do not apply to femoral hernias or hernias in women.

Surgical Options

Tissue Repairs

Surgical treatment of inguinal hernia dates back to the sixteenth century. The initial descriptions focused on repair of the anterior inguinal canal (external oblique) and tightening of the external ring. In 1887 Edoardo Bassini presented a paper to the Italian Surgical Society entitled "A Radical Cure of Inguinal Hernia," in which he described his technique for repairing the inguinal floor and internal ring. The tenets of the Bassini repair included division of the inguinal floor (transversalis fascia) and re-approximation of the superior/medial flap of the transversalis fascia and conjoined tendon to the inguinal ligament with interrupted permanent sutures. In the ensuing years, Bassini's tissue repair underwent numerous modifications; the most enduring has been the Shouldice repair. The Shouldice repair, similar to the Bassini, opens the inguinal floor and uses a running four-layer suture closure of the transversalis and approximation of the conjoined tendon to the inguinal ligament.

Currently, most groin hernias are repaired with either an open, tension-free, mesh technique or with a laparoscopic, preperitoneal mesh repair. Although most surgeons today have limited training and experience with primary, nonmesh, tissue repairs of the groin, this technique is invaluable when faced with strangulated hernias requiring repair in a contaminated field.

Open Mesh Repairs

In 1958 Sir Francis Usher reported a series of ventral hernia repairs with polypropylene mesh. This was the dawn of the mesh era in hernia surgery. However, for the next three decades primary tissue repair of the groin remained the norm. In 1989 Irvin Lichtenstein published a sentinel paper describing his series of 1000 inguinal hernia repairs. Lichtenstein was critical of the tension that was created by primary tissue repairs of the groin. The tension-free "Lichtenstein technique" used a 5- × 10-cm sheet of polypropylene mesh to bridge the gap between the conjoined tendon and inguinal ligament. The mesh was keyholed to allow passage of the spermatic cord through the mesh. It then was fixated medially to the pubic tubercle, inferiorly to Poupart's ligament, and superiorly to the internal oblique with permanent suture. Lichtenstein performed these procedures under local anesthesia, and there were no recurrences or mesh infections.

Despite his impressive results, Lichtenstein's technique was met with initial skepticism and critique within the surgical community. However, it soon became adopted widely and to this day remains the most common technique for inguinal hernia repair. The most common modifications to the Lichtenstein repair relate to variations in mesh material, weight, and fixation as well as the option of plugging the defect ("plug and patch" approach).

The "plug and patch" uses an anterior tension-free mesh repair similar to the Lichtenstein repair; however, it obliterates the defect with a mesh plug. The concept of adding a mesh plug to augment the Lichtenstein repair is conceptually appealing, but this technique has never been shown definitively to reduce recurrence rates. Importantly, the additional mesh plug can lead to complications such as chronic pain and is harder to remove if needed. Further, the intra-abdominal protrusion of the plug (Figure 4) may lead rarely to complications. The authors of this chapter do not recommend this technique for these reasons. Another option for open repair is posterior, preperitoneal placement of mesh as described by Stoppa (one

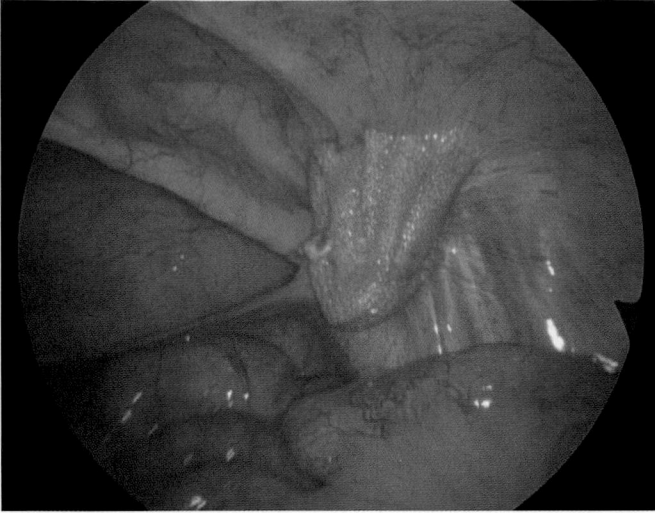

FIGURE 4 Intra-abdominal protrusion of mesh plug.

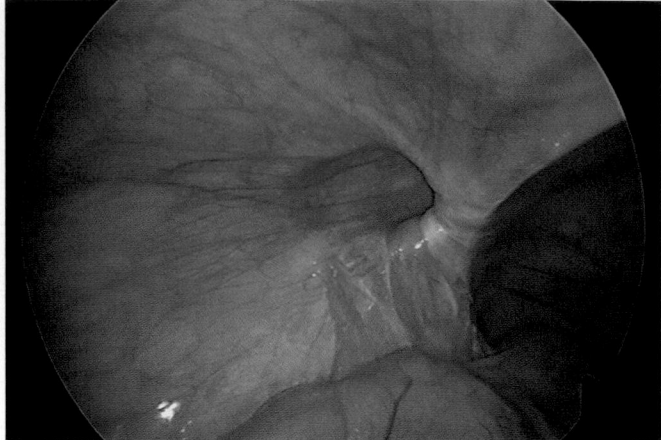

FIGURE 5 Visualization of the contralateral groin.

large mesh covering both groins). More recently the Kugel repair was popularized by the advent of a self-expanding mesh that facilitated positioning of the mesh through a small groin incision. However, there were problems with the rim of this mesh fracturing, and it ultimately was recalled. The adverse events with this mesh, coupled with a laparoscopic approach, which enables more direct visualization of the preperitoneum, have led to a decline in the popularity of this approach.

The Prolene Hernia System consists of an anterior oval polypropylene mesh connected to a posterior circular component. The posterior component is deployed in a bluntly created preperitoneal space through the internal ring. The anterior portion then is sutured above to the conjoined tendon and below to the shelving edge of the inguinal ligament and is tucked behind the external oblique aponeurosis (similar to the Lichtenstein approach). This technique has shown promising results in several trials with very low recurrence rates.

Laparoscopic Repairs

The first laparoscopic inguinal hernia repair with synthetic mesh was described by Schultz in 1990. His technique used a transabdominal preperitoneal (TAPP) approach to plug the defect with polypropylene mesh. In 1993 McKernan reported the first laparoscopic series employing a totally extraperitoneal (TEP) technique. As opposed to plugging the defect, McKernan placed the mesh in a preperitoneal, bridging position; he did not close the defect or obliterate it with mesh. To this day, TAPP and TEP with bridging mesh remain the two primary options for laparoscopic inguinal hernia repair.

The TAPP and TEP techniques use a bridging mesh that is placed in the preperitoneal space and covers the entire myopectineal orifice (see Figure 1). Although the TEP approach avoids violation of the peritoneum and its potential complications compared with TAPP, it is associated with a longer learning curve. Further, TAPP enables easy inspection of the contralateral side (without the need for dissection) and intra-abdominal organs. To avoid dissection of the contralateral side during TEP when suspicion for a hernia is small, we introduce a 5-mm trocar through the posterior rectus sheath at the umbilical trocar site and inspect directly the contralateral myopectineal orifice; this also allows for inspection of the repaired ipsilateral side to verify appropriate mesh positioning and lack of folding and ensure complete closure of any peritoneal defects that may have occurred during dissection. Overall, both techniques are considered equivalent in experienced hands. In both, it is imperative that a large preperitoneal pocket be created for placement of the mesh, particularly posterolaterally (and over the cord structures in men), where the mesh has a tendency to flip up and compromise coverage of the defect. There are a variety of options for mesh fixation, including tacks (both absorbable and permanent), suture, and adhesives, but controversy

exists even about the need for any fixation. If fixation is used, it should be limited to the region of Cooper's ligament, medial to the femoral space and the anterior abdominal wall. Tacks should not be placed posterior to the anterior superior iliac spine (ASIS) to avoid nerve injury.

There are several unique perioperative considerations when planning a laparoscopic inguinal hernia repair. The potential space created by the hernia sac is not obliterated during laparoscopic repair, thus the risk of seroma is higher than open surgery. Patients should be counseled on the possibility of a postoperative seroma that can mimic a recurrent hernia. However, patient and surgeon should be reassured that this is a self-limiting process that rarely requires drainage. Laparoscopy also affords visualization of the contralateral groin (Figure 5). It is important to clarify preoperatively the patient's desire for repair of an occult, contralateral hernia that is discovered during surgery. The benefits of repairing a small, asymptomatic, occult hernia must be weighed against the small but real risk of chronic pain from the repair.

Laparoscopic Versus Open Repair

Considerable debate still exists regarding the optimal approach to groin hernia repair (laparoscopic vs open), particularly for unilateral, primary hernias. A sentinel prospective study conducted at the Veterans Administration hospital system by Fitzgibbons and colleagues concluded that recurrence rates were significantly higher for the laparoscopic technique (10% laparoscopic vs 5% open). However, since the "VA Study" was published in 2004, there has been a growing body of evidence demonstrating equivalent or superior recurrence rates of laparoscopic compared with open technique, particularly when performed by surgeons with laparoscopic expertise. There are several potential advantages of the laparoscopic technique. First, it affords visualization of the entire groin, including the femoral and obturator spaces and the contralateral groin. The TAPP technique also enables the surgeon to assess the entire abdominal cavity, which may be particularly useful in identifying occult ventral hernias or compromised bowel that was reduced from an incarcerated inguinal hernia.

Laparoscopic repair tends to be less painful than open surgery and associated with earlier return to regular activities, particularly for bilateral repair. Laparoscopy avoids the more traumatic open exposure and is associated with a lower injury risk of the ilioinguinal, iliohypogastric, and genital branch of genitofemoral nerves. Posterior placement of mesh in the preperitoneal space covers the entire myopectineal orifice (internal ring, floor, and the femoral space). Mechanically, there also may be an advantage by allowing the intra-abdominal pressure to augment fixation of the mesh.

Despite these advantages, compared with other laparoscopic procedures (cholecystectomy, bariatric, appendectomy, and foregut surgery), laparoscopic herniorrhaphy has yet to be adopted widely. The small working space and potentially disorienting and unfamiliar posterior groin anatomy make it a challenging laparoscopic procedure with a long learning curve. Although rare, compared with the open approach, the risk of vascular and visceral injury is higher. In an era of cost containment, the relatively high operative cost of laparoscopy is an additional concern. Laparoscopy also requires general anesthesia, making it less appealing for high-risk patients who may be better served by an open repair under local anesthesia. Previous lower abdominal surgery, particularly preperitoneal procedures such as prostatectomy and vascular bypass, increase the complexity of a posterior approach. Finally, in the author's opinion, large inguinal scrotal hernias are better addressed with an open approach. Reducing a deep sac in the scrotum is tedious, and the large potential space that extends into the scrotum is at high risk for significant fluid accumulation (seroma) after surgery. The open approach is a more efficient technique for reduction of the scrotal peritoneal sac and associated with less seroma formation. In addition, if a patient develops a recurrent groin hernia after a laparoscopic repair, the anterior open technique affords virgin tissue planes. It would be significantly more difficult to approach such cases with repeat laparoscopy and ill-advised for the inexperienced surgeon.

Robotic Repair

With the increasing popularity of robotic surgery, a number of general surgeons have started using the currently available robotic system for inguinal hernia repair. Although the TAPP approach is applied typically with the robot, the newest generation robotic system makes TEP also feasible. The improved visualization (three-dimensional view, higher magnification), motion scaling, and enhanced dexterity that robotic surgery provides may be advantageous for the dissection and peritoneal closure during TAPP. Given that laparoscopic repair is associated with a well-recognized steep learning curve, these advantages of robotic surgery may translate to quicker achievement of competence with the technique. If this hypothesis proves true, it may allow larger penetration of minimally invasive techniques in the treatment of inguinal hernias. Nevertheless, robust outcome data with the technique are needed before the effectiveness of this approach can be judged reliably. In addition, in a financially strained health care system the cost effectiveness of this technique also must be demonstrated.

Mesh

Although technique is the major determinant of long-term outcomes in hernia surgery, it is critical that surgeons understand the important characteristics and relative cost of the various mesh materials. During the past decade there has been a dramatic increase in mesh options for hernia repair, including variations in weight, shape, material, and coating. The burgeoning class of biomesh materials further complicates the choice of mesh.

The most common material used in groin hernias is either polypropylene or polyester. Their macroporous configuration enhances tissue incorporation and subsequent fixation. This is particularly important when the mesh is placed in the preperitoneal space, where nerves and vasculature limit complete fixation with tacks or sutures. Because the mesh is not in direct contact with viscera, it does not have to be coated with antiadhesive barriers. The primary variable within this material group is weight (gm/m²). "Lightweight" mesh has been shown in some studies to reduce chronic inflammation, mesh rigidity, and mesh sensation, but systematic reviews and meta-analyses examining differences with regular-weight mesh have yet to demonstrate such differences. Expanded polytetrafluoroethylene (ePTFE) is another permanent synthetic option. However, its microporous construct inhibits incorporation and fixation and increases infection risk, thus it generally is not used in the groin.

Biomaterial options include allografts (human dermis), xenografts (bovine pericardium and porcine dermis and intestinal submucosa), and synthetic biomeshes. However, most inguinal repairs use a bridging mesh repair, and when biologics are used in this manner, the recurrence rate approaches 100%. Thus biologics are rarely, if ever, indicated in groin hernia surgery.

Chronic Postoperative Pain

Although the improvements in surgical techniques and technology for inguinal hernia repair have led to a significant decrease in hernia recurrence rates (in most series <5%), there is heightened appreciation for the risk of chronic postoperative pain. Defined as pain that persists for more than 3 months after surgery, chronic pain may affect up to one third of patients undergoing inguinal herniorrhaphy with a small subset of patients experiencing severe, disabling pain. Given the large number of patients undergoing inguinal hernia repair annually in the United States, many of whom have minimally symptomatic hernias, the number of patients affected by chronic pain is considerable. Severe pre-existing pain, young age, and female gender appear to be highest risk factors for chronic pain, and these patients should be counseled appropriately before surgery. Validated risk calculators (apps) for chronic postoperative pain allow surgeons to provide individual patients with a more precise risk assessment.

Chronic pain after groin surgery may be due to hernia recurrence, the presence of mesh, neuropathy, infection, or a combination thereof. When patients experience chronic pain after surgery, a thorough focused history and groin exam should be performed. The characteristics of the pain may point toward the underlying cause; recurrence of the patient's preoperative pain that is activity related and relieved when lying flat may point toward a recurrence of the hernia or a missed hernia at the time of the original repair. Women who undergo open inguinal repair are at the highest risk for a missed femoral hernia. Vague, dull groin pain that is accentuated with hip flexion and activities such as sitting, driving, or bending usually is related to the presence of the mesh. It typically does not radiate and is milder in intensity and rarely requires explantation of the mesh. Although discomfort related to the mesh can occur with a perfectly positioned mesh, it tends to be more common and intense if the mesh is contorted (the so-called "meshoma"). Patients with neuropathic pain typically have a burning or electrical shooting sensation in the dermatome of the affected nerve. Neuropathic pain can be caused by nerve injury or inflammation during the formation of the hernia (preoperative), injury of the nerve during surgery (entrapment of the nerve by suture or other fixation material), or ingrowth, entrapment, or impingement of the nerve by the mesh. The latter may explain why patients can have a delayed presentation of postoperative inguinodynia. Pain that is relieved temporarily with a local nerve block is indicative of neuropathic pain. Although very rare, mesh infection is another potential cause of inguinodynia; when present it typically is accompanied by wound drainage or local inflammatory signs, constitutional symptoms (fever, night sweats, or fatigue), or an elevated white blood cell count or C-reactive protein (CRP).

If the patient has an obvious recurrent hernia on exam, repair is indicated without further testing. If the exam is unrevealing, we recommend a CT scan of the pelvis with Valsalva specifically looking for recurrence, an occult femoral hernia, or a fluid collection deep to the mesh, which arouses suspicion regarding a mesh infection. Fluid anterior to the mesh usually represents a seroma, which is common in the first few months after surgery. If a mesh infection is suspected and the patient is not septic, a trial of antibiotics and drainage should be initiated. Macroporous mesh, such as polyester and polypropylene, may be salvaged by this approach, but removal of the mesh may be necessary.

The majority of patients presenting with chronic severe inguinodynia have a neuropathic cause, which is a vexing problem for patient and physician. Treatment should take a stepwise, multidisciplinary approach with initial referral to a pain specialist with expertise in chronic groin pain. In addition to nonsteroidal anti-inflammatory drugs, there are numerous non-narcotic pain-modulating medications that may offer some relief. Serial nerve blocks, nerve ablation, or steroid injections may relieve the patient's discomfort. Surgery, which usually consists of a triple neurectomy with mesh removal, should be the last resort. During this procedure, the surgeon should remove as much of the mesh as is safe and identify and divide the three groin nerves (ilioinguinal, iliohypogastric, and the genital branch of the genitofemoral nerve) proximally. Patients should be warned that removal of the mesh is likely to lead to a hernia recurrence, that the pain may not subside completely, and that numbness in the areas supplied by these nerves will occur. To avoid hernia recurrence, after prior open hernia repair, we prefer to place a mesh in the preperitoneal position laparoscopically before removing the old mesh and dividing the nerves; division of the nerves can be accomplished with an open or laparoscopic technique.

Regardless of the cause of the chronic pain, early treatment should be the goal to improve outcomes.

SUGGESTED READINGS

Alfieri S, Amid PK, Campanelli G, et al. International guidelines for prevention and management of post-operative chronic pain following inguinal hernia surgery. *Hernia*. 2011;15:239-249.

Burgmans JP, Voorbrood CE, Simmermacher RK, et al. Long-term results of a randomized double-blinded prospective trial of a lightweight (Ultrapro) versus a heavyweight mesh (Prolene) in laparoscopic total extraperitoneal inguinal hernia repair (TULP-trial). *Ann Surg*. 2016;263:862-866.

Fitzgibbons RJ Jr, Ramanan B, Arya S, Turner SA, Li X, Gibbs JO, Reda DJ; Investigators of the Original Trial. Long-term results of a randomized controlled trial of a nonoperative strategy (watchful waiting) for men with minimally symptomatic inguinal hernias. *Ann Surg*. 2013;258:508-515.

Poelman MM, van den Heuvel B, Deelder JD, et al. EAES Consensus Development Conference on endoscopic repair of groin hernias. *Surg Endosc*. 2013;27:3505-3519.

Simons MP, Aufenacker T, Bay-Nielsen M, et al. European Hernia Society guidelines on the treatment of inguinal hernia in adult patients. *Hernia*. 2009;13:343-403.

THE MANAGEMENT OF RECURRENT INGUINAL HERNIA

Iman Ghaderi, MS, MSc, and Leigh Neumayer, MD, MS

Inguinal hernia is a common general surgery problem and is one of the most frequently performed operations by general surgeons worldwide. The prevalence of inguinal hernias is about 1.5% in the United States, and more than 700,000 patients undergo hernia repair every year. Recurrent inguinal hernias have been reported in up to 15% of all inguinal hernia repairs. Although many studies report the recurrence rate of inguinal hernia repair to be less than 5%, evidence from large series and national registries show about 17% of inguinal hernia operations are for recurrent hernias. The true recurrence rate is unknown, which is due primarily to lack of long-term follow-up and varying definitions of recurrence. Therefore these must be considered estimates of the actual recurrence rate.

■ DEFINITION

A recurrent inguinal hernia is demonstrated by the presence of a bulge or defect in the abdominal wall in the groin area after previously repaired inguinal or femoral hernia. There are several factors that increase the chance of recurrence.

■ RISK FACTORS AND CAUSES OF RECURRENCE

The causes of recurrence after inguinal hernia repair can be categorized as follows: (1) technical issues (tissue repair vs repair with synthetic mesh; laparoscopic vs open repair), including surgeon's experience, (2) factors contributing to healing, and (3) genetics.

Technical Issues

Technical issues contributing to recurrence are due to either inadequate dissection and reduction of the indirect sac or failure to identify a direct or indirect hernia in either open or laparoscopic repair. Other common causes of recurrence are repair under tension in anterior approach, incorrect placement of mesh in laparoscopic repair, and inadequate overlap of mesh in the inferomedial side of inguinal canal near the pubic tubercle, where the medial recurrence classically occurs after open hernia repair. It also has been shown that a surgeon's experience and initial learning curve are elements that affect the recurrence rate.

Primary tissue repair techniques such as Bassini, Halstead, and McVay have a higher rate of recurrence (10% to 15%). This is due to significant tension at the repair site. The Shouldice repair is the only tissue repair technique that has been reported to have a low recurrence rate (1% to 2%) when it is performed in specialized clinics; otherwise, the recurrence rate is higher when compared with mesh repair in general practice. The reasons could be the complexity of dissection and repair and long learning curve without dedicated training. Therefore, unless there is a contraindication for placement of permanent mesh in situations such as strangulated hernia with perforation and contaminated field, repair of an inguinal hernia with mesh is the standard of care.

Mesh and Recurrence

The gold standard technique in inguinal hernia repair is the use of tension-free mesh to reduce recurrences. Use of mesh is associated with 50% to 75% reduction in the risk of recurrence. Heavyweight and lightweight mesh are two main mesh types that are used widely. The disadvantage of using heavyweight mesh results in a higher risk of postoperative pain and foreign body sensation. The concern with the use of lightweight mesh, however, has been possibility of a higher recurrence rate. In recent meta-analysis and systemic review, it was shown that there was no significant difference in recurrence between lightweight and heavyweight meshes either in open or laparoscopic repairs.

Laparoscopic Versus Open Hernia Repair and Recurrence

In contrast to the general agreement on necessity of mesh for primary inguinal hernia repair, there is no consensus on ideal technique for repair of recurrent inguinal hernia. There is still a controversy whether laparoscopic repair is as good as open inguinal hernia repair with respect to recurrence rate. In early experience with laparoscopic repair of inguinal hernia, Neumayer and colleagues in their VA Multicenter Trial showed recurrence was significantly higher with laparoscopic repair than after open repair of primary hernias (from 10.1% to 4.0%). The authors demonstrated that the recurrence was associated with surgeons' experience and the learning curve of the procedure. It has been shown that recurrence rate after laparoscopic repair can be reduced significantly with proper training, adequate experience, and technique and use of a larger size mesh.

Poor Healing

Common risk factors in poor healing such as malnutrition, immunosuppression, diabetes mellitus, and infection increase the risk of hernia recurrence. Obesity and smoking are two other important risk factors for recurrence. Obesity increases not only the chance of wound infection but also the tension on fixation site, which can predispose the patient to recurrence. Smoking plays an important role in hernia recurrence. It affects collagen metabolism, tissue remodeling, and tissue ischemia, resulting in poor healing. Smoker's cough is a known cause of increase in abdominal pressure, which also may increase the chance of recurrence. The recurrence rate after inguinal hernia repair is twice as high in patients who smoke.

Genetics

It is well documented that patients with collagen synthesis disorders such as Ehlers-Danlos syndrome and Marfan's syndrome have a higher chance of developing a hernia. This is true about patients who have poor tissue remolding, such as patients with aortic aneurysmal disease.

■ DIAGNOSIS

Similar to primary inguinal hernia, patients with a recurrent inguinal hernia usually have a bulge in the groin area. It could be small or large with scrotal extension of the hernia content. Loose closure of external ring in anterior repair should not be mistaken with recurrence. It is important to differentiate chronic groin pain from recurrence and not assume groin pain is always due to recurrence.

Role of Imaging

Physical examination is the main method in diagnosis of recurrence. However, in some situations imaging may be helpful: for example, if there is a very small defect with groin pain but no obvious bulge or if there is clinical doubt about presence of a hernia. Ultrasonography (US), computed tomography (CT) scan, and magnetic resonance imaging (MRI) can be used as adjunct to clinical assessment of patients with equivocal physical findings. US is a cheap and feasible modality, but it is operator dependent and has a low sensitivity. CT scan does not have a significant role in the diagnosis of primary or recurrent inguinal hernia, even though it has a sensitivity of 83% and a specificity of 67% to 83%. MRI, on the other hand, has high sensitivity and specificity and can be used to study any plane during Valsalva maneuver.

■ TREATMENT

To increase the success rate of repair in recurrent hernias, the possible risk factors, such as smoking, should be eliminated or modified. The patient also should be made aware of the higher risk of complications in redo operations. These include nerve injury and the possibility of chronic pain, injury to cord structures, and subsequent ischemic orchitis and testicular atrophy in male patients. The patient should be well informed that recurrence rate after the repair of recurrent hernia is even higher regardless of the type of repair, technique, and the type of mesh used. This is due to the fact that after recurrence the tissue is weaker than the initial repair.

Algorithm for Treatment

The cornerstones of recurrent inguinal hernia repairs are (1) re-enforcement of the entire inguinal canal, regardless of the size and location of the recurrence, and (2) to approach the hernia through the tissue that has not been violated previously when possible (Figure 1). If the previous repair with mesh was done from an anterior approach, the laparoscopic or open preperitoneal placement

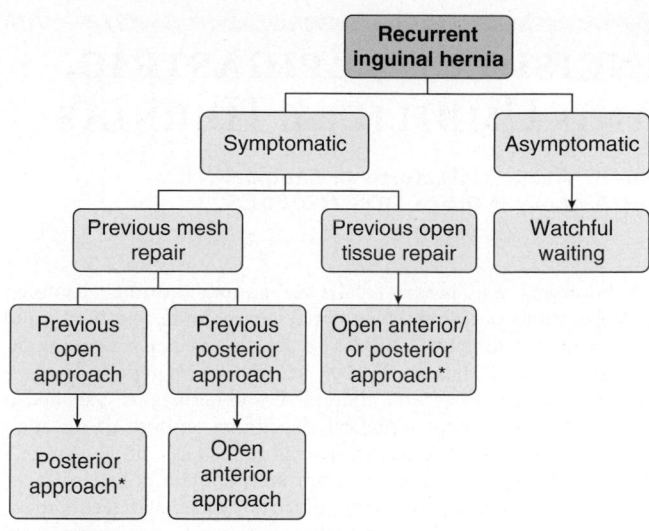

* Laparoscopic or open preperitoneal mesh placement

FIGURE I Algorithm for management of recurrent inguinal hernia.

mesh method (posterior approach) is preferable because it has been shown that the recurrent groin hernias were associated with the lowest risk of reoperation after these repairs. An anterior approach would be a reasonable choice after recurrence after laparoscopic or open posterior repair. This is especially appropriate if the preperitoneal space was once violated and there is significant scar tissue, making the dissection and exposure more difficult and unsafe by increasing the risk of injury to the cord structure and other structures, such as vessels and nerves in the vicinity of hernia. If the initial hernia repair was done without mesh, the same approach can be used. There is a general consensus that surgeon's experience and previous training have a definitive impact on the safety and success of repair in recurrent hernias.

In contrast to primary repair of inguinal hernia, in which there are extensive studies on various techniques and timing of repairs, there is limited literature regarding repair of recurrent hernias. Therefore most recommendations are based on expert opinions and extrapolation of data from studies on primary inguinal hernias. Given the challenges in repairing recurrent hernias, the surgeon must discuss carefully pros and cons of repair with the patient. It has been shown that the risk of recurrence increases with increasing number of hernia repairs. Therefore all possible options, including watchful waiting before any surgical repair, should be considered. Most experts consider the watchful waiting an acceptable alternative to repair because the risk of strangulation is very low. The surgical repair is a reasonable option if the patient becomes symptomatic or if there is a significant increase in the size of the hernia and concern for complications such as incarceration and strangulation.

SUGGESTED READINGS

Eker HH, Langeveld HR, Klitsie PJ, et al. Randomized clinical trial of total extraperitoneal inguinal hernioplasty vs Lichtenstein repair: a long-term follow-up study. *Arch Surg.* 2012;147:256-260.

Miserez M, Peeters E, Aufenacker T, et al. Update with level 1 studies of the European Hernia Society guidelines on the treatment of inguinal hernia in adult patients. *Hernia.* 2014;18:151-163.

Moesinger RC. Recurrent inguinal hernia. In: Cameron JL, Cameron AM, eds. *Current Surgical Therapy.* 11th ed. Philadelphia: Elsevier; 2013:536-539.

Neumayer L, Giobbie-Hurder A, Jonasson O, et al. Open mesh versus laparoscopic mesh repair of inguinal hernia. *N Engl J Med.* 2004;350:1819-1827.

Sajid MS, Leaver C, Baig MK, et al. Systematic review and meta-analysis of the use of lightweight versus heavyweight mesh in open inguinal hernia repair. *Br J Surg.* 2012;99:29-37.

INCISIONAL, EPIGASTRIC, AND UMBILICAL HERNIAS

Saïd C. Azoury, MD, Kurtis A. Campbell, MD,
and Anthony P. Tufaro, DDS, MD, FACS

Abdominal wall hernia repairs are among the most common operations performed by general, laparoscopic, and plastic and reconstructive surgeons worldwide. In the United States alone, approximately 250,000 to 350,000 ventral hernia repairs are performed each year. In general, abdominal wall hernias are classified as incisional, epigastric, or umbilical, depending on both the location and the underlying etiology. A hernia is defined as a protrusion of a structure through the tissues that normally contain it. Regardless of the type of hernia, each hernia results in a myofascial defect that can lead to serious complications such as intestinal incarceration and strangulation. Timely diagnosis of an abdominal hernia and related sequelae is crucial, as the presentation may be an elective, urgent, or emergent problem.

Incisional hernias are secondary to prior surgery and occur in 11% to 20% of patients after laparotomy. Epigastric and umbilical hernias are primary midline defects that are present in up to 50% of the population, thought to be a result of genetic predisposition or acquired structural abnormalities from mechanical strain. Epigastric and umbilical hernias account for 75% of all ventral hernia repairs performed annually in the United States. Epigastric hernias are typically acquired and related to attenuation of the midline fascia. Umbilical hernias are considered true congenital fascial defects and commonly are diagnosed and repaired in early childhood. The goal of repair of the aforementioned hernias is restoration of abdominal wall integrity and function in order to eliminate or prevent symptoms and complications that otherwise would occur. Surgical technique is usually via an open or laparoscopic approach, depending largely on the anticipated complexity of the case and medical/surgical history of the patient. Indications for repair include a symptomatic hernia that causes pain or change in bowel habits, significant risk of bowel obstruction, or significant protrusion that affects a patient's quality of life.

INCISIONAL HERNIA

Incisional hernias occur at the original surgical incision, a drain site, or a trocar site in the case of laparoscopy. A hernia through a port site occurs most often when a 10-mm or larger access incision is used. Incisional hernias may be either small, involving only a portion of the incision, or large, occupying the majority of the anterior abdominal wall with resultant loss of domain (Figure 1). Some of the more common patient-specific risk factors for developing an incisional hernia are obesity, diabetes, smoking, chronic obstructive pulmonary disease (COPD), connective tissue disorders (e.g., Ehlers-Danlos syndrome), advanced age, immunosuppression, history of prior surgeries or hernia operations at the same site, and wound infection or contamination. Incisional hernias are most often ventral in location (90%) but can be in the flank, subcostal, or lumbar area (Figure 2). Up to 50% of these hernias occur in the first 6 months after surgery, and the majority of them are diagnosed by 2 years after surgery.

EPIGASTRIC HERNIA

An epigastric hernia is a ventral hernia that occurs through the linea alba at the midline between the umbilicus and the xiphoid process. The majority of these hernias occur in young and middle-aged adults between 20 and 50 years of age, and they are more common in men. It is believed that these hernias form as a result of a gradual enlargement of the space where small blood vessels penetrate the linea alba (vascular lacunae) and/or as a result of a single, attenuated decussating layer of the fascial fibers of the linea alba rather than redundant aponeurotic fibers. The linea alba is wider in the upper part of the abdominal wall, and therefore there is a higher incidence of epigastric hernias at this location because of the weaker and attenuated decussating fibers when compared with the infraumbilical region. These hernias are often difficult to diagnose in morbidly obese or severely obese patients, as the surrounding fat makes the hernia protrusion less noticeable (Figure 3).

UMBILICAL HERNIA

An umbilical hernia is a ventral hernia located near or at the umbilicus. Umbilical hernias are very common in infancy, and approximately 80% of these defects will close by 5 years of age. When diagnosed in adulthood, these hernias occur more often in women and may be seen after periods of increased intra-abdominal pressure, such as with new-onset constipation, pregnancy, ascites, or COPD.

PREOPERATIVE ASSESSMENT

Diagnosis often is achieved though clinical patient interview and physical examination. Patients often may complain of discomfort and pain at the site. Physical examination may reveal a palpable bulge and fascial defect in the abdominal wall, which is exacerbated by increases in abdominal pressure, as with coughing. Furthermore, there may be associated changes of the overlying skin, including signs of ischemia, thinning, ulceration, and erythema. Although not always necessary, imaging may be pursued at the surgeon's discretion. Computed tomographic (CT) imaging remains the gold-standard preoperative imaging modality (Figure 4) and helps to detect herniation of abdominal structures other than the bowel (e.g., omentum, preperitoneal fat). Furthermore, CT imaging often will help to differentiate between diastasis recti (gap between left and right rectus abdominis muscles) and a true abdominal hernia, as the management of these entities may differ.

Patient optimization before surgery should focus on improved oxygenation in those with pulmonary disease, smoking cessation more than 3 to 4 weeks preoperatively, weight loss, adequate glucose control in patients with diabetes, improved nutritional status, and infection control if infection is present. These simple measures will help to optimize patients before surgery in order to minimize the risk of postoperative morbidity and surgical site occurrences (SSOs).

SURGICAL CONSIDERATIONS

Laparoscopic repair is a minimally invasive method that has gained popularity since the 1990s in an attempt to decrease postoperative morbidity. Despite major advances, only a quarter of ventral hernia repairs are performed laparoscopically. There are several situations in which a laparoscopic approach is preferable. Several studies have noted fewer wound infections and shorter hospital stays after laparoscopic repair compared with open hernia repair. Some surgeons may argue that laparoscopy can be used in the presence of acutely or chronically incarcerated hernias to allow for an assessment of bowel viability. It may be possible that, under general anesthesia, the hernia contents can be reduced more easily and adhesiolysis can proceed safely. However, if the patient is ill and there is a high suspicion for ischemic bowel, surgery should proceed in an open fashion. Furthermore, when preoperative assessment and imaging suggests multiple defects in the fascia, a laparoscopic approach will allow adequate visualization of the fascia to ensure proper prosthetic positioning and repair. Also, as long as trocar placement is not an issue, laparoscopic repair of larger defects will obviate the need for a large incision and the associated postoperative pain.

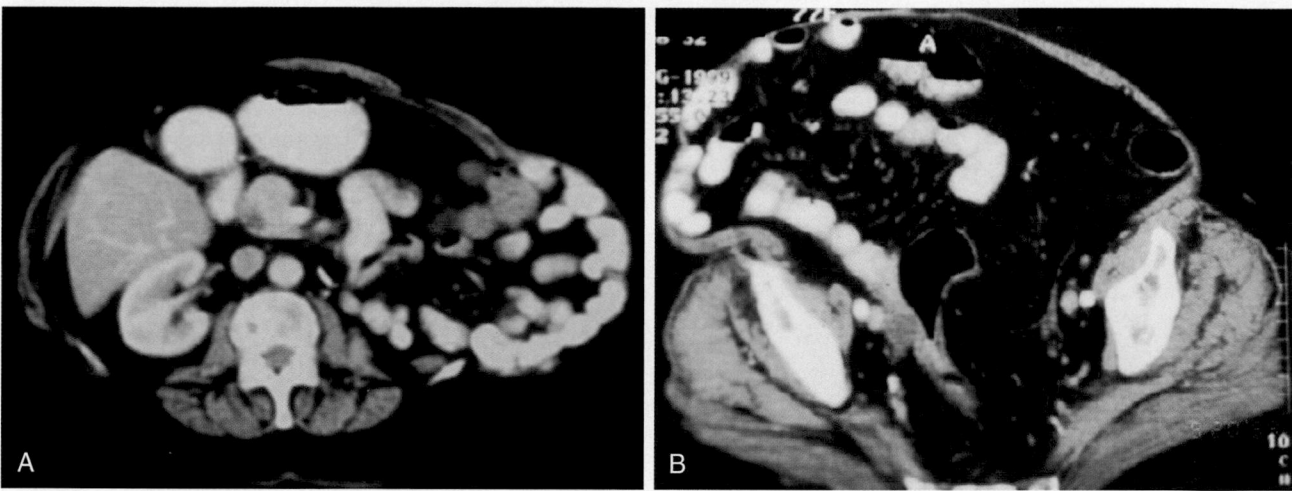

FIGURE 1 Lateral (**A**) and ventral (**B**) abdominal hernias resulting in significant loss of domain. Note the significant protrusion of intra-abdominal contents.

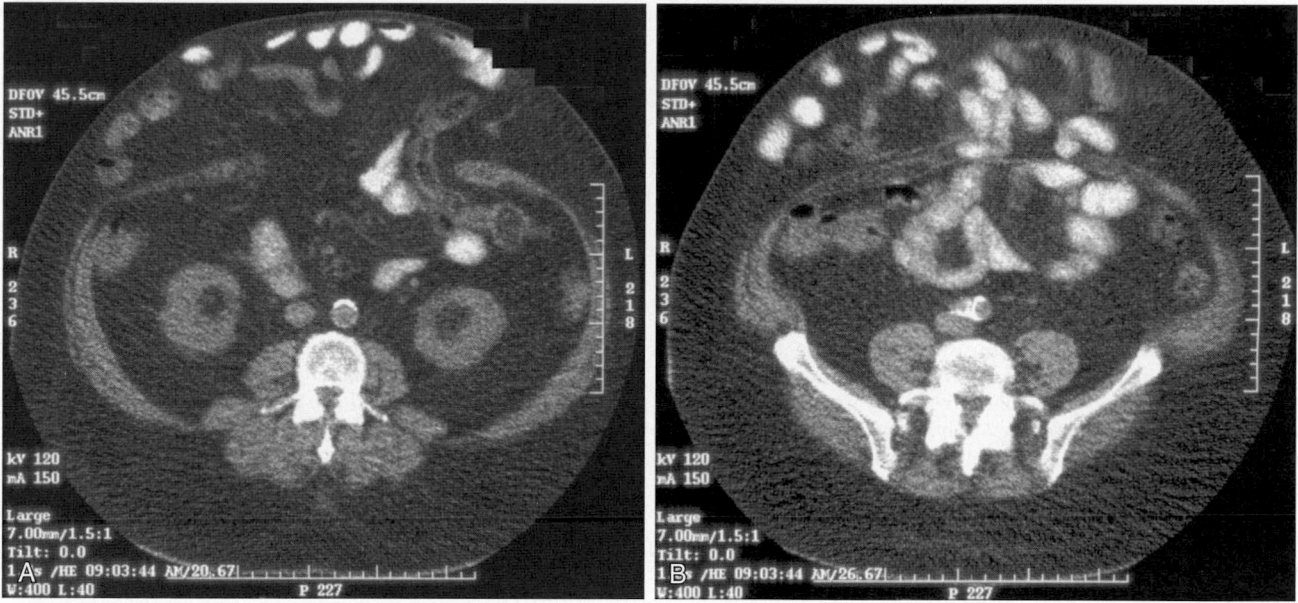

FIGURE 2 A and **B,** Computed tomography images of a large ventral hernia in the same patient with herniation of the small bowel through the abdominal fascia.

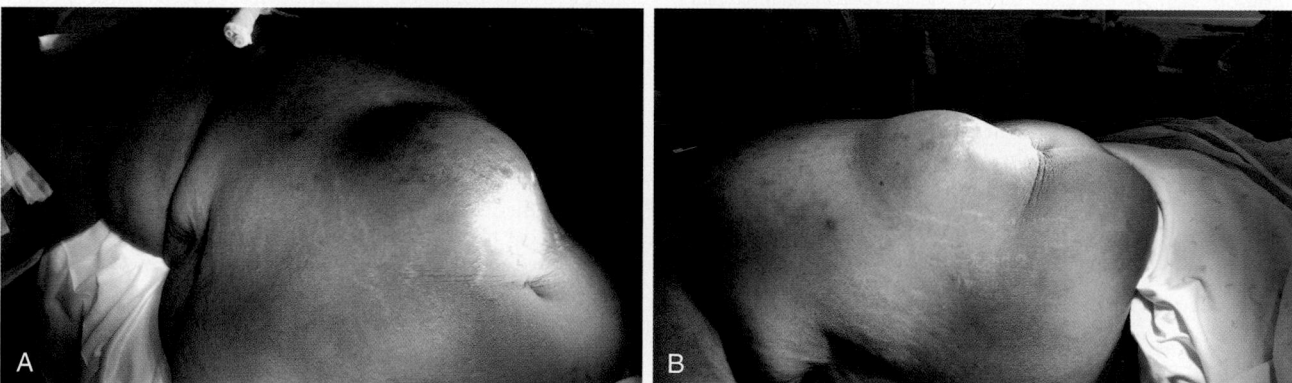

FIGURE 3 A, Morbidly obese individual with an epigastric hernia noted above the umbilicus. This patient did not have a prior history of abdominal surgeries. **B,** Note that the hernia is less obvious on the lateral view given the surrounding fat and folds.

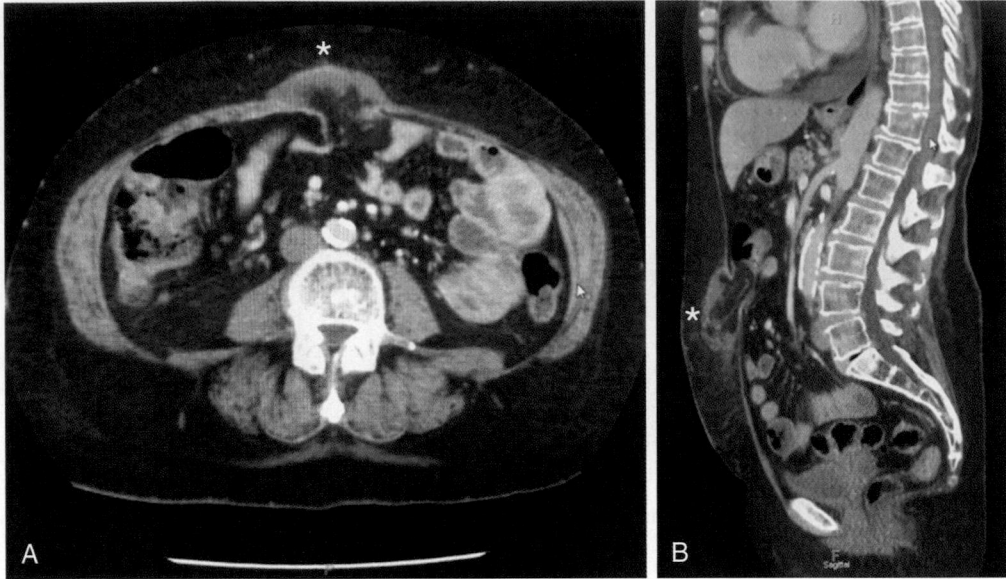

FIGURE 4 Example of axial (**A**) and sagittal (**B**) computed tomographic images of an umbilical hernia containing omentum. Note that the bowel is not present within the hernia. The hernia defect is marked with an asterisk (*) in each image.

An open approach is indicated for surgical emergencies, such as in the presence of acute incarceration or strangulation with the concern for bowel ischemia, for patients with uncontrolled coagulopathy, and for any patient with a hostile abdomen (e.g., enterocutaneous fistula, history of multiple prior abdominal operations or ventral hernia repairs). When there is a need for extensive adhesiolysis in the setting of multiple prior abdominal surgeries, laparoscopic surgery places the patient at an increased risk of undetected enterotomies. Often when an umbilical or epigastric hernia is small and easily identifiable in a thin patient, one incision above the defect will allow for an easy closure, either primarily or with a ventral patch. Laparoscopic repair in this clinical scenario is not necessary and will add to the operative morbidity with multiple incisions. Relative contraindications to laparoscopy include an infected or contaminated field with the potential for prior mesh explantation and a loss of domain such that the hernia defect is large enough to prevent proper placement of laparoscopic trocars. Open repair also allows for excision of excess or redundant and chronically thinned skin in obese patients, so that the closure can be approximated with healthy and well-vascularized tissue.

SURGICAL TECHNIQUE

Epidural catheters may be placed before large ventral hernia repairs, as their use may help in the early postoperative mobilization of the patient. On the day of surgery before the operation, subcutaneous heparin is administered for deep vein thrombosis prophylaxis. The patient is placed in a supine position with the arms extended outward at no more than 70 degrees on arm boards. Foley catheters are used in patients when an extensive adhesiolysis is anticipated and depending on the complexity of the surgery and the anticipated duration of the operation. The entire abdominal wall is prepped to the table in the standard sterile fashion.

Primary Closure

Umbilical hernias often have a small and narrow hernia neck, and therefore their repair is often performed on an outpatient basis. When the defect is small (e.g., 1-2 cm), a primary closure with simple apposition of the edges with sutures may be sufficient. Small epigastric and incisional hernias are managed similar to umbilical hernias.

First, an incision is made overlying the defect; if there is a scar overlying the hernia from a prior incision or trocar, an elliptical incision is used to excise the scar. Electrocautery is used to carefully dissect through the subcutaneous tissue, taking care to fully inspect for the presence of bowel. In the case of an umbilical hernia, care is taken to avoid unnecessary injury to the umbilical stalk during the dissection. Once the defect is located, contents are reduced within the abdominal cavity and the fascia should be inspected to ensure that there are no adherent loops of bowel in close proximity to the repair. Suture selection for closure often depends on a surgeon's preference, with the options being permanent or long-acting absorbable suture. The long-standing guiding principle for standard fascial closure is placement 1 cm from the fascial edge, ensuring a 1-cm space between each suture. After closure of the fascial defect, the subcutaneous layer is reapproximated with interrupted 3-0 absorbable sutures to decrease the area of dead space. Skin is then closed in a running fashion with 4-0 absorbable monofilament sutures. A sterile dressing is placed on the surgical wound and remains in place for 2 days after surgery.

Prosthetic Closure

When primary closure of an umbilical hernia is not possible and a prosthetic is to be used, the surgeon must decide if the hernia defect is best suited for a laparoscopic or open approach as described earlier. In adults, umbilical hernias occur as a result of increased intra-abdominal pressure; therefore many surgeons elect to place a ventral patch (e.g., Proceed Ventral Patch®; Ethicon, Somerville, NJ) or a plug (e.g., Gore Bio-A® Hernia Plug; W. L. Gore & Associates, Elkhart, DE) for additional reinforcement. Before the design of these products, incorporating a mesh via a small incision overlying an umbilical hernia was difficult. These new prosthetic designs allow the insertion of a prosthetic that is larger than the hernia defect into the peritoneum under the fascia. Size threshold for the use of prosthetic material should be smaller in patients with predisposing factors, such as smoking, steroid use, and obesity, or recurrence.

Unlike with most umbilical hernias, surgical repair of incisional and epigastric hernias should take into account that the fascia near the defect also may be weak, and so a ventral patch or plug may not be sufficient. Rather, a larger prosthetic may be needed to reinforce the area of weakness that exists beyond the identifiable hernia. It is our general practice to primarily repair incisional and epigastric hernias that are less than 5 cm in transverse dimension, in patients with well-vascularized and healthy fascia, as long as a tension-free repair is feasible. For defects larger than 5 cm, a synthetic/biologic prosthetic is often necessary. Prosthetic reinforcement can be coupled with component separation techniques (discussed briefly later) for even larger defect areas for additional fascial relaxation. Furthermore, prosthetic repair is favored for those patients who have higher baseline intra-abdominal pressures (e.g., COPD, strenuous or heavy lifting work), failed prior hernia repairs at the same site, higher risk of poor wound healing, and known collagen disorders. The use of a prosthetic in the repair does decrease recurrence rates compared with primary suture closure. However, prosthetics should be used only when necessary, as their use is associated with an increased risk of seroma and surgical site infections (SSIs). Many surgeons prefer the use of a biologic prosthetic to a synthetic mesh in patients at higher risk of developing postoperative SSI (contaminated wounds, smoking, history of infection at the site). However, recent data suggest that a synthetic mesh in a clean-contaminated or even contaminated wound may produce equally effective and durable results as a biologic alternative.

Open Hernia Repair With Prosthetic Reinforcement

For open umbilical hernia repairs with prosthetic mesh, after reduction of the hernia contents, an area large enough (at least 4-5 cm) is cleared around the fascial edges. The ventral patch is deployed within the abdominal cavity. These prosthetics often have fixation straps that are pulled up through the fascial defect and cut to an appropriate length. Closure of the fascia then incorporates these fixation straps into the repair. A long-acting absorbable suture is often used for these purposes. It is important to return the umbilicus to its original appearance, and this may require suture fixation of the umbilical skin to the underlying subcutaneous tissue or fascia in order to restore the original dimpling and folds. Laparoscopic repair for umbilical hernias would be performed in much the same way as for incisional and epigastric hernias (see Laparoscopic Hernia Repair section).

For larger incisional, umbilical, and epigastric hernias, an incision is made overlying the defect to allow for exposure of the most superior and inferior margins. For more complex incisional hernias with loss of domain in which a component separation in addition to prosthetic closure will be necessary, a full midline laparotomy incision is made. The lipocutaneous layer is mobilized and separated from the patient's native fascia with electrocautery. It is important to note that wide undermining has the potential to render the subcutaneous layer hypovascular and ischemic, and this eventually can lead to skin necrosis and the need for débridement. Therefore it is important to preserve abdominal wall perforators as they are encountered. Abdominal contents are reduced, and lysis of adhesions is performed as necessary so that the full extent of the hernia defect edges can be visualized easily and space can be created for transfascial sutures. The hernia sac is then dissected free, and the fascia is carefully palpated to inspect for additional defects. Any intervening fascial bridges are cut in order to create a single defect for closure. Traditionally, synthetic mesh is used in patients with clean wounds. Recent data do not support the superiority of biologic over synthetic nonabsorbable prosthetics in contaminated fields. We continue to use biologic prosthetics in patients at a higher risk of developing a postoperative SSI, which includes those with potentially contaminated or contaminated wounds as well as medical comorbidities (e.g., obesity, immunosuppression, diabetes). Underlay/intraperitoneal positioning of the prosthetic has been considered the gold standard by the American Hernia Society (Figure 5). Other commonly used configurations for mesh placement include a retrorectus underlay/sublay position (Figure 6), in which the mesh is placed within the posterior rectus sheath deep to the rectus abdominis muscle. The mesh is then secured to the linea semilunaris, followed by midline closure of the anterior rectus sheaths (Figure 7). An overlay placement also may be used; the mesh is placed superficial to the anterior rectus sheath and the external oblique aponeurosis. This is carried out after primary closure of the

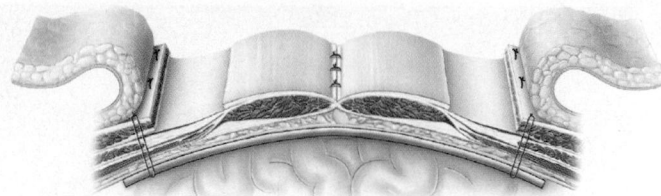

FIGURE 5 The prosthetic is placed in an intraperitoneal position and anchored to the abdominal wall. The anterior rectus sheath is then closed in the midline. *(From Losken A, Janis JE.* Advances in Abdominal Wall Reconstruction. *St. Louis, MO: Quality Medical Publishing; 2012.)*

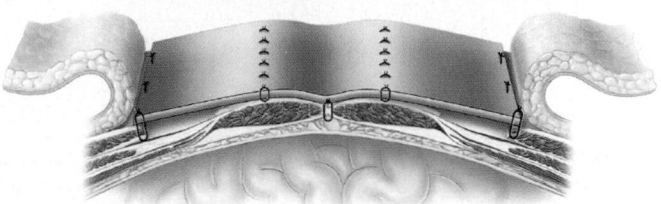

FIGURE 6 The prosthetic is placed within the posterior rectus sheath deep to the rectus abdominis muscle. It subsequently is anchored to the linea semilunaris, and the anterior rectus sheaths are closed in the midline. *(From Losken A, Janis JE.* Advances in Abdominal Wall Reconstruction. *St. Louis, MO: Quality Medical Publishing; 2012.)*

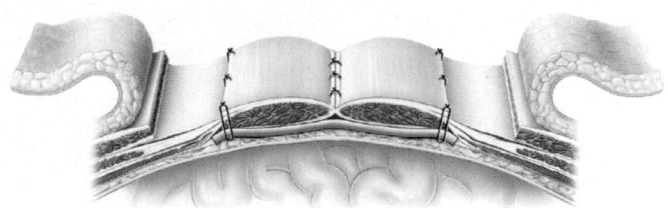

FIGURE 7 The prosthetic is placed superficial to the anterior rectus sheath and external oblique aponeurosis. *(From Losken A, Janis JE.* Advances in Abdominal Wall Reconstruction. *St. Louis, MO: Quality Medical Publishing; 2012.)*

midline fascia with or without the use of component separation. More recently, our experience with the use of a "sandwich technique" for complex abdominal incisional hernia repairs is growing. Examples of complex incisional hernia repairs include large defects with multiple prior failed repairs, in patients who are immunocompromised or have poorly vascularized fascia. This technique incorporates a biologic underlay and synthetic overlay. The biologic underlay creates a scaffold that facilitates vascular ingrowth and studies have shown that erosion into underlying structures (e.g., bowel and solid viscera) is less of a risk than with a synthetic mesh (Figure 8). We believe that the synthetic overlay renders long-term stability to the dynamic abdominal wall musculature and decreases the chances of failure at the margins of the interface between the dynamic abdominal wall and the adynamic biologic matrix.

At our institution, the "sandwich technique" recently has been shown to improve outcomes in high-grade hernia repairs (study in progress). Once mobilization and reduction of the hernia sac is complete and the fascial edges are freed, an acellular dermal matrix underlay extending at least 2 cm circumferentially beyond the fascial edge of the defect is placed. It is sutured in place using interrupted 2-0 polypropylene mattress sutures. These sutures are spaced 2 cm apart and 2 cm from the fascial edge. A polypropylene synthetic mesh

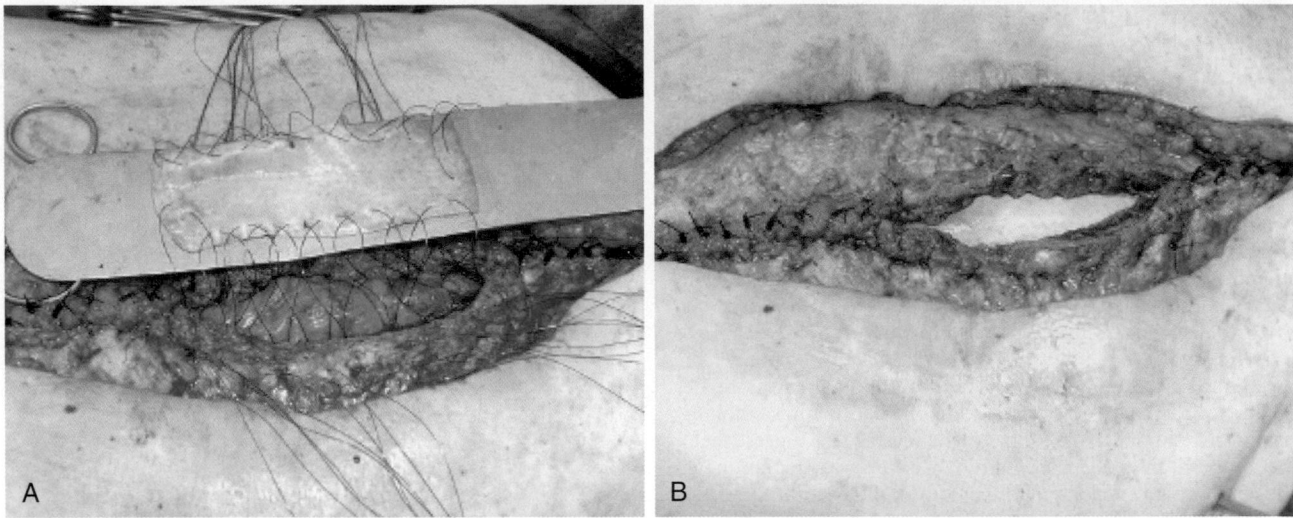

FIGURE 8 A, The acellular dermal matrix is sized appropriately and sutures are placed through the prosthetic to anchor it to the undersurface of the abdominal wall. **B,** The biologic graft is then placed in an intraperitoneal position and the overlying fascia is closed.

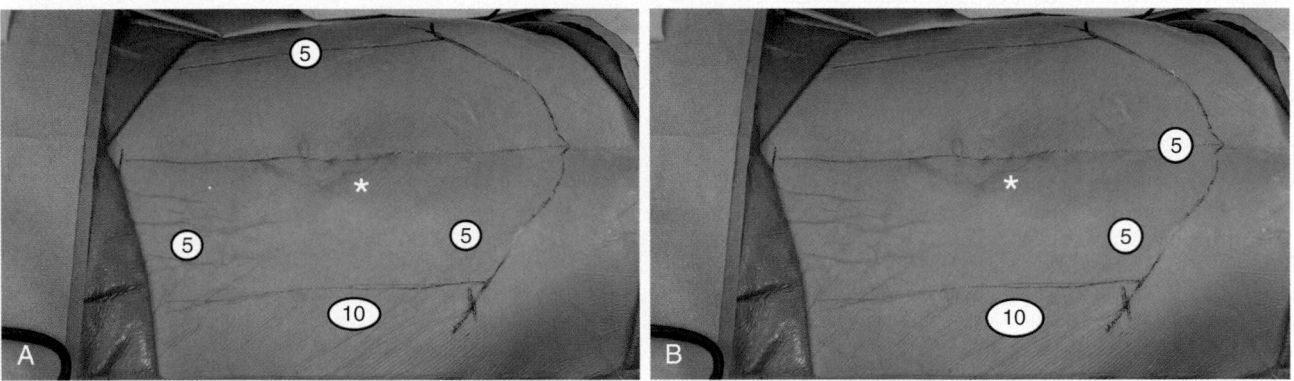

FIGURE 9 Options for port placement for a centrally located hernia. The numbers mark the size of the trocar in millimeters. Note that under general anesthesia, abdominal contents are reduced, making the midline hernia easily identifiable in this patient (*).

overlay is used in all cases to cover the abdominal wall. To secure the mesh to the abdominal wall, 2-0 long-term absorbable monofilament sutures are placed in a quilting fashion. Great care is used to take small bites of material and avoid crimping and creating folds in the prosthetic mesh. This avoids the potential of fluid accumulation under the mesh and encourages the early ingrowth of tissue, thereby stabilizing the mesh and avoiding infection. The mesh is then pulled tautly across the abdominal wall and fixed to the opposite side in a similar fashion. Multiple interrupted sutures are used to "quilt" the mesh to the abdominal wall as well as to the underlying acellular graft. The purpose of this "sandwich technique" is to create a "load sharing" construct that distributes forces of the abdominal wall from the biologic to the synthetic mesh. The mesh is fixed outside the zone of highest risk, the midline, and the forces are transmitted to this inherently more stable area. Often the lipocutaneous flaps are sutured to the mesh to decrease the dead space and facilitate rapid tissue ingrowth. Large bore fluted drains are placed and removed only when outputs drop below 30 cc for 24 hours. Recently some surgeons have been using incisional negative pressure wound care devices with good results. All of these maneuvers are done in an effort to reduce the potential dead space and fluid accumulation.

Laparoscopic Hernia Repair With Prosthetic Reinforcement

Trocars are positioned so that there is adequate space between each port site and the ports are far enough from the hernia defect to allow

for easy dissection and repair (Figure 9). The site of entrance into the abdomen should be chosen based on the location of the hernia, while avoiding areas expected to have dense adhesions from prior surgeries. For lower midline hernias, a right or left upper quadrant site is chosen initially, whereas for upper midline hernias, access via the right or left lower quadrants may be necessary. A Veress needle is used initially to create pneumoperitoneum, and an optical trocar is then used to enter the abdomen. Alternatively, an open cutdown technique can be used for the first trocar placement, and stay sutures are placed on either side of the fascia upon entering the peritoneal cavity to help facilitate identification of the fascia at termination of the case. A 30- or 45-degree laparoscope usually is used, and the abdomen is fully explored. The surgeon must ensure that inadvertent bowel or vessel injury did not occur either with the Veress needle or the first trocar placement. For midline defects, it is important to dissect the umbilical and falciform ligaments from the abdominal wall. This will allow for full inspection of the abdominal wall and fascia in order to identify any additional defects and to ensure adequate fascial overlap when placing the mesh in position. An additional three to four ports are placed under direct visualization. One of the ports should be either a 10-mm port or a 12-mm port for placement of the mesh.

Atraumatic graspers may be used to gently reduce the hernia contents after any necessary adhesiolysis. When applied, the prosthetic is placed intraperitoneally and should extend beyond the lateral border of the rectus muscles, in order to avoid injury to the epigastric vessels and to allow even distribution of intra-abdominal pressure along its surface. We prefer at least a 4- to 5-cm symmetric overlap of the mesh with the fascial edges. Our method for determining the size of the hernia defect is to introduce spinal needles percutaneously as the four edges of the defect and the distance between these holes is measured. This forms a template for sizing the mesh before its insertion into the peritoneal cavity, keeping in mind that an overlap of the fascial edges is prudent. The mesh subsequently is marked at four opposing edges to ensure adequate orientation on the undersurface of the abdomen. We prefer to use a permanent mesh with an antiadhesive barrier facing the underlying abdominal structures. Some surgeons prefer to reapproximate the edges of the fascial defect with a suture passer device through punctate incisions overlying the defect before placement of the mesh. This can be done using #1 monofilament absorbable sutures placed in a figure-of-eight fashion 1 to 1.5 cm lateral to the edge. Closing the hernia defect during the laparoscopic repair may prevent seroma formation in the space between the mesh and subcutaneous tissue. In our experience, closure of the fascia is not necessary. Four axial permanent sutures are placed in the mesh and tied, leaving adequate length before insertion into the abdomen, and these will be used for the initial suspension of the mesh on the undersurface of the abdominal wall. The mesh is then rolled and placed through the 10- to 12-mm trocar into the abdomen using a grasper. Once in the abdomen, the mesh is unrolled in proper orientation with the antiadhesive barrier positioned toward the underlying abdominal structures. Absorbable tacking devices are then used to fix the mesh to the abdominal wall, placed 2 to 3 cm around the perimeter and utilizing a "double crown" technique around the outer edge. Transfascial sutures have been associated with significant pain postoperatively and are used only in larger defects in which additional stabilization is deemed necessary.

Component Separation

Various component separation techniques have gained popularity over the past decade as an adjunct to closing complex abdominal wall hernias. The traditional open component separation technique was described by Ramirez in 1990. This technique, as it was originally described, is still widely used today. The external oblique muscle can be released from the underlying internal oblique muscle in a relatively avascular plane. The rectus abdominis muscle can be separated from the posterior rectus sheath. These muscles remain attached to the linea semilunaris, but the composite construct can be moved to the midline. This allows for 5-cm advancement in the epigastrium, 10 cm at the waistline, and 3 cm in the suprapubic region. This technique is often coupled with prosthetic reconstruction. Spigelian hernias and lateral bulges are a complication of the lateral dissection that occurs in the various component techniques, and many surgeons choose to place mesh laterally beyond these points of weakness in order to reduce such complications. Over the past decade, other minimally invasive component separation techniques have been described, including the endoscopic approach (Figure 10). These minimally invasive techniques have been shown to reduce the incidence of postoperative SSOs, and hernia repair outcomes are equally effective. However, this approach is associated with a significant learning curve and also may have a higher incidence of lateral bulges and Spigelian hernias postoperatively.

■ POSTOPERATIVE CARE

Sterile surgical dressings that are applied at the end of repair are removed on postoperative day 2, in order to prevent early surgical site contamination and subsequent infection. For small hernia repairs (e.g., primary closure, <3 cm), surgery may be performed on an outpatient basis and the patient may be discharged on the same day of operation. For larger hernias requiring prosthetic reinforcement and component separation techniques, patients are admitted for inpatient management and remain without oral intake until recovery of bowel function. Pain is managed initially with intravenous

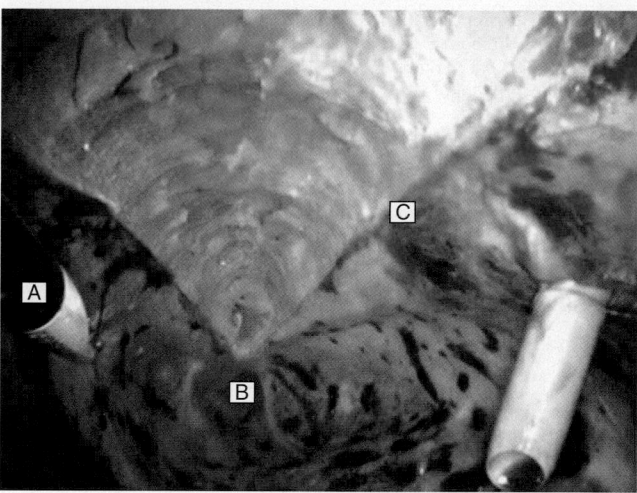

FIGURE 10 Endoscopic component separation. Hook cautery (A) is used to incise the fascia of the external oblique aponeurosis while preserving perforating blood vessels to the abdominal wall (B). This creates a relaxing incision in the fascia (C) that allows medial advancement of the abdominal wall. *(From Azoury SC, Dhanasopon AP, Hui X, De La Cruz C, Tuffaha SH, et al. A single institutional comparison of endoscopic and open abdominal component separation. Surg Endosc. 2014;28:3349-3358.)*

narcotics for as long as the patient is not eating. The patient is then transitioned to oral narcotic analgesia once he or she is tolerating a diet. Diet is then advanced as tolerated, and the patient is discharged once tolerating a diet and as long as oral pain medications provide adequate relief. After discharge, the first postoperative visit occurs 2 weeks after the date of surgery.

■ COMPLICATIONS

SSOs complicate the postoperative course in 24% to 34% of patients undergoing ventral hernia repairs. These occurrences include hernia recurrence, infection, seroma formation, enterocutaneous fistula, wound dehiscence, cellulitis, and others. Often these occurrences can be managed conservatively, yet at other times an intervention such as percutaneous drainage or reoperation may be necessary. Furthermore, several of these events, including the presence of infection or contamination at the wound site, increase the risk of hernia recurrence. Therefore close follow-up of these patients is prudent, and early management or treatment of any complication is necessary for long-term success.

SUGGESTED READINGS

Azoury SC, Dhanasopon AP, Hui X, De La Cruz C, Tuffaha SH, et al. A single institutional comparison of endoscopic and open abdominal component separation. *Surg Endosc.* 2014;28:3349-3358.

Breuing K, Butler CE, Ferzoco S, Franz M, Hultman CS, et al. Incisional ventral hernias: review of the literature and recommendations regarding the grading and technique of repair. *Surgery.* 2010;148:544-558.

Lee L, Mata J, Landry T, Khwaja KA, Vassiliou MC, et al. A systematic review of synthetic and biologic materials for abdominal wall reinforcement in contaminated fields. *Surg Endosc.* 2014;28:2531-2546.

Losken A, Janis JE. *Advances in Abdominal Wall Reconstruction.* St. Louis, MO: Quality Medical Publishing; 2012.

Nguyen MT, Berger RL, Hicks SC, Davila JA, Li LT, et al. Comparison of outcomes of synthetic mesh vs suture repair of elective primary ventral herniorrhaphy: a systematic review and meta-analysis. *JAMA Surg.* 2014;149:415-421.

Ramirez OM, Ruas E, Dellon AL. "Components separation" method for closure of abdominal-wall defects: an anatomic and clinical study. *Plast Reconstr Surg.* 1990;86:519-526.

Rogmark P, Petersson U, Bringman S, Ezra E, Osterberg J, et al. Quality-of-life and surgical outcome 1 year after open and laparoscopic incisional hernia repair: PROLOVE: a randomized controlled trial. *Ann Surg.* 2016;263:244-250. <http://dx.doi.org/10.1097/SLA.0000000000001305>.

Silecchia G, Campanile FC, Sanchez L, Ceccarelli G, Antinori A, et al. Laparoscopic ventral/incisional hernia repair: updated guidelines from the EAES and EHS endorsed Consensus Development Conference. *Surg Endosc.* 2015;29:2463-2484.

THE MANAGEMENT OF SEMILUNAR, LUMBAR, AND OBTURATOR HERNIAS

Hien T. Nguyen, MD, FACS

The three hernias covered in this chapter are relatively rare, which can lead to a misdiagnosis or delay in diagnosis. Patient presentation can be subtle because the exam can mimic other common conditions, or the patient may be too debilitated to allow a thorough examination. In addition, these hernias are difficult to diagnose by physical exam because they often manifest as herniation of abdominal contents through only part of the muscular abdominal wall. These defects can lead to a Richter's hernia, in which one side of bowel is incarcerated within the defect, which can lead to strangulated bowel without clinical signs of obstruction. Sliding hernias also can occur, leading to intermittent symptoms. For these reasons, use of imaging studies allows timely diagnosis and treatment planning (Figure 1). Surgery is the definitive treatment; a minimally invasive approach is associated with a shorter convalescence but reduced surgical exposure and a higher material cost.

▪ SEMILUNAR (SPIGELIAN) HERNIA

Anatomy

Adrian van der Spieghel first described the linea semilunaris, a curved line on the lateral side of the rectus abdominis extending between the ninth costal cartilage to the pubic tubercle. The Spigelian aponeurosis describes the aponeurosis of the transversus abdominis muscle, limited laterally by the linea semilunaris and medially by the lateral margin of the rectus abdominis. A Spigelian or semilunar hernia is a protrusion of intra-abdominal contents and peritoneal sac through a congenital or acquired defect in the Spigelian aponeurosis. Embryologically, Spigelian hernias may represent a weakness in fusion of the aponeuroses of layered abdominal muscles; the left side is more common if the result of a true congenital defect.

Also known as a *lateral ventral hernia*, Spigelian hernias most commonly occur as a protrusion between the Spigelian belt of Spangen, which describes the 6-cm transverse space above the anterior superior iliac spine. The lines of Monro extend from the umbilicus to each of the iliac crests, with a horizontal line between both iliac crests forming the base of the triangle. Within this space is the arcuate line of Douglas, which is where the posterior rectus sheath ends and the rectus abdominis muscle is covered only by transversalis fascia inferiorly. The majority of Spigelian hernias occur within this triangle below the arcuate line of Douglas. There are two subtypes of acquired hernias: interstitial, which describes a hernia sac posterior to the external oblique, and subcutaneous, in which the hernia has protruded through the obliques and the sac lies within the subdermal fatty tissue (Figures 2 through 4).

Clinical Indications

Spigelian hernias typically are acquired, occurring in 1% to 2% of all hernias with a slight female to male predominance, and most commonly in patients between the ages of 40 and 70 years. Common predisposing factors include advanced age, collagen disorders, obesity, prior abdominal surgery, and multiple pregnancies. The most common symptom is pain because of contraction of abdominal muscles, with a 2- to 5-cm palpable mass that may occur in only 35% of cases. Other common conditions such as hemangiomas and tumors can exhibit similar clinical findings, and physical examination alone fails to establish the diagnosis in 50% of cases. Ultrasound or computed tomography (CT) scan has high sensitivity for diagnosis and should be used frequently in the workup. Emergency surgery may be needed in up to 30% of cases because of incarceration and strangulation (Figure 5).

Surgical Tips

Because of the rare nature of these hernias, there is no universal consensus regarding guidelines. However, it is widely accepted that once the diagnosis has been made, surgical repair is indicated because of the high risk of complications, especially in obese patients. Postoperative complications range between 11% and 30%, depending on severity. The open anterior herniorrhaphy is most beneficial during urgent cases, allowing appropriate analysis of incarcerated tissue and repair with direct muscle reapproximation with or without mesh placement. In elective cases, the laparoscopic intraperitoneal mesh repair provides similar long-term outcomes with less postoperative pain, lower risk of wound infections, and shorter convalescence. For uncomplicated hernias, a laparoscopic repair should be attempted to allow sparing of the external oblique aponeurosis from being divided, and a shorter hospital length of stay.

The conventional open approach consists of a transverse skin incision over the protrusion with incision of the external oblique aponeurosis divided in the direction of its fibers in the case of the interstitial subtype. This exposes the peritoneal hernia sac, which is dissected down to the hernia neck. The external oblique is separated from the internal oblique in a 2- to 3-cm circumference. If there is low risk of ischemic strangulation, the hernia sac is inverted into the abdominal cavity without opening. Afterward a preformed synthetic mesh plug can be inserted into the defect and sutured into place with nonabsorbable suture. Otherwise, the hernia sac is opened and its contents examined and excised or reduced into the abdominal cavity. The hernia sac then is closed with absorbable running suture. Afterward the internal oblique defect is closed with running absorbable suture. If no bowel was removed, synthetic mesh can be used to reinforce the repair. In this case, the mesh is placed above the reapproximated internal oblique, overlapping the closed defect 3 to 4 cm in all directions. The mesh is sutured to the internal oblique laterally and rectus muscle medially with nonabsorbable mattress sutures. The external oblique is closed with running absorbable suture. In cases with necrotic bowel or spillage of intestinal contents, a biologic mesh should be used to minimize the risk of mesh infections.

In circumstances in which the patient is in shock or a large amount of intestine may be necrotic, a midline incision also can be performed (Figure 6).

The minimally invasive approach includes an intraperitoneal onlay mesh repair (IPOM), a transabdominal preperitoneal (TAPP), or a totally extraperitoneal (TEP) approach. The optimal laparoscopic approach depends on the size and location of the hernia. For easily reducible hernias less than 3 cm in diameter and positioned inferior to the umbilicus, the TEP approach allows direct access to the defect without exposure of gastrointestinal contents, thereby

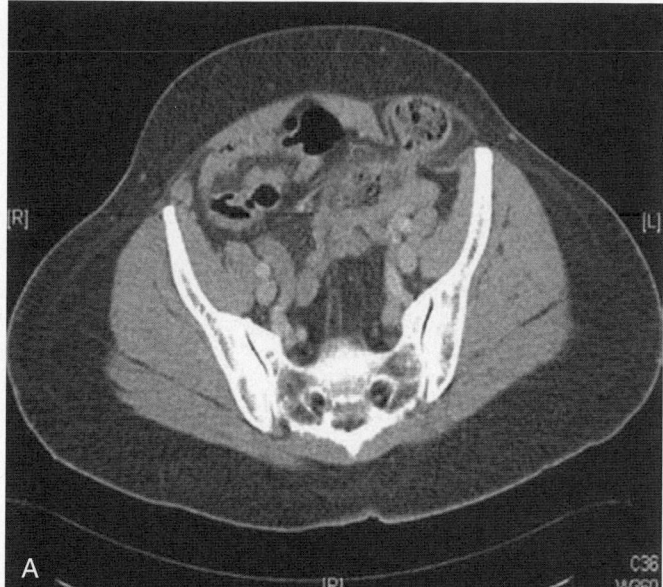

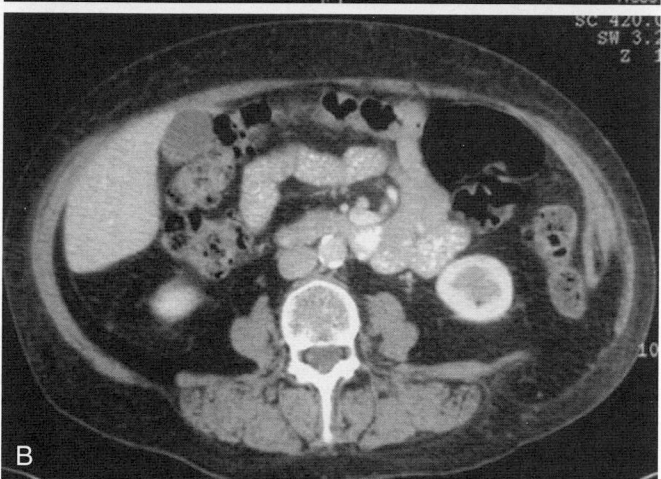

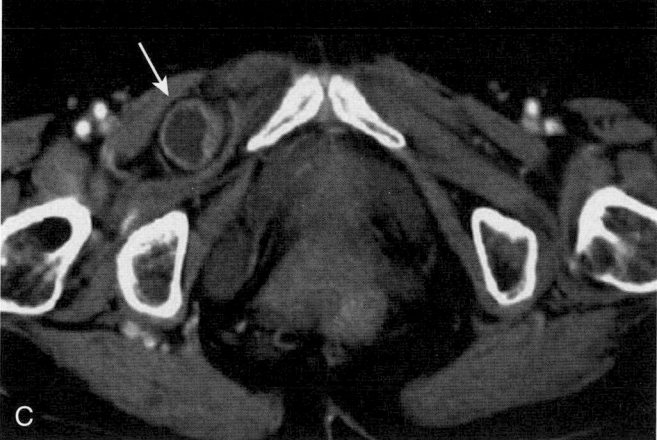

FIGURE 1 Computed tomography scans of the abdomen and pelvis showing a left-sided semilunar hernia containing sigmoid colon (**A**), a left lumbar hernia containing fat and a portion of descending colon (**B**), and a right obturator hernia containing a fluid-filled mass (**C**). (**A,** *From Sheu EG, Smink DS, Brooks DC. Spigelian hernia. In Jones DB, ed.* Mastery Techniques in Surgery: Hernia. *Philadelphia: Wolters Kluwer/Lippincott, Williams & Wilkins; 2013:385-392.* **B,** *From Cavallaro G, Sadighi A, Mecili M, et al. Primary lumbar hernia: the open approach.* Eur Surg Res. *2007;39:88-92.* **C,** *From Chang SS, Shan YS, Lin YJ, et al. A review of obturator hernia and a proposed algorithm for its diagnosis and treatment.* World J Surg. *2005;29:450-454.)*

allowing advantages similar to a TEP inguinal hernia repair. However, the TEP approach is minimally used because of limitations related to hernia access and higher disposable costs. For larger, nonreducible hernias above the umbilicus, a TAPP or IPOM approach allows easy location of the defect, safe reduction of the herniated contents, reapproximation of the fascial defect, and adequate space for mesh placement (Figure 7).

In a TEP approach, an infraumbilical incision extending through the anterior rectus sheath is made. The rectus muscles are identified and retracted laterally for a dissecting balloon to be placed superficially to the posterior rectus sheath. The balloon is advanced into the preperitoneal space and gradually insufflated with a 10-mm 45-degree camera inserted. The peritoneum is seen posterior to the balloon and should be intact. Both inferior epigastric vessels should be anterior to the balloon to avoid tearing of its branches during balloon insufflation. After the balloon has been used to adequately dissect the preperitoneal space, it is removed and insufflation of 12 mm Hg is established. A pair of 5-mm trocars are placed under direct vision in the midline between the umbilicus and the pubic symphysis to minimize risk of bleeding, with the inferior trocar placed 3 to 4 cm above the pubic symphysis. Care is taken to identify and protect the inferior epigastric vessels during the dissection process. After complete reduction of the hernia sac, the fascial edges can be reapproximated using a transfascial suture needle such as a Carter-Thomason and figure-of-8 monofilament absorbable suture. An uncoated synthetic mesh large enough to provide 3- to 5-cm extension from the hernia fascial defect is used to reinforce the repair. The mesh is grasped at the midpoint and placed through the 10-mm trocar site unrolled in the preperitoneal space, and tacks or fibrin glue is used to secure the mesh.

The TAPP or IPOM approach is ideal for larger hernias and begins with a 10-mm trocar entry on the contralateral side and is followed by standard intra-abdominal insufflation of 15 mm Hg. A pair of 5-mm trocars are placed through the contralateral flank, and the herniated tissue is reduced or resected appropriately. The most efficient repair is an IPOM approach, whereby the hernia can be measured with a ruler placed into the abdominal cavity, and the center of the hernia defect is identified with a needle. The fascia is first reapproximated with a transfascial suture passer and absorbable 0-monofilament suture, and the appropriate-sized coated synthetic mesh is chosen to allow a 3- to 5-cm overlap. Nonabsorbable U-stitch sutures are placed at the cardinal points on the edge of the mesh, which is positioned on the skin to estimate the center of the defect to the center of the mesh. The cardinal transfascial suture sites are marked on the skin with ink. The mesh is rolled up and placed through the 10-mm trocar site and unrolled intra-abdominally to allow the sutures to face anteriorly. The mesh is secured to extend 3 to 5 cm past the hernia defect using transfascial sutures at the four cardinal points and a double-crown tacking technique. The double-crown technique consists of two concentric rings of tacks. The outer ring tacks are placed close to the edge of the mesh at 1 cm apart to minimize the risk of bowel migration between the mesh and abdominal wall, whereas the inner ring tacks are placed to obliterate space between the mesh and the abdominal wall.

Although the IPOM is the preferred technique, one disadvantage is the risk of intra-abdominal adhesions and erosions resulting from the intraperitoneal location of the mesh. The TAPP approach has the advantage of allowing noncoated synthetic mesh placement in the preperitoneal space, thereby protecting it from the potential of erosion into intestine. Separation of the peritoneum should begin 5 to 7 cm medially from the edge of the hernia defect, and a flap of peritoneum is dissected laterally enough to allow mesh placement. The hernia defect is reapproximated in a similar method to the IPOM technique before mesh placement in the preperitoneal space. The mesh is secured with transfascial sutures and tacks are used sparingly. Afterwards, the peritoneum is reapproximated either with absorbable tacks with 1-cm spacing or running absorbable suture.

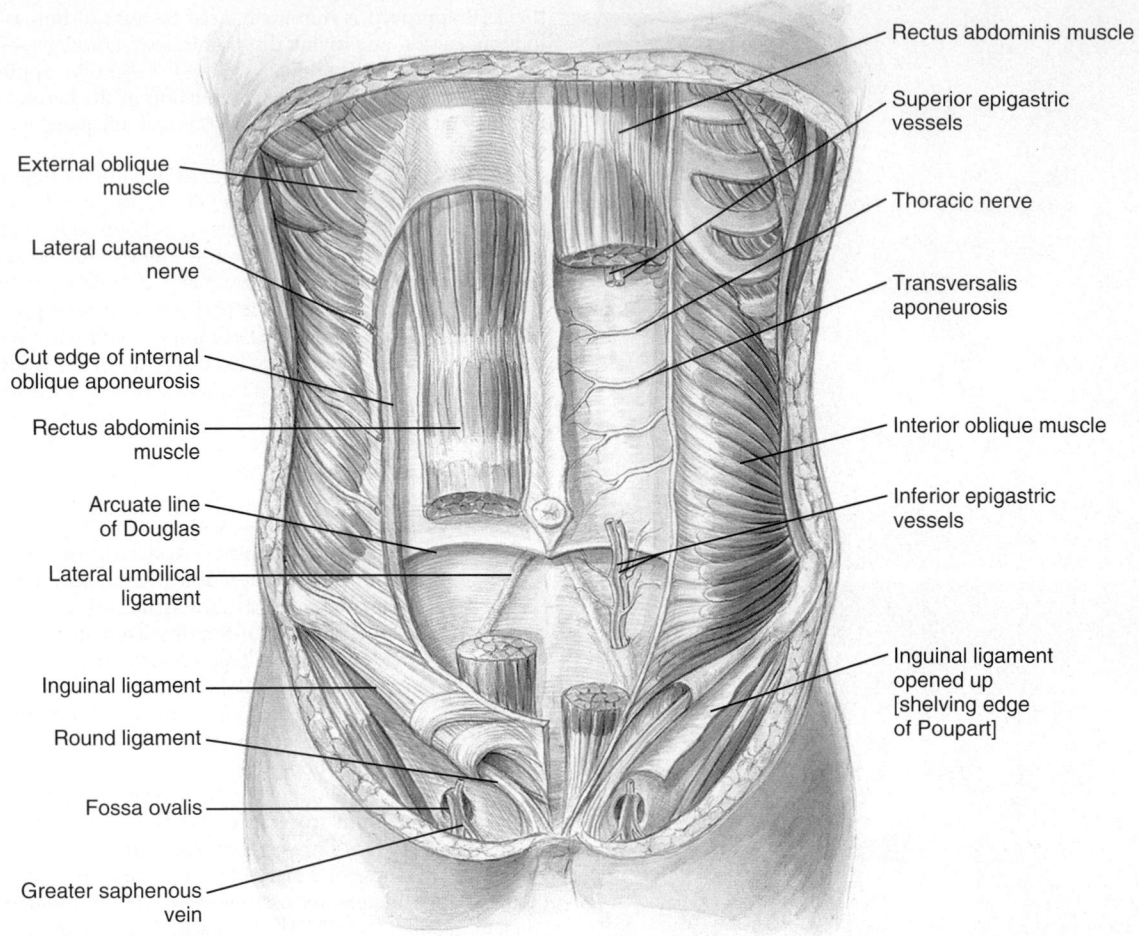

FIGURE 2 Anatomy of the anterior abdominal wall. *(From Richards A. Spigelian hernias. Oper Tech Gen Surg. 2004;6:228-239.)*

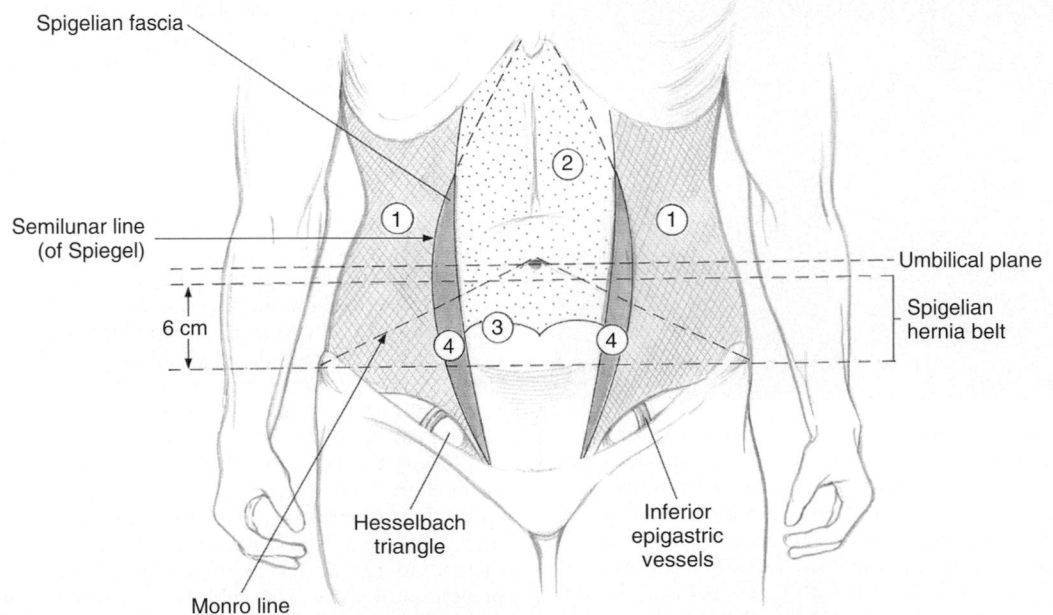

FIGURE 3 The Spigelian belt of Spangen. The area where most semilunar hernias occur. *(1)* Transversus abdominis, *(2)* dorsal rectus sheath, *(3)* arcuate line of Douglas, *(4)* Spigelian aponeurosis. *(From Richards A. Spigelian hernias. Oper Tech Gen Surg. 2004;6:228-239.)*

**Cross-section of abdominal wall
above the arcuate line**

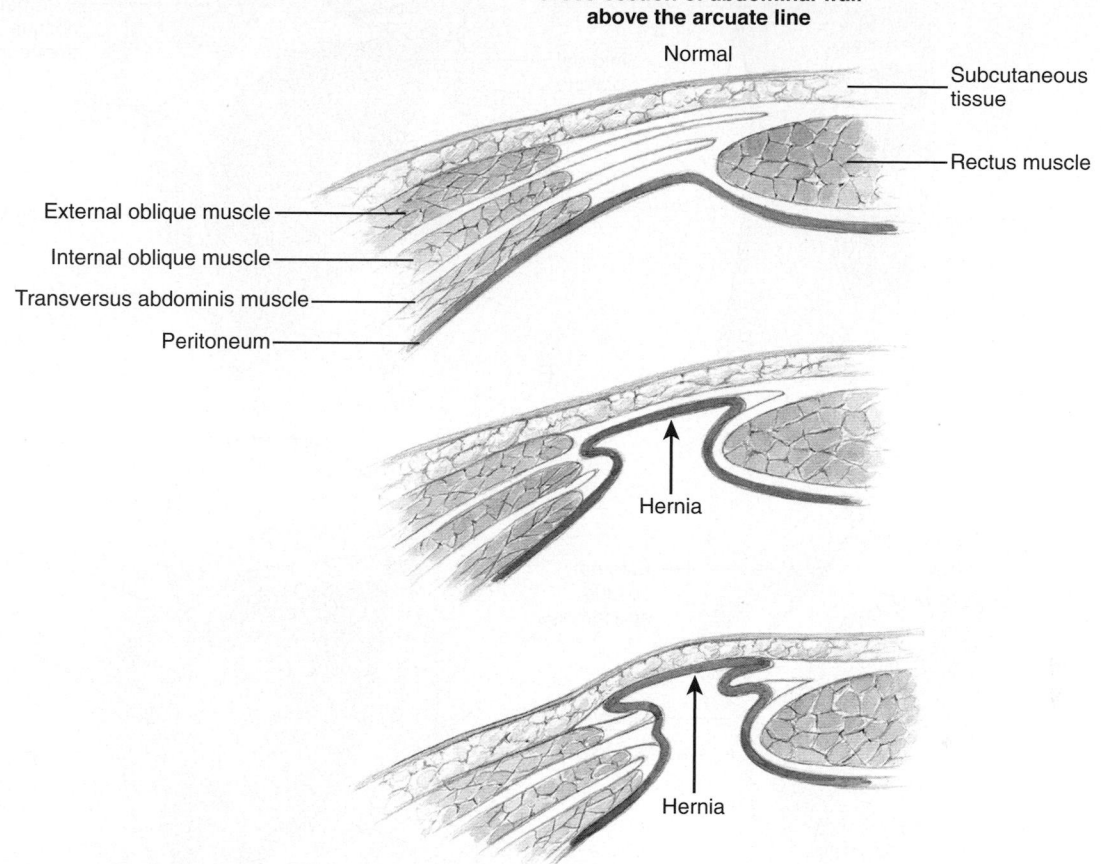

Normal

Subcutaneous
tissue

Rectus muscle

External oblique muscle

Internal oblique muscle

Transversus abdominis muscle

Peritoneum

Hernia

Hernia

FIGURE 4 Cross-sections of the abdominal wall. *Top,* Normal anatomy of abdominal wall above the arcuate line. Middle: interstitial hernia with sac posterior to the external oblique. *Bottom,* Subcutaneous hernia protruding through the obliques with sac in the subdermal fatty tissue. *(From Richards A. Spigelian hernias.* Oper Tech Gen Surg. *2004;6:228-239.)*

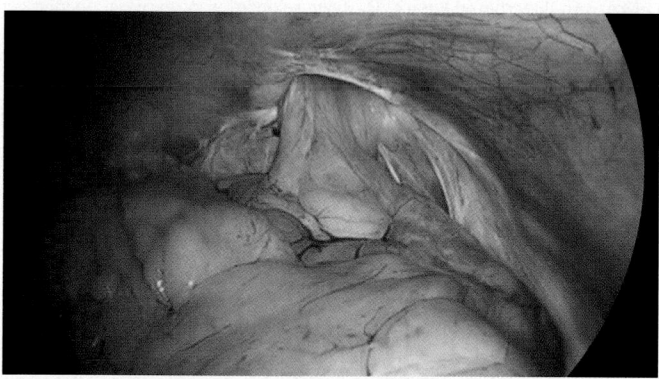

FIGURE 5 Intra-abdominal picture of semilunar hernia.

TABLE 1: Comparison of Anatomy Between Superior and Inferior Lumbar Hernias

Border	Superior (Grynfeltt-Lesshaft) Triangle	Inferior (Petit) Triangle
Superior	Twelfth rib	
Inferior		Iliac crest
Medial/posterior	Quadratus lumborum	Latissimus dorsi
Lateral/anterior	Internal oblique	External iliac
Roof	External oblique/ latissimus dorsi	
Floor	Transversus abdominis/ transversalis fascia	Transversalis/internal oblique fascia

LUMBAR HERNIA

Anatomy

The lumbar region is bordered superiorly by the twelfth rib, inferiorly by the iliac crest, medially by the erector spinae muscles, and laterally by the external oblique muscles. There are two spaces in which lumbar hernias occur, described as the *superior* and *inferior lumbar triangles.* The larger superior lumbar triangle was described independently by Joseph Grynfeltt and Peter Lesshaft as an inverted triangle formed by the edge of the twelfth rib and the edge of the quadratus lumborum muscle, the internal oblique laterally, and the external oblique forms

the roof. The floor of the superior lumbar triangle is formed by the aponeurosis of the transversus abdominis and transversalis fascia. The inferior lumbar space was described first by Jean Louis Petit and is bordered by the iliac crest inferiorly, the external oblique laterally, and the latissimus dorsi medially. The floor of the inferior lumbar space is made of the aponeurosis of the transversalis and internal oblique muscle and the lumbodorsal fascia (Figure 8, Table 1).

Most lumbar hernias are acquired, although 10% to 20% are congenital. Acquired hernias can be primary (spontaneous),

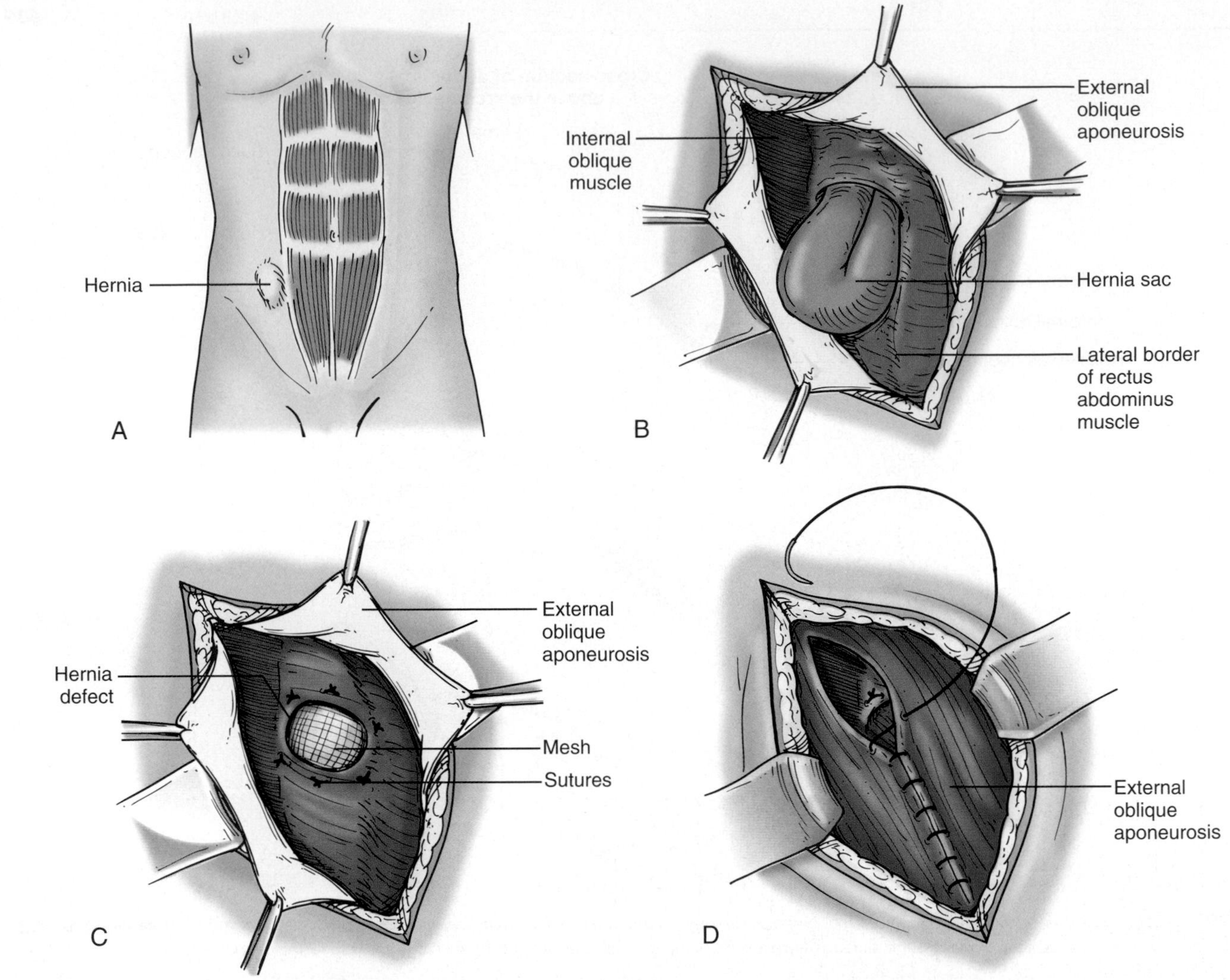

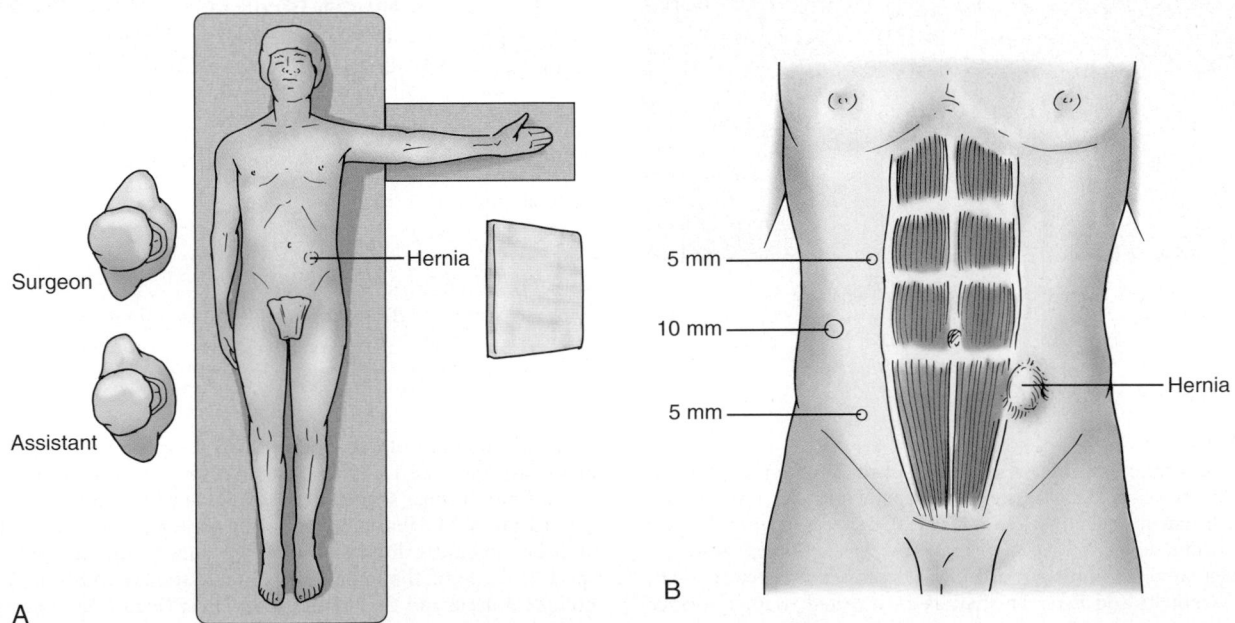

FIGURE 6 Open repair of semilunar hernia. **A,** Typical location of hernia. **B,** Exposure of hernia sac and fascial defect. External oblique aponeurosis has been divided. **C,** Placement of mesh to cover the hernia defect and secured into place with interrupted suture. **D,** Reapproximation of external oblique aponeurosis. *(From Sheu EG, Smink DS, Brooks DC. Spigelian hernia. In Jones DB, ed. Mastery Techniques in Surgery: Hernia. Philadelphia: Wolters Kluwer/Lippincott, Williams & Wilkins; 2013:385-392.)*

FIGURE 7 Laparoscopic repair of semilunar hernia. **A,** Patient positioning in supine, with contralateral arm tucked and surgeon standing on contralateral side. **B,** Typical trocar placement with 10-mm trocar at center. *(From Sheu EG, Smink DS, Brooks DC. Spigelian hernia. In Jones DB, ed. Mastery Techniques in Surgery: Hernia. Philadelphia: Wolters Kluwer/Lippincott, Williams & Wilkins; 2013:385-392.)*

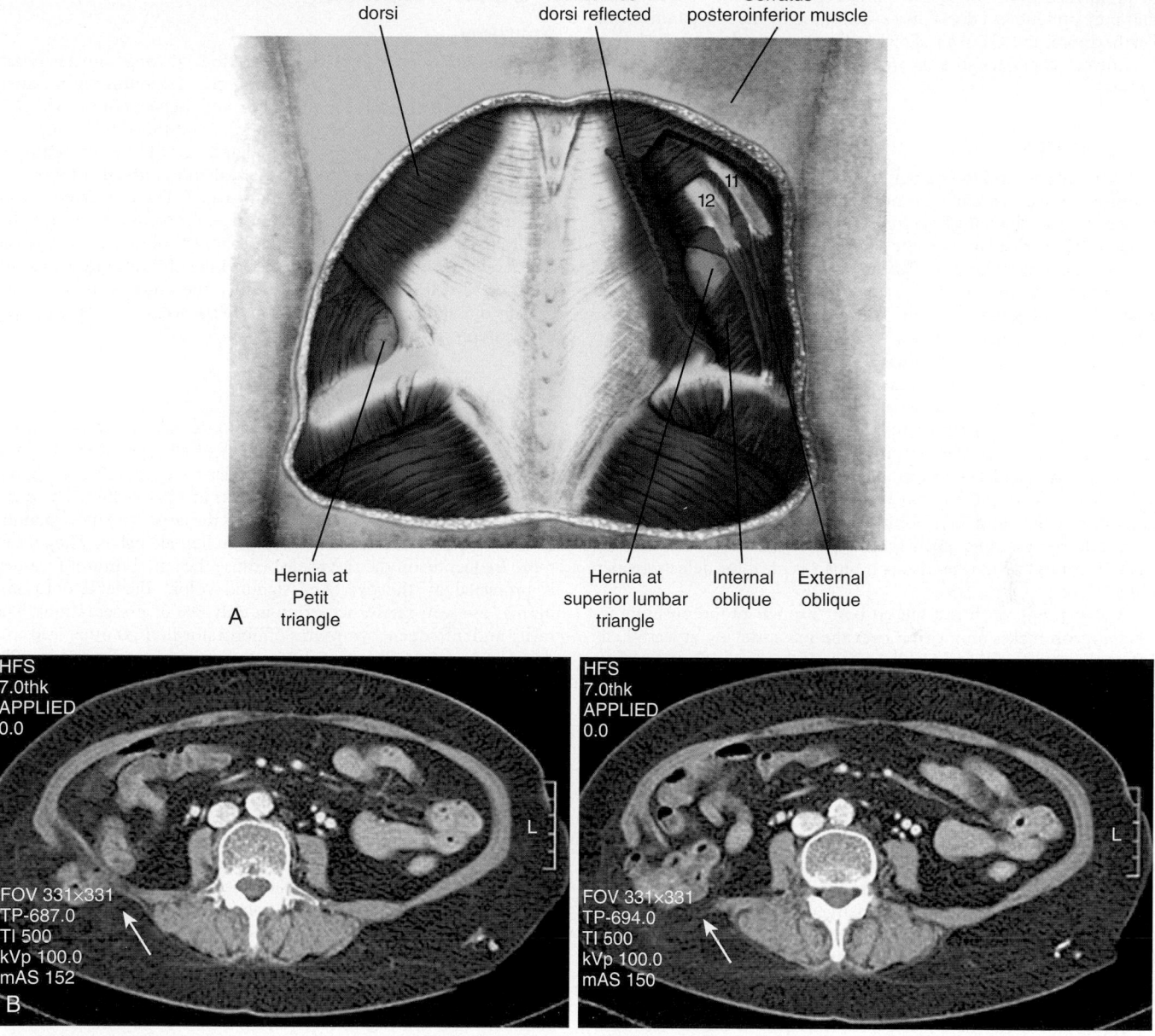

FIGURE 8 A, Anatomy of lumbar hernias, posterior view. Petit triangle on the left and Grynfeltt-Lesshaft hernia on the right. **B,** CT scan of right lumbar hernia involving fat and ascending colon. *(**A,** From Watson LF. Hernia, 3rd ed. St. Louis: Mosby, 1948. **B,** From Su Repair of lumbar hernia originating from autologous iliac bone graft with bilayer mesh. Formosan J Surg. 2012;45:59-62.)*

secondary resulting from trauma, or incisional from previous surgery such as those requiring a flank incision or an iliac bone graft. Primary hernias usually occur in the superior lumbar space and are caused by conditions that increase intra-abdominal pressures, such as chronic cough, pregnancy, or obesity. Secondary traumatic hernias often occur in the inferior lumbar space because of shearing force of weakened lumbar muscles against the iliac crest. Congenital defects appear in infancy and are associated with multiple malformations, including defects in the musculoskeletal system of the lumbar region. Predisposition to acquired hernias depends on various factors including the size and form of the muscles within the triangle, the length and angulation of the twelfth rib, and the size of the quadratus lumborum and serratus posterior muscles. Hernias occur more often through the superior lumbar space below the twelfth rib, where the subcostal neurovascular bundle penetrates a space in the region of the transversalis fascia. This area is weakened more commonly because it is not reinforced adequately by the external oblique. Fascial defects of the lumbodorsal or transversalis also create an area of weakness. These are seen more often in short, obese people with horizontal ribs and large triangles.

Clinical Indications

Most patients will be seen nonurgently, and approximately 9% are seen as acute surgical emergencies. Common complaints include nonspecific abdominal or back pain. Obstruction within the gastrointestinal or genitourinary tract can occur, leading to symptoms such as nausea/vomiting or urinary obstruction and hydronephrosis. Examination may reveal a palpable mass that becomes more protuberant with increased intra-abdominal pressure, such as Valsalva maneuver, commonly completely reducing in the recumbent position. CT scans have a 98% sensitivity for lumbar hernias and should be performed routinely to differentiate the multitude of conditions that may present as a dorsal mass, including tumors or panniculitis. Furthermore, the CT scan allows delineation of the muscle layers and defect characteristics as well as an assessment of herniated contents.

Surgical Tips

Lumbar hernias tend to be small and well-defined defects. However, because of the absence of clear musculoaponeurotic borders and the presence of nearby bony structures, these hernias can be technically challenging. Both a laparoscopic and an open technique are possible in repairing lumbar hernias. The laparoscopic approach has a higher cost but has a lower morbidity rate, shorter hospitalization, reduced analgesic requirements, and quicker convalescence. Furthermore, a laparoscopic approach permits visualization of the entire lumbar region as well as the abdominal contents. Laparoscopy should be preferred over the open technique except in cases of prior failed laparoscopic attempts, a very large defect, concern for acute bowel strangulation, or contraindications to laparoscopic surgery such as shock. Although there is greater postoperative morbidity after the open approach, the incidence of intraoperative complications are higher with the laparoscopic approach, commonly injury to the inferior epigastric artery and hematomas. In deciding the most optimal approach, laparoscopic repair should be considered for hernias less than 10 cm in width, whereas open repair is ideal for defects greater than 15 cm.

An open approach is achieved best through prone positioning. The surgeon makes an incision over the mass, staying at least 2 cm below the twelfth rib and paralleling the intercostal nerves to minimize the risk of injury to the neurovascular bundle. The hernia sac is identified and the contents reduced back into the abdominal cavity, potentially without opening the sac. Invagination of the sac is performed with absorbable suture, and the transversalis fascia is closed to obliterate the defect. In cases of incarceration, the sac is opened to evaluate the hernia contents for resection as needed. Afterwards, the fascial edge is reapproximated with interrupted figure-of-8 absorbable 0-monofilament suture. Synthetic mesh is placed as an overlay above the reapproximated fascia and secured to the surrounding muscle layers with 0-monfilament U-stitches. Afterward the mesh is covered with the overlying muscle. Larger incisional lumbar hernias may require a rotational flap repair to reapproximate the muscle defect and provide adequate mesh coverage but have been associated with a high incidence of recurrence, hematomas, seromas, and flap ischemia.

In the laparoscopic approach, a contralateral 45-degree decubitus position is obtained, and an umbilical Hasson entry is performed. A pair of 5-mm ports is placed in the ipsilateral upper and lower quadrants, usually adjacent to the subxiphoid and suprapubic position. The posterior abdominal wall is evaluated and the herniated contents are reduced. The fascial defects should be reapproximated with figure-of-8 absorbable 0-monofilament suture with a transfascial suturing device. IPOM techniques can be used to place a covered mesh in an underlay fashion to allow ideal mesh coverage of 3 to 5 cm from the fascial defect edge secured with judicious placement of transfascial sutures, tacks, or fibrin glue. Care is taken to avoid injury to the nerves running adjacent to the anterior-superior iliac spine or the subcostal neurovascular bundle. Securing mesh by tying it around the twelfth rib or drilling anchors to the iliac crest also has been described. Conversely, a TAPP approach can be performed, whereby three-sided peritoneal flaps are raised starting 5 to 7 cm anteriorly from the hernia defect. The fascia approximation is performed as described above, and the uncoated synthetic mesh is placed in the preperitoneal space and secured before peritoneal reapproximation with reabsorbable tacks or transfascial sutures. Afterwards, the peritoneum is reapproximated with running absorbable suture or absorbable tacks to cover the mesh (Figures 9 and 10).

▪ OBTURATOR HERNIA

Anatomy

The obturator canal is a 1 cm wide and 2 to 3 cm long tunnel between the obturator externus and internus muscles. The obturator foramen is the space between the pubic rami and ischial bones, which is covered by the obturator membrane in all but the anterior superior aspect. The obturator nerve, artery, and vein travel through the foramen and canal. The obturator nerve divides into an anterior and posterior branch within the obturator canal. The obturator hernia was first described by Arnaud de Ronsil as a protrusion through this obturator canal and foramen. The peritoneal obturator hernia sac can develop through a widening defect of the obturator externus and internus muscles, coursing along either the anterior or posterior branch of the obturator nerve. Symptoms occur more commonly with compression of the anterior nerve.

Clinical Indications

Obturator hernias are a rare cause of abdominal hernias, accounting for less than 1% of all hernias and 1.6% of all cases of small bowel obstruction. However, obturator hernias have one of the highest mortality rates of abdominal wall hernias at 13% to 40%. There is a female-to-male ratio of 6 : 1, explained by the larger and more oblique incline of the obturator canal seen in the female pelvis. They occur more frequently on the right side because the left obturator foramen is protected by the overlying sigmoid colon. Bilateral obturator hernias are seen rarely, occurring in only 6% of presentations. The rarity and infrequent symptoms of obturator hernias often lead to a delay in diagnosis and can lead to gangrenous bowel in up to 50% of repairs. Mortality is high largely because of poor physiologic reserve, malnutrition, pre-existing comorbidities, a high incidence of bowel strangulation, and delay in diagnosis. The typical patient is an emaciated, elderly woman with intermittent bowel obstruction and a history of recent weight loss. Patients often have increased pelvis laxity because of multiparity or causes of raised intra-abdominal pressure, such as chronic cough, ascites, or constipation. Weight loss leads to loss of the preperitoneal fatty tissue that usually inhabits the obturator canal, thereby increasing the risk of herniation. Tenderness may be elicited on palpation of the obturator foramen through a rectal or vaginal examination, but palpation of a mass occurs only in 20% of patients. The Howship-Romberg sign is referred pain down the medial thigh to the knee through compression of the obturator nerve with extension, abduction, and medial rotation that is relieved by flexion of the thigh. Although pathognomic, the Howship-Romberg sign is present in only 25% to 50% of patients.

A high index of suspicion should lead to early CT imaging to look for herniation through the obturator foramen between the pectineus muscle anteriorly and the obturator externus posteriorly. The CT scan has an accuracy of more than 90% and may decrease the rate of intestinal resection and improve survival by preventing a delay in diagnosis (Figures 11 through 13).

Surgical Tips

Obturator hernias require surgical repair shortly after diagnosis. Both minimally invasive and open techniques have been described. The open repair is used most commonly to allow evaluation of herniated contents as well as clear visualization of the structures within the obturator canal. The laparoscopic IPOM or TAPP approach is associated with less postoperative discomfort and shorter hospital stay but does not provide the same level of exposure as the open approach. A TEP approach should be avoided because of the inability to assess the viability of incarcerated contents and preventing necessary bowel resection. Synthetic mesh can be used to repair the obturator defect in circumstances when no resection is needed. In contaminated cases, biologic mesh or simple peritoneal closure or flaps should be considered.

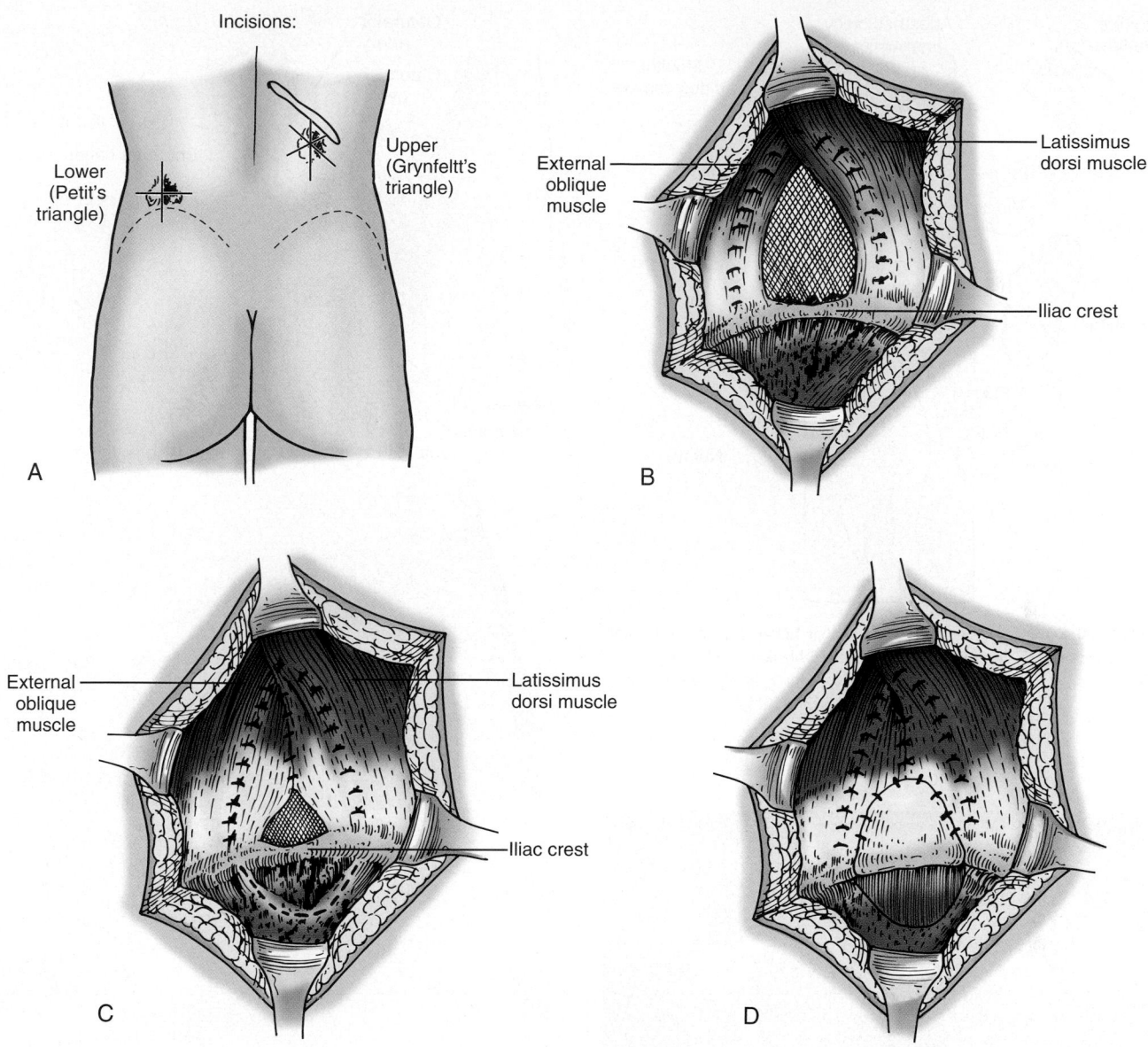

FIGURE 9 Open repair of lumbar hernia. **A,** Oblique incision over defect. **B,** Mesh repair of defect secured to muscles and periosteum. **C,** External oblique and latissimus dorsi muscles approximated to cover the mesh. *Dotted line* represents a flap of gluteal muscle which was divided. **D,** Rotational flap using gluteal fascia to completely cover mesh. *(From Skandalakis JE, Gray SW, Mansberger AR Jr, et al.* Hernia: Surgical Anatomy and Technique. *2nd ed. New York: Springer; 1989, with permission.)*

Open repair involves an intraperitoneal approach through a low midline incision. The herniated tissue tends to be well incarcerated and difficult to reduce. Steep Trendelenburg and gentle persistent retraction is often necessary. Otherwise, the obturator membrane can be incised to allow appropriate reduction of the incarcerated tissue, which is resected as needed. The hernia defect then can be closed primarily around the obturator vessels with nonabsorbable suture with approximation of the periosteum of the superior pubic ramus and the internal obturator muscle. A coated synthetic mesh is placed into the defect and secured with interrupted suture to the pectineal ligament and fascia overlying the pubic symphysis. In contaminated cases, simple peritoneal closure or biologic mesh has been described. Furthermore, local flaps using periosteum, uterine ligament, or aponeurosis can be used to patch the defect.

The laparoscopic TAPP or IPOM technique is performed with a periumbilical Hasson approach and insertion of two 5-mm trocars on each side of the umbilicus lateral to the semilunar line. Trendelenburg positioning can aid in identification of the obturator canal and its herniated contents. In certain circumstances when incarcerated bowel may be difficult to gradually retract, if a small catheter can be placed into the obturator foramen adjacent to the bowel, then gentle water pressure applied through the catheter may help reduce the incarcerated contents. In the TAPP repair, the peritoneum is incised from the ipsilateral anterior superior iliac spine toward the medial umbilical ligament and peeled towards the obturator foramen with enough space to allow placement of a 6 × 8 cm lightweight synthetic mesh. The mesh can be secured either by tacking laterally to the transversus abdominis muscle and medially to the rectus muscle superior to Cooper's ligament, or with fibrin glue. The peritoneum is then reapproximated with running absorbable suture or absorbable tacks. Bowel resection can be performed intra-abdominally, or through a minilaparotomy site by extending the umbilical incision.

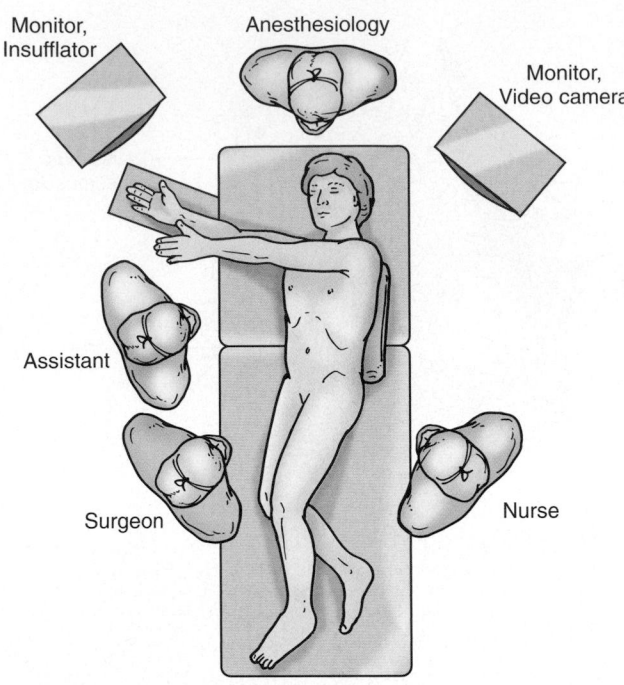

FIGURE 10 Patient positioning for left lumbar hernia repair. The patient is positioned at a 45-degree angle with a rolled blanket used as a posterior wedge. *(From Arca MJ, Heniford BT, Pokorny R, et al. Laparoscopic repair of lumbar hernias. J Am Coll Surg. 1998;187:147-152.)*

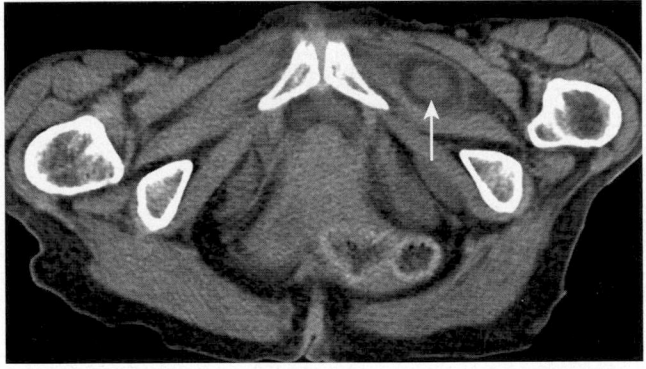

FIGURE 11 CT scan of incarcerated small bowel between external obturator and pectineal muscles (*arrow*). *(From Chen D, Fei Z, Wang X. Bowel obstruction secondary to incarcerated obturator hernia. Asian J Surg. 2015:S1015-9584. doi:10.1016/j.asjsur.2015.08.003. [Epub ahead of print].)*

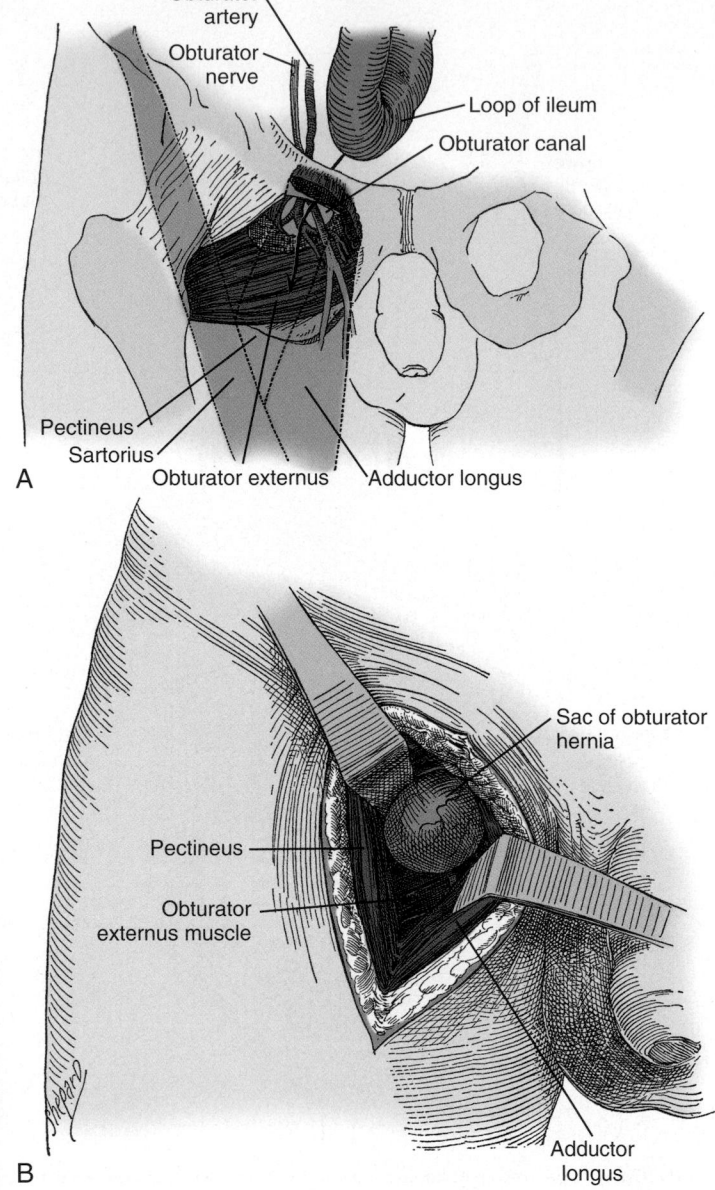

FIGURE 12 Anatomy of the obturator hernia. **A,** The structures passing though the obturator canal. **B,** Identification of hernia through an open approach. *(From Watson LF. Hernia, 3rd ed. St. Louis: Mosby, 1948.)*

In the IPOM technique the peritoneum is not incised, and simple peritoneal closure or coated mesh is used to repair the hernia defect. Biologic mesh is used in contaminated cases, even if it can be placed in the preperitoneal space (Figures 14 and 15).

SUMMARY

Hernias are a preventable cause of mortality, and the hernias covered in this chapter carry a high morbidity and mortality because of their rarity, subtle presentation, or difficult clinical diagnosis. The common use of CT scans in patients with abdominal discomfort can help diagnose these uncommon hernias. Unless the patient is a poor surgical candidate, surgical planning should follow diagnosis. Urgent or emergent surgery should be considered for obturator hernias, which have a higher risk of morbidity and mortality. In elective circumstances, the laparoscopic approach leads to faster recovery, although material cost is higher. Depending on the clinical expertise, a laparoscopic approach is still feasible in the setting of obstruction. However, an open approach is appropriate if there is preoperative evidence of shock.

ACKNOWLEDGMENT

The author would like to acknowledge the following people for their support of this chapter: Joanna Etra and Daniel Boyett.

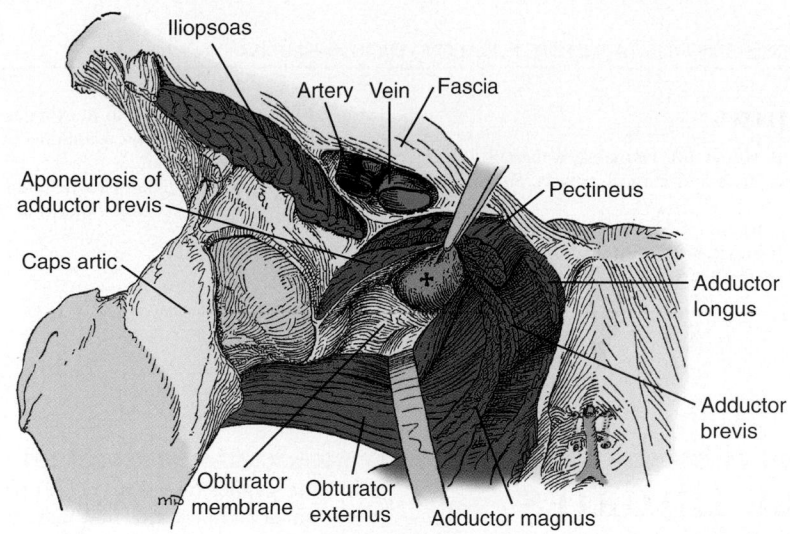

FIGURE 13 Dissection of obturator region to the level of the obturator canal and membrane. *(From Watson LF. Hernia, 3rd ed. St. Louis: Mosby, 1948.)*

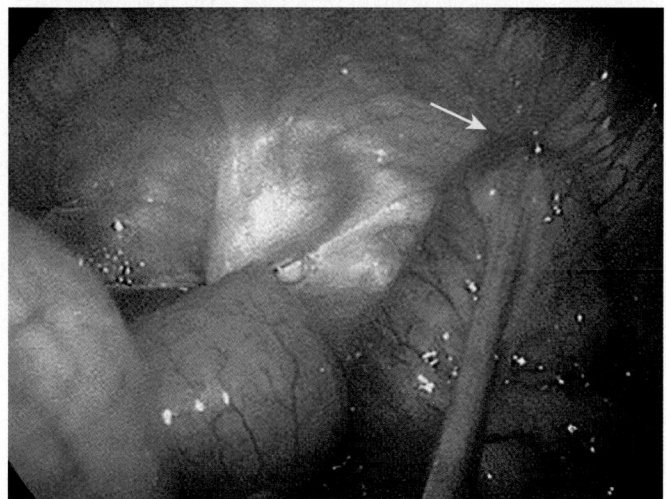

FIGURE 14 Intraoperative picture of incarcerated obturator hernia involving small bowel. *(From Yau KK, Siu WT, Fung KH, Li MK. Small bowel obstruction secondary to incarcerated obturator hernia. Am J Surg. 2006;192:207-208.)*

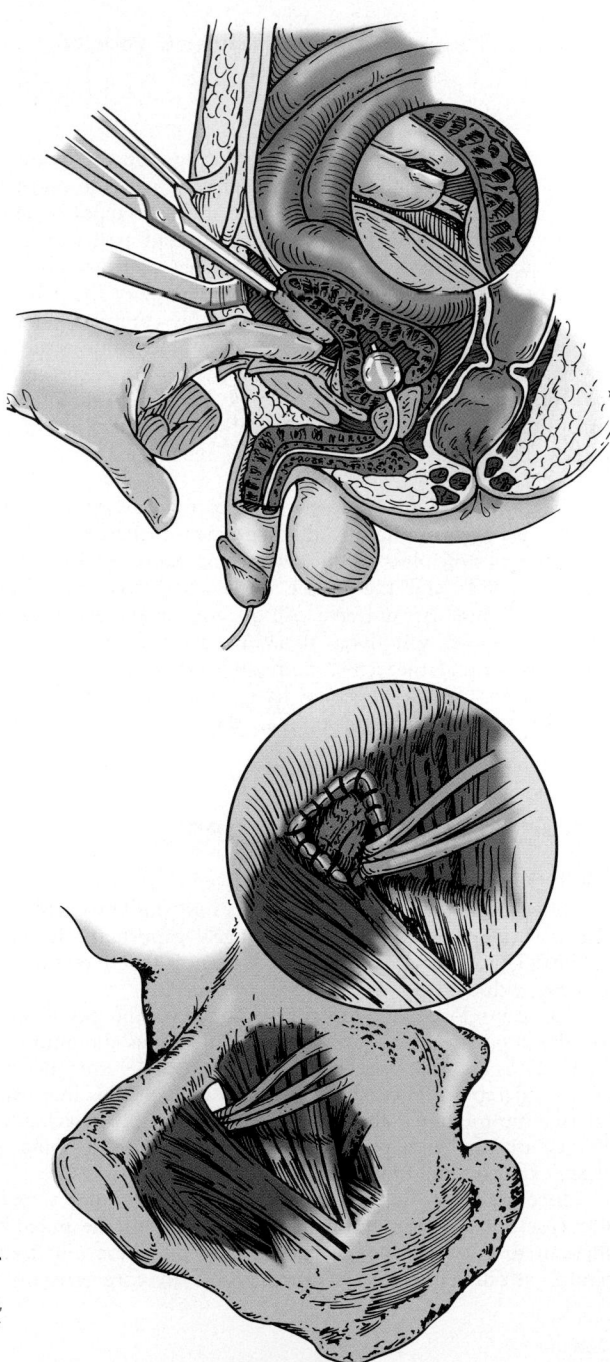

FIGURE 15 Closure of obturator defect using mesh. *(From Skandalakis LJ, Gadacz TB, Mansberger AR, et al. Modern Hernia Repair: The Embryological and Anatomical Basis of Surgery. New York: Parthenon Publishing Group; 1996:286-296, with permission.)*

SUGGESTED READINGS

Armstrong O, Hamel A, Grignon B, Ndoye JM, Hamel O, Robert R, Rogez JM. Lumbar hernia: anatomical basis and clinical aspects. *Surg Radiol Anat.* 2009;31:317.

Hayama S, Ohtaka K, Takahashi Y, Ichimura T, Senmaru N, Hirano S. Laparoscopic reduction and repair for incarcerated obturator hernia: comparison with open surgery. *Hernia.* 2015;19:809-814.

Moreno-Egea A, Campillo-Soto A, Morales-Cuenca G. Which should be the gold standard laparoscopic technique for handling Spigelian hernias? *Surg Endosc.* 2015;29:856-862.

Nasir BS, Zendejan B, Ali SM, Groenewald CB, Heller SF, Farley DR. Obturator hernia: the Mayo Clinic experience. *Hernia.* 2012;16:316-319.

CORE MUSCLE INJURIES (ATHLETIC PUBALGIA, SPORTS HERNIA)

William C. Meyers, MD, and Alexander E. Poor, MD

This chapter will help a surgeon treating someone with groin pain and no palpable hernia. The surgeon needs to understand details of core anatomy as well as the different types of injuries that occur there; otherwise, the patient should expect dissatisfaction. One of the most misunderstood subjects in medicine is the musculoskeletal physiology and pathophysiology of the pelvis. The term *sports hernia* not only understates this complexity, but also leads surgeons to think mistakenly that these pains result from tiny protuberances (i.e., occult hernias). Nothing is further from the truth. Most of these problems arise from real musculoskeletal disruptions and subsequent compensations. In 1 day in our clinic we saw 14 patients with failed "hernia" repairs for these types of problems.

While reading this chapter, assume that all groin pain in athletes can be explained by the anatomy. Furthermore, consider just two types of joints in the pelvis—the ball-in-socket hip joint without muscle and the "pubic bone joint"—as the center of the core's muscular universe. All of the surrounding muscles, bones, and other soft tissue structures arrange themselves symmetrically around the center point, the pubic bone. Perhaps for other reasons, people generally have considered the pubic bone to be the center of the universe. In the case of athletic injuries, this is particularly true.

■ BACKGROUND: THE CORE

Core Anatomy

The muscles that originate at or insert into the fibrocartilaginous plate covering the pubic bone play a hugely important role in pelvic stability. This complex constitutes the harness that allows the torso to move with the legs.

This central stability functionally anchors the pelvis so that peripheral parts of the body can move. The rectus abdominis flexes the trunk as it compresses abdominal viscera and forms the anchor for considerable abduction and adduction, as well as internal and external hip rotation. Laterally, the rectus abdominis attaches to the oblique muscles with pure fibrous connections, enveloping complexes of nerves and tiny vascular structures.

Three adductors—the pectineus, the adductor longus, and the adductor brevis—insert into the fibrocartilage of the pubic bone adjacent to the rectus abdominis attachment. These muscles with central attachments play a primary role in core stability. The adductor magnus inserts more laterally and the gracilis attachments are so small and posterior that these two muscles do not participate much in core stability. Interestingly, the anterior obturator nerve innervates all of the adductors except the magnus, consistent with the co-operative function of these muscles at this joint.

Basic experiments with this anatomy and fresh cadavers revealed the dynamic relationship of these structures. Cutting 30% of the rectus abdominis results in a huge shift in the balance across the pubic bone, and the adductors slam against the pubic bone with greater forces than one might expect, even with completely flaccid muscles. Dividing the rectus abdominis also causes pressure changes within the hip joint. These relationships are not subtle and are fundamental in understanding core injuries.

Pathophysiology

In athletes, tremendous torque occurs at the level of the pelvis. The anterior pelvis takes the brunt of most forces. The pubic bone functionally serves as a fulcrum around which many of the forces are connected. When one of these core muscles weakens, usually from fraying associated with hyperextension or hyperabduction, it results in an imbalance of forces on the pelvis. This imbalance causes disruption of the attachments to the fibrocartilaginous plate of the pubic bone, which can cause pain, weakness, and instability. Loss of stability leads to compensation from the other structures that cross the pubic bone (iliopsoas, rectus femoris, sartorius), which can then become additional sources of pain and injury.

Certain anatomic variants can predispose a person to certain injuries and should be recognized. For example, symptomatic femoroacetabular impingement results in spasm of the adductors (primarily adductor longus) and hip flexors (primarily rectus femoris) as a compensatory measure to limit range of motion in the hip joint. This places those muscles at increased risk for injury. In addition, the differences in the male and female pelvis probably explain why males more often develop central core muscle injuries at the pubic bone attachments whereas females are more likely to have hip and psoas problems. Men have thicker, heavier pelvises than women, causing greater shifts in force and a narrower subpubic angle, which leads to a different distribution of forces. In addition, men have a narrower pubic symphysis disc, which leads to less pelvic flexibility, and a narrower pelvis, which likely leads to less stability overall. The female hip is more prone to injury in part because the femoral head is 30% smaller than in the male hip, resulting in increased load on the articular surface.

The core is made up of everything from the chest to the midthigh (Figure 1). All of it must be considered when a patient has groin pain. There are four components of the core: the ball-and-socket hip joints, the back, all remaining skeletal muscles and bones, and everything else (all other muscles, ligaments, nerves, blood vessels, intestines, reproductive organs, genitourinary structures, lymphatic channels, etc.). This provides the basis for the differential diagnosis of exertional groin pain, which can be lumped grossly into the same four groups: hip, back, core muscles, and everything else.

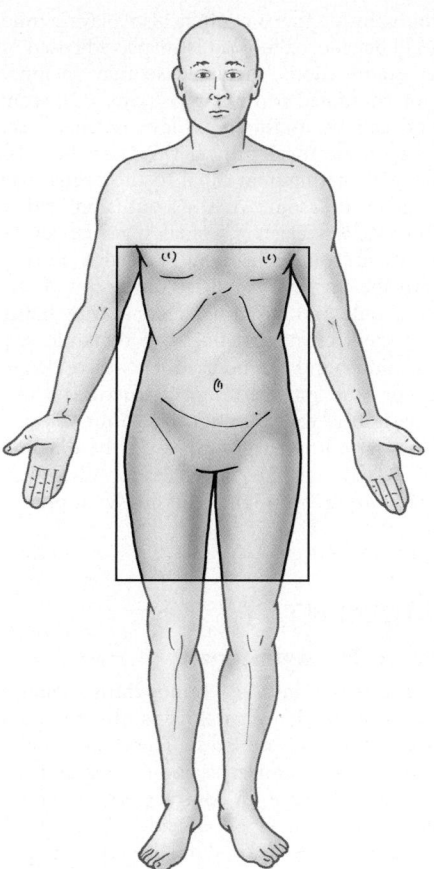

FIGURE I Anatomic location of the core.

■ DIAGNOSTIC APPROACH

History and Physical Examination

One must consider the muscles involved in the core; there are 29 muscles within the core, all of which have the potential to contribute to an injury. A compulsive history and physical examination and appropriate imaging are necessary to arrive at a complete diagnosis. Localized tenderness sometimes may help to confirm specific diagnoses, although tenderness from diffuse bony or soft tissue inflammation also may cause confusion. Resistance testing and compulsive attention to the location of elicited pain can help to identify the muscles involved.

Interpretation of each test involves three considerations: Does the test cause pain? Does the resulting pain correlate to the muscle being tested? And does the resulting pain re-create the pain that is causing the athlete's disability? One also must consider the potential for hip joint involvement. In the physical examination, this involves primarily range-of-motion tests without interference from contraction of muscles. These tests include the standard flexion–abduction–external rotation (FABER) test and the flexion–adduction–internal rotation (FADIR) test plus other rotational or hyperflexion/hyperextension tests that can isolate anterior, posterior, or lateral impingements, for example. In our practice, concurrent hip and core muscle injuries are seen in 16% of cases, and one must be prepared to work up and treat both conditions when evaluating a patient with groin pain.

Finally, one must consider that portions of the gastrointestinal, genitourinary, and gynecologic systems; lymphatics; blood vessels; and nerves also reside in the core. The importance of this final group cannot be overstated because some of these diagnoses can be life threatening, but it may be obvious from history and physical examination whether the problem is musculoskeletal in nature. Box 1 summarizes the differential diagnoses for groin pain in athletes.

Imaging

In a practical sense, history and physical examination, plain films, and magnetic resonance imaging (MRI) are generally the most useful modalities for diagnosing core injuries. Using specific MRI techniques ("athletic pubalgia protocol"; see Figure 1), core muscle injuries can be identified with sensitivity and specificity. A conventional MRI of the pelvis likely may be read as normal or as showing

---

BOX I: Differential Diagnosis of Groin Pain in Athletes

Hip-Associated Causes

Acetabular labral tear and femoroacetabular impingement
Osteoarthritis
Snapping hip syndrome and iliopsoas tendonitis
Avascular necrosis
Iliotibial band syndrome

Visceral Causes

Inguinal hernia
Other abdominal hernias
Testicular torsion

Infectious Causes

Septic arthritis
Osteomyelitis
Pelvic inflammatory disease
Prostatitis
Epididymitis and orchitis
Herpes infection

Inflammatory Causes

Endometriosis
Inflammatory bowel disease
Pelvic inflammatory disease
Primary osteitis pubis

Traumatic Causes

Stress fracture
Tendon avulsion
Muscle contusion
Baseball pitcher–hockey goalie syndrome

Developmental Causes

Apophysitis
Growth plate stress injury or fracture
Legg-Calvé-Perthes disease
Developmental dysplasia
Slipped capital femoral epiphysis

Neurologic Causes

Nerve entrapment syndromes
Referred pain
Sacroiliitis
Sciatic entrapment (piriformis syndrome)
Hamstring strain
Knee pain

Neoplastic Causes

Testicular carcinoma
Osteoid osteoma

some nonspecific changes in the pubic symphysis or edema patterns, leading to incorrect diagnoses such as stress fractures. Figure 2, in which a complete adductor longus avulsion is difficult to appreciate, demonstrates this point. Because of the high incidence of concomitant symptomatic hip pathology, magnetic resonance (MR) arthrography of the hip often also plays a role (Figure 3). Imaging should be tailored to what is suspected based on the history and physical examination. Imaging also may include plain films, ultrasound, or computed tomography scans (CT scans).

Ultrasound can be useful to achieve detailed visualization of structures, but its use to identify hernias can be misleading. The close proximity of the inguinal canal to the caudal rectus abdominis attachment creates some of the confusion and explains why the term *sports hernia* exists. Normal inguinal fat occurs in the spermatic cords or round ligament. Likewise, retroperitoneal fat extending into the inguinal canal is commonly observed on MRI but typically should not be considered a true hernia. If a true hernia is suspected, prone imaging and dynamic sequences with either MRI or ultrasound can be used. Definitive diagnosis requires the presence of true intraperitoneal structures (not simply fat) outside the peritoneal cavity or sliding within the inguinal canal. Bone scan does have limited usefulness in the diagnosis of osteitis pubis. Figure 4 outlines the categories of differential diagnoses associated with groin pain and the likely appropriate imaging modalities.

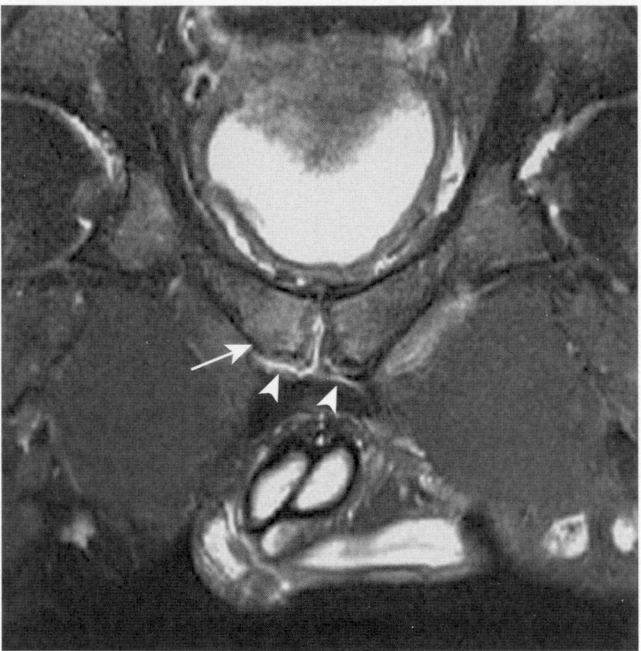

FIGURE 2 In this image obtained using magnetic resonance imaging, complete adductor longus avulsion (*arrow*) is difficult to appreciate (*arrowheads*).

■ MANAGEMENT

Nonoperative Management

For certain peripheral injuries, nonoperative management is a first-line treatment. In many cases, it is also required because of special considerations in athletes. These personal factors—the timing within a season, concerns about coaching or front office decisions, and the influence on contract negotiations—in addition to the clinical factors, must be considered in deciding when to use aggressive temporizing procedures versus permanent solutions. In general, the first treatment of groin pain involves rest; ice; anti-inflammatories; and, depending on the resources available, manual therapy, ultrasound, infrared, and the like. This treatment is often performed before surgical consultation, but increasingly astute athletic trainers and athletes are seeking treatment for

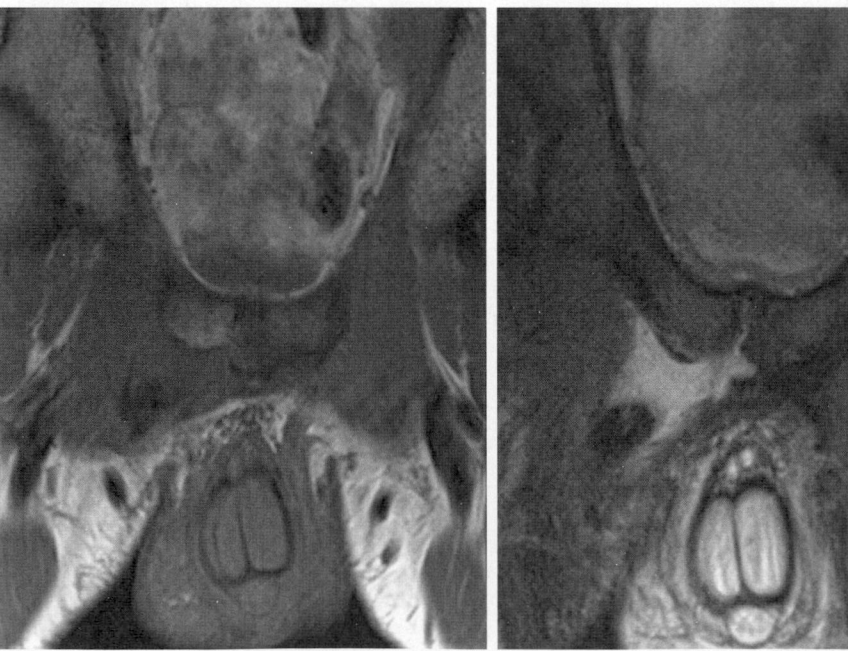

FIGURE 3 Magnetic resonance arthrography of the hip.

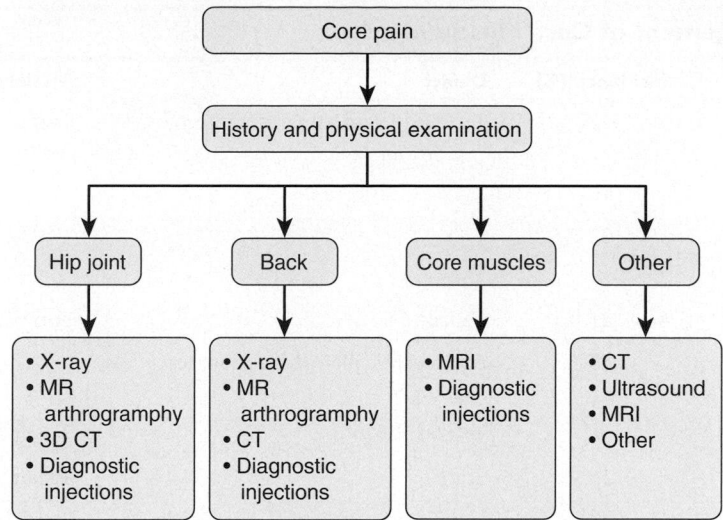

FIGURE 4 Differential diagnoses and imaging modalities for groin pain. *CT,* Computed tomography; *MR,* magnetic resonance; *MRI,* magnetic resonance imaging.

injuries earlier than has been the case historically. Classically, these injuries improve with rest, but the pain returns upon resuming activities. This period of rest is not a required component of the diagnostic workup, however, and a person with signs and symptoms of a core muscle injury need not wait for definitive repair. The mainstay of nonoperative treatment is physical therapy to strengthen the lateral and posterior core muscles to offload the injury and stabilize the pubic joint. This is analogous to strengthening the quadriceps and hamstrings after an injury to the anterior cruciate ligament (ACL).

Core muscle injuries involve a large number of muscles but fortunately tend to occur in predictable patterns (we often refer to 29 core muscles but, in reality, this number is too low). As a general rule, injuries that involve the central pubic bone attachments leave an athlete with instability that, as with an ACL tear, cannot be corrected until normal anatomy is restored. More peripheral injuries, however, often can be managed nonoperatively, and compensatory measures are more effective.

There are also percutaneous interventions, with varying degrees of evidence supporting their use for temporizing core muscle injuries. We prefer corticosteroid injections administered directly into the areas of injury and inflammation and recently reviewed this treatment. Overall, 79% of athletes with core injuries returned to high-level play for the duration of their seasons, and delaying definitive repair did not adversely affect postoperative outcomes. Other factors, however, such as the timing of the injection and the presence of clinically significant hip pathology, may play important roles. Some have been using platelet-rich plasma (PRP) as a form of temporizing treatment. We do not advocate its use because of its ineffectiveness and the newly identified risk of heterotopic ossification (HO).

Operative Management

Surgical management of core muscle injuries involves a number of procedures that mobilize the involved muscles to restore normal anatomy and balance without tension (Table 1). The procedures require the surgeon to expose, mobilize, and repair the injured muscles without damaging what remains intact and without tension. They do not involve simply dividing muscles or nerves or treating occult hernias. Mesh-related inguinodynia is becoming an increasingly recognized concern and should be reason enough to refrain

from placing mesh unless a true hernia is identified. If you are considering doing a hernia repair on a patient with inguinal pain in the absence of a palpable hernia, stop that line of thinking. Learn the different specific causes of pain and how they are fixed.

Postoperative Management

Surgery can be performed as an outpatient procedure, and early ambulation and activation of the repaired core muscles is key, as adhesions and scar tissue are the biggest hindrance to recovery. Carefully monitored resisted contraction of the repaired muscles begins on the day after surgery and should continue daily until the patient has returned to full activity. After the first week, massage also plays an important role. Depending on the muscles involved, the extent of injury and repair, and the degree of appropriate rehabilitation, most patients can expect a return to full activity in 3 to 6 weeks postoperatively.

Complications

Complications are uncommon. Wound infections and hematomas are the most serious complications. Hematomas may limit the patient's ability to return to full activity in a timely fashion; therefore they usually are treated aggressively with surgical evacuation and drain placement. Scar tissue is the most common postoperative problem and occasionally requires additional surgery. One must take care to identify any predisposing factors (such as symptomatic femoroacetabular impingement) that result in compensatory muscle damage before proceeding with surgery.

▪ RECOMMENDATIONS

1. Learn the anatomy.
2. Become familiar with the different types of procedures that can fix core muscle injuries.
3. Understand the roles of physical therapy, temporizing, and definitive interventions.
4. Beware the misnomers (sports hernia, sportsman's hernia, Gilmore's groin) associated with this large and diverse collection of injuries.

TABLE I: Surgical Management of Core Muscle Injuries

Structure or Syndrome	Incidence (%)	Defect	Possibly Indicated Procedure
Unilateral rectus abdominis/ unilateral adductor	22	Tear and compartment syndrome (CS)	Repair and compartmental decompression
Adductor longus	16		
Pectineus	22		
Adductor brevis	8		
Pure adductor syndromes	21	Usually CS	Compartmental decompression
Bilateral rectus abdominis/ bilateral adductor	17	Aponeurotic plate disruption; tear and CS	
Unilateral rectus abdominis	16	Tear	Repair
Bilateral rheumatoid arthritis	15	Tears	Repair
Severe osteitis variant	8	Usually tears, CS, and bone edema	Repair, compartmental decompression, and steroid injection
Unilateral/bilateral	7	Combination tear(s) and CS	Repair(s) and compartmental decompression(s)
Iliopsoas variant	4	Impingement and bursitis	Lengthening procedure
Baseball pitcher–hockey goalie syndrome	4	Adductor tear and adductor muscle belly CS	Compartmental decompression
Spigelian hernia	4	Tear	Repair
Rectus femoris variant	3	Impingement	Compartmental decompression
High rectus abdominis variant	2	Tear	Repair
Female variant	2	Medial disruption with lateral thigh compensation	Repair(s) and compartmental decompression(s)
Round ligament syndrome	1	Inflammation with tear	Repair and excision
Dancer's variants	<1	Obturator internus/externus	Compartmental decompression(s)
Rower's rib syndrome	<1	Subluxation	Excision and mesh
Avulsions		Usually acute adductor injury	Repair(s) and compartmental decompression(s)
Adductor/rectus abdominis calcification syndromes	<1	Chronic avulsion	Excision, compartmental decompression
Midline rectus abdominis variant	<1	Tears and muscle separation	Repair(s)
Anterior ischial tuberosity variant	<1	Posterior perineal inflammation, gracilis, hamstrings	Compartmental decompression
Adductor contractures	<1	Often associated with hip pathology	Compartmental decompression and hip repair
More uncommon variants	2	Eg, gracilis, quadratus, iliotibial band	Variable

Modified from Meyers WC, McKechnie A, Philippon MJ, et al. Experience with "sports hernia" spanning two decades. *Ann Surg.* 2008;248:656-665.

SUGGESTED READINGS

Byrd JWT. Gross anatomy. In: Byrd JWT, ed. *Operative Hip Arthroscopy.* New York: Springer; 2005:100-109.

Hammoud S, Bedi A, Magennis E, et al. High incidence of athletic pubalgia symptoms in professional athletes with symptomatic femoroacetabular impingement. *Arthroscopy.* 2012;28:1388-1395.

Meyers WC, Kahan DM, Joseph T, et al. Current analysis of women athletes with pelvic pain. *Med Sci Sports Exerc.* 2011;43:1387-1393.

Meyers WC, McKechnie A, Philippon MJ, et al. Experience with "sports hernia" spanning two decades. *Ann Surg.* 2008;248:656-665.

Meyers WC, Yoo E, Devon O, et al. Understanding "sports hernia" (athletic pubalgia): the anatomic and pathophysiologic basis for abdominal and groin pain in athletes. *Op Tech Sports Med.* 2007;15:165-177.

Palisch A, Zoga AC, Meyers WC. Imaging of athletic pubalgia and core muscle injuries: clinical and therapeutic correlations. *Clin Sports Med.* 2013;32:427-447.

Zoga AC, Kavanagh EC, Meyers WC, et al. MRI findings in athletic pubalgia and the "sports hernia." *Radiology.* 2008;247:797-807.

ABDOMINAL WALL RECONSTRUCTION

David M. Krpata, MD, and Michael J. Rosen, MD

Although hernia repair is not a new procedure in surgery, the growing complexity of patients and defects that require repairs has spawned the new field of abdominal wall reconstruction. Abdominal wall reconstruction surgeons recently have developed several innovative approaches to reconstructing complex hernia defects to expand the options for surgeons and patients. Refinements in our understanding of abdominal wall anatomy, preoperative optimization, and advanced surgical techniques have driven the field of abdominal wall reconstruction and are discussed in this chapter.

◼ ANATOMY

The foundation for successful abdominal wall reconstruction is a thorough understanding of the abdominal wall anatomy. The abdominal wall anatomy is misunderstood by most surgeons because the relationship of the linea semilunaris, lateral abdominal wall muscular contributions, and the posterior rectus sheath were depicted inaccurately in *Netter's Surgical Atlas*. For those who plan to perform abdominal wall reconstruction, an intricate understanding of the anatomy is required to fully appreciate the surgical techniques. Pertinent anatomic issues include a firm understanding of the functional myofascial and neurovascular anatomy. If the surgeon understands these anatomic planes and structures, safe complex operations can be performed. Without a complete understanding of these planes, major sections of the abdominal wall can become devascularized or defunctionalized, based on denervation injuries.

From a functional standpoint, the linea alba is a tendinous insertion point at which the abdominal muscles are under optimal tension to maximize function. However, there are key fascial interactions, between the lateral abdominal muscles and the rectus abdominis, including the linea semilunaris. This relationship can be manipulated to provide myofascial advancements when incised or released as performed in a components separation. The principle of a functional abdominal wall is the premise for abdominal wall reconstruction practices, such as components separation, that enable medialization of the rectus muscles with recreation of the linea alba and reloading of the abdominal muscles.

As surgical techniques are described later, surgeons performing abdominal wall reconstruction must think of these component separations as surgical flaps where they create a donor site and a recipient site. Surgeons must recognize that with these techniques they are stealing donor function to obtain recipient site tissue coverage and that this is a trade-off. Nonetheless, the reloading of the abdominal wall via recreation of the linea alba may have a net positive impact on function. Unfortunately, the implications of components separations are not understood fully, which is why decisions about approaches and techniques should not be taken lightly.

To better understand the myofascial relationships, the anterior abdominal wall can be broken down into upper, middle, and lower thirds. First, at all levels of the abdominal wall, the external oblique, internal oblique, and transversus abdominis come together to develop the linea semilunaris; however, at these different thirds of the abdominal wall these relationships vary and are not as once thought with just an anterior and posterior rectus sheath (Figure 1). In the upper third of the anterior abdominal wall the posterior lamellar of the internal oblique and the transversus abdominis muscle extend medial to the linea semilunaris. This relationship is critical to understanding

that lateral abdominal wall muscles can now be accessed in a retrorectus medial approach. Similarly, in the middle third of the abdominal wall the posterior lamellar of the internal oblique extends medial to the linea semilunaris; however, the transversus abdominis muscle ends lateral to the linea semilunaris, and the transversus abdominis fascia extends medial to the linea semilunaris with the posterior lamellar of the internal oblique forming the posterior rectus sheath. In the lower third, the contributions of the internal oblique and transversus abdominis muscle to the posterior rectus sheath end at the level of the arcuate line, leaving only peritoneum and transversalis fascia over the rectus abdominis muscle as it extends to the pubic tubercle. The importance of these relationships is emphasized further when describing the posterior components separation in the operative techniques section.

The neurovascular anatomy of the abdominal wall is intricate and is important to identify and preserve during complex abdominal wall reconstructions. First, the nerves that innervate the abdominal wall are from T7-L1, with T7-L1 making up the sensory innervation and T7-T12 making up the motor innervation of the rectus complex. The neurovascular bundles that innervate the rectus abdominis run between the internal oblique and transversus abdominis fascia before penetrating the posterior rectus sheath approximately 1 cm medial to the linea semilunaris. Second, the deep inferior epigastric artery provides the dominant blood supply to the medial abdominal wall. Along its longitudinal path as it runs inferior to the rectus abdominis muscle, it distributes a medial and a lateral row of musculocutaneous perforators. These perforators are in greatest concentration around the umbilicus. Preservation of these periumbilical perforators can maximize skin blood supply during abdominal wall reconstruction. In our practice, all abdominal wall neurovascular anatomy is preserved whenever possible.

◼ PATIENT EVALUATION AND PREHABILITATION

The initial evaluation of patients for abdominal wall reconstruction is critical for two reasons. First, it is an opportunity to intervene on modifiable risk factors that affect surgical outcomes and second, it is the point at which decisions on surgical technique must be considered.

With regard to surgical optimization for abdominal wall reconstruction, there are two main modifiable risk factors, obesity and smoking. Not only are these modifiable, they are in fact hard indications in our practice not to offer complex abdominal wall reconstruction to a patient. Obesity is a significant risk factor for postoperative wound morbidity, which may compromise the sterility of mesh prosthesis and increase hernia recurrence. As a result, any patient over a BMI of 40 kg/m² is counseled on weight loss. Appropriate candidates also are counseled about surgical weight loss options and, when interested, are referred to our bariatric surgeons for surgical weight loss procedures. Our center has collaborated with a medical weight loss specialist and has achieved meaningful weight loss preoperatively in certain patients. Other centers have started abdominal wall reconstruction prehabilitation programs, employing a multidisciplinary approach in which patients are evaluated and treated by a physical therapist, a dietician, and other appropriate practitioners (i.e., endocrinologist for diabetes mellitus).

Smoking cessation is an absolute necessity before any abdominal wall reconstruction. Patients are required to be smoke free for at least 4 weeks because there is ample evidence to suggest a significant reduction in wound morbidity with at least 4 weeks of smoking cessation. Patients are allowed to use nicotine replacement therapy, such as patches or chewing gum; however, electronic cigarettes are not acceptable because they are believed to have equivalent wound morbidity compared with regular cigarettes. For patients who agree to stop smoking, cessation is confirmed with a urine test before any operation being scheduled.

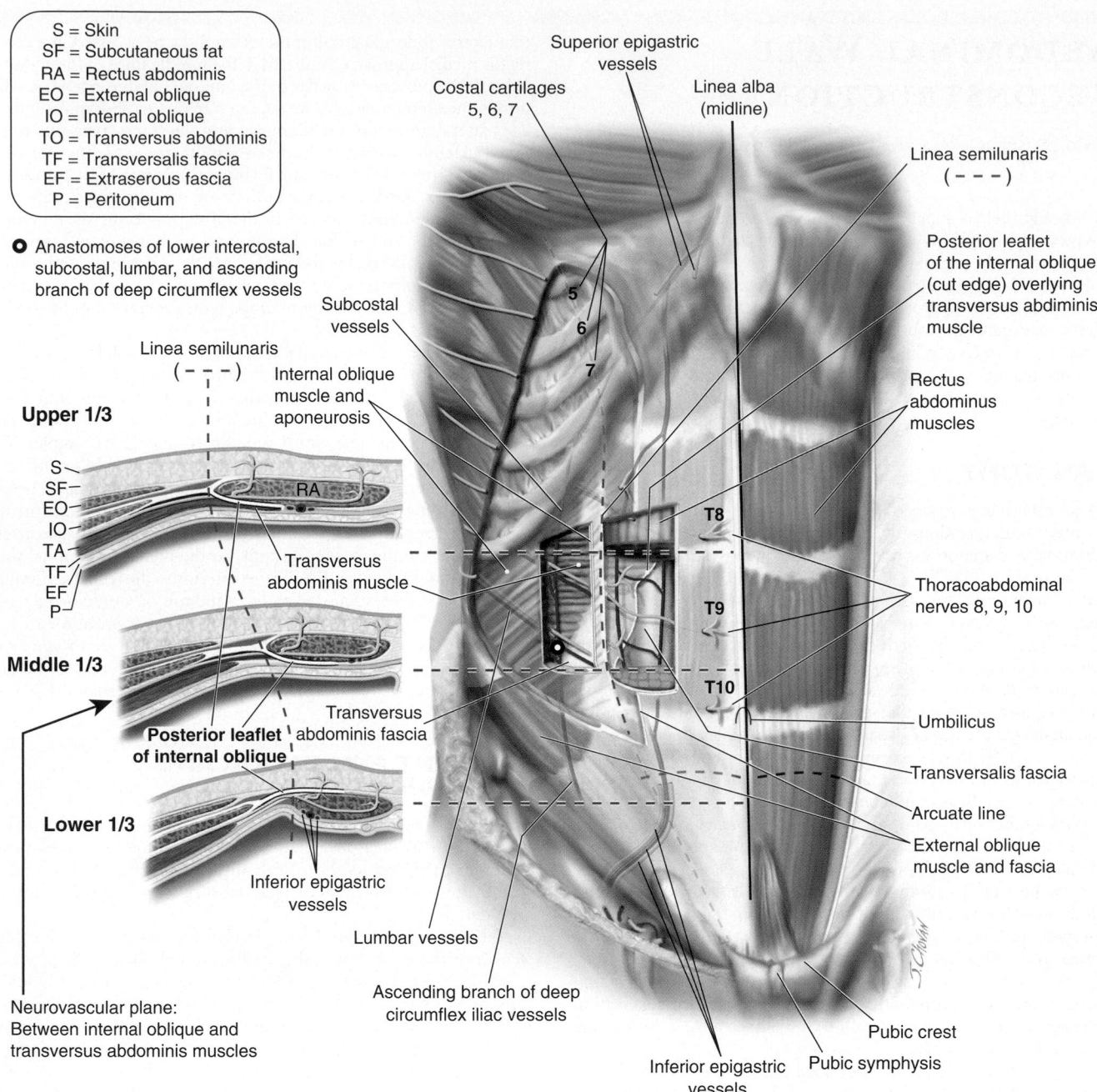

S = Skin
SF = Subcutaneous fat
RA = Rectus abdominis
EO = External oblique
IO = Internal oblique
TO = Transversus abdominis
TF = Transversalis fascia
EF = Extraserous fascia
P = Peritoneum

O Anastomoses of lower intercostal, subcostal, lumbar, and ascending branch of deep circumflex vessels

Upper 1/3

Linea semilunaris (– – –)

S
SF
EO
IO
TA
TF
EF
P

RA

Internal oblique muscle and aponeurosis

Transversus abdominis muscle

Middle 1/3

Posterior leaflet of internal oblique

Transversus abdominis fascia

Lower 1/3

Inferior epigastric vessels

Neurovascular plane: Between internal oblique and transversus abdominis muscles

Lumbar vessels

Ascending branch of deep circumflex iliac vessels

Inferior epigastric vessels

Costal cartilages 5, 6, 7

Superior epigastric vessels

Linea alba (midline)

Subcostal vessels

5
6
7

Linea semilunaris (– – –)

Posterior leaflet of the internal oblique (cut edge) overlying transversus abdiminis muscle

Rectus abdominus muscles

T8

T9

T10

Thoracoabdominal nerves 8, 9, 10

Umbilicus

Transversalis fascia

Arcuate line

External oblique muscle and fascia

Pubic crest

Pubic symphysis

FIGURE 1 Abdominal wall anatomy: myofascial relationships and neurovascular anatomy of the upper, middle, and lower thirds of the abdominal wall. *(From Rosen MJ. Atlas of Abdominal Wall Reconstruction. 2nd ed. Philadelphia: Elsevier; 2016.)*

All patients with a complex abdominal wall defect receive preoperative imaging with a CT scan of the abdomen and pelvis. Imaging provides information about prior mesh placement, defect characteristics, and myofascial anatomy, which may affect surgical planning. For example, a wide rectus abdominis muscle may indicate that a patient would require only a retrorectus dissection and mesh placement as opposed to a posterior components separation for a patient in whom the surgeon prefers sublay mesh. In addition, imaging, in combination with a physical exam, is used to assess the likelihood of fascial closure and soft tissue coverage. This is a critical point in the evaluation of these patients because failure to identify soft tissue coverage concerns in a patient who is not likely to achieve fascial closure and will require a bridge repair could compromise significantly any attempts at abdominal wall reconstruction. Those patients for whom fascial closure is unlikely and soft tissue coverage is of concern should be considered for alternative soft tissue flap coverage such as latissimus dorsi, rectus femoris, or anterolateral thigh flaps and, in some cases, tissue expanders.

OPERATIVE APPROACHES

There are multiple approaches to abdominal wall reconstruction, and it safely can be said that the field has yet to provide level 1 data to support or refute any specific technique. Deciding the approach for abdominal wall reconstructions involves answering four questions: (1) Is component separation required? (2) If so, what type of components separation will be used? (3) What type of mesh will be used? and (4) Where in the abdominal wall will the mesh be placed?

The decision to perform a component separation is based primarily on the ability to recreate the linea alba through medialization of the rectus abdominis muscles while maintaining appropriate physiologic tension on the repair. When the tension on the midline closure is too high, there is a greater risk of early hernia recurrence, tissue ischemia, and negative physiologic implications such as postoperative respiratory failure, renal failure, or venous thromboembolic events associated with high intra-abdominal compartment pressures. In these circumstances a separation of components should be considered.

There are two broad categories of components separations: anterior components separation and posterior components separation. Both approaches have potential benefits and pitfalls. Our preference is to perform a posterior components separation when possible because it provides the benefit of myofascial advancement similar to an anterior components separation; however, it also allows wide mesh overlap in a sublay position between the abdominal musculature and the peritoneum while eliminating large skin flaps. As such, the posterior components separation is described in detail.

Anterior Components Separation

The anterior components separation was introduced into practice by Dr. Oscar Ramirez in 1990 and has gained widespread acceptance (Figure 2). In its original description, this procedure requires large lipocutaneous flaps over the anterior rectus sheath to expose the external oblique fascia. Once exposed, the external oblique fascia and muscle are incised longitudinally along its medial border 1 to 2 cm lateral to its insertion into the linea semilunaris. The external oblique muscle is separated from the internal oblique fascia. Once completed, the anterior components release should provide approximately 5 cm of unilateral advancement at the upper portion of the abdomen, 10 cm at the middle of the abdomen, and 3 cm at the inferior portion of the abdomen. Bilaterally, this allows for as much as 20 cm of myofascial advancement to medialize the rectus abdominis and reduce tension of the linea alba. The major disadvantage to the anterior components separation is the large skin flaps that are required, which add significant wound morbidity, especially when combined with obesity, smoking, and diabetes.

Alternative approaches to the traditional anterior components separation have been described in an effort to reduce wound morbidity. These include (1) the periumbilical perforator sparing component separation, which preserves the anterior and medial rows of musculocutaneous perforators from the deep inferior epigastric, which have an increased concentration around the umbilicus, (2) the modified minimally invasive component separation, which attempts to preserve all the myocutaneous perforating vessels and reduce dead space by tunneling out to the external oblique fascia to perform the external oblique release, and (3) the endoscopic component separation, which uses minimally invasive surgical techniques to endoscopically divide the external oblique muscle and fascia without undermining the subcutaneous tissue at all.

Posterior Components Separation

The posterior components separation was introduced initially into the literature by the authors in 2012, although its development can be credited to many, as an alternative approach to an anterior components separation whereby myofascial advancement could be achieved without releasing the external oblique and creating large lipocutaneous skin flaps. Instead, the posterior lamellar of the internal oblique is incised to achieve myofascial advancement, while the transversus abdominis muscle is incised and released from the peritoneum to achieve wide mesh overlap of the preperitoneal abdominal cavity and advancement of the peritoneal flap. This technique has been a progression of surgeons' understanding of the abdominal wall, which began as a completely preperitoneal dissection with preperitoneal mesh placement. The preperitoneal approach remains a

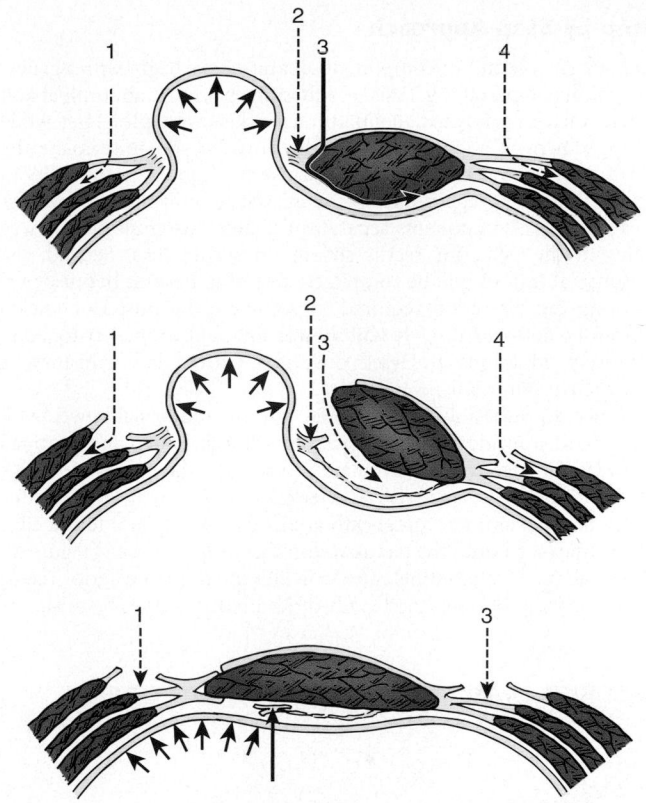

FIGURE 2 Component separation. *1,* Separation of the external oblique muscle from the underlying internal oblique. *2,* The internal oblique muscle is adherent to the transversus abdominis muscle. *3,* The rectus can be separated easily from the posterior rectus sheath. *4,* The anterior rectus sheath is adherent to the rectus muscle at the tendinous inscriptions above the umbilicus. The segmental neurovascular bundle of the rectus muscle travels in the deep surface of the internal oblique muscle, between this and the transversus muscle, not at its lateral margin but at a variable distance (10 to 25 mm) from the margin close to the axis formed by the deep superior and inferior epigastric arteries. The external oblique muscle alone can be advanced toward the midline 2 cm in the upper and lower, and 4 cm in the middle third in the midline around the waistline. Each rectus muscle with the overlying rectus sheath can be advanced 3, 5, and 3 cm, respectively, in the upper, middle, and lower thirds. For this advancement to occur, the muscle has to be removed from its encasement in the posterior rectus sheath. The rectus muscle with the overlying rectus sheath and its attached internal oblique and transversus muscles can be advanced 5 cm in the epigastrium, 10 cm at the waistline, and 3 cm in the suprapubic region. *(From Ramirez OM, Ruas E, Dellon AL. "Components separation" method for closure of abdominal wall defects: an anatomic and clinical study. Plast Reconstr Surg. 1990;86:519.)*

challenging dissection with little if any advancement of the midline fascia. Using an understanding of the Rives-Stoppa retromuscular approach, further iterations of the posterior release highlighted the transversus abdominis release, or TAR, while trying to gain access to the preperitoneal space through the posterior rectus sheath. At the time, it was felt the release of the transversus abdominis muscle offered the benefit of medialization of the rectus abdominis as a myofascial advancement flap. On closer inspection, it has become clear that it is actually the incision of the posterior lamellar of the internal oblique muscle that provides the advancement of the rectus abdominis muscle. In fact, the transversus abdominis muscle is cut only in the upper third of the abdomen and offers only a transition from the posterior rectus sheath to the preperitoneal plane.

Step-by-Step Approach

To perform a posterior component separation we begin with a generous midline laparotomy. Lysis of adhesions from the abdominal and pelvic walls is performed, maintaining two key principles. First, while taking down all abdominal wall adhesions, we do not violate the peritoneum and abdominal wall because this can cause difficulty in getting into the preperitoneal plane as well as limit the effectiveness of a posterior components separation if there are multiple or large holes in the posterior rectus sheath or peritoneum. Second, the abdominal wall should be completely free of adhesions because performing the dissection required to complete the posterior release cannot be performed safely with bowel adherent to the peritoneum. Interloop adhesions are lysed only if a patient has a history of obstructive symptoms.

Once the adhesiolysis is complete and no additional bowel work is required, a surgical towel is placed into the abdomen and wrapped from lateral edge of the peritoneum to seclude the bowel. One edge of the rectus is elevated with Kocher clamps (Figure 3). The peritoneum and posterior rectus sheath are incised just lateral to the edge of the linea alba until the rectus abdominis muscle is seen (Figure 4). Once the rectus abdominis muscle is identified, the posterior rectus sheath is incised along the length of its medial edge. The posterior

rectus sheath is dissected free from the rectus abdominis until the linea semilunaris is exposed. During this dissection the neurovascular bundles that innervate the rectus abdominis can be seen just medial to the linea semilunaris (Figure 5). These neurovascular bundles should be preserved. Under tension, the posterior lamellar of the internal oblique is incised just medial to the neurovascular bundles, which exposes the transversus abdominis muscle in upper third of the abdomen (Figures 6 and 7). After completely incising the posterior lamellar of the internal oblique, a right angle clamp is used to guide transection of the transversus abdominis muscle (Figure 8). This should expose the peritoneum. Once the posterior rectus sheath is incised completely along its length, the transversus abdominis muscle is separated from the peritoneum using appropriate traction-counter traction (Figures 9 and 10). A common pitfall at this point is making holes in the peritoneum. If this happens, the surgeon should begin to work lateral to the peritoneal defect and get behind the defect before it increases in size and significantly disrupts the peritoneum. The peritoneum can be freed from overlying muscle and fascia out to the psoas muscle if necessary. In the pelvis, Cooper's ligaments are exposed bilaterally, and the bladder is taken down,

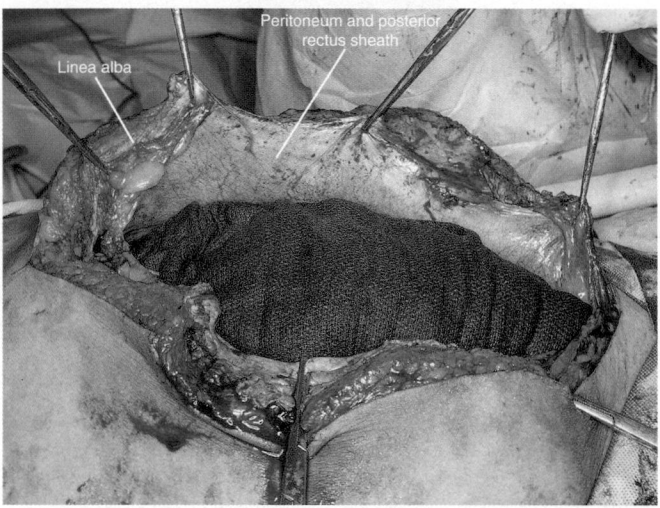

FIGURE 3 Posterior view of the abdominal wall.

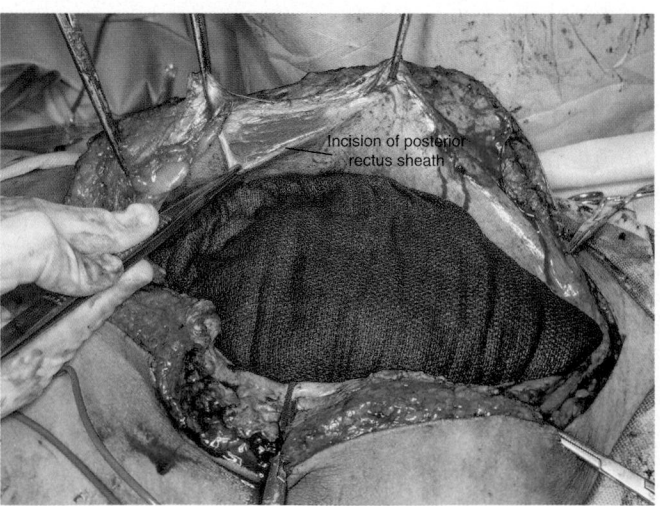

FIGURE 4 Posterior rectus sheath incised just medial to the linea alba.

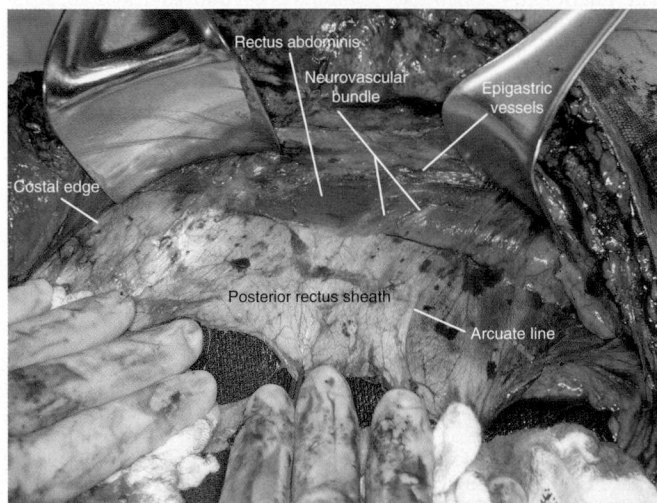

FIGURE 5 Neurovascular bundles 1 to 2 cm medial to the linea semilunaris.

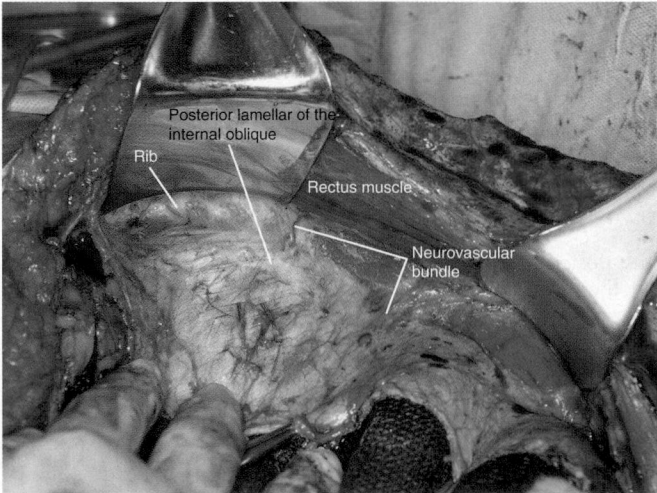

FIGURE 6 Along the upper third of the abdominal wall, the posterior lamellar of the internal oblique overlies the transversus abdominis muscle in the retrorectus space.

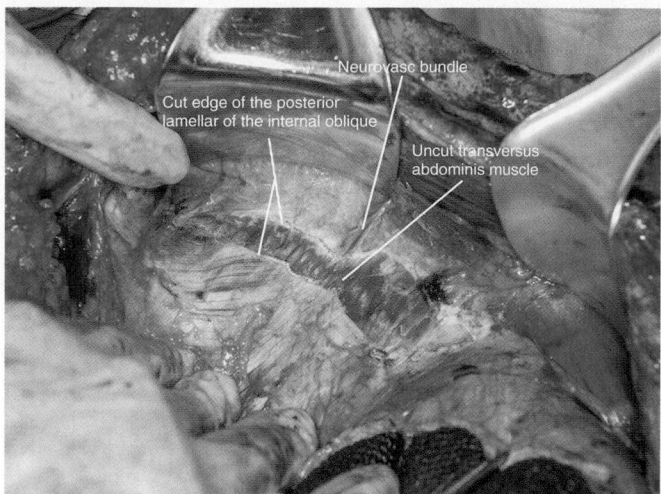

FIGURE 7 In a posterior components separation, the transversus abdominis is exposed after the posterior lamellar of the internal oblique is incised.

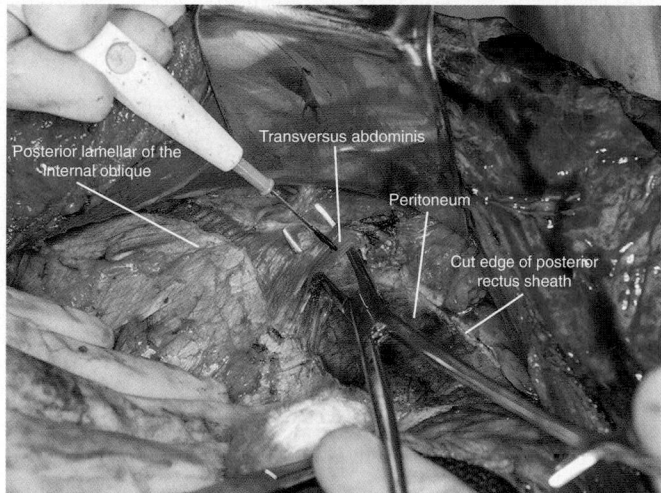

FIGURE 8 The transversus abdominis is incised after the posterior lamellar of the internal oblique is cut.

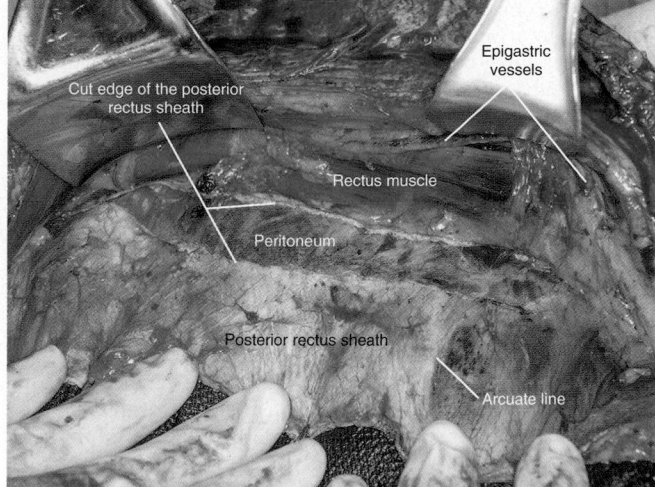

FIGURE 9 To expose the peritoneum, the posterior lamellar of the internal oblique and transversus abdominis muscle are incised in the upper third of the abdominal wall. In the middle third, the posterior lamellar of the internal oblique and transversus abdominis fascia are incised the length of the posterior rectus sheath to the arcuate line, exposing the peritoneum.

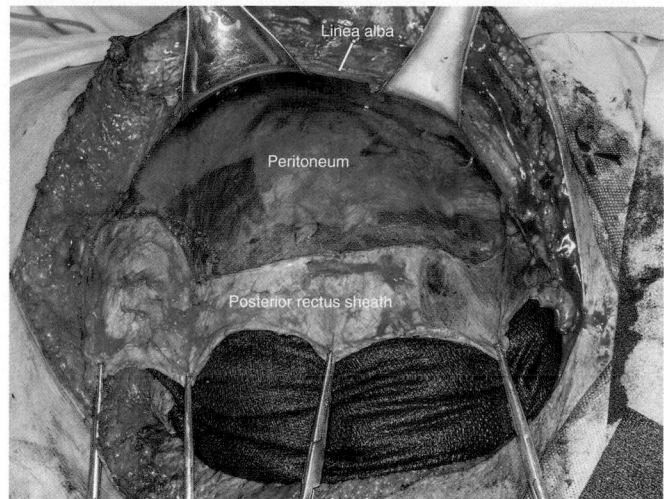

FIGURE 10 The peritoneum is separated from the transversus abdominis releasing the posterior rectus sheath for closure and creating a sublay pocket for mesh placement.

freeing the most inferior portion of the peritoneum from the anterior abdominal wall. At the xiphoid process, the medial edge of the posterior rectus sheath is incised in a cephalad fashion toward the diaphragm. Staying inferior to the xiphoid, the muscle fibers of the diaphragm are kept elevated off the peritoneum. This dissection will continue to the central tendon of the diaphragm, which may be necessary for abdominal defects that are primarily in the upper abdomen or subxiphoid.

After completing the posterior components separation and preperitoneal dissection, the surgeon removes the surgical towel, and the posterior rectus sheath is reapproximated with 2-0 absorbable suture. The mesh then is inserted into the preperitoneal pocket and fixated with eight slowly absorbable transfascial sutures, including one at the xiphoid, one at the pubis, bilaterally in the upper third of the abdomen just medial to the ribs, bilaterally in the lower third of the abdomen medial to the ASIS, and bilaterally in the middle third of the abdomen below the costal margin. The mesh should be taut so that when the abdomen is closed the mesh will not wrinkle. Two drains are placed over the mesh and below the fascial closure. Once the mesh is in place, the linea alba is reapproximated and skin closed.

For large abdominal wall defects in which the fascia will not reapproximate and a mesh bridge repair is required, we prefer to use a heavyweight synthetic mesh. Given this, it is imperative that the soft tissue coverage over the heavyweight mesh is reliable and at lowest risk for wound morbidity. As such, if there is too much tension on the skin or the skin is not healthy, we consider soft tissue flaps to ensure adequate soft tissue coverage of the mesh. The decision for a flap reconstruction should not be made at the end of the operation but rather planned well in advance to ensure the best possible outcome.

Prosthetic Materials

There are many prosthetic options for the reconstructive surgeon to choose from when reconstructing the abdominal wall. It is likely that each mesh has some place in abdominal wall reconstruction, but the paucity of comparative scientific data has led to the power of marketing to drive many mesh choices. Basically the reconstructive surgeon has three options: synthetic, bioabsorbable synthetic, and biologic mesh.

Synthetic Mesh

Various synthetic mesh materials, including polypropylene, polyester, polytetrafluoroethylene, and expanded PTFE, have played a significant role in hernia surgery since Luijendijk's landmark paper revealing the benefit of mesh repair over primary repair. The role of a mesh material is to provide a framework for scar formation while providing secondary stabilization and strength for hernia repair durability. These materials fit this role well; however, concerns about mesh infection either from mesh erosion or superficial or deep space surgical site infections have limited their use in patients at high risk for a wound infection, potentially contaminated, and contaminated surgical fields. As our understanding of mesh properties has improved, it has become clear that not all synthetic materials are created equal with regard to infection. Light and medium weight, macroporous, monofilament synthetic meshes have been used in high-risk comorbid patients, CDC wound class 2 and 3 cases, and even as prophylaxis around stomas without significant increase in mesh complications.

Biologic Mesh

Bioprosthetic hernia mesh, or biologic mesh, was introduced into abdominal wall reconstruction in the early 2000s. These materials were touted with the potential benefits of reduced mesh morbidity from infected mesh and its ability to regenerate into abdominal wall fascia, which aided in its popularity. Although it is clear now that these meshes have limited regenerative properties in their current form, they do provide an extracellular matrix for possible cellular infiltration and have limited morbidity if they become infected because they typically will be digested by bacterial collagenase and degrade. Several biologic materials are available, including extracellular dermal allografts and xenografts, porcine small intestinal submucosa, and bovine pericardium. Available data suggest that biologic mesh should not be used in a bridging fashion with the expectation of achieving a durable hernia repair. The primary limitation to biologic mesh use is its cost, which is difficult to justify in clean cases in which synthetic mesh can be used safely. Long-term data supporting the use of biologic mesh for abdominal wall reconstruction are limited. In addition, the largest series to date of biologic mesh use for abdominal wall reconstruction in contaminated fields has demonstrated a greater than 50% hernia recurrence rate at 3 years of follow-up.

Bioabsorbable Mesh

Bioabsorbable mesh offers an alternative material that handles and provides a framework for scar formation similar to synthetic mesh; however, it resorbs over a 6- to 18-month period, depending on the specific material. Although these materials may be safer to use in infected fields, the long-term durability of an abdominal wall reconstruction with a bioabsorbable material is still unknown. To date, no published trials exist defining the role of bioabsorbable mesh in abdominal wall reconstruction.

■ POSTOPERATIVE MANAGEMENT AND OUTCOMES

Although much has been made about enhanced recovery pathways in surgery, there are limited data to support its use in patients who require complex abdominal wall reconstruction. Our current practice is routine epidural placement for postoperative analgesia. Advancement from *nil per os* to clear liquids occurs on the morning of postoperative day 1 followed by advancement to ad lib dieting after return of bowel function defined by the presence of flatus. Nasogastric tubes are not placed routinely in patients undergoing abdominal wall reconstruction.

All patients have subfascial drains that are placed above the mesh. They are left in place until the drain output has reduced to less than 30 cc over a 24-hour period and subsequently removed. For synthetic mesh, the typical duration of drains is 3 to 5 days, and most patients have drains removed before discharge from the hospital. Patients with biologic or bioabsorbable mesh typically are discharged from the hospital with drains in place as the output tends to be greater initially for these mesh prostheses.

Although the majority of patients are extubated in the operating room after abdominal wall reconstruction, a small percentage will require prolonged mechanical ventilation from increased intra-abdominal pressure and underlying lung disease. These patients are identified most reliably by measuring the change in preoperative and postoperative plateau pressures. Patients with an increase in plateau pressure of greater than 6 cm H_2O are considered strongly for prolonged intubation for 24 to 48 hours after surgery. For an increase in plateau pressure of greater than 9 cm H_2O consideration is also given to 24 hours of postoperative paralysis.

Long-term outcomes after abdominal wall reconstruction are not well understood given the multiple variables including recent advancements in technique, addition of mesh prosthetics to the field, and a lack of follow-up on these patients. In an effort to improve knowledge of long-term outcomes, quality collaboratives such as the Americas Hernia Society Quality Collaborative (AHSQC.org) have begun as a platform for the reporting of patient outcomes in abdominal wall reconstruction with the aim of improving value for patients with hernias. Furthermore, the metric by which to define a quality outcome is not yet well defined because a quality outcome may appear different to different surgeons and different to different patients, depending on where the patient began physically and mentally before abdominal wall reconstruction. Nonetheless, hernia recurrence rate after components separation ranges from 5% to 10% based on technique and patient population. Surgeons who operate on smokers and morbidly obese patients should expect worse wound morbidity and higher hernia recurrence rates.

■ SUMMARY

The field of abdominal wall reconstruction has seen many recent advancements. A better understanding of anatomy has improved operative approaches while an increase in available mesh prosthesis has confused the market. Multiple methods of components separation exist, including anterior components separation and the various modifications that have been devised to try and reduce wound morbidity. Our preferred approach of a posterior component separation provides a reduction in wound morbidity and similar myofascial advancement while placing mesh in a retro-rectus preperitoneal sublay position. Limited data exist to guide surgeons on these methods of components separation as it relates to long-term outcomes and hernia recurrence, increasing the need for surgeon collaboration to ultimately improve patient care.

SUGGESTED READINGS

Carbonell AM, Criss CN, Cobb WS, et al. Outcomes of synthetic mesh in contaminated ventral hernia repairs. *J Am Coll Surg.* 2013;217:991-998.

Krpata DM, Blatnik JA, Novitsky YW, et al. Posterior and open anterior components separations: a comparative analysis. *Am J Surg.* 2012;203: 318-322.

Martindale RG, Deveney CW. Preoperative risk reduction: strategies to optimize outcomes. *Surg Clin North Am.* 2013;93:1041-1055.

Ramirez OM, Ruas E, Dellon AL. "Components separation" method for closure of abdominal-wall defects: an anatomic and clinical study. *Plast Reconstr Surg.* 1990;86:519-526.

Rosen MJ, Aydogdu K, Grafmiller K, et al. A multidisciplinary approach to medical weight loss prior to complex abdominal wall reconstruction: Is it feasible? *J Gastrointest Surg.* 2015;19:1399-1406.

Rosen MJ, Krpata DM, Ermlich B, et al. A 5-year experience with single-staged repairs of infected and contaminated abdominal wall defects utilizing biologic mesh. *Ann Surg.* 2013;257:991-996.

THE MANAGEMENT OF BENIGN BREAST DISEASE

Jieqiong Liu, MD, and Lisa K. Jacobs, MD, MSPH

Benign breast disease accounts for a significant number of referrals to a breast surgeon and is a source of substantial anxiety for patients. These conditions include mastalgia, nipple discharge, palpable solid masses and cysts, fibrocystic disease, and infections. These conditions must be managed appropriately to provide patients with the necessary care to either cure the disease or provide symptomatic relief, making them manageable. It is important to be able to discern when a coexisting suspicious disease develops and when further imaging and biopsy are indicated.

■ EVALUATION OF BENIGN BREAST COMPLAINTS

The evaluation of benign breast complaints begins with a focused history and clinical breast examination. The history should include a detailed assessment of the symptoms, aggravating and alleviating factors, duration of symptoms, and presence of associated symptoms. The goal of this history is to not only ascertain pertinent information to appropriately diagnose the patient but also help guide the selection of diagnostic testing that will have the most yield, especially taking into consideration the age of the patient. Furthermore, it will help to identify patients that are at high risk for development of breast cancer in the future and are high-risk screening candidates. Caution must be exercised to maintain clinical suspicion of atypical findings because patients with seemingly benign presentations could harbor findings suggestive of malignancy, and of course, some patients with benign disease may be at risk for later development of breast cancer.

The detailed history is followed by a thorough bilateral breast examination, including examination of regional lymph node basins. The physical examination should begin with visual inspection for asymmetries, skin or nipple changes, nipple inversion, breast edema, and breast erythema. This is followed by superficial and deep palpation in an orderly manner to carefully examine all quadrants of the breast, including the axillary tail. It is useful to ascertain if any nipple discharge is present and to characterize it in terms of color and location, especially noting if it involves a single duct or multiple ducts and if a trigger point can be identified.

Diagnostic imaging is selected based on clinical suspicion of the underlying cause of the patient's symptoms and includes the same studies available for evaluation of a patient suspected of breast cancer, including mammography, ultrasound (US), and magnetic resonance imaging (MRI), all of which have biopsy capability to help establish the diagnosis. It is important to consider the age of the patient as well. In a young patient with dense parenchyma who is experiencing typical benign symptoms suggestive of a cyst or fibroadenoma, a US may prove more useful than mammography, which would be less sensitive with dense parenchyma. As with patients suspected of having breast cancer, negative imaging should not deter the recommendation of aspiration or biopsy of suspicious palpable abnormalities detected on physical examination.

On occasion, women may experience abnormal imaging and no physical examination changes. These cases may require biopsy if there are features suspicious or indeterminate for malignancy. Abnormalities that can be visualized with US should have a US-guided biopsy because this is the most comfortable positioning for the patient. If visible only by mammography, a stereotactic biopsy would have to be considered. For abnormalities identified only by MRI, an MRI-guided biopsy is the only option. If the target lesion is deep in the breast along the chest wall, in a superficial location in proximity to the nipple, or if the patient cannot tolerate the positioning for an image-guided biopsy, then a needle-localized surgical excisional biopsy may be warranted.

■ BREAST MASSES

Palpable breast masses are one of the most common presenting complaints. In premenopausal women, most breast masses are benign, especially when present and stable over several months to years. However, any suspicious palpable breast mass requires additional imaging and diagnostic biopsy. Palpable abnormalities could represent dense breast parenchyma with fibrocystic changes, cysts, lipomas, or fibroadenomas. Based on the initial history and physical examination the differential diagnosis is usually evident. If a lesion is suspected to be cystic, this can be confirmed with US, and a cyst aspiration can be attempted if it is symptomatic. If the cyst expresses serous fluid and is collapsed completely at the end of the aspiration, no further biopsy is warranted. However, if the cyst fails to resolve completely or if it appears to be complex with a solid component, it warrants additional biopsy. If a lesion is felt to be solid, benign versus malignant characteristics can be determined based on imaging criteria. Benign fibroadenomas are well circumscribed and do not have spiculated, irregular margins typical of malignant lesions. These generally are identified with the aid of US and can undergo biopsy with US guidance. If the patient has a benign history with imaging findings supportive of a fibroadenoma and is asymptomatic, then close observation with short-term interval imaging remains an option.

■ FIBROADENOMAS

The majority of palpable breast masses are benign, especially in younger women, and the most frequently encountered solid benign mass is a fibroadenoma. These lesions are well circumscribed with smooth edges and are mobile with rubbery consistency. Many patients will have multiple fibroadenomas either synchronous or metachronous. They can be mildly symptomatic: patients complain of tenderness or pain at the site often worse at the time of menstruation. Fibroadenomas are believed to be hormonally sensitive and can increase in size or become more symptomatic at the time of menstruation or with hormonal changes associated with pregnancy or the use of oral contraception. They usually become less symptomatic with age and often calcify in postmenopausal women. A US is a useful diagnostic test for these lesions because they are more commonly diagnosed in younger women, and US-guided biopsy can confirm the diagnosis. These can be observed and followed if small and asymptomatic, but larger symptomatic lesions usually warrant excision, especially when more than 3 cm in diameter. Furthermore, if the lesion enlarges rapidly or if there is any suspicious pathologic condition associated with the fibroadenoma such as increased cellularity of the lesion, excision is warranted to exclude a more aggressive variant of a fibroepithelial lesion known as a *phyllodes tumor*. Phyllodes tumors can be locally aggressive and recurrent and require wide local excision. Of course, as with any growing palpable mass, excision also is warranted to ensure that a breast cancer was not misdiagnosed. In addition, studies have demonstrated that in addition to the traditional surgical resection, cryoablation is also a safe and effective primary therapy for selected breast fibroadenomas with durable results that can be reproduced in community practices. In summary, indications for resection include size greater than 3 cm, increasing size, pain associated with the lesion, increased cellularity on biopsy, or anxiety resulting from the presence of the mass.

BREAST CYSTS

Breast cysts also are a palpable abnormality or a cause of breast pain. The physical examination usually reveals benign findings of a lesion with well-circumscribed borders similar to a benign solid breast mass. US is a useful tool for diagnosis of a breast cyst. Cysts that are well circumscribed without septations or debris and are thin walled are referred to as *simple cysts*. An asymptomatic simple cyst with classic benign imaging features does not require intervention other than reassurance. If symptomatic, these can be observed or aspirated in the office using US or palpation guidance. However, we do not recommend aspiration for simple cysts. If the cyst aspirate is bloody in nature, it should be sent to the cytopathology laboratory to rule out possible malignant disease. If there are septations and the cyst is thought to be more complex with potentially a solid component or thick wall, then short interval follow-up or tissue biopsy is warranted. This can be done with US-guided core biopsy with a clip left in place to mark the location in the event that an excisional biopsy is warranted in the future.

BREAST PAIN

Breast pain remains a challenge to breast surgeons because the cause is not always clear and the symptoms can present along a spectrum from vague pain to debilitating pain. It also may be difficult to ascertain if there is an associated disorder contributing to the mastalgia, such as underlying bone disease, costochondritis, or fibromyalgia, all of which can contribute greatly to the sensation of mastalgia.

It is important to establish a timeline for the patient's symptoms, alleviating and aggravating factors, and associated symptoms and whether it is cyclic. The history should determine if the pain affects both breasts or if the symptoms are unilateral. Breast pain can be hormonally driven with escalation of symptoms during reproductive years or at the time of menses. Hormonally driven mastalgia also may be associated with fibrocystic breast disease. If cyclic, it tends to be bilateral and diffuse and often improves after the onset of menses. Noncyclic pain has no relation to the menstrual cycle, and therefore the patient does not experience the relief from breast pain at the start of menses. The most common causes of noncyclic breast pain include cysts, fibroadenomas, and chest wall syndromes such as costochondritis.

Breast pain may resolve on its own with little intervention. Conservative measures are often helpful, which include well-fitted, appropriately sized supportive bras, warm compresses, and dietary modifications to reduce high fat intake and lower caffeine intake. Nonsteroidal anti-inflammatory agents are very useful for persistent pain. Vitamin E, fish oil, and evening primrose oil may be helpful to women who have mastalgia. Topical nonsteroidal anti-inflammatory drugs are also a consideration for persistent, severe breast pain. In addition, in a meta-analysis of randomized trials that compared bromocriptine, danazol, evening primrose oil, and tamoxifen with placebo, it was concluded that tamoxifen should be the drug of choice, providing significant relief from mastalgia with the least side effects. It is important to realize that at times no further treatment is necessary other than reassurance and helping to reduce patient anxiety by explaining that breast pain is not a typical sign of breast cancer.

NIPPLE DISCHARGE

Nipple discharge is another common presenting complaint that can be worrisome to the patient. Benign physiologic nipple discharge is present in many women and often can be induced from several ducts by nipple manipulation and typically does not warrant any further evaluation. Nipple discharge that is spontaneous, recurrent, unilateral, and involving a single duct requires further diagnostic evaluation and on occasion surgical intervention. If pathologic discharge is present, it is useful to begin with diagnostic mammography and US. Cytology and occult blood testing of nipple discharge is often insufficient for accurate diagnosis and is misleading with low diagnostic yield. If a specific lesion is identified on imaging, then it warrants tissue biopsy for diagnosis. In some cases a ductogram is a useful diagnostic study. The fluid-producing duct is cannulated, and contrast material is injected. This is followed by a mammogram attempting to identify filling defects within the duct. The advantage of a ductogram is identification of lesions that are a greater distance from the nipple than would normally be excised by a resection of retroareolar tissue. If mammography and US fail to identify suspicious abnormalities, then an excisional biopsy of the duct in question is warranted. Cannulation of the offending duct with a lacrimal probe is often helpful. The other option would be subareolar ductal exploration with duct ligation and excision. It is important to discuss with the patient that she may be unable to breastfeed after this procedure. Nipple discharge is most commonly a result of benign intraductal lesions, specifically papillomas, duct ectasia, and fibrocystic breast disease, and it does not necessarily imply the presence of a malignancy. Of course, although rare, some patients have physiologic nipple discharge from hyperprolactinemia such as can occur with a primary pituitary tumor, hypothyroidism, or medication. Patients may experience copious, bilateral milky discharge, which typically is expressed from multiple ducts. No breast surgical intervention is required, and these patients should be referred to an endocrinologist for further evaluation.

In summary, a suspicious nipple discharge is unilateral and spontaneous, comes from a single duct, and is bloody or clear. These discharges require further evaluation because they may be the result of malignancy. However, even with these findings, the majority are benign.

BREAST INFECTION

Breast infections are more common in premenopausal women and those who are lactating. These infections are often very painful and demonstrate systemic symptoms such as fever, malaise, and leukocytosis. Mastitis in a lactating female often is caused by skin flora such as *Staphylococcus* infection. They respond to oral antibiotics and conservative measures, such as application of warm compresses, if diagnosed promptly. Lactating women should be encouraged to continue breastfeeding and ensure that the breast is emptied with each feeding. However, many women are seen later in the infection with fluctuant abscesses that require surgical incision and drainage. This can be very painful, and it is recommended to perform drainage procedures in the operating room with sedation if possible, especially for larger abscesses. Given the acidic environment of the abscess cavity, it is often difficult to attain adequate local anesthesia, which would significantly affect the ability to thoroughly drain the cavity. A US is useful to detect the true extent of the abscess cavity and for evaluation of recurrent abscesses because these may be caused by undrained pockets or retained debris that may require more formal débridement to prevent recurrence. It is important to send the exudate for Gram stain and culture to help direct antibiotic therapy. US also can be a useful therapeutic modality if the breast infection is caught in early stages of development with a free-flowing collection. US can be used to aspirate abscess cavities that have not organized into multiloculated collections, which are harder to drain completely. This conservative strategy in combination with antibiotic therapy may help to prevent the need for operative intervention. It is important, however, to document resolution of the cavity after the aspiration and to ensure that there are no residual cavity or undrained loculations, which would predispose to recurrent infection.

Breast infections in nonlactating women generally are caused by bacteria introduced through the nipple. These infections are typically retroareolar and sometimes recurrent and are managed with antibiotics and drainage if necessary as described earlier. Granulomatous mastitis (GM) is a rare chronic inflammatory breast disease with unclear cause. The patients often have a painful mass that often is associated with fistulas, abscesses, and inflammatory changes. The clinical presentation and radiologic findings of GM are similar to those of breast cancer; therefore diagnostic workup with biopsy often is warranted. A variety of treatments have been proposed, ranging from surgical excision, incision and drainage, antibiotics, steroids, prolactin-lowering medications, and observation with reassurance to the patient that the condition will resolve. With all treatment options, the time to resolution is usually several months, and recurrences are common. It is paramount to ensure inflammatory breast cancer is considered in the differential diagnosis from mastitis. Patients with mastitis should show some improvement in symptoms quickly with the initiation of treatment. If the symptoms are not improving with antibiotics, then biopsy of any underlying abnormality should be pursued. Inflammatory breast cancer always should be suspected in a nonlactating, postmenopausal woman without any precipitating factors or systemic signs of infection.

ABNORMAL SCREENING MAMMOGRAMS

As technology continues to improve with better mammographic imaging many women may be identified as having suspicious findings on mammography. These may include new microcalcifications, densities, architectural distortions, or developing masses. These mammographic abnormalities typically are not appreciated on clinical breast examination, and the patient is asymptomatic. In these cases, an image-guided biopsy is required to establish the diagnosis and rule out a malignancy. Often the findings are benign and warrant no additional intervention such as the finding of usual duct hyperplasia. On occasion, biopsy may demonstrate a benign but

indeterminate result. In these cases additional tissue is required to rule out a coexisting malignancy, which can occur in 10% to 15% of cases. Those women with these indeterminate lesions should have an excisional biopsy with needle localization performed. An excisional biopsy typically is recommended for patients found to have atypical ductal hyperplasia (ADH), atypical lobular hyperplasia (ALH), papillomas, or sclerosing adenosis with radial scar. Similarly, patients should have an excisional biopsy if they are identified as having lobular carcinoma in situ (LCIS), which is considered a marker for increased risk of developing breast cancer but not an early noninvasive breast cancer like its counterpart ductal carcinoma in situ (DCIS). The purpose of the excisional biopsy in all of these cases is to decrease the risk of sampling error. Although the biopsy specimen is considered benign, these women should be offered high-risk screening with the goal of early detection of any subsequent malignancies. These women also should be offered antiestrogen therapies for risk reduction. For patients with DCIS, the National Comprehensive Cancer Network (NCCN) guidelines recommend antiestrogen treatment for those with estrogen receptor (ER)–positive tumors, whereas for patients with ADH, ALH, or LCIS, the antiestrogen risk reduction therapy is recommended regardless of ER status. Some women do refuse to undergo excisional biopsy after image-guided biopsy with the previously mentioned findings. There have been studies showing that if a mammotome biopsy is performed instead of a core biopsy, in concert with an experienced and/or expert breast pathologist, then observation can be considered given that there is more tissue available for pathologic assessment and patients did not experience adverse outcomes. However, the standard of care is recommendation of excisional biopsy.

■ SUMMARY

Patients with benign breast problems commonly see surgeons for evaluation. The main goal is to establish the presence of a benign condition with appropriate history and physical examination, imaging, and, when necessary, biopsy. This also will help to ensure that the patients are not misdiagnosed, resulting in missed breast cancers, including inflammatory breast cancer, which masquerades as mastitis. Once the diagnosis is confirmed to be benign, then the decision regarding surgery is individualized to the patient according to the presence of symptoms amenable to surgical intervention. Patients will require scheduled follow-up to ensure that no interval problems develop. Those with benign biopsy results who pose an increased risk for the development of breast cancer in the future should be screened appropriately for breast cancer. Patient education and reassurance are vital.

SUGGESTED READINGS

Amin AL, Purdy AC, Mattingly JD, et al. Benign breast diseases. *Surg Clin North Am.* 2013;93:299-308.

Flynn GB, Tipton C. An algorithm for managing breast pain. *Clin Advisor.* 2011;47-54.

Pearlman M, Griffin J. Benign breast disease. *Obstet Gynecol.* 2010;116: 747-758.

Sheybani F, Sarvghad M, Naderi HR, et al. Treatment for and clinical characteristics of granulomatous mastitis. *Obstet Gynecol.* 2015;125:801-807.

Srivastava A, Mansel RE, Arvind N, et al. Evidence-based management of mastalgia: a meta-analysis of randomised trials. *Breast.* 2007;16:503-512.

SCREENING FOR BREAST CANCER

Megan Winner, MD, and Julie R. Lange, MD, ScM

Breast cancer is the most common noncutaneous malignancy diagnosed in women and in 2014 accounted for more than one in four new cancer cases and was the second most common cause of cancer death. In 1989 the American Cancer Society (ACS), the National Cancer Institute, and nine other organizations joined to issue a uniform set of guidelines for breast cancer screening; later, these organizations would add guidelines for screening of women at high to moderate risk. More recently, based on accumulated evidence from long-term follow-up of randomized controlled trials and observational studies of population-based screening, several organizations have published revisions, in some cases diverging significantly from prior recommendations and contemporary guidelines from other societies. This has been driven by a trend of placing a greater emphasis on estimating harm from screening and recognizing the interplay between published recommendations and an individual woman's values, preferences, and informed decision making.

In this chapter we review the advantages and limitations of screening modalities used to identify early breast cancer in asymptomatic women. This includes women without a personal history of breast cancer, a confirmed or suspected genetic mutation known to increase risk of breast cancer, or a history of previous radiotherapy to the chest at a young age. We then review the recommendations for screening generated by government-sponsored groups, medical societies, and coalitions in the United States.

■ SCREENING MODALITIES

There is more scientific evidence regarding screening for breast cancer than for any other cancer. As with all cancers, screening practices for breast cancer should be based on evidence regarding the prevalence of disease in the screened population, the effectiveness of the screening procedure, and any attendant harm, including the risks and costs associated with the screening test and any additional tests and procedures that follow a positive screen. In breast cancer, this translates into debates about who should be screened, at what age, and with what method. As more data have emerged regarding the frequency and consequences of false-positive test results (leading to unnecessary biopsy procedures) and overdiagnosis (i.e., the diagnosis of low-grade, nonaggressive tumors that likely would not have an impact on a person's life), and as breast cancer treatment becomes more effective, the trade-off between benefits and harm of screening have shifted.

Breast Palpation

Breast Self-Examination

Breast self-examination (BSE) once was advocated as an integral part of screening for breast cancer, and women were instructed routinely in BSE technique. However, large randomized trials have failed to show a reduction in breast cancer–specific or all-cause mortality from regular BSE in populations at average risk. As a consequence, BSE is deemphasized or absent in newer versions of screening guidelines. We share the opinion still held by many, however, that BSE has value. Some breast cancers are mammographically occult or develop between screening imaging. Some cancers are, first identified by a patient's self-examination and sometimes not in the setting of a

directed breast examination. Finally, teaching BSE and encouraging patients' familiarity with their self-examinations may assist in the detection or interpretation of more subtle findings on palpation and can help bring changes to clinical attention. The limitation of using BSE as a screening tool is the increased number of biopsies performed for benign breast disease, which comes at a financial and emotional cost.

Clinical Breast Examination

Because several randomized controlled screening trials included both clinical breast examination (CBE) and mammography, the contribution of CBE to the early detection of breast cancer is unclear. That said, 10% to 20% of breast cancers are not visible on screening mammography, and CBE performed by trained personnel has been shown to increase breast cancer detection over mammography alone. One limitation of CBE is that effectiveness depends on technique and time spent on the examination, and it is difficult to standardize. Another limitation is the expense of clinician availability and time, and of the high false-positive rate; there may be as many as 55 false-positive screens for each additional cancer detected by CBE. CBE remains an important screening tool globally, in places where mammography is not available but has become less emphasized in U.S. screening guidelines. We find it provides an important clinical opportunity to discuss breast health, to instruct patients on BSE technique, and to review findings with them that should prompt a clinical visit and clinical breast examination.

Mammography

Mammography is the primary imaging modality for the early detection of breast cancer among asymptomatic women because it is the only method of breast imaging that consistently has been found to decrease breast cancer-related mortality. Screening mammograms provide two views of each breast: the mediolateral oblique projection images the breast from an oblique medial to lateral approach, and the craniocaudal projection images the breast from a superior to inferior view. The use of two views allows physicians to localize an abnormality to a particular quadrant within the breast and increases the sensitivity of mammography. The mammography interpretation always is appended by an American College of Radiology Breast Imaging, Reporting, and Data System (BI-RADS) classification (Table 1). The BI-RADS categories classify mammographic findings by level of suspicion that the finding represents cancer. Each category is associated with guidelines for patient management to aid clinicians in their decision making about the need for a subsequent biopsy and follow-up recommendations. Screening mammograms are performed without a radiologist present, and suspicious findings are never classified as representing malignancy but prompt a call back for a diagnostic mammogram, which is performed with a radiologist present, who can decide whether additional spot- or magnification-views are necessary to interpret the positive finding on screening mammography. Diagnostic mammography (which is more expensive than screening mammography) should be the first test ordered in the cases of a palpable abnormality.

Nine randomized-controlled trials, including more than 650,000 asymptomatic, average-risk women have been conducted on screening mammography and have reported data on mortality. With long-term follow-up, pooled results from these studies found a 20% relative risk (RR) reduction for breast cancer mortality in women invited to screening as compared with controls, with the benefit most pronounced in older age groups (60 to 69 years). Pooled estimates from observational studies have demonstrated an even greater effect. The magnitude of these estimates is influenced by a number of factors, including whether they are based on invitation or exposure to screening and on the heterogeneity of the studied populations. Estimates of the number needed to invite (NNI) or number needed

TABLE 1: Breast Imaging-Reporting and Data System (BI-RADS) Classification

Category		Management	Likelihood of Cancer in the Mammographic Finding
0	Need additional imaging or prior examinations	Recall for additional imaging and/or await prior examinations	
1	Negative	Routine screening	
2	Benign	Routine screening	Essentially 0
3	Probably benign	Short interval follow-up (6 months)	>0 but ≤2%
4	Suspicious	Tissue diagnosis	4a. Low suspicion for malignancy (>2% to ≤10%) 4b. Moderate suspicion for malignancy (>10% to ≤50%) 4c. High suspicion for malignancy (>50% to <95%)
5	Highly suggestive of malignancy	Tissue diagnosis	≥95%
6	Known, biopsy-proven malignancy	Surgical excision when clinically appropriate	

to screen (NNS) to prevent a breast cancer death—increasingly cited as meaningful measures of benefit by organizations drafting guidelines—depends heavily on the RR reduction applied in the modeling, the underlying risk of mortality in the modeled population, and the duration of projected follow-up. As a result, they can be disparate (more information about NNI and NNS calculations can be found in the ACS and the United States Preventive Services Task Force guidelines). Further complicating interpretation of existing evidence is that most of the trials and observational studies were performed in the 1990s, before significant advances in the adjuvant treatment of breast cancer, and with the use of film mammography. Although the majority of breast cancers in the United States are in fact diagnosed as a result of an abnormal screening study, and death rates from breast cancer in the United States have decreased by 30% since the 1990s, it is estimated that approximately one third of that effect is due to screening, with the rest attributable to treatment advances.

There are several limitations specific to mammography as a screening tool. First is that mammography uses radiation, which is itself carcinogenic, although models suggest that the radiation risk from mammography is low enough to result in a net benefit from screening with respect to lives saved. Another limitation is that of overdiagnosis: the detection of disease by screening that would not have become clinically important in a woman's lifetime, including ductal carcinoma in situ (which may not progress to invasive cancer), a slow-growing cancer, or one that regresses. Results from randomized trials and cohort studies consistently demonstrate a higher rate of cancer diagnosed in a population screened by mammography versus an unscreened population, despite a long follow-up. Depending on method of estimation and definition (e.g., whether ductal carcinoma in situ is included as an event), estimates for overdiagnosis—and thus overtreatment—of breast cancer resulting from mammography range from less than 10% to more than 30%. Not unique to mammography but central to the controversy surrounding screening recommendations is the risk of false-positive screening tests, which result in additional imaging and procedures, potentially even surgical excision, all for a benign condition. False-positive screening tests are more common in younger women because mammography is less specific in this population and because cancer is less common.

Breast Density

The density of breast tissue reflects the relative amount of fibrous and glandular tissue in relation to fat and is important because mammographic sensitivity is lower in dense breasts. In addition,

there is suggestion that breast density is an independent risk factor for breast cancer. This importance tends to be overestimated in studies that compare women with the highest density to those with the lowest density, resulting in an estimated fourfold to sixfold increase in risk. With use of average breast density as a reference point, the risk among women with heterogeneously dense breasts is 1.2 times as great as the average, and with extremely dense breasts, 2.1 times as great. This is equivalent to the elevated risk of breast cancer associated with having a first-degree relative with unilateral, postmenopausal breast cancer. Breast density does not appear to be associated with increased mortality from breast cancer. It is not clear at this time whether breast density represents a modifiable risk factor for cancer, whether screening recommendations should be altered for women with dense breasts, or how women who have dense breasts should be counseled. Because breast density influences cancer risk and the performance of mammography as a screening tool, the American College of Radiology includes classification of breast density as a mandatory component of mammographic interpretation. In a development that some feel is premature, there also have been laws passed in 22 states mandating that women found to have dense breasts on mammography be notified in writing of the finding and be encouraged to consider additional testing. These policies have attracted criticism because there are no data that additional testing in women with dense breasts is effective in preventing breast cancer death and because they do not address insurance coverage for and reimbursement issues surrounding additional screening tests.

Digital Mammography

All of the randomized controlled trials addressing the effectiveness of screening used film mammography, and there is no direct evidence that digital mammography reduces breast cancer-related deaths. Nevertheless digital mammography has replaced film as the primary screening modality in the United States. In addition to facilitating remote reading and more efficient storage, the real advantage of digital image collection over film systems is higher contrast resolution and the ability to postprocess the image to enlarge it or change contrast and brightness, helping radiologists to more easily detect subtle abnormalities, particularly in a background of dense breast tissue. Most studies that have compared the performance of digital and film mammography have found little difference in cancer detection rates. There is a suggestion of an increase in detection of invasive cancer in premenopausal and perimenopausal women and in women with dense breasts but also an increase in false-positive findings.

Tomosynthesis

Tomosynthesis (or three-dimensional [3D] digital mammography) is a rapidly emerging technology that involves the acquisition of multiple images of the breast recorded at different angles while the detector is held stationary, providing the radiologist with a series of thin-slice (0.05-mm) images through the breast. There are limited data available as to the benefits and harm of tomosynthesis as a primary screening modality. Early data suggest that tomosynthesis may reduce the recall rates for false-positive tests and may increase the cancer detection rates over two-dimensional (2D) digital mammography; however, it is not clear whether these additional cancers detected would have become clinically significant (i.e., whether they represent over diagnosis). The disadvantages associated with tomosynthesis are that it exposes the woman to twice the amount of radiation of 2D digital mammography and generally is performed *in addition to* a 2D digital mammographic screening test. In 2013 the U.S. Department of Agriculture (USDA) approved a method to generate conventional 2D images from a 3D acquisition, obviating the need for double-screening tests. Tomosynthesis also is associated with a higher cost; however, this is common for most new technologies and there is usually some reduction in the incremental cost increase if and when a new technology moves in to the mainstream.

Magnetic Resonance Imaging

Nearly all invasive breast cancers are visible on gadolinium contrast-enhanced MRI, and the reported sensitivity of MRI is between 88% and 100%. Unfortunately, benign lesions can also enhance on MRI, and low specificity currently limits MRI as a screening tool. However, specificity can be improved somewhat by alterations in technique, and it is possible that overall specificity may continue to improve as technology advances. The positive predictive value of any test is enhanced as the prevalence of disease rises, and it follows that MRI would have higher utility in patients at higher relative risk for breast cancer. Indeed, the efficacy of MRI as a screening tool in patients at high risk has been validated in multiple studies. In 2007 the ACS recommended annual screening MRI as a supplement to screening mammography for women with high risk for breast cancer, based either on a known *BRCA* mutation, a first-degree relative of a known *BRCA* mutation carrier, or a predicted lifetime risk of 20% to 25% or greater according to risk modeling. On the basis of expert consensus opinion, the National Comprehensive Cancer Network (NCCN) also recommended annual MRI screening for those individuals who received radiation to the chest between the ages of 10 and 30 years; those with Li-Fraumeni, Cowden, or Bannayan-Riley-Ruvalcaba syndromes, and their first-degree relatives. Data are still insufficient for recommendation for or against MRI screening for individuals with a lifetime risk of 15% to 20%, those with lobular carcinoma in situ (LCIS), atypical ductal or lobular hyperplasia (ADH or ALH), and dense breast on mammography, and those with a personal diagnosis of breast cancer, including ductal carcinoma in situ. The downsides to MRI include the significant cost of the test, as well as discomfort on the part of the patient, which may be a limiting factor in a not-insignificant subpopulation.

Other Technologies and Adjuncts to Screening

Whole-Breast Ultrasound

Ultrasound scan is used primarily in diagnostic evaluation of abnormal findings on mammography, clinical examination, or MRI. Focused breast ultrasound scan characterizes palpable or screening-detected lesions and can be used to perform an image-guided needle biopsy of sonographically visible lesions. The role of whole-breast screening ultrasound scan was evaluated by the American College of Radiology Imaging Network National Breast Ultrasound Trial (ACRIN 6666). After screening 2809 women at very high risk, only 4 cancers per 1000 women were detected with ultrasound scan alone.

Considering the downside of ultrasound scan, including the increased numbers of false-positive findings, the length of time that it takes to perform, and its user-dependent variability, ultrasound is not currently a routinely useful screening tool.

Molecular Breast Imaging

Because screening mammography is recognized to have decreased sensitivity in women with denser breasts, several techniques are being considered that may supplement screening in this population, including molecular breast imaging (MBI). MBI is based on the observed preferential uptake of a radiopharmaceutical (such as ^{99m}Tc-sestamibi) in tumors relative to normal tissue, which is independent of breast density. In the setting of a single-institution prospective trial, the addition of MBI to screening mammogram increased the number of breast cancers identified by 7.5 per 1000 screened among a population with mammographically dense breasts. Although the addition of MBI increased the overall financial costs and the benign biopsy rate, the cost per detection of breast cancer was lower than with screening mammography alone. Currently there is not enough evidence to support MBI as a breast cancer screening tool, but it remains under investigation as a method that may mitigate limitations of mammography in women with dense breasts.

■ SCREENING GUIDELINES

The recommendations from the ACS, the U.S. Preventive Services Task Force (USPSTF), and the NCCN for asymptomatic women who do not have a pre-existing breast cancer or a previously diagnosed high-risk breast lesion and who are not high risk for breast cancer because of a known underlying genetic mutation or a history of chest radiation at a young age are summarized in Table 2.

Initial screening recommendations from the U.S. Preventive Services Task Force (USPSTF; http://www.uspreventiveservicestaskforce.org/Page/Document/UpdateSummaryFinal/breast-cancer-screening) included annual mammography starting at the age of 40; however, recent analyses of data pooled from screening trials have suggested that for women between the ages of 40 and 49, the elevated risk of false-positive results and the lower risk of breast cancer in this population translates into a low marginal benefit for screening. Specifically, in their recommendations, the USPSTF estimates that 1904 women ages 39 to 49 would need to be screened to prevent one death from breast cancer after at least 11 years of observation, compared with 1339 women in their 50s, and 377 women in their 60s. Additional analyses suggested that annual vs. biennial mammography did not carry a survival advantage. Thus in their 2009 update, the USPSTF raised the age at which they recommended initiating mammographic screening from 40 to 50, and revised their recommendations to include screening mammograms only every 2 years for women between the ages of 50 and 74 years of age. Critics of this decision pointed out that the false-positive rate and number needed to prevent a breast cancer death were not substantially different between women in their 40s and women in their 50s and that the decision to alter screening recommendations at that age cutoff was somewhat arbitrary. Moreover, it did not provide patients with the knowledge necessary to contribute to the decision. The USPSTF released a draft update to the 2009 recommendations for public comment in May of 2015, (http://www.uspreventiveservicestaskforce.org/Page/Document/RecommendationStatementDraft/breast-cancer-screening1). The draft softens the language of the recommendations surrounding screening among women 40 to 49, stating that the decision to perform mammography in this group should be an individual one based on considerations of the risks and benefits of screening in this population, and notes that women ages 40 to 49 with a first-degree relative with breast cancer may benefit potentially more than average-risk women in this age group.

The USPSTF feels that there is not enough evidence to support a mortality benefit in women ages 75 years and older and that

TABLE 2: Screening Guidelines for Asymptomatic Women of Average Risk for Invasive Breast Cancer From the ACS, the Current USPSTF, and the NCCN

	ACS	USPSTF	NCCN
≥25 but <40			CBE every 1-3 years (≥25 but <40) Breast awareness
40-44	Women should have the opportunity to begin annual screening between the ages of 40 and 44 years.*	The decision to start regular, biennial screening mammography before the age of 50 years should be an individual one and take patient context into account, including the patient's values regarding specific benefit and harm.	Annual CBE Annual screening mammogram Breast awareness
45-50	Women should undergo regular screening mammography beginning at age 45 years.† Screening should be annual.*		
51-54	Women should undergo regular screening mammography.† Screening should be annual.*	Biennial screening mammography Current evidence is insufficient to assess the additional benefit and harm of CBE beyond screening mammography	Annual clinical breast examination Annual screening mammogram Breast awareness
55-74	Women age 55 and older should transition to biennial screening or have the opportunity to continue screening annually.* Women should continue screening mammography as long as their overall health is good and they have a life expectancy of 10 years or longer.		
≥75		Current evidence is insufficient to assess the benefit and harm of screening in this age group.	Annual clinical breast examination Annual screening mammogram Breast awareness The upper age limit for screening is not yet established; consider life expectancy and whether therapeutic interventions are planned.
All women	CBE is not recommended for breast cancer screening among average-risk women at any age.* All women should become familiar with the potential benefits, limitations, and harm associated with breast cancer screening.	The USPSTF recommends against teaching BSE.	Women should be counseled regarding potential benefits, risks, and limitations of breast screening. Women should be familiar with their breasts and promptly report changes to their healthcare provider.

The USPSTF recommendations are currently under review for revision.

*Qualified Recommendation; qualified recommendations indicate that there is clear evidence of benefit of screening but less certainty about the balance of benefits and harms, or about patients' values and preferences, which could lead to different decisions.

†Strong recommendation; a strong recommendation conveys the consensus that the benefits of adherence to that intervention outweigh the undesirable effects that may result from screening.

ACS, American Cancer Society; *BSE*, breast self-examination; *CBE*, clinical breast examination; *NCCN*, National Cancer Comprehensive Network; *USPTSF*, United States Preventive Services Task Force.

screening decisions should be individualized in this group, a recommendation that was not changed in the 2015 draft. Furthermore, the USPSTF recommends against teaching breast self-examination and finds the evidence insufficient to make recommendations regarding clinical breast examination, language that remains in the 2015 draft version.

The American Cancer Society (ACS) recommendations for breast cancer screening are maintained on the ACS website (http://www.cancer.org/healthy/informationforhealthcareprofessionals/acsguidelines/breastcancerscreeningguidelines/index). The recommendations were updated in October of 2015 from earlier guidelines published in 2003. The major departure is that BSE and CBE,

TABLE 3: National Comprehensive Cancer Network and American Cancer Society Guidelines for Women With Elevated Risk for Breast Cancer

NCCN	Prior history of breast cancer	History and physical examination 1-4 times per year as clinically appropriate for 5 years after diagnosis, then annually Annual screening mammography starting at diagnosis
	5-year risk* ≥1.7% in women ≥35 years of age according to the Gail model	Annual screening mammogram and CBE every 6-12 months
	History of LCIS of ADH/ALH	Annual screening mammogram and CBE every 6-12 months, consider annual MRI Beginning at diagnosis but not earlier than age 30
	Lifetime risk* >20% according to models largely dependent on family history (e.g., Claus, BRCAPRO, BOADICEA, Tyrer-Cuzick)	Annual screening mammogram and CBE every 6-12 months, recommend annual MRI Beginning 10 years before youngest family member but not earlier than age 30 Referral to genetic counseling
	Prior thoracic RT (e.g., mantle irradiation) between ages 10 and 30 years old.	Age <25: annual CBE to start 8-10 years after RT Age ≥25: Annual screening mammogram and CBE every 6-12 months, recommend annual MRI Begin 8-10 years after RT
	Pedigree suggestive of or known genetic predisposition	Refer for genetic counseling; genetic testing as appropriate Screening recommendations depend on the cancer syndrome identified†
ACS‡	*BRCA* mutation First-degree relative of *BRCA* carrier but untested Lifetime risk ~20% or 25% of greater, as defined by BRCAPRO or other models that largely depend on family history	Annual MRI screening (based on evidence from nonrandomized screening trials and observational studies)
	Radiation to chest between ages 10 and 30 years Li-Fraumeni syndrome and first-degree relatives Cowden and Bannayan-Riley-Ruvalcaba syndrome and first-degree relatives	Annual MRI (based on expert consensus opinion)

*Of invasive breast cancer.

†See National Comprehensive Cancer Network. Genetic/familial high risk assessment: breast and ovarian (Version 2.2015). http://www.nccn.org/professionals/physician_gls/pdf/genetics_screening.pdf. Accessed August 29, 2015.

‡The ACS states that women at increased risk of breast cancer may benefit from additional screening strategies beyond those offered to women of average risk, such as earlier initiation of screening, shorter screening intervals, or the addition of screening modalities other than mammography and physical examination, such as ultrasound or magnetic resonance imaging, but that the evidence currently available is insufficient to justify recommendations for any of these screening approaches.

ADH, Atypical ductal hyperplasia; *ALH,* atypical lobular hyperplasia; *CBE,* clinical breast examination; *MRI,* magnetic resonance imaging; *RT,* radiation therapy.

previously suggested for all women starting at the age of 20, were eliminated from the recommendations entirely. The recommended age to start mammography also was raised, echoing changes in the USPSTF recommendations published in 2009. The reasoning for this change was the same, based on an analysis of the risks of false positives and overdiagnosis versus the small incremental benefits with respect to preventing breast cancer deaths in a relatively low-prevalence age group. Whereas previous recommendations suggested annual mammography start at the age of 40, the current expression qualifies this recommendation as a choice, and one that should be made with consideration of risks and benefits of screening. Strong recommendation for annual mammography starts at the age of 45

years. This decision was based on (1) clear data regarding the benefits of screening mammography in women between the ages of 50 and 75 and (2) the observation that the incidence of breast cancer and proportion of incident breast cancers in women 45 to 49 more closely resembled the 50 to 54 group than did the 40 to 44 group. Annual screening mammography should continue while a woman's life expectancy is at least 10 years, with the option to transition to biennial screening at the age of 55. There is no age after which the ACS recommends halting screening for breast cancer.

Concerns surrounding these new guidelines echoed some of the criticisms of the USPSTF guidelines, including the fact that the recommendations of the USPSTF and ACS focus primarily on the outcome of breast cancer lives saved. Other outcomes that may be important to patients were sparsely (if at all) addressed, and some may say undervalued. These include quality of life, although the ACS found the quality of evidence regarding the effect of screening on quality-adjusted life years to be too low to incorporate this outcome into their screening recommendations, and the stage at which a breast cancer is diagnosed, which may influence a woman's options for breast-conserving therapy. These issues and questions as to the magnitude of overdiagnosis that results from screening continue to pose a challenge to providing complete and accurate information to women about what to expect from breast cancer screening.

As of July 2015, the screening guidelines of the NCCN still recommends CBE every 1 to 3 years and states that women of all ages should be familiar with their breasts and promptly report changes to their healthcare provider. Annual screening mammogram begins at the age of 40 and is accompanied by annual CBE. The NCCN does not support an upper age limit for screening but does note that comorbidity, life expectancy, and the expectation that a positive examination finding would be followed by invasive treatment be incorporated into decision making in this age group. These recommendations are classified as evidence-level 2A, "based on lower-level evidence, [and] there is uniform NCCN consensus that the intervention is appropriate."

Many other organizations have issued recommendations about mammography screening of asymptomatic women not known to be at increased risk for breast cancer. The American College of Physicians recommends that clinicians should inform women ages 40 to 49 years about the potential benefits and harm of screening mammography and that screening decisions should be based on individualized assessment of risk for breast cancer and the benefits and harm of screening in this age group. They also should incorporate the woman's preferences and breast cancer risk profile. The American Congress of Obstetricians and Gynecologists recommends that mammography screening be offered annually to women beginning at age 40 years. The American College of Radiology and the Society for Breast Imaging, in a joint recommendation, advise screening continue until life expectancy is less than 5 to 7 years or when abnormal results of screening would not be acted on because of age or comorbid conditions. The Canadian Task Force on Preventive Health Care recommends routine screening mammography every 2 to 3 years in women ages 50 to 74 years and recommends against screening women ages 40 to 49 years.

Screening in High-Risk Individuals

Several national medical organizations have developed guidelines and recommendations for screening women at high risk. *BRCA1* or *BRCA2* mutation carriers are at the highest risk: 37% to 87% will be diagnosed with an invasive breast cancer by the age of 70. Women who have had a prior diagnosis of breast cancer or of atypical ductal or lobular hyperplasia or LCIS are also considered higher than average risk, as are women with a family history suggestive of familial breast and/or ovarian cancer, or a first-degree relative who has tested positive for a breast cancer–associated genetic mutation. Having received mantle cell irradiation between the ages of 10 and 30 years

of age qualifies a woman for a high-risk screening approach. Finally, special screening schedules apply to those women who are calculated to have an elevated lifetime risk of being diagnosed with invasive cancer according to a risk prediction model. A variety of models are available to predict risk, of which the most widely used is the Gail model, based on age, number of first-degree relatives with breast cancer, age of menarche, age of first live birth, number of previous biopsies (including presence of atypia), and race or ethnicity. The Claus model includes a more comprehensive family history. The BRCAPRO model is based on personal history and family history data, including breast and ovarian cancer and Jewish ancestry, and the BOA-DICEA model includes family history of prostate and pancreatic cancer in addition to breast and ovarian cancer family history. Finally, the Tyrer-Cuzick model incorporates family history and gynecologic history.

Table 3 contains a summary of screening recommendations based on high-risk category. Whereas NCCN guidelines are specific with respect to the age and modality of screening recommended, the ACS has only published guidelines for screening with MRI as an adjunct to mammography (see Table 3). In general, annual screening mammography is recommended for women of appropriately high risk beginning at 30 years, supplemental screening with breast MRI is recommended for a subset with very high risk, and screening ultrasound scan is recommended for women in whom MRI is unavailable. The results of a recent study with computer-simulated modeling concluded that annual MRI at age 25 years, alternating every 6 months with digital mammography beginning at age 30 years, may be the most effective screening strategy for mutation carriers.

SUGGESTED READINGS

Berg WA, Blume JD, Cormack JB, et al. Combined screening with ultrasound and mammography versus mammography alone in women at elevated risk of breast cancer. *JAMA*. 2008;299:2151-2163.

D'Orsi CJ, Newell MS. On the frontier of screening for breast cancer. *Semin Oncol*. 2011;38:119-127.

Independent UK Panel on Breast Cancer Screening. The benefits and harms of breast cancer screening: an independent review. *Lancet*. 2012;380:1778-1786.

Kerlikowske K, Hubbard RA, Miglioretti DL, et al. Comparative effectiveness of digital versus film-screen mammography in community practice in the United States: a cohort study. *Ann Intern Med*. 2011;155:493-502.

Lee CH, Dershaw DD, Kopans D, et al. Breast cancer screening with imaging: recommendations from the Society of Breast Imaging and the ACR on the use of mammography, breast MRI, breast ultrasound, and other technologies for the detection of clinically occult breast cancer. *J Am Coll Radiol*. 2010;7:18-27.

Miller AB, Wall C, Baines CJ, et al. Twenty five year follow-up for breast cancer incidence and mortality of the Canadian National Breast Screening Study: randomised screening trial. *BMJ*. 2014;348:g366.

Oeffinger KC, Fontman ETH, Etzioni R, et al. Breast cancer screening for women at average risk: 2015 guideline update from the American Cancer Society. *JAMA*. 2015;314:1599-1614.

US Preventive Task Force. Screening for breast cancer: US Preventive Services Task Force recommendation statement. *Ann Intern Med*. 2009;151:716-726.

THE ROLE OF STEREOTACTIC BREAST BIOPSY IN THE MANAGEMENT OF BREAST DISEASE

Catherine Parker, MD, Heidi Umphrey, MD, and Kirby Bland, MD

Breast cancer is the most frequently diagnosed non-skin cancer in women in the United States, and one in eight women will have breast cancer within her lifetime. It was estimated that there would be 231,840 new cases of and 40,290 deaths from breast cancer (women only) in the United States in 2015. Early and accurate detection of breast cancer is important for optimizing treatment and decreasing mortality. Screening mammography has improved early breast cancer detection drastically, as early-stage cancer is often nonpalpable and clinically occult. The stereotactic core biopsy technique offers a number of advantages compared with surgical excision. This chapter reviews the indications, technique, contraindications, and pathologic correlation of stereotactic breast biopsy.

HISTORY

Screening mammography detects nonpalpable abnormalities; however, a majority of these lesions are benign in nature. It is estimated that 1.6 million breast biopsies are performed each year in the United States. Historically, the only method for obtaining the breast tissue necessary for histopathologic diagnosis was surgical excision. However, the development of stereotactic biopsy offers a less invasive approach for mammographic-detected lesions without sonographic correlate. Stereotactic breast biopsy uses radiologic imaging to perform and guide the biopsy needle. The stereotactic method was developed by a neurosurgeon in 1908, but it was not until the late 1980s that Dr. Kambiz Dowlat introduced stereotactic breast biopsy technology to the United States. As breast biopsy tools became more advanced with spring-loaded and later vacuum-assisted core devices, the image-guided biopsy approach has become predominate for initial tissue diagnosis. This minimally invasive method offers a number of advantages, such as the need for only local anesthetic and a small incision with less scarring, surgery avoidance for benign lesions, and reliable identification of malignancies to facilitate a single definitive cancer operation that is cost effective. Today, image-guided percutaneous biopsy is the preferred method of diagnosis over surgical excision based on National Comprehensive Cancer Network (NCCN) guidelines, is endorsed by the American Society of Breast Surgeons (ASBS), and is a quality measure for National Accreditation Program for Breast Centers (NAPBC).

ACCURACY AND RISK

Stereotactic breast biopsy achieves an accuracy that makes it an acceptable alternative to surgical excision. A number of studies have analyzed the concordance with surgical biopsy, with results ranging from 91% to 98%. The false-negative rate of stereotactic percutaneous core biopsy also has been investigated and reportedly ranges from 11.8% to 28.6%. The most common cause of a false-negative result is inaccurate tissue sampling. Accurate tissue sampling is dependent on the lesion position, size, mobility, and type, as well as the size and density of the breast, operator experience, and patient compliance. For stereotactic core biopsy, diagnostic sensitivity is improved by increasing the number of cores taken to six or more. Accuracy of stereotactic core biopsy also can be increased with a larger needle size and the use of vacuum-assisted devices. The procedure is relatively safe. The risk of bleeding, hematoma, or infection at the biopsy site is rare (<1%).

INDICATIONS

As with any procedure, an understanding of which lesions are appropriate is crucial. A complete diagnostic workup is indicated. If a screening mammogram is abnormal, a woman should undergo a diagnostic mammogram, which consists of additional views of the suspicious area. Comparison with previous mammograms also assists in determining the role that breast biopsy may play. These additional steps assist with ruling out summation artifact caused by overlapping structures.

The American College of Radiology (ACR) Breast Imaging-Reporting and Data System (BI-RADS) developed a classification for mammograms in order to standardize reporting and interpretation and to facilitate outcome monitoring. Screening mammography may detect a finding that requires additional workup (BI-RADS assessment category 0) (Figure 1). A final assessment category based on the degree of suspicion for malignancy is assigned after a complete diagnostic workup. There are five BI-RADS categories: (1) negative, (2) benign finding, (3) probably benign finding, (4) suspicious, and (5) highly suggestive of malignancy. Lesions assigned BI-RADS 3, probably benign, typically undergo close follow-up with 6-month mammography; however, depending on clinical suspicion, patient anxiety, or physician preference, these cases may be referred for biopsy. BI-RADS 4 and 5 lesions require histologic sampling to rule out malignancy (Figure 2). A biopsy of suspicious lesions visible on both mammogram and ultrasound typically is performed under ultrasound guidance because this method is more easily tolerated by the patient, does not require exposure to additional radiation, is less costly, and often is readily accessible. Mammographic lesions occult on ultrasound most commonly are calcifications but also may include masses, developing asymmetries, and architectural distortion that may require stereotactic biopsy (Box 1).

PATIENT SELECTION

A thorough history and physical examination is warranted before performing a stereotactic core breast biopsy. Personal history of prior breast biopsies or breast surgeries, breast cancer risk factors, and family history of breast or ovarian cancer are important. The patient's allergies to local anesthetics, epinephrine, latex, or tape need to be determined in order to take necessary precautions. The patient's medical history and medication list also must be reviewed. To minimize bleeding, it is preferred that patients on anticoagulation and antiplatelet therapy either stop or adjust their medication before the biopsy in coordination with their treating physician, if possible. However, patients who must continue these therapies still may undergo a stereotactic biopsy, with some studies indicating a slight increase in bruising.

LIMITATIONS AND CONTRAINDICATIONS

A co-operative patient is imperative to performing a successful stereotactic biopsy. The procedure requires the patient to be immobile as the breast remains in compression for approximately 30 minutes. Therefore any physical limitations of the patient, such as movement disorders, limited range of motion, kyphosis, or weight, must be considered. Other important considerations include patient's breast size, compressed thickness of breast, and lesion depth and location. For example, there may not be enough breast tissue to compress to safely perform the biopsy without the needle penetrating through to the other side of the breast. On the other hand, if the breast is too large and the lesion is deep, using a stereotactic biopsy needle may not be technically feasible. If the lesion is too close to the nipple, superficial to the skin, or posterior near the chest wall or a breast implant, stereotactic biopsy may be contraindicated (Box 2). Stereotactic core biopsy also is not indicated in pregnant women.

■ TECHNIQUE

Stereotactic devices differ by imaging modality (analog vs digital), calculation of coordinates (manual or digital), and patient positioning (sitting or prone).

Patient Preparation

One of the most common causes of an unsuccessful stereotactic core biopsy is the patient's inability to tolerate the procedure. Anxiety

---

BOX 1: Indications for Stereotactic Core Biopsy

Certain probably benign lesions, BI-RADS 3, depending on clinical suspicion, patient or physician preference, or when short-term follow-up is not practical

Lesions suspicious, BI-RADS 4

Lesions highly suspicious, BI-RADS 5

New suspicious microcalcifications, developing asymmetries, or architectural distortions

Nonpalpable asymmetry, focal asymmetry, or solid mass on mammogram not seen on ultrasound

Mammographic lesions corresponding to suspicious areas of enhancement on MRI

BI-RADS, Breast Imaging-Reporting and Data System; *MRI*, magnetic resonance imaging.

BOX 2: Contraindications to Stereotactic Core Biopsy

Patient unable to lie prone or co-operate

Patient's weight

Lesion location near nipple, too superficial to skin, or too posterior to chest wall

Lesion mammographically occult

Patient has severe kyphosis or movement disorders

Lack of breast tissue thickness for adequate compression

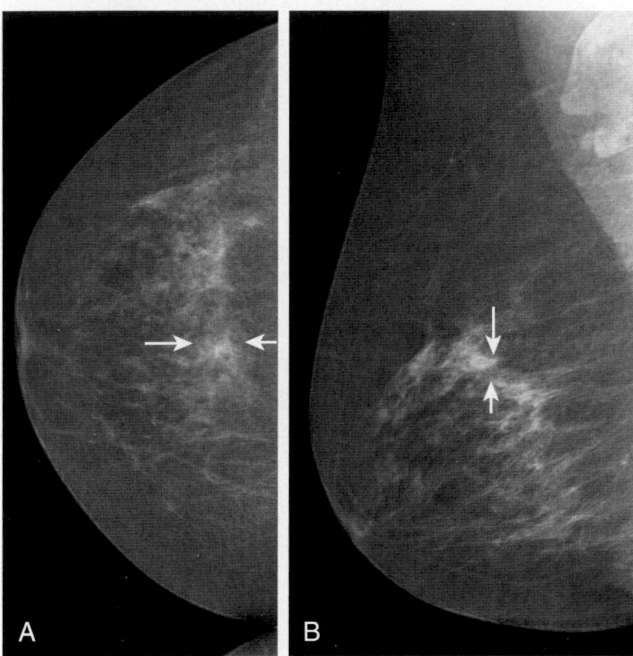

FIGURE 1 Screening mammogram (right craniocaudal view **[A]** and right mediolateral oblique view **[B]**) demonstrates fine pleomorphic calcifications (*arrows*) in a grouped distribution, Breast Imaging-Reporting and Data System (BI-RADS) 0, requiring additional evaluation.

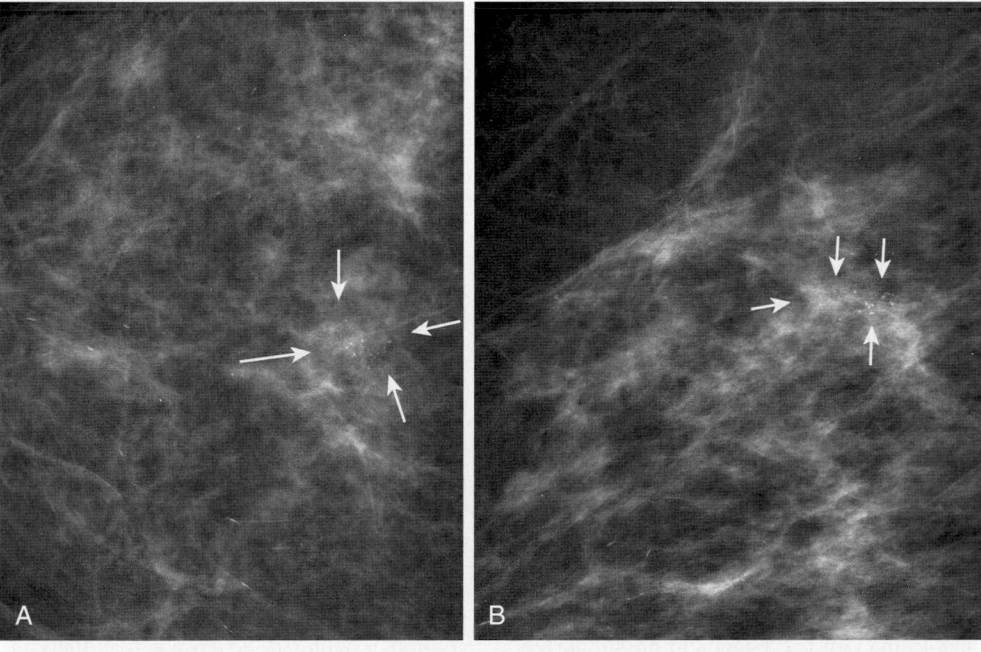

FIGURE 2 Right magnification mammogram views (craniocaudal **[A]** and lateral **[B]**)—reveal fine pleomorphic calcifications in a grouped distribution suspicious for malignancy, Breast Imaging-Reporting and Data System (BI-RADS) 4, requiring stereotactic biopsy for tissue diagnosis.

and vasovagal reactions are reported most commonly. Antianxiety medication given before the procedure may assist with patient co-operation. Also, it is important to ensure adequate pain control with local anesthesia for patient comfort and technical success.

Equipment

Stereotactic biopsy can be performed either prone with a traditional stereotactic biopsy table or upright with an add-on stereotactic biopsy unit that attaches to the standard mammography equipment. There are advantages and disadvantages to both systems. If a patient is wheelchair bound or obese, the traditional prone table may not be ideal. However, wheelchair-bound patients may be elevated on a stretcher and rolled onto the table, if this can be done safely. Otherwise, the biopsy must be performed with the add-on unit. The advantages of the prone position are that the patient is unable to view the needle, there is less patient anxiety resulting in less motion, and there is more room for the physician and technologist to maneuver because they can work under the table when the patient is prone. When an add-on unit is used, the patient can visualize the needle, which can result in more anxiety and motion. However, the advantage of the add-on unit is that the resolution and quality of the images acquired are similar to diagnostic workup.

Biopsy Needles

With the development of automatic, spring-loaded biopsy guns, stereotactic core biopsies became widely used. These devices use a double-action needle composed of an inner trocar with a sample notch and an outer cutting cannula. The needle is advanced rapidly into the breast when fired, sampling a core of tissue. Only one core of tissue is obtained and the sample must be removed from the needle each time the gun is fired, which requires multiple needle insertions into the breast. Therefore the standard for stereotactic biopsy is now the vacuum-assisted biopsy (VAB) needle devices. These are preferred and offer a number of advantages over spring-loaded biopsy guns. The vacuum-assisted devices can obtain multiple specimens in a 360-degree fashion, require only one needle insertion, and provide larger specimens. The needles are powered by a suction device and have a rotating cutter. The automated biopsy guns usually have 14- to 18-guage needles, whereas the VAB guns have 7- to 11-gauge needles.

Technique and Lesion Targeting

Once the patient is positioned and the device is chosen, another important part of a successful procedure is determining the needle's approach to the lesion. The ideal approach is the shortest distance from skin to targeted lesion. The breast is compressed, with the skin entrance exposed through an opening in the paddle. A scout view is obtained, and after the target is identified two additional images are obtained 30 degrees apart, at +15 degrees and −15 degrees. The basis of stereotactic localization is the principle of parallax, which is used to locate the lesion in the three dimensional (3D) breast from a pair of two-dimensional (2D) images. The scout view provides the x (horizontal) and y (vertical) coordinates of the lesion to be targeted in the breast. The two additional images are then used to determine depth (z coordinate). The amount of breast tissue compressed is important and, depending on the equipment used, must be at least 5 mm greater than the stroke of the needle (distance of fire). In addition, a positive stroke margin (distance from post-fire needle tip to image receptor plate) of 5 mm or more is suggested to avoid penetration of the image receptor plate and damage to the patient's skin (Figure 3). Once the lesion coordinates are calculated and confirmed, the skin is cleansed, local anesthetic is injected, and a small skin incision is made. The needle of the biopsy device is then introduced into the breast just proximal to the targeted lesion, and pre-fire images are obtained to confirm position (Figure 4). The needle is fired and then post-fire images are obtained to confirm position (Figures 5

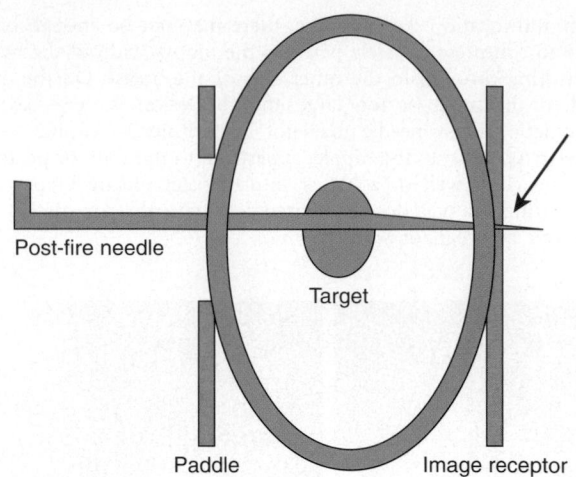

FIGURE 3 This figure demonstrates the possible consequences of a negative stroke margin, with skin and image receptor penetration by needle. The arrow denotes the negative stroke margin.

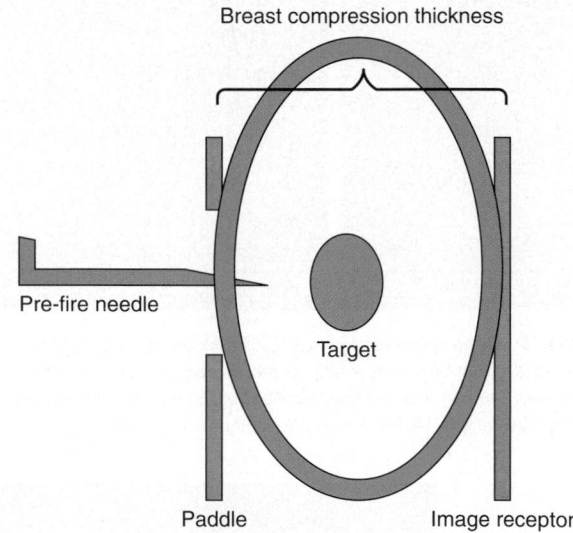

FIGURE 4 This figure demonstrates successful pre-fire positioning to target the lesion, with the needle near the lesion.

and 6). Then, when the VAB device is used, tissue sampling is performed in a 360-degree fashion.

Postprocedure: Core Specimen Handling, Imaging, and Patient Care

To ensure adequate sampling, a specimen radiograph is obtained of the histologic samples collected during core biopsy to document targeted lesion retrieval (Figure 7), especially microcalcifications. It is also the practice of certain centers to mark with ink the cores containing calcifications or to separate those cores with calcifications for submission to the pathology laboratory to assist the pathologists. The specimen cores are then preserved in formalin for histologic evaluation.

After the specimen cores have been retrieved, a postbiopsy marker (clip) should be placed at the biopsy site. This marker not only facilitates mammographic surveillance but also serves as a guide if surgical excision is required. To ensure that the clip is deployed at the biopsy site, a postprocedure mammogram should be performed; clip migration can occur in up to 20% of cases (Figure 8).

After the procedure, hemostasis is achieved with manual compression. Then the skin incision is closed, generally with thin adhesive strips. After the postprocedure mammogram is performed, a compression bandage and an ice pack may be used at the biopsy site.

■ OVERCOMING TECHNICAL CHALLENGES

Patient positioning is important for technical success. Therefore using pillows, cushions, or soothing music as necessary to ensure patient comfort, as well as engaging the patient in conversation for distraction, can be helpful. In the situation of a thin breast, different maneuvers may be used to allow for biopsy to be performed safely—for example, breast bolstering to increase the thickness of the compressed breast or use of the "double-paddle" approach, in which another biopsy paddle is placed in front of the image plate to allow the breast tissue to bulge anteriorly and posteriorly. Superficial lesions still may be accessed with a smaller biopsy aperture to avoid cutting the skin or a skin protection device. The lesion also can be pushed away from the skin by the expansion of subcutaneous tissue through injection of local anesthetic. The use of the "lateral arm" also can assist with accessing difficult lesions and allows for imaging to be performed through one approach while the biopsy needle is introduced parallel to the compression paddle. The technique of "arm through the hole" allows for full access to the posterior or upper breast, ensuring that this arm is well supported. Understanding that varying approaches may allow better access is important; for example, a lesion close to the chest wall is best visualized

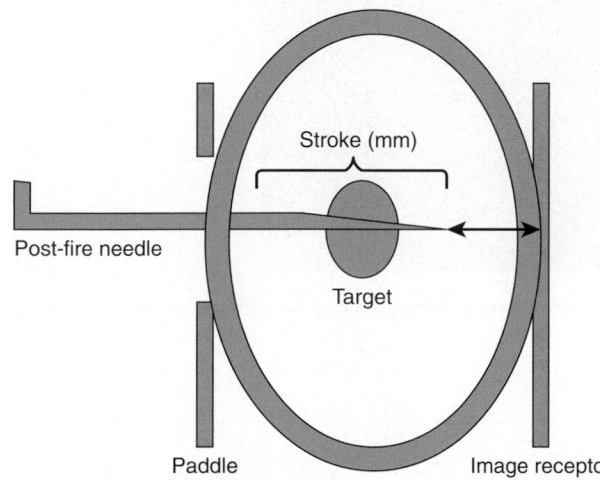

FIGURE 5 This figure demonstrates successful post-fire positioning to target the lesion, with the needle through the lesion. The distance traveled by the needle during the fire is the stroke (mm) and includes the needle aperture and needle tip (*bracket*). The stroke margin is the distance (mm) from the tip of the post-fire needle to the image receptor indicated by the double arrow.

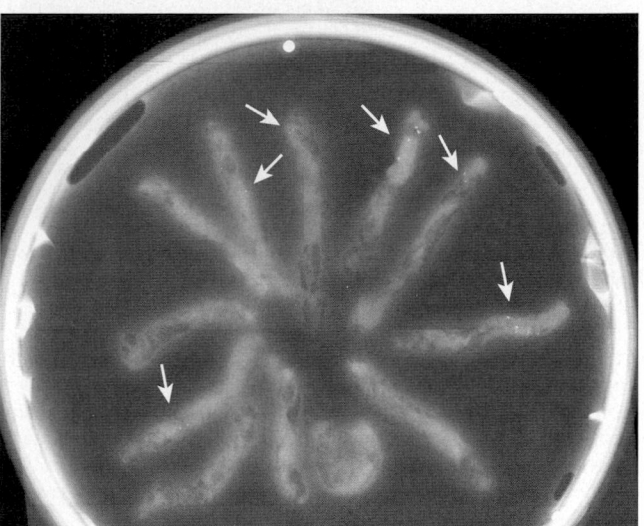

FIGURE 7 Specimen radiograph demonstrates successful retrieval of targeted calcifications (*arrows*).

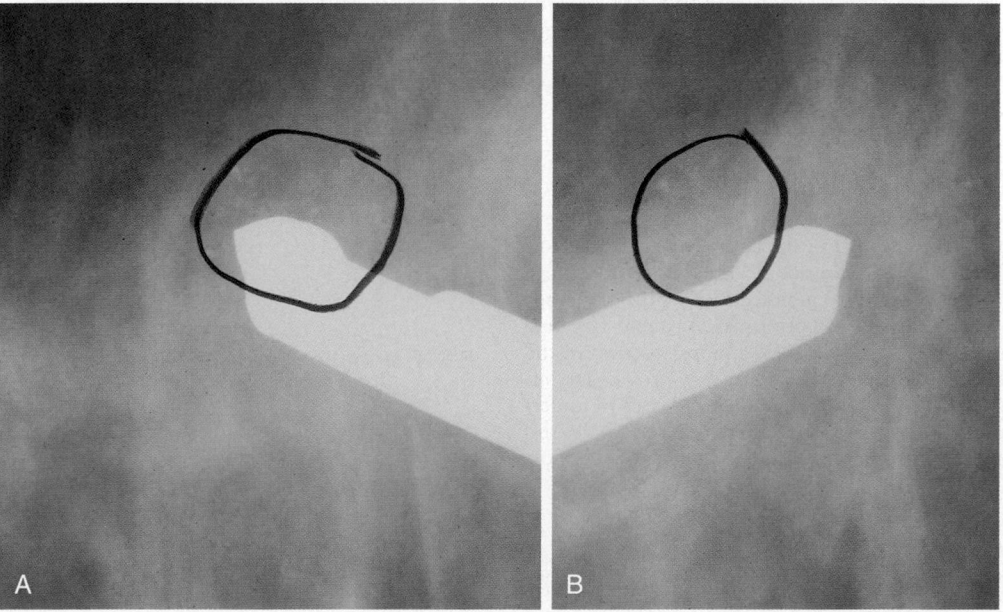

FIGURE 6 Post-fire stereo pair (+15 degrees **[A]** and −15 degrees **[B]**) shows optimal positioning with successful targeting of the suspicious fine pleomorphic calcifications (*circled*).

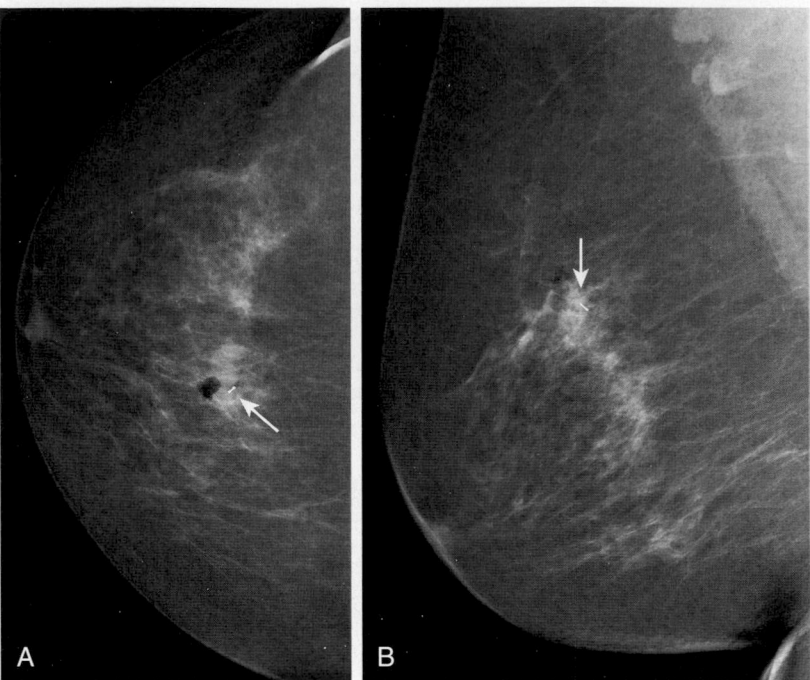

FIGURE 8 Right craniocaudal **(A)** and lateral **(B)** mammographic views obtained postprocedure demonstrate successful stereotactic biopsy of the right 12:00 suspicious calcifications and clip placement.

with mediolateral oblique (MLO) and lateral (LAT) views. On the other hand, in the setting of faint calcifications, the image will be improved if the lesion is closer to the image receptor. Therefore faint calcifications in the 6:00 position are best seen with a craniocaudal (CC) approach. To decrease radiation dose, calcifications initially may be identified with skin marking in a routine view in patients with faint calcifications or larger breasts.

▪ PATHOLOGIC CORRELATION

An important part of performing a biopsy is correlating the patho-logic findings with the radiologic findings that prompted the procedure. The pathologic findings should correlate with imaging findings; in other words, there should be radiology-pathology con-cordance (Figure 9). However, when pathologic findings do not cor-relate with imaging, there is discordance and excision is recommended. If, for example, the imaging has numerous calcifications but the pathology report lacks calcifications and indicates only benign breast tissue, the quality of the biopsy is suspect. If calcifications were noted in the specimen radiograph, the pathology blocks should be imaged to determine if calcifications remain unsampled in the block, prompting additional levels being cut for pathology review. Tissue also may be reviewed with polarization to determine if calcium oxalate is present. If no calcifications are identified by the pathology report, excisional biopsy should be performed. Accurate targeting and adequate tissue sampling are crucial for a biopsy procedure and can help to decrease discordance. A core biopsy may provide incom-plete characterization of the histologic findings and lead to under-estimation of the presence of disease. Therefore certain lesions require surgical excision in order to exclude a higher-grade lesion, malignancy (Box 3).

▪ CERTIFICATION

Whether surgeons or radiologists perform stereotactic biopsies, cer-tification is necessary to ensure standardization of care. Certification establishes the capability of the physician as well as the safety of the equipment. The ASBS has developed one of the most commonly used

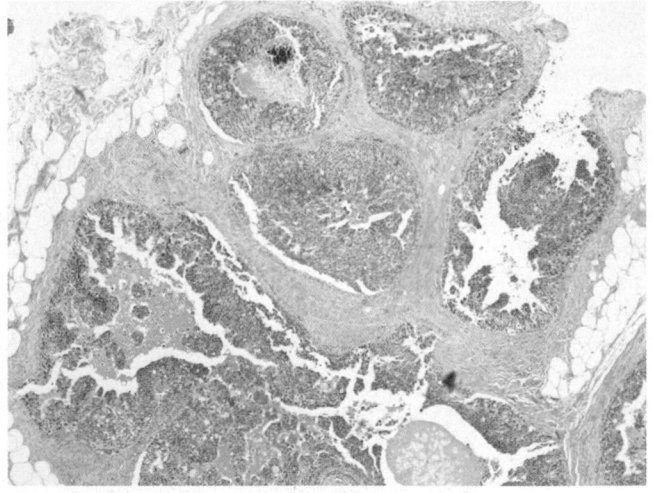

FIGURE 9 Ductal carcinoma in situ (DCIS), high nuclear grade with necrosis, is concordant with imaging findings.

BOX 3: Indications for Surgical Excision After Stereotactic Core Biopsy

---

Imaging findings and pathologic findings do not correlate (discordance)
Atypical ductal hyperplasia
Atypical lobular hyperplasia
Radical scar, complex sclerosing lesion
Papillary lesions
Cellular fibroepithelial lesions and Phyllodes tumors
Lobular carcinoma in situ
Mucocele-like lesions

certification programs. The process for successful certification includes prerequisites with a clinical application followed by a written and practical examination. The ACR has a stereotactic biopsy accreditation program as well.

CONCLUSIONS AND FUTURE DIRECTIONS

Percutaneous image-guided biopsy has emerged as the standard of care for initial diagnosis of breast lesions and is cost effective. Avoiding surgical excision by using less invasive diagnostic approaches for lesions found to be benign and adopting a coordinated approach to

malignant lesions are essential for excellent patient care. A multidisciplinary approach involving surgery, radiology, and pathology is an important part of management, especially with high-risk and malignant lesions.

SUGGESTED READINGS

Elmore JG, Longton GM, Carney PA, et al. Diagnostic concordance among pathologists interpreting breast biopsy specimens. *JAMA.* 2015;313:1122-1132. doi:10.1001/jama.2015.1405

Huang ML, Adrada BE, Candelaria R, et al. Stereotactic breast biopsy: pitfalls and pearls. *Tech Vasc Interv Radiol.* 2014;17:32-39. doi:10.1053/j.tvir.2013.12.006

MOLECULAR TARGETS IN BREAST CANCER

Catherine Parker, MD, Helen Krontiras, MD, and Marshall Urist, MD

Breast cancer is the most frequently diagnosed non–skin cancer in women. Although its name is based on a single tissue of origin, this cancer is heterogeneous with a multitude of presentations and prognoses. Advances in laboratory technology have expanded our knowledge of tumor biology. Understanding molecular profiling, breast cancer subtypes, and targeted drug therapies is key to providing personalized breast cancer care. This chapter focuses on the discovery of breast cancer subtypes, molecular targets, and the clinical relevance to surgeons.

MOLECULAR PROFILING

For many years, breast cancer heterogeneity was defined in terms of anatomic staging (American Joint Committee on Cancer [AJCC] tumor node metastasis [TNM]) and histologic appearances (ductal vs lobular, grade, lymphovascular invasion, etc.). These tumor characteristics were used to provide prognostic information on treatment response, risk of recurrence, and survival. Through advancements in technology and understanding of genetics, even more useful information is found at the molecular level.

In 2000 Perou and colleagues were the first to describe intrinsic breast cancer portraits, which are molecular classifications based on microarrays and hierarchal cluster analysis. Understanding these subtypes is crucial to the surgeon's management of breast cancer. The four major molecular portraits are (1) estrogen receptor (ER) positive; (2) basal-like; (3) human epidermal growth factor receptor–2 (HER2) enriched; and (4) normal-like. There are two subtypes of ER-positive tumors, luminal A and luminal B. Because complete molecular profiling is not feasible on individual patients, immunohistochemically defined surrogates were developed, and these generally are comparable with the genomic profile (Table 1).

LUMINAL SUBTYPES

The luminal subtypes account for approximately two thirds of all breast cancers and are generally low grade with a favorable prognosis. The term *luminal* is derived from the similar molecular expression of these tumors in comparison with the luminal epithelium of normal breast tissue. The two main ER-positive subtypes, luminal A

and luminal B, have different gene expressions, prognoses, and treatment responses.

Luminal A breast cancers typically have high expression levels of ER and therefore the best response rate to endocrine therapy. These are the most common subtype (40%) and have the best overall prognosis compared with the other breast cancer subtypes. Luminal B breast cancers are less common (20%) and have a worse prognosis in comparison with luminal A tumors. However, luminal B tumors still have a superior prognosis to basal-like and HER2-enriched tumors. Luminal B tumors have a higher grade, lower levels of ER, and higher expression of the proliferation cluster (Ki-67) in comparison with luminal A tumors. Luminal B tumors have a lower response to endocrine therapy but have an improved response rate to chemotherapy versus luminal A tumors.

Estrogen Receptor Signaling Pathways

In 1896 Beaston first reported the regression of advanced breast cancer by removing the ovaries in premenopausal patients with this disease. At that time it was also observed that not all breast cancers regressed with oophorectomy. In the 1970s, when the estrogen receptor was first described by Jensen, it was confirmed that not all breast cancers contain the estrogen receptor.

The ER is a member of the steroid hormone receptor superfamily and is a ligand-dependent transcription factor. It is composed of two receptors, the estrogen alpha receptor (ER-α) and the estrogen beta receptor (ER-β), both of which bind with high affinity to the ligand estrogen. When estrogen binds to the receptor, this results in dimerization and facilitates interaction of the receptor with promoter regions in the DNA.

In clinical practice, the assays used to define ER expression measure ER-α levels, referred to as the "classic ER." ER positivity is measured quantitatively with immunohistochemistry (IHC). About 65% of ER-positive tumors are also progesterone receptor (PR) positive. The level of expression of ER is used to predict response to endocrine therapy. Approximately 70% of ER/PR-positive breast cancers respond to endocrine therapy. A small percentage of breast cancers are ER negative/PR positive, and some of these tumors have shown a response with endocrine therapy, suggesting downstream endocrine pathway activation.

Endocrine therapy is administered with either selective estrogen receptor modulators (SERMs) or aromatase inhibitors (AIs) (Table 2). SERMs are competitive ER antagonists in breast tissue but act as partial agonists in other tissues. The most common and widely used SERM for breast cancer treatment is tamoxifen, which was introduced in 1977. Tamoxifen competitively inhibits the binding of estradiol to estrogen receptors in the breast but has agonist activity in endometrial tissue.

TABLE 1: Breast Cancer Intrinsic Subtypes

Subtype	Characteristics	Markers
Luminal A	Low grade High ER ~40% of all breast cancer Good prognosis	ER+, PR+, HER2– Low Ki-67 (<14%)
Luminal B	Higher grade Lower ER ~20% of all breast cancer Poorer prognosis than luminal A	ER+, PR+/–, HER2+/– High Ki-67 (>14%)
HER2-enriched	High grade Often node positive *P53* mutations ~10%-15% of all breast cancer	ER–, PR–, HER2+
Basal-like	High proliferation *BRCA* dysfunction ~15%-20% of all breast cancer Poor prognosis	ER–, PR–, HER2– CK5/6 Or EGFR+

CK, Cytokeratin; *EGFR*, epidermal growth factor receptor; *ER*, estrogen receptor; *HER2*, human epidermal growth factor receptor–2; *PR*, progesterone receptor.

TABLE 2: Treatment According to Breast Cancer Subtype

Subtype	Treatment Response and Prognosis
Luminal A	Respond to endocrine therapy • Premenopausal: SERMs (tamoxifen) • Postmenopausal: AIs (exemestane, anastrozole, letrozole)
Luminal B	Response to endocrine therapy lower Response to chemotherapy greater than luminal A
HER2-enriched	Respond to anti-HER2 agents (trastuzumab, pertuzumab, lapatinib)
Basal-like	No response to endocrine therapy or anti-HER2 agents Chemotherapy only treatment outside of a clinical trial

AIs, Aromatase inhibitors; *HER2*, human epidermal growth factor receptor–2; *SERMs*, selective estrogen receptor modulators.

Tamoxifen reduces the risk of breast cancer recurrence and death in premenopausal and postmenopausal women with ER-positive tumors. A number of landmark trials have investigated the safety and efficacy of tamoxifen in the adjuvant setting. The Early Breast Cancer Trialists' Collaborative Group meta-analysis included 10,645 patients from randomized trials and found that tamoxifen reduced the 15-year probability of breast cancer recurrence and breast cancer mortality. These results led to establishing the current standard of care: 5 years of adjuvant tamoxifen in premenopausal women with ER-positive breast cancers.

In 1982 the National Surgical Adjuvant Breast and Bowel Project (NSAPB B-14) performed a randomized, double-blind, placebo-controlled trial in 2800 patients with primary operable, ER-positive, and lymph node–negative breast cancer to determine the effectiveness of adjuvant tamoxifen therapy. Disease-free survival was prolonged significantly through 10 years of follow-up in women treated with tamoxifen (69%) versus placebo (57%). There was also a 37% relative reduction in the cumulative incidence of a second primary breast cancer in the contralateral breast at 10 years of follow-up, 3.8% for tamoxifen-treated patients versus 6.1% for those on placebo ($P = 0.007$).

Tamoxifen is an oral drug taken daily (20 mg) with side effects commonly including hot flashes and vaginal dryness or discharge. The rare but more severe side effects include thromboembolic events and development of endometrial cancer.

Because AIs work by a different mechanism of action than SERMs, they are indicated only for postmenopausal patients with ER-positive tumors. AIs block the conversion of adrenally synthesized androgens to estrogen, the final step in steroid conversion to the active form of the hormone. AIs do not interfere with the production of corticosteroids or mineralocorticoids. Estrogen production in the ovary is not suppressed; therefore AIs are indicated only for postmenopausal women. The AIs currently approved in the clinical setting include exemestane, anastrozole, and letrozole.

AIs are superior to tamoxifen for postmenopausal women because of improved effectiveness and a lower toxicity profile. Prospective randomized trials show that the risk of local recurrence is reduced and disease-free survival is improved with AIs compared with tamoxifen. The ATAC (Arimidex, Tamoxifen, Alone or in Combination) trial studied ER-positive breast cancers in postmenopausal women by comparing anastrozole with tamoxifen, alone or in combination. The trial evaluated 9366 postmenopausal women with localized breast cancer. Anastrozole significantly prolonged disease-free survival and time to recurrence, in addition to reduced distant metastases and contralateral breast cancers. Almost all patients completed their scheduled treatment, with fewer withdrawals from anastrozole than tamoxifen. Anastrozole was associated with fewer gynecologic and vascular events, but myalgia, arthralgia, and fractures were more common.

Extended Adjuvant Hormone Therapy

ER-positive breast cancers can have late recurrences (20 years or more after diagnosis) even after adjuvant endocrine therapy. Several studies have investigated and shown value in extending endocrine therapy from 5 to 10 years. Ongoing trials are analyzing the impact of an initial 5 years of tamoxifen or an AI followed by another 5 years of an AI, as well as the concept of continuous versus intermittent extended AI therapy. In the ATLAS (Adjuvant Tamoxifen: Longer Against Shorter) trial, 6846 women with ER-positive breast cancer who had completed 5 years of tamoxifen were randomly assigned to either stop tamoxifen or continue tamoxifen for another 5 years. A reduction in breast cancer recurrence and mortality was observed in the group that took tamoxifen for an additional 5 years. Although extended endocrine therapy in ER-positive breast cancers does reduce late recurrences, thus far investigators have been unable to identify a subgroup of high-risk patients who would benefit from extended therapy.

Endocrine Resistance

Although endocrine therapy is the most effective treatment for ER-positive breast cancers, the outcomes are limited by significant rates of both de novo resistance and resistance acquired during treatment. Methods of overcoming endocrine resistance include optimizing the schedule and dose of endocrine therapies, in addition to combining different agents. For example, the SWOG S0226 trial showed anastrozole plus fulvestrant to be superior to anastrozole alone in terms of progression-free survival and overall survival. Another method of addressing endocrine resistance is to understand, identify, and target crosstalk between ER and other signaling pathways, such as HER2, cyclin-dependent kinase (CDK), and phosphatidylinositol 3-kinase (PI3K/AKT)/mammalian target of rapamycin (mTOR). This has now become an important strategy in the setting of stage IV disease. Largely because of results from the BOLERO II phase III clinical trial, the U.S. Food and Drug Administration (FDA) has approved everolimus (mTOR inhibitor) in combination with exemestane for the treatment of ER-positive/HER2-negative women who have recurrence or progression after anastrozole or letrozole therapy.

Addressing Overtreatment

With a greater understanding of tumor biology and molecular signatures, the problem of overtreatment is being addressed. It is generally accepted that women with ER-positive, node-negative breast cancers treated with tamoxifen have a low likelihood of distant recurrence. Prognostic breast cancer tests based on gene expression profiling have been developed and are used in today's clinical setting to select which patients will obtain benefit from chemotherapy.

Genetic expression profile analysis is covered by most insurance carriers. These assays are typically used in ER-positive/HER2-negative, node-negative breast cancers as an adjunct to other prognostic markers. The 21-gene reverse transcriptase–polymerase chain reaction assay, Oncotype Dx (Genomic Health, Redwood City, CA), is performed on formalin-fixed, paraffin-embedded tissue. Paik and colleagues developed this assay with 16 cancer-related genes and 5 reference genes. An individualized risk estimate or recurrence score (RS) of 0 to 100 is provided for each tumor sample: low risk, less than 18; intermediate risk, 18 to 30; and high risk, 31 or greater. A low RS indicates that hormone therapy alone is considered adequate therapy. A high RS indicates a high-risk patient who would benefit from chemotherapy followed by hormonal therapy. Studies have shown that associations of RS with survival are independent from standard clinicopathologic factors. Current National Comprehensive Cancer Network (NCCN) breast cancer guidelines recommend the use of gene expression profiles in patients with ER-positive, node-negative breast cancers to assess the benefits of additional therapy. Trial Assigning IndividuaLized Options for Treatment (Rx) (TAILORx trial) is an ongoing phase III randomized trial of chemotherapy followed by hormonal therapy versus hormonal therapy alone in women with node-negative, ER-positive breast cancer with an Oncotype Dx RS of 11 to 25 (moderate risk). Investigators are also testing the value of the 21-gene assay in ER-positive, node-positive breast cancers. In the ongoing SWOG RxPONDER trial, women with ER-positive/HER2-negative breast cancers with 1 to 3 positive nodes and RS 25 or lower are randomly assigned to chemotherapy followed by hormonal therapy versus hormonal therapy alone.

Another commercially available genomic assay is PAM50 (Prosigna, Seattle, WA), which gives a Prosigna Score (0-100) with formalin-fixed, paraffin-embedded tissue. Prosigna is indicated for use in postmenopausal women with ER-positive, node-negative breast cancers. MammaPrint (Agendia, Amsterdam, Netherlands) is a 70-gene microarray assay performed originally only on freshly collected tissue, now also FDA-approved with formalin-fixed, paraffin-embedded tissue. It gives a low-risk or high-risk result to provide assistance with determining the benefit of adjuvant chemotherapy in selected patients with ER-positive or ER-negative disease.

■ HER2-ENRICHED

HER2-enriched tumors account for only 10% to 15% of all breast cancers. This subtype is characterized by high expression of HER2 and proliferation gene clusters but low expression of the luminal cluster. These tumors are typically HER2 positive and ER/PR negative. A few are also ER positive and included in the luminal B subtype. Before HER2-targeted therapy, this subtype was associated with a poor prognosis.

HER2-Targeted Therapy

Four receptors make up the epidermal growth factor receptor (EGFR) family: HER1 (ERBB1/EGFR), HER2 (ERBB2), HER3 (ERBB3), and HER4 (ERBB4). These receptors are transmembrane proteins, and the best characterized of the EGFR family is HER2. The HER2 gene, also known as *HER2/neu* or *ERBB2*, is a protooncogene located on chromosome 17q21 and encodes a transmembrane protein composed of a ligand-binding extracellular domain, an α-helical transmembrane segment, and an intracellular tyrosine kinase domain. Normally, HER2 is expressed at a low level on the surface of epithelial cells and is necessary for the development of many tissues. However, the amplification or overexpression of HER2 occurs in approximately 10% to 15% of breast cancers. These breast cancers often are associated with high-grade, axillary lymph node involvement and decreased expression of ER and PR, and these characteristics alone lead to increased risk of recurrence and decreased survival. However, HER2 overexpression is also an independent poor prognostic indicator.

Trastuzumab (Herceptin; Genentech, San Francisco, CA) is a recombinant humanized monoclonal antibody directed against the extracellular domain of the HER2 protein. Approved in 1998 for the treatment of metastatic breast cancer, trastuzumab significantly improved patients' outcomes and paved the way for developing targeted approaches in adjuvant breast cancer treatment. Several randomized controlled trials (NSABP B-31, NCCTG N9831, BCIRG 006, FinHer) using trastuzumab as adjuvant therapy have shown significantly improved disease-free and overall survival. As a result, current guidelines for patients with HER2-positive tumors include giving adjuvant trastuzumab with chemotherapy for tumors larger than 1 cm in diameter and node-positive disease. In addition, trastuzumab should be *considered* for patients with tumors between 5 and 10 mm and micrometastatic nodal disease.

Overcoming HER2 Resistance

Primary or acquired resistance to trastuzumab increasingly has been recognized as a major obstacle in the clinical management of HER2-positive breast cancers. Approximately 15% of patients relapse after therapy with trastuzumab. By understanding the mechanism of trastuzumab resistance, new anti-HER2 agents are emerging as treatment alternatives. Lapatinib (oral, reversible, small molecule dual inhibitor of both EGFR [HER1] and HER2 tyrosine kinases) for use in combination with capecitabine in trastuzumab-refractory, HER2-positive, metastatic breast cancers was approved in 2007. Pertuzumab (monoclonal antibody directed at a different site of the HER2 extracellular domain) was approved in 2012 for use in metastatic HER2-positive breast cancers in combination with docetaxel and trastuzumab. However, based on results from the NeoSphere phase II study demonstrating that pertuzumab increased pathologic complete response rate, the FDA subsequently approved the use of pertuzumab in combination with trastuzumab and chemotherapy for early-stage HER2-positive breast cancers in the neoadjuvant setting. Antibody-drug conjugates (T-DM1) consisting of the monoclonal antibody trastuzumab linked to the cytotoxic agent emtansine (DM1) are another emerging type of anti-HER2–targeted therapies. Current trials are investigating dual blockade, the potential synergistic effect of different combinations of both new and approved targeted HER pathway blockers, to determine if chemotherapy may be avoided, as well as the potential of decreasing the standard length of trastuzumab therapy to less than 1 year if benefit is reached with combination drugs.

■ BASAL-LIKE

The basal-like subtype has a gene cluster profile similar to basal epithelial cells and is characterized by low expression of the luminal and HER2 gene clusters. Basal-like breast cancers have a high expression of EGFR and basal epithelial cytokeratins (CK) CK5/6, CK14, and CK17. Typically these tumors are ER, PR, and HER2 negative and are termed triple-negative breast cancer (TNBC). The American Society of Clinical Oncology/College of American Pathologists (ASCO/CAP) guidelines used to define TNBC include lack of ER/PR (<1%) and HER2 expression (0 or 1+) by IHC and confirmation of HER2 status by fluorescent in situ hybridization (FISH) if indeterminate (2+) by IHC. The terms *basal-like subtype* and *TNBC* often are used interchangeably but they are not completely synonymous. For example, 20% of basal-like tumors are not triple negative, and 25% of TNBCs are composed of other mRNA subtypes. TNBC is the clinical surrogate for the basal-like subtype.

TNBC accounts for about 10% to 20% of all breast cancers and is biologically the most aggressive. TNBC more frequently affects younger patients (<40 years) and is more prevalent in African-American women than in other demographic groups. These tumors also tend to be larger, palpable, higher grade, and more often seen as interval cancers (between mammograms). Therefore TNBC is associated with a higher relapse rate and a poorer survival rate than non-TNBC. Distant metastases often occur at visceral sites and are seen within the first 3 years after diagnosis.

Triple-Negative Paradox

Because triple-negative tumors lack estrogen and HER2 expression, targeted therapies are currently unavailable. The standard of care for TNBC is anthracycline and taxane-based combination chemotherapy (see Table 2). Although patients with TNBC have a poor overall prognosis, their primary tumors are more sensitive to chemotherapy (higher pathologic complete response, or pCR) than luminal subtype breast cancers. This is termed the "triple-negative paradox." Although there is no overall survival advantage to receiving neoadjuvant versus adjuvant chemotherapy, it provides a surrogate marker for patients with TNBC who achieve pCR. Approximately, 20% to 45% of TNBCs achieve pCR after anthracycline or anthracycline/taxane-based treatments. Studies investigating the impact of pCR on overall survival in TNBC versus non-TNBC found that if pCR is achieved, patients with TNBC and non-TNBC have similar survival rates. However, TNBC patients with residual disease have a poor outcome, with a higher risk of relapse.

Potential Targets for Triple-Negative Breast Cancer

Though no specific therapies currently exist for TNBC, there is ongoing research to identify potential targets for therapy. The Cancer Genome Atlas (TCGA) network discovered that basal-like breast cancers are more similar to high-grade serous ovarian cancer on the genomic level than to other subtypes of breast cancer. Approximately 20% of basal-like tumors had germline or somatic *BRCA1/BRCA2* mutations, suggesting shared driving events of basal-like breast cancer and serous ovarian cancer. Therefore TNBC lacking functional *BRCA1/BRCA2* might benefit from poly(ADP-ribose) polymerase (PARP) inhibitors (olaparib, iniparib, veliparib). Given the clinical similarities between sporadic TNBC and *BRCA1* mutation–associated breast cancer, it has been suggested that sporadic TNBC also may possess underlying DNA repair defects and demonstrate similar chemosensitivity, resulting in renewed interest in platinum agents.

Triple-Negative Subtypes

Investigators recently have identified six different TNBC subtypes, and these subtypes have been found to be an independent predictor of pCR status. Analysis of distinct gene expression signatures and the results of current clinical trials will assist in the selection of initial neoadjuvant chemotherapy and ongoing treatment for those patients who do not achieve pCR.

■ CONCLUSIONS AND FUTURE DIRECTIONS

Through the discovery of cell receptors and molecular subtypes, we have a better understanding of tumor biology. Breast cancer subtypes provide prognostic information. Gene expression profiling assays in the clinical setting to address overtreatment provide personalized breast cancer care. New therapies are needed to address resistance to current targeted drugs and lack of tailored therapy for TNBC. Surgeons caring for breast cancer patients should be well versed in the importance of tumor subtypes and their impact on treatment.

SELECTED READINGS

Abramson VG, Lehmann BD, Ballinger TJ, Pietenpol JA. Subtyping of triple-negative breast cancer: implications for therapy. *Cancer*. 2015;121:8-16. doi:10.1002/cncr.28914.

Ignatiadis M, Sotiriou C. Luminal breast cancer: from biology to treatment. *Nat Rev Clin Oncol*. 2013;10:494-506.

Moasser MM, Krop IE. The evolving landscape of HER2 targeting in breast cancer. *JAMA Oncol*. Published online July 23, 2015. doi:10.1001/jamaoncol.2015.2286.

BREAST CANCER: SURGICAL THERAPY

David M. Euhus, MD

Breast surgery is the most dramatic component of breast cancer management, but there are no randomized prospective trials demonstrating an impact on survival. The breast surgeon's primary responsibility in the treatment phase of care is ensuring locoregional control. Zeal for avoiding locoregional recurrence must be balanced against the need to preserve physical, sexual, and psychologic health. Attention to final breast contour and symmetry is often important for achieving these goals. Patient preferences should weigh heavily into surgical planning.

Effective radiation and systemic therapies have caused a dramatic decline in locoregional recurrence rates. Breast cancer mortality is declining. Ample clinical trial data support less-intrusive surgical approaches for most breast cancer patients. The breast surgeon is positioned uniquely to help patients understand recent advances in breast cancer treatment as they collaboratively develop intelligent treatment plans essential for restoring health and well-being.

DIAGNOSING BREAST CANCER

Undiagnosed Breast Concerns

Breast cancer should be included in the differential diagnosis for any woman with a region of palpable concern, focal breast pain, skin change, or nipple discharge. Diagnostic imaging, including special mammography views and sonography, is indicated for most breast signs or symptoms. Failure to diagnose breast cancer is one of the most common medical malpractice complaints. The patients are usually under the age of 40, have a self-detected concern, and have normal breast imaging. Lobular cancers, in particular, often are associated with vague palpable findings and normal or indeterminate imaging. It is the breast surgeon's responsibility to persist in the evaluation of any patient concern.

Worrisome skin or nipple changes may need a punch biopsy, whereas palpable and imaging abnormalities should undergo core needle biopsy. Tissue core biopsy has replaced fine-needle aspiration biopsy because it distinguishes in situ from invasive cancer and usually provides ample material for biomarkers. It is preferable to diagnose breast cancer by core biopsy rather than incisional or excisional biopsy when possible. This permits comprehensive management planning and reduces the number of surgical procedures that will be required.

Inflammatory Breast Cancer

Inflammatory breast cancer should be considered in any woman with acute onset of breast swelling, erythema, and skin edema. Mastitis is a more likely diagnosis, especially for pregnant or lactating women, so a 1-week course of antibiotics is a reasonable first step. Failure to improve with antibiotics should prompt diagnostic breast imaging and a punch biopsy of the affected skin. Finding adenocarcinoma in the dermal lymphatics is diagnostic of inflammatory breast cancer in this setting, but a negative skin biopsy does not exclude the diagnosis. The surgeon must persist with additional investigations that could include breast magnetic resonance imaging (MRI) or other imaging modalities. Inflammatory breast cancer is a clinical and pathologic diagnosis. Rapid onset of the characteristic breast changes differentiates it from neglected primary breast cancer, which can look very similar but has a better prognosis. Finding carcinoma in the dermal lymphatics without the associated rapid onset of erythema and edema is not inflammatory breast cancer. Survival is better for inflammatory breast cancer patients who receive chemotherapy before surgery. Modified radical mastectomy is the appropriate surgical procedure after chemotherapy. Sentinel node biopsy is not accurate in this setting. Postmastectomy radiation is indicated.

INITIAL BREAST CANCER CONSULTATION

Defining Threats to Health and Life

Newly diagnosed breast cancer patients frequently want the tumor removed as quickly as possible and often request bilateral mastectomy because they mistakenly believe this will improve their chance of survival. Two threats must be assessed and addressed. (1) Untreated breast cancer will progress locally and regionally, eventually producing disabling symptoms that severely affect quality of life. Local modalities, such as surgery and radiation therapy, are very effective at addressing this threat. (2) Some tumors shed cells into the circulation even when they are small. These cells can seed into other organs later manifesting as metastatic breast cancer. This is a potentially lethal threat that is addressed with systemic therapies such as chemotherapy, antihormonal therapy, and targeted systemic therapies. After completing the history, physical examination, imaging review, and pathology review, the breast surgeon will have a good sense about how these two threats balance out. Communicating this information to the patient will put the disease in perspective and reinforce the importance of investing time in recruiting a treatment team capable of designing and executing the optimal multimodal treatment strategy. Understanding the disease and gaining a sense of what lies ahead is a potent antidote for the crippling anxiety that frequently follows a new breast cancer diagnosis.

PREOPERATIVE ASSESSMENTS AND DECISIONS

Initial Consultation

The initial evaluation should focus on precise clinical staging (Table 1), fitness for general anesthesia and surgery, contraindications to radiation therapy, life goals including fertility concerns, and estimation of contralateral breast cancer risk. Of particular importance are history of mantle radiation for lymphoma, a history of high-risk preneoplasia including atypical hyperplasia or lobular *carcinoma in situ*, and cancer family history. The personal and family cancer history, including cancer types and ages at diagnosis, should be obtained for three generations on both the maternal and paternal sides.

Clinical Staging

A careful examination of the breast and nodal basins (axillary, supraclavicular, infraclavicular, and cervical) and an imaging review are usually all that is required to establish the locoregional extent of the tumor. Routine breast MRI is not recommended because it has not been shown to affect re-excision rates, local recurrence rates, or survival but is associated with increased use of mastectomy. MRI should be considered for infiltrating lobular cancers and when tumor size and extent is still uncertain after clinical examination and imaging review. The value of routine axillary sonography is uncertain and not recommended. For patients who will be receiving neoadjuvant chemotherapy, axillary sonography and sonoguided needle biopsy of lymph nodes with thickened cortices (>3 mm) is useful because it establishes initial nodal stage and also provides valuable prognostic information when compared with post-chemotherapy nodal status. A review of systems is often all that is required to screen for metastatic disease with queries related to weight loss and fatigue, new onset back or bone pain, neurologic symptoms, respiratory symptoms, or abdominal pain or bloating. Whole-body scans such as computed tomography, positron emission tomography–computed tomography, or bone scans are recommended only for clinical stage III patients and patients with clinical signs or symptoms suspicious for metastatic disease.

Cancer Genetics

Fewer than 10% of newly diagnosed breast cancers are caused by mutations in major breast cancer predisposition genes, but genetic counseling and testing should be included in the preoperative assessment when indicated. Genetic test results can influence breast surgery decisions, radiation therapy decisions, and systemic treatment decisions (usually in the context of a clinical trial). Most of the inherited predisposition syndromes are associated with an increased risk for contralateral breast cancer, and these patients may wish to consider bilateral mastectomy. Simple family history screening tools are available for identifying patients who should be referred for genetic counseling (Table 2), but they are most relevant to inherited breast-ovarian cancer syndrome. *BRCA1* and *BRCA2* mutations are still the most frequently identified cause of inherited breast cancer predisposition; however, multigene panels are identifying *CHEK2*, *PALB2*, and *ATM* as the most frequent non-*BRCA* genes. Table 3 lists the key clinical features important for recognizing some of the rare syndromes.

Breast Conservation Versus Mastectomy

Randomized prospective trials have demonstrated consistently that breast cancer–specific and overall survival are the same for breast

TABLE 1: Breast Cancer Staging: *AJCC Cancer Staging Manual,* **Seventh Edition**

PRIMARY TUMOR (T)

TX	Primary tumor cannot be assessed
T0	No evidence of primary tumor
Tis	Carcinoma in situ
Tis (DCIS)	Ductal carcinoma in situ
Tis (LCIS)	Lobular carcinoma in situ
Tis (Paget's)	Paget's disease of the nipple NOT associated with invasive carcinoma and/or carcinoma in situ (DCIS and/or LCIS) in the underlying breast parenchyma. Carcinomas in the breast parenchyma associated with Paget's disease are categorized based on the size and characteristics of the parenchymal disease, although the presence of Paget's disease should still be noted.
T1	Tumor ≤20 mm in greatest dimension
T1mi	Tumor ≤1 mm in greatest dimension
T1a	Tumor >1 mm but ≤5 mm in greatest dimension
T1b	Tumor >5 mm but ≤10 mm in greatest dimension
T1c	Tumor >10 mm but ≤20 mm in greatest dimension
T2	Tumor >20 mm but ≤50 mm in greatest dimension
T3	Tumor >50 mm in greatest dimension
T4	Tumor of any size with direct extension to the chest wall and/or to the skin (ulceration or skin nodules)

Note: Invasion of the dermis alone does not qualify as T4.

T4a	Extension to the chest wall, not including only pectoralis muscle adherence/invasion
T4b	Ulceration and/or ipsilateral satellite nodules and/or edema (including peau d'orange) of the skin, which do not meet the criteria for inflammatory carcinoma
T4c	Both T4a and T4b
T4d	Inflammatory carcinoma

REGIONAL LYMPH NODES (N)

CLINICAL

NX	Regional lymph nodes cannot be assessed (e.g., previously removed)
N0	No regional lymph node metastases
N1	Metastases in ipsilateral level I, II axillary lymph node(s)
N2	Metastases in ipsilateral level I, II axillary lymph nodes that are clinically fixed or matted; or in clinically detected ipsilateral internal mammary nodes in the *absence* of clinically evident axillary lymph node metastases
N2a	Metastases in ipsilateral level I, II axillary lymph nodes fixed to one another (matted) or to other structures
N2b	Metastases only in clinically detected ipsilateral internal mammary nodes and in the absence of clinically evident level I, II axillary lymph node metastases
N3	Metastases in ipsilateral infraclavicular (level III axillary) lymph node(s) with or without level I, II axillary lymph node involvement; or in clinically detected ipsilateral internal mammary lymph node(s) with clinically evident level I, II axillary lymph node metastases; or metastases in ipsilateral supraclavicular lymph node(s) with or without axillary or internal mammary lymph node involvement
N3a	Metastases in ipsilateral infraclavicular lymph node(s)
N3b	Metastases in ipsilateral internal mammary lymph node(s)
N3c	Metastases in ipsilateral supraclavicular lymph node(s)

PATHOLOGIC (PN)

pNX	Regional lymph nodes cannot be assessed (e.g., previously removed, or not removed for pathologic study)
pN0	No regional lymph node metastasis identified histologically

Note: Isolated tumor cell clusters (ITC) are defined as small clusters of cells not greater than 0.2 mm, or single tumor cells, or a cluster of fewer than 200 cells in a single histologic cross-section. ITCs may be detected by routine histology or by immunohistochemical (IHC) methods. Nodes containing only ITCs are excluded from the total positive node count for purposes of N classification but should be included in the total number of nodes evaluated.

TABLE 1: Breast Cancer Staging: *AJCC Cancer Staging Manual*, Seventh Edition—cont'd

pN0(i−)	NO regional lymph node metastases histologically, negative IHC
pN0(i+)	Malignant cells in regional lymph node(s) no greater than 0.2 mm (detected by H&E or IHC including ITC)
pN0 (mol−)	No regional lymph node metastases histologically, negative molecular findings (RT-PCR)
pN0 (mol+)	Positive molecular findings (RT-PCR), but no regional lymph node metastases detected by histology or IHC
pN1	Micrometastases; or metastases in 1-3 axillary lymph nodes; and/or in internal mammary nodes with metastases detected by sentinel lymph node biopsy but not clinically detected
pN1mi	Micrometastases (greater than 0.2 mm and/or more than 200 cells, but none greater than 2.0 mm)
pN1a	Metastases in 1-3 axillary lymph nodes, at least one metastasis greater than 2.0 mm
pN1b	Metastases in internal mammary nodes with micrometastases or macrometastases detected by sentinel lymph node biopsy but not clinically detected
pN1c	Metastases in 1-3 axillary lymph nodes and in internal mammary lymph nodes with micrometastases or macrometastases detected by sentinel lymph node biopsy but not clinically detected
pN2	Metastases in 4-9 axillary lymph nodes; or in clinically detected internal mammary lymph nodes in the *absence* of axillary lymph node metastases
pN2a	Metastases in 4-9 axillary lymph nodes (at least one tumor deposit greater than 2.0 mm)
pN2b	Metastases in clinically detected internal mammary lymph nodes in the absence of axillary lymph node metastases
pN3	Metastases in 10 or more axillary lymph nodes; or in infraclavicular (level III axillary) lymph nodes; or in clinically detected ipsilateral internal mammary lymph nodes in the *presence* of one or more positive level I, II axillary lymph nodes; or in more than three axillary lymph nodes and in internal mammary lymph nodes with micrometastases or macrometastases detected by sentinel lymph node biopsy but not clinically detected; or in ipsilateral supraclavicular nodes
pN3a	Metastases in ten or more axillary lymph nodes (at least one tumor deposit greater than 2.0 mm); or metastases to the infraclavicular (level III axillary lymph) nodes
pN3b	Metastases in clinically detected ipsilateral internal mammary lymph nodes in the *presence* of one or more positive axillary lymph nodes; or in more than three axillary lymph nodes and in internal mammary lymph nodes with micrometastases or macrometastases detected by sentinel lymph node biopsy but not clinically detected
pN3c	Metastases in ipsilateral supraclavicular lymph nodes

DISTANT METASTASES (M)

M0	No clinical or radiographic evidence of distant metastases
cM0(i+)	No clinical or radiographic evidence of distant metastases, but deposits of molecularly or microscopically detected tumor cells in circulating blood, bone marrow, or other nonregional nodal tissue that are no larger than 0.2 mm in a patient without symptoms or signs of metastases
M1	Distant detectable metastases as determined by classic clinical and radiographic means and/or histologically proven larger than 0.2 mm

ANATOMIC STAGE/PROGNOSTIC GROUPS

Stage 0	Tis N0 M0
Stage 1A	T1 N0 M0
Stage 1B	T0 N1mi M0 T1 N1mi M0
Stage IIA	T0 N1 M0 T1 N1 M0 T2 N0 M0
Stage IIB	T2 N1 M0 T3 N0 M0
Stage IIIA	T0 N2 M0 T1 N2 M0 T2 N2 M0 T3 N1 M0 T3 N2 M0

Continued

TABLE 1: Breast Cancer Staging: AJCC Cancer Staging Manual, Seventh Edition—cont'd

Stage IIIB	T4 N0 M0
	T4 N1 M0
	T4 N2 M0
Stage IIIC	Any T N3 M0
Stage IV	Any T Any N M1

From Edge S, et al. *AJCC Cancer Staging Manual.* 7th ed. New York: Springer-Verlag; 2010.

TABLE 2: Pedigree Assessment Tool

Risk Factor	Score
Breast cancer at age ≥50 yr	3
Breast cancer at age <50 yr	4
Ovarian cancer at any age	5
Male breast cancer at any age	8
Ashkenazi Jewish heritage	4

A score ≥8 is the optimum referral threshold.

Adapted from Hoskins KF, et al. *Cancer.* 2006;107:1769-1775.

TABLE 3: Key Features of Some Predisposition Syndromes

Gene	Key Features
BRCA1	Basal type triple negative breast cancer; ovarian cancer
BRCA2	Hormone-sensitive breast cancer; male breast cancer; melanoma; pancreas cancer
CHEK2	Hormone-sensitive breast cancer
PALB2	Hormone-sensitive breast cancer; male breast cancer; pancreatic cancer; similar to BRCA2
ATM	Some truncating mutations, in some families associated with significantly increased risk.
CDH1	Hereditary diffuse gastric cancer; infiltrating lobular carcinoma
TP53	Very early onset high grade, hormone sensitive and HER2-positive breast cancer
RAD51C	Ovarian cancer families
PTEN	Cowden syndrome. Macrocephaly, tricholemmomas, extensive benign breast disease, thyroid and endometrial cancer
STK11	Peutz-Jeghers syndrome. Mucocutaneous pigmentation; hamartomatous polyps; early onset breast cancer; pancreas and GI cancer

GI, gastrointestinal; *HER2,* human epidermal growth factor receptor–2.

conservation as for mastectomy. Local recurrence rates after breast-conserving therapy are declining significantly. This is related most strongly to the use of effective adjuvant systemic therapies. Local recurrence risk is currently estimated at about 0.4% per year for older women with hormone receptor–positive breast cancer and about 1%

per year for young women with triple negative breast cancer. For patients who desire a smaller breast size, generous lumpectomy can be combined with breast reduction. This so-called *oncoplastic partial mastectomy* permits local excision of more extensive tumors with a greater probability of negative margins with one procedure. However, if initial margins are positive, there is a significantly higher rate of conversion to mastectomy.

Use of unilateral mastectomy is declining as more and more women, especially young women, are opting for bilateral mastectomy. Most women overestimate their risk for contralateral second primary breast cancer. This risk has been declining over the last decade and currently is estimated at about 0.3% per year but may be higher for younger women, women with hormone receptor–negative breast cancer, and women with deleterious mutations in breast cancer predisposition genes. It is not certain that bilateral mastectomy is not associated with improved disease-specific and overall survival. Observational data suggest that women younger than 50 years with hormone receptor–negative breast cancer may have a survival benefit if they opt for bilateral mastectomy. This is a group with increased risk for contralateral breast cancer.

Neoadjuvant Chemotherapy

The NSABP B-18 neoadjuvant chemotherapy trial found that, overall, breast conservation occurred 12% more frequently than had been planned before chemotherapy, but 175% more frequently for tumors initially larger than 5 cm. Tumors that lack estrogen and progesterone receptor expression are more likely to respond to neoadjuvant chemotherapy and if they also express HER2/neu, the probability of a pathologic complete response to neoadjuvant chemotherapy combined with dual HER2 blockade (trastuzumab plus pertuzumab) is about 65%. It is reasonable to consider neoadjuvant chemotherapy for any patient who would be receiving postoperative adjuvant chemotherapy because the degree of pathologic response in the breast and lymph nodes provides useful prognostic information.

Reimaging with mammography, sonography, and MRI is reasonable after the completion of neoadjuvant chemotherapy. Partial mastectomy in this setting should encompass any residual imaging abnormality.

■ SURGERY

Partial Mastectomy

It is always safe to plan the incision directly over the tumor, although some have described acceptable results with circumareolar, axillary, or inframammary incisions nearly irrespective of the tumor location. Some advocate curved incisions for every lumpectomy. This is certainly desirable for incisions superior to the 9 o'clock to 3 o'clock horizontal. Inferior to this, natural skin tension seems to preserve the breast contour better when radial incisions are used. When possible, 1-cm subcutaneous flaps should be raised in every direction over the tumor. This avoids dimpling even with fairly large excisions. For more superficial tumors it may be necessary to take an ellipse of skin over the tumor. It is acceptable to close the incision in layers, leaving the excision cavity to fill in with seroma fluid. Alternatively, the glandular breast tissue can be mobilized in every direction and then

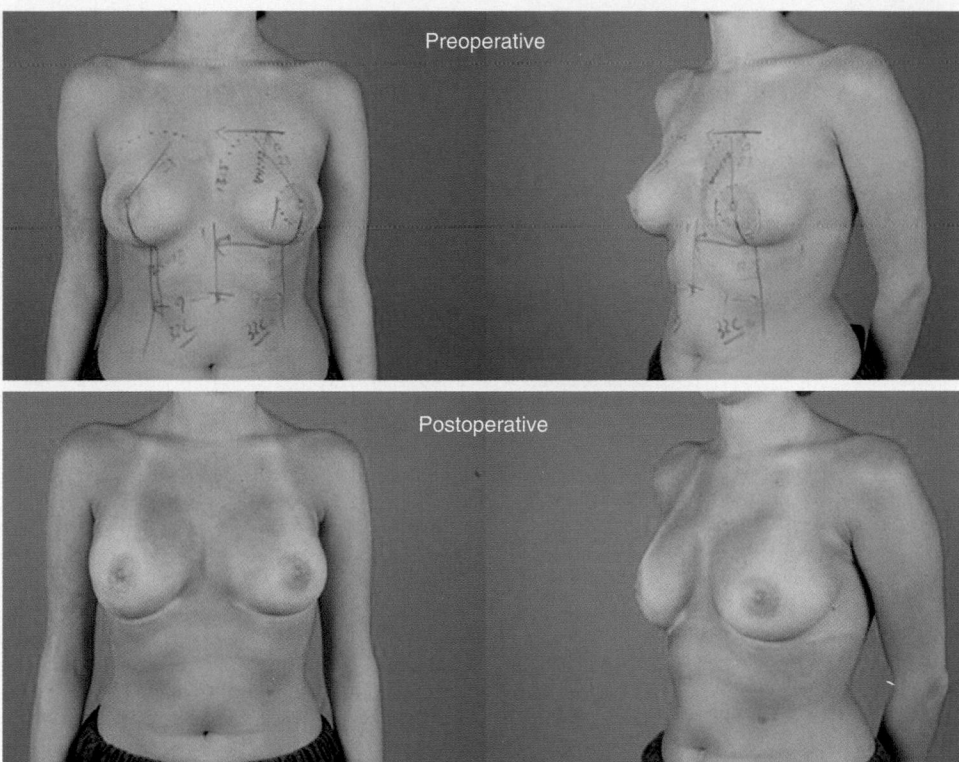

Preoperative

Postoperative

FIGURE I Approach for excising redundant axillary and lateral chest wall skin to eliminate bothersome "rolls" when mastectomy is performed without reconstruction.

sutured to obliterate the space. This aids in preservation of contour but can lead to a noticeably smaller breast.

The goal of partial mastectomy is to remove the entire tumor with a rim of normal tissue while preserving breast appearance. Wires, radioactive seeds, or intraoperative sonography are used to precisely localize the tumor, and a specimen mammogram is performed to ensure the lesion of interest has been excised with a radiographically negative margin. The specimen must be oriented in some way so that each of the surfaces can be inked for microscopic margin assessment. There is some evidence that margin assessment devices with optical coherence tomography, radiofrequency spectroscopy, or dielectric response can reduce re-excision rates, but it is currently unclear whether sensitivity and specificity are sufficient for general use. Some surgeons do targeted re-excisions at the time of lumpectomy according to clinical or radiographic suspicion; others routinely shave a thin margin from all six sides of the cavity. This has been shown to significantly reduce re-excision rates without compromising cosmesis.

A recent SSO-ASTRO consensus statement has recommended that "no ink on tumor" is the acceptable negative margin. This is based on a meta-analysis that showed similar local recurrence rates for 2-mm or 5-mm margins as compared with 1-mm margins. However, local recurrence was statistically significantly greater for margins classified as "close" compared with those classified as "negative," suggesting that there is some margin distance that would be associated with lower local recurrence risk than "no ink on tumor." Vagaries in the definitions of "close" or "negative" used in the different studies make it impossible to specify this value precisely. Historically, 11% to 59% of patients are returned to the operating room for re-excision of close or positive margins, but residual tumor is identified in only 23% to 68%. Re-excision decisions must be individualized even when the initial excision returns "no ink on the tumor." Multiple margins smaller than 1 mm for invasive cancer or even one margin smaller than 1 mm for ductal carcinoma in situ (DCIS) significantly increases the probability of finding residual cancer on re-excision.

Mastectomy

Total mastectomy, which removes most of the breast skin, including the nipple-areolar complex and all of the glandular tissue, often is required for patients with tumors involving the skin or nipple. For patients with extensive dermal involvement, generous skin excision is required and reconstruction should be postponed until after radiation therapy. For patients undergoing mastectomy without reconstruction, skin excisions must be designed to avoid bothersome skin folds especially in the axilla (Figure 1).

Nipple-sparing mastectomy removes all of the glandular tissue while retaining all of the breast skin, including the nipple-areolar complex. Modern nipple-sparing mastectomy is not the same procedure as subcutaneous mastectomy described in the 1960s. Subcutaneous mastectomy intentionally leaves breast tissue behind the nipple-areolar complex and any existing scars. Correctly performed nipple-sparing mastectomy results in a very thin areolar flap (Figure 2) and removes all of the breast tissue within the anatomic boundaries of the breast. Box 1 describes one approach to performing nipple-sparing mastectomy. Subareolar breast tissue is sampled and submitted separately. Extension of DCIS to this level should prompt excision of the nipple. Many incisions and reconstruction techniques have been described. A lateral inframammary incision provides excellent access to the entire breast and axilla with a relatively well-hidden scar. Two-staged reconstruction that starts with subpectoral expanders yields consistently good results. Immediate implant or autologous tissue reconstruction is associated with greater risk of skin or nipple necrosis especially when thin flaps are created.

Selection criteria for nipple-sparing mastectomy have been relaxing over the last several years and currently include: (1) the tumor does not involve the nipple or skin, (2) the tumor and glandular breast tissue can be removed with a negative margin, and (3) incision and reconstruction choices can bring the nipple to an aesthetically desirable level. Results are acceptable for large or small breasts, breasts that have been irradiated, breasts that will require radiation, and breasts that have previously undergone mastopexy or reduction.

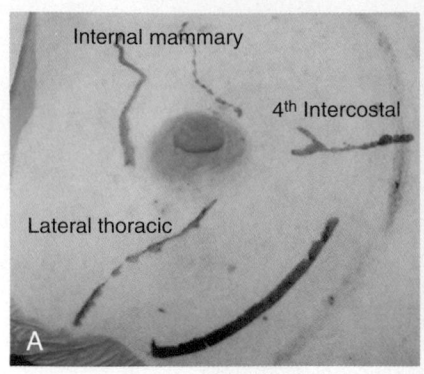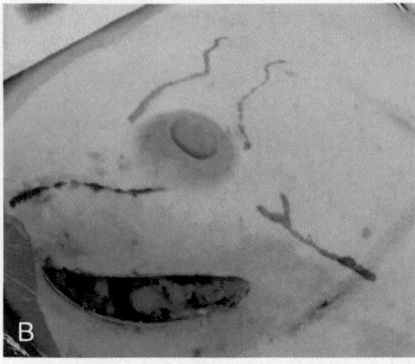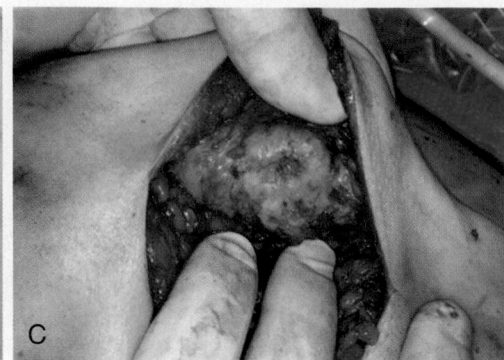

FIGURE 2 Nipple-sparing mastectomy. **A,** The major blood supply to the nipple has been marked out. **B,** A lateral inframammary incision provides excellent access to the entire breast and axilla. **C,** The skin flap should become thin behind the areola.

BOX 1: 10 Steps for Quickly Performing a Nipple-Sparing Mastectomy

1. Make a lateral inframammary incision just large enough to deliver the excised specimen through (see Figure 2).
2. Raise skin flaps (consider sharp dissection over electrocautery).
3. Create subdermal nipple-areolar flap (sharp dissection). Preserve the small vessels that are supplying the nipple and areola.
4. Sample the immediate subareolar tissue for separate pathology assessment.
5. Make a very short inferior flap and then separate the inferior pole of the breast from the subcutaneous tissue all of the way down to and through the pectoralis fascia.
6. Begin elevating the breast off of the pectoralis muscle from inferior to superior, taking care to retain the fascia with the specimen.
7. Pinch the inferior breast between two fingers and begin to separate it from the inframammary fold working from lateral to medial.
8. Do the same laterally taking care to free the entire axillary tail of the breast from the clavipectoral fascia.
9. Divide the medial attachments along the sternal border working from inferior to superior. Try to leave the internal mammary artery perforators (not always possible).
10. Alternating between medial and lateral as needed, free the superior attachments at the level of the clavicle (lighted retractors are invaluable).

Local recurrence rates after nipple-sparing mastectomy are about the same as after skin-sparing mastectomy. Nipple recurrence is rare, is treated with excision of the nipple, and has little if any impact on outcome.

Skin-sparing mastectomy is performed through a total circumareolar incision, which retains the nipple-areolar complex with the specimen. This is a desirable approach for patients with extreme nipple ptosis because a new nipple can be reconstructed at a more aesthetically pleasing level.

Management of the Axilla

Sentinel lymph node biopsy is the accepted axillary staging procedure for patients with clinically negative lymph nodes. Lymphatic mapping for identification of sentinel nodes can be done with ^{99m}Tc sulfur colloid, isosulfan blue dye, or both. Intraoperative pathologic assessment of sentinel nodes should not be performed routinely. Finding a positive sentinel node should trigger a multidisciplinary discussion incorporating all available clinical and pathologic data and directed at deciding about axillary dissection, radiation, or both. ACoSOG Z11 and IBCSG-23-01 reported axillary recurrence rates less than 1% and equivalent disease-specific and overall survival for patients with one or two positive sentinel nodes who did not undergo axillary dissection. These patients do need to receive postoperative adjuvant radiation and systemic therapies. It is currently not clear which patients benefit from the combination of axillary dissection and regional nodal irradiation. The AMAROS trial reported lymphedema in 11% of node-positive women treated with radiation and 23% in women treated with axillary dissection.

The place of sentinel node biopsy in patients receiving neoadjuvant chemotherapy is still debated, with some advocating for its use before chemotherapy and other's after. Proponents of nodal assessment before chemotherapy cite an increased false-negative rate after chemotherapy, which ranges from 8% to 11%, and also feel that the initial nodal status is required to make radiation decisions. The counter argument is that chemotherapy will reduce the pathologic node positive rate by 37%, potentially sparing axillary dissection in some women, and nodal status after neoadjuvant chemotherapy (not before) should dictate subsequent management. A good compromise is to perform axillary ultrasound and needle biopsy of any suspicious nodes before neoadjuvant chemotherapy. Performing sentinel node biopsy after chemotherapy in patients with a negative axillary assessment before chemotherapy should not engender controversy.

Axillary dissection is the current community standard of care for patients who have clinically apparent nodal metastases, but it is not certain that this is required in patients who achieve a complete clinical response to neoadjuvant chemotherapy. The currently accruing Alliance A011202 trial randomizes clinically node-positive patients with persistent pathologic positive nodes after neoadjuvant chemotherapy to axillary dissection plus axillary radiation versus axillary radiation only. The NSABP B-51/RTOG 1304 (NRG9353) trial randomizes clinically node-positive patients who are pathologic node-negative after neoadjuvant chemotherapy to regional nodal irradiation versus no axillary treatment. Data from the ACoSOG Z1071 and SENTINA trials suggest that the false-negative rate for sentinel node biopsy in the initial clinically node-positive patient is acceptably low if the patient achieves a complete clinical response to neoadjuvant chemotherapy, both ^{99m}Tc sulfur colloid and isosulfan blue dye are used for lymphatic mapping, at least three sentinel nodes are removed, and specimen radiography confirms that the initially clipped positive nodes have been removed. Repeating the axillary sonography after completion of neoadjuvant chemotherapy is a reasonable approach for assessing clinical response.

Male Breast Cancer

Male breast cancer is staged and treated nearly the same as female breast cancer. Total mastectomy usually is required because most of the tumors are subareolar. For more peripheral tumors, a nipple-sparing approach can be used, in which case a radiation therapy consult may be advisable. Sentinel lymph node biopsy is reliable in men. Nearly 90% of male breast cancers are hormone receptor positive. Tamoxifen is the adjuvant antihormonal therapy of choice because aromatase inhibitors can raise testosterone levels. Genetic counseling is indicated for any man diagnosed with breast cancer because 5% to 13% are due to *BRCA1* or *BRCA2* mutation, with *BRCA2* being more likely.

Breast Cancer in Pregnancy

Any breast lump discovered during pregnancy or lactation should be evaluated with sonography and undergo biopsy if it is solid. Surgery is safest for the fetus during the second trimester. Before this there is an increased risk for spontaneous abortion and after, an increased risk for pre-term labor. Mastectomy is the usual recommendation because radiation therapy cannot be administered at any time during pregnancy. Sentinel lymph node biopsy can be performed safely with ^{99m}Tc sulfur colloid for lymphatic mapping. Advanced breast cancer can be treated with neoadjuvant anthracycline-based chemotherapy beginning in the second trimester. No data suggest that subsequent pregnancies increase recurrence risk, but it is customary to recommend delaying conception for 2 years after initial treatment.

Breast Cancer Surgery in Stage IV Patients

Several retrospective studies have suggested that locoregional surgery improves survival in stage IV patients, especially for patients with oligometastatic, or bone-only, disease. All of these studies are confounded by selection bias; healthier patients are more likely to have surgery. Two international randomized prospective trials have been reported, and neither showed an advantage for primary breast surgery. ECOG E2108 is a U.S.-based randomized prospective trial that recently has completed accrual.

■ ADJUVANT THERAPY

Radiation Therapy After Breast-Conserving Surgery

The NSABP B-06 trial, conducted in the era before liberal use of adjuvant systemic therapy, reported a nearly threefold reduction in local recurrence with the use of postoperative adjuvant radiation therapy. A recent meta-analysis of randomized radiation therapy trials from the Early Breast Cancer Trialists Collaborative Group (EBCTCG) found that radiation therapy cuts the risk of any first recurrence in half and improved breast cancer–specific survival by 18%. This is the basis of the assertion that "about one breast cancer death [is] avoided by year 15 for every four recurrences avoided by year 10. …" Breast radiation is indicated for nearly any patient treated by partial mastectomy; however, data from the CALGB 9343 trial suggest that radiation therapy can be omitted safely for women age 70 years or older with stage I hormone receptor–positive breast cancer treated by partial mastectomy and postoperative adjuvant tamoxifen.

Accelerated Partial Breast Irradiation

Daily radiation treatments over 3 to 6 weeks can be burdensome, especially for patients who do not live close to a treatment center. In addition, true local recurrence occurs in the vicinity of the excision site, suggesting that this is where radiation is needed most. Radiation may be delivered in one fraction at the time of partial mastectomy (intraoperative radiation therapy), or in multiple fractions after surgery when the margin status is known. This later approach makes use of afterloading catheters (single or multiple) or external beams (e.g., 3D conformal or stereotactic body

radiation). Local recurrence rates appear similar to those observed with whole breast radiation, with higher rates in higher-risk women, but low rates in low-risk women. There has been concern that accelerated partial breast irradiation (APBI) is associated with more complications and worse cosmetic outcome (chronic seromas, fat necrosis, fibrosis, and skin changes) and a higher subsequent mastectomy rate. Available data are inconsistent on this point, but it is clear that patient selection and technical factors, such as tumor size, skin-spacing for balloon catheters, and treatment plans for external beam approaches, do influence cosmetic outcome. NSABP B-39 is a randomized prospective trial comparing postoperative APBI with whole-breast radiation. Follow-up data are not yet mature for this trial. It is anticipated that these results will help to resolve many of the controversies.

Radiation After Mastectomy

Historically radiation was recommended after mastectomy in women with four or more positive lymph nodes to reduce the high rate of local recurrence. A recent meta-analysis from the EBCTCG reported that for women with 1 to 3 positive nodes, radiation reduced local recurrence from about 2% per year to about 0.5% per year and was associated with an 8% reduction in breast cancer mortality. However, benefits from radiation therapy decrease as local recurrence risk decreases. More modern series estimate local recurrence risk at about 0.6% per year after mastectomy in patients with 1 to 3 positive nodes, making it unlikely that postmastectomy radiation would be associated with the same benefits observed in older trials.

Systemic Therapy

Most breast cancer patients, regardless of nodal status, receive some form of adjuvant systemic therapy, and this has been associated with significant reductions in local, regional, and distant recurrence risk. Dose-dense doxorubicin plus cyclophosphamide administered every other week for four cycles followed by weekly paclitaxel for 12 cycles is a common regimen for higher-risk tumors. Docetaxel plus cyclophosphamide every 3 weeks for four cycles is completed in about half the time and is appropriate for many patients. Docetaxel plus carboplatin frequently is administered with trastuzumab every 3 weeks for six cycles for *HER2/neu*–positive tumors. For these patients trastuzumab continues for 1 year.

Hormone receptor–positive breast cancer can be divided into low-risk tumors and higher-risk tumors. Low-risk tumors derive little benefit from chemotherapy but great benefit from antihormonal therapy. A 21-gene recurrence score (Oncotype DX) is ordered frequently on the primary tumor of node-negative, hormone receptor–positive patients to estimate recurrence risk and benefit of chemotherapy over tamoxifen alone. Antihormonal therapy for postmenopausal women usually consists of sequential tamoxifen and aromatase inhibition (anastrazole, letrozole, or exemestane), for at least 5 years, but accumulating data suggest benefit for 10 years of treatment. Use of an aromatase inhibitor at some point during treatment is associated with improved survival compared with tamoxifen-only strategies. Tamoxifen has been the dominant antihormonal therapy in premenopausal women for more than 30 years. There is some evidence that outcome is improved for certain higher-risk women when tamoxifen is combined with ovarian suppression (bilateral oophorectomy or goserelin, a gonadotropin-releasing hormone agonist). Data from the SOFT trial showed greatest benefit for the combination of aromatase inhibition (exemestane) combined with ovarian suppression in premenopausal, hormone receptor–positive breast cancers of great enough risk to require chemotherapy.

■ SURVIVORSHIP

There is no evidence that early detection of distant recurrence improves outcome. Consequently no imaging or blood tests are

BOX 2: Some Common Survivorship Issues

Emotional distress and depression
Menopausal symptoms
Fertility
Sexuality and intimacy
Weight gain
Bone health
Insomnia and fatigue
Lymphedema
Cognitive dysfunction

recommended for surveillance after breast cancer treatment apart from mammography to assess for local recurrence and second primary breast cancers. However, breast cancer survivors face a host of cancer-related and treatment-related issues (Box 2). The transition from breast cancer patient to survivor is the time to systematically assess for these issues and develop a management plan that can be shared with the primary care provider.

SUGGESTED READINGS

Canavan J, Truong PT, Smith SL, Lu L, Lesperance M, Olivotto IA. Local recurrence in women with stage I breast cancer: declining rates over time in a large, population-based cohort. *Int J Radiat Oncol Biol Phys*. 2014;88: 80-86.

Early Breast Cancer Trialists' Collaborative Group, Darby S, McGale P, Correa C, Taylor C, Arriagada R, Clarke M, Cutter D, Davies C, Ewertz M, Godwin J, Gray R, Pierce L, Whelan T, Wang Y, Peto R. Effect of radiotherapy after breast-conserving surgery on 10-year recurrence and 15-year breast cancer death: meta-analysis of individual patient data for 10,801 women in 17 randomised trials. *Lancet*. 2011;378:1707-1716. 3254252: 3254252.

Habermann EB, Abbott A, Parsons HM, Virnig BA, Al-Refaie WB, Tuttle TM. Are mastectomy rates really increasing in the United States? *J Clin Oncol*. 2010;28:3437-3441.

Moran MS, Schnitt SJ, Giuliano AE, Harris JR, Khan SA, Horton J, Klimberg S, Chavez-MacGregor M, Freedman G, Houssami N, Johnson PL, Morrow M. Society of Surgical Oncology-American Society for Radiation Oncology consensus guideline on margins for breast-conserving surgery with whole-breast irradiation in stages I and II invasive breast cancer. *Ann Surg Oncol*. 2014;21:704-716.

Rao R, Euhus D, Mayo HG, Balch C. Axillary node interventions in breast cancer: a systematic review. *JAMA*. 2013;310:1385-1394.

ABLATIVE TECHNIQUES IN THE TREATMENT OF BENIGN AND MALIGNANT BREAST DISEASE

Amy Rivere, MD, and V. Suzanne Klimberg, MD, FACS

As imaging has improved and more occult lesions are being detected, there is a growing interest in using image-guided percutaneous thermal ablation technologies to ablate benign and cancerous lesions as a replacement for resection. Many technologies have been developed in an effort to provide approaches to benign and malignant lesions that are both immediate and minimally invasive office-based procedures. Another distinct advantage of such approaches is the ability to treat multiple lesions at once. The hope is that these technologies could bring forth a new paradigm of immediate diagnosis and treatment that improves the cosmetic result and eventually may obviate the need for radiation. Further work is needed to prove the effectiveness of these modalities as well as real-time imaging of the various ablation processes. We review the most promising modalities, which include radiofrequency ablation, cryoablation, focused ultrasound, interstitial laser, and microwave ablation.

■ RADIOFREQUENCY ABLATION

Radiofrequency ablation (RFA) is accomplished through heat generated by high-frequency alternating currents that cause friction-generated heat from ion movement. The tissue is heated by gradually increasing the frequency of the currents until the desired temperature is reached or impedance occurs. RFA uses a percutaneously inserted electrode array placed into an area of interest under image guidance (Figure 1). Ablation results in increasing levels of cell damage with the rise in temperature above 42°C, and by 60°C protein denaturation and coagulation leads to necrosis and cell death. RFA is approved by the U.S. Food and Drug Administration (FDA) for liver and soft tissue ablation.

There have been a multitude of proof-of-concept ablate and resect protocols utilizing RFA, most involving fewer than 30 patients. RFA can be performed under local or general anesthesia. None of the studies involving ablation of intact tumor with more than 10 patients has achieved complete ablation of the tumor in breast cancer. Ductal carcinoma in situ (DCIS) is particularly problematic. Despite this, Japanese researchers have conducted quite a few thermal ablation studies in which the ablated tumor is left in situ and assessed for local recurrence using fine-needle aspiration (FNA) biopsies or core needle biopsies every 6 months. The outcomes have been fairly good. In the two largest trials, 12-month and 20-month follow-up revealed one recurrence and one death.

A different approach being studied is to percutaneously excise the tumor under image-guided needle core biopsy followed by percutaneous RFA (PeRFA) of the cavity. Our group has pioneered this technique and developed procedures to enhance it. The RFA electrode array is placed in the hematoma cavity utilizing the hematoma-directed ultrasound-guided (HUG) procedure. The advantage of this approach is that sufficient tissue can be obtained for tumor markers, genomics, and banking. In addition, the treatment is to the subcutaneous tissue surrounding the cavity and thus to a uniform tissue, usually fatty, that ablates very well. This is also an FDA-approved use of the device. Although further testing of this concept needs to be performed, with sufficient expertise and improved imaging this technique gets us closer to the goal of percutaneous treatment of breast cancer. This has been tested only in a small trial on lesions up to 1.5 cm, which is the limit of the stereotactic or ultrasound-guided percutaneous excisions. Magnetic resonance imaging (MRI) was used in this study to rule out multicentricity but was not very predictive of residual disease. Despite this, the ablation (PeRFA) had 100% success on whole mount reconstruction. The hematoma or seroma left in the percutaneous excision cavity was used to direct PeRFA. In addition, we developed a method using color Doppler to observe off-gassing of nitrogen, which allows for the extent of ablation to be observed as bubbling and movement during the procedure and can be measured and in the laboratory correlated with the zone or extent of ablation and also proximity to the skin. Follow-up studies are planned for percutaneous excision followed by ablation and follow-up with mammograms and FNA.

OPEN ABLATION (eRFA—EXCISION FOLLOWED BY RADIOFREQUENCY ABLATION)

Lumpectomy followed by radiation is widely utilized for the treatment of breast cancer. At least 75% to 90% of recurrences occur at the previous lumpectomy site and positive margins are found in 20% to 55% of lumpectomy specimens. Radiation effectively lowers the risk at the site of the lumpectomy but is not as important in reducing ipsilateral recurrences elsewhere in the breast, giving rise to the concept and the effective treatment of brachytherapy, which treats an approximately 1-cm area around the tumor bed with 100% radiation dose. In a similar way, excision followed by radiofrequency ablation (eRFA) utilizes the RFA to in effect extend the margins of the lumpectomy by 1 cm and ablate any undetectable residual disease. This procedure is designed to increase the margin in primary lumpectomy cavities without further excision, thereby avoiding additional tissue resection and maintaining optimum cosmesis in breast-conserving surgery (Figure 2). Re-excision can be avoided in 65% to 80% of patients.

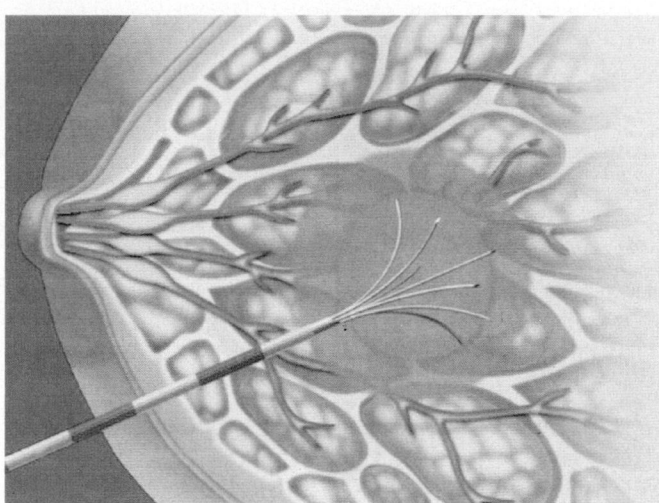

FIGURE 1 Representation of radiofrequency ablation showing star array probe with breast and surrounding frozen ablation zone. *(Courtesy RITA Medical Systems. From Simmons R. Ablative techniques in the treatment of benign and malignant breast disease. J Am Coll Surg. 2003;197:334-338. Copyright by the American College of Surgeons.)*

Significant preclinical and clinical data have demonstrated that RFA applied to a lumpectomy cavity can ablate a consistent centimeter around the cavity by heating to 100°C for 15 minutes. This concept has been demonstrated using whole mount reconstruction of simulated lumpectomies in mastectomy specimens treated with eRFA. A multi-institutional trial in Italy demonstrated that in vivo eRFA of invasive breast cancers followed by standard quadrantectomy showed at least a 1-cm circumferential ablation around the lumpectomy sites, again in whole mount sections. The procedure also has been shown to be effective in a pilot clinical trial in the United States to evaluate eRFA. One hundred patients underwent lumpectomy followed by intraoperative RFA. Biopsy of the cavity walls post-ablation demonstrated at least a 1-cm thick ablation in the initial patients. With a median 5-year follow-up, 3% of patients experienced recurrence while taking their prescribed hormonal therapy and 10% experienced recurrence if noncompliant with hormonal therapy, rates similar to those seen in partial breast and brachytherapy trials. A Phase II multicenter trial of 250 patients using eRFA has finished and is awaiting maturity.

CRYOABLATION

Cryoablation, as with most ablation procedures, is accomplished percutaneously through the same small incision used for core biopsy. Cryoablation uses argon gas and multiple freeze-thaw cycles to destroy cells. It can be performed in the office under local anesthesia or under general anesthesia. Cryoablation requires expertise in image-guided procedures in order to place the cryoprobe in the exact center of the lesion (benign or malignant). Unique to cryoablation is the formation of an "iceball" after at least two cycles at −40°C that can be used as a proxy for progression of the ablation and is visible by ultrasound scan (US) as a hypoechoic mass (Figure 3). Depending on the size of the ablation required, the procedure can take up to 20 to 40 minutes.

Initial studies with cryoablation were performed on fibroadenomas so as to avoid open excision. In one study of fibroadenomas, 95% of the ablated lesions (0.7 to 4.2 cm) regressed over 12 months both by palpation and by imaging. However, in those patients where palpable fibrosis remains, continued follow-up is necessary. Further, we believe that the need for such an ablative procedure on a benign lesion is obviated, as we published the first single-institution trial demonstrating simple removal via a vacuum-assisted device that is easy and had excellent results without the need for ablation. A multicenter trial demonstrated the same results, and this method is used routinely by us and others.

A multicenter trial also used cryoablation on breast cancer as a localization device to improve clear margin excision but this was not

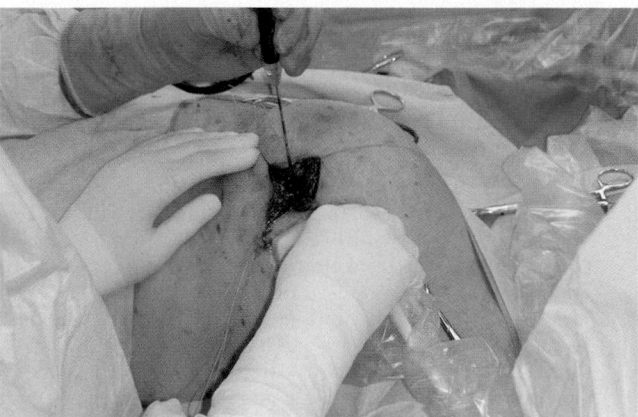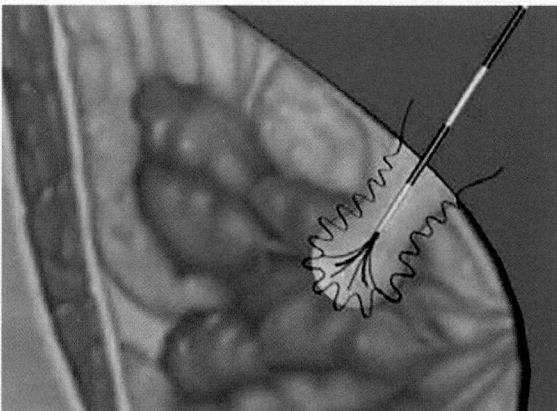

FIGURE 2 Concept of radiofrequency ablation for cavitary hyperthermia and ablation.

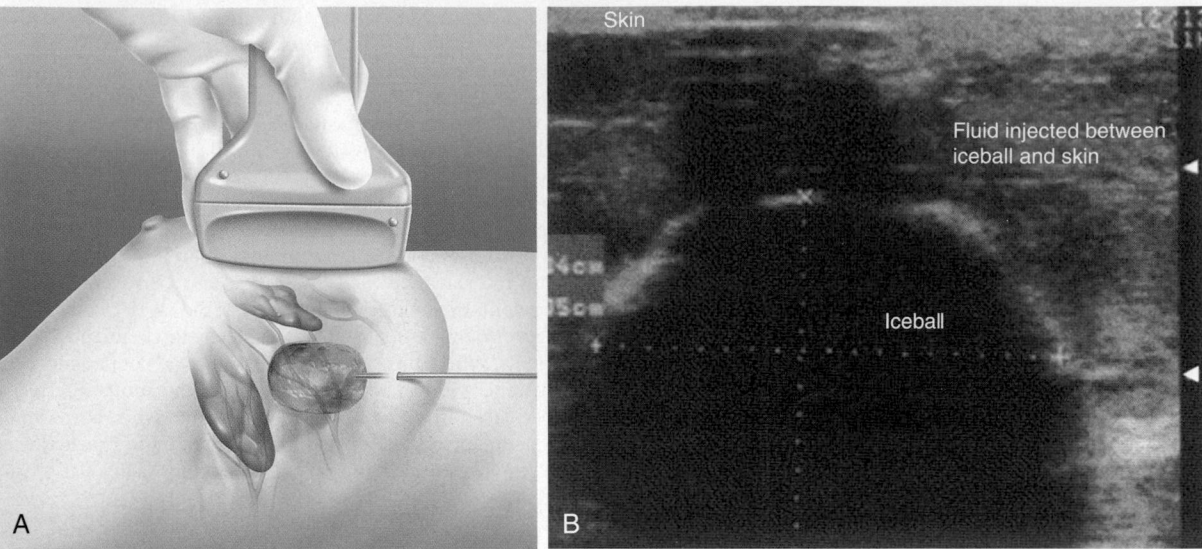

FIGURE 3 A, Ultrasonography is used to monitor the developing cryogenic zone created by the cryoprobe. **B,** Ultrasound image of hypoechoic iceball and protective saline injection. (**A,** *from Kaufman C, Littrup P, Freman-Gibb L, et al. Office-based cryoablation of breast fibroadenomas: 12 month follow-up.* J Am Coll Surg. *2004;198:914-923;* **B,** *from Kaufman C, Bachman B, Littrup P, et al. Office-based ultrasound-guided cryoablation of breast fibroadenomas.* Am J Surg. *2002;184:394-400.)*

found to be superior to needle localization breast biopsy. In a small Phase II "ablate and resect" cancer trial with cryoablation of intact T1 lesions (mean 1.2 cm), favorable results but not complete ablation (n = 27) were obtained. If lesions with associated DCIS were excluded, a subgroup analysis of those with only invasive carcinoma showed complete ablation. In another small study, 90% ablation was achieved. Most recently, Simmons and colleagues reported the initial results from ACOSOG Z1072 (Alliance) of an "ablate and resect" protocol of 87 breast cancer patients treated at 19 U.S. centers. As a part of this protocol patients underwent preablation and postablation MRI. In the overall analysis of the trial only 63% of patients achieved complete ablation. Subgroup analysis in this already small study demonstrated a 94% complete ablation rate in patients who had a tumor size of less than 1 cm. MRI did not accurately predict ablation. Further studies around cryoablation are ongoing, in particular around the possibility of cryoablation-induced lysing of tumor cell membranes that then may have a vaccination-like effect. Given the present-day knowledge of immunotherapy, any ablation technique likely will need to be combined with checkpoint inhibitors to be effective.

■ HIGH-INTENSITY FOCUSED ULTRASOUND

High-intensity focused ultrasound (HIFU) is the projection of ultrasound waves to deliver energy "transcutaneously," raising focal temperature to approximately 70°C and sonicating an area between $3 \times 3 \times 10$ mm^3 and $8 \times 8 \times 30$ mm^3 in 10 to 20 seconds (Figure 4). It is the only procedure of this type that can be performed without an incision but it requires spinal or general anesthesia. It does require much more time, expense, and dedicated space to perform. MRI before, during, and after HIFU ablation is used to follow the progress in real time. If target temperatures or complete ablation is not reached as determined by MRI, re-ablation of the same area can be performed. Because of the small ablation zone, HIFU has the disadvantage of needing multiple applications and longer time (2 to 3 hours) for complete ablation zone coverage. Assessment of the temperature change with MRI is valuable, as different tissues may require different sonication settings or time to achieve the target temperature, but not completely reliable. Peek

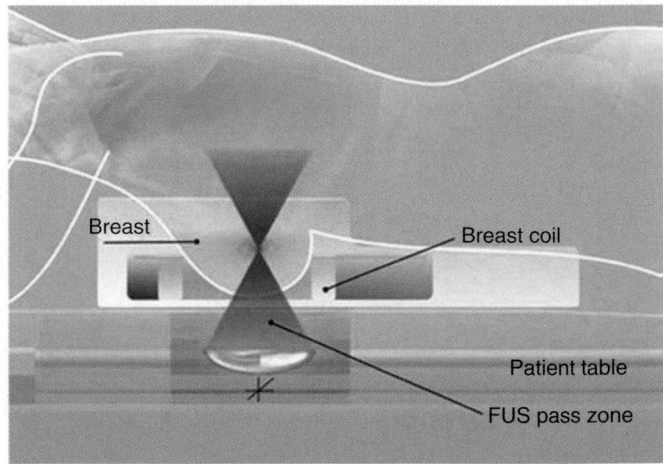

FIGURE 4 Schematic diagram of magnetic resonance imaging–guided high intensity focused ultrasound therapy for a breast cancer patient in prone position. *FUS,* focused ultrasound. (*From Zhou Y. Noninvasive treatment of breast cancer using high-intensity focused ultrasound.* J Med Imaging & Health Inform. *2013;3:141-156.)*

and colleagues published a systematic review of HIFU studies and found 9 studies with 167 patients with acceptable criteria for review—that is, HIFU was performed on breast cancer patients and there was at least one clinical outcome measure of response (e.g., imaging, histopathologic examination, cosmesis). No residual tumor was seen in only 46.2% of the studies, with only one study reporting complete ablation. Neither MRI nor US was reliable in predicting complete ablation of breast tumor. As with other ablation technologies, complications such as skin burns (first, second, and third degree), palpable fibrosis, and incomplete ablation can occur. Furusawa and colleagues have used MRI to follow 47 patients who have gone "excisionless" after ablation with HIFU, with low recurrence rates thus far. Peek and Doueck have started a study in England using HIFU for fibroadenomas and are recruiting patients at this time.

■ INTERSTITIAL LASER

Interstitial laser ablation for breast cancer involves placing a laser needle in the center of the tumor under stereotactic guidance while a second probe is placed in the periphery to measure temperature. It can be performed under local anesthesia. The laser energy is delivered to the center of the tumor until all thermal sensors in the periphery record 60°C. The average treatment time is 15 to 30 minutes for a T1 lesion at 6000 to 9000 joules, dependent on the vascularity of the breast. This requires that the patient be perfectly still and immobilized for quite some time on the stereotactic table. Because the breast is treated under compression, the procedure also requires a fairly ample breast. Despite this, the best report by Dowlatshai and colleagues is an overall complete tumor ablation of 70% in 50 patients with a mean diameter of 12 mm (5 to 23 mm). Incomplete tumor ablation was attributed to technical issues such as inadequate laser energy, patient motion, malfunctioning thermal probes and fluid pump, suboptimal target visualization, and tumors larger than 2 cm. Our group, led by Dr. Steve Harms, tried laser ablation under MRI as well as ultrasound guidance. This required multiple overlapping ablations with inconsistent success in a small group of patients.

As part of our National Cancer Institute (NCI) trial of percutaneous excision followed by ablation protocol, one arm of the trial underwent interstitial laser ablation. Unfortunately, laser of the percutaneous excision cavity (hematoma) was extremely unpredictable, showing wide variations in ablation on follow-up postablation pathologic testing. As a result of our experience we did not feel that with available laser fibers, laser was a fruitful line of investigation for percutaneous ablation of breast cancers.

■ MICROWAVE ABLATION

Microwave ablation is predicated on the fact that tumors have a higher content of water than most surrounding tissue, such as fat, and thus would absorb more heat than such tissues. Therefore delivering wide-field focused microwaves using a minimally invasive system can treat a fairly large area while sparing the bulk of normal breast tissue and fat. This will differ depending on the density of the breast. Microwave ablation uses a multiprobe catheter in the breast with temperature sensors on the skin. Patients are treated on a modified stereotactic table using opposing sensors with temperatures up to 50°C. The procedure can be performed under local anesthesia in an office setting and is estimated to take approximately 20 to 30 minutes in tumors up to 5 cm encompassing both the tumor and the margin. A small randomized trial was conducted using predictive thermal dose and comparing patients with microwave thermal therapy with those who had lumpectomy only. Pathologic testing revealed 10% positive margins in the lumpectomy-only group (n = 41) and zero positive margins in the ablation group. Small breast cancer treatment studies of focused microwave phased array thermotherapy show longer treatment times with lower temperatures and significant tumor size reduction but only 80% tumor kill and high complication rates. As of yet, no consistent way to calculate thermal heat and time necessary to ablate a specific size of tumor exists. Further human studies are needed.

■ IRREVERSIBLE ELECTROPORATION

Irreversible electroporation (IRE) uses a single-needle electrode to deliver short electric pulses (1000 V/cm field) across a cell membrane in order to create nanopores that will lead to cell death. The novelty of this method is that IRE affects only the cell membrane while sparing the extracellular matrix and tissues. Thus this method promises to be superior in reducing scar formation compared with traditional methods such as radiation but also the ablative methods already discussed. This is important when considering follow-up tumor surveillance and satisfaction with cosmesis.

■ SUMMARY

Cryoablation of benign breast lesions such as fibroadenomas is routine in some practices. In others, ablation has been superseded by percutaneous excision with large bore vacuum-assisted devices. Percutaneous excision really should be standard for benign lesions, as in our study 2% had undetected cancer and the procedure requires only routine follow-up and does not leave a mass from the ablated tissue. Ablation of breast cancer remains investigative and should be performed only as a part of clinical trial. Given our success with percutaneous excision followed by ablation for tumors smaller than 1.5 cm, we believe that percutaneous excision followed by RFA with real-time Doppler imaging is the ablation tool of choice and may obviate the need for excision and possibly radiation. We are planning further trials using this methodology. We also are planning a randomized trial of open excision followed by intracavitary RFA as the sole means of local treatment compared with traditional breast conservation therapy with radiation. We believe this is an important line of investigation, as nearly 85% of women treated for small, favorable tumors do not benefit from the addition of radiation therapy (NSABP B-21 trial). Development of ablation as a new alternative paradigm portends the future of breast cancer treatment.

SUGGESTED READINGS

Dooley WC, Vargas HI, Fenn AJ, Tomaselli MB, Harness JK. Focused microwave thermotherapy for preoperative treatment of invasive breast cancer: a review of clinical studies. *Ann Surg Oncol.* 2010;17:1076-1093.

Fornage BD, Hwang RF. Current status of imaging-guided percutaneous ablation of breast cancer. *AJR Am J Roentgenol.* 2014;203:442-448.

Klimberg VS, Boneti C, Adkins LL, et al. Feasibility of percutaneous excision followed by ablation for local control in breast cancer. *Ann Surg Oncol.* 2011;18:3079-3087.

Klimberg VS, Ochoa D, Henry-Tillman R. Long-term results of phase II ablation after breast lumpectomy added to extend intraoperative margins (ABLATE l) trial. *J Am Coll Surg.* 2014;218:741-749.

Knuttel FM, van den Bosch MA. Magnetic resonance-guided high intensity focused ultrasound ablation of breast cancer. *Adv Exp Med Biol.* 2016;880: 65-81.

Mackey A, Feldman S, Vaz A, Durrant L, Seaton C, Klimberg VS. Radiofrequency ablation after breast lumpectomy added to extend intraoperative margins in the treatment of breast cancer (ABLATE): a single-institution experience. *Ann Surg Oncol.* 2012;19:2618-2619.

Neal RE 2nd, Singh R, Hatcher HC, Kock ND, Torti SV, Davalos RV. Treatment of breast cancer through the application of irreversible electroporation using a novel minimally invasive single needle electrode. *Breast Cancer Res Treat.* 2010;123:295-301.

Peek MC, Ahmed M, Napoli A, ten Haken B, McWilliams S, Usiskin SI, Pinder SE, van Hemelrijck M, Douek M. Systematic review of high-intensity focused ultrasound ablation in the treatment of breast cancer. *Br J Surg.* 2015;102:873-882.

Zhou W, Zha X, Liu X, et al. US-guided percutaneous microwave coagulation of small breast cancers: a clinical study. *Radiology.* 2012;263:364-373.

LYMPHATIC MAPPING AND SENTINEL LYMPHADENECTOMY

Alexandra Gangi, MD, and Armando E. Giuliano, MD

Axillary staging is a critical component of breast cancer management and has evolved greatly in the last 20 years. Sentinel lymph node biopsy (SLNB), which was first investigated in the early 1990s, has replaced routine axillary lymph node dissection (ALND) for most clinically node-negative women. SLNB provides accurate assessment of nodal status and crucial staging information and even may replace ALND in some patients with early nodal metastases.

The concepts of the spread of metastatic cancer cells in reproducible patterns and the mistaken role of lymph nodes as barriers to distant metastatic spread were articulated more than a century ago by Virchow and investigated clinically in the 1940s. The understanding that a single draining lymph node may represent an entire nodal basin dates back more than half a century. In 1951 Gould and colleagues reported performing a frozen section of a single lymph node during a parotidectomy and completing a radical neck dissection only if metastatic disease was confirmed in this single lymph node. This concept of lymphatic drainage to a single node subsequently was reported in penile cancer and testicular cancer. Morton and colleagues developed lymphatic mapping and SLNB as a staging procedure for patients with early-stage melanoma and first proposed omission of complete lymphadenectomy if the sentinel lymph node (SLN) was tumor free. This technique was modified and applied to breast cancer in 1991. The initial experience, which defined the technical aspects, criteria for selecting patients for SLNB, safety, and feasibility, involved 174 patients with T1 to T3 breast cancers and included patients both with and without palpable axillary adenopathy. Using a peritumoral injection of 5 mL of 1% isosulfan blue dye (Lymphazurin), the technique identified SLNs in 114 of the 174 procedures (66%) and accurately predicted the tumor status of the axillary basin in 109 (96%) of the patients in whom an SLN was identified. The staging accuracy of SLNB then was evaluated prospectively by the same investigators in 162 clinically node-negative patients with T1 or T2 breast cancers who underwent SLNB followed by ALND compared with 134 patients who had only an ALND. By examining the SLN alone, a significantly higher rate of detection of metastases was shown in the group that had an SLNB followed by ALND than in the group that had only ALND (42% vs 29%). In addition, a nearly fourfold incidence of micrometastases was detected in the SLNB group compared with the ALND group, suggesting that a more focused examination of one or two SLNs could be more accurate than the histopathologic evaluation of the entire lymph node basin without SLNB. Other investigators subsequently validated the SLNB technique in breast cancer. Veronesi and colleagues performed the procedure using a subdermal injection of technetium 99m (^{99m}Tc)–labeled human serum albumin and reported a 98% success rate in 163 patients and accurately predicted the axillary status in 97% of the cases. These studies subsequently led to the first multicenter trial of 443 patients who had SLNB followed by ALND using radiotracer alone, which reported identification of the SLN in 93% of the cases, with a false-negative rate of 11.4%. A meta-analysis of 11 published studies was performed with 912 patients and compared injection techniques with lymphoscintigraphy or blue dye, or a combination of both, in patients who had SLNB followed by ALND for in situ and invasive cancer. This study reported a significantly higher rate of identification if radiocolloid and blue dye were used together or if radiocolloid was used alone than if blue dye was used

alone. Moreover, the SLN reflected the status of the axilla in 97% of the cases, with only a 5% false-negative rate. These studies confirmed that the status of the SLN accurately predicts the status of the axillary nodal basin. Veronesi and colleagues then performed the first randomized trial comparing the staging accuracy and recurrence rates in patients with tumor-free SLN. Five hundred sixteen patients with T1 clinically node-negative breast cancer were randomized to either SLNB followed by ALND or SLNB alone. ALND was performed if the SLN contained metastases. Both groups of patients had similar rates of SLN metastases. This early trial showed that SLNB alone could predict axillary nodal metastases with a false-negative rate of 8.8% in the group that underwent complete ALND. In addition, patients in the SLNB-only group had less pain and better arm mobility. Moreover, at a median follow-up of 46 months, patients treated with SLNB alone developed no axillary recurrence and had similar survival to patients who underwent ALND. Other randomized studies have confirmed these results (Table 1).

■ INDICATIONS FOR SENTINEL LYMPH NODE BIOPSY

The current literature supports SLNB in patients with clinically node-negative T1 to T2 invasive breast cancers who are undergoing partial mastectomy or total mastectomy. Most experts agree that SLNB is also suitable for patients with T3 cancers, multifocal/multicentric disease, prior radiation therapy, and prior breast or axillary surgery. However, there are limited data with respect to this cohort of patients. The available literature alluding to these situations has shown equivalent accuracy to ALND, but the decision to utilize SLNB in such situations requires good surgical judgment and a successful mapping procedure. In addition, SLNB should be performed for ductal carcinoma in situ (DCIS) whenever mastectomy is required or perhaps when there is a high suspicion for invasive disease such as high-grade, large (>5 cm), or palpable DCIS. Again, surgical judgment is required in these situations. Patients with T4 breast cancer, inflammatory breast cancer, or palpable biopsy-proven positive nodes are generally ineligible for SLNB. The American Society of Clinical Oncology (ASCO) guidelines were updated in 2014 (see Box 1 for indications for SLNB).

Patients with clinically positive axillary nodes should undergo axillary ultrasound and biopsy to evaluate for metastatic disease. If clinically positive nodes are found to harbor malignancy, a level I and II ALND is indicated. In those patients who are clinically node negative but have suspicious nodes on imaging and a needle biopsy that is positive for malignancy, some surgeons may recommend proceeding with full ALND. However, these patients with clinically negative but needle biopsy–proven positive nodes still may be eligible for SLNB and tangential whole breast irradiation if they meet the eligibility criteria of the American College of Surgeons Oncology Group (ACOSOG) Z0011 trial, which is discussed later.

■ TECHNICAL ASPECTS OF SENTINEL LYMPH NODE BIOPSY

The SLN can be localized by either lymphoscintigraphy or the intraoperative gamma counter without lymphoscintigraphy after injection of ^{99m}Tc-labeled sulfur colloid or intraoperative injection of vital blue dye (Lymphazurin or methylene blue), or both. The blue dye or radioisotope can be injected in a subareolar, subdermal, or peritumoral location. Radiocolloid may be injected intradermally, but blue dye should not be, as it may tattoo the skin. Also, only radiocolloid has been shown to be safe during pregnancy. If using radiocolloid, patients are injected preoperatively with 0.5 mL of 0.5 mCi of filtered ^{99m}Tc sulfur colloid. If lymphoscintigraphy is performed, imaging documents the drainage patterns from the tumor through the lymphatics to the regional lymph nodes. Intraoperatively, a gamma probe

TABLE 1: Comparison of Outcomes in Four Randomized Controlled Trials of Sentinel Lymph Node Biopsy Versus Axillary Lymph Node Dissection for Clinically Node-Negative Women

Study/Trial	Patient Number	F/u (months)	LRR: SLNB vs ALND	DFS: SLNB vs ALND	OS: SLNB vs ALND
Veronesi	516	102	2.3% vs 2.3%	88.8% vs 89.9%, 10 yr	93.5% vs 89.7%, 10 yr
Sentinella/GIVOM	697	56	4.6% vs 1.0%	87.6% vs 89.9%, 5 yr	94.8% vs 95.5%, 5 yr
NSABP B-32	5611	95.6	3.1% vs 3.1%	81.5% vs 82.4%, 8 yr	90.3% vs 91.8%, 8 yr
ACOSOG Z0011*	891	75.6	1.6% vs 3.1%	83.9% vs 82.2%, 5 yr	92.5% vs 91.8%, 5 yr

*SLN positive by hematoxylin and eosin (H&E) staining.

ACOSOG, American College of Surgeons Oncology Group; *ALND,* axillary lymph node dissection; *DFS,* disease-free survival; *F/u,* follow-up; *GIVOM,* Gruppo Interdisciplinare Veneto di Oncologia Mammaria; *LRR,* local-regional recurrence; *NSABP,* National Surgical Adjuvant Breast and Bowel Project; *OS,* overall survival; *SLN,* sentinel lymph node; *SLNB,* sentinel lymph node biopsy.

BOX 1: American Society of Clinical Oncology Guidelines: Indications for Sentinel Lymph Node Biopsy, 2005 and 2015

T1, T2
Unicentric or multicentric
Ductal carcinoma in situ with mastectomy
Any age
Any body mass index
Male or female
Prior excisional biopsy
Before or after neoadjuvant therapy
May omit axillary dissection for patients with one or two positive sentinel lymph nodes

emits a signal that guides the surgeon to the SLN. The blue dye typically is injected in the operating room after the induction of anesthesia and is followed by 5 to 10 minutes of breast massage. SLNs are located by visual identification of a blue lymphatic tract or blue-stained node after making a small axillary incision. If the SLN is not identified, regardless of the technique used, a level I and II ALND should be performed. Previous work has shown that for most surgeons, especially when first using the procedure, the combination of blue dye and radiocolloid has the highest success rate in SLN identification and the lowest false-negative rate. However, many experienced surgeons are comfortable with and highly successful at using a single agent, with some of the highest reported success rates.

Numerous multi-institutional randomized studies were conducted to validate the SLNB procedure and compare its accuracy and safety with that of ALND. The first study was from Milan by Veronesi and colleagues, followed by the larger National Surgical Adjuvant Breast and Bowel Project (NSABP) B-32 trial that included 5611 women and other international trials. All studies confirm that an SLN can be identified in nearly all patients with clinically node-negative stage I or II breast cancer. All studies had similar trial design, randomizing patients with clinically node-negative invasive breast cancer to either SLNB followed by ALND or SLNB alone if the SLN was tumor free. No large studies show a significant difference between ALND and SLNB alone with respect to overall survival, disease-free survival (DFS), or regional control. More than 2 decades of experience with SLNB and prospective randomized trials with long follow-up have shown that SLNB is as safe, accurate, and effective with less morbidity than ALND for early clinically node-negative breast cancer.

Several factors determine the success rate of SLNB. These factors include patient selection, age, body mass index (BMI), injection technique, addition of massage, timing of incision, and surgeon experience. There is no consensus on the optimal injection technique.

Although many groups are proponents of peritumoral injections, others support intradermal or subareolar injection. Although controversy exists regarding the most appropriate technique for injection of blue dye or radiocolloid, individual experience and comfort with a particular technique are perhaps the most important factors in successful SLNB.

In the multi-institutional ACOSOG Z0010 trial, 198 surgeons enrolled 5237 patients and used blue dye with radiocolloid in 79.4% of cases, blue dye alone in 14.8%, and radiocolloid alone in 5.7%, with a success rate of identifying SLNs of 98.7%, corresponding to a failure rate of 1.3%. The percentage of failed SLNB with blue dye alone was 1.4%, radiocolloid alone was 2.3%, and a combination was 1.2% ($P = 0.28$), supporting the observation that each of these techniques is highly successful in experienced hands and no real difference in accuracy exists. Reliable staging with SLNB depends on the success of SNL identification, a low false-negative rate, and reliable histopathologic assessment of SLNs. ACOSOG Z0010 specifically investigated the significance of SLN immunohistochemically detected small metastases. The significance of micrometastasis and isolated tumor cells had been debated. The SLN was evaluated in a central laboratory and the results blinded to the physician and patient. The study showed that immunohistochemically detected metastasis to the SLN had no adverse prognostic implications compared with patients without immunohistochemically detected nodal disease. A similar evaluation of NSABP B-32 showed a minimal (1.2%) decreased overall survival rate in patients with "occult" SLN metastasis, some of which were macrometastasis. Both studies recommended against routine immunohistochemistry (IHC) nodal evaluation and felt that differences in survival were not significant enough to influence further treatment decisions.

■ AMERICAN COLLEGE OF SURGEONS ONCOLOGY GROUP Z0011 TRIAL

Several small retrospective studies reported the outcomes of patients with SLN metastasis treated without completion ALND with low nodal recurrence rates. The appropriate management of the axilla after a tumor-positive SLN was addressed prospectively in the ACOSOG Z0011 trial. This prospective phase III noninferiority trial randomized women with clinical T1 or T2 N0M0 breast cancer who had a tumor-positive SLN to completion ALND or observation of the axilla. All patients were treated with breast-conserving surgery (BCS), whole breast radiotherapy (RT), and postoperative adjuvant systemic therapy. The primary endpoint of this study was overall survival and the secondary endpoints were morbidity and DFS. Despite suggestive evidence supporting the need to question the necessity of axillary dissection in the current era, ACOSOG Z0011 was considered a radical and potentially dangerous study. Many large institutions and prominent surgeons and oncologists declined to participate, which resulted in slow accrual and early closure of the study because of poor accrual and low event rate. Only 47% of the targeted 1900 patients were entered, and a very low event rate was observed. Despite the early closure, the findings were highly statistically significant favoring the SLNB alone group and were not likely to change with additional accrual.

In brief, 891 clinically node-negative women with T1 or T2 cancer and a hematoxylin and eosin–detected SLN metastasis were enrolled from 115 sites; 445 were randomized to completion ALND, and 446 were randomized to no further axillary treatment. There was no significant difference between the two groups with respect to patient age, tumor size, estrogen receptor (ER) status, lymphovascular invasion (LVI), grade, or histology of the primary. However, the SLN alone group had slightly more patients with micrometastasis in the SLN. Ninety-seven percent of patients received adjuvant systemic therapy, reflecting practice patterns in the United States at the time. The two groups varied naturally by number of lymph nodes removed, with a median of 2 axillary nodes removed in the SLNB-only group compared with 17 in the ALND group ($P < 0.001$). Additional tumor-positive axillary nodes were found in 27% of the ALND patients, suggesting that the SLNB-only group had a similar number of patients with retained nodes that were not removed surgically. At a median follow-up of 6.3 years, there was no significant difference between the SLNB-only and SLNB plus ALND groups with respect to nodal (0.9% vs 0.5%), in-breast (1.9% vs 3.6%), or overall local-regional recurrence (2.8% vs 4.9%; $P = 0.53$). Neither DFS (83.9% vs 82.2%) nor overall survival (92.5% vs 91.9%) differed significantly between the groups. For patients meeting study criteria, the routine use of ALND after a finding of metastasis in the SLN is no longer justified. Noninferiority between the two arms was achieved with high statistical significance ($P < 0.008$), showing that SLNB alone is not inferior to ALND for these patients. These results may be explained by the inclusion of women with only one or two proven nodal metastases, the use of opposing tangent whole breast RT, systemic therapy, or the biology of early breast cancer. The fact that about one quarter of the SLNB-only patients probably had retained nodal disease with only about a 1% nodal recurrence rate suggests that these patients were treated with the adjuvant RT or systemic therapy. However, in the NSABP B-04 study, in which nodal disease was neither resected nor treated with any adjuvant therapy, only about half the expected number of patients developed nodal recurrence as a first event, suggesting that even in untreated patients not all nodal metastases progress and perhaps the biology of early breast cancer is relevant to the low recurrence rate.

Results of the ACOSOG Z0011 study created controversy, and many questioned whether radiation oncologists irradiated the axillary nodes in the SLNB-only group, even though axillary irradiation was prohibited in the protocol. A recent analysis of those patients who had detailed RT records available (n = 228) showed that most patients received tangential field RT alone, with no significant differences in tangential field height between the two study arms, and that 18.9% of patients received directed nodal irradiation in both arms via a third field, which was prohibited by study protocol. In addition, there was a subgroup of patients who received no RT at all. These findings have prompted the need for additional studies to evaluate whether certain patients might safely avoid RT and others might benefit from more extensive treatment.

In summary, patients with SLN metastasis who may avoid ALND are those with clinical T1 to T2 N0 breast cancer with one or two tumor-positive SLNs without significant extracapsular extension (ECE) who are treated with lumpectomy, whole breast irradiation, and systemic therapy. Node-positive patients in whom completion ALND still should be recommended include those who receive neoadjuvant therapy, those who have a tumor-positive SLN and are treated with mastectomy, those with three or more tumor-positive SLNs, those who do not receive adjuvant systemic therapy, those who undergo partial breast irradiation, and those who have clinically palpable nodes preoperatively. The Z0011 trial represents level I data that should result in clinical practice changes in appropriately selected

---

BOX 2: Applicability of ACOSOG Z0011

ALND Is Not Required for Patients Who Meet All of the Following Criteria:

T1 or T2 tumors
Clinically node negative (even if ultrasound node positive)
One or two positive SLNs without evidence of significant extracapsular extension
Patient agreement to complete whole breast radiation therapy
Patient agreement to complete adjuvant systemic therapy (cytotoxic, hormonal, or both)

ALND May Be Required for Patients Who:

Have T3 tumors
Have more than two positive SLNs
Have been identified as having matted axillary nodes or preoperatively palpable nodes
Are receiving neoadjuvant chemotherapy

ACOSOG, American College of Surgeons Oncology Group; *ALND*, axillary lymph node dissection; *SLN*, sentinel lymph node.

---

patients. Studies show that in the United States, between 60% and 85% of SLN-positive patients could be treated appropriately without ALND (Box 2).

■ INTERNATIONAL BREAST CANCER STUDY GROUP 23-01

The International Breast Cancer Study Group (IBCSG) completed a phase III randomized controlled trial to determine whether SLNB with no ALND was noninferior to ALND in patients with one or more micrometastatic (≤2 mm) SLNs and tumors up to 5 cm. At a median follow-up of 5 years, Galimberti and colleagues found no difference between the axillary dissection and no axillary dissection groups with respect to DFS. The IBCSG 23-01 results supported those of the ACOSOG Z0011 study and show that with minimal SLN involvement, axillary dissection is not warranted.

Sentinel Lymph Node Biopsy and Neoadjuvant Systemic Therapy

Considerable controversy exists about the use of SLNB after preoperative systemic therapy because of the possibility of nonuniform, selective "sterilization" of lymph nodes and the observed low SLN identification rate and high false-negative rate of SLNB. A false-negative SLNB still may be associated with lymph nodes that harbor metastatic disease, resulting in reduced accuracy and unacceptably high false-negative rates. Studies to date, however, do not support this theory and, overall, demonstrate similar accuracy and false-negative rates in patients treated with neoadjuvant chemotherapy compared with those untreated preoperatively, especially in patients with a clinically negative axilla before systemic therapy. One of the largest published studies evaluating SLNB after preoperative chemotherapy is the NSABP B-27 trial, in which 428 patients had SLNB followed by completion axillary dissection. SLNs were identified successfully in 85% and the false-negative rate was 11%. These rates were not unlike the initial studies of SLNB but probably not as good as contemporary experience. A meta-analysis of 21 published studies, which included 1273 patients who underwent SLNB with subsequent axillary dissection after preoperative chemotherapy, reported an SLN identification rate of 90% and a false-negative rate of 12%. These results are similar to reported data from the NSABP B-32 trial, which compared SLN resection with conventional ALND for patients with node-negative breast cancer. However, these neoadjuvant studies involved women with clinically negative nodes. Retrospective analysis of node-positive women continues to support the observation of low identification rates and high false-negative rates. These discrepancies led to two large prospective studies of the value of SLNB after neoadjuvant chemotherapy.

AMERICAN COLLEGE OF SURGEONS ONCOLOGY GROUP Z1071 AND SENTINA

The accuracy of SLNB in patients with axillary metastasis undergoing induction chemotherapy was evaluated by the ACOSOG Z1071 trial. The study investigated SLNB after neoadjuvant chemotherapy for patients with stage II, stage IIIA, and stage IIIB breast cancer who had documented biopsy-proven axillary lymph node metastases before systemic therapy. The trial incorporated the use of pre–systemic therapy axillary ultrasound (US); in the event of a suspicious axillary US, a fine-needle aspiration (FNA) or core biopsy was performed to document the presence of metastasis. All patients underwent SLNB followed by completion ALND after neoadjuvant chemotherapy. A total of 701 patients were evaluated, all of whom had biopsy-proven N1/2 disease at presentation. Identification of at least one SLN was successful in 92% of patients. The false-negative rate, however, was 12.6% (39 of 310 patients); this included only patients with cN1 disease. The rate decreased to 10.8% when blue dye plus radiocolloid was used, compared with 20.3% for single-agent use ($P = 0.05$). The prespecified endpoint was a false-negative rate of less than 10% in order to support SLNB after neoadjuvant chemotherapy. Because this rate was not reached, widespread use of SLNB after neoadjuvant chemotherapy in node-positive patients was not recommended. One factor identified in ACOSOG Z1071 as contributing to a higher false-negative rate was increased axillary fibrosis after neoadjuvant chemotherapy, which makes lymphatic drainage and surgical dissection more challenging. The authors concluded that changes in approach and patient selection would be necessary to support the use of SLNB as an alternative to ALND in this patient population. However, evaluation of the data showed that if three or more SLNs were removed using both dye and tracer, the false-negative rate fell to 9.1%, and many have accepted the use of SLNB after neoadjuvant chemotherapy when tracer and dye are used together and three or more SLNs are removed. Others feel that a false-negative rate of 9.1% is too high in contemporary breast cancer management, especially among women who did not respond completely to chemotherapy.

The Sentinel-Lymph-Node Biopsy in Patients With Breast Cancer Before and After Neoadjuvant Chemotherapy (SENTINA) trial was a European prospective, multicenter study assessing the optimum timing and accuracy of SLNB in patients undergoing neoadjuvant chemotherapy. Patients with clinical N0 disease (identified via palpation and US) underwent SLNB, followed by neoadjuvant chemotherapy (n = 1022). If the preoperative SLN had evidence of metastatic disease, the patients received chemotherapy and a second SLNB and completion ALND after neoadjuvant chemotherapy (n = 455). Patients with clinical N1/2 disease at presentation received neoadjuvant chemotherapy; if they were clinically node negative after neoadjuvant chemotherapy, they then underwent SLNB and completion ALND (n = 642). Among clinically node-negative patients who did not undergo neoadjuvant therapy, an SLN was identified in 99.1%, with 35% of these SLNs harboring metastatic disease. In patients in whom nodal metastasis was detected before neoadjuvant chemotherapy, the post–neoadjuvant chemotherapy SLNB identified the SLN in only 60.8%, with a false-negative rate of 51% (33 of 64). Patients who were clinically node positive and who converted to clinically node negative after neoadjuvant chemotherapy had a SLN detection rate of 80.1%, with a false-negative rate of 14.2% (32 of 226 patients). On multivariate analysis of this group, the false-negative rate decreased from 18.5% when two SLNs were removed to less than 10% when three or more SLNs were removed. From these two studies, the authors concluded that selection of patients who can be spared further regional treatment after neoadjuvant chemotherapy remains a clinical challenge. However, many use the data from SENTINA and ACOSOG Z1071 to support the accuracy of SLNB after neoadjuvant chemotherapy if three or more nodes are removed during SLNB.

AFTER MAPPING OF THE AXILLA: RADIOTHERAPY OR SURGERY STUDY

The use of extensive nodal irradiation as an alternative to ALND has been evaluated in breast cancer patients with clinically negative axilla. Older trials have demonstrated no survival benefit between patients who undergo axillary irradiation versus ALND. Because of the inherent loss of staging information without ALND, axillary irradiation in lieu of ALND has not been adopted into clinical practice. Although axillary radiation may be an alternative to ALND in women with clinically node-negative breast cancer, there are limited data regarding its utility in patients with nodal metastasis and undissected axillae. The European Organisation for Research and Treatment of Cancer (EORTC) After Mapping of the Axilla: Radiotherapy or Surgery (AMAROS) study randomized patients with positive SLNs to ALND versus axillary radiation, regardless of breast procedure (mastectomy or BCS) or size and number of positive SLNs. This noninferiority trial randomly assigned more than 1000 patients with clinically node-negative T1 or T2 breast cancer with positive SLNB to either completion ALND or nodal radiation to the axilla, supraclavicular space, and internal mammary chain. The study reported no significant difference in DFS or overall survival between patients undergoing ALND and those undergoing axillary radiotherapy; DFS was 86.9% versus 82.7%, respectively ($P = 0.18$), and 5-year overall survival was 93.3% versus 92.5%, respectively ($P = 0.34$). Although this information is helpful, none of the patients in the trial received neoadjuvant chemotherapy, and 71% of patients undergoing ALND had only one positive SLN, making it difficult to correlate findings to patients with residual disease after neoadjuvant chemotherapy. The question remains from this study whether nodal irradiation is necessary in all patients because the nodal recurrence rate was similar to that in ACOSOG Z0011 with SLND alone. The AMAROS study lacked a nonirradiated arm, which may have answered this question.

Currently, two ongoing sister studies are looking at axillary management after neoadjuvant chemotherapy. Alliance A11202 is a prospective, randomized study evaluating the role of ALND in patients with T1 to T3 N1M0 breast cancer who have SLN-positive disease after neoadjuvant chemotherapy. Specifically, radiotherapy to the breast or chest wall and nodes plus ALND is being compared with radiotherapy only in this patient population. NSABP B-51/Radiation Therapy Oncology Group (RTOG) 1304 is evaluating patients with node-positive disease at presentation who have a pathologic complete response (pCR) after neoadjuvant chemotherapy. Patients are randomly assigned to either axillary radiation or no radiation after SLNB shows complete resection of nodal disease. The aim of this trial is to evaluate whether the addition of chest wall and regional nodal radiation after mastectomy or BCS will decrease recurrence in patients converting from node positive to node negative after neoadjuvant chemotherapy. The results of these studies will assist in clarifying appropriate axillary management after neoadjuvant chemotherapy. SLNB, a simple surgical procedure, has greatly altered the management of patients with early breast cancer by minimizing morbidity without compromising outcome.

SUGGESTED READINGS

Boughey JC, Suman VJ, Mittendorf EA, et al. Alliance for Clinical Trials in Oncology: sentinel lymph node surgery after neoadjuvant chemotherapy in patients with node-positive breast cancer: the ACOSOG Z1071 (Alliance) clinical trial. *JAMA*. 2013;310:1455-1461.

Giuliano AE, Hawes D, Ballman KV, et al. Association of occult metastases in
sentinel lymph nodes and bone marrow with survival among women with
early-stage invasive breast cancer. *JAMA*. 2011;306:385-393.

Giuliano AE, Hunt KK, Ballman KV, et al. Axillary dissection vs no axillary
dissection in women with invasive breast cancer and sentinel node metastasis: a randomized clinical trial. *JAMA*. 2011;305:569-575.

Giuliano AE, Jones RC, Brennan M, et al. Sentinel lymphadenectomy in breast
cancer. *J Clin Oncol*. 1997;15:2345-2350.

Hansen NM, Grube B, Ye X, et al. Impact of micrometastases in the sentinel
node of patients with invasive breast cancer. *J Clin Oncol*. 2009;27:
4679-4684.

Krag DN, Anderson SJ, Julian TB, et al. Sentinel-lymph-node resection compared with conventional axillary lymph node dissection in clinically node-
negative patients with breast cancer: overall survival findings from the
NSABP B-32 randomised phase 3 trial. *Lancet Oncol*. 2011;11:927-933.

Veronesi U, Viale G, Paganelli G, et al. Sentinel lymph node biopsy in breast
cancer: ten-year results of a randomized controlled study. *Ann Surg*.
2010;251:595-600.

Weaver DL, Ashikaga T, Krag DN, et al. Effect of occult metastases on survival
in node-negative breast cancer. *N Engl J Med*. 2011;364:412-421.

The Management of the Axilla in Breast Cancer

Damian McCartan, MD, and Mary L. Gemignani, MD

ANATOMY

Understanding the surgical anatomy of the axilla is critical to enabling
the surgeon to achieve a complete lymphadenectomy and in minimizing morbidity from injury to recognizable soft tissue structures.
The pectoralis major and minor muscles form the anterior boundary
of the axilla, whereas the posterior boundary is the subscapularis
muscle. Medially, the serratus anterior overlies the first four ribs and
intercostal muscles. The lateral boundary of the axilla is defined by
the anterior border of the latissimus dorsi muscle. The axilla is
covered by axillary fascia, which acts like a tent to cover the axillary
contents and overlies the insertion of the coracobrachialis and biceps
tendons.

The two important nerves in the medial axilla are the thoracodorsal nerve that supplies the latissimus dorsi and the long thoracic
nerve that innervates the serratus anterior. The thoracodorsal arises
medial to the subscapular vessels beneath the axillary vein. The nerve
crosses to lie in front of the thoracodorsal artery in its descent before
penetrating the latissimus dorsi muscle. Variants have described the
thoracodorsal nerve passing posterior to the subscapular vessels and
remaining posterior or medial until its insertion in up to 5% of
patients. The long thoracic nerve runs in a craniocaudal superficial
location on serratus anterior on the medial wall of the axilla. Injury
to the long thoracic nerve presents with severe burning or stabbing
shoulder pain that usually subsides, to be followed by evidence of
weakness resulting in the classical angel wing deformity.

For classification of lymph node stations within the axilla, the
description of three axillary levels defined by the pectoralis minor
muscle prevails. Level I nodes are those lateral to the lateral border
of pectoralis minor, whereas level II nodes lie behind the muscle and
level III nodes are medial to the medial border of pectoralis minor
to Halsted's ligament. Numerically, the largest proportion of lymph
nodes is found in levels I and II, with an average yield of 15 to
20 nodes, compared with an average of four nodes at level III. Axillary
nodes receive lymph from all quadrants of the breast.

HISTORICAL PERSPECTIVE

In the nineteenth century, Halsted described the importance of the
removal of the axillary contents in reducing rates of local recurrence. His influences included Kuster in Berlin, who systematically
resected even nonpalpable axillary nodes. This radical approach to
local-regional control persisted through the first half of the twentieth
century, with 5-year survival rates of 35% to 45% commonly
reported. One of the first challenges to this radical approach was
heralded in 1948 with a report from Scotland that substituted radiotherapy for surgery in axillary treatment, recognizing that when the
axilla is not involved with disease, it appears unnecessary to carry
out an axillary dissection.

IMPORTANCE TO STAGING

While Halsted and his contemporaries recognized the propensity for
axillary nodal involvement in patients with breast cancer, firm evidence for the prognostic significance of axillary nodal metastases was
provided in 1970. Follow-up of patients treated at the Mayo Clinic
identified axillary nodal involvement as the main determinant in
survival, with 5-year survival rates of 86% in node-negative patients
compared with 50% in node-positive patients.

SURGERY

Axillary Lymph Node Dissection

A standard axillary lymph node dissection (ALND) involves removal
of the level I and II axillary nodes. A level III lymphadenectomy may
be performed when gross disease is encountered at level II. The
patient should be positioned supine with the arm placed on a board
and abducted to 90 degrees. In patients undergoing mastectomy, the
axillary dissection can proceed through the mastectomy incision.
Nonetheless, increasing rates of both skin-sparing and nipple-sparing
mastectomy may necessitate a separate axillary incision to facilitate
adequate axillary access. A curved incision, convex upward, is made
just below the hair-bearing area of the axilla. The initial approach
should raise an anterior and posterior skin flap. As the flap is continued medially, the axillary contents are freed from the pectoralis
major and minor. The angular vein, a tributary of the subscapular
vein, is a constant finding in the majority of axillary dissections that
serves as a surrogate for the caudal extent of dissection. At this level,
the anterior muscle fibers of latissimus dorsi are seen, and the lateral
edge of the muscle can be freed in a cranial direction. The intercostobrachial nerve crosses the lateral border of latissimus dorsi 1 to
2 cm below the axillary vein. The clavipectoral fascia is divided followed by gentle dissection to expose the axillary vein.

Before commencing dissection of the level I or II nodes, the
surgeon must identify the thoracodorsal and long thoracic nerves.
Once the thoracodorsal nerve has been identified, the more antero-
laterally placed lateral thoracic vein can be ligated and divided. Dissection then can continue along the inferior surface of the axillary
vein, extending medially to identify the medial pectoral nerve. Elevation of the arm improves visualization of level II and allows nodes
at this level to be carefully swept down. Once freed from the tributaries of the medial pectoral vessels, the axillary contents can be mobilized caudally, observing at all times the thoracodorsal and long

thoracic nerves until reaching the already established point of distal dissection. After hemostasis has been secured, the cavity is irrigated and a suction drain (e.g., Jackson-Pratt) inserted. When performed as a modified radical mastectomy, the lymph node dissection is en bloc with the breast specimen. The same principles apply with regard to identification of latissimus dorsi and pectoralis muscles, followed by the axillary vein and then the long thoracic and thoracodorsal nerves.

Sentinel Lymph Node Biopsy

This technique allows for the identification of the first node(s) within a tumor's lymphatic basin. The lowest false-negative and nonidentification rates have been reported with the use of blue dye and a radiocolloid (technetium-99m) in combination. Recently, proponents of a single modality approach have reported success of each technique in isolation. The use of blue dye alone obviates the need for any additional equipment or procedures, albeit there is a risk of serious allergic reactions. A subareolar injection of either tracer has become the favored technique. Both superficial (subareolar, periareolar, deep dermal, and intradermal) and deep (peritumoral or intratumoral) injections of radiocolloid and blue dye are effective for identification of axillary sentinel nodes. The use of a deep injection technique is associated with a higher rate of identification of extraaxillary sentinel nodes.

■ INVASIVE BREAST CANCER, CLINICALLY NODE NEGATIVE

The accuracy and safety of sentinel lymph node biopsy (SLNB) in breast cancer patients with no clinical evidence of nodal metastases has been validated extensively through a wide range of studies, including six randomized trials. In clinically node-negative patients who have a negative SLNB, these trials all demonstrated low rates (≤1.2%) of axillary recurrence in patients with a negative SLNB who had no further surgery. The management of patients with pathologically confirmed sentinel node metastases has evolved, and a one-size-fits-all approach no longer applies.

The largest study to compare SLNB and ALND with regard to survival and regional control was the National Surgical Adjuvant Breast and Bowel Project (NSABP) B-32 trial. Clinically node negative women were assigned to SLNB plus ALND or to SLNB alone with ALND only if the sentinel node(s) were positive. The sentinel node was identified in 97% of patients. The study substantiated previous reports of reduced arm morbidity after SLNB alone when compared with ALND. The final outcomes data reported in 2010 concluded that the 8-year overall and disease-free survival did not differ substantially between the two groups. Axillary recurrence as a first disease relapse event was seen in less than 1% of both the SLNB followed by ALND dissection group and in patients who underwent SNLB only.

Micrometastases (N1m1), Isolated Tumor Cells (IHC Only) N0 [1+]

The advent of SLNB allowed more detailed pathologic assessment of the smaller number of removed nodes. The serial sectioning of individual nodes combined with the use of immunohistochemistry (IHC) stains in addition to routine hematoxylin and eosin (H&E) enabled identification of smaller tumor deposits. These smaller nodal deposits are classified in the seventh edition of the *American Joint Committee on Cancer Staging Manual* as:

■ pN0 (i+): Malignant cells in regional lymph node(s) no greater than 0.2 mm (H&E or IHC)
■ pN0(mol+): Positive pCR but no regional lymph node metastases detected by histology or IHC

■ pN1mi: Micrometastases (>0.2 mm and/or more than 200 cells, but none greater than 2.0 mm)

After recognition of these smaller nodal deposits, initial guidelines recommended a completion ALND. However, recent studies have shown that with modern adjuvant therapy regimens, additional surgical treatment of the axilla confers no advantage. Nodal specimens from initially SLNB negative patients from the NSABP B-32 trial were submitted for central pathology review. The nodes underwent further sectioning and were evaluated for occult metastases with H&E and IHC. Clusters of isolated tumor cells (ITCs) were identified in 11%, and a further 4% contained micrometastases. At 5 years' follow-up, the absolute reduction in overall survival in patients with occult metastases, although of statistical significance, was only 1.2%. The presence of micrometastases conferred a greater effect on this marginally worse outcome than the finding of ITCs. Women who underwent an SLNB plus ALND did not have any survival advantage over patients undergoing SLNB alone.

American College of Surgeons Oncology Group (ACOSOG) Z0010 Trial

The ACOSOG Z0010 study recruited women with clinical T1-T2, node-negative breast cancer undergoing breast-conserving surgery with SLNB followed by whole-breast irradiation. Occult sentinel node metastases were identified in 10.5% of patients. No difference in overall or disease-free survival was noted between patients with negative sentinel nodes compared with those with immunohistochemistry-positive occult metastases. Five-year overall survival rates exceeded 95% in both groups. The majority of patients received adjuvant systemic therapy in addition to whole-breast irradiation. In both the Z0010 study and the NSABP B-32 trials, decisions regarding adjuvant systemic therapy were taken independently of results of the sentinel node IHC analysis. This supports current practice, whereby decisions regarding adjuvant systemic therapy reflect consideration of biologic or molecular factors associated with the primary tumor rather than solely on the basis of occult sentinel nodal metastases.

International Breast Cancer Study Group Trial 23-01

In the International Breast Cancer Study Group (IBCSG) 23-01 trial, clinically node-negative patients with an SLNB containing micrometastases were randomized to completion ALND or no further axillary surgery. The majority of patients had small breast cancers (92% <3 cm), underwent breast-conserving surgery (91%), and received adjuvant systemic treatment (96%). Additional involved axillary nodes were found in 13% of patients who had a completion ALND. However, 5-year disease-free survival did not significantly differ in the SLNB alone (87.8%) versus the ALND (84.4%) group. In patients who did not undergo ALND, the rate of disease recurrence in the undissected axilla was less than 1%.

Taken in conjunction, the findings of these three multicenter trials confirm that patients in whom occult sentinel lymph node metastases (<2.0 mm) are identified do not require completion ALND and that decisions pertaining to further systemic therapy should not be based exclusively on the finding of sentinel node micrometastases or ITCs.

Macrometastases (N1)

Lymph node macrometastases are tumor deposits larger than 2.0 mm. Patients in whom macrometastases are identified traditionally have been treated by subsequent completion ALND or axillary radiotherapy. The observations in the above trials of excellent outcomes with a multimodal approach to breast cancer treatment with less emphasis on axillary surgery called into question the need for completion ALND in certain patients with sentinel node macrometastases.

This question underpinned the visionary ACOSOG Z0011 trial that recruited patients between 1999 and 2004. Eligible patients had T1 to T2, clinically node-negative breast cancer, and were undergoing breast-conserving surgery and SLNB. All patients had a positive SLNB by routine H&E staining (not IHC) and were randomized to completion ALND or no ALND and no further axillary-specific radiotherapy. Patients with three or more positive sentinel nodes were excluded. Lower-than-expected accrual and event rates resulted in the early closure of the trial, with a final cohort of 813 patients. All patients received whole-breast irradiation, and almost all received adjuvant systemic therapy (58% chemotherapy, 46% hormonal therapy). Forty-one percent of the study patients ultimately were determined to have small volume metastases (micrometastases or ITCs). In the completion ALND group, additional positive axillary nodes were found in 27% of cases. Discussion has focused on the radiotherapy field design. The trial authors acknowledged that the opposing tangential field whole-breast irradiation used in both groups culminated in a portion of the axilla receiving radiotherapy in patients on both study arms. Further analysis has shown that there was no significant difference between treatment arms in the use of protocol-prohibited nodal fields. After a 6-year median follow-up, there were no differences between the SLNB followed by completion ALND- and SLNB-only groups in the rates of axillary (0.5% vs 0.9%), breast (3.6% vs 1.9%), or overall locoregional recurrence (4.1% vs 2.8%). The ACOSOG Z0011 trial has had a major impact on contemporary breast surgical oncology. It has been accepted that in patients with tumors 5 cm or less and no clinically suspicious axillary lymph nodes, undergoing breast-conserving surgery with subsequent whole-breast irradiation and systemic therapy, omitting completion ALND in the setting of two or fewer metastatic lymph nodes on SLNB does not increase the risk of axillary recurrence. This is reflected in the most recent National Comprehensive Cancer Network (NCCN) guidelines, which allow for no further surgery in patients with a positive SLNB who meet all of the Z0011 criteria.

In patients undergoing a mastectomy who have a positive SLNB with macrometastases, no such strategy to omit further axillary treatment exists. It is worth revisiting the NSABP B-04, started in 1971, that examined clinically node-negative participants in one arm. Patients were randomized to receive radical mastectomy (removal of the breast, level I and II axillary nodes as well as pectoralis major and minor muscles), total mastectomy with axillary radiation, or total mastectomy alone. In the patients who did not undergo axillary dissection, the risk of developing axillary node metastases was 18.6%. Patients who subsequently developed palpable axillary node metastases underwent completion ALND with no inferior outcome in overall survival at 25 years ($P = 0.68$).

Radiotherapy Trials

AMAROS Trial

Radiotherapy has been validated as an effective primary therapeutic modality for treating the axilla in clinically node-negative patients. A number of studies that predate the routine use of SLNB for axillary staging reported rates of axillary recurrence of only 1% to 2% in clinically node-negative patients with long-term follow-up. The AMAROS trial was a noninferiority trial designed to determine if axillary radiotherapy resulted in comparable survival outcomes with ALND in patients with a positive SLNB. Patients with a unifocal primary tumor up to 3 cm (expanded to 5 cm in the final 2 years of enrollment) and no palpable lymphadenopathy were eligible. Patients were randomly assigned to ALND (level I and II clearance) or axillary radiotherapy (50Gy to axillary levels I to III and medial supraclavicular fossa) before SLNB was performed. The majority (82%) of the 1425 patients underwent breast-conserving surgery, and 60% of

patients in both arms had a sentinel node macrometastasis. The number of axillary recurrence events was lower than anticipated. Rates of lymphedema were lower in the axillary radiotherapy group, although no clinically relevant difference was noted in patient-reported arm symptoms between the two groups. Five-year axillary recurrence rates (0.4% ALND vs 1.2% axillary radiotherapy), disease-free survival (87% ALND vs 83% axillary radiotherapy), and overall survival (93% ALND vs 93% axillary radiotherapy) were comparable between the two groups. Accepting that 77% of patients in the AMAROS trial had only one positive sentinel lymph node, in light of the findings from the ACOSOG Z011 trial, it must be acknowledged that in these patients with low-volume disease many may not have required additional axillary specific treatment. Caution must be taken in extrapolating the findings to patients at higher risk of locoregional failure.

MA.20

The efficacy of nodal irradiation acted as the premise for the NCIC Clinical Trials Group MA.20 trial. In women with early stage breast cancer who completed breast-conserving surgery, investigators compared whole-breast irradiation plus regional nodal irradiation with whole-breast irradiation alone. The cohort included patients with positive axillary lymph nodes (majority with one to three nodes involved) or negative axillary nodes (10%), but with high-risk features such as large tumor size or lymphovascular invasion. The additional regional nodal irradiation targeted the ipsilateral internal mammary lymph nodes and the supraclavicular and axillary lymph nodes. Most patients received adjuvant chemotherapy (91%) and/or endocrine therapy (76%). Ten-year overall and breast-cancer–specific survival rates were equivocal. The nodal irradiation group had a marginally lower rate of isolated locoregional recurrence (4.8% vs 7.8%). The absolute regional recurrence rate was 2.5% in the group that did not undergo nodal irradiation. Regional nodal irradiation generally was well tolerated but did confer greater risks of lymphedema. Although some patients will benefit from comprehensive nodal irradiation after ALND, the challenge remains to accurately differentiate those at low risk of locoregional failure who do not stand to benefit from further nodal treatment from high-risk patients. Traditional clinic-pathologic factors such as metastases to four or more lymph nodes, extracapsular nodal extension, or substantial lymphovascular invasion may help these decisions, but it is likely that genomic profiling will serve as a more robust predictor of locoregional failure. Analysis of locoregional recurrence in pN0, ER positive patients recruited to the NSABP B-14 and NSABP B-20 trials whose tumors were characterized by the 21-Gene Recurrence Score Assay suggested that the efficacy of radiation therapy may not be uniform across the three recurrence score categories but that radiation may indeed be more effective with a higher recurrence score.

■ INVASIVE BREAST CANCER, CLINICALLY NODE POSITIVE

Multiple studies have shown that ALND provides excellent regional control, with reported long-term rates of isolated axillary recurrence of less than 4%. This excellent regional control does not necessarily translate to improvements in overall survival. Multiple trials of clinically node-negative patients beginning with NSABP B-04 and including the trials that validated SLNB did not demonstrate any overall survival benefit conferred by ALND. To date, no data are available assessing survival in women with clinically palpable nodes randomized to a no-axillary-intervention group.

A subset of the NSABP B-04 trial examined the outcomes for patients with clinically positive nodes. Patients were randomized to receive radical mastectomy or total mastectomy with radiation therapy and no ALND. The rate of axillary recurrence in the radical mastectomy group was 1% compared with 8% in the group with no ALND and axillary radiotherapy, but there was no statistically significant difference in overall rates of locoregional recurrence. The majority of breast cancer-related events were distant recurrences, even in women with node-positive disease.

Axillary surgery can result in postoperative shoulder and arm morbidity. Participants in the ALMANAC trial reported high rates of reduced shoulder flexion and abduction at 1 month postoperatively, but the majority had returned to near baseline at 1 year. Symptoms of arm pain or numbness are more persistent with almost one third of patients reporting some degree of pain or numbness at 1 year. These symptoms are severe in only a minority of cases. Lymphedema following ALND remains one of the most feared complications. Reported rates vary between 11% and 20% based on recent trial data from studies such as ACOSOG Z0011 and the ALMANAC study.

In identification of patients who are clinically node positive, the AJCC definition of clinically detected is "detected by imaging studies or by clinical examination." Increasingly, axillary ultrasound (US) combined with US-guided lymph node biopsy (core or FNA) is used as an adjunct in assessment of axillary lymph nodes. Establishing axillary nodal positivity preoperatively will select patients with axillary metastases who can proceed to ALND immediately without SLNB. The sensitivity of axillary US for identifying involved axillary nodes is 50%, with a false-negative rate of 25%. A judicious use of and interpretation of US-guided axillary staging is required when deciding on the subsequent surgical management of the axilla in light of results of the ACOSOG Z0011 trial, which established that further treatment is not required in certain patients with one or two positive axillary nodes.

NEOADJUVANT CHEMOTHERAPY

Initially introduced for locally advanced breast cancer, the indications for neoadjuvant chemotherapy have expanded, motivated by a steady rise in pathologic complete response (pCR) rates and the success of targeted treatments directed against HER2. In essence, neoadjuvant chemotherapy should be considered in any patient for whom adjuvant chemotherapy is indicated. The NCCN advocates a fundamental role for axillary US in patients selected for neoadjuvant systemic therapy both for clinically node-positive patients to allow confirmatory biopsy and for clinically node-negative patients recommending sampling by FNA or core biopsy of suspicious nodes. Feasibility has been proven for the use of US-guided placement of a clip to mark biopsy-confirmed metastatic axillary node(s) before the commencement of neoadjuvant therapy. This ensures removal of the biopsy-positive node at the time of surgery to confirm the presence or absence of a treatment response. A variety of localization techniques have been used to guide the surgeon in selectively removing these clip-containing lymph nodes at the time of axillary surgery.

Downstaging Axilla

There is ample evidence that neoadjuvant chemotherapy downstages involved axillary lymph nodes in a substantial proportion of patients. Up to 40% of patients will convert from biopsy-confirmed node positive to node negative (ypN0). In the NSABP B-18 trial, of whom one quarter of participants were initially clinically node positive, the rate of finding positive axillary nodes at time of surgery was 57% in the group who received adjuvant systemic therapy compared with 41% in the neoadjuvant cohort.

The NSABP B-27 trial contains the largest series examining the practicality of performing SLNB after neoadjuvant chemotherapy. This multicenter trial included clinically node-negative patients and those with positive but mobile axillary nodes (cN1). Eighteen percent of patients had an attempt at SLNB, and 75% of these were clinically node negative before therapy. An SLNB was successfully identified in 85% (false-negative rate: 11%). This trial accrued between 1995 and 2000, and a trend was noted toward improved identification rates in later study years and for surgeons who had performed a greater number of SLNB procedures. The results identified improved detection rates when both radiocolloid and blue dye were used in conjunction, findings that have been replicated in contemporary studies examining the feasibility and accuracy of SLNB post neoadjuvant therapy.

The ACOSOG Z1071 trial enrolled women with histologically proven clinical stage T0-T4, N1, or N2 breast cancer. The primary aim was to determine the false-negative rate of SLNB in patients with clinically node-positive disease who received neoadjuvant chemotherapy. The majority of patients had mobile (cN1) disease at presentation, and, after neoadjuvant treatment, more than 80% of these had no residual palpable axillary nodes. The study protocol stipulated that at least two sentinel nodes be removed, after which a completion ALND was performed. Although 93% of patients had at least one sentinel node identified, 79% met the criteria for removal of two sentinel nodes and had a completion ALND. The false-negative rate in cN1 patients who had at least two sentinel nodes removed was 12.6%. A reduction in the false-negative rate was evident as the number of sentinel nodes removed increased: 31%, one node; 21%, two nodes; dropping to a clinically acceptable 9% only when three or more nodes were removed. The false-negative rate was also lower (11%) when both blue dye and radiocolloid were used for mapping.

The SENTINA (sentinel neoadjuvant) trial enrolled both clinically node-negative and node-positive patients before neoadjuvant chemotherapy. One of the four arms examined initially clinically node-positive patients who reverted to clinically node negative after neoadjuvant treatment. These patients received a postneoadjuvant SLNB followed by completion ALND. Unlike the Z1071 trial, the most common modality for lymph node mapping was the use of radiocolloid alone. The overall sentinel node detection rate was only 80%, with a false-negative rate of 14%. Just like in ACOSOG Z1071, the false-negative rate varied according to the number of sentinel nodes removed: 24%, one node; 18%, two nodes; and less than 8% when three or more nodes were removed.

For SLNB after neoadjuvant chemotherapy to be considered a safe and viable strategy in the pretreatment of clinically node-positive patients, the current advice is to employ dual modality mapping and to attempt to identify three sentinel nodes, a challenge given that in the NSABP B-32 and other large prospective trials of SLNB, the median number of identified sentinel nodes was two.

Persistent Clinically Positive Axilla

Even with improvements in pCR rates, most patients with clinically positive axillary adenopathy will have residual axillary disease after neoadjuvant chemotherapy. Residual nodal disease outside of the sentinel node(s) was found in 39% of patients in the Z1071 trial and in 42% of pretreatment clinically node-positive patients who reverted to clinically node negative after chemotherapy in the SENTINA trial. In the absence of long-term data pertaining to survival and regional recurrence, the implications of residual axillary disease after neoadjuvant chemotherapy in clinically node-positive patients who do not receive a completion ALND are unknown. Outside of a clinical trial, the standard surgical approach to patients with residual axillary disease is completion ALND.

The prognostic implications of clinically node-positive patients who received neoadjuvant chemotherapy and who remain pathologically node positive have been demonstrated in an updated analysis of NSABP B-18 and B-27 neoadjuvant trials. These patients experienced high rates of locoregional recurrence after ALND: 15% to 22% after breast-conserving surgery and whole-breast irradiation, and 17% to 22% after mastectomy. This high locoregional failure rate suggests that these patients may benefit from adjuvant regional nodal radiotherapy in addition to any planned whole-breast or postmastectomy chest-wall radiotherapy. Additional nodal irradiation traditionally is recommended for all patients with at least four involved axillary lymph nodes and in selected patients with one to three involved nodes with additional adverse prognostic features, such as young age, high tumor grade, or extensive lymphovascular invasion. The targeted nodal areas are those of the nondissected axilla and supraclavicular nodes. Although reductions in rates of locoregional recurrence have been validated in a number of clinical trials, the results also reveal that the addition of regional nodal radiotherapy to planned whole-breast or chest wall radiotherapy increases the morbidity associated with ALND with rates of lymphedema of up to 28%.

Whether axillary radiotherapy will provide comparable regional control to ALND in patients who remain node positive after neoadjuvant chemotherapy is the focus for the Alliance for Clinical Trials in Oncology A11202 study. This randomized trial is evaluating the role of completion ALND in patients with clinical T1-T3 N1 M0 breast cancer who have a positive SLNB after neoadjuvant therapy. SLNB-positive patients are randomized to either completion ALND followed by nodal irradiation (undissected axilla, supraclavicular nodes, and internal mammary nodes) or to no further axillary surgery followed by radiotherapy to the full axilla, supraclavicular nodes, and internal mammary nodes. The primary outcome is breast cancer recurrence-free survival.

OCCULT BREAST CANCER PRESENTING WITH AXILLARY METASTASES

Extent of Disease Evaluation

Occult primary breast cancer, in which patients present with adenocarcinoma in axillary lymph nodes and have no evident primary breast lesion, accounts for 0.1% to 0.8% of all newly diagnosed breast cancers. Benign conditions account for many cases of palpable axillary nodes, and other malignancies such as lymphoma and melanoma can by accompanied by axillary adenopathy. The first step in evaluation of such a patient involves a biopsy of the involved node for pathologic assessment with a range of immunohistochemistry stains to confirm that the tumor is of breast origin (ER, PR, HER2, cytokeratins 7 and 20, mammaglobin, CEA, and CA125). Patients with axillary metastases should undergo a staging workup with a diagnostic chest, abdominal, and pelvis CT, and bone scan or fluorodeoxyglucose (FDG) positron emission tomography (PET)/CT to rule out distant metastases.

Magnetic Resonance Imaging

Before the introduction of breast magnetic resonance imaging (MRI), patients who proceeded to mastectomy on the premise of axillary nodal metastases with a mammographic and sonographic occult breast cancer, a breast primary was found in approximately 60% of cases on histologic review. Bilateral breast MRI is now the standard approach to breast evaluation in such patients and detects a primary breast cancer in approximately 75% of women with a normal breast clinical examination and mammogram. Because of the low specificity of lesions detected by breast MRI, these lesions should be subject to MRI or US guided—if a correlate is identifiable—biopsy for histologic confirmation. Accurate localization of the primary breast lesion may facilitate breast-conserving surgery in some of these patients.

Consideration for Completion ALND Versus Neoadjuvant Chemotherapy

The management of axillary disease in this setting is ALND. In patients with clinically fixed or matted axillary nodes (clinical stage N2), neoadjuvant systemic treatment should be considered, particularly taking into consideration the receptor profile. Optimal management of the ipsilateral breast in patients for whom, even after MRI, no primary breast lesion has been identified, is controversial. Trials have demonstrated lower rates of locoregional recurrence and

overall survival with mastectomy when compared with those who do not receive breast surgery. Whole-breast radiotherapy is a breast-conserving alternative to mastectomy with small retrospective reports reporting low rates of locoregional relapse and comparative survival to patients who underwent a mastectomy.

LOCALLY RECURRENT DISEASE TO AXILLA

Extent of Disease Evaluation

Long-term follow-up of both pathologically node-negative and pathologically node-positive patients has shown that overall isolated axillary recurrence rates are low. However, axillary recurrence can severely negatively affect a patient's quality of life. Overall survival rates from time of axillary recurrence of 60% at 5 years and 45% at 10 years have been reported. Any patient who presents with recurrent axillary disease should undergo full systemic staging (CT chest, abdomen, and pelvis plus bone scan or a FDG PET/CT) because of the risk of synchronous, clinically occult distant metastases.

Consideration for Completion Axillary Lymph Node Dissection

Core biopsy of the recurrent axillary disease, and assessment of ER, PR, and HER2 receptor status is required to examine for evidence of discordance when compared with the primary tumor because this may influence decisions regarding additional systemic therapy. If deemed amenable to surgical resection, isolated mobile axillary recurrences should be excised and combined with a level III axillary dissection if not already performed. Patients with inoperable axillary recurrence such as supraclavicular nodes may be considered for radiotherapy if not already administered as part of the primary treatment or systemic chemotherapy, or a combination of both. These nonoperative approaches rarely produce long-lasting control of disease but may help with palliation.

SPECIAL CASES AND MANAGEMENT OF THE AXILLA

Ductal Carcinoma in Situ

In patients with pure DCIS, there theoretically should be no risk of lymph node metastases and hence no role for axillary staging. However, in patients proceeding to surgery with a breast core-needle biopsy diagnosis of DCIS, there is a risk of being upstaged to invasive cancer upon pathologic assessment of the resected breast specimen. The current rate of upstaging to either microinvasion or invasive cancer is approximately 15%. There is a consensus that for patients undergoing a mastectomy for the surgical treatment of DCIS because of either disease extent or patient preference, an SLNB should be performed at the time of surgery in the event that final histology reveals invasive disease, at which point an SLNB would not be feasible. There is less agreement in selecting patients with DCIS who are undergoing breast-conserving surgery who may require an SLNB. A variety of nomograms have been proposed to stratify those at higher risk of upstaging to invasive disease after breast-conserving surgery. Factors such as the presence of a palpable mass with a diagnosis of DCIS are associated with higher rates of upstaging and accepted as an indication for an SLNB. Other cases should be managed on an individual basis remembering that although associated with lower rates of morbidity than ALND, the morbidity from SLNB is not zero. Even in patients upstaged to microinvasion, the risk of sentinel node metastases is only 1%.

Elderly

In certain patients with breast cancer, an SLNB can be omitted if the nodal information will not affect adjuvant treatment decisions. In medically fit older women, standard breast cancer surgery options should be offered. For older women with clinically positive axillary adenopathy who are deemed surgical candidates, ALND is appropriate, whereas axillary radiation can be considered for those felt not to be surgical candidates. In patients who are clinically node negative and who proceed to surgery for treatment of the breast, an SLNB is not always necessary. Ten-year follow-up of women more than 70 years of age with a stage T1, ER-positive breast cancer and clinically negative axilla who underwent lumpectomy and received adjuvant tamoxifen showed low rates of locoregional recurrence in both the groups that did receive radiotherapy (98%) and those that did not (90%).

Reoperative Sentinel Lymph Node Biopsy

In patients who develop an in-breast tumor recurrence after lumpectomy and SLNB, ALND commonly is still used as the standard axillary staging procedure in the belief that the initial surgery will alter the pattern of lymphatic drainage, rendering a repeat SLNB neither feasible nor accurate. Multiple case reports, small case series, and six retrospective studies with more than 15 reoperative cases have demonstrated a variable rate of success for reoperative SLNB ranging from 72% to 93%. Sentinel nodes outside of the ipsilateral axilla are identified in 8% of patients; therefore routine preoperative lymphoscintigraphy is advised. In patients who have had a previous ALND, attempts at axillary re-staging through use of SLNB demonstrate success rates of only 50%.

Pregnancy

Although some guidelines still suggest SLNB should not be performed during pregnancy, there are mounting clinical and preclinical data to suggest that the procedure can be performed safely.

Blue Dye Generally Avoided Because of Anaphylaxis

Blue dye as a mapping agent in pregnant patients is not an option because of the low (1%) but potentially very harmful underlying risk of a maternal anaphylactic reaction as well as very limited data on potential teratogenic effects of the agents used.

Multiple Newer Studies Looking at Safety of Technetium

Although the radiocolloids used for sentinel node mapping do emit a radiation dose, the administration of the agent is locoregional as opposed to systemic, and studies have demonstrated that the doses absorbed by the fetus are less than the limit for a pregnant woman. It is advisable to inject the technetium radiocolloid on the morning of surgery to minimize radiation exposure.

■ FUTURE DIRECTIONS

Buoyed by evidence from multi-institutional randomized clinical trials, the last two decades have witnessed remarkable and practice-changing advances in our approach to the axilla. However, the landscape continues to evolve. Surgery for the axilla for staging purposes is susceptible to improvements in preoperative imaging and more accurate predictive gene expression signatures, whereas the role of surgical treatment for confirmed nodal metastases may be assailable by advances in radiotherapy. Treatment selection for the individual patient is the key issue.

The introduction of national breast cancer screening programs, in various guises, across the globe has resulted in more breast cancer cases being diagnosed at an earlier stage. In patients with early breast cancer and a low probability of axillary nodal metastases coupled with excellent long-term survival outcomes based on current adjuvant therapy regimens, the need for SLNB to stage the axilla has been called into question. The SOUND trial (sentinel node vs observation after axillary US [commenced 2012]) hypothesizes that in patients with a low burden of axillary disease, the results of SLNB are unlikely

to alter adjuvant treatment decisions. Recruited patients with clinical T1 breast cancer and a negative axillary US will be randomized to either (1) SLNB ± axillary dissection or (2) no axillary surgical staging. The primary endpoint is distant disease-free survival.

The advent of validated gene expression profiles promises more accurate prognostication and better predictions of response to adjuvant therapy than conventional clinic-pathologic factors. The MINDACT (microarray in node-negative and 1 to 3 node-positive disease may avoid chemotherapy) and SWOG RxPONDER Trials (S1007) are assessing the ability of gene expression profiling to accurately identify patients with favorable tumor characteristics with excellent predicted long-term survival with adjuvant hormonal treatment in whom chemotherapy will not confer any additional benefit, even in the setting of lymph node positivity.

However, axillary surgery is far from obsolete, and the question of in which scenario a patient does not require axillary staging is currently under investigation. The results of the AMAROS trial show a clear role, in certain patients, for radiotherapy in treating the axilla with low morbidity. However, the data pertain to a select group of patients at low risk of locoregional failure similar to other reports of excellent locoregional control with axillary radiotherapy, but where recruitment was limited to clinically node-negative patients. The recently published NCIC MA.20 study and the EORTC 22922/10925 trials have shown a lower risk of locoregional recurrence with the use of extended radiation therapy in patients who have undergone ALND. It is as yet unknown whether comparable rates of locoregional control can be attained through treatment with axillary radiotherapy alone in patients with a higher burden of axillary disease than those recruited to the AMAROS trial.

As the indications for neoadjuvant chemotherapy expand, SLNB remains the standard for axillary staging post-treatment in the majority of patients. Imaging modalities such as PET or US lack sufficient sensitivity or specificity to accurately assess the status of axillary nodes after neoadjuvant chemotherapy. In patients with residual axillary disease, ALND is, for now, the standard of care for optimal locoregional control.

Innovative trials such as the Alliance A11202 study may add further options to the algorithms for axillary management, and the next generation of individualized treatment programs will reflect molecular characterization of tumor biology. However, axillary surgery will continue to play an important role in achieving locoregional control in selected breast cancer patients.

SUGGESTED READINGS

Boughey JC, Suman VJ, Mittendorf EA, et al. Sentinel lymph node surgery after neoadjuvant chemotherapy in patients with node-positive breast cancer. The ACOSOG Z1071 (Alliance) Clinical Trial. *JAMA.* 2013;310: 1455-1461.

Donker M, van Tienhoven G, Straver ME, et al. Radiotherapy or surgery of the axilla after a positive sentinel node in breast cancer (EORTC 10981-22023 AMAROS): a randomised, multicentre, open-label, phase 3 non-inferiority trial. *Lancet Oncol.* 2014;15:1303-1310.

Giuliano A, McCall L, Beitsch P, et al. Locoregional recurrence after sentinel lymph node dissection with or without axillary dissection in patients with sentinel lymph node metastases: the American College of Surgeons Oncology Group Z0011 Randomized Trial. *Ann Surg.* 2010;252:426-433.

Krag DN, Anderson SJ, Julian TB, et al. Sentinel lymph node resection compared with conventional axillary lymph node dissection in clinically node negative patients with breast cancer: overall survival findings from the NSABP B-32 randomized phase 3 trial. *Lancet Oncol.* 2010;11:927-933.

Lucci A, Mackie McCall L, Beitsch PD, et al. Surgical complications associated with sentinel lymph node dissection (SLND) plus axillary lymph node dissection compared with SLND alone in the American College of Surgeons Oncology Group Trial Z0011. *J Clin Oncol.* 2007;25:3657-3663.

Mamounas EP, Brown A, Anderson S, et al. Sentinel node biopsy after neoadjuvant chemotherapy in breast cancer: results from National Surgical Adjuvant Breast and Bowel Project Protocol B-27. *J Clin Oncol.* 2005;23: 2694-2702.

Rao R, Euhus D, Mayo HG, et al. Axillary node interventions in breast cancer. A systematic review. *JAMA.* 2013;310:1385-1394.

INFLAMMATORY BREAST CANCER

Jennifer K. Plichta, MD, MS, and Barbara L. Smith, MD, PhD

Inflammatory breast cancer (IBC) is an uncommon presentation of locally advanced breast cancer, observed in approximately 1% to 3% of new breast cancer diagnoses in the United States. IBC is a clinical diagnosis with no unique histologic subtype, molecular markers, or genetic signature that accounts for the inflammatory phenotype. The key feature of IBC is extensive tumor involvement of the breast and dermal lymphatics, which accounts for the clinical picture of a swollen breast with skin edema and erythema, with or without a discrete palpable mass. Regional lymph nodes frequently are involved by tumor at presentation, and rates of distant metastases are high. Although the prognosis of IBC has improved over time, survival rate remains poor compared with other breast cancers.

CLINICAL PRESENTATION AND DIAGNOSIS

The diagnosis of IBC is based on the overall clinical presentation and does not require a skin biopsy to document dermal lymphatic invasion. Based on current guidelines, the minimum criteria for a diagnosis of IBC include rapid onset (within 6 months) of breast edema or peau d'orange skin changes, erythema involving at least one third of the breast, and a biopsy consistent with invasive carcinoma.

Because of the rapid onset of symptoms, IBC often will be seen less than a year after a negative screening mammogram. Patients with IBC often will report breast swelling or redness developing over a period of several weeks to a few months. This may be accompanied by breast heaviness, burning or tenderness, nipple inversion or retraction, pitting of the skin (peau d'orange changes), or skin discoloration. These findings result from blockage of lymphatics in the breast and skin by tumor cells. Skin edema around hair follicles and skin pores creates tiny areas of skin pitting, termed "peau d'orange" or "orange peel" changes. Although generalized breast fullness and firmness without a focal mass is common, some patients will have a discrete palpable mass. Axillary lymph nodes frequently are involved and may be palpable on clinical examination. Supraclavicular nodes should be examined for possible involvement.

IBC initially may be misdiagnosed as an infection or mastitis. In contrast to an infection, IBC does not have associated fever, leukocytosis, or marked breast pain. A diagnosis of IBC should be considered in any patient with breast erythema that does not resolve completely with 7 to 10 days of antibiotic therapy.

BREAST IMAGING

Initial diagnostic breast imaging is performed to identify a possible primary breast tumor, evaluate the regional nodes, and enable image-guided biopsy for histopathologic diagnosis. All patients with signs and symptoms of breast cancer should undergo diagnostic mammography and ultrasound of the affected breast and ipsilateral axilla. The most common mammographic findings in IBC include skin thickening, unilateral diffusely increased breast density, a discrete mass, architectural distortion, suspicious calcifications, or enlarged axillary nodes. Breast ultrasound can identify masses in the breast and involved axillary nodes and guide diagnostic core biopsies at these sites. If no discrete mass is identified on mammography or ultrasound, breast tomosynthesis or magnetic resonance imaging (MRI) may be beneficial to identify an area appropriate for biopsy. A breast MRI may be obtained for evaluation of the contralateral breast in selected patients but will not change management of the affected breast, as mastectomy will be performed regardless of imaging results.

DIAGNOSTIC BIOPSY

Image-guided core biopsy is the standard of care for diagnosis of IBC. In the rare case where no target can be identified by any imaging modality, a freehand core biopsy guided by palpation usually can make the diagnosis. Open surgical biopsy is rarely required and should be avoided to minimize wound healing issues that may delay systemic therapy. Core biopsy or fine-needle aspiration of suspicious axillary or supraclavicular nodes also may be performed to determine the initial extent of regional disease.

HISTOPATHOLOGY

Most IBCs are found to be ductal histologic type, although lobular and other histologic types are also seen. IBC tumors are more likely to display aggressive histopathologic features, including high-grade nuclei and estrogen receptor (ER)–negative, HER2 (human epidermal growth factor receptor–2)-positive, and triple-negative phenotypes. Extensive involvement of lymphatics in breast parenchyma and skin is frequently present. IBC specimens often show diffuse involvement of breast tissue by tumor interspersed with normal tissue, making assessment of tumor size difficult even on gross pathologic examination.

INITIAL STAGING

Approximately 20% to 35% of patients with IBC have distant metastases at initial presentation, and the presence of metastatic disease will change treatment strategies (Figure 1). As a result, a full staging evaluation is performed at diagnosis. Standard staging includes a bone scan and computed tomographic (CT) scans of the chest, abdomen, and pelvis. Some centers prefer to use a positron emission tomography (PET)-CT scan for initial staging, although this may provide less fine resolution of small lesions and may have a higher cost. Brain MRI is performed in selected patients, often guided by symptoms suggestive of intracranial disease. When possible, biopsy of accessible suspicious lesions identified should be performed, to distinguish metastatic breast cancer from other benign or malignant conditions.

IBC is classified as T4d in the tumor node metastasis (TNM) staging classification. Patients with no metastatic disease will be classified as stage IIIB or IIIC based on the extent of regional node involvement. Patients with metastatic disease are classified as stage IV.

TREATMENT STRATEGY

Prior clinical experience has demonstrated the importance of combining medical systemic therapy, surgery, and radiation in treating patients with IBC who do not have metastatic disease at initial presentation. Omission of any one of these treatment modalities reduces survival. The inflammatory phenotype dictates the sequence of therapies: systemic therapy first, then modified radical mastectomy, post-mastectomy radiation therapy, and prolonged endocrine therapy in patients with ER-positive tumors. Prolonged use of other targeted therapies, such as anti-HER2 regimens, is also appropriate for some patients.

Although the inflammatory phenotype determines the overall treatment strategy, it is still the properties of the individual woman's tumor that guide the selection of systemic therapy regimens. At present, there is no IBC-specific molecular target for systemic therapy. ER, progesterone receptor (PR), and HER2 status are measured on the diagnostic core biopsy and used to select treatment regimens. Given the high recurrence rate of IBC with current standard systemic

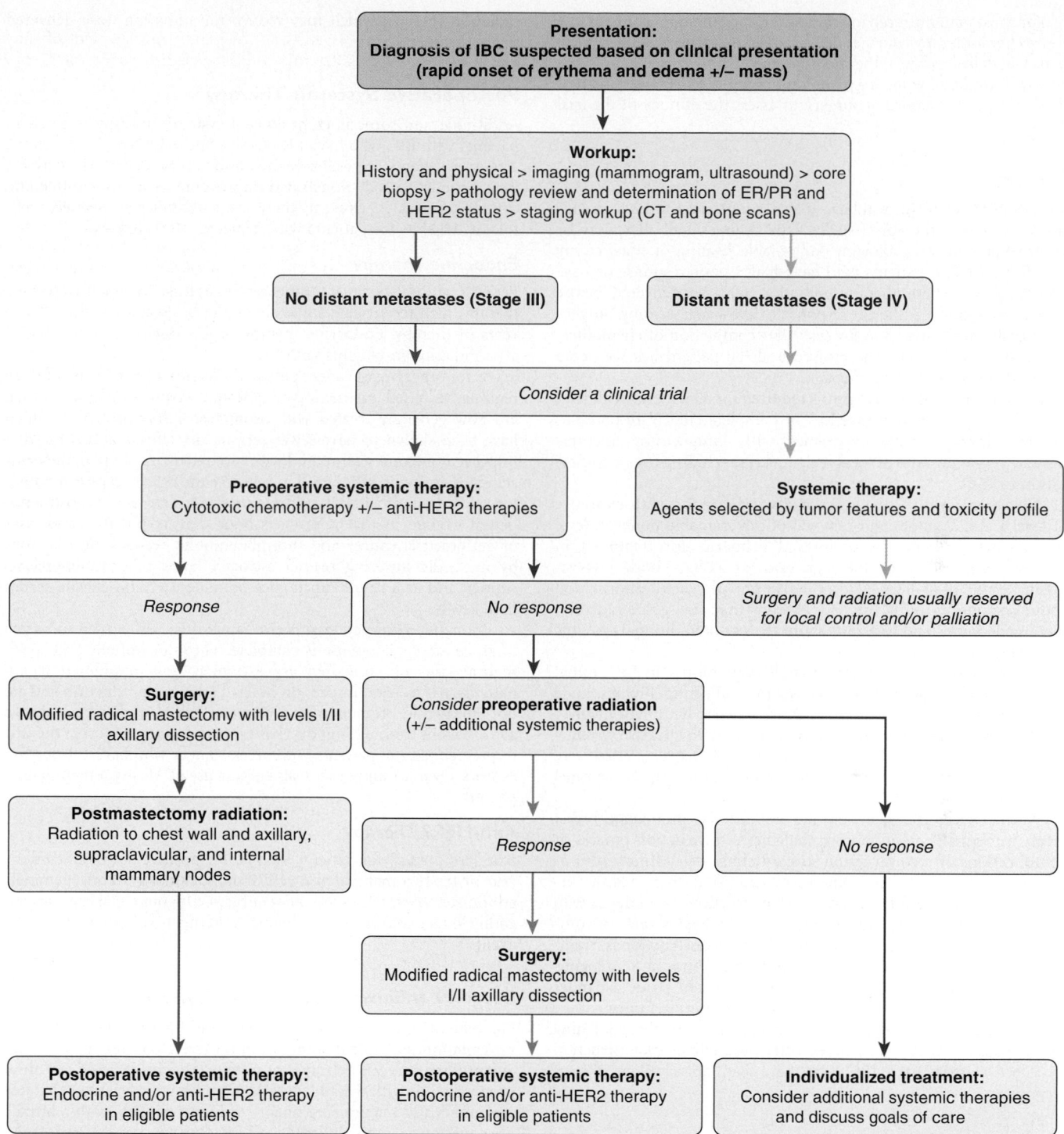

FIGURE 1 Inflammatory breast cancer (IBC) treatment algorithm. *CT*, Computed tomography; *ER*, estrogen receptor; *HER2*, human epidermal growth factor receptor–2; *PR*, progesterone receptor.

therapy regimens, use of novel therapies as part of a clinical trial should be considered whenever possible.

Preoperative Systemic Therapy

Cytotoxic chemotherapy is the initial therapeutic intervention for most patients with IBC. Use of endocrine therapy as the initial treatment is reserved for frail older patients with ER-positive tumors who are unable to tolerate chemotherapy.

Chemotherapy is tailored as specifically as possible to the individual patient's tumor. For patients with HER2 overexpression, initial regimens will include one or two anti-HER2 targeted therapies in addition to cytotoxic chemotherapy, often with a taxane and one or more other agents. Anthracyclines are used with caution in patients receiving anti-HER2 regimens because of an increased risk of cardiotoxicity when these agents are combined. Patients with HER2-negative tumors generally receive chemotherapy with an anthracycline and taxane, often combined with other agents.

For most patients receiving standard chemotherapy regimens, the entire chemotherapy course is delivered before surgery. Some clinical trials will deliver some of the chemotherapy before surgery and some postoperatively, allowing for pathologic and molecular assessment of residual tumor obtained at surgery to assess the efficacy of the trial therapy.

Surgery

Most patients with IBC will have at least a partial response to preoperative systemic therapy. Usually skin changes will disappear or improve significantly, allowing for reliable healing of mastectomy skin flaps. In rare patients who have had a poor response or have progressed on chemotherapy, radiation may be delivered before surgery to obtain a sufficient response to allow mastectomy. Surgery is generally performed 3 to 5 weeks after completion of chemotherapy, when neutropenia has resolved and the patient has recovered from other chemotherapy effects.

Modified radical mastectomy is required for all patients with IBC, even if they have had an excellent or complete clinical response to systemic therapy. Early experience with lumpectomy attempts showed very high rates of local recurrence, precluding breast conservation in IBC.

All patients with IBC require axillary dissection with clearance of level I and II nodes and removal of any palpable nodes in level III. Axillary dissection is performed primarily for treatment in patients with IBC given the high rates of axillary node involvement. Results of axillary dissection also provide useful information about response to initial systemic therapy that may guide radiation therapy decisions and decisions about the use of additional systemic therapies.

There is no role for sentinel lymph node biopsy in IBC. Initial sentinel lymph node trials found poor rates of sentinel lymph node identification in patients with IBC, likely related to lymphatic involvement by tumor and/or scarring of lymphatics with effective systemic therapy. When mapping was successful, false-negative rates were high. IBC currently is considered a contraindication to sentinel lymph node biopsy.

Women with IBC generally are not offered immediate breast reconstruction. There is concern that the reconstruction process or complications of reconstruction surgery might delay timely administration of needed radiation therapy. In addition, many plastic surgeons prefer to perform delayed reconstruction in patients who require postmastectomy irradiation, given the higher rates of complications and cosmetic issues when a breast reconstruction is irradiated. This delayed reconstruction approach requires an autologous tissue reconstruction, as outcomes are poor when tissue expander reconstruction of an irradiated mastectomy site is attempted.

In recent years, centers that are more comfortable irradiating reconstructed breasts sometimes offer immediate reconstruction to select women with IBC who have had an excellent clinical response.

Postmastectomy Radiation Therapy

Comprehensive chest wall and regional nodal irradiation after mastectomy is recommended for all patients with IBC to address the high risk of local and regional recurrence. Treatment fields include the ipsilateral chest wall, axillary and supraclavicular node areas, and internal mammary nodes. Radiation generally begins 4 to 6 weeks after surgery when incisions are healed and the patient is able to raise her arm above her head and out of the radiation field. Some patients may require physical therapy after axillary dissection to achieve the needed arm mobility and avoid delays in delivery of radiation.

Careful radiation planning is required to minimize cardiac and pulmonary effects of the comprehensive radiation required in IBC, particularly for left-sided cancers. Patients with left-sided IBC are being considered for trials of proton beam postmastectomy radiation therapy, which may reduce the radiation dose delivered to the heart.

Postoperative Systemic Therapy

Additional and sometimes prolonged systemic therapy is given to patients with IBC who have ER-positive and HER2-positive tumors. These treatments are well tolerated and can be delivered safely for long periods, with demonstrated improvements in disease-free and overall survival. At present, there are no similarly effective, well-tolerated agents for patients with triple-negative tumors.

Endocrine Therapy

Patients with ER-positive tumors receive at least 5 years of endocrine therapy, with recent data suggesting an even greater benefit with 10 years of therapy. Endocrine therapy begins during or immediately after radiation in patients with IBC.

As for other breast cancer patients, selection of endocrine therapy regimen is based on menopausal status. Postmenopausal women are now generally treated with aromatase inhibitors (AIs), which have been shown to have fewer serious side effects and somewhat improved outcomes compared with tamoxifen. Tamoxifen, the prior standard endocrine therapy, is a selective estrogen receptor modulator (SERM). Tamoxifen has effects similar to estrogen in postmenopausal women in that it protects bone density but increases risks of endometrial cancer and thromboembolic events. The AIs work by markedly lowering overall estrogen levels in postmenopausal women and as a result can reduce bone density and elevate serum lipid levels.

Premenopausal patients receive tamoxifen, with a plan to switch to an AI after menopause is complete. Thromboembolic and endometrial risks of tamoxifen are extremely low in premenopausal patients. AIs have no impact on ovarian estrogen production and are not effective in premenopausal women. Recent studies have shown some benefit from adding ovarian suppression to endocrine therapy in premenopausal patients with breast cancer who have ER-positive tumors. Ovarian suppression also allows use of AIs in premenopausal patients.

Anti-HER2 Therapy

Standard therapy for patients with HER2-positive tumors includes a year of trastuzumab, an anti-HER2 monoclonal antibody, generally administered every 3 weeks after surgery. Ongoing trials are investigating longer courses of trastuzumab and the use of other anti-HER2 agents.

Stage IV Inflammatory Breast Cancer

For patients with IBC found to have distant metastases at initial presentation, systemic therapy is administered to improve symptoms and prolong survival. Selection of systemic therapy is based on tumor properties but with the added goals of minimizing treatment-related symptoms and maximizing quality of life in patients with a limited life expectancy. Some patients with ER-positive tumors may receive endocrine therapy alone or a short course of chemotherapy followed by endocrine therapy. Patients with HER2-positive tumors will receive a course of chemotherapy plus targeted anti-HER2 therapy. Both endocrine therapy and targeted anti-HER2 therapy are given continuously until tumor progression is observed, at which time other therapies are instituted. Treatment in a clinical trial should be considered for patients with stage IV IBC at presentation or at the time of progression.

Although surgical resection of the primary tumor in the breast does not improve overall survival in women with stage IV breast cancer, it may be required for local control in patients with IBC who have well-controlled metastatic disease. For example, mastectomy may be performed for an enlarging primary tumor in a patient whose distant metastases are well controlled on an easily tolerated regimen such as endocrine therapy. In these cases, mastectomy allows the patient to continue her well-tolerated systemic therapy and avoid prolonged chemotherapy. Surgery also is sometimes performed for stage IV patients with triple-negative tumors and a good response to initial chemotherapy to prevent rapid growth of the primary tumor during planned breaks in chemotherapy. For patients with IBC who have well-controlled metastatic disease, postmastectomy radiation also may be considered given the risk of rapid chest wall recurrence after surgery alone.

■ PROGNOSIS

IBC was previously a lethal diagnosis with a 5-year overall survival rate of less than 5% and a median survival of only 15 months. With improved systemic therapies and consistent use of multimodality therapy, outcomes are markedly improved. A recent review of Surveillance, Epidemiology, and End Results (SEER) data noted that 2-year breast cancer–specific survival in women with IBC improved from 62% in 1990–1995 to 76% in 2006–2010.

At present, patients with stage III IBC have an approximately 40% 5-year survival rate, compared with an 11% 5-year survival rate in women with stage IV IBC. Overall 15-year survival rate for IBC is now approximately 20% to 30%.

An individual patient's prognosis is influenced by tumor subtype, receptor status, stage at presentation, and response to initial systemic therapy. Response to initial systemic therapy is an important predictor of prognosis, with improved survival in those with no residual invasive tumor found in the breast or nodes at surgery (pathologic complete response). Survival is higher among women who have ER-positive and HER2-positive tumors and can receive prolonged targeted therapy. African-American women with IBC tend to have a worse prognosis than other racial or ethnic groups, with an increased proportion of triple-negative tumors and other factors likely contributing to this result.

■ SURVEILLANCE AND SURVIVORSHIP

Patients with IBC have a high risk of local, regional, and systemic breast cancer recurrence. Recurrences may involve the ipsilateral breast, contralateral breast, local skin, regional nodes, or multiple distant sites. Standard follow-up includes a physical examination and review of symptoms every 3 to 6 months, with imaging studies performed to evaluate any abnormalities or symptoms identified. Routine scans and marker testing have not been associated with improvement in survival or quality of life.

As is the case for all breast cancer patients, women with IBC are at risk for early and late side effects and complications of the treatments received. Patients' survivorship concerns may include cardiac and pulmonary toxicity, neuropathy, anxiety and depression, impaired cognitive function, fatigue, pain, menopausal symptoms, decreased sexual function, and sleep disturbances. Given their intensive and multimodality treatment, patients with IBC may be at even higher risk for treatment-related complications than other breast cancer patients. In addition, intensive treatment and increased risk of recurrence in patients with IBC can increase rates of psychological side effects. Assessment and management of these concerns is now incorporated into most follow-up programs.

SUGGESTED READINGS

Bertuci F, Finetti P, Vermeulen P, Van Dam P, Dirix L, Birnbaum D, Viens P, Van Laere S. Genomic profiling of inflammatory breast cancer: a review. *Breast.* 2014;23:538-545.

Cristofanilli M, Valero V, Buzdar AU, Kau SW, Broglio KR, Gonzalez-Angulo AM, Sneige N, Islam R, Ueno NT, Buchholz TA, Singletary SE, Hortobagyi GN. Inflammatory breast cancer (IBC) and patterns of recurrence: understanding the biology of a unique disease. *Cancer.* 2007;110:1436-1444.

Dawood S, Lei X, Dent R, Gupta S, Sirohi B, Cortes J, Cristofanilli M, Buchholz T, Gonzalez-Angulo AM. Survival of women with inflammatory breast cancer: a large population-based study. *Ann Oncol.* 2014;25:1143-1151.

Dawood S, Merajver SD, Viens P, Vermeulen PB, Swain SM, Buchholz TA, Dirix LY, Levine PH, Lucci A, Krishnamurthy S, Robertson FM, Woodward WA, Yang WT, Ueno NT, Cristofanilli M. International expert panel on inflammatory breast cancer: consensus statement for standardized diagnosis and treatment. *Ann Oncol.* 2011;22:515-523.

Dawood S, Ueno NT, Valero V, Woodward WA, Buchholz TA, Hortobagyi GN, Gonzalez-Angulo AM, Cristofanilli M. Identifying factors that impact survival among women with inflammatory breast cancer. *Ann Oncol.* 2012;23:870-875.

Hance KW, Anderson WF, Devesa SS, Young HA, Levine PH. Trends in inflammatory breast carcinoma incidence and survival: the Surveillance, Epidemiology, and End Results program at the National Cancer Institute. *J Natl Cancer Inst.* 2005;97:966-975.

Li BD, Sicard MA, Ampil F, Abreo F, Lilien D, Chu QD, Burton GV. Trimodal therapy for inflammatory breast cancer: a surgeon's perspective. *Oncology.* 2010;79:3-12.

Matro JM, Li T, Cristofanilli M, Hughes ME, Ottesen RA, Weeks JC, Wong YN. Inflammatory breast cancer management in the national comprehensive cancer network: the disease, recurrence pattern, and outcome. *Clin Breast Cancer.* 2015;15:1-7.

National Comprehensive Cancer Network (NCCN). *NCCN Clinical Practice Guidelines in Oncology.* Breast Cancer. Version 3. <http://www.nccn.org>; 2015 Accessed 10.10.15.

Robertson FM, Bondy M, Yang W, Yamauchi H, Wiggins S, Kamrudin S, Krishnamurthy S, Le-Petross H, Bidaut L, Player AN, Barsky SH, Woodward WA, Buchholz T, Lucci A, Ueno NT, Cristofanilli M. Inflammatory breast cancer: the disease, the biology, the treatment. *CA Cancer J Clin.* 2010;60:351-375.

van Uden DJ, van Laarhoven HW, Westenberg AH, de Wilt JH, Blanken-Peeters CF. Inflammatory breast cancer: an overview. *Crit Rev Oncol Hematol.* 2015;93:116-126.

Yamauchi H, Woodward WA, Valero V, Alvarez RH, Lucci A, Buchholz TA, Iwamoto T, Krishnamurthy S, Yang W, Reuben JM, Hortobágyi GN, Ueno NT. Inflammatory breast cancer: what we know and what we need to learn. *Oncologist.* 2012;17:891-899.

DUCTAL AND LOBULAR CARCINOMA IN SITU OF THE BREAST

Melissa S. Camp, MD, MPH

Ductal carcinoma in situ (DCIS) and lobular carcinoma in situ (LCIS) sound very similar but are distinct entities that are managed and treated very differently. DCIS is regarded commonly as preinvasive breast cancer arising from within the ductal system of the breast, whereas LCIS develops in the lobules of the breast and typically is thought of as a marker of increased risk of developing breast cancer in the future. Both of these classic descriptions, however, are not without controversy. The classification of DCIS as cancer is an area of debate, as is whether LCIS should be considered a marker of increased risk versus a precursor lesion. Management and treatment of both DCIS and LCIS should involve a multidisciplinary approach to provide the best care for each patient.

■ DUCTAL CARCINOMA IN SITU

The incidence of DCIS has increased dramatically, from 5.8 per 100,000 women in the 1970s to 32.5 per 100,000 women in 2004. In 2015 approximately 60,000 women in the United States will be diagnosed with DCIS, representing 25% of all breast cancer diagnoses. The rise in the incidence of DCIS can be attributed to the increasing utilization of screening mammography as well as improvements in mammographic technology.

Diagnosis

DCIS most often presents as suspicious appearing calcifications visualized on mammography. The calcifications may appear as a new cluster, be pleomorphic in size and shape, or be arranged in a linear or segmental distribution. Rarely, DCIS can present as a palpable mass or as a mammographically detected mass. Paget's disease of the nipple or suspicious nipple discharge are also infrequent presentations of DCIS.

Stereotactic core needle biopsy is performed for tissue diagnosis of suspicious calcifications. The pathology from core needle biopsy provides information that can be used for appropriate surgical planning. DCIS with microinvasion on core needle biopsy, for example, indicates a need for sentinel lymph node evaluation. If the calcifications of interest are not amenable to stereotactic core needle biopsy (resulting from proximity to the chest wall, skin, or cosmetic breast implant), then wire localized excisional biopsy can be performed.

Once a diagnosis of DCIS is made, the role for evaluation of extent of disease with MRI is controversial. MRI does have an increased sensitivity for detecting DCIS compared with standard mammography. The use of MRI, however, has not been shown to decrease the rates of positive margins or the need for re-excision after lumpectomy for DCIS. Moreover, preoperative MRI has been associated with increased rates of initial mastectomy, increased rates of contralateral prophylactic mastectomy, and delay to surgery because of the need for additional imaging evaluation and/or biopsies of MRI findings. MRI is not necessary for all patients with a diagnosis of DCIS but can be useful in select patients in whom the extent of disease is difficult to define using standard imaging (mammography with or without ultrasound).

ECOG (Eastern Cooperative Oncology Group) E4112 is one ongoing trial evaluating the use of MRI in DCIS. A primary endpoint of this trial is the rate of conversion to mastectomy based on MRI results for patients who were deemed to be lumpectomy candidates according to standard imaging.

Treatment

The long-term prognosis of DCIS is excellent, with survival rates at 10 years greater than 95%. The goal of treatment for DCIS therefore is to prevent the development of invasive breast cancer and minimize any treatment-associated morbidity. Different types of DCIS have varying levels of risk associated with local recurrence or progression to invasive cancer. Multimodality therapy, including some combination of surgery, radiation, and hormonal therapy, typically is used in the treatment of DCIS. The treatment recommendations often are based on the perceived risk of local recurrence associated with the type of DCIS, the patient's comorbidities, and patient preference.

Historically, DCIS was treated with simple mastectomy or modified radical mastectomy. A randomized controlled trial for invasive breast cancer, the National Surgical Adjuvant Breast and Bowel Project (NSABP) B06 trial, demonstrated that long-term survival was equivalent for lumpectomy plus radiation (breast conservation) versus mastectomy. These results were extrapolated to the treatment of DCIS, although there was never a trial directly comparing mastectomy to breast conservation for DCIS. The early trials specifically focused on DCIS evaluated lumpectomy alone versus lumpectomy with radiation, and lumpectomy with radiation versus lumpectomy with radiation plus tamoxifen.

The NSABP B17 trial randomized 818 patients with DCIS to lumpectomy alone versus lumpectomy followed by radiation. There was no difference in survival between the two groups, but at 5 years the incidence of ipsilateral breast tumor recurrence was higher in women who underwent lumpectomy alone compared with those who underwent lumpectomy followed by radiation (16.4% vs 7.0%). Fifty percent of the local recurrences in the lumpectomy alone group were invasive compared with 28.6% in the lumpectomy plus radiation group. Radiation reduced both invasive and noninvasive breast cancer recurrences, but the magnitude of effect was greater for invasive breast cancer.

Taking the results from NSABP B17 into account, the NSABP B24 trial was designed to determine whether there would be any additional benefit to treatment with tamoxifen for women undergoing lumpectomy and radiation for DCIS. A total of 1804 women with DCIS who underwent lumpectomy followed by radiation were randomized to tamoxifen versus placebo daily for 5 years. With 5 years of follow-up, 9.7% of patients in the placebo arm experienced an ipsilateral breast tumor recurrence compared with 7.0% in the tamoxifen arm. Forty-six percent of all local recurrences in the placebo group were invasive compared with 36.5% in the tamoxifen group. The group receiving tamoxifen exhibited a 30% reduction overall in ipsilateral invasive and noninvasive breast cancers, with the reduction primarily attributed to a decrease in invasive breast cancers. In addition, contralateral breast cancers were reduced by 52% in women receiving tamoxifen compared with placebo.

With 15-year follow-up, the overall rates of local recurrence in the NSABP B17 trial were 35% in the lumpectomy alone arm compared with 19.8% in the lumpectomy plus radiation arm. Survival remained similar between the two groups. The 15-year follow-up of the NSABP B24 trial revealed overall rates of local recurrence of 16.6% in the lumpectomy with radiation plus placebo group compared with 13.2% in the lumpectomy with radiation plus tamoxifen group. Survival remained similar between the two arms.

Among patients in NSABP B17 and B24 who did develop a local recurrence within 15 years of follow-up, invasive ipsilateral breast tumor recurrence was shown to be associated with an increased risk of mortality (hazard ratio 1.75, 95% CI 1.45-2.96, $P < 0.001$). Local recurrence of DCIS, on the other hand, did not increase mortality. Specifically focusing on rates of invasive ipsilateral breast tumor recurrence, the cumulative incidence was 19.4% for lumpectomy alone (B17), 8.9% for lumpectomy plus radiation (B17), 10.0% for lumpectomy with radiation plus placebo (B24), and 8.5% for lumpectomy with radiation plus tamoxifen (B24).

The pervasive theme among all of these trials is that lumpectomy alone for DCIS results in higher rates of local recurrence. The addition of radiation to lumpectomy reduces the risk of local recurrence, and the addition of tamoxifen to lumpectomy plus radiation reduces the risk of local recurrence even further. The reduction in local recurrence afforded by radiation with or without tamoxifen has not been shown to result in a survival benefit. It is important to keep in mind, however, that up to 50% of local recurrences may represent invasive disease as opposed to DCIS, and ipsilateral invasive breast cancer recurrence has been shown to increase mortality.

Surgery

Surgical options for management of DCIS include both lumpectomy and mastectomy. Mastectomy is indicated for multicentric or extensive DCIS, persistently positive margins after lumpectomy for DCIS, or recurrence of DCIS after prior treatment with lumpectomy and radiation. Mastectomy can be performed in a skin-sparing or nipple-sparing fashion if reconstruction is desired. Appropriate candidates for nipple-sparing mastectomy should not have any evidence of disease on imaging or clinical exam in close proximity to the nipple areolar complex.

Wire localized lumpectomy can be performed for a localized area of DCIS in patients who desire breast conservation. The extent of DCIS visible on imaging must be taken into account relative to the size of the breast when determining which patients are appropriate candidates for breast conservation. It is always important to keep in mind that a greater extent of DCIS may be present on pathologic evaluation compared with the extent of calcifications visualized mammographically.

In the setting of lumpectomy for DCIS, the margin width considered acceptable for a negative margin is controversial. For invasive breast cancer, the Society of Surgical Oncology-American Society for Radiation Oncology margin consensus guidelines published in 2014 determined that no ink on tumor is adequate for a negative margin. These guidelines do not apply to DCIS, however. DCIS, unlike invasive breast cancer, typically does not form a discrete mass and can be discontinuous within a branching ductal system. Margins less than 2 mm for DCIS are associated with an increased risk of local recurrence, but margins of 5 mm or greater have not been shown to confer a significantly decreased risk of local recurrence in the setting of adjuvant radiation therapy. Therefore a margin of 2 mm often is considered adequate to declare a negative margin for DCIS.

Sentinel lymph node evaluation typically is not performed with lumpectomy for DCIS. If invasive disease is identified on final pathology of the lumpectomy specimen, it is possible to return to the operating room at a later date and perform a sentinel lymph node biopsy. Sentinel lymph node biopsy should be performed with lumpectomy for DCIS if the core needle biopsy revealed DCIS with microinvasion and strongly considered if the presentation of DCIS is suspicious for the presence of invasive disease (e.g., a palpable mass or a core needle biopsy with suspicion for microinvasion). In the setting of mastectomy for DCIS, sentinel lymph node biopsy should be performed just in case any areas of microinvasive or invasive disease are identified on final pathology of the mastectomy specimen. Once all of the breast tissue has been removed, returning to the operating room to perform a sentinel lymph node biopsy is not possible because there is no remaining breast tissue in which to inject the sentinel node tracer.

Radiation

As discussed above, radiation after lumpectomy for DCIS significantly decreases the risk of local recurrence but does not improve survival. Several trials have sought to answer the question whether all women undergoing lumpectomy for DCIS should receive radiation, or if there are select subgroups in which radiation can safely be omitted. The ECOG 5194 trial, published in 2009, reported a 5-year ipsilateral breast tumor recurrence risk of 6% among women who underwent lumpectomy alone for low to intermediate grade DCIS measuring 2.5 cm or smaller and excised with a minimum of 3-mm margins. In contrast, the 5-year ipsilateral breast tumor recurrence risk was 15% among women who underwent lumpectomy alone for high grade DCIS measuring 1.0 cm or less. Adjuvant hormonal therapy with tamoxifen was optional.

The RTOG (Radiation Therapy Oncology Group) 9804 trial, published in 2015, randomized 636 women with low- to intermediate-grade DCIS measuring 2.5 cm or less resected with margins 3 mm or more to lumpectomy alone versus lumpectomy plus radiation. Adjuvant hormonal therapy with tamoxifen was optional but was used as a stratification criteria before randomization. At 7 years, the ipsilateral breast tumor recurrence was 6.7% in the lumpectomy alone arm compared with 0.9% in the lumpectomy plus radiation arm. The authors concluded that in carefully selected patients with low risk DCIS, the risk of local recurrence was low if radiation was omitted but was decreased significantly by the addition of radiation. Longer-term follow-up is needed, however.

One of the newer tools to aid in the decision making process of whether to omit radiation is the Oncotype DX DCIS score. The Oncotype DX DCIS score is a 12-gene assay that was developed and validated using tissue blocks from patients enrolled in the ECOG 5194 trial. The score is derived from expression levels of 12 genes within the surgically resected DCIS and predicts 10-year risk of local recurrence (overall and invasive) for patients with DCIS undergoing lumpectomy without radiation. The score stratifies the risk of local recurrence into low risk, intermediate risk, and high risk. For patients whose Oncotype DX DCIS score falls into the low risk category, lumpectomy alone may be adequate. For scores that fall into the intermediate or high risk categories, omission of radiation may result in higher rates of local recurrence.

Decisions about adjuvant radiation therapy after lumpectomy for DCIS must be made in the context of many variables. The patient's age, comorbidities, estimated risk of local recurrence based on traditional clinical and pathologic factors (grade, size, hormone receptor status, margin width), estimated risk of local recurrence using tools such as the Oncotype DX DCIS score, ability of the patient to undergo additional treatment in the future if a local recurrence were to develop, and patient preference all must be taken into account.

Hormonal Therapy

For hormone receptor positive (estrogen receptor [ER] or progesterone receptor [PR] positive) DCIS, adjuvant hormonal therapy with tamoxifen daily for 5 years reduces both local recurrence and development of a contralateral breast cancer. In the NSABP B24 trial, women with DCIS were randomized to lumpectomy with radiation plus placebo versus lumpectomy with radiation plus tamoxifen. The 5-year cumulative incidence of all breast cancer events was 8.2% in the tamoxifen arm compared with 13.4% in the placebo arm. Tamoxifen reduced ipsilateral breast cancer recurrences by 30% overall (invasive recurrences by 44% and noninvasive recurrences by 18%). Tamoxifen reduced contralateral breast cancers by 52% overall (invasive breast cancers by 37% and noninvasive breast cancers by 78%). Although hormone receptor status of DCIS was not routinely collected at the time of the NSABP B24 trial, a retrospective analysis demonstrated that tamoxifen reduced the risk of invasive breast cancer recurrence in ER positive cases by 40%.

Despite decreasing risk of local recurrence and serving as chemoprevention for the contralateral breast, using tamoxifen for treatment of DCIS does not improve survival. Moreover, tamoxifen is not without side effects. Common side effects of tamoxifen that affect quality of life include hot flashes and menopausal-like symptoms. Far more rare but serious side effects include endometrial cancer and thromboembolic disease. Decisions about using tamoxifen for treatment of DCIS must be made in the context of the patient's age, comorbidities, tolerance of side effects, estimated risk of local recurrence based on clinical and pathologic factors (grade, size, hormone receptor status, margin width), estimated risk of developing a contralateral breast cancer, and patient preference.

For postmenopausal women with hormone-sensitive invasive breast cancer, aromatase inhibitors typically are used as first-line adjuvant hormonal therapy. Up until recently, however, there were no data available regarding the use of aromatase inhibitors for treatment of hormone sensitive DCIS. The NSABP B35 trial recently released results comparing the use of anastrozole to tamoxifen for postmenopausal women with hormone receptor positive DCIS. A total of 3104 women underwent lumpectomy and radiation for DCIS and were randomized to anastrozole and placebo or tamoxifen and placebo. Women in the anastrozole arm exhibited fewer ipsilateral breast cancer recurrences and fewer contralateral breast cancers (both nonstatistically significant) compared with women in the tamoxifen arm. A statistically significant difference was observed in contralateral invasive breast cancers, with fewer in the anastrozole arm. When stratified by age (younger than 60 vs 60 years old or older), disease-free survival was improved in the anastrozole arm for women younger than 60, but there was no difference for women 60 years of age or older. There was no difference in overall survival between the two arms. Based on the results of NSABP B35, anastrozole can be considered an effective alternative to tamoxifen for postmenopausal women with hormone sensitive DCIS.

■ LOBULAR CARCINOMA IN SITU

Diagnosis

LCIS often is found incidentally, when a breast biopsy is performed for another indication. LCIS traditionally has been considered to be a marker of increased risk for developing a future breast cancer, and this risk applies to both breasts. More recent studies suggest that LCIS may be both a risk factor as well as a possible precursor to invasive lobular cancer. LCIS is not considered to be preinvasive cancer, however, in the same way that DCIS is considered to be a preinvasive form of invasive ductal cancer. The management of LCIS therefore is different from the management of DCIS.

Treatment

For LCIS diagnosed on core needle biopsy, excisional biopsy is warranted to rule out the presence of any associated DCIS or invasive cancer. There is an approximately 20% upgrade rate to DCIS or invasive cancer when pathology from a core needle biopsy reveals LCIS. If DCIS or invasive cancer is identified, management with appropriate local therapy and systemic treatment is indicated. If pathology from excisional biopsy reveals LCIS (classic type), no further surgical intervention is necessary. Excision to negative margins and radiation are not indicated for treatment of LCIS.

Pathology from excisional biopsy may reveal pleomorphic LCIS, which is considered to be a rare but aggressive form of LCIS. Pleomorphic LCIS is often treated more like DCIS, with excision to negative margins.

Options for managing the increased risk of breast cancer associated with LCIS include surveillance, chemoprevention, and bilateral prophylactic mastectomy.

Surveillance

Close screening and surveillance should be implemented after a diagnosis of LCIS. For patients with LCIS, the estimated lifetime risk of developing breast cancer is 30% to 40%. Annual mammography should be performed, as well as consideration of annual breast MRI. Ideally, mammography and MRI should be alternated every 6 months.

LCIS is often multifocal (about 50% of patients will have additional foci of LCIS in the ipsilateral breast) and bilateral (in about 30% of patients). The future risk of developing breast cancer associated with LCIS applies to both breasts, but recent studies have shown the risk is higher in the ipsilateral compared with the contralateral breast. Both invasive ductal carcinoma and invasive lobular carcinoma occur after a diagnosis of LCIS, but the incidence of invasive lobular carcinoma is higher in patients with LCIS compared with those without. Therefore LCIS may be both a risk factor for developing breast cancer as well as a precursor lesion for invasive lobular carcinoma.

Chemoprevention

Because of the increased risk of breast cancer associated with LCIS, chemoprevention should be considered. Many trials have demonstrated a significant risk reduction with the use of tamoxifen, raloxifene, and aromatase inhibitors for prevention. The NSABP P-1 trial showed that 5 years of tamoxifen decreased invasive and noninvasive breast cancers by about 50% compared with placebo. For the subgroup of women with LCIS, risk was reduced by 56%. For postmenopausal women, the NSABP STAR trial demonstrated that raloxifene was almost as effective as tamoxifen, leading to a 38% reduction in invasive and noninvasive breast cancers. The MAP.3 trial revealed that exemestane decreased the development of breast cancer in postmenopausal women by 53% compared with placebo. A 65% risk reduction was observed for invasive breast cancer. The IBIS-II trial demonstrated a similar result with anastrozole in high-risk postmenopausal women, with a 53% reduction in invasive and noninvasive breast cancers compared with placebo. For the subgroup of women with LCIS or atypical hyperplasia in the IBIS-II trial, a 69% risk reduction was observed.

Tamoxifen is the only option for chemoprevention in premenopausal women with LCIS. Aromatase inhibitors, tamoxifen, and raloxifene are options for chemoprevention in postmenopausal women with LCIS. Selection of the most appropriate agent is based upon the patient's medical history and potential side effects of the various medications. Women who have undergone hysterectomy, for example, would not be at risk for endometrial cancer with tamoxifen. Women with osteopenia or osteoporosis, on the other hand, may experience worsening bone density with aromatase inhibitors but improved bone density with raloxifene or tamoxifen.

Prophylactic Mastectomy

Bilateral prophylactic mastectomy provides the maximal risk reduction, approximately 90% to 95%, for women at high risk for developing breast cancer. Although not routinely recommended for women with LCIS, bilateral prophylactic mastectomy can be considered for women with LCIS and additional risk factors (such as a strong family history of breast cancer) that place them at significantly elevated risk for developing breast cancer in the future.

SUGGESTED READINGS

Benson JR, Wishart GC. Predictors of recurrence for ductal carcinoma in situ after breast-conserving surgery. *Lancet Oncol.* 2013;14:e348-e357.

Coopey SB, Mazzola E, Buckley JM, et al. The role of chemoprevention in modifying the risk of breast cancer in women with atypical breast lesions. *Breast Cancer Res Treat.* 2012;136:627-633.

Cuzick J, Sestak I, Forbes J, et al. Anastrozole for prevention of breast cancer in high risk postmenopausal women (IBIS-II): an international, double-blind, randomized placebo-controlled trial. *Lancet.* 2014;383:1041-1048.

Lakhani SR, Audretsch W, Cleton-Jensen A-M, et al. The management of lobular carcinoma in situ (LCIS). Is LCIS the same as ductal carcinoma in situ (DCIS). *Eur J Cancer.* 2006;42:2205-2211.

McCormick B, Winter K, Hudis C, et al. RTOG 9804: a prospective randomized trial for good-risk ductal carcinoma in situ comparing radiotherapy with observation. *J Clin Oncol.* 2015;33:709-715.

Wapnir IL, Dignam JJ, Fisher B, et al. Long-term outcomes of invasive ipsilateral breast tumor recurrences after lumpectomy in NSABP B17 and B24 randomized clinical trials for DCIS. *J Natl Cancer Inst.* 2011;103:478-488.

ADVANCES IN NEOADJUVANT AND ADJUVANT THERAPY FOR BREAST CANCER

Kelly J. Rosso, MD, MS, and Lisa Newman, MD, MPH, FACS, FASCO

Advances in breast cancer early detection as well as systemic therapy have yielded improved survival rates over the past several decades. Surgery remains an essential component of care to optimize durable locoregional control, but medical/systemic therapies are necessary to eradicate the micrometastatic burden of disease. This risk of distant organ micrometastases exists even in the setting of early stage/node-negative breast cancer. Treatment guidelines established by the National Comprehensive Cancer Network (NCCN) therefore recommend systemic therapy in addition to surgical management for all women with node-positive breast cancer (which is a strong indication of micrometastatic disease) and in most cases of node-negative breast cancer, depending on the exact size of the invasive tumor as well as the molecular marker status. Ongoing expansion of the armamentarium of systemic therapy agents is largely responsible for reducing the breast cancer mortality risk among women with invasive disease; however, all of these agents are associated with toxicities that can affect quality of life, and in rare cases they may even be life threatening. Furthermore, micrometastatic disease is generally asymptomatic and occult on body imaging. The surgeon therefore also plays a critical role in assessing the clinicopathologic stage of disease so that the risk of overtreatment is minimized and in providing adequate tissue for evaluation of breast tumor phenotype/molecular markers so that the appropriate, most effective systemic therapy regimen is selected.

Most systemic therapies are delivered in the adjuvant setting (i.e., after primary breast and axillary surgery has been completed); in these cases the regimen is determined on the basis of the surgical pathology findings regarding size of the invasive tumor, nodal status, and molecular marker expression. The molecular markers that define currently available systemic therapy agents are the estrogen receptor (ER), the progesterone receptor (PR), and the *HER2/neu* marker *(HER2)*. The era of precision medicine also has generated tools that allow for selection of systemic therapy by genetic profiling of individual tumors. In cases in which the patient's clinicopathologic presentation feature characteristics that confirm the need for systemic therapy as well as the type of systemic therapy, this treatment sequence can be reversed, with delivery of the systemic therapy before surgery. This approach is referred to most commonly as *neoadjuvant systemic therapy* but also may be called *induction*, or *preoperative treatment*. Patients with inflammatory breast cancer and bulky, locally advanced or unresectable disease on the chest wall and/or axilla routinely are referred to receive neoadjuvant chemotherapy with the goal of improving operability. However, the tumor-downstaging benefits of the neoadjuvant sequence have made this approach an attractive option for many women with clinically early stage breast cancer as well.

One in eight women will develop invasive breast cancer at some point in her life. The surgeon is often the first member of the multidisciplinary team to interpret the biopsy results and discuss treatment options. Thus it is important for the surgeon to be familiar with the systemic therapy regimens available and indications for their use in the neoadjuvant and adjuvant settings. Multidisciplinary collaboration involving all specialists in the treatment of breast cancer allows for the comprehensive formulation of treatment plans, including optimal selection and timing of systemic therapy, surgery, and radiation to obtain the best possible outcome for the patient.

■ BASIC PRINCIPLES AND INDICATIONS FOR ADJUVANT SYSTEMIC THERAPY

Traditional cytotoxic chemotherapeutic agents used to empirically treat breast cancer and other cancers of epithelial origin disrupt ubiquitous cell cycle pathways. They are typically not specific to cancer cells and have toxic effects on body tissues that are hyperproliferative as part of their normal function, thereby accounting for the common adverse but generally temporary effects of chemotherapy on hair follicles (alopecia), gastrointestinal tract (nausea/vomiting), bone marrow (neutropenia), and brittle/fragile nails. Chemotherapeutic agents used in the treatment of breast cancer are divided into three basic groups: anthracyclines (doxorubicin, epirubicin), taxanes (docetaxel, paclitaxel) and antimetabolite-based regimens (cyclophosphamide, methotrexate, fluorouracil) (Tables 1 and 2). Advances in modern systemic therapy framed by the concept that breast cancer is a genetically heterogeneous disease have led to the identification of several unique molecular therapeutic targets and the development of effective individualized therapies that target hormone receptors (these are called *endocrine therapies*) and HER2 (trastuzumab and pertuzumab). The specific combination of cytotoxic, endocrine, and HER2-directed agents and timing of administration as it relates to surgical management and duration of treatment is based on many tumor- and patient-specific factors, including menopausal status. In general, the systemic therapy regimens offered in the adjuvant versus the neoadjuvant sequence are the same.

As noted above, systemic therapy to prolong survival from breast cancer is indicated in any patient deemed to have a significant risk of micrometastatic disease. Patients with metastatic disease that is apparent on body imaging (e.g., computed tomography scan, bone scan) and/or confirmed by biopsy of the metastatic focus are categorized as having stage IV breast cancer, in which management is with palliative/noncurative intent. Routine body imaging to identify stage IV breast cancer generally is reserved for patients with inflammatory breast cancer, locally advanced/bulky T3 or T4 tumors (involving skin and/or chest wall), and patients found to have four or more metastatic axillary lymph nodes. In these scenarios body imaging may reveal overt metastatic disease in at least 30% of patients. In all other cases of clinically early stage/resectable breast cancer among patients that have no symptoms of overt metastases, micrometastatic disease is likely to be occult on body imaging, and pathologic tumor features define the appropriateness of systemic/medical therapies for treatment with curative intent.

Regional metastatic disease to the axilla is one of the most powerful indicators of distant organ micrometastases requiring control with chemotherapy as well as targeted therapy based upon tumor phenotype/molecular marker expression. Among patients with node-negative breast cancer, young/premenopausal age, primary invasive tumor size, and molecular marker status determine systemic therapy needs. In general, hormone receptor–positive invasive breast cancer of any size (regardless of nodal status) will benefit from endocrine therapy. *HER2/neu* overexpressing cancers tend to be biologically more aggressive, and chemotherapy with targeted anti-*HER2* therapy is considered in this setting for node-negative disease associated with tumors of at least 6 to 10 mm. Tumors that are negative for ER, PR, and *HER2/neu* commonly are described as *triple-negative breast cancer (TNBC)*. Approximately 15% of all breast cancers are TNBC, but 75% to 80% of TNBC cases belong to the inherently virulent basal subtype as defined by gene expression studies. The TNBC phenotype is therefore another feature suggesting benefit from chemotherapy in the setting of node-negative disease measuring at least 6 to 10 mm. For T1a or T1b tumors that are node negative and either TNBC or *HER2*-overexpressing, the patient must have an in-depth discussion of the potential toxicity of

TABLE 1: Chemotherapeutic Agents

	Class	Mechanism of Action	Side Effects
TRADITIONAL CHEMOTHERAPY			
Doxorubicin (Adriamycin)	Anthracycline	Topoisomerase II inhibitor; directly binds and intercalates into deoxyribonucleic acid (DNA), causing breaks, inhibiting repair and impairing synthesis of DNA, ribonucleic acid (RNA), and proteins. It is a cytotoxic, antiproliferative, cell cycle–nonspecific agent	Nausea/vomiting, myocardial toxicity (dose dependent), acute myelogenous leukemia, myelodysplastic syndrome, hepatic impairment, mucositis, myelosuppression
Epirubicin (Ellence)	Anthracycline	Topoisomerase II inhibitor; directly binds and intercalates into DNA, causing breaks, inhibiting repair and impairing synthesis of DNA, RNA, and proteins. It is a cytotoxic, antiproliferative, cell cycle–nonspecific agent	Myocardial toxicity (dose dependent), acute myelogenous leukemia, myelodysplastic syndrome, hepatic function impairment, myelosuppression
Cyclophosphamide (Cytoxan)	Alkylating agent; nitrogen mustard	Prevents cell division by cross-linking DNA strands that leads to inhibition of DNA replication and subsequent cell death. It is a cytotoxic, antiproliferative, cell cycle–nonspecific agent.	Myelosuppression, hemorrhagic cystitis, electrolyte imbalances (hyponatremia), alopecia, gonadal suppression, nausea/vomiting
Docetaxel (Taxotere)	Taxane	Promotes the assembly and stabilization of microtubules from tubulin dimers and inhibits the depolymerization of tubulin, resulting in inhibition of cell replication and interruption of DNA, RNA, and protein synthesis. Most activity occurs during the M phase of the cell cycle	Myelosuppression (up to 20%, give granulocyte-colony stimulating factor (GCS-F), motor and sensory neuropathy, alopecia, fluid retention, stomatitis, hepatic impairment
Paclitaxel	Taxane	Promotes the assembly and stabilization of microtubules from tubulin dimers and inhibits the depolymerization of tubulin, resulting in inhibition of cell replication and interruption of DNA, RNA, and protein synthesis. Most activity occurs during the M phase of the cell cycle	Motor and sensory neuropathy, flushing, alopecia, myalgias, nausea, vomiting, diarrhea, myelosuppression, hepatic impairment, renal impairment
Carboplatin	Platinum-based alkylating agent	Covalently binds DNA to produce intrastrand cross-links that interfere with DNA conformation, function, and replication. It is a cytotoxic, cell cycle–nonspecific agent	Electrolyte imbalances (hyponatremia, hypomagnesemia, hypocalcemia, hypokalemia), vomiting, bone marrow suppression, increased alkaline phosphatase
Methotrexate	Antimetabolite	Irreversibly binds to and inhibits dihydrofolate reductase, the formation of reduced folates, and thymidylate synthetase, resulting in inhibition of purine and thymidylic acid synthesis, thus interfering with DNA synthesis, repair, and cellular replication. Activity occurs during the S phase of the cell cycle	Thrombosis; gastrointestinal (GI) upset: nausea, vomiting; pancytopenia; myelosuppression; interstitial pneumonitis; renal failure

TABLE I: Chemotherapeutic Agents—cont'd

	Class	Mechanism of Action	Side Effects
5-Fluorouracil (Adrucil)	Pyrimidine analog antimetabolite	Interferes with DNA and RNA synthesis by the intercellular conversion to several active metabolites (fluorodeoxyuridine monophosphate, fluorodeoxyuridine triphosphate, and fluorouridine triphosphate) that disrupt RNA synthesis and the action of thymidylate synthase. Activity occurs during the G1/S phase of the cell cycle	Angina, arrhythmia; GI upset; mucositis; agranulocytosis

COLONY-STIMULATING FACTORS

	Class	Mechanism of Action	Side Effects
Filgrastim (Neupogen)	GCS-F	Stimulates the production, maturation, and activation of neutrophils to increase both their migration and cytotoxicity	Chest pain, fatigue, thrombocytopenia, splenomegaly
Pegfilgrastim (Neulasta)	Colony-stimulating factor	Stimulates the production, maturation, and activation of neutrophils to increase both their migration and cytotoxicity	Ostealgia, limb pain

TARGETED CHEMOTHERAPY

	Class	Mechanism of Action	Side Effects
Trastuzumab (Herceptin)	Anti-HER2 monoclonal antibody	Binds to the extracellular domain of the human epidermal growth factor receptor 2–protein (HER2) and mediates antibody-dependent cellular cytotoxicity by inhibiting proliferation of cells which overexpress HER2 protein	Decreased left ventricular ejection fraction (LVEF), GI symptoms, weakness
Pertuzumab (Perjeta)	Anti-HER2 monoclonal antibody	Targets HER2 dimerization domain. Inhibits HER2 dimerization and blocks HER2 downstream signaling halting cell growth and initiating apoptosis. Binds a different epitope than trastuzumab.	Cardiotoxicity, birth defects
Lapatinib (Tykerb)	Anti-HER2; epidermal growth factor receptor (EGFR) inhibitor; tyrosine kinase (dual kinase) inhibitor	Reversibly binds to tyrosine kinase and inhibits EGFR (ErbB1) and HER2 (ErbB2), blocking phosphorylation and activation of downstream second messengers (Erk1/2 and Akt), regulating cellular proliferation and survival in ErbB1- and ErbB2-expressing tumors. Combination therapy with lapatinib and endocrine therapy may overcome endocrine resistance occurring in HER2+ and hormone receptor–positive disease	Nausea/vomiting, diarrhea, palmar-plantar erythrodysesthesia, rash, fatigue
Bevacizumab (Avastin)	Recombinant, humanized monoclonal antibody; VEGF inhibitor	Binds and neutralizes vascular endothelial growth factor (VEGF), preventing its association with endothelial receptors, Flt-1 and KDR. Inhibition of angiogenesis and microvascular growth to retard the growth of metastatic tissue.	GI perforation (0.3%-3.2%) Severe bleeding, venous thromboembolism, febrile neutropenia, mucositis, vomiting, abdominal pain, hypertension
Everolimus	Inhibitor of mammalian target of rapamycin (mTOR); macrolide immunosuppressant	Reduces protein synthesis and cell proliferation by binding to the FK binding protein 12, an intracellular protein to form a complex that inhibits activation of mTOR serine-threonine kinase activity. Reduces angiogenesis by inhibiting VEGF and hypoxia inducible factor (HIF-1) expression	Immunosuppression, nephrotoxicity, increased creatinine (Cr), hypertension, fatigue, GI symptoms, bone marrow suppression, angioedema, fertility effects

Continued

TABLE I: Chemotherapeutic Agents—cont'd

	Class	Mechanism of Action	Side Effects
ENDOCRINE THERAPY			
Tamoxifen	Selective estrogen receptor modulator (SERM); nonsteroidal agent	Competitively binds to estrogen receptors on tumors and other tissue targets, producing a nuclear complex that decreases DNA synthesis and inhibits estrogen effects; with potent antiestrogenic properties which compete with estrogen for binding sites in breast and other tissues; cells accumulate in the G0 and G1 phases; cytostatic agent	Endometrial cancer (<1%), deep venous thrombosis (<2%), pulmonary embolism, cataracts, vasomotor symptoms (hot flashes, sleep disturbance, headache, emotional lability irritability)
Raloxifene (Evista)	2nd generation SERM	Estrogenic effects on bone and lipids, but estrogen antagonist effects on the breast and uterus	Vasomotor symptoms, arthralgia
Anastrozole (Arimidex)	Aromatase inhibitor; selective nonsteroidal	Prevents conversion of androstenedione to estrone and testosterone to estradiol	Vasomotor symptoms, weakness, arthritis
Exemestane (Aromasin)	Aromatase inhibitor; irreversible, steroidal	Irreversibly blocks the active site of the aromatase enzyme, leading to inactivation and preventing conversion of androgens to estrogen in peripheral tissues	Hypertension, vasomotor symptoms
OVARIAN SUPPRESSION			
Goserelin (Zoladex) Leuprolide (Lupron) Triptorelin (Trelstar)	Gonadotropin-releasing hormone agonist	Causes in initial increase in luteinizing hormone (LH) and follicle-stimulating hormone (FSH) and subsequent sustained suppression of pituitary gonadotropins	Vasomotor symptoms, peripheral edema, decreased bone mineral density

chemotherapy and anti-HER2 therapy balanced against the limited clinical trials–based evidence of its benefits in the setting of such early stage disease. Patients with unusual but biologically favorable histology such as tubular or mucinous breast cancers (both of which are almost uniformly hormone receptor–positive) are less likely to require adjuvant chemotherapy compared with similar-stage invasive ductal and/or lobular cancers.

Neutropenia during the administration of chemotherapy can lead to hospitalization, fevers, life-threatening infections or cessation of chemotherapy. Granulocyte colony-stimulating factors (G-CSF, filgrastim, pegfilgrastim) have been shown to decrease the degree and duration of neutropenia. Prechemotherapy prophylaxis with G-CSF is recommended when the anticipated incidence of neutropenic fever is approximately 20% or higher, according to the American Society of Clinical Oncology and the NCCN.

■ ADJUVANT SYSTEMIC THERAPY

Adjuvant Endocrine Therapy

Systemic treatment for breast cancers that are positive for ER and/or PR represent the earliest forms of targeted therapy. Historically there has been inconsistency in methodology as well as interpretation of tests that identify hormone receptor–positive disease, but current guidelines established by the American Society of Clinical Oncology/College of American Pathologists (ASCO/CAP) define any tumor with at least 1% nuclear expression of ER and/or PR by immunohistochemistry as being hormone receptor–positive. The Early Breast Cancer Trialists Collaborative Group meta-analyses demonstrate that tamoxifen (the first approved endocrine agent) reduces breast cancer recurrence and mortality by 30% to 40% for both premenopausal and postmenopausal patients. The majority

(80%) of invasive breast cancers in adult American women are hormone receptor–positive. The extent of benefit from endocrine therapy is correlated directly with strength of hormone receptor expression. Premenopausal women, African Americans (at all ages), and *BRCA1* mutation carriers are less likely to have hormone receptor–positive breast cancer.

Options for endocrine therapy of breast cancer include the selective estrogen receptor modulator tamoxifen; aromatase inhibitors (Arimidex, exemestane, and letrozole); and ovarian ablation/suppression. Aromatase inhibitors are indicated only for postmenopausal patients (because they block production of estrogenic compounds from nonovarian pathways such as adipose tissues), and ovarian suppression/ablation is indicated only in premenopausal patients. Tamoxifen can be used in either premenopausal or postmenopausal breast cancer. It is therefore essential to document the menopausal status of breast cancer patients. Women whose ovaries have been surgically removed or are at least 60 years old and those younger than 60 that have been amenorrheic for at least 12 months (supported by postmenopausal follicle-stimulating hormone levels) are considered candidates for aromatase inhibition.

Adjuvant Endocrine Therapy for Premenopausal Hormone Receptor–Positive Breast Cancer

Tamoxifen is the only approved endocrine therapy for premenopausal women with hormone receptor–positive breast cancer. Tamoxifen is a selective estrogen receptor modulator; its ER antagonist activity on breast tissue results in its effectiveness as adjuvant therapy as well as chemoprevention. Tamoxifen reduces risk of new contralateral cancers by approximately 50%, establishing the basis for using tamoxifen in the National Surgical Adjuvant Breast and Bowel Project (NSABP) P-1 chemoprevention trial. Tamoxifen is not

TABLE 2: Common Traditional Regimens

AC-T	Doxorubicin (**A**driamycin), **C**yclophosphamide, **T**axane (Paclitaxel)
AC-T + CP	Doxorubicin (**A**driamycin), **C**yclophosphamide, **T**axane (Paclitaxel), **C**arboplatin
TAC	**T**axane (Docetaxel), Doxorubicin (**A**driamycin), **C**yclophosphamide
T-FAC	**T**axane (Paclitaxel), **F**luorouracil, Doxorubicin (**A**driamycin), **C**yclophosphamide
FEC-T	**F**luorouracil, **E**pirubicin, **C**yclophosphamide, **T**axane (Docetaxel)
CEF	**C**yclophosphamide, **E**pirubicin, **F**luorouracil
CAF	**C**yclophosphamide, **A**driamycin, **F**luorouracil
ACT	Doxorubicin (**A**driamycin), **C**yclophosphamide, **T**axane (Paclitaxel)
EP	**E**pirubicin, **P**aclitaxel
EC	**E**pirubicin, **C**yclophosphamide
TC	**T**axane (Docetaxel), **C**yclophosphamide
AC	Doxorubicin (**A**driamycin), **C**yclophosphamide
CMF	**C**yclophosphamide, **M**ethotrexate, **F**luorouracil

A, Doxorubicin (Adriamycin); *C*, Cyclophosphamide; *CP*, Carboplatin; *E*, Epirubicin; *F*, Fluorouracil; *M*, Methotrexate; *T*, Taxane (Paclitaxel, Docetaxel).

approved for use during pregnancy or in women planning to become pregnant. It can cause vasomotor symptoms (e.g., hot flashes, night sweats) in more than one third of patients, and as with other hormonally active medications (i.e., oral contraceptives and hormone replacement therapy), it increases the risk of venous thromboembolism. It should therefore be withheld for at least 2 weeks in women undergoing elective surgery. Tamoxifen also is associated with an increased risk of uterine hyperplasia and cancer, although this is seen primarily among postmenopausal women.

Tamoxifen generally is prescribed as 20 mg per day for at least 5 years. The worldwide Adjuvant Tamoxifen: Longer Against Shorter (ATLAS) trial, and the United Kingdom aTTOM (Adjuvant Tamoxifen: To Offer More?) trial each compared 5 versus 10 years of tamoxifen and found that prolonged therapy improved both recurrence and survival rates. The American Society of Clinical Oncology therefore currently recommends 10 years of adjuvant tamoxifen for hormone receptor–positive breast cancer. If the patient becomes postmenopausal after 5 years of tamoxifen, then aromatase inhibitors should be administered for the second 5 years, to complete 10 years of therapy.

Ovarian suppression/ablation via oophorectomy, ovarian irradiation, or gonadotropin-releasing-hormone agonist therapy (e.g., with leuprolide, goserelin, or triptorelin) is also effective as endocrine therapy for premenopausal breast cancer. Furthermore, if ovarian function is abolished, these patients become candidates for aromatase inhibition. The Suppression of Ovarian Function Trial (SOFT) and Tamoxifen and Exemestane Trial (TEXT) compared ovarian suppression plus aromatase inhibition with exemestane versus ovarian suppression plus tamoxifen; SOFT included a third randomization arm to tamoxifen without ovarian suppression. Both of these phase 3 trials demonstrated outcome advantages associated with ovarian suppression but at the cost of toxicities such as depression, osteoporosis, and vasomotor symptoms.

Adjuvant Endocrine Therapy for Postmenopausal Hormone Receptor–Positive Breast Cancer

Several prospective randomized clinical trials (Arimidex, Tamoxifen Alone or in Combination; Breast International Group study of tamoxifen versus exemestane; and the MA.17 study of tamoxifen versus letrozole) have all confirmed the superiority of aromatase inhibitors over tamoxifen for postmenopausal women with ER/PR-positive breast cancer. Aromatase inhibitors are prescribed for 5 years. Side effects include vasomotor symptoms and osteoporosis. Unlike tamoxifen, aromatase inhibitors do not increase significantly the risk of venous thromboembolism or uterine cancer.

Patients older than 70 years with T1 hormone receptor–positive/clinically node-negative breast cancer may be considered for omitting radiation after a margin-negative lumpectomy based upon results from a phase 3 trial conducted by the Cancer and Leukemia Group B. This study demonstrated equivalent survival for participants regardless of whether they received adjuvant radiation; however, these favorable results were dependent upon patients committing to 5 years of adjuvant endocrine therapy.

Adjuvant Chemotherapy for Breast Cancer

As noted above, generic and combination chemotherapy regimens for breast cancer in the adjuvant setting are prescribed most commonly for node-positive disease (regardless of hormone receptor status and/or primary invasive tumor size); HER2-overexpressing invasive cancers that are at least 1 cm (regardless of nodal status and in this setting chemotherapy is given concurrently with targeted anti-*HER2/neu* therapy as described below); and for triple-negative invasive tumors that are at least 1 cm (regardless of nodal status). Furthermore, adjuvant chemotherapy is considered strongly for medically fit adult women with *HER2/neu*-overexpressing or triple negative node-negative invasive cancers measuring 6 to 10 mm.

The most commonly used chemotherapy regimens include an anthracycline (doxorubicin or epirubicin) and a taxane (paclitaxel or docetaxel). Other possible components of these combination regimens are drugs such as fluorouracil, cyclophosphamide, and carboplatin.

Most chemotherapy regimens are given in cycles, so as to minimize toxicity, especially with regard to the bone marrow so that risk of immunocompromise is minimized. Historically, this resulted in most cycles being given at 3-week cycles (representing the time necessary for the bone marrow to recover). The advent of bone marrow-supporting agents has mitigated much of this risk, and dose-dense regimens therefore have increased in popularity. With dose-dense regimens, chemotherapy cycles can be shortened to every 1 to 2 weeks, resulting in a more aggressive and effective attack on the cancer.

Gene Expression Profiles to Individualize Adjuvant Therapy

Endocrine therapy is effective for hormone receptor–positive breast cancer, but chemotherapy is usually necessary as additional systemic treatment for cases of node-positive disease and cases of HER2-overexpressing breast cancer (regardless of nodal status). Among women with hormone receptor–positive, *HER2/neu*-negative breast cancer, it can be challenging to distinguish the patients who have biologically aggressive disease (in which chemotherapy as well as endocrine therapy are warranted) from those with more indolent disease (where endocrine therapy is adequate) on the basis of age and primary tumor size alone. Genetic analysis of tumor tissue on a molecular level can provide individual prognostic information and determine the value of adjuvant chemotherapy. Oncotype DX is a well-validated, commercially available 21-gene expression assay that reports a patient's disease in terms of low, intermediate, and high risk of recurrence. The recurrence score (RS) predicts the rate of distance recurrence at 10 years to be 7% for low (RS<18), 14% for intermediate (RS 18-30), and 31% for high (RS>30). The NSABP B-14 and B-20 trials revealed that RS was significantly predictive of chemotherapy benefit in tamoxifen-treated patients. Patients with low-risk scores can be treated with endocrine therapy alone; patients with high-risk scores should receive chemotherapy as well as endocrine therapy to improve their survival; and intermediate-risk cases require a balanced discussion of chemotherapy as an option.

Initial results from the Trial Assigning IndividuaLized Options for Treatment, a multicenter prospectively conducted international trial of more than 10,000 women with early stage breast cancer, have confirmed the safety of omitting chemotherapy in women with low-risk scores who receive endocrine therapy; future results from this trial will determine whether women with intermediate scores of 11 to 25 can avoid chemotherapy. The Southwest Oncology Group S1007 phase 3 clinical trial (commonly called the *RxPonder Trial*) recently has completed accrual and follow-up results will determine whether chemotherapy is necessary in addition to endocrine therapy for women with low-to-intermediate risk Oncotype Dx scores and limited node-positive disease (one to three metastatic nodes). Yet another ongoing phase 3 trial conducted in Europe and the United Kingdom, the Microarray In Node-negative and 1 to 3 positive lymph node Disease may Avoid ChemoTherapy (MINDACT) study will evaluate whether the 70-gene signature Mammaprint is appropriate for determining chemotherapy benefit among breast cancer patients, regardless of hormone receptor and HER2 status.

Adjuvant HER2 Targeted Therapy

Human epidermal growth factor receptor–2 (HER2) belongs to a family of transmembrane tyrosine kinase receptors involved in signal transduction pathways that promote cellular growth and differentiation. Amplification of the *HER2* proto-oncogene leading to protein overexpression occurs in approximately 20% of breast cancer and initially was viewed as a poor prognostic feature. In the era before HER2 targeted therapy, patients with HER2 overexpressing breast cancer experienced significantly shorter time to relapse and overall survival. Prolonged survival among patients receiving anti-HER2 therapy for metastatic breast cancer motivated studies of these targeted treatments in the setting of adjuvant therapy for clinically early stage breast cancer. The effectiveness of this therapy therefore also justifies repeated testing for HER2 overexpression among cancers exhibiting evidence of intratumoral heterogeneity. Conversely, microinvasive cancers associated with extensive ductal carcinoma in situ (DCIS) always should be scrutinized to ensure that the HER2 immunostaining is performed on the invasive component because the majority of DCIS lesions will overexpress HER2.

Targeted HER2 inhibition is achieved most commonly with monoclonal antibody therapies trastuzumab and pertuzumab. Trastuzumab given as monthly infusions for at least 1 year in combination with standard chemotherapy regimens has been shown to improve overall survival of HER2-overexpressing breast cancer patients by approximately 40% compared with chemotherapy alone. Current St. Gallen and NCCN guidelines therefore recommend 1 year of adjuvant trastuzumab concurrently with combination chemotherapy for all HER2-overexpressing invasive breast cancers that are larger than 1 cm, regardless of nodal status and hormone receptor expression. Single-agent trastuzumab has not been studied adequately in the adjuvant setting. A major risk of trastuzumab therapy is cardiotoxicity, especially when given in combination with anthracyclines.

Pertuzumab is another targeted anti-HER2 therapy, and based upon results of its effectiveness in neoadjuvant therapy as well as metastatic breast cancer, it was granted accelerated approval by the FDA in 2013 for preoperative treatment. NCCN guidelines suggest that it be considered as adjuvant therapy also, but long-term results from prospective adjuvant therapy trials involving this agent are pending. Pertuzumab and trastuzumab have different mechanisms of action and are therefore given as dual-agent anti-HER2 blockade for synergistic effect.

Ado-trastuzumab emtansine (Kadcyla, another monoclonal antibody, combined with a microtubular inhibitor) and lapatinib (Tykerb, an oral tyrosine kinase inhibitor) are alternative anti-HER2 therapies that currently are approved for advanced, metastatic breast cancer refractory to trastuzumab.

■ NEOADJUVANT SYSTEMIC THERAPY

Neoadjuvant Chemotherapy

Historically, the administration of systemic neoadjuvant chemotherapy was reserved for locally advanced or inflammatory breast cancer. In these settings preoperative downstaging of disease converted inoperable cancers to cases that could be managed with mastectomy surgery. A clinical response is seen in approximately 80% of cases, and fewer than 5% of patients will have evidence of disease progression during neoadjuvant treatment. Multiple prospective randomized clinical trials have been conducted internationally to compare outcomes in stage-matched patients receiving neoadjuvant versus conventional adjuvant (postoperative) chemotherapy, and these studies consistently have demonstrated equal overall survival rates for the two different sequences of treatment, thereby confirming the safety of deferring surgery while the chemotherapy is being delivered.

The NSABP B-18 trial randomized approximately 1500 women with operable, clinical stages I to III breast cancer to receive four cycles of doxorubicin and cyclophosphamide preoperatively versus postoperatively. The preoperatively treated patients were more likely to undergo breast-conserving surgery (68% vs 60%) and to be node negative (59% vs 43%). Overall survival rates at 9 years were the same (70% vs 69%).

Prospective as well as retrospective studies also have demonstrated several advantages and lessons associated with the neoadjuvant strategy:

1. Downstaging of the primary tumor improves eligibility for breast-conserving surgery, permitting resection of a smaller-volume lumpectomy.
2. Invasive tumors that tend to respond most briskly to neoadjuvant chemotherapy include tumors with ductal histology; high-grade cancers; hormone receptor negative and triple-negative breast cancers; HER-2 overexpressing tumors; and tumors with elevated Ki67. Conversely, invasive lobular cancers and hormone receptor–positive breast cancers tend to have a more indolent, difficult-to-monitor response.
3. Extent of clinical and pathologic response to neoadjuvant chemotherapy is an excellent surrogate marker for chemosensitivity of distant organ micrometastases, making neoadjuvant treatment a more rapid and less costly strategy for studying novel systemic therapy agents compared with prospective, randomized adjuvant therapy clinical trials. Furthermore, a theoretical clinical advantage is that patients with a suboptimal clinical response can be crossed over to an alternative chemotherapy regimen rather than continuing to be exposed to the toxicity of an ineffective regimen. In clinical practice, however, it can be difficult to distinguish patients that have a nonresponding residual mass from those that have an inflammatory response to treatment and a necrotic tumor mass. Patients with a questionable response therefore often are referred to undergo surgery so that definitive assessment of response and selection of subsequent chemotherapy regimen can be made on the basis of pathology findings.
4. The 3- to 4-month period during which neoadjuvant chemotherapy is being delivered provides patients with additional time to consider their breast surgery preferences and/or to pursue genetic counseling and testing (which often influences decisions regarding mastectomy/contralateral prophylactic mastectomy).

5. Doxorubicin-based chemotherapy regimens can be delivered safely during second- and third-trimester pregnancy, whereas breast radiation is contraindicated throughout pregnancy. Appropriately selected patients with pregnancy-associated breast cancer therefore may opt to receive neoadjuvant chemotherapy and then undergo breast-conserving surgery and adjuvant radiation therapy postpartum. These patients typically will undergo pre-planned, elective induced labor and delivery that is coordinated with the chemotherapy regimen so as to avoid any risk of spontaneous labor when the patient's blood counts are in chemotherapy-related nadir.

Several issues must be addressed in selecting patients for neoadjuvant chemotherapy at time of initial presentation and biopsy:

1. Percutaneous, image-guided biopsy of the tumor mass is preferable rather than open surgical/excisional biopsy so that a measurable focus of disease can be monitored during treatment.
2. Multiple diagnostic cores should be extracted so that the baseline extent of the invasive cancer can be assessed with confidence. Although unusual, some patients will present with bulky breast masses made up of extensive ductal carcinoma in situ associated with microinvasion only; neoadjuvant chemotherapy for these cases clearly would be considered overtreatment.
3. The multidisciplinary team should ensure that adequate and representative biopsy material is available on the invasive component so that hormone receptors and HER2 status can be assessed with confidence. Documenting these markers with multiple cores is especially important in cases of tumor heterogeneity or multifocality/multicentricity because they will guide selection of the neoadjuvant as well as postoperative systemic regimen, including endocrine therapy.
4. Radio-opaque clip(s) should be left in place at the sites of image-detected disease because these will serve as the target(s) for subsequent definitive lumpectomy in breast-conserving surgery.
5. As with any newly diagnosed breast cancer patient, bilateral mammography is essential to rule out coexisting breast abnormalities. Contralateral and/or ipsilateral lesions should be biopsied before initiation of neoadjuvant therapy so that molecular marker status can be established and other foci of disease can be accounted for in the final surgical plan. Patients with diffuse cancerous-appearing or difficult-to-monitor microcalcifications, and patients with multiple widely spaced tumors that cannot be reasonably excised through a single margin-negative lumpectomy should be informed up front that they will require mastectomy regardless of how well their tumor appears to respond to neoadjuvant treatment.
6. Pretreatment breast ultrasound is valuable for accurate measurement of the baseline tumor mass, and axillary ultrasound with sonoguided biopsy of any morphologically abnormal-appearing nodes is also helpful in assessing stage at diagnosis.

Comprehensive breast imaging should be repeated after delivery of neoadjuvant chemotherapy to facilitate final surgical planning. Some patients will have "unmasking" of microcalcifications previously obscured by the pretreatment tumor mass, and others can have microcalcifications deposited as an inflammatory response to treatment. Either circumstance will have to be taken into account in planning the final extent of surgery. Prechemotherapy and post-chemotherapy magnetic resonance imaging also is being used increasingly to monitor chemotherapy response.

Postchemotherapy surgical specimens from the breast and axilla should be assessed for extent of residual invasive tumor, DCIS, and treatment response (fibrosis, ghost cells, necrosis). A complete pathologic response (pCR) is defined as no residual viable cancer in both breast and axillary tissue. Patients with a pCR have 5-year overall survival rates of approximately 90% even when they present with initially locally advanced disease, thereby confirming the prognostic value of this metric. It is important for patients to understand that the clinical response tends to overestimate the final pathologically

defined extent of residual disease and surgery is therefore necessary for durable locoregional control of disease.

Approximately 13% of patients receiving conventional doxorubicin-based neoadjuvant chemotherapy will experience a pCR, and the addition of a taxane to the neoadjuvant regimen will double this rate. Patients with HER2+ cancers have a relatively high pCR regardless of hormone receptor status. The Investigation of Serial studies to Predict your Therapeutic response with Imaging and Molecular Analysis (I-SPY 1) Trial demonstrated a pCR of 60% when trastuzumab was added to the traditional neoadjuvant chemotherapy regimen of ACT.

In the multicenter, randomized NeoSphere trial, dual-agent anti-HER2 neoadjuvant therapy with pertuzumab and trastuzumab plus docetaxel resulted in significantly higher rates of pCR than for those treated with trastuzumab plus docetaxel alone. The benefit of dual HER2-targeted therapy with the addition of lapatinib also was demonstrated in the NeoALTTO study, resulting in a 51% pCR rate.

The recent randomized multicenter GeparSixto and CALGB 40603 (Alliance) trials demonstrated that the addition of carboplatin and/or bevacizumab to standard neoadjuvant chemotherapy improved pCR rates in this population. Carboplatin is an option for the neoadjuvant treatment of early stage TNBC in the neoadjuvant setting. Improved disease-free and overall survival with the addition of these newer agents has yet to be firmly demonstrated.

Neoadjuvant Endocrine Therapy

Neoadjuvant endocrine therapy usually is reserved for postmenopausal women with ER-positive tumors. The administration of aromatase inhibitor is preferred over tamoxifen in this setting. This is based on studies that suggest a higher tumor response rate and breast conservation rate. Hormonal therapy is used approximately 3 to 4 months.

Surgery After Neoadjuvant Chemotherapy

Successful breast conserving surgery after neoadjuvant chemotherapy requires a margin-negative lumpectomy with inclusion of any sites of residual disease as well as sites of radio-opaque clip(s) placed pretreatment at sites of biopsy-proven cancer. Patients with suspicious microcalcifications should have a postlumpectomy mammogram to ensure complete resection.

Patients that were proven definitively to have node-negative disease based upon prechemotherapy SLN biopsy do not require any further axillary surgery. Conversely, patients with documented node-positive disease at time of diagnosis (prechemotherapy) generally will require completion ALND at the time of their definitive breast surgery. Several oncology groups perform the SLN biopsy after delivery of neoadjuvant chemotherapy in patients that present with a clinically negative axilla. The accuracy of the SLN biopsy in this setting, however, remains uncertain, with reported false-negative results ranging from 0 to 33% in retrospective studies.

Recent prospective studies have sought to evaluate the accuracy of SLN biopsy after neoadjuvant chemotherapy and specifically as a strategy for identifying patients with axillary nodal downstaging. The European SENTINA study (Sentinel Lymph Node Biopsy in patients with breast cancer before and after neoadjuvant chemotherapy) found a higher false-negative rate and lower detection rate of SLN in patients who received chemotherapy versus those who did not. Results from the ACOSOG Z1071 trial, conducted to evaluate the utility of SLN biopsy in patients with node-positive disease who received chemotherapy, demonstrated a false-negative rate of 12.6%, which exceeded the a priori–defined acceptable rate. However, a decrease in the false-negative rate to 7.4% and 10.8% was observed when a preoperative biopsy clip was placed and dual tracer technique was used, respectively. New NCCN recommendations include placing a clip in a biopsied lymph node and removing all clip-containing axillary nodes during definitive axillary surgery.

Results from the SENTINA and Z1071 trials are being incorporated into ongoing clinical studies via the targeted axillary dissection (TAD). TAD allows for biopsy-proven lymph node–positive patients treated with neoadjuvant chemotherapy to have the biopsied nodes selectively removed at the time of their definitive breast surgery. Preoperative image guided wire or I^{125} radioactive seed localization allows the biopsy-proven positive axillary node to be identified and removed at the time of definitive axillary surgery after neoadjuvant chemotherapy. Early results are promising, but the false-negative rate and correlation between the previously biopsied (clipped) node versus the operative SLN continue to be evaluated. TAD therefore typically is accompanied by complete axillary dissection and considered investigational. TAD offers a less invasive approach to restaging the axilla after neoadjuvant chemotherapy, and randomized studies are needed to determine its impact on outcomes.

■ SUMMARY

As the study of breast cancer as a heterogeneous genetic disease continues to advance, novel targeted agents will be discovered and individualized therapy invented to further drive down mortality rates. Additional biologic markers and unique cell cycle pathways constantly are being discovered, and future challenges in the medical management of breast cancer will involve the translation of the vast breast cancer genome into meaningful individualized therapies. Surgeons are essential in coordinating these medical advances with optimal locoregional care.

SUGGESTED READINGS

Boughey JC, Suman VJ, Mittendorf EA, et al. Sentinel lymph node surgery after neoadjuvant chemotherapy in patients with node-positive breast cancer: the ACOSOG Z1071 (Alliance) clinical trial. *JAMA.* 2013;310: 1455-1461.

Mathew A, Davidson NE. Adjuvant endocrine therapy for premenopausal women with hormone-responsive breast cancer. *Breast.* 2015;24(suppl 2):S120-S125.

National Comprehensive Cancer Network. *Management of breast cancer guidelines.* <www.nccn.org>.

Rastogi P, Anderson SJ, Bear HD, et al. Preoperative chemotherapy: updates of National Surgical Adjuvant Breast and Bowel Project Protocols B-18 and B-27. *J Clin Oncol.* 2008;26:778-785.

Schramm A, De Gregorio N, Widschwendter P, et al. Targeted Therapies in HER2-Positive Breast Cancer—a Systematic Review. *Breast Care (Basel).* 2015;10:173-178.

Sparano JA, Gray RJ, Makower DF, et al. Prospective Validation of a 21-Gene Expression Assay in Breast Cancer. *N Engl J Med.* 2015 Sep 27 (epub ahead of print).

Telli ML, Sledge GW. The future of breast cancer systemic therapy: the next 10 years. *J Mol Med.* 2015;93:119-125.

THE MANAGEMENT OF RECURRENT AND METASTATIC BREAST CANCER

Carlos A. Puig, MD, and Judy C. Boughey, MD, FACS

About 10% to 20% of stage I to III breast cancers will recur locally, with the risk of recurrence being higher with lymph node–positive disease and higher T stage. Despite this fact, no significant differences in disease-free survival (DFS), distant DFS, or overall survival have been demonstrated by multiple randomized controlled trials between mastectomy and breast-conserving therapy (BCT). BCT is known to be associated with higher rates of ipsilateral breast tumor recurrence (IBTR) compared with mastectomy. Isolated IBTR rates range from 8.8% at 20 years in the Milan study, to 14.3% at 20 years in the National Surgical Adjuvant Breast and Bowel Project (NSABP) B-06 trial, to 22% at 18 years in the National Cancer Institute (NCI) study. The differences in IBTR rates across the studies is explained by the differing inclusion criteria and methods, specifically tumor sizes, margin status, and length of follow-up. More recently, studies have shown lower rates of IBTR, with one study from Japan reporting a 10-year cumulative IBTR rate of 8.5% and a Dutch study reporting a 5-year overall IBTR rate of 2.9%. Advances in our understanding of tumor biology and improvements in early detection, operative techniques, systemic therapies, and radiation delivery have resulted in improvement in the local-regional control rates over historical studies.

■ RELAPSE AND RECURRENCE PATTERNS AND DEFINITIONS

1. **Local recurrence:** Recurrence in the breast (IBTR) or chest wall, including preserved skin, nipple-areolar complex, subcutaneous tissues, remaining breast, pectoral muscle, fascia, ribs, or intercostal muscles.

2. **Regional recurrence:** Recurrence in the draining lymph nodes: axillary, infraclavicular, supraclavicular, or internal mammary nodes.

Local and regional recurrence rates and management vary based on prior breast surgery (lumpectomy +/− radiation vs mastectomy) and prior axillary surgery (sentinel lymph node [SLN] surgery vs axillary lymph node dissection [ALND]).

3. **Metastatic disease:** Disease occurring at distant sites, such as bone or visceral organs (brain, lung, liver, abdominopelvic cavity). This can exist at presentation or develop during follow-up after management of the index breast cancer.

IBTRs can be divided further into:

1. **True recurrence:** Recurrence at the original lumpectomy site or within the boost volume of the preserved breast.

2. **Marginal miss:** Recurrence close to but not within the boost volume.

3. **Elsewhere recurrence:** Recurrence in quadrants other than the quadrant previously involved by the original breast cancer.

True recurrences and marginal misses constitute about 80% of IBRTs. True breast cancer recurrence and new ipsilateral primary breast cancer have different natural histories and prognoses. These two entities can be distinguished based on differing histologic subtype, hormone receptor status, human epidermal growth factor receptor–2 (HER2) overexpression, tumor location, and discordant DNA flow cytometry. True recurrence has been defined as a tumor located within 3 cm of the primary tumor bed or whose histologic subtype or estrogen receptor/progesterone receptor (ER/PR) and HER2 status is consistent with the primary tumor. New ipsilateral primary breast cancer has been defined as a tumor located more than 3 cm from the primary tumor site (by breast imaging or clinical examination) and of different tumor histology or whose ER/PR or HER2 status is different from the primary tumor.

■ THERAPEUTIC PRINCIPLES AND STRATEGIES

Ipsilateral Breast Tumor Recurrence After Breast-Conserving Therapy

Preoperative Considerations

IBTR after BCT is resectable in up to 85% of cases. Mastectomy remains the standard of care for patients with localized IBTR that is amenable to operative intervention and where distant metastatic disease has been ruled out by computed tomography (CT), positron emission tomography (PET), and/or bone scan. Repeat BCT is an option but has been associated with higher re-recurrence rates, especially if the disease-free interval (DFI) is less than 5 years. Recurrences that occur more than 5 years after primary tumor resection are more likely to be second primary cancers.

BCT generally is not recommended in IBTR given that the recommendation for radiation and re-irradiating may not be feasible. However, early results from a recent prospective phase II trial suggest that BCT may be a possibility for some patients. Radiation Therapy Oncology Group (RTOG) 1014 used 3D conformal external beam partial breast reirradiation after lumpectomy for IBTR in patients with previous lumpectomy and whole breast irradiation. This study of 55 eligible patients with 1 year of follow-up demonstrated that it is a safe and feasible approach with acceptable treatment quality. Skin, fibrosis, and breast pain toxicity were acceptable (grade 1 or 2), and grade 3 toxicity was rare (<2%) at the 1-year follow-up interval.

About 10% to 20% of patients with recurrent disease are classified as inoperable because of locally advanced tumors or extensive regional recurrences or synchronous distant metastases. Patients with locally advanced tumors (large or fixed tumors, skin or chest wall involvement, or inflammatory carcinomas) or regionally advanced disease should undergo neoadjuvant systemic therapy before any surgical intervention (Figure 1).

Choice of Operation

Mastectomy is the standard treatment recommended for operable IBTR after BCT. Often a standard total mastectomy is recommended, as these patients have had previous breast radiation, which complicates options for immediate reconstruction. For patients who wish to pursue immediate reconstruction, discussion with a plastic and reconstructive surgeon and counseling of the patient regarding potential risks and complications associated with reconstruction in a radiated field are needed. Use of an autologous tissue flap, such as

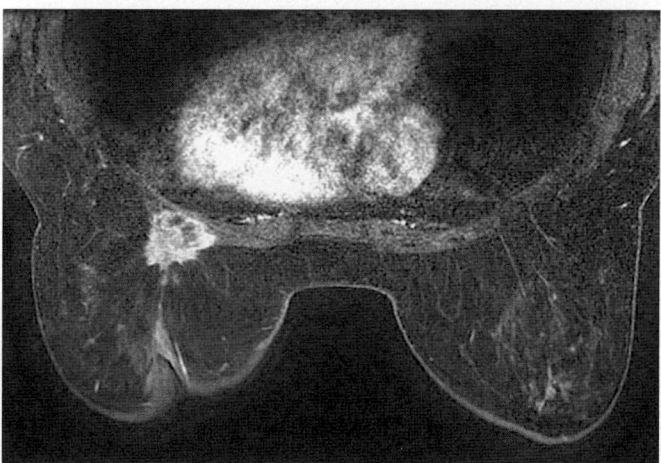

FIGURE 1 Magnetic resonance imaging scan showing ipsilateral breast tumor recurrence involving the chest wall after prior right breast cancer treated with lumpectomy.

deep inferior epigastric (DIEP) flap or transverse rectus abdominis myocutaneous (TRAM) flap, is recommended in these situations. Implant-based reconstruction can be used but has a higher failure rate. The choice of reconstruction type depends on patient preference, extent of tumor and any skin involvement, and timing of breast reconstruction. Skin-sparing mastectomy can be considered as long as there is no skin involvement. Use of nipple-sparing mastectomy in patients with IBTR and previous radiation has not been studied and lacks oncologic safety and outcome data.

The choice of incision depends on the type of mastectomy, location of the tumor, previous surgical scars, and skin involvement by tumor. In most cases a standard simple mastectomy incision can be used. Care should be taken when designing the incision so that the old surgical incision and any involved skin are incorporated into the mastectomy incision where possible to avoid multiple scars on the chest wall.

Occasionally, patients treated with lumpectomy decline adjuvant radiation therapy at the time of their initial breast cancer diagnosis, and some of these patients subsequently are seen with recurrent disease in the breast. In these cases, the lack of previous radiation simplifies the management. Mastectomy remains the standard recommendation. However, depending on breast size, tumor size, and the extent of the previous lumpectomy, a second lumpectomy in the same breast may be considered if feasible to resect and obtain reasonable cosmetic outcome. If lumpectomy is performed for recurrence, clips should be placed in the lumpectomy bed to mark the cavity for the delivery of the radiation boost. Adjuvant whole breast radiation is strongly recommended, and patients who remain unprepared to consider adjuvant radiation would be better served with mastectomy.

Technical Factors During Mastectomy for Ipsilateral Breast Tumor Recurrence

In patients who have previously undergone breast-conserving surgery (BCS) and adjuvant breast radiation, extra care should be taken during the dissection of the skin flaps because of radiation-associated microvascular changes that result in a tenuous blood supply to the skin, thus predisposing the flaps to a higher risk of flap ischemia and necrosis. Because of the fibrosis secondary to the previous radiation, the plane between the breast tissue and subcutaneous tissue may be harder to visualize. If the prior lumpectomy scar is not incorporated into the mastectomy incision, special care is required when performing the flap dissection in the area of the previous lumpectomy scar to avoid skin flap necrosis. Attention is also required in the area of the recurrent tumor to ensure that adequate margins are achieved, resecting the skin overlying the tumor and/or the underlying muscle if necessary. When dissecting the breast from the underlying pectoralis muscle, this plane is often fibrosed from the previous radiation and requires additional attention to avoid leaving breast tissue behind or damaging the underlying muscle.

Complications and Their Prevention

There is an increased risk of seroma and wound healing complications in patients who have had prior breast radiation. The surgeon should attempt to minimize the risk of these complications. The risk of seroma formation after total mastectomy may be reduced by the use of quilting sutures (which involves mastectomy flap fixation to the muscle with absorbable sutures). Because of the microvascular changes that occur after breast radiation, there is an increased risk of skin flap necrosis. Meticulous surgical technique during mastectomy should be maintained to minimize this risk. SPY angiography (SPY Elite; Novadaq Technologies, Concord, Canada) may be performed preoperatively to evaluate cutaneous blood flow to assist in planning the surgical incision or intraoperatively to evaluate mastectomy flap perfusion after mastectomy and before reconstruction. SPY angiography is performed by injecting 5 mL of indocyanine green intravenously and then using the SPY camera to evaluate the perfusion of the mastectomy flaps. Preoperative SPY images usually will show decreased blood flow to the mastectomy flaps on the radiated side compared with blood flow on the contralateral nonradiated side. In addition, this technology can be used to guide the volume of fluid placed in a tissue expander to minimize risk of skin flap necrosis. SPY angiography can direct attention to areas with poor blood flow, and surgeons can consider excising this skin and/or decreasing the volume of the expander and then repeat the angiography.

Recurrence After Mastectomy

Preoperative Considerations

Breast cancer recurrence after mastectomy is less common than recurrence after BCS. However, local recurrences after mastectomy can be more difficult to manage and are associated with a higher rate of distant metastasis and a worse prognosis. Feasibility of resection should be assessed with physical examination, ultrasound, and magnetic resonance imaging (MRI) or CT scan. Local recurrence may involve the skin, chest wall, muscle, or ribs and requires wide local excision of the involved structures. Preoperative evaluation should include a multidisciplinary team discussion including medical and radiation oncology, breast surgery, and plastic surgery. The patient should be evaluated for distant disease with use of PET scan and additional imaging as indicated.

Systemic neoadjuvant chemotherapy or hormonal therapy should be considered for large recurrences to decrease the extent of surgery required. After systemic therapy, if there is no evidence of distant disease, curative resection should be considered if complete resection is feasible. Surgery should occur about 4 to 6 weeks after the last dose of chemotherapy. These patients often end up with large wound defects after excision of the recurrence and may require input from a plastic surgeon to close the resulting wounds. Therefore, preoperatively, the surgeon should estimate carefully the extent of resection that will be required. A thoracic surgeon should be involved if the

tumor involves the bony chest wall and if it is anticipated that resection of involved rib cage may be necessary.

Technical Tips

Patients with skin or chest wall recurrence can require wide resections to obtain negative margins, and it may be difficult to close the resulting wound primarily depending on the size of the lesion, the laxity of the skin at the mastectomy site, and any prior radiation to the area. Often the recurrent disease, especially recurrence in the skin, extends further histologically than can be seen with visual and imaging evaluation of the chest wall. In planning the incision either preoperatively or intraoperatively, multiple punch biopsies of skin areas that are hyperemic or contain petechiae or other suspicious skin change may be performed with pathologic analysis to determine the extent of resection required. After resection to grossly normal margins, intraoperative pathologic analysis is helpful to guide the intraoperative decision making regarding further resection of the adjacent tissue and skin as well as evaluation of the deep margin.

In patients where resection results in large skin defects, different options exist for achieving wound closure. The ideal goal is to achieve closure of the wound with skin to allow for possible subsequent adjuvant radiation in many cases. Options include local skin primary closure, local advancement flaps, DermaClose device-assisted delayed primary closure, skin grafts, local vascularized pedicle flaps, and free flaps. Local advancement skin flaps can be created by undermining the skin and subcutaneous tissues to the clavicle superiorly, the sternal border medially, the posterior axillary line posteriorly, and the abdomen inferiorly (Figure 2). After this mobilization, the wound edges may be approximated temporarily with clamps. If there is concern for too much tension during this maneuver, the skin flap perfusion may be assessed with the SPY angiography as described earlier; tense areas of skin with poor perfusion should be identified

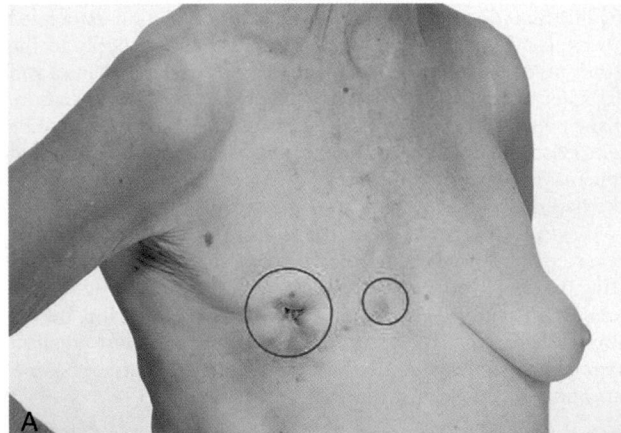
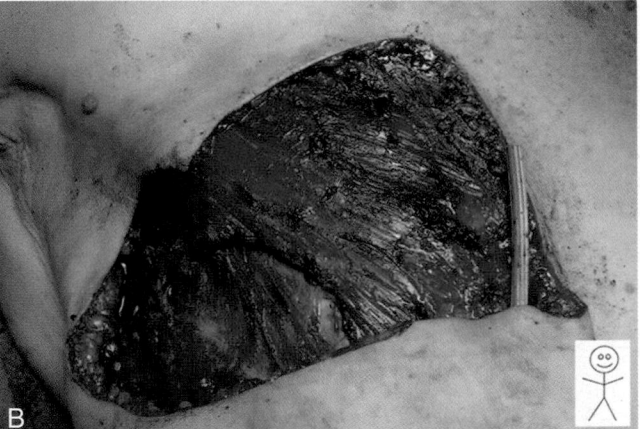
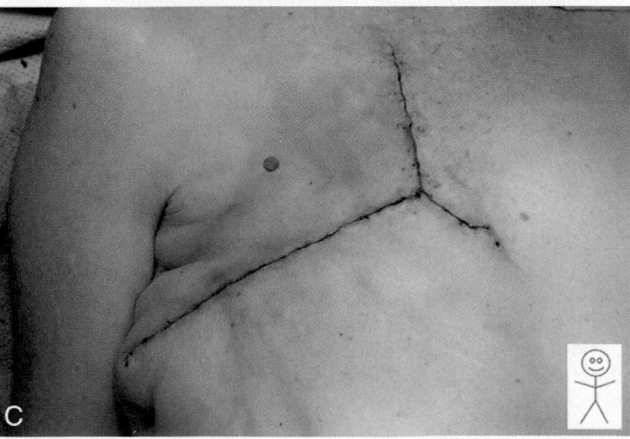

FIGURE 2 A, A patient with recurrent disease involving the skin after prior mastectomy. Note that in addition to the large primary area, a satellite skin recurrence is seen more medially (circles indicate areas of recurrence). **B,** Disease was more extensive pathologically than anticipated based on preoperative examination. Surgical bed after mastectomy with multiple intraoperative resections of skin to achieve negative margins. **C,** Local advancement flap allowed for primary closure of skin defect. *(Courtesy James Jakub, MD.)*

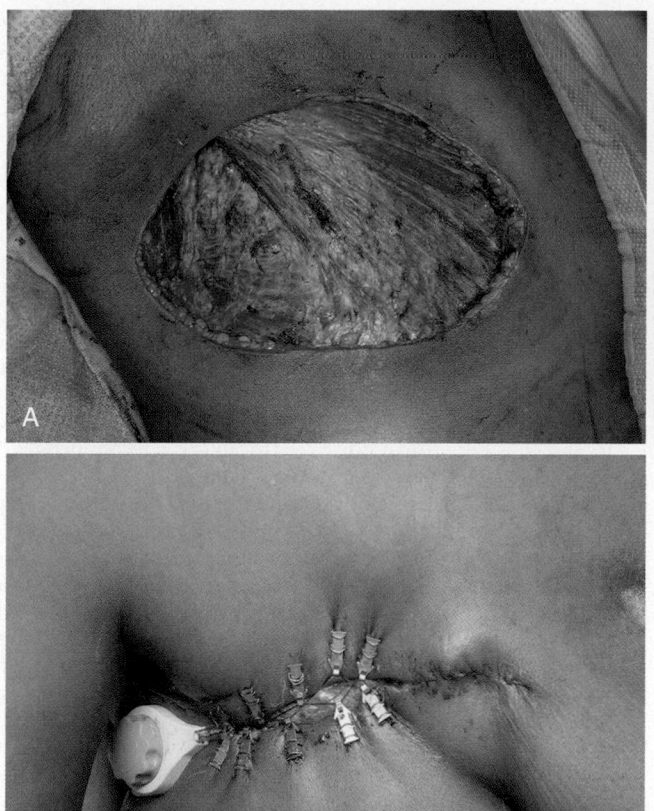

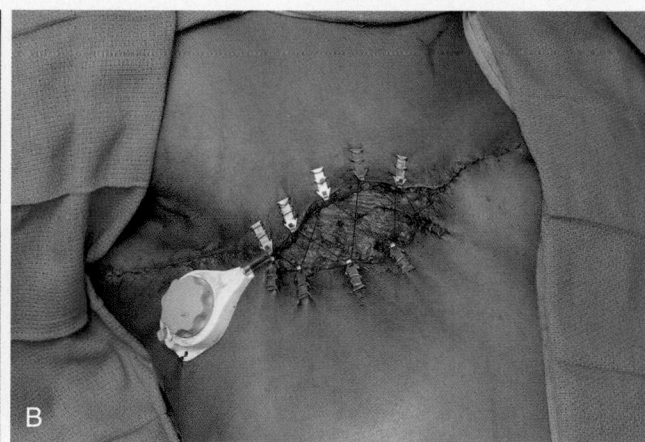

FIGURE 3 A, Surgical bed after mastectomy with resection of involved skin. The image demonstrates the exposed pectoralis major muscle and lack of sufficient overlying or adjacent skin for primary closure. **B,** DermaClose device placement to apply tension and try to pull together residual skin defect after local advancement flap and primary closure of medial and lateral aspects. **C,** Progressive increase in tension of the DermaClose device over the course of days brings the skin edges together and ultimately can allow primary wound closure.

and tension decreased in these areas. Well-perfused areas then may be approximated with interrupted vertical mattress sutures starting at the peripheries. Often a defect that cannot be approximated safely remains in the center of the wound. In this case, a DermaClose device may be applied to the defect, and appropriate tension is applied (Figure 3). SPY angiography may be used again to reassess the perfusion of the skin flaps and the wound edges. The tension of the DermaClose may be increased progressively over several days (see Figure 3, C) to approximate the wound edges and facilitate subsequent delayed primary closure. If primary closure cannot be achieved, split-thickness skin grafts can be considered.

When there is a positive deep margin at the level of the ribs, rib resection may be necessary. This is associated with a high rate of pneumothorax, usually from parietal pleural disruption. It also may be associated with hemothorax. In this case, however, the pneumothorax is caused by external atmospheric air gaining entry into the pleural space and not a visceral pleural leak, unless a visceral pleural disruption is known to have occurred. Therefore airtight closure and dressing will help to prevent persistence of the pneumothorax. If there is visceral pleural disruption, chest tube thoracostomy is performed. The resulting chest wall defects after en bloc resection of ribs with exposed lung may be closed with mesh, typically a biologic mesh, and subsequently covered with local advancement flaps, a pedicled TRAM flap, or a free flap.

Nodal Staging of Recurrent Breast Cancer After Breast Conservation or Mastectomy

The ability to perform repeat nodal staging at the time of recurrence depends on the extent of the previous nodal surgery performed for the index breast cancer as well as the prior breast surgery and radiation therapy received. Physical examination and ultrasound examination of the regional nodal basins to include ipsilateral and

contralateral axilla, supraclavicular nodal basin, and internal mammary nodes is recommended with fine-needle aspiration (FNA) or core needle biopsy of any suspicious lymph nodes. Patients with positive axillary lymph nodes should undergo ALND.

In patients with clinically negative lymph nodes (i.e., no palpable lymph nodes and sonographically negative nodes), SLN mapping should be considered and has been demonstrated to be feasible, although there are limited data on the false-negative rate in this situation. SLN mapping can provide valuable information to assist in planning adjuvant therapy and potentially avoid the morbidity of ALND. However, previous breast surgery and radiation with SLN surgery or ALND may have interfered with the native lymphatic drainage patterns, resulting in contralateral axillary drainage or extra-axillary drainage to the internal mammary or other nodal basins (Figure 4). Therefore a preoperative lymphoscintigraphy with imaging should be performed to map out the lymphatic drainage of the current tumor, even in patients who have previously undergone an ipsilateral ALND. Blue dye injection in addition to radiolabeled colloid should be used intraoperatively to assist in lymph node mapping.

Studies have demonstrated that SLNs could be identified in 65% of patients with IBTR after BCT with SLN surgery. SLNs were identified in 70% of patients in whom fewer than 10 lymph nodes had been removed during their initial surgery and in 67% of those in whom more than 10 lymph nodes had been removed during their initial surgery. The incidence of alternative lymphatic drainage (extra-axillary or internal mammary) increased as the number of axillary lymph nodes removed during the initial surgery increased, or if mastectomy or radiation was part of the initial treatment. A similar study from Memorial Sloan Kettering Cancer Center (MSKCC) reported success in identifying an SLN in 75% of patients who had fewer than 10 lymph nodes removed at their initial surgery and in 44% of those who had more than 10 lymph nodes removed. SLN identification

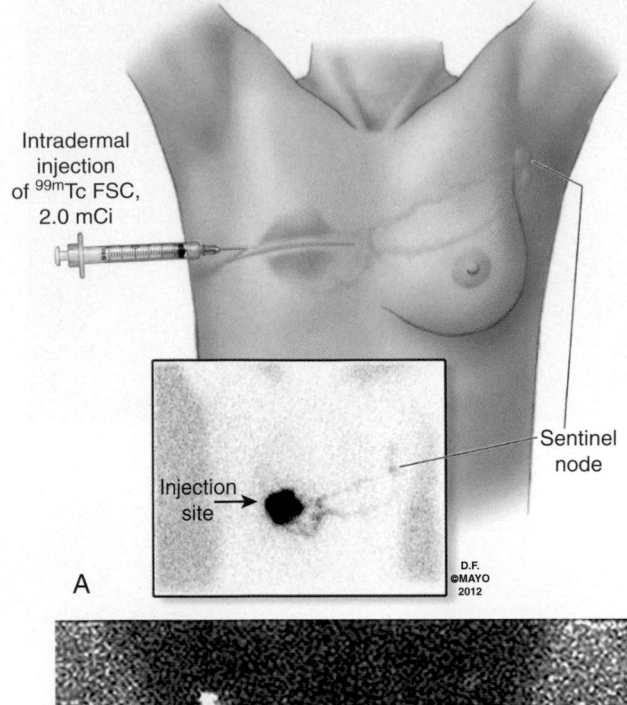

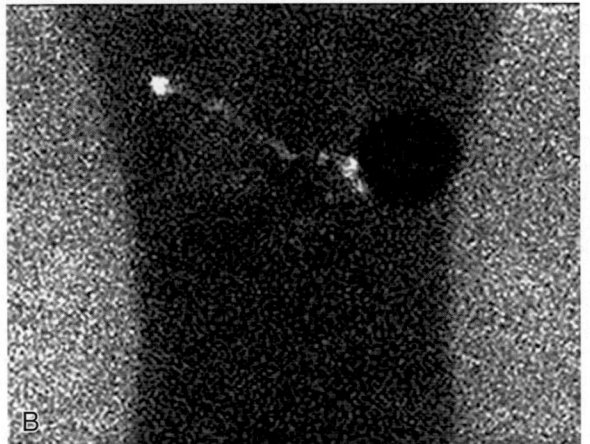

FIGURE 4 A, Injection site and lymphoscintigraphic mapping for patient with recurrence in the right breast after mastectomy showing drainage to the contralateral (left) axilla. **B,** Injection site and lymphoscintigraphic mapping for patient with recurrence in the left breast after mastectomy showing drainage to the contralateral (right) axilla. ^{99m}Tc, technetium 99m; *FSC*, filtered sulfur colloid.

rates in literature in patients with local recurrence after initial mastectomy range from 40% to 50%. In patients with a previously undissected axilla with large tumors and high-risk disease, ALND can be considered given the lack of false-negative data on SLN surgery in this situation.

Lymph Node Recurrence

The incidence of axillary and supraclavicular lymph node recurrences in patients who have undergone previous ALND is 0.7% and 1.3%, respectively, at 7 years. In the pre-SLN era, the incidence of axillary nodal recurrences in patients who did not undergo ALND was about 20%. In the current SLN sampling era, SLN-negative patients develop nodal recurrences less than 1% of the time.

Patients who are seen with axillary recurrence and who were previously SLN negative or those who did not undergo ALND should undergo ALND. For patients with axillary recurrence treated with a prior ALND, a redo axillary dissection should be done to excise the recurrent disease and any residual axillary tissue. Patients with nodal recurrence benefit from subsequent adjuvant systemic therapy and radiation therapy if not contraindicated based on previous radiation fields.

Technical Tips for Axillary Lymph Node Dissection

Use the incision from the previous SLN surgery or previous axillary dissection if present, and extend it as needed for adequate exposure in the axilla. If no prior scar exists, use a curvilinear or a lazy S incision 1 cm below the hair-bearing portion of the axilla. The extent of the previous axillary surgery and amount of scar tissue present will affect the complexity of dissection. Avoid paralytics so that the nerves can be identified easily, and perform dissection slowly and meticulously to avoid damage to the nerves. The nerves can be difficult to identify and may not be in their usual anatomic location, depending on scarring from prior surgery and any prior radiation. Use of scissors and clips rather than Bovie electrocautery is recommended.

Superior and inferior subcutaneous flaps are created, and the axilla is entered by incising the clavipectoral fascia. Adequate exposure is obtained by medial and cephalad retraction of the pectoralis major muscle. Two other retractors are used to triangulate the wound. The next step should be to define the axillary dissection borders and identify the important structures. The borders of axillary dissection are the axillary vein superiorly, the pectoralis muscles superomedially, the latissimus dorsi posterolaterally, and the serratus anterior and fascia medially. Initial dissection of the axilla should begin with identification of the axillary vein superiorly. The medial pectoral nerve is then identified and preserved. The surgeon should avoid dissection cephalad to the inferior border of the axillary vein. Dissection begins along the inferior border of the axillary vein, ligating or clipping small venous or lymphatic vessels. The thoracoepigastric vein then should be identified because it is a very important landmark to identify and protect the thoracodorsal neurovascular bundle, which usually lies deep to this vein. The thoracoepigastric vein invariably may be ligated. The thoracodorsal neurovascular bundle is isolated and preserved. Dissection continues along the pectoralis minor muscle to the chest wall, identifying and protecting the medial pectoral nerve. Dissection along the pectoralis minor muscle to the chest wall with retraction of this muscle medially allows the level II lymph nodes to be dissected away and the intercostobrachial nerves to be identified coursing from the chest wall laterally. The long thoracic nerve of Bell enters the axilla deep to the axillary vein and courses posterior to the intercostobrachial nerves and along the lateral border of the serratus anterior deep to the superficial fascia. It is identified deep to the serratus anterior fascia on the medial chest wall and should be preserved. Sometimes in the lower axilla, a small vein that is a tributary of the thoracodorsal vein may course from the long thoracic nerve and help in identifying it. Once these major structures have been identified, the surgeon is then ready to proceed to removing the axillary nodal tissue. While keeping the thoracodorsal neurovascular bundle and the long thoracic nerve visible at all times, the fibrofatty tissue between them that contains the axillary nodes is dissected from the axilla, starting at the inferior border of the axillary vein proceeding caudally and off the subscapularis muscle while skeletonizing the thoracodorsal neurovascular bundle and ligating the multiple arterial and venous branches from and into the fibrofatty tissue, respectively. All visible and palpable lymph nodes, normal and abnormal, should be removed, taking care to clip the small lymphatic channels to minimize lymphocele formation. The specimen is amputated and submitted for pathologic analysis.

In cases where there is significant scarring, an alternative approach is to dissect laterally to identify the latissimus dorsi muscle first. From there, enter the axilla and identify the thoracodorsal nerve, vein, and artery. Accessing from this direction can be helpful if there is scarring around the axillary vein and less scarring laterally in the axilla. From there, the thoracodorsal bundle can be followed cephalad to where the thoracodorsal vein enters the axillary vein, taking care to preserve the adjacent thoracodorsal nerve. Inferior in the axilla, a tributary of the thoracodorsal vein crosses over to the serratus muscle, enters the muscle at the level of the long thoracic nerve of Bell, and can aid identification of the long thoracic nerve.

■ METASTATIC DISEASE

A multidisciplinary team including a medical oncologist, breast surgical oncologist, radiation oncologist, palliative care specialist, psychosocial support worker, pathologist, and plastic surgeon, where appropriate, should manage patients with metastatic breast cancer.

Therapy for metastatic disease can be divided into local and systemic. The selection of appropriate candidates for surgical intervention should include consideration of factors such as performance status, comorbidities, risks versus benefits, number of metastatic sites and location of metastatic disease, feasibility of R0 resection, and DFI.

Intact Primary Tumor in Patients With Metastatic Breast Cancer

Approximately 5% to 10% of women in the United States have stage IV breast cancer at diagnosis. Historically, women with metastatic breast cancer were not offered surgical treatment. Current literature on resection of the breast primary in patients with stage IV disease is mixed. Multiple retrospective studies have indicated benefit from surgical resection of the primary breast tumor. Data from MSKCC of 186 patients with stage IV disease and intact breast primary showed that 37 had surgery and there was a trend to improved survival in patients who had surgery. ER positivity, PR positivity, and *HER2/neu* amplification were predictive of improved survival, and no survival benefit was seen in patients with triple-negative breast cancer. Another study reported that the median survival of patients treated surgically was 27.1 months versus 16.8 months for patients without surgical resection. In multivariate analysis, which included surgical treatment, age, race, ER and PR status, number of metastatic sites, and presence of visceral metastases, surgery remained an independent factor associated with improved survival. In a review of the literature, Ruiterkamp and colleagues reported that younger patients and patients with a single metastatic site benefit the most from surgery and also that lumpectomy or mastectomy can be performed as long as the intention is R0 resection.

Conversely, a randomized controlled trial from India published in 2015 reported that local-regional treatment (mastectomy or BCS + ALND) in patients with stage IV breast cancer and an intact primary tumor should not be part of routine practice in patients who have responded to front-line chemotherapy because of lack of benefit in terms of overall survival. Median survival was 19.2 months in the local-regional treatment group versus 20.5 months in the no local-regional treatment group (only systemic chemotherapy). However, a significant limitation is that patients in this study did not have the benefit of targeted hormonal or anti-HER2 therapy.

Bone Metastasis

Bone is the most common site of metastatic involvement in breast cancer, and this metastasis can be associated with significant morbidity and mortality. Despite modern cancer therapy, up to two thirds of patients with bone metastasis subsequently will develop a skeletal-related event, defined as any pathologic fracture, requirement for surgical intervention or palliative radiotherapy (RT) to bone lesions, hypercalcemia of malignancy, or spinal cord compression. Bone-confined metastatic breast cancer usually is characterized by an indolent course and good response to systemic therapy. Surgery, RT, and radiofrequency ablation (RFA) can provide effective pain relief and prevent fracture. In addition, surgical intervention and RT are used for the palliative treatment of epidural spinal cord or nerve compression. Bisphosphonates and other osteoclast inhibitors have been shown to reduce the morbidity of metastatic bone disease, in particular skeletal-related events.

Hepatic Metastasis

About 10% to 15% of patients with newly diagnosed metastatic breast cancers have hepatic metastases, with about 5% of these having isolated hepatic metastases as the only site of distant metastasis. Systemic chemotherapy is the standard treatment, often with a palliative intent. However, recent studies have shown a survival benefit of hepatic resection in selected patients. In a study from MD Anderson Cancer Center (MDACC), in 86 patients who underwent resection of breast cancer hepatic metastases with 62-month median follow-up, the DFS and overall survival were 14 months and 57 months, respectively. On multivariate analysis, ER-negative primary breast disease and preoperative progressive disease were associated with decreased overall survival. Other factors that convey poorer overall survival are age less than 50 years, the presence of extrahepatic metastases, hormone receptor negativity of the primary tumor, and an overall hepatic metastasis diameter of 3.5 cm or greater. The ideal candidate for consideration of hepatic metastasectomy has a solitary metastasis, no evidence of extrahepatic metastatic disease, normal liver function, a good performance status, and a long DFI. Given that these patients are usually undergoing systemic chemotherapy and/or hormonal therapy in some cases, the exact survival benefit from metastasectomy may be difficult to discern from that achieved from systemic therapy only, without a randomized controlled trial.

For patients in which liver resection is not an option, other local therapies, such as radiofrequency ablation (RFA) (especially in lesions smaller than 3 cm), percutaneous ethanol injection, stereotactic body RT, selective internal RT, cryotherapy, hepatic arterial infusion chemotherapy, transhepatic arterial chemoembolization, and interstitial laser therapy, can be considered. Data comparing these therapies with systemic chemotherapy are lacking.

Pulmonary Metastasis

Lung is one of the most common sites of breast cancer metastasis, along with bone. About 15% to 25% of patients have isolated lung metastases. A select number of patients may benefit from metastasectomy along with systemic therapy (chemotherapy +/− hormonal therapy). A meta-analysis of 16 studies showed that the pooled 5-year overall survival rates after pulmonary metastasectomy was 46%. The poor prognostic factors were DFI less than 3 years, incomplete resection of metastasis, higher number of pulmonary metastases (>1), and hormonal receptor–negative status of metastasis.

SUGGESTED READINGS

Abbott DE, Brouquet A, Mittendorf EA, et al. Resection of liver metastases from breast cancer: estrogen receptor status and response to chemotherapy before metastasectomy define outcome. *Surgery*. 2012;151:710-716.

Badwe R, Hawaldar R, Nair N, et al. Locoregional treatment versus no treatment of the primary tumour in metastatic breast cancer: an open-label randomised controlled trial. *Lancet Oncol*. 2015;16:1380-1388.

Briasoulis E, Karavasilis V, Kostadima L, et al. Metastatic breast carcinoma confined to bone: portrait of a clinical entity. *Cancer*. 2004;101:1524-1528.

Fan J, Chen D, Du H, et al. Prognostic factors for resection of isolated pulmonary metastases in breast cancer patients: a systematic review and meta-analysis. *J Thorac Dis*. 2015;7:1441-1451.

van der Heiden–van der Loo M, Siesling S, Wouters MWJM, et al. The value of ipsilateral breast tumor recurrence as a quality indicator: hospital variation in the Netherlands. *Ann Surg Oncol*. 2015;22:522-528. doi:10.1245/s10434-015-4626-9.

THE MANAGEMENT OF MALE BREAST CANCER

Hiram S. Cody III, MD

Male breast cancer (MBC) is rare, comprising about 1% (2350 of 234,190) of all incident breast cancers diagnosed in the United States this year and corresponding to a lifetime risk of about 1 in 1000. The risk of MBC is increased by those conditions that increase the effects of estrogen (cirrhosis, obesity, exogenous estrogens) or decrease the effects of testosterone (testicular nondescent, infection, trauma, 5α-reductase inhibitors, or Klinefelter's syndrome [XXY]) and is especially increased by genetic predisposition. The estimated proportion of MBC associated with *BRCA* mutations varies widely (4% to 40%), but for men with *BRCA* mutations the cumulative absolute risk of MBC by age 70 is estimated to be 1.2% for *BRCA1* (a relative risk 12 times that of nonmutation carriers) and 6.8% for *BRCA2* (a relative risk 42 times that of nonmutation carriers). The evidence linking MBC to other gene mutations (*CHEK2*, *AR*, *CYP17*, *PTEN*) is suggestive but inconclusive.

Virtually all MBC is ductal in origin. Most MBCs are invasive but about 5% are in situ, and more than 90% are hormone receptor (HR)–positive. The prognosis of MBC appears to be worse than for female breast cancer but when corrected for stage of disease (most MBC is detected as a mass, not by mammography) is comparable. Historically, more than half of MBCs were seen as advanced disease (stages III to IV), but with a trend toward earlier diagnosis in the more recent series, about 90% of MBCs have been seen with local-regional disease.

■ DIAGNOSIS

Most male breast masses are gynecomastia, which typically occurs as sudden onset of a unilateral *tender* mass; if mammography and ultrasound (US) are consistent with a benign diagnosis, observation alone is sufficient, a hormonal workup is not required, and most masses will resolve spontaneously over a 2- to 3-month period. Core biopsy need not be routine but makes sense for persistent masses or suspicious physical findings.

The most common presentation of MBC is a painless breast mass, but a minority of patients may have bloody nipple discharge, skin changes in the nipple and areola, or (rarely) suspicious axillary adenopathy as the first sign of disease. Both mammography and US are appropriate, with core biopsy of the breast lesion, punch biopsy of the nipple and areola, or US-guided fine-needle aspiration of suspicious axillary nodes. Excisional biopsy is required for no more than 5% to 10% of patients, mainly those in whom the core biopsy is non-diagnostic or discordant with imaging characteristics. All biopsy diagnoses of MBC should include determination of estrogen receptor (ER), progesterone receptor (PR), and human epidermal growth factor receptor–2 (HER2). As with female breast cancer, a preoperative workup for distant metastases (by positron emission tomography/computed tomography [PET/CT] or CT and bone scan) is indicated only for locally advanced disease (stage III) or suspicious symptoms.

■ TREATMENT

Preoperative Considerations

Although surgery is the appropriate initial treatment for most MBC, neoadjuvant chemotherapy or hormonal therapy should be considered. The indications for neoadjuvant chemotherapy are the same as for women—advanced T or N stage: T3 to T4 tumors, including inflammatory cancer, or N2 to N3 nodes. The main limitation of neoadjuvant chemotherapy is that almost all MBC is ER-positive, and

this tumor subtype is not particularly responsive to neoadjuvant chemotherapy, with rates of pathologic complete response of 10% or less. For the same reason, neoadjuvant hormonal therapy makes sense for locally advanced MBC, especially in the setting of advanced age or significant comorbidities. Most patients respond to hormonal management with tamoxifen or aromatase inhibitors; the typical duration of response is in the range of 1 to 2 years, and those who progress often will respond to a change in hormonal agent.

Breast Conservation

Although breast-conserving surgery (BCS) is possible at least in theory for those MBCs that are not directly adjacent to the nipple and areola, there are no data to support this approach and there are legitimate concerns. The extent of excision required to obtain negative margins for BCS in women is significant and for most men could easily approach the volume of the entire breast. Further, the delivery of tangential-field radiotherapy (RT) to the much smaller male breast raises concerns about exposure to the chest wall, lung, and heart; although these concerns are substantially reduced by contemporary techniques of CT-guided treatment planning, they are eliminated altogether by the performance of mastectomy, after which RT is required only for locally advanced disease. Finally, even for men who wish to preserve the nipple as part of a nipple-sparing mastectomy, the proximity of most MBC to the nipple and areola renders this approach unsound from both a cosmetic and an oncologic perspective.

Mastectomy

Mastectomy remains standard care for virtually all MBC. The incision is dependent on body habitus. For most men, separate breast and axillary incisions will give the best cosmetic result, but for those with a laterally placed nipple and areola, a single oblique elliptical incision encompassing both breast and axilla is also reasonable (Figure 1). For certain bulky or locally advanced cancers, a single incision will allow en bloc resection of the breast in continuity with the intervening soft tissues, lymphatics, and axillary nodes, but because these patients will all receive postmastectomy RT (PMRT), the benefit of this approach in local control is debatable.

The mastectomy is done through a transversely oriented elliptical incision sufficient to encompass all of the breast and tumor tissue. The incision should widely encompass any areas of skin, nipple, or areolar involvement. For men with marked obesity or gynecomastia, the incision will be comparable to that required for a female mastectomy, whereas for those who are thin, the incision barely needs to encompass the nipple and areola but should be long enough to avoid "dog ears" at the time of skin closure.

Skin flaps are elevated peripherally sufficient to remove all breast tissue and any gynecomastia. The extent of this dissection again varies widely and is highly dependent on body habitus, but in general the skin flaps in MBC do not need to be as thin as for women. In obese patients, as one nears the edges of the breast the skin flaps should be thickened gradually to avoid a sharp "drop-off" deformity at the periphery of the operative defect. The breast is dissected from the underlying pectoralis major muscle, removing the pectoral fascia and, if muscle invasion is found, the adherent portion of the pectoral muscle. The surgical specimen is oriented with sutures for inking of the margins by the surgical pathologist and handed off. Resection of the entire pectoralis major (i.e., radical mastectomy) is almost never required in the current era, but PMRT is indicated for all patients with muscle invasion.

Axillary Management

Management of the axilla in MBC is comparable to that in female breast cancer. Sentinel lymph node (SLN) biopsy is appropriate for

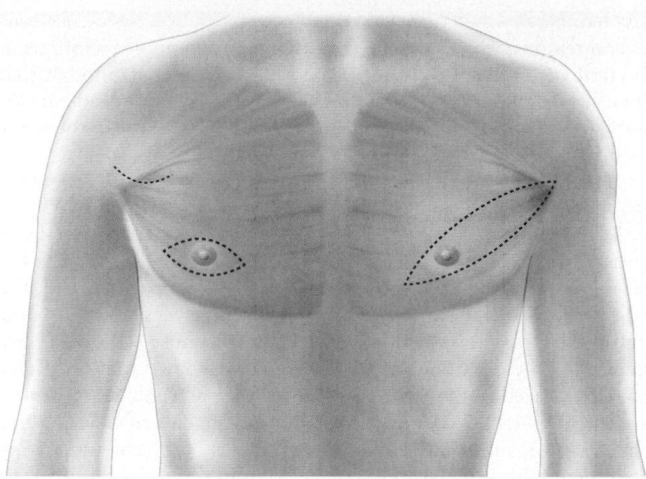

FIGURE 1 Suggested incisions for mastectomy with axillary staging in male breast cancer.

all operable invasive MBC with clinically negative axillary nodes (cT1-3N0). Because most men with a core biopsy diagnosis of ductal carcinoma in situ (DCIS) also have a palpable mass, invasion cannot be ruled out and SLN biopsy makes sense for them as well. Because patients with MBC do not fall within the eligibility of the American College of Surgeons Oncology Group (ACOSOG) Z0011 trial (which showed that patients with one or two positive SLNs having BCS *with whole breast RT* do not require axillary lymph node dissection [ALND]), we recommend intraoperative pathologic assessment of the SLN and ALND for patients who are SLN positive. For patients who are clinically node positive we recommend a stepwise approach. First, if metastasis is confirmed preoperatively by fine-needle aspiration or core biopsy, we recommend ALND. Second, if metastasis cannot be confirmed by preoperative needle biopsy, we recommend SLN biopsy with intraoperative assessment and, if positive, ALND. Finally, when metastasis cannot be confirmed at the time of SLN biopsy, surgical judgment prevails, and it is reasonable to proceed to ALND on the basis of intraoperative suspicion alone, recognizing that the possibility of a false-positive clinical and intraoperative lymph node examination must be balanced against the consequences of leaving gross axillary disease behind.

For men who will receive neoadjuvant chemotherapy for locally advanced disease, we recommend axillary staging upfront by US-guided fine-needle aspiration, not SLN biopsy. Because about 40% of patients with positive axillary nodes will convert to node negative, we recommend SLN biopsy with intraoperative assessment after chemotherapy at the time of definitive surgery and ALND for those with positive SLN.

Perioperative Management

Wound closure is straightforward. Even for tumors that have required an extensive skin excision, primary wound closure is virtually always possible by elevating the skin flaps superiorly toward the clavicle and inferiorly onto the abdomen. We recommend closed suction drainage for mastectomy and ALND but not for SLN biopsy, and we instruct all patients in shoulder exercises to maintain or restore range of motion. There is no evidence to support any of the "standard" recommendations for the avoidance of lymphedema, and patients are encouraged to use their arms as normally as possible.

■ POSTOPERATIVE MANAGEMENT

Postoperative consultations should include referral to genetic counseling (*BRCA* testing is appropriate for all patients with MBC and especially appropriate if there is a family history of breast or ovarian cancer), to medical oncology (the criteria for adjuvant hormonal therapy and chemotherapy in MBC are the same as with female breast cancer), and to radiation oncology (for patients with more locally advanced disease requiring PMRT). Plastic surgical consultation is also reasonable for the small minority of men who are bothered by loss of the nipple; nipple reconstruction by a local skin flap and tattooing gives excellent results in appropriate patients.

Postoperative follow-up for MBC, as for female breast cancer, should include regular physical examination. Unlike female breast cancer, contralateral MBC is very rare and there are no data to support screening of the contralateral breast by mammography; however, patients may be unconvinced of this and mammography every 2 to 3 years is a reasonable compromise. As with female breast cancer, there are no data to support routine screening for distant metastases, but further workup is indicated for all new and persistent complaints suspicious for metastatic disease. ER-positive breast cancers in women have a long natural history, with as many breast cancer events in years 5 to 10 as in years 0 to 5, and relapses beyond 10 years are not rare. The same is probably true for men, and because 90% of MBC is ER-positive there is a strong rationale for lifelong surveillance of all MBC.

SUGGESTED READINGS

Cemal Y, Pusic A, Mehrara BJ. Preventative measures for lymphedema: separating fact from fiction. *J Am Coll Surg*. 2011;213:543-551.

Donegan WL, Redlich PN, Lang PJ, et al. Carcinoma of the breast in males: a multi-institutional survey. *Cancer*. 1998;83:498-509.

Giordano SH, Buzdar AU, Hortobagyi GN. Breast cancer in men. *Ann Intern Med*. 2002;137:678-687.

Giuliano AE, McCall L, Beitsch P, et al. Locoregional recurrence after sentinel lymph node dissection with or without axillary dissection in patients with sentinel lymph node metastases: the American College of Surgeons Oncology Group Z0011 randomized trial. *Ann Surg*. 2010;252:426-432.

Gómez-Raposo C, Zambrana Tévar F, Sereno Moyano M, et al. Male breast cancer. *Cancer Treat Rev*. 2010;36:451-457.

Houssami N, Macaskill P, von Minckwitz G, et al. Meta-analysis of the association of breast cancer subtype and pathologic complete response to neoadjuvant chemotherapy. *Eur J Cancer*. 2012;48:3342-3354.

Ottini L, Palli D, Rizzo S, et al. Male breast cancer. *Crit Rev Oncol Hematol*. 2010;73:141-155.

Tai YC, Domchek S, Parmigiani G, et al. Breast cancer risk among male *BRCA1* and *BRCA2* mutation carriers. *J Natl Cancer Inst*. 2007;99: 1811-1814.

BREAST IMAGING

Nagi Khouri, MD

There are many issues that are considered unsettled or controversial in the field of breast imaging. This is not unusual in any domain that has undergone a revolution. So it has been for breast imaging in the past 25 years. This chapter addresses issues that have been raised in these years and recently regarding the validity of the mammographic screening data and the screening recommendations, the indications and impact of the newer technologies, and the transformation of the organization of care for the newly diagnosed breast cancer patient.

■ BREAST CANCER SCREENING

Breast cancer is the most common cancer in women in the United States as well as worldwide, accounting for 30% of malignancies affecting women. Breast cancer is also the second leading cause of cancer death in women in the United States.

Although 75% of women who develop breast cancer have no known predisposing factor for breast cancer other than being a woman and entering the age category in which breast cancer becomes prevalent (≥40 years), known additional risk factors include family history, personal history of breast cancer, prior biopsies showing high-risk lesions, reproductive factors, hormonal factors, alcohol consumption, obesity in postmenopausal women, exposure to ionizing radiation, and genetic inheritance.

In 2015 it is estimated that there will be 231,840 new cases of invasive breast cancer in the United States, plus 50,040 new cases of ductal carcinoma in situ (DCIS) and 40,730 deaths resulting from breast cancer.

Before 2002 there was a gradual increase in the number of new breast cancer cases per year in the United States, which was accounted for by an increasing number of women entering the age category in which they become at risk of breast cancer. Between 2002 and 2003 the breast cancer incidence dropped by 7%, attributed to the large number of women who discontinued hormone replacement therapy after it was reported that the combined estrogen and progesterone was associated with an increased risk of breast cancer and coronary artery disease. Concomitantly, the mortality from breast cancer decreased 35% between 1990 and 2008. This is believed to be because of early detection with mammographic screening and improvements in the treatment of breast cancer (including surgery, chemotherapeutic and hormonal therapies, and radiation therapy). It is difficult to determine which of these two factors contributed the most to mortality reduction. Needless to say, there are proponents at both ends of the spectrum as well as proponents for close to equal contributions. Regardless, early detection remains critical for improved breast cancer survival. Mammography, magnetic resonance imaging (MRI), and breast ultrasound are the most common tools used for breast cancer screening and the workup of detected abnormalities (Euhus et al., 2015).

Mammographic Screening

Eight randomized clinical trials of screening mammography, "invited to screening" versus controls, starting in the 1960s and continuing through the 1980s have shown mortality reduction from breast cancer between 19% and 31% in women in the study group between the ages of 40 and 69. More than half a million women participated in those trials, which varied in many ways, such as age of enlistment, duration of the study and years of follow-up, and single view versus two view mammograms. The mortality reduction achieved in those trials is believed to underestimate the benefit of mammography for several reasons, which include that the mammographic technique at the time of those trials would be considered inadequate today, that the interpretation skills of the breast imagers have improved considerably, and a noncompliance rate of 20% to 35% in some of the study groups.

A study from Sweden examining more than 20 years of follow-up has shown a mortality reduction among screened women of 45%.

Despite most of the trials showing mortality reduction from breast cancer screening, there has been ongoing controversy from the earliest days of the trials about the interpretation of the data, the validity of the results, and the harms from mammography (anxiety from callbacks, false-positive biopsies, overdiagnosis). Women have recognized these limitations but studies have shown that they have not discouraged women from continuing their screening. Regardless, there is abundant evidence supporting the benefits of mammography. Most organizations in the United States had been supporting mammographic screening every year beginning at the age of 40, with the recent exception of the U.S. Preventive Services Task Force (USPSTF) in 2009. More recently, in 2015, the American Cancer Society released a new set of guidelines for women to start annual mammographic screening at age 45 until the age of 55 and then adopt biannual screening with the option to continue annually. Screening should continue as long as a woman would be able to be treated for breast cancer and have a lifetime expectancy of more than 10 years. The USPSTF recommends biannual screening between the ages of 50 and 74 and screening for women in their 40s only if they are at higher risk and has no recommendations for women aged 75 and older. The American College of Radiology (ACR) and the Society of Breast Imaging (SBI) have restated their recommendations for annual breast cancer screening with mammography for all women as of age 40, emphasizing that this strategy saves the most lives. This disagreement regarding mammographic screening has confused women and health care professionals. Women and their referring physicians should be well informed of the pros and cons of every strategy they consider. See Table 1, which compares the various recommendations.

The incidence of breast cancer increases around the age of 40. For women aged 40 to 44, the incidence is twice that for women aged 35 to 39, and for women aged 45 to 49, it is three times that for women aged 35 to 39. Sixteen percent of all cancers occur in women in their 40s. So, cancer is not rare in this age group.

Screening mammography is the only test that has been shown to be associated with decreased mortality in all age categories from 40 to 69 years compared with women who are not screened. However, mammography is far from perfect. An important factor that affects the sensitivity of mammography is breast density. There is an inverse relationship between breast density and sensitivity. The sensitivity of mammography in fatty breast is close to 98% whereas the sensitivity of mammography in very dense breasts varies between 45% and 60%. Breast density is part of a spectrum between the two extremes.

Another factor that affects the performance of screening mammography is the variable skills among breast imagers and general radiologists. Although the standardization of the terminology and the adoption of the Breast Imaging-Reporting and Data System (BI-RADS) have led to better communication of the findings (Tables 2 and 3), there are still issues related to the quality of the interpretation of breast imaging examinations. Studies have shown greater sensitivity and overall accuracy in fellowship-trained radiologists. We are not yet at the stage where mammography is always interpreted by experts, but we are gradually moving in that direction.

Magnetic Resonance Imaging Screening

Breast MRI has a very high sensitivity for invasive breast carcinoma and slightly less sensitivity for DCIS. An important drawback is that MRI has many false-positive calls. One of the major uncontested indications for breast MRI is screening in high-risk women.

TABLE 1: Comparison of American Cancer Society (ACS), U.S. Preventive Services Task Force (USPSTF), and American College of Radiology (ACR) and Society of Breast Imaging (SBI) Guidelines

Variable	ACS Guidelines	USPSTF Guidelines	ACR and SBI Guidelines
Age to begin mammograms	45 years 40 to 44 years to be discussed	50 years	40 years
Frequency of mammograms	45-55 annual >55 should switch to every 2 years with option for annual As long as life expectancy >10 years	Every 2 years	Annually
Clinical breast examination	Not recommended	Insufficient evidence	Annually
Breast self-examination (BSE)	Not recommended	Against BSE	Optional

TABLE 2: Breast Imaging-Reporting and Data System (BI-RADS) Classification of Breast Imaging

Category	Assessment	Recommendation
0	Incomplete	Need additional imaging or prior studies for comparison
1	Negative	Resume routine screening mammography
2	Benign	Resume routine screening mammography
3	Probably benign	Risk of malignancy <2%; short-term follow-up recommended in 6 months
4	Suspicious abnormality	Intermediate risk of malignancy; biopsy recommended
5	Highly suggestive of malignancy	Chance of malignancy >95%; appropriate action should be taken
6	Known biopsy-proven malignancy	Treatment of known malignancy

TABLE 3: Subdivisions of Category 4 (Suspicious Abnormality)

Category 4A	Low suspicion for malignancy (>2%-10% likelihood of malignancy)
Category 4B	Moderate suspicion for malignancy (>10%-50% likelihood of malignancy)
Category 4C	High suspicion for malignancy (>50%-<95% likelihood of malignancy)

Women with breast cancer lifetime risk greater than 20% should be considered for supplemental screening with MRI in addition to mammography (Figure 1). The various risk models used to estimate short-term and long-term risks are based on age, ethnicity, family history of breast cancer on maternal and paternal sides, and personal history of biopsy or atypia. They include Gail, BRCAPRO, Claus, and Tyrer-Cuzick models. All of the models have some limitation and variation in their predictability. There is a benefit sometimes in simultaneously using more than one model. Breast cancer risk evaluation is done most comprehensively in high-risk clinics that include trained professionals and geneticists. Individuals with several family members affected by breast or ovarian cancer should be referred to these clinics for counseling and testing.

The American Cancer Society recommends annual mammography and MRI screening for all *BRCA* carriers and untested first-degree relatives, women with a very strong family history of breast or ovarian cancer with lifetime risk greater than 20%, women who underwent chest radiation treatment between the ages of 10 and 30, and women with one of a variety of syndromes (Li-Fraumeni, Cowden, Bannayan-Riley-Ruvalcaba). Typically, annual breast cancer MRI screening should start 10 years before the youngest breast cancer in the family but not younger than age 25. Annual mammography is also recommended at the same time, though some physicians may hesitate to recommend mammography between ages 25 and 30, as the breasts are more sensitive to radiation in that period. Once mammography and MRI are used for surveillance, the patient has the option to alternate the MRI and the mammogram every 6 months.

Supplemental MRI screening has been suggested for women with biopsy-proven atypia (ductal or lobular), as a recent study has shown a 30% incidence of invasive cancer within 25 years from biopsy. On the other hand, recent data suggest that these individuals' cancers actually may be phenotypically different than the ones that develop in genetic carriers and that they may not be as readily detectable by MRI. Concomitantly more than 10% of the cancers were detected only on physical examination. There is a need for a prospective controlled study of MRI screening of patients who have had biopsies of high-risk lesions.

Currently most breast screening MRIs are done using a standard protocol.

The recent introduction of an abbreviated breast MRI protocol allows the examination to be performed in a much shorter time and shortens the reading time by a factor of more than 50%. The immediate benefits are that of greater speed of the examination and its interpretation and greater throughput. Several screening studies have shown the shortened protocol to be as accurate as the standard protocol. In a prospective study, 443 women at mild to moderate risk for breast cancer, with dense breasts and a negative mammogram, underwent 606 screening MRIs over a period of 18 months. Eleven cancers were detected (7 invasive cancers and 4 DCIS), for an additional cancer yield of 18.2 per 1000. Interpretation of the standard protocol as well as the abbreviated protocol identified all 11 cancers. In addition, the specificity and positive predictive value (PPV) were equivalent for both protocols.

The adoption of an abbreviated protocol for breast MRI screening allows a faster examination and interpretation time with the same accuracy as the standard protocol. This results in greater throughput, allowing a larger number of women to be screened in a shorter

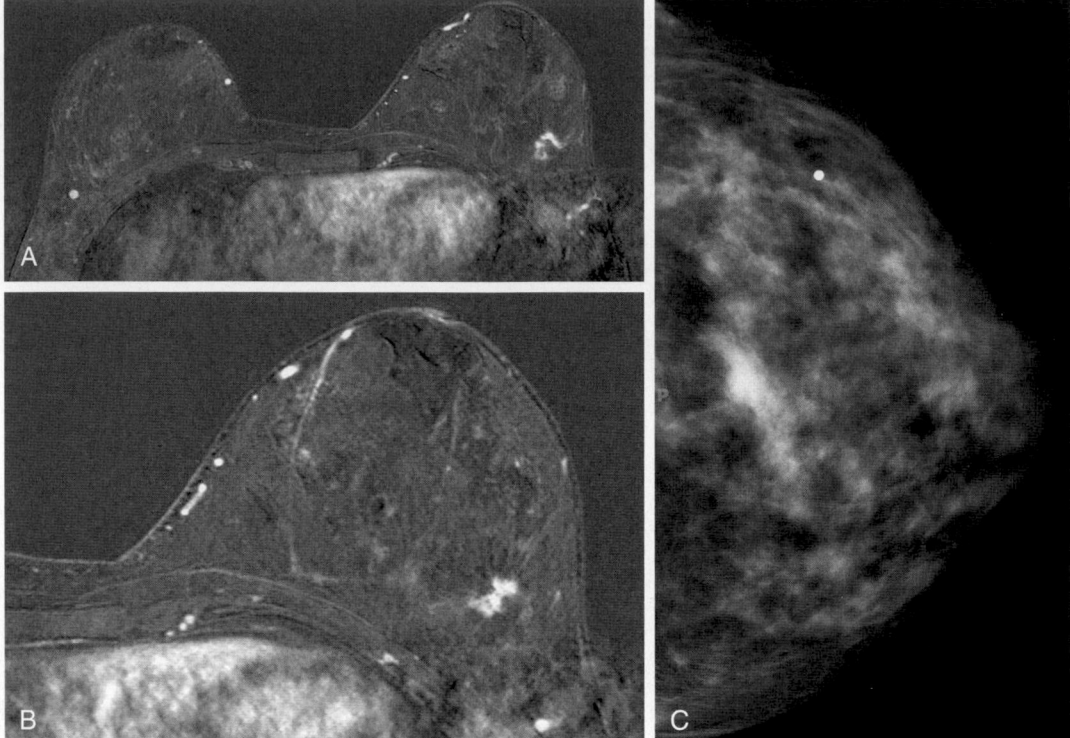

FIGURE 1 A 42-year-old woman with *BRCA2* mutation. Magnetic resonance imaging (MRI) screening showed a 1.2-cm invasive ductal cancer in the lower outer left breast seen only on MRI (**A** and **B**) and subsequently on second look ultrasound. **C,** The mammogram showed only dense breast tissue.

period of time, potentially opening the door to lowering the cost of the examination, and possibly including women at lower risk to be screened with MRI, somewhat edging toward competing with the cost of the standard screening modalities.

Ultrasound Screening

A number of studies have shown that whole breast ultrasound screening in high-risk individuals with dense breasts can detect small cancers not visible on standard mammography. Results of the American College of Radiology Imaging Network (ACRIN) 6666 study showed 4.2 additional cancers per 1000, a 55% increase in addition to mammography. This study confirmed several single-institution studies that reported the discovery of an additional 3 cancers per 1000 examinations, not visible mammographically or suspected clinically. Almost all cancers found on screening ultrasound are invasive, and most are lymph node negative, with a median size of 9 to 11 mm. There are several drawbacks to screening ultrasound, which include operator dependence, the long time it takes to perform the study, frequent short-term follow-up (8.6%), and an uneven reimbursement. In addition the low PPV of 9.5% compared with about 30% for mammography is an important limitation to a wider adoption. Nevertheless, there has been a large increase in the number of ultrasound screening studies performed in the United States because of the increased awareness of the limitations of mammography in dense breasts (40% to 60% of women have dense breasts), resulting in physicians and women asking for it, state legislation conducive to greater use of ultrasound screening for women with dense breasts (Hooley et al., 2012), and its use as an option for women at an intermediate risk (15% to 20%) for breast cancer. Ultrasound screening can be used for high-risk women who do not have access to MRI or who are not able to have MRI screening. None of the medical societies have formally endorsed ultrasound screening. The drawbacks of ultrasound screening could be lessened by any of the following: an increase in the performance of high-quality breast ultrasound by

well-trained technologists, improvement in the technology of automated whole breast ultrasound (ABUS) and a resultant greater adoption by breast imagers, the careful modification of the criteria and threshold for intervention, the development of technologies that would allow greater sensitivity and specificity for the characterization of benign and malignant lesions by noninvasive techniques, and the adoption of reimbursement more appropriate to cover the cost of the examination and its interpretation. All of these factors can diminish some of the drawbacks, leading to a wider application of ultrasound screening.

■ DIGITAL BREAST TOMOSYNTHESIS

Digital breast tomosynthesis, commonly known as 3D mammography, is an advanced mammographic technique that enhances the detection of breast cancer by markedly decreasing the masking of cancer by overlying breast tissue and simultaneously decreasing the creation of pseudolesions from overlapping tissues, phenomena that are well known in women with denser breasts. The technology involves the acquisition of multiple mammographic images by a digital detector from a mammography tube that moves over a limited arc while the breast is compressed in the standard craniocaudal and mediolateral projections. It does not involve any changes from the patient's perspective. The breast is compressed in the same manner as for a standard 2D mammogram for about the same length of time. The result is that tomosynthesis simultaneously increases the cancer detection rate and reduces the callback rate in screening mammography.

In a retrospective study to evaluate the impact of breast tomosynthesis (Friedewald et al., 2014), 454,850 examinations were reviewed (281,187 digital mammograms and 173,663 digital mammograms plus tomosynthesis) from 13 different sites, academic and nonacademic, geographically diverse, and including specialist and nonspecialist radiologists. A 27% relative increase in the cancer detection rate and a 15% relative decrease in the callback rate were noted. Two prospective single-site European studies have demonstrated similar results: 40% to 51% increase in the cancer detection rate and 15% to 17% decrease in the callback rate. Some studies in the United States have shown a drop of 30% to 37% in the callback rate. The wide variation in the drop of the callback rate is probably a reflection of how high or low the original callback rate is. The callback rate in the United States is on average significantly higher than the callback rate in Europe. In a study published in 2005, comparing the performance of 2D mammographic screening in the United States and the United Kingdom, the recall rate was twice as high in the United States as in the United Kingdom. The number of cancers detected was also higher in the United States, and most of the increase was in the detection of small invasive and in situ cancers; the number of large cancers detected (>2 cm) were very similar between the two countries. This raises questions as to what the ideal callback rate should be while achieving the highest sensitivity. An acceptable callback rate in the United States seems to be between 6% and 9%.

Drawbacks of tomosynthesis include an increase in the time for interpretation of the studies by 50% to 150% and a marked increase in storage space needs, as 3D images are very large, with resulting information technology challenges.

The technology of tomosynthesis is still in its infancy. There are several manufacturers of tomosynthesis units. Most of the published data involve almost exclusively a single manufacturer (Hologic) that was the first to receive approval from the U.S. Food and Drug Administration (FDA). There is currently a second manufacturer (GE) approved by the FDA for tomosynthesis on the market and three others who have applied for approval. Their units differ in many ways, including the type of tube and detector; the angle of travel of the x-ray tube (11 to 60 degrees); the way the images are acquired, whether while the tube is stationary or in motion (pulsed or continuous); whether there is stability or movement of the detector; and the reconstruction algorithms. These variables may affect the degree of visibility of mammographic pathology. Hologic was approved for tomosynthesis using the 3D study in combination with a 2D mammogram. A recent development was the approval of a reconstructed 2D image from the 3D set of images, allowing a shorter exposure as well as a 50% decrease in the radiation dose. It is not yet clear whether there are only advantages to this change and whether the reconstructed 2D image has similar sensitivity and specificity for masses and calcifications compared with the standard 2D image. There is not yet widespread adoption of the reconstructed 2D image alone in conjunction with the 3D set of images.

Tomosynthesis definitely appears to be superior to standard mammography in the demonstration of noncalcified lesions such as architectural distortion in particular, masses, and asymmetries. Masses sometimes may be less dense and less contrasted against the surrounding tissues on the 3D image when compared with the standard 2D image, compensated by greater distinction and visibility of their borders. It is also not definite whether tomosynthesis is as sensitive as 2D mammography in the detection and characterization of microcalcifications. There are few and conflicting reports in the literature. Further research is needed on the detection and evaluation of microcalcifications with 3D images, on the performance of the reconstructed 2D image, and on the performance of units produced by other manufacturers.

The discovery of subtle architectural distortion exclusively seen on tomosynthesis frequently can be seen on ultrasound. If not, some of these lesions can be seen and biopsied under stereotactic guidance. They frequently turn out to result from cancer or radial scar frequently retrospectively recognizable on studies performed many years before, for both diagnoses. Stability in such lesions should not deter from performing a biopsy. In a recent study, 36% of such lesions turned out to be malignant.

There are lesions, however, that are seen exclusively on tomosynthesis and not visible on ultrasound or under stereotaxy. A recent study showed a promising role for digital breast tomosynthesis–

guided, vacuum-assisted breast biopsy, which can be performed with an add-on to the tomosynthesis unit.

In addition, in a recent review in Korea, 54% of cancers detected by ultrasound not evident on a 2D mammogram were detectable on digital tomosynthesis. Additional studies are warranted to evaluate the relationship of lesions seen exclusively on the 3D versus 2D image in relation to the ones detected on ultrasound screening with a negative 2D mammogram.

◾ CONTRAST-ENHANCED DIGITAL MAMMOGRAPHY (CEDM)

Based on the knowledge that most breast malignancies have neoangiogenesis and on the experience acquired with breast MRI, several investigators have explored the field of contrast-enhanced mammography with the use of injection of iodinated contrast material. Initially, temporal contrast-enhanced mammography was tried. It consisted of injecting an iodinated contrast agent while a breast was compressed in one projection after a scout film, taking several sequential films, and subtracting them from the scout film. Because the films were obtained only in one projection, several limitations were apparent, such as the need to have the breast in compression during the injection of contrast, decreasing the blood and contrast flow to the breast, lack of information on the exact location of a lesion and comparison with the other breast, and motion artifacts resulting from the length of time the breast was compressed.

In dual-energy contrast-enhanced digital mammography (CEDM) both breasts are imaged 2 minutes after the injection of an iodinated contrast agent, with one image at a low kilovolt (26 to 30) and another image at a high kilovolt (45 to 49), obtained simultaneously in a split second. A subtracted image is then obtained using a recombination algorithm. It takes less than 7 minutes to take all four standard sets of images from two breasts. The total procedure time is around 10 minutes (Figure 2). The radiation dose does not exceed 20% more than that of a mammogram.

As with MRI, not only malignant lesions enhance with CEDM. Benign lesions like fibroadenomata and inflamed cysts also can enhance. In a study of 120 women with abnormalities on mammography 74/80 cancers enhanced (92%) and 13/50 benign (26%) lesions.

The diagnostic performance of CEDM is remarkable in that it is significantly more sensitive for cancer than standard digital mammography, in the range of 92% for CEDM and 78% for digital mammography. Several of the studies have confirmed similar performance. CEDM also has improved specificity and better positive and negative predictive values.

Several studies have shown that CEDM approaches the sensitivity of MRI for invasive carcinoma. In addition, whether the CEDM study is conducted in the context of a screening examination or a diagnostic one, studies have shown that the low-energy image obtained in CEDM is comparable to the image obtained in standard digital mammography, with no statistical difference found in the technical parameters or in the measured size and conspicuity of the mammographic findings (masses or calcifications). Therefore there is no need to perform a standard mammogram and a CEDM. Because the low-energy exposure (26 to 30 kV) is below the K-edge of iodine (33 keV), the low-energy CEDM image obtained after injection of contrast is similar to a standard digital mammogram. Because CEDM is able to stand alone, providing the full information from a standard digital mammogram as well as the information from vascular enhancement, one can see a potential role of CEDM in the screening of higher-risk individuals and the diagnostic workup of patients with a breast problem.

Currently, there is no biopsy guidance for CEDM-detected lesions. If a mass is suspected or seen, an ultrasound examination and possibly an MRI would be recommended.

CEDM is superior to standard digital mammography. It also may play a role in the screening of moderate to high-risk individuals and

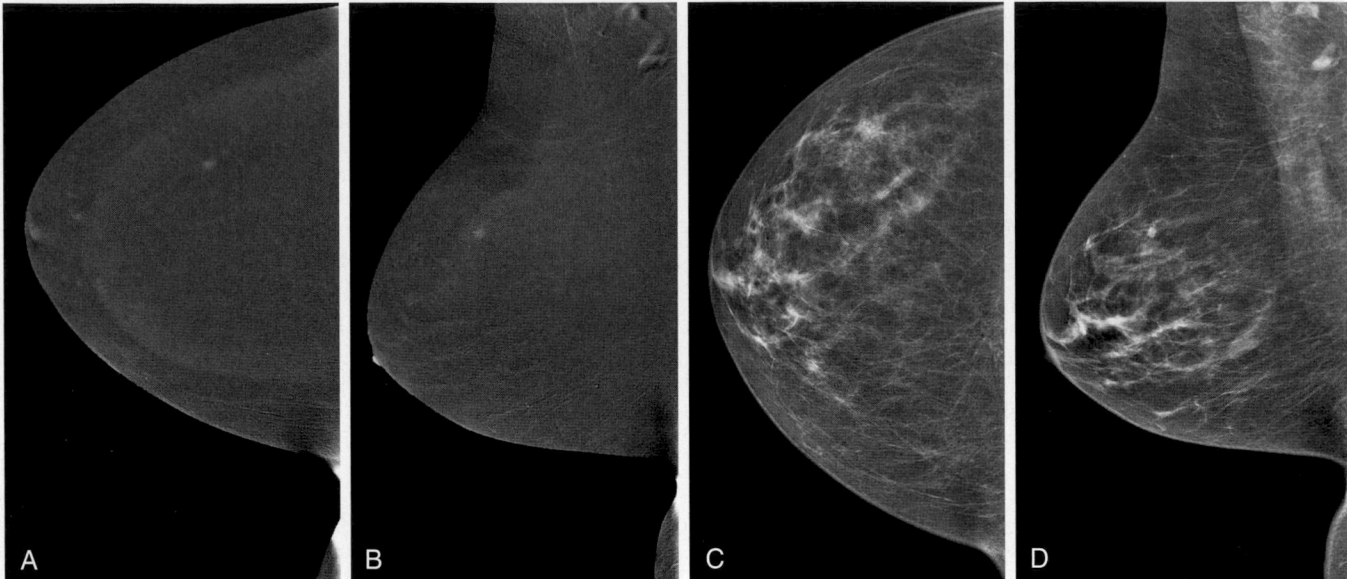

FIGURE 2 Incidental tiny cancer seen with contrast-enhanced digital mammography (**A** and **B**) not seen on standard 2-D mammography (**C** and **D**). Very subtle on ultrasound screening (not shown). (*Courtesy Maxine Jochelson MD, MSKCC.*)

has a potential role for all indications of breast MRI, keeping in mind its easier access and lower cost in both the developed and the underdeveloped world. A well-recognized drawback is the injection of iodinated contrast material and associated potential reactions. Additional prospective studies are warranted.

■ BREAST MAGNETIC RESONANCE IMAGING: DIAGNOSTIC INDICATIONS

Breast MRI is well known to have a high sensitivity for breast cancer (94% to 100%). Unfortunately it also has a high false-positive rate, which leads to many biopsies and a delay in initiating treatment for the newly diagnosed breast cancer patient. The newly diagnosed breast cancer is probably the most utilized indication for breast MRI, to evaluate the extent of the cancer, to evaluate its unifocality versus multifocality or multicentricity, to assess the suitability of breast conservation, and to better plan breast-conserving surgery. Concomitantly it helps to rule out another cancer in the contralateral breast.

There are controversial and noncontroversial indications for breast MRI in the patient with newly diagnosed breast cancer.

Noncontroversial Indications

Occult Primary Breast Cancer

Isolated unilateral axillary adenopathy with a negative mammogram and physical breast examination is an occasional presentation of malignant conditions (metastatic breast cancer; metastases from other malignancies, known or unknown; lymphoproliferative disorders) and nonmalignant conditions (reactive, inflammatory, granulomatous). In that setting, a core biopsy, not a fine-needle biopsy, is the appropriate procedure. One percent of breast cancers are seen that way. If a diagnosis of carcinoma is established even without any further specific characterization, breast MRI is the next test that needs to be performed. The primary lesion is identified 70% of the time with MRI and frequently confirmed by second-look focused ultrasound.

Considering Neoadjuvant Chemotherapy

Patients with newly diagnosed breast cancer, locally advanced or not, may be considered for preoperative systemic therapy depending on the type and size of the tumor, the relative size of the breast, and the

presence of metastatic lymph nodes. Patients considered for preoperative therapy may benefit from tumor downstaging and from in vivo assessment of tumor response or resistance. Shrinking the primary tumor also may make the surgical definitive procedure easier as well as allow consideration of breast conservation when it may not have been considered at presentation. MRI is more sensitive than conventional imaging in delineating the type and possible extent of the cancer before systemic therapy and in assessing the response to neoadjuvant chemotherapy along with mammography, which is essential for visualization of microcalcifications.

Controversial Indication

The routine evaluation of extent of disease in the newly diagnosed breast cancer is probably the most common application for breast MRI in most settings. Breast cancer is seen most frequently as a unifocal disease by standard imaging. In 1985 Holland and colleagues found unsuspected significant multifocal disease in 63% of mastectomy specimens of T1 and T2 tumors extending up to 4 cm away from the primary lesion. It is therefore not surprising to have frequent demonstration of more extensive disease by MRI (16% to 34%), frequently not proven, that most often leads to additional biopsies—some benign, some malignant—and a delay in surgical planning and intervention, resulting in a greater number of women choosing mastectomy for their treatment, not infrequently bilateral. In a larger meta-analysis that included 10,011 women in 50 studies, similar results were found, with an average of 20% of cases where additional lesions were discovered. The problem is that there are no data showing improvement in surgical outcomes or reduction in re-excision rates in patients who have a preoperative MRI versus patients who do not. Long-term outcomes manifested by in-breast tumor recurrence have decreased tremendously over the past 20 years, down to 1% to 5% because of improvements in surgery, medical oncology, and radiation therapy. In-breast tumor recurrence appears to be related more to the biology of the tumor and less to the tumor burden. In summary, there is currently no evidence to support the routine use of MRI for the preoperative evaluation of a patient newly diagnosed with breast cancer.

The current National Comprehensive Cancer Network (NCCN) guidelines include a recommendation that breast MRI be considered for patients with newly diagnosed breast cancer to evaluate the extent of disease in the affected breast and to screen for the contralateral breast. In addition, the guidelines stress the importance of high quality for the MRI examination to obtain its full potential.

Ordering a breast MRI on every patient diagnosed with breast cancer is widely practiced in the community. Academic institutions have attempted to be more selective in view of data that question any impact from performing preoperative MRI on patients' outcomes. In a recent published study to evaluate which category of patients with breast cancer might benefit from preoperative MRI, 1102 consecutive patients were reviewed retrospectively. Additional malignant disease was found in 32% of the patients. Premenopausal women, invasive lobular carcinoma, and women with dense breasts were significantly associated with additional malignant findings in the ipsilateral breast, each category being independently significant.

Various guidelines are developed at large institutions through the collaborative efforts of breast imagers and breast surgeons. An example of the criteria that influence the decision to order a breast MRI in the context of breast cancer is that used at our institution:

1. Specific tumor types for which it is traditionally harder to define the full extent of disease on mammography (e.g., invasive lobular carcinoma)
2. Cases where mammography or ultrasound suggests multifocality or multicentricity
3. Patients with dense breast tissue
4. Young patients (e.g., patients in their 40s and younger)
5. Patients who will be undergoing neoadjuvant therapy
6. BRCA-positive patients or patients with family history suggestive of a genetic mutation
7. Patients planning for bilateral mastectomy (i.e., to assess the contralateral breast for malignancy); this is especially true for those breast surgeons who do not routinely do sentinel lymph node biopsies on the side of prophylactic mastectomy.

Alliance A011104/ACRIN 6694 is a current multi-institutional study being conducted to assess the benefits of MRI in patients selected for breast conservation. The main objective of this trial is to compare the rates of local-regional recurrence after attempted breast-conserving therapy in a cohort of women with triple-negative or human epidermal growth factor receptor–2 (HER2) amplified breast cancer (two groups at the highest risk for local recurrence) randomized to preoperative staging with mammography (control arm) or mammography plus breast MRI (MRI arm). Randomization of the patients may be challenging, as preoperative MRI is the standard of care in many practices and increasingly requested by patients.

It will be a while before we know which patients actually might achieve a better outcome because of the preoperative MRI, all else being equal. At our institution the decision to order a breast MRI study in the context of a newly diagnosed breast cancer is left to the surgeon rather than the breast imager. Not infrequently there is a joint discussion on the issue.

■ AXILLARY ULTRASOUND IN PATIENTS WITH BREAST CANCER

The role of axillary ultrasound (AUS) has undergone many changes in the past 10 years and is currently uncertain. Axillary lymph node dissection (ALND) used to be the standard procedure in the management of the patient with invasive carcinoma of the breast until the advent of sentinel lymph node biopsy (SLNB) in the early 2000s. ALND then became the standard procedure for patients whose SLNB showed metastatic disease, including micrometastases.

AUS and image-guided biopsy of axillary nodes has gained popularity since that time to identify patients with positive lymph nodes in order to spare them the surgical procedure of SLNB, the additional cost, and the added wait time associated with intraoperative frozen section of sentinel lymph node and to possibly offer the patient the option of preoperative chemotherapy. The morphologic characteristics of suspicious lymph nodes include cortical thickening greater

than 3 mm; asymmetric bulge of the cortex of the lymph node; a longitudinal to transverse ratio of less than 2; and the absence of a fatty hilum, suggesting a totally replaced lymph node. The most reliable signs are a totally replaced lymph node and an eccentric cortical bulge. The evaluation of the axilla is preferably performed at the same time as a suspicious mass is discovered in the breast before a biopsy. Lymph nodes not infrequently will enlarge and look suspicious as early as 10 days after a breast biopsy. A diagnosis of a reactive abnormal lymph node on biopsy is more frequently encountered when lymph nodes undergo biopsy sometime after the initial biopsy of the cancer.

Image-guided biopsy of axillary nodes can be performed using fine-needle aspiration biopsy (FNAB) or core biopsy. The yield is similar for both procedures, with each having advantages and disadvantages. The advantages of FNAB are that it is relatively inexpensive, easier to perform a biopsy on more than one node, and less traumatic to the axilla and to the patient. Great precision can be achieved, enabling one to sample a tiny abnormality as well as the upper and lower poles and the ventral portion of a node. The disadvantages are the need to acquire the meticulous skills required to perform an FNAB and how to smear the slides. The advantages of a core biopsy are the larger sample and the ability to differentiate limited from extensive intranodal disease. The disadvantages are the relative greater cost, greater limitation of access, possible greater complication rates with the adjacent neurovascular bundle, and more invasive nature of the procedure. Both procedures require necessary additional skills from the biopsy operator and the pathologists for cytologic and surgical pathologic interpretation.

The sensitivity and specificity of FNAB of axillary nodes are high, particularly in the setting of clinically suspicious nodes and abnormal ultrasound. In a study carried out at our institution, 65 axillae were analyzed by FNAB; 60% were positive, 6% were nondiagnostic, and 34% were negative. FNAB had 89% sensitivity, 100% specificity, and 100% PPV in patients with palpable or ultrasound sonographically suspicious nodes. FNAB's sensitivity drops very significantly for nonpalpable, normal nodes on ultrasound (54%). FNAB in all patients has a moderate sensitivity and excellent specificity. Many other studies have confirmed that. The high specificity and PPV can allow definitive management of the patient without SLNB if the FNAB is positive for cancer.

The surgical management of the axilla is evolving. The Z0011 study is allowing patients with a clinically node-negative axilla, T1 or T2 tumors, and one or two positive sentinel lymph nodes with macrometastases without gross extracapsular extension to forgo ALND, provided they are candidates for breast conservation and will undergo whole breast radiation therapy. Patients with clinically node-positive axilla should undergo ultrasound evaluation and biopsy of abnormal lymph nodes. If the needle biopsy is positive, surgical management is axillary dissection. If the needle biopsy is negative, SLNB is performed.

In my practice, clinically node-negative patients who have an abnormal AUS are managed based on the number of abnormal lymph nodes identified. If there are less than three, the patient undergoes SLNB. If more than three abnormal nodes are identified, image-guided biopsy is performed, with the results determining the management.

Because a negative axilla on clinical examination is not reliable enough, it seems reasonable that the initial approach for a patient diagnosed with cancer or with a highly suspicious lesion in the breast is to perform an ultrasound examination of the axilla with careful evaluation of the presence and number of abnormal nodes and with comparison to the contralateral axilla in case of uncertain findings. If the axilla shows multiple abnormal lymph nodes (≥3), biopsy of one or multiple nodes is performed. If the axilla is entirely negative, no image-guided procedure is done, and if fewer than three nodes are affected, a discussion with the surgeon is warranted.

In a recent study in which 513 patients were evaluated with preoperative ultrasound, 113 of them were found to have a suspicious axilla. The sensitivity and specificity of AUS for predicting more than three node metastases were 71% and 83%, respectively. The false-negative rate for detecting more than three metastatic nodes was 4% and higher in infiltrating lobular carcinoma. AUS can be used for preoperative identification in patients with a high nodal disease burden and can identify candidates for preoperative chemotherapy. Increasingly, a clip is placed in the node that was biopsied for patients likely to undergo preoperative chemotherapy. At the time of surgery one could place a wire under ultrasound guidance through the node that was biopsied, as the clip is frequently visible in those instances, ensuring its resection.

MULTIDISCIPLINARY BREAST CANCER CARE (MDBCC)

In the world of fragmented care, the woman who is told that she needs a biopsy because of an abnormal breast imaging finding develops a high degree of anxiety. When a diagnosis of cancer is established by core biopsy, the patient is soon overwhelmed by what she faces, as she has to digest the news and undertake the different steps before her while trying to listen, understand, and make decisions. She needs to schedule consultations with the various specialists and possibly undergo additional tests, waiting several days between one and the next. This process often takes several weeks before a treatment plan is fully established.

The multidisciplinary approach to breast cancer care is now considered the gold standard of breast cancer care. It has been shown to facilitate prompt management of the issues, to improve the process and clinical outcomes, to lower mortality, and to improve the quality of life. It also reduces health care costs and improves the academic experience.

Concentrating expertise in breast cancer care with a multidisciplinary approach is a model that brings together all disciplines that are involved in the care of patients with breast cancer, which include breast imaging, oncologic surgery, pathology, medical oncology, radiation therapy, nursing, plastic surgery, genetics, psychology, and physical therapy. As each specialty has increased in complexity, each member of the team can focus on his or her own area of expertise while providing the patient with the benefit of that expertise and collaboration with various colleagues.

The delivery of coordinated and efficient care is greatly enhanced by the presence of nurse navigators who provide valuable support to the enterprise and education for patients and help to ensure the success of the multidisciplinary breast cancer care (MDBCC). Their dedication is to the patient, and their responsibility is to the clinicians dealing with the patient. They are indispensable, particularly for patients with complex problems.

The primary goals of MDBCC are to improve the care management of the breast cancer patient, increase the standardization of care, improve the communication between different disciplines, improve the patient experience, and increase participation in clinical trials.

Although the organization of MDBCC may vary, so does the patient's experience. As the approach to MDBCC is being developed by an institution, it is critical that the key members from the various disciplines meet on a regular basis to discuss organizational issues and how to improve the patient's experience (Box 1).

All patients seen in our institution benefit from the multidisciplinary approach. For patients who have been worked up and biopsied at our institution the process is faster compared with patients who have had their imaging and biopsy performed at outside institutions, most commonly a community hospital. For those patients, a second opinion review of the imaging studies and pathologic slides is mandatory.

In a study of 1970 breast pathology referral cases at a major cancer center, there was an 11.5% disagreement in the interpretation that affected patient care. Almost 60% of those disagreements had to do with histologic category or biomarker reporting. In addition, 32% of

BOX 1: Multidisciplinary Breast Cancer Care (MDBCC)

The Gold Standard

1. Core Disciplines: breast imaging, oncologic surgery, pathology, medical oncology, radiation oncology, plastic surgery
2. Patient-Centered Care
3. Team Communication
4. Efficient Navigation
5. Multidisciplinary Conference
6. Standard Protocols for Investigation and Treatment
7. Quality Assurance

Outcomes

Improved clinical outcomes, improved patient experience and satisfaction, increased participation in clinical trials, greater professional satisfaction

the total cases reviewed had specific required information missing from the College of American Pathologists checklist.

On the imaging side, in a recent review of 380 patients whose imaging studies were submitted for second opinion, there was a 47% distinct variance in the radiologic impression, and 53% had a recommendation for change in management plan with additional imaging or biopsies. The rate of additional recommended biopsies was 17%. Thirty-three percent of these biopsies were high-risk lesions or malignant lesions. In total, this resulted in a change of the overall surgical management for 27% of patients.

Large institutions with a large volume of breast cancer patients stand the best chance to have optimal MDBCC. The volume of patients ensures that they can recruit the top specialists in the various fields.

OUTLOOK

There has been a large transformation in the past 30 years in the way that breast cancer is detected, diagnosed, evaluated, and treated. These changes have been accompanied in the world of breast imaging by the development of new technologies as well as the refinement of older ones, allowing the breast imager to play a central role in the care of the breast cancer patient with direct responsibilities to the patient, the breast surgeon, and the members of the "breast team." Optimization of the care provided necessitates expanding the knowledge that all disciplines have of each other's fields and maintaining that interest as the understanding of the facets of breast cancer increases.

SUGGESTED READINGS

Boland M, Prichard R, Daskalova I, et al. Axillary nodal burden in primary breast cancer patients with positive pre-operative ultrasound guided fine needle aspiration cytology: management in the era of ACOSOG Z011. *Eur J Surg Oncol.* 2015;41:559-565.

Conant E. Clinical implementation of digital breast tomosynthesis. *Radiol Clin N Am.* 2014;52:499-518.

Debald M, Abramian A, Nemes L, et al. Who may benefit from preoperative breast MRI? A single-center analysis of 1102 consecutive patients with primary breast cancer. *Breast Cancer Res Treat.* 2015;153:531-537.

Elmore J, Kramer B. Breast cancer screening. *JAMA.* 2014;311:1298-1299.

Euhus D, Di Carlo P, Khouri N. Breast cancer screening. *Surg Clin N Am.* 2015;95:991-1011.

Friedewald S, Rafferty E, Rose S, et al. Breast cancer screening using tomosynthesis in combination with digital mammography. *JAMA.* 2014;311: 2499-2507.

Harvey S, Di Carlo P, Lee B, et al. An abbreviated protocol for high-risk screening breast MRI saves time and resources. *J Am Coll Radiol.* 2015; in press.

Hooley R, Greenberg K, Stackhouse R, et al. Screening US in patients with mammographically dense breasts: initial experience with Connecticut Public Act 09-41. *Radiology.* 2012;265:59-69.

Jackson R, Mylander C, Rosman M, et al. Normal axillary ultrasound excludes heavy nodal disease burden in patients with breast cancer. *Ann Surg Oncol.* 2015;22:3289-3295.

Jain A, Haisfield-Wolfe M, Lange J, et al. The role of ultrasound-guided fine-needle aspiration of axillary in the staging of breast cancer. *Ann Surg Oncol.* 2008;15:462-471.

Khazai L, Middleton L, Goktepe N, et al. Breast pathology second review identifies clinically significant discrepancies in over 10% of patients. *J Surg Oncol.* 2015;111:192-197.

Kuhl C, Schrading S, Strobel K, et al. Abbreviated breast imaging magnetic resonance imaging (MRI): first postcontrast images and maximum-intensity projection—a novel approach to breast cancer screening with MRI. *J Clin Oncol.* 2014;32:2304-2310.

Lehman C, DeMartini W, Anderson B, et al. Indications for breast MRI in the patient with newly diagnosed breast cancer. *J Natl Compr Canc Netw.* 2009;7:193-201.

Mallory M, Losk K, Lin N, et al. The influence of radiology image consultation in the surgical management of breast cancer patients. *Ann Surg Oncol.* 2015;22:3383-3388.

Morris E. Rethinking breast cancer screening: ultra FAST breast magnetic resonance imaging. *J Clin Oncol.* 2014;32:2281-2283.

Morrow M. Progress in the surgical management of breast cancer: present and future. *Breast.* 2015;24(suppl):S2-S5.

Morrow M, Schnitt S, Norton L. Current management of lesions associated with an increased risk of breast cancer. *Nat Rev Clin Oncol.* 2015;12:227-238.

Pace L, Keating N. A systematic assessment of benefits and risks to guide breast cancer screening decisions. *JAMA.* 2014;311:1327-1335.

Pilewskie M, King T. Magnetic resonance imaging in patients with newly diagnosed breast cancer. *Cancer.* 2014;120:2080-2089.

Pilewskie M, Morrow M. Management of the clinically node-negative axilla: what have we learned from the clinical trials? *Cancer Network.* 2014;1-8.

Pisano E, Yaffe M. Breast cancer screening: should tomosynthesis replace digital mammography? *JAMA.* 2014;311:2488-2489.

Spivey T, Carlson K, Janssen I, et al. Breast imaging second opinions impact surgical management. *Ann Surg Oncol.* 2015;22:2359-2364.

GENETIC COUNSELING AND TESTING

Kevin S. Hughes, MD, FACS

Although the mapping of the human genome was completed in 2001, this achievement has yet to be fully integrated into mainstream clinical medicine. Widespread genetic testing finally is becoming common in clinical practice, and the potential to identify high-risk patients before they develop cancer has never been greater. More than 100 genes have been identified with activating or inactivating mutations that can increase the risk of cancer, and many more are likely to be found in the near future.

The majority of these genes are tumor suppressor genes, in which the protein produced by the gene actively works to prevent the development of cancer. Tumor suppressor genes tend to be organ specific, each preventing cancer in a subset of organs (or leading to cancer in that subset when inactivated through mutation), thus establishing a spectrum of susceptible organs for each syndrome.

The responsible gene (or genes) has been identified for the major hereditary cancer syndromes (Table 1). These genes tend to be dominantly inherited in that a single mutation of one of the two paired genes causes cancer susceptibility, but they tend to behave recessively at the cellular level. Therefore not every cell of the specific organ will become cancerous. As humans, we have two sets of genes, one from each parent. When a germline tumor suppressor gene has an inactivating mutation, the other copy of the gene continues to produce the cancer-preventing product. It is only when the second gene loses function that the cell begins to accumulate other mutations, eventually leading to cancer. This is known as the *Knudson two-hit hypothesis* and helps to explain why most patients with a mutation develop cancer, often in multiple organs, whereas some never develop cancer, or develop it only in a single organ.

A small number of genes, such as the *RET* gene, which causes multiple endocrine neoplasia type 2 (MEN2), are oncogenes. Oncogenes are the mutant form of proto-oncogenes, the genes that regulate cellular proliferation and apoptosis. In cancers involving oncogenes, such as MEN2, a single germline mutant gene can drive cancer development without a second hit, causing the cancer to develop at a very young age. This helps explain the need for thyroidectomy in children under the age of 5 in some cases of MEN2.

MECHANISM OF CANCER DEVELOPMENT

How these genes cause cancer development is interesting and has implications for how they should be managed. Normally, in sporadic colon cancer, the original mutation leads to an overgrowth of cells that develops into a polyp. Given the large number of cells in a polyp, the chance that one cell will accumulate an additional mutation, leading it toward cancer, is more likely. The *APC* gene mutation, associated with familial adenomatous polyposis, causes innumerable cells in the colon to overgrow, forming innumerable polyps, and each polyp, with its rapidly dividing cells, has a high likelihood of progressing to cancer. Thus the rate of cancer approaches 100% in the patient's lifetime, and the best approach is prophylactic removal of the colon.

MLH1 (one of the Lynch syndrome genes) is a tumor suppressor gene that acts by helping to maintain the integrity of the genome. Loss of function in that gene hastens the accumulation of mutations in the cell, thus leading to colon cancer without the need for a precursor polyp. (Because a single cell with this mutation has a high likelihood of accumulating additional cancer-causing mutations, large numbers of cells are not a prerequisite.) This explains the other name for this syndrome, *hereditary nonpolyposis colorectal cancer syndrome.* Because the progression to cancer is rapid and often skips the polyp stage, colonoscopy every 1 to 2 years is needed to catch the cancer early. The penetrance of this gene is lower, with a lifetime risk of about 70% to 80%.

IDENTIFICATION OF THOSE AT RISK

To identify patients with a hereditary predisposition to cancer, it is critical to take a thorough family history. The key thing to look for among family members is a pattern of multiple cancers associated with a specific syndrome occurring in a single bloodline. For example, multiple relatives with breast and/or ovarian cancer in a single bloodline may suggest a hereditary breast/ovarian cancer syndrome, whereas multiple relatives with colon and/or endometrial cancer in a single bloodline may suggest a hereditary colon cancer syndrome (e.g., Lynch syndrome). The second hallmark of hereditary cancer is young age at diagnosis. Cancers diagnosed in young adults are more

TABLE I: Examples of Hereditary Cancer Syndromes and Their Associated Genes

	Breast Cancer	Ovarian Cancer	Colorectal Cancer	Uterine Cancer	Melanoma	Pancreatic Cancer	Stomach Cancer	Prostate Cancer	Leukemia
HEREDITARY BREAST OVARIAN CANCER SYNDROME									
BRCA1	*	*				*		*	
BRCA2	*	*			*	*		*	
LYNCH SYNDROME									
MLH1		*	*	*		*	*		
MSH2		*	*	*		*	*		
MSH6		*	*	*		*	*		
PMS2		*	*	*		*	*		
FAMILIAL ADENOMATOUS POLYPOSIS SYNDROME									
APC			*			*	*		
LI-FRAUMENI SYNDROME									
TP53	*	*	*	*	*	*	*	*	*
COWDEN'S SYNDROME									
PTEN	*		*	*	*				
PEUTZ-JEGHERS SYNDROME									
STK11	*	*	*	*		*	*		
HEREDITARY DIFFUSE GASTRIC CANCER SYNDROME									
CDH 1	*		*				*		

likely to be hereditary because the first mutation is already present at birth and thus is more likely to indicate the presence of a hereditary syndrome in other family members. Multiple cancers in a single individual are a third indicator, and an unusual cancer, such as male breast cancer or medullary thyroid cancer, is the fourth indicator of hereditary cancer. In addition, the threshold required for testing drops significantly in groups with a high probability of mutation, such as Ashkenazi Jewish individuals, who may be eligible for testing even without one of these indicators.

If any of these indicators are observed in the family history, genetic testing should be considered. Guidelines, such as those established by the National Comprehensive Cancer Center (NCCN) or the United States Preventive Services Task Force, provide examples of testable patterns, whereas risk models (e.g., BRCAPRO, Tyrer-Cuzick) can be helpful for quantitating risk and setting thresholds for testable families.

■ POPULATION-BASED SCREENING

The current approach to cancer screening limits genetic testing to a small number of patients with extreme family histories. This approach is primarily an outgrowth of the high cost of testing and our lack of comfort with and understanding of hereditary cancer. As costs have come down and practitioners have become more accepting of genetic testing, there has been greater acceptance of this approach, further decreasing the threshold for testing. There is now discussion of population-level screening, in which whole populations are targeted, with or without indicators of high risk. This trend toward population-level screening is not unprecedented. Newborn screening for genetic diseases has been practiced for decades.

It is now commonplace to screen all young-onset colon cancers with microsatellite instability testing or immunohistochemical staining to identify tumors characteristic of hereditary cancer. Although it remains controversial, population screening for common, highly penetrant gene mutations among selected populations (e.g., Ashkenazi Jews) has been suggested, as has screening of all women over age 30 for BRCA mutations. In addition, whole genome sequencing and whole exome sequencing have the potential to reveal mutations incidentally when cancer-causing genes are screened in patients with minimal or no family history.

Widespread population screening is certain to raise new issues. Although we have a fairly good idea of how to manage a patient with a gene mutation and a very strong family history, the question arises, should that same management be applied to a patient with an incidentally discovered mutation and no family history? Currently the answer tends toward yes, but much remains to be learned.

■ IDENTIFICATION OF INDIVIDUALS AT HIGH RISK

Identifying individuals who are at risk for hereditary cancer is critical and may occur at multiple stages in the patient's care. Within your practice, you will find potential mutation carriers among (1) patients who do not have cancer, (2) patients with newly diagnosed cancer, and (3) patients being followed for past cancers. It is critical to have a system in place to identify high-risk individuals in each of these categories.

Patients Who Do Not Have Cancer

Ideally, mutation carriers should be identified before the development of cancer. As surgeons, we see a large number of women and men in our offices for a variety of problems. It is good medical practice to take a family history for each of these individuals, not just the ones who have or potentially have a cancer diagnosis. A strong family history, as defined earlier, should indicate the need for genetic testing. If testing is positive, the patient can be placed on a management strategy that either prevents cancer or finds it at an earlier, more treatable stage. In the past, it was recommended that a living affected relative be tested first, to identify the family-specific mutation. If testing of a relative can be accomplished expeditiously, this remains the ideal approach because it provides the entire family with clinically actionable information. However, because the cost of testing has decreased and our comfort with testing has increased, it is becoming more common to test the patients in front of us, whether or not they have cancer.

Patients With Newly Diagnosed Cancer

Among patients with a newly diagnosed cancer, immediate identification of the mutation status is critical because this can have implications for treatment. For example, a small breast cancer in a 40-year-old woman can be managed easily by lumpectomy with radiation unless she is a *BRCA1* carrier. If she carries the *BRCA1* gene mutation, bilateral mastectomy may be the better choice of therapy. *BRCA* carriers also may be better served by different chemotherapy regimens. For example, a *BRCA1* carrier may receive adjuvant platinum therapy, whereas a patient who is not a mutation carrier may be better served by taxane-based therapy. In terms of radiation, *TP53* carriers (i.e., with Li-Fraumeni syndrome) should not receive radiation therapy owing to their extreme sensitivity to this modality.

Patients Being Followed for a Past Cancer

As surgeons, we routinely follow a large number of cancer patients. Many in this group will have been missed as potential mutation carriers at the time of their original diagnosis and may never have been tested. Even those tested may have undergone less comprehensive testing than is available today. These patients need to be identified as potential carriers, and testing must be done to help avoid future cancers. The follow-up of mutation carriers will be more intensive and potentially will involve different screening methods. For example, patients with Lynch syndrome would benefit from colonoscopy every 1 to 2 years and may benefit from a hysterectomy with bilateral salpingo-oophorectomy, whereas *BRCA* carriers would benefit from magnetic resonance imaging (MRI) screening of the breasts (if mastectomies have not been done). For those who tested negative on screening, even within the last few years, updating their testing with new gene panels or new testing methods may be worthwhile if the family history is extensive.

Relatives of Mutation Carriers

When a patient with a hereditary syndrome is identified, it is extremely important to inform and test as many family members as possible. Because physicians are limited to dealing with the patient in front of them, it is critical to make the patient aware of the need to inform other family members. Close to half of the patient's close relatives, and a high proportion of more distant relatives, will have the mutation and be at extremely high risk yet will be unaware of the risk. Although informing other family members can be difficult for patients dealing with a new and potential deadly diagnosis, and although it may seem to fall outside the surgeon's purview, the implications are so great, it cannot be ignored. Testing these relatives will deliver the highest yield of positive tests. Gene mutations are rare, and the majority of families have only a single cancer-causing mutation. Thus, if an individual does not carry the family mutation, the result is considered a true negative, and that person can be assumed to be back at the population risk. Unfortunately, most relatives of mutation carriers remain untested. If a patient in your practice has a positive relative, encourage testing. If you identify a mutation carrier, encourage that patient to tell his or her family members that testing is critical.

■ TIMING OF TESTING

Genetic testing usually is recommended when the individual is of the age when a positive finding will result in a change in clinical management. For potential *BRCA* carriers, that would be around age 25, but for potential carriers of the *APC* gene mutation that age may be as young as 10 to 12 years. In general, testing before the age of 18 is discouraged, unless a positive result would lead to a change in clinical management at a younger age.

■ HOW TO ARRANGE OR UNDERTAKE GENETIC TESTING

Once the patient has been identified as being at risk of having a mutation, genetic testing is a very appropriate approach. The American College of Surgeons Commission on Cancer requires that any certified cancer center have access to a genetic testing resource. Surgeons should be involved intimately in genetic testing, either referring the patient to a genetics expert for testing or doing the testing themselves. Regardless, the surgeon must have expertise in interpreting the test results and organizing the proper clinical management.

For surgeons who choose to do their own genetic testing, it is important to provide pretest and post-test counseling, in keeping with the recommendations of the American Society of Clinical Oncology (ASCO). This entails carefully reviewing the ASCO elements of informed consent with patients before testing and counseling patients regarding the implications of their results after testing is completed.

■ SELECTION OF GENETIC TESTING

Once a patient has been identified as appropriate for genetic testing, the next consideration is which test to order. In the recent past, a physician, a nurse practitioner, or a genetic counselor would evaluate the family history and make an educated guess as to which syndrome was most likely, and the genetic test for that syndrome would be ordered. If the result was negative, the provider then had to decide if other syndromes may be possible and order additional tests. This approach (also known as the *diagnostic odyssey*) was time consuming and expensive. It is now no longer necessary. The advent of a new approach to deoxyribonucleic acid (DNA) analysis called *next-generation sequencing* has decreased markedly the cost of genetic testing. Labs can now test multiple cancer genes simultaneously at a fraction of the cost of sequencing a single gene.

The advent of this technology has led to the creation of cancer panels that contain a number of cancer-associated genes. These panels may be organ directed, representing multiple genes that are related to a single organ system, or they may be pan-cancer panels, sometimes covering all cancer genes known to man. The advantage of these panels is that it is no longer necessary to limit the test to a small subset of genes, and it is far less likely that the wrong gene will be tested. The disadvantage of these panels is that many include less well-studied genes with management issues that are still up for debate and mutations that remain unclassified.

Keeping these limitations in mind, it is now more common to move directly to panel testing unless a gene mutation is known to exist in a family. In the latter case, single site mutation testing remains a reasonable option.

INTERPRETATION OF RESULTS

Mutations or variants in cancer susceptibility genes can be classified in one of five categories: benign, likely benign, variant of uncertain significance (VUS), likely pathogenic, and pathogenic. Benign or likely benign variants basically should be ignored. Pathogenic mutations should be treated aggressively, whereas mutations that are likely pathogenic should be managed based on the family history and the clinical situation, although a low threshold for action is reasonable. The results that are most frustrating for patients and clinicians are the variants of uncertain significance. A VUS means that although there is indeed a change in the DNA sequence of the gene, the change may or may not be cancer causing. These variants are seen more commonly in newer, less well studied genes, such as *PALB2*, but can still be found, although less commonly, even in extensively tested genes, such as *BRCA1* or *BRCA2*. Patients with a VUS should be managed based on the family history and the clinical situation, as if the VUS had not been found. Over time, most VUS mutations will be reclassified, at which time the lab involved usually will notify you and you, in turn, should inform the patient.

INTERPRETING THE RESULTS

When a patient has a pathogenic mutation in a cancer susceptibility gene, what does it mean for that patient? As in all of medicine, much depends on the patients' current circumstances: What are their ages? Do they have a newly diagnosed cancer, were they diagnosed with cancer in the past, or have they never had cancer? If they have cancer or had cancer in the past, which cancer did they have and what was the clinical stage? One must consider the penetrance and clinical spectrum of that specific gene mutation and then determine the management options that apply to the individual patient.

The number and variety of genes that cause cancer, together with our rapidly accumulating knowledge of cancer genetics, has made it virtually impossible for anyone to know what every gene mutation in every gene means in terms of cancer risk or how it should be managed. In most instances, expect to carefully read the penetrance and suggested management that the laboratory provides and then to go to the literature to learn more, including identifying whether management guidelines exist. The NCCN and many specialty societies have produced excellent guidelines for many of the major cancer syndromes. Once you understand the disease spectrum, be prepared to apply it to your specific patient. Determining management often requires a multidisciplinary approach. It is important to identify a set of consultants in your area on whom you can depend. For *BRCA* mutations, experts in gynecologic oncology, medical oncology, and breast surgery will be critical to assembling your team, whereas for Lynch syndrome, look for experts in gynecologic oncology, medical oncology, gastroenterology, and colorectal surgery.

RISK AND MANAGEMENT

Although we cannot review the recommended management of every gene in this limited chapter, we can provide some general rules and give a few examples. Each gene, when mutated, will place the person at risk for a different spectrum of diseases at different levels of risk.

In general, genes with high penetrance tend to be rare, whereas syndromes with low penetrance tend to be relatively common, and those with intermediate penetrance tend to be uncommon but not rare.

For example, a woman with a *BRCA2* mutation has a lifetime risk of 70% for breast cancer but less than 5% risk for pancreas cancer. A woman with a *CHEK2* mutation (which is much more common than *BRCA*) has an elevated risk of developing breast cancer, but that risk is only slightly greater than the general population. A young woman with a *CHEK2* mutation and a minimal family history is likely to be best managed with screening mammography, whereas a woman with a *BRCA1* mutation should undergo either mammography plus MRI screening or prophylactic mastectomy. Because screening with MRI and mammography is very likely to catch a breast cancer early, the use of prophylactic surgery is optional. On the other hand, a *BRCA1* carrier should undergo prophylactic oophorectomy at age 35 or as soon after as possible, once childbearing is complete, because ovarian screening is almost useless, and the chance of catching an early ovarian cancer is small.

In addition, the stage of the patient's cancer also should be considered. A *BRCA* carrier with a newly diagnosed stage 4 ovarian cancer will likely not benefit from prophylactic mastectomy, whereas a carrier with a stage one breast cancer may be treated best with bilateral mastectomy.

SUMMARY

Genetic testing is a critical part of medical practice today, especially among specialists who treat cancer. It is imperative that we identify patients at risk and facilitate their testing as soon as possible. Whether surgeons opt to test their own patients or refer them to a genetic counselor, the surgeon must be involved intimately in the management of the genetic syndrome that ultimately is revealed. Changes in management prompted by the results of genetic testing can save lives and markedly decrease the morbidity of cancer for these individuals and their families. As the noted human geneticist and *BRCA* pioneer, Dr. Mary-Claire King, has stated, "Every mutation carrier identified after a cancer has developed is a failure of cancer prevention."

ACKNOWLEDGMENT

I wish to acknowledge the writing and editorial support of Ann S. Adams.

SUGGESTED READINGS

Desmond A, Kurian AW, Gabree M, et al. Clinical actionability of multigene panel testing for hereditary breast and ovarian cancer risk assessment. *JAMA Oncol.* 2015;1:943-951.

Easton DF, Pharoah PD, Antoniou AC, et al. Gene-panel sequencing and the prediction of breast-cancer risk. *N Engl J Med.* 2015;372:2243-2257.

Evans DG, Howell A. Breast cancer risk-assessment models. *Breast Cancer Res.* 2007;9:213.

Foulkes WD, Knoppers BM, Turnbull C. Population genetic testing for cancer susceptibility: founder mutations to genomes. *Nat Rev Clin Oncol.* 2015.

Robson ME, Bradbury AR, Arun B, et al. American Society of Clinical Oncology Policy Statement update: genetic and genomic testing for cancer susceptibility. *J Clin Oncol.* 2015;33:3660-3667.

CONTRALATERAL PROPHYLACTIC MASTECTOMY

L. Mark Knab, MD, and Swati A. Kulkarni, MD

Contralateral prophylactic mastectomy (CPM) is defined as a risk-reducing mastectomy of the contralateral breast in a woman with unilateral breast cancer. In the United States, CPM rates have increased dramatically since 1998. Tuttle and colleagues used the Surveillance, Epidemiology, and End Results (SEER) database to review the treatment of patients with unilateral breast cancer from 1998 to 2003. The overall rate of CPM rose from 1.8% to 4.5% (a 150% increase). The study found that young patient age, lobular-type histology, and non-Hispanic Caucasian race were associated with higher CPM rates. This trend has persisted in more recent studies and is driven largely by the increase of CPM in women under the age of 40 years (Box 1).

■ INDICATIONS: CONTRALATERAL BREAST CANCER RISK

Suggested guidelines for CPM have been put forth by a number of national organizations and clinical societies to help guide patients and physicians. However, there are no absolute indications for CPM. CPM most frequently is recommended for women with unilateral breast cancer who are at high risk for a contralateral breast cancer. This group includes *BRCA1* and *BRCA2* mutation carriers, women with mutations in other genetic susceptibility genes, those with a strong family history of breast cancer without an identified mutation, and those with a history of supradiaphragmatic radiation during puberty. Contraindications for CPM include the presence of serious medical comorbidities, distant metastases, synchronous or recently treated advanced stage malignancies, and pregnancy-associated breast cancer.

BRCA1 and *BRCA2* Mutation Carriers

Women with a mutation in *BRCA1* or *BRCA2* are at increased risk for developing a contralateral breast cancer. A multicenter study by Graeser and others included 2020 women with unilateral breast cancer who were found to have *BRCA1* or *BRCA2* mutations. The cumulative risk of developing contralateral breast cancer was 47.4% at 25 years. *BRCA1* carriers had a risk 1.6 times higher than *BRCA2* carriers of developing a contralateral breast cancer, and women under 40 years of age were at a much greater risk of developing a contralateral breast cancer compared with women over 50 years of age (62.9% vs 19.5%, respectively). The 10-year cumulative risk of developing contralateral breast cancer in *BRCA1* and *BRCA2* mutation carriers varies according to study but ranges from 16.6% to 29.5%, or a 3% risk per year.

Other Breast Cancer Susceptibility Genes Associated With Contralateral Breast Cancer

In addition to *BRCA1* and *BRCA2*, autosomal dominant germline mutations in *PTEN* and *P53* are known to confer a significant risk of contralateral breast cancer. Patients who carry a germline mutation in the tumor suppressor gene *P53* (Li-Fraumeni syndrome) are at increased risk of developing multiple malignancies before the age of 46 years. Breast cancer is the most common malignancy identified in adult mutation carriers. These cancers are characterized by early age of diagnosis, human epidermal growth factor receptor–2 (HER2) overexpression, and the presence of synchronous or metachronous contralateral breast cancers. In some cohorts up to one third of women develop a contralateral breast cancer. Cowden syndrome is associated with a mutation in the tumor suppressor *PTEN*. Germline mutations in *PTEN* are characterized by multiple benign hamartomas and carcinomas of the breast, thyroid, kidney, and endometrium. The lifetime risk of breast cancer in women with *PTEN* mutations has been reported to be as high as 85% and the 10-year risk of developing a second breast cancer is approximately 25%. Benign breast disease also affects about two thirds of mutation carriers and can result in additional imaging and breast biopsies.

Advances in gene sequencing technology have allowed for examination of multiple breast cancer susceptibility genes simultaneously through panel testing (commonly tested genes include *CDH1*, *CHEK2*, *STK11*, and *PALB2*). However, at present insufficient data exist on the risk that these gene mutations confer on contralateral breast cancer. Identification of germline mutations in these genes should not be an indication for prophylactic surgery.

History of Therapeutic Radiation for Hodgkin's Lymphoma

The risk for breast cancer is significant in women diagnosed with Hodgkin's lymphoma (HL) who are treated with supradiaphragmatic radiation. Age of treatment and type of treatment (radiation alone vs radiation plus chemotherapy) are key for determining the level of risk. A study that included 5002 women under the age of 36 years who received supradiaphragmatic radiation for HL demonstrated a relative risk of 5.0, with the highest risk among those women who received radiation at age 14 years (relative risk of 47.2, which translates into a cumulative risk of about 50% at 40 years). It is believed that the risk is highest at this age because of the effects of radiation on dividing breast cells during puberty. There was a reduced risk of breast cancer in those women older than 20 years of age who received a combination of radiation therapy and chemotherapy because of chemotherapy-induced early onset menopause. Because the radiation fields for HL generally encompass both breasts, the risk is bilateral. A discussion about CPM should be included for those women who are diagnosed with an ipsilateral breast cancer in the setting of radiation for HL.

Histology

Several retrospective studies have reported certain histologies that are associated with an increased risk of contralateral breast lesions. In a series of 239 patients, Goldflam and others found that in the index tumor, lobular histology, additional moderate- to high-risk lesions, and estrogen receptor/progesterone receptor (ER/PR) positivity were predictors of malignant or moderate- to high-risk lesions in the contralateral breast. In a study including 542 patients, multivariate analysis demonstrated that ipsilateral invasive lobular histology, an ipsilateral multicentric tumor, and a 5-year Gail risk score greater than 1.67 were all independent predictors of contralateral breast cancer. Findings from these studies potentially could be used to justify additional imaging of the contralateral breast before surgical intervention to determine whether there is an invasive breast cancer present in the contralateral breast that could alter surgical or medical management. However, the presence of these characteristics alone should not prompt the surgeon to recommend CPM.

General Population

The dramatic increase in the CPM rate is driven largely by women with an average risk of contralateral breast cancer. However, for the general population the annual incidence of developing contralateral

BOX 1: Characteristics of Women Associated With Contralateral Prophylactic Mastectomy

- Use of preoperative magnetic resonance imaging
- Availability of immediate breast reconstruction
- History of prior breast biopsy
- Estrogen receptor–negative breast cancer
- Invasive lobular cancer
- *BRCA* mutation testing
- Family history of breast cancer
- Younger age
- Higher education level
- Caucasian ethnicity
- Private insurance

breast cancer is very low and remains constant over time at about 0.5% to 0.7% per year. Gao and colleagues conducted a study using the SEER database and found that the cumulative risk of developing contralateral breast cancer at 10, 15, and 20 years was 6.1%, 9.1%, and 12%, respectively. More recent analysis of the SEER database shows the contralateral breast cancer rate declining, specifically after diagnosis of ER-positive cancer. The decrease to about 3% over 10 years likely is driven by the widespread use of adjuvant endocrine therapy that has been shown to significantly reduce the incidence of contralateral breast cancer.

BREAST SURVEILLANCE

Digital mammography, magnetic resonance imaging (MRI), tomosynthesis, and screening ultrasound techniques are excellent tools that are now available for surveillance of the contralateral breast. These tools are particularly useful for screening women with mammographically dense breasts. Therefore CPM should not be recommended for women on the basis of increased mammographic density. In very rare cases CPM can be considered in those patients for whom surveillance is difficult or challenging, such as those with extensive dystrophic calcifications from prior trauma or radiation to the breast.

Because of the extensive surveillance needed for women in high-risk groups, the question of long-term cost is raised often. One study examined cost effectiveness of CPM compared with routine surveillance using a Markov model. The study determined that for women of average risk with unilateral breast cancer, the mean costs of CPM and routine surveillance for a woman 45 years old were comparable. CPM is not cost effective over the age of 70 years. The study did demonstrate cost effectiveness of CPM in all ages for those patients who carry a *BRCA* mutation. A related study used software to model the costs and effects of CPM compared with a unilateral mastectomy in women less than 50 years of age with sporadic, unilateral breast cancer. It showed that CPM is cost saving in women younger than 50 years of age but did not improve the quality or quantity of life. The study concluded that CPM was not ultimately cost effective in this group of women.

OUTCOMES OF CONTRALATERAL PROPHYLACTIC MASTECTOMY

Complications

The operative risks associated with a bilateral mastectomy are greater than those associated with a unilateral mastectomy. In a study with 600 patients with unilateral breast cancer, 65% underwent a unilateral mastectomy and 35% underwent a bilateral mastectomy. There were significantly more complications in the bilateral mastectomy group compared with the unilateral mastectomy group (41.6% vs 28.6%, respectively). After risk adjustment, women who underwent CPM were 1.5 times more likely to have any complication and 2.7 times more likely to have a major complication compared with those

who underwent a unilateral mastectomy. A different study used the National Surgery Quality Improvement Program (NSQIP) database to identify women who underwent a unilateral or bilateral mastectomy and determine their 30-day complication rates. Women who underwent a bilateral mastectomy had a significantly higher wound complication rate (5.8% vs 2.9%) and an overall 30-day complication rate of 7.6% versus 4.2% compared with those who underwent a unilateral mastectomy.

Risk Reduction

CPM confers a 90% to 95% risk reduction for the development of a new breast cancer. The efficacy of CPM in women with a personal and family history of breast cancer was studied by McDonnell. The study included 745 women with a first breast cancer and a family history of breast or ovarian cancer who were treated with CPM. It demonstrated a 94.4% risk reduction in premenopausal women and a 96% risk reduction in postmenopausal women. Overall, the benefit of CPM in reducing the incidence of a contralateral breast cancer is greatest in those women at highest risk for developing contralateral breast cancer.

Survival

Although it is well established that CPM confers a risk reduction in developing breast cancer in those women who are at high risk, it is not clear if this risk reduction translates into a clear survival benefit. As more women undergo genetic testing and there is longer follow-up, the effect of CPM on survival in high-risk patients should become clearer.

Several retrospective studies on women who are *BRCA1* and *BRCA2* mutations carriers have shown no difference in overall survival after CPM. Van Sprundel and colleagues studied a cohort of 148 women with a mutation in *BRCA1* or *BRCA2* in which 79 women underwent CPM and 69 did not. After 5 years of follow-up, the overall survival of the CPM group was 94% and of the surveillance group was 77%, although after multivariate analysis accounting for bilateral prophylactic oophorectomy the CPM effect on survival was not significant. Several other studies have shown a significant improvement in overall survival after CPM, although it is difficult to interpret the results given selection biases in the studies. It is likely that survival improvements in the women who undergo CPM result from the fact that women who choose CPM tend to be younger, healthier, and have more favorable tumors. Lostumbo and colleagues conducted a Cochrane review of the data including 39 studies and a total of 7384 women who were at high risk for breast cancer (not necessarily limited to *BRCA1* and *BRCA2* mutation carriers). The study concluded that although CPM reduces the risk of a contralateral breast cancer, there was no definitive evidence that CPM improved survival in high-risk women.

There have been a number of studies evaluating the effect of CPM in women with average risk factors. Although a few studies do demonstrate an overall survival benefit for women who undergo CPM, selection bias is an inherent confounding factor. As with women at high risk, the women at average risk who undergo CPM are more likely to be young, insured, and diagnosed with earlier stage disease. In summary, there are no clear overall survival benefits for women who undergo CPM. In select high-risk patient populations in which CPM is being considered, the theoretic survival benefit must be weighed against the increased operative risk of a mastectomy.

COUNSELING

Perceived Risk Versus Actual Risk

A patient's actual risk versus perceived risk of developing a contralateral breast cancer often can be disparate. It has been documented in both prospective and retrospective studies that patients significantly overestimate their risk of developing a second breast cancer.

BOX 2: Counseling Points for Women With Average Risk Interested in Contralateral Prophylactic Mastectomy (CPM)

- There is a low annual contralateral breast cancer risk in women with average risk factors.
- Risk of contralateral breast cancer is decreasing with use of adjuvant therapy.
- Removing the contralateral breast does not decrease the risk for developing distant metastases.
- Breast cancer does not commonly metastasize from one breast to the other.
- CPM does not improve breast cancer–specific survival.
- CPM does not decrease local recurrence.
- Contralateral breast cancers tend to be at a lower stage than the initial primary cancer.
- CPM increases the surgical complication risk.
- Choice of CPM may influence reconstruction options.
- There are alternatives to CPM, including chemoprevention and surveillance.

One study evaluated the perceptions of contralateral breast cancer risk and showed that women with newly diagnosed breast cancer estimated their 10-year risk of contralateral breast cancer to be about 30%. They also did not associate their perceived risk with age, cancer stage, family history, or CPM. In a similar study, women at average risk estimated that 10% of women would have a contralateral breast cancer within 5 years without a CPM. This underscores the need for patient education and counseling to delineate the actual risk of developing of contralateral breast cancer (Box 2).

Surgical Decision Making

Approximately half of women diagnosed with breast cancer come to their initial consultation with the surgeon wanting or considering CPM. As part of surgical consultation for a newly diagnosed breast cancer, in addition to discussing the treatment options and risk for ipsilateral breast cancer recurrence and distant recurrence, the surgeon should address contralateral breast cancer risk and provide actual numbers to patients. Women with *BRCA1* or *BRCA2* mutations or other gene mutations that predispose them to contralateral breast cancer should be counseled about their elevated risk for contralateral breast cancer and the potential benefits of CPM as part of the surgical consultation. Likewise, women without risk factors for contralateral breast cancer should be informed of their annual risk for developing a contralateral breast cancer and the additional benefit of adjuvant therapy on reducing breast cancer risk.

General concepts about the risks and benefits of CPM with respect to outcomes also should be addressed, including additional operative risks of CPM and the fact that removing the contralateral breast prophylactically does not reduce the risk for local or distant recurrence. Also, some patients may not understand that breast cancer does not spread from one breast to the other and may believe that removing the healthy breast will prevent breast cancer from recurring. Finally, it is important to explain to patients that CPM is not associated with a survival benefit. Survival generally is determined by the stage of the known diagnosed cancer. If a subsequent breast cancer develops, it likely will be detected by imaging and be at a lower stage.

The majority of women who choose CPM are younger. Because the diagnosis is often unexpected in this group of women, fear and anxiety play a significant role in the decision-making process. Peace of mind is often cited as a reason why young women undergo CPM. Women also often say that they do not want to go through the experience again. If possible, a second surgical consultation should be offered to give the patient time to process all information before

making a final decision. Asking the patient to defer the decision about undergoing CPM until genetic counseling and testing are completed can provide the patient with additional information about her risk for contralateral breast cancer. Referral for counseling with a social worker or psychologist may be beneficial, as may be meeting with other breast cancer survivors. For the surgeon, it is key to provide as much information as possible so that women are making an informed decision about CPM. Patient and physician decision aids currently under development may further assist the education and decision-making process. Despite counseling and patient education, a number of women with average risk factors will still request CPM. In this scenario the surgeon should feel confident that, to the extent possible, the patient is making a well-informed decision.

■ SURGICAL CONSIDERATIONS

Types of Mastectomy

The most common types of mastectomies that are performed for CPM include simple mastectomy, skin-sparing mastectomy, and nipple and areola–sparing mastectomy. In general, when performing a therapeutic mastectomy and CPM it is recommended that the therapeutic mastectomy be performed as the first procedure and the CPM as the second. Some surgeons recommend using bowel technique to prevent spread of tumor cells to the unaffected breast, but there are no data to suggest that breast cancer cells can spread through operative instruments to the unaffected breast, and the use of a second operative setup adds unnecessary cost and time to the procedure.

Simple mastectomy can be performed when the woman does not wish to undergo immediate reconstruction. Care should be taken to ensure that the incisions are approximately the same length and level in the breast. The skin-sparing mastectomy and nipple and areola–sparing mastectomy are generally the two approaches used for CPM when reconstruction is involved. In a skin-sparing approach, the breast parenchyma is excised generally through a circular incision around the nipple-areolar complex. This approach has the advantage of allowing for a reconstructive procedure that better preserves the natural breast contour and shape. A skin-sparing mastectomy is oncologically acceptable in patients with ductal carcinoma in situ (DCIS) and stages I to III breast cancer. It is contraindicated in those with inflammatory breast cancer.

The nipple and areola–sparing mastectomy, or nipple-sparing mastectomy (NSM), preserves the dermis and epidermis of the nipple but removes the major ducts from the nipple. The use of NSM has expanded significantly in recent years for surgical treatment of women with invasive breast cancer and for CPM. It is considered oncologically safe. Inframammary incisions can be used for optimal cosmetic results. Implant-based reconstruction is used most frequently in this setting.

A study by Coopey and colleagues involving 645 breasts in 370 patients who underwent NSM demonstrated the oncologic safety of this operative approach as well as the low incidence of nipple necrosis. Local recurrence was reported in 2.6% of breasts operated on for cancer, none of it involving the nipple. Total nipple necrosis occurred in 1.7% of breasts, and the nipple was removed in 3.7% of breasts because of positive nipple or subareolar margins.

Absolute contraindications for NSM include clinical or imaging evidence of nipple-areolar complex involvement, inflammatory breast cancer, locally advanced breast cancer with skin involvement, and bloody nipple discharge.

Sentinel Lymph Node Biopsy

Sentinel lymph node (SLN) biopsy of the contralateral axilla is not recommended in the setting of CPM given the increased incidence of seroma formation, infection, and lymphedema. The incidence of occult synchronous contralateral breast cancer is less than 5%. The incidence of contralateral lymph node metastasis is less than 2%.

Most of the occult cancer identified is DCIS. MRI may be beneficial in identifying contralateral disease, but this must be weighed against the low specificity and additional biopsies that may result.

Breast Reconstruction

Some patients undergo CPM to improve symmetry. Women who are small breasted, have little mammary fat, and have ptosis may be difficult to match with unilateral implant-based reconstruction. Likewise, women with very large, pendulous breasts may face similar challenges. However, for many women CPM is not necessary. Other procedures are available to achieve breast symmetry, including reduction mammoplasty and mastopexy of the contralateral breast. Many women are not aware of these options and may wish to pursue these alternative procedures that allow them to keep their breasts once they weigh the risks and benefits of CPM. In these cases, close coordination with the reconstructive surgeon is essential.

There are two basic options for breast reconstruction: prosthetic implants and autologous tissue reconstruction, which involves the transfer of tissue from a donor site to the chest wall. Implantable prostheses with silicone gel or saline are a popular option and result in shorter operative times and shorter hospital lengths of stay compared with autologous reconstructions. Autologous reconstruction with procedures such as a transverse rectus abdominis myocutaneous (TRAM) flap or a deep inferior epigastric artery perforator (DIEP) flap have notable advantages, including the creation of a soft, naturally textured, and ptotic breast that usually does not change with time. One limitation of autologous reconstruction is that occasionally there is not enough autologous tissue available for bilateral reconstruction. Additional disadvantages include increased operative times and postoperative complications.

The choice of breast reconstruction is an individualized decision involving a variety of factors, including body habitus, comorbidities, shape and contour of the contralateral breast, quality of the tissue, smoking habits, and personal preference.

ALTERNATIVES TO CONTRALATERAL PROPHYLACTIC MASTECTOMY

The main alternatives to CPM include enhanced surveillance and chemoprevention. Ultrasound, breast MRI, and mammography all can be used to screen high-risk women. There is debate about the ideal screening protocol, but ultrasound and breast MRI have been shown to increase the sensitivity of screening for women at high risk for breast cancer. Chemopreventive agents approved for use in high-risk women include tamoxifen, raloxifene, and exemestane. These agents are effective in ER-positive breast cancers but may not prevent ER-negative breast cancers.

CONCLUSION

Over the past several decades there have been significant advances in understanding the biology of breast cancer, which in turn has affected breast cancer treatment, both medically and surgically. Simultaneously, the rates of CPM recently have increased dramatically without good evidence to suggest that women are enjoying a survival advantage from the operation. Because of the retrospective nature of the evidence available, there is no risk factor threshold that can be used definitively to counsel patients about CPM. It is clear that CPM reduces the risk for developing a contralateral breast cancer, although the survival implications are less clear. The surgeon must be willing to enter a dialogue with the patient and clearly explain the benefits and risks of the surgical options.

SUGGESTED READINGS

Coopey SB, et al. Increasing eligibility for nipple-sparing mastectomy. *Ann Surg Oncol.* 2013;20:3218-3222.

Gao X, Fisher SG, Emami B. Risk of second primary cancer in the contralateral breast in women treated for early-stage breast cancer: a population-based study. *Int J Radiat Oncol Biol Phys.* 2003;56:1038-1045.

Goldflam K, et al. Contralateral prophylactic mastectomy: predictors of significant histologic findings. *Cancer.* 2004;101:1977-1986.

Graeser MK, et al. Contralateral breast cancer risk in *BRCA1* and *BRCA2* mutation carriers. *J Clin Oncol.* 2009;27:5887-5892.

Lostumbo L, et al. Prophylactic mastectomy for the prevention of breast cancer. *Cochrane Database Syst Rev.* 2004;(4):CD002748.

Osman F, et al. Increased postoperative complications in bilateral mastectomy patients compared to unilateral mastectomy: an analysis of the NSQIP database. *Ann Surg Oncol.* 2013;20:3212-3217.

Rosenberg SM, et al. Perceptions, knowledge, and satisfaction with contralateral prophylactic mastectomy among young women with breast cancer: a cross-sectional survey. *Ann Intern Med.* 2013;159:373-381.

Tuttle TM, et al. Increasing use of contralateral prophylactic mastectomy for breast cancer patients: a trend toward more aggressive surgical treatment. *J Clin Oncol.* 2007;25:5203-5209.

van Sprundel TC, et al. Risk reduction of contralateral breast cancer and survival after contralateral prophylactic mastectomy in *BRCA1* or *BRCA2* mutation carriers. *Br J Cancer.* 2005;93:287-292.

Yi M, et al. Predictors of contralateral breast cancer in patients with unilateral breast cancer undergoing contralateral prophylactic mastectomy. *Cancer.* 2009;115:962-971.

MARGINS: HOW TO AND HOW BIG?

Richard J. Gray, MD, FACS

Achieving negative margins of excision is an important component of breast surgery. The first question a surgeon is asked by the patient and family after an operation is: "Did you get it all?" Local recurrence (LR) rates are significantly higher for patients who have positive margins of excision. Therefore how to assure negative margins and what constitutes an adequate margin of excision are important factors for surgeons to consider. Achieving adequate margins of excision, and ultimately local control, does not simply involve awaiting a measurement on a pathology report. Rather, it requires careful operative planning, precise operative technique, appropriate handling of the specimen, intraoperative evaluation of the margins, coordinated pathologic processing, an understanding of the implications of histologic margin findings, and multidisciplinary planning of adjuvant therapies.

OPERATIVE PLANNING

High-quality management of breast cancer margins begins with the surgeon's appreciation of the lesion's location and configuration within the intact breast. One must have good breast imaging that demonstrates the extent of disease. For most patients with ductal carcinoma in situ (DCIS), mammography is adequate for planning purposes, whereas for most patients with invasive breast cancer, mammography and ultrasonography are adequate for planning purposes.

The use of magnetic resonance imaging (MRI) of the breast has been shown in a prospective randomized trial to *not* decrease the rates of inadequate margins or the rates of ipsilateral breast tumor recurrence. Therefore adjunctive imaging techniques such as MRI as well as contrast-enhanced mammography, molecular breast imaging, or positron emission mammography are not routinely indicated in planning breast surgery. Indications for MRI and/or these other adjunct imaging modalities include the need to trouble-shoot complex conventional imaging, a mammographically occult primary tumor with lymph node metastasis, extensive or multifocal disease that is not well appreciated on conventional imaging, Paget's disease of the nipple with no additional primary lesion demonstrated on conventional imaging, and invasive lobular carcinoma that is difficult to define on conventional imaging.

Patient selection for breast-conserving surgery (BCS) is another important influence on margin management. The more aggressive the surgeon and patient are in attempting to achieve breast conservation with extensive or multifocal disease, the more likely are inadequate margins of excision. There is no fixed cut-off for the size of a lesion at which BCS is no longer feasible. The surgeon must consider the ratio of breast tissue that would be removed to breast tissue that would be preserved and therefore the expected cosmetic outcome. LR rates are known to be higher when BCS is performed in patients with DCIS larger than 4 cm, so BCS should be done in such cases only with a well-informed patient who is motivated to achieve breast conservation despite this higher risk. BCS for multifocal disease likewise should be used for patients who are motivated to achieve breast conservation and in whom the disease can be removed in a single specimen with a reasonable cosmetic result. Oncoplastic techniques such as combined reduction mammoplasty with BCS can facilitate such resections with adequate margins and a good cosmetic outcome.

■ EXCISION TECHNIQUE

For BCS, the technique of lesion localization can have a major influence on the rates of achieving adequate margins of excision. Traditionally, lumpectomies for palpable tumors have been performed with palpation guidance, and lumpectomies for nonpalpable tumors have been performed with wire localization. Some trials have demonstrated lower rates of reoperation for inadequate margins when ultrasound guidance is used as an adjunct for lumpectomies

of palpable tumors. Some trials have demonstrated lower rates of reoperation for inadequate margins using alternatives to wire localization such as radioactive seed localization (RSL), hematoma-directed ultrasound-guided (HUG) localization, and radioguided occult lesion localization (ROLL). Each surgeon should know his or her rate of inadequate margins of excision and be engaged in continuous quality improvement, which may include the institution of one or more of these techniques.

For patients with large (i.e., >3 cm) nonpalpable lesions, especially DCIS or invasive tumors with an extensive in situ component, bracketing localization devices may facilitate complete excision (Figure 1). In such cases, the surgeon should request that localization wires or radioactive seeds be placed at two or more edges of the lesion. Typically it is more important to localize the radial margins, so the medial to lateral extent, the superior to inferior extent, or both should be delineated by the localization devices. This facilitates both the surgeon's dissection around the entire lesion and the radiologist's and surgeon's perception of the lesion within the specimen radiograph. Close communication between the surgeon and localizing radiologist is always important but particularly so when performing such bracketing.

The surgeon should review the preoperative and, if applicable, localization imaging contemporaneously with the operation to assure a clear understanding of the position of the targeted disease and position(s) of the localization device(s). These images should be on display in the operating room throughout the procedure to allow reference to them as needed.

The position of and type of incision should take into account the distance from the lesion to the skin. For superficial lesions in thin women undergoing BCS, it may be best to excise an ellipse of skin overlying the lesion to assure an adequate anterior margin. For similar patients and lesions in whom a skin-sparing or nipple-sparing mastectomy is being performed, an ellipse of skin likewise may need to be resected overlying the tumor. A frozen section or imprint cytologic analysis of such margins may be performed before the decision to resect the skin ellipse if such an excision will compromise the cosmetic result. Once the incision is made, it is important that the surgeon maintain smooth, consistent margins of dissection. This

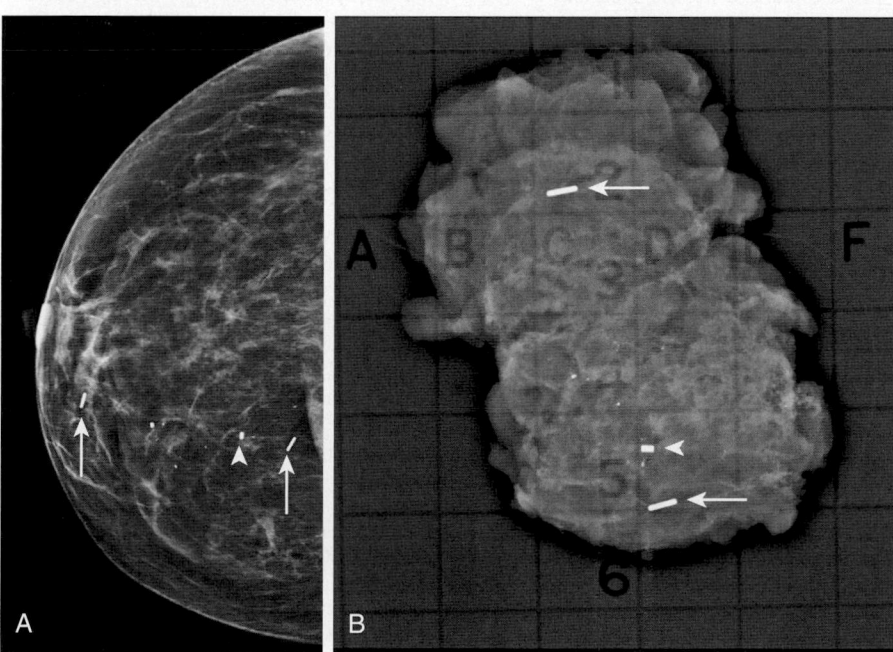

FIGURE 1 A, Localization mammogram demonstrating bracketing radioactive seeds (*arrows*) around an area of extensive ductal carcinoma in situ with biopsy clip (*arrowhead*). **B,** Specimen radiograph after oncoplastic resection demonstrating bracketing radioactive seeds (*arrows*) around an area of extensive ductal carcinoma in situ with biopsy clip (*arrowhead*).

avoids creating crevices in the surface of the breast specimen into which ink may run when applied to the margins. Such migration of ink may confuse the pathologic assessment of the margin status.

The surgeon must maintain a consistent distance from the margin of dissection to the carcinoma. In mastectomies this is achieved by carefully following the plane between the subcutaneous fat and the breast tissue (except in instances of superficial tumor near the subcutaneous fat), whereas in BCS this is achieved by maintaining orientation to the position of the tumor. Such orientation is maintained by ongoing palpation of the tumor, frequent assessment with intraoperative ultrasound of the distance from the plane of dissection to the tumor, frequent assessment with a gamma probe of the distance from the plane of dissection to the tumor with RSL by the gamma counts detected, or maintaining a three-dimensional mental image of the position of the lesion in relationship to the wire in the case of wire localization. If a tumor approaches the underlying pectoralis or other muscular fascia, the surgeon should not hesitate to include a portion of the underlying musculature to assure an adequate posterior margin. If the surgeon recognizes that a portion of the dissection was close to the tumor, that site on both the specimen side and the patient side should be marked with clips, sutures, or ink. Such marking facilitates accurate assessment of the margin by the pathologist and precise re-excision of the margin if it is found to be inadequate. This is especially valuable during mastectomies for extensive disease where it is more difficult to assess the position of a close or positive margin within the operative cavity.

In multiple studies, including prospective randomized trials, the use of cavity shave margins in BCS (excising an additional 3 to 10 mm of breast tissue at each of the margins of excision) has been associated with lower rates of inadequate margins. Although the use of shave margins by definition results in the removal of more breast tissue than occurs with a conventional lumpectomy, it allows accurate assessment of which margins are and are not negative and lowers the rates of positive margins. Again, each surgeon must know his or her rate of inadequate margins and perform continuous quality improvement; therefore if this rate is not already low from the use of other techniques, the addition of shave margins should be considered. This may be particularly valuable where intraoperative pathology is unavailable or for patients with DCIS or extensive in situ components where the rates of positive margins are elevated and a gross assessment of margins is more difficult. Among patients who have residual disease found at re-excision for inadequate margins, nearly three quarters have only DCIS remaining.

HANDLING OF THE BREAST SPECIMEN

The specimen must be oriented by the surgeon, and the institution must maintain a consistent protocol so that the orientation is well understood by all clinicians and pathologists. Six ink colors for each of the six margins should be applied to the specimen by the surgeon or via guidance from the surgeon in the form of suture markings, clips, or direct show-and-tell. If additional margins are excised intraoperatively as a result of assessing one or more margins to be inadequate or because of routine shave margin excision, the "new" or true margin must be marked clearly and inked. Likewise, mastectomy specimens should have all margins marked with ink. We prefer to use six ink colors, as with BCS specimens, whereas others use one color throughout or two colors for anterior and posterior. Again, a consistent institutional protocol well understood by all is important. In addition, the surgeon should mark the nipple and subareolar site of a nipple-sparing mastectomy specimen to aid pathologic assessment and to allow the measurement from the nipple site to the position of the lesion and any potential close margins. This can facilitate identifying the site of a positive mastectomy margin to facilitate re-excision if it is deemed necessary.

A specimen radiograph should be obtained during BCS when a localization device has been placed. Orthogonal views may facilitate margin assessment. There is no clear evidence that specimen radiography improves the rate of adequate margins of excision, but the surgeon and/or breast imager should nonetheless assess the relationship of the lesion or calcifications to the margins of excision on each specimen radiograph obtained. Compression of the specimen for specimen radiograph should be avoided, as it is unnecessary for adequate imaging and can distort the margins.

■ PATHOLOGIC PROCESS

Intraoperative pathologic margin assessment is associated with lower rates of reoperation for inadequate margins of excision. Any margins considered close or positive can be re-excised without the need for a second operation. This requires close coordination of the surgical, breast imaging, and pathology teams and may not be feasible in all practice settings. Such assessment can be as simple as gross evaluation of a sectioned specimen after inking. Frozen section analysis and imprint cytology also have been shown to reduce the rate of second operations for inadequate margins.

Sectioning the specimen perpendicular to the margins allows for the most accurate measurement of the distance from tumor to inked margin, whereas shaving or peeling the inked surface allows for a broader portion of the margin to be evaluated per section. Peeled margins may overestimate the rate of positive margins if shaved too thickly. We prefer perpendicular sectioning, but neither method has been proven superior to the other.

■ WHEN TO PERFORM RE-EXCISION OF MARGINS

The decision to re-excise breast margins for close or positive margins of excision should balance the risk of residual disease and LR with the morbidity, cosmetic effect, and cost of re-excision. Such decisions are best made by a multidisciplinary team, preferably one including more than just the treating team members themselves. Adjuvant therapy decisions must integrate with margin re-excision decisions rather than making each decision in isolation. For example, a surgeon avoiding a re-excision to maintain cosmesis may cause the addition of a radiation boost dose that could do as much or more to worsen the cosmetic outcome. Multidisciplinary group review of final margin status improves consistency through accountability and helps to take into account not just a single data point (margin width) but also the patient and tumor characteristics, the planned adjuvant therapies, and the imaging findings from preoperative and intraoperative studies. See Table 1 for a summary of recommended criteria for margin width thresholds for re-excision.

Breast-Conserving Surgery for Invasive Cancer

A consensus statement from the Society of Surgical Oncology and American Society for Radiation Oncology, endorsed by the American Society of Clinical Oncology, states that for patients with stage I or stage II breast cancer undergoing whole breast radiation, a margin criterion of no ink on tumor "is associated with low rates of IBTR [ipsilateral breast tumor recurrence] and has the potential to decrease re-excision rates, improve cosmetic outcomes, and decrease health care costs." In the meta-analysis on which the statement was based, the odds ratio (OR) for LR was 2.44 for positive versus negative margins and 1.74 for close versus negative margins. LR was not associated with margin distance when the analysis was limited to those studies using a criterion of 1 mm, 2 mm, or 5 mm or more for an adequate margin. The assessment of margin widths used for this analysis is an oversimplification because the studies did not report margin distance by increments, simply as positive or negative with a given threshold definition. Thus a study with a 2-mm threshold for "negative" margins may have had many patients in the negative category who had margins larger than 5 mm, and other studies with a threshold of no ink on tumor may have had a similar number of patients with margins larger than 5 mm. Therefore detecting a

TABLE 1: Summary Recommendations for Margin Re-excision

Disease Type	Routine Re-excision	Multidisciplinary Review	No Re-excision
BCS for invasive cancer	Positive margin ("ink on tumor")	Negative but <2-mm margins	≥2-mm margins
BCS for DCIS	<2-mm margins	Patients foregoing adjuvant RT	≥2-mm margins
Mastectomy for invasive cancer	Positive margin ("ink on tumor")	–	Negative margins
Mastectomy for DCIS	Positive margin ("ink on tumor")	–	Negative margins

BCS, Breast-conserving surgery; *DCIS,* ductal carcinoma in situ; *RT,* radiation therapy.

difference based on measured margin threshold would be extremely difficult in such a meta-analysis. The guidelines panel chose to ignore the increased LR risk with "close" margins because it couldn't be quantified, but this may be a more reliable indicator of margin width effect than measured margin distance because of the factors discussed earlier. For these reasons, we recommend that patients with positive margins (ink on tumor) routinely undergo re-excision of margins, that those with negative but close (<2 mm) margins undergo multidisciplinary assessment and counseling but *not* routine re-excision, and that those with margins larger than 2 mm not undergo re-excision except in unusual circumstances identified by the multidisciplinary team. For patients with stage III or stage IV breast cancer, similar thresholds are appropriate. For patients not undergoing whole breast radiation, multidisciplinary management decisions are warranted for each patient's unique plan.

Breast-Conserving Surgery for Ductal Carcinoma in Situ

There is currently no specific guideline for defining adequate or ideal margins for patients with DCIS. National Comprehensive Cancer Network guidelines state that for patients undergoing adjuvant radiation therapy (RT) a margin less than 1 mm from DCIS is inadequate and that any margin from 1 to 10 mm is controversial. One meta-analysis of those undergoing adjuvant RT has reported a standard margin of 2 mm or more to have superior LR rates for DCIS as compared with no ink on tumor with no advantage to wider margins. Another meta-analysis reported superiority of a threshold of 10 mm or more.

Patients and clinicians both often desire to avoid RT for DCIS, and therefore the potential advantage of wide margins of excision for DCIS reducing the need for adjuvant radiation has been studied widely. Prospective trials have consistently demonstrated lower LR rates with adjuvant RT, even with margins 10 mm or larger as the threshold. However, LR risks can be reasonable without adjuvant radiation: patients in Intergroup E5194 trial Group 1 with margins of 3 mm or more and low-grade to intermediate-grade DCIS of less than 2.5 cm had a 5-year LR rate of 6%.

We currently recommend that patients with DCIS with margins of less than 2 mm routinely undergo re-excision of margins. For patients not undergoing whole breast radiation, multidisciplinary management decisions are warranted for each patient's unique plan, but well-informed, motivated patients who meet E5194 criteria or other reasonable thresholds, such as those based on the Van Nuys criteria, may be offered the option of foregoing adjuvant RT. Re-excisions specifically to meet these thresholds are discouraged but may be used on a case-by-case basis.

Mastectomy Margins

There are also no guidelines for what constitutes an adequate margin of excision for patients undergoing mastectomies. Positive margins of excision have been associated with an increased recurrence risk among mastectomy patients, as has been the case for BCS patients. One must not, however, extrapolate the guidelines for BCS patients

undergoing adjuvant RT to mastectomy patients who usually do not undergo adjuvant RT. We recommend that patients with positive mastectomy margins (ink on tumor) routinely undergo re-excision of mastectomy margins if the site of the positive margin can be assessed based on a combination of preoperative imaging, specimen inking, measurement of the distance from the nipple or nipple and subareolar site, and marking of close margin sites intraoperatively. An exception to this is a positive posterior margin for DCIS, in which case there is no risk of invasion into the underlying musculature and should be no risk of residual breast tissue. Adjuvant RT should be used only for positive mastectomy margins if the site cannot be identified and re-excised using these tools. Patients with close but negative mastectomy margins usually do not require re-excision unless an unusual concern is identified on multidisciplinary review.

Other Margin Issues

Lobular carcinoma in situ (LCIS), atypical ductal hyperplasia, and atypical lobular hyperplasia are not of significance at or near margins. These entities are not associated with LR rate. The significance of pleomorphic LCIS at or near a margin has yet to be defined, as this may be a precursor lesion akin to DCIS. We currently favor re-excision to negative margins for pleomorphic LCIS when doing so does not produce substantial morbidity.

■ RE-EXCISION TECHNIQUES

Re-excision of inadequate margins is facilitated by viewing the gross examination of the specimen with the pathologist, so this should be done whenever feasible. If one must re-excise margins after having not seen the gross margin in question, and if the inking of margins was done by pathology personnel, consider overlapping the re-excision onto surrounding margin(s) to account for some mismatch where one margin borders another. This is especially true of anterior and posterior margins in relation to the radial margins because of gravity effects on the ex vivo specimen when inking. If a mastectomy margin is to be re-excised, the location of the margin must be identified through a combination of measuring the distance from the nipple site or nipple on the gross specimen, any margin sites marked at the initial dissection, the preoperative imaging, and the ink color of the positive margin.

When re-excising a margin, an additional 0.5 to 1 cm of tissue is usually appropriate. For an anterior margin, one may have to excise a portion of skin if little subcutaneous tissue remains. Each re-excised margin must be submitted separately for pathologic analysis, with the "new" margin clearly identified.

■ EXPECTED OUTCOMES

Recent reports of LR risk are much better than those in the historical randomized trials conducted in the 1980s. This is because of improvements through all phases of care: imaging, patient selection, surgical technique and margin management, pathologic processing, biologic understanding of tumor types, adjuvant systemic therapies, and radiation techniques. Margin management is only important insofar as it influences LR risk and/or survival. Each institution and clinician should engage in continuous quality improvement by ongoing study of one's rate of inadequate margins, rate of reoperation for margins, rate of altering adjuvant RT because of margin findings, and rate of 5-year LR.

SUGGESTED READINGS

Dunne C, et al. Effect of margin status on local recurrence after breast conservation and radiation therapy for ductal carcinoma in situ. *J Clin Oncol.* 2009;27:1615-1620.

Garvey EM, et al. Rates of residual disease with close but negative margins in breast cancer surgery. *Breast.* 2015;24:413-417.

Houssami N, et al. The association of surgical margins and local recurrence in women with early-stage invasive breast cancer treated with breast-conserving therapy: a meta-analysis. *Ann Surg Oncol.* 2014;21:717-730.

Hughes LL, et al. Local excision alone without irradiation for ductal carcinoma in situ of the breast: a trial of the Eastern Cooperative Oncology Group. *J Clin Oncol.* 2009;27:5319-5324.

Moran MS, et al. Society of Surgical Oncology–American Society for Radiation Oncology consensus guideline on margins for breast-conserving surgery with whole-breast irradiation in stages I and II invasive breast cancer. *Ann Surg Oncol.* 2014;21:704-716.

INTRAOPERATIVE RADIATION FOR BREAST CANCER

Courtney A. Vito, MD, and Melvin Silverstein, MD

Surgical therapy for the cure of breast cancer has been a mainstay of treatment, even predating the Halsted radical mastectomy popularized in the late nineteenth and early twentieth centuries. However, less invasive surgical procedures are preferred now. The National Surgical Adjuvant Breast and Bowel Project (NSABP) B-06 trial validated breast conservation as the preferred approach to early-stage breast cancers. Breast conservation is a multiple modality treatment encompassing surgical extirpation of the tumor with negative margins followed by whole breast irradiation. With this approach, a woman is able to achieve equivalent overall survival compared with treatment via mastectomy and minimize long-term morbidity. However, there is implied acceptance of a small increased risk of local recurrence. Further research has shown that the risk of local recurrence varies based on host and tumor characteristics, and some studies have called into question the need for full course, whole breast irradiation when favorable host and tumor characteristics exists. One such method to limit morbidity and inconvenience associated with whole breast irradiation is delivery of a single dose of irradiation to the tumor bed intraoperatively with a combined team of surgeons and radiation oncologists. Intraoperative radiation therapy (IORT) is a relatively young, novel procedure gaining traction to treat small breast cancer in appropriately selected candidates.

■ REVIEW OF EXISTING LITERATURE

Two recent large randomized controlled studies explored single-dose IORT as a component of breast conservation. The ELIOT Trial, published by Veronesi and colleagues in *Lancet Oncology* in 2013, included 1305 patients with early-stage breast cancer, randomized to whole breast irradiation or single-dose IORT after quadrantectomy. Inclusion criteria included female sex, age range of 48 to 75 years, and a unifocal tumor less than 2.5 cm on preoperative imaging. IORT was delivered via intraoperative electron radiotherapy via linear accelerator, delivering a 21 Gy fraction as previously published in multiple case series from the European Institute of Oncology in Milan, Italy. The groups were well matched, with the majority of patients in each group 60 years of age or older, with node-negative, estrogen receptor/progesterone receptor–positive, invasive ductal tumors that were well or moderately differentiated. The majority of patients on study received endocrine treatment alone. However, the inclusion criteria did not eliminate higher-risk women with aggressive subtypes of breast cancer, T2 tumors up to 2.5 cm, and node-positive women. Despite the aggressive inclusion criteria, statistically

there was no difference observed between the groups in overall survival and breast cancer–specific survival. However, the rate of local-regional recurrence was significantly worse in the IORT group (5.4%) compared with the whole breast irradiation group (0.8%) ($P < 0.0001$). Silverstein and colleagues reviewed the recurrence data and found that the majority of recurrences occurred in a small subset of higher-risk patients, with a greater than 10% local-regional recurrence rate in those with tumors larger than 2 cm, with four or more nodes involved with tumor, who were estrogen receptor (ER)–negative, and with poorly differentiated tumors. Removing these patients from the cohort likely would have shown IORT recurrence rates closer to those seen with patients receiving traditional whole breast irradiation.

The second trial (TARGIT) by Vaidya and colleagues was published initially in *The Lancet* in 2010 and updated in 2014. This was a large, international, multicenter, randomized controlled clinical trial that initially accrued 2232 patients. It was designed as a noninferiority trial with an allowable margin of up to a 2.5% greater local recurrence in the IORT treatment group compared with controls treated with whole breast irradiation. Two schemas for enrollment existed. The first schema enrolled patients age 45 years or older with unifocal invasive ductal carcinoma suitable for lumpectomy. Patients then were randomized to receive whole breast irradiation or IORT at 20 Gy tumor bed dosing via Intrabeam (Carl Zeiss Meditec, Oberkochen, Germany) after enrollment. Final pathology then was examined. Patients with positive margins were relegated to re-excision plus whole breast irradiation, eliminating boost doses. Patients found to have either extensive intraductal component (EIC) or lobular tumors on final pathologic testing but who had adequate resection also were relegated to whole breast irradiation. Further, each center was allowed to agree on any other adverse pathologic features (e.g., nodal involvement, poorly differentiated grading) that would allow reflexing to whole breast irradiation, but this was not standardized among centers. The second schema enrolled patients "postpathology," whereby the patient underwent lumpectomy and, after final pathologic testing confirmed good candidacy for IORT, was taken back to the operating room (OR) for a second procedure to reopen the lumpectomy cavity and deliver the IORT. The groups were well matched, with the majority of patients age 55 years or older, with node-negative, low- to intermediate-grade, ER-positive, *HER2/neu*-negative invasive ductal tumors that were 2 cm or smaller. The majority of patients received antihormonal therapy alone.

At the initial report, there was no statistical difference between overall survival or local-regional recurrence. As data have matured, the authors continue to report results and accrue additional patients. The overall survival is actually superior in the IORT group, but there has been an increasing number of local-regional recurrences. Regardless, the IORT cohort in total has not breached the 2.5% noninferiority benchmark originally set by the authors. Subset analysis reveals only one group, those in the postpathology arm whose IORT was applied at a second surgery after lumpectomy, to have breached the 2.5% noninferiority standard. The authors caution against using

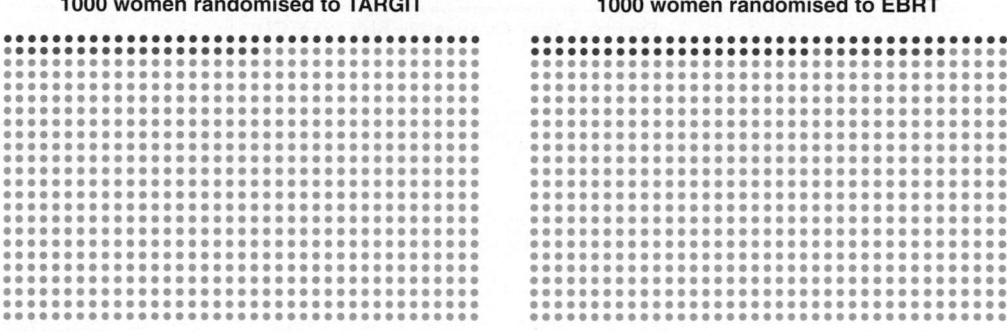

WHAT HAPPENED TO WOMEN WITH EARLY BREAST CANCER,
TREATED WITH TARGIT DURING LUMPECTOMY COMPARED WITH THOSE TREATED WITH EBRT,
OVER THE FIRST 5 YEARS?

1000 women randomised to TARGIT

1000 women randomised to EBRT

1 dot = 1 woman

There was no statistically significant difference in survival without local recurrence

- 939 women alive without local recurrence
- 20 women alive after treatment of local recurrence
- 1 woman died after local recurrence
- 40 women died

- 925 women alive without local recurrence
- 10 women alive after treatment of local recurrence
- 1 woman died after local recurrence
- 64 women died

FIGURE 1 Pictogram to help patients and doctors make a shared, well-informed decision. *(From Vaidya JS, et al. Pride, prejudice, or science: attitudes towards the results of the TARGIT-A trial of targeted intraoperative radiation therapy for breast cancer. Int J Radiat Oncol Biol Phys. 2015;92:491-497.)*

this strategy but continue to endorse IORT in conjunction with lumpectomy as noninferior to whole breast irradiation, noting that events in both groups remain very low (Figure 1). In 2014 Vaidya and colleagues published an updated TARGIT-A cohort with risk-adapted strategy. A total of 3451 patients were randomized to receive either IORT or whole breast irradiation. For those in the IORT arm, if adverse criteria, including margins 1 mm or less, lobular cancer, or extensive intraductal component, were seen on final pathologic testing, the addition of whole breast irradiation was mandatory. Centers also were allowed to add breast irradiation on a case by case basis for other adverse criteria such as nodal involvement, margins less than 1 cm, and extensive lymphovascular invasion. Postpathology enrollment still was permitted, though all postpathology IORT recipients required additional whole breast radiotherapy. With this individualized approach, the authors reported an overall 2% increase in local recurrence with IORT versus whole breast irradiation, not breaching the previously set 2.5% inferiority benchmark. Also seen are similar wound complication rates in the two groups but statistically fewer grades 3 and 4 skin toxicities from radiation in the IORT group. Again, the IORT group had fewer deaths because of fewer cardiovascular events and events from other cancers (Table 1).

■ PATIENT SELECTION AND PRECAUTIONS

As noted previously, patient selection and eligibility criteria were broad and unrefined initially within both the TARGIT-A and ELIOT trials, and certain subgroups have seen unacceptably high rates of local recurrence after lumpectomy and IORT. Appropriate patient selection is critical to the success of IORT. Vaidya and colleagues reported that patients who underwent lumpectomy as an initial operation and then, after confirming negative margins on final pathologic testing, underwent a second operation to apply radiation to the lumpectomy cavity had unacceptably higher rates of recurrence compared with those who underwent lumpectomy with concomitant IORT. In 2009 the American Society of Therapeutic Radiology and Oncology (ASTRO) set forth consensus guidelines for patient eligibility to undergo any form of accelerated partial breast irradiation (APBI). This applies not only to IORT but also

to other brachytherapy techniques such as interstitial radiation, balloon-based brachytherapy, and external beam three-dimensional (3D) conformal radiation. The consensus guidelines break down patients as suitable, cautionary, and unsuitable (Table 2). The ideal or suitable candidate is older, with a small, unifocal, ER-positive, node-negative invasive ductal tumor without lymphovascular invasion or EIC and negative margins of 2 mm or more. Herein lies the importance of preoperative patient selection. The ELIOT trial incorporated 26% with positive nodes and 44% with age younger than 60 years, making a large portion of the study population considered cautionary or unsuitable candidates for IORT per ASTRO guidelines. The TARGIT-A trial has similar selection bias issues, as only 32% of patients would have been considered suitable per ASTRO guidelines, with the remaining subjects considered cautionary (27%) or unsuitable (41%). This distinction should be addressed clearly when discussing data with patients as they make informed decisions regarding IORT.

Imaging

When evaluating a patient's candidacy for IORT, the clinician must review all imaging, including mammograms, ultrasounds, and (if available) breast magnetic resonance imaging (MRI). Pertinent considerations on mammogram include any associated calcifications. Extensive surrounding calcifications may indicate EIC and, if not resected, may lead to positive margins on final pathologic testing. If the span is greater than 3 cm, a biopsy of these calcifications may elucidate candidacy. The planned resection should include all suspicious or involved calcifications with a span no greater than 3 cm. On ultrasound, one should carefully review for any satellite lesions and confirm the size of the index tumor. Also, one should consider distance from the tumor to skin to ensure adequate tissue to resect an anterior margin of 2 mm or more plus have room for a 1-cm bridge of tissue from the lumpectomy cavity to the skin. In cases where the skin bridge is close but inadequate, intraoperative techniques discussed later still may allow successful placement of the device, and thus this preoperative criterion is not absolute. Finally, ultrasound evaluation of the axillary nodal basin may help to identify those candidates with axillary metastases not palpable on clinical

TABLE 1: Results of Primary (Local Recurrence in the Conserved Breast), Secondary (Death), and Exploratory (Any Other Recurrence) Outcomes for All Patients and the Two Strata as Per Timing of Randomization and Delivery of TARGIT

| | Events; 5-Year Cumulative Risk (95% CI) | | |
	TARGIT	EBRT	Absolute Difference*
ALL PATIENTS			
Local recurrence (n = 3375)	23; 3.3% (2.1-5.1)	11; 1.3% (0.7-2.5)	12 (2.0%)
Any other recurrence (n = 3375)	46; 4.9% (3.5-6.9)	37; 4.4% (3.0-6.4)	9 (0.5%)
Death (n = 3451)	37; 3.9% (2.7-5.8)	51; 5.3% (3.9-7.3)	−14 (−1.4%)
PREPATHOLOGY†			
Local recurrence (n = 2234)	10; 2.1% (1.1-4.2)	6; 1.1% (0.5-2.5)	4 (1.0%)
Any other recurrence (n = 2234)	29; 4.8% (3.1-7.3)	25; 4.7% (3.0-7.4)	4 (0.1%)
Death (n = 2298)	29; 4.6% (1.8-6.0)	42; 6.9% (4.3-9.6)	−13 (−2.3%)
POSTPATHOLOGY‡			
Local recurrence (n = 1141)	13; 5.4% (3.0-9.7)	5; 1.7% (0.6-4.9)	8 (3.7%)
Any other recurrence (n = 1141)	17; 5.2% (3.0-8.8)	12; 3.7% (1.9-7.0)	5 (1.5%)
Death (n = 1153)	8; 2.8% (1.3-5.9)	9; 2.3% (1.0-5.2)	−1 (0.5%)

From Vaidya JS, et al. Risk-adapted targeted intraoperative radiotherapy versus whole-breast radiotherapy for breast cancer: 5-year results for local control and overall survival from the TARGIT-A randomized trial. *Lancet.* 2014;383:603-613.

*In Kaplan-Meier point estimate at 5 years (TARGIT minus EBRT).

†TARGIT given at same time as lumpectomy.

‡TARGIT given after lumpectomy, as separate procedure.

CI, Confidence interval; *EBRT*, external beam radiotherapy; *TARGIT*, targeted intraoperative radiotherapy.

TABLE 2: ASTRO Guidelines (2009) for Candidates Suitable to Receive Accelerated Partial Breast Irradiation After Lumpectomy

	Suitable	Cautionary	Unsuitable
Definition	Off clinical trial	Limited data	On trial only
Age	≥60 years	50-60 years	<50 years
Tumor size	≤2 cm	2-3 cm	>3 cm or inflammatory
Nodes	Negative	—	Positive or not yet evaluated
Histology	IDCA	ILCA, DCIS	—
Margins	>2 mm	≤2 mm	Positive
Path features	No EIC nor LVI	EIC or focal LVI	Extensive LVI
Grade	Any	—	—
Multicentricity	Clinically unifocal	—	Any multifocality or centricity
ER status	Positive	Negative	—
Neoadjuvant therapy	None	—	If any used
BRCA status	Negative	—	Positive or suspected

ASTRO, American Society of Therapeutic Radiology and Oncology; *DCIS*, ductal carcinoma in situ; *EIC*, extensive intraductal component; *ER*, estrogen receptor; *IDCA*, International Classification of Disease Adapted; *ILCA*, International Lactation Consultant Association; *LVI*, lymphovascular invasion.

examination. The decision to perform a biopsy on an axillary node is dependent on patient and clinician desires. If a suspicious node is found, the patient should be informed fully of the implications of biopsy.

■ EQUIPMENT

Previous attempts at IORT were hampered by the need for either intraoperative patient transport from the OR to a radiation suite or cost- and staff-prohibitive machines installed in the OR with extensive shielding similar to a radiation vault. Currently three devices that are commercially available in the United States can be used to deliver IORT to the breast without such extensive measures. Each device delivers radiation in a different manner.

The Mobetron, developed in 1997 by IntraOp Medical Corporation, is a large but portable, self-shielded linear accelerator that delivers radiation via electrons. Electron beam radiation is most similar to radiation delivered via external beam, has the most precise tissue targeting, and requires the shortest treatment time compared with other IORT machines. The Mobetron is also the most costly of all IORT machines available. It is available at a limited number of sites in the United States, mainly tertiary referral centers. It has broad intraoperative application for use not only in breast cancer but also in many other types of cancers within the abdominal cavity and the pelvis as well as sarcomas and head and neck cancers. One drawback is the size of the cylindrical applicators used to dock the machine to the lumpectomy cavity. The radiation must be delivered to the lumpectomy cavity from directly above it. There is very limited opportunity to tunnel the device, and thus the surgical approach can be limited to a larger incision immediately over or very near the lumpectomy cavity (Figures 2 and 3).

The Intrabeam by Zeiss is an IORT machine that delivers low-energy x-ray radiation emitted by a gold source. The gold source is introduced via a rigid applicator shaped like a cone with a sphere at its tip. The sphere houses the gold source during treatment and is embedded into the breast tissue. Because of the size and shape of the applicators, smaller incisions can be utilized, but often tunneling is difficult or impossible, thus necessitating an incision over the tumor bed as opposed to a more cosmetic approach. The machine is portable and does not require room shielding. It is smaller and less costly than the Mobetron (Figures 4 to 6).

The Xoft Axxent Electronic Brachytherapy (eBx) System by Xoft, a subsidiary of iCAD, Inc., is an IORT machine that delivers low-energy, high-dose radiation via an x-ray source (Figure 7) introduced into the breast via a balloon applicator (Figures 8 and 9). The main advantage to this delivery system is that the balloon catheter can be tunneled through the breast, allowing the surgeon to use a

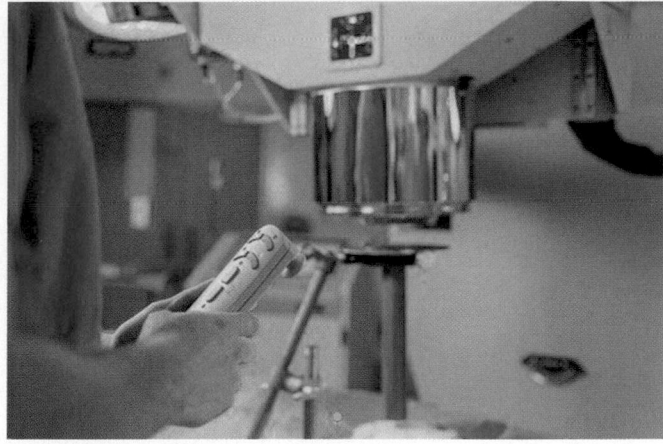

FIGURE 3 The Mobetron docking onto the cylindrical applicator in the breast. *(Courtesy IntraOp Medical Corporation.)*

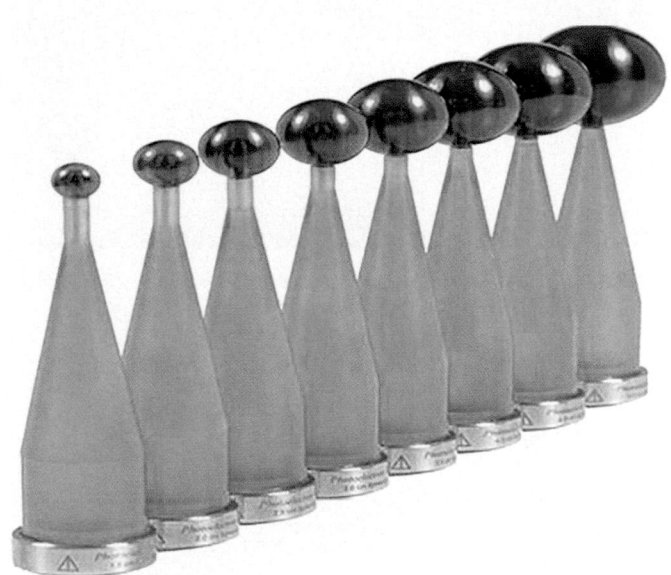

FIGURE 4 Intrabeam (Carl Zeiss Meditec) intraoperative radiation therapy applicators.

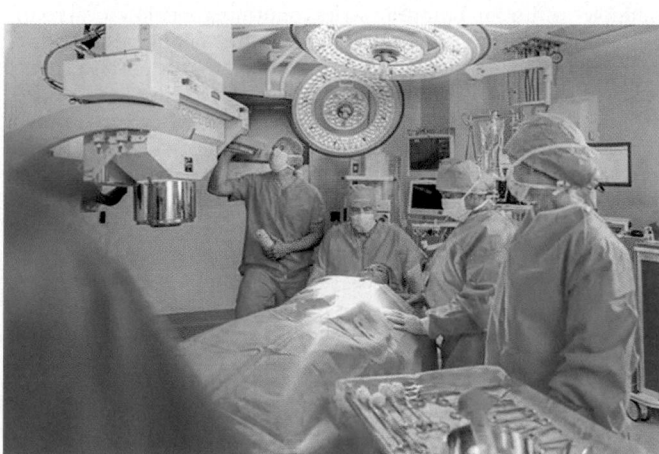

FIGURE 2 The Mobetron in the operating room as the patient is prepared for surgery. *(Courtesy IntraOp Medical Corporation.)*

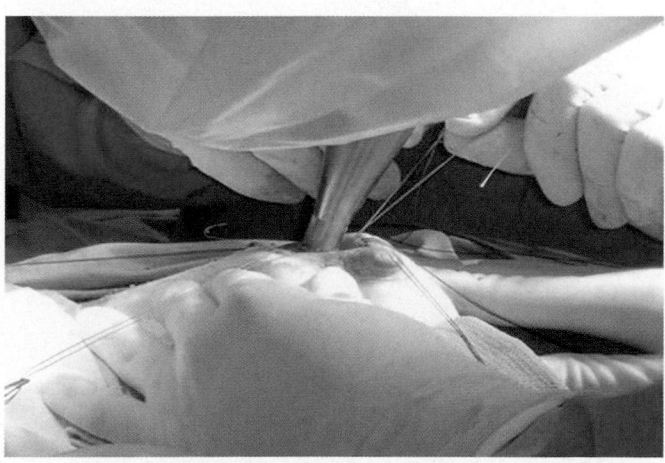

FIGURE 5 Intrabeam applicator surgically placed within the breast.

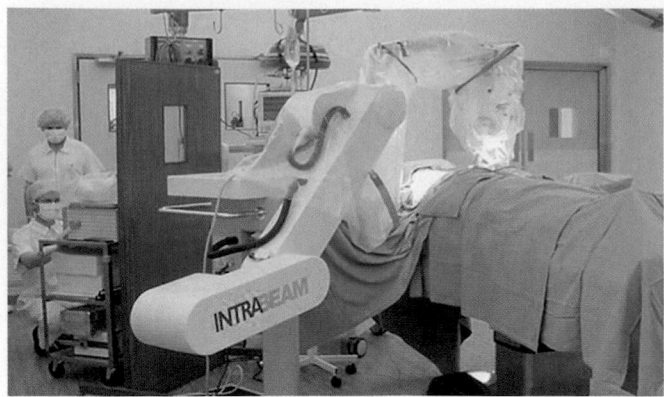

FIGURE 6 Intraoperative delivery of radiation with the Intrabeam machine. *(Courtesy Melvin Silverstein.)*

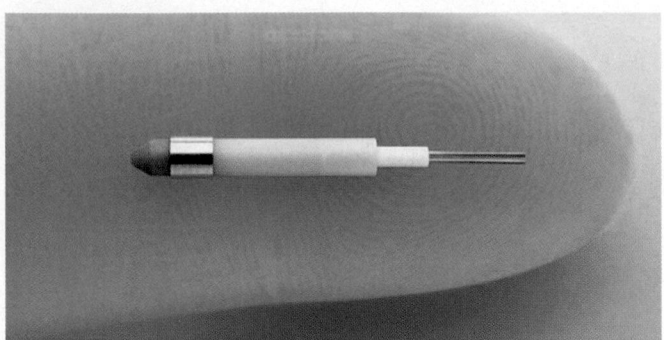

FIGURE 7 X-ray generator source for the Xoft system. *(Courtesy Xoft, a subsidiary of iCAD, Inc.)*

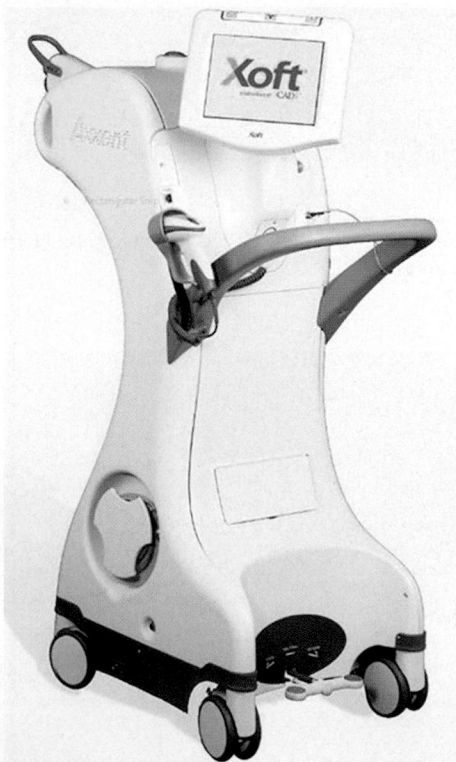

FIGURE 8 The Xoft system. *(Courtesy Xoft, a subsidiary of iCAD, Inc.)*

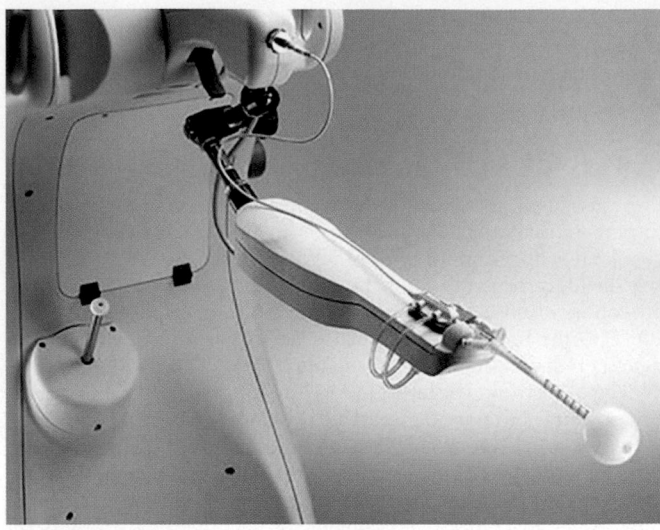

FIGURE 9 Balloon applicator loaded on the Xoft system. *(Courtesy Xoft, a subsidiary of iCAD, Inc.)*

much wider range of approaches to the lumpectomy. The applicator is often inserted through a stab incision separate from the lumpectomy incision. Like the other machines, the Xoft System does not require a shielded OR. It is the smallest and least costly of the three machines. However, the disposable costs are higher for the balloon applicators, whereas the other delivery systems used reusable applicators. Also, unlike the other delivery systems, the Xoft System has not yet been validated in a randomized, controlled clinical trial.

■ INTRAOPERATIVE TECHNIQUES

Regardless of the device being used, the primary goal of the operation should be extirpation of the tumor with negative margins and retrieval of sentinel lymph nodes. Margins should be assessed intraoperatively with at least specimen radiography to ensure adequate tumor removal as well as removal of all suspicious calcifications and a normal-appearing rim of tissue. Consideration should be given to further assessment such as rapid gross assessment by the pathology team. Attainment of negative margins is crucially important, as failure to do so, seen on final pathologic testing, commits the patient to a second operation and many treatment teams then will recommend the addition of whole breast radiation, counting the IORT dose as the boost dose alone. Although this is the frequent fallback position, IORT as a boost dose has never been validated in a prospective randomized clinical trial (although there are many good single- and multiple-institution European series confirming very low local recurrence rates for IORT as a boost) and is the focus of ongoing investigation. Sentinel node biopsy with frozen section analysis also should be performed. IORT has been found to be less effective in those with positive sentinel nodes, and thus it is not the preferred treatment modality. Intraoperatively positive sentinel nodes should be treated as a contraindication to IORT unless IORT is performed on trial as a planned boost dose. However, the patient remains eligible under ACOSOG Z0011 criteria to avoid axillary dissection if fewer than three sentinel nodes are positive; thus a positive intraoperative node should lead to abortion of IORT plans but not to immediate reflection to axillary dissection.

Once negative margins and sentinel nodes are assured, the last intraoperative criterion is appropriate placement of an applicator for IORT. In cases of full-thickness resection from skin to chest wall, shielding should be placed on the floor of the lumpectomy bed to protect underlying structures such as ribs, lung, and heart from IORT. Shielding is available in multiple sizes. The appropriate size of shielding should be chosen based on lumpectomy bed dimensions. The breast, ideally with fascia, then can be mobilized off of the

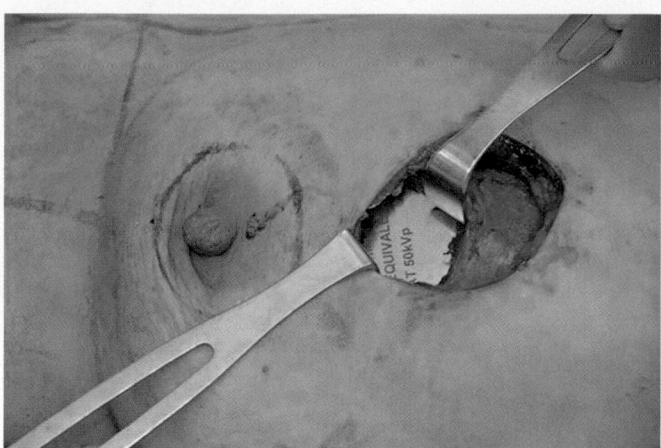

FIGURE 10 Chest wall shield in place below the pectoralis major muscle. *(Courtesy Melvin Silverstein.)*

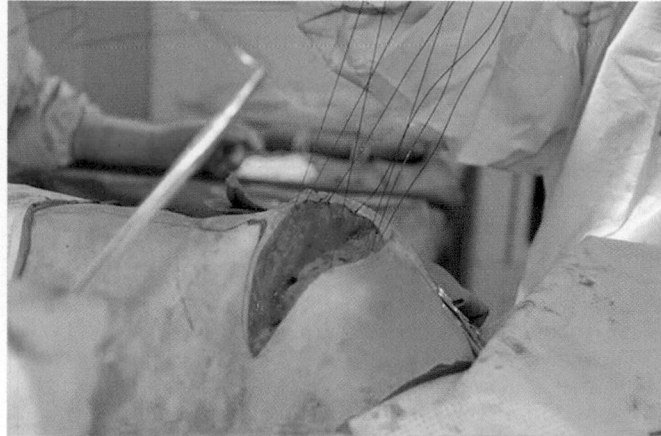

FIGURE 11 Retention sutures used to reapproximate the breast tissue around the intraoperative radiation therapy applicator. *(Courtesy Melvin Silverstein.)*

pectoralis major muscle and reapproximated over the shield if desired, but this is not required. Alternatively, the shielding can be placed below the pectoralis major. In cases where the resection is not taken down to the pectoralis major, ultrasound should be used to ascertain the distance from the lumpectomy cavity to the chest wall. If sufficient tissue exists, as the treatment field encompasses only tissue 1 cm from the lumpectomy cavity, shielding may be omitted depending on the comfort level of the treating radiation oncologist and surgeon. If the tissue thickness is not sufficient to protect the chest wall, the tissue should be divided and a pocket should be created beneath the fascia or pectoralis major to house the chest wall shielding (Figure 10).

From here, intraoperative technique varies based on the equipment used. For the Mobetron machine, the diameter of the cavity is measured and the appropriate-size cylindrical applicator or collimator for docking is chosen. The glandular breast tissue is mobilized both off of the pectoralis major muscle and from the overlying skin. A Lucite chest wall shield is placed, and the gland is reapproximated with a purse-string suture. The applicator then is placed through the incision. Tissue at the base of the applicator will receive the radiation (similar to how a flashlight would light the field directly at the targeted base of its beam). Appropriate tissue targeting is confirmed either by direct visualization if possible or with a laparoscope inserted through the applicator. Via laser guidance, the linear accelerator is docked and treatment commences.

Unlike the Mobetron, the Zeiss Intrabeam and the Xoft systems require temporary implantation of a delivery catheter. The Intrabeam delivers electron radiation from a gold source through a rigid applicator with a spherical tip. The Xoft system's high–dose rate (HDR) x-ray source is introduced through a balloon applicator. In both cases, the spherical portion of the applicators is buried within the glandular tissue of the breast. Sutures are used to reapproximate the parenchyma around the applicators. This can be done with internal purse-string sutures or external retention sutures (Figure 11). In addition to ensuring that all tissue margins are appropriately situated around the applicator, the surgeon also must ensure good tissue conformance without air pocketing around the applicator and a distance 1 cm or greater at all points from the applicator to the skin. Both conformance and skin bridge thickness must be confirmed after applicator placement via intraoperative ultrasound. Many surgeons express concern about achieving the 1-cm skin bridge, especially in superficial tumors. Several techniques exist to assist with this. In cases where at least a few millimeters of tissue exist, tumescence with injectable saline can be used to thicken the tissue and achieve a 1-cm margin. In cases where this is not possible, the skin can be mobilized off of the breast tissue and reflected back with stay stitches away from the applicator (Figure 12). Alternatively, a moist 4 × 4 gauze can be

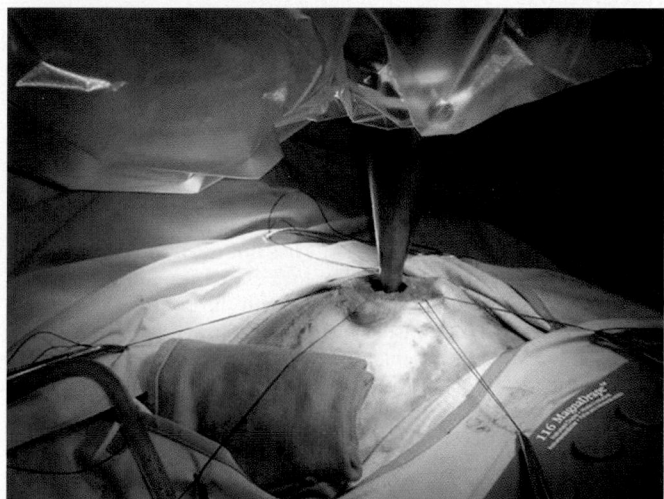

FIGURE 12 Intrabeam applicator in the breast, with skin edges everted to avoid the radiation field. *(Courtesy Dennis Holmes.)*

packed between the skin and the anterior margin of the gland to move the skin out of the radiation field. Finally, if all of these techniques fail, the surgeon can consider excising skin and using an oncoplastic closure. Nonetheless, a tumor situated less than 1 cm from the skin at diagnosis should not be considered an absolute contraindication to the use of IORT.

▪ UNIQUE ADVANTAGES

Toxicity

In almost every instance, confirmed by ELIOT and TARGIT trial data, skin toxicity is significantly less with IORT versus whole breast irradiation. Further, IORT offers lower rates of pulmonary fibrosis. At the last update of the TARGIT trial, it was noted that the IORT arm had fewer deaths related to coronary artery disease. This relationship has been hypothesized to suggest that perhaps IORT is safer than whole breast irradiation, which can accelerate coronary atherosclerosis. In essence, collateral damage is minimized. This frequently is one of the most appealing features of IORT for patients.

Convenience

IORT offers a host of unique advantages over traditional whole breast irradiation. The most obvious benefit to the patient is convenience.

Whereas whole breast irradiation can require as many as 30 to 35 daily, consecutive visits to a radiation center lasting one and a half months, intraoperative radiation is completed at the time of operation and, barring any unexpected complications, does not extend a patient's recovery period compared with lumpectomy alone. This may well factor into a patient's decision when choosing between lumpectomy and mastectomy for early-stage breast cancer, with the former being the least morbid and medically advisable choice. It is known that barriers to accessing radiation, such as time commitment and distance to a radiation center, increase the likelihood that a woman will choose to sacrifice her breast despite being a candidate for breast conservation. Because we now have more women than ever in the workforce and with the delay of retirement beyond the age of 65 years, there are more breast cancer survivors in active treatment with less flexible schedules than ever before. If IORT allows a patient to choose breast conservation over mastectomy, with or without reconstruction, the patient is spared the potential higher morbidity of a more aggressive surgical procedure with mastectomy and without the gains of increasing her overall survival.

Recurrence

Although it is known based on experiences from both the TARGIT-A and the ELIOT trials that there is a small increase in local recurrence with IORT, the absolute difference between the IORT and whole breast irradiation groups is small. However, treatment of the recurrence may vary widely. Whereas the standard of care for a patient who received whole breast irradiation in the past is to undergo mastectomy and not receive any further irradiation to her breast, the standard of care after lumpectomy and IORT failure remains debatable. The majority of the breast tissue has not received radiation after IORT, and thus if the site of recurrence allows for full resection of the previous lumpectomy cavity along with the 1-cm rim of treated tissue, it is feasible to consider resection followed by whole breast irradiation. Although a viable option, this technique would be considered outside the realm of traditional treatment and should be offered only when the patient is fully aware of the risks, the surgeon feels that adequate cosmetic and oncologic outcomes can be attained, and the radiation oncologist feels confident about the treatment planning and avoidance of excess radiation to the tissues.

Cosmesis

Cosmetic outcome is often a leading concern for patients when choosing a surgical approach to breast cancer treatment. Whole breast irradiation can lead to permanent thickening and darkening of the skin. Wound contracture also can worsen, deforming the contour of the breast. Intraoperative radiation offers distinct advantages in this regard. The skin should be at least 1 cm from the device and thus outside of the treatment field. Therefore with appropriate surgical technique and applicator placement, the skin ideally should not be prone to cosmetic changes. It is rare to see induration or color change in the skin when IORT is administered appropriately.

In regard to contour deformity, IORT offers surgeons the unique opportunity to close the lumpectomy cavity and rearrange tissue as necessary to reshape the gland after the completion of radiation treatment. This is a clear advantage over other types of breast brachytherapy where catheters are removed percutaneously in the office after several days of treatment. When the catheter is removed in an office setting without opening the cavity, this can lead to unaddressed, radiated dead space and then to cavity collapse or chronic seroma formation. These two problems can be minimized with IORT if the cavity is closed after the applicator is removed but before the skin is closed at the end of the case. In this capacity, IORT is uniquely appealing in the case of oncoplasty, not only from the cosmetic standpoint of closing the cavity but also oncologically to ensure appropriate tissue targeting. In cases where oncoplastic approaches are planned, the oncologic surgeon can remove the tumor, and IORT then can be applied directly to the lumpectomy cavity. Once the radiation treatment is complete, the cosmetic surgeon can rearrange the tissue via local flaps or more advanced plastic surgery techniques such as reduction mammoplasty. With these techniques, the original lumpectomy cavity will be obliterated and rearranged, which creates difficulties in planning external beam radiation boost dosing. IORT allows for direct targeting of the tissue at the site of the tumor.

Another common concern related to radiation and cosmesis of the breast is seen in the case of a woman with pre-existing breast implants. Many centers will not radiate a breast with an implant in place because of risks related to capsular contracture and poor cosmesis. This damage is often difficult for the plastic surgeon to correct without autologous flap. IORT offers the advantage of minimal risk for capsular contracture because such a small amount of tissue is targeted for therapy. In these cases it can be difficult to place the applicator with an implant in place. The best approach is combined with the oncologic surgeon performing lumpectomy first. The implant then is removed, relaxing the glandular tissue and facilitating applicator placement. The IORT dose is delivered, and the plastic surgeon then can replace the implant.

■ COMPLICATIONS AND PITFALLS

Intraoperative Abortion

Intraoperatively a patient should achieve (1) negative margins with intraoperative assessment of at least specimen radiograph, (2) negative sentinel lymph nodes, and (3) appropriate placement of the radiation applicator. If any of these criteria cannot be met, IORT should not proceed. Many patients who choose IORT do so for very specific reasons, wishing to avoid whole breast irradiation. There can be significant disappointment when a patient awakens to learn that she could not receive IORT safely and then is committed to whole breast irradiation. Therefore rigorous preoperative evaluation of the breast and axilla are imperative to minimize intraoperative failures.

Chronic Seroma

Chronic seroma is the most widely reported complication of IORT. It can be minimized by reapproximating the cavity at the time of surgery, but this is not a complete safeguard. Chronic seroma can lead to distortion of the breast, tenderness, and palpable abnormality, which may cause the patient distress and impair physical examination. It also can obscure mammography. Seromas can be managed by serial aspiration as needed for symptom control. If the mammogram is sufficiently obscured, augmentation of screening with ultrasound should be considered.

Positive Margins Postoperatively

An unexpected positive margin on final pathologic testing can be the most disappointing outcome of IORT. Positive margins require re-excision in a radiated field that inherently has increased risks of infection and poor wound healing. Furthermore, patients should be considered for a course of whole breast irradiation with the IORT taking the place of the boost doses. In cases where margins are less than 2 mm but negative, re-excision and whole breast irradiation must be considered on a case by case basis. Whole breast irradiation after IORT carries significant risks of poor cosmesis and fibrosis of the breast, more so than IORT or whole breast irradiation alone. The shorter the time interval from IORT to whole breast irradiation, the worse the complications will be. Waiting at least 6 weeks from IORT to initiation of whole breast irradiation is advisable.

■ BOOST DOSING

The use of IORT to provide a boost dose of radiation followed by whole breast irradiation is a topic of ongoing investigation. The TARGIT-B trial, using the Intrabeam device to deliver a planned boost dose of radiation followed by whole breast irradiation, is already underway. A similar trial is under development by a group of investigators using the Xoft system. The patient inclusion criteria in both trials are much wider and include patients with less favorable host and tumor characteristics. As of now, this approach is considered experimental only.

■ CONCLUSIONS

Single-dose IORT as a modality to complete breast conservation is a relatively immature technique that lacks robust, long-term follow-up in clinical trials. Nonetheless, the current literature indicates that when used in a highly selective manner for appropriately chosen patients, this technique offers distinct advantages over whole breast irradiation. A successful treatment program relies heavily on a coordinated, multidisciplinary team that includes breast radiologists to help identify appropriate candidates correctly, both preoperatively and intraoperatively; pathologists to intraoperatively assess margin and nodal status quickly and accurately; surgeons to select patients preoperatively after rigorous assessment, to perform adequate surgical resection, and to place the device of choice safely; and radiation oncologists to, along with surgical colleagues, identify appropriate patients preoperatively and deliver the radiation in conjunction with the surgery. Each patient receiving IORT requires close, long-term follow-up by a coordinated, multidisciplinary breast cancer treatment team to survey for local recurrence. Because this is an emerging technology, giving strong consideration to performing this technique within the bounds of a clinical trial is most prudent.

SUGGESTED READINGS

Fisher ER, Anderson S, Redmond C, Fisher B. Ipsilateral breast tumor recurrence and survival following lumpectomy and irradiation: pathological findings from NSABP protocol B-06. *Semin Surg Oncol.* 1992;8:161-166.

Silverstein MJ, Fastner G, Maluta S, Reitsamer R, Goer DA, Vicini F, Wazer D. Intraoperative radiation therapy: a critical analysis of the ELIOT and TARGIT trials. Part 1—ELIOT. *Ann Surg Oncol.* 2014;21:3787-3792.

Smith BD, Arthur DW, Buchholz TA, Haffty BG, Hahn CA, Hardenbergh PH, Julian TA, Marks LB, Todor DA, Vicini FA, Whelan TJ, White J, Wo JY, Harris JR. Accelerated partial breast irradiation consensus statement from the American Society for Radiation Oncology (ASTRO). *Int J Radiat Oncol Biol Phys.* 2009;74:987-1001.

Vaidya JS, et al. Targeted intraoperative radiotherapy versus whole breast radiotherapy for breast cancer (TARGIT-A trial): an international, prospective, randomised, non-inferiority phase 3 trial. *Lancet.* 2010;376: 91-102.

Vaidya JS, et al. Risk-adapted targeted intraoperative radiotherapy versus whole-breast radiotherapy for breast cancer: 5-year results for local control and overall survival from the TARGIT-A randomised trial. *Lancet.* 2014;383:603-613.

Vaidya JS, Bulsara M, Wenz F, Joseph D, Saunders C, Massarut S, Flyger H, Eiermann W, Alvarado M, Esserman L, Falzon M, Brew-Graves C, Potyka I, Tobias J, Baum M. Pride, prejudice, or science: attitudes towards the results of the TARGIT-A trial of targeted intraoperative radiation therapy for breast cancer. *Int J Radiat Oncol Biol Phys.* 2015;92:491-497.

Veronesi U, et al. Intraoperative radiotherapy versus external radiotherapy for early breast cancer (ELIOT): a randomized controlled equivalence trial. *Lancet Oncol.* 2013;14:1269-1277.

BREAST RECONSTRUCTION AFTER BREAST CANCER TREATMENT: GOALS, OPTIONS, AND REASONING

Mark S. Burke, MD, FACS, and Dennis K. Schimpf, MD, FACS

According to the American Cancer Society, the United States alone will see nearly 250,000 new diagnoses of invasive breast cancer and 60,000 diagnoses of carcinoma in situ, resulting in more than 40,000 deaths, in 2016. Treatment for this disease typically includes surgery and also may require radiation or chemotherapy (or both). In addition to their function in childrearing, in many cultures breasts have a significant social and sexual role. Some women may see their breasts as part of their identity and what makes them a woman. Although the loss of milk production after mastectomy cannot be replaced with current breast reconstructive techniques, improvement in psychosocial and sexual satisfaction, resulting in a better quality of life after breast reconstruction, is a reasonable and reliably achievable goal.

■ SURGICAL OPTIONS FOR BREAST CANCER

Mastectomy

Mastectomy involves the removal of nearly all breast tissue while preserving varying amounts of the skin envelope. Skin-sparing mastectomy preserves a larger amount of breast skin relative to standard mastectomy, with an elliptical incision made around the nipple. The preservation of a larger amount of healthy skin aids in subsequent reconstruction. Nipple-sparing mastectomy preserves the entire skin envelope as well as the nipple and is gaining popularity in the United States. Mastectomy is performed in less than 40% of early stage breast cancers in the United States and in even less than that number in other industrialized nations around the world. Mastectomy is the standard of care for recurrent, multifocal, and larger or more advanced cancers. Patients who are diagnosed with breast cancer during pregnancy, those who do not wish to undergo radiation, those who do not wish to undergo the follow-up necessary for breast conservation treatment, and *BRCA*-positive patients may opt for mastectomy as primary surgical treatment.

Breast Conservation (Lumpectomy) With Radiation

This technique involves removal of the tumor with a small margin of normal breast tissue, typically followed by whole or partial breast radiation. This technique is chosen more than 60% of the time by patients with stages I and II breast cancers. Lumpectomy with radiation peaked in popularity in the 1990s and 2000s after the National Cancer Institute declared this method "preferable" to mastectomy for early stage breast cancers. Advantages include preservation of the majority of the native breast with associated sensation and potential for eventual resumption of milk production on the affected side. Disadvantages include the nearly universal requirement for radiation and a recurrence risk of approximately 0.5% per year, requiring close follow-up (a 40-year-old woman who could expect to live another 40 years after treatment would have a 20% recurrence risk). Some patients who undergo this treatment method still develop post-treatment breast defects that they may be unhappy with. Severity of post-treatment deformity depends in part on the tumor size and location, breast size, and type of radiation used (whole breast radiation vs partial breast radiation with either high-dose radiation utilizing a balloon catheter or intraoperative intralesional radiation).

Oncoplastic Resection

This method refers to the blending of oncologic resection with plastic surgical breast resection techniques. This allows for a breast-conserving approach to the resection of breast cancer in cases where standard lumpectomy likely would create an unsatisfactory defect. The goal of this method is to remove the tumor using skin and parenchyma resection patterns that allow for adequate surgical margins (and in some cases better margins than with standard lumpectomy) around the cancer, while at the same time leaving an aesthetically pleasing breast volume and contour after resection. Disadvantages include the combined need for plastic surgical and oncologic expertise to plan and execute the operation. In addition, as with standard lumpectomy, the majority of these patients still will require adjuvant radiation.

■ RECONSTRUCTIVE CONSIDERATIONS

Smoking

Patients who are active smokers clearly have much higher rates of complications after breast reconstruction, and the results can be disastrous. Most complications involve wound infections, delayed wound healing, and necrosis if breast skin flaps or other skin flaps are raised for autologous tissue reconstructions. Patients should be encouraged to quit smoking for at least 4 weeks before and 4 weeks after reconstruction to reduce their risk of suffering smoking-related complications. Many surgeons refuse to perform reconstructions on patients who are unable or unwilling to quit smoking. If one chooses to perform a breast reconstruction on an active smoker, efforts to get her to quit and a thorough explanation of the increased risks associated with breast reconstruction in smokers should be documented carefully in the patient's chart.

Obesity

Patients with a body mass index (BMI) greater than 25 have been shown to have increased risk for postoperative complications after breast reconstruction as well as higher rates of reconstructive failure. These risks increase with increasing BMI. In morbidly obese patients (BMI >35) it is difficult to achieve a breast mound with adequate volume and definition, especially at the inframammary crease. This is especially true with implant-based reconstructions and results from the thick soft tissue of the chest wall and abdomen.

Postmastectomy Skin Flaps

The blood supply to the skin of the breast runs in the subdermal plexus and is bolstered segmentally by multiple perforators that traverse the breast tissue. During mastectomy these perforators are removed with the breast tissue, leaving the only blood supply to the skin flaps via the subdermal plexus. This remaining blood supply is tenuous, and the larger the amount of skin left after mastectomy, the more concerning the blood supply to the remaining skin becomes. The most worrisome situation would be a large breast on which a major skin-sparing or nipple-sparing mastectomy was performed. The ablative surgeon is faced with the task of performing an oncologically sound operation while preserving the subdermal plexus and minimizing trauma to the skin flaps to avoid tissue ischemia. Whereas problems with the native breast skin flaps can be compensated for when autologous tissue is being used for reconstruction, healthy skin flaps are vital to the success of a purely implant-based reconstruction. All complications regarding postmastectomy skin flaps are significantly higher in smokers.

■ BREAST RECONSTRUCTION

Reconstruction after surgery for breast cancer differs from the oncologic portion of patient care in many ways, not the least of which is the number of decisions a patient must make. When patients are diagnosed with breast cancer, they are staged and treatment recommendations are made regarding the cancer treatment. There are not many oncologic choices for a patient to make, and the patient is more or less swept along into the treatment regimen. The reconstructive part of breast cancer care is very different, with many choices needing to be made regarding both the timing and the method of reconstruction. The many options regarding reconstruction may be empowering for some women, giving them back part of the control they lost to their cancer. At the same time, having to make so many decisions regarding reconstruction may be frustrating to other women who agonize over these choices at such a stressful time in their lives. Patients may try to shift the burden of reconstructive decisions back to their reconstructive surgeon, stating that they "just want whatever reconstruction is best." To combat this, it is important to spend time explaining the reasonable options for reconstruction, the differences between them, and the potential complications from each in order to create an informed patient. All too often the options explained to a patient reflect the operations that a particular reconstructive surgeon is capable of doing or personally wishes to do, rather than a true explanation of all of the patient's options. A thoughtful and well-organized discussion of breast reconstruction with a patient, and ideally with the patient's loved ones, will allow her to understand that there is not one technique or method that is "best." However, when patients' goals for reconstruction, timing, tolerance for complications, and prior medical and surgical history are all taken into account, we can help them to discover not the "best" reconstruction but the "best reconstruction for them."

Reconstructive Timing Options

Timing of breast reconstruction can be either immediate (at the time of the mastectomy) or delayed (at some later date after mastectomy). Timing of reconstruction is an important consideration for both the patient and the physicians involved in her care. For the patient, this is a personal decision, and there can be a wide range of opinions on the matter. On one end of the spectrum, some patients complain that they "would die" if they woke up without breasts after mastectomy, and they cannot conceive of spending one day without a reconstruction. On the other end of the spectrum, some patients say that although they eventually would like to have a reconstruction, they cannot think about something that they perceive as so "trivial" as reconstruction while they are being treated for breast cancer and would like to wait until all of their therapy is complete.

Immediate Breast Reconstruction

Immediate breast reconstruction refers to performing (or starting) the reconstruction at the time of mastectomy. Immediate reconstruction provides a quicker route to completion of the reconstructive process, with fewer operations required. Disadvantages to immediate reconstruction include the need to coordinate two or more surgeons for the operation and a longer operative time. Care must be taken not to inappropriately delay the oncologic resection while trying to plan and coordinate a simultaneous reconstruction. Delays in scheduling can be especially problematic when a patient chooses autologous reconstruction, as these operations tend to be longer and may involve more than one reconstructive surgeon.

Delayed Breast Reconstruction

With delayed breast reconstruction the patient undergoes mastectomy and the skin is closed. This route has the advantages of greatest ease of scheduling, shortest operative times, and fewest postoperative complications. In addition, this method allows the patient to complete any additional therapy, especially radiation, which could cause an immediate reconstruction to be less than optimal. This may be the best option for patients who are unsure of what type of reconstruction they would like, those who are expected to require radiation, and those who continue to struggle with smoking cessation.

Immediate-Delayed Breast Reconstruction

This method involves placement of a tissue expander at the time of mastectomy, with plans to return to the operating room for autologous reconstruction either when it is certain that radiation will not be required or when radiation is completed.

■ RECONSTRUCTIVE TECHNIQUE OPTIONS

Implant-Based Reconstruction

Implant-based reconstruction uses silicone or saline implants to recreate the breast parenchyma, typically after first expanding the space with a tissue expander (two-stage reconstruction), but a straight-to-implant (one-stage) reconstruction is becoming more popular in selected patients (Figure 1).

Two-Stage Reconstruction

A two-stage implant-based reconstruction is by far the most common breast reconstruction performed in the United States after mastectomy. The first stage entails placement of a tissue expander. Tissue expanders come in a variety of shapes and sizes, but in general they consist of a shaped, silicone-shelled balloon with a magnetic access port designed for needle access and filling. The appropriate tissue expander size is chosen to fit the patient's breast footprint, and a submuscular pocket deep to the pectoralis major muscle is dissected to the dimensions of the breast footprint. The tissue expander is placed in the submuscular pocket, and the skin is closed. The surgeon may choose to start filling the expander just enough to minimize laxity in the breast space without placing undue stress on the breast skin flaps and suture lines. The reconstruction then is allowed to heal for several weeks before the start of expansion. Once adequate healing has been allowed, the expansion process begins. Expansion involves the patient coming in for weekly "fills" during which the injection port is identified beneath the skin and muscle (either by manual palpation or using a magnet), the port is accessed with a needle, and normally 30 to 75 mL of saline are injected into the implant. This

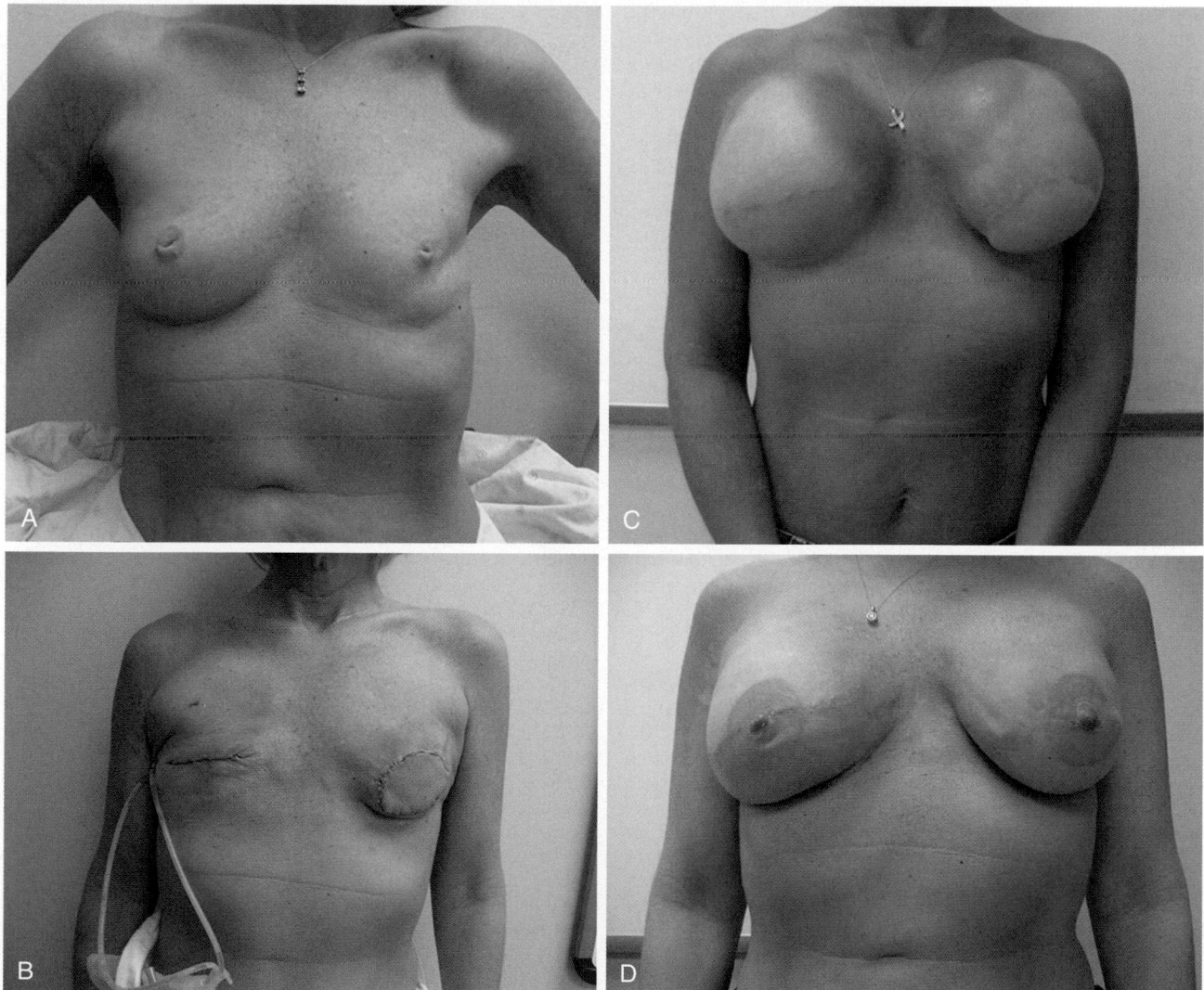

FIGURE 1 Immediate bilateral breast reconstruction with expander-implant technique, utilizing a latissimus myocutaneous flap on the left secondary to radiation to neoadjuvant radiation. **A,** Preoperative. **B,** Immediately postoperative after mastectomies, tissue expanders, and latissimus rotation. **C,** After expansion. **D,** After conversion to permanent implants and nipple reconstruction.

process typically takes 2 to 3 months to reach the desired volume, which is determined by both the desired final breast volume and the type of permanent implant to be used. The patient should be counseled during this process that as the tissue expanders are inflated, they will be high on the chest wall, very firm, and will not resemble a natural breast during this phase. After the completion of expansion, several months are allowed to elapse to create a better stretch of the tissues before returning the patient to surgery for expander to permanent implant exchange. At the time of exchange, a portion of the existing breast scar is reopened, the expander is removed, the permanent implant is positioned, and the skin is meticulously closed. Advantages of two-stage over one-stage reconstruction include less stress on fresh mastectomy skin flaps and suture lines and more control over the final size of the breast. Disadvantages compared with one-stage reconstruction include more discomfort postoperatively secondary to the submuscular dissection, frequent physician visits, prolongation of the reconstruction process, and the need for a second surgery to complete the reconstruction.

One-Stage Reconstruction

One-stage "straight-to-implant" breast reconstruction is gaining popularity in the United States. This method involves immediate placement of the permanent implant in the subcutaneous space (above the pectoralis major muscle) at the time of mastectomy (skin-sparing or nipple-sparing). This method of reconstruction may be appropriate in well-selected patients with minimal risk factors (non-smoking, nonradiated, nonobese patients) and healthy-appearing skin flaps after mastectomy. Advantages compared with its two-stage counterpart include less pain postoperatively because of the lack of submuscular dissection and a quicker completion of the reconstruction by avoiding need for tissue expansion and subsequent surgery for expander-implant exchange. Disadvantages include the absolute need for an adequate amount of healthy skin to cover the implant, more stress on the breast suture line from the weight of the implant, and less control over the final size and shape of the breast.

Types of Implants

Breast implants in use today break down into variations of either saline or silicone. Despite a moratorium on their use from 1992 to 2006 in the United States, silicone breast implants are considered safe for both breast reconstruction and cosmetic breast augmentation. Highly cohesive gel implants (third-generation silicone implants) have more extensively cross-linked silicone molecules, resulting in a thicker gel than the second-generation implants while still providing a soft feel. Very highly cohesive gel (fourth-generation or "gummy-bear") implants have an even thicker gel compared with the third generation, which allows for these to be available as anatomically shaped implants that can provide a more natural shape to the reconstructed breast, especially in thinner women.

Biologic Tissue Matrices

Biologic tissue matrix is commonly used to complete the submuscular tissue expander pocket, creating a "sling" from the infralateral pectoralis major edge to the chest wall at the desired location of the inframammary crease of the reconstructed breast. The most common tissue matrices used for this purpose are acellular dermal matrices, but silk-derived matrices are now available as well. The alternative method to this technique is to lift the ipsilateral serratus anterior muscle along with the pectoralis major muscle to complete the pocket for the tissue expander. Proponents of using tissue matrices to complete the pocket report more control over the pocket shape and a better ability to define the inframammary crease. Disadvantages to this technique include seroma formation, requiring placement of drains that may lead to increased infection complications.

Implant Advantages and Disadvantages

Standard two-stage implant reconstruction is a slower, more drawn-out process (often 6 months or more) from start to finish, involving shorter, lower-risk operations with frequent office visits during the expansion phase but little to no time admitted to the hospital. Whether this reconstructive course is an advantage or disadvantage depends on the patient's outlook, and this is why thorough discussion of the reconstructive process during preoperative consultation is so vital. Clear advantages to implant reconstruction include the lack of a donor site (which avoids a scar, pain, and potential complications at the donor site) and the potential for the patient to be included in decision making regarding the final volume of the reconstructed breast during the tissue expander fill process. Disadvantages of this method include the presence of a foreign body, which makes infection a major concern. If the implant becomes exposed or otherwise contaminated, rarely can it be salvaged with antibiotics alone. Minor, nonpurulent infections in some cases may be treated by operative removal of the prosthetic device, pocket washout, and placement of a new device in the same setting, although this method carries a high reinfection rate of 25%. Placement of a new device in a contaminated field should not be attempted with major infections or in the setting of purulence; in these cases all foreign material should be removed and another attempt at reconstruction planned weeks later. Additional disadvantages of implant reconstruction include the potential for complications requiring additional surgeries years after reconstruction for such problems as capsular contracture, implant rupture, or implant malposition.

Autologous Reconstruction

Autologous reconstruction refers to the use of the patient's own tissue to replace the resected breast parenchyma. By far the most common donor site for autologous breast reconstruction in the United States is the abdomen. There are multiple additional sites from which to obtain tissue for breast reconstruction, with the most commonly described being the upper trunk (latissimus flap), thigh (transverse upper gracilis flap), and gluteus (superior and inferior gluteal artery flaps).

Abdominal Donor Site

The abdomen is the most common donor site for autologous reconstruction of the breast. The most common operation utilizing the abdomen is the transverse rectus abdominis myocutaneous (TRAM) flap. This flap includes a transversely oriented section of skin and fat from the lower abdomen, which is left attached to the underlying rectus muscle, thereby preserving the vascular perforators of the inferior epigastric vessels that traverse the muscle and perfuse the flap. This tissue can be transferred as a "pedicled TRAM," where it is left attached via the superior epigastric vessels and simply rotated via a subcutaneous tunnel into the breast defect, never detaching the flap from its blood supply. Alternatively, it can be transferred as a "free TRAM," basing the flap on the inferior epigastric vessels, which are disconnected near their origin, and then transferring the flap to the breast pocket and anastomosing flap vessels to recipient vessels (typically either internal mammary or axillary vessel branches in the axilla), re-establishing a blood supply to the flap. Muscle-sparing TRAM flaps have been described, where a column of native rectus muscle is preserved while still including the majority of the rectus muscle and the associated vascular perforators with the flap. A further evolution of the TRAM flap known as the deep inferior epigastric artery perforator (DIEP) flap was popularized by Dr. Robert Allen and is our technique of choice for autologous breast reconstruction (Figures 2 and 3). This technique involves the same skin and fat harvest as the TRAM flap, but bases the blood supply off the inferior epigastric vessels without the removal or destruction of rectus muscle or fascia, carefully opening and preserving these structures and dissecting one or more perforators through them to the inferior epigastric vessels. This flap then is transferred as a free flap (as described for free TRAM). Advantages of the TRAM technique include a greater ease of harvest, faster operative times, and the potential to avoid the need for microvascular skills if a pedicled

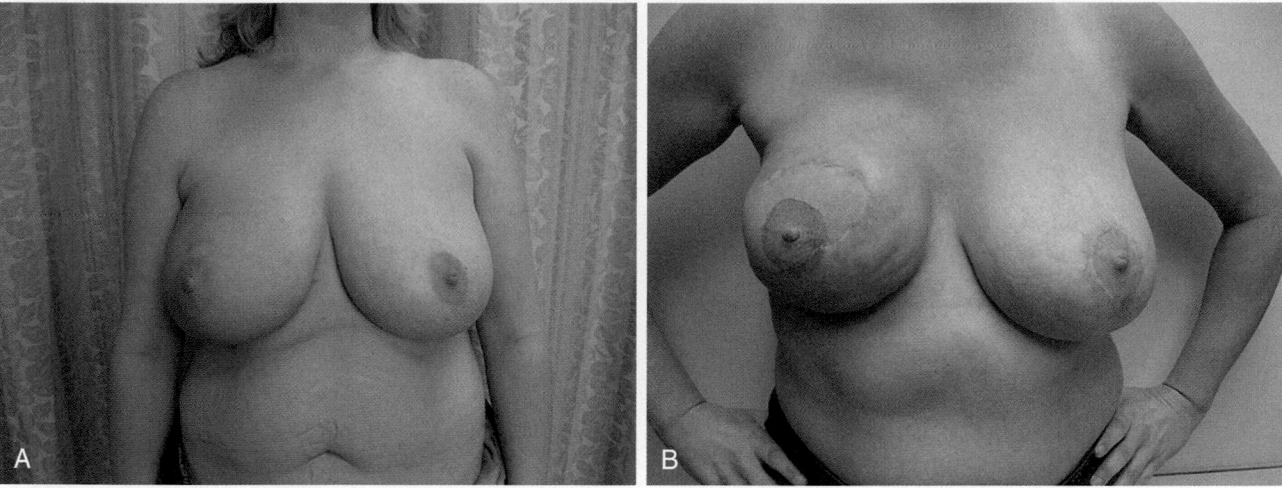

FIGURE 2 Unilateral immediate right breast reconstruction with a deep inferior epigastric artery perforator flap, followed by nipple reconstruction and left breast mastopexy. **A,** Preoperative. **B,** Postoperative.

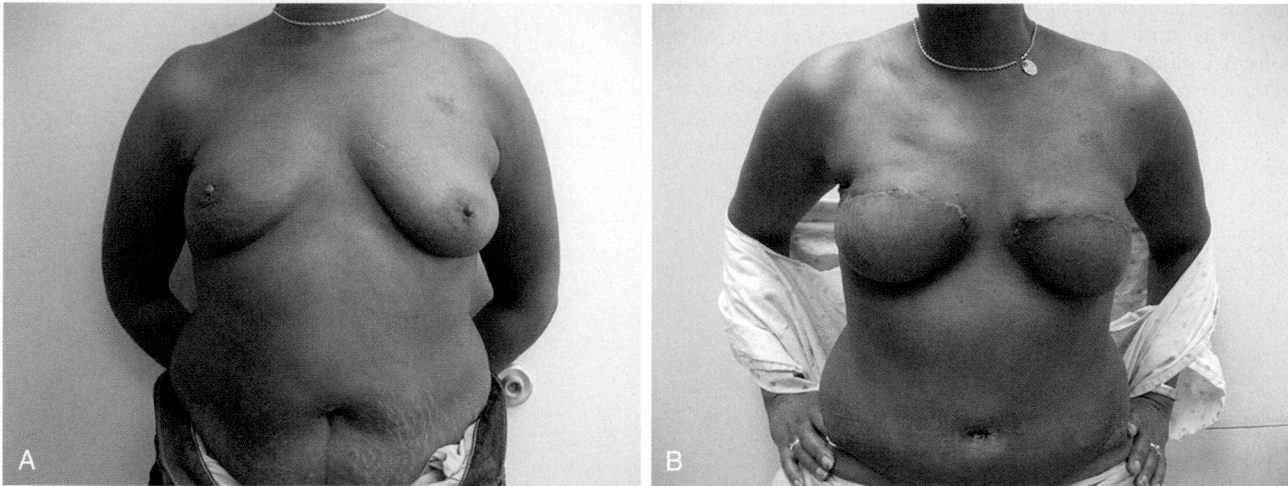

FIGURE 3 Bilateral delayed breast reconstruction utilizing deep inferior epigastric artery perforator flaps. **A,** Preoperative. **B,** Postoperative.

TRAM is utilized. Advantages of a DIEP flap include lower risk for abdominal wall weakness or abdominal "bulging" postoperatively and not needing mesh implantation to reconstruct the abdominal wall intraoperatively because no fascia is removed. In addition, in selected patients with adequate vessels, a similar lower abdominal flap can be harvested based on the superficial inferior epigastric artery (SIEA) flap. Advantages of this flap versus a TRAM or DIEP flap include the lack of any violation of the patient's fascia or muscle, resulting in greater ease of dissection for the surgeon; no risk for abdominal wall weakness or bulging; and less pain postoperatively. Disadvantages of the SIEA flap include the fact that there is a limited number of patients with adequate vessels to support this flap, resulting in higher failure rates.

Trunk Donor Site

The latissimus myocutaneous flap is a workhorse flap in breast reconstruction. This flap involves an ellipse of skin and fat from the back with the underlying latissimus dorsi muscle based on the thoracodorsal vessels that is harvested and "tunneled" in a subcutaneous plane through the axilla to the ipsilateral breast defect. This flap is almost always used as a "hybrid" reconstruction along with an implant because of a paucity of soft tissue available in this area. This flap is used commonly to provide additional coverage over implants in

patients who have or will undergo radiation treatment and as a salvage operation after complications from previous reconstruction attempts. Some surgeons use this flap routinely as part of implant reconstruction to provide a more natural feel and look over implants (Hammond flap). Advantages of this technique include ease of dissection, very high flap reliability, and lack of microsurgical anastomosis. The main disadvantage is the typical need for an implant to get adequate volume for a reconstructed breast. Also described is the thoracodorsal artery perforator (TDAP) flap utilizing only skin and fat from over the latissimus muscle, based on the dissection of a single perforator from the thoracodorsal vessels that is dissected through the latissimus muscle while sparing the entire muscle. This flap is more difficult to dissect and lacks the muscle that may be desired in some reconstructive scenarios.

Thigh Donor Site

The most common operation for breast reconstruction using the thigh is the transverse upper gracilis (TUG) flap. This technique utilizes the skin and fat of the upper medial thigh and harvests with it a section of the gracilis muscle, where the medial femoral circumflex vessel perforates it. This technique has the advantages of an inconspicuous donor site and relative ease of harvest. Disadvantages include the need for microsurgical skills and the relatively small amount of tissue available, allowing reconstruction of only a small breast without use of an implant or additional flap. Use of anterolateral thigh (ALT) perforator flap based on the lateral femoral circumflex vessels is less common but has been described for breast reconstruction.

Gluteal Donor Site

Superior gluteal artery perforator (SGAP) and inferior gluteal artery perforator (IGAP) flaps can be harvested for use in breast reconstruction and utilize skin and fat from the buttocks without sacrificing the underlying muscle. Advantages of these techniques include inconspicuous donor site location with minimal donor site morbidity. Disadvantages include difficulty of harvest and need for microsurgical ability, the ability to create only a small to moderate-sized breast, and the need to turn the patient prone intraoperatively for flap harvest.

Autologous Advantages and Disadvantages

The most prominent advantage of purely autologous breast reconstruction is the absence of a prosthetic device, which minimizes concerns of infectious complications. In addition, autologous tissue tends to feel and age more like a natural breast and even will gain and lose weight with the patient. Autologous tissue is much more compatible with previous or future radiation and provides a much shorter time from the beginning to the end of reconstruction. After the initial healing process, new problems with autologous flaps are rare, and in fact patient satisfaction tends to increase with time, minimizing the chance that revision procedures will be required years after initial reconstruction. Disadvantages for the patient include scarring, pain, and potential complications at the chosen donor site and longer hospital admission time. Disadvantages for the surgeon include longer operative times and more complicated operations with the possible need for microsurgical expertise.

SUGGESTED READINGS

Alderman A, Gutowski K, Ahuja A, Gray D. ASPS clinical practice guideline summary on breast reconstruction with expanders and implants. *Plast Reconstr Surg.* 2014;134:648e-655e.

Berry T, Brooks S, Sydow N, Djohan R, Nutter B, Lyons J, Dietz J. Complication rates of radiation of tissue expander and autologous tissue breast reconstruction. *Ann Surg Oncol.* 2010;17(suppl 3):202-210.

Haloua M, Krekel N, Winters H, Rietveld D, Meijer S, Bloemers F, van den Tol M. A systematic review of oncoplastic breast-conserving surgery: current weaknesses and future prospects. *Ann Surg.* 2013;257:609-620.

Jagsi R, Li Y, Morrow M, Janz N, Alderman A, Graff J, Hamilton A, Katz S, Hawley S. Patient-reported quality of life and satisfaction with cosmetic outcomes after breast conservation and mastectomy with and without reconstruction: results of a survey of breast cancer survivors. *Ann Surg.* 2015;261:1198-1206.

Kamali P, Koolen P, Paul MA, Medin C, Shermerhorn M, Lin SJ. Regional and national trends over 20 years in one-stage vs two-staged implant based breast reconstruction. *Plast Reconstr Surg.* 2015;136:122.

Rossi C, Mingozzi M, Curcio A, Buggi F, Folli S. Nipple areola complex sparing mastectomy. *Gland Surg.* 2015;4:528-540.

Sullivan SR, Fletcher DR, Isom CD, Isik FF. True incidence of all complications following immediate and delayed breast reconstruction. *Plast Reconstr Surg.* 2008;122:19-28.

Warren PA, Foster RD, Stover AC, et al. Outcomes after total skin-sparing mastectomy and immediate reconstruction in 657 breasts. *Ann Surg Oncol.* 2012;19:3402-3409.

ADRENAL INCIDENTALOMA

L. Michael Brunt, MD and Arghavan Salles, MD, PhD

Because of the widespread use of cross-sectional imaging in clinical practice, the most common adrenal lesion that surgeons are asked to evaluate today is the adrenal incidentaloma. Incidentally discovered adrenal lesions have been estimated to be found in anywhere from 1% to 5% of patients undergoing abdominal computed tomography (CT) for other reasons. This purported incidence has been challenged in an analysis of the incidence of adrenal incidentalomas in more than 3000 chest and abdominal CT scans performed over 2 years. In this study, adrenal incidentalomas were found on 0.98% of abdominal CTs and 0.81% of chest scans (Davenport et al). Most adrenal incidentalomas are clinically silent and nonfunctioning.

There are three steps that the surgeon should take when faced with an adrenal incidentaloma: (1) verify that the lesion is in the adrenal gland; (2) determine if the lesion is hypersecreting adrenal hormones; and (3) assess whether it is potentially malignant. If there is biochemical evidence of increased production of adrenal hormones or if the imaging characteristics are concerning for malignancy, then adrenalectomy is indicated. It is important for surgeons who evaluate patients with adrenal incidentalomas to understand the biochemical and diagnostic evaluation and to be familiar with the imaging characteristics of various benign and malignant adrenal lesions to properly select patients for adrenalectomy. For a detailed evidence-based review of this topic, the American Association of Clinical Endocrinologists and American Association of Endocrine Surgeons medical guidelines for the management of adrenal incidentalomas are recommended.

■ DIFFERENTIAL DIAGNOSIS

The differential diagnosis of adrenal incidentalomas is shown in Box 1. Broadly, these lesions can be categorized into three groups: functional benign, nonfunctional benign, and malignant. The most common functional benign lesions detected incidentally are pheochromocytomas and subclinical cortisol-producing tumors (subclinical Cushing's syndrome). Aldosteronomas are less likely to be seen as an incidentaloma because of their small size (less than 1 to 2 cm). The most common nonfunctional benign lesion is a cortical adenoma, which is by far the most common lesion encountered as an incidentaloma. Myelolipoma is the second most common nonfunctioning adrenal lesion (6% of cases in one series) and may be referred for surgical evaluation because of their larger size and concern for possible adrenal malignancy. Other benign lesions include adrenal cysts, hemorrhage, and ganglioneuromas.

Malignancies that may be seen as incidentalomas include primary adrenocortical carcinomas or metastatic disease from other primary tumors. Adrenocortical carcinomas are usually large tumors (>6 cm) that can be recognized by their imaging features and typically are associated with clinical symptoms. Adrenal metastases most commonly occur in the setting of other metastatic disease or a history of known primary malignancy. Patients also may have bilateral incidentalomas, which may be cortical adenomas or hyperplasia, bilateral pheochromocytomas, myelolipomas, metastases, lymphoma, or infection. Infection (e.g., tuberculosis) is an uncommon cause of incidentaloma in North America and often results in bilateral adrenal abnormalities. The following sections describe the management of the most common types of incidentalomas.

■ BENIGN FUNCTIONING ADRENAL LESIONS

Pheochromocytoma

Pheochromocytoma (pheos) always should be considered in the differential diagnosis of an adrenal incidentaloma. In recent years, up to 30% to 40% of all pheochromocytomas in reported series originally were detected as incidentalomas. Incidentally discovered pheochromocytomas may be completely silent clinically, although most patients have some degree of hypertension. For that reason, it is important to inquire about history of hypertension in every incidentaloma case. Specifically, the patient should be asked whether he or she has experienced any difficulty with hypertensive control medically or has any associated spell-like symptoms such as palpitations, headache, sweating, or anxiety. The risk of occurrence of a hypertensive crisis from operating on an undiagnosed pheochromocytoma mandates that every adrenal incidentaloma be screened for this possibility.

The simplest screening test to rule out pheochromocytoma is measurement of plasma fractionated metanephrines (metanephrines and normetanephrines). False-positive results, primarily with the normetanephrine component of the assay, can occur. If either the metanephrine or normetanephrine is elevated mildly, then further testing with 24-hour urine for catecholamines and metanephrines should be done to confirm or rule out this diagnosis. Pheochromocytomas also have a characteristic appearance on imaging. On CT they often appear heterogeneous and have higher attenuation values (Figure 1). They are typically relatively large tumors (greater than 3 to 4 cm). On magnetic resonance imaging (MRI) sequences, pheochromocytomas have a bright appearance on T2-weighted sequences.

Adrenalectomy is indicated for any patient with an incidentally discovered pheochromocytoma. Pharmacologic preparation for surgery should occur with an alpha-adrenergic receptor blocking with phenoxybenzamine. The goal is to control hypertension and tachycardia. Alternatively, some groups have used selective alpha-1 blocking agents and/or calcium channel blockers. Beta blockade should be reserved for patients who have predominantly epinephrine-secreting tumors or hypertension and/or tachycardia that persists after alpha blockade.

Subclinical Cushing's Syndrome

Subclinical Cushing's syndrome (SCS) refers to autonomous cortisol secretion in the absence of overt signs of Cushing's syndrome. In one

BOX 1: Differential Diagnosis for Adrenal Incidentaloma

Functional Tumors

Pheochromocytoma
Cortisol-producing adenoma/subclinical Cushing's syndrome
Aldosteronoma
Primary adrenal hyperplasia

Nonfunctional Lesions

Nonfunctioning cortical adenoma
Myelolipoma
Adrenal hemorrhage
Adrenal cyst
Ganglioneuroma

Malignant

Adrenocortical carcinoma
Metastases to the adrenal gland

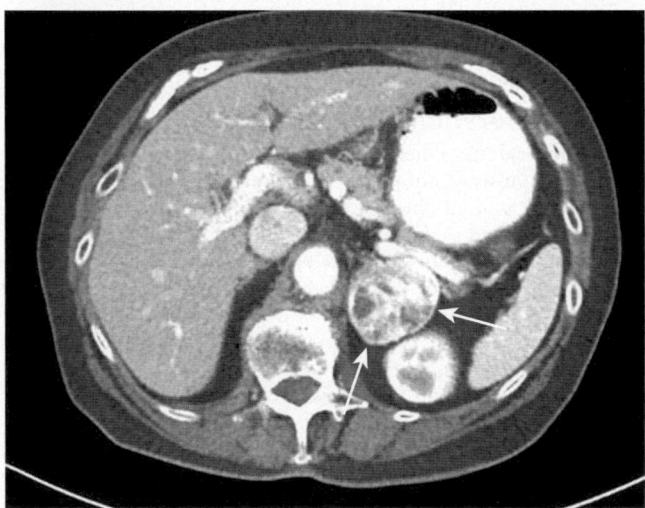

FIGURE 1 Incidentally discovered 5.5-cm mass on contrast enhanced CT scan done for the evaluation of back pain *(arrows)*. The lesion is heterogenous and well circumscribed. Biochemical evaluation was positive for a pheochromocytoma.

review of more than 1400 patients with adrenal incidentalomas, 7.8% were found to have SCS. The biochemical abnormalities that define SCS include failure to suppress cortisol with dexamethasone, a loss in the diurnal variation of cortisol secretion, and low or suppressed plasma adrenocorticotropin hormone (ACTH). The 24-hour urine free cortisol levels may or may not be elevated and when elevated usually are associated with emerging clinical signs of Cushing's syndrome. Patients with SCS do have a higher incidence of hypertension, diabetes, and obesity compared with other patients with adrenal incidentalomas. In one review, hypertension was present in 76% of patients, diabetes in 30%, and obesity in 52%.

Screening for SCS should consist of an overnight dexamethasone suppression test. In this test, 1 mg of dexamethasone is given at 11 PM and a plasma cortisol level is collected the following morning at 8 AM. In normal individuals, the cortisol level should suppress to less than 3 μg/dL. Patients who fail to suppress cortisol after dexamethasone should undergo further testing with a 24-hour urine free cortisol measurement and plasma ACTH levels. A low or suppressed plasma ACTH is supportive of this diagnosis.

The natural history of SCS has not been studied widely, but in one series the rate of progression to overt Cushing's syndrome at 1 year was 12.5%. The role of surgery versus conservative management of these patients has not been well defined, but most endocrine surgeons recommend adrenalectomy for patients with SCS provided they are suitable candidates for surgery. One group (Toniato et al) has carried out a prospective randomized trial of surgical versus conservative management for SCS in patients with adrenal incidentalomas. This study was carried out over a 15-year period, and 45 SCS patients were randomized to undergo either surgery (23 patients) or conservative management (22 patients). Patients were followed for a mean of 7.7 years. In the surgical group, diabetes normalized or improved in 62.5%, hypertension improved in 67%, hyperlipidemia improved in 37.5%, and obesity improved in 50% of patients. In contrast, none of the patients in the conservatively managed group improved, and some had worsening of diabetes, hypertension, and hyperlipidemia. Of note, none of the patients in the conservatively managed group progressed from subclinical to overt Cushing's syndrome during the course of follow-up. However, three patients crossed over to surgical management because of an increase in adrenal mass size to more than 3.5 cm. All cases were completed laparoscopically, and there were no major complications reported from adrenalectomy. The conclusion from this study was that adrenalectomy for SCS provides superior outcomes compared with conservative management.

A second study compared outcomes in 35 consecutive patients with SCS, 20 of whom underwent adrenalectomy and 15 of whom were managed conservatively (Iacobone et al). Although the two groups were comparable in terms of all baseline parameters, improvements in blood pressure, glucose control, and BMI occurred only in the adrenalectomy group, and these parameters either did not improve or worsened in the conservatively managed group. These studies argue for surgical management in patients with SCS who are deemed suitable candidates for operation.

Patients with SCS may undergo a period of adrenal insufficiency after adrenalectomy and therefore should be given supplemental glucocorticoids postoperatively. In uncertain cases, a morning plasma cortisol level on postoperative day 1 may be obtained and glucocorticoid replacement therapy initiated if the cortisol level is low.

Aldosteronoma

Aldosterone-producing adenoma (aldosteronoma) is the most common hypersecretory adrenal lesion overall and is the most common cause of secondary hypertension, accounting for 8% to 12% of hypertensive patients. Because these lesions are small (1.0 to 1.5 cm or smaller), they are not often discovered as or referred to as incidentalomas. Primary hyperaldosteronism should be suspected in any patient who is hypertensive and hypokalemic or with difficult-to-control or refractory hypertension. These patients typically have hypertension that is refractory to medical management and is predominantly diastolic.

Biochemical screening for hyperaldosteronism should consist of measurement of plasma aldosterone and renin activity. No special preparation is required for testing except that patients should be upright and not on spironolactone or an ACE inhibitor. An aldosterone-to-renin ratio greater than 20 to 25 in conjunction with a plasma aldosterone concentration greater than 15 mg/dL and a plasma renin concentration less than 0.5 is suggestive of the diagnosis. Confirmation should be obtained by collection of a 24-hour urine for measurement of aldosterone, sodium, and potassium levels while on a high-salt diet or during saline loading. The 24-hour urine aldosterone level after salt loading should be greater than 12 μg/dL. Before proceeding to adrenalectomy in a patient with primary hyperaldosteronism, it is important to differentiate idiopathic hyperaldosteronism from bilateral cortical hyperplasia. Adrenal vein sampling for aldosterone and cortisol is recommended for all patients with bilateral adrenal nodularity, a unilateral nodule less than 1 cm, normal-appearing glands, or age older than 45 to determine if there is a unilateral source of increased aldosterone production.

BENIGN NONFUNCTIONING ADRENAL LESIONS

Nonfunctioning cortical adenoma is the most common lesion to be seen as an incidentaloma and may account for up to 60% of incidentalomas in major series. These lesions are diagnosed by their imaging appearance as described later (see the section on radiographic assessment) and a normal biochemical evaluation. Most adenomas are smaller than 4 cm, but they may be up to 6 cm in diameter. Adrenalectomy is indicated for those larger than 4 cm or with imaging characteristics that are atypical for an adenoma.

Myelolipomas are benign adrenal lesions that are made up of fat and bone marrow elements. They can become large (up to 10 to 15 cm in diameter) and can be bilateral. They are recognizable by the presence of macroscopic fat on CT or MRI imaging (Figure 2). Myelolipomas are typically asymptomatic and should not be removed unless they have an atypical imaging appearance (i.e., uncertain diagnosis) or are suspected to be causing local symptoms.

A number of other lesions may be seen as incidentalomas, including adrenal cysts, hemorrhage, and ganglioneuromas. In most cases, these lesions can be differentiated according to their imaging characteristics. Adrenal cysts may be endothelial cysts or pseudocysts from prior hemorrhage or infarction. Adrenal cysts are usually readily recognizable, although there may be evidence of hemorrhage within them. They usually do not require adrenalectomy, unless they are large in size and the patient is having symptoms. Adrenal hemorrhage can occur from past trauma or may be a spontaneous event in patients who are anticoagulated, especially in the setting of an adrenal tumor. If adrenal hemorrhage is suspected, that patient should be followed with serial imaging and, in most cases, will not require adrenalectomy. Ganglioneuromas are benign tumors that arise from the sympathetic nerve fibers and therefore may be immediately adjacent to the adrenal and be seen as an incidentaloma. They are not functionally active and do not have to be removed unless the diagnosis is uncertain.

MALIGNANT ADRENAL LESIONS

Adrenocortical Carcinoma

Most adrenocortical carcinomas cause clinical signs and symptoms. These tumors are typically large (greater than 6 to 8 cm in diameter)

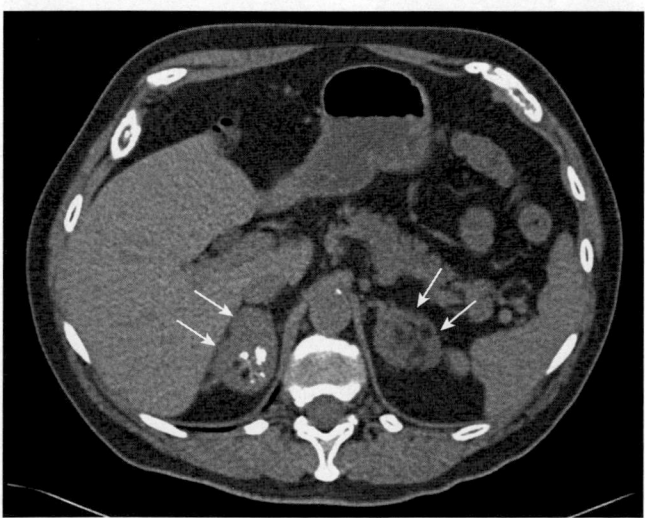

FIGURE 2 CT scan of bilateral adrenal myelolipomas *(arrows)*. Note the areas of macroscopic fat (hypodense areas) that are typical for this lesion.

and have imaging characteristics typical for malignancy: irregular borders and higher attenuation values. Most patients present with advanced (stage III or IV) disease. Adrenal cancers also may be associated with increased steroid hormone secretion with biochemical features of Cushing's syndrome, virilization, or both.

The incidence of primary adrenocortical carcinoma in series of adrenalectomies for incidentalomas has averaged in the 8% to 9% range, although the incidence is lower in North American series. In one large study from the Mayo Clinic of 342 adrenal incidentalomas, only 4 (1.2%) were nonfunctioning adrenal cancers. Another large study from Italy, of 380 incidentalomas in a national database, identified 44 patients with primary adrenal carcinomas for an overall incidence of 12.4%. Small adrenal cancers (<5 cm in size) do occur but are distinctly uncommon. Suspicion in such cases should be based on the imaging characteristics as described subsequently.

Adrenal Metastases

Adrenal incidentalomas are sometimes identified during cross-sectional imaging done for tumor staging and should be differentiated from potential metastasis on the basis of their imaging characteristics. An adrenal metastasis that occurs as part of imaging follow-up and screening for a patient with a known primary malignancy should not be considered a true incidentaloma, and it would be unusual for an adrenal metastasis to be the initial presenting manifestation of an extra-adrenal malignancy. Adrenal metastases usually occur in the setting of other extra-adrenal metastatic disease. Typically, adrenal metastases have higher attenuation on CT, demonstrate no loss of signal on MRI chemical shift imaging, and show increased metabolic activity on positron emission tomography (PET) scanning. Adrenalectomy may be indicated for a patient with an isolated adrenal metastasis or occasionally for staging purposes. Fine-needle aspiration (FNA) biopsy should be done *only* for patients in whom a tissue diagnosis will alter therapy. If the lesion is appropriate for surgical resection, adrenal biopsy is *not* recommended because of the potential risk for tumor seeding. False-positive imaging can occur in patients with underlying malignancy and an adrenal mass. In one recent study of 49 adrenalectomies performed for metastatic disease, PET imaging had been done preoperatively in 30 cases. The PET-positive imaging rate in this group was 20%, and there was only one false-negative PET-CT. However, there were five false-positive lesions, all of which proved to be cortical adenomas. Therefore other features of the adrenal lesion, including size and other imaging characteristics, should be used to determine the appropriateness of adrenalectomy in this setting.

DIAGNOSTIC EVALUATION

The diagnostic algorithm for the evaluation of adrenal incidentalomas is outlined in Figure 3. The first step in the evaluation is to rule out a hypersecretory lesion. Patients should be questioned for possible adrenal-related symptoms that include hypertension, spells (headaches, palpitations, anxiety), weight gain, and hypokalemia. All adrenal incidentalomas should be screened for pheochromocytoma with plasma fractionated metanephrines and/or a 24-hour urine collection for measurement of catecholamine and metanephrines. In most centers, plasma fractionated metanephrines are done initially because they are much easier to obtain, and 24-hour urine testing is reserved for patients with elevated or abnormal plasma metanephrines. Urine vanillylmandelic acid is no longer used for screening for pheochromocytoma because of the lower specificity of this test. Subclinical hypercortisolism should be evaluated with an overnight dexamethasone test as described previously. For patients who fail to suppress cortisol levels to less than 3 μg/dL with dexamethasone, further testing is warranted with plasma ACTH levels and a 24-hour urine free cortisol. Screening for hyperaldosteronism is done only if the patient is hypertensive or hypokalemic and consists simply of measuring plasma aldosterone and renin levels. Adrenal androgen

DIAGNOSTIC AND MANAGEMENT ALGORITHM

```
                          ┌─────────────────────────┐
                          │  Adrenal incidentaloma  │
                          └─────────────────────────┘
                    ┌──────────────┴───────────────────┐
          ┌───────────────────────┐          ┌──────────────────────────┐
          │ Biochemical evaluation │          │ Radiographic assessment  │
          └───────────────────────┘          └──────────────────────────┘
```

| Plasma fractionated metanephrines or 24-hr urine catecholamines and metanephrines | Overnight Dexamethasone (DM) test (1 mg DM at 11 PM, 8 AM plasma cortisol) | PAC:PRA* (only if hypertensive and/or hypokalemic) |

Imaging review (lesion size, attenuation, homogeneity)

| Nonfunctioning lesion | Functioning lesion |

MRI if CT is indeterminate

– Repeat imaging at 3–6 mos and yearly for 1–2 yrs
– Biochemical reassessment at 12 and 24 months

Laparoscopic adrenalectomy

| Adenoma <4 cm | Myelolipoma | Size >4.5 cm or atypical appearance |

| Observe | Observe—unless atypical appearance or symptoms | Adrenalectomy |

*PAC = plasma aldosterone concentration; PRA = plasma renin activity

FIGURE 3 Diagnostic and management algorithm for adrenal incidentaloma.

testing should be considered in patients in whom a primary adrenal malignancy is suspected. Typically, this would consist of a DHEA-sulfate level, although plasma testosterone could be measured if the patient has clinical features of virilization.

■ RADIOGRAPHIC ASSESSMENT

By definition, because adrenal incidentaloma is an unsuspected finding on radiologic investigation done for other reasons, the initial first step in the evaluation of these patients is to carefully review the imaging studies. If the initial imaging modality was ultrasound, then either a CT or MRI should be done to further characterize the adrenal lesion depending on the suspected nature of the underlying mass. If a pheochromocytoma is suspected, then MRI would be the preferred imaging test, whereas CT should be the initial modality for most other lesions. MRI is reserved for differentiation of lesions that are nondiagnostic on CT. An important initial step is also to confirm that the mass is in the adrenal gland itself and not in an adjacent retro-peritoneal structure (e.g., pancreas or kidney). Imaging assessment is also an important determinant in the management algorithm for whether adrenalectomy is indicated. In the vast majority of cases, differentiation of benign from malignant can be made with a high degree of sensitivity and specificity by imaging alone. In a study of 196 consecutive adrenalectomies, the specificity of imaging in pre-dicting a benign lesion was 100% (Yim et al). In this group there were 17 patients with malignant adrenal lesions, and the sensitivity of imaging in predicting malignancy was also 100%.

Benign adrenal adenomas (both functioning and nonfunction-ing) are lipid-rich lesions that are typically smooth and homogenous in appearance. Because of the abundance of intracellular lipid, they are low in attenuation on unenhanced CT scans (<10 Hounsfield units). This means they are lower in attenuation than liver or kidney but higher attenuation than retroperitoneal fat (Figure 4). About 30% of adenomas are lipid poor, which can make them difficult to distinguish from other adrenal masses. For these lesions, a washout value of greater than 50% on contrast CT may help confirm the

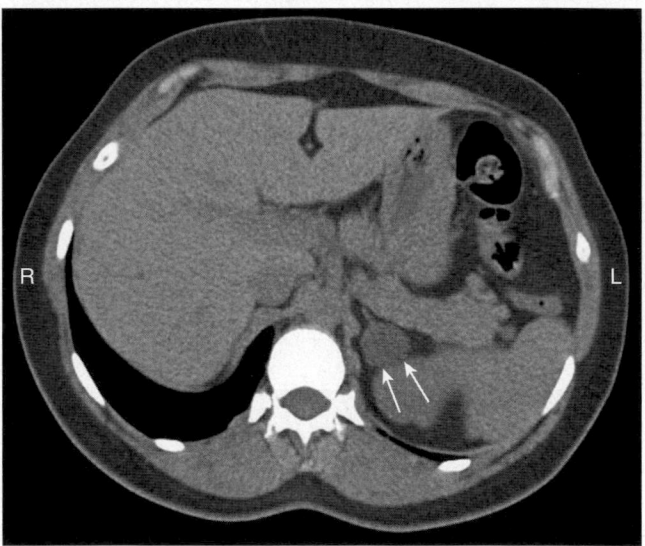

FIGURE 4 Noncontrast CT scan that demonstrates a left adrenal cortical adenoma (arrows). Note the lesion is low attenuation with a lower density than adjacent kidney and spleen, which is due to its high fat content.

diagnosis. The abundance of intracellular lipid also results in a loss in signal intensity in the adenoma on MRI opposed-phase chemical shift imaging. Chemical shift imaging sequences make use of the differential processing of proton signals in fat and water. With in-phase chemical shift imaging, the fat and water proton signals are aligned, whereas in opposed-phase imaging the water and fat signals are diametrically opposed. This results in the cancellation of the signal and a drop in signal intensity if the lesion has both water and fat in it. Because pheos and malignant adrenal lesions have less fat and higher water content, they do not incur a loss of signal on opposed-phase chemical shift imaging. Figure 5 shows the typical appearance of an adrenal adenoma on chemical shift imaging with a loss of signal on opposed-phase sequences.

Pheochromocytomas tend to be larger than adenomas. Smaller pheos may be homogenous in appearance, whereas larger pheos typically have areas of heterogeneous attenuation resulting from hemorrhage, cystic degeneration, or necrosis. Calcification can be present in up to 10% of cases. On MRI, pheochromocytomas typically have a high T2 signal intensity and appear bright, although lesions with a heterogeneous signal for the reasons mentioned previously can have a low T2 signal. On enhanced CT, there often is evidence of contrast retention rather than washout. Since confirmation of the diagnosis of a pheo is biochemical and, by definition, in the setting of an incidentaloma there is an obvious adrenal mass present, there is no role for nuclear imaging with metaiodobenzylguanidine (MIBG) in this setting.

Myelolipomas can be diagnosed reliably on imaging by the presence of macroscopic fat. On imaging, these lesions, in addition to macroscopic fat, have interspersed areas of denser myeloid tissue. Other adrenal lesions that may be detected by imaging include cysts and adrenal hemorrhage. Both CT and MRI are able to identify cystic lesions with a high level of sensitivity, but it is important to differentiate them from cysts of the kidney, pancreas, or liver. Adrenal hemorrhage may be due to prior trauma and can occur spontaneously in the setting of anticoagulation or coagulopathy. Adrenal hemorrhage typically appears as a high attenuation adrenal mass and may be associated with an underlying neoplasm. If adrenal hemorrhage is suspected by imaging, the patient should be followed with subsequent reimaging until resolution or near resolution. If there is an associated underlying lesion that is suspicious at all, then adrenalectomy is appropriate once the acute event has resolved.

Adrenocortical carcinomas, in addition to their large size, are high in attenuation on unenhanced CT and tend to have irregular borders and a heterogeneous appearance with areas of necrosis, hemorrhage, or calcification. On MRI chemical shift imaging, there is no loss of signal on opposed phase sequences (Figure 6). There also may be associated local invasion or regional lymphadenopathy.

Adrenal metastases have the typical imaging features associated with malignancy: higher attenuation values on CT (Figure 7) and no loss of signal intensity on chemical shift MRI imaging sequences. Adrenal metastases are also often hypermetabolic on FDG-PET imaging and therefore PET positive. The broader role of FDG-PET imaging in evaluation of adrenal incidentalomas has not been well defined and is not recommended except in the setting of a patient with a known extra-adrenal malignancy. In such cases, PET imaging

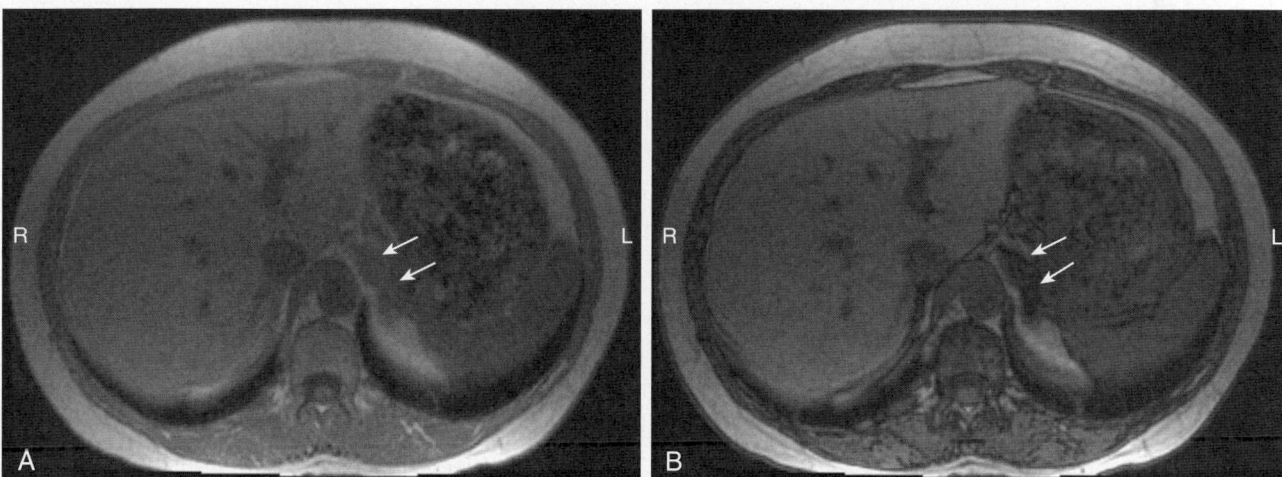

FIGURE 5 Chemical shift MRI in a patient with a benign cortical adenoma in phase sequences (**A**) and opposed phase sequences (**B**). Note the drop in signal intensity *(arrows)* on opposed phase images.

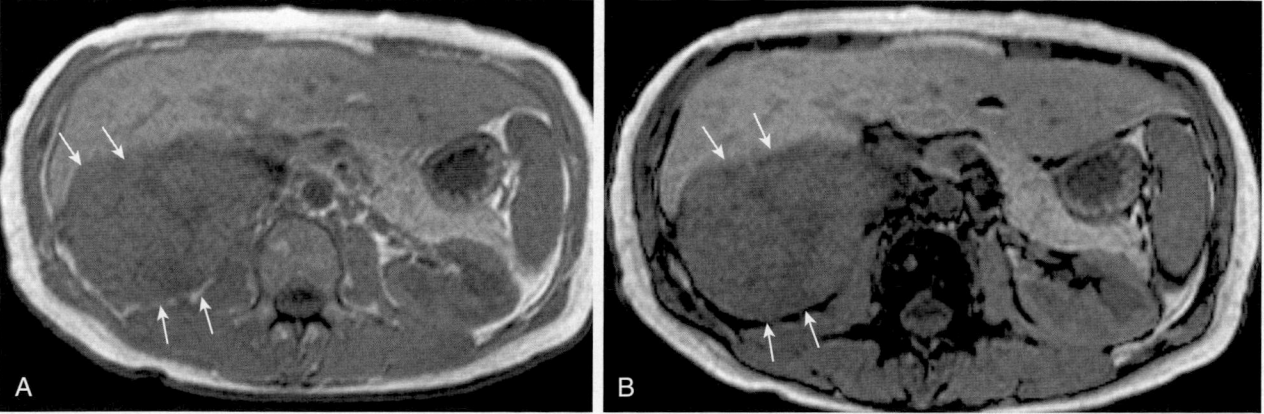

FIGURE 6 Chemical shift MRI in a patient who presented with right upper quadrant pain and was found to have a 12-cm right adrenal mass that was an adrenocortical cancer. Note no change in signal intensity from in phase (**A**) to opposed phase (**B**) gradient-recalled echo sequences. *(Courtesy Dr. Sanjeev Bhalla, Mallinckrodt Institute of Radiology, Washington University School of Medicine, St. Louis.)*

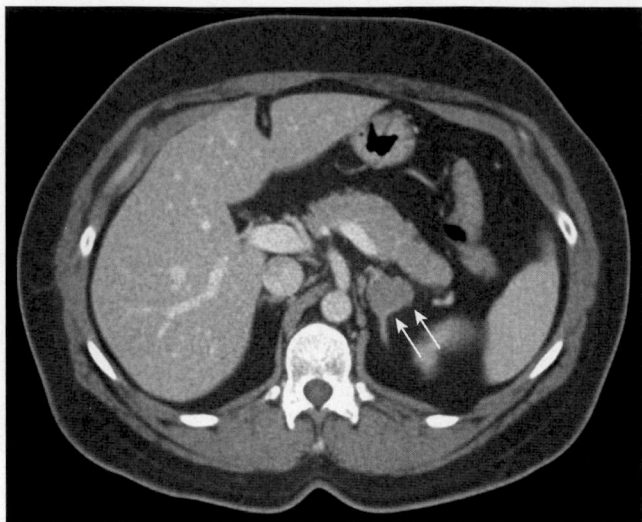

FIGURE 7 CT scan that shows a solitary right adrenal metastasis *(arrows)* in a patient with a history of lung cancer. Note the higher attenuation of the lesion that approaches that of liver and spleen.

may be useful for extra-adrenal metastatic disease before considering adrenalectomy for a potentially resectable primary tumor or metastasis.

■ TUMOR SIZE

The size of an adrenal incidentaloma is an important consideration in the management of an adrenal incidentaloma. The primary concern regarding size is the risk of adrenocortical carcinoma, which increases in lesions more than 4 to 5 cm in diameter. In a national Italian series of adrenal incidentalomas, a size cut-off of 4 cm for performing adrenalectomy resulted in a 90% sensitivity for detecting adrenal carcinoma. Adrenal metastases also may be large but are more likely to overlap with adenomas in terms of size.

In making the decision regarding adrenalectomy, size must be taken into consideration in conjunction with the radiographic appearance of the lesion. For example, a 4.5-cm adrenal lesion that has imaging characteristics diagnostic of an adenoma may be observed depending on the clinical scenario, such as in an older patient. The recommendations from the American Association of Clinical Endocrinologists and American Association of Endocrine Surgeons guidelines for the management of incidentaloma are that any adrenal mass with concerning radiographic characteristics as well as most lesions 4 cm or larger should be resected because of the increased cancer risk. An exception to this rule would be adrenal myelolipomas, which tend to be larger, have a very characteristic radiographic appearance, and generally do not require excision.

■ FINE-NEEDLE ASPIRATION BIOPSY

Fine-needle aspiration (FNA) biopsy has a very limited role in the evaluation of the adrenal incidentaloma. FNA biopsy does not differentiate benign from malignant primary adrenal tumors, and biopsy is associated with certain risks. The decision regarding adrenalectomy instead should be based on lesion size, functional state, and imaging characteristics. Several prior studies have analyzed the role of adrenal biopsy in the evaluation of adrenal neoplasms. In these reports, the biopsy rarely changed management and was associated with a significant risk of complications. In particular, biopsy of undiagnosed pheochromocytomas occurred in a number of circumstances and was associated with a high biopsy-related complication rate leading to hematoma and/or severe hypertension with subsequent increased difficulty of adrenalectomy. The primary role of

adrenal biopsy should be to exclude unresectable metastatic disease. In patients who have a solitary lesion of the adrenal gland that is suspicious for malignancy and no other extra-adrenal metastatic disease, the decision to proceed with adrenalectomy almost always can be based on clinical and radiologic assessment alone.

■ MANAGEMENT

A management algorithm for adrenal incidentaloma is presented in Figure 3. The ability to remove the adrenal gland in a minimally invasive fashion should not result in an overly liberal approach to adrenalectomy for incidentalomas. Surgery is indicated for any patient who has evidence of secretion of excess adrenal hormones and for those who have imaging characteristics suspicious for malignancy or atypical for a benign lesion. Adrenal myelolipomas should not be removed unless they have atypical imaging features or are symptomatic, which is uncommon. Adrenal incidentalomas that do not meet these criteria should be followed with repeat imaging and biochemical testing as outlined later.

Laparoscopic adrenalectomy is the preferred approach for most patients with incidentaloma who require adrenalectomy. The exception is the patient with a large suspected adrenocortical carcinoma (greater than 6 to 7 cm) because of a greater difficulty in removing these lesions laparoscopically and also the potential increased risk for local recurrence. Both transabdominal lateral approaches and a retroperitoneal endoscopic approach can be considered for incidentalomas depending on local surgical expertise. The retroperitoneal endoscopic approach has the advantages of avoiding entry into the abdominal cavity and provides the most direct route to the adrenals. It is more difficult in patients with larger tumors (>4 to 5 cm) and obese subjects (BMI >35), however. A laparoscopic or retroperitoneal endoscopic approach appears to be appropriate for selected patients with adrenal metastases, provided the surgeon has substantial experience in performing laparoscopic adrenalectomy. Long-term follow-up studies of resection of adrenal metastases are lacking, however, so these patients should be approached with caution. Removal of an intact specimen with negative surgical margins should be the primary goal regardless of the nature of the underlying lesion.

Patients with pheochromocytomas should be adequately prepared pharmacologically for surgery with alpha receptor blockade as discussed previously. Patients with subclinical Cushing's syndrome should receive perioperative supplemental corticosteroids and may require several weeks to months of replacement before recovery of the hypothalamic-pituitary-adrenal axis. Patients with primary hyperaldosteronism should have monitoring of potassium and renal function as well as hypertension postoperatively until these have stabilized. Most patients can be discharged within 1 day of the procedure.

■ FOLLOW-UP

The recommended follow-up of a nonfunctioning adrenal incidentaloma that has benign radiographic features and is smaller than 4 to 5 cm is to repeat cross-sectional imaging with CT at 3 to 6 months and then annually for the next 1 to 2 years. Biochemical screening, the primary goal of which is to test for the subsequent development of subclinical Cushing's, is recommended yearly for up to 5 years. Surgical excision should be considered for lesions that increase in size or that have emerging evidence of hormonal hypersecretion.

Suggested Readings

Davenport C, Liew A, Doherty B, Win HH, Misran H, Hanna S, Kealy D, Al-Nooh F, Agha A, Thompson CJ, Lee M, Smith D. The prevalence of adrenal incidentaloma in routine clinical practice. *Endocrine.* 2011;40: 80-83.

Iacobone M, Citton M, Viel G, et al. Adrenalectomy may improve cardiovascular and metabolic impairment and ameliorate quality of life in patients with adrenal incidentalomas and subclinical Cushing's syndrome. *Surgery.* 2012;152:991-997.

Taffel M, Haji-Momenian S, Nikolaidis P, Miller FH. Adrenal imaging: a comprehensive review. *Radiol Clin North Am.* 2012;50:219-243.

Toniato A, Merante-Boschin I, Opocher G, et al. Surgical versus conservative management for subclinical Cushing syndrome in adrenal incidentalomas: a prospective randomized study. *Ann Surg.* 2009;249: 388-391.

Yim L, Tublin ME, Falcone JA, et al. The adrenal mass: correlation of histopathology with imaging. *Ann Surg Oncol.* 2010;17:846-852.

Zeiger MA, Thompson GB, Duh Q-Y, Hamrahian AH, Angelos P, Elaraj D, Fishman E, Kharlip J. American Association of Clinical Endocrinologists and American Association of Endocrine Surgeons medical guidelines for the management of adrenal incidentalomas. *Endocr Pract.* 2009;15:1-20.

THE MANAGEMENT OF ADRENAL CORTICAL TUMORS

Konstantinos Makris, MD, and Alan P. B. Dackiw, MD, PhD, MBA

The adrenal glands consist of an inner core, the medulla, which derives embryologically from the neural crest, and an outer shell, the adrenal cortex, which is mesenchymal in origin during the fetal life and is later replaced by mesothelium. The adult adrenal cortex consists of three concentric layers: (1) the zona reticularis (deep), (2) the zona fasciculata, and (3) the zona glomerulosa (superficial), which secrete sex hormones, cortisol, and aldosterone, respectively.

Pheochromocytomas arise from the neuroendocrine cells of the medulla (discussed in Chapter 140), whereas the cortex gives rise to benign and malignant neoplasms, which can be either hormonally active (functional) or hormonally inactive (nonfunctional). These tumors are diagnosed during the workup of signs and symptoms of excessive hormonal production by them, symptoms from local tumor growth (with or without invasion), and frequently as incidental findings on cross-sectional imaging performed for other reasons (adrenal incidentalomas are discussed in a Chapter 138).

■ PREOPERATIVE EVALUATION

Initial evaluation of adrenal cortical tumors consists of detailed history and physical examination directed at the signs of the related endocrine syndrome (Cushing's, hyperaldosteronism, virilization/feminization) and the personal history of other malignancy. Family history can reveal rare familial syndromes involving the adrenal cortex. Biochemical workup includes a variety of screening and confirmatory tests intended to describe the hormonal profile of the tumor. The diagnosis of pheochromocytoma should be excluded, usually with plasma metanephrine levels. Computed tomography (CT) with specifically timed contrast administration and multiphase scanning (adrenal protocol) is the mainstay of adrenal pathology imaging, which provides information on the size, heterogeneity, contrast uptake and washout, regularity of border, and local invasion of the adrenal tumors. This may accurately suggest the tumor's benign or malignant nature. Magnetic resonance imaging (MRI) also can distinguish benign from malignant lesions, and it also can reveal local tumor invasion in great detail. Positron emission tomography (PET), most commonly with fluorodeoxyglucose (FDG), is used only selectively, for example, in the staging of adrenocortical carcinoma (ACC). Percutaneous biopsies of adrenal lesions generally are avoided as both unnecessary (since required information can be gathered in noninvasive manner) and possibly harmful (i.e., malignant seeding of biopsy needle tract, hypertensive crisis in undiagnosed pheochromocytoma, adrenal hemorrhage). Biopsy may be considered, if confirmation of metastatic lesion to the adrenal is needed before treatment. Overall, differentiation between benign and malignant

lesions is based heavily on imaging findings, and this is crucial because it affects perioperative management and surgical approach.

Indications for surgical intervention are dictated by (1) the functionality of the adrenal cortical tumor and (2) the suspicion of malignancy by clinical evaluation and imaging. Tumors with excessive hormone production leading to hypercortisolism, hyperaldosteronism, or virilization/feminization should be considered for resection. Moreover, imaging findings suspicious for adrenocortical carcinoma or adrenal metastasis are indications for adrenalectomy. Adrenal incidentalomas of 4 to 6 cm carry a risk of malignancy of about 6%, whereas those larger than 6 cm have a risk of greater than 25%. Therefore AACE/AAES guidelines suggest consideration of adrenalectomy for adrenal incidentalomas larger than 4 cm, when surgical risk is appropriate.

■ BENIGN CORTICAL TUMORS

Hyperaldosteronism

Primary aldosteronism (PA) is caused by the autonomous overproduction of aldosterone by the adrenal glands and is not suppressed by sodium loading. Underlying pathology includes aldosterone-secreting adrenal adenoma (aldosteronoma), unilateral or bilateral adrenal hyperplasia, and the rare, inherited disorder of glucocorticoid-remediable aldosteronism (which is treated medically). Surgical intervention is indicated only in unilateral disease, either adenoma or hyperplasia.

PA is believed to account for more than 10% of hypertensive patients and is particularly prevalent in the severely hypertensive, those recalcitrant to medical therapy, and younger patients with hypokalemia. Classically, PA patients have Conn's syndrome, which is characterized by hypertension, polyuria-polydipsia, and hypokalemia (which leads to muscle cramps and palpitations). In most recent studies, the majority of patients with PA are found to have normal serum potassium, and hypokalemia is noted in less than 40% of the patients.

The ratio of plasma aldosterone concentration (PAC) to plasma renin activity (PRA) is the main screening tool, with a PAC/PRA ratio of equal or greater than 20 being highly suggestive of PA. The combination of a PAC/PRA ratio of 20 or greater with a PAC of 15 ng/dL or more increases the specificity for PA diagnosis. Testing should be performed with the patient on an unrestricted sodium intake diet, with avoidance of medications that may confound the results (e.g., beta-blockers, ACE inhibitors, diuretics). Antihypertensives without major effect on aldosterone levels (e.g., terazosin, hydralazine, prazosin, verapamil) can be maintained. The diagnosis must be verified with one of four confirmatory tests, which are expected to detect nonsuppression of aldosterone levels in PA patients: oral sodium loading, saline infusion, fludrocortisone suppression, and captopril challenge. Caution should be paid when using the sodium loading tests in patients with severe hypertension and congestive heart failure.

CT imaging of PA patients may reveal (1) normal-appearing glands, (2) unilateral or bilateral adrenal nodules (microadenomas or macroadenomas; typically aldosteronomas are less than 2 cm in size; aldosterone-producing carcinomas are almost always larger than 4 cm), (3) unilateral or bilateral adrenal hyperplasia, or (4) minimal unilateral adrenal limb thickening. CT cannot determine the functionality of each lesion and detect the source of hyperaldosteronism.

MRI does not add any more information. However, determining laterality of aldosterone hypersecretion is crucial to substantiate the indication for surgery (only unilateral disease should prompt surgical consideration) as well as to identify which adrenal gland should be resected. CT does not suffice to determine laterality of the disease. For instance, a normal-appearing or only mildly thickened adrenal gland may be the source of hyperaldosteronism, in a patient with an obvious contralateral adrenal nodule, which may be an incidental, nonfunctional cortical adenoma.

Adrenal venous sampling (AVS) is the gold standard test that helps identify lateralization of aldosterone hypersecretion. It is recommended for all patients with PA older than 40 years (because the incidence of nonfunctional incidentalomas increases with age), regardless of previous cross-sectional imaging. AVS can be omitted in younger patients with indisputable unilateral adrenal nodule on CT. An experienced interventional radiologist is needed to obtain reliable AVS results. Both adrenal veins are cannulated and sampled either sequentially or simultaneously, via a transfemoral vein access. Various AVS protocols exist, but most centers use either continuous or bolus cosyntropin (synthetic adrenocorticotrophic hormone [ACTH]) infusion during AVS to increase hormone levels and the accuracy of the test. Blood samples are obtained from each adrenal vein, the inferior vena cava, and a peripheral vein and are analyzed for aldosterone and cortisol levels. Aldosterone levels from each site are divided by the corresponding cortisol level to correct for the dilutional effect of the left inferior phrenic vein flow, which joins the left adrenal vein before emptying into the left renal vein. This correction also helps with malpositioned catheters on the right side (it is more challenging to cannulate the short right adrenal vein, which branches off from IVC in right angle), which end up sampling the diluted blood of the IVC. Interpretation of the results may vary by protocol, but a side-to-side ratio of at least 4:1 for the cortisol-corrected aldosterone concentrations is accepted widely as indicative of unilateral hypersecretion. In contrast, a ratio of 3:1 or less suggests bilateral hypersecretion (and thus disease that should be managed medically).

Unilateral adrenalectomy should be offered to patients with unilateral primary aldosteronism who are medically fit for surgery. Patients with prohibitive comorbidities and those who are unwilling to undergo surgery should be treated with mineralocorticoid-receptor antagonists (spironolactone or eplerenone). Preoperative preparation should include hypertension control (including spironolactone use) and correction of electrolyte abnormalities. Adrenalectomy corrects hypokalemia in all patients, and potassium supplementation is discontinued. Blood pressure is improved in almost all patients, but hypertension is corrected fully in only 33% of patients.

Hypercortisolism: Cushing's Syndrome

Cushing's syndrome (CS) is caused by high levels of glucocorticoids, which have resulted from exogenous iatrogenic glucocorticoid administration, pituitary or suprapituitary tumors causing ACTH excess, ectopic sources of ACTH (e.g., lung cancer, head and neck squamous cell cancer), or primary adrenal pathology in the zona fasciculata. Cortisol-secreting adrenal adenomas account for 15% of patients with CS.

Clinical presentation varies widely between classic CS and mild cases with subtle abnormal clinical findings. Relevant symptoms and signs include weight gain, depression, insomnia, menstrual irregularities, truncal obesity with proximal muscle wasting and weakness, facial plethora, acne, dorsocervical fat pad ("buffalo hump"), hypertension, striae, easy bruising, hirsutism, glucose intolerance, and others. Normalization of cortisol levels is recommended by the Endocrine Society for patients with overt CS.

Biochemical testing for diagnosis of CS suggested by the Endocrine Society includes the 1-mg dexamethasone suppression test (DST), late-night salivary cortisol measurement (performed twice), 24-hour urine free cortisol levels (at least twice), longer low-dose DST (2 mg/day for 2 days; used only for certain populations). The 1-mg DST is a fairly widely accepted screening tool for CS, which also is suggested by AACE/AAES as one of the three screening biochemical tests for adrenal incidentalomas. For this test, 1 mg of dexamethasone is given orally to the patient at 11 PM and a serum cortisol level is checked early in the next morning (7 AM). CS patients have a deranged hypothalamus-pituitary-adrenal axis, and therefore their morning cortisol level will be insufficiently suppressed by the exogenous dexamethasone. The exact cut-off value may be somewhat disputable, but a morning serum cortisol of 5 µg/dL or more is an acceptable cut-off, suggestive of hypercortisolism with a sensitivity of 85% and specificity of 95% (sensitivity increases to 95% with a cut-off of 1.8 µg/dL, which many centers support, but more false positives may result because specificity drops to 80%). These abnormal DST findings must be confirmed with at least one of the other tests. Unrevealing test results should be interpreted with the knowledge of the caveats of each test and the cyclic (over days) variation of excess cortisol secretion, which may require repeat testing if clinical suspicion is high. Serum ACTH also should be checked, and a level of less than 10 pg/mL excludes an extra-adrenal cause of CS.

Cortisol-secreting adenomas are better treated by adrenalectomy over medical management. Depending on the cortisol levels, preoperative preparation may include a short course of ketoconazole, metyrapone, mifepristone, or mitotane to decrease cortisol levels. Attention should be given to the side effects of these medications, and the treatment should be discontinued postoperatively. Postoperative administration of glucocorticoids is indicated to prevent adrenal insufficiency, and a slow taper should be planned until the hypothalamus-pituitary-adrenal axis is restored (ACTH stimulation testing may be required to confirm restoration in ambiguous cases), a process that may take up to 6 months.

Patients with adrenal incidentalomas are identified with abnormal biochemical results suggestive of hypercortisolemia, but no overt clinical findings of CS in 5% to 24% of all cases. This condition, called *subclinical Cushing's syndrome (SCS)*, evolves into florid CS in only 12.5% of these patients. Despite the absence of the classic CS findings, there is a higher prevalence of obesity, diabetes, and hypertension in patients identified with SCS. Biochemical workup and identification of SCS is recommended to include the combination of all three tests: DST, 24-hour UFC, and serum ACTH. The need for surgical treatment of an adrenal nodule with concomitant SCS is controversial. Endocrine Society guidelines currently recommend against treatment to reduce cortisol levels or action, if there is not an established diagnosis of CS. However, several small studies, recently meta-analyzed by Iacobone and colleagues, have shown improvement in body weight, hypertension, and blood glucose levels of SCS patients treated with adrenalectomy. Results on the effects on hyperlipidemia have been conflicting. Given the absence of overt clinical findings (by the definition of SCS), direct clinical benefits of treatment may be difficult to demonstrate. However, it is disputed that benefit may be inferred by the improvement noted in several of the aforementioned risk factors (diabetes, hypertension, obesity) for cardiovascular disease and metabolic syndrome. Consideration for surgical resection may be given for patients with SCS, particularly when associated with an adrenal mass greater than 4 cm. Perioperative glucocorticoids are advised for these patients as well.

Virilizing and Feminizing Tumors

Virilizing and feminizing tumors are rare adrenal tumors and carry a high risk of malignancy. Most feminizing adrenal tumors are malignant, and half of androgen-secreting adrenal tumors are malignant. Estrogen-secreting tumors cause precocious puberty or postmenopausal vaginal bleeding in women and signs of feminization in men (gynecomastia, testicular atrophy). Increased levels of estrogens (estradiol, estrone) and decreased levels of gonadotropins (FSH, LH) are found, along with the imaging finding of an adrenal mass. Androgen-secreting adrenal tumors are accompanied by hirsutism and menstrual irregularities in women. Biochemical diagnosis is based on elevated levels of serum testosterone, dehydroepiandrosterone sulfate (DHEA-S), and androstenedione. Surgical resection is the treatment for both these adenomas and adrenocortical carcinomas.

Nonfunctional Cortical Adenomas and Other Adrenal Tumors

Nonfunctional benign cortical adenomas are the most common adrenal masses: they make up about 85% of all adrenal incidentalomas. These are lipid-rich cortical lesions with low attenuation in the nonenhanced phase of CT, and prompt washout of contrast in delayed images. They are usually smaller than 4 to 5 cm. Given the absence of hormone secretion, these benign cortical adenomas do not cause specific symptoms and do not require excision. All small (<4 cm), benign-appearing, hormonally inactive adrenal tumors that do not merit surgical excision should undergo follow-up imaging at 3 to 6 months and then annually for 1 or 2 years. The risk of enlargement at 1 and 2 years is 6% and 14%, respectively. Annual hormonal evaluation also is recommended for 5 years, with the risk of the tumor becoming active at 5 years being as high as 47%. Subclinical CS is the most common hormonal conversion in previously inactive adrenocortical adenomas. The risk of transformation of a benign adrenal adenoma into adrenocortical carcinoma is not well known but seems to be extremely low. Hormonal conversion or tumor growth of more than 1 cm should prompt consideration of excision. There are no clear recommendations for follow-up beyond 5 years.

Other benign adrenal tumors include myelolipomas, angiomyolipomas, oncocytic neoplasms, and others. Surgical indications include symptoms from local growth, rapid enlargement, or size greater than 4 cm, and adrenal hemorrhage (i.e., in large myelolipomas).

■ MALIGNANT CORTICAL TUMORS

Adrenocortical Carcinoma

Adrenocortical carcinoma (ACC) is a rare endocrine malignancy, but it confers a very poor prognosis. Its incidence is two cases per million persons per year, and the overall 5-year survival ranges between 32% to 50% for patients with resectable disease. Patients with metastatic disease have a median survival of 1 year. The inherent biologic aggressiveness and the retroperitoneal location of the tumor lead to delayed diagnosis and are accountable for this poor prognosis. More than 40% of patients have metastases at the time of diagnosis, and they are not candidates for curative resection. Even after resection, local recurrence or metastases develop in 85% of patients. Most ACCs are sporadic, but they also can be part of familial syndromes, such as the Li-Fraumeni syndrome, multiple endocrine neoplasia type 1, and Beckwith-Wiedemann syndrome. The incidence of ACCs peaks at the ages of 5 and 60 years.

As with all adrenal masses, ACCs are found either incidentally on CT and MRI or after workup for signs and symptoms of adrenal hormone excess or local tumor growth. About 40% to 60% of ACCs are hormonally active, and patients may have symptoms related to the hormone hypersecreted. About 45% have glucocorticoid excess alone and 25% have combined glucocorticoid and androgen excess. About 20% of patients have androgen hypersecretion alone, and less than 10% of ACCs are accompanied by hyperaldosteronism or feminization. However, any adrenal mass with associated androgen or estrogen excess should raise the suspicion of ACC.

Imaging with CT and/or MRI is the cornerstone of diagnosis and surgical planning. Suspicion for ACC increases with adrenal masses larger than 6 cm, with attenuation of more than 10 Hounsfield units in the unenhanced phase and poor washout of contrast (<50% to 60%) of adrenal-protocol CT. Heterogeneous appearance, calcifications, central necrosis, irregular borders, and invasion of the adrenal mass to adjacent structures, adjacent venous thrombus (left renal

vein, IVC) and lymphadenopathy also are highly suspicious findings for malignancy. PET-CT avidity of more than 3.4 SUV increases the risk of adrenal malignancy. MRI suggests ACC when there is higher signal intensity in T2-weighted images and heterogeneous enhancement in gadolinium-enhanced T1-weighted images. The MRI technique of chemical shift imaging offers more information, with a malignant lesion maintaining high signal intensity between in-phase and opposed-phase imaging. MRI also can assess resectability of the adrenal mass by depicting adjacent structures and dissection planes in detail.

Preoperatively, clinical staging (Tables 1 and 2) requires CT of the chest, abdomen, and pelvis because the most common of sites of metastases for ACC include the lung, liver, and bones. FDG-PET-CT also can be used in the same direction. Brain metastases are rare, but brain imaging should be obtained in the proper clinical setting. Patients with functional ACCs additionally should be prepared for possible hypercortisolism or hyperaldosteronism. The diagnosis of pheochromocytoma should be excluded preoperatively, as for all adrenal masses, with plasma metanephrines. As previously discussed, FNA of the adrenal mass is discouraged.

Surgical resection is the only potentially curative treatment for ACC. Complete resection (R0) of nonmetastatic (stages I through III) ACC is the main predictive factor of longer survival and may require en bloc resection of adjacent organs, such as part of the liver, kidney, colon, and stomach. Extension in and thrombosis of the adjacent large veins (renal/IVC) is not prohibitive of complete resection, and thrombectomy should be performed. Venovenous or cardiopulmonary bypass may be required. The need for locoregional lymphadenectomy is not clear in the literature. A retrospective study by Reibetnaz and colleagues suggested improved outcomes with lymphadenectomy, likely because of more accurate staging of the disease and more aggressive use of adjuvant therapies. Miller and Doherty commented that improved outcomes with increased number of nodes removed may have been a reflection of more aggressive, wider resections (to include all periadrenal fat and invaded adjacent organs), whereas the true value of prophylactic lymphadenectomy by itself is still to be elucidated. Controversy exists as to whether minimally invasive surgical approaches are adequate for ACC, but the current guidelines support open adrenalectomy for ACC.

Adrenal Metastases

Metastases to the adrenal glands from distant primary sites are the second most common cause of adrenal masses, after benign adrenal cortical adenomas. Although almost any malignancy spreading hematogenously or via the lymphatics can metastasize to the richly vascularized adrenal glands, the most common primary sites include the lungs (non–small cell cancer), breasts, kidneys (renal cortical carcinoma), skin (melanoma), and the gastrointestinal tract. The prevalence of adrenal metastases in patients with known history of cancer ranges between 10% and 25%. In contrast, the possibility of an adrenal mass representing metastasis from a previously unknown primary malignancy is very low. It is reported that almost half of adrenal masses excised from patients with known history of other malignancy were metastases, although this may have been affected by selection bias (not accounting for adrenal masses that may not have been excised based on benign results of preoperative workup).

The standard biochemical workup of adrenal nodules should be performed, even if the suspicion of adrenal metastases is high. For example, in a series of patients with history of cancer undergoing adrenalectomy, almost 25% of adrenal masses were pheochromocytomas. Imaging includes CT, MRI, and FDG-PET. MRI can provide more detailed information regarding local invasion for surgical planning and can help discern metastatic adrenal lesion from primary renal cell carcinoma invading the adjacent adrenal gland. PET demonstrates hypermetabolic state of adrenal metastases (although genitourinary [GU] cancers can be hypometabolic) and can exclude other distant metastatic disease. Previous imaging can help

TABLE 1: TNM Classification of Adrenocortical Carcinoma

Primary Tumor (T)		Regional Lymph Nodes (N)		Distant Metastasis (M)	
Tx	Primary tumor cannot be assessed	Nx	Regional lymph nodes cannot be assessed		
T0	No signs of primary tumor	N0	No regional lymph node metastasis	M0	No distant metastasis
T1	Tumor ≤5 cm, no extra-adrenal invasion	N1	Metastasis in regional lymph node(s)	M1	Distant metastasis
T2	Tumor >5 cm, no extra-adrenal invasion				
T3	Any size of tumor with local invasion, not invading surrounding organs*				
T4	Any size of tumor with invasion of surrounding organs*				

From AJCC. Adrenal. In: Edge SB, Byrd DR, Compton CC, et al., eds. *AJCC Cancer Staging Manual.* 7th ed. New York, NY: Springer; 2010:515-520.

*Liver, spleen, pancreas, great vessels, diaphragm.

TNM, Tumor-node-metastasis.

TABLE 2: AJCC and ENS@T Staging Systems for ACC

Stage	AJCC*	ENS@T†
I	T1 N0 M0	T1 N0 M0
II	T2 N0 M0	T2 N0 M0
III	T1-2 N1 M0 T3 N0 M0	T1-2 N1 M0 T3-4 N0-1 M0
IV	T3 N1 M0 T4 N0-1 M0 Any T Any N M1	Any T Any N M1

*From American Joint Committee on Cancer. Adrenal. In: Edge SB, Byrd DR, Compton CC, et al., eds. *AJCC Cancer Staging Manual.* 7th ed. New York: Springer; 2010:515-520.

†From Miller BS, Doherty GM. Surgical management of adrenocortical tumours. *Nat Rev Endocrinol.* 2014;10:282-292.

ACC, Adrenocortical carcinoma; *AJCC,* American Joint Committee on Cancer; *ENS@T,* European Network for the Study of Adrenal Tumors.

differentiate new from pre-existing adrenal lesions. FNA of suspected adrenal metastases could be attempted after pheochromocytoma is ruled out, only if the information obtained is expected to change the management. The diagnosis of malignancy on FNA is helpful, but negative results are not confirmatory given the low sensitivity of the test. FNA-related complications include adrenal hemorrhage, hematuria, and pancreatitis.

Surgical resection of adrenal metastases appears to confer a survival benefit, which varies based on the underlying pathology. The presence of a single adrenal metastasis, with or without a small number of additional resectable metastases, is associated with more favorable prognosis. Multidisciplinary evaluation should guide the decision for surgical intervention, taking into account the overall tumor burden. Similarly to ACC, controversy exists regarding whether laparoscopic approach is adequate. Several series have shown comparable results and rates of local recurrence between laparoscopic and open approach, and therefore laparoscopic adrenalectomy can be considered for smaller adrenal metastases (<4.5 cm).

In select patients, who are poor surgical candidates, the option of stereotactic ablative body therapy of adrenal metastasis can be considered. Percutaneous catheter ablation with either radiofrequency ablation or microwave ablation is also available, but oncologic outcome data are scarce.

■ SURGICAL APPROACH

Laparoscopic Transabdominal Adrenalectomy

The patient is placed in the right or left lateral decubitus position, depending on the adrenal gland targeted. A beanbag and axillary roll are used for securing the patient on the operating bed and protect the axillary structures. The upper arm is kept parallel to the lower one with or without the use of an overhead armrest. The bed is flexed to increase the distance between the upper costal margin and the iliac crest to allow for more operative space and to bring the adrenal gland more superficial. The use of the "kidney rest" that many operating beds have, or an additional roll under the lower flank, can further increase the desired lateral flexion of the torso. The surgeon is positioned on the opposite side of the targeted adrenal, whereas the assistant can stay on the same side or opposite to the operating surgeon. It is helpful for the scrub nurse to stand opposite to the surgeon for efficient communication and handing of the instruments. The monitors are placed on both sides of the patient for the surgeons and the nurse.

Pneumoperitoneum is established, either with a Veress needle or the Hasson trocar, along the anterior axillary line, about 2 cm caudal to the costal margin. This port is used for the camera, and the trocar size depends on the size of the camera. A working port is placed medial to the camera port, 10 cm apart, close to the costal margin, and is used for the laparoscopic retractor (snake, paddle, or other), which helps with medial rotation of the liver or spleen. Two additional working ports are placed lateral to the camera port, close to the rib cage, keeping them 10 cm apart from each other for maximum triangulation of the instruments in the abdomen. The placement of the fourth port may require mobilization of the hepatic or splenic flexure of the colon first for proper positioning of the trocar. The size of the trocars can vary depending on the size of the instruments used and the possible need to change the position of the camera.

Right adrenalectomy starts with division of the posterior peritoneum along the lower edge of the liver and division of the right triangular ligament to allow elevation and medial rotation of the liver with the laparoscopic retractor. Extended division of the ligament far posteriorly is key to proper mobilization of the liver and exposure of the right adrenal gland, which is located high, under the liver. Mobilization of the hepatic flexure of the colon may or may not be required. The IVC is identified, and dissection is performed between the medial edge of the right adrenal gland and the posterolateral aspect of the inferior vena cava. Dissection can be performed with hook electrocautery or other vessel-sealing devices (e.g., Harmonic, LigaSure, Enseal), with the assistance of laparoscopic Kittner dissectors or even the tip of the laparoscopic sucker, as needed. Surgeons' preferences vary, but we find that hook electrocautery allows for more accurate dissection, whereas the vessel-sealing devices have the tendency to fuse the tissues and obscure the dissection planes, particularly between the adrenal gland and the perinephric fat, which are only slightly different in their yellow-orange color. The short right adrenal vein is identified usually close to the upper end of the medial edge of the right adrenal, entering the IVC at a right angle. The vein is divided between clips or with a vessel-sealing device. Dissection is continued inferiorly to separate the adrenal gland from the right kidney. The adrenal arteries, which are not always identified separately, are divided with the vessel-sealing device. Lateral dissection is usually easier and is performed with the energy devices. The adrenal gland is lifted off of the underlying psoas and kidney. Attention is paid to avoiding injuring the right hemidiaphragm posteriorly. Dissection is completed superiorly, where the superior adrenal artery is divided. We prefer keeping the lateral and superior attachments of the adrenal intact until the end of the dissection, to take advantage of the retraction they offer by not allowing the gland to drop inferiorly. During dissection, retraction of the adrenal should be gentle and usually consists of gentle pressure and rolling of the gland with a blunt instrument or Kittner to avoid even minor disruptions of the capsule that cause brisk oozing by the highly vascularized gland. The specimen is removed in a bag.

Left adrenalectomy starts with mobilization of the spleen by dividing the peritoneum lateral to the spleen, about 1 to 2 cm from the line of attachment of the peritoneum to the spleen. Leaving this cuff of peritoneum attached to the spleen aids with avoiding injury to the splenic hilum and with providing a cuff of tissue for initial medial retraction of the spleen, without exerting force on the splenic parenchyma. The line of peritoneal division is extended cephalad, all the way to the left crus, allowing full medial rotation of the spleen. The back of the gastric fundus is visualized in that area. The spleen is retracted medially with a laparoscopic retractor and the pancreatic tail is identified. Dissection is continued between the pancreas, which is also gradually rotated medially with the retractor, and the left kidney. This dissection is described as "opening a book," with the dissection plane resembling the spine of a book, the pancreas and spleen staying on the left page and the left kidney and adrenal staying on the right page of the book. Mobilization of the splenic flexure of the colon is undertaken as needed to access the left adrenal, which is located superiorly and mostly medially to the upper pole of the kidney. The Gerota's fascia is incised to access the adrenal gland. Attention is directed initially to the inferior edge of the adrenal gland, where the left adrenal vein is encountered coursing vertically to drain into the left renal vein. When the adrenal vein is not readily identifiable, the left inferior phrenic vein can be found along the medial edge of the adrenal and followed caudally, where it joins the left adrenal vein, before entering the renal vein. The inferior phrenic vein frequently is divided to facilitate the medial dissection of the adrenal. The adrenal vein is dissected and divided; the left renal vein does not have to be visualized. Circumferential dissection of the adrenal is completed as described earlier.

Minimally Invasive Retroperitoneal Adrenalectomy

Although the open retroperitoneal approach to the adrenal glands rarely is performed anymore, the retroperitoneal minimally invasive adrenalectomy has emerged as an alternative minimally invasive approach to the transabdominal laparoscopic technique. This approach, which has been popularized by Waltz and others, and requires positioning of the patient in a modified prone position and placement of the trocars in the back of the patient, in proximity to the twelfth and eleventh ribs. The technique provides benefit when bilateral adrenalectomies are planned (i.e., for familial pheochromocytoma, Von Hippel–Lindau disease, recalcitrant Cushing's disease) by avoiding repositioning of the patient, as well as when access through the peritoneal cavity is not desired (i.e., previous laparotomy). Although the proponents of the technique support it as an easier access to the adrenal glands, familiarity with the dorsal view of the retroperitoneal anatomy is required. Experts suggest that surgeons should use either of the minimally invasive techniques based on their personal experience because no data show a clear superiority of one technique over the other.

Robotic assistance with both transabdominal and retroperitoneal minimally invasive adrenalectomies has been reported as feasible and safe.

Open Adrenalectomy

Open adrenalectomy currently is reserved for larger adrenal masses (because of the increased risk of ACC and the greater difficulty of the minimally invasive technique in larger masses) or when malignancy is suspected regardless of the size of the tumor. The patient is placed supine or in a modified lateral (45-degree) position (the pelvis can remain in supine position). The steps of the procedure are similar to the transabdominal laparoscopic approach. Attention should be paid to the dissection, avoiding disruption of the adrenal capsule, which can compromise the oncologic completeness of the excision. En bloc resection of locally invaded adjacent structures, which are identified preoperatively or intraoperatively, should be performed. Partial hepatectomy is needed for R0 resection of locally advanced right-sided ACC.

Extension of the tumor in the neighboring large vein (IVC or left renal) does not preclude excision. Intravenous extension of tumor and related thrombus can be removed from the veins. Even in the presence of distant metastases, which generally preclude any surgical intervention, experts have suggested that palliative adrenalectomy can be attempted if there is tumor thrombus in the vena cava because this can occlude the IVC with subsequent severe lower body edema and poor quality of life. Depending on the degree of vascular involvement, the vein can be opened and the tumor thrombus can be removed, whereas sometimes partial vein resection with graft reconstruction is required. Occasionally, resection of a large right ACC with IVC invasion requires cardiopulmonary bypass.

■ POSTOPERATIVE COMPLICATIONS

Adrenalectomies are generally well tolerated by the patients, particularly with minimally invasive approaches. However, morbidity and mortality can occur with open and laparoscopic adrenalectomies. Bleeding, superficial or deep surgical site infection, incisional hernia, and injury to surrounding organs (i.e., spleen, colon, liver) can complicate an adrenalectomy. More complex resections can be complicated by bile leak, pancreatic leak, and diaphragmatic injury. The risk of postoperative adrenal insufficiency always should be considered in patients with hypercortisolism, and adequate replacement therapy should be instituted promptly and continued until the hypothalamic-pituitary-adrenal axis is restored.

SUGGESTED READINGS

Bradley CT, Strong VE. Surgical management of adrenal metastases. *J Surg Oncol.* 2014;109:31-35.

Funder JW, Carey RM, Fardella C, et al. Case detection, diagnosis, and treatment of patients with primary aldosteronism: an endocrine society clinical practice guideline. *J Clin Endocrinol Metab.* 2008;93:3266-3281.

Iacobone M, Citton M, Scarpa M, et al. Systematic review of surgical treatment of subclinical Cushing's syndrome. *Br J Surg.* 2015;102:318-330.

Miller BS, Doherty GM. Surgical management of adrenocortical tumours. *Nat Rev Endocrinol.* 2014;10:282-292.

Nieman LK, Biller BM, Findling JW, et al. The diagnosis of Cushing's syndrome: an Endocrine Society clinical practice guideline. *J Clin Endocrinol Metab.* 2008;93:1526-1540.

Nieman LK, Biller BM, Findling JW, et al. Treatment of Cushing's syndrome: an Endocrine Society clinical practice guideline. *J Clin Endocrinol Metab.* 2015;100:2807-2831.

Ranvier GG, Inabnet WB 3rd. Surgical management of adrenocortical carcinoma. *Endocrinol Metab Clin North Am.* 2015;44:435-452.

Reibetanz J, Jurowich C, Erdogan I, et al. Impact of lymphadenectomy on the oncologic outcome of patients with adrenocortical carcinoma. *Ann Surg.* 2012;255:363-369.

Zeiger MA, Thompson GB, Duh QY, et al. The American Association of Clinical Endocrinologists and American Association of Endocrine Surgeons medical guidelines for the management of adrenal incidentalomas. *Endocr Pract.* 2009;15(suppl 1):1-20.

THE MANAGEMENT OF PHEOCHROMOCYTOMA

Dhaval Patel, MD, Naris Nilubol, MD, and Electron Kebebew, MD

Pheochromocytomas and paragangliomas are rare tumors that arise from chromaffin cells and may secrete catecholamines and metabolites. Approximately 80% to 85% of these tumors arise from the adrenal medulla and are referred to as pheochromocytomas. The remaining 15% to 20% arise from extra-adrenal chromaffin tissue and are referred to as paragangliomas. In patients with hypertension, the incidence and prevalence of pheochromocytoma and paraganglioma is one to six cases per million and 0.1% to 0.6%, respectively. In autopsy studies, the prevalence has been noted to be about 0.05%, indicating that some of these tumors are undiagnosed, which may lead to premature death. Patients with functional pheochromocytomas and paragangliomas may have cardiovascular and metabolic complications, such as hypertension, myocarditis, cardiomyopathy, arrhythmias, impaired glucose tolerance, and diabetes. With the increasing use of imaging studies, adrenal incidentalomas are increasingly being discovered and can be functionally active pheochromocytomas. In recent years, advancements in genetic analyses have revealed that about one third of patients with pheochromocytomas and half of patients with paragangliomas have a genetic predisposition to developing these tumors. A patient with this genetic predisposition has an increased likelihood of developing bilateral adrenal and extra-adrenal tumors, and this information should be considered when selecting the optimal surgical treatment for such patients. More accurate localizing studies that better define the extent of disease in patients with pheochromocytomas and paragangliomas also have emerged, and this information has important implications when making surgical management decisions. Malignant pheochromocytomas, estimated to be between 5% and 40% of cases depending on the presence or absence of genetic susceptibility genes, require evidence of metastatic disease at nonchromaffin sites distant from the tumor, gross local invasion, or regional lymph node metastasis. In this chapter, we highlight the important clinical features, diagnostic tests, syndromic features and susceptibility genes, imaging studies, and key perioperative measures that are essential for the optimal surgical management of patients with pheochromocytomas and paragangliomas.

■ CLINICAL PRESENTATION

Patients with pheochromocytomas and paragangliomas who have excessive secretion of catecholamines and metabolites commonly experience symptoms of headache, excessive sweating, and palpitations. These symptoms may be provoked by a variety of stimuli, including postural changes, exercise, anxiety, trauma, pain, or certain medications. Hypertension can be sustained, with episodes of orthostatic hypotension, or it can be paroxysmal. These paroxysmal hypertensive episodes can occur weekly but may occur even daily or every few months. Patients also may experience other symptoms, such as warmth, pallor, tremors, paresthesia, weight loss, anxiety and fear of death, vision changes, dyspnea, chest pain, abdominal pain, nausea, vomiting, and grand mal seizures. Patients with these symptoms, as well as patients with an adrenal incidentaloma with or without hypertension, patients with hypertensive episodes during surgery or anesthesia without a previous diagnosis of pheochromocytoma, and patients with a genetic predisposition to or history of pheochromocytoma or paraganglioma, should undergo screening. Approximately 10% of patients with adrenal incidentalomas discovered by abdominal imaging will have pheochromocytomas, and 40% of patients with pheochromocytomas initially are identified as having an adrenal incidentaloma, highlighting the importance of screening this group of patients who may or may not have hypertension.

Pheochromocytomas can be hereditary in nearly one third of patients and have a distinct clinical and family history. Patients with hereditary forms of pheochromocytomas and paragangliomas commonly have a familial history, multiple and bilateral lesions, a younger age at presentation, and extra-adrenal disease. Pheochromocytomas and paragangliomas can occur in hereditary syndromes associated with germline mutations, such as von Hippel–Lindau (VHL) syndrome, multiple endocrine neoplasia type 2 (MEN 2), neurofibromatosis type 1 (NF1), and hereditary paraganglioma-pheochromocytoma syndrome (resulting from mutations in succinate dehydrogenase B [*SDHB*], D [*SJHD*], *SDHC*, *SDHA*, and *SDHAF2* subunits). More than 14 genes with germline or somatic mutations have been identified, so patients with pheochromocytomas or paragangliomas should be sent for genetic counseling when hereditary disease is suspected. This information is important when surgeons select the optimal surgical approach and treatment (Table 1).

■ DIAGNOSIS

Biochemical Testing

Patients with suspected catecholamine-secreting pheochromocytomas or paragangliomas should undergo biochemical testing. Once a diagnosis of pheochromocytoma is confirmed by biochemical testing, the tumor is localized with imaging studies. The initial biochemical screening tests include 24-hour urinary fractionated metanephrine and normetanephrine, and plasma-free fractionated metanephrine and normetanephrine. The sensitivities and specificities of these biochemical tests are dependent on the cutoff value used (greater than twofold to fourfold of the upper limit of normal) and whether the patient has a hereditary predisposition for pheochromocytoma. The specificity is lower for serum-fractionated metanephrine and normetanephrine. Plasma metanephrine should be drawn in a supine

TABLE 1: Clinical Features of Genetic Syndromes or Mutations Associated With Pheochromocytomas and Paragangliomas.*

Gene	SDHD	SDHC	SDHB	SDHA	SDHAF2	VHL	RET	NF1	TMEM127	MAX	HIF2α†	PHD1†	PHD2†	FH
Single PCC	+	+/−	++	−	−	++	++	+	+++	++	++	+	+	+
Chest/ abdomen/ pelvic PGL	++	+	+++	+	−	+	−	−	+/−	−	++	+/−	+/−	+/−
Head and neck PGL	+++	++	++	+	+++	+/−	−	−	+/−	−	+/−	−	−	−
Multiple PGL	+++	+	++	−	++	+	−	−	+/−	−	+	++	++	++
Bilateral PCC	+	−	+	−	−	+++	++		++	++	++	+	+	+
Malignant PGL/PCC	+	+/−	+++	+/−	+/−	+	−	+	+/−	+	+	+/−	+/−	+

*Patients who have bilateral or multiple pheochromocytomas/paragangliomas or extra-adrenal paragangliomas, who are younger than 40 years at presentation, or who have a family history of pheochromocytoma/paraganglioma should undergo genetic testing for *SDHx, VHL,* and *RET* mutations. Patients with a history of any of the tumors present in MEN 2 (medullary thyroid cancer, hyperparathyroidism) and VHL syndrome (central nervous system and retinal hemangioblastomas, renal cell carcinoma and cysts, pancreatic tumors and cysts, and epididymal cystadenomas) should also undergo genetic testing.

†Occur as somatic mutations and have been associated with polycythemia and require aggressive hydration perioperatively. Most of these patients are on aspirin therapy. Patients with *HIF2α* mutation are also at risk of developing neuroendocrine tumors such as somatostatinomas.

+/−, Not enough data; *MEN 2,* multiple endocrine neoplasia type 2; *PCC,* pheochromocytoma; *PGL,* paraganglioma; *VHL,* von Hippel–Lindau.

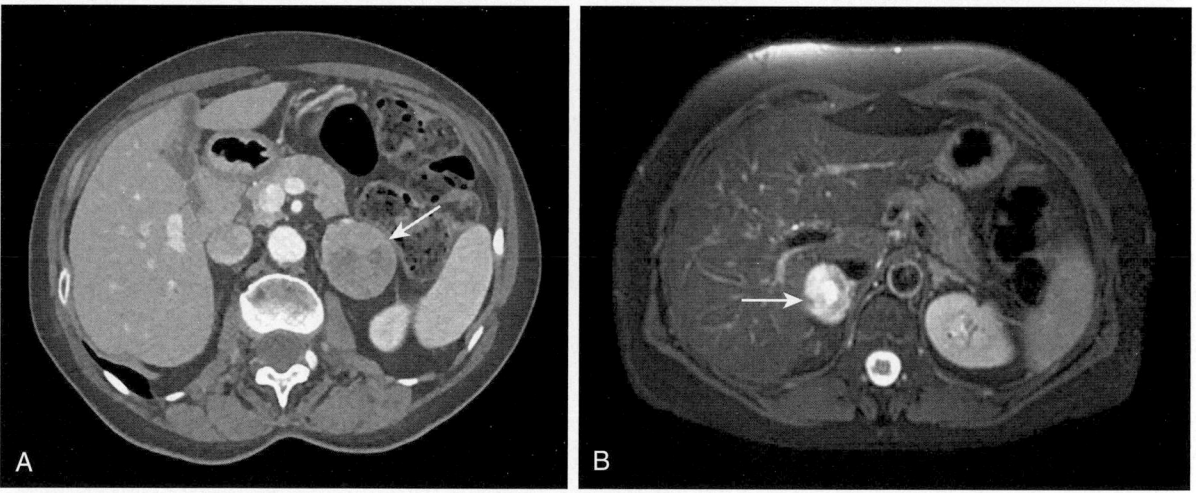

FIGURE 1 Anatomic imaging of pheochromocytoma. **A,** Computed tomographic scan of the abdomen with intravenous contrast of a 74-year-old woman diagnosed with a left pheochromocytoma (*arrow*) that has a Hounsfield unit greater than 10 and is heterogeneous with areas of necrosis. **B,** Magnetic resonance imaging scan of the abdomen on fat-suppressed T2-weighted imaging of a 59-year-old woman diagnosed with a right-sided pheochromocytoma (*arrow*) that is heterogeneous and hyperintense.

position and after an overnight fast to reduce the likelihood of false-positive results from increased levels resulting from upright posture or caffeine and nicotine use. In patients with borderline elevation, measuring chromogranin A and urinary-fractionated metanephrine in combination has been proposed as an adjunctive test to reduce false positives. In addition, there are a number of medications, including acetaminophen, labetalol, sotalol, alpha-methyldopa, tricyclic antidepressants, buspirone, phenoxybenzamine, monoamine oxidase (MAO) inhibitors, sympathomimetics, cocaine, sulfasalazine, and levodopa, that can cause falsely elevated levels of plasma and urinary metanephrine and normetanephrine.

Imaging

With biochemical evidence of pheochromocytoma confirmed, the precise location of the tumor(s) must be identified. Computed tomography (CT) and magnetic resonance imaging (MRI) are the most commonly used imaging modalities (Figure 1). On noncontrast

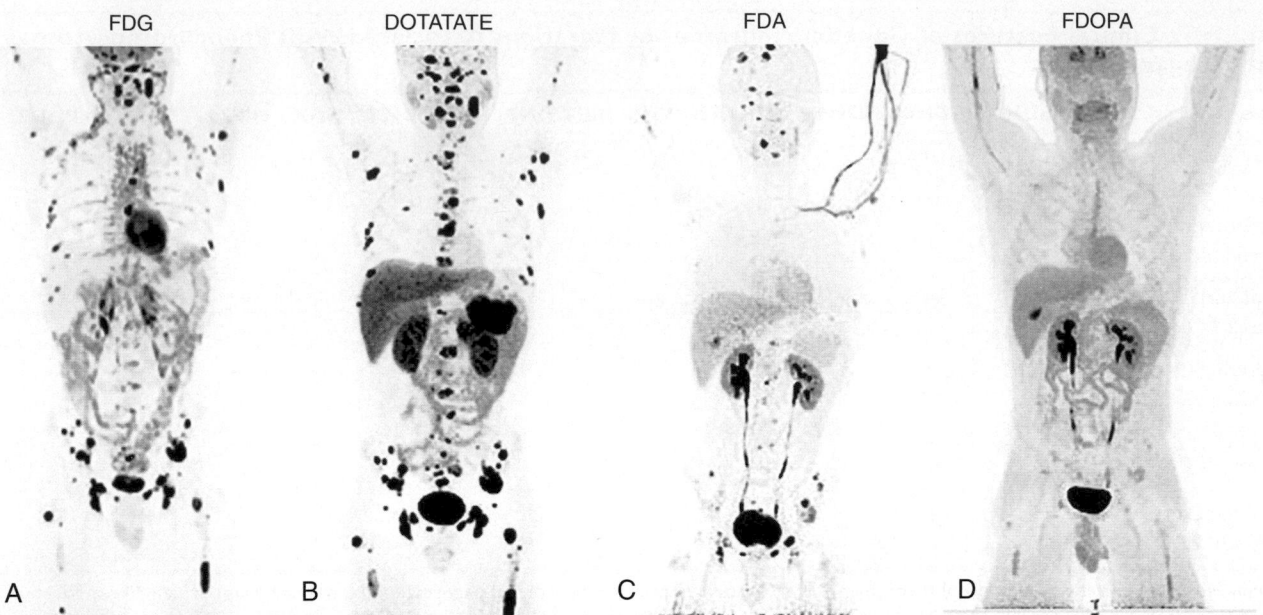

FIGURE 2 Functional imaging in a patient with metastatic and recurrent pheochromocytoma. **A**, ^{18}F-fluorodeoxyglucose (FDG). **B**, ^{68}Ga-DOTATATE. **C**, ^{18}F-fluorodopamine (FDA). **D**, ^{18}F-3,4-dihydroxyphenylalanine (FDOPA). The DOTATATE imaging shows the most number of metastatic lesions, followed by FDG and FDA; only one site of disease is seen on FDOPA.

CT scans, pheochromocytomas commonly have Hounsfield units (HUs) greater than 10. The tumors may appear homogeneous or heterogeneous, necrotic with some calcification, solid, or cystic. CT scans show excellent sensitivity, ranging from 90% to 100% for the detection of both pheochromocytomas and paragangliomas. CT scans of the neck, chest, abdomen, and/or pelvis, with and without contrast, should be performed to exclude extra-adrenal paragangliomas, using a section thickness of 2 to 2.5 mm in the neck and 5 mm through the chest, abdomen, and pelvis, especially in young patients (<40 years) and in those who have germline *SDHx* mutations or a family history of pheochromocytomas and paragangliomas (see Table 1).

MRI is the imaging test of choice in pediatric and pregnant patients. Other patient groups that would benefit from this modality include patients with documented allergies to CT contrast agents and patients who refuse radiation exposure. On MRI scans, pheochromocytomas may have pathognomonic high signal intensity on T2-weighted images (see Figure 1). However, this is not always the case, and the pheochromocytomas can appear homogeneous with intermediate intensity, diffusely heterogeneous with swirl-like areas of high and low signal intensity, and heterogeneous with multiple pockets of high signal intensity (cystic lesions).

Anatomic imaging methods such as CT and MRI have excellent sensitivity but suffer from poor specificity. Functional imaging studies, such as nuclear scintigraphy with ^{123}I-metaiodobenzylguanidine (MIBG), ^{18}F-fluorodeoxyglucose (FDG), ^{18}F-3,4-dihydroxyphenylalanine (FDOPA), ^{18}F-fluorodopamine (FDA), and ^{68}Ga-DOTA (DOTATATE, DOTATOC, DOTANOC) peptide positron emission tomography (PET)/CT, can be helpful in localizing additional tumor sites (Figure 2). For ruling out metastatic disease and localizing the primary tumor, ^{18}F-FDG PET/CT and ^{68}Ga-DOTA peptide PET/CT are most accurate (see Figure 2). ^{123}I-MIBG scanning is not as sensitive as the other functional imaging modalities and should be used when planning radiotherapy with ^{131}I-MIBG for patients with metastatic disease. Table 2 summarizes the anatomic and functional imaging studies that can be used to localize pheochromocytomas and paragangliomas, with their advantages and disadvantages, and the clinical settings in which their use can facilitate the selection of the optimal surgical management strategy.

PREOPERATIVE MANAGEMENT

Hypertension and elevated levels of circulating catecholamines predispose patients with pheochromocytomas and paragangliomas to compromised cardiovascular function, which commonly manifests as a tachyarrhythmia. These patients may have had concomitant, long-lasting hypertension, which predisposes them to cardiomyopathy and aseptic myocarditis. A preoperative cardiac evaluation is prudent, regardless of blood pressure levels, to assess cardiac function, optimize perioperative management, and risk-stratify patients for perioperative cardiovascular events.

Preoperative antihypertensive medications to reduce intraoperative hemodynamic instability are required for all patients with catecholamine-producing pheochromocytomas and paragangliomas. Alpha-adrenoreceptor antagonists are usually the first choice because of their ability to lower blood pressure, reverse volume depletion, and reduce peripheral vascular resistance. Patients who are normotensive should start taking alpha blockers to counter any potential activity from dormant tumors that may release catecholamines during intraoperative tumor manipulation. Adrenergic blockade should start 7 to 14 days preoperatively to normalize the blood pressure and heart rate. We normally initially place patients on phenoxybenzamine (10 mg twice a day). Other options include a selective alpha antagonist such as doxazosin (2 mg once a day), prazosin (2 mg twice a day), or terazosin (2 mg once a day). The goal should be to achieve a preoperative blood pressure of 130/80 mm Hg or less while sitting and approximately 100 mm Hg while standing. If the patient continues to have high blood pressure, the dose is increased in increments of 10 to 20 mg every 2 to 3 days. In addition, medications are titrated for a heart rate of about 60 to 70 beats per minute (bpm) while sitting and 70 to 80 bpm while standing.

Many patients with pheochromocytoma have chronic vasoconstriction secondary to high levels of catecholamines. Normalization of blood volume reduces the risk of hypotension during or after removal of the tumor. A high-salt diet 3 days after initiation of alpha

TABLE 2: Anatomic and Functional Imaging Studies That Can Be Used to Localize Pheochromocytomas and Paragangliomas

Imaging Modality	MRI	CT	^{18}F-FDG	^{68}Ga-DOTA Peptide	^{18}F-FDA	^{18}F-DOPA	MIBG
Advantages	Anatomic detail	Anatomic detail	Widely available, preferred functional imaging test	Most sensitive functional imaging study for all sites of disease, potential for therapy with avid disease	Sensitive functional imaging for primary tumor (except skull base and neck)	Most sensitive functional imaging study for skull base and neck paragangliomas	Potential for therapy if disease avid tumor is not resectable
Disadvantages	Lower specificity	Lower specificity	Lower sensitivity and higher false-positive rate as compared with other functional imaging studies	Not widely available	Not widely available	Not widely available	Lower sensitivity than other functioning imaging studies
Best clinical setting to use imaging studies	Initial localization of tumor	Initial localization of tumor	Rule out metastatic disease or multiple primary	Rule out metastatic disease or multiple primary; *SDHx* mutation carriers; when planning treatment with peptide receptor radionuclide therapy	Rule out metastatic disease or multiple primary	Patients with primary skull base and neck paragangliomas; multiple and metastatic disease	When planning treatment with ^{131}I-MIBG

CT, Computed tomography; *DOPA*, dihydroxyphenylalanine; *FDA*, fluorodopamine; *FDG*, fluorodeoxyglucose; *MIBG*, metaiodobenzylguanidine; *MRI*, magnetic resonance imaging.

blockers and 1 to 2 liters of normal saline starting the evening before surgery can reduce the risk of hypotension after removal of the tumor. With the appropriate alpha-adrenergic blockade, patients may experience tachyarrhythmias. A beta-blocker should be added to control the heart rate 2 to 3 days after initiation of alpha blockers. Most important, a beta-blocker should never be used in the absence of alpha blockers. The use of a beta-blocker without alpha blockers will exacerbate vasoconstriction by blocking its vasodilator component. Beta-selective drugs such as atenolol or metoprolol are started for a target heart rate of 60 to 70 bpm. Labetalol, a nonselective beta-blocker, should not be used as first-line therapy because the beta effect is seven times more potent than the alpha effect. If the patient continues to have high blood pressure, at our institution a calcium channel blocker or metyrosine therapy is initiated.

■ INTRAOPERATIVE CONSIDERATIONS

Although patients may be blocked adequately by preoperative adrenergic blockade, they still may have hypertensive crises or tachyarrhythmias during manipulation of the tumor. Therefore intra-arterial monitoring is required and appropriate access, including a central venous catheter for monitoring the volume status, is imperative. It is also vital to provide the patient with vasoactive agents. Patients may have fluctuations in blood pressure during the operation, requiring vasoactive drugs, so these should be ready and premixed. Hypertensive episodes can be treated with sodium nitroprusside (0.5 to 3 μg/kg/min), which will reduce cardiac preload. After dividing the adrenal vein, patients may have sudden hypotension, necessitating crystalloids, which should be used initially. If adequate volume resuscitation has been performed, treatment with vasopressors such as norepinephrine, phenylephrine, or vasopressin can be initiated.

■ OPERATIVE TECHNIQUE

The surgical approaches to the resection of pheochromocytomas and paragangliomas include open, laparoscopic, or robotic approaches, which can be performed with either a transabdominal or retroperitoneal approach. Minimally invasive surgery for the removal of pheochromocytomas has been shown to be associated with significant advantages compared with open resection: decreased blood loss, decreased blood transfusion requirement, shorter intensive care unit and postoperative hospitalization, and decreased analgesic requirements. Conversion to an open procedure may be required because of intraoperative suspicion of malignancy. Robotic-assisted removal of pheochromocytomas and paragangliomas is also safe and feasible, but it does not appear to afford any significant advantages over laparoscopic resection with either the transabdominal or the retroperitoneal approach.

The surgical approach and extent of resection we use depends on (1) whether the tumor is unilateral or bilateral, (2) whether there are any additional paragangliomas or possible sites of metastatic disease, (3) tumor size, (4) patient body habitus and body mass index, (5) whether the tumor is sporadic or familial relative to the risk of malignancy, and (6) the risk of developing metachronous pheochromocytoma in the contralateral and remnant adrenal gland. We most commonly use a transabdominal laparoscopic approach in patients who have unilateral tumors and sporadic disease and who have no evidence of extra-adrenal tumors. In patients with bilateral tumors and familial disease with a low risk of malignant pheochromocytoma, such as the MEN 2 or VHL syndromes, we perform a cortical-sparing adrenalectomy using a transabdominal or retroperitoneal laparoscopic approach. When patients have unilateral or recurrent tumors, possible site(s) of lymph node metastasis or local invasion, and the *SDHB* gene mutation, we perform a complete adrenalectomy and retroperitoneal lymph node dissection with an open approach. Even when the tumor is large, we usually begin the operation using a laparoscopic approach until we encounter evidence of local invasion or features suspicious for malignancy. We believe that a complete resection is most important and, whatever the surgical approach, there should be no fracturing of the tumor or violating the tumor capsule, as there have been two reports of pheochromocytomatosis (peritoneal implants with local-regional recurrence) in a series of patients in the United States and France who underwent laparoscopic resections.

TRANSABDOMINAL LAPAROSCOPIC ADRENALECTOMY AND PARAGANGLIOMA RESECTION

Transabdominal laparoscopic adrenalectomy is the most common laparoscopic approach used by most surgeons. The main advantage of this approach is a larger working space than that afforded by the retroperitoneal approach. The procedure is performed by placing the patient in the lateral decubitus position, with the operating table flexed. An incision is made 1 fingerbreadth below the costal margin in the midclavicular line. We use a 0-degree videoscope to enter the peritoneal cavity under direct visualization. Then a 30-degree videoscope is used to place additional trocars and for the dissection. The tumor should not be manipulated, or manipulation should be kept to a minimum, until the venous drainage is divided, as severe hypertension can result otherwise. Clear communication with the anesthesia team is important to anticipate and treat hemodynamic instability during manipulation of the tumor and division of the adrenal vein. The key steps and intraoperative images of a transabdominal laparoscopic adrenalectomy (right and left) are summarized in Figure 3.

For a right adrenalectomy, we use four trocars, with two trocars lateral in the anterior and midaxillary lines, one trocar at the midclavicular line, and one trocar medial to this, with a distance of approximately 2 fingerbreadths between the trocars. The initial dissection consists of dividing the triangular ligament of the liver to mobilize the right lobe of the liver medially and expose the right adrenal gland. Once this has been completed, a fan, paddle, or snake retractor is placed on the right lobe of the liver to maintain the working space. The dissection from the triangular ligament is

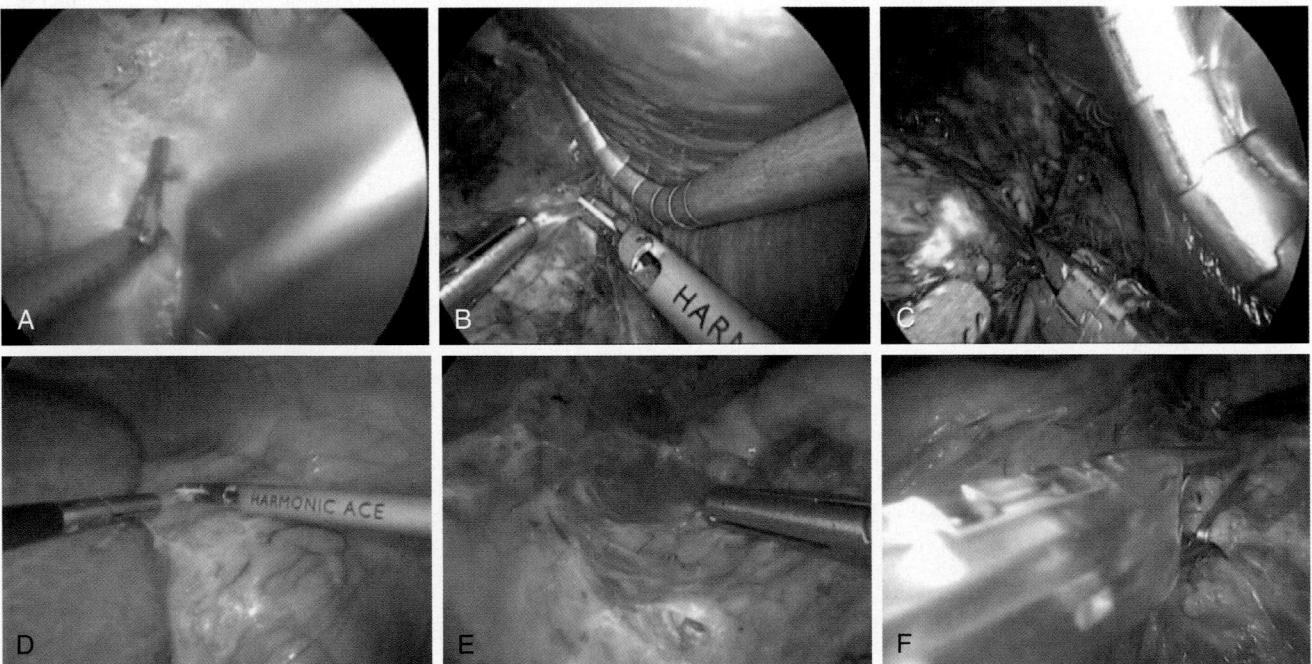

FIGURE 3 Key steps in lateral approach laparoscopic adrenalectomy. On the right side, **(A)** the triangular ligament is divided to mobilize the right lobe of the liver medially, **(B)** the adrenal gland and tumor are dissected from the top down along the medial edge after opening Gerota's fascia, and **(C)** the adrenal arteries (usually small) and the adrenal vein are encountered during this dissection and the vein is clipped and divided. Pheochromocytoma may have multiple parasitic vessels. The inferior limb of the gland is carefully dissected free from the renal hilum and the renal vessels. The gland is then mobilized free from the kidney and retroperitoneal fat. The adrenal gland is placed in a bag and removed without morcellization. On the left side, **(D)** the splenic flexure of the colon is mobilized free as well as the lateral attachments of the spleen along the avascular space, **(E)** Gerota's fascia is divided superior and medial to the adrenal gland and the dissection continued inferior, and **(F)** often the inferior phrenic vein is identified along the medial aspect of the adrenal gland and can be traced downward to the adrenal vein. The vein is clipped and divided. The inferior limb of the gland is carefully dissected free from the renal hilum and the renal vessels. The gland is then mobilized free from the kidney and retroperitoneal fat. The adrenal gland is removed in a bag.

extended downward inferiorly, dividing the peritoneum and Gerota's fascia along the liver down to the infrahepatic inferior vena cava. Commonly, the adrenal vein is encountered during this top-down dissection and is circumferentially dissected, clipped, and divided. Any accessory veins or arteries, which are usually more prominent in patients with pheochromocytoma, are clipped and transected along this medial dissection. The inferior pole of the gland is then mobilized free from the renal hilum, taking care to not injure the renal artery and vein. The attachment to the superior pole of the kidney and posterior musculature is then divided, and the dissection is extended upward to the diaphragm, removing the periadrenal fat along with the gland. We usually detach the attachment to the diaphragm last, as it keeps the adrenal gland in place, allowing good visualization of the adrenal hilum and inferior limb of the gland.

For a left adrenalectomy, we usually use three trocars because the spleen and the tail of the pancreas are retracted by gravity. The first subcostal trocar is placed in the midclavicular line at Palmer's point, and the lateral two are placed approximately 2 fingerbreadths apart and 1 fingerbreadth from the costal margin. The lateral attachment of the spleen (approximately 1 cm from the lateral edge of the spleen) and the splenic flexure of the colon are released up to the diaphragm until visualization of the gastric fundus occurs. This dissection allows the spleen and the tail of the pancreas to be retracted medially by gravity. At the medial aspect, the adrenal gland is dissected from the top down, along with the periadrenal fat, and then the dissection is carried posteriorly to the psoas muscle and continued inferiorly. Often the inferior phrenic vein is encountered during this medial dissection and can be traced to the left adrenal vein. The adrenal vein is then clipped and divided above the renal vein into which it drains.

The inferior pole is carefully dissected free from the renal hilum without injury to the renal vein and artery, from the superior pole of the kidney, and from the posterior musculature.

■ POSTERIOR RETROPERITONEAL ADRENALECTOMY

We commonly use the posterior retroperitoneal approach in patients who require bilateral total or partial adrenalectomy and in patients who have undergone previous abdominal operations and have significant intra-abdominal adhesions. The key steps of a posterior retroperitoneal adrenalectomy (left and right), including intraoperative images, are outlined in Figure 4. Once there is adequate general anesthesia and intravenous and intra-arterial lines are placed and secured, the patient is placed in a prone jackknife position. The hips and knees are flexed at 90 degrees and all pressure points are padded. Cushions are used to support the hips and lower chest, allowing the anterior abdominal wall to hang unconstrained between the cushions. This helps to expand the retroperitoneal space. The tip of the twelfth rib is palpated, and a 1.5-cm transverse incision is made below the tip of the rib and extended into and through the posterior musculature and fascia to enter the retroperitoneum. A working space is created initially by blunt digital separation of the posterior abdominal wall fascia and the retroperitoneal fat. A lateral 5-mm trocar is inserted 4 to 5 cm from the initial incision, beneath the eleventh rib, under finger guidance. Next, a medial 10-mm trocar is inserted 4 to 5 cm medially from the initial incision, 2 to 3 cm below the twelfth rib, under finger guidance. Finally, a 10-mm, blunt-tip trocar with an inflatable balloon is inserted and secured in the initial

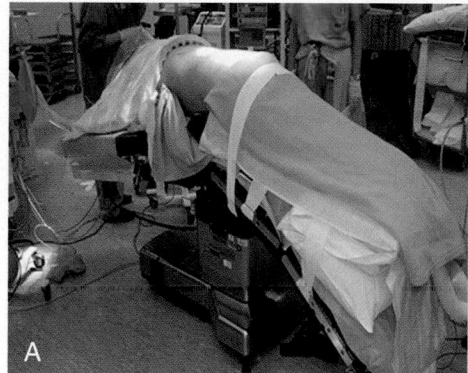

The patient is supported in a modified prone jackknife position

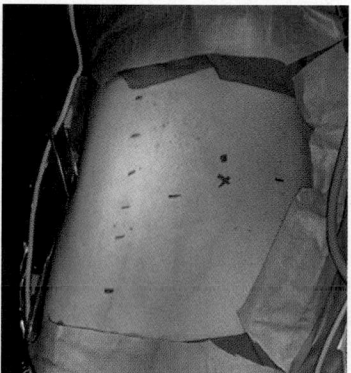

Port sites are marked using the twelfth rib as a landmark

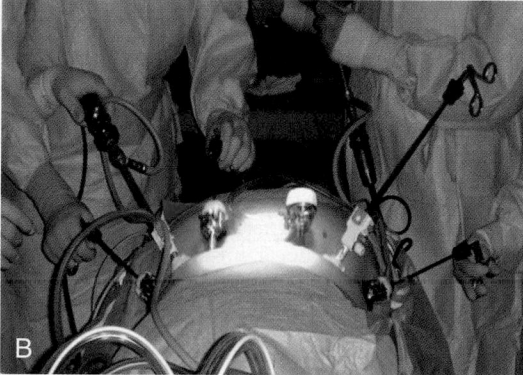

Port placement for the bilateral synchronous laparoscopic posterior retroperitoneal adrenalectomy

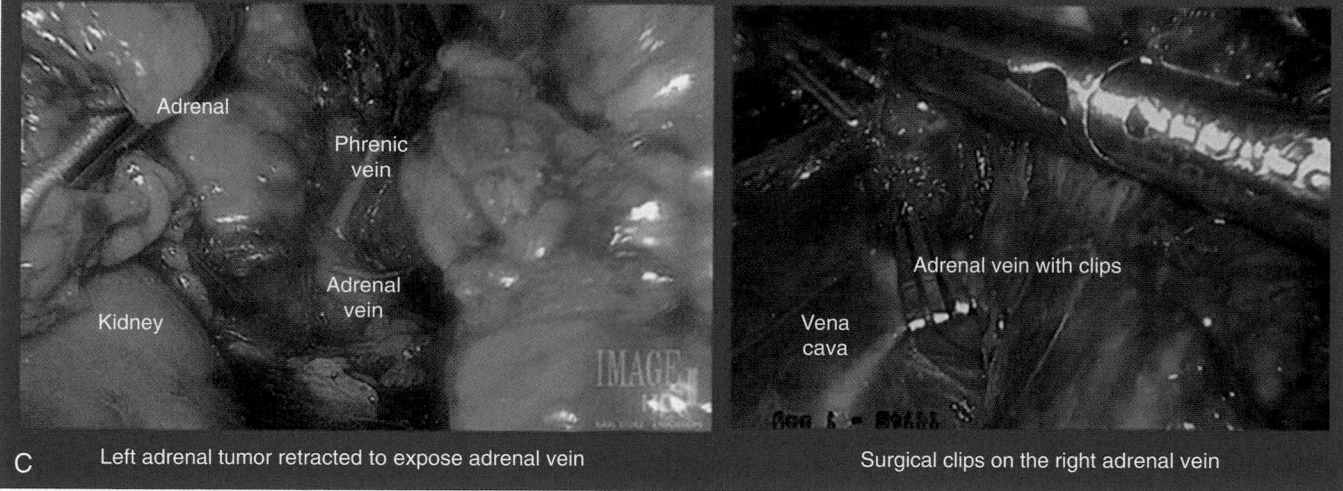

Left adrenal tumor retracted to expose adrenal vein

Surgical clips on the right adrenal vein

FIGURE 4 Retroperitoneal approach for adrenalectomy. **A,** Patient positioning and trocar placement. **B,** Operative image of simultaneous bilateral adrenalectomy. **C,** Operative field after blunt dissection of the retroperitoneal fat downward with visualization of the adrenal vein.

incision, followed by insufflation with carbon dioxide. The pressure should be maintained around 20 mm Hg. The retroperitoneal fat is pushed down and away medially from the posterior musculature and diaphragm. Retroperitoneal fat and the adrenal gland are dissected free from the diaphragm superiorly. The superior pole of the kidney is retracted and the adrenal gland is mobilized from the medial and inferior aspects. The right adrenal gland is dissected gently from the inferior vena cava to identify the right adrenal vein; the left adrenal gland is also dissected at the medial aspect to identify the left adrenal vein. Once the adrenal vein is clipped and divided, the gland, along with the retroperitoneal fat, is lifted and retracted laterally and superiorly to divide the remaining small vessels and attachments. Hemostasis is checked after the carbon dioxide pressure is reduced.

■ LAPAROSCOPIC CORTEX-SPARING ADRENALECTOMY

In patients who have MEN 2 and VHL syndromes and who also have bilateral pheochromocytomas, there is an indication to perform cortex-sparing adrenalectomy to avoid the need for long-term steroid replacement and the risk of an addisonian crisis if a bilateral total adrenalectomy were to be performed. Furthermore, patients with MEN 2 and VHL syndromes who have unilateral pheochromocytoma also may need to have cortical-sparing adrenalectomy because of the risk of developing a contralateral pheochromocytoma, which would require an adrenalectomy. Laparoscopic cortex-sparing adrenalectomy can be performed in a similar fashion to laparoscopic adrenalectomy in terms of port placement and mobilization of surrounding organs. Intraoperative ultrasound is beneficial in identifying smaller tumors and helping the surgeon to identify the margins of resection. The adrenal gland parenchyma can be transected with electrocautery or Harmonic and LigaSure scissors. The remnant adrenal gland is left in situ and not dissected. This is critical, especially if the adrenal vein cannot be spared, to maintain adequate blood flow and drainage of the remnant adrenal gland.

■ OPEN ADRENALECTOMY

We use an open adrenalectomy approach in patients who may have malignant tumors, a diagnosis based on a sufficiently large tumor size, the presence of local invasion, or presentation with local-regional recurrence, and who are positive for a germline *SDHB* mutation or other less common susceptibility gene mutations, such as *FH* and *HIF2α*, which are associated with a high rate of metastatic disease. We use a subcostal incision for our open adrenalectomies, but a thoracoabdominal incision may be necessary in patients with large, locally invasive tumors. In addition to resecting the primary tumors or site of recurrent disease, we routinely perform a prophylactic retroperitoneal local-regional lymph node dissection. There are several key steps in an open right adrenalectomy for malignant or potentially malignant pheochromocytomas and paragangliomas. An extended Kocher's maneuver is essential for adequate exposure and to allow vascular control of the infrahepatic inferior vena cava. The triangular ligament should be divided routinely, and the right lobe of the liver mobilized medially. When resecting locally invasive tumors, it is essential to gain vascular control over the suprahepatic and infrahepatic inferior vena cava before dissecting the tumor free from the vena cava or dissecting the right adrenal vein. Depending on the extent of local disease, adjacent organs may need to be resected (nephrectomy, nonanatomic liver resection, right hepatic lobectomy). For a left open adrenalectomy, division of the gastrocolic ligament and mobilization of the tail of the pancreas and spleen may be necessary if an en bloc resection of the tail of the pancreas and spleen is planned. If not, the left adrenal gland is exposed by medial rotation of the spleen, pancreas, and left colon. Vascular control of the renal vessels is important for a right or a left open adrenalectomy when removing a locally invasive tumor. For negative margins, a cuff of the posterior musculature or diaphragm, or a full-thickness resection of the diaphragm

may be necessary and should be reconstructed primarily or with a Gore-Tex patch graft and an angled chest tube left above the diaphragm. Although it is rare for a patient to require such aggressive surgical treatment for locally advanced pheochromocytomas and paragangliomas, most patients who have cardiovascular complications associated with their tumors benefit from such an approach to functioning tumors, especially when an R0/R1 resection can be performed.

■ POSTOPERATIVE MANAGEMENT

Postoperatively, patients should be monitored for blood pressure fluctuations in an intensive care unit or a stepdown unit for the first 24 hours. Patients may have hypotension resulting from the continued effects of the alpha adrenergic blockade or withdrawal of catecholamine and metabolites and may require intravenous fluids. There have been reports of hypoglycemia resulting from rebound secretion of insulin after removal of a pheochromocytoma, and therefore blood sugars should be monitored. Plasma metanephrine levels should be evaluated at 6 weeks and at 6 months to confirm the patient's biochemical response.

■ MALIGNANT PHEOCHROMOCYTOMA

Currently there are no histologic, biochemical, or molecular markers that can differentiate patients with benign and malignant pheochromocytomas in the absence of local-regional invasion or distant or lymph node metastasis. A metastatic pheochromocytoma may be present at the time of diagnosis or (commonly) become evident within 5 years of diagnosis. However, there are reports in the literature of recurrences up to 42 years after pheochromocytoma resection, which emphasizes the importance of annual biochemical screening in both sporadic and hereditary pheochromocytomas and paragangliomas. Features that have been associated with malignant pheochromocytomas and paragangliomas include a tumor size greater than 5 cm, the presence of necrosis and hemorrhage, and a high mitotic index. Patients with *SDHB* gene mutation have a high rate of malignancy, reported to be up to 40%, whereas patients with *SDHD*, *VHL*, and *RET* mutations have a low risk of malignancy.

In patients with malignant pheochromocytomas and paragangliomas, surgical resection of recurrent or metastatic disease is the best treatment option. This is especially true in patients for whom an R0 or R1 resection can be achieved. However, some patients who have widely metastatic disease with elevated catecholamine and metabolites may still benefit from cytoreductive surgery to palliate symptoms or control cardiovascular events associated with the presence of excess catecholamine and their metabolites. The prognosis of patients with metastatic pheochromocytomas and paragangliomas is variable, with some patients developing stable disease and some developing rapidly progressive disease, including debilitating symptoms and difficult-to-control cardiovascular complications from the presence of excess catecholamine and metabolites. Overall, the 5-year, 10-year, and 20-year survival rates are approximately 77.2%, 61.3%, and 39.5%, respectively.

Patients with unresectable disease may benefit from cytotoxic chemotherapy, such as treatment with a combination of cyclophosphamide, vincristine, and dacarbazine, or ^{131}I-MIBG therapy. Unfortunately, only two thirds of metastases are avid on MIBG scanning, which can limit the efficacy of this therapy. Up to two thirds of patients can have an objective response, with complete response, partial response, or stable disease with ^{131}I-MIBG therapy. Pheochromocytomas and paragangliomas have been localized using newer imaging modalities such as ^{68}Ga-DOTA peptide PET/CT, which shows superior localization capability in metastatic disease compared with other anatomic and functional imaging studies. For tumors that are ^{68}Ga-DOTA peptide-avid, peptide receptor radionuclide therapy with ^{177}Lu or ^{90}Y may result in a partial or complete response and symptomatic relief.

SUGGESTED READINGS

Ellis RJ, Patel D, Prodanov T, Sadowski S, Nilubol N, Adams K, Steinberg SM, Pacak K, Kebebew E. Response after surgical resection of metastatic pheochromocytoma and paraganglioma: can postoperative biochemical remission be predicted? *J Am Coll Surg.* 2013;217:489-496.

Janssen I, Blanchet EM, Adams K, Chen CC, Millo CM, Herscovitch P, Taieb D, Kebebew E, Lehnert H, Fojo AT, Pacak K. Superiority of [68Ga]-DOTATATE PET/CT to other functional imaging modalities in the localization of SDHB-associated metastatic pheochromocytoma and paraganglioma. *Clin Cancer Res.* 2015;21:3888-3895.

Lenders JW, Duh QY, Eisenhofer G, Gimenez-Roqueplo AP, Grebe SK, Murad MH, Naruse M, Pacak K, Young WF Jr, Endocrine S. Pheochromocytoma and paraganglioma: an endocrine society clinical practice guideline. *J Clin Endocrinol Metab.* 2014;99:1915-1942.

Young WF, Kaplan NM, Kebebew E. *Treatment of Pheochromocytoma in Adults. UpToDate.* Waltham, MA: Wolters Kluwer Health; 2012-2016. <http://www.uptodate.com>.

THE MANAGEMENT OF THYROID NODULES

Jesse D. Pasternak, MD, and Quan-Yang Duh, MD

There has been a substantial increase in the detection of thyroid nodules and thyroid cancer over the past decades in the United States and other developed countries, most likely because of the availability of neck ultrasound. Almost all the additional diagnoses are for small (less than 2 cm) papillary thyroid cancer, and deaths from thyroid cancer have remained rare and relatively constant. Some are concerned about overdiagnosis and overtreatment of thyroid nodules and cancer, and the controversy has been popularized in the mainstream press. Because death from thyroid cancer is rare and morbidities from overtreatment can affect quality of life substantially, it is very important to risk stratify these patients to receive appropriate treatment to achieve optimal outcomes.

Thyroid nodules are very common, affecting as many as one in seven adults. Most thyroid nodules are asymptomatic. They may be detected incidentally from imaging studies ("thyroid incidentalomas"). Some patients have a palpable neck mass or symptomatic goiter. Although most thyroid nodules are not cancerous (fewer than 5%), some patients are at higher risk for developing thyroid cancer. These risk factors include being exposed to ionizing radiation at a young age or having a first-degree relative with thyroid cancer. In contrast, thyroid nodules causing hyperthyroidism are rarely cancerous. Patients with suppressed thyroid-stimulating hormone (TSH) (hyperthyroid) and a thyroid nodule usually first are evaluated by scintigraphy to establish the diagnosis (e.g., solitary or multiple hyperfunctioning nodules [Plummer's disease] or hypofunctioning nodules in Graves' disease).

ULTRASONOGRAPHY

Ultrasonography is safe and the most efficient first-line evaluation for thyroid nodules. Multiple large cohort studies have identified ultrasound characteristics of thyroid nodules that are associated with risk of cancer. The high-risk characteristics include nodules that are large, are hypoechoic, contain microcalcifications, have irregular borders, or are taller than they are wide. Ultrasound characteristics associated with a low risk of thyroid cancer include nodules with more cystic components and those that have clear borders or are spongiform. Ultrasound characteristics help to stratify the risk of thyroid cancer and are used to determine when fine-needle aspiration (FNA) biopsy is indicated. The 2015 American Thyroid Association (ATA) guidelines recommend FNA for thyroid nodules larger than 1 to 2 cm depending on their ultrasound characteristics, 1 cm for those classified at highest risk by ultrasound, and 2 cm for those classified at the lowest risk (Figure 1).

NONULTRASOUND THYROID INCIDENTALOMAS

Occasionally, thyroid nodules are found on imaging modalities other than ultrasound, such as computed tomography scans and magnetic resonance imaging. These still should be investigated by ultrasound, and further workup should proceed accordingly. Hypermetabolic thyroid nodules incidentally found on fluorodeoxyglucose positron emission tomography (FDG-PET) scan are at higher risk for cancer, thus FNA is recommended at the lower threshold of more than 1 cm.

OTHER TESTS IN EVALUATION OF THYROID NODULES

Serum levels of thyroglobulin are useful in the follow-up of patients with differentiated thyroid cancer but not in the diagnosis of whether a thyroid nodule is cancerous, because serum thyroglobulin can be elevated in many patients with benign thyroid disease. Although routine serum calcitonin measurement has been advocated in some European countries, as a screening test for medullary thyroid cancer in patients with thyroid nodules, it is not done routinely in the United States. Furthermore, of studies showing that calcitonin screening is helpful, most used pentagastrin stimulation, which is not available in the United States or Canada. Without a known risk for medullary thyroid cancer (such as family history or other manifestation of multiple endocrine neoplasia type 2), routine measurement of serum calcitonin has low yield and high false-positive risk and is not cost effective.

SIZE OF THYROID NODULE

Current guidelines generally recommend further evaluation only for thyroid nodules larger than 1 cm. Nodules smaller than 1 cm in patients with previous radiation exposure, family history of thyroid cancer, or other high-risk clinical findings, such as hoarseness or rapid growth, may warrant biopsy. Evaluation of multinodular goiters follows similar criteria for biopsy as for solitary thyroid nodules. Rapidly growing goiters or those causing compressive symptoms, such as dysphagia, dysphonia or dyspnea, have independent indications for thyroidectomy and may not need biopsy.

BIOPSY

FNA biopsy can be done by palpation, but ultrasound-guided biopsy is associated with fewer nondiagnostic aspirates. To address variability in the reporting of FNA results for thyroid nodules, the National Cancer Institute developed the *Bethesda Classification* of thyroid cytopathology in 2009. In this system there are six categories that represent a spectrum for the risk of thyroid cancer. Category I is nondiagnostic, and categories II and VI are benign and malignant, respectively. Benign FNA cytology (category II) has a malignancy rate of 3%. A small subset of thyroid nodules with very high-risk ultrasound characteristic will likely have a much higher

ATA nodule sonographic pattern risk of malignancy

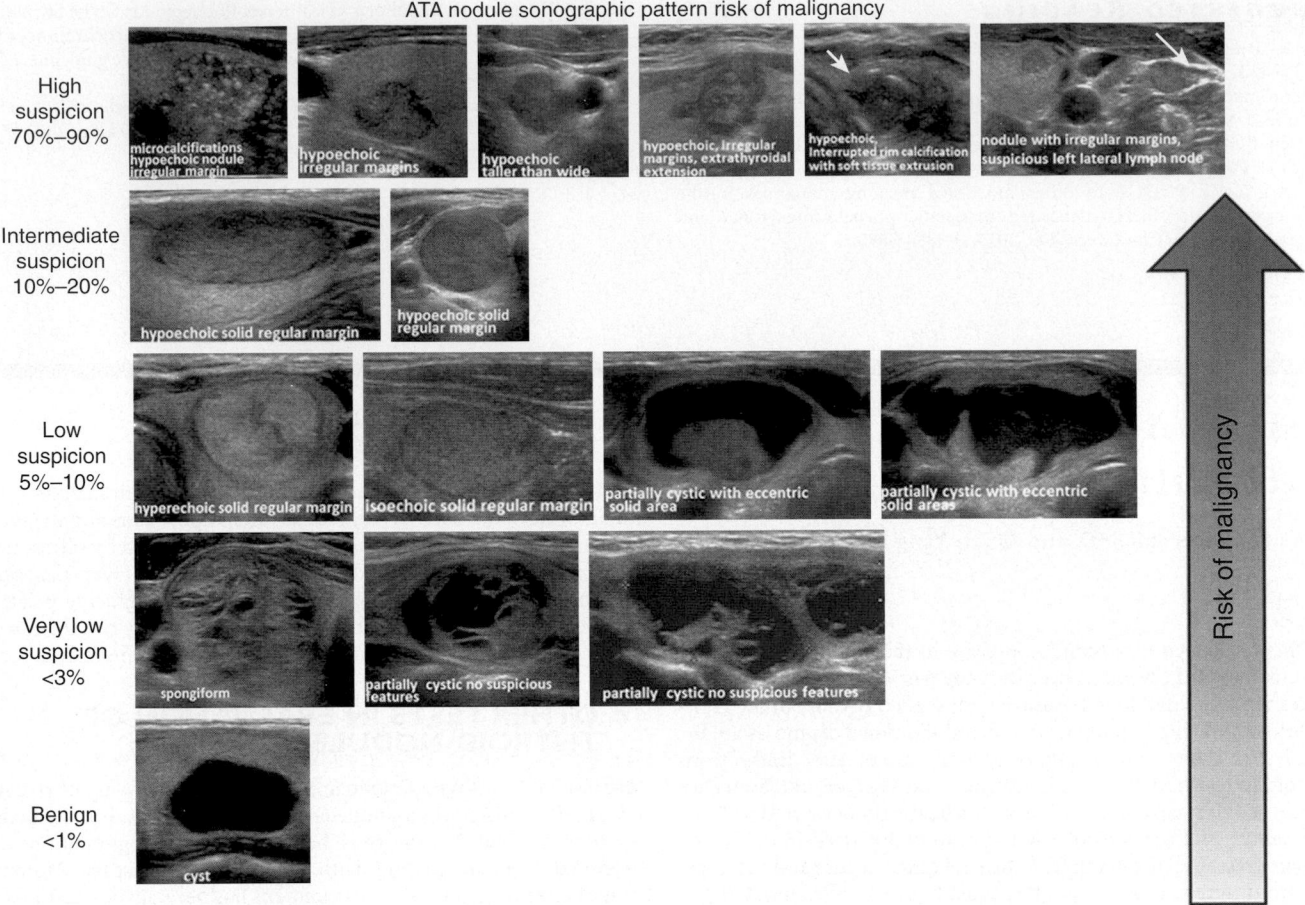

FIGURE 1 American Thyroid Association (ATA) nodule sonographic pattern risk of malignancy. *(From Haugen BR Md, Alexander EK, Bible KC, et al. 2015 American Thyroid Association Management Guidelines for Adult Patients with Thyroid Nodules and Differentiated Thyroid Cancer. Thyroid. 2015;14:26, Fig 2.)*

risk of malignancy even with a benign FNA cytology. Malignant biopsies (category VI) have an accuracy rate of close to 99%. Categories III through V nodules have a spectrum of risk that varies by centers and depends also on the malignancy rates of the population ("pretest probability"). Category III nodules include nodule with atypia of undetermined significance (AUS) and follicular lesion of undetermined significance (FLUS). Category IV nodules include follicular neoplasm (FN)/suspicious for a follicular neoplasm. Hurthle cell neoplasms are included in this category. Category V nodules are those suspicious for malignancy. The reported rates of cancer in these categories are 5% to 15% for AUS/FLUS, 15% to 30% for FN, and 60% to 75% for suspicious for malignancy lesions (Table 1).

■ INDETERMINATE NODULES

For patients with benign or malignant nodules there is usually a clear treatment plan. For FNA cytology indeterminate nodules, Bethesda categories III and IV, the decision for operation versus observation is more complex because of the uncertainty for risk of malignancy. Over the past decade there has been an explosion of research into molecular analysis of these thyroid nodules with indeterminate cytology. Molecular testing adds significant cost and may improve the accuracy of diagnosis over that of cytology alone but may or may not change the treatment plan. Knowing when and whether to use which molecular tests and how to interpret their results has become an important prerequisite for a modern thyroid surgeon.

TABLE 1 The Bethesda System for Reporting Thyroid Cytopathology: Implied Risk of Malignancy

Diagnostic Category	Risk of Malignancy (%)
I Nondiagnostic or unsatisfactory	1-4
II Benign	0-3
III Atypia of undetermined significance or follicular lesion of undetermined significance	~5-15*
IV Follicular neoplasm or suspicious for a follicular neoplasm	15-30
V Suspicious for malignancy	60-75
VI Malignant	97-99

From Cibas ES, Ali SZ. The Bethesda System for reporting thyroid cytopathology. *Am J Clin Pathol.* 2009;132:658-665.

*Estimate extrapolated from histopathologic data from patients with "repeated atypicals."

FNA, Fine-needle aspiration.

■ MOLECULAR TESTING

Molecular testing may be used for patients with indeterminate nodules to help with the decision to operate (or to perform a more aggressive operation) or to observe. It is important to know that molecular testing rarely gives a simple yes and no answer but usually returns a probability for risk of cancer for the nodule tested. For some molecular testing a positive test can increase significantly the probability of cancer, a high positive predictive value (PPV). For others a negative test can lower significantly the probability of cancer, a high negative predictive value (NPV). Which test to choose depends on what clinical decision is being made. In addition to the sensitivity and specificity of the tests, the interpretation of the test (PPV and NPV) is affected significantly by the pretest probability of cancer. A very sensitive test used in a population with low pretest probability may generate many false-positive results. On the other hand, a very specific test used in a population with high risk of cancer would risk false negatives.

■ MUTATIONAL ANALYSIS

Deoxyribonucleic Acid Genotyping

Most differentiated thyroid cancer appears to have only a single driver mutation that causes the cancer. Mutational analysis tests for specific gene mutations (point mutations or rearrangements) that are present in some thyroid cancers but not in normal or benign thyroid tumors. It can be performed on FNA material even in the case of a few hundred cell yields. Earlier panels analyzed for seven gene mutations in *BRAF, RAS, RET/PTC,* and *PAX8/PPARγ* and found excellent PPV of 88% to 95%. However, a negative result could not definitively rule out malignancy. Therefore the test had a risk of false negative and missing a cancer of 5.9% to 28%, depending of the pretest risk of cancer according to the Bethesda category. Current panels of mutational analysis (ThySeq II) improved the sensitivity by testing for additional mutations (including 60 point mutations, 13 rearrangements, and 42 fusions) and lowered the false-negative rate to about 5%, but at the same time increased the risk of false positive to about 20%.

Messenger RNA Microarray

Gene Expression Classifier

Cancer and benign thyroid nodules have different profiles of gene expression when analyzed by messenger RNA (mRNA) microarray. FNA material of indeterminate nodules can be tested for gene expression and reclassified to higher or lower risk for cancer (gene expression classifier, GEC). Currently, the most commonly used GEC test analyzes the expression profile of 142 genes. A large multicenter study showed that GEC is excellent in ruling out cancer for nodules that were Bethesda category III (5% to 15% cancer risk) or IV (15% to 30% cancer risk). A negative GEC test dropped the risk of cancer to 5% and 6%, respectively. However, for Bethesda category V (suspicious for malignancy, 70% cancer risk) a negative GEC test still carried a cancer risk of 15%. Thus GEC is useful for patients with Bethesda III or IV thyroid nodules who wish to defer surgery if possible. Because the test was designed to have high sensitivity, the positive predictive value of GEC is only about 40% in Bethesda III and

IV nodules. Again, the PPV and NPV are influenced significantly by cancer rate in the population tested so that the test results should be interpreted appropriately to aid surgical decision.

■ COMBINATION OF MUTATIONAL ANALYSIS AND MICRORNA ANALYSIS

Another commercially available test uses a combination of mutational analysis and gene expression classifier and supported by only a single study. The original panel of seven-gene mutational analysis is performed first. If mutational analysis is positive (which identified 69% of the cancers), it is reported as cancer. If mutational analysis is negative, a 10 microRNA (miRNA) (gene expression classifier is applied (which identified another 20% of the cancers) with an overall sensitivity of 89% and specificity of 85%.

■ SURGICAL MANAGEMENT

Although surgery is not the main focus of this chapter, it is obvious that diagnostic testing for thyroid nodules has significant implications for thyroid surgery. Current guidelines have trended toward more conservative surgery (lobectomy instead of total thyroidectomy with no routine central neck node dissection) for smaller, low-risk thyroid cancers. If a diagnostic lobectomy is also the definitive treatment for low-risk small cancer, preoperative confirmation of thyroid cancer may become less useful. On the other hand, if molecular characteristic of cancer (e.g., *BRAF* mutation) should influence the aggressiveness of treatment, then molecular testing may become more relevant. Indications other than risk of cancer may be present for patients with thyroid nodules. In these patients, extensive workup for the possibility of thyroid cancer may not be necessary or useful.

■ CONCLUSION

As more thyroid nodules are being found, it is important for a thyroid surgeon to have a clear algorithm for their evaluation. Ultrasound is the primary imaging test for a thyroid nodule. Size and ultrasound characteristics are used to determine the need for FNA. Cytology should be reported based on Bethesda classification, which stratifies the risk of cancer. Advances in molecular testing, including mutational analysis and gene expression classifier, are potentially useful for surgical decision in patients with Bethesda category III and IV indeterminate nodules. Clinical judgment remains paramount in deciding when to use these tests and how to interpret them.

Suggested Readings

Alexander EK, Kennedy GC, Baloch ZW. Preoperative diagnosis of benign thyroid nodules with indeterminate cytology. *N Engl J Med.* 2012;367:705-715.

Cibas ES, Ali SZ. The Bethesda System for reporting thyroid cytopathology. *Am J Clin Pathol.* 2009;132:658-665.

Haugen BR, Alexander EK, Bible KC, et al. 2015 American Thyroid Association management guidelines for adult patients with thyroid nodules and differentiated thyroid cancer. *Thyroid.* 2015.

National Comprehensive Cancer Network. Thyroid carcinoma. (version 2.2015). <http://www.nccn.org/professionals/physician_gls/pdf/thyroid.pdf>.

NONTOXIC GOITER

Stacie A. Kahan, MD, and Martha A. Zeiger, MD, FACS

The term *goiter* is derived from the French (*goiter*) and Latin (*guttur*), both meaning throat. A goiter refers to a thyroid gland that is enlarged to twice its normal size or weighs more than 40 g. Goiters have existed since the beginning of humankind and commonly have been depicted in artwork over the ages. Indeed, images of goiters were included in illustrations by Leonardo da Vinci and in Michelangelo's Sistine Chapel; however, the function of the thyroid gland and the cause of goiter remained elusive until the nineteenth century. Influenced by Theodor Billroth and the father of thyroid surgery, Theodor Kocher, William Stewart Halsted standardized the technique of thyroidectomy and wrote of his utmost respect for the gland and of the artful skill necessary for its "extirpation."

■ PATHOGENESIS

Classically, the cause for the development of a goiter is dietary iodine deficiency, which leads to hypothyroidism, an increase in thyroid-stimulating hormone (TSH), and, in turn, thyroid gland hypertrophy. This disorder is especially found in mountainous regions such as the Himalayas and the Andes and in lowland regions far from the ocean. Goiters in endemic areas also have been attributed to goitrogens found in food such as maize, bamboo shoots, and sweet potatoes. Most of the surgical literature, however, relates to nonendemic goiters. Other causative factors of goiter development include genetic factors, smoking, autoimmune thyroid disease (Graves' or Hashimoto's disease), malignancy, dyshormonogenesis, and infiltrative diseases. Rare causes include TSH-secreting pituitary tumors and thyroid hormone resistance. Patients with goiters may be euthyroid, hypothyroid, or hyperthyroid. The goiter may be associated with simple or diffuse gland enlargement without nodules or may have a uninodular or multinodular pattern. The focus of this chapter is the evaluation and surgical management of the nontoxic goiter.

■ CLINICAL PRESENTATION

Goiters may be completely asymptomatic or may give rise to locally compressive symptoms. A complete history should ascertain whether the patient is experiencing compressive symptoms of the upper respiratory or alimentary tracts, including cough, stridor, shortness of breath, hoarseness, choking sensation (especially when supine), dysphagia, aspiration, the presence of a globus sensation (a lump in one's throat), or pain. Other conditions in the differential diagnosis with similar symptoms can include aerodigestive tract neoplasms, gastroesophageal reflux, dysmotility disorders, esophageal diverticulum or stricture, and asthma. In general, symptoms develop gradually, as most goiters demonstrate slow growth patterns. Acute regional and airway symptoms may develop secondary to spontaneous hemorrhage into an existing nodule or occasionally after fine-needle aspiration (FNA) biopsy. Symptoms associated with hypothyroidism and hyperthyroidism also should be elicited from the patient. Finally, a family history of thyroid disease and risk factors for malignancy, such as exposure to ionizing radiation, should be obtained.

Physical examination should assess the size, consistency, and mobility or fixation of the mass. The examiner should determine if the gland has unilateral or bilateral nodularity, diffuse enlargement, tracheal deviation, or substernal extension. It is important to determine if the caudal aspect of the gland can be palpated and if the gland rises with swallowing. The central and lateral compartments of the neck also should be evaluated for cervical lymphadenopathy. Preoperative laryngoscopy to assess laryngeal nerve function should be considered in patients undergoing thyroidectomy for goiter, especially in the setting of prior anterior neck surgery or subjective symptoms of hoarseness or dysphonia.

■ LABORATORY AND RADIOLOGIC EVALUATION

TSH, free thyroxine (T4), and triiodothyronine (T3) levels should be obtained to evaluate for subclinical or overt thyrotoxicosis, hypothyroidism, or euthyroidism. Thyroid ultrasound should be used to assess gland architecture, to determine the size and number of nodules and the need for FNA biopsy. Nodules larger than 1 cm or with suspicious features should be biopsied preferentially. Ultrasonographic features such as microcalcifications, irregular margins, hypoechogenicity, extrathyroidal extension, hypervascularity, and suspicious lymph nodes are associated with an increased likelihood of malignancy and would warrant further evaluation with FNA; however, the incidence of thyroid cancer within a multinodular goiter is no different than with solitary thyroid nodules (5% to 10%). A chest radiograph is not routinely used to image the thyroid gland but is recommended for a substernal goiter and may demonstrate tracheal narrowing, tracheal deviation, and the degree of mediastinal extension. Routine computed tomographic (CT) scan of the neck and chest can be very helpful in preoperative assessment of large cervical or substernal goiters (Figures 1 and 2). With contrast, the extent of the goiter can be defined accurately, and its exact relationship to the trachea, esophagus, and great vessels can be determined. One must be cognizant of the rare intrathoracic or aberrant thyroid, a congenital abnormality in which the blood supply arises from the intrathoracic vessels and a thoracic thyroid separate from the cervical thyroid. In these rare cases, the surgeon may have to perform a median sternotomy to gain access to the blood supply originating from the thyroid ima, subclavian, or internal mammary artery.

■ INDICATIONS FOR TREATMENT

Surgery is the mainstay and most rational and definitive treatment for nontoxic goiter. Indications for surgery include regional aerodigestive tract symptoms without other cause, tracheal compression, nodules larger than 4 cm, suspected or proven malignancy, and substernal goiters. The extent of the surgery should be tailored to the extent of the disease as determined by preoperative imaging. For dominant unilateral goitrous enlargement without any nodularity of the contralateral lobe, a thyroid lobectomy may be appropriate. Total thyroidectomy is appropriate for patients with evidence of bilateral goiter, patients with a positive family history of thyroid disease or thyroid cancer, and patients who are on thyroid hormone supplementation before surgery.

■ SURGERY

The surgical management of goiters is well tolerated, even in those who are older and infirm, and outcomes can be optimized, especially when performed by an experienced surgeon along with an excellent anesthesia team. An experienced anesthesiologist who is familiar with complex airway management can easily intubate the majority of patients with large goiters, even those with tracheal deviation. Fiber optic intubation may be necessary to safely secure the airway in cases of marked tracheal deviation or compression but is rarely required.

The patient should be placed in the supine position with the neck hyperextended. A generous Kocher's incision extending to the medial edge of the sternocleidomastoid muscles is performed, and superior and inferior subplatysmal flaps are created, extending to the thyroid cartilage and the sternal notch for optimal exposure. The strap muscles are divided in the midline and reflected laterally. It is sometimes helpful to transversely divide the sternothyroid muscle near the upper pole to increase exposure of the upper pole vessels. The muscle(s) can be reapproximated with an absorbable suture at the

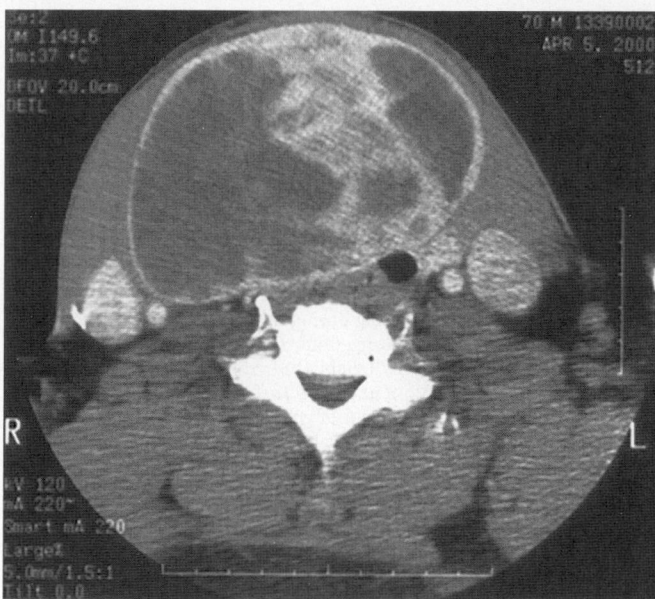

FIGURE 1 Axial section of computed tomographic scan with contrast demonstrating a massively enlarged goiter with marked tracheal deviation.

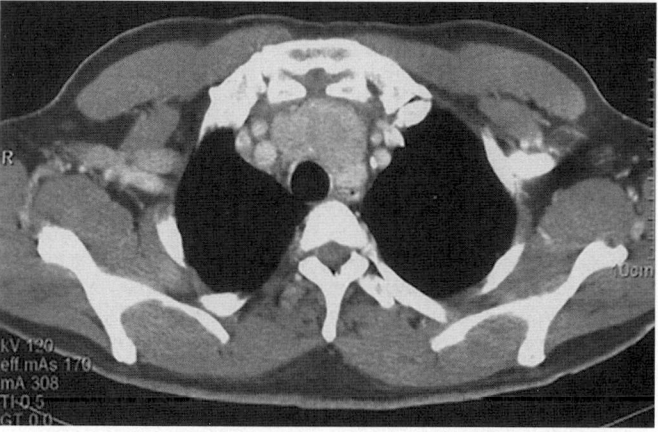

FIGURE 2 Goiter with significant substernal component.

end of the case. In large goiters, the anterior jugular veins as well as the vessels of the inferior and superior poles may be congested. It is imperative to obtain prompt and direct control of all vasculature with ties, clips, or commercial hemostatic devices. The superior and inferior vascular pedicles are typically in their normal anatomic locations. Large goiters may have additional enlarged arteries and veins that require hemostatic control.

It is important to recognize that the recurrent laryngeal nerve (RLN) is usually in its normal position in the tracheoesophageal groove. The mass of the goiter, however, will obstruct initial visualization of the nerve and thus one should try to obtain a vagal signal within the carotid sheath to document nerve integrity. Identification of the vagus nerve allows for intermittent stimulation to confirm the integrity of the RLN during the dissection, although often even this is impossible, because of the size of the goiter, until the goiter is delivered into the neck. Of note, one does not need to open the carotid sheath in order to test the vagus nerve. When utilizing a nerve monitor, its signal is only useful with the presence of both a positive and a negative signal and documented with any tissue that is to be divided and is suspected of including the RLN.

The normal steps of routine thyroidectomy, including middle thyroid vein division, inferior thyroid vein division, and identifica-

tion of the inferior thyroid artery, are performed. The inferior thyroid artery might not be identified at this time, depending on the size of the goiter, but the branches of the artery may be taken directly on the thyroid capsule in order to help preserve the inferior parathyroid gland. Attention should then be turned to the superior pole where the plane between the larynx and the upper pole is opened (Jolles space), exposing the branches of the superior thyroid artery, the superior thyroid vein, and the external branch of the superior laryngeal nerve. Often, however, the superior laryngeal nerve cannot be identified during dissection. Nerve stimulation can be used to trace the path of the external branch of the superior laryngeal nerve to avoid injury during ligation of the superior pole vessels. The vessels should be ligated individually on the thyroid capsule, minimizing the risk of incorporating the external nerve in the vascular ligature.

At this point, gentle finger dissection in the capsular plane can allow for the goiter, be it cervical or partially substernal, to be delivered into the wound in its entirety. The blood supply to substernal goiters is almost always cervical through the inferior thyroid artery. Fascial bands produced during digital dissection can be cauterized if transparent. Thicker pedicles of tissue should be approached with more caution and after testing them with the nerve monitor.

Finally, the RLN is identified and traced to its insertion point caudal to the cricoid cartilage and deep to the inferior constrictor muscle. With anteriorly displaced goiters, the RLN and parathyroid glands often are displaced posteriorly, safely out of harm's way. In rare instances, the nerve can be splayed over the surface of the goiter or even pass over the gland between nodules. The nerve should be dissected carefully away from the thyroid tissue with both blunt and sharp dissection. Electrocautery should be used cautiously during this meticulous dissection around the nerve. To avoid inadvertent injury or stretching of the nerve, it may be wise to leave a small remnant of thyroid tissue at the insertion point. The dissected nerve may appear significantly redundant but will stimulate normally and function postoperatively. A capsular dissection also decreases the chances of parathyroid gland devascularization. Devascularized parathyroid glands should be cut into small (1-mm) pieces and autotransplanted into pockets of the sternocleidomastoid muscle at the end of the case, after documentation of parathyroid tissue by frozen section. These pockets should be marked with either a nonabsorbable suture or a clip. Unfortunately, the massive thyroid gland surface may obscure the parathyroid glands and make them extremely difficult to identify. Parathyroid glands may be subcapsular or even intrathyroidal and thus impossible to preserve.

The contralateral thyroid lobe is dissected and removed in the same manner. Before passing the specimen off the field, it should be examined carefully in an attempt to identify subcapsular parathyroid glands that should be autotransplanted after confirmation by frozen section (Figure 3). When utilizing a nerve monitor, a normal and audible signal from the RLN bilaterally at completion of the dissection indicates intact RLN function.

For closure, the strap muscles and platysma are reapproximated using an absorbable suture and the skin is closed with a running absorbable 4-0 subcuticular stitch. Surgical glue may be used in place of a dressing. Drains usually are not required, and the placement of a drain has never been shown to reduce the risk of life-threatening neck hematoma.

■ POSTOPERATIVE MANAGEMENT

Complications related to surgery for nontoxic goiter are essentially the same as those for routine thyroid surgery. These include bleeding, infection, RLN injury, voice hoarseness, superior laryngeal nerve injury, and temporary or permanent hypoparathyroidism. All patients generally are admitted overnight after total thyroidectomy for goiter. They are observed for development of hematoma or symptomatic hypoparathyroidism, and calcium levels are checked in the postoperative period. Patients are treated with calcium supplementation upon discharge if calcium levels are low on the first

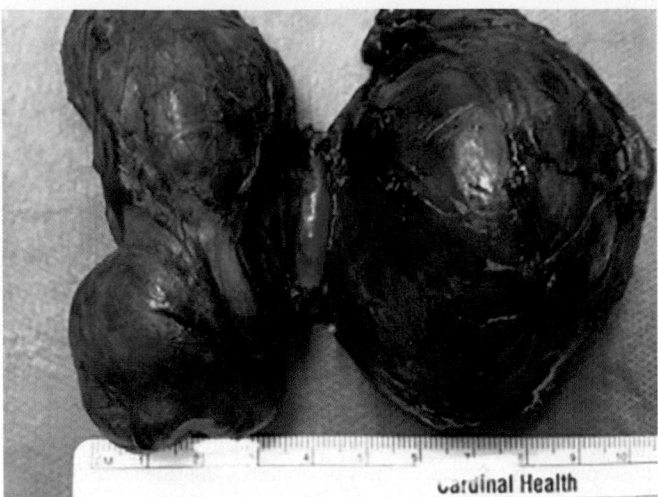

FIGURE 3 Surgical specimen of an enlarged multinodular goiter.

postoperative day. Thyroid hormone replacement is initiated on the third postoperative day. TSH levels are checked 4 to 6 weeks after surgery, with titration of thyroid hormone replacement as necessary.

SUGGESTED READINGS

Angelos P. Recurrent laryngeal nerve monitoring: state of the art, ethical and legal issues. *Surg Clin North Am*. 2009;89:1157-1169.

Baloch ZW, LiVolsi VA. Current role and value of fine-needle aspiration in nodular goitre. *Best Pract Res Clin Endocrinol Metab*. 2014;28:531-544.

Barczynski M, Randolph GW, Cernea CR, et al. External branch of the superior laryngeal nerve monitoring during thyroid and parathyroid surgery: International Neural Monitoring Study Group standards guideline statement. *Laryngoscope*. 2013;123(suppl 4):S1-S14.

Chen AY, Bernet VJ, Carty SE, et al. American Thyroid Association statement on optimal surgical management of goiter. *Thyroid*. 2014;24:181-189.

Lee KC, Zeiger MA. William Stewart Halsted and goiter: from "horrid butchery" to "supreme triumph." In: Zeiger MA, Shen WT, Felger EA, eds. *The Supreme Triumph of the Surgeon's Art: A Narrative History of Endocrine Surgery*. San Francisco: University of California Medical Humanities Press; 2013:60-74.

THE MANAGEMENT OF THYROIDITIS

Christopher R. McHenry, MD, FACS

The term *thyroiditis* refers to inflammation of the thyroid gland. Thyroiditis consists of a diverse group of acute, subacute, and chronic conditions that are characterized by inflammation of the thyroid gland (Box 1). Thyroiditis may be manifested by neck pain and tenderness, enlargement of the thyroid gland, thyroid dysfunction, and rarely fever. Patients may be thyrotoxic, euthyroid, or hypothyroid. Patients may be asymptomatic. Patients may develop hypothyroidism after a large iodine load, which occurs with administration of intravenous contrast material or iodine-containing drugs.

Evaluation consists of a history and physical examination; laboratory evaluation, including free thyroxine (T4), free triiodothyronine (T3), thyrotropin (thyroid-stimulating hormone, or TSH) levels with or without an antimicrosomal antibody titer, erythrocyte sedimentation rate, and radioiodine uptake; and thyroid scintigraphy. Ultrasound may be used for evaluation of thyroid enlargement or associated nodular thyroid disease. Computed tomography has a role for evaluation of large goiters to determine the extent of substernal extension (Figure 1) and mass effect, primarily tracheal impingement (Figure 2).

Various agents are used for treatment of thyroiditis, including acetylsalicylic acid, nonsteroidal anti-inflammatory drugs, corticosteroids or other immunosuppressive agents, beta-blocker therapy for thyrotoxicosis, and thyroid hormone replacement for hypothyroidism. Surgical therapy is indicated for patients with large goiters and compressive symptoms. The clinical entities, which account for most cases of thyroiditis (see Box 1), are reviewed in more detail, emphasizing their unique characteristics and specific treatment.

◼ HASHIMOTO'S THYROIDITIS

Hashimoto's thyroiditis is a chronic, progressive autoimmune disorder characterized by diffuse lymphocytic infiltration of the thyroid gland with formation of germinal centers, follicular cell atrophy, Hürthle cell metaplasia, Hürthle cell nodules, and fibrosis. There is a familial predisposition and it tends to occur in association with other autoimmune diseases. Patients with Hashimoto's thyroiditis also have an increased risk of thyroid lymphoma. Hashimoto's thyroiditis is the most common cause of goiter and hypothyroidism in the Unites States and in other countries with high iodine intake. It has been reported to affect approximately 2% of the population in the United States. Increased antimicrosomal or antithyroglobulin antibody titers are present in 10% of the population and in 25% of women over the age of 60.

Most patients are seen with an asymptomatic diffuse goiter, which can enlarge over time. Some patients complain of neck pressure or fullness and less commonly of neck pain. Approximately 20% to 25% of patients will be hypothyroid at the time of presentation and may have symptoms of hypothyroidism (Box 2). Patients also may have mild thyrotoxicosis, referred to as Hashitoxicosis, which occurs as a result of immunoglobulins that increase thyroid hormone synthesis. Patients with large goiters may complain of dysphagia, dyspnea, hoarseness, cough, and a choking sensation.

On physical examination, patients have a nontender, diffusely firm, bumpy, or bosselated thyroid gland. Associated thyroid nodules may be present but are not typical. An associated thyroid nodule is usually a benign Hürthle cell nodule; however, all nodules 1 cm or larger or smaller nodules with abnormal sonographic features should be evaluated with fine-needle aspiration (FNA) biopsy to exclude cancer. Enlarged lymph nodes may be present and are usually benign reactive lymph nodes. Ophthalmopathy may occur rarely in patients with Hashimoto's thyroiditis. A rapidly enlarging goiter in a patient with Hashimoto's thyroiditis should raise suspicion for lymphoma, and FNA biopsy and flow cytometry should be performed to help establish a diagnosis.

The diagnostic evaluation for a patient suspected of having Hashimoto's thyroiditis should consist of measurement of antimicrosomal and antithyroglobulin antibody titers, a screening serum TSH level to evaluate the functional status of the thyroid gland, and an ultrasound evaluation of the neck. Almost all patients have elevated antimicrosomal antibodies (90%) and less often antithyroglobulin antibodies (20% to 50%) and TSH receptor blocking antibodies (10%). The diagnosis of Hashimoto's thyroiditis also can be made by FNA biopsy, which reveals a predominance of lymphocytes with histiocytes, plasma cells, and Hürthle cells. Rare patients may have a normal antimicrosomal and antithyroglobulin antibody titer and are diagnosed with Hashimoto's thyroiditis based on an ultrasound examination that demonstrates diffuse heterogeneous

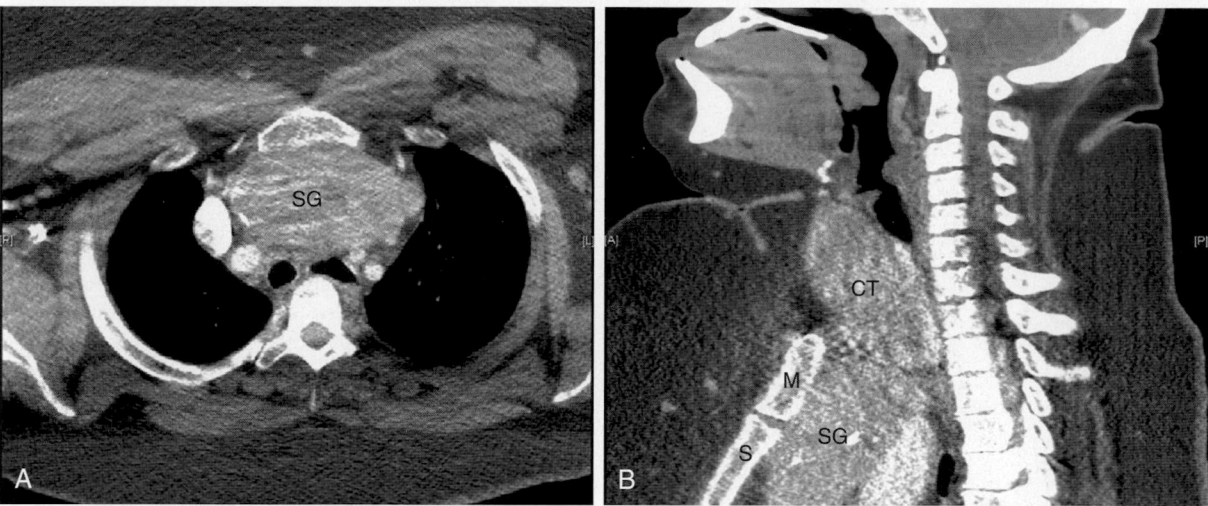

FIGURE 1 A large substernal goiter from Hashimoto's thyroiditis. **A,** Anterior-posterior view of the substernal goiter. **B,** Coronal view demonstrating the cervical thyroid (CT), the substernal goiter (SG), and its relationship to the manubrium (M) and the sternum (S).

BOX 1: Various Forms of Thyroiditis

1. Hashimoto's thyroiditis (chronic lymphocytic or autoimmune thyroiditis)
2. Subacute granulomatous or de Quervain's thyroiditis
3. Painless or silent thyroiditis (lymphocytic thyroiditis)
4. Drug-induced thyroiditis
5. Radioiodine-induced thyroiditis
6. Riedel's thyroiditis
7. Acute suppurative thyroiditis

BOX 2: Symptoms of Hypothyroidism

Weight gain
Fatigue
Coarse, dry skin
Constipation
Cold intolerance
Menstrual irregularity
Muscle cramps
Hair loss
Decreased libido

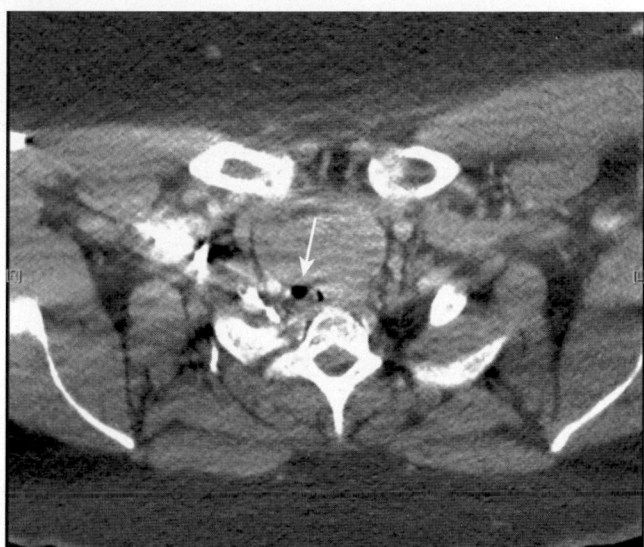

FIGURE 2 A substernal goiter that is compressing the trachea (*arrow*) in a patient with thyroiditis.

hypoechogenicity of the thyroid gland or incidentally based on pathologic evaluation of the thyroid gland removed for some other reason.

Hashimoto's thyroiditis is usually asymptomatic and requires no treatment. In patients with hypothyroidism, treatment consists of thyroid hormone replacement. Patients start taking a replacement dose of levothyroxine (1.6 µg/kg, once daily). The goal of therapy is to have the serum TSH level in the normal range. Thyroxine has a half-life of approximately 7 days. As a result, steady-state hormone levels are not achieved for 4 to 6 weeks. A serum TSH level is obtained 6 weeks after initiating therapy to ensure that the patient is on the appropriate dose of levothyroxine. Thyroid hormone replacement results in a decrease in goiter size.

Patients with Hashimoto's thyroiditis are followed long term for the potential development of hypothyroidism, thyroid enlargement, compressive symptoms, and lymphoma. Hashimoto's thyroiditis is often associated with a defect in organification of iodine and, as a result, patients with euthyroid goiter are at risk for hypothyroidism

after the administration of a large iodine load that occurs with intravenous contrast or iodine-containing drugs. Patients with Hashimoto's thyroiditis have a higher incidence of lymphoma than the general population. It is most commonly a B-cell variant of non-Hodgkin's lymphoma. Up to 80% of patients with thyroid lymphoma will have associated Hashimoto's thyroiditis.

Thyroidectomy is indicated for patients with a large goiter (Figure 3) and compressive symptoms and for associated nodular thyroid disease when there is suspicion of cancer. When physical examination, ultrasound, and intraoperative palpation confirm that disease is limited to one lobe, a thyroid lobectomy and isthmusectomy is adequate therapy. Total thyroidectomy is preferable for bilateral disease.

Thyroidectomy is effective in relieving compressive symptoms in patients with Hashimoto's thyroiditis, but it can be challenging because chronic inflammation makes the anatomic dissection more difficult. The firmness of the thyroid gland makes it difficult to retract anteromedially and difficult to remove without excessive

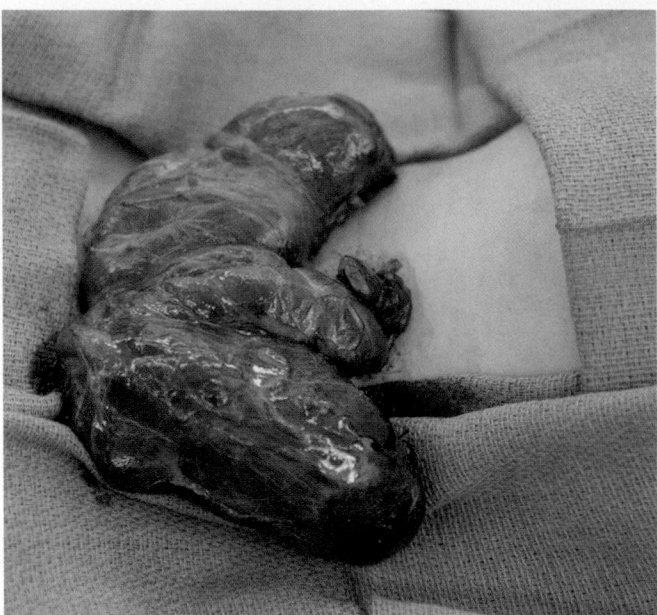

FIGURE 3 Intraoperative photograph of a patient with a large goiter from Hashimoto's thyroiditis that was causing compressive symptoms.

BOX 3: Symptoms of Thyrotoxicosis

Palpitations
Anxiety
Tremor
Heat intolerance
Thinning of hair and hair loss
Frequent loose bowel movements
Irritability
Insomnia
Increased sweating
Muscle weakness
Menstrual irregularities
Infertility

traction on the recurrent laryngeal nerves. It also makes the identification of the recurrent laryngeal nerves more difficult. In some series, the complication rates are higher.

■ SILENT AND POSTPARTUM THYROIDITIS

Silent and postpartum thyroiditis are variants of an autoimmune-mediated, self-limited, destruction-induced thyroiditis characterized by a thyrotoxic phase followed by a euthyroid phase, a hypothyroid phase, and a recovery phase. They are also known as lymphocytic thyroiditis because of the characteristic histopathology, which includes diffuse lymphocytic infiltration with focal or diffuse follicles and follicular cell degeneration. Fibrosis, germinal centers, and Hürthle cell metaplasia, which characteristically are seen in Hashimoto's thyroiditis, are usually absent. Patients with silent or postpartum thyroiditis often have a personal or family history of other autoimmune diseases, which suggests that there is some inherited susceptibility.

Patients usually are seen with the acute onset of symptomatic thyrotoxicosis (Box 3) and nontender thyroid enlargement without neck pain. The thyrotoxic phase is related to autoimmune-induced destruction of the follicular cells of the thyroid gland with release of

thyroid hormone stores and usually lasts for a few months until the thyroid hormone stores have been depleted. The thyrotoxic phase in patients with postpartum thyroiditis occurs 2 to 8 weeks after delivery. The thyrotoxic phase is followed by a euthyroid phase, which can last for a few months, and then by a hypothyroid phase with symptomatic hypothyroidism (see Box 2), which can last for up to 1 year. Most patients recover and become euthyroid, but 20% of patients develop permanent hypothyroidism.

During the thyrotoxic phase, free T4 levels, free T3 levels, or both are increased and the serum TSH level and radioiodine uptake are low. Thyroid-stimulating immunoglobulin levels, which are elevated in patients with Graves' disease, are negative. Patients have elevated antimicrosomal and antithyroglobulin antibody titers. Ultrasound examination of the thyroid gland reveals diffuse hypoechogenicity, which resolves with resolution of the thyroiditis.

Patients are followed with serial thyroid function tests to determine the clinical progression through the various phases of silent or postpartum thyroiditis. The thyrotoxic phase of silent or postpartum thyroiditis can be treated with a beta-blocker agent when necessary. Antithyroid drugs and radioiodine therapy are not effective for treatment of thyrotoxicosis in patients with silent or postpartum thyroiditis. The thyrotoxicosis occurs as a result of increased release of thyroid hormone stores, not as a result of increased synthesis of thyroid hormone. A beta-blocker agent may be of value for control of symptoms related to excess sympathetic nervous system activity such as palpitations, tremor, heat intolerance, and diaphoresis. During the hypothyroid phase, levothyroxine therapy is started in patients who are symptomatic and may need to be continued for 6 to 12 months. This therapy eventually will need to be discontinued to determine transition to the recovery phase. Lifelong thyroid hormone replacement will be necessary for the 20% of patients who develop permanent hypothyroidism. Recurrences are common after subsequent pregnancies and also are not unusual after silent thyroiditis, warranting long-term follow-up.

■ SUBACUTE THYROIDITIS

Subacute thyroiditis also is referred to as subacute granulomatous thyroiditis and de Quervain's thyroiditis. It is a self-limited inflammatory condition of the thyroid gland that usually occurs after a viral upper respiratory infection and lasts for 1 to 3 months. Patients are seen with acute onset of neck pain and tenderness, often with fever, myalgias, generalized malaise, and symptoms of thyrotoxicosis (see Box 3). The neck pain may radiate to the jaw, ear, and upper chest. Neck tenderness can be severe, such that patients are unable to tolerate palpation or tight-fitting clothing. Most patients have an asymmetrically enlarged, tender goiter.

Patients typically develop transient thyrotoxicosis, which usually is followed by euthyroidism and then transient hypothyroidism. Fifteen percent of patients may develop permanent hypothyroidism. Thyrotoxicosis occurs as a result of inflammatory destruction of the follicular epithelial cells, which release preformed thyroid hormone. As a result, free T4 levels, free T3 levels, or both are elevated and TSH level is suppressed. The erythrocyte sedimentation rate, C-reactive protein level, and white blood cell count are elevated. TSH suppression inhibits iodine uptake by the thyroid gland. Radioiodine uptake measurements, which are used to help determine the cause of thyrotoxicosis, are typically less than 1% in patients with subacute thyroiditis during the thyrotoxic phase. The thyrotoxic phase lasts until the thyroid hormones that are stored by the follicular epithelial cells are depleted, usually in 2 to 8 weeks. The hypothyroid phase also can last 2 to 8 weeks. Most patients recover without any residual thyroid dysfunction.

Ultrasound examination and FNA or core needle biopsy are rarely necessary, although patients with a thyroid nodule and acute hemorrhage may mimic subacute thyroiditis. The sonographic features in a patient with subacute thyroiditis are a heterogeneous hypoechoic gland with a diffuse decrease in vascularity. Needle biopsy, which may be used to differentiate subacute thyroiditis from suppurative thyroiditis, reveals neutrophils, lymphocytes, histiocytes, and giant cells.

The treatment of patients with subacute thyroiditis depends on the severity of the symptoms. When symptoms are mild and tolerable, patients may not need treatment. Most patients benefit from an anti-inflammatory agent for analgesia, acetylsalicylic acid, or a nonsteroidal anti-inflammatory drug such as ibuprofen or naproxen. For severe neck pain or persistent pain after 2 to 3 days of nonsteroidal anti-inflammatory therapy, 40 mg of prednisone once daily is started and other analgesics are discontinued. Most patients experience rapid pain relief with prednisone therapy. After resolution of the pain, the prednisone is tapered. Recurrent pain may occur with dosage reduction, necessitating renewal of higher doses. Subacute thyroiditis is self-limited and most patients experience resolution in 8 weeks.

Short-term beta-blocker therapy may be of value for symptomatic thyrotoxicosis, particularly for patients with palpitations, increased nervousness and anxiety, and tremor. Propranolol, atenolol, or metoprolol may be used, and thyroid function tests should be monitored to establish resolution of thyrotoxicity, for detection of hypothyroidism, and for documentation of eventual euthyroidism or permanent hypothyroidism. Thioamide drugs, propylthiouracil and methimazole, are not indicated because the thyrotoxicosis is not from increased thyroid hormone synthesis but instead from increased release of thyroid hormone from damaged follicular epithelial cells. Iodine-131 therapy is not indicated nor is it effective because radioiodine uptake in patients with subacute thyroiditis is suppressed. The hypothyroidism that ensues is usually transient and subclinical and does not require therapy. Thyroid hormone therapy is usually necessary only for patients with permanent hypothyroidism.

ACUTE SUPPURATIVE THYROIDITIS

Acute suppurative thyroiditis (AST) is a rare, potentially life-threatening disease characterized by neck pain, dysphagia, and odynophagia with fever, a tender goiter, and often systemic toxicity. Patients are usually euthyroid, although transient symptomatic thyrotoxicosis or transient hypothyroidism may occur. Some patients may develop permanent hypothyroidism. In the absence of appropriate intervention, mortality may exceed 10%.

The thyroid gland is an uncommon site of infection, which is thought to be related to multiple factors, including high iodine content, a rich blood supply, extensive lymphatic drainage, and a capsule. Adults who develop AST are often immune compromised, older, or debilitated. The cause of infection is most commonly hematogenous spread, although it also may occur from lymphatic spread, direct extension of the pre-existing abscess, esophageal perforation, neck trauma, or direct inoculation. In children, direct extension from a pyriform sinus fistula is the most common cause.

An initial evaluation includes a complete blood count with differential, thyroid function studies, and blood cultures. In adults, *Staphylococcus aureus* and *Streptococcus pyogenes* are the most common causative organisms. Serial thyroid function studies are recommended because patients may develop thyrotoxicosis related to the release of T3 and T4 from follicular cell destruction. In the setting of thyrotoxicosis, patients have a radioiodine uptake that is usually less than 1%. An ultrasound examination of the thyroid gland and FNA are helpful in establishing the diagnosis and in differentiating AST from subacute thyroiditis and, rarely, thyroid cancer. Gram stain and culture of the thyroid aspirate and antimicrobial susceptibility testing are helpful in directing antibiotic therapy. Computed tomography of the neck and chest is of value to assess for pyriform sinus fistula as well as abscess formation and extrapharyngeal or mediastinal involvement.

The treatment of AST consists of prompt empiric antibiotic therapy and abscess drainage. Antibiotics are modified based on antimicrobial susceptibility data. Abscess drainage is accomplished by ultrasound-guided needle aspiration or open drainage when necessary. Open drainage or thyroidectomy is indicated for patients who undergo clinical deterioration despite antibiotic therapy and ultrasound-guided aspiration or for patients with persistent abscess despite appropriate antibiotic therapy and ultrasound-guided drainage.

RIEDEL'S THYROIDITIS

Riedel's thyroiditis is a rare, chronic, idiopathic inflammatory disease characterized by inflammatory cell infiltration followed by dense fibrous tissue replacement of the thyroid gland, which extends beyond the thyroid gland to involve adjacent structures in the neck. Patients are seen with an enlarging, nontender goiter. They also may have neck pressure, dyspnea, hoarseness, stridor, airway obstruction, and dysphagia from compression of the trachea and esophagus. Patients are often suspected of having anaplastic thyroid cancer. Hypothyroidism occurs in 30% of patients and hypoparathyroidism also may occur from fibrotic replacement of the parathyroid glands. Riedel's thyroiditis is a systemic disease in which one third of patients have fibrosis involving other sites, including the retroperitoneum, mediastinum, lungs, lacrimal and parotid glands, bile ducts (sclerosing cholangitis), and orbits (orbital pseudotumor). It is not uncommon for Riedel's thyroiditis to occur in association with autoimmune diseases such as Addison's disease, diabetes mellitus, and pernicious anemia.

On examination, patients have a firm, fixed mass in the neck that is rock hard in consistency and involves one or both lobes of the thyroid gland. Diagnostic evaluation should include a screening serum TSH level, a serum calcium level, and an ultrasound examination of the neck. Ultrasound examination typically demonstrates diffuse hypoechogenicity, reduced vascularity throughout the entire thyroid gland, and absence of demarcation of the thyroid gland from other surrounding structures. There also may be encasement of the carotid arteries. Computed tomography of the chest, abdomen, and pelvis has a role in evaluating patients for extracervical sites of fibrosis, mainly in the mediastinum and retroperitoneum. FNA biopsy often is not able to be completed because of the hardness of the mass. When successful, FNA biopsy of the mass reveals a paucity of follicular epithelial cells and extensive fibrotic change, findings that cannot be distinguished from the fibrotic change that occurs in patients with poorly differentiated or anaplastic thyroid cancer. Definitive diagnosis requires open biopsy. Riedel's thyroiditis is distinguished from invasive thyroid cancer using immunohistochemistry.

Riedel's thyroiditis may stabilize, resolve spontaneously, or progress over time. It may be a self-limited condition, although in most patients it is a progressive disease. The mainstay of treatment is high-dose corticosteroids, which reduce inflammation and inhibit cytokines, which are involved in the induction of fibrosis. Corticosteroids reduce goiter size and are important in relieving compressive symptoms. Tamoxifen also has been shown to reduce goiter size and relieve compressive symptoms. It works by inducing transforming growth factor beta, an inhibitor of fibroblast proliferation. In patients with symptoms of airway obstruction, an isthmusectomy can be performed to relieve airway compression and make a definitive diagnosis of Riedel's thyroiditis. More extensive surgery can be dangerous because of the loss of normal tissue planes, which is associated with a higher risk for injury to important structures.

Mycophenolate mofetil, an immunosuppressive agent used to prevent transplant rejection; rituximab, a monoclonal antibody directed against the protein CD20 on B cells; and methotrexate, an antimetabolite and antifolate drug, also have been used to treat Riedel's thyroiditis. Patients with hypothyroidism start levothyroxine replacement therapy. Calcium and calcitriol are used for treatment of hypoparathyroidism.

DRUG-INDUCED THYROIDITIS

Drug-induced thyroiditis is a significant adverse side effect that may occur in patients receiving interferon alpha, amiodarone, and tyrosine-kinase inhibitors. Five to ten percent of patients receiving interferon alpha therapy may develop painless or Hashimoto's thyroiditis. Up to 40% of patients with hepatitis C infection receiving interferon alpha develop symptomatic or subclinical thyroiditis. It is thought to occur more often in patients with pre-existing autoimmune dysfunction. When symptoms are severe, interferon alpha is discontinued.

Amiodarone has a molecular structure similar to T3 and T4. One third of its molecular weight is made up of iodine. Amiodarone-induced thyrotoxicosis (AIT) occurs in 3% to 5% of patients on chronic amiodarone therapy. Amiodarone can have a direct toxic effect on the thyroid gland, causing thyroiditis and inflammatory-induced destruction of follicular epithelial cells that results in increased release of stored thyroid hormone, a condition referred to as type II AIT. It is often followed by transient hypothyroidism. This differs from type I AIT, which occurs as a result of an iodine-induced increase in thyroid hormone synthesis, especially in patients with a pre-existing multinodular goiter. It is less common than type II AIT.

The treatment of type II AIT is complicated. In the absence of life-threatening arrhythmias, amiodarone may be discontinued and an alternative antiarrhythmic agent started. However, because of its high lipid solubility, plasma levels of amiodarone decrease very slowly. High-dose prednisone, 40 to 60 mg per day, is first-line therapy for AIT. Beta adrenergic receptor antagonists may be used, but with caution because, in combination with amiodarone, they may cause bradycardia and sinus arrest. Potassium perchlorate, which inhibits iodine uptake and release by the thyroid gland, also has been used to treat AIT, often in combination with a thioamide agent. However, perchlorate is currently not available for use in the United States. Patients with type II AIT who respond to medical therapy, including discontinuation of amiodarone, may develop transient or, less commonly, permanent hypothyroidism requiring thyroid hormone replacement. In patients with persistent AIT despite medical therapy, near total or total thyroidectomy is indicated. Near total or total thyroidectomy results in rapid resolution of thyrotoxicosis and allows for continued use of amiodarone. Subtotal thyroidectomy is not a good option because of the potential for recurrent thyrotoxicosis in patients requiring long-term amiodarone treatment.

Patients with underlying Hashimoto's thyroiditis are more likely to develop amiodarone-induced hypothyroidism. This can be treated with amiodarone withdrawal or thyroid hormone replacement when amiodarone is continued. If amiodarone is discontinued, hypothyroidism usually resolves. However, patients with underlying Hashimoto's thyroiditis may develop permanent hypothyroidism and require lifelong thyroid hormone replacement.

Tyrosine-kinase inhibitors also may cause thyrotoxicosis, possibly from destructive thyroiditis; however, hypothyroidism is the most common abnormality, occurring in 50% to 70% of patients. Thyroid function should be determined before initiation of a tyrosine-kinase inhibitor and at least every 3 months thereafter. Thyroid hormone should be given for patients with hypothyroidism. Discontinuation or dosage reduction of the tyrosine-kinase inhibitor is typically not necessary.

■ RADIOIODINE-INDUCED THYROIDITIS

Patients receiving radioiodine therapy for thyroid cancer, Graves' disease, and toxic and nontoxic multinodular goiter may experience mild to severe neck pain and tenderness and symptomatic thyrotoxicosis from radioiodine-induced follicular cell destruction and release of thyroid hormone stores. This is a rare adverse effect of radioiodine that occurs in less than 1% of patients. The symptoms occur 5 to 10 days after radioiodine administration and are transient, usually resolving within a week. Anti-inflammatory agents and, rarely, steroid therapy are indicated for symptomatic relief.

SUGGESTED READINGS

Farwell AP, Braverman LE. Thyroiditis. In: Randolph GW, ed. *Surgery of the Thyroid and Parathyroid Glands.* Philadelphia: Elsevier; 2003:41-51.

Mulligan D, McHenry CR, Kinney W, Esselstyn CB. Amiodarone-induced thyrotoxicosis: clinical presentation and expanded indications for thyroidectomy. *Surgery.* 1993;114:1114-1119.

Paes JE, Burman KD, Cohen J, Franklyn J, McHenry CR, Shoham S, Kloos RT. Acute bacterial suppurative thyroiditis: a clinical review and expert opinion. *Thyroid.* 2010;20:247-255.

Wormer BA, McHenry CR. Hashimoto's thyroiditis: outcome of surgical resection for patients with thyromegaly and compressive symptoms. *Am J Surg.* 2011;201:416-419.

HYPERTHYROIDISM

Clive S. Grant, MD

Hyperthyroidism has a prevalence of 2% in women and 0.2% in men and refers to thyroid gland hyperfunction—inappropriately high synthesis and secretion of thyroid hormone. Typical of all endocrine gland function, regulation is characterized by a servomechanism. In this case, thyroid-stimulating hormone (TSH) is secreted by the pituitary gland, which stimulates thyroid gland secretion of thyroxine (T4) and triiodothyronine (T3, the active form of thyroid hormone), which in turn negatively feedbacks on the pituitary to regulate TSH secretion. Hyperthyroidism can have many causes, and determining the cause is essential to formulating a rationale treatment plan. Whereas thyrotoxicosis due to Graves' disease most commonly develops during the second to fourth decades of life, nodular goiter with hyperthyroidism evolves with increasing age and most commonly in regions where dietary iodine is insufficient.

Medical options for definitive treatment of hyperthyroidism include antithyroid drugs and radioactive iodine administration.

Surgical management of hyperthyroidism, which should be extremely safe and highly effective, is considered for the following conditions:

■ Graves' disease
■ Toxic nodular goiter, either solitary thyroid nodule (STN) or multinodular goiter (MNG, Plummer's disease)
■ Amiodarone-induced thyrotoxicosis

■ SYMPTOMS AND DIAGNOSIS

Patients with overt thyrotoxicosis may have a multitude of symptoms indicative of hypermetabolism (Table 1) that if left untreated could progress to cardiac arrhythmias and cardiac failure, thyroid storm, and even death.

In overt thyrotoxicosis, the serum level of TSH is decreased, often to below 0.1 mU/L, and the serum levels of free T4 or free T3 are elevated. In subclinical hyperthyroidism, TSH levels are decreased but T4 and T3 levels remain normal. Radioactive iodine uptake is elevated in Graves' disease and may be either elevated or normal in nodular goiter with hyperthyroidism. In contrast, the uptake is low or undetectable in thyroiditis or amiodarone-associated thyrotoxicosis. A thyroid scan may be helpful to distinguish Graves' disease—diffuse uptake—from toxic multinodular goiter—focal areas of increased uptake with intervening suppressed uptake. In addition, elevated levels of thyroperoxidase (TPO) antibodies are characteristic of autoimmune thyroiditis (Hashimoto's disease). Table 2 provides a summary of disease states related to hyperthyroidism.

TABLE 1: Thyrotoxicosis: Signs and Symptoms

Symptoms	Signs
Palpitations	Tremor
Fatigue	Tachycardia; congestive heart failure
Weight loss	Goiter
Diaphoresis	Lid lag
Muscle weakness	Proptosis
Anxiety or nervousness	Exophthalmos
Irritability	Periorbital edema
Emotional lability	Chemosis
Insomnia	Hyperreflexia
Diarrhea	Warm, moist skin
Hair loss	Dermopathy
Psychosis	Pretibial edema
Irregular menses	Bone demineralization

■ DISEASE STATES

Graves' Disease

Graves' disease, the most common cause of hyperthyroidism in the United States, is an autoimmune systemic disorder, and hyperthyroidism is caused by thyrotropin receptor antibody (TRAb) binding to and stimulating the TSH receptor, resulting in excessive synthesis and secretion of thyroid hormone. The thyroid gland usually is diffusely and symmetrically enlarged and firm. If nodules are present in conjunction with Graves' disease, they should be evaluated in the usual fashion—often necessitating ultrasound and fine-needle aspiration (FNA).

Antithyroid Drugs

Thioamides, including propylthiouracil (PTU, given three times daily) and methimazole (given once daily), decrease thyroid hormone synthesis and control hyperthyroidism in 90% of patients within several weeks. The intent is to induce remission, but despite continuous treatment for 12 to 18 months, relapse occurs after discontinuing the drug in 60% to 80% of patients. Minor side effects occur in 5%; agranulocytosis occurs in 0.5% and severe hepatotoxicity may occur with PTU, prompting the U.S. Food and Drug Administration (FDA) to recommend limiting the use of PTU to patients in their first trimester of pregnancy or to those allergic or intolerant to methimazole. In the United States, these drugs are seldom favored for definitive treatment but commonly utilized for preoperative preparation or for temporary management of pregnant patients with Graves' disease.

Radioactive Iodine (^{131}I)

Treatment with iodine-131 (^{131}I) is highly effective in Graves' disease, resulting in relief of hyperthyroidism in more than 90% of patients with a single dose. It is the treatment chosen for the majority of Graves' patients in the United States. These patients commonly if not

TABLE 2: Summary of Hyperthyroid Disease States

Disease	Diagnostic Features	Preoperative Preparation	Operation
Graves' disease	↑ T4, T3, TSI, TPO ↓ TSH ↑ Symmetric radioiodine uptake, scan Diffuse goiter Eye signs	Antithyroid drugs Beta-blockers Iodine drops	Bilateral near-total or total thyroidectomy
Unilateral toxic nodule	↑ T4, T3 ↓ TSH Single "hot" nodule on scan; remaining thyroid suppressed	None	Unilateral thyroid subtotal or total lobectomy
Multinodular goiter	↑ T4, T3 ↓ TSH Multiple "hot" nodules on scan; remaining thyroid suppressed	None	Bilateral near-total or total thyroidectomy (conservative)
Amiodarone-induced thyrotoxicosis	↑ T4, T3 ↓ TSH Taking amiodarone Minimal or no uptake on thyroid scan	Cardiac evaluation relative to the use of amiodarone	Bilateral near-total or total thyroidectomy
Autoimmune thyroiditis	↑ T4, T3, TPO ↓ TSH Minimal or no uptake on thyroid scan	None	Nonsurgical

T3, Triiodothyronine; *T4,* thyroxine; *TPO,* thyroperoxidase; *TSH,* thyroid-stimulating hormone; *TSI,* thyroid-stimulating immunoglobulin.

intentionally become hypothyroid, which usually is managed easily with replacement T4. Side effects include neck pain from radiation thyroiditis, especially in larger goiters; sialadenitis and dry mouth; temporary worsening of thyrotoxicosis; and sometimes worsening of Graves' ophthalmopathy. Prophylactic simultaneous administration of glucocorticoids may ameliorate the neck pain and worsening eye signs. Return to euthyroidism is delayed for several weeks. Some patients have significant fear of any radioactivity, even though the frequencies of major genetic or carcinogenic effects are not increased in more than 25 years of follow-up experience with adults. Conflicting studies still exist, however. ^{131}I is contraindicated during pregnancy or in lactating mothers and has been used in relatively few children and adolescents because of lack of data regarding very long-term effects. Recurrence and need for more than a single dose of ^{131}I in young patients seem more prevalent.

Surgery

Bilateral near-total or total thyroidectomy is virtually 100% effective in permanently curing hyperthyroidism. It predictably results in the need for replacement T4 treatment that is inexpensive, is free of side effects in proper doses, and can be precisely managed with minimal blood testing. Thyroidectomy rapidly resolves hyperthyroidism and can be performed within 10 days of establishing the diagnosis, usually requiring only a single night of hospitalization. It is equally effective for all age groups, establishes definitive pathology for any accompanying suspicious nodules or thyroid cancer (5%), precludes any fear of radiation, and may be utilized safely during the second trimester of pregnancy and in the lactating mother. Whether total thyroidectomy predictably improves the eye signs of Graves' disease remains an unresolved debate.

The risk of permanent recurrent laryngeal nerve (RLN) damage ranges from 0% to 5%, and transient neurapraxia may occur in a similar number. Permanent hypoparathyroidism is thought to occur more frequently than other bilateral thyroidectomy operations in Graves' disease but should not exceed 1% to 4%. Careful identification and preservation of even a single, well-vascularized parathyroid gland is sufficient for eventual normal parathyroid function. Auto-transplantation of excised parathyroid glands, minced into 1-mm fragments and placed in muscular pockets of the sternocleidomastoid muscle, should function in weeks to months in 95% of patients. Normal parathyroid function based solely on transplanted parathyroid tissue is not recommended and probably requires at least two parathyroid glands.

A few technical points that may be of help include the following (Figure 1):

- After the thyroid gland has been mobilized and elevated out of its bed, the RLN can be detected beneath fat and other soft tissue by palpating it against the trachea, below the level of the thyroid gland.
- The vascular supply to both superior and inferior parathyroid glands, derived from the inferior thyroid artery, enters from the anterior aspect. Therefore transecting soft tissue just barely anterior to these glands will threaten devascularization.

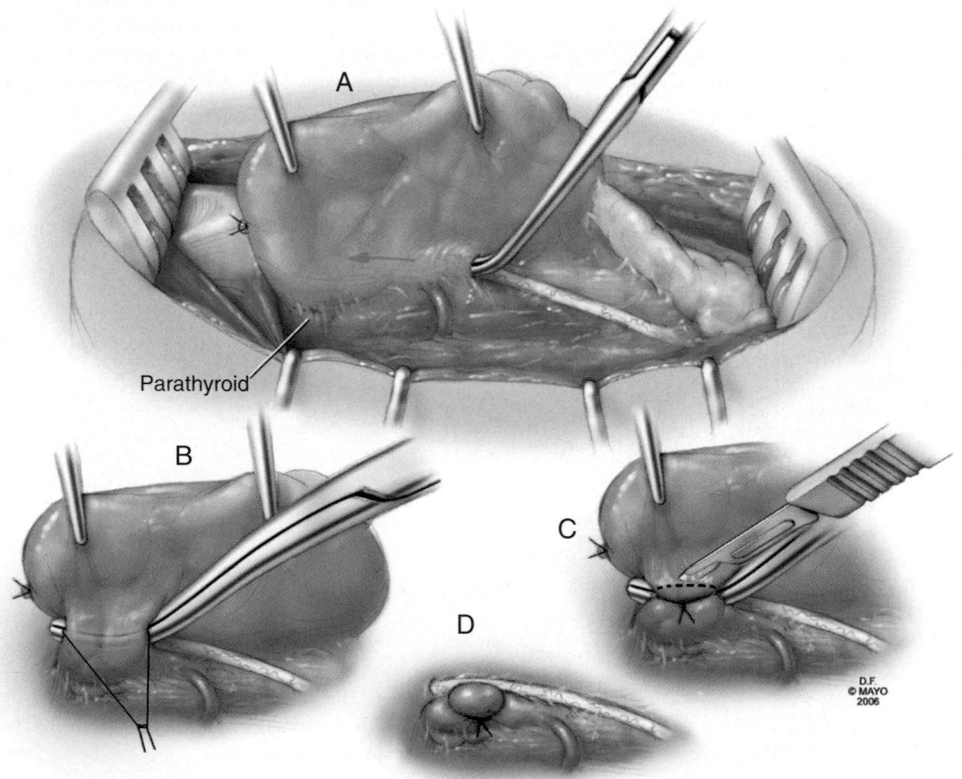

FIGURE 1 Method for preserving the superior parathyroid gland in near-total thyroidectomy. **A,** An Adson right-angle clamp is advanced immediately adjacent to and on top of the recurrent laryngeal nerve (RLN; areolar space along the RLN allows easy, nonforceful opening of this plane) until the tip of the clamp can be seen medial and superior to the remaining attached superior aspect of the thyroid lobe. **B,** A tie is passed through the dissected opening, anterior to the RLN, which is confirmed through this maneuver to be safe from ligation or transection. **C,** After the ligature is tied with a small remnant of thyroid preserved anterior to the superior parathyroid gland (visible posterior to the small thyroid remnant), the bridge of thyroid tissue is transected with a scalpel, protecting the RLN with the clamp. **D,** After the bridge is transected, the RLN is fully exposed, the tiny thyroid remnant retracts posteriorly with the protected superior parathyroid gland, and the remaining thyroid lobe can be excised easily and safely. *(Copyright David Factor, Mayo Clinic, 2006.)*

■ The superior parathyroid gland and the RLN can be visualized and, if necessary, may be saved by preserving a small remnant of thyroid tissue just anterior to the parathyroid gland together with its blood supply, by developing the areolar space adjacent to the RLN as illustrated in Figure 1. The amount of thyroid tissue preserved should be no more than 100 to 200 mg.

The surgical scar ranges up to 7 cm, depending on the patient's body habitus, and initially may represent the single most important concern for a surgical approach when consulting on a young female patient. Nevertheless, either the necessity of prolonged daily antithyroid medication or the perceived specter of radioactive treatment often ultimately outweighs this issue.

Preoperative preparation is absolutely required. For most patients, antithyroid drugs (discussed earlier) are instituted for 3 to 6 weeks with a goal of nearly normalizing the T3 and T4. The addition of beta-blockers such as propranolol or atenolol rapidly controls the adrenergic side effects of excess T4 and T3, such as tachycardia, tremor, and diaphoresis. The administration of iodine in the form of potassium iodide (SSKI) or Lugol's solution frequently has been used as the sole means of preoperative preparation in the past. It rapidly but temporarily restores normal thyroid function and reduces thyroid gland vascularity.

Toxic Single Adenoma

Toxic adenomas are single, benign, monoclonal thyroid tumors that autonomously oversecrete thyroid hormone. The nodule is usually 3 cm or larger, evolves through a course of subclinical to overt hyperthyroidism, and is virtually never malignant.

Antithyroid Drugs

Whereas hyperthyroidism can be controlled with antithyroid drugs (thioamides), remission does not occur, recurrence inevitably develops when the medication is discontinued, and lifelong treatment is unacceptable. Therefore these drugs are seldom if ever chosen as definitive treatment.

Radioactive Iodine

Iodine-131 is effective, with little risk to surrounding structures or of causing radiation-induced tumors. The nodules may shrink to some extent but rarely disappear. Euthyroidism is re-established in at least 80% of patients with a single dose. However, variability in size of the nodule, uptake, and dose of ^{131}I administered may lead to either recurrence or hypothyroidism. Pregnancy and lactation are contraindications to ^{131}I.

Surgery

Subtotal or total lobectomy to resect the hot nodule is virtually 100% effective in controlling hyperthyroidism. Most patients are restored to euthyroidism if the remaining thyroid gland is normal. The risk of RLN paralysis is 1% or less, hypoparathyroidism is not a concern, and other surgical complications are rare. The surgical scar, hospitalization and anesthesia, and cost are the principal deterrents to a surgical approach.

Toxic Multinodular Goiter (Plummer's Disease)

First described by H.S. Plummer in 1913, this condition is unremitting and often develops slowly, with more subtle symptoms than Graves' disease (and without the eye signs). A long phase of subclinical hyperthyroidism can precede the appearance of overt symptoms. Cardiac symptoms such as tachycardia, heart failure, or arrhythmia and atrial fibrillation are most frequent. In addition, unexplained, asymptomatic weight loss may occur in older patients with toxic MNG. Patients also may experience local pressure complications of large nodular goiters, such as tracheal, esophageal, or jugular venous compression (Pemberton's sign: facial plethora, inspiratory stridor, and venous congestion when arms are raised above the head).

Antithyroid Drugs

For the same reasons as for single toxic adenoma, thioamides are virtually never used as definitive treatment but rather as preoperative preparation.

Radioactive Iodine

Increasingly, ^{131}I has been advocated in the treatment of toxic MNG. Iodine-131 offers an attractive alternative to thyroidectomy in patients who have high operative risk. In addition, it is often used for smaller goiters without local pressure symptoms. Cardiac symptoms are more prevalent in patients treated with ^{131}I. Resolution of hyperthyroidism with ^{131}I takes 5 to 6 months on average, the goiter size is reduced by about 40%, and treatment with ^{131}I is associated with subsequent hypothyroidism in about 10% of patients. A second dose of ^{131}I may be necessary in 15% to 25% of patients. Complications, however, are rare, with the exception of radiation-related thyroiditis causing neck pain.

Surgery

The advantages of surgical treatment include prompt, permanent resolution of hyperthyroidism; removal of the goiter, resolving any associated compressive or cosmetic problems; and treatment of associated malignancy. With conservative bilateral near-total thyroidectomy, virtually all patients have their hyperthyroidism resolved within a month postoperatively. All start taking replacement T4, as surgically induced hypothyroidism is the desired operative goal.

Because of the size of MNG, the surgical risks are often higher than with bilateral thyroidectomy for either cancer or Graves' disease. Bleeding and postoperative hematoma are more likely because of the markedly enlarged and plentiful thyroid vasculature. The RLNs may be more difficult to identify because of anatomic displacement by nodules or difficulty with exposure from the sheer size of the goiter. Equally difficult to identify may be the parathyroid glands in large MNG. For these reasons, a few technical hints may be of help:

■ A larger incision is usually necessary to gain adequate exposure.
■ Reverse Trendelenburg position reduces venous pressure and bleeding.
■ Careful dissection and preservation of the sternohyoid strap muscles is valuable to protect the trachea at the time of closure. However, the sternothyroid muscles are often thin and splayed over the surface of the goiter and may be sacrificed (Figure 2).
■ Even though the goiter may be large, the isthmus is still often narrow. Early transection of the isthmus with careful control of the paired inferior thyroid veins and control of the confluence of three veins along the superior border of the isthmus yields an exposed trachea, which serves as a useful landmark in later dissection.
■ Early ligation of the superior thyroid artery along the anterior superior surface of the superior pole may be easier than expected, as it is often elongated by the goiter extending substernally (Figure 3). This reduces the inevitable bothersome bleeding associated with mobilization and resection of the large nodular lobe.
■ Blunt finger dissection on the surface of the thyroid lobe, carried posteriorly and inferiorly immediately under the strap muscles, facilitates mobilization of the inferior pole of the lobe out of its bed (Figure 4).
■ As the lobe is mobilized, it is helpful to recall that no anatomic structure of importance crosses transversely across the carotid artery from the base of the neck to the thyroid cartilage (except the middle thyroid vein, which is sacrificed). To expose the carotid over this length facilitates further dissection, particularly identification of the RLN.
■ With a large goiter elevated out of its bed, the trachea and esophagus often are rotated anteriorly, exposing the RLN to potential

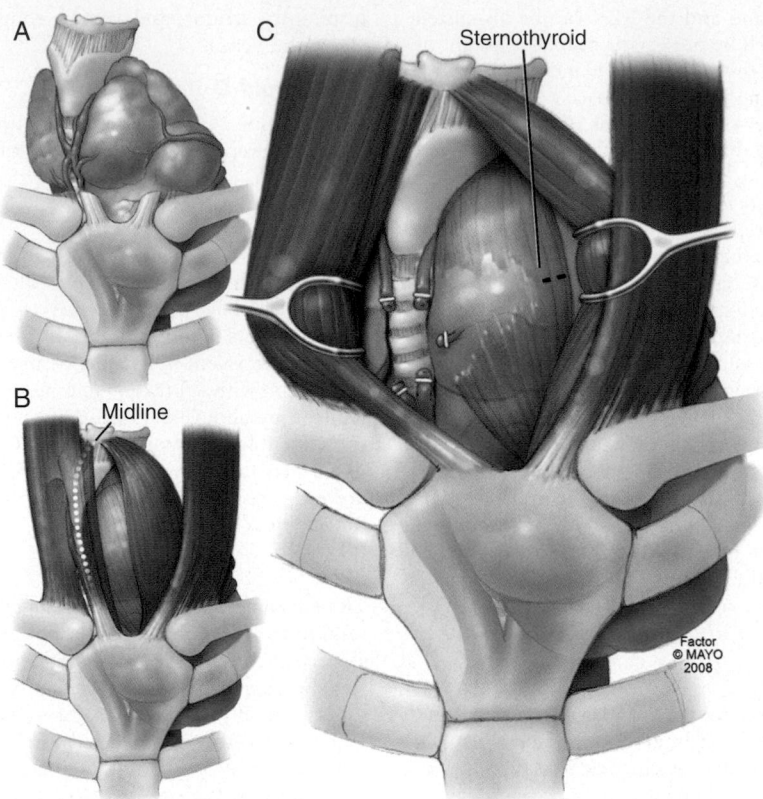

FIGURE 2 **A,** Large multinodular goiter extending behind the manubrium and sternum into the anterior mediastinum. **B,** The midline is shifted to the patient's right by the large goiter deviating the trachea (dotted line depicts the incision line to separate strap muscles). **C,** Inferior thyroid veins have been transected, the sternohyoid muscle has been retracted, and the sternothyroid muscle is thin and transected transversely with no ill effects. *(Copyright David Factor, Mayo Clinic, 2008.)*

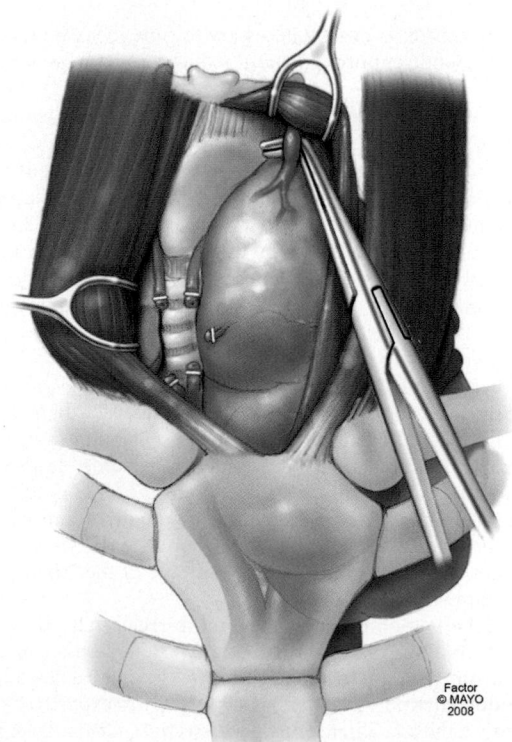

FIGURE 3 The large multinodular goiter has caused elongation of the superior thyroid artery, facilitating its sacrifice early in the procedure. *(Copyright David Factor, Mayo Clinic, 2008.)*

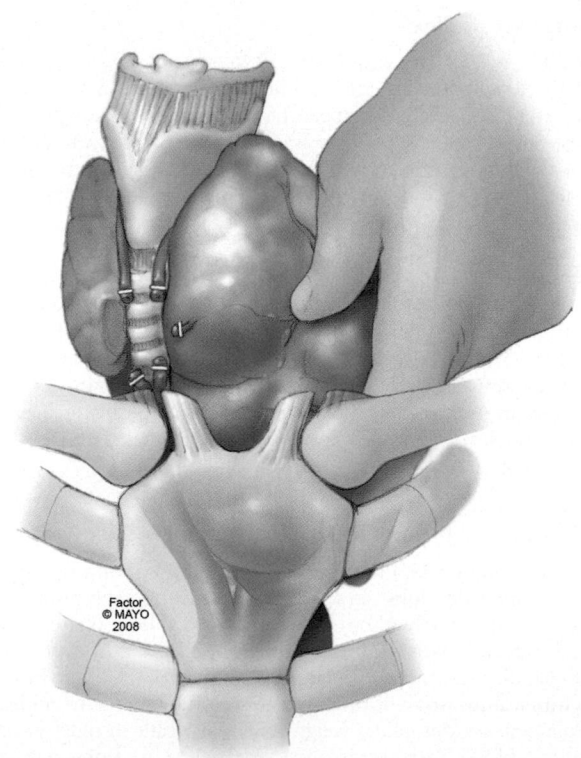

FIGURE 4 Blunt finger dissection is undertaken, immediately on the smooth surface of the thyroid gland, deep just to the thin sternothyroid muscle. A clamp may be necessary to help withdraw the large goiter from the superior mediastinum. *(Copyright David Factor, Mayo Clinic, 2008.)*

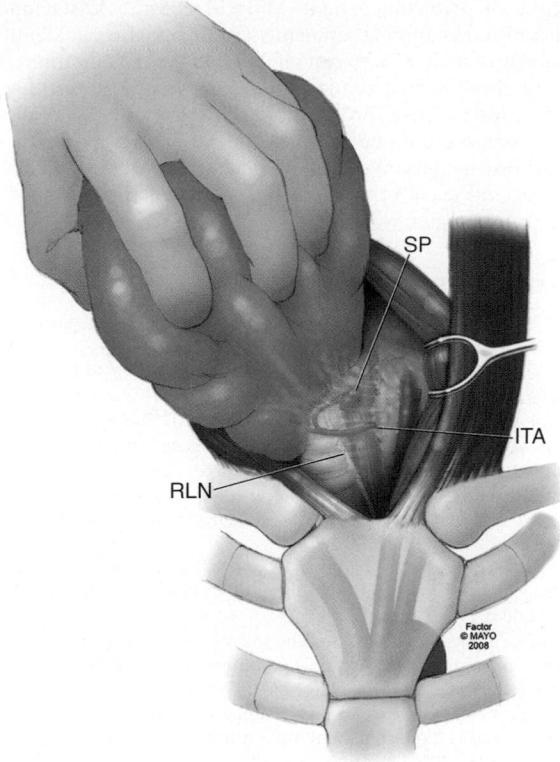

FIGURE 5 The large left lobe of the multinodular goiter has been delivered from the superior mediastinum and rotated to the patient's right. This must be performed gently, as it will put the recurrent laryngeal nerve (RLN) on stretch, which facilitates palpation of the nerve against the trachea. The blood supply from the inferior thyroid artery (ITA) to the superior parathyroid gland (SP) is demonstrated. Safe resection of the lobe can now be undertaken, as the key anatomic landmarks and structures have been exposed and protected. *(Copyright David Factor, Mayo Clinic, 2008.)*

danger. With the lobe so elevated, however, the nerve is usually taut and rather easily palpated. Once the RLN is exposed and protected, resection may begin (Figure 5).

- The inferior parathyroid seems more variable in location because of the distortion caused by the large goiter. However, the cervical extension of the thymus (and associated vein) to the inferior pole of the thyroid often will lead to this parathyroid gland. Less variable is the deep, posterior position of the superior parathyroid gland. The inferior parathyroid gland may be excised, undergo biopsy for identity confirmation, and be autotransplanted into the sternocleidomastoid muscle, whereas the superior parathyroid gland can be protected in situ more easily.
- If the inferior parathyroid has been excised, there is nothing of importance to save anterior to the RLN, inferior to the lower pole of the thyroid, or around to the midline surface of the trachea; this soft tissue may be sacrificed.
- Lobectomy is undertaken by circumferential dissection facilitated by earlier isthmic transection.

Amiodarone-Associated Thyrotoxicosis (AAT)

Amiodarone is an iodine-rich (37% by molecular weight) antiarrhythmic agent that initially was introduced for refractory arrhythmias but has seen increasing usage because of its effectiveness. Even conventional doses of this drug result in large expansion of the iodine pool. Often amiodarone-associated thyrotoxicosis (AAT) occurs in patients with significant cardiac dysrhythmias who do not tolerate

the cardiac effects of hyperthyroidism. Two forms of AAT have been described. Type 1 develops in patients with pre-existing goiter, resulting in excessive hormone production from the marked iodine excess. Type 2 occurs without pre-existing thyroid disease from a chemical-induced thyroiditis and resultant release of hormone. Type 2 is more common in the United States, occurring in 2% of patients treated with amiodarone. AAT is notoriously refractory to medical management, with low radioactive iodine uptake, thereby precluding use of ^{131}I for treatment. Discontinuation of amiodarone may help, but often that is a poor choice in patients with life-threatening arrhythmias. In addition, the long half-life of the drug requires weeks to months for the hyperthyroidism to resolve.

Antithyroid Drugs

Although thioamides have been utilized with some success, inadequate results are the rule. Only if hyperthyroidism is mild and amiodarone can be discontinued do antithyroid drugs have the likelihood of prolonged success.

Radioactive Iodine

Because the iodine uptake is low in the usual patients with type 2 AAT, ^{131}I is not an option.

Surgery

Thyroidectomy offers many of the same benefits discussed in previous sections: prompt and permanent control of hyperthyroidism, low risk of RLN damage or hypoparathyroidism, short hospitalization, and quick recovery. However, this is the highest-risk group of patients undergoing thyroidectomy, and almost all of the risk is related to the severity of these patients' cardiac disease. These patients may have severe cardiac failure, life-threatening arrhythmias, and ejection fractions of 10% to 30%. Despite their very high operative risk, thyroidectomy is efficacious in treating AAT, and most patients ultimately recover well.

■ POSTOPERATIVE MANAGEMENT AND COMPLICATIONS

The postoperative care of these patients varies considerably, influenced by surgeon preference and tradition, specific cause of hyperthyroidism, conduct and difficulty of the operation, and facilities and practice management algorithms. Even though literature evidence supporting different management patterns may exist, these patterns depend on specific areas of expertise. Nevertheless, several general aspects of postoperative care and complications should be addressed.

- Outpatient thyroidectomy. There has been more enthusiasm and even a white paper from the Surgical Affairs Committee of the American Thyroid Association (ATA) on this topic—specifically referring to patient dismissal on the same day as the operation. Because thyroidectomy for Graves' disease or large MNG with hyperthyroidism may be significantly more difficult and demanding, these patients might not be good candidates for outpatient surgery. The thoughtful advice and criteria in the ATA review are valuable. However, the topic remains controversial and largely depends on motivated surgeons, patients, favorable situations, and careful adherence to all components of the management algorithm.
- RLN function. The evolution and popularity of intraoperative nerve monitoring (IONM), although not considered a standard of care as yet, have given surgeons added confidence that, if verified intraoperatively to be normal, the vocal cords will function normally postoperatively. IONM is not a substitute for confident and careful visual identification and protection of the RLN. IONM has not reduced statistically rates of vocal cord paralysis. If unilateral cord paresis is noted postoperatively and the nerve was clearly intact and not damaged intraoperatively, return of function is highly likely. Function usually returns to normal

within 6 weeks, but 6 to 12 months may be required for full return of function. Voice improvement may be helpful in the interim and can be achieved with temporary injections. Permanent paralysis may require subsequent surgical intervention.

■ Hematoma. Postoperative hematoma is rare and, if evaluated carefully, usually apparent by 6 hours postoperatively (but it also may develop later—by 24 hours or even after a few days). However, it represents the most feared and potentially lethal complication and is not prevented by a surgically placed drain. In contrast to operations in the thorax or abdomen, only a relatively small amount of blood in the confined thyroid bed is required to cause airway obstruction or spasm. The immediate solution to a hematoma is opening the incision and the strap muscles to evacuate the hematoma and relieve the pressure. This is performed in conjunction with intubation if the airway has been compromised, with subsequent return to the operating room for definitive management of the hematoma and incision. Again, Graves' disease and large MNG are precisely the settings that demand meticulous hemostasis to prevent this complication.

■ Hypocalcemia. Parathyroid function can be maintained over the long term even with only a single, well-vascularized parathyroid gland. However, early postoperative hypocalcemia is common, occurring in up to one third of thyroidectomy patients, and can be distressing and potentially dangerous to the patient if left unrecognized and untreated. Many surgeons routinely dismiss patients on calcium and vitamin D supplementation, with subsequent serum calcium monitoring on variable schedules. As an alternative, when available, rapid parathyroid hormone testing approximately 2 to 6 hours postoperatively not only is highly accurate in predicting patients who will require at least temporary calcium and vitamin D supplementation, but also can identify the majority of patients who can safely avoid these medications. Early symptoms of hypocalcemia include paresthesias of the fingertips and perioral regions. Progression to frank tetany and respiratory compromise should not occur if the patient has received appropriate instructions on symptom management, early evaluation by the surgical team, or adherence to either of the two previously detailed strategies.

SUGGESTED READINGS

Bahn R, Burch HB, Cooper D, Garber J, Greenlee M, et al. Hyperthyroidism and other causes of thyrotoxicosis: management guidelines of the American Thyroid Association and American Association of Clinical Endocrinologists. *Thyroid*. 2011;21:593-646.

Houghton S, Farley D, Brennan M, van Heerden J, Thompson G, Grant C. Surgical management of amiodarone-associated thyrotoxicosis: Mayo Clinic experience. *World J Surg*. 2004;28:1083-1087.

O'Brien T, Gharib H, Suman V, van Heerden J. Treatment of toxic solitary thyroid nodules: surgery versus radioactive iodine. *Surgery*. 1992;112:1166-1170.

Porterfield J, Thompson G, Farley D, Grant C, Richards M. Evidence-based management of toxic multinodular goiter (Plummer's disease). *World J Surg*. 2008;32:1278-1284.

Sherman J, Thompson G, Lteif A, Schwenk W, van Heerden J, et al. Surgical management of Graves' disease in childhood and adolescence: an institutional experience. *Surgery*. 2006;140:1056-1062.

Terris D, Snyder S, Carneiro-Pla D, Inabnet W, Kandil E, et al. American Thyroid Association statement on outpatient thyroidectomy. *Thyroid*. 2013;23:1193-1202.

SURGICAL APPROACH TO THYROID CANCER

Glenda G. Callender, MD, and Robert Udelsman, MD, MBA

Thyroid cancer accounts for only 3.8% of all new cancer cases; however, the incidence of thyroid cancer is rising more rapidly than that of any other malignancy. According to the National Cancer Institute (NCI) Surveillance, Epidemiology, and End Results (SEER) database, approximately 62,450 people in the United States will be diagnosed with thyroid cancer in 2015, and 1950 people will die from their disease. The rising incidence of thyroid cancer in the United States is largely attributable to the rising incidence of papillary thyroid carcinoma (PTC), the most common endocrine malignancy. In 1990 the annual incidence of PTC was 5.50 per 100,000 people per year; by 2010 the annual incidence was 13.83 per 100,000 people per year. Increased detection of papillary thyroid microcarcinoma (PTMC; PTC ≤1 cm) related to increasingly sensitive diagnostic studies and medical surveillance accounts for much of the rising incidence of PTC; however, increased diagnosis cannot completely explain the observed increase in the incidence of PTC. The incidence of larger PTCs and the other histologic subtypes of thyroid cancer (follicular thyroid carcinoma [FTC], medullary thyroid carcinoma [MTC], and anaplastic thyroid carcinoma [ATC]) also have increased modestly over the past 40 years.

The surgical management of the patient with thyroid cancer is usually more complex and extensive than the surgical management of the patient with benign thyroid disease. As the epidemiology of thyroid cancer has changed, there exists an increased need for surgeons with a thorough understanding of thyroid cancer management. Data have shown that high-volume thyroid surgeons (>100 cases over a 6-year period) experience lower hospital lengths of stay, lower costs, and complication rates at least two-thirds lower than those of low-volume surgeons (1 to 9 cases over a 6-year period) when operating for thyroid cancer. To provide optimal care for the patient with thyroid cancer, the surgeon must not serve as a mere "technician"; the surgeon must understand how to incorporate new technology and emerging data into his or her practice.

■ INDICATIONS

Surgery for thyroid cancer typically is performed in one of the following settings: (1) diagnostic resection of a nodule suspected to be a thyroid cancer; (2) treatment of a known primary or recurrent thyroid cancer; or (3) prophylactic thyroidectomy in a patient with a genetic mutation conferring high risk for future development of thyroid cancer.

Thyroid cancer usually is seen as a thyroid nodule discovered because it is palpated, creates compressive symptoms, or is discovered incidentally on an imaging study performed for another reason. According to American Thyroid Association (ATA) management guidelines for adult patients with thyroid nodules and differentiated thyroid cancer published in 2015, evaluation with ultrasound-guided fine-needle aspiration (FNA) biopsy is recommended for thyroid nodules 1 cm or larger, unless the ultrasound features are completely benign (e.g., purely cystic or spongiform). FNA biopsy may be considered for subcentimeter thyroid nodules with features suspicious for cancer (e.g., hypoechoic, solid, calcifications) or for a nodule not otherwise meeting criteria for biopsy in a patient at increased risk of thyroid cancer because of either radiation exposure early in life or a family history of thyroid cancer.

Thyroid cytopathology is notoriously difficult to interpret because the cytologic features of thyroid cancer overlap with those of thyroid

TABLE 1: Bethesda Classification System for Thyroid Cytopathology

Category	Risk of Malignancy	Recommended Initial Management
1: Nondiagnostic/ unsatisfactory	1%-4%	Repeat FNA
2: Benign	0-3%	Clinical follow-up
3: Follicular lesion (atypia) of uncertain significance	5-15%	Repeat FNA, clinical follow-up, or diagnostic thyroid lobectomy*
4: Follicular neoplasm	20%-30%	Diagnostic thyroid lobectomy
5: Suspicious for malignancy	60%-75%	Diagnostic thyroid lobectomy with frozen section and formal thyroid cancer operation if frozen section positive; or up-front formal thyroid cancer operation*
6: Malignant	97%-99%	Formal thyroid cancer operation

From Cibas ES, Ali SZ. The Bethesda System for reporting thyroid cytopathology. *Am J Clin Pathol.* 2009;132:658-665.

*Depending upon institutional rates of malignancy; *BRAF* and other molecular markers may be useful in interpretation of risk of malignancy in these categories.

FNA, Fine-needle aspiration.

inflammation. The wide variability in reporting historically has led to frustration for clinicians and patients. The Bethesda classification system for reporting thyroid cytopathology was published in 2009 in order to standardize thyroid FNA reporting. Under the Bethesda System, cytopathologists are required to assign thyroid cytology to one of six categories based on the adequacy of the specimen and the risk of malignancy (Table 1). This standardized approach allows clinicians to determine appropriate management based on the patient's predicted risk. However, there remains considerable variability between institutions; therefore each institution should determine its own rate of malignancy in each category. For example, according to published literature, the diagnostic category "suspicious for PTC" is associated with a 50% to 75% risk of cancer, suggesting that diagnostic thyroid lobectomy may be appropriate initial management for most patients. However, in our institution, the true risk of malignancy in patients assigned to this category is greater than 90%, and therefore a formal oncologic operation is preferred.

The diagnostic accuracy of FNA biopsy can be improved by the use of molecular markers, and a variety of panels that test for mutations in an array of markers are being developed and validated. The *BRAF* V600E mutation is the most commonly used marker. It is present in 40% to 70% of PTCs and, if identified on a thyroid nodule FNA biopsy, confers a nearly 100% risk of PTC. However, absence of a *BRAF* mutation cannot be used reliably to exclude cancer in an indeterminate FNA biopsy. When *BRAF* was first characterized in the context of PTC, it was thought to signify a more aggressive phenotype of PTC and confer worse prognosis; however, recent studies have not supported this hypothesis. In general, more data are needed before molecular markers will add substantially to the information generated by cytopathology alone.

■ PREOPERATIVE EVALUATION

The patient history should focus on symptoms of mass effect, such as difficulty swallowing or breathing, globus sensation, stridor, or pressure in the neck when lying supine or turning the head. Subjective voice changes or hoarseness could indicate involvement of the recurrent laryngeal nerve with tumor. Patients with MTC should be asked about symptoms of hypercalcitoninemia suggestive of advanced disease, such as flushing and diarrhea. They also should be asked about symptoms suggesting pheochromocytoma or primary hyperparathyroidism. Patients should be asked about the details of any prior surgery, especially procedures in the neck or mediastinum, as well as a history of radiation to the head or neck.

A personal or family history of thyroid cancer and other cancers should be elicited. Up to 25% of cases of MTC occur in the setting of germline *RET* proto-oncogene mutations resulting in the inherited autosomal-dominant syndrome multiple endocrine neoplasia type 2 (MEN 2, described in more detail later in this chapter). Nonmedullary thyroid cancers (PTC and FTC) appear to be hereditary in up to 5% of cases, although a specific mutation has not been identified.

Physical examination should include a general assessment of the patient and focused palpation of the thyroid and lymph node basins of the neck. Benign nodules are usually smooth and mobile. Cancers may be irregular and hard and may be fixed to neck structures if advanced and locally invasive. Regional lymph nodes grossly involved with metastatic disease may be identified by palpation of the lymph node basins of the neck. If the inferior aspect of the thyroid gland cannot be palpated, cross-sectional imaging with noncontrast computed tomography (CT) may be warranted to evaluate the extent of substernal goiter. It is important to auscultate the carotid arteries to detect a bruit because lateral retraction of the carotid arteries during thyroidectomy can lead to intraoperative stroke in patients with untreated severe carotid atherosclerotic disease.

Preoperative laryngoscopy to evaluate vocal cord function is essential in a patient whose voice is impaired or in a patient who has previously undergone neck or mediastinal surgery with a risk of laryngeal nerve injury, even if the voice is normal. Preoperative evaluation of the vocal cords may be performed using direct (flexible fiber optic or rigid) or indirect (mirror) laryngoscopy. Formal laryngoscopy may contribute little to the preoperative evaluation of a patient with a normal voice and in whom there is no reason to suspect an immobile vocal cord; however, preoperative laryngoscopy is routine for all patients in our practice because it has the potential to provide useful information while adding little time to the physical examination and creating minimal risk or discomfort to the patient.

Preoperative laboratory evaluation must include blood tests to verify that the patient is euthyroid. A serum calcium level should be obtained to screen for co-existing undiagnosed parathyroid disease that should be addressed during thyroidectomy. In a patient with MTC, preoperative *RET* proto-oncogene genetic testing is essential because the specific *RET* mutation predicts whether the patient is likely to also develop pheochromocytoma or primary hyperparathyroidism (PHPT). If the patient has hereditary MTC, failure to diagnose a pheochromocytoma preoperatively may lead to life-threatening consequences; in addition, the intraoperative management of the parathyroid glands may differ for a patient with hereditary disease and a patient with sporadic MTC.

According to current ATA guidelines, patients with known or suspected thyroid cancer should undergo preoperative staging of the lateral neck lymph node basins by ultrasound, with FNA biopsy of any abnormal lymph node. The sensitivity of ultrasound to detect metastatic thyroid cancer in lateral neck lymph nodes is 90% to 100%. Biopsy-proven disease in the lateral neck is an indication for modified radical neck dissection; prophylactic modified radical neck dissection is virtually never indicated in PTC and indicated only rarely in a patient with MTC.

■ SURGERY FOR DIFFERENTIATED THYROID CANCER

Surgery is the primary treatment for patients with differentiated thyroid cancer (PTC and FTC). The goals of surgery are to (1) resect the primary tumor and involved regional lymph nodes; (2) minimize morbidity; (3) provide accurate staging; (4) minimize the risk of local-regional disease recurrence; (5) facilitate adjuvant treatment with radioactive iodine (RAI), if appropriate; and (6) facilitate accurate long-term surveillance for recurrence. The standard treatment for most patients with differentiated thyroid cancer is total or near-total thyroidectomy, with dissection of involved lymph node basins.

The optimal extent of thyroidectomy for patients with PTC is controversial. It is important to note that the excellent overall prognosis of patients with PTC means that most studies comparing treatment strategies for PTC are underpowered: several thousand patients would be required in each study arm in order to exclude a type II error and determine that no difference exists between groups. Within the context of that limitation, retrospective data demonstrate that total or near-total thyroidectomy results in lower recurrence and improved survival rates than thyroid lobectomy for patients with primary tumors larger than 1 cm. Total thyroidectomy also allows postoperative use of RAI scintigraphy to screen for metastatic disease and thyroglobulin as a tumor marker to detect recurrence. According to ATA guidelines, thyroid lobectomy may be considered for patients with single, small tumors up to 1 cm (PTMC). In addition, a longitudinal study from Japan demonstrated that observation may be an acceptable option for patients with cytologically proven PTMC in the absence of worrisome features.

Therapeutic central neck dissection should be performed for clinically involved central neck lymph nodes. The boundaries of the central neck (level VI) extend to the medial aspect of the carotid arteries laterally, the hyoid bone superiorly, and the sternal notch/brachiocephalic vessels inferiorly (Figure 1). At the time of diagnosis,

PTC is metastatic to central neck lymph nodes in 20% to 90% of patients, but ultrasound detects central neck lymph node metastasis in approximately only half of patients who ultimately have histopathology-proven involved lymph nodes. Thus central neck disease usually is not diagnosed by preoperative FNA biopsy. Central neck dissection usually is performed because of clinical suspicion of involved central neck lymph nodes or for prophylactic reasons, particularly in the setting of a larger primary tumor.

The role of prophylactic central neck dissection in PTC is controversial. No data exist to definitively guide management. Because of the overall excellent prognosis of PTC, existing retrospective data are underpowered and an adequately powered randomized trial is unrealistic because a large number of patients and long follow-up time would be required in order to detect a meaningful difference in survival. However, the following line of reasoning argues in favor of routine prophylactic central neck dissection: (1) metastasis to central neck lymph nodes cannot be detected reliably preoperatively by ultrasound or intraoperatively by the surgeon; (2) central neck dissection improves accuracy in staging, with a substantial proportion of patients upstaged from Nx to N1a disease, which may be their only indication for RAI; (3) central neck dissection results in decreased postoperative thyroglobulin levels, allowing greater utility of thyroglobulin to detect recurrence; (4) central neck dissection leads to reduced recurrence rates; (5) reduced recurrence rates decrease the need for central neck reoperation with the associated morbidity; and (6) central neck dissection can be performed with essentially the same morbidity as thyroidectomy alone in the hands of a high-volume endocrine surgeon. Arguments against routine prophylactic central neck dissection include (1) absence of randomized trial data demonstrating that central neck dissection leads to lower recurrence and mortality rates; (2) the fact that less than a quarter of thyroidectomies in the United States are actually performed by high-volume surgeons; and (3) the resulting potential for increased rates of recurrent laryngeal nerve injury and hypoparathyroidism. Therefore the

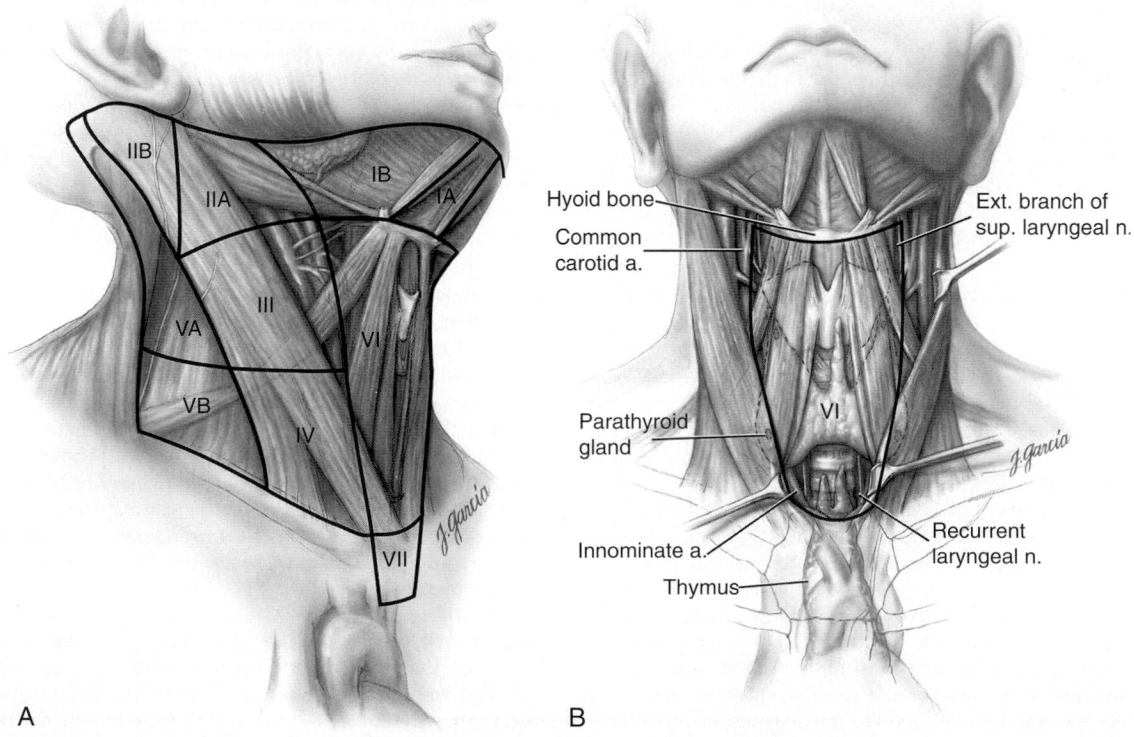

A   B

FIGURE 1 Anatomy of the central neck (level VI). **A,** The boundaries of the central neck extend to the medial carotid artery bilaterally, from the hyoid bone to the sternal notch/brachiocephalic vessels. **B,** A central neck lymph node dissection includes the precricoid laryngeal (Delphian), pretracheal, paratracheal, intrathymic, retropharyngeal, and retroesophageal lymph nodes. *(Reprinted with permission from Mary Ann Liebert Publishers. From Carty SE, Cooper DS, Doherty GM, et al. Consensus statement on the terminology and classification of central neck dissection for thyroid cancer. Thyroid. 2009;19:1153-1158.)*

patient's overall prognosis (based on patient age and size of the primary tumor), the findings on preoperative ultrasound and careful intraoperative inspection of the central neck lymph nodes, and the experience of the surgeon all play into the risk/benefit ratio of prophylactic central neck dissection for PTC.

Modified radical neck dissection should be performed for biopsy-proven metastatic disease in the lateral neck (Figure 2); there is no role for prophylactic modified radical neck dissection for PTC. Modified radical neck dissection preserves the sternocleidomastoid muscle, internal jugular vein, and spinal accessory nerve with much less morbidity than the radical neck dissection first described by George Crile in 1906 for the treatment of head and neck squamous cell carcinoma. The definition and extent of modified radical neck dissection remains controversial; in the literature, the terms *functional neck dissection*, *lateral neck dissection*, and *compartment-oriented neck dissection* may be used interchangeably with *modified radical neck dissection*. Some centers advocate dissection of only those levels of the neck documented to contain biopsy-proven disease or at highest risk of containing disease (i.e., levels III–IV or levels II–IV); however, dissection of levels IIA to VB offers patients the best opportunity for removal of macroscopic disease that could result in recurrence. In expert hands, the morbidity of modified radical neck dissection is low; potential complications include hematoma, seroma, wound infection, chylous leak, pneumothorax, and nerve injury (spinal accessory, hypoglossal, vagus, phrenic, marginal mandibular, sympathetic trunk, brachial plexus, and cutaneous cervical plexus).

FTC and Hürthle cell carcinoma (generally considered to be a subtype of FTC) differ from PTC in that they do not have the same

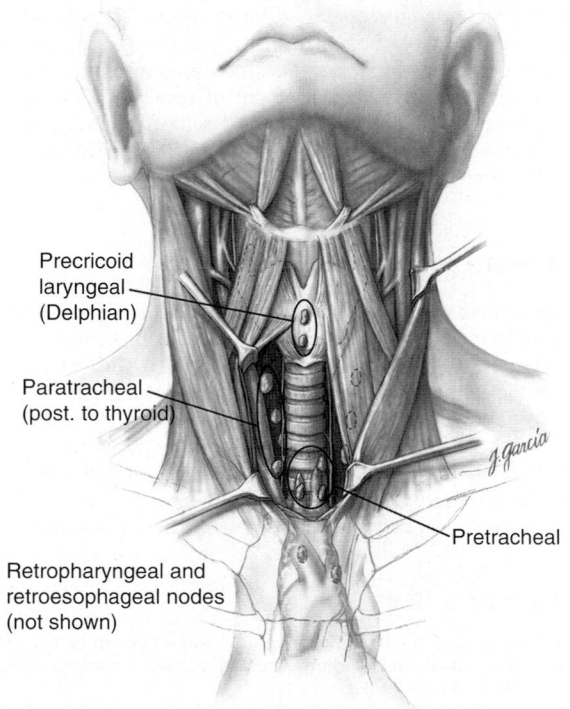

Precricoid laryngeal (Delphian)

Paratracheal (post. to thyroid)

Pretracheal

Retropharyngeal and retroesophageal nodes (not shown)

FIGURE 2 Anatomy of the lateral neck (levels II to V). The boundary between the central and lateral neck is the medial aspect of the carotid artery. The spinal accessory nerve delineates the boundary between levels IIA and IIB. The boundary between levels IIA and III occurs at the level of the hyoid bone. The boundary between levels III and IV and levels VA and VB occurs at the level of the cricoid cartilage. *(Reprinted with permission from Mary Ann Liebert Publishers. From Carty SE, Cooper DS, Doherty GM, et al. Consensus statement on the terminology and classification of central neck dissection for thyroid cancer. Thyroid. 2009;19:1153-1158.)*

propensity for lymph node metastasis and their diagnosis cannot be made reliably by preoperative FNA biopsy. FTC or Hürthle cell carcinoma is diagnosed by documenting vascular or capsular invasion; thus surgery usually is performed for FNA findings of follicular neoplasm, Hürthle cell neoplasm, or follicular lesion of undetermined significance. Diagnostic thyroid lobectomy is often appropriate, with subsequent completion thyroidectomy if cancer is confirmed on final pathology. The risk of cancer is increased in follicular or Hürthle cell neoplasms larger than 4 cm; therefore up-front total thyroidectomy may be preferred. Frozen section is rarely useful for the intraoperative diagnosis of FTC.

■ SURGERY FOR MEDULLARY THYROID CARCINOMA

MTC originates from the calcitonin-producing C cells in the thyroid and accounts for 1% to 2% of adult thyroid cancers and 5% of pediatric thyroid cancers. It is critically important to distinguish from the outset whether disease is sporadic or hereditary. Approximately 25% of cases of MTC result from a *RET* proto-oncogene mutation inherited in an autosomal-dominant fashion; affected individuals develop primary C-cell hyperplasia that progresses to invasive MTC. Three syndromes are observed: (1) MEN 2A, characterized by MTC in 100%, pheochromocytoma in 40%, and PHPT in up to 30%; (2) MEN 2B, characterized by early onset, aggressive MTC in 100%, pheochromocytoma in 40%, and characteristic physical features (Marfanoid habitus, mucosal neuromas, ganglioneuromatosis of the gastrointestinal tract, and megacolon); and (3) familial MTC (FMTC), which is likely a reduced-penetrance variant of MEN 2A in which only MTC is seen.

The surgical management of sporadic and hereditary MTC differs; failure to identify inherited MTC means that the index patient may not be treated appropriately and members of the patient's family may remain undiagnosed. ATA guidelines for the management of MTC published in 2015 recommend that all patients with a cytologically confirmed diagnosis of MTC undergo genetic testing to evaluate for the presence of a germline *RET* proto-oncogene mutation. Serum calcitonin and carcinoembryonic antigen (CEA) levels should be measured as baseline tumor markers and to indicate extent of disease and to guide decisions regarding the need for additional staging studies to identify distant metastatic disease. Finally, biochemical testing should be performed to evaluate for the presence of PHPT and pheochromocytoma (i.e., serum calcium and intact parathyroid hormone levels and plasma free metanephrine or 24-hour urinary catecholamine levels). It is critical that pheochromocytoma be diagnosed preoperatively if it is present; the patient should be appropriately medically blocked before administration of an anesthetic so that the potentially catastrophic cardiovascular consequences associated with massive catecholamine release can be avoided. When pheochromocytoma is present in a patient with newly diagnosed MTC, adrenalectomy should be performed before thyroidectomy.

In addition to preoperative staging of the lateral neck lymph node basins by ultrasound, ATA guidelines recommend additional imaging to detect distant metastatic disease if the patient has extensive neck disease, signs or symptoms of distant metastasis, or a serum calcitonin level greater than 500 pg/mL. The presence of metastatic disease may influence the aggressiveness of surgical management of the neck disease. Evaluation should include chest CT to evaluate for metastases to the lung and mediastinal lymph nodes, three-phase contrast-enhanced multidetector liver CT or contrast-enhanced magnetic resonance imaging (MRI) to evaluate for liver metastases, and both bone scintigraphy and axial MRI to detect bone metastases.

Surgery for MTC is performed in two distinct contexts: (1) therapeutic (i.e., to treat clinically evident disease) or (2) prophylactic (i.e., to prevent development of MTC in a patient with a *RET* proto-oncogene mutation). Clinically evident MTC is treated with thyroidectomy and bilateral central neck dissection; modified radical neck dissection is performed for biopsy-proven lateral neck disease.

Prophylactic modified radical neck dissection may be considered rarely in cases in which metastatic disease to the lateral compartment is likely but not confirmed by FNA biopsy (e.g., for a large primary tumor with extensive central neck disease or in a patient with MEN 2B who did not undergo prophylactic thyroidectomy before the development of disease). Surgical treatment of local-regional MTC is often more aggressive than the surgical management of differentiated thyroid cancer because no other truly effective therapy exists for MTC. Unlike differentiated thyroid cancer for which adjuvant RAI often can treat residual microscopic disease effectively, RAI has no effect on MTC, as the cell of origin is not the thyroid follicular cell.

Patients with MEN 2A who have biochemically confirmed PHPT should undergo concurrent parathyroidectomy at the time of thyroidectomy, although PHPT typically develops later in life than MTC and thus usually involves parathyroidectomy in the setting of a reoperative neck. At the time of thyroidectomy, most endocrine surgeons leave normal parathyroid glands in situ; enlarged parathyroid glands should be resected, even in a patient who is eucalcemic. Total parathyroidectomy with autotransplantation at the time of initial thyroid surgery is recommended in a very few centers to reduce the risk that PHPT will develop in residual cervical parathyroid tissue, requiring reoperation. In patients with MEN 2A, normal parathyroid glands that are inadvertently devascularized during thyroidectomy should be autotransplanted into the forearm musculature, as they are at risk of developing PHPT; in patients with sporadic MTC or MEN 2B, parathyroid glands that are inadvertently devascularized may be autotransplanted into the neck (usually the sternocleidomastoid muscle).

The timing of prophylactic thyroidectomy for a patient identified as carrying a *RET* proto-oncogene mutation is guided by genotype-phenotype correlations. The specific *RET* mutation dictates the age of onset and the aggressiveness of MTC. Based on this information, the ATA has developed risk levels to guide the timing of surgery in children with inherited MTC. For patients with the highest-risk mutations (MEN 2B), prophylactic total thyroidectomy and bilateral central neck dissection should be performed in infancy, ideally before 1 year of age. Patients with a mutation leading to MEN 2A or familial MTC should undergo initial screening with thyroid ultrasound and serum calcitonin measurement between the ages of 3 and 5 years. Patients with MEN 2A and higher-risk mutations (i.e., codon 634) should undergo prophylactic thyroidectomy before age 5; bilateral central neck dissection should be performed if nodules larger than 5 mm are visible on ultrasound or if the serum calcitonin level is elevated. Patients with lower-risk mutations may be monitored with serial ultrasound and serum calcitonin levels, with prophylactic thyroidectomy delayed until they are older and surgery is safer, as long as the monitoring remains reassuring.

■ SURGERY FOR ANAPLASTIC THYROID CARCINOMA

Anaplastic thyroid carcinoma (ATC) is rare and accounts for approximately 1% of thyroid cancers but is a highly lethal undifferentiated cancer that leads to more than half of all deaths attributed to thyroid cancer annually in the United States. At presentation, disease is usually locally advanced and metastatic, and life expectancy ranges from 2 to 6 months. The majority of patients are not candidates for surgery; the mainstays of therapy are chemotherapy and radiation. Several studies have evaluated surgical debulking followed by chemotherapy and radiation versus chemotherapy and radiation alone. In general, there is no survival benefit with surgical debulking unless complete microscopic tumor resection can be achieved. Therefore surgery is reserved for specific situations: (1) open biopsy if FNA biopsy is insufficient to differentiate ATC from thyroid lymphoma; (2) tracheostomy to provide an airway in patients with advanced and rapidly progressive local disease; and (3) complete tumor resection in the limited number of patients who are discovered to have resectable ATC confined to the thyroid.

■ THYROID LYMPHOMA

Thyroid lymphoma is rare and accounts for 1% to 2% of thyroid cancers. Hashimoto's thyroiditis appears to be a predisposing factor. The most common histologic subtype to affect the thyroid is non-Hodgkin's B-cell lymphoma, and overall survival is 50% to 70%. Most patients have symptoms similar to those for ATC, with a rapidly enlarging neck mass that can progress to serious compressive symptoms and a compromised airway within a matter of weeks. FNA biopsy may be able to provide sufficient tissue for diagnosis, but core needle biopsy or an open surgical biopsy is sometimes necessary. Chemotherapy and radiation are the mainstays of therapy.

■ REOPERATIVE THYROID SURGERY

After initial surgical treatment with curative intent, disease recurs in 10% to 30% of patients with differentiated thyroid cancer. The majority of recurrences are local-regional (i.e., in the thyroid bed or in central or lateral neck lymph nodes). Reoperative neck surgery is associated with increased complications, particularly temporary or permanent hypoparathyroidism if the central neck is re-explored. As the quality of ultrasound has improved and assays to detect serum thyroglobulin levels have become more sensitive, PTC recurrences of ever-smaller clinical significance are now being identified routinely. Considering the usual indolent course of PTC, the zealousness of physicians, and the anxiety of patients, the morbidity of reoperation must be balanced against the overall low morbidity of recurrent PTC in most cases.

Surgery may not be the ideal management strategy for all patients with recurrent PTC in the central or lateral neck. Approximately 75% of patients who undergo reoperation for recurrent PTC still will not achieve an undetectable postoperative thyroglobulin, and surgery fails to remove the target disease recurrence in up to 10% of patients. Additional options for the management of recurrent PTC include RAI, percutaneous ethanol injection, and radiofrequency ablation. Careful observation alone may suffice in some cases, particularly for very small recurrences (i.e., <1 cm).

■ SUMMARY

The surgical management of patients with thyroid cancer is more challenging than the management of patients with benign thyroid disease. Because of the increased risks associated with reoperative surgery in the central and lateral neck, it is important to perform an optimal initial operation for thyroid cancer. The surgeon must be familiar with the details of genetics, pathology, endocrinology, surgery, and radiology that specifically pertain to thyroid cancer and be able to incorporate emerging technology into clinical practice in order to provide ideal care for this complex patient population.

SUGGESTED READINGS

Carty SE, Cooper DS, Doherty GM, et al. Consensus statement on the terminology and classification of central neck dissection for thyroid cancer. *Thyroid.* 2009;19:1153-1158.

Cibas ES, Ali SZ. The Bethesda System for reporting thyroid cytopathology. *Am J Clin Pathol.* 2009;132:658-665.

Haugen BR, Alexander EK, Bible KC, et al. 2015 American Thyroid Association management guidelines for adult patients with thyroid nodules and differentiated thyroid cancer. *Thyroid.* 2016;26:1-133.

Udelsman R, Zhang Y. The epidemic of thyroid cancer in the United States: the role of endocrinologists and ultrasounds. *Thyroid.* 2014;24:472-479.

Wells SA Jr, Asa SL, Dralle H, et al. Revised American Thyroid Association guidelines for the management of medullary thyroid carcinoma: the American Thyroid Association Guidelines Task Force on Medullary Thyroid Carcinoma. *Thyroid.* 2015;25:567-610.

PRIMARY HYPERPARATHYROIDISM

Faris K. Azar, MD, and Jason D. Prescott, MD, PhD

The parathyroid glands are endoderm-derived endocrine organs responsible for synthesis and secretion of parathyroid hormone, an 84 amino acid polypeptide that acts to increase blood calcium levels. Parathyroid gland function is required for normal blood calcium homeostasis and, under normal circumstances, parathyroid hormone synthesis is controlled tightly by feedback mechanisms involving blood calcium and vitamin D levels. Most commonly, there are four parathyroid glands, one gland near the posterior superior surface of the thyroid lobe on each side (superior glands) and the remaining glands near the inferior posterior thyroid lobe surface bilaterally (inferior glands). These glands are redundant, and, in general, only one functional gland is required for normal calcium homeostasis. The parathyroid glands receive arterial blood via one or more very fine vessels derived from the ipsilateral inferior thyroid artery, which branches from the thyrocervical trunk on the same side.

Hyperparathyroidism refers to a frank or inappropriate elevation in blood parathyroid hormone level, and this condition is categorized into three subtypes: primary, secondary, and tertiary disease. Primary hyperparathyroidism (PHPT) is the result of inappropriate parathyroid hormone production by one or more intrinsically abnormal parathyroid glands and is the most common cause of hypercalcemia. The incidence of PHPT in the United States is approximately 30 per 100,000 person years, with a female gender bias of 3:1. Roughly 80% of PHPT results from clonal expansion of parathyroid hormone–secreting cells (Chief cells) within a single gland, whereas 10% to 15% of cases are due to four-gland hyperplasia, and 4% are the product of adenomatous expansion in two or three of the four glands. Parathyroid carcinoma is responsible for approximately 1% of PHPT and generally is characterized by very high blood calcium and parathyroid hormone levels (total serum calcium >14 mg/dL, with blood parathyroid hormone levels >300 pg/mL). A careful family history is critical to the workup of PHPT because a number of familial syndromes feature this disease and, if present, necessitate evaluation for additional syndromic manifestations. These syndromes include multiple endocrine neoplasia type 1 (MEN 1, PHPT penetrance 100%), multiple endocrine neoplasia type 2A (MEN 2A, PHPT penetrance 20% to 30%), and jaw tumor syndrome (PHPT penetrance 80%).

The diagnosis of PHPT is entirely biochemical and depends on the presence of both inappropriate blood calcium and parathyroid hormone level elevations, in the context of normal blood vitamin D levels. Vitamin D plays an important role in normal blood calcium homeostasis, and low vitamin D levels may result in an appropriate compensatory elevation in blood parathyroid hormone, leading to an incorrect diagnosis of PHPT. Thus blood vitamin D levels should be normalized using vitamin D supplementation before assigning a diagnosis of PHPT. In addition, biochemical testing for familial hypocalciuric hypercalcemia (FHH), an autosomal dominant syndrome resulting from loss-of-function mutation(s) in the calcium sensing receptor gene, is necessary before diagnosing PHPT. This condition is characterized by mild elevations in blood-intact parathyroid hormone level, with associated relative hypercalcemia, and is diagnosed by 24-hour urine calcium level testing. A value of less than 100 mg in 24 hours is diagnostic of FHH and rules out PHPT. In contrast, hypercalciuria will be present in up to 80% of PHPT patients. Finally, it is important to note that imaging studies are neither sensitive nor specific for parathyroid disease and thus play no role in the diagnosis of hyperparathyroidism.

■ INDICATIONS FOR SURGERY

Elevated blood parathyroid hormone levels and associated hypercalcemia may be asymptomatic or may produce any of a myriad of nonspecific, but significant, symptoms. These include neurocognitive complaints, such as irritability, depression, short-term memory deficits, and difficulty concentrating; constitutional symptoms, including fatigue and insomnia; gastrointestinal complaints such as dyspepsia, abdominal pain, and constipation; musculoskeletal symptoms, including muscle pain, bone pain, and joint pain; and genitourinary complaints, such as polydipsia/polyuria. Signs of hyperparathyroidism include osteoporosis/osteopenia (parathyroid hormone stimulates osteoclast activity, thus liberating bone calcium stores), with possible associated pathologic fracture and bone deformities (osteitis fibrosa cystica/brown tumors), pseudogout, nephrolithiasis, hypertension, peptic ulcer disease, and pancreatitis. These signs and symptoms classically have been summarized by the mnemonic "stones, bones, abdominal groans, and psychiatric overtones."

Parathyroidectomy remains the only curative intervention for hyperparathyroidism and, although associated symptoms are generally nonspecific, such symptoms often improve after successful surgery. Thus symptomatic disease should prompt surgical referral. Management guidelines for asymptomatic PHPT recently were updated during the Fourth International Workshop on Asymptomatic Primary Hyperparathyroidism, and asymptomatic patients meeting these guidelines should be referred for parathyroidectomy (Table 1). Asymptomatic patients who do not meet criteria for parathyroidectomy should undergo annual reassessment for the development of symptoms, annual blood testing to reassess whether the magnitude of their hypercalcemia has reached levels meriting parathyroidectomy, and bone mineral density scanning every 1 to 2 years to evaluate for the development of osteoporosis. Medical therapy for primary hyperparathyroidism, including use of Cinacalcet (Sensipar) and bisphosphonates, is currently less efficacious than parathyroidectomy and should be limited to patients who are not operative candidates.

■ PREOPERATIVE LOCALIZATION

After a diagnosis of primary hyperparathyroidism is made and an indication for parathyroidectomy has been established, the next step in management is localization of the offending parathyroid gland(s). Successful disease localization allows targeted resection of the abnormal gland(s), thus minimizing both the extent of surgery necessary and risk of incurring an operative complication. A number of imaging techniques have been described for abnormal parathyroid gland localization, including neck ultrasonography, technetium-99m sestamibi scanning, with or without single-photon emission computed tomography (SPECT), four-dimensional computed tomography (4D CT) scanning, magnetic resonance imaging (MRI), and venography with venous sampling (generally performed only in reoperative cases for which localization using less-invasive imaging techniques has been unsuccessful). At our institution, all patients diagnosed with PHPT undergo both preoperative sestamibi-SPECT scanning and neck ultrasonography (Figures 1 and 2). When hyperparathyroidism is mediated by a single hyperfunctioning parathyroid gland, these studies individually will localize the responsible gland in 80% to 90% of cases. Concordant sestamibi-SPECT and ultrasound findings raise the sensitivity of preoperative localization to 94% to 99% in high-volume endocrine surgical centers, whereas multigland disease decreases the sensitivity of these techniques. Sestamibi-SPECT scanning also can localize ectopic disease (present in up to 20% of cases) that is not readily identified by other imaging modalities, especially abnormal inferior parathyroid glands that have descended into the mediastinum and are thus not accessible via a cervical incision. Neck ultrasonography also can identify concomitant surgical thyroid pathology that can be resected at the time of parathyroidectomy, thus avoiding progression of otherwise unidentified thyroid disease and the need for subsequent neck surgery. In cases in which both sestamibi-SPECT scanning and neck ultrasonography fail to localize the causative gland(s), we reattempt preoperative disease localization using 4D CT scanning (Figure 3). This technique involves fine-cut (1- to 3-mm) imaging of the neck and upper chest using noncontrast, arterial contrast, and venous contrast phases. Comparison between images obtained using these three different phases allows differentiation of enlarged parathyroid glands from adjacent structures, including thyroid tissue and cervical lymph nodes. We do not use MRI for disease localization because we have found this modality to offer relatively poor localization results, with associated costs exceeding those of ultrasound, sestamibi, and CT scanning, respectively.

We strongly recommend that parathyroid surgeons review all parathyroid imaging with the reading radiologist before proceeding with surgery. In our experience, such review has led to development of critical expertise in localizing pathologic parathyroid glands. This expertise is particularly important when interpreting the results of sestamibi scanning, which may be extremely subtle. We define such subtle localization findings as "shadows," which are evident as

asymmetry of the thyroid gland from the anterior view and/or posterior thyroidal extension from the lateral view (Figure 4). These "shadows" are present in more than 40% of otherwise nonlocalizing sestamibi scans and have led to a successful minimally invasive surgical approach for more than 90% of such patients at our institution (see Suggested Readings). Finally, the sensitivity of sestamibi scanning and of ultrasonography for parathyroid disease localization is dependent on the skill of the performing provider, with more experienced providers generally achieving the best localization accuracy. For this reason, these imaging studies should be performed at high-volume centers whenever possible.

Successful preoperative localization should prompt minimally invasive parathyroidectomy. Patients with PHPT for whom preoperative localization fails often have multigland disease and should undergo bilateral neck/four gland exploration.

TABLE 1: Indications for Parathyroidectomy in Patients With Asymptomatic Primary Hyperparathyroidism

Age	<50 years
Serum calcium	1.0 mg/dL (0.25 mmol/L) above upper limit of normal
24-hour urinary calcium	>400 mg/day (10 mmol/day)
Renal involvement	Creatinine clearance <60 mL/min or nephrolithiasis/nephrocalcinosis
Bone mineral density	T-score <-2.5 at the lumbar spine, total hip, femoral neck, or distal ⅓ radius, or documented vertebral fracture

Adapted from the 2013 Fourth International Workshop on Asymptomatic Primary Hyperparathyroidism Guidelines.

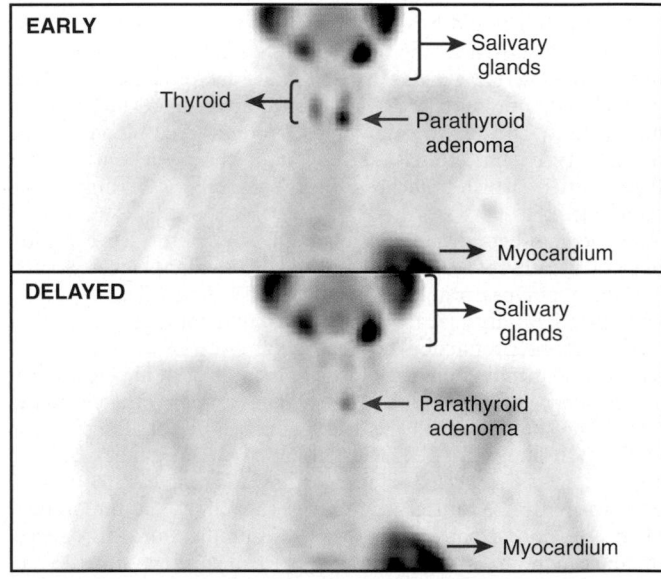

FIGURE 1 Sestamibi-SPECT scanning for parathyroid adenoma localization in PHPT. Early *(top)* and delayed/washout *(bottom)* coronal images are shown for the same lesion. A left lower parathyroid adenoma is identified *(red arrow)*. *Blue arrows* show spurious sestamibi uptake in the salivary glands, the thyroid gland (early/washout images only) and the myocardium.

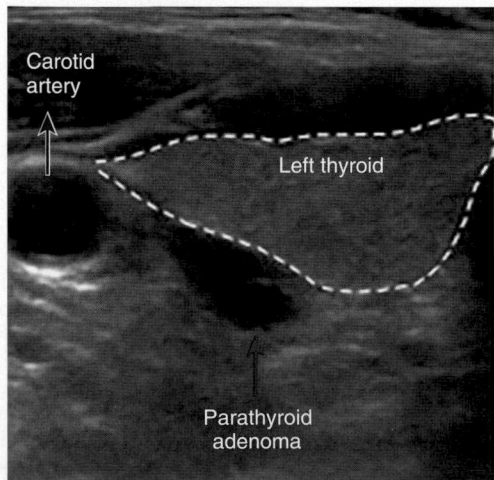
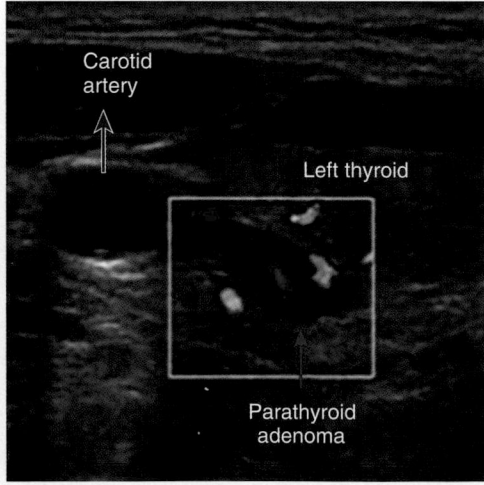

FIGURE 2 Ultrasound scanning for parathyroid adenoma localization in PHPT. Standard *(left)* and Doppler *(right)* transverse orientation images are shown for the same lesion. A left upper parathyroid adenoma is identified *(red arrow)*. This demonstrates hypoechoic echotexture relative to surrounding tissues and areas of internal vascularity are seen when Doppler imaging is employed. The left thyroid lobe is outlined in white and left carotid artery is shown by a blue arrow.

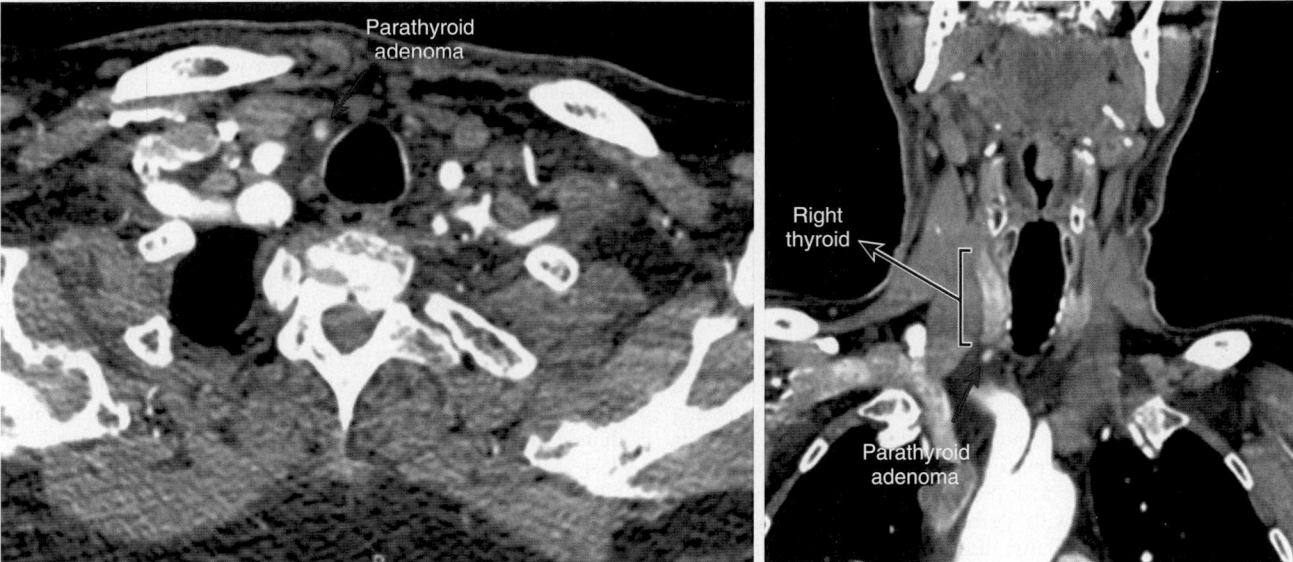

FIGURE 3 4D CT scanning for parathyroid adenoma localization in PHPT. Arterial phase axial *(left)* and coronal *(right)* orientation images are shown for the same lesion. A right lower parathyroid adenoma is identified *(red arrow)*. This demonstrates increased contrast enhancement relative to the adjacent thyroid tissue *(blue arrow)*.

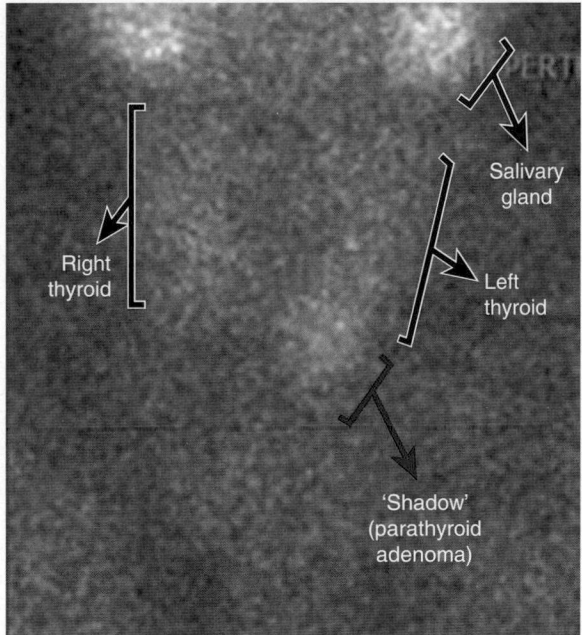

FIGURE 4 Sestamibi-SPECT scanning for parathyroid adenoma localization in PHPT. A delayed/washout coronal image is shown. The thyroid is asymmetric, with a left lower prominence ("shadow") noted. This prominence proved to correspond to a left lower parathyroid adenoma *(red arrow)*. *Blue arrows* show spurious sestamibi uptake in the salivary and thyroid glands.

■ INTRAOPERATIVE ADJUNCTS

Intraoperative Blood Parathyroid Hormone Level Testing

Intraoperative blood-intact parathyroid hormone level testing, developed by Dr. George Irvin at the University of Miami in the early 1990s, allows intraoperative verification of cure after parathyroidectomy. This technique is based on the following premises:

1. Successful preoperative disease localization, leading to focused excision of a single parathyroid gland, will not always result in cure because a fraction of such cases will involve additional foci of unidentified parathyroid disease.
2. Blood-intact parathyroid hormone has a short half-life of 2 to 4 minutes, and the levels of this hormone thus should drop rapidly after successful excision of hyperfunctional parathyroid tissue.
3. Failure of the blood-intact parathyroid hormone level to decrease appropriately after excision of an enlarged parathyroid gland indicates the presence of additional disease and should prompt additional surgical exploration.
4. An appropriate drop in the intraoperative blood-intact parathyroid hormone level after excision of enlarged parathyroid gland(s) is indicative of cure, allowing the surgeon to forgo additional surgical exploration and thus decrease both the operative time and the risk of incurring a surgical complication.

This technique has been shown to improve cure rates, and we use intraoperative parathyroid hormone level testing for all patients undergoing surgery for PHPT.

Recurrent Laryngeal Nerve Monitoring

The recurrent laryngeal nerves are paired structures coursing through the central neck on each side, traveling from the thorax inlet, deep to carotid/innominate arteries, superiorly to the larynx, where they innervate all but one of the intrinsic laryngeal muscles. Intraoperative injury to these subtle and delicate structures, which often are situated immediately adjacent to the parathyroid glands, can produce devastating symptoms, including severe hoarseness, thin liquid aspiration, and/or airway compromise requiring tracheostomy. Recurrent laryngeal nerve monitoring allows intraoperative evaluation of nerve function and has been shown to improve recognition of nerve injury. Anecdotally, this technique also may facilitate intraoperative nerve localization. Recurrent laryngeal nerve monitoring requires specialized equipment, including a specialized electrode integrated into, or affixed to, the endotracheal tube (thus necessitating use of general anesthesia).

Gamma Probe-Mediated Intraoperative Parathyroid Adenoma Localization

Technetium 99m (^{99m}TC) sestamibi is a pharmaceutical agent preferentially absorbed by thyroid tissue and, in particular, by hyperfunctional parathyroid glands. The rate of ^{99m}TC sestamibi tissue clearance is greater for thyroid tissue than for parathyroid glands, leading to preferential parathyroid ^{99m}TC sestamibi retention. Some parathyroid surgeons have reported successful intraoperative parathyroid disease localization using a radioisotope (gamma) probe to guide intraoperative exploration after preoperative ^{99m}TC sestamibi injection. Despite the differential in ^{99m}TC sestamibi clearance between tissues, however, we have found the accuracy of this technique to be confounded by background signal from normal thyroid tissue, and we therefore do not employ this intraoperative adjunct.

■ PARATHYROIDECTOMY

Minimally Invasive Parathyroidectomy

Focused parathyroidectomy using a small cervical incision (minimally invasive parathyroidectomy, or MIP) has become the standard surgical approach for PHPT when preoperative localization is successful. This approach can be performed under general anesthesia or using superficial cervical plexus nerve blockade and local anesthesia (regional anesthesia). MIP performed using regional anesthesia has been associated with decreased postoperative care unit recovery time/faster postoperative discharge, decreased postoperative nausea, decreased postoperative narcotic pain control requirements, and, as a result, decreased overall cost. On the other hand, regional anesthesia requires an experienced anesthesia team capable of intraoperative conversion to general anesthesia, if necessary, and a compliant patient capable of tolerating neck surgery while awake. Intraoperative recurrent laryngeal nerve monitoring, which requires a specialized endotracheal tube electrode, is also not possible using regional anesthesia.

Our practice uses general anesthesia, with placement of a neural integrity monitor electromyogram endotracheal tube, allowing for intraoperative recurrent laryngeal nerve monitoring. A baseline venous blood parathyroid hormone level is obtained in the preoperative holding area, and a large-bore intravenous catheter is placed for intraoperative blood sampling (intraoperative blood-intact parathyroid hormone levels also may be acquired through direct cannulation of the ipsilateral internal jugular vein, which courses along the lateral border of the dissection field). The patient is positioned in the semi-Fowler's position on the operating table, with the arms tucked and appropriately padded. The neck is placed into extension by inflating a pressure bag positioned along the upper back, and we verify that the head is resting on the operating table (rather than floating/suspended by the cervical spine). After standard sterile preparation, the operation begins with a symmetric, transverse Kocher incision, 2 to 4 cm long and one or two fingerbreadths above the sternal notch, in a pre-existing skin crease, if possible. The platysma is divided using electrocautery, and subplatysmal flaps are raised. The superior flap is carried to the level of the cricoid cartilage, whereas the inferior flap is freed to the level of the sternal notch/clavicles. The midline raphe between the strap muscles then is divided, and the plane between these muscles (anterior) and the ipsilateral thyroid lobe (posterior) is dissected. Bridging vessels are ligated using silk suture, hemoclips, and/or a vessel-sealing device. The dissection plane is maintained strictly at the level of the thyroid capsule so as to avoid damaging the recurrent laryngeal nerve and normal parathyroid gland(s) on the ipsilateral side. The thyroid is rotated medially to expose the targeted parathyroid adenoma, which will be attached to the posterior capsule of the thyroid in more than 80% of cases. The superior parathyroid glands are located most commonly posterior relative to the recurrent laryngeal nerve and superior to the inferior thyroid artery, whereas the inferior glands are generally anterior to the nerve and inferior to the inferior thyroid artery. Care must be taken during dissection to avoid rupturing the capsule of an enlarged parathyroid gland because potential associated cell spillage may lead to diffuse cervical implantation and growth of these abnormal cells, causing a rare but generally incurable form of disease recurrence called *parathyromatosis*. Nonetheless, dissection should be carried out at the level of the parathyroid capsule to avoid injury to adjacent structures and to

allow skeletonization and ligation of the associated blood supply. Upon gland excision, we confirm tissue identity by frozen section analysis and verify that the specimen weight is consistent with an enlarged parathyroid gland (exceeding the normal parathyroid gland weight range of 20 to 40 mg).

Blood-intact parathyroid hormone levels are assessed immediately after excision of an enlarged gland (time zero) and again 5, 10, and 20 minutes later. The probability of cure is estimated concomitantly on the basis of the Miami criteria, which stipulate a drop in blood-intact parathyroid hormone level of 50%, or more, relative to either the preoperative baseline value obtained on the day of surgery or to the highest value obtained intraoperatively before gland excision. A 97% cure rate has been reported when blood-intact parathyroid hormone levels fulfill the Miami criteria, and we therefore cease operative exploration under this circumstance. Blood samples acquired via aspiration from a peripheral intravenous line may be diluted by saline within the associated tubing, leading to false decreases in blood-intact parathyroid hormone levels. Accurate blood testing therefore requires initial aspiration of all intravenous line contents before acquiring blood samples for testing. Alternatively, blunt dissection may be used to expose the ipsilateral internal jugular vein, just lateral to the carotid artery, which then may be cannulated directly with a small-gauge needle for sample acquisition. We then carefully inspect the wound beds and obtain total hemostasis to minimize the risk of potentially life-threatening postoperative neck hematoma formation. Any normal parathyroid glands identified during exploration are inspected for viability, and the anatomic integrity of the recurrent laryngeal nerve(s), if exposed, is verified. Hemostatic agents then may be placed in the wound bed(s); in our case, we cover the wound bed base with polymeric oxidized cellulose, which acts to nucleate blood clot formation. The operation concludes with vertical midline closure of the strap muscles using absorbable 3-0 suture, reapproximation of the platysma using 3-0 suture, and skin closure with a 4-0 running absorbable monofilament suture. Careful attention to dermal edge apposition during skin closure and minimization of skin edge trauma during the procedure generally lead to excellent cosmetic outcomes and minimal scar formation.

■ BILATERAL NECK EXPLORATION

Patients for whom preoperative localization studies are negative require conventional bilateral neck exploration. This also is required for patients in whom four gland disease is expected, including those diagnosed with MEN 1 or familial hyperparathyroidism and for those MEN 2A patients diagnosed with hyperparathyroidism. Failure of blood-intact parathyroid hormone levels to decrease appropriately after excision of a preoperatively localized enlarged parathyroid gland also necessitates exploration, which should continue until additional enlarged gland(s) are resected, with the subsequent blood parathyroid hormone level decrement fulfilling the Miami criteria or, in cases of four gland involvement, subtotal parathyroidectomy or total parathyroidectomy with autotransplantation is performed. The parathyroid glands are notorious for ectopic localization, that supernumerary glands (additional parathyroid glands beyond the typical four gland scenario) may be present in up to 13% of patients, and that approximately 5% of patients will have only three glands. When present, these circumstances generally necessitate neck exploration. Operative exploration for ectopic abnormal parathyroid gland(s) requires clear understanding of parathyroid embryologic development because such knowledge informs on the most probable anatomic location(s) of ectopic glands. Inferior parathyroid glands are derived from the third pharyngeal pouch and thus descend with the thymus during embryologic development. Ectopic inferior glands thus often are located within the thyrothymic ligament or within the thymus itself. Ectopic superior glands, in contrast, are more likely to localize within the carotid sheath or in the retroesophageal space. Additional sites of ectopic localization include the paraesophageal space, within the thyroid itself and in the tracheoesophageal groove.

TABLE 2: Locations, by Frequency, of Ectopic Enlarged Parathyroid Glands in Primary Hyperparathyroidism

ECTOPIC INFERIOR GLANDS

Intrathymic	55%
Intrathyroidal	20%
Superior mediastinal	20%
Submandibular	5%

ECTOPIC SUPERIOR GLANDS

Tracheoesophageal groove	40%
Periesophageal	30%
Superior mediastinal	20%
Intrathyroidal	5%
Carotid sheath	5%

Sites of disease localization outside of the usual cervical operative field include the mediastinum, requiring sternotomy or thoracotomy, and high in the neck, potentially necessitating a high cervical incision (Table 2).

Bilateral neck exploration requires a longer, 5- to 6-cm, Kocher incision, although the subsequent initial dissection is carried out as previously described. All four glands are inspected visually. Normal parathyroid glands should be preserved carefully, peeled away from the thyroid, and left in situ on their native vascular pedicles. If the identity of a normal parathyroid gland is unclear, we will sharply resect a small fragment of this tissue at a site distant from the gland's blood supply for intraoperative frozen section analysis. In the setting of two or three enlarged parathyroid glands, all diseased glands should be excised. When four gland enlargement is present, a subtotal (3½-gland) or total (4-gland) parathyroidectomy with autotransplantation is performed. The goal of subtotal parathyroidectomy is to leave the approximate equivalent volume of a normal parathyroid gland in situ on the gland's native vascular pedicle. To accomplish this, we place a large titanium hemoclip across the width of the unresected gland at a position that is distal to both the gland's vascular pedicle and a normal associated volume of parathyroid tissue. We then sharply resect the tissue on the other side of the clip, leaving the clip, a normal volume of parathyroid tissue, and the associated vascular supply intact.

When performing a total parathyroidectomy with autotransplantation, we transplant into the nondominant brachioradialis muscle rather than the ipsilateral sternocleidomastoid muscle because the former practice allows avoidance of potential complications associated with reoperative neck surgery should the transplanted tissue subsequently grow to produce recurrent disease. Autotransplantation involves harvesting, by sharp dissection, a volume of parathyroid tissue approximately equivalent to that of a normal parathyroid gland from the most normal-appearing/least enlarged of the four glands resected. This tissue then is minced sharply into a fine slurry (1- to 2-mm fragments). The nondominant brachioradialis muscle then is exposed, and three or four pockets are made in the muscle belly using blunt dissection. Equal volumes of the prepared parathyroid slurry then are placed into each respective muscle pocket, and the pockets are closed with nonabsorbable suture. We leave the suture ends long, to facilitate future operative localization, if necessary, and also place a hemoclip on each suture end to allow subsequent radiographic localization. Whenever possible, we favor subtotal parathyroidectomy over total parathyroidectomy with autotransplantation because we find that parathyroid tissue viability is maximized when residual tissue is maintained on its native blood supply, thus

minimizing the risk of postoperative hypoparathyroidism. Further, autotransplanted parathyroid tissue will not function adequately to maintain serum calcium levels for at least 2 weeks after surgery, during which time aggressive calcium replacement therapy, including treatment with calcitriol (Rocaltrol/activated vitamin D), will be required. These patients also may require hospitalization for intravenous calcium gluconate infusion.

Because of potential involvement of hyperfunctional supernumerary parathyroid glands, we employ intraoperative blood parathyroid hormone level testing whenever performing parathyroidectomy for PHPT. On occasion, parathyroid hormone levels will not decrease appropriately, despite excision of all enlarged glands encountered and performance of a thorough neck exploration (including opening and exploring the carotid sheaths, bilateral exploration of the paraesophageal and retroesophageal spaces, and performing bilateral cervical thymectomies). Under such circumstances, the causative gland may be intrathyroidal. The laterality of such intrathyroidal hyperfunctional parathyroid glands will be apparent if both glands on the contralateral side have been identified. In addition, direct comparison of blood-intact parathyroid hormone levels obtained from each internal jugular vein may allow disease lateralization. Under such circumstances, we perform an ipsilateral thyroid lobectomy (the possible need for cervical thymectomy and for thyroid lobectomy should be discussed thoroughly with all PHPT patients before surgery). If, after these maneuvers, blood parathyroid hormone levels have not decreased appropriately, we will stop the operation and plan for subsequent additional localization attempts and possible reoperation (discussed elsewhere in this volume). Sternotomy and/or thoracotomy should never be performed in the absence of clear mediastinal disease localization.

Parathyroid carcinoma is a rare cause of PHPT (approximately 1% of cases) and usually is heralded preoperatively by very high blood-intact parathyroid hormone and calcium levels, as described above. Unlike benign parathyroid disease, parathyroid carcinoma often is appreciated during preoperative physical exam because the causative gland is generally very firm and often is fixed to the adjacent thyroid lobe. Appropriate treatment requires en bloc resection of the tumor with the adjacent thyroid lobe and all additional involved structures, as well as ipsilateral central neck dissection. Extreme caution must be exercised during this procedure to avoid damaging the tumor capsule because this will result in implantation of spilled tumor cells, with subsequent, likely incurable, parathyromatosis.

■ OPERATIVE COMPLICATIONS AND POSTOPERATIVE OUTCOMES

The two primary complications associated with parathyroidectomy are recurrent laryngeal nerve injury and hypoparathyroidism. The overall complication rate is approximately 4% among patients who undergo bilateral neck exploration, and between 1% and 3% among patients undergoing MIP. Unilateral recurrent laryngeal nerve injury produces either temporary ipsilateral vocal cord dysfunction, if the nerve is damaged but not transected, or permanent cord paralysis if the nerve is cut. Unilateral injury may be asymptomatic or may produce severe hoarseness, dyspnea, and thin liquid aspiration, depending on the relative position of the paralyzed cord, whereas bilateral nerve injury may result in airway compromise requiring emergent tracheostomy. Temporary hypoparathyroidism is common after parathyroidectomy because the preoperatively suppressed synthetic function of normal parathyroid tissue often requires several days for reinitiation. Permanent hypoparathyroidism occurs when all parathyroid tissue is resected or damaged inadvertently during bilateral neck exploration or if autotransplantation is unsuccessful. Associated signs and symptoms are primarily the result of hypocalcemia and most commonly manifest as paresthesias (usually perioral and/or involving the distal extremities) and muscle spasms. Severe hypocalcemia may present with tetany and seizures. Blood calcium levels should be monitored if symptoms develop, and oral calcium supplementation should be titrated to achieve normal serum total calcium levels. Normal blood vitamin D levels usually are needed to maximize gastrointestinal calcium absorption, and oral vitamin D supplementation is important if blood levels are low. Severe cases of postoperative hypoparathyroidism may require intermittent intravenous calcium gluconate administration. Postoperative neck hematoma formation and wound infection are rare, although the former is a surgical emergency and, because of associated risk of airway compromise, requires immediate bedside opening of the surgical wound for clot evacuation.

The benefits of parathyroidectomy for PHPT patients who meet criteria for surgery are well established and include resolution of preoperative symptoms and improvement in renal function and bone mineral density. Surgical cure is achieved in greater than 95% of cases when bilateral exploration is required, with comparable results among patients undergoing MIP (cure rates as high as 98%). We evaluate blood-intact parathyroid hormone, calcium, and vitamin D levels 1 to 2 weeks after surgery to establish postoperative baseline levels. It is common for blood parathyroid hormone levels to be elevated mildly at that time, with low normal blood total calcium levels. These findings are virtually always the result of vitamin D deficiency and will normalize with initiation of oral vitamin D

supplementation. Blood testing subsequently is reperformed 6 months after surgery, and normal blood parathyroid hormone and calcium values at that time rule out persistent disease. Approximately 2% of patients develop recurrent HPTH after initially curative surgery, and thus blood parathyroid hormone and calcium levels should be assessed annually to identify disease recurrence.

SUGGESTED READINGS

Bilezikian JP, Brandi ML, Eastell R, et al. Guidelines for the management of asymptomatic primary hyperparathyroidism: summary statement from the Fourth International Workshop. *J Clin Endocrinol Metab.* 2014;99: 3561-3569.

Callender GG, Udelsman R. Surgery for primary hyperparathyroidism. *Cancer.* 2014;120:3602-3618.

Laird AM, Libutti SK. Minimally invasive parathyroidectomy versus bilateral neck exploration for primary hyperparathyroidism. *Surg Oncol Clin N Am.* 2016;25:103-118.

Neychev VK, Kouniavsky G, Shiue Z, et al. Chasing "shadows": discovering the subtleties of sestamibi scans to facilitate minimally invasive parathyroidectomy. *World J Surg.* 2011;35:140-146.

Solorzano CC, Carneiro-Pla D. Minimizing cost and maximizing success in the preoperative localization strategy for primary hyperparathyroidism. *Surg Clin North Am.* 2014;94:587-605.

EVALUATION AND MANAGEMENT OF PERSISTENT OR RECURRENT HYPERPARATHYROIDISM

Ioannis A. Christakis, MD, MSc, MSc(surg), PhD, FRCS(eng), and Nancy D. Perrier, MD, FACS

Primary hyperparathyroidism (PHPT) can be diagnosed with relative ease and cured surgically in up to 96% of cases. Patients with PHPT are considered biochemically cured if they maintain eucalcemia 6 months after parathyroidectomy; patients who do not achieve or maintain eucalcemia in this period are considered to have persistent disease (incidence ranges from 1% to 6%). If the patient has an apparently successful operation (with temporary normalization of serum calcium and parathyroid hormone [PTH] levels) but then develops hypercalcemia with inappropriately elevated PTH levels after having cure for 6 months, the patient is diagnosed with recurrent disease.

This chapter discusses the etiology of persistent HPT, the preoperative evaluation of patients, surgical indications and contraindications, risk factors, surgical planning, surgical techniques, and technical adjuncts.

■ ETIOLOGY

Causes of persistent or recurrent HPT include missed glands, multigland disease incorrectly diagnosed as a single adenoma, incomplete resection of a single gland, and implantation of disease from a ruptured parathyroid cyst. Multigland disease is always present in secondary HPT (SHPT) because of the nature of the disease. Supernumerary glands occur in 7% to 10% of the general population, and disease in a supernumerary gland can account for persistent or recurrent HPT (Figure 1).

The most common cause of persistent HPT is a missed diseased parathyroid gland. Anatomic locations that can harbor missed glands are commonly the deep trachea-esophageal groove, the thyroid gland, the thymus, the posterior mediastinum, the base of the skull,

and the carotid sheath; glands that are in a high cervical undescended position also are commonly missed. Most missed abnormal parathyroid glands are found in the usual anatomic locations; hence the surgeon should have a thorough knowledge and understanding of the anatomy and embryology of the cervical and mediastinal regions.

■ DIAGNOSTIC AND PREOPERATIVE EVALUATION

The evaluation of suspected persistent or recurrent HPT is complex but follows the general principles of managing HPT (see Figure 1). HPT should be confirmed biochemically; documentation of inappropriately elevated PTH confirms the diagnosis of PHPT, but in the postoperative setting this finding can be confused with elevated PTH due to an appropriate response to hungry bone syndrome, low vitamin D, or renal failure. A 24-hour urinary calcium level measurement also should be performed to exclude familial hypocalciuric hypercalcemia. A young patient should raise the suspicion of multiple endocrine neoplasia syndromes and familial endocrinopathies. Physical examination can reveal anatomic details (e.g., a short or long neck, the location of previous neck incision, the presence of a goiter) that will be helpful as the surgeon plans the operative strategy.

For reoperative parathyroidectomy, a minimum of two concordant imaging studies are required for proper operative planning. If preoperative localization is concomitant and independently supports localization, the rate of cure is greater than 90%. In case of nonlocalization, this success rate drops to between 60% and 70%. Neck ultrasonography, technetium (^{99m}Tc) sestamibi scintigraphy (sestamibi), and four-dimensional multidetector computed tomography (4D CT) are the preferred initial imaging modalities for reoperative cases.

Ultrasonography is highly operator dependent, and an expert with a designated interest in parathyroid disease is important for reoperative success. Cervical ultrasonography provides excellent anatomic information; however, this modality cannot assess the hypersecretory status of any lesion that is identified. A fine-needle aspiration (FNA) biopsy of a suspicious lesion can be obtained at the time of ultrasonography, and the samples can be sent for cytologic confirmation and PTH biochemical assay to confirm the presence of PTH and to differentiate it from other structures (e.g., thyroid nodules or lymph nodes). The combination of cytologic and

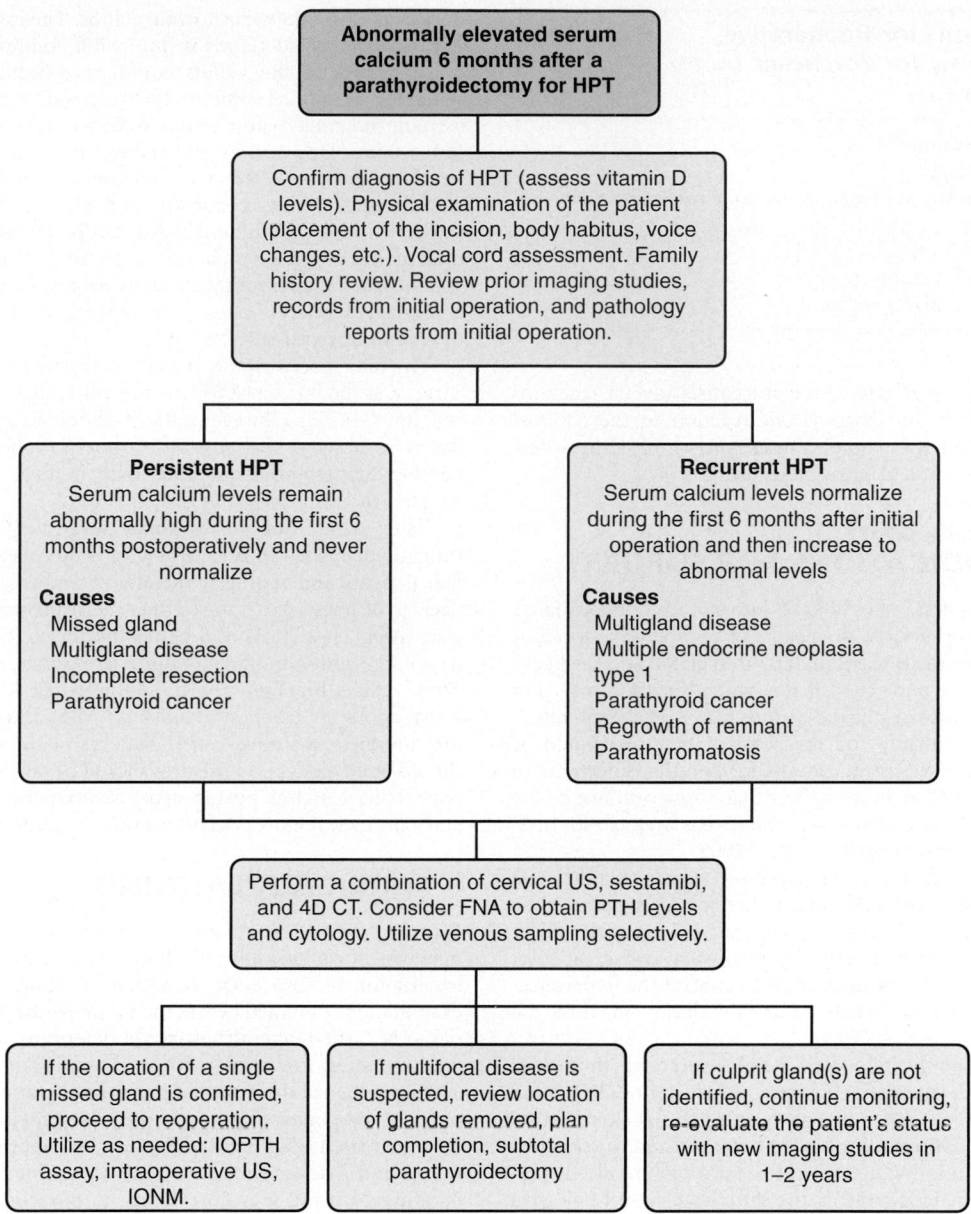

FIGURE 1 Algorithm for managing persistent or recurrent hyperparathyroidism (HPT). *4D CT*, Four-dimensional computed tomography; *FNA*, fine-needle aspiration; *IONM*, intraoperative neurophysiologic monitoring; *IOPTH*, intraoperative parathyroid hormone; *PTH*, parathyroid hormone; *sestamibi*, technetium (^{99m}Tc) sestamibi imaging; *US*, ultrasonography.

biochemical confirmation improves the accuracy of ultrasonography alone from 65% to more than 80% and the sensitivity from 75% to 90%.

Single-photon emission computed tomography (CT) or magnetic resonance imaging often is used as a second-line modality to identify an ectopic gland. The CT study should include mediastinal views to locate an ectopic gland in the thorax as well as jaw views to locate an undescended gland. CT is most valuable for identifying an adenoma in an ectopic, hyperfunctioning gland that was not identified during the initial surgery.

4D CT is a powerful modality for identifying missed parathyroid glands. The study should include axial views from jaw to aortic arch and perfusion. In addition to generating detailed multiplanar images of the neck, 4D CT allows visualization of differences in perfusion characteristics between hyperfunctioning parathyroid glands (i.e., rapid uptake and quick washout) and normal parathyroid glands and other structures in the neck. The images generated by 4D CT

therefore provide both anatomic information and a correlate for function (perfusion) in a single study.

In very selected cases, invasive methods to localize persistent or recurrent HPT can be utilized only when all other imaging studies have failed to provide sufficient information. One such technique is selective venous sampling (SVS), which involves catheterization of the internal jugular vein for lateralization and if necessary multiple veins in the neck and mediastinum, including the superior, middle, and inferior thyroid veins as well as the subclavian vein. A limitation of this approach is that the source of PTH overproduction often is only roughly regionalized. Furthermore, the venous drainage pattern for each parathyroid gland often is altered by previous neck operations, making exact localization of the gland challenging. With SVS, venograms are obtained in two planes to delineate the precise anatomic location of the vessel being sampled, and the PTH assay results direct the angiographer to site-specific locations. SVS is highly operator dependent, and there is always a risk of technical failure. Other

---

BOX 1: Indications for Reoperative Parathyroidectomy for Persistent or Recurrent Disease

Worrisome hypercalcemia
Ongoing nephrolithiasis
Worsening bone disease, as evidenced by bone mineral density
   scores
Worsening renal function
Associated psychiatric symptoms
Associated neuromuscular symptoms

---

limitations include the high cost of the procedure, adverse reactions (including renal failure and anaphylactic reaction to the contrast medium), and rare operative complications (such as bleeding, infection, pseudoaneurysm, and arteriovenous fistula).

■ INDICATIONS AND CONTRAINDICATIONS FOR SURGERY

The decision to reoperate should take into account the patient's symptoms and disease severity, the results of preoperative localization studies to identify the diseased parathyroid gland, and the likelihood of achieving cure and relief of the patient's symptoms. After confirmation of HPT disease, the indications for surgical exploration should be reviewed critically and the risk/benefit ratio should be weighed. The criteria used as indications for parathyroidectomy in the reoperative setting (Box 1) are stricter than those outlined by the National Institute of Health consensus conference statement for first-time parathyroidectomies (Bilezikian et al., 2002).

Hypercalcemia usually can be managed conservatively (although this is not a long-term solution), and life-threatening hypercalcemia is encountered very rarely. In general, reoperative surgery should be considered for all symptomatic HPT patients when conservative or pharmacologic treatments are inadequate to control the hypercalcemia symptoms and for patients with progressive decline in end organ disease (e.g., osteoporosis).

An absolute contraindication to reoperative surgery is the lack of confirmation of the diagnosis of persistent or recurrent PHPT. Blind explorations should not be performed. Inconclusive localization studies are a relative contraindication, and the decision to reoperate should be made on an individual basis. Reoperations should be performed only by experienced surgeons in a setting where technological adjuncts are available.

■ RISK ASSESSMENT

The decision to reoperate should take into account the patient's functional status, comorbidities, any sequelae of previous neck operations, and the anesthetic risks. Compared with initial surgery, reoperative surgery is associated with more operative complications.

Reoperations are associated with a greater incidence of vocal cord paralysis, with a recurrent laryngeal nerve (RLN) injury rate of approximately 2% to 15% (compared with 0.5% to 1% in initial operations). Before undertaking reoperative parathyroidectomy, the patient should undergo videostroboscopy to assess vocal cord status. Unilateral paralysis may already be present yet unnoticed, especially if the length of time between the initial operation and recurrence has been extensive. If there is a documented unilateral injury of the RLN with associated symptoms, the benefits and risks of reoperating on the contralateral side should be considered. The implications of bilateral RLN palsy for quality of life should be explained. Hypoparathyroidism may be permanent in 10% to 16% of patients.

Patients must be counseled about the risk for aparathyroidism, particularly if they had a previous four-gland exploration with resection of multiple glands or if an extensive previous operation

devascularized otherwise normal glands. The exact number of functioning parathyroid glands is impossible to know preoperatively, as one or more of the glands could have been devascularized but remained in situ. Therefore the reoperative surgeon should use extreme judgment before removing any gland, as it could be the only functioning gland and its removal would render the patient permanently aparathyroid. Patients should be advised that such an outcome would require lifelong calcium and vitamin D supplementation. With planning, parathyroid tissue can be cryopreserved in patients undergoing reoperative parathyroidectomy. If the patient becomes aparathyroid, the cryopreserved tissue can be defrosted and autotransplanted. Success rates are acceptable after autotransplantation of cryopreserved tissue.

Thyroid lobectomy is rarely performed during parathyroid surgery, as the incidence of true intrathyroidal parathyroid glands is very low (~0.7%). However, patients should be aware of this possibility, as a subset of patients who undergo lobectomy (~15%) will develop hypothyroidism and may require lifelong thyroxine supplementation.

Using data from the National Surgical Quality Improvement Program database (2008 to 2011), Kuo and colleagues (2014) showed that patients undergoing reoperative parathyroidectomy were more likely to be obese, to belong to the American Society of Anesthesiologists (ASA) class III, and to be readmitted to the hospital within 30 days compared with patients undergoing initial parathyroidectomy. These results highlight the need for increased vigilance from the anesthesiologist, as obesity and high ASA class are also risk factors for anesthetic complications. Patients with many comorbidities should be advised, and measures should be taken to ensure that these patients have a clear postoperative safety network and clinical plan and can reach the hospital after hours if needed.

■ SURGICAL PLANNING

Planning for the reoperation should begin by reviewing previous operative imaging and pathology reports. Independent review of localization studies such as sestamibi scans or ultrasonography examinations obtained before the initial parathyroidectomy is essential to help the reoperative surgeon determine whether the intraoperative findings correlated with preoperative imaging.

Knowledge of the extent of previous operations is crucial to planning the reoperative approach. Because previously dissected areas have increased scarring and fibrosis, complications such as RLN injury and inadvertent removal or devascularization of a normal parathyroid gland are more frequent. Surgeons should review the report from the initial operation to determine whether a unilateral or bilateral exploration was performed, the location of parathyroid glands that were identified, and the pathologic confirmation of glands removed. Accurate documentation of the glands' size and appearance is important. A thorough operative report will identify areas that were evaluated and whether a thymectomy was performed for a missing inferior gland. Factors that could complicate the identification of parathyroid glands, such as co-existing thyroid abnormalities (e.g., Hashimoto's thyroiditis, multinodular goiter, or the presence of reactive lymph nodes), should be ascertained from the report.

The pathology report from the initial surgery should be reviewed meticulously. This report will provide details regarding the size, weight, and cellularity of the pathologic tissue that was removed as well as information about any normal tissue that was resected. Multiple biopsies can be informative about the difficulty of gland identification. In case of uncertainty about the histopathologic diagnosis, the slides from the initial operation should be reviewed.

The reoperative surgeon should have a clear strategy for the remaining parathyroid glands when there is a risk that the patient will become aparathyroid. If the suspected diseased gland is the only viable parathyroid gland (three documented glands at pathology report), autotransplantation should be considered to avoid permanent hypoparathyroidism. A small portion of the gland also should be cryopreserved for future use in case the transplanted gland is not functional or is inadequate. Patients should be counseled about the risks of future repeat hyperfunction of autotransplantation tissue and the potential, albeit exceedingly rare, of debulking a portion of the autotransplanted tissue.

■ SURGICAL TECHNIQUES

The intraoperative localization of parathyroid glands during reoperation for persistent or recurrent HPT can be hindered significantly by scar tissue, the loss of normal anatomic planes, and anatomic modifications that resulted from the initial operation. Critical to technical success is a thorough knowledge of the embryology and anatomy. The lateral incision approach is an excellent option in reoperative cases to avoid scar tissue in the central compartment of the neck if the initial operation used a central approach.

A nomenclature system proposed by Perrier and colleagues (2009) classifies parathyroid glands as type A to type G, with a "+" sign used to designate superior glands that have not descended and a "−" sign used to designate glands that appear inferior to the usual position (Figure 2). This nomenclature system emphasizes the anterior-posterior location of enlarged parathyroid glands in relation to the thyroid parenchyma, trachea, and esophagus. Superior parathyroid glands usually are found on a vascular pedicle that is lateral and posterior to the RLN; when adenomatous, these glands may fall posterior to the thyroid tissue or into the tracheoesophageal groove (Figures 3 and 4). Glands that are derived embryologically from the inferior pedicle are classified as type E or F glands; the pedicles of these glands are medial and slightly more anterior to the RLN. Such a standardized system allows for efficient surgical planning. For example, hyperextension may be necessary for a posteriorly located type C gland lying deep in the tracheoesophageal groove (Figure 5).

The reoperative surgical approach selected is guided by two factors: preoperative localization studies and the initial operation. If there is adequate localization and the surgeon is experienced, a unilateral focused approach is possible; this approach helps to reduce operative morbidity by minimizing dissection in a challenging area.

Strategies for reoperative parathyroidectomy include the central approach and the lateral approach. If the initial operation was performed via a collar incision, reoperative surgery through a central approach usually requires incision of the pre-existing Kocher's incision. The central approach takes the surgeon through the previously dissected operative field (via separation of the strap muscles and medial-to-lateral dissection) and has obvious disadvantages, but this

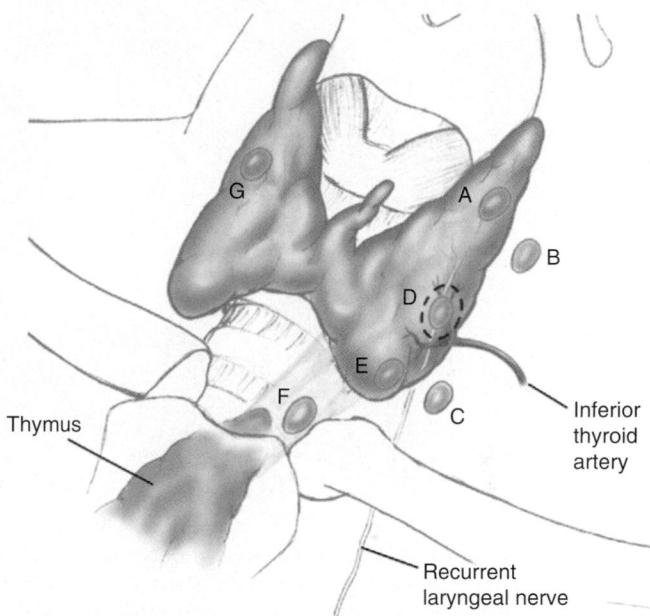

FIGURE 2 The position of type A to G glands in the nomenclature system of Perrier and colleagues (2009). Type A, B, and C glands are superior glands and type E, F, and G glands are inferior glands. Type D glands are difficult to discern if they are superior or inferior glands; the origin of the vascular pedicle of the gland should be assessed intraoperatively.

FIGURE 3 Cross-sectional drawing of the cervical region. The dissection plane is lateral to the strap muscles for a minimally invasive parathyroidectomy. Retracting the thyroid lobe superiorly and medially allows the identification of a left superior parathyroid gland (type A gland) attached to the undersurface of the left thyroid parenchyma. *Int. jugular vein*, Internal jugular vein; *SCM*, sternocleidomastoid muscle.

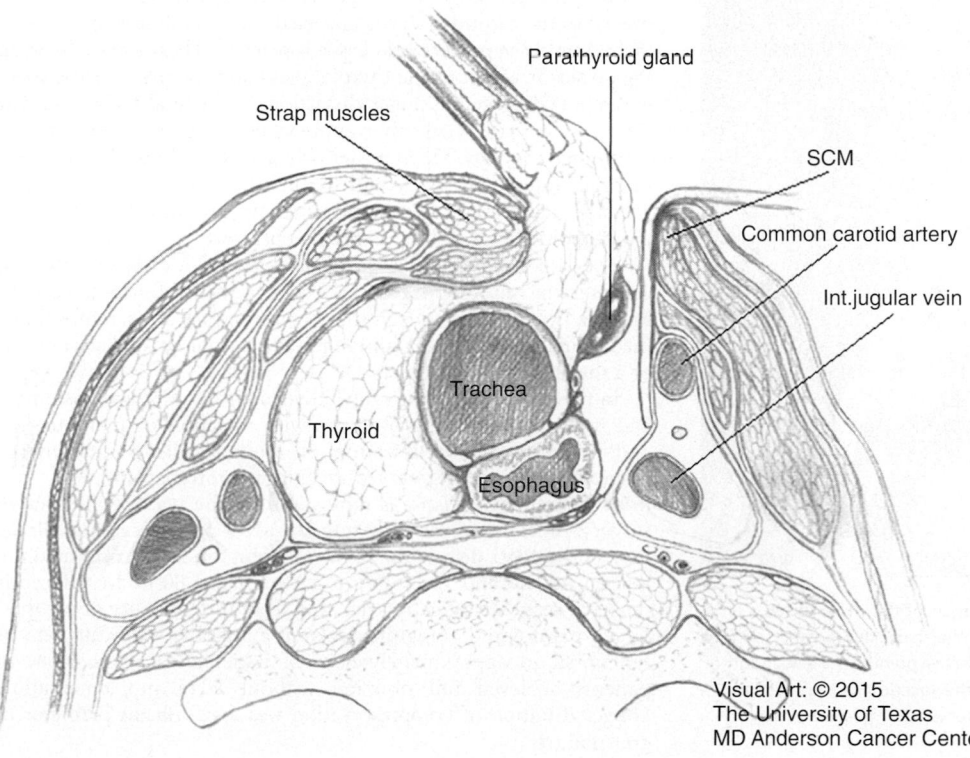

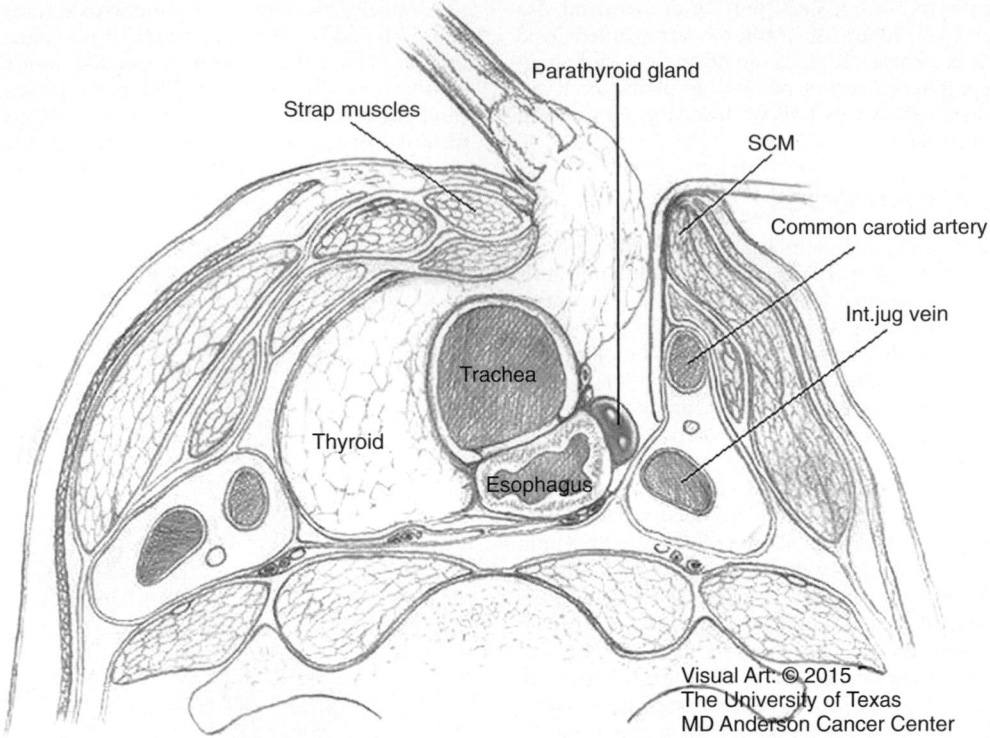

FIGURE 4 Cross-sectional drawing of the cervical region. The dissection plane is lateral to the strap muscles for a minimally invasive parathyroidectomy. Retracting the thyroid lobe superiorly and medially allows the identification of a left superior parathyroid gland (type B gland) residing in the deep left-sided tracheoesophageal groove. *Int.jug vein*, Internal jugular vein; *SCM*, sternocleidomastoid muscle.

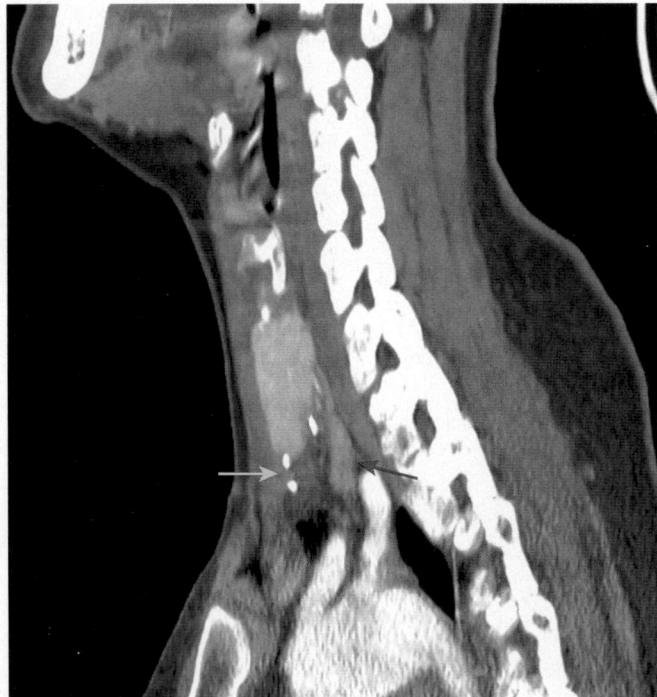

FIGURE 5 Sagittal computed tomography scan of the neck shows a missed parathyroid adenoma (type C gland) that has fallen posteriorly into the tracheoesophageal groove. The orange arrow points to the location of the missed gland. The blue arrow points to the location of the metallic clips from the initial unsuccessful surgical intervention (placed anteriorly to the actual location of the missed gland).

approach may provide a direct route to the inferior glands (type E and F glands).

The lateral technique approaches the gland between the strap muscles (retracted medially) and the sternocleidomastoid muscle (with the medial edge of this muscle retracted laterally). The space medial to the carotid artery is dissected, and the pretracheal fascia is incised until the prevertebral fascia is reached. Then a space between the posterior aspect of the thyroid gland and the prevertebral space is developed by gentle finger dissection. The lateral technique may offer easier access than other approaches and can expose superior glands that may have fallen posteriorly. The RLN should be protected to avoid injury. The RLN and the inferior thyroid artery provide valuable landmarks for orienting the surgeon and identifying the parathyroid glands in their expected positions.

The lateral approach is particularly useful for missed superior glands in the retroesophageal space or in the carotid sheath. A central incision is ideal for glands in the thymus. In rare cases, removal of a mediastinal parathyroid gland requires a partial or total sternotomy or a thoracoscopic approach.

In patients undergoing reoperative parathyroidectomy who have had multiple previous procedures with resection or manipulation and potential devascularization of multiple glands, parathyroid tissue should be cryopreserved for future autotransplantation. Confirmed parathyroid tissue is removed from the neck at the time of surgery, morcellated carefully into 20- to 30-mm pieces, and placed in a sterile Petri dish with Tis-U-Sol solution. A freezing medium is then added, and the mixture is frozen at −80°C. In a recently reported series investigating the long-term functionality of cryopreserved parathyroid autografts, delayed autografts were found to be functional in approximately 60% of patients. Of these, 40% of patients achieved full function without PTH supplementation. Longer duration of cryopreservation was a significant predictor of graft failure.

In contrast, the success rate for fresh parathyroid autografts has been reported to exceed 80%. For this reason, in patients who have already had multiple glands removed, autotransplantation into the nondominant brachioradialis muscle at the time of reoperative surgery is preferred. This site is preferred over the sternocleidomastoid muscle in the neck because the forearm is easier to explore if the patient experiences persistent or recurrent disease owing to the autotransplanted tissue. However, immediate autotransplantation adds extra time, limits the operating space because the arm needs to be extended, can create technical challenges if the gland must be removed at a later time, and poses a potential risk for nerve and muscle injury in the forearm.

We prefer to use the pectoralis major muscle just inferior to the clavicle as a site for autotransplantation. This approach allows quick and easy access to an area close to the operating field, prevents recurrence of disease in the area of the neck, and potentially reduces morbidity if reoperation is necessary after the autotransplantation. The transplanted gland is placed in a small pocket of the pectoralis major muscle through a mini-incision, and the wound is closed with Steri-Strips. On the first postoperative day, the patient's PTH level is measured; a detectable PTH level indicates that there is functioning parathyroid tissue in the neck (as the transplanted graft has not started producing PTH yet). In this case, the pectoralis major wound can be opened at bedside, and the transplanted graft, now proven unnecessary, can be removed with the help of gentle suction. If PTH is undetectable, the patient and physician can expect function in 8 to 12 weeks. Most parathyroid glands located in the superior mediastinum can be removed by gentle manipulation and retraction of the ipsilateral thymic tissue with the help of digital dissection and the use of a right-angle instrument. In rare cases in which the parathyroid gland is located inferiorly in the mediastinum, the use of video-assisted thoracoscopy can prevent the need for a sternotomy to excise the gland. This procedure is performed on patients under general anesthesia and in a supine position; patients receive ventilation through a double-lumen endotracheal tube, and carbon dioxide is insufflated through a Veress needle to collapse the ipsilateral lung (to the site of the parathyroid gland), which is selectively nonventilated. Then a 12-mm camera port is inserted in the fourth intercostal space along the midaxillary line, and the procedure is performed with two 5-mm working ports inserted under direct vision.

■ TECHNICAL ADJUNCTS

Intraoperative Neurophysiologic Monitoring

Intraoperative neurophysiologic monitoring (IONM) in reoperative parathyroid surgery can be useful to confirm nerve function if the contralateral nerve is going to be placed at risk.

Intraoperative Histologic Analysis

When abnormal parathyroid glands are identified during surgery, frozen section analysis can confirm histologically that the removed parathyroid tissue is cellular parathyroid tissue. Direct aspiration of the gland with a 25-gauge needle can be useful for biochemical confirmation of PTH levels. PTH values greater than 1900 pg/dL confirm that the tissue is of parathyroid origin, although this does not confirm cellularity; hence aspiration of the gland for PTH measurement can be a useful tool to complement histologic evaluation.

Intraoperative Ultrasonography

Intraoperative ultrasonography can facilitate incision placement in patients with ectopic glands. After the patient is anesthetized and in position, an on-the-table ultrasonographic examination is performed to identify and confirm the location of the gland.

Intravenous Methylene Blue

Ultrasound-guided instillation of methylene blue to stain the targeted tissue can be useful. With precise injection with a small tuberculin needle, stained tissue can be targeted more easily.

■ POSTOPERATIVE MANAGEMENT

The postoperative management for reoperative parathyroidectomy follows the same principles as for first-time parathyroidectomy. Patients may begin a regular oral diet immediately after nausea from the anesthetic resolves. Vigilance is needed to detect early signs and symptoms of hypocalcemia. In general, serum calcium and PTH levels should be measured on the evening of the procedure and on the morning of the first postoperative day. Confirmation of detectable PTH ensures viability of residual parathyroid gland function. Interpretation of the biochemistry along with the clinical status of the patient should drive the decisions regarding hospital discharge.

In our practice, we do not favor prophylactic calcium supplementation; medical therapy is given only in the presence of clinical symptoms and/or calcium levels lower than 8.0 mg/dL. If the patient has a calcium level lower than 8.0 mg/dL and a PTH level lower than 5 pg/mL, we administer calcium carbonate supplements (0.5 µg orally, twice daily) and vitamin D supplements (0.25 µg/day). If the calcium level is lower than 7.5 mg/dL, the patient can be treated with calcium carbonate supplements (two 0.5-µg tablets, three times daily) and vitamin D supplements. If the calcium level is lower than 7.0 mg/dL, we administer 10 mL of 10% calcium gluconate intravenously over 10 minutes and then 20 mL of 10% calcium gluconate in 1 L of 0.9% normal saline over 6 hours. After discharge, the patient returns for a blood test 2 to 3 days postoperatively and then 10 days postoperatively to check the serum calcium and PTH levels; medical treatment is adjusted accordingly.

■ CONCLUSION

Reoperative parathyroid surgery can be complex. Confirmation of the diagnosis and understanding of the etiology of the initial procedure are important. For suspected single-gland disease concomitant, concordant imaging suggesting a single area of uptake should direct the minimally invasive plan. If multigland disease is suspected, an operation to accomplish a 3.5 gland resection is necessary.

SUGGESTED READINGS

Bilezikian JP, et al. Summary statement from a workshop on asymptomatic primary hyperparathyroidism: a perspective for the 21st century. *J Clin Endocrinol Metab.* 2002;87:5353-5361.

Kuo LE, et al. Reoperative parathyroidectomy: who is at risk and what is the risk? *J Surg Res.* 2014;191:256-261.

Perrier ND, et al. A novel nomenclature to classify parathyroid adenomas. *World J Surg.* 2009;33:412-416.

SECONDARY AND TERTIARY HYPERPARATHYROIDISM

Tracy S. Wang, MD, MPH, and Julie Ann Sosa, MD, MA

The parathyroid gland was the last major organ to be recognized in mammals, discovered in an Indian rhinoceros in 1834 by Sir Richard Owen and in humans in the late 1870s by a Swedish medical student, Ivar Sandström. It was not until 1906, however, that the physiology of the parathyroid gland was recognized, when a Viennese pathologist, Jacob Erdheim, first theorized about an association between the parathyroid glands, bone disease, and calcium metabolism. Through the early twentieth century other physicians and scientists, including Friedrich Schlagenhaufer, William MacCallum, and Adolph Hanson, began to realize that the parathyroid gland was responsible for bone disease and calcium metabolism; this was in conjunction with the experience of early thyroid surgeons such as William Stewart Halsted, Theodor Kocher, Charles Mayo, and George Crile, who were discovering that preservation of the parathyroid glands reduced postoperative tetany in patients undergoing thyroidectomy. In 1934 Fuller Albright suggested a relationship between chronic renal disease and hyperparathyroidism (HPT), and in 1971 Richard Wilson and colleagues first reported their experience with subtotal parathyroidectomy as a means to retard the progression of osteitis fibrosa cystica in patients with severe secondary hyperparathyroidism (SHPT) and renal failure.

In contrast to primary hyperparathyroidism (PHPT), in which an intrinsic abnormality of the parathyroid glands leads to overproduction of parathyroid hormone (PTH), SHPT is characterized by increased PTH production in response to external stimuli, most commonly chronic kidney disease. Tertiary hyperparathyroidism (THPT) refers to the autonomous hypersecretion of PTH even after causes of SHPT have been corrected (e.g., after resolution of chronic kidney disease in patients who have undergone kidney transplantation) or when patients with SHPT develop hypercalcemia refractory to medical management. This chapter focuses on the pathophysiology and current strategies for the medical and surgical management of SHPT and THPT.

■ PATHOPHYSIOLOGY

The most common cause of SHPT is chronic kidney disease, although the pathologic mechanisms are complex and incompletely understood. The kidneys have a key role in the regulation of mineral metabolism; therefore renal failure is associated with altered metabolism of calcium, phosphorus, vitamin D, PTH, and fibroblast growth factor 23 (FGF23). Multiple interdependent factors lead to the subsequent development of hypocalcemia in patients with chronic kidney disease. Limited renal excretion of phosphorus stimulates production of FGF23; this in turn leads to a reduction in the renal production of 1,25-dihydroxyvitamin D_3 (1,25[OH]$_2$D; calcitriol, the active metabolite of vitamin D) and decreased serum calcium levels. High serum phosphorus and low 1,25(OH)$_2$D levels also directly stimulate the production of PTH, which in turn stimulates production of FGF23. Uremic hyperplastic parathyroid glands also have been shown to demonstrate reduced expression of calcium, 1,25(OH)$_2$D, and FGF23 receptors, making the parathyroid cell even less sensitive to the inhibitory actions of these three compounds. This combination of factors leads to continuous overstimulation of the parathyroid glands and the development of diffuse parathyroid hyperplasia (Figure 1). SHPT is characterized by low to normal serum calcium levels and significant elevation of PTH levels. In contrast, THPT, in which there is autonomous function of the parathyroid gland as a response to prolonged compensatory stimulation, is characterized by elevated serum calcium levels and elevated PTH levels.

SHPT also can occur in the setting of vitamin D deficiency in patients with normal renal function. Vitamin D primarily is obtained from exposure to sunlight, diet, and dietary supplements and subsequently is metabolized in the liver to 25-hydroxyvitamin D (25[OH]D). Measurement of this form of vitamin D is the primary determinant of a patient's vitamin D status; patients are vitamin D deficient with levels lower than 20 ng/mL and vitamin D insufficient with levels lower than 30 ng/mL. 25(OH)D is metabolized in the kidneys to its active form, 1,25(OH)$_2$D. As discussed previously, deficiency in 1,25(OH)$_2$D levels leads to stimulation of the parathyroid glands to increase PTH production; patients subsequently may have normal serum calcium levels and elevated PTH levels. However, in contrast to SHPT caused by chronic kidney disease, patients have normal renal function and a lower degree of PTH elevation. Vitamin D deficiency and SHPT often are seen in the obese and may be exacerbated by bariatric surgery and its associated reduction in gastric volume, reduced caloric intake, and alterations in the gastrointestinal absorption of minerals and nutrients.

■ MEDICAL MANAGEMENT

In patients with SHPT due to vitamin D deficiency and normal renal function, aggressive vitamin D supplementation is recommended; 25(OH)D levels are inversely associated with PTH levels until supplemented to 30 to 40 ng/mL. Current recommendations from the Institute of Medicine for adequate daily intake of vitamin D are 200 IU for adults up to age 50 years, 400 IU for adults ages 51 to 70 years, and 600 IU for adults age 71 years and older. Patients with vitamin D deficiency can take vitamin D_2 (50,000 IU weekly for 8 weeks, or 3000 IU daily) or vitamin D_3 (1000 IU daily); both have been shown to be effective and cost-conscious methods of supplementation.

In patients with SHPT due to chronic kidney disease, medical management is dependent on the severity of renal disease; treatment algorithms published by the National Kidney Foundation (Kidney Disease Outcomes Quality Initiative [KDOQI]) and Kidney Disease: Improving Global Outcomes (KDIGO) are aimed at minimizing cardiovascular-related and skeletal-related morbidity and mortality, respectively. In general, in patients with stage 3 or 4 chronic kidney disease (glomerular filtration rate of 30–59 and 15–29 mL/min/1.73 mol/L^2, respectively), therapies are aimed at preventing hyperphosphatemia and maintaining 1,25(OH)$_2$D levels. In patients with more advanced chronic kidney disease, including those on dialysis, goals of treatment are to reduce serum phosphorus levels and decrease PTH secretion.

In patients with early stage renal disease, dietary restriction of phosphorus, primarily achieved by eating foods that are low in protein, may be adequate in controlling serum phosphorus levels. In patients with more advanced disease, phosphate-binding medications may be required. Aluminum salts were highly effective in reducing hyperphosphatemia but led to significant toxicity to the skeletal and nervous systems. As a result, calcium-containing phosphate binders, such as calcium carbonate and calcium acetate, became widely utilized; however, use of these products can lead to hypercalcemia, bone disease, and vascular and extraosseous calcifications. More recently, calcium-free binders, such as sevelamer hydrochloride and lanthanum carbonate, increasingly have been utilized, and iron-based compounds are being developed as another alternative. Vitamin D supplementation can help to suppress the synthesis of PTH and inhibit the evolution of parathyroid hyperplasia, although high doses can lead to hypercalcemia. This led to the development of vitamin D analogues such as paricalcitol (19-nor-1,25-[OH]$_2$-vitamin D_2) and doxercalciferol (1α[OH]D_2), which are less likely to cause hypercalcemia.

The identification of the calcium-sensing receptor (CaSR) in the 1990s led to the development of a new class of drugs, calcimimetics,

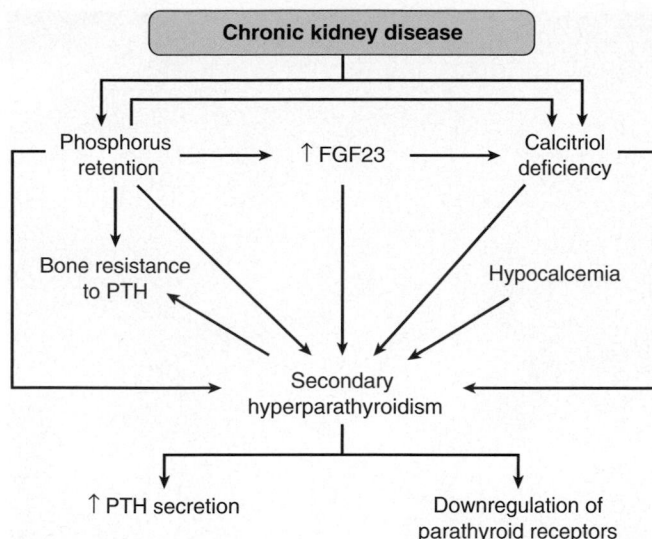

FIGURE 1 Schematic view of the pathophysiology of hyperparathyroidism secondary to chronic kidney disease. *FGF23*, fibroblast growth factor 23; *PTH*, parathyroid hormone. *(Reprinted with permission from Rodriguez M, Rodrigue-Ortiz ME. Advances in pharmacotherapy for secondary hyperparathyroidism. Expert Opin Pharmacother. 2015;16:1703-1716.)*

BOX 1: Indications for Parathyroidectomy in Patients With Secondary and Tertiary Hyperparathyroidism

Indications for Parathyroidectomy in Patients With Secondary Hyperparathyroidism (SHPT)

SHPT refractory to medical therapy:
- Parathyroid hormone >600-800 pg/mL
- Calcium × Phosphorus product >55

Renal osteodystrophy

Calciphylaxis

Other retractable symptoms, including uremic pruritus, persistent anemia, bone pain, muscle pain, abdominal pain, fatigue, and weakness

Indications for Parathyroidectomy in Patients With Tertiary Hyperparathyroidism

Severe hypercalcemia (calcium >12.5 mg/dL)

Persistent hypercalcemia ≥2 years after renal transplantation, associated with:
- Decline in renal function, without graft rejection
- Nephrolithiasis
- Progressive bone disease
- Pancreatitis

which act on the CaSR and increase the sensitivity of the parathyroid glands to extracellular calcium, thereby suppressing PTH secretion. Cinacalcet remains the only calcimimetic approved for treatment of patients with SHPT and has been shown in multiple studies to reduce serum concentrations of PTH, calcium, and phosphorus. Cinacalcet reaches peak plasma levels within 2 to 3 hours of oral administration, and it can lower circulating PTH levels within this same period. Studies examining the use of cinacalcet in combination with vitamin D have been performed and suggest greater reductions in PTH, although rates of hypercalcemia are higher when vitamin D analogues are utilized. A new calcimimetic, AMG 416, is in development; in contrast to cinacalcet, which is an allosteric activator of the CaSR, AMG 416 stimulates the CaSR directly. Administered intravenously, it is more potent and long acting than cinacalcet, and initial studies have shown dose-dependent reductions in serum PTH and calcium levels with few adverse effects.

■ INDICATIONS FOR PARATHYROIDECTOMY

Parathyroidectomy has been shown to be an effective method of achieving control of SHPT in patients who fail medical therapy. In recent years rates of parathyroidectomy for SHPT have decreased because of the increased effectiveness of medical therapies, including calcimimetics. However, because persistent elevation of serum phosphorus and PTH levels has been shown to be associated with an increased risk of cardiovascular morbidity, fractures, and mortality in patients with chronic kidney disease, failure of medical therapies to control biochemical parameters of SHPT remains an indication for parathyroidectomy (Box 1). In patients with SHPT, parathyroidectomy has led to durable reductions in serum PTH, phosphorus, calcium, and FGF23 levels, with resultant decreases in patient morbidity and mortality.

Other indications for parathyroidectomy in patients with SHPT include renal osteodystrophy and calciphylaxis (see Box 1). Renal osteodystrophy includes osteitis fibrosa cystica, osteomalacia, and adynamic bone disease. Osteitis fibrosa cystica is caused by high levels of PTH, increased cytokine production, and low $1,25(OH)_2D$ levels.

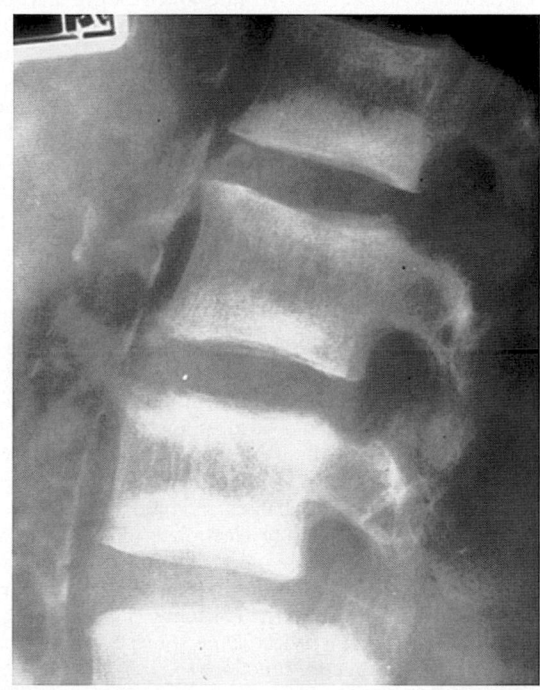

FIGURE 2 Lateral radiograph of the thoracic spine in a patient with end-stage renal disease showing bandlike regions of increased opacity at the superior and inferior margins of the vertebral bodies. This is typical of the "rugger jersey spine" sign.

It is associated with osteopenia, long bone fractures, and reduced bone strength and is improved by parathyroidectomy (Figure 2). Osteomalacia develops secondary to vitamin D deficiency and/or accumulation of aluminum in bone; with decreased use of aluminum-based phosphate binders, there has been a decrease in the occurrence of osteomalacia in patients with SHPT. Calciphylaxis (also referred

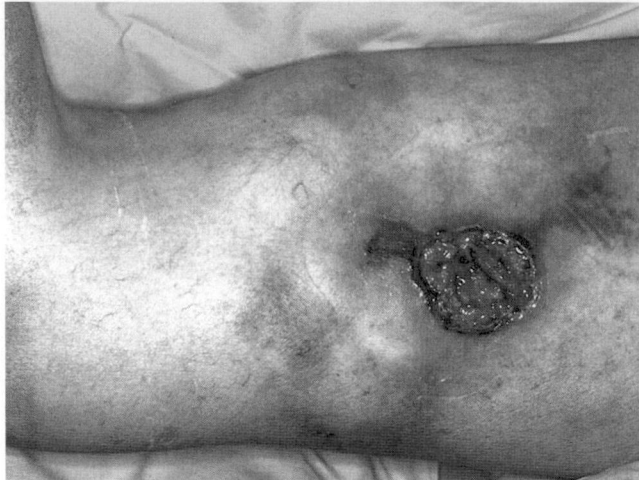

FIGURE 3 Eschar formation with central ulceration in a patient with end-stage renal disease and calciphylaxis.

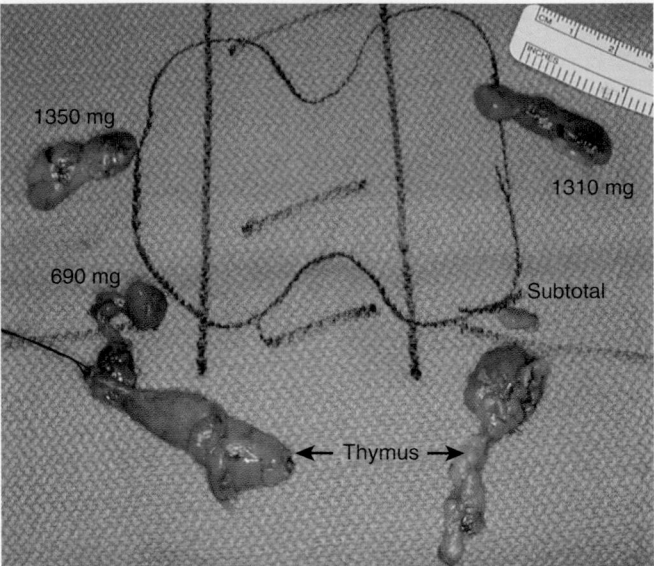

FIGURE 4 Intraoperative photo of subtotal parathyroidectomy and cervical thymectomy.

to as calcific uremic arteriolopathy) is characterized by calcification of the media layer of small- to medium-sized arteries, resulting in ischemic damage to dermal and epidermal structures. Patients develop violaceous, erythematous, painful skin lesions that can progress to ulceration and gangrene (Figure 3). Definitive diagnosis of calciphylaxis requires a skin biopsy, preferably a punch biopsy, which allows for differentiation from other similar skin conditions, such as cholesterol embolization, nephrogenic systemic fibrosis, vasculitis, and warfarin necrosis. Parathyroidectomy can slow progression of lesions and allow for proper wound healing; because calciphylaxis is associated with a greater than 50% rate of mortality, it remains an indication for parathyroidectomy.

■ PREOPERATIVE MANAGEMENT

Patients with SHPT and THPT are chronically ill patients who often have multiple comorbid conditions, including cardiovascular disease, hypertension, and diabetes mellitus. Patients should undergo a comprehensive medical evaluation with communication and coordination of care between treating providers in surgery, anesthesiology, and nephrology. Surgery should be coordinated with dialysis; the optimal timing for hemodialysis is the day before surgery, and patients should be evaluated in the immediate postoperative period for the need for an additional dialysis session. Particular attention should be paid intraoperatively to electrolyte imbalances, volume status, and the possibility of uremic platelet dysfunction. Patients with subjective voice changes or who have had prior anterior neck surgery, including previous thyroidectomy, parathyroidectomy, carotid endarterectomy, or cervical spine surgery, should undergo formal evaluation of vocal cord function.

Because SHPT and often THPT are associated with parathyroid hyperplasia, in contrast to the single parathyroid adenoma most often found during parathyroidectomy for sporadic PHPT, bilateral exploration is always indicated, and preoperative imaging studies for localization of abnormal glands is usually unnecessary. However, ultrasound of the cervical region can allow careful assessment of the thyroid gland for any thyroid nodules that may warrant additional evaluation with fine-needle aspiration before planned parathyroidectomy. In addition, sestamibi imaging may be used to identify ectopic or supernumerary parathyroid glands that are not in the usual anatomic location and may alter the surgical approach. Imaging with computed tomography (CT), namely four-dimensional CT, would be relatively contraindicated, given that the majority of patients will have compromised renal function.

■ EXTENT OF SURGERY

Subtotal Parathyroidectomy Versus Total Parathyroidectomy (Usually With Heterotopic Parathyroid Autotransplantation)

Subtotal parathyroidectomy for patients with SHPT was first described in 1960 and subsequently has become the procedure of choice. In 1975, with the description of parathyroid autotransplantation by Samuel Wells, total parathyroidectomy with heterotopic parathyroid autotransplantation became a popular technique. However, debate continues as to the optimal surgical approach for patients with SHPT.

Subtotal parathyroidectomy is the resection of three (or more, if supernumerary glands are present) glands and 50% to 75% removal of the last gland, with preservation of a viable, histologically confirmed remnant (Figure 4). Preservation of a well-vascularized, orthotopic gland will maintain function better than an autotransplanted gland can regain function, which requires neovascularization and may prolong postoperative hypoparathyroidism. This is particularly important in the postoperative management of patients who may require prolonged supplementation with calcium and/or calcitriol. In addition, there is always the risk that an autografted parathyroid gland may not develop an adequate vascular supply, leading to permanent hypoparathyroidism. Subtotal parathyroidectomy also precludes the need for an incision in the forearm for autotransplantation and may allow for easier hemodialysis access in the future. Disadvantages include the potential need for reoperative cervical surgery if HPT recurs and the possibility of inadvertently devascularizing the in situ parathyroid remnant.

Total parathyroidectomy removes all identified parathyroid glands, including supernumerary glands. In patients who develop recurrent HPT, reimplantation into the forearm allows for easier debulking, avoiding the need for reoperative surgery in the neck, and easier confirmation of graft-related recurrence, as opposed to an ectopic or supernumerary gland within the neck, by comparison of PTH levels drawn from both arms (downstream from the graft). Disadvantages of total parathyroidectomy include the need for much more aggressive postoperative management of hypocalcemia to avoid complications, especially because autograft failure can lead to persistent, potentially profound hypoparathyroidism and significantly compromised quality of life. Total parathyroidectomy without autotransplantation also has been described but is performed less commonly.

In patients undergoing total parathyroidectomy, cryopreservation of excised tissue is critical, especially because the parathyroid autograft could prove to be nonfunctional. The resected parathyroid gland is minced into 1- to 2-mm pieces and placed on ice. Fragments are stored in sterile RPMI solution with 10% autologous serum and 10% dimethyl sulfoxide, frozen to −80°C, and kept in liquid nitrogen in a tissue bank. Cryopreservation is not available at all centers, and data on the long-term function of reimplanted, cryopreserved parathyroid tissue are scarce, but to date it has demonstrated low rates of successful transplantation.

Two meta-analyses have compared subtotal parathyroidectomy and total parathyroidectomy with autotransplantation. Chen and colleagues compared five studies in patients undergoing initial surgery, including 100 patients who underwent subtotal parathyroidectomy and 597 patients who underwent total parathyroidectomy with autotransplantation. The rate of recurrent HPT was similar between the two groups (odds ratio = 0.825; 95% confidence interval = 0.368–1.846; $P = 0.639$). Secondary outcomes examining changes in serum calcium, PTH, and phosphorus also were not different between the two treatment groups, suggesting that the optimal approach could be dependent on surgeon or patient preference. Richards and colleagues performed a meta-analysis of 53 publications and 501 patients who underwent surgery for persistent or recurrent SHPT; the initial operation was subtotal parathyroidectomy in 36% of patients and total parathyroidectomy with autotransplantation in 64% of patients. At reoperation, 49% of patients had autograft hyperplasia, 20% had supernumerary glands, 17% had remnant hyperplasia, 7% had a missed in situ gland, and 5% had a negative exploration.

Overall, subtotal parathyroidectomy appears to be the preferred surgical approach, given lower rates of transient and permanent hypoparathyroidism, with minimal differences in long-term rates of recurrent HPT, which vary from 5% to 17% in the published literature. Furthermore, difficulty with forearm debulking after recurrences may require en bloc resection of muscle and involve a higher risk of long-term hypoparathyroidism.

In patients with THPT, subtotal parathyroidectomy is the preferred approach. A retrospective analysis of 74 patients with THPT demonstrated a greater than five times increased risk of persistent or recurrent HPT with less than subtotal parathyroidectomy. Patients with THPT typically have normal renal function after successful renal transplantation, decreasing the likelihood of recurrent disease from chronic overstimulation and parathyroid hyperplasia. As a result, the risk of permanent hypoparathyroidism after total parathyroidectomy is unacceptably high.

Cervical Thymectomy

Cervical thymectomy during parathyroidectomy in patients with SHPT or THPT should be considered, given the likelihood of there being supernumerary parathyroid glands (reported to be as high as 13%) and parathyroid rests in thymic tissue, which can become hyperplastic in the context of ongoing stimulus from renal failure (see Figure 4). Both supernumerary glands and parathyroid rests can be a source of persistent and recurrent HPT after initial parathyroid surgery. Use of intraoperative adjuncts, such as intraoperative PTH monitoring, can be useful in determining the need for cervical thymectomy during parathyroidectomy.

■ SURGICAL TECHNIQUE

Parathyroidectomy for SHPT and THPT should be performed under general anesthesia. Patients should be placed in a beach chair position, with arms tucked and adequate protection placed at pressure points. A shoulder roll (we use an inflatable intravenous bag) should be inserted under the upper back to facilitate slight extension of the neck. We favor use of a traditional Kocher's incision (transverse, symmetric, slightly curved incision approximately two fingerbreadths above the sternoclavicular joint) measuring 3 to 5 cm in length. The subcutaneous tissues and platysma are divided transversely, and subplatysmal skin flaps can be raised using electrocautery. The median raphe should be identified, and the strap muscles divided vertically in the midline and separated from the thyroid gland.

The thyroid lobe on the initial side of exploration should be mobilized, with ligation of the middle thyroid vein, if needed, for adequate exposure. The superior parathyroid glands, derived from the fourth pharyngeal pouch, typically are located posterior to the recurrent laryngeal nerve and posteromedial to the superior thyroid lobe; ectopic glands may be located in a retroesophageal location. The inferior parathyroid glands, derived from the third pharyngeal pouch, are more variable in location but typically located anterior to the recurrent laryngeal nerve and lateral to the inferior pole of the thyroid lobe. Inferior parathyroid glands also may be present within the thyrothymic ligament, and ectopic glands can be located within the anterior mediastinum or carotid sheath.

Systematic examination of all four parathyroid glands should be performed; all four parathyroid glands should be identified before resection, particularly if subtotal parathyroidectomy is planned. The most normal appearing gland is preferentially chosen to become the partial remnant gland; ideally, this gland also would be a eutopic, inferior parathyroid located in a relatively anterior position, as this would facilitate reoperative parathyroidectomy, if required. Subtotal resection of the gland should be performed before resection of at least one of the remaining parathyroid glands, to ensure viability of the remnant. A titanium clip or a Prolene suture can be placed on the remnant to facilitate future identification of the gland during potential reoperation. Resection of the remaining glands then should be performed. Intraoperative confirmation of parathyroid tissue can be performed via intraoperative frozen section or ex vivo aspiration of the parathyroid glands. For the latter technique, a 25-gauge needle attached to a syringe with a small amount of saline is used to aspirate tissue from the parathyroid. The sample is then run with intraoperative PTH serum samples. PTH levels significantly above the serum PTH or the upper limit of detection on the laboratory machine (typically >5000 pg/mL) are confirmatory for parathyroid tissue.

In patients undergoing total parathyroidectomy, heterotopic parathyroid autotransplantation should be performed with a 40- to 50-mg remnant of the most normal appearing parathyroid gland. An easily accessible and well-vascularized area, most commonly the forearm (brachioradialis muscle) or sternocleidomastoid muscle, is identified for the site of implantation; if placed within the forearm, the nondominant arm should be chosen. The parathyroid gland is then minced into small (1 to 2 mm) pieces, which are inserted directly into the muscle within either a single pocket or multiple pockets. An alternative technique for heterotopic parathyroid autotransplantation involves mincing the parathyroid remnant into small pieces in 1 to 2 cc of a saline solution; the minced parathyroid gland is then aspirated into a 3-cc syringe and injected into the muscle. With either technique, the site of autotransplantation is marked with a nonabsorbable suture or titanium clip for ease of future identification.

During parathyroidectomy, several technical considerations should be noted. Although ligation of thyroid arteries and/or veins may be required to obtain adequate exposure and maintain a bloodless surgical field, this should be minimized if possible in order to avoid the risk of postoperative hypothyroidism or hypoparathyroidism. Care must be taken at all times to fastidiously protect the recurrent laryngeal nerve, which typically runs within the tracheoesophageal groove; its location may be slightly more variable on the right side. Once identified, electrocautery and suction irrigation within the vicinity of the nerve should be used with the utmost caution. Parathyroid tissue should be manipulated as little as possible in order to prevent rupture of the parathyroid capsule and possible seeding of parathyroid cells that would result in parathyromatosis. If a parathyroid gland is ruptured, the parathyroid bed should be irrigated with hypotonic solution (water) before closure. Finally, hemostasis is critical at all times, and a small amount of an absorbable hemostatic agent may be placed in the parathyroid bed before closure.

The use of intraoperative adjuncts, such as intraoperative PTH monitoring and the radioguided gamma probe, has been described in parathyroidectomy for patients with SHPT or THPT. Advantages to the use of intraoperative adjuncts include the ability to guide the extent of resection and determine if supernumerary or ectopic parathyroid glands are present, as they are more prevalent in these patients. Unlike for PHPT, the appropriate decline of intraoperative PTH levels that lead to durable biochemical cure has not been well defined for SHPT and THPT, although use of intraoperative PTH monitoring may serve as a relative guide to the extent of parathyroidectomy. In addition, intraoperative PTH levels can help to prevent postoperative hypoparathyroidism, as autotransplantation could be performed should intraoperative PTH levels become too low or undetectable. Use of the radioguided gamma probe, though not routine, also may facilitate identification and resection of parathyroid tissue autografted in the forearm, particularly if this tissue was not marked previously.

■ POSTOPERATIVE MANAGEMENT

Patients undergoing subtotal parathyroidectomy or total parathyroidectomy with heterotopic parathyroid autotransplantation are at high risk for postoperative hypocalcemia. This is particularly pronounced in patients with SHPT or THPT, who also have a high risk of postoperative hungry bone syndrome, secondary to increased skeletal calcium deposition. Patients should start taking oral calcium supplementation (1 to 3 g of elemental calcium daily) and calcitriol (0.5 to 4.0 μg daily) immediately after surgery and be monitored closely for development of symptomatic hypocalcemia. Symptoms include numbness or paresthesias periorally or in the distal extremities; more severe symptoms include muscle cramps or carpopedal spasm. Severe hypocalcemia can lead to tetany and convulsions. Patients with profound hypocalcemia may require intravenous calcium administration, typically calcium gluconate (10 g in 1 L of normal saline, initiated at 30 mL/hr and titrated for symptoms and serum calcium levels). For patients requiring intravenous calcium, consideration should be given to continuous cardiac monitoring; electrocardiogram changes associated with hypocalcemia include a prolonged QT interval. Dialysis patients should be administered high-calcium dialysate during the postoperative period. In patients with significant hypocalcemia, serum magnesium levels should be corrected because low levels may aggravate and potentiate hypocalcemia; serum phosphorus levels also should be evaluated to prevent hyperphosphatemia. The nadir for hypocalcemia typically occurs 24 to 48 hours after surgery, although patients should be maintained on oral calcium and calcitriol for at least several weeks postoperatively. All patients should have serum calcium measurements at least annually, to evaluate for potential persistent or recurrent HPT.

■ SUMMARY

Significant advances in the medical management of patients with SHPT or THPT with the development of calcimimetic agents have reduced the need for parathyroidectomy. Parathyroidectomy remains the preferred management approach in patients with SHPT who have elevated calcium, phosphorus, and/or PTH levels refractory to medical therapies and who develop other sequelae of SHPT. Subtotal parathyroidectomy is the preferred surgical approach, as it minimizes the risk of long-term hypoparathyroidism and has similar rates of recurrent HPT as total parathyroidectomy with heterotopic parathyroid autotransplantation.

SUGGESTED READINGS

Chen J, Zhou QU, Wang JD. Comparison between subtotal parathyroidectomy and total parathyroidectomy with autotransplantation for secondary hyperparathyroidism in patients with chronic renal failure: a meta-analysis. *Horm Metab Res.* 2015;47:643-651.

Kidney Disease: Improving Global Outcomes (KDIGO) CKD-MBD Work Group. KDIGO clinical practice guideline for the diagnosis, evaluation, prevention, and treatment of chronic kidney disease–mineral and bone disorder (CKD-MBD). *Kidney Int Suppl.* 2009;113:S1-S130.

Madorin C, Owen RP, Fraser WD, et al. The surgical management of renal hyperparathyroidism. *Eur Arch Otorhinolaryngol.* 2012;269:1565-1576.

Moffett JM, Suliburk J. Parathyroid autotransplantation. *Endocr Pract.* 2011;17(suppl 1):83-89.

Richards ML, Wormuth J, Bingener J, et al. Parathyroidectomy in secondary hyperparathyroidism: is there an optimal operative management? *Surgery.* 2006;139:174-180.

Rodriguez M, Rodriguez-Ortiz ME. Advances in pharmacotherapy for secondary hyperparathyroidism. *Expert Opin Pharmacother.* 2015;16:1703-1716.

METABOLIC CHANGES FOLLOWING BARIATRIC SURGERY

Daniel Boyett, MD, Thomas Magnuson, MD, and Michael Schweitzer, MD

■ METABOLIC CONSEQUENCES OF OBESITY

Obesity is a syndrome resulting from an excess accumulation of body fat that may impair health, often termed *metabolic syndrome*. There are multiple ways to define obesity, each with benefits and limitations. Body mass index (BMI), a ratio of weight to height, is the most commonly used measurement of obesity, especially in the world of medicine and biostatistics, because it is easy to calculate and a reproducible and accurate population level indicator. BMI is calculated by dividing a person's weight in kilograms by the square of the height in meters (kg/m^2), and BMI of more than 30 kg/m^2 indicates obesity. One limitation of BMI is that it was designed to describe populations (distributions of individuals) and not to diagnose an individual. This can be seen in that world class athletes can be classified as overweight or obese because BMI does not differentiate between fat and lean muscle mass. An alternative method for defining obesity is body fat: more than 32% in women and 25% in men. Body fat calculations require specialized measurements or devices such as calipers or body composition analysis and thus may be less reproducible, especially in unskilled hands. Furthermore, neither of these methods addresses regional distribution of fat or weight; central adiposity is of chief concern. A simple measurement of waist circumference or waist-to-hip ratio can address central adiposity but does not accurately address height and fat content. A waist circumference of more than 35 inches in women or 40 inches in men indicates higher risk of metabolic syndrome and obesity-related comorbidities, and a waist-to-hip ratio above 0.85 for females or 0.90 for males can be used to classify obesity.

Body fat distribution is important because abdominal or visceral fat is a highly active endocrine organ, which may lead to a chronic inflammatory state caused in part by the release of free fatty acids and cytokines from this adipose tissue. Visceral obesity (also referred to as *android obesity*) is more common in men and is associated with increased risk of insulin resistance, hyperlipidemia, hypertension, cardiovascular disease (CVD), and stroke. The gynecoid pattern of obesity is characterized by an excess accumulation of subcutaneous fat in the hips and thighs, typically seen in women. Gynecoid obesity is associated less frequently with adverse metabolic effects. The importance of central obesity is highlighted in populations who, despite relatively low BMI, have high levels of visceral obesity (e.g., Asians) and are prone to adverse effects of obesity at a lower BMI. Conversely, central adiposity is less prevalent in some populations even at higher BMI (e.g., African Americans), resulting in lower risk of metabolic syndrome than BMI would indicate.

The obesity epidemic has been well publicized in the United States: 33.7% of the adult population was classified as obese in 2014. The most recent statistics from the World Health Organization indicate that, in fact, this is a global problem. In 2014 more than 1.9 billion adults (39% of the world population) 18 years and older were overweight, and of these, more than 600 million (13%) were obese. Worldwide obesity has more than doubled since 1980, and now most of the world's population live in countries where overweight and obesity kills more people than underweight. The obesity epidemic also extends to children: 42 million children under the age of 5 were overweight or obese in 2013. Some of the highest rates of obesity among adults are observed in some South Pacific islands such as Samoa (43.4%) and Cook Islands (50.8%). The global epidemic of obesity is multifactorial with genetic, environmental, cultural, and economic roots.

Adipose tissue is not simply a quiescent storage medium for excess calories but has a metabolically and hormonally active role in cell signaling. In severe obesity, excess lipid accumulates in adipocytes, hepatocytes, and muscle cells. Excess accumulation of nutrients, especially fat, within these cells leads to increased secretion of adipocyte-derived peptides (e.g., leptin, adiponectin, resistin) and cytokines (e.g., tumor necrosis factor-α [TNF-α], interleukin-6 [IL-6]), collectively referred to as *adipokines*. The paracrine and endocrine actions of these adipokines contribute to a state of chronic low-grade inflammation, which in turn interferes with many physiologic cellular processes (e.g., insulin signaling) and leads to the metabolic derangements seen in obesity (e.g., insulin resistance and type 2 diabetes mellitus [T2DM]). Our center has conducted the first studies showing the relevance of C1q/TNF-related protein family, a family of novel adipokines, in humans as it relates to obesity, metabolic syndrome, insulin resistance, and T2DM.

The obesity-induced inflammatory state adversely affects organ systems in the body and contributes to a shortened life expectancy. Each five-unit increase in BMI is associated with a 30% increase in all-cause mortality, with BMIs of more than 40 associated with a reduced life expectancy of 8 to 10 years, similar to that of regular cigarette smoking. Obesity is characterized by poor quality of life with increased risk of many life-threatening conditions. These include cancers, heart disease, T2DM, hypertension, stroke, GERD, hyperlipidemia, and sleep apnea. The prevalence of these comorbidities often increases with the severity of obesity (Table 1). This is most evident with T2DM. At age 18 years, women with a BMI of 30 to 35 have a 54.6% lifetime risk of development of diabetes, which is increased to 74.4% for those with BMI of more than 35.

Although modest weight loss (5% to 10% excess weight) can lead to reductions in the risk of these chronic diseases, nonsurgical weight loss is often unsuccessful or short lived in 90% to 95% of patients. As a result, bariatric surgery (weight loss surgery) has become the standard of care in the treatment of medically complicated or severe obesity.

■ METABOLIC IMPROVEMENTS AFTER WEIGHT LOSS SURGERY

Weight Loss

The term *excess body weight loss (EBWL)*, calculated by subtracting ideal body weight from current weight, is used commonly to describe

TABLE 1: Risks of Cardiovascular and Metabolic Disorders With Obesity

Life expectancy	30% increase in mortality rate for each 5-unit increase in BMI. At BMI > 40, life expectancy reduced by 8-10 years
Hypertension	Fivefold risk of hypertension in obesity. 85% of patients with hypertension have a BMI > 25
Cardiovascular disease	A 9% increase in cardiovascular mortality rate with each unit increase in BMI
Type 2 diabetes mellitus	Men with BMI > 35 have forty-two–fold increase in risk of diabetes compared with men with BMI < 23. At BMI > 35 patients have a 74% lifetime risk of T2DM

BMI, Body mass index; *T2DM*, type 2 diabetes mellitus.

weight loss. Not surprisingly, the degree of EBWL varies between procedures. At 2 years postprocedure, mean EBWL is 70% to 80% for biliopancreatic diversion (BPD) with or without duodenal switch, 60% to 70% for Roux-en-Y gastric bypass (RYGB), 50% to 60% for sleeve gastrectomy (SG), and 40% to 45% for laparoscopic adjustable gastric banding (LAGB). In general, procedures with higher EBWL also are associated with increased short-term and long-term complications. The balance between the desired weight loss and surgical risk influences the patient and surgeon when deciding upon the optimal procedure.

The mechanisms underlying postprocedure weight loss are multifactorial and vary by procedure, the proposed mechanisms of which are summarized in Table 2. Of critical importance are long-term changes in appetite and hunger after surgery. In contrast, nonsurgical weight loss leads to increased hunger and reduced energy expenditure, which presumptively contribute to the ultimate failure of dieting in achieving long-term weight reduction. Weight loss surgery prevents such physiologic responses and maintains hunger control despite limited caloric intake.

Long-term follow-up studies such as the Swedish Obesity Study show significant long-term weight loss in surgical patients compared with control subjects, with up to 20 years of follow-up. The durability of postsurgical weight loss is a concern for patients and clinicians. Definition of successful weight loss for bariatric surgery varies depending on the procedure; for RYGB, success often is described as losing and maintaining 50% or more EBWL. Most patients regain some weight after reaching their nadir weight, with pathologic weight regain (>20% of the maximal weight loss) reported in 15% to 20% of patients. This observation highlights the fact that bariatric surgery is not a replacement for long-term lifestyle changes, which are needed to help maintain weight loss. A commitment to changes in diet and exercise are critical for long-term success. The importance of such lifestyle changes and the need for regular (at least annual) postoperative follow-up with the bariatric team should be discussed with patients before surgery.

Nonalcoholic Fatty Liver Disease

Nonalcoholic fatty liver disease (NAFLD) is a spectrum of clinical disease that ranges from simple accumulation of liver fat (steatosis) to the resultant inflammation, nonalcoholic steatohepatitis (NASH), fibrosis, and cirrhosis. Hepatic steatosis and NASH, markers of central adiposity, are thought to be important in the pathogenesis of obesity-related metabolic disorders, often referred to as the *metabolic syndrome* (visceral adiposity, insulin resistance,

TABLE 2: Proposed Mechanisms for Weight Loss After Bariatric Procedures

Physical restriction of food intake	Although a common belief, especially in the case of LAGB, few data support this as a mechanism for weight loss. Food transit through the stomach is only minimally altered after LAGB, and the supraband compartment is empty of food within 1-2 min after ingestion. BPD has a large gastric reservoir and yet leads to the best weight loss results.
Malabsorption	Although a degree of this occurs after BPD, little malabsorption is seen after LAGB, SG, or RYGB as measured with stool calorimetry and nitrogen balance.
Decreased hunger signals and reduced food intake	This is true for all bariatric procedures and the result of altered hormonal expression (e.g., leptin, ghrelin, GLP-1, PYY) along the gut-brain axis after surgery.
Increased energy expenditure and diet induced thermogenesis	RYGB surgery has been shown to increase respiratory quotient and energy expenditure during food intake.
Changes in food preference	Changes in food preference have been documented and are related in part to alterations in reward and taste, as well as concerns about physiologic implications of ingestion of certain foods that may lead to dysphagia or dumping syndrome.
Changes in gut microbiota	Animal studies show a potential role for the gut microbiome in obesity and diabetes. Definitive human data are currently lacking, but this is an area of significant scientific interest.

BPD, Biliopancreatic diversion; *GLP-1,* glucagon-like peptide 1; *LAGB,* laparoscopic adjustable gastric banding; *RYGB,* Roux-en-Y gastric bypass; *SG,* sleeve gastrectomy; *PYY,* peptide YY.

hyperinsulinemia, hypertension, and hyperlipidemia). NASH now ranks among the top three conditions for terminal liver failure and inclusion on the waiting list for liver transplantation. In patients undergoing bariatric surgery, the prevalence of simple steatosis may be greater than 95%, NASH often is reported from 20% to 30% (prospective data from our center shows a prevalence of NASH of 54.5%), and fibrosis between 10% and 14%. Accumulation of fat in the liver is the result of an imbalance between lipid deposition and removal, where the hepatic synthesis of triglycerides can be considered a partially protective mechanism, aimed at storing cytotoxic free fatty acids as inert components. Hepatic FFAs arise from diet, lipolysis of visceral fat, and de novo lipogenesis; the last two components are mostly dependent on insulin resistance and are associated with obesity and T2DM. The development of NAFLD has been linked to lipid overload in the liver resulting from an increased release of free fatty acids from adipocytes triggered by insulin resistance. Weight loss surgery leads to a near universal improvement in the severity of hepatic steatosis with most studies reporting more than 75% of patients with no evidence of steatosis after weight loss. In addition, bariatric surgery induces the disappearance of NASH in around 85% of cases and is associated with significant reductions in lobular inflammation. Overall RYGB has greater improvement in liver disease compared with primarily restrictive procedures such as SG.

Lipid Profiles

Dyslipidemia is seen in up to 50% of patients who undergo bariatric surgery and has been linked not only to obesity but also to obstructive sleep apnea. It has been found that patients who have chronic intermittent hypoxia associated with sleep apnea have higher plasma triglyceride and low-density lipoprotein cholesterol levels. Of these patients with preoperative dyslipidemia, more than 70% have improvement or resolution of this comorbidity within 2 years of surgery. Bariatric surgery patients, at 2 years postoperation, have significant beneficial improvements in triglycerides (−27.2%) and HDL-C (+22%) concentrations. By contrast, a small effect is observed for total cholesterol concentration (−2.9%). Overall RYGB has a greater effect than primarily restrictive procedures. At 10 years, RYGB led to improvements in triglycerides by −28%, HDL-C by +47.5%, and total cholesterol by −12.6%. Significant changes in lipid profiles can be seen as early as 1 month postoperation.

Hypertension

Hypertension (HTN) can be defined as currently taking antihypertensive medications, or by mean blood pressure parameters of systolic blood pressure greater than or equal to 140 mm Hg or diastolic blood pressure greater than or equal to 90 mm Hg. HTN is common in obese individuals and is increasingly prevalent in patients with increasing BMI. In the normal weight population (BMI < 25), HTN is present in 15% to 20%, rising to 30% to 40% in the obese population (BMI > 30). When compared with normal weight controls, the odds ratio for HTN is 1.7 for BMI 25 to 29.9 kg/m^2, 2.6 for BMI 30 to 34.9 kg/m^2, 3.7 for BMI 35 to 39.9 kg/m^2, and 4.8 for BMI 40 kg/m^2 or more. Furthermore, a 10-kg (22-lb) higher body weight is associated with 3.0 mm Hg higher systolic and 2.3 mm Hg higher diastolic blood pressure.

The mechanism that links obesity with HTN is not understood fully. It is thought to involve a combination of enhanced renal reabsorption of sodium (possibly resulting from insulin resistance), expansion of intravascular volume, activation of the renin-angiotensin-aldosterone system, activation of the sympathetic nervous system, release of angiotensinogen from adipose tissue, and insulin resistance. The chronically increased intra-abdominal pressure seen with central obesity has been shown to significantly upregulate the hormonal output of the renin-angiotensin-aldosterone system and may play an important role in obesity-induced hypertension. Weight loss has been shown to be associated with a reduction in vascular resistance, total blood volume and cardiac output, an improvement in insulin resistance, a reduction in sympathetic nervous system activity, and suppression of the activity of the renin-angiotensin-aldosterone system.

HTN is seen in up to 50% of patients who undergo bariatric surgery. Of these, 50% to 60% have remission and 60% to 70% show improvement after bariatric surgery. One study of patients undergoing RYGB or intensive medical therapy showed the rate of hypertension remission was 49% for the surgical group versus 23% for the medical therapy group. BPD also has been shown to resolve hypertension in 60% to 80% of patients.

Cardiovascular Risk and Mortality

CVD remains the leading cause of mortality in the United States. The Framingham Heart Study (FHS) is a long-running prospective cohort study, initiated in 1948, that has contributed to our understanding of obesity, its associated diseases, and to how these conditions relate to overall and cardiovascular-related mortality. Long-term data show a relative risk for cardiovascular disease of 1.38 in obesity compared with normal weight. This study also has been used to create a cardiovascular risk score, and weight loss procedures have been shown to reduce the 10-year risk of a cardiac event by 40%. Serum and laboratory risk predictors, such as C-reactive protein (CRP), also have been shown to decline after surgery by about 60%. The Swedish Obesity Study has shown at 10 years a 23.7% unadjusted (30.7% adjusted) overall reduction in overall mortality in well-matched patients who underwent weight loss surgery when compared with those who did not. A retrospective study of gastric bypass patients shows an adjusted long-term mortality decrease of 40% over that of controls.

Polycystic Ovary Syndrome

Polycystic ovary syndrome (PCOS) is a common endocrine disorder of unknown cause characterized by menstrual abnormalities with hyperandrogenism and is a common cause of infertility, especially in severe obesity. Up to 50% of those with PCOS are overweight or obese, and phenotypic severity of PCOS is reported to correlate with severity of insulin resistance and to worsen with increased weight. Small studies report resolution of regular menstrual cycle in 82% of PCOS patients after RYGB, correlating to a 100% postoperative conception rate in infertile PCOS patients seeking pregnancy.

Type 2 Diabetes

"Diabesity" is a term describing diabetes in the context of obesity, and it recently has been recognized as a major public health problem that is evolving to become an epidemic. Over the last 25 years, the prevalence of diabetes has doubled in the United States and multiplied by three to five times in India, Indonesia, China, Korea, and Thailand. The global prevalence of diabetes in 2010 was 284 million people (6.4%), and projections for 2030 predict the prevalence to reach 439 million individuals (7.7%) worldwide. Diabesity represents a substantial economic burden as reflected by diabetes and obesity consuming 14% and 5.7% of the total U.S. health expenditure, respectively.

Improvements in glycemic control after gastrointestinal surgery were reported in the 1960s, and the durable effect of bariatric surgery in controlling T2DM was reported in 1995. This gave way for the development of metabolic surgery, or the operative manipulation of a normal organ or organ system to achieve a biologic result for a potential health gain. Despite recent advancements of medical management for obesity-induced T2DM, most patients with diabetes do not reach the therapeutic goals set by the American Diabetic Association and other endocrine societies (glycosylated hemoglobin [HbAlc], <7%).

Several studies and meta-analyses have confirmed that all bariatric procedures lead to significant improvements in glucose control and diabetes remission. The Swedish Obese Subjects data show that of the patients who underwent bariatric surgery with T2DM at baseline, 72% were in remission at 2 years postoperation compared with 21% in the medical treatment group. At 10 years this decreased to 36% in the surgery group and 13% in the control group. In addition, bariatric surgery reduced the risk of developing T2DM by 96%, 84%, and 78% after 2, 10, and 15 years, respectively, when compared with medical management. The 3-year STAMPEDE (Surgical Therapy And Medications Potentially Eradicate Diabetes Efficiently) data show similar results with 38% remission rate in the RYGP group, 24% in the SG group, and 5% in the medical therapy group.

These impressive data have prompted many of the diabetes societies to alter their treatment guidelines for management of diabesity. For instance, the International Diabetes Federation's guidelines state that bariatric surgery should be considered earlier in the treatment of eligible patients to help stem the serious complications that can

TABLE 3: Weight Changes and Metabolic Improvements 2 Years After Bariatric Procedures

	Excess Weight Loss	Dyslipidemia	Hypertension	Type 2 Diabetes
BPD	70%-80%	90%	80%	90%
RYGB	60%-70%	60%-70%	60%	80%
SG	50%-60%	50%-60%	60%	70%
LAGB	40%-45%	60%	58%	50%-60%

BPD, Biliopancreatic diversion; *LAGB*, laparoscopic adjustable gastric banding; *RYGB*, Roux-en-Y gastric bypass; *SG*, sleeve gastrectomy.

result from diabetes. Eligible patients include those who have T2DM and a BMI of 35 kg/m^2 or more; or with a BMI between 30 and 35 kg/m^2 when diabetes cannot be controlled adequately by optimal medical regimen, especially in the presence of other major CVD risk factors.

As the metabolic effects of weight loss surgery become more defined through research, surgical outcomes will be judged not only on successful weight reduction but also on amelioration of detrimental metabolic changes associated with obesity (summarized in Table 3).

■ METABOLIC SURGERY AND FUTURE DIRECTIONS

Low Body Mass Index Metabolic Surgery

Effective and reliable medical therapy for T2DM traditionally has been a challenge both clinically and in terms of research. With the increasing prevalence of the disease, and the success with surgical treatment, there is a progressively strong push to lower the BMI threshold for surgical intervention in patients with diabetes to 30 kg/m^2 or even lower.

The current National Institutes of Health consensus statement recommends bariatric surgery in patients with BMI of more than 40 kg/m^2 or BMI of more than 35 kg/m^2 with concomitant comorbidities. Although most patients with T2DM are overweight or obese, around 70% have a BMI of less than 35 kg/m^2 and fail to qualify for surgical intervention on the basis of BMI alone. There has been some momentum to lower the BMI requirement to 30 kg/m^2, with this number lowered further to 27 kg/m^2 for those of Asian descent, in whom adverse metabolic effects are seen at a lower BMI. Several small studies have confirmed the safety of bariatric procedures in this patient population. Although long-term data are currently lacking, this will likely come in due time. In this lower BMI range, diabetic remission was seen after RYBG and SG in 93% and 47%, respectively. Importantly, the mean postoperative BMI remained within the normal range, meaning these lower BMI patients did not lose excessive weight after RYGB. However, data are sparse in these lower BMI ranges, so more studies will be needed to confirm success, safety, and durability of surgical outcomes before metabolic surgery for low BMI patients can be considered a treatment of choice.

Pediatric Bariatric and Metabolic Surgery

The use of BMI as a measure for childhood obesity is more problematic than its use in adults because of the additional complications of growth patterns, age, and sex in a growing child. Special BMI growth charts have been devised to correct for these variables and are used when assessing the pediatric population. These define the BMI range of 85th to 94th percentile as overweight, and 95th percentile or higher as obese. This has been further clarified by the American Academy of Pediatrics who propose a BMI of 30 to 32 kg/m^2 for youths 10 to 12 years old and of 34 kg/m^2 for youths 14 to 16 years old as the 99th percentile. The Bogalusa Heart Study showed that 84% of children with a BMI in the 95th to 98th percentile had a BMI of greater than 30 kg/m² as adults, showing that childhood BMI was associated strongly with adult BMI in this BMI range.

Childhood obesity has more than doubled in children and quadrupled in adolescents in the past 30 years. The percentage of obesity in children aged 6 to 11 years in the United States increased from 7% in 1980 to nearly 18% in 2012. Similarly, the percentage of obesity in adolescents aged 12 to 19 years increased from 5% to nearly 21% over the same period. In addition, obese youth are more likely to have risk factors for cardiovascular disease, such as high cholesterol or high blood pressure. In a population-based sample of 5- to 17-year-olds, 70% of obese youth had at least one risk factor for cardiovascular disease. Current estimates predict a decrease in life expectancy in obese adolescents of 5 to 20 years depending on additional risk factors such as race and sex.

Although studies are limited, current data suggest that bariatric surgery is at least as safe in adolescents as it is in adults, having similar success in both weight reduction and resolution of metabolic derangement. Because of the paucity of long-term outcome data, the role of bariatric surgery in the pediatric patient remains controversial, which may account for the hesitancy on the part of pediatricians and pediatric specialists to consider surgery, even for adolescents with life-threatening comorbidities and of polled pediatricians, half of the respondents would not refer their patients who are younger than 18 years of age for bariatric surgery.

Alternative Surgical Procedures

Research into defining the physiologic mechanisms that underlie the antidiabetic effects of the current bariatric procedures is of particular interest because of the opportunity to develop less invasive alternative techniques that can reproduce the results of current surgical options. Isolation of duodenum and proximal bowel from nutrient exposure and early exposure of distal bowel and ileum to undigested food are thought to be critical to the metabolic success of bariatric surgical procedures. New surgical procedures such as duodenal-jejunal bypass and ileal interposition may offer less invasive options for metabolic surgery targets, especially in patients with low BMI. More studies would be required to assess the safety and efficacy of these proposed surgical options.

Endosurgical Options and Devices

An area of heavy development at this time, in part because it is the least invasive option, is endoscopically delivered gastrointestinal manipulation. The goal of these endoscopic procedures is to replicate the metabolic or weight loss success of bariatric surgery without an abdominal incision, making for a less invasive procedure. These options range from implantable neurostimulators to modify vagal or gastric tone, to barrier devices that stent through the proximal bowel to block nutrient contact, to intragastric balloons designed to provide gastric volume restriction and therefore potentially increased satiety. The efficacy of these minimally invasive options must be further studied, but endoscopic procedures will be an ongoing target for development in the near future.

SUGGESTED READINGS

Adams TD, Gress RE, Smith SC, et al. Long-term mortality after gastric bypass surgery. *NEJM*. 2007;357:753-761.

Buchwald H, Avidor Y, Braunwald E, et al. Bariatric surgery–a systematic review and meta-analysis. *JAMA*. 2004;292:1724-1737.

Dixon JB, le Roux CW, Rubino F, et al. Bariatric surgery for type 2 diabetes. *Lancet*. 2012.

Hsia DS, Fallon SC, Brandt ML. Adolescent bariatric surgery. *Arch Pediatr Adolesc Med*. 2012;166:757-766.

Long MT, Fox CS. The Framingham Heart Study – 67 years of discovery in metabolic disease. *Nat Rev Endocrinol*. 2016;12:177-183.

Schauer PR, Bhatt DL, et al. Bariatric surgery versus intensive medical therapy for diabetes–3 year outcomes. *N Engl J Med*. 2014;370:2002-2013.

Sjöström L, Peltonen M, Jacobson P, et al. Bariatric surgery and long-term cardiovascular events. *JAMA*. 2012;307:56-65.

GLYCEMIC CONTROL AND CARDIOVASCULAR DISEASE RISK REDUCTION AFTER BARIATRIC SURGERY

Britney L. Corey, MD, and Richard D. Stahl, MD, FACS

Obesity continues to be prevalent in the United States and other industrialized countries. It is associated with serious comorbid conditions, including cardiovascular disease (CVD) and type 2 diabetes mellitus (T2DM). It also represents a significant economic burden on the healthcare industry: the Centers for Disease Control and Prevention (CDC) estimate an annual increased healthcare cost of greater than $1400 for those with obesity. Bariatric surgery is clearly the most effective treatment for class II and III obesity. The aim of this chapter is to review the current literature on obesity, its relationship to CVD and T2DM, and the effect of bariatric surgery on these conditions. The discussion is focused on the most common current surgical therapies: Roux-en-Y gastric bypass (RYGB), vertical sleeve gastrectomy (VSG), and laparoscopic adjustable gastric banding (LAGB).

Obesity as an Epidemic

Data released by the CDC from the National Health and Nutrition Examination Survey in 2012 examined the prevalence of obesity in the United States. Their research revealed that more than one third of adults and 17% of youth in the United States are obese. The World Health Organization (WHO) estimates that more than 1.9 billion adults worldwide were overweight in 2014; more than 600 million of these were obese. The WHO and the CDC classify obesity based on body mass index (BMI). Although BMI is a useful tool, it is limited by the fact that it cannot distinguish between body fat and lean body mass, is not as accurate at predicting body fat in the elderly, and does not account for the fact that, for the same BMI, females and Asians have more body fat than males and Caucasians, respectively (Table 1).

Fat as an Endocrine Gland

Adipose tissue previously was thought to be simply an energy storage depot; however, translational research in the last 2 decades has revealed that adipose tissue also plays an important role as an endocrine gland that secretes more than 600 adipokines. These metabolically active factors influence adipocytes and other adipose tissue cells, the immune system, and the brain, pancreas, liver, and cardiovascular system (Figure 1). Although much is still to be learned in this area, current research as reviewed by Bluher and Mantzoros (2015) reveals obesity is associated with dysfunction of adipose tissue and subsequent dysregulation of adipokines. Adipose tissue plays an important role in the regulation of appetite, satiety, energy expenditure, insulin

TABLE 1: Body Mass Index, Calculation, and Interpretation*

BMI CALCULATION

Kilograms and meters	Formula: Formula: weight (kg)/ [height (m)]^2
Pounds and inches	Formula: weight (lb) / [height (in)]^2 × 703

BMI INTERPRETATION, FOR ADULTS 20 AND OLDER

Below 18.5	Underweight
18.5-24.9	Normal or healthy weight
25-29.9	Overweight
30-34.9	Class I obesity
35-39.9	Class II obesity
≥40	Class III obesity

*As defined by the World Health Organization.

sensitivity, inflammation, blood pressure, hemostasis, and endothelial function. However, excess and dysfunctional adipose tissue is associated with insulin resistance, hyperglycemia, dyslipidemia, hypertension, and induces proinflammatory and prothrombotic states. As adipose tissue excess decreases because of weight loss, adipocyte function normalizes back toward baseline. This may contribute to the improvement in CVD risk and glycemic control after weight loss.

The Metabolic Syndrome, Diabetes, and Cardiovascular Disease Risk

The National Cholesterol Education Program's Adult Treatment Panel III (ATP III) defines metabolic syndrome as the presence of any three of the following five conditions: abdominal obesity, hypertriglyceridemia, low HDL cholesterol, hypertension, and hyperglycemia (Box 1). ATP III considers the metabolic syndrome to be a direct result of excess adipose tissue, particularly abdominal obesity. According to a 2009 joint statement released by the International Diabetes Federation, National Heart, Lung, and Blood Institute, American Heart Association (AHA), World Heart Federation, International Atherosclerosis Society, and International Association for

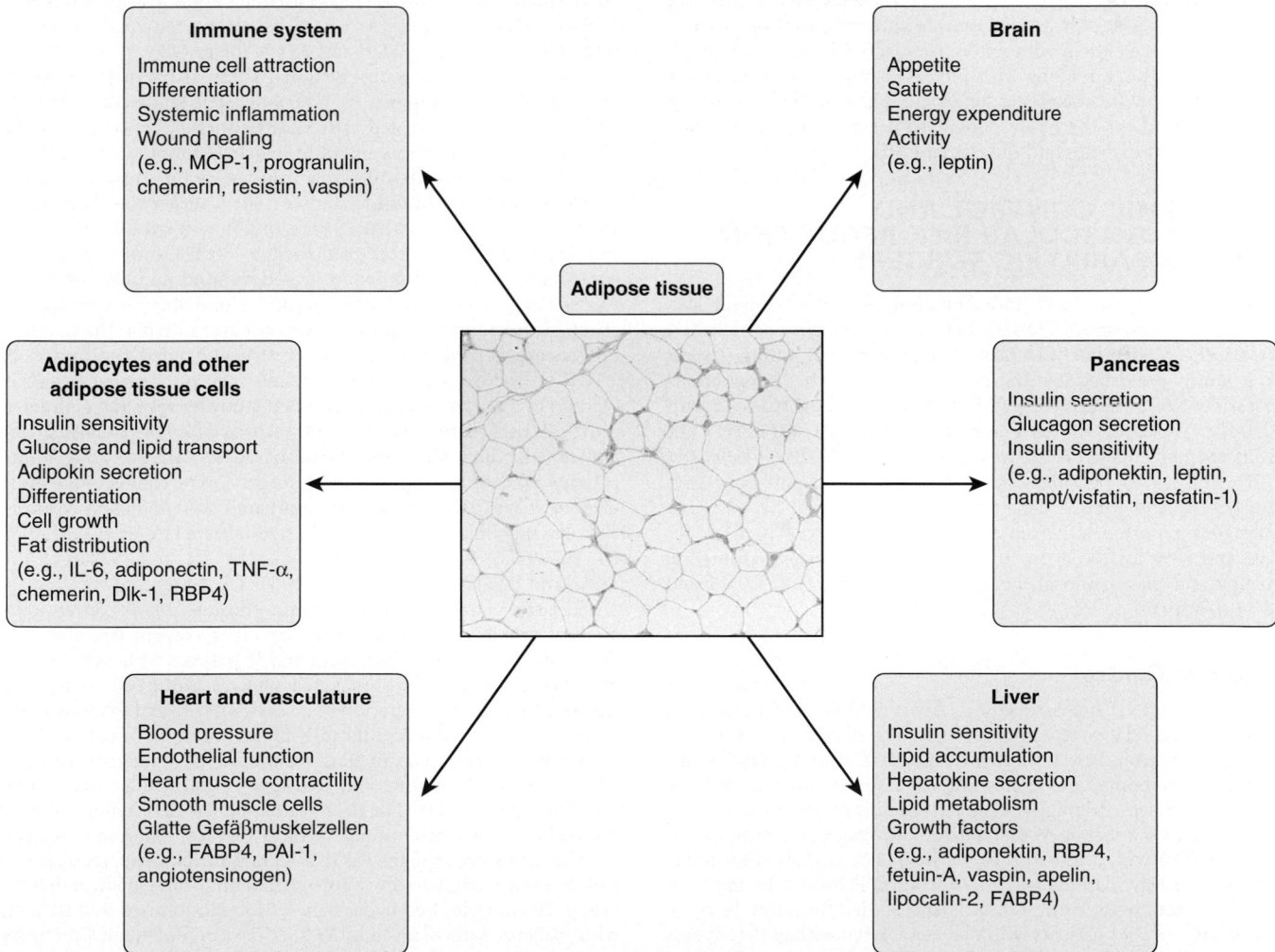

FIGURE 1 Secreted factors from adipose tissue (representative histologic slide of human subcutaneous adipose tissue, hematoxylin and eosin staining; magnification: 20×) play an important role in the regulation of appetite and satiety, energy expenditure, insulin sensitivity and insulin secretions, inflammation, blood pressure, hemostasis, endothelial function, and others. *(From Bluher M, Mantzoros CS. From leptin to other adipokines in health and disease: facts and expectations at the beginning of the 21st century. Metabolism. 2015;64:131-145.)*

BOX 1: Diagnostic Criteria for the Metabolic Syndrome*

Diagnostic Criteria for the Metabolic Syndrome

Three or more of the following five cardiovascular risk factors:
Central obesity (waist circumference): ≥102 cm in men; ≥88 cm in women
Hypertriglyceridemia: triglyceride levels ≥1.7 mmol/L (≥150 mg/dL)
Low levels of high-density lipoprotein (HDL): <1.03 mmol/L (<40 mg/dL) in men; <1.29 mmol/L (<50 mg/dL) in women
Systemic hypertension: blood pressure ≥130/85 mm Hg or necessity for medication
Elevated fasting plasma glucose level: ≥5.5 mmol/L (≥100 mg/dL)

*As defined by the National Cholesterol Education Program's Adult Treatment Panel III (ATP III).

BOX 2: Diagnostic Criteria for Type II Diabetes Mellitus*

Any one of the following, verified on subsequent day with any of the other criteria:
Symptoms of diabetes (i.e., polyuria, polydipsia, unexplained weight loss), and plasma glucose concentration 200 mg/dL (11.1 mmol/L), or
Fasting plasma glucose of 126 mg/dL (7.0 mmol/L), or
Plasma glucose ≥ 200 mg/dL (11.1 mmol/l) 2 hours after a 75 g glucose load or
HgbA1c ≥ 6.5%.

*As defined by the American Diabetes Association.

the Study of Obesity, the diagnosis of metabolic syndrome confers a twofold increased risk of developing CVD over the next 5 to 10 years, and a fivefold increased risk of developing T2DM. Of patients with T2DM 90% are overweight or obese, and diabetes itself confers the same risk of coronary heart disease as a known history of ischemic heart disease in a patient without diabetes. The ATP III recommends that weight reduction along with increased physical activity be the first-line therapy for metabolic syndrome. Thus weight reduction is a laudable goal for the obese patient to decrease the severity and implications of diabetes and the risk of CVD.

■ GLYCEMIC CONTROL AND CARDIOVASCULAR RISK REDUCTION AFTER BARIATRIC SURGERY

Bariatric surgery is a safe and efficacious means of weight loss, glycemic control, and CVD risk reduction. It is also cost effective for healthcare systems, with cost effectiveness seen within 2 years in a study published by Boriensko in 2015. The Longitudinal Assessment of Bariatric Surgery (LABS) Consortium study showed a 30-day mortality of 0.3% for RYGB and LAGB (2009). The estimated percentage of excess weight loss for RYGB is 61.6% and 47.5% for LAGB per meta-analysis by Buchwald and colleagues (2004). There are fewer data available for VSG, but Schauer and colleagues reported a percentage excess weight loss of 81% for VSG and 88% for RYGB in 2012. These results far exceed medical therapy and place surgical therapy at the forefront of T2DM and CVD treatment.

Glycemic Control

The American Diabetes Association (ADA) defines T2DM as insulin resistance and relative insulin deficiency. The diagnostic criteria for T2DM are listed in Box 2. It often is associated with obesity, specifically central obesity, and excess adipose tissue is known to cause insulin resistance. Although the benefits of losing weight for diabetes was not a new concept, Walter Pories and colleagues published a paper in 1995 with a title as provocative as it was ground breaking: Who Would Have Thought It? An Operation Proves to Be the Most Effective Therapy for Adult-Onset Diabetes Mellitus. Over 14 years, 121 of 146 (82.9%) patients with diabetes treated with gastric bypass experienced resolution of their diabetes. No treatment ever described came close to that degree of success. Bariatric surgery was no longer seen simply as a weight loss procedure. It was truly metabolic surgery, and a disease relegated to chronic management with expected gradual deterioration now had a potential for reversal.

Multiple other observational studies have supported these findings. A meta-analysis performed by Buchwald and colleagues in 2009 evaluated 621 studies with 888 treatment arms and 135,246 patients undergoing bariatric surgery (LAGB, vertical banded gastroplasty, RYGB, and biliopancreatic diversion/duodenal switch) and found an overall T2DM remission rate of 78.1%. Courcoulas and the LABS-2 Consortium published a more recent observational cohort study looking at 3-year outcomes on patients who underwent an RYGB or LAGB (2013). This was a large study across 10 U.S. hospitals with 2458 patients and showed 31.5% baseline weight loss for RYGB and 15.9% baseline weight loss for LAGB. They reported a diabetes remission rate of 67.5% for RYGB and 28.6% for LAGB.

The longest-running observational study of bariatric surgery is the Swedish Obese Subjects (SOS) cohort. The study compared 343 patients with T2DM treated with bariatric surgery between 1987 and 2001 with 260 contemporaneously matched cohorts treated medically. The 2-year results from this trial showed a remission rate of 72.3% in patients who underwent bariatric surgery, as opposed to 16.4% in control patients. At 15 years of follow-up, the T2DM remission rates for the surgical group fell to 30.4% and 6.5% for the control group. They also demonstrated reduced numbers of microvascular and macrovascular complications of diabetes in the surgical group. This improvement in diabetes occurred despite the majority of the surgical patients having either vertical banded gastroplasty or LAGB, procedures known to have results inferior to gastric bypass in relation to diabetes (Figure 2). A recent study by Yska and colleagues (2015) evaluated the primary care records of 2978 patients in the United Kingdom who underwent bariatric surgery. They found patients who underwent bariatric surgery were eighteenfold more likely to have T2DM remission compared with matched controls. This was more likely for RYGB (adjusted relative rate [RR], 43.1, 95% CI, 19.7-94.5), followed by VSG (adjusted RR, 16.6; 95% CI, 4.7-58.4), and LAGB (adjusted RR, 6.9; 95% CI, 3.1-15.2).

Bariatric surgery remains more effective than conventional medical therapy for T2DM in randomized control trials as well. Dixon and associates (2008) compared 30 patients with diabetes who underwent LAGB with a matched control group of 30 patients treated medically over a period of 2 years. They found that remission of diabetes occurred in significantly higher numbers of patients who underwent surgery than in those who received standard treatment (73% vs 13%). Mingrone and colleagues published a single-center randomized control trial in 2012 evaluating RYGB or biliopancreatic diversion versus conventional medical therapy. They saw diabetes remission rates of 75% for RYGB and 95% for biliopancreatic diversion at 2 years, compared with 0% remission for the medical therapy group. Ikramuddin and colleagues (2013) randomized 120 patients with diabetes with BMI 30 to 39.9 kg/m^2 to RYGB versus intensive medical therapy and achieved the predefined composite triple end point (HgbA$_{1c}$ <7.0%, LDL <100 mg/dL, and systolic blood pressure <130 mm Hg at the 12-month visit) in 49% of the surgery patients versus 19% of the controls. The Surgical Treatment and Medications Potentially Eradicate Diabetes Efficiently (STAMPEDE) trial (Schauer

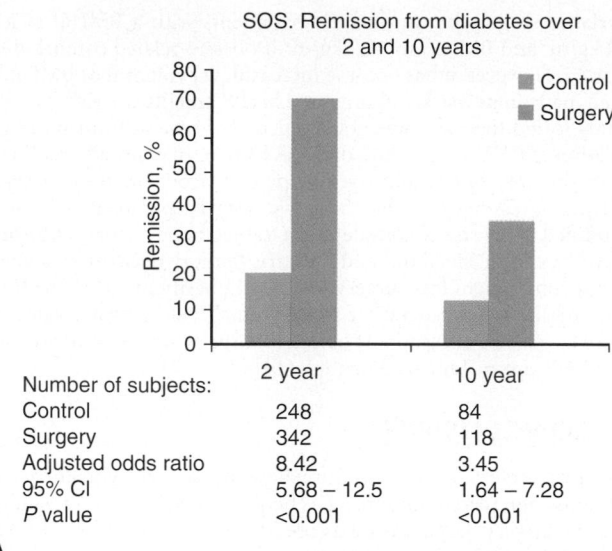

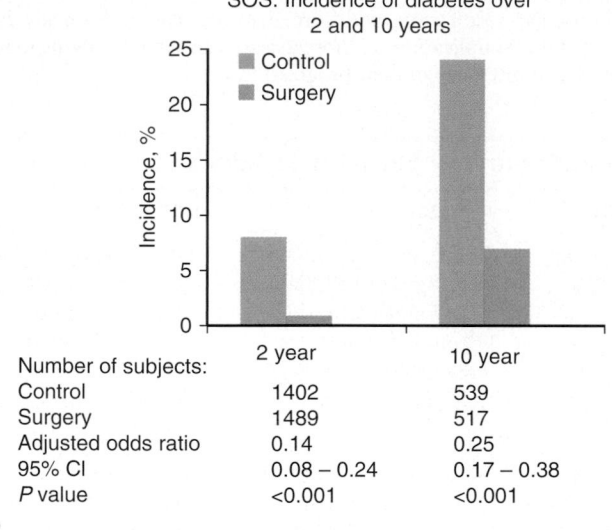

FIGURE 2 Diabetes remission and prevention during follow-up for 2 and 10 years in the control and surgery groups of the Swedish Obese Subjects study. *Upper panel:* Diabetes remission in 248 controls and 342 surgery patients with type 2 diabetes at baseline. *Lower panel:* Diabetes incidence in 1402 controls and 1489 surgery patients without diabetes at baseline. *(Data from Sjöström L, Lindroos AK, Peltonen M, Torgerson J, Bouchard C, Carlsson B, Dahlgren S, Larsson B, Narbro K, Sjöström CD, Sullivan M, Wedel H. Swedish Obese Subjects Study Scientific Group. Lifestyle, diabetes, and cardiovascular risk factors 10 years after bariatric surgery. N Engl J Med. 2004;23;351:2683-2693.)*

et al, 2014) published 3-year outcomes for RYGB and VSG versus medical therapy. T2DM remission was seen in 38% of RYGB and 24% of VSG versus 5% in the medical therapy group. Notably in both the STAMPEDE trial and the Swedish Obesity Study Group, remission was predicted by shorter duration of diabetes before surgery, supporting the contention of the bariatric surgery community that weight loss surgery should not be a therapy of last resort for obese patients with T2DM. Waiting for years of medical management to fail only diminishes the benefits of surgical treatment.

Since Pories' notable paper, much research has been devoted to understanding the mechanism of T2DM remission and reversal of insulin resistance. The mechanism remains unclear but is likely multifactorial. Certainly reduced caloric and carbohydrate intake play a role. In a well designed study by Lingvay and colleagues (2013), 10 patients with T2DM scheduled to undergo gastric bypass surgery

were placed on a diet identical to their postsurgery diet for 10 days 6 weeks before their operation. Glucose homeostasis measures were performed during the 10-day preoperative diet and compared with the same measures performed for 10 days in the postoperative period. Glycemic control was as good or better in the preoperative period. Others have implicated changes in the neural and hormonal pathways of the gut, glucose metabolism by enterocytes themselves, bile acid receptors, alteration of the gut microbiome, and other complex mechanisms beyond the scope of this chapter, but nonetheless fascinating, and an area of active research.

Cardiovascular Disease Risk Reduction

According to the AHA, independent modifiable risk factors for CVD in general and coronary heart disease in particular include cigarette smoking, hypertension, dyslipidemia, diabetes, and obesity. Furthermore, obesity also is linked to hypertension, dyslipidemia, and a proinflammatory state, which increase cardiovascular risk (Box 3). Therefore it is logical to hypothesize that weight loss through surgical means would decrease cardiovascular risk. In 2004 the meta-analysis of bariatric surgery by Buchwald and colleagues indeed showed a remarkable decrease in CVD risk factors with hyperlipidemia resolution in 70% of patients, and resolution of hypertension in 61.7%. Similarly, in 2004 the SOS group showed 2- and 10-year rates of recovery from diabetes, hypertriglyceridemia, low levels of high-density lipoprotein cholesterol, and hypertension were more favorable in the surgery group than in the control group, and the degree of improvement was more pronounced in the RYGB patients. Habib and colleagues published data in 2009 that showed significant improvement in mean carotid intima-media thickness and mean flow-mediated dilation and significant decrease in mean high-sensitivity C-reactive protein at 6, 12, and 24 months after

RYGB. Likewise, Appachi and colleagues (2011) demonstrated favorable improvements in the proinflammatory profile (adiponectin, leptin, and tumor necrosis factor-α levels) of patients who underwent RYGB, LABG, or VSG. These improvements were associated strongly with improvement in triglycerides and lipid profiles. Vest and colleagues (2012) pooled data from 16 studies evaluating cardiac imaging and saw an improvement in diastolic dysfunction after bariatric surgery. Other studies have suggested cardiac remodeling and improved cardiac function as well (Ashrafian et al, 2008).

More important, bariatric surgery not only reduces CVD risk factors but also decreases the number and mortality of cardiovascular events. In 2012 the SOS published 10-year data showing bariatric surgery reduced the number of cardiovascular events by one third, (adjusted hazard ratio [HR] 0.67) and cardiovascular deaths by one half (HR 0.47) versus the control group. Likewise, Pontiroli and Morabito published a meta-analysis in 2011, which showed reduced long-term overall mortality and cardiovascular specific mortality in patients undergoing RYGB and LAGB, with greater effect on cardiovascular mortality in the RYGB group.

The Future of Bariatric Surgery

Ideally, morbidly obese patients should undergo bariatric surgery at a time that will allow for the greatest risk reduction and most benefit. The original 1991 NIH Consensus Statement recommended that bariatric surgery be considered for patients with a BMI of at least 40 kg/m^2 and BMI 35 to 39.9 kg/m^2 if obesity-related comorbidities existed. However, it has become increasingly evident that BMI alone is an inadequate marker of impaired health and disease risk. The SOS study found that BMI was not predictive of benefit from surgery in relation to CVD, cancer, and diabetes (2012). In contrast, insulin use and impaired fasting glucose did predict a benefit from bariatric surgery. This suggests that bariatric surgery parameters must be modified to give more consideration to metabolic factors. The American Society for Metabolic and Bariatric Surgery released a statement supporting weight loss surgery for class I obesity in 2012. The International Diabetes Federation and National Institute for Health and Care Excellence also support bariatric surgery for class I obesity and T2DM if optimal medical therapy fails (Table 2).

■ CONCLUSION

Bariatric surgery remains a continually evolving field with an increasing body of research supporting its benefits. It is an inherently unique area of surgery because it treats obesity and chronic medical conditions that have long been considered outside of the realm of surgical intervention. Indeed, few surgeons have ever set out to modify cardiovascular risk factors and cure diabetes. We traditionally have treated the complications of those diseases, and it is gratifying to now be able to intervene in their progression.

TABLE 2: American and International Guidelines for Bariatric Surgery Eligibility in Adults

Guideline	ASMBS (2012)*	ADA/AHA (2015)†	IDF (2011)‡	NICE (2014)¶
Prioritization for surgery *recommended*	BMI ≥ 40 kg/m^2 or BMI ≥ 35 kg/m^2 with one serious weight loss–responsive comorbid condition	Not prioritized for any group	BMI ≥ 40 kg/m^2 or BMI ≥ 35 kg/m^2 when diabetes and other comorbid conditions not controlled by optimum medical treatment	BMI ≥ 40 kg/m^2 or BMI ≥ 35 kg/m^2 when diabetes and other comorbid conditions not controlled by optimum medical treatment
Eligibility for surgery can be *considered*	BMI ≥ 30 kg/m^2 when substantial and durable weight loss and comorbidity improvement are unachievable with nonsurgical methods	BMI ≥ 40 kg/m^2 or BMI ≥ 35 kg/m^2 with T2DM or other obesity-related comorbidity who have not responded to other treatments§	BMI ≥ 35 kg/m^2, or BMI ≥ 30 kg/m^2 when diabetes and other comorbid conditions are not controlled by optimum medical treatment	BMI 30-34.9 kg/m^2 with onset of T2DM in last 10 years
Comment	LAGB, VSG, and RYGB have been shown in randomized controlled trials to be safe and effective in patients with BMIs of 30-35 kg/m^2 in short and medium term follow-up	Further research needed on durability of weight loss, HgbA$_{1c}$ improvement, and CVD risk reduction	Adjustment of BMI down 2.5 kg/m^2 for patients of Asian or higher risk ethnic origin is advised	Consider bariatric surgery for Asian origin with recent onset T2DM at lower BMI than other populations

*From ASMBS statements/guidelines: Bariatric surgery in class I obesity (body mass index 30–35 kg/m^2). *Surg Obes Relat Dis.* 2012;9 (2013):e1-e10.

†From Fox CS, Golden SH, Anderson C, et al. Update on prevention of cardiovascular disease in adults with type 2 diabetes mellitus in light of recent evidence: a scientific statement from the American Heart Association and the American Diabetes Association. *Circulation.* 2015;132:691-718.

‡From Dixon JB, Zimmet P, Alberti KG, et al. Bariatric surgery: an IDF statement for obese type 2 diabetes. *Diabet Med.* 2011;28:628-642.

§Adapted from the 2013 American Heart Association/American College of Cardiology/The Obesity Society guidelines.

¶From Stegenga H, Haines A, Jones K, et al. Identification, assessment, and management of overweight and obesity: summary of updated NICE guidance. *BMJ.* 2014;349:g6608.

ADA/AHA, American Diabetes Association/American Heart Association; *ASMBS,* American Society for Metabolic and Bariatric Surgery; *BMI,* body mass index; *IDF,* International Diabetes Foundation; *LAGB,* laparoscopic adjustable gastric banding; *NICE,* National Institute for Health and Clinical Excellence; *RYGB,* Roux-en-Y gastric bypass; *T2DM,* type 2 diabetes mellitus; *VSG,* vertical sleeve gastrectomy.

Suggested Readings

Buchwald H, Estok R, Fahrbach K, et al. Weight and type 2 diabetes after bariatric surgery: systematic review and meta-analysis. *Am J Med.* 2009;122:248-256.

Knop FK, Taylor R. Mechanism of metabolic advantages after bariatric surgery. *Diabetes Care.* 2013;36:S287-S291.

Schauer PR, Bhatt DL, Kirwan JP, et al. Bariatric surgery versus intensive medical therapy for diabetes–3-year outcomes. *N Engl J Med.* 2014;370: 2002-2013.

Sjostrom L, Peltonen M, Jacobson P, et al. Bariatric surgery and long-term cardiovascular events. *JAMA.* 2012;307:56-65.

Vest AR, Heneghan HM, Agarwal S, Schauer PR, et al. Bariatric surgery and cardiovascular outcomes: a systematic review. *Heart.* 2012;98:1763-1777.

NONMELANOMA SKIN CANCERS

Michele A. Shermak, MD

Nonmelanoma skin cancer (NMSC) is the most common malignancy in the United States, with more than 1 million NMSCs occurring in the United States each year. Basal cell and squamous cell carcinoma are the most common NMSCs. One in five Americans develops skin cancer in a lifetime. Incidence rates of skin cancer continue to rise dramatically, with a 100% increase from 1992 to 2012 in the Medicare fee-for-service population and a 35% increase in NMSC in the overall U.S. population from 2006 to 2012. The average annual cost of treating NMSC in the United States was $4.8 billion from 2007 to 2011, making skin cancer the fifth most costly malignancy to treat in the United States.

■ PRESENTATION

An individual may arrive at a surgeon's office with a concern about a specific skin lesion or more often through referral by a dermatologist or primary care provider who requests definitive removal of a suspicious lesion and who may have performed a diagnostic biopsy of that lesion. Clinically, NMSCs range from red, tan, or off-white plaques to smooth or ulcerative papules, nodules, subcutaneous nodules, or deep ulcerations. Their biological behavior is also variable, with some following a relatively benign course and others progressing to mutilation, metastasis, and death.

Basal cell carcinoma (BCC) is slow growing and rarely metastasizes. Eighty-six percent of BCC occur on the head, and 7% occur on the trunk and extremities. BCC is rare on the hand, penis, and lower lip; cutaneous malignancies at these sites are more likely squamous cell carcinoma (SCC). Cutaneous malignancies of the upper lip are almost always BCC whereas those of the lower lip are usually SCC. BCC is the most common malignant eyelid tumor, with 67% on the lower lid and 10% at the inner canthus. The major risk factors include cumulative exposure to ultraviolet (UV) light, fair skin phototype (Fitzpatrick type I and II), tanning bed visits, smoking, blistering sunburns, and immunosuppression, particularly in transplant patients.

The three most common subtypes of BCC are nodular, superficial, and morpheaform, a high-risk subtype of BCC. A large retrospective analysis demonstrated that almost 79% of BCC are nodular, 15% are superficial, and 6% are morpheaform. Classical nodular BCC appears dome shaped, with well-defined borders, a "pearly" appearance, telangiectasias, and possibly ulceration (Figure 1). Histologically, BCCs may contain focal areas of individual dyskeratotic cells to keratin pearls. If a predominance of this mature, atypical keratinizing squamous component is seen, the tumor is termed basosquamous carcinoma. This tumor may have a capacity to metastasize more similar to that of a SCC. When predicting tumor behavior and hence optimizing treatment, histologic growth pattern is more relevant than type of differentiation.

Squamous cell carcinoma, unlike BCC, has premalignant precursors and an in situ variant. Actinic keratoses are SCC "precursor" lesions. Subtypes of SCC include squamous cell carcinoma in situ, which is confined to epidermis; invasive SCC; and keratoacanthoma, a subtype of invasive SCC (Figure 2). SCC most frequently occurs on the face, hands, and forearms. SCC arising in chronically sun-exposed skin behave in a relatively indolent manner with a lower than 5% risk of metastases; however, SCC arising in mucocutaneous interfaces such as the lips, genitalia, and perianal areas are more aggressive, with a higher risk of metastases. Two thirds of SCC develop in non–sun-exposed sites such as the legs, anus, and areas of chronic ulceration and scarring, known as Marjolin's ulcer (Figure 3). Lesions developing at these sites have a worse prognosis, with more aggressive behavior and more frequent metastases than those in sun-exposed skin. External ear, lips, nose, scalp, and genitals are high-risk locations as well.

SCCs appear as hyperkeratotic, flesh-colored, and raised, with possible associated ulceration or erythema. Clinically, the in situ form of SCC often is seen as solitary, sharply demarcated, pink to red scaly plaques that may resemble superficial BCCs or small patches of psoriasis or eczema. Most arise in sun-exposed skin. Typically the lesions grow slowly over years, seldom progressing to invasive carcinoma.

Merkel cell carcinoma (MCC) is a rare tumor of the skin of neuroendocrine origin, probably developing from neuronal mechanoreceptors. The tumor is a red-pink to violaceous, firm, solitary, rapidly growing nodule, typically on the head and neck. Other sites include extremities and buttock. It is characterized by its aggressive behavior, with 40% of patients developing distant metastases and 30% of patients dying of the disease within 5 years. The diagnosis is made by histopathology testing, and an incisional or excisional biopsy is mandatory. Immunohistochemical staining contributes to clarification of the diagnosis. Initial workup comprises ultrasound of the local-regional lymph nodes and total body scanning examinations.

■ MANAGEMENT

Incisional biopsy of a suspicious skin lesion is recommended. If the lesion has pigmentation, the diagnosis of melanoma must be considered, and, accordingly, this type of lesion should undergo full-thickness biopsy in case histologic depth influences treatment and prognosis. In general, complete excision may be performed in lieu of diagnostic biopsy if the wound created will be closed easily in a region of straightforward reconstruction. For those patients who have had a prior biopsy, the biopsy report must be reviewed and addressed accordingly.

Surgery is the optimal treatment for skin cancer, including Mohs' surgery. Surgical excision offers overall cure rates of greater than 90%. Recommended margins for excision of BCC and SCC are 4 mm extending into subcutaneous fat, according to the National Comprehensive Cancer Network (NCCN). When possible, excision of NMSC of the face should be performed in relaxed skin tension lines in which

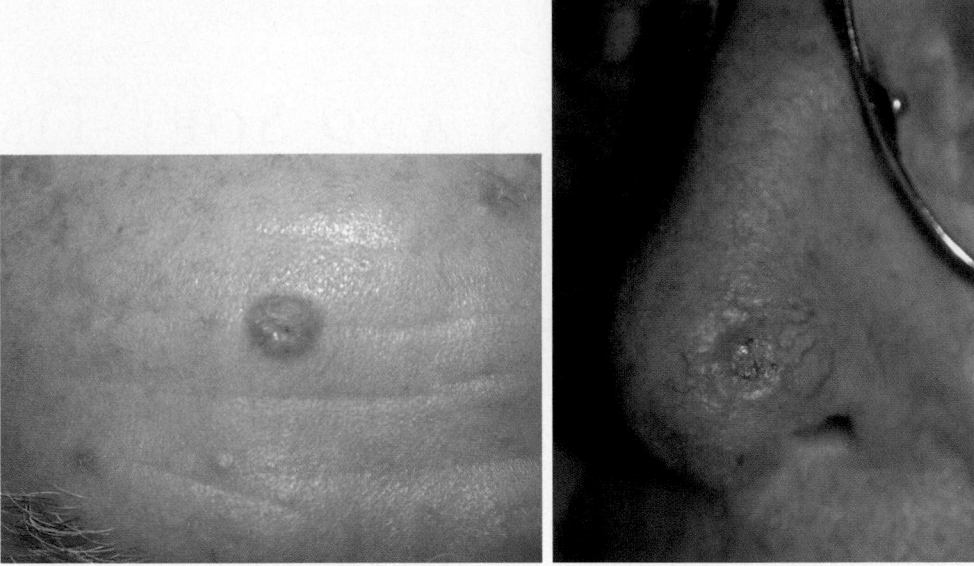

FIGURE 1 Basal cell cancer typically is seen as a pearly, raised, well-circumscribed skin lesion, often on the face, sometimes with ulceration and associated telangiectasias.

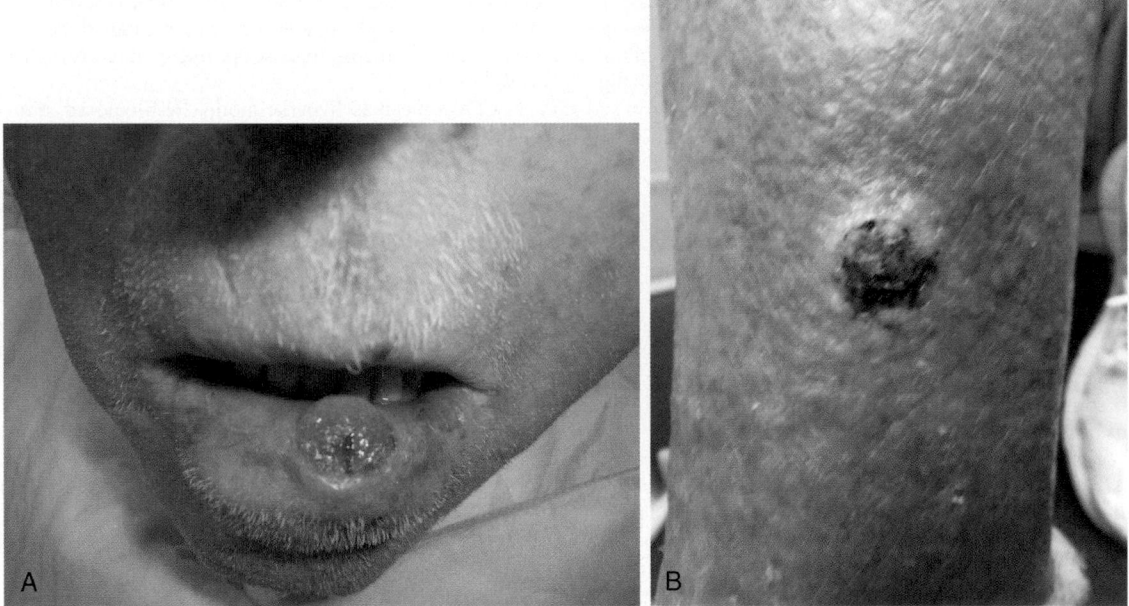

FIGURE 2 A, Cutaneous malignancy of the lower lip is most likely squamous cell carcinoma (SCC), with ulceration. **B,** Keratoacanthoma is a subtype of SCC that is seen as a cutaneous horn.

the scar will heal imperceptibly within dynamic facial lines (Figure 4). Directionality of the incision also must be planned with the possibility of malignancy in mind in case re-excision will be necessary. For higher-risk NMSC, with characteristics including poorly defined borders, recurrent disease, immunosuppression, site of prior radiation therapy, perineural involvement, or aggressive histologic subtype on biopsy (e.g., morpheaform BCC, Marjolin's ulcer, MCC), recommended margins increase to 1 cm. To evaluate completeness of excision, frozen sections of margins are recommended for high-risk SCC and BCC in high-risk areas, lesions larger than 2 cm, and any morpheaform BCC. An alternative to frozen section is to dress the open wound or temporarily graft the wound until the final pathology

report returns, allowing for reconstruction with definitively clear margins (Figure 5). Complete excision also may be confirmed through Mohs' surgery, with satisfactory results. Indications for Mohs' surgery include tumors larger than 2 cm, recurrent tumors, tumors in high-risk areas, tumors with indistinct clinical margins, and tumors in cosmetically sensitive regions. When positive margins are identified after excisional biopsy, re-excision with either Mohs' surgery or excision until negative complete circumferential margins are obtained is required.

In patients diagnosed with MCC without clinical evidence of regional lymph node involvement, sentinel lymph node biopsy is recommended in addition to excision of gross tumor with 1-cm margins. In patients with regional lymph node involvement, radical lymphadenectomy is recommended. Adjuvant radiotherapy should be considered in patients with excision margins of less than 1 cm and multiple affected lymph nodes of extracapsular extension.

Radiotherapy is a primary treatment option for patients in whom excision of NMSC is not possible. Such scenarios include frail patients, patients with large lesions, and patients with medical comorbidities that complicate surgery. Five-year recurrence for primary BCC treated with radiotherapy is 8.0% to 15.8%, and the rate for SCC is similar at 5% to 10%. Radiotherapy also can be used for adjuvant treatment of NMSC, such as incompletely excised large tumors or tumors at high risk for metastasis (e.g., large or deep SCCs, tumors with perineural invasion).

Perineural invasion, typically asymptomatic and diagnosed on histology testing, is a poor prognostic sign for both recurrence and metastasis and an indication for postexcision radiation therapy. It is associated with 47% local recurrence, 35% metastasis to regional nodes, and 15% distant metastasis. Referral to a radiation oncologist is recommended with perineural invasion.

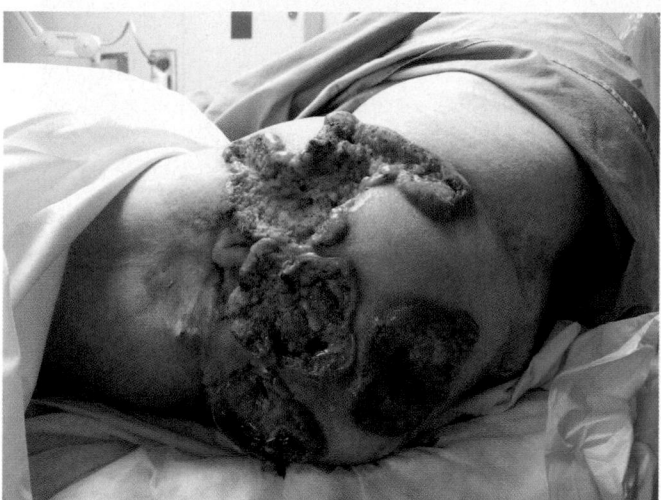

FIGURE 3 Marjolin's ulcer is an aggressive form of squamous cell carcinoma developing in chronic wounds such as this trochanteric pressure sore.

■ CLOSURE AND RECONSTRUCTION

Reconstructive consideration first includes delayed versus immediate reconstruction. Most often, wounds are closed primarily at the time of extirpation. In some cases, wounds may be left to heal secondarily, such as for cutaneous defects smaller than 2 cm and for wounds on concave surfaces like the medial canthal area or supra-alar crease that predictably heal with excellent color match and contour. Purse-string suture also may be considered to close circular defects, particularly on the face. Local wound care or temporary coverage with allograft and delayed reconstruction are recommended if margins may be inadequate when primary closure or full-thickness skin grafting with good donor resources is not possible (see Figure 5).

When thinking about the reconstructive approach, plastic surgeons consider the reconstructive ladder (Figure 6). The lowest rungs of the reconstructive ladder include primary closure, ascending to grafts and flaps, local and microvascular. Grafts may be partial thickness through dermis or full thickness including the deep dermis. Split-thickness skin grafts heal more easily than full-thickness skin grafts but result in greater contracture and a less cosmetic result. Full-thickness skin grafts are better for cosmetically important regions like the face or areas that cannot withstand contraction, such as the fingers (Figure 7). Retroauricular, preauricular, forehead, and supraclavicular regions are excellent donor sites for skin grafts. Composite grafts including skin and cartilage or bone are optimal for ear, nose, and eyelid recipient defects that are missing components beyond skin alone and require structural support.

Local flaps are composed of skin adjacent to the extirpation defect with random vascular pattern that may be moved into the defect to reconstruct the site with "like" tissue. Such flaps include advancement flaps and rotation flaps. Advancement flaps involve release of tissue along cosmetically amenable landmarks, with sliding of tissue forward into the defect, including V-Y flaps and cervicofacial flaps (Figure 8). Rotation flaps involve movement into the defect analogous to moving along the circumference of a circle, with the leading edge rotated along the circle's radius to close the defect. The bilobed flap is a type of rotation flap (Figure 9). The rhomboid flap is another type of local flap involving precise geometric shifting of single or multiple rhomboid-shaped skin flaps to cover adjacent defects (Figure 10). Z-plasty also may be performed as a stand-alone technical maneuver or in conjunction with flaps to effectively recruit additional length to release tight closures, particularly longitudinal closures across joints.

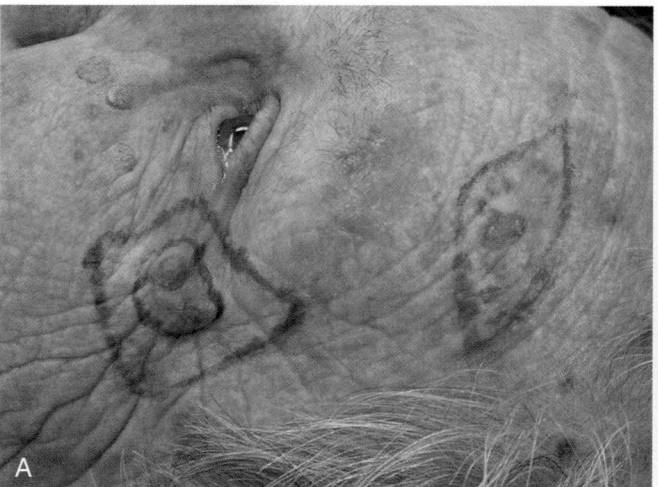
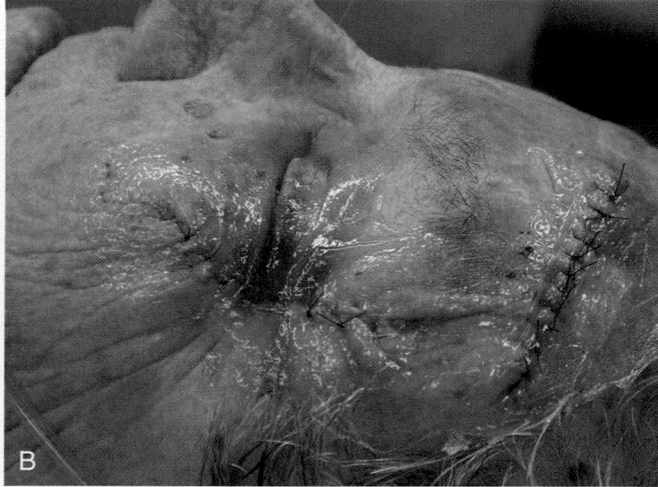

FIGURE 4 A, This patient has a basosquamous carcinoma in the lateral orbicularis region and a lentigo on the forehead. **B,** Both skin lesions were excised with 5-mm margins, and the forehead was closed along relaxed skin tension lines. The lateral orbicularis was not, in light of tension if both wounds were closed in parallel fashion.

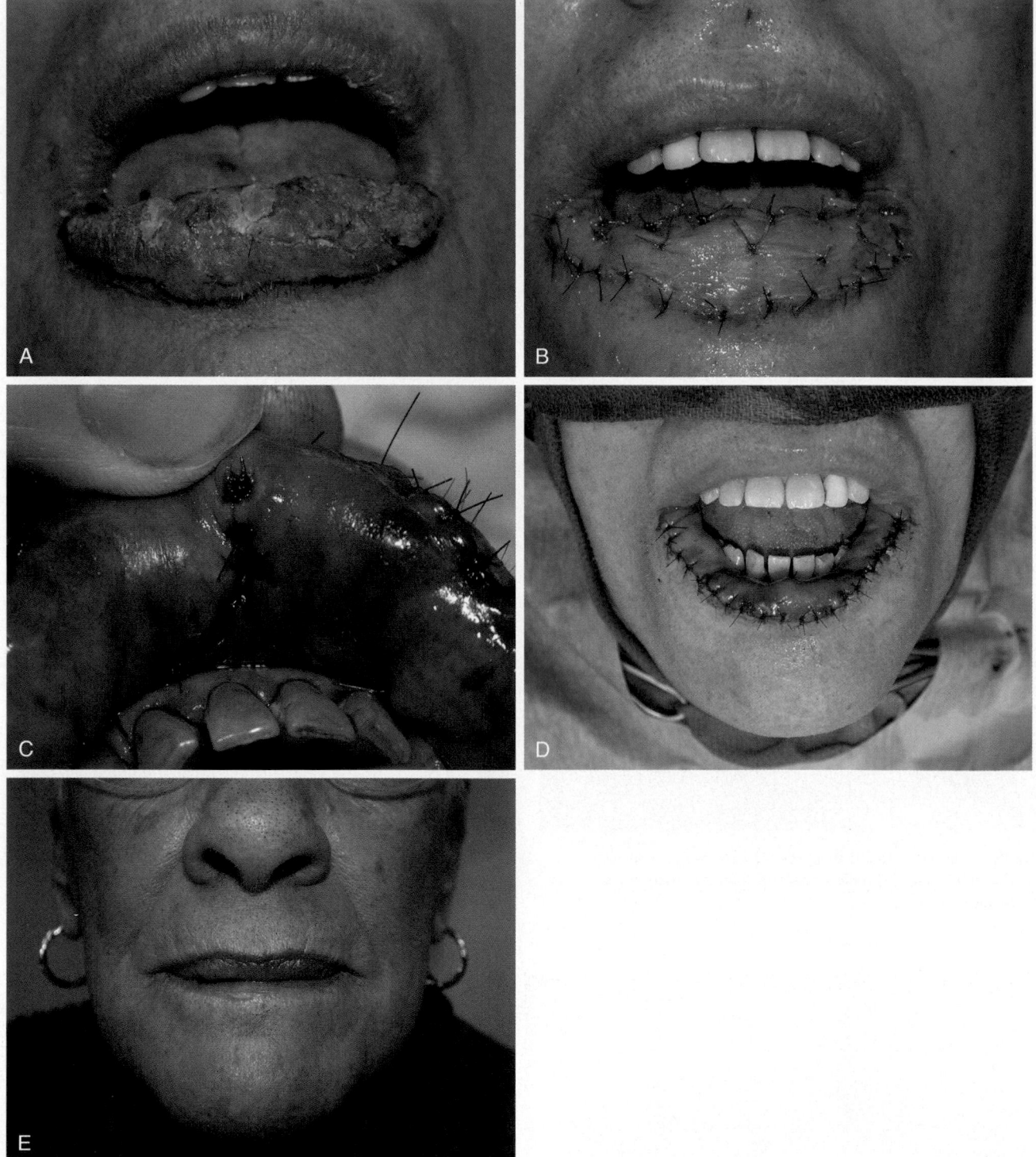

FIGURE 5 A, This patient had squamous cell carcinoma in situ of the lower lip. **B,** It was excised and dressed with allograft to protect the wound and allow time for the final pathology report on margins to return. **C** and **D,** The patient returned to the operating room, and the allograft was removed. A V-Y advancement flap composed of mucosa from the gingivobuccal sulcus was created to reconstruct the dry vermilion of the lower lip. **E,** The postoperative healed result.

Pedicled flaps have a defined vascular supply and therefore may be larger in dimension with the known vascular anatomy. Pedicled flaps include skin, muscle, nerve, fascia, cartilage, and/or bone. Pedicled flaps provide excellent coverage for grafts required to provide structural support, such as in the nose or lower eyelid. Forehead flaps are an example of this (Figure 11). Pedicled flaps also may be shaped

after a healing period through scar reduction, dermabrasion, or liposuction.

The most complex form of flap reconstruction, seen at the top of the reconstructive ladder, is free flap reconstruction, in which a remote segment of vascularized tissue is moved to a wound defect, with the arterial and venous blood supply completely disconnected

RECONSTRUCTIVE LADDER

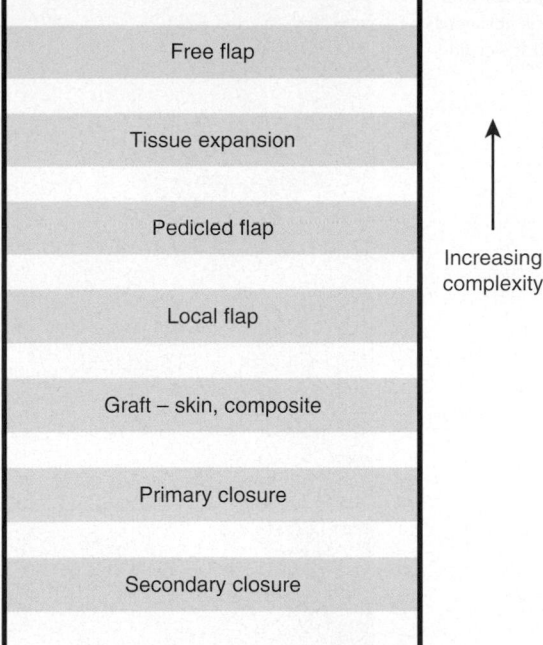

Free flap

Tissue expansion

Pedicled flap

Local flap

Graft – skin, composite

Primary closure

Secondary closure

Increasing
complexity

FIGURE 6 The reconstructive ladder. The lowest rung is secondary wound healing, working up to primary closure, grafts, and flaps, from local to pedicled to microvascular free flaps. Plastic surgeons follow this model and opt for the least morbidity and lowest level of complexity when possible.

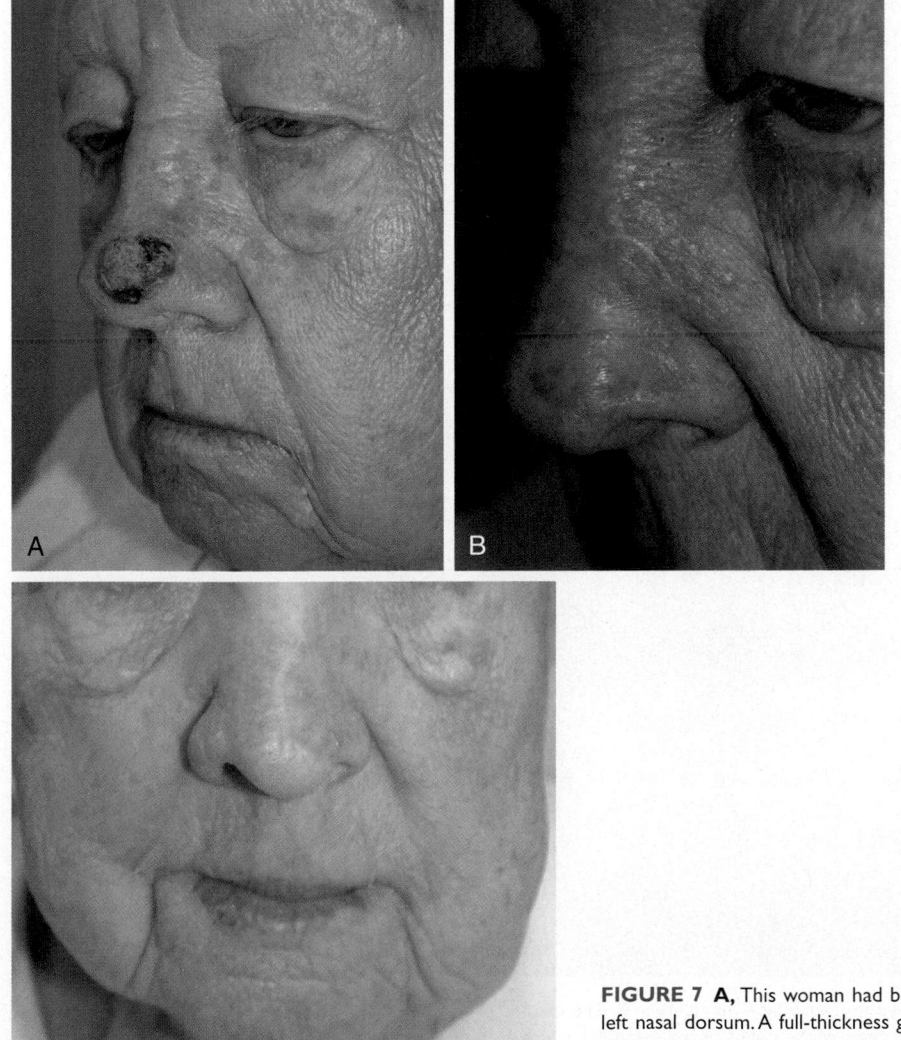

FIGURE 7 A, This woman had biopsy-proven squamous cell carcinoma in situ of the left nasal dorsum. A full-thickness graft was the reconstruction method of choice, with donor site being the clavicle skin. Lateral (**B**) and frontal (**C**) views demonstrate an acceptable cosmetic result without any nasal alar retraction or architectural deformity.

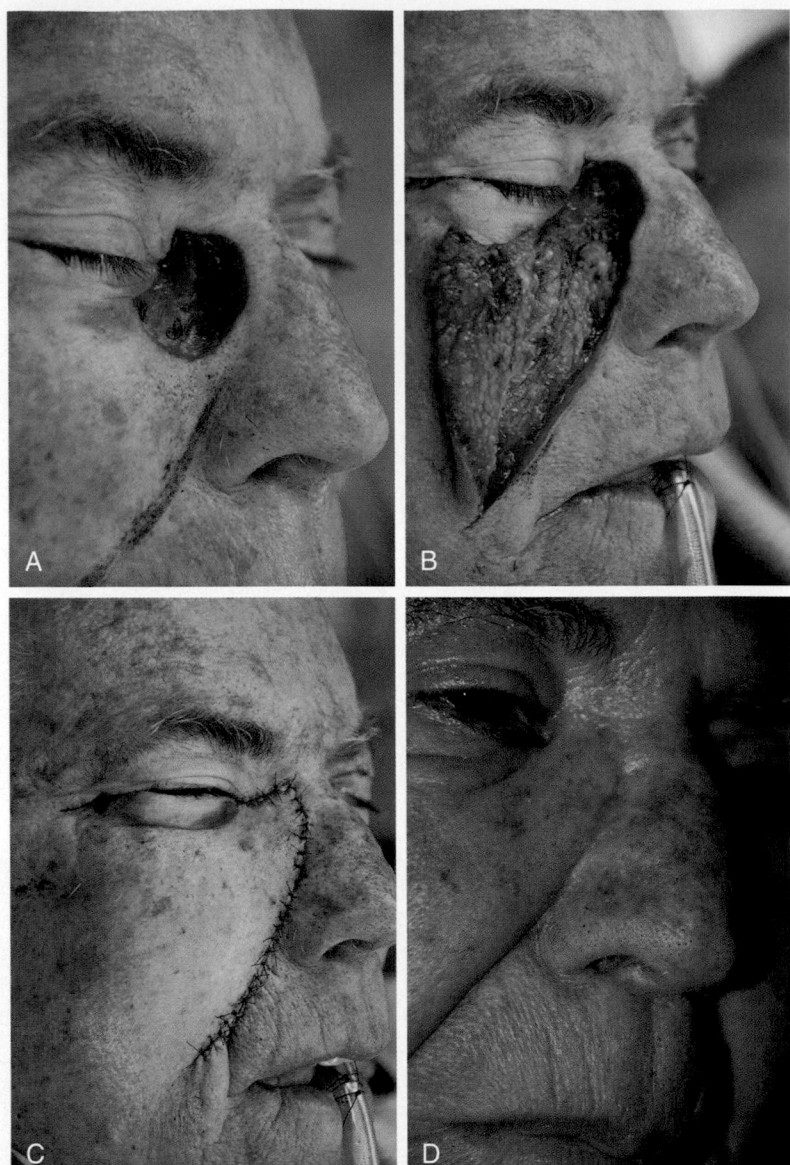

FIGURE 8 A, Large Mohs' defect involving the right medial canthal region. **B,** Facial advancement flap is designed with incisions in aesthetically acceptable skin folds and based on random blood supply to the facial skin. **C,** Flap is advanced and closed. **D,** Postoperative result with normal lower lid position and protection of underlying bone.

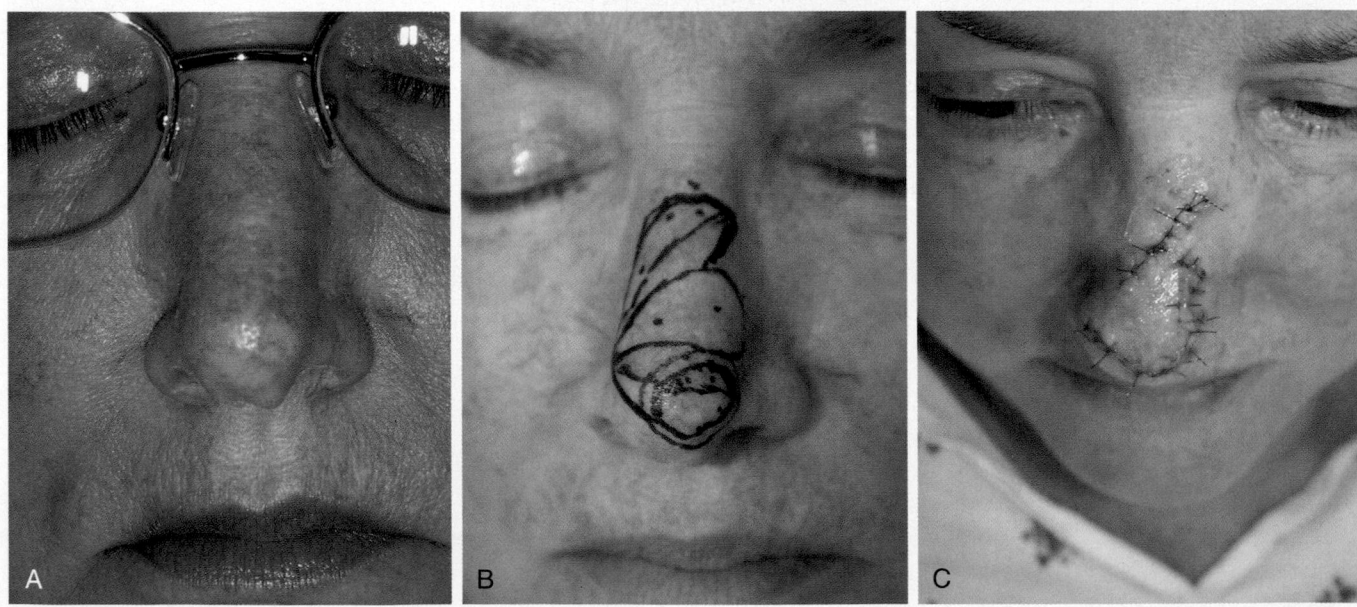

FIGURE 9 A, Squamous cell carcinoma in situ of nasal tip, requiring 4-mm margin. **B,** The closure plan includes a bilobed flap. Three lobes of skin of the same length are designed within 100 degrees of the axis of the radius of the first lobe, which is the surgical defect. **C,** The remaining two lobes are rotated: the first of these two flaps fills C, the defect, and the second somewhat smaller lobe is rotated into the defect of the first lobe rotated, with primary closure of this last donor defect.

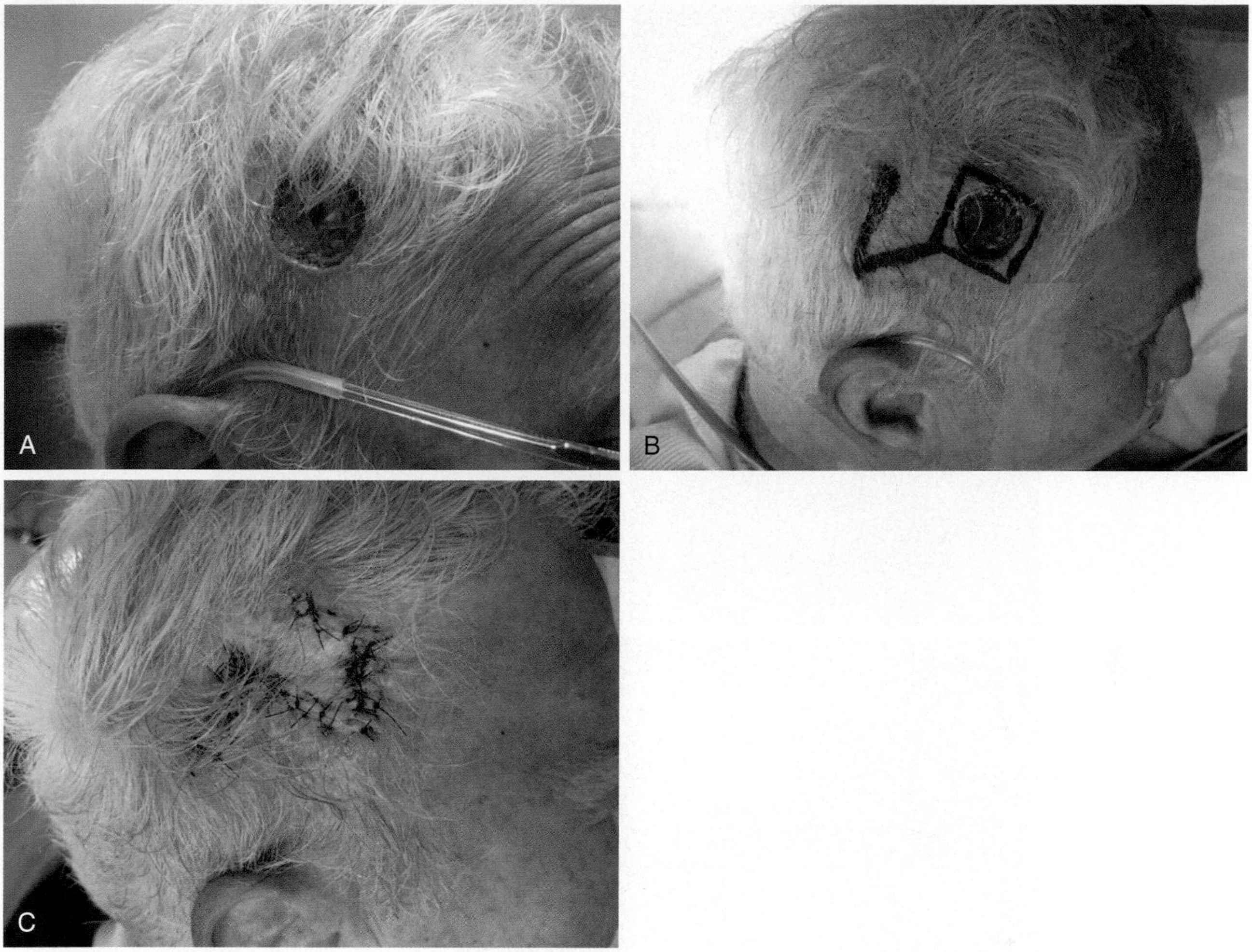

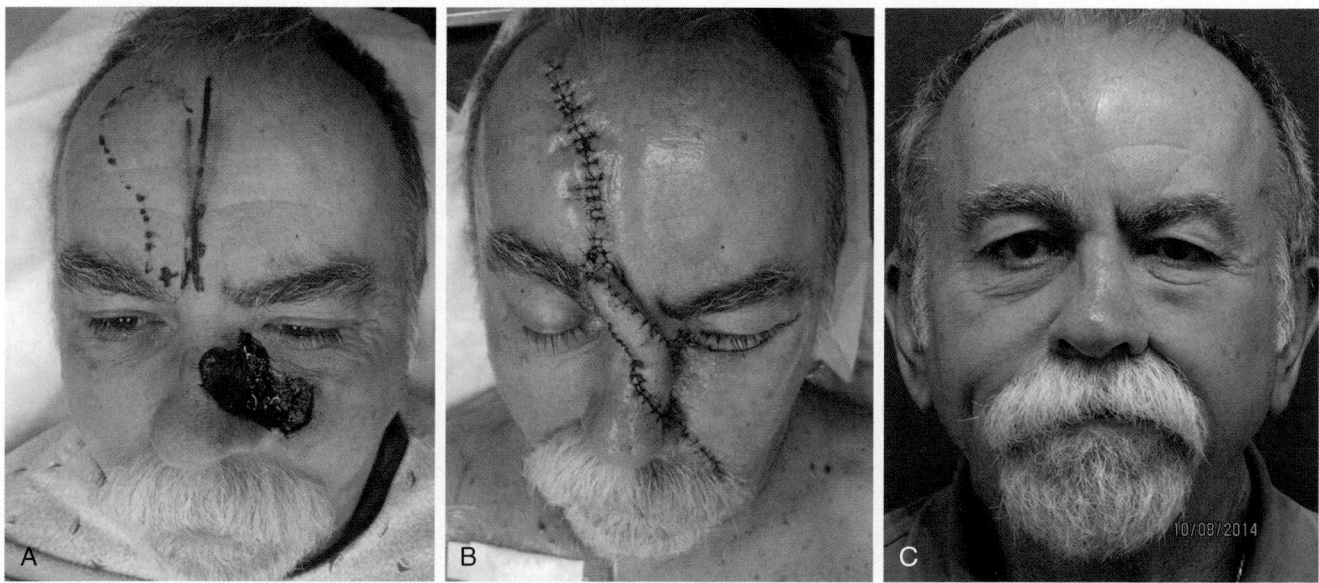

FIGURE 10 **A,** Large Mohs' defect of the right lateral scalp. **B,** The defect is converted to a rhomboid shape, and a rhomboid flap with the same dimensions of the wound defect is designed. **C,** The flap is advanced and closed.

FIGURE 11 **A,** This man had a generous Mohs' defect of his medial left cheek extending to the dorsal nose and left nasal sidewall, with exposed nasal bone. **B,** He was reconstructed with a forehead flap to cover the nose and a left cheek advancement flap based laterally to close the cheek to the nasal sidewall. **C,** Postoperatively he has a satisfactory result, lacking pull on the lower lid and with undisturbed nasal architecture.

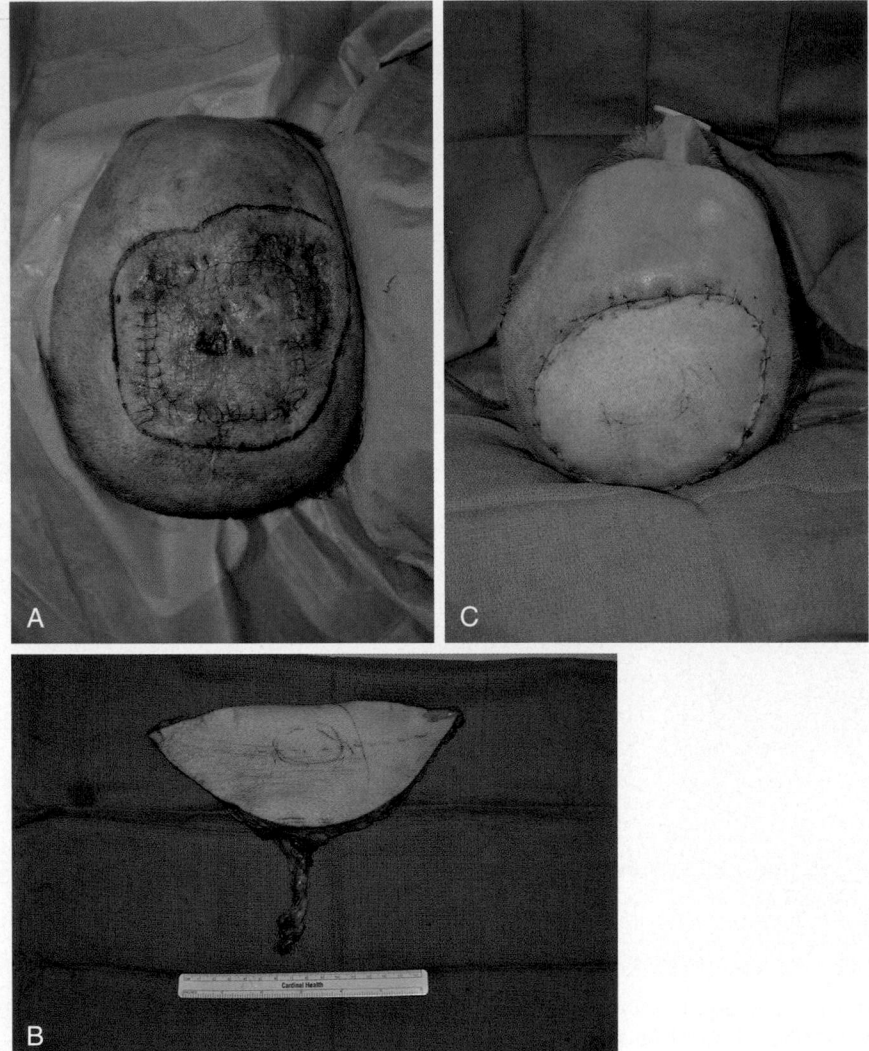

FIGURE 12 A, Diffuse scalp involvement with recurrent basal cell carcinoma. Computed tomographic scan revealed likely periosteal involvement of underlying cranial bone. **B,** With exposed bone and a large defect size, a microvascular tissue transfer is necessary. The anterolateral thigh (ALT) flap is dissected out of its donor region with its feeding artery, the descending branch of lateral circumflex femoris artery, and vein. The lateral femoral cutaneous nerve may be used to improve sensation at the recipient site. **C,** The flap is sutured into place on the upper scalp defect with exposed cranium.

at its recipient site and reattached with the assistance of magnifying loupes or microscope to the vascular supply near the wound defect. This flap may be composed of skin, fascia, nerve, muscle, cartilage, and/or bone. Examples of free flaps include latissimus and anterolateral thigh (ALT) flaps (Figure 12).

■ CONCLUSION

NMSC is more prevalent than any other malignant neoplasm, so understanding the presentation, proper excision, and closure of the wounds created at extirpation are important tools in the surgeon's armamentarium.

SUGGESTED READINGS

Ibrahim O, Gastman B, Zhang A. Advances in diagnosis and treatment of nonmelanoma skin cancer. *Ann Plast Surg.* 2014;73:615-619.

Jackson IT. *Local Flaps in Head and Neck Reconstruction.* 2nd ed. Valencia, CA: Quality Medical Publishers; 2007.

Lebbe C, Becker JC, Grob JJ, Malvehy J, Del Marmol V, Pehamberger H, Peris K, Saiag P, Middleton MR, Bastholt L, Testori A, Stratigos A, Garbe C, European Dermatology Forum (EDF), European Association of Dermato-Oncology (EADO), European Organization for Research and Treatment of Cancer (EORTC). Diagnosis and treatment of Merkel cell carcinoma: European consensus-based interdisciplinary guideline. *Eur J Cancer.* 2015;51:2396-2403.

Netscher DT, Leong M, Orengo I, et al. Cutaneous malignancies: melanoma and nonmelanoma types. *Plast Reconstr Surg.* 2011;127:37e-56e.

Rogers-Vizena CR, Lalonde DH, Menick FJ, Bentz ML. Surgical treatment and reconstruction of nonmelanoma facial skin cancers. *Plast Reconstr Surg.* 2015;135:895e-908e.

Zbar RI, Canady JW. MOC-PSSM CME article: nonmelanoma facial skin malignancy. *Plast Reconstr Surg.* 2008;121(suppl 1):1-9.

THE MANAGEMENT OF CUTANEOUS MELANOMA

Charles M. Balch, MD, Keith Delman, MD, and Glen C. Balch, MD

The current guidelines for surgical management of cutaneous melanoma are based on multiple prospective clinical trials and database analysis that use the staging characteristics of the primary melanoma (tumor thickness, ulceration, mitotic rate), the status of the regional lymph nodes (presence or absence of nodal metastases, tumor burden, and number of metastatic nodes), and the clinical/radiologic evidence of distant metastases (including the site and the number of distant metastases).

■ BIOPSY TECHNIQUE

A suspicious skin lesion should undergo biopsy with either complete excision for smaller lesions, an incisional biopsy for larger lesions, or a shave biopsy to rule out melanoma for borderline lesions. An excisional biopsy is performed with a 1- to 2-mm clinical lateral margin and a deep margin in the subcutaneous fat, underneath all epithelial appendageal structures. This can be performed on most lesions up to 1.5 cm in diameter. The biopsy scar should be oriented to be compatible with a subsequent wide local excision should the lesion prove to be melanoma. On the extremities a longitudinal or oblique incision is preferred. On the trunk or the head and neck the biopsy should be oriented parallel to the skin lines. A full-thickness biopsy should be undertaken to accurately interpret the maximum tumor thickness, the presence or absence of ulceration, and the level of invasion.

An incisional biopsy taken from the most raised or the most darkly pigmented area may be appropriate for lesions that are large or located at a difficult anatomic site. Because it removes only part of the tumor, a repeat biopsy may be necessary if the initial histologic diagnosis does not agree with the clinical impression. An incisional biopsy involves removal of a portion of a skin lesion, in which the lateral margins are incomplete, and therefore, by definition, positive, but the deep margin should be in the subcutaneous fat, underneath all epithelial appendageal structures. Final determination of the tumor thickness cannot be made until the entire lesion has been excised and examined by the pathologist. For suspicious lesions beneath nail beds, the biopsy approach is more problematic. Although digital tumors usually arise from the proximal nail fold from which the biopsy must be procured, biopsies of subungual pigmented lesions necessitate splitting of the nail plate.

Shave biopsies may be considered for small, flat lesions, in which the likelihood of melanoma is considered to be low, but are inappropriate when a melanoma is suspected, because it could result in an incomplete Breslow thickness measurement. However, it is a useful biopsy technique when performed by an experienced clinician, in the specific setting in which melanoma in situ is being considered in the differential diagnosis along with, perhaps, a benign lentigo or flat seborrheic keratosis.

■ SURGICAL EXCISION OF THE PRIMARY MELANOMA

Most wide local excisions can be performed as an elliptic excision with a primary closure (Figure 1). The deep excision incorporates the superficial fascia and is carried down to (but not through) the underlying deep fascia in most patients. In extremely obese patients the depth need not be all the way to the deep fascia but should be at least to the superficial fascia. Primary closure often is facilitated by a length-to-width ratio of approximately 3:1. The closure usually is accomplished by a standard simple advancement flap, although occasionally either a rotational flap or a split-thickness skin graft may be necessary to cover the defect. On the trunk and the head and neck, the direction of the long axis of the wide local excision usually should be parallel to the skin lines. On an extremity the orientation should be either longitudinal or somewhat oblique to facilitate closure and cosmesis. Excision of melanomas on the head and neck is more complicated because of the functional and cosmetic features of structures such as the eyelid, ear, and nose. Nevertheless, appropriate surgical margins should be used and reconstruction of the defect accomplished with skin flaps or grafts. Whenever a split-thickness skin graft is used to cover the defect after wide excision of a melanoma, the skin graft donor site should be chosen preferentially outside the area of any potential in transit metastases. Guidelines for wide local excision of a primary melanoma are based on six randomized surgical trials that provide the basis for current recommendations for the extent of surgical margins for cutaneous melanoma according to tumor thickness (see Table 1).

Overall, recommendations must, of course, be individualized for a given patient. The importance of other prognostic factors, the anatomic location of the primary tumor, specific factors related to wound healing, and associated medical risk factors must be considered. If these general guidelines are followed, however, overall local recurrence rates should be minimized to acceptable risk levels (less than 3%), with the overwhelming majority of patients effectively treated by relatively simple operations, usually on an outpatient basis with minimal morbidity.

For melanoma in situ, excision of the lesion or biopsy site with a 0.5- to 1-cm border of clinically normal skin and a layer of subcutaneous tissue is sufficient. Although these lesions are noninvasive, a local recurrence may be seen as an invasive melanoma with the potential for metastasis. Margin recommendations for melanomas in situ are based on a consensus of the available data demonstrating excellent local control with the use of such margins. Most in situ melanomas are excised completely and easily with 0.5- to 1-cm margins under local anesthesia, and the surgical defect most often is closed primarily.

For invasive melanomas of 1 mm thickness or less, the World Health Organization Melanoma Program suggests that excision with a 1 cm margin of clinically normal skin and underlying subcutaneous tissue is adequate. The use of this narrow margin for these low-risk patients yields excellent cosmetic and functional results in any anatomic location without compromising therapeutic efficacy. Except for the occasional lesion arising on the distal extremities, scalp, or face, essentially all 1-cm excisions can be closed primarily.

The appropriate margin of excision to be used for melanomas between 1 and 2 mm in thickness cannot be resolved by the prospective trials noted previously. In the absence of data from a randomized controlled trial, it is reasonable to perform a 2-cm surgical margin for these melanomas whenever it is anatomically feasible and where the surgical defect can be closed primarily without a skin graft. However, in anatomic locations where a proposed 2-cm margin may compromise adjacent functional or cosmetic structures, or require the use of complex wound reconstruction techniques or a split-thickness skin graft, a surgical margin less than 2 cm but greater than 1 cm may be used preferentially.

For melanomas between 2 and 4 mm, a 2-cm surgical margin is currently the recommended standard based on the Intergroup data. The U.K. trial, which included a 2- to 4-mm subset that overlapped with the Intergroup trial, demonstrated improved local/regional control with a 3-cm margin vs. a 1-cm margin. In a recent report with a mean follow-up of 8.8 years, patients with a 1-cm margin had a higher melanoma-specific death rate ($P = 0.039$) and a worse melanoma-specific survival rate ($P = 0.05$) compared with those

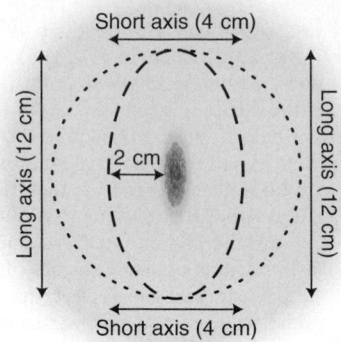

FIGURE 1 Schematic of melanoma excisions. *(From Ross MI. Excision of primary melanoma. In: Balch CM, et al, eds. Cutaneous Melanoma. 5th ed. St Louis: QMP; 2009.)*

TABLE 1: Recommended Surgical Margins of Excision for Melanomas Based on Randomized Surgical Trials and Tumor Thickness

Tumor Thickness (in mm)	Excision Margin (in cm)
In situ	0.5-1.0
0.1 to 1.0	1.0
1.01-2.0	1.0 or 2.0
2.01-4.0	2.0
>4.0	2.0

having a 3-cm surgical margin (Hayes et al., 2016). In a multivariate analysis, surgical margin was an independent predictor of a worse outcome ($P = 0.036$). Although a 3-cm margin may be superior to a 1-cm margin in terms of local control (as seen in the U.K. trial), 4 cm has not been demonstrated to be superior to 2 cm (as seen in the Intergroup trial). The recently reported Swedish trial, which focused on melanomas 2 mm or greater in thickness provided convincing evidence that a 2-cm margin of excision is safe. In addition, the narrower margin of excision can be closed primarily in the majority of patients without a skin graft, thus reducing morbidity and costs of care. Consequently there are no data to support any surgical approach for this group of patients that would include margins greater than 2 cm (Figure 2).

How deep should a melanoma excision extend? In general, sun-induced cutaneous melanomas do not cross fascial barriers, so an excision that extends deep to the superficial fascia of the skin but not through the deep fascia is appropriate for all but the thickest tumors. In contrast, desmoplastic melanomas can invade across fascia. For this reason, we would excise both the superficial and the muscular fascia for desmoplastic melanomas and also consider adjuvant radiation to the excision site after the wounds have healed.

Primary melanomas on the sole of the foot require wide local excision down to the plantar fascia, with either skin graft, healing by secondary intention, or soft tissue coverage. When primary melanoma occurs on non–weight-bearing surfaces, such as the instep, a split-thickness skin graft can provide adequate coverage. However, on weight-bearing surfaces such as over the calcaneus and over the head of the first metatarsal, standard split-thickness skin grafts do not provide durable soft tissue coverage, but thick split skin grafts taken from the instep of the contralateral foot are more robust. Soft tissue defects created over the ball of the foot can be covered by

MELANOMA-SPECIFIC SURVIVAL – NODE+

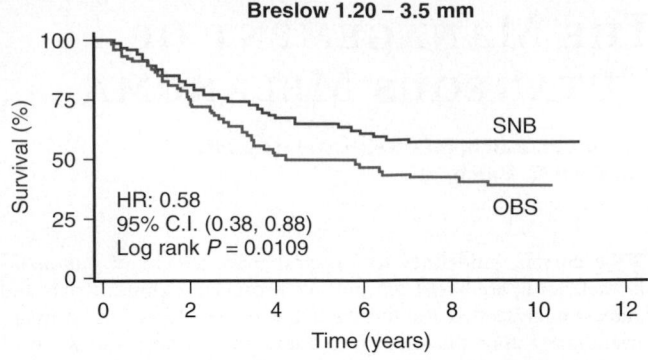

Group	# Event /	Estimate S(t) ± SE %	
	Total N	5-year	10-year
OBS, had nodal recur.	47 / 85	56.5 ± 5.5	41.8 ± 5.7
SNB+	40 / 122	69.6 ± 4.4	60.9 ± 5.1

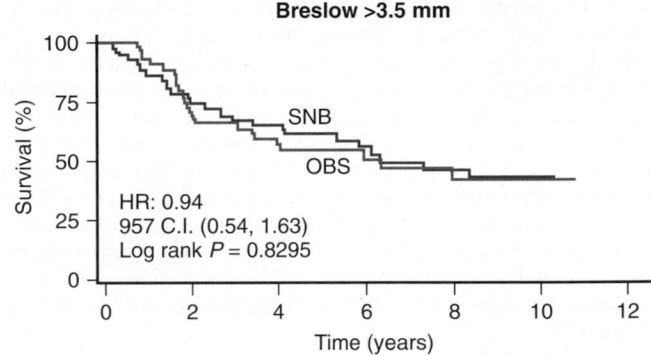

Group	# Event /	Estimate S(t) ± SE %	
	Total N	5-year	10-year
OBS, had nodal recur.	23 / 44	53.8 ± 7.6	41.2 ± 8.7
SNB+	28 / 57	60.6 ± 6.6	41.4 ± 8.0

FIGURE 2 Melanoma-specific survival in a randomized surgical trial (Multicenter Selective Lymphadenectomy Trial 1). Among the 1687 patients with melanomas of at least 1.2-mm thickness, the sentinel node status was the strongest predictor of disease recurrence or death from melanoma (<0.001). Among the 325 patients with regional nodal metastases, those patients who had early lymphadenectomy based on the sentinel node staging had a better survival (56% vs. 41%, HR 0.66, $P = 0.0117$) compared with those patients who had observation *(OBS)* without a sentinel node staging and had clinically detectable nodal metastases requiring a delayed lymphadenectomy. As shown in the figure, the survival benefit occurred in those patients whose melanoma was intermediate thickness, whereas those with thick melanomas did not have a survival benefit with early nodal intervention. In both groups, there was a prognostic and staging value. *C.I.,* confidence interval; *SNB,* sentinel node biopsy. *(Data from Morton DL, Thompson JF, Cochran AJ. Final trial report of sentinel-node biopsy versus nodal observation in melanoma. N Engl J Med. 2014;370:599-609.)*

amputating the great toe but preserving full-thickness skin and soft tissue on the dorsum of the toe to be used as a rotational flap to cover the defect on the plantar surface of the ball of the foot. Lesions on the heel that require significant soft tissue excisions are more problematic but often can be closed by a rotational flap from the arch of the foot based on the posterior tibial artery. This full-thickness soft tissue flap can cover the surgical defect on the heel, and the defect created at the non–weight-bearing donor site can be covered with a skin graft. In some situations the defect is too large or positioned too far posteriorly to allow adequate coverage with this type of flap, and a myocutaneous transfer from a distant site with microvascular reconstruction provides an excellent alternative.

Digital melanoma often requires amputation at the midphalanx proximal to the melanoma and follows the same margin recommendations as other sites. The great toe is the most common site of melanoma of the digits and generally requires amputation at the midproximal phalanx. Sufficient skin and soft tissue usually can be saved on the plantar surface to allow soft tissue coverage of the stump. A significant functional deficit rarely is produced by the total amputation of a single digit from the foot. Because the metatarsal head of the great toe is a critical structure for ambulation, its removal (i.e., a ray amputation) should be avoided when performing amputations of the great toe. Primary melanoma of the distal second through fifth toes usually requires amputation at the midproximal phalanx. Amputation of fingers and thumb can give rise to significant functional impairment. When excising melanomas on the fingers, the surgeon should preserve as much length as possible without compromising margins. The digit is preferentially amputated proximal to the distal interphalangeal joint, if the extent of nail bed involvement or parenchymal involvement and the proximal location of the lesion's border allow this.

■ SENTINEL LYMPH NODE BIOPSY: INDICATIONS AND TECHNICAL ISSUES

The sentinel lymph node biopsy (SLNB) procedure (including preoperative lymphoscintigraphy and intraoperative lymphatic mapping) provides valuable staging information for melanoma patients. The use of SLNB has enabled clinicians to identify patients with occult nodal metastases that would otherwise take months or years to become clinically palpable. In particular, the pathologic evaluation of the sentinel lymph node (SNL) allows for the detection of micrometastatic disease through a combination of serial sectioning and immunohistochemical staining. The latter technique has been incorporated into the guidelines of the Society of Surgical Oncology/American Society of Clinical Oncology (SSO/ASCO), the National Cancer Center Network guidelines, and in the seventh edition of the American Joint Committee on Cancer (AJCC) melanoma staging system. These recommendations are consistent with the landmark randomized surgical trial (Multicenter Selective Lymphadenectomy Trial 1, MSLT1) demonstrating the important role of the SLNB in a defined group of patients, with staging value for those with intermediate thickness (1.0 to 4.0 mm or T2/T3 melanomas) and thicker (T4 melanomas), as well as a survival benefit for those patients with a metastatic sentinel node (SN) arising from an intermediate thickness melanoma (T2/T3 melanomas).

The minimally invasive SLNB procedure should be discussed with and recommended to patients when at least one of the following indications is present: (1) the risk of clinically occult nodal metastasis is considered sufficient to justify the procedure (approximately 10% or greater); (2) the prognostic information provided by SLNB would be of value to the patient and their treating physicians; (3) the tumor status of the sentinel node would be useful in guiding decisions regarding completion lymphadenectomy and adjuvant therapy; and/or (4) nodal staging information will be required for entry into clinical trials in which the patient is interested.

Thus the SLNB procedure should be discussed with and offered to all patients with primary melanomas at least 1.0 mm thick and clinically normal regional lymph nodes by physical examination when the criteria described previously are met, and when the morbidity and risks of SLNB are considered acceptable to the physician and the patient.

Most experienced melanoma surgeons would also offer SLNB to patients with T1 melanomas (i.e., not thicker than 1.0 mm) that have characteristics that substantially increase the likelihood of regional

node micrometastasis. This would include patients with T1 melanomas with primary tumor ulceration, a mitotic rate *of at least* $1/mm^2$ and/or Clark level IV/V invasion, especially if tumor thickness exceeds 0.75 mm. Ulceration, mitotic rate, and Clark level would be especially relevant in patients who have no significant comorbidity, who are younger than 40 to 45 years, or whose primary tumor depth is uncertain because of tumor-positive deep margins in the biopsy specimen.

The staging information provided by SLNB is of particular value because it reliably identifies patients with nodal micrometastases. Used in conjunction with Breslow thickness and other prognostic features of the primary melanoma, accurate predictions of metastatic risk and survival outcome can be obtained. Information based on SN status is also valuable for counseling SLNB-positive patients about the need for completion lymphadenectomy to improve regional disease control, reduce operative morbidity (as compared with the morbidity associated with possibly more radical regional surgery and often radiation therapy for palpable nodal recurrence), reduce the relative risk of recurrence by 26%, and potentially improve survival if nodal metastases are present. In addition, the information about their SLN status can be used to counsel patients regarding enrollment into melanoma clinical trials and can serve as the basis for discussing a screening and follow-up regimen based on risk for subsequent development of metastases. Patients who are SLN negative can be reassured that their prognosis is relatively improved; these patients are less likely to require adjuvant treatments and/or frequent follow-up.

■ THERAPEUTIC OR COMPLETION LYMPHADENECTOMY FOR REGIONAL NODAL METASTASES

Complete lymphadenectomy is currently the standard treatment for melanoma patients with identified regional nodal metastases. As a general principle, lymphadenectomy should be anatomic. The contents of the nodal basin are excised in a single block of tissue, preserving motor nerves and muscle whenever possible. Perioperative antibiotics are used routinely.

The goals of surgery include staging, regional control of disease, and possibly improved survival for some patients with clinically occult metastases identified by sentinel node biopsy. Indeed, the majority of patients who undergo lymphadenectomy today are now those who have histologically positive sentinel nodes. According to evidence-based SSO/ASCO guidelines, "completion lymph node dissection (CLND) is recommended for all patients with a positive SLN biopsy and achieves good regional disease control. CLND should be performed until there is convincing evidence that it does *not* improve regional disease control or survival."

Patients with clinically suspicious nodes should be evaluated by fine-needle biopsy if possible, with excisional biopsy done only if the results of fine-needle biopsy are indeterminate. Patients with bulky, biopsy-proven, nodal disease should be evaluated with baseline computed tomography (CT) scans, a full blood count, and measurement of liver enzymes, including LDH, to rule out identifiable distant disease before proceeding with nodal surgery.

■ AXILLARY NODAL DISSECTION

The goal of axillary lymph node dissection for melanoma is complete resection of all lymph nodes at levels I, II, and III. The long thoracic nerve and the thoracodorsal neurovascular bundle are left intact unless they are directly invaded by tumor. Although division of the pectoralis minor muscle rarely is considered necessary for breast cancer, it sometimes is used for melanoma patients to obtain complete exposure of level II and III nodes. After removal of the axillary contents, a closed-suction drain is placed. Further details about surgical technique are described elsewhere. Patients undergoing a radical axillary lymphadenectomy should have no appreciable loss of range of motion or motor function. After a complete axillary dissection for melanoma, there is approximately a 5% to 10% risk of symptomatic lymphedema of the upper extremity.

■ INGUINAL AND ILIAC NODAL DISSECTION

For patients with metastatic nodes in the groin, an anatomically complete subinguinal (inguinofemoral) dissection is performed. In most cases a vertical incision is used, often with wide excision of an ellipse of skin over the femoral vessels, an area inevitably devascularized to some degree by the subsequent dissection. Flaps are then raised. The boundaries of the dissection extend superiorly to approximately 5 cm above the inguinal ligament, medially to the pubic tubercle and the midbelly of adductor longus, laterally to the anterior superior iliac spine and the lateral border of sartorius, and inferiorly to the apex of the femoral triangle. In patients with clinically detected nodal metastases, the femoral canal is explored from below, and Cloquet's node is removed. This step can be omitted in patients undergoing completion node dissection after detection of clinically occult or microscopic nodal disease. If there is concern about the possibility of wound breakdown, the sartorius muscle may be taken down from its insertion into the anterior superior iliac spine, rotated over the femoral vessels to cover and protect them, and tacked in place to the edge of the inguinal ligament and the fascia of the adductor longus. A closed-suction drain is placed in the inguinofemoral area before closure. Although prophylactic antibiotics usually are given, inguinal dissection wounds have an infection rate of up to 15%. The risk of symptomatic lymphedema of the lower extremity is approximately 20%. Routine measures aimed at reducing the risk of lymphedema include a program of wearing a fitted compression garment at 20 to 30 mm Hg during the day for the first 3 to 6 months postoperatively, and leg elevation when possible.

Indications for iliac and obturator node dissection include the finding of a positive Cloquet's node intraoperatively or the detection of enlarged iliac or obturator nodes on preoperative CT scans, or fluorodeoxyglucose (FDG)–avid iliac or obturator nodes on a positron emission tomography (PET) scan. The boundaries of the dissection are from the bifurcation of the common iliac vessels superiorly to the inguinal ligament inferiorly and to the obturator vessels medially. Technical details of iliac and obturator node clearance are given elsewhere.

The minimally invasive or "videoscopic" approach to inguinal lymphadenectomy should be anatomically and pathologically identical to the technique a surgeon uses in an open approach. This feasibility of this procedure for melanoma was first reported in 2010 and subsequently has found increased use among surgical oncologists. Briefly, the anatomic boundaries remain the same as those described previously. The saphenous vein may be preserved or sacrificed; however, for facilitating dissection the fascia of both the sartorius and the adductor muscles are routinely included in the specimen.

For a unilateral groin dissection, patients are positioned on a split-leg table with the operative leg flexed at the knee and the hip externally rotated. The boundaries of the femoral triangle are marked and ports are placed 3 cm below the femoral apex and 2 cm lateral and medial to the boundaries of the triangle. A 15-mm balloon port is used at the apex and two 10-mm ports at each working site, which should lay transversely across the extremity at the level of the apex. The initial working space, inferior to the femoral triangle is made with a Metzenbaum scissors or digital blunt dissection. The flap is raised just superficial to the superficial fascia of leg, leaving approximately 5 to 7 mm of fat on the dermis. The space is insufflated and a zero degree scope used for the predominance of the surgery. An auto-sealing energy device is used to raise the flaps to create the space identical to that used for the open procedure. Lymph node biopsy scars are left intact. The dissection then is carried out to include the tissue on the external oblique aponeurosis, both muscular fascial boundaries as mentioned, and then to skeletonize the femoral artery and vein to the level of the femoral canal. If indicated, or desired, Cloquet's node may be undergo biopsy at this point. The specimen is placed in a standard retrieval bag and removed from the apical port site. A drain is left in the lateral trocar site.

This approach has demonstrated a marked reduction in complications compared with the open approach (Table 2). It is worth noting that modern analyses, likely in an effort to diligently report all potential complications, appear to over-report the morbidity from both open and minimally invasive approaches to inguinal lymphadenectomy (Figure 3). As such, the data in the table included, which reflect similar reports published elsewhere, overestimate the incidence of clinically significant complications from either approach by nearly 30%.

■ CERVICAL NODAL DISSECTION

The extent of cervical lymphadenectomy depends on the location of the metastatic node or nodes and whether there is evidence of direct invasion into the structures of the neck. When a metastatic sentinel node is found, a functional neck dissection preserving the internal jugular vein, spinal accessory nerve, and sternal head of sternocleidomastoid is appropriate. These structures should be sacrificed only if they are invaded directly by tumor. When there is clinical involvement of the parotid lymph nodes, the lymph nodes more inferiorly in the neck are also at risk of harboring metastatic disease, even if they are clinically negative. For this reason, a neck dissection generally is performed in addition to a therapeutic parotidectomy. Conversely, patients with clinically evident cervical node metastases arising from a melanoma located on the ipsilateral face, anterior scalp, or ear should have a superficial parotidectomy performed at the time of a comprehensive neck dissection, even if the parotid

---

TABLE 2: Data From a Series of Melanoma Patients Undergoing Open and Minimally Invasive Approaches (Video-Assisted Inguinal Lymphadenectomy or VIL) to Open Lymphadenectomy

In modern series of analyses, there has been a tendency toward over reporting of complications, including uncomplicated erythema and other clinically trivial outcomes to be comprehensive in the reporting. As such, we believe that our own analysis overstates the incidence of true complications. A more accurate reflection of the data is likely from the two groups of patients with flap necrosis and seroma, totaling approximately 40% in the open group and 25% in the minimally invasive group. Of significance, the minimally invasive approach markedly reduces the incidence of complications compared with the open approach.

	VIL (n = 40)	Open (n = 40)	P Value
Complications	47.5%	80.0%	0.002
Infection	40.0%	65.0%	0.025
Flap necrosis/ dehiscence	2.5%	15.0%	0.047
Seroma	22.5%	35.0%	0.217

Data from Martin BM et al. Oncologic outcomes of patients undergoing videoscopic inguinal lymphadenectomy for metastatic melanoma. *J Am Coll Surg.* 2014;218:620-626.

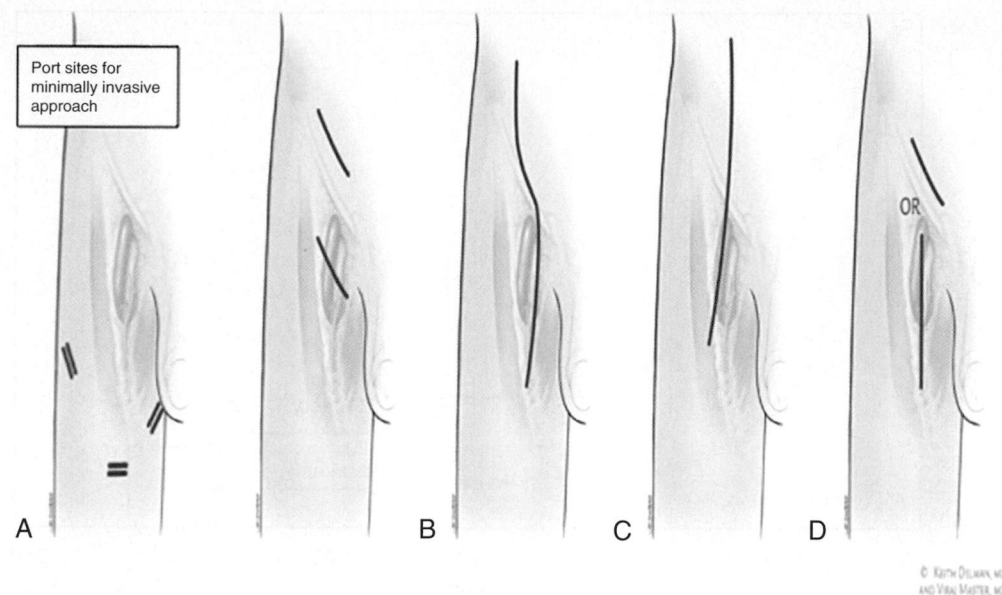

Port sites for minimally invasive approach

A   B   C   D

© KEITH DELMAN, MD
AND VIRAJ MASTER, MD

FIGURE 3 Difference incisions for inguinal or inguinal-iliac lymphadenectomy.

nodes are clinically negative, because there is a high risk of clinically occult nodal disease in the parotid area.

A therapeutic neck dissection is associated with a 20% to 30% recurrence rate in the neck. Patients with multiple metastatic nodes, especially those with gross extracapsular invasion into surrounding tissues, have a particularly high risk of neck recurrence, even after a thorough neck dissection. When this occurs, there can be severe morbidity. Many centers therefore recommend adjuvant postoperative radiation therapy after a neck dissection for clinically palpable nodal metastases in the neck, especially when the nodes are large or multiple and when there is extranodal extension of tumor. This has been shown in a randomized trial to reduce substantially the risk of node field recurrence.

SURGICAL CONSIDERATIONS FOR STAGE IV MELANOMA

Surgery for advanced melanoma is most effective when disease is limited to a few sites, and there are a small number of metastases. Surgical excision of isolated melanoma metastases can provide effective and quick palliation and, in some instances, a survival exceeding 5 or 10 years. In general, prognosis depends on the initial site of metastasis. Median and 5-year survival times decrease progressively for involvement of the skin and subcutaneous tissue, distant lymph nodes, gastrointestinal tract, lung, bone, liver, and brain. The number of organ and tissue sites containing metastasis is also an important prognostic factor: median survival is 7 months for patients with metastasis to one site, 4 months for those with metastasis to two sites, and only 2 months for those with metastatic disease to three or more sites.

Even in the modern era where effective systemic agents for stage IV melanoma are available, surgery should be considered in the multimodality management of patients with stage IV metastatic disease. Surgical treatment to relieve symptoms caused by metastases is generally worthwhile, especially when the anticipated benefit from palliation exceeds the morbidity of the procedure (e.g., resection of small bowel metastases to relieve bowel obstruction or gastrointestinal bleeding). Expectant (or prophylactic) palliation is used for control of disease that is otherwise likely to cause disabling symptoms.

There are several strong theoretical arguments for more frequent use of surgery as the initial treatment for distant melanoma. First is the development of sophisticated imaging techniques such as CT, PET/CT, and magnetic resonance imaging (MRI), which better differentiate between single and multiple metastatic sites and allow the planning of a surgical procedure that resects tumor at all metastatic sites. Second is the fact that most patients initially have metastasis confined to a single organ. Resection of the initial organ metastasis may delay or abort the metastatic cascade to secondary metastatic sites. A third argument is the dramatic reduction in the morbidity and mortality of major surgical operations that has resulted from improved anesthetic and surgical techniques, allowing most patients to return to normal performance status very quickly. Fourth, if all metastatic disease can be resected, patients have the highest chance of prolonged survival and high-quality life. It is important to emphasize that patients who have an incomplete resection will have little or no improvement in their survival rates. Fifth, a patient who has recurrence after initial metastasectomy may benefit from secondary resection of asynchronous metastases. Finally, if surgical therapy is not successful, the patient is still a candidate for systemic therapy, either before or after the surgical excision.

Possibly the best surgical outcomes data available are from MSLT1 patients who were followed prospectively for relapse at distant sites. Of the 291 patients with a stage IV recurrence, 161 (55%) underwent surgery, with or without systemic medical therapy (SMT). Median survival was 15.8 versus 6.9 months, and 4-year survival was 20.8 versus 7.0% for patients receiving surgery with or without SMT versus SMT alone (P < 0.0001l HR 0.406) (Figure 4). Patients who had one or two metastasis(es), regardless of site, had a significant survival advantage compared with patients undergoing best medical therapy without surgical excision (Figure 5). It was concluded that approximately half of patients who progress to stage IV disease may be candidates for surgical excision, especially those with a single metastasis, and those with distant metastases to skin, subcutaneous, or distant lymph node sites (M1a metastases) or to the lungs (M1b metastases). The results of these studies cannot distinguish between the relatively more favorable biology of limited metastases and the treatment impact of surgical excision in the absence of randomized studies. In general, however, they consistently demonstrate the importance of completely resecting all distant metastases (compared with incomplete resection) with regard to survival outcome.

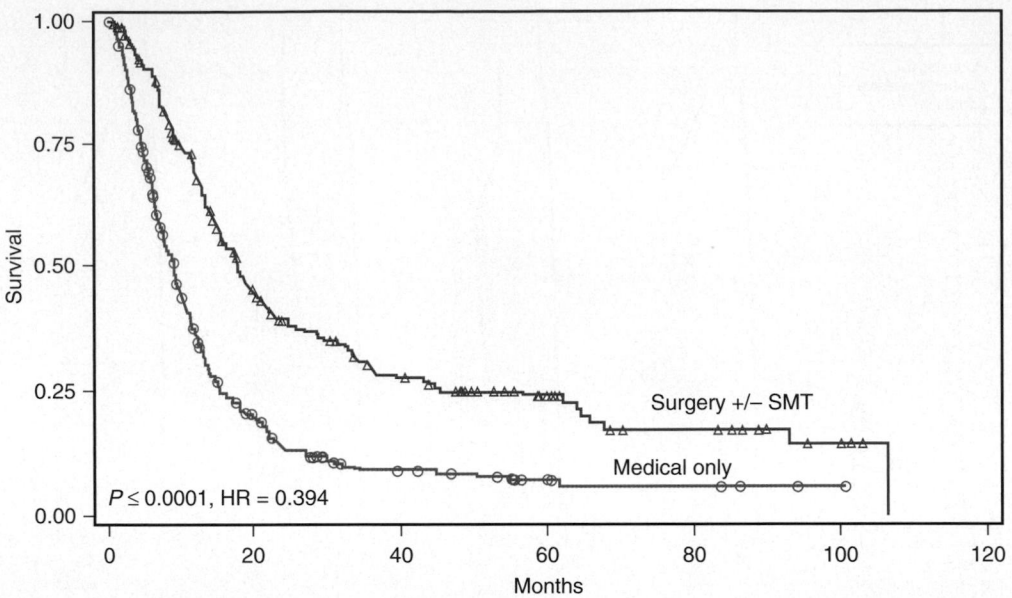

FIGURE 4 Survival for Multicenter Selective Lymphadenectomy Trial I patients treated surgically with or without standard medical treatment (SMT) and medically for stage IV melanoma recurrence P<0.0001, HR = 0.394. *(From Howard JH, Thompson JF, Mozzillo N, et al. Metastasectomy for Distant Metastatic Melanoma, Analysis of Data from the First Multicenter Selective Lymphadenectomy Trial [MSLT-1]. Ann Surg Oncol. 2012;19:2547-2555.)*

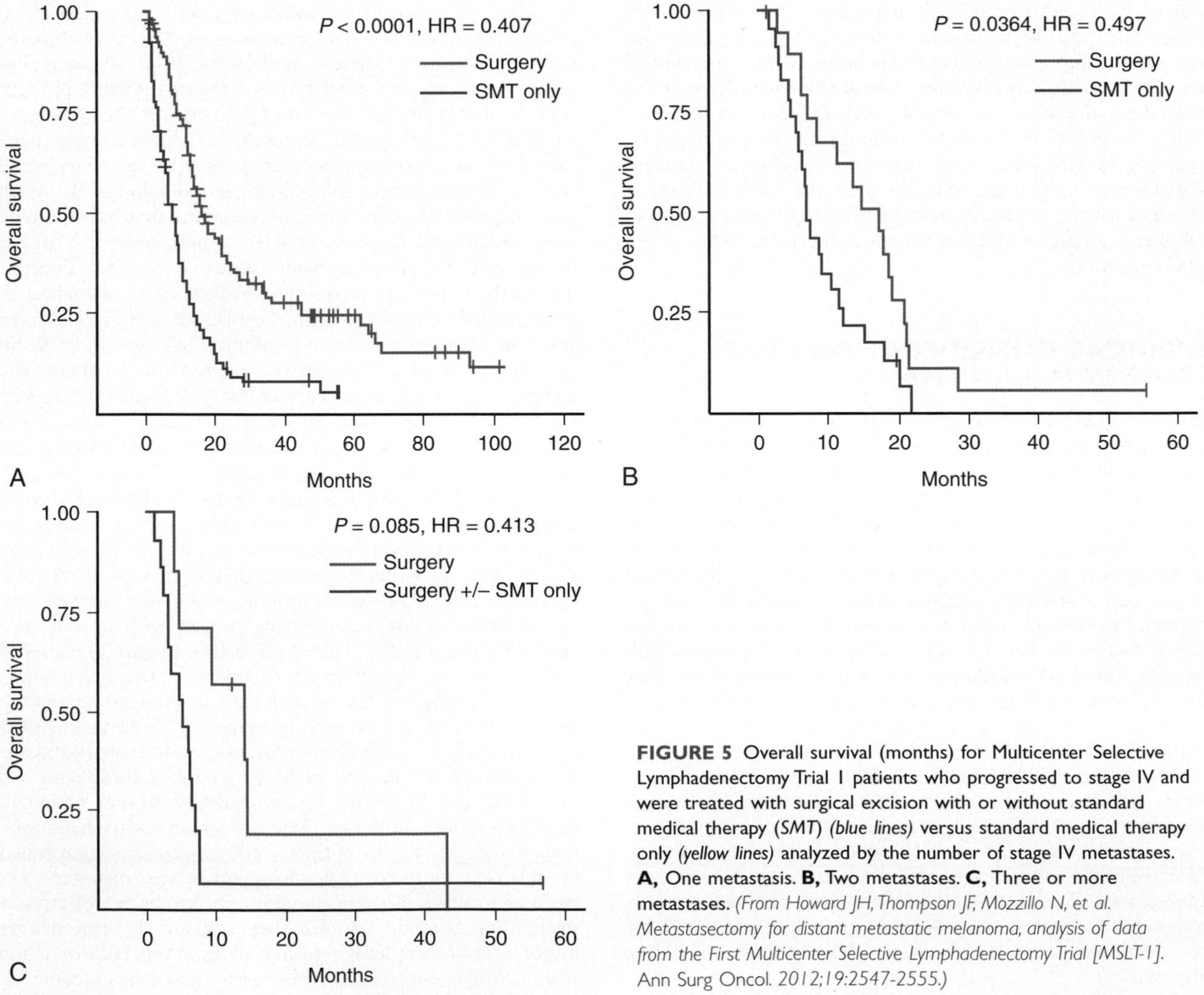

FIGURE 5 Overall survival (months) for Multicenter Selective Lymphadenectomy Trial I patients who progressed to stage IV and were treated with surgical excision with or without standard medical therapy *(SMT)* *(blue lines)* versus standard medical therapy only *(yellow lines)* analyzed by the number of stage IV metastases. **A,** One metastasis. **B,** Two metastases. **C,** Three or more metastases. *(From Howard JH, Thompson JF, Mozzillo N, et al. Metastasectomy for distant metastatic melanoma, analysis of data from the First Multicenter Selective Lymphadenectomy Trial [MSLT-1]. Ann Surg Oncol. 2012;19:2547-2555.)*

Suggested Readings

Balch CM, Balch GC, Thompson JF. Surgical management of metastatic melanoma (Stages III and IV). In: Morita S, Balch CM, Klimberg VS, Pawlik T, Tanabe K, Posner M, eds. *Complex Surgical Oncology Textbook*. New York: McGraw Hill; 2017.

Balch CM, Gershenwald JE, Soong SJ, et al. Final Version of 2009 AJCC Melanoma Staging and Classification. *J Clin Oncol*. 2009;27:6199-6206.

Balch CM, Soong SJ, Smith T, et al. Long-term results of a prospective surgical trial comparing 2 cm vs. 4 cm excision margins for 740 patients with 1-4 mm melanomas. *Ann Surg Oncol*. 2001;8:101-108.

Grotz TE, Markovic SN, Erickson LA, et al. Mayo Clinic consensus recommendations for the depth of excision in primary cutaneous melanoma. *Mayo Clin Proc*. 2011;86:522-528.

Hayes AJ, Maynard L, Coombes G, et al. Wide versus narrow excision margins for high-risk, primary cutaneous melanomas: long-term follow-up of survival in a randomised trial. *Lancet Oncol*. 2016;15:482-489.

MacKenzie Ross A, Haydu L, Quinn M, et al. The association between excision margins and local recurrence in 11,290 thin (T1) primary cutaneous melanomas. A case control study. *Ann Surg Oncol*. 2015 Sept.

Martin BM, Etra JW, Russell MC, et al. Oncologic outcomes of patients undergoing videoscopic inguinal lymphadenectomy for metastatic melanoma. *J Am Coll Surg*. 2014;218:620-626.

Morton DL, Thompson JF, Cochran AJ. Final trial report of sentinel-node biopsy versus nodal observation in melanoma. *N Engl J Med*. 2014;370:599-609.

Sladden MJ, Balch C, Barzilai DA, et al. Surgical excision margins for primary cutaneous melanoma. *Cochrane Database Syst Rev*. 2009;CD004835.

Veronesi U, Cascinelli N, Adamus J, Balch CM, et al. Thin stage I primary cutaneous melanoma: comparison of excision with margins of 1 or 3 cm. *N Engl J Med*. 1988;318:1159-1162.

Wong SL, Balch CM, Hurley P, et al. Sentinel lymph node biopsy for melanoma: American Society of Clinical Oncology and Society of Surgical Oncology joint clinical practice guideline. *Ann Surg Oncol*. 2012;19:3313-3324.

The Management of Soft Tissue Sarcoma

Amanda Kirane, MD, and Murray F. Brennan, MD

Soft tissue sarcomas (STSs) are tumors of mesenchymal origin that broadly describe nearly 100 histopathologic subtypes with a variable spectrum of clinical behavior and prognosis. Treatment strategy is highly individualized based on tumor location, size, grade, and histology (Figure 1). The majority of STSs in the adult (50%) are seen in the extremity and to a lesser extent in the retroperitoneum (15%). In the United States there are approximately 15,000 cases per year, comprising 1% of all adult malignancies and 15% of pediatric cancers, with equal gender distribution. The American Joint Committee on Cancer (AJCC) staging system stratifies risk by size, grade, and depth, although this may not be consistently accurate as a prognosticator given the absence of histology as a categoric variable. In an effort to better predict disease-specific outcomes, many groups have developed complementary staging systems or nomogram models that reflect additional factors of tumor location and subtype (Figure 2). The most crucial prognostic factor remains surgical control of primary and, in selected cases, metastatic disease, with quality of surgery significantly affecting local and distant failure and overall survival (Figure 3). Pattern of recurrence is largely determined by site of origin and tumor grade, with low-grade tumors typically occurring with local-regional disease and high-grade tumors more likely to exhibit distant failure. The extent of surgery and indications for adjuvant therapy critically rely on accurate histologic diagnosis, and referral to a specialty center for multidisciplinary management is strongly encouraged.

■ DIAGNOSTIC EVALUATION

Although most STSs are sporadic, several associated genetic syndromes and environmental exposures are associated with the development of sarcoma. Li-Fraumeni syndrome, a germline mutation in the p53 tumor suppressor gene, is associated with increased risk of STS in addition to leukemia, breast, brain, germ cell, and adrenocortical tumors. Gardner's syndrome describes a propensity for the development of desmoid tumors in the setting of familial adenomatous polyposis. Neurofibromatosis type 1, or von Recklinghausen's disease, is an autosomal disorder of multiple neurofibromas that predisposes to the development of malignant peripheral nerve sheath tumors (MPNSTs) and other malignancies.

The development of lymphangiosarcoma in the setting of chronic lymphedema after mastectomy and axillary lymph node dissection, Stewart-Treves syndrome, or parasitic infection is a known but uncommon risk factor. Exposure to radiation confers significant predilection for developing several STS subtypes with a median onset 10 to 12 years after radiation therapy (RT). These tumors are generally more virulent than those of identical histopathology arising de novo and have become a worrisome although rare complication of modern breast cancer treatment. Although no definitive relationship is established with chemical exposures, various herbicides and compounds such as vinyl chloride have been listed as risk factors. Patients often describe a traumatic injury before the observation of STS; however, this is rarely causal.

Clinical evaluation and treatment of STS are tailored by location. Thorough history and physical examination of patients with a palpable mass of the extremity should include elicitation of any neurovascular complaints. STS of the extremity generally warrants cross-sectional magnetic resonance imaging (MRI) to assess depth and anatomic relationship to critical neurovascular bundles. Complete staging should include imaging of the chest with x-ray for low-grade lesions and computed tomographic (CT) scan for large high-grade lesions. In visceral locations, preoperative imaging by CT scan is usually sufficient, with selective use of MRI. Positron emission tomography (PET) is rarely of value in sarcoma evaluation.

Apart from small (<5 cm) extremity lesions, pretreatment biopsy by Tru-cut core needle biopsy is preferred and should be planned carefully in the longitudinal axis of the extremity in anticipation of subsequent re-excision. Results of core biopsy are sufficient to confirm presence of sarcoma and accurately reflect grade and histology in 80% and 75% of cases, respectively, as well as to make definitive molecular diagnosis, such as with the presence of *SYT-SSX* fusion gene in synovial sarcoma. For visceral or retroperitoneal lesions, biopsy is reserved for situations that clearly would change management, as imaging characteristics are often adequate for presumptive diagnosis.

The primary treatment for most histologic subtypes of STS is wide surgical resection. Radical resection is indicated to achieve negative margins with the tumor resected en bloc with a cuff of healthy tissue circumferentially. Adequacy of resection is often defined by the presence of an intact biologic barrier such as fascia, epineurium, periosteum, or adventitia. Although surgery provides the only potentially curative therapy, multidisciplinary team planning is essential to the total management of these patients. Referral to specialty centers is encouraged not only for individualized management but also for confirmation of histology. Review of pathology slides by sarcoma specialists has been demonstrated to find incorrect histologic diagnosis in up to 25% of specimens, with 15% suggested

DISEASE-SPECIFIC SURVIVAL BY HISTOLOGY

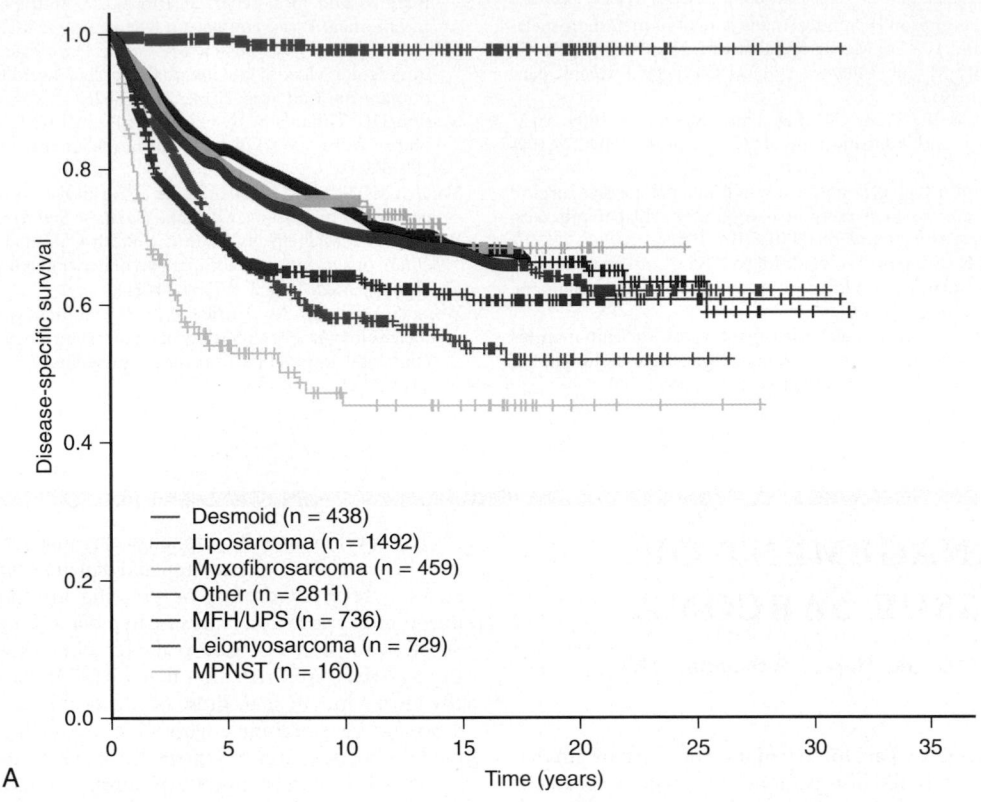

A

DISEASE-SPECIFIC SURVIVAL BY PRIMARY TUMOR SITE

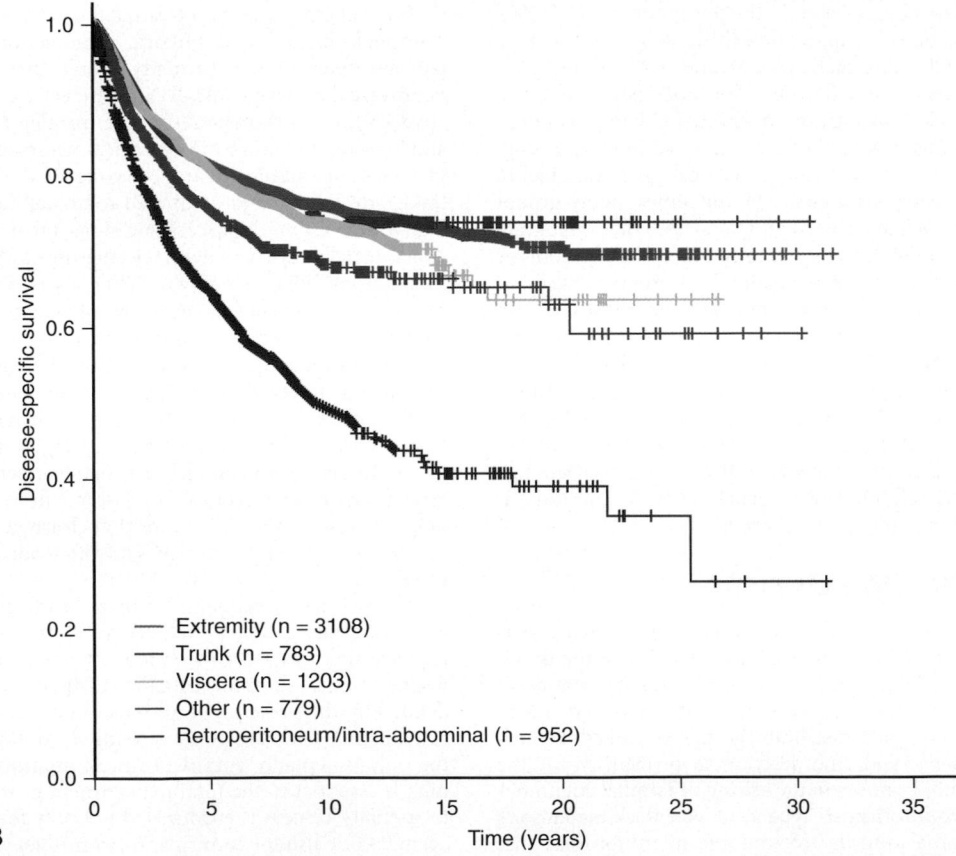

B

FIGURE 1 Disease-specific survival by (**A**) histology and (**B**) location. Data describe soft tissue sarcoma followed prospectively at Memorial Sloan Kettering Cancer Center over a 32-year period from July 1, 1982, to December 31, 2014, n = 6825. *MFH*, Malignant fibrous histiocytoma; *MPNST*, malignant peripheral nerve sheath tumor; *UPS*, undifferentiated pleomorphic sarcoma.

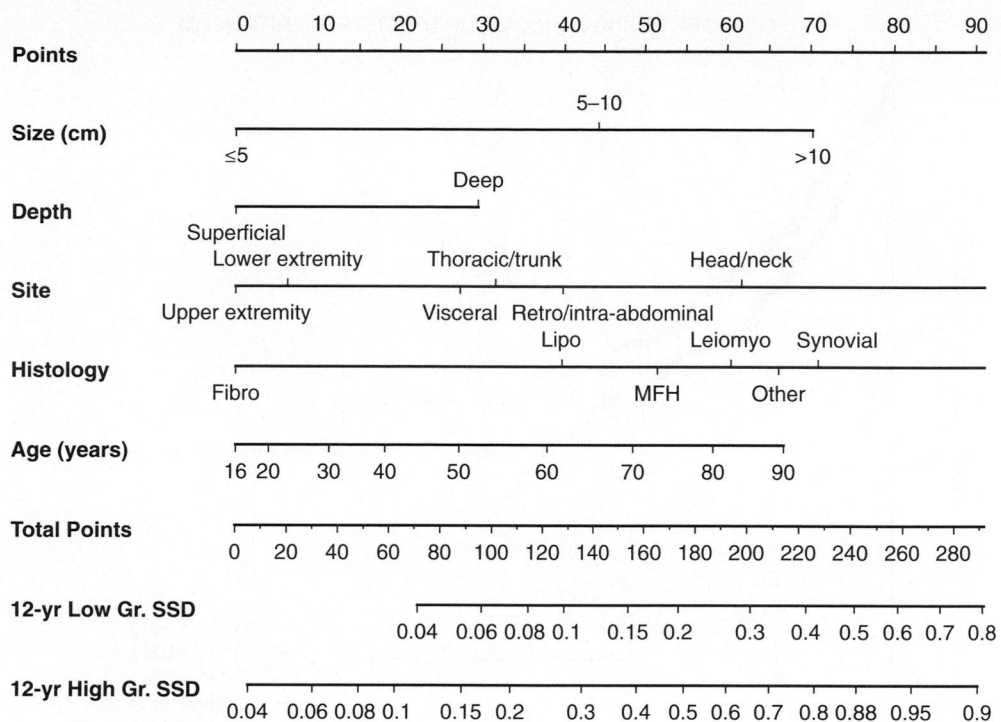

FIGURE 2 Soft tissue sarcoma nomogram for prediction of sarcoma-specific death (*SSD*) at 12 years after resection. Points are assigned to each variable by drawing a straight line from variable axis. Total points determine probability of disease-specific death. *Fibro*, Fibrosarcoma; *Gr.*, grade; *Leiomyo*, leiomyosarcoma; *Lipo*, liposarcoma; *MFH*, malignant fibrous histiocytoma. (*With permission from Kattan MW, Leung DH, Brennan MF. Postoperative nomogram for 12-year sarcoma-specific death. J Clin Oncol. 2002;20:791-796.*)

to affect designated treatment strategy. Co-evaluation with additional surgical specialties, including reconstructive, vascular, and thoracic surgery and urology, is often necessary.

■ TECHNICAL CONSIDERATIONS IN EXTREMITY SARCOMAS

Therapeutic aim has evolved greatly in the management of extremity tumors, with avoidance of major morbidity and functional preservation of the limb being paramount goals of care. Previously, radical resection often led to significant impairment and morbidity necessitating amputation. Randomized data have demonstrated equivalent oncologic outcomes in disease-free survival (DFS) and overall survival for patients undergoing limb salvage compared with amputation, with radiation applied in selected cases. Although most sarcomas are surrounded by an appreciable pseudocapsule, it is understood that microscopic disease extends beyond this perimeter, especially in selected histologies such as undifferentiated pleomorphic sarcoma, and failure to take an additional rim of healthy tissue increases the risk of local recurrence (LR). The resection margin ideally should be targeted at normal non-neoplastic tissue 1 to 2 cm beyond this plane. Adequacy of margin may be limited by functional or anatomic constraints such as neurovascular bundle or bony involvement. Adjuvant radiation can reduce the risk of LR in these cases by 10% to 20%. Amputation rates at most specialty centers are less than 5%, and amputation typically is limited to disease-compromising function or very distal tumors.

Positive resection margins are associated with an increased risk of LR. Recurrence often can be salvaged with additional surgery; however, LR of high-grade lesions is often a harbinger of systemic disease. Primary tumors do not commonly violate fascial planes, but involvement is more common in recurrent disease. Closure over drains is generally performed, and drain sites are oriented so that they can be included in any adjuvant radiation or future resections

for recurrent disease. Marking sutures should be used to orient the specimen.

Resection of STS abutting bone may include periosteum, which serves as a natural biologic barrier, most often preventing the need for bone resection. However, when periosteal stripping of irradiated bone is performed, thought may be given to prophylactic plating or rodding because of risk of fracture. In cases of vascular or nerve encasement, preoperative radiation should be considered to minimize further injury. Tumors abutting major vascular structures may be safely dissected free in most cases, but encasement may require arterial reconstruction that typically can be achieved with good result. Venous reconstruction is rarely necessary and often unsuccessful. The inferior vena cava can be sacrificed with minimal overall consequence because of the development of collateral circulation; however, attempts are made to preserve venous flow when possible, such as with the greater saphenous when the superficial femoral vein also will be taken. Limb-sparing surgery can be heavily reliant on pedicled or free flap reconstruction for wound closure, and preoperative evaluation by a reconstructive surgeon is often indicated.

A causal relationship has not been determined between LR and survival, with randomized trials of wide local excision versus amputation demonstrating no measurable difference in overall survival despite a 20% to 30% difference in LR. Subsequent survival is associated with time interval to LR and grade and size of tumor. Survival advantage has been demonstrated for successful re-excision. Neoadjuvant chemotherapy should be considered for patients with large primary tumors and LR of high-grade pathologic lesions. Isolated metastases should be resected as long as complete resection is possible; survival at 5 years in this setting ranges from 15% to 30%. Mortality is usually related to distant disease, with highest risk occurring in tumors larger than 5 cm with high-grade histology. Lymph node involvement is rare given predilection for hematogenous spread by STS, and lymph node sampling generally is not indicated. Rare subsets (epithelioid, synovial sarcoma, and rhabdomyosarcoma) may have metastases to regional lymph nodes and are at most risk for LR.

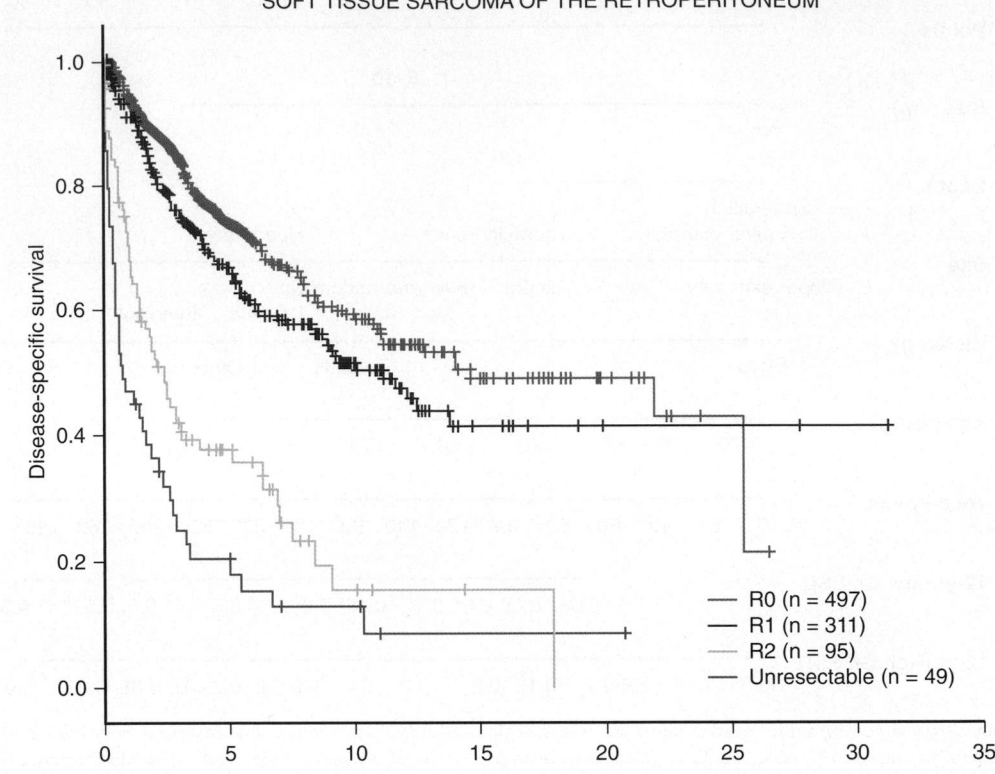

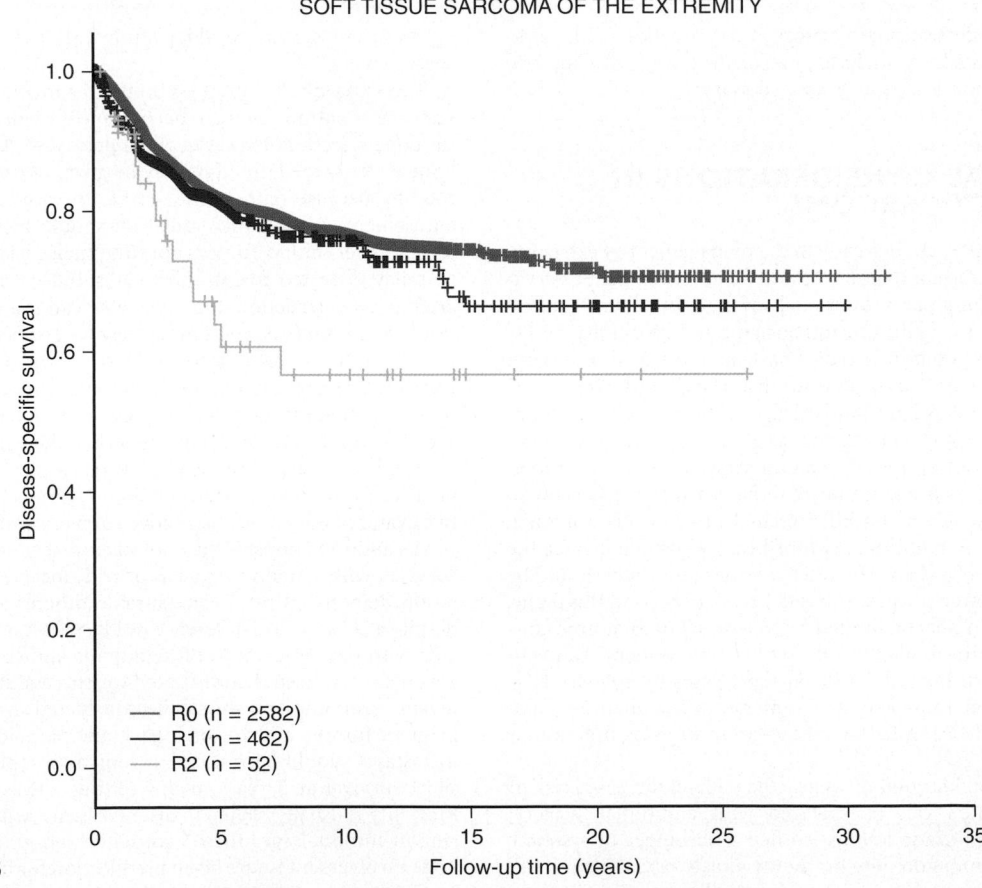

FIGURE 3 Disease-specific survival according to extent of resection among patients with retroperitoneal sarcoma (**A**) and extremity sarcoma (**B**) treated at Memorial Sloan Kettering over a 25-year period. Outcomes are similar in patients undergoing incomplete (R2) resection to those in patients with unresectable disease; survival is significantly decreased when compared with macroscopically complete resection.

■ TECHNICAL CONSIDERATIONS IN RETROPERITONEAL SARCOMAS

Retroperitoneal sarcomas (RPSs) comprise 15% of all STSs. Typical presentation of RPS involves an abdominal mass and pain, although many RPSs are identified incidentally. A rare subset may have a paraneoplastic syndrome, such as hypoglycemia associated with solitary fibrous tumors. In most cases, CT of the abdomen and pelvis can sufficiently diagnose liposarcomas and leiomyosarcomas arising from vascular structures based on image characteristics, which together comprise the vast majority of RPSs, 50% and 25%, respectively. Excepting extremely well-differentiated liposarcomas, which metastasize in fewer than 3% of patients, staging imaging of the chest with CT should be obtained preoperatively. Biopsy is indicated when imaging is not clearly diagnostic and the differential may include nonsarcomatous disease such as lymphoma and germ cell tumors.

Surgery remains the mainstay of treatment for RPS, although wide resection can be limited by anatomic constraints that similarly limit the application of adjunct RT. Local control remains a major challenge in the management of RPS, with even low-grade tumors demonstrating significant mortality related to relentless recurrence. Large RPSs often displace and encase viscera, necessitating resection despite lack of direct invasion. The definition of adequate extent of resection to minimize LR is controversial. Some authors advocate aggressive adjacent organ resection, but this has not been shown to consistently alter outcome beyond complete gross resection. Major determinants of oncologic outcome relate to size, multifocality, grade, type of presentation (primary vs recurrent), and adequacy of initial surgery. Complete resection is a clear predictor of disease-specific survival (DSS) and should be the therapeutic goal of operation. An R2 resection is rarely, if ever, of value in the asymptomatic patient. In the case of liposarcoma, failure to distinguish very well-differentiated tumor areas from normal retroperitoneal fat is the most common cause of residual and recurrent disease (Figure 4). High-grade histology of tumors does correlate with significantly poorer overall survival (33 vs 149 months). Distant recurrence is usually found in the lung (38%) or liver (44%).

Although the majority (>90%) of initial operations for RPS will achieve macroscopically negative margins, up to 20% ultimately will demonstrate positive microscopic margins. Clearing the entire ipsilateral compartment of fat is advocated to eliminate residual or discontiguous disease. Quality of resection will be limited by the closest margin, so it is hard to justify removal of uninvolved normal organs such as spleen, pancreas, colon, and kidney when the limiting margin involves a major neurovascular structure. Extended resection may not be justifiable unless indicated for complete gross resection. Frozen section is generally not of benefit in the assessment of margin analysis, as fatty tissue by frozen section is challenged by significant artifact.

Advocates of the en bloc extended technique specify that it is intended for primary presentation only. Improvements in LR by extended compartmental resection have not been translated clearly to improvement in overall survival. In published data of liposarcoma from Memorial Sloan Kettering Cancer Center (MSKCC), 72% of R1 resections did not develop recurrence in the follow-up period (median 44 months). Patients with contiguous organ resection demonstrated 55% probability of 3-year local recurrence–free survival (LRFS) versus 45% for standard surgery ($P = 0.06$), yet a twofold increase in risk of disease-specific death. This suggests that the need for contiguous resection is indicative of invasive biology associated with increased recurrence both locally and distally.

Definite goals of surgery include optimal systematic exposure with circumferential dissection, macroscopic clearance of disease, and meticulous avoidance of rupture, as outcomes for ruptured tumors are no different from unresectable disease. Low-grade tumors, specifically well-differentiated liposarcoma (WDLPS), displace rather than involve local organs and typically can be dissected free without sacrifice (Figure 5). The practice of dissecting under the renal capsule and reserving nephrectomy for instances of circumferential hilar involvement has not been associated with a reduction in DSS, with 5-year survival at 92%. The most commonly resected organ is the ipsilateral kidney, although parenchymal invasion is seen in less than 10% of specimens. Renal scan should be considered in the preoperative evaluation of patients with borderline renal function.

Many instances of recurrent disease are amenable to repeat resection, but this should be undertaken only when complete excision is anticipated, as rates of successful R0 resection diminish progressively with each repeat resection, reaching <20% by a fourth operation. Timing of operation should be considered thoughtfully, as many recurrent lesions can be observed while asymptomatic to allow for assessment of progression. Outcomes in recurrent disease have been reviewed extensively, and consensus opinion defines growth rate of more than 1 cm/month as well as sarcomatosis (defined as >7 sites of discontiguous disease) as demonstrating no benefit from surgical intervention. In unresectable disease, debulking should be undertaken only for palliation. Although distant sites of recurrence portend worsened overall survival, isolated metastases should be considered for metastasectomy.

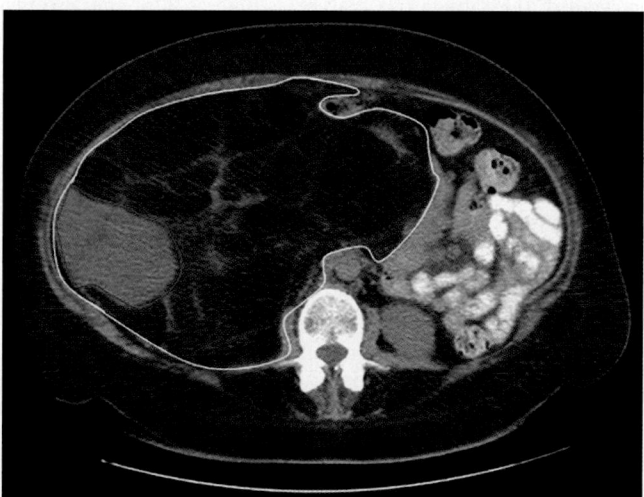

FIGURE 4 Computed tomographic image of right retroperitoneal liposarcoma with dedifferentiated (*red*) and well-differentiated (*yellow*) components. Residual well-differentiated disease frequently is mistaken for normal retroperitoneal fat; complete excision of ipsilateral fat is recommended.

■ ADJUVANT THERAPY

Use of radiation is integral to limb-sparing strategy to treat microscopic margins and minimize recurrence. Risk of LR is reduced from 30% or greater to less than 10% in most series but has not demonstrated an impact on overall or distant recurrence–free survival (DRFS). Lesions greater than 5 cm, particularly with close margins (<1 cm), should be considered for additional radiotherapy, which may be administered before, during, or after surgery. In comparing preoperative and postoperative RT in extremity STS, neoadjuvant treatment may be advantageous and result in a smaller field and lower dose. Although no difference in LR and survival are seen, a greater rate of wound complications has been observed with use of radiation in the neoadjuvant setting. However, further analysis of this finding implicated that complications were more pronounced in the lower extremity, and it is our practice to reserve adjuvant radiation for tumors in this location. Neoadjuvant therapy is used frequently in upper extremity and truncal cases in which large size may carry unacceptable morbidity or complicate wound closure. It should be

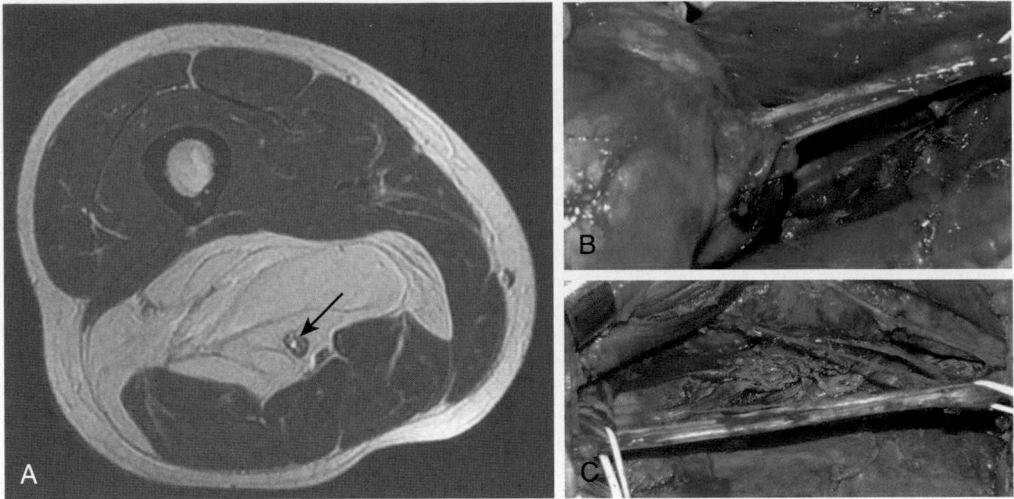

FIGURE 5 A, Well-differentiated liposarcoma encasing sciatic nerve (*arrow*). **B** and **C,** Tumor peels easily from nerve, with the resection bed showing skeletonized nerve.

noted that tumors may not decrease in size by imaging, making size a poor correlate of histologic response.

External beam radiation therapy (EBRT) and brachytherapy (BRT) have been compared, with no difference in LR rates for high-grade tumors but improved LR with EBRT in low-grade tumors. EBRT may be given in the preoperative setting, which is associated with lower rate of late complications of tissue fibrosis and functional impairment. To minimize wound complications with BRT, treatment is delayed until at least postoperative day 5.

Small (<5 cm) tumors in superficial location resected with an adequately wide (>1 cm) margin of healthy tissue should be followed by no additional radiation. Patients with large (>10 cm) tumors in deep location with high-grade histopathologic diagnosis are at risk for having distant metastases (25% to 50%) and may be considered for chemotherapy. Further controversy exists regarding the role of radiation in the retroperitoneum, and no randomized controlled data currently exist. As in the extremity, radiation reduces risk of LR, but anatomic field limitations compromise application. BRT and intraoperative radiation have been explored and shown to increase complication rate without demonstrating improved survival. The role of neoadjuvant radiotherapy is under investigation by a large phase III international trial by the European Organisation for Research and Treatment of Cancer (EORTC).

Randomized trials in chemotherapy are few, with minimal conclusive data regarding neoadjuvant therapy. Individualized trials in the adjuvant setting failed to reveal significant improvement but meta-analysis of previous randomized trials shows statistically significant improvement in LR, distant recurrence, and DFS with 10% absolute benefit at 10 years for patients on doxorubicin-based regimens. Overall survival indicated a 4% improvement and failed to reach statistical significance. Combination doxorubicin (Adriamycin)–ifosfamide appears to have improved antitumor activity in large, high-grade sarcoma, yet toxicity is substantial. Current second-line regimens include combination gemcitabine-docetaxel, with numerous trials of targeted therapy ongoing. Given the high risk of recurrence in tumors larger than 10 cm, patients with these tumors generally are considered candidates for therapy, particularly neoadjuvant administration in subtypes demonstrating high-risk distal recurrence such as Ewing's sarcoma, rhabdomyosarcoma, osteosarcoma, and leiomyosarcoma. Chemotherapy in the preoperative setting additionally allows for assessment of tumor responsiveness. It is our preference to use a neoadjuvant strategy due to better compliance rates, specifically in the case of large leiomyosarcomas and undifferentiated pleomorphic sarcomas. Chemotherapy is always administered in the case of rhabdomyosarcoma and Ewing's sarcoma. Additional consideration is given in cases of synovial cell sarcomas larger than 5 cm and myxoid liposarcomas with more than 5% round cell component. Systemic chemotherapy may palliate patients, resulting in tumor regression and improved progression-free survival in 30% to 50%, but rarely will be curative.

Hyperthermic isolated limb perfusion (ILP) and isolated limb infusion (ILI), in which vascular access catheters are placed to perfuse the extremity with high-dose chemotherapy, have been investigated as a means to preserve limb function in locally advanced extremity tumors. Currently no randomized trials have been performed in comparison with aggressive surgical resection or salvage radiation, but this strategy generally is used in patients who are not candidates for other therapies. Although reports are small, good result with even complete response has been observed with melphalan and tumor necrosis factor alpha under hyperthermic conditions. The latter is not currently approved for use in the United States but is continuing investigation internationally. This technique addresses only local disease and has been largely limited to cases where amputation is to be avoided. ILP salvage rate may be as high as 80% and also may palliate unresectable stage IV disease by improved quality of life and local wound control.

SPECIAL CONSIDERATIONS IN HISTOLOGY

Because histology has been discussed to be critical to outcomes, a surgeon approaching STS must understand the pathologic subtypes. Accuracy of diagnosis and multidisciplinary evaluation are necessary to devise an appropriate treatment plan, and as such it is advocated repeatedly that many cases be evaluated at specialty centers. Historically, malignant fibrous histiocytoma (MFH) was the most common type of sarcoma. However, this classification is used rarely and has been replaced by numerous more specific pathologic subtypes that delineate very different clinical behaviors and treatment strategies. Those falling outside of these pathologic subtypes are now typically diagnosed as unclassified pleomorphic sarcoma (UPS). In this section we aim to highlight key points of the major subtypes.

Liposarcoma

Atypical lipomatous tumors (ALTs) and well-differentiated liposarcomas (WDLPSs) of the extremity are at sufficiently low risk of recurrence that radiation is not used, even in large tumors with positive microscopic margins. These tumors grow slowly and have a relatively low risk of recurrence in the extremity and virtually no risk of distant spread in the absence of dedifferentiation. Dedifferentiation carries a 20% risk of metastatic presentation. ALTs may be difficult to distinguish from intramuscular lipoma, but given their deep location, they generally should be excised with a small margin of muscle to reduce recurrence. Retroperitoneal location of WDLPS portends a poorer outcome, with 50% local-regional failure and associated higher mortality. Myxoid/round cell liposarcomas are at significantly higher risk for distant failure if greater than 5% round cell component is found. These tumors, unlike WDLPS, are uniquely radiation sensitive and chemosensitive and should be referred for systemic treatment.

Leiomyosarcoma

Leiomyosarcoma is a tumor originating in smooth muscle cells and comprises 10% of all STSs, although it is the second most common subtype in the retroperitoneum. Most commonly, these tumors occur in the uterus or vascular smooth muscle cells and frequently arise from venous structures such as the vena cava. Overall, distant recurrence rates are higher for leiomyosarcoma (>30%), with LR in the absence of distant recurrence occurring in less than 4% of cases. As such, systemic chemotherapy is commonly administered and radiation may be indicated less often. Biopsy should be considered preoperatively if leiomyosarcoma is within the differential in order to determine the need for systemic neoadjuvant therapy as well as obtaining CT of the chest.

Synovial Sarcoma

Synovial sarcomas represent a unique subset of STS with identified chromosomal translocations composed of the *SYT-SSX1* or *SYT-SSX2* genes. These tumors also may be relatively chemosensitive with doxorubicin (Adriamycin)–ifosfamide–based therapy providing survival benefit in select patients. Patient age and tumor size, location, and grade have been shown to be significant prognostic factors, which may guide decision for use of chemotherapy. *SYT-SSX1* fusion type may be predictive of early (<3 year) distant recurrence.

Malignant Peripheral Nerve Sheath Tumors

MPNSTs can be observed in neurofibromatosis undergoing sarcomatous degeneration or sporadically from major peripheral nerves. High-grade tumors tend to metastasize early but may spread along the nerve bundle proximally as well. Associated nerve of origin

generally can be macroscopically identified, and a wide margin (up to 4 cm) is indicated to reduce LR. Frozen section may be of benefit in these cases to assess nerve margin.

Desmoid-Type Fibromatosis

Desmoid-type fibromatosis describes exceedingly rare tumors that lack the ability to metastasize but can be very locally aggressive, with most complications arising in the setting of repeated and morbid surgical or radiation intervention. Many are sporadic abdominal wall lesions associated with pregnancy, but they also can occur in the setting of Gardner's syndrome with familial adenomatous polyposis. Pregnancy-associated tumors frequently regress when hormonal stimulation is withdrawn. Small (<5 cm) abdominal wall desmoids may be removed with low recurrence rates, particularly if symptomatic, but extremity and deep intra-abdominal tumors can be particularly difficult. Cryotherapy for small tumors or radiation may be a reasonable alternative; large or symptomatic tumors in challenging locations are frequently referred for systemic therapy. Both sorafenib and salvage doxorubicin–based therapy are effective in controlling disease. In many cases, these tumors eventually "burn out," evidenced by decreased cellularity on radiographic evaluation, and the morbidity of operation can be avoided (Figure 6).

Solitary Fibrous Tumors

Solitary fibrous tumors (SFTs) represent a spectrum of STS of fibroblastic differentiation, with most common sites of occurrence being the visceral pleura and retroperitoneum. These tumors are of intermediate biologic potential, with fewer than 10% metastasizing. SFTs may be seen uniquely with neoplastic syndrome similar to clinical findings in insulinoma. Doege-Potter syndrome describes a condition in which production of insulin-like growth factor 1 (IGF-1) by SFTs results in symptomatic hypoglycemia that resolves with tumor resection. Patient age, tumor size, and mitotic index have been shown as predictive of outcome, with specifically tumor size greater than 15 cm, age older than 55, and greater than 4/10 high-power field (HPF) mitoses deserving closer follow-up because of risk for metastases and disease-specific mortality.

Fibrosarcoma and Variants

Low-grade fibromyxosarcomas are fairly indolent neoplasms but like other fibrosarcomas tend to recur locally. Recurrence is seen even after very long disease-free intervals beyond 5 years, and long-term follow-up is necessary. Dermatofibrosarcoma protuberans

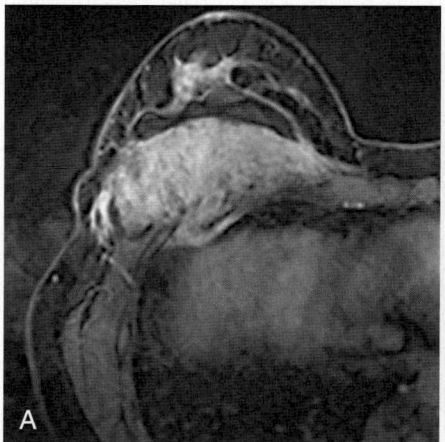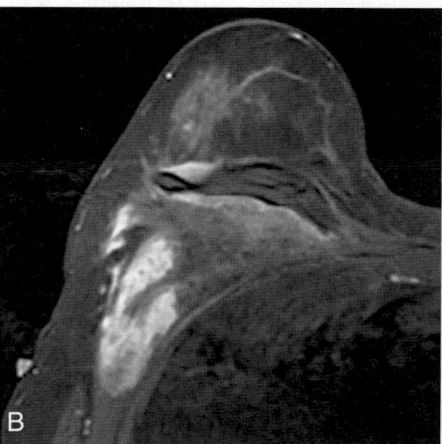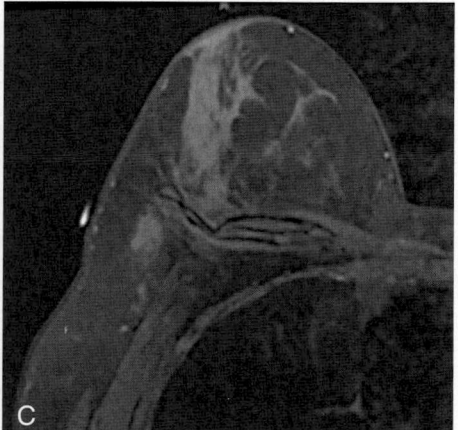

FIGURE 6 Axial imaging of desmoid fibromatosis before (**A**) and after (**B** and **C**) chemotherapy demonstrating decreased active cellularity and increasing gelatinous component.

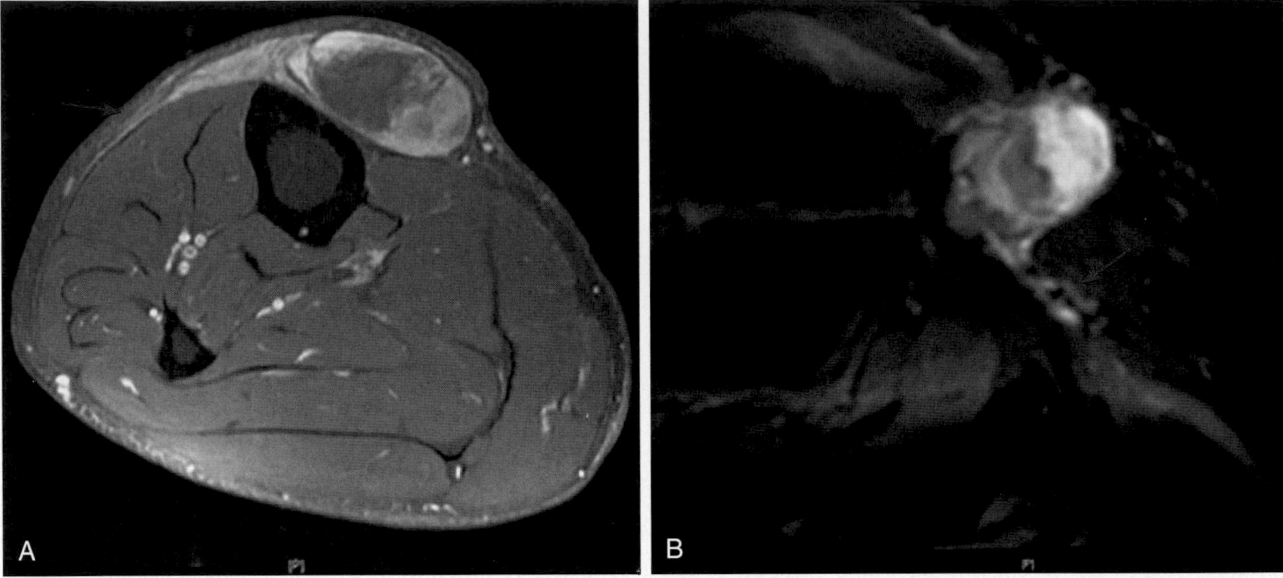

FIGURE 7 **A** and **B,** Myxofibrosarcomas on axial imaging demonstrating "myxoid tail" (*arrow*) characteristic of peripheral infiltration away from mass.

(DFSP) is a superficial tumor that typically projects radially via infiltrative extensions from the main mass and should be excised with wider margins (at least 2 cm) with inclusion of deep fascia. DFSP carries no risk of metastases unless fibrosarcomatous degeneration is observed on pathology testing (<10%), and radiation is usually unnecessary. Positive margins should be resected aggressively, and any use of skin graft or flap reconstruction should be delayed until final negative margins are demonstrated. If cosmesis is of concern, the indolent nature of these tumors may allow for use of a tissue expander or smaller margins with anticipation of wider resection at time of recurrence. Despite concern for marginality, as with other STS, frozen section is not generally helpful, as fatty tissue is poorly preserved in the freezing process. Follow-up with physical examination is sufficient excepting in cases of sarcomatous degeneration, which necessitate imaging and treatment as conventional sarcoma.

Myxofibrosarcoma

Myxofibrosarcomas, like DFSP, represent tumors with microscopic infiltration and require wider resection with at least 2-cm margins (Figure 7). Recurrence rate is as high as 30%, and as such, aggressive wide resection is critical to control of disease. These tumors, although generally contained by natural biologic barriers, do show higher incidence of local infiltration when compared with other STS. Radiation generally may be avoided in initial recurrence with very low-grade pathologic diagnosis; however, it should be noted that recurrences tend to be of higher grade with second and subsequent presentations. As such, radiation is generally indicated for recurrent disease. Any closure by means of reconstruction with graft or flap should be delayed until final negative pathologic diagnosis is achieved.

Angiosarcoma

Angiosarcomas should be recognized, as very commonly multifocal tumors and failure to recognize satellite lesions may result in a high rate of recurrence outside the original resection bed (Figure 8). Surgery often is not curative, but these tumors are relatively chemosensitive and radiosensitive; systemic treatment generally should be explored before radical surgery. Any preoperative evaluation and subsequent surveillance should involve high-quality axial imaging.

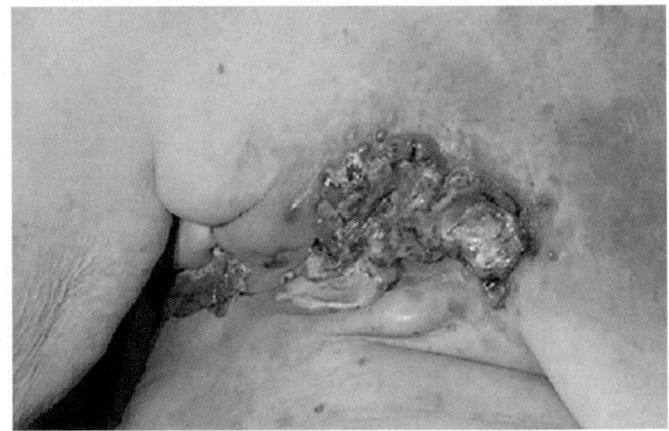

FIGURE 8 Multilobulated angiosarcoma with satellite lesions.

Radiation-Induced Sarcomas

Radiation-induced sarcomas present a unique challenge, with high recurrence rates resulting from both difficulty in determining healthy tissue in a radiation field and multifocal disease in the presence of a field defect. Histologic subtypes may include UPS, angiosarcoma, MPNST, and leiomyosarcoma, but given the poorer clinical behavior than their subtype counterparts, excision should be as wide as possible and systemic chemotherapy should be considered. Reconstruction with plastic surgery and sacrifice of neurovascular structures are frequently necessary.

Epithelioid Sarcoma

Epithelioid sarcomas are rare tumors of mixed histogenesis differing in behavior from both mesenchymal tumors and epithelial carcinomas. They are slow-growing tumors with peak incidence in young men and extremity location. Recurrence rate is high, and unlike most sarcomas, up to 50% will metastasize, specifically in a lymphatic basin and by direct local extension. The role of sentinel lymph node biopsy remains controversial and may be of largely prognostic utility only.

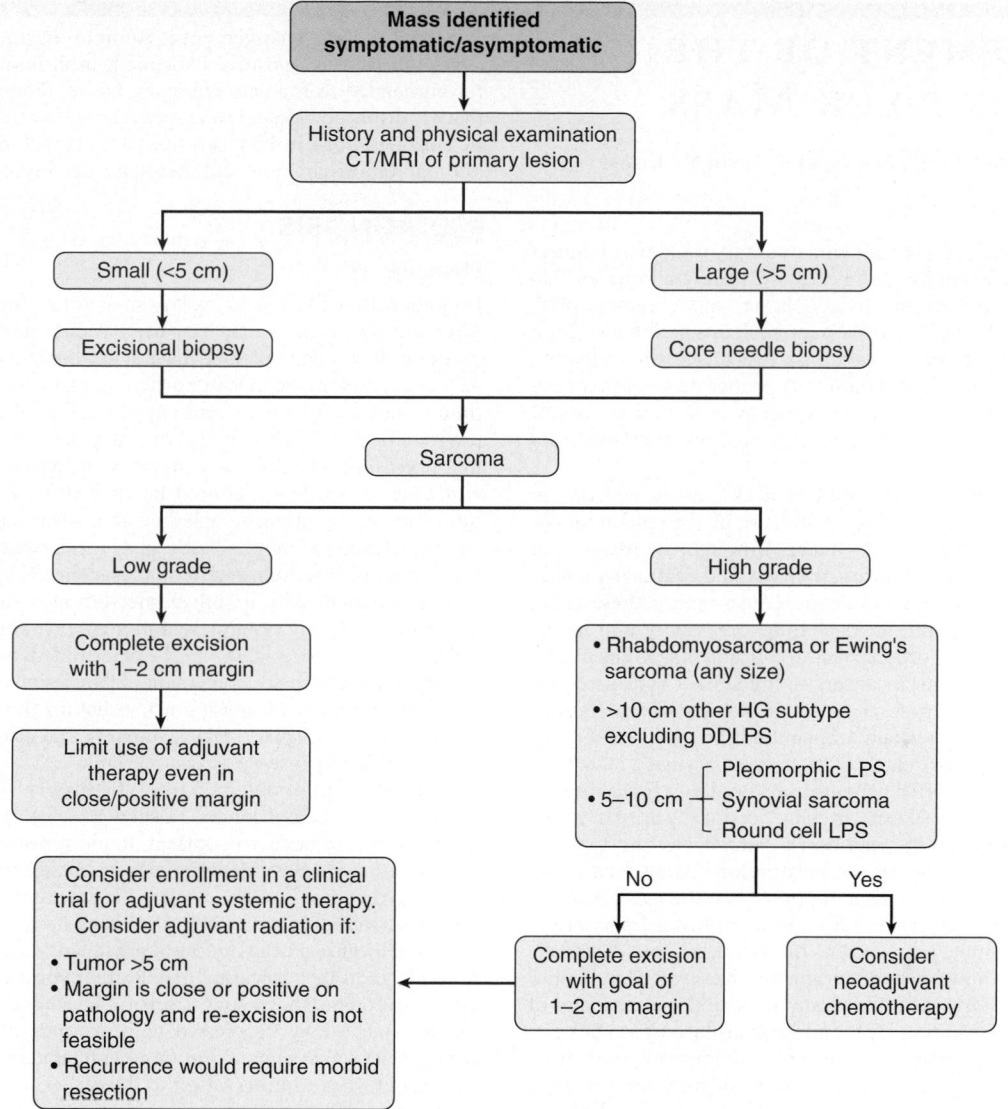

FIGURE 9 Management strategy for soft tissue sarcoma. *CT*, Computed tomography; *DDLPS*, dedifferentiated liposarcoma; *HG*, high-grade; *LPS*, liposarcoma; *MRI*, magnetic resonance imaging.

■ CONCLUSIONS

Surgery remains the dominant effective form of treatment. Complete gross resection should always be the goal. Adjuvant RT can limit LR but has not improved survival. A prospective randomized controlled trial of preoperative RT for intra-abdominal tumors is ongoing and should be encouraged. Recurrent local and metastatic disease continues to be a major challenge in the long-term treatment of STS, with rates as high as 10% to 30% in the extremity and as high as 50% in the retroperitoneum. Selected patients should be offered investigative trials based on molecular profiling. Our approach to patients with STS is summarized in the algorithm shown in Figure 9.

SUGGESTED READINGS

Bonvalot S, Chandrajit PR, Pollock RE, Rutkowski P, Strauss DC, Hayes AJ, Van Coevorden F, Fiore M, Stoeckle E, Hohenberger P, Gronchi A. Technical consideration in surgery for retroperitoneal sarcomas: position paper from E-Surge, a master class in sarcoma surgery, and EORTC-STBSG. *Ann Surg Oncol.* 2012;19:2981-2991.

Brennan MF, Antonescu CR, Maki RG. *Management of Soft Tissue Sarcoma.* New York: Springer; 2012.

Brennan MF, Antonescu CR, Moraco N, Singer S. Lessons learned from the study of 10,000 patients with soft tissue sarcoma. *Ann Surg.* 2014;260: 416-422.

Crago A, Brennan MF. Principles in management of soft tissue sarcoma. *Adv Surg.* 2015;49:107-122.

Dalal KM, Kattan MW, Antonescu CR, Brennan MF, Singer S. Subtype specific prognostic nomogram for patients with primary liposarcoma of the retroperitoneum, extremity or trunk. *Ann Surg.* 2006;244:381-391.

MANAGEMENT OF THE SOLITARY NECK MASS

Carole Fakhry, MD, MPH, FACS, and David W. Eisele, MD, FACS

Proper management of a patient with a solitary neck mass requires a thorough understanding of head and neck anatomy and an appreciation of the heterogeneous neoplastic, inflammatory, infectious, and congenital conditions that may result in a neck mass. Given the diverse causes that result in a neck mass, the diagnostic evaluation of the solitary neck mass is paramount. A proper diagnosis requires the rational synthesis of a patient's demographic factors, history of present illness, social history, physical examination, and laboratory and imaging studies.

The diagnostic approach of a solitary neck mass has evolved in the past several decades in large part because of the epidemiologic shifts observed in head and neck cancer. Although the majority of head and neck cancers were previously larynx and oral cavity malignancies related to tobacco use and alcohol consumption, these trends have reversed with a significant decline in oral cavity and larynx malignancies and a rise in oropharyngeal cancers. Indeed the majority of incident head and neck cancers in the United States are now oropharyngeal cancers. These changes are attributable to human papillomavirus (HPV), a sexually transmitted infection. HPV is the causative agent for approximately 80% of oropharyngeal malignancies in the United States. HPV patients have a unique clinical profile. HPV-positive oropharyngeal cancers characteristically arise in young men without exposure to the traditional carcinogens and typically cause small primary tumors in the palatine or lingual tonsils and large nodal metastases. In the contemporary era, the overwhelming majority of squamous cell cancer (SCC) of unknown primary origin is HPV-related oropharynx cancer. In addition, the diagnostic workup of SCC unknown primary origin also has evolved in light of the availability of biomarkers for virally mediated malignancies of the head and neck, including HPV and Epstein-Barr virus (EBV).

Although the diagnostic evaluation of a therapeutic neck mass can converge on therapeutic efforts, excisional biopsies and neck dissections should be approached with caution. Excisional biopsy may be appropriate for diagnosing and treating select solitary neck masses; however, this approach is ill advised for some masses, most notably parotid neoplasms and cervical lymph nodes involved with metastatic cancer from head and neck primaries. The decision to perform excisional biopsy of a solitary neck mass should be incorporated into the overall evaluation and treatment plan for the patient. As such, it should be guided by an appropriately thorough history, physical examination, and the use of diagnostic tests, including imaging studies, laboratory tests, and cytopathologic evaluation from fine-needle aspiration biopsy (FNAB).

■ CAUSES

Solitary neck masses can be from neoplastic, congenital, inflammatory, or traumatic causes. Most solitary neck masses in children are benign; cervical lymphadenitis is the most common cause. Congenital neck masses, including thyroglossal duct cysts and branchial cleft cysts, are the second most common pediatric neck masses. Malignant pediatric neck masses, although uncommon, are most commonly lymphoma, rhabdomyosarcoma, and neuroblastoma, in that order.

Conversely, most adult solitary neck masses are malignant, with the majority representing metastatic carcinoma from a head and neck primary. Thus a solitary neck mass in an adult requires an appropriate evaluation to exclude malignancy. Table 1 lists common causes of solitary neck masses.

Cervical nodal enlargement is common in human immunodeficiency virus (HIV)-positive patients. Lymph node biopsy usually is recommended to evaluate enlarging nodes, tender nodes, or nodes that are disproportionately enlarged relative to other nodes. Diagnostic considerations in HIV-positive patients include infections, lymphoma, Kaposi sarcoma, and metastatic carcinoma.

■ DIAGNOSIS

History

Patients with solitary neck masses may notice the mass themselves. Alternatively, the mass may have been found during a routine physical examination. Patients may have symptoms related to the mass or may be asymptomatic. It is important to query patients regarding the time of onset of the mass and any changes in the size (fluctuation, progressive growth, or stability) or character of the mass since it was first noted. Associated local symptoms, including pain, sensory loss, erythema, or weakness, should be elicited. In addition, associated head and neck symptoms, including nasal obstruction, epistaxis, dysarthria, trismus, odynophagia, dysphagia, hoarseness, otalgia, hearing loss, airway obstruction, and hemoptysis, should be sought. A history of recent dental, skin, or other infection also should be obtained. The presence of any systemic symptoms, such as fever, night sweats, weight loss, or anorexia, should be determined. A thorough medical history, including prior malignancy, skin lesions (previously treatment or regression of any lesion), radiation therapy, immunosuppression (e.g., transplant, HIV), smoking and alcohol consumption, travel, and family history, is also relevant.

The information obtained from the history is invaluable to formulate a differential diagnosis. A slow-growing mass suggests a congenital lesion or benign neoplasm. Rapid growth is consistent with inflammatory masses or progression of malignant neoplasms. Pain related to the mass is rather nonspecific for cause but indicates irritation of surrounding structures. Associated head and neck symptoms may help localize a head and neck malignancy. For example, hoarseness may indicate a laryngeal neoplasm or vocal cord paralysis. Dysphagia and odynophagia suggest an oropharyngeal or hypopharyngeal lesion. Otalgia may be present with an underlying pharyngeal or laryngeal lesion, causing irritation of cranial nerves IX and X, which also supply sensory innervation to the ear.

A high index of suspicion is advised for a solitary neck mass arising from SCC of the upper aerodigestive tract in users of tobacco, alcohol, or marijuana. A solitary neck mass in a nonsmoker is highly suspicious for malignancy arising from the cryptic lymphoepithelium of the oropharynx. Prior low-dose radiation therapy is a causative factor for developing salivary gland and thyroid neoplasms. Associated systemic symptoms or symptoms related to other organ systems, as determined by a thorough review of systems, may provide information suggesting an infraclavicular primary. Fever and rapid onset of a neck mass may accompany an infectious process (e.g., lymphadenitis). The constellation of fevers, night sweats, and diffuse lymphadenopathy, however, can be suggestive of lymphoma.

Physical Examination

A complete head and neck examination should always be performed. The scalp, face, ear, and neck skin should be inspected for lesions. The external ear canal, tympanic membrane, nasal cavity, nasopharynx, oral cavity, oropharynx, hypopharynx, and larynx should be examined visually, directly, and with a mirror or fiberoptic endoscope. Inspection with fiberoptic endoscopes supplements indirect visualization of the upper aerodigestive tract if mirror examination is inadequate. A topical anesthetic (e.g., lidocaine, benzocaine) may facilitate the pharyngeal and laryngeal examination in patients with active gag reflexes. Vocal cord mobility should be determined. The function of all cranial nerves should be assessed. The face, parotid glands, and neck should be palpated carefully. Also, the oral cavity,

TABLE 1: Common Causes of Solitary Neck Masses

Benign Neoplasms	Malignant Neoplasms	Other
Salivary gland	Metastatic	Traumatic
Thyroid	Upper aerodigestive	Hematoma
Lipoma	tract	Fibroma
Paraganglioma	Skin	Neuroma
Schwannoma	Thyroid	Pseudoaneurysm
Neurofibroma	Salivary gland	Arteriovenous
Congenital	Infraclavicular primary	malformation
Thyroglossal duct	site (breast, lung,	
cyst	gastrointestinal,	
Branchial cleft cyst	genitourinary,	
Dermoid cyst	gynecologic)	
Lymphangioma	Unknown primary	
Hemangioma	Salivary gland	
Inflammatory	Thyroid	
Lymphadenitis	Sarcoma	
Sialadenitis	Lymphoma (Hodgkin's,	
Thyroiditis	non-Hodgkin's)	

TABLE 2: Cervical Lymph Node Levels

Level	Lymph Node Group
I	Submental, submandibular, prevascular, and retrovascular facial nodes
II	Upper jugular nodes
III	Midjugular nodes (hyoid bone to cricothyroid membrane)
IV	Lower jugular nodes
V	Posterior triangle nodes
VI	Prelaryngeal, pretracheal, and paratracheal nodes

TABLE 3: Major Differential Diagnosis of Neck Masses Relative to Anatomic Areas of the Neck

Neck Area	Diagnoses
Submental triangle	Lymph node* Plunging ranula Dermoid cyst
Submandibular triangle	Submandibular gland mass Lymph node*
Carotid triangle	Branchial cleft cyst Lymph node* Carotid body tumor
Posterior triangle	Lymph node* Neurogenic tumor Lipoma
Supraclavicular fossa	Lymph node*
Central neck	Thyroglossal duct remnant Thyroid nodule Lymph node* Laryngeal neoplasm Laryngocele

*Includes reactive hyperplasia, metastatic lymphadenopathy, and lymphoma.

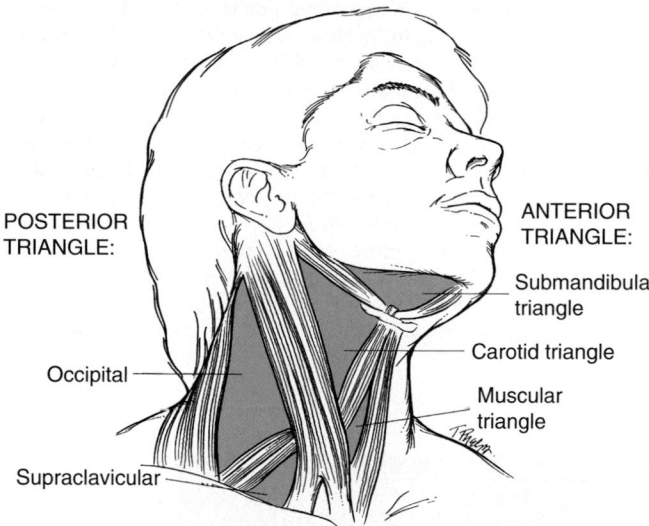

POSTERIOR TRIANGLE:

ANTERIOR TRIANGLE:

Submandibular triangle

Carotid triangle

Muscular triangle

Occipital

Supraclavicular

FIGURE 1 Triangles of the neck. (*Modified from Lingeman RE. Surgical anatomy. In: Cummings CW, et al, eds.* Otolaryngology—head and neck surgery. *3rd ed. St Louis: Mosby; 1998.*)

tonsil, and base of the tongue should be palpated with a gloved finger. In addition, a pertinent general physical examination should be performed.

The location of the neck mass should be documented with standard nomenclature. One useful anatomic designation relates to the triangles of the neck formed by the neck muscles, the mandible, and the clavicle (Figure 1). Each side of the neck is divided into two major triangles by the sternocleidomastoid muscle (SCM). The *anterior triangle* is formed by the vertical midline of the neck, the inferior border of the mandible, and the SCM. The *posterior triangle* is bordered by the SCM, the clavicle, and the anterior border of the trapezius muscle.

The anterior triangle consists of smaller triangles, including the *submandibular triangle,* bordered by the mandible and the anterior and posterior bellies of the digastric muscle. The *carotid triangle* is bounded by the posterior belly of the digastric muscle, the SCM, and

the superior belly of the omohyoid muscle. The *submental triangle* is bounded by the anterior bellies of the digastric muscles and the hyoid bone. The *supraclavicular fossa* is defined by three points: the sternal end of the clavicle, the lateral end of the clavicle, and the point where the neck meets the shoulder.

Another useful neck region schema to document the location of a neck mass is the Memorial Sloan-Kettering system, which designates cervical lymph nodes by levels (Table 2).

The location of the mass in the neck may be informative regarding differential diagnoses to consider (Table 3). Each anatomic triangle comprises specific types of tissue (e.g., nervous structures) that can result in a specific pathologic entity and therefore provide clues regarding primary origin. In addition, the location of a metastatic cervical lymph node suggests the site of the primary tumor from which the metastasis is arising because the patterns of lymphatic spread are generally predictable (Table 4).

Supraclavicular masses are most commonly malignant and are typically either metastatic carcinoma or lymphoma. Metastatic supraclavicular nodes are usually from infraclavicular primaries; adenocarcinoma is the most common tumor type, followed by SCC. The usual infraclavicular primaries are breast and lung. Pelvic and abdominal malignancies have a predilection to present as a left supra-clavicular mass (Virchow's node). This is the result of spread via the thoracic duct, which receives lymphatic drainage from the abdomen and pelvis and drains into the left subclavian and internal jugular veins. In contrast, the right lymphatic duct does not drain these pelvic and abdominal sites.

Variants of normal anatomic structures also may be misinterpreted as an abnormal neck mass. For example, masseter or omohyoid muscle hypertrophy, a prominent carotid bulb, an elongated lateral process of the C1 vertebra (atlas), a ptotic submandibular gland, a prominent hyoid bone cornu, or mandibular bony processes may be confused with neck mass.

The size and mobility of the mass relative to adjacent structures should be determined. Masses in the submental and submandibular triangles of the neck also can be assessed by bimanual palpation with a gloved finger. The consistency of the mass often can be determined

by palpation. The degree of firmness and the presence of fluctuance or tenderness should be determined.

In addition to location, specific physical examination characteristics of the mass may provide useful information regarding the origin of the mass. Hard masses, masses with fixation to adjacent structures, and multiple masses are worrisome signs of malignancy. Some metastatic nodes, particularly those from tonsil or base of tongue primaries, may be cystic. Multiple cystic parotid masses or bilateral parotid enlargement suggests an HIV infection. Carotid body tumors classically can be moved horizontally but not vertically and may be pulsatile. Masses in the central neck that elevate with swallowing are consistent with a laryngeal or thyroid mass. Elevation of a central neck mass with tongue protrusion suggests a thyroglossal duct cyst or mass.

Imaging Studies

Imaging studies, including computed tomography (CT) scan, magnetic resonance imaging (MRI), and ultrasound can provide additional useful diagnostic information, including the character of a neck mass (e.g., solid, cystic, vascular), its relationship to surrounding structures, and the presence of additional nonpalpable masses or nodes. CT and MRI have the advantage of providing information regarding concomitant disease of the upper aerodigestive tract and head and neck. Lymph nodes suspicious of harboring metastatic malignancy are those with central necrosis, larger than 1.5 cm, and with irregular borders. For metastatic malignancy, imaging studies also can provide information about the location of the primary tumor and extent of disease. In cases of metastatic carcinoma from a known or suspected head and neck primary origin, chest imaging should be obtained to rule out concomitant lung lesions. Metastatic carcinoma from a suspected infraclavicular source should prompt appropriate diagnostic and imaging studies to search for the infraclavicular primary and to determine the extent of disease. For lymphoma evaluation, a chest and abdominal CT scan or MRI is obtained for disease staging. In addition, a bone marrow aspiration biopsy may be necessary to further evaluate lymphoma. PET imaging can be used in the evaluation of metastatic disease, with the caveat that it has high sensitivity and physiologic uptake in the palatine and lingual tonsils (Figure 2).

TABLE 4: Potential Primary Sites for a Solitary Cervical Lymph Node Metastasis

Cervical Node Level	Potential Primary Sites
I	Skin, lip, oral cavity, submandibular gland, parotid gland, paranasal sinuses
II	Parotid, oral cavity, oropharynx, larynx, hypopharynx, nasopharynx, thyroid
III	Oral cavity, oropharynx, hypopharynx, larynx, thyroid, cervical esophagus
IV	Oropharynx, hypopharynx, larynx, thyroid, infraclavicular primary, cervical esophagus
V	Nasopharynx, skin, thyroid, infraclavicular primary
VI	Thyroid, larynx, hypopharynx, cervical esophagus

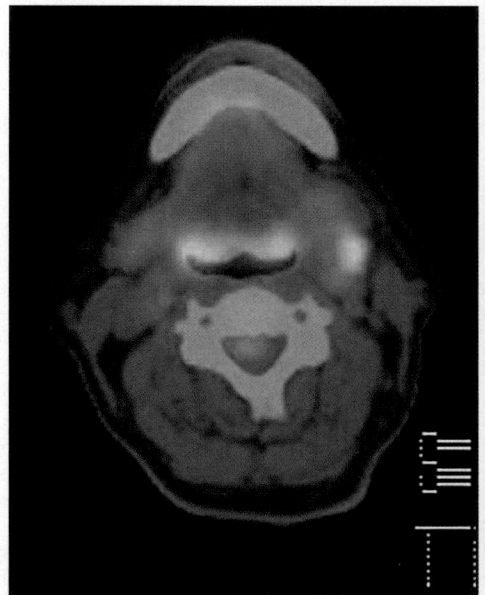
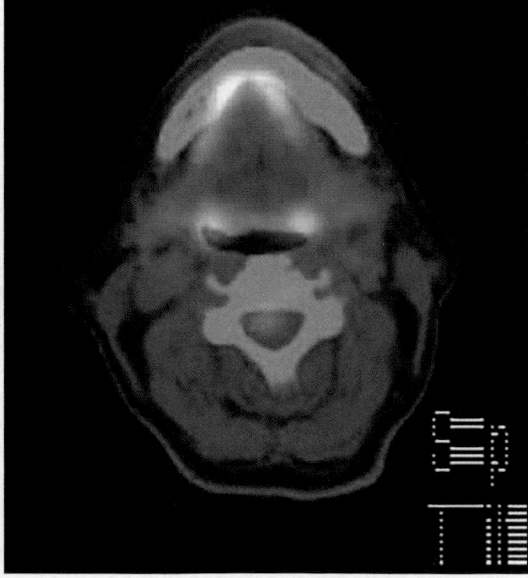

FIGURE 2 PET/CT axial images of left cervical squamous cell carcinoma metastasis with occult primary. Physiologic uptake is observed in the lingual tonsils. Palatine tonsils are absent. Despite uptake in the lingual tonsils, the primary is not necessarily in the base of tongue.

Laboratory Tests

In general, laboratory tests provide little additional information. Blood counts may aid in the workup of the patient with an infectious neck mass or suspected lymphoma. A serum calcitonin level should be obtained if medullary carcinoma of the thyroid is a diagnostic consideration.

Fine-Needle Aspiration Biopsy

FNAB is a simple, and the preferred, technique for diagnosing neck masses. FNAB often is used as the first diagnostic study for patients with a solitary neck mass, especially if no obvious cause is evident on initial head and neck examination. The FNAB technique is accurate and safe. Unlike Tru-cut and core-needle biopsies, FNAB does not risk tumor spread into the surrounding tissues. In addition, FNAB does not violate the neck skin or subsequent surgical planes if surgery is necessary.

FNAB of head and neck masses is simple to perform. The necessary equipment includes 20-mL syringes, 22-gauge disposable needles, a syringe pistol, alcohol swabs, sterile gauze pads, glass slides, and fixatives, including 95% ethyl alcohol and Hank's solution (Figure 3). The mass is palpated, and the skin overlying the mass is cleansed with an alcohol swab. The mass is immobilized between the thumb and forefinger of the nondominant hand. The needle, attached to the syringe and syringe pistol, is inserted into the mass (Figure 4, *A*). The mass is aspirated by creating negative pressure in the syringe (Figure 4, *B*). The needle is passed back and forth within the mass in different directions (Figure 4, *C*). The needle plunger then is released and the needle withdrawn from the patient (Figure 4, *D*). Pressure with a sterile gauze is applied to the puncture site for several minutes.

The needle containing the specimen then is detached from the syringe and the syringe filled with air. After reapplication of the needle to the syringe, the aspirated material is expressed onto a slide. A second slide then is used to smear the aspirated material, and the two slides are placed into 95% ethyl alcohol. A needle washing then is obtained by drawing 5 to 10 mL of Hank's solution through the needle into the syringe. The solution then is expressed back into the Hank's solution container. This needle-washing solution later is subjected to cytocentrifugation, and smears of the collected cellular material are prepared. FNAB of cystic masses may yield fluid, which should be submitted for cytologic evaluation. Any residual solid mass should be reaspirated in the standard fashion.

An inadequate specimen is the most common reason for a nondiagnostic FNAB. Synchronous on-site determination of the adequacy of the FNAB specimen by a cytologist reduces the frequency of inadequate specimens. Repeat FNAB can be performed until an adequate cytopathologic specimen is obtained, as determined by immediate microscopic examination of the procured specimen. Immediate microscopic evaluation of the specimen also allows for specimens to be set aside for special stains and studies, such as flow cytometry, when appropriate (e.g., for suspected lymphoma).

FNAB can be guided by ultrasound if the mass is nonpalpable. Masses as small as 5 mm can undergo biopsy with ultrasound-guided FNAB. Masses in difficult locations, which are inaccessible to ultrasound-guided FNAB, can undergo biopsy by CT guidance with good accuracy.

Complications of head and neck FNAB are rare but include hemorrhage and infection. A relative contraindication to FNAB of a neck mass is suspicion of a carotid body tumor because of reported hemorrhagic complications and cerebrovascular accidents after FNAB of these neoplasms. The diagnosis of carotid body tumor usually is suggested by physical examination and confirmed with imaging studies, including contrast-enhanced CT scan and MRI.

Accuracy of FNAB depends on the experience of the cytopathologist. Disadvantages of FNAB include occasional interpretation difficulty or error. In addition, FNAB can be problematic in typing certain carcinomas and lymphomas. Inadequate specimens can result because of sampling difficulties related to tumor necrosis, partial lymph node involvement, cystic content, and fibrosis.

When FNAB is unsuccessful or inconclusive, core biopsy or excisional biopsies may be considered. In general, excisional biopsies should be avoided unless other less invasive diagnostic measures have been unsuccessful and the patient consents to concurrent definitive surgical management if malignancy is confirmed intraoperatively.

Biopsy materials (FNA, core or excisional) can be tested for the presence of HPV or EBV. If positive, both are biomarkers for anatomic site of origin. HPV-positive tumor status points to a primary tumor arising from the oropharynx. In the context of solitary neck mass and no obvious primary lesion, in situ hybridization testing for HPV is more specific for a tumor arising from the oropharynx, whereas p16 immunohistochemistry is less specific. Skin primaries have been shown to be associated with p16-positivity, and therefore caution must be exercised in the interpretation and treatment-related decision making in this case. EBV testing, which comprises EBER immunohistochemistry, is a surrogate for nasopharyngeal cancer.

■ MANAGEMENT

Diagnostic information obtained from history, physical examination, imaging studies, and FNAB guides definitive treatment of the solitary neck mass. If the head and neck examination is unrevealing and an inflammatory lymph node enlargement is suspected, a course of antibiotics and close observation over several weeks is reasonable. Further diagnostic assessment is necessary for masses that enlarge or persist during this observation period.

Benign lesions and benign neoplasms are resected surgically. Benign and malignant submandibular neoplasms are managed by submandibular gland resection. Similarly, benign and malignant parotid neoplasms are managed by complete resection with a parotidectomy. The facial nerve is preserved in all cases, unless the nerve is invaded by a malignant neoplasm. Enucleation of parotid neoplasms is to be avoided and carries the risk of incomplete tumor removal because of poor tumor encapsulation.

Other benign neoplasms, such as dermoid cysts, lipomas, and branchial cleft cysts, are excised for definitive treatment. Thyroglossal duct cysts and thyroglossal duct neoplasms are resected by a Sistrunk

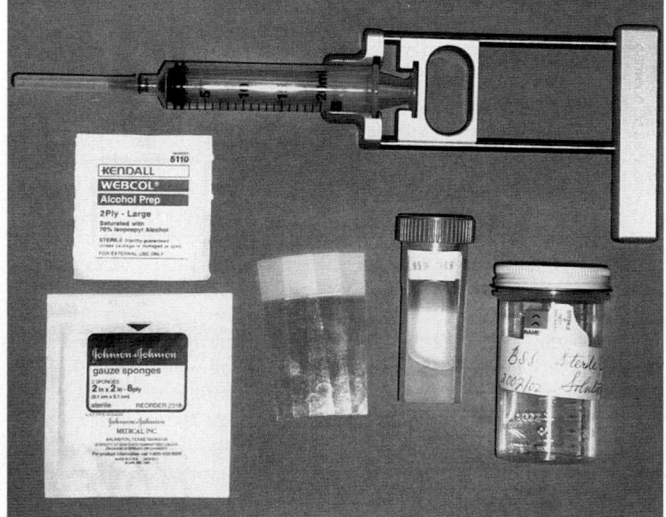

FIGURE 3 Equipment for fine-needle aspiration biopsy.

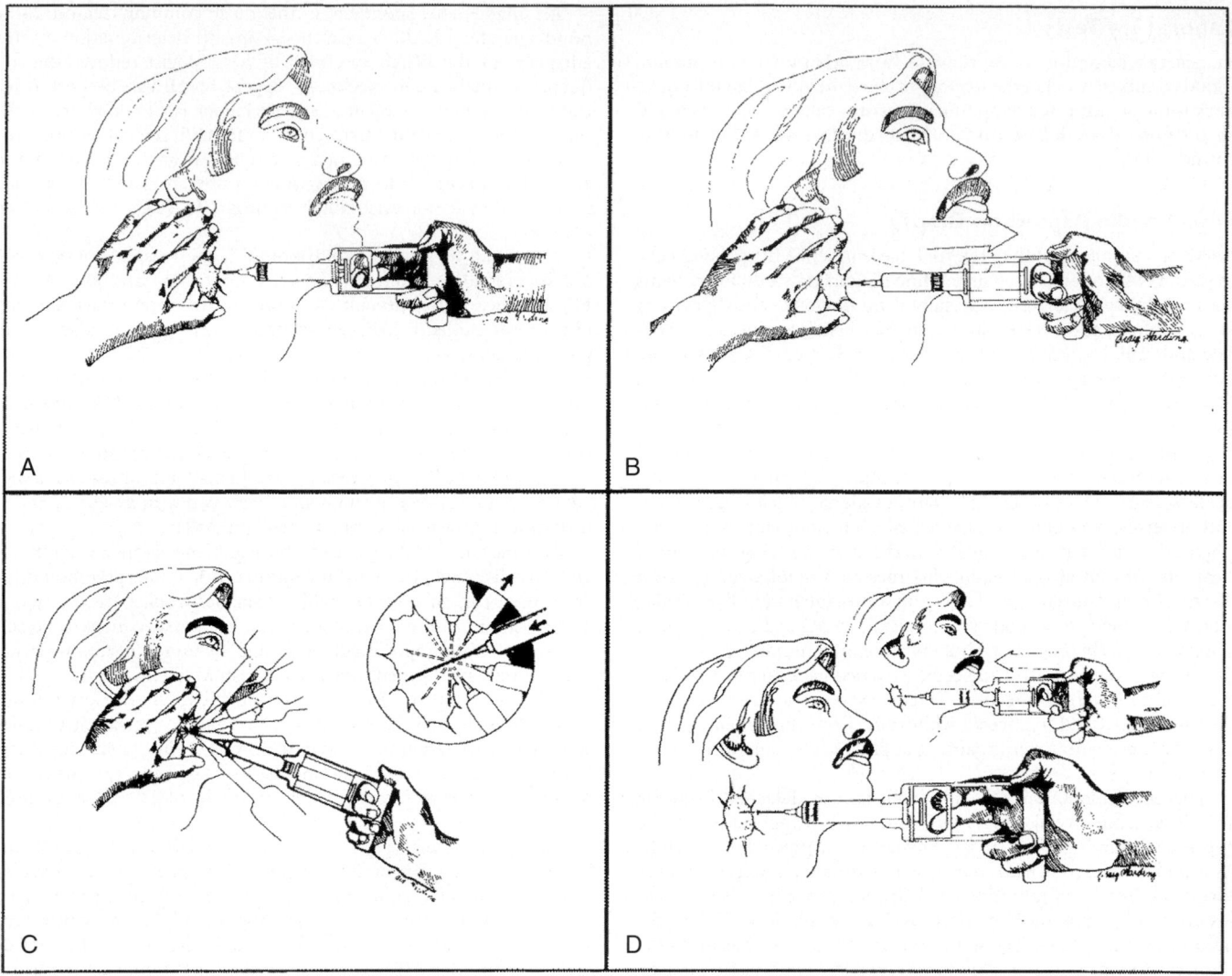

FIGURE 4 A, The needle is inserted into the mass. **B,** Aspiration of the mass is performed to create negative pressure. **C,** On each pass the needle is moved in multiple directions within the mass to optimize cell count. **D,** Before the needle is withdrawn, the plunger is released. *(From Feldman PS, et al, eds. Fine needle aspiration cytology. Chicago: ASCP Press; 1998.)*

procedure, which entails complete resection of the mass and thyroglossal duct tract to the tongue base with the central portion of the hyoid bone. Carotid body tumors are treated by total excision with or without preoperative embolization. A few carotid body tumors or paragangliomas are vasoactive, which should be ruled out preoperatively by urine catecholamine screening.

Malignant thyroid neoplasms are managed by total thyroidectomy or hemithyroidectomy in select cases of small papillary thyroid cancer. Follicular and Hürthle cell neoplasms and suspicious thyroid nodules are resected by thyroid lobectomy for definitive diagnosis and completion total thyroidectomy if the neoplasm is determined to be malignant by permanent histopathology. If medullary carcinoma of the thyroid is diagnosed, concomitant pheochromocytoma should be ruled out with abdominal CT scan or MRI preoperatively.

Lymph nodes diagnosed as reactive hyperplasia by FNAB can be observed safely. Further enlargement requires repeat FNAB or surgical excision. Infectious lymphadenitis is managed by appropriate antimicrobial therapy. Lymphoma diagnosed by FNAB may require lymph node biopsy for definitive lymphoma typing to guide therapy.

The management of metastatic cervical lymphadenopathy is guided by the tumor type. Metastatic thyroid carcinoma is managed by selective lateral neck dissection, central neck dissection, and total thyroidectomy. The management of metastatic SCC depends on the location and size of the primary tumor, which usually is identified during the initial head and neck examination. Upper aerodigestive tract endoscopy and imaging studies (MRI or CT scan) aid in evaluating the extent of disease at the primary site and in the neck.

If the FNAB of a neck mass suggests malignancy but is inconclusive regarding tumor type, complete endoscopic evaluation of the upper aerodigestive tract is performed. If the primary tumor is not identified during endoscopy, only then is excisional biopsy indicated for definitive diagnosis. The neck biopsy incision should be planned so that it may be incorporated into an appropriate neck dissection incision. Neck dissection is performed if frozen-section pathologic evaluation confirms SCC or melanoma. The patient should be counseled preoperatively regarding the possibility of the need for a neck dissection. If a definitive frozen-section diagnosis cannot be rendered, the wound is closed and a plan is developed on the basis of permanent histopathology results. Inflammatory or granulomatous nodes should be cultured immediately after excision. A resected node suspected of harboring lymphoma should be sent fresh for pathologic evaluation.

Carcinoma metastatic to a cervical lymph node without an identifiable primary tumor by physical examination or imaging studies is unusual and requires further diagnostic workup. SCC metastatic to cervical lymph nodes is almost always from a head and neck primary site; therefore thorough examination of the upper aerodigestive tract to identify the primary tumor is warranted. The presence of HPV in the cervical metastasis is indicative of a primary in the oropharynx. Similarly, an EBV-positive lymph node suggests metastasis from the nasopharynx. The patient should undergo a careful examination under general anesthesia of the nasopharynx, oropharynx, hypopharynx, and larynx with appropriate endoscopes. If no primary tumor is visible during examination under anesthesia, bilateral tonsillectomy should be performed (if the tonsils are present) because this procedure reveals a primary tonsil carcinoma in approximately 40% of patients. Flexible bronchoscopy and esophagoscopy also are performed to identify the primary tumor or a synchronous malignancy. The base of the tongue, tonsils, and other structures should be palpated carefully. Any mucosal lesions, friable areas, or palpable masses should be appropriately biopsied. Frozen-section evaluation may be helpful to confirm the presence of a suspected neoplasm and adequacy of the biopsy. In the case of HPV-positive cervical metastases and absence of palatine tonsils or primary in the palatine tonsils, an ipsilateral lingual tonsillectomy, performed robotically or by transoral laser excision, also may be considered. Identification of an upper aerodigestive tract malignancy precludes the need for excisional biopsy of the neck mass as a diagnostic intervention, and the neck mass should be considered a metastatic node.

Definitive treatment of the neck for metastatic SCC is a modified radical neck dissection. Important pathologic information obtained from the neck dissection specimen includes the number and location of metastatic lymph nodes as well as the presence or absence of extracapsular nodal spread of tumor. In most instances radiation therapy is delivered postoperatively to the neck to provide adjuvant therapy. In general, radiation therapy is administered to the neck if the neck specimen includes more than one metastatic node, large nodes, or extracapsular nodal tumor spread.

Management of the primary tumor depends on tumor location and size. Oral cavity and select oropharyngeal carcinomas can be resected surgically. Other oropharyngeal and hypopharyngeal carcinomas can be treated definitively with radiation therapy. A multidisciplinary treatment plan designed for the individual patient is recommended.

Most patients with metastatic SCC to the neck have a primary tumor identified. In approximately 10% of patients, however, a primary tumor is not identified, which is referred to as the *unknown primary*. The unknown primary is managed with a modified radical neck dissection and radiation therapy to the neck postoperatively. In addition, radiation therapy is administered to the upper aerodigestive tract, including the nasopharynx, to include the presumed occult primary tumor within the radiation therapy portals. In the setting of HPV-positive unknown primary, radiation of the mucosal sites can be restricted to the oropharynx.

Patients with head and neck SCC should have long-term follow-up for tumor recurrence surveillance and to screen for new primary tumors. Most recurrences become clinically apparent within several years after treatment. An annual chest radiograph is performed. Patients who smoke and consume significant quantities of alcohol should be counseled to abstain from these substances to reduce their risk of metachronous malignancy.

Diagnosis of metastatic carcinoma from an infraclavicular primary should guide an appropriate search for the primary tumor. Appropriate therapy is based on the tumor type and extent of disease. A chest, abdominal, and pelvic CT scan or MRI typically is used for initial evaluation, with other studies guided by the tumor type. The patient may benefit from palliative excision of the metastatic neck node to prevent further growth and tumor-related compromise of neck structures. Such an approach should be incorporated carefully into the overall treatment plan for the patient.

■ POSTERIOR TRIANGLE OF NECK

Extreme caution should be exercised during the surgical excision of neck masses involving the posterior triangle of the neck. The posterior triangle of the neck is bounded anteriorly by the posterior border of the SCM, posteriorly by the anterior border of the trapezius muscle, and inferiorly by the clavicle. The spinal accessory nerve, which innervates the trapezius muscle, courses obliquely through the posterior triangle of the neck and is often superficial in location. Identification and protection of the spinal accessory nerve during excisional biopsy of a posterior triangle neck mass minimizes the risk of injury to the spinal accessory nerve. Nerve identification is performed easily with a battery-powered nerve stimulator. Stimulation of the spinal accessory nerve results in trapezius contraction, which confirms identification of the spinal accessory nerve.

General anesthesia should be considered for surgical excision of posterior triangle neck masses because local anesthetics may render nerve identification difficult because of the local anesthetic effects on the nerve. Numerous cutaneous sensory nerves from the cervical plexus also course through the posterior triangle of the neck, adding to the difficulty of spinal accessory nerve identification. Spinal accessory nerve injury resulting in trapezius denervation can be a debilitating surgical complication. If spinal accessory nerve injury is suspected after surgery in the posterior triangle of the neck, the patient should undergo neck exploration and accessory nerve repair to reestablish trapezius muscle innervation.

SUGGESTED READINGS

Batsakis JG. The pathology of head and neck tumors: the occult primary and metastases to the head and neck. *Head Neck Surg.* 1981;3:409.

Eisele DW, et al. Utility of immediate on-site cytopathological procurement and evaluation in fine needle aspiration biopsy of head and neck masses. *Laryngoscope.* 1992;102:1328.

Galloway TJ, Ridge JA. Management of squamous cancer metastatic to cervical nodes with an unknown primary site. *J Clin Oncol.* 2015;33: 3328-3337.

McQuone SJ, et al. Occult tonsillar carcinoma in the unknown primary. *Laryngoscope.* 1998;108:1605.

Mehta V, Johnson P, et al. A new paradigm for the diagnosis and management of unknown primary tumors of the head and neck: a role for transoral robotic surgery. *Laryngoscope.* 2013;123:146-151.

Reddy SP, Marks JE. Metastatic carcinoma in the cervical lymph nodes from an unknown primary site: results of bilateral neck plus mucosal irradiation vs. ipsilateral neck irradiation. *Int J Radiat Oncol Biol Phys.* 1997;37: 797-802.

Robbins KT, et al. The violated neck: cervical node biopsy prior to definitive treatment. *Otolaryngol Head Neck Surg.* 1986;94:605.

Wang RC, et al. Unknown primary squamous cell carcinoma metastatic to the neck. *Arch Otolaryngol Head Neck Surg.* 1990;116:1388.

HAND INFECTIONS

Christopher L. Forthman, MD

Hand infections are common and often managed by a wide range of medical professionals. These infections can range from isolated and simple to complex with great potential for extensive damage, particularly in select patient populations, including those who are diabetic or immunocompromised. Early recognition of these infections with implementation of treatment is imperative to avoid more complex sequelae and tissue destruction. As with most infections, antibiotic therapy has a central role; however, if there is more than just superficial cellulitis, these infections often require surgical therapy for complete eradication (Table 1).

Any patient with a possible hand infection should undergo a thorough history and complete hand examination, including neurovascular status and evaluation of motion. In addition, specific attention should be paid to hand and finger posture, swelling, skin changes, focal pain, and tenderness, and an examination both proximal and distal to the area of concern should be performed. Comparison should be made between the adjacent nonaffected tissue (e.g., the other fingers) and the contralateral hand.

Hand x-rays should be performed to evaluate for skeletal abnormalities such as bony destruction and the presence of any gas formed by bacteria and to rule out a foreign body. Routine laboratory studies, including complete blood cell count (CBC), erythrocyte sedimentation rate (ESR), and C-reactive protein (CRP), may be performed. The physician should be reminded that laboratory studies often may be indeterminate and clinical judgment ultimately will decide which patients require surgical intervention regardless of specific laboratory results. When possible, cultures should be taken to help tailor antibiotic coverage.

■ MICROBIOLOGY

By far the most common pathogen cultured in hand infections is *Staphylococcus aureus*, which accounts for up to 80% of hand infections in some series. Anaerobes or mixed flora typically make up the remainder of the cultures and are more common in select patient groups, such as those who are diabetic or immunocompromised (e.g., those with human immunodeficiency virus [HIV]). Human bites often contain oral flora such as *Eikenella corrodens*, whereas dog and cat bites may contain *Pasteurella multocida*. Cat scratches may be associated with *Bartonella henselae* and regional lymphadenopathy. Infections resulting from interactions with marine animals may contain *Vibrio* species or *Mycobacterium marinum*.

Methicillin-Resistant *Staphylococcus aureus*

The rate of methicillin resistance in *S. aureus* hand infections ranges from 34% to 78%. Community-acquired methicillin-resistant *Staphylococcus aureus* (MRSA) infections are becoming more common, and patients with MRSA infections often experience a delay in appropriate antibiotic treatment. In urban areas, empiric coverage for MRSA is warranted (Figure 1). When intravenous antibiotics are needed, MRSA is almost always sensitive to vancomycin, daptomycin, and linezolid. Effective oral agents include trimethoprim-sulfamethoxazole, tetracycline, and moxifloxacin. Of note, clindamycin resistance is increasing markedly and may preclude use of this drug for empiric therapy.

Patients Who Are Diabetic or Immunocompromised

The rising populations of patients who are diabetic or immunocompromised mandate that physicians be aware of the rapid downward course that these patients can encounter once infected. These patients may develop polymicrobial abscesses or abscesses with especially virulent bacteria, such as pseudomonas or other gram-negative bacteria. This fact should be considered when choosing antibiotic coverage. In addition, infection spread can be rapid in these patient populations, leading to challenges in treatment and greater morbidity and mortality. Even the simplest infections can lead to devastating complications and impairment in these individuals. These factors necessitate swift evaluation and require a low threshold for surgical exploration to prevent progressive tissue damage.

Bite Wounds

Bite wounds, most commonly from domesticated pets or other humans, contribute significantly to hand infections. With the vast amount of bacteria found in the animal or human mouth, these wounds have the propensity to produce serious infections. There are approximately 2 million cases of animal bite wounds accounting for 1% of emergency room visits each year in the United States. Although the majority of these bites are from dogs, only a small amount of dog bites result in infection, in part because of the destructive nature of canine teeth that leave open wounds. In contrast, cat bites more frequently become infected because feline teeth cause small puncture wounds that are able to inoculate the deeper structures of the upper extremity. These small puncture-type wounds can be the source of a flexor tenosynovitis, dorsal abscesses, or other deep hand infections.

Human "bites" are more often associated with an altercation that involves a direct blow to a person's mouth with a hand. The so-called "fight bite" can result in septic arthritis if the injury inoculates bacteria into an underlying joint. Septic arthritis is seen as a swollen joint that is painful with limited motion. Suspected septic arthritis, particularly after a "fight bite," requires immediate surgical drainage aimed at preventing damage to the articular cartilage.

High-Pressure Injection Injuries

High-pressure injection injuries occur in laborers when fluid is inoculated into the finger from a device such as a paint or grease gun. Amputation is sometimes necessary depending on the substance injected, the pressure of the injection, and the time to treatment. The liquid infiltrates the subcutaneous tissues and spreads along the neurovascular bundles and sometimes through the flexor tendon sheath. The typical punctate skin wound is misleading, as these injuries must be recognized and treated early to minimize tissue necrosis and secondary infection. Extensive surgical débridement and broad-spectrum antibiotics are the mainstays of treatment (Figure 2).

■ FINGER INFECTIONS

Many finger infections that require surgical drainage can be treated under local anesthesia using a digital block. Care should be taken to critically evaluate the patient to be certain that the infection is localized to only the finger. If there is an indication of a more proximal infection (such as flexor tenosynovitis), a wrist block or general anesthesia should be considered.

A digital block is performed by inserting a 25-gauge needle through the skin and into the subcutaneous tissues at the level of the palmar digital crease of the affected digit. Three milliliters of 2% lidocaine or 0.5% Marcaine without epinephrine is injected. A digital tourniquet then can be made by clamping a Penrose drain around the base of the digit. Care must be taken to remove the tourniquet at the completion of the drainage procedure.

Paronychia
Diagnosis

A paronychia is an infection involving the tissue surrounding the lateral fingernail (paronychial fold) or the proximal nail fold (eponychial fold), or extending into the nail matrix. Risk factors include nail

TABLE I: General Recommendations for Hand Infections

Infection	Likely Organism(s)	Initial Antibiotic Therapy*	Surgical Therapy
Cellulitis	*Staphylococcus* or *Streptococcus*	Cephalexin. Use clindamycin or trimethoprim-sulfamethoxazole (Bactrim) for suspected MRSA.	Only indicated for associated abscess
Abscess	*Staphylococcus*	Vancomycin. Add piperacillin-tazobactam (Zosyn) for diabetic or immunocompromised patients.	Immediate drainage (no closure), soaks, and motion the day after surgery
Flexor tenosynovitis	*Staphylococcus*, anaerobes, polymicrobial	Ampicillin-sulbactam (Unasyn). Replace Unasyn with Zosyn for diabetic or immunocompromised patient and add vancomycin if possible MRSA.	Consider 12-24 hours observation for early signs; otherwise, drainage of flexor sheath (no closure), soaks, and motion the day after surgery
Septic arthritis	*Staphylococcus*	Vancomycin. Add ceftriaxone if *Neisseria gonorrhoeae* is suspected.	Immediate drainage (no closure), soaks, and motion the day after surgery
Animal bite	*Pasteurella multocida* is classic, but staphylococcus, streptococcus, and anaerobes are common	Unasyn or PO equivalent. If penicillin allergic, consider fluoroquinolone and clindamycin.	Clean thoroughly in ED and observe closely for signs of a deep infection. Cat teeth inoculate the deep tissues, so consider incising the puncture site to facilitate drainage. Dog teeth tear local tissues and usually will drain spontaneously.
Human bite	*Eikenella corrodens* is classic, but staphylococcus, streptococcus, and anaerobes are common	Unasyn or PO equivalent. If penicillin allergic, consider fluoroquinolone and clindamycin.	Clean thoroughly in ED and observe closely for signs of a deep infection (e.g., abscess, FTS). "Fight bites" require immediate drainage, even in the absence of overt infection.
Necrotizing fasciitis	*Streptococcus* or polymicrobial	Vancomycin *and* clindamycin *and* piperacillin-tazobactam (Zosyn)	Emergent radical débridement(s), hemodynamic monitoring, possible amputation
Gas gangrene	*Clostridium perfringens*, *Streptococcus pyogenes*, *Staphylococcus aureus*, *Vibrio vulnificus*, polymicrobial	Vancomycin *and* clindamycin *and* piperacillin-tazobactam (Zosyn). Consider high-dose penicillin.	Emergent radical débridement(s), hemodynamic monitoring, possible amputation

*Antibiotic coverage should be adjusted once cultures are back from the laboratory to decrease the creation of antibiotic-resistant organisms and to minimize drug side effects to the patient.

ED, Emergency department; *FTS*, flexor tendon sheath; *MRSA*, methicillin-resistant *Staphylococcus aureus*; *PO*, oral.

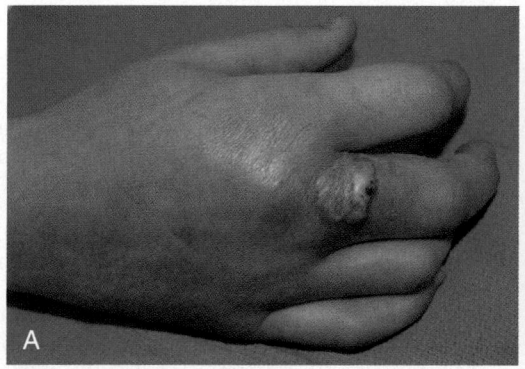
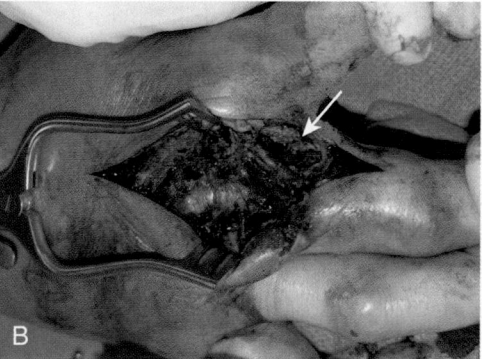

FIGURE I **A,** Methicillin-resistant *Staphylococcus aureus* abscess. The red, swollen region with central necrosis or "spider-bite appearance" is typical. **B,** Infection has entered the web space (*arrow*), a "collar-button" abscess, and will require a palmar incision for adequate drainage.

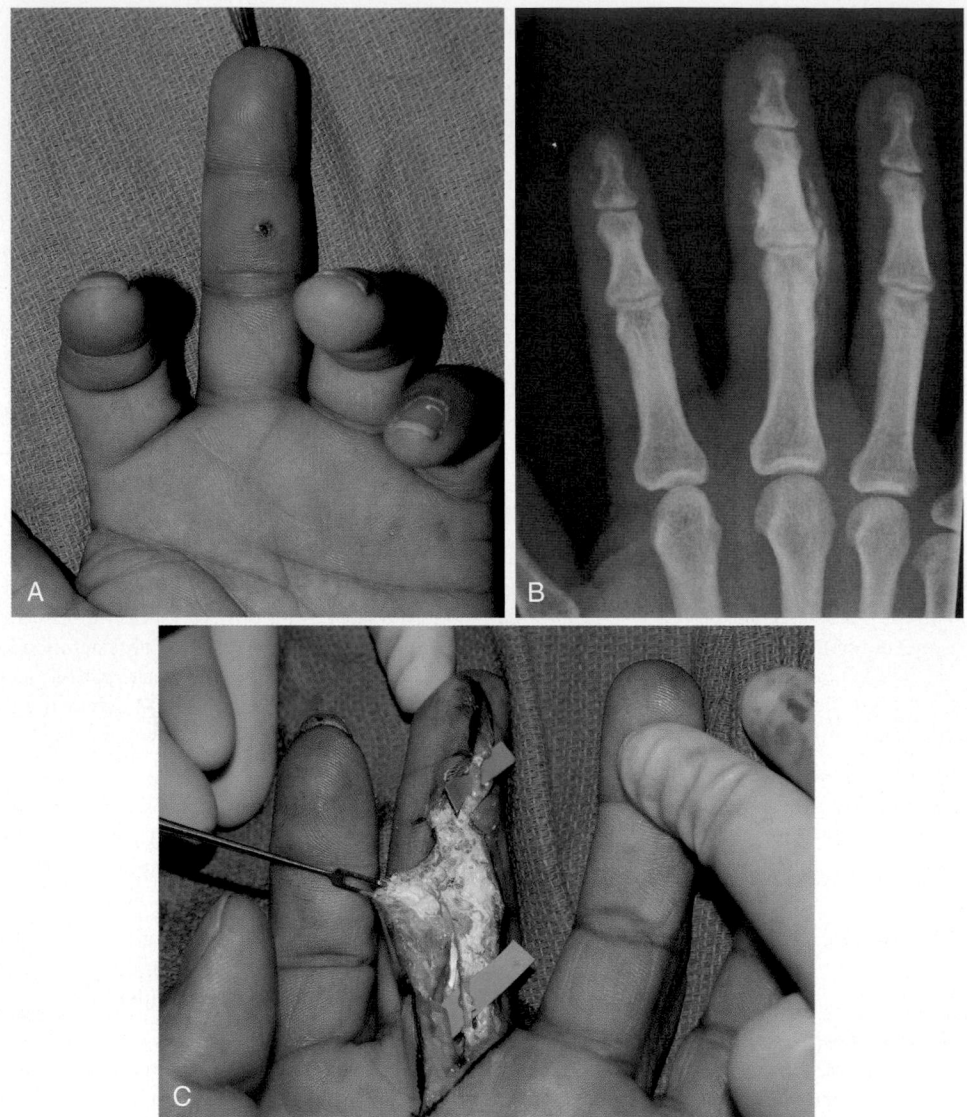

FIGURE 2 A, Red, swollen finger with innocuous appearing punctate wound after high-pressure paint injection injury. **B,** Radiographic appearance. **C,** Intraoperative view with the digital nerve identified proximally and distally.

biting, hangnails, and manicures. The most common inciting organism is *S. aureus*, but inciting organisms also can include oral flora. Typically, a painful swollen area with erythema along the lateral border of the fingernail or beneath the proximal nail fold is the hallmark of an acute paronychia (Figure 3). Purulent drainage or failed conservative therapy with warm soaks necessitates surgical drainage.

Treatment

Early paronychia can be treated with warm soaks several times a day. If a visible or palpable abscess has developed, incision and drainage are needed. The procedure can be done at the bedside or in the office with a digital block. Superficial paronychia can be treated by elevating the nail fold off of the nail plate with an elevator or scalpel to drain the abscess. Infections that have spread below the nail plate require removal of at least part of the nail plate. The nail fold is elevated and a longitudinal strip of nail is cut away on the affected side (Figure 4). If necessary, the entire nail is removed. The wound is irrigated, and daily soaks in warm, soapy water are continued at home. Empiric antibiotic treatment should be initiated with either cephalexin or amoxicillin-clavulanate (Augmentin) to cover the most common pathogens. In areas with frequent community-acquired MRSA,

trimethoprim-sulfamethoxazole (Bactrim) or clindamycin should be used.

Felon

Diagnosis

In the pulp of the fingertip, vertical septa extend from the distal phalanx to the dermis, forming numerous potential spaces. Once inoculated with bacteria, an abscess may develop. The patient usually has a swollen fingertip, throbbing pain, and erythema. The swelling is mostly distal to the distal interphalangeal (DIP) joint, and any extension proximally should raise the suspicion of a flexor tendon sheath infection.

Care should be taken to distinguish a felon from herpetic whitlow, which can have a similar appearance when present at the fingertip (Figure 5). Herpetic whitlow is a viral lesion caused by herpes simplex virus. Whitlow is common in children, dental workers, and other populations frequently exposed to saliva. The disease appears as clear vesicles and mild finger swelling that may resemble a felon. Although the fluid may be turbid or hemorrhagic, it is not purulent and unlike a felon the pulp space does not have increased tension.

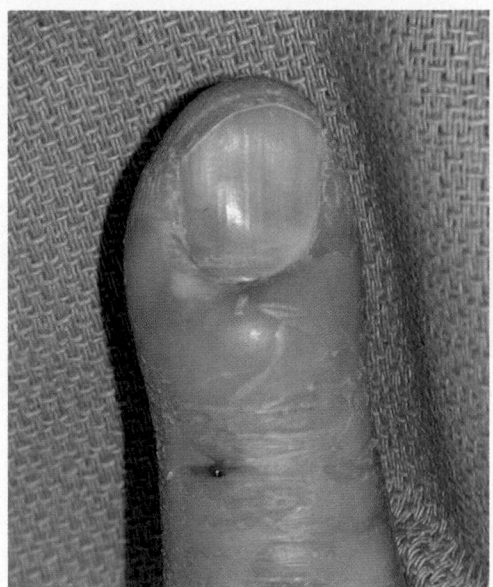

FIGURE 3 Paronychia with pus visible at the paronychial fold and a collection extending below the eponychial fold.

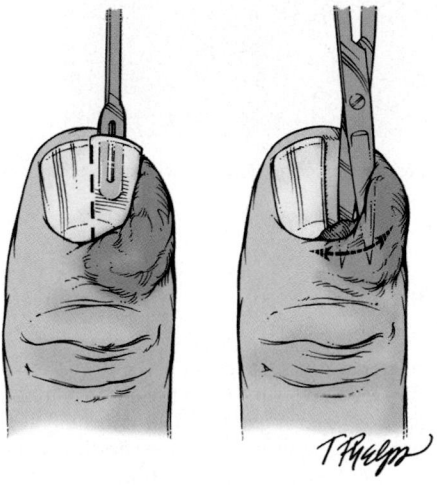

FIGURE 4 Surgical drainage of acute paronychia. The lateral nail on the affected side is elevated gently from the nail bed, and a longitudinal strip of nail is removed. If this does not decompress the infection adequately, the margins of the nail fold are opened gently to drain the adjacent soft tissues.

The diagnosis can be made by sending scrapings from an open vesicle for a Tzanck smear.

Treatment

In the earliest stages of a felon, a trial of warm soaks, elevation, and antibiotics may be initiated; however, surgical decompression is often necessary. Surgical drainage requires a thoughtful skin incision and then blunt dissection with disruption of the pulp septa. Multiple incisions have been described. If the felon is located along the volar midline, a volar longitudinal incision can be made. Otherwise a high lateral incision just below the nail can be performed, avoiding the digital artery or nerve (Figure 6). This incision should be placed on the noncontact side of the affected digit (radial for the thumb and ulnar for the remaining digits) to avoid painful scarring that interferes with pinch. Once careful disruption of the septa has been performed and the fingertip is adequately decompressed, it should be

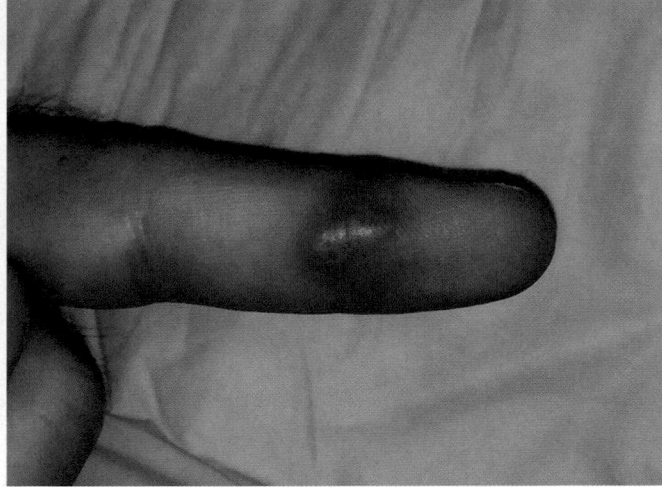

FIGURE 5 Herpetic whitlow may be confused with a felon if the characteristic vesicles of viral infection are overlooked.

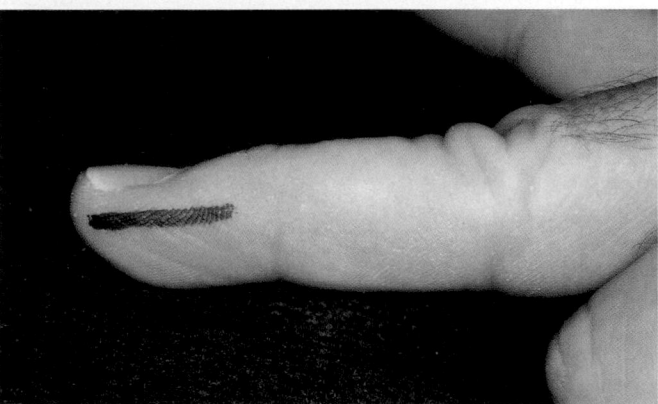

FIGURE 6 A felon can be drained safely through a lateral incision with blunt spreading dorsal to the neurovascular bundle and through the fibrous septa of the pulp.

packed and dressed. Empiric antibiotics are started, followed by soaks and dressing changes the next day.

Pyogenic Flexor Tenosynovitis

Diagnosis

The flexor sheath runs from the distal interphalangeal joint crease to the distal palm crease. Penetrating trauma (e.g., a cat bite) anywhere along this course may allow bacteria to enter the sheath and cause pyogenic flexor tenosynovitis. Failure to institute treatment in a timely manner can have devastating consequences, ranging from tendon adhesions to finger necrosis. Kanavel described four cardinal signs of flexor tenosynovitis: tenderness along the course of the sheath, fixed flexed position of the finger, extreme pain with passive extension of the finger, and fusiform swelling of the affected digit (Figure 7). All of these signs may not be present, but the clinician should evaluate for each and have a low threshold to begin treatment. Early infections (<24 hours) in healthy individuals may be managed with a trial of antibiotics; however, failure to respond or delayed presentation is an indication for surgical débridement.

Treatment

Surgical treatment of pyogenic flexor tenosynovitis includes operative exploration, débridement of necrotic tissue, and flushing of the

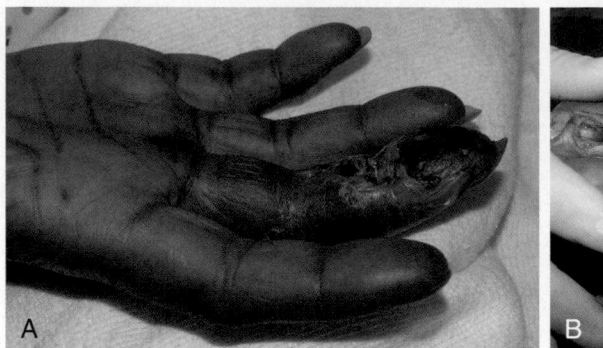
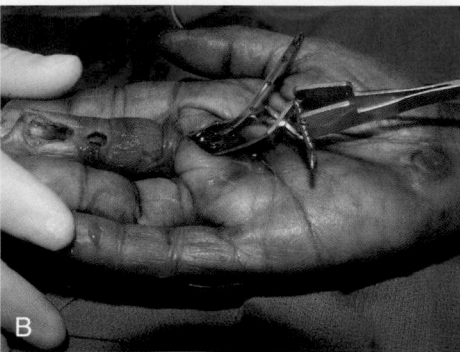

FIGURE 7 A, Late pyogenic flexor tenosynovitis in a patient who is diabetic and immunocompromised. Swelling and a slightly flexed posture are evident. **B,** Necrotic tissue has been débrided, and the sheath is irrigated in a closed fashion.

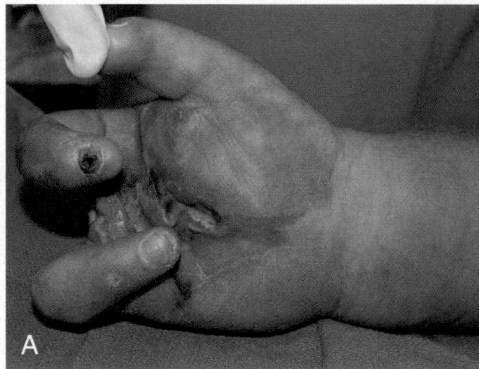
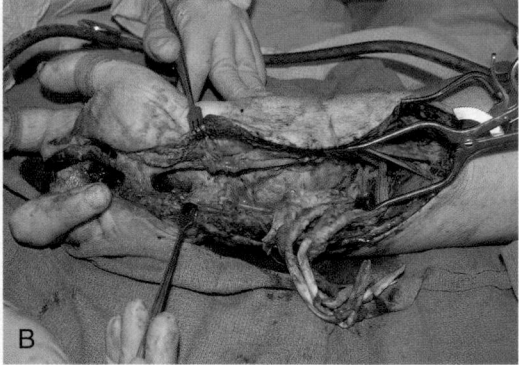

FIGURE 8 A, Inadequate treatment of "finger infections" is manifest as generalized hand and forearm swelling. **B,** Bacterial extension through the carpal tunnel and Parona's space results in a severe, generalized deep volar forearm infection.

tendon sheath. Surgery should be performed in the operating room and may consist of either open or closed sheath irrigation. In open sheath irrigation, the flexor sheath is exposed using either a Brunner-type or a midlateral incision, taking care to not injure the digital neurovascular bundles that reside laterally. The tendon sheath is opened in order to remove all infectious material. Care should be taken to preserve the critical annular pulleys of the digit, with the A2 pulley being located over the proximal part of the proximal phalanx and the A4 pulley located over the middle portion of the middle phalanx. The sheath is irrigated copiously with sterile saline until all purulent material is removed. Any large incisions should be closed loosely.

The alternative method is the closed sheath technique, which involves limited incisions located proximally and distally to allow access to the sheath. The proximal incision is located at the level of the A1 pulley volarly, and the distal incision is placed either midlateral or volar at the distal interphalangeal crease. The sheath is then accessed at both sites, and a pediatric feeding tube or other small intravenous catheter is introduced to allow antegrade irrigation.

After tendon sheath irrigation, the hand should be splinted and elevated, and a course of antibiotics should be prescribed. Wound soaks are then performed several times a day. The wounds can be dressed with gauze and allowed to heal secondarily.

■ HAND INFECTIONS

Some hand infections, such as a dorsal abscess, may be treated in the emergency room with a local field block. The patient requires débridement in the operating room when the infection involves volar spaces or joints.

Bursal Infections

Diagnosis

The flexor tendon sheath of the thumb is continuous with the radial bursa, a thin envelope extending from the flexor pollicis sheath at the level of the metacarpophalangeal (MP) joint through the carpal canal into the forearm. The small finger flexor sheath is continuous with the ulnar bursa, another fine envelope tracking ulnar to the flexor tendons and into the carpal canal and forearm. Infections of the thumb and small finger flexor tendons may propagate along these bursa and into the distal forearm. "Parona's space," a potential space that lies between the pronator quadratus and flexor tendons, may communicate infections between the radial and ulnar sides of the hand. This space also may communicate with the thenar and mid-palmar spaces deep in the palm. Bacterial extension through this communication is generally associated with a severe, generalized deep volar infection. Sometimes the result is a more limited but nonetheless serious radial and ulnar bursal space infection referred to as a "horseshoe" abscess. It is important for the surgeon to be aware of the potential spaces and communications when treating the infected hand. Failure to recognize bacterial extension into these spaces can lead to an incomplete débridement and increased morbidity (Figure 8).

Treatment

Infections that spread along bursa require aggressive débridement in the operating room under general anesthesia. The infected digits should be débrided thoroughly, as previously described for flexor tenosynovitis. Often the extent of the disease is not recognized until the time of surgery. As the infection is followed proximally, care should be taken to avoid making large continuous incisions across

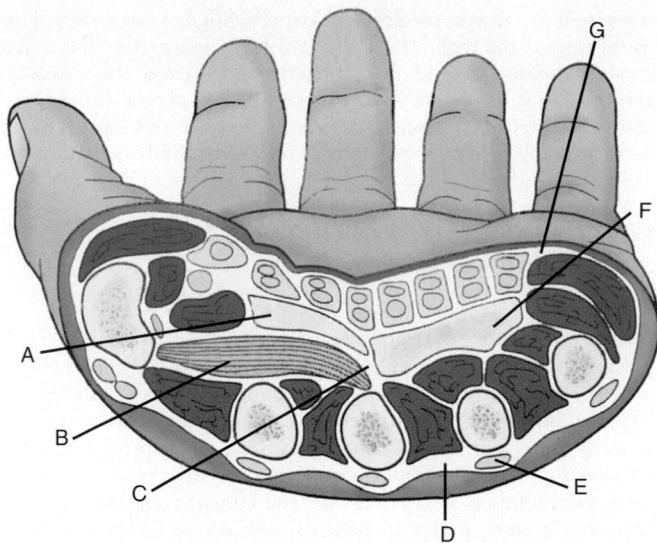

FIGURE 9 Cross-section anatomy of the hand. **A,** Thenar space. **B,** Adductor pollicis. **C,** Midpalmar septum. **D,** Dorsal subaponeurotic space. **E,** Extensor tendon. **F,** Midpalmar space. **G,** Hypothenar space.

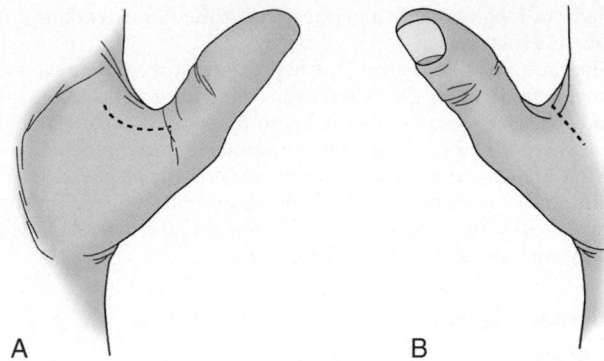

FIGURE 10 Surgical approach for incision and drainage of a thenar space infection. **A,** Transverse incision. **B,** Dorsal longitudinal incision.

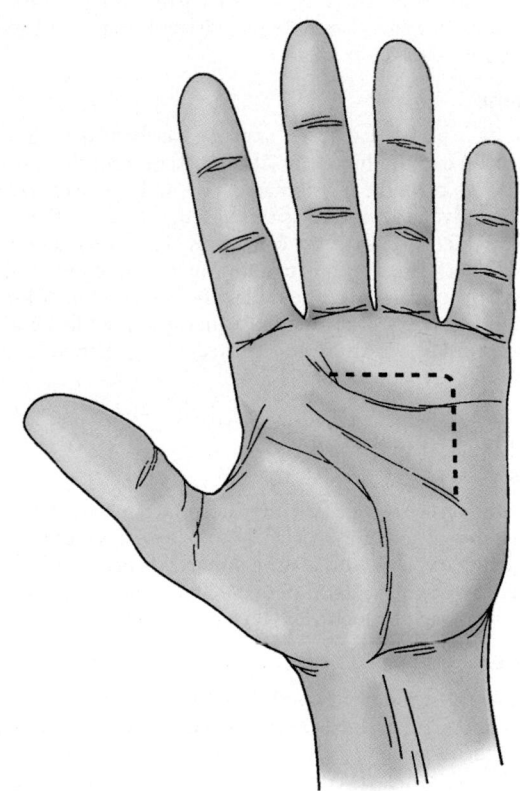

FIGURE 11 Combined longitudinal and transverse incision for drainage of a midpalmar space abscess.

the hand. Separate thenar or hypothenar incisions can be made in the palm, in line with skin creases, and another incision can be placed on the distal volar forearm to inspect for infection in Parona's space. The most severe infections will require an extended carpal tunnel release in order to adequately débride necrotic tissue and infected tenosynovium. After copious irrigation, the wounds can be closed loosely over a drain and the hand splinted. Postoperative care includes appropriate antibiotics, daily dressing changes and soaks, and hand therapy.

Deep Space Infections of the Hand

Thenar, Hypothenar, and Midpalmar Space Abscess

Diagnosis

Three potential spaces that can become infected, with resultant abscess formation, exist in the palm. The interosseous muscles are deep to these spaces and the flexor tendons are superficial (Figure 9).

The thenar space is bordered by the adductor pollicus dorsally, the index finger flexor volarly, the adductor pollicis insertion on the proximal phalanx radially, and the midpalmar septum ulnarly. Infections are often the result of penetrating trauma. The first web space area becomes swollen and exquisitely tender to palpation as the potential space becomes filled with purulent fluid. The thumb may come to rest in an abducted position and have extreme pain on passive adduction or opposition.

The midpalmar space lies between the thenar and hypothenar eminences. The floor is the fascia of the second and third volar interosseous, and the superficial border is the flexor sheaths of the long, ring, and small fingers. The radial and ulnar borders are defined by septa running from the third and fifth metacarpals to the dermis. These septa are termed the oblique septum and hypothenar septum. Infections are most often a result of penetrating trauma or extension from an adjacent infection.

The hypothenar space lies between the hypothenar septum and the hypothenar muscles with the periosteum of the fifth metacarpal as the floor. Infection of this space is rare, as is spread of infection to adjacent areas. The patient may have localized pain and swelling along the hypothenar eminence with absence of swelling elsewhere in the palm or fingers.

Treatment

The thenar space can be approached either dorsally or volarly (Figure 10). The volar approach typically involves an incision along the thenar crease approximately 1 cm proximal to the web space and proceeding proximally. Blunt dissection is then carried out to the adductor pollicis, and the abscess is drained. Care should be taken proximally where the motor branch from the median nerve may be encountered. Dorsal incisions may be transverse or longitudinal, and blunt dissection is then performed to the interval between the first dorsal interosseous and adductor pollicis where the abscess should be encountered. The radial artery may be encountered in this region.

The midpalmar space is approached volarly with a transverse incision at or about the distal palmar crease, a longitudinal incision, or a combination of the two (Figure 11). Blunt dissection is again used to avoid damage to the palmar neurovascular bundles and then carried out longitudinally on either side of the flexor tendons until the abscess is expressed.

Similar to the thenar space, the hypothenar space can be accessed with an incision along the hypothenar eminence, parallel to the fifth metacarpal. The dissection is carried to the level of the hypothenar fascia where the abscess should be encountered and drained.

After drainage and irrigation, all wounds should be closed loosely over drains or packing, and the hand should be splinted. Dressing changes, soaks, or irrigation should begin the next day along with therapy attempts to restore hand function.

Web Space Abscess

Diagnosis

Often referred to as "collar-button" abscesses because of their hour-glass shape, these infections may result from a fissure in the skin between adjacent fingers or from a distal palmar callus or may track from dorsal to volar. There is localized pain and swelling in the affected web space and classically the adjacent fingers are abducted away from the abscess.

Treatment

Drainage of a web space abscess can be performed with a single dorsal incision or a combined dorsal and volar approach. Care should be taken not to place the incision across the web space or to connect the dorsal and volar incisions, as this will decrease the ability of the fingers to abduct because of the contracting scar. After skin incision, dissection is performed bluntly to allow full egress of purulent material. After irrigation, a drain should be placed in each incision, but a through-and-through drain for both incisions should be avoided. The hand should be splinted and daily dressing changes and soaks should begin the following day.

Dorsal Hand Abscesses

Diagnosis

Dorsal hand abscesses can be either deep, occupying the so-called "subaponeurotic" potential space below the extensors, or subcutaneous. The depth of the abscess may be difficult to distinguish clinically. The patient typically has focal pain, swelling, and erythema. Dorsal abscesses also may develop in the fingers (Figure 12).

Treatment

Although simple cellulitis responds favorably to antibiotics, fluctuant infections must be drained. Most dorsal hand abscesses may be drained in the emergency department under a local field or regional block. If the clinician is certain that the abscess is in the subcutaneous tissue, a simple longitudinal incision can be made over the most prominent part of the abscess in order to fully express the infectious

material. If the abscess seems deep, a longitudinal incision should be biased toward the region over the second metacarpal or the space between the fourth and fifth metacarpal to avoid the extensor tendons. Blunt dissection is then performed to expose the abscess below the extensor tendons and fully express the pus. Irrigation is performed, followed by loose closure and a splint. Early hand motion is initiated when possible.

■ NECROTIZING FASCIITIS OF THE UPPER EXTREMITY

Diagnosis

Necrotizing fasciitis is a rapidly progressive, potentially fatal bacterial infection that most commonly spreads along the fascial planes of the muscles (Figure 13). In the upper extremity it is most common in diabetics, alcoholics, and intravenous drug users, with some reports showing more than half of these infections being precipitated by self-injection. The presentation may be delayed several days after initial symptoms. It is essential that the clinician maintain a high suspicion for this disease in patients with severe upper extremity infections. Symptoms may include extreme pain, blistering and bullae, skin hemorrhage or loss, rapid progression, and crepitus. If there is any suspicion for necrotizing fasciitis, immediate resuscitation and empiric intravenous antibiotics should be initiated, followed

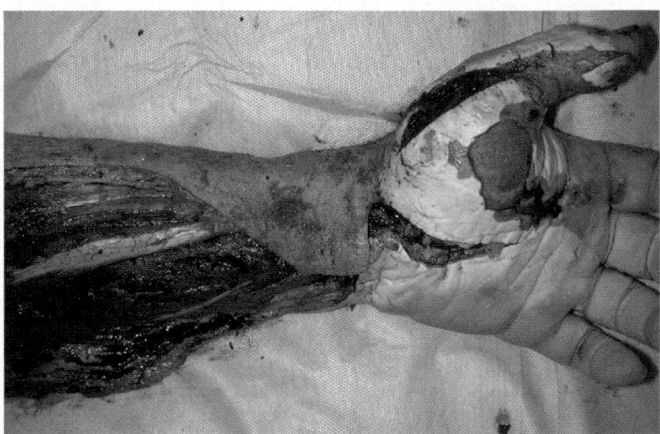

FIGURE 13 A 78-year-old patient had systemic illness and a rapidly progressing dominant arm soft tissue infection. Early and aggressive management with serial wide surgical débridement, negative pressure therapy, and subsequent delayed closure allowed for preservation of the limb. Tissue sample confirmed the diagnosis of necrotizing fasciitis. *(From McDonald LS, et al. Hand infections,* J Hand Surg Am. *2011;36:1403-1412.)*

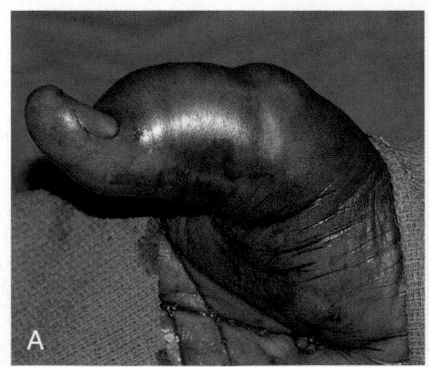 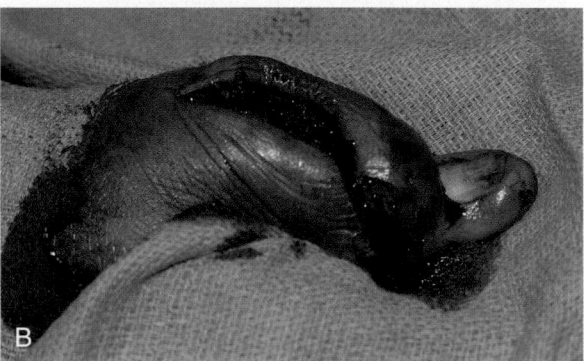

FIGURE 12 **A,** A large dorsal abscess is anatomically separated from the palmar tissues by finger ligaments (Cleland and Grayson). **B,** The abscess is drained by a linear incision made over the path of greatest fluctuance.

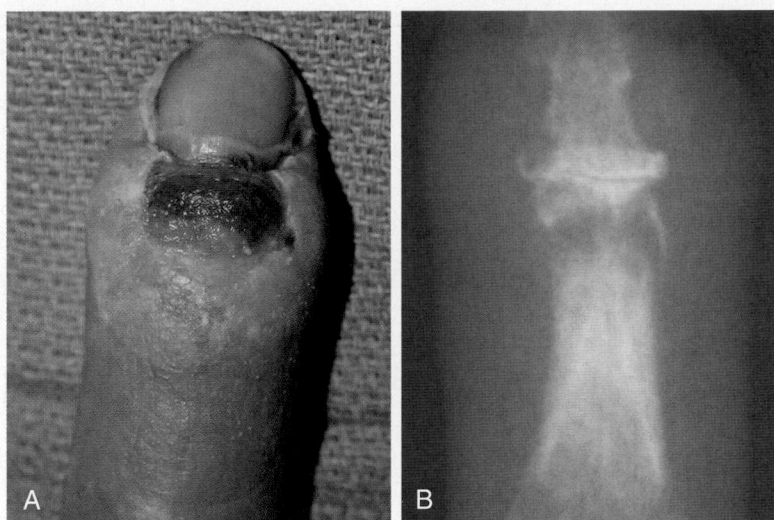

FIGURE 14 Osteomyelitis of the middle finger as a complication of pyarthrosis of the distal interphalangeal (DIP) joint. **A,** Granulation tissue overlying the DIP joint. **B,** Radiograph shows characteristic metaphyseal rarefaction and osteopenia. *(From Wolfe S, et al. Green's Operative Hand Surgery. 6th ed. Philadelphia: Churchill-Livingstone; 2010.)*

immediately by surgical débridement. The most common pathogen is *Streptococcus pyogenes* (Group A streptococcus), although some cases may be polymicrobial or contain other bacteria such as anaerobes. With the rising incidence of MRSA, more MRSA-related necrotizing fasciitis cases are being encountered.

Treatment

After resuscitation, the patient should be taken urgently to the operating room. Patient outcomes for necrotizing fasciitis are directly linked to adequacy and timing of débridement. Exsanguination of the extremity should be avoided so as to not milk the bacteria proximally. Débridement requires longitudinal incisions along the affected extremity with liberal removal of infected and devitalized tissue. Amputation may be necessary. Tissue samples should be taken for culture. The classic finding is "dishwater pus," a thin, foul-smelling fluid along the fascial planes, along with thrombosis of the microvasculature in the affected area. The fascia may appear gray or grayish-green and swollen. The surgeon should have a low threshold for extending incisions and further débridement because the possibility of missing large pockets of purulent material can have devastating consequences. After removal of all infected tissue, the wounds should be irrigated copiously and left open. Dressing changes should be started within 24 hours and be done 2 to 3 times a day. The patient likely will require multiple débridements occurring every couple of days until it is certain that all infectious and devitalized tissue has been removed. These patients may require soft tissue reconstruction once the infection is eradicated.

■ OSTEOMYELITIS

Diagnosis

Osteomyelitis in the hand can result from penetrating trauma, septic arthritis, other deep infections, or seeding of the bone from bacteremia. Injured bones, either from trauma or surgery, are particularly susceptible because of the damaged cortex, which allows pathogen penetration. Plain x-rays may show signs of bony destruction, although this typically appears several weeks after the infection has begun (Figure 14). Magnetic resonance imaging or bone scan will help with early detection. The gold standard for diagnosis is tissue culture and bone biopsy with pathologic confirmation.

Treatment

Although it is possible for early cases of osteomyelitis to be treated with intravenous antibiotics alone, treatment often requires surgery. Draining wounds, abscess, and areas of necrotic bone should be washed out and débrided to a margin of healthy bone and soft tissues. Necrotic soft bone is easily débrided with a rongeur or osteotome until firm, hard bone is encountered. The presence of hardware may make eradication of the infection difficult. Any implantable hardware should be considered for removal, especially if it is loose or no longer needed for stability. External fixators can provide provisional fixation during the interim. Antibiotics should be culture driven when possible and should be administered intravenously for 4 to 6 weeks. The surgeon should have a low threshold for an infectious disease consultation to aid with antibiotic tailoring and duration.

SUGGESTED READINGS

Osterman M, Draeger R, Stern P. Acute hand infections. *J Hand Surg Am.* 2014;39:1628-1635.

Sunderland IR, Friedrich JB. Predictors of mortality and limb loss in necrotizing soft tissue infections of the upper extremity. *J Hand Surg Am.* 2009;34:1900-1901.

Tosti R, Samuelsen B, Bender S, et al. Emerging multidrug resistance of methicillin-resistant *Staphylococcus aureus* in hand infections. *J Bone Joint Surg Am.* 2014;96:1535-1540.

NERVE INJURY AND REPAIR

Marie-Noëlle Hébert-Blouin, MD,
and Robert J. Spinner, MD

Nerve lesions can be traumatic, iatrogenic, neoplastic, or inflammatory in origin; they can be partial or complete, can involve any part of the body, and may lead to significant impairment and disability. The management of nerve injuries involves principles and techniques that differ from those used to treat other injuries. Answering five simple questions related to nerve injuries—what, when, how, why, and who—gives a medical care provider a platform on which to approach nerve injuries.

▪ WHAT IS THE NERVE INJURY?

The first step in the treatment of nerve injuries is to determine *what* nerve injury has been sustained by the patient; this in turn will dictate the right treatment. The nerve injury is defined by the mechanism of injury, the degree of injury, and the nerve components affected by the injury. The mechanism of injury may be penetrating, such as a sharp or ragged laceration, or nonpenetrating, such as occurs with overstretching, blunt, or compressive trauma. Nerve injuries caused by gunshot wounds are considered nonpenetrating injuries because the nerve damage is generally due to the shock wave along the tract of the projectile and not the tract itself; contrary to common belief, the affected nerves are rarely severed.

The extent of nerve injury is determined by a careful neurologic assessment done by clinical and often electrophysiologic examinations to determine the severity of the injury. A detailed knowledge of the anatomy and expected deficits for each nerve or plexus element involved is therefore essential to document complete or partial motor or sensory loss of function in the nerve distribution. Finally, determining the degree of injury—as neurapraxia, axonotmesis, or neurotmesis using Seddon's or Sunderland's classification of nerve injuries—may help to determine if and when a nerve injury requires a surgical intervention (Table 1).

Nerves (Figure 1) are composed of axons, myelin sheaths, and supporting connective tissues (endoneurium, perineurium, and epineurium). The endoneurium surrounds the axons, which are grouped into fascicles. Each fascicle is surrounded by a thin perineurium, which in turn is surrounded by interfascicular epineurium. The main nerve is surrounded by an external epineurial sheath, and blood supply to the nerve travels through a final layer of connective tissue, referred to as the paraneurium or mesoneurium, that also allows nerve gliding during normal range of motion. Injuries involve these components to variable degrees. If the injury is limited, neurologic function may recover—for example, if only the myelin is injured, recovery will occur. In contrast, if the injury involves all components, surgical repair is needed. It is sometimes difficult to assign a classification to a particular injury; the mechanism of injury, the degree of deficit, and the presence or absence of recovery over time helps to classify the injury and to determine if a surgical intervention would be beneficial.

▪ WHAT ARE THE TREATMENT OPTIONS?

Various options are available for the treatment of nerve injury and include observation; neurolysis; direct nerve repair; nerve graft; nerve transfer, which may be direct or via interpositional graft; nerve reimplantation; tendon or muscle transfer, including free functioning muscle transfer; and bone or joint procedures. Each repair option has its own indications (Table 2). Inherent limitations include (1) speed of regeneration (1 mm/day or 1 inch/month); (2) distance from repair site; (3) muscle atrophy or neuromuscular junction degeneration; (4) limited availability of functional donors or graft materials; and (5) expected outcomes, which may determine best use of resources. These limitations are reflected in the differences between the management of an individual injured nerve and the management of multiple injured nerves. Although a single nerve injury in the distal part of an extremity can be reconstructed effectively, multiple nerve injuries, such as from a brachial plexus lesion, may be only partially reconstructed, in which case functions requiring reconstruction must be prioritized and expectations must be limited. For example, in severe injuries, reconstructive efforts are aimed at restoration of elbow flexion, shoulder stability, shoulder abduction and external rotation, hand sensibility, grasp, wrist and finger extension, and intrinsic hand function, in that order.

▪ WHEN IS SURGERY INDICATED?

Deciding if and *when* a patient with a nerve injury would benefit from a surgical intervention is crucial. The window of opportunity for repair of a nerve injury is limited; early surgery or early referral is important.

Pathophysiology

Understanding the pathophysiology of nerve injury underscores the importance of the timing of nerve repair and therefore will be discussed briefly. Three broad scenarios are possible. The first scenario occurs when there is focal or segmental demyelination with preservation of the axon (neurapraxia), the neurologic deficit being secondary to a conduction block. As the myelin heals, functional recovery occurs spontaneously, often within days. Usually by 6 weeks, recovery is complete. In this scenario, no surgical intervention is indicated. A common example is a wrist drop from radial nerve palsy caused by pressure from prolonged compression in one position, so-called *Saturday night palsy*.

The second scenario is characterized by axonal injury (axonotmesis). When an axon is injured, its proximal portion, the part connected to the neuron cell body, remains intact and viable. The distal portion of the axon, now disconnected from the neuron cell body, will undergo Wallerian degeneration (the myelin sheath and cellular debris will be phagocytized). The proximal axon will attempt to regenerate by sprouting (generating multiple growth cones) and growing approximately 1 mm per day or 1 inch per month. If the supporting tissues of the nerve—the endoneurium, perineurium, and epineurium—are sufficiently intact, the regenerating axons will be guided appropriately and will reach the distal target, the neuromuscular junctions or sensory receptors, within months or even years, depending on the distance from the zone of injury. If and when spontaneous recovery occurs, it usually gives better results than any surgical intervention could.

The third scenario occurs when the axon and its surrounding tissues are injured, either partially (axonotmesis) or completely (neurotmesis), such as damage that occurs after a transection injury. The regenerating axon sprouts will not be able to be guided toward the end organ. They will create a neuroma, if the nerve is transected, or a neuroma-in-continuity, if the nerve is significantly injured but in continuity, such as in more severe axonotmetic injuries. In these cases, surgery is required for return of function.

It is important to highlight that the distal nerve segment will still have viable axons, which can transmit electrical stimulation for up to 72 to 96 hours. This may be important when repairing a mixed or predominantly motor nerve acutely because the distal nerve endings when stimulated can still result in motor contraction; this can help to map motor fascicles.

Regeneration starts at the time of repair and proceeds at a rate of 1 mm per day from the repair site. However, with time, generally 18 to 24 months after the injury, the neuromuscular junctions undergo

TABLE 1: Classification and Expected Recovery of Nerve Injuries

Classifications		Nerve Component Injured					Expected Recovery		
Seddon	Sunderland Degree (Modified)	Myelin	Axon	Endoneurium	Perineurium	Epineurium	Extent	Rate	Surgery Indicated
Neurapraxia	First	X					Complete	Fast	No
Axonotmesis	Second	X	X				Good	Slow	Not usually
	Third	X	X	X			Variable	Slow	Variable
	Fourth	X	X	X	X		None	None	Yes
Neurotmesis	Fifth	X	X	X	X	X	None	None	Yes
	Sixth	Combination of injury					Variable	Variable	Variable

X, Injury.

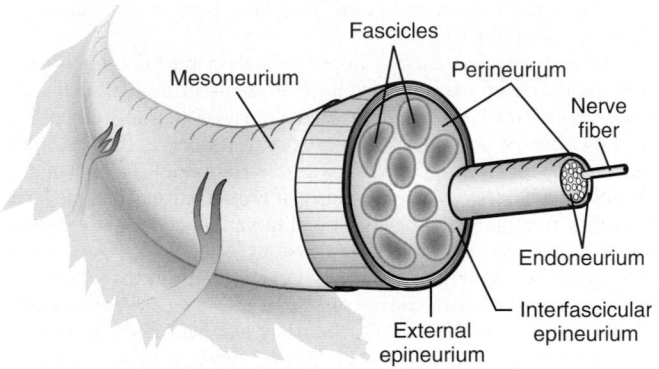

FIGURE 1 The normal anatomy of the peripheral nerve.

Labels: Fascicles, Perineurium, Mesoneurium, Nerve fiber, Endoneurium, Interfascicular epineurium, External epineurium

irreversible damage, and the muscles undergo irreversible atrophy and fibrosis. After this period, even if a functional axon would reach the muscle, little meaningful function will return. This explains why repair of nerve injury must occur early and why some injuries, if very proximal, may not recover significantly, even if repaired immediately (e.g., ulnar nerve injury in the proximal upper arm, supplying the distal hand muscles). Because sensory receptors do not undergo degeneration, sensory recovery theoretically can occur longer after injury, even after 5 years.

Timing

Optimal surgical timing is an essential factor for successful nerve repair. The timing of surgery is based on the scenarios discussed earlier and can be simplified by the "3 plus 1" rule (Table 3), with early repair occurring within 3 days, subacute repair around 3 weeks, delayed repair within 3 to 6 months, and late repair after 1 year.

Early repair, occurring within 3 days after the injury or at presentation if evaluated after 3 days, is indicated in cases of suspected transection with sharp injuries, when the transected nerve will not recover function spontaneously (Figure 2). It is also indicated in situations with vascular (e.g., hematoma, pseudoaneurysm) or bony injuries causing acute nerve compression, especially if they occur in the vicinity of a closed compartment. If a neurologic examination worsens acutely under close observation, the nerve damage potentially can be reversed or reduced by immediate surgical intervention.

Subacute repair, occurring around 3 weeks after injury, is advocated by some for blunt or ragged transections (e.g., by propeller blades or chainsaw), but others still treat these injuries acutely. Again,

TABLE 2: Treatment Options and Indications for Repair of Nerve Injuries

Options	Indications
Observation	Recovering nerve injury Partial nerve injury
Neurolysis	Neuroma-in-continuity with positive NAP
Direct repair	Laceration Short gap after resection of a neuroma-in-continuity with negative NAP
Nerve graft	Laceration with retracted stumps (delayed repair) Larger gap after resection of a neuroma-in-continuity with negative NAP Direct repair without tension not possible
Nerve conduits (autogenous or synthetic)	Short gaps (<3 cm) of small diameter, usually sensory nerves (e.g., digital nerves)
Nerve transfer	Avulsions (brachial plexus avulsion) Specific cases of nerve injury for which nerve transfer may lead to a more rapid and reliable recovery (i.e., because of proximity to end organ) than proximal nerve grafting Innervation of free functioning muscle transfers
Direct neurotization	Under investigation for direct muscle reinnervation after severe trauma
Nerve reimplantation	Under investigation
Tendon or muscle transfers	Delayed (>1 year) for improvement of function
Bony or joint procedures	Delayed (>1 year) for improvement of function
Amputation	Rarely indicated; sometimes desired by patients

NAP, Nerve action potential.

TABLE 3: "3 Plus 1" Rule for Timing of Nerve Repair

Timing	Time	Injury Type	Injury Classification
Early	3 days	Sharp laceration or transection Acute nerve compression resulting from vascular (e.g., hematoma, pseudoaneurysm) or bony injuries Acute neurologic worsening under close observation	Neurotmesis
Subacute	3 weeks	Blunt transection Ragged transection	Neurotmesis
Delayed	3 months	Lesions-in-continuity (nonpenetrating injuries such as stretch injuries, contusive injuries, gunshot wounds)	Axonotmesis
Late	>1 year	Salvage procedures	Neurotmesis or axonotmesis

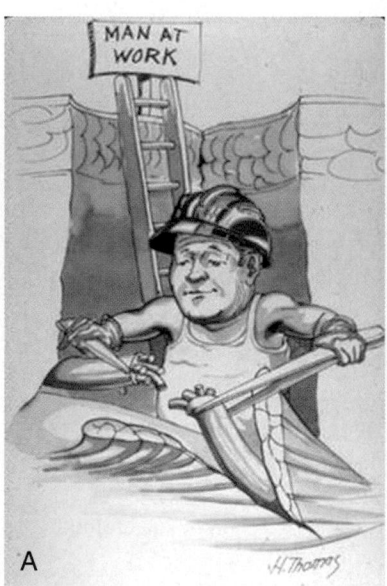
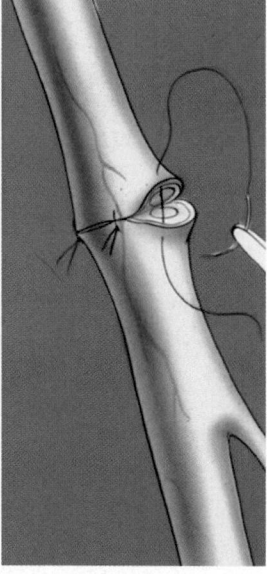

FIGURE 2 **A,** A transected or ruptured nerve cannot recover function spontaneously. This type of neurotmetic injury, a Sunderland grade 5 injury, requires surgical repair. **B,** If possible, direct nerve repair with end-to-end suture is the preferred technique. Epineurial sutures are shown; epineurial vessels are used to align nerve ends.

this situation is clearly one of neurotmesis. Those who advocate waiting for several weeks stress the importance of allowing the zone of injury to define itself with time, manifested by changes caused by Wallerian degeneration that occur during this period. At the time of repair, the nerve endings can be resected back to healthy tissue, which would be difficult to evaluate if the injured nerves were explored immediately after the injury.

In contrast, advocates for earlier surgery feel that surgery is easier and more practical at an earlier time, especially if done at the same time that surgical intervention is performed by another team, such as a general, vascular, or orthopedic surgical team. Furthermore, the additional technical challenges of dealing with spontaneous or postoperative scarring can be avoided. For example, if a patient with a fracture and associated nerve palsy is being explored by an orthopedist, it would be reasonable to explore the nerve at the same time. If the nerve is found to be in continuity but nonfunctional, observation for several months is indicated (note that intraoperative electrophysiologic testing would not be reliable or helpful in predicting recovery or acutely determining the grade of injury). If the nerve is found to be ruptured, some would repair it at the same time.

Others would perform the surgery at a second stage, when the zone of injury can be better defined; nerve ends are tacked down under tension so they do not retract, using radiopaque clips or staples so that they can be identified easily. At a later time, a subacute nerve repair can be done.

Delayed repair, occurring approximately 3 months but up to 6 months after injury, is indicated for lesions-in-continuity, such as the majority of stretch injuries, contusive injuries, and gunshot wounds. In these cases, it is difficult to predict with certainty which path the nerve injury will follow from those described previously and whether the injury will recover spontaneously or require surgical repair. Nonoperative treatment can be continued in patients with early signs of spontaneous recovery or in partial lesions. Note that 90% of nerves that recover do so within 4 months. Surgery is indicated when there has been no evidence of clinical or electrical recovery after this period of observation. In these cases, the delay also will allow lesions-in-continuity to be evaluated intraoperatively with nerve action potential (NAP) testing, described later, to distinguish between recovering lesions and nonrecovering lesions that require repair.

Late surgery, occurring more than 1 year after injury, may be considered a salvage procedure in patients who are seen in a delayed fashion or in those who either have not recovered or have recovered incompletely after spontaneous recovery or previous nerve surgery. Nerve repair and reconstruction typically does not work well after this period, which can be considered to be as short as 9 months by some surgeons, because of permanent changes at the muscular level. The one exception might be distal nerve transfers (those performed close to the end organ), which can be performed in select cases even up to 18 months after injury. However, reconstructive options addressing muscles, tendons, bones, and joints may be useful.

■ TREATMENT FOR NERVE INJURY

The management and surgical treatment of nerve injury involves the application of general principles that are relevant to all nerve surgeries and of specific nerve repair techniques particular to each situation.

General Principles
Preoperative Assessment

Preoperative assessment of the nerve injury should include a detailed history of the mechanism of the injury and onset of the deficit; a physical examination (i.e., neurologic, vascular, and musculoskeletal assessment); electrodiagnostic studies, such as electromyogram and nerve conduction studies; and appropriate imaging, which may include radiographs, ultrasound, computed tomography, magnetic resonance imaging, and/or myelogram.

A sensory and motor function grading system, such as the Medical Research Council (MRC) muscle grading system, should be used to document the initial physical examination and each subsequent

TABLE 4: Key Operative Principles of Nerve Repair

Preparation for repair	Know the anatomy.
	Plan adequate exposure and plan for the possible need for additional exposure.
	Plan for nerve graft harvest.
	Expose normal segment of nerve first, then find pathologic segment.
	Dissect down to the nerve, then dissect along it.
	Dissect between the muscle groups.
	Preserve vascular structures.
Repair	Use nerve action potential to evaluate neuroma-in-continuity.
	Prepare nerve endings.
	Use microsurgical technique.
	Perform a tension-free nerve repair.
	Simpler is better.

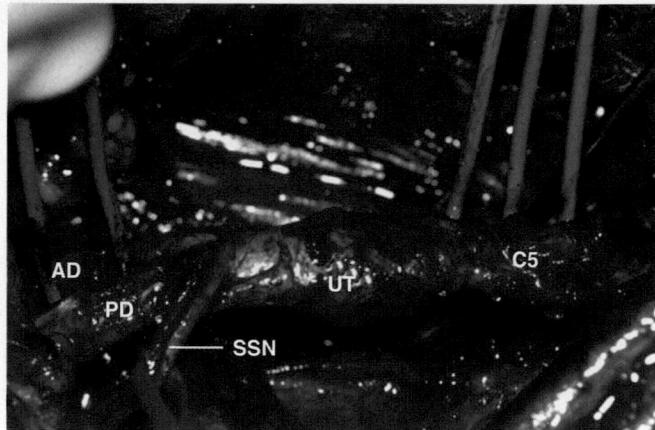

FIGURE 3 Intraoperative photograph showing a nerve action potential (NAP) being recorded. The NAP is tested across a neuroma-in-continuity at the level of the upper trunk (UT) of the brachial plexus. The C5 spinal nerve, the UT, the anterior (AD) and posterior (PD) divisions of the UT, and the suprascapular nerve (SSN) are seen. The C6 spinal nerve contributing to the UT is not seen in this view. The stimulating electrode (three prongs) is seen proximal to the neuroma-in-continuity; the recording electrode (two prongs) is seen distal to it.

examination. The grading system will help to measure the outcomes of observation and surgical interventions. After determining the type of nerve injury and that surgery is indicated, patients should be adequately informed. Making patients aware of the limitations of nerve reconstruction surgery can produce more realistic expectations and more satisfied patients.

Key Operative Principles

At surgery, the steps taken to expose the injured nerve before the nerve repair itself are important (Table 4). Knowledge of the anatomy is crucial, especially when scarring from the injury is expected and likely will distort the anatomy. Adequate exposure should be planned, including the possibility of harvesting nerve grafts. Dissection usually is done between two muscle groups parallel to the long axis of the nerve. Ideally, a normal segment of the nerve is identified first, both proximally and distally, before dissection is carried toward the injured segment. If the injured segment is near a compression site, such as the median nerve near the carpal tunnel, then the site of compression should be released at this time. For practical purposes, there are two possibilities: the identification of a neuroma-in-continuity or nerve stumps.

If there is a neuroma-in-continuity (Figure 3), intraoperative NAP recordings can be performed to assess the degree of injury (recovery or no recovery). In our opinion, these are helpful because gross inspection or palpation of a neuroma-in-continuity does not predict histology, recovery, or outcomes. Furthermore, NAP can determine recovery across a short segment of nerve (i.e., proximal and distal to an injury) before recovery can be seen by physical examination or conventional electromyogram. When a NAP is present (+) across a lesion, the lesion should not be resected, as the outcome generally will be better with neurolysis alone. If a NAP is absent (–) across a lesion, the outcomes are generally poor if the lesion is left intact; therefore surgical repair is indicated.

If two nerve ends suggestive of a rupture or transection are identified or if a nerve end suspicious for an avulsion is found, a nerve repair or reconstruction is indicated. The use of NAP recordings still can be helpful in these situations and can allow identification of the proximal location at which nerve grafting can be performed. Some use NAP in brachial plexus avulsion injuries to define preganglionic responses. Others use other techniques, including somatosensory evoked potential (SSEP) and motor evoked potential (MEP), to assess whether the proximal nerve stump is intact and can be used for reinnervation.

For the nerve repair, microsurgical techniques, which involve the use of micro instruments and of a microscope or magnifying loupes

(Figure 4), should be used. The nerve ends on both sides should be prepared by removing sharply the neuroma and scar tissue, until normal fascicular structures are obtained. The fascicles that protrude past the cut nerve ending should be divided further until all of the fascicles lie flush with the epineurial sheath. This is critical so that the fascicles do not overlap once the epineurium is sutured. Optimal microsurgical technique will cause minimal surgical trauma and permit an end-to-end repair (see Figure 2) or interpositional grafting; it is further recommended that 8-0, 9-0, or 10-0 sutures be used, and using the fewest number of sutures to approximate the nerve accurately is preferred. The repair must be without tension to obtain good results. Fibrin glue may be used to reinforce the suture line, but other methods involve the use of fibrin glue alone or with a variety of nerve conduits (entubulation).

Postoperative Management

Postoperatively, the nerve repair should be protected for 3 weeks. After this period, early protected mobilization is started to promote neural gliding. During the observation period, physical therapy should be continued. Careful sequential clinical and electrophysiologic examinations should be performed to assess neurologic function, and these can be compared with baseline examinations. The Tinel's sign, which consists of a sensation of tingling in the distribution of the nerve caused by percussion over the nerve, is indicative of nerve regeneration. Percussion should be performed from a distal site to a more proximal one, and the exact location of the Tinel's sign should be recorded using topographic landmarks. The Tinel's sign should advance (move distally) in cases of recovery; with time, the Tinel's sign at the distal site should be stronger than the one at the suture line.

Once reinnervation has started, sensory and motor re-education can improve functional recovery. Occasionally patients have paresthesia and dysesthesia in the neurosensory territories. These can be treated with neuropathic pain medications, such as gabapentin or pregabalin, and patients can undergo a desensitization program. Patients who underwent nerve repairs should be followed for at least 2 years in children and for up to 5 years in adults, because the regeneration distance is longer in adults. However, in some pediatric cases, such as with brachial plexus injuries, even longer follow-up is needed to ensure that secondary deformities (e.g., shoulder deformities) that could be addressed are not developing.

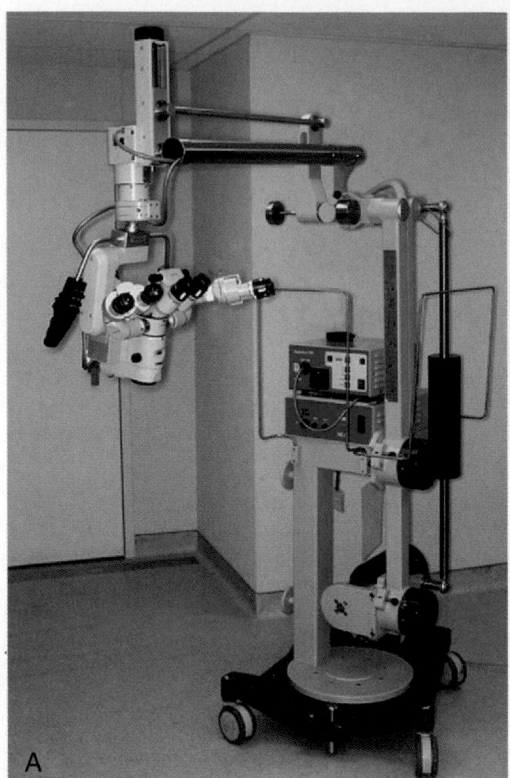
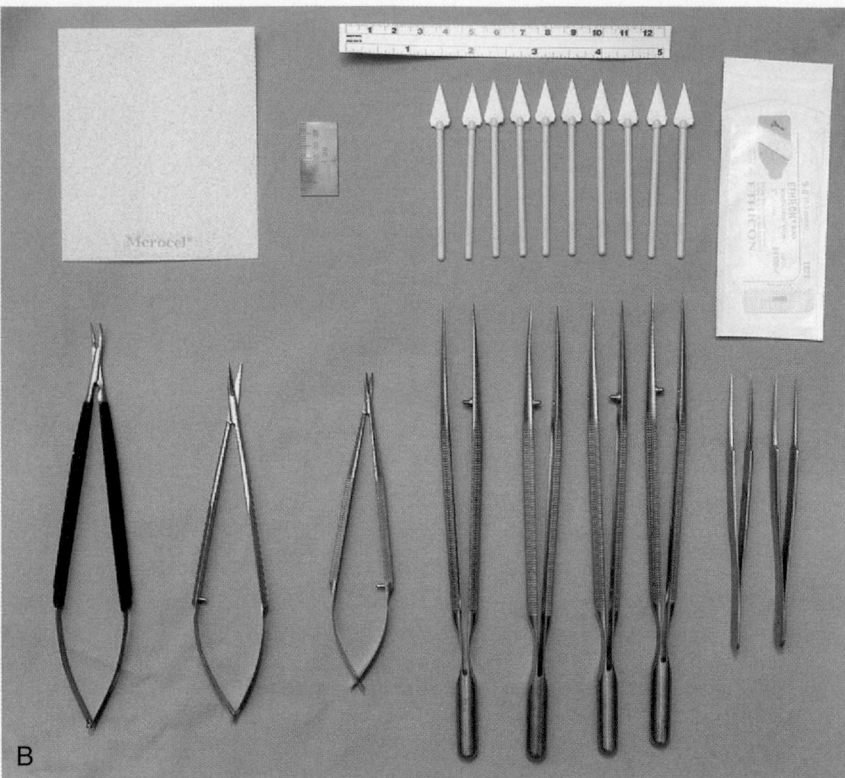

FIGURE 4 **A,** Microscope used for the repair of nerve injury. **B,** A basic microsurgical instrument tray for repair of nerve injuries.

Techniques for Nerve Surgery

Neurolysis

Neurolysis, defined as releasing scar tissue surrounding the injured nerve, is indicated when a neuroma-in-continuity conducting a NAP is found. In general, external neurolysis, which is completed during the nerve exposition, is sufficient. In select instances, some advocate limited internal neurolysis, or removal of the scar tissue between the various nerve fascicles.

Direct Repair

Direct nerve repair is the end-to-end suture of nerve stumps (see Figure 2). It is indicated when a short nerve gap exists, either from a sharply transected nerve—such as a cut from glass, a knife, or a razor—or after removing a focal neuroma-in-continuity that did not conduct a NAP (Figures 5 and 6). Direct repair is the preferred method of nerve repair whenever possible, assuming that the damaged segment of the nerve has been resected and that the sutures are without tension. This method allows direct delivery of proximal axons to the distal stump via a single suture line. It also usually permits fascicular alignment, which increases matching between motor and sensory axons and their targets (Figure 7).

Both epineurial repair and grouped fascicular repair can achieve fascicular alignment. If a small nerve gap is present, several methods can be used to reduce the gap and achieve a direct repair. Commonly used methods include nerve mobilization (see Figure 6); nerve transposition, as with the ulnar and radial nerves; and joint positioning, such as repair and immobilization of a joint in some degree of flexion with gradual postoperative extension beginning at about 3 weeks. In some cases, bone shortening, as with comminuted fracture, may offer an opportunity for decreasing a nerve gap. Some innovative surgeons have applied nerve elongation techniques. Intraoperatively, restoration of fascicular orientation can be facilitated by (1) epineurial alignment of the vessels; (2) knowledge of the

serial cross-sectional topography; and (3) gross fascicular matching. Some surgeons use other techniques, such as fascicular stimulation and histochemical stains. Fascicular stimulation of the stumps allows mapping of motor and sensory fascicles: distally, motor fascicles can be identified by stimulation that produces muscle contraction if early exposure is done before Wallerian degeneration occurs; proximally, sensory fascicles can be identified by stimulation that produces dysesthesia, but the technique requires the patient to be awake, although sedated, and may be painful. Histochemical stains may be used to identify motor fascicles. When performing nerve repairs, it is important to understand the difference between the fascicular topography in the proximal nerve trunk and the fascicular topography in the distal nerve. Most nerves have a significant intermingling of sensory and motor fibers with plexus formation proximally, whereas more distally they usually become groups of sensory or motor fibers. This partially explains why more distal nerve repairs have better long-term functional outcomes.

Nerve Graft

Nerve graft repair is performed when nerve stumps on either side of a gap cannot be apposed for a direct end-to-end repair without tension (Figure 8). Often this technique is necessary for neuromas-in-continuity of moderate or longer lengths with unrecordable (negative) NAP or for transected nerves with retracted stumps, which occurs when the initial surgery is delayed. Nerve grafts are not indicated for brachial plexus injuries in which the nerves are avulsed because there is no "functional" proximal nerve stump (Figure 9).

The most frequent source of nerve graft is the sural nerve (Figure 10). However, the medial or lateral antebrachial cutaneous nerves, superficial sensory radial nerve, superficial peroneal nerve, distal posterior interosseous nerve, great auricular nerve, and cervical plexus nerves are alternatives. The disadvantage of nerve grafting is related to the minor sequelae associated with donor morbidity from the

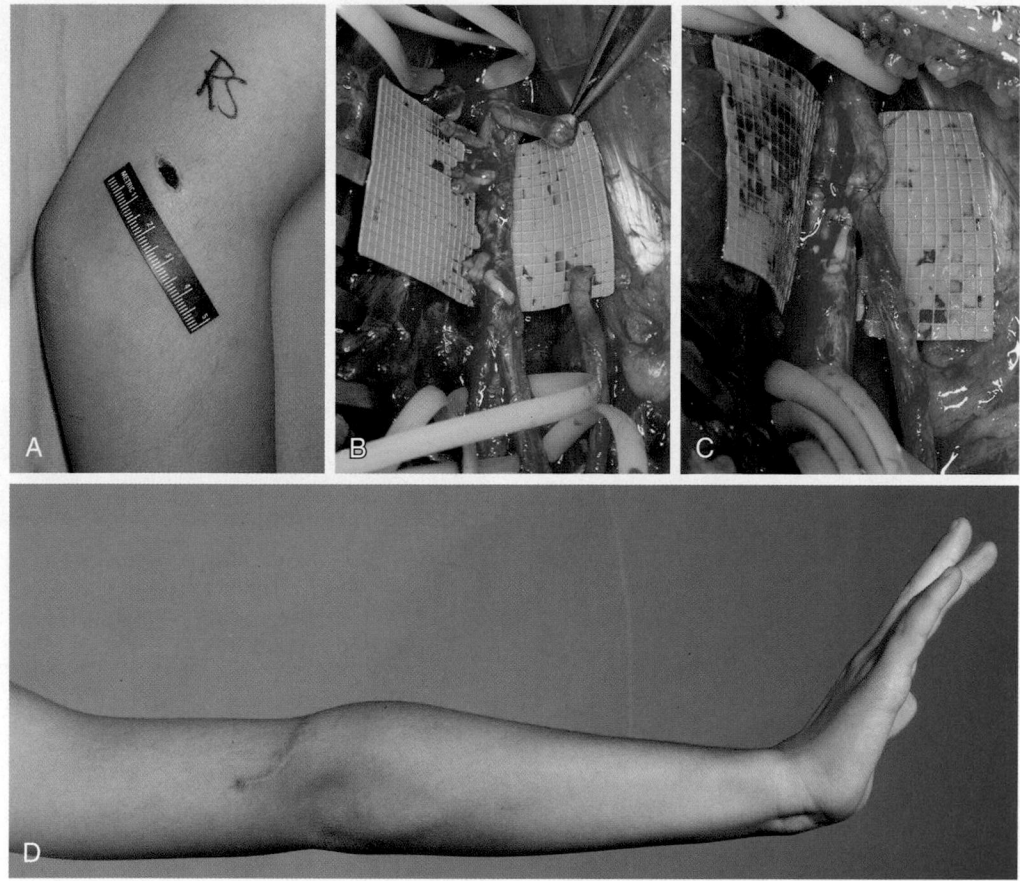

FIGURE 5 Patient with a partial laceration of the radial nerve treated at presentation 1 week after injury. **A,** The open knife-entry wound is seen in the right arm, slightly proximal to the elbow, near the interval between the brachioradialis and triceps. The knife blade had penetrated the arm to a depth of approximately 5 cm (2 inches). The patient had no thumb extension, partial weakness of the finger extensors and wrist extensors, and decreased sensation in the dorsum of the hand. **B,** At exploration, the radial nerve was found to be partially lacerated at its bifurcation into the deep and superficial radial nerve. The complete laceration of the superficial (sensory) radial nerve is seen, as is the partial injury to multiple fascicles of the deep (motor) branch of the radial nerve. **C,** The direct repair of the superficial sensory radial nerve and the fascicles of the deep branch of the radial nerve are shown; a 9-0 suture was used to perform this repair. **D,** After 6 months, the patient had already regained good (Medical Research Council [MRC] grade 4) finger and wrist extension. Thumb extension (the most distal motor target) improved to MRC grade 3, although the patient still had sensory abnormality in the dorsum of the hand.

nerve harvest, such as expected permanent sensory loss and small chance of neuropathic pain.

The graft length is calculated by measuring the nerve gap and adding 10% to account for some desiccation of the graft and to avoid tension. One graft or several "cable" grafts are placed to maximize the surface area at the repair sites and to prevent mismatch (Figure 11). Interposed grafts may be sutured individually at both ends or may be glued together and then sutured as a single unit.

Vascularized nerve grafts have been advocated by some to improve the speed and quality of regeneration compared with standard, non-vascularized nerve grafts; however, this practice is controversial. Autogenous or synthetic conduits may be used for short gaps (<3 cm) of small diameter, usually sensory nerves (e.g., digital nerves). Using a nerve conduit requires an entubulation technique. The nerve conduit must be the correct diameter to accommodate the nerve and should be approximately 10 mm longer than the nerve gap. The entubulation technique involves placing the proximal nerve ending 5 mm within one end of the nerve tube and the distal nerve ending 5 mm within the distal end of the nerve tube, with horizontal mattress sutures tied on the outside of the nerve conduit. Nerve transplants and decellularized nerve allografts have been reported, and the specific indications and outcomes are still evolving.

Nerve Transfers

Nerve transfers, also known as *neurotizations*, consist of the transfer of an expandable or redundant working nerve, branch, or fascicle to a nonfunctioning nerve. The donor functional nerve may be intraplexal or extraplexal, motor or sensory. Preferably, the donor nerve should be synergistic to the recipient, and relearning of a new function with independence is possible in many situations. The indications for nerve transfers include (1) irreparable brachial plexus nerves (avulsions); (2) specific cases of nerve injury, for which nerve transfer may lead to a more rapid or reliable recovery because of proximity of the end organ (an alternative to nerve grafting); and (3) innervation of free functioning muscle transfers.

The two main advantages of nerve transfers are that they are often closer to the end organ, thereby decreasing the distance and, by extension, the time to reinnervation, and that they typically have a large number of relatively "pure" (motor or sensory) axons because they are more distal. The cost-benefit ratio of neurotization needs to be evaluated for each patient and for each nerve transfer. Standard examples of extraplexal donor nerves are the spinal accessory nerve and the intercostal nerves; intercostal motor nerves are separate from intercostal sensory nerves, and each may be used separately. Examples of intraplexal donor nerve branches are

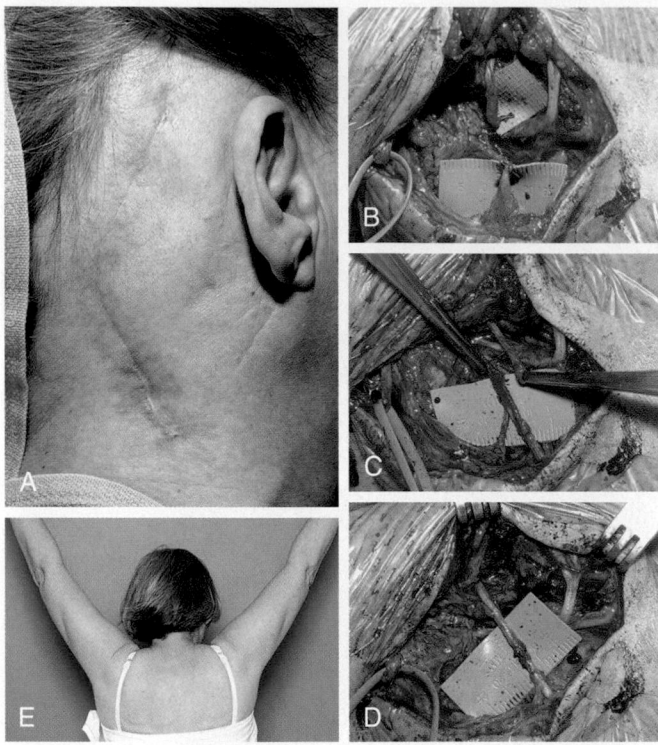

FIGURE 6 Patient with a spinal accessory nerve injury after a right retrosigmoid craniotomy for removal of a vestibular schwannoma. **A,** Photograph of the surgical incision used for the resection of the right vestibular schwannoma. Postoperatively, the patient developed prominent scapular winging, atrophy of the right trapezius muscle, and significant difficulty in abducting the right arm. Electromyography 3 months after surgery confirmed a right spinal accessory neuropathy affecting the motor branch to the trapezius (normal sternocleidomastoid) without evidence of reinnervation. **B,** At exploration soon thereafter, the great auricular nerve (at the right of the nerve stump) and the greater occipital nerve (in the blue vasoloop) were identified. The proximal and distal stumps (seen here clipped to a green background) of the spinal accessory nerve were found within the scar of the prior surgical exposure. **C,** To achieve a direct repair, the two nerve stumps were mobilized proximally and distally. **D,** A direct end-to-end repair was performed using an 8-0 suture. **E,** The patient regained excellent function, scapular stability, and range of motion, shown here at 15 months after the repair.

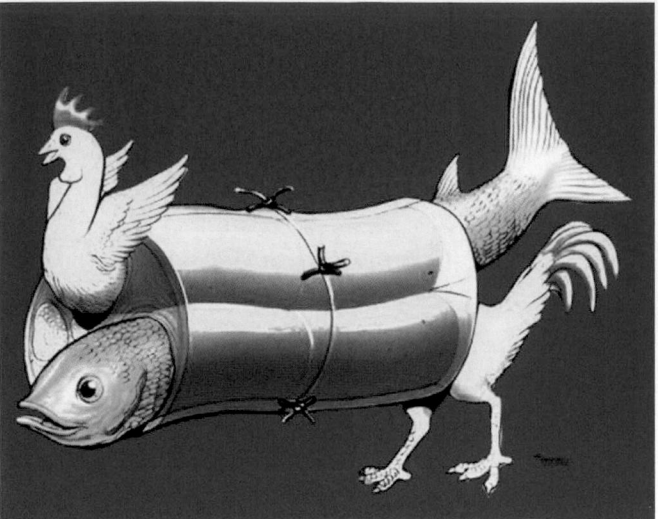

FIGURE 7 This schematic depicts fascicular mismatch. When a nerve is repaired, an attempt is made to restore the fascicular alignment to allow matching between motor and sensory axons and their targets. Restoration of fascicular orientation is easier in direct repair, but as the nerve gap increases, restoration becomes more difficult.

medial pectoral branches and triceps branches, and examples of intraplexal donor nerve fascicles are fascicles from the ulnar and median nerves (Figure 12). In the past decade, novel nerve transfers have been developed and utilized because of increased interest in this technique.

Less common and potentially more risky examples of extraplexal nerve transfers include the use of the phrenic nerve, contralateral C7 nerve, and hypoglossal nerve. Because of improvements in techniques and outcomes with newer nerve transfers, many surgeons are advocating nerve transfer in cases where more conventional nerve grafting could be done. Furthermore, wherever possible and feasible, many are advocating distal nerve transfers closer to the end organ rather than proximal nerve transfer farther from the end organ.

Muscle and Tendon Transfer and Bone and Joint Procedures

These various procedures usually are performed in a delayed fashion, sometimes more than a year after the injury. Muscle or tendon transfer is the transfer of a muscle or tendon that is working and is expendable to achieve a new function. This technique, similar to

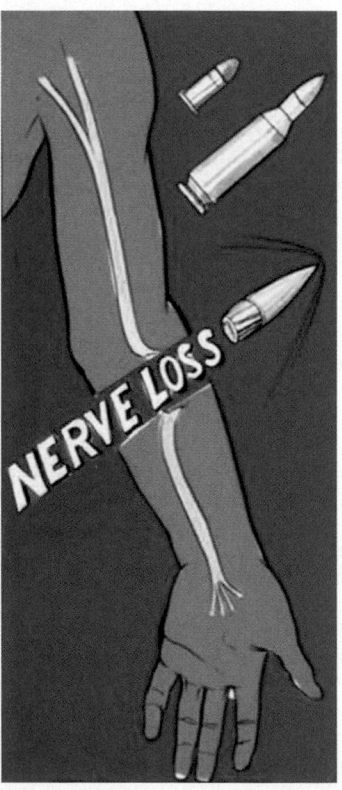

FIGURE 8 Some injuries may cause nerve tissue loss and create a nerve gap, which can occur in blunt or ragged transection, in sharp transection if the repair is done late, in nerve rupture (as can occur in brachial plexus injuries), and after resection of a nonconducting neuroma-in-continuity. In these instances, a graft is needed to bridge the gap and repair the nerve.

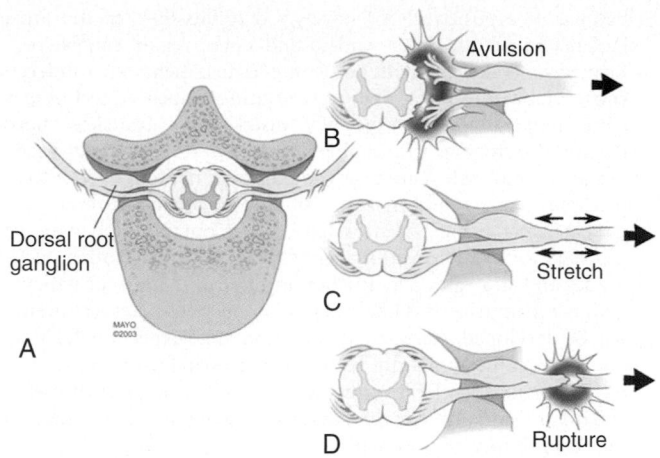

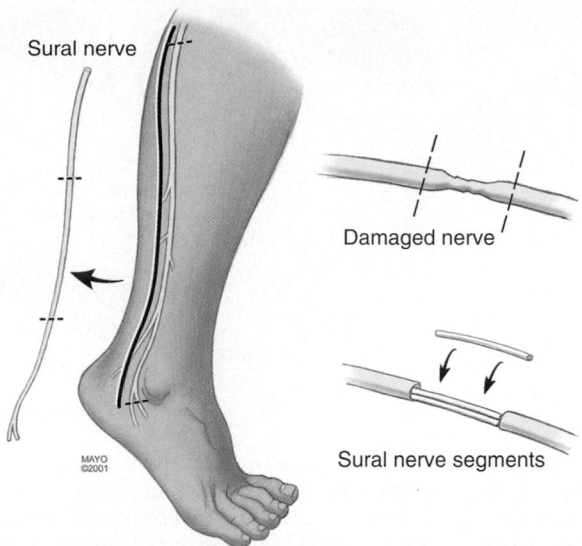

FIGURE 9 This schematic illustration depicts the different types of spinal nerve injuries seen in closed/traction injuries of the brachial plexus. **A,** Axial cross-section of a vertebral body showing the normal anatomy of the spinal cord, giving rise to the anterior and posterior spinal rootlets, which combine to form the spinal nerve. The dorsal root ganglion is seen in the intervertebral foramen. **B,** In brachial plexus injuries, the spinal roots can be avulsed directly from the spinal cord. These lesions are characterized as preganglionic. In this injury, the spinal nerves cannot be used and grafted, as there is no "functional" proximal nerve stump, and the reconstruction consists of nerve transfers. **C,** Spinal nerves and brachial plexus elements may be stretched by trauma. Although the nerve is in continuity, the nerve injury may be variable (axonotmesis, Sunderland's grades 2 to 4). Some of these nerve injuries will recover function spontaneously, but others will not. At surgery, a neuroma-in-continuity (postganglionic) will be found, and nerve action potential (NAP) recording may help to evaluate whether the nerve is recovering or if it will require repair. If repair is needed, the spinal nerve proximal to the lesion is generally available for grafting. **D,** The spinal nerves and brachial plexus elements can be ruptured by trauma and may be found in discontinuity at surgery (neurotmesis, Sunderland's grade 5). In these cases, spontaneous recovery is not possible; these lesions require repair. The rupture is generally postganglionic. The proximal spinal nerve stump found at surgery can be used for grafting; NAP, somatosensory evoked potentials, and/or motor evoked potentials can help to assess its integrity (i.e., its connection to the spinal cord). *(Courtesy Mayo Foundation for Medical and Educational Research. All rights reserved.)*

FIGURE 10 The sural nerve is the most common source of nerve graft. A purely sensory nerve, it supplies sensation to a small area of the dorsolateral aspect of the foot. The sural nerve is up to 40 cm long in each leg; nerve grafts may be harvested bilaterally, and sural nerve segments are used to bridge the nerve gap. *(Courtesy Mayo Foundation for Medical and Educational Research. All rights reserved.)*

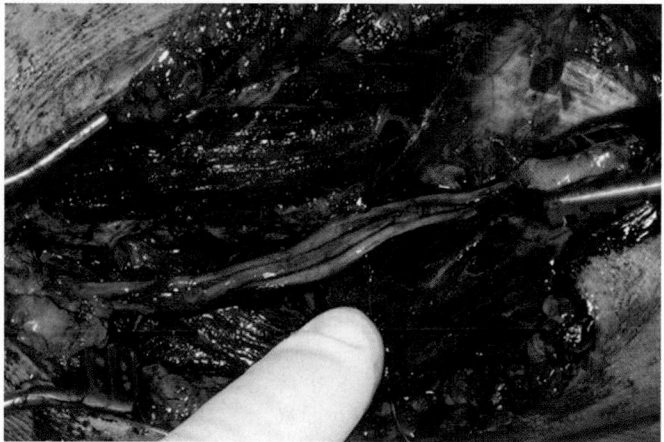

FIGURE 11 Intraoperative photograph of three sural nerve segments bridging a radial nerve gap in the distal arm after a humeral fracture.

nerve transfer, requires a functional expendable innervated muscle in the vicinity. Examples of reliable tendon transfers include opponensplasty, anticlaw procedure, thumb adductorplasty, flexor to extensor transfers, elbow flexorplasty, transfers for shoulder external rotation, antiwing (scapular) transfers, transfers for pronation, and extensor to flexor transfers. An alternative is the transfer of a free functioning muscle, such as the gracilis muscle from the lower extremity, which can be transferred at a late stage for elbow flexion or finger flexion. This requires the presence of an arterial and venous supply as well as a functioning nerve to reinnervate the muscle. Bone and joint procedures, such as osteotomies and arthrodesis, also may improve function. Shoulder fusion may be an option for patients with brachial plexus palsy and refractory instability with pain.

■ EXPECTED OUTCOMES FROM REPAIR AND RECONSTRUCTION

The main reason *why* surgeons perform nerve repair and reconstruction procedures is to improve outcomes for patients with nerve injuries. In general, the goals of surgical intervention, which include motor function, sensibility, sudomotor function, pain relief, patient satisfaction, and return to work, often can be achieved to varying extents. However, it is difficult to predict the outcome for an individual patient with a nerve injury because multiple factors influence nerve recovery (discussed later). It is also difficult to analyze and study these patients' outcomes because of several issues: (1) definition of a "good result" is lacking; (2) multiple variables exist, and data from a single surgeon using the same technique at the same time postinjury in the same population of patients with the same pattern of injury are often unavailable; and (3) examination and analysis unfortunately is often performed by the surgical team alone, creating a potential for bias.

Despite these issues, generalizations can be made. The best outcomes are achieved when spontaneous neural recovery occurs (i.e., when surgery is not indicated). Other factors influencing the recovery of nerve repair and reconstruction include the following:

1. Patient age: The younger the patient, the better the recovery because of inherent physiologic factors related to regeneration, limb length, and capacity for cortical reorganization and re-education.

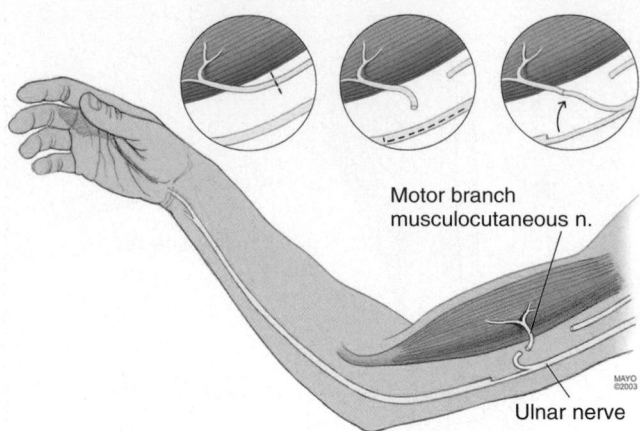

Motor branch
musculocutaneous n.

Ulnar nerve

FIGURE 12 Example of an intraplexal nerve transfer technique used for the repair of injury to the brachial plexus or musculocutaneous nerve leading to loss of biceps motor function. To perform this transfer, called Oberlin's procedure, the ulnar nerve function must be preserved. At the level of the middle or proximal third of the arm, a functioning ulnar nerve fascicle is used to reinnervate the biceps motor branch originating from the musculocutaneous nerve. In general, ulnar motor function is preserved (deficit in <1%), but the patient may experience transient sensory changes in the distribution of the ulnar nerve. A case series using this technique reports that 85% of patients recovered good elbow flexion after surgery. *(Courtesy Mayo Foundation for Medical and Educational Research. All rights reserved.)*

2. Level of injury: Distal injuries fare better because of the shorter distance to the end organ.
3. Type of nerve injured: Pure nerves fare better than mixed nerves because there is less chance of fascicular mismatch.
4. Specific nerve involved: Radial nerve recovers better than median nerve, which recovers better than ulnar nerve; nerves C5 and C6 and those of the upper trunk recover better than nerves C8 and T1 and those of the lower trunk; and tibial nerve recovers better than peroneal nerve.
5. Mechanism of injury: Lacerations have better outcomes than low-velocity gunshot injuries, which in turn have better outcomes than high-velocity gunshot injuries; transections have better outcomes than crush or avulsions injuries; and stretch injuries generally have better outcomes than ruptures, which fare better than avulsions. These variations in outcomes are related to the zone of injury and associated soft tissue and vascular damage.
6. Timing of repair and reconstruction: The earlier the better; outcomes are typically best before 6 months, but they depend on the size of the gap, the status of the end plate, and the status of the alpha motor neurons.
7. Type of repair or reconstruction: Patients in whom exploratory surgery is indicated, but in whom only neurolysis is performed

because of a positive NAP, have good results 90% of the time. Patients in whom direct end-to-end nerve repair can be performed generally have better outcomes than patients who undergo conventional interpositional nerve grafting. Improved techniques with nerve transfers, especially distal nerve transfers, have improved outcomes in peripheral nerve surgery in recent years. Distal nerve transfers are now thought by some to be better than proximal nerve grafts in some situations, but controversy still exists. Direct nerve transfers have better outcomes than nerve transfers with interpositional grafts. In the future, other techniques and strategies may further improve outcomes for patients with nerve injuries. It is likely that other nerve transfer techniques will be developed. Nerve reimplantation, now experimental, may one day become an option. Techniques, growth factors, and materials that could accelerate growth, promote regeneration, preserve end organs, and improve the interface between the nerve ends also may lead to improved outcomes.

WHO SHOULD OPERATE

By extrapolation based on data related to other surgical techniques, it seems reasonable to expect improved outcomes in centers performing high-volume practice. Timely referral to centers specializing in evaluation and management of nerve injuries is important and should be considered.

SUMMARY

The treatment and management of nerve injuries requires thorough knowledge of anatomy, of the nerve injury process, and of the available repair and reconstructive options. It also requires specific microsurgical skills in the context of a multidisciplinary team able to address the peripheral nerves and associated muscles, tendons, and joint problems as well as concomitant injuries to the central nervous system (spinal cord and brain) and other systems.

SUGGESTED READINGS

Kline DG, Happel LT. Penfield lecture: a quarter century's experience with intraoperative nerve action potential recording. *Can J Neurol Sci.* 1993;20:3-10.

Midha R, Lee P, Mackay M. Surgical techniques for peripheral nerve repair. In: Wolfa CE, Resnick DK, eds. *Neurosurgical Operative Atlas: Spine and Peripheral Nerves.* 2nd ed. New York: Thieme; 2007:402-408.

Midha R, Serrano-Almedia C, Mackay M. Harvesting techniques of sural and other cutaneous nerves for cable graft repair. In: Wolfa CE, Resnick DK, eds. *Neurosurgical Operative Atlas: Spine and Peripheral Nerves.* 2nd ed. New York: Thieme; 2007:409-413.

Oberlin C, Durand S, Belheyar Z, et al. Nerve transfers in brachial plexus palsies. *Chir Main.* 2009;28:1-9.

Robert EG, Happel LT, Kline DG. Intraoperative nerve action potential recordings: technical considerations, problems, and pitfalls. *Neurosurgery.* 2009;65(4 suppl):A97-A104.

Spinner RJ, Kline DG. Surgery for peripheral nerve and brachial plexus injuries or other nerve lesions. *Muscle Nerve.* 2000;23:680-695.

EXTREMITY GAS GANGRENE

Robert Sheridan, MD, and Yuk Ming Liu, MD, MPH

Clostridial myonecrosis, commonly referred to as gas gangrene, is a devastating soft tissue infection that progresses rapidly. Gaseous cellulitis and gaseous fasciitis are pathognomonic for clostridial myonecrosis. The progression from superficial skin infection

to rapid extension deep into the soft tissues, fascial planes, and muscle distinguishes it from a generic cellulitis. Historically, it has been common during all wars. The presentation of gas gangrene is not limited to traumatic wounds. Early recognition of gas gangrene has important implications for the patient's outcome. Delayed diagnosis may lead to overwhelming systemic infection followed by shock and death. The most common organism responsible is *Clostridium perfringens,* but several other species of clostridia have been identified. Exotoxins from the organism generate a cascade of physiologic derangements that contribute to its local invasiveness, morbidity, and mortality.

BOX 1: Known Settings for Clostridial Myonecrosis

Trauma

Penetrating wounds
Blast injuries
Natural disasters
Industrial injury

Procedural

Gynecologic surgery
Gastrointestinal surgery
Subcutaneous injections
Intramuscular injections

Spontaneous

Diabetes mellitus
Leukemia
Gastrointestinal malignancies
Drug-induced immunosuppression

BOX 2: Clostridial Species

Clostridium perfringens
C. septicum
C. sordellii
C. novyi

■ EPIDEMIOLOGY

With an estimated incidence of 1000 cases per year, gas gangrene is a rare infection in the United States. Before the twentieth century, gas gangrene was a common cause of limb loss and death in wartime. As the pathophysiology was elicited during these earlier conflicts, incidence declined and mortality improved in subsequent years. Current management is founded on early evacuation of injured soldiers with prompt surgical débridement and effective antibiotics.

Gas gangrene can be classified in three categories: traumatic, postprocedural, and spontaneous. A shift in the epidemiology of gas gangrene has occurred in recent decades, from traumatic injuries to postoperative wounds and sites of intravenous drug administration (Box 1). *Clostridium* colonization of the gut has been identified as a potential source for nontraumatic cases of spontaneous clostridial myonecrosis. These patients often have a hematologic or occult malignancy as their underlying predisposition to gastrointestinal seeding, leading to a distant myonecrosis.

Traumatic causes include penetrating wounds from gunshots and stab injuries, crush injuries, and fractures, especially those injuries contaminated by soil. Natural disasters like the Sichuan earthquake are associated with gas gangrene infection, with associated delay in care worsening prognosis. Nontraumatic cases are seen in postoperative wounds and in intravenous drug users. Spontaneous or nontraumatic cases have been reported in patients who have hematologic disorders and malignancies. Mortality rates have decreased considerably in recent decades, but case fatality rates of 25% are still reported.

■ PATHOGENESIS

C. perfringens was discovered in 1892 by George Nuttall and William Welch. Originally named *C. welchii*, this gram-positive, spore-forming bacillus is ubiquitous in the environment, especially in soil. The spores are heat resistant and can survive in a dormant state in unfavorable environments for long periods. Clostridial spores are routinely found on skin surfaces and are also a part of the normal flora of human gastrointestinal, biliary, and genitourinary tracts. The clinical spectrum of clostridial infections includes cellulitis, bacteremia, and invasion of tissue and muscle planes. The progressive destruction of intact muscle tissue is termed clostridial myonecrosis or gas gangrene.

C. perfringens is commonly the organism associated with traumatic wounds and myonecrosis. Reports of other clostridial species are associated with certain groups of myonecrosis presentations (Box 2). *C. septicum* is the causative agent in cases related to dissemination from a colonic source. *C. novyi* has been characterized in intravenous drug users with gas gangrene originating from their injection sites. *C. sordellii* induces a toxic shock–like myonecrosis after gynecologic procedures, caesarean sections, and black tar heroin injections known as "skin popping."

The virulence of clostridial infection is dependent on the exotoxin production. In general, these exotoxins target the plasma membrane and lead to tissue destruction. The typical setting for gas gangrene to manifest begins with a break in the skin and inoculation of the wound with clostridial spores from a penetrating source or soilage from the environment.

Although many exotoxins have been identified, the alpha and theta toxins are the virulence factors responsible for myonecrosis from the various clostridial species. Alpha toxin is a lecithinase, and its activity comes from phospholipase C (PLC) and sphingomyelinase. Theta toxin, also known as perfringolysin O (PFO), is a cholesterol-dependent cytolysin that is similar to the streptococcal streptolysin found in necrotizing soft tissue infections. PFO binds cholesterol in the host plasma membrane, forms pores, and causes cell lysis. PFO also contributes to the gas production associated with its clinical presentation. Myonecrosis happens from the inside out as the clostridial bacteria multiply and continue to produce exotoxin. Alpha toxin was shown in animal models to directly and indirectly affect myocardial contractility, thereby causing hypotension and eventually shock. Theta toxin additionally reduces systemic vascular resistance and induces endogenous mediators such as prostacyclin to cause vasodilation.

■ CLINICAL PRESENTATION AND DIAGNOSIS

Early diagnosis is critical and should be suspected in the correct historical and clinical settings, such as patients with contaminated soft tissue wounds. Gram stains and wound cultures can aid in the diagnosis. Radiographic imaging with x-rays, computed tomographic (CT) scans, and magnetic resonance imaging (MRI) is also a valuable adjunct to physical examination. Clinically, the patient will have pain that is disproportionate to physical findings of cellulitis, erythema, and edema. The skin at the site of injury may be pale and slowly turn a purple-red hue (Figure 1, *A*). In many cases, hemorrhagic bullae will develop (Figure 1, *B*). Crepitus is often a late finding and indicates the urgency for surgical débridement as well as aggressive resuscitation with fluids, pressors, and antibiotics. When in doubt as to the diagnosis, it is often wise to proceed to the operating room for exploration of muscle compartments at risk. In the event of a negative exploration, the exposures required rarely cause major morbidity.

Of concern is the increasing incidence of spontaneous clostridial myonecrosis. As early as the 1960s, these cases were described in the gynecologic and oncologic literature. They can be highly lethal. Leukocytosis, pain, and edema are nonspecific symptoms and signs that do not facilitate early diagnosis of spontaneous gas gangrene. Physical change in the skin and tissue with discoloration and crepitation are late manifestations. The earliest manifestation may be altered mental state such as confusion. For the general surgeon, the diagnosis should be considered even in the absence of local trauma or incision. Blood cultures and imaging should be utilized in addition to careful physical examination looking for early local signs of deep infection.

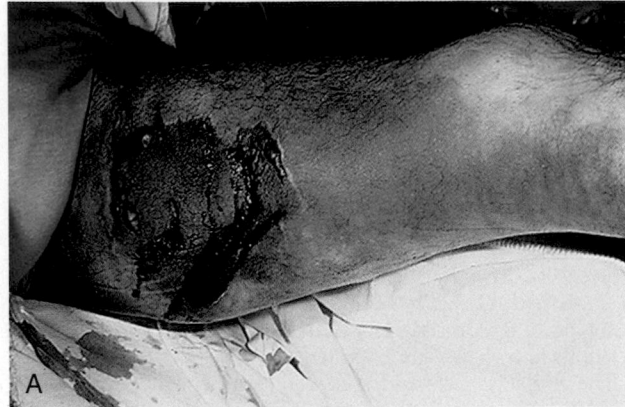

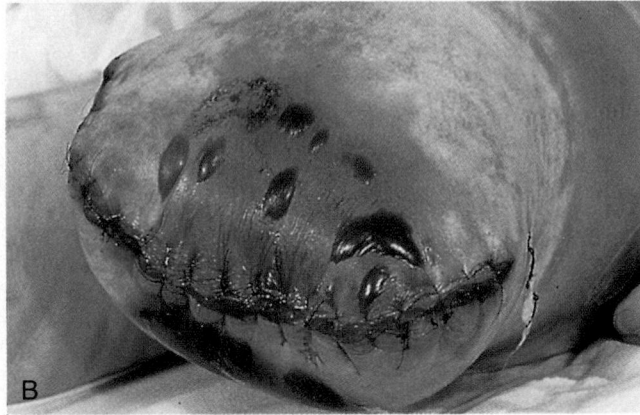

FIGURE 1 A, Gas gangrene with hemorrhagic bullae, edema, erythema, and necrotic skin changes. **B,** Postoperative gas gangrene with edema, erythema, and hemorrhagic bullae. (**A,** From Spicer WJ. Clinical Microbiology and Infectious Disease. London: Churchill Livingstone; 2008; **B,** From Goering RV, Dockrell HM, Zuckerman M, Ciodini PL, Roitt IM. Mims' Medical Microbiology. Philadelphia: Saunders; 2013.)

■ MANAGEMENT AND TREATMENT

Timely management affects mortality. If the diagnosis is suspected based on clinical presentation, fluid resuscitation should be initiated and antibiotics administered after blood and wound cultures are obtained. In addition, routine blood work includes complete blood count, electrolytes, blood urea nitrogen, creatinine, glucose, and creatine phosphokinase. Suspicious wounds should be explored in the operating room. Penicillin G is the antibiotic of choice for clostridial infections. This is administered at 4 million units intravenously every 4 hours. However, with the more common polymicrobial nature of wounds and the possibility of drug-resistant bacteria, empiric broad-spectrum antibiotics such as piperacillin-tazobactam can be started until culture data definitively identify specific clostridium species. Later-generation cephalosporins are utilized for penicillin allergies. Clindamycin may inhibit exotoxin production. Duration of antibiotic treatment has not been standardized and is tailored to the individual patient's disease burden. The patient's physiologic response to débridement and wound inspection serves as a guide to determining the course of antibiotic treatment. Tetanus immunization should be updated and tetanus immune globulin administered in those patients not vaccinated previously.

Patients suspected to be suffering from gas gangrene need prompt surgical intervention for diagnosis and treatment. Suspicious wounds originating from trauma should be thoroughly explored operatively. Postsurgical wounds may be opened at bedside for evaluation, with likely definitive exploration in the operating room. Muscle compartments at risk should be opened widely to enable adequate visualization of the involved tissues (Figure 2). Involved tissues should

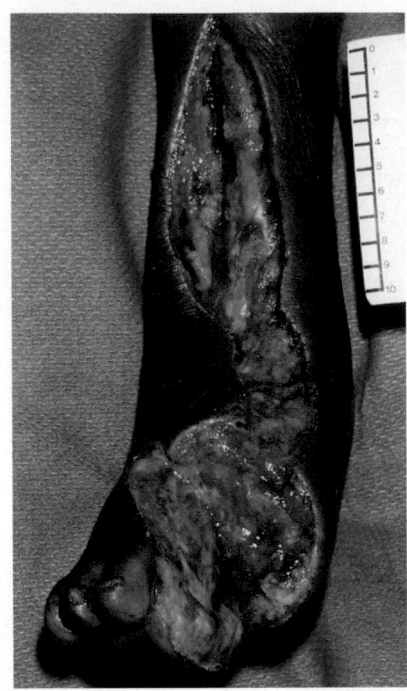

FIGURE 2 Wide débridement of gas gangrene that included amputation of two medial toes. (Reprinted from Riley TV. Medical Microbiology. Elsevier; 2012.)

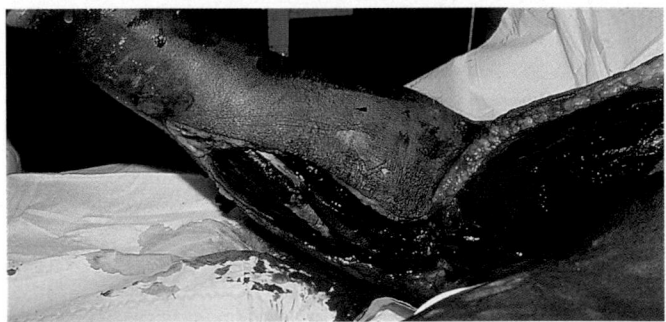

FIGURE 3 Initial débridement of gas gangrene that required repeat débridement and eventual amputation of the limb. (Reprinted from Stevens D, et al. Necrotizing fasciitis, gas gangrene, myositis, and myonecrosis. In Cohen J, Powderly W, Opal S, eds. Infectious Diseases, 3rd ed. Elsevier; 2010, Fig. 10.9.)

be excised to healthy margins. Infected muscle may be dark or pale in appearance and may not contract when stimulated mechanically or with electrocautery. Under appreciation of this, rapidly progressive infection is common. Therefore planned repeat operation is important at 12- to 24-hour intervals to ensure complete eradication of infected tissue (Figure 3). Major débridement and amputation may be required to gain control. All wounds should be left open and treated topically as a burn. Late closure often requires a creative combination of flaps and skin grafts.

■ HYPERBARIC OXYGEN THERAPY

Hyperbaric oxygen therapy (HBOT) remains controversial as a therapeutic strategy for gas gangrene. HBOT was introduced in 1960 by Boerema and Brummelkamp (Figure 4). Theoretically, enhanced delivery of oxygen through the bloodstream can be lethal to the clostridial bacteria. However, dormant spores of clostridium are unaffected by the high arterial PO_2 of 800 to 1000 mm Hg. Although in vitro studies demonstrated HBOT to be effective, in vivo data are

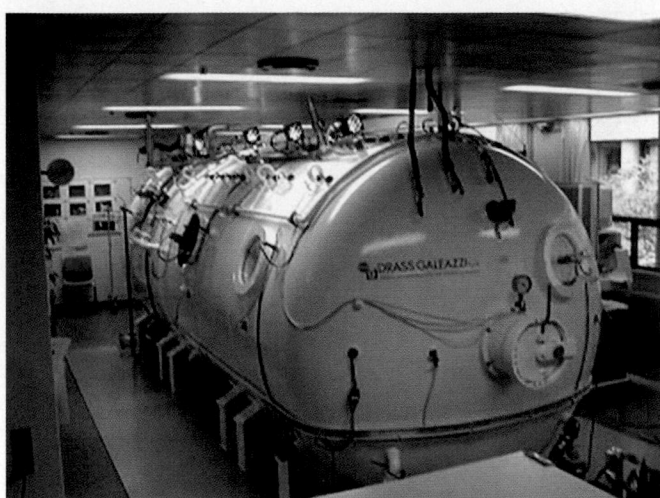

FIGURE 4 Multiplace hyperbaric oxygen treatment chamber. *(From Mortensen CR. Hyperbaric oxygen therapy. Curr Anaesth Crit Care. 2008;19:333-337.)*

inconclusive. A few case series have reported good treatment outcomes with use of HBOT. However, there is a lack of evidence supporting routine adjunctive use. Surgical débridement and antibiotics are the cornerstone of care. HBOT is not recommended as solo or first-line treatment in unstable patients with progressive infection. The dangers and logistic difficulties associated with treating an unstable patient in a hyperbaric chamber may outweigh the putative adjunctive benefits.

■ PROGNOSIS

Gas gangrene is recognized as a morbid infection with a mortality averaging 25%. Prognosis varies by location, with gas gangrene of the extremities having a more favorable outlook than cases involving the torso and its contents. Gas gangrene involving an extremity is easier to recognize, débride, and isolate. Delayed operative débridement has been shown to be an independent predictor of mortality. Functional outcomes vary with the extent of resection required to achieve control. Again, early surgery may enhance outcomes.

■ CONCLUSIONS

Gas gangrene is a fatal infection that progresses rapidly without early débridement and antibiotics. Infections most commonly follow local trauma or surgery, but nontraumatic spontaneous gas gangrene is seen increasingly and requires a high index of suspicion to make a timely diagnosis. The infections can be caused by several clostridial species, with *C. perfringens* being most common. Outcomes are improved with early intervention. Early diagnosis is facilitated by a high index of suspicion and may require operative exploration to confirm or exclude diagnosis. Initial management requires antibiotics and surgical débridement. Vigilant evaluation of the wound bed after initial débridement is important to recognize and address progression of infection. Antibiotic coverage should be adjusted to final culture isolates, but mixed infection should be assumed initially. HBOT may have an adjunctive role but should not be used as primary therapy. Both survival and functional outcomes likely are enhanced by early intervention.

SUGGESTED READINGS

Brummelkamp WH, Boerema I, Hoogendyk L. Treatment of clostridial infections with hyperbaric oxygen drenching: a report on 26 cases. *Lancet.* 1963;1:235-238.

Chen E, Den L, Liu Z, et al. Management of gas gangrene in Wenchuan earthquake victims. *J Huazhong Univ Sci Technol Med Sci.* 2011;31:83-87.

Collier PE, Diamond DL, Young JC. Nontraumatic *Clostridium septicum* gangrenous myonecrosis. *Dis Colon Rectum.* 1983;26:703-704.

Demello FJ, Haglin JJ, Hitchcock CR. Comparative study of experimental *Clostridium perfringens* infection in dogs treated with antibiotics, surgery, and hyperbaric oxygen. *Surgery.* 1973;73:936-941.

Elliott D, Kufera JA, Myers RA. The microbiology of necrotizing soft tissue infections. *Am J Surg.* 2000;179:361-366.

Katlic MR, Derkac WM, Coleman WS. *Clostridium septicum* infection and malignancy. *Ann Surg.* 1981;193:361-364.

Kizer KW, Ogle LC. Occult clostridial myonecrosis. *Ann Emerg Med.* 1981;10:307-311.

Lehner PJ, Powell H. Gas gangrene. *BMJ.* 1991;303:240-242.

McGuigan CC, Penrice GM, Guer L, et al. Lethal outbreak of infection with *Clostridium novyi* type A and other spore-forming organisms in Scottish injecting drug users. *J Med Microbiol.* 2002;51:971-977.

Pitt M, Purser NJ. Gas gangrene. *Lancet.* 1996;347:1116.

Ray D, Cohle SD, Lamb P. Spontaneous clostridial myonecrosis. *J Forensic Sci.* 1992;37:1428-1432.

Schexnayder SM, Klein SG. Images in clinical medicine: gas gangrene. *N Engl J Med.* 2004;350:2603.

Stevens DL. The pathogenesis of clostridial myonecrosis. *Int J Med Microbiol.* 2000;290:497-502.

Stevens DL, Aldape MJ, Bryant AE. Life-threatening clostridial infections. *Anaerobe.* 2012;18:254-259.

Stevens DL, Bisno AL, Chambers HF, et al. Practice guidelines for the diagnosis and management of skin and soft tissue infections: 2014 update by the infectious diseases society of America. *Clin Infect Dis.* 2014;59:147-159.

Stevens DL, Musher DM, Watson DA, et al. Spontaneous, nontraumatic gangrene due to *Clostridium septicum. Rev Infect Dis.* 1990;12:286-296.

NECROTIZING SKIN AND SOFT TISSUE INFECTIONS

Diane A. Schwartz, MD, Amir Mehdi Ansari, MD, Aerielle E. Matsangos, BS, Christopher Ng, BS, Louis J. Born, BS, Frank Lay, BS, Ali Karim Ahmed, BS, Guy P. Marti, MD, Stephen M. Milner, MS, BS, BDS, DSc, FRCS(Ed), and John W. Harmon, MD, FACS

Necrotizing soft tissue infections (NSTIs) represent a spectrum of skin, subcutaneous, fascial, and muscular diseases of variable morbidity and mortality. These infections have transcended time and are relatively unchanged in their devastation when compared with early reports.

Hippocrates documented, "Many were attacked by the erysipelas all over the body when the exciting cause was a trivial accident or a very small wound ... many even while undergoing treatment suffered from severe inflammations, and the erysipelas would quickly spread widely in all directions. Flesh, sinews and bones fell away in large quantities ... the bones were bared and fell away, and there were copious fluxes. Fever was sometimes present and sometimes absent."

In 1871 Dr. Joseph Jones, a Confederate military surgeon, described gangrene in 2642 military casualties with a mortality rate of 46%. He noted that victims of blast injury succumbed to subsequent infection, in which skin and soft tissue were affected notably.

He labeled this phenomenon a virtual "melting" of the surrounding area followed by quick death. Jean Alfred Fournier applied his eponym to the condition now known as *Fournier's gangrene* in a series of lectures in Paris in 1883.

In the 1990s the concept of NSTIs was introduced to the general public by the media as "flesh-eating infections." Since then, NSTIs have gained widespread attention. Although treatment modalities have improved, it is still imperative to recognize and débride these infections because the untreated infectious process remains almost identical to that described by Hippocrates. As the field of critical care has developed, mitigation of end-organ dysfunction has emerged as adjunctive to débridement and antibiotics. This chapter describes what is understood about NSTI causes, treatments, and outcomes.

■ PATHOPHYSIOLOGY

These infections spread rapidly, involve bacterial load, and destroy end-organ perfusion. Once the pathogen gains entry past the skin barrier, remote release of cytokines induces widespread third spacing and inability of the vasculature to maintain its volume. Microorganisms produce toxins that promote destruction of surrounding and distant tissue. On the microscopic level a variety of microorganisms infect susceptible soft tissues, promoting polymorphonuclear cell infiltration of the dermis and fascia. The microorganisms and inflammatory cells also invade blood vessels of the soft tissue, leading to obliterative endarteritis and necrosis of blood vessel walls and thrombosis of the small vessels passing through the soft tissue. Liquefactive necrosis of the fascia ensues, with concomitant necrosis and breakdown of skin, muscle, and surrounding tissues. Macroscopically, cellulitic skin often represents the "tip of the iceberg" in terms of the extent of underlying soft tissue necrosis.

The effect on the permeability of the vasculature and alteration in blood flow prevents an immunologic response from the host. Ability of the host to fight off virulent soft tissue infection is weakened by the inciting organism in many cases. Antibiotics given intravenously do not reach affected tissue well because of the derangement in blood flow and vascular integrity. The toxicity of the pathogen, the abnormal host response, and the difficulty in intravenous medication delivery to affected areas result in organ malperfusion and more diffuse soft tissue disruption than what is appreciated at the level of skin. Source control is key in almost all cases, requiring a combination of surgical débridement of all involved tissue and antibiotics against the bacteria and their destructive products or toxins.

Bacteroides and *Streptococcus* spp. are the most frequently cultured organisms. In cases attributable to single microorganisms, anaerobes such as *Clostridium* spp. (most commonly *Clostridium perfringens*) are twice as likely as aerobes such as group A beta-hemolytic *Streptococcus*. The severity of presentation in monomicrobial infections often results from the toxins produced by the pathogen (i.e., hemolysin, streptolysins O and S, and leukocidin by group A streptococci and alpha-toxin by *C. perfringens*). Infections of the skin without deeper involvement are most likely monomicrobial.

The typical described "flesh-eating" soft tissue infections reported by the press are caused by marine organisms such as *Vibrio* spp. and *Aeromonas hydrophila*. They result after seawater contamination of wounds, injuries involving fish fins or stings, and raw seafood consumption. They can be extremely devastating, particularly in patients with chronic liver disease. The term "flesh-eating" is misleading, however, because these bacteria destroy tissue via toxins.

■ DIAGNOSIS

Because the disease is a spectrum, it can have infinite manifestations. True necrotizing fasciitis is rare and its consequences are deadly, so clinical cues are key in determining the diagnosis in a timely fashion. Any clinical concern regarding the possibility of necrotizing fasciitis should prompt further investigation and action. In general, anyone with pain to the skin and a global ill appearance out of proportion

TABLE 1: Laboratory Risk Indicator for Necrotizing Fasciitis

WBC COUNT (×10³/mm³)	HEMOGLOBIN (g/dL)
<15: 0 points	>13.5: 0 points
15-25: 1 point	11-13.5: 1 point
>25: 2 points	<11: 2 points
CRP (mg/L)	**SODIUM (mmol/L)**
≥150: 4 points	<135: 2 points
GLUCOSE (mg/dL)	**CREATININE (mg/dL)**
>180: 1 point	>1.6: 2 points

Score ≥6 suggests diagnosis of necrotizing fasciitis; a score <6 does not rule out the diagnosis.

to what is visualized by exam could be affected. The skin typically has a normal to red appearance, can have crepitus, and is exquisitely tender. There may be an appearance of cellulitis, bruising, bullae, or abnormal pigmentation with definitive breech of skin integrity. The Laboratory Risk Indicator for Necrotizing Fasciitis (Table 1) is a beneficial scoring system that can help with differentiating necrotizing fasciitis from other soft tissue infections. Although patients with a score of 6 or more should be considered seriously for necrotizing fasciitis, a score of less than 6 should not rule out the diagnosis.

Hyponatremia, hypochloremia, and derangements in renal function often are seen and are indicators of more advanced disease with surgical urgency. Scoring systems that employ measurement of end-organ function such as the Fournier's Gangrene Severity Index (Table 2) can be useful in determining predicted mortality. Mortality is increased in patients with scores greater than 9. Imaging may be additive but is not universally indicated if the diagnosis can be made clinically. In fact imaging should not be pursued in cases in which the diagnosis is readily evident because obtaining imaging can delay timing to treatment.

Certain patient populations may be more vulnerable than others to necrotizing infections. Patients with diabetes or in an immunocompromised state should be examined carefully for soft tissue infected sources any time they have toxicity, acidosis, new-onset end-organ failure, or shock, when other source is not readily identifiable. This is especially critical in patients with diabetic ketoacidosis or diabetic coma because the history may not indicate soft tissue infection as the inciting event, and treatment could be delayed consequently.

An estimated 20% of patients affected by NSTIs are evaluated as immunologically normal. In many cases, however, a prior event can explain the infection. Examples of shaving prior to saltwater exposure or traumatic injury to the skin have been described as potential culprits of disease.

The infections are polymicrobial, with a number of culpable instigating organisms, including staphylococcus, streptococcus, and clostridium species, being most common. Because not all of these are gas producers not all cases of soft tissue infection or fasciitis have evidence of crepitus. Furthermore, these organisms differ in their virulence and the timing of their spread. *Streptococcus* species are typically slow to cause end-organ failure; thus diagnosis in these cases has the luxury of time before widespread damage or need for aggressive surgical débridement. This is in comparison to clostridial disease, in which spread is rapid, often becoming evident in the short amount of time it takes to travel from an emergency department to an operative theater.

■ TREATMENT

In cases in which the diagnosis is in question and the patient is unstable, quick diagnostic surgical interrogation can be performed

TABLE 2: Fournier's Gangrene Severity Index

Physiologic Variable/ Point Assignment	High Abnormal Values				Normal	Low Abnormal			
	+4	+3	+2	+1	0	+1	+2	+3	+4
Temperature (C)	More than 41	39-40.9	—	38.5-38.9	36-38.4	34-35.9	32-33.9	30-31.9	Less than 29.9
Heart rate	More than 180	140-179	110-139	—	70-109	—	55-69	40-54	Less than 39
Respiratory rate	More than 50	35-49	—	25-34	12-24	10-11	6-9	—	Less than 5
Serum sodium (mmol/L)	More than 180	160-179	155-159	150-154	130-149	—	120-129	111-119	Less than 110
Serum potassium (mmol/L)	More than 7	6-6.9	—	5.5-5.9	3.5-5.4	3-3.4	2.5-2.9	—	Less than 2.5
Serum creatinine (mg/100 mL, ×2 for acute renal failure)	More than 3.5	2-3.4	1.5-1.9	—	0.6-1.4	—	Less than 0.6	—	—
Hematocrit (%)	More than 60	—	50-59.9	46-49.9	30-45.9	—	20-29.9	—	Less than 20
White blood count (total/mm^3 × 1000)	More than 40	—	20-39.9	15-19.9	3-14.9	—	1-2.9	—	Less than 1
Serum bicarbonate (venous, mmol/L)	More than 52	41-51.9	—	32-40.9	22-31.9	—	18-21.9	15-17.9	Less than 15

Score 9 is the threshold of mortality rate. Scores >9 are associated with 75% mortality rate. Survival rate is 78% for a score ≤9.

at bedside. Surgical consultation should be immediate, and surgeon judgment dictates whether ambiguity in the diagnosis exists. In situations in which bedside evaluation is warranted, local anesthetic administration is recommended, followed by incision and investigation of the underlying soft tissue and fascial plane. If NSTI is present, then the underlying tissue will be discolored and separate with minimal finger pressure from the fascia. There may be odor or the classic "dishwater fluid," turbid, foul smelling, nonpurulent effluent. Any of these findings should prompt a more thorough débridement in the operating room. Cultures can be used to confirm the bacterial cause, but antibiotics should not be withheld awaiting results because antibiotics are an integral adjuvant to treatment.

Wound evaluation and surgical débridement should be carried out at frequent serial intervals; the frequency should match clinical parameters. If the clinical situation worsens, the wound should be investigated immediately because it is the prime source and must be controlled. When the initial diagnosis is made, débridement may be frequent, even occurring hours apart. The patient's clinical course should determine the frequency of débridement, and débridement is not to be withheld if clinical deterioration is noted because surgical source control is imperative to survival (Figures 1 through 3).

Patients diagnosed with NSTI should be maintained in an intensive care setting during the initial resuscitation. In concert with surgical excision, broad-spectrum antibiotics are essential and may be tailored as culture data become available. The standard regimen includes penicillin G (18 to 24 million units/day divided into 4 or 6 doses) or ampicillin (500 mg to 2 g every 4 to 6 hr) to treat gram-positive organisms such as clostridia, enterococci (not covered by penicillin G), and peptostreptococci; vancomycin for other gram-positive organisms such as resistant *Staphylococcus aureus* (15 mg/kg/dose every 12 hr); clindamycin (600 to 900 mg every 8 hr) or metronidazole (1 g intravenous load then 0.5 g every 6 hr or 1 g every 12 hr) for anaerobic coverage; and gentamicin (2 mg/kg intravenous load then 5 mg/kg/day or 1.7 mg/kg every 8 hr) or another aminoglycoside to cover gram-negative organisms. Use of extended-spectrum pharmaceuticals (imipenem/cilastatin, piperacillin/tazobactam, and ampicillin/sulbactam) may be used as monotherapy if resistance is not likely, reducing the number of individual drugs received by the patient. Given the high concurrent rate of systemic toxicity in NSTI patients, intensive monitoring, hemodynamic resuscitation, and nutritional support are also critical and have been shown to decrease mortality.

There is some argument in the literature regarding the utility of hyperbaric oxygen and wound healing. There is no high-quality evidence supporting the use of hyperbaric oxygen treatment. If it is to be used, it should not be instituted until débridement is completed. These wounds can be well managed in centers that do not offer hyperbaric therapy.

Because these wounds tend to be large and extend down to the fascia or muscle there is a practical advantage in using vacuum-assisted dressings. These dressings require less frequent changes than the wet-to-dry dressings and enable granulation. There is no high-quality evidence supporting the idea that vacuum dressings improve outcome. Regardless of the type of dressing used, the skin around the débrided site should be monitored for progression, and any clinical deterioration should first prompt investigation and further débridement of the wound.

Another treatment modality that has been suggested is serial culture of wound margins. The purpose of serially culturing the wound would be to direct antibiotic therapy when serial débridement is completed and to ensure that there is resolution of the disease at the margin. Wound margin disease can prevent healthy granulation tissue from forming. The routine implementation of this approach should await the completion of clinical trials supporting this approach.

Morbidity is affected by the size and location of the wound. Coverage options include grafts and flaps but should not be pursued until débridement is completed, all margins are clean, and physiologic normalcy is reestablished.

■ CONCLUSION

Successful management of NSTIs is predicated on having a high level of suspicion for the condition. Prompt and complete débridement is necessary to achieve source control. These are the features of care that are lifesaving. Excellent critical care and surgical reconstruction complete the spectrum of care required for this complex condition.

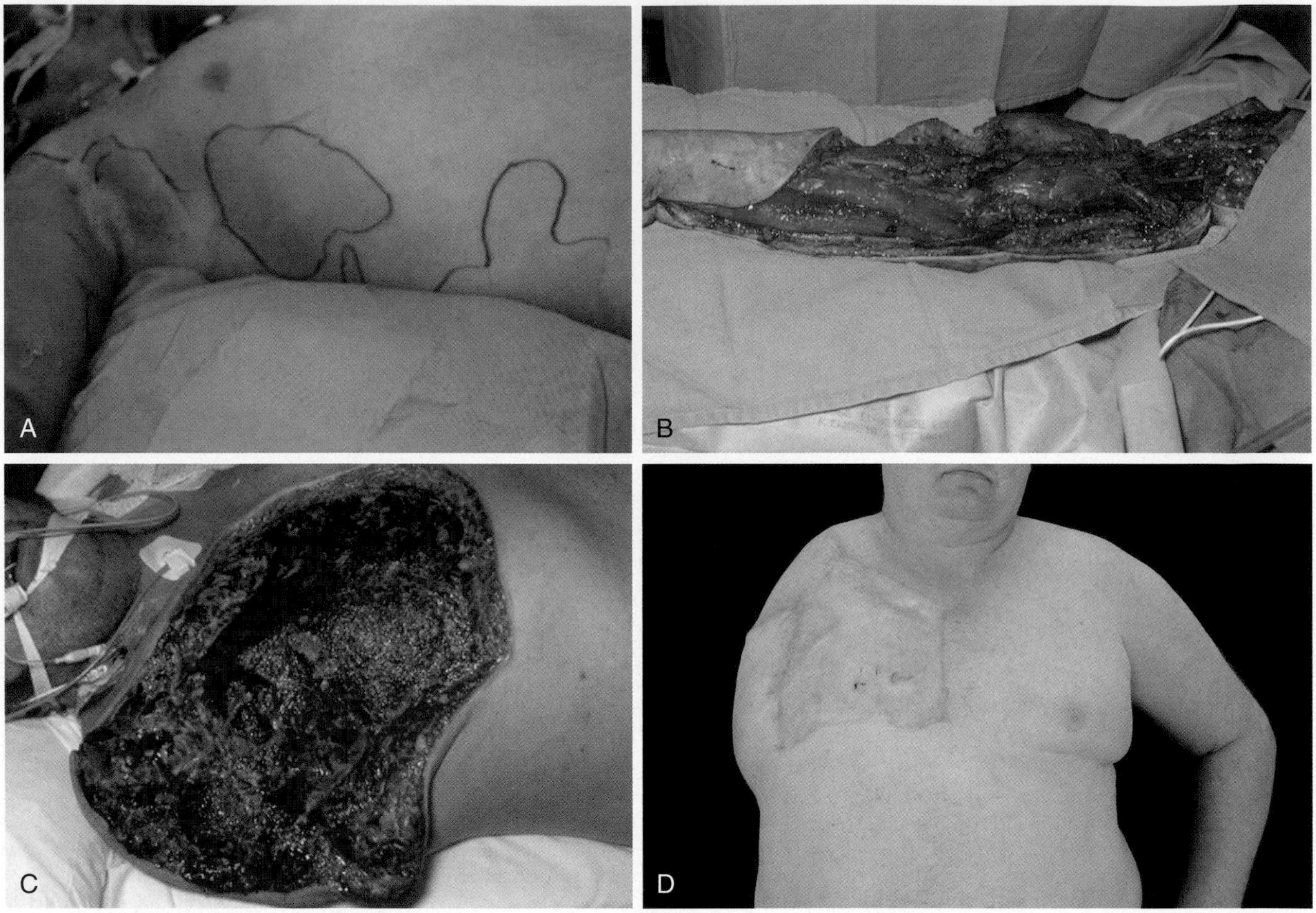

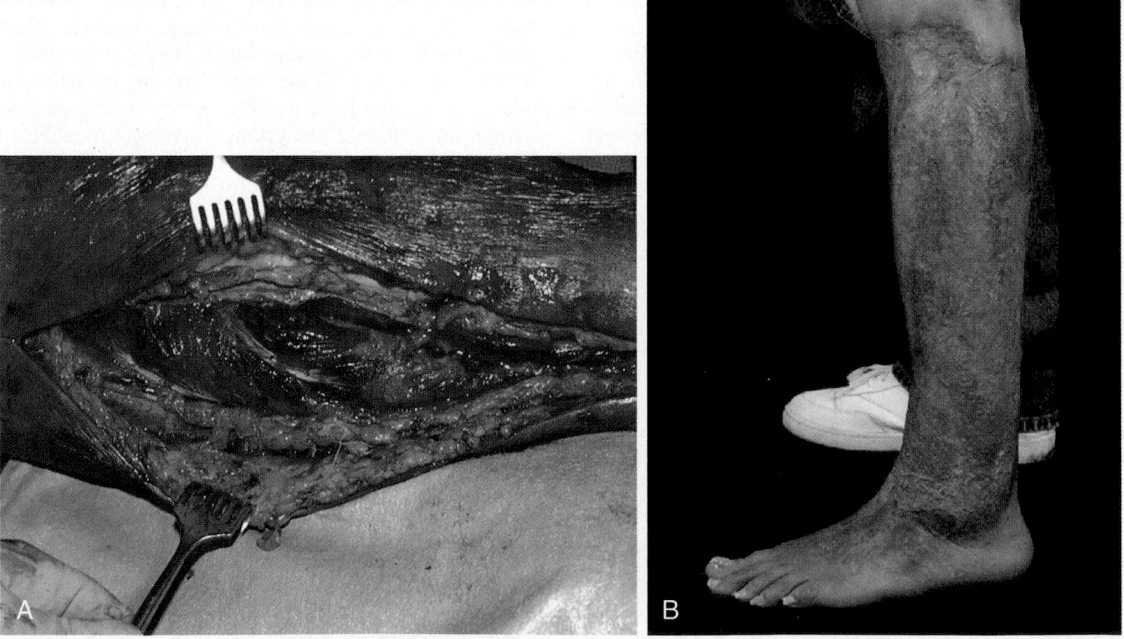

FIGURE 1 A, Erythematous intact skin in a patient diagnosed with necrotizing soft tissue infection. **B,** Postdébridement of severe underlying necrotizing infection in the same patient. **C,** Right arm amputation resulting from severity of the infection. **D,** Patient after skin grafting and reconstruction.

FIGURE 2 A, Image of a deep necrotizing fasciitis in lower limb. **B,** Same patient after débridement, skin grafting, and reconstruction.

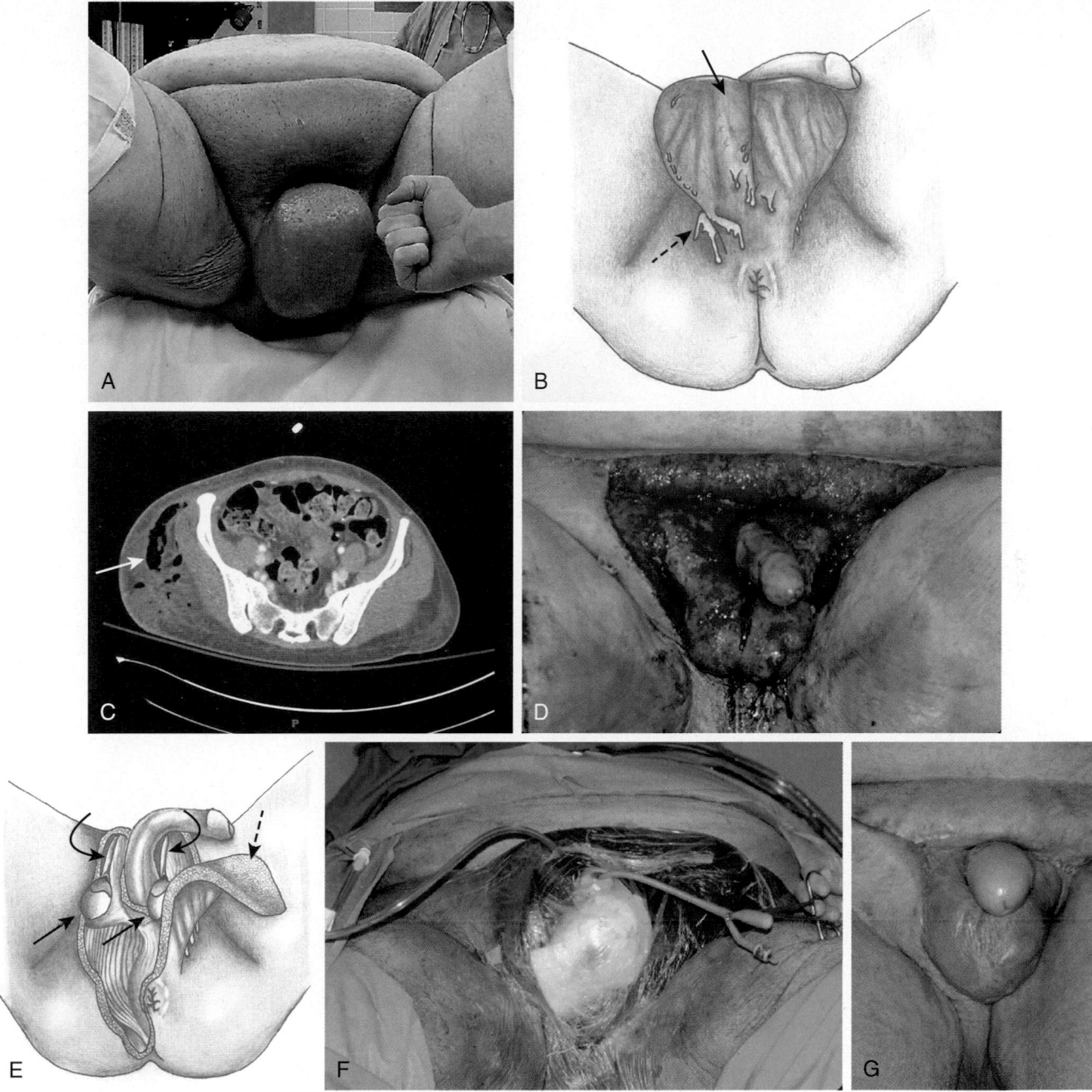

FIGURE 3 A, Discolored skin and swelling of genitalia suggestive of necrotizing soft tissue infection of perineum, Fournier's gangrene. **B,** Schematic illustration of Fournier's gangrene. Swollen necrotic scrotum *(solid arrow)* with purulent drainage *(dashed arrow).* **C,** Pelvis tomography of a patient diagnosed with Fournier's gangrene. Note the swollen soft tissue along with subcutaneous emphysema on the right side *(white arrow).* **D,** Surgical débridement of necrotic tissue has been performed. The testes are spared, as is the usual circumstance. **E,** Postdébridement illustration of the Fournier's gangrene. Testicles *(solid arrows)* hanging from the spermatic cords *(curved arrows)* underneath the partially débrided necrotic scrotum *(dashed arrow).* **F,** Vacuum dressing after surgical débridement. **G,** Appearance after skin grafting and reconstruction.

SUGGESTED READINGS

Descamps V, Aitken J, Lee MG. Hippocrates on necrotizing fasciitis. *Lancet.* 1994;344:556.

Hakkarainen TW, Kopari NM, Pham TN, et al. Necrotizing soft tissue infections: review and current concepts in treatment, systems of care, and outcomes. *Curr Probl Surg.* 2014;51:344-362.

Hippocrates. *Epidemics: (Translated by WHS Jones).* Vol. I. London: Heinemann, for Harvard University Press; 1957:24-43.

Jones J, United States Sanitary Commission. *Surgical Memoirs of the War of the Rebellion.* New York, NY: Hurd and Houghton; 1871 Investigation upon the nature, causes and treatment of hospital gangrene as prevailed in the Confederate armies 1861–1865; 142-580.

Laor E, Palmer LS, Tolia BM, et al. Outcome prediction in patients with Fournier's gangrene. *J Urol.* 1995;154:89-92.

Massey PR, Sakran JV, Mills AM, et al. Hyperbaric oxygen therapy in necrotizing soft tissue infections. *J Surg Res.* 2012;177:146-151.

Vacuum assisted wound closure therapy (2011). Stockholm: Swedish Council on Health and Technology Assessment (SBU). Alert Report Number: 2011-09.

Wong CH, Khin LW, Heng KS, et al. The LRINEC (Laboratory Risk Indicator for Necrotizing Fasciitis) score: a tool for distinguishing necrotizing fasciitis from other soft tissue infections. *Crit Care Med.* 2004;32:153.

THE MANAGEMENT OF PRIMARY CHEST WALL TUMORS

Jennifer L. Wilson, MD, and Richard I. Whyte, MD, MBA

Although chest wall masses are relatively uncommon, many surgeons will encounter them at some point in their practices. The differential diagnosis of primary chest wall masses is broad and includes primary and secondary tumors as well as benign processes. Primary chest wall tumors are rare and constitute only 1% to 2% of all primary tumors and 5% of all thoracic neoplasms. They can be categorized into two dominant types based on their tissue of origin: (1) bony and cartilaginous tumors, and (2) soft tissue tumors. Nearly half of primary chest wall tumors are benign lesions. The most common benign lesions are chondromas and fibrous dysplasia (which is seen as a mass but is not technically a neoplasm), whereas the most common malignant lesions are chondrosarcoma in the adult population and Ewing's sarcoma in the pediatric population. Secondary neoplasms of the chest wall comprise nearly half of chest wall tumors and include metastatic lesions from primary carcinomas as well as direct extension from adjacent breast or lung neoplasms. A survey of benign and malignant primary chest wall tumors is provided in Box 1. The mean age at presentation is 26 years for benign tumors and 40 years for malignant tumors. With the exception of desmoid tumors, primary chest wall tumors are twice as frequent in males as in females. In most cases, the paradigm of diagnosis, followed by staging, followed by treatment is applicable. In some cases, a multidisciplinary approach is critical in determining the optimal treatment strategy, and in cases in which a wide chest wall resection is necessary, careful preoperative planning is necessary to guarantee a successful reconstruction.

■ INITIAL EVALUATION

History and Physical Examination

Chest wall tumors generally are seen in one of three ways: as a painless, enlarging mass; as a painful mass; or as an incidental finding on a radiologic study done for other reasons. The history should focus on whether the mass is symptomatic or asymptomatic, with symptoms such as pain or a history of rapid enlargement suggesting malignancy. Associated symptoms such as sensory or motor deficits, weight loss, fatigue, dyspnea, and hoarseness may be clues to the underlying pathology or extent of the lesion. A history of a malignancy should lead one to consider metastatic disease as a likely diagnosis, whereas a history of a hematologic disorder may lead one to consider multiple myeloma.

On physical examination the surgeon should assess the size and mobility of the lesion relative to overlying or underlying structures. Also important is the presence or absence of skin changes, as these may indicate how much skin needs to be removed in the case of a future resection.

Imaging

After physical examination, imaging is critical in assessing any chest wall mass. The primary imaging modalities are computed tomography (CT) and magnetic resonance imaging (MRI). Although plain films often are obtained as part of an initial evaluation of a chest wall mass, these studies will provide little information regarding purely soft tissue lesions and information that is generally inadequate for either diagnosis or surgical planning regarding bony or cartilaginous lesions. Although perhaps diagnostic for multiple myeloma (multiple punched-out rib lesions), plain films almost invariably will be followed by CT or MRI—CT being better for bony lesions and MRI being better for soft tissue lesions. In many cases, both CT and MRI are necessary. CT is used to evaluate tumor extent and identify pulmonary metastases, whereas MRI is particularly useful for identifying invasion into contiguous structures. Many primary bony and cartilaginous tumors have highly characteristic radiographic features. Bone scans, rarely performed nowadays, have a limited role but are helpful in the differentiation of solitary plasmacytoma from multiple myeloma and in the identification of polyostotic fibrous dysplasia. For secondary chest wall tumors, positron emission tomography (PET) may be important to fully stage the primary tumor.

Biopsy

Once identified, primary chest wall tumors require a histologic diagnosis. Excisional biopsies are preferred for tumors less than 4 to 5 cm in diameter, whereas incisional biopsies may be performed for larger tumors. Several principles must be followed when performing incisional biopsies. One should avoid raising skin flaps because seeding of malignant cells has been reported. Moreover, the biopsy incision should be positioned in a manner that allows for re-excision if pathologic analysis demonstrates malignancy. A needle biopsy may be an alternative to an incisional biopsy, although seeding of the biopsy tract may occur and tissue may be insufficient for diagnosis. Fine-needle aspiration usually is not adequate for anything other than diagnosing metastatic disease from a distant primary site. On the other hand, a core needle biopsy is far more likely to be diagnostic for a primary chest wall mass. Some cartilaginous tumors, such as chondrosarcoma, have a heterogeneous histologic picture, and a limited biopsy, either incisional or core needle, may misrepresent the histologic degree of differentiation.

Finally, as with other tumors, an indeterminate biopsy, or the presence of a benign diagnosis, does not rule out malignancy, and therefore resection often remains indicated.

BOX 1: Primary Chest Wall Tumors

Benign

Chondroma
Fibrous dysplasia
Osteochondroma
Lipoma
- Fibroma
- Neurilemmoma

Eosinophilic granuloma
Aneurysmal bone cyst
Osteoid osteoma
Osteoblastoma
Giant cell tumor

Malignant

Chondrosarcoma
Osteosarcoma
Liposarcoma
Malignant fibrous histiocytoma
Rhabdomyosarcoma
Angiosarcoma
Fibrosarcoma
Neurofibrosarcoma
Ewing's sarcoma, primitive neuroectodermal tumor (PNET),
    small round blue cell tumor
Plasmacytoma

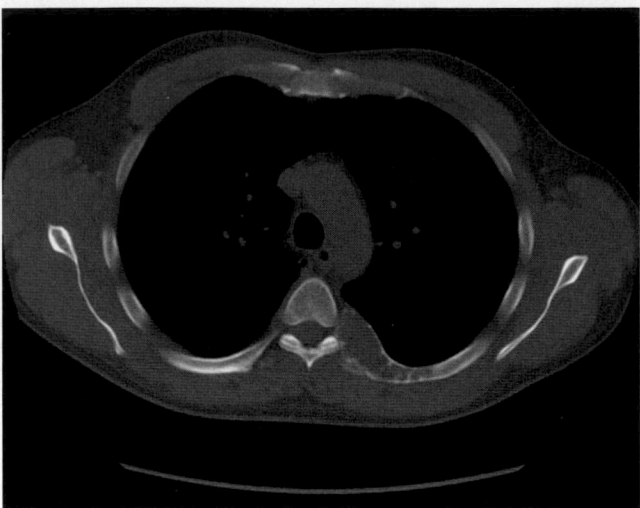

FIGURE 1 Chest computed tomographic scan demonstrating fibrous dysplasia of the posterior left sixth rib.

Radiographic features include a pedunculated osseous protuberance with cortical and medullary continuity with the bone of origin. Osteochondromas may lead to pathologic fractures or nerve compression. Malignant degeneration is rare but should be suspected in patients with new onset of pain at the lesion site and thickening of the characteristic cartilage cap documented on imaging studies. Treatment of osteochondromas is with local excision.

■ COMMON BENIGN CHEST WALL TUMORS

Chondroma

Chondromas are benign cartilaginous tumors that typically arise anteriorly from cartilage at the costochondral junction and are the most common benign chest wall tumor. Radiographically, they appear as lobulated, well-demarcated osteolytic lesions with well-defined sclerotic margins. There is a 1% to 2% incidence of malignant transformation to chondrosarcoma. Radiographically, it may be difficult to differentiate between chondromas and chondrosarcomas; consequently, treatment is local excision.

Fibrous Dysplasia

Fibrous dysplasia is a disorder in which osteoblasts fail to undergo normal differentiation and maturation. The result is a benign tumor that is monostotic in 70% to 80% of cases and polyostotic in 20% to 30% of cases. Fibrous dysplasia constitutes approximately 30% of benign chest wall tumors. Lesions usually occur in the posterior or lateral aspect of the rib and may be associated with a prior history of trauma. Most cases occur in the second and third decades of life. Most patients are asymptomatic, although occasionally the tumor may lead to a pathologic fracture and resultant pain. Radiographic findings include a fusiform mass with amorphous or irregular calcification and cortical thickening (Figure 1). Ground-glass appearance in the central aspect of the rib is characteristic. Local excision is performed for symptomatic painful, enlarging masses and is curative. Excision of an asymptomatic rib lesion generally is not necessary. However, it may be appropriate in other locations to prevent deformity or pathologic fracture.

Osteochondroma

These tumors are cartilage-capped bony growths that usually occur anteriorly at the costochondral junction. Peak incidence is in the second decade of life, and these lesions are most common in males.

■ MALIGNANT PRIMARY CHEST WALL TUMORS

Surgery is the mainstay of treatment for localized sarcomas, whereas multimodality therapy is the standard for small round cell tumors. Plasmacytomas are treated with high-dose radiation therapy.

Chondrosarcoma

Chondrosarcomas are the most common malignant primary chest wall tumor. These tumors constitute 50% of all malignant primary chest wall tumors and 25% of all primary chest wall tumors. They typically are seen between ages 30 and 60 and may develop de novo or in previously benign cartilaginous tumors. They arise anteriorly from the ribs in 80% of cases and from the sternum in 20% of cases. Radiographically, the typical appearance of a chondrosarcoma is one of a lobulated mass arising from the medullary portion of a rib or the sternum, often with associated cortical bone destruction (Figure 2). Treatment consists of wide local excision. For tumors that originate in the sternum, sternectomy with excision of bilateral costal arches is indicated.

Chondrosarcomas are relatively resistant to chemotherapy and radiation, although postoperative radiation therapy has been used for local control for resections with positive margins. Five-year survival after surgical resection is 60% for all patients and 80% for those without evidence of metastatic disease. Local recurrence rate for all patients is approximately 20%. Recurrence in one series was reported as 10% in patients with adequate surgical margins compared with 75% in those with inadequate margins. Furthermore, mortality at 5 years was twice as high in the patients with local recurrence in this series. Metastatic disease is present at the time of diagnosis in 10% of patients and most frequently involves the lung. Poor prognostic factors for chondrosarcomas include high tumor grade, large tumor size, incomplete resection, local recurrence, presence of metastatic disease, and age older than 50 years.

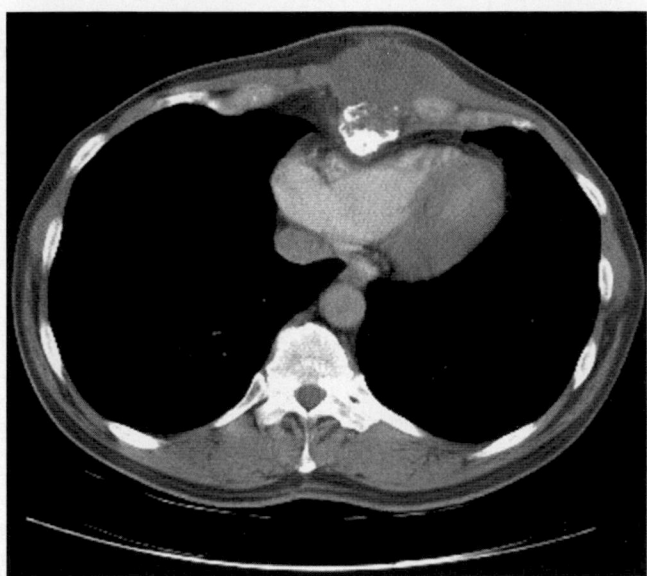

FIGURE 2 Computed tomographic scan demonstrating a chondrosarcoma of the lower sternum and xyphoid.

Osteosarcoma

Although osteosarcomas commonly originate from the metaphysis of long bones, occasionally they originate from a rib, scapula, or clavicle. Most chest wall osteosarcomas are seen in young adults as a painful mass. Less often, they may be seen in older persons in association with prior irradiation, Paget's disease, or chemotherapy. Radiographic findings include a classic sunburst pattern of new periosteal bone formation. A multimodality treatment strategy is used, beginning with preoperative chemotherapy followed by wide local excision. Long-term survival for patients with chest wall osteosarcomas is poor, with only a 15% reported 5-year survival. Of the 70% of patients who have metastases, the majority of which occur in the lung, 5-year survival is near zero. Poor prognostic factors include poor response to preoperative chemotherapy and multifocal disease.

Soft Tissue Sarcoma

Fifty percent of primary chest wall sarcomas are soft tissue sarcomas. This diverse group of tumors includes liposarcomas, malignant fibrous histiocytomas, rhabdomyosarcomas, angiosarcomas, and fibrosarcomas. Wide local excision is the mainstay of treatment, although adjuvant radiation therapy may be useful for inadequate margins of resection and recurrences. Chemotherapy also is used in the treatment of rhabdomyosarcoma, in which protocols of neoadjuvant chemotherapy followed by surgical excision confer a survival advantage of 70% at 5 years compared with 25% for surgical excision alone. Poor prognostic factors for chest wall soft tissue sarcomas include high tumor grade, positive surgical margins, and presence of metastatic disease.

Desmoid Tumors

Desmoid tumors, also known as aggressive fibromatoses, may be considered low-grade fibrosarcomas, but their unique characteristics warrant further discussion. Desmoids are seen most often in women of reproductive age and, although 50% of these lesions arise in the abdomen, the chest wall is the most common extra-abdominal site of origin (10% to 20%). Predisposing factors include a history of trauma (present in 25% of cases), Gardner's syndrome, and estrogen exposure. These tumors are characterized by local invasion and frequent recurrences; they do not metastasize. Wide local excision is the primary treatment. Radiation may be used as an adjunct for incomplete resection. Anecdotal studies on the use of antiestrogen therapy also have been reported. A report from the Mayo Clinic demonstrates a 37.5% 5-year probability of local recurrence after resection. Of the recurrences, 89% occurred in cases with positive margins of excision and 18% occurred in cases with negative margins.

Ewing's Sarcoma and Primitive Neuroectodermal Tumor

Ewing's sarcoma and primitive neuroectodermal tumor (PNET or Askin's tumor) are small round cell tumors with local and systemic manifestations. Both are associated with a translocation between chromosomes 11 and 22 and occur predominantly in children and young adults. Ewing's sarcoma arises from the chest wall in 15% of cases and is the most common primary chest wall malignancy in children. Presentation is with a painful mass and associated systemic signs, including fever and malaise. Characteristic radiographic findings are a chest wall mass with bony destruction and an onion-peel appearance due to multiple layers of new periosteal bone formation. Treatment requires a multidisciplinary approach including neoadjuvant multidrug chemotherapy followed by wide surgical excision. Radiation often is used for additional local control, and adjuvant chemotherapy may prevent or treat metastases. A recent study found a 5-year event-free survival (defined as freedom from disease progression, death, or diagnosis of second malignant neoplasm) of 56% with a multimodality treatment strategy. Overall 5-year survival has been reported as 50% to 65% in various single-institution studies.

Plasmacytoma

Solitary plasmacytomas, tumors of plasma cell origin, constitute 10% to 30% of primary chest wall malignancies. They occur most frequently in the rib, followed by the clavicle and sternum. Evaluation includes excisional biopsy, imaging studies, and serum and urine electrophoresis to rule out multiple myeloma. The radiographic appearance is of a multicystic expansile mass or an osteolytic mass without expansion. Once the diagnosis is established, treatment consists of high-dose irradiation to 5000 cGy. Late progression to multiple myeloma occurs in 35% to 55% of cases and correlates with a worse prognosis. Overall 5-year survival after treatment is 25% to 37%.

■ TREATMENT OF PRIMARY CHEST WALL TUMORS

Most primary chest wall tumors are treated with wide local excision. Acceptable margins of excision for benign lesions are 2 cm or less, whereas acceptable margins of excision for most malignant chest wall tumors are 4 cm. Many of these tumors are locally aggressive, and the incidence of tumor recurrence correlates with the presence of positive surgical margins. Negative margins of 4 cm are associated with significantly lower local recurrence rates than margins of 2 cm. One study reported a 56% 5-year freedom from recurrence in patients with malignant primary chest wall tumors resected with 4-cm margins, compared with 29% in a cohort resected with 2-cm margins. Given the location of chest wall tumors, it may be difficult to obtain wide surgical margins circumferentially. Adjuvant external beam irradiation or intraoperative radiation therapy has been used in these cases to improve local control.

A small group of malignant chest wall tumors are treated nonoperatively—that is, with chemotherapy or radiation—or with combined modality therapy consisting of chemotherapy, surgery, and radiation therapy. These include plasmacytomas, which are treated with radiation, and the small round cell tumors (Ewing's sarcoma and PNETs), which are treated with a combination of chemotherapy and radiation.

■ OPERATIVE TECHNIQUES

Chest Wall Resection

The goals of the operation are complete en bloc excision with negative margins, preservation of uninvolved tissue for coverage, and restoration of chest wall mechanics. With appropriate planning and preoperative evaluation, chest wall resection can be performed with limited morbidity and mortality to the patient. Preoperative evaluation should include pulmonary function assessment, cardiac evaluation, and appropriate imaging studies. In the current era, respiratory failure secondary to paradoxic ventilation can be avoided with appropriate skeletal reconstruction.

Careful planning preoperatively can allow the surgeon to perform the resection without violating the tumor capsule and potentially causing tumor spread. Surgery for malignant chest wall tumors proceeds in three phases: resection, skeletal reconstruction, and soft tissue reconstruction.

For the chest wall resection, single lung ventilation is helpful but not essential, and placement of an epidural catheter should be considered. The patient typically is positioned in either supine or lateral decubitus position, depending on tumor location. For tumors that do not involve the skin, an incision is made overlying the tumor mass; skin flaps are raised, and skeletal and soft tissue resections are performed. If a prior biopsy scar is present, the scar is excised. Preoperative planning is essential if a muscle flap will be used for postexcision reconstruction. For example, sparing the serratus anterior and latissimus muscles during thoracotomy or the pectoralis during anterior chest wall resection will preserve these muscles for subsequent chest wall reconstruction (see Box 1). Before reconstruction, frozen sections may be helpful to evaluate for negative margins. The specimen should be oriented carefully and the margins marked clearly for pathology testing; it is helpful to orient the pathologist in person when possible. For anterior rib tumors, the anterior costal cartilage also should be excised, and because of the possibility of extension of the tumor within the bone marrow, resections for malignant rib tumors should include all involved ribs in their entirety—as well as what is necessary to obtain an adequate margin and one rib above and below the tumor.

Malignant sternal tumors require either partial or total sternectomy along with excision of the contiguous bilateral costal cartilages. For tumors in the lower sternum, the manubrium can be preserved. A subtotal sternectomy with preservation of the upper 2 cm of the manubrium and clavicles is performed for tumors of the sternal body. For tumors in the manubrium, preservation of the lower sternum is feasible. Tissues adherent to the tumor, including lung, thymus, pericardium, and diaphragm, should be resected en bloc with the tumor.

In cases of vertebral involvement, preoperative evaluation by an experienced spine surgeon is important. An MRI must be obtained to better visualize the area of suspected invasion and to rule out intradural extension. Disarticulation of the ribs can be performed by reflecting the paraspinous ligament posteriorly and dividing the cartilage between the transverse process and the rib. The rib then can be lifted off the foramen with a curved osteotome with any force directed away from the spinal cord, taking care to avoid intercostal nerve avulsion, which could cause a cerebrospinal fluid leak as a result of a dural sheath injury. If disarticulation of the rib is required, ligation of the intercostal bundle should be performed at the level of the neural foramen. Depending on tumor involvement, partial or total laminectomy or vertebrectomy may be required. Bleeding can be controlled with bipolar cautery to avoid thermal injury to the spinal cord. In addition, expanding hemostatic agents (i.e., Surgicel or gel foam) should not be used, to avoid spinal cord compression.

Chest Wall Reconstruction

Skeletal reconstruction is the next phase of the procedure. The goals of skeletal reconstruction are to re-establish stability of the rib cage and maintain adequate lung function. A general principle of chest wall reconstruction is that defects of up to two ribs do not require specific reconstructive efforts. Furthermore, larger posterior resections beneath the scapula may not require reconstruction, as lung herniation is prevented by the scapula. An important point about posterior resections involving the fifth rib is that painful entrapment of the scapula may occur unless either the rib is notched or the tip of the scapula is removed. Smaller defects (<5 cm) may be covered with autologous tissue alone, whereas larger defects (>5 cm) require chest wall stabilization in order to preserve respiratory mechanics and prevent paradoxical respiration.

In general, skeletal reconstruction is achieved by suturing prosthetic mesh to the chest wall under tension, creating a drum-tight chest wall prosthesis. A variety of materials have been used to achieve this effect. These include Marlex mesh, Prolene mesh, and polytetrafluoroethylene (PTFE) patches. Rigid Marlex-methyl methacrylate prostheses, although associated with an excellent cosmetic appearance, are often associated with an uncomfortable subjective sense of chest wall rigidity and noncompliance and have fallen out of favor. Use of flexible mesh is now more popular, as the mesh can be attached quickly and provides for prevention of lung herniation, and resultant cosmetic issues can be dealt with later. Prosthetic (metal) ribs and sternum have been used in chest wall reconstructions; however, their use has not become routine. Prosthetic reconstruction is contraindicated in infected wounds; in these cases, either skeletal reconstruction is delayed or acellular dermal matrix (AlloDerm or Strattice) can be used in place of the prosthetic material.

Reconstruction of the anterior chest wall after complete sternal resection requires a rigid prosthesis for chest wall stabilization (i.e., prevention of paradoxical respiration and protection of underlying mediastinal structures). Reconstruction is accomplished with a rigid prosthesis and free or rotational muscle flap coverage. Rigid reconstruction is not necessary in cases of partial resection (when less than one third of the sternum or the manubrium only is removed), but soft tissue flap coverage still may be necessary in order to cover the defect.

Various materials have been used, including mesh supported by moldable titanium metal plates, sandwiched Marlex and stainless steel mesh, and Marlex mesh–methyl methacrylate composites. For partial sternal resections, a flexible patch alone may be sufficient to prevent paradoxic respiration. Resection of the manubrium and its associated costal cartilages typically does not result in paradoxic respiration, so soft tissue reconstruction alone (without prosthetic reconstruction) is sufficient.

There are many options for free or rotational flaps (Table 1) depending on the location and size of defect to be covered, local

TABLE 1: Commonly Used Autologous Flaps for Chest Wall Reconstruction

Tissue	Arterial Supply	Location of Defect
Latissimus	Thoracodorsal	Anterolateral and posterior
Pectoralis major	Thoracoacromial	Anterior
Serratus anterior	Lateral thoracic	Intrathoracic
Rectus abdominis	Superior epigastric	Anterior and midline
External oblique	Deep circumflex iliac, posterior intercostal arteries	Inframammary fold
Omentum	Gastroepiploic	Anterior and midline

wound conditions (including prior irradiation and residual tumor), nutritional status, and overall prognosis. In general, rotational flaps based on an axial blood supply are used most often. Latissimus dorsi is the largest flat muscle on the thorax and can cover defects antero-laterally as well as posteriorly. A previous non–muscle-sparing pos-terolateral thoracotomy will compromise the ability to use a latissimus dorsi flap. The pectoralis major is well suited for coverage of anterior chest wall defects. The rectus abdominis can be used for coverage of lower sternal wounds, and the harvest site can be closed primarily. Other muscle sources that are used include serratus anterior, external oblique, and trapezius. When rotational flaps are not adequate, soft tissue reconstruction can be achieved with a free flap or omentum. The omentum is an excellent flap as well, especially when the chest wall has been irradiated and wound healing is a concern. If a pedicled or advancement flap is not an option, free flaps with microvascular anastomoses or transverse rectus abdominis myocutaneous (TRAM) flaps can be used.

■ SUMMARY

In summary, chest wall tumors comprise a heterogeneous group of lesions that require a consistent diagnostic approach, a thorough preoperative evaluation, and detailed operative planning. A histologic diagnosis must be obtained without compromising future treatment. The most common lesions are treated surgically, with such operations comprising both ablative and reconstructive com-ponents. Appropriate excisional margins must be obtained so as to minimize the chance of local recurrence, and subsequent recon-structions may use simple prosthetic replacement or more complex tissue transposition techniques.

SUGGESTED READINGS

Abbas AE, Deschamps C, Cassivi SD, et al. Chest-wall desmoid tumors: results of surgical intervention. *Ann Thorac Surg.* 2004;78:1219-1223.

Butterworth JA, Garvey PB, Baumann DP, et al. Optimizing reconstruction of oncologic sternectomy defects based on surgical outcomes. *J Am Coll Surg.* 2013;217:306-316.

Chapelier A. Resection and reconstruction for primary sternal tumors. *Thorac Surg Clin.* 2010;20:529-534. doi:10.1016/j.thorsurg.2010.06.002.

De Perrot M. Resection of superior sulcus tumors: anterior approach. *Op Tech Thorac Cardiovasc Surg.* 2011;16:138-153.

Gaspar N, Hawkins DS, Dirksen U, et al. Ewing sarcoma: current management and future approaches through collaboration. *J Clin Oncol.* 2015;33:3036-3046. doi:10.1200/JCO.2014.59.5256.

Thomas PA, Brouchet L. Prosthetic reconstruction of the chest wall. *Thorac Surg Clin.* 2010;20:551-558.

MEDIASTINAL MASSES

Douglas E. Wood, MD, and Edo K. S. Bedzra, MD

Mediastinal masses are a wide range of neoplasms, with unique characteristics, that are uncommon, represent only 3% of tho-racic tumors, and are divided equally between primary mediastinal neoplasms and secondary (metastatic) lesions. This spectrum includes an array of benign and malignant lesions, which are divided into three separate classes (anterior, middle, and posterior) by virtue of location (Box 1). Incidences in the general population vary by age, with most reports quoting a range in the third to fifth decades of life with a peak in the fifth.

Primary tumors generally arise from neurogenic and thymic tissues that together make up 50% of all such lesions but also do arise, not uncommonly, from lymphoid and mesenchymal tissues. Secondary mediastinal masses usually represent lymphatic spread from extramediastinal primary tumors, particularly of the gonads or lungs. Neurogenic tumors make up the preponderance of medi-astinal masses in the pediatric population, whereas thymic tumors are more prevalent in the adult population. This explains the varying incidence of mediastinal tumors by location; in adults, 54% to 68% of tumors are anterior mediastinal, about 18% to 20% are middle mediastinal, and 15% to 25% posterior mediastinal. In the pediatric population, these incidences are 35%, 12% to 15%, and 50%, respectively.

The mainstays of therapy for mediastinal masses are surgical exci-sion and chemotherapy, and the great majority of these neoplasms have favorable treatment outcomes, particularly when discovered early. However, most mediastinal masses are associated with no symptoms and are found incidentally on workup of unrelated condi-tions. This can lead to delays in diagnosis and affect choice of therapy and outcomes. Malignant lesions, which form 25% to 50% of medi-astinal lesions, with their aggressive biology are more likely to be symptomatic and result in compression or direct invasion of adjacent structures. Neoplasms such as thymomas and mediastinal parathy-roid tumors may have associated paraneoplastic syndromes such as myasthenia gravis.

A combination of history, imaging, and serology usually can suggest a diagnosis, but definitive management usually is guided by tissue biopsy.

■ ANATOMY

It generally is agreed that the mediastinum is bordered superiorly by the thoracic inlet, inferiorly by the diaphragm, and laterally by the medial reflections of the visceral pleura and extends posteriorly to the paravertebral sulci. Beyond this, however, consensus is hard to find within the radiologic and surgical realms. Some texts describe four mediastinal compartments, including superior, anterior, middle, and posterior divisions, whereas others note three compartments and exclude the superior compartment. For the thoracic surgeon, the most useful division is that proposed by Shields in 1972. It divides the mediastinum into anterior, middle or visceral, and posterior compartments. The anterior compartment is bordered by the innominate vessels, the anterior surface of the great vessels and peri-cardium, the posterior surface of the sternum, and the diaphragm. The middle mediastinum extends from the thoracic inlet to the dia-phragm and includes the innominate vessels and pericardium and all structures posterior to them but anterior to the vertebral column. Finally, the posterior mediastinum is located within the paravertebral sulci bilaterally and contains the proximal portions of the intercostal vessels and nerves, the sympathetic trunk, and the distal azygos vein, among others.

■ CLINICAL PRESENTATION AND DIAGNOSIS

Signs and Symptoms

It is unusual for a mediastinal mass to be seen with symptoms. In fact, only a third of these masses are symptomatic. To produce symp-toms, they have to enlarge to adequate size to compress adjacent structures or be aggressive enough to invade other structures. Malig-nant masses are thus more likely to be symptomatic. Consequently, the presence of symptoms is an important diagnostic clue in the management of mediastinal masses. Typical symptoms include shortness of breath, cough, and chest pain, whereas other presenta-tions may include physical examination findings of facial plethora

BOX 1: Mediastinal Masses

Anterior

Thymic neoplasms
Lymphoma
Substernal thyroid
Parathyroid adenoma
Germ-cell tumor

Middle

Bronchogenic cyst
Lymphoma
Pericardial cyst
Neuroenteric cyst
Lymphangioma
Fibroma

Posterior

Schwannoma
Neurofibroma
Ganglioneuroma
Ganglioneuroblastoma
Neuroblastoma
Pheochromocytoma
Chemodectoma

from superior vena cava (SVC) compression, Horner's syndrome with involvement of the sympathetic chain, diaphragmatic paralysis from phrenic nerve invasion, and hoarseness from involvement of the recurrent laryngeal nerve. Systemic manifestations of mediastinal tumors include paraneoplastic syndromes such as myasthenia gravis as well as the direct activity of tumor hormonal secretions such as hypercalcemia from parathyroid adenomas or gynecomastia from germ-cell tumors.

Imaging

The first hint of a mediastinal abnormality usually is found on a plain chest film obtained for an unrelated reason. This can be of some use in grossly localizing the lesion to one of the mediastinal compartments, particularly if a lateral image is obtained. Because pathology and incidence of different masses varies by compartments, the differential diagnoses can be narrowed. However, chest x-ray is not specific for diagnosis. A more sensitive and specific imaging modality is computed tomographic (CT) scanning, which can provide information on size, cystic versus solid composition of tumor, and involvement of nearby structures. In some cases, such as thymoma, CT scanning is practically diagnostic even without biopsy. Magnetic resonance imaging (MRI) can be helpful when involvement of the neural foramen is suggested in posterior mediastinal tumors but is rarely necessary otherwise. Likewise, positron emission tomographic (PET) scanning may be useful for evaluation of extrathoracic disease or extent of lymph node disease but does not have routine utility for the evaluation of most mediastinal masses.

Serology

Systemic tumor markers are important clinical tools in the evaluation and management of mediastinal tumors. Many different markers, including thyroid hormone, adrenocorticotropic hormone, catecholamines, and vasoactive intestinal polypeptide, are expressed by variant tumors. Levels of these hormones can correlate with presence of pathology, response to treatment, and recurrence. In particular, alpha-fetoprotein (AFP), beta human chorionic gonadotropin (beta-hCG), and lactate dehydrogenase (LDH) can diagnose malignant nonseminomatous germ-cell tumors and are used to differentiate such tumors from seminomatous germ-cell tumors and to guide therapy.

Biopsy Techniques and Surgical Approaches

The resolution of CT scans is so high now and available serologic testing is so improved that characteristics and behavior of mediastinal masses often can be ascertained by these tests alone and can obviate the need for pretreatment biopsy or guide the modality used for such biopsies. In fact, in certain instances biopsy may carry risks for seeding mediastinal structures and the chest wall and increasing the stage of disease. Therefore the general recommendation is that for small masses (<5 cm) with characteristic features like encapsulation in thymomas and heterogenous calcification in teratomas or for cases involving cysts, surgical resection can be performed for definitive diagnosis without a preceding biopsy.

For larger masses, those showing evidence of invasion, or those suspicious for lymphoma where no surgical resection is warranted, biopsy is performed. CT-guided needle biopsy is the standard choice. However, endobronchial ultrasound and endoesophageal ultrasound also provide avenues for obtaining fine-needle samples, especially in the middle mediastinum. Fine-needle aspiration with cytometric evaluation is sensitive and can provide diagnostic yields in excess of 90% in carcinomatous lesions. However, in cases where architecture of the tumor is important in diagnosis, such as lymphoma or thymomas, or where there is intratumoral heterogeneity, the yield can be much lower and a core needle or incisional biopsy becomes a more accurate modality. Reports from Europe suggest that core needle biopsy alone with histologic analyses can result in a diagnostic yield in excess of 95% in lymphomas.

Many surgical approaches can be used to perform biopsy on or to resect mediastinal tumors. It is important that biopsies are planned with anticipation of future surgical resection. A critical anesthetic issue of which the surgeon must be aware is airway compromise on induction, especially in cases of large masses. Surgical approaches include cervical mediastinoscopy, anterior mediastinoscopy (Chamberlain's procedure), median sternotomy, thoracotomy, unilateral and bilateral thoracosternotomy, and minimally invasive techniques such as video-assisted thoracoscopic surgery (VATS) and robotic surgery.

Cervical Mediastinoscopy

Cervical mediastinoscopy is a minimally invasive and helpful tool for diagnosis of mediastinal lesions that is used mostly for assessment of lymphadenopathy, particularly in the staging of lung cancer. Sampling of lymph node stations 2, 4, and 7 is accomplished fairly easily. A common error is to consider mediastinoscopy for large anterior mediastinal masses. In general, these tumors lie anterior to the great vessels and therefore are not accessible by mediastinoscopy, which is most useful for middle mediastinal tumors cephalad to the subcarinal space, most commonly lymphomas or mediastinal nodal involvement of other benign or malignant processes.

An understanding of the three-dimensional anatomy of the mediastinum is critical to safety during this procedure. Particularly, one should be acutely aware of the azygos vein and SVC to the right, the right pulmonary artery anterior to the carina, the recurrent laryngeal nerve in the tracheoesophageal groove on the left, and the innominate vessels and aortic arch just anterior to the trachea. Careful palpation of anatomy and correlation to preoperative imaging before insertion of the scope will alert the operator to high-riding innominate arteries and areas of significant pathology to guide mediastinoscopy. Dissecting onto the airway as opposed to away from the airway and eliminating cautery on the left will minimize pneumothoraces and injury to the SVC, azygos, and recurrent laryngeal nerve.

Anterior Mediastinoscopy

One of the limitations of cervical mediastinoscopy is an inability to access prevascular or aortopulmonary window lesions or lymphadenopathy for biopsy. In these cases, an anterior mediastinoscopy, the so-called Chamberlain's procedure, can be a useful tool. It is described classically as an incision through the left second interspace. Splitting the pectoral muscle fibers reveals the intercostal muscles, which can be incised, and the chondral cartilage, a piece of which can be resected if necessary to provide access to the anterior mediastinum. If necessary, the pleura can be incised to perform lung biopsy or assess the pulmonary hilum.

Median Sternotomy

Median sternotomy is the procedure of choice for thymectomy and other tumors in the anterior mediastinum. It provides excellent exposure, allowing for safe and complete resection. A partial sternotomy can be performed for cosmesis but provides little advantage over a full sternotomy.

Thoracotomy, Thoracosternotomy, and Bilateral Thoracosternotomy

Thoracotomy can provide access to tumors in all three mediastinal compartments but mostly is utilized for tumors in the posterior mediastinum. An open approach provides excellent exposure for complete resection. However, where anterior tumors extend to or involve hilar structures, a unilateral thoracosternotomy incorporating a sternotomy and an anterior thoracotomy is a versatile incision that allows anteromedial dissection to provide intrapericardial hilar control. First, the thoracotomy is made through the fourth interspace to evaluate resectability. Then a partial sternotomy is completed through an adjoining incision extended to the anterior border of the sternocleidomastoid.

A bilateral (clamshell) thoracosternotomy is even more versatile, as it provides access to the anterior mediastinum and bilateral hemithoraces. It involves bilateral thoracotomies through the fourth interspace extending to the midaxillary line that are connected with a transverse sternotomy. This incision is used classically in bilateral lung transplantation but can be very helpful in resection of large anterior mediastinal masses, particularly when they extend to the pleura on both sides.

Video-Assisted Thoracoscopic Surgery and Robotic Surgery

Minimally invasive videoscopic techniques are established paradigms in thoracic surgery and can be used for thymectomy, resection of smaller masses, and mediastinal cysts. For selected masses they actually may provide better visualization than open procedures and have similar outcomes. They are highly specialized, however, and should be utilized only by surgeons who use them frequently for other procedures. Here again we urge caution in adapting these approaches for resection of thymomas and other malignant lesions, as port site and pleural seeding have been reported, resulting in conversion of stage I thymomas to stage IV disease because of failures in surgical technique.

■ ANTERIOR MEDIASTINUM

The anterior mediastinum contains the largest proportion of mediastinal masses. About 95% belong to the so-called four Ts of anterior mediastinal tumors: thymic tumors, thyroid goiters, teratomas, and "terrible" lymphoma.

Thymic Tumors

Thymic tumors are the most common anterior mediastinal masses. Historically they have been classified by histologic characteristics into two categories: thymoma, typically neoplasms with well-differentiated features, and thymic carcinoma, with abundant mitotic figures and features of aggression and poor differentiation. However, to further improve this classification's prognostic usefulness, the World Health Organization (WHO) developed a classification system (Table 1) that correlates to prognosis and tumor biology.

TABLE 1: World Health Organization Classification of Thymic Epithelial Tissues

Tumor Type	Histology
A	Medullary
AB	Mixed, normal thymic tissue with lymphocyte-rich foci
B1	Predominantly cortical, appears like normal thymic tissue
B2	Cortical, lymphocyte-rich
B3	Well-differentiated thymic carcinoma, epithelial cells with mild or no atypia
C	Thymic carcinoma with histologic atypia

Thymomas are the most common thymic neoplasms and are the type most often associated with myasthenia gravis. The syndrome is present in approximately 50% of all patients with thymomas. However, only 15% to 20% of patients who have myasthenia gravis have a thymoma. One half to two thirds of patients with thymoma are symptomatic at presentation, with symptoms caused by locoregional mass effects such as pain, dyspnea, and cough and by parathymic syndromes such as myasthenia gravis, aplastic anemia in 5%, and hypogammaglobulinemia in 1%. The patient's age at presentation varies based on whether the patient has myasthenia gravis. Patients with the syndrome usually are seen at younger ages, with the peak being 30 to 40 years, whereas those without myasthenia gravis are seen later, at 60 to 70 years.

CT scan typically shows a well-defined anterior mediastinal soft tissue mass in early stage disease but may show a mass with irregular borders exhibiting invasion of adjacent structures such as mediastinal pleura and encasement of vasculature in advanced disease. A common area of confusion on interpretation of imaging is the important differentiation of thymoma from lymphoma, particularly because treatment is markedly different. Lymphoma nearly always is seen with extensive unresectable mediastinal disease or more widespread lymphadenopathy, whereas most thymomas are seen as discrete anterior mediastinal masses in the thymic bed. The latter characteristics on imaging allow a strong presumptive diagnosis of thymoma and a choice of direct surgical excision without biopsy. A more extensive or apparently unresectable anterior mediastinal mass is one that does warrant biopsy, by either core needle or anterior mediastinoscopy, in order to obtain a tissue diagnosis and plan appropriate therapy, including possible multimodal therapy for an advanced stage thymoma.

Thymic carcinomas make up less than 10% of thymic neoplasms and are usually symptomatic at presentation. Prognosis is considerably worse because of a high degree of systemic disease, with median survival pegged at 2 years. These tumors are not associated with paraneoplastic syndromes, with the exception of thymic carcinoids, which do cause syndromes such as Cushing's syndrome and the syndrome of inappropriate antidiuretic hormone secretion. In all cases, myasthenia gravis has not been described.

Staging of resected thymic tumors most commonly is done with the Masaoka staging system (Table 2). It is a pathologic staging system because microscopic invasion of the capsule can be determined only in resected specimen. This system and completeness of resection are the main predictors of survival in the treatment of thymic neoplasms.

The underpinning of definitive treatment for thymoma is complete surgical resection. If the tumor is small and amenable to resection, this is the preferred approach and a biopsy to guide management is not warranted. The only tumors warranting needle

TABLE 2: Masaoka Staging of Thymic Neoplasms

Stage	Criteria	5-Year Disease-Free Survival
I	Macroscopically completely encapsulated and microscopically no capsular invasion	100%
II	Macroscopic invasion into surrounding fatty tissue or mediastinal pleura, or microscopic invasion into capsule	100%
III	Macroscopic invasion into neighboring organ (i.e., pericardium, great vessels, or lung)	59.6%
IVa	Pleural or pericardial dissemination	53.7%
IVb	Lymphogenous or hematogenous metastasis	41.7%

or open biopsy are large, invasive tumors that are not amenable to resection.

Because more than 90% of these neoplasms are localized at presentation, margin-negative resection can be achieved in most early stage disease. Even for advanced stage disease, resection of vascular structures, pericardium, or lung can enable complete resection. Where tumors are too large and for advanced stage disease, neoadjuvant chemotherapy using cisplatin-based regimens can lead to a decrease in tumor size and extent, thus facilitating surgical resection. It is unclear whether adjuvant radiotherapy in the management of thymic neoplasms in the absence of microscopic residual disease after resection is of benefit. As well, it is unclear if incomplete resection is better than no resection. However, where there is incomplete resection of tumor, adjuvant radiotherapy is associated with decreased recurrence rates and is considered for stage II and stage III tumors after resection.

Special preoperative planning is necessary in the management of patients with the presence of myasthenia gravis. In this instance, thymectomy is indicated in all cases where there is a thymoma or in cases where the nonthymomatous myasthenia is refractory to medical management with anticholinesterases, immunosuppressives, or short-term immunotherapy like plasmapheresis. Thymectomy results in significant improvement of symptoms, with remission mostly experienced between 5 and 10 years. Anesthetic management should be based on inhaled anesthetics with no neuromuscular blockade or depolarizing agents, and consideration should be given to plasmapheresis where disease is severe or there is significant reduction in pulmonary function preoperatively.

For both thymoma and nonthymomatous myasthenia, we recommend complete resection of thymic tissue extending laterally from phrenic nerve to phrenic nerve and extending from the lower pole of the thyroids to the diaphragm. This is best achieved through a median sternotomy. As described previously, however, videoscopic approaches have been used in specialized centers for the management of thymic disease.

Germ-Cell Tumors

Extragonadal germ-cell tumors are believed to arise from embryonic cells left behind during cellular division and migration. There are three different types: teratomas and seminomatous and nonseminomatous germ-cell tumors. Diagnosis usually can be established with a combination of CT scanning and serologic testing of AFP and beta-hCG levels, although tissue biopsy is still commonly performed.

Mature Teratomas

Mature teratomas are benign germ-cell neoplasms that account for 5% to 10% of all mediastinal masses but 50% to 70% of all mediastinal germ-cell tumors. They have equal prevalence in males and females but occur with more frequency in the pediatric population. Mature teratomas routinely contain tissue from all three germ-cell lines of mesoderm, ectoderm, and endoderm, with ectoderm predominance. They thus have a heterogenous appearance on CT scans, with images revealing a mass with fluid, fat, and calcification. Diagnosis often can be made on cross-sectional imaging, and AFP and beta-hCG levels are routinely obtained and are normal. Surgical resection remains the standard treatment, as these tumors have not shown susceptibility to systemic or radiation therapy. Management can be complicated by infected or ruptured cysts. Recurrence rates are low in mature teratomas. Rare immature teratomas that contain fetal tissue are malignant and should be followed with imaging for recurrence or metastasis after resection.

Seminomas

Primary mediastinal seminomatous germ-cell tumors, seminomas, account for one third of malignant mediastinal germ-cell tumors. They are found almost exclusively in young adult males in the third to fourth decades of life and are often asymptomatic, discovered coincidentally on chest imaging for other reasons. This is because they are slow-growing tumors. However, because of the absence of symptoms until advanced disease, 60% to 70% of seminomas have metastasized to such sites as local lymph nodes, lung, and bone by the time of presentation. Diagnosis is by a combination of CT imaging and CT-guided biopsy. Imaging reveals large, lobulated, but homogenous anterior mediastinal lesions. Given their cell line of origin, it is imperative that clinical evaluation include evaluation for a gonadal primary. Though historical treatment was predicated on mediastinal radiation, concerns for radiation toxicity and subsequent studies showing high efficacy of cisplatin-based chemotherapy have changed practice patterns. Now treatment is predominantly systemic, with a regimen of bleomycin, etoposide, and cisplatin often combined with adjuvant radiation, yielding an 85% survival at 5 years.

Residual masses are usually bland with no active tumor and deserve no further management. However, a small percentage of these will enlarge on follow-up. A second line of systemic therapy or radiation is used if this situation arises.

The only time that surgical resection plays a role in the management of seminomas is when an excisional biopsy of a small, isolated mediastinal mass indicates seminoma with negative margins. Surveillance then is pursued postoperatively.

Nonseminomatous Germ-Cell Tumors

Primary mediastinal nonseminomatous germ-cell tumors (PMNSGCTs) share a similar demographic with seminomatous tumors. Prognosis is considerably worse and only approaches 50% at 5 years. Patients have symptoms of SVC syndrome and dyspnea and signs of compression and invasion of surrounding structures such as lung and SVC. Unlike with seminomas and teratomas, AFP and beta-hCG levels are elevated on presentation, and that along with radiographic appearance of a heterogenous anterior mediastinal mass is sufficient for diagnosis. In cases of nonsignificant tumor marker elevation, CT-guided needle biopsy is useful in confirming diagnosis and guiding therapy. There are cases where a biopsy of a heterogenous mass may reveal a benign cell line such as teratoma in the presence of significant elevation of serologic markers. When this occurs, it is generally because malignant portions of the tumors were not sampled. Patients thus are treated as if they have PMNSGCTs.

Treatment, as with seminomas, is primarily systemic, with a cisplatin-based regimen. Residual masses in PMNSGCTs do warrant resection, as microscopic tumor cells exist in close to one half of pathologic specimens. Normalization of serum markers and a decrease in tumor size with chemotherapy are correlated to improved prognosis after surgical resection. Surgical resection frequently includes excision of mediastinal structures such as phrenic nerve, lung, and great veins. Should pulmonary resection be anticipated, bleomycin is eliminated from the chemotherapy regimen because of its toxicity.

A recent report has raised the possibility of radiotherapy with or without surgical resection for local tumor control after chemotherapy. Patients who received radiation between 55 and 60 Gy as part of their treatment regimen achieved significantly higher 5-year overall and progression-free survival when compared with those who did not. This benefit did not extend to patients with extensive disease.

Lymphomas

Lymphomas are malignant tumors of lymphocytes that make up 20% of mediastinal masses. They are usually multicentric and rarely are found limited to the thorax. The current classification is the system proposed by the WHO, but a useful broad categorization is into Hodgkin's lymphoma (HL) and non-Hodgkin's lymphoma (NHL). NHL is more common than HL in the United States by a factor of 8:1, mainly because the incidence of NHL has risen in the United States whereas that of HL has remained essentially flat over several decades. Both lymphoma types are staged using the Ann Arbor system, which ascribes higher stages to an increasing number of nodal and extralymphatic involvement as well as presence of disease on both sites of the diaphragm. Presenting symptoms usually are caused by mass effect and include chest pain, dyspnea, and cough. So-called B symptoms, including fevers, night sweats, and weight loss, may be the first indicators of disease. However, some symptoms are more prevalent in certain lymphomas. For example, patients with NHL are more likely to have SVC syndrome, whereas those with HL are more likely to have no symptoms at presentation.

Diagnosis includes PET and CT scanning, which shows a large homogenous mass in the anterior mediastinum. Biopsy via anterior mediastinoscopy or core needle can provide a diagnosis. Open biopsy obtains a large specimen that includes the tumor periphery. Thus it previously was thought that needle biopsy could not provide enough architectural information to determine the subtype of lymphoma. However, reports from Europe suggest that core needle biopsy alone with histologic analyses can result in a diagnostic yield in excess of 95% in lymphomas. Yields can be improved by targeting peripheral lymph nodes with high levels of fluorodeoxyglucose (FDG) avidity.

The mainstay of treatment of lymphoma is chemotherapy and radiation, with different regimens for varying histologic types. Radiographic response is rapid and can occur in a matter of days. There is residual mass and radiographic abnormality in up to 88% of patients. These do not predict relapse in patients who are treated with combined modality therapy and thus should not be biopsied routinely. Although lack of uptake in these residual masses on PET scanning has been shown to have a high negative predictive value for relapse, FDG avidity exhibits a poor positive predictive value. Thus patients with a positive PET scan should undergo a biopsy to evaluate residual masses.

Surgical extirpation has no role in the management of lymphoma at any stage.

HL is caused by proliferation of Reed-Sternberg cells (large cells) in lymph nodes and exhibits a bimodal age prevalence, with the peak in ages 15 to 40 years. Two thirds of patients have mediastinal disease at presentation. HL is subclassified into classic HL and nodular lymphocyte-predominant HL, with the latter being more common. HL, in contrast to NHL, is seen with severe pruritus and leukocytosis with neutrophilia. Alcohol-induced pain in affected lymph nodes is pathognomonic. Nonbulky disease usually is treated with an ABVD (adriamycin, bleomycin, vinblastine, and dacarbazine) regimen followed by radiation. A 94% 12-year survival rate can be achieved with this combination in early stage disease. Complications of this treatment can arise and include cardiomyopathy and reversible

pulmonary disease. Special mention must be made of an increased risk for breast cancer in women under the age of 30 years.

NHL of the mediastinum includes primary mediastinal large B-cell lymphomas (PMLBLs), which comprise 3% of all NHL, and lymphoblastic lymphomas, which make up another 5% of adult NHL. PMLBLs can be difficult to distinguish from HL by histology, and thus diagnosis is made by the presence of B cell CD20 and the absence of T cell CD3 on immunohistochemistry. These lymphomas originate in the thymus and spread aggressively. They are most common in women in their 30s.

In comparison, lymphoblastic lymphomas are twice as common in males as in females, with a bimodal age distribution in the second and seventh decades of life. Because of their increased susceptibility to chemotherapy, risk for tumor lysis is high. Vigorous hydration and prophylactic allopurinol are often necessary with initiation of therapy.

Thyroid Lesions

Thyroid lesions comprise up to 15% of mediastinal masses. Rare presentation of ectopic thyroid tissue is defined as mediastinal thyroid tissue, with entirely separate mediastinal blood supply, associated with a normal or absent cervical thyroid in a patient with no prior thyroid surgery and no shared pathology with a cervical thyroid. They can be symptomatic because of compression of airways and esophagus and thus manifest as dyspnea, dysphagia, and chest pain.

More common presentations are extensions of cervical thyroid tissue into the mediastinum or mediastinal spread secondary to malignancy or surgical seeding. The most common of them are benign multinodular goiters, with up to 15% of cervical goiters exhibiting mediastinal extension. To be classified as mediastinal goiters, they must have more than half of the thyroid mass below the sternal body. Their risk of malignant degeneration approaches 1 in 5, and medical management is only marginally effective but delays and complicates definitive surgery. Surgical resection of substernal thyroids can be performed through a cervical incision in most cases, with an upper manubriotomy as needed for safe and complete resection. Preoperative planning should include CT scanning and thyroid-stimulating hormone testing to ensure that hyperthyroidism is medically managed before surgery. Thyroid tissue appears enhanced on noncontrast imaging and demonstrates early enhancement on contrast CT.

Parathyroid Adenomas

The incidence of ectopic parathyroid adenoma is 6% to 25%, and most of these are found in the mediastinum associated with the thymus, although some reports suggest a higher predilection for the retrotracheal space. In the general population, 6% of people have supernumerary parathyroid glands. These also are found mostly in the mediastinum. Thus investigation for a parathyroid adenoma in the setting of hypercalcemia must be thorough and include CT and sestamibi scanning to decrease the likelihood of negative cervical explorations. As in cervical parathyroidectomies, intraoperative parathyroid hormone level testing to ensure a greater than 50% drop with resection is warranted. Resection usually is achieved via a median sternotomy, although more recently discrete mediastinal parathyroids have been resected using both VATS and robotic techniques.

■ MIDDLE MEDIASTINUM

Castleman's Disease

Castleman's disease is a rare lymphoproliferative disease, first described in 1965, that affects young people with a mean age of 35 years. It is also known as angiofollicular hyperplasia. Although first described in immunocompetent patients, now it is found frequently in immunocompromised patients such as those with human immunodeficiency virus (HIV). Its etiology is unknown, but some cases are associated with the human herpesvirus-8. There are three subtypes: hyaline vascular (90% of described cases), plasma cell type, and mixed. It is seen as an asymptomatic mass in the neck (10% to 15%), mediastinum (70%), or pelvis (10% to 15%) and can occur in any of the three mediastinal compartments, though it favors the middle and anterior parts. Tumors are either multicentric or unicentric, which has implications for management. Unicentric lesions are treated with resection, and recurrence is low. However, multicentric forms require multimodal therapy including radiation, chemotherapy, and immunomodulation. Unicentric lesions are more common in the mediastinum and have a better prognosis. CT imaging shows a solitary mass, a mass with lymphadenopathy, or lymphadenopathy without a mass. These masses are enhancing and isointense on MRI.

Mediastinal Lymphadenopathy

Mediastinal lymphadenopathy is the most common mass of the middle mediastinum. There are three main types: malignant, inflammatory, and infectious. It can be difficult to differentiate pathology by imaging alone. Serology may aid clinical diagnosis, but surgical pathology is most accurate and tissue for this can be obtained via cervical or anterior mediastinoscopy or via endoscopic biopsies.

In patients without previous malignancy, malignant mediastinal lymphadenopathy is caused by metastatic lung cancer in more than 80% of cases. Lymphadenopathy usually is found during clinical staging of lung cancer, although tissue diagnosis is the gold standard. Positive metastasis is prognostic of poor outcomes.

Sarcoidosis is a multisystem disease with noncaseating granulomas and hilar lymphadenopathy seen in the third and fourth decades of life. Prevalence is higher in African Americans, and less than half of patients are asymptomatic on presentation. When present, symptoms include cough and dyspnea, whereas polyarthralgia and erythema nodosum exists in advanced disease. Sarcoid tumors express parathyroid-related peptide and thus can cause hypercalcemia. Serum angiotensin-converting enzymes are generally high. Early stage disease frequently regresses, but advanced stage disease requires treatment with immunosuppressive agents.

Infectious lymphadenopathy is caused by fungal agents, including histoplasmosis and coccidiomycosis, which produce caseating granulomas on histology. Antifungal agents are indicated with exacerbations of disease.

Mediastinal Cysts

Mediastinal cysts comprise 20% of all middle mediastinal masses and are named for their tissues of origin: bronchogenic, enteric duplication, and pericardial cysts. Diagnosis is made by determining with which structure the cyst is associated. CT scan with intravenous contrast is required to show fluid content that does not enhance. If this is equivocal, MRI can confirm the diagnosis. Resection is often amenable to thoracoscopic approaches. However, fibrotic reactions may necessitate conversion to open resection.

Bronchogenic cysts are the most common mediastinal cysts, making up 60% of cases. They are located mostly at the carina and, though asymptomatic at presentation, two thirds eventually will develop symptoms, including compression and obstruction of airways. Secondary infection can lead to abscess formation, marked by air in the cyst, and difficult resection. As well, these cysts have the potential for malignant degeneration. Therefore resection is indicated once diagnosis is confirmed. Care is taken to protect the airway during resection. In the event of incomplete resection, remaining epithelium is cauterized to prevent recurrence.

Enteric duplication cysts in the mediastinum abut the esophagus or are present within its wall. They occasionally communicate with the lumen. The epithelial lining can arise from any gastrointestinal tract tissue, including esophageal, gastric, and even colonic tissue. They are located predominantly in the distal third of the esophagus and on the right of the esophagus. Like their bronchogenic counterparts, these cysts become symptomatic, causing dysphagia. Gastric mucosal lining frequently bleeds and complicates resection. Thus resection is recommended on diagnosis.

Neuroenteric cysts frequently are associated with vertebral abnormalities and can mimic the appearance of bronchogenic cysts but may be more tubular when in contact with the esophagus. Measuring up to several centimeters in length, they can extend into the spinal canal and require a combined neurosurgery and thoracic surgery effort during resection. MRI is mandated if the cyst is posterior mediastinal.

Pericardial cysts arise from the right anterior cardiophrenic angle in the fourth to fifth decades of life and are generally asymptomatic. They are said to have a "spring water" appearance. Unlike esophageal duplication and bronchogenic cysts, pericardial cysts have no potential for malignant degeneration. Development of symptoms or enlargement on radiography is an indication for resection.

■ POSTERIOR MEDIASTINUM

The posterior mediastinum is a limited space with neural tissue composed of ganglions and the sympathetic chain. Neurogenic tumors make up 60% of neoplasms within the compartment. They are made up of nerve sheath and ganglionic and paraganglionic cells. Each cell type has benign and malignant lines, but they are mostly benign except for a high incidence of malignancy in the pediatric population. These tumors are generally asymptomatic, but symptoms such as back pain, neurologic deficits, and Horner's syndrome can occur with involvement of the intercostal nerves, spinal canal, or sympathetic chain, respectively. CT scanning is usually sufficient to diagnose these well-defined paraspinal lesions, but MRI is usually necessary to evaluate foraminal extension, as is the case with dumbbell tumors. Treatment is generally via primary resection, with thoracoscopic resection being appropriate for smaller tumors. In cases with classic radiologic presentation, preoperative biopsy usually is not needed, and patients can proceed directly to surgical resection. In the special case of dumbbell tumors, paravertebral tumors extending into the foramen and at times into the contralateral sulcus, a truly posterolateral thoracotomy combined with neurosurgical exposure is needed for resection. These particular tumors require thoracic and neurosurgical expertise with simultaneous thoracic resection and neurosurgical excision.

Schwannomas and Neurofibromas

Schwannomas and neurofibromas are nerve sheath tumors that together make up more than 90% of adult neurogenic tumors. They are benign but have malignant counterparts in malignant schwannomas and neurofibrosarcomas. Schwannomas appear white on imaging arising from intercostal nerve sheaths and may have large blood vessels intrinsic to them. Neurofibromas frequently are seen as part of von Recklinghausen's disease and may have a plexiform appearance that is pathognomonic. Although surgical resection often is advocated for schwannomas, it is rarely applied to neurofibromas unless there is invasion of the spinal canal causing symptoms.

Their malignant counterparts are highly aggressive, with local invasion and distant metastasis common. They are often symptomatic and recur after primary surgical therapy. Advanced disease may be treated with chemotherapy, but prognosis is poor.

Ganglion Cell Tumors

Ganglion cell tumors include ganglioneuromas, ganglioneuroblastomas, and neuroblastomas that are of adrenal origin. Ganglioneuromas are benign lesions found along the sympathetic chain of children and in adults in their 20s and 30s. They are well-defined, benign lesions that are asymptomatic but may erode into adjacent structures and secrete vasoactive intestinal peptide, causing diarrhea.

Neuroblastomas are highly malignant lesions, the most common extracranial malignancy of the pediatric population, that occur in the first 2 years of life. They frequently have calcifications on imaging. These lesions can produce catecholamines, vanillylmandelic acid (VMA), and homovanillic acid (HMA) and may cause Cushing's syndrome. Treatment involves resection and adjuvant radiation as needed for local disease and systemic therapy for metastasis. Prognostic factors include age, extent of disease, tumor histology, and completeness of resection. There are reports of neuroblastomas transforming into benign ganglioneuromas. Ganglioneuroblastomas have a better prognosis than neuroblastomas.

Paraganglionic Cell Tumors

Pheochromocytomas and chemodectomas are rare neurogenic cells, with the former being hormonally active and producing catecholamines. Mediastinal pheochromocytomas may cause the classic symptoms of headache, palpitations, and hypertension. [131I]metaiodobenzylguanidine scans may be needed to localize tumors if CT or MRI are nondiagnostic. Resection is indicated when diagnosed, and preoperative management with alpha and then beta blockade will prevent a sympathetic crisis intraoperatively.

■ UNUSUAL TUMORS

Mesenchymal Tumors

Mesenchymal tumors arise in and make up 6% of all mediastinal masses and have equal incidence in males and females. They are located predominantly in the anterior mediastinum. Approximately 55% of these tumors are malignant in adults, though this can reach 85% in the pediatric population. Progenitor cells include vascular and lymphatic, muscular, adipose, and connective tissue. Lymphatic and vascular tumors account for more than half of mediastinal mesenchymal lesions, but lipomas are the most common tumor. Treatment is usually surgical for benign lesions and multimodal therapy for malignant cases. We discuss representative lesions in this section.

Lipomas and Liposarcomas

Lipomas represent 2% of all mediastinal tumors and are located mostly in the anterior mediastinum. They are well-encapsulated lesions that grow to remarkable sizes before causing symptoms. Rarely, they extend into the spinal canal, causing neurologic symptoms. The larger majority are seen with symptoms such as chest pain and dyspnea, at which point resection mandates an open procedure. Definitive therapy is surgical resection, and recurrence is rare. Lipomas have no potential for malignant transformation.

Liposarcomas are rare mediastinal masses that invade local structures, have a bad prognosis, and have no recourse to resection. They are mostly posterior mediastinal and cause weight loss in addition to the symptoms of lipomas. Radiation provides little benefit.

Hemangiomas

Mediastinal hemangiomas are anterior mediastinum predominant neoplasms (50% to 75%) that usually are seen as well-encapsulated

tumors and can occur at any age. There are at least three histologic variants: cavernous, capillary, and venous, in order of incidence. They can grow to large sizes and are frequently friable. However, surgical resection is frequently curative. Some have reported embolization of feeding vessels or induction chemotherapy with interferon-alpha2 (INF-2α) to decrease size and bleeding risk before surgery.

Lymphangiomas

Lymphangiomas are malformations of lymphatic network leading to obstruction of lymphatic drainage and subsequent cystic degeneration. They often are located in the cervical area, with extension into the anterior mediastinum. Only about 17% are primarily mediastinal. They are classified into two types—cystic hygromas and cavernous lymphangiomas—based on appearance. Because of a similar appearance as hemangiomas on histology, the content of cysts (chyle or blood) is used to determine final pathology. Where diagnosis is inconclusive, intracytoplasmic factor VIII staining can be useful, as it is reactive with vascular but not lymphatic endothelium. Lymphangiomas can cause symptoms by compression of adjacent structures and can rupture, causing pleural effusions.

Fibromas and Fibrosarcomas

Tumors with fibroblastic origin are seen as nebulous tumors with a predilection for invasion of adjacent structures. Fibromas are benign, slow-growing tumors with no metastatic potential. Thus symptoms are absent until advanced stages, when complete resection is difficult. Incomplete resection is associated with high rates of local recurrence.

Fibrosarcomas, on the other hand, are aggressive lesions that grow to be large and invade mediastinal structures to cause symptoms. They sometimes may have associated hypoglycemia, which may be caused by increased glucose use or insulin-like metabolite secretion. Although they rarely metastasize, prognosis is poor because fibrosarcomas, not uncommonly, are unresectable. Radiation has no role in management.

SUGGESTED READINGS

Den Bakker MA, Marx A, Mukai K, et al. Mesenchymal tumors of the mediastinum—parts I and II. *Virchows Arch.* 2015;467:487-517.

Detterbeck FC, Parsons AM. Thymic tumors. *Ann Thorac Surg.* 2004;77:1860-1869.

Hamlin P. Evolving treatment paradigms for primary mediastinal diffuse large B-cell lymphoma. *J Clin Oncol.* 2014;32:1751-1753.

Masaoka A. Staging system of thymoma. *J Thorac Oncol.* 2010;5:S304-S312.

Skelton E, Jewison A, Okpaluba C, et al. Image-guided core needle biopsy in the diagnosis of malignant lymphoma. *Eur J Surg Oncol.* 2015;41:e852-e858.

Talat N, Belgaumkar AP, Schulte KM. Surgery in Castleman's disease: a systematic review of 404 published cases. *Ann Surg.* 2012;255:677-684.

Wang J, Bi N, Wang X, et al. Role of radiotherapy in treating patients with primary malignant mediastinal non-seminomatous germ cell tumor: a 21-year experience at a single institution. *Thorac Cancer.* 2015;6:399-406.

Primary Tumors of the Thymus

Hugh G. Auchincloss, MD, MPH,
and Christopher R. Morse, MD

Primary thymic tumors are an infrequent and challenging clinical problem. The incidence in the United States is estimated to be 0.15 cases per 100,000 person-years. Roughly half of all mediastinal tumors in adults are thymic in origin. The term *primary thymic tumor* encompasses a variety of histologies, including thymoma, thymic carcinoma, and neuroendocrine tumor of the thymus. Other entities such as thymolipoma and thymic lymphoma are rare. Thymic tumors may be asymptomatic or be seen with local or systemic symptoms. Thymoma is strongly associated with myasthenia gravis. Patients with thymoma-associated myasthenia gravis are seen in the third or fourth decade of life, whereas those without myasthenia gravis are seen in the sixth or seventh decade. There is no gender predominance. The treatment of thymic tumors is complete surgical resection through an open or minimally invasive approach. Adjuvant radiation and chemotherapy are useful when a tumor is histologically aggressive or when surgical resection is incomplete. Neoadjuvant treatment and targeted therapies are becoming increasingly common in the management of locally advanced thymic tumors. The long-term prognosis for most thymic tumors is good. More than 90% of patients with early-stage tumors are alive at 5 years.

■ OVERVIEW OF THE NORMAL THYMUS

The thymus is a lobular gland located in the anterior mediastinum. It originates from the third and fourth pharyngeal pouch and descends in the anterior mediastinum during embryologic development. These embryologic origins explain the close association between the thymus and the thyroid gland. The thymus grows to a maximum of 30 to 40 grams during puberty and then begins a process of involution such that the adult gland weighs between 5 and 25 grams. The thymus gives the appearance of being divided into left and right lobes but it is more accurately described as a fusion of multiple lobes of tissue. The anatomic boundaries are the innominate vein superiorly and the phrenic nerves laterally. However, extension beyond these boundaries is the rule rather than the exception. Ectopic thymic tissue is similarly common. Approximately 75% of people will have foci of thymic cells in the surrounding mediastinal fat, cardiophrenic angle, thyroid gland, or pulmonary parenchyma. This observation has implications for the complete resection of thymic tumors.

The arterial blood supply to the thymus is primarily from branches of the bilateral internal mammary arteries with some contribution from the thyrocervical trunk and the pericardiophrenic arteries. Venous drainage is largely to the innominate vein.

Histologically, the thymus is composed of lobes covered in a fibrous capsule. This capsule extends within the lobes and further divides them into lobules. Each lobule is made up of an outer cortex consisting of densely packed lymphocytes ("thymocytes") mixed with epithelial and mesenchymal cells and an inner medulla containing glandular cells important for the differentiation of cortical thymocytes. As the thymus involutes after puberty, the majority of thymocytes and thymic epithelial cells are replaced by lipid-laden macrophages.

The thymus functions as an immunologic organ, primarily in the pathway of cellular immunity but also indirectly in humoral immunity. Surgical extirpation of the neonatal thymus has a significant detrimental effect on the developing immune system; however, the pediatric and adult thymus can be removed without obvious consequence.

■ STAGING AND CLASSIFICATION OF THYMIC TUMORS

Several methods of classifying and staging thymic tumors have been proposed. The topic remains controversial. A formal tumor node metastasis (TNM) staging system is expected in 2016. Currently, thymic tumors are classified by histology according to the guidelines introduced by the World Health Organization (WHO) and staged using the Masaoka-Koga staging system.

World Health Organization Classification

Primary thymic tumors, also called *thymic epithelial tumors*, historically have been recognized as falling into three categories: (1) tumors with no mitotic activity or atypia, referred to as *thymoma*, (2) tumors with features closely resembling thymoma but with some features of malignancy, referred to as *well-differentiated thymic carcinoma*, and (3) tumors with atypia, mitoses, and aggressive behavior, referred to as *thymic carcinoma*. A subgroup of thymic tumors of neuroendocrine origin, sometimes called thymic carcinoid tumors or *neuroendocrine tumors of the thymus (NETTs)*, is included under the definition of thymic carcinoma. However, the histology and behavior of NETTs are similar to those of bronchial carcinoid tumors, leading some authors to consider these tumors separately from thymic carcinoma.

The WHO classification schema (Table 1) incorporates tumor histology into the historical understanding of thymic tumors. The current system was introduced in 2004 and updated in 2015 to reflect improved methods of tissue staining and immunohistochemistry. Type A thymic tumors are derived from medullary cells, type B tumors arise from cortical cells, and type AB tumors contain a mixture of both cells. Type B tumors are further divided into types B1, B2, and B3 based on the degree of lymphocytic involvement. Type A, AB, B1, and B2 histologic tumors all fall under the general term *thymoma*. Similarly, type B3 covers what has previously been understood as well-differentiated thymic carcinoma. Type C tumors represent thymic carcinoma.

The clinical value of the WHO classification has been debated. It is useful as a research tool in that it produces good agreement among pathologists at different institutions. It does appear to identify distinct cohorts of patients. For example, type A and AB tumors tend to be early-stage tumors and are associated with myasthenia gravis, whereas type B and C tumors tend to be more advanced and lack associated parathymic syndromes. It is important to note that WHO type appears to be an independent predictor of survival, although it is a less important predictor than either Masaoka-Koga stage or the completeness of surgical resection. It has been suggested that the prognostic power of WHO type is explained mostly by the separation of thymic carcinoma from other types of thymic tumors. Thymic carcinoma is known to have a poor prognosis akin to that seen with primary lung cancer.

The chief limitation of the WHO classification system is that it is difficult to ascertain prospectively and therefore has a limited role in clinical decision making. However, improvements in imaging and histologic techniques soon may make it easier to determine the WHO type of a thymic tumor before surgical resection, which in turn may guide decisions about neoadjuvant therapy.

Masaoka-Koga Staging System

The Masaoka-Koga staging system (Table 2), introduced by Akira Masaoka in 1981 and modified by Kenji Koga in 1994, is currently the most practical tool for staging thymic tumors. The system is based on local behavior of the tumor. Early-stage tumors (Masaoka-Koga stages I and II) are either well encapsulated or have local invasion only into the surrounding thymus or mediastinal fat. Locally advanced tumors (Masaoka-Koga stage III) have invasion into surrounding structures such as the lung, pericardium, or great vessels. Masaoka-Koga stage IV tumors are metastatic, by virtue of either distant pericardial or pleural implants (stage IVa) or lymphatic or hematogenous spread to extrapleural sites (stage IVb). The Masaoka-Koga staging system has several advantages that have led to its widespread adoption, namely that its prognostic significance has been demonstrated in multiple studies. In addition, it is usually possible to have a reasonable estimate of the stage preoperatively based on available imaging. This in turn guides decisions regarding surgical approach and use of neoadjuvant therapy and helps to manage patient expectations.

Tumor Node Metastasis Staging System

The International Thymic Malignancy Interest Group (ITMIG) was formed in 2009 with a goal of creating a coherent TNM staging system for primary thymic tumors. This system is expected to be formally announced in 2016, but most details are available already (Tables 3 to 5). The system borrows directly from the Masaoka-Koga staging system with regard to the T component of the TNM staging system. The WHO classification system is also represented, albeit obliquely, by the inclusion of criteria for stratifying nodal and metastatic disease. Because only type C thymic carcinoma and occasionally type B3 well-differentiated thymic carcinoma have a real propensity for lymphatic or hematogenous spread, the N and M components of the new staging system differentiate these histologic types.

■ APPROACH TO THE PATIENT WITH A MEDIASTINAL MASS

Differential Diagnosis

The differential diagnosis for an anterior mediastinal mass includes primary thymic tumor, lymphoma, mature teratoma, immature germ cell tumor, substernal thyroid tumor, ectopic parathyroid adenoma, and benign thymic pathology such as thymic hyperplasia. Of these, primary thymic tumors are most common.

Clinical Presentation

Anterior mediastinal masses are symptomatic in about half of patients with them. The remaining masses are discovered incidentally on imaging studies. Among symptomatic patients, half will have symptoms related to local effect of the mass, including chest pain, dyspnea, cough, and rarely superior vena cava syndrome. The other half will develop systemic symptoms related to a constellation of autoimmune parathymic syndromes, most commonly myasthenia gravis. Between 40% and 50% of patients with a thymoma will have associated myasthenia gravis, whereas 10% of patients with myasthenia gravis will be found to have a thymoma. In contrast, thymic carcinoma is not associated with myasthenia gravis. Other common parathymic syndromes include red cell aplasia and hypogammaglobulinemia, both of which are seen in 2% to 5% of patients with thymoma. NETT—like thymic carcinoma—is not associated with myasthenia gravis but can be associated with neuroendocrine phenomena such as Cushing's syndrome. NETT associated with Cushing's syndrome portends a poor prognosis. Laboratory tests play little role in the evaluation of a patient with a mediastinal mass. Serum alpha-fetoprotein and beta-human chorionic gonadotropin should be checked to exclude a germ-cell tumor. Serum antibodies against acetylcholine receptors also may be checked, but in the absence

TABLE 1: World Health Organization Staging: Histologic Categories

A	Spindle cell or medullary thymoma
AB	Mixed thymoma
B1	Lymphocyte-rich or predominately cortical thymoma
B2	Cortical thymoma
B3	Epithelial thymoma
C	Thymic carcinoma

TABLE 3: T Descriptors

Category	Definition (Involvement of)*†
T1	
a	Encapsulated or unencapsulated, with or without extension into mediastinal fat
b	Extension into mediastinal pleura
T2	Pericardium
T3	Lung, brachiocephalic vein, superior vena cava, chest wall, phrenic nerve, hilar (extrapericardial) pulmonary vessels
T4	Aorta, arch vessels, main pulmonary artery, myocardium, trachea, or esophagus

*Involvement must be pathologically proven in pathologic staging.

†A tumor is classified according to the highest T level of involvement that is present with or without any invasion of structure of lower T levels.

TABLE 2: Masaoko-Koga Staging System and Survival

Stage	Definition	Frequency at Presentation	5-Year Survival Rate	10-Year Survival Rate
I	Macroscopically encapsulated, no microscopic invasion of the capsule	40%	92%	88%
II	IIa: Macroscopic invasion into mediastinal fat or pleura IIb: Microscopic invasion of the capsule	25%	82%	70%
III	Invasion into neighboring organs	25%	68%	57%
IVa	Pleural or pericardial metastasis	10%	61%	38%
IVb	Lymphatic or hematogenous metastasis	1%-2%	0%	0%

Data summarizing the results from multiple large studies from Detterbeck FC, Parsons AM. Thymic tumors. *Ann Thorac Surg.* 2004;77:1860-1869.

TABLE 4: N and M Descriptors

Category	Definition (Involvement of)*
N0	No nodal involvement
N1	Anterior (perithymic) nodes
N2	Deep intrathoracic or cervical nodes
M0	No metastatic pleural, pericardial, or distant sites
M1 a b	Separate pleural or pericardial nodule(s) Pulmonary intraparenchymal nodule or distant organ metastasis

*Involvement must be pathologically proven in pathologic staging.

TABLE 5: Stage Grouping

Stage	T	N	M
I	**T1**	N0	M0
II	**T2**	N0	M0
IIIa	**T3**	N0	M0
IIIb	**T4**	N0	M0
IVa	T any T any	**N1** N0,1	M0 **M1a**
IVb	T any T any	**N2** N any	M0,1a **M1b**

of clinical myasthenia gravis their presence is of questionable significance.

Imaging

The radiologic assessment of the mediastinum is the most important component of the workup of a patient with a mediastinal mass. Imaging modalities include computed tomography (CT), magnetic resonance imaging (MRI), and positron emission tomography (PET). Imaging provides valuable clues to the cause of a mediastinal mass and its relationship to surrounding structures.

Typically, initial evaluation is with contrast-enhanced CT. Frequently this study alone is sufficient to determine both that surgical excision of a mediastinal mass is indicated and that complete resection is possible. A discrete, smooth-contoured mass arising from the thymus is likely to be an early-stage thymoma, and surgery can proceed without further evaluation. Alternatively, CT may identify calcifications or internal necrosis suggestive of thymic carcinoma or demonstrate a bulky mass with associated adenopathy suspicious for lymphoma. CT is also useful for evaluating the pleural space for drop metastases that would qualify the patient as Masaoka-Koga stage IVa. MRI is a useful adjunct for determining the character of a mass (i.e., cystic vs solid) and whether there is local invasion into vascular structures. The role of PET in the evaluation of a mediastinal mass has not been established, and substantial variation in practice between centers exists. Currently, PET is most useful for diagnosing nodal and metastatic disease in patients with known or suspected thymic carcinoma. However, as imaging techniques improve it may be possible to use PET in conjunction with other diagnostic modalities to make reliable predictions about the histology of a mediastinal tumor of presumed thymic origin. As such, the role of PET in the management of thymic tumors is evolving.

Tissue Diagnosis

The role of tissue biopsy in the evaluation of a mediastinal mass is controversial. Historically, biopsy has been avoided partly because of fear of seeding the biopsy tract but more importantly because the majority of mediastinal masses require resection regardless of histology. Currently, tissue biopsy is used to guide medical therapy for patients with a mediastinal mass that is unresectable based on imaging findings or when a diagnosis of lymphoma is suspected. However, recent innovations in the histologic classification of thymic tumors have focused primarily on the differentiation between thymic tumor subtypes based on limited tissue sampling. Histology increasingly is seen as both a prognostic factor and a determinant of the need for neoadjuvant treatment, even in the absence of advanced disease. Routine biopsy of thymic tumors is therefore certain to increase.

If a biopsy is indicated, several approaches are acceptable. CT-guided core needle biopsy may be sufficient to establish a diagnosis. Alternatively, a left or right anterior mediastinotomy provides excellent exposure to the anterior mediastinum and yields a large amount of tissue. Thoracoscopic transpleural biopsy should be avoided because it may promote spread of the tumor to the pleural space.

■ PRINCIPLES OF TREATMENT

Surgery

The treatment for an early-stage (Masaoka-Koga stages I and II) primary thymic tumor is complete surgical resection. Resection includes the entire thymus and a generous margin of surrounding mediastinal fat to clear all foci of ectopic thymic tissue. Incomplete resection of normal thymic tissue increases the likelihood of local recurrence and may put the patient at risk for postoperative myasthenia gravis even in the absence of preoperative symptoms. Most studies report successful complete resection in almost all stage I tumors and the vast majority (~85%) of stage II tumors.

The treatment of locally advanced disease (Masaoka-Koga stage III) depends on the likelihood of complete surgical resection. If imaging suggests resectability, it is reasonable to proceed with upfront surgery. Complete surgical resection is achieved in approximately half of patients with stage III tumors. The majority of structures susceptible to local invasion, including lung, pericardium, and phrenic nerve, can be resected en bloc with the thymus. Conventional wisdom holds that it is acceptable to sacrifice one phrenic nerve but that bilateral resection places the patient at prohibitive risk for respiratory insufficiency. Some surgeons would avoid sacrificing even one phrenic nerve in a patient with myasthenia gravis. Diaphragmatic plication concurrent with phrenic nerve resection is theoretically beneficial; however, the technical challenge associated with plicating the diaphragm through any of the standard thymectomy approaches seldom makes this a feasible option. Pericardiectomy usually requires reconstruction with a synthetic patch to prevent cardiac herniation. Extension of the tumor into the great vessels is a more challenging scenario. Resection of venous structures, including the superior vena cava and innominate vein, with or without reconstruction may be indicated in some patients, particularly if these structures are occluded preoperatively and collateralization has occurred. Radical resection and reconstruction of the aortic arch, pulmonary artery, and heart have been described, but such approaches are prohibitively risky and seldom indicated. Most surgeons instead would accept a positive resection margin and mark the area with surgical clips for postoperative radiation. Ideally, though, invasion into an unresectable structure is suspected on the basis of imaging. Such patients should be treated with neoadjuvant radiation or chemoradiotherapy followed by restaging. Doing so has been shown to increase the odds of complete resection and freedom from local recurrence.

Surgery has an important role in the management of Masaoka-Koga stage IVa disease. If stage IVa disease is diagnosed prospectively, neoadjuvant chemoradiotherapy followed by surgery has been shown to increase the likelihood of complete resection. As much as a quarter of such patients ultimately will undergo complete surgical resection. Alternatively, if distant pleural or pericardial metastases are discovered unexpectedly at the time of surgery, it is reasonable to perform maximum debulking followed by postoperative radiation and chemotherapy.

Lymph node dissection traditionally has not been considered part of the surgical management of primary thymic tumors. However, the new ITMIG guidelines recommend routine clearance of all N1 (anterior perithymic) nodes for accurate staging of all thymic tumors and clearance of both N1 and N2 (deep intrathoracic and cervical) nodes for curative-intent resection of known thymic carcinoma.

Radiation

Thymic tumors are generally radiosensitive, and external beam radiation therapy may be used as a neoadjuvant or adjuvant therapy in the management of locally invasive disease. There is general agreement that adjuvant radiotherapy should be used after surgical resection with positive margins. However, significant institutional variation exists regarding the routine use of postoperative radiation for completely resected Masaoka-Koga stage II or III disease. There is a little evidence that radiation in this setting decreases local recurrence. Neoadjuvant radiation for locally advanced tumors is becoming more common and, as discussed earlier, may improve the odds of complete resection and long-term survival.

Chemotherapy

Systemic chemotherapy is used for inoperable, incompletely resected, or recurrent thymic tumors and for histologically aggressive tumors (i.e., thymic carcinoma and some WHO type B tumors). Several chemotherapy regimens have been studied and found to be comparably effective. Platinum-based chemotherapy is central to all regimens. Most thymic tumors show some response to polychemotherapy. Unfortunately this response is less consistent with thymic carcinoma.

Targeted Therapy

Targeted therapies for thymic tumors remain in their infancy owing to a lack of available models and limited understanding of the biologic pathways responsible for tumorigenesis. Several targeted therapies have been tried in practice and have provided the anecdotal evidence to support ongoing clinical trials. These include inhibitors of stem cell factor receptor, vascular endothelial growth factor (VEGF), epidermal growth factor receptor (EGFR), insulin-like growth factor 1 receptor (IGF-1R), somatostatin receptors, histone deacetylase (HDAC), sarcoma protein (Src), and mammalian target of rapamycin (mTOR). To date, response to these targeted therapies has been mixed.

Recurrent Disease

Local recurrence refers to all disease occurring in the mediastinum or pleural space after resection of a thymic tumor. Unfortunately, local recurrence is relatively common, even when the initial resection was thought to be complete. Fewer than 5% of Masaoka-Koga stage I thymic tumors will recur, but this increases to approximately 15% and 25% for stages II and III, respectively. Recurrence may take many years to become apparent, reflecting the indolent nature of most thymic tumors. Although distant recurrence is managed with systemic therapy, most experts advocate an aggressive surgical approach to local recurrence. This is based on the observation that when disease recurs locally and reoperation is attempted, it is successful in achieving complete resection more than half the time. Patients who undergo complete resection of recurrent disease have 5- and 10-year

survival rates of around 70% and 60%, respectively. This is far superior to patients who undergo incomplete resection and significantly better than those for whom recurrence is managed medically.

Prognosis

Thymic tumors are generally associated with a good prognosis. Even with advanced-stage tumors, most patients can expect reasonable long-term survival. Ten-year survival for patients with stages III and IV disease is approximately 55% and 35%, respectively, compared with 90% and 70% for stage I and II disease, respectively.

Most tumors are indolent and grow locally over a period of many years without distant spread. The factors associated with long-term and disease-free survival are—overwhelmingly—the stage of disease and the completeness of surgical resection. All other factors, including young age, the presence or absence of a parathymic syndrome, and the use of multimodality therapy, seem to be significant only as they relate to those two chief determinants. Histologic type is an independent predictor of survival in that thymic carcinoma is associated with a far worse prognosis than other subtypes of thymic tumor.

■ SURGICAL MANAGEMENT OF PRIMARY THYMIC TUMORS

The operation of choice for primary tumors of the thymus is total thymectomy. This may be accomplished through an open (transsternal) or minimally invasive approach. Transcervical thymectomy is reserved for nonthymomatous myasthenia gravis and should be avoided in patients with primary thymic tumors. Thymectomy is generally a well-tolerated procedure, and most patients are appropriate operative candidates.

Patients with myasthenia gravis should have their symptoms medically managed before resection. Thymectomy does not result in immediate improvement in symptoms and should be deferred in the setting of a myasthenic crisis. Patients with myasthenia gravis also deserve special anesthetic consideration given their sensitivity to neuromuscular blockade. Some surgeons and anesthesiologists recommend managing all patients undergoing thymectomy as if they were at risk for myasthenia gravis and avoiding neuromuscular blockade whenever possible.

Transsternal Thymectomy

Transsternal thymectomy is a safe, technically straightforward operation. It allows the surgeon maximum ability to dissect the tumor and thymus free from surrounding structures and should be the approach of choice when local invasion is suspected. Several variations of the transsternal thymectomy exist. Most commonly the operation is performed through a standard median sternotomy, but other options include partial sternotomy, bilateral thoracosternotomy (clamshell thoracotomy), or some combination of sternotomy with thoracotomy for improved access to one or the other pleural spaces. "Maximal thymectomy" with extension of the incision into the neck for access to the anterior cervical triangles is probably unnecessary. For patients with nonthymomatous myasthenia gravis or Masaoka-Koga stage I disease, it is possible to perform a satisfactory thymectomy without entering either pleural space. Patients with more advanced disease require inspection of both pleural spaces to look for drop metastases. After opening the pleura, resection of the thymus proceeds from caudad to cephalad with clearance of all thymic tissue from the anterior surface of the pericardium. The lateral resection borders are the phrenic nerves bilaterally. Frequently there are small branches of the pericardiophrenic arteries in this area that can be clipped or divided with ultrasonic shears. Superiorly the gland is removed from the inferior border of the innominate vein. Multiple small veins drain into the innominate vein and must be clipped and divided. At the level of the innominate vein, the phrenic nerves can be deceptively medial and are at risk for injury. Care should be taken when using electrocautery in this area. The superior horns of the thymus can extend anterior or posterior to the innominate vein into the neck and should be bluntly dissected free from their avascular attachments. Branches of the thyrocervical trunk may provide some arterial supply to the superior horns and should be clipped and divided. The specimen is then removed intact. A drain is left in each entered pleural space and a mediastinal tube is placed in the resection bed to prevent hematoma. The sternum is approximated with wires and the fascia overlying the sternum is closed.

Patients should be extubated in the operating room. Monitoring in an intensive care setting is reasonable on the first postoperative night. If pain control is adequate and pulmonary complications are avoided, most patients make a rapid recovery. In the absence of excessive or bloody drainage, the pleural and mediastinal drains may be removed on the first postoperative day, and an overall hospital stay of 3 to 4 days is expected. Sternal wound precautions should be observed for the first few weeks of recovery.

Minimally Invasive Thymectomy

Several thoracoscopic and robotic approaches to thymectomy have been described. Advocates of the minimally invasive approach argue that it shortens hospital stay, decreases postoperative pain, and improves cosmetic result without sacrificing completeness of resection. Long-term studies demonstrating the efficacy of minimally invasive thymectomy for treatment of thymic tumors are lacking, but most experts agree that a small (<4 cm) well-encapsulated thymoma may be approached in minimally invasive fashion by a surgeon skilled in this approach.

Minimally invasive thymectomy can be performed thoracoscopically or robotically from either the left or the right chest. Operative strategy depends on surgeon preference and the laterality of the tumor. The right chest provides better exposure to the confluence of the superior vena cava and the left innominate vein and facilitates identification of the more inconstant right phrenic nerve. Access from the left chest allows for better visualization of the aortopulmonary window and the deep left lateral cardiophrenic angle. In both cases the patient is placed in the appropriate lateral decubitus position with the operating table flexed. Three or four ports are placed with the camera port at the anterior axillary line. The addition of carbon dioxide insufflation (to 6 to 8 mm Hg) or elevation of the sternum with hooks are techniques for creating more working space. They are not always necessary for thoracoscopic approaches but are useful when operating robotically. A combination of blunt dissection and electrocautery is used to mobilize the thymus from inferior to

superior between the phrenic nerves in the same fashion as with transsternal thymectomy. Clips are applied to the veins draining into the innominate vein. The thymus is placed in an endoscopic retrieval bag and removed from the chest. A single chest tube is placed and can be removed the following day. Most patients can be discharged on the first or second postoperative day.

An alternative to the left or right minimally invasive approach is video-assisted thoracoscopic extended thymectomy (VATET), which is performed using bilateral thoracoscopic exposure. The addition of a cervical incision facilitates clearance of the superior horns of the thymus. Advocates of this approach argue that it allows for maximum clearance of all thymic tissue while avoiding the morbidity of an open operation.

■ CONCLUSION

The management of primary tumors of the thymus is poised to change in coming years. Multimodality therapy in the neoadjuvant setting is likely to occupy a larger role as improvements in imaging techniques and tissue diagnosis help to reliably identify patients who will benefit. Targeted therapies will mature and become an established part of the medical management. Complete surgical resection, though, will remain the core of the treatment strategy for this uncommon and challenging disease.

SELECTED READINGS

Detterbeck FC. Clinical value of the WHO classification system of thymoma. *Ann Thorac Surg.* 2006;81:2328-2334.

Detterbeck FC, Nicholson AG, Kondo K, Van Schil P, Moran C. The Masaoka-Koga stage classification for thymic malignancies: clarification and definition of terms. *J Thorac Oncol.* 2011;6(7 suppl 3):S1710-S1716.

Detterbeck FC, Parsons AM. Thymic tumors. *Ann Thorac Surg.* 2004;77:1860-1869.

Detterbeck FC, Stratton K, et al. The IASLC/ITMIG Thymic Epithelial Tumors Staging Project: proposal for an evidence-based stage classification system for the forthcoming (8th) edition of the TNM classification of malignant tumors. *J Thorac Oncol.* 2014;9(9 suppl 2):S65-S72.

Marx A, Chan JK, et al. The 2015 World Health Organization classification of tumors of the thymus: continuity and changes. *J Thorac Oncol.* 2015;10:1383-1395.

Ruffini E, Venuta F. Management of thymic tumors: a European perspective. *J Thorac Dis.* 2014;6(suppl 2):S228-S237.

Serpico D, Trama A, et al. Available evidence and new biological perspectives on medical treatment of advanced thymic epithelial tumors. *Ann Oncol.* 2015;26:838-847.

THE MANAGEMENT OF TRACHEAL STENOSIS

Andrea L. Axtell, MD, and Douglas J. Mathisen, MD

Tracheal stenosis is the most common postintubation injury to the trachea and is usually the result of endotracheal tube cuff ischemic necrosis of the underlying trachea or tracheostomy stomal injury. Injury at the stomal level can lead to side to side contraction and an A-shaped stenosis sparing the membranous wall. Tracheostomy can have a combined stenosis with stomal and cuff injury. Patients with tracheal stenosis have signs and symptoms of upper airway obstruction: dyspnea on exertion, wheezing, stridor, and obstructive pneumonia. The presentation of tracheal stenosis often

is confused with adult-onset asthma; therefore steroid therapy often is initiated before the correct diagnosis is ascertained.

■ INDICATIONS FOR TRACHEAL RESECTION

In general, any patient who has airway stenosis as a result of tracheal injury should be considered for a tracheal resection and reconstruction. Absolute contraindications are few and include a nonreconstructible airway (usually because of an excessive length of damaged airway), severe comorbidities, or a prolonged need for mechanical ventilation. Relative contraindications include a history of radiation to the trachea, which limits tracheal mobility and impairs microvascular blood supply; active trachea mucosal inflammation; and active steroid therapy. Steroids should be weaned before tracheal reconstruction because they play no role in the amelioration of postintubation stenosis and interfere with healing of the tracheal anastomosis.

If necessary, tracheal dilation can be performed until inflammation subsides and steroids are discontinued.

■ PREOPERATIVE ASSESSMENT

Before tracheal resection and reconstruction is undertaken, the definitive diagnosis of the underlying pathology of the airway must be established. A preoperative assessment should include a history and physical, radiologic imaging, and bronchoscopy. Relatively simple radiologic techniques can delineate most pathologic conditions of the trachea. X-rays can demonstrate the location of a lesion, its linear extent, extratracheal involvement, and the amount of normal trachea. High-resolution computed tomography with 3D reconstruction has become the preferred method of imaging and allows measurement of the length and configuration of tracheal stenosis as well as its relationship to surrounding structures (Figure 1).

Bronchoscopy is invaluable in determining the extent of airway disease and the quality of the mucosa. The initial evaluation is best performed in the operating room with a rigid bronchoscope carefully inserted through the vocal cords just proximal to the point of stenosis. The rigid bronchoscope then can be used to measure the length of a stenotic segment of trachea as well as to assess the mucosa for inflammatory changes and granulation tissue. Crucial to the management of tracheal stenosis is the ability to control the airway. Control of the airway is best accomplished in the operating room with an assortment of rigid bronchoscopes. Attempting to pass a large rigid bronchoscope beyond a tight inflammatory stricture is usually difficult and can result in tracheal rupture or total airway obstruction from bleeding and edema. Graduated rigid bronchoscopes (pediatric to adult) are preferred to dilatate postintubation strictures serially. Balloon dilators are used by some but not preferred by us. Racemic epinephrine and steroids often are administered for 24 to 48 hours to minimize postdilatation edema.

■ ANESTHESIA AND AIRWAY MANAGEMENT

Anesthesia for tracheal resection is best administered as total intravenous anesthesia (TIVA). This process provides satisfactory

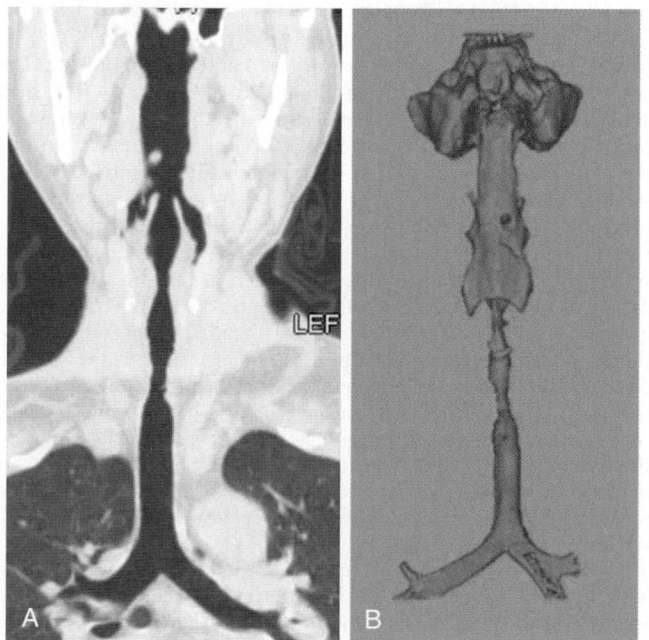

FIGURE 1 Computed tomography (**A**) with 3D reconstruction (**B**) of a patient with tracheal stenosis.

anesthesia and muscle relaxation before intubation, decouples ventilation and the delivery of anesthesia, and avoids environmental contamination of volatile anesthetics during the case. It also blunts airway reflexes, and its effects wear off quickly at the completion of the operation. Remifentanil and propofol are delivered by infusion and are excellent agents commonly used with TIVA.

The surgeon should be available with an array of rigid bronchoscopes during induction of anesthesia to control the airway. A stricture less than 6 mm in diameter is dilatated under direct vision with rigid pediatric bronchoscopes. If the stricture is more than 6 mm in diameter, a small endotracheal tube (5.5 mm) may be placed through the lesion. If the tracheal stenosis is located in the subglottic area, the lesion usually requires dilatation to allow passage of a small endotracheal tube. During resection of the trachea, the airway is divided, and the distal end of the trachea can be intubated directly with an armored, flexible endotracheal tube (Tovell tube). Sterile connecting tubes are passed off the surgical field to the anesthesiologist. The Tovell tube can be removed intermittently for brief periods of apnea to allow careful and precise placement of sutures. This technique allows ventilation during reconstruction of the trachea. Before completion of the tracheal anastomosis, the oral endotracheal tube is retrieved from the proximal trachea and passed distal to the suture line. Ideally the patient should be extubated and breathe spontaneously at the conclusion of the operative procedure. This requires close coordination between surgeon and anesthesiologist. It is not desirable to have even a low-pressure cuff in close contact with the anastomosis for any period of time. If the patient does require intubation after surgery, a small, uncuffed endotracheal tube is preferred. The tube should be removed within 24 to 48 hours. If the airway is still a concern, a small tracheostomy should be placed two rings below the anastomosis. The innominate artery and the tracheal anastomosis should be separated by a strap muscle flap that is carefully sutured to the trachea.

■ SURGICAL TECHNIQUE FOR TRACHEAL RESECTION

The patient is placed supine on the operating table with a roll or inflatable bag underneath the shoulders to extend the neck. A cervical or upper cervicomediastinal approach is used for benign strictures of the trachea at any level. The trachea is explored through a collar incision, which may encompass an existing tracheal stoma (Figure 2, *A*). Skin flaps are raised with platysma to the cricoid cartilage superiorly and the sternal notch inferiorly. The medial margins of the strap muscles are elevated and the anterior surface of the trachea is bluntly exposed from the cricoid cartilage to the carina. The thyroid isthmus is divided, dissected from the trachea, and retracted laterally with sutures. It is essential to keep the dissection absolutely close to the trachea to avoid injury to the recurrent laryngeal nerves, esophagus, and back wall of the innominate artery. If the innominate artery is adherent to the trachea and requires dissection, a strap muscle flap should be interposed between the artery and the tracheal anastomosis at the completion of reconstruction. For lesions that are too far below the sternum to be accessible through a collar incision, the exposure can be increased by making a T incision in which the vertical arm extends downward to a point 1 cm below the sternal angle (see Figure 2, *A*). The sternum is divided to that point and separated with a pediatric chest spreader (Figure 2, *B*). No additional useful exposure is obtained by full median sternotomy because the carina lies at the level of the angle of Louis and the great vessels obstruct access from an anterior approach. The upper sternal division provides access to the lower trachea. The innominate vein, which lies anterior and caudal to the dissection, is not divided. The innominate artery is dissected away from the trachea without exposing the wall of the artery. The anterior carina and the right and left tracheobronchial angles can be exposed as needed.

In cases of tracheal stenosis, the dissection is made meticulously along the lateral borders of the involved trachea and posteriorly

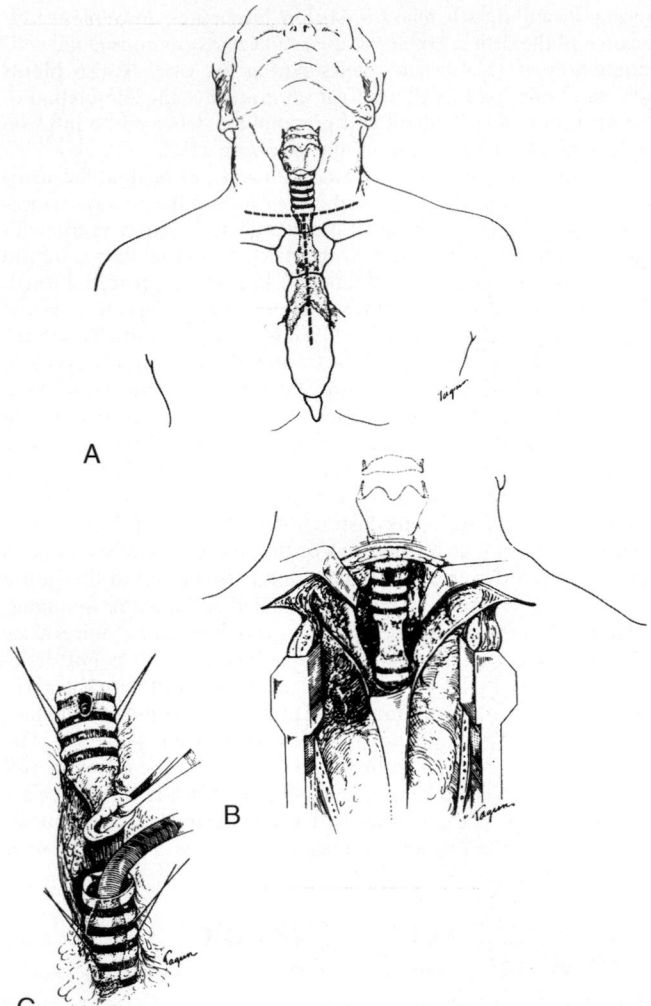

A

B

C

FIGURE 2 Tracheal resection and reconstruction for postintubation stenosis. **A,** A collar incision provides access for many upper tracheal lesions. For wider access to the upper thoracic inlet and the mediastinum, a partial sternotomy is performed. Usually the incision is not carried more than 1 to 2 cm below the angle of Louis. This provides exposure even for the supracarinal benign stenosis. **B,** Partial sternotomy with retraction of innominate vein and artery without their exposure. The pretracheal plane is dissected only. Circumferential dissection is performed only just below the lesion. **C,** After placement of lateral traction sutures above and below the points of the tracheal transection and after circumferential dissection around the distal trachea just below the lesion, the specimen is divided from the trachea. Upward traction on the specimen permits safe dissection of the esophagus and lateral tissues away from the specimen without injury to esophagus or recurrent laryngeal nerves. Eventually the specimen is transected above the level of stenosis. *(From Mathisen DJ. Surgery of the trachea.* Curr Probl Surg. *1998;35:453-542.)*

approximately 1 cm below the lesion (Figure 2, *C*). If it is difficult to identify the level of the lesion, intraoperative bronchoscopy can help to localize the lesion. After carefully pulling the endotracheal tube back under bronchoscopic control, the position of the bronchoscope light is identified at the upper and then the lower end of the lesion while an assistant inserts a 25-gauge needle through the tracheal wall for precise localization. These levels are marked with fine sutures. Dissection close to the tracheal wall avoids injury to the recurrent laryngeal nerves, which lie in the tracheoesophageal groove on either side. The recurrent laryngeal nerves are vulnerable to injury

and are best not exposed by keeping the dissection close to the tracheal wall. This is particularly important if the stenosis lies just below the cricoid cartilage because the recurrent laryngeal nerves enter the larynx just medial to the inferior cornua of the thyroid cartilages. As the trachea is dissected circumferentially, great care must be taken to avoid perforation of the esophagus or the membranous wall of the trachea posteriorly. After the circumferential dissection of the trachea is completed, a tape is passed beneath the trachea for traction on the airway.

Before the division of the trachea, sterile anesthesia equipment is assembled on the field, and sterile corrugated tubing is passed off the table to the anesthesiologist. Lateral traction sutures of 2-0 Vicryl (Ethicon, Somerville, NJ) are placed on either side of the trachea in the midlateral position approximately 1 cm below the anticipated level of transection. These sutures pass vertically through the full thickness of the tracheal wall and around one or more rings (see Figure 2, *C*). The trachea is opened anteriorly just distal to the lesion, staying close to the lesion if it is a benign stricture. Healthy cartilage should be present at the cut edge of the trachea. Transection of the trachea is generally above the ring, but it is acceptable to make the incision in the cartilage. When the airway is open, continuous suctioning prevents seepage of blood into the distal airway. After transection, an assistant holds tension on the two lateral traction sutures and holds the flexible armored Tovell tube in the distal trachea. This maneuver draws the distal trachea and the ventilating tube away from the dissection. Circumferential dissection of the remaining proximal and distal trachea is limited to no more than 1 cm to protect the segmental blood supply, which enters laterally. Devascularization of healthy trachea that will be anastomosed invites possible necrosis and anastomotic dehiscence.

To test the ease with which the tracheal ends can be brought together, the anesthesiologist flexes the patient's neck, and the surgeons draw on the crossed proximal and distal traction sutures, bringing the tracheal ends together. The surgeon should be able to judge whether the tension is excessive. The length of trachea that may be removed safely should be determined before division of the trachea. The feasibility of resection is based on radiologic and bronchoscopic examinations made before the operation. The length of trachea that can be removed safely is influenced by the patient's age and body habitus, by the anatomy of the trachea, and by previous treatments. After it has been demonstrated that the tracheal ends will come together without excessive tension, the neck is hyperextended again. The first anastomotic suture (4-0 coated Vicryl) is placed in the posterior midline with the knots on the outside. The sutures are clipped carefully to the drapes (Figure 3, *A*). The next suture is placed anterior to this and clipped to the drapes just caudad to the previous one. The sutures are placed serially until a point is reached at the midlateral tracheal traction suture (Figure 3, *B*). The same placement of sutures is now carried out on the opposite side, from the posterior midline to the midlateral traction suture. Serial sutures are similarly placed anteriorly, proceeding from the lateral traction sutures to the midline. The sutures are placed through the cartilage approximately 4 mm from the cut edge of the trachea and 4 mm apart. When all of the sutures are placed, the oral endotracheal tube is advanced from above until the tip is visible in the wound. The distal trachea is suctioned, and the endotracheal tube is advanced further, resuming ventilation through the original oral endotracheal tube. Care must be taken not to entangle the endotracheal tube in the anastomotic sutures. The patient's head is supported firmly on blankets in flexion. The crossed lateral traction sutures are pulled together on either side and tied with surgeon's knots opposing the tracheal ends.

The anterior anastomotic sutures are tied first without tension, and the ends are cut after each suture is tied. The assistant then rotates the trachea by carefully drawing medially on the traction sutures on the surgeon's side of the table. The surgeon ties the suture just behind the lateral traction suture and ties sutures in the direction

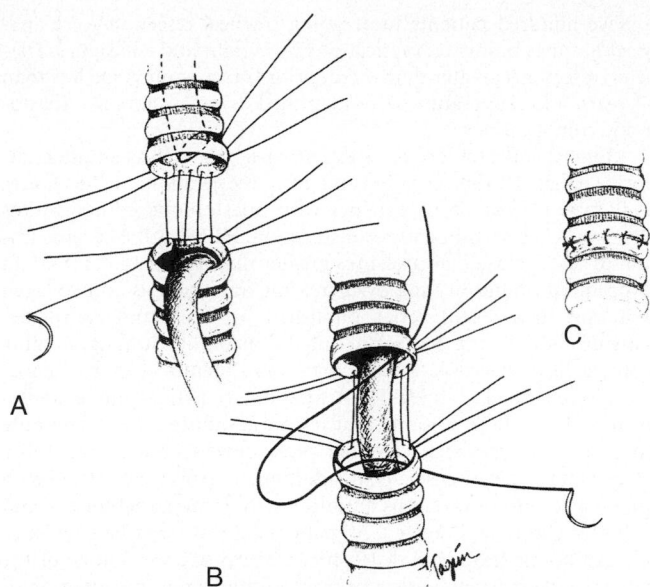

FIGURE 3 Tracheal anastomosis. **A,** Sutures are placed individually beginning in the midline posteriorly and ranging anteriorly on either side. **B,** After the sutures are placed on either side up to the level of the midlateral traction sutures, the anterior sutures are placed. Frequently the endotracheal tube is not advanced from above until after all sutures are placed. **C,** The neck is placed in the flexed position, and the lateral traction sutures are tied on either side (not shown) to remove tension from the anastomotic sutures. After this, anastomotic sutures are tied from anterior to posterior on either side. The completed anastomosis is airtight. *(From Mathisen DJ. Surgery of the trachea.* Curr Probl Surg. *1998;35:453-542.)*

of the posterior midline. This technique is repeated on the opposite side (Figure 3, *C*). The cut traction sutures are left in place to guard against tension on the anastomotic sutures. The integrity of the anastomosis is checked by submersing the wound in saline solution, deflating the tube cuff, and insufflating to pressures between 20 and 30 cm H₂O. All anastomoses must be airtight, and a patient should not leave the operating room with an air leak. A leak must be repaired, even if it means taking the anastomosis down and redoing it again. The sternohyoid muscle or the thyroid isthmus is then used to cover all suture lines. This serves as a buttress, an adjunct to healing, and a barrier to superficial wound infections. If there is any concern regarding dissection of the innominate artery, a pedicled strap muscle should be interposed between the innominate artery and the trachea. Flat suction drains are placed in the pretracheal and substernal spaces, and the strap muscles are approximated in the midline. After the incision is closed, a heavy suture is placed through the submental skin crease beneath the chin and through the presternal skin. This suture is tied with the patient's neck in moderate flexion to prevent sudden hyperextension of the neck in the first week after the operation.

If it is determined after neck flexion that excessive anastomotic tension exists, maneuvers should be performed to reduce tension. The most helpful maneuver for the upper and middle trachea is Montgomery's suprahyoid release. This can be performed by exposing the hyoid through a small horizontal incision just over the hyoid. The muscles inserting on the superior aspect of the hyoid between the lesser cornu are divided. The hyoid bone is divided just lateral to the lesser cornu on both sides. This release maneuver usually gives between 1 and 2 cm of additional mobility of the trachea.

After tracheal resection, patients usually are extubated in the operating room. If the airway is not satisfactory at this point, it is not likely to improve later unless the problem is caused by laryngeal edema. A small endotracheal tube with the cuff deflated can be left in place for 24 to 48 hours while the laryngeal edema resolves. The patient should be given 24 to 48 hours of steroids (Decadron [dexamethasone; Merck, Whitehouse Station, NY], 4 mg intravenously every 6 hours) and diuretics, be placed on fluid restriction, and have the head elevated in bed to reduce edema. We prefer to return to the operating room at the end of 48 hours and extubate the patient under anesthesia. If there is still a problem, a small tracheostomy tube is placed two rings below the anastomosis. A pedicled strap muscle flap should be used to cover the anastomosis if not already performed.

■ COMPLICATIONS OF TRACHEAL SURGERY

Complications after tracheal surgery are similar regardless of the problem for which resection and reconstruction are performed. Avoiding anastomotic tension and devascularization are the keys to minimizing complications. In general, resections greater than 4 cm should include additional maneuvers to avoid anastomotic tension. Standard techniques include dissection of the pretracheal plane, neck flexion, traction sutures, and suprahyoid laryngeal release in extreme cases.

One of the most common complications in the immediate postoperative period is edema, especially after subglottic resection. Edema generally manifests after 24 to 72 hours and is the most likely culprit for reduced airflow in the first few days after surgery if an adequate airway was demonstrated in the operating room. Separation and secretions are other explanations that must be considered. Edema is treated as previously described.

If an air leak develops postoperatively, as manifested by subcutaneous emphysema, this could be a harbinger of separation and is a surgical emergency. The patient should be returned to the operating room immediately and the airway secured. In cases of separation, repair is unlikely and tracheostomy or a T-tube should be used to secure the airway. Local muscles can be used to buttress the tracheostomy or T-tube. If the airway is stable and the subcutaneous air is minimal, CT imaging may be helpful in the initial assessment. Either way, the patient should undergo bronchoscopy to assess the competency of the airway. If a dehiscence is found, surgical exploration and securing the airway with a tracheostomy or T-tube are preferable. If the airway is secure and only a small leak from a suture or a small area of necrosis is identified, attempted local repair buttressed by muscles utilizing suction to press the flaps securely in the damaged area is often successful. Alternatively, hyperbaric oxygen therapy (HBOT) has been used to enhance angiogenesis, improve wound healing, and avoid reoperation.

The most in-depth analysis of complications after tracheal surgery in patients with postintubation stenosis was reported by Grillo and colleagues. The complications reported in this series of 503 patients are summarized in Table 1. Granulation tissue formed at the site of tracheal anastomosis in 49 patients in the series. After 1978, when the suture material was switched from nonabsorbable Tevdek (Deknatel, Mansfield, MA) to absorbable Vicryl, only five such cases occurred. Thirty-eight of these patients were treated with bronchoscopic removal of granulation tissue, and five patients required reoperation with a second tracheal resection. Four patients required tracheostomy, and two patients were treated with T-tubes.

A total of 25 patients had varying degrees of laryngeal dysfunction (aspiration or vocal cord dysfunction) after tracheal resection and reconstruction. Fourteen of these patients had temporary laryngeal dysfunction that required no specific intervention. Eleven cases had more severe laryngeal dysfunction requiring either tracheostomy or T-tube. Two patients in this series required gastrostomy tube feedings for persistent aspiration as a result of glottic dysfunction.

A total of 29 patients had anastomotic dehiscence or restenosis. Seven patients with this complication died. Two patients had erosion into the innominate artery, resulting in death. Eight patients with anastomotic dehiscence were treated with repeat tracheal resection with either good or satisfactory results. Four patients were treated with permanent tracheostomy, and another five patients were treated with T-tubes, three of which were temporary. Three patients developed a dehiscence of a small portion of the anastomosis. Two patients required reoperation and primary closure, and one patient was treated with cervical wound drainage and antibiotics. An additional two patients required serial dilatations. Other complications included tracheal malacia, hemorrhage, and infectious complications, including 15 wound infections and 19 cases of pneumonia or bronchitis. In total there were 12 perioperative deaths, 7 of which were related to the complication of anastomotic dehiscence.

Five hundred patients undergoing tracheal resection were analyzed for anastomotic complications by Wright and colleagues. Diabetes, resections greater than 4 cm, prior tracheostomy, age less than 17 years, and reoperation were identified as risk factors for anastomotic complications.

More recently, the use of HBOT has been studied as an intervention to enhance wound healing and avoid reoperation, tracheostomy, or T-tube placement in patients with anastomotic complications after tracheal resection and reconstruction. HBOT is the administration of 100% oxygen at pressures greater than 1 atm and is thought to promote wound healing by increasing angiogenesis and collagen synthesis. In a recent series published by Stock and colleagues, patients with varying degrees of failed anastomotic healing, ranging from cartilage necrosis to mild separation identified by bronchoscopy, were treated with HBOT. A total of five patients underwent a mean of 13.2 HBOT sessions, which were administered in 90-minute intervals in a hyperbaric chamber pressurized to 2 atm with 100% oxygen one or two times daily. In addition, patients were treated with broad-spectrum intravenous antibiotics, tobramycin nebulizers, and Heliox as clinically indicated. All patients in this series had evidence of anastomotic healing within a mean of 9.6 days, and none of the patients required reoperation or tracheostomy after the initiation of HBOT. Complications were minor and included inner ear discomfort requiring tympanostomy tube placement, temporary blurry vision, and one patient who developed tracheal granulation tissue requiring bronchoscopic débridement.

■ RESULTS

The results of tracheal resection and reconstruction have proven to be successful. In a series spanning 1965 to 1995, a total of 503 patients underwent 521 tracheal resections for postintubation stenosis, 13 of which were done for restenosis after the initial repair. The amount of trachea resected ranged from 1.0 to 7.5 cm and was most commonly between 2 and 4 cm. Laryngeal release was performed in 9.7% of cases. Overall results are summarized in Table 2. Results were good (defined as an anatomically intact airway in a functionally normal patient) in 440 patients (87.5%) and satisfactory (defined as patients able to perform normal activities but with abnormalities such as stress with exercise, a paralyzed vocal cord, or bronchoscopic evidence of narrowing) in 31 patients (6.0%). There were 20 failures (4.0%) and 12 deaths (2.4%). Failures were treated with tracheostomy in 11 patients, with T-tubes in 7 patients, and with dilations in 2 patients. Prior resection and reconstruction increased the failure rate from 3.6% to 5.6% and the mortality rate from 2.1% to 3.8%. The level of the airway anastomosis also was found to be a predictor of success. Trachea to trachea anastomoses were the most successful with failure rates of only 2.2%. Trachea to cricoid anastomoses had a failure rate of 6%, and trachea to thyroid cartilage anastomoses had a failure rate of 8.1%. Minor complications also became more prevalent with each level. Risk factors for anastomotic failure have been shown to include length greater than 4 cm, diabetes, age less than 17 years, preoperative tracheostomy, reoperation, and laryngeal anastomosis.

TABLE 1: Complications of Operations for Postintubation Tracheal Stenosis

	Major	Minor	Total
Granulations	11	38	49
Before 1978	11	34	44
After 1978	1	4	5
Dehiscence	28	1	29
Laryngeal dysfunction	11	14	25
Malacia	10	0	10
Hemorrhage	5	0	5
Edema (anastomosis)	3	1	4
Infection	12	22	34
Wound	7	8	15
Pulmonary	5	14	19
Myocardial infarction	1	0	1
Tracheoesophageal fistula	1	0	1
Pneumothorax	0	3	3
Line infection	0	1	1
Atrial fibrillation	0	1	1
Deep venous thrombosis	0	1	1
Totals	82	82	164

From Grillo HC, Donahue DM, Mathisen DJ, et al. Postintubation tracheal stenosis: treatment and results. *J Thorac Cardiovasc Surg.* 1995;109:486-492.

TABLE 2: Results of Surgical Treatment of Postintubation Tracheal Stenosis

	No. of Patients	Good		Satisfactory		Failure		Death		Reoperation	
		No.	%	No.	%	No.	%	No.	%	No.	%
Initial operation	503	427	84.9	27	5.3	19	3.8	12	2.4	18	3.6
Reoperation	18	13	72.2	4	22.2	1	5.6	0	–	–	–
Overall	503	440	87.5	31	6.2	20	3.9	12	2.4	–	–

From Grillo HC, Donahue DM, Mathisen DJ, et al. Postintubation tracheal stenosis: treatment and results. *J Thorac Cardiovasc Surg.* 1995;109:486-492.

SUGGESTED READINGS

Ashiku SK, Grillo HC, Mathisen DJ, et al. Idiopathic laryngotracheal stenosis: effective definitive treatment with laryngotracheal resection. *J Thorac Cardiovasc Surg.* 2004;127:99-107.

Gaissert HA, Grillo HC, Mathisen DJ, et al. Long-term survival after resection of primary adenoid cystic and squamous cell carcinoma of the trachea and carina. *Ann Thorac Surg.* 2004;78:1889-1896.

Grillo HC, Donahue DM, Mathisen DJ, et al. Postintubation tracheal stenosis: treatment and results. *J Thorac Cardiovasc Surg.* 1995;109:486-492.

Montgomery WW. Suprahyoid release for tracheal anastomosis. *Arch Otolaryngol.* 1974;99:255-260.

Stock C, Gukasan N, Muniappan A, et al. Hyperbaric oxygen therapy for the treatment of anastomotic complications after tracheal resection and reconstruction. *J Thorac Cardiovasc Surg.* 2014;147:1030-1035.

Wright CD, Grillo HC, Wain JC, et al. Anastomotic complications after tracheal resection: prognostic factors and management. *J Thorac Cardiovasc Surg.* 2004;128:731-739.

THE MANAGEMENT OF ACQUIRED ESOPHAGEAL RESPIRATORY TRACT FISTULA

Cameron D. Wright, MD

Acquired esophageal respiratory tract fistulas are commonly separated into two types: malignant and benign. Their presentation is similar, with coughing while eating or drinking, aspiration pneumonia, and difficulty ventilating a patient when on mechanical ventilation. Small fistulas may be difficult to diagnose and are usually not life threatening. Large fistulas (>1 cm) are often life threatening and are readily diagnosed. Suspected small fistulas are best diagnosed with a barium swallow. Suspected large fistulas usually are best diagnosed with bronchoscopy and esophagoscopy.

■ MALIGNANT ESOPHAGEAL RESPIRATORY TRACT FISTULA

Esophageal and lung cancers are the most common tumors that cause airway fistulas because of their proximity to each other. These fistulas cause the rapid demise of the patient from aspiration pneumonia. Patients characteristically have a constant cough resulting from ongoing aspiration. The cough is not suppressed by usual measures and requires palliation. The survival of patients with malignant fistulas in a report by Dubecz and colleagues was 1 to 3 months. These dismal survival results indicate that quick and effective palliation is required in these patients, as their limited life expectancy precludes large operations that have substantial risk of major complications. Esophageal diversion and exclusion are largely historical operations that have little role today given their high operative mortality and morbidity.

■ ESOPHAGEAL STENTS

Thin-walled, expandable covered metallic stents that are easy to place endoscopically are now available. They effectively palliate dysphagia and fistulas caused by esophageal cancer. Ideally there is a stricture present at the fistula site so that the stent can be seated securely to prevent migration (which there usually is).

Placement of Expandable Esophageal Stents

Although local anesthesia with sedation can be used, I prefer general anesthesia because it is most comfortable for the patient. Fluoroscopic guidance is used, so a proper fluoroscopic bed must be used as well. Endoscopy is performed to obtain landmarks and delineate the fistula. If the stricture is tight, I dilate it first so that the stent can readily pass through the stricture. It should be underdilated, however,

as the stricture helps to hold the stent in place. I place radioopaque markers (commonly large safety pins on the patient's gown) to mark the distal and proximal extent of the fistula under direct endoscopic and fluoroscopic guidance. A long guidewire is then placed in the stomach, and the endoscope is removed. The stent and applicator are threaded over the guidewire and inserted distally so as to span the fistula. The radioopaque markers are key here, to ensure that the middle of the covered portion (the center) of the stent exactly spans the fistula. The stent is then deployed, and the applicator and guidewire are removed. Repeat endoscopy confirms proper stent placement and fistula coverage. Alternatively, the stent can be placed under direct endoscopic guidance without fluoroscopy by deploying the stent over the guidewire while watching and controlling the proximal portion of the stent to ensure its proper placement. If needed, balloon dilation of the stent is performed to reduce luminal narrowing. Again, it is better to underdilate, as quick, large dilations are more prone to perforate and are more likely to lead to pain. Stent expansion continues to occur as the stent warms to body temperature. I commonly perform a bronchoscopy at the conclusion of the procedure, as patients invariably have a large amount of inspissated secretions. If possible, I prefer to obtain a barium swallow to confirm fistula occlusion before allowing the patient to eat.

■ TRACHEOBRONCHIAL STENTS

Thin-walled, expandable covered metallic stents that are easy to place endoscopically are now available. They are commonly placed if the fistula is not associated with esophageal cancer that produces a malignant stricture. These stents often cause troublesome granulation tissue at the two ends, which is of concern in patients with benign disease but not usually of concern in those with advanced malignant disease who only have months to live. These stents also can be placed as a second stent in difficult-to-close fistulas where the esophageal stent has not occluded the fistula completely. Like esophageal stents, they also can palliate airway narrowing caused by the associated cancer.

Placement of Airway Stents

There are many possibilities in placing airway stents. Again, local anesthesia with sedation or general anesthesia may be used, but I prefer general anesthesia. Fluoroscopy can be used, but I rarely find it necessary, as I deploy stents under direct endoscopic control. If desired, the airway can be controlled with a rigid bronchoscope and the stent deployed through the lumen (as well as the flexible bronchoscope, to help guide the placement of the stent). Alternatively, intermittent apneic spells can be used to place a stent if the procedure can be done expeditiously under bronchoscopic control. A preliminary bronchoscopy is done to map the location of the fistula and clean up the airway. The airway is dilated if there is a tight stenosis. A guidewire can be used if desired, but I rarely find it necessary, as I place the stent under direct bronchoscopic control. When the stent is in proper position, it is deployed. It is best to adjust the position of the stent partway through deployment rather than waiting until full deployment, as it is easier to move when it is only partially deployed. I usually try to firmly seat the stent by performing balloon dilation of the stent once it is deployed. A chest x-ray is obtained at the conclusion of the procedure to search for pneumothorax and document the position of the stent. Again, I prefer to obtain a barium swallow to confirm occlusion of the fistula by the stent.

■ RESULTS OF PALLIATIVE TREATMENT WITH COVERED EXPANDABLE METALLIC STENTS

Success rates of 80% to 100% have been reported with sealing of malignant fistulas. Fistulas may reopen after initial successful closure because of stent migration or fistula enlargement. Successful fistula occlusion is associated with longer survival. Complications include migration, perforation, erosion into a vascular structure, recurrent fistulization, and food impaction with esophageal stents.

■ BENIGN ESOPHAGEAL RESPIRATORY TRACT FISTULA

Most tracheoesophageal fistulas (TEFs) result from long-term ventilation with either an endotracheal tube or more commonly a tracheostomy tube. The mechanism of injury is usually ischemic necrosis from an overinflated cuff. TEFs also may result from injudicious oral intubation or placement of a tracheostomy tube (either by the traditional technique or by percutaneous dilation) with perforation of the posterior tracheal wall. Other causes include trauma, iatrogenic injury, caustic ingestion, infection, granulomatous inflammation, and impacted esophageal foreign bodies. Essentially all benign fistulas should be closed, as spontaneous closure is very rare.

■ POSTINTUBATION TRACHEOESOPHAGEAL FISTULAS

Most postintubation TEFs are diagnosed while the patient is still receiving mechanical ventilation. The most common sign is a loss of returned tidal volume with a resultant difficulty in maintaining satisfactory ventilation. The cuff is commonly inflated more, which temporarily improves the situation but also enlarges the fistula. Other signs are an increase in secretions, distension of the stomach, and aspiration of tube feeds. Many patients have an indwelling hard nasogastric tube rather than a soft feeding tube or a gastrostomy. The diagnosis is made easily by bronchoscopy with the tracheostomy tube removed. The fistula size should be measured, the position of the fistula in relation to the rest of the airway should be measured, and the status of the surrounding trachea should be ascertained. In almost all cases, the patient should be weaned from ventilation before definitive repair to maximize the possibility of success. It makes no sense to ventilate a fresh tracheal suture line if spontaneous ventilation is possible. A long tracheostomy tube usually can be inserted so that the cuff is well below the fistula, which effectively excludes the fistula. I prefer tracheostomy tubes that can be custom made in different lengths (Bivona) with large foam cuffs that seal the airway very well yet do not cause further tracheal damage. The nasogastric tube should be removed, and a draining gastrostomy and feeding jejunostomy should be performed. When the patient is in reasonable shape, a definitive repair should be undertaken. Several techniques have been used to close a TEF: lateral division and closure, methods that involve esophageal division and exclusion, various muscle flaps, and an anterior approach with tracheal resection. The anterior approach is most common and usually leads to good results.

Tracheal Resection and Reconstruction With Esophageal Fistula Closure

Grillo popularized the anterior approach to repair postintubation TEFs in large part because of the frequent presence of concomitant

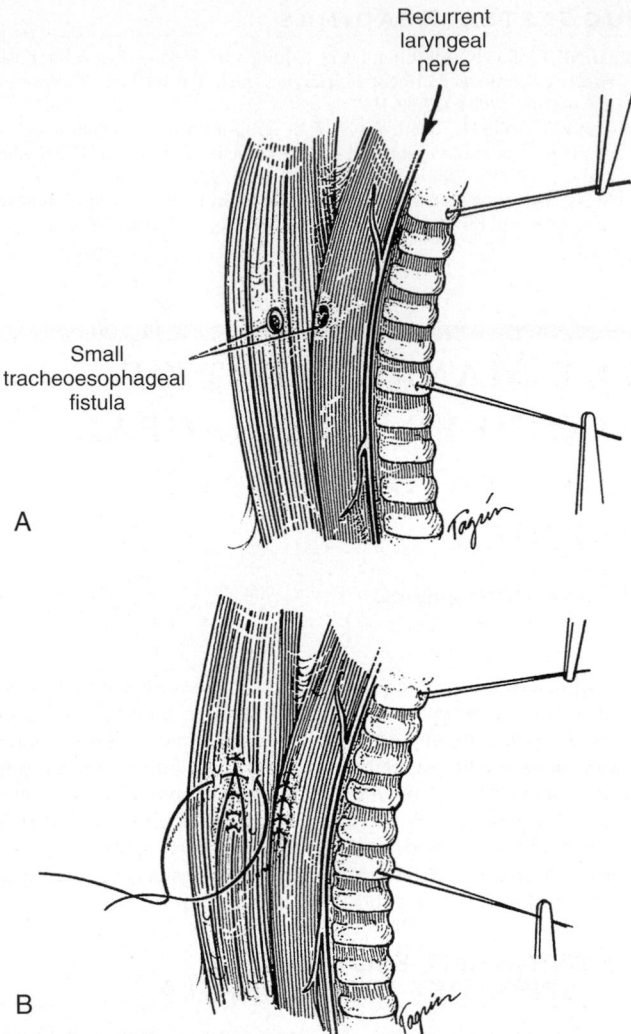

FIGURE 1 Small high tracheoesophageal fistulas can be repaired by a lateral approach in the neck when there is no significant tracheal stenosis. **A,** The trachea is rotated off the front of the esophagus to expose the fistula. **B,** The fistula is repaired with fine interrupted sutures. A strap muscle flap is interposed between the two repairs to separate the suture lines. *(From Mathisen DJ, Grillo HC, Wain JC, et al: Management of acquired nonmalignant tracheoesophageal fistula. Ann Thorac Surg. 1991;52:759.)*

tracheal stenosis and malacia at the fistula site. The anterior approach has been extended to include patients with a normal trachea, as division of the trachea at the fistula site provides the best exposure to a satisfactory esophageal repair. The trachea is then reapproximated in the standard fashion (Figures 1 to 5).

The patient is placed supine with the back elevated and the head extended as far as possible. A low collar incision, usually encompassing the stoma, is performed. Subplatysmal flaps are elevated. The strap muscles are separated in the midline. The thyroid isthmus is divided. The anterior aspect of the airway is exposed from the cricoid to the carina. The fistula site is identified, usually by bronchoscopy done on the field to precisely mark the limits of the fistula. This is easily done with a 25-gauge needle placed through the trachea under bronchoscopic control. A decision needs to be made about the stoma—will it be resected with the fistula or, if too far away, will it be closed or left open to close at a later date? Circumferential dissection is then done at the resection site staying right on the tracheal wall to avoid injury to the recurrent nerve. The nerve should never

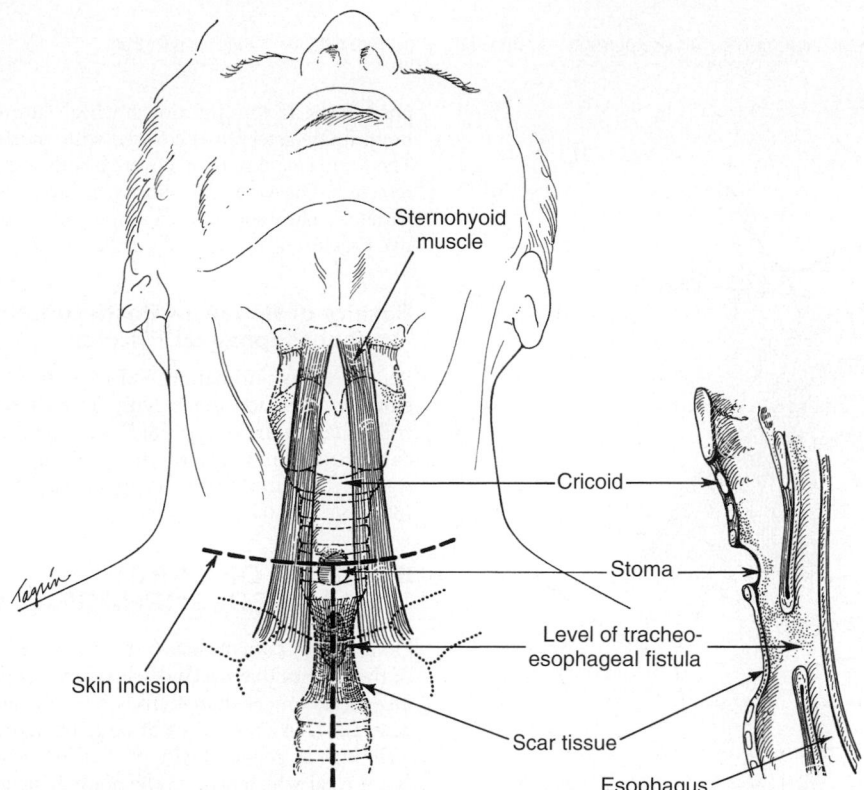

FIGURE 2 Anterior approach for postintubation tracheoesophageal fistula. Most high fistulas can be repaired through a simple collar incision. For lower fistulas, the manubrium can be divided in the midline to give excellent exposure. *(From Mathisen DJ, Grillo HC, Wain JC, et al. Management of acquired nonmalignant tracheoesophageal fistula. Ann Thorac Surg. 1991;52:759.)*

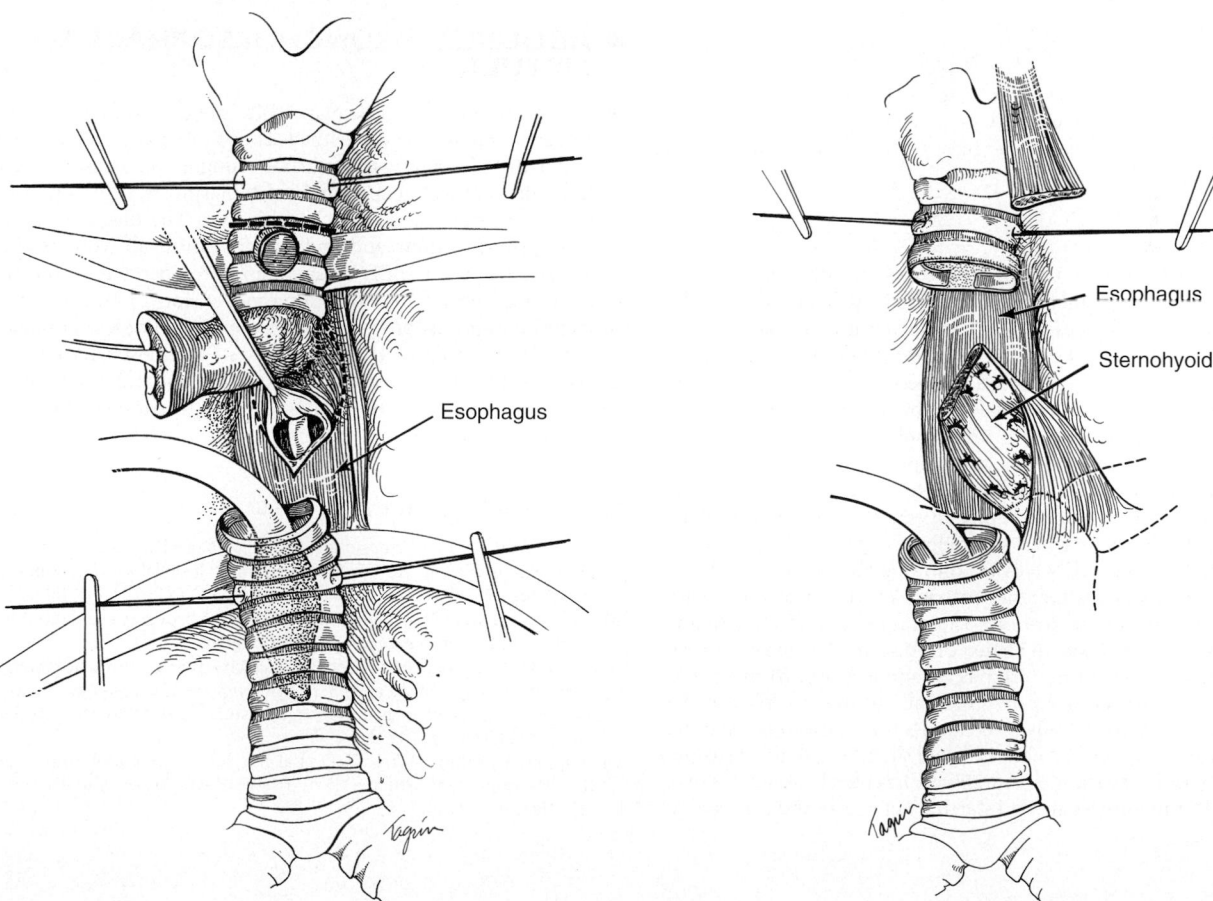

FIGURE 3 The trachea is divided below the fistula, providing excellent exposure to the esophageal fistula. The distal trachea is intubated with a sterile endotracheal tube for ventilation. *(From Mathisen DJ, Grillo HC, Wain JC, et al. Management of acquired nonmalignant tracheoesophageal fistula. Ann Thorac Surg. 1991;52:759.)*

FIGURE 4 The esophagus is closed in two layers with fine sutures, and a pedicled strap muscle is sutured carefully around the edges to provide a reinforcing layer and to separate the two suture lines. Circumferential sutures are then placed between the two ends of the trachea. *(From Mathisen DJ, Grillo HC, Wain JC, et al. Management of acquired nonmalignant tracheoesophageal fistula. Ann Thorac Surg. 1991;52:759.)*

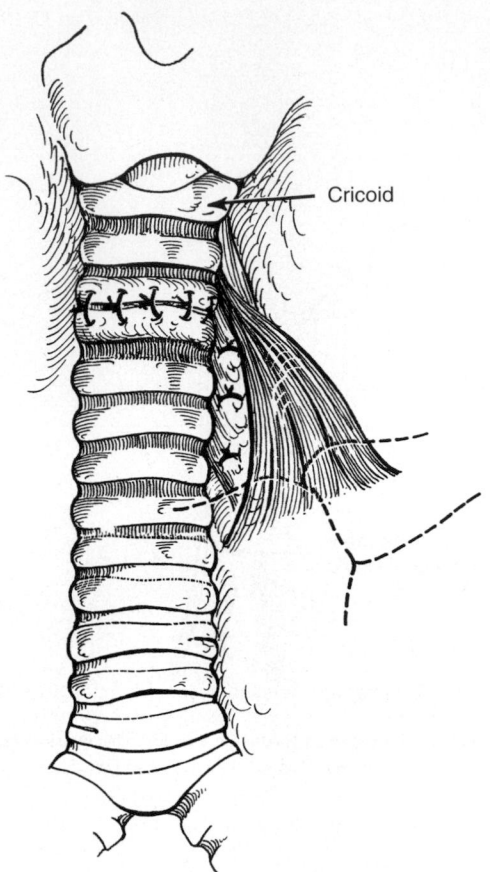

Cricoid

FIGURE 5 The tracheal repair is complete and the pedicled strap muscle is seen separating the two suture lines. *(From Mathisen DJ, Grillo HC, Wain JC, et al. Management of acquired nonmalignant tracheoesophageal fistula. Ann Thorac Surg. 1991;52:759.)*

be sought in the dense scar around the fistula site, as the risk of injury is high. The trachea is then divided above and below the fistula. Intermittent ventilation is carried out with a sterile endotracheal tube inserted in the distal trachea while the native endotracheal tube is pulled back in the proximal trachea. The esophagus is dissected off the undersurface of the trachea above and below the tracheal transection site to allow ready closure of the esophagus. The esophagus is then closed in two layers with fine interrupted sutures, with the first layer inverting with knots on the inside. A pedicled strap muscle is then sutured over the repair site along all edges to buttress the repair and separate it from the tracheal suture line. Stay sutures (2-0 Vicryl) are placed at 3 o'clock and 9 o'clock, one ring back and around one ring to reduce tension on the finer sutures. The tracheal sutures are then placed starting at the posterior membranous wall in a circumferential fashion, with knots to be tied on the outside. Fine 4-0 Vicryl sutures are used. The sutures are placed about 4 mm from the cut edge and are about 5 mm apart. Once all sutures are placed, the native endotracheal tube is advanced across the anastomosis and the stay sutures are tied after the neck is flexed slightly to reduce tension. If there is excessive tension, a suprahyoid laryngeal release is done. Thereafter the fine sutures are tied starting anteriorly and proceeding

posteriorly. If the anterior tracheal suture line is adjacent to the innominate artery, it is covered with another pedicled strap muscle. The stoma is closed or covered with a strap muscle if it was not resected. The wound is closed in layers over a suction drain. The patient is always extubated at the end of the procedure so that positive pressure is not placed on the suture line.

Results of Repair of Postintubation Tracheoesophageal Fistulas

Repair of postintubation TEFs has been very successful with the anterior approach along with tracheal resection. Muniappan and colleagues recently reported their results with 36 patients. Tracheal resection was required in 53% of patients. Fistula closure was successful in 94% of patients. There was only one death (3% mortality).

■ REPAIR OF LARGE TRACHEOESOPHAGEAL FISTULAS

Occasionally patients have very large defects in the membranous wall of the trachea that preclude closure by tracheal resection (commonly any fistula longer than 4 cm is not amenable to repair with tracheal resection). In these cases of large benign fistulas, the membranous wall must be replaced with an alternative. Many options exist, and it is not clear which is best. The options include pericardium, intercostal muscle, free myocutaneous flaps such as a free radial forearm flap, decellularized dermis, and aortic homograft. If devascularized tissue is used I prefer to augment the repair with an omental flap to hopefully augment the blood supply to the grafted material.

■ ACQUIRED BRONCHOESOPHAGEAL FISTULA

Most bronchoesophageal fistulas (BEFs) are due to lung or esophageal cancer and are treated with stents. Rarely patients have benign acquired BEF, usually with a chronic cough. The causes of a BEF include postsurgical, congenital, histoplasmosis, silicosis, foreign body, lye ingestion, and bronchogenic cyst. The diagnosis is made with a barium swallow and endoscopy. Almost all patients should undergo repair of the BEF. Most patients are operated on through a right thoracotomy with exposure and division of the fistula. The bronchus and the esophagus are then closed and covered (and separated) with local tissue transposition. An intercostal muscle is the favored tissue flap because of its ease of harvest and ready location. Mangi and colleagues recently reported on 13 patients with benign BEF, with success in 12.

SUGGESTED READINGS

Dubecz A, Watson TJ, Raymond DP, et al. Esophageal stenting for malignant and benign disease: 133 cases on a thoracic surgical service. *Ann Thorac Surg.* 2011;92:2028-2033.

Mangi AA, Gaissert HA, Wright CD, et al. Benign broncho-esophageal fistula in the adult. *Ann Thorac Surg.* 2000;73:911-915.

Mathisen DJ, Grill HC, Wain JC, et al. Management of acquired nonmalignant tracheoesophageal fistula. *Ann Thorac Surg.* 1991;52:759-765.

Morse CR. Repair of bronchial esophageal fistula using Alloderm. *Ann Thorac Surg.* 2009;88:1018-1019.

Muniappan A, Wain JC, Wright CD, et al. Surgical treatment of nonmalignant tracheoesophageal fistula: a thirty-five year experience. *Ann Thorac Surg.* 2013;95:1141-1146.

CONGENITAL CHEST WALL DEFORMITIES

Laura Martin, MD, and David Hackam, MD, PhD

Congenital chest wall deformities encompass a spectrum of disorders that include pectus carinatum and pectus excavatum, with a range of variants in between. Other congenital chest wall abnormalities include Poland's syndrome and cleft sternum. In all cases, the severity of the deformity falls along a continuum. In some cases, deformities may be barely perceptible and cause no problem throughout life. Other deformities are severe enough to impair quality of life, and in the most severe of cases surgical correction may be necessary to restore quality of life. This chapter reviews the most common chest wall deformities seen by pediatricians and surgeons and discusses current approaches to management.

■ POLAND'S SYNDROME

Poland's syndrome is rare, with an incidence estimated between 1 in 30,000 and 1 in 80,000 births, and consists of unilateral pectoral aplasia and dysdactylia. The syndrome ranges in severity, from mild cases characterized by superficial defects such as aplasia or hypoplasia of the nipple and breast tissues to more severe forms that may include absence of the costosternal portion of the pectoralis major muscle, absence of the pectoralis minor or serratus anterior muscle, aplasia or deformity of the second through fourth ribs, spinal abnormalities, and brachysyndactyly. In severe cases there may be hypoplasia of the latissimus dorsi and deltoid muscles as well as severe rib and diaphragmatic defects resulting in lung herniation. The severity and type of deformities vary widely, and it is uncommon for all features to be present in the same individual. The vast majority of cases are sporadic, with an increased incidence in males and right-sided predominance. Familial cases are rare and without gender or laterality predominance. The etiology of the condition is poorly understood but is thought to relate to disruption of subclavian artery flow during embryogenesis, with hypoplasia or transient disruption of flow in branches of the internal thoracic artery leading to hypoplasia of the breast and sternocostal tissues and disruption of flow in brachial artery branches causing the hand abnormalities. In accordance with this theory, there is no correlation between severity of chest and hand abnormalities. In some cases there may be no apparent abnormality in the vessels, suggesting that a transient disruption of flow in the critical period of development may be responsible for some cases. Reconstruction is complex and highly individualized and typically focuses on soft tissue reconstruction with musculocutaneous flaps and silicone prostheses for chest wall abnormalities, with orthopedic repair of hand abnormalities. There are reported cases of use of the Nuss procedure (discussed later) as a temporizing operation to improve chest wall structure and allow normal pulmonary function and development while preserving bone and soft tissue for later cosmetic repair.

■ CLEFT STERNUM

Cleft sternum, also known as sternum bifidum, is a rare chest wall abnormality resulting from failure of fusion of the two sternal halves during development. It is classified by its location and severity (superior or inferior, subtotal or complete). Symptoms are related to paradoxical chest wall motion, with deepening on inspiration and bulging on expiration, which may result in poor respiratory function and frequent infections as well as compression or displacement of the heart and great vessels. There are frequently associated midline abnormalities such as umbilical hernia or omphalocele; less commonly and somewhat surprisingly, there may be an associated midline defect in the mandible. For unknown reasons, cleft sternum is associated with hemangiomas and other cardiac and vascular abnormalities and therefore requires a thorough evaluation for these associated abnormalities after diagnosis of the chest wall deformity. The etiology of cleft sternum is still under investigation but is believed to involve abnormal migration of mesenchymal progenitor cells to the midline chest during development. In support of this hypothesis, the absence of profilin 1, an actin-binding protein involved in control of actin fiber structure and cellular migration, causes an absence of trabecular bone in the marrow space of appendicular long bone as well as retardation of osteoblastic cell migration, resulting in complete cleft sternum in mice. Repair of cleft sternum focuses on improvement of cardiorespiratory function as well as protection from trauma to the unprotected thoracic structures. When diagnosed prenatally, repair may be performed primarily in the neonatal period. Later repair or repair of more extensive defects may be achieved by approximation of the sternal halves with bone graft or synthetic mesh and may require a staged approach.

■ PECTUS CARINATUM

Pectus carinatum is defined as a congenital chest wall disorder resulting in bowing of the sternum and rib cage. It is the second most common chest wall abnormality after pectus excavatum (discussed later), comprising 5% to 10% of cases. The majority of patients with this condition are asymptomatic. When patients are symptomatic, the most common complaint is pain, likely related to abnormal bone and cartilage growth at the costochondral junction. Pectus carinatum typically does not affect cardiopulmonary function or limit physical activity and as such rarely requires surgical intervention. However, there may be significant body image issues that motivate many patients to seek repair. Etiology is not clearly defined, although as in pectus excavatum, abnormal costochondral growth is thought to be involved. Presently the favored treatment in motivated patients seeking repair is external bracing. The brace is composed of anterior and posterior steel-enforced plates connected by an adjustable strap that is tightened gradually over time to achieve repair. Compliance is the primary obstacle to this treatment, as the brace must be worn for at least 16 hours a day during the most intensive stage of treatment and then continued nightly for at least 2 years or until growth is complete. The vast majority of patients who are compliant with treatment achieve satisfactory results with orthotic bracing. In patients who fail orthotic bracing and in whom symptoms are severe enough to limit quality of life, an open repair may be performed to correct the defect.

■ PECTUS EXCAVATUM

Pectus excavatum is a congenital depression of the chest wall, is the most common chest wall deformity (representing 90% of all deformities), and has an incidence of approximately 1 in 300 to 1 in 400 live births. Males are more frequently affected than females, with a predominance noted in multiple series ranging from 2:1 to 12:1. The inheritance appears to be multifactorial, and the genetics are difficult to assess because of its association with multiple syndromes and disorders that appear to involve a wide variety of genetic aberrations. The most commonly seen cases occur spontaneously, without any evidence of family history, suggesting possible de novo mutations. Pectus excavatum may be seen with other connective tissue abnormalities, but some cases appear to be isolated. Up to 42% of cases are found to have a positive family history. Of those, many are associated with heritable genetic syndromes such as Marfan's, Noonan's, and Loeys-Dietz syndromes, each of whose inheritance is associated with well-described genetic aberrations. However, pectus excavatum also has been linked with an array of mild to severe connective tissue abnormalities collectively known as heritable disorders of connective tissue (HDCTs), a group of genetic disorders that affect proteins of the connective tissue matrix, such as collagens, proteoglycans, elastins, fibrillins, and laminins. As with de novo cases, familial pectus excavatum also may be inherited as an isolated abnormality without evidence of an underlying connective tissue disorder. Many studies have attempted to elucidate a genetic source for isolated pectus excavatum, but these studies are difficult because of small sample size as well as inclusion of nonisolated pectus cases associated with other soft tissue disorders. One recent familial study of isolated pectus excavatum abnormality with an autosomal dominant inheritance pattern suggested that a missense mutation in the first exon of *GAL3ST4*, a member of the sulfotransferase family responsible for sulfation of galactoses in O-linked glycoproteins, may be responsible for the familial isolated pectus defect.

Etiology of Pectus Excavatum

The etiology of pectus excavatum is not yet entirely clear, although it appears to be related to abnormal growth of the sternocostal cartilage, with leading hypotheses focusing on abnormal metabolism within the cartilage, causing biomechanical weakness and overgrowth. Functional alterations that have been observed include decreased activity of chondrocytes, inadequate degradation, and premature aging of the cartilage. Histologic evaluation reveals disorganization of the cellular matrix, although no studies have been able to elucidate the exact means by which these abnormalities in the matrix result in the pectus defect. Studies repeatedly have failed to show a significant difference in cartilage length between the more severely affected side and the opposite side, suggesting that the defect results instead from poor function and integrity of the cartilage.

Physiologic Consequences of Pectus Excavatum

The extent of cardiopulmonary limitation relating to pectus excavatum remains difficult to quantify. Most patients with pectus excavatum do not complain of significant symptoms at rest but rather experience dyspnea with exertion and exercise intolerance. Right axis deviation and depressed ST segments are common in severe pectus excavatum, reflecting rotation and compression of the heart. Patients with clinically significant pectus excavatum are noted to have diminished cardiac filling, stroke volume, cardiac index, and maximum oxygen consumption with exertion when compared with matched controls, suggesting that sternal rotation and compression limit the heart's ability to compensate for increased cardiac requirements during exercise, possibly explaining symptoms on exertion.

In addition, pectus excavatum limits respiratory function because of decreased thoracic expansion and respiratory muscle contraction resulting from the mechanical disadvantage. Further, there is a high association with scoliosis, which contributes to a limitation in thoracic expansion and respiratory function. The most commonly observed abnormalities in preoperative functional evaluation are reduced forced vital capacity (FVC), forced expiratory volume during the first second (FEV1), and maximal inspiratory and expiratory pressures, which are often on the low end of normal or slightly reduced. In resting individuals with healthy lungs, these differences typically are not functionally limiting. However, during exercise or in the case of physiologic processes that decrease lung compliance, patients with pectus excavatum develop disproportionately more severe symptoms and functional limitations.

■ PREOPERATIVE EVALUATION OF THE PATIENT WITH PECTUS EXCAVATUM

History, Physical Examination, and Functional Assessment

Patients with pectus excavatum typically are seen during adolescence with an onset most frequently occurring during puberty. The most common complaints are exercise intolerance, dyspnea, and psychologic distress. Consideration of operative repair is determined by the severity of disease as suggested by patient symptoms, physical examination, physiologic testing abnormalities, and radiologic evaluation.

A detailed history, physical examination, and functional assessment are critical in order to rule out comorbidities and associated connective tissue disorders. Cardiac comorbidities are particularly common in patients with pectus excavatum, and up to 10% of cases have associated mitral valve prolapse. Pulmonary limitations, spinal deformities, and multiple other congenital abnormalities also are associated with pectus excavatum and may require attention before consideration of surgical repair of the chest wall. In addition, patients should be screened for any pertinent allergies, particularly to nickel and titanium, as these metals often are implanted as part of the treatment. Nickel allergy, found in 5% to 15% of individuals, was reported commonly in early minimally invasive repairs that resulted in a high rate of pericarditis and bar removal after surgical repair (discussed later). Chromium allergy also may preclude placement of the standard stainless steel bar, and any history of possible metal allergy should prompt further investigation.

Anatomic considerations include localization of the deformity (localized and deep vs shallow and diffuse), length and symmetry of the defect, and sternal torsion (typically an angle >30 degrees is considered significant). Physical examination and history also should include evaluation for evidence of scoliosis or stigmata of connective tissue diseases.

Preoperative cardiopulmonary assessment should include, at a minimum, electrocardiogram (ECG) to evaluate for arrhythmias; echocardiogram to evaluate stroke volume and cardiac function and to rule out any concomitant valvular disease; pulmonary function tests including spirometry, maximal inspiratory pressure (MIP), and maximum expiratory pressure (MEP); and cardiopulmonary exercise testing. Screening for other abnormalities, including further cardiac evaluation, ophthalmologic evaluation, or genetic testing, also may be indicated, particularly in cases where there is concern for a possible associated connective tissue disorder.

Radiologic Evaluation

Radiologic evaluation is useful to characterize the nature of the deformity for preoperative planning. In addition, the literature demonstrates a statistically significant association between more severe disease as quantified by radiologic evaluation and worse performance on cardiopulmonary physiologic testing, including exercise tolerance, stroke volume, maximal inspiratory volume (MIV), maximal expiratory volume (MEV), and FVC. As such, radiologic imaging has become a useful tool for quantifying the severity of pectus excavatum. Historically, the Haller index has been used to quantify the severity of the pectus defect and predict the response to surgical correction of the deformity. In this regard, significant progress was made by Dr. Alex Haller of Johns Hopkins University to define the severity of disease based on radiographic findings. The Haller index is defined as the ratio of the transverse thoracic diameter to the anteroposterior diameter at the narrowest point of the defect. A ratio less than 2.5 is considered to be normal, and a ratio greater than 3.5 is considered an indication for repair. The Haller index is limited by variability in transverse thoracic diameter that may confound its ability to quantify severity of defect in a standardized manner. More recently, the correction index has been introduced as an alternative to the Haller index. The correction index is defined as the ratio of the difference in anteroposterior diameter from the level of the anterior spine at the maximum diameter of the chest to the anteroposterior diameter from the level of the anterior spine to sternum at the narrowest point of depression. Both measurements can be attained from preoperative chest x-rays, and both are still commonly used.

■ SURGICAL CONSIDERATIONS IN THE APPROACH TO THE CHILD WITH PECTUS EXCAVATUM

Open Repair

In the 1920s Sauerbruch performed the first open pectus repair using the bilateral costal cartilage resection and sternal osteotomy, a technique later refined and popularized by Dr. Mark Ravitch of Johns Hopkins University. In 1956 Wallgren and Sulamaa introduced the concept of internal support by using a slightly curved stainless steel bar. Since its introduction, the procedure has been modified extensively, with progressively less extensive tissue resection.

In the modified Ravitch procedure, a midline sternal incision is performed and skin flaps are elevated to expose the sternum and the costal cartilages. In females, a transverse inframammary incision at the level of the fourth interspace with the creation of subpectoral flaps may be preferred for improved cosmetic results (Figure 1, *A*). In all cases, the abnormal cartilage is elevated from the perichondrium and divided at the sternocostal junction in the subperichondrial plane (Figure 1, *B*). An anterior sternal osteotomy allows elevation of the sternum to a normal position (Figure 1, *C*). A metal strut usually is placed retrosternally to reinforce the fixation (Figure 1, *D*). The strut typically is removed after 1 or more years.

Although the Ravitch procedure largely has been replaced by minimally invasive approaches for repair of primary and even recurrent pectus excavatum (discussed later), there are instances in which Ravitch repair still may be indicated. The force required to elevate the sternum in adults is significantly higher than that in adolescents because of decreased cartilage flexibility after completion of pubertal growth. Complete and durable repair may require costochondral resection in some adult cases, although several minimally invasive studies include adult cohorts with positive outcomes. Other considerations for open repair include complex asymmetric cases in which sternal angle is prohibitive to satisfactory cosmetic result with minimally invasive repair, complicated revisions of previous surgeries, and simultaneous repair of cardiac defects. Minimally invasive approaches are being used increasingly during complicated surgical revisions, but in some cases the degree of inflammation and scarring may be prohibitive to simple correction with a bar without resection of tissue. In cases of concomitant repair of cardiac defects and pectus excavatum, surgeons may forgo extensive costochondral resection, instead placing a Nuss bar via the lateral incisions and passing it under direct visualization before closure of the sternum; positive results have been reported in small series. However, the use of the Nuss bar in cardiothoracic surgery continues to be a source of debate, as opponents point out concerns related to sternal healing, limitation to rapid re-entry, and inability to perform effective cardiopulmonary resuscitation (CPR) compressions in the event of postoperative complications. One final consideration for open repair is nickel or chromium allergy, which can be prohibitive to standard stainless steel bar placement in minimally invasive repair.

Minimally Invasive Repair: The Nuss Procedure

In the late 1980s Donald Nuss began to practice minimally invasive repair of pectus excavatum, relying on the flexibility of the costal cartilage to facilitate retrosternal repair without resection. Initial attempts at the minimally invasive approach involved the use of a titanium bar, which was found to be too malleable and therefore was replaced with a stainless steel bar, and a longer medial incision that

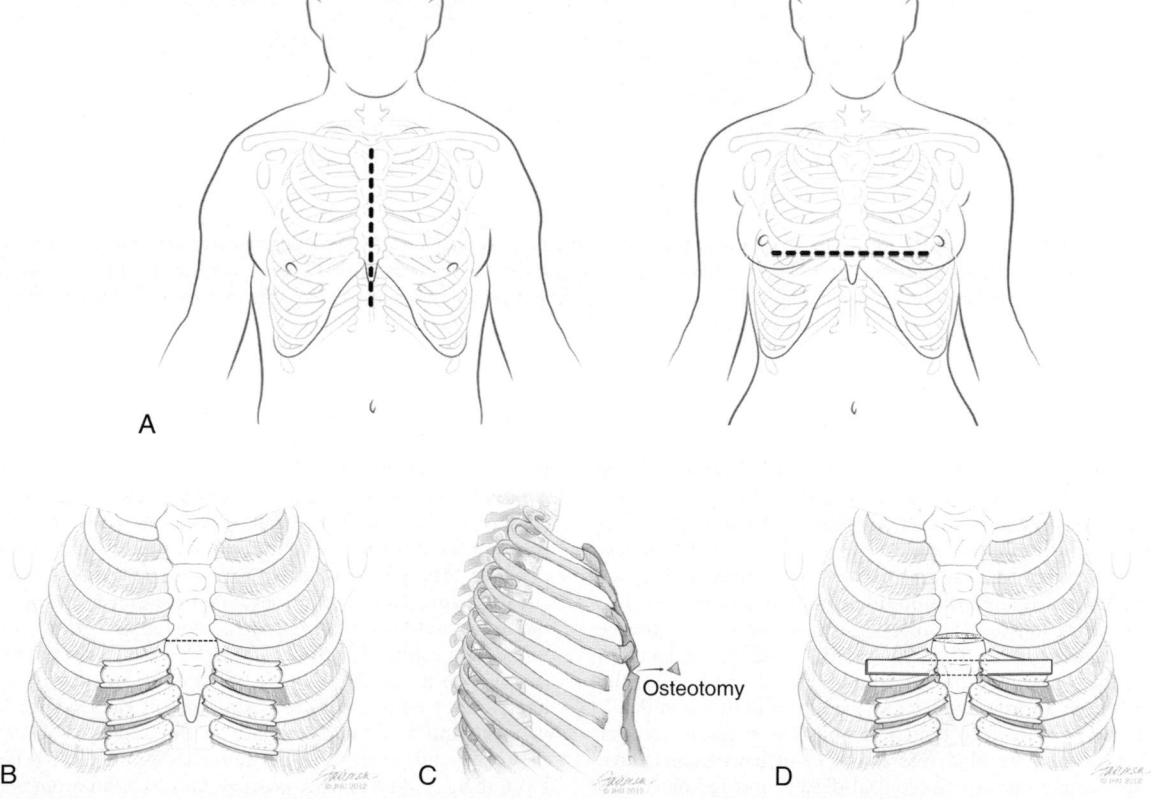

FIGURE 1 Open repair of pectus excavatum. **A,** *Left,* Standard midline sternal incision. *Right,* Alternative inframammary incision for improved cosmetic appearance in females. **B,** Abnormal cartilage is elevated from the perichondrium and divided at the sternocostal junction in the subperichondrial plane. **C,** Anterior sternal osteostomy allows elevation of the sternum to a normal position. **D,** Retrosternal strut position. *(Courtesy Jennifer E. Fairman, CMI, FAMI, Johns Hopkins University Illustrations.)*

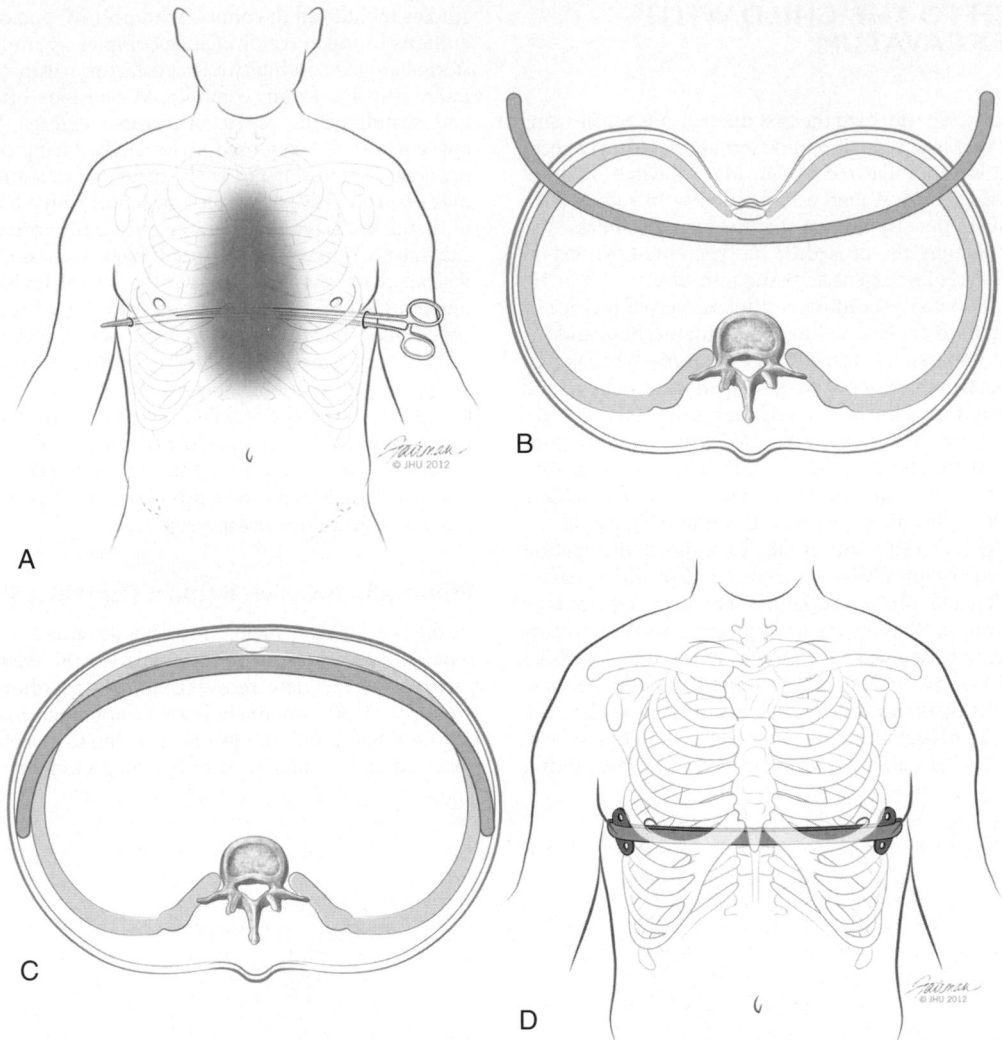

FIGURE 2 Minimally invasive approach for pectus excavatum repair. **A,** Schematic of curved introducer passing retrosternally through bilateral intercostal incisions. **B,** Initial position of the pectus bar traversing the mediastinum with convexity facing posteriorly. **C,** Position of the pectus bar after rotation. **D,** Final position of the pectus bar with stabilizers in place. The pectus bar initially is passed through the mediastinum with the convexity facing posteriorly.
(*Courtesy Jennifer E. Fairman, CMI, FAMI, Johns Hopkins University Illustrations.*)

was later modified to two small lateral incisions for improved cosmetic result.

The details of the Nuss repair, as described in 1997, are as follows: The patient is placed supine with arms abducted for optimal chest wall exposure. The intercostal level at which the bar is passed is selected based on the level of maximal severity of the defect, as determined by physical examination and preoperative imaging. The bar must lie 2 to 3 cm above the xyphoid in order to minimize the likelihood of slippage or rotation. A malleable sizer is used to measure the anticipated size and curvature of the bar that will be necessary to correct the defect. Typically the bar should extend just beyond the edge of the rib cage, approximately 2.5 cm shorter than the midaxillary diameter, and conform to the chest wall. The surgical steel bar of appropriate length is molded accordingly using bar benders. Each bar is bent to compensate for individual defects and to correct for depth and symmetry of the deformity. It is adjusted as necessary until it is well conformed to the lateral chest wall with appropriate convexity of the central portion to correct the defect. Occasionally an additional bar may be necessary to correct diffuse defects.

Two transverse inframammary incisions are made at the level of the midclavicular line and extended for 3 to 4 cm laterally. A skin

tunnel is raised medially, and a curved introducer is used to enter the previously selected intercostal space lateral to the sternum, traverse the anterior mediastinum immediately beneath the sternum, and exit the corresponding intercostal space on the other side (Figure 2, *A*). The introducer is used to pass an umbilical tape through the retrosternal tunnel, which then is used to pass the prebent bar through the mediastinum with the convexity facing posteriorly (Figure 2, *B*). Bar turners then are placed on each end of the bar and simultaneously rotated 180 degrees in order to bring the bar into final position (Figure 2, *C*). Bar benders then are used for final contouring to ensure that the bar is conformed snugly against the lateral chest wall. A stabilizer is placed on each side to lock the bar in place and is secured in place to the adjacent rib or connective tissue, depending on surgeon preference (Figure 2, *D*). The muscular layer then is closed, with positive end-expiratory pressure applied before securing the final suture in order to prevent air trapping. A rib block frequently is performed at this time, before closure of the skin. The remainder of the incision is approximated in layers and standard subcuticular closure.

Although the principles of the minimally invasive technique are largely standardized, the placement of incisions, bar passage technique, stabilizer placement, and means of securing the bar vary according to surgeon preference. One of the more widely used modifications involves the use of thoracoscopic guidance to pass the introducer through the mediastinum, with a recent National Surgical Quality Improvement Program (NSQIP) cross-sectional study indicating use of thoracoscopy in more than 80% of cases. Proponents suggest that direct visualization reduces the risk of cardiac injury, although direct cardiac injury has been noted both with and without thoracoscopic guidance. In addition, thoracoscopic guidance may allow somewhat more lateral incisions to be made safely because of direct visualization. Opponents argue that a more medial intercostal entry with direct visualization of the mediastinum and use of the sternum to pass the bar provide the same safety without the additional risks and operative times associated with thoracoscopy. Multiple studies have demonstrated no significant difference in complications with or without thoracoscopy, possibly related to the low incidence of such complications with both techniques.

Timing of Repair of Pectus Excavatum

Historically, the Ravitch procedure often was performed in children as young as 4 or 5 years. However, papers by Pena and Haller in the early 1990s drew attention to a small subset of patients who underwent such early repair and developed acquired Jeune's syndrome (i.e., constrictive dystrophy of the chest wall). They hypothesized that this complication occurred because of damage to sternal growth centers. This realization led to a shift in the age of repair to puberty. In more recent years, studies have suggested that recurrence rates are higher when performed in early adolescence, prompting a shift toward later adolescence and young adulthood. We prefer to perform minimally invasive repair after 15 years of age, when the cartilage is more flexible than in adulthood but after the majority of pubertal growth, in order to decrease the likelihood of recurrence. Open repair also typically is performed in later adolescence now because of higher rates of failure and recurrence when performed before completion of pubertal growth. Open repair also may be used in adulthood with similar success rates as in adolescents, but minimally invasive repair may be more difficult because of decreased cartilage flexibility.

Postoperative Course After Repair of Pectus Excavatum

Days 1 and 2

Most patients do extremely well after the Nuss repair or the open repair. In the acute postoperative period the most common complications are pain, pneumothorax, and urinary retention (typically resulting from pain or overly aggressive fluid administration). To avoid this last complication, the Foley catheter is left in place until postoperative day 2, at which point the majority of patients can void spontaneously. Hemothorax and ongoing postoperative bleeding are less common but significant complications.

Often the most significant challenge in the immediate and later postoperative period is pain control. Postoperative pain can be persistent and difficult to manage, and preoperative counseling is essential to prepare patients and parents for what to expect and to discuss management options. Preoperative epidural placement is used routinely in many centers now and has been reported to improve subjective pain scores in the immediate postoperative period. When epidural catheter placement is compared with patient-controlled analgesia (PCA) alone, there is no difference in hospital length of stay, time to regular diet, or transition to oral pain medications. Epidural failure rate and associated complications must be weighed against potential benefits. Intraoperative rib block also has been shown to reduce postoperative narcotic use and can be performed easily at the end of the procedure with minimal risk of complications. Ketorolac has demonstrated efficacy in postoperative pain management, with improved subjective pain scores and reduced use of narcotics. PCA is essential in all cases without contraindication, and the

addition of ketamine may augment analgesic effects. We utilize rib block, routine ketorolac, and PCA with a low basal rate of ketamine for 24 hours, followed by continued PCA until the patient is tolerating a diet, and have found that most patients can achieve adequate pain control with oral medication 2 to 3 days postoperatively.

In centers where routine chest x-ray is performed postoperatively, the rate of pneumothorax has been reported to be between 20% and 65%. However, multiple large series have demonstrated the rate of clinically significant pneumothorax and hemothorax to be less than 4%, and more recent series suggest a rate of intervention for pneumothorax to be less than 1%. Although the rate of pneumothorax is low, in rare cases intervention is required for ongoing bleeding or significant pneumothorax. Patients must be monitored in the postanesthesia care unit for any evidence of respiratory distress or blood loss. Although routine postoperative chest x-ray is not mandatory, it is preferred by us to rule out pneumothorax and document appropriate placement of the bar.

Days 3 to 5

In the subacute postoperative period, potential complications of both open and closed repair of pectus excavatum include pain, missed persistent pneumothorax or hemothorax, pericarditis, seroma, surgical site infection, and bar infection.

By day 3 the vast majority of patients have achieved successful pain control with a combination of oral nonsteroidal anti-inflammatory drugs (NSAIDs) and narcotics. However, patients and families should be counseled that pain can be prolonged, and most patients require oral narcotics for several weeks postoperatively, slowly weaning with the use of NSAIDs. Up to 5% of patients may require ongoing narcotic use 2 months after surgery. Given the prolonged use of narcotics, risk for constipation is high but can be avoided easily with routine use of bowel regimens.

Seroma is one of the more common complications with both minimally invasive and open repair, with a reported incidence ranging from 3% to 5% in most series. Most resolve spontaneously and do not require drainage.

Clinically significant pneumothorax or hemothorax typically is seen in the acute postoperative period but also may be seen in subacute fashion. Difficulty weaning from oxygen or failure of blood counts to stabilize must prompt radiologic evaluation. The majority of patients with subacute presentation resolve spontaneously, and less than 1% require intervention.

Pericarditis is a rare but feared complication in the subacute postoperative period. Although rates with minimally invasive repair initially were reported to be higher, current series suggest an incidence of approximately 0.5%, similar to open repair. The majority of cases respond to treatment with NSAIDs and steroids, though drainage may be required on a case-dependent basis. Some correlation between pericarditis and nickel allergy has been noted, which further reinforces the importance of preoperative screening before placement of a bar or strut.

Published rates of superficial site infections and bar infections range from 1% to 6.8% and 0.5% to 4.2%, respectively. The rate of surgical site infection is similar with open and minimally invasive repair. Although there are no official guidelines for perioperative antibiotic use in noncardiac thoracic surgery, preoperative chlorhexidine scrub followed by chlorhexidine preparation of the site and a single preoperative dose of a first-generation cephalosporin are used by us. Surgical site infections may be treated with antibiotics for superficial infections or with surgical drainage where indicated for more extensive infections. Deeper surgical site infections may be associated with bar or retrosternal strut infection, with approximately 0.3% of infected bars requiring removal.

Days 5 to 10

Prolonged chest pain is a common complaint, with 5% of patients requiring ongoing narcotic management at 2 months postoperatively. Ongoing evaluation must continue to optimize pain management regimens and allow weaning from narcotics as soon as pain may be controlled by other means.

Bar displacement was a frequently reported complication of the Nuss procedure in early series, with a reported rate up to 10% to 15%. After the introduction of stabilizers, more recent studies suggest a rate closer to 2%, with a reoperative rate of only 0.5% to 1%.

Rates of recurrence and failure are exceptionally low with both minimally invasive and open repair. Historically, risk of recurrence has been associated most closely with early age of repair. Costochondral resection or Nuss repair with bar removal before or during pubertal growth was associated with failure rates of up to 15%, likely because of ongoing remodeling and growth in adolescence. Recent studies of repairs performed later in adolescence, near the end of pubertal growth, suggest much lower recurrence rates. Mild recurrent depression is reported in approximately 5% of cases in both open and minimally invasive repair, with severe or full recurrence requiring operative intervention in less than 1% of patients. Rates of early failure in minimally invasive repair typically were associated with the high rate of bar displacement and have decreased dramatically as the incidence of bar displacement declined with use of lateral stabilizers. The currently reported rate of early failure is around 0.5%.

■ BAR REMOVAL AFTER REPAIR OF PECTUS EXCAVATUM

After Nuss repair, the bar is left in place for a minimum of 2 years in order to allow remodeling of cartilage. Additional recommendations are to remove the bar once pubertal growth has been completed and near maximal height has been achieved.

Bar removal is performed as an outpatient procedure, 2 to 4 years after placement, according to surgeon preference. The patient is placed supine with arms abducted, prepared, and draped. The previous incision sites are reopened in order to expose the stabilizer and wires. Frequently scar tissue encases the entirety of the stabilizer, and the stabilizer must be dissected circumferentially in order to free it. Wire cutters are used to cut the wire and free the stabilizer, and both are removed. Bar benders are used to straighten the curve of the bar bilaterally, and a clamp can be used to remove the bar through one of the chest entry sites. The wound is closed in layers, and as described for the initial procedure, Valsalva's maneuver is performed on final closure of the muscular layer in order to evacuate any air. The scar may be revised as necessary for improved cosmesis and then is closed with a standard subcuticular closure. A postoperative chest x-ray may be performed if clinical suspicion is high but is not mandatory. The patient should be monitored carefully for a suitable period in the postanesthesia care unit for any signs of respiratory distress and can be discharged home once the patient is ambulatory on room air and pain is controlled with oral medications.

Strut removal after open repair is also an outpatient procedure performed between 6 months and 2 years after repair. The patient is positioned, prepared, and draped in similar fashion as for Nuss bar removal. Fluoroscopy or preoperative chest x-ray is used to located the tip of the strut for guidance of incision placement. A small 2-cm midline incision within the previous incision is made for removal of the wire securing the strut to the sternum. A small 2-cm lateral incision is used to remove the strut. Location of the incisions may vary dependent on the surgical technique used when placing and securing the bar. The patient should be monitored postoperatively in the postanesthesia care unit for any signs of complications and can be discharged home once ambulation and an oral pain management regimen have been achieved.

■ LONG-TERM OUTCOMES AFTER REPAIR OF PECTUS EXCAVATUM

Rates of failure and recurrence after repair of pectus excavatum are extremely low, with rates of reoperation less than 1%. Outcomes more frequently are measured by patient satisfaction with improvement of symptoms and physical appearance. The most common indications prompting patients to seek surgical intervention for pectus excavatum are subjective exercise intolerance compared with peers and psychological distress. Additional physiologic parameters suggesting need for repair because of impaired cardiopulmonary function also play a role. Successful outcomes generally are measured by improvement in each of the following factors.

Cosmetic Outcomes

More than 97% of patients report that they are happy with their appearance postoperatively, rating their repair as "good or excellent." Surgeon satisfaction with repair is also extremely high, with 95% to 97% of repairs rated "good or excellent" by their surgeon, although the rate of "good" versus "excellent" is higher among surgeons than patients. The most common causes for decreased satisfaction with appearance are related to undercorrection, overcorrection, and scars. The rate of undercorrection is highly variable, dependent largely on the extent of the defect and sternal rotation as well as the type of surgical repair. In some patients it may not be possible to achieve the ideal degree of uniform sternal elevation. However, the majority of patients in whom the cosmetic reversal of the defect is incomplete still report improvement in symptoms and satisfaction with their appearance compared with preoperative appearance. Overcorrection is a potential complication of minimally invasive repair that is not seen after open repairs. It is reported by surgeons in 3% to 5% of cases, with an increased incidence in cases of highly asymmetric pectus excavatum. Although overcorrection does not affect physiologic outcome, poor cosmetic outcome may result in decreased patient satisfaction postoperatively. Overcorrection is particularly bothersome in females, as bowing of the sternum may cause breast asymmetry or eversion, leading to dissatisfaction with appearance. Surgeon-reported rates of overcorrection are higher than patient-reported rates, and the majority of patients report satisfaction with their postoperative appearance. Overcorrection and undercorrection are best avoided by careful preoperative physical examination and review of imaging and precise manipulation of the bar for repair of the individual defect. One final consideration in cosmetic outcome is the incisional scar. In the open technique, the scar is placed in the inframammary fold in females in order to minimize scar appearance. Some surgeons also prefer this incision in males. With more minimal cartilage resection, incision size has decreased in recent years. In minimally invasive repair, the incisions are shorter and more lateral. With thoracoscopic guidance, incisions may be placed further laterally and aligned with rib curvature to minimize their appearance. Without thoracoscopic guidance, incisions typically are placed more medially and often are hidden in the inframammary fold when possible. Overall, patients who have undergone minimally invasive repair report higher rates of satisfaction with their cosmetic appearance than those who have undergone an open repair, but cosmetic benefit must be weighed on an individual basis when considering the optimal approach for repair.

Cardiopulmonary Function

The effect of repair on cardiovascular and pulmonary performance remains difficult to quantify by objective measurement because of the heterogeneity of study populations and variation in methods of indirect cardiopulmonary evaluation. However, there does appear to be an early improvement in cardiac function after both open and minimally invasive repair, as evidenced by improvement in one or more of the following: stroke volume, cardiac index, and maximal aerobic capacity (VO_2 max). In the acute period and up to 1 year after repair, multiple pulmonary parameters, including total lung capacity (TLC), FVC, and FEV1, decline, which is noted in both open and minimally invasive repair and likely because of decreased compliance. Longer-term follow-up shows variable but mild improvement in TLC, FVC, and FEV1, which is comparable between open repair and minimally invasive repair while the bar remains in place. However, after bar removal, long-term series have shown statistically significant improvement in FVC, TLC, and FEV1 as compared with open repair cohorts, likely because of further improvement in pulmonary compliance after removal of the inflexible bar.

Perhaps the most important indicator of successful treatment of cardiopulmonary limitations is subjective improvement in symptoms as reported by the patient. The vast majority of patients report an immediate improvement in exercise tolerance and endurance, with more than 95% of patients reporting improvement in symptoms in the first 6 months after surgery. Early symptom relief is noted after both open and minimally invasive repair, although after the Nuss procedure patients often report an earlier, more dramatic improvement because of the immediate nature of correction of the defect with no requirement for sternocostal healing. This improvement continues throughout the first year in both cohorts and is comparable at 1 year. However, after removal of the bar placed during minimally invasive repairs, Nuss patients report even further improvement beyond that reported after open repair, likely corresponding to the improvement in lung function that is observed after bar removal. In addition, Nuss patients report higher average ratings of subjective improvement in overall health as compared with patients who received open repair.

Quality of Life

Improvement in quality of life as reported by patients and parents is correlated directly with satisfaction with cosmetic result and symptomatic improvement. Preoperative counseling is imperative to prepare patients for what to expect postoperatively, including pain management, incisional scar, duration of treatment, and timeline of expected improvements. Patients who are undergoing open repair must be prepared that cartilage remodeling and ultimate cosmetic appearance may take more than a year for full effects to be achieved. Patients who are undergoing minimally invasive repair should be counseled that improvement in symptoms may continue over the course of years and even after bar removal. Although few studies have compared quality of life improvement in minimally invasive and open repair, some series suggest that adolescent quality of life scores improve more after minimally invasive repair than after open repair.

Open Versus Minimally Invasive Approach

After the introduction of the Nuss procedure there was significant debate about whether an open or minimally invasive repair provides the best outcomes. Today, most pediatric surgeons offer the Nuss procedure as the first line of treatment if surgery is indicated. However, it should be noted that although improvement in cardiopulmonary performance and satisfaction with appearance appear to be higher on average after minimally invasive repair, both surgical approaches are associated with greater than 95% success rates with regard to correction of physical appearance and subjective cardiopulmonary limitations. In addition, studies comparing outcomes are clouded by differences in preoperative and postoperative evaluation, surgical technique, and variability in severity of defect.

Early reports of minimally invasive series describe relatively high rates of complications requiring surgical intervention, including a high rate of bar displacement ranging from 10% to 15%. Upon introduction of stabilizers, the rate of bar displacement dropped drastically, and general complications also dropped dramatically as the procedure became more widely used. It is therefore likely that the high complication rate early in the use of minimally invasive surgery was associated with a learning curve. This complicates the use of meta-analyses as a reference for general outcomes and incidence of complications. Recent meta-analysis suggested a displacement rate of 6.3%, which includes the earliest reported cases. However, the rate of bar displacement in recent years is closer to 1% to 2%, and a recent cross-sectional analysis of the NSQIP database reports a rate

of only 1.1% in 2012. The rates of complications, including prolonged pain, superficial and deep infection, need for bar or strut removal, incomplete or poor cosmetic results, and recurrence, are low and comparable with open and minimally invasive repair. Ultimately the approach for repair requires consideration of the individual patient with regard to severity and morphology of defect, type and severity of symptoms, patient age, physiologic evaluation, and comorbidities, as well as an open dialogue with patient and family members about their goals and expectations.

■ CONCLUSIONS

The patient who has a chest wall deformity requires a careful and thorough evaluation and a full and frank discussion of the necessity of treatment and the timing of surgery should operative repair be indicated. Although the vast majority of patients have a superb outcome, the fact that severe and potentially life-threatening complications may occur requires that an extremely thoughtful approach be undertaken before surgery is offered. To manage postoperative pain and impaired mobility, the surgical team should carefully manage expectations preoperatively and make clear that there is significant discomfort in the short term associated with surgical correction of chest wall deformities. However, patients ultimately should be reassured by the overall safety of the operative approach and the tremendous satisfaction that most patients report with the operative result.

SUGGESTED READINGS

Chen Z, Amos AB, Luo H, et al. Comparative pulmonary functional recovery after Nuss and Ravitch procedures for pectus excavatum repair: a meta-analysis. *J Cardiothorac Surg.* 2012;7:1-9.

Croitoru DP, Kelly RE, Goretsky MJ, et al. The minimally invasive Nuss technique for recurrent or failed pectus excavatum repair in 50 patients. *J Pediatr Surg.* 2005;40:181-187.

Fokin AA. Thoracic defects: cleft sternum and Poland syndrome. *Thorac Surg Clin.* 2010;20:575-582.

Fokin AA, Steuerwald NM, Ahrens WA, Allen KE. Anatomical, histologic, and genetic characteristics of congenital chest wall deformities. *Semin Thorac Cardiovasc Surg.* 2009;21:44-57.

Fonkalsrud EW. 912 open pectus excavatum repairs: changing trends, lessons learned: one surgeon's experience. *World J Surg.* 2009;33:180-190.

Haller JK, Colombani PM, Humphries CT, et al. Chest wall constriction after too extensive and too early operations for pectus excavatum. *Ann Thorac Surg.* 1996;61:1618-1625.

Johnson JN, Hartman TK, Pianosi PT, Driscoll DJ. Cardiorespiratory function after operation for pectus excavatum. *J Pediatr.* 2008;153:359-364.

Kelly RE, Goretsky MJ, Obermeyer R, et al. Twenty-one years of experience with minimally invasive repair of pectus excavatum by the Nuss procedure in 1215 patients. *Ann Surg.* 2010;252:1072-1081.

Koizumi T, Mitsukawa N, Saiga A, Satoh K. Clinical application of Nuss procedure for chest wall deformity in Poland syndrome. *Kardiochir Torakochirurgia Pol.* 2014;11:421-423.

Kotzot D, Schwabegger A. Etiology of chest wall deformities: a genetic review for the treating physician. *J Pediatr Surg.* 2009;44:2004-2011.

Koumbourlis AC. Pectus deformities and their impact on pulmonary physiology. *Paediatr Respir Rev.* 2015;16:18-24.

Lam MW, Klassen AF, Montgomery CJ, et al. Quality-of-life outcomes after surgical correction of pectus excavatum: a comparison of the Ravitch and Nuss procedures. *J Pediatr Surg.* 2008;43:819-825.

Lawson ML, Mellins RB, Paulson JF, et al. Increasing severity of pectus excavaum is associated with reduced pulmonary function. *J Pediatr.* 2011;159:256-261.

Lesbo M, Tang M, Nielsen H, et al. Compromised cardiac function in exercising teenagers with pectus excavatum. *Interact Cardiovasc Thorac Surg.* 2011;13:377-380.

Lukosiene L, Rugyte D, Macas A, et al. Postoperative pain management in pediatric patients undergoing minimally invasive repair of pectus excavatum: the role of intercostal block. *J Pediatr Surg.* 2013;48:2425-2430.

Majdak-Paredes EJ, Shfighi M, Fatah F. Integrated algorithm for reconstruction of complex forms of Poland syndrome: 20-year outcomes. *J Plast Reconstr Aesthet Surg.* 2015;68:1-9.

Miyajima D, Hayata T, Suzuki T, et al. Profilin 1 regulates sternum development and endochondral bone formation. *J Biol Chem*. 2012;287: 33545-33553.

O'Keefe J, Byrne R, Montgomery M, et al. Longer term effects of closed repair of pectus excavatum on cardiopulmonary status. *J Pediatr Surg*. 2013;48: 1049-1054.

Papandria D, Arlikar J, Sacco-Casamassima MG, et al. Increasing age at time of pectus excavatum repair in children: emerging consensus? *J Pediatr Surg*. 2013;48:191-196.

Poston PM, McHugh MA, Rossi NO, et al. The case for using the correction index obtained from chest radiography for evaluation of pectus excavatum. *J Pediatr Surg*. 2015;50:1940-1944.

Rousse N, Hysi I, Juthier F, et al. Combined repair of pectus excavatum and cardiopulmonary bypass surgery: what is the best strategy? *Ann Thorac Surg*. 2013;96:1525-1527.

Sacco-Casamassima MG, Goldstein SD, Gause CD, Karim O, et al. Minimally invasive repair of pectus excavatum: analyzing contemporary practice in 50 ACS NSQIP-pediatric institutions. *Pediatr Surg Int*. 2015;31:493-499.

Sacco-Casamassima MG, Goldstein SD, Salazar JH, et al. Perioperative strategies and technical modifications to the Nuss repair for pectus excavatum in pediatric patients: a large volume, single institution experience. *J Pediatr Surg*. 2013;49:575-582.

Sacco-Casamassima MG, Papandria D, Goldstein SD, et al. Contemporary management of recurrent pectus excavatum. *J Pediatr Surg*. 2015;50: 1726-1733.

Sacco-Casamassima MG, Wong LL, Papandria D, et al. Modified Nuss procedure in concurrent repair of pectus excavatum and open heart surgery. *Ann Thorac Surg*. 2013;95:1043-1049.

Schmidt J, Redwan B, Koesek V, et al. Pectus excavatum and cardiac surgery: simultaneous correction advocated. *Thorac Cardiovasc Surg*. 2014;62: 238-244.

Sigalet DL, Montgomery M, Harder J, et al. Long term cardiopulmonary effects of closed repair of pectus excavatum. *Pediatr Surg Int*. 2007;23: 493-497.

Tocchioni F, Ghionzoli M, Messineo A, et al. Pectus excavatum and heritable disorders of the connective tissue. *Pediatr Rep*. 2013;5:58-63.

Wu A, Sun X, Zhu W, et al. Evidence for GAL3ST4 mutation as the potential cause of pectus excavatum. *Cell Res*. 2012;22:1712-1715.

Wurtz A, Rousse N, Benhamed L, Conti M, et al. Simplified open repair for anterior chest wall deformities: analysis of results in 205 patients. *Orthop Traumatol Surg Res*. 2012;98:319-326.

OPEN REPAIR OF ABDOMINAL AORTIC ANEURYSMS

R. Todd Lancaster, MD, MPH, and Richard P. Cambria, MD

Aneurysmal dilation of the abdominal aorta is defined as a 1.5-fold increase in the normal aortic diameter or an aortic diameter greater than 3 cm. In most cases (>80%), such aneurysmal degeneration is isolated to the infrarenal aorta. An increase in the incidence and prevalence of abdominal aortic aneurysms (AAAs) has been noted in recent years, with rates as high as 10% to 15% in high-risk populations. Individuals at highest risk include older patients, white patients, males, those with a family history of aneurysms, and those with cardiovascular risk factors and concomitant cardiovascular and peripheral vascular disease. The natural history of aneurysmal disease is that of progressive enlargement leading to increased risk of rupture, with approximately 15,000 deaths occurring annually resulting from rupture of AAAs. The risk of rupture is increased in patients with chronic obstructive pulmonary disease (COPD), hypertension, family history of AAA, and rapid AAA expansion and most notably with aneurysm size. As such, the effective management of AAAs relies on early diagnosis, serial observation, and treatment with open surgical reconstruction or endovascular aneurysm repair (EVAR).

The open repair of AAA entered the modern era in 1951 with the first successful repair by Dubost using an aortic homograft. Subsequently, Juan Parodi's initial report of endovascular therapy again dramatically altered the management of AAAs. The less invasive nature, improvement in perioperative morbidity and mortality, rapid recovery to normal function, and beneficial intermediate and long-term outcomes of EVAR have resulted in stent graft repair increasingly being used for repair of infrarenal AAAs. This is reflected in our own practice, wherein up to two thirds of infrarenal AAAs are repaired with stent grafts. Open surgical repair is used for repair of aneurysms in patients with anatomy unfavorable for stent graft repair, in emergency situations wherein stent grafts or endovascular capabilities may not be readily available, in young patients for whom EVAR durability is in question, and in patients with complex aortic neck anatomy such as pararenal and suprarenal aneurysms. Pararenal AAAs are defined by an infrarenal aneurysm neck of up to 1 cm and the term *pararenal* is often used interchangeably with *juxtarenal*. Suprarenal aneurysm occurs when one or both main renal arteries arise from the aneurysm itself, implying that separate renal artery reconstruction will be required. In instances of complex proximal anatomy, the cross-clamp will need to be applied in a suprarenal or supraceliac position to permit the proximal aortic reconstruction (Figure 1). This chapter therefore emphasizes the cognitive and technical repair of infrarenal, pararenal, and suprarenal aortic aneurysms.

■ INDICATIONS FOR REPAIR

Symptomatic Aneurysms

The majority of AAAs are asymptomatic, but some may be seen with signs and symptoms of thrombosis, embolization of mural debris, compression of adjacent organs, aortic dissection, rapid expansion or impending rupture, and frank rupture. The presence of associated symptoms necessitates early repair independent of aneurysm size. Mural debris, which accumulates along the aneurysmal aortic wall, may contribute to progressive aortic thrombosis, resulting in symptoms of lower extremity ischemia. This ischemia will manifest as claudication, rest pain, or gangrene, depending on the time course of development and on the presence of collateral circulation. Alternatively, distal embolization may be seen with digital ischemia or gangrene, often referred to as "trash foot" or "blue toe syndrome." Compression of the duodenum and stomach, albeit rare, results in gastric outlet obstruction and occurs along a spectrum from early satiety and fullness to nausea and vomiting with dehydration and malnutrition. Compression of other surrounding structures may be seen with symptoms referable to the structure involved (e.g., hydronephrosis with ureteral compression). Dissection within aneurysmal aorta is seen with acute onset severe abdominal or back pain, often described as tearing in nature, and is associated with a significant increase in rupture risk. Acute dissection within AAA therefore should be repaired promptly. Up to a quarter of abdominal aneurysms are seen with symptoms of rapid expansion or impending rupture, including mild to severe abdominal, back, or flank pain; in cases of frank rupture, abdominal aneurysms are seen with hemodynamic instability. On spiral computed tomographic angiography (CTA), heterogeneous mural thrombus with intraplaque hemorrhage, loss of fat planes around the aorta, periaortic inflammation, and retroperitoneal hematoma are suggestive findings, and urgent AAA repair should be undertaken. Hemodynamic instability suggestive of rupture in patients with known AAA should prompt emergent exploration and repair; however, in our practice, wherein a variety of complex aortic pathologies are routinely treated, patients undergo rapid resuscitation with permissive hypotension and rapid CTA if no recent imaging is available to facilitate operative planning and patient positioning (if, for example, a flank approach is used).

Asymptomatic Aneurysms

Natural history data aid in balancing risk of aneurysm rupture with that of surgical morbidity and mortality. Rupture risk correlates directly with aneurysm size and is very low for aneurysms smaller than 5 cm in diameter. On the basis of such data, an aneurysm diameter of 5.5 cm typically is used as a threshold for open repair, at least in male patients. Other predictors of rupture include female gender, family history of AAA, smoking status, hypertension, and COPD. Two randomized controlled trials have been performed to evaluate the role of early repair of small aneurysms.

The UK Small Aneurysm Trial randomized 1090 patients to early elective AAA repair or surveillance. All patients were 60 to 76 years

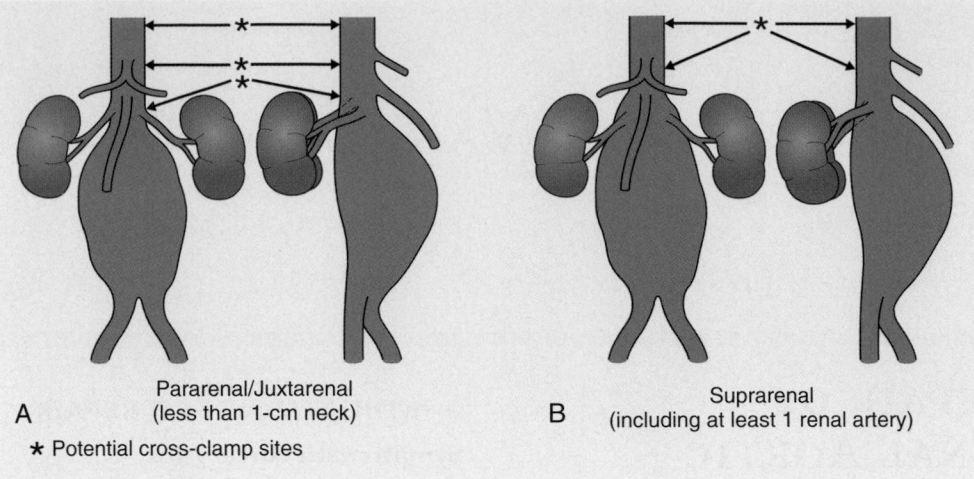

FIGURE 1 Classification of complex abdominal aortic aneurysms. **A,** Pararenal aneurysms with an infrarenal neck of less than 1 cm. **B,** Suprarenal aneurysm with at least one renal artery involved in the aneurysm.

old and were found to have an aneurysm between 4.0 and 5.4 cm in diameter. The early elective surgery group included 563 patients, of which 520 (92%) underwent AAA repair by the end of the study, with an operative mortality of 5.8%. The annual rupture rates in the surveillance group were 1% overall, 0.3% for AAAs smaller than 4 cm, 1.5% for AAAs between 4.0 and 4.9 cm, and 6.5% for AAAs between 5.0 and 5.4 cm. The surveillance group included 527 patients, of which 389 (73%) underwent AAA repair by the end of the study. The results of the study showed no significant improvement in survival for patients who underwent elective repair of a small AAA. The study authors concluded that patients should undergo surveillance of AAA until the diameter exceeds 5.5 cm. Women were more likely to die as a result of AAA rupture; hence the aneurysm repair threshold of 5.5 cm should be lowered in women.

The Aneurysm Detection and Management (ADAM) trial was performed within the Veterans Affairs (VA) medical system and presented similar results. A total of 1136 patients ages 50 to 79 years with aneurysms 4.0 to 5.4 cm in diameter were randomized to undergo immediate open surgical repair or routine surveillance. Surveillance was performed with ultrasound or computed tomography every 3 to 6 months, and aneurysm repair was performed for AAA size of 5.5 cm or larger, symptoms attributed to the AAA, or annual increase in size greater than 1 cm. The immediate repair group consisted of 569 patients, of whom 93% underwent aneurysm repair, with a 30-day mortality rate of 2.7%. The annual aneurysm rupture rate in the surveillance group was 0.6% and was not stratified on the basis of aneurysm size. A total of 350 patients (61.6%) in the surveillance group underwent aneurysm repair during a mean follow-up of 4.8 years. Aneurysm repair rates increased as aneurysm diameter at enrollment increased, with 27% of AAAs between 4.0 and 4.4 cm requiring repair compared with 81% of AAAs between 5.0 and 5.4 cm requiring repair. Long-term survival was similar in both groups, and the study authors concluded that elective AAA repair should be reserved for aneurysms that are at least 5.5 cm in diameter.

The decision to proceed with AAA repair is complex and involves assessment of the patient's health status and personal preferences. Aneurysm repair is most effective if the risk of rupture and aneurysm-related death outweighs the operative risk to the patient, with consideration given to the patient's life expectancy. Current clinical data support open aneurysm repair at a threshold size of 5.5 cm in male patients and 5.0 cm in female patients. The natural history of patients under surveillance is such that 70% to 80% of patients eventually undergo aneurysm repair; thus in many patients the issue is timing rather than ultimate necessity of intervention.

OPERATIVE PLANNING

Accurate and complete preoperative imaging is of utmost importance to assess the extent of proximal and distal aortic resection and the need for concomitant visceral and renal artery reconstruction. In contemporary practice, the detail available with contrast-enhanced fine-cut CTA provides the surgeon with an adequate preoperative map. As the proximal aortic anatomy becomes more complex or the need to investigate potential renovascular or aortoiliac occlusive disease arises, arteriography may be added, and the information from these two studies is complementary with respect to important operative decisions. With the use of three-dimensional reconstructions from fine-cut CT scans, the need for aortography is rare in our practice. We currently use such reconstructions for both EVAR planning and precise anatomic delineation before open repair. A thorough evaluation of preoperative imaging aids in the development of an operative plan, which must include (1) the extent of resection; (2) location of aortic cross-clamp application; (3) qualitative assessment of the aorta; (4) evaluation of visceral vessel topography and patency; (5) identification of aneurysmal or occlusive iliac disease; and (6) the need for concomitant renovisceral reconstructions. On the basis of careful examination of a contrast-enhanced CT, the extent of resection necessary and how best to achieve it should be formulated by the operating surgeon.

PREOPERATIVE PATIENT PREPARATION

Because of the high-risk nature of aortic surgery and the frequent existence of comorbid conditions in these patients, a thorough medical workup is necessary. Patients undergoing elective aneurysm repair should be appropriately risk stratified from a cardiovascular standpoint in accordance with published American College of Cardiology guidelines. If operative reconstruction is necessary without delay, patients with significant cardiovascular risk can safely undergo aortic reconstruction with optimal medical therapy as highlighted by the Coronary Artery Revascularization Prophylaxis (CARP) trial. The CARP trial showed no significant benefit of preoperative revascularization in patients with coronary disease, excluding patients with left main coronary artery, low ejection fraction (<20%), and valvular disease. CARP trial patients were noted to have similar rates of cardiovascular complications and cardiovascular mortality at 30 days and 2 years in both revascularized and nonrevascularized patients undergoing major elective vascular surgical procedures.

Patients who are seen acutely require rapid surgical intervention; for such patients, preoperative preparation is bypassed in favor of expeditious repair. In such cases, preparation entails ensuring adequate intravenous (IV) access (large bore antecubital IVs), availability of blood products for intraoperative and perioperative resuscitation, and preoperative resuscitation with permissive hypotension. Intraoperatively, prepping and draping of the patient should be performed before induction of general anesthesia in case a need for rapid proximal aortic control arises.

■ OPEN SURGICAL REPAIR

Surgical Approaches

Abdominal aortic surgery can be performed readily with a transperitoneal/transabdominal (TP) approach or a left flank approach, which is often referred to as the retroperitoneal (RP) approach (Figure 2). The merits of both approaches have been espoused by randomized and uncontrolled studies. The TP approach may be performed with a longitudinal midline (xiphoid to pubis) incision or alternatively with a generous transverse incision extending from flank to flank. The latter has the advantage of keeping the incision away from the epigastrium, possibly decreasing postoperative pain and respiratory compromise.

The RP approach is performed through the left flank and can vary from a total RP (eleventh interspace) to thoracoabdominal (ninth interspace) exposure. Depending on body habitus, aneurysm anatomy, a number of other anatomic factors, and surgeon's experience, either approach can be used for the majority of infrarenal and juxtarenal AAAs, whereas suprarenal aneurysms are best approached using one of the left flank approaches. Irrespective of the benefit or use of either approach, there are clearly certain anatomic and clinical circumstances that dictate preferential use of a particular approach in individual patients. These variables are considered in the individual description of surgical techniques.

Transperitoneal Approach

The TP, anterior midline approach performed through a vertical xiphoid to pubis incision is used commonly and remains favored by most surgeons because of familiarity and expediency. Exposure for the majority of infrarenal AAAs is satisfactory and allows the surgeon the ability to explore the remainder of the abdomen and provide superior exposure for dealing with the vagaries of iliac aneurysmal or occlusive disease. With the usual inframesocolic exposure, the root of the mesentery and small bowel is retracted to the right, and the transverse colon is retracted superiorly. After division of the ligament of Treitz and the RP tissues over the aneurysm itself, exposure and mobilization of the left renal vein is straightforward. Division of the inferior mesenteric vein generally allows for lateral retraction of the left mesocolon and superior retraction of the pancreas. The latter should be well padded to minimize the chance of perioperative pancreatitis.

Depending on the length of the aneurysm neck, wide mobilization of the left renal vein may be desirable by ligation of its adrenal, gonadal, and lumbar branches, thus allowing cephalad retraction of the left renal vein (Figure 3). Division of the left renal vein should be avoided, as it may increase the risk of postoperative renal failure and more importantly will contribute to local venous hypertension leading to increased local bleeding. Additional proximal exposure on the aneurysm neck or visceral aortic segment can be obtained by sharply dissecting off the dense neural/splanchnic tissue enveloping the aorta at the level of the origin of the superior mesenteric artery (SMA). This frequently will allow placement of a suprarenal clamp below the origin of the SMA without needing to resort to the supraceliac aorta.

In circumstances of prior aortic surgery, suprarenal aneurysms, and extensive juxtarenal aortic atherosclerotic disease, modifications of the transabdominal approach will be needed for more proximal aortic cross-clamp placement or partial exposure of the visceral aortic segment. Modifications of the anterior transabdominal approach are discussed later and include (1) transcrural supraceliac aortic control and clamping; (2) supplementation with a right-sided medial visceral rotation; and (3) supplementation with a left-sided medial visceral rotation.

Transperitoneal Approach With Supraceliac Clamping

TP supraceliac clamping is most useful in the setting of ruptured AAA, juxtarenal aortic aneurysm, or infected aortic graft or tissue or when the AAA neck is heavily involved with atheromatous debris

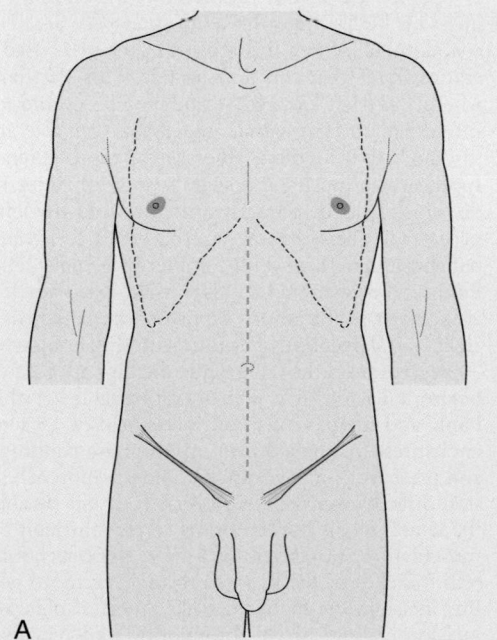
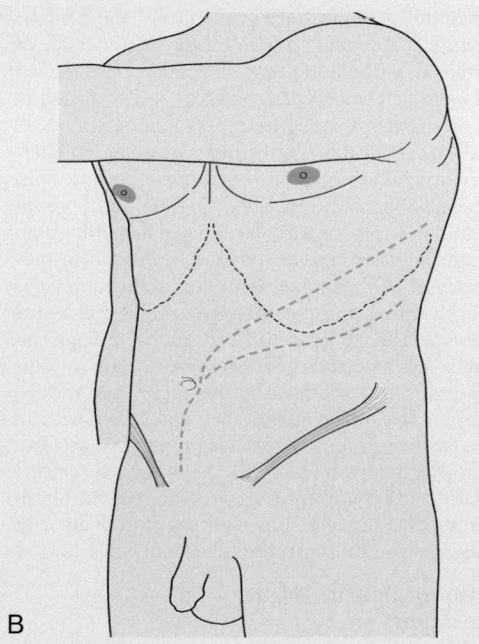

FIGURE 2 Surgical approaches for abdominal aortic aneurysm repair. **A,** The anterior transabdominal approach via a midline (xiphoid to pubis) incision (*dashed line*). **B,** The lateral approach with low thoracoabdominal (*upper dashed line*) or retroperitoneal (*lower dashed line*) incision.

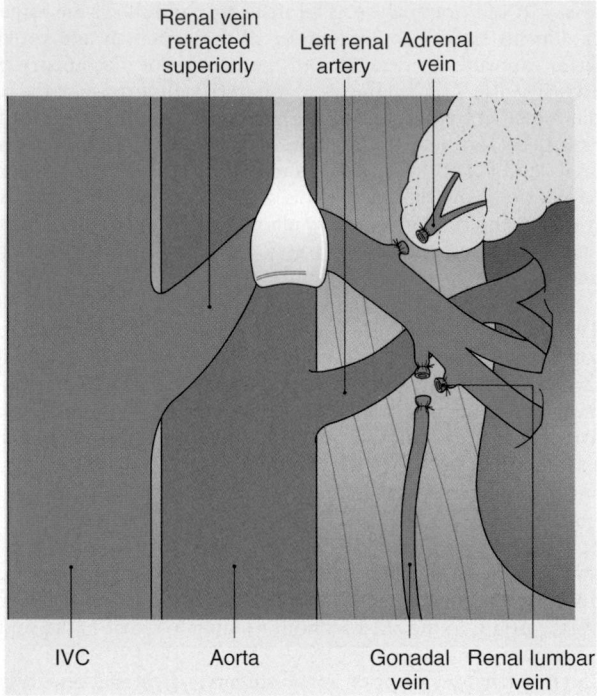

FIGURE 3 Left renal vein mobilization. Ligation of the left adrenal, gonadal, and renal-lumbar veins results in exposure of the left renal artery and suprarenal aorta. *IVC,* Inferior vena cava.

such that clamping in the infrarenal or suprarenal location poses a significant threat of atheroembolism. Unlike a RP approach, this maneuver does not permit continuous exposure of the visceral aortic segment for direct operation. A number of important technical steps are crucial to achieving control of the supraceliac aorta from the midline approach. The proximal extent of the abdominal incision must be carried well onto the xiphoid. Depending on the anatomy of the costal arch, it may be necessary to split the lower sternum in its cartilaginous portion. The triangular ligament of the left lobe of the liver must be taken down to facilitate retraction of the left lobe for the majority of patients. Adequate retraction of the underside of the diaphragm on either side of the midline is necessary, and the left hepatic lobe should be folded upon itself, padded, and retracted to the right of midline along with the diaphragm. A nasogastric (NG) tube should be placed, and its location confirmed within the stomach. With gentle traction on the stomach and gastroesophageal (GE) junction, the gastrohepatic ligament is divided. Evaluation of preoperative imaging for the existence of a replaced right hepatic artery (which travels beneath the gastrohepatic ligament) will aid in preventing injury to this vessel. With tactile orientation of the esophagus by palpating for the NG tube, the esophagus is mobilized to the patient's left at the level of the GE junction, and the right diaphragmatic crus is divided to facilitate access to the aorta (Figure 4). This is mandatory if the aorta is to be clamped in this region but may be unnecessary if temporary proximal control is being obtained with an aortic compressor. In elective circumstances, we prefer to dissect out the aorta in this region and surround it with a vessel tape for easy subsequent manipulation and clamping. One should avoid the temptation to incise the median arcuate ligament from the anterior approach, as this may result in injury to the celiac axis.

Transperitoneal Approach With Right Medial Visceral Rotation

This technique is one that is underused but can be very helpful for juxtarenal aneurysm repair or in circumstances in which right renal artery bypass or transaortic renal endarterectomy are necessary. The

usual midline incision in the RP tissues is extended over the right pelvic rim, and the entire right colon is mobilized in continuity with the duodenum. The small bowel, right colon, and transverse colon are eviscerated and placed superiorly on the patient's chest. The root of the mesentery and the origin of the SMA are thus exposed, and the orientation of the SMA is now straight up and down at 90 degrees to the aorta rather than the usual 45 degrees (Figure 5). The dense splanchnic autonomic nervous tissue that envelops the aorta at and onto the origin of the SMA is sharply dissected away. Posteriorly, it will be necessary to divide the insertions of the diaphragmatic crus to achieve exposure of the posterolateral aspects of the aorta. After all of these maneuvers have been performed, suprarenal clamping is easily achieved, or if the SMA and renal origins are close together, clamping above the SMA can be carried out.

Transperitoneal Approach With Left Medial Visceral Rotation

Left medial visceral rotation allows for continuous exposure of the entire abdominal aorta (Figure 6); however, when continuous exposure of visceral aortic segments is required, we opt for a lateral approach. The small bowel is wrapped in moist towels and reflected superiorly and to the patient's right. The left colon is mobilized by dividing the left peritoneal reflection (line of Toldt). This is continued on to divide the splenorenal and phrenocolic ligaments proximally and the RP attachments of the sigmoid colon distally. The sigmoid colon, descending colon, splenic flexure, distal transverse colon, stomach, spleen, and pancreas are then mobilized in continuity, and this mobilization can include the left kidney, which is facilitated by incision of Gerota's fascia. Mobilization of the kidney allows for unimpeded access to the visceral aorta. Alternatively, if extensive dissection and exposure of the superior mesenteric or right renal artery is necessary, the left kidney is left in situ. The decision as to whether the left kidney is reflected anteriorly also depends on the anatomic variants of the left renal vein. Splenic or pancreatic injury is a potential complication of this exposure.

Retroperitoneal and Thoracoabdominal (Lateral) Approaches

There are two ways to perform a lateral approach to the abdominal aorta (see Figure 2). The term *retroperitoneal approach* has been used to refer to incisions at the level of the eleventh rib or below, and incisions higher than the tenth interspace are referred to as thoracoabdominal. When this type of exposure is used, the main considerations are what the necessary level of the flank incision is and whether the left kidney is to be mobilized anteriorly or left in situ. Infrarenal and pararenal aneurysms can be approached readily through a RP incision, whereas for more extensive aneurysms or supraceliac exposure, an eighth or ninth interspace incision with division of the diaphragm and entry into the left thoracic cavity is necessary. These lateral approaches are advantageous in obese patients and in those with complex proximal aortic anatomy, but the limitation is restricted access to right-sided aortic branches.

For a truly RP aortic exposure, the patient is positioned in the right lateral decubitus position with the shoulders and torso at 60 to 70 degrees from the table while the hips are rotated back, as close to horizontal as possible. The operating table is jackknifed to open the flank, and the patient's position is held by a vacuum bean bag and an armrest for the left arm. Appropriate padding of the legs, arms, and pressure points is applied. The RP approach starts with an incision directly over the eleventh rib from the posterior axillary line to the lateral rectus border and is carried through the abdominal wall musculature onto the rib. The eleventh rib is mobilized and the distal 6 to 8 inches of the rib are excised. The more posterior one brings this incision, the higher the likelihood of pleural cavity entry. The incision is then carried through the transversalis fascia and the RP space is entered laterally. The peritoneal sac is swept anteromedially, further defining the RP space. This is continued medially until the aneurysmal aorta is identified. As noted earlier, a plane anterior or

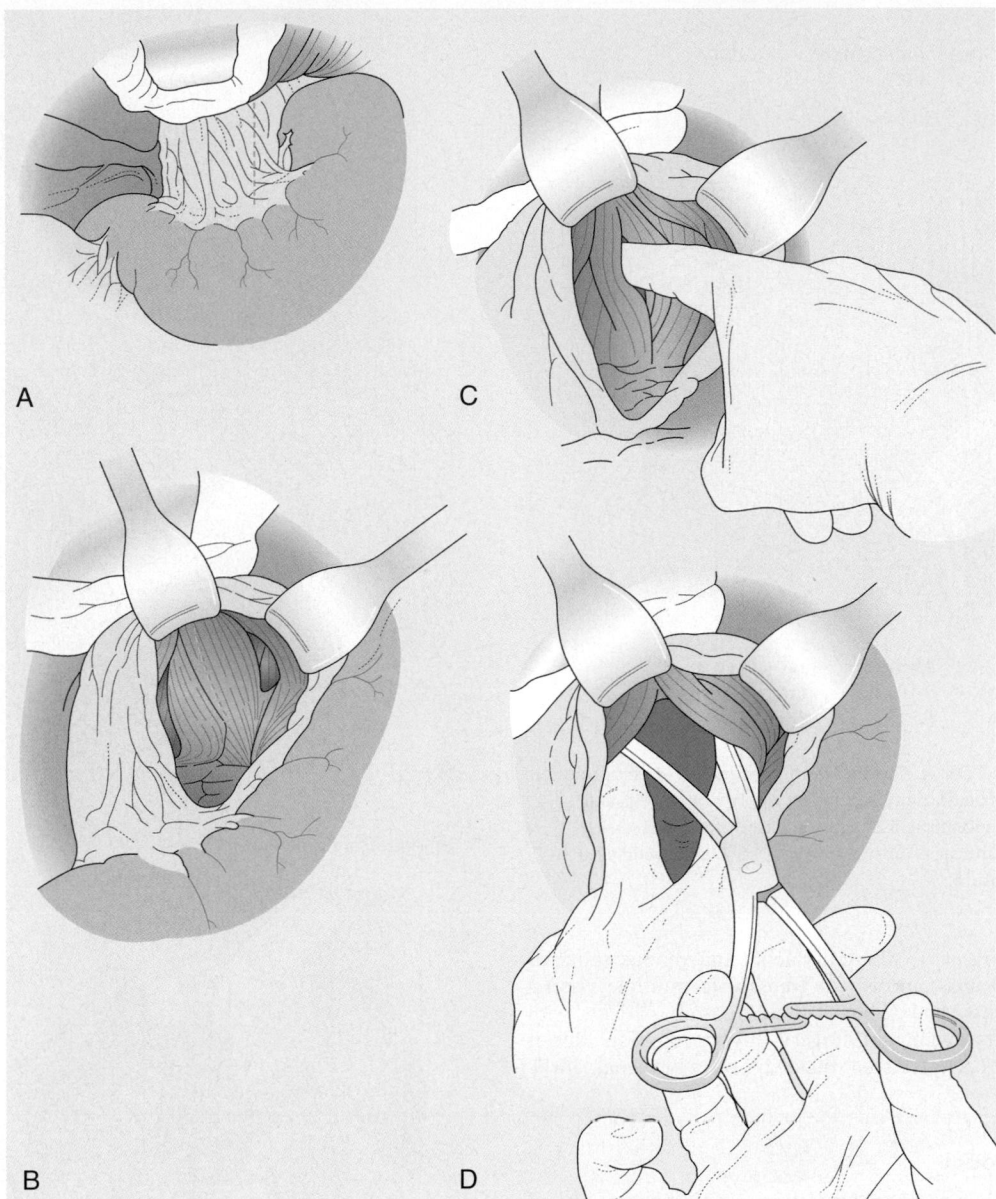

FIGURE 4 Exposure and supraceliac aortic clamping. **A,** Appropriate retraction of the diaphragm and liver adequately expose the gastrohepatic ligament. **B,** After division of the gastrohepatic ligament, the right crus of the diaphragm is exposed. **C,** Division of the crus or dissection with a fingertip identifies the aorta. **D,** Further dissection on either side of the aorta allows for placement of a clamp with tips against the vertebral body.

posterior to the left kidney may be developed, and in most circumstances anterior mobilization of the left kidney is chosen. The aorta is thus approached on its left posterolateral aspect, and the aortic origin of the left renal artery is an important point of anatomic reference. Depending on the patient's body habitus and the nature of the pathology, it is possible to carry the dissection proximally, divide the median arcuate ligament and left diaphragmatic crural muscular fibers, and expose and control the supravisceral aorta.

There is great overestimation in the literature regarding the undue morbidity of a two-cavity, thoracoabdominal approach. We believe that a formal thoracoabdominal approach with pleural and peritoneal cavity entry and sharp division of the costal margin is the preferred approach for the majority of lesions where the surgeon will be working on the visceral aortic segment. The proximal extent of the incision is dictated by the nature of the pathology, the patient's body habitus, and the nature of the surgery to be carried out. We have found no specific advantage to keeping the abdominal portion of the

incision in the RP plane. Rather, the inability to directly inspect intestinal contents or palpate visceral vessel pulses on the other side of the transverse mesocolon is a valid reason to enter the peritoneal cavity.

After entry into the left thoracic and abdominal cavities, the costal margin is divided sharply, and a limited radial, lateral incision in the diaphragm will allow the surgeon to preserve the phrenic nerve and to retract and work entirely below the diaphragm. The abdominal dissection proceeds as described for left medial visceral rotation. Although the entire operation is conducted in the retroperitoneum, patient positioning is such that evisceration generally is not necessary. The position and handling of the left kidney is as previously discussed, and in the majority of cases the left kidney is elevated out of its bed. Direct and continuous exposure of the aorta from the posterior mediastinum to the bifurcation is therefore possible with this approach. We have found this approach most useful in the following circumstances: (1) suprarenal aneurysms; (2) extensive redo

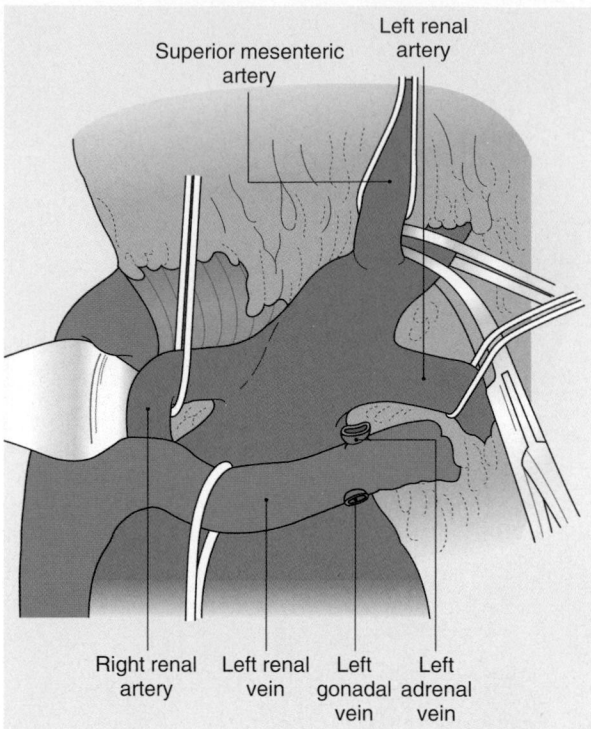

FIGURE 5 Suprarenal aortic exposure with right medial visceral rotation. After medial visceral rotation, mobilization of the left renal vein, and division of periaortic splanchnic tissue, the suprarenal aorta is easily accessible. Note that the superior mesenteric artery is perpendicular to the aorta in this exposure.

(difficult) aortic surgery; (3) Linton splenorenal venous shunt or splenorenal arterial anastomosis; (4) transaortic multiple visceral vessel endarterectomy; and (5) ruptured AAAs in patients with extensive prior intra-abdominal surgery. In our opinion, this is the preferred approach for the majority of suprarenal aortic aneurysms.

Operative Conduct

For elective AAA repair, preoperative planning should dictate patient positioning and approach such that a complete resection of the aneurysm and occlusive disease is achieved, rather than partial resection of a more diffuse disease process, in order to prevent late aneurysmal degeneration and the need for subsequent reintervention. Limited dissection designed to confine either clamping or resection to the infrarenal aorta is inappropriate when this represents a compromise in resection of the aneurysmal process. However, in case of emergent surgery with patient instability and extensive comorbidities, surgical objectives must be tailored to fit the clinical circumstances.

Aside from technical considerations, perioperative bleeding complications may occur as a result of dilutional coagulopathy resulting from large blood turnover and inadequate repletion of blood products. Blood turnover by necessity may be excessive, especially in circumstances of complex aneurysm repair; therefore a cell saver is used during all aortic reconstructions, except in cases of suspected infection. Blood component replacement with fresh frozen plasma and platelets during surgery alleviates coagulopathic bleeding. Infusion lines and monitoring lines appropriate for the anticipated complexity of aneurysm repair and planned level of aortic cross-clamping should be placed in conjunction with the anesthesia team. Fluid and external warmers should be applied with the intention of maintaining normothermia throughout the procedure. Use of an epidural for intraoperative anesthesia and postoperative analgesia has been associated

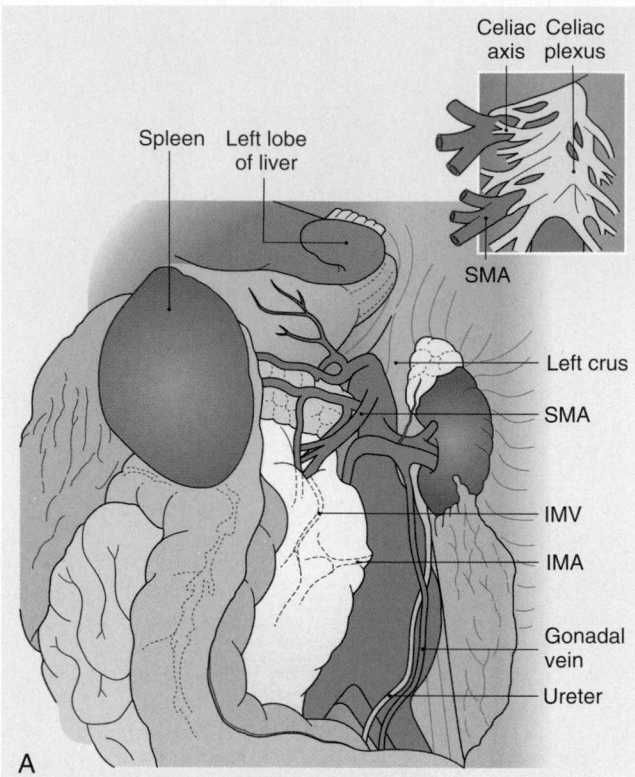

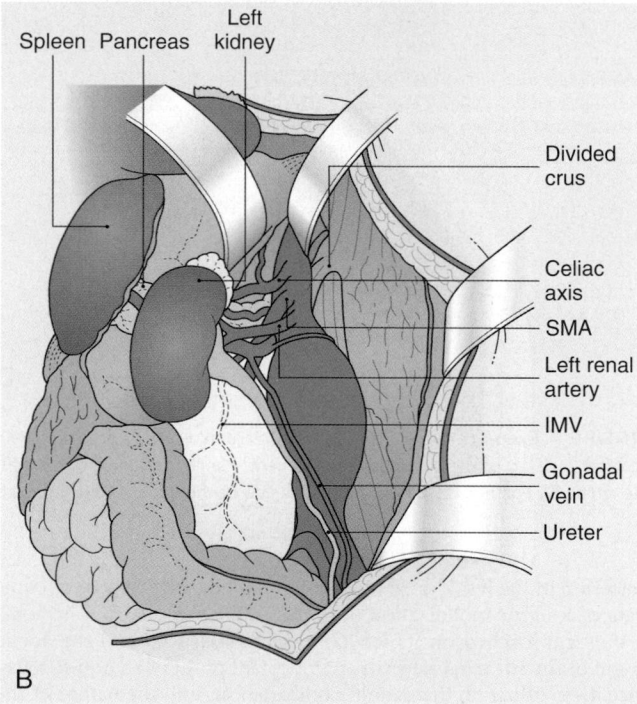

FIGURE 6 Left lateral retroperitoneal or thoracoabdominal approach. **A,** Various levels of incision depend on the extent of aneurysmal disease. The abdominal portion is not carried to midline so as to keep the viscera intraperitoneal, to decrease evaporative and heat losses. In this example, the left kidney is left in situ. **B,** With the left kidney mobilized anteriorly, excellent contiguous exposure to the visceral aortic segment is obtained, as division of the left crus at the aortic hiatus facilitates supraceliac aortic exposure. Note the renal lumbar vein at the level of the left renal artery. Identification of the left renal artery serves as a point of reference for further dissection of the visceral aorta. *IMA,* Inferior mesenteric artery; *IMV,* inferior mesenteric vein; *SMA,* superior mesenteric artery.

with improved pain control, decreased ileus, and improved pulmonary toilet and aids in rapid recovery.

During the operation, a number of key principles aid surgical efficiency and success.

1. Continuous and adequate exposure of the involved portions of the aorta is necessary, implying the routine use of a fixed, self-retaining retractor system.
2. Gentle dissection on and around an AAA should be performed, as atheroembolism is equally likely to occur during dissection of the aneurysm as during application of cross-clamps. This concern is particularly appropriate in patients with a preoperative history of "blue toe syndrome."
3. Careful conduct of dissection with emphasis on hemostasis reduces blood turnover and decreases the likelihood of bleeding complications.
4. Except in cases of rupture, all patients are anticoagulated judiciously before application of cross-clamps or occlusion of branch vessels, and systemic anticoagulation is reversed after completion of all distal anastamoses.
5. Locations for aortic clamping should be such that an adequate aortic "cuff" is available for anastomosis. In addition, in planning the location of proximal or distal cross-clamps it is imperative to avoid clamping a heavily diseased aorta, particularly where extensive mural atherothrombotic debris is demonstrated on preoperative imaging studies. This principle is specifically intended to avoid atheromatous embolization to renal, visceral, or outflow vessels. Accordingly, visceral vessel and distal outflow vessel clamps are applied before proximal aortic cross-clamping.

After clamp application, the aortic sac is opened longitudinally and mural thrombus and debris is evacuated with care such that mobilization of debris into outflow iliac vessels is avoided. Retrograde bleeding from lumbar vessels is controlled by suture ligatures and may require local endarterectomy and removal of calcific plaque for successful control of the bleeding vessels. Aortic reconstructions typically are performed with appropriately sized Dacron or polytetrafluoroethylene (PTFE) tube grafts, with use of bifurcated grafts in instances where distal reconstruction should require iliac or femoral level outflow anastamoses (Figures 7 and 8). The main body of a bifurcated graft should be cut short (~4 cm) to prevent kinking of the iliac limbs.

More proximal clamp placement is associated with increased cardiac strain, hemodynamic compromise, and the potential for coagulopathy. However, with appropriate exposure and planning the proximal reconstruction can be performed with clamp times of less than 30 minutes in most instances. Aortic grafts can be prefashioned with side arms for visceral vessel reconstruction before cross-clamp application to expedite reperfusion of the reconstructed vessels. In instances of suprarenal clamp application, renal preservation is achieved through direct instillation of cold renal preservation fluid (4°C Lactated Ringer's solution with 25 g of mannitol per liter and 1 g of methyl prednisolone per liter) into the renal artery ostia after opening of the aorta. After completion of the distal anastomosis, hemodynamic shifts associated with reperfusion should be coordinated and managed in conjunction with the anesthesia team. Reimplantation of the inferior mesenteric artery (IMA) should be considered in patients with occluded hypogastric arteries, poor back bleeding from the IMA, and previous colon surgery such that normal collateral pathways have been significantly altered.

After aortic reconstruction, coverage of the graft by closing the aneurysm sac over the reconstruction—and in cases of TP exposure, closure of the retroperitoneum augmented with omental flap coverage—reduces the likelihood of late graft-enteric erosion and attendant graft infection or fistulae (Figure 9). Before wound closure, inspection of the viscera, Doppler evaluation and palpation of reconstructed vessels, and pulse volume recording analysis of the lower extremity circulation are performed. Postoperative splenic bleeding and undetected bleeding from intercostal or lumbar vessels are

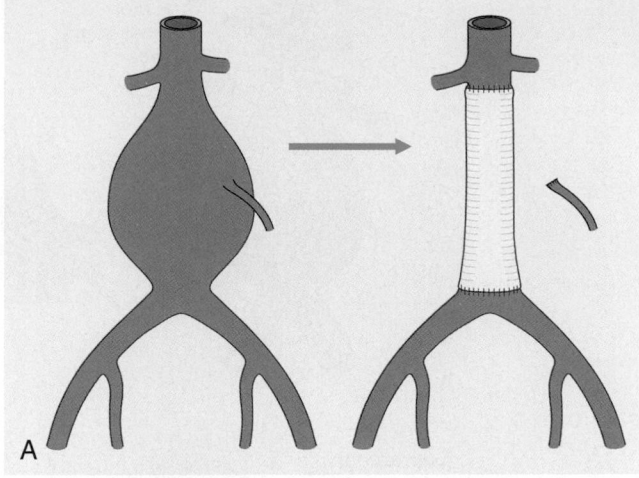

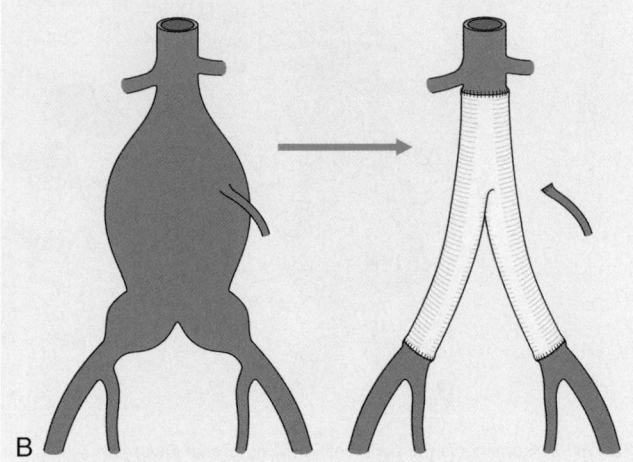

FIGURE 7 Constructs for infrarenal aneurysm repair. Infrarenal aneurysms are most commonly repaired with tube grafts (**A**) or bifurcated grafts (graft neck <4 cm in length) (**B**).

principle sources of postoperative hemorrhage. Accordingly, a careful search for bleeding vessels after reperfusion and an aggressive posture toward splenectomy limit such complications. All patients with repaired AAAs are transferred to the surgical intensive care unit for postoperative monitoring and treatment.

An expeditious operation is to be emphasized in all patients. We reviewed a series of 200 consecutive aortic operations at our institution (80% conducted for AAA) and evaluated a variety of preoperative and intraoperative technical variables to assess their impact on operative complications and mortality. Among these, only a prolonged operation (>5 hours) was associated independently with death or major cardiopulmonary complications after abdominal aortic surgery (odds ratio [OR] 5.11; 95% confidence interval [CI] 1.69-15.52]; P <0.004). Technical factors of significance in predicting perioperative complications also include urgency of procedure, body core temperature (≤35°C), volume of blood loss, perioperative fluid requirements, location of surgery (intraperitoneal and intrathoracic), and location of aortic clamping.

■ RESULTS

Independent of operative conduct, perioperative morbidity and mortality after AAA repair are influenced by patient characteristics and circumstances of clinical presentation. Patient age, extent of comorbid conditions, and complexity of aneurysm repair all have been reported to increase operative risk. Mortality rates associated

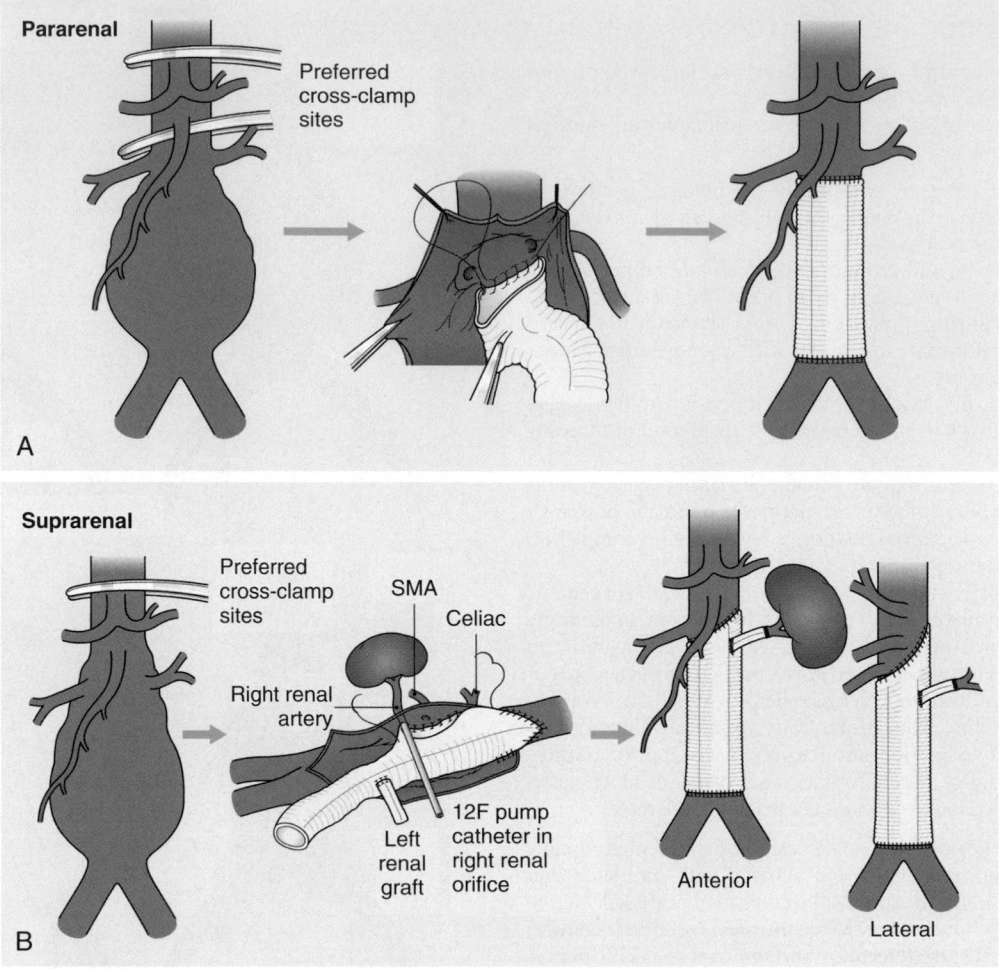

FIGURE 8 Constructs for pararenal and suprarenal aneurysm repair. Our preferred methods: **A,** Pararenal aneurysm. Cross-clamp: supraceliac or suprarenal inframesenteric depending on aortic disease and renovisceral artery spacing. Inset: Sewing proximally to the cuff of aorta at the renal artery orifices. **B,** Suprarenal aneurysm. Cross-clamp: supraceliac. Inset: Beveled proximal anastomosis with 12F perfusion catheter used to stent open the right renal artery to inhibit orificial compromise during suture placement. Left renal artery reconstruction with 6-mm polytetrafluoroethylene tube graft preattached to aortic prosthesis. *SMA,* Superior mesenteric artery.

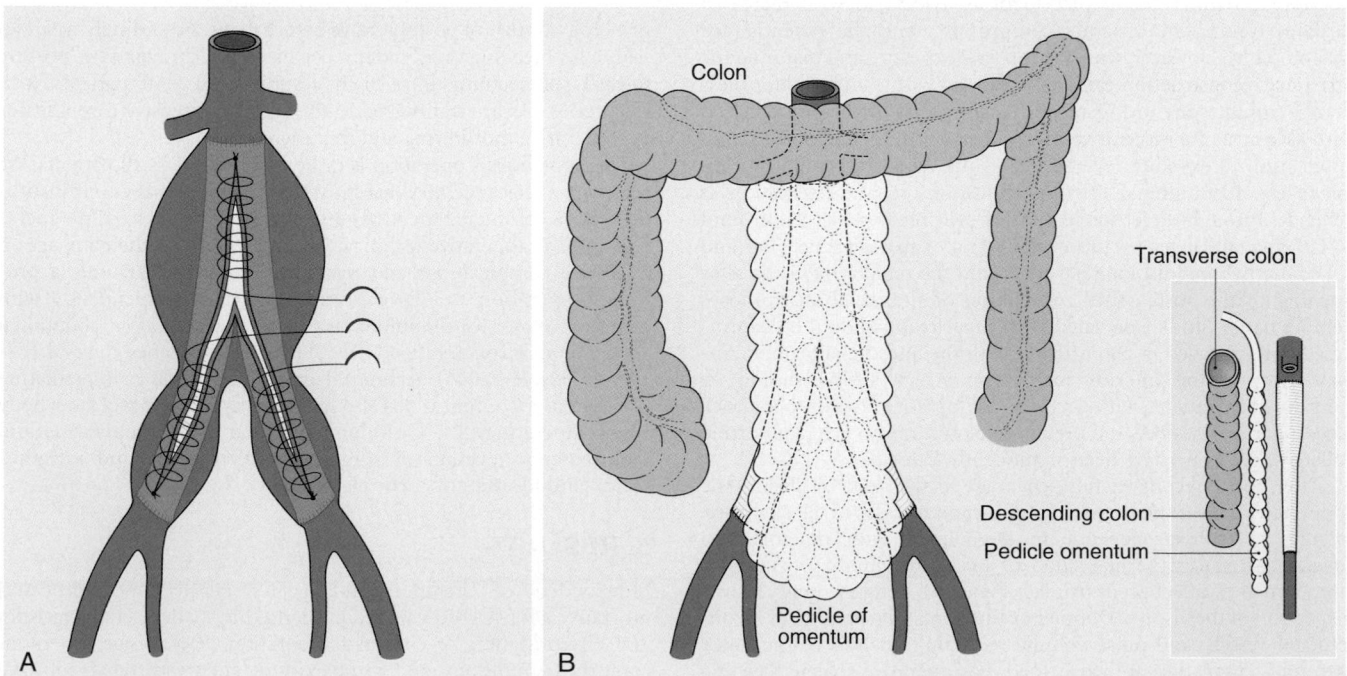

FIGURE 9 Aneurysm sac closure and coverage. After aneurysm repair, closure of the aneurysm sac over the aortic graft (**A**) or use of an omental pedicle flap (**B**) help to separate the synthetic graft material from the gastrointestinal tract.

with elective pararenal or suprarenal AAA repair approach 5% to 10%, whereas mortality rates associated with infrarenal AAA repair are less than 5%. In circumstances of symptomatic or ruptured AAA repair, mortality rates ranging from 20% to 70% have been reported, with an equally high incidence of major morbidity. In a previous report of our own experience with open AAA repair in the era predating the widespread use of EVAR, we reported an operative mortality rate of 3% and major morbidity of 10%. In this series of 540 patients, 25% of patients required suprarenal clamp application for AAA repair. Independent predictors of both perioperative morbidity and mortality included previous myocardial infarction (MI) (OR 2.0 [95% CI 1.2–3.6]; $P = 0.01$) and renal insufficiency (OR 2.5 [95% CI 1.2–5.3]; $P = 0.02$).

Many series demonstrate increased operative risk in patients with coronary artery disease, COPD, and renal insufficiency, with dysfunction in these respective organ systems increasing the risks of organ-specific postoperative complications. Variables predictive of cardiac complications include recent MI, advanced age, diabetes, poor functional status, history of arrhythmia, and congestive heart failure. Cardiac complications can be prevented with appropriate risk stratification and optimizing of perioperative medical management such that patients are treated with statin medications, aspirin, and beta-blockers (goal heart rate <60 beats per minute and systolic blood pressure <100 mm Hg).

Variables predictive of postoperative pulmonary complications include active cigarette smoking, COPD, urgent clinical presentation, and extent of operation. Respiratory complications are avoided by preoperative smoking cessation and can be managed in the postoperative setting with optimal bronchodilator therapy and aggressive pulmonary toilet in conjunction with a pulmonary specialist.

Variables predictive of postoperative renal complications include preoperative renal insufficiency, duration of renal ischemia, failure of renal artery reconstruction, and cholesterol embolization from surgical manipulation. Transient decreases in renal function are inevitable as a result of the obligatory periods of ischemia, resulting in nonoliguric renal insufficiency that is easily managed with maintenance of intravascular volume and hemodynamic support. The use of adjuncts such as cold crystalloid renal perfusion may prevent postoperative renal insufficiency, but minimizing renal ischemia time is the most important factor in avoiding this complication.

In addition to predicting perioperative morbidity, the presence of cardiopulmonary and renal comorbidities is associated with significant decreases in long-term patient survival. Five-year survival in patients after complex AAA repair is reported to be 40% to 75%. The majority of late mortality is related to cardiovascular events, and some groups have reported improved late outcomes in patients who have undergone previous coronary revascularization. Our own experience noted late survival of 71 ± 2% and 44 ± 2% at 5 and 10 years, respectively. Predictors of late mortality included advanced age at operation, history of MI, congestive heart failure, and preoperative renal insufficiency. In the same patient cohort, freedom from aneurysm-related mortality was 95% at 5 and 10 years. Graft-related complications were identified in 2% of patients. Additional aneurysmal disease in noncontiguous aortic segments was found in 13% of patients at a mean follow-up of 7.2 years. Thus patients undergoing open AAA repair are afforded good long-term survival and excellent durability of the reconstruction.

SUGGESTED READINGS

Cambria RP, Brewster DC, Abbott WM, et al. Transperitoneal versus retroperitoneal approach for aortic reconstruction: a randomized prospective study. *J Vasc Surg.* 1990;11:314-325.

Cambria RP, Brewster DC, L'Italien G, et al. Simultaneous aortic and renal artery reconstruction: evolution of an eighteen-year experience. *J Vasc Surg.* 1995;21:916-925.

Conrad MF, Crawford RS, Pedraza JD, et al. Long-term durability of open abdominal aortic aneurysm repair. *J Vasc Surg.* 2007;46:669-675.

Patel VI, Lancaster RT, Conrad MF, et al. Comparable mortality with open repair of complex and infrarenal aortic aneurysm. *J Vasc Surg.* 2011;54: 952-959.

Patel VI, Lancaster RT, Mukhopadhyay S, et al. Impact of chronic kidney disease on outcomes after abdominal aortic aneurysm repair. *J Vasc Surg.* 2012;56:1206-1213.

Tsai S, Conrad MF, Patel VI, et al. Durability of open repair of juxtarenal abdominal aortic aneurysms. *J Vasc Surg.* 2012;56:2-7.

ENDOVASCULAR TREATMENT OF ABDOMINAL AORTIC ANEURYSM

Michael J. Osgood, MD, and James H. Black III, MD

The Society for Vascular Surgery defines abdominal aortic aneurysm (AAA) as a 50% increase over the baseline diameter of this vessel, or an aneurysm exceeding 3 cm in diameter. AAA is a common entity that affects up to 8% of people over 60 years of age and up to 15% of men over 65 years of age. The average age of affected individuals is 75 years, and there is a strong male predominance of this condition, with a male to female ratio of 6 : 1. Risk factors for this condition have been evaluated extensively, and smoking is by far the most significant risk factor. Other risk factors include hyperhomocysteinemia, history of hernia, advancing age, family history of aneurysm, history of atherosclerosis, and hypercholesterolemia. Factors demonstrated to be protective against AAA include Caucasian race, presence of diabetes mellitus, and female gender.

The natural history of AAA is growth and eventual rupture, and AAA rupture accounts for approximately 15,000 deaths annually in the United States. The average rate of growth of AAA is 2 to 3 mm/year. Current smoking status accelerates the growth rate by 20% and doubles the rupture risk. It has been well established that the rupture risk increases significantly when AAA diameter increases from 5 to 6 cm. AAAs measuring 5 cm have a 5-year rupture risk less than 2.5%, whereas AAAs measuring 6 cm have a 5-year rupture risk exceeding 20%. Many trials have established AAA diameter of 5.5 cm in males and 5 cm in females as appropriate size thresholds for repair, regardless of technique utilized (open or endovascular), and these sizing recommendations are supported by guidelines from the Society for Vascular Surgery.

Endovascular aneurysm repair (EVAR) was first performed in 1990 in Buenos Aires by Drs. Juan Parodi and Julio Palmaz in a patient who had been deemed an unsuitable candidate for open AAA repair. The aneurysm was excluded endoluminally with a Dacron graft that was anchored at the proximal infrarenal neck with a stainless steel balloon-expandable stent. The system was assembled by affixing (with sutures) the Dacron graft to an undeployed Palmaz stent mounted on a large-diameter angioplasty balloon. The contraption then was sheathed inside a large bore catheter that served as the delivery system. Access to the aorta for delivery and deployment was achieved in a retrograde transluminal fashion through the surgically exposed common femoral artery. It worked, resulting in exclusion and depressurization of the large aneurysm. This revolutionary new technique was destined to change the management of AAA and signaled the beginning of a new era in aortic surgery and vascular surgery overall.

In the 25 years since this technique was first described, EVAR devices and techniques have been refined, and the technique has become the preferred treatment for infrarenal AAA. Indeed, EVAR supplanted open repair in 2003, with increasing volume of EVAR cases performed every year. EVAR is now used as the method of repair in 80% of patients with infrarenal AAA in the United States. EVAR also has broadened the population of patients amenable to AAA repair, as the technique avoids the invasive nature and physiologic stress of the open operation and is associated with a more rapid recovery, shorter hospital length of stay, and lower rates of early complications.

Trials comparing EVAR with open AAA repair include the EVAR 1 trial, the DREAM trial, and the Open Versus Endovascular Repair (OVER) trial. These prospective randomized controlled trials yielded remarkably similar results, with several consistent findings. First, EVAR is associated with significantly lower rates of perioperative morbidity and mortality compared with open AAA repair. Second, the short-term survival advantage of EVAR diminishes over time and equalizes at approximately 2 years of follow-up such that survival is similar. Third, EVAR is associated with significantly higher rates of procedure- and device-related complications that require reintervention. Therefore successful long-term results after EVAR require accurate up-front technical execution with respect to device selection and placement and subsequent close follow-up with long-term surveillance after the procedure for optimal outcome.

■ PREOPERATIVE PLANNING

Performing EVAR with successful and durable results relies on precise sizing and preoperative planning. Successful EVAR must fulfill a few basic principles: (1) achieving adequate iliofemoral access for delivery of the device, (2) achieving an adequate seal zone proximally between the graft and nonaneurysmal aorta, (3) achieving an adequate seal zone distally between the graft limbs and nonaneurysmal common or external iliac arteries, and (4) achieving adequate seal between the graft components.

Adequate assessment of the patient's anatomy in preparation for a proposed endovascular repair requires a preoperative computed tomographic angiography (CTA) scan with fine cuts (3 mm or less) and three-dimensional (3D) reconstructions. Several software programs are available for reformatting of CTA images and facilitate length and diameter measurements of the aorta and its branches to aid in device selection. These software programs include the TeraRecon Aquarius 3D Workstation (TeraRecon Inc., San Mateo, CA) and 3mensio Vascular (Pie Medical Imaging, Bilthoven, Netherlands). The reconstructions generated by these programs show the contrast-filled lumen of the aorta and its branches and allow inspection of the morphology and composition of the aneurysm and the aortic wall, including calcification and intraluminal thrombus. The software generates a centerline pathway through the aorta and extending into both of the external iliac arteries. The software allows precise measurements of distances between branch vessels to aid in planning of device size in relation to critical branch vessels, typically renal and internal iliac arteries. Using preoperative imaging, a decision needs to be made regarding which iliofemoral access site will be used for delivery of the main body of the device (ipsilateral side), with the other iliofemoral access site being used for delivery of the contralateral limb (contralateral side). The length of the main body and the corresponding ipsilateral iliac limb is determined using the centerline path on the ipsilateral side. In general, the length of the main body and ipsilateral iliac limb needs to be less than the distance between the lowest renal artery and the ipsilateral internal iliac artery, a distance that ideally is measured along the centerline path. The length of the contralateral iliac artery extension is likewise calculated by measuring the centerline path until the contralateral iliac artery.

The decision regarding side of introduction of the main body (ipsilateral) and the contralateral iliac extension is based on the size and tortuosity of the iliofemoral access and the feasibility of introduction of the larger main body sheath. The software also allows determination of the appropriate angle to place the image intensifier to correct for parallax when deploying the main body relative to the renal arteries. In the event of renal insufficiency, a noncontrast computed tomographic (CT) scan may be obtained and selectively may be supplemented with intravascular ultrasound to define the luminal anatomy of the patient's aorta and iliac arteries.

Assessing Iliofemoral Access

Existing EVAR grafts require bilateral iliofemoral access for device delivery. The most common site of access for delivery of an endovascular aortic device is the bilateral common femoral arteries. Important in assessment of the iliofemoral vessels is confirming adequate patency, luminal diameter, presence of calcification and intraluminal thrombus, and tortuosity. Luminal diameter furthermore must be of sufficient caliber to accommodate the proposed device sheaths. Common femoral artery disease may be significant and may require concomitant thromboendarterectomy. Significant iliac stenosis should be managed with angioplasty before introduction of the device. Patients with small external iliac vessels may require placement of an iliac conduit, which is created by anastomosis of a 10-mm Dacron graft end-to-side to the distal common iliac artery through direct retroperitoneal exposure of the vessel. Introduction of the EVAR devices is achieved over stiff wire access, and iliac tortuosity is usually straightened during deployment; however, iliofemoral segments with severe tortuosity may preclude safe device delivery.

Iliofemoral access can be achieved by direct surgical exposure of the vessels or by percutaneous techniques. When we perform direct surgical exposure, we prefer to utilize bilateral oblique incisions (4 to 6 cm) inferior to the inguinal ligament and superior to the groin crease. The location of arterial access should be the common femoral artery, ideally 1 to 2 cm cephalad to the femoral bifurcation. Percutaneous EVAR (PEVAR) is a technique that avoids surgical incisions by utilizing percutaneous arterial closure devices, which deploy sutures in full-thickness bites through the wall of the vessel that subsequently are cinched down and tied after sheath removal in order to achieve hemostasis. In the "preclose" technique, a closure device is introduced into the vessel over a guidewire placed through percutaneous access, which then deploys the suture materials, which can be clipped temporarily with a hemostat to aid in subsequent sealing of the large arteriotomy remaining after sheath removal at completion of EVAR. Available closure devices include the Perclose ProGlide and the ProStar XL (both Abbott Vascular, Santa Clara, CA). Relative contraindications to percutaneous access for EVAR include obesity, severely scarred groin, high or suprainguinal femoral bifurcation, need for frequent introducer sheath exchanges, significant proximal iliac occlusive disease, small iliofemoral arteries, and significant anterior or circumferential calcific femoral disease.

Achieving Proximal Aortic Seal

Appropriate seal between the EVAR device and the aorta at this proximal level relies on an adequate zone of apposition between nonaneurysmal aorta and the stent-graft. The length of minimum adequate seal zone varies between devices and ranges from 10 to 15 mm (Table 1). Assessment of the seal zone involves measurement of the aortic neck diameter at the level of the lowest renal artery and also 10 to 15 mm caudally, depending on the indications for use (IFU) specifying minimal neck length for the device. This "seal zone" should be assessed for angulation relative to adjacent aorta, tortuosity, and presence of mural thrombus. Measurements of the diameter of the aorta in this location should be obtained. Important to accurate measurement is assessing the diameter perpendicular to the aorta, rather than tangential to it, which is a frequent and easily made

TABLE 1: Current Endovascular Aneurysm Repair (EVAR) Devices and Indications for Use (IFU) Specifications With Regard to Aortic Neck Sizing, Aortic Neck Morphology, Neck Angle, Proximal and Distal Seal Zones, Design Attributes, and Presence of Suprarenal Stent

Device/Type (avg # pieces)	Manufacturer	Main Body Diameter (mm)	Aortic Treatment Diameter (mm)	Main Body Delivery Size (F)	IFU Neck Length/Angle	Iliac Treatment Diameter (mm)	Distal Iliac Fixation Length (mm)	Other Design Attributes	Suprarenal Stent
Zenith Flex/Modular (2-3)	Cook Medical (Bloomington, IN)	22-36	18-32	20-24 OD	≥15 mm ≤60°	7.5-20	>10	Standard configuration includes bilateral iliac limb extensions (ipsilateral and contralateral)	Yes
AFX/Unibody (1-3)	Endologix (Irvine, CA)	25-34	18-32	19 OD	≥15 mm ≤60°	10-23	≥15	Stent endoskeleton with fabric on outside; main body of device designed to seat on aortic bifurcation; can extend proximally and extend contralateral iliac limb	Optional
Excluder C3/Modular (2-3)	W. L. Gore (Flagstaff, AZ)	23-35	19-32	18-20 OD	≥15 mm ≤60°	8-25	≥10	Can recapture graft neck and redeploy if malpositioned; standard configuration includes contralateral iliac extension only; ipsilateral limb extension optional	No
Endurant II/modular (2-3)	Medtronic (Minneapolis, MN)	23-36	19-32	18-20 OD	≥10 mm and ≤60° or ≥15 mm and ≤75°	8-25	≥15	Standard configuration includes contralateral iliac extension only; ipsilateral limb extension optional	Yes
Ovation Prime/Modular (3)	Trivascular (Santa Rosa, CA)	20-34	16-30	14-15 OD	≥10 mm and ≤60° or <10 mm and ≤45°	8-25	≥10	Injectable polymer ring at aortic seal zone; standard configuration includes bilateral iliac limb extensions (ipsilateral and contralateral)	Yes
Aorfix/modular (2-3)	Lombard Medical (Didcot, United Kingdom)	24-36	19-33	22 OD	15 mm ≤90	9-19	≥15	Standard configuration includes contralateral iliac extension only; ipsilateral limb extension optional	No

OD, Outer diameter.

error on axial cuts. Most devices are measured relative to adventitia-to-adventitia dimensions, whereas the Excluder device (W. L. Gore & Associates, Flagstaff, AZ) is measured relative to intima-to-intima dimensions. Proximal endograft diameter is typically oversized by 10% to 20% relative to the neck diameter measurement described earlier. Aggressive oversizing should be avoided, as the excess fabric forms pleats that can generate a type Ia endoleak. Type Ia (proximal) endoleak can be minimized by intraoperative balloon angioplasty to fully expand the stent components and achieve adequate seal in the proximal aortic neck.

Achieving Distal Iliac Seal and Junctional Seal

A nonaneurysmal iliac artery segment is required to achieve an adequate distal seal zone for successful EVAR. Current devices require a 10- to 15-mm length of nonaneurysmal iliac artery to achieve adequate seal. The seal zone typically is placed in the distal common iliac artery. If the common iliac artery is aneurysmal or otherwise inappropriate for achieving adequate seal, the iliac limb seal zone can be accomplished in the external iliac artery. In this instance, the internal iliac artery orifice is covered by the device, and therefore it is necessary to perform preoperative or concomitant embolization of this vessel. It is our preference to perform embolization 2 to 4 weeks before planned EVAR, as this procedure typically is associated with transient or occasionally permanent pelvic ischemia. If the internal iliac artery is chronically occluded, embolization is unnecessary. As with measurement of the aortic neck, the iliac artery measurement typically is performed perpendicular to the axis of the vessel from adventitia to adventitia, or from intima to intima in the case of the Excluder device. As with the proximal aortic seal zone, the iliac limbs should be oversized by 10% to 20%. Type Ib (distal) endoleak can be minimized by intraoperative balloon angioplasty to fully expand the stent components and achieve adequate seal in the iliac seal zones. Adequate junctional seal generally requires a 3-cm length of graft overlap between graft components, depending on the device. Balloon angioplasty also should be performed intraoperatively to dilate the sites of junctional graft overlap in order to minimize type III (junctional) endoleak.

Endovascular Device Selection and Deployment

The process of regulatory approval of endograft devices in the United States requires rigorous and extensive preclinical assessment and clinical study results to validate the specific anatomic features and constraints to guide EVAR placement in patients. These collective features are designated IFU and include aortic neck diameter, aortic neck length, aortic neck angle, and iliac artery morphology. Manufacturers are required to publish the IFU criteria and include them with the device packaging. There are currently six EVAR devices approved by the U.S. Food and Drug Administration (FDA) and available in the United States, and their IFU criteria vary slightly. Most devices require an aortic neck angle of 60 degrees or less relative to the long axis of the aneurysm. The exception to this is the Aorfix device (Lombard Medical, Didcot, United Kingdom), which may be placed in aortic neck angles of 90 degrees or less (see Table 1).

Vascular surgeons vary in adherence to IFU in selecting and placing EVAR devices. In a recent review of a multicenter imaging database, Schanzer and colleagues evaluated adherence to IFU among 10,228 patients who underwent EVAR over a 10-year period. They found a relatively low rate of adherence to device IFU (42%), and this cohort had a corresponding high rate of AAA sac enlargement at 5 years post-EVAR (41%). Factors predictive of AAA sac enlargement were as follows: endoleak, age of 80 years or older, aortic neck diameter of 28 mm or more, aortic neck angle greater than 60 degrees, and common iliac diameter greater than 20 mm. The findings of this landmark study highlight the importance of performing EVAR within IFU criteria in order to avoid complications, endoleaks, reinterventions, and postprocedure AAA rupture.

Contraindications to Endovascular Aortic Aneurysm Repair

There are several additional factors that should be considered when evaluating patients for EVAR. Relative contraindications are as follows. Renal insufficiency, depending on the degree of renal dysfunction, may preclude safely performing EVAR. Although efforts can be made to minimize contrast load and to identify aortic branch vessels to avoid intraoperative coverage using intravascular ultrasound (IVUS), it is not technically possible to perform the procedure without using at least a small amount of contrast to identify the renal arteries to facilitate precise deployment and perform a completion angiogram to evaluate for endoleak. Some patients with chronic renal insufficiency are extremely intolerant of even the slightest contrast load, which can lead to end-stage renal disease that requires dialysis. Iliofemoral access, when inadequate, may preclude EVAR. Common femoral or external iliac artery access, when too small to accommodate the necessary sheath, can be solved by placement of an external iliac or common iliac access conduit, depending on the device configuration and the necessary distal iliac seal zone. Inadequate iliofemoral access may preclude safe EVAR, especially in women. Absolute contraindications to EVAR are as follows. Patients with connective tissue disorders, patients with infected aneurysms, and patients whose anatomy is not compatible with currently available endografts are more appropriate candidates for open repair. Table 1 summarizes the sizing and anatomic restrictions particular to each graft. Patients with extremely narrow (<16-18 mm) aortic necks or distal aortic diameters, extremely large (>32 mm) aortic necks, or extremely small distal iliac seal zones (<7.5 mm) do not have anatomy amenable to EVAR using currently available devices. Patients whose intestinal circulation is supplied by a large or dominant inferior mesenteric artery (IMA) should not undergo EVAR because it is impossible to perform the procedure without interrupting flow to this vessel. In addition, patients with a pelvic kidney with the renal artery emanating off the infrarenal aorta (Figure 1) or other anatomic abnormality placing an important branch vessel in the aortic region being covered by the

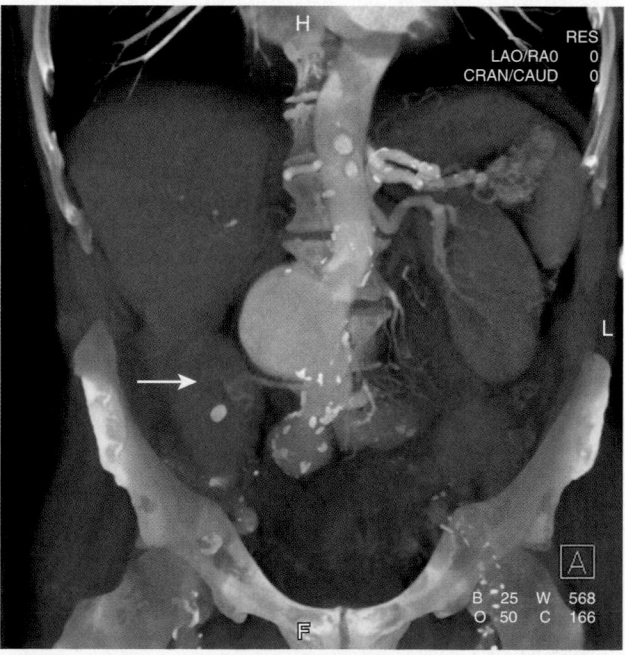

FIGURE 1 Computed tomography angiography (CTA) of a patient with a right pelvic kidney (*arrow*) with renal artery arising from the distal infrarenal abdominal aorta. This patient was deemed an unacceptable candidate for conventional endovascular aneurysm repair because of inevitable coverage of the right renal artery without the ability to preserve the right renal artery.

endograft should not undergo EVAR. In addition, patients who are unwilling or incapable of undergoing annual postoperative surveillance imaging should not be considered for EVAR.

Procedural Steps

The basic procedural steps in graft deployment will be described for modular bifurcated grafts, which constitute the majority of currently available devices. Once femoral access has been achieved, a catheter and Glidewire are introduced into the descending thoracic aorta and the Glidewire is exchanged for a stiff wire (Amplatz or Lunderquist) on the ipsilateral side. The patient is systemically heparinized. Through the contralateral femoral access, a pigtail catheter is advanced to a position overlying the L1 vertebral body, and an abdominal aortogram is then performed with the image intensifier angled cranially approximately 10 degrees. Power injection is then performed to identify the location of the renal arteries and internal iliac artery on the ipsilateral side. If there is uncertainty regarding appropriate length of the main body of the device, the marking pigtail catheter can alternatively be introduced on the ipsilateral side with injection performed to measure the length from the low renal artery to the ipsilateral internal iliac artery. The position of the renal arteries is then marked on the screen. A main body of appropriate length is selected, introduced over the stiff wire, and deployed through but not beyond the contralateral gate, reserving the ipsilateral limb deployment for later. The contralateral gate must then be selected from the contralateral femoral access with a wire and catheter to allow placement of a stiff wire (Amplatz or Lunderquist) through the device into the descending thoracic aorta. A marking pigtail catheter should be advanced over the contralateral stiff wire and positioned to allow measurement of the distance from the contralateral gate to the internal iliac artery. Contrast is then injected retrograde from the contralateral sheath under digital subtraction angiography, and the position of the internal iliac is noted and marked on the screen and the distance from graft to internal iliac artery is measured. A contralateral iliac limb of appropriate length is then selected, introduced, and deployed with adequate graft-graft overlap (typically 3 cm) and positioned in a cephalad location relative to the internal iliac artery. At this point, deployment of the ipsilateral iliac limb is completed. Once this limb has been deployed, it may be necessary to extend the device on this side with an ipsilateral iliac limb, depending on the type of endograft being used. After complete deployment of all device components, balloon angioplasty is performed to fully expand the stent components and achieve adequate seal in the proximal, distal, and graft-graft seal zones. This can be achieved with the Coda Balloon Catheter (Cook Medical, Bloomington, IN) or the Q50 Balloon Catheter (W. L. Gore & Associates, Inc., Flagstaff, AZ) inflated manually with a 30-cc syringe filled with dilute contrast. Balloon insertion is required bilaterally, and gentle angioplasty should be performed of the iliac limb seal zones and proximal aortic neck because overdistension can cause rupture. More force can be applied when ballooning graft-graft junctions. After balloon angioplasty, a pigtail catheter is reintroduced into position cephalad to the renal arteries for completion angiogram. The following factors should be specifically evaluated on the completion angiogram: (1) filling of the renal and visceral vessels; (2) the position of the proximal endograft with respect to the renal arteries and evaluation for the presence of a type IA (proximal) endoleak; (3) blood flow through the main body and the iliac limbs; (4) distal flow into the iliac vessels, internal iliac arteries, and runoff vessels, including evaluation for the presence of a type IB (distal) endoleak; and (5) delayed flow into the aneurysm sac via lumbar collaterals and the inferior mesenteric artery, leading to a type II endoleak. When the surgeon is satisfied with the result, femoral artery closure can then be accomplished. When surgical femoral artery access is used, the sheaths and wires are removed under direct visualization. Vascular clamps are placed proximal and distal to the arteriotomy, and the defect is repaired transversely using running 5-0 Prolene suture.

When the PEVAR technique is used, the sheaths are removed, leaving wires in place to maintain access, and the femoral arteriotomies are closed by cinching down the sutures previously placed by the femoral closure device. Once satisfied with adequate hemostasis, the wires are withdrawn.

Postoperative Care and Follow-Up

Patients routinely are admitted to the floor postoperatively. It is our practice to advance the diet as tolerated and remove the Foley catheter at midnight after the procedure, and we prepare patients for discharge home the next day. Patients return to clinic 6 weeks postoperatively for CTA of the abdomen and pelvis. This serves as their baseline study against which future surveillance imaging is assessed. We obtain repeat CTA at 1 year. Aneurysm sac regression or progression dictates the frequency of follow-up and the type of imaging obtained. After the 1-year follow-up, in general it is appropriate to image patients annually. Patients with shrinking aneurysm sacs are managed appropriately with duplex ultrasound, and imaging can be spaced out to every 2 years if the aneurysm sac is stable or shrinking at 5 years of follow-up. Patients with enlarging aneurysm sacs or endoleaks need to be followed with more frequent imaging with CTA.

■ COMPLICATIONS

Endoleak

Endoleak, a complication unique to endovascular aneurysm repair, is defined as persistent blood entry into the aneurysm sac after EVAR. This complication results in continued pressurization of the

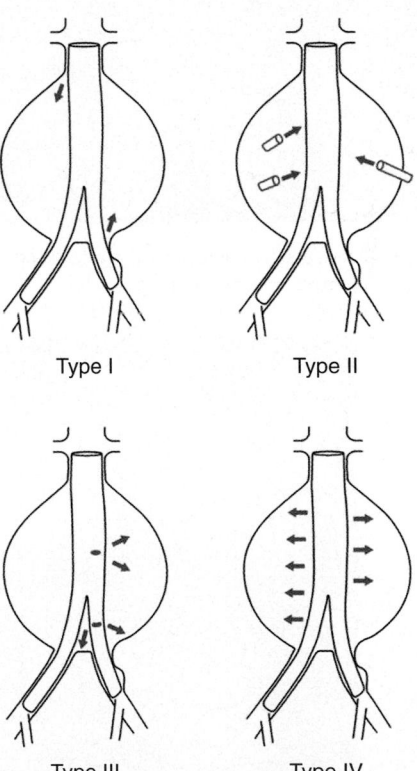

FIGURE 2 Endoleak types I to IV are shown here. Type I endoleaks originate from incomplete seal at the proximal (type Ia) and distal (type Ib) seal zones of the endograft. Type II endoleaks result from backbleeding from patent branch vessels of the abdominal aorta, including inferior mesenteric artery and lumbar arteries. Type III endoleaks originate from tears in the graft fabric, from junctional leaks at sites where graft components separate or incompletely seal. Type IV endoleaks result from porosity in the graft fabric.

aneurysm sac, placing the patient at risk for continued aneurysm growth and rupture. Endoleaks are classified into five categories, types I through IV (Figure 2) and endotension (sometimes referred to as type V endoleak); the categories aid in determining the appropriate treatment and its urgency.

Type I Endoleak

Type I endoleak occurs when there is an incomplete seal between the stent-graft device and the native vessel, either at the proximal (type Ia) or distal (type Ib) attachment site, resulting in continued blood flow into the aneurysm sac and concomitant sac growth (Figures 2 and 3). Type I endoleaks typically are encountered at the time of EVAR placement and in the early postprocedure period, although they can develop later. These represent a continued risk for aneurysm rupture, and treatment generally is mandated. Initial treatment of either type Ia or Ib endoleaks usually consists of balloon angioplasty. If that fails, type Ia endoleaks can be treated with placement of a proximal aortic cuff or Palmaz stent (Cordis Corporation, Miami

Lakes, FL), and type Ib endoleaks can be remedied by deploying an iliac extension limb.

Type II Endoleak

Type II endoleaks are frequent, can be seen at any point after EVAR, and affect up to 30% of EVAR patients. Type II endoleak results from persistent retrograde blood flow into the aneurysm sac secondary to branch vessels of the infrarenal abdominal aorta, usually the inferior mesenteric artery or patent lumbar arteries (see Figure 2). Their management remains controversial. Many surgeons approach these endoleaks using a conservative approach because 60% to 80% will resolve spontaneously and permanently, only 1% are associated with aneurysm sac enlargement, and the presence of a type II endoleak does not alter survival at 48 months. For those type II endoleaks that are apparent immediately at the time of the procedure, the discontinuation of anticoagulation at the end of the procedure frequently will cause a spontaneous resolution of the leak. However, persistent type II endoleaks, defined as those lasting for more than 6 months, may require reintervention, as they are associated with a significantly higher rate of sac expansion and are a significant predictor of rupture. In addition, treatment is indicated for symptoms (abdominal or back pain) or in the setting of continued aneurysm growth. Interventions range from embolization to open exploration with ligation of the culprit vessel (Figure 4).

Type III Endoleak

Blood flow through a tear or rupture in the fabric of the graft or flow between separated components of the graft causes a type III endoleak (see Figures 2 and 5). The natural history of continued aneurysm sac growth and increased risk for rupture is similar to that of type I endoleak, necessitating an intervention. Treatment entails the placement of a cuff or relining the stent-graft using a new stent within the stent-graft to cover the tear in the fabric. Devices such as the Renu (Cook Medical, Bloomington, IN) are designed specifically to address this type of endoleak and involve placement of an aortouniiliac limb with contralateral common iliac artery embolization and femoral-femoral bypass (see Figure 9).

Type IV Endoleak

Type IV endoleak, a rather rare finding, especially in contemporary stent-graft devices, is the passage of blood through the graft fabric

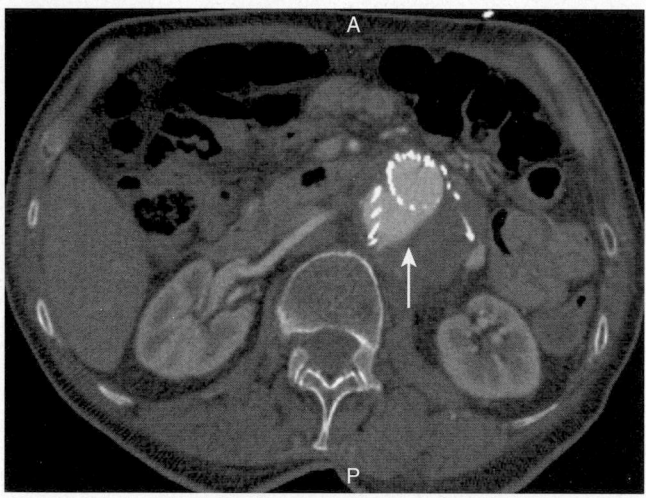

FIGURE 3 Type Ia (proximal) endoleak (*arrow*) originating from the superior seal zone of an abdominal endograft.

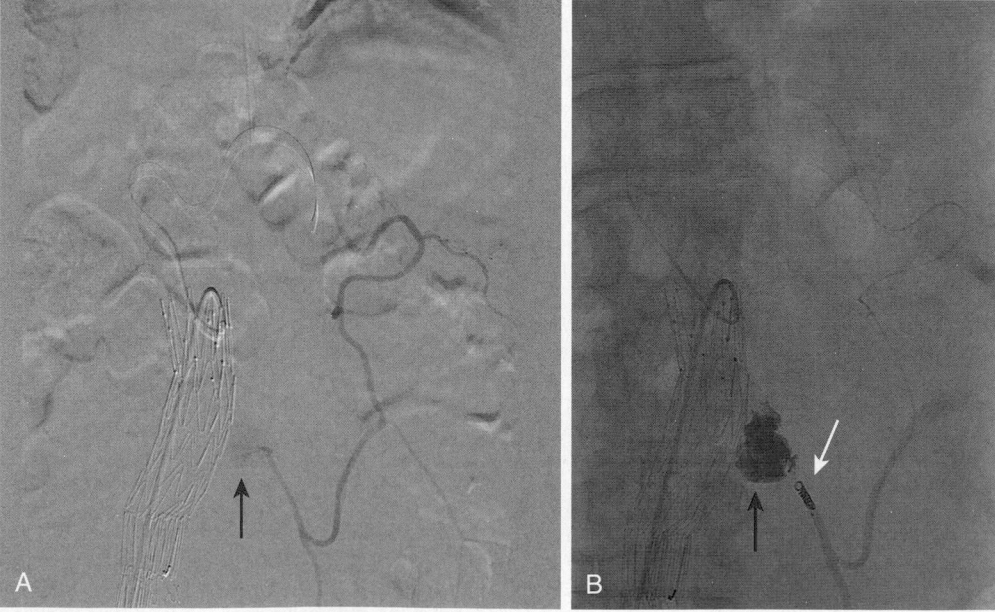

FIGURE 4 Type II endoleak from the inferior mesenteric artery (IMA). **A,** Angiogram performed via selective catheter placement in the superior mesenteric artery demonstrates blush (*arrow*) at the ostium of the IMA feeding an enlarging abdominal aortic aneurysm sac. **B,** Coil embolization of the endoleak using Onyx glue (red arrow) and coil embolization (*white arrow*) of the IMA.

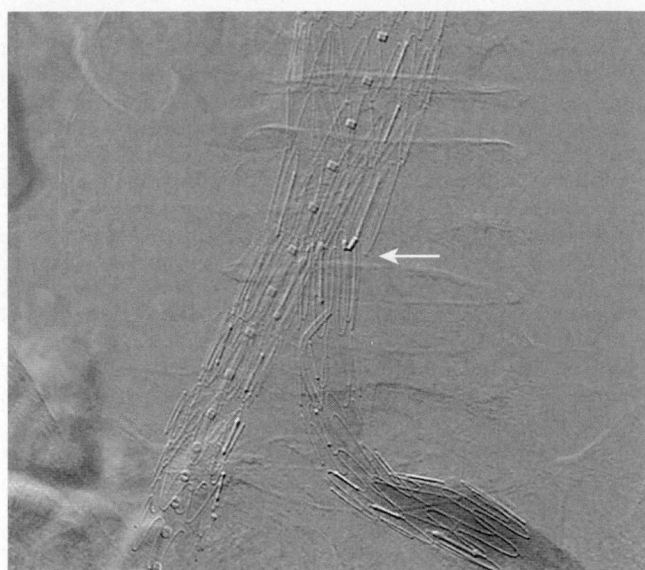

FIGURE 5 Type III endoleak from component separation at the junction of the iliac limb and contralateral gate (*arrow*).

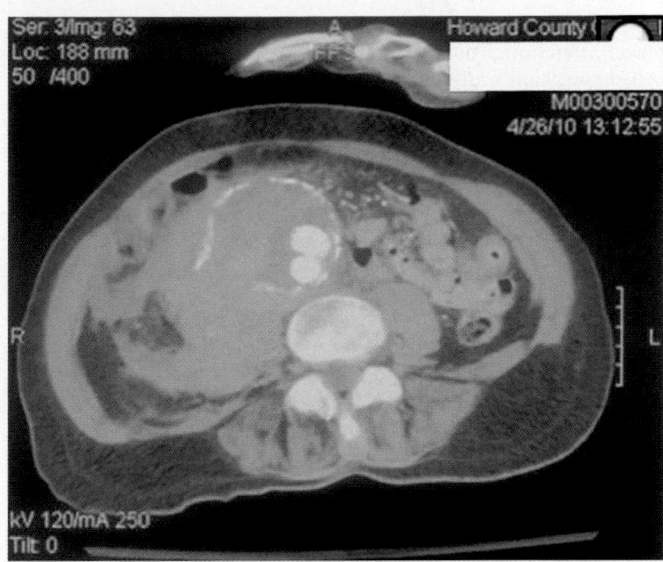

FIGURE 6 Abdominal aortic aneurysm (AAA) rupture in a patient previously treated with endovascular aneurysm repair (EVAR) seen with Type V endoleak, which had been followed for 2 years for ongoing AAA sac growth without definable focal endoleak. This patient then was seen with acute onset of abdominal and back pain after experiencing several weeks of flank pain and malaise and computed tomographic angiography demonstrated AAA rupture. The patient was successfully converted to open AAA repair.

and is related to the graft's porosity (see Figure 2). It is most apparent in fully anticoagulated patients and, as with type II endoleak, often will resolve once the anticoagulation has been discontinued. Type IV endoleak was mostly seen with the earlier generation Excluder device, which has higher porosity graft fabric, but this problem has been solved in later versions of the graft.

Type V Endoleak (Endotension)

Type V endoleak, more commonly called endotension, refers to persistently elevated intra-aneurysmal sac pressure in the absence of an endoleak on delayed contrast CT scan. A number of theories exist to explain the etiology of endotension, which underscores the uncertainty surrounding this phenomenon and the appropriate methods of diagnosing and treating it. For example, it has been proposed that endotension results from endoleak that is so slow in nature as to be invisible to current radiographic techniques. Others advocate that aneurysm growth results from pressure transmitted across a thrombus, whether the thrombus is within occluded vessels that communicate with the sac or a clot that sits between the aortic wall and the stent-graft. Patients with Type V endoleak need to be followed closely with surveillance imaging, as this condition predisposes to rupture risk (Figure 6).

Graft Occlusion

Stent-graft occlusion, whether by limb thrombosis or kinking of the stent, may be seen with buttock, thigh, or calf claudication; rest pain; or acute ischemia. According to one prospective series conducted over 10 years, limb occlusion occurred in 3.1% of EVAR cases. This study looked exclusively at supported stent-grafts, though the incidence of limb occlusion is known to be significantly higher—as high as 44%—in unsupported grafts. Most of these events occur in the intraoperative and early postoperative period, although graft kinking and thrombosis can occur years after EVAR. The fact that many of these problems were observed and subsequently managed at the time of the procedure underscores the importance of completion angiography to ensure limb patency and to avoid a return to the endovascular suite or operating room in the postoperative period. Contributing factors include pre-existing iliac artery stenosis, heavily angulated vessels, and tortuous anatomy. Small iliac arteries are a recognized risk factor for limb occlusion, which may explain why women are at an increased risk for this complication.

As with many of the complications of this emerging technology, no consensus exists as to the optimal treatment for stent-graft limb

occlusion or thrombosis. A variety of approaches have been used, including further stent placement to provide support to the iliac limbs, pharmacologic or mechanical thrombolysis, and angioplasty. Surgical approaches include femoral-femoral bypass, axillary-femoral bypass, axillary-bifemoral bypass, or surgical thrombectomy. Care needs to be taken when performing thrombectomy, as this may result in damage to the stent-graft, component separation, or stent-graft migration.

Ischemic Complications

The recognized ischemic complications of EVAR result from one or a combination of several possible mechanisms: direct vessel occlusion by the stent-graft or occlusion of the stent-graft itself, atheroembolic events during catheter manipulation or device deployment, and inadequate collateralization of the mesenteric or pelvic circulation.

Pelvic Ischemia

Pelvic ischemia broadly refers to a range of ischemic complications: sexual dysfunction, buttock claudication or necrosis, and colon ischemia or infarction. These complicate 2% to 3% of EVARs. Sexual dysfunction, likely an under-reported complication of EVAR, has been reported to be as high as 82% after EVAR (from a preoperative baseline incidence of 74%); however, this is not different from open AAA repair, and both groups tended to return to their baseline after approximately 3 months. Buttock ischemia can be seen as claudication or frank necrosis of the skin and muscle. Claudication occurs in as many as one third of patients who have internal iliac artery embolization of occlusion during EVAR. Typically this is managed conservatively, as most cases improve with time. Although exceedingly rare, the presence of myonecrosis requires prompt recognition, surgical débridement, and institution of renal protective mechanisms.

Mesenteric Ischemia

In the DREAM trial, patients were randomized to either EVAR or open AAA repair, and colon ischemia was a rare event in both groups (0.6% and 1.1%, respectively), with no significant difference between the two approaches. The severity can range from ischemic colitis to bowel infarction. The former can be managed with bowel rest and broad-spectrum antibiotics, whereas the latter requires colectomy. Patients may have diarrhea, rectal bleeding, leukocytosis, hypotension, fever, sepsis, or multisystem organ failure. Because the mortality rate is exceedingly high (>50%), any suspicion of colon ischemia mandates early endoscopic evaluation, close monitoring, serial laboratory testing and abdominal examinations, and a low threshold for operative intervention.

Spinal Cord Ischemia

Spinal cord ischemia, which can result in paraplegia, is a dreaded complication of aortic aneurysm repair. Patients can have a variety of neurologic symptoms, from urinary or fecal incontinence, to sensory or motor deficits, to frank paralysis. Proposed etiologies include intraprocedural and postprocedural hypotension, prolonged deployment that causes temporary aortic occlusion, poor collateral blood flow of the spinal cord, disruption of the pelvic circulation, and embolic events. Open surgical repair is associated with a 0.25% rate of paraplegia, and analysis of the Eurostar database of patients who underwent EVAR reveals a comparable rate of 0.21%.

Renal Insufficiency and Renal Artery Occlusion

Postoperative renal insufficiency is a common complication of open AAA repair, occurring in more than 10% of cases according to one large, population-based study. Postoperative renal insufficiency is a problem that plagues EVAR as well. Greenberg and colleagues reported that patients undergoing EVAR using suprarenal fixation of the graft had an attenuated rise in serum creatinine at the time of discharge compared with patients undergoing open repair, but following those patients out to 12 months revealed no difference in serum creatinine based on the operative approach undertaken. There tends to be a 10% decline in creatinine clearance at 1 year post-EVAR. The exact etiology of this phenomenon is unknown, but it has prompted some to recommend minimization of preprocedure and postprocedure contrast-enhanced radiographic studies, alternative radiographic studies that do not utilize contrast when feasible, the institution of measures to mitigate contrast-induced nephropathy, and minimization of the amount of contrast utilized during EVAR.

Renal artery occlusion by the stent-graft at the time of the operation is a technical error and should be caught at the latest by the end of the operation when a completion angiogram is performed (Figure 7); however, a more nuanced discussion is warranted in the

case of accessory renal arteries and late renal artery occlusion. Accessory renal arteries are a frequent anatomic variant, being present in more than 15% of the population. Some clinicians are reluctant to offer EVAR to patients with accessory renal arteries for fear of causing segmental renal infarction and a subsequent decline in renal function, as well as creating a possible source of endoleak. It would be unfortunate to deny such a large subset of the population the benefits of EVAR, but the long-term effects of accessory renal artery coverage are unknown. Karmacharya and colleagues reviewed their experience with EVAR in this patient population and found that an accessory renal artery was not implicated in any of their endoleaks. In follow-up, 20% of the patients who had accessory renal arteries had renal infarcts found on CT imaging; however, they did not observe any long-term effect on patients' blood pressure, serum creatinine, or creatinine clearance. The mean follow-up for these patients was 16 months. These findings suggest that patients with this frequent anatomic variant still can be candidates for EVAR; however, these results must be interpreted with caution given the known decline in renal function as part of the normal aging process and the relatively frequent use of contrast-enhanced imaging for surveillance in these patients.

Late Complications

Late conversion to open repair is infrequently necessary after EVAR, required in 1.6% of patients in a cohort of more than 1600 EVAR procedures performed at the Cleveland Clinic. Late conversion may be necessary in the event of persistent endoleaks refractory to embolization attempts, endotension, migration, rupture, aortoenteric fistula, infection, or limb thrombosis or stenosis. There are a variety of other conditions that can occur after EVAR that may require a secondary surgical intervention. As mentioned previously, a variety of surgical bypass options exist for graft limb occlusion that cannot be managed utilizing an endovascular approach. Clinically significant renal artery narrowing, whether by graft migration or atherosclerotic disease, may require aortorenal or iliorenal bypass, though the need for this is relatively uncommon.

Because the most important objective of aortic aneurysm repair is the prevention of sac rupture, late rupture of the aneurysm, defined as rupture at least 30 days after EVAR, represents absolute treatment failure. The prospectively collected EUROSTAR Registry demonstrated a 1% per year rate of late rupture, with a nearly 60% associated mortality rate. Type I and type III endoleaks are significant risk factors for late rupture, underscoring the importance of expeditiously treating these findings. Stent-graft migration and endograft kinking are also risk factors. Late rupture occurs at a median of 20 months post-EVAR. The most common symptoms are abdominal or back pain, hypovolemia and hypotension, syncope, and shock.

Infections involving aortic stent-grafts are not well described in the literature and fortunately are a rare occurrence (Figure 8). Vogel and colleagues reported 2-year rates of graft infection of 0.2%, irrespective of an open or endovascular approach to aneurysm repair based on data from a large administrative database. A different group reported an incidence of graft-related sepsis in EVAR of 6.2 per 1000 person-years. Advanced age and an immunocompromised state are likely risk factors. An additional possible risk factor for aortic stent-graft infection that is relevant to the EVAR population is the need for secondary endovascular interventions, such as coil embolization, which as mentioned earlier is rather common. Aortoenteric fistula (AEF) is a dreaded complication of aortic surgery. Classically, these patients have upper gastrointestinal bleeding, and the presence of AEF can often be confirmed with esophagogastroduodenoscopy. A number of mechanisms for this fistulization process have been proposed: continued aneurysm growth secondary to endoleak, inflammatory aortic aneurysm, inflammatory bowel disease, graft migration or erosion, and injury to bowel from fixation hooks. Treatment involves graft excision, aortic reconstruction, and bowel resection and reanastomosis.

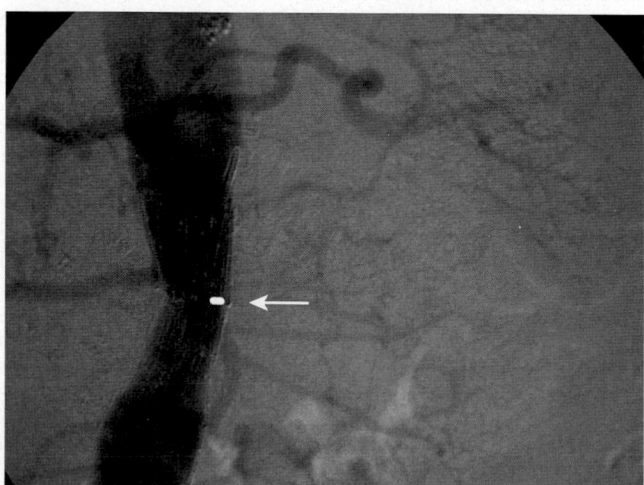

FIGURE 7 Inadvertent coverage of the left renal artery during endovascular aneurysm repair (EVAR). Completion angiogram demonstrated nonfilling of the left renal artery ostium (*arrow*) after EVAR.

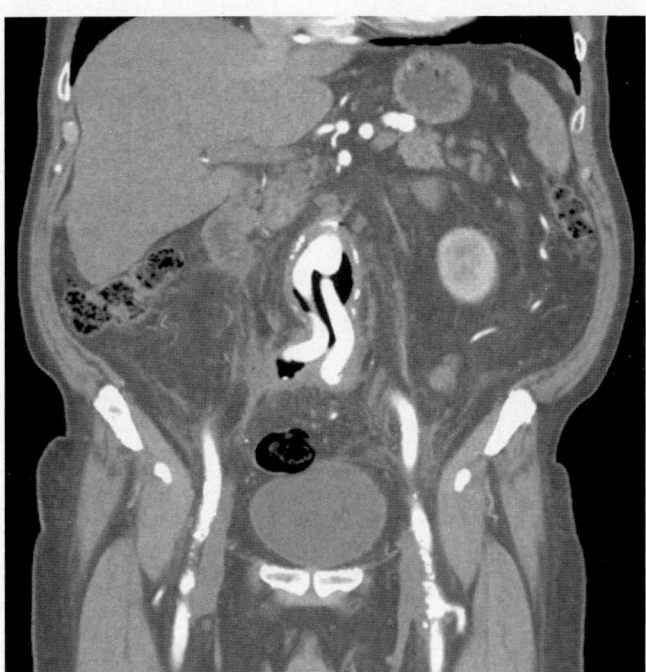

FIGURE 8 Infected abdominal aortic aneurysm (AAA) graft with air and stranding around the graft.

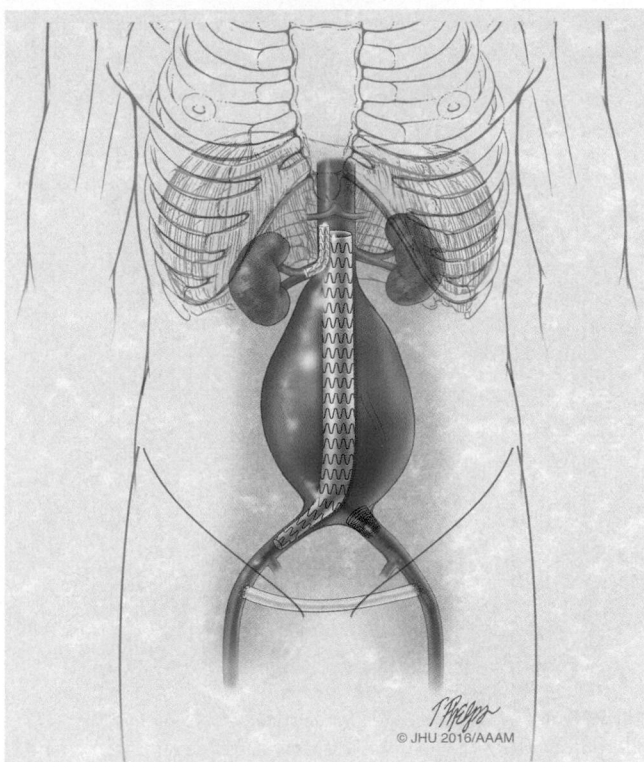

© JHU 2016/AAAM

FIGURE 9 Depiction of a snorkel and chimney technique utilized to maintain flow to the right renal artery using a covered stent placed in parallel to an aortic endograft, in this case an aortouniiliac graft with contralateral common iliac artery embolization and femoral-femoral bypass.

■ COMPLEX AND FENESTRATED ENDOVASCULAR ANEURYSM REPAIR TECHNOLOGY

Over the past decade, EVAR techniques have been expanded to facilitate repair of juxtarenal, pararenal, and even suprarenal AAAs that do not meet IFU for repair using conventional EVAR devices. Up to 40% of patients with AAA do not have anatomy acceptable for performing EVAR because of short neck length or involvement of visceral vessels. In these patients, open AAA repair traditionally has been considered the only option for repair. However, many patients have significant comorbidities precluding safe open AAA repair. The chimney and snorkel techniques use existing on-the-shelf endovascular technology available in most centers and allow preservation of flow to important visceral aortic branches while moving the seal zone proximally into the visceral segment of the abdominal aorta. Similarly, fenestrated EVAR is an FDA-approved technology and allows preservation of flow to visceral vessels through side fenestrations or scallops in the fabric of the main body of the graft, although these grafts require custom ordering and fabrication. These techniques can facilitate EVAR in patients who are unsuitable for open AAA repair.

Snorkel and Chimney Techniques

The chimney and snorkel techniques are achieved by placing covered stents in the renal arteries, and possibly the superior mesenteric and celiac arteries and directing these stents in parallel to an aortic stent graft. Stents most commonly used for the visceral vessels in this technique include the Viabahn (W. L. Gore & Associates, Flagstaff, AZ) and the iCast (Atrium Medical Corp., Hudson, NH). These stents are introduced from a transbrachial or transaxillary approach and deployed partially inside the visceral target vessels with extension into the aortic lumen in a cephalad orientation. An aortic stent-graft then is introduced via iliofemoral access and expanded in parallel against the visceral stents. The stents are oriented such that the visceral stents emerge at the same level as the aortic stent (Figure 9). Aortic devices that have been utilized for this technique include the Endurant, Zenith, and Excluder.

The PERICLES Registry collected the world experience with chimney and snorkel EVAR for patients with juxtarenal or suprarenal AAA at high risk for open AAA repair and published the results of these techniques in a 517-patient cohort. The average proximal aortic neck length in this registry was 4.8 mm. The utilization of the chimney and snorkel techniques allowed an increase in the seal zone at the neck by an average of 21.1 mm. This procedure was demonstrated to have acceptable 30-day mortality of 4.9%; when patients with ruptured AAA were excluded, the 30-day mortality was 3.7%.

Fenestrated Endovascular Aneurysm Repair Technology

Endograft technology also has been developed with fenestrations to accommodate and preserve flow to visceral arteries. Similar to the chimney and snorkel technique, the fenestrated technique allows proximal extension of the seal zone into nonaneurysmal visceral aorta. This technique increasingly has been utilized to repair juxtarenal AAA in patients who are unsuitable for conventional EVAR or open AAA repair. The Zenith Fenestrated device (Cook Medical, Bloomington, IN) is an FDA-approved device that is customized to a specific patient's anatomy and consists of bilateral renal artery fenestrations and a scallop at the superior margin of the graft fabric for the superior mesenteric artery to incorporate the visceral aorta into the seal zone (Figure 10). IFU criteria require an infrarenal neck measuring 4 to 15 mm in length. Performing fenestrated EVAR with this device requires a significant degree of preoperative planning using TeraRecon in order to precisely place fenestrations and scallops in the graft fabric to accommodate the visceral vessels. In addition, the device takes 4 to 6 weeks for custom fabrication and therefore is not available for urgent treatment of symptomatic or ruptured AAA.

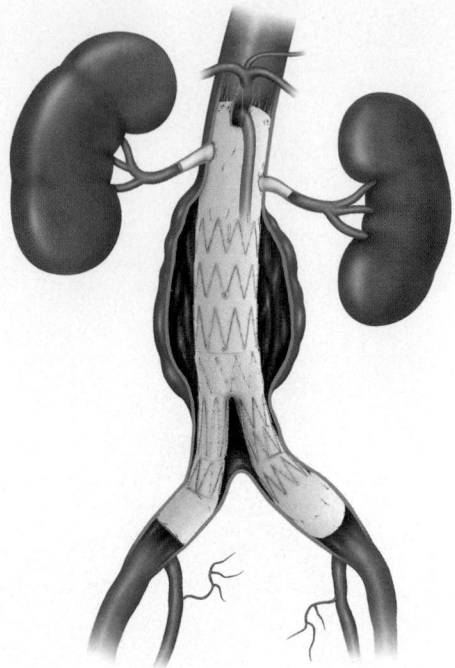

FIGURE 10 Zenith Fenestrated aortic endograft (Cook Medical, Bloomington, IN) with bilateral renal artery fenestrations, covered renal artery stents, and a superior mesenteric artery scallop.

Published results from a prospectively enrolled cohort of patients who underwent fenestrated EVAR using the Zenith Fenestrated device demonstrated excellent results, with technical success of 100%, mean hospital length of stay of 3.3 days, type I endoleak in 1.5%, renal stent patency of 97%, with 30-day mortality of 1.5%, and 5-year survival of 91%. These results demonstrate that this procedure can be performed safely in appropriately selected patients with results comparable with conventional EVAR. With time, this technology will increase in use and become more broadly available for mainstream application.

SUGGESTED READINGS

Chaikof EL, Brewster DC, Dalman RL, Makaroun MS, Illig KA, Sicard GA, Timaran CH, Upchurch GR, Veith FJ. The care of patients with an abdominal aortic aneurysm: The Society for Vascular Surgery practice guidelines. *J Vasc Surg.* 2012;50(suppl 4):S2-S49.

De Bruin JL, Baas AF, Buth J, Prinssen M, Verhoeven EL, Cuypers PW, van Sambeek MR, Balm R, Grobbee DE, Blankensteijn JD. DREAM Study Group. Long-term outcome of open or endovascular repair of abdominal aortic aneurysm. *N Engl J Med.* 2010;362:1881-1889.

Donas KP, Lee JT, Lachat M, Torsello G, Veith FJ. Collected world experience about the performance of the snorkel/chimney endovascular technique in the treatment of complex aortic pathologies. *Ann Surg.* 2015;262:546-553.

Greenberg RK, Chuter TA, Lawrence-Brown M, Haulon S, Nolte L. Analysis of renal function after aneurysm repair with a device using suprarenal fixation (Zenith AAA Endovascular Graft) in contrast to open surgical repair. *J Vasc Surg.* 2004;39:1219-1228.

Greenhalgh RM, Brown LC, Powell JT, Thompson SG, Epstein D, Sculpher MJ, United Kingdom EVAR Trial Investigators. Endovascular versus open repair of abdominal aortic aneurysm. *N Engl J Med.* 2010;362:1863-1871.

Karmacharya J, Parmer SS, Antezana JN, Fairman RM, Woo EY, Velazquez OC, et al. Outcomes of accessory renal artery occlusion during endovascular aneurysm repair. *J Vasc Surg.* 2006;43:8-13.

Kelso RL, Lyden SP, Butler B, Greenberg RK, Eagleton MJ, Clair DG. Late conversion of aortic stent grafts. *J Vasc Surg.* 2009;49:589-595.

Lederle FA, Freischlag JA, Kyriakides TC, Padberg FT Jr, Matsumura JS, Kohler TR, Lin PH, Jean-Claude JM, Cikrit DF, Swanson KM, Peduzzi PN, Open Versus Endovascular Repair (OVER) Veterans Affairs Cooperative Study Group. Outcomes following endovascular vs open repair of abdominal aortic aneurysm: a randomized trial. *JAMA.* 2009;302:1535-1542.

Lee AW. Endovascular abdominal aortic aneurysm sizing and case planning using the TeraRecon Aquarius workstation. *Vasc Endovasc Surg.* 2007;41:61-67.

Oderich GS, Greenberg RK, Farber M, Lyden S, Sanchez L, Fairman R, Jia F, Bharadwaj P. Results of the United States multicenter prospective study evaluating the Zenith fenestrated endovascular graft for treatment of juxtarenal abdominal aortic aneurysms. *J Vasc Surg.* 2014;60:1420-1428.

Schanzer A, Greenberg RK, Hevelone N, Robinson WP, Eslami MH, Goldberg RJ, Messina L. Predictors of abdominal aortic aneurysm sac enlargement after endovascular repair. *Circulation.* 2011;123:2848-2855.

Vogel TR, Symons R, Flum DR. The incidence and factors associated with graft infection after aortic aneurysm repair. *J Vasc Surg.* 2008;47:264-269.

THE MANAGEMENT OF RUPTURED ABDOMINAL AORTIC ANEURYSM

Patrick J. Phelan, MD, and K. Craig Kent, MD

Rupture of an abdominal aortic aneurysm (AAA) is a catastrophic event, with a mortality of 80% to 90%. Two thirds of these individuals die before reaching a hospital and many more before reaching the operating room. For individuals with rupture who are treated surgically, mortality has diminished over the past decade from approximately 50% to 30%. The cost associated with treating ruptured aneurysms is staggering, with the average expense exceeding that of elective repair by more than $90,000. Over the past two decades there has been increased emphasis on screening with the goal of identifying large, asymptomatic aneurysms that can be treated electively. The risk factors for AAA have been well established; the three most prominent are age, male gender, and smoking. Several countries, including the United States and the United Kingdom, have screening policies. In the United States, Medicare offers screening to ever-smoking males age 65 to 75 years. The incidence of rupture is decreasing; this may be related partially to screening but more likely is the result of lower rates of smoking.

▪ PRESENTATION

The classic triad of symptoms and findings for ruptured AAA includes hypotension, abdominal or back pain, and a pulsatile abdominal mass. This triad is moderately specific but highly insensitive for the diagnosis of a ruptured AAA. Abdominal, back, or flank pain in any patient with a known aneurysm should warrant a thorough investigation for rupture. Nevertheless, aneurysms can produce a wide array of symptoms, including duodenal obstruction, gastrointestinal hemorrhage with erosion into the gastrointestinal tract, femoral neuropathy, dysuria, congestive heart failure with an aortocaval fistula, and many others. Symptoms usually are related to pressure from a gradually or rapidly expanding aneurysm. With rupture (rather than slow expansion) pain is typically severe and unrelenting. Abdominal, back, or flank pain commonly radiates to the pelvis or groins. Nevertheless, at times the only manifestation of rupture is shock. Diagnosing a ruptured aneurysm can be difficult, particularly

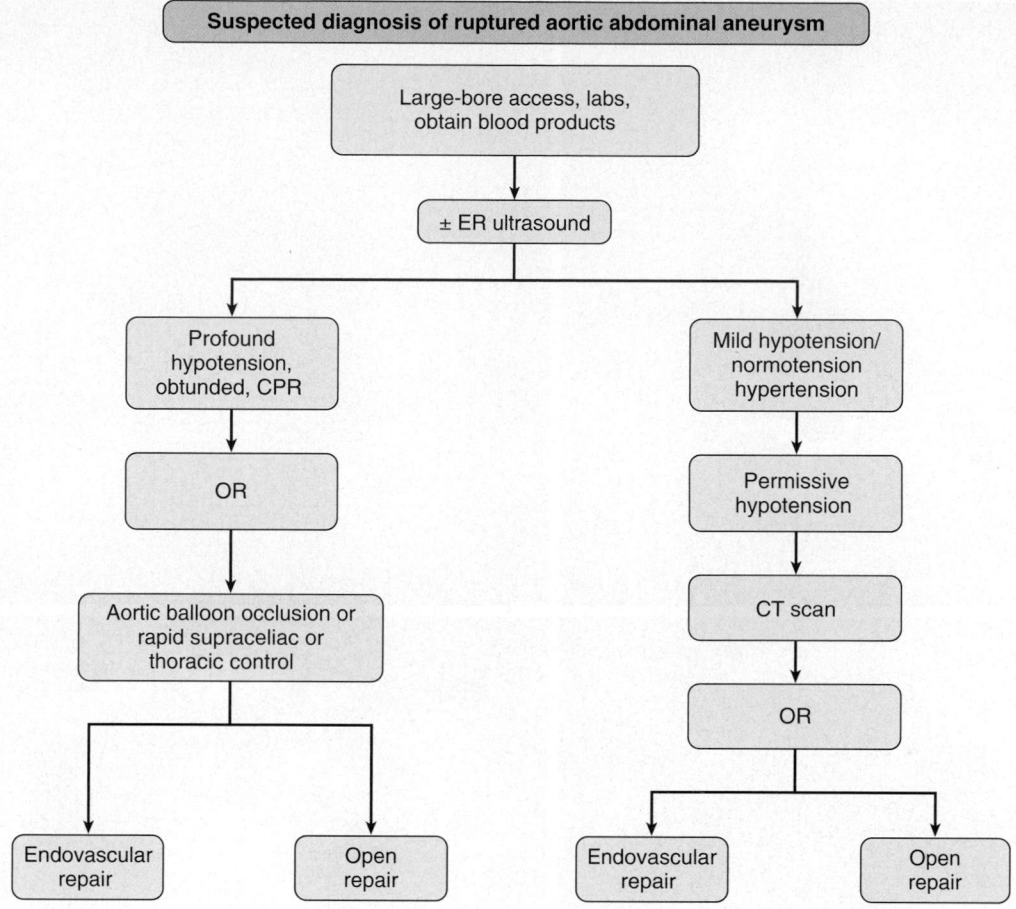

FIGURE 1 Algorithm for suspected diagnosis of ruptured aortic abdominal aneurysm. *CT,* Computed tomography; *OR,* operating room.

for a physician without vascular training. However, a history of an aneurysm or a pulsatile abdominal mass in a patient with new onset of any symptoms should prompt a rapid evaluation for rupture.

INITIAL MANAGEMENT

If the diagnosis of ruptured AAA is suspected, management must be expeditious (Figure 1). Patients who die before reaching medical attention most often experience free rupture of the aneurysm into the peritoneal cavity with profound hypotension followed by death. Those who reach medical attention likely have achieved some degree of tamponade. The stability of this tamponade, however, is unpredictable. Free rupture always could be seconds away. Alternatively many ruptured aneurysms remain stable for significant periods of time. This uncertainty makes the acute management of these patients challenging. One of the goals of early management is to minimize further hemorrhage through permissive hypotension. Large-bore venous access should be obtained. Fluid resuscitation should be gauged to produce systolic blood pressures in the 80 to 100 mm Hg range with the goal of maintaining consciousness and preventing myocardial and renal ischemia but without normotension or hypertension that may propagate further hemorrhage. The drugs associated with intubation result in the interruption of sympathetic tone, which can hasten cardiopulmonary collapse. Consequently, intubation should be avoided in patients who can protect their airway until aortic control is imminent. Patients who are unstable should be taken directly to the operating room, even if the diagnosis is not confirmed. If there is time and an accessible scanner and expertise, an expeditious ultrasound can be obtained in the emergency room so that the presence of abdominal aortic aneurysm can be confirmed. A computed tomography angiogram (CTA) is extremely useful not only for

diagnosis but also for operative planning. Periaortic stranding on a computed tomography (CT) scan suggests rupture or impending rupture, whereas a retroperitoneal hematoma or contrast extravasation confirms that rupture has occurred (Figure 2). If open surgery is being contemplated, a CT scan will identify the location of the proximal neck and extent of the aneurysm including iliac involvement, as well as the presence or absence of occlusive disease in the mesenteric, renal, or iliac circulation. This information will help with determining the location of the incision and the arteries that require treatment. A CT scan also will determine if an endovascular approach can be used and, if so, the dimensions of the graft to be used. One of the most dreaded outcomes for a patient with a ruptured aneurysm is to expire in the CT scanner. Thus a patient who is persistently hypotensive despite active resuscitation should be taken directly to the operating room without further imaging. Alternatively, if a patient is stable at the time of presentation or has achieved stability after resuscitation, a CT scan should be performed. A final caveat is that patients with severe abdominal, back, or flank pain and a large aneurysm without CT evidence of rupture should be presumed to have impending rupture and taken for expeditious repair. The only exception would be in a patient for whom another definitive source of pain has been identified.

PREPARATION FOR OPERATION

Once the patient is in the operating room, permissive hypotension is maintained until proximal aortic control is obtained. A high level of communication is required between the surgical, anesthesia, and nursing teams. It is important for these teams to work in parallel: anesthesia placing an arterial line and central access, surgeons positioning the patient and prepping, nursing preparing the necessary

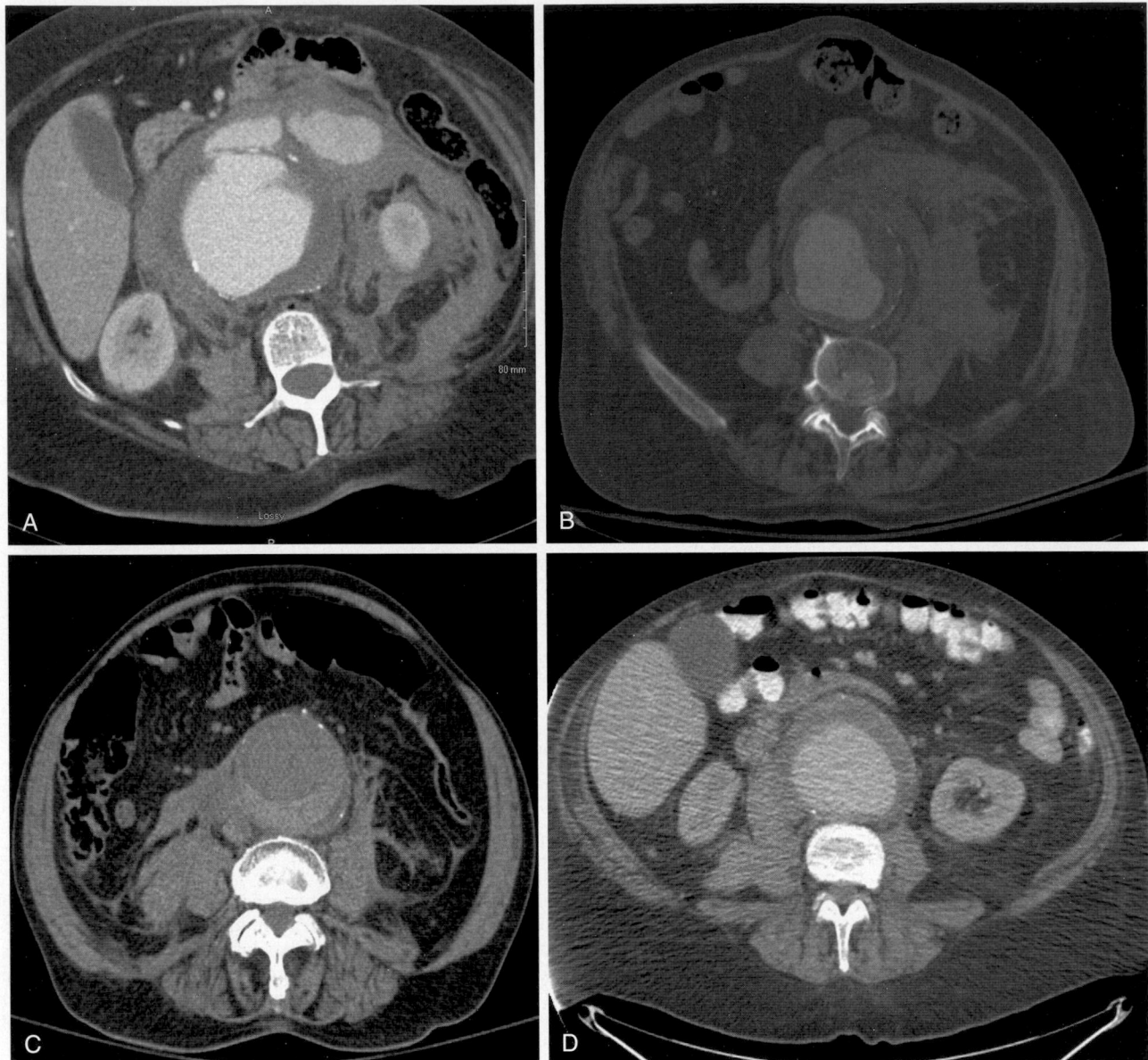

FIGURE 2 Computed tomographic (CT) imaging of ruptured abdominal aortic aneurysm: **A,** Free rupture. **B,** Retroperitoneal stranding. **C,** Crescent sign on noncontrast CT. **D,** Drape sign with posterior aortic contour "draped" on vertebra.

instrumentation. The operating room should be warm to prevent hypothermia. For open surgery, the timing of intubation is critical; patients should not be intubated until they are completely prepped and draped and the surgical team is ready for incision. Nasogastric tube placement is necessary for open operations because the tube aids in identification of the esophagus if supraceliac aortic control is required. Many of these complexities can be avoided by endovascular repair, which can be performed entirely under local anesthesia.

OPEN VERSUS ENDOVASCULAR REPAIR

Endovascular stent grafts have revolutionized the repair of elective aortic aneurysms. In the United States, endovascular aneurysm repair (EVAR) has become the standard of care for nonruptured aortic aneurysms with appropriate anatomy. This technology also has been applied to ruptured aneurysms with significant enthusiasm. There are numerous theoretical advantages of endovascular repair, including the ability to intervene without a general anesthetic. The aneurysm can be repaired without relieving abdominal tamponade, and

thus stability is maintained throughout the intervention. Fluid shifts, temperature changes, and the ileus associated with a laparotomy can be avoided.

Despite these theoretical advantages, the superiority of EVAR versus open repair has been difficult to demonstrate. There are numerous single-institutional series, meta-analyses, and analyses of administrative databases that have shown the superiority of EVAR in the prevention of early mortality in patients with ruptured aneurysms. However, three randomized controlled trials (RCTs) have failed to confirm an advantage of EVAR in patients with rupture. The difference in these findings may be related to a selection process that is inherent in nonrandomized studies. For example, in practice more stable patients may be offered EVAR and those with less stability treated with open repair. Also patients with more favorable anatomy likely will be offered EVAR, and those with more complex anatomy will be subject to open repair. IMPROVE, the largest of these RCTs, did demonstrate a shortened hospital stay with EVAR but no improvement in mortality. A large retrospective study of prospectively collected data from National Surgical Quality Improvement Program (NSQIP) demonstrated a substantial mortality benefit for EVAR versus open surgery for patients with unstable ruptured aneurysms (36% vs 53%) (Kent). This benefit was similar with regard to myocardial infarction (19% vs 29%), renal failure (13% vs 19%), and respiratory failure (36% vs 45%). Unfortunately, NSQIP data do not provide the level of anatomic detail to analyze how physicians selected EVAR versus open surgery. Undeterred by the conflicting data, some practitioners have advocated a dramatically broadened approach to endovascular management of ruptured aortic aneurysm, including the use of adjuncts, such as snorkels, periscopes, and fenestrations, for difficult anatomy. Despite the controversy and uncertain data, the role of endovascular techniques in treatment of ruptured aneurysms is certain to expand. Level of preparedness and expertise play a significant role. Centers that have appropriate imaging, endovascular teams, a broad array of grafts, as well as surgeons with significant experience are well positioned to achieve favorable outcomes with EVAR. Alternatively, in centers without this expertise, open repair may remain a better alternative.

■ OPERATIVE TECHNIQUE

Proximal Aortic Control

A successful outcome with a ruptured aneurysm hinges on timely and effective cessation of hemorrhage, achieved through proximal aortic control. Several strategies, open and endovascular, can be employed. A CTA can guide the decision regarding the type of repair and the design of the graft to be used. A CT also informs the operating surgeon of the options for proximal aortic control.

If open repair is planned, in most circumstances after laparotomy rapid control of the supraceliac aorta should be gained. This is particularly important in an unstable patient or if there is a large retroperitoneal hematoma that extends to the base of the mesentery. A midline incision is made from xiphoid to pubis without entering the peritoneal cavity. The peritoneum then is incised and the left hepatic lobe mobilized and retracted to the right. The stomach is retracted firmly inferiorly and to the right, placing the gastrohepatic ligament on tension. This ligament then is divided, taking care to avoid injury to the left gastric artery. The esophagus is identified anterior to the aorta by palpation of the nasogastric tube and retracted leftward, and the right crux is divided to allow access to the aorta. A finger is advanced along each side of the aorta until the spine is palpated. An aortic clamp then is slid in place using the fingers as a guide. Control at this level is lifesaving but results in visceral ischemia, and thus the clamp should be moved distally as soon as possible. An alternative to the full dissection is to use an aortic occluder, which is an instrument that blindly places pressure on the supraceliac aorta. In an extremely unstable patient who develops free hemorrhage once the peritoneum has been incised, this approach can be lifesaving. In a relatively stable patient in whom the hematoma does not extend up to the base of the mesentery, the initial clamp can be placed on the infrarenal aorta; however, it is important not to enter and decompress the hematoma. This exposure usually is confined to ruptures that are more distal and/or involve the iliac arteries. If retroperitoneal exposure is performed hastily or blindly, in the presence of acute hemorrhage, there is risk of damaging the duodenum, vena cava, or the left renal vein.

In rare circumstances an anterolateral thoracotomy will allow the most expeditious proximal control. An incision is made to the fifth interspace, the lung is retracted cephalad, the spine is palpated posteriorly, and the pleura is divided. A nasogastric tube facilitates identification of the esophagus, and the aorta is finger dissected anteriorly and posteriorly. Manual pressure can be applied until there is definitive control. This technique allows for control of the aorta before opening of the abdomen and release of the tamponade. This approach should be used rarely because the cost is an additional incision, violation of the thoracic cavity with pulmonary consequences, and often a prolonged supraceliac clamp.

Endovascular balloon occlusion of the suprarenal aorta is an option for proximal control before either open or endovascular repair. Percutaneous access of the common femoral artery is obtained

through the groin. After placement of a stiff wire, a 12F to 14F sheath is inserted into the proximal aneurysm. An aortic balloon (usually compliant) then is inserted through the sheath, centered in the neck above the aneurysm, and inflated until proximal control is obtained. Unfortunately, these balloons are often occlusive of the renal and mesenteric circulation and thus should be left in place for the least amount of time possible. In open operations, the balloon should be replaced with an infrarenal clamp once the proximal neck is exposed. In endovascular repairs, the balloon is deflated once the main body of the graft is in place and reintroduced into the main body along an ipsilateral wire, allowing maintenance of proximal control during placement of the contralateral limb (Figure 3).

Open Repair

The general surgical principles are similar for elective and emergent aneurysm repair. For a ruptured aneurysm, the surgeon should attempt to perform the simplest and most efficient adequate repair, thereby minimizing the physiologic insult. When possible, tube grafts are preferred over anastomoses to the iliac or femoral vessels. Treatment of mild to moderate iliac pathology should be deferred. Systemic heparinization should be avoided unless the cross-clamp is prolonged. Alternatively, local heparin administration to the iliac arteries and copious intra-arterial flushing and irrigation can prevent thrombus formation and embolization. Care must be taken when dissecting the proximal and distal necks. A large hematoma can obscure adjacent anatomy, leading to injuries to the vena cava, renal vein, duodenum, and the mesentery of the left colon. Although excessive blood loss is inevitable, this should be minimized by expeditious proximal, distal, and lumbar control. Astute management of blood pressure, fluids, temperature, and blood products by the anesthesiology team is just as critical to patient survival as the skill of the operating surgeon.

When a suprarenal aneurysm is identified preoperatively, a thoracoabdominal approach via a ninth interspace incision greatly facilitates repair. Rapid aortic control is achieved in the descending thoracic aorta before opening the retroperitoneal hematoma. Visceral arteries can be controlled directly, preventing excessive blood loss, and cold renal perfusion can be employed for renal protection. Although a suprarenal aneurysm can be addressed through a midline laparotomy, supraceliac control, and a medial visceral rotation, a thoracoabdominal incision allows for a more expeditious repair.

Endovascular Aneurysm Repair

EVAR is initiated through bilateral groin access. In many institutions, this is performed percutaneously under ultrasound guidance. Preclosure devices are placed so that when sheaths are removed, hemostasis can be achieved without the need for a femoral cut down. In unstable patients, proximal aortic occlusion should be performed through the side contralateral to that chosen for placement of the main body of the graft. An angiogram can be performed with the aortic balloon inflated to delineate the renal arteries and identify the landing zone. Immediately before deployment of the graft, the aortic occlusion balloon is withdrawn to prevent entanglement in the graft's fixation mechanism. The balloon can be reintroduced into the center of the graft via the ipsilateral limb if necessary. The contralateral limb is deployed, and an angiogram then is performed to confirm a complete seal (see Figure 2). Type 1 endoleaks can be ignored occasionally in elective EVAR repair; however, after rupture, a complete proximal and distal seal is essential. As in the open repair, simplicity is optimal. All that is necessary is exclusion of the ruptured portion of the aorta; large iliac arteries or short seal zones can be addressed at a later date. With the appropriate expertise, repair of a juxtarenal or pararenal aneurysm can be undertaken using endovascular techniques. One approach is to modify a traditional graft by creating fenestrations for the renal arteries. Another option is to land the main body of the graft above the renal/mesenteric vessels, bringing in parallel to the main body additional covered stents to maintain patency of the renal

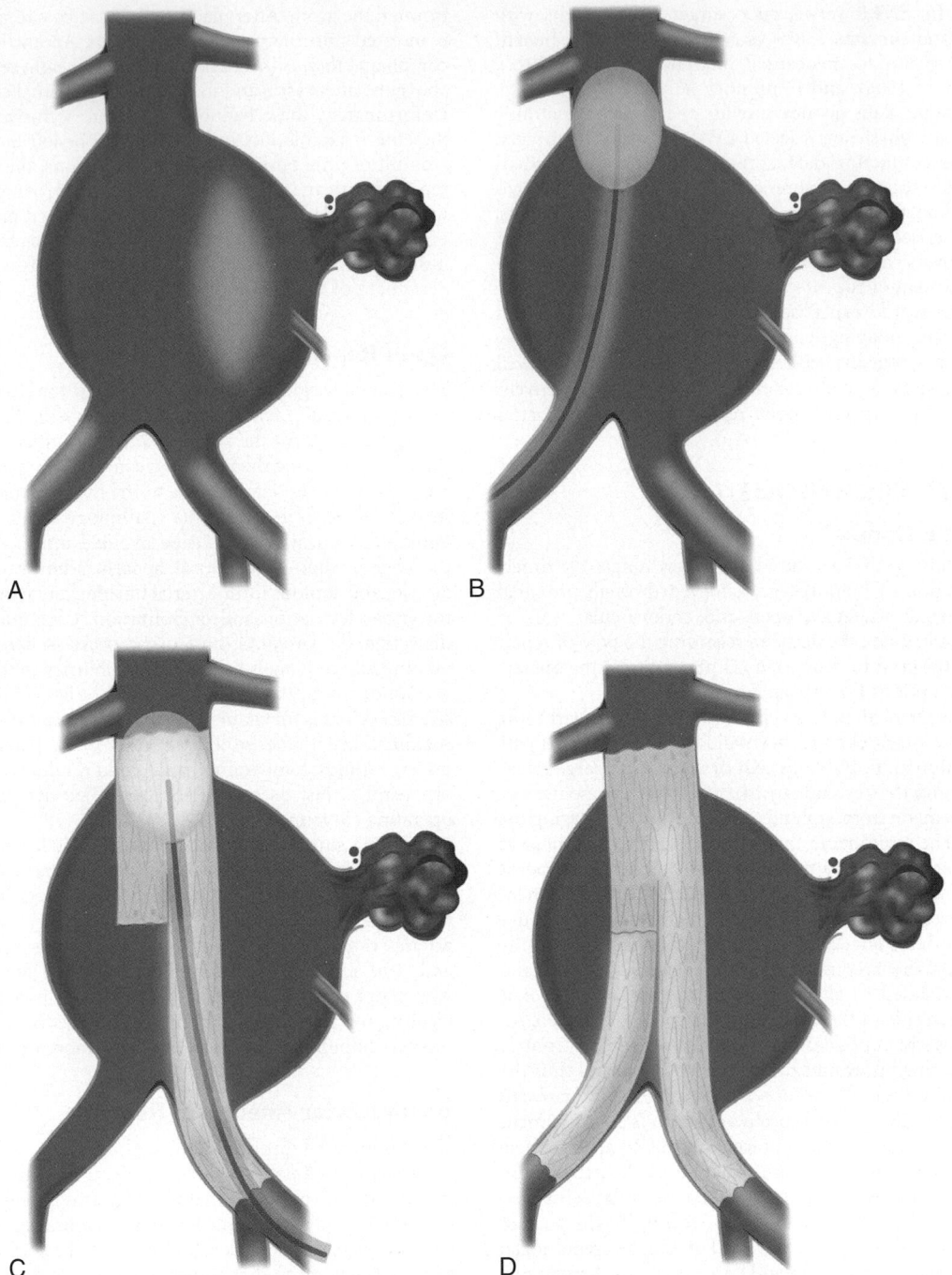

FIGURE 3 **A,** Free rupture of infrarenal abdominal aortic aneurysm. **B,** An aortic occlusion balloon is advanced into the visceral segment above the aneurysm. This requires support with a long 12F sheath to prevent distal displacement. **C,** The graft is deployed and the balloon can be transferred to the ipsilateral side if the patient remains unstable. **D,** The remainder of the graft is built out. *(Courtesy University of Wisconsin Hospitals and Clinics.)*

and mesenteric arteries (snorkels, sandwiches, and periscopes). Advanced techniques such as these should be reserved for surgeons comfortable with their use and for those well versed in the treatment of ensuing complications.

■ COMPLICATIONS OF OPEN AND ENDOVASCULAR REPAIR

General

A ruptured aneurysm with or without associated shock produces a tremendous physiologic stress, leading to multiple systemic compli-

cations. In an analysis of the NSQIP data from unstable patients with rupture, myocardial infarction occurred in 26%, renal failure requiring dialysis in 11.5%, and respiratory failure (defined by mechanical ventilation for more than 48 hours) in 40% of patients. Excessive hemorrhage can lead to an ongoing coagulopathy, making control of bleeding impossible. For patients treated for rupture, death can occur early usually from hemorrhage, or days or weeks later, related to sepsis, multiple organ failure, or one of the various complications outlined below. It is not unusual that patients who survive the initial operation appear stable the first morning after surgery, leading to early celebration of success. However, by day 2 this initial optimism is replaced by insidious onset of bowel ischemia, sepsis, renal failure, and other complications, leading to the patient's eventual demise.

Lower Extremity Ischemia

Lower extremity ischemia can occur after either open or endovascular repair. Causes are either distal embolization or occlusion of the proximal reconstruction. For patients treated with EVAR, proximal occlusion often is related to kinking or compression of the graft as it passes through a diseased aortic bifurcation or the iliac circulation. This is a much more frequent event in patients with tortuous, diseased, or heavily calcified iliac arteries. For open repair, the groins always should be prepped into the field, and for endorepair and open repair, distal pulses should be assessed before leaving the operating room. Absence of distal pulses should lead to an angiogram followed by embolectomy as indicated. Absence of a femoral pulse should likewise lead to investigation of the cause with an angiogram. Options when there is absence of inflow include repair of the proximal source of obstruction; however, an expeditious solution, particularly for open repair, can be a cross-femoral bypass.

Abdominal Compartment Syndrome

Abdominal compartment syndrome can occur after open and endovascular repair. With endovascular repair the large retroperitoneal hematoma is purposely not decompressed. In most circumstances the hematoma just resolves over time. However, occasionally if there has been significant hemorrhage, pressure can result in a compartment syndrome. After open repair, edematous bowel, the residual hematoma, and/or ongoing bleeding also can lead to compartment syndrome, particularly if the abdomen has been closed. This syndrome manifests most often with renal failure secondary to renal vein obstruction. Untreated, compartment syndrome will progress to renal and respiratory failure and eventually shock. Clinical suspicion should be high in any patient who is not recovering appropriately after a ruptured aneurysm repair. Bladder pressure measurements can be used to make the diagnosis, and treatment should be initiated immediately with an urgent decompressive laparotomy.

Ischemic Colitis

Sacrifice of the inferior mesenteric artery can result in impaired colonic perfusion. This can be enhanced further by the hypotension and global malperfusion that often accompany aortic rupture. In the vast majority of patients, these issues are tolerated and the colon remains adequately perfused via collateral circulation. A bloody stool, abdominal pain, or unexplained hypotension necessitates assessment of the colon for ischemia. The left colon is at greatest risk, and therefore flexible sigmoidoscopy should be used for evaluation. If an ischemic colon is identified but there is not full-thickness necrosis, patients can be managed by optimizing perfusion, antibiotics for colonic flora, and observation. Extensive necrosis by sigmoidoscopy, or in patients demonstrating peritonitis or signs of early sepsis, urgent exploration is the necessary next step. A thorough assessment of the inferior mesenteric artery should be performed at the time of aneurysm repair. Vigorous back bleeding from the artery is a sign that adequate collaterals exist. Patency of the hypogastric arteries is another positive sign. After endovascular repair, colonic ischemia is rare and, when it does occur, is often the result of microembolization of the colonic or small bowel circulation.

Infection

Graft infection is a rare but devastating consequence of open or endovascular repair. Urgent repair increases the opportunity for contamination or misuse of antibiotics. Local infections in the abdominal incision or the groins should be treated aggressively in all patients. Treatment of infection often requires complete excision of the graft and carries a high mortality.

Groin Access Complications

Femoral pseudoaneurysms, groin or retroperitoneal hematomas, and access artery dissection can occur after endovascular repair. Gaining access with the use of ultrasound guidance can reduce the incidence of these complications.

■ CONCLUSION

Ruptured abdominal aortic aneurysms are devastating and highly lethal. The incidence appears to be decreasing related to more readily available screening as well as diminished rates of smoking. Early diagnosis is critical, and suspicion should be high for any patient with a known aneurysm or a pulsatile mass and the new onset of symptoms. Unstable patients should be taken directly to the operating room, but for others a preoperative CT is invaluable (see Figure 1). Preoperative permissive hypotension and a well-coordinated operating team can improve outcomes. The most important task is to gain proximal aortic control, which can be achieved through a variety of approaches. Open and endovascular repair are acceptable strategies; randomized trials have not been able to demonstrate an advantage of either. Postoperative complications are frequent, and their early recognition and management are essential to obtaining excellent long-term outcomes. The longevity of patients that have recovered from a ruptured aneurysm is excellent and parallels that of age-matched individuals (vs certain death without treatment). Thus salvage of a patient with ruptured aneurysm can be a gratifying experience for the treating surgeon.

SELECTED READINGS

Ascher E, et al. Ruptured versus elective abdominal aortic aneurysm repair: outcome and cost. *Ann Vasc Surg.* 1999;13:613-617.

Boyle JR, et al. Existing delays following the presentation of ruptured abdominal aortic aneurysm allow sufficient time to assess patients for endovascular repair. *Eur J Vasc Endovasc Surg.* 2005;29:505-509.

Dick F, Erdoes G, Opfermann P, et al. Delayed volume resuscitation during initial management of ruptured abdominal aortic aneurysm. *J Vasc Surg.* 2013;57:943.

Gupta PK, Ramanan B, Engelbert TL, Tefera G, Hoch JR, Kent KC. A comparison of open surgery versus endovascular repair of unstable ruptured abdominal aortic aneurysms. *Vasc Surg.* 2014;60:1439-1445.

Malina MM, Veith F, Ivancev K, et al. Balloon occlusion of the aorta during endovascular repair of ruptured abdominal aortic aneurysm. *J Endovasc Ther.* 2005;12:556-559.

Powell JT, Thompson SG, et al. The Immediate Management of the Patient with Rupture: Open Versus Endovascular repair (IMPROVE) aneurysm trial—ISRCTN 48334791 IMPROVE trialists. *Acta Chir Belg.* 2009;109:678.

ABDOMINAL AORTIC ANEURYSM AND UNEXPECTED ABDOMINAL PATHOLOGY

Jeniann Yi, MD, MS, and David Kuwayama, MD, MPA

Abdominal aortic aneurysm (AAA) is a common, typically asymptomatic, potentially life-threatening condition. Management revolves around replacing or depressurizing the dilated segment of aorta from blood flow to prevent further growth and eliminate the risk of rupture. Currently two major approaches exist for treating AAA: open surgical repair, via anterior or retroperitoneal approaches, and minimally invasive endovascular aneurysm repair (EVAR).

Open repair remains the gold standard for treating AAA, with proven long-term efficacy. However, EVAR is quickly replacing open repair as the first-line treatment in suitable candidates because of the significantly decreased risk of perioperative morbidity and mortality. Continued evolution of stent-grafts and delivery systems has made EVAR feasible in progressively more unfavorable aneurysm anatomy. As EVAR grows in popularity, fewer patients are undergoing laparotomy for repair of their aneurysms; thus the discovery of unexpected, coincident intra-abdominal pathology at the time of operation has become less common. Furthermore, the frequent preoperative use of noninvasive imaging modalities, including computed tomography (CT), Doppler ultrasound, and magnetic resonance imaging (MRI), has increased the likelihood of discovering co-existing conditions well before the patient ever sees the operating room. Nevertheless, indications for open repair still exist, and surgeons who subsequently make unexpected discoveries at the time of repair still must know how to prioritize their findings so as to develop an operative strategy that minimizes the overall risk to the patient.

Clinical scenarios involving aortic aneurysms and coincident intra-abdominal pathology generally may be separated into four distinct categories: (1) elective operation for aortic pathology with incidental finding of asymptomatic nonvascular pathology, (2) emergent operation for presumed symptomatic aortic pathology with incidental finding of nonvascular pathology, (3) emergent operation for abdominal pathology with incidental finding of an aortic aneurysm, and (4) elective operation for abdominal pathology with incidental finding of an aortic aneurysm.

This chapter describes each of these scenarios, focusing on those clinical entities most commonly encountered.

ELECTIVE ABDOMINAL AORTIC ANEURYSM REPAIR AND ASYMPTOMATIC ABDOMINAL DISEASE

Virtually every patient undergoing an elective aneurysm repair, either EVAR or open repair, has undergone a preoperative CT scan. Unsurprisingly, patients with AAA, who typically are older and often have a history of smoking, are prone to the discovery of additional non-vascular findings on preoperative imaging. Indes (2002) reviewed CT scans of 176 patients undergoing EVAR and found that 89% had additional incidental findings, with 19% of these being clinically significant and requiring further workup. Morris and Colquitt (1988) reviewed records of 158 consecutive AAA patients and found that 12.7% had co-existent histologically proven malignancies, most of which were prostate, colorectal, and lung cancers.

When concomitant intra-abdominal disease is discovered on imaging before planned EVAR, the surgeon generally is able to choose whether to proceed with EVAR or treat the nonvascular pathology first. Because EVAR is so well tolerated and usually causes minimal physiologic derangement, the aneurysm typically can be repaired without significantly delaying the subsequent treatment of other time-sensitive pathology, such as cancer. Furthermore, the peritoneal cavity is left untouched by EVAR, permitting a subsequent clean laparotomy for other intra-abdominal interventions.

In the event that a patient with co-existent intra-abdominal pathology is being considered for open repair, a retroperitoneal approach to the aorta should be strongly considered. Such an approach provides superb exposure to the perivisceral and infrarenal aorta while leaving the midline fascia intact and the peritoneal cavity and its contents undisturbed, thereby preserving future laparotomy or laparoscopy options. However, certain technical considerations, such as extensive right common iliac aneurysmal involvement, still may make midline laparotomy the preferred approach to aortic exposure, and such considerations should take priority over concerns about subsequent bowel adhesion formation.

More commonly, pathology that went unrecognized during the prescreening process is discovered while approaching the aorta through a midline laparotomy. Frequently this discovered pathology either will have been too small to appear on CT scan or will have been of a nature that made it unlikely to appear. At this point the surgeon has three options: (1) continue the open AAA repair without any other concomitant surgical procedure, (2) abandon the AAA repair and treat the concomitant condition first, or (3) attempt simultaneous treatment of both the AAA and the unexpected pathology. The decision depends on the type and severity of abnormality found.

If the surgeon elects to continue the AAA repair without synchronous treatment of concomitant disease, it must be recognized that the patient may not have another opportunity for the secondary disease process to be addressed safely for some time because of the need for the patient to first recover from the physiologic insult of a major open vascular procedure, followed by the well-recognized risks of subsequent reoperative laparotomy (e.g., adhesion formation, potential bowel injury, poor fascial integrity).

If the surgeon elects to treat only the concomitant pathology without treating the AAA, the increased risk of aneurysm rupture caused by the delay in repair must be accepted. Because open AAA repair is almost always reserved for those aneurysms large enough to exhibit an elevated risk of rupture, this risk should not be considered insignificant. A 5.5-cm AAA is associated with an annual rupture risk of at least 10%, whereas AAAs larger than 7.0 cm have an annual rupture risk of at least 35%. Therefore each month of delay in AAA repair exposes the patient to a 1% to 3% risk of rupture. Furthermore, several small series have documented an increased risk of rupture of previously asymptomatic, sizable AAAs after unrelated laparotomies, with rupture incidence ranging between 6% and 10% in the 30-day postoperative period. The exact causes for this phenomenon are unclear, but possibilities include elevated aortic wall stress from postoperative tachycardia and hypertension and a trauma-related decrease in aortic wall collagen content because of matrix metalloproteinase activation.

If the surgeon chooses to address both problems simultaneously, he or she must be willing to accept the potentially increased morbidity of putting a patient through two procedures instead of one, lengthening anesthetic time and increasing blood loss. Furthermore, resection of the concomitant pathology may require opening the gastrointestinal (GI) or biliary tracts, thereby risking the potentially devastating complication of an aortic prosthetic graft infection, with an associated mortality as high as 65%.

The most commonly encountered intra-abdominal issues include cholelithiasis, GI malignancies, genitourinary malignancies, solid organ tumors, and the presence of the appendix or a Meckel's diverticulum.

Cholelithiasis

Cholelithiasis is found in up to 20% of AAA laparotomies. When it is noted, the surgeon must choose whether to leave the gallstones alone, as simultaneous treatment may increase the chances of graft infection, or to perform a cholecystectomy to avoid the risk of postoperative cholecystitis or choledocholithiasis. Since cholecystectomy generally can be performed quickly with a minimum of blood loss, the greatest factor at play is the elevated risk of graft infection associated with opening the biliary tract.

This topic was once a subject of much debate in the literature, with some citing an elevated risk of cholecystitis in the postoperative period. However, as advances in minimally invasive and interventional radiologic techniques have improved our ability to treat gallbladder disease, the weight of opinion has shifted away from synchronous cholecystectomy. Laparoscopic cholecystectomy, percutaneous cholecystostomy, transhepatic biliary stenting, and endoscopic retrograde cholangiopancreatography (ERCP) have permitted symptomatic cholelithiasis and choledocholithiasis to be safely treated almost always without the need for a second laparotomy.

Patients with known gallstone disease should be monitored in the postoperative period for any signs or symptoms suggestive of symptomatic cholelithiasis and referred for interventional therapy only if they meet traditional indications. Postoperative education on dietary modification should be provided, and consideration should be given to ursodiol therapy.

Gastrointestinal Malignancies

GI malignancies are notoriously difficult to identify on CT scans. Furthermore, aortic aneurysms and GI malignancies tend to occur in the same patient populations: in smokers and in those older than age 50 years. Thus the discovery of previously unrecognized colorectal or small bowel malignancies at the time of laparotomy for AAA repair is a relatively common occurrence. Colorectal cancers (CRCs) are most common, with an estimated frequency of concurrence with AAA between 0.5% and 1.4%. Therefore the occasional discovery of synchronous GI malignancies most certainly would be encountered in high-volume vascular centers.

Concomitant surgical correction of both GI malignancy and AAA is considered controversial because of both the magnitude of a combined operation and the general taboo against placing an aortic prosthetic graft in a potentially contaminated field. A staged procedure generally is recommended, with the order of treatment depending on the judged severity of each condition; a 4- to 6-week period of convalescence between operations is required to maximize the patient's physiologic reserve. Unfortunately, during this period the untreated pathology may worsen or become symptomatic. Repairing the AAA first postpones bowel resection and risks cancer metastasis or obstruction, whereas starting with bowel resection leaves the patient at risk of death from rupture of the aneurysm.

Baxter and colleagues (2002) published a retrospective review of 83 patients with AAA and concomitant CRC. Among the patients with AAAs larger than 5 cm in which CRC was treated first, the authors observed an alarming aneurysm rupture rate of 10% in the postoperative period. Just as disheartening, however, among those who underwent AAA repair first, the time to subsequent colectomy averaged more than 4 months, a prolonged window during which cancers may have progressed or spread. The authors' results support the idea of concomitant AAA repair and colorectal resection in patients with large aneurysms and CRC.

Velanovich and Andersen (1991) performed an applied decision analysis and concluded that patients with aneurysms larger than 5 cm, a colonic tumor that has a greater than 75% chance of obstruction or perforation, and a projected mortality of less than 10% would benefit from a combined operation rather than a staged one. Conversely, in patients with small aneurysms, tumors unlikely to perforate or obstruct in the near term, or a poor American Society of Anesthesiologists classification, the authors recommended a staged approach.

Shalhoub and colleagues (2009) published a review of prospectively collected data on 24 patients with concurrent CRC and AAA. In their series, patients with large aneurysms (greater than 7 cm) underwent EVAR first, with a median interval to subsequent colectomy of only 2 months. Those with smaller aneurysms (5.5 to 7 cm) underwent colectomy first, followed by either open repair or EVAR, with no aneurysm ruptures during the median interval period of 8 months. The authors concluded that staged management that addresses the most pressing pathology first is a reasonable approach, with a low risk of aneurysm rupture if colectomy is performed first. However, an EVAR-first strategy minimized overall time to treatment of both conditions. The authors suggested that the relatively modest physiologic insult from EVAR therefore may make it the preferred first step in staged management of synchronous disease.

Similar support for an EVAR-first strategy was provided by Lin and colleagues (2008), who published a retrospective review of 108 patients with concomitant AAA and CRC. Only 8 patients underwent synchronous open repair; the remainder were split evenly between a colectomy-first approach and an aneurysm-first approach (either open repair or EVAR). No aortic graft infections were identified in any of the patients. The patients with the shortest treatment delay were those who underwent EVAR first (median 12 days), whereas the patients with the longest delay were those who underwent open repair first (median 115 days). Patients who underwent colectomy first had a median delay of 35 to 42 days. Furthermore, survival analysis over the mean follow-up period of 43 months found a significant advantage for patients who underwent EVAR before staged CRC resection. In all treatment groups, regardless of the order of procedures, a postoperative morbidity and mortality reduction was noted with EVAR versus open repair.

While an EVAR-first strategy may seem to be clearly preferable in suitable endovascular candidates, an important potential drawback is that EVAR by necessity covers the inferior mesenteric artery (IMA). In patients with a chronically occluded IMA or a robust marginal artery of Drummond, this is not of concern. However, in as much as 48% of patients the marginal artery is absent or diminutive. In these patients a patent IMA may be important to healing of colonic anastomoses, particularly when the zone of resection involves the descending or sigmoid colon. IMA angiography, with visualization of the robustness of superior mesenteric artery (SMA) to IMA collateralization, may be useful in risk stratifying questionable patients with left-sided tumors. Absence of good collateral flow may suggest that a colectomy-first strategy, an open repair with IMA reimplantation, or a synchronous repair may be best.

Should a surgeon opt to proceed with synchronous open repair and colorectal excision, excellent surgical technique with meticulous control of peritoneal contamination is a must if graft infection is to be avoided. Intraoperatively, the aneurysm should be repaired first, with the prosthetic aortic interposition graft covered as well as possible using remaining aortic sac, retroperitoneal tissue, a pedicled omental flap, or bovine pericardium. Bowel resection then can proceed, with abundant packing used to isolate the periaortic retroperitoneum from any bowel contents. Serious consideration should be given to a Hartmann's procedure, with stoma maturation after abdominal wall closure, as the safest way to minimize intraperitoneal contamination. If synchronous AAA and CRC management is planned preoperatively, administration of bowel-specific antibiotics and aggressive bowel preparation (if not obstructed) should be performed.

Discoveries of small bowel and gastric tumors also have been reported, with patients undergoing simultaneous enterectomies or gastrectomies. In such cases, we feel that a management algorithm similar to that described earlier for colorectal malignancies is best followed. Patients should be staged when possible, unless the acuity of each condition individually is felt to be so high as to mandate synchronous intervention.

Genitourinary Malignancies

Renal carcinoma, unless large or invasive, may go unrecognized if aneurysms are approached via midline laparotomy. The chance of discovering a synchronous (left-sided) renal mass is increased with the retroperitoneal approach. Synchronous repair of AAA and nephrectomy has been described, with a low risk of bacterial graft contamination. Although synchronous treatment avoids the need for a second retroperitoneal exploration, a staged approach should be used if the AAA repair is particularly difficult or if intraoperative blood loss is significant.

When renal tumors are recognized preoperatively, it may help to guide the surgical approach. For left kidney tumors, a retroperitoneal approach to the aorta provides adequate exposure for both procedures. For right kidney tumors, a midline laparotomy is preferred. Important considerations when planning whether to perform synchronous resection are the need for a suprarenal clamp, baseline reduced kidney function, or both. Such patients are at elevated risk for acute tubular necrosis and transient renal insufficiency after aneurysm repair; simultaneous nephrectomy in such patients could result in temporary or permanent dependence on dialysis. These patients likely would benefit from a staged approach, with sufficient time after aneurysm repair for recovery of renal function.

Bladder or prostate cancer and AAA are challenging to manage concomitantly, but simultaneous resections and aneurysm repairs have been reported. A prospective study by Grego and colleagues (2003) compared simultaneous and staged aneurysm repair and radical cystoprostatectomy and found no statistically significant difference in clinical outcome, although a trend toward increased mortality was found in patients with baseline stage 3 or higher chronic renal insufficiency. Nevertheless, lower genitourinary tract malignancies are associated with a significant risk of urinary bacterial contamination, and transient bacterial translocation may occur during surgical manipulation or instrumentation. Synchronous repair therefore presents the theoretical risk of an aortic prosthetic graft infection from hematogenous seeding. Any combined procedure should be performed with preoperative and sustained intraoperative administration of antibiotic prophylaxis targeted at potential genitourinary pathogens.

A staged management approach must weigh the risk of aneurysm rupture versus malignancy. The oncologic priority for prompt resection and tumor staging, as well as the presence of low-grade urinary tract infection, argues for staging with resection of the genitourinary malignancy first. Conversely, in addition to the ever-present risk of aneurysm rupture, the untreated aneurysm also may present a technical obstacle to the urologic surgeon performing an extended retroperitoneal lymph node dissection, particularly when the aneurysm involves the aortic bifurcation and common iliac arteries.

Staging with aneurysm repair first addresses rupture risk, but does so at the expense of ongoing metastasis risk. Open aortic repair through a midline laparotomy risks causing subsequent adhesions between loops of small bowel and the dome of the bladder, which may complicate later cystectomy. Therefore if open repair is necessary, a retroperitoneal approach is preferable if feasible. EVAR is tolerated more easily than open repair and similarly avoids causing intra-abdominal adhesions. However, EVAR does not lead to an immediate change in aneurysm shape or size. As such, retroperitoneal lymph node dissections after EVAR still will be hampered by distortion of the retroperitoneal tissues.

Solid Organ Tumors

Solid tumors of the spleen, liver, and adrenal gland also have been documented and resected successfully at the time of AAA repair. Given the typically sterile nature of these organs, simultaneous resection appears reasonable, as long as the patient can tolerate the blood loss and the additional anesthetic time associated with the second procedure.

Appendix and Meckel's Diverticulum

Because of the significant risk of aortic prosthetic infection associated with opening the GI tract, asymptomatic appendices and Meckel's diverticula unequivocally should be left alone during an open repair. Incidental discovery of acute appendicitis during an open repair would be a rare occurrence, but if discovered, the appendix certainly would need to be resected. A more challenging dilemma arises if evidence of a chronically inflamed appendix or Meckel's diverticulum is discovered. In our opinion, the risk/benefit ratio still would argue against synchronous resection, unless the inflammation clearly appears to be acute. Advances in laparoscopic management of the appendix and Meckel's diverticula have made resection after AAA repair, even in the immediate postoperative period, feasible, with a low likelihood of the need for repeat laparotomy.

◼ EMERGENT ABDOMINAL AORTIC ANEURYSM REPAIR AND CONCOMITANT DISEASE

Emergent AAA repair is indicated in two situations: with symptomatic AAA and with ruptured AAA (rAAA). Imaging studies are usually available in the first case but not necessarily available in the second case because of the extreme urgency of the condition and the need for prompt transport to the operating room. In either case, the first priority is aneurysm repair, after which the major goal should be prompt and aggressive resuscitation in the intensive care unit (ICU). Pursuing other intra-abdominal findings at this time would be ill advised unless they were deemed to be life threatening in nature.

Among patients with a symptomatic but unruptured AAA and a synchronous intra-abdominal lesion, the prioritization of conditions should depend on the severity and related mortality risk of each. Symptomatic AAAs are felt to represent aneurysms in the initial stages of rupture, suggesting that the risk of leaving them untreated would be significant. However, if a concomitant intra-abdominal condition is considered life threatening or extremely urgent, aneurysm repair conceivably could be delayed temporarily, with interval close observation and blood pressure management in a monitored setting. If the AAA is massive or is demonstrating early signs of rupture on visual inspection, synchronous open repair would be necessary. Thankfully, the concurrence of two such unrelated yet life-threatening conditions is a rare event.

The treatment of ruptured AAAs is shifting gradually away from open repair toward EVAR when technically possible, with studies indicating a 30% mortality rate reduction in EVAR cohorts. Unexpected concomitant disease may be evident on preoperative imaging conducted for EVAR planning, but otherwise it is unlikely to be discovered. Even if other pathology is noted preoperatively, treatment of the aneurysm always is the first priority. However, if suspicion of a synchronous intra-abdominal catastrophe develops during EVAR, aneurysm repair may need to be followed by diagnostic laparoscopy or exploratory laparotomy before transport to the ICU.

Unfortunately, patients in whom control of aneurysmal bleeding has been achieved and aortic continuity restored nevertheless may have suffered enough visceral ischemia during the procedure to develop bowel necrosis. In such cases, clearly nonviable bowel should be resected before returning the patient to the ICU for resuscitation, and the abdomen should be left open for marginal bowel to be inspected 24 to 48 hours later.

◼ EMERGENT LAPAROTOMY FOR SYMPTOMATIC ABDOMINAL PATHOLOGY WITH INCIDENTAL ASYMPTOMATIC ABDOMINAL AORTIC ANEURYSM

A broad spectrum of emergent intra-abdominal pathologies may bring a patient to the operating room without prior CT imaging.

Possible scenarios are blunt or penetrating abdominal trauma, severe lactic acidosis of suspected intra-abdominal origin, obvious bowel obstruction in a virgin abdomen, or clear perforation with peritonitis, to name only a few.

Clearly, acute intra-abdominal pathology must be prioritized and treated first, and any life-threatening conditions should be addressed promptly. If the aneurysm is found to be exceedingly large or at imminent risk for rupture, either an intraoperative or a prompt postoperative vascular surgical consult should be sought.

Operations for intra-abdominal infectious conditions, such as perforated viscus or infected necrotizing pancreatitis, make open aneurysm repair in the near term prohibitively dangerous given the high likelihood of graft infection. If at all possible, such patients should be considered for EVAR, as this prevents infected peritoneal contents from coming into contact with prosthetic material. In the very rare patient with disseminated intra-abdominal infection and an aortic aneurysm not amenable to an endovascular approach but mandating immediate repair, secondary options for open aortic reconstruction include a rifampin-soaked Dacron graft covered with omentum, cryopreserved aorta or paneled cryopreserved femoral vein, autogenous femoral vein harvest for construction of a neoaortoiliac system (NAIS) interposition graft, and aneurysm resection and ligation of the infrarenal aortic stump followed by immediate extra-anatomic bypass (bilateral axillofemoral or axillobifemoral bypass grafting).

If the patient did not undergo preoperative imaging or was taken for laparotomy based solely on clinical impression, it is important to ascertain whether the patient's acute presentation (e.g., abdominal pain) actually was a result of the anticipated nonvascular pathology or rather stemmed from the aneurysm. If laparotomy is otherwise negative for findings explaining severe abdominal pain, a symptomatic aneurysm in the early stages of rupture should be added to the differential diagnosis, and a vascular surgeon should be consulted intraoperatively for prompt assessment.

Necrotic small bowel with SMA compromise in the setting of AAA also should prompt an urgent vascular surgical consultation. Aneurysmal thrombus or dissection could account for a sudden SMA ostial thrombosis. This life-threatening condition would require emergent revascularization, with or without concomitant aneurysm repair, if the patient is to survive.

ELECTIVE LAPAROTOMY FOR ABDOMINAL PATHOLOGY WITH INCIDENTAL ASYMPTOMATIC ABDOMINAL AORTIC ANEURYSM

Because of the frequent use of preoperative imaging studies in preparation for elective intra-abdominal surgeries, the unexpected discovery of AAA at laparotomy is rare. However, the discovery of an unexpected aneurysm may be alarming, especially to an operating surgeon who in all likelihood is not a vascular specialist. Unless the aneurysm is exceedingly large or appears to be at imminent risk for rupture (irregular morphology, discoloration or inflammation of the adjacent retroperitoneum), it is probably reasonable for the surgeon to proceed with the planned abdominal operation. A vascular surgeon should be consulted either intraoperatively or promptly after the conclusion of the operation to assess the aneurysm and the patient's suitability for repair. Given the need for high-quality preoperative CT angiography, as well as specialized equipment including fluoroscopy and a fluoroscopy compatible bed, synchronous EVAR in such a situation generally is not feasible. However, patients with aneurysms larger than 5 cm may be considered for prompt EVAR in the perioperative period. Patients who need open repair of an aneurysm may do better with an extended convalescent interval. When the patient

has recovered sufficiently, open repair then can be performed, preferably through a retroperitoneal approach so as to avoid intraperitoneal adhesions.

SUMMARY

Although several case series and theoretical models that address the topic of AAA repair and synchronous disease management do exist in the literature, much of the decision making boils down to basic surgical principles of infection control and minimization of patient morbidity. Several general recommendations may be followed:

1. Emergent AAA repair takes priority over any concomitant disease.
2. Any nonlethal, nonvascular pathology discovered during elective AAA repair may be left alone at that time.
3. Incidental AAA found during emergent or elective laparotomy should be evaluated promptly by a vascular surgeon in the perioperative period; if the aneurysm is large enough to represent a rupture risk, it should be addressed soon thereafter, preferably via EVAR.
4. Meticulous surgical technique must be followed if the GI or biliary tracts are to be violated during a synchronous aneurysm repair, as aortic prosthetic graft infection is a highly lethal complication.

SUGGESTED READINGS

Baxter NN, Noel AA, Cherry K, et al. Management of patients with colorectal cancer and concomitant abdominal aortic aneurysm. *Dis Colon Rectum.* 2002;45:165-170.

Bickerstaff LK, Hollier LH, Van Peenen HJ, et al. Abdominal aortic aneurysm repair combined with second surgical procedure. *Surgery.* 1984;95: 487-491.

Grego F, Lepidi S, Bassi P, et al. Simultaneous surgical treatment of abdominal aortic aneurysm and carcinoma of the bladder. *J Vasc Surg.* 2003;37: 607-614.

Indes JE, Lipsitz EC, Veith FJ, et al. Incidence and significance of nonaneurysmal-related computed tomography scan findings in patients undergoing endovascular aortic aneurysm repair. *J Vasc Surg.* 2002;48: 286-290.

Lin PH, Barshes NR, Albo D, et al. Concomitant colorectal cancer and abdominal aortic aneurysm: evolution of treatment paradigm in the endovascular era. *J Am Coll Surg.* 2008;206:1065-1073.

McDougal JL, Valentine RJ, Josephs S, et al. Computer tomographic angiography has added value in patients with vascular disease. *J Vasc Surg.* 2006;44:998-1001.

Morris DM, Colquitt J. Concomitant abdominal aortic aneurysm and malignant disease: a difficult management problem. *J Surg Oncol.* 1988;39: 122-125.

Ouriel K, Ricotta JJ, Adams JT, et al. Management of cholelithiasis in patients with abdominal aortic aneurysm. *Ann Surg.* 1983;198:717-719.

Prusa AM, Wolff KS, Sahal M, et al. Abdominal aortic aneurysms and concomitant disease requiring surgical intervention: simultaneous operation versus staged treatment using endoluminal stent grafting. *Arch Surg.* 2005;140:686-691.

Shalhoub J, Naughton P, Lau N, et al. Concurrent colorectal malignancy and abdominal aortic aneurysm: a multicentre experience and review of the literature. *Eur J Vasc Endovasc Surg.* 2009;37:544-556.

String ST. Cholelithiasis and aortic reconstruction. *J Vasc Surg.* 1984;1: 664-669.

Swanson RJ, Littooy FN, Hunt TK, et al. Laparotomy as a precipitating factor in the rupture of intra-abdominal aneurysm. *Arch Surg.* 1980;115: 299-304.

Thomas JH, McCroskey BL, Iliopoulos JI, et al. Aortoiliac reconstruction combined with nonvascular operations. *Am J Surg.* 1983;146:784-787.

Velanovich A, Andersen CA. Concomitant abdominal aortic aneurysm and colorectal cancer: a decision analysis approach to the therapeutical dilemma. *Ann Vasc Surg.* 1991;5:449-455.

THE MANAGEMENT OF THORACIC AND THORACOABDOMINAL AORTIC ANEURYSMS

Bryan A. Ehlert, MD, and James H. Black III, MD

Descending thoracic aortic aneurysms (DTAAs) and thoracoabdominal aortic aneurysms (TAAAs) are uncommon when compared with isolated infrarenal abdominal aortic aneurysms (AAAs), accounting for only 2% to 5% of all aortic aneurysms. DTAAs are defined as those that involve the thoracic aorta between the origin of the left subclavian artery (LSA) and the diaphragmatic hiatus, whereas TAAAs can involve varying degrees of the visceral aortic segment along with the thoracic and infrarenal aorta. TAAAs are classified by anatomic definitions as devised by Dr. Stanley Crawford (Figure 1).

Although pathologies of the abdominal aorta are commonly degenerative, those affecting the thoracic and visceral aorta include a more diverse range of predisposing conditions, such as connective tissue disorders (e.g., Marfan's syndrome, Loeys-Dietz syndrome), dissections, aortitis, and trauma. Open repair of DTAAs and TAAAs, first described in 1952 by Bahnson and later mastered by Crawford, initially was plagued by increased morbidity and mortality rates as a result of renovisceral and spinal cord complications. Although adjuncts have been developed to decrease the incidence of these devastating complications at high-volume centers, these aneurysms continue to pose technical challenges to cardiac and vascular surgeons. The advent of thoracic endovascular aortic repair (TEVAR) has diminished further the morbidity associated with surgical repair. TEVAR is a well-established modality for the treatment of degenerative aneurysms of the thoracic aorta and traumatic transections; however, its use in patients with connective tissue disorders and for acute and chronic dissections continues to be the subject of ongoing study.

In a majority of patients, DTAAs or TAAAs are diagnosed incidentally while undergoing radiographic imaging for workup of unrelated diagnoses. For the approximately 40% of patients who do have symptoms, these are often the result of compression or erosion of nearby structures (esophagus, recurrent laryngeal nerve, trachea, or vertebral bodies) or from mediastinal pleura inflammation. Aneurysmal dilatation also may be accompanied by back pain and in extreme circumstances, rupture. As has been in seen in patients with infrarenal abdominal aortic aneurysm (AAA), those who have symptoms are associated with an increased rupture risk.

INDICATIONS FOR SURGERY

The mean rate of growth for thoracic aneurysms has been found to be 0.1 cm per year. Similar to infrarenal AAA, increasing aneurysm size is associated with a higher rupture risk. Originally, the size threshold for elective repair of aneurysms in DTAA populations was maintained at 7 cm; however, rupture rates as high as 23% were observed using this criterion, with up to an additional 20% of patients with symptoms of impending rupture. In a separate study on the natural history of thoracic aneurysms, a 30% 5-year rupture risk was observed when aneurysm size exceeded 6 cm. Rupture risk was negligible in aneurysms less than 5 cm and equivalent to morbidity risk of surgical repair at the 5- to 6-cm range. Given these findings, 6 cm or larger has been accepted as the size threshold to consider elective repair in acceptable risk patients.

As aneurysms of the thoracic aorta become larger, they also begin to expand at more accelerated rates. This increased expansion has been found to correlate with higher rupture rates. As such, patients with aneurysm growth rates of 10 mm or more per year also should be considered for surgical repair. Additional risk factors for rupture have been identified and include increasing patient age, female gender, chronic pain, history of chronic obstructive pulmonary disease, compression of surrounding structures, and development of a dissection within a degenerative aneurysm. Chronic type B aortic dissections and presence of connective tissue disorders have been found to be independent risk factors for rupture proclivity at smaller aneurysm sizes. In these settings, the size threshold to consider surgical repair is reduced to 5 cm. Furthermore, these populations tend to seek medical attention at younger ages compared with patients with degenerative aneurysms, potentially resulting in better comorbidity profiles and decreased operative risk.

The advent of improved techniques and devices in the endovascular treatment of thoracic aneurysms, particularly DTAAs, eventually may lead to further revisions of the aforementioned size thresholds. The emergence of stent-graft repair has resulted in decreased perioperative morbidity and mortality rates compared with traditional open surgical repair. Intermediate and long-term results from pivotal TEVAR trials show significantly decreased aneurysm-related mortality. Lower-profile devices and continued stent-graft innovation, including branched and fenestrated devices, have resulted in fewer anatomic limitations and increased the number of patients who are candidates for endovascular treatment. As such, one may consider intervening in aneurysms of smaller sizes, particularly in patients possessing other risk factors that may constitute a higher rupture risk.

PATIENT SELECTION AND PREOPERATIVE RISK ASSESSMENT

The approach and extent of operative repair required for DTAAs and TAAAs vary greatly depending on the Crawford classification; however, consistent themes exist regarding clinical variables that influence overall morbidity and ischemic spinal cord injury (SCI). Each patient's associated comorbid conditions, particularly those affecting cardiac, renal, and pulmonary function, require an accurate assessment to appropriately steer operative decision making. Aortic aneurysms are considered markers of coronary atherosclerotic disease, and because a majority of patients possess additional atherosclerotic risk factors, preoperative cardiac testing is mandatory in the elective setting. Echocardiography, either transthoracic or transesophageal, should be used to rule out valvular or ventricular dysfunction that may result in hemodynamic compromise from increased cardiac afterload after aortic cross-clamping. In addition, nuclear stress testing can identify major areas of myocardium potentially at risk for significant ischemia. In patients with abnormal noninvasive workup, further evaluation via cardiac catheterization should be considered as a definitive diagnostic and potentially therapeutic intervention. Nonreversible ischemic cardiomyopathy resulting in significantly decreased left ventricular function generally precludes open surgical repair.

A baseline serum creatinine is used commonly to assess renal function. If renal dysfunction is noted by elevated serum creatinine levels, patients may benefit from preoperative revascularization via percutaneous stenting or by surgical bypass or endarterectomy at the time of aneurysm repair. Up to 15% of TAAA patients have significant renal insufficiency, defined as a serum creatinine at least 1.8 mg/dL, and this has been shown to correlate with perioperative renal failure and mortality. Patients with renal insufficiency requiring extensive repairs, especially those with type II, type III, or type V TAAAs, have relative contraindications to open repair given the strong correlation with poor outcomes in these populations. Indeed, acute renal failure can have devastating effects on many other systems,

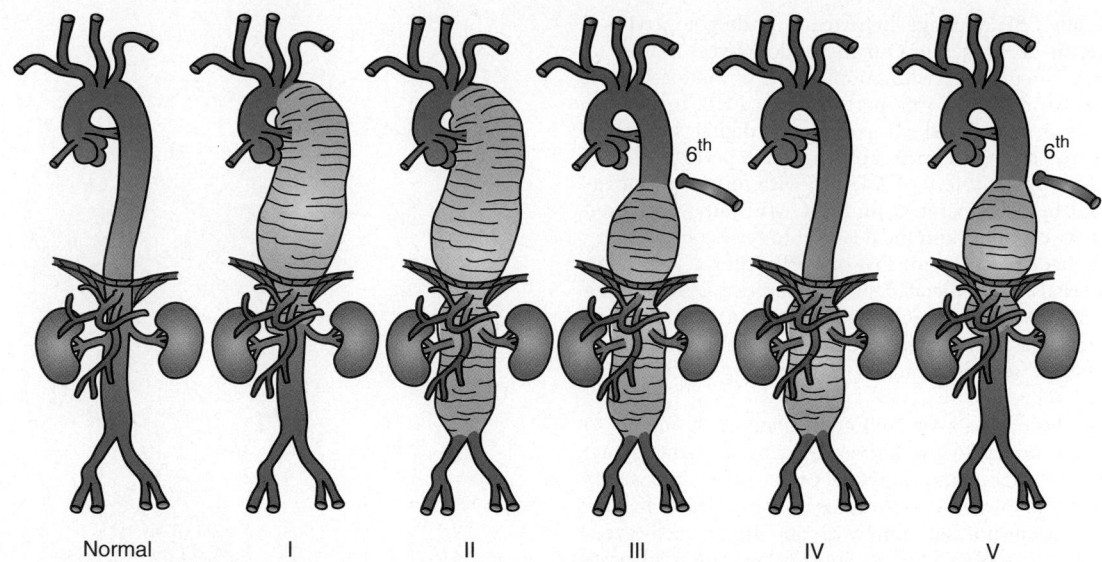

Normal   I   II   III   IV   V

FIGURE 1 Crawford classification of thoracoabdominal aortic aneurysms, types I through V. Type I, distal from origin of left subclavian artery to above renal arteries. Type II, distal from the left subclavian artery to the infrarenal aorta. Type III, from the sixth intercostal space to the infrarenal aorta. Type IV, from the thirteenth intercostal space to the aortic bifurcation. Type V, below the sixth intercostal space to the renal arteries. *(From* Rutherford's Vascular Surgery. *7th ed., Figure 131-8.)*

such as fluid overload and electrolyte disturbances promoting malignant arrhythmias.

Patients with aneurysms involving large portions of the thoracic aorta, DTAAs and types I through III TAAAs, should undergo preoperative pulmonary function tests. These patients often require single-lung ventilation, and without the necessary pulmonary reserve, may not tolerate such technique. A forced expiratory volume in 1 second (FEV1) of at least 1.0 L or a PCO_2 of 45 mm Hg or less generally represents appropriate pulmonary function to accept single-lung ventilation. Patients who fail to meet these criteria should undergo aggressive medical therapy with subsequent re-evaluation or evaluation for possible endovascular repair. Patient age is not a contraindication to open repair; however, overall functional status should be evaluated as part of the preoperative risk assessment. Previous series have shown that the elderly with appropriate functional status have acceptable perioperative morbidity and mortality rates. Patients with overall fragility probably should not be offered open surgical repair, although they may be candidates for endovascular repair or hybrid procedures, depending on their anatomy.

Along with the above physiologic assessments, patients being considered for endovascular repairs have independent anatomic criteria that must be assessed. High-quality imaging is necessary to ensure that there are appropriate proximal and distal seal zones to prevent endoleaks that may result in late aneurysm rupture. Patients with thoracic aneurysms may have extreme tortuosity of the aorta that prohibits the delivery and accurate placement of a stent-graft. Likewise, these aneurysms also commonly require larger diameter devices compared with isolated infrarenal AAA, making femoral and iliac artery access evaluation a priority. Patients with diffuse iliofemoral disease may not allow for passage of the larger sheaths that are necessary to deliver the stent-graft. Inadequate evaluation of the iliofemoral access can result in disastrous complications resulting from iliac artery disruption or avulsion. The presence of difficult access can be circumvented by using iliac conduits, which are further described later in the chapter.

Standard central venous access and invasive hemodynamic monitoring should be employed for all cases, including the use of pulmonary artery catheter placement when indicated. Double-lumen intubation is often necessary to provide single-lung ventilation for aneurysms with extensive thoracic components. Systemic hypothermia can be avoided by using fluid warmers along with passive external warming after completion of aortic reconstruction. Washed red blood cells (Cell Saver; Haemonetics, Braintree, MA) and transfusion of banked packed red blood cells and fresh frozen plasma should be applied liberally as opposed to large volume crystalloid infusions. Given the extensive nature of the reconstructions and long graft surfaces, platelet consumption is common and platelets should be administered to prevent significant thrombocytopenia.

STRATEGIES FOR THORACIC AND THORACOABDOMINAL AORTIC RECONSTRUCTION

Two surgical techniques that are used commonly to repair DTAAs and TAAAs are the "clamp-and-sew" technique and the use of distal aortic perfusion through a left heart bypass (LHB) circuit. Each technique has been found to be efficacious and is often surgeon and center dependent. Both techniques often are paired with other adjuncts to decrease complications related to spinal cord and visceral and renal ischemia. Operative technique variations and ongoing research have been centered on preventing the dreaded complications of renal failure and SCI. The judicious application of adjuncts for organ protection have been supported by the literature and include cerebrospinal fluid (CSF) drainage, intercostal revascularization, renal hypothermic perfusion, and distal aortic perfusion.

Organ Protection Adjuncts

SCI after DTAA or TAAA repair is the most feared morbid complication after DTAA and TAAA reconstruction. Placement of spinal drains to allow CSF drainage has been the best studied and widely accepted strategy employed to prevent paraplegia after thoracic aortic surgery. Early studies suggested that proximal aortic cross-clamping results in elevated CSF pressures that may compromise perfusion of the spinal cord. Preoperative placement of drainage catheters to allow efflux of CSF during the perioperative period functions to preserve the spinal cord circulation. In a randomized trial comparing types I and II TAAAs with and without CSF drainage, paraplegia rates were reduced from 13.0% to 2.6% with the use of CSF drainage. Both patient populations had similar aortic cross-clamp times, LHB use and intercostal artery revascularizations. An 80% overall risk reduction of postoperative SCI complications was observed with CSF drainage in patients undergoing types I and II TAAA repair in this series. Our institution favors the use of CSF drainage in conjunction with monitoring of motor evoked potentials (MEPs) and distal aortic perfusion via LHB. In patients thought to be at increased risk of paraplegia, digital subtracted angiography (DSA) of the thoracic aorta may be performed preoperatively to identify the artery of Adamkiewicz for revascularization if mandated by intraoperative findings. MEPs are monitored during aortic cross-clamping and the decision to revascularize intercostal arteries is made based on the loss of MEPs, clinical inspection of patent intercostals, or as dictated by preoperative DSA imaging of the artery of Adamkiewicz. Other adjuncts include epidural cooling to decrease neuronal energy requirement and continuous infusion of naloxone as a free radical scavenger and inhibitor of excitatory amino acids.

Cold renal perfusion has been well established as an adjunct to minimize ischemic injury to the kidneys. Perfusion catheters are placed into the renal orifices, and cold renal preservation fluid is used to flush the kidneys followed by continuous infusion. At our institution, we use 1 L bags of normal saline with 500 mg of methylprednisolone added and then placed on ice. Some other centers advocate the use of 25 g of mannitol as part of their protocol. A fenoldopam infusion, a selective dopamine agonist (D_1 receptor), also has been described as an adjunct to minimize the ischemic effects on renal function. Preservation of renal function is paramount to successful outcomes, as evident from a study that found postoperative renal failure to result in an eightfold increase in mortality risk ([odds ratio {OR}, 7.8]; 95% CI, 3.4-17.9; $P <0.01$).

Operative Technique

A double-lumen endotracheal tube is often necessary for single-lung ventilation for patients with types I through III TAAA to facilitate exposure to the thoracic aorta and inferior pulmonary vein for partial LHB. In patients with type IV TAAA, LHB is not often necessary and the chest not opened widely enough to require single-lung ventilation. All patients with DTAA and TAAA are positioned in a modified right lateral decubitus position, with the left chest rolled upward between 70 and 90 degrees and the pelvis rotated only approximately 30 degrees. The patient is placed on an adjustable beanbag to support the position, and an axillary roll is placed to protect the brachial plexus. The rib spaces then are identified and counted to mark the proper intercostal space for the necessary exposure (Figure 2). The patient then is prepped and draped, to include the left chest, left flank, and both groins.

The Johns Hopkins approach employs a thoracoretroperitoneal approach to all TAAA repairs to minimize the convective fluid and temperature losses incurred by an open peritoneum. The transversalis muscle is identified at the costal margin, and the fibers are split to identify the peritoneal sac. This then is bluntly swept medially out of the left retroperitoneal space. The anterior abdominal wall then is divided with electrocautery to the distal extent of the incision. Blunt mobilization of the retroperitoneum is continued medially to expose the left psoas muscle, where the left common iliac artery often is identified. The left ureter then is found commonly on the back of the peritoneal sac, and at this point a static self-retaining retraction system is placed. For type I TAAA, we recommend the use of two separate thoracotomies at the fifth and eighth interspace, through a single skin incision, as depicted in Figure 2. This allows for sufficient exposure to the proximal descending thoracic aorta (DTA) while also allowing diaphragm mobilization and identification of visceral branches for distal clamp location. The left renal artery then is identified to further guide the remainder of the visceral dissection. A prominent left lumbar vein normally is encountered coursing along the left aorta as it empties into the left renal vein. This structure can be ligated and divided to allow for safe medial retraction of the left kidney. The diaphragm can be mobilized in a circumferential fashion to further expose the DTA and suprarenal aorta (Figure 3). We do

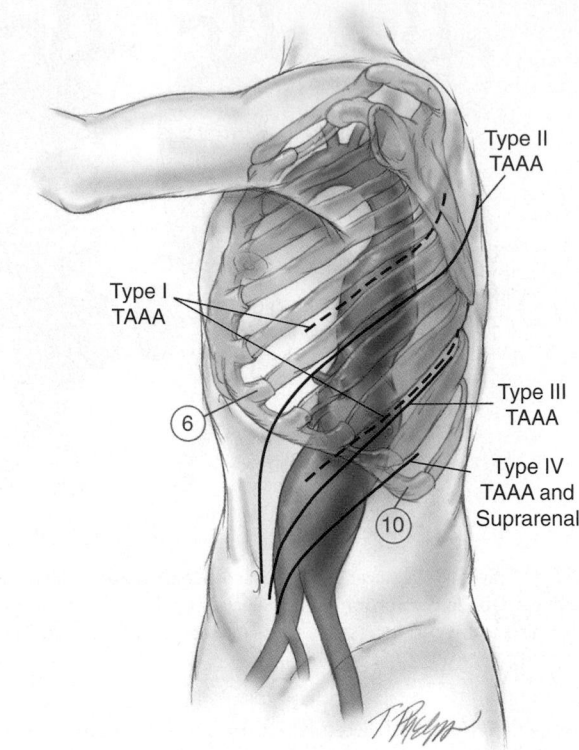

FIGURE 2 Illustration depicting the different incisions based on patient anatomy and aneurysm classification. For type I thoracoabdominal aortic aneurysm repairs, two separate thoracotomies are made at the fifth and eighth intercostal spaces through a single skin incision.

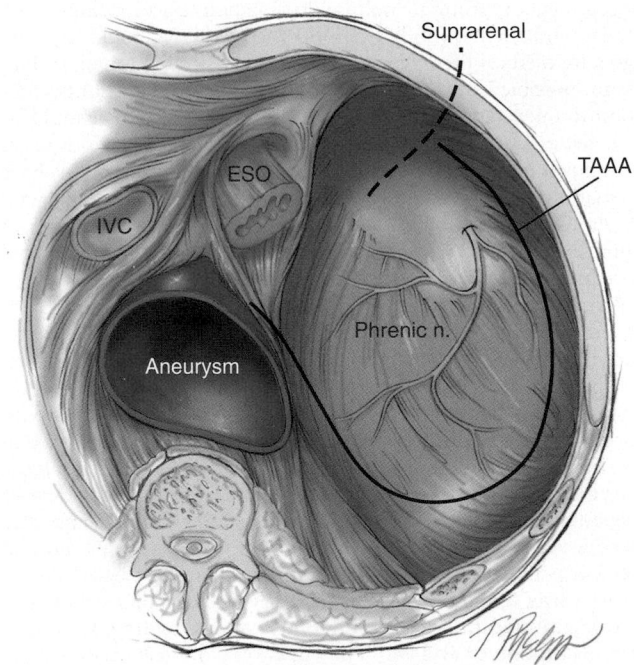

FIGURE 3 For thoracoabdominal aortic aneurysm (*TAAA*) repairs, the diaphragm is taken down in a circumferential fashion to allow for exposure of the DTA and suprarenal aorta. This method prevents sacrifice of phrenic nerve branches, which may contribute to postoperative pulmonary complications. In patients with suprarenal aneurysms in which the DTA does not have to be completely exposed, a partial division of the medial diaphragm can be used. *ESO*, esophagus; *IVC*, inferior vena cava.

not endorse radial division of the diaphragm because this sacrifices branches of the phrenic nerve, which may predispose to pulmonary complications postoperatively. Once the left kidney and retroperitoneum have been mobilized completely, they can be retracted safely to provide complete exposure to the thoracic and abdominal aorta. For types I and II TAAA and proximal DTAA, the left vagus nerve is identified, crossing the distal aortic arch and giving rise to the left recurrent laryngeal nerve as it courses around the arch at the ligamentum arteriosum. If the anatomy dictates a proximal clamp between the left common carotid artery and LSA, the ligamentum arteriosum usually is ligated and divided.

If LHB is to be used for distal aortic perfusion for types I through III TAAAs, the left inferior pulmonary ligament is taken down to expose the left inferior pulmonary vein. A purse-string 4-0 polypropylene suture then is placed before sharply performing a venotomy to place a 24F venous cannula. An 8-mm Dacron graft then is sewn in an end-to-side fashion onto the left common femoral or left iliac artery to avoid leg ischemia from direct cannulation that may confound MEP monitoring. Distal aortic perfusion then is initiated along with moderate hypothermia at 32° to 34° C. Sequential aortic cross-clamping then is used to isolate the proximal DTA while the proximal anastomosis is performed, followed by the lower thoracic aorta if intercostal revascularization via an inclusion patch anastomosis is to be done, then the abdominal aorta during visceral revascularization, and finally the iliac vessels for the distal anastomosis (Figure 4). Before placing the initial cross-clamp, emphasize to the anesthesia team to maintain lower systolic blood pressures to avoid complications from the increased afterload created from the aortic cross-clamp. Our institution strives to maintain bypass circuit flows of 2.0 to 3.5 L/min to provide 60 to 80 mm Hg for distal pressures. Once the visceral reconstruction has begun, the rewarming process is started.

For the aortic reconstruction, after appropriate exposure and proximal and distal control, the aorta is entered posterior to the left renal artery and the aortotomy extended as necessary. Figure 4 demonstrates the sequence of steps used to perform the aortic reconstruction for a type II TAAA. Depending on the type of DTAA or TAAA and the anatomy of the patient, the sequence of clamping and anastomotic sites can be modified. During the visceral revascularization, cold renal perfusion is maintained as described above. The patient body temperature should be monitored during cold renal perfusion to avoid excessive hypothermia that can result in heart arrhythmias or poor myocardial performance. We advocate for left aortorenal bypass versus direct Carrel patch of the left renal artery because this prevents thinning of the artery and potential for kinking if a renal endarterectomy is to be performed. Furthermore, the left renal bypass graft can be constructed onto the main conduit before cross-clamping to avoid unnecessary additional renal ischemia. The distal anastomosis then is completed at the appropriate level based on the patient's anatomy. The aneurysm sac should be closed over the reconstruction if possible. The retractors then are released and the retroperitoneal contents returned to their appropriate position.

The thoracoabdominal incision closure then is begun with the purpose to secure the chest wall and abdominal musculature to promote return to baseline function. A large axiom drain is placed routinely in the left retroperitoneal space that can be brought through the abdominal wall. The diaphragm then is reconstructed with interrupted figure-of-eight 0-silk sutures. The final several centimeters of the lateral diaphragm can be closed after the chest closure and can be done from the abdomen. For types I through III TAAAs, pleural chest tubes are placed to drain any effusions resulting from the chest dissection and proximal suture line. The rib interspaces are reapproximated using #2 looped absorbable sutures, and any residual cartilaginous joint at the costal margin is excised to provide stabilization and to prevent overriding of the adjacent ribs. The chest and abdominal musculature then is closed in multiple layers along with the subcutaneous tissues and skin.

Outcomes

Postoperative outcomes after DTAA and TAAA repair depend on the level of disease. Patients with DTAA are more prone to neurologic complications, whereas those undergoing TAAA repair are more susceptible to renal failure. As mentioned above, the evolution of adjuncts for end organ protection has made a considerable impact on patient mortality and significant morbidity. Likewise, the acuity at the time of patient presentation also affects patient outcomes because those with need for emergent repair have a higher incidence of morbidity and mortality.

A review of our experience with 300 patients undergoing open TAAA repair or open DTAA demonstrated a perioperative mortality rate of 7.5%. Furthermore, our rate for SCI was only 2.5% with the judicious use of LHB for distal aortic perfusion, moderate hypothermia, and CFS drainage and selective use of intercostal revascularization based on MEP monitoring. Acute renal failure, using the definition of many clinical series that is more than doubling of the baseline creatinine or an absolute value of more than 3.0 mg/dL, occurred in 12.5% of patients with dialysis dependence in 2% to 3%. However, in most of this subset of patients, they had return to their baseline renal function over the course of their follow-up. These findings are comparable to and have been replicated by other large-volume studies at centers of excellence.

The experience at other centers of expertise again has emphasized the importance of end organ adjuncts on perioperative morbidity and mortality. It has been reported that in patients undergoing types I through III TAAA repair in which LHB and MEP monitoring was used, the postoperative paraplegia rate was 0 compared with 5% in the clamp-and-sew cohort. Furthermore, the composite death/ paraplegia rate was decreased significantly from 9% to 2% in the LHB/MEP group ($P = 0.01$). LHB and MEP monitoring also resulted in improved long-term survival. At 4 years, there was an increased survival in this cohort compared with clamp-and-sew patients (73 ± 6% vs 60 ± 3%; $P = 0.004$). Safi and colleagues reported a greater than sevenfold decrease in SCI rates in those patients at highest risk, patients with type II TAAA. Using similar adjuncts as our institution, they saw the incidence of SCI drop from 31% during the clamp-and-sew era down to 4% with modern techniques. Their overall rate for SCI in non–type II cases was only 1.1%.

Postoperative renal function is most affected in those patients whose aneurysm pathology requires prolonged renal ischemia, such as types II through IV TAAA. The strongest predictor for postoperative renal failure is preoperative renal insufficiency, especially in those patients with a glomerular filtration rate less than 40 mL/min. Although the utilization of cold renal perfusion and other adjuncts has led to a decrease in the incidence of postoperative renal failure, it has not been as profound a resolution as seen with SCI. Other measures to improve postoperative renal function have included sequential clamping to reduce renal ischemia time and fenoldopam infusions. Despite these maneuvers, most studies have found anywhere between 2% and 9% of patients require hemodialysis for postoperative renal failure. After 2286 open TAAA repairs, Coselli and colleagues observed that hemodialysis was needed in 5.6% of all patients, with the incidence increasing to 8.3% in those with type II TAAA. Postoperative renal failure has been observed repeatedly to be a predictor of perioperative mortality. Patients that develop postoperative renal failure have been found to have a tenfold increase in risk of mortality.

ENDOVASCULAR MANAGEMENT OF DESCENDING THORACIC AORTIC ANEURYSM

TEVAR has emerged as an exciting new technology to treat thoracic aortic pathologies as an alternative to the significant morbidity and mortality associated with traditional open repair. TEVAR offers decreased operative risk by minimizing aortic manipulation,

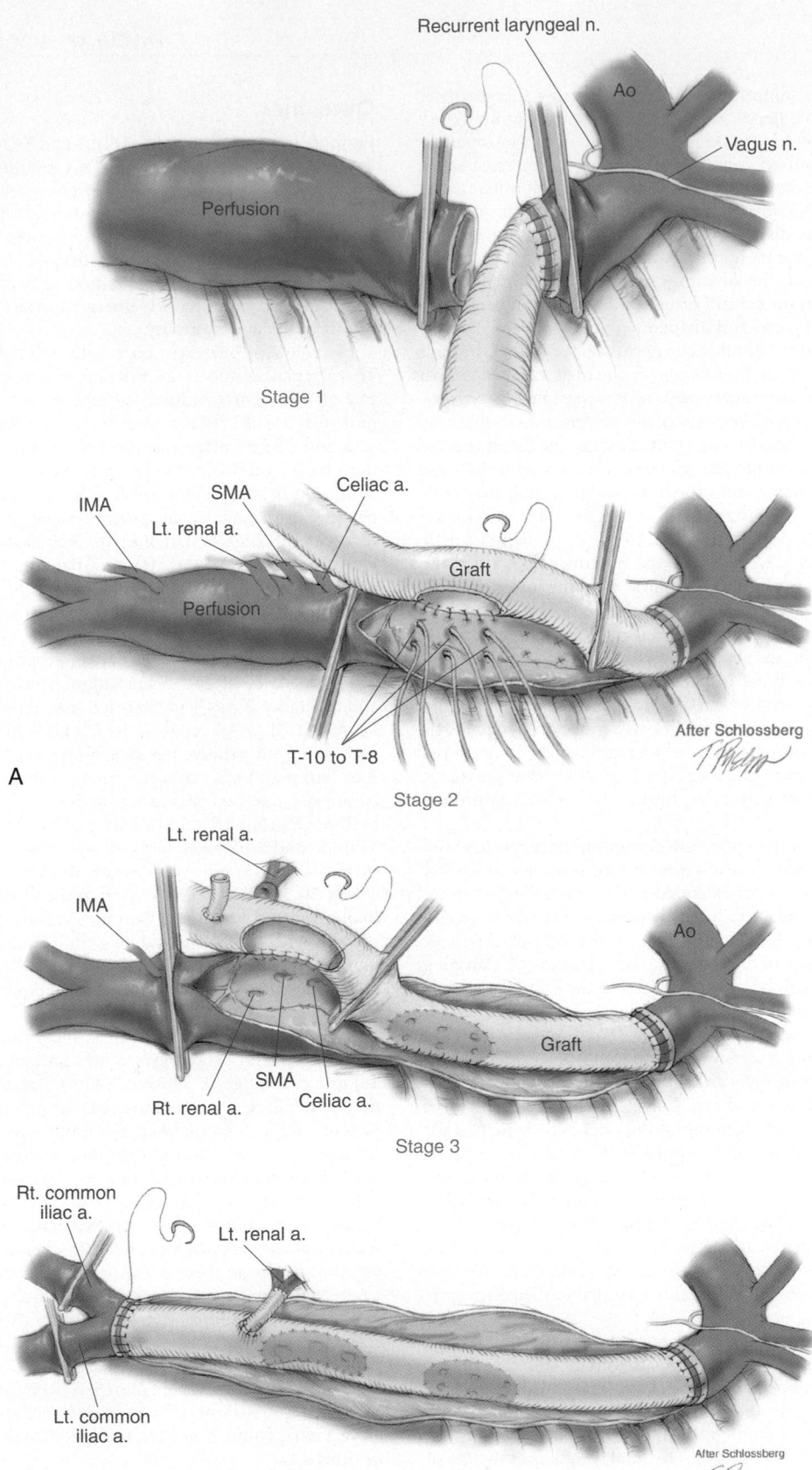

FIGURE 4 A, To minimize the risk of end-organ ischemic complications, we advocate for distal aortic perfusion and sequential aortic cross-clamping. The first stage includes proximal aortic cross-clamping with a distal clamp on the DTA to allow for completion of the proximal anastomosis. Next, the graft is clamped while a supraceliac clamp is placed distally to allow for either intercostal reimplantation or ligation. Balloon occluders can be placed to temporarily control intercostal arteries to be reimplanted. **B,** The next clamp is placed on the infrarenal aorta to allow for reconstruction of the visceral segment. This is accomplished with either a Crawford visceral inclusion patch to revascularize the right renal, superior mesenteric, and celiac arteries; or, in the case of patients with connective tissue disorders, with separate bypass grafts to each vessel to reduce the risk of patch aneurysms in the follow-up period. Finally, clamps are placed on bilateral common iliac arteries for the distal anastomosis and reimplantation of the left renal artery. We prefer aortorenal bypass to a Carrel patch so as not to cause thinning of the artery or kinking if a renal endarterectomy is necessary. *IMA,* inferior mesenteric artery; *SMA,* superior mesenteric artery.

hemodynamic shifts resulting from large volume hemorrhage, and complications associated with LHB. Next-generation devices have provided improved flexibility with lower profile delivery systems compared with first-generation stent grafts, which were bulky and necessitated large diameter sheaths (up to 26F) that often required iliac or abdominal aortic conduits to permit delivery of the device. Since the U.S. Food and Drug Administration's first device was approved in 2004 for degenerative thoracic aorta aneurysms, multiple devices and additional indications, such as traumatic injuries, penetrating ulcers, and aortic dissections, have been approved.

Preoperative Planning

High-resolution imaging is imperative for all patients being considered for TEVAR. The tortuous nature of the thoracic aorta and potential for involvement of the distal aortic arch mandate precise preoperative planning to prevent immediate treatment failures. Computed tomography angiography (CTA) is the most commonly used diagnostic test for patients with suspected aortic pathology. Of the many benefits of CTA, perhaps the most important is the multiple reconstructions that can be created from the original images that are vital for preoperative planning. Magnetic resonance angiography is another option, particularly in patients with renal insufficiency; however, this modality includes long examination times, higher expenses, and lack of immediate availability and is almost prohibitive in patients with pacemakers or other implants. Possessing accurate preoperative imaging allows for the appropriate device selection and operative planning in regard to proximal and distal seal zones. A classification system has been created to better define proximal seal zones based on anatomic landmarks (Figure 5). The distal seal zone is typically proximal to the celiac axis.

The location of the proximal seal zone dictates the potential need for additional interventions. Pathologies involving the proximal DTA or distal arch may require coverage of the LSA. The most recent literature suggests that patients undergoing LSA coverage have improved outcomes with preservation of flow to the LSA. This can

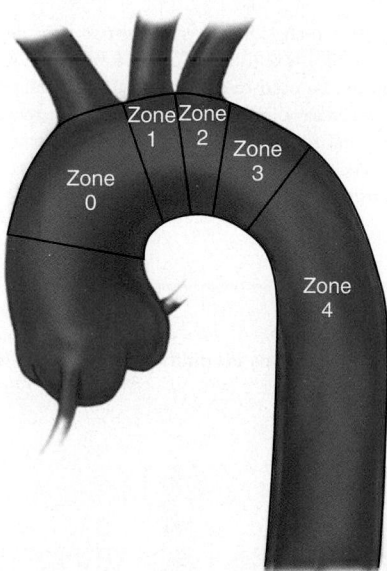

FIGURE 5 Depiction of the proximal seal zones depending on patient anatomy. Patients with proximal seal zones between zones 0 to 2 often require debranching procedures to preserve cerebral and upper extremity perfusion. In patients requiring zone 2 proximal seal zone, we recommend staged left subclavian artery (SCA) revascularization for elective cases. *(From Cameron JL.* Current Surgical Therapy. *11th ed. Chapter 169, Figure 18.)*

be done either in a staged approach with a carotid-subclavian bypass or transposition; or, at the time of TEVAR with creation of a fenestration to the LSA. Patients who mandate preservation of flow to the LSA include prior left internal mammary-coronary bypass, dominant left vertebral artery, incomplete circle of Willis, and presence of a functioning left upper extremity arteriovenous fistula or graft. Another critical element of preoperative planning is evaluation of the access vessels for delivery of the device, particularly the iliofemoral system. Although the evolution of devices has resulted in lower profile delivery systems, absence of appropriate access is a contraindication to TEVAR. An alternative to circumvent poor access vessels is to create an iliac or aortic conduit. Inadequate access vessel evaluation can lead to catastrophic consequences, including dissection, perforation, or frank rupture, which can result in patient mortality.

Operative Technique

In our Johns Hopkins approach to TEVAR, we advocate for preoperative placement of a lumbar drain for CSF drainage to reduce the risk of paraplegia, as well as LSA revascularization. CSF drainage is particularly important in cases in which coverage of the entire thoracic aorta is planned or the patient has previously undergone prior AAA repair. We recommend the drain be placed preoperatively because rapid placement of a lumbar drain after the onset of neurologic deficit is not practical in most settings. Furthermore, in our experience a limited time frame of 1 to 2 hours exists to initiate CSF drainage before irreversible ischemia to the spinal cord occurs. As such, delaying CSF drainage until the completion of the procedure and reversal of general anesthesia may place the patient at unnecessary risk. In addition, the LSA should not be covered by the stent graft in the absence of a first stage revascularization. For elective procedures, it is our practice to admit patients in advance of TEVAR to undergo either LSA-carotid transposition or bypass. Although our preference is for LSA transposition, LSA-carotid bypass may be necessary for situations unsuitable for transposition, such as prohibitive distance between the LSA and left carotid or an early take-off of the left vertebral artery just distal to the LSA origin. After a recovery period of 2 to 3 days, they return to the operating room for TEVAR during the same hospitalization.

The patient is placed in a supine position, and bilateral groins and abdomen are prepped and draped. General anesthetic is used commonly in these patients; however, the advent of percutaneous closure devices has resulted in the possibility of local anesthetic and moderate sedation for patients thought to be a prohibitive risk for general anesthesia based on cardiopulmonary comorbidities. Another option for high-risk patients includes epidural anesthesia.

A groin cutdown is performed on the intended access vessel that is identified on preoperative imaging. Percutaneous access is obtained on the contralateral common femoral artery (CFA) if there is no anatomic contraindication, and a 5F sheath is introduced. After the surgical exposure of the CFA for delivery of the device, the patient is systemically heparinized. An angiographic pigtail catheter then is introduced over a guidewire through the 5F sheath and into the thoracic aorta. The device then is introduced through the exposed CFA over a stiff wire to the approximate position of the pathology. Aortic arch or thoracic aorta angiography then is performed using DSA to delineate the aortic anatomy and determine the appropriate positioning of the stent graft (Figure 6). After deployment of the stent graft, a large-diameter compliant balloon can be used for improved fixation of the stent graft to the aortic wall at the proximal and distal landing zones, or at sites of overlap if multiple devices are deployed (Figure 7).

The access sheath from the device then is removed while concurrently monitoring the patient's hemodynamics to evaluate for any signs of access vessel disruption. If there are any indications of iatrogenic access injury, the sheath can be reinserted over the stiff wire to obturate the injury. In instances in which the sheath cannot be replaced, the large-diameter compliant balloon can be placed proximal to the site of injury to occlude the aorta and provide vascular control. Depending on the degree of vessel injury, repair options include a flank incision to access the retroperitoneum for reconstruction of the vessel in cases of frank disruption versus endovascular covered stent placement for less severe injuries. The contralateral 5F sheath can be removed with hemostasis obtained via manual pressure for 15 to 20 minutes or other commercially available closure assist devices. The access vessel arteriotomy is closed after appropriate flushing maneuvers. The femoral sheath is reapproximated, and the incision then closed in multiple layers to reduce the risk of seroma formation.

Outcomes

The application of endovascular therapies for pathologies of the thoracic aorta was pioneered by Dake and colleagues in 1994. Their initial series of 13 patients undergoing TEVAR demonstrated 100% technical success with the absence of mortality and paraplegia. This initial report was followed by the first long-term outcomes as part of the midterm follow-up results of the Gore TAG trial. The trial compared 191 patients undergoing TEVAR for DTAA to 94 patients who received traditional, open surgical repair. Their findings demonstrated that patients undergoing TEVAR had decreased rates of

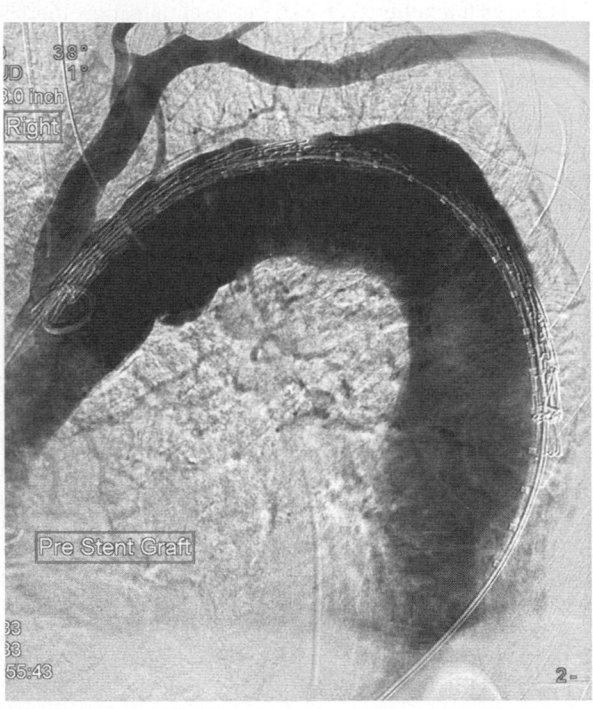

FIGURE 6 Thoracic aorta digital subtraction angiography is used once the thoracic stent graft has been introduced through the femoral vessels. After appropriate imaging and positioning, the stent graft is then ready to be deployed.

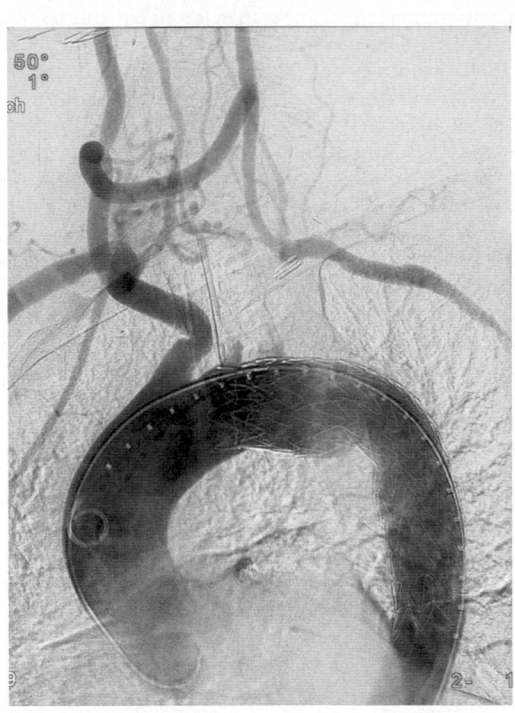

FIGURE 7 Completion angiography is performed after deployment of the stent graft to confirm exclusion of the aneurysm sac. A large-diameter compliant balloon can be used to improve fixation at the proximal or distal seal zone if necessary. In this case, the aneurysm anatomy dictated a zone 1 proximal seal zone, and completion imaging demonstrates preoperative debranching with a carotid-carotid bypass and left carotid-subclavian transposition.

TABLE 1 Comparison of TEVAR With Open Surgical Repair*

	Gore TAG	Cook TX2	Medtronic Talent	Johns Hopkins Hospital	Open Repair
Patients	140	160	195	90	353
Mean age (yr)	71	72	70	67	68
Mortality	1.5%	1.9%	2.1%	3.3%	7.1%
SCI (paraplegia/paraparesis)	2.8%	5.6%	8.7%	1%	13.0%
Stroke	3.5%	2.5%	3.6%	1%	6.7%
1-year reintervention	2.1%	4.4%	10.7%	NR	3.7%
Aneurysm-related survival	83%	91.6%	83.9%	NR	82%

*Summary of outcomes among the three multicenter regulatory trials, as well as The Johns Hopkins Hospital experience, comparing TEVAR to open surgical repair. Patients undergoing TEVAR had decreased rates of perioperative mortality, SCI and stroke compared with those having traditional open repairs.

SCI, Spinal cord injury; *TEVAR,* thoracic endovascular aortic repair.

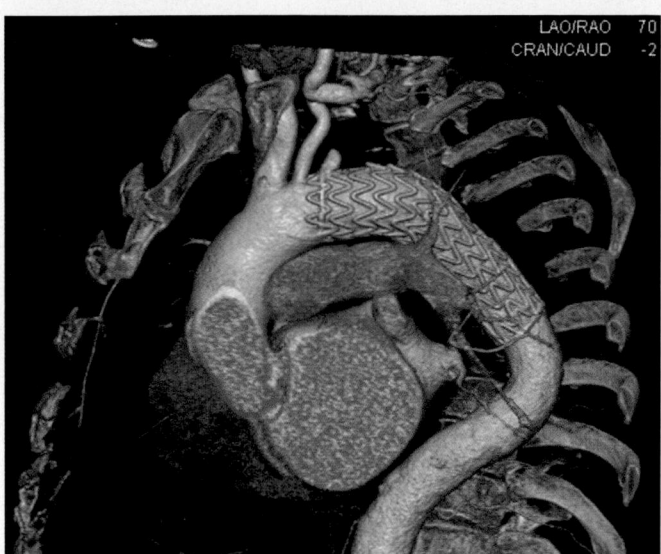

FIGURE 8 Postoperative computed tomography angiography after thoracic endovascular repair for a descending thoracic aortic aneurysm. Three-dimensional reconstructions in the sagittal plane confirm appropriate positioning of the stent graft with exclusion of the aneurysm sac without evidence of migration or endoleak. Previous ligation of the proximal left subclavian artery (SCA) with a patent left carotid-subclavian transposition to allow for zone 2 deployment also is demonstrated.

aneurysm-related mortality (2.8% vs 11.7%, $P = 0.008$) but similar rate of all-cause mortality (68% vs 67%, $P = 0.433$) at 5-year follow-up. TEVAR also was associated with lower rates of major adverse events during the first postoperative year (42% vs 77%, $P < 0.001$). However, 3.6% of TEVAR patients were subjected to secondary interventions, and 21% were found to have endoleaks, or

persistent communication between the previously sealed aorta and the aneurysm sac. During the follow-up period, there were no reported ruptures or stent graft collapse, and only one incidence of significant stent graft migration. Trials using additional devices have since been performed and again were found to be at least comparable with, if not superior to, open surgical repair (Table 1). Walsh and colleagues published a meta-analysis of 17 studies and found significant reductions in mortality and major neurologic complication rates when comparing TEVAR with open surgical repair. Although prospective, randomized trials comparing TEVAR to open surgical repair are lacking, most mid-term and long-term follow-up data suggest that TEVAR is superior to traditional open surgical repair in regard to perioperative mortality and SCI. TEVAR is particularly of benefit in patients thought to be unfit for open surgical repair because of pre-existing comorbidities or baseline functional status (Figure 8).

SUGGESTED READINGS

Arnaoutakis DJ, Arnaoutakis GJ, Beaulieu RJ, et al. Results of adjunctive spinal drainage and/or left subclavian artery bypass in thoracic endovascular aortic repair. *Ann Vasc Surg.* 2014;28:65-73.

Cambria RP, Davison JK, Zannetti S, et al. Thoracoabdominal aneurysm repair: perspectives over a decade with the clamp-and-sew technique. *Ann Surg.* 1997;226:294-303.

Coselli JS, LeMaire SA, Koksoy C, et al. Cerebrospinal fluid drainage reduces paraplegia after thoracoabdominal aortic aneurysm repair: results of a randomized clinical trial. *J Vasc Surg.* 2002;35:631-639.

Crawford ES, Crawford JL, Safi HJ, et al. Thoracoabdominal aortic aneurysms: preoperative and intraoperative factors determining immediate and long-term results of operations in 605 patients. *J Vasc Surg.* 1986;3: 389-404.

LeMaire SA, Price MD, Green SY, et al. Results of open thoracoabdominal aortic aneurysm repair. *Ann Cardiothorac Surg.* 2012;1:286-292.

Makaroun MS, Dillavou ED, Wheatley GH, Cambria RP. Five-year results of endovascular treatment with the Gore TAG device compared with open repair of thoracic aortic aneurysms. *J Vasc Surg.* 2008;47:912-918.

Safi HJ, Miller CC 3rd, Huynh TT, et al. Distal aortic perfusion and cerebrospinal fluid drainage for thoracoabdominal and descending thoracic aortic repair: ten years of organ protection. *Ann Surg.* 2003;238:372-380.

THE MANAGEMENT OF ACUTE AORTIC DISSECTIONS

Karen M. Kim, MD, and Thomas E. MacGillivray, MD

Acute aortic dissection is the most common catastrophe of the human aorta. With a reported incidence of 3 out of 100,000 patients each year, aortic dissections are a deadly disease with an early mortality of 1% to 2% per hour. Without appropriate treatment, the 2-week mortality of aortic dissections involving the ascending aorta is approximately 90%. Although the presentation may be classic, symptoms can be nonspecific and can occur in patients with no evident risk factors. Misdiagnosis leading to even a slight delay in treatment is associated with increased mortality. Therefore proper diagnosis and expeditious therapy are essential for improved survival.

■ CLASSIFICATION

Acute aortic dissection can manifest in several different patterns, which have different therapeutic and prognostic implications. There

are two classification schemes in use worldwide to describe aortic dissection: the DeBakey and Stanford systems (Figure 1). The DeBakey system categorizes the dissection based on the origin of the intimal tear and the extent of the dissection. Aortic dissections involving the ascending, arch, and descending aorta are DeBakey type I. Dissections confined only to the ascending aorta are DeBakey type II. Aortic dissections that originate and propagate distal to the left subclavian artery are DeBakey type III (IIIa is limited to the descending thoracic aorta, IIIb extends below the diaphragm).

The Stanford classification system divides dissections into two categories: those that involve the ascending aorta (proximal to the innominate artery) and those that do not. Stanford A dissections include all dissections involving the ascending aorta (DeBakey types I and II) regardless of the site of origin. Stanford B dissections describe dissections not involving the ascending aorta, including those involving the aortic arch.

Historically, "acute" dissections are those present for 14 days or less, whereas "chronic" dissections describe those present for greater than 2 weeks. Recently, the nomenclature has been modified to include a "subacute" phase between 2 to 6 weeks from the initial presentation. This subacute phase can be a time of potential instability of the remaining dissected aortic segment. Acute Stanford A dissections account for greater than 60% of all dissections and are considered surgical emergencies requiring immediate operation. Acute Stanford B dissections are further classified as "complicated" and "uncomplicated." Complicated Stanford B dissections include

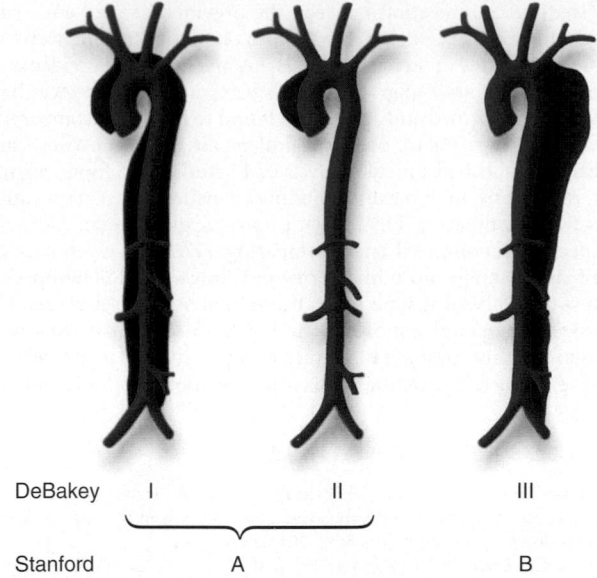

FIGURE 1 Anatomy and classification of aortic dissection: DeBakey and Stanford systems. *(Modified from Cambria RP, Brewster DC, Gertler J, et al. Vascular complications associated with spontaneous aortic dissection, J Vasc Surg. 1988;7:199-209.)*

approximately 20% of patients with rupture or impending rupture, malperfusion, and/or refractory pain or hypertension for whom open surgical or endovascular therapy is recommended. Uncomplicated Stanford B dissections are effectively managed with aggressive medical therapy.

Intramural hematoma (IMH) comprises approximately 10% to 20% of patients who have the clinical picture of acute aortic dissection but on imaging have no blood flow in the false lumen or any identifiable intimal lesions. IMH may result from a microscopic intimal tear, hemorrhage of the vasa vasorum, or a penetrating aortic ulcer. IMH is sometimes inappropriately referred to as a dissection with a thrombosed false lumen. Although it is a matter of discussion and debate, we manage IMH the same as acute aortic dissection.

PRESENTATION AND DIAGNOSIS

An acute aortic dissection results from a sudden aortic intimal disruption, which leads to the pressurized propagation of blood flow plowing through the false lumen within the media of the aorta. Circulatory collapse and death can occur within seconds because of aortic rupture frequently misdiagnosed as a massive myocardial infarction. The classic presentation is acute, severe, "10/10," "tearing," or "ripping" chest pain radiating to the back between the scapulae. Occasionally, patients have little or no pain. Afflicted patients often appear listless and possess a sense of impending doom.

Because blood flow in the false lumen can disrupt and occlude branch vessels of the aorta, patients can have symptoms and signs of malperfusion. A new neurologic deficit or a pulseless extremity can distract the unsuspecting clinician. Electrocardiogram changes or a new diastolic murmur can occur from retrograde dissection into the coronary arteries or the aortic valve resulting in myocardial ischemia or congestive heart failure. Acute paralysis, abdominal pain, renal insufficiency, and syncope are well-recognized atypical presentations of acute dissection. Difficult-to-control hypertension can be a risk factor and a presenting sign in patients with aortic dissection. Hypotension and shock are concerning signs of tamponade, cardiac dysfunction, or ongoing hemorrhage. A high index of suspicion for aortic dissection is imperative for any patient with asymmetric pulses or differential blood pressures in the extremities.

High-resolution contrast-enhanced computed tomographic angiography (CTA) has replaced conventional aortography as the gold standard diagnostic study to confirm or exclude the diagnosis of acute aortic dissection. CTA has a diagnostic sensitivity and specificity of 90% to 100% and is readily available in most hospitals. False-positive diagnoses can occur as a result of artifactual lines resulting from mistiming of contrast boluses or inappropriate gating with the cardiac cycle. Although scans limited to the thoracic aorta can confirm the diagnosis, it is helpful to scan the entire aorta and iliofemoral vessels to assess for subclinical malperfusion and to assist in planning the surgical strategy.

Transesophageal echocardiography (TEE) is a valuable tool to diagnose and manage patients with acute aortic dissection. Although TEE does require special expertise, it can assess rapidly for tamponade, valvular dysfunction, and cardiac wall motion abnormalities, particularly in the hemodynamically unstable patient transported directly to the operating room. Magnetic resonance imaging (MRI), conventional aortography, and coronary angiography have a very limited role in the acute management of aortic dissection patients.

MANAGEMENT

Once the diagnosis of acute aortic dissection is suspected, invasive hemodynamic monitoring and aggressive anti-impulse therapy should be instituted without delay. A radial or femoral arterial monitoring cannula should be placed in the extremity with the best pulse and blood pressure. Intravenous beta-blockade should be the medication of first choice to decrease the aortic dP/dT, titrating the infusion to a goal heart rate of 60 to 70 beats per minute and a systolic blood pressure of 100 to 110 mm Hg. Once adequate beta-blockade is achieved, vasodilators can be added to further control hypertension. Initial blood pressure control with vasodilators such as nitroprusside or hydralazine should be avoided. Although vasodilators will lower the blood pressure, they can increase the dP/dT and shear forces in the aorta, thereby increasing the risk of rupture. Acute Stanford A dissection patients with a diastolic murmur or TEE evidence of significant aortic valve regurgitation should not be managed with beta-blockers because of the high risk of exacerbating congestive heart failure.

Acute aortic dissection can be a dynamic disease with a rapidly evolving clinical course. Patients diagnosed with acute type A aortic dissection should be transferred emergently to a cardiac surgical center for immediate surgical repair. Time is critical. Unnecessary testing or optimizing medical therapy should not be allowed to delay definitive treatment, which is surgery. Even patients with cerebral, renal, visceral, and/or extremity malperfusion should be managed with central aortic reconstruction as a first step, which frequently will correct the malperfusion syndrome. Although nonoperative management carries a very high risk of death, good clinical judgment always has an important role in the management of very high-risk patients.

Surgical Management of Stanford A Dissections

The goal of surgical therapy for acute type A aortic dissection is to prevent imminent death from aortic rupture (causing exsanguination or tamponade), acute aortic insufficiency, or malperfusion to the coronary, cerebral, and systemic circulations. The principal technique to accomplish these goals is to replace the tenuous ascending aorta with a tube interposition graft and to re-establish blood flow in the true lumen of the aorta.

Invasive arterial and central venous pressure monitoring are helpful for the induction and conduct of general anesthesia. Temperature monitoring of the nasopharynx, central venous or pulmonary arterial blood, and bladder can ensure uniform perfusion and cooling. TEE, electroencephalogram, and cerebral oximetry are useful adjuncts for monitoring.

Cardiopulmonary bypass is required for ascending aortic replacement; therefore the surgeon must determine the site of arterial cannulation and perfusion. Traditionally, the common femoral artery has been the most common approach for arterial cannulation given its size, easy accessibility, and surgeons' familiarity. In recent years, experienced aortic surgeons have been using the right axillary/subclavian artery as the preferred site for arterial perfusion. The arterial cannula can be connected to an 8- or 10-mm Dacron graft that is anastomosed in end-to-side fashion to the axillary artery. This approach allows for antegrade systemic perfusion and the option of selective antegrade cerebral perfusion during circulatory arrest should extensive arch reconstruction be required. Some experienced surgeons advocate the use of direct central ascending aortic cannulation with the use of TEE guidance. This approach can be challenging, but central aortic cannulation can be lifesaving in the management of an unstable patient.

Through a median sternotomy the heart and ascending aorta are readily exposed. The right atrium is cannulated easily for venous drainage to initiate cardiopulmonary bypass. Most aortic surgeons recommend deep hypothermia in preparation for an open distal aortic anastomosis, although recent reports of using moderate hypothermia with antegrade cerebral perfusion have been successful. During cooling, it is imperative that the surgical, anesthesia, and perfusion teams monitor the patient to ensure uniform perfusion and cooling. Occasionally, cannulation strategies must be altered to manage malperfusion during cardiopulmonary bypass. Given the increased frequency of aortic insufficiency and coronary malperfusion, the surgeon should be prepared to vent the left ventricle on bypass and meticulously protect the myocardium with direct antegrade coronary ostial and/or retrograde coronary sinus cardioplegia strategies.

Although there is considerable debate about the optimal temperature for profound hypothermia and circulatory arrest, we achieve 18° C in the nasopharynx before turning off the circulation. With the patient in Trendelenburg position, the entire ascending aorta from the sinotubular junction up to the innominate artery is resected. The aortic tissues are extremely fragile, and they should be handled delicately. Without an aortic cross-clamp, the aortic arch can be inspected for complex intimal disruptions and to confirm that the brachiocephalic branches are intact and arising from the true lumen. All of the layers of the proximal aortic arch then are reconstructed, thereby obliterating the false lumen, which will then allow blood flow through the true lumen once central perfusion is re-established. Some surgeons reconstitute the aortic wall between two Teflon felt strips and anastomose a Dacron graft to the aortic-felt sandwich (Figure 2, *A*). We prefer to insert Teflon felt into the false lumen and then sew the Dacron graft to the reconstituted aorta buttressed with a strip of Dacron around the adventitia. We avoid the use of glues during these operations. Although glues allow for easier tissue handling, they can be destructive to the aorta and promote late pseudoaneurysm formation.

With the distal anastomosis completed, the aortic arch is de-aired, the proximal end of the graft is clamped, and cardiopulmonary bypass is resumed through the Dacron graft to promote true lumen flow (Figure 2, *B* and *C*). Generally, aortic arch replacement is not routinely necessary for managing most patients with acute type A aortic dissection. Arch replacement increases the complexity and length of the procedure, which can add to the already high-risk operation. Situations when the aortic arch should be considered for replacement in acute dissection patients include complex intimal disruptions in the arch, arch aneurysms larger than 5 cm, or connective tissue syndromes (e.g., Marfan, Loeys-Dietz, Ehlers-Danlos). Arch replacements should be performed with the use of selective antegrade cerebral perfusion, which has been demonstrated to improve outcomes.

During rewarming the aortic root and proximal ascending aorta are assessed and reconstructed (Figure 2, *D*). Often, the aortic root is involved minimally with the dissection, and the sinotubular junction can be reconstructed in a similar sandwich-type fashion as the distal anastomosis. Aortic dissections extending into the sinus portion of the aortic root can be reconstructed using a "neo-media" technique by obliterating the false lumen with Teflon felt. Attention is required in patients with aortic regurgitation and in those who have complex aortic root dissections approaching the coronary ostia. Aortic regurgitation is the most common cardiac complication associated with acute type A dissection. There are three possible dissection-related mechanisms that can contribute to aortic regurgitation. Acute dilation of the sinotubular junction and root caused by the expanding false lumen can result in incomplete coaptation of the valve cusps. The dissection also can extend into the aortic root, disrupting the commissural posts, resulting in prolapse of the valve cusps. In addition, an aortic flap can prolapse through the valve in diastole, preventing appropriate valve function. In most patients, the sinotubular junction can be reconstructed, the aortic valve commissures resuspended, and the aortic root preserved. Situations when composite aortic root replacement with coronary button reimplantation should be considered include patients with aneurysms of the aortic root exceeding 5 cm, complex aortic valve pathology, dissection approaching the coronary ostia, and connective tissue syndromes (e.g., Marfan, Loeys-Dietz, Ehlers-Danlos). Valve-sparing aortic root replacement should be reserved for highly experienced aortic surgeons in this setting.

Surgical Results With Acute Type A Dissections

According to the International Registry of Acute Aortic Dissection (IRAD) database, the overall surgical mortality of acute type A aortic dissection is 25%. In unstable patients (preoperative presence of tamponade, shock, congestive heart failure, stroke, coma, myocardial ischemia/infarction, acute renal failure, or mesenteric ischemia) the surgical mortality is 31%. Postoperatively, aortic dissection patients are at risk for coagulopathic bleeding, requiring transfusions and re-exploration. Transient neurologic dysfunction, stroke, renal insufficiency, acute lung injury, new malperfusion syndromes, multiorgan system failure, and refractory hypertension are some of the possible early postoperative complications requiring intensive care and prolonged hospital care of these complicated patients. There is variability of outcomes reported from different centers, but the fact remains that acute type A aortic dissection is a highly lethal condition that, even when appropriately managed, has a high risk of morbidity and mortality.

Management of Acute Type B Dissections

Medical management of patients with "uncomplicated" type B dissections with anti-impulse therapy remains the preferred treatment, resulting in reported in-hospital mortality rates of less than 10%. Approximately 25% of patients with acute type B dissections are "complicated" by refractory hypertension (at least three different classes of drugs), malperfusion syndromes, increasing periaortic hematomas, bloody pleural effusions, and/or shock. Patients with complicated acute type B aortic dissection have a high risk of early death if not appropriately treated. Historically, the results of open surgical therapy for acute type B dissection have been associated with a higher mortality rate than medical therapy, perhaps because of patient selection or complications requiring surgery. For patients with complicated type B dissections, thoracic endovascular aortic repair (TEVAR) largely has replaced open surgery with improved results. The 5-year survival of patients with chronic type B aortic dissection is 60% to 80%. Whether TEVAR is superior to medical management in high-risk patients with uncomplicated type B dissection remains to be proven. There are reports that TEVAR improves aortic remodeling over time, which may translate to decreased aortic complications and improved long-term survival.

cerebral infarction and its extent. MRI is more accurate in the early hours after a stroke. Previous studies have demonstrated that as much as 10% of asymptomatic patients and 30% of patients who have experienced TIAs will have evidence of cerebral infarctions on CT or MRI studies.

INDICATIONS FOR CAROTID ENDARTERECTOMY

The indications for CEA have been established by level I evidence derived from several randomized prospective clinical trials (Table 1). The North American Symptomatic Carotid Endarterectomy Trial (NASCET) demonstrated a clear benefit of CEA and best medical management compared with best medical management alone for symptomatic patients with high-grade (70% to 99%) carotid stenoses. In the same year the European Carotid Surgery Trial (ECST) demonstrated a similar but smaller benefit in symptomatic patients with 70% to 99% stenoses. Analysis of a second cohort of symptomatic patients with moderate (50% to 69%) stenoses in the NASCET demonstrated a smaller but statistically significant benefit as well. Interim and late analysis of patients in the ECST did not show benefit of treating patients with moderate stenoses, owing to higher perioperative morbidity and mortality rates.

The Asymptomatic Carotid Atherosclerosis Study (ACAS) demonstrated a significant benefit of CEA and best medical management compared with best medical management alone for patients with asymptomatic stenoses of 60% to 99%. These findings have been confirmed in the Asymptomatic Carotid Surgery Trial (ACST) in Europe.

The most recent published clinical practice guidelines of the Society for Vascular Surgery recommend CEA and optimal medical therapy for patients with symptomatic disease (stroke or TIA) and a 50% or greater internal carotid stenosis, and state that CEA should be "considered" for asymptomatic patients with a 60% or greater internal carotid stenosis, assuming that the patient has reasonable life expectancy (3 to 5 years) and that the operation can be performed with a stroke/death rate less than 3%. These recommendations mirror earlier guidelines from the American Heart Association (AHA). Specifically, the AHA recommends CEA for patients who have experienced a TIA or stroke within 6 months and have ipsilateral 70% to 99% internal carotid stenoses if the surgeon has a perioperative stroke/death rate of 6% or less. For symptomatic patients with a 50% to 69% ipsilateral internal carotid stenosis, CEA is recommended after consideration of patient-specific factors such as age, comorbidity, and severity of symptoms. For asymptomatic patients, the AHA recommends CEA for patients with a 60% to 99% stenosis if the surgeon's perioperative stroke/death rate is 3% or less.

Despite this level I evidence, the role of CEA in the management of patients with asymptomatic carotid disease has been challenged recently by a small number of international opinion leaders. This argument is predicated on the observation that the natural history of asymptomatic carotid disease in contemporary practice is better than what was observed in the medically managed patients in the randomized trials because of recent improvements in medical management. However, it is also true that the outcome of CEA today is superior to what was observed in the trials as well. Therefore I believe that there is no logical evidence to dismiss the findings of the ACAS and ACST investigations and that the recommendations for CEA in the currently published guidelines remain appropriate. The ongoing CREST-2 trial is designed to address this issue.

CAROTID ENDARTERECTOMY: OPERATIVE TECHNIQUE

Anesthesia

CEA may be performed under general anesthesia, regional anesthesia with deep or superficial cervical block, or even pure local anesthesia. Although early reports suggested a reduced length of stay associated with CEA performed under regional anesthesia, comparable lengths of stay are routinely documented today among patients who undergo operation under general anesthesia. The majority of studies comparing the two techniques have reported improved perioperative cardiac stability with regional anesthesia, but this does not necessarily result in a reduced incidence of myocardial infarction. Disadvantages of regional anesthesia include potential patient discomfort or anxiety, risk of seizure or allergic reaction, anxiety for the operating surgeon, and compromise of technique.

Patient Positioning

Careful positioning of the patient is important to ensure patient comfort and adequate operative exposure. Positioning begins with placing a roll behind the scapula to achieve some extension of the neck. A padded ring is placed under the head to prevent neck injury from hyperextension. If general anesthesia is used, the endotracheal tube should be taped to the corner of the mouth opposite to the surgical field. If local or regional anesthesia is used, a Mayo stand is placed over the patient's head to suspend the surgical drapes away from the patient's face to prevent sensations of claustrophobia.

Skin Incision

The standard incision used is a longitudinal incision parallel to the medial border of the sternocleidomastoid muscle. The upper portion of the incision is angled posterior to the earlobe if cephalad exposure above the angle of the jaw is required. An alternative is to place the incision transversely in an appropriately located skin crease, usually 1 to 2 cm inferior to the angle of the jaw. This incision provides excellent cosmesis postoperatively. However, if the transverse incision is made in a suboptimal location, it may be more difficult to obtain more cephalad or caudal exposure in the wound.

TABLE 1: Carotid Endarterectomy: Randomized Trials

Trial	Indication	Perioperative CVA/Death	Risk Reduction	P
NASCET	Sx: >70%	5.8%	16.5% / 2 years	<0.001
	Sx: 50%-69%	6.7%	10.1% / 5 years	<0.05
ECST	Sx: 70%-99%	7.5%	9.6% / 3 years	<0.01
ACAS	Asx: >60%	2.3%	5.9% / 5 years	0.004
ACST	Asx: >60%	3.1%	5.4% / 5 years	<0.0001

ACAS, Asymptomatic Carotid Atherosclerosis Study; *ACST*, Asymptomatic Carotid Surgery Trial; *Asx*, asymptomatic; *CVA*, cerebrovascular accident; *ECST*, European Carotid Surgery Trial; *NASCET*, North American Symptomatic Carotid Endarterectomy Trial; *Sx*, symptomatic.

Operative Exposure

Meticulous surgical technique is paramount to a successful operation. Manipulation of the carotid artery should be minimized, as intraoperative embolization can result from careless handling. The dissection is begun by dividing the platysma and mobilizing the medial border of the sternocleidomastoid muscle. The external jugular vein lies deep to the platysma and should be sought out in this plane to avoid injury or in the event that it is needed for patching. It is more commonly encountered with an oblique skin crease incision than with a longitudinal incision. The other structure located at this level is the greater auricular nerve; injury to this nerve leads to numbness of the earlobe. The carotid sheath is entered, and the medial border of the internal jugular vein is dissected. The facial vein is identified crossing medially in the base of the wound and divided; sometimes it has an early bifurcation or trifurcation, and multiple branches need to be ligated. The jugular vein is then retracted laterally. The vagus nerve is identified at this point in the carotid sheath, usually located posteriorly between the jugular vein and carotid artery, although in a minority of patients it may lie anteriorly. The common carotid artery (CCA) is controlled circumferentially with an umbilical tape and Rummel's tourniquet if a shunt is to be used. At this point the ansa cervicalis nerve should be identified; it usually lies medial to the distal CCA. Identifying this nerve facilitates the safe dissection of the carotid bifurcation and avoids injury to the hypoglossal nerve, which crosses medially from a superior to inferior location. The superior thyroid artery is identified coming off the medial border of the carotid bifurcation or proximal external carotid artery (ECA) and controlled with a tie or vessel loop. The ECA and ICA are encircled with vessel loops, making certain to control the latter beyond the disease process. During the dissection of the carotid bifurcation and its branches, one should avoid dissecting in the crotch of the carotid bifurcation to avoid injuring the carotid body because this can result in hemodynamic instability and troublesome bleeding. If hemodynamic instability results, the carotid body can be injected gently with 1% lidocaine.

Before clamping, the patient is administered 70 to 100 units/kg of heparin, and it is allowed to circulate for 3 minutes. The ICA is clamped first to prevent embolization that can result when the CCA or ECA is clamped. Care should be taken to make sure the ICA is clamped on a normal portion of the artery distal to the plaque.

If local anesthesia or intraoperative EEG is used for selective shunting, a test clamp on the distal ICA should be applied for at least 3 minutes to check for changes in the neurologic examination or electroencephalogram (EEG) pattern. If such changes occur, the artery should be unclamped to allow for reperfusion before reclamping and opening the carotid bifurcation because opening the bifurcation and placing a shunt may take 2 to 3 minutes and should not be performed while the brain is already ischemic. However, unclamping the ICA introduces the potential for embolization from a disrupted plaque.

If carotid stump pressure is to be measured, clamps are placed on the CCA and ECA and a needle connected to a pressure line is placed into the distal CCA artery below the carotid bifurcation. A stump pressure higher than 50 mm Hg is generally indicative of adequate perfusion, but this is not foolproof. Clamping the CCA and placing the needle into the artery does introduce the potential for embolization.

Conventional Endarterectomy

The conventional technique for CEA consists of a vertical arteriotomy and, today, closure with a patch angioplasty. The arteriotomy is begun in the CCA and continued through the carotid bifurcation into the ICA. One should avoid making the incision too close to the flow divider at the ECA origin because this can distort the anatomy and make the closure more difficult. If a shunt is used, it is first placed in the distal ICA and back bled before the proximal end is placed into the CCA. Two commonly used shunts are the Pruitt-Inahara and Javid shunts. A third shunt, preferred by me, is a simple vinyl tube. Because this shunt lies entirely within the artery, it allows the surgeon to almost completely finish closing the arteriotomy before the shunt is removed. Its small diameter allows atraumatic placement in even small ICAs, whereas its short length offers less resistance to blood flow such that physiologic flow in the ICA is maintained.

The endarterectomy is begun in the CCA in the plane between the media and the adventitia. The proximal endpoint in the distal CCA is established and the plaque is trimmed at that location in a beveled manner. The endarterectomy is continued into the orifice of the ECA, first with a Freer elevator and then with a fine clamp that is passed up into the ECA in the plane of the endarterectomy. The vessel loop on the ECA is released transiently while the plaque is everted from within the ECA. The endpoint of the plaque is inspected; an ideal endpoint is a gradually tapering, feathered endpoint.

Then the endarterectomy is continued upward into the ICA. A technically perfect endpoint in the ICA is absolutely critical to avoid perioperative stroke and recurrent stenosis. It is virtually always possible to achieve a satisfactory endpoint in the ICA, although this may require special maneuvers to expose the distal ICA with extension of the arteriotomy to facilitate extraction of a long endarterectomy specimen. Tacking sutures at the distal endpoint should be avoided unless absolutely necessary; these are associated with increased perioperative stroke and are indicative of a problematic endpoint. The endarterectomy should be terminated in normal ICA with a gradual, tapered transition to normal intima. This is best accomplished by pulling the plaque transversely away from the artery with lateral traction. One should avoid pulling out or down on the plaque, which is more likely to result in a step-off that can be difficult to correct.

The preponderance of evidence indicates that the arteriotomy should be closed with a patch. A variety of patch materials are available for use, including autologous vein, polytetrafluoroethylene (PTFE), woven polyester (Dacron), and bovine pericardium. I prefer Dacron and running 6-0 polypropylene suture. The vessels are bled and then the endarterectomy site is irrigated vigorously with heparinized saline and inspected again for debris or intimal flaps before the arteriotomy is finally closed. The clamp on the ICA is released briefly to fill the vessel with blood. It then is replaced while the clamps on the CCA and ECA are released so that any remaining air or debris will be flushed up the territory of the ECA rather than the ICA. At this point the ICA clamp is removed.

Eversion Endarterectomy

Eversion endarterectomy represents an excellent alternative technique. The ICA is amputated obliquely at the carotid bifurcation and the adventitia is rolled back until normal intima is encountered at the distal endpoint. Residual plaque in the common and external carotid arteries is endarterectomized, and the ICA is reanastomosed to the CCA with 6-0 polypropylene suture. The advantage of this technique is that the anastomosis can be performed rapidly and is not prone to restenosis, and therefore patching is not required. The disadvantages are that a more extensive dissection is sometimes necessary to mobilize the vessels during the eversion, the procedure does not lend itself readily to shunting (although shunting is not precluded by this technique), and it can be difficult to visualize the endpoint in the ICA after the plaque has been removed (the artery tends to retract as soon as the plaque pulls away from the adventitia, and it can be difficult to expose and reinspect this area of the artery).

Cerebral Protection and Monitoring

One of the long-standing debated issues related to the performance of CEA concerns the use of intravascular shunts: routine nonuse of shunts, selective use of shunts, and routine use of shunts. The simplest way to perform CEA is to just clamp the carotid bifurcation and perform CEA without a shunt, and several large series document excellent results of CEA without shunts. However, all of these studies demonstrate at least a small incidence of stroke, and in at least some cases the cause of the stroke is intraoperative cerebral ischemia during carotid artery clamping.

Alternatively, some routinely shunt in all cases of CEA, and excellent results have been reported in several large series. However, all of these studies document an incidence of stroke, and in some of these cases the cause of the stroke was attributed to technical problems related to the use of the shunt.

A third option is to shunt selectively. Several techniques have been utilized to identify the patient who truly needs a shunt. In the patient who is under general anesthesia, these techniques include intraoperative measurement of carotid "stump pressure" after the CCA and ECA have been clamped, intraoperative neurologic monitoring of the patient's EEG or somatosensory evoked potential (SSEP), measurement of middle cerebral artery (MCA) flow by transcranial Doppler (TCD), and monitoring of cerebral oximetry. The most accurate method is to perform CEA under regional anesthesia, whereby the selection of patients for shunting is based on alterations in the neurologic examination that develop after the carotid artery is clamped.

Completion Studies

Although there are several potential causes of perioperative stroke among patients who undergo CEA, a preventable cause is thromboembolism or carotid artery thrombosis resulting from technical imperfection in the carotid artery repair. To minimize this risk, intraoperative completion studies, including continuous wave Doppler, duplex ultrasound, and intraoperative angiography, have been utilized.

Continuous wave Doppler analysis is a purely qualitative method by which an experienced operator also can identify areas of stenosis by the high pitch associated with a stenosis. However, it is insensitive to small intimal flaps or more subtle stenoses and is operator dependent. Duplex ultrasound is a much more sensitive tool that provides detailed anatomic imaging as well as real-time physiologic information regarding blood flow through the carotid vessels and is my preference. However, although the ICA endpoint should be visualized directly before closing the arteriotomy, the CCA clamp site is a relative blind spot so that duplex examination allows one to rule out unsuspected plaque injury that can be repaired before completing the arteriotomy closure. The data yielded from duplex examination are somewhat operator dependent, and there can be technical limitations with placing the Doppler probe in the wound to achieve an adequate examination. Intraoperative angiography has been considered the gold standard of completion studies.

Exposure for High Lesions

Several methods can be used to gain additional cephalad exposure of the high carotid bifurcation (Box 1). The easiest of these, and the initial approach, is to start the operation with nasotracheal intubation; with the patient's mouth closed, the vertical ramus of the mandible is displaced anteriorly 1 to 2 cm compared with when the mouth is open with an oral endotracheal tube. The additional few millimeters of distal ICA exposure afforded by this maneuver often will be the difference in achieving a suitable endarterectomy

---

BOX 1: Options to Facilitate High Carotid Exposure

Nasotracheal intubation
Division of posterior belly of digastric muscle
Resection of styloid process
Anterior subluxation of mandible
Vertical osteotomy ramus of mandible

---

endpoint in the distal ICA. The next step to enhance distal exposure is to divide the posterior belly of the digastric muscle. This muscle takes the same diagonal course through the wound as the hypoglossal nerve, but it is located superficial to the nerve. Therefore this nerve should be identified carefully and protected before the muscle is divided. Two other nerves that can be injured high in the neck are the spinal accessory nerve, which enters the tendinous portion of the sternocleidomastoid muscle, usually in the upper third of the muscle, and the glossopharyngeal nerve, which lies deep to the digastric muscle. The next maneuver that can be extremely effective in gaining cephalad exposure is resection of the styloid process. The insertions of the muscles on the styloid process are excised and it is carefully resected with a rongeur. This maneuver will permit exposure of the ICA all the way to the skull base.

There are two other options for improving distal exposure of the high bifurcation, both of which require preoperative planning and coordination with the oral or plastic surgeon. Anterior subluxation of the mandible requires placing the mandible in temporary intermaxillary fixation. An even more aggressive approach utilizes a complete vertical osteotomy through the vertical ramus of the mandible, with separation of the mandible to expose the ICA.

■ PERIOPERATIVE MEDICAL MANAGEMENT

In addition to risk factor control, the patient should be on an antiplatelet medication (aspirin or clopidogrel) at the time of the CEA. Furthermore, there is compelling evidence that all patients undergoing CEA should be on a statin medication. In my series of nearly 1600 CEAs, the 30-day rate of stroke and death was significantly lower among patients taking a statin medication at the time of operation compared with nonusers. There was also a trend toward a lower rate of perioperative myocardial infarction among statin users. I prefer a continuous infusion of low-molecular-weight dextran for the first 24 hours postoperatively or until hospital discharge. Antiplatelet and statin therapy should be continued long term in the patient who has undergone a CEA.

■ RESULTS

Perioperative mortality has become exceedingly uncommon after CEA, averaging less than 1% and generally around 0.5%. Cardiac disease is the most common cause. The incidence of perioperative stroke ranges from 1% to 5% in contemporary practice and correlates directly with the clinical indication for operation. The perioperative stroke incidence should be no more than 1% to 2% among asymptomatic patients and ranges from 2% to 6% among symptomatic patients.

Carotid artery disease is an excellent marker for underlying coronary artery disease, and perioperative myocardial infarction occurs in 2% to 4% of patients in practice today. Systemic blood pressure instability is seen in at least 60% of patients after CEA and generally resolves within 4 to 8 hours in most patients, although it often requires close hemodynamic monitoring and aggressive pharmacologic treatment. The incidence of postoperative bleeding requiring re-exploration is 1% to 4%. Wound infections are extremely uncommon after CEA and have been reported in less than 1% of cases.

One of the most frequent complications of CEA is cranial nerve injury. This relates to the anatomic location of these nerves with respect to the carotid arteries. The incidence ranges from 5% to 17% in reported series (Table 2). The majority of these injuries result from traction or minor trauma and are transitory, often resolving in a few days or weeks.

Recurrent Carotid Stenosis

The incidence of recurrent stenosis has been estimated to range from 5% to 22% of patients in several published institutional series,

TABLE 2: Incidence of Cranial Nerve Injury

Nerve	Incidence (%)
Hypoglossal	4.4-17.5
Recurrent laryngeal	1.5-15.0
Superior laryngeal	1.8-4.5
Marginal mandibular	1.1-3.1
Glossopharyngeal	0.2-1.5
Spinal accessory	<1.0

although only approximately 3% of these lesions were symptomatic. Within the first 36 months after CEA, recurrent stenosis usually results from intimal hyperplasia. Evidence from serial duplex evaluations suggests that at least some of these lesions regress with time, and in part this may be responsible for some variability in the reported rates of recurrent stenosis. An occasional "recurrent" stenosis in fact represents residual arteriosclerotic disease after the endarterectomy. Lesions that develop more than a few years after CEA usually result from progressive or new arteriosclerotic disease. Recurrent stenoses develop more frequently in women; patients who continue to smoke; and hypercholesterolemic, diabetic, and hypertensive individuals. It also has been suggested that intraoperative injury secondary to arterial clamping, the placement of an intraluminal shunt, or the placement of tacking sutures within the vessel also may predispose to early myointimal hyperplasia lesions. As noted previously, there is compelling evidence that closure of the arteriotomy with a patch will reduce the incidence of recurrent stenosis, although the optimal patch material remains to be identified.

■ REDO CAROTID ENDARTERECTOMY

Reoperative CEA presents additional challenges with dissection and reconstruction that can increase the risk compared with a primary procedure, but with careful planning and technique excellent results can be achieved in this situation as well. An early recurrent stenosis usually develops within 2 years of CEA; typically results from intimal hyperplasia, an inflammatory response that produces a firm, rubbery plaque rich in fibroblasts and smooth muscle cells surrounded by dense accumulations of collagen and acid mucopolysaccharide; and typically develops within the endarterectomy bed. Later restenoses

typically have features of atheromatous plaques and are more widely distributed along the carotid artery. There are no prospective randomized trials to support repeat CEA, but most available evidence supports treating symptomatic and very high-grade asymptomatic recurrent stenoses.

Scarring typically makes the dissection more technically difficult, such that a higher incidence of cranial nerve injury and hematoma can be anticipated. In addition, the more extensive disease within the carotid artery may necessitate carotid artery replacement with an interposition graft. This is technically more difficult, may preclude shunting, and may be associated with longer periods of cerebral ischemia, possibly leading to higher perioperative stroke rates. However, endarterectomy is often possible, even with eversion endarterectomy.

SUGGESTED READINGS

Barnett HJM, Taylor DW, Eliasziw M, Fox AJ, Ferguson GG, Haynes RB, et al. Benefit of carotid endarterectomy in patients with symptomatic moderate or severe stenosis. *N Engl J Med.* 1998;339:1415-1425.

Endarterectomy for asymptomatic carotid artery stenosis. Executive Committee for the Asymptomatic Carotid Atherosclerosis Study. *JAMA.* 1995;273:1421-1428.

European Carotid Surgery Trialists' Collaborative Group. Endarterectomy for moderate symptomatic carotid stenosis: interim results from the MRC European Carotid Surgery Trial. *Lancet.* 1996;347:1591-1593.

Halliday A, Mansfield A, Marro J, Peto C, Peto R, Potter J, et al. Prevention of disabling and fatal strokes by successful carotid endarterectomy in patients without recent neurological symptoms: randomised controlled trial. *Lancet.* 2004;363:1491-1502.

McGirt MJ, Perler BA, Brooke B, Woodworth GF, Coon A, Jain S, et al. HMG CoA-reductase inhibitors reduce the risk of perioperative stroke and mortality after carotid endarterectomy. *J Vasc Surg.* 2005;42:829-836.

MRC European Carotid Surgery Trial: interim results for symptomatic patients with severe (70-99%) or with mild (0-29%) carotid stenosis. European Carotid Surgery Trialists' Collaborative Group. *Lancet.* 1991;337:1235-1243.

North American Symptomatic Carotid Endarterectomy Trial Collaborators. Beneficial effect of carotid endarterectomy in symptomatic patients with high-grade carotid stenosis. *N Engl J Med.* 1991;325:445-453.

Perler BA. Carotid endarterectomy: the "gold standard" in the endovascular era. *J Am Coll Surg.* 2002;194(suppl 1):S2-S8.

Perler BA. The effect of statin medications on the perioperative and long-term outcomes following carotid endarterectomy or stenting. *Semin Vasc Surg.* 2007;20:252-258.

Ricotta JJ, Aburahma A, Ascher E, Eskandari M, Faries P, Lal BK. Updated Society for Vascular Surgery guidelines for management of extracranial carotid disease. *J Vasc Surg.* 2011;54:e1-e31.

THE MANAGEMENT OF RECURRENT CAROTID ARTERY STENOSIS

Michael J. Osgood, MD, and Christopher J. Abularrage, MD

Carotid endarterectomy (CEA) is the gold standard treatment for high-grade symptomatic and asymptomatic carotid artery stenosis in appropriate candidates. Several prospective randomized trials demonstrated that CEA significantly reduces the risk of stroke and death in comparison with best medical treatment alone. The North American Symptomatic Carotid Endarterectomy Trial (NASCET) established the role of CEA for treatment of symptomatic

carotid stenosis, whereas the Asymptomatic Carotid Atherosclerosis Study (ACAS) and Asymptomatic Carotid Surgery Trial (ACST) established the role of CEA for treatment of asymptomatic carotid stenosis. These trials demonstrated that CEA is a durable procedure with minimal perioperative morbidity and mortality when performed by qualified practitioners. Despite the excellent long-term results after CEA, a minority of patients develop recurrent carotid stenosis that requires reintervention.

Over the past 2 decades, carotid angioplasty and stenting (CAS) has emerged as an acceptable and effective endovascular treatment alternative to CEA in certain populations. The role of endovascular therapy in the management of primary carotid stenosis has been investigated by several randomized trials comparing this modality with CEA. As with CEA, a minority of patients undergoing CAS may progress to high-grade restenosis that requires reintervention.

In this chapter we review the literature on recurrent carotid stenosis after CEA and CAS, the risk of cerebrovascular ischemia with recurrent stenosis, and indications for intervention and methods of revascularization for recurrent stenosis.

DEFINITION OF RECURRENT CAROTID STENOSIS

A broad definition of recurrent carotid stenosis implies any narrowing of the carotid artery occurring at or adjacent to the site of a revascularization procedure to manage an atherosclerotic stenosis. Some practitioners suggest that an evaluation for recurrent carotid stenosis cannot be made without the presence of a baseline assessment performed at or immediately after the initial revascularization procedure in order to exclude residual abnormalities that persist immediately after the procedure. This may be especially true after CAS, where the goal is to prevent embolism by tacking the plaque with a stent rather than to improve luminal diameter. The degree of luminal narrowing constituting restenosis varies among studies examining this entity, but the most commonly used definition of restenosis is the presence of a 50% or greater diameter reduction as determined by duplex ultrasonography, which corresponds to a 75% or greater reduction in cross-sectional area. According to the Strandness criteria, a 50% or greater reduction in luminal diameter of the carotid artery is identified by a peak systolic velocity greater than 125 cm/sec with marked spectral broadening throughout systole.

INCIDENCE OF RESTENOSIS AFTER CAROTID ENDARTERECTOMY

The incidence of recurrent carotid stenosis after CEA has been reported to range from 1.3% to 37% and varies widely based on method of surveillance, duration of follow-up, and definition of recurrent disease. The ACAS examined the incidence of recurrent carotid stenosis after CEA. Among 720 patients followed prospectively after CEA in the ACAS, 12.7% developed recurrent stenosis. In the early postoperative period (<3 months), 4.1% developed recurrent stenosis; in the 3- to 18-month time frame, 7.6% developed recurrent carotid stenosis; and in the late time period (18 to 60 months), 1.9% developed recurrent carotid stenosis (Figure 1). A systematic review of studies examining recurrent carotid stenosis similarly noted overall rates of recurrent stenosis of 10% within the first year, 3% in the second year, and 2% in the third year after CEA. The cumulative long-term risk of recurrent stenosis is approximately 1% per year in the late term after CEA. Patients who develop recurrent carotid stenosis after CEA are more likely to be asymptomatic than symptomatic; between 8% and 25% of patients who develop recurrent carotid stenosis will be symptomatic.

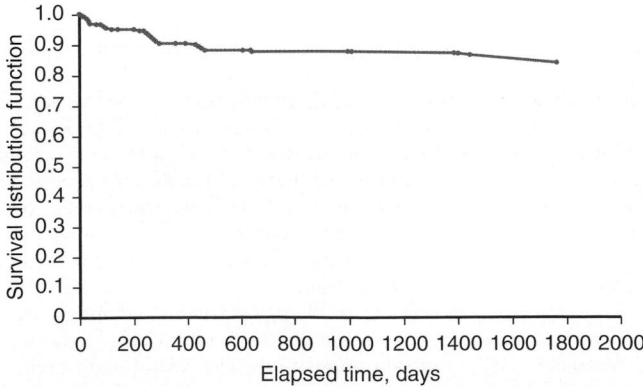

FIGURE 1 Probability of nonrecurrence of carotid stenosis after carotid endarterectomy in the Asymptomatic Carotid Atherosclerosis Study. *(Adapted from Moore WS, Kempczinski RF, Nelson JJ, Toole JF. Recurrent carotid stenosis: results of the asymptomatic carotid atherosclerosis study. Stroke. 1998;29:2018-2025).*

PATHOGENESIS AND TIME FRAME OF RESTENOSIS AFTER CAROTID ENDARTERECTOMY

Intimal hyperplasia is the primary pathologic lesion responsible for recurrent carotid stenosis in the first 2 years after surgery. The intimal hyperplastic lesion in these patients has been noted to occur primarily in the endarterectomy bed. After 2 years, recurrent atherosclerosis is the primary process accounting for recurrent stenosis. In these patients, the recurrent lesion occurs diffusely throughout the artery, outside the confines of the endarterectomy bed. Of interest, in patients who are followed with serial imaging, regression of restenosis of the carotid artery occurs in up to 40% after endarterectomy. Thus asymptomatic carotid restenosis generally should not be treated immediately.

Technical imperfections, when not detected, may predispose to restenosis and include residual atheroma, myointimal flaps, intraluminal thrombi, kinks, proximal shelves of atheroma, patch irregularities, and focal trauma from surgical forceps or clamps. Vascular injury caused by surgical manipulation, clamp injury, placement of tacking sutures, and shunt trauma may predispose to a vigorous hyperplastic response leading to restenosis. Several demographic, comorbid, and anatomic features have been identified as risk factors for the development of recurrent carotid stenosis after CEA (Box 1). Regarding plaque morphology, patients with stable plaques characterized by low macrophage content have been associated with increased risk of restenosis in comparison with those with unstable plaques with inflammatory characteristics. As a result, asymptomatic patients undergoing CEA have been observed to have an increased risk of restenosis at 1 year when compared with patients undergoing CEA after transient ischemic attack (TIA) or stroke.

MEDICAL MANAGEMENT AFTER CAROTID ENDARTERECTOMY TO PREVENT RESTENOSIS

It is important to continue aggressive medical management with antiplatelet and lipid-lowering therapy after CEA in order to optimize results and reduce the incidence of restenosis. It is important to remember that the randomized trials that established CEA as standard therapy for asymptomatic and symptomatic carotid stenosis compared best medical treatment alone with best medical treatment in addition to CEA in the surgical arms of these studies. In the NASCET, medical therapy consisted of antiplatelet therapy (usually aspirin) in addition to antihypertensive and nonstatin lipid-lowering drugs when indicated. In the ACAS, medical management consisted of daily aspirin administration and management of modifiable medical risk factors. In the ACST, antiplatelet therapy, antihypertensive therapy,

---

BOX 1: Risk Factors Associated With Development of Recurrent Carotid Stenosis After Carotid Endarterectomy (CEA)

Continued smoking
Hyperlipidemia
Young age
Diabetes mellitus
Female sex
Primary carotid closure without patch use
Hypertension
Small internal carotid artery diameter
Contralateral 80% or greater internal carotid artery stenosis
Dialysis
Elevated serum creatinine
Elevated serum lipids and cholesterol
History of ipsilateral carotid surgery

and nonstatin lipid-lowering therapy were widely but not universally used in the surgical arm. Therefore the results established by these trials reflect the combination of best medical management in addition to CEA and should be interpreted in this context.

Serum lipid and cholesterol levels have been observed by several authors to modulate the development of recurrent carotid stenosis. The importance of lipid-lowering therapy was emphasized by the findings of a large retrospective review of 2127 CEA procedures performed in 1853 patients at Massachusetts General Hospital. In this large series, serum cholesterol levels correlated with the development of recurrent carotid stenosis. Moreover, the use of lipid-lowering drugs in general and statin therapy in particular was independently associated with reduced rates of early restenosis (<2 years), early failure (severe recurrent stenosis or occlusion), late progression, and late failure (severe recurrent stenosis or occlusion). It is our practice to continue aspirin and moderate- to high-dose statin therapy indefinitely in all patients after CEA or CAS.

METHOD OF RECONSTRUCTION AND INFLUENCE ON RESTENOSIS AFTER CAROTID ENDARTERECTOMY

Many studies have examined patch angioplasty versus primary closure of the carotid artery and its association with restenosis. Although older studies demonstrated mixed results, they consist primarily of small retrospective series that are now dated because they were performed before medical management with aspirin and statin therapy were utilized widely. Prospective data from the ACAS demonstrated a 4.5% restenosis rate with patch closure versus a 16.9% restenosis rate with primary closure. Additional prospective data from the Carotid Revascularization Endarterectomy Versus Stenting Trial (CREST) demonstrated a significant reduction in restenosis with patch closure but no difference in stroke rate. A more recent Cochrane systematic review examining 1307 CEA procedures in 1127 patients supports patch angioplasty after CEA preferentially over primary closure, as there was a more than 50% reduction in occlusion or restenosis at 1 year, in addition to reductions in stroke at 30 days and 1 year, perioperative arterial occlusion, return to the operating room, and any stroke at 1 year. A retrospective review of 3014 CEAs performed on 2644 patients at Massachusetts General Hospital similarly identified primary closure as an independent risk factor for development of restenosis. Moreover, patch angioplasty closure after CEA is supported by a recent analysis of the Vascular Study Group of New England (VSGNE) vascular registry from 2003 to 2008. Based on the sum total of this evidence, patch angioplasty closure is recommended over primary closure by the Society for Vascular Surgery (SVS) in its practice management guidelines for CEA in order to decrease the risk of restenosis.

Regarding type of patch material, there is no definitive evidence supporting a type of patch material preferentially for primary CEA, and as such the SVS endorses patch use without a preference offered for patch type. A single small trial comparing collagen-impregnated Dacron (Hemashield) with polytetrafluoroethylene (PTFE) noted a reduced rate of recurrent carotid stenosis as well as perioperative stroke and TIA in the PTFE group. A recent large analysis of the VSGNE noted a steady increase in use of bovine pericardium from 50% to 86% between 2003 and 2008 and a corresponding decline in the use of Dacron from 32% to 9% for 4465 CEA procedures. This correlated with a decline in the restenosis rate from 11% to 7% over the same time period. The overall rate of patch use also increased from 87% to 96% over the study period, which may account for the reduced rate of restenosis observed during the same time frame.

Eversion endarterectomy is a technique for CEA utilized preferentially by some surgeons. This technique involves dividing the vessel at the carotid bulb–internal carotid artery level and performing eversion endarterectomy of the distal segment. In the Eversion Carotid Endarterectomy Versus Standard Trial (EVEREST), eversion CEA demonstrated comparable rates of restenosis compared with conventional CEA. A recent review of 2365 eversion CEA procedures and 17,155 conventional CEA procedures from the Vascular Quality Initiative (VQI) database demonstrated similar freedom from reintervention at 1 year between the two groups. Assessment of restenosis rates was confounded by limited follow-up data. In its practice management guidelines, the SVS recommends eversion CEA or conventional CEA with patch closure preferentially over CEA with primary closure in order to decrease the risk of restenosis.

SURVEILLANCE FOR RESTENOSIS AFTER CAROTID ENDARTERECTOMY

Duplex ultrasound is the method of choice for surveillance after CEA. This technique is noninvasive and cost effective. For detection of recurrent stenosis, this methodology carries a sensitivity and specificity of 91% and 87%, respectively, for detection of a 50% restenosis of the carotid artery. In addition to developing ipsilateral recurrent stenosis, patients undergoing CEA are at risk for contralateral progression of stenosis. In fact, progression of contralateral stenosis is more common than ipsilateral restenosis. The SVS recommends obtaining a duplex ultrasound after CEA within 30 days postoperatively. The SVS recommends continued surveillance imaging beyond this point in the following subsets of patients: those with 50% or greater ipsilateral or contralateral stenosis, those with primary endarterectomy closure, and those with multiple risk factors for progression of atherosclerosis. The subsequent frequency of duplex ultrasonography after CEA has been debated extensively, and there is currently no consensus regarding frequency or duration of postoperative surveillance. Because restenosis occurs with highest frequency in the first 2 years after CEA, surveillance is particularly important in this early postoperative time frame. Based on the fact that the majority of patients have multiple risk factors for progression of atherosclerosis, it is our practice to perform postoperative duplex imaging at 30 days, 6 months, and 1 year. In the absence of any technical abnormalities or evidence of recurrent stenosis, the surveillance interval subsequently can be spread out on a case-by-case basis depending on the patient's risk factors and medical comorbidities.

IMPLICATIONS OF RESTENOSIS AFTER CAROTID ENDARTERECTOMY: RISK OF CEREBROVASCULAR ISCHEMIA

When all patients are followed after CEA, symptomatic carotid restenosis occurs in up to 8% of patients. The risk of cerebrovascular ischemia is increased in patients with recurrent carotid stenosis. In the setting of recurrent carotid stenosis, symptoms (including stroke) occur in 8% to 25% of patients. Up to 50% of ipsilateral strokes occurring after CEA are attributable to recurrent stenosis. The risk of stroke after CEA is greatest in the first 2 years after the operation, coincidental with the overall increased incidence of carotid restenosis during this time frame. The risk of stroke then decreases over time, corresponding with the decrease in the incidence of recurrent stenosis. The primary pathophysiologic mechanism causing cerebrovascular ischemic events is flow obstruction in the first 2 years when intimal hyperplasia predominates. After 2 years from CEA, with the gradual progression of recurrent atherosclerosis, thromboembolism is the primary mechanism accounting for stroke.

MANAGEMENT OF RECURRENT STENOSIS AFTER CAROTID ENDARTERECTOMY

Reoperative CEA traditionally has been associated with higher surgical risk compared with primary endarterectomy. Periprocedural stroke rates may be as high as 7%, with cranial nerve injury rates up to 19%. Several recent analyses have indicated that reoperative CEA can be performed with perioperative morbidity approaching that of the primary procedure, with acceptable rates of cranial nerve injury and perioperative neurologic events. Overall, however, the risks of death, stroke, and myocardial infarction (MI) are increased compared with the primary procedure. A meta-analysis of studies investigating CEA for recurrent carotid stenosis noted a perioperative stroke rate of 3.9% for reoperative CEA. A recent analysis of the VSGNE registry noted a 3.3% rate of stroke and death with reoperative CEA versus a 1.2% rate of stroke and death after primary CEA. Compared with primary CEA, reoperative CEA has been associated with an increased rate of late occlusion, TIA, and stroke. This increased failure rate probably is explained by an aggressive biology leading to recurrent intimal hyperplasia in these patients.

There is general consensus that symptomatic recurrent stenosis after CEA warrants treatment in patients with stenosis of 50% or greater. Intervention for asymptomatic recurrent stenosis is more controversial. In asymptomatic patients, the risk of intervention (CEA or CAS) may outweigh the risk of observation. Because both CEA and CAS have been associated with measurable risks of stroke, death, and MI in the reoperative scenario, a key determination in the evaluation of patients for management of recurrent stenosis is to assess their perioperative risk and weigh it against the risk of stroke with medical (nonoperative) management. The SVS and European Society for Vascular Surgery (ESVS) recommend against intervention when the postinterventional combined stroke and death rate exceeds 6% for patients with symptomatic carotid restenosis and 3% for those with asymptomatic carotid restenosis. For example, for asymptomatic stenosis, a recent SVS vascular registry analysis of 529 patients undergoing CAS for recurrent carotid stenosis observed a 3.8% rate of combined stroke and death at 30 days. This number slightly exceeds the recommended 3% maximum postinterventional combined stroke and death rate considered acceptable for asymptomatic patients in the SVS and ESVS recommendations. Any interventions on asymptomatic patients should be considered carefully, and patient factors should be re-evaluated in the reintervention setting in order to avoid excessive perioperative morbidity and mortality. It is our practice to initially treat asymptomatic restenosis with maximal statin dosing, in addition to antiplatelet therapy. Surgical intervention is warranted for restenosis that progresses despite such medical management.

Surgical Management of Recurrent Stenosis After Carotid Endarterectomy

Many techniques of reoperative CEA have been described, but there are insufficient data to support the use of one technique over another. Options that have been described include endarterectomy alone, patch angioplasty alone without endarterectomy (saphenous vein, PTFE, or Dacron), endarterectomy with patch angioplasty (saphenous vein, PTFE, or Dacron), and excision of the carotid artery with graft interposition (saphenous vein, PTFE, or Dacron; Figure 2). Our approach to reoperative CEA includes repeat endarterectomy, excision of the previous patch, and replacement with Dacron or bovine pericardium. In the event that a satisfactory endarterectomy plane cannot be established, our approach is resection of the involved artery and replacement with a reversed saphenous vein graft preferentially. If the patient does not have suitable saphenous vein, PTFE is utilized (see Figure 2). Studies of reoperative CEA report largely durable results, with 85% freedom from recurrent restenosis 50% or greater at 5 years when patch angioplasty is utilized.

It should be noted that a small number of patients whose biology predisposes them to an aggressive intimal hyperplasia develop recurrent restenosis and may require tertiary carotid interventions at follow-up. Our approach to the management of recurrent restenosis is similar to the management of patients with restenosis. Intervention is reserved for those with symptomatic lesions exceeding 50% and for those with high-grade (70% to 80%) asymptomatic lesions. For tertiary carotid interventions, our preferred surgical approach is resection of the involved artery and replacement with a reversed saphenous vein graft or PTFE (see Figure 2).

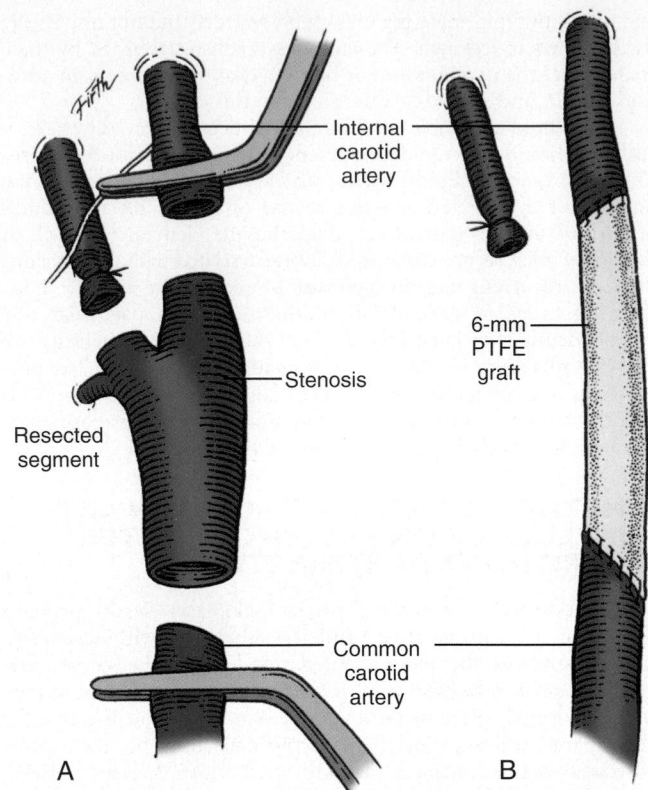

FIGURE 2 A, Resection of a diseased segment of the common and internal carotid arteries with ligation of the external carotid artery. **B,** Placement of an interposition graft for revascularization of the internal carotid artery circulation, in this case using polytetrafluoroethylene (PTFE). Reversed saphenous vein graft (rSVG) or Dacron additionally may be utilized. This is our preferred technique for management of tertiary recurrent carotid stenosis and for management of recurrent in-stent stenosis when endovascular options are not technically feasible.

Because of the perceived risks associated with reoperative CEA, CAS has been advocated by some as the first-line management for recurrent carotid stenosis. CAS avoids the need for reoperative neck dissection and therefore decreases the risk of cranial nerve injury. Several studies have investigated the application of CAS for management of post-CEA restenosis and have established CAS as an acceptable technique for this indication. Reoperative CEA and CAS have been compared retrospectively and have been observed to have similar outcomes in the endpoints of death, stroke, and MI. However, for reintervention for recurrent stenosis, some studies suggest that CAS is associated with higher rates of restenosis compared with reoperative CEA. One study noted 50% or greater restenosis rates of 5% for reoperative CEA versus 28% for CAS. However, because this was not associated with any differences in clinical outcomes (death, stroke, and MI), current evidence does not support the preferential application of CEA or CAS for recurrent stenosis after CEA, as clinical endpoints are roughly equivalent. Therefore the decision regarding best technique for reintervention should be addressed individually. Standard anatomic features and comorbidities should be evaluated, and intervention should be tailored to the patient. If patient characteristics confer increased perioperative risk for MI from reoperative CEA, then CAS should be utilized preferentially. Our practice is to perform CAS for management of recurrent carotid stenosis in anatomically suitable candidates. If CAS is not feasible based on anatomy or issues related to technical execution (i.e., excessive tortuosity of the internal carotid and/or common carotid arteries, severe atherosclerosis and/or calcification of ICA/CCA, severe atherosclerosis and/or calcification of the aortic arch or Type III aortic arch, and complex or long lesions of the ICA/CCA), reoperative CEA is performed.

PATHOGENESIS AND TIME FRAME OF RESTENOSIS AFTER CAROTID ANGIOPLASTY AND STENTING

Several randomized controlled trials conducted over the past 2 decades have prospectively evaluated CAS outcomes, including progression to carotid in-stent restenosis (ISR). These trials include the Carotid and Vertebral Artery Transluminal Angioplasty Study (CAVATAS), Stenting and Angioplasty with Protection in Patients at High Risk for Endarterectomy (SAPPHIRE), Endarterectomy versus Angioplasty in Patients with Symptomatic Severe Carotid Stenosis (EVA-3S), Carotid Revascularization Endarterectomy versus Stenting Trial (CREST), and Stent-Protected Angioplasty versus Carotid Endarterectomy (SPACE). The patients included in these trials constituted heterogeneous populations: the CAVATAS enrolled primarily symptomatic patients, and only 25% of the patients treated with endovascular means underwent placement of a carotid stent (the remaining 75% were managed with angioplasty only); the SAPPHIRE trial enrolled both asymptomatic and symptomatic patients who were deemed to have increased surgical risk for CEA; the CREST enrolled both asymptomatic and symptomatic patients; and the EVA-3S and SPACE trials enrolled only symptomatic patients. These trials used different criteria to identify ISR and had variable follow-up. ISR after CAS occurred in 3% of patients at 3 years in the SAPPHIRE trial, 3.3% of patients at 3 years in the EVA-3S trial, 6% of patients at 2 years in the CREST, 11.1% of patients at 2 years in the SPACE trial, and 16.6% of patients at 5 years in the CAVATAS. This variation in ISR is accounted for in part by duration of follow-up (5 years for the CAVATAS) and also by the diagnostic criteria used to define ISR (peak systolic velocity [PSV] >210 cm/sec in the CAVATAS, PSV >300 cm/sec in the CREST and EVA-3S trial, repeat revascularization procedure in the SAPPHIRE trial). Another analysis evaluated the incidence of ISR at 5 years and observed 40% or greater diameter reduction in 42.7% of patients, 60% or greater diameter reduction in 16.4%, and 80% or greater diameter reduction in 6.4%. In contrast to CEA, where the entire plaque is endarterectomized, CAS simply tacks the plaque with the stent. The goal is not increased luminal diameter but prevention of distal embolism. Thus many patients have a residual stenosis at completion of the procedure that should be accounted for when determining ISR during follow-up.

Risk factors for ISR after CAS are similar to those for restenosis after CEA. In the prospective trials evaluating CAS, the following factors have been identified as conferring increased risk for development of ISR: increased age, female sex, diabetes mellitus, dyslipidemia, and smoking (Box 2). The pathophysiology of ISR is primarily related to the occurrence of intimal hyperplasia. This lesion is a nearly universal occurrence after stent placement in a variety of vascular beds. Intimal hyperplasia plays an important role in the development of early ISR within the first year after stent placement, particularly within the first 3 months. Some individuals have been observed to have especially unfavorable biology and rapid development of intimal hyperplasia. These individuals exhibit short durations of time between intervention and time to initial ISR, and they are particularly prone to restenosis after repeat interventions. Therefore they are at risk for recurrent ISR after CAS as well as recurrent stenosis after CEA. Subsequent delayed or late progression of stenosis

occurs gradually over time in some individuals and eventually may involve recurrence of atherosclerosis.

The geographic pattern of ISR within the stent has been described and characterized. A classification system for ISR has been adapted from a similar classification scheme utilized for the coronary circulation and introduced for use in the carotid circulation (Figure 3; Table 1). The advantage of this classification scheme is its ease of application through use of duplex ultrasonography as a diagnostic modality. Type I lesions are the most common after CAS. Type IV lesions have been identified as the highest risk for target vessel failure and progression to requiring subsequent reintervention, similar to what has been observed in the coronary circulation. The presence of diabetes mellitus was found to be predictive of Type IV ISR and subsequent stent failure and progression to reintervention.

SURVEILLANCE FOR IN-STENT RESTENOSIS AFTER CAROTID ANGIOPLASTY AND STENTING

Overall, restenosis is more common after CAS than it is after CEA. The majority of ISR is mild to moderate in nature, and a minority of patients will develop severe ISR. The incidence of 40% or greater ISR after CAS has been reported to occur in up to 42.7% of patients at 5 years, whereas only 6.4% develop 80% or greater ISR. ISR occurs over a wide time frame after CAS. Although typically occurring within the first year, carotid ISR has been described as occurring as late as 6 years after the procedure. Therefore surveillance imaging is indicated postoperatively to monitor for restenosis and to identify those lesions that will lead to significant hemodynamic compromise requiring reintervention. Surveillance using duplex ultrasound is recommended, but there is no consensus regarding timing, duration, and interval of postoperative imaging. It is our practice to follow patients after CAS in a similar manner to those who have undergone CEA. Follow-up duplex ultrasounds are obtained at 30 days, 6 months, and 1 year. In the absence of any technical abnormalities, the surveillance interval is subsequently spread out.

Use of established duplex ultrasound criteria traditionally used to determine degree of stenosis secondary to atherosclerosis cannot be applied to ISR after CAS. Duplex ultrasound evaluation for ISR is altered by stent-induced alterations in the velocity measurements, including loss of elastic recoil, thereby precluding application of standard duplex ultrasound diagnostic criteria. Standard duplex criteria tend to overestimate the degree of restenosis. Metallic stent artifact during computed tomographic angiography (CTA) and magnetic resonance angiography similarly limit the application of these methodologies in patients after CAS, and the results obtained from these studies should be interpreted with caution, as they tend to overestimate the degree of ISR present. Thus any suspected hemodynamically significant restenosis identified on noninvasive imaging should be confirmed with digital subtraction angiography.

The goal of surveillance duplex ultrasound imaging after CAS is to identify the patients at risk for developing hemodynamically significant (>70% to 80%) restenosis. Patients identified as having normal luminal diameters (<20% stenosis) probably do not warrant intensive surveillance. Those identified as having residual stenosis (20% to 50%) should be followed more closely with surveillance imaging, as there are few data available regarding the natural history of these lesions. Patients who are identified to have moderate (50% to 70%) ISR probably warrant intensive monitoring with duplex ultrasound every 6 months to evaluate for progression to severe (>70% to 80%) ISR. Those identified as having a high-grade restenosis (>70% to 80%) by duplex ultrasound are at increased risk for stroke and warrant confirmatory digital subtraction catheter angiography. A longitudinal comparison of duplex ultrasound and CTA identified a PSV of 220 cm/sec or higher and an internal carotid artery/common carotid artery (ICA/CCA) ratio of 2.7 or greater as an appropriate threshold predictive of 50% or greater (moderate) ISR. Most of the trials evaluating CAS utilize a higher PSV threshold

---

BOX 2: Risk Factors Associated With the Development of In-Stent Restenosis (ISR) After Carotid Angioplasty and Stenting (CAS)

Increased age
Female sex
Diabetes mellitus
Dyslipidemia
Smoking

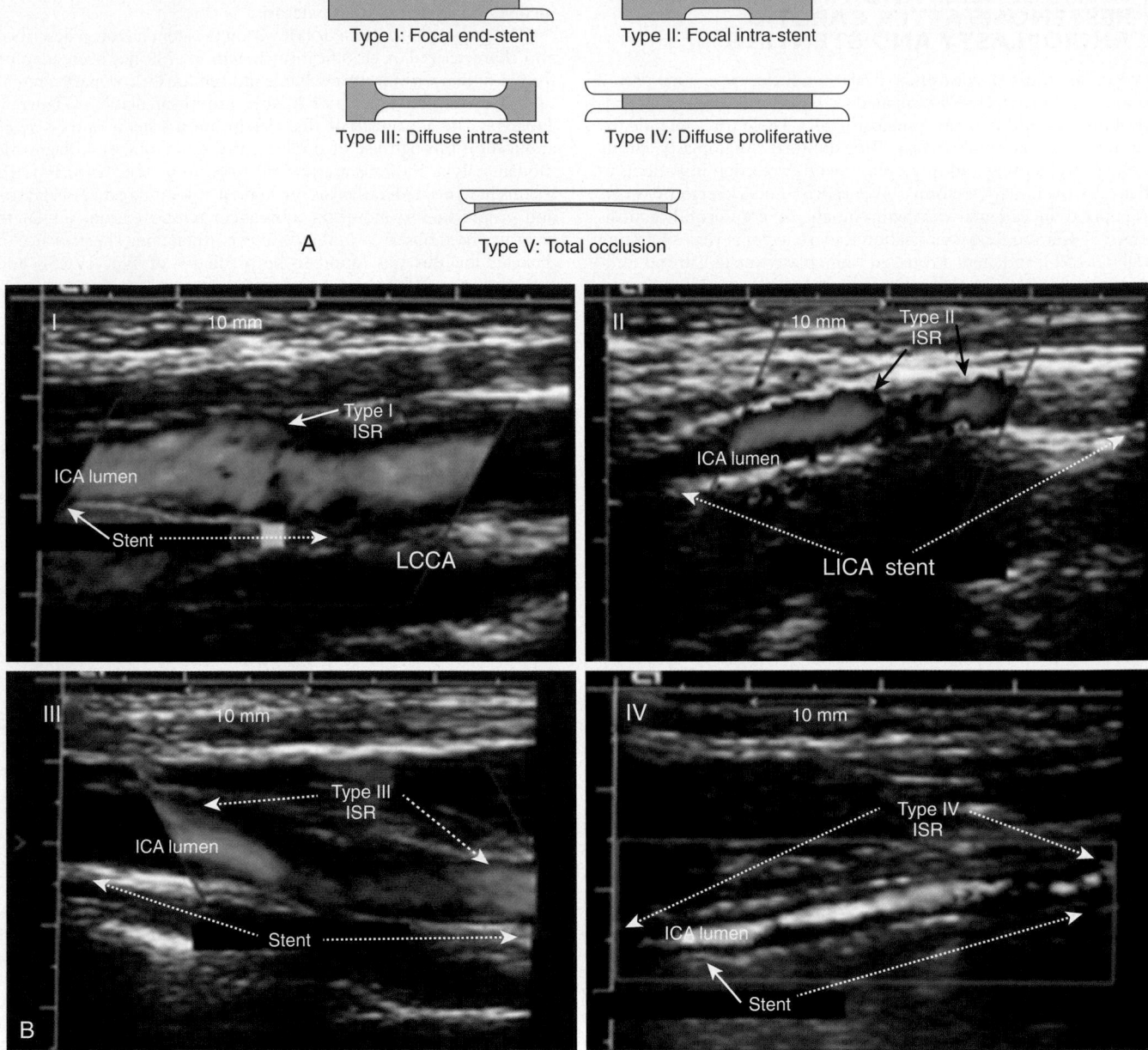

FIGURE 3 A, Schematic depicting different patterns (types I to V) of carotid in-stent restenosis (ISR). **B,** Representative B-mode ultrasound images of ISR correspond to types I to IV of post-CAS ISR. *LCCA,* Left common carotid artery; *LICA,* left internal carotid artery. *(Adapted from Lal BK, et al. Patterns of in-stent restenosis after carotid artery stenting: classification and implications for long-term outcome. J Vasc Surg. 2007;46:833-840).*

TABLE 1: Different Patterns of Carotid In-Stent Restenosis (ISR)

Type	Description and Characteristics of ISR Lesion
I (Focal end-stent group)	Lesions are ≤10 mm long and are positioned at the proximal or distal margin (but not both) of the stent. Lesions ≤10 mm long at both ends of the stent are defined as type I, multifocal end-stent.
II (Focal intra-stent group)	Lesions are ≤10 mm long and are confined to within the stent(s) without extending outside the margins. Two or more discrete lesions ≤10 mm long located within the stent are defined as type II, multifocal intra-stent.
III (Diffuse intra-stent group)	Lesions are >10 mm long and are confined to within the stent(s) without extending outside the margins.
IV (Diffuse proliferative group)	Lesions are >10 mm long and extend beyond the margin(s) of the stent(s).
V (Occlusion group)	Lesions have no prograde flow and no lumen is identified.

(>300 cm/sec) to diagnose severe (>70% to 80%) ISR. A number of authors have identified a PSV higher than 300 to 340 cm/sec, an end diastolic velocity (EDV) higher than 90 cm/sec, and an ICA/CCA ratio greater than 4 to 4.5 as predictive of greater than 70% to 80% ISR (Table 2). Accepted velocity criteria for evaluation of post-CAS ISR are depicted in Table 2, and we have adopted these criteria for use in our vascular lab.

IMPLICATIONS OF IN-STENT RESTENOSIS AFTER CAROTID ANGIOPLASTY AND STENTING: RISK OF CEREBROVASCULAR ISCHEMIA

The CAVATAS demonstrated that severe (>70%) carotid restenosis or occlusion portended an increased risk for subsequent ipsilateral TIA or stroke at 5 years. Similarly, the CREST demonstrated that restenosis greater than 70% after CAS conferred increased risk for stroke. The EVA-3S trial of CAS additionally demonstrated a 10.3% incidence of stroke or TIA in patients with restenosis, versus 5.3% in patients without restenosis, but this difference was not statistically significant. The overall number of ischemic events was small, which precluded a meaningful analysis. Similarly, in the SPACE trial, recurrent stenosis was not associated with a significantly increased risk of cerebrovascular ischemic events.

MANAGEMENT OF IN-STENT RESTENOSIS AFTER CAROTID ANGIOPLASTY AND STENTING

The management of patients with ISR after CAS is an area in evolution, as there are no prospective data guiding reintervention. Based

TABLE 2: Duplex Ultrasonography Velocity Criteria to Establish the Presence of Recurrent Carotid Stenosis in the Native Carotid Artery Post-CEA Compared With Established Velocity Criteria to Establish the Presence of In-Stent Restenosis Post-CAS

Degree of Stenosis	Native Carotid Artery	Stented Carotid Artery
0%-19%	PSV <130 cm/sec	PSV <150 cm/sec and ICA/CCA ratio <2.15
20%-49%	PSV 130-189 cm/sec	PSV 150-219 cm/sec
50%-79%	PSV 190-249 cm/sec and EDV <120 cm/sec	PSV 220-339 cm/sec and ICA/CCA ratio ≥2.7
80%-99%	PSV ≥250 cm/sec and EDV ≥120 cm/sec, or ICA/CCA ratio ≥3.2	PSV ≥340 cm/sec and ICA/CCA ratio ≥4.5

CAS, Carotid artery stenosis; *CEA,* carotid endarterectomy; *EDV,* end diastolic velocity; *ICA/CCA,* internal carotid artery/common carotid artery; *PSV,* peak systolic velocity.

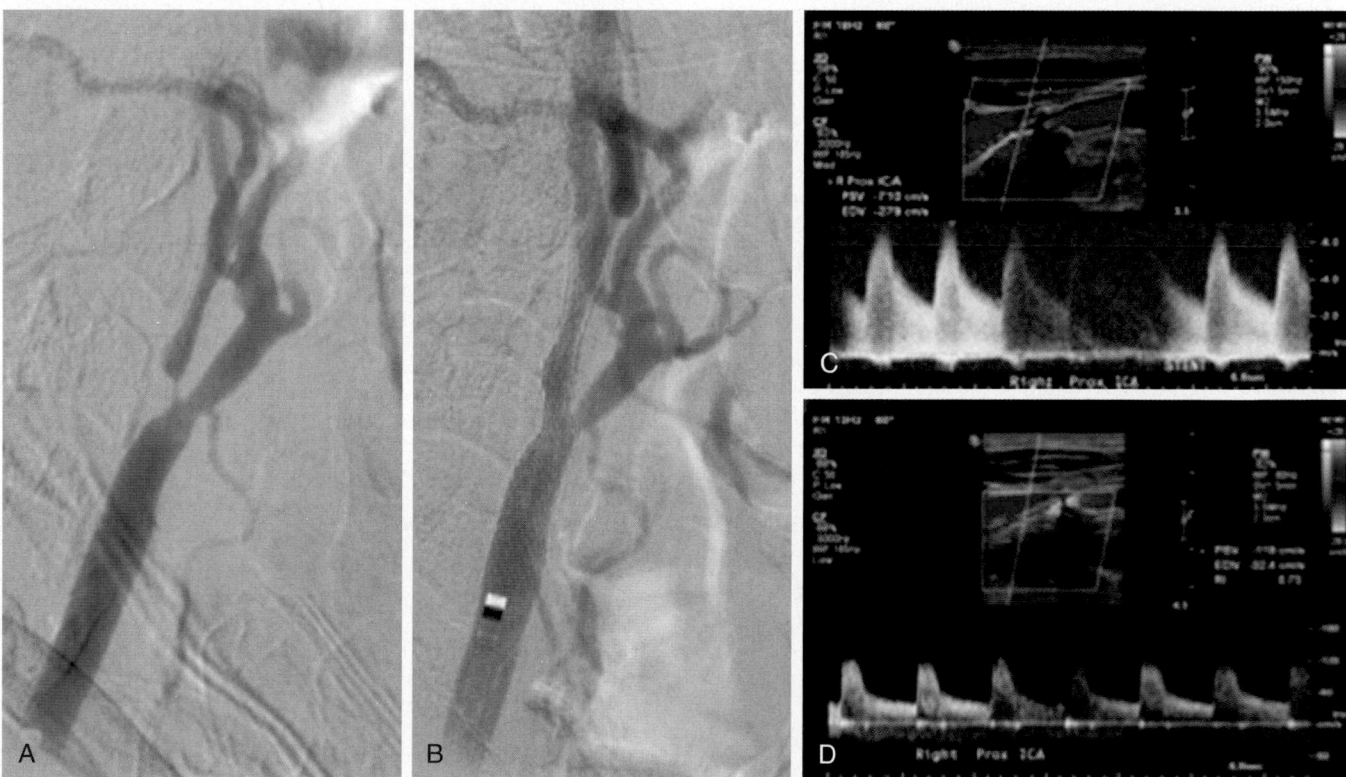

FIGURE 4 Focal (type II) carotid in-stent restenosis (ISR) in a 78-year-old male with high-grade asymptomatic ISR 6 years after initial CAS. **A,** Carotid angiography demonstrated a string sign of the proximal internal carotid artery (ICA) with approximately 99% stenosis. **B,** This restenosis was managed with carotid angioplasty with embolic protection followed by placement of a self-expanding 7- × 30-mm stent. Postprocedural angiogram is demonstrated. **C,** Preoperative duplex ultrasound demonstrated severe ISR with peak systolic velocity (PSV) of 710, end diastolic velocity (EDV) of 279, and ICA/common carotid artery (CCA) ratio of 12.2. **D,** Duplex ultrasound obtained 1 month postoperatively demonstrated PSV of 128, EDV of 33, and ICA/CCA ratio of 2.5.

on available retrospective data, the consensus among most authors is to consider reintervention in symptomatic patients with ISR of 50% or greater. Reintervention for asymptomatic patients is more controversial, and most authors believe that reintervention should be considered only for high-grade (>70% to 80%) ISR. Intervention for asymptomatic carotid ISR should be entertained on a case-by-case basis and should take into consideration the likelihood of technical success based on the anatomic characteristics of the lesion as well as patient characteristics, including perioperative risk of stroke and death.

Various endovascular approaches have been described for the treatment of carotid ISR. These include balloon angioplasty alone, balloon angioplasty using a drug-eluting balloon, cutting balloon angioplasty alone, CAS alone, angioplasty with CAS, and CAS using a drug-eluting stent. Currently there are no prospective data supporting use of one technique over another. Because these lesions are caused by intimal hyperplasia, many authors prefer cutting balloon angioplasty for treatment of carotid ISR. The lowest rates of recurrent ISR after endovascular treatment for ISR have been described with cutting balloon angioplasty and angioplasty with repeat CAS (Figure 4). These techniques are associated with recurrent restenosis rates of 4.2%, as opposed to higher restenosis rates of 15% to 23% with balloon angioplasty alone. In addition, open surgical options have been described for management of ISR. CEA with stent removal has been described and may need to be utilized in heavily calcified lesions with inadequate primary stenting results, preocclusive lesions unable to be traversed with conventional endovascular techniques, stent technical failure, and primary stent thrombosis. In addition, carotid artery bypass and interposition grafting utilizing either reversed greater saphenous vein or PTFE have been described. Our preference is to manage carotid ISR using angioplasty and repeat CAS when anatomically feasible. For patients in whom an endovascular technique is not a viable option based on previously described anatomic features (i.e., excessive tortuosity of the internal carotid and/or common carotid arteries, severe atherosclerosis and/or calcification of ICA/CCA, severe atherosclerosis and/or calcification of the aortic arch or Type III aortic arch, and complex or long lesions of the ICA/CCA), we prefer to manage carotid ISR using endarterectomy with stent removal and patch angioplasty. In cases where the stent is heavily incorporated or a clean endarterectomy endpoint cannot be achieved, we perform resection of the involved segment with interposition grafting using reversed saphenous vein graft, PTFE, or Dacron (see Figure 2).

■ SUMMARY

CEA and CAS are commonly performed for treatment of both symptomatic and asymptomatic carotid stenosis. Although these procedures have been demonstrated to be durable, a small proportion of patients will progress to develop recurrent stenosis after CEA or

ISR after CAS. Medical therapy with antiplatelet and lipid-lowering drugs is indicated in all patients after carotid interventions in order to reduce the risk of recurrent stenosis. Surveillance imaging using duplex ultrasound is the technique of choice to identify patients with recurrent stenosis and may be supplemented selectively with CTA or catheter angiography in the reoperative scenario. Patients with symptomatic disease and restenosis of 50% or greater should be evaluated for reintervention. CEA and CAS are both appropriate methods of treating restenosis and should be considered in the context of the patient's anatomy and comorbidities. Asymptomatic patients with high-grade (>70% to 80%) recurrent stenosis should be medically optimized with antiplatelet and lipid-lowering drugs, and reintervention should be considered individually. Although reintervention carries acceptable rates of periprocedural morbidity and mortality, the risks are higher compared with the primary procedure for both CEA and CAS. The patient's degree of cerebrovascular symptoms, medical comorbidities, and anatomic characteristics all should be evaluated when reintervention is contemplated. A small proportion of patients will progress to develop recurrent restenosis and may require more aggressive tertiary intervention, such as internal carotid resection with interposition grafting or bypass.

SUGGESTED READINGS

AbuRahma AF, Abu-Halimah S, Hass SM, et al. Carotid artery stenting outcomes are equivalent to carotid endarterectomy outcomes for patients with post-carotid endarterectomy stenosis. *J Vasc Surg.* 2010;52:1180-1187.

Fokkema M, de Borst GJ, Nolan BW, et al. Carotid stenting versus endarterectomy in patients undergoing reintervention after prior carotid endarterectomy. *J Vasc Surg.* 2014;59:8-15, e1-2.

Frericks H, Kievit J, van Baalen JM, et al. Carotid recurrent stenosis and risk of ipsilateral stroke: a systematic review of the literature. *Stroke.* 1998;29:244-250.

Kang J, Conrad MF, Patel VI, et al. Clinical and anatomic outcomes after carotid endarterectomy. *J Vasc Surg.* 2014;59:944-949.

Lal BK, Hobson RW 2nd, Tofighi B, et al. Duplex ultrasound velocity criteria for the stented carotid artery. *J Vasc Surg.* 2008;47:63-73.

Lal BK, Kaperonis EA, Cuadra S, et al. Patterns of in-stent restenosis after carotid artery stenting: classification and implications for long-term outcome. *J Vasc Surg.* 2007;46:833-840.

Lattimer CR, Burnand KG. Recurrent carotid stenosis after carotid endarterectomy. *Br J Surg.* 1997;84:1206-1219.

Liapis CD, Bell PR, Mikhailidis D, et al. ESVS guidelines. Invasive treatment for carotid stenosis: indications, techniques. *Eur J Vasc Endovasc Surg.* 2009;37(suppl 4):1-19.

Moore WS, Kempczinski RF, Nelson JJ, et al. Recurrent carotid stenosis: results of the asymptomatic carotid atherosclerosis study. *Stroke.* 1998;29:2018-2025.

van Lammeren GW, Peeters W, de Vries JP, et al. Restenosis after carotid surgery: the importance of clinical presentation and preoperative timing. *Stroke.* 2011;42:965-971.

BALLOON ANGIOPLASTY AND STENTS IN CAROTID ARTERY OCCLUSIVE DISEASE

Jeffery B. Dattilo, MD, and Evan R. Brownie, MD

No discussion of carotid artery occlusive disease can begin without at least mentioning the impact of stroke, both worldwide and in the United States. Globally, stroke is the second leading cause of

mortality, and it remains the third most common cause of death domestically. In the United States, the annual incidence of new or recurrent stroke is about 795,000, and stroke is the leading cause of permanent disability. Up to 40% of strokes can be attributed to atherosclerosis of the internal carotid artery (ICA), therefore making prevention and treatment of carotid artery stenosis an important health care opportunity.

Michael DeBakey first performed carotid endarterectomy (CEA) in the 1950s, with an initial reported durability that spanned nearly 2 decades. In the late 1990s two large multicenter randomized trials, the North American Symptomatic Carotid Endarterectomy Trial (NASCET) and the Asymptomatic Carotid Atherosclerosis Study (ACAS), compared CEA with medical therapy alone and showed benefit of surgery in comparison with best medical therapy (BMT). Fast forwarding to the modern era, percutaneous transluminal

TABLE 1: Randomized Multicenter Trials Comparing Carotid Artery Stenting (CAS) and Carotid Endarterectomy (CEA)

Trial	Year	No. of Patients	MAE Rate for CAS	MAE Rate for CEA	Length of Follow-Up
CAVATAS	2001	504	10.0%	9.9%	3 years
SAPPHIRE	2008	334	24.6%	26.9%	3 years
SPACE	2008	1214	9.5%	8.8%	2 years
EVA-3S	2008	527	11.1%	6.2%	4 years
ICSS	2010	1713	8.5%	4.7%	120 days

CAVATAS, Carotid and Vertebral Artery Transluminal Angioplasty Study; *EVA-3S*, Endarterectomy Versus Angioplasty in Patients with Symptomatic Severe Carotid Stenosis; *ICSS*, International Carotid Stenting Study; *MAE*, major adverse event (stroke, death, or myocardial infarction, varied by trial); *SAPPHIRE*, Stenting and Angioplasty with Protection in Patients at High Risk for Endarterectomy; *SPACE*, Stent-Protected Angioplasty versus Carotid Endarterectomy.

balloon angioplasty of the carotid artery is performed with success in patients with carotid stenosis, and by 1990 embolic protection devices (EPDs) were developed. In 2004 the U.S. Food and Drug Administration (FDA) approved carotid angioplasty and stenting (CAS) systems, and therefore this therapy was thrust into the forefront as a legitimate alternative to CEA.

The potential for CAS was recognized quickly, and funding was directed toward performing randomized controlled trials (RCTs) comparing CAS with CEA. Early trials in the 1990s resulted in a wide range of results and were criticized for inconsistent operator skill, nonuniform use of EPDs, and lack of complete antiplatelet therapy. Because of advances in CAS systems, including EPDs and periprocedural management, the question of comparison with endarterectomy was inevitable (Table 1). The results of several of these comparisons fell short of determining with certainty which patients would benefit from stenting versus endarterectomy.

The National Institutes of Health (NIH) funded the Carotid Revascularization Endarterectomy versus Stenting Trial (CREST), performed in 2010. It is the most recent and largest RCT designed to compare the efficacy of CAS and CEA. The trial included 2502 patients. The 477 surgeons and 224 interventionalists who were allowed to perform procedures within the trial each met a set of standards for training and experience. Endovascular therapy was standardized in the CAS arm, performed with the RX Acculink Carotid Stent System (Abbott Vascular, Abbott Park, IL) and a distal EPD (RX Accunet Embolic Protection System, Abbott Vascular) in 96.1% of cases. The rate of achieving the primary composite endpoint of any stroke, myocardial infarction (MI), or death during the periprocedural period or ipsilateral stroke at 4-year follow-up was insignificant: 7.2% for CAS compared with 6.8% for CEA (Table 2). However, there are important differences between the groups worth mentioning. Periprocedural stroke rate was significantly higher with CAS at 4.1% versus 2.3% with CEA, and MI was significantly higher with CEA at 2.3% versus 1.1% with CAS.

Critics of CREST point to the inclusion of MI as a component of the primary endpoint and argue that the use of only stroke and death as the primary endpoint would clearly favor CEA. Proponents of CAS argue that the statistical similarity in achieving the primary composite endpoint establishes CAS as an alternative to CEA for treating carotid artery occlusive disease. Regardless, the results of CREST are encouraging and represent level 1 data establishing both procedures as effective in long-term stroke prevention (see Table 2).

■ PATIENT SELECTION

With regard to reducing periprocedural morbidity and mortality of CAS, one can argue that judicious patient selection is equipoise to technical prowess. At present, the Centers for Medicare and Medicaid

TABLE 2: Results of Carotid Revascularization Endarterectomy Versus Stenting Trial (CREST; 2502 patients)

Endpoint	CAS	CEA	P value
Primary composite endpoint of periprocedural stroke, death, or MI or ipsilateral stroke in 4 years	7.2%	6.8%	0.51
Periprocedural death	0.7%	0.3%	0.18
Any periprocedural stroke	4.1%	2.3%	0.01*
Periprocedural MI	1.1%	2.3%	0.03*
4-year rate of stroke or death	6.4%	4.7%	0.03*
Ipsilateral stroke after periprocedural period	2.0%	2.4%	0.85

*Statistically significant difference.

CAS, Carotid artery stenting; *CEA*, carotid endarterectomy; *MI*, myocardial infarction.

Services (CMS) provides reimbursement only for patients who are at high risk for CEA and who also have symptomatic carotid artery stenosis of 70% or more outside of its clinical trials policies and regulations. Coverage is limited to procedures performed using FDA-approved CAS systems and EPDs. Patients deemed at high risk include those with congestive heart failure (CHF) class III or IV, left ventricular ejection fraction less than 30%, recent MI, unstable angina, previous CEA or recurrent carotid stenosis, prior neck irradiation, and contralateral carotid occlusions. The aforementioned high-risk patients are all reasonable for consideration to select CAS over CEA; however, it has been my experience that CEA can be performed safely and remains superior in regard to stroke risk and durability when compared with CAS despite many of the CMS-labeled comorbidities. There is strong evidence to suggest that if given the data, furthermore, patients will choose a cardiac complication over an increased risk of stroke.

A history of prior cervical surgery, radiation, or a stoma alone does not prohibit CEA. A hostile neck, rather, is defined by the anticipated local tissue change that would preclude safe dissection and visualization of key structures. There are multiple retrospective studies supporting the safety of CEA both in the irradiated neck and in recurrent carotid stenosis after initial CEA. Although we prefer to perform CEA when possible for recurrent carotid stenosis after CEA, the local wound complication after cervical radiation and/or the presence of a stoma tends to sway decision making toward CAS in that specific patient population.

Another key clinical consideration in patient selection for CAS is age. In the Cochrane meta-analysis of pooled RCTs, the odds ratio of CAS versus CEA for 30-day death or any stroke risk was 1.16 (95% confidence interval [CI]: 0.80 to 1.67) in patients younger than 70 years of age and 2.20 (95% CI: 1.47 to 3.29) in patients 70 years or older. Further data from CREST suggested that octogenarians did poorly with CAS compared with CEA. The hypothesis of this difference has to do with plaque morphology of the carotid disease process and is somewhat contradictory to the supposition that an endovascular procedure with conscious sedation should have better outcomes than an open vascular reconstruction in these older patients.

The two predominant societal guidelines for the management of patients with carotid stenosis in the United States, published by the American Heart Association (AHA) and Society for Vascular Surgery (SVS), are noteworthy for subtle yet key semantic differences in recommended therapy. The AHA recommends CEA for symptomatic patients with 50% to 99% carotid stenosis, with CAS as an *alternative* in patients at an average or low risk of CAS-associated complications. Also recommended by the AHA is CEA for asymptomatic patients with 60% to 99% carotid stenosis, and CAS might be considered. The position of the AHA emphasizes equivalence in major adverse cardiovascular events as demonstrated by CREST and notes that the effectiveness of CAS in asymptomatic patients is not well established. In contrast, the SVS holds the position that CEA is *preferred* in symptomatic patients with 50% to 99% carotid stenosis, with CAS reserved for patients with a hostile neck and severe, uncorrectable cardiac conditions. For patients with asymptomatic disease, the SVS supports CEA if there is a normal risk and a 3- to 5-year life expectancy, but does not support CAS outside trials. In asymptomatic patients, CAS may be offered in centers that demonstrate periprocedural stroke and death rates lower than 3%. For the high-risk patient with asymptomatic carotid stenosis, the SVS recommends BMT because of the relatively benign nature of asymptomatic benign disease. The position of the SVS assumes that the primary role of carotid intervention is to *reduce stroke*, and to do so with minimal mortality and non-neurologic morbidity. The SVS, therefore, weighs heavier the symptomatic stroke trials, particularly the International Carotid Stenting Study (ICSS), and weighs less the reduction of cardiovascular events seen in CREST, many of which were not clinically apparent.

Finally, patients with contraindications to anticoagulation, especially antiplatelet agents, generally are not considered candidates for stenting. Those patients include anyone allergic to antiplatelet agents or at high risk of hemorrhagic complications from prolonged antiplatelet therapy.

RELEVANT ANATOMY

When selecting and performing CAS, anatomic variations and pathology, specifically in the carotid arteries and aorta, can predict difficulty with catheter guidance and exchange. Analysis from the Endarterectomy Versus Angioplasty in Patients with Symptomatic Severe Carotid Stenosis (EVA-3S) trial found that the risk of stroke or death in CAS was higher in patients with internal carotid artery (ICA) to common carotid artery (CCA) angulation of 60 degrees or more (relative risk [RR]: 4.96; 95% CI: 2.29 to 10.74). A systematic review of literature by the same authors that included 34,398 patients with CAS confirmed that the risk of 30-day stroke or death was higher in patients with increased carotid vessel angulation (RR: 3.41; 95% CI: 1.52 to 7.63) and when the target ICA lesion was more than 10 mm in length (RR: 2.36; 95% CI: 1.28 to 3.38). In addition, distal ICA kinking may limit distal EPD positioning, manifesting as an insufficient landing zone for stent deployment. Furthermore, extensive calcification in the area of carotid stenosis may lead to insufficient stent expansion after deployment.

Variations in aortic arch anatomy are present in roughly one quarter of patients and must be accounted for during the procedure. Aortic arch morphology can be graded using two lines drawn across the highest point of the outer and inner curvatures of the aortic arch. The great vessels arise above or in the same horizontal plane as the outer curvature of a type I aortic arch. The origin of the innominate artery in a type II aortic arch lies between the horizontal planes of the outer and inner curvatures. In a type III aortic arch, the origin of the innominate artery lies inferior to the horizontal plane of the inner curvature of the arch. More inferior origins of the great vessels (aortic arch types II and III) may be associated with prolonged catheter manipulation and difficulty maintaining sheath access, increasing the possibility of aortic plaque embolization. We consider great vessel origination past the lesser curve of the arch on the ascending aorta to be prohibitive (Figure 1).

The risk of potentially catastrophic aortic plaque embolization is further increased in the presence of extensive aortic wall irregularities with multiple atheromas (shaggy aorta) and severe aortic calcification (eggshell aorta). The eggshell aorta poses the additional risk of intimal disruption. Both shaggy and eggshell aortas are potential contraindications to proceeding with CAS.

TECHNICAL CONSIDERATIONS

Procedural Technique

The use of dual antiplatelet agents is now considered to be routine during the perioperative period for CAS. In those patients who are not on clopidogrel, we begin therapy 1 week ahead of surgery; if that is not possible, a 300-mg loading dose at the time of the procedure is administered. Patient positioning should be supine and comfortable on the table with access to either femoral artery. The patient is typically awake and given a noise-making device in the contralateral hand to squeeze during the procedure. Venous access is required to manage possible bradycardia or hypotension that can occur with manipulation of the carotid sinus. We routinely use ultrasound to identify the common femoral artery and use a 4F micropuncture set for arterial access. After access to the iliac system is gained, we use a Kumpe

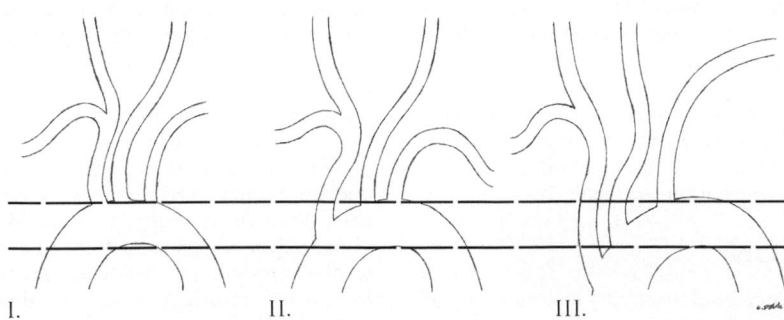

FIGURE 1 Aortic arch anatomy: types I, II, and III. *(Illustrations courtesy Stephanie Dziezyk, 2015. Under the copyright of St. Thomas Health.)*

catheter to negotiate our way past the visceral segment of the aorta and then insert a long marker pigtail or Omni Flush catheter into the midascending aorta. Once the marked catheter is in place, the patient is anticoagulated. An activated clotting time (ACT) of more than 275 seconds (>200 seconds if using a glycoprotein [GP] IIb/IIIa inhibitor) should be maintained to prevent thrombus formation on any device within the arch. Omnipaque is our preferred contrast agent because of its low cost and minimal documented adverse renal consequences. Because of the high flow through the aortic arch, we routinely inject at 30 mL/min for a volume delivered of 30 mL. For patients with renal insufficiency, dilution of the contrast material is often utilized. The image intensifier should be at least 30 degrees left anterior oblique (LAO), with attention directed toward opening up the view of the arch to its maximum. This is accomplished by looking at the marks on the catheter while moving the image intensifier to dynamically assess the marks becoming even in the projection.

No manipulation of any wire or catheter is done unless visualized with fluoroscopy. To minimize the introduction of air into the system it is imperative to maintain tight catheter connections and to thoroughly flush the delivery system. There should be no rapid pulling back of wires or catheters because of the concern of introducing air via a vaccum phenomenon. Selection of the innominate artery usually can be accomplished with an H1 catheter and the use of a floppy Glidewire. The technique of slowly turning the catheter counterclockwise as you withdraw the catheter usually accomplishes this task readily. Other catheters that are helpful in type II or type III aortic arches are the Cobra series of catheters, JB-2, or Slip catheter configurations. Once in the CCA, the catheter is advanced over a 0.035-inch wire past the clavicle, and additional imaging is performed. Use of high-quality biplane imaging is very helpful in reducing the contrast administered. Once the carotid bifurcation is identified, wire access into the external carotid artery (ECA) is achieved with a 0.035-inch stiff Glidewire. This gives us adequate support for our sheath exchange to a 6F 90-cm sheath. We deliver this to the level of the CCA approximately 5 cm below the carotid bifurcation. The wire in the ECA subsequently is removed. Baseline intracranial imaging is then performed in both lateral and anterior posterior projections. Our anterior projections are in a Towne's view (slightly craniocaudal). Additional images are obtained to provide three essential components: (1) visualization of the distal end of the sheath, (2) adequate splay of the carotid bifurcation, and (3) target area for landing of the distal protection device (4 to 5 cm above the target for the distal-most aspect of the stent).

We routinely have used a distal filter EPD in our center for cerebral protection, but there are other options. The 0.014-inch EPD is then prepped according to the manufacturer's recommendations to avoid air being introduced during insertion. At this time we usually prepare all balloons and stents, laying them out in the order of insertion. This can help with efficiency, limiting the time that the EPD is in place. Care is taken to insert the wire of the EPD with appropriate protection for the tip of the wire, which is very delicate and prone to irrevocable bends or kinks. We set up a continuous flow bag of heparinized saline going through the sheath using a three-way stopcock after the EPD is deployed. Once placed appropriately past the lesion, the EPD is deployed according to the manufacturer's directions. After deployment, someone in the room is assigned to keep watch on its location during all other manipulations.

Typically, we predilate the lesion with at least a 3-mm balloon of sufficient length to avoid multiple dilations. This provides a channel for safely traversing the lesion with the stent. Monorail balloons and stents are very advantageous to facilitate rapid exchanges and shorter access wires. Maintain the stent delivery system on a clear field and discuss with the team to keep the system as straight as possible, avoiding any slack in the system. Using the 6F sheath allows for additional arteriography if the patient moves or is uncooperative. Make certain that the location of the lesion within nondiseased artery is understood completely before deployment of the stent. Stent size is based on the diameter of the largest artery to be stented adjacent to the

stenosis and length of the stenotic segment. The diameter of the stent should be 1 to 2 mm larger than the diameter of the largest artery to be covered by the stent. The stent should overlap nondiseased artery by 5 mm on either side of the stenosis. These parameters help to prevent stent migration. It is common practice to partially deploy the stent distal to the target and move the stent proximally into its ideal location. Once the stent is fully deployed, the conformity of the stent is assessed and postdilated with a 5- or 6-mm balloon of at least the length of the inserted stent (Figures 2 and 3). This facilitates avoiding multiple dilations if a shorter balloon is used. We perform diagnostic arteriography at this time and assess. Often there will be some spasm of the carotid artery, but this can be treated with 50 to 100 µg injections of nitroglycerine. The EPD then is removed according to the directions for use supplied. Completion arteriography then is performed to compare with the preprocedural films—both lateral and Towne's views. The long sheath is removed over a stiff wire and usually replaced with a short 6F sheath. A closure device or manual pressure can be used.

The patient then is allowed to recover fully in an appropriate stepdown unit with personnel adept at assessing for cardiovascular or neurovascular compromise. It is our practice to watch these patients overnight for neurologic complications or access complications and discharge them in the morning.

Stent Selection and Embolic Protection Devices

Carotid arterial stents are no different than other peripheral endovascular stents and can be divided into two categories: balloon expandable and self-expanding. The advantage of balloon-expandable stents is their ability to be carefully positioned at their proximal landing zone. They are well suited for lesions at the orifice of the great vessels. Generally speaking, self-expanding stents are less rigid than their counterparts and are ideal for cervical carotid lesions to allow for neck mobility or tortuosity of the vessel.

Self-expanding stents can be further classified into two configurations: closed cell and open cell. All stent struts are interconnected in closed-cell stents, allowing for application of greater radial force but less flexibility. Open-cell stents, on the other hand, have more flexibility, permitting better wall apposition, but lack the radial force of closed-cell stents. This may limit self-expansion as a result of recoil and contribute to in-stent restenosis. At present, there is no consensus as to which self-expanding stent configuration is best suited for the carotid territory.

The use of EPDs during CAS is required by CMS to qualify for reimbursement, and their use has been one of the largest advances in the evolution of CAS. Three conceptually different methods for extracranial protection presently exist (Figure 4). The first method, a distal occlusion balloon, generally has been abandoned but remains available. The major disadvantages of distal occlusion balloons include the need to cross the lesion without protection, the potential inability to remove all embolic material, and the risk for intimal damage and spasm as a result of inflation in the distal ICA. Distal filter devices have the advantage of maintenance of cerebral blood flow and angiographic control during the procedure, with reduced need for device manipulation. Distal filters are the most commonly used EPD, largely attributable to their wide availability and utility. It is easy for a single operator to insert, deploy, and retrieve a filter device, with obvious advantages in efficiency in time. Like distal occlusion balloons, distal filters also have the disadvantage of having to cross the lesion without protection. Additional disadvantages include the uncertainty of capturing all debris and risk of incomplete wall apposition.

Reversal of flow, the third method of extracranial protection, differs significantly in its principle and application from the two methods previously discussed. This strategy relies on balloon occlusion of the proximal common and external carotid arteries via a single delivery catheter and on flow reversal created in the distal CCA with active inspiration or shunting to an additional introducer in the

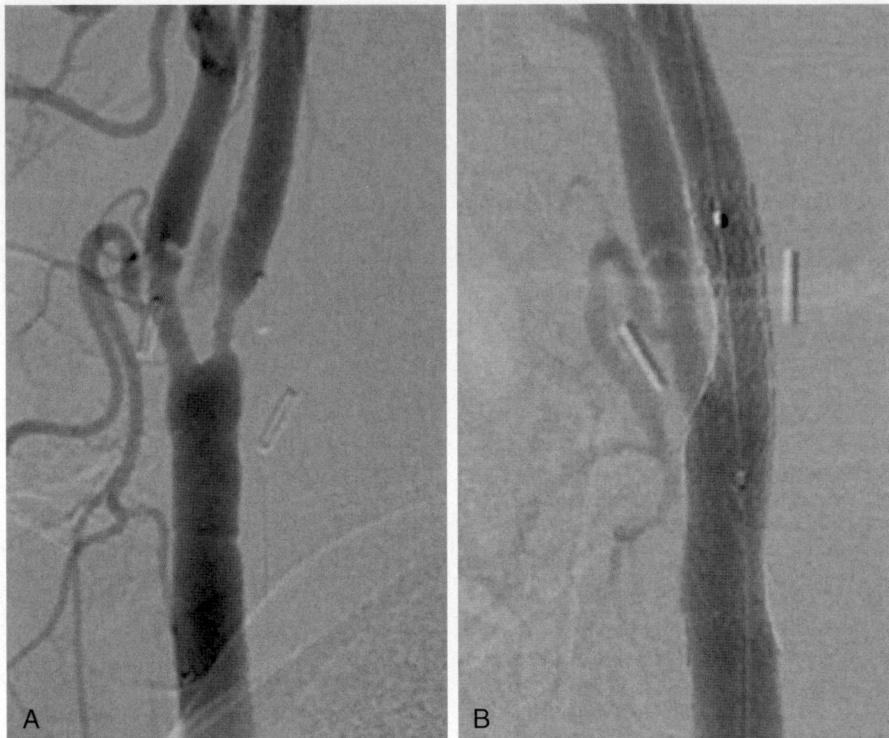

FIGURE 2 Digital subtraction arteriogram demonstrating severe internal carotid artery (ICA) stenosis before (**A**) and after (**B**) stenting.

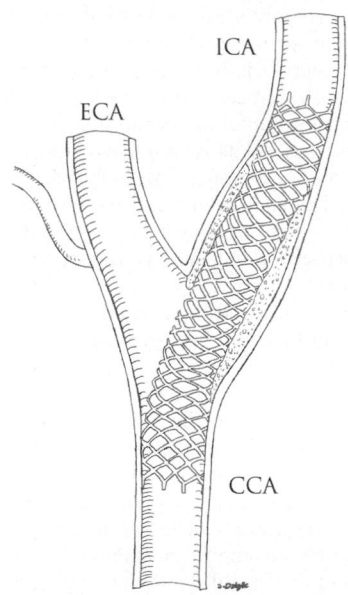

FIGURE 3 Sketch of a deployed stent within the carotid artery in proper position spanning the internal carotid artery (ICA) to the common carotid artery (CCA). *ECA*, External carotid artery. *(Illustrations courtesy Stephanie Dziezyk, 2015. Under the copyright of St. Thomas Health.)*

femoral vein. The principal advantage of this method is that no plaque interaction occurs until after reversal of flow is established, with the disadvantages being increased device manipulation near the target lesion, a larger access sheath, and a potential for neurologic intolerance. The ENROUTE Transcarotid Neuroprotection System (Silk Road Medical Inc, Sunnyvale, CA) uses reversal of flow in addition to directly accessing the common carotid artery, thus bypassing the need to traverse a complicated aortic arch.

Complications and Management

Access Complications

Most CAS procedures are done via a transfemoral approach. With use of dual antiplatelet agents and aggressive anticoagulation, bleeding is not a rare complication. Quality centers report a less than 5% access complication rate, nevertheless. Bleeding at the puncture site, subcutaneously, or into the retroperitoneum are the usual sites. Hypotension, hematoma, or a combination should alert the practitioner. When discovered, pressure should be applied at the site while the patient is stabilized. Reassessment is often helpful with imaging, such as computed tomographic angiography (CTA) or duplex ultrasound. Continued bleeding should be handled promptly with open repair as deemed necessary. Closure devices have led to ischemic complications after femoral access, an additional means of access complication. Prompt assessment and diligent management in the operating room is indicated if a limb-threatening situation should exist.

Carotid Dissection

Carotid dissection can be caused by overdilating the artery, lifting a plaque distal to the bifurcation not covered by the stent, or injury to the artery from the distal protection device. If minimal, angiographic presence of carotid dissection alone may not warrant repair. Regulation of blood pressure and heart rate can be attempted, with a repeat of the arteriogram in a few moments, and progression can be assessed. If the patient's vital signs remain unsatisfactory or if the lumen of the vessel is compromised, extension of the stent to include that segment is recommended. Assuring that anticoagulation is therapeutic is also encouraged.

Thrombosed Filter

If the EPD filter thromboses, we leave it in place and deploy an aspiration catheter. A 5F angled Glide catheter is then typically placed in the stent until no further debris is retrievable; then, an attempt is made to remove the filter. If there is a need for additional treatment

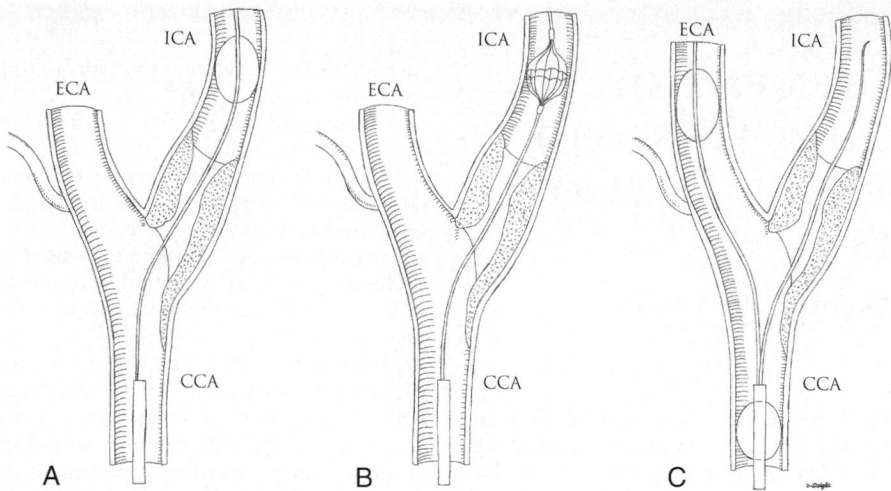

FIGURE 4 Schematic of embolic protection options. **A,** Distal internal occlusion. Flow and debris are interrupted from proceeding distally into the internal carotid artery (ICA). **B,** Filter device. Flow is allowed to continue during all manipulations and stent deployment. The filter is retrieved after postdilation of the stent is performed. **C,** Flow reversal. Flow is allowed and encouraged to reverse by taking advantage of back bleeding from the ICA. The flow is directed back into the patient via a passive vein. A filter is used within this system to catch any debris from the manipulations. *CCA,* Common carotid artery; *ECA,* external carotid artery. *(Illustrations courtesy Stephanie Dziezyk, 2015. Under the copyright of St. Thomas Health.)*

to the carotid lesion after removal, another filter can be inserted. We reassess, and again make certain that anticoagulation is therapeutic.

Stent Thrombosis

The first assessment is to assure proper anticoagulation. With the EPD in place, aspiration can be performed as stated earlier. If a clot is present, it can be lysed with 1 to 2 mg of tissue plasminogen activator (tPA) in 5 mL of saline. A Possis Anjiojet Catheter (Boston Scientific, Marlborough, MA) could be considered here as well.

Follow-Up

At our institution, the patient recovers for 24 hours in the hospital. A select nursing team trained in neurologic assessment monitors the patient for signs of neurologic insult. We ensure that the patient is on dual antiplatelet therapy along with a statin. The patient typically follows up in 1 month with a carotid duplex. If no issues are discovered at the time of the initial follow-up, the patient then returns 6 months later for continued surveillance with duplex ultrasonography. Typically we discontinue Plavix within 90 days after the procedure, and the patient remains on a statin for life.

■ CONCLUSIONS

Both CAS and CEA are effective in long-term stroke prevention, as demonstrated by multiple clinical trials. Although the equivalence of CAS and CEA in periprocedural prevention of stroke and death is not definitively established, CAS certainly has its place in certain clinical situations. As stent delivery systems and EPDs continue to advance along with proceduralist experience and formal training programs, one can only expect continued improvement of CAS outcomes with time.

In addition to increased periprocedural stroke risk, other key concerns about CAS include reimbursement restrictions and higher procedural costs, thus keeping CEA the standard in the management of carotid artery occlusive disease. At present, CAS should be performed only in high-risk, symptomatic patients with significant carotid stenosis by experienced interventionalists with high center volumes to optimize patient outcomes. The role of CAS in asymptomatic disease is not well established, and in these cases CAS should be performed only as part of a clinical trial.

A combination of antiplatelet agents, statins, dietary restriction with regular exercise, and abstaining from tobacco continues to offer promise in the medical management of carotid artery occlusive disease, suggesting the increasing role of BMT, especially in asymptomatic patients. With new data and advancing technique, the vascular surgeon will continue to offer patients the best personalized care for carotid artery occlusive disease encompassing medical therapy, endovascular procedures, and open operative techniques.

SUGGESTED READINGS

Abbott AL, Paraskevas KI, Kakkos SK, et al. Systematic review of guidelines for the management of asymptomatic and symptomatic carotid stenosis. *Stroke.* 2015;46:3288-3301.

Bonati LH, Dobson J, Featherstone RL, International Carotid Stenting Study investigators, et al. Long-term outcomes after stenting versus endarterectomy for treatment of symptomatic carotid stenosis: the International Carotid Stenting Study (ICSS) randomised trial. *Lancet.* 2015;385:529-538.

Bonati LH, Lyrer P, Ederle J, et al. Percutaneous transluminal balloon angioplasty and stenting for carotid artery stenosis. *Cochrane Database Syst Rev.* 2012;(9):CD000515.

Brott TG, Hobson RW, Howard G, et al. Stenting versus endarterectomy for treatment of carotid artery stenosis. *N Engl J Med.* 2010;363:11-23.

Naggara O, Touzé E, Beyssen B, et al. Anatomical and technical factors associated with stroke or death during carotid angioplasty and stenting: results from the endarterectomy versus angioplasty in patients with symptomatic severe carotid stenosis (EVA-3S) trial and systematic review. *Stroke.* 2011;42:380-388.

The Management of Extracranial Carotid and Vertebral Artery Aneurysms

Gregory A. Stanley, MD, and Charles S. O'Mara, MD, MBA

Only a small percentage of arterial aneurysms involving the head and neck vasculature reside in the extracranial circulation of the carotid and vertebral arteries. Contemporary reviews of invasive treatment for extracranial carotid artery aneurysm (ECAA) estimate that 0.1% to 2% of all carotid interventions are performed for aneurysmal disease. The rarity of ECAA is substantiated by the relative paucity of literature on the natural history, clinical decision making, and long-term outcomes of available treatment options. Current management guidelines stem largely from historical case reports or small series. Only recently have single-center retrospective reviews and meta-analyses been published to provide further insight into treatment algorithms that are currently appropriate for managing patients with ECAA.

Extracranial vertebral artery aneurysm (EVAA) is even rarer than ECAA, and as expected the experience and data to support management decisions for this entity are limited. However, a review of published case reports and series offers guidelines for treatment of this clinical entity, albeit with incomplete follow-up.

■ EXTRACRANIAL CAROTID ARTERY ANEURYSM

Etiology

In the past, mycotic aneurysms were the most common form of ECAA encountered. These aneurysms were seen primarily in young patients with locally untreated or uncontrolled infections of the head and neck, including peritonsillar abscess, mastoiditis, and pharyngeal infection. The historical predominance of infectious cause is attributed to the lack of effective antibiotic medication, poor healthcare access, and late presentation of the disease process. With advances in antibiotic regimens and healthcare delivery, mycotic aneurysms now comprise less than 5% of aneurysms in the extracranial circulation, even including patch angioplasty infection after carotid endarterectomy (CEA).

The incidence of post-CEA patch angioplasty infection remains extremely low at 0.025% to 0.85%. In a modern single-center retrospective review of more than 1300 CEAs, no significant difference was found in the rate of postoperative infection between primary closure, Dacron patch angioplasty, and bovine pericardium angioplasty. Other studies have failed to show that the use of a prosthetic (Dacron or polytetrafluoroethylene [PTFE]) or xenograft (bovine pericardium) patch has a risk of infection that is higher than using autogenous vein for patch angioplasty. The offending organism in patch infections is usually a *Staphylococcus* species, but *Streptococcus* and gram-negative bacteria have been reported as well.

Atherosclerotic disease and trauma are now the most common causes of ECAA, representing nearly half of all identified aneurysms in a contemporary review. Poststenotic dilatation and degeneration associated with atherosclerosis and plaque ulceration create saccular rather than fusiform aneurysms, which involve the carotid bifurcation and proximal internal carotid artery (ICA) in at least two thirds of cases. Extracranial carotid artery aneurysms have been reported in patients with fibromuscular dysplasia, collagen vascular disorders

such as Marfan's syndrome and Ehlers-Danlos syndrome, and other connective tissue diseases.

Trauma-related aneurysms arise from both penetrating and blunt mechanisms, in addition to an increasing number of iatrogenic injuries during the last decade. Penetrating injuries that result in pseudoaneurysm formation may occur in neck zones I to III, but they most frequently involve the common carotid artery. Blunt force trauma, usually associated with extreme cervical hyperextension that causes carotid artery dissection, accounts for approximately 0.08% of ECCAs. Although the distal ICA near the skull base (zone III) is most prone to this type of injury, any segment of a dissected and weakened carotid artery may progress to aneurysm formation. External iatrogenic injury with pseudoaneurysm formation is associated with errant attempts at central line placement and tends to occur in the proximal and middle common carotid artery. Conversely, internal iatrogenic injury associated with endovascular manipulation can occur at any location in which a wire, catheter, or device has been placed intentionally or unintentionally; such injury typically is caused by arterial wall perforation or dissection with subsequent aneurysmal degeneration at that site.

Presentation and Diagnosis

Given the atherosclerotic nature of most ECAAs, the representative patient is a male in the seventh or eighth decade of life. Women are afflicted half as often as their male counterparts. Typical cardiovascular risk factors such as hypertension, smoking history, hyperlipidemia, and diabetes are frequent comorbid conditions. Younger patients with ECAA are likely to have a local-regional infection, a history of trauma to the head and/or neck, or manifestations of fibromuscular dysplasia or connective tissue disease. Inquiries into recent hospitalizations or procedures may reveal an underlying iatrogenic traumatic injury to the extracranial circulation, sometimes initially unsuspected. Not surprisingly, the association with atherosclerotic disease is reinforced by the most common ECAA locations: ICA, nearly 50%; carotid bifurcation, approximately 20%; common carotid artery, less than 10%; and external carotid artery, less than 1%.

The presence of a pulsatile neck mass is a common early finding that initiates the diagnostic and treatment algorithm depicted in Figure 1. The neck mass may range from a subtle prominent carotid pulse to an obvious ipsilateral neck enlargement with pulsatility. A neck mass may be the only abnormal finding, as up to 35% of patients are asymptomatic at presentation. The remaining patient cohort is symptomatic secondary to local compressive symptoms, arterial thromboembolism, or aneurysmal rupture.

The constellation of symptoms related to compression varies with aneurysm location, size, and orientation. Cranial nerve dysfunction is present in approximately 10% of patients; involvement of the hypoglossal, glossopharyngeal, facial, or vagus nerves may result in dysphagia, facial muscle paralysis, or hoarseness. Disruption of the ipsilateral sympathetic chain with development of Horner's syndrome (ptosis, miosis, enophthalmos, and anhidrosis) also has been reported. Headache, neck pain, or facial pain may be present but is observed in less than 5% of patients. In contrast to local compressive symptoms, thromboembolic events such as temporary monocular blindness (amaurosis fugax), transient ischemic attack (TIA), and ipsilateral ischemic stroke are present in one third to one half of patients. The presence of intraluminal thrombus within the aneurysm cavity is variable and related to aneurysm size and morphology; however, when present, the risk of distal thromboembolism is significantly increased.

Finally, rupture of ECAA, a once familiar and somewhat predictable complication of untreated mycotic carotid aneurysms, is a relatively uncommon event in the current era of modern antibiotic therapy. Infectious causes continue to pose the highest risk of rupture,

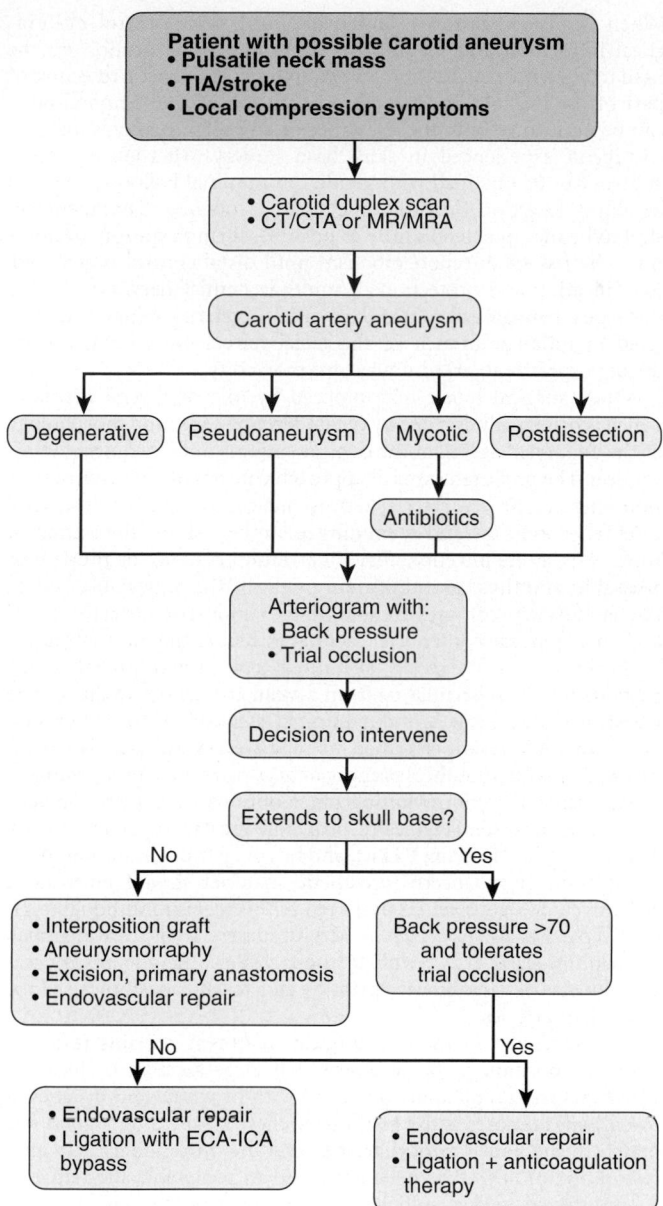

FIGURE 1 Algorithm for diagnosis and treatment of carotid aneurysms. *CT*, Computed tomography; *CTA*, computed tomographic angiography; *ECA*, external carotid artery; *ICA*, internal carotid artery; *MR*, magnetic resonance; *MRA*, magnetic resonance angiography; *TIA*, transient ischemic attack. *(Modified from Rothstein J, Goldstone J: Carotid artery aneurysm. In: Cronenwett JL, Rutherford RB, eds.* Decision Making in Vascular Surgery. *Orlando, FL: WB Saunders; 2001:54.)*

both internally (i.e., erosion into pharynx) and externally (e.g., via a draining sinus tract). An important distinction should be made between ECAA rupture and carotid blowout syndrome, which typically is associated with hemorrhage secondary to invasive head and neck cancers, despite their similar presentation.

Because of its accessibility, low cost, and reliability, the first-line diagnostic test for ECAA is duplex ultrasound (DUS; see Figure 1). Ultrasound images detailing the anatomic location, diameter, flow characteristics, presence of intraluminal thrombus, and presence of dissection provide valuable diagnostic and treatment information. Noted limitations of DUS are operator experience and ability and anatomic inaccessibility, particularly as visualization generally becomes more difficult and less reliable above the mandible and below

the clavicles. Aneurysms in these restricted locations may be missed altogether by DUS; thus a strong index of suspicion must be maintained to investigate further with additional imaging studies. Computed tomographic angiography (CTA) or magnetic resonance angiography (MRA) now have emerged as the investigative modalities of choice because both offer detailed three-dimensional information of the arterial anatomy and surrounding structures that is critical for appropriate treatment planning. Catheter-based angiography largely has been supplanted by CTA and MRA because of the latter's widespread availability, noninvasive nature, and negligible stroke risk compared with invasive angiography. Carotid angiography maintains the specific and sometimes crucial role of measuring carotid back pressure or performing ICA balloon occlusion testing, especially when carotid ligation is being considered as a possible treatment option.

Indications for Intervention

Unlike their visceral or infrarenal aortic counterparts, general consensus is lacking regarding the specific size at which ECAAs warrant repair. Many authors reason that a carotid artery diameter that is 1.5 times larger than the adjacent normal artery or expected artery size is grounds for aneurysm diagnosis. The argument is also made that, similar to aortic aneurysms, ECAA diameter exceeding twice that of the adjacent normal artery indicates need for repair, although supporting data for this contention are lacking. Although little is known of the natural history of asymptomatic ECAA, historical publications document mortality rates exceeding 70% with nonoperative management secondary to thrombotic or embolic cerebrovascular events or carotid artery rupture. Multiple contemporary retrospective reviews report a 50% or greater risk of TIA, stroke, or death in asymptomatic patients with ECAA. These studies suggest that an aggressive treatment approach for asymptomatic ECAA is indicated, regardless of aneurysm size, to prevent a future potentially fatal cerebrovascular event. Decision about intervention for asymptomatic ECAA must be individualized and is strongly influenced by factors such as size, configuration, growth pattern, and location of the aneurysm, along with interventional risk and age of the patient.

Certainly symptomatic patients should be considered strongly for definitive treatment to reduce or relieve compressive complications, prevent progression of cranial nerve dysfunction, minimize the risk of recurrent cerebral ischemic insults, and reduce or eliminate the risk of rupture. Pain is an uncommon finding in patients with ECAA and should prompt suspicion for contained or impending rupture. Although rare, carotid aneurysm rupture is associated with considerable blood loss, transfusion requirements, and high rates of morbidity and mortality secondary to cerebral ischemia. A mycotic aneurysm with adjacent abscess or carotid patch infection requires urgent diagnosis and initiation of multispecialty care to address concomitant issues involving multiple regional organ systems.

Treatment Methods

Simply stated, the treatment goals of ECAA repair are to prevent new or recurrent cerebrovascular thromboembolic events, to exclude the aneurysm from the pressurized arterial circulation to prevent expansion and rupture, and to relieve compressive symptoms. The three options for treatment familiar to vascular specialists certainly apply to ECAA, namely nonoperative (medical) management, open surgical repair, and endovascular therapy. The literature largely has supported open surgical repair, but endovascular options are becoming more common as familiarity and comfort with carotid interventions increases. Despite the potentially malignant natural history of ECAA, isolated reports disclose treatment algorithms using various antiplatelet and anticoagulant regimens in small asymptomatic aneurysms and surgically high-risk patients. Thus there is no one-size-fits-all approach to treating ECAA; rather, a customized approach that considers the clinical, anatomic, and diagnostic factors of each patient is likely to produce the best outcomes.

Evaluation Before Treatment

Consideration for intervention must begin with a thorough assessment of the presentation and accompanying symptoms. Compressive symptoms often necessitate surgical repair depending on the severity, whereas asymptomatic patients and those with thromboembolic symptoms may be treated variably. A detailed cranial nerve examination and neurologic evaluation is mandatory to establish the baseline functionality of the patient. Neck extension and rotation, as well as body habitus and neck size, should be considered. Bilateral saphenous vein mapping (and arm vein mapping, as necessary) should be completed if interposition grafting is planned. In the setting of infection, soft tissue coverage of the carotid repair may be a concern, and plastic surgery consultation is appropriate. With the preponderance of atherosclerotic aneurysms, cardiac risk stratification should be completed in applicable patients. General anesthesia is preferred for surgical repair because prolonged procedure time, more extensive dissection, and extended carotid clamp time are expected compared with standard CEA. For the same reasons, cerebral perfusion monitoring in the form of either electroencephalography, transcranial Doppler, or evoked potentials should be utilized intraoperatively.

An extensive study of the CTA or MRA, including three-dimensional reconstructions, may offer valuable insights to enhance decision making. The location, size, and shape of the aneurysm are vital variables that will guide potential treatment options. Larger aneurysms may distort typical anatomic relationships significantly, and cranial nerves may be displaced or closely adherent to the aneurysm wall. Proximal common carotid and distal ICA aneurysms can present exposure challenges that result in increased morbidity and therefore may be better treated by an endovascular approach. Vessel tortuosity or aortic arch anatomy (especially a type III arch) adds considerable complexity to an endovascular approach, and the presence of significant intraluminal plaque or heavy calcification poses additional stroke risk because of possible intraoperative embolism.

A careful examination of intracranial collaterals on preoperative imaging is required to identify perfusion deficits that might arise during repair because of carotid occlusion. However, preoperative physiologic cerebral perfusion testing is recommended in all patients being considered for elective open repair to determine the neurologic impact of temporary or permanent carotid occlusion. This test is accomplished by temporary balloon occlusion with carotid stump pressure measurement. After full heparinization and selective angiography of the involved carotid artery, an occlusive balloon is inflated in the ICA distal to the aneurysm to halt ipsilateral antegrade cerebral blood flow for 30 minutes, during which time the patient is carefully monitored for neurologic or mental status changes. Carotid stump pressure measurement greater than 70 mm Hg (i.e., the pressure measured in the ICA during occlusion of the common and external carotid arteries) suggests that intracranial collaterals are adequate to maintain satisfactory cerebral perfusion without neurologic compromise in the setting of carotid occlusion. Patients unable to tolerate carotid occlusion on preoperative testing require the use of a carotid shunt during surgical repair. Even if a carotid occlusion test suggests adequate intracranial collaterals, shunting is recommended for added stroke risk mitigation given the limited experience of most surgeons with ECAA repair. It is worth noting that carotid balloon occlusion testing carries a small but acceptable risk of neurologic complication similar to that of cerebral angiography in the range of 0.4% to 2.0%.

Open Surgical Repair

Open surgical repair can be accomplished through a standard neck incision along the anterior border of the sternocleidomastoid muscle. Common carotid aneurysms below the level of the clavicle may require extension to a mini- or full sternotomy for proximal control. Distal ICA aneurysm exposure is achieved by lengthening the cervical incision behind the ear and may necessitate uncommon maneuvers such as dividing the posterior belly of the digastric muscle, ligating external carotid artery branches, and excising the styloid process.

When far distal exposure is anticipated for arterial control, nasotracheal intubation and mandible subluxation or dislocation can be used to aid with visualization. In extreme circumstances, resection of part of the mastoid and the petrous portion of the temporal bone can be performed with the assistance of an otolaryngologist or neurosurgeon experienced in skull base surgery. Alternatively, distal control can be obtained with gentle intraluminal balloon occlusion or shunt insertion once the aneurysm is opened. The aneurysm should be manipulated as little as possible during exposure to minimize the risk of thromboembolism until distal control is achieved. Identification and protection of multiple cranial nerves, including the vagus, hypoglossal, glossopharyngeal, accessory spinal, and marginal mandibular branch of the facial nerve, must be a priority during exposure to avoid injury and morbidity.

Open surgical repair may proceed by one of several methods, which is principally dictated by the underlying cause and morphology of the aneurysm as well as the clinical circumstances requiring intervention. The preferred surgical approach consists of aneurysm exclusion with concurrent arterial reconstruction to maintain ipsilateral cerebral blood flow and to minimize stroke risk. In the setting of rupture or severe infection, revascularization may not be prudent or advisable, and thus carotid ligation might be the only viable option. For patients with compressive symptoms, removal of mural thrombus and aneurysm sac contents is essential to relieve the mass effect.

Primary repair generally is limited to traumatic or iatrogenic pseudoaneurysms originating from a small arterial defect that can be reapproximated easily without luminal stenosis. More commonly, patch angioplasty is performed to repair eccentric saccular aneurysms and wide-mouthed pseudoaneurysms related to a traumatic or iatrogenic dissection. Multiple patch options are available, including autologous vein (typically proximal greater saphenous vein), prosthetic graft (Dacron, PTFE), and bovine pericardium (Figure 2). If infection is a concern, prosthetic material should be avoided ardently; autologous vein is preferred in this scenario, although pericardial patches also have been used with success. In the case of a small or medium-sized ECAA with tortuous vessels, the aneurysm occasionally may be resected with primary end-to-end anastomosis of the redundant arteries.

The preferred method of surgical treatment remains resection with interposition graft placement. For large saccular or fusiform ECAA, reversed saphenous vein graft with proximal and distal end-to-end anastomoses is the conduit of choice, providing a good size match to the native carotid arteries and low thrombogenicity after restoration of flow. Prosthetic grafts are an acceptable alternative in a noninfected field if sufficient autologous vein conduit does not exist. When carotid infection is present and autologous vein is otherwise inadequate, a segment of proximal superficial femoral artery (SFA) may be translocated for use as an interposition autograft, followed by replacement of the donor artery with a prosthetic graft in the noninfected leg. Of course, any significant atherosclerotic plaque in the donor SFA segment should be removed with endarterectomy before grafting. Previous authors have described the successful use of an occluded SFA segment as an interposition autograft after it has been recanalized by performing endarterectomy before integration into the carotid circulation.

Carotid artery ligation remains an alternative surgical treatment option for ECAA and has the advantages of technical ease and shorter procedure duration. These benefits are outweighed, however, by the extraordinarily high risk of stroke (up to 60% in some studies). Thus this technique is used sparingly in cases of trauma, rupture, or severe infection or as a bailout option when previously described maneuvers fail to provide adequate exposure for distal control of the aneurysm. Patients who cannot tolerate carotid occlusion based on preoperative testing should be considered for extracranial-intracranial (EC-IC) bypass before aneurysm ligation. Once carotid ligation is performed, therapeutic anticoagulation should be initiated in the early postoperative period to minimize the risk of thrombus propagation or embolism into the cerebral circulation from the stagnant column of

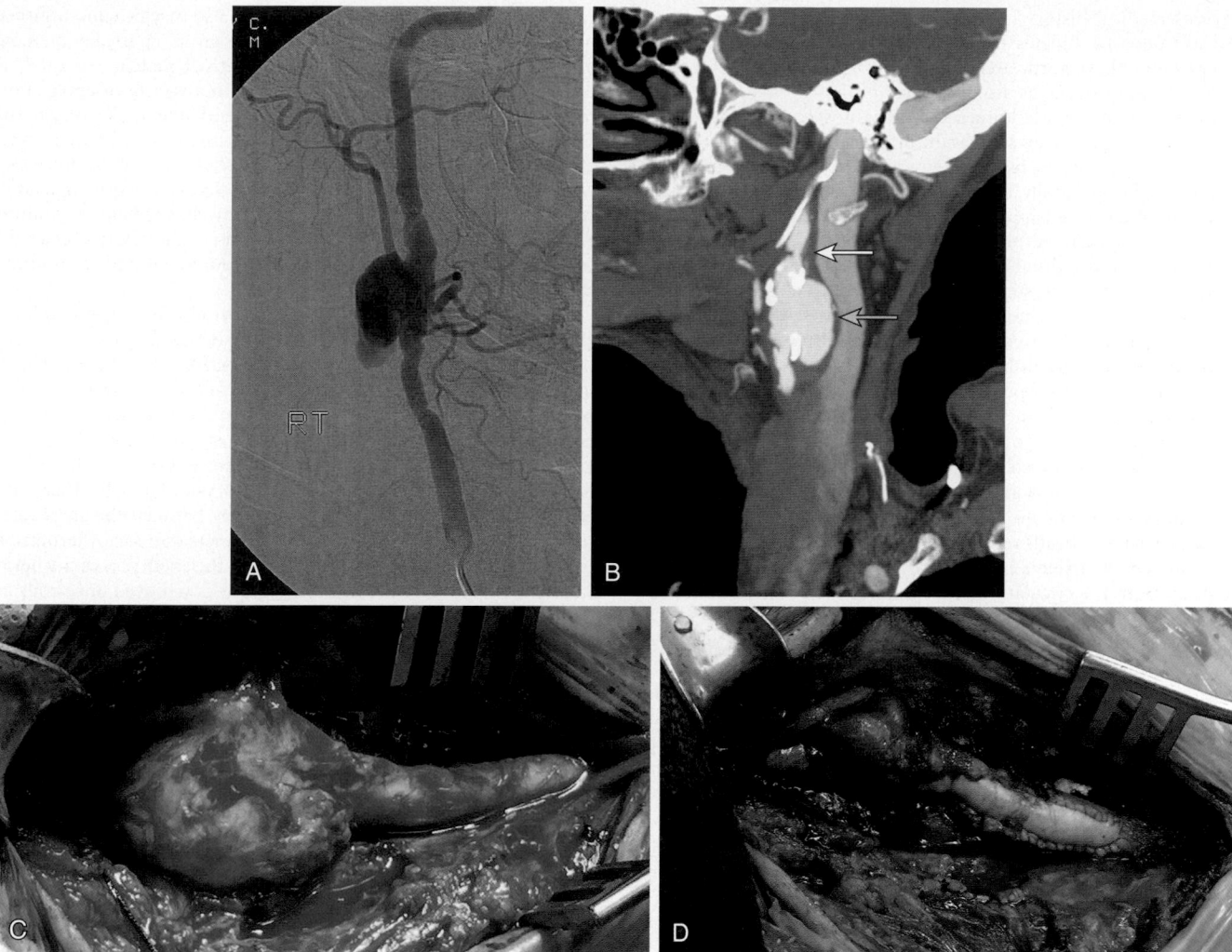

FIGURE 2 A, Digital subtraction angiography of a right carotid artery aneurysm at the site of carotid endarterectomy done 26 years previously. **B,** Computed tomographic angiography done 4 years later showing further enlargement of the aneurysm (*gray arrow*) and development of severe stenosis (*white arrow*) in the internal carotid artery distal to the aneurysm. Operative photographs showing (**C**) exposure of the aneurysm and (**D**) bovine pericardial patch angioplasty repair. *(Photographs courtesy Dr. Daniel Ramirez.)*

blood distal to the site of ligation. Oral anticoagulation should be continued for at least 12 weeks postoperatively, and lifelong aspirin is recommended.

In the setting of infection, preoperative broad-spectrum antibiotics should be initiated at presentation and tailored to culture results. Patients with a punctate draining sinus after CEA would suggest infection with a low virulence organism, and repair can be performed expediently in a semielective fashion. Gross purulence, significant surrounding cellulitis, and a herald bleed are ominous signs and warrant urgent repair. Intraoperatively, cultures are imperative to direct postoperative antibiotic therapy, and a reasonable attempt should be made to remove all prosthetic material from the infected field. Devitalized or otherwise infected surrounding tissue should be débrided sharply and irrigated with a pulse irrigation system as needed, and all suture lines, patches, and grafts must be covered with healthy vascularized tissue, preferably the adjacent sternocleidomastoid muscle. In certain circumstances, such as previous neck radiation or a history of radical neck dissection, tissue coverage is inadequate and a myofascial or myocutaneous flap may be required.

Endovascular Repair

Modern endovascular techniques have emerged as a viable and sometimes preferred treatment option for ECAA. A growing body of literature supports several endovascular options for ECAA, including embolization, stent and stent graft placement, and a combination thereof. The risk of cranial nerve injury is negligible compared with open repair, and rates of bleeding and postoperative infection are significantly less. In addition, most endovascular efforts are approached with the goal of maintaining cerebral blood flow during and after intervention. However, a different complication profile is associated with endovascular intervention, including access site complications, stent thrombosis, stent fracture, in-stent restenosis, and failure to achieve aneurysm thrombosis. The stroke risk may be slightly higher with endovascular procedures, as atheroembolism from existing occlusive disease and thromboembolism from the aneurysm itself is possible and in some cases likely during wire access and sheath placement in preparation for treatment.

Attempting endovascular repair requires an appropriate setup, including a modern fluoroscopic imaging suite, dedicated staff with substantial training, familiarity and experience with endovascular procedures, carotid-specific equipment (sheaths, stents, embolic protection devices), and an endovascular specialist who has experience performing carotid interventions with at least moderate annual case volume. Primary consideration for endovascular treatment is appropriate for surgically inaccessible aneurysms (especially those involving the distal ICA), for patients with unfavorable neck anatomy or previous medical history (e.g., surgery, radiation), and for patients who are poor candidates for general anesthesia. In addition, the patient should have aortic arch and carotid anatomy amenable to an endovascular approach as discussed previously.

Standard retrograde femoral access is the most common approach, but alternative access sites such as the brachial, axillary, and proximal carotid arteries can be used. After therapeutic heparin has been administered systemically, the common carotid artery is catheterized selectively, and then an appropriately sized sheath is advanced over a supportive guidewire. A full cervical and cerebral carotid angiogram is performed, and a distal embolic protection filter is placed in the ICA distal to the aneurysm. A variety of stents have been implanted for aneurysm repair, including bare metal stents (self-expanding and balloon expandable), overlapping or layered stents, and covered stents. A proximal and distal landing zone of healthy nonaneurysmal artery is required for proper stent performance, and stent size selection should be based on diameter measurements of the landing zones. Postdilatation is not performed routinely but may be necessary if inadequate stent wall apposition is present. Completion angiography of the cervical and cerebral circulation is mandatory to assess for possible embolic events.

Despite larger sheath requirements, covered stents are the most frequently selected stents because they provide complete aneurysm exclusion from the circulation and eliminate the potential for aneurysm growth or rupture. In addition, the PTFE covering prevents distal thromboembolism once the stents are deployed. As expected, covered stent placement across the carotid bifurcation will block antegrade flow into the external carotid artery; this typically is well tolerated without noticeable sequela. Bare metal stents occasionally are selected over covered stents when attempting to secure a dissection flap or to disrupt flow into a small pseudoaneurysm neck that cannot be catheterized. Bare metal stents also may be chosen instead of covered stents for distal ICA aneurysms given the smaller diameter of the native artery and better vessel-stent size match.

Coil embolization has been reported in a variety of applications related to endovascular ECAA repair. Pseudoaneurysms originating from a narrow-mouthed arteriotomy (as might be seen after a penetrating injury) may be candidates for isolated coil embolization. Direct catheterization of the aneurysm sac is performed using a coaxial microcatheter system, followed by deployment of multiple thrombogenic coils to achieve thrombosis of the cavity. Detachable coils are preferred to assure controlled placement and to minimize the risk of coil migration.

In a slight variation, coil embolization also has been combined with bare metal stent placement to broaden applicability to larger saccular aneurysms. Such coiling can be performed at the time of the index stenting procedure or remotely in follow-up. Delay in coiling offers the possible benefit of allowing spontaneous closure of initially persistent flow into the aneurysm after stenting alone (Figure 3). When completed concurrently, a closed-cell stent is selected and deployed first as a scaffold across the aneurysm. Then the microcatheter is advanced into the aneurysm cavity between the stent interstices, and coils are deployed to fill the aneurysm sac. Alternatively, these steps are reversed to secure access to the aneurysm cavity before stent placement; the microcatheter simply is removed once coils are inserted. The stent inhibits coil migration to the brain after deployment and creates a pathway through which antegrade cerebral blood flow can continue. This technique also can be used if the aneurysm sac has failed to thrombose completely after bare metal stent placement alone. Several alternative embolization materials are currently available, including a variety of microparticles and liquid embolics; however, the uncontrolled nature of these injections and the extremely

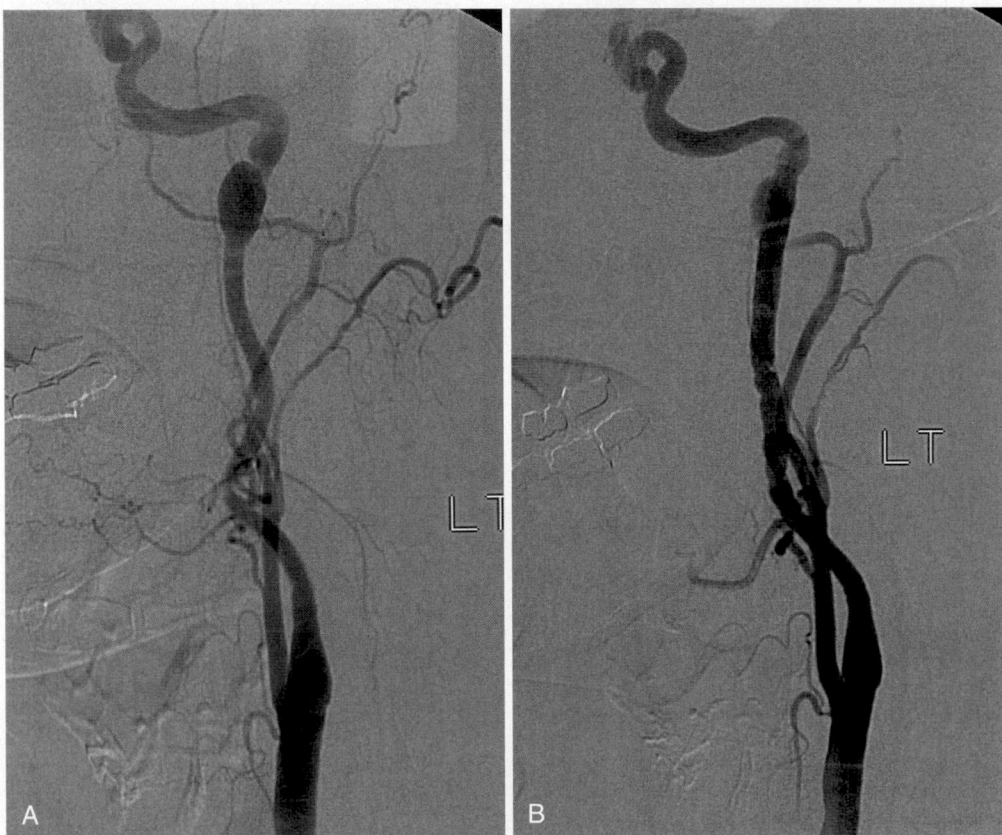

FIGURE 3 Digital subtraction angiography of a left internal carotid aneurysm at the skull base with associated weblike stenosis. **A,** Before treatment by bare metal stent placement. **B,** After treatment. Note the absence of residual stenosis and presence of a small residual aneurysm sac, which subsequently closed completely.

high risk of distal embolization and resultant stroke have thus far precluded use of these products for ECAA repair.

Coil embolization is an effective tool for achieving carotid artery occlusion. It has been used in the elective setting as primary treatment of an aneurysm as well as for rapid hemorrhage control in the setting of acute rupture or carotid blowout. Proper embolization technique involves placing coils distal to, within, and proximal to the aneurysm and requires embolization of any significant branches that originate from the aneurysm sac. As expected with this treatment modality that is akin to open surgical aneurysm ligation, similar stroke rates are observed.

Hybrid techniques are likely to emerge as viable therapeutic options in the future. A recently published case report describes a hybrid technique combining endovascular coil embolization followed by surgical resection of an infected ICA aneurysm as a means to gain arterial control and decrease intraoperative blood loss in a hostile surgical field. Another case report demonstrated the use of the Gore Hybrid Vascular Graft (Gore Medical, Flagstaff, AZ) to treat a distal ICA aneurysm by deploying the covered stent portion of the graft into the distal ICA and creating a surgical end-to-end anastomosis to the native artery proximal to the aneurysm. Although still considered experimental and lacking long-term follow-up, these creative solutions offer a glimpse into the many possible hybrid treatment options that have yet to be realized.

Results of Treatment

Given the rarity of ECAA, no randomized controlled trials are available to compare treatment options or to dictate an optimal clinical algorithm. An international registry, the Carotid Aneurysm Registry (CAR; www.carotidaneurysmregistry.com), has been established to prospectively enroll patients via an Internet-based platform with the hope that additional insights can be gained into the natural history, diagnostic and practice patterns, intervention outcomes, and long-term follow-up of ECAA. The results of this registry are scheduled to be published at 1-year and 5-year time points. Recently published single-center retrospective reviews and comprehensive literature reviews highlight the outcomes of various treatment strategies currently in practice around the world.

Nonoperative medical therapy, including observation alone, antiplatelet agents, anticoagulation medication, or a combination thereof, historically has been an undesirable treatment option for ECAA, with rates of TIA, stroke, and rupture ranging up to 60%. However, a recent retrospective review by Fankhauser and colleagues at the Mayo Clinic revealed that nearly half of the 141 patients with ECAA included in the study were treated nonoperatively using medical therapy with either antiplatelets, anticoagulants, or serial imaging studies. The vast majority of these patients were asymptomatic with stable ECAA, and notably none of these patients developed symptoms requiring intervention during a mean follow-up of 77 months. These results suggest that nonoperative management with medical therapy and close follow-up may be appropriate for highly selected patients, but confirmation of these outcomes by additional authors is required.

Surgical repair remains the recommended treatment modality at present. Contemporary results regarding open surgical intervention with arterial reconstruction appear to be consistent with historical controls. Recent data demonstrate 30-day stroke rates between 0.7% and 10% and 30-day mortality less than 2%. Cranial nerve injury remains the most common morbidity, with historical rates as high as 30%. Modern studies demonstrate a lower incidence of permanent cranial nerve injury ranging from 2.4% to 12.5%, which could be a reflection of patient selection bias because of the emergence of endovascular treatment options. Surgical ligation of ECAAs continues to be associated with high stroke rates in excess of 30%. Preoperative balloon occlusion testing has demonstrated good reliability and predictive value; however, approximately 12% of patients who tolerate the balloon occlusion test will suffer a perioperative neurologic insult after carotid ligation. Long-term data after surgical reconstruction continue to be favorable with 83% to 95% survival, and more

than 85% of deaths were non–aneurysm related. Patency rates after arterial reconstruction cannot be stated accurately, as the follow-up imaging reporting is poor. Nevertheless, most series identify excellent arterial patency, and the patients remained asymptomatic in several instances of bypass graft occlusion or carotid artery thrombosis.

Results of endovascular treatment continue to be encouraging. Technical success repeatedly has been reported to be greater than 90%. Perioperative stroke rates are consistent with open repair, ranging from 2% to 6% in larger reviews. Expected low rates of cranial nerve injury and arterial access complications are observed. Although not accurately quantifiable, endovascular "failures," primarily involving endoleaks and incomplete aneurysm thrombosis, are estimated to be less than 10%. Nearly all reported endoleaks were identified at the time of the index procedure and resolved with post-dilatation angioplasty or additional stent placement. Reintervention was required in several patients with incomplete aneurysm thrombosis at 12-month follow-up; typical reintervention involved placement of additional coils within the aneurysm sac.

The advantages and successes of endovascular interventions for ECAA have made the treatment algorithm less obvious. The patient's ability to tolerate surgical repair is a principal factor in the decision; however, aneurysm location and anatomy may prove to be equally important. To aid in clinical decision making, a classification system for ECAA has been proposed by Attigah and colleagues based on the anatomic location and extent of the aneurysm (Figure 4). A review of complication rates using this aneurysm classification scheme identifies a significantly elevated risk of cranial nerve injury during surgical repair of aneurysm types I, II, and IV, the common thread being involvement of the distal ICA. As more data are published, additional recommendations based on this classification system may become apparent to help guide management decisions for ECAA.

■ VERTEBRAL ARTERY ANEURYSM

Aneurysms involving the posterior cervical arterial circulation are exceedingly rare. The limited understanding of EVAA from the medical literature is based on numerous case reports and a selection of case series, from which it is difficult to determine appropriate management guidelines. The majority of EVAAs are the result of trauma to the head and neck in the form of either penetrating injuries that result in focal pseudoaneurysms or blunt injuries that produce dissection with subsequent aneurysmal dilatation. Rapid flexion-extension injuries and medical manipulation also have been reported to cause vertebral artery dissection. As much as 20% of vertebral artery dissections progress to aneurysm requiring intervention. Spontaneous vertebral dissection also has been increasingly reported. Other known causes of EVAA include iatrogenic dissection from endovascular interventions, arterial dysplasia, collagen vascular disorders, and prior radiation treatment of the head and neck.

These patients are often asymptomatic but may have unilateral headache and neck pain. A pulsatile neck mass is not as commonly observed as with ECAA. Multiple reports have documented visual changes such as transient blurred vision and lateral hemianopsia, in addition to signs of vertebrobasilar ischemia. The incidence of TIA or stroke as the presenting symptom is not entirely known; however, in recently published studies of trauma patients with extracranial vertebral artery dissection the stroke rate was less than 5%. Rupture of EVAA has been reported but is also extremely rare. Aneurysms of the intracranial vertebral artery appear to be slightly more common than those in the cervical circulation; rupture in this location results in subarachnoid hemorrhage.

Diagnosing EVAA is accomplished mainly by CTA or MRA. DUS is extremely limited in this clinical situation because of the tortuosity and visual inaccessibility of the vertebral artery. A determination of the patency and direction of flow in the vertebral artery is possible, but little else. Cerebral angiography also has been largely replaced as a diagnostic modality by CTA or MRA because of their ease of access,

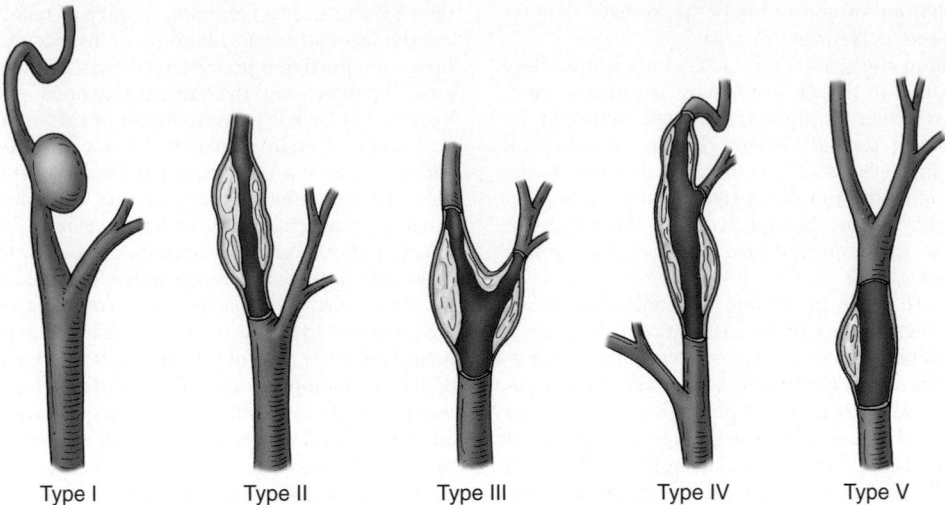

| Type I | Type II | Type III | Type IV | Type V |

FIGURE 4 Extracranial carotid artery aneurysm (ECAA) classification system proposed by Attigah and colleagues. Type I: aneurysm of the middle to distal internal carotid artery (ICA); Type II: aneurysm of the proximal to middle ICA; Type III: aneurysm of the carotid bifurcation; Type IV: aneurysm of the common carotid artery and ICA; Type V: aneurysm of the common carotid artery. *(From Nordanstig J, et al. National experience with extracranial carotid artery aneurysms: epidemiology, surgical treatment strategy, and treatment outcome.* Ann Vasc Surg. *2014;28:882-886.)*

rapid results, and image quality that offers valuable anatomic information to guide intervention.

Strong evidence now suggests that close to 80% of vertebral artery dissections will resolve with medical treatment alone. Randomized controlled trials demonstrate no significant difference in stroke rate, bleeding events, or progression to surgery between treatments with antiplatelet versus anticoagulant therapy. Similar data for EVAA are not known, but an aggressive treatment algorithm has been recommended historically. Intervention typically is warranted in patients with ongoing pain, neurologic symptoms, aneurysm growth, significant contralateral vertebral occlusive disease, or aneurysm rupture.

Once again, both open surgical and endovascular treatment options are available. Surgical repair of EVAA remains a complicated and involved procedure, stemming primarily from the challenge of adequately exposing the vertebral artery. The V1 segment is the most familiar and perhaps the easiest portion to access, as it courses from the subclavian artery and enters the vertebral foramen of C6. A transverse supraclavicular incision will provide adequate visualization at this location. The subsequent intraosseous V2 segment travels along the transverse processes from C6 to C2 and is a relatively hostile surgical field secondary to bony impediments and the extensive venous plexus that accompanies the artery along this path. The V3 segment exits the C2 foramen, courses around the transverse process, and ultimately enters the foramen magnum as the V4 segment. This territory can be accessed appropriately via a posterior approach, but such exposure is generally a task best attempted with the guidance of a neurosurgeon.

For aneurysms of the V1 segment, surgical repair can be accomplished in one of a variety of ways, including the following: resection with primary repair, resection with transposition onto the carotid artery, or bypass from the subclavian or carotid arteries. Also, in the presence of an adequate contralateral vertebral artery, ligation can be performed. Given the small working space and challenging exposure, ligation may be the most desirable option, especially in the setting of rupture. However, both proximal and distal ligation must be achieved to adequately exclude the aneurysm from retrograde flow originating from the contralateral vertebral artery. Surgical options in the V2-4 segments become increasingly limited and consist of bypass from the subclavian or carotid arteries and interposition grafting using a local autograft of the external carotid artery.

Because of the technical challenges and limited options to open surgical repair, endovascular treatment has become the preferred therapeutic modality for EVAA. Similar to carotid aneurysms, intervention proceeds with the use of embolization coils to occlude the vertebral artery or with stent placement to exclude the aneurysm from active circulation. Covered stents are again preferred for similar reasons as in the carotid vasculature. Although embolization and subsequent thrombosis of the vertebral artery typically is well tolerated in the presence of a normal contralateral vertebral artery, pre-intervention balloon occlusion can be performed to identify patients who will require a strategy to maintain posterior perfusion throughout the procedure and in the postoperative period. Limitations to successful endovascular intervention include severe tortuosity or significant occlusive disease of the proximal vertebral artery. To maximize chances of success, it is advisable to place the sheath at or in the origin of the vertebral artery for additional support and to be prepared to use advanced wire skills such as buddy wire techniques for stent delivery. If unsuccessful, attempts at retrograde access via the contralateral vertebral artery might be considered. Current published data suggest that both surgical repair and endovascular interventions are viable treatment options with satisfactory initial and long-term results.

SELECTED READINGS

Bush RL, Lin PH, Dodson TF, et al. Endoluminal stent placement and coil embolization for the management of carotid artery pseudoaneurysms. *J Endovasc Ther.* 2001;8:53-61.

Choudhary AS, Evans RJ, Naik DK, et al. Surgical management of extracranial carotid artery aneurysms. *ANZ J Surg.* 2009;79:281-287.

Fankhauser GT, Stone WM, Fowl RJ, et al. Surgical and medical management of extracranial carotid artery aneurysms. *J Vasc Surg.* 2013;57:291.

Garg K, Rockman CB, Lee V, et al. Presentation and management of carotid artery aneurysms and pseudoaneurysms. *J Vasc Surg.* 2012;55:1618-1622.

Nordanstig J, Gelin J, Jensen N, et al. National experience with extracranial carotid artery aneurysms: epidemiology, surgical treatment strategy, and treatment outcome. *Ann Vasc Surg.* 2014;28:882-886.

BRACHIOCEPHALIC RECONSTRUCTION

Ali F. AbuRahma, MD, Patrick A. Stone, MD, and Zachary T. AbuRahma, DO

The most common anatomic configuration of the supra-aortic trunks (brachiocephalic vessels) off the transverse aortic arch is three separate vessels: the innominate artery (which gives rise to the right subclavian and right common carotid artery), the left common carotid artery, and the left subclavian artery. The three most common variants of the supra-aortic trunks have implications in terms of the technique that is chosen for reconstruction. These variants are a shared ostium (16%) or a common origin (bovine, 8%) for the innominate and left common carotid arteries (Figure 1), a left vertebral artery with a separate origin from the aortic arch (between the left common carotid artery and the left subclavian artery (6%; Figure 2), and a right retroesophageal subclavian artery (arising distal and posterior to the left subclavian artery, 0.5%; Figure 3). A retro-esophageal right subclavian artery is associated with a thoracic duct that drains in the right jugulo-subclavian confluence, a nonrecurrent right inferior laryngeal nerve, and, in half of these patients, a common carotid trunk giving origin to both common carotid arteries. A separate origin of the left vertebral artery is associated with an abnormally high entry of this artery (C4 or C5) into the transverse foramina of the cervical spine.

Atherosclerosis predominates as the most frequent indication for supra-aortic intervention (Figures 4 and 5). All of the nonatherosclerotic pathologies of the supra-aortic trunk—including Takayasu's arteritis; aneurysmal degeneration; aortic dissection; and complication of radiation to the head, neck, and mediastinum for varying cancers—account for less than 20% of those requiring surgical therapy.

Debranching procedures of the brachiocephalic trunks also have become an important adjunct in endovascular therapy of aortic aneurysmal disease or aortic dissections involving the transverse aortic arch or proximal descending thoracic aorta.

Occlusive disease of the origin (proximal) of the great vessels of the aortic arch rarely require intervention, compared with the number of extracranial carotid arterial procedures performed annually. Although the need for revascularization of the supra-aortic vessels is infrequent, it has been a challenging area for most surgeons. The Joint Study of Extracranial Arterial Occlusion of more than 6000 patients demonstrated that only 17% had more than 30% luminal reduction of the innominate or subclavian arteries. In addition, the indications for interventions are less clear than the indications for extracranial carotid interventions. Furthermore, the management strategy is more complex because multiple routes of revascularization, such as direct intrathoracic, reconstruction and bypass, cervical or extrathoracic bypasses, and endovascular treatment, can be used.

Surgery historically has been the treatment of choice for supra-aortic vessel disease. However, over the past 10 years, there has been a growing trend toward endovascular intervention. Therefore, with the increased use of endoluminal therapy, transposition and bypass procedures for these vessels have declined at most institutions.

■ DIAGNOSTIC EVALUATION

An evaluation of a patient with symptoms in the cerebrovascular system or upper extremities may identify pathology of the innominate, subclavian, vertebral, or proximal carotid arteries. Although cerebrovascular symptoms typically occur as a result of bifurcation disease, ostial lesions can produce identical symptoms because of both flow reduction and atheroemboli. Vertebrobasilar insufficiency may be seen with symptoms including vertigo, ataxia, binocular visual symptoms, and drop attacks. Upper extremity ischemia may manifest as absent, diminished, or asymmetric pulses in the arm and with limb fatigue with exercise or routine activities. Also, embolic complications may be seen as ulcerations or nonhealing wounds of the digits. Rarely, patients with aneurysmal disease of an aberrant right subclavian artery aneurysm may have dysphagia. History and physical examination is the backbone of diagnosing pathology of the brachiocephalic vessels. Palpation and auscultation of the carotids and evaluation of the upper extremity pulses should be performed at the initial evaluation. Inspection of the upper extremity for signs of embolic insult, including digital ulcerations and ischemic changes of the hand and digits, should be performed. Brachial artery blood pressures should be measured and compared, with a difference of more than 15 to 20 mm Hg between the two extremities considered a significant finding.

Severe stenosis or occlusion of the proximal subclavian arteries may produce reversal of flow in the ipsilateral vertebral artery, leading to the condition known as subclavian steal syndrome. Reversal of flow in the vertebral artery noted on duplex ultrasound examination of the neck is not an uncommon finding and is frequently asymptomatic. However, in the classic clinical subclavian steal, the patient will experience typical symptoms of vertebrobasilar insufficiency associated with arm exercise. Complaints of arm fatigue secondary to proximal subclavian atherosclerotic occlusive disease are uncommon because of the extensive capacity of collateral flow to the upper extremity combined with the decreased physical demands inherent in the atherosclerotic age group and therefore rarely require intervention. Patients with severe stenosis or occlusion of the left subclavian artery with internal mammary to coronary artery bypass grafts may experience angina on left arm exertion (coronary steal syndrome), which is relieved by correcting the stenotic lesion.

A complete neurologic examination also should be performed to evaluate for previous stroke. In addition, if patient history suggests vasculitis or collagen vascular disease, a comprehensive examination should include serologic testing.

Duplex examination should be the first line of investigation. With suspected carotid artery lesions, a standard evaluation of the extracranial carotid vessels should be performed. A dampened common carotid waveform with low velocities suggests proximal disease. The vertebral arteries also should be evaluated for antegrade and retrograde flow. Reversal of flow suggests high-grade subclavian or innominate disease. Transcranial Doppler also can provide additional data, leading one toward a diagnosis of disease of the supra-aortic arteries.

Computed tomographic angiography (CTA) and magnetic resonance arteriography continue to improve in their ability to diagnose supra-aortic disease, but conventional catheter arteriography continues to be used before endovascular therapy and should include arch views in both left and right obliques and four-vessel selective injections (Figure 6). In patients with concomitant coronary artery disease, these evaluations also should be performed during the workup. In addition, if arch reconstruction is planned, a combined approach will prevent a redo sternotomy.

■ INDICATIONS FOR TREATMENT

There have not been any prospective randomized trials to compare medical, endovascular, and surgical treatment modalities for supra-aortic disease. Therefore the indications for the treatment of brachiocephalic disease are not as readily defined as those for carotid bifurcation disease. Patients with classical hemispheric symptoms with corresponding lesion or lesion of the innominate or origin/proximal common carotid artery or upper extremity ischemic symptoms with subclavian artery lesions can be treated by the appropriate

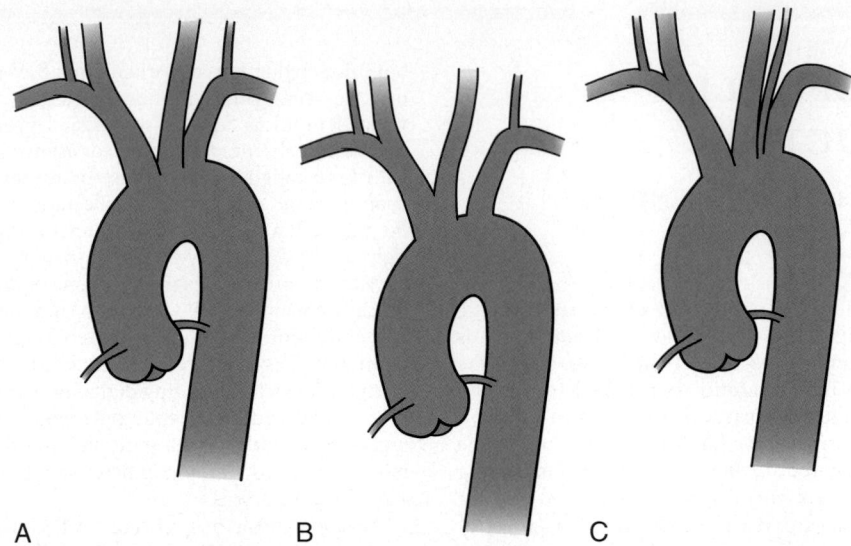

A   B   C

FIGURE 1 Normal arch (**A**), bovine arch (**B**), and arch origin (**C**) of the left vertebral artery. *(From Cronenwett JL, Johnston KW, eds.* Rutherford's Vascular Surgery. *8th ed. St Louis: Elsevier Saunders; 2014.)*

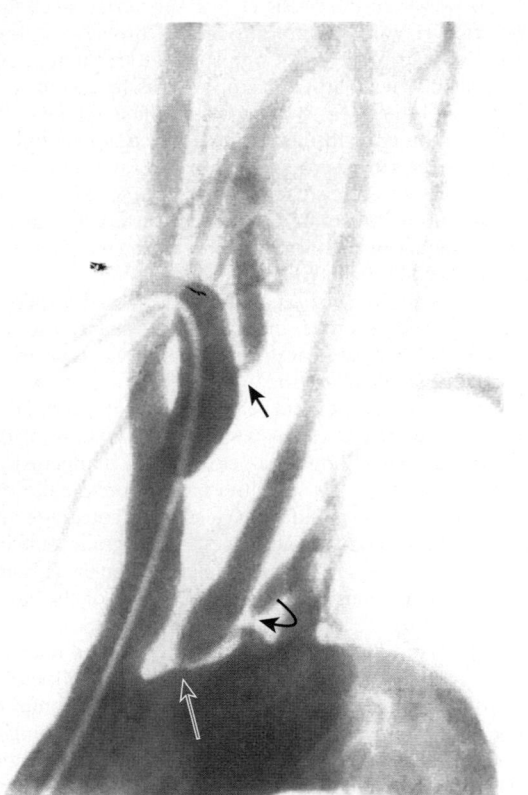

FIGURE 2 Arch aortogram showing the left vertebral artery originating from the arch of the aorta with tight stenosis at its origin (*curved arrow*) and the right vertebral artery (coming off the right subclavian artery) with a tight stenosis at the origin of the left common carotid artery (*white arrow*). *(From AbuRahma AF, Bandyk DF, eds.* Noninvasive Vascular Diagnosis: A Practical Guide to Therapy. *3rd ed. London: Springer-Verlag; 2013.)*

hypoperfusion, multivessel brachiocephalic involvement, bilateral carotid disease, or tandem lesions should be suspected and confirmed with a thorough workup. Intervention in these patients may be justified for lesions causing 75% or more stenosis or occlusion. When combined carotid bifurcation and proximal disease (severe ≥75% stenosis) is present, carotid endarterectomy and proximal repair are recommended, including carotid-subclavian transposition, bypass, or retrograde proximal stenting at the time of endarterectomy.

If atheroembolism is the suspected source in lesions involving the proximal vertebral arteries, stenosis greater than 75% should be treated. If, however, vertebrobasilar insufficiency is suspected as the source of symptoms, assessing the status of the contralateral vertebral artery is imperative, including a unilateral greater than 75% stenosis and the contralateral vertebral artery that has similar luminal narrowing or is hypoplastic or absent.

It is not uncommon for patients with diffuse atherosclerotic disease to also have subclavian artery stenosis or occlusion with associated vertebral flow reversal (i.e., subclavian steal). However, in the absence of symptoms of subclavian steal syndrome, these lesions should not be treated. Rarely, a patient with bilateral proximal subclavian artery occlusion may need transposition or carotid-subclavian bypass. This mainly would be done in order to ensure accurate measurement of central arterial pressure for hypertension management or in patients with planned coronary artery revascularization in which the internal mammary artery is to be used as a conduit.

In patients with nonatherosclerotic conditions affecting the brachiocephalic vessels, treatment should be reserved for symptomatic patients. For patients with inflammatory arteritis (Takayasu's arteritis), the acute inflammatory phase should be treated medically to quiescence, and intervention should be reserved for symptomatic stenotic lesions.

■ TECHNICAL PRINCIPLES AND TREATMENT OPTIONS

The goal of brachiocephalic reconstruction is to normalize arterial perfusion. This can be achieved by several surgical and endovascular methods, including endarterectomy, transpositions, bypasses, or endoluminal stent placement.

Brachiocephalic vessels can be reconstructed through direct routes (the chest) or indirect extra-anatomic routes (cervical incisions). Direct repairs are usually preferred in younger patients who have complex lesions (e.g., innominate artery lesions or multiple

arterial reconstruction. Treatment for asymptomatic patients is controversial at the least. For patients with proximal carotid artery disease, and not carotid bifurcation disease, treatment is recommended for lesions with luminal encroachment greater than 75%. Patients with nonlateralizing symptoms secondary to global cerebral

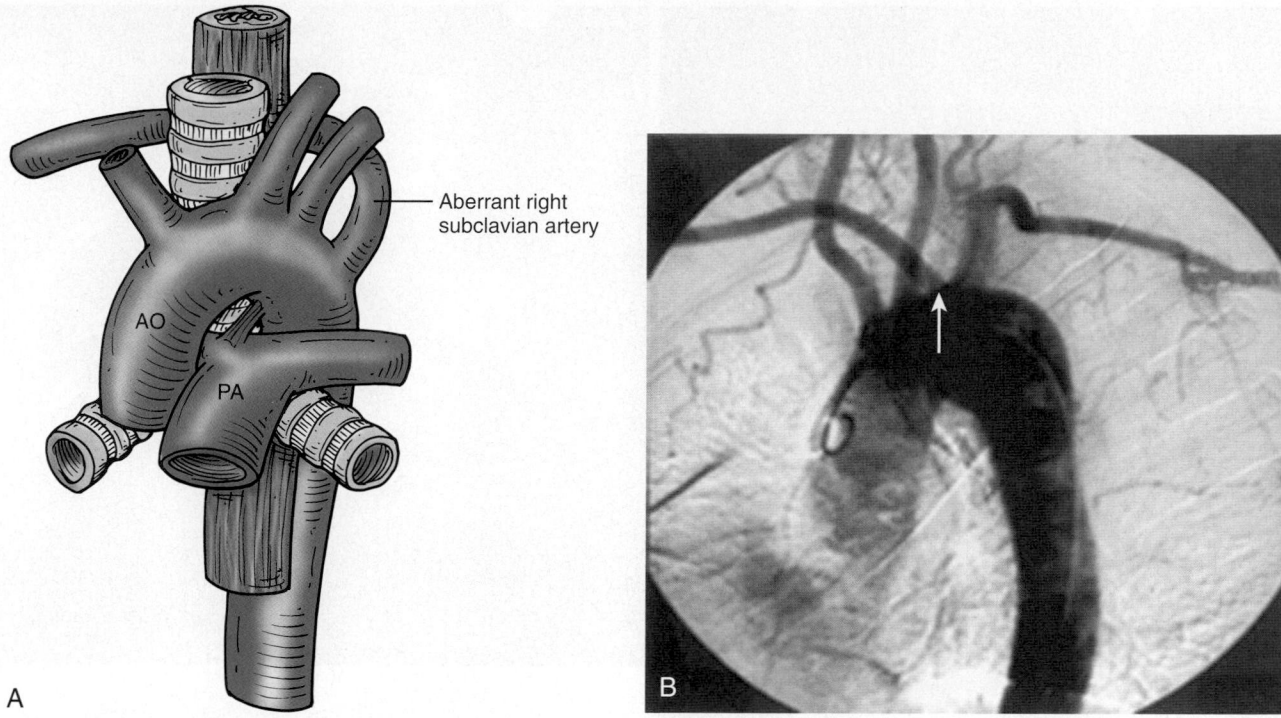

Aberrant right
subclavian artery

AO

PA

A

B

FIGURE 3 Drawing (**A**) and digital subtraction arteriogram (**B**) demonstrating the anatomic configuration of an aberrant right subclavian artery (*arrow*). *AO*, Aorta; *PA*, pulmonary artery. *(From Pearl GJ. Brachiocephalic reconstruction. In: Cameron J, Cameron A, eds.* Current Surgical Therapy. *11th ed. Philadelphia: Saunders; 2013:837-843.)*

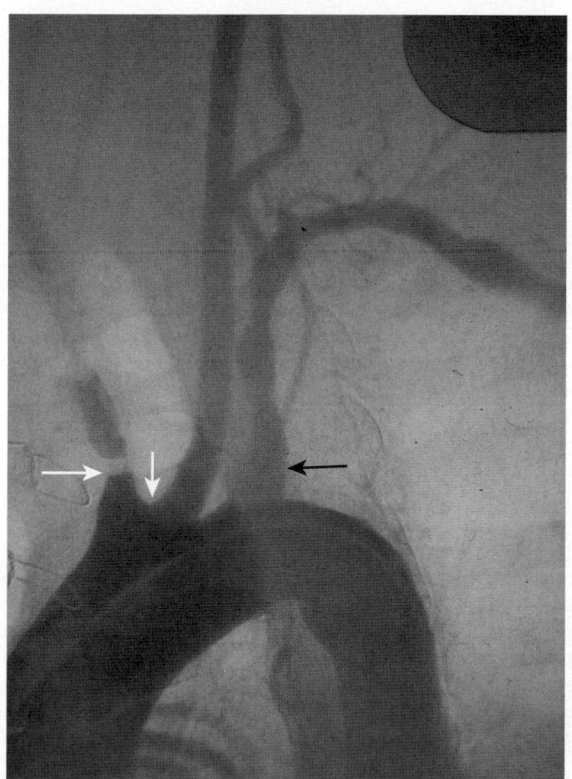

FIGURE 4 Digital subtraction angiogram showing multivessel atherosclerosis involving brachiocephalic (*white horizontal arrow*), left common carotid (*short arrow*), and left subclavian (*thin black arrow*) arteries. *(From Pearl GJ. Brachiocephalic reconstruction. In: Cameron J, Cameron A, eds.* Current Surgical Therapy. *11th ed. Philadelphia: Saunders; 2013:837-843.)*

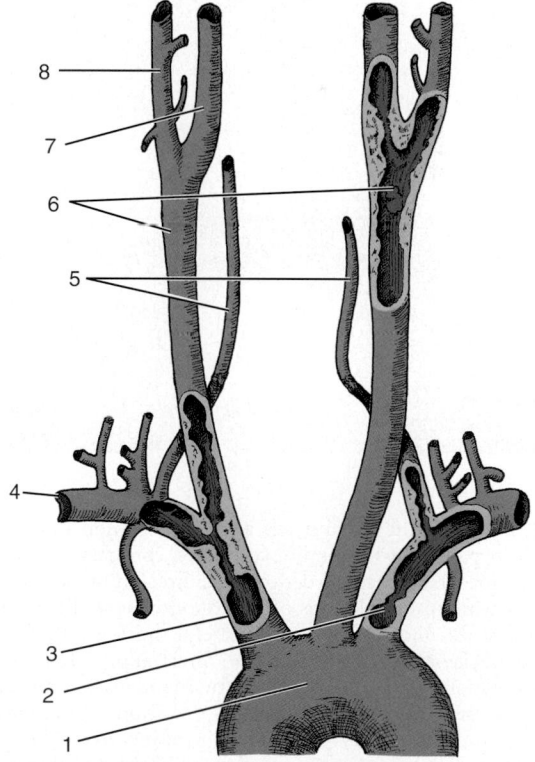

FIGURE 5 Sites of atherosclerosis of brachiocephalic vessels. (1) Aortic arch, (2) left subclavian artery, (3) innominate artery, (4) right subclavian artery, (5) right and left vertebral arteries, (6) right and left common carotid arteries, (7) right internal carotid artery, and (8) right external carotid artery. Note atherosclerosis at left subclavian, left vertebral, and innominate with proximal right common carotid and subclavian arteries and left carotid bifurcation. *(From AbuRahma AF, Bandyk DF, eds.* Noninvasive Vascular Diagnosis: A Practical Guide to Therapy. *3rd ed. London: Springer-Verlag; 2013.)*

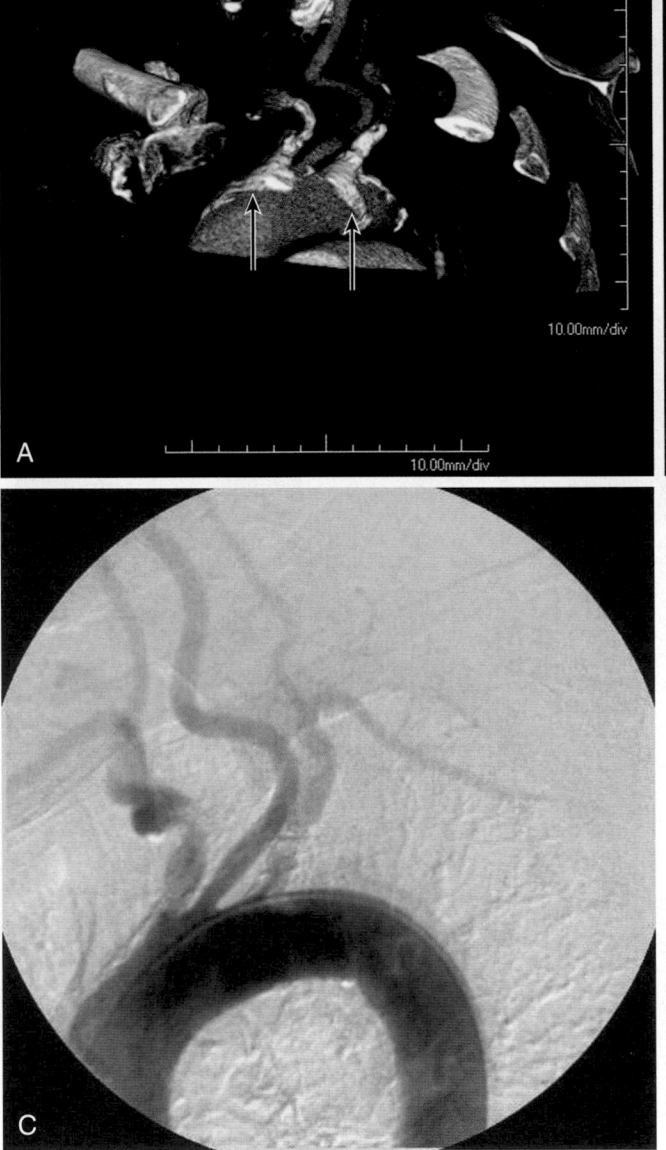

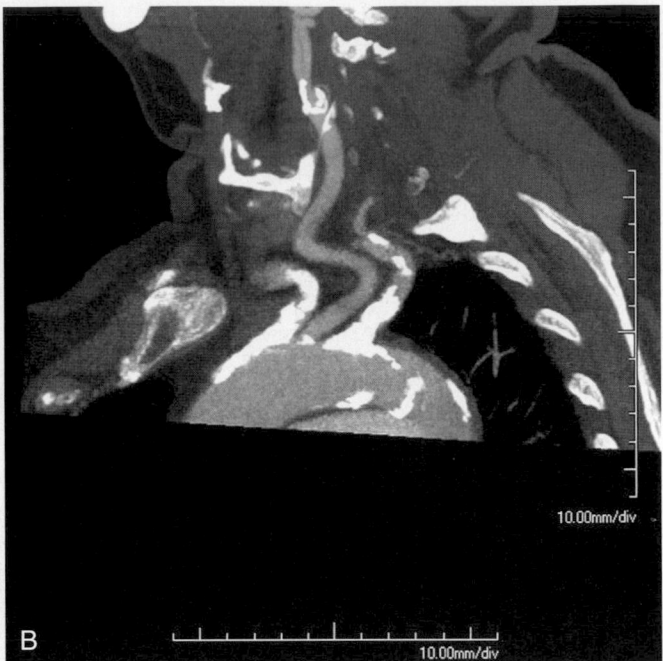

FIGURE 6 A, Computed tomographic (CT) three-dimensional surface rendering of the aortic arch showing severe calcific disease of the origins of the innominate and left subclavian arteries (*arrows*). **B,** Maximum intensity projection images of the same patient reconstructed from the CT scan. **C,** Arteriogram of the same patient. Note the extensive calcification at the origins of the innominate and proximal left subclavian arteries. *(From Cronenwett JL, Johnston KW, eds. Rutherford's Vascular Surgery. 8th ed. St Louis: Elsevier Saunders; 2014.)*

lesions, including the innominate and left common carotid arteries) and in patients who require combined coronary artery bypass and brachiocephalic reconstruction. The direct approach requires a median sternotomy for lesions of the innominate and left common carotid arteries, and a left posterior lateral thoracotomy for proximal left subclavian artery disease. The direct approach also is indicated for patients with aneurysms or traumatic disruptions of these major vessels. These direct procedures include endarterectomy of the innominate artery and bypass grafting from the ascending aorta to the innominate artery or to carotid and subclavian arteries.

Cervical repairs are usually selected in older patients who are at high risk of thoracotomy and in those who have had previous transsternal procedures or radiotherapy. They also are recommended for patients with single arterial lesions, other than in the innominate artery.

The cervical approach also is recommended in patients with severe calcific disease of the ascending aorta, where cross-clamping the aorta would be impossible or hazardous. These indirect or cervical operations can be performed through transverse supraclavicular or cervical incisions, which are easily tolerated, even in high-risk patients. Although the cervical procedures have excellent results and low morbidity and mortality rates, advances in perioperative management, including contemporary surgical and anesthetic techniques, have made direct transthoracic repair nearly as safe as cervical repairs.

Shunting during proximal repair usually is not required, unless the contralateral carotid artery has hemodynamically significant stenosis. Transcranial Doppler and cerebral oximetry or stump pressure can aid in identifying patients who are at risk for cerebral malperfusion during surgical repair.

Advances in endovascular therapy of fairly complex brachiocephalic disease have gained wider acceptance. With appropriate techniques, excellent results have been achieved with low morbidity. Endovascular principles for the treatment of proximal common carotid lesions should be similar to those widely used for bifurcation disease, including the use of a filter wire for embolic protection when approaching from the femoral artery. When using a retrograde approach with concomitant endarterectomy, the common carotid artery can be controlled during proximal endovascular treatment. Most centers use balloon-expandable stents for more accurate placement and place the proximal stent 1 to 2 mm in the aortic arch.

Innominate Artery Reconstruction

The direct transthoracic approach generally is recommended for certain innominate artery lesions, including aneurysms and traumatic disruptions or dissections, and usually is done through a full-length sternotomy. If the innominate lesion is suspected to be embolizing, as shown by grossly irregular ulcerative plaque, the distal innominate artery should be ligated or excluded at the completion of the remote bypass procedure.

Although the most widely accepted direct surgical route to either the innominate or the proximal left common carotid artery is a full median sternotomy, a minimally invasive approach for aortic branch reconstruction can be accomplished with a mini-sternotomy with inverted T transaction. In this approach, a limited skin incision of approximately 7 to 8 cm is made in the midline; the incision extends from the sternal notch to just past the angle of Louis. The manubrium and upper sternum are divided in the midline down to the third intercostal space using a narrow blade mounted on a redo sternotomy oscillating saw (Stryker, Kalamazoo, MI). The sternum is then transected transversely at the third intercostal space, creating an upside-down T incision (Figure 7, *A*). A small or pediatric sternal retractor is placed to open the upper sternum, which allows good exposure of a piece of the heart and arch vessels (Figure 7, *B*). Innominate or left common carotid artery reconstruction then can be done by either endarterectomy or bypass grafting in the usual fashion.

Endarterectomy

Endarterectomy is considered for focal lesions involving the middle portion of the proximal innominate artery. When the lesion is located at the orifice of the brachiocephalic trunk, the transverse arch is usually involved. In this setting, endarterectomy can be fraught with dangers of incomplete endarterectomy, embolization, and aortic dissection. Endarterectomy is also unsuitable for patients with disease involving a bovine arch variant because clamping of the innominate artery would cause ischemia in both cerebral hemispheres.

Extensive calcification of the ascending aorta or the aortic arch at the base of the innominate is a relative contraindication for an endarterectomy because of the risk of fracturing the plaque and producing distal embolization. It is also necessary to have space between the left common carotid artery and the innominate during clamping to prevent clamping of the left carotid artery, which may cause left cerebral ischemia.

Innominate Bypass Graft

Overall, bypass grafting is done more often than an endarterectomy of the innominate because revascularization of two or more distal arteries can be done. These grafts usually originate from the lateral aspect of the ascending aorta. A bifurcation or single limb graft can be used for the distal anastomosis made to the innominate, common carotid, or subclavian arteries. Clamping of the innominate artery usually does not require shunting for cerebral perfusion.

To avoid kinking or graft compression in the retrosternal space when the sternum is closed, proper sizing and positioning of the graft are necessary. The grafts are tunneled posterior to the innominate vein to avoid compression, which can lead to left brachiocephalic vein occlusion or postprocedure left arm swelling. When both the

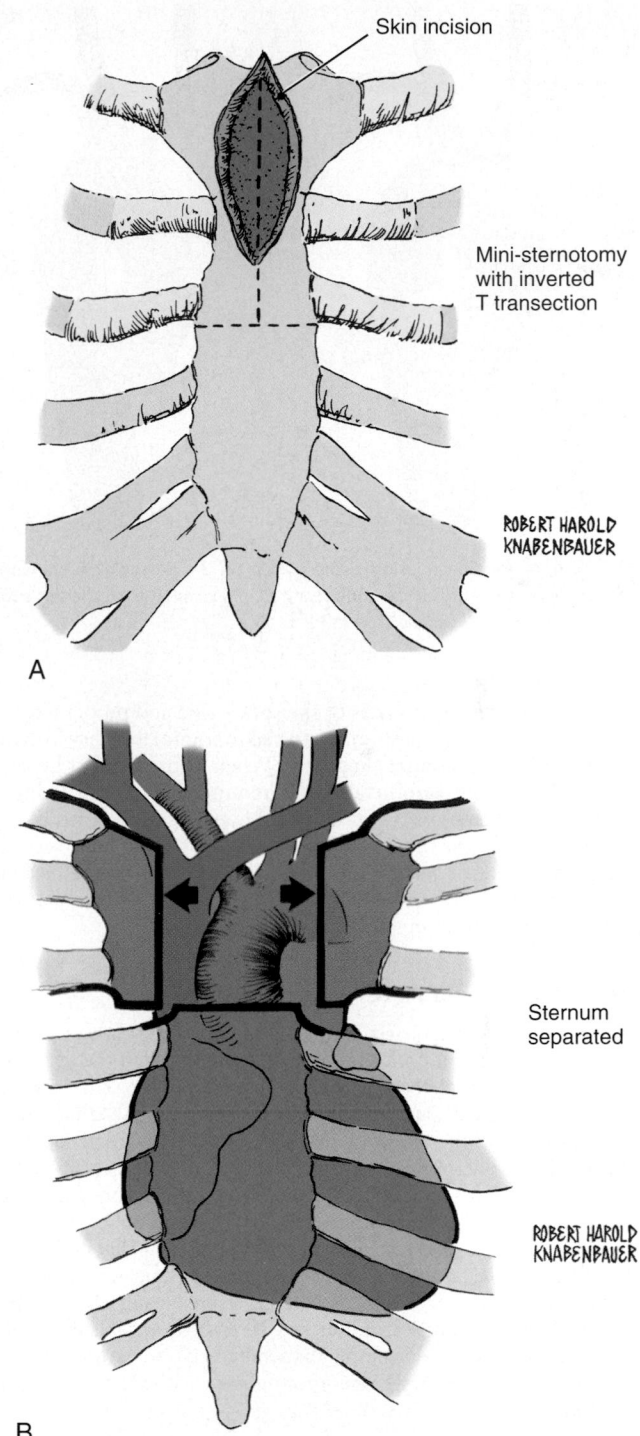

FIGURE 7 A, Artist's rendering of skin incision and mini-sternotomy sternal division. **B,** The upper sternum is divided and separated (*arrows*), exposing the ascending aorta and arch vessels. (*From Sakopoulos AG, Ballard JL, Gundry SR. Minimally invasive approach for aortic arch branch vessel reconstruction. J Vasc Surg. 2000;31:200-202.*)

innominate and the left common carotid arteries are bypassed, a bifurcated graft should be avoided because of the limited space. A partially occluding clamp is applied on the ascending aorta after systemic heparinization and a 10- to 12-mm woven Dacron tube graft is anastomosed to the ascending aorta in an end-to-side fashion with a 4-0 Prolene suture. The graft is then clamped and distended

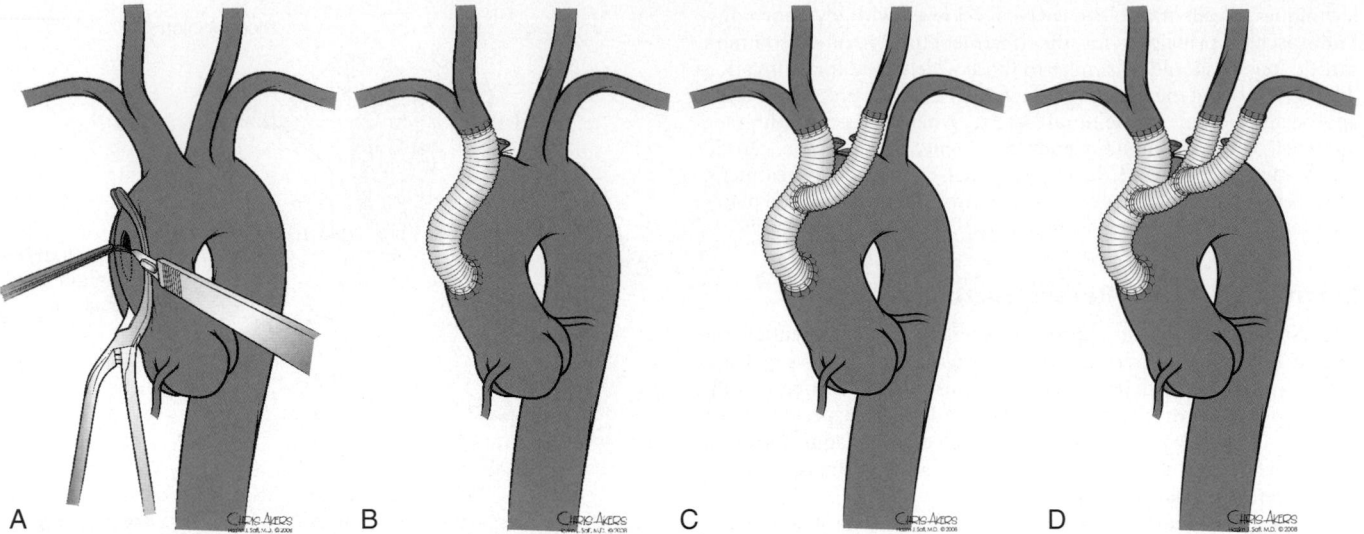

FIGURE 8 A, Partial occlusion clamp placed on the ascending aorta with creation of a punch arteriotomy. **B,** Creation of an aortoinnominate bypass. **C,** Sidearm graft to the left carotid artery. **D,** Sidearm graft to the left subclavian artery. *(From Cronenwett JL, Johnston KW, eds. Rutherford's Vascular Surgery. 8th ed. St Louis: Elsevier Saunders; 2014.)*

with blood to assess hemostasis of the suture line and proper length of the graft. The distal anastomosis to the innominate artery is then done in end-to-end fashion (Figure 8). When a concomitant bypass to the left common carotid artery is required, an 8-mm knitted Dacron graft is taken off the innominate bypass graft in an end-to-side fashion above the thoracic inlet and left brachiocephalic vein to avoid graft kinking or compression. The distal anastomosis to the left common carotid artery then may be performed in an end-to-side or end-to-end configuration with a 5-0 Prolene suture.

Common Carotid Artery Reconstruction

Stenoses of the proximal left common carotid artery are relatively common and the second most common lesions beyond the left subclavian artery. Most of these lesions are asymptomatic. They can be approached by direct transthoracic approach through a median sternotomy, similar to the innominate lesions, or preferably by indirect cervical repairs. The common carotid artery can be revascularized by means of subclavian or carotid bypass grafts, preferably from the ipsilateral side; however, the procedure also can be done from the left subclavian artery to the right carotid artery or even by left carotid to right carotid cervical arterial bypass. If the stenotic lesion of the common carotid artery is at its origin, transposing the middle portion of the common carotid artery, if healthy, to the subclavian artery may be a better alternative than subclavian to carotid bypass grafting. This requires only one anastomosis, without the need of prosthesis.

Subclavian Artery Stenosis or Occlusion

Subclavian artery reconstruction generally is indicated to correct a symptomatic subclavian steal or arm ischemia secondary to a proximal subclavian lesion, to revascularize the subclavian artery before an internal mammary to coronary artery bypass grafting, or to transpose the left subclavian artery to the left common carotid artery before extending a thoracic stent graft across its origin. This can be accomplished by carotid-subclavian bypass or carotid-subclavian transposition. If the subclavian lesion is the source of thromboembolization, the prevertebral subclavian artery must be ligated at the time of the bypass. In certain high-risk patients, axillary to axillary artery bypass can be a simple alternative. Subclavian to subclavian artery bypass also can be used for patients with symptomatic subclavian artery disease.

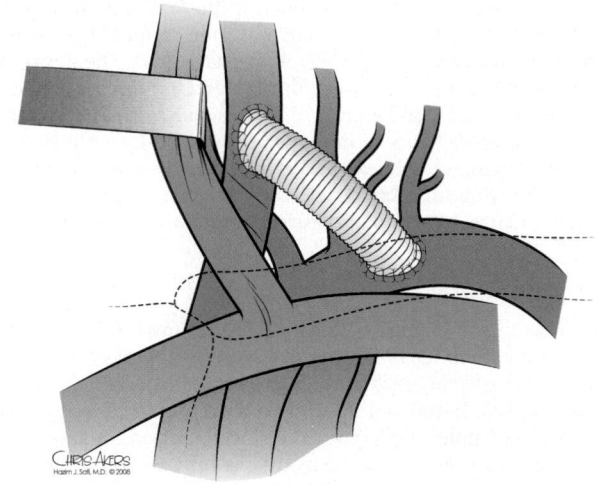

FIGURE 9 Carotid-subclavian bypass. *(From Cronenwett JL, Johnston KW, eds. Rutherford's Vascular Surgery. 8th ed. St Louis: Elsevier Saunders; 2014.)*

Brief Technical Notes on Commonly Performed Cervical Procedures

Carotid-Subclavian Bypass Grafts

A transverse supraclavicular incision is made. The subcutaneous tissue, platysma, and clavicular head of the sternocleidomastoid muscle are incised. The sternal head of the sternocleidomastoid muscle is retracted medially, and the common carotid artery is exposed and isolated. The scalenus anticus muscle is transected after isolation of the phrenic nerve. The vagus and internal jugular veins should be identified and gently retracted laterally. On the left side, great care also should be taken to avoid injury to the thoracic duct. The subclavian artery is exposed and isolated. The graft is tunneled under the internal jugular vein and sutured to the subclavian artery in end-to-side fashion. The distal end of the graft is then anastomosed end to side of the common carotid artery (Figure 9).

Prosthetic polytetrafluoroethylene (PTFE) grafts generally are preferable to autogenous vein grafts in this location and usually have

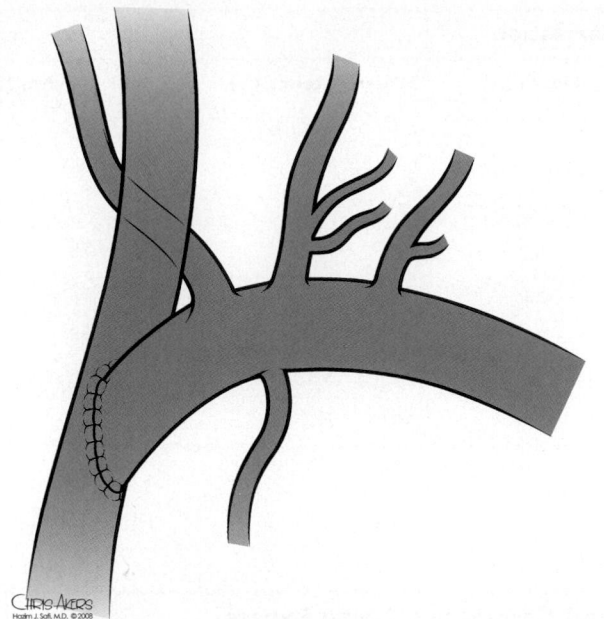

FIGURE 10 Carotid-subclavian transposition. *(From Cronenwett JL, Johnston KW, eds. Rutherford's Vascular Surgery. 8th ed. St Louis: Elsevier Saunders; 2014.)*

higher long-term patency rates. Kinking is less likely with prosthetic grafts than with autogenous vein grafts. This bypass can be combined with carotid endarterectomy, if indicated. The carotid bifurcation endarterectomy is done in the usual fashion, and the distal end of the subclavian to carotid bypass graft is fashioned to cover the arteriotomy in the form of a patch.

Carotid-Subclavian Transposition

An alternative approach to common carotid to subclavian bypass is transposition of the subclavian artery into the left common carotid artery. This technique requires more extensive mobilization of the common carotid artery and the subclavian artery (Figure 10). One major advantage of this technique is the avoidance of prosthetic grafts and the potential small risk of infection. The proximal portions of the vessels require retrosternal exposure, and particular attention must be paid to visualizing and exposing the vertebral and internal mammary arteries for transposition of the subclavian artery. The procedures are performed through a transverse supraclavicular incision. Then the dissection is carried along the anterior border or between the heads of the sternocleidomastoid muscle down to the internal jugular vein. The vagus nerve and internal jugular vein then are mobilized and gently retracted laterally, exposing the proximal common carotid artery. Then the vertebral vein is identified and ligated, and the subclavian artery is exposed and carefully dissected proximal to the takeoff of the vertebral and internal mammary arteries. During the subclavian to carotid transposition, the proximal subclavian artery is clamped, transected, and carefully sutured. Control of the proximal stump is crucial because the stump is placed with tension to facilitate exposure in the upper mediastinum, and loss of the stump into the thoracic cavity before suture ligation would be disastrous. Then the common carotid artery is cross-clamped proximally and distally, and the subclavian artery is transposed and sewn in an end-to-side fashion with 6-0 Prolene suture. During the transposition, special care must be taken to avoid kinking of the vertebral artery.

Subclavian-Subclavian Artery Bypass

This technique is rarely done, but it can be considered for patients with an innominate lesion who may be at high risk for other repairs. The incision is supraclavicular on both sides, and the second, or rarely the third, portion of the subclavian artery is exposed in a manner similar to that described earlier. The graft is placed behind the sternocleidomastoid muscle and as low as possible.

Axillary to Axillary Artery Bypass Grafting

Two transverse incisions are made over the deltopectoral grooves. The incision is deepened to expose the axillary artery, axillary vein, and brachial plexus. The second portion of the axillary artery is isolated. An 8-mm Gore-Tex graft is sutured in place in end-to-side fashion. The graft is placed underneath the pectoralis major and then through a tunnel made in the presternal subcutaneous tissue to the contralateral axilla. The contralateral end of the graft also is placed under the pectoralis major. The distal end of the graft is then sutured to the other axillary artery in end-to-side fashion.

Carotid to Carotid Artery Bypass

In this technique, one carotid artery is used to revascularize the contralateral carotid artery, whose origin is in the mediastinum or which is severely diseased proximally. The common carotid artery is exposed in the usual fashion bilaterally. The bypass usually lies low in the midline, partially hidden by the upper edge of the manubrium. The bypass can be tunneled across the neck through the retropharyngeal space, which is a shorter and straighter path. A nasopharyngeal tube or temperature probe can facilitate palpation of the pharynx, ensure dissection in the proper plane, and avoid skin erosion and the feeling of strangulation that sometimes occur with subcutaneous tunneling of grafts in the anterior neck. When these grafts are tunneled anteriorly, they can present a cosmetic issue in a patient with a very slender neck.

■ CLINICAL EXPERIENCE AND RESULTS OF BRACHIOCEPHALIC RECONSTRUCTION (OPEN REPAIR)

Several studies have reported very satisfactory outcomes for various brachiocephalic reconstruction procedures. Tables 1 through 3 summarize the results of various methods of brachiocephalic reconstruction (open repair). Berguer and colleagues reported on one of the largest series in which they analyzed their experience of 282 cases (182 cervical repairs and 100 transthoracic repairs) involving supra-aortic trunk reconstruction from 1982 to 1998. The most frequent indication for cervical repair in the authors' practice was single trunk disease (carotid or subclavian artery) or history of myocardial revascularization. All innominate artery lesions were approached through a direct chest incision. The authors reported a 3.8% incidence of transient ischemic attack (TIA) or stroke and a 0.5% death rate for patients with cervical repairs, in contrast to an 8% incidence of TIA or stroke and an 8% death rate for those with thoracic repairs.

Takach and colleagues reported on the results of a large series of brachiocephalic reconstruction, operative versus endovascular management of single-vessel disease. Their study included 391 consecutive patients with single-vessel brachiocephalic disease that were treated with either operative bypass (group A; n = 229) or percutaneous transluminal angioplasty (PTA)/stenting (group B; n = 162). All patients were asymptomatic after surgery or endovascular intervention. Both groups had similar operative mortality (0.9% vs 0%) and stroke rates (1.3% vs 0%). However, 5 years after the procedure, group A had significantly better freedom from graft or intervention failure (92.7% ± 2.1%) than did group B (83.9% ± 3.7%; $P = 0.03$). The authors reported that endovascular intervention involved less initial cost (mean savings of $8787 per procedure), was less invasive, and did not necessitate general anesthesia. They concluded that both operative bypass and endovascular intervention for single-vessel brachiocephalic disease were associated with acceptably low operative morbidity and mortality. However, operative bypass had significantly better midterm freedom from graft or intervention failure than endovascular intervention and had excellent long-term freedom from failure. Meanwhile, endovascular intervention had

TABLE 1: Results of Open Repair: Transthoracic Revascularization

Author/Year	No. of Patients	Stroke (%)	MI (%)	Death (%)	5-Year Patency (%)	5-Year Survival (%)
Crawford et al./1962	67	2.9	NA	7.5	NA	NA
Crawford et al./1969	122	NA	NA	13.0 (11.0)*	NA	NA
Crawford et al./1983	43	6.9	NA	4.7	NA	NA
Kieffer et al./1995	135	2.9	1.5	5.2	98	78
Berguer et al./1998	100	8.0**	3.0	8.0	94	87
Rhodes et al./2000	92	7.0	3.0	3.0	80	88
Sigala et al./2015	16	6.0	NA	0	NA	NA
All series combined	575	5.6	2.5	6.6	91	84

*11% for bypasses alone.

**Transient ischemic attack (TIA) or stroke.

MI, Myocardial infarction; NA, not/applicable.

TABLE 2: Results of Open Repair: Extrathoracic or Cervical Carotid-Subclavian Bypass

Author/Year	No. of Patients	Stroke (%)	MI (%)	Death (%)	5-Year Patency (%)	5-Year Survival (%)
Diethrich et al./1967	125	1.6	2.4	4.8	NA	NA
Crawford et al./1969	177	NA	NA	2.2	NA	NA
Perler et al./1990	28	NA	NA	0	92	88
Salam et al./1994	28	0	0	0	82	NA
Vitti et al./1994	124	NA	NA	0.8	95	83
Law et al./1995	51	2.0	0	0	88	100
AbuRahma et al./2000	51	0	2.0	0	96	86
Cinar et al./2004	66	1.5	NA	1.5	83	93
Takach et al./2011	287	2.1	NA	1.0	94	88
Sigala et al./2015	91	NA	NA	0	95	75
All series combined	1028	1.2	2.2	1.0	90	88

MI, Myocardial infarction; NA, not applicable.

tangible benefits regarding cost, level of invasiveness, and subjective patient satisfaction.

Takach and colleagues also reported on their experience of brachiocephalic reconstruction, operative and long-term results for complex disease. One hundred and fifty-seven consecutive patients with innominate artery or multivessel brachiocephalic disease underwent operative reconstruction using either a transthoracic approach (group A, n = 113) or a less invasive extrathoracic approach (group B, n = 44). Reconstruction required multiple distal anastomoses in 70 patients (45%), concomitant coronary artery bypass grafting (CABG) in 36 patients (24%), and concomitant carotid endarterectomy in 26 patients (17%). They found no significant differences between both groups in operative mortality (2.7% vs 2.3%) and stroke rates (2.7% vs 6.8%). However, 10 years after surgery, freedom from graft failure was significantly better in group A (94.4% ± 4.4%) than in group B (60.3% ± 13.4%, P = 0.002). They concluded that transthoracic arch reconstruction for complex brachiocephalic disease can be done with acceptably low morbidity and mortality similar to those of a less invasive extrathoracic approach. Furthermore, the transthoracic approach was associated with significantly better long-term freedom from graft failure, possibly because it preserves aortic inflow to the great vessels.

More recently, Takach and colleagues reported on their experience with 287 patients with carotid-subclavian bypass over 5 decades, with an operative mortality of 1% and a total stroke rate of 2% (ipsilateral 1% and contralateral 0.7%). They reported primary patency rates at 5, 10, and 15 years of 94%, 89%, and 87%, respectively, and concluded that carotid-subclavian bypass had excellent long-term patency and provided extended symptom relief with low operative morbidity and mortality rates. The durability of these grafts may offer extended symptom relief in younger patients and survival advantage associated with preservation of the internal mammary artery in patients at risk for myocardial revascularization.

Sigala and colleagues reported on their experience with 107 patients: 81 patients operated on for subclavian lesions, 14 operated on for innominate lesions, and 12 operated on for common carotid lesions. The patients underwent either extrathoracic reconstruction (91 patients) or transthoracic reconstruction (16 patients). The authors reported a 0% perioperative mortality rate and a 17% morbidity rate with cumulative primary patency rates of 95% at 5 years and 91% at 10 years, with no difference between transthoracic and extrathoracic reconstructions (P = 0.278).

We reported on our 20-year experience with carotid-subclavian bypass procedures in 51 patients (40 occlusions and 11 stenoses)

TABLE 3: Results of Open Repair: Extrathoracic or Cervical Carotid-Subclavian Transposition, Carotid-Carotid Bypass, and Axilloaxillary Bypass

Author/Year	No. of Patients	Stroke (%)	MI (%)	Death (%)	5-Year Patency (%)	5-Year Survival (%)
CAROTID-SUBCLAVIAN TRANSPOSITION						
Edwards et al./1994	178	1.0	0	2.2	NA	NA
Schardey et al./1996	108	0	1.0	0	100	83
Cina et al./2002	27	0	0	0	NA	NA
All series combined	313	0.3	0.3	0.7	100	83
CAROTID-CAROTID BYPASS						
Berguer et al./1994	16	6.2	0	0	94	88
Ozsvath et al./2003	24	4.1	0	0	70	NA
All series combined	40	5.2	0	0	82	–
AXILLOAXILLARY BYPASS						
AbuRahma et al./1992	31	0	0	3.0	NA	NA
Chang et al./1997	39	0	0	0	NA	NA
Mingoli et al./1999	61	0	0	1.6	90	NA
All series combined	131	0	0	1.5	90	87

MI, Myocardial infarction; *NA*, not applicable.

using PTFE grafts for symptomatic subclavian artery stenosis or occlusion, with a mean follow-up of 7.7 years. The 30-day morbidity rate was 6%, with no perioperative stroke or mortality. Immediate relief of symptoms was achieved in 100% of patients; however, four patients (8%) had late recurrent symptoms. The primary patency and secondary patency rates at 1, 3, 5, and 10 years were 100%, 98%, 96%, and 92% and 100%, 98%, 98%, and 95%, respectively. The symptom-free survival rates at 1, 3, 5, and 10 years were 100%, 96%, 82%, and 47%, respectively. The overall survival rates at 1, 3, 5, and 10 years were 100%, 98%, 86%, and 57%, respectively. We concluded that carotid-subclavian bypass using PTFE grafts for subclavian artery disease is safe, effective, and durable and should remain the procedure of choice, particularly in good-risk patients.

ENDOVASCULAR TREATMENT

In contrast to excellent reported results with open surgical revascularization in the setting of brachiocephalic disease by either direct reconstructions or indirect revascularization routes, endovascular intervention for this vascular bed has not been studied as thoroughly or evaluated for long-term durability. Despite the lack of solid data, pursuit of minimally invasive procedures to treat brachiocephalic disease has been inevitable. Early reports of endovascular intervention in the arch vessels consisted mainly of lesions treated with angioplasty alone, and follow-up was limited. These studies revealed that endovascular intervention was feasible, and, as expected, use of endovascular techniques has increased with improvements in balloon and stent technology and maturation of technical skills in the treatment of cerebrovascular disease. In skilled hands, excellent technical success rates of approximately 95% and 5-year patency rates exceeding 80% have been achieved. A major limitation of examining patency is the location of these interventions within the thoracic cavity and outside direct insonation by duplex imaging in most cases. In addition, in comparison with surgical revascularization, many interventions are performed in the setting of stenosis and not complete occlusion, which likely could affect a direct comparison of these two techniques. Also of note, most methods using endovascular techniques do not alter the intended surgical reconstruction, making an endovascular attempt as initial revascularization appealing.

Anatomic considerations are important in the planning of any treatment of brachiocephalic disease but especially if endovascular therapy is being considered. The anatomic characteristics of the lesions to be treated are imperative to determine in the assessment for feasibility of management with catheter-based tools. Endovascular intervention is preferable for stenosis rather than total occlusion and for nonostial, nonulcerative, and minimally calcified concentric lesions. Endovascular treatment is less favorable for severely eccentric lesions and lesions that extend contiguous to or into a major branch vessel, such as the vertebral artery when treating subclavian artery pathology, the left common carotid artery arising off the innominate artery in the bovine configuration, or minimal separation of the origins of the innominate and left common carotid artery off the aortic arch. These anatomic configurations carry the added risk of compromising the origin of an adjacent artery in the treatment of another. In addition, aortic arch degenerative disease poses increased risk of embolization with catheter manipulation and increasing great vessel angulation from the aortic arch (i.e., type 3 aortic arches).

INNOMINATE ARTERY ENDOVASCULAR INTERVENTIONS

Endovascular treatment of innominate lesions exposes the patient to potential embolization to both the right carotid and the right vertebral artery distributions and therefore must be performed with great precision and caution. Accurate localization of the origins of the right common carotid and right subclavian artery branches in relation to the disease process is imperative. A right anterior oblique imaging pattern typically is needed to appropriately identify the takeoff of the right common carotid and subclavian arteries. A kissing balloon technique is necessary to treat innominate lesions that extend directly proximate to or into the primary branches to ensure that the origin of the left common carotid is not compromised by angioplasty and stenting of a proximately calcific lesion of the innominate artery (Figures 11 and 12).

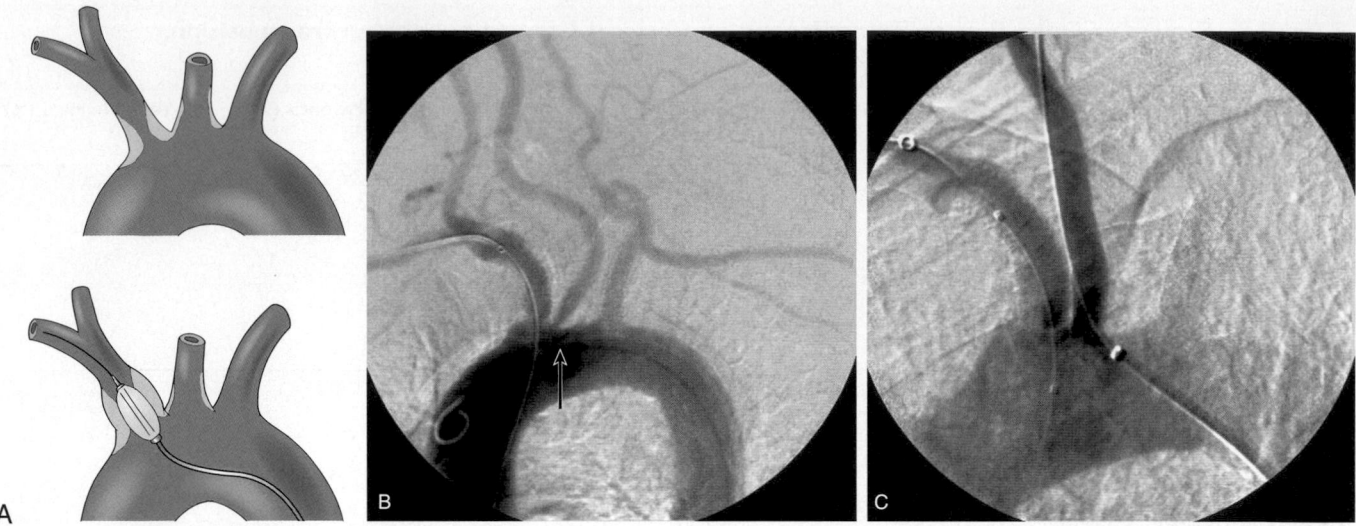

FIGURE 11 A, Treatment of a neighboring arch vessel can force treatment of an adjacent arch branch. After treatment of the innominate artery, the left common carotid can be impinged on by a shift of aortic plaque, thus necessitating intervention in the left common carotid origin. **B,** A successfully treated innominate artery has shifted aortic plaque, which resulted in stenosis at the origin of the left common carotid artery (*arrow*). **C,** Treatment of the common carotid origin and simultaneous protection of the innominate artery's stented origin. *(From Cronenwett JL, Johnston KW, eds. Rutherford's Vascular Surgery. 8th ed. St Louis: Elsevier Saunders; 2014.)*

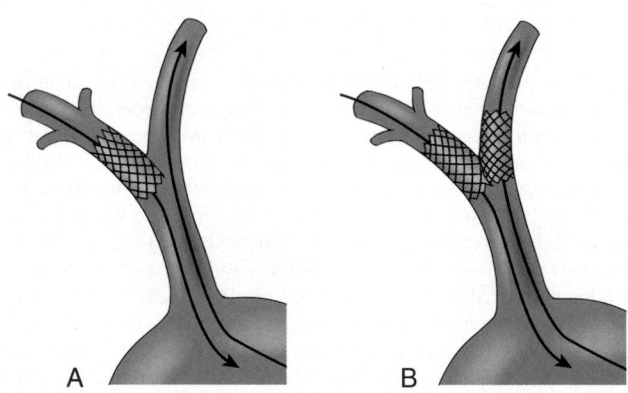

FIGURE 12 A, Treatment of the right subclavian artery origin can result in "jailing" the origin of the right common carotid artery, by the proximal end of the stent projecting into the common carotid lumen, as shown. **B,** Treatment of the innominate artery branch origins with a kissing balloon stent technique to preserve both origins. *(From Cronenwett JL, Johnston KW, eds. Rutherford's Vascular Surgery. 8th ed. St Louis: Elsevier Saunders; 2014.)*

The innominate artery has the most challenging angulation extending off the aortic arch for cannulation through an antegrade transfemoral approach. Prolonged attempts at cannulation should not be pursued from this approach because of the risk of trauma and consequent embolization from the associated atherosclerotic disease in the aorta. In this situation, a retrograde brachial access may be performed and safe traversal of the innominate lesion accomplished. The innominate lesion then may be treated over the wire placed from the retrograde brachial approach, or the retrograde brachial wire can be snared from below and brought down with a through-and-through technique for greater stability for passage of the sheath angioplasty system.

For ostial lesions, 1 to 2 mm of the stent should protrude into the aortic lumen. If the angioplasty and stent are being performed through the retrograde right brachial approach, it may be difficult to inject adequate contrast to visualize the exact position of the innominate orifice relative to the aortic arch. It is helpful to have an angiographic pigtail in place for arteriography and facilitation of better imaging. The transfemoral guidewire or angiographic catheter itself can act as a marker around the greater curvature of the aortic arch abutting the innominate orifice. With the brachial approach, the guidewire should be directed into the ascending aorta rather than into the descending thoracic aorta because this facilitates deployment of the stent.

The risk of embolization with primary angioplasty and stenting of innominate lesions appears to be low, and therefore the requirement for cerebral protection in these procedures remains unclear. In most instances, the simplest, most straightforward approach without protection is best unless a "high-risk" lesion with a worrisome potential for embolization is to be treated. Some small series have advocated dual embolic protection of the vertebral and common carotid arteries during innominate stenting, but the risk versus benefit of this more advanced technique has not been studied enough to be routinely advocated.

■ LEFT COMMON CAROTID ARTERY ENDOVASCULAR INTERVENTION

Endovascular treatment of left common carotid artery lesions at the level of the aortic arch is feasible and safe and may be performed using an antegrade transfemoral approach similar to that described for the innominate artery intervention. In the situation of an angulated takeoff of the left common carotid artery from the arch and when better stability of the angioplasty system is required, a "buddy wire" may be positioned in the external carotid artery to facilitate maintenance of the guidewire and sheath position at the origin of the vessel, as is done in the treatment of more distal carotid disease (Figure 13). A protection device (see Figure 13) frequently is used with the antegrade transfemoral approach for endovascular interventions on "high-risk" lesions and requires either two 0.014-inch wires or one 0.014-inch and one 0.018-inch wire to provide smooth transition of 0.035-inch balloon-expandable stents that are best suited for ostial calcified lesions. In addition, the use of a guide catheter in the aorta (not crossing the lesion) potentially reduces distal embolization.

Again, when transfemoral access to the origin of the vessel proves difficult, a retrograde approach from the distal common carotid artery may be performed, particularly in situations where a concomitant ipsilateral carotid endarterectomy is to be performed. The carotid branches are thus readily controlled with application of a distal clamp protection.

Transfemoral-based access for treatment of ostial common carotid lesions is associated with low perioperative neurologic events and satisfactory patency. Paukovits and colleagues reported ipsilateral neurologic events in less than 3% of patients and primary patency and secondary patency of 82% and 88%, respectively, even in a large series of 147 patients with less than 10% use of embolic protection.

A meta-analysis of 13 studies by Sfyroeras and colleagues, including 133 patients using combined retrograde angioplasty alone or angioplasty/stenting with concomitant carotid endarterectomy, reported less than 2% perioperative neurologic events and less than 10% 3-year significant restenosis of the common carotid lesion, with the majority of restenosis occurring in those treated with plain old balloon angioplasty (POBA).

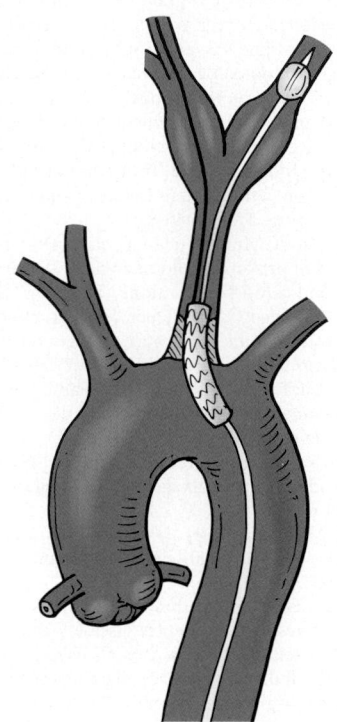

FIGURE 13 Use of a "buddy wire" into the external carotid artery to stabilize the guide at the origin of the carotid artery. *(From Cronenwett JL, Johnson JW, eds.* Rutherford's Vascular Surgery, *8th ed. St. Louis: Elsevier Saunders, 2014, pg 1635.)*

◼ LEFT SUBCLAVIAN ARTERY ENDOVASCULAR INTERVENTION

The left subclavian artery ostium is the most frequently treated of the proximal great vessels.

Antegrade transfemoral access to the left subclavian artery off the arch is the easiest of the three arch vessels. After accessing the origin of the vessel, a 0.035-inch guidewire is passed across the lesion into the distal subclavian artery. The guidewire then may be exchanged for a stiffer wire if this is deemed necessary. A long 6F or 7F sheath is then positioned just across the origin of the vessel at the level of disease. Predilation with a 4-mm angioplasty balloon may be necessary to facilitate crossing the lesion with a balloon-mounted stent. After angioplasty the sheath should be advanced with the dilator past the lesion (Figure 14). The balloon-expandable stent then should be positioned across the lesion and the sheath withdrawn to avoid the hazard of the lesion stripping the stent off the balloon. A guidewire also can be placed in the aorta, not crossing the lesion, and then after predilation advanced across the lesion as the predilation balloon is deflated. Correct sizing of the stent is essential to ensure that the area of disease is treated completely and that the vertebral artery origin is not entrapped or compromised. For ostial lesions, the stent should extend 1 to 2 mm into the aortic lumen to assure adequate treatment of the ostium. However, too much extension into the aorta may lead to future issues when catheter manipulations are required (i.e., coronary angiography).

If the subclavian lesion approaches the origin of the vertebral artery, it may be important to protect the vertebral artery origin. This may be accomplished after placement of a larger sheath into the origin of the subclavian artery and exchange of the 0.035-inch guidewire for two separate 0.014-inch wires, one placed antegrade out into the axillary artery and the other placed antegrade in the vertebral artery. A balloon-expandable stent may be placed accurately over both 0.014-inch wires immediately at the takeoff of the vertebral

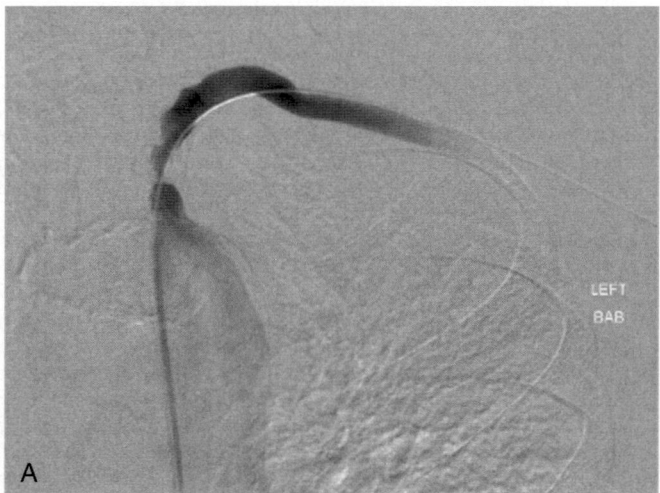

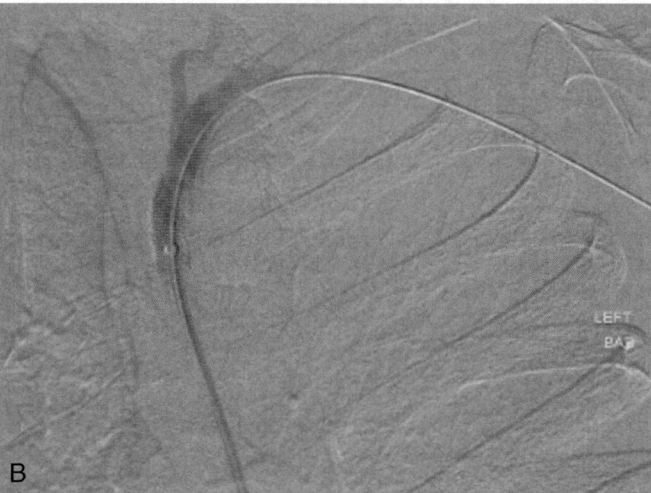

FIGURE 14 A, Proximal subclavian artery stenosis before treatment. **B,** Selective left subclavian angiogram: sheath advanced to lesion. *(From Stanley JC, Veith FJ, Wakefield TW, eds.* Current Therapy in Vascular and Endovascular Surgery. *5th ed. Philadelphia: Elsevier Saunders; 2014.)*

artery. In another approach in which both antegrade transfemoral access and retrograde brachial access into the subclavian artery are obtained, the 0.014-inch wire is placed through the retrograde transbrachial sheath into the vertebral artery, and the angioplasty and stenting are performed across the 0.035-inch guidewire from the antegrade transfemoral approach. The retrograde transbrachial or radial access can facilitate the imaging of the vertebral artery at the time of the intervention. Embolic protection of the vertebral artery has been described, but its routine use cannot be advocated because of the exceedingly low risk (<1%) of emboli to the vertebral basilar system during subclavian artery intervention, as well as the risk of dissection of the vertebral artery with instrumentation. Again, for emphasis, the simplest, most straightforward approach with the least amount of guidewire and catheter manipulation is generally best.

Soga and colleagues reported on the perioperative and long-term outcomes of endovascular treatment for subclavian artery disease from a large multicenter registry. Perioperative events are rare, with risk of combined neurologic events being less than 2%, including less than 1% ipsilateral posterior circulation neurologic events. Longer procedure times (114 min vs 70 min) and need for blood transfusions were associated with increased risk of perioperative stroke. A large multicenter registry of more than 500 patients reported primary patency of approximately 80% and secondary patency of 98% at 5 years. Multivariate analysis revealed lesion length by 1-cm increments, current smoking, cerebrovascular disease, and critical hand ischemia as negative independent predictors of patency, whereas the use of intravascular ultrasound showed a positive predictor of patency. In this large registry, stenosis compared with occlusions was comparable in terms of patency.

Our group also compared carotid-subclavian bypass with primary stenting for isolated subclavian artery disease in 121 patients treated with endovascular techniques and 51 patients with carotid-subclavian prosthetic bypass grafts. The early 30-day primary patency rate was 100% for the bypass group and 99% for the PTA and stent group. The 5-year patency rate was 96% for the carotid-subclavian bypass graft and 70% for PTA and stenting (*P* <0.0001). Major complications in the surgical patients were limited to two phrenic nerve injuries that recovered over a 2-month period and one nonfatal myocardial infarction. In comparison, complications in the endovascular group included two embolic complications and one death after coronary artery bypass grafting within 30 days of the stenting procedure. There was no significant difference in survival between both groups at 3 and 5 years.

SUGGESTED READINGS

AbuRahma AF, Bates MC, Stone PA, et al. Angioplasty and stenting versus carotid-subclavian bypass for the treatment of isolated subclavian artery disease. *J Endovasc Ther.* 2007;14:698-704.

AbuRahma AF, Robinson PA, Jennings TG. Carotid-subclavian bypass grafting with polytetrafluoroethylene grafts for symptomatic subclavian artery stenosis or occlusion: a 20-year experience. *J Vasc Surg.* 2000;32:411-419.

Bates MC, Broce M, Lavigne PS, et al. Subclavian artery stenting: factors influencing long-term outcome. *Catheter Cardiovasc Interv.* 2004;61:5-11.

Berguer R, Morasch MD, Kline RA. Transthoracic repair of innominate and common carotid artery disease: immediate and long-term outcome for 100 consecutive surgical reconstructions. *J Vasc Surg.* 1998;27:34-41.

Paukovits TM, Haasz J, Molnar A, et al. Transfemoral endovascular treatment of proximal common carotid artery lesions: a single center experience of 153 lesions. *J Vasc Surg.* 2008;48:80-87.

Sfyroeras GS, Karathanos C, Antoniou GA, et al. A meta-analysis of combined endarterectomy and proximal balloon angioplasty for tandem disease of the arch vessels and carotid bifurcation. *J Vasc Surg.* 2011;54:534-540.

Sigala F, Galyfos G, Coutelle AG, et al. Open reconstructions for symptomatic atherosclerotic lesions of the supra-aortic vessels: thirty years results from two university hospitals. *Ann Vasc Surg.* 2015;29:404-410.

Soga Y, Tomoi Y, Fujijara M, et al. Perioperative and long-term outcomes of endovascular treatment for subclavian artery disease from a large multicenter registry. *J Endovasc Ther.* 2015;22:626-633.

Takach TJ, Duncan JM, Livesay JJ, et al. Brachiocephalic reconstruction II: operative and endovascular management of single-vessel disease. *J Vasc Surg.* 2005;42:55-61.

Takach TJ, Duncan M, Livesay JJ, et al. Contemporary relevancy of carotid-subclavian bypass defined by an experience spanning five decades. *Ann Vasc Surg.* 2011;25:895-901.

Takach TJ, Reul GJ, Cooley DA, et al. Brachiocephalic reconstruction I: operative and long-term results for complex disease. *J Vasc Surg.* 2005;42:47-54.

van de Weijer AK, Vonken EJ, de Vries JP, et al. Technical and clinical success and long-term durability of endovascular treatment for atherosclerotic aortic arch branch origin obstruction: evaluation of 144 procedures. *Eur J Vasc Endovasc Surg.* 2015;50:13-20.

UPPER EXTREMITY ARTERIAL OCCLUSIVE DISEASE

Mitchell R. Weaver, MD, and Alexander D. Shepard, MD

Symptomatic arterial occlusive disease of the upper extremity (UE) is seen by the vascular surgeon significantly less frequently than its lower extremity counterpart. Extensive collateral networks around the shoulder, elbow, and wrist, along with the lack of heavy load repetitive use activities of the UE compared with the lower extremity, allow many patients to remain asymptomatic despite significant occlusive lesions. However, when ischemic symptoms of the hands and digits do manifest, the loss of function can lead to significant disability and limitation. Although atherosclerosis is the most common cause of clinically significant arterial ischemia of the UE, many cases of UE ischemia are caused by nonatherosclerotic disease states. These factors make the diagnosis and treatment of UE ischemia more complex than the management of lower extremity ischemia.

ETIOLOGY

A wide variety of disease states may lead to UE ischemia. Box 1 offers a broad, conceptual categorization that is far from exhaustive. The most common cause of symptomatic UE ischemia is vasospasm involving the digital vessels, but this is rarely severe and is almost always managed medically (see chapter on Raynaud's phenomenon). Large artery vasospasm is rare but can be caused by ergot poisoning, most often from migraine medications containing ergotamine (Figure 1).

Intrinsic Arterial Disease

Atherosclerosis of the UE vasculature is usually limited to the more proximal brachiocephalic arteries. The origin of the left subclavian artery is the most frequently involved segment. Prior radiation exposure may accelerate this process. Atherosclerosis involving the distal extremity vasculature is seen most often in patients with end-stage renal disease, of which a particularly virulent form, azotemic arteriopathy, frequently leads to critical limb ischemia and is associated with a poorer prognosis.

A number of inflammatory diseases also can affect the upper extremity arteries. Takayasu's disease and giant cell arteritis (GCA)

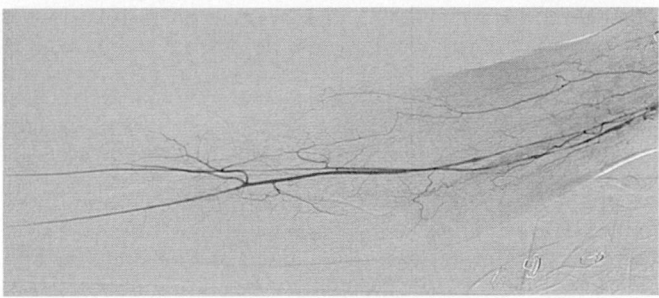

FIGURE 1 Right upper extremity angiogram demonstrating severe brachial artery vasospasm in a 65-year-old woman taking an ergotamine-containing medication for treatment of migraine headaches.

BOX 1: Causes of Upper Extremity Ischemia

Vasospasm

Raynaud's phenomenon (palmar digital)
Drug induced: ergotomines, beta-blockers, vasopressors

Intrinsic Arterial Disease

Atherosclerosis (innominate-subclavian)
Radiation arteritis (innominate-axillosubclavian)
Azotemic arteriopathy (radial/ulnar, palmar, digital)

Inflammatory Diseases

Connective tissue disorders (palmar digital)
Hypersensitivity angiitis (palmar digital)
Thromboangiitis obliterans (Buerger's disease; radial/ulnar, palmar, digital)
Takayasu's arteritis (innominate, subclavian)
Temporal arteritis (axillobrachial)

Medical Diseases

Thrombophilic states (palmar and digital arteries)
Myeloproliferative disorders (palmar and digital arteries)
Hepatitis-associated vasculitis (palmar and digital arteries)
Cryoglobulinemia (palmar and digital arteries)

Environmental

Cold injury
Vinyl chloride exposure

Embolism

Cardiac (brachial)
Arterial Source
  • Arterial thoracic outlet syndrome (subclavian artery source)
  • Peripheral aneurysm
  • Atheroembolism

Trauma

Blunt or penetrating trauma
Iatrogenic
  • Angioaccess (brachial, radial)
Hypothenar hammer syndrome (ulnar)
Vibration (palmar, digital)
Sports or athletic injury (axillosubclavian)

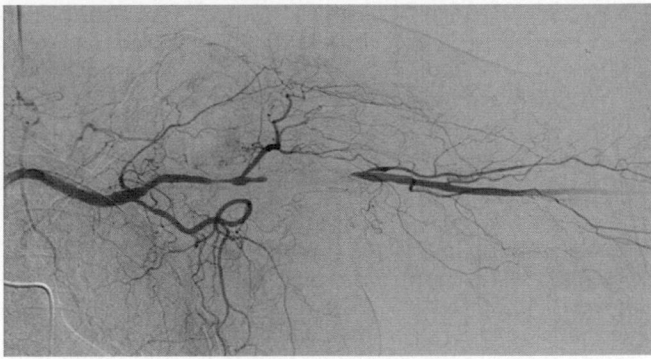

FIGURE 2 Left upper extremity angiogram demonstrating an area of smooth tapering stenosis and adjacent occlusion in the brachial artery of a 57-year-old woman with giant cell arteritis who experienced effort fatigue of the hand and forearm.

loss of vision develop. Angiographic findings typically reveal a smooth tapering stenosis resulting from inflammation involving all three layers of the vessel wall. Takayasu's disease typically involves the carotid and subclavian arteries in women age 20 to 40 years. GCA usually affects older women (>50 years), most commonly involving the extracranial carotid artery. When GCA involves the UE it affects the distal subclavian artery, axillary artery, and brachial artery (Figure 2). Thromboangiitis obliterans, or Buerger's disease, is a segmental, inflammatory, obliterative disease of the medium and small arteries of the extremities seen in heavy smokers (see chapter on Buerger's disease). It frequently affects the forearm and palmar digital arteries, sparing the more proximal arteries.

A number of connective tissue disorders can cause small vessel disease affecting the palmar digital vessels. These include scleroderma, CREST (calcinosis, Raynaud's phenomenon, esophageal dysmotility, sclerodactyly, and telangiectasia) syndrome, lupus, and rheumatoid arthritis. A similar small vessel disease pattern can be seen with a variety of relatively rare medical disorders (e.g., cryoglobulinemia or hepatitis-associated vasculitis), which should be looked for only after connective tissue diseases have been excluded. In the absence of an identifiable cause, which occurs in approximately one third of cases, such small artery occlusive disease is termed hypersensitivity angiitis.

Embolism

Most emboli to the UE are of cardiac origin and are macroemboli that typically lodge in the brachial artery just proximal to the takeoff of the deep brachial artery or at its bifurcation into the ulnar and radial arteries. These emboli usually result in acute episodes of forearm or hand ischemia in patients with an underlying cardiac condition but may be seen more chronically in older or debilitated patients who do not use their UE enough to induce symptoms. However, up to 30% of UE emboli have an arterial site of origin and tend to be microemboli that lodge in more distal arterial segments (palmar digital). The most common culprit is an aneurysm or ulcerative lesion within the distal subclavian artery associated with thoracic outlet syndrome (see chapter on thoracic outlet syndrome). In this situation, repetitive compression of the subclavian artery by anomalous myofascial bands attached to a cervical rib (or other osseous anomaly) leads to a focal stenosis. Poststenotic dilatation (aneurysm) or intimal ulceration results in mural thrombus formation. Subsequent embolization of luminal debris can produce both large and small artery occlusions distally. Unilateral Raynaud's phenomenon is a common presentation. Degenerative aneurysms of the subclavian artery or posttraumatic aneurysms of other UE arteries (e.g., crutch-induced axillary artery aneurysms) are other rare causes

are large vessel vasculitides. These diseases are associated with an initial inflammatory phase, which may have symptoms of fever, arthritis, and myalgias, along with laboratory findings of elevated erythrocyte sedimentation rate, before ischemic symptoms such as effort fatigue, asymmetric blood pressures, and in the case of GCA of ischemia and produce symptoms either through distal emboli or, less commonly, by in situ thrombosis. Ulcerative atherosclerotic plaques within the aorta or proximal brachiocephalic arteries also can lead, rarely, to emboli.

Trauma

Undiagnosed or neglected arterial injuries are a well-recognized cause of UE occlusive disease. Although bleeding and significant ischemia are obvious manifestations of arterial injury requiring treatment in the acute setting, intimal injuries from both penetrating and blunt trauma may lead to delayed arterial thrombosis with less dramatic symptomatology. Iatrogenic injuries are particularly common. Brachial artery injuries are a well-recognized complication of cardiac catheterization procedures performed via this approach. Such occlusions may go undetected in the acute setting because of the abundant collaterals around the elbow. The only manifestation may be the development of effort fatigue in the forearm on resumption of normal activities. Cumulative occupational trauma also can lead to significant vascular injury. Hypothenar hammer syndrome results from repetitive blunt trauma to the terminal portion of the ulnar artery in ulnar tunnel (formed by the pisiform, the hook of the hamate, and the transverse carpal ligament in the proximal palm). This injury is caused by repetitively striking objects with the base of the palm. Segmental occlusion or aneurysm formation of the ulnar artery, with or without distal digital artery embolism, can result (Figure 3). Vibration-induced injury to the digital arteries occurs after prolonged exposure of the hands to vibratory tools or machinery. The tools most commonly implicated are pneumatic tools and chainsaws. Patients initially report neurologic complaints (i.e., numbness or paresthesia) in the affected hand and digits. As the syndrome progresses, Raynaud's phenomenon develops. Tissue loss is rare. Sports-related trauma is a rare cause of ischemia but can occur in individuals who use a fixed, repetitive UE motion in competitive athletic endeavors. Axillary and subclavian artery injuries in baseball pitchers are the most frequently encountered.

■ EVALUATION

Performing a thorough history and physical examination is the first step in narrowing down the multiple causes of UE arterial occlusive disease to come to the appropriate diagnosis and thus be able to formulate a comprehensive treatment plan. Symptoms can range

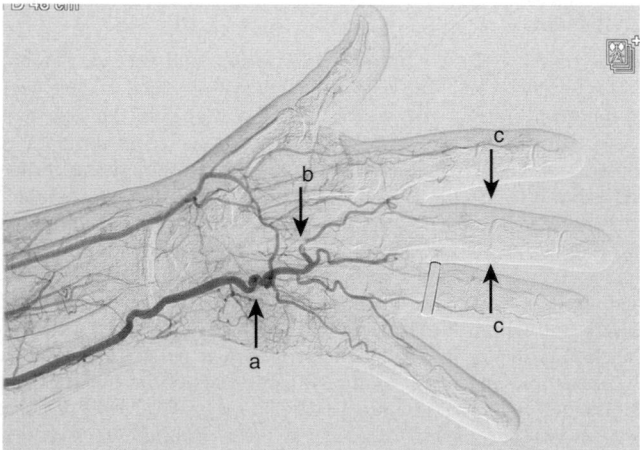

FIGURE 3 Angiogram of the left hand of a patient with hypothenar hammer syndrome seen with color changes and pain in the fingers, specifically the middle finger. Note the irregularity of the distal ulnar artery (*arrow a*), embolic filling defect in the superficial palmar arch (*arrow b*), and occlusion of digital arteries of the middle finger (*arrows c*).

from the incidental finding of a blood pressure differential in the UE by a patient's primary care physician on physical examination; to color changes, coolness, numbness, weakness, effort-induced fatigue, and ischemic rest pain; and all the way to tissue loss. Raynaud's phenomenon, which may result from pure vasospasm, is also a frequent manifestation of fixed occlusive lesions. Most patients will note only one or two of the classic tricolor digital changes: pallor (white) to cyanosis (blue) to hyperemic rubor (red). Exercise-induced fatigue in the arm musculature is brought on by repetitive use and, like its lower extremity counterpart claudication, is relieved quickly by a short period of rest. This phenomenon usually results from large vessel occlusive disease. Symptoms manifested in the hand or digits may result from large vessel disease, small vessel disease, or multilevel disease. Digital tissue loss is nearly always associated with small artery occlusive disease, with or without more proximal involvement.

Laterality of symptoms should be assessed. Bilateral UE symptoms suggest the presence of a systemic cause, such as a connective tissue or inflammatory disease. Patients also should be questioned about possible underlying connective tissue disorders or associated symptoms—tight skin or dysphagia in scleroderma, facial rash in lupus, or joint complaints in rheumatoid arthritis. The patient also should be interrogated for other systemic symptoms such as weight loss and myalgias. Unilateral complaints suggest localized arterial pathology such as arterial thoracic outlet syndrome, arterial aneurysm, or hypothenar hammer syndrome.

Because atherosclerotic disease is the most common cause of UE arterial occlusive disease, pathology should be evaluated thoroughly in all cases and associated risk factors identified (i.e., tobacco use, dyslipidemia, hypertension, diabetes mellitus, renal insufficiency, and family history). Symptoms or history of arterial occlusive disease in other vascular beds, including the coronary arteries, lower extremities (claudication), and cerebrovascular circulation, should be sought. Specifically, if concomitant posterior cerebral circulation symptoms such as dizziness, ataxia, or diplopia are identified, possible involvement of the subclavian or innominate arteries proximal to the takeoff of the vertebral artery should be investigated.

In the medical history, one should inquire about hypercoagulable states, renal insufficiency, cardiac arrhythmias and disorders, medication and supplement use, and drug abuse. A history of prior trauma to the neck or UE should be sought. The history also should include any catheter-based procedures in the UE as well as catheters placed for invasive hemodynamic monitoring. Patients with renal failure should be evaluated for prior vascular access procedures. Social history includes occupational or environmental exposures, athletic activities, and hobbies that may be important. The family history should focus on connective tissue disorders, hypercoagulable states, and premature atherosclerotic disease.

The physical examination includes measurement of blood pressure in both upper extremities. A complete pulse examination of the neck, upper extremities, and lower extremities is essential and remains the primary modality for diagnosing UE occlusive disease. A decreased or absent pulse indicates a proximal high-grade stenosis or occlusion; however, the presence of a pulse does not completely exclude proximal disease, particularly in the setting of a chronic occlusion, given the rich collateral pathways present in the upper extremity. An irregular pulse should prompt a more detailed cardiac examination to identify atrial fibrillation or other arrhythmias that may predispose to cardioembolism. Auscultation for bruits over all major arteries should be performed. The skin envelope of the digits is examined for signs of color or temperature differences, tissue loss, or trophic changes. In patients with unilateral complaints, the asymptomatic extremity should be examined carefully for occult disease. Allen's test can be used to assess patency of the palmar arch. In this test the patient's radial and ulnar arteries are occluded with digital pressure while the patient opens and closes the hand. Once the hand is pale, the ulnar artery is released and reperfusion of the hand is assessed; then the maneuver is repeated, except the radial artery is released first.

Noninvasive Vascular Laboratory Assessment

All patients with ischemic symptoms should undergo bilateral UE arterial segmental pressure testing. This testing provides objective and reproducible data that may identify fixed obstructions as well as inducible vasospasm and also quantify the degree of arterial insufficiency. Serial examinations allow for objective assessment of disease status and evaluation of the effectiveness of therapeutic interventions. Bilateral brachial, upper forearm, and wrist systolic pressures are obtained along with associated Doppler waveforms. The normal pressure differential between arms should not exceed 15 mm Hg, and a pressure drop of 20 mm Hg or more between levels indicates an intervening hemodynamically significant lesion. Reduced brachial pressures bilaterally, particularly when associated with blunted or monophasic Doppler waveforms, should prompt high thigh pressure measurements to exclude the possibility of bilateral proximal UE arterial disease. Although digital pressures and waveforms are notoriously temperature dependent, they can be extremely helpful in documenting the presence of small artery occlusive disease or vasospasm. An absolute digital pressure less than 70 mm Hg, a wrist/digital gradient greater than 30 mm Hg, and an interdigital gradient greater than 15 mm Hg are all considered abnormal. The finding of normal or near-normal digital pressures with vasospastic waveforms is helpful in establishing a diagnosis of Raynaud's phenomenon. Arterial duplex scanning may provide even more information than segmental pressures but has limited utility proximally because of the bony structures of the thoracic outlet. We have found it most useful when dealing with suspected lesions in the axillary, brachial, and forearm arteries.

Imaging

Advanced imaging usually is reserved for patients with critical limb ischemia or debilitating symptoms with evidence of proximal disease amenable to intervention. Significant improvements in imaging equipment and technique have increased the use of both computed tomographic angiography (CTA) and magnetic resonance angiography (MRA) in the evaluation of UE arterial diseases. Both are valuable in evaluating the aortic arch and larger, more proximal vessels. The use of postprocessing techniques and three-dimensional (3D) reconstruction also is useful in planning invasive intervention. However, these modalities do have limits, specifically in providing adequate detailed imaging of the distal forearm, hand, and fingers. When such imaging is required, conventional catheter angiography remains the gold standard, using digital subtraction technology to minimize the radiocontrast load. Angiography also allows for concomitant administration of vasodilators, such as tolazoline or nitroglycerin, which are often necessary to adequately visualize the arteries of the hand and fingers. Selective studies of both UEs should be obtained because many disease processes affect both UEs. With the proliferation of endoluminal treatment modalities, catheter angiography also provides the opportunity for simultaneous therapeutic intervention.

Laboratory Testing

Specific laboratory studies are obtained based on the index of suspicion and are most useful when dealing with distal small artery occlusive disease. Routine chemistries, blood counts, and coagulation profiles should be drawn when the diagnosis is unclear. If a hypercoagulable state is considered, patients should be checked for factor V Leiden, antithrombin III deficiency, protein C and S deficiencies, antiphospholipid antibodies, the prothrombin gene mutation, and hyperhomocysteinemia. Testing for connective tissue disorders should include rheumatoid factor, antinuclear antibodies, complement levels, and a sedimentation rate. Additional tests looking for cryoglobulinemia, hepatitis, or myeloproliferative disorders may be helpful if the other, more common causes of small artery occlusive

disease have been excluded. When a cardioembolic source is suspected, electrocardiography is obtained to evaluate for arrhythmia, and echocardiography may be obtained to evaluate for a cardiac structural abnormality or residual cardiac thrombus. Similarly, plain films of the neck looking for a cervical rib or other osseous abnormalities are useful to exclude most arterial thoracic outlet problems.

■ MANAGEMENT

Appropriate treatment of UE occlusive disease depends on both its etiology and its degree of symptomatology. Medical therapy is frequently the first-line treatment, as invasive intervention is neither indicated nor helpful for many of the causes of UE ischemia.

Patients with vasospasm are advised to abstain from tobacco and to avoid cold. Vasodilators, primarily calcium-channel blockers, have been used with varying degrees of success to treat severely symptomatic Raynaud's phenomenon. Patients with atherosclerotic lesions should undergo aggressive risk factor modification implemented in the same way as occurs when atherosclerosis is identified in other vascular beds.

Patients with a large to medium vessel systemic vasculitis (i.e., Takayasu's arteritis or GCA) generally have an initial inflammatory phase for which corticosteroid treatment should be initiated. Alternative immunosuppressive and immunomodulating agents such as cyclophosphamide, methotrexate, and azathioprine also can be used. These patients benefit from well-coordinated multidisciplinary care. Invasive intervention should be avoided during the active inflammatory phase because of the high risk for recurrence and failure.

Revascularization for chronic occlusive disease is limited to limb salvage situations for patients with critical ischemia (tissue loss or rest pain) or debilitating symptoms of effort fatigue secondary to large or medium vessel occlusive disease. Acute arterial occlusions resulting from arterial emboli or trauma generally should be addressed when diagnosed, as operative intervention is easiest in the acute setting and ischemic symptoms frequently develop once the patient recovers from the acute event.

Regardless of the indication, great care is necessary when operating on the UE vasculature. The proximal UE arteries lack the thick muscular layer of the femoral artery and are torn easily if handled roughly. The forearm arteries are also problematic because of their extreme vasoreactivity. Avoidance of excessive manipulation is critical. Operative intervention is most useful for treating atherosclerotic occlusive disease of the proximal arteries. Intrathoracic procedures to treat innominate and subclavian artery occlusive disease are discussed in the chapter on brachiocephalic reconstruction.

Endovascular Therapy

Endovascular techniques most commonly are used to treat short segment occlusive lesions found in the proximal vessels of the upper extremity, specifically in the proximal left subclavian artery. Standard endovascular techniques typically are used with an antegrade approach via femoral access or if necessary a retrograde approach via brachial artery. Typically, long sheaths are used to give adequate support. Because of the larger sheaths that are required (6F and larger), we prefer open exposure of the brachial artery to limit access site complications when a retrograde approach is used. If primary stenting is not performed, it should be added to the procedure if there is residual stenosis greater than 30% after balloon angioplasty, a flow limiting dissection, a heavily calcified lesion, or a complete occlusion. Excellent technical success rates have been reported, though success rates are somewhat lower in cases of chronic total occlusions compared with stenotic lesions. This procedure is associated with low morbidity and mortality. Short and midterm patency rates are comparable with open surgical reconstruction. Longer term open repairs have superior patency compared with endovascular interventions. However, given the low complication rates, the minimally invasive nature, and the often frail patient population that requires such interventions, endoluminal therapy is assuming its place as first-line therapy for many of these lesions.

The use of endovascular techniques for other lesions of the UE is as yet not well defined. Traumatic disruptions of the subclavian-axillary artery, which can be difficult to repair surgically, have been treated successfully with stent grafts. Catheter-directed thrombolysis has been used for thrombotic occlusions of the upper extremity. Technically successful balloon angioplasty of arterial occlusive lesions in the arm, forearm, and hand has been described. The infrequency of the UE pathology and the lack of long-term follow-up make it difficult to establish the role of these interventions.

Open Surgical Revascularization

Subclavian

Provided that the ipsilateral common carotid artery is disease free, both carotid subclavian bypass and subclavian transposition can be considered for the treatment of proximal subclavian artery occlusive disease. Although bypass is technically simpler, we prefer transposition whenever feasible because of its superior long-term patency. Although endovascular techniques have reduced our reliance on these operations for the treatment of occlusive disease, these operations have in fact become more commonly performed as part of "debranching" the aortic arch in preparation for endovascular repair of thoracic aortic pathology.

The procedure is performed as follows. The patient is placed on the operating table in a semi-Fowler's position, with the head of the table elevated 20 to 30 degrees. A roll is placed under the shoulders to allow for moderate extension of the neck, and the head is rotated slightly toward the contralateral side. The ipsilateral arm is placed at the side with the shoulder depressed as much as possible. A transverse incision is made approximately one fingerbreadth (2 cm) above the clavicle, extending from the edge of the sternocleidomastoid muscle to the midportion of the clavicle. Subcutaneous tissues and platysma are divided, and the clavicular head of the sternocleidomastoid is transected. The omohyoid is identified and divided. The underlying scalene fat pad is mobilized along its medial and inferior aspects and retracted superiorly and laterally. During this dissection one must be alert for lymphatic structures, which are carefully ligated before division. However, the thoracic duct or right lymphatic duct is not routinely ligated if encountered unless it is injured. After retraction of the scalene fat pad, the anterior scalene muscle is exposed. The phrenic nerve is identified (coursing lateral to medial along the surface of the anterior scalene) and carefully mobilized and retracted to allow division of the anterior scalene from its tubercle on the first rib. Care is taken not to injure the underlying subclavian artery and adjacent brachial plexus. The subclavian artery is gently dissected free. Exposure of the carotid artery is accomplished through the medial portion of the incision. Injury to the vagus nerve and internal jugular vein is avoided by retracting them laterally. If exposure of the carotid bifurcation is necessary (e.g., for concomitant endarterectomy), a separate incision can be made along the medial border of the sternocleidomastoid. For both bypass and transposition, we create a tunnel posterior to the internal jugular vein, and systemic heparin is administered.

Transposition of the subclavian artery to the carotid artery is suitable only when plaque extends no more than a few centimeters beyond the subclavian artery origin. Transposition requires mobilization of the subclavian artery as proximally as possible. Small branches are divided, but an effort should be made to preserve the vertebral and internal mammary arteries. However, if additional mobilization of the subclavian artery is required to avoid kinking, it may be necessary to divide the internal mammary branch. To minimize the risk of embolization, the distal subclavian, vertebral, and internal mammary arteries are clamped before ligating the proximal subclavian artery. The subclavian is transected proximally with very careful ligation of the proximal stump. A 4- to 5-cm segment of the common carotid artery is clamped proximally and distally, and a short vertical arteriotomy is made along the lateral wall of the carotid, appropriately sized to accept the diameter of the subclavian artery. An end-to-side anastomosis is fashioned with running Prolene sutures. Flow is restored after appropriate venting. We do not routinely monitor cerebral perfusion with an electroencephalogram (EEG) during this procedure.

If a bypass is planned, only a short segment (4 to 5 cm) of the subclavian artery just distal to the thyrocervical trunk must be exposed. Small branches can and should be ligated to improve exposure. As outlined previously, care should be taken when retracting the subclavian artery to avoid inadvertent injury. A 7- to 8-mm prosthetic graft or a large-caliber saphenous vein graft typically is chosen as the conduit. It is technically easier to perform the subclavian artery anastomosis first. After systemic heparinization, the subclavian artery is clamped proximally and distally, and a short longitudinal arteriotomy is made along the superior surface of the artery at the highest point of its arc above the clavicle. The graft should be beveled to promote a slightly downward course of the graft. An end-to-side anastomosis then is constructed with 5-0 Prolene sutures. Then the graft to the carotid artery anastomosis is performed in an end-to-side fashion with running Prolene sutures as described for the transposition. We routinely leave a small closed suction drain in place; this is removed only after the patient has resumed normal oral intake.

Both carotid subclavian bypass and subclavian transposition have low morbidity and excellent long-term patency (75% to 80% at 5 years for bypass and almost 100% for transposition). Complications include injury to adjacent nerves (brachial plexus, phrenic nerve, and sympathetic chain) and lymphatic structures (thoracic and accessory thoracic ducts). Nerve injuries are usually self-limited. Lymphatic injuries can be problematic, and if drainage is significant or persistent, early re-exploration and thoracic duct ligation is advised.

Axillary Artery

Occlusive lesions of the axillary artery are extremely unusual. Trauma or neglected emboli are the most common causes. Bypass procedures originating from or terminating on the axillary artery also are relatively rare. In the past, axilloaxillary bypass was advocated as an alternative procedure for dealing with subclavian disease when the ipsilateral carotid was an unsuitable inflow site. This bypass largely has been abandoned, however, because of its superficial location and reduced patency. Carotid axillary bypass has been used to manage extensive subclavian disease, whereas axillobrachial bypass has been implemented for distal axillary or proximal brachial occlusions. To expose the first and second portions of the axillary artery, the arm should be positioned at the patient's side (a narrow arm board is helpful). Significant abduction must be avoided because this position stretches the axillary artery. A transverse incision is made one fingerbreadth below the clavicle, extending from the midclavicular line to the deltopectoral groove. The fibers of the pectoralis major muscle are split, and the underlying clavipectoral fascia is incised. Tributaries of the axillary vein are divided and traced back to the axillary vein, which lies inferior and slightly anterior to the artery. If encountered, the crossing medial and lateral pectoral nerves should be preserved to avoid postoperative atrophy of the pectoralis muscles. It is usually necessary to divide a branch or two of the thoracoacromial artery to gain exposure. The artery is located just above the vein, with the cords of the brachial plexus lying superiorly and posteriorly. As with the subclavian artery, care should be taken when mobilizing this thin-walled artery, which frequently has small posterior branches. The head of the pectoralis minor can be divided to facilitate exposure laterally (second portion of the axillary artery). Saphenous vein is the conduit of choice for bypasses originating from or terminating on the axillary artery. Bypasses from the carotid to the axillary (or brachial) artery are best tunneled under the clavicle.

Brachial Artery

Brachial artery lesions are rare and most commonly caused by emboli and trauma. GCA is a rare cause of proximal brachial occlusive disease. For brachial artery exposure, the arm is abducted and the hand supinated on an arm board. The proximal brachial artery is exposed through a longitudinal incision along the medial aspect of the upper arm in the bicipital groove. Dissection along the posterior aspect of the muscle belly reveals the artery, accompanied by the median and ulnar nerves. The proximal brachial–distal axillary artery can be exposed through a hockey stick–shaped extension of this incision along the lateral border of the pectoralis major. Brachial exposure immediately proximal to the elbow is achieved through an incision along the bicipital groove extended laterally across to the antecubital fossa. The median nerve lies immediately medial to the artery at this level. Alternatively, the distal brachial artery and its bifurcation into the radial and ulnar arteries can be exposed by making a longitudinal incision in the antecubital fossa just distal to the elbow crease and dividing the bicipital aponeurosis. If more distal exposure is required, the incision can be carried inferiorly along the volar aspect of the forearm. If the entire brachial artery at the elbow requires exposure, a lazy S incision is used to avoid scar contracture across the elbow crease. Autogenous vein is the only conduit suitable for bypasses involving the brachial and more distal arteries

Radial and Ulnar Arteries

Bypass to the forearm arteries is rarely necessary and is most often used for trauma and neglected embolic occlusions (Figure 4). In dialysis patients, these arteries can be affected by a particularly aggressive form of atherosclerosis (azotemic arteriopathy) that is rarely amenable to revascularization. Buerger's disease is another cause of forearm occlusive disease that usually is not reconstructable. Exposure of these arteries at the wrist is relatively straightforward, but more proximal exposure requires a thorough understanding of forearm anatomy. Topical papaverine or nitroglycerin is helpful to combat dissection-induced vasospasm. Hypothenar hammer syndrome can be treated by an interposition vein graft of the involved segment of ulnar artery in the proximal hand. A dorsal foot vein provides the best size match.

Embolism

The management of large artery embolism is discussed in more detail in the chapter on peripheral arterial embolism. Because of increased vasoreactivity and the inevitable resulting vasospasm, multiple passages with balloon embolectomy catheters should be avoided with UE emboli. For this reason, we have a lower threshold for obtaining preoperative imaging when dealing with acute arterial occlusions of the UE, even with a good clinical story for embolism. Imaging confirms the diagnosis and allows a more directed approach, a particularly important concept when dealing with emboli in the axillary and subclavian arteries.

Although retrograde removal of such proximal clots usually can be performed through a brachial approach, we sometimes prefer to expose the occluded segment directly if there is significant clot burden. This approach minimizes the number of catheter passages necessary to extract the embolus and avoids stripping off clot into patent branches of the segment between the arteriotomy and the occlusion. Although most macroemboli originate from the heart, an arterial source sometimes can be responsible and, if identified, must be addressed. Treatment of arterial thoracic outlet syndrome requires not only excision of the compressive thoracic outlet elements but also some type of arterial reconstruction (discussed in more detail in the chapter on thoracic outlet syndrome).

Trauma

As outlined previously, most traumatic occlusions should be fixed at the time of diagnosis. Isolated radial or ulnar artery occlusions are an exception because they are usually well tolerated. Iatrogenic occlusions usually can be relieved with local exploration, thrombectomy, and repair of associated vessel wall injury. For more significant injuries, formal arterial reconstruction is required. Resection with end-to-end anastomosis can be performed rarely, but in the vast majority of cases interposition grafting with saphenous vein of appropriate caliber is required. A more detailed description of how to manage traumatic occlusions is provided in the chapter on management of vascular injuries.

Small Artery Occlusive Disease

Treatment of occlusive disease affecting the small arteries of the digits and hands can be challenging. After a proximal embolic source has been ruled out, attention is focused on identification and treatment of any underlying causative diseases. Patients with Buerger's disease frequently experience significant improvement with successful tobacco abstinence. Vibration-induced injury will respond to avoidance of the causative vibratory machinery. The rare patient with cryoglobulinemia or hepatitis-associated vasculitis will respond to appropriate

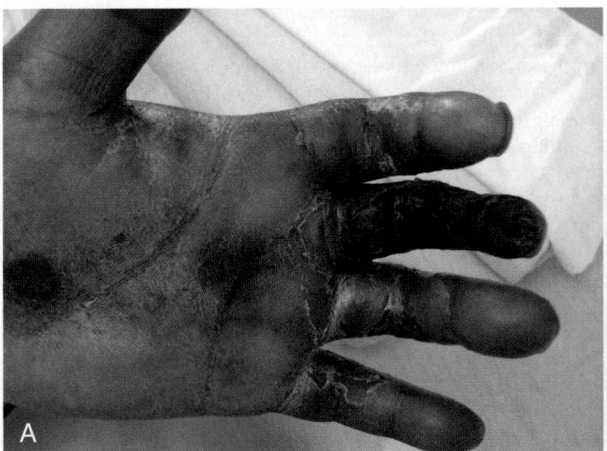
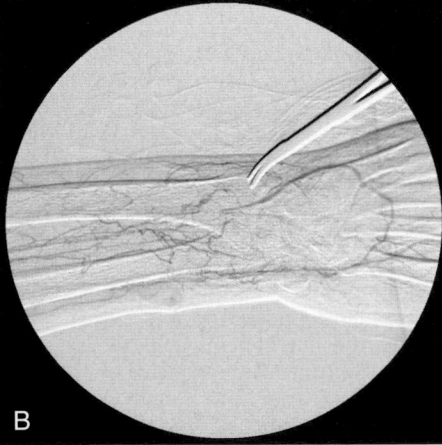
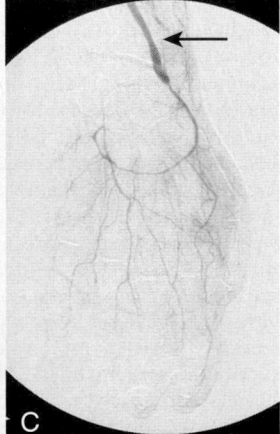

FIGURE 4 **A,** Ischemic left hand with gangrene of the middle finger in a patient with end-stage renal disease and neglected thromboembolization of the forearm after percutaneous dialysis access graft thrombectomy. **B,** Angiography demonstrating occlusion of the ulnar and radial arteries with reconstitution of the radial artery at the wrist. **C,** Angiogram demonstrating distal anastomosis and runoff of brachial artery to radial artery bypass with reversed great saphenous vein (*arrow*).

therapy. Unfortunately, in the majority of cases, no specific therapy is available. In our practice, these are patients with an associated connective tissue disorder, hypersensitivity angiitis, or renal failure. For these individuals, care is focused on supportive measures. Abstinence from tobacco and avoidance of cold are routinely advised. Antiplatelet therapy (aspirin or clopidogrel) and hemorrheologic agents (cilostazol) usually are prescribed. Vasodilators, primarily calcium-channel blockers, can be used to treat associated vasospasm with variable success. Areas of tissue loss are treated with local wound care and débridement as indicated. Sympathectomy, both cervicothoracic and digital, can lead to a temporary improvement in skin blood flow but has such limited durability (approximately 6 months) that most authorities have abandoned it except in highly selected patients with residual ischemia after revascularization.

CONCLUSIONS

UE arterial occlusive disease is an uncommon problem with diverse causes. Accurate diagnosis depends on a thorough history and physical examination supported by noninvasive vascular testing. Angiography remains the primary modality of diagnosis. Treatment depends on the nature of the disease process and the severity of the ischemia. Patients with embolic or traumatic occlusions and significantly symptomatic proximal large artery disease usually can undergo vascular intervention with good results. On the other hand, revascularization options for patients with distal small artery occlusive disease are extremely limited. In this setting, after a careful search for treatable causes, management is primarily supportive. Fortunately, progression to limb loss is rare.

SUGGESTED READINGS

AbuRahma AF, Bates MC, Stone PA, Dyer B, Armistead L, Scott Dean L, Scott Lavigne P. Angioplasty and stenting versus carotid-subclavian bypass for the treatment of isolated subclavian artery disease. *J Endovasc Ther.* 2007;14:698-704.

Aiello F, Morrissey NJ. Open and endovascular management of subclavian and innominate arterial pathology. *Semin Vasc Surg.* 2011;24:31-35.

Deguara J, Ali T, Modarai B, Burnand KG. Upper limb ischemia: 20 years experience from a single center. *Vascular.* 2005;13:84-91.

Ferraresi R, Palloshi A, Aprigliano G, Caravaggi C, Centola M, Sozzi F, Danzi GB, Manzi M. Angioplasty of below-the-elbow arteries in critical hand ischaemia. *Eur J Vasc Endovasc Surg.* 2012;43:73-80.

Hughes K, Hamdan A, Schermerhorn M, Giordano A, Scovell S, Pomposelli F Jr. Bypass for chronic ischemia of the upper extremity: results in 20 patients. *J Vasc Surg.* 2007;46:303-307.

Klitfod L, Jensen LP. Treatment of chronic upper limb ischaemia is safe and results are good. *Dan Med J.* 2014;61:A4859.

Soga Y, Tomoi Y, Fujihara M, Okazaki S, Yamauchi Y, Shintani Y, Suzuki K, SCALLOP Investigators. Perioperative and long-term outcomes of endovascular treatment for subclavian artery disease from a large multicenter registry. *J Endovasc Ther.* 2015;22:626-633.

Spinelli F, Benedetto F, Passari G, La Spada M, Carella G, Stilo F, De Caridi G, Lentini S. Bypass surgery for the treatment of upper limb chronic ischaemia. *Eur J Vasc Endovasc Surg.* 2010;39:165-170.

AORTOILIAC OCCLUSIVE DISEASE

Dean J. Arnaoutakis, MD, and Mahmoud B. Malas, MD, MHS

Atherosclerotic disease of the infrarenal aorta and iliac arteries is a common cause of lower extremity ischemia. The identification of this disease process at the aortic bifurcation dates to the eighteenth century with cadaveric dissections created by John Hunter. The clinical sequelae of obliteration of the aortic bifurcation—namely impotence, claudication, lower extremity pallor, and absent femoral pulses—was described in the 1940s by René Leriche and is known as Leriche's syndrome. The initial modern treatment for aortoiliac occlusive disease (AIOD) was based on thromboendarterectomy, a technique championed by dos Santos and Wylie. Ultimately endarterectomy was surpassed by one of the most durable operations that vascular surgeons undertake, the aortobifemoral bypass (AFB). To this day, this procedure is based on the use of prosthetic grafts, a key discovery made by Blakemore and Voorhees in the 1950s.

Atherosclerotic disease typically begins at the aortic bifurcation and extends both superiorly and inferiorly. Often disease is multisegmental, affecting the femoropopliteal arterial system, which may exacerbate symptoms and complicate treatment decisions. Patients with multilevel disease are typically older and suffer from hypertension and diabetes. Symptoms can vary from intermittent claudication to critical limb ischemia (CLI). This spectrum can be explained by the degree to which the patient develops collateral circulation reconstituting the infrainguinal system, by the presence of concomitant multilevel peripheral arterial disease (PAD), or by the development of large thromboemboli. The goal of intervention in those patients with intermittent claudication is improving quality of life. In contrast, patients with CLI should undergo revascularization to reduce rest pain, heal open wounds, and ultimately salvage their limbs.

INITIAL EVALUATION AND INDICATIONS FOR INTERVENTION

A thorough history and physical examination remains paramount during the initial evaluation for patients with PAD. AIOD typically affects older smokers who suffer from hypertension, hyperlipidemia, and diabetes. Nonatherosclerotic disease processes, such as Takayasu's disease and radiation arteritis, can involve the aortoiliac vessels. These less common causes are beyond the scope of this chapter. Patients often are seen with hip, thigh, or buttock claudication along with absent femoral pulses. In addition, pelvic ischemia in men can lead to Leriche's syndrome, mentioned previously. Tissue loss and rest pain is less common, as many patients develop a rich network of collaterals from the lumbar and hypogastric arteries to the circumflex iliac, femoral, and profunda vessels. Connections also can develop between the mesenteric arteries, which can supply the pelvis through the hemorrhoidal vessels.

Noninvasive testing with segmental Doppler pressures and pulse volume recordings can help to confirm the diagnosis of AIOD and also can suggest the presence of concomitant infrainguinal disease. A 20 mm Hg or greater difference between the brachial pressure and the proximal thigh pressure represents a significant stenosis in the aorta or iliac arteries. Duplex assessment of the aortoiliac segment is not ideal because of overlying bowel gas, obesity, and vessel tortuosity or calcification. Axial imaging with computed tomographic angiography (CTA) or magnetic resonance angiography (MRA) has become the most common modality used to view the aortoiliac system. CTA is particularly useful for operative planning because this imaging modality readily identifies the location of calcific disease (Figure 1). If endovascular therapies are not possible based on CTA or MRA, direct reconstruction typically can be planned without the use of arteriography. Angiography, previously deemed the "gold standard," is also useful if the patient has previous stents or implanted orthopedic hardware because these items compromise the quality of axial imaging. If performing angiography, multiple projections of the iliac and femoral bifurcations are needed to identify disease burden, which may dictate treatment options. In

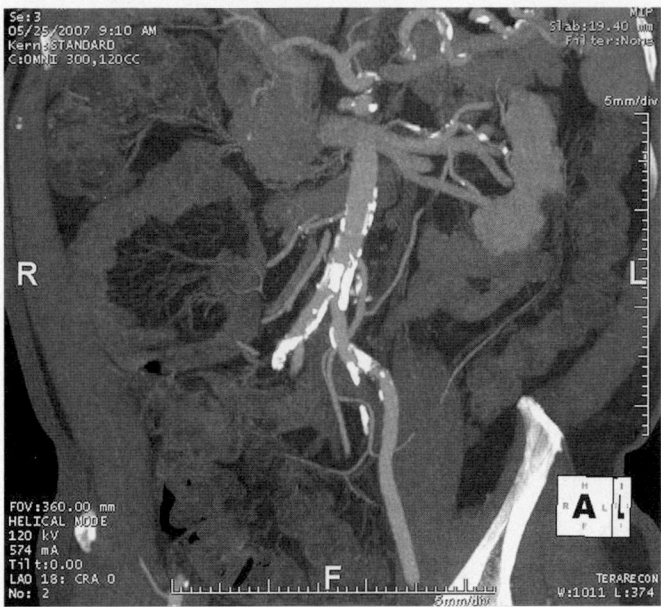

FIGURE 1 Preprocedure imaging. Computed tomographic angiography is an excellent imaging modality for evaluating aortoiliac occlusive disease. Not only is it informative regarding the degree and length of stenosis or occlusions, but the location and distribution of calcified atheroma also are revealed. Understanding both is important in selecting the appropriate revascularization strategy. In this maximum intensity projection, heavy calcification of the aortoiliac segment is evident, with occlusion of the right external iliac artery.

addition, identification of the inferior mesenteric artery (IMA) is essential because preservation of a large IMA in the setting of severely diseased superior mesenteric artery (SMA) or hypogastric arteries is critical for preventing catastrophic bowel or pelvic ischemia. Finally, distal angiographic runoff views also are obtained to detect the presence of femoropopliteal or tibial disease. Ultimately the most cost-effective imaging approach remains controversial and often is based on whether the patient is thought to be an endovascular candidate. Our current practice is to first obtain cross-sectional imaging with a CTA in order to obtain an anatomic roadmap and to create a treatment strategy.

Indications for intervention include disabling symptoms of intermittent claudication that significantly affect a patient's daily lifestyle despite optimal medical therapy, as well as ischemic rest pain or tissue loss. Initial interventions for those with lifestyle-limiting claudication should include smoking cessation; weight loss; initiation of antiplatelet therapy; treatment of hypertension, hyperlipidemia, and diabetes; and a trial of an organized exercise program. Evidence has shown that routine exercise may be as effective as revascularization procedures in certain patients with claudication. Results from the CLEVER (Claudication: Exercise Versus Endoluminal Revascularization) trial, a randomized controlled trial comparing supervised exercise therapy with endovascular treatment of AIOD, showed that the exercise therapy group had better objective short-term improvements in walking performance. Similar results have been shown for PAD of the infrainguinal segment. As such, surgical intervention for intermittent claudication should be offered only after medical therapy has been optimized. In contrast, treatment for CLI, via either open or endovascular approach, should be offered more aggressively in an attempt to minimize the chance of limb loss. However, before undergoing any invasive intervention, the patient's functional status before disease exacerbation, life expectancy, and concomitant medical problems must be evaluated in order to gauge the risk and benefit of the procedure.

When selecting the operative strategy, direct open repair or endovascular therapy, one must consider the safety and benefit of the procedure. Perhaps more important, the durability of the procedure for the given atherosclerotic lesion must be evaluated. Understanding the anatomic disease pattern is critical when making these decisions. The TransAtlantic Inter-Society Consensus (TASC) guidelines, presented by a multidisciplinary, international consensus statement, provide an anatomic classification system to help guide selection of open versus endovascular repair (Figure 2). In general, endovascular options are offered first to patients with focal lesions (TASC classes A and B), given the relatively decreased periprocedural morbidity of a percutaneous approach. In contrast, more advanced, diffuse disease (TASC class D) typically is best treated with open revascularization unless comorbid conditions preclude such intervention. However, as endovascular technologies evolve and improve, TASC class C and even TASC class D patients can be treated percutaneously, as made evident in the BRAVISSIMO trial, a nonrandomized trial comparing the endovascular treatment of TASC class A/B lesions with that of TASC class C/D lesions. Early results show no difference in outcomes at 2 years between the groups; however, some argue that this trial harbors inclusion bias, which explains the results. Despite these optimistic outcomes, the long-term implications and durability of such an intervention remain unclear. In the setting of advanced disease, we reserve endovascular treatment for those who are young or who have medical contraindications to open surgery.

■ DIRECT SURGICAL REVASCULARIZATION

Given its superior long-term patency rates, direct surgical revascularization is considered the "gold standard" for the treatment of AIOD. There are several historical treatment options, including aortoiliac endarterectomy and aortobiiliac bypass, but AFB grafting is the preferred open approach given its 10-year patency rate that approaches 85% (Figure 3). However, with improvements in the endovascular arena, the AFB procedure is now reserved for those with advanced AIOD yet acceptable operative risk. Besides comorbid conditions, several additional factors must be considered when selecting patients for open repair. First, studies have shown that female smokers have the worst outcomes, mostly attributed to the small caliber or hypoplastic nature of their native aorta and iliac vessels. Second, those with multilevel disease have decreased patency rates; consequently, they should be considered for concomitant or staged infrainguinal bypass procedures. Finally, several series have shown that young age (<50 years) portends a significantly worse outcome. We feel that younger patients should exhaust all medical options and even endovascular modalities before embarking on AFB grafting.

Preoperative preparation should begin with evaluating and optimizing cardiac, pulmonary, renal, cerebrovascular, and hematologic disease. Fluid status also should be optimized, especially in patients with chronic renal insufficiency. In patients with chronic kidney disease, surgical reconstruction should be delayed, if their vascular disease status permits, after completion of the diagnostic angiogram to allow for recovery from the nephrotoxic contrast load. When treating patients with AIOD, one must assume that they have some degree of coronary artery disease. As such, identification of those with critical coronary lesions, who would first benefit from coronary revascularization, is critical. In addition, all patients with AIOD should receive routine prophylactic measures such as perioperative beta-blockade and continuation of aspirin. Mechanical bowel preparations are not used routinely. Minimizing postoperative narcotics with the use of epidural analgesia can promote earlier return of bowel function and potentially reduce hospital stay. Placement of adequate intravenous access, intra-arterial pressure monitoring, and Foley catheter are routine. Finally, preoperative antibiotics, typically cefazolin, should be administered to minimize the risk of wound or graft infection.

Type A lesions

- Unilateral or bilateral stenoses of CIA
- Unilateral or bilateral single short (≤3 cm) stenosis of EIA

Type B lesions

- Short (≤3 cm) stenosis of infrarenal aorta
- Unilateral CIA occlusion
- Single or multiple stenosis totaling 3-10 cm involving the EIA not extending into the CFA
- Unilateral EIA occlusion not involving the origins of internal iliac of CFA

Type C lesions

- Bilateral CIA occlusions
- Bilateral EIA stenoses 3-10 cm long not extending into the CFA
- Unilateral EIA stenosis extending into the CFA
- Unilateral EIA occlusion that involves the origins of internal iliac and/or CFA
- Heavily calcified unilateral EIA occlusion with or without involvement of origins of internal iliac and/or CFA

Type D lesions

- Infrarenal aortoiliac occlusion
- Diffuse disease involving the aorta and both iliac arteries requiring treatment
- Diffuse multiple stenoses involving the unilateral CIA, EIA, and CFA
- Unilateral occlusions of both CIA and EIA
- Bilateral occlusion of EIA
- Iliac stenoses in patients with AAA requiring treatment and not amenable to endograft placement or other lesions requiring open aortic or iliac surgery

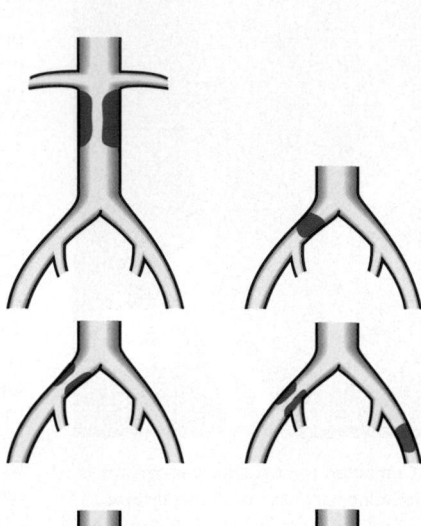
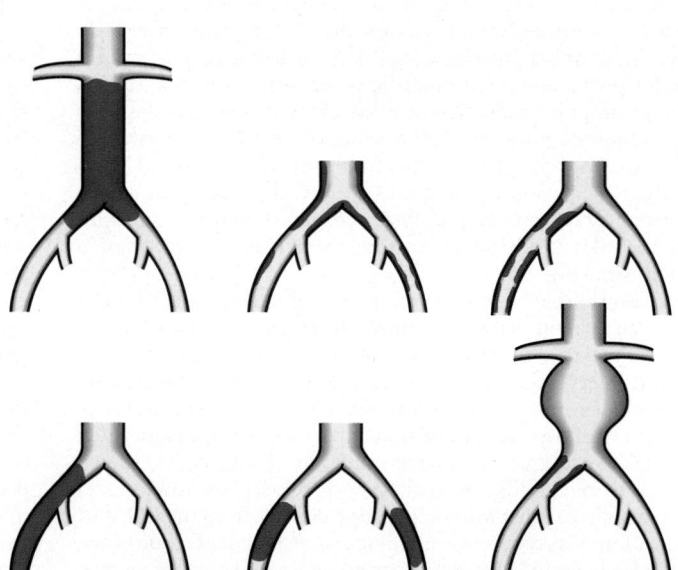

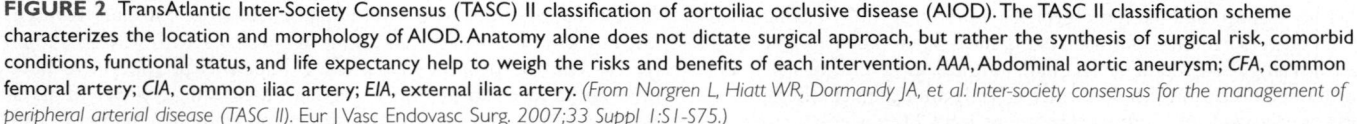

FIGURE 2 TransAtlantic Inter-Society Consensus (TASC) II classification of aortoiliac occlusive disease (AIOD). The TASC II classification scheme characterizes the location and morphology of AIOD. Anatomy alone does not dictate surgical approach, but rather the synthesis of surgical risk, comorbid conditions, functional status, and life expectancy help to weigh the risks and benefits of each intervention. *AAA,* Abdominal aortic aneurysm; *CFA,* common femoral artery; *CIA,* common iliac artery; *EIA,* external iliac artery. *(From Norgren L, Hiatt WR, Dormandy JA, et al. Inter-society consensus for the management of peripheral arterial disease (TASC II). Eur J Vasc Endovasc Surg. 2007;33 Suppl 1:S1-S75.)*

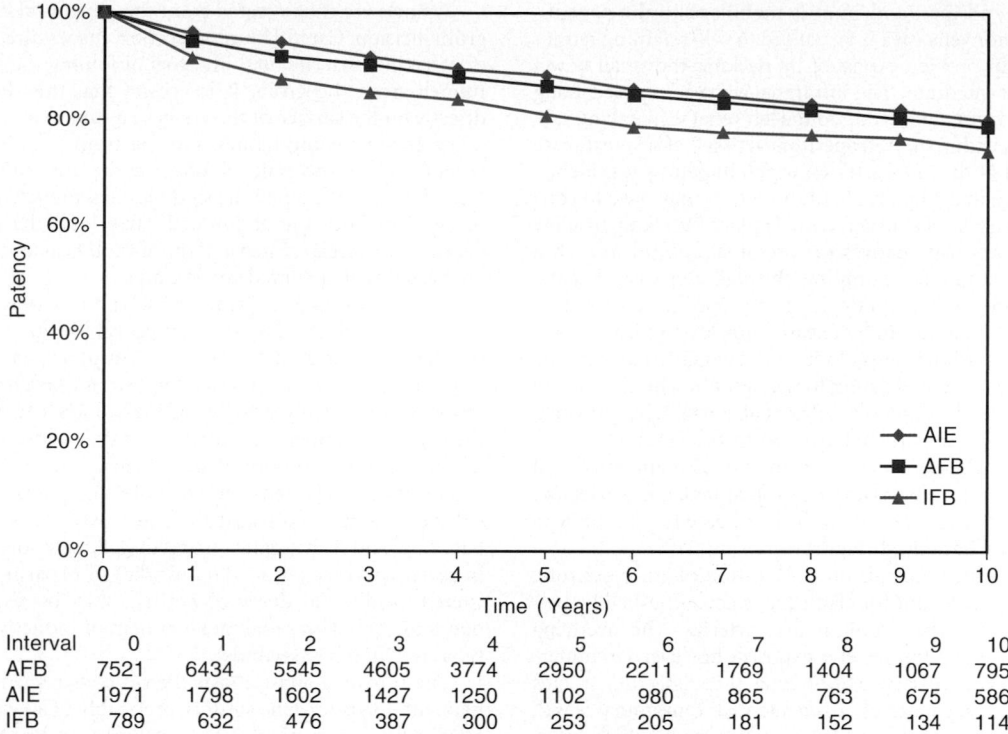

Interval	0	1	2	3	4	5	6	7	8	9	10
AFB	7521	6434	5545	4605	3774	2950	2211	1769	1404	1067	795
AIE	1971	1798	1602	1427	1250	1102	980	865	763	675	586
IFB	789	632	476	387	300	253	205	181	152	134	114

FIGURE 3 Long-term patency for direct revascularization. A review of 51 studies of direct surgical revascularization spanning 4 decades of compiled long-term patency data from 8006 patients. Durability of each type of procedure was excellent. *AFB*, Aortofemoral bypass; *AIE*, aortoiliac endarterectomy; *IFB*, iliofemoral bypass. *(Adapted from Chiu KW, Davies RS, Nightingale PG, et al. Review of direct anatomical open surgical management of atherosclerotic aorto-iliac occlusive disease. Eur J Vasc Endovasc Surg. 2010;39:460-471.)*

Aortobifemoral Bypass

Preoperative planning is just as essential for a successful AFB as is the exposure and anastomotic technique. Several issues should be determined before surgery, many of which can be answered by reviewing the cross-sectional preoperative imaging. First, one should determine a suitable level of aortic and iliac artery control for clamping based on the extent of disease calcification. In addition, the presence of concomitant renal or visceral artery disease should be recognized, as reimplantation of a patent IMA may be required in the setting of significant SMA disease. The location of the left renal vein should be documented because aortic mobilization or clamping can be hazardous if a retroaortic or circumaortic left renal vein is present. Determining the configuration of the proximal anastomosis should be given careful thought. Most favor an end-to-end configuration because it allows for a more comprehensive thromboendarterectomy of the proximal native aorta; a better in-line flow pattern with theoretically less intraluminal turbulence; and an easier closure of the retroperitoneum over the graft, which arguably minimizes graft infection and aortoenteric fistulae rates. In the presence of concomitant aneurysmal degeneration of the infrarenal aorta, an end-to-end anastomosis unquestionably should be used. This configuration, however, is predicated on the presence of patent external iliac arteries because the pelvis will be mostly perfused in a retrograde fashion from the external iliac vessels. In comparison, the proximal anastomosis should be fashioned in an end-to-side manner when there is severe disease or occlusion of bilateral external iliac arteries yet patent common and internal iliac arteries. In this scenario, pelvic ischemia (hip and buttock claudication, erectile dysfunction, and cauda equina syndrome) is prevented by the maintenance of forward flow through the native aorta.

The procedure begins with exposure of the femoral arteries, typically via bilateral oblique incisions. Often the proximal extent of the dissection must be carried to the level of the inguinal ligament, if not further superiorly, in order to identify a soft segment of the vessel that will be amenable to clamping. A portion of the inguinal ligament may need to be divided in order to achieve this exposure. The deep circumflex iliac vein, which overlies the distal external iliac artery, should be divided to prevent injury during graft tunneling. During this exposure, care must be taken to control the inferior epigastric and circumflex iliac arteries because they likely will have developed into formidable vessels from years of receiving collateral flow and thus can generate substantial backbleeding.

The extent to which the distal common femoral artery and its bifurcation are dissected and controlled depends on the severity of disease, the level to which reconstruction is planned, and whether femoral endarterectomy or profundaplasty is required. Regardless, the origins of the superficial femoral and profunda femoris arteries are exposed, which often requires ligation of the crossing lateral circumflex femoral vein. The vessels should be assessed to determine whether endarterectomy or patch angioplasty will be necessary for reconstruction. It has been widely established that providing adequate flow through the profunda femoris artery (PFA) is critical for achieving durable long-term patency of the inflow graft. In fact, the hood of the distal anastomosis is often carried onto the origin of the PFA. If the proximal portion of the PFA has extensive calcific disease, the secondary branches of this vessel are dissected free. After completion of the dissection, the inferior portion of the retroperitoneal tunnels is created with blunt dissection anterior to the external iliac artery. Once this is complete, the incisions are packed with moistened gauze sponges and attention is turned to the abdomen.

The abdominal aorta is exposed, typically through a midline transperitoneal incision, after completing the groin dissections in an effort to minimize insensible fluid losses and hypothermia. A retroperitoneal approach via a left flank incision can be utilized in the setting of a hostile abdomen, but creating the tunnel for the right limb of the graft can be difficult with this approach. Upon entering the peritoneal cavity, the abdomen is explored for any abnormalities and the nasogastric tube placement is confirmed. The ligament of

Treitz is dissected, and the duodenum is mobilized to the patient's right until the inferior vena cava is visualized. A self-retaining retractor is placed to help provide exposure by packing the small bowel into the right lower quadrant. The infrarenal aorta is exposed along its anterior surface from the IMA up to the left renal vein, taking care to ligate lymphatics within this retroperitoneal tissue. If severe disease extends to the level of the renal arteries, which hopefully was identified on preoperative imaging, proximal dissection may have to continue to the suprarenal level in order to safely place the clamp to allow for an endarterectomy. Alternatives for proximal control in such a situation include supraceliac clamping through the gastrohepatic ligament or intraluminal balloon deployment. Once the endarterectomy is complete, the clamp can be released quickly to flush thrombotic debris. Before flushing, vessel loops can be secured around the renal arteries to prevent embolization to the kidneys. The clamp then can be moved inferiorly onto the infrarenal aorta. The proximal anastomosis should be constructed as close to the renal arteries as possible to prevent disease progression in the remnant infrarenal aortic neck. If an end-to-side anastomosis is planned, more extensive aortic mobilization is necessary to control or ligate lumbar arteries that would otherwise backbleed (Figure 4).

Distal aortic exposure depends on the location of atherosclerotic disease. Identifying a soft spot for clamping is accomplished by palpating the distal aorta and common iliac arteries. The overlying peritoneum is incised and the vessel is exposed; however, circumferential control is not necessary. Minimizing the dissection in this region will decrease the chance of iatrogenic iliac vein injury as well as injury to hypogastric plexus and presacral nerves, which travel anterior to the aortic bifurcation. Damage to these nerves can result in impotence and retrograde ejaculation. To avoid damaging these nerves, the common iliac arteries are approached laterally and the overlying nerve plexus is swept upward and toward the midline.

Tunnels are then created from the peritoneal cavity toward each groin incision. Careful blunt dissection ensues directly anterior to the external iliac arteries, with the goal of joining the previously created tunnels from the groin. It is critical that this dissection proceeds directly on the surface of the vessel so as not to incorporate the ureter or its encompassing tissues into the tunnel. Doing so could cause renal failure, as the graft can obstruct the ureter. On the left side, the tunnel is created deep to the sigmoid mesentery. Working simultaneously from both the abdominal cavity and the groin incisions, a common tunnel is created and moist umbilical tape or Penrose drains are passed with a curved aortic clamp.

After controlling the critical vessels and creating tunnels, the aorta is palpated carefully for soft, compressible segments in preparation for clamping. Atraumatic vascular clamps are selected carefully and typically applied in an anterior to posterior fashion because the posterior wall is usually heavily calcified. Such a technique minimizes the chance of emboli. A bifurcated graft is chosen to match the size of the aorta and femoral vessels; usually an 18- × 9-mm or 16- × 8-mm graft is selected. Knitted polyester grafts (Dacron) that are collagen coated or presealed are used most often, given their excellent handling and hemostatic properties. Finally, before clamping, an intravenous bolus (70 to 100 units/kg) of heparin sodium is administered. Additional doses of heparin may be required during the operation based on serial measurement of the activated clotting time (goal is 250 to 350 seconds).

The proximal anastomosis then is constructed using 3-0 monofilament polypropylene sutures, preferably in an end-to-end fashion, after excising a portion of the aorta (2 to 4 cm) that is superior to the IMA. This provides space for the main body of the graft to lie flat in the retroperitoneum and permits for retrograde perfusion of the IMA. The distal segment of the aorta is oversewn or stapled, although stapling can malfunction if the aorta is heavily diseased. The graft

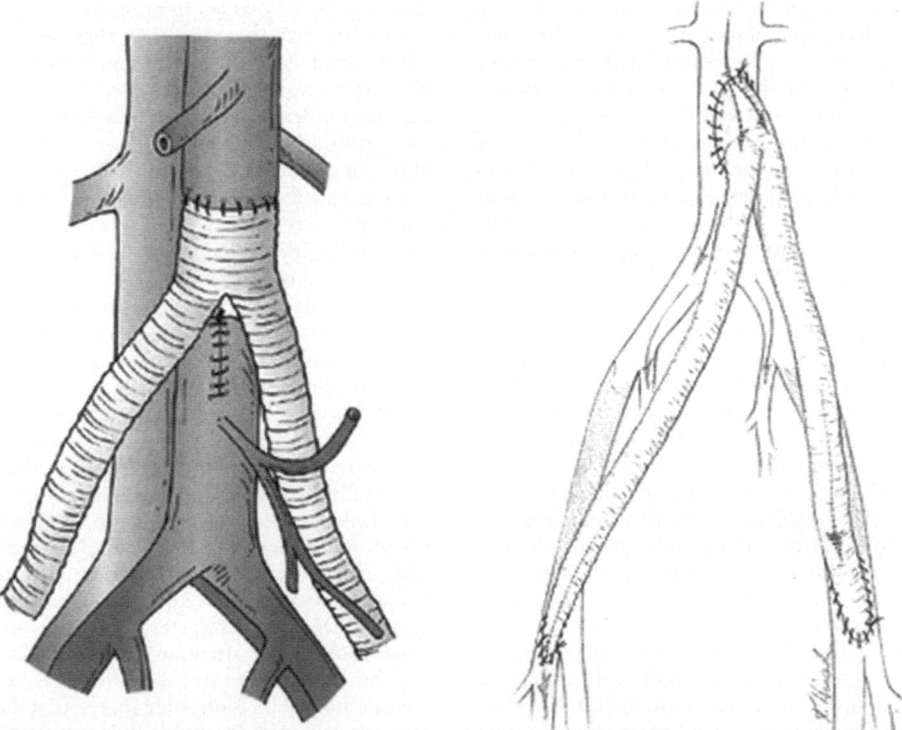

FIGURE 4 The proximal anastomosis. By resecting a short segment of aorta, the end-to-end proximal anastomosis lies flat along the retroperitoneum. This configuration ensures nonturbulent flow at the proximal anastomosis and simplifies the retroperitoneal closure at the completion of the reconstruction. In situations where antegrade flow to the pelvis needs to be preserved, an end-to-side anastomosis is favored. *(Adapted from Cronenwett JL, Johnston, KW. Rutherford's Vascular Surgery. 7th ed. Philadelphia: Saunders; 2010; and Zarins CK, Gewertz BL. Atlas of Vascular Surgery. St. Louis: Elsevier; 2005.)*

thus may require clamping of the aorta and contralateral common iliac artery. Once the proximal anastomosis is complete, the graft is passed through the tunnel and the remainder of the operation is completed similarly to the AFB. It is important to stress that this operation is done rarely today because aortoiliac disease is typically bilateral and progresses with time.

Extra-Anatomic Bypass

Extra-anatomic bypass procedures were developed to treat patients with excessively high operative risk due to concomitant cardiopulmonary disease or those with a "hostile" abdomen or infected prosthetic vascular grafts. These procedures, namely the femorofemoral bypass (FFB), can minimize pulmonary complications by being performed under local or regional anesthesia. In general, postoperative complications are less frequent with extra-anatomic bypass procedures, but their long-term patency is not as durable as the AFB. Multiple extra-anatomic techniques can be used, but this chapter focuses only on the two most common procedures: the FFB and the axillobifemoral bypass (AxBF).

Femorofemoral Bypass

FFB traditionally has been an option only in patients who have unilateral iliac occlusive disease because its function is dependent on the patency and inflow of the contralateral limb. This principle has evolved over time, however, given the increased application of endovascular therapies. Now, hybrid procedures can be performed whereby focal stenoses in the donor iliac system are first stented, followed by creation of a FFB graft.

The operation begins with bilateral longitudinal groin incisions because this orientation provides the best exposure of the femoral arteries, which usually is required when treating occlusive disease. Oblique incisions, albeit associated with fewer wound complications, are less versatile. Once proximal and distal control of the femoral vessels is obtained, a tunnel is created using both blunt dissection and a curved clamp in the prefascial subcutaneous plane overlying the pubis. Tunneling anterior to the fascia eliminates the chance of injury to the bowel or bladder. Several graft configurations have been described, with the "inverted C" (also termed the "inverted U") being the most common. Regardless of the configuration, it is critical to ensure that the graft does not become kinked. Allowing some redundancy in the length of the graft, making the tunnel a continuous curve, and sewing the toe of the anastomosis distally on the common femoral artery are various techniques to prevent graft kinking. After administering intravenous heparin and keeping in mind the aforementioned strategies, the femoral vessels are clamped, an end-to-side anastomosis is created, and the graft is passed through the tunnel and trimmed to length with it fully distended. Then the contralateral anastomosis is fashioned in an end-to-side manner.

Axillobifemoral Bypass

The AxBF is used almost always in ill, older patients with infrarenal aortic or iliac occlusive disease resulting in critical limb ischemia. In addition, this procedure can be used in patients with secondary disease processes such as "hostile" abdomens, previous radiation therapy, intestinal stomas, infected prosthetic arterial grafts, or aortoenteric fistulae. Unlike the FFB, general anesthesia typically is required.

Ability to perform an AxBF is predicated on a healthy axillary artery that can provide sufficient inflow to both the ipsilateral arm and both legs. The right axillary artery usually is used, but blood pressure measurements should be obtained in both arms preoperatively. Outflow, albeit somewhat controversial, is of particular importance with regards to graft patency. Many argue that the durability of AxBF is superior to that of axillounifemoral graft because of increased blood flow in the former. Although this theoretically makes sense, some authors have found no significant difference between the two procedures.

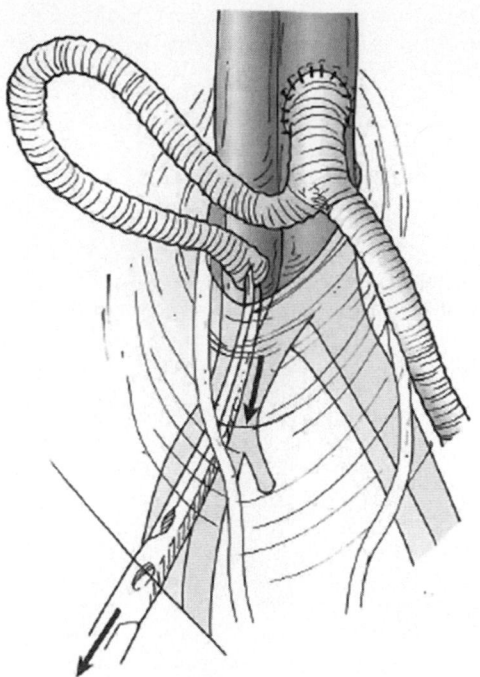

FIGURE 5 Tunneling of the graft limbs. The retroperitoneal tunnel is developed by blunt manual dissection under direct vision, taking care to establish a plane posterior to the ureter. After completion of the proximal anastomosis, the graft limb is passed through the tunnel with a curved aortic clamp. *(Adapted from Cronenwett JL, Johnston, KW. Rutherford's Vascular Surgery. 7th ed. Philadelphia: Saunders; 2010.)*

limbs then are flushed, rinsed with heparinized saline, clamped, and passed through the tunnels with an aortic clamp (Figure 5). Then attention is turned to the distal anastomoses, where an arteriotomy is made on the common femoral artery once clamps have been applied. Often the longitudinal arteriotomy extends onto the PFA and may mandate a profundaplasty (Figure 6). In cases where the SFA is occluded, it is crucial that the PFA is wide enough to accommodate a 4-mm coronary dilator. The anastomoses are constructed with 5-0 polypropylene sutures in a beveled end-to-side fashion, and before completion typical flushing maneuvers are used. Before unclamping the vessel, the anesthesia team should be notified of impending hypotension with reperfusion.

Assessing the adequacy of distal perfusion must occur before the reversal of heparinization with protamine sulfate (1 mg/100 units of circulating heparin). The quality of Doppler signals in the target artery as well as at the pedal level should be determined, along with the color and temperature of the feet. Once satisfied, hemostasis is achieved, the abdomen is irrigated, and the retroperitoneum is approximated over the graft to minimize the chance of developing a graft-enteric fistula. If the retroperitoneum cannot be closed primarily, a pedicle of omentum can be mobilized and secured over the graft instead. The fascia is closed and the groin wounds are irrigated and closed in multiple layers.

Iliofemoral Bypass

An iliofemoral bypass (IFB) begins in the same way as an AFB. After obtaining adequate femoral artery exposure and satisfactory clamping points, attention is turned to the iliac vessel. However, unlike the AFB, a retroperitoneal approach is almost always used for the IFB given the unilateral nature of the procedure. An oblique lower abdominal incision avoids potential injury to the presacral nerves and theoretically minimizes postoperative ileus. The proximal anastomosis can be complicated, depending on the extent of disease, and

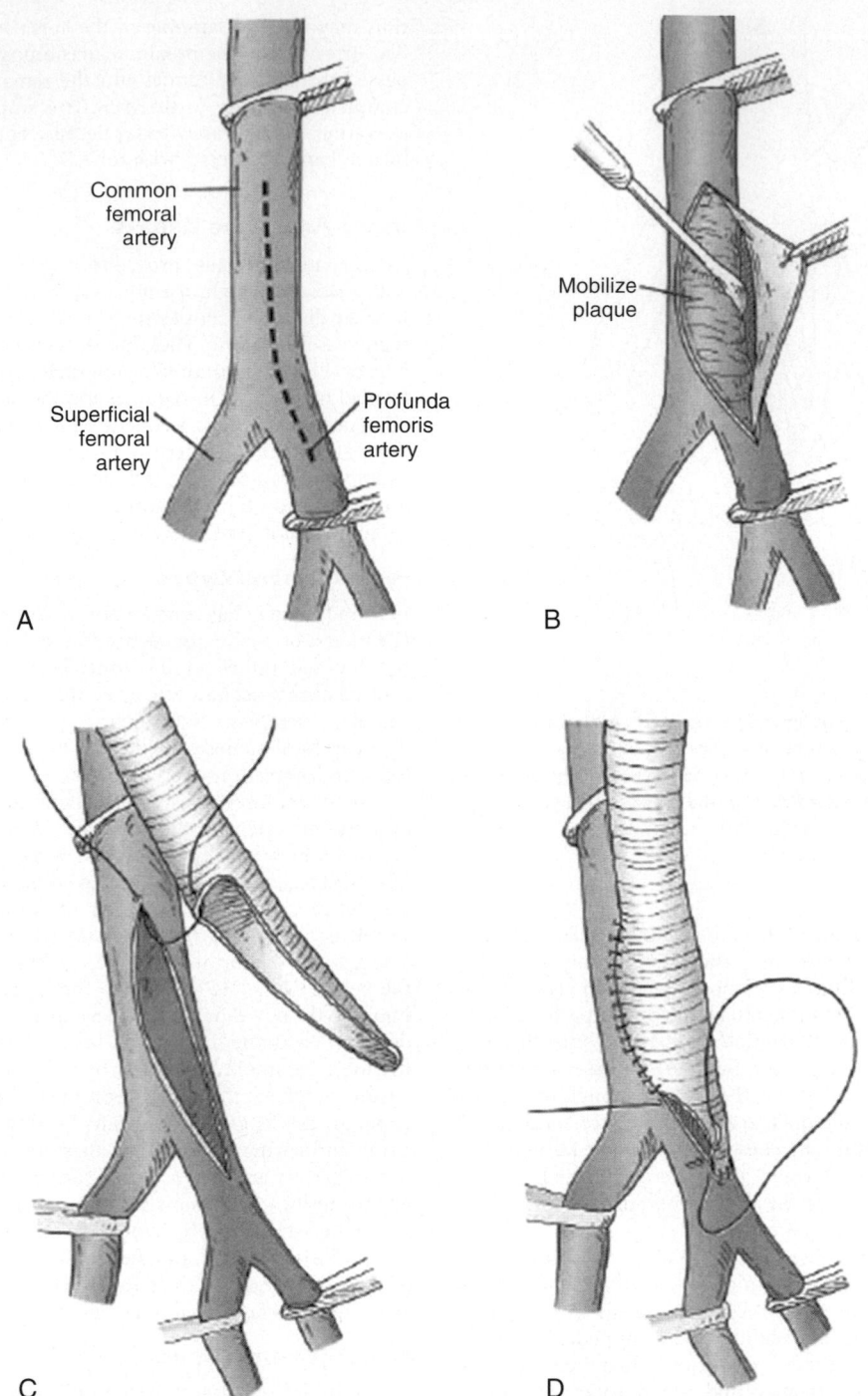

FIGURE 6 A to **D,** Adjunctive profundaplasty. Graft patency is optimized by maximizing the graft limb outflow. Concomitant disease of the profunda femoris orifice should be treated with limited endarterectomy and a profundaplasty using the toe of the aortofemoral graft limb. *(Adapted from Cronenwett JL, Johnston, KW. Rutherford's Vascular Surgery. 7th ed. Philadelphia: Saunders; 2010.)*

With the patient supine, a shoulder roll is placed between the scapulas and the arm is tucked to the side. After widely prepping and draping, an infraclavicular incision directed over the insertion of the pectoralis minor is made. The clavipectoral fascia is divided and then a muscle-splitting technique is used to dissect through the pectoralis major in order to divide the deep pectoral fascia and pectoralis minor. The axillary artery and vein then are encountered deep to this plane. The axillary artery is exposed from the clavicle medially to the pectoralis muscle laterally in order to deliver the artery into a more anterior position so that the anastomosis is not performed in a deep hole. Great care must be taken during the dissection and anastomosis because the axillary artery is very fragile and thus prone to laceration, dissection, and tearing (Figure 7). The common femoral arteries are exposed in the typical fashion, and a tunnel is created between the two as was described for the FFB. A tunnel then is created from the axillary artery to the femoral artery. The course is typically posterior to the pectoralis major muscle, then along the fascia of the abdominal wall in the midaxillary line, and anterior to the anterior superior iliac

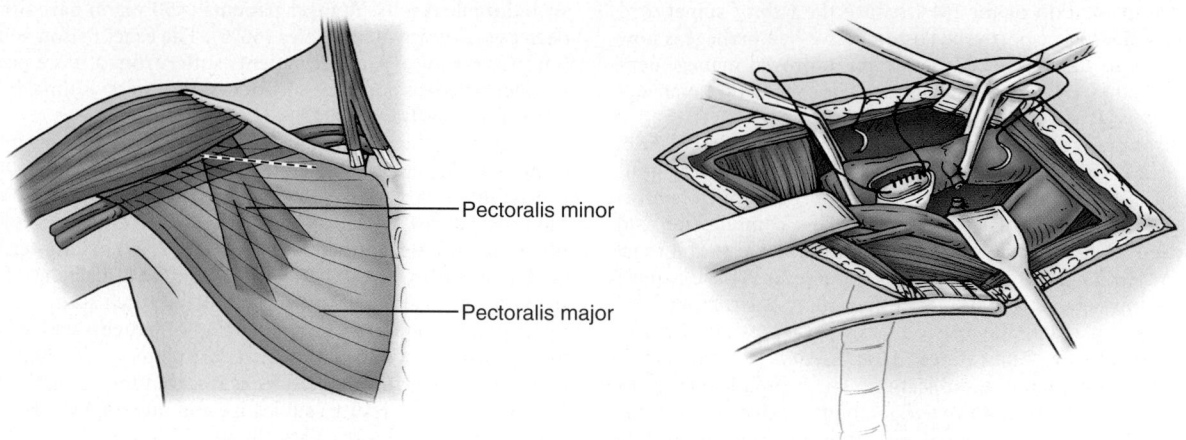

— Pectoralis minor

— Pectoralis major

FIGURE 7 Axillofemoral bypass. An infraclavicular incision overlying the insertion of the pectoralis minor is used to expose the axillary artery. The pectoralis minor is divided, exposing the second portion of the axillary artery. Dividing the deep thoracic artery allows for a generous mobilization and helps to deliver the artery upward into the surgical field, simplifying the anastomosis. *(Adapted from Zarins CK, Gewertz BL.* Atlas of Vascular Surgery. *St. Louis: Elsevier; 2005.)*

TABLE 1: Results of Direct Surgical Revascularization

Procedure	5-Year Patency	Perioperative Morbidity	Operative Mortality
Aortofemoral bypass	80% to 95%	10% to 30%	2% to 4%
Iliofemoral bypass	80% to 90%	10% to 25%	1% to 3%
Femorofemoral bypass	55% to 85%	10% to 25%	1% to 3%
Axillobifemoral bypass	50% to 75%	10% to 40%	1% to 4%
Axillofemoral bypass	45% to 70%	10% to 40%	1% to 4%
Iliac endarterectomy	80% to 90%	10% to 20%	1% to 3%

spine. An externally supported prosthetic graft (ringed polytetrafluoroethylene [PTFE]) usually is selected to prevent compression when lying on the side. The axillary anastomosis is created in an end-to-side fashion as far medially on the axillary artery as possible. A medially located anastomosis and building slight redundancy into the graft length minimize anastomotic tension when the arm is abducted. The femoral anastomosis is created in an end-to-side manner, and then the femorofemoral component may be placed by "piggybacking" the femorofemoral graft on the distal anastomotic hood of the axillofemoral graft. This configuration represents an inverted "C" or "U" that mimics the most common orientation seen in the FFB. Of note, preconfigured AxBF grafts are available, which eliminates an anastomosis and thus decreases operative time.

Other Surgical Revascularization Options

Aortoiliac endarterectomy was the earliest standard therapy for AIOD. Despite its excellent results, its use diminished once prosthetic grafts were popularized and the long-term durability of AFB was demonstrated. Nonetheless, this technique has some advantages, including the avoidance of prosthetic material, which eliminates future concerns of infectious complications, and arguably improved flow to the hypogastric vessels. As such, patients with erectile dysfunction may be better served with this operation. Finally, some propose that an endarterectomy should be used in young patients with focal lesions in relatively small-caliber vessels. In reality, however, endarterectomy is now mostly of historical concern given the high

success rates of endovascular therapy for focal lesions and AFB for more diffuse disease.

Rarely, a patient may be a candidate for direct surgical revascularization, but the patient's infrarenal abdominal aorta is inaccessible. In this situation, and as long as the patient can tolerate the physiology of a thoracotomy, a thoracofemoral bypass can be used. This technique is challenging but yields excellent long-term results on par with AFB.

Complications of Surgical Revascularization

Improved perioperative management and more careful patient selection have made AFB a reliably safe procedure. In modern series, the perioperative mortality rate is as low as 1% (Table 1). However, the overall morbidity rate ranges from 17% to 35%. Wound complications (infection, hematoma, lymphocele) are some of the most common early complications, reported in up to 15% of patients. Cardiac complications, although less frequent (1% to 5%), are the most common cause of mortality. These events can be minimized with appropriate use of beta-blockers, statins, and aspirin. Chronic obstructive pulmonary disease and smoking are risk factors for the development of postoperative pulmonary complications, which develop in 7% of patients. Acute renal failure is relatively uncommon because clamps usually are placed in an infrarenal position. Injury to the ureters during dissection or graft tunneling is rare (<1%). Atheroemboli can be generated during clamping and flushing, which can lead to spinal cord or bowel ischemia. Preserving hypogastric artery flow and reimplantation of the IMA reduce the risk of spinal cord and colonic ischemia, respectively. Postoperative hemorrhage is now rare, occurring in 1% to 2% of cases, given improved management of bleeding diatheses, better intraoperative anticoagulation management, and superior prosthetic graft properties.

Graft thrombosis is the most common late complication of AFB, reported in 5% to 30% of patients. Occlusion of the entire graft is uncommon, but its development suggests progression of infrarenal aortic disease proximal to the graft. This complication can be minimized by placing the graft as close as possible to the renal arteries. Unilateral graft limb thrombosis is the more typical pattern seen. Its development usually results from outflow obstruction from neointimal hyperplasia at the anastomosis or progression of native femoral artery disease. Anastomotic false aneurysm formation is another late yet infrequent complication. These pseudoaneurysms arise from suture fracture, graft material fatigue, undue anastomotic tension, weakened recipient arterial wall after endarterectomy, and chronic infection. Graft infection occurs in less than 3% of cases but is a feared late complication given its high associated morbidity. The diagnosis usually is made based on examination findings (draining sinus tract, cellulitis, induration, abdominal tenderness), radiographic features seen on CTA, or leukocyte scanning. Another feared late complication associated with AFB is an aortoenteric fistula. The most common pattern occurs when the proximal aortic suture line erodes through the duodenum, which may result in catastrophic gastrointestinal bleeding. Ensuring that there is adequate tissue coverage between the graft and the overlying bowel at the time of the index operation is essential to prevent this devastating complication.

Most of the aforementioned early and late complications also can occur after extra-anatomic bypass procedures. Bowel and bladder perforations have been reported if creating a subfascial crossfemoral tunnel during FFB and AxBF procedures. Injury to the brachial plexus and showering of atheroemboli to the hand have been reported during AxBF. Finally, the graft can avulse off the axillary artery with abduction of the arm. As mentioned previously, this rare complication can be avoided by medial placement of the graft on the axillary artery and planning some redundancy in the graft length.

Result of Surgical Revascularization

The short-term and long-term results of AFB grafting are excellent, with modern series reporting 5-year and 10-year graft patency rates of 90% and 85%, respectively (see Table 1). These outcomes remain true regardless of indication (disabling claudication vs CLI), approach (transperitoneal vs retroperitoneal), or proximal anastomosis technique (end-to-end vs end-to-side). However, not all patients have

such durable results. Younger patients (<50 years) have dramatically decreased 5-year patency rates (66%). The exact reason is unknown, but perhaps these younger patients suffer from a more potent form of atherosclerosis and have a tendency to develop intimal hyperplasia more aggressively.

In general, the long-term results after extra-anatomic bypass procedures are acceptable but not as durable as with AFB. Often these procedures are reserved for critically ill patients who have shortened life expectancies, which can bias long-term results. A review of the literature indicates a broad range (45% to 75%) in long-term patency rates after AxBF. The wide-ranging results are likely a reflection of the varying patient population included in each study. For instance, series that include a greater proportion of patients with claudication as opposed to patients with CLI report better graft patency rates. In addition, typically AxBF grafting is reserved for "high-risk" patients, but this definition is often subjective and therefore patient comorbid conditions can differ dramatically in each series.

ENDOVASCULAR INTERVENTIONS

With the advent of higher resolution imaging, lower profile deployment systems, and self-expanding stents, the majority of patients with AIOD now can be treated safely with endovascular procedures. Indications for intervention include both patient-specific (claudication, CLI, atheroembolization) and lesion-specific (TASC classification) factors. Typically, percutaneous endovascular therapies are indicated for TASC class A and B lesions and progressively more for TASC class C disease. As mentioned previously, endovascular techniques can be applied cautiously to TASC class D lesions. Preprocedure noninvasive imaging is critical to identify the extent of disease, degree of calcification, and quality of access vessels. Such information will enable the operator to determine the best approach: ipsilateral retrograde, contralateral antegrade, transbrachial, or open femoral. Most commonly, common iliac artery disease is treated via an ipsilateral retrograde approach, whereas external iliac artery disease is best approached in a contralateral antegrade fashion.

Under ultrasound guidance, the common femoral artery is accessed using Seldinger's technique, taking care to avoid areas of calcified disease so as to minimize the chance of postprocedure retroperitoneal hematoma, pseudoaneurysm, or arteriovenous fistula development. A 5F sheath is inserted and an angled-tip, hydrophilic guidewire is advanced into the abdominal aorta. After heparinizing, a flush catheter (Omni Flush, pigtail) is inserted to the level of renal arteries and connected to a power injector, and aortoiliac arteriography is performed (Figure 8). Anteroposterior (AP) projections are obtained first, followed by oblique views of the pelvis to

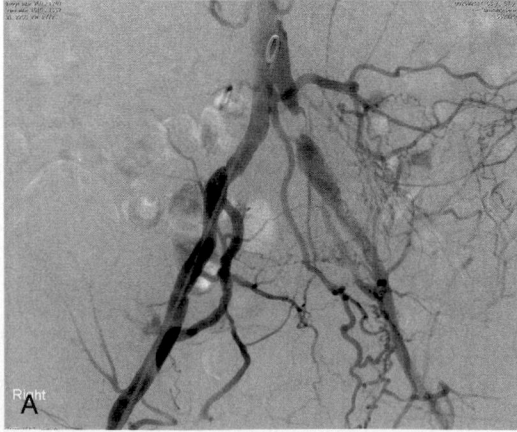 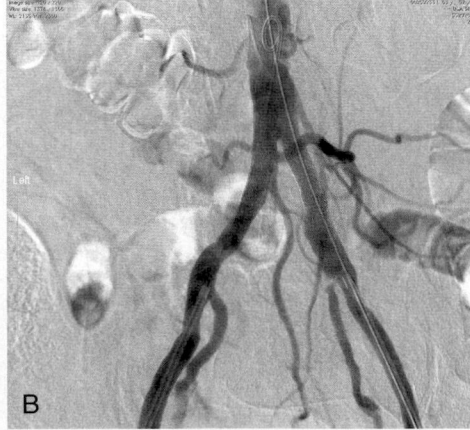

FIGURE 8 Diagnostic angiography and percutaneous intervention. A diagnostic angiogram shows a left common iliac stenosis, with extensive collateralization from the middle sacral and segmental lumbar arteries. **A,** Focal lesions are excellent candidates for endovascular interventions. **B,** Note the absence of collateralized vessels after the left common iliac lesion is treated with a stent.

better visualize the iliac bifurcation. A 50% stenosis is considered hemodynamically significant. If there is concern about the physiologic significance of a lesion, direct pressure measurements across the lesion can be used to more accurately estimate the degree of stenosis. When using the "pullback method," an end-hole catheter is withdrawn across a lesion. A resting systolic pressure gradient of at least 10 mm Hg is considered significant.

The lesion(s) of concern usually can be crossed with hydrophilic guidewires and catheters. However, recanalizing chronically occluded iliac vessels can be a challenge. A retrograde approach through the ipsilateral femoral artery permits "pushability" because the guidewires and catheters are not hindered by working around a curve. With this approach, however, the guidewire frequently finds a subintimal path, which can be problematic. Re-entry catheters, which aid in directing the guidewire back into the vessel lumen, have been developed and consequently have increased technical success rates. Re-entry into the aorta is not an issue when accessing the lesion in an antegrade fashion from the contralateral femoral artery; instead, "pushability" is lost at the bifurcation, and thus engaging the subintimal plane at the occlusion is difficult. Given these limitations, a transbrachial approach can be helpful in the setting of flush common iliac artery occlusion. This approach, albeit with better "pushability" and decreased dissection risk, has shortcomings as well. Specifically, an open brachial cutdown often is required given the relatively large sheath size necessary for stenting, and navigating the aortic arch has mechanical disadvantages and atheroembolic risk.

The lesion's length, location, and degree of calcification determine whether angioplasty is performed alone or in conjunction with the insertion of either a balloon-expandable or a self-expanding stent. Balloon-expandable stents have high radial strength and can be deployed with superior precision. However, these stents are less flexible and can become deformed by external force; thus self-expanding stents are used if they need to traverse a tortuous path. Stents are usually oversized by 10%, except when intervening on heavily calcified vessels that can rupture. Ballooning only one common iliac artery orifice can be hazardous, as this can cause the plaque to shift, thereby obstructing the contralateral iliac origin, or even dislodge, with distal embolization. As such, even in the presence of unilateral disease, simultaneous angioplasty of bilateral common iliac arteries is recommended. Ostial lesions of bilateral common iliac arteries or disease at the aortic bifurcation typically are treated with balloon-expanding "kissing" stents, taking care to not extend a generous portion of the stents into the distal aorta, as this may promote thrombus formation or hemolysis (Figure 9).

Because the external iliac artery is more mobile than the common iliac artery, balloon angioplasty alone is often sufficient when treating low-grade lesions. If stenting is necessary, self-expanding stents are selected because their flexibility minimizes the chance that they will be crushed if deployed in close proximity to the inguinal ligament. Covered self-expanding stents should be considered if the vessel is heavily calcified because such arteries are at high risk for rupture with aggressive angioplasty.

Finally, a hybrid technique is worth mentioning given its utility in patients with concomitant femoral artery disease. If preoperative imaging suggests significant femoral artery disease in conjunction with AIOD, an open femoral endarterectomy can be combined with endovascular iliac therapy. Most commonly, endarterectomy and patch angioplasty is completed first in order to not temporarily require inflow occlusion of the stent. Then either the patch is punctured directly or a sheath is introduced in the patch suture line before securing the patch. A wire is passed retrograde, taking care to not create a dissection plane, and iliac stenting proceeds.

Complications of Endovascular Interventions

Overall complication rates after percutaneous endovascular therapies are low. Most complications are related to contrast administration,

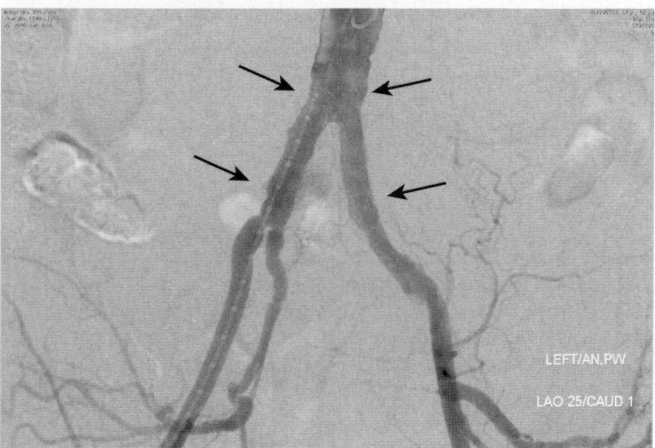

FIGURE 9 "Kissing" stents. Endovascular treatment of bilateral common iliac disease originating at or near the aortic bifurcation requires "kissing" stents. Simultaneous deployment of balloon-expanding stents avoids complications related to plaque shift during angioplasty. Well-positioned and appropriately sized stents do not encroach on the distal abdominal aorta or the contralateral limb.

sheath insertion, or some remote arterial process. Contrast-induced nephropathy is of particular concern in those patients who have baseline renal insufficiency. These patients should receive intravenous fluid hydration preprocedure and postprocedure, and contrast should be used sparingly during the procedure. Carbon dioxide angiography is another option for patients with chronic renal disease. Complications related to sheath insertion, including pseudoaneurysm and retroperitoneal hematoma, occur in 1% to 3% of cases. These complications can be mitigated by avoiding high or low punctures and properly using percutaneous closure devices. Arterial dissection, distal embolization, and arterial rupture are uncommon complications that typically arise from aggressive balloon dilatation of small, calcified vessels. If vessel rupture occurs, rapid reinflation of the balloon can be a life-saving maneuver while the correctly sized covered stent is selected and deployed.

Results of Endovascular Interventions

Although several factors, such as diabetes and renal failure, may influence outcome, long-term durability ultimately depends on the underlying burden of disease (Figure 10). As such, the TASC classification is important. For instance, TASC class A and B lesions have reported 5-year primary patency rates of 75% to 85%, whereas TASC class C and D lesions have reported 5-year primary patency rates of 65% to 75% (Table 2). Ongoing surveillance after percutaneous intervention with ankle-brachial indices or ultrasound is critical to maintaining long-term patency because many patients will require some form of reintervention. Patients who undergo angioplasty alone as opposed to primary stenting are more likely to have an early recurrence and require reintervention. Therefore many argue that it is more cost effective to treat with primary stenting at the time of the index procedure.

■ SUMMARY

AIOD is a frequent cause of claudication and CLI for which there are multiple safe and durable treatment options. Over the past 2 decades, endovascular interventions have become the initial treatment choice for many patients with AIOD, but their application can be limited by disease burden. As such, the AFB, especially in light of its excellent durability, should remain an essential surgical skill. Preoperative planning is fundamental to both direct surgical revascularization and

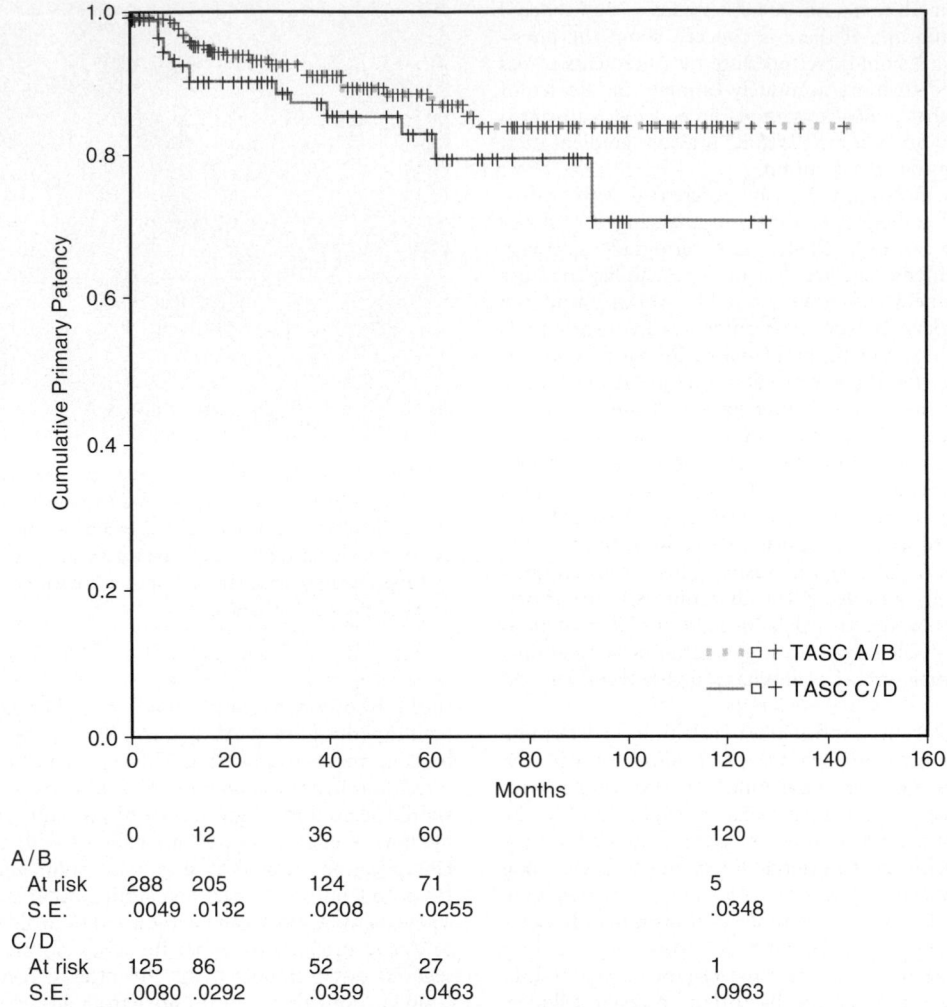

	0	12	36	60	120
A/B					
At risk	288	205	124	71	5
S.E.	.0049	.0132	.0208	.0255	.0348
C/D					
At risk	125	86	52	27	1
S.E.	.0080	.0292	.0359	.0463	.0963

FIGURE 10 Long-term patency of endovascular interventions. A retrospective review of 413 patients with aortoiliac occlusive disease treated with primary stenting was performed. Cumulative primary patency was 83% at 5 years. Long-term primary patency lessens with advancing patterns of disease. *S.E.,* standard error; *TASC A/B,* TransAtlantic Inter-Society Consensus II classes A and B; *TASC C/D,* TransAtlantic Inter-Society Consensus II classes C and D. *(Adapted from Ichihashi S, Higashiura W, Itoh H, et al. Long-term outcomes for systematic primary stent placement in complex iliac artery occlusive disease classified according to Trans-Atlantic Inter-Society Consensus [TASC]-II. J Vasc Surg. 2011;53:992-999.)*

TABLE 2: Results of Endovascular Interventions

TASC II Classification	Technical Success	Procedural Complications	5-Year Patency
TASC A or B	98%	5% to 10%	80%
TASC C	95%	5% to 10%	65%
TASC D	90%	5% to 10%	65%

TASC, Trans-Atlantic Inter-Society Consensus.

endovascular therapy because a successful outcome requires substantial forethought for each step of the procedure. Regardless of whether one proceeds with open or endovascular techniques, the treatment of AIOD ultimately will be unsuccessful unless risk factor reduction is emphasized preprocedure and postprocedure. In addition, it must be emphasized that atherosclerosis is a lifelong disease process, and thus these patients require frequent and close surveillance.

SUGGESTED READINGS

Leville CD, Kashyap VS, Clair DG, et al. Endovascular management of iliac artery occlusions: extending treatment to TransAtlantic Inter-Society Consensus class C and D patients. *J Vasc Surg.* 2006;43:32-39.

Norgren L, Hiatt WR, Dormandy JA, et al. Inter-society consensus for the management of peripheral arterial disease (TASC II). *J Vasc Surg.* 2007;45(suppl S):S5-S67.

Passman MA, Taylor LM, Moneta GL, et al. Comparison of axillofemoral and aortofemoral bypass for aortoiliac occlusive disease. *J Vasc Surg.* 1996;23:263-269.

Reed AB, Conte MS, Donaldson MC, et al. The impact of patient age and aortic size on the results of aortobifemoral bypass grafting. *J Vasc Surg.* 2003;37:1219-1225.

Sharafuddin MJ, Hoballah JJ, Kresowik TF, et al. Kissing stent reconstruction of the aortoiliac bifurcation. *Perspect Vasc Surg Endovasc Ther.* 2008;20:50-60.

FEMOROPOPLITEAL OCCLUSIVE DISEASE

Joseph-Vincent V. Blas, MD, Mark P. Androes, MD, and Spence M. Taylor, MD

Peripheral arterial occlusive disease (PAOD) affects more than 202 million people worldwide, with an estimated 27 million people affected in Europe and North America. Atherosclerosis is the cause in the vast majority of cases of PAOD. Other, less common causes include fibromuscular dysplasia, inflammatory arteritides, entrapment syndromes, cystic adventitial disease, congenital vascular anomalies, and chronic compartment syndromes. Risk factors for PAOD are similar to those for other atherosclerotic conditions (e.g., coronary artery disease) and include age, tobacco use, gender, ethnicity, diabetes, hypertension, dyslipidemia, a family history of PAOD, renal disease, and hyperhomocysteinemia. The prevalence of PAOD increases progressively with age, with up to 15% of patients older than age 70 affected. PAOD historically has been cited as having a male gender predilection; however, some studies have shown higher disease prevalence in women. Tobacco use is a powerful risk factor for PAOD. It has a dose-related association with development and severity of PAOD. The clinical manifestations of PAOD depend on the location(s) and severity of the disease. PAOD may be asymptomatic and discovered incidentally or may range from activity-induced pain (e.g., claudication) to critical limb ischemia (CLI). The natural history of PAOD depends on the severity of disease. PAOD remains a strong predictor of future adverse cardiovascular outcomes and death. All-cause mortality and cardiovascular mortality in patients with PAOD at 5 years was 19% and 7.3%, respectively, in asymptomatic patients, and 24% and 7.7%, respectively, in symptomatic patients. Patients with asymptomatic PAOD or intermittent claudication show little to no progression to a state of CLI. The estimated risk of major amputation in patients with intermittent claudication is 7% over a 5-year period and 12% over a 10-year period (~1% per year). CLI is defined as ischemic rest pain, ulceration, or gangrene. Twenty-five percent of patients with CLI die of a cardiovascular event within 1 year of diagnosis. Limb amputation occurs in 25% of patients with CLI. Premature atherosclerosis deserves mention. It is defined as PAOD developing before age 50 years. Amputation rates and mortality are worse for this group compared with older patients with PAOD. This chapter focuses on PAOD specifically in the femoropopliteal artery distribution.

■ DIAGNOSTIC EVALUATION

A thorough history and physical examination is paramount. Identification of risk factors associated with PAOD is crucial, as risk factor modification is a cornerstone of treatment for PAOD. The femoropopliteal segment is defined as beginning at the common femoral artery (at the inguinal ligament) and ending in the popliteal artery (at the origin of the tibial vessels). Femoropopliteal PAOD may be seen in three different ways: asymptomatic (incidentally diagnosed), intermittent claudication, or CLI. Intermittent claudication (from the Latin *claudicare*, meaning "to limp") manifests as stereotypical, reproducible calf pain or cramping with activity. Patients will report aching, cramping calf pain at a certain distance, which readily abates with rest. The patient is then able to walk the same distance before the pain begins again. *Pseudoclaudication* is typified by pain that is position dependent, not stereotypically associated with or reproducible with activity. Causes of pseudoclaudication include spinal stenosis or neurogenic issues (e.g., sciatic nerve impingement or diabetic neuropathy). CLI includes ischemic rest pain, ulceration, or gangrene. Ischemic rest pain is manifest as forefoot pain occurring at rest resulting from the severe lack of blood flow. Patients often will report a history of dangling the extremity to allow gravity to assist blood flow to the foot. The foot and lower leg may be edematous and ruborous (dependent rubor). Typical ulcers secondary to arterial insufficiency appear on the distal toes and over bony prominences. They may be exquisitely painful and have irregular margins with a pale, necrotic base.

In many cases, a clinical history and thorough physical examination are sufficient to diagnose femoropopliteal PAOD. Supportive diagnostic and potentially therapeutic tests can help to quantify the degree of ischemia and to plan an interventional strategy. The ankle-brachial index (ABI) is the calculated ratio of the ankle systolic pressure in each leg divided by the highest brachial artery systolic pressure. A normal ABI is between 0.9 and 1.1. With a compatible history, ABIs less than 0.9 are diagnostic of PAOD. In general, the ABI correlates to symptoms and severity of disease:

- Claudication ABI typically is between 0.4 and 0.9.
- Rest pain or tissue loss ABI is less than 0.4.

An ABI greater than 1.1 may be seen in cases where the lower extremity arteries are calcified (such as in patients with diabetes or end-stage renal disease). Other tests used in this scenario include digital toe pressures, transcutaneous oximetry, and pulse volume recordings.

■ MEDICAL TREATMENT

Treatment options are divided into medical, endovascular, open surgical, a combination of endovascular and open surgical (hybrid approach), and primary amputation. Medical management is the cornerstone of treatment of PAOD to reduce future cardiovascular morbidity and mortality. Risk factor modification includes smoking cessation, treatment with antiplatelet medication (e.g., aspirin, clopidogrel), statin therapy, antihypertensive medication, and diabetic blood sugar control. In addition to risk factor modification, cilostazol (a phosphodiesterase inhibitor) or naftidrofuryl (a 5-hydroxytryptamine$_2$ receptor antagonist; not available in the United States) may provide symptomatic improvement in patients with claudication. Finally, exercise programs have been proven effective for improving walking distance in those with claudication, with supervised exercise programs being more effective than unsupervised programs. In general, exercise should be performed at least three times a week for a duration of 30 to 45 minutes. Patients should be encouraged to exercise to a point where their claudication symptoms appear.

Medical management should be used in all patients with femoropopliteal PAOD. However, intervention beyond medical management should be undertaken on a case-by-case basis, taking into account the presenting symptom(s) and the natural history of the stage of disease of each patient. The goals of revascularization differ between patients with claudication and those with CLI and should be factored into the decision to undergo intervention.

■ ENDOVASCULAR TREATMENT

The endovascular options for treatment of femoropopliteal PAOD continue to evolve, and the armamentarium of the interventionalist continues to expand. To date, landmark studies to assist in patient selection and/or treatment algorithms have not been published. The BEST-CLI (Best Endovascular Versus Best Surgical Therapy in Patients with Critical Limb Ischemia) trial is a multicenter, randomized clinical trial comparing best endovascular therapy with best surgical therapy in patients eligible for both. The objective is to provide clinical guidance for treatment in patients with CLI. The landmark BASIL (Bypass Versus Angioplasty in Severe Ischaemia of the Leg) trial, published in 2005, showed that endovascular therapy (angioplasty alone) was associated with reduced early mortality and morbidity when compared with open surgical therapy (bypass). Currently, the Inter-Society Consensus for the Management of Peripheral Arterial Disease (TASC II) classifies disease in the femoropopliteal distribution into four groups based on anatomic complexity (Figure 1). The guidelines recommend endovascular therapy first for relatively short and simple type A and type B lesions. Surgery-first treatment is recommended for more complex type C lesions, though endovascular-first revascularization can be considered. Finally, surgery is recommended as the preferred approach to treat type D lesions: long, chronic total occlusions of the common femoral, superficial femoral, and popliteal arteries. However, modern endovascular techniques allow all TASC lesions to be approached with a percutaneous strategy.

Endovascular therapy typically is performed with intravenous sedation and local anesthesia. The general approach to an endovascular intervention involves the following steps:

- Establishing arterial access
- Diagnostic arteriogram
- Identifying the culprit lesion(s)
- Successful traversal of the lesion(s)
- Balloon angioplasty with or without the adjunctive use of stents
- Completion arteriogram to assess result
- Successful closure of the arterial access site

Establishing Arterial Access

Successful endovascular intervention begins with appropriate, safe establishment of intra-arterial wire access. Anatomic site for access is dictated by the anticipated site of intervention. In general, the contralateral groin is chosen as the site of access. From this point, the entire contralateral femoropopliteal artery segment can be intervened upon successfully. When intervention is planned more distally, alternative access may be needed. The contralateral common femoral

Type A Lesions

- Single stenosis ≤10 cm in length
- Single occlusion ≤5 cm in length

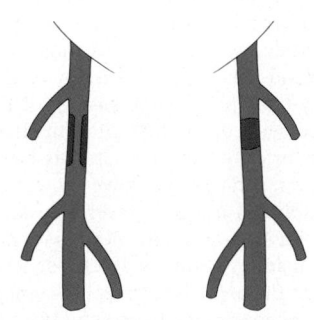

Type B Lesions

- Multiple lesions (stenosis or occlusions), each ≤5 cm
- Single stenosis or occlusion ≤15 cm not involving the infrageniculate popliteal artery
- Single or multiple lesions in the absence of continuous tibial vessels to improve inflow for a distal bypass
- Heavily calcified occlusion ≤5 cm in length
- Single popliteal stenosis

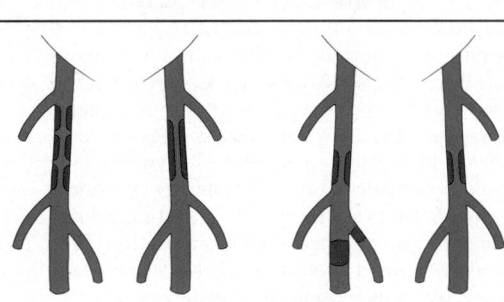

Type C Lesions

- Multiple stenosis or occlusions totaling >15 cm with or without heavy calcification
- Recurrent stenosis or occlusions that need treatment after two endovascular interventions

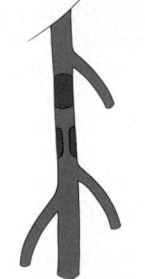

Type D Lesions

- Chronic total occlusions of CFA or SFA (>20 cm, involving the popliteal artery)
- Chronic total occlusion of popliteal artery and proximal trifurcation vessels

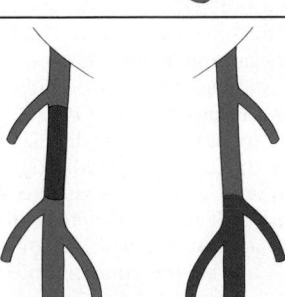

FIGURE 1 TransAtlantic Inter-Society Consensus (TASC II) classification of femoropopliteal lesions. *CFA*, Common femoral artery; *SFA*, superficial femoral artery. *(From Norgren L, Hiatt WR, Dormandy JA, Nehler MR, Harris KA, Fowkes FGR, TASC II Working Group. Inter-Society Consensus for the Management of Peripheral Arterial Disease (TASC II). J Vasc Surg. 2007;45 Suppl S:S5-S67.)*

artery (CFA) is chosen because of its caliber, consistent anatomic location, and ability to successfully close the puncture site. The CFA is located angiographically overlying the medial two thirds of the femoral condylar head. This allows for manual compression, should it be necessary. The CFA may be accessed by manual palpation of the arterial pulse, angiographically in the area of calcifications, or with the use of ultrasound. The technique chosen should take into account patient factors and the technical expertise of the interventionalist. Two forms of access needles exist: a standard 18-gauge puncture needle and a "micropuncture" small-caliber access needle. Once arterial access is accomplished, a 0.035-inch guidewire can be advanced into the iliac system and the aorta.

Diagnostic Arteriogram

After the guidewire is advanced into the aorta, a 5F 10-cm sheath can be placed into the CFA over the wire. A flush catheter then can be advanced over the wire to sit within the aorta for a diagnostic arteriogram. Arteriography of the lower extremities can be obtained by positioning the flush catheter above the iliac bifurcation and using a "bolus chase" technique. Traversing the bifurcation then can be accomplished with a variety of catheters to feed the wire into the contralateral iliac and femoral artery system.

Identifying the Culprit Lesion

Careful review of the diagnostic arteriogram helps to identify the culprit lesion and localize the area for intervention. Once a decision has been made for intervention, the patient should receive 50 to 80 U/kg of intravenous heparin. To perform intervention, we prefer exchanging the access 5F 10-cm sheath for a longer (45- or 55-cm) 5F or 6F sheath positioned at the level of the external iliac or CFA on the side of intervention. This allows for wire and catheter support for the intervention, magnified images, and more judicious use of contrast.

Traversing the Lesion

Stenoses and occlusions are different and should be approached in a different manner. In cases of stenosis, typically a steerable tip, angled, hydrophilic guidewire is chosen. The strategy should be to gently and delicately steer the guidewire tip through the stenosis. After traversal, an exchange or support catheter can be advanced over the wire through the stenosis. The wire then can be removed, and a small contrast injection can be done to confirm successful traversal.

Crossing an occlusion can be accomplished with several techniques. We prefer an angled support catheter in combination with a straight, stiff hydrophilic wire as the initial strategy for luminal traversal. At the proximal end of the occlusion is a firm, fibrous cap. The combination of a support catheter and hydrophilic guidewire allows for more penetration power to pass the cap. Once the occlusion has been traversed successfully with the wire, the catheter can be advanced past the lesion. Again, confirmation of successful traversal is done with a small contrast injection.

Subintimal traversal may be necessary. It involves passing a hydrophilic angled glidewire into the subintimal plane with a "loop" orientation. Again, catheter support is essential. Toward the end of the occlusion, the "loop" is shortened to provide a smaller profile to re-enter the luminal space. In addition, re-entry into the lumen may be accomplished with the use of a re-entry catheter (e.g., Outback [Cordis, Hialeah, FL] or Pioneer [Volcano, San Diego, CA]).

Balloon Angioplasty With or Without Adjunctive Interventions

Balloon angioplasty is performed with a balloon diameter that approximates the normal diameter of the reference vessel. The length of angioplasty is dictated by the length of the diseased segment,

taking care to avoid ballooning normal adjacent artery. In general, balloon angioplasty should be performed slowly and deliberately. This affords the best angiographic result and minimizes the potential risk for dissection. In general, angioplasty is most successful for short, focal lesions. After angioplasty, contrast injection is performed to assess the result. Evidence of suboptimal angioplasty result (e.g., elastic recoil, dissection, residual stenosis) should prompt stent placement. Self-expanding nitinol stents are preferred for the superficial femoral artery (SFA). A stent-to-artery ratio of 1.4 has been deemed optimal. Balloon angioplasty after stent placement is necessary for complete expansion. Then additional contrast injection is performed to document and assess the result.

Stenting in the popliteal artery segment deserves special mention. The popliteal artery is highly mobile because of its location across a joint. Stenting of this artery has been complicated by stent fractures and restenosis rates that are notoriously higher than rates in the SFA. Therefore placing a stent in this region should be undertaken with special consideration. The Supera stent (Abbott Vascular, Abbott Park, IL) has been shown to have favorable results in this highly mobile segment.

Viabahn (W. L. Gore and Associates, Flagstaff, AZ) is a self-expanding nitinol covered stent-graft lined with expanded polytetrafluoroethylene (PTFE). It is approved by the U.S. Food and Drug Administration (FDA) for use in the femoropopliteal artery segment. It contains a proprietary heparin-bonded technology lined on the luminal surface. Results from the VIASTAR trial comparing Viabahn with bare metal stents in long SFA lesions (>20 cm) show improved patency at 1 year in lesions treated with Viabahn. This technique sometimes is referred to as "endoluminal bypass."

An alternative to standard balloon angioplasty and stenting is the excision and removal of luminal plaque by atherectomy devices. Atherectomy may be done using several methods: ablation of atherosclerotic plaque (laser), longitudinal excision of the plaque (directional), or rotational excision of the plaque (orbital or rotational). The premise, however, is the same: removal of obstructive atherosclerotic or intimal hyperplasia to improve luminal caliber and vessel compliance. These techniques can be used alone or in combination with balloon angioplasty and/or stents. To date, there are no studies comparing efficacy of the FDA-approved atherectomy devices. Available data do not support the use of atherectomy alone, and studies to refine the role of atherectomy in modern practice are needed.

Successful Closure of the Arterial Access Site

The most common complications associated with endovascular interventions are access related. Therefore meticulous access site care is paramount for a successful endovascular intervention. There are a variety of closure devices at the disposal of the interventionalist. Choice is influenced by operator familiarity, size of access sheath, and the state of the access vessel. Refer to each device's manual for information regarding instructions for use and exceptions to its use. Manual pressure may be appropriate in certain situations (e.g., highly scarred groin, densely calcific access artery).

New and Emerging Technologies

Drug-coated balloons deliver paclitaxel, a chemotherapeutic agent, to the walls of the reference vessel during the angioplasty procedure. Recent studies have shown significant improvement compared with plain balloon angioplasty. One study has shown similar results to drug-eluting stents in long femoropopliteal lesions.

Drug-eluting stents have a chemotherapeutic agent mounted on the stent struts. Previous experience with sirolimus-eluting stents did not show improvement in the femoropopliteal region when compared with bare metal stents. Recently, Zilver PTX (Cook Medical, Bloomington, IN), a paclitaxel-eluting self-expanding stent, has been approved for use in the femoropopliteal segment. It has shown superior results when compared with angioplasty alone or with nitinol self-expanding stents.

Bioabsorbable scaffolds or stents are currently under investigation. The ongoing ESPRIT 1 trial was developed to evaluate the safety and efficacy profile of the Esprit BVS bioresorbable vascular scaffold system (Abbott Vascular, Santa Clara, CA) in patients with claudication and SFA or iliac lesions (ClinicalTrials.gov Identifier NCT01468974). Preliminary reported results show significant symptomatic improvement at 6 months and indicate improvement in rates of restenosis.

■ SURGICAL TREATMENT

Few studies exist comparing endovascular therapy with open surgical therapy to aid in decision making. Although the BASIL trial suggested an early improvement in morbidity and mortality in patients treated with endovascular therapy, in patients expected to live for more than 2 years, bypass with single-segment saphenous vein was superior to angioplasty alone. Again, the BEST-CLI trial may provide guidance in making treatment decisions.

The decision to perform open surgical revascularization should be based on the patient's comorbidities, long-term prognosis, severity or degree of ischemia, and anatomic complexity. Open surgical therapy is still considered the gold standard for ischemic rest pain or tissue loss. Surgical options in the femoropopliteal artery segment include endarterectomy and bypass.

We have published the Lower Extremity Grading System (LEGS) to assist in decision making for patients with CLI (Table 1). It was devised from specific anatomic and clinical factors in order to propose treatment using open surgery, endovascular intervention, or primary amputation. Cumulative scores between 0 and 9 recommend open surgical therapy, scores between 10 and 19 recommend endovascular intervention, and scores of 20 or more recommend primary amputation. The LEGS score appropriately predicted the actual treatment received in 90.6% of cases, indicating that creation of a standardization tool was feasible. Outcomes at 6 months demonstrated acceptable results for all patient cohorts with respect to patency, limb salvage, and quality of life measures. Finally, when the LEGS score was used to drive patient treatment compared with a nonstandard algorithm, our results (patency, limb salvage, and survival) indicated that patients treated with a standardized approach fared better than those who were not.

Endarterectomy of the common femoral and profunda (deep) femoral arteries (i.e., profundaplasty) can be utilized in certain situations. For successful bypass, adequate inflow site, adequate outflow site, and adequate conduit are necessary. When any one of these factors is not adequate, endarterectomy and profundaplasty may be a useful alternative. Furthermore, disease limited to the common femoral or profunda femoral artery is best approached with this strategy. CFA disease should be addressed at the time of bypass if the CFA will serve as the origin of the bypass. Older studies on isolated profunda femoral artery reconstruction showed improvement over a 1- to 2-year period in patients with claudication but not in those with rest pain or tissue loss. The success of isolated profundaplasty can be estimated using the profunda popliteal collateral index (PPCI), with indices less than 0.19 indicative of a good outcome with the procedure.

Superficial femoral endarterectomy largely has been supplanted by endovascular procedures and bypass procedures because of the well-established superior results of vein bypasses. It remains a viable option in certain situations, however. Open endarterectomy involves a longitudinal arteriotomy through which a standard endarterectomy is performed (similar to a carotid endarterectomy). The artery is closed with a saphenous vein patch, bovine pericardial patch, or some alternative patch material to increase the vessel's luminal diameter. Results are better for short lesions (<15 cm).

Remote superficial femoral artery endarterectomy (RSFAE) is a hybrid superficial endarterectomy procedure. The procedure involves the use of a wire loop ring stripper positioned in the subintimal plane. The stripper is advanced down the SFA, the specimen is removed, and the distal endpoint is tacked endovascularly with a stent. The REVAS (Remote Endarterectomy Versus Above-knee Bypass Surgery) trial compared RSFAE with above-knee femoropopliteal vein bypass. There were no significant differences in outcomes between the two groups. The conclusion was that RSFAE should be considered in patients with inadequate venous conduit.

Lower extremity bypass requires a good inflow source of blood, a good outflow target, and a suitable conduit. Single-segment autologous saphenous vein is the conduit of choice. Adequate saphenous vein should not have evidence of sclerosis and should be at least 3 mm in diameter. Alternative conduits include spliced autologous vein grafts (upper or lower extremity veins), polyester grafts (Dacron), PTFE grafts (with or without heparin bonding), and cryopreserved vein graft. Inflow source can be any artery without hemodynamically significant stenosis. The CFA most commonly is chosen as the source of inflow; however, if limited conduit length is an issue, the profunda femoral artery or the SFA may serve as the inflow source. If the CFA is chosen, hemodynamically significant CFA disease should be addressed at the time of bypass (e.g., common femoral endarterectomy). A good outflow target should be the least diseased vessel with contiguous flow to the foot. If ulceration is present, an effort should be made to revascularize the target artery that supplies the area where the ulceration is present (angiosome concept; Figure 2). Whether revascularization is done using the angiosome concept or not, the objective is to have direct blood flow to the foot.

Femoropopliteal artery bypass usually is performed under general anesthesia. Before the patient is prepared for surgery, the vein is identified and marked with an ultrasound. The patient is then prepped from umbilicus to the toes and circumferentially around the legs. The first priority is the vein harvest. A "bump" is placed beneath the ipsilateral knee. This allows the medial aspect of the thigh and lower leg to be approached with ease. Vein harvest can be done with one contiguous longitudinal incision or with skip incisions. Endoscopic vein harvest also can be done, but comparative results with open vein harvest have been disappointing. The saphenous vein should be handled meticulously. Tributaries are ligated with silk ties and divided sharply. Attention must be paid to the position of the silk ties on the saphenous vein tributaries. Placement too close to the vein will result in a purse-string effect of the adventitia, potentially causing a focal stenosis. After the appropriate length of vein has been dissected, it is transected sharply both proximally and distally and placed into a solution of heparinized saline. We prefer to transect the vein distally, approximately 2 cm distal to a sizable vein tributary. This allows us to use an "origin branch" technique at the proximal anastomosis (Figure 3). The vein stumps are ligated with silk sutures. Orientation of the proximal and distal parts of the vein should be maintained and marked. The vein then should be gently hydrostatically dilated. Small tributaries that were not previously ligated are repaired with fine polypropylene sutures.

Next, attention is turned to dissection of the inflow and outflow arteries. The CFA is dissected using either a longitudinal or an oblique incision. The dissection should carry to the inguinal ligament proximally. Silastic vessel loops are used to encircle the CFA, the profunda femoral artery, and the SFA. Additional smaller branches should be controlled with Silastic vessel loops or Potts vessel ties.

The distal target artery can be the above-knee popliteal artery or the below-knee popliteal artery. Dissection of the above-knee popliteal artery begins with a longitudinal incision placed along the anterior border of the sartorius muscle. The incision is deepened through the subcutaneous tissue and the muscular fascia between the vastus medialis anteriorly and the sartorius posteriorly. Division of the adductor tendon, which forms the border of the adductor hiatus, aids in exposure of the artery. The popliteal artery lies medial to its accompanying vein upon entry into the vascular sheath. An additional vein may lie on the lateral aspect of the artery, so care should be taken when dissecting the artery circumferentially. Small arterial

TABLE 1: LEGS (Lower Extremity Grading System) Score

Arteriographic Findings		Presentation		Functional Status		Comorbidities*		Technical Factors	
		Claudication	5	Ambulatory	2	Obesity	0	Redo surgery	2
AORTIC									
<3 cm aortic stenosis/occlusion or 3-5 cm stenosis of aorto-iliac bifurcation	8	Limb threatening ischemia	2	Ambulatory/At home only	3	High-risk coronary artery disease	2	Redo angioplasty	−2
>3 cm aortic stenosis/occlusion or 3-5 cm stenosis of aorto-iliac bifurcation	0			Non-ambulatory/transfer only	5	Age		Blind segment target	2
ILIAC				Non-ambulatory	20	>70	1	No venous conduit	6
TASC A or B	8					>80	2	No vein w/foot infection	8
TASC C	2								
TASC D	0								
or									
FEM-POP-TIB									
<5 cm occlusion/stenosis	5								
>5 cm occlusion w/distal target	0								
Isolated common/deep femoral stenosis	0								
>5 cm occlusion w/out distal target	6								
Possible score	0-8	Possible Score	2-5	Possible Score	0-20	Possible Score	0-7	Possible Score	−2-12

RECOMMENDED TREATMENT (SUM OF TOTAL SCORE FROM EACH COLUMN)

0-9: Open surgery
10-19: Endovascular
≥20: Primary amputation

From Taylor SM, Kalbaugh CA, Gray BH, et al. The LEGS score: a proposed grading system to direct treatment of chronic lower extremity ischemia. *Ann Surg.* 2003;237:812-818, discussion 818-819.

*If a heel ulcer and ESRD are present, double the score.

ESRD, End-stage renal disease; *Fem-pop-tib*, femoral-popliteal-tibial; *TASC*, TransAtlantic Inter-Society Consensus (type of lesion).

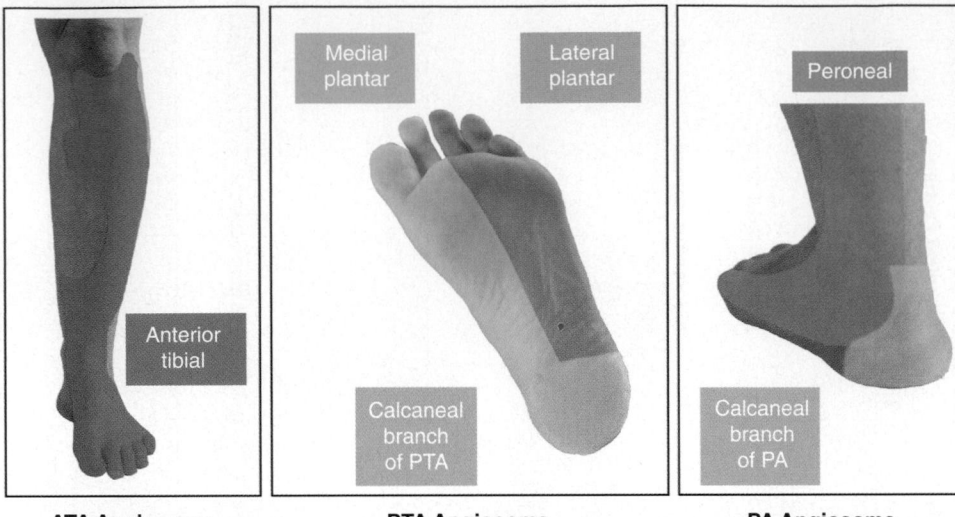

ATA Angiosome   **PTA Angiosome**   **PA Angiosome**

FIGURE 2 Angiosome concept. Six angiosomes of the foot and ankle are supplied by three main arteries. *Left,* The anterior tibial artery (ATA) becomes the dorsalis pedis artery that supplies the dorsum of the foot and dorsum side of the toes. *Middle,* Three main branches of the posterior tibial artery (PTA) supply distinct portions of the sole: the calcaneal branch to the heel, the medial plantar artery to the medial foot, and the lateral plantar artery to the lateral midfoot and the forefoot. The PTA supplies the plantar side of the toes, the web spaces between the toes, the sole of the foot, and the inside of the heel. *Right,* The peroneal artery (PA) supplies the lateral border of the ankle and the outside of the heel. *(Iida O, Soga Y, Hirano K, Kawasaki D, Suzuki K, Miyashita Y, Terashi H, Uematsu M. Long-term results of direct and indirect endovascular revascularization based on the angiosome concept in patients with critical limb ischemia presenting with isolated below-the-knee lesions. J Vasc Surg. 2012;55:363-370.e5.)*

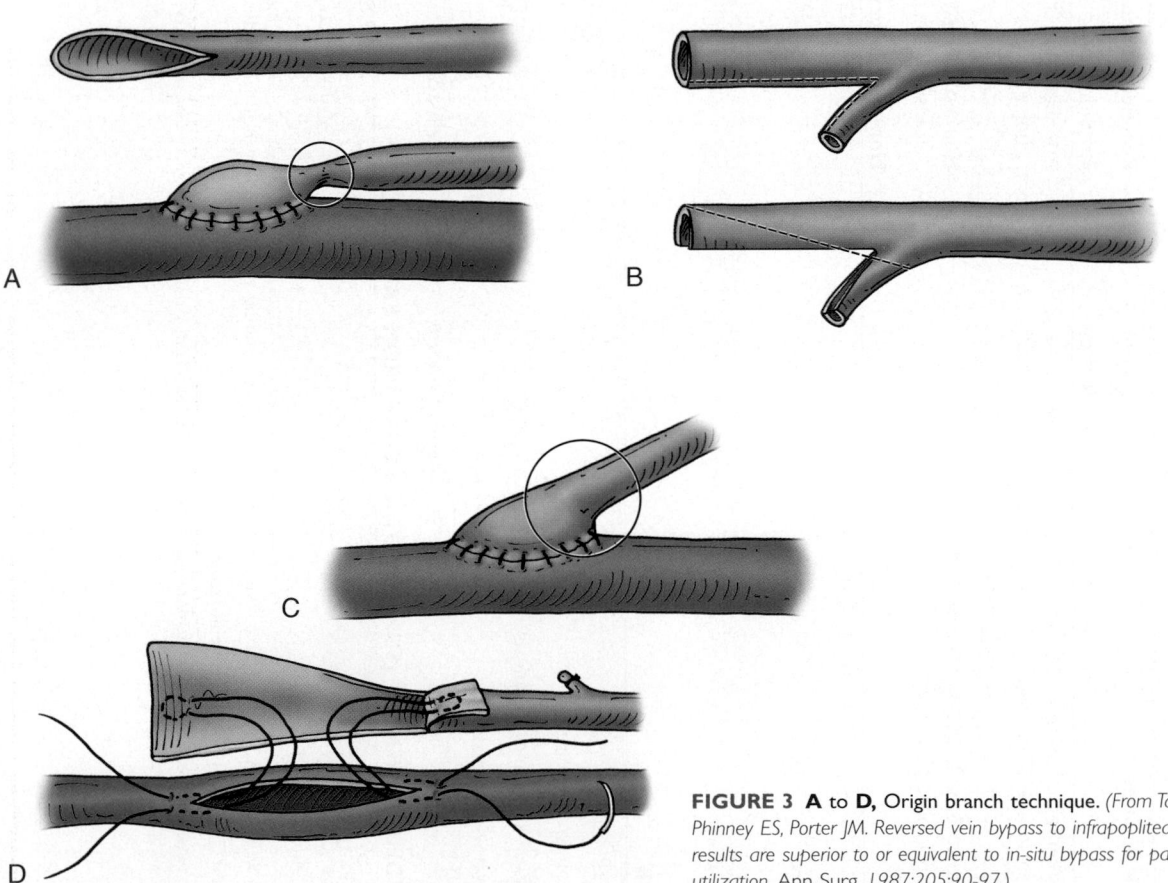

FIGURE 3 A to **D,** Origin branch technique. *(From Taylor LM Jr, Edwards JM, Phinney ES, Porter JM. Reversed vein bypass to infrapopliteal arteries: modern results are superior to or equivalent to in-situ bypass for patency and for vein utilization. Ann Surg. 1987;205:90-97.)*

branches should be controlled and not divided, if possible. Once the artery has been dissected circumferentially, it is controlled with Silastic vessel loops. Tunneling to the above-knee popliteal artery segment most commonly is done in an anatomic, subsartorius fashion. A blunt tip tunneler is passed from the distal incision toward the proximal incision in the avascular subsartorius plane. Care should be taken to ensure that the tunnel does not pierce the muscle, as this could lead to bleeding or compression of the vein graft.

If the below-knee popliteal artery is the intended distal target, the incision is positioned below the knee along the medial aspect. If this was anticipated before the vein harvest, the same incision can be utilized for both purposes. The incision should be placed 1 fingerbreadth posterior to the tibia and carried through the muscular fascia. After incising the muscular fascia, the gastrocnemius is identified and retracted posteriorly. Then dissection into the popliteal space is done bluntly. Further proximal exposure of the popliteal space can be obtained by dividing the tendinous attachments of the sartorius, gracilis, and semitendinosus muscles (the pes anserinus) in the superior aspect of the incision. These tendons may be marked with suture for eventual reattachment, although functional impairment after division is seldom seen. In this position, the popliteal vein(s) are encountered first. Dissection of the popliteal artery should be of sufficient length to accommodate the proximal and distal vessel loops or clamps and the eventual anastomosis. Tunneling to this position can be done in an anatomic or subcutaneous fashion. For anatomic tunneling, the blunt tip tunneler should be directed between the heads of the gastrocnemius and into the subsartorius plane in a distal to proximal direction. For a subcutaneous tunnel, care must be taken to ensure a gradual descent from the tunnel into the popliteal space, as often the entry can be made too acute and predispose to early graft failure from kinking.

Once the tunnel has been completed, the patient should be heparinized systemically with 80 to 100 U/kg of intravenous heparin. After adequate heparin circulation time is allowed (approximately 3 minutes), the common femoral, profunda femoral, and superficial femoral arteries and all other branches are occluded sequentially. A longitudinal arteriotomy is made in the CFA with a #11 blade and extended using angled Potts scissors. Endarterectomy is performed, if needed. Vein bypass may be performed in reversed or nonreversed fashion. Outcomes are equivalent. We prefer a reversed orientation. The "origin branch" technique is done using angled Potts scissors, with one tine placed through the distal end of the vein and advanced through the side branch allowing the cut to extend into the crotch of the branch (see Figure 3). Using double-armed 5-0 polypropylene sutures, the proximal anastomosis is done bidirectionally. The vein is allowed to distend with blood after loosening the vessel loops or clamps. It then is marked along one side to maintain orientation during tunneling. Then the vein is tunneled down to the distal incision in a distended state, and the tunneler is removed. Care is taken to ensure that the vein graft has not twisted or kinked. The distal anastomosis then is performed. Similar to the proximal anastomosis, the artery is occluded. A longitudinal arteriotomy is made and extended. The vein is measured for appropriate length and tension. It is spatulated along the wall to be used for the anastomosis. In this case, double-armed 6-0 polypropylene sutures are used for this anastomosis. Before completion, the artery and the vein graft are allowed to flush. Hemostasis is then assessed.

It is imperative to assess for graft patency. Direct assessment of distal pulses by palpation or continuous wave Doppler is a simple method of assessment. Otherwise, completion ultrasound or on-table arteriography can be performed for assessment of graft patency. Both completion ultrasound and arteriography can identify factors associated with early graft failure and can be used to aid in decision making for immediate graft revision.

Incisional closure is a particularly important step. Incisions should be made with as minimal blood loss as possible. Likewise, closure should be done meticulously. A layered closure is preferred, but there have been no studies assessing the optimal closure technique.

Negative wound pressure therapy may contribute to a lower incidence of groin wound infections.

Primary amputation may be appropriate in certain situations. A patient with long-standing functional impairment, with significant tissue loss, and who is not likely to return to ambulatory status may be best served by a primary amputation. Similarly, patients with a paralyzed limb, severe sepsis, contractures, short life expectancy, dementia, or end-stage renal disease *with* significant functional impairment also may be best served by primary amputation.

GRAFT SURVEILLANCE

A graft surveillance protocol for vein bypasses has been shown to be effective in maintaining graft patency. It is well documented that nearly one third of vein grafts will develop lesions that threaten patency. Loss of graft patency within the first 30 days typically implies a technical issue. Graft failure or impending graft failure within 1 to 2 years is usually the result of myointimal hyperplasia. Graft failure after 2 years is typically from progression of atherosclerotic disease, usually at the distal bed. Other factors associated with vein graft failure include young patient age, ethnicity (African American or Hispanic), a hypercoagulable state, redo bypass, CLI, ongoing tobacco use, and dyslipidemia. A graft surveillance protocol uses ABI and duplex ultrasound. The first study is usually done within 1 month of the index operation. Serial studies then are done every 3 months for 1 year, then every 6 months for 2 years, and annually thereafter. Grafts with evidence of impending failure may demonstrate:

- Focal elevated peak systolic velocity greater than 300 cm/s
- A peak systolic velocity ratio of 3 to 4 (PSV at the lesion: PSV proximal to the lesion) compared with an adjacent segment
- Low-flow velocities throughout the graft (<40 cm/s)
- A drop in the ABI of 0.15 or more from the previous study

Intervening on failing bypass vein grafts can be done via an endovascular or open surgical approach. Open surgical revision has been shown to be more effective for longer lesions (>2 cm), failures within 3 months of graft placement, multiple stenosis, or graft thrombosis. Focal stenoses are amenable to localized patch angioplasty. Tandem stenoses or longer segment stenoses are amenable to local excision and interposition graft placement. Stenotic lesions at the distal anastomosis may be amenable to either patch angioplasty or sequential ("jump") bypass grafting to a more suitable downstream target. The optimal conduit for these revisions is not standardized, and either autologous or prosthetic conduits may be used.

Balloon angioplasty is a low-morbidity procedure used to improve graft patency. It has been shown to be effective for select lesions; however, to date the outcomes remain inferior to open surgical revision. There is a higher rate of repeat interventions to maintain patency in vein grafts treated with balloon angioplasty. Cutting balloon angioplasty has not been shown to remarkably improve vein graft patency compared with simple balloon angioplasty alone. Drug-coated angioplasty currently is being investigated for vein graft stenoses.

Regardless of the technique chosen for vein graft revision, continued graft surveillance is imperative.

RESULTS

Previous comparisons of autologous vein and prosthetic femoropopliteal artery bypass to the above-knee popliteal artery were similar with respect to patency. More recently, a meta-analysis has shown that saphenous vein bypasses are superior to prosthetic bypasses in the above-knee segment (Figure 4). There is no doubt, however, that patency of autologous vein bypasses is far superior to prosthetic bypasses in the below-knee segment (Figure 5). In cases where autologous vein is not available for below-knee bypass, a PTFE graft with distal anastomotic vein cuff has proven superior to prosthetic distal anastomosis alone.

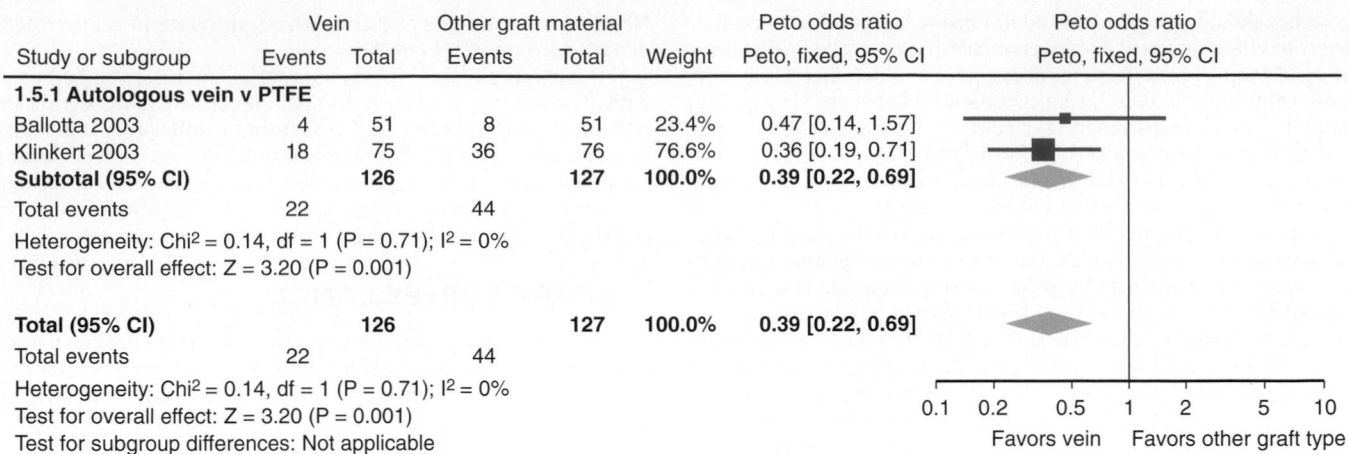

FIGURE 4 Meta-analysis of patency data in above-knee bypasses. *CI*, Confidence interval; *PTFE*, polytetrafluoroethylene. *(From Twine CP, McLain AD. Graft type for femoro-popliteal bypass surgery. Cochrane Database Syst Rev. 2010:CD001487.)*

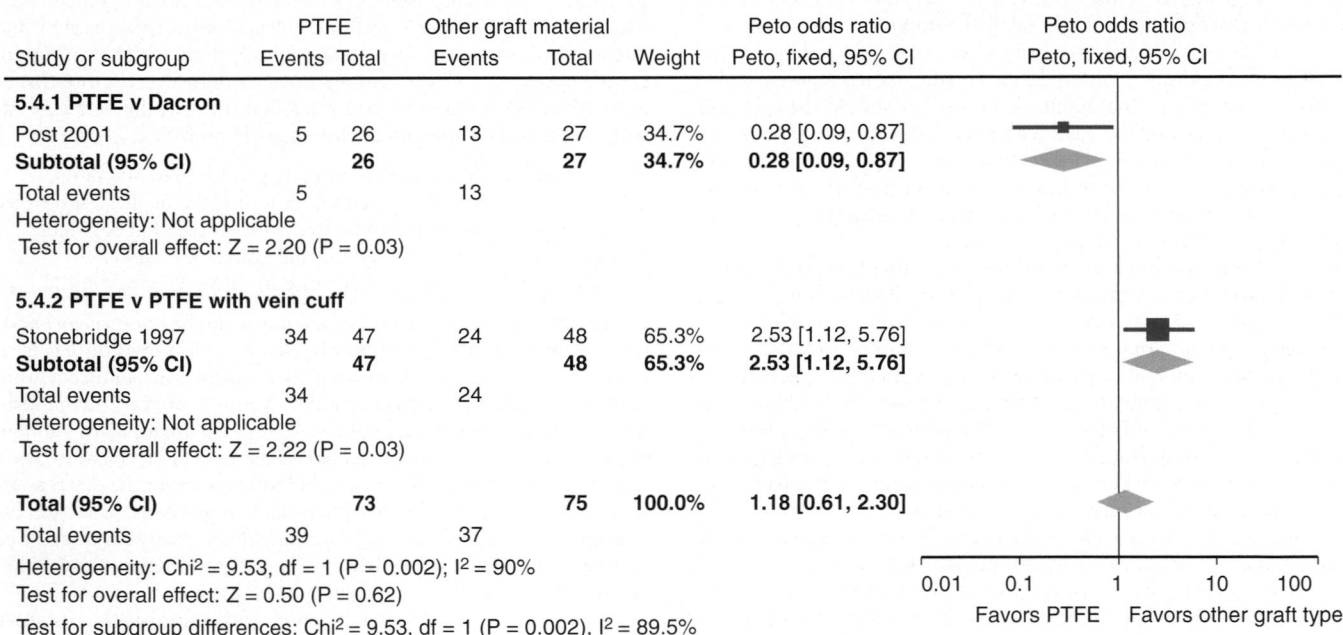

FIGURE 5 Meta-analysis of patency data in below-knee bypasses. *CI*, Confidence interval; *PTFE*, polytetrafluoroethylene. *(From Twine CP, McLain AD. Graft type for femoro-popliteal bypass surgery. Cochrane Database Syst Rev. 2010:CD001487.)*

■ SUMMARY

Femoropopliteal PAOD is defined by disease in the infrainguinal region to the popliteal artery. Patients may have no symptoms with intermittent claudication or with CLI. A thorough history and physical examination is paramount for diagnosis and may be aided by the use of noninvasive vascular laboratory studies, including ankle-brachial indices and duplex ultrasound examination. The cornerstone of treatment is risk factor modification. Symptomatic improvement may be accomplished with cilostazol and an exercise program. Intervention can be divided into endovascular, open surgical, or hybrid approaches. Sound judgment should be exercised when choosing the type of intervention and should be dictated by patient comorbidities, anatomic complexity, and disease severity. Endovascular therapy includes balloon angioplasty with or without stenting, and newer alternative treatments are available at the operator's disposal. As such, the endovascular options continue to expand and evolve. Surgical options include endarterectomy or bypass, and

surgery remains the gold standard for patients with ischemic rest pain or tissue loss. The ongoing BEST-CLI trial is attempting to answer questions regarding an optimal treatment strategy.

SUGGESTED READINGS

Adam DJ, Beard JD, Cleveland T, et al. Bypass versus angioplasty in severe ischaemia of the leg (BASIL): multicentre, randomised controlled trial. *Lancet.* 2005;366:1925-1934.

Androes MP, Kalbaugh CA, Taylor SM, et al. Does a standardization tool to direct invasive therapy for symptomatic lower extremity peripheral arterial disease improve outcomes? *J Vasc Surg.* 2004;40:907-915.

Attinger CE, Evans KK, Bulan E, Blume P, Cooper P. Angiosomes of the foot and ankle and clinical implications for limb salvage: reconstruction, incisions, and revascularization. *Plast Reconstr Surg.* 2006;117:261S-293S.

Hirsch AT, Haskal ZJ, Hertzer NR, et al. ACC/AHA 2005 Practice Guidelines for the management of patients with peripheral arterial disease (lower extremity, renal, mesenteric, and abdominal aortic): a collaborative report from the American Association for Vascular Surgery/Society for

Vascular Surgery, Society for Cardiovascular Angiography and Interventions, Society for Vascular Medicine and Biology, Society of Interventional Radiology, and the ACC/AHA Task Force on Practice Guidelines (Writing Committee to Develop Guidelines for the Management of Patients With Peripheral Arterial Disease): endorsed by the American Association of Cardiovascular and Pulmonary Rehabilitation; National Heart, Lung, and Blood Institute; Society for Vascular Nursing; TransAtlantic Inter-Society Consensus; and Vascular Disease Foundation. *Circulation.* 2006;113:e463-e654.

Kalbaugh CA, Taylor SM, Cull DL, et al. Invasive treatment of chronic limb ischemia according to the Lower Extremity Grading System (LEGS) score: a 6-month report. *J Vasc Surg.* 2004;39:1268-1276.

Menard MT, Farber A. The BEST-CLI trial: a multidisciplinary effort to assess whether surgical or endovascular therapy is better for patients with critical limb ischemia. *Semin Vasc Surg.* 2014;27:82-84.

Norgren L, Hiatt WR, Dormandy JA, et al. Inter-Society Consensus for the Management of Peripheral Arterial Disease (TASC II). *J Vasc Surg.* 2007;45(suppl S):S5-S67.

Taylor LM Jr, Edwards JM, Phinney ES, Porter JM. Reversed vein bypass to infrapopliteal arteries: modern results are superior to or equivalent to in-situ bypass for patency and for vein utilization. *Ann Surg.* 1987;205:90-97.

Taylor SM, Kalbaugh CA, Gray BH, et al. The LEGS score: a proposed grading system to direct treatment of chronic lower extremity ischemia. *Ann Surg.* 2003;237:812-818, discussion 818-819.

Twine CP, McLain AD. Graft type for femoro-popliteal bypass surgery. *Cochrane Database Syst Rev.* 2010;CD001487.

TIBIOPERONEAL ARTERIAL OCCLUSIVE DISEASE

John C. Eun, MD, and Natalia O. Glebova, MD, PhD

Approximately 8 to 12 million people suffer from peripheral arterial disease (PAD) in the United States, which rivals the prevalence of coronary artery disease. In 2001 U.S. Medicare spent more than $4.3 billion on PAD treatment; in the United States an estimated total of $21 billion was spent on vascular-related treatment, with the majority being treatment for PAD. PAD is a systemic inflammatory process that affects the entire arterial tree; however, the anatomic patterns of distribution are associated with specific patient demographics, medical risk factors, and symptoms. The symptoms of PAD are caused by inadequate blood flow to a skeletal muscle bed resulting from a more proximal flow-limiting arterial stenosis. Lower extremity claudication is defined as pain with exercise in the thigh or calf muscles that is relieved at rest. Typically patients with claudication symptoms alone do not have a greatly increased risk of limb loss. Critical limb ischemia (CLI) occurs when there is such limited blood flow to the leg that, even at rest, the metabolic demands of the tissue are not met. CLI is characterized by pain at rest or tissue loss (ulceration or gangrene). Patients with CLI are at risk of limb loss if interventions to restore arterial perfusion are not performed. Patients with a predominant distribution of athero-occlusive disease in the tibial and peroneal arteries are more likely to initially have signs and symptoms of CLI than are patients with proximal femoropopliteal disease secondary to the absence of collateral vessel flow to the foot. Revascularization in these patients is often challenging because of anatomic factors, disease severity, and patient comorbidities. Patients with tibioperoneal occlusive disease (TPOD) have a higher frequency (>60%) of diabetes mellitus and renal insufficiency as compared with patients with PAD in more proximal arterial distribution. These patients are also at significant risk for vascular disease of the coronary, cerebral, and renal arteries; thus when an intervention is planned, the surgeon must consider the patient's comorbidities in order to weigh the risks and benefits of the planned intervention.

■ PATIENT ASSESMENT

In the assessment of a patient with TPOD, a complete history and physical examination are critical for planning treatment. This evaluation should include an assessment of the patient's functional status with regard to current ability to ambulate, the patient's expectations of therapy, risk stratification for major adverse cardiac events (MACE), and the patient's social and home support. The 2014 American College of Cardiology/American Heart Association (ACC/AHA) guidelines outline the recommended perioperative cardiovascular evaluation. For patients who have less than a 1% chance of MACE, based on combined surgical and patient characteristics, no further cardiac workup is required. Several risk calculators are available online for convenient determination of a patient's cardiac risk, including one developed by the American College of Surgeons. Unfortunately the majority of vascular patients and vascular procedures are classified in the "elevated risk" category, in which there is a 1% or greater risk of MACE. If a patient has moderate or greater functional capacity, defined as four or more metabolic equivalents (classically described as being able to "walk up a flight of stairs"), then typically no further workup is required. In patients with CLI, such symptomatic evaluation is often limited, as patients often are unable to walk for any significant distance secondary to leg pain from critically poor blood flow, and this may preclude the identification of significant cardiac disease that would become apparent symptomatically if the patient was able to walk. If a patient has poor or unknown functional capacity and the results of further testing would influence decision making or perioperative care, pharmacologic stress testing is warranted, with subsequent coronary revascularization if an abnormality is found.

A thorough examination of the leg and foot helps to determine the likelihood of functional salvage. The examiner should note the patient's ability to walk, evidence of flexion contractures, or other neuromuscular disabilities that may affect ambulation. The presence of local infection, soft tissue edema, venous disease, and prior surgical incisions can influence the choice of intervention. Physical examination also should focus on the arterial perfusion of the symptomatic limb. The ankle-brachial index (ABI) is one of the most sensitive and reproducible tests used to diagnose PAD. An ABI of 0.9 or less signifies a hemodynamically significant stenosis. The ABI can be falsely elevated with calcified vessels; if the ABI is found to be 1.4 or greater, it is likely unreliable. In this case, the toe-brachial index (TBI) may be a more accurate tool to determine the presence of PAD (a TBI of 0.7 or less is indicative of a significant arterial stenosis). In general, CLI occurs at an ABI less than 0.4 or a TBI less than 0.5, but this is patient dependent. The examiner should note the presence and quality of the femoral, popliteal, posterior tibial, and dorsalis pedis pulses. The quality of femoral pulses is a crucial aspect of the examination because diminished femoral pulses reveal concomitant suprainguinal occlusive arterial disease, for which an inflow revascularization procedure would be indicated. Inflow disease involving the common and external iliac arteries should be addressed before or during distal revascularization. Likewise, an atherosclerotic common femoral artery can be reconstructed with endarterectomy at the time of bypass. A palpable pulse in the popliteal artery usually indicates absence of flow-limiting proximal stenosis or occlusion in the femoral artery. This is a common finding in young diabetic patients who have disease predominantly in the tibial and peroneal arteries. Dorsalis pedis and posterior tibial pulses often are not palpable in patients with TPOD, and Doppler assessment with a handheld probe is most helpful. Triphasic signals indicate normal arterial wall transduction of systolic and diastolic pressures; transduction signals become attenuated to a biphasic pattern with mild to moderate disease and become monophasic with severe disease. Absence of hair and shiny tone of the skin on the lower leg reflect chronic arterial insufficiency, and evidence of ulceration is a sign of severe ischemia and potential limb loss. Along with a thorough physical examination, preoperative laboratory tests are conducted, with particular attention to renal function, in anticipation of imaging studies with contrast materials that may be nephrotoxic.

The vascular laboratory is a crucial adjunct to the preoperative evaluation. Not only can the vascular laboratory provide ABIs and TBIs, but arterial perfusion also can be estimated from segmental blood pressures measured at the upper thigh, middle thigh, calf, and ankle. A pressure change greater than 30 mm Hg between each segment indicates an intervening flow-limiting stenosis and is helpful to determine the level of disease. Critical levels of ischemia are evidenced by an ABI less than 0.4 or an absolute pressure lower than 50 mm Hg as well as by toe pressures lower than 30 mm Hg. If a venous conduit is to be considered for surgical bypass, a duplex ultrasound of bilateral lower extremities should be ordered to ensure that the proposed vein is adequate, with a diameter of at least 3 mm throughout its length.

Once a patient is determined to have CLI, it is imperative to plan a revascularization procedure with endovascular techniques or surgical bypass because the risk of limb loss within 1 year of diagnosis is 40%. Although the perception is that amputation is a less morbid procedure in the patient with CLI who is at high operative risk, current data reveal that the 30-day mortality rates for endovascular intervention (2% to 8%) and surgical bypass (2% to 6%) in CLI are similar, whereas the rate is generally higher for primary amputation (6% to 12%). High-resolution imaging is essential for planning revascularization, regardless of whether a surgical or endovascular approach is being considered. Although computed tomographic angiography (CTA) is excellent in evaluating proximal arterial disease of the aorta, iliac arteries, and femoral arteries, it is limited in assessment of tibial disease because of the small caliber of vessels and frequent presence of arterial calcifications interfering with one's ability to distinguish between contrast and calcification. Digital subtraction angiography (DSA) with iodinated contrast material delivered via an intra-arterial catheter is considered the gold standard for evaluation of TPOD. DSA image quality is not compromised by calcification of the arterial wall, and selective catheter placement in the external iliac or femoral arteries can provide high-quality images of the tibial vessels, which can be difficult to evaluate with other modes of imaging. If a tibial bypass is planned, we recommend a diagnostic angiogram, which can be done either before the day of surgery or concomitantly with the planned bypass to verify the suitability of the bypass target. In diabetic patients and patients with renal insufficiency, nephrotoxicity of iodinated contrast material can be minimized with preprocedure and postprocedure hydration with normal saline, administration of acetylcysteine, and selection of a nonionic contrast agent. Carbon dioxide gas also can be used as a contrast agent during angiography; although it is adequate to visualize the abdominal and thigh vasculature, it typically has low resolution to visualize the tibial vessels. Multiple-slice spiral CTA is a noninvasive technique for imaging the entire arterial tree from the abdominal aorta to the level of the foot; it provides superb spatial and temporal resolution with a single bolus infusion of contrast agent. The accuracy of CTA in visualizing lumen patency is restricted by calcification in the vessel wall, a frequent occurrence in the tibial arteries of patients with diabetes. Magnetic resonance angiography (MRA) has poorer resolution compared with CTA but is not affected by calcification. Use of gadolinium-based contrast helps to increase image quality but cannot be used in patients with renal failure (glomerular filtration rate ≤60 mL/min/1.73 m^2) because of the risk of nephrogenic systemic fibrosis. Time-of-flight MRA can be used without contrast and can yield high-quality imaging.

In the initial planning for intervention for the patient with TPOD, noninvasive testing should be performed first; this includes ABIs and segmental pressures with toe pressures, and if abnormal is followed by arterial duplex ultrasound of the symptomatic extremity. If on physical examination the patient has symmetric femoral pulses and there is no evidence of inflow disease on noninvasive vascular studies, the next step in imaging should be diagnostic angiography for possible endovascular intervention or to obtain high-resolution images of a potential bypass target. If there is evidence of inflow disease, a CTA or MRA of the abdomen and pelvis with lower extremity runoff should be ordered. In planning a surgical bypass, the target artery chosen for the distal anastomosis should have continuous unimpeded flow to the plantar arches of the foot, especially in patients with tissue loss. In many patients with diabetes, the peroneal artery is the only remaining patent artery below the knee; however, either the anterior branch to the dorsalis pedal artery or the posterior branch to the posterior tibial artery (and ideally both) must be intact to provide perfusion to the foot, as the artery terminates above the ankle. In patients with occlusion of the tibial and peroneal arteries throughout the lower leg, the plantar and tarsal arteries should be examined as possible sites of a distal anastomosis for limb salvage. In the angiosome model of revascularization, if multiple tibial vessels are available for bypass, the artery that provides the majority of blood flow to the wound should be revascularized. Typically the anterior tibial artery supplies the anterior ankle and dorsum of the foot, the posterior tibial artery supplies the plantar aspect of the foot, and the peroneal artery supplies the anterolateral ankle.

■ SELECTION OF INTERVENTION

Patients who are seen only with claudication initially should be managed nonoperatively, as fewer than 5% of such patients progress to CLI and limb loss. Treatment should focus on modification of cardiac risk factors. Patients should stop using all tobacco products, be placed on aspirin and a statin, and have medication adjustments for optimal blood pressure and glycemic control. A supervised exercise program of 30 to 60 minutes of exercise, such as walking three times a week, should be instituted, and treatment with cilostazol may be considered to improve exercise tolerance in patients with claudication.

Patients with rest pain or tissue loss should be offered an intervention to prevent limb loss. The primary objectives in treating patients with TPOD are to relieve pain, promote healing of ulcers, preserve a functional limb, and restore or maintain the ability to ambulate. These objectives must be tempered by the patient's general medical condition, current ambulatory status, and previous operations. In general, the success of surgical bypass depends on the availability of a single segment of autogenous vein of suitable diameter, whereas the success of endovascular treatment is determined by the extent of atherosclerotic disease, as quantified by the TransAtlantic Inter-Society Consensus (TASC) II Working Group. Infrapopliteal lesions are categorized in severity from classes A to D (Figure 1). The Bypass versus Angioplasty in Severe Ischaemia of the Leg (BASIL) trial is the only randomized trial (452 patients) in which outcomes of surgical bypass and percutaneous transluminal angioplasty (PTA) were compared for treatment of severe infrainguinal PAD, and it provides level I evidence in the field. At 1 year, the amputation-free survival (AFS) rates were equivalent; however, at 2 years, AFS rates were better among the patients who underwent bypass. The BASIL authors concluded that bypass with autogenous vein is the best treatment for patients with severe limb ischemia who are expected to survive more than 2 years and that bypass with prosthetic grafts in patients

TASC A lesions

Single focal stenosis, ≤5 cm in length, in the target tibial artery with occlusion or stenosis of similar or worse severity in the other tibial arteries.

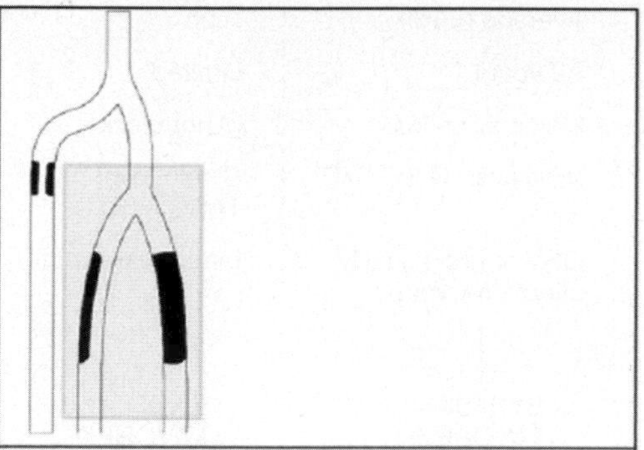

TASC B lesions

Multiple stenoses, each ≤5 cm in length, or total length ≤10 cm or single occlusion ≤3 cm in length, in the target tibial artery with occlusion or stenosis of similar or worse severity in the other tibial arteries.

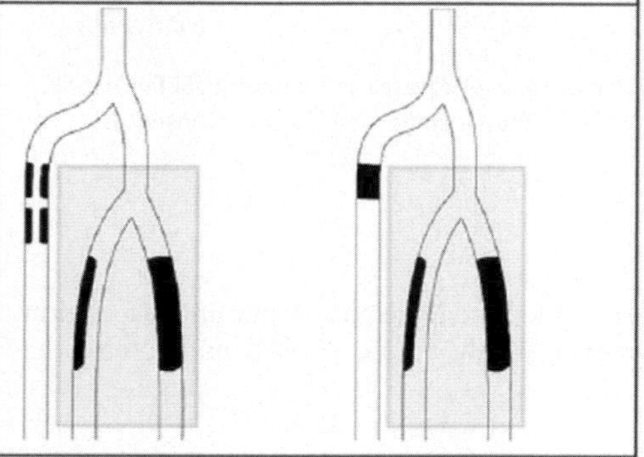

TASC C lesions

Multiple stenoses in the target tibial artery and/or single occlusion with total lesion length >10 cm with occlusion or stenosis of similar or worse severity in the other tibial arteries.

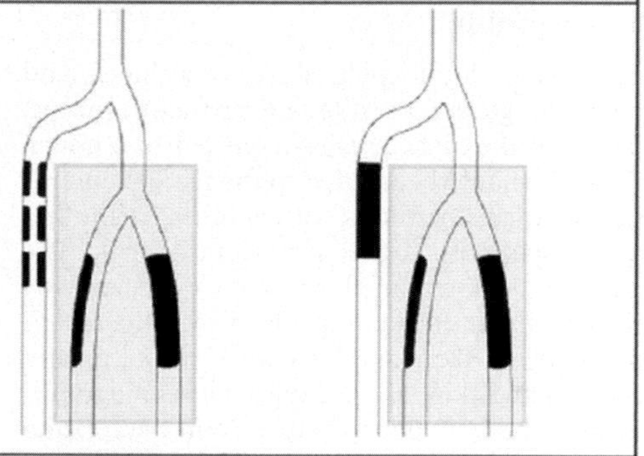

TASC D lesions

Multiple occlusions involving the target tibial artery with total lesion length >10 cm or dense lesion calcification or nonvisualization of collaterals. The other tibial arteries are occluded or have dense calcification.

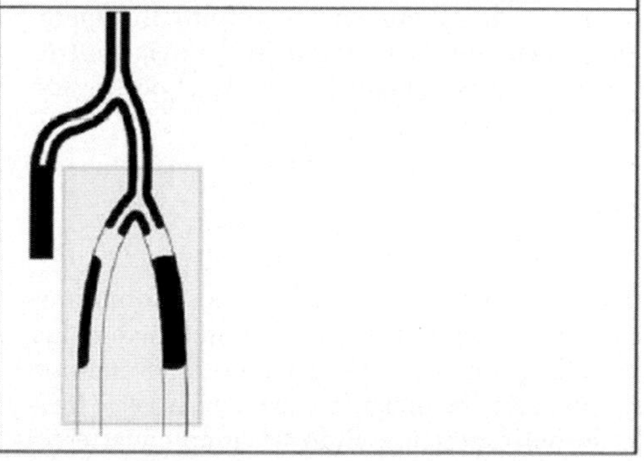

FIGURE 1 Inter-Society Consensus for the Management of Peripheral Arterial Disease (TASC II) classification of infrapopliteal lesions. The unshaded areas represent the target lesions; the areas inside the shaded rectangles represent typical background disease. *(From Jaff MR, White CJ, Hiatt WR, et al. An update on methods for revascularization and expansion of the TASC lesion classification to include below-the-knee arteries: a supplement to the Inter-Society Consensus for the Management of Peripheral Arterial Disease [TASC II]. Vasc Med. 2015;20:465-478.)*

without sufficient autogenous vein is associated with poor results. Endovascular interventions are the preferred option for TASC classes A, B, and single-level C lesions, whereas surgical bypass is recommended for multilevel TASC classes C and D lesions in a patient with average surgical risk. Bypass is the first choice with significant tissue loss (ulcer larger than 1 cm or gangrene involving the foot; Figure 2). The surgeon should be both flexible and creative. A patient with an open wound over the anticipated distal anastomosis site or without adequate single segment vein would be served best with PTA.

SURGICAL BYPASS

All patients are maintained on aspirin before the surgical procedure. Clopidogrel therapy can be continued if the patient is on this medication preoperatively. Unless it is contraindicated, warfarin (Coumadin) as well as the newer oral anticoagulants need to be stopped several days before elective open operations. Typically warfarin is held for 5 days before the surgery, and the newer oral anticoagulants are held for 2 to 3 days before the surgery. If limb ischemia is acute,

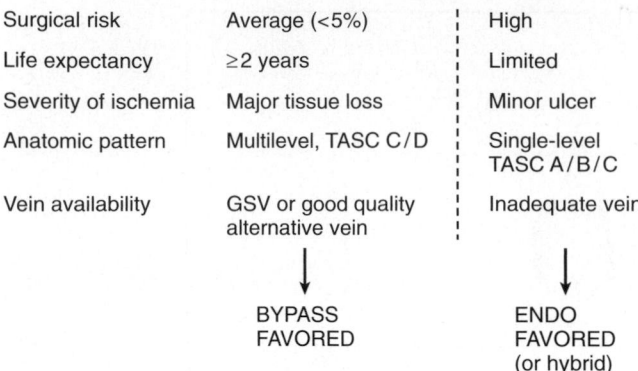

Surgical risk	Average (<5%)	High
Life expectancy	≥2 years	Limited
Severity of ischemia	Major tissue loss	Minor ulcer
Anatomic pattern	Multilevel, TASC C/D	Single-level TASC A/B/C
Vein availability	GSV or good quality alternative vein	Inadequate vein

BYPASS FAVORED

ENDO FAVORED (or hybrid)

FIGURE 2 Schema for bypass or endovascular treatment (ENDO). *GSV*, Greater saphenous vein; *TASC*, TransAtlantic Inter-Society Consensus **(class)**. *(From Conte MS: Critical appraisal of surgical revascularization for critical limb ischemia.* J Vasc Surg. *2013;57:2).*

however, patients are admitted and undergo systemic anticoagulation with intravenous heparin, which can be stopped en route to the operating room.

Anesthesia and Positioning

Options for anesthesia include local, epidural, regional block, and general anesthesia. We prefer general anesthesia for patient comfort, as most surgical bypasses to the tibial arteries require 4 to 6 hours, but the choice of anesthesia should be tailored to the patient and his or her associated risks. Regional anesthesia with epidural is another excellent choice for a patient with higher perioperative risk. The patient is placed supine on the operating fluoroscopy table, and any open wounds are covered with an Ioban drape. Hair over the anticipated incisions sites is clipped. We mark the course of the greater saphenous vein (GSV) on the skin using duplex ultrasonography guidance before the start of the operation to help prevent the creation of skin flaps. The skin of the lower abdomen, both groins, the operative leg(s), and feet is painted with ChloraPrep. Two Bovie electrocautery devices are used to enable simultaneous arterial exposure and vein harvest.

Operative Exposures

Inflow Vessels

The common femoral artery (CFA) is the artery most commonly used for the proximal anastomosis and is easily exposed with either a transverse incision in the groin crease or a longitudinal incision centered over the femoral pulse. We prefer to use the transverse incision, as it heals better in our experience. Even when an endarterectomy of the inflow artery is necessary, we find that with appropriate retraction, exposure may be attained via a transverse groin incision such that endarterectomy from the external iliac to the CFA bifurcation and even the profunda femoris artery (PFA) is possible. Subcutaneous dissection is performed with the help of Bovie electrocautery, and obvious lymph nodes and lymphatics are controlled with ties. The proximal CFA, PFA, and superficial femoral arteries (SFAs) are controlled circumferentially with vessel loops. If conduit length is limited and there are no flow-limiting lesions in the CFA or SFA, alternative inflow sites for the proximal anastomosis include the PFA, middle and distal SFA, and popliteal artery above and below the knee. A lateral approach to the PFA is a useful approach for inflow when the patient has a normal CFA in order to avoid a redo groin operation or to stay away from an infected field. Patients with diabetes frequently have no significant arterial occlusive disease above the knee, and a popliteal-tibial bypass is a reasonable choice in such situations when available conduit length is limited.

Outflow Vessels

When a tibial bypass is necessary, the anterior or posterior tibial arteries are the first choice for the distal outflow anastomosis because they are more accessible and are in direct continuity with the arterial arches of the foot. The peroneal artery is selected if the anterior tibial and posterior tibial arteries are diffusely diseased. The target for the distal anastomosis must be free of calcified plaque, as this may lead to dissection of the intima and compromise graft patency. Preoperative imaging with DSA is utilized to help determine the most suitable distal target.

Proximal Posterior Tibial and Peroneal Arteries

To expose the tibioperoneal trunk and the proximal segments of the posterior tibial and peroneal arteries, an incision is made approximately 2 cm posterior to the medial edge of the tibia, starting just below the knee joint and extending distally for 10 to 15 cm. If the ipsilateral GSV is being used as conduit, one can make the incision directly over the course of the vein, which is marked on the skin preoperatively. The fascia of the gastrocnemius muscle is incised, and the medial head is retracted posteriorly with a Weitlaner retractor with dull prongs. The popliteal fossa is entered, and the popliteal vein is encountered medial and anterior to the artery and usually has several large tributary branches at the level of the tibioperoneal trunk that should be ligated and divided. The popliteal vein is then mobilized with sharp dissection and retracted posteriorly with a vessel loop, which exposes the distal popliteal artery. The soleus muscle is detached as close as possible to the tibia, and a second Weitlaner retractor is placed. Meticulous dissection with Metzenbaum scissors exposes the distal popliteal artery and is continued distally to expose the tibioperoneal trunk, which then bifurcates to the posterior tibial and peroneal arteries usually approximately 2.5 cm from the origin of the anterior artery. Care must be taken because there are multiple vein branches that tear easily; thus these should be ligated and divided when encountered to avoid bleeding, as the transected vein will retract into the muscle if inadvertently torn. The two concomitant veins that usually run parallel to each artery are equally friable and send branches that cross the arteries at frequent points; these branches should be ligated.

The middle segment of the posterior tibial artery is exposed with a longitudinal incision approximately 2 cm posterior to the medial edge of the tibia (Figure 3, *A*) and extended for 10 cm. The fascia is incised longitudinally, and the soleus is divided off the tibia. Once the soleus is retraced posteriorly, the posterior tibial artery can be found in the plane between the flexor digitorum longus and soleus muscles. The artery is dissected sharply on the anterior surface with Metzenbaum scissors, again taking care to ligate and divide venous branches that cross the artery anteriorly (Figure 3, *B*). When isolating tibial arteries, we avoid circumferential dissection and clear only the artery on the most anterior surface facing the surgeon. This avoids inadvertent damage to the artery from sharp dissection. Circumferential dissection of tibial arteries is unnecessary, as we use tourniquet control for the distal anastomosis (described later) and never clamp the tibial arteries in order to avoid damaging these fragile vessels.

This distal posterior tibial artery can be exposed at the medial ankle with an incision 1 cm posterior to the distal tibia; this may be extended posterior to the medial malleolus. The flexor retinaculum is divided, and the artery is found between the tendons of the flexor digitorum longus and flexor hallucis longus muscles. The bifurcation of the posterior tibial artery into the medial and lateral plantar branches can be found by creating a 5-cm curvilinear incision from behind the medial malleolus to the instep of the foot. Division of the abductor hallucis muscle is usually necessary to facilitate exposure. The lateral plantar artery takes a slightly more inferior course to the medial plantar artery and is often larger. Usually a segment suitable for bypass can be exposed before it courses laterally across the sole of the foot.

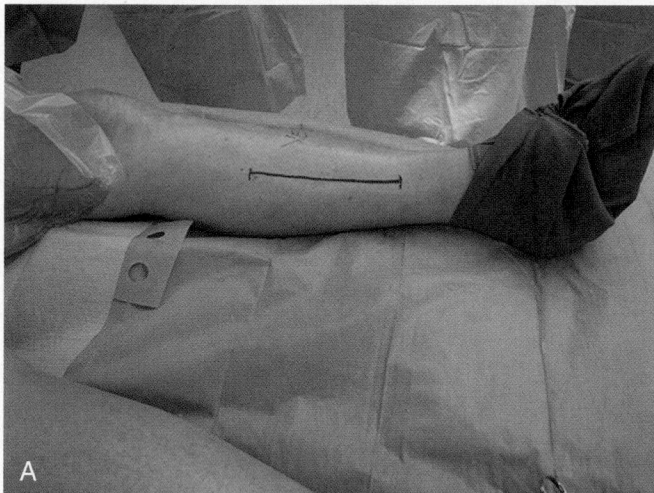

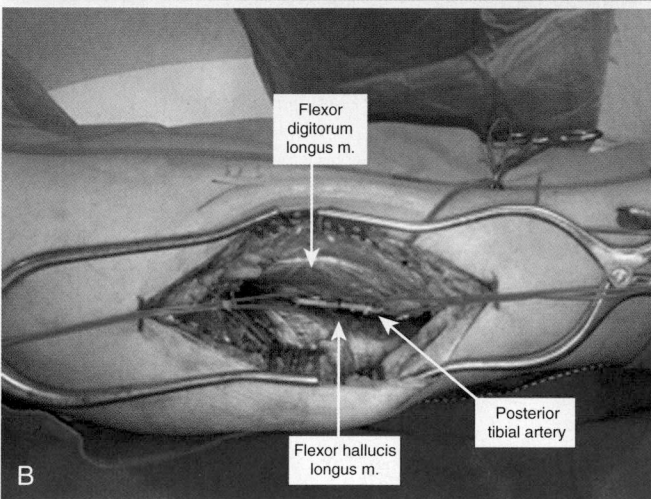

FIGURE 3 Exposure of the posterior tibial artery. **A,** An incision is made on the middle third of the medial portion of the leg. **B,** The posterior tibial artery lies between the flexor digitorum longus and flexor hallucis longus muscles, which are separated with sharp and blunt dissection.

The middle segment of the peroneal artery can be exposed through the same incision used to expose the posterior tibial artery (2 cm posterior to the tibia). Once the fascia is incised, the soleus is divided off the tibia and retracted posteriorly, taking the posterior tibial neurovascular bundle with it. The fascia over the flexor digitorum longus muscle is divided, and the plane of dissection is carried deeper, where the peroneal artery can be found. The distal peroneal artery can be exposed via a lateral incision and partial fibulectomy. The skin incision is placed laterally over the fibula, and the bone is cleared of all muscular and tendinous attachments (Figure 4, *A* and *B*). The bone is then gently resected for a distance of at least 8 cm, and the peroneal artery is found medially on the flexor hallucis longus muscle (Figure 4, *C* and *D*).

Anterior Tibial Artery and Dorsalis Pedis Artery

The anterior tibial artery is exposed through a longitudinal incision placed between the tibia and fibula (Figure 5, *A*). The fascia overlying the tibialis anterior and the extensor digitorum longus muscles is opened, and the groove between these two muscles is separated (Figure 5, *B*), which exposes the anterior tibial artery, its concomitant veins, and the deep peroneal nerve (Figure 5, *C*). The dorsalis pedal artery is the continuation of the anterior tibial artery onto the dorsum of the foot and is exposed by an incision made between the

first and second metatarsal bones. The incision is made off to the side of the artery, not directly over it; this allows for the creation of a skin flap to provide tissue coverage for the bypass graft. After the deep fascia is incised, the extensor hallucis longus and brevis muscles are separated to expose the artery.

Conduit

For patients with TPOD, bypass grafting with single-segment GSV remains the gold standard of revascularization; 1-year and 5-year limb salvage rates exceed 90% and 80%, respectively. If the ipsilateral portion of the GSV is inadequate or was previously used for bypass, the GSV from the contralateral leg should be used. If no GSV is available and endovascular attempts for revascularization are unsuccessful, the lesser saphenous vein or the basilic and cephalic veins from the arms are other options, if they are of adequate diameter. The basilic and cephalic veins, if not damaged by repeated venipuncture, can be harvested as a single continuous graft of significant length. Splicing of multiple vein segments is sometimes required to obtain the required conduit length. We splice vein segments over a pediatric feeding tube to facilitate the creation of the conduit with two 7-0 polypropylene sutures to prevent purse stringing of the venovenous anastomosis that can occur with a single running stitch. A distal origin bypass from the profunda or distal SFA/popliteal artery can be considered if no proximal stenosis is identified to minimize the conduit length needed. Bypass to the tibial vessels should be with autogenous conduit. If no leg or arm vein is available (which is rare), bypasses with heparin-bonded expanded polytetrafluoroethylene (ePTFE) with a distal vein patch or cryopreserved vein may be considered, although we strongly advise against the use of prosthetic conduits or cryopreserved vein in infrapopliteal revascularization, as 2-year patency with such conduits is as low as 20%, with even lower limb salvage rates, when compared with native vein conduits.

The GSV can be procured with either open or endoscopic techniques. For open vein harvests, a long continuous incision can be used, or multiple skip incisions of 10 cm in length separated by a 3- to 5-cm skin bridge may be made (Figure 6). It is crucial that the GSV be exposed and extracted with meticulous technique because injury and repair may compromise patency. The vein side branches should be ligated approximately 1 to 2 mm distal to their origin from the GSV to prevent crimping and luminal narrowing of the GSV. The final harvesting of the conduit should be done after exposure of the proximal and distal arterial targets, which allows estimation of the length of conduit necessary and helps to minimize ischemia of the vein. The GSV can be used in a reversed, nonreversed, or in situ manner. For bypass to the tibial arteries, the best lumen size match typically is found with a nonreversed GSV, which will require valvulotomy. To facilitate valvulotomy, we recommend completing the proximal anastomosis, allowing distension of the vein, and using a Mills valvulotome to lyse the valves that can be visualized through the dilated vein. If size mismatch is not significant, the GSV may be used in a reversed fashion. In situ GSV bypasses are limited by proximity of the GSV to the inflow and outflow vessels and typically are used for femoral to proximal tibial bypasses in patients who are at low risk for wound infection that could expose the nontunneled GSV (and thus usually are not used in patients who are diabetic or who smoke because they are at high risk for wound infection in general).

Inflow Anastomosis

The distal external iliac artery, CFA, PFA, and SFA are exposed as previously described. Tunnels for the bypass graft are created (described later), and the patient undergoes systemic anticoagulation with heparin at an initial dose of 100 units/kg, followed by periodic boluses to maintain an activated clotting time greater than 250 seconds. The CFA is palpated to determine the site that is most free of atherosclerosis. Atraumatic clamps are placed on the SFA, PFA,

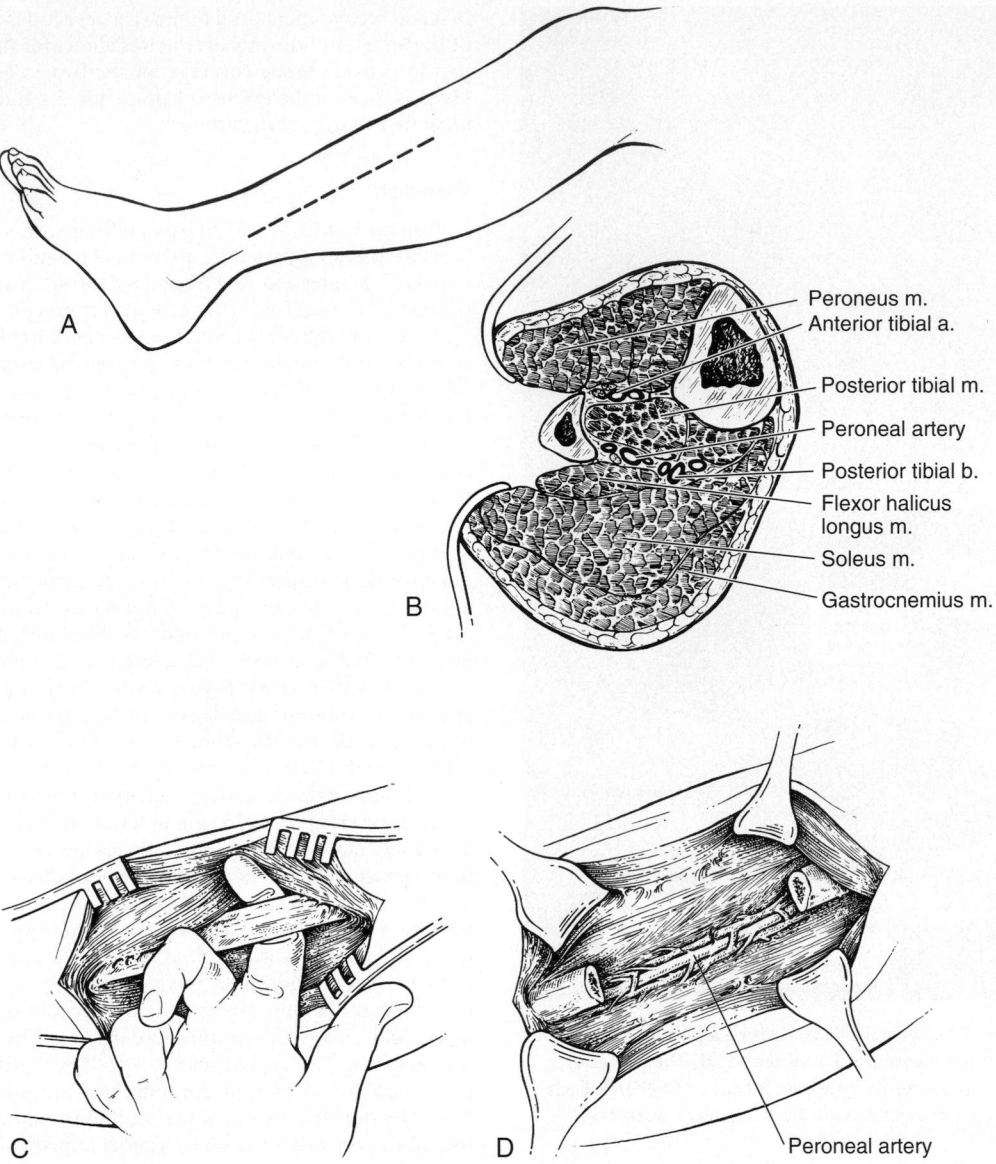

Peroneus m.
Anterior tibial a.

Posterior tibial m.

Peroneal artery

Posterior tibial b.
Flexor halicus longus m.

Soleus m.

Gastrocnemius m.

FIGURE 4 Lateral exposure of the peroneal artery. **A,** The incision is made longitudinally over the fibula. **B,** Cross-section of the lower leg, illustrating the lateral approach with fibula resection. **C,** The muscle and fascia are stripped from the fibula, and an 8-cm section is removed. **D,** The peroneal artery is exposed and seen to lie on the surface of the hallucis longus muscle. *(Copyright Herbert Dardik, 2001).*

Peroneal artery

and proximal portion of the CFA, and an arteriotomy is created with a #11 blade. The arteriotomy is extended with Potts scissors to 25 to 35 mm, depending on the diameter of the GSV. The proximal portion of the GSV is beveled to accommodate the arteriotomy, and the anastomosis is created with 5-0 or 6-0 polypropylene sutures in a continuous manner. In patients without proximal flow-limiting lesions, more distal sites can be used for the proximal anastomosis, including the profunda and popliteal arteries.

Tunnels for Bypass Grafts

Before the patient receives heparin for the proximal anastomosis, a tunnel for the bypass graft is created by advancing a tunneling device or a large aortic clamp in either an anatomic or a subcutaneous fashion. We prefer an anatomic tunnel, as it requires less conduit length, the vein graft has a less acute angle as it turns to the distal anastomosis, and it is protected by the soft tissues of the leg

and distanced from the skin and wounds in patients with TBOD who are usually poor healers because of diabetes and tobacco use. To reach the proximal third of the posterior tibial and peroneal arteries, the graft is tunneled from the adductor hiatus through the popliteal fossa to maintain a straight path. One must ensure that the vein passes between the heads of the gastrocnemius muscle at the popliteal fossa to avoid compression of the vein. The main advantage of the subcutaneous tunnel is that the graft is close enough to the skin to allow for percutaneous access for future endovascular procedures if needed as well as easier access to the graft for open revisions. If the ipsilateral vein is harvested, subcutaneous tunneling is still possible, but one must stay away from the harvest site to avoid possible exposure of the bypass graft to a wound infection involving the vein harvest site. Once the proximal anastomosis is completed, the vein graft is clamped distally and inflated with blood. The vein is marked longitudinally on its anterior surface to prevent twisting and passed through the tunnel. Vein flow is then checked; any

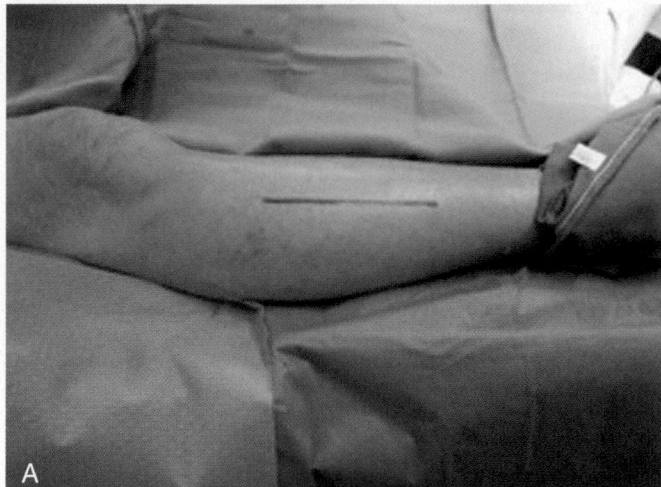

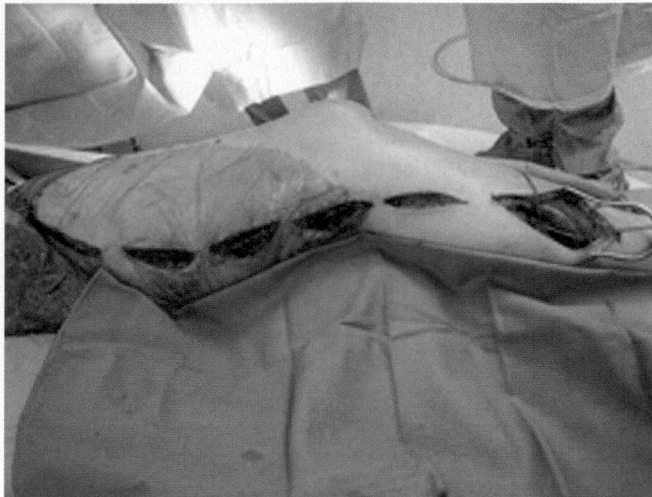

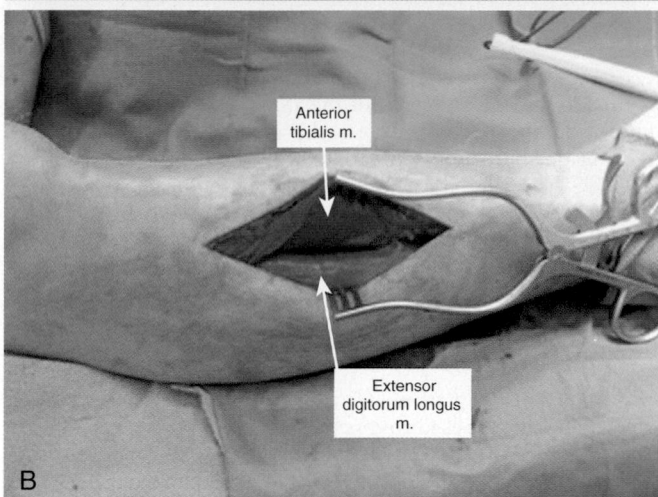

FIGURE 6 The greater saphenous vein (GSV) is exposed with a series of incisions along its course on the medial aspect of the leg. Skin bridges are left in place to minimize tension on the incision closure and prevent wound dehiscence. Alternatively, a continuous incision may be made along the entire length of the GSV.

Outflow Anastomosis

Creation of the outflow anastomosis requires adherence to meticulous technique and gentle manipulation of arteries, many of which are calcified. Loupe magnification is essential. We do not control tibial vessels with vessel loops or clamps. We do not dissect tibial vessels circumferentially. Instead, we use a pneumatic tourniquet placed on the thigh and inflated after the leg is exsanguinated with an Esmark elastic bandage. An arteriotomy is initiated with a Beaver Blade, taking care not to lacerate the posterior wall of the artery. In general, the arteriotomy should be approximately 1.5 times the diameter of the vein graft because longer anastomoses tend to flatten the hood of the vein and create a sharp angle at the heel, which lead to flow turbulence and consequently a nidus for intimal hyperplasia. A 7-0 polypropylene suture is used to create the distal anastomosis. The tibial artery is handled minimally; it is touched with fine pickups only when necessary and very gently.

■ ENDOVASCULAR REVASCULARIZATION

Indications for Intervention

With lower rates of perioperative morbidity and mortality, high rates of technical success, and equivalent rates of limb salvage, PTA of the tibial and peroneal arteries is a critical skill of the vascular surgeon. Evidence of long-term efficacy was provided by the Beth Israel Deaconess Medical Center, which demonstrates that PTA of the tibial and peroneal arteries results in 1-year and 5-year primary patency rates of 57% and 38% and limb salvage rates of 84% and 81%, respectively. According to the TASC II classification for infrapopliteal lesions, PTA is recommended for TASC classes A, B, and single-level C lesions in the tibial or peroneal arteries. In general, lesions that are more amenable to successful endovascular interventions are stenoses shorter than 4 cm or segments of occlusion shorter than 2 cm. Extensive disease that involves trifurcation, numerous stenoses, a diffusely diseased tibioperoneal artery, or long occlusions is best treated with surgical bypass. In these situations, endovascular therapies may be used as an adjunct to open surgical bypass to improve inflow or outflow during bypass procedures or for patients who are poor candidates for open surgical bypass because of either a lack of conduit or significant medical comorbid conditions.

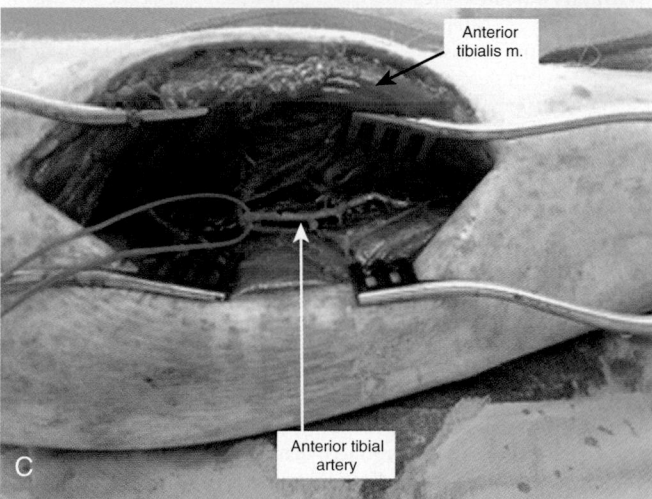

FIGURE 5 Exposure of the anterior tibial artery. **A,** A longitudinal incision is placed lateral to the anterior border of the tibia. **B,** The groove between the tibialis anterior and the extensor digitorum longus muscles is separated. **C,** The anterior tibial artery is exposed.

twisting in the tunnel will result in reduced blood flow after tunneling as compared with the strength of the blood flow before tunneling of the vein. We prefer to use the Oregon tunneler, as it allows for creation of the tunnel from either the distal or the proximal aspect of the wound.

Vascular Access and Imaging

Preprocedure imaging with CTA is most helpful in planning the point of arterial access and locations of critical stenoses and occlusions. For tibioperoneal interventions, the contralateral CFA is the preferred access site. If this is not a suitable option, either because of extensive atherosclerosis or because of the presence of an aortobifemoral graft, the left brachial artery or ipsilateral CFA can be accessed with an antegrade approach. The contralateral CFA is accessed with a 21-gauge needle with ultrasound guidance, and a micro wire is advanced under fluoroscopic guidance. Then a 5F transitional dilator is placed. Over a stiff wire, a 5F or 6F sheath is placed in the artery. A diagnostic catheter is advanced into the abdominal aorta and exchanged for a catheter designed to go over the bifurcation. As with open surgical bypass, inflow and outflow must be considered in maintaining perfusion throughout the infrapopliteal system. The advantage of contralateral retrograde access is that it allows for access to the aortoiliac and femoropopliteal regions; stenoses in these areas can be addressed at the same time as the infrapopliteal intervention in many cases. Once the aortic bifurcation is crossed, the short sheath is then exchanged for a longer and stiffer sheath that is placed in the ipsilateral femoral or distal external iliac artery for diagnostic imaging. The sheath then can be advanced into the SFA for stable access to support the various devices and catheters used in infrapopliteal interventions. A crossing catheter is used to provide adequate support to cross tibial arterial occlusions. We tend to use 0.014-inch or 0.018-inch wires with added weight at the tip, which provide pushability to cross the infrapopliteal lesions. If this route is unsuccessful, pedal arteries can be cannulated under ultrasound guidance, and a wire can be advanced in a retrograde direction. A snare device then can be used to grasp the proximal wire and navigate it through the tibial arteries (Figure 7). Careful consideration is necessary if one decides on retrograde tibial access, as one does not want to damage the distal outflow and eliminate a possible bypass target.

Precise mapping of infrapopliteal anatomy is crucial for proper intervention. In more proximal arterial imaging, diluted contrast material or carbon dioxide can be used to reduce the contrast load. However, for imaging below the knee, full-strength contrast material allows for the best resolution. Imaging of the trifurcation usually is performed with a zero-degree anterior-posterior view. A 30-degree ipsilateral oblique or 90-degree true lateral view may be utilized to properly detail the anterior and posterior tibial arteries. Although tibial vessels are imaged, the catheter ideally should be positioned in the distal popliteal artery.

Balloon Angioplasty and Stent Placement

The mainstay of endovascular treatment of the tibioperoneal vessels has been PTA. Balloons suitable for these interventions range from 1.5 to 4 mm in diameter and up to 20 cm in length. Currently available tibial arterial balloons are delivered in shaft lengths of up to 170 cm. It is better to use a balloon length that will cross the entire lesion in a single pass. These balloons are noncompliant and low profile, and a long inflation time of 1 to 3 minutes reduces the risk of dissection of the artery. If disease is still present, the balloon can be inflated for 3 to 4 minutes, or a cutting balloon can be utilized.

The use of stents previously was a bailout technique after PTA if there was greater than 30% stenosis or flow-limiting dissection after balloon inflation. The stents used in these situations were classically bare metal, and the restenosis rate was approximately 50% at 6 months. There has been a growing trend toward placement of drug-eluting stents (DES) in the hope of improving patency rates similar to those observed with the use of DES in coronary revascularization. Because of the comparable caliber of coronary and tibioperoneal arteries, researchers in several studies have used coronary DES in the infrapopliteal arteries. There are now four randomized trials with four meta-analyses to show that DES have better

patency, reduced reintervention rates, reduced amputation rates, and improved event-free survival over PTA alone or with bare metal stent placement. Drug-eluting balloons (DEB) are a new development in the field and have been studied in several industry-sponsored trials that seem to show favorable outcomes, particularly in longer lesions; however, more studies are needed to determine long-term benefit. Currently, DEB sizes are not small enough for tibial intervention. Once the decision has been made to perform an intervention, the patient should be heparinized systemically with an initial dose of 100 units/kg followed by periodic boluses to maintain an activated clotting time greater than 250 seconds. All lesions should be treated if possible, and completion angiography should be performed to evaluate distal runoff. At the end of the procedure, several arterial closure devices are available. Protamine can be administered at the physician's discretion to reverse the anticoagulation. Closure devices have a similar complication rate as manual pressure but decrease the time needed to hold pressure and shorten the time to patient ambulation.

■ OTHER TECHNOLOGIES

Mechanical atherectomy devices, both rotational and directional, can be used to remove a portion of the atheromatous plaque from the luminal surface. The advantage of this method is an actual decrease in the plaque burden in comparison with PTA and stent placement; however, there is concern for distal embolization of plaque when using these devices, and the use of a distal embolic protection device is encouraged. For occluded lesions, several crossing devices are available if a wire and support sheath are not adequate to cross a lesion.

■ POSTINTERVENTION MANAGEMENT AND SURVEILLANCE

After intervention, patients are placed in a monitored setting in which pulses are checked routinely every 1 to 2 hours. Patients who received an endovascular intervention with percutaneous access to the groin are kept on strict bed rest with the hip in a neutral position for 6 hours if manual pressure was held for hemostasis and no closure device was used. After observation for 6 hours and if no hematoma is present at the access site, discharge may be considered for patients who underwent percutaneous endovascular intervention. Those who undergo an open surgical bypass are kept in a monitored setting overnight or longer to assess for hemodynamic stability and fluid shifts. After this period, the focus can shift to physical therapy and mobility. The leg after a bypass typically becomes swollen; this may increase patient discomfort and result in problems with wound healing. We routinely use a multilayer compressive dressing of cast padding and 3M Coban Self-Adherent Wrap. Limitation of intravenous fluids and diuresis once hemodynamically stable are also important in postoperative care. All patients should be maintained on aspirin regimen after their intervention. Dual antiplatelet therapy of aspirin and clopidogrel is prescribed to recipients of endovascular therapy. Statin therapy has been shown to improve the patency rate in bypass recipients, and this is routinely started or continued.

Patients who have undergone bypass grafting should have stringent outpatient follow-up. Particular attention should be paid to symptoms (return of claudication, development of new wounds or nonhealing older wounds) and physical examination. Bypass surveillance should be performed. Noninvasive vascular imaging is performed with measurement of the ABI and arterial bypass duplex ultrasound before discharge and then at 1 month, 3 months, and then every 6 months, for up to 2 years, followed by yearly evaluation in clinic. Increasing focal velocities within the bypass or at the anastomoses or a decrease in the ABI of more than 0.15 should prompt further investigation with angiography and angioplasty of any hemodynamically significant stenoses in order to prevent graft failure. Patients with endovascular interventions are monitored at similar intervals.

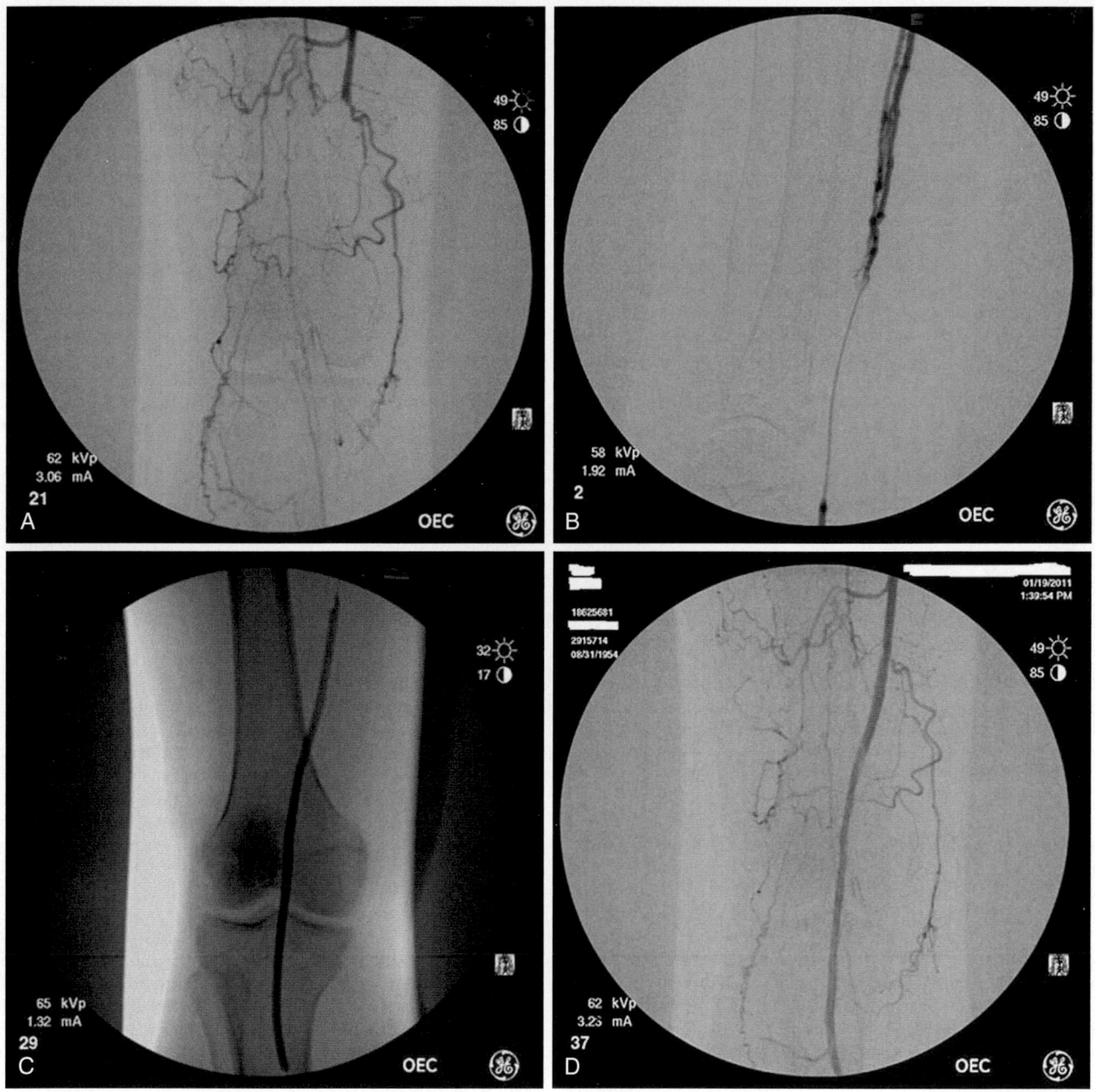

FIGURE 7 Retrograde access of the posterior tibial artery in a patient with critical limb ischemia and previously harvested great saphenous vein. **A,** Chronic total occlusion that could not be traversed with subintimal dissection with a guidewire. **B,** Retrograde access of the posterior tibial artery with a 0.014-inch guidewire and Quick-Cross catheter that is snared from the ipsilateral common femoral artery access. **C,** Inflation of 3 mm × 20 cm balloon placed in an antegrade manner after wire exchange. **D,** Completion arteriogram demonstrating unrestricted flow to the ankle. *(Courtesy George A. Akingba, MD, PhD.)*

■ COMPLICATIONS

Immediate complications include hemorrhage or graft thrombosis and necessitate reoperation. Hemorrhage manifests as an expanding hematoma in the groin or leg and possibly hemodynamic instability. Affected patients should be taken back to the operating room for exploration and evacuation of the hematoma in order to prevent shock, infection, or formation of a pseudoaneurysm. Early graft thrombosis is almost always the result of a technical error but can arise from compression of the graft, twisting of the graft, undiagnosed inflow disease, or an unknown hypercoagulable state. Affected patients should undergo thrombectomy and arteriography to evaluate for technical problems related to anastomoses, twisting of the graft, an intimal flap, or inadequate outflow. Late complications include infection, pseudoaneurysm formation, and graft thrombosis. Graft thromboses up to 24 months after the initial operation probably result from neointimal hyperplasia at the distal anastomosis, whereas those that occur after this period typically are caused by recurrent atherosclerotic disease. For endovascular treatment, the most common complication is access related, complicating up to 4% of all catheter-based treatment. A high puncture is associated with a retroperitoneal hematoma that may require arterial repair in the operating room, and low punctures are associated with arteriovenous fistula development or thigh hematoma and pseudoaneurysm formation.

■ FUTURE TREATMENT: CELL-BASED THERAPIES

Although revascularization with either surgical bypass or endovascular techniques can result in exceptional improvements in patients to TPOD with acceptably low rates of morbidity and mortality, approximately 20% to 40% of patients with CLI are not candidates for these interventions because of lack of conduits or extensive disease within the outflow tibial vessels. For these patients with historically unsalvageable disease, stem cell therapies are emerging as a potential option. A prospective case study evaluated 49 patients (56 limbs) with severe limb-threatening PAD and without other revascularization options who were injected with bone marrow mononuclear cells harvested from the iliac crest. Five amputations needed to be performed before the 3-month follow-up evaluation. Of the remaining 49 limbs that made it to the 3-month evaluation, 4 limbs needed minor amputations; rest pain was still present in 8 limbs (16.3%) but was absent in 39 limbs (79.6%). ABIs did improve but did not meet statistical significance. There was an improvement in wound healing in 26 limbs (59.1%). Overall freedom from major adverse limb events was 91.1% at 3 months and 75.6% at 12 months. These results are encouraging, but any conclusions regarding cell-based therapies for CLI await the results of a much broader randomized study.

SUGGESTED READINGS

Dobrow EM, Mittleider D. Retrograde tibiopedal access for the treatment of critical limb ischemia. *Tech Vasc Interv Radiol.* 2015;18:66-75.

Fleisher LA, Fleischmann KE, Auerbach AD, et al. 2014 ACC/AHA guideline on perioperative cardiovascular evaluation and management of patients undergoing noncardiac surgery. *J Am Coll Cardiol.* 2014;64:e77-e137.

Holzenbein TJ, Pomposelli FB Jr, Miller A, et al. The upper arm basilic-cephalic loop for distal bypass grafting: technical considerations and follow-up. *J Vasc Surg.* 1995;21:586-592.

Jaff MR, White CJ, Hiatt WR, et al. An update on methods for revascularization and expansion of the TASC lesion classification to include below-the-knee arteries: a supplement to the Inter-Society Consensus for the Management of Peripheral Arterial Disease (TASC II). *Vasc Med.* 2015;20:465-478.

Norgren L, Hiatt WR, Dormandy JA, et al. Inter-Society Consensus for the Management of Peripheral Arterial Disease (TASC II). *J Vasc Surg.* 2007;45(suppl S):S5-S67.

Wind GG, Valentine RJ. *Anatomic Exposures in Vascular Surgery.* 3rd ed. Philadelphia: Lippincott Williams and Wilkins; 2013.

Zarins CK, Gewertz BL. *Atlas of Vascular Surgery.* 2nd ed. New York: Elsevier Churchill Livingstone; 2005.

PROFUNDA FEMORIS RECONSTRUCTION

Luke X. Zhan, MD, PhD, and Addi Z. Rizvi, MD

The profunda femoris artery (PFA)—also called the deep femoral artery or deep artery of the thigh—serves critical functions in the perfusion of the lower extremity. It provides the majority of blood flow to the thigh muscles, supplemented by the obturator artery and descending branches of the superior and inferior gluteal arteries. In addition, it provides rich collateral flow to the tibial arteries in the setting of significant arterial occlusive disease of the superficial femoral artery (SFA) or popliteal artery and collateral flow to the pelvis in the setting of iliac arterial occlusive disease (Figure 1). The PFA plays an important role in lower extremity revascularization procedures. It frequently is relatively spared of significant atherosclerosis disease compared with the common femoral and superficial femoral arteries. Thus it can serve as a bypass target for outflow or as a source vessel for inflow in infrainguinal arterial bypass procedures. A stand-alone profundaplasty with open endarterectomy or endovascular angioplasty also can be a main source of leg perfusion in selected patients (Figure 2; Mills, 2014).

■ SURGICAL ANATOMY

Basic Anatomy

The common femoral artery (CFA) bifurcates into the PFA and the SFA 3 to 5 cm inferior to the inguinal ligament. The PFA usually arises from the posterolateral aspect of the CFA and travels in a posterior direction deep to the SFA. A visible change in caliber in the CFA usually marks the femoral bifurcation. An important anatomic relationship in surgical exposure is that the lateral circumflex femoral vein travels between the SFA and PFA. The PFA travels down the thigh close to the femur, running between the pectineus and the adductor longus muscles and on the posterior surface of adductor longus muscle. The PFA typically gives off three branches. The lateral circumflex femoral artery arises from the lateral side of the PFA,

passing horizontally between the division of the femoral nerve and posteriorly to the sartorius and rectus femoris muscles. It divides into ascending, transverse, and descending branches. The medial circumflex femoral artery arises from the medial and posterior aspect and winds around the medial side of the femur. The lateral and medial circumflex femoral arteries can originate directly from the CFA 14% to 20% of the time. They can provide collateral branches to pelvic and tibial vessels. The PFA continues as the perforating arteries, so named because they perforate the tendon of the adductor magnus muscle to reach the posterior and medial compartments of the thigh. The perforating arteries usually have three branches. The first perforating artery passes posteriorly between the pectineus and adductor brevis muscles. The second branch, usually the largest branch, perforates the tendon of the adductor brevis and magnus muscles. The third branch arises below the adductor brevis and pierces the adductor magnus to supply the posterior compartment. These three branches have rich anastomoses with each other.

The PFA is divided into three zones. Zone 1 (proximal) begins at the origin of the artery and extends to the lateral circumflex femoral artery. Zone 2 (middle) begins at the lateral circumflex artery and extends to the second perforating branch. Zone 3 (distal) continues beyond the secondary perforating branch to the segment posterior to the adductor longus muscles. The sartorius muscle serves as an important landmark to aid the surgical exposure of zones 1 to 3 of the PFA (see Figure 1; Figures 3 and 4).

Surgical Exposure of the Profunda Femoris Artery

Proximal Zone Exposure

The most common surgical exposure of the PFA is via an upper anterior thigh incision. It allows access to the CFA and the proximal PFA and SFA. The patient is placed in the supine position. Arms may be tucked to facilitate intraoperative angiography. A longitudinal incision that starts approximately two fingerbreadths lateral to pubic tubercle, directly over the course of the common femoral artery, is created. Palpation of the inguinal ligament and the femoral pulse or direct visualization with duplex ultrasound can demonstrate the course of the common femoral artery and its bifurcation and can be used as an additional guide for incision placement. Even when the

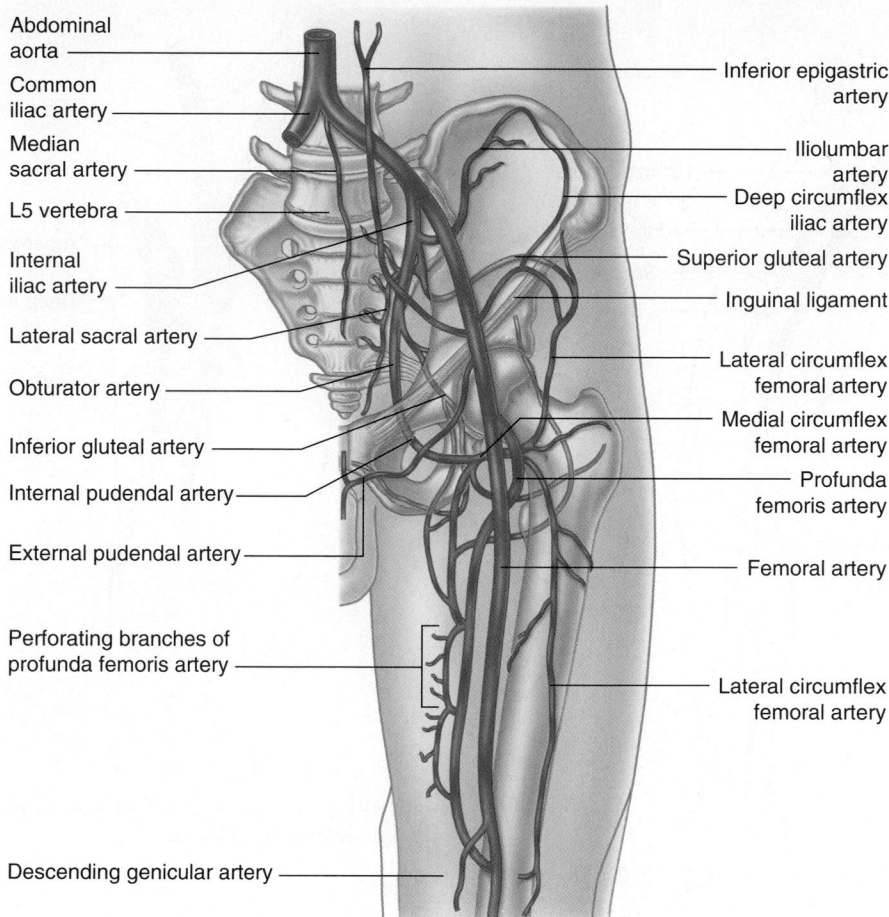

Abdominal aorta

Common iliac artery

Median sacral artery

L5 vertebra

Internal iliac artery

Lateral sacral artery

Obturator artery

Inferior gluteal artery

Internal pudendal artery

External pudendal artery

Perforating branches of profunda femoris artery

Descending genicular artery

Inferior epigastric artery

Iliolumbar artery

Deep circumflex iliac artery

Superior gluteal artery

Inguinal ligament

Lateral circumflex femoral artery

Medial circumflex femoral artery

Profunda femoris artery

Femoral artery

Lateral circumflex femoral artery

FIGURE 1 Vascular anatomy of the thigh depicting the rich collateral network between the internal iliac artery, profunda femoris artery, and popliteal artery.

CFA is pulseless because of excessive calcification or occlusive disease, it can be localized by anatomic landmarks and is usually palpable as a firm tubular structure when rolled beneath the examiner's fingers. Incision usually begins just proximal to the inguinal crease and is carried distally, inclining slightly toward the medial aspect of the knee. The incision can be extended superiorly or inferiorly to expose the distal external iliac, proximal superficial femoral, or profunda femoris artery. Alternatively, especially in the obese, a curvilinear incision can be made 1 cm below and parallel to the inguinal ligament, distal to the abdominal panniculus so as to avoid potential skin maceration and wound complications associated with vertical incisions. Although the proximal superficial femoral and profunda femoris arteries can be exposed via this incision, such a curvilinear or oblique incision limits further distal arterial exposure. It therefore would not be selected if an extensive common and profunda femoris artery endarterectomy were planned. The dissection is extended more deeply in vertical fashion (even when the initial incision is oblique). It is important to remain directly over the arteries as dissection is carried down deep to the femoral sheath. Encountering venous structures indicates that one is too medial, whereas encountering underlying iliopsoas muscle, femoral nerve fibers, or lymphatics suggests that dissection is too lateral. Dissection is carried directly along the CFA both superiorly and distally. Proximal dissection along the artery allows exposure of the entire CFA, with the cephalad extent being inguinal ligament. Caution is necessary when dissecting the CFA segment at or beneath the inguinal ligament. There is usually a vein beneath the inguinal ligament that crosses directly anteriorly

over the CFA, nicknamed the "vein of misery" or "vein of sorrow," as its inadvertent transection produces troublesome bleeding. The medial and lateral femoral circumflex arteries are often near the level of the inguinal ligament and should be identified, spared, and controlled with small Silastic vessel loops. As the dissection proceeds distally, an abrupt change in caliber marks the femoral bifurcation and indicates the origin of the PFA, usually oriented more deeply and posterolaterally. After encircling the common and superficial femoral arteries with Silastic vessel loops, gentle upward traction on either of these loops can help to bring the PFA into view. The lateral circumflex femoral vein may cross under the SFA and course over the PFA near its origin. Division of this vein allows one to mobilize and further expose the first segment of the PFA, which is typically necessary when performing a profunda endarterectomy (zone 1; Figure 5; Wind & Valentine, 2013).

Middle and Distal Segments of Profunda Femoris Artery Exposure

The middle (zone 2) and distal (zone 3) segments of the PFA can be exposed with either anterolateral or anteromedial incisions. This exposure for the PFA is useful regardless of whether the PFA is an inflow vessel or outflow target vessel, and the sole goal is to expose the PFA in "virgin" territory. These two exposures are common in the setting of multiple prior proximal groin exposures, infection in the groin region, or prior irradiation to the groin region. The skin incision is placed along either the medial border (anteromedial approach) or the lateral border (anterolateral approach) of

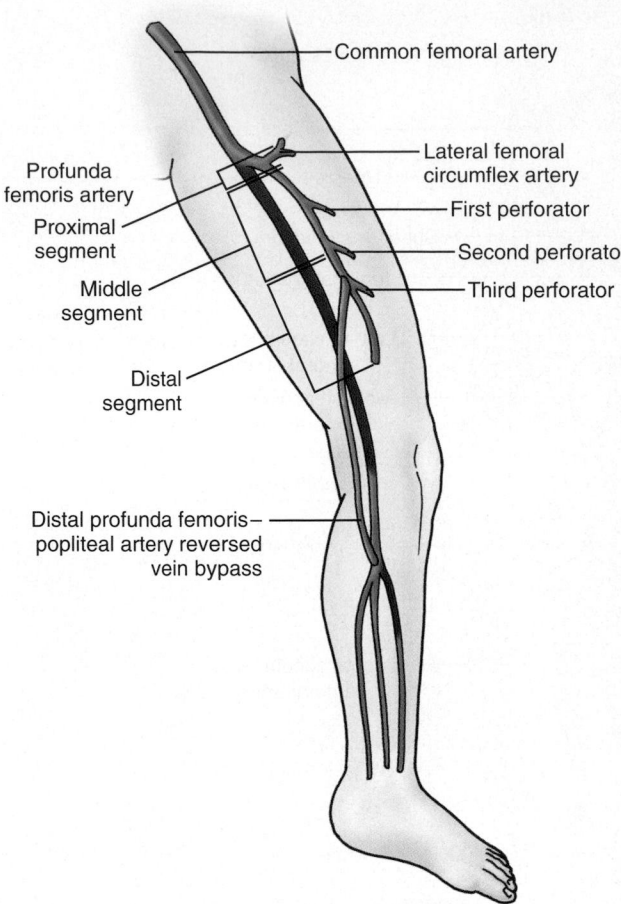

FIGURE 2 Schematic of the profunda femoris artery used as an inflow source for an infrainguinal bypass.

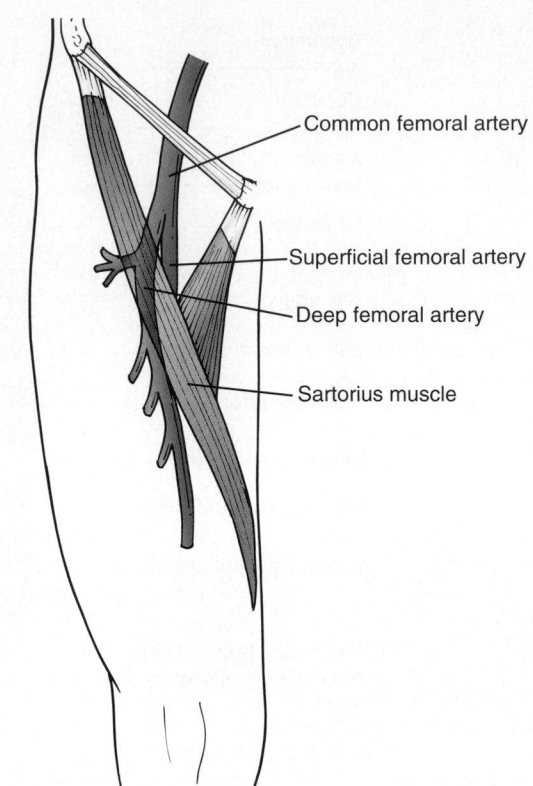

FIGURE 3 The course of the sartorius muscle is represented in relation to the profunda femoris artery.

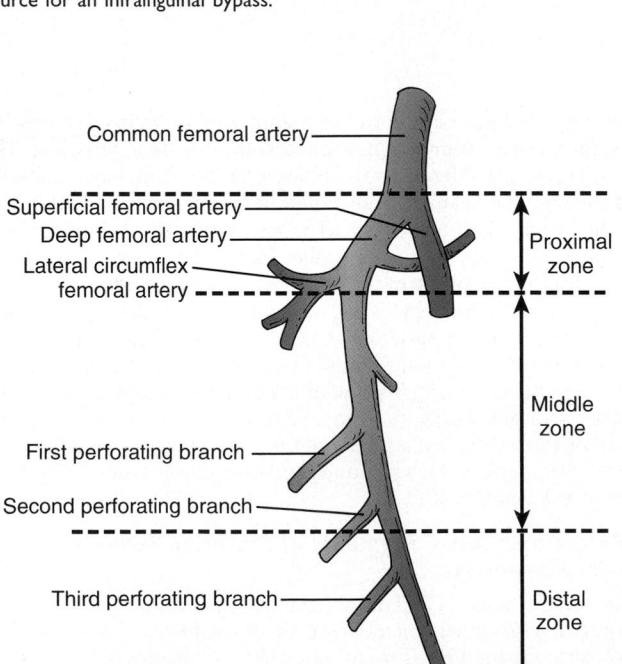

FIGURE 4 The branches and zones of the profunda femoris artery.

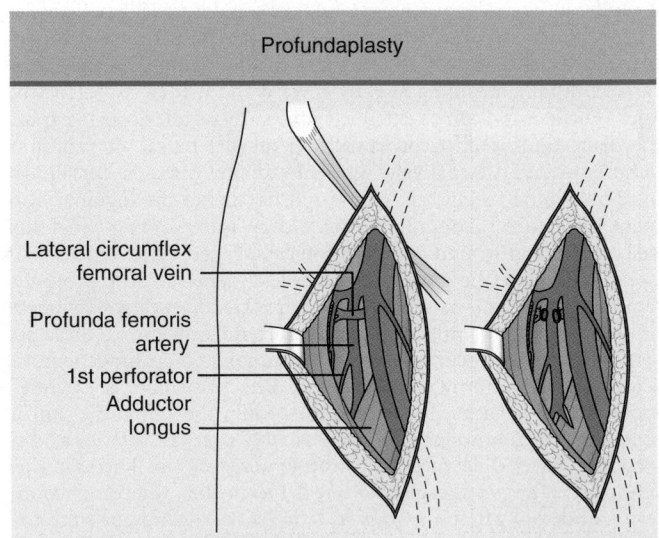

FIGURE 5 Standard anterior approach to the profunda femoris artery.

the sartorius muscle. Carry the dissection deeply through the subcutaneous tissue and fascia, passing alongside the lateral or medial edge of the sartorius muscle to the deep layer, respectively. Once you are deep behind the sartorius muscle, mobilize and retract the sartorius muscle laterally or medially, depending on approach. Continue the dissection deeply, passing lateral to the superficial femoral vessels and accompanying nerve, to the valley formed between the adductor longus muscle (medially) and vastus medialis (laterally). The PFA and the profunda femoris vein reside directly underneath. Next one dissects between the adductor longus and vastus medialis muscles to expose the PFA. It may be necessary to ligate and divide the crossing venous tributaries to isolate and control the middle and distal segments of the artery. Alternatively, an incision can be made between the adductor longus (anteriorly) and gracilis muscle (posteromedially). Dissect between the adductor longus and adductor magnus muscles to approach the PFA medially from the distal thigh (Figures 6 to 8; Wind & Valentine, 2013).

Posterior Medial Approach

The posterior medial approach is also used in the setting of prior groin surgery, groin infection, or a previously irradiated groin. The middle and distal zones of the PFA can be exposed via this incision, and it is a useful exposure in the setting of an iliofemoral obturator bypass if the PFA is the outflow target vessel. With the knee flexed and the hip rotated externally, a medial thigh incision is placed. The fascia is incised and the dissection is continued along the posterior surface of the adductor longus muscle and anterior to the adductor brevis muscle. At the deep aspect of this exposure before encountering the femur, the PFA should be identified and isolated (see Figures 6 and 8).

■ PROFUNDA FEMORIS ARTERY RECONSTRUCTION

Bypass

Often the PFA is used as a source of inflow, particularly in the setting of a distal bypass if there is inadequate vein length or if exposure of the CFA is challenging (i.e., multiple prior groin dissections, infection, or prior irradiation; see Figure 2). The PFA is an excellent outflow target vessel and is used often in the setting of an aortofemoral, axillofemoral or femorofemoral bypass. Often, when utilizing the PFA as an outflow target, the CFA and PFA will require an endarterectomy, and the hood of the bypass is sewn to both the CFA and the proximal PFA. Once the PFA is exposed, proximal and distal vessels and branches are occluded with small vascular clamps or Silastic vessel loops, the patient is systemically heparinized, and a longitudinal arteriotomy is created extending onto the PFA. Regardless of whether the PFA is the inflow or outflow vessel, the hood of the graft can be anastomosed to the profunda in a standard end-to-side fashion using fine polypropylene sutures. If there is significant atherosclerotic disease involving the PFA, it may be necessary to perform a concomitant extended profunda endarterectomy. After an extended endarterectomy, particularly if the PFA is the inflow vessel, it may be necessary to close the arteriotomy with a patch, and the graft then can be sewn onto the patch.

Isolated Profundaplasty

The PFA is essential for maintaining limb viability when severe occlusive arterial disease affects the extremity. It provides the primary

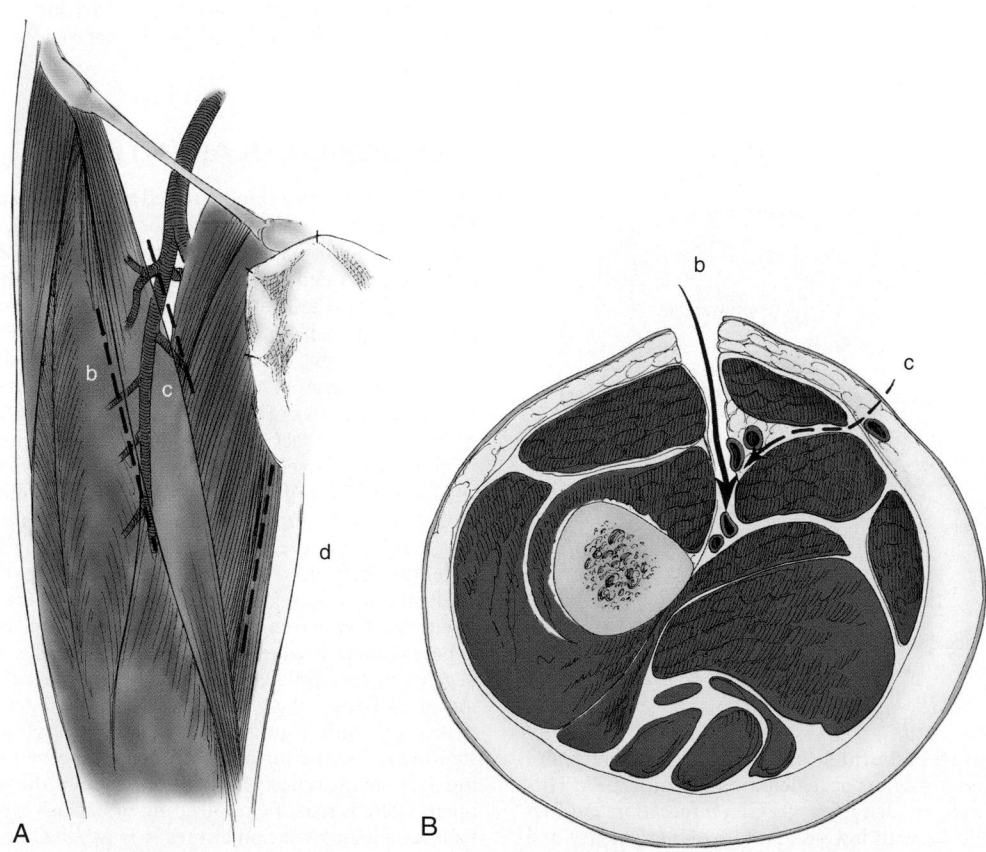

FIGURE 6 A, Incisions to expose the middle and distal profunda femoris artery: (b) arterolateral approach, (c) arteromedial approach, and (d) posteromedial approach. **B,** Cross-section of the right thigh: (b) arterolateral approach and (c) arteromedial approach.

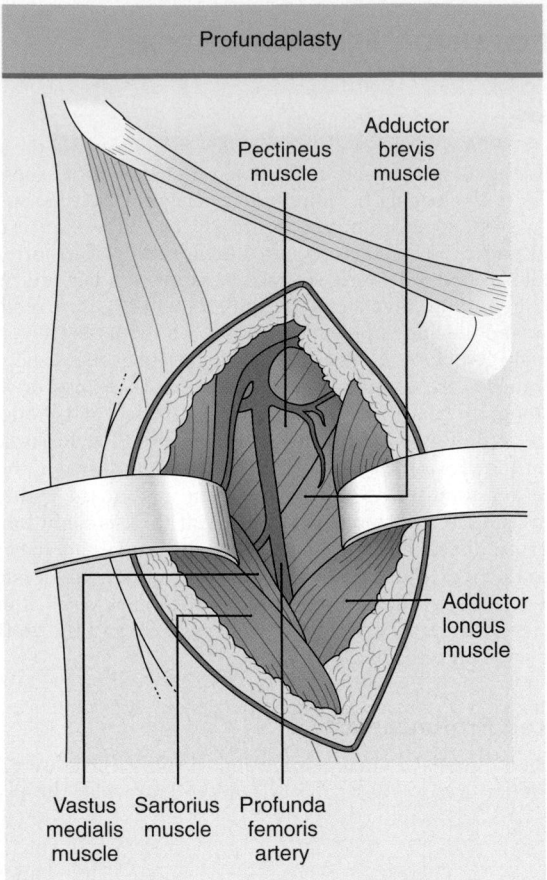

FIGURE 7 Schematic depicting a view of the profunda femoris artery through the anteromedial approach.

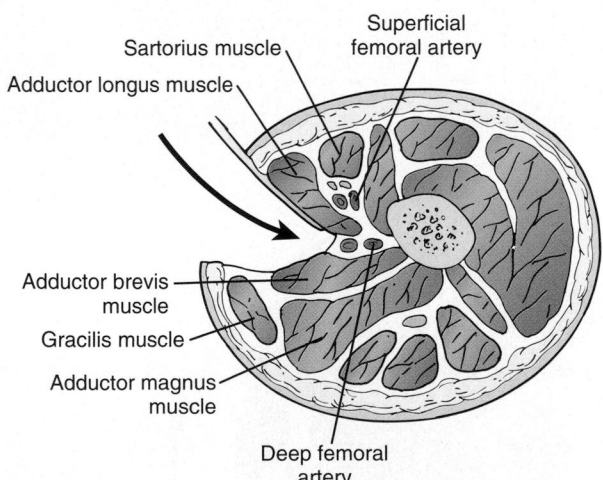

FIGURE 8 Schematic depicting posteromedial approach to the left profunda femoris artery.

blood supply to the tissues of the thigh and is also the most important collateral vessel for bypassing an obstructed or occluded SFA. Historically, significant occlusive disease of the CFA bifurcation and PFA has been treated surgically with low risk and sustained patency and clinical benefit. However, atherosclerosis of the PFA is usually focal, preferentially involving the origin and the very proximal portion of the artery in the majority of limbs; this is essential to consider during

strategic planning of an ostial or proximal SFA intervention. An isolated profundaplasty is indicated when the PFA is the only vessel perfusing the thigh directly and the distal leg via geniculate collaterals. The PFA also can prove useful in removal of an infected prosthetic graft from the groin, in salvage of a nonhealing above-knee or below-knee amputation, and as primary treatment for critical limb ischemia when other surgical or endovascular options are limited (Savolainen et al., 2008; Koscielny et al., 2010).

The success of an isolated profundaplasty in improvement of distal flow can be estimated with the profunda popliteal collateral index (PPCI):

$$PPCI = (AKSP - BKSP)/BKSP$$

where AKSP is above-knee segment pressure and BKSP is below-knee segment pressure. A PPCI greater than 0.5 indicates poor collateral development and likely failure of a stand-alone profundaplasty. A PPCI less than 0.19 indicates significant collateral formation and likely a good response to stand-alone profundaplasty. However, it is generally accepted that profundaplasty alone without concomitant distal bypass is not sufficient to provide pulsatile in-line flow to the foot with significant tissue loss (Boren et al., 1980).

A profundaplasty typically is performed with a CFA endarterectomy. After systemic anticoagulation, the femoral vessels are occluded. A longitudinal arteriotomy is initiated in the mid-CFA and extends proximally toward the external iliac artery and distally veering toward the profunda. A deep medial plane is entered with a plaque elevator proximally in the CFA. The plaque is divided, and the endarterectomy is continued into the PFA to the distal extent of disease. Sometimes eversion is necessary to terminate the PFA plaque with a thin, feathered endpoint in the PFA. Any loose flap is trimmed sharply or tacked down with 7-0 tacking sutures. The arteriotomy is closed with a patch fashioned from bovine pericardium, Dacron, autogenous vein, or a piece of endarterectomized occluded SFA segment. The latter two are the preferred patch materials in the setting of an infected field (Figure 9).

ENDOVASCULAR INTERVENTION

The PFA disease also can be treated with endovascular interventions. This serves as a viable option for patients who are poor surgical candidates because of severe systemic comorbidities or prohibitive challenges to open surgical reconstruction resulting from a hostile groin. It is also indicated as a secondary intervention to maintain the assisted patency of a bypass graft when the PFA was used either as a bypass target or as an inflow source (Donas et al., 2010; Poi et al., 2012; Davies et al., 2013). The access of the PFA for endovascular intervention can be approached from a contralateral retrograde common femoral access in an "up-and-over" the aortic bifurcation fashion. Alternatively, it can be approached via a retrograde brachial access. The indication for brachial access includes contralateral iliofemoral occlusion, history of aortobifemoral bypass, or presence of a modular bifurcated endograft, as crossing in an up-and-over technique may be challenging in the latter two settings. The left brachial artery access generally is preferred because it allows access to either lower extremity without crossing the aortic arch. The PFA is best visualized with the imaging intensifier set at an angle of 30 degrees in the ipsilateral oblique view. This offers the best splaying of PFA from the CFA and SFA on angiography. Once the PFA is accessed with a guidewire, balloon angioplasty with or without stenting can be performed. Caution should be used when performing balloon angioplasty at the PFA ostium if the proximal SFA is still open. There is risk of embolization or occlusion of the SFA from the balloon angioplasty. Sometimes it is worthwhile to place a "buddy wire" into the SFA to maintain access to the SFA for rescue interventions if any of these events occur. The value of PFA angioplasty was demonstrated in a small case series in which PFA angioplasty was the

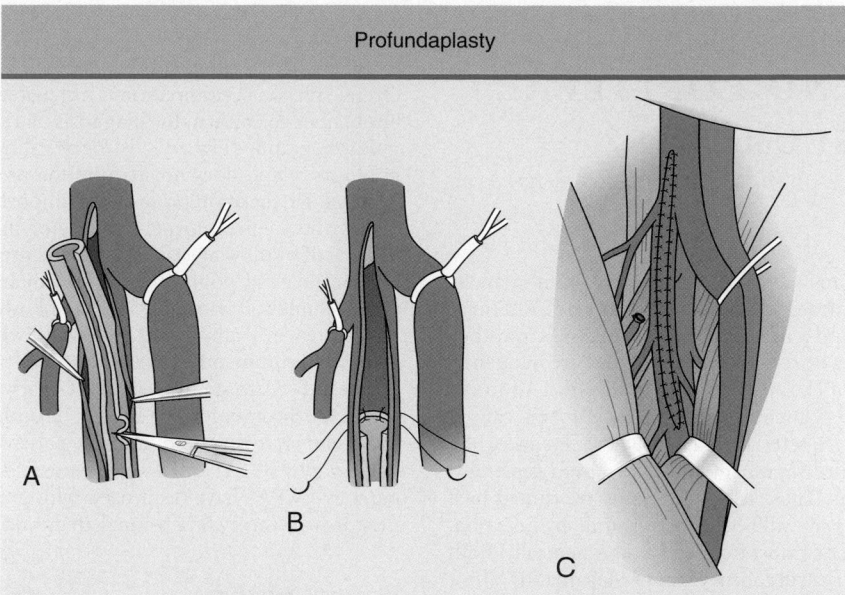

FIGURE 9 Profundaplasty. **A,** Endarterectomy of the profunda femoris artery. **B,** Tacking sutures placed on the distal endpoint. **C,** Vein patch angioplasty.

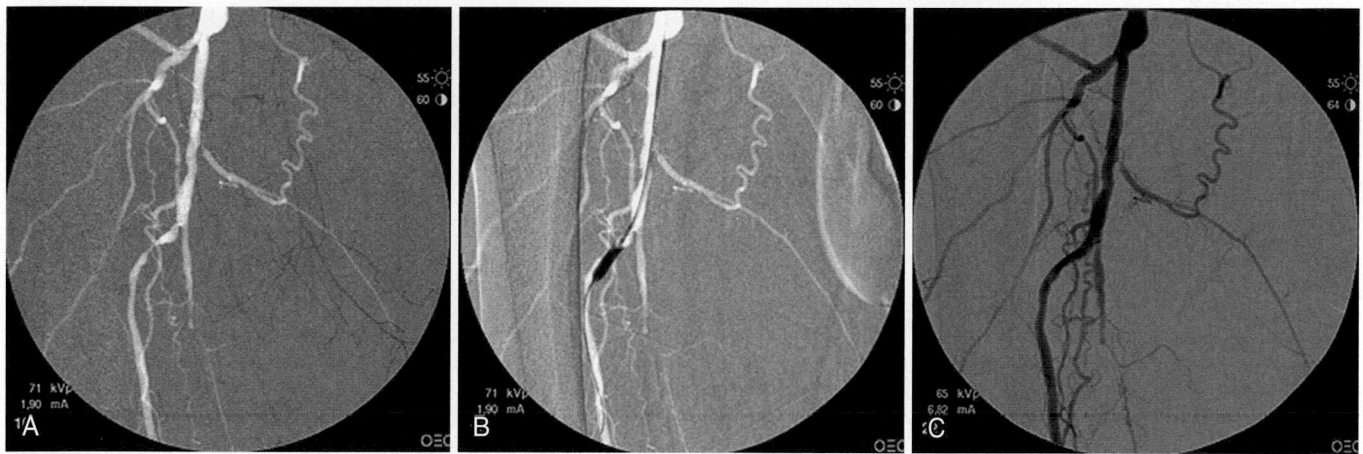

FIGURE 10 Arteriograms. **A,** Profunda femoris artery stenosis. **B,** Angioplasty of profunda femoris artery stenosis. **C,** Profunda femoris artery after angioplasty.

primary treatment in patients with critical limb ischemia and technically demanding open profunda reconstruction and in patients with amputation stump ischemia at risk of hip disarticulation (Figure 10).

■ CONCLUSION

The PFA plays a crucial role in maintaining the viability of the lower extremity. It is a versatile vessel that can serve as an outflow target for suprainguinal bypass as well as an inflow source for infrainguinal bypass. Dedicated profunda angioplasty by either an open surgical or an endovascular approach also may be useful in improving lower extremity perfusion. For vascular specialists involved in lower extremity revascularization, it is a critical skill to possess in preserving the patency of the PFA and utilize in lower extremity vascular reconstruction procedures.

SUGGESTED READINGS

Boren CH, Towne JB, Bernhard VM, et al. Profundapopliteal collateral index: a guide to successful profundaplasty. *Arch Surg.* 1980;115:1366-1372.

Davies RSM, Rashid SH, Adair W, et al. Isolated percutaneous transluminal angioplasty of the profunda femoris artery for limb ischemia. *Vasc Endovascular Surg.* 2013;47:423-428.

Donas KP, Pitoulias GA, Schwindt A, et al. Endovascular treatment of profunda femoris artery obstructive disease: nonsense or useful tool in selected cases? *Eur J Vasc Endovasc Surg.* 2010;39:308-313.

Koscielny A, Pütz U, Willinek W, et al. Case-control comparison of profundaplasty and femoropopliteal supragenicular bypass for peripheral arterial disease. *Br J Surg.* 2010;97:344-348.

Mills JL. Infrainguinal disease: surgical treatment. In: Cronenwett JL, Johnston KW, eds. *Rutherford's Vascular Surgery.* Philadelphia: Saunders; 2014.

Poi MJ, Pisimisis G, Barshes NR, et al. Percutaneous profunda femoris artery revascularization to prevent hip disarticulation: case series and review of the literature. *Am J Surg.* 2012;204:649-654.

Savolainen H, Hansen A, Diehm N. Small is beautiful: why profundaplasty should not be forgotten. *J Vasc Surg.* 2008;47:1119.

Wind GG, Valentine RJ. *Anatomic Exposures in Vascular Surgery.* Philadelphia: Lippincott Williams & Wilkins; 2013.

FEMORAL AND POPLITEAL ARTERY ANEURYSMS

David P. Franklin, MD

Lower extremity aneurysms are the second most common aneurysm after those of the infrarenal aorta and iliac arteries. Although the incidence of popliteal and femoral artery aneurysms is low, they are the most common lower extremity aneurysms and are frequently associated with concomitant abdominal aortic aneurysms. Although the majority of popliteal artery aneurysms are true aneurysms, caused by degeneration of the entire arterial wall, many aneurysms of the femoral arteries that require treatment are false aneurysms, also known as pseudoaneurysms. These false aneurysms are caused by a focal disruption of the arterial wall because of trauma, by infection, by anastomotic disruption, or (most frequently) iatrogenically. Both popliteal and femoral artery true aneurysms predominantly affect older males and typically are symptomatic, and their repair involves excluding the aneurysm via interposition or bypass grafting, although select popliteal cases often are amenable to endovascular approaches.

■ POPLITEAL ARTERY ANEURYSMS

Clinical Presentation

Although the normal diameter of the popliteal artery varies, a popliteal artery with a 1.5- to 2-cm external diameter is considered aneurysmal. Although popliteal artery aneurysms are uncommon, they are the most common lower extremity true aneurysm (80% to 85%) and are found almost exclusively in men (95% to 100%). Patients with a popliteal artery aneurysm frequently have a history of tobacco use, hypertension, and coronary artery disease. Although the exact pathogenesis of popliteal aneurysm formation remains unclear, it is thought to be a result of inflammatory and atherosclerotic degeneration of the arterial wall.

Popliteal aneurysms frequently are identified as an asymptomatic pulsatile mass behind the knee or as an incidental finding on imaging studies performed for other reasons. However, 40% to 60% of patients with a popliteal aneurysm eventually will be symptomatic. Acute limb ischemia, resulting from thrombosis or embolism, is the feared complication of an untreated popliteal artery aneurysm, as up to a quarter of these patients will require limb amputation. Patients also may be seen with chronic symptoms of claudication due to recurrent thromboembolism or with "blue toe syndrome" due to digital artery embolization. Less commonly, patients will be seen with symptoms from compression of adjacent structures, such as venous compression resulting in deep venous thrombosis or edema or nerve compression causing tibial or peroneal neuropathy. Rupture of a popliteal artery aneurysm is a rare event (~2%) and infrequently life threatening, as hemorrhage usually is confined to the popliteal space. Because half of patients with a popliteal aneurysm are asymptomatic, a high index of suspicion is necessary to make the diagnosis. This is especially important in patients with a known popliteal artery aneurysm, as bilateral aneurysms occur in up to 40% of patients, and in patients with an abdominal aortic aneurysm, as the incidence of a popliteal artery aneurysm has been reported to be as high as 14%.

Diagnosis

During physical examination, a popliteal artery aneurysm should be suspected whenever there is a prominent pulse in the popliteal space, as the popliteal artery can be somewhat difficult to palpate in many unaffected individuals. In contrast, if the popliteal artery aneurysm has thrombosed, there may be an absent popliteal pulse and only a firm mass behind the knee may be apparent, masquerading as a Baker's cyst. Overall, physical examination is unreliable and imaging studies must be obtained to confirm the diagnosis of a popliteal aneurysm. Duplex ultrasonography (Figure 1) is the first-line imaging modality, as it is noninvasive and does not require the use of radiation or iodinated contrast. Furthermore, it provides important information about the size of the aneurysm, the presence of intraluminal thrombus, and patency of outflow arteries and can be used to simultaneously screen for contralateral popliteal or concomitant abdominal aortic aneurysms. Duplex ultrasound is used to follow patients after repair. Before repair, greater anatomic detail, beyond what duplex ultrasound provides, is recommended. Catheter-based arteriography traditionally has been used to define suitable targets for surgical bypass. It also allows for thrombolysis of acutely thrombosed arteries or for definitive stent graft repair in suitable patients. Computed tomography angiography (CTA) and, to a lesser extent, magnetic resonance angiography (MRA) have been used with greater frequency recently, as they provide three-dimensional anatomic information (Figure 2).

Natural History

Unlike for aortic aneurysms, there is not widespread screening for popliteal aneurysms, and therefore the natural history of this disease process is poorly understood. Furthermore, most large series analyzing patients with a popliteal aneurysm include only those patients who underwent surgical repair. On average, a third of patients undergoing observation of a popliteal aneurysm will develop thromboembolic complications at 3 years, with an associated amputation rate of 25%. On the basis of these outcomes, it is recommended that popliteal aneurysms 2 cm or greater in diameter and any symptomatic popliteal aneurysm undergo repair. In patients who have simultaneous abdominal aortic and popliteal aneurysms, the more life-threatening problem should be addressed first. It is important to remember, however, that treatment of the abdominal aortic aneurysm before the popliteal aneurysm may increase the risk of popliteal aneurysm thrombosis.

Management

Any symptomatic patient with a popliteal aneurysm, especially one who has acute limb ischemia, should undergo repair; otherwise the likelihood of limb loss is high. The options for repair include surgical bypass or endovascular stent graft placement. Alternatively, even large asymptomatic popliteal aneurysms may be observed in patients with limited life expectancy and a high operative risk. In general, a threshold size of 2 cm warrants repair in good-risk asymptomatic patients. Proponents of this approach cite the excellent graft patency and limb salvage rates when treating popliteal aneurysms early and the small but definite risk of thromboembolism seen even with small aneurysms. Alternatively, others have demonstrated that popliteal aneurysms can be observed safely up to 3 cm if the estimated risk of thromboembolic complications is low (no evidence of distal embolization, minimal intraluminal thrombus, and little anatomic distortion proximal and distal to the aneurysm). In patients with a thrombosed popliteal aneurysm and compensated collateral arterial flow (i.e., no critical limb ischemia), surgical repair is not required, and these patients should be managed similarly to patients with peripheral arterial occlusive disease and claudication. With no prospective randomized controlled clinical trials, the management strategy for patients with a popliteal aneurysm must be individualized.

Operative Technique

Emergency Surgical Treatment

When patients with a popliteal aneurysm have acute limb ischemia, it is of utmost importance to determine limb viability. If there is no

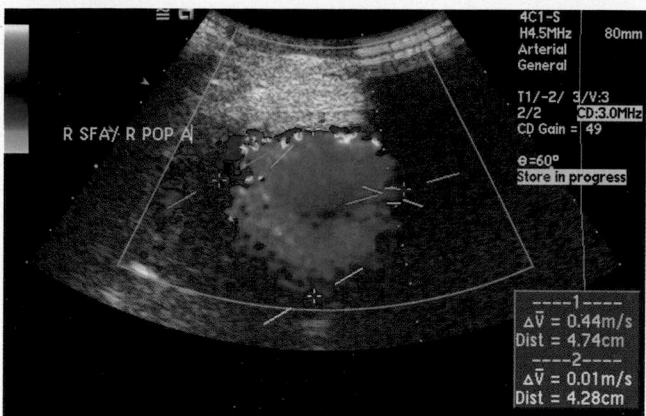

FIGURE 1 Transverse image of a fusiform popliteal aneurysm on color duplex scan.

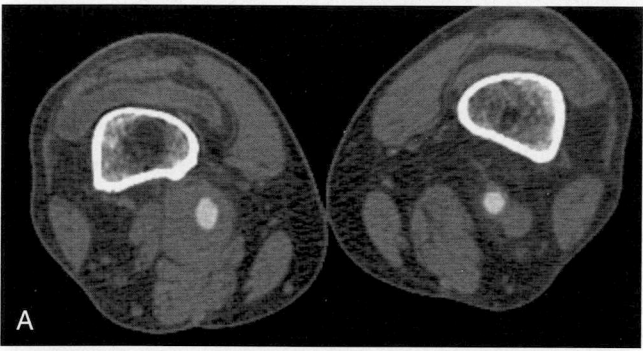

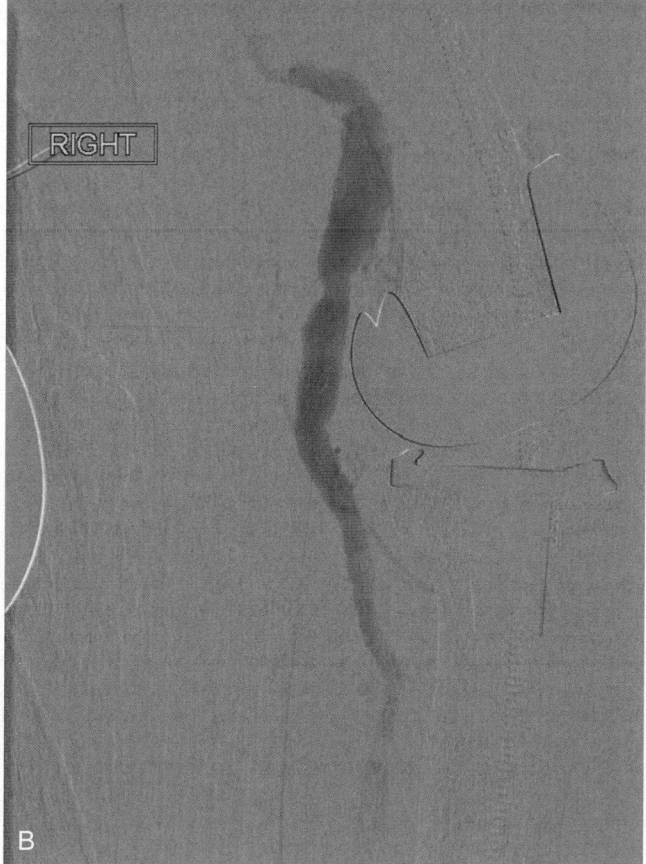

FIGURE 2 Computed tomography angiography (*top*) and contrast arteriogram (*bottom*) showing the right popliteal artery.

motor or sensory deficit, it is appropriate to begin systemic anticoagulation and proceed with diagnostic angiography on an urgent basis. If a suitable outflow vessel for surgical bypass is identified, a medial approach, proximal and distal ligation of the aneurysm, and surgical bypass with saphenous vein (described later) is the most reasonable approach. If there is no suitable outflow artery for bypass, the patient should undergo catheter-directed thrombolysis with tissue plasminogen activator for 12 to 24 hours, possibly in conjunction with the use of a mechanical thrombectomy catheter such as the AngioJet device (Boston Scientific, Marlborough, MA). The goal is to establish a suitable outflow vessel (distal target) for subsequent surgical bypass. Any patient with progression to a motor or sensory deficit during thrombolysis should return immediately to the operating room. If there is a motor or sensory deficit at presentation, the patient's limb is threatened and requires immediate revascularization. In this situation, begin systemic anticoagulation and perform emergent angiography. If there is a suitable outflow vessel, a medial approach, ligation of the aneurysm, and surgical bypass with saphenous vein remains the best approach. If there is no suitable outflow artery for bypass on angiography, operative tibial thrombectomy should be performed. This requires isolation of the below-knee popliteal artery and the origin of all three tibial arteries. After securing proximal and distal control, a Number 2 thrombectomy catheter is directed sequentially down all three tibial vessels. Follow-up arteriography is necessary to identify the optimal distal target for surgical bypass.

Elective Open Surgical Repair

The operative plan for elective surgical repair of popliteal artery aneurysms must consider the arterial inflow and outflow, availability of venous conduit, extent of preoperative embolization, compression of adjacent structures requiring decompression, and degree of aneurysmal degeneration. Most commonly, elective surgical management of a popliteal aneurysm is approached by a medial incision, proximal and distal ligation of the aneurysm, and great saphenous vein bypass grafting. With this technique, the patient is positioned supine. The great saphenous vein is mobilized and harvested for a sufficient length. The same incision can be used to expose the above-knee and below-knee popliteal artery. If the distal nonaneurysmal popliteal artery, proximal posterior tibial artery, or peroneal artery is the distal target of the bypass, this incision, extended distally, will suffice. If the more distal anterior tibial artery or peroneal artery is the outflow target, a separate incision is required. In the majority of cases, a subfascial tunnel or an anatomic tunnel between the heads of the gastrocnemius muscles is used for the bypass. After the administration of 80 to 100 U/kg of intravenous heparin, an arterial bypass is performed in a standard fashion with either an end-to-end or end-to-side configuration sewn in place with monofilament polypropylene suture. The saphenous vein conduit can be reversed or nonreversed, the latter obviously requiring vein valve lysis. In general, the bypass should be kept as short as possible while being performed from a nonaneurysmal inflow artery to the most suitable distal target. After completing the proximal and distal anastomoses, ligatures are secured proximal and distal to the aneurysmal segment, and a completion study (either arteriography or duplex ultrasonography) should be performed to ensure the absence of a technical error.

In contrast to the medial approach, a posterior approach (Figure 3) is favorable when a large aneurysm is causing compressive symptoms. Although it allows for decompression, this approach limits the arterial exposure and access to the great saphenous vein. The patient is positioned prone, and an S-shaped incision is made starting medially on the thigh and extending laterally across the flexion crease. The incision ends laterally over the proximal small saphenous vein. The great saphenous vein in the medial thigh or small saphenous vein can be used as the conduit for this approach. Once the conduit is obtained, the popliteal artery is identified by palpation and exposed in its proximal portion by separating the

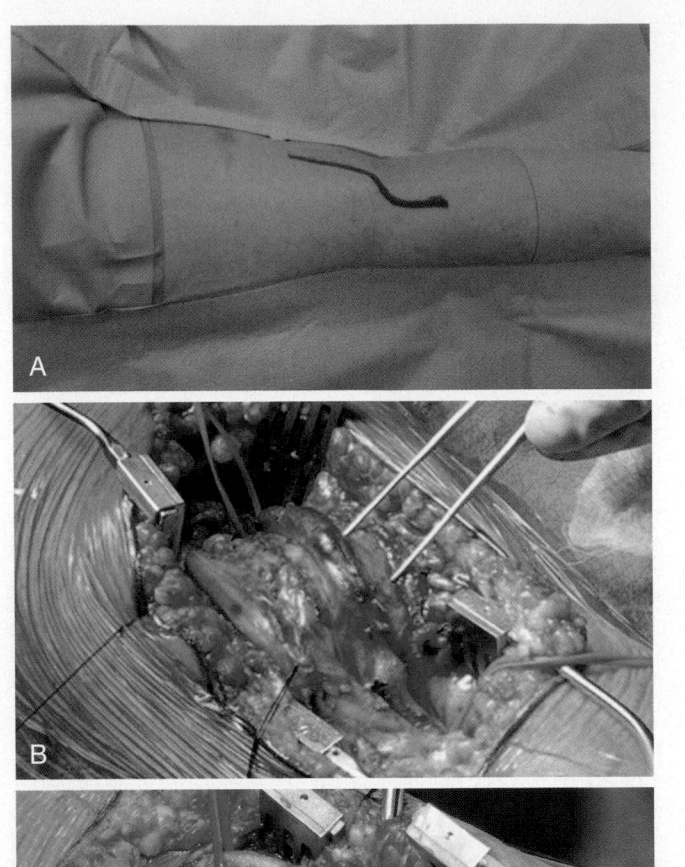

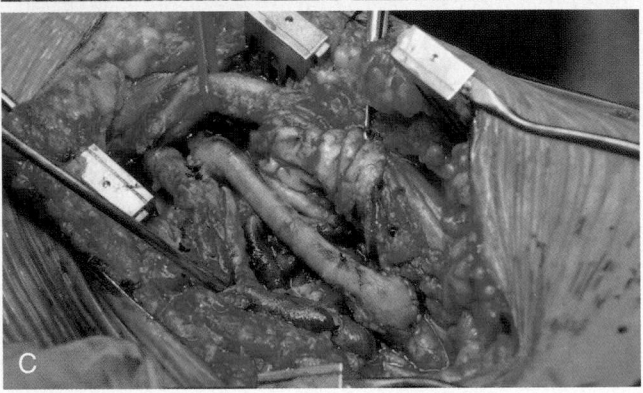

FIGURE 3 Intraoperative photos from a posterior approach for repair of a popliteal artery aneurysm. **A,** An S-shaped incision is made starting medially on the thigh and extending laterally across the flexion crease. **B,** The adjacent popliteal vein and tibial nerve adherent to the aneurysm sac. **C,** Completed great saphenous vein interposition graft before closure of the residual popliteal aneurysm sac.

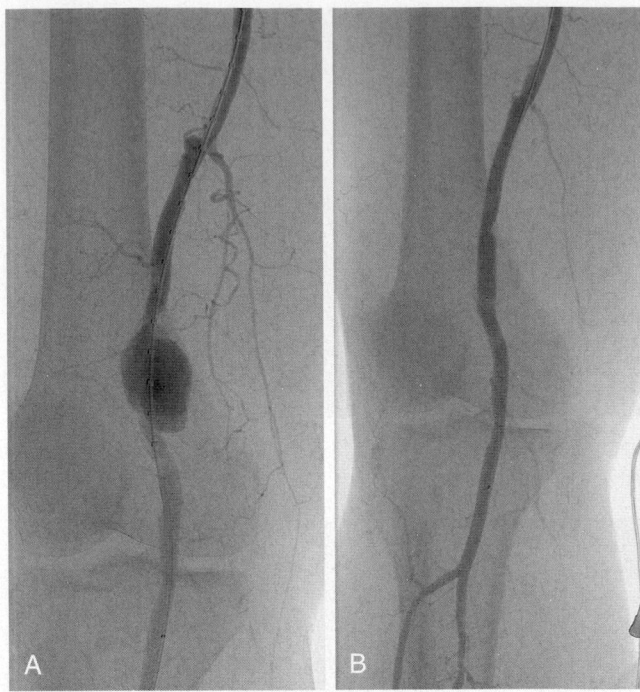

FIGURE 4 Contrast arteriogram before (**A**) and after (**B**) endovascular stent graft repair of a popliteal artery aneurysm.

semimembraneous and semitendinosus muscles from the biceps femoris. After obtaining proximal control, the dissection is carried distally, taking care not to injure the tibial and peroneal nerves, which are often adherent to the aneurysm sac. Next, the distal nonaneurysmal popliteal artery is dissected free and controlled in a fashion similar to the proximal artery. After the administration of intravenous heparin, proximal and distal control is secured and the aneurysm sac is incised. Thrombus is removed and geniculate collaterals are oversewn from within. Analogous to the technique of abdominal aortic aneurysm repair, a beveled vein graft is sewn end to end to the popliteal artery. If there is a significant size discrepancy between the native popliteal artery and the venous conduit or if venous conduit is not available, a prosthetic conduit (i.e., polytetrafluoro-

ethylene [PTFE]) is acceptable and demonstrates excellent intermediate results.

Endovascular Popliteal Aneurysm Repair

The indications for endovascular popliteal aneurysm repair are identical to those of open surgery. Although endovascular repair provides some short-term benefit in terms of reduced perioperative morbidity and decreased length of hospital stay, long-term results are still unknown. Endovascular repair generally is reserved for patients who are of high operative risk, have suitable anatomy, and are free from multiple embolic tibial artery occlusions. Analogous to endovascular abdominal aortic aneurysm repair, the arterial anatomy should be defined with a preprocedure CTA. To be a suitable candidate, the popliteal aneurysm should not be extensive in length and have at least 2 cm of normal artery proximal and distal to the aneurysm to ensure stent graft exclusion of the aneurysm. The procedure can be performed under general, regional, or local anesthesia. The patient should start taking an antiplatelet medicine, ideally clopidogrel, preoperatively. After anesthesia, the common femoral artery (contralateral or ipsilateral) is accessed percutaneously or with open exposure. After systemic heparinization, arteriography is performed and the aneurysm is traversed with a guidewire. Repeat angiography ensures the selection of stent(s) with appropriate diameter and length, along with precise selection of proximal and distal landing zones. The stent diameter should be oversized by 10% to 15% in comparison with the nonaneurysmal proximal and distal artery, and multiple stents may be needed if the popliteal aneurysm is more extensive. Next, a nitinol stent(s) lined with PTFE, such as the Viabahn endoprosthesis (W. L. Gore & Associates, Flagstaff, AZ), is deployed. After stent deployment, balloon angioplasty should be performed to ensure sealing proximally and distally as well as overlap of multiple stents. Completion angiography should be performed to exclude endoleak (Figure 4). Clopidogrel is continued indefinitely, and surveillance duplex ultrasound is performed every 3 months for the first year and biannually thereafter.

Results

Outcomes after popliteal artery aneurysm repair depend on the clinical presentation. Asymptomatic patients can expect a perioperative mortality of less than 1% and patency rates superior to those of arterial reconstructions performed for peripheral arterial occlusive disease. Specifically, average 5-year patency and limb salvage rates are approximately 85% and 95%, respectively. In contrast, emergent operations on symptomatic patients demonstrate 5-year patency and limb salvage rates that are inferior and average 60% and 70%, respectively. It is also important to highlight that the amputation rate in patients with acute limb ischemia is as high as 25%. Endovascular repair of popliteal artery aneurysms continues to evolve, and long-term follow-up data remain limited. Although initial technical success with endovascular repair approaches 100%, secondary patency ranges from 75% to 100% at 12 months and from 80% to 85% at 36 months. In addition to surveillance directed at optimizing bypass or stent graft patency, patients with a popliteal artery aneurysm require ongoing observation, as they are at significant risk for developing additional aneurysms (thoracoabdominal, aortoiliac, femoral, and contralateral popliteal).

◼ ARTERIOSCLEROTIC (TRUE) FEMORAL ARTERY ANEURYSMS

Clinical Presentation

Although relatively uncommon, arteriosclerotic (or true) femoral artery aneurysms are the second most common peripheral artery aneurysm. Although the rate of complications associated with femoral artery aneurysms is much lower than that attributed to popliteal artery aneurysms, femoral artery aneurysms are more commonly associated with the presence of life-threatening and limb-threatening aneurysms in other locations. For instance, approximately 60% of patients with a true femoral artery aneurysm will have a concomitant abdominal aortic aneurysm and approximately 50% will have a popliteal artery aneurysm. True femoral aneurysms most commonly involve the common femoral artery. Aneurysmal degeneration of the deep femoral (or profunda femoris) artery occurs in approximately half of cases, whereas involvement of the proximal superficial femoral artery is rare. Similar to popliteal artery aneurysms, the pathogenesis of femoral artery aneurysm formation is unclear but is again thought to relate to inflammation and atherosclerotic degeneration of the arterial wall. Furthermore, the relationship of femoral artery aneurysms to other aneurysms points toward a systemic cause.

Femoral artery aneurysms are much more common in men, with a male-to-female ratio of 20:1. The typical patient with a femoral artery aneurysm is a male in the sixth or seventh decade of life with a history of cigarette smoking, hypertension, and coronary artery disease. Patients may be seen with a pulsatile mass (30%), pain (10%), or compressive symptoms leading to edema or neuropathy (3%). Most patients, approximately 40% to 60%, will be asymptomatic at the time of their initial diagnosis. Complications such as embolization, thrombosis (~1%), and rupture (2%) are seen at a lower rate than with aortic or popliteal artery aneurysms.

Diagnosis

The majority of femoral artery aneurysms are identifiable on physical examination. Duplex ultrasound is an excellent confirmatory test and provides important information about aneurysm diameter, luminal thrombus, and extension into the deep or superficial femoral arteries. CTA provides additional detailed anatomic information and has largely supplanted angiography as the imaging modality of choice before surgical reconstruction (Figure 5).

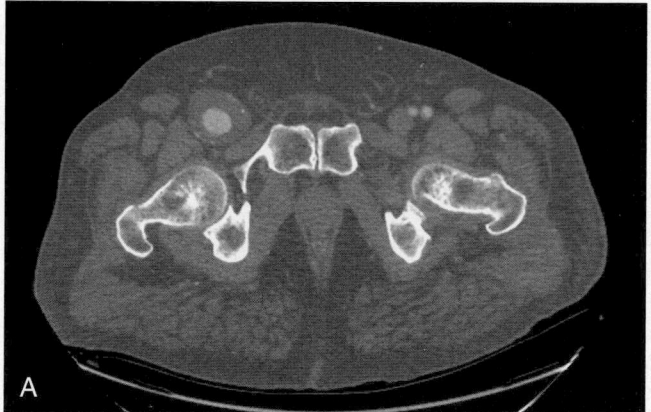

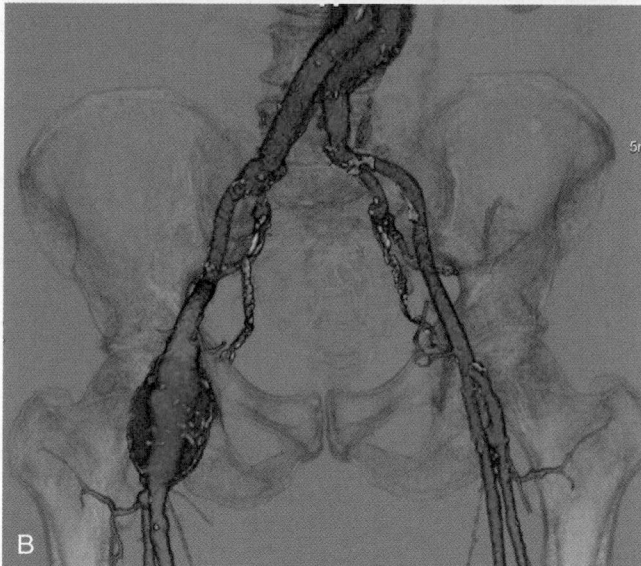

FIGURE 5 Axial image (*top*) and three-dimensional volume-rendered image (*bottom*) from computed tomography angiography demonstrating a large right common femoral artery true aneurysm. Note the previous open repair of a concomitant abdominal aortic aneurysm.

Natural History

The natural history of arteriosclerotic femoral aneurysms is not well defined, as most information is gathered from surgical case series. However, it is generally agreed upon that the natural history of femoral artery aneurysms is more benign than that of popliteal artery aneurysms.

Management

Operative repair is indicated in all symptomatic, complicated, or rapidly enlarging femoral artery aneurysms. Furthermore, emergent repair is indicated in acute limb ischemia due to thromboembolism or in the event of aneurysm rupture. The optimal diameter threshold for repair of asymptomatic femoral artery aneurysm is less clear and appears to be evolving. Historical recommendations called for repair of all femoral artery aneurysms with a diameter greater than 2.5 cm. These recommendations, however, were based on surgical series from an era predating current imaging and surgical techniques. A recent series of isolated arteriosclerotic femoral artery aneurysms, and the largest to date, has demonstrated that acute complications in isolated true femoral artery aneurysms did not occur in those with a diameter of less than 3.5 cm. With this in mind, these authors have called for a change in the repair criteria to be a diameter greater than 3.5 cm. This study also demonstrated that the presence of intraluminal thrombus correlated to the development of thromboembolic complications and should reduce the size threshold for elective repair. With this mind, we recommend repair in good-risk patients with a femoral artery aneurysm greater than 3 cm, especially if there is evidence of substantial intraluminal thrombus.

Operative Technique

The approach to an isolated femoral artery aneurysm is dictated by the involvement of the deep or superficial femoral arteries and the extent of peripheral artery occlusive disease. In the majority of cases, the surgical approach is through a standard vertical groin incision. Proximal control is obtained by isolating the uninvolved distal external iliac artery. This may require partial division of the inguinal ligament and infrequently requires a retroperitoneal approach via a transverse lower quadrant incision. After obtaining proximal control, distal control of normal-caliber superficial and deep femoral arteries is obtained. Aneurysms isolated to the common femoral artery are best treated with an interposition graft of PTFE or Dacron (8- to 10-mm diameter) anastomosed end to end from the distal external iliac to the distal common femoral artery. Given the high flow and large-caliber vessels involved, there is no disadvantage (in the absence of infection) to using prosthetic material rather than saphenous vein in this reconstruction. The aneurysm sac is seldom excised, as this can result in injury to adjacent structures. If the aneurysm involves the deep femoral artery, repair is dictated by the patency of the superficial femoral artery. If the superficial femoral artery is patent, an interposition graft from the common femoral artery to the deep femoral or superficial femoral artery may be constructed. This configuration then requires reimplantation or a graft side limb to the other artery. In patients with an occluded superficial femoral artery and without significant ischemia, an interposition graft to the deep femoral artery is sufficient. If the superficial femoral artery is occluded and lower extremity ischemia is significant, an interposition graft to the deep femoral artery followed by a standard femoral popliteal or femoral tibial bypass is needed. Currently, endovascular repair (i.e., stent graft) is not recommended because of the anatomic constraints of the femoral artery as well as the concern for stent fracture secondary to frequent hip flexion.

Results

Elective operative repair of asymptomatic femoral artery aneurysms is associated with low perioperative morbidity and mortality. Furthermore, long-term patency and limb salvage rates approach 100%. For repairs performed on an urgent or emergent basis, results are less favorable. Common perioperative complications include wound infection, seroma, and hematoma (~10%); renal insufficiency (~2%); acute limb ischemia (~2%); compartment syndrome (~1%); and deep venous thrombosis (~1%). Recurrent aneurysmal degeneration is rare.

◼ ANASTAMOTIC FEMORAL ARTERY ANEURYSMS

Anastomotic femoral artery aneurysms occur when there is disruption of an inflow or outflow femoral artery anastomosis. Most commonly, the anastomotic suture line has dehisced and the anastomosis is held together by the fibrous capsule of a pseudoaneurysm. Although this usually is seen with prosthetic bypass grafts, these aneurysms also can occur with an autologous conduit. Although this pathology is less frequently encountered in modern-day vascular surgery practice because of improvements in technique and graft and suture materials, these cases still pose a challenge for those who care for vascular surgery patients. It is important to keep in mind that these aneurysms are often (~60%) caused by infections with low-virulence

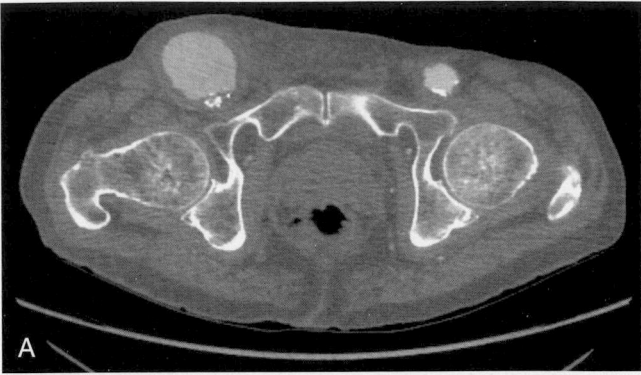
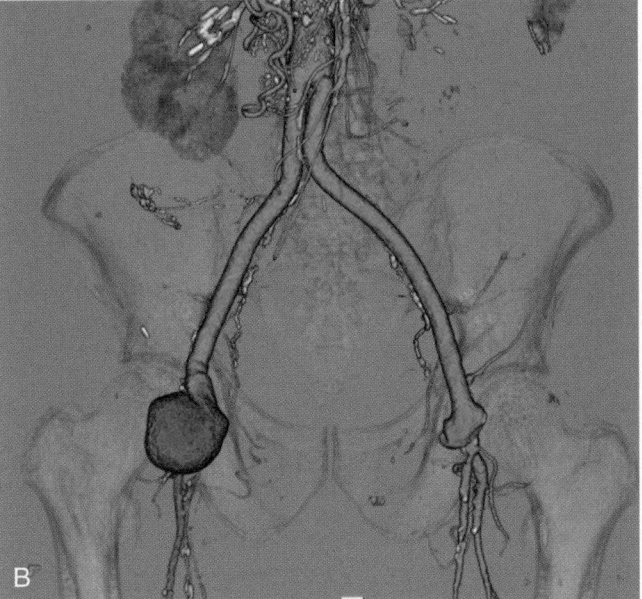

FIGURE 6 Axial image (*top*) and three-dimensional volume-rendered image (*bottom*) from computed tomography angiography demonstrating bilateral anastomotic aneurysms after aorta bifemoral bypass graft.

gram-positive organisms, such as *Staphylococcus epidermidis.* Despite this, serial duplex ultrasound surveillance is sufficient for most patients until symptoms develop or the aneurysm reaches a diameter greater than 2 to 3 cm. Once large or symptomatic, all anastomotic aneurysms require reconstruction. Because of the reoperative surgical field, these cases may be tedious. Preoperative CTA is useful for surgical planning (Figure 6). Moreover, adjunct techniques such as intraluminal vascular control with balloon catheters and remote incisions for proximal or distal control may be helpful. Rarely, débridement of the affected artery and simple re-anastomosis of the old graft are sufficient. More frequently, the affected portion of the old graft is excised and a new interposition graft is sewn into place. This requires that the affected artery is of good quality after débridement. Lastly, because infection is common, graft, tissue, and intraluminal thrombus should be sent for microbiology evaluation, and an all-autologous reconstruction should be considered when feasible.

◼ INFECTED FEMORAL PSEUDOANEURYSMS

An infected femoral artery aneurysm with subsequent pseudoaneurysm can result in hemorrhage, limb loss, or death. The majority of cases are a result of inadvertent intra-arterial injection of illicit drugs. Infection after percutaneous arterial procedures is much less common. A tender, pulsatile groin mass is often present. Other associated findings include cellulitis; an open, draining punctate skin lesion; signs of systemic infection; and sequelae of arterial embolization or occlusion. *Staphylococcus aureus* (with ~50% methicillin resistance) followed by *Pseudomonas aeruginosa* are the most common responsible organisms, although other more rare pathogens have been isolated from these patients. Arterial ligation with monofilament suture, débridement of all devitalized tissue, and 6 weeks of intravenous antibiotic therapy is appropriate for most infected femoral artery pseudoaneurysms. Intraoperative test clamping and Doppler interrogation of the extremity can help to determine how safely ligation of the femoral artery will be tolerated. Multiple reports have documented that this approach is generally well tolerated and that revascularization usually is not required in patients without pre-existing arterial occlusive disease. When ligating the femoral artery, it is important to preserve the proximal deep and superficial femoral artery branches, as these collaterals are necessary to optimize distal arterial perfusion. When limb viability is questionable, extra-anatomic reconstruction through clean surgical fields (i.e., obturator foramen bypass) or autologous reconstruction with contralateral saphenous or femoral vein may be required.

FEMORAL PSEUDOANEURYSM AFTER PERCUTANEOUS ARTERIAL ACCESS

There are conflicting data regarding the natural history of pseudoaneurysms after percutaneous access of the femoral artery. Some investigators have reported a very benign natural history, with up to 90% of iatrogenic femoral artery pseudoaneurysms undergoing spontaneous closure at 1 month. In contrast, others have found that approximately one third of iatrogenic femoral pseudoaneurysms will require surgical repair, with a greater risk in those who require ongoing anticoagulation or dual antiplatelet agents. Given these discordant natural history data, it is important for the clinician to individualize treatment. For the majority of small, uncomplicated pseudoaneurysms, nonoperative management with serial evaluations is safe and effective. In contrast, patients with large (>3 cm in diameter) or symptomatic pseudoaneurysms should undergo treatment. In addition, those with a need for ongoing anticoagulation or those with a questionable ability to follow up may benefit from intervention. Initial treatment of iatrogenic femoral artery pseudoaneurysms involves either ultrasound-guided compression or thrombin injection. In most investigations, percutaneous thrombin injection has proven to be more effective and less painful than ultrasound-guided compression in achieving primary pseudoaneurysm thrombosis. Nonetheless, we will provide a brief overview of both approaches.

Ultrasound-guided compression involves the use of a duplex ultrasound probe and concurrent ultrasound imaging to compress the pseudoaneurysm and eliminate flow into the aneurysm cavity while simultaneously maintaining flow in the native artery. Compression usually is applied for 20 to 30 minutes, and multiple sessions may be required to achieve thrombosis. Because of a high recurrence rate (~10%) and the associated patient discomfort, most regard this as a second-tier treatment option.

In comparison, ultrasound-guided thrombin injection is a safe, effective, and rapid method to induce femoral pseudoaneurysm thrombosis. Thrombin injection is performed via 20- or 22-gauge spinal needle directed into the pseudoaneurysm cavity with the aid of ultrasound scanning. After confirming proper needle placement and the return of pulsatile blood, less than 1 mL of a recombinant thrombin solution (1000 U/mL) is injected slowly over 2 to 3 seconds until flow into the pseudoaneurysm ceases on color Doppler. Care must be taken to avoid spillage of thrombin solution into the native artery by excessive volume injection. Pseudoaneurysms with short or wide necks are not suitable for this technique.

In patients who fail or who are not candidates for either of these techniques, surgical repair through a standard vertical groin incision is indicated. Because of overlying hematoma, vascular control may be difficult. The initial focus of the surgeon should be to expeditiously obtain proximal arterial control at the inguinal ligament. After obtaining proximal vascular control, distal control can be obtained via traditional methods or with finger compression. The responsible arterial injury is usually small and identifiable after hematoma evacuation. The majority of cases can be repaired primarily with monofilament vascular suture.

SUGGESTED READINGS

Antonello M, Frigatti P, Battocchio P, et al. Open repair versus endovascular treatment for asymptomatic popliteal artery aneurysm: results of a prospective randomized study. *J Vasc Surg.* 2005;42:185-193.

Diwan A, Sarkar R, Stanley JC, et al. Incidence of femoral and popliteal artery aneurysms in patients with abdominal aortic aneurysms. *J Vasc Surg.* 2000;31:863-869.

Huang Y, Gloviczki P, Noel AA, et al. Early complications and long-term outcome after open surgical treatment of popliteal artery aneurysms: is exclusion with saphenous vein bypass still the gold standard? *J Vasc Surg.* 2007;45:706, 713, discussion 713-715.

Kang SS, Labropoulos N, Mansour MA, et al. Percutaneous ultrasound guided thrombin injection: a new method for treating postcatheterization femoral pseudoaneurysms. *J Vasc Surg.* 1998;27:1032 1038.

Lawrence PF, Harlander-Locke MP, Oderich GS, et al. The current management of isolated degenerative femoral artery aneurysms is too aggressive for their natural history. *J Vasc Surg.* 2014;59:343-349.

Ravn H, Bjorck M. Popliteal artery aneurysm with acute ischemia in 229 patients: outcome after thrombolytic and surgical therapy. *Eur J Vasc Endovasc Surg.* 2007;33:690-695.

THE TREATMENT OF CLAUDICATION

Margo Hoyler, MD, and Glenn M. LaMuraglia, MD

Claudication, defined as muscular impairment due to exercise-induced ischemia, is the earliest and most frequent presentation of lower extremity peripheral arterial disease (PAD). It is commonly experienced as pain, discomfort, or weakness of the extremities on exertion, and claudication symptoms may range from mild to debilitating. Although unlikely to progress to critical limb ischemia (CLI) or limb loss, claudication is a marker of systemic atherosclerosis and is associated with increased rates of cardiovascular complications such as myocardial infarction, stroke, and death. Short of these associations, claudication can be a significant source of morbidity, disability, and impaired quality of life for the millions of people it affects.

Appropriate treatment of claudication can alleviate symptoms, slow local disease progression, and reduce systemic cardiovascular risk. This chapter summarizes the clinical approach to claudication, including diagnosis, medical and behavioral management, and the indications and strategies for vascular reconstruction.

PATHOPHYSIOLOGY AND INITIAL EVALUATION

Claudication is caused by an imbalance in circulatory peripheral oxygen supply and muscular metabolic demand. Atherosclerotic occlusive disease leads to diminished muscle perfusion and oxygen reserves that cannot accommodate increased local oxygen requirements during exercise. Classic claudication symptoms include fatigue, aching, and cramping of the buttock, hip, or leg during exercise. Less commonly, affected individuals may experience muscular weakness, with resultant instability that can cause imbalance or falling while walking. Symptoms are highly reproducible, occur only during exercise of the hypoperfused muscle groups, and promptly resolve with rest. Nerve compression, venous congestion, arthritis, and other processes may produce similar symptoms. However, a careful history usually will differentiate atherosclerotic ischemic impairment from other causes of limb pain and weakness. Indeed, the diagnosis of claudication often can be made solely on the basis of an appropriately focused patient interview.

On initial evaluation, particular attention is paid to symptom reproducibility and the impact of claudication on activities of daily living. Patients are screened for symptoms of CLI, most notably rest pain, and prior diagnoses of coronary artery and cerebrovascular disease. Clinicians also must identify and address all cardiovascular risk factors, such as hypertension, hyperlipidemia, chronic kidney disease, diabetes, and tobacco use, in an attempt to arrest the progression of the atherosclerotic disease process. Finally, it is important to assess at the initial evaluation what the patient's rehabilitation potential is, and to identify any major comorbid conditions, such as age, significant arthritis, cardiac failure or stroke, that could pre-empt major attempts at improvement in symptoms.

Physical examination consists of a full vascular assessment of the cardiac, carotid, and peripheral systems. This includes deep abdominal palpation for possible aortic aneurysm and careful evaluation of all peripheral pulses. The lower extremities are inspected for early skin breakdown and wounds and for atrophy, pallor, and rubor suggestive of chronic ischemia. Musculoskeletal deformities, especially of the foot or toes, may be indicative of significant neuropathy. Evaluation of the presence and amplitude of peripheral pulses is valuable, although pulse quality may not truly reflect muscle perfusion, particularly in the setting of diffuse vessel calcification. Instead, perfusion of the lower extremities is most accurately assessed through vascular laboratory studies.

Ankle-brachial index (ABI), a ratio of upper and lower extremity systolic blood pressures, should be measured in any patient with suspected claudication or PAD. A decreased ABI reflects a hemodynamically significant compromise in blood flow between the upper and lower body. A resting ABI less than 0.9 is diagnostic of PAD, and a resting ABI between 0.5 and 0.7 is a reliable predictor of claudication, though not necessarily symptom severity. Exercise testing often is required to delineate severity and verify the diagnosis. If a patient with compelling history and risk factors has a normal ABI on initial evaluation, exercise ABI is warranted. Of note, ABIs also may be falsely elevated because of vessel wall calcifications, particularly in patients who are diabetic or who undergo hemodialysis. Other methods for assessing perfusion include segmental limb pressures including the toes, duplex evaluation, and volume plethysmography. Duplex analysis identifies vessel stenosis and rigidity through progressive arterial waveform deterioration. Volume plethysmography measures global lower extremity perfusion through changes in limb volume across the cardiac cycle. These studies are useful both on initial evaluation and on subsequent assessment of disease progression but may be confounded by edema, obesity, or technical considerations. Finally, although laboratory studies are not necessary for a diagnosis of claudication, hemoglobin A_{1c} (HbA$_{1c}$), serum creatinine, and fasting lipid profiles may provide additional valuable information regarding a patient's overall cardiovascular risk profile. Once diagnosed, a patient with claudication should be evaluated at least annually by a vascular specialist.

Several staging systems have been developed to describe the severity of PAD, most notably the Fontaine and Rutherford classifications (Tables 1 and 2). In patients with claudication, these severity scales have been shown to correspond to degrees of global physical disability. Furthermore, severity score on presentation can help to

TABLE 1: Fontaine Symptom Classification System for Peripheral Arterial Disease

Stage	Symptoms
I	No symptoms
IIa	Intermittent claudication; symptoms occur at distances >200 m (650 ft)
IIb	Intermittent claudication; symptoms occur at distances <200 m (650 ft)
III	Rest pain
IV	Tissue necrosis; gangrene

TABLE 2: Rutherford Symptom Classification System for Peripheral Arterial Disease

Stage	Symptoms
1	No symptoms
2	Mild claudication
3	Moderate claudication
4	Severe claudication
5	Ischemic ulceration confined to digits of the foot
6	Ischemic ulceration not limited to digits of the foot; gangrene

predict which patients will fall into the 10% to 20% of those with claudication who experience significant deterioration of symptoms over time or into the 5% to 10% who ultimately develop CLI.

◼ MEDICAL MANAGEMENT OF ATHEROSCLEROTIC RISK AND DISEASE

Appropriate management of intermittent claudication has two central aims: (1) reduction of overall cardiovascular risk and (2) improvement of specific claudication symptoms with a resultant increased physical function. This includes aggressive management of comorbidities and risk factors, smoking cessation and focused exercise therapy, and potentially vascular reconstruction. The following discussion of medical therapies addresses long-term treatment goals. It is summarized in Figure 1.

Hypertension

Data from the Framingham Heart Study indicate that patients with stage 2 hypertension are more than twice as likely as normotensive patients to have PAD. The association between hypertension and cardiovascular disease (CVD) is similarly well established, as are the benefits of angiotensin-converting enzyme (ACE) inhibitors and beta-blockers. Hypertension in claudicants should be managed as it would be in any patient with atherosclerotic disease: goal blood pressure (BP) less than 140/90 mm Hg for nondiabetics or less than 130/80 mm Hg for diabetics. There is a theoretical concern that beta-blockers can exacerbate claudication and lower extremity ischemia, but clinical data have not substantiated this correlation. Beta-blockers and ACE inhibitors should be prescribed if otherwise indicated.

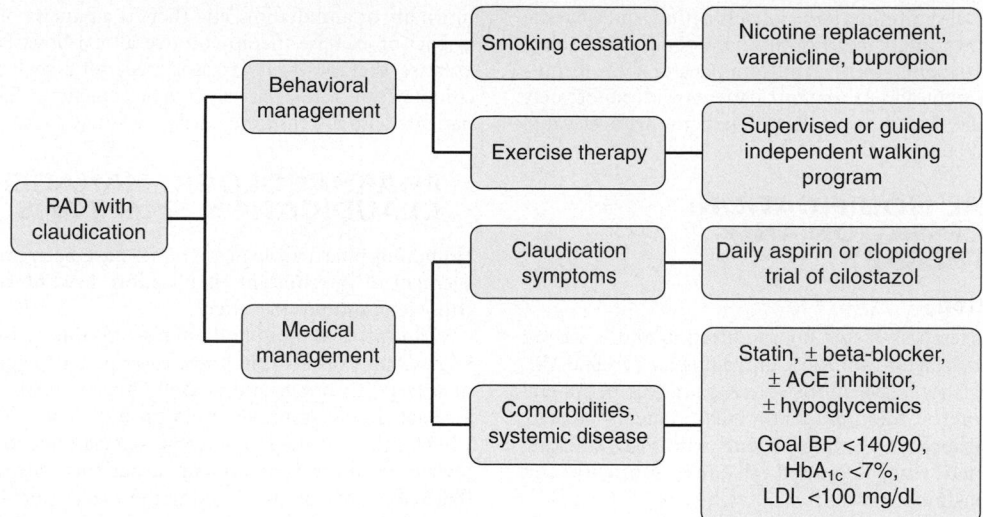

FIGURE 1 Algorithm for revascularization in the management of claudication. *ACE,* Angiotensin-converting enzyme; *BP,* blood pressure; *HbA$_{1c}$,* hemoglobin A$_{1c}$; *LDL,* low-density lipoprotein; *PAD,* peripheral arterial disease.

Diabetes

Diabetes is the strongest risk factor for PAD, with roughly 29% of diabetics identified as having the condition. When compared with nondiabetics with similar risk factors, patients with diabetes are twice as likely to suffer from intermittent claudication. Insulin requirement, compared with oral hypoglycemic and diet-driven management, repeatedly has been correlated to decreased survival in patients with lower extremity ischemia. In patients with PAD, appropriate glucose control has been associated with trends toward decreased rates of myocardial infarction (MI) and stroke but has not been shown to reduce the risk of death or limb loss. More aggressive glucose control—for instance, targeting normal glucose levels—is not necessarily beneficial. The Action to Control Cardiovascular Risk in Diabetes (ACCORD) trial found lower rates of nonfatal cardiovascular events in patients with type 2 diabetes assigned to intensive glucose-lowering therapy (goal HbA$_{1c}$ <6%). On the other hand, this group was found to have a higher rate of all-cause and cardiovascular mortality, resulting in a premature termination of the trial. As a result, current evidence does not support overly aggressive glucose management; the goal in patients with PAD should be HbA$_{1c}$ less than 7.0%, as it is with other patients with CVD.

Hyperlipidemia

Statin therapy is indicated in all patients with hyperlipidemia and symptomatic PAD, with a goal low-density lipoprotein (LDL) level less than 70 mg/dL in patients with a history of acute coronary syndrome and less than 100 mg/dL in patients with no history of acute coronary syndrome. Treatment is indicated primarily because of the high likelihood of coronary or cerebral atherosclerosis in patients with PAD and the documented benefit of statin therapy in reducing cardiovascular risk in patients with systemic atherosclerotic disease. However, statins also may have additional benefit for patients with PAD, as studies have shown decreased risk of new-onset claudication, decreased image-based disease progression, and improved pain-free walking time in patients with PAD who are treated with statins.

Ezetimibe and niacin may be considered as adjunct lipid-lowering therapies or as alternative therapies in statin-intolerant patients. Indeed, recent data suggest that lower LDL levels may yield significant clinical benefits, regardless of the medical therapy involved. The Improved Reduction of Outcomes: Vytorin Efficacy International Trial (IMPROVE-IT) found that treatment ezetimibe and simvastatin, compared with simvastatin alone, was associated with significantly decreased LDL levels and reduced risk of cardiovascular events in patients with a history of acute coronary syndrome. A similar effect has not been specifically demonstrated in patients with PAD and claudication.

Coagulation

Among patients with CVD, antiplatelet therapy is known to reduce the risk of nonfatal MI and stroke and mortality from vascular causes. Across hundreds of studies, low-dose aspirin therapy has been shown to be an effective antiplatelet regimen. Among patients with documented coronary artery disease (CAD), CVD, or PAD, the CAPRIE (clopidogrel versus aspirin in patients at risk of ischemic events) trial found that treatment with clopidogrel was associated with an 8.7% relative risk reduction for stroke, MI, and vascular death relative to treatment with aspirin (95% confidence interval [CI]: 0.3 to 16.5; $P = 0.043$). In the subgroup of patients with moderate to severe PAD, clopidogrel was associated with a 23.8% relative risk reduction (95% CI: 8.9 to 36.2; $P = 0.0028$). Of note, the latter analysis was not limited to patients with intermittent claudication but also included patients with CLI and a history of revascularization procedures.

The Society for Vascular Surgery (SVS) currently recommends 81 to 325 mg of aspirin daily as the primary antiplatelet regimen for these patients, with 75 mg of clopidogrel as an acceptable alternative. Combined aspirin-clopidogrel treatment is not recommended because of risk for bleeding and lack of data showing superior outcomes on a dual regimen. Most notably, the MATCH (management of atherothrombosis with clopidogrel in high-risk patients) trial demonstrated a small but significant increased risk for major or life-threatening bleeding in cerebrovascular patients treated with both aspirin and clopidogrel, with no significant reduction in risk of cardiovascular events.

Hyperhomocysteinemia

Hyperhomocysteinemia is an independent predictor of PAD. Homocysteine promotes oxidation of LDL cholesterol and through production of free radicals may predispose to endothelial dysfunction and accelerated atherosclerosis. Vitamin B$_{12}$ and folic acid supplementation can be used to decrease serum levels of homocysteine and has been associated with increased ABIs in short-term trials of patients with PAD. It is unclear, however, if there is a corresponding improvement in clinical symptoms and global function, and what the durability of this effect might be. Routine vitamin B_{12} and folate supplementation in patients with claudication cannot be recommended based on current clinical data in patients with moderately elevated homocysteine, but it is unclear if patients with elevated homocysteine should be treated.

◼ BEHAVIORAL MODIFICATION: SMOKING CESSATION AND EXERCISE THERAPY

Smoking Cessation

Smoking is the strongest risk factor for claudication and is second only to diabetes as a risk factor for PAD. Controlling for baseline ABI, smokers with claudication have more severe pain, less peripheral circulation, and poorer cardiopulmonary measurements at peak exercise than do nonsmokers. Among patients with PAD, smoking cessation is associated with decreased all-cause mortality and improved amputation-free survival.

Smokers with claudication should be counseled extensively regarding the risks of smoking and its association with lower extremity symptoms. Patients should be offered smoking cessation aids and counseling whenever possible. Nicotine replacement therapy (NRT) has been shown to increase quit rates by 50% to 70%; bupropion is equally effective and varenicline may be even more effective. Data suggest that NRT combined with varenicline is the most effective smoking cessation regimen overall.

Exercise Therapy

Patients with intermittent claudication have impaired peak physiologic responses to exercise as well as lower levels of physical activity overall. Focused physical activity of the affected limbs is thus a mainstay of claudication management. A 2014 Cochrane review of exercise therapy for patients with claudication found that exercise therapy increased maximal walking time by nearly 5 minutes, on average, and pain-free walking distance by more than 80 meters. Exercise therapy also improves patients' ability to carry out activities of daily living and has been shown to increase function for up to 2 years after the termination of therapy. These benefits of exercise therapy also extend to patients who have diabetes and are active smokers.

It is important to note that supervised exercise therapy effects greater functional improvements than unsupervised exercise, with a demonstrated dose-response relationship according to the degree of supervision. A recent Cochrane review of supervised exercise therapy found a statistically significant improvement in pain-free walking distance relative to unsupervised exercise regimens, with an increased walking distance of approximately 180 meters in the supervised group. In the absence of supervised programs, structured and goal-oriented exercise programs are critical. Clinicians should recognize that encouraging patients to "walk more" is unlikely to yield significant improvement. Instead, patients should be "prescribed" a specific exercise regimen. Exercise plans studied in the medical literature typically include 3 to 5 exercise sessions per week for approximately 2 hours total, or 35 to 50 minutes per session. During these sessions, patients are instructed to exercise to a point of significant discomfort, recover through a brief period of rest, and then resume the exercise activity. Treadmill and track walking are the most effective in improving claudication symptoms; resistance training may supplement but should not replace walking therapy.

The mechanisms by which exercise therapy improves claudication symptoms have not been identified. However, demonstrated responses to exercise training include increased efficiency in walking, induction of angiogenesis and formation of collateral blood vessels, increased metabolic efficiency of myocytes, and overall improved conditioning. It is likely that each of these mechanisms contributes to the clinical improvement of claudication symptoms. Of note, exercise therapy has not been shown to increase ABI or decrease rates of mortality or amputation, and there is a paucity of data regarding the impact of exercise therapy on overall cardiovascular risk. Although exercise therapy itself is associated with very low cardiovascular complication rates, routine cardiac screening may be considered in patients with a significant cardiac history.

◼ PHARMACOLOGIC MANAGEMENT OF CLAUDICATION SYMPTOMS

Numerous pharmacologic therapies have been proposed in the management of intermittent claudication. Few, however, have shown a consistent and positive effect.

Cilostazol, a phosphodiesterase inhibitor, is a smooth muscle relaxant and vasodilator. It decreases platelet aggregation, formation of arterial thrombi, and smooth muscle proliferation and is also associated with improved lipid profiles. The drug was approved in 1999 for the treatment of intermittent claudication. A 2014 Cochrane review of cilostazol treatment in patients with claudication found that across eight double-blind randomized controlled trials, pain-free and maximum walking distances were increased significantly in participants who were taking cilostazol 100 mg and 50 mg twice daily, compared with placebo. A single study reported improvement in both metrics for patients taking 150 mg twice daily. The 100-mg dose also correlated to an improvement in ABI.

Cilostazol has not been shown to reduce all-cause mortality or cardiovascular events or increase quality of life. Furthermore, several early studies found that it was associated with trends toward increased rates of nonfatal MI as well as cardiovascular death; however, the increased risk was not statistically significant. Subsequent research has not found significantly different rates of morbidity or mortality in patients taking cilostazol compared with placebo, and the drug generally is considered safe for most patients with claudication. Because of its pharmacologic similarities to milrinone, however, cilostazol carries a black box warning against use in patients with heart failure. Of note, a postmarketing clinical study of cilostazol found no increased risk of bleeding in patients treated simultaneously with clopidogrel and cilostazol. Cilostazol is also contraindicated in patients with moderate to severe renal or hepatic impairment. Finally, patients taking cilostazol are at increased risk of headache, diarrhea, dizziness, and palpitations. These side effects are generally mild and treatable and can be dose dependent.

Propionyl carnitine and propionyl levocarnitine (PLC) may improve the exercise capacity of ischemic muscles by moderating the accumulation of oxidative metabolism intermediates. A recent meta-analysis of six phase III trials found that PLC increased walking distance by an average of 16 meters compared with placebo. The clinical significance of this effect is unclear, and this drug is not approved for intermittent claudication in the United States.

Finally, numerous vasodilators also have been proposed in the management of claudication. These include prostaglandins, ACE inhibitors, and calcium-channel blockers. To date, none of these drugs has been evaluated for this indication in large, high-quality trials.

◼ REVASCULARIZATION FOR INTERMITTENT CLAUDICATION

For many decades, the management of claudication was strictly noninvasive. This paradigm reflected both the relatively benign clinical course of the disease and the significant morbidity and mortality associated with open surgery. With the advent and refinement of endovascular techniques, nearly 30% of claudication patients now undergo revascularization procedures.

Endovascular techniques for revascularization include percutaneous transluminal angioplasty (PTA) and stenting; surgical approaches include endarterectomy and arterial reconstructions via anatomic or extra-anatomic bypass. Choice of treatment modality depends largely on the location and morphology of atherosclerotic disease, as identified on preoperative imaging, as well as the patient's comorbidities and overall operative risk profile. Endovascular therapies are typically more appropriate for focal lesions, whereas surgery may be indicated in patients with advanced, diffuse, and more complex lower extremity disease. A detailed discussion of revascularization indications and techniques is beyond the scope of this chapter, but a brief overview is in order (Figure 2).

There is broad consensus that revascularization should be offered only to patients with claudication who have optimized their risk factors and failed to show significant improvement from medical and exercise therapy. In addition, these patients should have work- or lifestyle-limiting symptoms and must not have comorbidities that would significantly impair walking in the absence of claudication (e.g., severe chronic obstructive pulmonary disease, arthritis). Revascularization also should be offered only if there is a high likelihood of durable symptomatic improvement. Finally, patients must be acceptable revascularization candidates in terms of cardiovascular risk. Before these interventions, all patients should be evaluated for untreated cardiac disease, including but not limited to unstable or severe angina, decompensated congestive heart failure, significant arrhythmias, and valvular disease. These conditions must be addressed appropriately before pursuing an elective intervention for claudication.

High-quality anatomic imaging is essential in determining lesion location, morphology, and suitability for intervention. However, clinicians may disagree regarding the amount and kinds of imaging to obtain. Duplex ultrasonography and magnetic resonance (MR) or computed tomographic (CT) angiography are increasingly common as preliminary or even definitive imaging modalities to determine suitability for an intervention. However, catheter-based angiography remains the "gold standard" and is necessary as part of any percutaneous intervention. The risk associated with angiography in experienced hands is exceedingly low, though notable complications include contrast-induced kidney injury, access site complications, and arterial dissection. Vein mapping is also a consideration for patients when surgical bypass is considered.

Benefits, Complications, and Costs

There is mounting evidence in favor of revascularization for intermittent claudication in appropriate candidates. The Claudication: Exercise Versus Endoluminal Revascularization (CLEVER) trial randomized patients with claudication and aortoiliac disease to a 6-month supervised exercise program, angioplasty and stenting, or optimal medical management and demonstrated that supervised exercise and stent revascularization each led to comparable increases in total walking time and time to symptom onset. These improvements were significantly greater than those achieved by optimal medical management alone and persisted at 18-month follow-up. The SUPER trial, currently underway, will compare exercise therapy with angioplasty in patients with claudication and iliac disease.

Similarly, a 2015 systematic review, commissioned by the SVS, concluded that revascularization was strongly superior to medical management alone in terms of walk performance and blood flow parameters. The same review also reported that revascularization and supervised exercise therapy together were superior to either approach in isolation. It cited a low level of evidence indicating that revascularization was superior to supervised exercise therapy alone, noting that some evidence suggested that blood flow parameters improved to a greater degree and more quickly after revascularization. Finally,

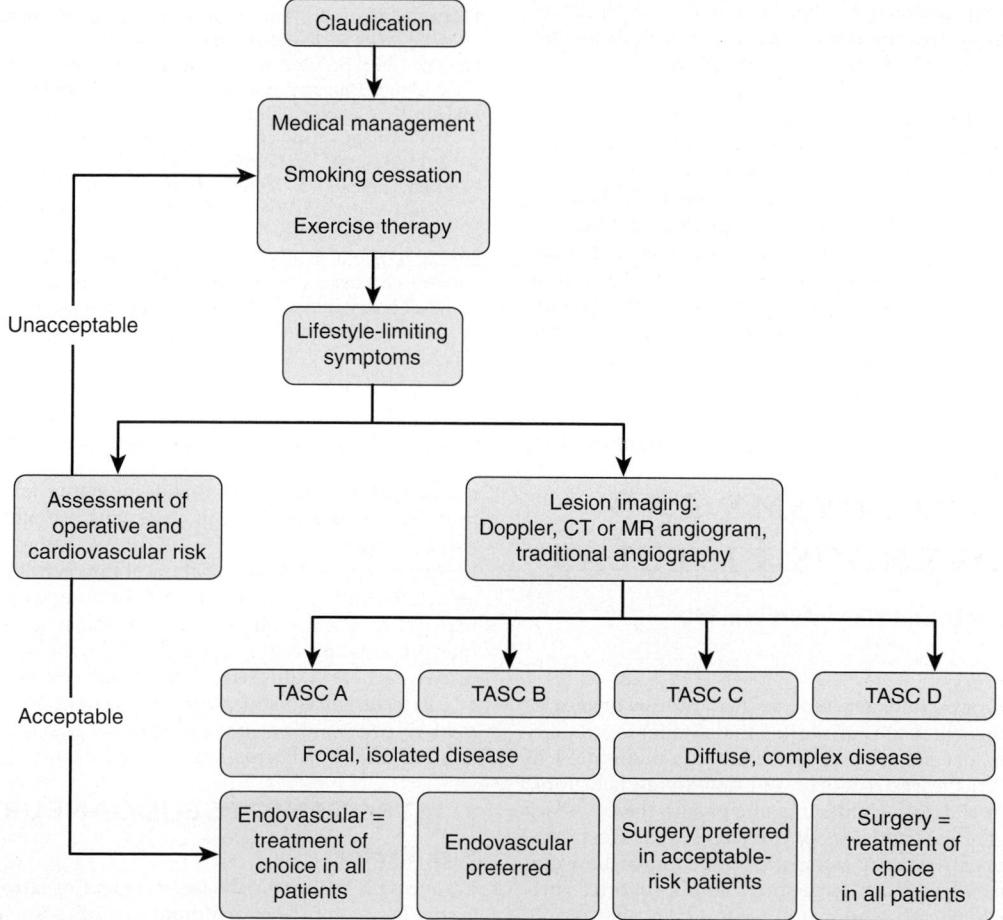

FIGURE 2 Nonoperative management of claudication. *CT,* Computed tomographic; *MR,* magnetic resonance; *TASC,* TransAtlantic Inter-Society Consensus class.

the report referenced moderate-quality evidence to indicate that endovascular therapy was favorable to open surgery, with lower endovascular patency rates counterbalanced by a decreased risk of perioperative complications and a shorter length of hospital stay compared with recipients of open surgery.

Revascularization in patients with claudication remains an elective procedure, the goal of which is lifestyle improvement and not limb salvage. Potential lifestyle improvements must be carefully balanced against the risks for periprocedural morbidity and mortality. Although endovascular intervention has a favorable morbidity and mortality profile compared with open surgery, complications include contrast-induced renal failure, arterial dissection and perforation, pseudoaneurysm, and embolism. Stents can fracture, migrate, and re-stenose. Furthermore, patency rates for endovascular treatments are generally inferior to those of open surgery; therefore the need for eventual reoperation should be discussed with patients. Stent placement also can constrain and possibly compromise subsequent bypass procedures, should they be necessary. These considerations may be especially relevant for young patients with early-onset, aggressive disease. In that population, intervention should be deferred for as long as possible and ample time allowed for the development of collateral flow. Perhaps most notably, in rare circumstances stent or graft occlusion can be acutely limb threatening. In this uncommon scenario, the "treatment" for claudication seems incomparably more dangerous than the original condition.

As these concerns illustrate, there is reason to think critically and carefully about the shift toward aggressive revascularization for claudication symptoms. At the very least, data indicate that revascularization should be used as a supplement to, not a replacement for, exercise therapy. Revascularization does not address the full range of factors, including muscle weakness, biomechanical strain, and poor balance, that contribute to exercise impairment in those with claudication. Patients likely derive important benefits from exercise therapy that are not easily captured by measuring total and pain-free walking distances.

Cost is another important consideration. Both open and endovascular procedures are dramatically more expensive than supervised walking programs, but the outcomes may not be materially better. A randomized controlled trial by Spronk and colleagues (2008) found no significant difference in the effectiveness of endovascular and exercise therapies, although endovascular treatments cost an additional 75,000 euros per quality-adjusted life-year. A similar trial by Mazari and colleagues concluded that supervised exercise therapy was the most cost-effective first-line intervention for patients with femoral-popliteal disease and that exercise therapy also increased the cost effectiveness of PTA when offered in conjunction with that intervention. Finally, the CLEVER trial found that stenting increased total costs by approximately $5000 compared with exercise, with an "uncertain" incremental clinical benefit. Studies also have shown significant savings from a "stepped" healthcare model for claudication, in which patients are offered supervised exercise therapy before revascularization. The importance of these data is magnified by the already tremendous costs associated with PAD and claudication in the United States. As of 2001 Medicare expenditures for PAD totaled more than $4.3 billion, with 6.8% of enrollees receiving PAD treatment. Clearly, further data are needed to guide cost-effective and maximally effective management of claudication.

CONCLUSION

Intermittent claudication is a significant cause of morbidity and disability and a powerful marker of systemic cardiovascular risk. Primary treatment includes atherosclerotic risk factor reduction and supervised or guided exercise therapy. Patients who have work- or lifestyle-limiting claudication despite appropriate medical and behavioral management may benefit from revascularization. The benefits of such procedures must be balanced carefully against their risks, cost, and limitations.

SUGGESTED READINGS

Conte MS, Pomposelli FB, Clair DG, et al. Society for Vascular Surgery practice guidelines for atherosclerotic occlusive disease of the lower extremities: management of asymptomatic disease and claudication. *J Vasc Surg.* 2015;61(suppl 3):2S-41S.

Hiatt WR. Medical treatment of peripheral arterial disease and claudication. *N Engl J Med.* 2001;344:1608-1621.

Lane R, Ellis B, Watson L, et al. Exercise for intermittent claudication. *Cochrane Database Syst Rev.* 2014;(7):CD000990.

Malgor RD, Alahdab F, Elraiyah TA, et al. A systematic review of treatment of intermittent claudication in the lower extremities. *J Vasc Surg.* 2015;61(suppl 3):54S-73S.

Norgren L, Hiatt WR, Dormandy JA, et al. Inter-Society Consensus for the Management of Peripheral Arterial Disease (TASC II). *J Vasc Surg.* 2007;45(suppl S):S5-S67.

Spronk S, Bosch JL, den Hoed PT, Veen HF, Pattynama PM, Hunink MG. Cost-effectiveness of endovascular revascularization compared to supervised hospital-based exercise training in patients with intermittent claudication: a randomized controlled trial. *J Vasc Surg.* 2008;48:1472-1480.

PSEUDOANEURYSMS AND ARTERIOVENOUS FISTULAS

M. Libby Weaver, MD, and Ying Wei Lum, MD

A false aneurysm, or pseudoaneurysm, refers to rupture of an arterial wall contained by a fibrous capsule that develops secondary to a local inflammatory response to persistent communication of arterial flow between the vessel lumen and developing hematoma adjacent to the arterial defect. Unlike true aneurysms, there is a lack of involvement of the normal layers of the artery wall. Most commonly, pseudoaneurysms develop as an iatrogenic complication after vascular access for endovascular procedures, with a reported incidence in 0.2% to 6% of interventional procedures. Other causes of pseudoaneurysm formation include blunt or penetrating trauma, anastomotic aneurysms, infection from bacterial seeding or direct needle injection, and congenital or idiopathic false aneurysm formation, particularly in those patients with vasculitides or connective tissue diseases.

Arteriovenous fistulas are atypical connections that occur between an arterial and venous structure. Like pseudoaneurysms, these may materialize as a complication after vascular access for diagnostic or interventional procedures, which will be the primary focus of their discussion here. In this setting the incidence is believed to be less than 1%. Arteriovenous fistulas also can occur as a result of trauma, particularly penetrating trauma; as a postsurgical complication; or rarely as a congenital malformation.

IATROGENIC PSEUDOANEURYSMS

Risk Factors

Various risk factors for the development of iatrogenic pseudoaneurysms exist. Improper anatomic identification of the appropriate access site during femoral cannulation for endovascular interventional or diagnostic procedures may lead to puncture of the external

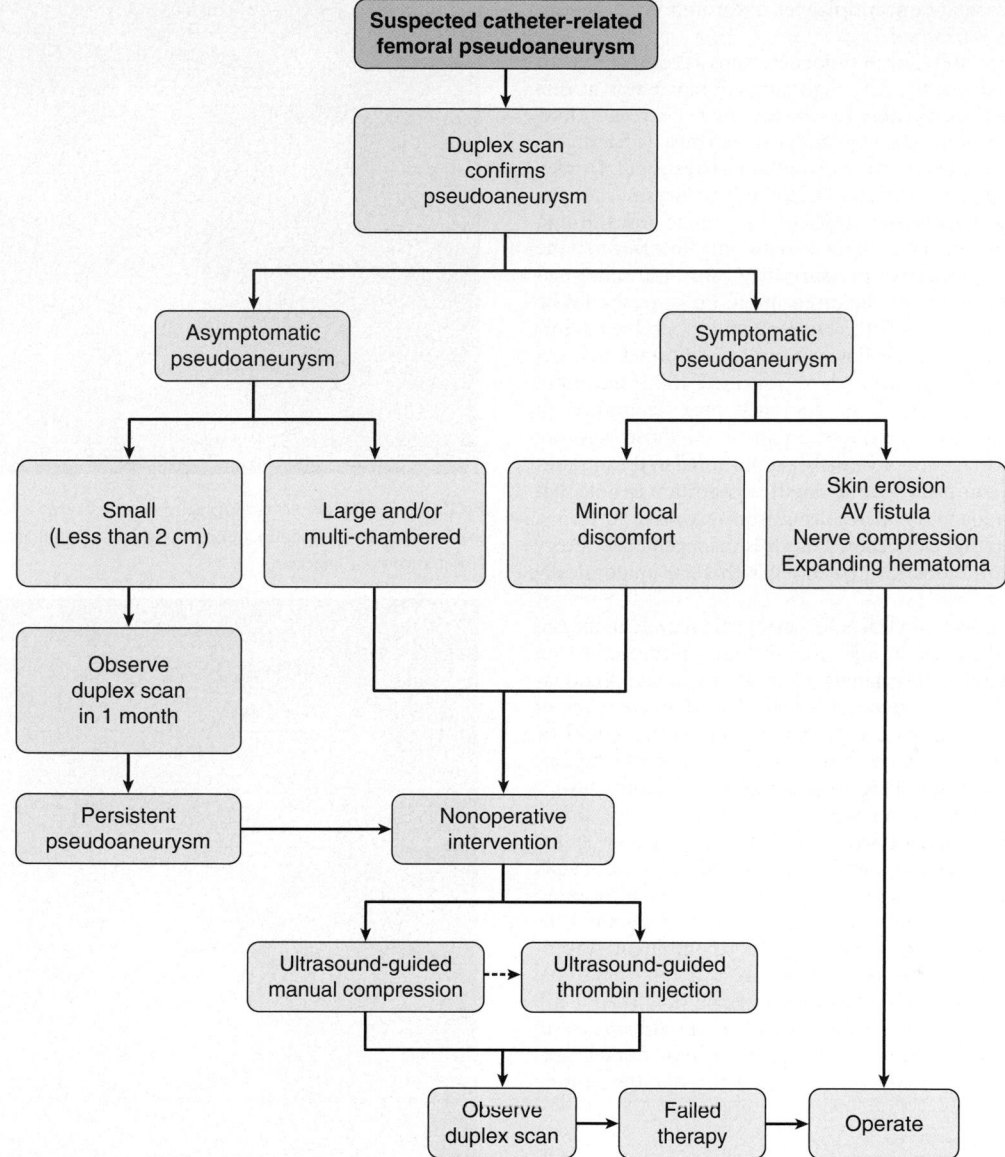

FIGURE 1 Algorithm for treatment of iatrogenic femoral artery pseudoaneurysms. AV, Arteriovenous. *(From Hirsch AT, Haskal ZJ, Hertzer NR, et al. Peripheral arterial disease: ACC/AHA 2005 guidelines for the management of patients with peripheral arterial disease [lower extremity, renal, mesenteric, and abdominal aortic]. J Am Coll Cardiol. 2006;47:1239-1312.)*

common iliac or superficial femoral arteries, which may be difficult to compress after sheath removal, leading to an increased risk of pseudoaneurysm development. The appropriate anatomic puncture site typically can be determined by identifying the center of the femoral head, which correlates with the midpoint of the common femoral artery, or by using ultrasound guidance for vascular access. Other risk factors include multiple puncture attempts, inadequate compression of the puncture site, use of anticoagulation (with a dose-related increase in risk), large sheath size, older age, hypertension, female gender, left-sided puncture, obesity, hemodialysis, heavily calcified vessels, and steroid use.

Clinical Presentation and Diagnosis

Iatrogenic pseudoaneurysms may be seen incidentally in the immediate postprocedure period by detection of a bruit on physical examination. They also may be seen as a pulsatile mass, severe groin pain, ecchymosis underlying the puncture site, or any combination of these. In severe cases there also may be overlying skin necrosis.

Diagnosis is confirmed with duplex ultrasonography. It is important to examine flow using color duplex to differentiate a pseudoaneurysm from a simple hematoma. A to-and-fro motion of blood flow within the aneurysmal sac is considered pathognomonic for pseudoaneurysm. It is important to determine both the length and the width of the neck of the pseudoaneurysm when evaluating with duplex ultrasonography, as these dimensions will play a role in determining the appropriate management strategy.

Treatment

The treatment algorithm for iatrogenic pseudoaneurysm is dependent on several factors and is summarized in Figure 1.

The majority of lesions measuring less than 2 cm in diameter can be managed expectantly. Nearly 90% of these lesions are likely to undergo spontaneous thrombosis over the course of several weeks in those patients who are not anticoagulated. These patients may be followed with serial duplex ultrasonography. In contrast, for those patients with pseudoaneurysms greater than 2 cm in diameter or for those receiving anticoagulation, antiplatelet, or thrombolytic therapy, prompt treatment is warranted.

The treatment principles for pseudoaneurysms as compared with true aneurysms differ greatly. Although surgical repair was at one time a mainstay of treatment, other less invasive management options are now preferred in appropriately selected patients. Ultrasound-guided compression can be an effective method of treatment. Duplex ultrasonography is used to identify the pseudoaneurysm, and the appropriate amount of pressure is applied to eliminate flow through the neck of the pseudoaneurysm while maintaining flow through the native arterial lumen. Excessive pressure may cause the unwanted complication of thrombosis of the artery itself. Pressure should be applied for at least 10 minutes with reassessment for persevered flow through the pseudoaneurysm. If flow continues, additional cycles of 20 minutes of compression should be executed until successful thrombosis occurs. This treatment approach may be limited in patients who are experiencing extreme pain or in those who are obese. Chronicity of the lesion is directly proportional to the amount of time required for complete thrombosis. It is important to note that rupture of the pseudoaneurysm resulting from excessive force is a serious complication that can occur. Thus this management strategy should be limited to lesions located in areas that are anatomically easy to access.

The current treatment of choice for iatrogenic pseudoaneurysm is ultrasound-guided thrombin injection. A duplex ultrasound scan should be performed first to evaluate the anatomy of the pseudoaneurysm in relation to the femoral artery. The characteristics of the neck, including its visualization, length, and width, should be taken into consideration because short, wide necks have the highest risk for distal thromboembolism as a complication from thrombin injection. After infiltration with local anesthetic, we prefer to puncture the pseudoaneurysm cavity with a 22-gauge spinal needle. The tip of the needle may be scored with a sterile scalpel to increase echogenicity and assist with visualization by ultrasound scan. Once the needle is visualized using ultrasound scan and centered in the pseudoaneurysm cavity, topical recombinant thrombin (1000 IU/mL) is infused percutaneously through the spinal needle with color Doppler visualization. Typically less than 1 mL is required to cause complete thrombosis of the pseudoaneurysm almost instantaneously (Figures 2 through 6). Repeat duplex scan examination then is performed to evaluate flow through the femoral artery and vein.

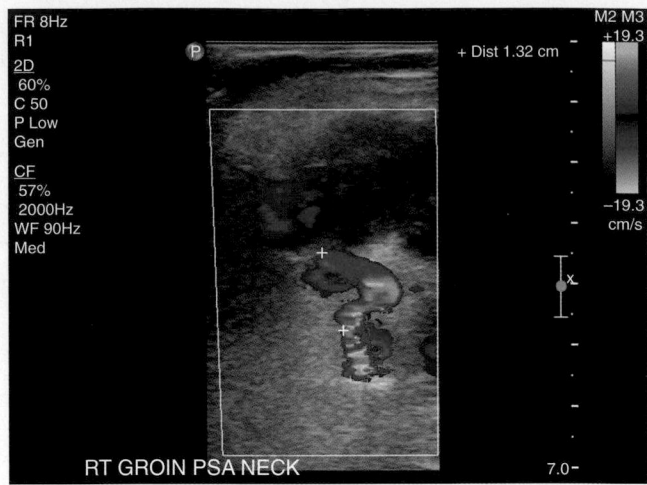

FIGURE 3 Duplex ultrasonography demonstrates a long, narrow neck of the femoral artery pseudoaneurysm, which is adequate for treatment with direct thrombin injection.

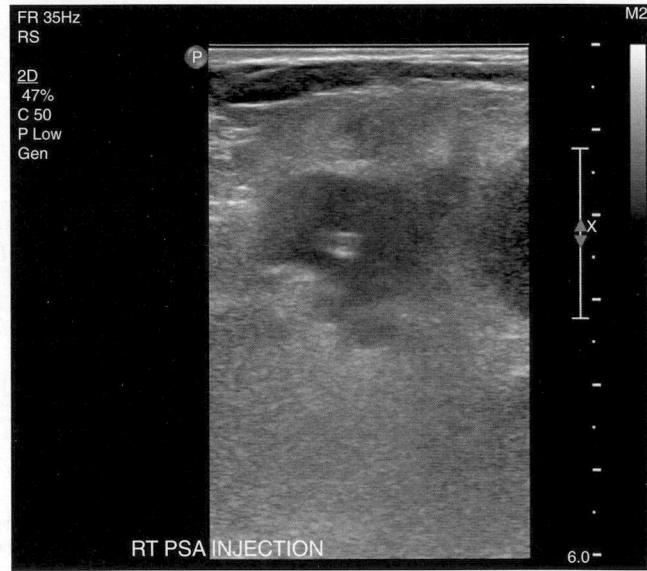

FIGURE 4 Ultrasonography demonstrates direct thrombin injection of a femoral artery pseudoaneurysm with a needle tip located in the center of the pseudoaneurysm sac.

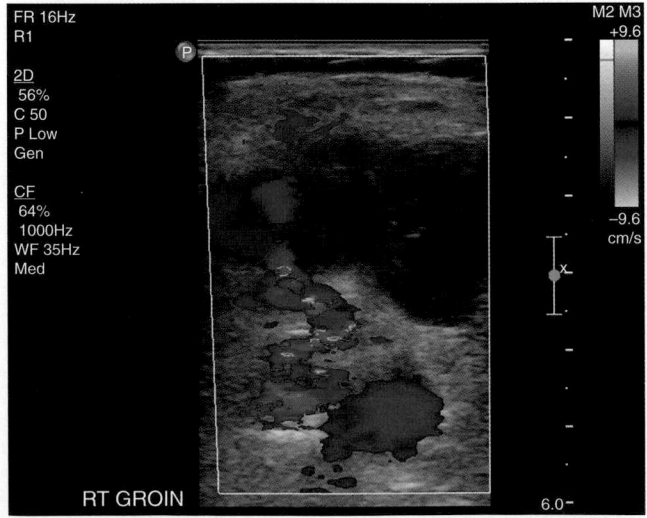

FIGURE 2 Duplex ultrasonography demonstrates a femoral artery pseudoaneurysm with a neck, active component within the pseudoaneurysm cavity, and surrounding hematoma.

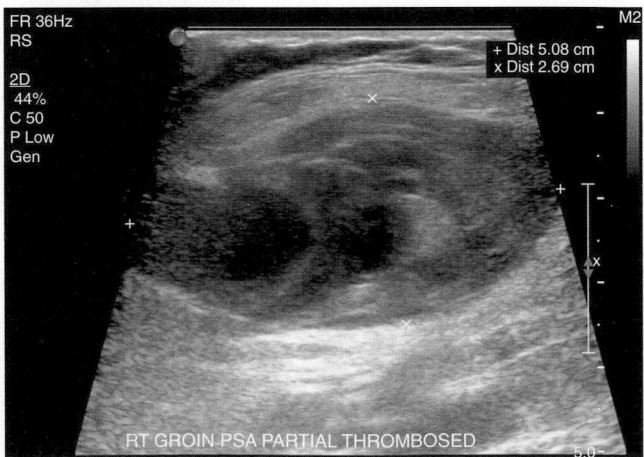

FIGURE 5 Ultrasonography demonstrates a partially thrombosed femoral artery pseudoaneurysm directly after direct thrombin injection.

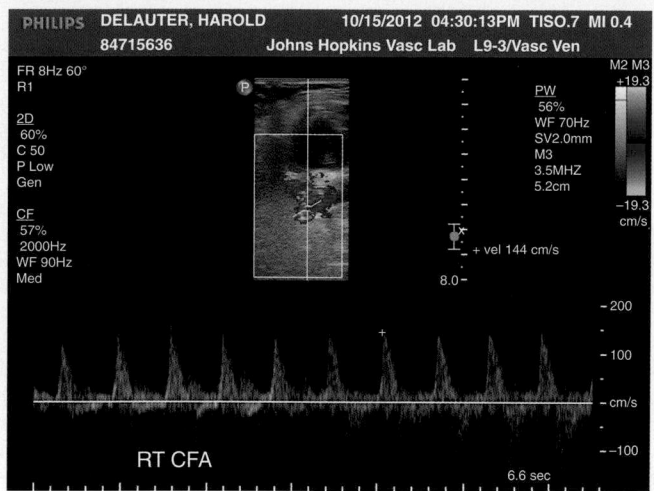

FIGURE 6 Duplex ultrasonography demonstrates complete thrombosis and resolution of the femoral artery pseudoaneurysm after direct thrombin injection with preservation of flow in the common femoral artery.

After both ultrasound-guided compression and direct thrombin injection, patients are required to remain on bed rest for 6 hours postprocedure. A repeat duplex examination should be performed 24 hours later to confirm thrombosis of the pseudoaneurysm.

Certain presenting factors indicate a need for open surgical repair. Those who have failed the therapies mentioned earlier, as well as those who have hemorrhage, expanding hematoma, unsuitable anatomy of the neck of the pseudoaneurysm, ischemic necrosis of the overlying skin, and compression neuropathy of the femoral nerve are appropriate candidates for open repair. The surgical dissection occasionally can be troublesome given the presence of the overlying pseudoaneurysm above the femoral vessels that bleed profusely once it is encountered. A peanut sponge is often useful and can be placed over the underlying arterial puncture site to assist in controlling hemorrhage while proximal and distal control is obtained. A distal retroperitoneal dissection sometimes may be necessary to obtain more proximal control of the distal external iliac artery in difficult circumstances. Simple surgical repair with horizontal stitches is usually sufficient once the arterial puncture site is visualized clearly and dissected free from the surrounding femoral sheath. The femoral sheath should be approximated to prevent further complication in the event of a wound breakdown, particularly in cases with extensive undermining of the skin from the hematoma cavity. A closed suction drain should be left in place in these circumstances. In some instances in which extensive skin necrosis is present, wide débridement followed by placement of a wound vacuum device has been used with success.

Results

Although ultrasound-guided compression is effective in appropriately selected patients, some limitations are present, such as discomfort to the patient. In addition, the length of the procedure may be impractical in terms of resources and availability of the vascular laboratory. In those patients receiving anticoagulation, success rates of this strategy are poor (<40%). Direct thrombin injection avoids these limitations and is associated with a success rate of 92% to 100%. Less than 2% of patients undergoing direct thrombin injection experience the complication of distal arterial thromboembolism. There is an approximate 5% recurrence rate, but previous attempts at direct thrombin injection do not preclude subsequent repeated attempts. Open surgical repair is effective but invasive and limited mainly by complications related to poor wound healing.

Prevention

There is some debate regarding the use of percutaneous vascular closure devices after catheterization. For arteriotomy closure, vascular closure devices are an alternative to manual compression after percutaneous vascular access. When manual compression is used, depending on the sheath size, sometimes up to 20 to 45 minutes of compression should be applied, and the patient must remain supine for at least 6 hours after sheath removal. Vascular closure devices provide advantages to manual compression such as early ambulation and elimination of the discomfort associated with prolonged compression. The use of these devices also mitigates the need for coagulopathy reversal, which generally is required for successful manual compression without resulting complications. Vascular closure devices come in various forms, including collagen-based occlusive devices, suture-based closure devices, and metal clip or disk-based closure devices. Some studies suggest that there is an increased risk of pseudoaneurysm formation with the use of these devices. However, a recently published Cochrane systematic review included 52 controlled trials in which patients who underwent procedures requiring femoral access were randomized to closure with one type of vascular closure device as compared with another device type or manual compression. The results revealed a lower rate of pseudoaneurysm formation with the use of collagen-based vascular closure devices as compared with manual compression. No difference in pseudoaneurysm formation was observed when comparing other types of vascular closure devices with manual compression. A limiting factor in the use of vascular closure devices is cost, which proponents argue may be offset by earlier ambulation times and thus earlier discharge from hospitalization.

■ ARTERIOVENOUS FISTULAS

Risk Factors

Arteriovenous fistula formation after percutaneous access is a complication less commonly observed than pseudoaneurysm formation. In this setting the fistula forms between the femoral artery and vein, particularly if the puncture is not anatomically optimal and occurs "low" (i.e., more distal than the common femoral artery). Low punctures may involve the common femoral bifurcation or the profunda femoris artery and profunda femoral vein. Like pseudoaneurysm formation, risk factors for arteriovenous fistula formation include anticoagulation, female gender, hypertension, and left groin puncture.

Arteriovenous fistula formation in the setting of trauma has been studied for decades, particularly in the military population, with one report by Elkin and Debakey in 1955 describing treatment of 593 arteriovenous fistulas incurred in World War II combat alone. In civilian trauma, the highest risk of developing an arteriovenous fistula occurs in victims of penetrating trauma by stab wounds, followed by gunshot wounds and, rarely, blunt trauma.

Clinical Presentation and Diagnosis

Arteriovenous fistulas are detected on physical examination by the presence of a palpable thrill or audible bruit. Like pseudoaneurysms, fistulas also may be seen as a pulsatile mass. In those patients who have chronic fistulas, ischemic symptoms of the distal extremity may be present because of steal syndrome. Signs and symptoms of steal may include diminished pulses, claudication, pain, and pallor of the affected extremity. Alternatively, patients may be seen with signs and symptoms of venous insufficiency. In cases of long-standing presence of arteriovenous fistulas, patients can be seen with high-output heart failure because of shunting of blood from the arterial to venous circulation. This in turn causes an increase in preload and subsequently in cardiac output, leading to cardiac hypertrophy and eventual failure. Although rare, presence of the Nicoladoni sign (also known as Branham's sign or Nicoladoni-Israel-Branham sign) also may be elicited on physical examination. This refers to a decrease in heart rate and pulse pressure with proximal compression of the arteriovenous fistula because of a sudden decrease in shunting and therefore in preload.

It is important to note that nearly half of all trauma patients who develop arteriovenous fistulas are undiagnosed on initial presentation and thus may be more likely to present with chronic symptoms of arteriovenous fistula. Obtaining a thorough history in these patients is critical for proper diagnosis.

Arteriovenous fistulas may be diagnosed through history and physical examination findings alone. As with pseudoaneurysms, color-flow duplex imaging confirms the diagnosis. Ultrasonographic findings demonstrate a stream of flow maintaining communication between the affected artery and vein with a patchy array of color representing turbulence. An increase in diastolic flow velocity with continuous forward arterial flow replaces the expected absence or reversal of diastolic flow that otherwise creates the triphasic waveform associated with normal laminar flow. Distal arterial flow is decreased, and venous flow is increased proximally with high-velocity flow because of shunting of blood through the fistulous connection. Other imaging modalities, particularly computed tomographic angiography (CTA), may be useful for operative planning.

Treatment

In asymptomatic patients who have postcatheterization femoral arteriovenous fistulas, conservative management with observation only may be appropriate, as studies indicate that anywhere from 38% to 81% of these fistulas spontaneously resolve within 1 year. Endovascular treatment is not generally adequate for patients with iatrogenic femoral arteriovenous fistulas, as the stent-graft is at risk of fracture because of its location and the mechanical stress caused by repeated hip flexure. In those patients who are symptomatic, who show evidence of hemodynamic instability, or whose iatrogenic arteriovenous fistulas do not self-resolve, management proceeds with surgical repair by ligation of the fistula. Ligation is accomplished by first gaining proximal and distal control of the involved artery, dividing the fistulous channel, and performing primary repair of the remaining arterial and venous defects with interrupted polypropylene suture, or with patch angioplasty or interposition graft when primary repair without stenosis cannot be achieved.

Endovascular repair with stent placement across the fistula may be appropriate for arteriovenous fistulas in locations in which stent durability is not of concern. Coil or gelatin embolization also may be effective in arteriovenous fistulas, particularly when treating visceral arteriovenous fistulas.

Results

Both surgical and endovascular management of femoral arteriovenous fistulas are associated with high morbidity and mortality. This is largely attributable to the underlying medical condition and comorbidities of those patients undergoing cardiac catheterization. Surgical repair is associated with 8% mortality and 25% morbidity rates. Alternatively, endovascular repair has a reported in-hospital mortality of 10% and 1-year mortality of 20% and subsequently requires total leg revascularization in 17% of cases and lower extremity amputation in 3.3% of cases. Surgical treatment of acquired arteriovenous fistulas in other locations, such as visceral arteriovenous fistulas, is associated with an estimated 5% mortality rate with elective repair. The use of endovascular techniques in the management of visceral arteriovenous fistulas is promising, but the long-term success rate is not yet clear.

■ OTHER PSEUDOANEURYSMS

Anastomotic Pseudoaneurysms

Anastomotic pseudoaneurysms are a widely recognized complication after revascularization in which prosthetic graft material is utilized

to re-establish arterial flow. The incidence of anastomotic pseudoaneurysm is highest at femoral anastomotic sites, and these pseudoaneurysms complicate as many as 13.6% of these anastomoses. Overall incidence of anastomotic pseudoaneurysm is an estimated 1.4% to 4%. They most frequently are associated with aortobifemoral bypass, in which both femoral anastomoses may be affected in at-risk patients. Any factor that causes disruption of the established anastomosis puts patients at risk of pseudoaneurysm formation. In those patients who are seen acutely, technical errors or infection should be suspected culprits of pseudoaneurysm formation. Even in patients who are seen with anastomotic pseudoaneurysms and without clinical evidence of local or systemic infection, bacterial colonization of the graft is present at a very high rate of up to 80%. In those patients who are seen many months or years after surgical repair, arterial wall degeneration is the most common cause of this complication. Other risk factors include any circumstance that puts a patient at risk for compromising the integrity of the anastomosis, including graft failure, suture line disruption, mechanical stress, tobacco use, hypertension, hyperlipidemia, vasculitides, and use of anticoagulation.

Anastomotic pseudoaneurysms may be detected incidentally on postoperative surveillance imaging, or patients may have any of the clinical findings previously described for postcatheterization pseudoaneurysms. Diagnosis is confirmed in the same manner as previously described for pseudoaneurysms of any etiology (Figures 7 and 8).

Prompt intervention is necessary when anastomotic pseudoaneurysms are detected, as they are associated with a high rate of rupture. In general, particularly in the case of femoral pseudoaneurysms, open surgical repair is the treatment of choice and involves resection of the false aneurysm and repair with interposition graft placement.

Postsurgical Pseudoaneurysms

Although rare, postsurgical pseudoaneurysms are important to mention, as they can present with nebulous signs or symptoms and failure to identify this complication in a timely manner is often fatal. Most notably, gastroduodenal artery pseudoaneurysms are a rare but serious complication after pancreaticoduodenectomy. Pseudoaneurysm formation in this setting generally is associated with pancreatic fistulas, which can occur in as many as a third of those patients undergoing pancreaticoduodenectomy. In this setting, leakage of pancreatic enzymes leads to degeneration of the arterial wall, causing a defect that allows for pseudoaneurysm formation. Gastroduodenal artery pseudoaneurysm in these patients may be seen with new onset gastrointestinal hemorrhage, abdominal pain, or a precipitous drop in hemoglobin or as an incidental finding on surveillance imaging. In

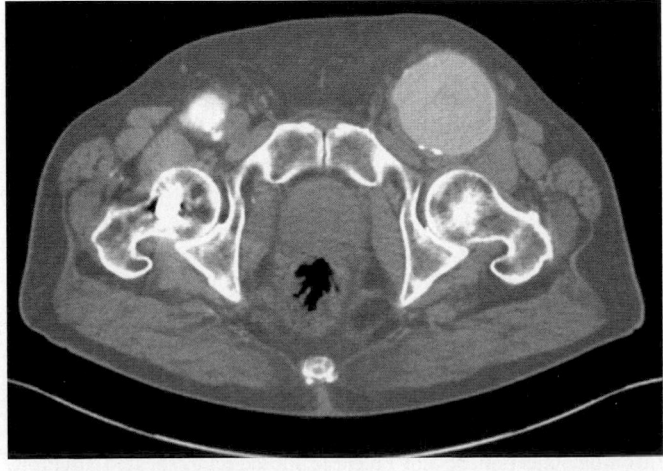

FIGURE 7 Computed tomographic imaging demonstrates bilateral anastomotic pseudoaneurysms in a patient after aortobifemoral bypass.

hemodynamically stable patients, CTA is an appropriate diagnostic tool. Patients who are hemodynamically unstable should proceed directly to interventional radiology for coil embolization of the pseudoaneurysm, which is the treatment of choice for this complication.

Infected Pseudoaneurysms

Infected pseudoaneurysms may arise from several sources, including intravenous or intra-arterial injection in drug users, contamination associated with instrumentation after catheterization, or bacterial seeding from systemic infection, particularly endocarditis. The term *mycotic aneurysm* often is used to describe any pseudoaneurysm with an infectious etiology, although this term originally was coined to describe those pseudoaneurysms arising strictly from distal emboli occurring in patients with endocarditis. Most commonly, patients with infected pseudoaneurysms will be seen with bacteremia. Staphylococcus and salmonella species are the most commonly associated pathogens. Patients may be frankly septic or may have vague symptoms associated with an underlying smoldering infectious process.

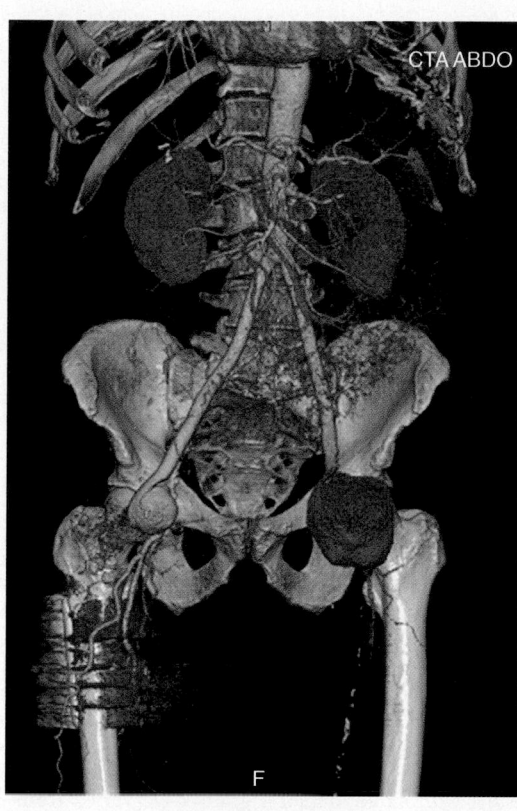

FIGURE 8 Computed tomographic angiography three-dimensional reconstruction demonstrates bilateral anastomotic pseudoaneurysms in a patient after aortobifemoral bypass.

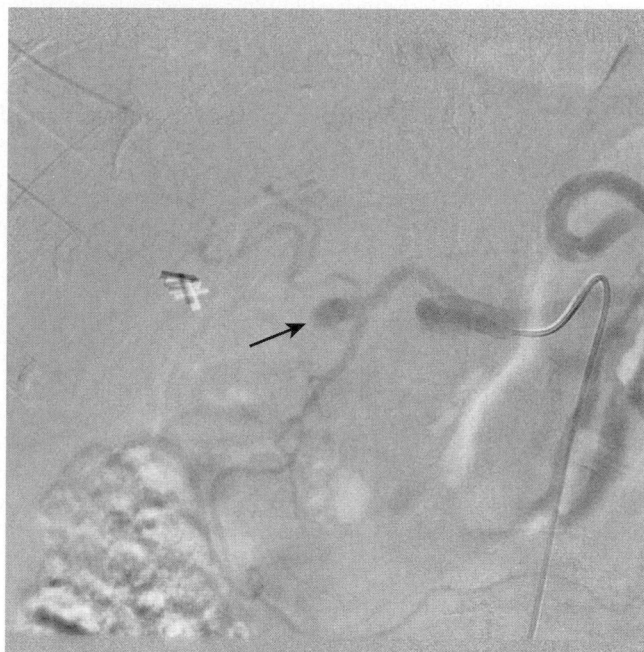

FIGURE 10 Angiography demonstrates an idiopathic pseudoaneurysm (*arrow*) off the hepatic artery–gastroduodenal artery junction.

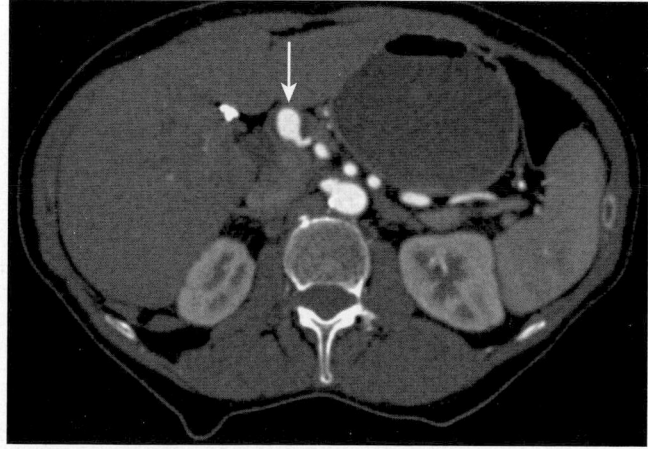

FIGURE 9 Computed tomography demonstrates an idiopathic hepatic artery pseudoaneurysm (*arrow*) in a patient who is seen with abdominal pain.

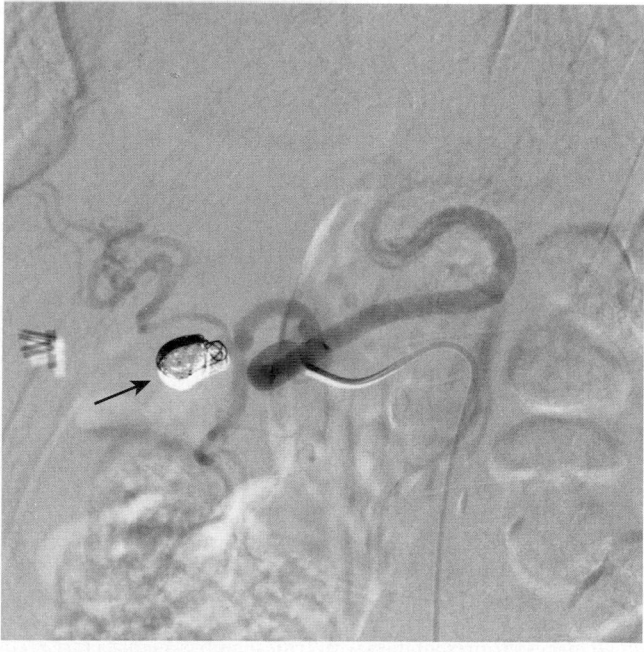

FIGURE 11 Angiography demonstrates successful coil embolization (*arrow*) of an idiopathic hepatic artery pseudoaneurysm.

Physical examination may reveal a pulsatile mass with overlying cellulitis. Depending on the location and etiology of the infected pseudoaneurysm, diagnosis may be confirmed with duplex ultrasonography, CTA, or echocardiogram in the setting of signs of infection such as leukocytosis or positive blood cultures. Treatment requires complete source control. Broad-spectrum intravenous antibiotic therapy should be initiated in a timely manner but is generally not successful as a measure of definitive management. Operative repair is necessary to allow for total source control. Ultrasonography-guided compression and direct thrombin injection techniques are contraindicated in the setting of infected pseudoaneurysms. Surgical repair is as described previously for pseudoaneurysms of other etiologies. However, operative management of infected pseudoaneurysms also requires complete excision of surrounding tissue that displays evidence of infection or necrosis. Extra-anatomic revascularization then is required to restore arterial blood flow within unaffected tissue planes. It is best to avoid reconstruction with prosthetic grafts and preferable to utilize autogenous tissue as a conduit. Muscle flaps may be used to cover and protect the newly created anastomoses. In the case of intra-abdominal repair of infected aneurysms, this same protection may be attained with the use of an overlying omental flap.

Idiopathic Pseudoaneurysms

Idiopathic pseudoaneurysms arising spontaneously, particularly in visceral arteries, also can be managed with coil embolization or covered stent placement if there are not too many side branches. Strategies include placing coils proximally and distally to exclude vascular flow or coil packing of the pseudoaneurysm cavity itself (Figures 9 through 11).

SUGGESTED READINGS

Belli A-M, Markose G, Morgan R. The role of interventional radiology in the management of abdominal visceral artery aneurysms. *Cardiovasc Intervent Radiol*. 2011;35:234-243. doi: 10.1007/s00270-011-0201-3.

Deipolyi A, Rho J, Khademhosseini A, Oklu R. Diagnosis and management of mycotic aneurysms. *Clin Imaging*. 2015;40:256-262.

Dzijan-Horn M, Langwieser N, Groha P. Safety and efficacy of a potential treatment algorithm by using manual compression repair and ultrasound-guided thrombin injection for the management of iatrogenic femoral artery pseudoaneurysm in a large patient cohort. *J Vasc Surg*. 2015;61:281. doi: 10.1016/j.jvs.2014.11.052.

AXILLOBIFEMORAL BYPASS GRAFTING IN THE TWENTY-FIRST CENTURY

Sean J. English, MD, and Michael T. Watkins, MD

The axillobifemoral bypass operation is an alternative to direct arterial reconstruction, specifically aortobifemoral or aortobiiliac grafting with prosthetic or venous tissue. This procedure is performed in patients with aortic graft sepsis or a mycotic aneurysm and in patients with a totally occluded abdominal aorta with a high operative risk. The advantage of the axillobifemoral operation is that it is a less invasive operation compared with a total reconstruction of the infrarenal aorta when surgical replacement of the infected aortobifemoral graft is required, or bypass of the aortoiliac segment is desired in the setting of a "hostile" abdomen (Figure 1). Extra-anatomic axillofemoral construction to revascularize the lower extremity was proposed first in the early 1960s.

Atherosclerotic occlusive disease of the abdominal aorta and iliac arteries and its clinical manifestation is a common therapeutic challenge encountered by vascular surgeons. It is one subset of peripheral arterial disease, which affects 8 to 10 million people in the United States per year. Aortoiliac occlusive disease ultimately starts at the terminal aorta and the origin of the iliac arteries. Often, there is slow progression proximally and distally over time to end in complete occlusion of the aorta and iliac arteries.

There is no consensus regarding the natural history of aortoiliac occlusive disease. Some surgeons suggest that the natural history is not always benign and report that in a third of their patients the aortic occlusive disease extends to show thrombosis of the renal arteries over a period of 5 to 10 years. Others suggest that renal arteries remain open with no incidence of extension of the thrombosis proximally to involve the renal or the mesenteric vessels. Aortoiliac atherosclerotic occlusive disease is characterized by abundant collateralization between abdominal, pelvic, and infrainguinal arteries, which makes the presentation with critical limb ischemia a rare event. A more common presentation is of claudication of varying severity and levels. The two exceptions to this observation are a large thrombus lodged at the narrow aorta, causing acute limb ischemia, and blue toe syndrome, in which microemboli target the small vessels in the toes or the heel.

■ INDICATIONS

Substantial changes have occurred in the surgical management of occlusive aortoiliofemoral occlusive disease during the past 40 years, all of which reflect an ongoing evolution of prosthetic materials and alternate forms of intervention. Large series that were reported during the 1970s and early 1980s dealt almost exclusively with open abdominal procedures using Dacron aortoiliac and aortofemoral replacement grafts that for the most part had supplanted aortoiliac and femoral endarterectomy. Although reported 5-year patency rates after aortobifemoral grafts consistently have exceeded 80%, long-term results with axillobifemoral grafts have varied from 10% to more than 70% at 5 years. This variation has led to a perception of axillobifemoral construct as a "compromised" procedure with a limited clinical role. After the introduction of externally supported prostheses by Sauvage in 1978, however, patency rates of axillobifemoral grafts dramatically improved. Dacron extra-anatomic grafts subsequently were replaced by polytetrafluoroethylene (PTFE) grafts, external ring reinforcement, or both, in an attempt to improve their durability.

The widespread adoption of percutaneous transluminal angioplasty for iliac atherosclerosis now has eroded the number of candidates for open abdominal or extra-anatomic procedures to the point that traditional operations may remain necessary only in the few patients who either have exceptionally severe aortoiliac occlusive disease or represent failures of previous catheter-based intervention. The Trans-Atlantic Inter-Society Consensus for the Management of Peripheral Arterial Disease (TASC) published a document authored by a working group of representatives from 14 surgical vascular, cardiovascular, and radiologic societies, and an upgraded document (TASC II) was published in January 2007. These important works interpreted evidence-based data concerning the treatment of lower extremity PAD and offered a series of treatment recommendations based on presentation. Whereas percutaneous treatment of the aorta and iliac arteries was limited previously to short-segment, TASC type A or B iliac lesions, wire-based technology has now been applied successfully to even long-segment (TASC type D) occlusions extending for the length of the iliac arteries.

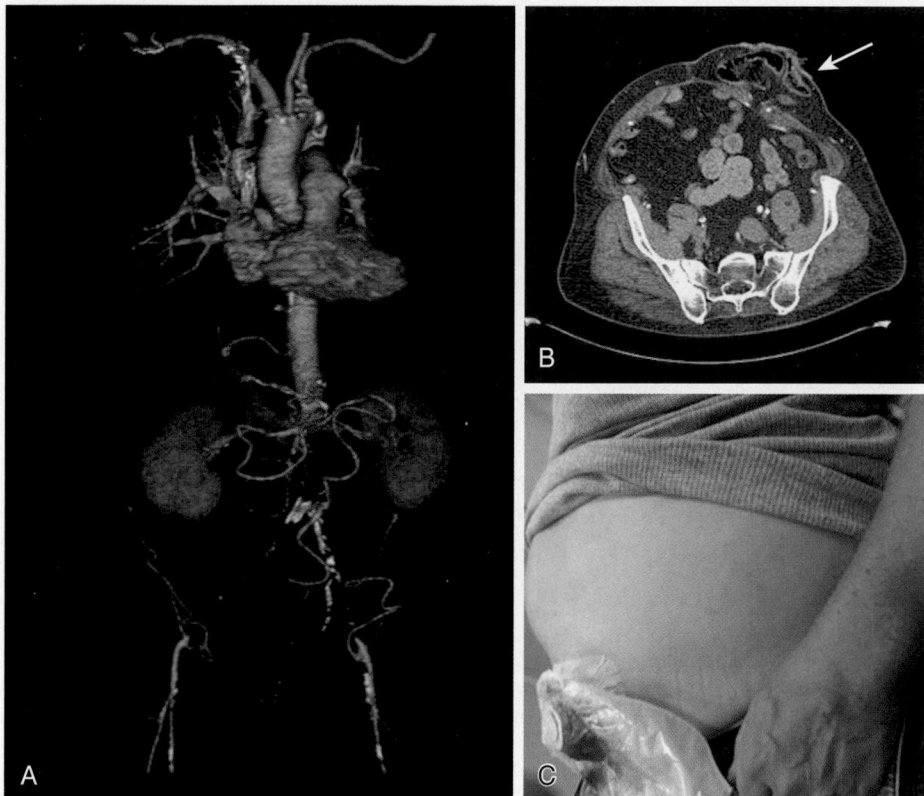

FIGURE 1 Candidate for axillobifemoral bypass for aortoiliac occlusive disease because of hostile abdomen. **A,** CT angiogram showing infrarenal aortic occlusion and runoff at the groin level. **B,** CT axial image through the abdomen demonstrating colostomy (for Crohn's) with large parastomal hernia *(arrow).* **C,** Picture of protuberant abdomen in an obese patient and low abdominal stoma.

In a high-risk patient with a combination of aortic and proximal iliac occlusive disease; need for peritoneal dialysis; severe cardiopulmonary, renal, hepatic disease; and those with other comorbidities such as multiple prior abdominal operations, abdominal stomas, or prior radiation therapy, axillofemoral bypass is a valuable alternative for distal revascularization. Axillofemoral bypass has been an essential tool for the treatment of many patients with infected aortic or prosthetic arterial grafts or aortoenteric fistulae. A staged approach to resecting infected aortic aneurysms or prosthetic grafts has been preferred after axillobifemoral grafting. Axillobifemoral bypass has been a bail-out procedure for symptomatic thrombosis or infection of an infrarenal aortic endograft or as a temporary adjunct to decrease lower extremity ischemia time during placement of a fenestrated aortic endograft or for visceral and renal artery perfusion during complex thoracoabdominal aortic reconstruction. Axillobifemoral bypass constructs also have been used to manage infrarenal blunt aortic occlusion.

A small subset of patients with aortoiliac occlusive disease also may have aortic aneurysms. Axillofemoral bypass is not the preferred treatment for this group of patients. These patients require either open aortofemoral bypass or endovascular angioplasty to allow an aortounilateral reconstruction to be followed by a femorofemoral bypass.

In patients in whom the axillary arteries may not be suitable for inflow, another alternative for direct reconstruction is to use the supraceliac or distal thoracic aorta for inflow. Exposure via medial visceral rotation, a retroperitoneal incision, or a thoracotomy may be necessary. In patients with combined aortoiliac and infrainguinal occlusive disease, the aortoiliac segment should be restored first and the infrainguinal disease treated subsequently as needed. When the common femoral artery is occluded, patients undergoing axillofemoral bypass require outflow to the profunda femoris artery, the superficial femoral, or the popliteal artery.

PREOPERATIVE EVALUATION

Although it is clear that patients are selected for axillobifemoral bypass, most often on the basis of their comorbid conditions their medical condition should be optimized. The choice of the donor artery can be made by invasive and noninvasive methods. If there is a significant blood pressure gradient between both arms, the arm with the higher pressure is chosen for inflow. Upper extremity pulse volume recordings or Doppler waveform analysis can be useful to identify proximal occlusive disease. Abnormal noninvasive testing requires subsequent noninvasive imaging with computed tomographic angiography or magnetic resonance angiography. If a significant proximal stenosis is identified on noninvasive imaging, digital subtraction angiography and possible angioplasty/stenting should be considered. Grafts should not be based off limbs where there is evidence of distal arm ischemia or dialysis access. The donor artery position should take into consideration the presence of thoracic outlet syndrome, breast cancer, presence of an ostomy, abdominal hernias, or other previous surgery. In patients undergoing axillofemoral bypass for intra-abdominal aortic sepsis who may be candidates for subsequent inline reconstruction via a left retroperitoneal approach, the right axillary artery should be used for inflow to avoid interference of a left-sided graft with a retroperitoneal procedure.

OPERATIVE CONSIDERATIONS

Axillofemoral bypass nearly always is performed with general anesthesia in the supine position. Although the procedure can be performed with local anesthesia and sedation, large volumes of anesthetic are required. A rolled towel is placed between the scapulae to facilitate exposure of the medial most portion of the axillary artery. The donor artery arm is prepped circumferentially to facilitate passive movement of the arm during the procedure to confirm by direct inspection that

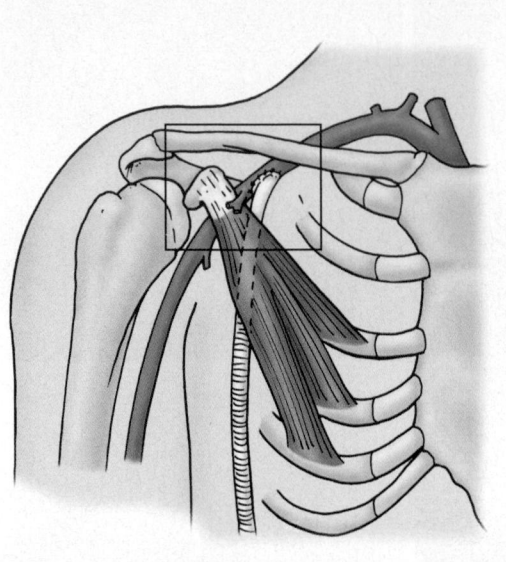
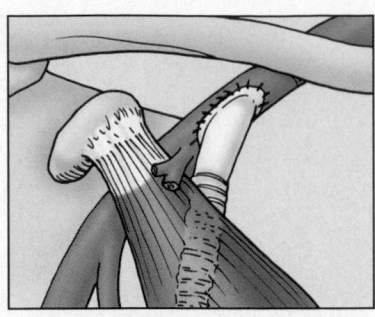
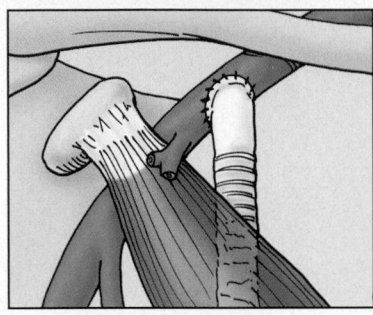

FIGURE 2 Operative findings in cases of graft disruption. Force producing disruption occurs with arm abduction/shoulder elevation as illustrated. *Upper inset,* Combined disruption with "heel" of graft tear and sutures pulling out of "toe" of graft. *Lower inset,* Complete circumferential graft disruption adjacent to anastomosis. Blaisdell and Hall in their initial description of the procedure, carefully recommend placing the axillary anastomosis on the first portion of the axillary artery, to avoid undue tension with arm movement. *(From Taylor LM, Jr., Park TC, Edwards JM, et al. Acute disruption of polytetrafluoroethylene grafts adjacent to axillary anastomoses: a complication of axillofemoral grafting. J Vasc Surg. 1994;20:520-526; discussion 526-528.)*

undue tension is not placed on the axillary anastomosis. A transverse infraclavicular incision is carried through the clavipectoral fascia, exposing the pectoralis major muscle. The pectoralis major muscle fibers are pushed superiorly and inferiorly, exposing the deep fascia and, beneath that, the fat containing the axillary vein, artery, and brachial plexus elements. The axillary artery is exposed from the clavicle medially to the pectoralis minor muscle laterally, often requiring the ligation of crossing veins or small arterial branches. Often division of the pectoralis minor muscle will be needed to avoid tension on the axillofemoral graft. It is very important to place the axillary graft anastomosis as medially as possible to avoid tension on the axillary anastomosis when the arm is abducted (Figure 2).

A modified technique for the proximal anastomosis to alleviate tension on the proximal anastomosis involves performing the proximal anastomosis on the anterior surface of the axillary artery medial to the thoracoacromial artery. It is essential to ensure adequate blood flow in the donor arm beyond the axillary anastomosis. The course of the graft may be modified where the graft initially is routed adjacent and parallel to the axillary artery for a distance of 8 to 10 cm, into the axilla, and then directed in a gentle and redundant curve inferiorly to the chest wall (Figure 3). By this technique, tension along the graft is concentrated on the area of the curve in the axilla, instead of at the anastomosis.

The axillofemoral graft should be tunneled in the midaxillary line to prevent kinking of the graft. The anastomosis of the proximal end of the graft to the side of the axillary artery generally is performed first. Conventional longitudinal or oblique groin incisions are used for femoral artery exposure. The distal anastomosis is performed conventionally end to side to an appropriate artery in the groin. It is important to ensure adequate outflow. The crossover femoral to femoral graft should be sewn as close to the axillofemoral anastomosis to maximize outflow through the axillofemoral graft.

■ RESULTS

Patency rates with axillofemoral bypass vary widely between 30% to as high as 85%. The reason for this variability is due in part to

patient selection, indication, and status of the outflow arteries. Patients with claudication do better than limb salvage patients because of the inherent outflow restriction in the latter group. Patients with a previous distal bypass often have longer patency rates. In some series, the estimated survival after axillofemoral bypass may be as low as only 43% at 28 months because of medical comorbidities. For patients whose initial presentation was critical limb ischemia, the 3-year limb salvage estimates range from 69% to slightly more than 80%.

Significant differences have been found between patient groups that underwent aortobifemoral bypass versus axillobifemoral bypass. Patients who underwent axillobifemoral bypass in a study were on average a decade older, and a greater number had heart disease, renal failure, and previous intra-abdominal or aortic surgery than those who underwent aortofemoral bypass. The frequency of complications associated with axillobifemoral bypass versus aortofemoral bypass occurred less frequently after axillobifemoral bypass (9.2%) than after aortobifemoral bypass (19.4%) ($P < 0.05$). Myocardial infarction, graft occlusion, and bleeding that required reoperation occurred with similar frequency for both procedures. Pulmonary failure, acute renal failure, and stroke occurred more frequently in patients undergoing aortobifemoral bypass. Wound complications (including superficial infection, hematoma, or lymphocele) occurred after axillobifemoral bypass and after aortobifemoral bypass at an equivalent rate. Despite these differences in complication rate between aortobifemoral bypass and axillobifemoral bypass, there is ongoing and increasing use of in situ aortic reconstructions for septic aortic grafts or aneurysms with antibiotic soaked grafts or venous composite grafts. These in situ approaches for aortoiliac reconstruction in the setting of sepsis have variable track records and durability.

■ COMPLICATIONS

Aside from issues related to graft patency, axillofemoral constructions are associated with several infrequently reported complications, such as graft avulsion/anastomotic pseudoaneurysm, acute or chronic

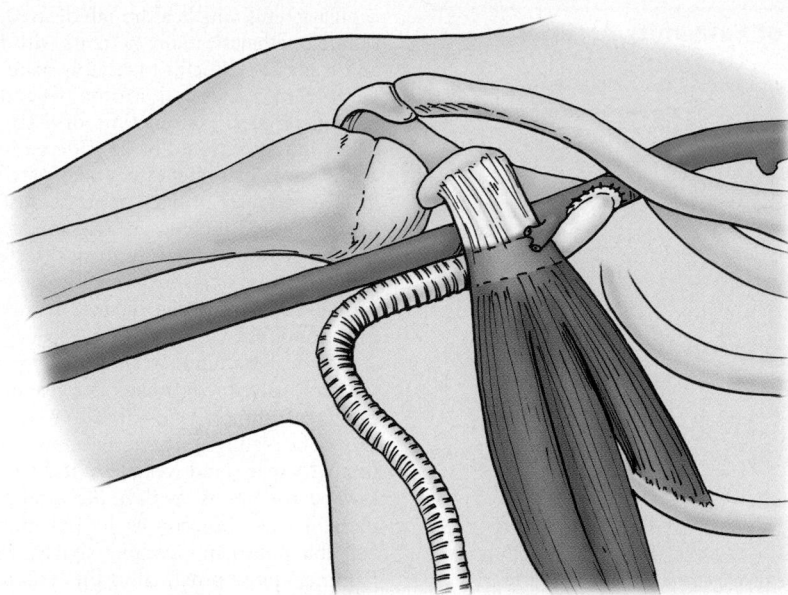

FIGURE 3 Modified technique of axillofemoral graft proximal anastomosis. Graft is anastomosed in end-to-side fashion to first portion of axillary artery and routed parallel and adjacent to artery beneath pectoralis minor for 8 to 10 cm before being directed in gentle and redundant curve in axilla to lie against chest wall in subcutaneous position. *(From Taylor LM, Jr., Park TC, Edwards JM, et al. Acute disruption of polytetrafluoroethylene grafts adjacent to axillary anastomoses: a complication of axillofemoral grafting. J Vasc Surg. 1994;20:520-526; discussion 526-528.)*

thrombosis of the axillary artery, upper extremity steal phenomenon, and thromboembolism of the brachial artery resulting from stump syndrome when graft occlusion occurs. These complications are rarely limb threatening and often are managed by standard open or endovascular approaches. Strategies to avoid graft avulsion have been alluded to earlier in this report, but in instances where this has occurred and a large pseudoaneurysm is present at the proximal anastomoses, proximal control can be obtained with balloon occlusion. There are reports in which supraclavicular approach has facilitated repair of the axillary artery pseudoaneurysm associated with an axillobifemoral graft. Acute thrombosis of the axillary artery often is associated with a technical problem such as a clamp injury or kinking of the native axillary artery. Thrombectomy with patch angioplasty is often the solution to this problem. Upper extremity steal often is associated with proximal subclavian disease, which can be treated with transfemoral or transbrachial balloon angioplasty with or without stent. Thromboembolism related to stump syndrome is seen when the axillofemoral graft has thrombosed. Thrombectomy of the brachial artery with flush ligation of the axillofemoral graft at the anastomoses or exclusion of the occluded graft using a stent is the recommended approach to this problem. Although the stenting procedure is described in the literature, we would use it with caution

because the risk of stent fracture in the mobile axillary artery in the thoracic outlet is not insignificant.

SUGGESTED READINGS

Armstrong PA, Back MR, Wilson JS, et al. Improved outcomes in the recent management of secondary aortoenteric fistula. *J Vasc Surg.* 2005;42:660-666.

Fatima J, Duncan AA, de Grandis E, et al. Treatment strategies and outcomes in patients with infected aortic endografts. *J Vasc Surg.* 2013;58:371-379.

Harris DG, Drucker CB, Brenner ML, et al. Patterns and management of blunt abdominal aortic injury. *Ann Vasc Surg.* 2013;27:1074-1080.

Kim KH, Choi JB, Kuh JH. Simultaneous relief of acute visceral and limb ischemia in complicated type B aortic dissection by axillobifemoral bypass. *J Thorac Cardiovasc Surg.* 2013;147:524-525.

Lotun K, Schainfeld RM, Razvi S, et al. An unusual late complication of axillobifemoral bypass graft: a case report. *Ann Vasc Surg.* 2006;20:830-833.

O'Connor S, Andrew P, Batt M, Becquemin JP. A systematic review and meta-analysis of treatments for aortic graft infection. *J Vasc Surg.* 2006;44:38-45.

Taylor LM Jr, Park TC, Edwards JM, et al. Acute disruption of polytetrafluoroethylene grafts adjacent to axillary anastomoses: a complication of axillofemoral grafting. *J Vasc Surg.* 1994;20:520-526, discussion 526-528.

PERIPHERAL ARTERIAL EMBOLISM

Madhukar S. Patel, MD, MBA, ScM, and Elliot L. Chaikof, MD, PhD

Rudolph Virchow is credited with coining the term *embolia* in 1856, to describe lower extremity venous thrombi that ultimately lodged in the pulmonary arteries. Over the past century, numerous types of emboli have been described based on composition, including thrombus, cholesterol, air, fat, septic matter, tissue, foreign body, and amniotic fluid, as well as location in the arterial and venous circulation. Anatomically, peripheral arterial emboli of the extremities lodge at bifurcations, with the lower extremities being affected more commonly than the upper extremities (Table 1). Regardless of type and location, if not diagnosed early and managed expeditiously, peripheral arterial emboli will result in severe morbidity or mortality.

Arterial emboli most often originate in the left atrium among patients with atrial fibrillation (AF) or from a left ventricular

TABLE 1: Distribution of Extremity Arterial Emboli

Site of Emboli	Approximate Frequency
Lower Extremity	**84.0%**
Aortoiliac	25.7%
Common femoral	34.0%
Superficial femoral	4.5%
Popliteal	14.2%
Tibial	5.6%
Upper Extremity	**16.0%**
Brachial	9.1%
Axillary	4.5%
Radial and ulnar	2.4%

Adapted from Tan T, Farber A. The management of peripheral arterial emboli. In: Cameron JL, Cameron AM, eds. *Current Surgical Therapy.* 11th ed. Philadelphia: Elsevier; 2014:903-909.

thrombus in the setting of a recent myocardial infarction. Specifically, 0.5% of patients with AF will suffer clinically significant noncerebrovascular systemic embolic events, with an incidence in contemporary reviews of 0.24 per 100 patient-years. Approximately two thirds of these events will affect the extremities and one third will affect the visceral-mesenteric circulation. Risks are significantly higher among patients with permanent rather than paroxysmal AF and with AF of longer duration (>2 years). In these patients, anticoagulation use has been associated with a lower incidence of systemic emboli, with direct oral anticoagulants being at least as effective as vitamin K antagonists. Thirty-day mortality in this patient population after a systemic embolic event is 25% and has changed little over the past 3 decades. Other cardiac sources of emboli include atrial myxomas, valvular heart disease due to rheumatic fever or endocarditis, and prosthetic heart valves. Notably, the thromboembolic risk for prosthetic heart valves is between 0.6% and 2.3% per patient year, with patients with bioprosthetic valves not on anticoagulation having similar risks to those with mechanical valves on therapeutic anticoagulation. Further, owing to changes in hemodynamic flow depending on valve position, mitral prosthetic valves generally are associated with two to three times greater risk of thromboembolic complication as compared with aortic valves. In addition to cardiogenic sources, emboli may arise from an arterial aneurysm, atherosclerotic plaque or ulcer, traumatically injured vessel, recently thrombosed bypass graft or native artery, or lower extremity deep venous thrombosis in the case of paradoxic emboli that traverse into the arterial circulation through an intracardiac septal defect.

CLINICAL PRESENTATION

An acute peripheral artery embolism most often leads to lower extremity ischemia characterized by the "six Ps": pain, pulselessness, poikilothermia, paresthesias, pallor, and paralysis. History and physical examination may help to differentiate an acute embolism from rest pain or acute arterial thrombosis of progressive atherosclerotic peripheral arterial disease (PAD). Patients with established PAD who have an acute thrombosis will describe a history of claudication that often has been present for months or years, as well as rest pain that has been present for weeks or months. Although rest pain can be severe and persistent, the presence of an established collateral circulation typically will limit the magnitude of ischemia, and

capillary refill, which, although delayed, is often present on examination. Nonetheless, many patients with PAD may have associated AF, and it may be difficult to reliably distinguish between an "acute-on-chronic" in situ arterial thrombosis and an acute embolism based on history, physical examination, or even imaging studies. Acute aortic dissection also should be considered in the differential diagnosis of acute lower extremity ischemia, particularly among patients who have acute onset of back pain. Because presentations may vary, the history should include an assessment of the patient's cardiovascular risk profile, with an inquiry directed at elucidating a history of prior embolic episodes, arrhythmia, valvular heart disease, aneurysmal disease, arterial dissection, recent vascular intervention, or thrombophilia.

Physical examination should compare the affected extremity with the uninvolved contralateral extremity, as profound differences, ranging from pallor to livedo reticularis and cyanotic mottling, should be readily apparent. Diminished sensation, particularly of the first web space, and weakness of dorsiflexion may be present in the lower extremity, as the deep peroneal nerve in the anterior compartment is most susceptible to ischemia. Asymmetric loss of distal palpable pulses and Doppler signals, with an accompanying "waterhammer" pulse proximal to the level of arterial obstruction, should be noted. These changes often are accompanied by delayed or absent capillary refill of the distal vascular bed.

CLASSIFICATION AND DIAGNOSIS

To decrease limb loss, as well as ischemia-reperfusion–related local and systemic injury, prompt diagnosis and treatment of peripheral artery emboli is necessary. A classification system to grade acute limb ischemia (ALI) and stratify urgency of intervention has been developed (Table 2). In addition to a complete history and physical examination, preintervention imaging may be of value to help exclude dissection, a thrombosed aneurysm, or an acute thrombosis of an atherosclerotic vessel. However, given the irreversible muscle and peripheral nerve damage associated with persistent ischemia, intervention should not be delayed unduly in order to obtain an imaging study in a patient with profound ischemia. Current imaging modalities include duplex ultrasonography, magnetic resonance angiography (MRA), computed tomographic angiography (CTA), and conventional angiography. Of these, CTA of the chest, abdomen, and pelvis with lower extremity runoffs is preferred, as it can be performed expeditiously at most centers and may provide insight into etiology and assist in operative planning. Because CTA imaging requires a large volume load of iodinated contrast, patients with renal insufficiency require prehydration; therefore if renal insufficiency is sufficiently severe, direct intraoperative assessment using a limited volume of contrast dye or carbon dioxide angiography may be a preferred approach.

MANAGEMENT STRATEGY

When a peripheral artery embolism is suspected (Figure 1), initial management includes intravenous fluid resuscitation as well as heparin anticoagulation with intravenous bolus loading (100 U/kg) followed by an infusion (15 U/kg) to reach an activated partial thromboplastin time (aPTT) of 60 to 80 seconds, assuming that contraindications to anticoagulation are not present. Patients who are intolerant to heparin should receive a direct thrombin inhibitor, such as lepirudin or argatroban, with a similar aPTT goal. Intravenous fluids should be isotonic and ideally not contain potassium until baseline renal function has been assessed. Depending on underlying renal function, intravenous mannitol for diuresis and alkalinization of the urine with bicarbonate should be considered in the setting of myoglobinuria or likely compartment syndrome. Laboratory examination should include a basic metabolic panel, complete blood count, coagulation studies, creatinine phosphokinase (CPK), lactic acid level, and a blood bank sample for type and screen.

TABLE 2: Stratification of an Ischemic Extremity

| Category | Description/ Prognosis | Findings | | Doppler Signals | |
		Sensory Loss	Muscle Weakness	Arterial	Venous
I. Viable	Not immediately threatened	None	None	Audible	Audible
II. Threatened					
a. Marginally	Salvageable if promptly treated	Minimal (toes) or none	None	Inaudible	Audible
b. Immediately	Salvageable with immediate revascularization	More than toes, associated with rest pain	Mild, moderate	Inaudible	Audible
III. Irreversible	Major tissue loss or permanent nerve damage inevitable	Profound, anesthetic	Profound, paralysis (rigor)	Inaudible	Inaudible

From Rutherford RB, Baker JD, Ernst C, et al. Recommended standards for reports dealing with lower extremity ischemia: revised version. *J Vasc Surg.* 1997;26:517-538.

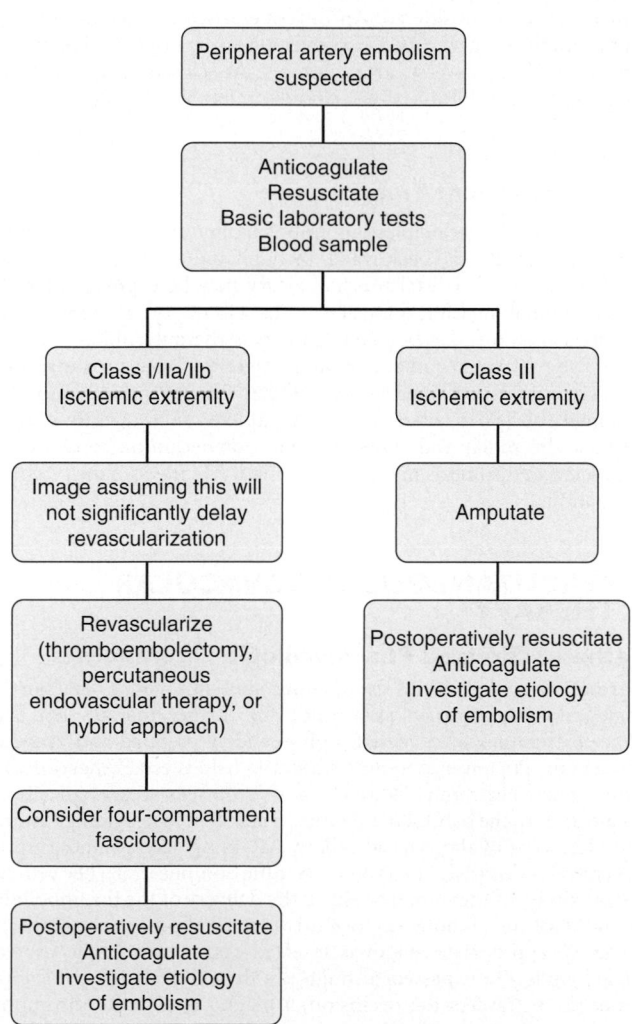

FIGURE 1 General management strategy for a patient with suspected peripheral artery embolism.

The two primary approaches for treatment of peripheral artery embolism are thromboembolectomy and percutaneous endovascular therapy, which may consist of catheter-directed pharmacologic thrombolysis or pharmacomechanical thrombectomy. A Cochrane meta-analysis of five prospective randomized controlled trials with a total of 1283 patients compared peripheral artery thrombolysis using tissue plasminogen activator (tPA) or urokinase with surgery. There was no advantage for either modality with regards to preventing major amputation or death within 1 year. However, significantly higher rates of stroke (1.3% vs 0%), major bleeding (8.8% vs 3.3%), and distal embolization (12.3% vs 0%) were observed for patients who underwent thrombolysis. This meta-analysis was limited in that only a small proportion of patients in these studies had motor and sensory deficits of class IIb or III ischemia, and current methods of percutaneous management such as mechanical thrombolysis were not evaluated. A subsequent single-institution series, in which most patients had class IIa (mild) or IIb (moderate) ischemia and endovascular treatment was largely mechanical thrombolysis, observed similar technical success and amputation rates for both open and endovascular revascularization.

A critical factor to consider is time to reperfusion. Ideally, arterial inflow should be re-established as soon as possible and preferably within 6 hours of symptoms, thus making emergent surgical thromboembolectomy more appealing than catheter-directed pharmacologic thrombolysis. Within the last decade, however, a growing experience with pharmacomechanical thrombectomy has demonstrated that in many instances rapid revascularization may be achieved, with an opportunity for continued catheter-directed pharmacologic thrombolysis for lysis of thrombus that has propagated or embolized within vessels that are too small to access by embolectomy. Contraindications to pharmacologic thrombolysis include active bleeding, stroke, trauma or a surgical procedure within 3 months, an intracranial tumor, severe hypertension, end-stage liver disease with associated coagulopathy, and active peptic ulcer disease with recent gastrointestinal bleeding.

In the rare patient who is seen at a very late stage with profound ischemia of duration greater than 12 hours, complete loss of motor and sensory function, and livedo reticularis, revascularization and an attempt at limb salvage may cause more harm than benefit. Although the absolute inability to salvage an ischemic extremity is often difficult to discern, establishing flow to nonviable tissue can disseminate toxic metabolic byproducts that can induce multisystem organ failure. Such patients would be better served with a primary amputation.

Lastly, given these considerations, patients with peripheral artery embolism often are best served in a hybrid operating room with angiographic equipment so that even if a predominantly open approach is pursued, completion angiography can be obtained in order to assess the completeness of embolus removal and re-establishment of inline flow. Most patients have significant underlying comorbidities, which substantially increases the risk of any emergent procedure. Thus regardless of the selected approach, patients and families should be counseled on the risk of morbidity and mortality as well as limb loss.

■ OPEN SURGICAL TREATMENT

Surgical Embolectomy

Surgical embolectomy typically involves the removal of a clot through an open arteriotomy. During the 1950s, surgical embolectomy was attempted by flushing saline through proximal and distal arteriotomies, above and below the site of the presumed embolism, as well as by passing pigtail metal wire extraction devices. The results using these approaches were often unsatisfactory, and embolectomy was greatly simplified by the introduction of a balloon embolectomy catheter by Thomas J. Fogarty and colleagues in 1963 (Figure 2). In brief, after systemic heparinization, a balloon-tipped catheter is passed distal to an area of occlusion, with subsequent balloon inflation and withdrawal leading to removal of the occlusive material. Although resistance to balloon withdrawal may be related to the presence of an embolism, it also may be related to the existence of an atherosclerotic plaque, and a degree of balloon deflation may be required to avoid arterial injury. Likewise, overinflation of an inappropriately large balloon or inadvertent passage of the catheter into a branch vessel may cause arterial dissection or rupture. Two to three passes of an embolectomy catheter without retrieval of additional embolic material is usually sufficient. Submission of the thrombus for pathologic examination may be considered should a myxomatous or tumor thrombus be a possibility. The availability of "over-the-wire" Fogarty catheters allows the catheter to be passed into all major branch vessels of an extremity under fluoroscopic guidance.

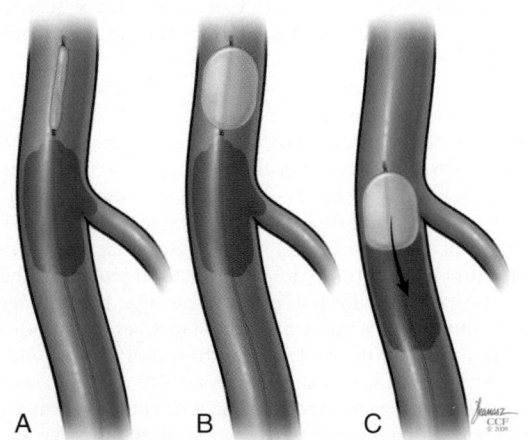

FIGURE 2 Technique of balloon embolectomy. **A,** Pass a balloon-tipped catheter distal to an area of occlusion. **B,** Inflate the balloon, being cautious not to cause damage to the unaffected vessel wall. **C,** Withdraw the inflated balloon and remove the embolic material. *(From Arthurs Z, Lyden S. Management of peripheral arterial emboli. In: Cameron JL, Cameron AM, eds. Current Surgical Therapy. 10th ed. Philadelphia: Elsevier; 2011:812-816.)*

Otherwise, if a standard Fogarty catheter has been used, upon completion of an embolectomy an intraoperative angiogram should be considered, as the presence of backbleeding alone does not confirm complete thrombus retrieval. Intraoperative angiography is mandatory should Doppler signals not be restored.

Aortic and Lower Extremity Emboli

When an aortic embolus is suspected, bilateral groin cutdowns should be performed and the common, superficial, and deep femoral arteries exposed in order to obtain proximal and distal control. After systemic heparinization, a 5F or 6F embolectomy catheter is passed cranially, approximately 25 cm into the infrarenal aorta through transverse femoral arteriotomies in each vessel. The contralateral femoral artery should be occluded during the passage of the balloon catheter to minimize inadvertent embolization from the aorta down the opposite limb. After achieving appropriate prograde flow, distal embolectomy of the superficial femoral and popliteal arteries is performed using a 3F or 4F catheter, followed by embolectomy of the deep femoral artery with a 3F catheter.

If an initial attempt at distal embolectomy is unsuccessful, exposure of the below-knee popliteal artery should be performed with control of the proximal peroneal, anterior tibial, and posterior tibial arteries. A 2F or 3F embolectomy catheter may be passed through a longitudinal arteriotomy in the popliteal artery to remove emboli in the runoff vessels. If unsuccessful, embolectomy of the dorsalis pedis or posterior tibial arteries at the ankle using a 2F catheter may be considered. An intraoperative completion angiography should be performed if distal pulses or Doppler signals are not restored. Transverse arteriotomies are closed primarily and longitudinal arteriotomies are closed preferably through the use of a patch.

Upper Extremity Emboli

Following similar principles, an embolectomy for upper extremity ischemia typically is performed through an arteriotomy in the brachial artery. The distal brachial artery may be exposed through a longitudinal incision just above the elbow, or, if needed, an S-shaped incision may be extended across the antecubital fossa to expose the proximal radial and ulnar arteries. Once proximal and distal control is obtained, a 4F catheter can be passed into the proximal subclavian artery and a 3F catheter subsequently passed through the radial and ulnar arteries. Some caution is required, as subclavian thrombus may embolize inadvertently into the cerebral circulation.

■ PERCUTANEOUS ENDOVACULAR THERAPY

Catheter-Directed Pharmacologic Thrombolysis

Ultrasound-guided access is obtained initially, and a diagnostic angiogram is performed as a guide for further therapy. For the upper extremities the affected limb is widely prepped and draped, whereas for the lower extremities a sterile field is established for the entire affected extremity as well as both groins, as access typically is obtained from the contralateral limb. In addition to providing a more complete view of the arterial inflow, obtaining access remote from the embolus decreases the risk of bleeding complications because of the proximity of the puncture site to the delivery of the thrombolytic agent. Once the embolic occlusion is identified on arteriography, a sheath of appropriate length is inserted and a hydrophilic coated angled guidewire is passed through the thrombus. If the guidewire is unable to traverse the occlusion, a diagnosis of acute thrombosis of an atherosclerotic plaque or a critical collateral vessel in a patient with PAD should be considered. Once the thrombus has been traversed by the guidewire, a multiple sidehole catheter is advanced over the guidewire and a lytic agent is delivered directly into the thrombus.

Although streptokinase and urokinase continue to be used worldwide, the current lytic agent of choice in the United States is tPA. Typically a pulse spray bolus of 10 mg of thrombolytic is delivered into the thrombus, followed by continuous infusion at approximately 0.5 mg/hr. Heparin is administered through the side port of the sheath at 500 units/hr to prevent catheter-associated thrombus. Reimaging is performed in 12 to 24 hours to assess thrombus dissolution.

Percutaneous Mechanical Thrombectomy

Percutaneous mechanical thrombectomy was introduced to decrease the need for prolonged infusion times and decrease the need for the multiple procedures often required for successful catheter-directed thrombolysis. Under ideal circumstances percutaneous mechanical thrombectomy expeditiously reduces overall clot burden and increases the surface area of exposed clot to enable more effective pharmacologic lysis. Various devices have been designed to use suction, rotational infusion, ultrasound, or a high-velocity rheolytic jet to achieve mechanical thrombectomy. Pharmacomechanical thrombolysis refers to using the percutaneous device to lace the thrombus with thrombolytic agent, which after a brief dwell time is followed by mechanical thrombectomy. The AngioJet Thrombectomy System (Boston Scientific, Marlborough, MA) is an example of a rheolytic device that works on the premise of Bernoulli's effect (Figure 3). Specifically, circumferentially oriented pressurized saline jets fragment the thrombus with creation of a low-pressure zone, which facilitates the removal of the resultant thrombotic debris through catheter sideholes. In a large multicenter registry of 283 patients, successful outcome was obtained in 83% of patients without a requirement for adjunctive catheter-directed thrombolysis in 52% of patients.

■ POSTPROCEDURE MANAGEMENT AND CONSIDERATIONS

Hemodynamic monitoring, routine laboratory analysis with correction of acidosis or electrolyte imbalance, and serial neurovascular examinations are necessary. Despite successful revascularization, limb loss may occur should the development of acute compartment syndrome go unrecognized. The diagnosis of compartment syndrome should be considered in the presence of a tensely swollen extremity with pain on passive motion. In patients who are sedated, uncooperative, or neurologically impaired, physical examination will be unhelpful. Elevated CPK levels and myoglobinuria are late markers of tissue destruction and should not be used to establish the diagnosis. Direct compartment pressure measurements can be obtained and fasciotomy considered if pressures are elevated (>30 mm Hg), but even in the presence of normal compartment pressures, fasciotomies should be performed if clinical suspicion exists. In patients with a history of prolonged ischemia (>6 hours), a four-compartment fasciotomy should be performed prophylactically through medial and lateral lower extremity incisions or dorsal and volar upper extremity incisions and the degree of viable muscle assessed by electrocautery stimulation. The wound should be left open and a vacuum-assisted closure device applied in the postoperative period to reduce muscle edema. Systemic effects of muscle ischemia include rhabdomyolysis, which may cause acute tubular necrosis and renal failure. To minimize this risk, intravenous mannitol and bicarbonate should be administered to aid in excretion of myoglobin and alkalization of the urine.

For patients undergoing catheter-directed thrombolysis, close monitoring of the access site is imperative. Of note, patients may report an increase in distal extremity pain because of embolization of thrombus that is being lysed by tPA. Continued thrombolytic infusion and analgesia are recommended with continued close monitoring, as symptoms should eventually improve. All patients

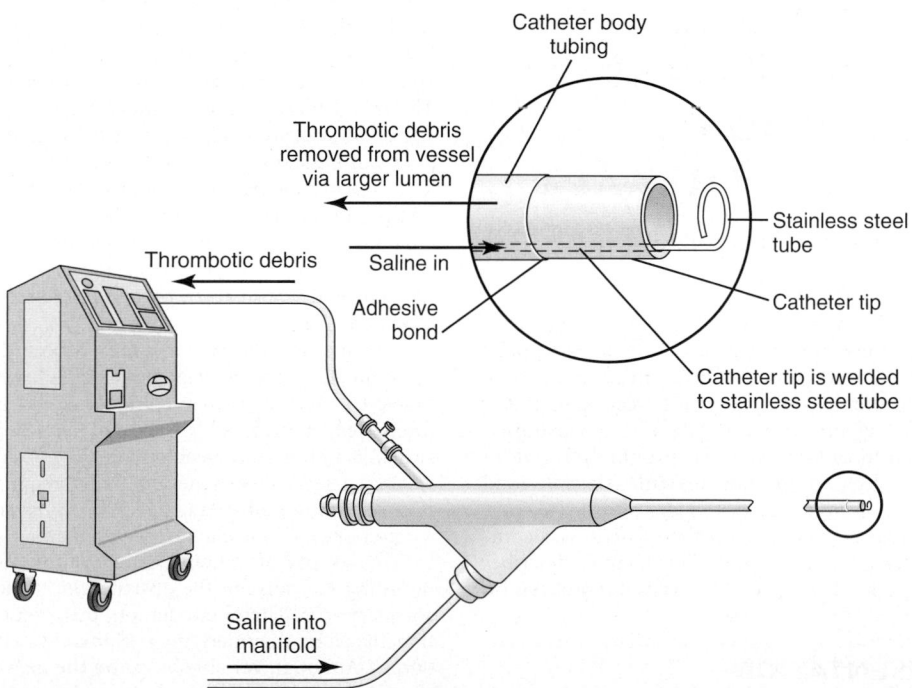

FIGURE 3 Diagram of the AngioJet Thrombectomy System (Boston Scientific, Marlborough, MA) that is often used for percutaneous mechanical thrombectomy. *From Kwolek CJ, Shuja F. Acute ischemia: treatment. In: Cronenwett JL, Johnston KW, eds. Rutherford's Vascular Surgery, 8th ed. Philadelphia: Elsevier; 2014: 2535.)*

undergoing continued thrombolysis should have fibrinogen levels and aPTT monitored every 4 to 6 hours. If fibrinogen levels are 150 mg/dL or less, thrombolytic infusion should cease. As low-dose heparin is administered to prevent catheter-associated thrombotic complications, the aPTT is titrated to 30 to 50 seconds.

Nearly all patients will require long-term systemic anticoagulation to decrease the chance of a recurrent event. In the initial postoperative period, this typically is achieved with heparin or a direct thrombin inhibitor, such as lepirudin or argatroban, until bridging to an oral vitamin K antagonist is complete. Once the acute ischemic episode and its sequelae have been managed, the underlying etiology should be investigated thoroughly. A general approach includes a transesophageal echocardiogram to evaluate the heart for vegetations, thrombus, or the presence of right-to-left shunt; a CTA of the chest, abdomen, and pelvis with bilateral lower extremity runoff to evaluate for the presence of an aneurysm, atherosclerotic lesion or ulcer, or areas of organized thrombus; a hypercoagulable workup; and bilateral lower extremity ultrasonography to assess for deep venous thrombosis if the possibility of a paradoxic embolism has been raised.

■ CONCLUSIONS

In the past decade, the incidence of acute limb ischemia has decreased significantly, possibly because of an improvement in the management of AF. As percutaneous techniques have evolved, there has been a significant decrease in the proportion of patients undergoing open embolectomy and a concomitant increase in those treated by catheter interventions. Notwithstanding these changes, 1-year amputation-free survival after a peripheral arterial embolism remains low at 52%, with an attendant risk-adjusted mortality of 42%. Early diagnosis and treatment of peripheral artery emboli remain essential.

SUGGESTED READINGS

Baril DT, Ghosh K, Rosen AB. Trends in the incidence, treatment, and outcomes of acute lower extremity ischemia in the United States Medicare population. *J Vasc Surg.* 2014;60:669-677.e2.

Bekwelem W, Connolly SJ, Halperin JL, et al. Extracranial systemic embolic events in patients with nonvalvular atrial fibrillation: incidence, risk factors, and outcomes. *Circulation.* 2015;132:796-803.

Berridge DC, Kessel DO, Robertson I. Surgery versus thrombolysis for initial management of acute limb ischaemia. *Cochrane Database Syst Rev.* 2013;(6):CD002784.

Blecha MJ. Critical limb ischemia. *Surg Clin North Am.* 2013;93:789-812, viii.

Creager MA, Kaufman JA, Conte MS. Clinical practice: acute limb ischemia. *N Engl J Med.* 2012;366:2198-2206.

Leung DA, Blitz LR, Nelson T, et al. Rheolytic pharmacomechanical thrombectomy for the management of acute limb ischemia: results from the PEARL registry. *J Endovasc Ther.* 2015;22:546-557.

Mumoli N, Cei M, Vitale J, et al. Are direct oral anticoagulants effective in reducing systemic embolism in patients with atrial fibrillation? A systematic review and meta-analysis of the literature. *Int J Cardiol.* 2015;180:192-195.

Rutherford RB, Baker JD, Ernst C, et al. Recommended standards for reports dealing with lower extremity ischemia: revised version. *J Vasc Surg.* 1997;26:517-538.

Taha AG, Byrne RM, Avgerinos ED, et al. Comparative effectiveness of endovascular versus surgical revascularization for acute lower extremity ischemia. *J Vasc Surg.* 2015;61:147-154.

Vesey JM, Otto CM. Complications of prosthetic heart valves. *Curr Cardiol Rep.* 2004;6:106-111.

ACUTE PERIPHERAL ARTERIAL AND BYPASS GRAFT OCCLUSION: THROMBOLYTIC THERAPY

Elizabeth Ann Ignacio, MD, and Robert P. Liddell, MD

Acute limb ischemia (ALI) is a vascular emergency caused by arterial embolism or thrombosis of native vessels or bypass grafts. Timely management of ALI requires expedited clinical evaluation, diagnostic workup, and initiation of appropriate treatment. Today, advances in thrombolytic agents, infusion catheters, and endovascular techniques have led to catheter-directed thrombolysis (CDT) becoming the treatment of choice for patients with relatively mild ALI. Patients with severe ALI need emergent surgical revascularization. However, CDT should be considered if the relative risks compared with primary operation are favorable. This chapter describes how to select the appropriate therapy for ALI, with an emphasis on the role of CDT.

■ PATIENT PRESENTATION AND WORKUP

Clinical Assessment

The clinical assessment of a patient with ALI should begin with a thorough history, focusing on the patient's presenting symptoms and current overall health. A history of rest pain, claudication, myocardial infarction, stroke, hypertension, diabetes mellitus, atrial fibrillation, aneurysmal disease, smoking, high cholesterol, vasculitis and prior vascular or endovascular surgery is important to obtain. The initial physical exam should assess for the dominant clinical signs and symptoms of ALI, which traditionally include the six Ps: *p*ain, *p*ulselessness, *p*allor, *p*oikilothermy, *p*aresthesias, and *p*aralysis. The presence of one or more of these findings and the abruptness of their onset also may aid in determining the underlying cause. Obvious neurologic deficits suggest an advanced state of ischemia, with sensory deficits preceding motor deficits. Fixed mottling of the skin with muscle necrosis and induration implies irreversible limb ischemia.

A formal stratification system has been developed to help guide the evaluation and management of ALI, while defining prognosis (Table 1). Acutely ischemic limbs should be described as viable, threatened, or irreversibly ischemic. Threatened limbs are reversibly ischemic and are salvageable with appropriate, timely intervention, whereas irreversibly ischemic limbs require amputation because major neuromuscular damage has occurred and is not reversible with surgical or endovascular revascularization.

The severity of ischemia is determined by a number of factors, including the cause of the obstruction, the level of obstruction, the adequacy of collateral circulation, the extent of thrombus propagation, the patient's underlying peripheral vascular disease, and cardiac output. Although variable based on the network of existing collaterals, a period of 6 hours generally is accepted as the window in which revascularization is absolutely necessary for ALI. However, in practice, the degree of ischemia is more important than the absolute duration of ischemia; therefore patients must be assessed on an individual basis and in a timely fashion.

TABLE 1: Clinical Categories of Acute Limb Ischemia

| Category | Description/Prognosis | Findings | | Doppler Signals | |
		Sensory Loss	Muscle Weakness	Arterial	Venous
I. Viable	Not immediately threatened	None	None	Audible	Audible
II. Threatened					
a. Marginally	Salvageable if promptly treated	Minimal (toes) or none	None	Inaudible	Audible
b. Immediately	Salvageable with immediate revascularization	More than toes, associated with rest pain	Mild, moderate	Inaudible	Audible
III. Irreversible	Major tissue loss or permanent nerve damage inevitable	Profound, anesthetic	Profound, paralysis (rigor)	Inaudible	Inaudible

From Rutherford RB, Baker JD, Ernst C, et al. *J Vasc Surg.* 1997;26:517-538.

Imaging Assessment

Imaging is done to evaluate the extent of blood flow compromise, localize culprit flow limiting lesions, and identify other sequelae of peripheral vascular disease (dissection, aneurysmal disease, thrombi, vasculitis). An acutely ischemic limb may be imaged with Doppler ultrasound (DUS), computed tomography angiography (CTA), magnetic resonance angiography (MRA), or digital subtraction angiography (DSA) before treatment. When choosing an imaging modality for native vessel disease, clinicians should take into account whether the patient has underlying renal insufficiency, diabetes, or implanted metal devices. For patients who have normal renal function and are not diabetic, initial evaluation with either CTA or MRA is reasonable based on their similar excellent diagnostic capabilities. Overall, DUS is a less sensitive technique for imaging native vessel stenosis than CTA or MRA. However, DUS is suited more ideally for post-lower extremity arterial bypass surgery surveillance. Asymptomatic vein graft stenosis can result in acute thrombosis and ultimately graft failure if not detected early. In contrast, DUS is not well established for evaluating long-term patency of synthetic conduit bypass grafts.

DSA remains the gold standard for imaging of patients with acute limb ischemia (Figure 1). The chief benefit of DSA is that endovascular therapies may be initiated in the same setting as diagnostic angiography because arterial access already is achieved. Although DSA is a more invasive technique when compared with MRA and CTA, the risks associated with arterial access are minimal.

▪ SELECTION OF THERAPY

The clinical and imaging assessment of a patient with ALI should be completed as quickly and efficiently as possible. Once the diagnosis of ALI is made, treatment should be initiated as soon as possible. Regardless of the cause, all patients without contraindications should receive IV fluids, supplemental oxygen, an 81-mg dose of aspirin and a 100 U/kg bolus of IV heparin followed by a continuous infusion to keep the partial thromboplastin time at 2.0 to 2.5 times normal. As described earlier, the length of time a limb can endure ischemia varies with the cause and severity. The previously described SVS/ISCVC (Society for Vascular Surgery/International Society for Cardiac Vascular Surgery) classification based on sensory motor and Doppler evaluation is used to triage initial limb treatments. Level I patients should be treated with heparin and observation, followed by more definite therapy once comorbidities, functional status, and activity level are determined. Level II patients should be treated soon (IIa) or immediately (IIb) after imaging. Endovascular or operative interventions are equally efficacious in these patients, the choice being contingent on the skill and availability of the interventional radiologist or vascular surgeon. Patients with more severe ischemia (IIb) traditionally had been sent to surgery, but the recent advent of fast-acting lytic drugs, spray-pulse infusion techniques, and pharmacomechanical thrombolysis allow endovascular techniques to have a wider application. Level III patients who seek care shortly after symptom onset are candidates for surgical revascularization and fasciotomy; those seeking care some time after symptom onset require amputation. Attempts to revascularize ischemic limbs late in the progression of disease are not only likely to fail but also frequently result in severe pain, myoglobinemia, renal failure, and sepsis.

▪ RECOMMENDED INTERVENTIONS FOR DISEASE IN NATIVE ARTERIES

Catheter-directed thrombolysis first was described by Dotter in 1974. When compared with high-dose systemic intravenous thrombolysis CDT, it resulted in significantly better outcomes with significantly fewer adverse bleeding events. During the mid 1990s, a number of randomized, multicenter trials compared CDT with surgery for ALI. The Surgery versus Thrombolysis for Ischemia of the Lower Extremity (STILE) trial showed that CDT produces outcomes similar to surgery when used to treat thrombosed native arteries presenting within 2 weeks of the onset of symptoms. In patients seeking care more than 2 weeks from the onset of symptoms, surgery showed better outcomes. The Thrombolysis or Peripheral Arterial Surgery (TOPAS) trial showed that CDT may be attempted and then abandoned when unsuccessful in favor of more localized surgery, without increasing mortality or amputation rate. A number of retrospective studies also have demonstrated that performing CDT and angioplasty before attempting surgery can reduce the number of patients who ultimately will require surgical bypass or amputation. Although these studies do not provide definitive answers to a preferred treatment in all cases, they do suggest that CDT may improve outcomes without compromising the efficacy of subsequent surgery. Therefore, if readily available, CDT should be the first-line therapy for acute native artery occlusion, with endovascular or surgical intervention to treat underlying disease once unmasked.

Before initiating CDT, one should assess the extent of disease in the affected limb, not only in the thrombosed segment but also in the vasculature proximal and distal to the occlusion. The assessment of distal runoff sometimes is hindered by the fact that outflow distal to an occlusion often is limited significantly. If prior studies are available, their review is often helpful in identifying possible causative underlying stenoses as well as defining distal runoff. If prior studies are not available, it is important to attempt to cross the occlusion and directly assess distal runoff without causing distal embolization. According to the Trans-Atlantic Inter-Society Consensus Document

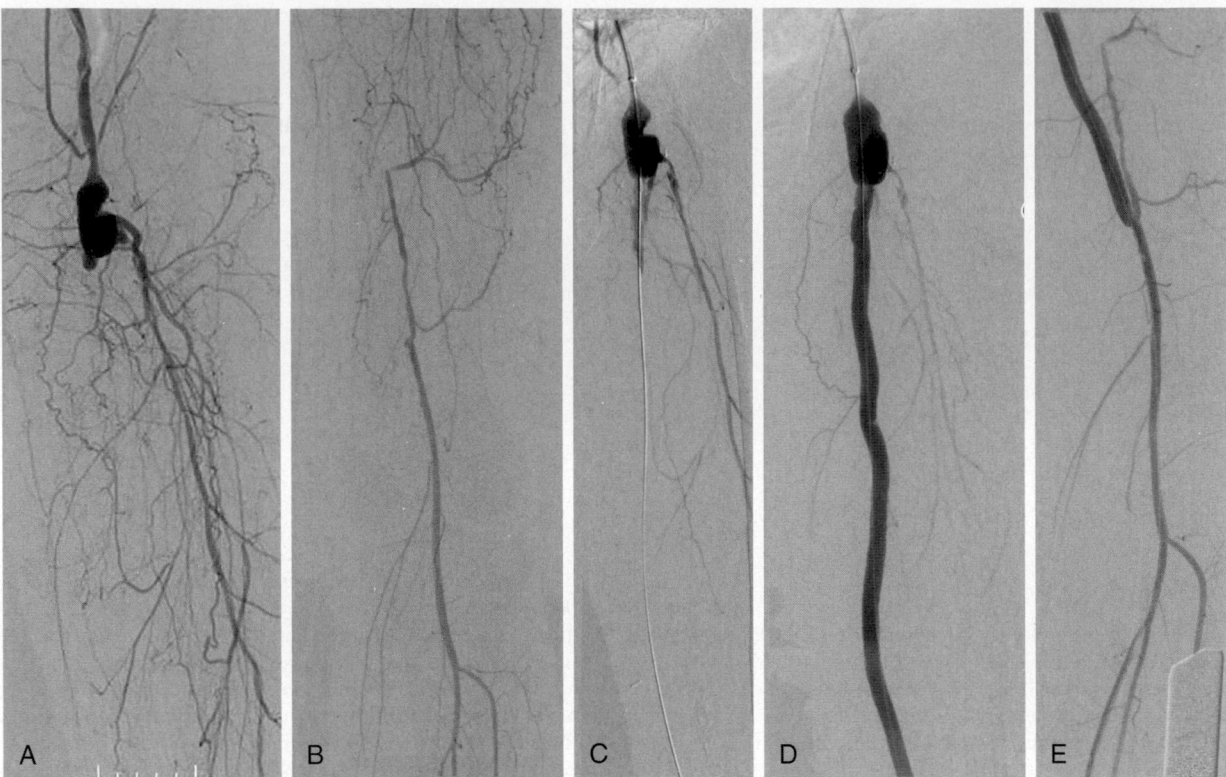

FIGURE 1 DSA of a 69-year-old male with femoropopliteal bypass who presented with acute ischemia. Proximal (**A**) and distal (**B**) occlusion of the bypass. Overnight thrombolysis using a 40-cm long infusion catheter followed angioplasty of the distal anastomosis (**C**). Catheter-directed thrombolysis and angioplasty resulted in a widely patent bypass graft with excellent runoff (**D** and **E**).

on Management of Peripheral Vascular Disease (TASC II) guidelines, focal stenoses are best treated with percutaneous balloon angioplasty (PTA) and stenting once the native artery is opened with CDT. In contrast, long-segment stenosis, diffuse disease, or limited runoff from the affected vessel should dissuade one from initiating CDT. In diffusely diseased vessels thrombolysis serves to only consume time while exposing the patient to potential bleeding complications; therefore these patients often will be triaged directly to surgical bypass.

In patients with native vessel occlusions resulting from embolic disease, lack of well-developed collaterals often results in dramatic, poorly tolerated symptoms very early in the course of ischemia. When initial assessments suggest minimal baseline atherosclerotic disease, or when history points to an embolic occlusion, these patients should undergo surgical embolectomy. CDT in combination with mechanical or aspiration embolectomy is also an option. These endovascular techniques are especially efficacious below the knee, where angiographic guidance allows for evaluation and selective interventions in small arteries.

■ RECOMMENDED INTERVENTIONS FOR DISEASE IN BYPASS GRAFTS

The STILE trial demonstrated lower amputation rates with CDT compared with surgery for thrombotic occlusions of bypass grafts. In patients with thrombosed bypass grafts, timing of the graft failure determines the appropriate treatment. If the patient seeks care within the first 30 days after bypass, graft failure is most often a result of technical problems with the graft, assuming the patient is not hypercoagulable. If the bypass is partially open, imaging usually reveals the causative lesion: the most common finding is a distal anastomosis stenosis. In native vessel conduits, occasionally a stenosis will be seen that results from the use of too small a caliber venous conduit, or

even more uncommonly, a perivascular hematoma, resulting from improper vein preparation. Patients with early bypass failure should undergo surgical revision. An endovascular approach is recommended only in the rare case of an isolated angiographic lesion that appears amenable to PTA. More often, thrombolysis alone serves only to open the bypass temporarily. The underlying technical problem quickly reasserts itself, and the limb once again becomes ischemic.

If the bypass goes down beyond the 30-day perioperative period one first should consider the severity of the ischemia and the indications for the original surgery. If the ischemia does not threaten the viability of the limb, as it did in 30% of the patients in the STILE trial, and the original bypass was performed to treat life-threatening ischemia, a watch-and-wait approach may be warranted. It is unlikely that any revision of the graft will provide long-term improvement in limb perfusion, but it is possible that further surgery could make things worse. In these cases, noninvasive imaging and DSA are appropriate to assess whether distal target vessels are available for the secondary bypass and to assess whether endovascular treatments could improve outflow from the poorly functioning bypass.

In cases of life-threatening ischemia occurring beyond the 30-day perioperative window, the most common causative lesion is focal intimal hyperplasia, typically at a valve or anastomosis. CDT is the treatment of choice in these instances because it allows for identification of the treatable lesion. CDT also restores flow through the thrombosed collaterals, thus reperfusing the threatened limb. Thrombolysis should be followed by PTA once the focal lesion is identified. If a causative lesion can be identified and treated, the 1-year patency is more favorable than if there had been no lesion. Grafts maintained exclusively by CDT and PTA have been found to have excellent long-term patency rates, especially if ankle-brachial indices (ABIs) immediately after treatment are high. There are, however, two caveats: first, the outcomes of thrombolysis are generally much better in venous grafts than in synthetic grafts; second, the beneficial effect of CDT is short-lived in patients with diabetes, with 1-year patencies being very low. In these patients, if imaging reveals suitable distal target vessel, secondary bypasses are a superior treatment choice because of their higher patency rates.

Patients with vein grafts more than 1 year old are excellent candidates for CDT because the mature conduit has proven itself over time. The failure is usually a result of progressive atherosclerotic disease in the inflow or outflow vessels. CDT often unmasks a normal-appearing graft with poor inflow or outflow vessels, which themselves can be treated via endovascular means to maintain graft function.

Catheter-Directed Thrombolysis

Over the last 20 years CDT has supplanted completely systemic intravenous thrombolysis. The role of CDT is to (1) restore flow, (2) reveal any underlying causative lesion, and (3) improve perfusion of the outflow vessels. The unmasked lesion then should be treated via endovascular or open surgery.

PREOPERATIVE PLANNING

If CDT is to be used as part of the ischemic limb treatment plan, the preprocedural consent should describe the risk of hemorrhage, limb loss, renal failure, anaphylaxis, stroke, and death. Bleeding is the most frequent significant complication associated with CDT. Intracranial hemorrhage often can be devastating but is fortunately rare, having been reported in 1.2% (STILE) to 2.1% (TOPAS-1) of patients undergoing CDT. Absolute contraindications to CDT include active/life-threatening bleeding, aortic dissection, recent intracranial or intraspinal surgery or trauma, and intracranial arteriovenous malformations or aneurysms. Relative contraindications include major surgery within the past 4 weeks, uncontrolled hypertension, gastric ulcers, recent eye surgery, recent stroke, pregnancy or the first 10 days postpartum, and intracranial neoplasms.

TECHNIQUE

Patients should be given aspirin and heparin as they are being worked up for CDT. Any previous noninvasive imaging should be made available and reviewed. Pulses in both limbs should be documented, and an operating room suite should be available in the event that conversion to open surgery is necessary. Iso-osmolar contrast should be used throughout, and the procedure should be performed under conscious sedation.

Retrograde contralateral access should be obtained with arterial puncture occurring over the femoral head. Ultrasound guided 21-gauge micropuncture access is recommended to minimize the risk of hematoma and dissection. A 5F vascular sheath then should be placed. A 5F Omni flush (AngioDynamics, Latham, NY) or pigtail catheter then should be advanced to the level of the renal arteries. An aortogram and bilateral lower extremity runoff then should be performed.

Once the thrombosed vascular segment is identified, the wire-catheter combination should be advanced up and over the iliac bifurcation to the levels of the contralateral (affected side) external iliac artery. After a wire is placed in the contralateral external iliac artery the access catheter and 5F sheath should be exchanged for a 6F or 7F "up and over" sheath such as a Felxor Balkin (Cook Medical, Bloomington, IN) into the contralateral common iliac or external iliac artery. A heparin bolus then usually is administered (100 U/kg), and an activated clotting time (ACT) is checked (goal ACT >250 seconds).

An attempt then should be made to cross the thrombosed segment. We prefer a combination of a 4F straight or 5F angle taper Glide catheter (Terumo, Somerset, NJ) and a hydrophilic guidewire (e.g., Glidewire [Terumo] or Roadrunner [Cook]). This combination imparts excellent maneuverability and easily crosses most occlusions.

In cases with significant underlying atherosclerotic disease, a combination of a 4F straight Glide catheter and a Rosen wire (Cook) can be used to traverse the thrombus. This combination ensures that the blunt tip of the wire leads in the lumen of the diseased vessel, minimizing the risk of dissection. Gentle, controlled attempts to cross the thrombus should be made, with injections of dilute contrast whenever the wire-catheter combination does not easily advance. The goal is to carefully advance through the soft thrombus, avoiding embolization while staying intraluminal. Rarely, a microwire (<0.018 inch) and microcatheter (<3F) may be advanced coaxially to aid in successful crossing of thrombus in heavily diseased vessels with tight stenoses.

Once the thrombosed segment is crossed, the length of the occlusion should be defined and measured. An appropriate multiple side-hole infusion catheter (Pulse Spray infusion system [AngioDynamics Inc., Queensbury, NY], Katzen infusion wire [Boston Scientific, Natick, MA]) then should be advanced over the wire through the occlusion. The infusion length should be as close to possible to the length of the occlusion, erring on the side of a shorter infusion length. If some side holes are outside the thrombus, the infused drug will take the path of least resistance and will escape out the holes in the patent artery. After the infusion catheter is in position, the guidewire is removed, and the end hole of the infusion catheter is plugged with an occlusion wire (Pulse Spray infusion system) or infusion wire (Katzen infusion wire). The sheath and catheter are sutured to the skin, while the infusion catheter is secured to the sheath with Steri-Strips and suture to prevent catheter displacement. Before the patient leaves the angiography suite we initiate a 150 to 300 U/hr intra-arterial infusion of heparin via the up and over sheath, to prevent thrombus from forming on the tip of the sheath or along the non-infusion portion of the infusion catheter.

INFUSION

Very limited data are available that compare the efficacy of fibrinolytic agents for use in CDT. In the United States, streptokinase, anistreplase, alteplase (recombinant tissue plasminogen activator [tPA]), reteplase, and tenecteplase are available. Lysis and bleeding rates are comparable among the various agents, with very few direct comparison trials available and no clear-cut evidence of superiority of one agent over another for CDT.

There are a number of different thrombolysis techniques described in the literature. The simplest and most often employed technique is continuous infusion. In this technique, thrombolysis is performed via an infusion catheter placed after diagnostic angiography. The patient subsequently returns for follow-up angiography until a procedure end point (successful lysis) is reached. The bolus method involves delivery of a single highly concentrated dose of thrombolytic agent throughout the occlusion and then initiation of continuous infusion. The pulse spray technique refers to repeated forceful injection of small aliquots of thrombolytic, thus distributing the thrombolytic agent rapidly throughout the thrombus as well as mechanically disrupting the thrombus. Pulse spray is initiated and continued in the angiography suite until antegrade flow is restored. In the graded infusion technique, the rate of drug infusion is diminished over time. Stepwise infusion differs from the other methods in that it employs an end hole catheter that is imbedded in the proximal portion of the thrombus. There is no evidence of significant differences in amputation-free survival between the methods. Continuous infusion requires the least procedure time and is an appropriate choice for relatively mild ALI. If an infusion is begun late in the day, the infusion rate can be set relatively low for a 12- to 15-hour overnight infusion. However, studies have shown faster thrombolysis times when bolus or pulse-spray methods are combined with continuous infusion. Therefore bolus and pulse-spray methods often are used when time is limited for reestablishing antegrade flow, which is often the case in ALI. Some reports, however, show an increased risk of bleeding complications compared with continuous infusion, whereas others do not. There is concern with both bolus and pulse-spray infusion techniques that there may be an increase in distal embolization because of thrombus fragmentation.

We typically lace the thrombus with an initial 5- to 10-g bolus of tPA then initiate a 0.5 to 1.0 mg/hr continuous infusion (10 mg tPA in 1 L of normal saline, infused at a rate of 50 to 100 mL/hr). A recent study has shown similar positive results using an ultra-high–dose infusion CDT protocol. The ultra-high–dose technique employed an initial pulse spray technique delivering 1 mg/min for 15 minutes, followed by an infusion of 35 mg over 2 hours. An angiogram then is performed, and if there was residual thrombus present, a further 10 mg of alteplase is infused over an additional 2 hours.

Patients should be admitted to a monitored bed, where checks of the treated limb, Doppler pulses, groin checks, and neurologic checks should be performed at regularly prescribed intervals (every 2 hours). Fibrinogen, hematocrit, hemoglobin, platelets, and partial thromboplastin time should be checked at baseline and every 4 to 6 hours, with the tPA infusion rate halved when the fibrinogen level falls below 150 mg/dL. If the fibrinogen level falls below 100 mg/dL, the infusion should be discontinued because of the increased of bleeding demonstrated in the STILE-1 trial. However, there is no prospective evidence that this practice lowers bleeding risk, and consequently, many other practices do not monitor fibrinogen levels. Alternatively, cryoprecipitate can be given to raise the fibrinogen level and allow for continued infusion of tPA.

Increased pain in the treated limb may indicate successful thrombolysis, with pain occurring as a result of distal emboli showering and washout of cytokines. Other clinical variables such as temperature, color, pulse, and capillary refill should point toward improving perfusion. If at any point the treated limb appears to be more ischemic, the infusion setup and catheter position should be checked. If the limb becomes critically ischemic, CDT should be aborted and surgical revascularization should be attempted. If the limb ischemia is stable or improving, reevaluation with angiography is indicated every 6 to 24 hours until flow is restored.

A number of devices have been developed in an effort to accelerate the thrombolytic process, therefore decreasing the risk of hemorrhage and other complications. Pulse-spray catheters, mechanical lysis catheters, aspiration catheters, rheolytic catheters, and ultrasound-accelerated devices are all currently available. These devices have been developed to facilitate disruption and penetration of the thrombus by the thrombolytic agent. In theory this allows less thrombolytic to be used and shortens the infusion time necessary to achieve thrombolysis. A recent study showed that there was a significant improvement in complete thrombolysis, lower 30-day amputation rate, and fewer bleeding complications with ultrasound-accelerated CDT (EKOS [EKOS, Bothell, WA]) when compared with standard CDT. The study also reported a significant decrease in thrombolysis time and volume of lytic agent required for successful thrombolysis in native arteries and bypass grafts.

■ ADJUNCTIVE PHARMACEUTICALS

The addition of glycoprotein IIb/IIIa (GP IIb/IIIa) platelet-receptor inhibitors reduce platelet aggregation and reduce thrombolytic resistance of platelet-bound fibrin. There are several drugs in clinical use that bind GP IIb/IIIa receptors. These include abciximab (Reopro, [Janssen Biotech, Horsham, PA]), a monoclonal antibody fragment; eptifibatide (Integrilin, [Shering-Plough, Kenilworth, NJ]); and tirofiban (Aggrastat [Merck, Kenilworth, NJ]). Studies comparing adjunctive use of abciximab during peripheral arterial CDT to CDT alone have shown no difference in technical success (PROMPT and APART trials). Infusion time was either shorter or equivalent. The frequency of bleeding was either equivalent or higher. Experience with tirofiban and eptifibatide is limited. Use of these agents in peripheral arterial CDT has not been adopted widely given the clinical results so far.

■ FOLLOW-UP

The goal of CDT is to provide timely, safe, effective, and durable revascularization of the affected limb. After successful revascularization, the patient should be placed on an 81-mg daily dose of aspirin for life. Underlying vascular risk factors should be addressed with antihypertensives, glycemic control, statins, and smoking cessation. Additional antithrombotic drugs may be administered, depending on the nature of the revascularization procedure. The value of dual antiplatelet therapy comprising aspirin plus clopidogrel or ticlopidine, which is well established in coronary stenting, remains controversial in peripheral revascularizations, and evidence-based guidelines do not recommend routine use. ABIs should be used to monitor patency after revascularization. If the ABI decreases by more than 0.2, angiography or noninvasive imaging is indicated.

SELECTED READINGS

Berridge DC, Kessel DO, Robertson I. Surgery versus thrombolysis for initial management of acute limb ischemia. *Cochrane Database Syst Rev.* 2013;(6):CD002784.

Creager MA, Kaufman JA, Conte MS. Acute limb ischemia. *N Engl J Med.* 2012;366:2198-2206.

Kuoppala M, Franzen S, Lindblad B, et al. Long-term prognostic factors after thrombolysis for lower limb ischemia. *J Vasc Surg.* 2008;47:1243-1250.

Mills JL, Conte MS, Armstrong DG, et al. The Society of Vascular Surgery lower extremity threatened limb classification system: risk stratification based on wound, ischemia, and foot infection (WIfI). *J Vasc Surg.* 2014;59:220-234.

Norgen L, Hiatt WR, Dormandy JA, et al. TransAtlantic Inter-Society consensus for the management of peripheral vascular disease (TASC II). *J Vasc Surg.* 2007;45:S5.

Patel NH, Krishnamurthy VN, Kim S, et al. Quality improvement guidelines for percutaneous management of acute lower-extremity ischemia. *J Vasc Interv Radiol.* 2013;24:3-15.

Rooke TW, Hirsch AT, Misra S, et al. 2011 ACCF/AHA Focused update of the guideline for the management of patients with peripheral artery disease (Updating the 2005 Guideline). *Circulation.* 2011;124:2020-2045.

Rutherford RB. Clinical staging of acute limb ischemia as the basis for choice of revascularization method: when and how to intervene. *Semin Vasc Surg.* 2009;22:5-9.

Schernthaner MB, Samuels S, Biegler P, et al. Ultrasound-accelerated versus standard catheter-directed thrombolysis in 102 patients with acute and subacute limb ischemia. *J Vasc Interv Radiol.* 2014;25:1149-1156.

Thukkani AK, Kinlay S. Endovascular intervention for peripheral artery disease. *Circ Res.* 2015;116:1599-1613.

ATHEROSCLEROTIC RENAL ARTERY STENOSIS

Ryan S. Watson, MD, and Thomas H. Cogbill, MD, FACS

Atherosclerosis is the most common cause of renal artery stenosis (RAS), accounting for 90% of cases. Atherosclerotic RAS has been implicated as a significant contributor to systemic hypertension and impaired renal function. However, RAS is rarely the sole cause of these two multifactorial clinical entities. Although the incidence of RAS may be as high as 43% in certain high-risk groups, no data are available to justify prophylactic treatment of asymptomatic patients. In fact, the majority of patients with symptomatic RAS are managed medically; endovascular and open surgical interventions are required in only a select subset of patients. As in other areas of vascular surgery, the explosion of catheter-based endovascular interventions has revolutionized the procedures used to treat RAS, relegating open surgery to a small number of cases with specific indications.

■ INCIDENCE

The incidence of atherosclerotic RAS is approximately 5.4% in patients with resistant hypertension, and it may affect as many as 6.8% of adults over 65 years of age. It is even more prevalent in those with vascular disease, with estimates between 22% and 60%. Risk factors associated with atherosclerotic RAS include older age, hyperlipidemia, peripheral arterial disease (PAD), cerebrovascular disease (CVD), and coronary artery disease (CAD), with the severity of atherosclerotic RAS often paralleling the severity of CAD.

■ NATURAL HISTORY

Although RAS often is implicated as a cause of systemic hypertension and worsening renal function, RAS is more frequently discovered as an incidental finding on abdominal ultrasound, computed tomography angiography (CTA), magnetic resonance angiography (MRA), or angiography performed for another reason. In studies using sequential angiography, atherosclerotic RAS lesions progressed in 11% to 44% of subjects. Progression to complete occlusion occurred in only 10% to 16% of patients with more than 60% stenosis. In patients studied by ultrasound, complete occlusion occurred in only 7% of patients with a stenosis greater than 60%. Progression of these lesions may be even less common, as a significant increase in RAS was seen annually in only 0.5% of patients with cardiovascular risk factors. These observations have led to a shift in the paradigm of RAS treatment.

The underlying pathophysiology is complex but likely related to a combination of renal ischemia and activation of the renin-angiotensin-aldosterone (RAA) system. Activation of the RAA system results in the release of the vasopressor angiotensin II and plasma expansion via the effects of aldosterone. In most cases, the resultant hypertension can be managed medically. The ultimate endpoint of the disease process is hypertension resistant to medical therapy and progressive renal dysfunction due to ischemia, with renal atrophy being documented in 5.5%, 11.7%, and 20.8% of patients with normal renal arteries, renal arteries with less than 60% stenosis, and renal arteries with more than 60% stenosis, respectively.

■ EVALUATION

Symptomatic RAS patients are seen with resistant hypertension (uncontrolled hypertension on three medications) or progressive renal failure. Current guidelines suggest screening for RAS as part of a secondary hypertension etiology workup for those with resistant hypertension, severe hypertension (systolic blood pressure >180 mm Hg, diastolic blood pressure >110 mm Hg), elevated nighttime blood pressures during 24-hour monitoring, malignant hypertension, onset of hypertension at age less than 30 years, sudden worsening of previously well-controlled hypertension, or discrepant kidney length on imaging. Patients with sudden worsening of renal function or recurrent flash pulmonary edema also should undergo evaluation for RAS. Individuals in whom renal function acutely worsens after the initiation of an angiotensin converting enzyme (ACE) inhibitor have an increased incidence of bilateral RAS.

Duplex ultrasound is the initial method of choice for RAS screening. The degree of stenosis is best determined by measurement of each renal artery peak systolic velocity (PSV). Normal renal arteries have a PSV of 60 to 100 cm/sec. Renal artery PSV greater than 180 cm/sec is indicative of RAS greater than 60%. The ratio of renal artery PSV to aortic PSV also is calculated, with a value higher than 3.5 being indicative of RAS with luminal stenosis greater than 60%. Other signs of RAS include intrarenal vascular tardus-parvus and renal atrophy. CTA and MRA are more sensitive and specific modalities for delineating the precise anatomy and degree of RAS. Conventional arteriography remains highly accurate for identification and quantification of RAS and has the added advantage of providing access for therapeutic interventions, if indicated.

Patients with RAS often have concomitant CAD, PAD, and CVD and should undergo evaluation as indicated by history and physical examination. Baseline serum creatinine, hemoglobin, lipid panel, and glucose are checked routinely.

■ TREATMENT

Although atherosclerotic RAS is associated with increased cardiovascular morbidity and mortality, there is no current evidence to support revascularization of asymptomatic patients or patients with well-controlled hypertension. Numerous randomized controlled studies, including the Cardiovascular Outcomes in Renal Atherosclerotic Lesions (CORAL) trial, comparing the results of endovascular interventions versus medical management have demonstrated no benefit of stenting in patients with atherosclerotic RAS who are treated with antiplatelet therapy, statins, and blood pressure control with an ACE inhibitor or angiotensin receptor blocker (ARB).

Revascularization of patients with atherosclerotic RAS currently is reserved for renovascular hypertension that is not responsive to maximal medical therapy and for patients with worsening excretory renal function. Young patients in whom flash pulmonary edema is caused by atherosclerotic RAS also may benefit from revascularization.

Medical Therapy

Because all patients with atherosclerotic RAS are at increased risk for cardiovascular morbidity and mortality, hypertension should be controlled aggressively, as should factors known to be associated with progression of atherosclerosis.

Hypertension Control

Hypertension control should start with an ACE inhibitor or ARB. Calcium-channel blockers, beta-blockers, chlorothiazide, or hydralazine may be added for better control. There is good evidence that ACE inhibitors and ARBs are helpful in patients with underlying cardiac disease and nephropathy. Most patients are able to tolerate ACE inhibitor or ARB therapy. However, ACE inhibitors can decrease glomerular filtration rate (GFR) by blocking efferent arteriolar constriction, and therapy must be monitored closely to ensure that the decrease in GFR is minimal.

Lipid-Lowering Agents

Hyperlipidemia should be treated with a statin. Statin therapy decreases rates of myocardial infarction; prevents progression of CAD, PAD, and CVD; and decreases cardiovascular mortality. Although few studies have directly correlated statin use to outcomes in patients with RAS, reduction in angiographic progression of RAS has been demonstrated.

Antiplatelet Therapy

Although no study has focused specifically on patients with atherosclerotic RAS, antiplatelet therapy with aspirin or clopidogrel has been associated with decreased adverse cardiovascular events and mortality in patients with CAD, PAD, and CVD. Antiplatelet therapy is also an important adjunct after endovascular RAS revascularization. Patients who receive renal artery stents are treated with clopidogrel for at least 30 days, followed by low-dose aspirin indefinitely. Antiplatelet therapy in these instances is meant to reduce early thrombotic complications as well as to reduce the chance of restenosis.

Smoking Cessation

As in all patients with atherosclerosis, smoking cessation is essential. Smoking has been implicated in arterial endothelial cell damage, increased levels of low-density lipoprotein cholesterol, and increased platelet aggregation. Smoking also causes vasoconstriction, increased heart rate, and increased blood pressure. Smoking cessation has been shown to improve survival in patients with CAD and PAD. Patients who are able to quit smoking enjoy a 13% reduction in all-cause mortality.

Glycemic Control

Patients with diabetes and concomitant atherosclerosis are at increased risk for progression of vascular disease. Good glycemic control (hemoglobin A_{1C} <7.0%) should be attained via either oral hypoglycemic agents or insulin therapy to prevent microvascular complications.

Renal Artery Stenosis Surveillance and Follow-up

Although there are no quality data on RAS surveillance, we recommend duplex ultrasound initially every 6 to 12 months for patients with RAS greater than 60% to assess for progression of stenosis and renal atrophy. Blood pressure must be monitored carefully along with measurement of serum creatinine or estimated GFR. An abrupt change in control of hypertension or renal function may prompt earlier reimaging of the renal arteries.

Revascularization

Based on the results of the Angioplasty and Stenting for Renal Artery Lesions (ASTRAL) and CORAL trials, revascularization for atherosclerotic RAS currently is reserved for patients with recalcitrant hypertension or worsening kidney function despite optimal medical management and young patients with flash pulmonary edema caused by RAS. It is important to note that entry criteria for these studies excluded patients most likely to benefit from revascularization. For example, during the CORAL trial, enrollment was broadened to include patients with well-controlled hypertension, and patients with a recent history of congestive heart failure were excluded.

Revascularization can be accomplished by endovascular procedures or by open surgery. Endovascular approaches are preferred in most cases because of their minimally invasive nature, excellent early results, and lower periprocedural morbidity and mortality when compared with open surgery. Angioplasty alone has lower success rates than angioplasty with stent placement. Open renal artery surgery is reserved for urgent salvage of endovascular technical failures resulting in hemorrhage or renal ischemia, revascularization of renal artery branches that are not amenable to endovascular repairs, and renal artery revascularization in combination with elective aortic reconstructions that require an open approach.

Endovascular Therapy

The endovascular approach begins with percutaneous femoral artery access. Using standard Seldinger technique, a diagnostic catheter is inserted into the aorta, and an aortogram is obtained (Figure 1). If the renal artery is angled steeply from the aorta, access via the radial artery or brachial artery is helpful for cannulation and stent deployment. Unfractionated intravenous heparin is administered. After identification of the lesion, a selective catheter is used with wire guidance to enter the affected renal artery. Use of distal embolic protection devices is controversial; small trial evidence supports their use and should be considered in patients at high risk for renal failure. After selection of the renal artery and deployment of an embolic protection device, percutaneous balloon angioplasty is performed, followed by deployment of a balloon-expandable stent (Figure 2). Because aortic wall plaque is often contiguous with proximal renal artery stenosis, it is important to place the stent such that 1 to 3 mm of the proximal end of the stent is free within the aortic lumen (Figure 3). Repeat aortogram with evaluation of the renal arteries should be performed for confirmation of the anatomy after intervention. Closure of the access sites may be accomplished with a closure device or simple removal of the sheath followed by manual pressure for 20 minutes.

Medical Management After Revascularization

Patients start taking clopidogrel for at least 30 days, followed by low-dose aspirin therapy indefinitely. Systemic blood pressures are controlled assiduously and risk factors for progression of atherosclerosis are managed aggressively.

Complications

Complications include rapid postintervention decline in renal function, which can result from atheromatous embolization or

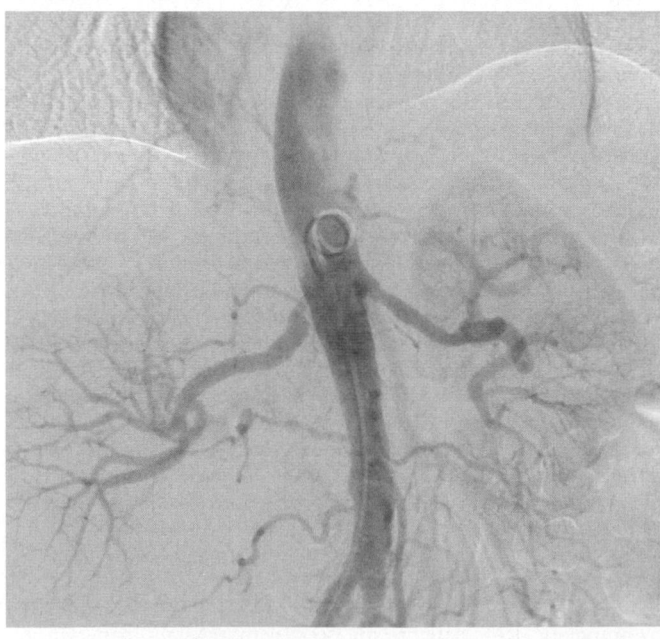

FIGURE 1 Aortogram illustrating right renal artery stenosis.

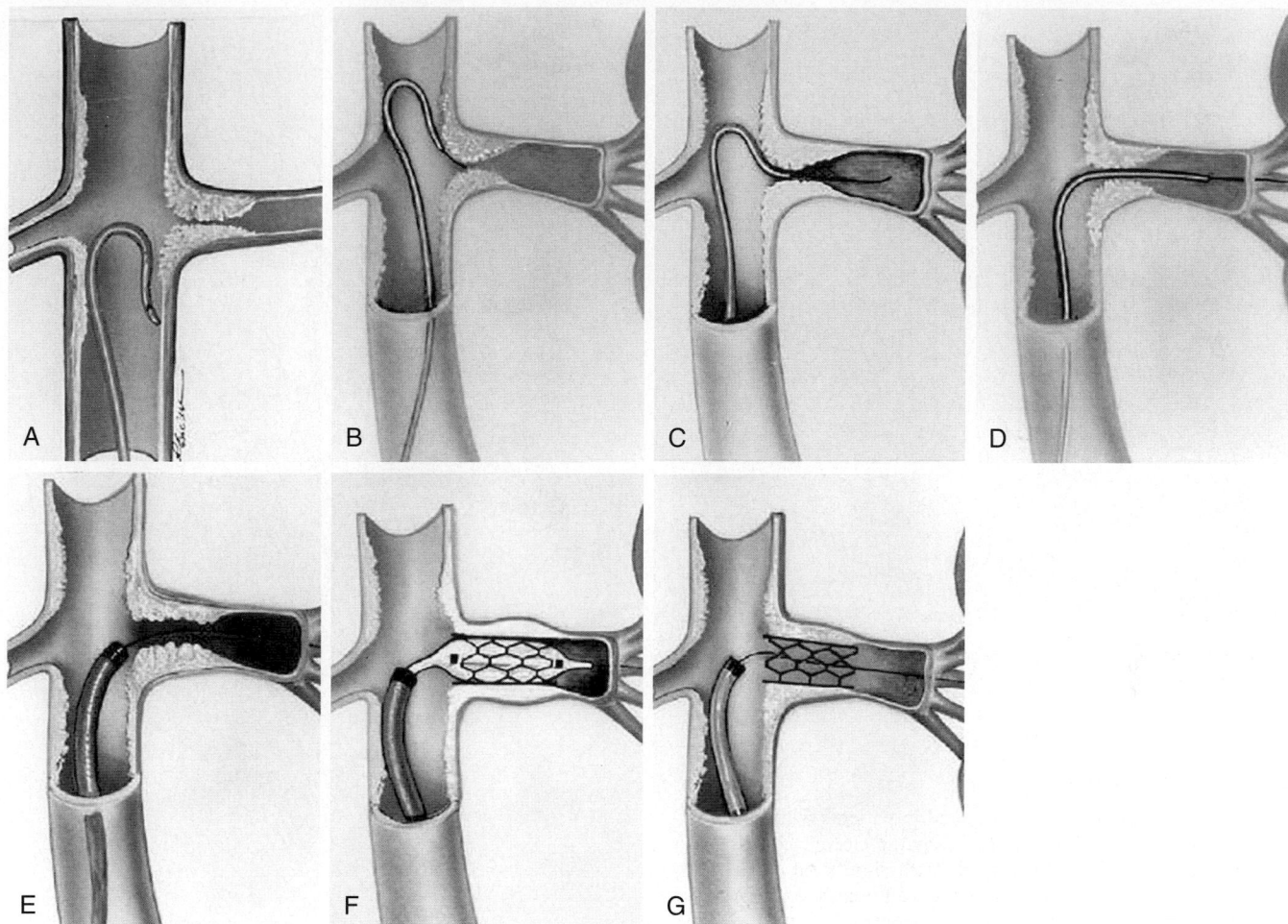

FIGURE 2 **A,** Pigtail diagnostic catheter is placed to obtain an aortogram. **B,** Pigtail catheter is advanced to the origin of the left renal artery. **C,** A guidewire is positioned across the stenosis. **D,** Therapeutic catheter is advanced along the guidewire. **E,** Contrast is used to visualize the stenosis. **F,** A balloon-expandable stent is positioned, and the balloon is inflated. **G,** The balloon and catheter are withdrawn, leaving the stent in place. *(From Carr TM, Sabri SS, Turba UC, et al. Stenting for atherosclerotic renal artery stenosis. Tech Vasc Interv Radiol. 2010;13:134-145.)*

contrast-induced nephropathy. We routinely hydrate patients with normal saline while in the periprocedural area.

Renal artery rupture is a rare but serious complication during percutaneous balloon dilation and stent deployment; it is critical to maintain wire selection of the vessel until satisfied with postintervention anatomy. In the event of rupture of the renal artery, an additional stent may be placed to control the site of perforation. Endovascular access to a ruptured vessel may be exceedingly difficult if wire selection is lost before repair, necessitating an urgent open salvage procedure.

Access site complications, including femoral pseudoaneurysm, hematoma with potentially significant blood loss, lymphatic leak, and femoral artery dissection, are possible. To mitigate percutaneous access site complications, we use fluoroscopy to ensure that access is overlying the femoral head, enhancing the ability to control bleeding with postprocedure pressure, and ultrasound guidance to locate the common femoral artery.

Outcomes

Control of hypertension, measured by number of antihypertensive medications, has been demonstrated to improve in up to 80% of RAS patients treated by angioplasty and stenting. Renal dysfunction, measured by serum creatinine or estimated GFR, has been shown to stabilize or improve in 60% of RAS patients.

Surveillance and Follow-up

Although there are no quality data on RAS surveillance after angioplasty and stenting, we recommend a duplex ultrasound within 1 to 2 weeks after the procedure to document the postprocedural change in renal artery PSV and in the renal artery PSV to aortic PSV ratio. Several additional duplex ultrasounds are performed every 6 to 12 months to assess for recurrent stenosis and renal atrophy. Blood pressure must be monitored carefully along with measurement of serum creatinine or estimated GFR. An abrupt change in control of hypertension or renal function may prompt earlier reimaging of the renal vasculature.

Endovascular Management of Restenosis

Restenosis rates are as high as 50% at 12 months and 60% at 18 months. Unfortunately, the impact of restenosis has been addressed poorly in the randomized controlled trials comparing stenting and medical management. Postintervention statins and antiplatelet medications are beneficial for prevention of restenosis. Patients with progressively worsening restenosis on follow-up duplex studies and all symptomatic patients with worsening renal function or blood pressure control who have imaging evidence of restenosis should undergo reintervention if no contraindications exist. Endovascular reintervention has modest success with a 47% rate of hypertension improvement and 99% renal function stabilization or improvement in several small studies.

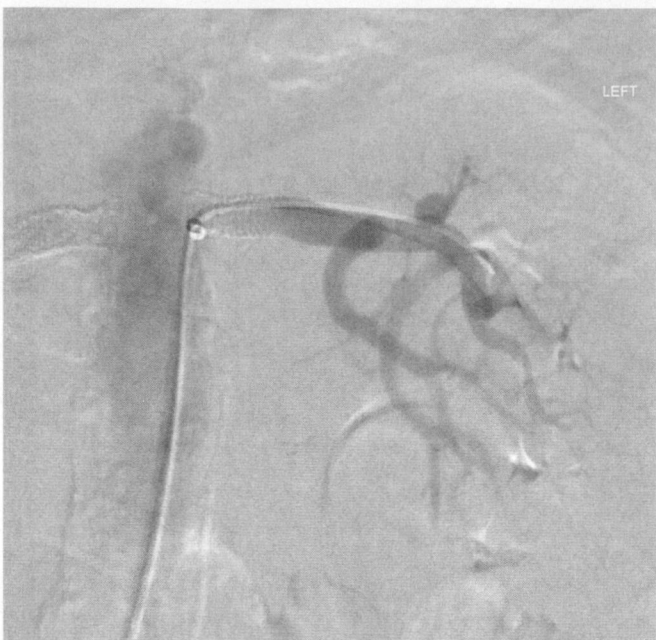

FIGURE 3 Poststent placement arteriogram confirming proper position of the stents with the proximal ends of the stents extending within the aortic lumen.

Open Surgical Repairs

Open surgical repair may be considered in patients with symptomatic atherosclerotic RAS who are undergoing elective open surgery for aortic disease. Those individuals with significant renal artery branch disease also should be considered candidates for open repair, as stenting may not be feasible in these patients. Urgent open renal artery surgery is also occasionally necessary for renal artery hemorrhage or occlusion during endovascular revascularization.

For elective open renal artery revascularization, careful preoperative risk assessment is essential. RAS is a marker for generalized atherosclerosis, and these patients must be screened for CAD, PAD, and CVD. Preoperative cardiac and pulmonary assessments are paramount to assess perioperative risk and initiate therapy to mitigate risk.

Aortorenal Artery Bypass

The patient should be positioned with the umbilicus at the level of the bed break, with the table angled at 15 degrees. The most versatile approach for open repair is the midline incision from xiphoid to pubis. After mobilization of the small bowel, the retroperitoneum is incised to expose the aorta (Figure 4). The duodenum is subsequently reflected to the patient's right. The left renal vein may be retracted to expose the underlying aorta and the left renal artery. Several left renal vein branches (gonadal, adrenal, lumbar) may need to be divided to permit mobilization. The proximal right renal artery can be accessed through this same exposure. Access to the entire right renal artery is best accomplished by medial mobilization of the right colon and duodenum (Cattell-Braasch maneuver). Mannitol (12.5 mg) is administered before clamping the arteries and after release of vascular control. Mannitol may help to prevent the development of acute renal failure by renal vasodilation, flushing of renal tubules, and scavenging free radicals. The patient is systemically heparinized before clamping the arteries. Consideration should be given to perfusion with cold preservation solution if the renal ischemia time is expected to be more than 1 hour.

Autologous saphenous vein or synthetic grafts are used to create the aortorenal artery bypass. A Satinsky or Ochsner side-biting vascular clamp is applied to a suitably soft portion of the aorta. An arteriotomy is made with a #11 blade or an aortic punch. An end-to-side

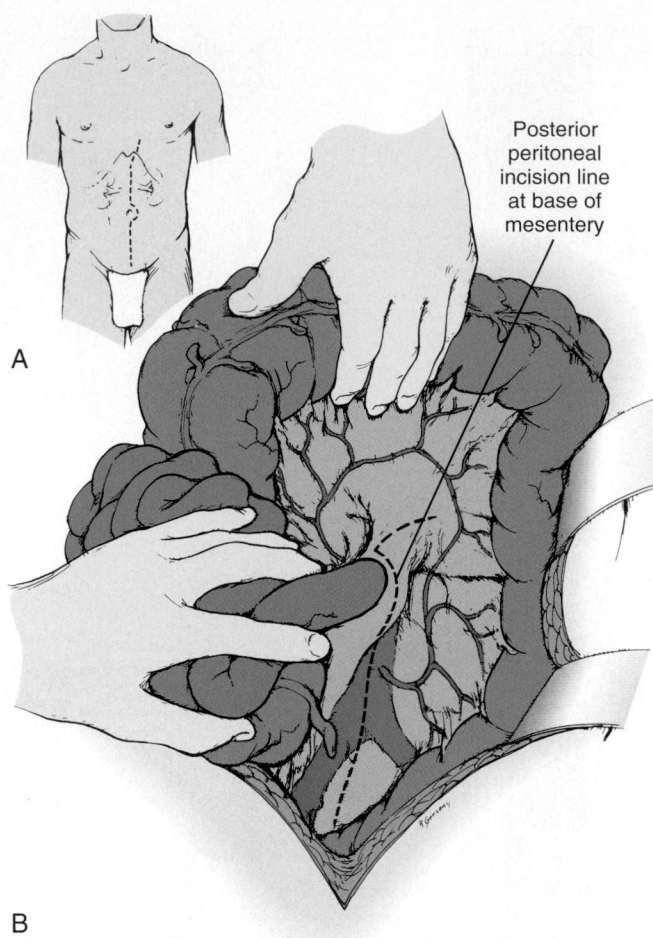

Posterior peritoneal incision line at base of mesentery

FIGURE 4 A, The midline laparotomy incision from xiphoid to pubis (*dotted line*). **B,** The retroperitoneum is opened to the left of the ligament of Treitz and carried inferiorly along the aorta (*dotted line*). *(Adapted from Benjamin ME, Dean RH. Techniques in renal artery reconstruction: part I. Ann Vasc Surg. 1996;10:306-314.)*

anastomosis is then fashioned using running 5-0 polypropylene sutures. The graft is measured to length after the renal artery has been transected distal to the stenosis; graft length is critical to ensure that there is no tension but the graft is not so long that a kink will be present. The proximal end of the renal artery is oversewn with running 4-0 polypropylene sutures. The distal end of the graft and the distal end of the renal artery are spatulated (Figure 5). An end-to-end anastomosis is then fashioned using 6-0 polypropylene sutures (Figure 6). After vascular clamps are removed, flow within the distal renal artery is interrogated with a handheld Doppler ultrasound. The retroperitoneum is closed and the abdominal incision is closed in layers.

Extra-Anatomic Renal Artery Bypass

When the aorta is heavily diseased by hard, atherosclerotic plaque and aortic bypass is not feasible, there are several options for extra-anatomic bypass. The splenic artery may be anastomosed to the left renal artery. To obtain access to the splenic artery, the retroperitoneal exposure described earlier is carried cephalad, and the pancreas is mobilized anteriorly to expose and mobilize the splenic artery. Intravenous unfractionated heparin is administered, and the splenic artery is controlled proximally and distally with DeBakey clamps and then ligated distally with #0 silk ties. The renal artery is then controlled proximally and distally with vascular clamps and transected distal to the stenosis. The proximal end of the renal artery is oversewn

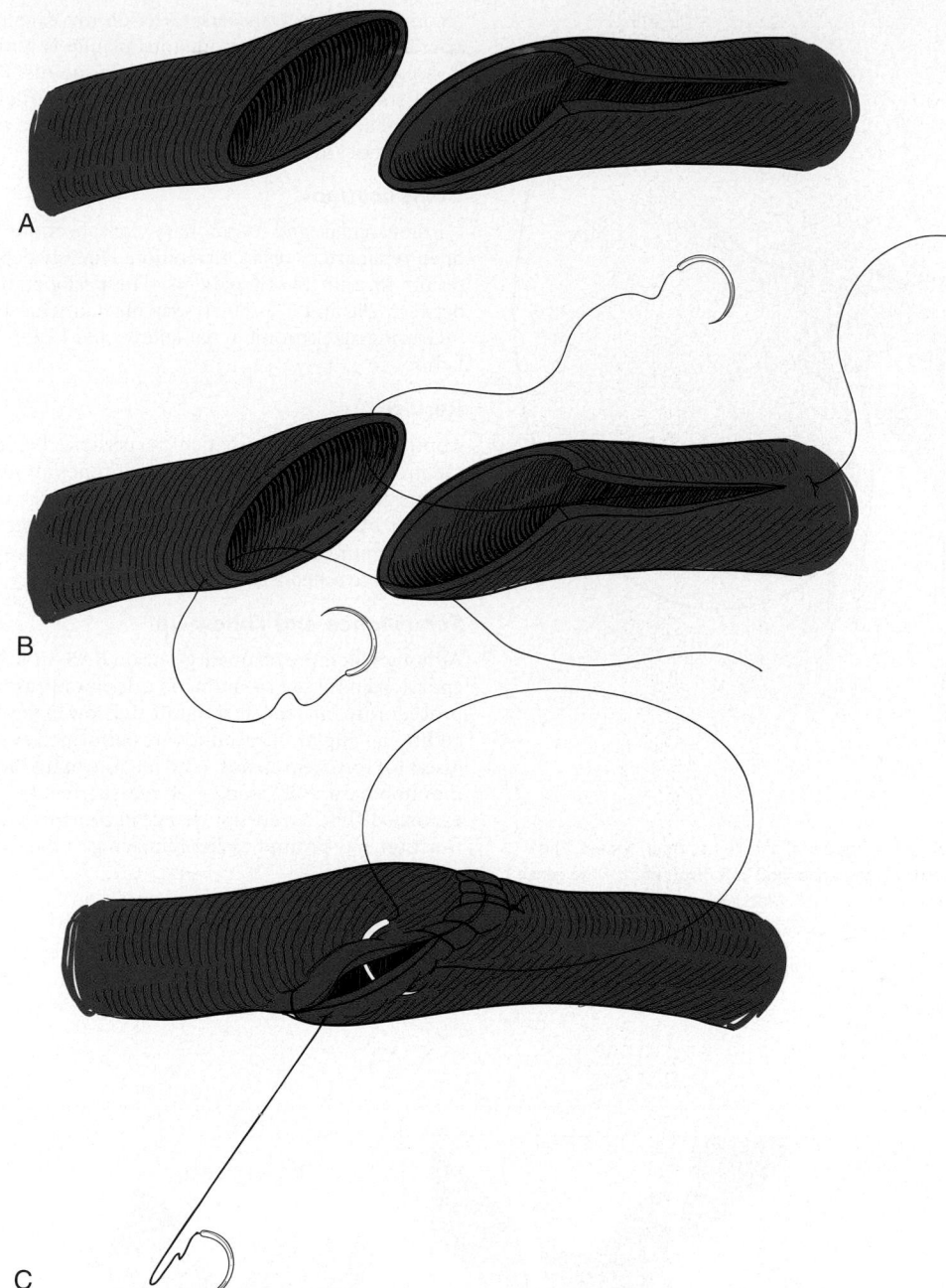

FIGURE 5 A, A longitudinal cut is made on the renal artery to lengthen the arteriotomy. **B,** Sutures are placed from the toe of the graft to the heel of the renal arteriotomy and from the heel of the graft to the toe of the renal arteriotomy. **C,** Running sutures complete the spatulated anastomosis. *(From Riles TS. General principles of vascular surgery. In: Chaikof EL, Cambria RP, eds. Atlas of Vascular Surgery and Endovascular Therapy. Philadelphia: Saunders; 2014:2-16.)*

with 4-0 polypropylene sutures. The proximal end of the splenic artery then may be sewn to the distal end of the left renal artery in spatulated fashion with running 6-0 polypropylene sutures. The spleen is left in situ if collateral circulation is intact.

The right renal artery may be bypassed similarly from the common hepatic artery. However, the common hepatic artery is left intact and a polytetrafluoroethylene (PTFE) or saphenous vein interposition graft will be needed to bridge the distance with an end-to-side proximal anastomosis and an end-to-end distal anastomosis to the right renal artery (Figure 7).

The left and right renal arteries also may be revascularized with PTFE or vein interposition grafts originating from the iliac arteries. Whenever a graft is used, graft length is critical to ensure that there is no tension but the graft is not so long that a kink will be present.

Aortorenal Endarterectomy

A midline incision is made and the retroperitoneum is opened overlying the infrarenal aorta, with exposure obtained as outlined previously. The left and right renal arteries are dissected free, and vascular loops are placed around each of the renal arteries. The aorta is circumferentially freed above and below the renal artery origins. Intravenous unfractionated heparin is administered. Vascular loops are used to control the renal arteries. Sidewinder or Satinsky clamps are placed on the infrarenal aorta. The suprarenal aorta is controlled with a Cherry clamp. Aortorenal endarterectomy can be

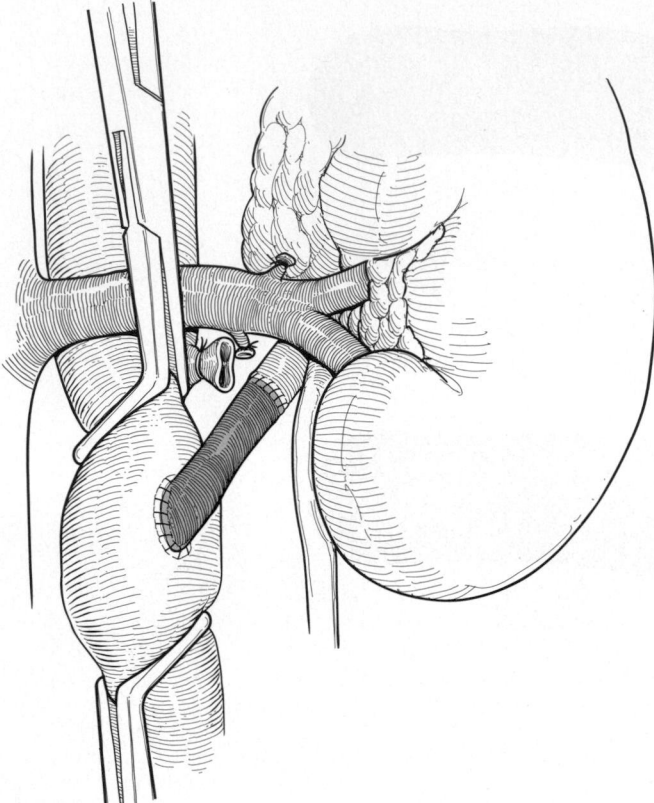

FIGURE 6 The proximal end of the renal artery has been ligated. The vein graft is interposed between the aorta and the distal end of the renal artery. *(Adapted from Benjamin ME, Dean RH. Techniques in renal artery reconstruction: part I. Ann Vasc Surg. 1996;10:306-314.)*

accomplished via transverse arteriotomy extending onto the renal arteries (Figure 8). Atheromatous plaque is removed carefully with a vascular freer to achieve tapered endpoints. Occasionally a small distal shelf will require placement of a 7-0 polypropylene tacking suture. The arteriotomy is closed with either a synthetic patch or bovine pericardium.

Complications

Cardiovascular and pulmonary complications are common after open renal artery revascularization. Dialysis-dependent renal failure occurs in only 1% of patients. The perioperative mortality rate is between 2% and 6%. Thirty-day mortality has been associated with increasing age, chronic renal failure, and history of congestive heart failure.

Results

Approximately 85% of patients experience blood pressure improvement or cure postoperatively. Renal function improves or stabilizes in approximately 60% of patients who undergo open repair. As many as 70% of selected patients who recently started dialysis may no longer require dialysis after open renal artery revascularization. Early postoperative stenosis occurs in only 1% to 2% of patients.

Surveillance and Follow-up

Although there are no quality data on RAS surveillance after bypass or endarterectomy, we recommend a duplex ultrasound 30 days after the procedure to interrogate the graft and flow in the renal arteries. Several additional duplex ultrasounds are performed every 6 to 12 months to assess for recurrent stenosis and renal atrophy. Blood pressure must be monitored carefully along with measurement of serum creatinine or estimated GFR. An abrupt change in control of hypertension or renal function may prompt earlier reimaging of the renal vasculature.

■ SUMMARY

Atherosclerotic RAS may cause systemic hypertension or impaired renal function. The vast majority of patients with symptomatic RAS

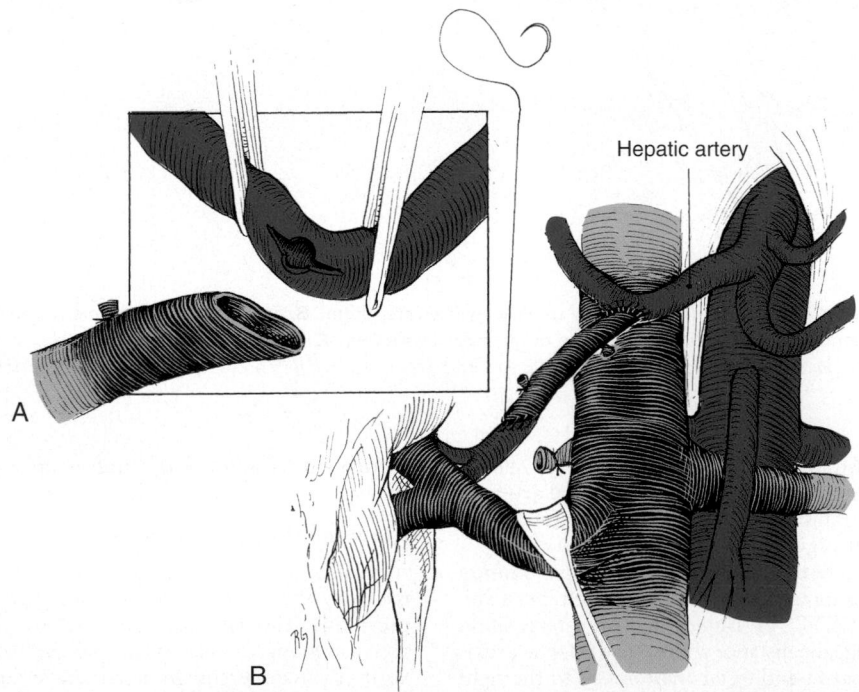

Hepatic artery

FIGURE 7 A longitudinal arteriotomy is made on the side of the common hepatic artery. **A,** The end of the interposition vein graft is fashioned to match the arteriotomy. **B,** The distal end of the vein graft is anastomosed in end-to-end spatulated fashion to the right renal artery. *(Adapted from Benjamin ME, Dean RH. Techniques in renal artery reconstruction: part I. Ann Vasc Surg. 1996;10:306-314.)*

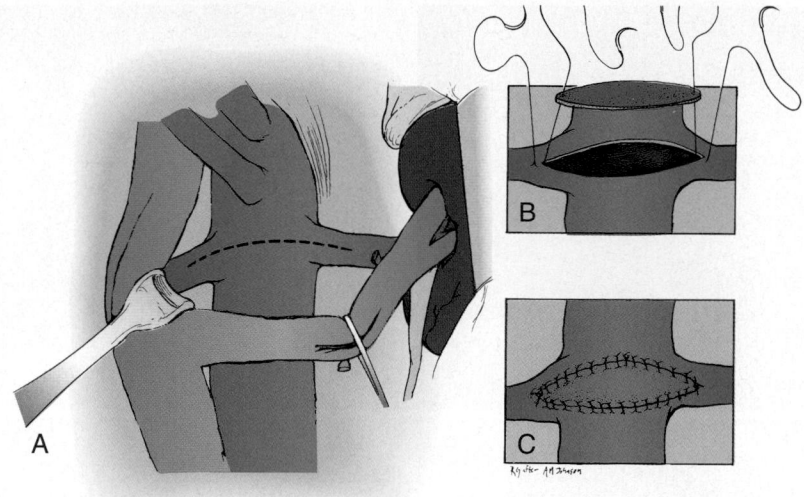

FIGURE 8 A, Exposure of the juxtarenal aorta and renal arteries is achieved. Vessel loops (not shown) are placed around each renal artery. **B,** A transverse aortotomy is made with extensions onto each renal artery to a point beyond the stenoses. **C,** After completion of the endarterectomy, the arteriotomy is closed with a prosthetic or bovine pericardial patch angioplasty. *(From Benjamin ME, et al. Techniques in renal artery reconstruction: part I. Ann Vasc Surg. 1996;10:306-314.)*

are managed successfully by careful control of hypertension and risk factors associated with the progression of arteriosclerosis. Revascularization is recommended for RAS patients with renovascular hypertension that is not responsive to maximal medical therapy, those with worsening excretory renal function, and young individuals in whom flash pulmonary edema is caused by RAS. Revascularization by renal artery angioplasty and stenting has largely supplanted open renal artery surgery because of its minimally invasive nature, excellent early renal artery patency, and decreased periprocedural morbidity and mortality when compared with open surgery. Open renal artery bypass and endarterectomy currently are reserved for urgent salvage after technical endovascular failures and procedures in combination with elective aortic reconstructions that require an open approach.

SUGGESTED READINGS

Cooper CJ, Murphy TP, Cutlip DE, CORAL Investigators, et al. Stenting and medical therapy for atherosclerotic renal-artery stenosis. *N Engl J Med.* 2014;370:13-22.

Hirsch AT, Haskal ZJ, Hertzer NR, American Association for Vascular Surgery; Society for Vascular Surgery; Society for Cardiovascular Angiography and Interventions; Society for Vascular Medicine and Biology; Society of Interventional Radiology; ACC/AHA Task Force on Practice Guidelines; American Association of Cardiovascular and Pulmonary Rehabilitation; National Heart; Lung; and Blood Institute; Society for Vascular Nursing; TransAtlantic Inter-Society Consensus; Vascular Disease Foundation, et al. ACC/AHA 2005 guidelines for the management of patients with peripheral arterial disease (lower extremity, renal, mesenteric, and abdominal aortic): executive summary a collaborative report from the American Association for Vascular Surgery/Society for Vascular Surgery, Society for Cardiovascular Angiography and Interventions, Society for Vascular Medicine and Biology, Society of Interventional Radiology, and the ACC/AHA Task Force on Practice Guidelines (Writing Committee to Develop Guidelines for the Management of Patients With Peripheral Arterial Disease) endorsed by the American Association of Cardiovascular and Pulmonary Rehabilitation; National Heart, Lung, and Blood Institute; Society for Vascular Nursing; TransAtlantic Inter-Society Consensus; and Vascular Disease Foundation. *J Am Coll Cardiol.* 2006;47:1239-1312.

Mousa AY, AbuRahma AF, Bozzay J, Broce M, Bates M. Update on intervention versus medical therapy for atherosclerotic renal artery stenosis. *J Vasc Surg.* 2015;61:1613-1623.

RAYNAUD'S PHENOMENON

Joseph S. Giglia, MD

Raynaud's phenomenon (RP) is a condition characterized by episodic excessive vasoconstriction of small arteries of the digits and appendages after cold or emotional stimuli. Maurice Raynaud initially described the condition in his classic paper published in 1862.

RP characteristically involves progression from a period of pallor secondary to intense vasospasm, to cyanosis related to pooling of deoxygenated blood, to hyperemia due to vasorelaxation.

The nomenclature of this entity is confusing, misleading, and often wrong. The terminology has changed over time. Raynaud's syndrome, Raynaud's disease, Raynaud's phenomenon, primary Raynaud's, and secondary Raynaud's have all been used.

In 1992 LeRoy and Medsger addressed the issue and proposed the following solution: primary RP refers to the characteristic findings without evidence of an underlying medical or surgical condition. Secondary RP describes the characteristic findings related to an underlying medical or surgical condition. This chapter follows the language suggested by LeRoy and Medsger and emphasizes secondary RP related to surgical conditions.

▇ PRIMARY RAYNAUD'S PHENOMENON

RP is seen worldwide, with the incidence higher in colder climates. The median age at onset of primary RP is 14 years, and only 27% of cases begin at the age of 40 or later. Symmetric events involving both hands are common. Gangrene or tissue necrosis is never associated with primary RP. Diagnostic tests, including nail fold capillary examination (discussed later), erythrocyte sedimentation rate, and serologic markers, are normal (Figure 1; Table 1).

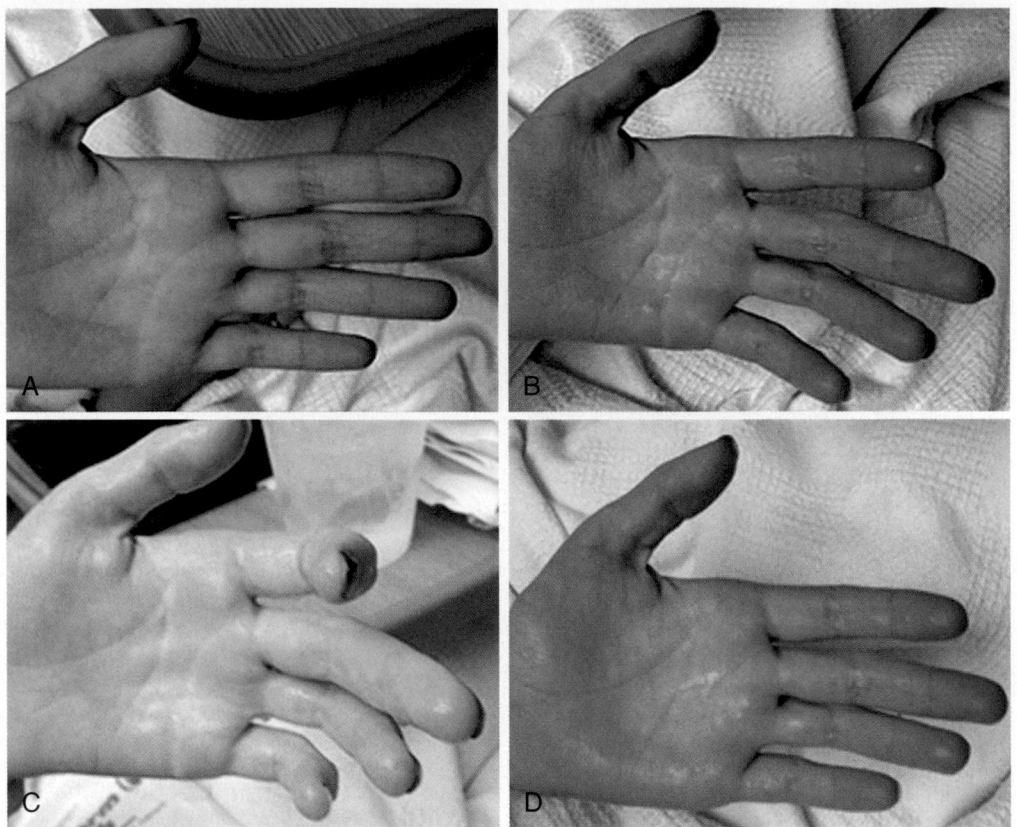

FIGURE 1 Raynaud's phenomenon in a patient with Ehlers-Danlos syndrome to illustrate the color changes associated with stressful stimuli. **A,** Normal-appearing hand. **B,** After cold stimuli, the pallor from vasoconstriction can be seen. **C,** After 30 seconds, the hyperemic red appears in fingers with blood reperfusion. **D,** Hand after 3 minutes exposed to stimuli.

TABLE 1: Characteristics of Primary and Secondary Raynaud's Phenomenon

	Primary	Secondary
Age	Younger (<30 years)	Older (>30 years)
Gender preference	Female	Male (depending on secondary cause)
Incidence	Most common	Less common
Familial predisposition	Yes	Yes
Combination with other disease	No, idiopathic	Associated with systemic disease
Vascular defect	Functional dysregulation of autonomic nervous system	Structural changes in connective tissue or vessels
Associated signs	None	Arthritis, sclerodactyly, cardiopulmonary abnormality, rash
Frequency	Precipitated by stimuli	Periodic and stimuli trigger
Severity of symptoms	Long history of mild attacks	Severe and disabling pain
Distribution	Symmetric	Asymmetric
Duration	Self-limited	Need for additional treatment (pharmacologic, surgery)
Critical complications	None	Ischemia and ulcers
Capillaroscopy	Normal (symmetric, thin, and uniform)	Abnormal (dilated, irregular, elongated, and tortuous vessel)
Vascular examination	Normal pulses	Abnormal pulses
Erythrocyte sedimentation rate	Normal	Elevated
Serologic studies	Negative	Antinuclear antibody, autoantibodies
C-reactive protein	Normal	Elevated

■ SECONDARY RAYNAUD'S PHENOMENON

Secondary RP more commonly is seen after the age of 30. Unlike primary RP, it is associated with severe attacks that may be isolated to one extremity. Gangrene and ischemic ulceration are possible. Common systemic diseases associated with secondary RP include certain rheumatologic, autoimmune, endocrine, and hematologic disorders. Secondary RP also can be associated with vascular conditions, including atherosclerosis, arterial thoracic outlet syndrome, and thromboembolic events. Patients with signs and symptoms isolated to a single digit and those with abnormal pulse examinations should undergo an evaluation for arterial disease (Box 1).

■ PATHOGENESIS

The pathogenesis of RP is not completely defined. The underlying abnormality is an imbalance between the normal vasodilation and vasoconstriction of the digital arteries. Decreased production of endothelial nitric oxide and prostacyclin has been implicated in impaired vasodilation. Alteration in the metabolism of endothelin-1 and angiotensin II has been associated with abnormal vasoconstriction. Chronic inflammation can lead to structural changes, including intimal fibrosis. Abnormally increased sympathetic tone can contribute to the condition. In addition, an imbalance between coagulation and fibrinolysis has been observed in both primary and secondary RP.

■ DIAGNOSIS

It is critical to differentiate between primary and secondary RP to correctly manage and treat patients, as management is significantly different for the two conditions. A correct diagnosis is especially important for surgeons, since a subset of patients with secondary RP require surgical intervention.

A detailed clinical history with special emphasis on the location, severity, and frequency of symptoms is required. Seasonal variation and association with the stressful situation are important to elicit. The physical examination should include bilateral brachial blood pressure measurements and a thorough pulse examination.

Nail bed video capillography is a simple, noninvasive test that is highly sensitive and specific for patients with RP. With practice, a patient's cutaneous capillaries can be examined at the bedside with just a drop of grade B immersion oil and a handheld ophthalmoscope.

The first diagnostic test chosen is usually a noninvasive upper arterial study (Figure 2). The study should include evaluation of both upper extremities with segmental pressures, Doppler waveforms, and wrist-brachial ratios.

Plain radiographs are of limited utility, but they may demonstrate heterotopic calcification, cervical ribs, or excessive vascular calcification. Computerized axial tomography with three-dimensional reconstruction is helpful to screen for arterial disease. Invasive catheter digital subtraction angiography is reserved for those cases where noninvasive testing has suggested the presence of disease.

BOX 1: Secondary Causes of Raynaud's Phenomenon

Rheumatologic

Systemic sclerosis (CREST syndrome)
Sjögren's syndrome
Systemic lupus erythematosus
Ehlers-Danlos syndrome
Rheumatoid arthritis
Dermatomyositis
Polymyositis
Mixed connective tissue disease

Autoimmune

Reiter's syndrome
Vasculitis (polyarteritis nodosa, Henoch-Schönlein purpura)
Antiphospholipid syndrome
Primary pulmonary hypertension

Endocrine

Hypothyroidism
Pheochromocytoma
Carcinoid

Infectious

Hepatitis B and C infection
Mycoplasma pneumonia

Medications

Cyclosporine
Ergotamine
Beta-blockers
Cytotoxic (bleomycin, cisplatin, vinblastine)
Bromocriptine
Nicotine
Cocaine
Sulfasalazine
Interferon-alpha and interferon-beta

Clonidine
Sympathomimetics
Estrogen in oral contraceptives
Caffeine

Occlusive Vascular

Arteriosclerosis
Vascular trauma (hypothenar hammer syndrome)
Buerger's disease
Thoracic outlet syndrome
Thromboembolism

Hematologic Proliferative

Leukemia
Lymphoma
Polycythemia vera
Multiple myeloma
Disseminated intravascular coagulation
Cryoglobulinemia
Cold agglutinin disease

Neurologic

Migraines
Carpal tunnel syndrome
Polyneuropathy

Environmental

Emotional stress
Frostbite
Repetitive trauma or injuries to hand

Malignancy

Lung, stomach, small bowel
Paraneoplastic syndrome
Neurofibromatosis

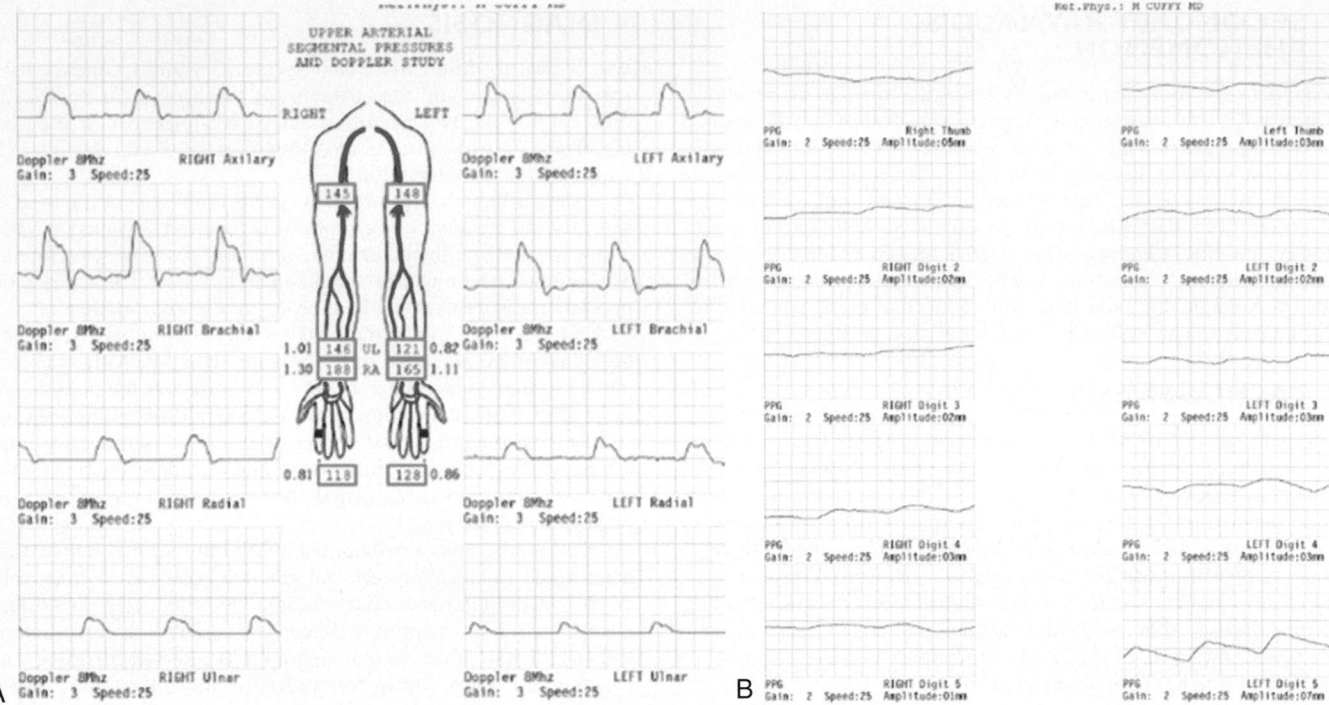

FIGURE 2 **A** and **B,** An example of an abnormal upper extremity noninvasive arterial study. Note the blunted waveforms proximally and the flat digital tracings.

Angiography has the added benefit of being therapeutic if an appropriate lesion is detected.

Serologic tests are appropriate when secondary RP is suspected unless an anatomic vascular condition is present. This is especially true when systemic symptoms such as myalgias, arthralgias, fever, weakness, and rash are present. A complete blood count, routine blood chemistry panel, antinuclear antibodies test, rheumatoid factor, and complement levels should be drawn (see Box 1).

■ MANAGEMENT

Primary RP patients can be reassured that their symptoms most likely will not progress to tissue loss and gangrene. In a cohort of patients who met the criteria for primary RP and were followed for 2 years, only 12.6% were diagnosed with a secondary disorder. Secondary RP requires further investigation and treatment of any underlying arterial pathology or any systemic disease.

Nonpharmacologic

Avoidance of triggers is the first-line treatment of primary RP. Cold exposure should be limited to brief periods, and the use of mittens should be encouraged. Caffeine and cigarette smoking should be avoided. The severity and frequency of symptoms determines how drastic the lifestyle modification should be.

Pharmacologic

The first-line pharmacologic treatment of RP is a long-acting calcium-channel blocker. Typically, sustained-release nifedipine is initiated at a dose of 30 mg/day. Dose escalation to 120 mg/day may be attempted. Phosphodiesterase inhibitors (e.g., sildenafil, tadalafil) may be tried if calcium-channel blockers are ineffective.

There are multiple second-line agents for the treatment of RP, including prazosin, losartan, and prostaglandins. These drugs are reserved for recalcitrant cases and usually are utilized by subspecialists in the field.

Surgical Treatment

Surgical treatment for secondary RP is almost only necessary when it is associated with occlusive vascular conditions (Box 1). Local wound care is initiated, with limited débridement of most necrotic tissue and dressing changes. Limited digital amputation may be required with the treatment goal of alleviating pain and preserving function.

Cervical or lumbar sympathectomy (chemical or surgical) can provide temporary relief of pain and ulcer healing, but long-term results are variable. A thoracoscopic approach mostly has replaced an open procedure for cervical sympathectomy.

Atherosclerosis and Atheroembolic Renal Disease

Atherosclerosis can mimic RP. Unilateral symptoms and the usual lack of association with cold exposure can be helpful in making the the distinction. Patients with systemic atherosclerosis will have risk factors such as an extensive smoking history or end-stage renal disease (Figure 2).

Compression-Related Conditions

Arterial thoracic outlet syndrome can be seen as secondary RP. Repetitive trauma to the subclavian artery at the thoracic outlet can lead to a stenosis or a lesion prone to embolize (Figures 3 to 7).

Neurocompression syndrome, such as cervical spine disease or carpal tunnel syndrome, can lead to secondary RP. Localized tenderness and history of trauma can be helpful in making the correct diagnosis.

■ KEY POINTS

Primary Raynaud's Phenomenon

Usually benign
Rarely involves the thumb
Rarely leads to gangrene

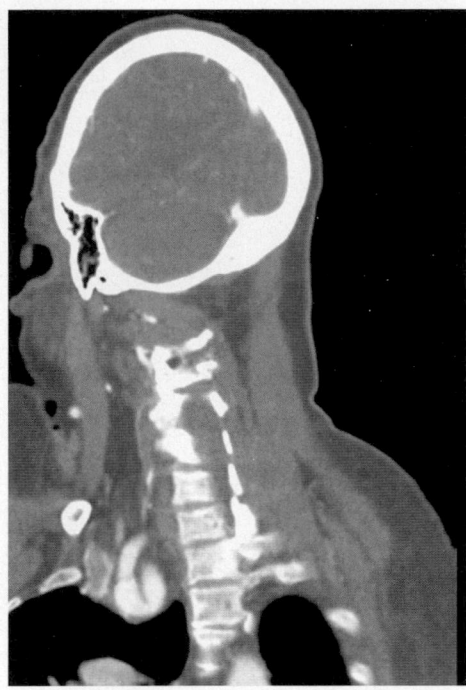

FIGURE 3 Computed tomography scan (sagittal view of the upper chest and neck) of a patient with secondary Raynaud's phenomenon related to arterial kink. Note the proximal right subclavian artery.

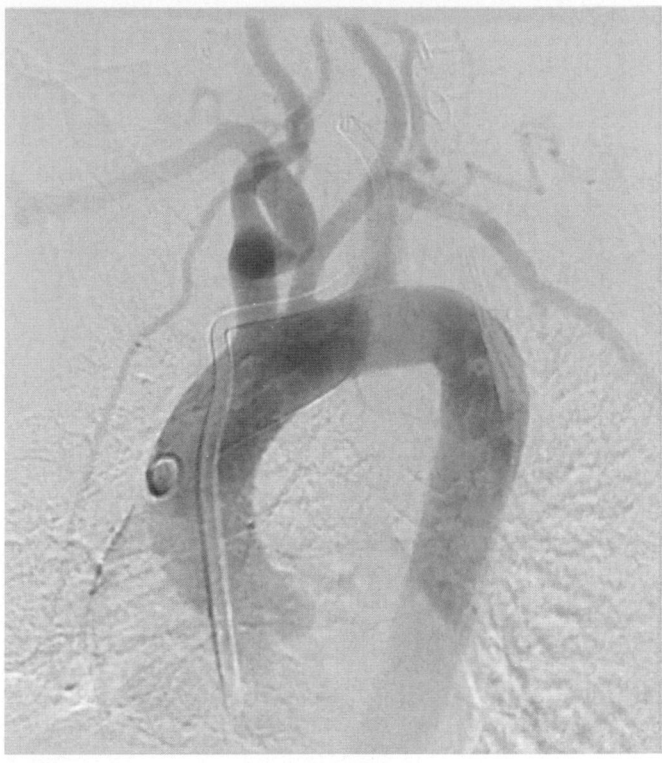

FIGURE 4 Arch aortogram image of a patient with secondary Raynaud's phenomenon related to kink of the proximal right subclavian artery.

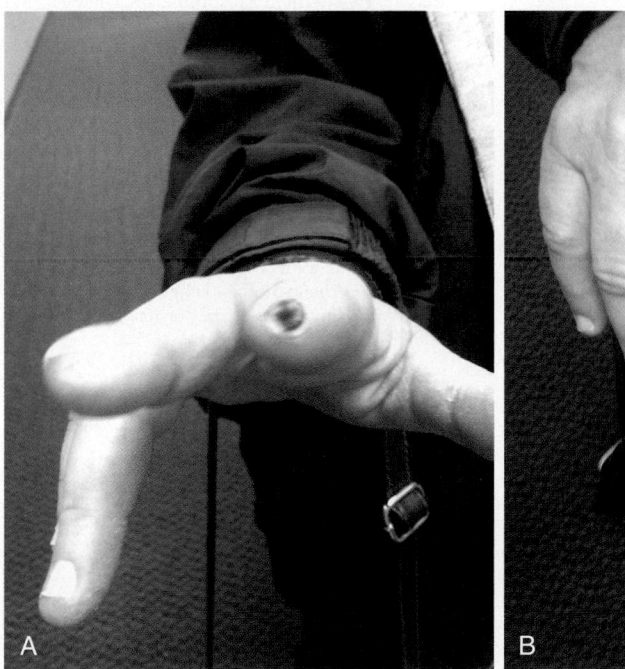

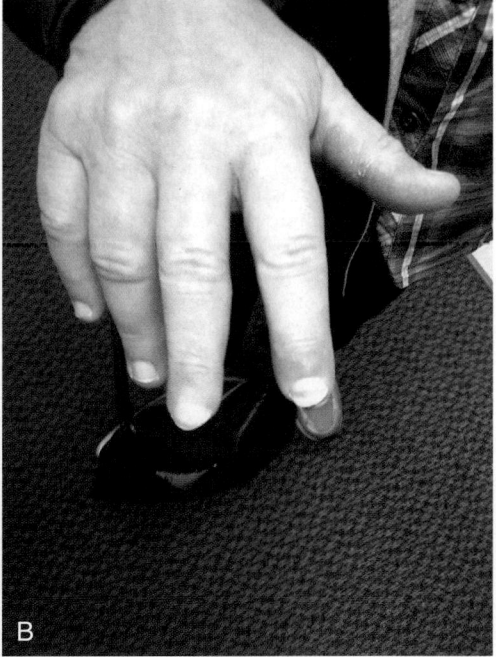

FIGURE 5 A and **B,** Images of digits in a patient with secondary Raynaud's phenomenon related to arterial thoracic outlet syndrome.

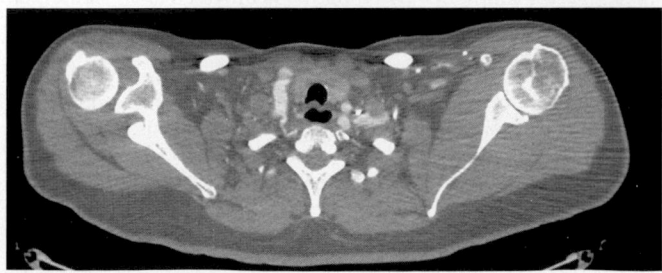

FIGURE 6 Preoperative computed tomography scan of a patient with secondary Raynaud's phenomenon with bilateral arterial thoracic outlet syndrome.

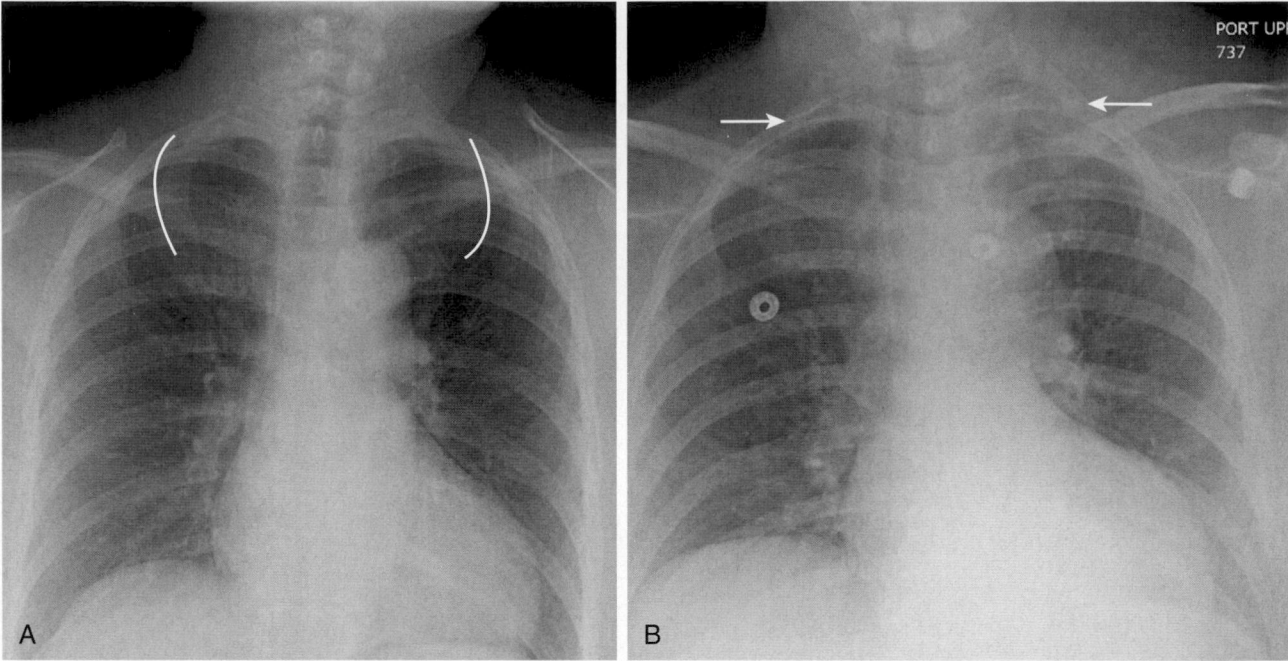

FIGURE 7 Preoperative (**A**) and postoperative (**B**) chest radiographs of a patient with secondary Raynaud's phenomenon related to arterial thoracic outlet syndrome. Curved lines outline the first rib. Arrows indicate the edges of the transected first ribs.

Secondary Raynaud's Phenomenon

Usually more severe
May be associated with gangrene
Systemic disease
Anatomic problem

■ SUMMARY

RP is a condition characterized by periodic vasoconstriction of digital arteries. Primary RP is associated with environmental and emotional triggers but not systemic disease. Secondary RP is associated with systemic disease or an anatomic abnormality. Making the correct diagnosis is critical for the surgeon confronted with a patient with RP, as secondary RP requires specific treatment of the underlying condition and primary RP usually requires only supportive care and reassurance. Several of the causes of secondary RP are surgical diseases (e.g., thoracic outlet, atherosclerotic disease) that can be addressed and corrected.

SUGGESTED READINGS

Chikura B, Moore T, Manning J, Vail A, Herrick AL. Thumb involvement in Raynaud's phenomenon as an indicator of underlying connective tissue disease. *J Rheumatol.* 2010;37:783-786.

LeRoy EC, Medsger TA Jr. Raynaud's phenomenon: a proposal for classification. *Clin Exp Rheumatol.* 1992;10:485-488.

Maverakis E, Patel F, Kronenberg D, Chung L, Fiorentino D, Allanore Y, Guiducci S, Hesselstrand R, Hummers L, Duong C, Kahaleh B, Macgregor A, Matucci-Cerinic M, Wollheim F, Mayes M, Gershwin ME. International consensus criteria for the diagnosis of Raynaud's phenomenon. *J Autoimmun.* 2014;48-49:60-65.

Planchon B, Pistorius MA, Beurrier P, De Faucal P. Primary Raynaud's phenomenon: age of onset and pathogenesis in a prospective study of 424 patients. *Angiology.* 1994;45:677-686.

Ratchford EV, Evans NS. Raynaud's phenomenon. *Vasc Med.* 2015;20:269-271.

Raynaud M. *De l'asphyxie locale et de la gangrene symetrique des extremites.* Thesis. L Leclerc, libraire-éditeur. Paris; 1862.

Thompson AE, Pope JE. Calcium channel blockers for primary Raynaud's phenomenon: a meta-analysis. *Rheumatology (Oxford).* 2005;44:145-150. doi:10.1093/rheumatology/keh390.

Wigley FM. Clinical practice: Raynaud's phenomenon. *N Engl J Med.* 2002;347:1001-1008.

THORACIC OUTLET SYNDROME

Caitlin W. Hicks, MD, MS, and Ying Wei Lum, MD

Thoracic outlet syndrome (TOS) describes a constellation of symptoms that arise from compression of the neurovascular bundle located in the thoracic outlet, which is a confined space located posterior to the clavicle and superior to the first rib (Figure 1). TOS is estimated to affect 80 in 1000 patients overall but in reality comprises three separate conditions based on the neurovascular structure that is involved. Neurogenic TOS (NTOS), which accounts for approximately 95% of all TOS cases, involves compression of the brachial plexus. Venous TOS (VTOS) accounts for approximately 4% of all TOS cases and involves compression of the subclavian vein, which can lead to acute or chronic subclavian vein thrombosis. Arterial TOS (ATOS) is the rarest form of TOS, accounting for only about 1% of all cases. ATOS is a condition in which there is arterial occlusion or embolization (usually with aneurysmal degeneration) resulting from

TABLE I: Preliminary Criteria for the Clinical Diagnosis of Neurogenic Thoracic Outlet Syndrome

Unilateral or bilateral upper extremity symptoms that:
(1) Extend beyond the distribution of a single cervical nerve root or peripheral nerve
(2) Have been present for at least 12 weeks
(3) Have not been explained satisfactorily by another condition
(4) Meet at least one criterion in at least four of the following five categories:

1. Principal symptoms	1A. Pain in the neck, upper back, shoulder, arm, or hand
	1B. Numbness; paresthesias; or weakness in the arm, hand, or digits
2. Symptom characteristics	2A. Pain, paresthesias, or weakness exacerbated with elevated arm positions
	2B. Pain, paresthesias, or weakness exacerbated by prolonged or repetitive arm or hand use or by prolonged work on a keyboard or other repetitive strain
	2C. Pain or paresthesias radiate down the arm from the supraclavicular or infraclavicular space
3. Clinical history	3A. Symptoms began after occupational, recreational, or accidental injury of the head, neck, or upper extremity, including repetitive upper extremity strain or overuse activity
	3B. Previous clavicle or first rib fracture or known cervical rib(s)
	3C. Previous cervical spine or peripheral nerve surgery without sustained improvement
	3D. Previous conservative or surgical treatment for thoracic outlet syndrome
4. Physical examination	4A. Local tenderness on palpation over scalene triangle or subcoracoid space
	4B. Arm, hand, or digit paresthesias on palpation over scalene triangle or subcoracoid space
	4C. Weak handgrip, intrinsic muscles, or digit 5 or thenar or hypothenar atrophy
5. Provocative maneuvers	5A. Positive upper limb tension test (ULTT)
	5B. Positive 1- or 3-min elevated arm stress test (EAST)

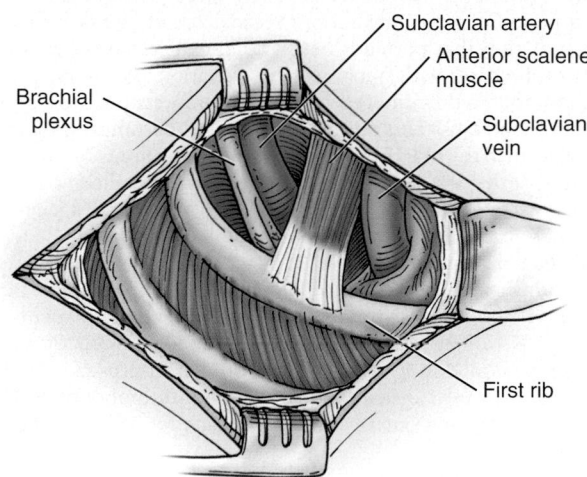

FIGURE I Anatomy of the thoracic outlet. *(Adapted from Propper BW, Freischlag JA. Thoracic outlet syndrome. In: Cameron JL, Cameron AM, eds. Current Surgical Therapy. 11th ed. Philadelphia: Elsevier Saunders; 2013:924-927.)*

compression of the subclavian artery or an ancillary artery within the thoracic outlet space. The diagnosis of each of the different forms of TOS is important because the workup and management of NTOS, VTOS, and ATOS vary greatly.

■ DIAGNOSIS AND TREATMENT

Neurogenic Thoracic Outlet Syndrome

NTOS involves compression of the brachial plexus leading to upper extremity pain, paresthesias, dysesthesia, numbness, and weakness classically in an ulnar distribution but frequently in a nonspecific peripheral nerve distribution as well. Raising the arms overhead, classically reported as weakness when patients try to brush or wash their hair, tends to aggravate symptoms. NTOS occurs most commonly in women, with a female-to-male ratio of 9:1. Presenting complaints, including back pain, neck pain, and shoulder pain, tend to be varied and often can be difficult to distinguish from alternative pathologies. Symptom onset can be temporally related to a traumatic event (e.g., motor vehicle accident) or to repetitive upper extremity activities (e.g., throwing a baseball).

The Consortium for Outcomes Research and Education on Thoracic Outlet Syndrome (CORE-TOS) recently developed a preliminary set of diagnostic criteria for NTOS, which are summarized in Table 1. In brief, patients must have unilateral or bilateral extremity symptoms lasting longer than 12 weeks that cannot be explained by an alternative diagnosis and are associated with a set of established symptom characteristics, clinical history, physical examination findings, and positive upper limb tension test (ULTT)* or elevated arm stress test (EAST).†

Although NTOS is primarily a clinical diagnosis of exclusion, electromyography (EMG) and imaging studies can be helpful in some cases. EMG can be used to exclude other entrapment syndromes. A chest x-ray should be obtained in all patients to determine the presence of a cervical rib (Figure 2), which should raise suspicion for TOS. Imaging studies such as chest computed tomography (CT) or shoulder magnetic resonance imaging (MRI) can be useful in distinguishing NTOS from cervical or muscular pathologies. Recently, magnetic resonance neurography has been shown to be potentially valuable for identifying the source of nerve compression in patients with NTOS, although this is not commonly used at most centers as part of a standard patient workup.

---

*ULTT (upper limb tension test). A series of provocative maneuvers designed to create tension on components of the brachial plexus in an effort to reproduce a patient's symptoms.

†EAST (elevated arm stress test). A provocative test in which the hands are repetitively clenched and unclenched while the patient is standing with the elbows flexed and the shoulders abducted to 90 degrees. The test is positive if the exercise produces symptoms of pain, paresthesias, weakness, or fatigue (1-minute test), or the patient cannot continue the exercise because of symptoms (3-minute test).

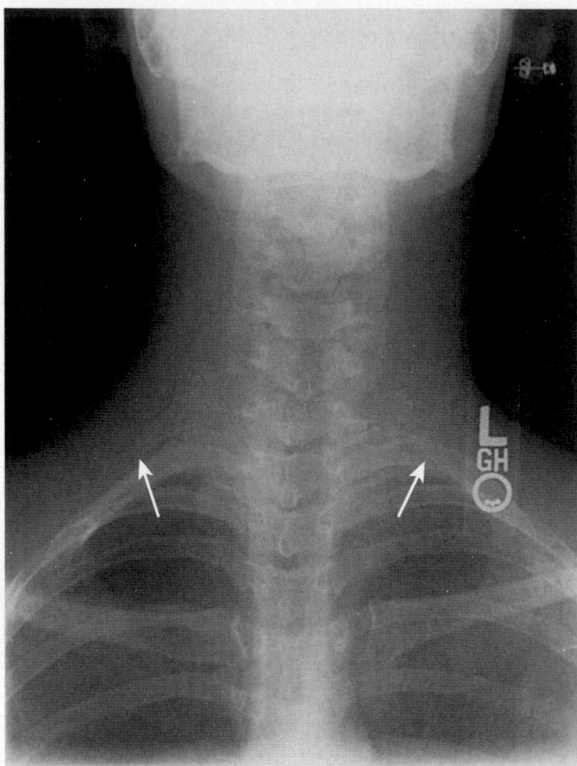

FIGURE 2 Appearance of a cervical rib on chest x-ray. Arrows denote the presence of bilateral cervical ribs. *(Adapted from Kirkwood ML, Valentine RJ. Thoracic outlet syndrome. In: Cronenwett JL, Johnston KW, eds. Rutherford's Vascular Surgery. 8th ed. Philadelphia: Elsevier Saunders; 2014:1969-1976.e1.)*

Perhaps the most useful test among patients with possible NTOS is the scalene muscle block, which can be both diagnostic and therapeutic. Recent data show that patients who experience symptom relief with a scalene block (with local anesthetic) are more likely to experience pain relief after surgery for TOS, and thus this test can be useful in determining which patients may be appropriate surgical candidates. In addition, patients also can undergo a trial of a scalene injection with botulinum toxin (Botox) for longer relief. Other treatment options for NTOS include physical and occupational therapy, workplace modifications, activity restrictions, and weight loss. Adjuvant medical treatment with muscle relaxants or anti-inflammatory and analgesic agents also is considered a standard of care. In the majority of cases, conservative management is appropriate for a trial of at least 6 to 8 weeks before more aggressive modalities such as surgery are considered.

Venous Thoracic Outlet Syndrome

VTOS involves compression of the subclavian vein and is the second most common form of TOS. Because the compartment of the costoclavicular space through which the subclavian vein runs is tight even in normal patients, any trigger involving expansion of one of the surrounding structures, such as muscular hypertrophy or scar formation as a result of repetitive trauma, can create an environment that is prone to venous inflammation, scarring, stenosis, and thrombosis (also known as Paget-Schroetter syndrome). Patients presenting with acute VTOS usually have swelling and congestion consistent with acute subclavian deep venous thrombosis. Patients may describe their symptoms as a feeling of heaviness, pressure, or fatigue. Paresthesias may be present, but pain is uncommon. Patients with a more chronic presentation may describe symptoms of venous hypertension that are usually worse after exercise. Patients with intermittent

positional (nonthrombotic) VTOS (McCleery's syndrome) usually complain of these symptoms during activity, with resolution afterward, when the affected arm is left to relax in an adducted position.

Unlike with NTOS, the diagnosis of VTOS is usually fairly straightforward. Patients are usually young, athletic males who engage in activities that involve repetitive overhead upper arm motions (e.g., pitching, swimming) that lead to subclavius and scalene muscle hypertrophy. Physical examination usually demonstrates well-developed upper body musculature and an unusual prominence of superficial veins in the upper arm; among patients with thrombosis, swelling, plethora, and engorgement of the affected arm and its collateral vessels are noted.

Despite the accuracy of clinical presentation for diagnosing VTOS, diagnostic imaging nearly always is obtained, preferentially in the form of duplex ultrasonography. A chest x-ray should be obtained to assess for the presence of a cervical rib, and a hypercoagulability workup can be considered to rule out the presence of a prothrombotic disorder (especially in cases with a strong family history of thrombosis), which occurs in approximately 8% of VTOS patients.

Treatment of VTOS involves initiation of anticoagulation and surgery with or without thrombolysis, depending on the situation. For patients with acute thrombosis, catheter-directed thrombolysis of the subclavian vein has been shown to be beneficial when performed within 2 weeks of the onset of symptoms. After this time, surgery is essential to release external compression and restore normal venous flow. The optimal timing for surgery in patients with acute thrombosis is controversial. Some surgeons argue that waiting for a period of time after venous recanalization allows for reduced inflammation that portends better healing. These physicians advocate for discharge with systemic anticoagulation after venous recanalization, followed by interval surgical decompression 1 to 3 months later. In contrast, others suggest that surgical decompression should be performed during the same hospital stay as venous recanalization because of the risk for recurrent thrombosis. Regardless, all patients with acute venous thrombosis should start taking therapeutic anticoagulation as soon as they are seen; the medication can be temporarily halted perioperatively.

Among patients with chronic subclavian vein thrombosis, preoperative thrombolysis is less effective. For these patients, our practice is to start systemic anticoagulation, followed by surgical decompression 2 to 4 weeks later. A similar approach is used for patients with intermittent obstructive (nonthrombotic) VTOS. A flowchart depicting our treatment approach for VTOS is shown in Figure 3.

Arterial Thoracic Outlet Syndrome

ATOS is the least common form of TOS. ATOS is frequently associated with a cervical or anomalous first rib. Similar to VTOS, patients prone to ATOS tend to be younger individuals who engage in activities involving repetitive upper extremity motion. This causes repetitive damage to the subclavian artery as it crosses over the cervical rib or anomalous first rib, leading to poststenotic subclavian artery dilatation and subsequent aneurysmal degeneration. Such arterial pathologies are prone to thrombus formation, putting these patients at high risk for acute thromboembolic events.

Although symptoms can be subtle, including hand fatigue with exercise, color changes, or temperature sensitivity, patients with ATOS more commonly are seen after acute embolic events. As a result, presenting symptoms typically are similar to the 6 Ps classically found in critical limb ischemia: pain, pallor, paresthesias, poikilothermia, pulselessness, and paralysis. Rarely, retrograde embolization causing a transient ischemic attack or posterior circulation stroke can occur. On physical examination, evidence of finger discoloration or ischemia may be present. There may be discrepant blood pressure measurements in addition to diminished

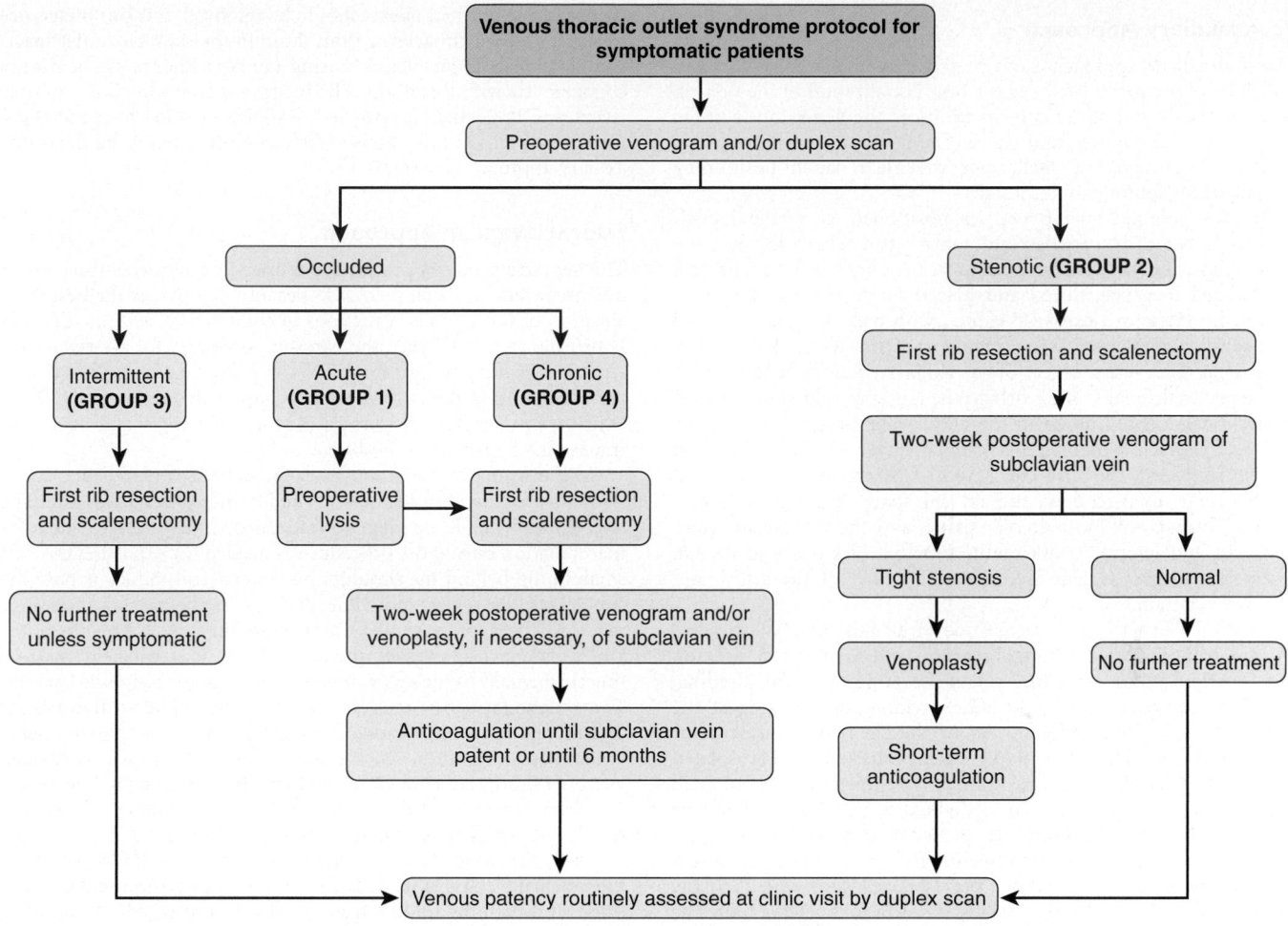

FIGURE 3 Flowchart depicting our treatment algorithm for venous thoracic outlet syndrome. The "occluded" branch (Groups 1, 3, 4) represents those with Paget-Schroetter syndrome. The "stenotic" branch (Group 2) represents those with McCleery's syndrome. *(Adapted from Moore R, Lum YW. Venous thoracic outlet syndrome. Vasc Med. 2015;20:182-189.)*

distal pulses. A subclavian artery bruit occasionally can be heard, and in patients with poststenotic aneurysms a pulsatile mass in the supraclavicular fossa may be palpated. Provocative maneuvers such as Adson's test can be performed but should not be used as the sole basis of diagnosis, as this test is neither sensitive nor specific for ATOS.*

A chest x-ray is indicated in all patients with ATOS to evaluate for a cervical rib. Dynamic duplex ultrasonography can show aneurysmal degeneration, poststenotic dilatation, mural thrombus, intimal flaps, and evidence of distal thromboembolism; in more subtle cases, it may demonstrate arterial flow changes with abduction and adduction of the arm. Ultimately, either computed tomographic angiography (CTA) or arteriogram is usually necessary to assess the extent and location of arterial disease, including the presence or absence of aneurysm and proximity of disease to the proximal subclavian artery. Either of these tests also can be performed dynamically (i.e., with the arm abducted and adducted) if needed to elicit arterial compression. A good understanding of the arterial anatomy is essential in order to allow for surgical planning, especially when surgical decompression with complex vascular reconstruction will be required.

Treatment of ATOS is almost always surgical. In cases where patients have minor degrees of acute upper extremity ischemia, catheter-directed thrombolysis can be attempted, followed by systemic anticoagulation and surgical decompression within the same hospital stay. However, more severe degrees of ischemia warrant urgent surgical embolectomy with or without upper extremity fasciotomy. Surgical decompression of the thoracic outlet should be performed concurrently to mitigate the risk of recurrent thromboembolic events. In many cases, vascular reconstruction with a native (great saphenous vein, femoral vein) or synthetic (ringed polytetrafluoroethylene [PTFE], polyester) conduit, or a distal bypass for chronic lesions, may be required.

■ SURGICAL APPROACHES

Surgical decompression of the thoracic outlet can be performed using a transaxillary, supraclavicular, or infraclavicular approach depending on patient anatomy and surgeon preference. Our preference, in general, is to use a transaxillary approach for NTOS and VTOS patients and a supraclavicular approach for ATOS patients. The infraclavicular approach is used when more distal exposure is needed for complex vascular reconstructions in ATOS cases.

---

*Adson's maneuver test: a provocative maneuver designed to reproduce symptoms of positional subclavian artery compression. Patients extend their neck and rotate their heads to the contralateral side while extending and externally rotating the affected arm. A positive Adson's sign occurs when the radial pulse of the affected arm is diminished or lost after deep inspiration.

Transaxillary Approach

The transaxillary approach is our preferred approach for NTOS and VTOS cases because it provides the best visualization of the first rib both anteriorly and posteriorly. In addition, the dissection required for the case is minimal, and the incision is cosmetically pleasing. However, because of the smaller operative field, patient positioning and adequate lighting are imperative.

In this approach the patient is positioned in a lateral position using a suction beanbag and axillary pad. The complete arm, axilla, and chest wall are prepped into the surgical field. The arm is wrapped in gauze, flexed and placed on top of padding in a Machleder retractor (Koros USA, Inc., Moorpark, CA), and secured with self-adherent elastic wrap (Figure 4). A transverse skin incision is made at the inferior aspect of the axillary space from the border of the pectoralis major anteriorly to the latissimus dorsi posteriorly. Dissection is carried down to the chest wall, taking care to avoid the long thoracic and intercostal brachial nerves. Once the chest wall is identified, the first and second ribs can be palpated, and a retractor is used to open the axillary space. Blunt dissection is used to free up any loose areolar tissue, and the subclavian artery and vein and inferior trunk of the brachial plexus are identified. Then the anterior scalene is dissected bluntly off the artery and vein with caution.

Next, the first rib is dissected free of all muscular attachments using a combination of blunt dissection and a periosteal elevator. This portion of the procedure can cause some muscular bleeding, which is best dealt with by periodic packing and lowering of the retractor. Once the inferior border of the rib is free, the anterior scalene muscle and then the middle scalene muscle should be isolated and divided sharply (Figure 5, A and B). At this point, the first rib should be mostly clear and can be divided using a bone cutter. The anterior side of the rib should be cut first, taking care not to injure the subclavian vein. Any remaining muscle attachments are removed, again by blunt dissection and a periosteal elevator, and then the posterior side of the rib is divided just anterior to the nerve root. The rib then can be removed from the field, and the remaining rib can be cut further posteriorly with the bone cutter or removed in pieces with a rongeur (Figure 5, C). Scalene muscle fibers interdigitating the

trunks of the brachial plexus should be removed. It is our preference to leave a 3/16-inch Jackson-Pratt drain in the thoracic outlet space. Any small tears in the pleura causing a pneumothorax can be treated concurrently with this drain. The incision is then closed in multiple layers, and the patient is returned to supine position for extubation. Cervical ribs also can be excised concurrently when using the transaxillary approach (Figure 6).

Supraclavicular Approach

The supraclavicular approach for thoracic outlet decompression is our preferred approach for ATOS because it provides the best visualization of the vascular structures in conjunction with the first rib. It also allows for the space and exposure necessary for arterial reconstruction, making it ideal for ATOS cases. Brachial neurolysis can be performed using the supraclavicular approach for cases of NTOS, which we prefer only in redo cases when scarring would make the transaxillary approach prohibitive.

In the supraclavicular approach the patient is placed in a semi-Fowler's position with the head turned to the contralateral side. The affected arm should be prepped into the operative field to allow for manipulation during the procedure as needed for exposure. Use of a small bump behind the shoulder blades can also to help expose the supraclavicular region more effectively. A transverse skin incision is made in the supraclavicular fossa approximately 2 fingerbreadths above the clavicle, extending from the lateral sternocleidomastoid muscle medially to the anterior edge of the trapezius muscle laterally. The scalene fat pad is retracted laterally after dividing the inferior and medial edges with cautery or ligature. After the phrenic nerve is identified (Figure 7, A), the anterior scalene muscle is divided sharply from its attachment to the first rib (exposing the underlying subclavian artery) and then at its origin on the transverse process of the cervical spine, removing it completely (Figure 7, B).

Next, the middle scalene muscle is exposed by gently retracting the brachial plexus forward. The long thoracic nerve should be identified, and then the middle scalene muscle is dissected on top of it, leaving the inferolateral portion of the muscle below intact in order to avoid nerve injury. This defines the lateral border of the muscle resection. The middle scalene muscle then is detached from the top of the first rib using a combination of sharp dissection, cautery, and a periosteal elevator (Figure 7, C).

Finally, the first rib is cleared from its attachments to the surrounding tissue using blunt dissection, taking care not to enter the pleural space. A right angle clamp is placed below the rib at the medial border, and the subclavian artery is elevated to expose the middle and anterior portions of the rib. A bone cutter is inserted as posteriorly as possible on the rib, taking care to avoid the brachial plexus (Figure 7, D). The rib is cut first posteriorly and then anteriorly and is removed from the field. Then a rongeur is used to remove any remaining posterior rib all the way to the level of the transverse process. The first rib cannot be removed completely anteriorly because the subclavian artery limits visualization of the costosternal junction in this approach but should be resected as far anteriorly as the artery will allow (usually about 1 cm).

Infraclavicular Approach

The infraclavicular approach for thoracic outlet decompression is reserved primarily for VTOS cases to allow for more medial resection of the first rib or as an extension for cases that require distal arterial reconstructions. It provides exposure of the central vasculature and can allow for open venous reconstruction for VTOS as well.

In the infraclavicular approach the patient should be positioned similar to the manner described earlier for the supraclavicular approach. A transverse incision is made 1 fingerbreadth below the clavicle, extending from the medial third of the clavicle to the deltopectoral groove laterally as necessary. The pectoralis major muscle is identified and spread using blunt dissection, exposing the

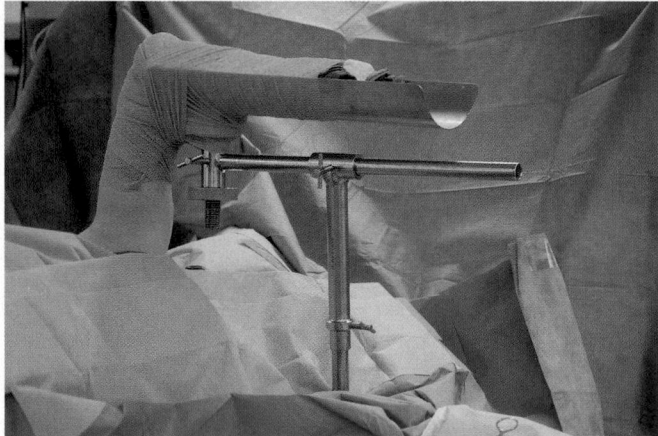

FIGURE 4 Patient positioning for a transaxillary approach for thoracic outlet decompression. The patient is placed in a lateral position using a suction beanbag and axillary pad. The complete arm, axilla, and chest wall are prepped into the surgical field. The arm is wrapped in gauze, flexed and placed on top of padding in a Machleder retractor, and secured with self-adherent elastic wrap. *(Adapted from Propper BW, Freischlag JA. Thoracic outlet syndrome. In: Cameron JL, Cameron AM, eds. Current Surgical Therapy. 11th ed. Philadelphia: Elsevier Saunders; 2013:924-927.)*

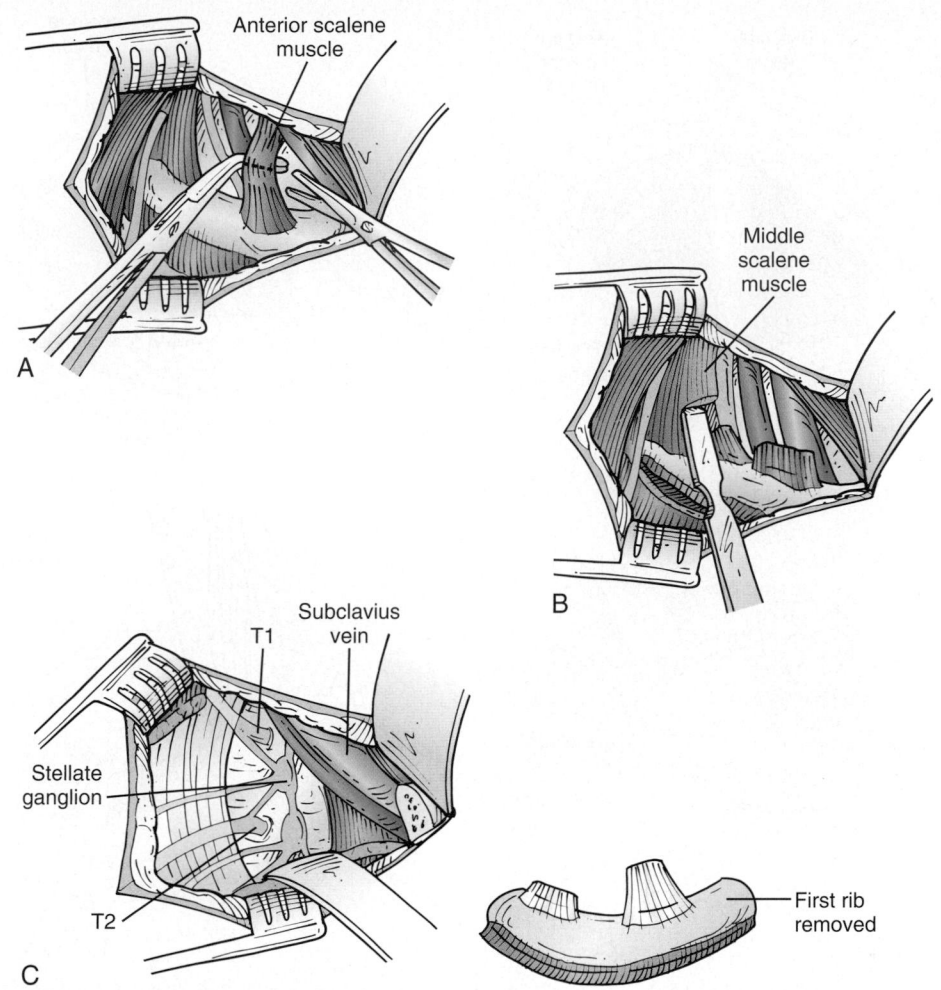

FIGURE 5 Transaxillary approach to thoracic outlet decompression. **A,** Once the inferior border of the rib is freed using a combination of blunt dissection and a periosteal elevator, the anterior scalene muscle should be isolated and divided sharply. **B,** Then the middle scalene muscle attachment is removed sharply. **C,** At this point, the first rib should be mostly clear and can be divided using a bone cutter. The posterior side of the rib should be divided just anterior to the nerve root, and any remaining rib can be cut further posteriorly or removed in pieces with a rongeur. *(Adapted from Lee JT. Thoracic outlet syndrome. In: Cronenwett JL, Johnston KW, eds.* Rutherford's Vascular Surgery. *8th ed. Philadelphia: Elsevier Saunders; 2014:1951-1968.e2.)*

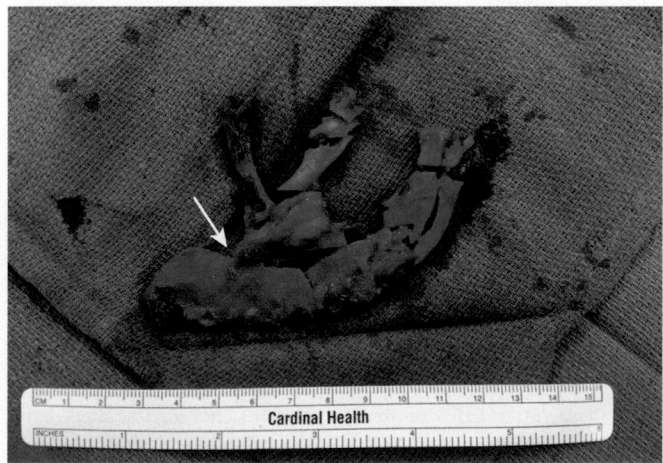

FIGURE 6 Cervical and first rib with corresponding attached anterior scalene muscle. A sizable portion of the first rib and cervical rib can be removed successfully via the transaxillary approach. The cervical rib frequently articulates with the first rib to form a large bony prominence (*arrow*).

clavipectoral fascia and pectoralis minor, which can be transected using electrocautery to expose the axillary sheath. This is opened sharply, and the axillary vein is retracted gently caudally to expose the axillary artery, which can be dissected for whatever length necessary to perform an appropriate vascular reconstruction. If distal axillary artery exposure is required, the incision can be extended onto the upper arm to the intersection of the deltoid muscle and biceps muscles. All three segments of the axillary artery can be exposed using the infraclavicular approach, making it ideal for cases that require complex vascular reconstruction.

SURGICAL OUTCOMES

Approximately 3000 surgeries for TOS are performed annually in the United States. The efficacy of surgical decompression varies from 64% to 95% depending on the type of TOS being treated and the length of time being reported.

For patients with NTOS, surgical success is as high as 93% immediately postoperatively but tends to decrease over time. At 10 years postoperatively, surgical success rates for NTOS are reported to be approximately 64% to 71%. Psychologic factors, chronicity, diffuse symptoms, and lack of response to anterior scalene muscle block are all predictive of surgical failure. One ongoing challenge

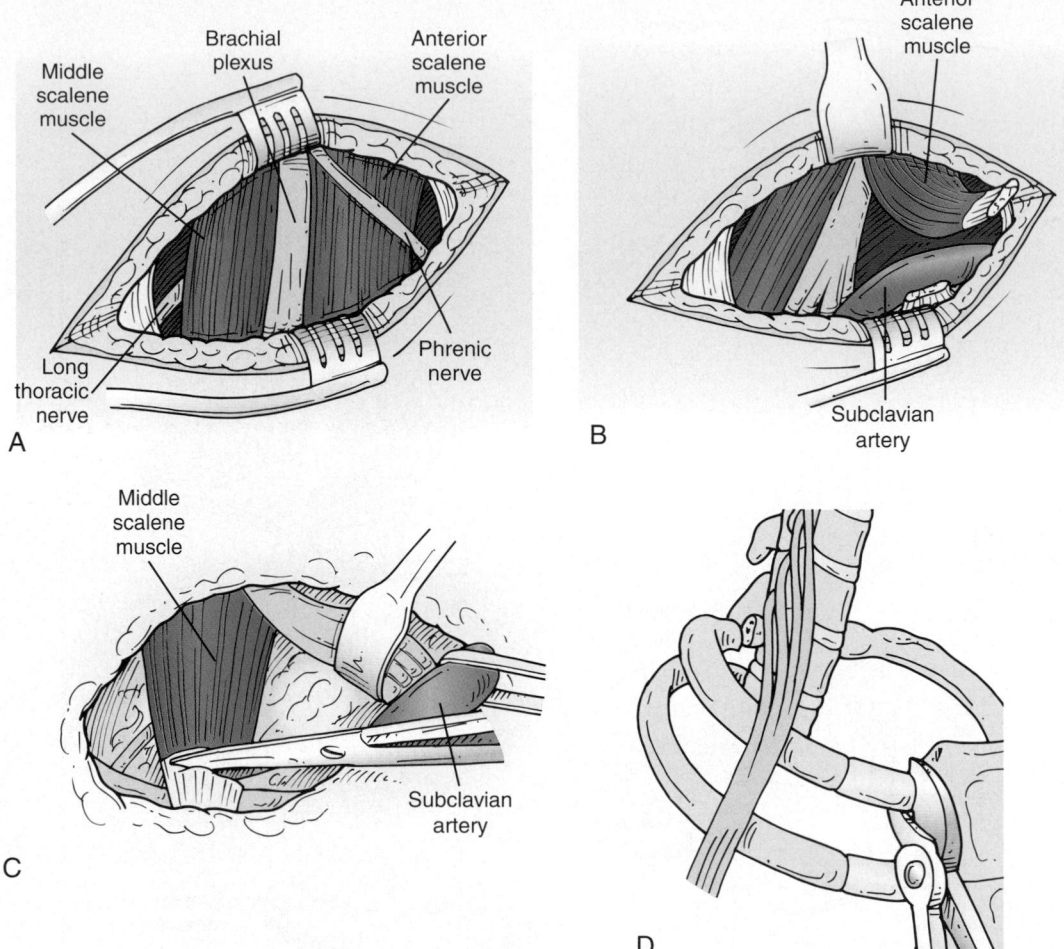

FIGURE 7 Supraclavicular approach to thoracic outlet decompression. **A,** After making an incision 2 fingerbreadths above the clavicle, the skin, subcutaneous tissue, and platysma are transected and the supraclavicular fat pad is reflected superiorly and laterally to expose the anterior scalene muscle, phrenic nerve, middle scalene muscle, and long thoracic nerve. **B,** The anterior scalene muscle is divided sharply and lifted upward to expose the underlying subclavian artery before it is divided at its origin on the cervical spine. **C,** Next, the middle scalene muscle is exposed by gently retracting the brachial plexus forward and is dissected to the level of the long thoracic nerve before being sharply detached from the first rib. **D,** Finally, after ensuring that the subclavian artery is protected, the first rib is divided with a bone cutter as posteriorly as possible without disrupting the brachial plexus. *(Adapted from Messina LM, Thoracic outlet syndrome. In: Cronenwett JL, Johnston KW, eds. Rutherford's Vascular Surgery. 8th ed. Philadelphia: Elsevier Saunders; 2014:1977-1987.e2.)*

in determining success in this population is that the definition of success is largely subjective; most studies report changes in patient-perceived disability preprocedure versus postprocedure.

For patients with ATOS or VTOS, success rates are more easily defined. Arterial and venous patency rates are reported to be 92% and 95% after thoracic outlet decompression with vascular reconstruction and thrombolysis, respectively.

In our practice, systemic anticoagulation is continued postoperatively in all patients with VTOS for 3 to 6 months. Approximately 80% to 90% of all VTOS cases are amenable to venoplasty performed 2 to 3 weeks after surgical decompression. There is a small number of patients who have chronic occlusion of their subclavian vein that is not amenable to venoplasty; most of these patients will have some degree of recanalization or further development of collaterals by 6 months of anticoagulation, after which it can be discontinued.

■ CONCLUSION

The diagnosis and treatment of TOS can be controversial. Careful selection of patients appropriate for surgical decompression for NTOS is key. Excellent surgical outcomes for VTOS can be achieved with a methodical algorithm for treatment (see Figure 3). The treatment for ATOS should be tailored depending on patient presentation.

SUGGESTED READINGS

Freischlag J, Orion K. Understanding thoracic outlet syndrome. *Scientifica (Cairo).* 2014;2014:248163.

Illig KA, Thompson RW, Freischlag JA, Donahue DM, Jordan SE, Edgelow PI, eds. *Thoracic Outlet Syndrome.* London: Springer-Verlag; 2013.

Likes KC, Orlando MS, Salditch Q, Mirza S, Cohen A, Reifsnyder T, Lum YW, Freischlag JA. Lessons learned in the surgical treatment of neurogenic thoracic outlet syndrome over 10 years. *Vasc Endovascular Surg.* 2015;49:8-11.

Lum YW, Brooke BS, Likes K, Modi M, Grunebach H, Christo PJ, Freischlag JA. Impact of anterior scalene lidocaine blocks on predicting surgical success in older patients with neurogenic thoracic outlet syndrome. *J Vasc Surg.* 2012;55:1370-1375.

Moore R, Wei Lum Y. Venous thoracic outlet syndrome. *Vasc Med.* 2015;20:182-189.

Orlando MS, Likes KC, Mirza S, Cao Y, Cohen A, Lum YW, Reifsnyder T, Freischlag JA. A decade of excellent outcomes after surgical intervention in 538 patients with thoracic outlet syndrome. *J Am Coll Surg.* 2015;220:934-939.

Povlsen B, Hansson T, Povlsen SD. Treatment for thoracic outlet syndrome. *Cochrane Database Syst Rev.* 2014;(11):CD007218.

Schrijver AM, De Borst GJ, Van Herwaarden JA, Vonken EJ, Moll FL, Vos JA, De Vries JP. Catheter-directed thrombolysis for acute upper extremity ischemia. *J Cardiovasc Surg (Torino).* 2015;56:433-439.

THE DIABETIC FOOT

Joshua C. Grimm, MD, Robert J. Beaulieu, MD,
and Heitham T. Hassoun, MD

Diabetic foot wounds confer considerable morbidity and mortality and burden the healthcare system with significant costs. Approximately 1 in 4 patients with diabetes will develop a foot complication during their lifetime. Risk factors include poor glycemic control, impaired immune function, peripheral neuropathy, and vascular insufficiency. Up to 50% of all diabetic patients suffer from some degree of sensory neuropathy, which can lead to the inability to detect traumatic insults because of blunting of both pain and thermal receptors. Motor neuropathies promote often unrecognized deformities in the plantar surfaces of the foot, thus exposing certain areas to skin breakdown and injury. In addition, dysregulation of the autonomic nervous system disrupts the natural protective function of sweat glands, resulting in potential points of entry for bacteria and other pathogens. Some level of neuropathy is present in more than 80% of patients with diabetic ulcers. Host defenses are further affected by the deleterious effect of hyperglycemia on neutrophil chemotaxis and the poor regional perfusion associated with concomitant small vessel disease. Although the exact pathogenesis of peripheral vascular disease is unclear, endothelial cell dysfunction and disturbances in vascular regulation undoubtedly contribute to the proinflammatory cascade that culminates in the formation of atheromatous plaques. These lesions typically affect the tibial and peroneal arteries and can result in long-segment stenoses.

It is important to determine whether a diabetic ulcer is complicated by infection. If it is not, the management strategy consists of serial débridement; nonadherent, occlusive dressings; and pressure offloading with a variety of casts and specialty shoes. Infected ulcers and wounds, however, can be an operative emergency, and thus every surgeon must be familiar with their clinical manifestation and management. Accordingly, that is the focus of the remainder of this chapter.

MICROBIOLOGY

In an antibiotic-naive patient with an acute, superficial infection, Staphylococcus aureus and beta-hemolytic streptococci are implicated most commonly. Conversely, in patients with chronic wounds at risk for loss of limb, aerobic gram-negative and anaerobic organisms likely are accountable. Because methicillin-resistant Staphylococcus aureus (MRSA) is common in this demographic, the clinician always must be cognizant of its potential influence, especially in individuals with recalcitrant or recurrent infections. In this setting, initiating empiric broad-spectrum antibiotics while awaiting culture results is encouraged and can diminish the risk for progression of the infection, both within the foot and systemically.

CLINICAL PRESENTATION

Diabetic foot infections exist on a spectrum, ranging from minor abrasions to extensive soft tissue destruction with underlying muscle or bone involvement. Although many of these lesions also manifest with signs of local and systemic inflammation (pain, purulent drainage, fever, or frank shock), these cardinal symptoms are not uniformly present. Sensory neuropathies can minimize much of the pain associated with these wounds, even in the context of a severe, necrotizing infection. The latter typically harbors additional physical examination findings such as cutaneous blistering, gas formation, skin discoloration, and malodorous discharge. An additional ailment, Charcot's arthropathy, in which chronic neuropathy leads

to join and bone degeneration, has an insidious onset, eventually resulting in foot deformation with increased likelihood of ulceration.

DIAGNOSIS

The accurate and prompt diagnosis of a diabetic foot wound or infection can be challenging. The updated guidelines from the Infectious Diseases Society of America have sought to simplify the process and recommend the following algorithmic approach: (1) determine the extent of involvement (superficial vs deep), (2) appreciate patient-specific risk factors, and (3) identify the causative organism. The diagnosis is based largely on clinical examination findings (erythema, warmth, purulent drainage) and a detailed history (fever, chills, labile blood glucose).

To determine the extent of infection, the wound should be irrigated copiously, and all necrotic tissue and foreign bodies should be removed. In general, wounds lacking purulence and erythema in a patient without systemic signs of infection can be presumed to be "uninfected." The presence of fever, hypotension, or bacteremia should alert the physician to a severe infection or an immunocompromised host. The wound base should be probed to evaluate for sinus tracts or exposed bone. Factors that raise the suspicion for the presence of osteomyelitis include an ulcer greater than 2 cm^2 or 3 mm deep, the presence of a "sausage toe," an erythrocyte sedimentation rate greater than 70 mm/hr, a nonhealing ulcer after appropriate conservative management, and radiographic evidence of bony destruction below the ulcer (Figures 1 and 2).

In cases of grossly exposed bone or wounds that probe to obvious bony structures, there is minimal clinical benefit in obtaining supportive imaging of the foot. However, if the diagnosis is uncertain, a conventional radiograph can demonstrate signs of chronic destruction and provide a baseline for future examinations. When there is still doubt, magnetic resonance imaging (MRI), which is highly sensitive and specific, should be obtained.

Superficial cultures should be sent to the pathology department only when the probability of an infection is high or there is concern for a multidrug resistant organism. Because most of these wounds are colonized chronically, there is no utility in obtaining routine samples. Moreover, although the definitive test to diagnose osteomyelitis is a bone biopsy, the risk of bacterial translocation typically precludes this intervention.

To quantify the extent of baseline vascular disease, a thorough pulse examination should be performed. In addition, obtaining an ankle-brachial index (ABI) can provide valuable information regarding the patient's burden of arterial insufficiency. Given the prevalence of arterial calcification in these patients, it is not uncommon for diabetics to have ABIs greater than 1.30, thereby necessitating additional studies (pulse volume recordings, toe-brachial index [TBI], toe pressure) to gauge arterial perfusion. It is critical that any significant arterial disease be mitigated to facilitate an appropriate response to local wound therapy.

TREATMENT

Most centers now use multidisciplinary teams to address the multitude of factors affecting the diabetic patient, a strategy that has resulted in improved outcomes among these patients. Nutritionists can provide insight into meals with low glycemic indices while general practitioners optimize medication regimens to target a hemoglobin A$_{1C}$ between 6.5% and 7.5%. Conservative strategies, including offloading of the affected area of the foot to minimize pressure and shear forces, are also critical. A timely referral to an occupational therapist to fit the patient with a specialized orthotic, cast, or boot can assist in this therapeutic goal. It is equally important that this relationship persist even after the wound has healed in order to prevent future tissue loss and recurrent infection.

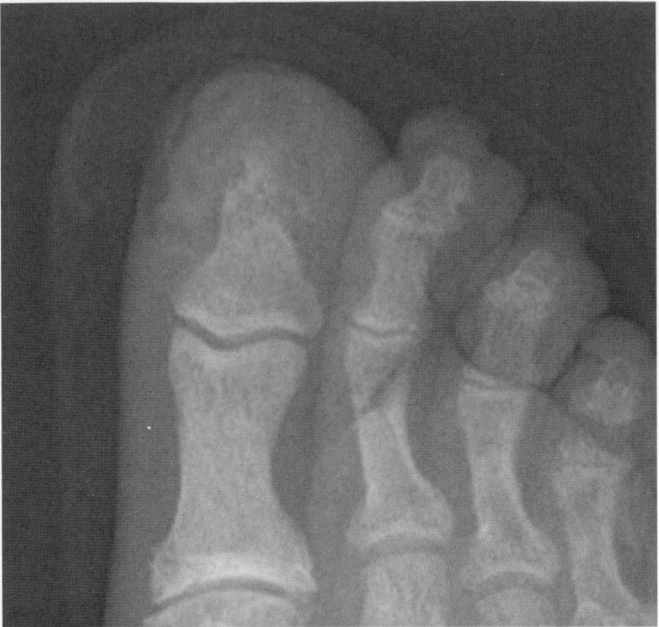

FIGURE 1 Oblique view radiograph of right foot demonstrating erosion and destruction of the first distal phalanx with soft tissue changes, consistent with osteomyelitis.

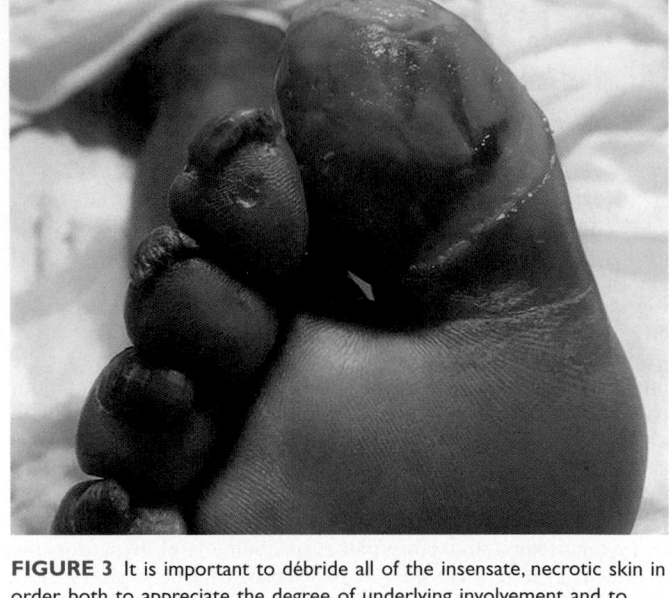

FIGURE 3 It is important to débride all of the insensate, necrotic skin in order both to appreciate the degree of underlying involvement and to readily drain all infectious fluid below the skin's surface.

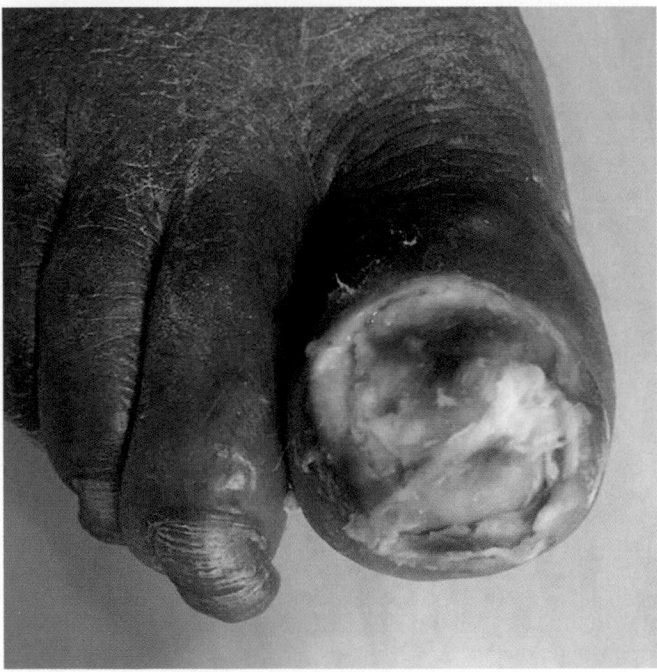

FIGURE 2 Clinical presentation of a patient with right first toe osteomyelitis and significant soft tissue destruction. The edema and purulent fluid present are indicative of a severe infection.

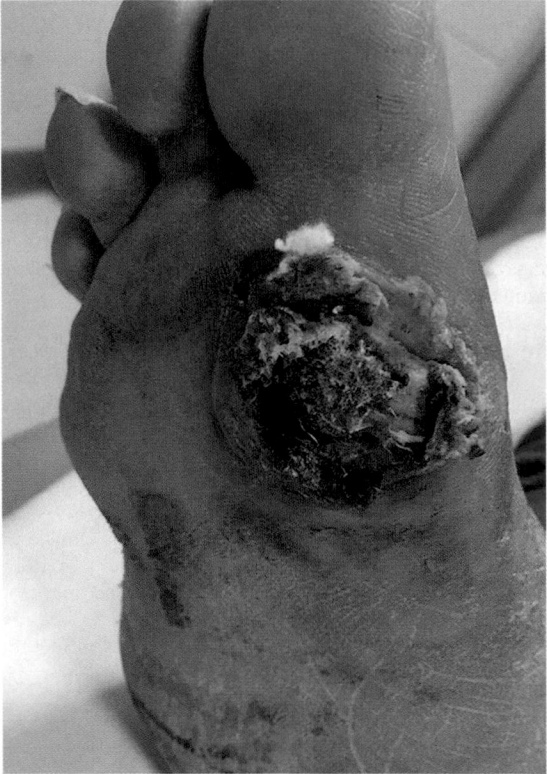

FIGURE 4 Patient with a malum perforans ulcer. These painless lesions can probe deep below the surface and require aggressive treatment to avoid subsequent limb loss.

Involvement of a surgeon in the multidisciplinary care of diabetic feet is critical. Early débridement is an important component in the treatment paradigm and has been associated with limb salvage in multiple studies. As mentioned previously, the wound bed should be washed out thoroughly and all necrotic tissue removed. In addition, abscess cavities should be incised and drained completely.

Digital ulcers and gangrene are managed with amputation with or without extension to include the metatarsal head. If multiple toes are infected, a more extensive procedure, such as a transmetatarsal amputation, may be required to clear all of the affected tissue and avoid a chronically nonhealing wound. Delayed, definitive closure often is used to allow for serial débridements and antibiotic therapy to reduce the bacterial burden in the remaining healthy tissue (Figures 3 and 4).

Correction of underlying vascular disease should be pursued aggressively if the aforementioned strategies fail to achieve an appropriate recovery or as a primary strategy in patients with critical limb ischemia (i.e., ABI or TBI <0.4). Appropriate patient selection, especially in the immobile or severely debilitated patient with gangrene extending past the midfoot, is essential in such strategies. Moreover, these interventions should be attempted only once the acute infection has been addressed with local débridement and antibiotic therapy. Restoration of perfusion is best achieved via revascularization of the tibial or pedal vessels, as the peroneal artery has no direct braches below the ankle. It is important to note that although direct flow to the plantar arch is not always required to relieve claudication or rest pain, it is preferred to meet the high metabolic demands of a healing diabetic ulcer.

The decision to utilize either endovascular therapies or more conventional open techniques depends on the patient's overall condition as well as the characteristics of the target lesions. The small vessel disease most common in diabetic patients typically is not amenable to percutaneous intervention; however, perfusion occasionally can be augmented by improving inflow at the iliofemoral level in patients with multivessel arterial occlusions or by relieving short-segment, focal stenoses. If targets are present, an autologous vein conduit can be used to bypass longer segments or distal, tibial or peroneal disease. Although the primary and secondary patencies are undoubtedly higher in the latter, limb salvage rates are no different. Hybrid approaches that combine both modalities also can be used in select situations.

The defect present after débridement can be substantial and prove difficult to cover with the remaining local soft tissue. Negative-pressure, vacuum-assisted dressings can lead to a reduction in the defect size and assist in primary closure or subsequent tissue transfer. Patience throughout the entire process is paramount, as up to 75% of these wounds remain unhealed at 6 months.

■ CONCLUSIONS

Diabetic foot infections can be challenging to diagnose and manage. A multidisciplinary approach consisting of early débridement, medical optimization, and offloading of pressure and shear forces is critical in ensuring wound regression. These strategies should not be uniform but rather should be dictated by unique, patient-specific factors.

SUGGESTED READINGS

Bowling FL, Rashid ST, Boulton AJ. Preventing and treating foot complications associated with diabetes mellitus. *Nat Rev Endocrinol.* 2015;11: 606-616.

Elraiyah T, Domecq JP, Prutsky G, et al. A systematic review and meta-analysis of debridement methods for chronic diabetic foot ulcers. *J Vasc Surg.* 2016;63(suppl 2):37S-45S.

Jeffcoate WJ, Harding KG. Diabetic foot ulcers. *Lancet.* 2003;361:1545-1551.

Singh N, Armstrong DG, Lipsky BA. Preventing foot ulcers in patients with diabetes. *JAMA.* 2005;293:217-228.

GANGRENE OF THE FOOT

Peter Beaulieu, DO, MPH, and M. Ashraf Mansour, MD, FACS

Gangrene is defined as the death and putrefaction of a body tissue. Most commonly it is the result of irreversible ischemia. In the lower extremity, decreased perfusion to the skin and soft tissue, if not reversed in time, will lead to gangrenous changes. The most vulnerable areas tend to be in the peripheral circulation and end arteries, such as the toes. Prolonged bed rest may cause pressure necrosis in the heel fat pad. Trauma, sepsis, prolonged use of peripheral vasoconstrictors, or exposure to cold may lead to gangrene. However, in the lower extremity, peripheral arterial disease (PAD) is the most common cause.

Three types of gangrene are recognized: *dry*, *wet*, and *gas gangrene*. In dry gangrene, the soft tissue becomes dry and desiccated, and usually a line of demarcation between viable and dead tissue can be defined. In wet gangrene, the affected tissue still may be partially perfused and retains some turgor; a line of demarcation is not readily apparent (Figure 1). Gas gangrene occurs when anaerobic bacteria, such as the *Clostridia* species, invade the tissue and muscle and release gas and toxins locally and systemically. If not treated promptly, gas gangrene can spread rapidly and be fatal. The clinician's role is to recognize gangrene as a potentially serious problem and initiate a management plan. Surgical treatment of the gangrenous area ranges from simple débridement of necrotic tissue to a major lower extremity amputation. If blood supply to the limb is inadequate, revascularization to improve blood flow needs to be part of the management plan.

■ EPIDEMIOLOGY

It is estimated that 10 to 12 million individuals in the United States have PAD. Critical limb ischemia (CLI) is said to be present if the patient has rest pain, ischemic ulceration, or gangrene. In a recent study the annual incidence of PAD in patients over the age of 40 years was 2.35%, and CLI had an annual incidence of 0.35%. Every year, 11% of patients progress from PAD to CLI. Risk factors for developing PAD include smoking, hypertension, hyperlipidemia, and diabetes mellitus. Although the number of smokers has decreased over the years, 17.8% of the U.S. population (42.1 million people) still smoked in 2013. The Centers for Disease Control and Prevention (CDC) also estimates that there are 29.1 million diabetics (9.3% of the population) in the United States. Patients with diabetes are especially vulnerable to the complications of PAD because they often have decreased sensation from neuropathy, making their feet more prone to injury, and their wounds are more susceptible to infection. More than 100,000 amputations are performed yearly in the United States, with more than 55,000 considered major, defined as above the ankle. The most common indication for amputation is gangrene.

■ CLINICAL EVALUATION

When examining a patient with gangrene of the foot, a detailed history and physical examination are required. The physician should ask directly about risk factors, and in many cases a thorough past medical and surgical history will provide clues about the disease process and whether previous revascularization was attempted. Patients with long-standing PAD harbor symptoms for months to years and a slow progression of the disease process can be elicited. A complete physical examination should be performed, paying particular attention to the presence or absence of bruits or pulses. A diminished or absent popliteal pulse will inform the examiner that a superficial femoral or popliteal artery stenosis or occlusion may be present. Conversely, a large pulsatile mass behind the knee is a clue for a popliteal aneurysm that could be the source of distal atheroemboli ("trash foot"), causing a black toe. After a thorough examination, an experienced clinician should be able to distinguish whether the cause of gangrene is occlusive disease or atheroembolization, although less commonly these

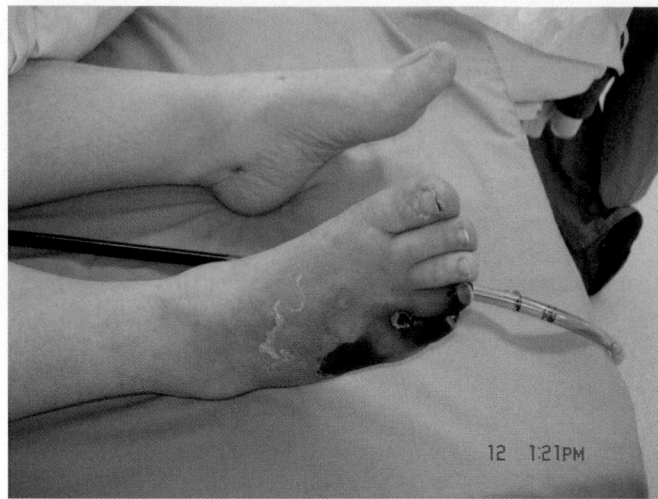

FIGURE 1 Wet gangrene of the right fourth and fifth toes. Note the ill-defined border of necrotic tissue.

two conditions may co-exist. Other less common causes of gangrene include myeloproliferative disorders, vasculitides, disseminated intravascular coagulation, and prolonged use of vasoconstrictors.

PAD frequently co-exists with coronary artery and cerebrovascular disease. The clinical evaluation of the patient should address the potential presence of comorbid conditions that may complicate treatment. A patient with angina or a recent myocardial infarction may require a thorough cardiac evaluation before embarking on a lower extremity bypass. The clinician also should assess the patient's reserve potential and ability to participate in rehabilitation. A bedridden patient who cannot ambulate is better served by a lower extremity amputation than a complicated or futile attempt at saving the foot.

Finally, soft tissue infection may be present with gangrene. Antibiotics, tailored to attack the causative organisms, should be used. However, treatment should not be delayed if the infection does not respond to medical treatment. The surgeon should be vigilant in examining the wound and especially the sole of the foot, where an occult deep space infection may be present. A patient with diabetic neuropathy may not have a normal pain response to infection.

■ DIAGNOSTICS

Noninvasive Tests

Even with an experienced clinician, the pulse examination can be inaccurate 40% of the time. Therefore an objective and repeatable noninvasive test is essential to making the diagnosis of PAD. The vascular laboratory testing should be considered an extension of the physical examination. The objective of noninvasive testing is to identify the cause of gangrene and help to formulate a rational and expeditious management plan.

Ankle-Brachial Index

The ankle-brachial index (ABI) is the simplest test used to assess the peripheral circulation. It consists of recording the systolic blood pressure in both arms and at both ankles. A proper blood pressure cuff of appropriate size (diameter) should be selected to fit around the arm and the ankle. This is an important detail because an improper cuff will yield a falsely elevated measurement. Using a continuous Doppler probe, the examiner locates the arterial signal, inflates the cuff until the signal disappears, and then allows the cuff to deflate. The systolic pressure is recorded when the first audible signal is detected as the pressure in the cuff is released slowly.

A normal adult with no vascular disease will have a normal ABI of 1.0. An ABI less than 0.9 is indicative of PAD, an ABI less than 0.5 correlates with severe disease, and an ABI of less than 0.3 is consistent with a threatened limb (Figure 2). A ratio above 1.3 suggests calcification of the vessels, commonly seen in long-term diabetics or advanced atherosclerosis. A patient may have a normal ABI with toe gangrene in a case of distal embolization. The vast majority of patients with PAD will have an abnormal ABI. Patients who have milder PAD and claudication may have an ABI that is normal at rest but drops after a few minutes of exercise.

Toe-Brachial Index

The toe-brachial index (TBI) is calculated in a similar fashion to the ABI, except that a photoelectrode is placed on the toe instead of continuous wave Doppler. The photoelectrode is used to record an arterial waveform that then can be obliterated by inflating the small cuff and signal the return of flow with deflation. There is a natural gradient between the toe and ankle pressures of 20 to 30 mm Hg so that a TBI of 0.7 to 0.8 is considered normal. An absolute toe pressure of 30 mm Hg is the minimum required for healing, and in cases involving diabetics, a toe pressure of 40 mm Hg or greater is needed.

Segmental Limb Pressures

A ratio of the systolic blood pressure compared with the brachial pressure can be obtained at different levels of the lower extremity (thigh, calf). Often an arterial waveform also is recorded at these levels, allowing the clinician to compare pressure and waveforms at different levels and sides. In general, a gradient of 20 mm Hg is considered abnormal and can point to the location of significant vascular occlusive disease.

Fluorescence Angiography

Fluorescence angiography, used extensively for eye examinations, is a relatively new technique applied to the evaluation of soft tissue perfusion. It has been used to aid in breast reconstruction and assessing tissue flaps. The viability of tissue flaps is critical for planning the level of amputation. Using a charge-coupled device camera and a low-power laser with indocyanine green (ICG), tissue perfusion can be assessed. Known as ICG fluorescence angiography (Novadaq's SPY system), this technique is being trialed in patients who are undergoing vascular reconstruction and amputations to guide surgeons in planning revascularization and extent of tissue resection.

Transcutaneous Oxygen Measurement

Measurement of transcutaneous partial pressure of oxygen ($TcPO_2$) is a noninvasive method of determining local tissue perfusion using small sensors on the skin of the extremity. The rationale is that in order to heal, tissues need an adequate oxygen level. Sensors can be placed in multiple areas of the body and either the absolute value of the oxygen tension can be recorded or a ratio between the area of interest and the chest can be calculated. $TcPO_2$ measurements have been shown to have an accuracy of 87% to 100% at predicting wound healing. Values greater than 60 mm Hg are necessary for absolute wound healing and values lower than 20 mm Hg are associated with complete failure. Many studies have reported mixed results, and reliance on $TcPO_2$ alone should not supersede clinical examination and other objective testing.

■ IMAGING

The objective of imaging is to reach the correct diagnosis and plan proper treatment. The diagnostic process should proceed in an orderly fashion, beginning with noninvasive tests and finishing with

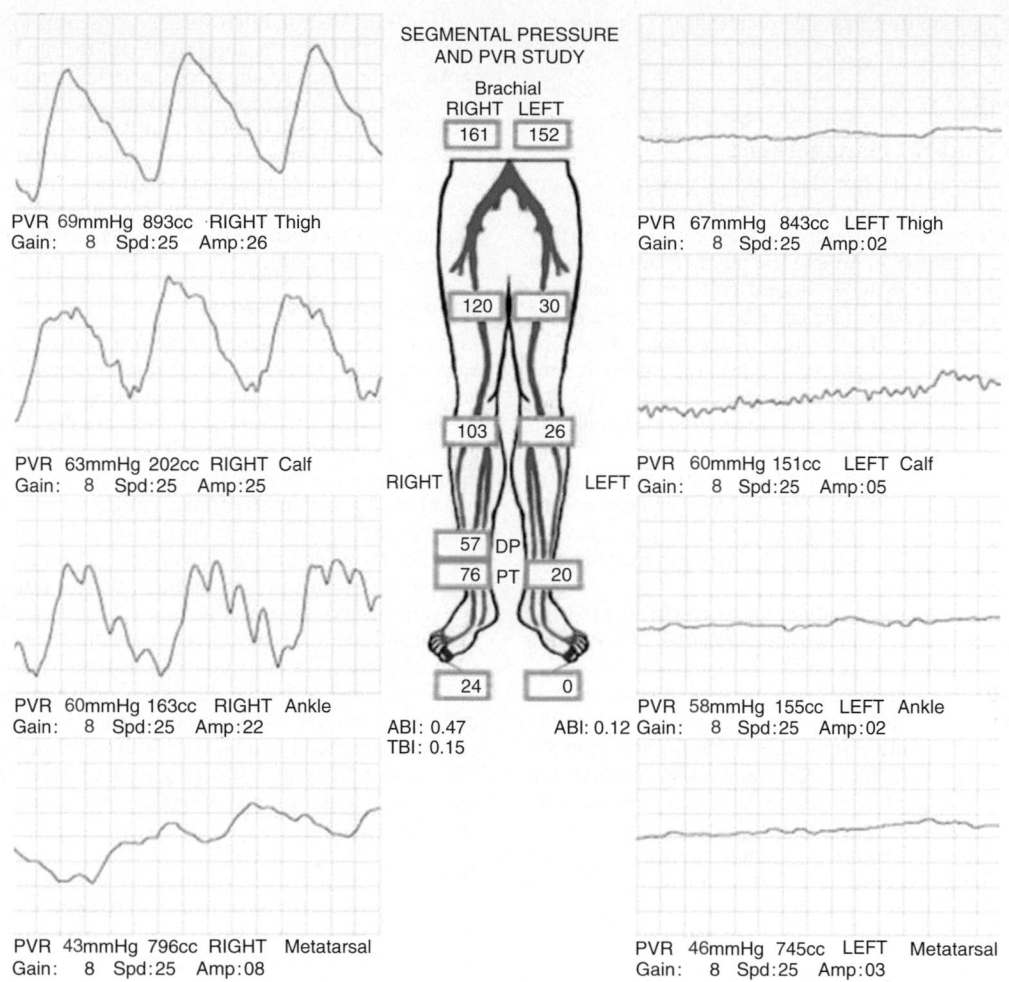

FIGURE 2 Ankle-brachial index in a patient with severe left leg ischemia. Note that toe pressure on the left is zero and the segmental waveforms are all flattened, consistent with severe multilevel ischemia. *ABI,* Ankle-brachial index; *DP,* dorsalis pedis; *PT,* posterior tibial; *PVR,* pulsed volume recording; *TBI,* toe-brachial index.

more invasive tests, if necessary. To plan revascularization, a more extensive imaging protocol may be required.

Duplex Ultrasonography

Duplex ultrasonography combines grayscale imaging (B-mode), Doppler, and color-flow assessment. Initially used to assess carotid arteries, duplex ultrasonography now is used widely to evaluate all vascular beds, including the brain (transcranial Doppler). The ability to assess the diameter of a blood vessel, detect whether it is patent, and measure the speed of the blood flowing through it provides a wealth of information to the examiner. Although not used widely because it is tedious, arterial duplex mapping of the lower extremities can yield a correct diagnosis in more than 90% of cases in experienced hands.

Multidetector Computed Tomographic Angiography

Multidetector computed tomographic angiography (CTA) now is replacing digital subtraction angiography (DSA) as the primary modality to image abdominal and lower extremity arteries. The scanner is programmed to acquire images in the arterial phase after a bolus of intravenous contrast is administered. CTA is accurate, with a sensitivity and specificity of 95% and 96%, respectively, when a lesion is greater than 50%. Drawbacks include increased cost when compared with other noninvasive imaging modalities, the requirement for ionizing radiation exposure, and intravenous contrast having the potential to cause contrast-induced nephropathy.

Magnetic Resonance Angiography

Magnetic resonance angiography (MRA) uses radio waves and magnetic fields in conjunction with gadolinium contrast to opacify the vessels and produce detailed three-dimensional images. MRA has not been adopted fully for general use in vascular surgery for a number of reasons. Typically it is more expensive than CTA, and it does not provide the spatial resolution necessary to assess small vessels. In addition, it is time consuming, and many patients cannot tolerate being in the magnet because of claustrophobia or other medical conditions. Furthermore, gadolinium is contraindicated in patients with chronic kidney disease. Newer magnets are being introduced that use 4 Tesla, potentially improving the visualization of small vessels.

Digital Subtraction Angiography

Before CTA, intra-arterial injection of contrast agents was the primary invasive diagnostic modality used to evaluate the arterial tree. DSA now is used predominantly in combination with an endovascular intervention, such as angioplasty or atherectomy. Less frequently it is used diagnostically to clarify the runoff status when the

CTA is inadequate or extensive vascular calcifications obscure the runoff status.

■ MANAGEMENT

Antibiotic and Medical Management

The extent of gangrene can vary, from localized toe gangrene to more extensive involvement of the whole foot or distal leg. If a soft tissue infection is present, systemic antibiotics are used to prevent further spread and attempt to control it. An empiric regimen can be started after obtaining appropriate tissue or wound cultures. In diabetics, mixed aerobic and anaerobic organisms may be present, and a broad coverage is usually necessary. The duration of treatment should be as short as possible, as prolonged courses will lead to resistant organisms or other untoward sequelae. Débridement of necrotic infected tissues and drainage of purulent material are the first steps taken to control infection.

Antibiotic-resistant bacteria, including methicillin-resistant *Staphylococcus aureus* and resistant forms of *Pseudomonas aeruginosa*, now are being seen with increasing frequency. Any unnecessary delay in revascularization will complicate the patient's recovery and timely elimination of infection.

Surgeons now are paying more attention to enhanced recovery protocols that have the benefit of improving outcomes and reducing perioperative complications. Although the primary surgical objectives to treating gangrene are removing necrotic tissue and re-establishing adequate blood flow and tissue oxygen perfusion, the patient's nutritional status and physical-mental condition should not be neglected. Initiation of early physical therapy is very important in helping patients to return to ambulation as quickly as possible. Appropriate precautions to prevent bedsores, deep venous thrombosis, urinary tract infections, falls, and inadvertent trauma to amputation stumps should be exercised.

Débridement

The role of débridement is to get rid of devitalized tissue and promote rapid healing. It is important to have a conservative mindset (i.e., preserving viable tissue while excising necrotic material). Aggressive débridement before proper revascularization should be avoided if possible. Sharp débridement using the knife and cautery, and occasionally a curette, is all that is necessary. Hydroresection or jet lavage can be used to wash out deeper spaces. If the wound is clean and the edges are viable, primary closure can be attempted. However, if the wound is left open for drainage and granulation, a vacuum dressing is very helpful and more comfortable for the patient. If the débrided site needs frequent inspection, wet-to-dry dressings with saline can be used. The wet-to-dry dressing will draw immune cells into the tissues and promote healing while acting to débride the tissue when it is removed. A variety of topical enzymes, protease scavengers, and biologic wound matrices have been used. However, none has been shown to be superior to surgical débridement and proper revascularization.

Revascularization

The common path to the development of gangrene is inadequate blood flow to keep tissues viable. Therefore the goal of treatment is to restore blood flow to premorbid levels or to an adequate level to sustain normal tissue perfusion and healing, as much as possible. Most patients who develop foot gangrene have some pre-existing arterial pathology. It is imperative to evaluate the vascular tree, from proximal to distal, lest the examiner miss a subtle lesion. In the planning of treatment, proximal arterial occlusive lesions should be addressed first and then more distal ones tackled. Many patients with PAD have multilevel disease and frequently require multilevel interventions or hybrid interventions, such as an endovascular procedure combined with a bypass.

The TransAtlantic Inter-Society Consensus (TASC) has classified arterial lesions from the aorta to the ankles into four categories: A to D. An A lesion is typically a focal arterial stenosis that is very likely to respond to balloon angioplasty, whereas a D lesion is a long arterial occlusion. In general, TASC A and B lesions can be addressed with an endovascular approach, whereas C and D lesions respond best to a surgical bypass. Many clinicians will attempt an endovascular procedure for a TASC C or D lesion in a frail patient who is not a good candidate for an open bypass. However, long-term patency rarely is achieved in such cases.

Endovascular Procedures

Percutaneous endovascular techniques range from simple balloon angioplasty to complex intentional subintimal dissection of occluded vessels. Balloon angioplasty and stenting is a durable procedure in the iliac arteries. This technique is less durable for superficial femoral and popliteal artery stenosis and occlusion. Drug-eluting stents and drug-coated balloons have been shown to improve the 1-year patency of femoropopliteal interventions. Longer-term outcomes are awaited. Another endovascular technique is subintimal dissection. In cases of superficial femoral or popliteal artery occlusions, a Glidewire is used to cross the lesion and then re-enter the true lumen, with or without a re-entry device, beyond the lesion. The diseased vessel can be ballooned and stented. Some interventionalists have added atherectomy, a device that shaves or grinds the plaque to re-establish an adequate arterial channel or lumen. In all percutaneous endovascular procedures performed in the superficial femoral artery and more distally, outcomes are predicated on the diameter of the vessel and the length of the lesion. In general, shorter lesions in larger vessels have the best long-term patency and, conversely, longer lesions in smaller vessels have the worst patency.

Bypass Procedures

Surgical bypass, with prosthetic material or autogenous conduit, has stood the test of time. The patency of aortobifemoral bypass for occlusive disease is more than 80% at 5 years. Similarly, femoropopliteal bypass with adequate size autogenous saphenous vein can have a patency of 75% at 5 years. If no vein is available, a prosthetic bypass can be attempted, accepting a less favorable long-term patency. Older, frail patients are poor candidates for a prolonged open surgical bypass operation. Many patients with PAD do not have an adequate autogenous conduit, especially if they have undergone a previous coronary or leg bypass. In these cases the clinician is left to choose between inferior options.

Patients with multilevel occlusive disease can undergo hybrid procedures (i.e., a combination of an endovascular balloon and stent with an open bypass). A frequent occurrence is iliac balloon angioplasty with a femorofemoral bypass or femoropopliteal bypass.

Amputations

Amputations for gangrene in the lower extremity can range from a simple partial toe amputation to a most aggressive hip disarticulation. The goal of amputation is to remove necrotic and infected tissue and allow tissue healing and weight-bearing as soon as possible. Often the patient who requires an amputation is evaluated by a multidisciplinary team that includes the surgeon, physiatrist, physical therapist, orthotist, nutritionist, visiting nurse, and social worker, among others. Involving the patient's family members for moral support and coordinating the discharge process is no less important. This team participates in planning for the operation and the postoperative recovery period, which is often prolonged and complicated in an older frail patient with many medical and psychosocial issues.

Toe Amputation

If gangrene is confined to the tip or part of the toe, a partial toe amputation preserving the proximal phalanx can be done. This procedure should have the least impact on the patient's recovery and

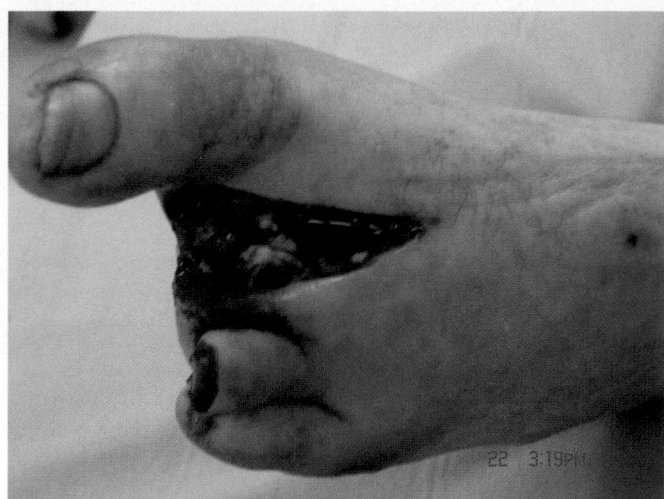

FIGURE 3 Left second and third toe amputation and partial amputation of the fourth toe for gangrene. The wound is left open to heal.

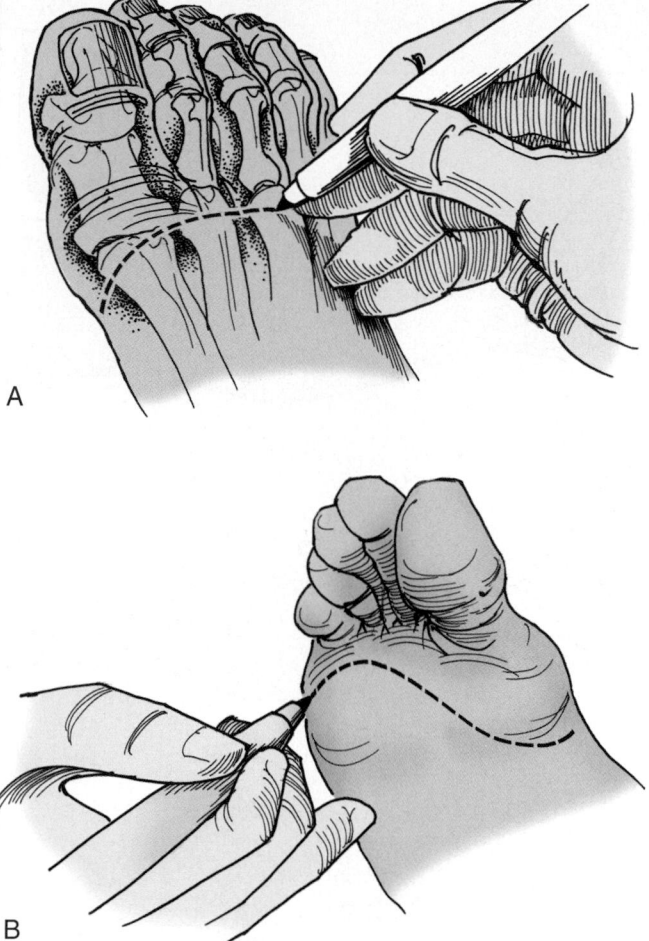

FIGURE 4 Transmetatarsal amputation. A transverse dorsal incision is made proximal to the metatarsal heads (**A**), and a curvilinear plantar incision is made at the base of the toes (**B**) to create a long plantar flap. *(Modified from Barnes RW, Cox B. Amputations: An Illustrated Manual. Philadelphia. Hanley & Belfus, 2000:39.)*

ambulation. When gangrene affects the entire toe, the surgeon must decide whether there is enough viable tissue to perform an adequate wound closure with or without taking the metatarsal head (Figure 3). The first metatarsal head plays an important role in gait and balance and should be preserved if possible.

Toe amputation preserving the metatarsal head can be done with a simple curvilinear incision at the base of the toe, either in antero-posterior or mediolateral fish-mouth or racquet-like fashion. The metatarsophalangeal joint is identified easily by flexing the toe and can be disarticulated after sharply incising the joint capsule. A rongeur is used to remove cartilage. Wound closure is done loosely with nylon sutures. In ray amputations, the proximal extent involves the removal of the metatarsal head. The sesamoid bones of the first metatarsal head also are removed. An oscillating saw can be used to transect the bone. Nerves and tendon sheaths should be cut sharply under tension so that they retract. Primary closure is done in clean wounds. Occasionally when there is not enough skin for a tension-free closure, healing by secondary intention can be initiated with a vacuum dressing. Sutures can be left in for 2 or more weeks or until the wound is healed completely. If the patient is allowed to bear weight shortly after the procedure, proper wound protection and padding is desirable. A plastic "ski boot" is helpful in protecting the foot from soiling and unnecessary trauma. Often toe and foot amputations can be performed with a toe or ankle block, and a tourniquet is not needed.

Transmetatarsal Amputation

In the event of forefoot gangrene or multiple toe involvement, it is not practical to save any toes. In this case, a transmetatarsal amputation is performed. The incision is planned near the heads of the metatarsals on the dorsal aspect and taken in a curvilinear fashion on the plantar aspect to create a flap (Figure 4). The plantar flap is slightly longer to allow easy approximation once the bones are removed. The oscillating saw is used to cut across the metatarsals one by one, progressively shortening the bones proceeding laterally. The toes with the metatarsal heads are peeled away after the tendons have been cut. Hemostasis can be achieved with the cautery, but larger digital arteries are ligated or sutured. The plantar flap has to be thinned in order to close the wound without undue tension.

Transtibial Amputation

When the entire foot and heel are involved and foot salvage is not possible, a leg amputation is necessary. In emergent cases, where infection is poorly controlled or spreading and the patient is septic,

a guillotine amputation can be done rapidly. Here the objective is to remove the necrotic infected tissue as quickly as possible without worrying about wound closure. Guillotine should be done as distal as possible so as not to compromise the definitive amputation procedure. The bleeding vessels are ligated and either a vacuum or a gauze dressing is placed. The most common indication for this is gas gangrene of the foot. This is a temporary and often lifesaving maneuver, and formal amputation usually follows in the next few days.

A formal transtibial amputation, commonly referred to as a below-knee amputation (BKA), can be technically challenging. It is very important to properly construct the myocutaneous flap so that the wound heals and the patient can use a prosthesis. The most commonly performed type is the posterior flap. The incision is started anteriorly about 10 cm below the tibial tuberosity. The anterior circular incision is roughly two thirds the circumference of the calf at its largest girth. This can be measured easily using an umbilical tape or suture (Figure 5). The medial and lateral incisions extend down roughly one third the circumference, or about 9 to 12 cm. A Gigli or oscillating saw is used to cut the tibia, and the fibula should be at least 1 cm shorter than the tibia. The tibia edge by the shin is beveled so that it does not protrude when the patient is ready for a prosthesis. The tibial arteries and veins are suture ligated, and the nerve is cut sharply and foreshortened to avoid a neuroma. The crural flap can

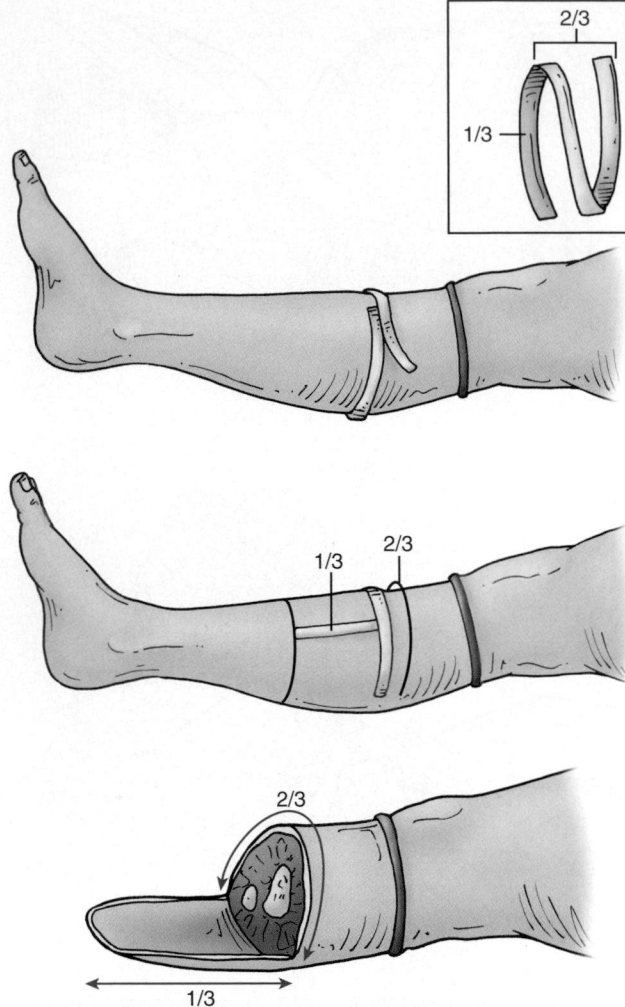

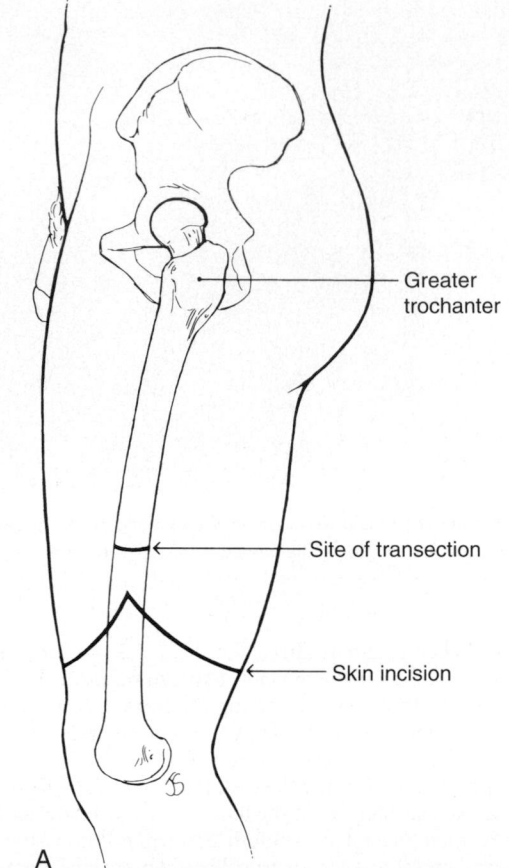

FIGURE 5 Using tape to obtain the measurement for a transtibial amputation with a posterior flap. *(From Sanders RJ, Augspurger R. Skin flap measurement for below-knee amputation. Surg Gynecol Obstet. 1977;145:740-742.)*

be thinned or debulked so that wound approximation is tension free. Interrupted fascial closure is done with an absorbable suture. The skin can be closed with nylon or staples, which are usually left for at least 3 weeks or until the wound is healed. A closed suction drain may be used at the surgeon's discretion. A posterior splint is used to avoid a knee flexion contracture. A variety of options are available to keep the knee straight and the wound protected from trauma but accessible for inspection (e.g., plastic mold, posterior splint). The posterior flap is the most commonly used flap for a BKA; however, skew flaps can be configured when the viability of the posterior tissue is in question. The most common local complications after a BKA are wound breakdown and infection. If not properly recognized and managed, these problems invariably lead to a transfemoral amputation.

Transfemoral Amputation

Amputation of the lower extremity above the knee (above-knee amputation; AKA) is indicated when the ischemia extends proximally enough so that it is not possible to get adequate viable tissue for closing a BKA. A fish-mouth type of incision is planned just above the knee (Figure 6). The femur is transected with a Gigli or oscillating saw. The popliteal vessels are suture ligated. The nerve is cut and ligated as well. The fascia is approximated with interrupted sutures,

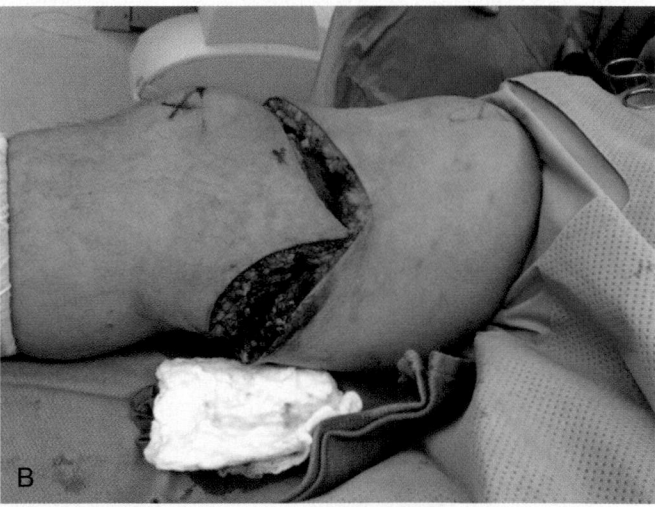

FIGURE 6 A, Schematic of a fish-mouth incision for above-knee amputation (AKA). **B,** Operative picture of right AKA.

and the skin is closed with nylon or staples. A protective dressing with gauze and compression with Ace bandage is often helpful. The most challenging postoperative problem is to keep the dressing on and the wound protected from soilage. As in BKA, wound breakdown and infection are the most common complications.

The energy required to ambulate with a BKA prosthesis is 40% more than normal bipedal ambulation; after an AKA, it is 60% more.

Other Amputations

Many modified foot amputations have been devised to address amputations that are more extensive than a transmetatarsal but less extensive than a transtibial. These include the Lisfranc, Chopart, and Syme amputations. They are indicated in very select patients and performed infrequently. Similarly, through-knee amputations, such as the Gritti-Stokes, are performed less often. In very rare situations a complete hip disarticulation is required. This is a morbid procedure, and long-term survival is questionable.

SUMMARY

Lower extremity gangrene occurs when the normal blood supply is disrupted because of vascular disease, trauma, or prolonged use of vasoconstrictors. The aim of the surgeon is to remove the devitalized tissue that will not heal and ensure that an adequate blood supply is present for healing. Formal evaluation of the blood flow to the extremity can be performed with a variety of noninvasive and invasive diagnostic tests. Vascular reconstruction is planned to maximize blood flow to the limb. Rapid recovery from this insult is assured when the patient is managed by a multidisciplinary team that addresses, among other things, nutritional status, rehabilitation potential, and psychosocial support of the patient.

SUGGESTED READINGS

Bradbury AW, Adam DJ, Bell J, et al. Multicentre randomized controlled trials of the clinical and cost-effectiveness of a bypass-surgery-first versus balloon-angioplasty-first revascularization strategy for severe limb ischaemia due to infrainguinal disease. The Bypass versus Angioplasty in Severe Ischaemia of the Leg (BASIL) trial. *Health Technol Assess.* 2010;14:1-252.
Connolly PH, Meltzer AJ, Spector JA, Schneider DB. Indocyanine green angiography aids in prediction of limb salvage in vascular trauma. *Ann Vasc Surg.* 2015;29:1453.e1-1453.e4.
Egorova NN, Guillerme S, Geljins A, Morrisssey N, Dayal R, et al. An analysis of a decade of experience with lower extremity revascularization including limb salvage, lengths of stay, and safety. *J Vasc Surg.* 2010;51:878-885.
Hirsch AT, Haskal ZA, Hertzer NR, et al. ACC/AHA 2005 practice guidelines for the management of patients with peripheral arterial disease: a collaborative report from the American Association for Vascular Surgery/Society for Vascular Surgery, Society for Cardiovascular Angiography and Interventions, Society for Vascular Medicine and Biology, Society for Interventional Radiology, and the ACC/AHA task force of the practice guidelines. *Circulation.* 2006;113:e463-e654.
Krishnan SA, Nash F, Baker N. Reduction of diabetic amputations over 11 years in a defined UK population: benefits of multidisciplinary team work and continuous prospective audit. *Diabetes Care.* 2008;31:99-101.
Nehler MR, Duval S, Diao L, Annex B, et al. Epidemiology of peripheral arterial disease and critical limb ischemia in an insured national population. *J Vasc Surg.* 2014;60:686-695.
Norgren L, Hiatt WR, Dormandy JA, Nehler MR, et al. Inter-society consensus for the management of peripheral arterial disease (TASC II). *J Vasc Surg.* 2007;45:S5A-S67A.
Siracuse JJ, Gill HL, Cassidy SP, Messina MD, et al. Endovascular treatment of lesions in the below-knee popliteal artery. *J Vasc Surg.* 2014;60:356-361.

BUERGER'S DISEASE (THROMBOANGIITIS OBLITERANS)

Palma Shaw, MD, Ian B. Bailey, BA, and Vivian Gahtan, MD

Thromboangiitis obliterans (TAO), or Buerger's disease, is a segmental nonatherosclerotic occlusive inflammatory condition of arteries and veins characterized by thrombosis and recanalization of small and medium-sized vessels. TAO more commonly affects the upper and lower extremities, seen with distal extremity ischemia, ischemic ulcers, or gangrene; however, mesenteric and cerebral involvement has been reported as well. Although cases have been reported worldwide, the greatest prevalence is in Eastern European, Mediterranean, and Asian countries. Characteristically, TAO is seen in males who have a history of long-term, heavy tobacco use; however, the incidence in women has increased and is up to 20%. The exact etiology is unknown and felt to be multifactorial, but any tobacco use (in any form, including smokeless tobacco) generally is agreed to perpetuate active disease. The pathogenesis involves impaired vasorelaxation and function of the sympathetic system. An ensuing inflammatory process often leads to vessel thrombosis.

PRESENTATION

TAO usually is seen in heavy smokers who are less than 40 to 45 years old, with symptoms affecting two or more extremities.

Digit ischemia is the most common presentation, with patients often reporting pain and discoloration. Later manifestations include ischemic ulcers, gangrene, sensory abnormalities, Raynaud's phenomenon, and distal claudication in the upper and lower extremities. Of note, instep claudication, which frequently is mistaken for an orthopedic issue, also is found in this disease process. This distal claudication can provide some differentiation between patients with TAO and those with peripheral arterial disease (PAD), as the latter group commonly has claudication of the calves. Superficial thrombophlebitis, which appears as tender nodules or cords with venous distribution in patients with TAO, is another contrasting feature that can predate ischemic symptoms.

Signs of more proximal vessel involvement can be seen with disease progression, which can include claudication of the calf and thigh that is indistinguishable from that seen in PAD. Rare reports of cerebral, coronary, pulmonary, internal thoracic, renal, and mesenteric vessel involvement also have been made. Mesenteric TAO, although rare, is associated with a poor prognosis and warrants prompt evaluation and surgical intervention for bowel ischemia. Aortic and iliac artery involvement is also rare and more likely because of PAD in these vessels.

DIAGNOSIS

TAO is often a diagnosis of exclusion derived after extensive workup for causes of occlusive vascular disease. The Olin criteria use disease onset before age 45 years, history of tobacco use, distal extremity ischemia signs, and arteriographic findings as key diagnostic features. In addition, other causes of limb ischemia such as embolization, diabetes, atherosclerosis, connective tissue disease, and autoimmune disorders must be ruled out. Although there are no specific laboratory tests used for the diagnosis of TAO, Table 1 summarizes clinical, laboratory, and imaging studies that should be included in this evaluation. Some of these are helpful to exclude other causes of limb ischemia. Imaging studies are helpful to quantitate the degree of ischemia, help to assess tissue perfusion, and characterize the arterial anatomy. Arteriographic findings that are classic for patients with TAO are shown in Figure 1.

PATHOLOGY

TAO is mainly a clinical diagnosis, and definitive diagnosis via arterial or venous biopsy is performed rarely. TAO is distinguished from other vasculitides, as the segmental intraluminal thrombi of small and medium-sized arteries and veins are composed largely of inflammatory cells before the disease becomes chronic. Furthermore, this inflammation does not extend beyond the intima of the vessel wall (Figure 2). In addition, the pathogenesis demonstrates an impaired endothelium-dependent and endothelium-independent vasorelaxation and decreased peripheral sympathetic outflow, and pathology reveals segmental infiltration of inflammatory cells in the vessel wall, leading to thrombotic occlusion of the vessel.

■ TREATMENT

Paramount to successful therapy is the patient's cessation of tobacco use or smoking. In fact, smoking cessation generally is accepted as the only proven therapy. Even the use of smokeless tobacco or nicotine replacement has been found to exacerbate this disease. Other treatments, either medical or invasive, are adjunctive and part of a multimodal approach often required in managing these patients. A summary of adjunct treatment is provided in Box 1.

Medical Therapy

A number of medications have been used in combination with smoking cessation. Nicotine gum and other approaches that facilitate smoking cessation are available. Some investigators advocate that the most effective drugs used to manage TAO are prostacyclin (PGI2) or its analogues (iloprost, beraprost, treprostinil sodium), aspirin, and streptokinase (as a thrombolytic). Other medications reported to have some benefit also are included in Box 1. Three reported cases of Buerger's disease have been treated successfully with phosphodiesterase type 5 (PDE5) inhibitors (sildenafil or tadalafil) in combination with other agents such as clopidogrel, alprostadil, and pentoxifylline. There is a small pilot study that looked at the use of oral Bosentan, a dual endothelin-1 receptor antagonist. Its antiinflammatory, antifibrotic, and selective vasodilatory properties have been shown to alleviate pain at rest and reduce the size of ischemic ulcers caused by damage to the microcirculation.

Invasive Modalities

Historically, limb revascularization has not been as helpful in this patient population. Endovascular therapy can be attempted if the lesion can be crossed; however, loss of the distal runoff may result. A more proximal lesion should be treated, if possible, in an effort to improve perfusion. For those patients who have anatomy permitting extended angioplasty of each tibial or foot artery lesion, this option can be considered.

Surgical revascularization with distal arterial bypass for these patients with rest pain or tissue loss can be utilized if angiography reveals a suitable target and adequate conduit is available. Reported outcomes in this population demonstrate poor long-term outcomes, in part because these distal vessels tend to be diminutive and the venous conduit may not be optimal because at times it is affected by the inflammatory condition and more so if the patient continues to use tobacco. If a bypass is feasible, the limb salvage rates may exceed graft patency. Most authors advocate for an initial attempt at conservative measures and reserve bypass for those cases in which these measures fail.

Other nonvascular adjunctive surgical procedures include sympathectomy with or without adrenalectomy, which has been used primarily or as an adjunct with variable results, and omental transfer, which has been reported as successful in several case series. Kirschner wire placement in the medullary canal of the tibia (see Box 1) has been reported in patients for whom medical and surgical therapy failed. In this small series, relief of pain and a decrease in major amputations were demonstrated in patients with Buerger's disease. Ultimately, these patients may progress to gangrene and require major amputation in a non–limb salvage situation.

TABLE 1: Diagnostic Evaluation for Thromboangiitis Obliterans

Clinical	Laboratory	Imaging and Physiologic Testing
Digit ulcers	Complete blood cell count	Echocardiography
Gangrene	Liver function tests	Arteriography
Venous nodules or cords	Serum creatinine	Segmental pressures
Sensory deficits	Fasting blood glucose	Arterial waveform analysis
Allen's test	Sedimentation rate	
Ankle-brachial index	Antinuclear antibody Rheumatoid factor Complement CREST serology Scleroderma serology Hypercoagulability Toxicology screen	

CREST, Calcinosis, Raynaud's phenomenon, esophageal dysmotility, sclerodactyly, and telangiectasia.

BOX 1: Treatment Options for Thromboangiitis Obliterans

Tobacco cessation*

Medical

Prostacyclin and its analogues
Aspirin
Selective low-dose intra-arterial streptokinase
Bosentan, a dual endothelin-1 receptor antagonist
Cyclophosphamide
Guanethidine sympathetic blocks
Serotonin blockers
Sarpogrelate
Intramuscular injections of vascular endothelial growth factor
Phosphodiesterase type 5 (PDE5) inhibitors

Endovascular Therapies

Extended angioplasty of each tibial and foot artery obstruction

Surgical Treatment

Sympathectomy
Arterial reconstruction
Omental transfer
Kirschner wire in medullary canal of tibia

Experimental Therapies

Intramuscular injection of vascular endothelial growth factor
Autologous whole bone marrow stem cell transplantation by fenestration
Immunoadsorption
Beperminogene perplasmid use

*Only known, proven, established, and effective therapy.

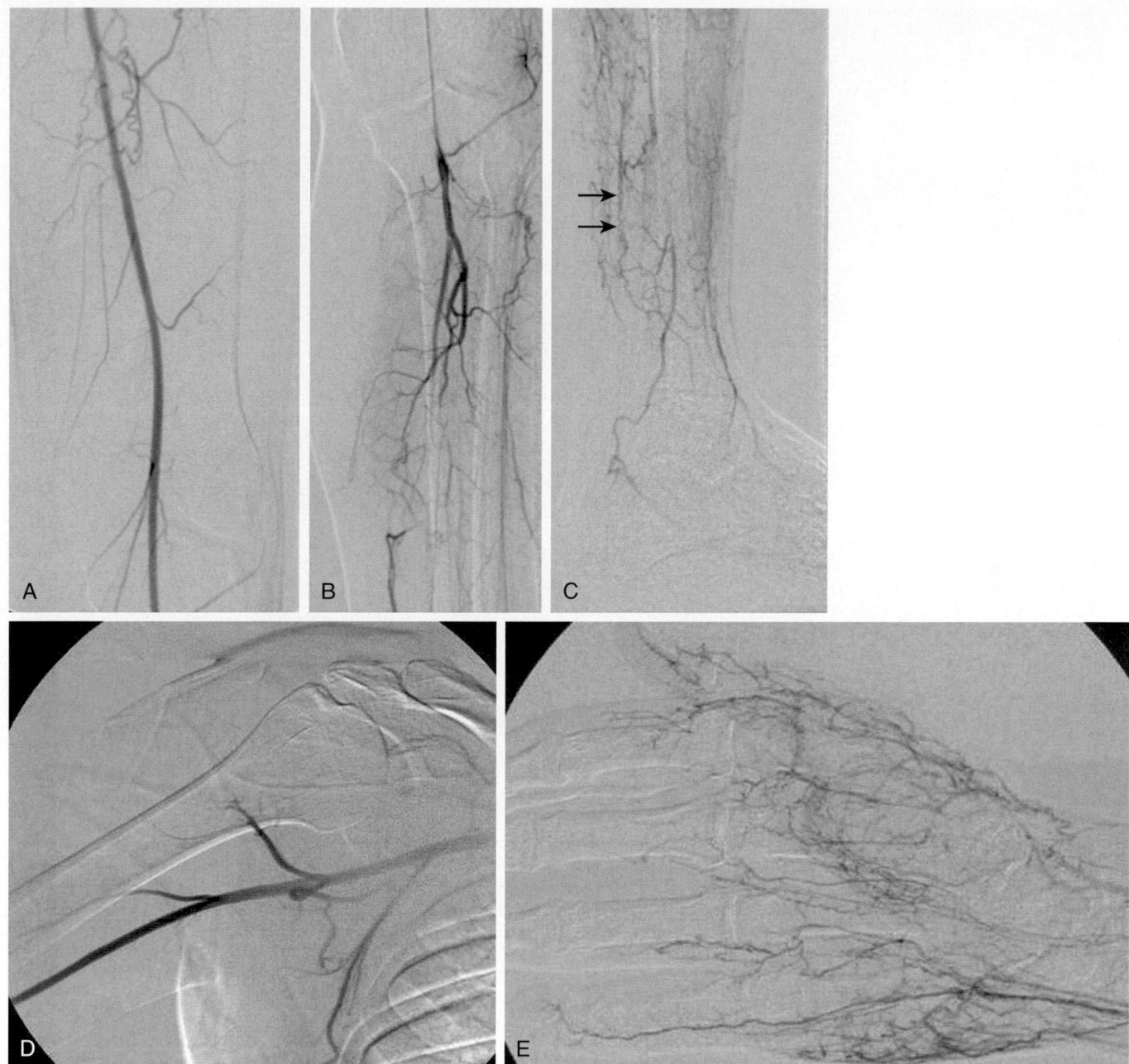

FIGURE 1 Angiogram of patient with Buerger's disease. **A,** The appearance of proximal lower extremity vessels is unremarkable. **B,** Distal runoffs show severe peripheral occlusive disease with corkscrew-appearing collaterals. **C,** Corkscrew collaterals (*arrows*) magnified. **D,** Upper extremity angiogram also reveals normal proximal vasculature. **E,** Distal occlusive disease with many collaterals. (*C,* *Courtesy Dr. Michael Costanza;* *E,* *Courtesy Dr. Thomas Reifsnyder.*)

Adjunctive Measures

Pain control and local wound care are standard measures. Other adjuncts, such as autologous bone marrow transplantation, autologous peripheral blood mononuclear cell implantation, hyperbaric oxygen therapy, and electrical spinal cord stimulation and subsequent permanent cervical epidural spinal cord stimulator implantation, have been used.

Experimental Therapies

The theory that TAO has an immunopathology related to autoantibodies has led to treatment with immunoadsorption. Other approaches involving gene therapy through intramuscular injection of vascular endothelial growth factor, performance of autologous whole bone marrow stem cell transplantation by fenestration, and introduction of a beperminogene perplasmid (the naked plasmid DNA encoding the complementary DNA of human hepatocyte growth factor) have been used in an effort to enhance angiogenesis (see Box 1). Although some progress has been suggested, larger randomized trials are necessary to evaluate the effectiveness of these therapies.

■ PROGNOSIS

Patients who stop tobacco use can avoid disease progression, but those who continue to use tobacco, smokeless tobacco, or

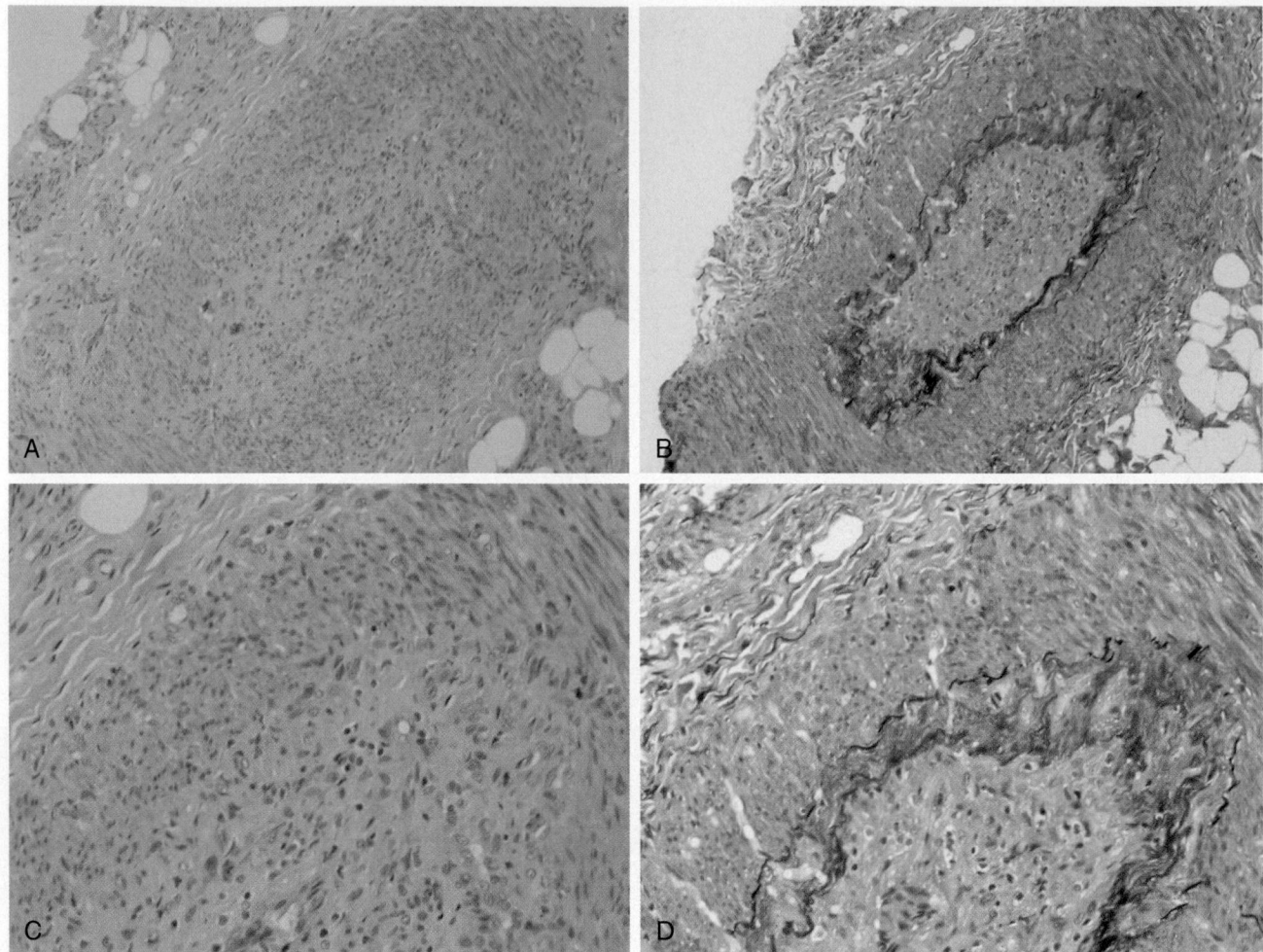

FIGURE 2 Arterial lesions in a case of Buerger's disease. **A,** The low magnification hematoxylin and eosin (H&E) staining shows an organizing inflammatory thrombus along with minor inflammatory infiltrate in the tunica media in a small artery. **B,** Low power elastic stain shows maintenance of the internal elastic lamina within the thrombus (50×). **C,** High power H&E stain demonstrates a thrombus largely composed of fibroblasts and chronic inflammatory cells obliterating the vascular lumen. **D,** Elastic stain at high power (200×). *(Images courtesy Tiffany Caza, MD, Department of Pathology, Upstate Medical Center, Syracuse, NY.)*

nicotine-containing products likely will have active disease and may progress to subsequent amputation. The risk of amputation is highly correlated with continuation of smoking. One review of 112 patients demonstrated that of the 43 patients who quit smoking, only 2 had amputations, whereas 22 patients who continued smoking required amputation. There may be periods of exacerbation and improvement over time. These patients need to be followed. Retrospective analysis of TAO patient outcomes demonstrated a cumulative survival rate of 84% up to 25 years from initial diagnosis.

■ CONCLUSION

TAO, or Buerger's disease, is a segmental nonatherosclerotic occlusive inflammatory condition of arteries and veins characterized by thrombosis and recanalization of small and medium-sized vessels. TAO is a disease found most often in young smokers and is affected by active use of tobacco. Other causes of limb ischemia such as embolization, atherosclerosis, and autoimmune disorders must be ruled out. Smoking cessation can be used in conjunction with other approaches to achieve limb salvage. A multimodal approach is used most often in advanced cases, with some benefit. Vascular and endovascular therapies have mixed results and depend mostly on the

ability to recanalize the tibial or plantar vessels. The goal is pain relief and healing of trophic lesions while also reducing the risk of amputation. Abstinence from tobacco is paramount to success in managing this disease. Ultimately, major amputation affects the patient's quality of life and long-term outcome.

SUGGESTED READINGS

Fujita Y. Classification of corkscrew collaterals in thromboangiitis obliterans (Buerger's disease). *Circ J*. 2010;74:1684-1688.

Jorge VC, Araujo AC, Noronha C, et al. Buerger's disease (thromboangiitis obliterans): a diagnostic challenge. *BMJ Case Rep*. 2011; bcr0820114621.

Ketha SS, Cooper LT. The role of autoimmunity in thromboangiitis obliterans (Buerger's disease). *Ann N Y Acad Sci*. 2013;1285:15-25. doi:10.1111/nyas.12048.

Mills JL Sr. Buerger disease in the 21st century: diagnosis, clinical features, and therapy. *Semin Vasc Surg*. 2003;16:179-189.

Mohler ER III, Olin JW. *Thromboangiitis obliterans (Buerger's disease)*. UpToDate. 2013;Available at: <http://www.uptodate.com/contents/thromboangiitis-obliterans-buergers-disease>.

Olin JW, Shih A. Thromboangiitis obliterans (Buerger's disease). *Curr Opin Rheumatol*. 2006;18:18-24.

Puechal X, Fiessinger JN. Thromboangiitis obliterans or Buerger's disease: challenges for the rheumatologist. *Rheumatology*. 2007;46:192-199.

ACUTE MESENTERIC ISCHEMIA

Mohammad H. Eslami, MD, FACS, FACC

Acute mesenteric ischemia (AMI) is an uncommon life-threatening clinical entity with a reported incidence rate of 0.09% to 0.2% per patient-year at tertiary referral centers. The main presentation of AMI is abdominal pain that is vague, varied, and similar to other pathologic abdominal conditions. In addition, there are no pathognomonic laboratory tests specific for AMI. Therefore it is often difficult to distinguish AMI from other pathologic conditions with any clinical certainty, and diagnostic confirmation invariably requires radiographic studies. These factors often lead to a significant delay in diagnosis and the institution of treatment. Because rapid diagnosis and revascularization are paramount to improving outcomes in patients with AMI, the delay in diagnosis and revascularization leads to persistently high mortality rates in patients with AMI. Because no significant advances have been made to more quickly diagnose this significantly morbid condition, the 30-day mortality rate remains high (32% to 80%). Accordingly, the index of suspicion for AMI should be high whenever a patient has acute onset of severe abdominal pain that is *out of proportion* to the physical findings. Once the diagnosis is made, prompt intervention is required to minimize morbidity and mortality.

AMI can result from any of four distinct processes: (1) embolic occlusion of the mesenteric circulation (usually the superior mesenteric artery [SMA]); (2) acute thrombosis of the mesenteric circulation; (3) intense splanchnic vasoconstriction—so-called nonocclusive mesenteric ischemia (NOMI)—which is usually associated with a low flow state or profound hypovolemia; or (4) mesenteric venous thrombosis (MVT). In older publications, arterial embolism of the SMA was noted to be the most common cause of AMI, accounting for 40% to 50% of AMI, followed by thrombotic causes (20% to 30%), NOMI (10% to 20%) and MVT (10%). In more contemporary studies from the Mayo Clinic and the Cleveland Clinic, however, arterial thrombosis was the most common cause (50% to 56%) of AMI. It is possible that the epidemiology of AMI has changed consistent with contemporary changes in the U.S. population, which is becoming older with higher rates of atherosclerosis.

■ CLINICAL PRESENTATION AND DIAGNOSIS

The classical presentation for patients with embolic disease of the mesenteric vessels is sudden onset of midabdominal pain that is described as being *out of proportion* to the physical findings and is associated with immediate bowel evacuation. In fact, only about one third of patients have the triad of classical symptoms, and this presentation is particularly classical for AMI due to SMA embolism. A study that considered all causes of AMI found that 95% of patients were seen with abdominal pain, 44% with nausea, 35% with vomiting, and 35% with diarrhea; however, only 16% were seen with blood per rectum. Patients with embolic occlusion of the mesenteric circulation typically have a history of recent cardiac events (e.g., myocardial infarction, atrial fibrillation, mural thrombus, mitral valve disease, or left ventricular aneurysm). In addition, a history of prior embolization to other arterial trees should raise the suspicion of mesenteric emboli significantly in patients with acute onset of abdominal pain.

Patients with thrombotic mesenteric occlusion also have sudden onset of severe midabdominal pain that is out of proportion to the physical findings, but unlike patients with acute embolic occlusion,

they typically have a history of chronic mesenteric ischemia (postprandial abdominal pain, history of food avoidance leading to significant weight loss) as well as other manifestations of diffuse atherosclerotic disease such as coronary or peripheral artery disease. In these patients, any clinical scenario leading to low flow or hypotension can result in thrombosis of SMA stenosis and mesenteric ischemia.

Patients with NOMI are seen somewhat differently. The pain reported is usually not as sudden as that noted with embolic or thrombotic occlusion; it is generally more diffuse and tends to wax and wane depending on the patient's hemodynamic stability in contradistinction to the progressively worsening abdominal pain associated with embolic or thrombotic causes of AMI. If abdominal pain is absent or if the patient in the intensive care unit is unresponsive, the diagnosis may be suggested by progressive abdominal distension with worsening acidosis. There should be a high index of suspicion among older patients with these symptoms who have a recent history of cardiogenic, hypovolemic, hemorrhagic, or septic shock.

Patients with MVT often have various nonspecific abdominal complaints; accordingly, this diagnosis may be especially challenging. Common complaints include nausea, vomiting, diarrhea, abdominal cramping, and nonlocalized abdominal pain. As a rule, these symptoms are *not acute*. The risk factors for MVT include a history of previous venous thrombosis or pulmonary embolism, a known or suspected hypercoagulable state, oral contraception, and estrogen supplementation. In a study of 31 patients who were seen with MVT at Northwestern University, 13 (42%) were diagnosed with a hypercoagulable state, 6 (19%) had a history of previous thrombotic episodes, and 4 (13%) had a history of cancer. The underlying ischemia in MVT is from vascular congestion due to poor venous outflow, which may be precipitated also by intra-abdominal inflammatory processes such as appendicitis, pancreatitis, or diverticulitis.

The diagnosis of AMI is made definitively using radiographic studies. There is no pathognomonic laboratory finding of mesenteric ischemia, and laboratory abnormalities seen with AMI are common to many other disease processes. Complete blood cell count may show hemoconcentration with increased hemoglobin and hematocrit. There is also typically a leukocytosis with "left shift." With advanced ischemia and bowel necrosis, metabolic acidosis occurs, and amylase, lactic dehydrogenase, and alkaline phosphatase levels are elevated. Neither plain abdominal radiographs nor duplex ultrasound is very helpful in establishing the diagnosis of AMI. Upper endoscopy and colonoscopy do not provide any useful information, and barium contrast evaluation is contraindicated. (Intraluminal barium can limit the visualization of the mesenteric arteries.) Computed tomographic (CT) scans are the most common studies used to establish the diagnosis of AMI. With the advent of helical multislice multiarray (spiral) CT scanning, the visceral arterial anatomy can be accomplished with three-dimensional (3D) spatial resolution (Figure 1). This technology allows much more rapid acquisition of data and has 96% accuracy in diagnosing AMI. Thus multidetector CT angiography (CTA) is the most useful and rapid tool for the fast and accurate diagnosis of AMI. Given the significant ease of obtaining a multidetector CTA, this study has become the most important radiologic study used to establish a diagnosis. Arterial and venous phase CTA can readily reveal SMA occlusion or thrombosis of the superior mesenteric vein (SMV), as well as associated bowel abnormalities (Figure 2).

Although angiography is considered the gold standard, given the current state of imaging technology, it is possible to confirm the diagnosis of AMI with CTA alone and proceed to operative intervention without conventional angiography. Angiography is still used if the diagnosis is not clear, endovascular interventions are contemplated, or further details of SMA anatomy are required for SMA revascularization. In modern operating rooms with fixed or mobile angiographic capabilities, intraoperative angiogram is feasible provided

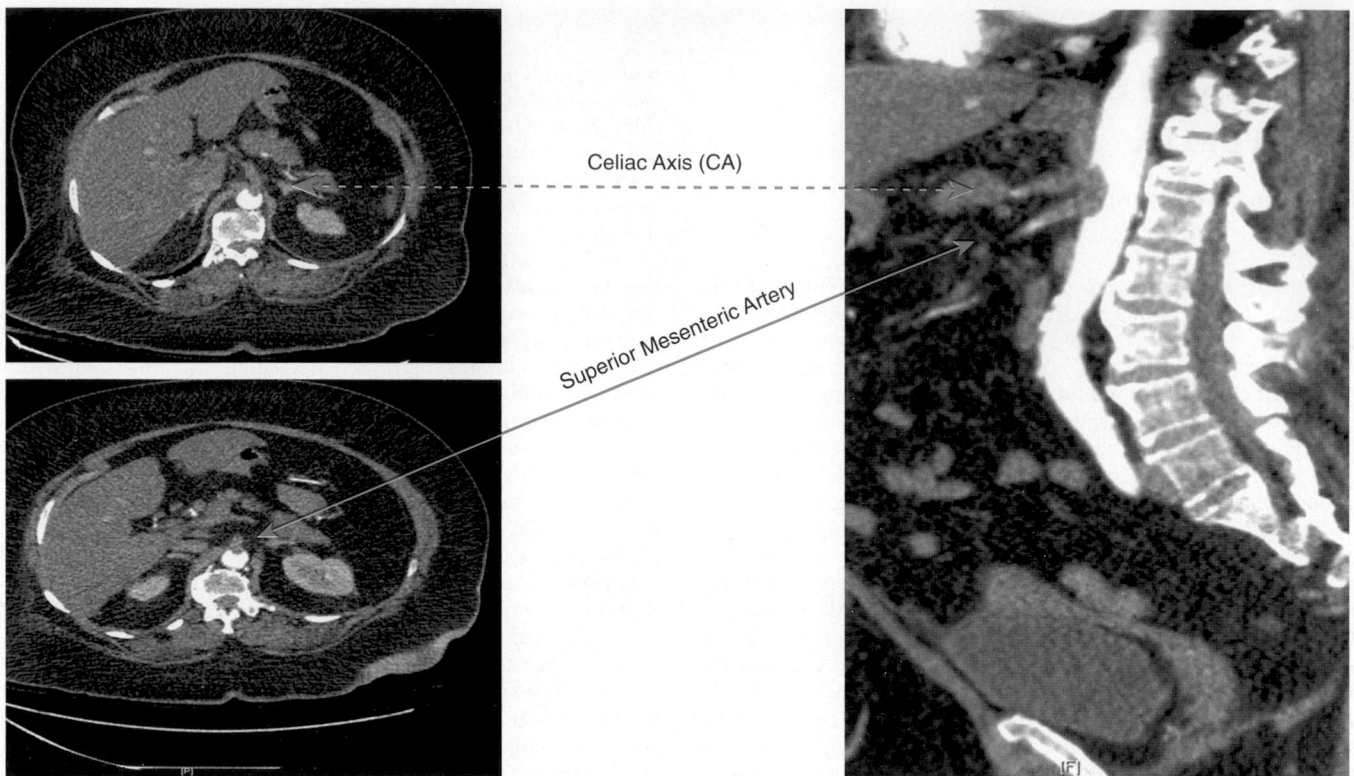

FIGURE 1 An unusual embolization to both the superior mesenteric artery and the celiac axis.

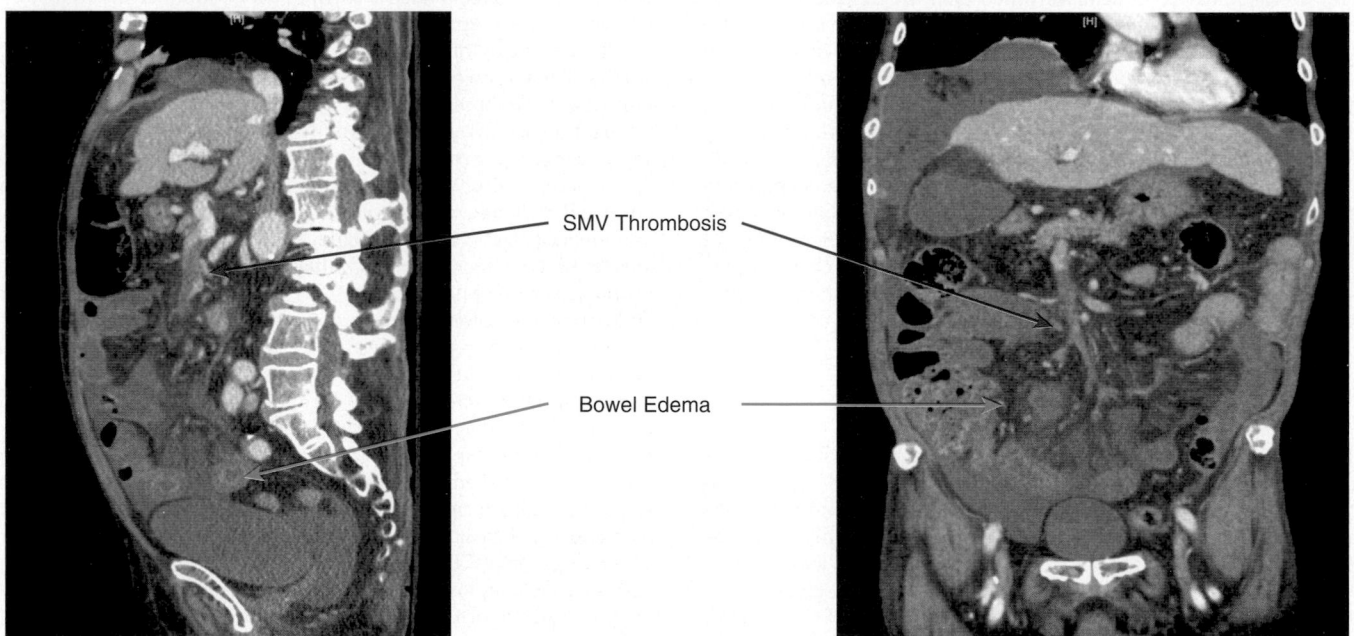

FIGURE 2 Superior mesenteric vein (SMV) thrombosis with bowel edema.

the patient is on a table where fluoroscopy is possible. Angiography with multiple views is needed for the adequate evaluation of the SMA and celiac artery (CA). The lateral views (Figure 3, *A*) are used to assess the origin of the CA and the SMA, whereas the circulation of the distal CA and SMA is best evaluated with the anteroposterior views (Figure 3, *B*). Selective catheterizations of the CA and the SMA also are needed for complete visualization of the anatomy and to define the pathophysiologic process. In mesenteric embolization (usually involving the SMA), the emboli that lodge at branch points create a "meniscus sign," with an abrupt occlusion of a normal proximal SMA several centimeters from its origin. In contrast, with mesenteric thrombosis, the lesion occurs near the origin and tapers off 1 to 2 cm distally. Usually patients with thrombosis have a history of chronic mesenteric ischemia, and collateral circulations such as

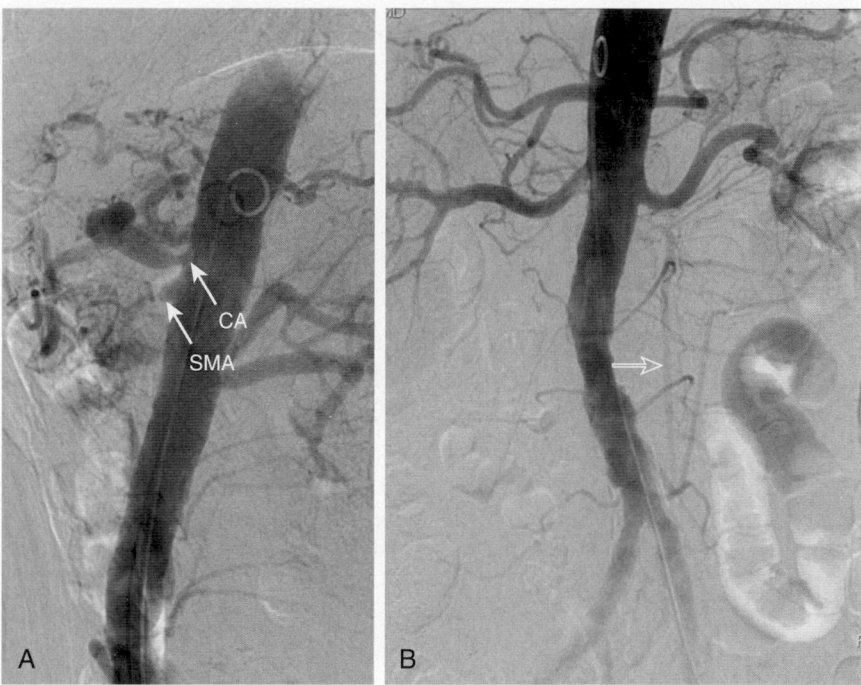

FIGURE 3 Acute-on-chronic mesenteric ischemia. Both lateral (**A**) and anteroposterior (**B**) images are needed to make the correct diagnosis. Hollow arrow points to a major collateral from the inferior mesenteric artery to the superior mesenteric artery–marginal artery of Drummond. *CA*, Celiac axis stenosis; *SMA*, superior mesenteric artery occlusion.

the arch of Riolan and the marginal arteries of Drummond can be visualized (see Figure 3, *B*). In NOMI, angiography shows a normal-appearing SMA with segments of vasospasm. In MVT, arterial circulation is intact but there are no delayed images of mesenteric veins (discussed later).

■ TREATMENT

Initial treatment of all patients with AMI includes fluid resuscitation, correction of metabolic acidosis with sodium bicarbonate, and administration of antibiotics. Anticoagulation with heparin is used to prevent further propagation of thrombus. Patient hemodynamic status is monitored carefully in the intensive care unit. Mesenteric angiography or abdominal CTA is performed immediately to confirm the diagnosis and to plan for appropriate intervention according to the cause of the ischemia. The goals in the surgical treatment of AMI are (1) to restore normal pulsatile flow to the SMA, (2) to resect any nonviable intestine, and (3) to restore intestinal continuity once mesenteric revascularization is achieved. In general, revascularization precedes resection because this will lead to improvement of partially ischemic intestine that might not need resection after revascularization. The therapeutic approach varies, depending on the specific underlying pathophysiologic causes of AMI (Table 1; Figures 4 to 6). Exposure of the SMA and CA is critical in the operative plan for embolic and thrombotic causes of AMI, and the surgeon must be familiar with the exposure of these vessels as well as of the suprarenal and infrarenal aorta, which may serve as the inflow vessel.

Embolism of Mesenteric Artery

In acute embolic mesenteric ischemia, the treatment is surgical or endovascular removal of the embolus to restore arterial blood flow. A midline incision is made, and the extent of the mesenteric ischemia and bowel necrosis is assessed. There is usually variable bowel ischemia from the midjejunum to the transverse colon. Bowel resection usually is delayed until revascularization of the mesenteric artery.

There are two intraperitoneal methods for the exposure of the SMA. In the lateral approach to expose the SMA, the transverse colon is reflected superiorly and the small bowel is retracted to the right upper quadrant. The ligament of Treitz is divided to mobilize the fourth portion of the duodenum. The SMA is palpated at the root of the mesentery over the junction of the third and fourth portions of the duodenum. In the anterior approach, after superior retraction of the transverse colon, small intestines are retracted to the right. The middle colic artery is traced proximally, and a horizontal excision at the root of the mesentery is made. The SMA is identified medial to the SMV after careful dissection of surrounding lymphatic and autonomic nerve fibers. Proximal and distal vascular control of the proximal SMA segment is obtained in the standard manner. A longitudinal arteriotomy, rather than transverse arteriotomy, is made, and an embolectomy balloon catheter is passed proximally and distally to ensure complete removal of the embolus. When proximal inflow and distal backflow are adequate, an autogenous or cryopreserved vein patch is used for closure of the arteriotomy. If embolectomy is unsuccessful in re-establishing blood flow, this longitudinal arteriotomy can be used for distal anastomoses of the bypass graft (Figure 7).

An alternative to open surgical technique is percutaneous embolectomy. In this technique, which should be used very selectively and only in patients without peritoneal signs, an infusion catheter is placed in the SMA and thrombolytic agents are infused while the patient is observed closely in the intensive care unit. There are reports of successful use of thrombolytic therapy with or without percutaneous mechanical thrombectomy catheters. At the current time, this should be performed only very selectively among patients with AMI with minimal abdominal pain at the time of presentation and should be abandoned for open repair if the patient develops worsening of abdominal symptoms.

After restoration of mesenteric blood flow, the viability of the bowel is assessed. Segments of bowel whose viability was equivocal previously may improve after revascularization. Intravenous fluorescein injection followed by Wood's lamp inspection and Doppler imaging can assist in assessing the viability of the bowel. If bowel

TABLE 1: Pathophysiology of the Four Different Causes of Acute Mesenteric Ischemia (AMI)

Cause	Pathophysiology
Embolism	• Often in patients with atrial fibrillation • Emboli lodge 3-10 cm distal to origin of SMA (see Figure 4), often past branching of middle colic artery (see Figure 5) • Proximal midjejunum is spared
Thrombosis	• Typically these patients have a history of symptomatic stenosis of mesenteric arteries (see Figure 6) • Any clinical scenario that leads to low flow or hypotension can result in acute-on-chronic arterial thrombosis • Affects the orifice of the SMA (see Figure 6) • Flush occlusion of the SMA and the entire middle gut is involved during the initial presentation
Nonocclusive	• Low flow state resulting from any type of shock or the use of vasoconstrictors • The entire bowel may be involved
Mesenteric venous thrombosis	• Thrombosis of the veins draining the intestines; SMV, IMV, splenic and portal veins among hypercoagulable patients with cancer or hypercoagulable state • Decreased venous outflow, bowel edema, distension, and decreased mesenteric perfusion

IMV, Inferior mesenteric vein; *SMA,* superior mesenteric artery.

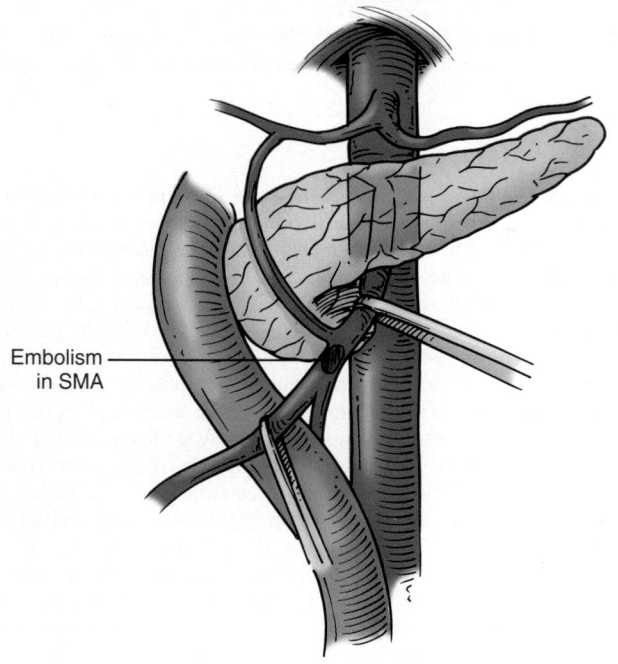

FIGURE 4 Embolization of the superior mesenteric artery (SMA).

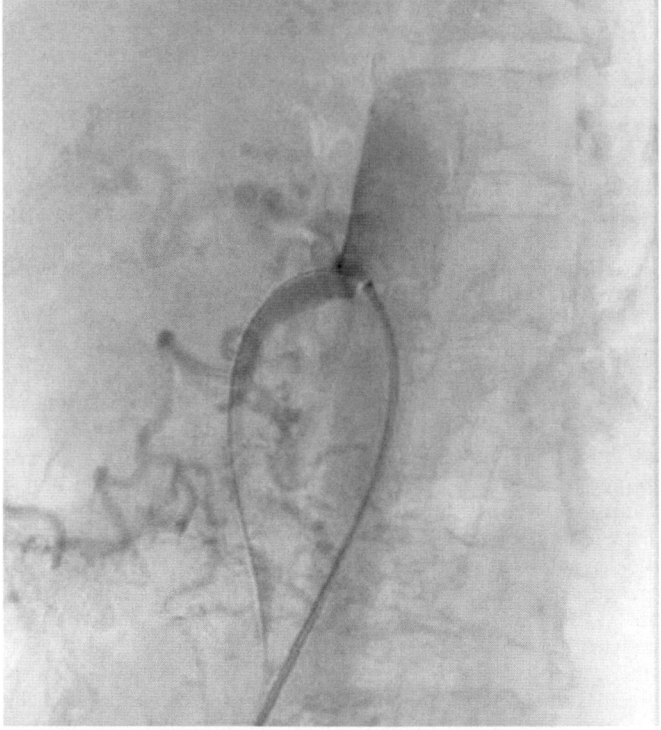

FIGURE 5 Angiogram of acute mesenteric ischemia related to superior mesenteric artery emboli, often sparing the jejunal branches.

viability remains questionable, a second-look operation can be performed in 24 to 36 hours. This allows for bowel resection to be limited and ensures that bowel anastomoses are performed with viable bowel. Many authors recommend performing a second-look operation within 24 to 36 hours on all patients with AMI because second-look laparotomy is the most reliable means of determining the viability of marginally perfused bowel after revascularization. A second-look laparotomy should be preceded by adequate fluid resuscitation and correction of the acid-base imbalance. Occasionally, even though the patient is in better physical condition 24 to 48 hours after revascularization, there is still some necrotic bowel that must be resected. Accordingly, I adhere to a strict policy of planned re-exploration for patients with AMI who require any bowel

resection during the initial operation or who have areas of marginally viable bowel after revascularization.

Thrombosis of Mesenteric Artery

Surgical treatment is more challenging with AMI due to thrombosis of the mesenteric artery than with AMI due to SMA embolism, as these visceral vessels are often abnormal. The treatment consists of a bypass procedure to a distal normal visceral artery, which may be done in either an antegrade manner (Figure 8) from the proximal supraceliac abdominal aorta or in a retrograde manner (Figure 9) from the distal abdominal aorta or iliac artery. The conduit of choice is a reversed autologous greater saphenous vein graft, as these patients often require bowel resection and the operative field is often contaminated because of transmural bowel infarction and perforation. If native vein is not available, the alternative choice is cryopreserved vein or rifampin-soaked Dacron grafts. Another surgical technique is trapdoor thromboendarterectomy of the aorta and endarterectomy of the proximal SMA and CA with patch angioplasty with autogenous patch material. This technique leads to very limited exposure of the proximal SMA and CA and is rarely performed in an emergent fashion.

As noted, there are several different inflow options for revascularizing the SMA that must be considered carefully. The main choices for inflow are the supraceliac aorta, the infrarenal aorta, and the iliac artery. The choice of inflow should be selected carefully and is based mainly on the familiarity of the surgeon with the specific exposures and how quickly each can be performed to establish inflow. If the

surgeon is not familiar with the supraceliac exposure, he or she should perform a retrograde bypass from the infrarenal aorta or the iliac artery. If the surgeon is familiar with the supraceliac aorta, this is a better choice of inflow because of lack of atherosclerotic changes of the proximal abdominal aorta. Another advantage of antegrade bypass is that an antegrade graft from the suprarenal aorta to the SMA is often shorter, will lie better, and is less susceptible to kinking than a retrograde graft once the bowel is restored to its correct anatomic position. This exposure is challenging in obese patients, and it requires supraceliac aortic occlusion that may cause significant hemodynamic instability in these patients during clamping and declamping of the proximal abdominal aorta. The advantage of retrograde bypass (see Figure 9) is the ease of exposure of the infrarenal aorta and iliac, but there is high likelihood of kinking in the retrograde bypass, and the donor vessels are frequently involved with atherosclerotic disease.

In antegrade bypass (see Figure 8), the initial exposure of the supraceliac aorta is accomplished by dividing the gastrohepatic ligament and mobilizing the left lobe of the liver. The esophagus is retracted to the left, and division of the diaphragmatic crura and median arcuate ligament provides exposure of the distal 10 cm of thoracic aorta without division of the diaphragm. Often the origin of the CA has been dissected already during exposure of the aorta, and dissection is continued distally until a soft, patent distal target is reached. The SMA is dissected at the root of the mesentery, as described previously. The vein graft is bypassed first to the CA and then sequentially to the SMA via a tunnel behind the pancreas. In patients without bowel infarct, a synthetic graft can be used very cautiously. If a bifurcated synthetic graft is used, the proximal aortic graft is beveled and sutured to the supraceliac aorta. The limbs are cut into appropriate lengths and anastomosed to the CA and the SMA.

In retrograde bypass, the most proximal SMA segment that is patent is exposed as it exits from behind the pancreas. This decreases the risk of kinking in the bypass graft. This anastomosis is completed first, and the bowel is returned to its anatomic position. The bypass graft is then pulled and placed adjacent to the aorta. A soft spot on the infrarenal aorta or the iliac artery is located and used for the proximal anastomosis. Tension is maintained on the vein graft during anastomosis to avoid graft laxity and kinking (see Figure 9, *A*). Revascularization to the CA usually is performed via the common hepatic artery (see Figure 9, *B*) or, less commonly, via the splenic artery. The distal anastomosis is again performed first, and the graft is pulled taut behind the duodenum and the head of pancreas. The graft is tunneled behind the tail of the pancreas and, if the distal anastomosis is to the splenic artery, anterior to the left renal vein.

A percutaneous approach to revascularization and thrombectomy of occluded SMA can be successful (Figure 10). In patients with

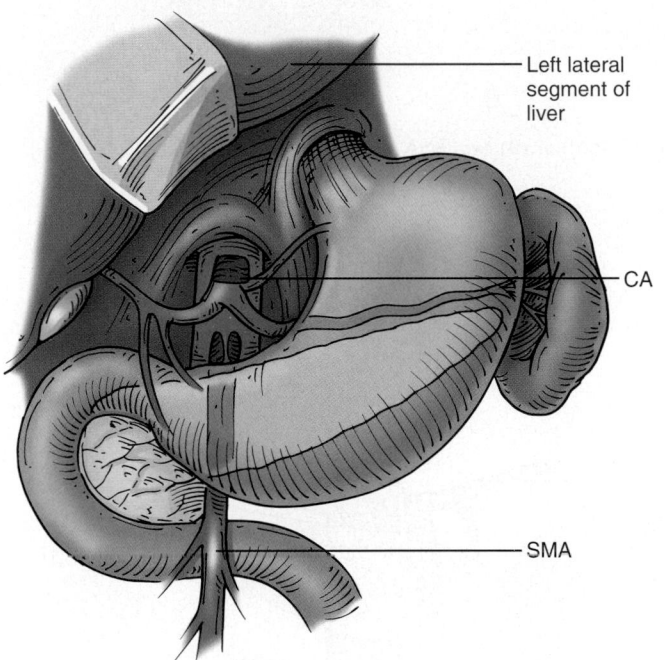

Left lateral segment of liver

CA

SMA

FIGURE 6 Stenotic narrowing at the orifice of the superior mesenteric artery (SMA) and celiac axis (CA).

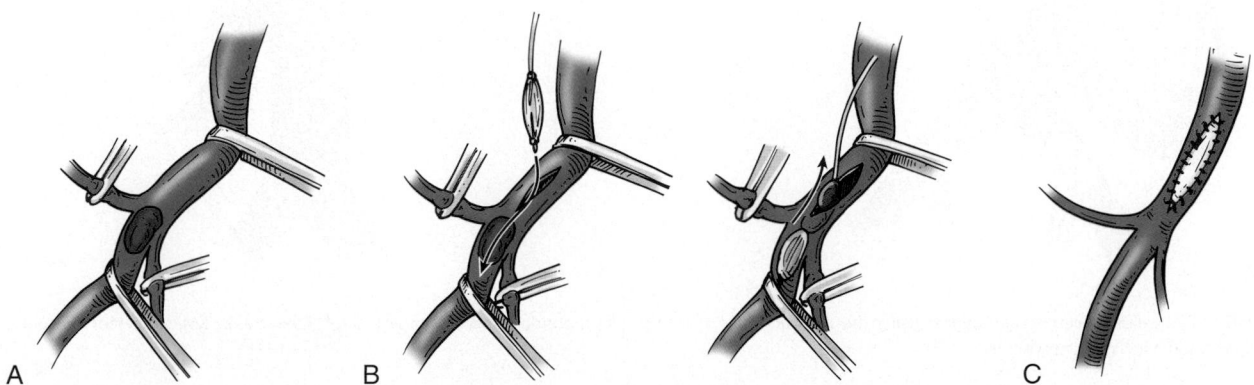

A   B   C

FIGURE 7 Open embolectomy and patch angioplasty. Either autogenous or cryopreserved vein should be used. **A,** Vessel control. **B,** Embolectomy. **C,** Patch angioplasty.

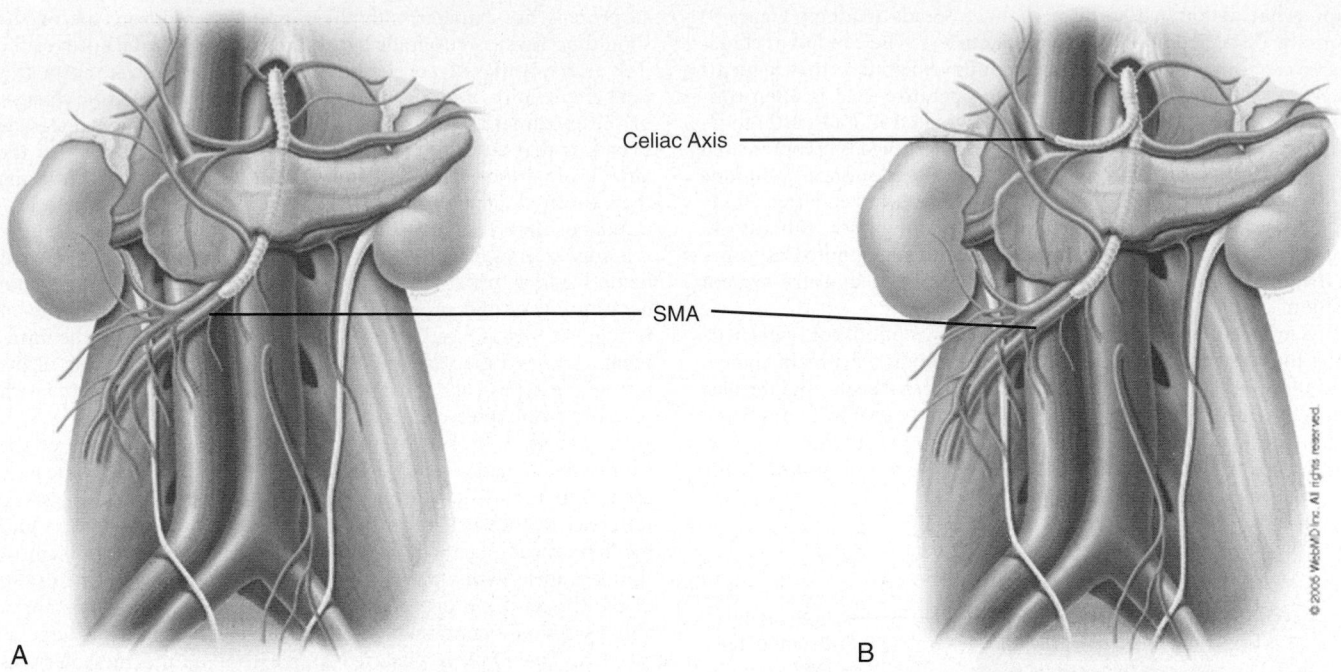

FIGURE 8 Antegrade bypass using either (**A**) one (superior mesenteric artery [SMA]) or (**B**) two (SMA and celiac axis) vessels. *(© WebMD, 2006.)*

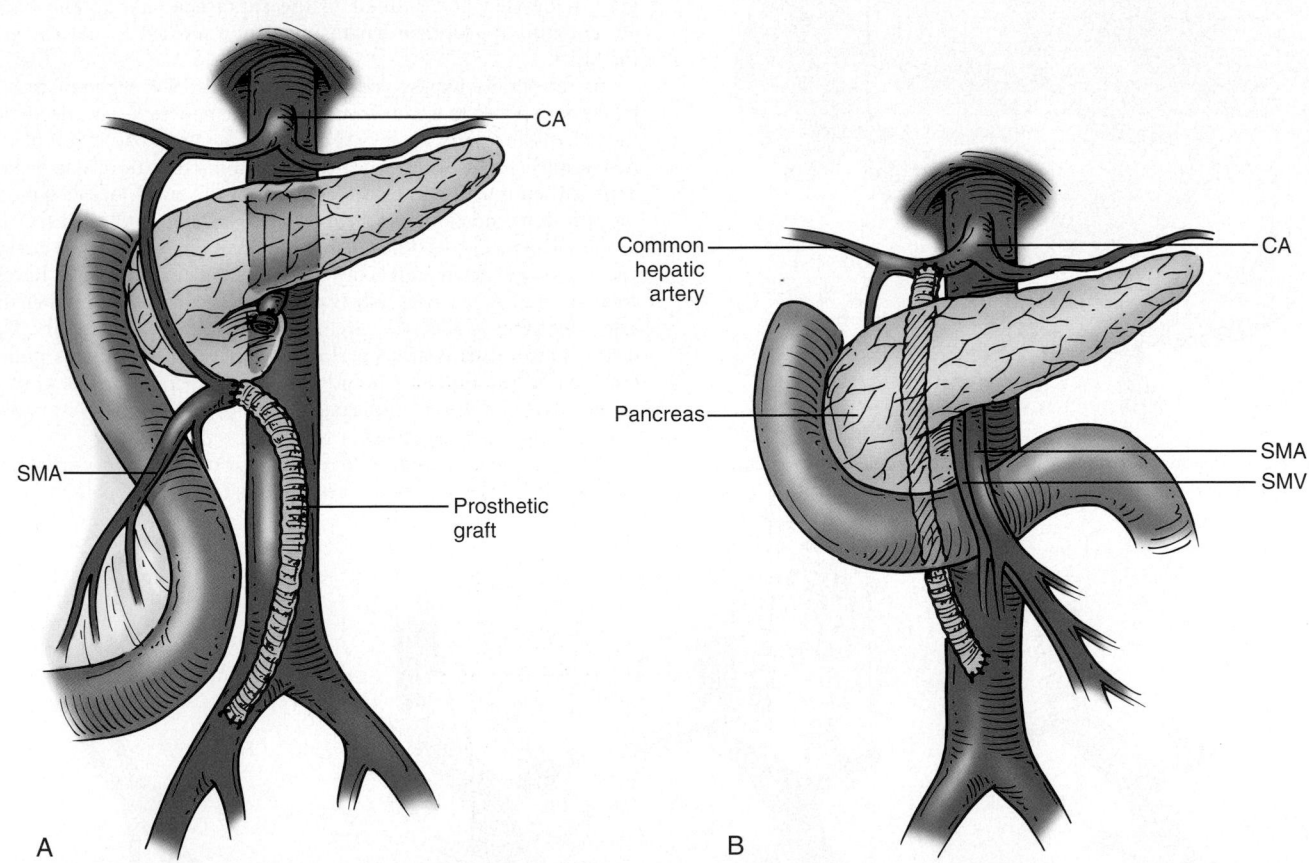

FIGURE 9 Examples of retrograde bypass using the common iliac artery as (**A**) a conduit and (**B**) an aorta. *CA*, Celiac axis; *SMA*, superior mesenteric artery; *SMV*, superior mesenteric vein.

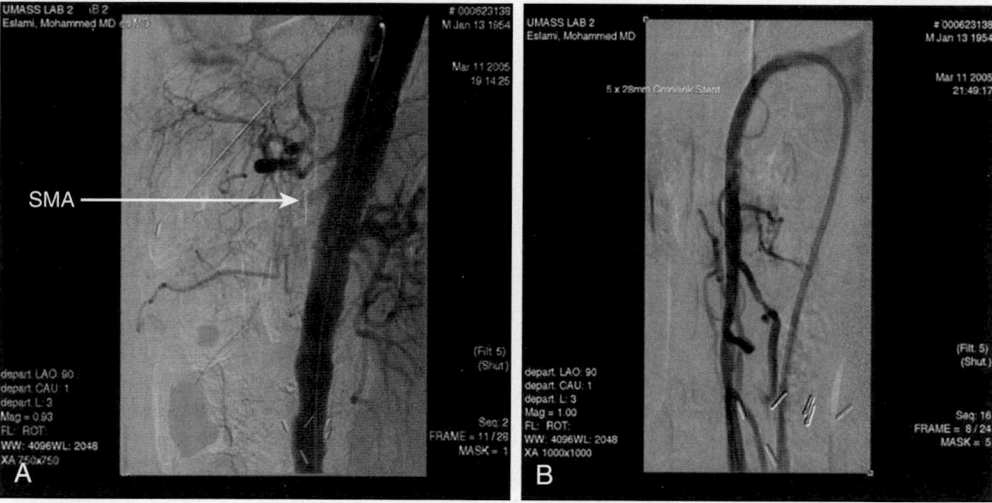

FIGURE 10 Endovascular revascularization of (**A**) a completely occluded superior mesenteric artery (SMA), which (**B**) was traversed and stented.

medical comorbid conditions who are at high risk for open surgical interventions, endovascular therapy is a useful, less invasive treatment modality. Arterial access is obtained in a common femoral artery. Left brachial arterial access may be needed in mesenteric arteries that branch in an acute angle from the aorta. A diagnostic catheter is placed in the proximal abdominal aorta below the diaphragm. Lateral aortography is used to assess the origin of the CA and the SMA (see Figure 10, *A*), and anteroposterior mesenteric angiography is used to assess the distal mesenteric circulation. An angled catheter is used to catheterize the CA and SMA, and selective mesenteric angiography is performed. When the location of the lesion is identified, a 6F or 7F working sheath is placed with the tip at the origin of the mesenteric artery, and the lesion is crossed with a wire. For occlusive lesions, a trial of lytic therapy is undertaken, whereby a thrombolytic agent is given via an infusion catheter that is placed across the length of the occluded arterial segment. Any residual stenotic lesion identified on angiography can be treated with balloon angioplasty. Postangioplasty angiography is performed to assess for evidence of possible suboptimal angioplasty results, such as dissection or residual stenosis. If any are observed, the lesion is best treated by placement of covered or uncovered stents (see Figure 10, *B*).

More recently, a hybrid technique that successfully combines open laparotomy and endovascular approach for the treatment of thrombotic occlusion of an atherosclerotic SMA lesion has been described. In this approach, the infracolic SMA is exposed (discussed earlier), and after thrombectomy and patch angioplasty a 10-cm 6F or 7F sheath is placed in the infracolic SMA through the distal end of the patch for retrograde cannulation and stenting of the proximal SMA lesion. Once the proximal lesion is crossed, the stenosis is angioplastied and stented as described earlier. This hybrid technique is an attractive alternative to the traditional surgical approach because it combines open laparotomy and bowel assessment with a rapid approach to revascularization that limits ischemic time and does not require aortic clamping. Initially this technique was described using mobile fluoroscopy units, but with the rapid acquisition of hybrid operating rooms with fixed fluoroscopic units, this hybrid technique may and should supplant open revascularization. Reporting their results on 68 patients, Blauw and colleagues reported excellent results using this technique. Given the advantages noted earlier and further familiarity of vascular surgeons with endovascular techniques, this hybrid technique may replace open thromboendarterectomy.

Nonocclusive Mesenteric Ischemia

Management of NOMI is largely nonoperative and supportive. Once the diagnosis has been established with angiography, treatment of the underlying precipitating cause is the key therapeutic intervention. Optimization of fluid resuscitation, improvement of cardiac output, and elimination of vasopressors are the measures that have the greatest impact on outcome. Selective catheterization of the SMA with direct intra-arterial infusion of vasodilators such as papaverine (30 to 60 mg/hr) may be used as adjunctive therapy. The infusion is continued for at least 24 hours, with repeat angiography performed at regular intervals to determine the effectiveness of this therapy. Other local vasodilator agents used with some success include intra-arterial administration of a combination of tolazoline and glycerol trinitrate or prostaglandin E1. System anticoagulation is achieved with heparin, given via peripheral intravenous catheter, to prevent thrombosis in the catheterized vessels. Vasoconstricting agents also should be stopped. The hemodynamic status of the patient is monitored for any hypotension that may signify systemic infusion of the vasodilator with migration of the infusion catheter into the aorta. The patient's response and clinical status are observed closely. If abdominal symptoms improve, mesenteric angiography is repeated to ensure resolution of the vasospasm and perfusion of the bowel. If the patient has or develops peritoneal signs on physical examination, an exploratory laparotomy will be required for resection of frankly necrotic or gangrenous bowel. If an intra-arterial infusion of papaverine has been initiated, it should be continued throughout the exploratory laparotomy. Given the known propensity of this disease process for waxing and waning, a second-look laparotomy is also imperative.

Mesenteric Vein Thrombosis

In addition to the initial management with fluid resuscitation and anticoagulation (described previously), patients need to be evaluated for hypercoagulopathy and hypercoagulable states such as cancer. Surgical exploration is indicated in a patient with signs of bowel ischemia and infarction. Surgery should be limited to bowel resection because venous thrombectomy has not been shown to be effective. Bowel resection is generous, and repeated surgical explorations may be necessary to ensure adequate bowel resection.

In patients who do not have peritonitis but continue to have abdominal pain despite resuscitation and anticoagulation, catheter-directed thrombolytic therapy is potentially useful. The thrombolytic agent is delivered to the mesenteric venous circulation via catheter-directed infusion of the splenic artery and the SMA (Figure 11). Bilateral common femoral arterial access is obtained for placement of two catheters for the infusion of the two mesenteric arteries. The thrombolytic agent is infused slowly overnight, and angiography is repeated in 24 hours to assess for progress of lytic therapy. If there is residual thrombus, slow thrombolytic therapy is continued for

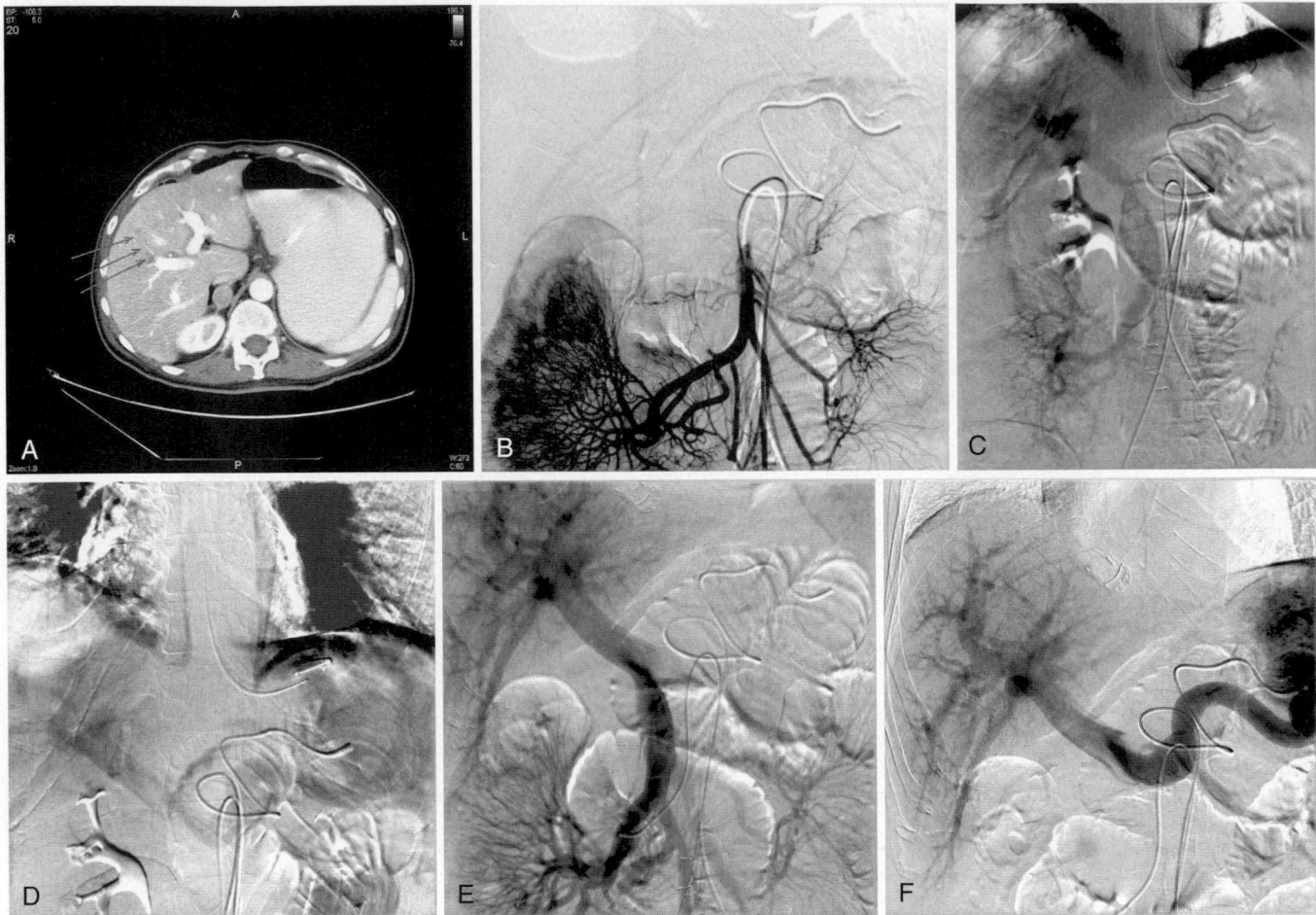

FIGURE 11 Hepatic venous thrombosis. **A,** Computed tomographic scan showing thrombus. **B,** Angiogram of the superior mesenteric artery (SMA). **C,** Catheter in the SMA, delayed imaging showed patent mesenteric venous outflow. **D,** Catheter in splenic artery, delayed imaging showed patent splenic and portal veins, with poor visualization of hepatic veins. **E,** After thrombolytic therapy, angiogram from the SMA catheter showed patent mesenteric and hepatic veins. **F,** Angiogram from the splenic catheter showing patent splenic, portal, and hepatic veins.

another 24 hours. After a maximum of 48 hours of lytic therapy, sheaths and catheters are removed, and the patient starts taking anticoagulants while being monitored closely for any peritoneal signs that may require laparotomy.

Outcome After Surgical Treatment

Most studies that include a large number of patients with AMI report perioperative mortalities ranging from 32% to 69% and 5-year survival rates ranging from 18% to 50%. In a recent meta-analysis, Cudnik and colleagues reported a pooled mortality rate of 47% among the patients who had surgical revascularization (range, 22% to 72%). These authors observed a mortality rate of 100% when no revascularization was attempted in 23 case series studies they evaluated. A retrospective study in 2012 reviewed the institutional experience at the Mayo Clinic over a 20-year period starting in 1990, with an overall 30-day perioperative mortality of 23%. The authors divided their series into 2 decades and although they noted a slightly lower mortality rate in the 2000s (17% vs 27% in 1990s), the differences were not statistically significant ($P = 0.28$). The relatively stable mortality rates have been observed in other studies and most recently reported by us, using a large administrative database and evaluating outcomes among patients who were seen with AMI and underwent a revascularization procedure. In most studies the most significant factor associated with mortality was bowel resection at the time of

initial operation. In our large administrative retrospective analysis, we observed a similar trend, with bowel resection increasing the odds of mortality by 2.88-fold (95% confidence interval [CI]: 2.01 to 4.12, $P < 0.001$) regardless of the type of revascularization procedures. In addition, the specific cause of the ischemia affects mortality rates differently. Within the category of arterial causes, mortality was 54.1% after treatment of arterial embolic disease, 77.4% after treatment of arterial thrombotic disease, and 72.7% after treatment of NOMI. The difference in mortality between embolic and thrombotic disease may be accounted for by the tendency of thrombosis to occur more proximally and thus to be associated with a greater degree of bowel infarction than embolic disease, as well as by the fact that patients with thrombotic disease have a greater burden of underlying cardiovascular comorbidity.

Independent predictors of survival include age less than 60 years, bowel resection, and the absence of a recent major cardiovascular procedure. In our recent analysis using a large administrative study, in addition to bowel resection (as noted earlier), advanced age and a history of congestive heart failure and open operations (vs endovascular interventions) independently led to increased odds of postoperative mortality. Despite significant increases in the use of endovascular revascularization, however, the mortality rate for AMI remains unchanged, as the most important factors predicting mortality are the duration of ischemia and delayed diagnosis (as noted previously).

SUGGESTED READINGS

Arthurs ZM, Titus J, Bannazadeh M, et al. A comparison of endovascular revascularization with traditional therapy for the treatment of acute mesenteric ischemia. *J Vasc Surg.* 2011;53:698-704, discussion 704-705.

Blauw JTM, Meerwaldt R, Brusse-Keizer M, et al. Retrograde open mesenteric stenting for acute mesenteric ischemia. *J Vasc Surg.* 2014;60:726-734.

Cudnik MT, Darbha S, Jones J, Macedo J, et al. The diagnosis of acute mesenteric ischemia: a systematic review and meta-analysis. *Acad Emerg Med.* 2013;20:1087-1100.

Eslami MH, Rybin D, Doros G, et al. Mortality of acute mesenteric ischemia remains unchanged despite significant increase in utilization of endovascular techniques. *Vascular.* 2016;24:44-52.

Park WM, Gloviczki P, Cherry KJ Jr, et al. Contemporary management of acute mesenteric ischemia: factors associated with survival. *J Vasc Surg.* 2002;35:445-452.

Ryer EJ, Kalra M, Oderich GS, et al. Revascularization for acute mesenteric ischemia. *J Vasc Surg.* 2012;55:1682-1689.

Schoots IG, Koffeman GI, Legemate DA, et al. Systematic review of survival after acute mesenteric ischemia according to disease etiology. *Br J Surg.* 2004;91:17-27.

Wind GG, Valentine RJ. Celiac and mesenteric arteries. In: *Anatomic Exposures in Vascular Surgery*. Philadelphia: Lippincott; 2013:273-295.

Wyers MC, Powell RN, Nolan BW, et al. Retrograde mesenteric stenting during laparotomy for acute mesenteric ischemia. *J Vasc Surg.* 2007;45:269-275.

THE MANAGEMENT OF CHRONIC MESENTERIC ISCHEMIA

Dennis F. Bandyk, MD

Chronic mesenteric ischemia (CMI) results from inadequate arterial perfusion of the abdominal viscera. Postprandial pain is the hallmark of CMI, also termed *intestinal angina*, and caused by episodic gut ischemia induced by eating as a result of multivessel visceral artery stenosis or occlusion. In the fasting state, gut and organ perfusion is normal, but the fixed occlusive lesion limits the increase in visceral blood flow required in the postprandial state. Patients with this gastrointestinal (GI) condition are seen with sitophobia (fear of eating because of abdominal pain), which prevents adequate nutrition and causes progressive and potentially life-threatening weight loss. In symptomatic patients the superior mesenteric artery (SMA) is always diseased, either occluded or severely stenotic (i.e., >70% diameter reduction). CMI is a precursor to intestinal infarction, which is a lethal event when visceral involvement is extensive or the diagnosis is delayed. Therefore the goal of treatment is to restore gut perfusion by either endovascular intervention or open visceral artery bypass. Revascularization relieves symptoms, results in weight gain, and provides durable protection from intestinal infarction. Like most disorders of arterial hypoperfusion, visceral blood flow may be diminished by conditions other than arterial obstruction, such as venous obstruction or systemic conditions that produce global hypoperfusion of the gut, but these conditions typically produce *acute* mesenteric ischemia.

Atherosclerosis of the aorta involving the origins of the SMA and celiac artery is the most common cause of CMI. Dissection of the SMA or arteritis of the visceral arteries also may cause CMI but is less common. Asymptomatic occlusive disease involving the visceral arteries is commonplace in older patients (observed in up to 20% of those over 65 years of age) because of the abundant collateral routes between the celiac artery, SMA, and inferior mesenteric artery (IMA). In general, symptomatic CMI requires hemodynamically significant occlusive disease that involves at least two of the three visceral arteries and that always involves the SMA. The most common disease pattern is involvement of the SMA and celiac artery, but CMI can result from SMA occlusion with the IMA developing into a major collateral (meandering mesenteric artery). The occlusive lesions typically involve the origins of the visceral arteries, often with concomitant aortic plaque (i.e., coral reef atherosclerosis). Least common are stenotic lesions involving long segments of the SMA and its branches. The anatomic disease pattern dictates which treatment option is most appropriate. For example, atherosclerotic lesions limited to 1 to 2 cm

of a proximal visceral artery segment is best treated by stent angioplasty (Figure 1). By contrast, arterial dissection (fibromuscular dysplasia) and arteritis (Takayasu's disease, polyarteritis nodosa) generally affect long segments involving both the main trunk and its branches and may require bypass grafting. Compression of the celiac artery by the median arcuate ligament of the diaphragm is an uncommon cause for postprandial abdominal pain. The abdominal pain in this syndrome in part may be neurologic in origin because of celiac ganglion compression and not be associated with reduced stomach perfusion.

■ DIAGNOSTICS

Duplex ultrasound testing has evolved to be a clinically useful modality for the evaluation of CMI due to visceral artery origin atherosclerosis. Patients with known or suspected CMI can be scanned to identify stenosis or occlusion of the celiac, superior mesenteric, and inferior mesenteric arteries. Testing requires expertise in abdominal ultrasound imaging and arterial duplex scan interpretation as well as a fundamental understanding of visceral artery hemodynamics and collateral pathways created as a result of occlusive lesions. Duplex imaging of the pararenal aorta is best performed in the morning after an overnight fast, which minimizes presence of bowel gas to optimize conditions for the vascular technologist to identify and interrogate the visceral arteries. A slight reverse Trendelenburg or head elevated position can be helpful for para-aortic segment imaging. Renal arteries and the left renal vein anterior to the aorta are reliable landmarks to then image the origins of the SMA and celiac artery. Both transverse and sagittal scan planes should be used to image the celiac trunk and SMA origins and to acquire Doppler angle correction velocity spectra from the origin and mid-SMA, celiac artery trunk, hepatic artery, and (if possible) splenic artery. Often a Doppler angle of less than 30 degrees is required to acquire velocity spectra from the celiac artery origin. Disease classification is based on measurements of peak systolic velocity (PSV), end diastolic velocity (EDV), and changes in the SMA velocity spectral waveform from a fasting to postprandial state (Box 1). Significant ($\geq$70% diameter reduction [DR]) stenosis (i.e., pressure- or flow-reducing lesion) is associated with color power Doppler lumen reduction on imaging with elevated blood flow velocity, PSV greater than 275 to 300 cm/s, and EDV greater than 45 to 55 cm/s (Figure 2). The spectral waveform at and immediately distal to the stenosis should demonstrate turbulence that abates farther downstream when damping of the velocity waveform occurs (Figure 3). A mesenteric-aortic PSV ratio greater than 3 is also predictive of more than 50% DR stenosis. Aburahma and colleagues reported a PSV threshold of 400 cm/s for more than 70% stenosis of the SMA (overall accuracy of 85%) and of 320 cm/s for more than 70% stenosis of the celiac artery origin (overall accuracy of 85%). An interpretable study is possible in more than 80% of individuals, with excessive bowel gas being the primary reason for a suboptimal study. Visceral duplex testing should be considered a screening diagnostic modality that complements clinical assessment of patients with suspected CMI, and when abnormal it should prompt additional arterial imaging such as computed tomographic angiography (CTA) to confirm disease severity and plan intervention.

■ RECONSTRUCTION OPTIONS

Reconstruction options for visceral arterial occlusive disease take three forms: endovascular intervention by stent angioplasty, endarterectomy, and open bypass grafting.

Endovascular Therapy

Intraluminal stent angioplasty is best suited for the treatment of focal arterial lesions (Figure 4, *A* and *B*). Unfortunately, visceral occlusive lesions are rarely truly focal because aortic involvement is common and contributes to limited durability of endoluminal treatments.

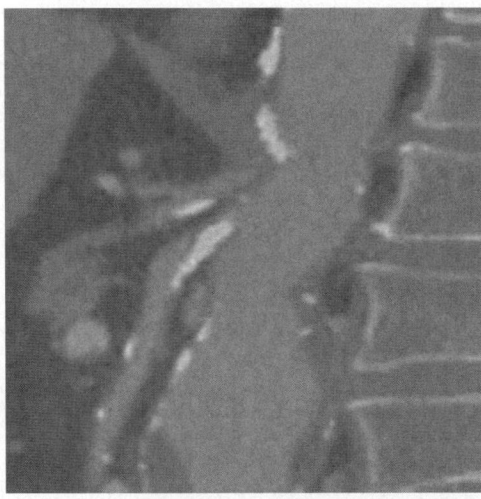

FIGURE 1 Lateral angiogram of the aorta showing atherosclerotic plaque involving the origin of the celiac and superior mesenteric arteries.

BOX 1: Visceral Duplex Ultrasound Criteria for Normal and Stenotic Celiac Artery, SMA, and IMA Flow

Normal

Celiac: PSV 90-110 cm/s; low resistance flow pattern
SMA: PSV 95-150 cm/s; high resistance flow pattern in fasting state with EDV >0 after meal
IMA: PSV 90-180 cm/s; high resistance flow pattern

Diagnostic Testing (Fasting)

<70% Stenosis

Celiac: PSV <200 cm/s, EDV <55 cm/s; resistive index <0.75
SMA: PSV <300 cm/s, EDV <45 cm/s with diastolic flow reversal in distal SMA
IMA: PSV <200 cm/s, antegrade resistive flow (like SFA)

>70% Stenosis

Celiac: PSV >200 cm/s, EDV >55 cm/s with retrograde common hepatic artery flow with severe stenosis or celiac artery occlusion
SMA: PSV >300 cm/s, EDV >45 cm/s with loss of diastolic flow reversal
IMA: PSV >200 cm/s, antegrade flow with loss of diastolic flow reversal
Mesenteric-aorta ratio >3

Velocity Spectra Changes With Test Meal

Increase in PSV at sites of stenosis with damping of distal waveform; used most frequently to assess the significance of SMA occlusive disease

EDV, End diastolic velocity; *IMA,* inferior mesenteric artery; *PSV,* peak systolic velocity; *SFA,* superficial femoral artery; *SMA,* superior mesenteric artery.

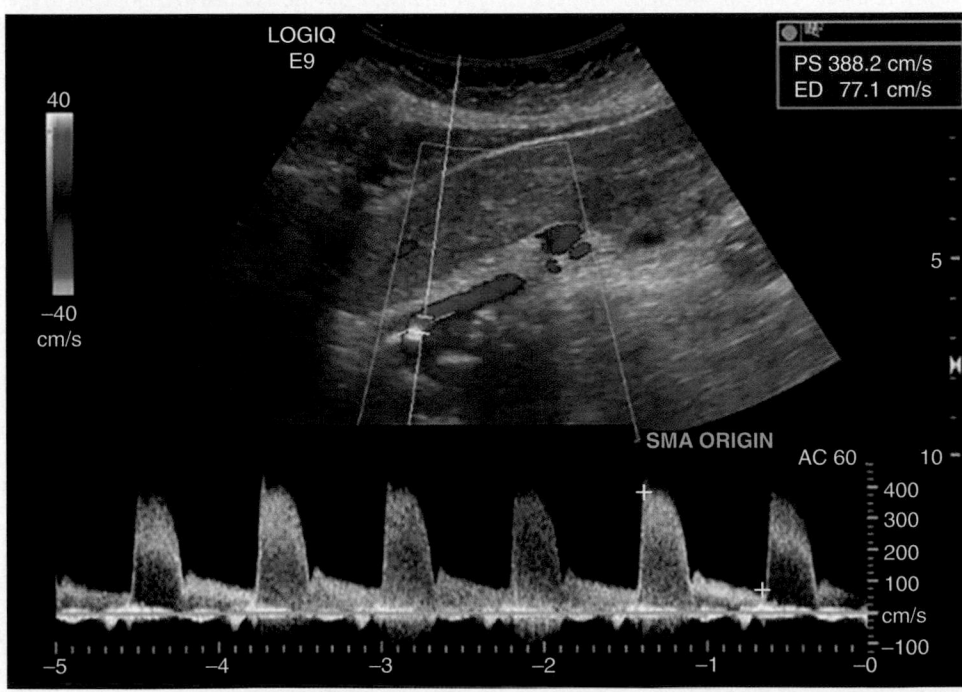

FIGURE 2 Duplex image and velocity spectra recorded from the origin of the superior mesenteric artery with a greater than 70% diameter-reducing stenosis based on a peak systolic velocity of 388 cm/s and end diastolic velocity of 77 cm/s.

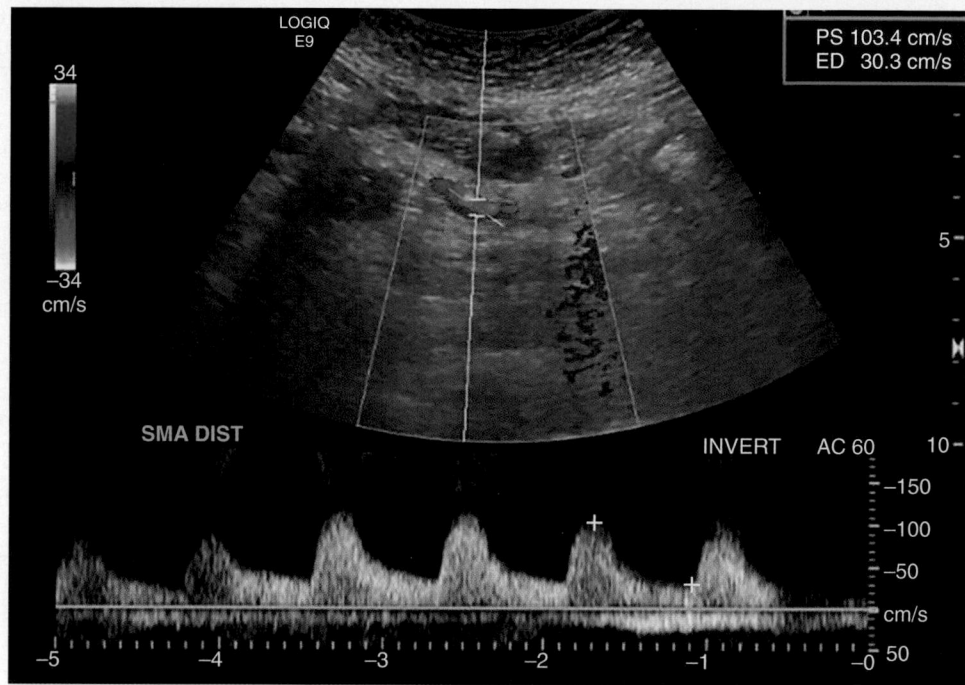

FIGURE 3 Duplex image and velocity spectra recorded from the distal superior mesenteric artery with an origin greater than 70% diameter-reducing stenosis. Note damped waveform configuration with slow acceleration time and flow throughout the pulse cycle in a fasting state.

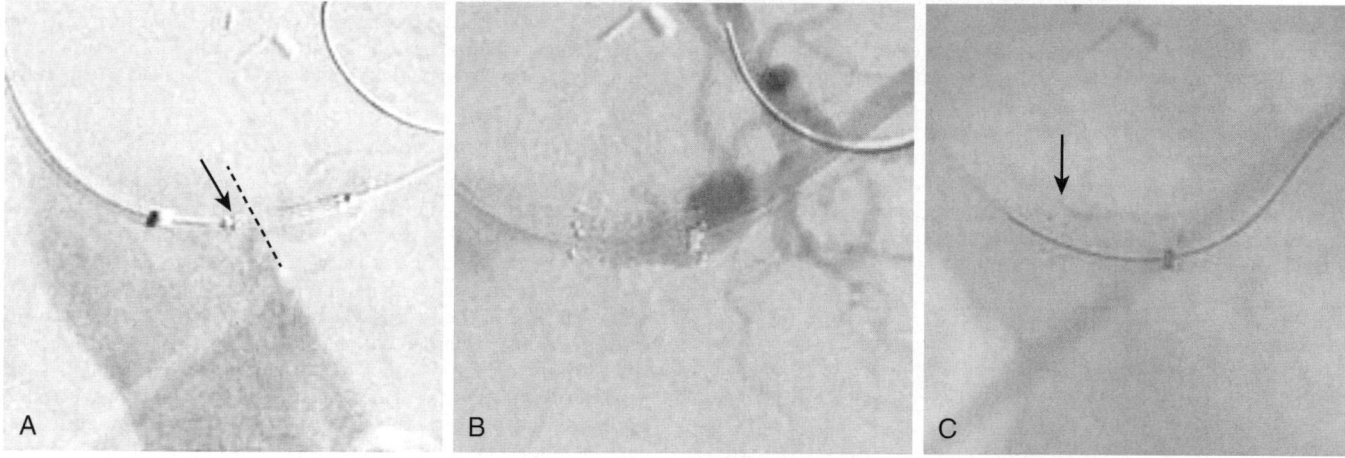

FIGURE 4 Intraprocedure fluoroscopic images of visceral artery stent angioplasty. **A,** Image demonstrating the optimal position of the celiac stent extending 1 to 2 mm into the aortic lumen. The *arrow* represents the proximal end of the stent; the *dotted line* represents the aortic wall. **B,** Image of the celiac stent after pressure-monitored deployment of a balloon-mounted stainless steel stent. **C,** Image of the deployed celiac stent, showing a flared proximal end *(arrow)*. The stent "waist" represents the location of the aortic wall.

Balloon angioplasty is not recommended for the treatment of atherosclerotic stenosis because of recoil potential of the calcified plaque, which is better dilated by stent angioplasty. In addition, the firm median arcuate ligament surrounding the celiac axis and (to a lesser extent) the SMA can be a mechanical barrier to achieving and maintaining an adequate lumen with endovascular treatment, even with placement of balloon-expandable stainless steel stents with increased radial force. Residual extrinsic compression may be managed effectively by placement of one stent inside the other, so as to create a rigid artery segment. Stent fracture produced by extrinsic compression and aorta motion is an etiologic factor, as in development of myointimal hyperplasia within the stent in angioplasty restenosis and failure. Several procedural points are pertinent to endovascular treatment of visceral arterial occlusive disease. First is the choice of percutaneous access site: femoral versus brachial artery. The common

femoral artery access site is more familiar to interventionalists, but cannulation of the visceral artery origin involves at best a right angle and more commonly an acute backward turn, resulting in unfavorable catheter force vectors. In contrast, brachial access, although less familiar and carrying a slightly greater risk, provides an optimal angle of approach as well as the support that might be needed to cross tightly stenotic lesions, heavily calcified lesions, or total occlusions. In fact, a parallel brachiofemoral wire may be necessary in some cases to provide sufficient sheath stabilization to allow the considerable guidewire pushing needed to cross a high-grade stenosis or an occlusion. The risk for embolization during the treatment of visceral occlusive disease, particularly when total occlusions are recanalized, has prompted the use of distal embolic protection devices (i.e., filters) to catch dislodged plaque fragments or thrombus during guidewire and catheter manipulations.

A covered stent provides protection against inadvertent visceral branch or aortic injury during the high pressure inflation required to efface a calcified plaque, and it also traps the atherosclerotic plaque against the vessel wall, avoiding distal embolization. The visceral arteries are unique in the difference between the orifice segment and the rest of the artery. The diseased artery origin is fixed and involves calcified plaque that necessitates stents with high radial force (balloon-expandable stents). The more distal celiac artery and SMA segments, however, are flexible and mobile, and thus a flexible (self-expanding) stent with lower radial force is a better choice. Despite the challenges associated with endovascular treatment of visceral arterial occlusive disease, technical success rates approach 100%, anatomic results are good, and initial clinical outcomes are comparable with or better than open surgical treatment. However, the lower rates of mortality and morbidity and high rate of technical success come at the price of less durability, with 1-year failure rates of approximately 30%.

Endarterectomy

Plaque excision via the endarterectomy technique was the initial approach to the treatment of visceral artery occlusive disease. The operative technique evolved from a transarterial *retrograde approach*, through either the celiac artery or the SMA, or through both, to a *transaortic approach* to the origins of the visceral vessels, including the renal arteries. Plaque excision via an aortotomy allows plaque excision from the aorta and each involved arterial branch using the eversion endarterectomy technique. Aorta exposure can be achieved via a transperitoneal (midline incision) or retroperitoneal left flank approach. For each approach, the left kidney remains in its anatomic position while the plane behind the left colon, spleen, pancreas, and stomach is developed to allow medial visceral displacement toward the midline (Figure 5). If necessary, the entire aorta from the distal thoracic level to the aortic bifurcation can be exposed completely. After aorta clamp occlusion, a U-shaped trapdoor aortotomy circumscribes the orifices of the celiac and superior mesenteric arteries, and an endarterectomy is performed to remove the aortic plaque and its extensions into the visceral orifices. If diffuse aortic disease is present, extension of the aortotomy caudally is performed to expose the renal arteries and allow a sleeve aortic endarterectomy to be performed when the disease includes renal artery origins. The resulting

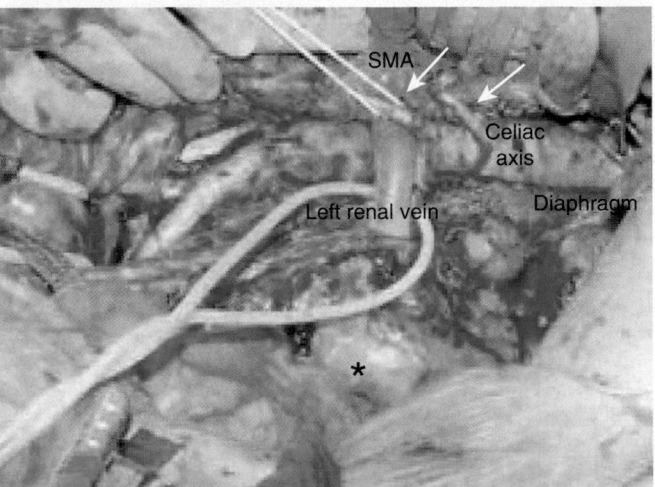

FIGURE 5 Operative photo of the aortic exposure provided by the transabdominal approach with medial rotation of the viscera from the left to perform endarterectomy. Note that the entire abdominal aorta from the diaphragm (under the narrow retractor blades at the right) to the bifurcation of the iliac arteries is dissected, and the left kidney *(asterisk)* remains in its anatomic position. The large vessel loop encircles the left renal vein, which usually can be left intact. *SMA*, Superior mesenteric artery.

hockey stick–shaped aortotomy is then closed with a running Prolene suture with or without a prosthetic polyester patch.

A limitation of endarterectomy is its ability to remove visceral artery plaque extending beyond 2 cm from the origin. If inspection of the distal endarterectomy endpoint reveals a residual obstructing plaque, a stent can be deployed across this region under direct vision. Transmural calcification of the involved portions of the aorta or visceral artery generally is considered a contraindication to endarterectomy because plaque removal requires a deep endarterectomy plane, which can compromise the integrity of the remaining media and adventitia. Bleeding due to reduced wall strength is difficult to repair; if it results in shock and prolonged visceral ischemia, this is invariably a fatal combination. Endarterectomy is particularly appealing when occlusive disease involves the entire para-aortic visceral segment because plaque excision and aortotomy closure are much faster than bypasses to each artery. Similarly, endarterectomy is the preferred technique to address occlusive disease involving accessory renal arteries and the IMA because of their smaller caliber. Typically the transaortic endarterectomy procedure can be completed with a visceral-renal ischemia time of less than 45 minutes. Longer aortic clamp occlusion times produce hepatic ischemia injury, which leads to coagulopathy, a condition that is difficult to reverse despite administration of blood component products (platelets, fresh frozen plasma, coagulation factors).

Arterial Bypass Grafting

The technique of bypass grafting for visceral artery occlusive disease is applicable to all disease patterns and is selected for patients with long segment stenosis or occlusion that is not amenable to endovascular stent angioplasty. Bypass grafts to the mesenteric arteries can originate from a nondiseased supraceliac portion of the aorta (antegrade bypass) or from the infrarenal aorta or the iliac artery (retrograde bypass).

Antegrade Mesenteric Bypass

Aortic exposure for antegrade bypass is achieved through a transabdominal, transcrural approach (Figure 6) or via a medial visceral rotation from the left as previously detailed for transaortic endarterectomy. The transcrural exposure of the supraceliac aorta can be performed via midline or bilateral subcostal incision. The attachment of the left lobe of the liver is divided to expose the aortic hiatus for division of the median arcuate ligament and dissection of the aorta and its branches. Exposure of the aorta for cross-clamping is facilitated by careful retractor blade placement. Bypass grafting with either a polyester or a polytetrafluoroethylene (PTFE) conduit is performed with focal aorta endarterectomy at the proximal anastomosis if necessary. Graft length and alignment are easy to determine with the transcrural approach, with retropancreatic tunnel of the SMA graft as shown in Figure 6. In selected patients, an endarterectomy of the origin of the celiac artery can be performed and used as the proximal anastomosis of the bypass to the SMA.

The proximal anastomosis of an antegrade aortomesenteric bypass should be placed in a disease-free supraceliac or distal thoracic portion of the aorta. Total aortic cross-clamping is preferred to construct this anastomosis unless the aortic segment is of large caliber and suitable for a side-biting clamp placement. Circumferential supraceliac aortic mobilization is not performed routinely unless there is an intervening pair of intercostal arteries that need to be exposed for temporary control. Typically aortic clamp occlusion time is less than 30 minutes to complete the proximal anastomosis. The anastomosis to the celiac artery is end-to-end and to the SMA is end-to-side.

Retrograde Mesenteric Bypass

The infrarenal portion of the aorta, the right iliac artery, or a previously placed prosthetic aortic or aortoiliac graft all can provide inflow for a retrograde mesenteric bypass. Exposure of the aorta is

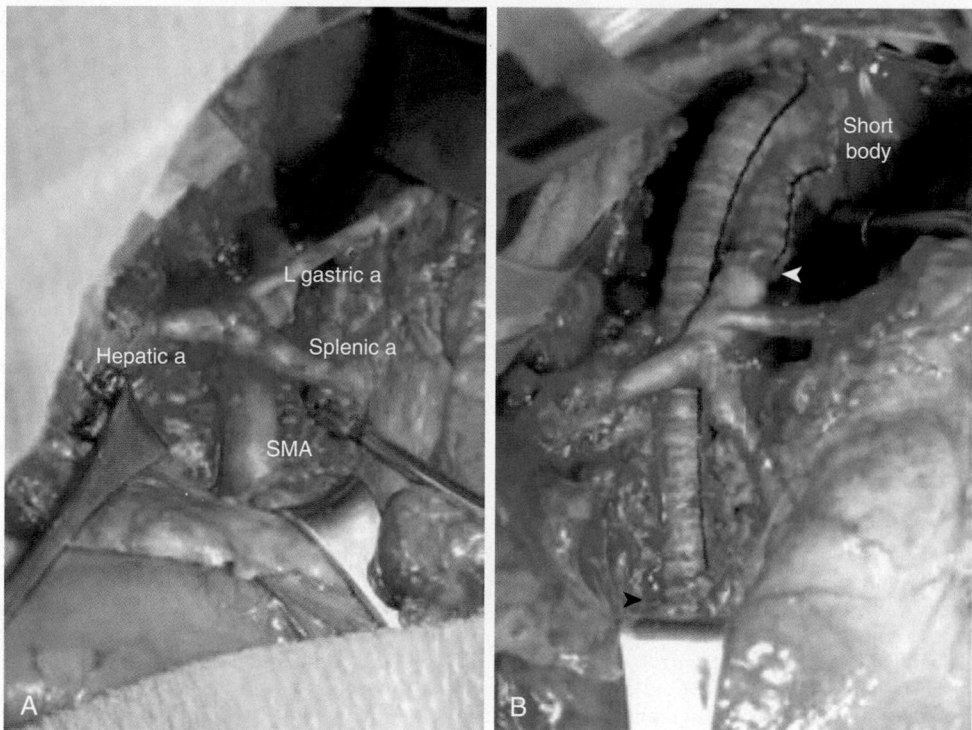

FIGURE 6 A, Operative photo showing transcrural exposure of the celiac axis and its branches (left gastric, hepatic, and splenic arteries) and the superior mesenteric artery (SMA). Note the caudal retraction of the stomach and pancreas and the complete division of the median arcuate ligament, including the celiac ganglion and plexus on the anterior aortic wall. **B,** Photo of completed antegrade polyester bifurcated aortic bypass graft to the celiac axis and SMA. The *white arrowhead* indicates the celiac artery anastomosis; the *black arrowhead* indicates the SMA anastomosis.

performed via a standard infracolic approach, and both the inflow (aortic, iliac, or graft) and outflow (visceral branch) anastomoses are performed end-to-side. If the SMA is the revascularization target, it is exposed beyond the diseased areas in the root of the mesentery. The celiac axis is selected infrequently for the distal anastomosis of a retrograde bypass because of disease involvement, and bypass to the common hepatic artery requires less dissection and the graft alignment is easier. To avoid graft torsion and kinking, use of a ringed PTFE conduit in C-shaped configuration is recommended. The advantages of retrograde bypass are a less complex exposure, no supraceliac aortic occlusion, and the preferred repair for isolated SMA occlusion in patients with minimal aortoiliac occlusive disease.

■ EXTENT OF VISCERAL ARTERY RECONSTRUCTION

Because of multivessel visceral artery disease in CMI, it generally is agreed that at least two visceral arteries should be treated by either angioplasty or open repair to provide symptom relief, weight gain, and protection for gut infarction. The controversy of "complete" versus "SMA revascularization alone" exists regarding both endovascular and open repair for CMI. Some vascular groups have reported a correlation between durable symptom relief and "complete" visceral revascularization, whereas others have reported equivalent results after single-vessel revascularization. The guiding principle is always to revascularize the SMA; if this is not technically feasible, the goal is to repair occlusive lesions of both the celiac artery and the IMA. There are collateral pathways between the three main visceral arteries, including the gastroduodenal artery (Figure 7) and the meandering mesenteric artery from the IMA to the SMA. Treatment of a celiac artery stenosis alone in the presence of an SMA occlusion may not resolve CMI symptoms. Single-vessel reconstruction to the IMA should be performed only if neither the celiac artery nor the SMA can be repaired.

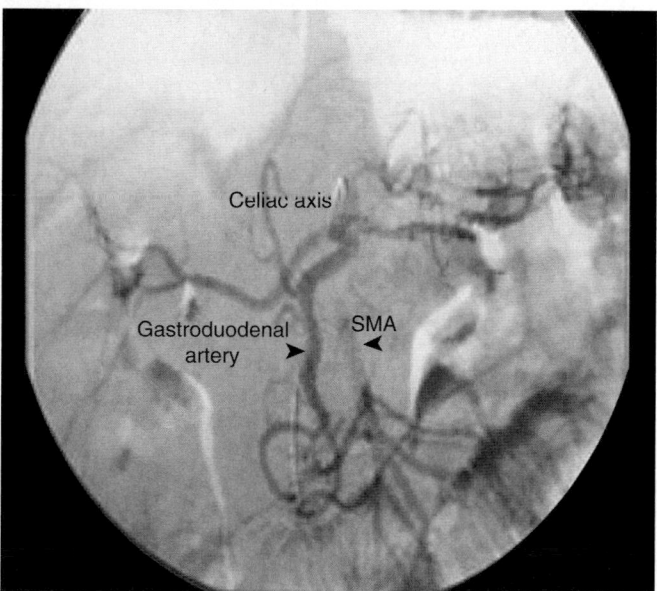

FIGURE 7 Angiogram by selective contrast injection into the celiac axis with opacification of the superior mesenteric artery (SMA) via a large gastroduodenal artery. In this case, reconstruction of either the celiac axis or the SMA could provide perfusion to the entire visceral circulation.

■ OUTCOME OF REVASCULARIZATION

The clinical outcomes of endovascular and open treatment for CMI are not equivalent (Table 1). The morbidity of open repair is higher than that of endovascular intervention, but endovascular interventions are less durable and treated patients require more secondary procedures for angioplasty failure. The results of both endovascular and open therapies have improved, with mortality rates after endarterectomy or bypass of less than 10% and reintervention after endovascular angioplasty in one quarter of patients. It is important to note that the incidence of death due to gut infarction is low (<5%) in both treatment groups, and long-term symptom relief is achieved in more than 80% of patients. Factors that have correlated with increased probability of recurrent symptoms include very early age at time of first diagnosis, greater weight loss at initial presentation, and intraoperative modification of the planned reconstruction technique because of more extensive visceral occlusive disease. It is important to note that patients who develop recurrent CMI symptoms because of endovascular or bypass stenosis can be rendered symptom free again by repeat visceral artery intervention.

■ DUPLEX SURVEILLANCE AFTER MESENTERIC REVASCULARIZATION

Duplex ultrasound testing is a useful technique to evaluate functional patency after visceral artery bypass grafting procedures or endovascular stent angioplasty. Repair site stenosis can be identified reliably, which assists in decision making regarding the need for reintervention to treat or prevent recurrent gut ischemia. Visceral duplex testing of a bypass graft or stent angioplasty site that shows PSV greater than 300 cm/s with EDV greater than 50 to 70 cm/s (Figure 8) or a damped velocity spectra within a bypass graft and low PSV (<40 cm/s) should be considered for interrogation by visceral angiography to confirm or exclude severe stenosis (>70%). In a patient with questionable recurrent CMI symptoms, both preprandial and postprandial visceral duplex testing should be performed.

To induce a postprandial state, the patient is asked to drink 8 oz of a protein calorie supplement as a test meal, with duplex testing repeated within 30 minutes to identify changes in the SMA velocity spectra (i.e., PSV and EDV increase). If an SMA stenosis is present, further damping of the mid-downstream SMA spectral waveform will occur and indicates that an increase in the systolic pressure gradient across the stenosis has developed. A test meal produces no change in IMA flow and minimal elevation in celiac artery PSV, unless that artery is providing compensatory collateral flow. Using this protocol, visceral duplex testing has the ability to verify hemodynamic changes associated with eating and provide justification for additional visceral artery imaging, including angiography with pressure gradient measurement across imaged stenosis. Although postprandial testing with administration of a test meal is not performed routinely, this maneuver is helpful in study interpretation and particularly relevant after endovascular intervention when elevated PSV (>200 cm/s) is recorded from the stent angioplasty site. The presence of in-stent stenosis based on duplex PSV threshold criteria is common (20% to 50% incidence) because of incomplete stent expansion, myointimal thickening, or compensatory collateral flow if the celiac artery occlusive disease is present. The higher rate of SMA stent stenosis compared with other artery stents (celiac, renal) makes duplex scanning an ideal, noninvasive monitoring technique after endovascular therapy.

Duplex scanning of bypass grafts to the SMA is facilitated by knowing the origin of the conduit from the supraceliac aorta (antegrade bypass) or iliac artery (retrograde bypass). Once identified, the bypass graft is imaged along its length for lumen or color Doppler flow abnormality, with particular attention to proximal and distal anastomotic sites. Recording a midgraft spectral waveform and volume flow measurement can facilitate the diagnosis of graft stenosis and disease progression, as often complete graft imaging is difficult. The blood flow characteristics in retrograde and antegrade visceral bypass grafts are similar: PSV in the graft in the range of 150 to 200 cm/s for a 6-mm diameter PTFE conduit. The volume flow is in the range of 1 to 1.5 L/min for retrograde iliac-SMA bypasses.

TABLE 1: Outcome of Endovascular and Open Interventions for Chronic Mesenteric Ischemia

Study	No. of Patients/No. of Vessels	Mortality	Morbidity	Symptom Relief	Primary Patency
ENDOVASCULAR TREATMENT					
Aburahma et al. (2013)	83/105	2.0%	2.0%	65% (5 yr)	68% (1 yr)
Tallarita et al. (2013)	156/173	2.6%			
Pecoraro et al. (2013)	786/1007	3.6%	13.2%		49.1% (5 yr)
Turba et al. (2012)	166				
Tallarita et al. (2011)	157/170				
Schoch et al. (2011)	107/130	0.0%	7.0%	54.0%	44% (1 yr)
Gupta et al. (2010)	776/1018	3.1%-4.1%	4%-14%	53%-88% (2 yr)	79%-89% (3 yr)
Oderich et al. (2009)	409	6.0%	15.0%	75.0%	74% (1 yr)
Schermerhorn et al. (2009)	3455	3.7%	20.2%		
OPEN SURGICAL TREATMENT					
Tallarita et al. (2013)	187/327	2.7%			
Pecoraro et al. (2013)	1009/1593	7.2%	33.1%		80.9% (5 yr)
Davenport et al. (2012)	156	7.7%	40.0%		
Ryer et al. (2011)	116/203	2.6%	50.0%		80.5% (5 yr)
Gupta et al. (2010)	1163/1995	4.5%-7.5%	29%-35%	83%-88% (5 yr)	78%-80% (5 yr)
Oderich et al. (2009)	992	11.0%	47.0%	93.0%	89% (1 yr)
Schermerhorn et al. (2009)	2128	15.4%	39.7%		

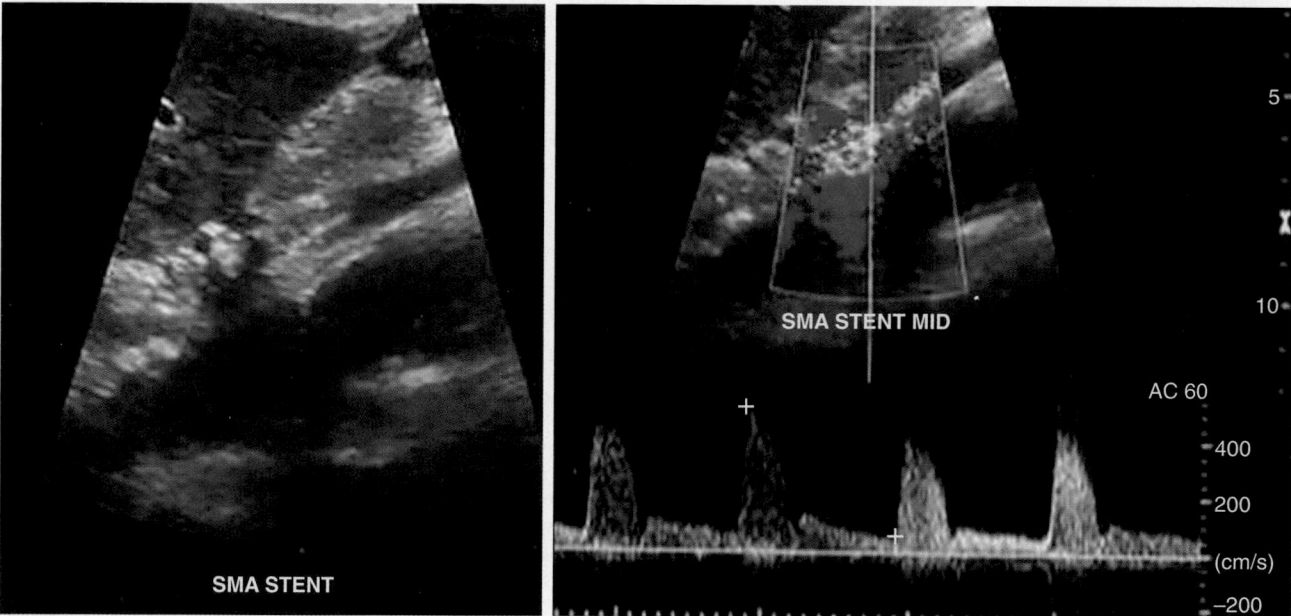

FIGURE 8 The duplex scan images of the superior mesenteric artery (SMA) after stent angioplasty demonstrating greater than 70% in-stent stenosis with peak systolic velocity greater than 400 cm/sec.

Currently there is no consensus on which velocity criteria should be used to define high-grade recurrent visceral artery stenosis. Published vascular case series recommend periodic clinical reassessment of the patient with a focus on uncovering recurrent symptoms of intestinal angina, such as meal intolerance, pain, diarrhea, dyspepsia, and weight loss, before considering a need for reintervention. Although intuitively this seems like a rational course of action, the danger of complacency must be considered, as most investigators have reported high mortality rates in individuals who develop acute mesenteric ischemia after revascularization. Among reported series of mesenteric revascularizations, clinical follow-up alone inaccurately predicted graft occlusion and was associated with a sensitivity as low as 33%.

The management of asymptomatic high-grade stenosis after both open and endovascular repair remains undefined. Fortunately, the embolic potential of myointimal hyperplasia associated with surgical or endovascular intervention is uncommon. Progressive stenosis of the original atherosclerotic lesion or restenosis/occlusion of the splanchnic repair remains the most common cause of recurrent symptoms among treated patients. Because recurrent symptoms are associated with intervention failure and increase the risk for gut necrosis, a more aggressive approach toward treating endovascular stent stenosis is appropriate in these patients. In asymptomatic patients, intervention should be limited to vessels showing progressive repair site stenosis greater than 70% DR as shown by duplex ultrasound, followed by confirmatory angiographic imaging with pressure gradient measurement. Reintervention using endovascular therapy is usually successful, reduces PSV at the stenosis site, and is associated with continued relief of gut ischemia.

Testing at 6-month intervals has been sufficiently frequent to detect developing stenosis after intervention. A retrospective audit performed by the vascular group at the University of South Florida identified no occurrence of asymptomatic SMA occlusion developed using biannual surveillance. Asymptomatic celiac artery repair occlusion was observed and confirms that duplex surveillance is primarily a screening study. Any recurrence of CMI symptoms combined with elevated in-stent or mesenteric bypass velocities (SMA: PSV >300 cm/s, EDV >50 cm/s; celiac artery: PSV >250 cm/s, EDV >45 cm/s) should prompt angiographic confirmation of restenosis (see Figure 8). For patients with asymptomatic CMI with elevated in-stent or graft anastomotic velocities, serial studies are compared, with attention given to changes in stent structure, development of intimal hyperplasia, and changes in collateral or downstream mesenteric velocities. In the asymptomatic patient, the finding of a lesion with poststenotic turbulence, a PSV greater than 300 cm/s, and an EDV greater than 50 cm/s in the SMA is an indication to consider angiographic evaluation. Angiography also is recommended when stent migration or changes in mesenteric bypass volume flow or graft PSV are identified. A PSV increase of more than 150 cm/s on serial testing was associated with the development of either clinical symptoms or an angiographic stenosis with a resting systolic pressure gradient greater than 15 mm Hg. Stenosis in a celiac artery or IMA repair also may be clinically important, especially in patients with SMA occlusion or stenosis. Duplex surveillance after mesenteric revascularization resulted in 3-year primary patency rates of 62% after endovascular therapy and 82% after surgical bypass ($P < 0.01$). Secondary interventions for duplex-detected stenosis produced similar primary-assisted patency rates (95% and 92%) in surviving patients. The benefit of duplex surveillance was most evident after endovascular therapy, with 25% of stent angioplasty sites developing progressive in-stent stenosis necessitating a secondary endovascular reparative procedure.

The finding of a PSV in the range of 300 cm/s or higher has been observed after angiographically successful SMA stent angioplasty. Because duplex testing is a screening study, when there is a progressive increase in PSV and EDV suggesting in-stent stenosis, it remains a clinical decision whether to proceed with confirmatory angiography and potential secondary intervention. Treatment options are limited for some patients with stent stenosis because of medical comorbidities, disease location, and patient preferences.

SUGGESTED READINGS

Aburahma AF, Campbell JE, Stone PA, et al. Perioperative and late clinical outcomes of percutaneous transluminal stentings of the celiac and superior mesenteric arteries over the past decade. *J Vasc Surg.* 2013;57:1052-1061.

Aburahma AF, Mousa AY, Stone PA, et al. Duplex velocity criteria for native celiac/superior mesenteric artery stenosis vs in-stent stenosis. *J Vasc Surg.* 2012;55:730-738.

Cunningham CG, Reilly LM, Rapp JH, et al. Chronic intestinal ischemia: three decades of surgical progress. *Ann Surg.* 1991;214:276-288.

Davenport DL, Shivazad A, Endean ED. Short-term outcomes for open revascularization of chronic mesenteric ischemia. *Ann Vasc Surg.* 2012;26:447-453.

Foley MI, Moneta GL, Abou-Zamzam AM Jr, et al. Revascularization of the superior mesenteric artery alone for treatment of intestinal ischemia. *J Vasc Surg.* 2000;32:37-47.

Gupta PK, Horan SM, Turaga KK, et al. Chronic mesenteric ischemia: endovascular versus open revascularization. *J Endovasc Ther.* 2010;17:540-549.

Hodgkiss-Harlow KD. Interpretation of visceral duplex scanning before and after intervention for chronic mesenteric ischemia. *Sem Vassc Surg.* 2014;26:127-132.

Mitchell EL, et al. Duplex criteria for native superior mesenteric artery stenosis overestimate stenosis in stented superior mesenteric arteries. *J Vasc Surg.* 2009;50:335-340.

HEMODIALYSIS ACCESS SURGERY

Bonnie E. Lonze, MD, PhD, and Thomas Reifsnyder, MD

For the past decade, the overall prevalence of end-stage renal disease in the United States has increased at a rate of approximately 2% per year. In 2012, 111,818 new patients initiated dialysis treatment, bringing the total number of Americans living on dialysis to more than 450,000. For the vast majority of these patients, hemodialysis is the preferred mode of renal replacement therapy. The ability to deliver this lifesaving therapy depends on the creation and maintenance of adequate vascular access.

■ HISTORICAL NOTES

Over the course of approximately a century, end-stage renal failure went from a universally fatal disease to a tolerable chronic illness with reasonable long-term survival. In the United States a series of events involving science, medicine, and politics led to universally available and undeniable renal replacement therapy.

The concept of dialysis was introduced by the Scottish physical chemist Thomas Graham, whose experiments in the 1850s characterized the movement of water across semipermeable membranes and led to an understanding of the principle of osmosis. It was, in fact, Graham himself who first applied the term *dialysis* to describe the phenomenon of exploiting osmotic gradients to move solutes across a membrane separating two solutions.

Fifty years later, John Jacob Abel, a pharmacologist at the Johns Hopkins Hospital, first explored the application of dialysis in a clinical setting. Abel, working with Leonard Rowntree and B. B. Turner, described in 1914 the construction of the "artificial kidney," an apparatus that consisted of 32 tubes connected in series and encased in a large glass container filled with a dialysate solution. Using hirudin as an anticoagulant to prevent clotting in the tubes, they tested the invention on anesthetized animals. Using arterial cannulae to channel blood into the narrow tubes of the circuit, they demonstrated that indeed blood could be dialyzed.

The first successful human use of dialysis is credited to Willem Kolff, a Dutch physician who had studied Abel's work. During the German occupation of the Netherlands in the 1940s, he designed and built, mainly from household items, a dialysis device he named the "rotating drum kidney." This device consisted of a large drum, covered with thin tubing that sat partly submerged in a large tank of dialysate. Blood passed through the series of tubes affixed to the drum that then rotated within the tank, facilitating dialysis of the blood across the tubing. Kolff's first surviving patient was a 67-year-old woman with acute renal failure secondary to sepsis. She endured an 11-hour dialysis session, in which a measured 60 g of urea was removed. He foresaw many possible applications of hemodialysis and was astutely aware that its implementation for chronic renal failure would require durable vascular access.

The first solution to the access problem was developed by Belding Scribner at the University of Washington. Having been introduced to a newly engineered material called polytetrafluoroethylene or PTFE (Teflon), and recognizing its inert and noninflammatory properties, he conceived of using a U-shaped Teflon tube to create an external arteriovenous connection that could be accessed for dialysis. On March 9, 1960, the first dialysis by way of the "Scribner shunt" was performed. Although this did establish an important proof of principle, Scribner shunts had unacceptably high rates of infection, thrombosis, and hemorrhage, and their functional patency rarely exceeded a few months. Seeking to improve upon this, James Cimino and Michael Brescia invented the radiocephalic arteriovenous fistula and described the technique in their landmark *New England Journal of Medicine* manuscript in 1966.

With safe and reliable vascular access technically feasible, widespread availability of hemodialysis had a final major obstacle: its prohibitive cost. Lobbying at local and national levels resulted in government funding for improvements in dialysis machine technology and the construction of more dialysis units. However, because of its cost, most people believed that without federal government support, access would remain limited to the privileged few. In November 1971, a chronic dialysis patient named Shep Glazer and his nephrologist demonstrated a dialysis session before a congressional committee in Washington, DC. This had a tremendous impact on the committee members, which led Congress to act. In October 1972, President Nixon signed into law a bill authorizing Medicare coverage of dialysis.

In this chapter, we review and summarize our current practices for the evaluation, placement, and maintenance of hemodialysis access. In 2002 the Society for Vascular Surgery and the American Association for Vascular Surgery published recommendations for standardized reporting of dialysis access techniques, procedures, and configurations. For purposes of brevity, however, we preferentially use common nomenclature throughout the following discussion.

■ NATIONAL PRACTICES AND GUIDELINES

In 2009 the End-Stage Renal Disease Program alone consumed 6% of the overall Medicare budget, a total of $29 billion, and this staggering sum is rising annually. As health care cost containment has become a major national focus, there has been great motivation within the dialysis community to identify best practices that minimize costs and maximize patient benefit. Until recently, the majority of arm accesses placed had been prosthetic grafts. Certainly some of these grafts were placed out of necessity. Unfortunately, convenience, lack of surgeon experience, and the higher reimbursement rate for prosthetic grafts undoubtedly played a role in their preferential placement. Specifically, in 1990 ePTFE grafts were placed twice as frequently as autogenous arteriovenous fistulae. According to the Centers for Disease Control, in 1995 just more than 20% of patients on dialysis were using autogenous access. Clear evidence has since emerged that autogenous fistulas are associated with better outcomes and lower costs, and this has drawn attention to the unacceptably low proportion of patients in the United States dialyzing through autogenous accesses. The disproportionate and often inappropriate use of prosthetic grafts fueled the National Kidney Foundation's Kidney Disease Outcomes and Quality Initiative (KDOQI). This is a comprehensive analysis of the best practices with regard to the management of end-stage renal disease. An offspring of KDOQI was The Centers for Medicare and Medicaid Services' Fistula First Breakthrough Initiative, which aimed to promote awareness among patients and physicians of the superiority of autogenous access. The current national goal is to place autogenous access in at least 65% of new dialysis patients.

Currently, the three main avenues for hemodialysis access are tunneled central venous catheters, arteriovenous prosthetic grafts, and autogenous arteriovenous fistulae. Clearly, the worst outcomes are associated with catheter usage, and therefore every effort should be made to avoid them. To this end, current KDOQI guidelines stipulate that all patients should be referred to a surgeon for the placement of autogenous access when they reach stage 4 chronic kidney disease (glomerular filtration rate [GFR] < 30). This allows sufficient time for fistula placement and maturation before the commencement of dialysis. The caveat to this scenario is that not all patients have a suitable vein for autogenous fistula creation. Only those with suitable veins should have their access placed far in advance of the initiation of dialysis, and this access should be an autogenous fistula. The most common cause of prosthetic graft failure is stenosis at the venous anastomosis because of neointimal hyperplasia. This worsens with time, so if a prosthetic graft is required, it should be placed only when dialysis is imminent or already has begun.

The options for dialysis access frequently are affected by treatment options instituted years before the patient reaches end-stage renal disease. Patients and physicians must be aware that for those with any degree of renal dysfunction, subclavian vein central lines and ports, peripherally inserted central catheter (PICC) lines, and even forearm intravenous catheters ("intern's vein" or distal cephalic vein) should be avoided whenever possible. PICC lines are the curse of the dialysis access surgeon. Not only do they frequently ruin a typical good access vein, the basilic vein, but also they are associated with rates of central venous stenosis or thrombosis estimated up to 85%, which renders the arm unsuitable for the most common and durable access types.

The algorithm for selecting which fistula to place is fairly straightforward. One should begin distally and work proximally in the nondominant arm: radiocephalic (Figure 1), brachiocephalic, then upper arm basilic transposition. We believe that the benefits of autogenous access are so great that many exceptions to the standard algorithm are permitted. Although use of the nondominant arm is preferable, frequently the veins are better in the more active dominant arm. In this circumstance, the dominant arm is used without hesitation for fistula placement. If a patient has no suitable vein for autogenous access, then a prosthetic graft may be used. A good prosthetic graft is better than a bad vein. Although prosthetic grafts may be placed between any artery with sufficient flow and any suitable vein with unobstructed outflow, it is best to begin as far distally as possible and reserve more proximal sites for the future. For example, we would consider these configurations in the following order: distal radial artery to brachial vein straight graft, distal brachial artery to distal brachial vein forearm loop graft, and finally, distal brachial artery to proximal brachial vein, or distal axillary vein straight graft.

With education and careful attention to best practices, autogenous accesses can be placed preferentially, and the use of prosthetic grafts can and should be limited.

■ PREOPERATIVE EVALUATION

End-stage renal disease is rarely an entity that exists in isolation, and dialysis patients have a higher incidence of significant comorbid conditions. According to the United States Renal Data System, among the cohort of new dialysis patients who were registered in 2006 to 2009, 84% had hypertension, 21% coronary artery disease, 32% congestive heart failure, 35% insulin-dependent diabetes, 14% peripheral vascular disease, 9% had a history of previous stroke or transient ischemic attack, and 7% were unable to ambulate. Briefly stated, these patients are poor operative candidates. The preoperative evaluation revolves around assessing cardiopulmonary reserve and selecting the anesthetic with the least risk.

Aside from a history of events relevant to cardiopulmonary status and prior dialysis access attempts, it is imperative to inquire as to all previous venous access procedures, including dialysis catheters, subclavian lines or ports, PICC lines, pacemakers, and defibrillators. Prior trauma to the upper extremities or clavicles should be noted. The physical exam should include auscultation of the heart and lungs and an evaluation of the extremities to determine the patient's best option for dialysis access. The radial, ulnar, and brachial pulses should be palpated bilaterally. Uncommonly, a radial pulse is present with an occluded brachial artery. An Allen's test to confirm adequacy of ulnar flow to the hand should be performed if a radiocephalic fistula is contemplated. It cannot be overemphasized that the preoperative physical examination is incomplete unless a venous tourniquet is used to assess the superficial veins. To end up with a successful radiocephalic fistula, the forearm cephalic vein should be palpable from the wrist to the antecubital fossa. Otherwise, attention should be directed to the upper arm veins.

Duplex ultrasound–based vein mapping before dialysis access surgery essentially was mandated by the KDOQI guidelines. We strongly disagree with this blanket recommendation. Although vein mapping at times may be helpful for operative planning, it is frequently unnecessary, adds cost, and may not always give valid information. In patients already on dialysis via a catheter, we rarely request a vein map. If no suitable vein is found at surgery (see operative techniques below), then the patient will require a prosthetic graft. In patients referred before the initiation of dialysis, vein mapping may be helpful in those who are obese, intravenous drug abusers, or have had prior PICC lines. It also may be helpful in patients with normal-size arms, in whom neither an adequate basilic nor cephalic vein is palpable with a tourniquet in place. Last, with the ubiquity of portable ultrasound machines, surgeon-performed vein mapping in the preoperative area or intraoperatively is becoming more routine, and this option generally obviates the need for a formal vein mapping study.

Venography is an important component of successful dialysis access surgery. Its primary use is not to roadmap the arm veins, but rather to confirm central vein patency. Our practice is to use it liberally in any patient with a history of arm swelling or prior central venous cannulation on the side of proposed access. In predialysis patients, carbon dioxide may be used as a contrast agent, thereby avoiding the risks of iodinated contrast-induced nephrotoxicity. If a hybrid endovascular operative suite is available, the venogram may be done at the beginning of the access case, allowing for a combined procedure that is more convenient for the patient.

Last, for the safety of the surgical team, any patient with a history of intravenous drug use should have a plain radiograph of the upper extremity to evaluate for the presence of foreign bodies.

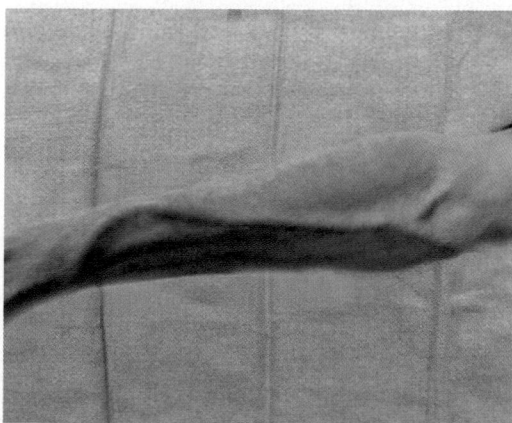

FIGURE 1 Mature radiocephalic arteriovenous fistula 6 weeks postoperatively.

Before surgery, standard blood chemistries and a complete blood count are all that are necessary. The surgeon can assume that uremic platelet dysfunction will always be present, and we have found no utility in checking bleeding times preoperatively. Uncommonly, DDAVP (arginine vasopressin) at a dose of 0.3 μg/kg will be needed intraoperatively to control oozing. In addition, aspirin use does not seem to affect bleeding significantly, and considering the cardiovascular risk profile of these patients, we routinely administer a dose of 81 mg in the preoperative area. Clopidogrel does seem to increase oozing in some patients, so this should be held for 5 to 7 days unless the patient has recently undergone coronary artery stenting. Many patients are also on warfarin. In general, we do not advocate holding warfarin and feel comfortable proceeding with access surgery with an international normalized ratio (INR) up to 2.5.

■ OPERATIVE TECHNIQUES

The best option for anesthesia depends upon the patient's comorbid conditions, the anesthesiologist, and the proposed surgery. Although local anesthesia is a viable option for many patients, it works best for patients undergoing radiocephalic or nontransposed brachiocephalic fistulas. Although we have used it successfully for upper arm basilic transpositions, it tends to be somewhat less than ideal for both patient and surgeon because of the relatively large area that must be anesthetized. More recently, we have used infraclavicular regional nerve blocks. The blocks are placed in the preoperative area by a dedicated block team while the preceding case is under way. This helps to maximize efficiency and shorten turnover time. If the skin incision approaches the deltopectoral groove or the axilla, supplementation of the regional block with local anesthetic will be necessary. Our experience with supraclavicular blocks has been less satisfactory. In the past we have had to cancel several cases because of shortness of breath secondary to phrenic nerve paresis after this more proximal nerve block.

Autogenous Arm Fistulae

The patient is positioned supine with the shoulder of the operative side near the edge of the bed. The arm board should be positioned such that the arm rests in the center of the board. A standard skin preparation including the shoulder and axilla is performed. If available, an arm board drape is most convenient; otherwise an extremity drape will suffice.

Radiocephalic Fistula

A 3- to 4-cm incision is placed just proximal to the wrist along the lateral or radial aspect of the arm. Once the skin is incised, the surgeon and assistant both lift the skin with Adson forceps, facilitating easy identification of the cephalic vein after some gentle blunt dissection. The vein is encircled with a vessel loop and then sharply dissected out, tying all branches with 4-0 or 5-0 ties. The radial artery is dissected out circumferentially in a standard fashion and controlled with vessel loops. Any side branches are tied but not divided, which helps to maintain its orientation. The cephalic vein is divided distally, gently dilated with sequential coronary dilators, and then flushed with heparinized saline. After the radial artery is flushed, a spatulated end-to-side anastomosis is performed using 6-0 or 7-0 polypropylene suture. Any large proximal vein branches are ligated through separate 1-cm incisions. Closure consists of 3-0 interrupted absorbable dermal sutures and a 4-0 running absorbable subcuticular suture.

Upper Arm Fistula

If there is a potentially good cephalic vein, then a transverse incision is made in the antecubital crease (Figure 2, A) and the cephalic vein is identified (Figure 2, B). If of suitable size, it is dissected out to its confluence with the median cubital vein, ligated distally, and divided.

Sequential coronary dilators are passed gently cephalad and should pass easily if there is no intraluminal scarring. Although a sufficient length of vein can be mobilized at this point to easily reach the brachial artery, we frequently convert the incision into a hockey stick–shaped incision (with the handle of the stick along the cephalic vein; Figure 2, C) and mobilize 10 to 15 or more cm of the vein (Figure 2, D and E). Not only does this allow ligation of the accessory cephalic vein and other small branches, but also it allows superficial tunneling of the vein (Figure 2, F), which is necessary in all but the thinnest of arms. With the vein transposed, accessing the fistula can be performed earlier (as soon as 4 weeks depending on vein size), easier, and more consistently, enabling earlier removal of dialysis catheters.

Dissection of the distal brachial artery through the medial aspect of the antecubital incision is done in a standard fashion with control obtained with vessel loops. If the brachial artery appears smaller than expected, the patient most likely has a high brachial bifurcation. In these cases, the more suitable donor artery almost always is the deeper of the two vessels and should be evaluated before proceeding with the anastomosis. The vein is tunneled just beneath the skin, making sure that there is no kink or twist at the most proximal site of mobilization (Figure 2, G). Once an arteriotomy is made and the artery flushed with heparinized saline, the vessel loops are replaced with baby bulldog clamps. This eliminates any vessel stretching and makes the end-to-side anastomosis easier to perform. Closure consists of 2-0 absorbable suture in the subcutaneous tissue and 3-0 nylon vertical mattress skin sutures (Figure 2, H). In our experience, subcuticular closures in the upper arm have been associated with postoperative wound problems much more frequently than with interrupted nylon closures. In addition, patients are much more apt to keep their follow-up appointment if they have sutures that must be removed. If the cephalic vein is not of adequate size or quality, then the median cubital vein is identified near the medial aspect of the incision. If the median cubital vein is adequate, it is ligated distally, divided, and flushed with heparinized saline. We then extend the medial end of our skin incision in a hockey-stick fashion along the medial aspect of the arm nearly to the axilla. The vein is dissected circumferentially over its course toward the axilla as it joins the basilic vein, which subsequently joins the proximal brachial vein. If the median cubital vein is not adequate, then the basilic vein is used. In this instance we place two surgical towels under the upper arm to improve positioning and then make a new incision just anterior to the medial epicondyle of the humerus. Once the basilic vein is identified and found to be of appropriate size and quality, the incision is extended proximally and distally until enough vein for a transposition has been exposed. The brachial artery is then dissected out at the antecubital fossa either through a separate incision or through the medial aspect of the antecubital incision if that incision already had been made to inspect the cephalic vein. The vein is then tunneled and the anastomosis prepared and performed as described above. The fascia and subcutaneous layers are reapproximated with running 2-0 absorbable suture. The skin is closed with interrupted 3-0 nylon vertical mattress sutures. At the end of the case there should be a palpable thrill in the fistula. If there is not, then there is a technical problem and the incision should be reopened.

Prosthetic Arteriovenous Grafts

If there is no suitable vein, then a prosthetic graft must be placed. Although the most commonly used graft is 6-mm ePTFE, bovine carotid artery, *bovine mesenteric vein*, and polyurethane-urea (Vectra, BARD Peripheral Vascular, Inc., Tempe, AZ) grafts also may be used. A transverse incision is made over the brachial artery in the antecubital fossa. The brachial artery and vein (if at least 5 mm in diameter) are isolated and encircled with vessel loops. The vein should be dissected out generously to allow a long venous anastomosis. A second smaller counterincision is made on the volar surface of the mid-forearm on the radial side. Placement of the counterincision in this fashion skews the graft toward the radial aspect of the forearm,

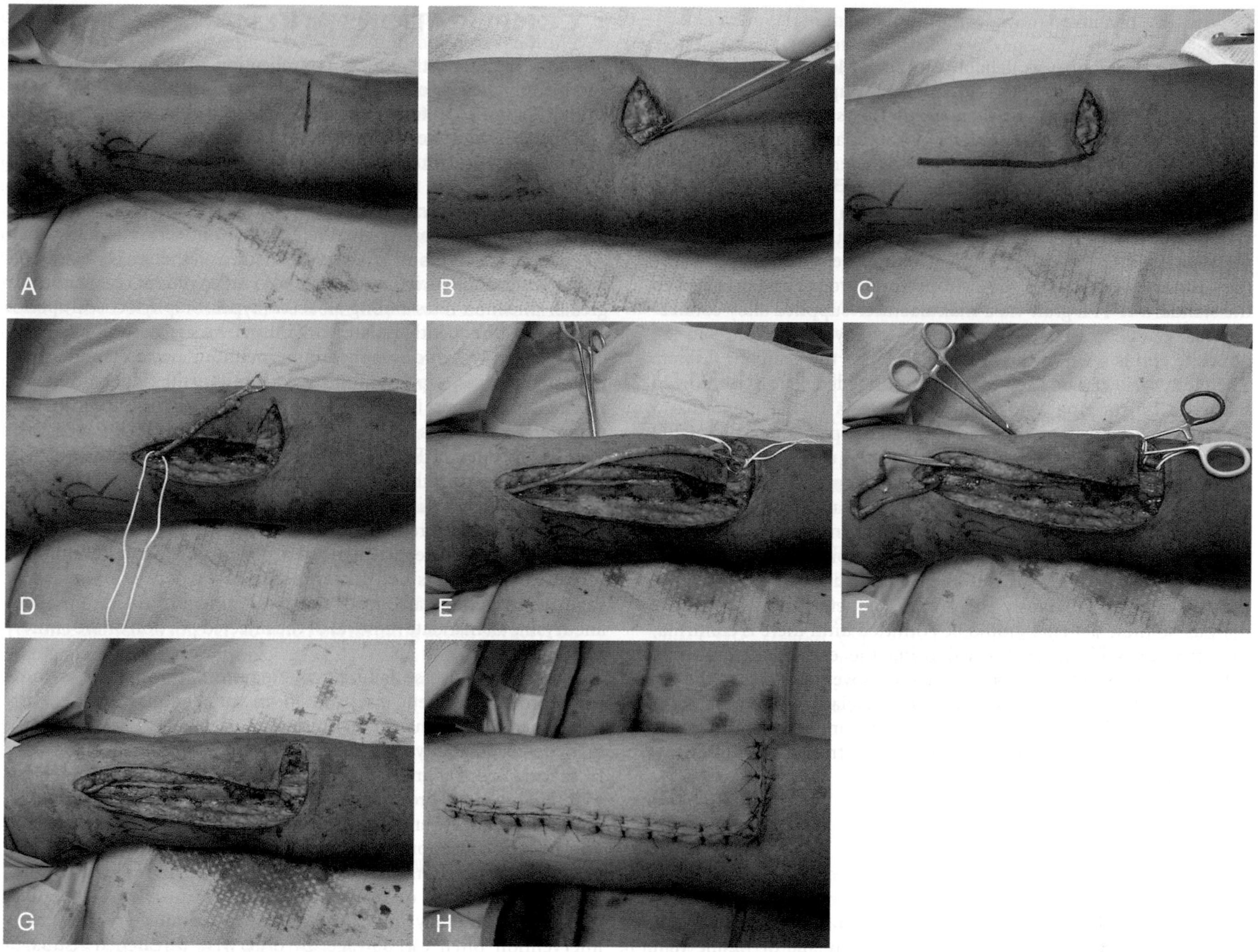

FIGURE 2 Brachiocephalic arteriovenous fistula creation. **A,** Antecubital incision. **B,** Identification of cephalic vein in antecubital fossa. **C,** Hockey-stick incision. **D,** Proximal dissection of cephalic vein. **E,** Ligation of cephalic vein branches, dissection of brachial artery in antecubital fossa. **F,** Superficial tunneling of mobilized cephalic vein. **G,** Completed arteriovenous anastomosis. **H,** Closure of skin with vertical mattress nylon sutures.

and this allows the patient's arm to be in a comfortable position during a dialysis session. The venous anastomosis is performed first (when using ePTFE; however, if using a biologic graft, the arterial anastomosis is performed first), particularly if the graft has a premade flared end. The graft is tunneled in a gentle arc to the counterincision and then back to the antecubital fossa. Tunneling is accomplished best with a Kelly-Wick tunneler (IMPRA, Tempe, AZ), although an aortic clamp may be used. The arterial anastomosis is then performed and the incisions are closed. If the brachial vein is too small at the antecubital fossa, then a second incision is made on the proximal medial aspect of the upper arm, and the proximal brachial or distal axillary vein is used for the venous outflow. Although this describes the two most common graft configurations, in reality any suitable artery and vein may be used. We strongly believe in fistula first and therefore do not agree with the use of forearm grafts to help mature upper arm cephalic or basilic veins.

■ OPTIONS FOR NONCONVENTIONAL ACCESSES

Not uncommonly patients are seen for dialysis access after many months of catheter usage and have developed upper extremity central vein occlusion or stenosis (Figure 3). Placing brachial artery–based access ipsilateral to this problem will lead to significant arm edema

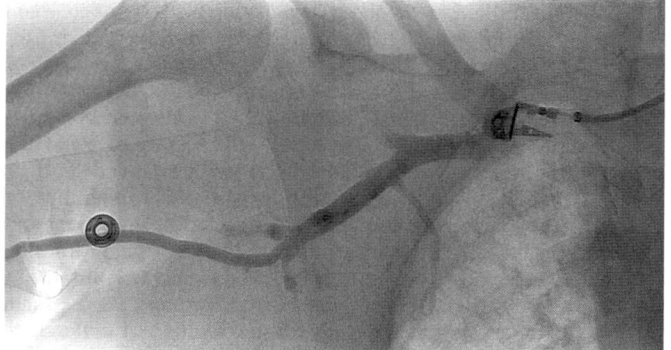

FIGURE 3 Superior vena cava occlusion as demonstrated by upper extremity venogram in a dialysis patient with history of multiple prior dialysis catheters and failed upper extremity accesses.

and an unusable access. Longstanding dialysis patients with central vein stenosis or thromboses pose a particular challenge. Options must be considered carefully in these cases, and there is no room for error. Failure to establish access quickly can turn into a life-threatening situation.

costs relative to norms, with an estimated total annual cost of VTE at $15.4 to $34.4 billion in the United States.

Despite an overall trend toward increasing VTE diagnoses, overall rates of death from VTE appear to be decreasing. The upward trend in VTE diagnosis may be due to improved diagnostic accuracy of various imaging modalities, or a heightened awareness of the clinical issue by the entire healthcare team. The fact that surgeons are now able to operatively manage an older, more obese, and less mobile cohort means that the incidence of VTE is unlikely to decrease in the near future, as has been validated by the population-based studies.

■ RISK FACTORS

There are a host of commonly accepted intrinsic (i.e., genetic) and acquired (i.e., "secondary"; either temporary or persistent) risk factors for VTE (Box 1) and additional stratification variables (Box 2). However, provoked VTE is typically multifactorial in nature, with an estimated incidence of idiopathic VTE in approximately 50% of cases. The pathophysiology of VTE is rooted in Rudolph Virchow's triad, initially described in the mid-nineteenth century. In Virchow's triad, thrombosis was postulated to be a result of at least one of a triumvirate of factors, including endothelial injury, hypercoagulability, and stasis of flow. Prior retrospective reviews have demonstrated that much of Virchow's postulation remains true, with more than 90% of patients with diagnosed VTE having at least one of the three risk factors.

Commonly accepted high-risk factors for VTE include, but are not limited to, trauma, major general/orthopedic surgical procedures, paralysis, spinal cord injuries, long bone fractures, and a prior history of VTE. A history of VTE portends a particularly high risk for future VTE, with one study demonstrating that 21.5% of patients will have a recurrent VTE within 5 years after the diagnosis of initial DVT and a 2.6% incidence of fatal PE. This serves as not only an important concept clarifying the incidence of VTE but also a harrowing predictor by which the surgeon must risk-stratify patients carefully in the management of perioperative prophylactic and therapeutic anticoagulation. High-risk factors should be accounted for and potentially addressed with a dose of VTE chemoprophylaxis in the preoperative setting (given an acceptable intraoperative bleeding risk), as discussed later in this chapter.

Although much of the stratification of VTE events into different criteria may seem arbitrary, studies have demonstrated differences in the risks and incidence of recurrent VTE after anticoagulation, with patients with unprovoked VTE having a higher risk for recurrence than those with provoked VTE.

■ PREVENTION AND PROPHYLAXIS OF VENOUS THROMBOEMBOLISM

Although it is apparent from population studies that the total incidence of mortality resulting from VTE events appears to be decreasing, the rate of detection of VTE undoubtedly is increasing given improvements in imaging modalities and increased awareness of the clinical issue. Before the institution of prophylactic measures to prevent VTE, a thorough risk assessment of the individual patient, as discussed previously, must be undertaken. As such, a multitude of risk assessment models for medical, orthopedic, and nonorthopedic surgical patients have been proposed, relying heavily on many of the aforementioned risk factors, with the Rogers and Caprini scores serving as the most up-to-date nonorthopedic surgical models. However, widespread acceptance of many of these perioperative predictive models has been limited despite validation. Criticisms of these models include skewing of data by an increased presence of comorbid/predisposing conditions, which confer "higher risk" of VTE events, such as neoplastic processes.

Despite the utility of these risk scores, all surgical patients should be evaluated thoroughly for VTE risk factors and given strong consideration for aggressive VTE prophylaxis. Virtually all surgical patients are at increased risk for VTE given a multitude of factors, including the actual surgical procedure ("provoked" VTE), with its resultant aberrations in physiology and the inflammatory response;

BOX 1: Risk Factors for Venous Thromboembolism

Unprovoked (Inherited)

Family history of thrombophilia
Factor V Leiden
Prothrombin G20210A mutation
Protein C deficiency
Protein S deficiency
Antithrombin deficiency
Sickle cell trait
Antiphospholipid antibody syndrome
May-Thurner syndrome

Provoked (Acquired)

Age
Obesity
Smoking
Cancer
Heart failure (NYHA class III or IV)
Pregnancy or postpartum period
Trauma
Immobility
Surgery
Hospitalization
Oral contraception
Personal prior history of VTE
Inflammatory bowel disease
Central venous catheter

NYHA, New York Heart Association; *VTE*, venous thromboembolism.

BOX 2: Stratification of Common Risk Factors for Venous Thromboembolism

High Risk

Long bone fracture
Major general surgery
Trauma
Spinal cord injury
Major orthopedic surgery (major joint replacement)
Active malignancy

Moderate Risk

Indwelling central venous catheter
Congestive heart failure
Oral contraceptives
Paralysis after stroke
Pregnancy or postpartum period
Known thrombophilia

Low Risk

Laparoscopic surgery
Obesity
Smoking
Varicose veins
Immobility or bed rest > 3 days

limitations in mobility conferred upon the patient as a result of the surgical procedure; as well as the cause of the disease surgically intervened upon (e.g., neoplastic). Evidence-based guidelines from the American College of Chest Physicians (ACCP) are published and updated regularly to address the subject of VTE prevention, prophylaxis, and management in medical and surgical patients, with the most recent guidelines published in 2012 and subsequent guidelines due in 2016. Additional organizations in subspecialty areas such as trauma (Eastern Association for the Surgery of Trauma; EAST) and orthopedics (American Academy of Orthopaedic Surgeons) likewise publish evidence-based guidelines for VTE prevention and prophylaxis in these patient subpopulations.

Regardless of predictor scores, the clinical decision of if and when to institute pharmacologic VTE prophylaxis must be undertaken by and is at the discretion of the surgeon. Not only is this because of the nature of the surgeons' relationship with the patients and their role as the responsible provider during perioperative management, but also the surgeon is the individual best qualified to discern the risk of operative bleeding given knowledge of the procedure at hand and direct visualization of the tissues and cut surfaces at the time of operation. In addition, the timing and necessity for pharmacologic VTE prophylaxis is a decision that is based upon weighing the risks of bleeding versus the risks of incurring a VTE event,

both of which have the potential for high morbidity and even mortality. As such, there have been a variety of schema/guidelines for tailoring VTE chemoprophylaxis in the perioperative period, one of which we demonstrate in Figure 1 (based on the recommendations of the ACCP). Traditionally, patients at high risk for bleeding sequelae in this schema are those with recent gastrointestinal (GI) bleeding, intracranial bleeding/hemorrhagic stroke, indicators of hematologic derangement (such as thrombocytopenia), as well as patients whose surgical procedure resulted in high blood volume loss and/or places them at some resultant risk for postoperative rebleeding.

Nonpharmacologic VTE prophylaxis measures are well established and integrated into virtually all postoperative units. General strategies such as early postoperative ambulation encourage lower extremity venous blood flow. Additional nonpharmacologic, "mechanical," VTE prophylaxis methods are available and include intermittent pneumatic and graduated compression devices and stockings, which have been shown in studies to reduce the risk of VTE events in postsurgical patients by approximately 50%. Similar to early ambulation, mechanical VTE prophylaxis improves blood flow, reduces venous stasis, and is thought to result in locoregional production of endogenous anticoagulant compounds, reducing the risk of VTE in postoperative patients. Limitations of these nonpharmacologic

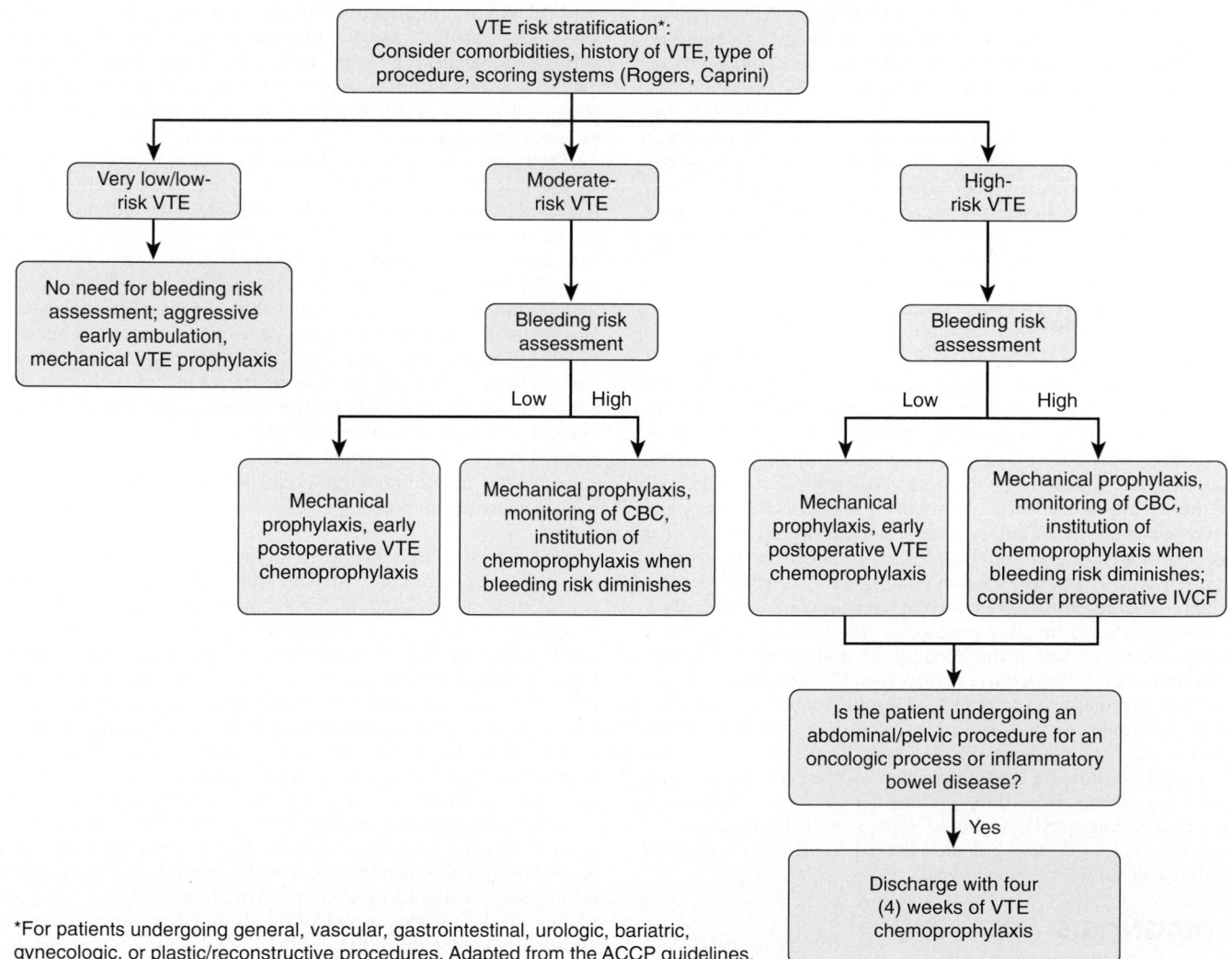

*For patients undergoing general, vascular, gastrointestinal, urologic, bariatric, gynecologic, or plastic/reconstructive procedures. Adapted from the ACCP guidelines.

FIGURE 1 Example of perioperative venous thromboembolism prophylaxis guidelines, adopted in part from American College of Chest Physicians recommendations. *CBC,* Complete blood count; *IVCF,* inferior vena cava filter; *VTE,* venous thromboembolism.

VTE prophylactic measures, despite their efficacy in targeting the venous stasis limb of Virchow's triad and serving as vital adjuncts to pharmacologic VTE prophylaxis, include difficulties with patient adherence and an increased incidence of VTE versus VTE chemoprophylaxis alone.

Given these limitations in mechanical VTE prophylaxis, the most consistent and adequate VTE prophylaxis is achieved via pharmacologic means in patients at low to moderate risk for postoperative bleeding. As such, VTE pharmacoprophylaxis is administered typically through subcutaneous injections of either unfractionated or low-molecular-weight heparin (UFH or LMWH, respectively), with a host of additional available agents, including aspirin, dalteparin, or fondaparinux. Limitations apply to UFH and LMHW in terms of efficacy, patient compliance/satisfaction, bleeding risk, induction of heparin-induced thrombocytopenia (HIT), as well as bioavailability. In general, UFH must be administered every 8 hours owing to its shorter half-life and confers a higher risk of HIT, whereas other agents are dosed in a weight-based fashion and administered once daily (exception: LMWH in trauma patients is administered every 12 hours), which may increase patient satisfaction and adherence, especially with postdischarge treatment regimens. Despite the increased frequency of use, UFH remains the least expensive option for VTE prophylaxis and may be administered to patients with chronic kidney disease, whereas the more readily bioavailable LMWH cannot. The bleeding risks of UFH and LMWH are under constant scrutiny and frequently are compared to one another. A recent meta-analysis demonstrated an overall lower risk for major bleeding in LMHW with no differences in the incidence of VTE between groups. It should be noted that bleeding events consistently have been shown to be increased versus controls and most frequently occur at operative sites.

The utilization of inferior vena cava (IVC) filters for VTE prophylaxis is not currently accepted as a modality in low- or moderate-risk patients. IVC filters likewise do not prevent the formation or propagation of thrombus but instead serve as a salvage means by which VTE events from the iliofemoral system can be "caught" by a variety of different types of devices. IVC filters, which remain controversial, are discussed in more detail later in the chapter.

Special Populations

Certain patient populations warrant brief but special mention in terms of VTE prophylaxis. Because the risk for hemorrhage into the pleural space is high, patients undergoing cardiac surgery with routine postoperative courses are not prescribed VTE pharmacoprophylaxis regularly but instead are encouraged to ambulate early and given mechanical means of VTE prophylaxis, regardless of VTE risk. For these same cardiac surgical patients who appear to suffer postoperative complications and require prolonged hospitalization, it is suggested that VTE pharmacoprophylaxis be added to the prophylactic regimen. For patients undergoing thoracic surgery, often for the purpose of resecting tumor, recommendations are for VTE pharmacoprophylaxis to be given postoperatively if the bleeding risk is appropriate. Conversely, if the bleeding risk in these patients is high in the immediate postoperative period, then VTE chemoprophylaxis should be instituted as soon as deemed feasible and safe by the operative team. Similar to this last cohort of patients, those who have suffered major trauma immediately should be started on VTE chemoprophylaxis, unless a contraindication such as bleeding or injury pattern (e.g., splenic laceration, subdural hematoma) precludes such. VTE pharmacoprophylaxis should subsequently be employed in these patients regardless of risk after the risk to heparin exposure or bleeding risk subsides.

▪ DIAGNOSIS

For any patient with a clinical suspicion for VTE, prompt diagnosis is critical, especially when the potentially fatal consequence of PE is considered. Initial diagnosis by history and physical exam is useful but must be confirmed by prompt imaging to guide management because the differential diagnoses for shortness of breath and lower extremity swelling (both clinical signs of PE and VTE, respectively) are broad. Symptoms of DVT include but are not limited to erythema, swelling, pain, skin discoloration, and dilatation of superficial leg veins. DVT can progress to phlegmasia cerulea dolens or phlegmasia alba dolens, the latter of which is a surgical emergency because arterial inflow to the lower extremity is compromised secondary to total occlusion of the deep (initial) and superficial (subsequent) venous outflow. However, postoperative DVT typically is not accompanied by dramatic symptomatology and is often asymptomatic. Symptoms of PE, which may be the first clinical manifestation of DVT, include dyspnea, pleuritic chest pain, hemoptysis, tachycardia, desaturation on pulse oximetry, and dramatic and sudden cardiopulmonary compromise and even new-onset atrial fibrillation. With respect to the duration of symptoms, although in some regard the physiology of VTE is a chronic or subacute process, symptoms of VTE typically have an acute onset.

The utility of laboratory or serum tests, such as the D-dimer level, a marker of endogenous fibrinolysis, has been debated for some time. D-dimer utility is limited in the postoperative setting because of false-positive results (aberrant elevations), and the measurement and reporting of D-dimer itself is hindered by heterogeneity in test results and specificity. Regardless, for medical patients being seen for evaluation of VTE, D-dimer has proven a useful diagnostic adjunct. Additional testing such as genetic screens for certain polymorphisms, anticardiolipin antibodies, and functional endogenous anticoagulant levels (i.e., proteins C and S, antithrombin levels) are of diagnostic and management utility in the long term. However, obtaining and interpreting these studies should not delay further treatment and imaging diagnosis as the timeframe for results can range from days to weeks and activity and protein measurements are not accurate during an acute thromboembolic event, nor during anticoagulation.

The diagnosis of DVT, although simplified in recent years by the increased availability and resolution of duplex ultrasound (US), has certain limitations. These include morbidly obese patients, patients with excessive pain precluding venous compression with the US probe, aberrant venous anatomy, interoperator variability, and iliofemoral thrombus, which typically cannot be visualized by routine US. Hence, imaging adjuncts such as magnetic resonance imaging (MRI) or computed tomography (CT) may be used for further diagnostic clarity in this situation, with the utility of each modality enhanced with contrast administration and accurate venous phase imaging. Conventional catheter-based, two-dimensional (2D) venography is not used frequently to diagnose DVT because of the invasive nature of the study, although it has demonstrated utility in diagnosing and subsequently treating proximal iliofemoral venous occlusive disease.

Undoubtedly, the gold standard for the diagnosis of PE is contrast-enhanced imaging of the chest, with filling defects of the pulmonary arterial tree readily visible (Figure 2), and perfusion artifacts limited by improved scanner resolution and timing. Given the improvements in CT technology, such as multidetector scanners, increased scanning speed, higher-resolution imaging, and complete electronic integration of imaging, the American College of Radiology has endorsed CT angiography as the imaging modality of choice for PE diagnosis.

Intermittently, patients will be precluded from receiving pulmonary CT angiograms because of renal insufficiency or an allergy to intravenous contrast dye, and thus other imaging modalities must be sought. Ventilation-perfusion (V/Q) scintigraphic scanning is another imaging modality employed for detection of pulmonary embolism, and although the test is highly specific, it is not particularly sensitive, with other pulmonary pathology resulting in a potential positive V/Q scan. Current V/Q scanning diagnostic criteria are as delineated in the PISAPED and PIOPED II studies. Other imaging modalities, such as MRI-based pulmonary angiography, have not gained widespread use, whereas conventional angiography has diminished in use but remains useful as a diagnostic and therapeutic

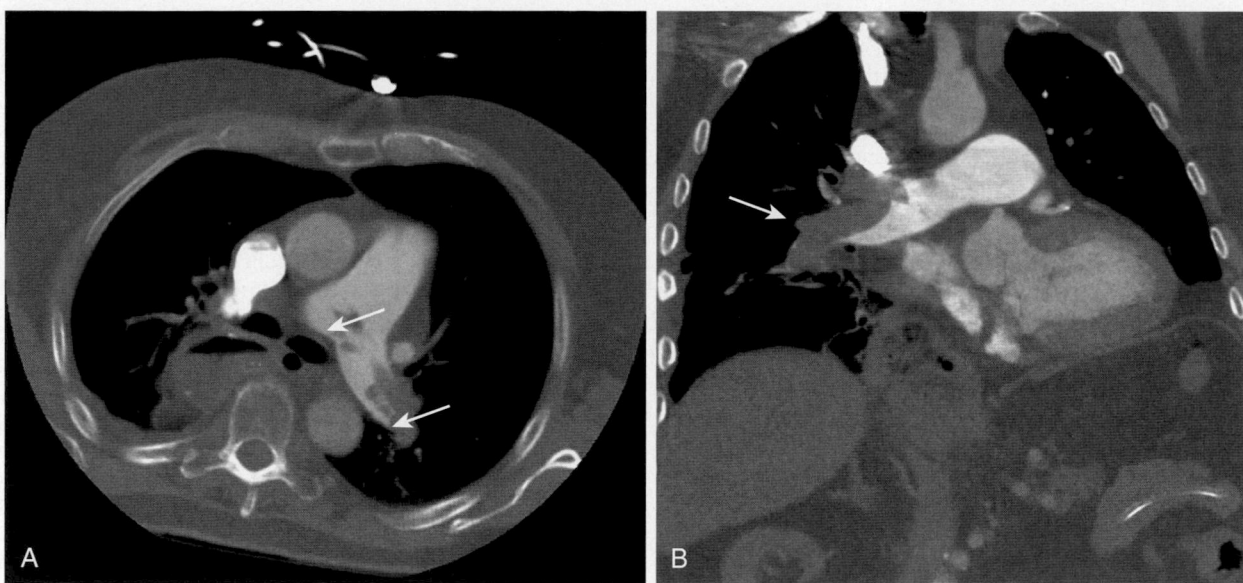

FIGURE 2 Pulmonary embolism (PE), as demonstrated by computed tomography (CT) scan. The arrow indicates the PE.

modality in certain instances (see the section on Treatment). Conventional plain-film imaging of the chest, although able to demonstrate certain characteristics of the pulmonary vasculature (prominence of the pulmonary arterial tree), is not an adequate diagnostic imaging modality for PE and should not be used for definitive diagnosis, although it is useful for ruling out other pathology.

Likewise, high-risk patients who are critically ill and unable to be transported from the intensive care unit (ICU) with high clinical suspicion of PE may be diagnosed with bedside transthoracic or transesophageal echocardiography. Echocardiography can demonstrate right ventricular strain or overload and, in rare instances, visualize thrombus in the right heart. Patients with shock or hemodynamic instability with a high suspicion of PE should be diagnosed with CT angiography only if it is immediately available, with echocardiographic confirmation of PE leading to subsequent imaging with CT angiography upon patient stabilization, or directed treatment for PE otherwise. There are specific echocardiographic signs that can assist in the diagnosis of PE as well.

■ TREATMENT

The treatment of VTE is aimed at addressing the underlying cause of the thrombus as well as preventing future, more devastating thromboembolic events, the most feared of which is PE. In this section, we aim to discuss separately the treatment schema for DVT and PE, as well as more controversial treatment adjuncts in patients with potential contraindications to anticoagulation.

Superficial Venous Thrombosis

Although the focus of this chapter is not in the discussion of superficial venous thrombosis (SVT), this seemingly benign venous pathology can, in a similar fashion to DVT, lead to morbidity such as inflammation, infection, extension into the deep venous system (creating a DVT), as well as PE, hence meriting brief mention. SVT often is seen as a tender, palpable superficial cord with associated erythema and edema of the affected extremity. Moreover, SVT is thought to be more common than DVT, shares many of the same risk factors with DVT, can present concomitantly with DVT, and, when present, has been demonstrated to have an association with symptomatic and asymptomatic VTE. Despite these serious

implications for SVT, there appear to be no true consensus guidelines published in a similar vein to those for DVT or PE. In general, it is advocated that treatment of local symptoms should be instituted through administration of anti-inflammatory medications such as nonsteroidal anti-inflammatory drugs (NSAIDs), which appear to reduce the extension and/or recurrence of SVT in combination with LMWH or fondaparinux for approximately 45 days. SVT that extends to the saphenofemoral junction can be treated by ligation or anticoagulation.

Deep Venous Thrombosis

The open surgical era for DVT treatment is bygone, with current efforts aimed at medically managing patients through effective therapeutic (as opposed to prophylactic) anticoagulation, treating the potential underlying cause for DVT, and determining the risk for recurrence or propagation of the thrombus. All of these considerations must be made within the context for the individual patients' bleeding risk, especially given factors such as poor patient compliance, postoperative or post-traumatic states, recent GI bleeding, or recent intracranial hemorrhage. In addition, when formulating treatment duration, one must take into consideration the phases of VTE treatment—acute, long-term, and extended treatment—and whether the VTE event was provoked or unprovoked. The overarching goals of DVT treatment in the short and long term are to stabilize the thrombus, prevent PE, reduce recurrence, and minimize DVT-related morbidity.

Initial ("acute-phase") treatment of DVT is guided at thrombus stabilization and prevention of propagation of thrombus and prevention of thrombus embolism to PE, and typically is performed through combination of knee-high compression stockings (30 to 40 mm Hg) with weight-based parenteral or subcutaneous dosing of UFH, LMWH, fondaparinux, or rivaroxaban, which should not be delayed upon initial diagnosis or reasonable clinical suspicion of DVT. Although any of these medications may be employed in the treatment of DVT, recent studies have demonstrated that LMWH may demonstrate a lower overall associated mortality, bleeding risk, and recurrence of VTE when compared with UFH. In addition, UFH should be used preferentially in instances in which patients have chronic renal insufficiency (creatinine clearance < 30 mL/min). Subsequent efforts to transition patients in the acute DVT treatment phase to longer-term oral anticoagulation regimens typically is done with vitamin K antagonists such as warfarin, with therapeutic effect of the drug monitored through the international normalized ratio (INR) in the 2.0 to 3.0 range.

More recently, new oral factor Xa inhibitors (apixaban, rivaroxaban) and direct thrombin inhibitors (dabigatran) have garnered FDA approval for treatment of VTE and do not require monitoring of therapeutic effect via INR. However, these new oral anticoagulant agents appear to be more difficult to reverse in times of acute need (i.e., emergency surgery) when compared with vitamin K antagonists. In terms of treatment duration, the decision is based largely upon risk and whether the DVT was provoked. In general, 3 months is the shortest acceptable period for DVT treatment in situations in which it was provoked, with unprovoked DVT commonly treated between 3 and 6 months. There are several high-risk features, which may predispose patients to recurrent DVT or even PE (such as malignancy, thrombophilia, or recurrence of prior VTE), at which point extended treatment to greater than 6 months or lifetime treatment are considered.

In the special circumstance of acute iliofemoral DVT (in young patients) or venous gangrene, early thrombolysis has been employed as an attractive therapy owing to its efficacy in treating the thrombus and permitting for recanalization of the affected venous segment through pharmacologic, mechanical, or pharmacomechanical means. This contrasts with "conventional" noninvasive treatment, which prevents thrombus propagation and recurrence but does not allow for the removal of thrombus and potential venous salvage, placing patients at high risk for development of the post-thrombotic syndrome (PTS). This syndrome, which may affect up to 50% of patients after an episode of DVT up to 2 years after diagnosis, is characterized by chronic valvular disruption and venous occlusion resulting in pain, cramping, swelling, and a sensation of heaviness in the affected lower extremity, which can progress to skin ulceration if not treated adequately. Studies have demonstrated that PTS places tremendous socioeconomic burdens and quality of life restrictions on patients, which has served as the foundation for the ATTRACT (Acute venous Thrombosis: Thrombus Removal with Adjunctive Catheter-direct Thrombolysis) trial. The ATTRACT trial hypothesizes that pharmacomechanical catheter-directed thrombolysis significantly reduces the proportion of patients who suffer from PTS within a 2-year timeframe. Results of the ATTRACT trial, which is currently in Phase III testing, are pending. Initial attempts at percutaneous treatment of thrombus, it should be noted, were limited by the bleeding risk conferred by the systemic administration of thrombolytic or fibrinolytic agents, which subsequently have been minimized with the advent of percutaneous catheter-directed therapy. Current Society for Vascular Surgery guidelines have evolved to recommend pharmacomechanical thrombolysis over catheter-directed therapies, if available. Although some individuals routinely have employed IVC filter use at the time of percutaneous treatment for DVT, this currently is not recommended except as a PE preventative measure in patients with DVT and too high of a risk for bleeding, precluding them from parenteral and oral anticoagulation. However, if bleeding risk is transient and anticoagulation may be started when this risk subsides, a host of IVC filters have been developed that are retrievable through percutaneous means.

Pulmonary Embolism

The more feared and potentially lethal complication of DVT is that of PE. It can be the initial presentation of VTE in many patients, especially in the postoperative setting. The treatment strategy for PE is guided by the hemodynamic or cardiopulmonary state of the patient, which serves to risk-stratify those with acute PE. Massive PE in low-bleeding-risk patients with hypotension or systemic shock are classified as high-risk PE, and upon confirmation of the diagnosis with imaging or echocardiography, these patients should be treated preferentially with systemic antifibrinolytic agents

(i.e., pharmacologic thrombolysis) or "primary reperfusion" therapy. In the instance of a high-bleeding-risk patient or one with a contraindication to thrombolysis, those with intracranial or uncontrolled hemorrhage or recent surgery/trauma, consideration of surgical or percutaneous embolectomy (without concurrent catheter-directed pharmacologic thrombolysis) must be given in addition to placement of an IVC filter for future PE prophylaxis. Otherwise, patients should be given immediate therapeutic doses of UFH or LMHW with subsequent administration of an antifibrinolytic agent or percutaneous catheter-directed therapy (with concurrent pharmacologic thrombolysis). Surgical embolectomy also serves as a backup treatment strategy should thrombolysis fail to rescue.

In the situation in which the diagnosis of PE is made without the presence of cardiopulmonary collapse (low- to intermediate-risk PE) and in the absence of contraindications to anticoagulation (as discussed above), therapeutic anticoagulation is started as either intravenous UFH or subcutaneous LMWH in the acute phase. The subsequent transition to long-term oral anticoagulation (or continuation of LMHW) is performed after approximately 24 hours of acute therapy, the duration of which is incumbent on the nature of the thrombus and is similar to that described for DVT, as trials for efficacy of varying durations of post-PE only anticoagulation are limited.

Inferior Vena Cava Filters

As has been described, IVC filter use most frequently occurs in those with risk factors for or contraindications to acute bleeding on initiation of therapeutic anticoagulation, or in the instance of recurrent VTE despite adequate anticoagulation. Notably, these filters neither prevent the formation of DVT nor are they resistant to the formation of additional thrombus on the struts of the filter (in the most severe cases resulting in caval occlusion), nor are they without complications such as filter migration, filter fracture, and filter erosion through the caval wall into adjacent viscera. Instead, IVC filters are thought to serve as salvage mechanisms by which a large embolus from the deep veins of the lower extremity or iliofemoral region is prevented physically from reaching the pulmonary arterial circuit. Despite recommendations for their use by subspecialty organizations such as EAST, current ACCP guidelines recommend against the use of IVC filters for VTE prophylaxis even in the cohort of high-risk patients. IVC filters are instead indicated in those with iliofemoral DVT and a contraindication to anticoagulation or with an impending surgical procedure. Notably, no society guidelines have advocated for or recommend IVC filter placement in those receiving percutaneous procedures or systemic thrombolysis, and the Prévention du Risque d'Embolie Pulmonaire par Interruption Cave (PREPIC) and subsequent PREPIC2 trials have demonstrated that anticoagulation is far superior to IVC filter placement alone in patients eligible for therapeutic anticoagulation and that filter placement does not confer a long-term mortality benefit, at the cost of increased recurrent DVT events. In particular, the PREPIC2 trial used retrievable IVC filters, which can serve as a means of "bridging" high-risk bleeding patients to oral anticoagulation when the bleeding risk expires.

IVC filters represent a potential bedside solution to the problem of addressing PE prophylaxis in those with absolute and relative indications for anticoagulation. Typically placed in an infrarenal location, filters are placed by a variety of subspecialists, and technology has evolved to the point where intravascular ultrasound can be used for filter placement, as opposed to more traditional venography.

■ SUMMARY AND CONCLUSIONS

Venous thromboembolism includes DVT and PE and is a common condition in medical and surgical patients. The incidence of VTE is rising, and the ability to diagnose an often clinically silent, but potentially fatal, condition in a timely fashion is improving owing to enhanced awareness of the condition, imaging modalities, and predictor models. There are a host of established risk factors for VTE, which must be taken carefully into consideration when risk-stratifying surgical patients, virtually all of whom are at least at an intermediate risk for VTE events in the perioperative period and hence must be prophylaxed appropriately. If a VTE event is detected, in the acute setting immediate therapeutic anticoagulation, and in some instances, thrombolysis, remains the mainstay of treatment, although in surgical patients in particular, bleeding risk must be weighed against the risk of recurrent thrombosis. The eventual duration of therapy subsequently is determined by the nature of the thrombotic event ("provoked" vs "unprovoked"), and individual risk factors. New oral medications are emerging that do not require monitoring of therapeutic effect or efficacy, and IVC filters are used in specific patient subpopulations given certain criteria. Regardless, individual patient characteristics must be weighed to formulate an appropriate therapeutic modality.

Suggested Readings

Anderson FA Jr, Spencer FA. Risk factors for venous thromboembolism. *Circulation.* 2003;107(23 suppl 1):I9-I16.

Anderson FA Jr, Wheeler HB. Physician practices in the management of venous thromboembolism: a community-wide survey. *J Vasc Surg.* 1992;16:707-714.

Anderson FA Jr, Zayaruzny M, Heit JA, et al. Estimated annual numbers of US acute-care hospital patients at risk for venous thromboembolism. *Am J Hematol.* 2007;82:777-782.

Bahl V, Hu HM, Henke PK, et al. A validation study of a retrospective venous thromboembolism risk scoring method. *Ann Surg.* 2010;251:344-350.

Barbar S, Noventa F, Rossetto V, et al. A risk assessment model for the identification of hospitalized medical patients at risk for venous thromboembolism: the Padua Prediction Score. *J Thromb Haemost.* 2010;8:2450-2457.

Bergqvist D, Jaroszewski H. Deep vein thrombosis in patients with superficial thrombophlebitis of the leg. *Br Med J (Clin Res Ed).* 1986;292:658-659.

Blumenberg RM, Barton E, Gelfand ML, et al. Occult deep venous thrombosis complicating superficial thrombophlebitis. *J Vasc Surg.* 1998;27:338-343.

Boutitie F, Pinede L, Schulman S, et al. Influence of preceding length of anticoagulant treatment and initial presentation of venous thromboembolism on risk of recurrence after stopping treatment: analysis of individual participants' data from seven trials. *BMJ.* 2011;342:d3036.

Casciano JP, Dotiwala Z, Kemp R, et al. Economic burden of recurrent venous thromboembolism: analysis from a U.S. hospital perspective. *Am J Health Syst Pharm.* 2015;72:291-300.

Chopra N, Doddamreddy P, Grewal H, et al. An elevated D-dimer value: a burden on our patients and hospitals. *Int J Gen Med.* 2012;5:87-92.

Cohen AT, Tapson VF, Bergmann JF, et al. Venous thromboembolism risk and prophylaxis in the acute hospital care setting (ENDORSE study): a multinational cross-sectional study. *Lancet.* 2008;371:387-394.

Cohoon KP, Leibson CL, Ransom JE, et al. Direct medical costs attributable to venous thromboembolism among persons hospitalized for major operation: a population-based longitudinal study. *Surgery.* 2015;157:423-431.

Collins R, Scrimgeour A, Yusuf S, et al. Reduction in fatal pulmonary embolism and venous thrombosis by perioperative administration of subcutaneous heparin. Overview of results of randomized trials in general, orthopedic, and urologic surgery. *N Engl J Med.* 1988;318:1162-1173.

Decousus H, Leizorovicz A, Parent F, et al. A clinical trial of vena caval filters in the prevention of pulmonary embolism in patients with proximal deep-vein thrombosis. Prevention du Risque d'Embolie Pulmonaire par Interruption Cave Study Group. *N Engl J Med.* 1998;338:409-415.

Di Nisio M, Wichers IM, Middeldorp S. Treatment for superficial thrombophlebitis of the leg. *Cochrane Database Syst Rev.* 2013;(4):CD004982.

Erkens PM, Prins MH. Fixed dose subcutaneous low molecular weight heparins versus adjusted dose unfractionated heparin for venous thromboembolism. *Cochrane Database Syst Rev.* 2010;(9):CD001100.

Fedullo PF, Tapson VF. Clinical practice. The evaluation of suspected pulmonary embolism. *N Engl J Med.* 2003;349:1247-1256.

Flanc C, Kakkar VV, Clarke MB. The detection of venous thrombosis of the legs using 125-1-labelled fibrinogen. *Br J Surg.* 1968;55:742-747.

Group PS. Eight-year follow-up of patients with permanent vena cava filters in the prevention of pulmonary embolism: the PREPIC (Prevention du Risque d'Embolie Pulmonaire par Interruption Cave) randomized study. *Circulation.* 2005;112:416-422.

Guyatt GH, Akl EA, Crowther M, et al. Executive summary: Antithrombotic therapy and prevention of thrombosis, 9th ed: American College of Chest Physicians evidence-based clinical practice guidelines. *Chest.* 2012;141(2 suppl):7S-47S.

Hansson PO, Sorbo J, Eriksson H. Recurrent venous thromboembolism after deep vein thrombosis: incidence and risk factors. *Arch Intern Med.* 2000;160:769-774.

Iannuzzi JC, Young KC, Kim MJ, et al. Prediction of postdischarge venous thromboembolism using a risk assessment model. *J Vasc Surg.* 2013;58:1014-1020 e1.

Kahn SR, Ducruet T, Lamping DL, et al. Prospective evaluation of health-related quality of life in patients with deep venous thrombosis. *Arch Intern Med.* 2005;165:1173-1178.

Kahn SR, Shbaklo H, Lamping DL, et al. Determinants of health-related quality of life during the 2 years following deep vein thrombosis. *J Thromb Haemost.* 2008;6:1105-1112.

Kahn SR, Shrier I, Julian JA, et al. Determinants and time course of the postthrombotic syndrome after acute deep venous thrombosis. *Ann Intern Med.* 2008;149:698-707.

Kearon C, Akl EA, Comerota AJ, et al. Antithrombotic therapy for VTE disease: antithrombotic therapy and prevention of thrombosis, 9th ed: American College of Chest Physicians evidence-based clinical practice guidelines. *Chest.* 2012;141(2 suppl):e419S-e494S.

Konstantinides SV, Torbicki A, Agnelli G, et al. 2014 ESC guidelines on the diagnosis and management of acute pulmonary embolism. *Eur Heart J.* 2014;35:3033-3069, 69a-69k.

Kucher N, Koo S, Quiroz R, et al. Electronic alerts to prevent venous thromboembolism among hospitalized patients. *N Engl J Med.* 2005;352:969-977.

Kurzyna M, Torbicki A, Pruszczyk P, et al. Disturbed right ventricular ejection pattern as a new Doppler echocardiographic sign of acute pulmonary embolism. *Am J Cardiol.* 2002;90:507-511.

Mahan CE, Borrego ME, Woersching AL, et al. Venous thromboembolism: annualised United States models for total, hospital-acquired and preventable costs utilising long-term attack rates. *Thromb Haemost.* 2012;108:291-302.

Meissner MH, Gloviczki P, Comerota AJ, et al. Early thrombus removal strategies for acute deep venous thrombosis: clinical practice guidelines of the Society for Vascular Surgery and the American Venous Forum. *J Vasc Surg.* 2012;55:1449-1462.

Mismetti P, Laporte S, Pellerin O, et al. Effect of a retrievable inferior vena cava filter plus anticoagulation vs anticoagulation alone on risk of recurrent pulmonary embolism: a randomized clinical trial. *JAMA.* 2015;313:1627-1635.

Mismetti P, Laporte-Simitsidis S, Tardy B, et al. Prevention of venous thromboembolism in internal medicine with unfractionated or low-molecular-weight heparins: a meta-analysis of randomised clinical trials. *Thromb Haemost.* 2000;83:14-19.

Nasr H, Scriven JM. Superficial thrombophlebitis (superficial venous thrombosis). *BMJ.* 2015;350.

Nordstrom M, Lindblad B, Bergqvist D, et al. A prospective study of the incidence of deep-vein thrombosis within a defined urban population. *J Intern Med.* 1992;232:155-160.

Office of the Surgeon General (US) NH, Lung, and Blood Institute (US). *The Surgeon General's Call to Action to Prevent Deep Vein Thrombosis and Pulmonary Embolism.* Rockville (MD): Office of the Surgeon General (US); 2008.

Park B, Messina L, Dargon P, et al. Recent trends in clinical outcomes and resource utilization for pulmonary embolism in the United States: findings from the nationwide inpatient sample. *Chest.* 2009;136:983-990.

Pesavento R, Villalta S, Prandoni P. The postthrombotic syndrome. *Intern Emerg Med.* 2010;5:185-192.

Quenet S, Laporte S, Decousus H, et al. Factors predictive of venous thrombotic complications in patients with isolated superficial vein thrombosis. *J Vasc Surg.* 2003;38:944-949.

Rogers SO Jr, Kilaru RK, Hosokawa P, et al. Multivariable predictors of postoperative venous thromboembolic events after general and vascular surgery: results from the patient safety in surgery study. *J Am Coll Surg.* 2007;204:1211-1221.

Sachdeva A, Dalton M, Amaragiri SV, et al. Graduated compression stockings for prevention of deep vein thrombosis. *Cochrane Database Syst Rev.* 2014;(12):CD001484.

Silverstein MD, Heit JA, Mohr DN, et al. Trends in the incidence of deep vein thrombosis and pulmonary embolism: a 25-year population-based study. *Arch Intern Med.* 1998;158:585-593.

Sostman HD, Miniati M, Gottschalk A, et al. Sensitivity and specificity of perfusion scintigraphy combined with chest radiography for acute pulmonary embolism in PIOPED II. *J Nucl Med.* 2008;49:1741-1748.

Spencer FA, Emery C, Lessard D, et al. The Worcester Venous Thromboembolism study: a population-based study of the clinical epidemiology of venous thromboembolism. *J Gen Intern Med.* 2006;21:722-727.

Tan M, Bornais C, Rodger M. Interobserver reliability of compression ultrasound for residual thrombosis after first unprovoked deep vein thrombosis. *J Thromb Haemostasis.* 2012;10:1775-1782.

Urbankova J, Quiroz R, Kucher N, et al. Intermittent pneumatic compression and deep vein thrombosis prevention. A meta-analysis in postoperative patients. *Thromb Haemost.* 2005;94:1181-1185.

Vedantham S, Goldhaber SZ, Kahn SR, et al. Rationale and design of the ATTRACT Study: a multicenter randomized trial to evaluate pharmacomechanical catheter-directed thrombolysis for the prevention of postthrombotic syndrome in patients with proximal deep vein thrombosis. *Am Heart J.* 2013;165:523-530 e3.

Verlato F, Zucchetta P, Prandoni P, et al. An unexpectedly high rate of pulmonary embolism in patients with superficial thrombophlebitis of the thigh. *J Vasc Surg.* 1999;30:1113-1115.

Wells PS, Anderson DR, Rodger M, et al. Evaluation of D-dimer in the diagnosis of suspected deep-vein thrombosis. *N Engl J Med.* 2003;349:1227-1235.

Wells PS, Forgie MA, Rodger MA. Treatment of venous thromboembolism. *JAMA.* 2014;311:717-728.

White RH, Zhou H, Murin S, et al. Effect of ethnicity and gender on the incidence of venous thromboembolism in a diverse population in California in 1996. *Thromb Haemost.* 2005;93:298-305.

White RH. The epidemiology of venous thromboembolism. *Circulation.* 2003;107(23 suppl 1):I4-I8.

Yazdani M, Lau CT, Lempel JK, et al. Historical evolution of imaging techniques for the evaluation of pulmonary embolism: RSNA Centennial Article. *Radiographics.* 2015;3:1245-1262.

VENA CAVA FILTERS

Maria Tsitskari, MD, and Christos Georgiades, MD, PhD, FSIR, FCIRSE

The objective of vena cava filtration is to reduce the risk of clinically significant pulmonary embolic events by means of inferior (or, rarely, superior) vena cava interruption.

The rationale is that because the majority of pulmonary emboli (PE) originate in the deep veins of the pelvis or lower extremities, effective inferior vena cava (IVC) filtering will reduce the frequency, mortality, and morbidity associated with PE.

EPIDEMIOLOGY OF PULMONARY EMBOLI

The reported incidence of deep venous thrombosis (DVT; the primary risk factor for PE) in the United States is approximately 125 new cases per 100,000 population per year (Belohlavec, 2013). Some authors put the true number of new DVT events (diagnosed and undiagnosed DVT) at 2 million (Lopez, 2004). The conservative estimates translate to nearly 375,000 patients diagnosed with DVT per year, a number that represents only the reported or clinically significant cases. Of those patients, approximately 200,000 (Belohlavec, 2013) subsequently will develop venous thromboembolism (VTE), most commonly a PE, yielding an incidence of approximately 70 new PE per 100,000 population per year. The overall mortality of all patients with PE (treated and untreated) approaches 18%, or 35,000 deaths per year in the United States (Figure 1; Belohlavec, 2013; Lopez, 2004). Irrespective of the exact incidence, PE is a major healthcare burden, being the third most common type of vascular disease after coronary disease and stroke. If untreated, PE has a 30% mortality rate, with most patients (2 out of 3) dying within 2 hours of symptom onset. Prompt and effective treatment of PE (anticoagulation with or without IVC filtration when indicated) reduces the risk for mortality from 30% to 8% (Figure 2; Belohlavec, 2013). Overall, 10% of hospital deaths are related to PE, and 1% of patients admitted die as a result of a PE (Lankei, 2011).

INDICATIONS AND CONTRAINDICATIONS FOR PLACEMENT OF AN INFERIOR VENA CAVA FILTER

There are instances when the standard of care, systemic anticoagulation, is either ineffective or contraindicated. In such instances, placement of an IVC filter is indicated absolutely, as it provides an additional layer of protection against PE. The IVC filters currently available in the United States are shown in Figure 3. In addition to the two absolute indications, there are a number of relative indications for placing an IVC filter (Kaufman, 2006); both types of indications are outlined in Table 1.

Contraindications to IVC filter placement are rare. A thrombosed, intrahepatic, infra-atrial IVC is an absolute contraindication, as there is no room for filter placement. A thrombosed IVC is a relative contraindication if there is no infrarenal space for filter placement. In this case, a suprarenal filter can be placed, being cognizant of the risk for renal vein thrombosis. A megacava (diameter >32 mm) precludes the use of most IVC filters; however, filtration still can be provided by the Bird's Nest filter (Cook Medical, Bloomington, IN). Bacteremia is a relative contraindication, with studies showing a low risk of seeding and subsequent septic emboli. Finally, a prothrombotic state requires careful review of the possible risks and benefits of IVC filtration, as the filter itself may cause thrombosis. In such cases, hematology consultation can help to guide appropriate treatment.

INDICATIONS AND CONTRAINDICATIONS FOR FILTER REMOVAL

Any filter that can be retrieved and is no longer needed or effective should be retrieved. If the patient's underlying risk for PE has returned to baseline or if the patient has become a candidate for effective anticoagulation, serious consideration should be given to filter removal. If the filter itself is ineffective (migrated, kinked, fractured), retrieval and replacement, if necessary, also should be considered. Active bacteremia is a relative indication for filter removal. The filter should be suspected as a source of infection or septic emboli if no other definitive source of the recurrent infection or septic emboli is found. In such cases, the filter can be removed if not needed or replaced once the bacteremia has resolved.

Frequently, patient safety concerns may prevent filter removal. A clotted filter cannot be removed for fear of sending the clot to the lungs. Technical issues include the filter being imbedded in the wall of the IVC, preventing safe removal. A variety of methods have been developed that allow retrieval in such cases (even in cases of permanent filters); however, retrieval should be attempted only by experienced interventionalists, as the IVC may be traumatized.

TECHNIQUE

The role of an IVC filter is to minimize the risk of a PE. Optimum performance requires catheter expertise, proper venous access

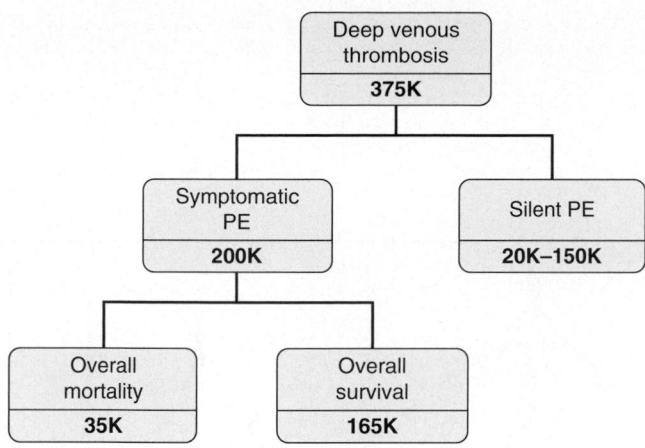

FIGURE 1 Conservative estimates place the incidence of deep venous thrombosis in the United States at 375,000. Of these, at least 200,000 will be seen with pulmonary thromboembolism. The overall mortality of patients from pulmonary embolism (PE) in the United States is 35,000, or 18% overall (treated and untreated). *K*, Thousand.

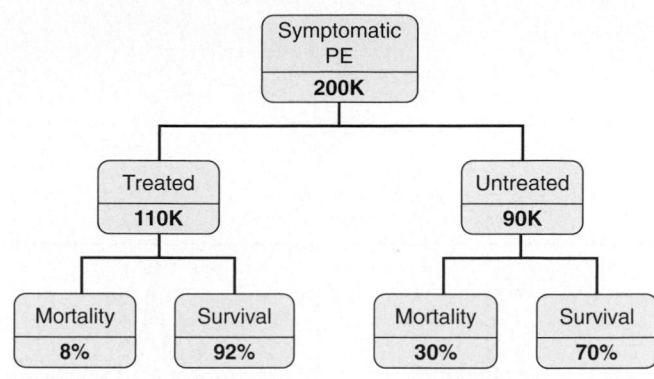

FIGURE 2 Prompt and effective treatment (systemic anticoagulation with or without inferior vena cava filtration if indicated) is crucial in reducing the morbidity and mortality related to pulmonary embolism (PE). Of the 200,000 new symptomatic patients with PE per year in the United States, only 55% receive prompt and effective treatment. This reduces their mortality to 8%, compared with 30% for those who are not treated. *K*, Thousand.

TABLE 1: Indications for IVC Filter Placement

	Indications for IVC Filter Placement	Examples
1.	DVT and contraindication to anticoagulation (A)	Hemorrhage while on anticoagulation.
2.	DVT and failure of anticoagulation (A)	Recurrent DVT or PE despite anticoagulation, inability to achieve or maintain adequate anticoagulation.
3.	DVT and low cardiopulmonary reserve or high mortality risk from possible PE (R)	Severe pulmonary hypertension, right heart failure, known large right-to-left shunt.
4.	Populations with very high risk for PE (R)	Some postbariatric, orthopedic or neurosurgical patients or multitrauma patients. Patients with expected prolonged immobilization.
5.	High risk for life-threatening PE (R)	Large, unstable (free-floating) IVC clot
6.	DVT and high fall risk (R)	
7.	Prophylaxis during catheter-directed thrombolysis of DVT (R)	

There are two absolute indications for IVC filter placement. First, if the patient is at risk for PE (i.e., DVT) but for whatever reason he/she is not a candidate for systemic anticoagulation (i.e., hemorrhage) and second, if the patient developed a PE or new/extension of DVT while on proper anticoagulation. There is a number of relative indications for filter placement. They are presented in rows 3 through 7. In every case the decision to place a filter compels careful consideration of the risks and benefits and may require multidisciplinary input.

(A), Absolute; *DVT*, deep vein thrombosis; *IVC*, inferior vena cava; *PE*, pulmonary embolism; *(R)*, relative.

selection, appropriate filter type selection, and proper location and orientation of filter. First, the clinical indication and appropriateness criteria for IVC filter placement should be confirmed. Then a review of imaging studies and physical examination of the patient will dictate appropriate venous access selection. For example, common femoral vein thrombosis precludes use of this vein for access, lest an iatrogenic PE is caused. Then the choice of filter becomes crucial. If permanent anticoagulation is required, one may place a permanent or retrievable filter. If there is any question as to the future need to retrieve the filter, a retrievable filter should be placed. The sooner a retrieval attempt is made, the more likely it is to be successful.

Filter Placement Steps (Figures 4 and 5)

1. Venous access. This most commonly is obtained in the common femoral vein or jugular vein. Other sites include the popliteal, subclavian, or brachial vein if an appropriately long filter catheter is available. The operator must avoid using a thrombosed vein as access, if possible. Ultrasound use (if no preprocedure imaging exists) is useful in this regard.
2. An IVC venogram before filter placement in order to ensure the following:
   a. The IVC is not thrombosed or, if it is, the filter is placed above the clot (Figure 6)

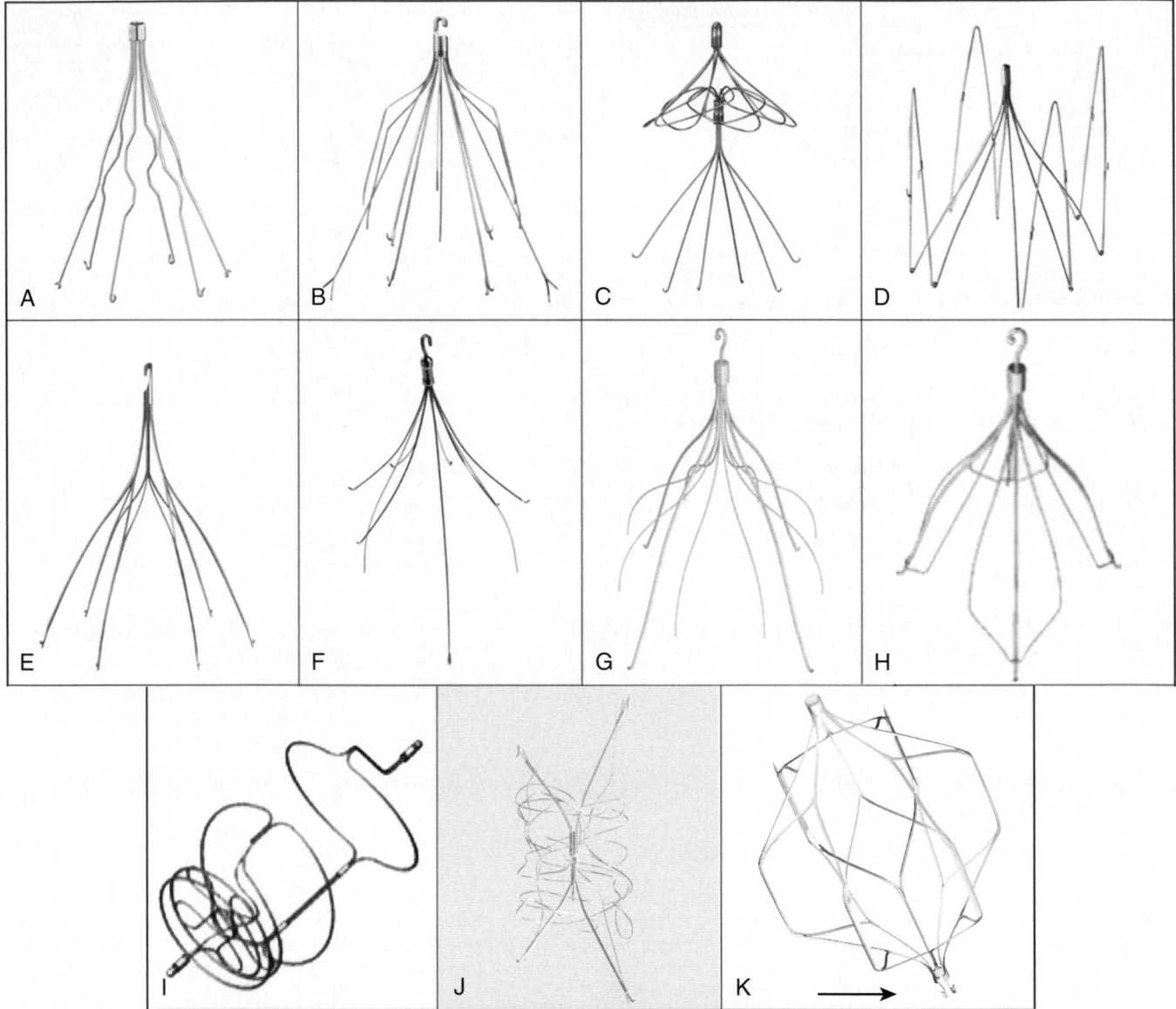

FIGURE 3 Filter types currently available in the United States. **A,** Greenfield (Boston Scientific, Marlborough, MA). **B,** Denali (Bard Medical, Covington, GA). **C,** Simon Nitinol (Bard Medical, Covington, GA). **D,** Vena Tech (B. Braun, Bethlehem, PA). **E,** Option (Rex Medical, Conshohoken, PA). **F,** ALN Optional (ALN International, Miami, FL). **G,** Celect (Cook Medical, Bloomington, IN). **H,** Günther Tulip (Cook Medical, Bloomington, IN). **I,** SafeFlo (Rafael Medical Technologies, Dover, DE). **J,** Bird's Nest (Cook Medical, Bloomington, IN). **K,** OptEase. The TrapEase is the permanent counterpart to the OptEase lacing the caudal hook (*arrow*) (Cordis, Fremont, CA). All filters are at least magnetic resonance imaging (MRI) conditional, which means that patients can be imaged safely with standard magnetic field MRI. Filters **A, C, D, I, J,** and the TrapEase (see **K**) are permanent filters. Filters **B, E, F, G, H,** and **K** have retrievability approval.

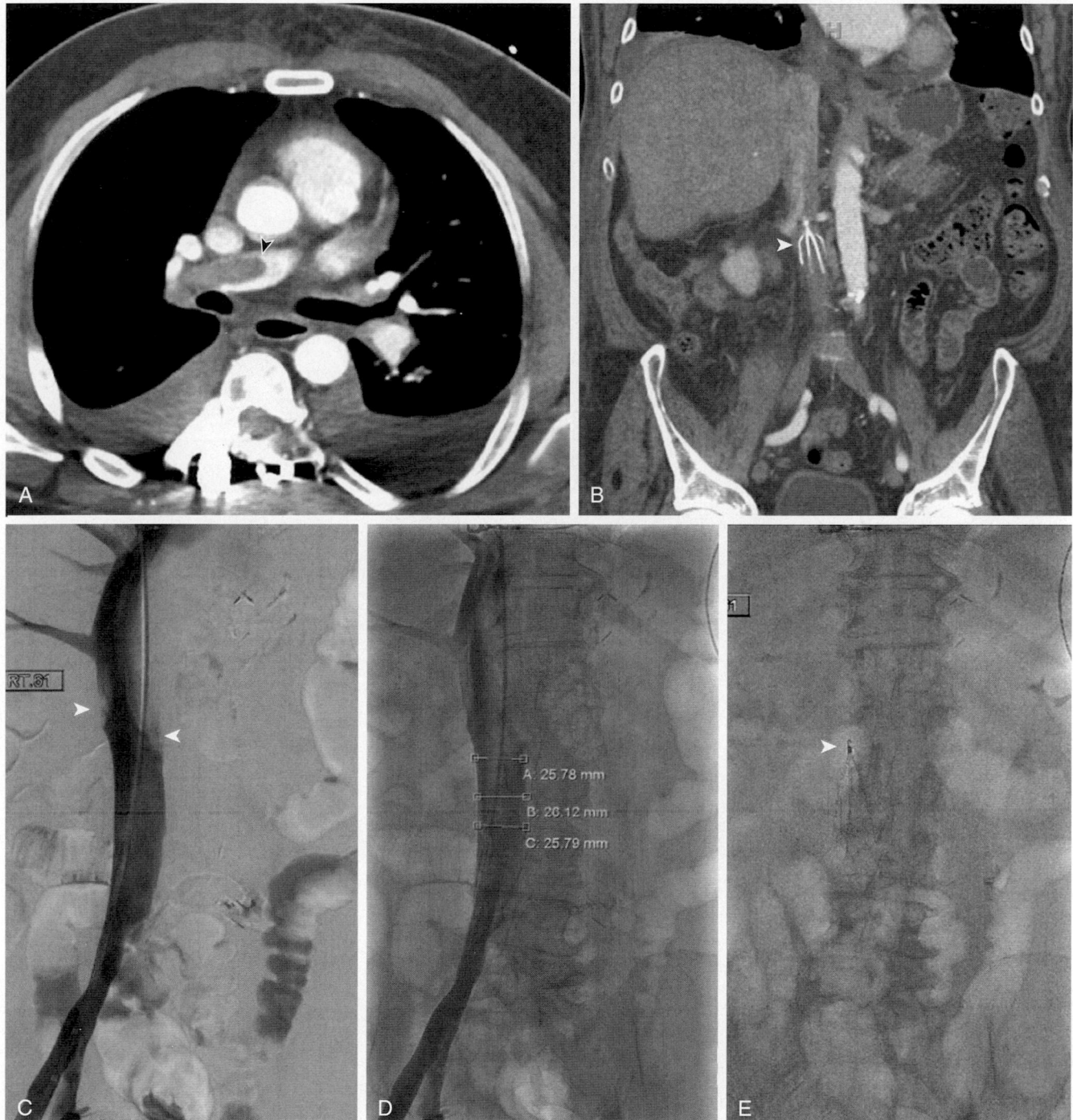

FIGURE 4 Placement of an inferior vena cava (IVC) filter. A 52-year-old patient who had undergone spinal fixation surgery was seen with severe shortness of breath and tachycardia. **A,** Axial pulmonary embolism (PE) protocol contrast-enhanced computed tomography is performed because of suspicion of PE. A large thrombus (*arrowhead*) is noted occluding the main right pulmonary artery. **B,** Because of evidence of right heart strain on echocardiography and concerns about the patient surviving another PE, an IVC filter is placed (*arrowhead*). **C,** An IVC venogram is performed from a jugular approach and excludes thrombus in the IVC. The level of the renal veins is revealed by the inflow of the unopacified blood into the IVC (*arrowheads*). **D,** Using the same venogram, the diameter of the IVC is measured to ensure that it is within the filter manufacturer's specifications. **E,** The filter is deployed with its tip (*arrowhead*) at or just below the renal vein inflow level.

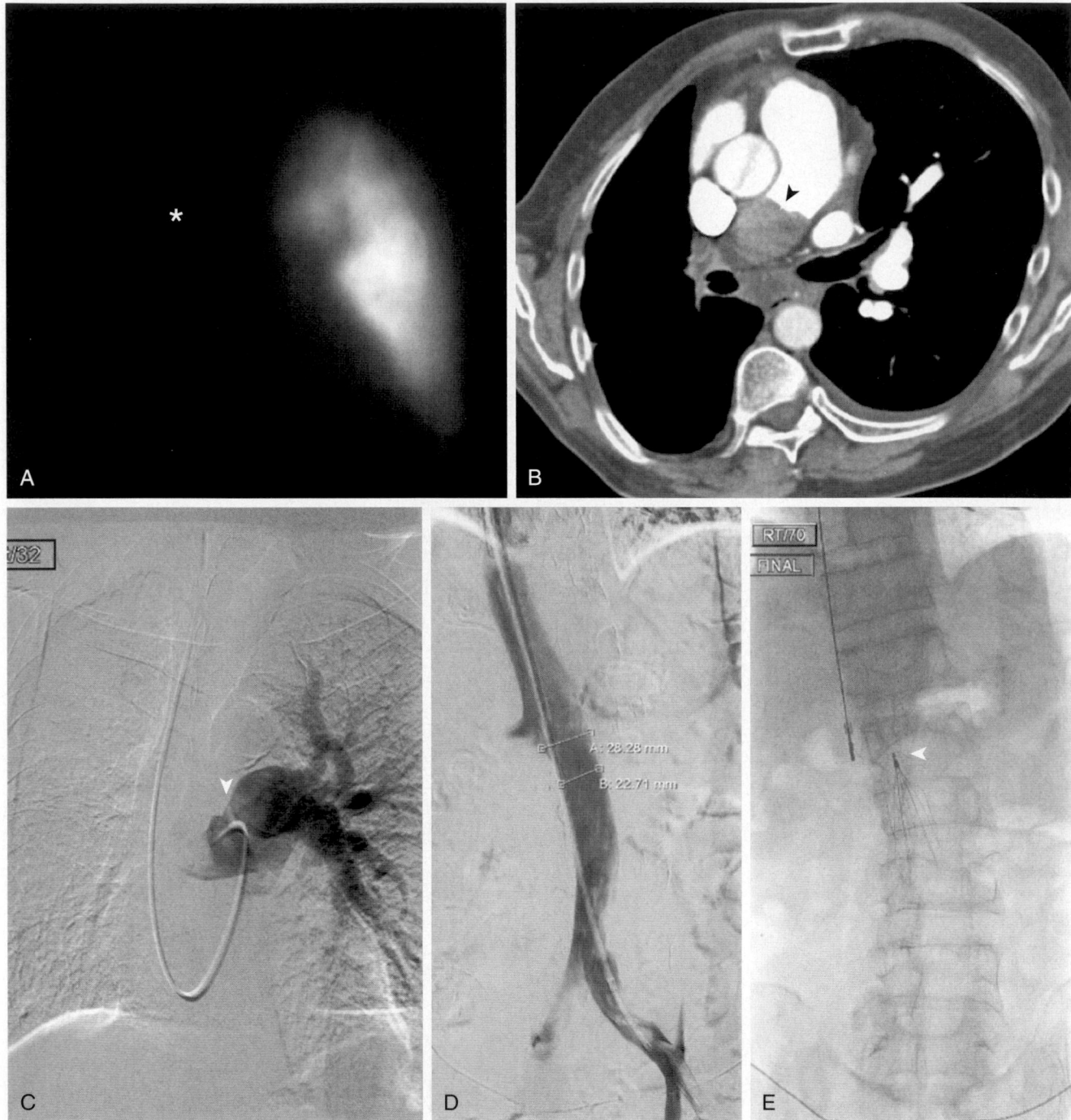

FIGURE 5 A 49-year-old patient with chronic pulmonary hypertension with acute onset was seen with worsening shortness of breath. **A,** Frontal view of the perfusion phase of the ventilation-perfusion scan shows complete lack of blood flow to the right lung (*asterisk*). **B,** Pulmonary embolism (PE) protocol contrast-enhanced computed tomography shows a large occlusive thrombus in the right main pulmonary artery (*arrowhead*). Because of severe right heart strain and hemodynamic instability, catheter-directed thrombolysis of the right pulmonary artery is initiated. **C,** The pulmonary arteriogram performed via a catheter in the main pulmonary artery (*arrowhead*) shows lack of flow in the right pulmonary artery. In addition, centrally dilated and peripherally pruned left pulmonary arteries are noted, characteristic of pulmonary hypertension. **D,** An inferior vena cava (IVC) venogram is performed and shows an IVC free from clot, delineates the level of the renal veins, and determines the diameter of the IVC. **E,** The filter is deployed with its tip at the renal vein inflow level (*arrowhead*).

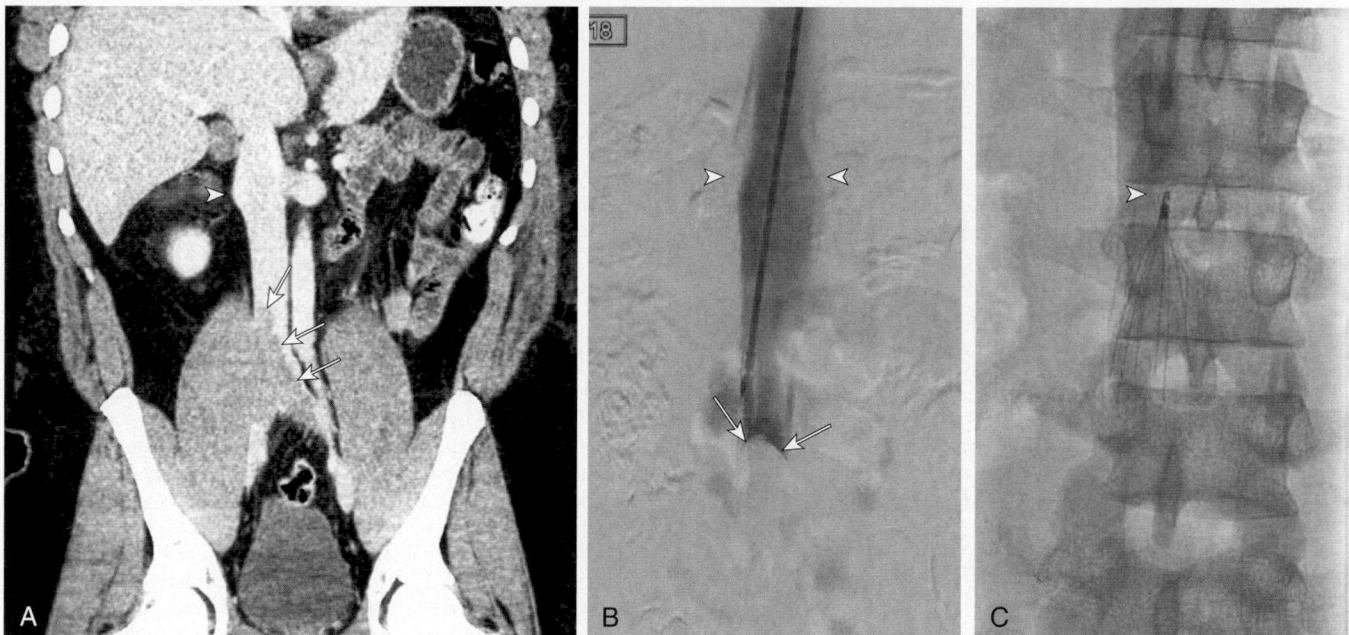

FIGURE 6 Inferior vena cava (IVC) filter placement in a patient with IVC clot. **A,** Coronal reformatted contrast-enhanced computed tomographic image shows a large, nearly occlusive clot in the IVC (*arrows*). The level of the renal veins is also shown (*arrowhead*). **B,** Digital subtraction IVC venogram shows the level of the renal veins (*arrowheads*) indicated by the inflow of the unopacified blood from the kidneys. The outline of the clot obstructing the retrograde flow of contrast is indicated by the arrows. **C,** Post–filter deployment image shows the filter with its tip (*arrowhead*) just below the renal vein inflow and above the location of the clot.

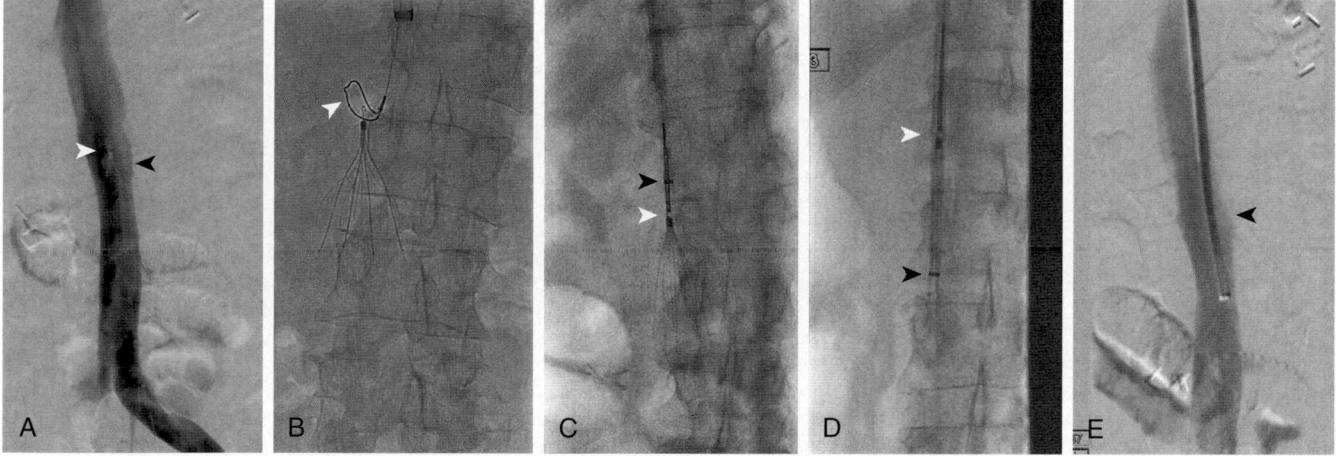

FIGURE 7 Filter retrieval steps. The patient was diagnosed with symptomatic deep venous thrombosis and initially was unable to be anticoagulated. He is now able to be anticoagulated, thus the filter is no longer required. **A,** Inferior vena cava (IVC) venogram from a jugular approach shows a properly centered filter with its tip (*white arrowhead*) placed at the level of the left renal vein inflow (*black arrowhead*). **B,** After sheath insertion, a looped wire (*arrowhead*) is advanced and used to snare the hook of the filter. **C,** The snared filter (*white arrowhead*) is pulled into the sheath (*black arrowhead*), which is advanced slowly to cover the filter. **D,** The tip of the sheath (*black arrowhead*) is advanced further to cover the filter, whose tip is still hooked by the snare (*white arrowhead*). **E,** A post–filter removal IVC venogram is performed via the sheath once the filter is removed completely to ensure an intact IVC (*arrowhead*). After removal the filter is examined visually to ensure that it has been removed completely.

b. The IVC diameter is within the filter manufacturer's specifications
c. There is no duplicated IVC
d. The renal veins, including the occasional left retroaortic renal vein, are identified
3. Deployment of the filter: stable, centered, and just below the renal vein inflow
4. Documentation of appropriate position of the filter
5. Sheath removal and hemostasis

Filter Retrieval Steps (Figure 7)

1. Venous access. This is determined by the type of filter. Some are retrieved via a cephalad approach requiring jugular access, whereas others are retrieved via a caudal approach requiring common femoral vein access. During this process, a sheath long and large enough to accommodate the filter (and other retrieval hardware that will be utilized) should be used, usually 10F or higher.

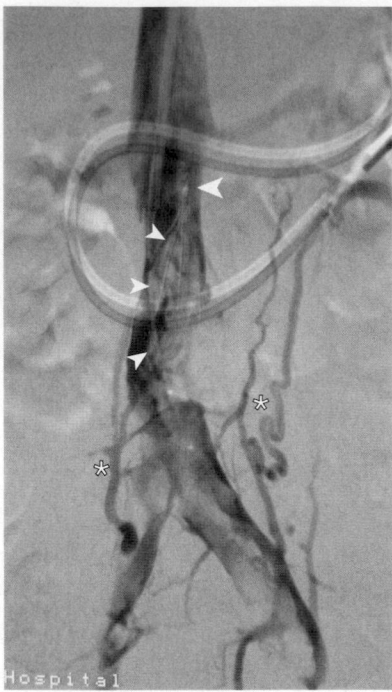

FIGURE 8 Attempted inferior vena cava (IVC) filter removal. Frontal digital subtraction IVC venogram shows a filter with its tip (*white arrowhead*) just below the renal veins. However, a large amount of clot is noted filling the filter and extending below it (*small white arrowheads*). This is a contraindication to filter removal, as the clot may dislodge and result in a pulmonary embolism. The entrapped clot is causing partial IVC flow obstruction, indicated by the retroperitoneal collaterals (*asterisks*).

2. IVC venogram. This is a crucial step and cannot be bypassed. The purpose of the IVC venogram is to exclude clot entrapped in the filter. Although some authors set 1 to 2 cc of clot as not being an absolute contraindication to filter removal, anything more than that should result in aborting the retrieval attempt (Figure 8).
3. The filter is ensnared. This can be achieved using a variety of techniques. Commonly these techniques include a snare, a clam-shell type of forceps, or a looped wire.
4. The filter is pulled gently into the sheath, which at the same time is advanced to cover the filter. The filter collapses and is covered by the sheath. Overzealous attempts to remove an imbedded filter can result in IVC rupture. It is important that the operator have a developed tactile sense of resistance against pulling.
5. The filter is removed completely via the sheath (which remains in place) and examined on the table to ensure that it has been removed in toto.
6. An IVC venogram via the sheath is performed. This is to ensure that the IVC has not been traumatized during the retrieval process.
7. Sheath removal and hemostasis

COMPLICATIONS

Complications related to IVC filters (placement or retrieval) are either periprocedural or delayed. Periprocedural complications include filter malpositioning, migration, iatrogenic pulmonary embolism, IVC perforation or groin hematoma, and (extremely rarely) infection. All of these complications are avoidable. Meticulous technique and experience can prevent malpositioning and IVC trauma, choice of appropriate filter can prevent migration, and proper technique and patient care can prevent hematoma and infection. The reported rates of these complications range between 0%

and 6% (Caplin, 2011; Linsenmaier, 1998). Complications are more likely during difficult filter retrievals than during filter insertion, especially if the filter is imbedded in the wall of the IVC. A number of methods and tools have been developed to improve safe retrieval in such cases (Figures 9 and 10). Delayed complications of IVC filtration include filter or IVC thrombosis with subsequent IVC occlusion and possible PE. IVC thrombosis after filter placement is reportedly between 2% and 19% (Caplin, 2011; Stein, 2004). The risk increases with time, and long-term risk is unknown. On the other hand, the newer, lower profile, flexible filters likely have a lower risk of long-term thrombosis; however, this is still unknown.

SPECIAL CONSIDERATIONS

The conventional wisdom that PE arise from pelvic or lower extremity DVT (LEDVT) has been challenged recently, with authors postulating the formation of de novo PE (DNPE) (Van Gent, 2014; Velmahos, 2009). However, although DNPE surely account for a small portion of clinical PE (especially in patients with direct pulmonary trauma), their epidemiologic significance is likely very small.

Upper extremity DVT (UEDVT) as a cause of PE is rare and less significant than LEDVT. Patients with symptomatic UEDVT have a 9% risk for PE and a 6% mortality from PE (Lee, 2012), compared with about 50% and 30%, respectively, in patients with LEDVT. In situations where protection from UEDVT is required, a superior vena cava filter can be placed.

Occasionally a patient who requires an IVC filter is either allergic to intravenous (IV) contrast or cannot receive IV contrast because of renal function limitations. In such cases the use of carbon dioxide is a safe and effective alternative.

CONCLUSIONS

The standard of care for the treatment of DVT and prevention of PE is systemic anticoagulation. Despite that, over the last few years there has been an explosive increase in the use of IVC filtration as a means to reduce the mortality and morbidity from PE. Indeed, IVC filters have a demonstrated efficacy in preventing PE and related morbidities and saving lives. It is instructive to note that the presence of DVT in patients who already have a PE increases their mortality risk. Specifically, patients with a PE and DVT have an overall 13% mortality risk, compared with only 4.6% for patients with a PE but no DVT (Sevestre, 2010). The increased mortality risk from presumed recurrent PE can be mitigated by IVC filtration. Another positive development is the fact that despite the incidence of DVT being fairly stable over the years, the PE-related mortality has decreased dramatically (Søgaard, 2014), which is a testament to the efficacy of treatment (systemic anticoagulation and, when indicated, IVC filtration).

However, as with any other medical device, there are risks associated with IVC filters, both immediate and long term. It is therefore prudent to properly select patients and ensure that placing an IVC filter is truly indicated. The clinical scenario for each patient is different, which affects the need, choice and location of filter, possibility of future retrievability, indwell duration, and associated risks. The development of new, low profile, efficient, retrievable filters (which can be left in the IVC indefinitely) has all but eliminated the need for permanent filters, save for the occasional megacava for which only a permanent filter is available. Any filter that is no longer serving its intended purpose—whether because the underlying risk for PE has returned to baseline or the filter is ineffective—should be removed if possible.

In conclusion, the appropriate use of IVC filtration has contributed to the reduction in morbidity and mortality related to VTE and PE. Systemic anticoagulation remains the standard of treatment, and IVC filters should be used only when indicated. Despite the development of newer, lower profile filters with fewer long-term complications, physicians should consider filter removal as soon as the risk/benefit analysis so dictates.

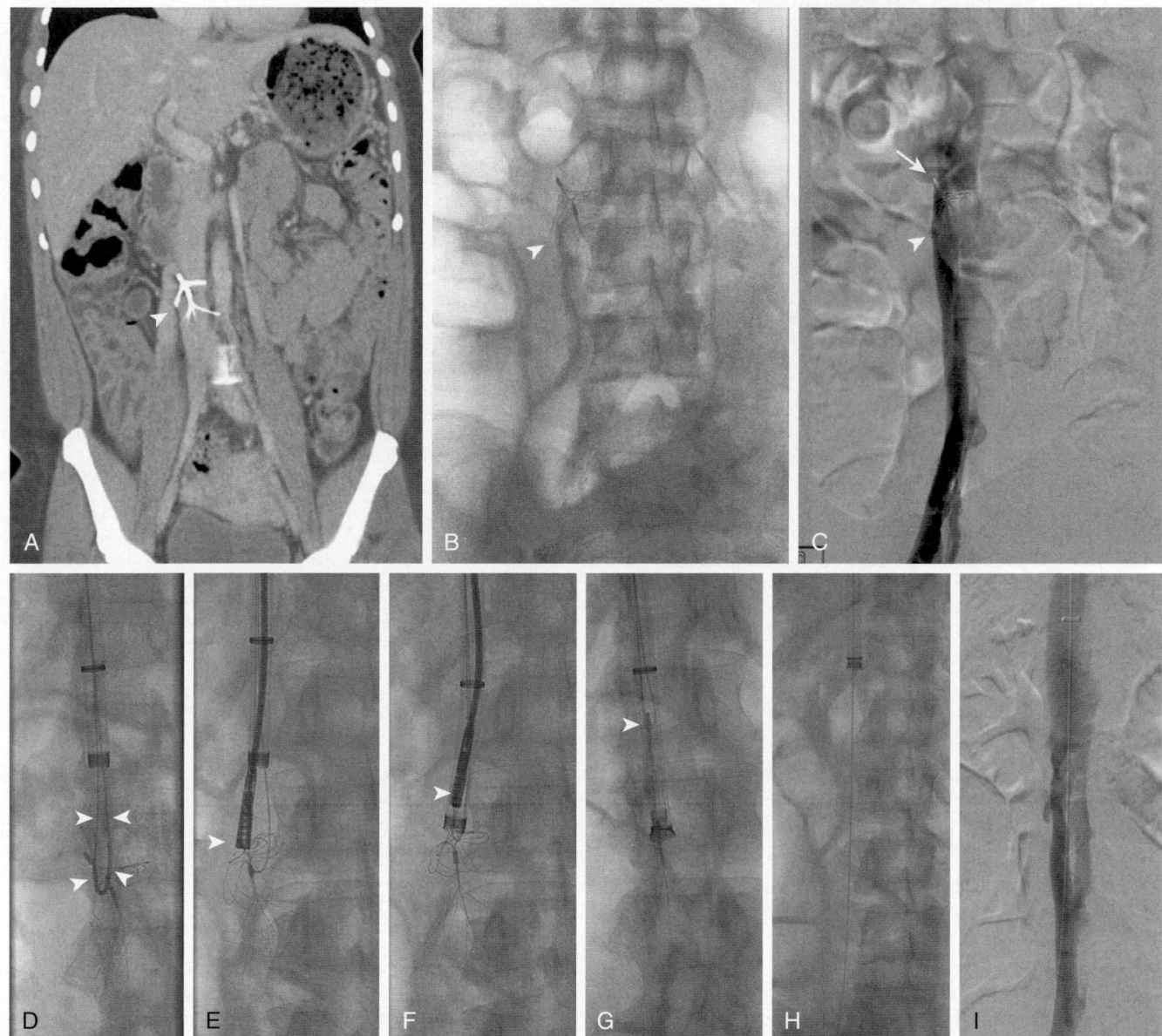

FIGURE 9 Complex filter removal 5 years after placement. Coronal reformatted contrast-enhanced computed tomographic image (**A**) and frontal fluoroscopic image (**B**) show a filter (*arrowheads*) slanted in the inferior vena cava (IVC). **C,** An IVC venogram shows tines (*arrowhead*) and the tip (*arrow*) imbedded in the IVC wall. Attempts to snare the tip failed. **D,** A wire was placed via a jugular sheath, looped under the filter tip (*arrowheads*), and returned via the sheath. **E,** With the filter gently pulled away from the IVC wall using the looped wire, a pair of clamshell forceps (*arrowhead*) was used to securely grab the filter tip. **F,** Simultaneously, the forceps and wire were used to pull the filter, and the sheath was advanced to cover them (*arrowhead*). **G,** Further traction and sheath advancement pulled the filter (*arrowhead*) securely into the sheath. **H,** A spot film was obtained to ensure that no filter fragments remained. **I,** After the filter was examined in vitro to ensure complete removal, an IVC venogram was performed to ensure no IVC extravasation.

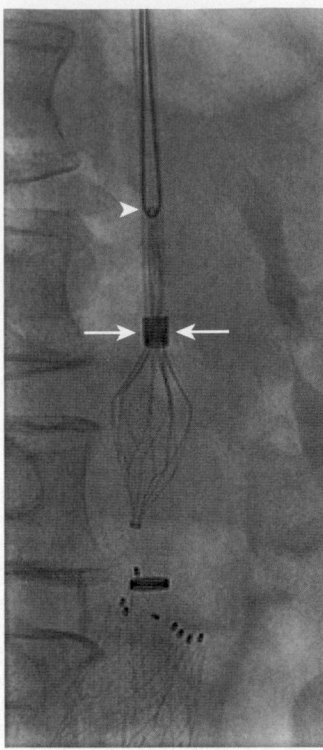

FIGURE 10 Retrieval of a "permanent" TrapEase filter (Cordis, Freemont, CA). The cephalad tip of the filter has been snared by a looped wire (*arrowhead*) and partially pulled into a sheath. During the procedure, retrieval was difficult because the filter was embedded in the inferior vena cava (IVC) wall. The sheath was exchanged for a laser sheath emitting energy at its tip (*arrows*), and the filter was freed from the IVC wall. Special expertise is advised lest the use of laser results in serious IVC trauma.

SUGGESTED READINGS

Belohlavec J, Dytrych V, Linhart A. Pulmonary embolism, part I: epidemiology, risk factors and risk stratification, pathophysiology, clinical presentation, diagnosis and nonthrombotic pulmonary embolism. *Exp Clin Cardiol.* 2013;18:129-138.

Caplin DM, Nikolic B, Kalva SP. Quality improvement guidelines for the performance of inferior vena cava filter placement for the prevention of pulmonary embolism. *J Vasc Interv Radiol.* 2011;22:1499-1506.

Kaufman JA, Kienny TB, Streiff MB. Guidelines for the use of retrievable and convertible vena cava filters: report from the Society of Interventional Radiology multidisciplinary consensus conference. *J Vasc Interv Radiol.* 2006;17:449-459.

Lankei M, Konstantinides S. Mortality risk assessment and the role of thrombolysis in pulmonary embolism. *Crit Care Clin.* 2011;27: 953-967.

Lee JA, Zierler BK, Zierler RE. The risk factors and clinical outcomes of upper extremity deep vein thrombosis. *Vasc Endovasc Surg.* 2012;46: 139-144.

Linsenmaier U, Rieger J, Schenk F, Rock C, Mangel E, Pfeifer KJ. Indications, management, and complications of temporary inferior vena cava filters. *CardioVasc Inter Rad.* 1998;21:464-469.

Lopez JA, Kearon C, Lee AY. Deep venous thrombosis. *Hematology Am Soc Hematol Educ Program.* 2004;439-456.

Sevestre MA, Quashie C, Genty C, Rolland C, Quere I, Bosson JL. Clinical presentation and mortality in pulmonary embolism: the Optimev study. *J Mal Vasc.* 2010;35:242-249.

Søgaard KK, Schmidt M, Pedersen L, Horvath-Puho E, Sorensen HT. 30-year mortality after venous thromboembolism: a population based cohort study. *Circulation.* 2014;130:829-836.

Stein PD, Kavali F, Olson RE. Twenty-one year trends in the use of inferior vena cava filters. *Arch Intern Med.* 2004;164:1541-1545.

Van Gent J-M, Zander AL, Olson EJ, Shackford SR, Dunne CE, Sise CB, Badiee J, Schechter MS, Sise MJ. Pulmonary embolism without deep venous thrombosis: de novo or missed deep venous thrombosis? *J Trauma Acute Care Surg.* 2014;76:1270-1274.

Velmahos GC, Spaniolas K, Tabbara M, Abujudeh HH, de Moya M, Gervasini A, Alam HB. Pulmonary embolism and deep venous thrombosis in trauma: are they related? *Arch Surg.* 2009;144:928-932.

LYMPHEDEMA

Ricardo J. Bello, MD, MPH, Damon S. Cooney, MD, PhD, and Gedge D. Rosson, MD

Lymphedema is a chronic condition that develops over months to years of an increasing lymphatic load that exceeds the lymphatic system's transport capacity. Impairment of lymphatic transport leads to interstitial accumulation of a protein-rich fluid that includes excess water, plasma proteins, extravascular blood cells, and cell products that are normally transported by the lymphatic system from the interstitium into the circulation.

Progressively, lymphatic impairment leads to dilation of the remaining functional lymphatics, causing vascular incompetence and reversal of flow. Lymphatic walls become fibrotic, and fibrinoid thrombi ultimately obliterate the remaining patent channels. Stasis of interstitial proteins leads to an inflammatory response, with macrophages and fibroblasts replacing supple, elastic interstitium with fibrosclerotic, thickened, congested tissues. Soft, pitting edema gives way to induration, hypertrophy and deposition of adipose tissue, acanthosis, hyperkeratosis, and skin breakdown. Infectious complications follow, with recurrent episodes of cellulitis and lymphangitis. In rare severe cases, chronic lymphedema can degenerate into a highly aggressive lymphangiosarcoma known as Stewart-Treves syndrome. The International Society of Lymphology (ISL) updated the staging guidelines for lymphedema in 2013 (Box 1).

◼ ETIOLOGY

Lymphedema can be primary or secondary. Primary cases result from a developmental abnormality, often with delayed manifestations. Primary lymphedema can be subdivided further into congenital lymphedema, lymphedema praecox, and lymphedema tarda. Congenital lymphedema (10% to 25% of primary cases), or Milroy's disease, is seen within the first 2 years of life. It usually affects females (female to male ratio is 2:1), is bilateral, and involves the lower extremities. It often is not progressive and may improve spontaneously with age. Lymphedema praecox (65% to 85% of primary cases), or Meige disease, is seen before 35 years of age, typically at puberty. It predominantly affects females (female to male ratio is 4:1), is unilateral, and involves the lower extremities. Lymphedema tarda occurs spontaneously after 35 years of age and is the rarest form of primary lymphedema. It also tends to affect females more than males.

Secondary lymphedema is an acquired dysfunction of normally developed lymphatics. It results from disease, trauma, or iatrogenic causes. Worldwide, the most common cause is infection by the microfilaria *Wuchereria bancrofti*, transmitted by various mosquito vectors. Adult filarial worms reside in and obstruct lymphatic channels, causing irreversible scarring and fibrosis and often massive

BOX 1: Lymphedema Staging

Stage 0: Latent or Subclinical

- Impaired lymphatic transport
- No evident edema, subtle changes in tissue fluid/composition
- Changes in subjective symptoms
- May last months or years before progression

Stage I: Spontaneously Reversible

- Early accumulation of protein-rich fluid
- Pitting edema
- Subsides with elevation

Stage II: Spontaneously Irreversible

- Accumulation of protein-rich fluid
- Pitting edema may progress to nonpitting as excess fat and fibrosis develop
- Does not resolve with elevation alone

Stage III: Lymphostatic Elephantiasis

- Nonpitting
- Significant fibrosis
- Trophic skin changes

Data from the International Society of Lymphology. The diagnosis and treatment of peripheral lymphedema: 2013 Consensus Document of the International Society of Lymphology. *Lymphology.* 2013;46:1-11.

BOX 2: Diagnostic Workup for Lymphedema

1. Thorough history and physical examination
2. Rule out causes of edema (basic laboratory tests for renal and liver function)
3. Infectious disease workup (in patients with travel history or exposure)
4. Lymphatic imaging (lymphoscintigraphy, magnetic resonance lymphatic mapping, indocyanine green imaging)

edema. In the United States and most higher-income countries, however, nearly all cases of secondary lymphedema are related to cancer therapy. Tumor extirpation, radiation therapy, and lymphadenectomy can cause lymphedema. Other factors such as trauma, infection, and obesity contribute to secondary lymphedema. Chronic edema also may deteriorate lymphatic function gradually, causing a mixed form of lymphedema that can be specially challenging to treat.

DIAGNOSIS

The workup for lymphedema starts with a thorough history and physical examination (Box 2). Other causes of edema must be ruled out, including cardiac, venous, renal, and hepatic causes and compressive or occlusive vascular syndromes.

Lymphoscintigraphy and indocyanine green (ICG) fluorescence lymphography are useful techniques to map lymphatic vessels, which may aid in diagnosis and help to plan surgical management. Findings from both techniques have been found to be correlated with clinical severity. The advantage of ICG lymphography is that the dye used is nonradioactive and thus is more suitable for repeated follow-up. Magnetic resonance imaging and computed tomography are also useful in lymphatic visualization and may help to rule out suspicions of associated malignancy. Ultrasound imaging can help to examine secondary lymphedema, especially if it is associated with filarial infection, or to describe tissue changes. However, most patients can be diagnosed without additional testing.

TREATMENT

Treatment of lymphedema is determined by the etiology and stage of the disease. When parasitic infection is the cause of lymphedema, the infection must be treated appropriately; this is outside the scope of this chapter. In general, the mainstay of lymphedema treatment is conservative management, of which several modalities are available. Surgical treatment historically has been considered an adjunct to conservative therapy in severe cases. However, recent advances in microsurgical procedures have broadened indications for surgery to include earlier stages of lymphedema.

Conservative Management

Conservative therapies are directed at reducing interstitial fluid accumulation and preventing development of further edema, inflammation, and fibrosis. Conservative treatment is often consuming and inconvenient. It requires lifelong care and includes hygiene, compression, elevation, and physical therapy. A multidisciplinary team, which may include a physiotherapist, an occupational therapist, and a social worker, should be involved in lymphedema treatment. Psychosocial support also may be required, which can be important for long-term compliance with any regimen.

Basic lifestyle modifications should be started early and are essential in managing the sequelae of lymphedema. Meticulous hygiene and skin care are important to reduce skin breakdown and infection. Patients should be encouraged to lose weight if they are obese, to address minor skin traumas and breakdown appropriately, and to avoid constrictive clothing.

Compression therapies range widely and include graduated compression garments, multilayered inelastic bandaging, and controlled compression therapy. Compression garments are refitted as swelling decreases. These methods reduce volume of edema by 30% to 45%, approximately. External sequential compressive devices also have been used with variable success. Basic range-of-motion exercises can be a useful strategy as a complement to limb compression and elevation. Contraindications for compression include arterial disease, painful post-phlebitic syndrome, and occult visceral malignancy.

Physical therapy, specifically complex decongestive lymphatic therapy, is a more time-intensive strategy. This modality involves manual lymphatic drainage via massage, compressive therapy, exercise, skin care, self-management, and use of compression garments. Studies have found mixed results as to whether lymphatic massage leads to improved outcomes compared with compression garments or bandaging alone. Massage alone does not appear to be beneficial.

The success of conservative strategies varies widely, in part because of a heterogeneous patient population. Patient compliance generally plays a significant role in outcomes. Discomfort or embarrassment associated with compression garments or the inconvenience of physical therapy may limit outcomes. It is important to discuss compliance with patients, stressing that individual investment and long-term compliance are central to managing this chronic, lifelong condition.

Antibiotics are valuable in treating recurrent infections. Beyond antibiotics, pharmacologic therapy plays a limited role in the management of lymphedema. Benzopyrenes are thought to increase lymphatic uptake of peptides through proteolysis of interstitial proteins, but results have been mixed and documented hepatotoxicity limits long-term therapy. Historically, diuretics have been used, but with only limited benefit. Diuretics actually may lead to increased interstitial protein accumulation and fibrosis. Studies examining the use of nutritional supplements, such as sodium selenite or vitamin E with pentoxifylline, have not demonstrated any significant benefit in patients with lymphedema.

Surgical Treatment

Surgery is usually complementary to primary conservative therapy, historically indicated only in refractory cases, but it also has been shown to be effective for earlier stages of the disease. Surgical indications for lymphedema are not absolute. Relative indications include size and weight of the patient, extent and stage of lymphedema, recurrent cellulitis or lymphangitis, lymphorrhagia, abscess, fistula, diminished quality of life, worsening comorbidities, and failure of conservative management. Documentation with photographs, limb measurements, functional assessments, and radiology is paramount. Preoperative imaging studies such as lymphoscintigraphy and ICG lymphography can help to assess the severity of lymphedema and thus decide among surgical options. Patient compliance and overall health are crucial to the success of any operation.

There is no single surgical procedure for all classifications of lymphedema. The two general categories for surgical therapy are physiologic procedures and debulking procedures. Conservative therapy should be continued immediately after any surgical procedure.

Physiologic Procedures

Physiologic or lymphatic reconstructive procedures aim to improve lymphatic flow and drainage. Omental flaps, enteromesenteric bridging, dermal flaps, myocutaneous flaps, and lymphangioplasty have been attempted with limited to no success.

However, lymphovenous bypass and vascularized lymph node transfer (VLNT) have been shown to be effective treatment options for patients with lymphedema, especially in earlier stages, before the onset of fibrosis.

Lymphovenous Bypass

Also known as lymphaticovenular anastomosis, this procedure was introduced in 1953 by Sherman and colleagues. To relieve postobstructive lymphedema, subdermal lymphatic vessels are anastomosed with adjacent venules using supermicrosurgical techniques (Box 3). This creates an artificial shunt to drain lymphedematous fluid into the circulation.

ICG lymphography can be performed before surgical planning to help determine patient eligibility for lymphovenous bypass and map suitable lymphatic vessels for anastomosis. Yamamoto and colleagues described ICG mapping patterns for upper and lower extremities, indicating lymphovenous bypass for patients with stardust or diffuse dermal backflow patterns as opposed to earlier stages with splash pattern. However, if lymphatic vessel damage is found to be too advanced to allow anastomosis, other surgical options may be more suitable than this procedure.

Campisi's experience with lymphovenous bypass showed improvement in more than 80% of patients, with significant reduction of excess volume (67% on average) and an even greater

reduction in incidence of cellulitis. Kochima reported 88.5% effectiveness by anastomosing one to three vessels per patient under local anesthesia. These results were consistent at long-term follow-up. Chang and colleagues reported a series of 100 lymphovenous bypasses, showing improvement in symptoms in 96% of patients and improvements in volume differential in 74% of patients. Volume differential was reduced, on average, by 42% at 12 months postoperatively. Interestingly, this reduction was significantly larger in patients with earlier stages of lymphedema compared with those with later stages (61% vs 17%, respectively, at 12 months postoperatively). The drawbacks of this procedure are that it is difficult to perform and it requires training and equipment for supermicrosurgical techniques, given that the vessels involved are 0.5 to 0.8 mm in diameter.

Vascularized Lymph Node Transfer

VLNT was first demonstrated in rats by Shesol in 1979 and used for a human patient by Clodius in 1982. An advantage in the case of postmastectomy lymphedema is that VLNT can be combined with autologous flaps for simultaneous breast reconstruction and VLNT.

This procedure harvests healthy fat tissue and lymph nodes and transfers these into the affected site (Box 4). Two mechanisms have been proposed for the effectiveness of VLNT. The first theory is that VLNT induces lymphangiogenesis and bridges healthy lymphatic vessels, which is stimulated by growth factors produced by transplanted lymph nodes (including prolymphoangiogenic vascular endothelial growth factor C [VEGF-C] and antifibrotic interleukin-10 [IL-10]). The second theory is that the graft acts as a lymphatic pump in the affected site.

The most common donor site used for VLNT is the groin. The lymph nodes used in this technique are located at the level of the muscular aponeurosis and subcutaneous fat medial to the femoral artery. Preoperatively, magnetic resonance angiogram has been used to identify lymph nodes, and Doppler imaging can confirm the location of superficial circumflex vessels. Care must be taken not to dissect farther caudally from the inguinal ligament or deep from the muscular aponeurosis, which risks damaging the lymphatic drainage to the lower limb and causing donor site lymphedema.

Reverse lymphatic mapping has emerged as a promising technical refinement in VLNT to reduce the incidence of donor site morbidity. This technique was described by Dayan and colleagues and involves mapping the lymphatic drainage of the extremity using technetium injected into the web spaces of the hand or foot and identifying lymph nodes that are to be avoided during flap harvest with a gamma probe. Lymph nodes that drain the trunk, which are targeted for the

---

BOX 3: Lymphovenous Bypass

1. Begin with lymphatic lymphangiography.
2. Inject 0.01 to 0.02 mL of indocyanine green into the web spaces in the extremity.
3. Visualize fluorescent images and mark visible lymphatic pathways and incision sites.
4. Inject local anesthetic with epinephrine.
5. Inject 0.1 to 0.2 mL of Lymphazurin into the web spaces in the extremity.
6. Take subdermal postobstruction dissection down to venous and lymphatic channels.
7. Use microsurgical connection to re-establish lymph flow with end-to-end anastomoses. End-to-side anastomoses can be used when veins are larger than the lymphatic channel.
8. Confirm that shunts are patent by observing passage of Lymphazurin into the vein.
9. Evaluate postoperative flow and imaging studies.

BOX 4: Vascularized Groin Lymph Node Transfer

Donor Site

1. Palpate femoral pulse and design elliptical skin paddle lateral to pulse, inferior and parallel to the inguinal ligament.
2. Incise skin superiorly.
3. Dissect from distal to proximal, use fascia of sartorius muscle as deep plane.
4. Harvest the superficial circumflex iliac vessels, lymph nodes, and surrounding fatty tissue.

Recipient Site

1. Make a transverse incision on the recipient site (e.g., wrist).
2. Transfer flap onto the recipient site.
3. Perform microvascular anastomosis to the radial artery and cephalic vein.
4. Consider need for extra coverage of the flap with a split-thickness skin graft.
5. Use a skin paddle for monitoring.

flap, also are mapped using ICG and near-infrared fluorescence lymphangiography. Dayan and colleagues report no cases of donor site morbidity in a series of 35 patients treated with VLNT and reverse lymphatic mapping with follow-up between 1 and 30 months postoperatively. However, long-term follow-up is still needed to confirm the benefits of this technique, especially given the added costs of these two procedures.

The groin is an ideal donor site in terms of scar concealment and provision of large skin paddles when needed. However, there is increased risk for donor site lymphedema. Other donor sites, such as submental and supraclavicular locations, carry lower risks of donor site lymphedema, but scars may be more evident, particularly in submental VLNTs. Submental lymph node harvest also carries the risk of injuring the marginal mandibular nerve.

Cheng and colleagues performed groin VLNT for postmastectomy lymphedema in patients with total occlusion on lymphoscintigraphy and increased limb circumference (15% or more than the unaffected limb).

VNLT has demonstrated good results. These include decreased size, increased skin elasticity, decreased infection rates, increased lymphatic flow, increased lymphatic pathways toward the flap site, discontinued need for physiotherapy, and an anti-inflammatory and antifibrotic response. Donor site morbidity remains a concern.

Debulking Procedures

More advanced cases of lymphedema require treatment with debulking procedures. Liposuction is a useful technique to address adipose tissue deposits in later stages (ISL stages II and III). Older, more aggressive treatments, such as the Charles and Sistrunk procedures, are reserved for severe and refractory cases of lymphedema.

Liposuction was first used for brachial lymphedema in 1987. This technique was refined in 1993 (Box 5). Controlled trials and long-term follow-up have demonstrated that liposuction is a useful adjunct to treatment. It is particularly useful to address adipose tissue deposits in later stages of lymphedematous limbs. It is safe, quick, and allows for an immediate decrease in volume and pressure of the lymph fluid, promoting better lymphatic flow.

According to Brorson, liposuction should be indicated only for cases where conservative therapy has been maximized without achieving desired outcomes. Relative indications are subjective discomfort of a heavy extremity and chronic, large lymphedema (1 L in excess volume). Contraindications include presence of more than minimal pitting, metastatic disease, open wounds, coagulation disorders, and reluctance to wear compression garments after surgery.

Brorson reports complete reduction with no recurrence in a cohort of 116 women with 15-year follow-up. Boyages and colleagues recently reported a mean reduction of volume differential of 89.6% by 6 months postoperatively. Risks include lidocaine toxicity, thrombotic and fat emboli, hematoma, seroma, and contour irregularities. Liposuction has been used alone or in addition to other debulking or physiologic procedures.

Among more aggressive treatments, the Charles procedure (described by Charles in 1912) is a radical excision technique that removes all skin and subcutaneous tissue down to the muscle fascia (Figure 1; Box 6). Excised skin is used for grafting on the fascia. The van der Walt modification allows for negative-pressure dressing with grafting to be done in a delayed fashion. Surgery is indicated for severe cases and carries a high risk of complications, including destruction of the remaining lymphatics, infection, ulceration, hyperpigmentation, dermatitis, unstable scars, and a severely altered aesthetic outcome.

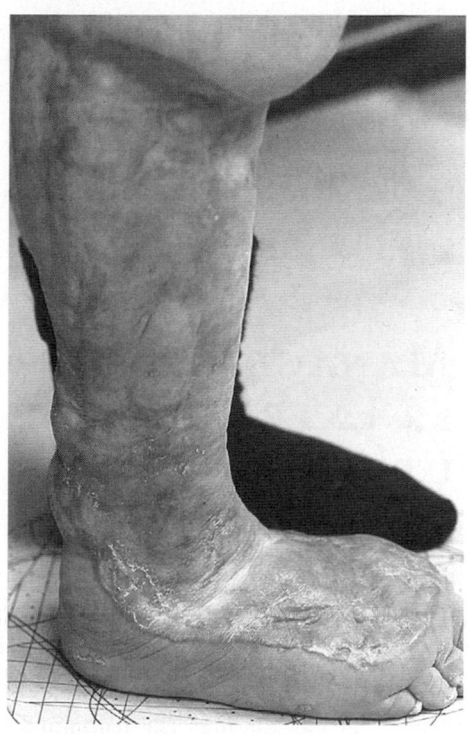

FIGURE 1 Lower extremity after the Charles procedure.

BOX 5: Liposuction

1. Mark out the affected area and 2 cm beyond.
2. Choose port sites to effectively reach all areas, both proximally and distally.
3. Inject tumescent solution (1 L Lactated Ringer's solution mixed with 1 mL ampule of epinephrine 1:1000 and 30 mL of 1% lidocaine) until blanching is achieved and a moderate amount of turgor is seen.
4. Wait 30 to 45 minutes.
5. Suction with a 4- to 6-mm cannula in a deep plane in all areas, followed by a 2- to 3-mm cannula in a more superficial plane for a smoother contour.
6. Close port sites with absorbable suture.
7. Apply sterile dressings and a pressure garment.
8. Advise the patient not to shower or remove the pressure garment for 72 hours, and encourage the patient to walk at least three times a day.
9. After 3 days, the patient can shower daily and may begin massaging the affected areas.
10. The pressure garment should be worn for 6 to 10 weeks.

BOX 6: Charles Procedure

1. Mark the lymphedematous area both proximally and distally.
2. Make an incision both medially and laterally down to the muscle fascia.
3. Excise all tissue superficial to this plane.
4. Remove the skin of the affected area with a dermatome for a split-thickness graft or with a knife for a full-thickness graft. If a full-thickness graft, make sure to remove all fat from the skin.
5. Use this graft to cover the exposed area.
6. Apply petroleum gauze or other nonadherent dressing over the graft.
7. Apply a pressure dressing via a vacuum-assisted device, bolster, or cotton.
8. Splint the extremity in the proper anatomic position.
9. Remove dressing after 3 to 5 days for a split-thickness graft or after 7 to 12 days for a full-thickness graft.

The Sistrunk procedure (1918) is a planned, staged excision of affected subcutaneous tissues. This technique has been modified over the last 80 years and involves burying dermal flaps within skin flaps (Box 7). Long-term results include a reduction of at least half of the affected tissue in 75% of patients. The Sistrunk procedure is safe, reliable, and predictable. Complications include nerve damage in the affected area, epidermolysis secondary to poor blood supply, wound dehiscence, and infection.

SUMMARY

Lymphedema is a challenging clinical problem that produces significant morbidity in a large population worldwide. All treatment modalities include long-term conservative measures along with support from a multidisciplinary team. Surgical procedures can be a useful adjunct to treatment according to disease progression; physiologic procedures appear to be more successful in earlier stages of the disease, and debulking procedures are used only for later stages. Regardless of the treatment strategy chosen, patient commitment and lifestyle modifications are central to achieving improvement in symptoms and quality of life.

BOX 7: Sistrunk Procedure

1. Mark out the affected area.
2. Plan to excise and debulk sufficient tissue, leaving dermal flaps to bury beneath the skin in the closure. A variation of this is carried out in the Thompson procedure, in which dermal flaps are buried beneath the muscle.
3. Close the incision over drains.
4. Allow 12 weeks to heal before the next serial excision.

SUGGESTED READINGS

Chang DW, Suami H, Skoracki R. A prospective analysis of 100 consecutive lymphovenous bypass cases for treatment of extremity lymphedema. *Plast Reconstr Surg.* 2013;132:1305-1314.

Cheng MH, Chen SC, Henry SL, Tan BK, Lin MC, Huang JJ. Vascularized groin lymph node flap transfer for postmastectomy upper limb lymphedema: flap anatomy, recipient sites, and outcomes. *Plast Reconstr Surg.* 2013;131:1286-1298.

Gharb BB, Rampazzo A, Spanio di Spilimbergo S, Xu ES, Chung KP, Chen HC. Vascularized lymph node transfer based on the hilar perforators improves the outcome in upper limb lymphedema. *Ann Plast Surg.* 2011;67:589-593.

International Society of Lymphology. The diagnosis and treatment of peripheral lymphedema: 2013 Consensus Document of the International Society of Lymphology. *Lymphology.* 2013;46:1-11.

Koshima I, Narushima M, Yamamoto Y, Mihara M, Iida T. Recent advancement on surgical treatments for lymphedema. *Ann Vasc Dis.* 2012;5:409-415.

Raju A, Chang DW. Vascularized lymph node transfer for treatment of lymphedema. *Ann Surg.* 2015;261:1013-1023.

THE MANAGEMENT OF LOWER EXTREMITY AMPUTATIONS

Robert F. Cuff, MD, FACS, and Justin M. Simmons, DO

Lower extremity amputations are one of the oldest surgical procedures performed in the medical field, and Hippocrates is credited with performing the first therapeutic amputation. Major amputations of the leg were performed for any degree of tissue loss, including that present on the foot and toes. This remained the mainstay of therapy for nontraumatic problems with the leg until Leland McKittrick published his technique of transmetatarsal amputation in 1949.

There are an estimated 140,000 amputations performed in the United States yearly, with an estimated cost of $3.1 billion annually. More than half of these amputations are performed on the lower extremity. Although the surgical technique itself has not changed for some time, advancements in perioperative care, prosthetic development, and rehabilitation medicine have led to significant improvements in the success and quality of life for patients who undergo amputations. Conversely, poor selection of the amputation level or suboptimal postoperative care can lead to significant physical and psychologic impairment for patients and a significant financial burden for healthcare systems and society through complications, readmissions, and the need for re-amputation.

As treating physicians, it is important to not think of these procedures as a failure of prior revascularization strategies but instead as another therapeutic option in a person's global rehabilitation, especially in those individuals who suffer from critical limb ischemia. The goals of amputation should be to preserve life and improve quality of life through relief of pain, prevention of infection, return to a functional life, and decreased hospitalizations. These are the same goals used when treating patients with peripheral arterial disease via endovascular interventions or bypass surgery.

INDICATIONS

The primary indications for major amputation are the preservation of life through prevention of ascending infection and tissue loss, relief of ischemic pain, or removal of a neurologically nonfunctioning foot that may lead to decreased function and increased risk of wound development. The majority of patients requiring a lower extremity amputation have underlying peripheral arterial disease, diabetes mellitus, or both of these disease processes. Often they have had a steady progression toward the need for an amputation over several years despite interventions to save the limb. Some patients are seen with an acute life-threatening ascending infection that requires an emergent amputation for source control followed by a staged amputation closure once the infection is resolved. Other less common indications include frostbite, trauma, chronic nonischemic pain, neuroma, distal arterial embolization, and venous insufficiency.

AMPUTATION TYPES

Amputations of the lower extremities can be classified as either minor or major. A minor amputation of the lower extremity can be thought of one confined to the foot. This includes any digit amputation or transmetatarsal amputation as well as more complex amputations of the foot such as Lisfranc, Chopart, or Syme amputations. Major amputations consist of any amputation proximal to the ankle, including transtibial, transfemoral, through-knee, and hip disarticulation amputations (Table 1).

Minor Amputations

A simple digital amputation generally is indicated in the setting of a gangrenous process or chronic osteomyelitis. This disease process should be confined to the distal phalanx, and in the setting of a more proximal problem a ray amputation may be indicated. In general,

TABLE 1: Types of Amputations

Minor Amputation	Major Amputation
Digit	Transtibial amputation, below-knee amputation (BKA)
Ray amputation	Through-knee amputation
Transmetatarsal amputation	Transfemur amputation, above-knee amputation (AKA)
Chopart amputation	Hip disarticulation
Syme amputation	

patients will tolerate the loss of a toe very well with the exception of the great toe, which is responsible for propulsion during ambulation. The most tolerable digital amputation involves the third digit of the foot.

A ray amputation is a more involved procedure resulting in removal of the entire phalanx. The indications are the same as with a simple digital amputation. The difference is that the disease process is more proximal in the toe, with involvement of the web space or metatarsal head. When faced with the need to perform a ray amputation of the great toe or fifth toe, it is necessary to extend the incision over the medial or lateral border of the foot, respectively.

Transmetatarsal amputations are reserved for those scenarios in which the infectious process or tissue loss is more extensive into the forefoot or when multiple toes are involved and leaving a patient with one or two toes is not beneficial. The infectious process or tissue loss should be confined to the distal aspects of the forefoot, however, because success of this amputation relies on the ability to create a viable posterior flap.

The Syme amputation is a less common amputation of the foot in today's practice. It was designed to preserve as much limb length as feasible while also leaving the growth plates intact. An added benefit of this approach is the ability to ambulate without a prosthesis. Typically this procedure has been used in the setting of severe foot trauma and is relatively contraindicated in patients with neurotrophic ulcers or ischemic vascular disease.

The Chopart amputation is also referred to as a midtarsal joint amputation and offers some advantages over the Syme amputation. This procedure is performed at the level of the calcaneocuboid-talonavicular bones and preserves the talus and calcaneus, resulting in less limb shortening. Unfortunately, this also places these amputees at risk for future problems resulting from equinus deformities and a limited weight-bearing surface leading to continued breakdown.

Major Amputations

Transtibial amputation, also referred to as a below-knee amputation (BKA), is one of the most common major lower extremity amputations performed and offers improved rehabilitation potential secondary to knee joint preservation and prosthetic options. In general, this is the preferred level of amputation if the patient is relatively healthy and has good potential for ambulation with a prosthetic.

Transfemoral amputation, also referred to as an above-knee amputation (AKA), usually is reserved for patients who cannot have a transtibial amputation because of tissue loss, muscle ischemia, or poor rehabilitation potential based on their general medical condition.

Through-knee amputations are rarely performed as a definitive amputation in patients with dysvascular limbs but are sometimes used as a primary amputation level in patients who require emergent intervention for an ascending infection. These are often converted to transfemoral amputations once the infection has cleared.

Hip disarticulation amputations are reserved for patients with proximal thigh ischemia or trauma and carry a high risk of mortality and morbidity without options for prosthetic rehabilitation. Few surgeons have the experience and expertise to perform this amputation safely and successfully.

SELECTION OF AMPUTATION LEVEL AND PREOPERATIVE MANAGEMENT

The most critical decision regarding lower extremity amputation is the selection of the appropriate level. The ideal amputation level will heal without need for readmission and reoperation while preserving the best options for rehabilitation for the individual patient. In general, the higher the level of amputation, the greater the chance of healing without complication but also the greater the amount of energy required to achieve ambulation with a prosthetic. The energy expenditure at various levels of amputation can vary considerably between patients. In general, there is minimal increase in energy expenditure to ambulate with any of the minor amputations discussed earlier. The variability comes into play with the major amputations. For a BKA, the patient will need roughly a 30% to 60% increase in energy to ambulate with a prosthetic. In comparison, those who receive an AKA often will require a 60% to 100% increase in total energy expenditure. This is because of the loss of the functional knee joint and the need to use muscle groups poorly suited for ambulation needs. The increase in energy can be overcome easily in young, motivated patients, but in the older patient population with multiple chronic comorbidities ambulation with a prosthetic will not be achieved even with a BKA.

Overall clinical assessment of the likelihood of an amputation to heal is achieved through a combination of physical examination findings and some type of diagnostic imaging study. Usually the presence of a palpable pulse proximal to the level of amputation is a reliable indicator that the site will heal. Assessment of the soft tissue integrity, joint mobility, and muscle strength should be performed as part of the physical assessment. Significant calf soft tissue loss or infection, knee contractures, or muscle wasting would indicate a high likelihood that a transtibial (BKA) amputation would be at risk of failing or of limited value because of an inability to ambulate. Unfortunately, there is no single definitive imaging test that can determine what level of amputation will heal. Several noninvasive tests have been used to help determine the amount of perfusion and the potential to heal at a specific level and must be interpreted in the setting of the overall health and status of the patient and the surgeon's experience.

One of the most widely used diagnostic adjuncts in patients with peripheral arterial disease is lower extremity Doppler in conjunction with ultrasound. When used appropriately, it can provide the clinician with both an anatomic and a physiologic assessment of the limb. These studies are not without their limitations, however, and usually are hampered by the inability to compress the tibial vessels because of medial calcinosis, especially in diabetic patients. In those situations, the clinician still can obtain usable information usually in the form of toe pressures or waveforms because these vessels typically are spared from noncompressibility even in the worst diabetic patients. It has been suggested that absolute pressures of 60 mm Hg or higher at the level of the ankle can accurately predict the healing potential of a BKA in more than 50% of cases.

Another commonly used adjunct is the transcutaneous partial pressure of oxygen ($TcPO_2$) measurement. Unfortunately, this modality may not be available to all clinicians. In general, values of 40 mm Hg or higher are strong predictors of wound healing, whereas values of 20 mm Hg or lower almost universally predict failure of healing. To date, there is no measurement that can reliably predict healing 100% of the time.

Computed tomography, magnetic resonance imaging, and invasive angiography may all be of help in assessing for underlying infection, vascular supply, and potential for intervention to improve perfusion.

Recently, a few groups have reported success in predicting the level of amputation using tissue scintigraphy either preoperatively or during surgery. This may be of benefit for patients with marginal perfusion and hopefully may prevent the need for reoperation after a failed initial surgery. Further studies are needed to assess the ideal timing and benefits of this promising technology.

In addition to the assessment of the amputation level, significant time and effort should be spent preoperatively to prepare the patient physically and mentally for the procedure and for life after amputation. If at all possible, nutritional assessment and support should be initiated before amputation to help with healing of wounds and ability to participate in rehabilitation. Involvement of the patient's family in discussions with physical therapy, occupational therapy and rehabilitation specialists, prosthetists, and current amputees can increase the chance of acceptance, understanding, and support for the patient's recovery. Information on local and national support groups for amputees should be made available to help with the transition to amputee living and as a resource for future questions. By starting this dialogue before surgery, many patients will be less fearful and more motivated for their postoperative management.

■ POSTOPERATIVE MANAGEMENT AND COMPLICATIONS

Patients who undergo amputations have risks for postoperative complications similar to those of other patients who undergo major surgery. Patients who undergo a major lower extremity amputation carry estimated mortality risks of 19.2%, 48.7%, and 61.3% at 1, 3, and 5 years, respectively. Overall 30-day mortality after a major lower extremity amputation is approximately 9%. When looked at individually, a BKA carries an estimated 12% mortality, whereas an AKA carries a 6.5% mortality. Independent risk factors for mortality are similar to those associated with a perioperative cardiac event, as this is one of the more common causes of death. These risk factors include a history of congestive heart failure, cerebrovascular disease, high-risk surgery, and a creatinine level greater than 2. Beyond these factors, a history of myocardial infarction, postoperative respiratory complications, hemodialysis, preoperative pneumonia, American Society of Anesthesiologists (ASA) class IV or greater, and preoperative total dependence all carry significant risk for early perioperative mortality. It should be noted that diabetes mellitus itself does not confer a higher perioperative mortality risk but does contribute significantly to long-term mortality.

Postoperative deep venous thrombosis (DVT), wound infection, and trauma to the amputation site secondary to falls are a few of the more common complications after major lower extremity amputation. DVT or pulmonary embolism can have devastating consequences in a patient population with minimal physiologic reserve at baseline. Both of these problems have been reported in as many as 50% of patients undergoing lower extremity amputation in some series. For this reason, it is imperative that these patients start taking prophylaxis with either subcutaneous heparin or a low-molecular-weight heparin within the first 24 to 48 hours.

Trauma in the immediate postoperative setting is commonplace and can have very deleterious effects on the patient. It has been estimated that 1 in 5 patients with a new unilateral amputation will fall as they become accustomed to their new life as an amputee. This trauma is often in the form of a direct blow to the stump itself. Hematoma formation or dehiscence of the wound can occur. Depending on the severity of the trauma and the effect it has on the stump, these inadvertent falls can result in the need for revision or a more proximal amputation in upward of 16% of patients, which can convert some from a below-knee to an above-knee situation. The choice of postoperative dressings can play a significant role in reducing risk of injury as well as promoting healing and reducing discomfort. Soft dressings are composed of a nonadhesive barrier to the staple line, which then is covered with gauze and finally an elastic wrap. They allow easy access to view the limb and evaluate ongoing healing in addition to being relatively inexpensive and easy to apply. However, overzealous application of the elastic wrap can result in ischemia of the staple line, which may result in wound dehiscence or failure. It also can be detrimental if the elastic wrap is applied too lightly, resulting in slippage of the dressing and exposure of the staple line before epithelialization when it is most vulnerable to bacterial invasion. Also, it has been suggested that softer dressings may lead to contracture formation or lengthen the time before ambulation can occur and that they provide no protection to the stump itself in the event of a trauma (e.g., fall), which occurs not infrequently in new amputees.

Rigid dressings use all of the same components as soft dressings but then are covered with plaster. They are gaining popularity among surgeons who perform amputations for multiple reasons. In addition to providing protection to the stump itself should the patient suffer a fall in the immediate postoperative period, these dressings also aid in preventing joint contractures and have been shown to decrease the length of time to ambulation with a prosthetic. Decreased healing time resulting in earlier fitting of a patient's prosthesis and quicker time to ambulation can have a profound positive impact on the patient's overall psychologic state. The downside to such a dressing is the inability to readily access and visualize the staple line to evaluate wound healing and the technical knowledge needed to place one of these dressings without compromising the stump, which most surgeons lack initially. As an alternative to plaster, there are some commercially available removable rigid dressings, such as the KIWI, supplied by many prosthetic companies (Figure 1).

Some commercially prefabricated rigid removable dressings provide the benefits of a rigid dressing but are removed more easily for wound assessment and care. For example, the adjustable postoperative prosthesis (APOP) is composed of a hard plastic that is designed to protect the residual limb while simultaneously preventing a flexion contracture of the knee. These dressings typically are applied by the prosthetist in the immediate postoperative setting in conjunction with a stump shrinker to decrease residual edema. These devices are held in place with Velcro, providing the clinician with easy accessibility to the stump for continued evaluation of healing. If these commercially available devices are used, whoever takes the dressing off should have a complete understanding of how to reapply it. Placing the APOP in the wrong configuration could have deleterious

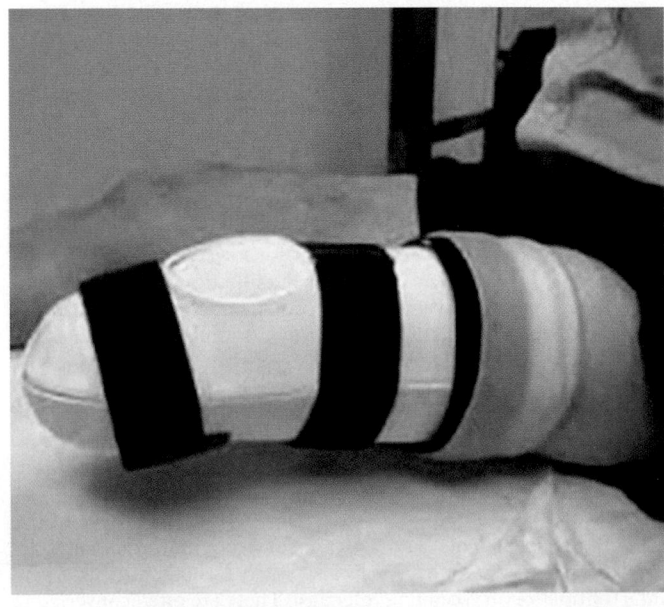

FIGURE 1 KIWI rigid removable dressing.

effects on the stump and not provide the patient with the intended benefits of its usage.

It cannot be emphasized enough that postoperative rehabilitation therapy must be instituted early in the postoperative course. Close coordination with your hospital's physical and occupational therapists is invaluable in the overall rehabilitation of amputees. These therapists are able to work closely with the patients to aid them in learning to manage their activities of daily living (ADLs) and adjust to the life of an amputee. In addition, therapy is geared toward prevention of flexion contractures of the knee in the below-knee amputee and improvement of upper body conditioning in all postoperative lower extremity amputees.

Postoperative pain after a major lower extremity amputation is one of the most important morbidities in the eyes of the patient. This pain can be grouped into either residual stump pain or phantom limb pain. Phantom limb pain can be a very debilitating problem for the treating physician. The exact cause is unknown at this time, and the true incidence varies among published reports. It has been suggested that those individuals who suffered from prolonged preoperative pain are at increased risk of suffering from phantom limb pain. Some patients describe episodic discomfort but as many as 25% may suffer from chronic, unrelenting pain. Various treatment strategies, including pharmacotherapy, nerve stimulation, and behavioral therapy, have been utilized in an effort to manage this debilitating phenomenon. Each patient responds differently to each modality, and treatment should be individualized.

■ OUTCOMES

Postoperative Ambulation

The preservation of one's ability to ambulate is integral to the preservation of one's overall independence. Any minor amputation carries a nearly 100% ambulation rate. Patients who undergo BKA have about a 75% chance of ambulating postoperatively with a prosthetic, whereas those who undergo AKA have a 40% or less chance of ambulating.

ADLs consist of those tasks constituting one's ability to provide even the most basic care to self, including eating, dressing, cooking, and overall mobility with or without assistance. Baseline function includes variables such as age, medical comorbidities, and independence status. Impairment in these simple tasks has been suggested to lead to poorer health, repeated hospitalization, and even death. Advanced age, prolonged hospitalization, history of a stroke, end-stage renal disease, and diabetes all lead to poorer performance of ADLs upon discharge, primarily in the nursing home population. Residents who undergo BKA exhibit better performance on ADLs, emphasizing the benefit of limb preservation even in older patients. This may support attempts at a BKA in any individual who was performing basic ADLs independently preoperatively.

Contralateral Amputation

One of the greatest fears an amputee experiences is the risk to the remaining lower extremity after any type of amputation, and this fear is not without merit. It has long been identified that those individuals who undergo an amputation are at risk for subsequent amputations or revisions on the ipsilateral leg, in addition to amputations of the contralateral leg. The latter can have overwhelming debilitating consequences for the patient. Independent factors that place the contralateral extremity at risk have been identified and include chronic renal insufficiency or end-stage renal disease, atherosclerosis of the native vasculature with or without diabetic neuropathy, and history of a major lower extremity amputation. Diabetes also has been recognized and is associated with a significantly higher percentage of contralateral major lower extremity amputation. The greatest risk comes from a combination of diabetes mellitus and chronic renal insufficiency. It has been estimated that patients who undergo an initial major lower extremity amputation carry upward

of 12% risk for a contralateral major amputation within 5 years, compared with roughly 8.5% risk in patients undergoing an initial minor amputation.

Prosthesis

Not everyone who undergoes an amputation will ambulate successfully with a prosthesis, mainly because of their underlying condition and functional capabilities. For those who are able to rehabilitate successfully, the advancement in prosthetic limbs makes it possible to resume almost all activities. Specialized limbs for athletic competition have led to amputee athletes competing at the highest levels against athletes with two human limbs. Computerized controllers (Figure 2) for prosthetics allow amputees to navigate uneven terrain, stand safely on boats at sea, and resume many of their presurgical activities that would have been impossible in previous decades. The costs of tailoring even a basic prosthesis for a patient are not insignificant, and so it is important to attempt to identify those patients who are likely to ambulate before proceeding with prosthetic development, especially for the more advanced limbs. One tool developed to help in patient selection is the Medicare K-level scale (Table 2), which assesses functional ability and rehabilitation potential to help guide prosthetic choice. In general, the higher the K-level, the more likely the patient is to benefit from a sophisticated prosthetic limb. Those patients who succumb to an amputation because of vascular disease are typically K1 to K3, in contrast to those with traumatic amputations, which tend to be K4. Patients with higher K-levels are most likely to benefit from advanced prosthetics.

Prosthetic preparation begins in the immediate postoperative period through use of rigid removable dressings, early physical therapy, and rehabilitation assessments. Some physicians are proponents of an immediate postoperative prosthesis (IPOP), which allows patients to ambulate within a few days. These devices typically are applied in the operating room at the completion of surgery and suspend the limb within the device to avoid pressure on the stump. They are usually cumbersome to don and may increase the risk for falls as patients attempt to use them. Others prefer patients

TABLE 2: K-Level Scale

K-Level	Description
0	Lacks ability or potential to ambulate or transfer safely with or without assistance and therefore a prosthesis does not enhance quality of life or mobility
1	Ability or potential to use a prosthesis for transfers or ambulation on level surfaces at fixed cadence and is typical of a household ambulatory individual, or a person who walks about only in the home
2	Ability or potential for ambulation with ability to traverse low-level environmental barriers and is typical of a limited community ambulatory individual
3	Ability or potential for ambulation with variable cadence and is typically someone who can traverse most environmental barriers and have additional demands on the prosthetic beyond simple locomotion
4	Ability or potential for prosthetic ambulation exceeding basic skills and typical of a child, active adult, or athlete

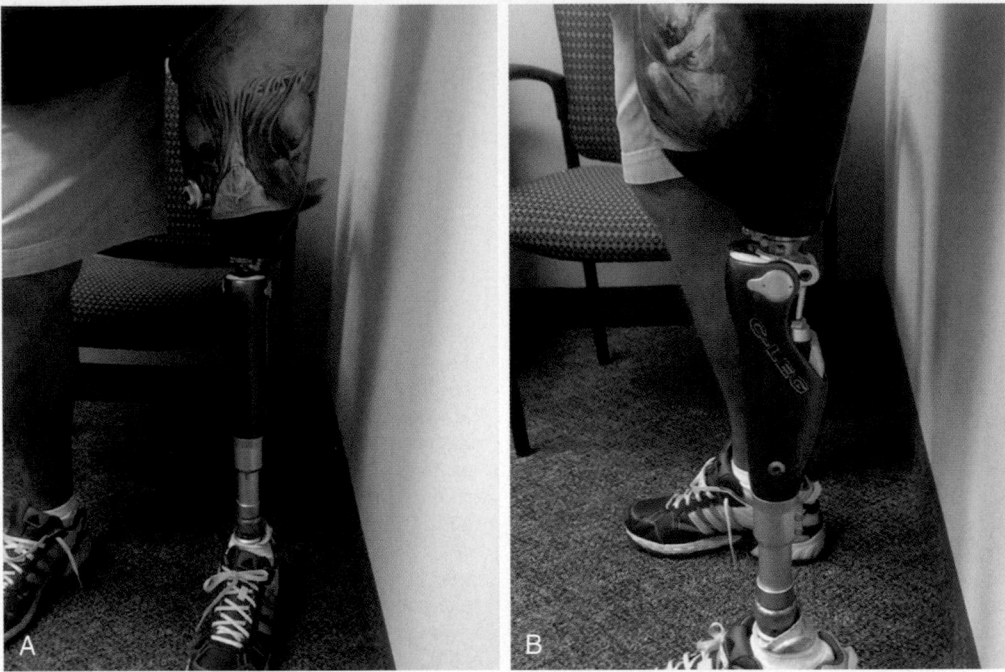

FIGURE 2 Computerized "C-Leg" for above-knee amputation.

to recover for a longer period and move more toward a traditional prosthetic path.

In the traditional prosthetic path, the amputee undergoes a series of "stump shrinker" applications, rehabilitation, and wound care before being fitted for the initial prosthesis. It may take up to 3 months before the patient begins the initial prosthesis training, and the initial prosthesis may be used for up to 6 months. After this, the permanent prosthesis is fitted and has an overall durability of 3 to 5 years on average before it needs to be replaced. While wearing the temporary (or preparatory) prosthesis, the patient needs continued physical therapy with the ultimate goal of ambulation without the use of any gait aids, including walkers and crutches. As part of this rehabilitation process, the patient is exposed to a schedule of progressive prosthetic wearing time, leading to continuous wearing of the prosthetic. This focuses on learning balance, coordination, weight shifting, and ambulation. As the program progresses, the therapist needs to work with the patient on overcoming common obstacles, including curbs, stairs, and uneven terrain, in addition to falling in a safe manner and recovering after a fall. Patients also are counseled on weight maintenance. Weight loss is an easy problem to overcome and usually entails padding within the prosthetic, whereas weight gain can lead to problems with the socket fitting and increases the energy requirements to ambulate.

■ CONCLUSION

Although little has changed in the surgical procedures for lower extremity amputations, dramatic advances have been made in perioperative wound management, prosthetics, and rehabilitation. Appropriate patient assessment for amputation level selection and multidisciplinary involvement should minimize the need for reoperation and allow patients to achieve a better quality of life free from infection, ischemic pain, and dysfunction.

SUGGESTED READINGS

Curran T, Zhang J, Lo R, et al. Risk factors and indications for readmission after lower extremity amputation in the American College of Surgeons National Surgical Quality Improvement Program. *J Vasc Surg.* 2014;60:1315-1324.

Glaser J, Bensley R, Hurks R, et al. Fate of the contralateral limb after lower extremity amputation. *J Vasc Surg.* 2013;58:1571-1577.

Karam J, Shepard A, Rubinfeld I. Predictors of operative mortality following major lower extremity amputations using the National Surgical Quality Improvement Program public use data. *J Vasc Surg.* 2013;58:1276-1282.

Sumpio B, Shine SR, Mahler D, et al. A comparison of immediate postoperative rigid and soft dressings for below-knee amputations. *Ann Vasc Surg.* 2013;27:774-780.

INITIAL ASSESSMENT AND RESUSCITATION OF THE TRAUMA PATIENT

**L.D. Britt, MD, MPH, FACS, FCCM,
and Jessica Burgess, MD**

Medical and surgical disciplines, which are responsible for the emergency assessment and management of critically ill and severely injured trauma patients, have adopted a two-tier system in the evaluation of this category of patients. This approach has been labeled the "initial assessment" (Box 1). In trauma management, the first-tier evaluation process of the initial assessment is the primary survey, followed by the second-tier evaluation, which is a detailed secondary survey. The secondary evaluation can be initiated only after the primary survey is completed. An adequately conducted initial assessment phase of trauma management should expeditiously detect and treat what has been labeled the "deadly dozen" (Box 2).

In the critically ill and severely injured trauma patient, a systematic approach of the entire patient always must be conducted—without exception. An initial assessment of the entire patient is imperative before focusing on the specific anatomic region where an obvious traumatic injury exists. The concept of initial assessment includes the following components: (1) rapid primary survey, (2) resuscitation, (3) detailed secondary survey (evaluation), and (4) re-evaluation. Such an assessment is the cornerstone of the Advanced Trauma Life Support® (ATLS®) program. Integrated into primary and secondary surveys are specific adjuncts. Such adjuncts include the application of electrocardiographic monitoring and the use of other monitoring modalities such as arterial blood gas determination; pulse oximetry; measurement of ventilatory rate and blood pressure; insertion of urinary and gastric catheters; and obtaining necessary x-rays and other diagnostic studies, when applicable, such as focused assessment with sonography for trauma (FAST) and others (plain radiography of the spine, chest, and pelvis and computed tomography [CT]). The initial assessment essentially underscores the prioritization of patient management. Determination of the status of an airway and optimal oxygenation (airway [A] and breathing [B]) are inevitably the top priorities, followed by assessing the adequacy of blood flow—circulation (C). For example, when an airway is believed to be inadequate, the establishment of a rapid sequence translaryngeal endotracheal intubation might be indicated. If circulation is deemed suboptimal and bleeding is suspected, an expeditious search for an external or cavitary (peritoneum, thorax) source is conducted. Following the "ABCs" of the primary survey, a rapid assessment of the neurologic status for gross disability (D)—including determining (1) the level of consciousness; (2) motor function (extremity movement); (3) sensory function; and (4) the presence of reflexes (pupillary, bulbocavernosus)—is the next priority. This rapid neurologic assessment allows for the calculation of a Glasgow Coma Score (GCS). The final component of the primary survey is ensuring that full exposure (E) of the patient is achieved, along with environmental control, in order to lessen the chance of the patient becoming hypothermic.

The focus of the primary survey is to both identify and rapidly address immediate life-threatening injuries. In addition to resuscitation, the necessary adjuncts to the primary survey (and secondary evaluation) include electrocardiographic monitoring; placement of urinary and gastric catheters (when appropriate and not contraindicated); and close monitoring of physiologic parameters such as respiratory rate, pulse rate, blood pressure, pulse pressure, arterial blood gases, body temperature, and urinary output. Only after the primary survey is completed (including the initiation of resuscitation) and hemodynamic stability is addressed should the secondary survey be conducted, which entails a head-to-toe (and back-to-front) physical examination, along with a more detailed history. Normalization of all vital functions should be evident before proceeding to the secondary survey.

■ PRIMARY SURVEY

As highlighted earlier, the primary survey is designed to quickly detect life-threatening injuries. Therefore a universal approach has been established with the following prioritization:

- Airway maintenance (with protection of the cervical spine)
- Breathing (ventilation)
- Circulation (including hemorrhage control)
- Disability (neurologic status)
- Exposure and environmental control

Such a systematic and methodical approach (better known as the ABCDEs of the initial assessment) greatly assists the surgical and medical team in the timely management of those injuries that could result in a poor outcome.

Airway Assessment Management (Along With Cervical Spine Protection)

Because loss of a secure airway could be lethal within 4 minutes, airway assessment and management always has the highest priority during the primary survey of the initial assessment of any injured patient, irrespective of the mechanism of injury or the anatomic wound. The chin lift and jaw thrust maneuvers are occasionally helpful in attempting to secure a patient airway. However, in the trauma setting, the airway management of choice is often translaryngeal endotracheal intubation (Box 3). If this cannot be achieved because of an upper airway obstruction or some technical difficulty, a surgical airway (needle or surgical cricothyroidotomy) should be the alternative approach. No other management can take precedence over obtaining an appropriate airway control. Until adequate and sustained oxygenation can be documented, administration of 100% oxygen is required.

BOX 1: Initial Assessment and Management of the Injured Patient

Primary Survey
    Airway
    Breathing (ventilation)
    Circulation
    Disability
    Exposure/Environmental Control
Resuscitation*
Secondary Evaluation
Definitive Care

*Although the assessment process and management interventions are appropriately sequenced and prioritized, resuscitation is initiated as soon as possible and integrated throughout the entire initial assessment and management process, as indicated.

BOX 2: "Deadly Dozen" Potentially Lethal Airway and Torso Injuries

"Lethal Six"
    airway obstruction
    tension pneumothorax
    massive hemothorax
    cardiac tamponade
    open pneumothorax (or "sucking" chest wound)
    flail chest
"Hidden (Occult) Six"
    thoracic aortic disruption
    tracheobronchial injury
    blunt cardiac injury
    diaphragmatic injury
    esophageal injury
    pulmonary contusion

From American College of Surgeons Committee. *Advanced Trauma Life Support Instructor Manual.* 6th ed. Chicago: American College of Surgeons; 1997.

Breathing (Ventilation Assessment)

An adequate airway can be established and optimal ventilation still not be achieved. For example, such is the case when there is an associated tension pneumothorax (other examples include a substantial hemothorax, open pneumothorax, or large flail chest wall segment). Worsening oxygenation and an adverse outcome would ensue unless such problems are emergently addressed. Therefore assessment of breathing is imperative, even when there is an established and secure airway. A patent airway, but poor gas exchange, still will result in a less than optimal outcome. Tachypnea, absent breath sounds, percussion hyperresonance, distended neck veins, and tracheal deviation are all consistent with inadequate gas exchange. Decompression of the pleural space with a needle or chest tube insertion should be the initial intervention for a pneumothorax or hemothorax that compromises a patient's respiratory or cardiovascular status. A large flail chest, with underlying pulmonary contusion, likely will require endotracheal intubation and the administration of positive pressure ventilation.

Circulation Assessment (Adequacy of Perfusion Management)

The most important initial step in determining adequacy of circulatory perfusion is to quickly identify and control any active source of bleeding. The patient's blood volume is then restored with crystalloid fluid resuscitation and blood products, if required. The estimation of blood loss, based on a patient's initial presentation, has been

BOX 3: Airway Management and Indications for Endotracheal Intubation

Absolute Indications

Airway obstruction
Apnea
Severe respiratory distress (e.g., stridor, dyspnea, cyanosis, tachypnea, hypoxemia, hypercardia)
Decreased level of consciousness (e.g., comatose, Glasgow Coma Score ≤8)

Strong Indications

Hemodynamic instability
Chest wall injury or deformity that compromises ventilation
Risk of aspiration

Relative Indications

Facial trauma
Documented pulmonary contusion
Agitated or sedated patient who is at risk for airway compromise
Pre-emptive for the patient who will be undergoing diagnostic or therapeutic interventions and will be unable to undergo close surveillance

classified into levels (Class I to IV) (Table 1). Decreased levels of consciousness, pale skin color, slow (or nonexistent) capillary refill, cool body temperature, tachycardia, or diminished urinary output are all suggestive of inadequate tissue perfusion. Optimal resuscitation requires the insertion of two large bore intravenous lines and infusion of warmed crystalloid fluids. Adult patients who are severely compromised will require a fluid bolus (two liters of Lactated Ringer's or saline solution). Children should receive a 20 mL/kg fluid bolus. Blood and blood products are administered, as required. Along with the initiation of fluid resuscitation, emphasis must remain on identifying the source of active bleeding and stopping the hemorrhage. For a patient in hemorrhagic shock, the source of blood loss could be an open wound with profuse bleeding, or within the thoracic or abdominal cavity, or from an associated pelvic fracture with venous or arterial injuries. Disposition (operating room, angiography suite, etc.) of the patient depends on the site of bleeding. For example, a FAST that documents substantial blood loss in the abdominal cavity in a patient who is hemodynamically labile dictates an emergency celiotomy. However, if the quick diagnostic workup of a hemodynamically unstable patient who has sustained blunt trauma demonstrates no blood loss from an open wound in the abdomen or chest, the source of hemorrhage likely would be a pelvic injury, necessitating angiography and embolization of a probable arterial injury if external stabilization (e.g., a commercial wrap or binder) of the pelvic fracture fails to stop the bleeding. Profuse bleeding from open wounds usually can be addressed by application of direct pressure or occasionally ligating torn arterial vessels that can be identified and isolated easily.

Disability Assessment and Management

Only a baseline neurologic examination is required when performing the primary survey in order to determine neurologic function deterioration that might necessitate surgical intervention. It is inappropriate to attempt a detailed neurologic examination initially. Such a comprehensive examination should be done during the secondary survey or evaluation. This baseline neurologic assessment could be the determination of the GCS, with an emphasis on the best motor or verbal response, and eye opening. An alternative approach for a rapid neurologic evaluation is the assessment of the pupillary size and reaction, along with establishing the patient's level of consciousness (alert, responds to visual stimuli, responds only to painful

TABLE 1: Estimated Blood Loss Based on Patient's Initial Presentation

	Class I	Class II	Class III	Class IV
Blood loss (mL)	Up to 750	750-1500	1500-2000	>2000
Blood loss (% blood volume)	Up to 15%	15%-30%	30%-40%	>40%
Pulse rate (BPM)	<100	100-120	120-140	>140
Systolic blood pressure	Normal	Normal	Decreased	Decreased
Pulse pressure (mm Hg)	Normal or increased	Decreased	Decreased	Decreased
Respiratory rate	14-20	20-30	30-40	>35
Urine output (mL/hr)	>30	20-30	5-15	Negligible
CNS/mental status	Slightly anxious	Mildly anxious	Anxious, confused	Confused, lethargic
Initial fluid replacement	Crystalloid	Crystalloid	Crystalloid and blood	Crystalloid and blood

From American College of Surgeons, Committee on Trauma. *ATLS—Advanced Trauma Life Support: Student Manual.* Chicago: American College of Surgeons; 2012.

BPM, beats per minute; *CNS,* central nervous system.

stimuli, or unresponsive to all stimuli). The caveat that must be highlighted is the fact that neurologic deterioration can occur rapidly and that a patient with a devastating injury (e.g., epidural hematoma) can have a lucid interval. Because the leading causes of secondary brain injury are hypoxia and hypotension, adequate cerebral oxygenation and perfusion are essential in the management of a patient with neurologic injury.

Exposure and Environmental Control

To perform a thorough examination of a patient, the patient must be completely undressed. This often requires cutting off the patient's garments to safely expedite such exposure. However, care must be taken to maintain normothermia and prevent the patient from becoming hypothermic. Adjusting the room temperature and infusing warmed intravenous fluids can help to establish an optimal environment for the patient.

Secondary Survey

As underscored earlier, the secondary survey should not be done until the primary survey has been completed and resuscitation has been initiated, with some evidence of normalization of vital signs. It is imperative that this head-to-toe (front-to-back) evaluation be performed in a detailed and systematic fashion in order to detect less obvious or occult injuries. This is particularly important in the unevaluable patient (e.g., head injury, severely intoxicated). The management of blunt abdominal trauma continues to evolve more toward the nonoperative arena rather than surgical intervention. The workup has shifted largely from the use of physical examination, plain x-ray, laboratory findings, and diagnostic peritoneal lavage to the extensive use of CT and ultrasonography. Treatment for visceral injury traditionally has been surgical, but many forms of solid organ injury can now be successfully managed nonoperatively or with minimally invasive and interventional radiology techniques. Nonoperative management of the multiple injured trauma patient at level I trauma centers, with state-of-the-art techniques, has now conclusively shown significantly improved patient outcomes and survival.

Diagnostic and Imaging Adjuncts

Diagnostic peritoneal lavage (DPL) has now been essentially supplanted by the adoption and new popularity of abdominal sonography. The use of DPL has diminished substantially. Originally

TABLE 2: Diagnostic Criteria for a Positive Diagnostic Peritoneal Lavage

Any Viscus	Bowel
10 mL gross blood	Bacteria
>100,000 red blood cells/mm^3	Bile
>500 white blood cells/mm^3	Food particles
>75 IU/L amylase	

described by Root in 1965, DPL was a mainstay in the management of blunt abdominal trauma for more than 4 decades. Before the era of routine CT scanning, DPL was used as a screening tool to evaluate patients with blunt or penetrating abdominal trauma, with an accuracy rate reported between 92% and 98%. CT scans and FAST are now the diagnostic modalities of choice for the assessment of the injured patient. However, DPL remains an excellent tool for further workup of occult bowel injury or in unstable patients when FAST is not available or has questionable findings. In the workup for occult bowel injury, traditional parameters (Table 2) should be used to guide therapy. In unstable patients and when FAST is not an option, a diagnostic tap is usually all that is necessary, and exploration is indicated when there is aspiration of greater than 10 mL of gross blood.

The pitfalls of DPL are a relatively high false-positive rate, risk of creating visceral injury, and poor sensitivity for detecting injury to retroperitoneal structures such as the pancreas and duodenum. Iatrogenic events are minimized if a Foley catheter and nasogastric tube are placed before the procedure. Patients with pelvic fractures and suspected retroperitoneal hematoma or pregnant females should undergo a supraumbilical approach. Visceral injury is less likely with an open approach but more time consuming and invasive. Checking amylase or lipase in the lavage sample, concomitant use of CT scan, and high index of suspicion are necessary to avoid missed retroperitoneal injury.

■ FOCUSED ASSESSMENT WITH SONOGRAPHY FOR TRAUMA

In the diagnostic assessment of the acutely injured patient, bedside ultrasonography for detection of cardiac and intra-abdominal injury

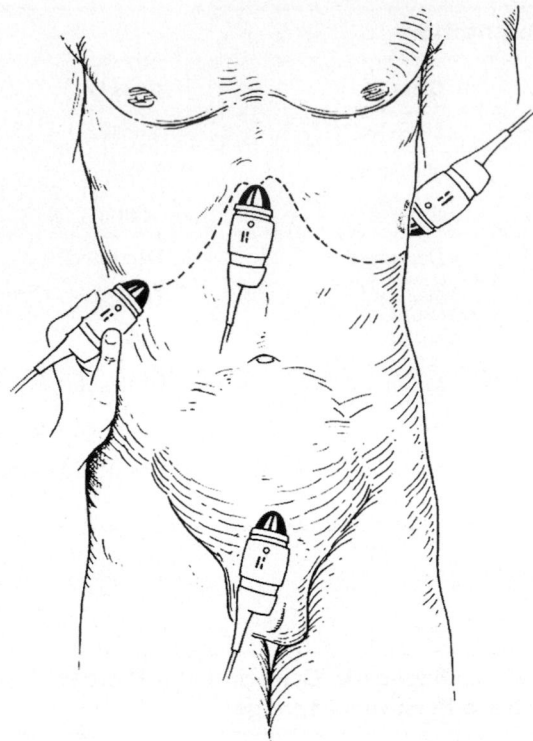

FIGURE 1 Schematic showing sonographic windows for subxyphoid, left subcostal, right subcostal, and suprapubic areas. Distension of the urinary bladder either before Foley catheter placement or by installation of 150 to 200 mL normal saline will enhance sensitivity. *(From Rozycki GS, Ochsner MG, Schmidt JA, et al. A prospective study of surgeon-performed ultrasound as the primary adjuvant modality for injured patient assessment. J Trauma. 1995;39:492-498; discussion 498-500.)*

is considered the standard of care. Because FAST is noninvasive, this diagnostic modality allows the operator to perform an examination simultaneously during the initial resuscitation and stabilization of a multiple injured trauma patient. Because of the relative insensitivity of abdominal examination in the severely injured patient, FAST may provide evidence of significant hemorrhage early in the course of an evaluation. An ultrasound probe is used to examine four key windows for fluid: the subxiphoid area permits visualization of the pericardium, the left subcostal area visualization of the splenorenal recess, the right subcostal area visualization of Morison's pouch, and the suprapubic area visualization of the pelvic cul de sac (Figure 1). The presence of fluid may indicate presence of cardiac tamponade (fluid in the pericardial space), intra-abdominal hemorrhage, hollow viscus perforation, hemoperitoneum, or ascites. False-positive results secondary to pre-existing ascites or false-negative results because of operator error or body habitus are the main limitations. Scanning the suprapubic area with distension of the urinary bladder will enhance the sensitivity of the examination for the detection of pelvic fluid.

A threshold of at least 200 mL of fluid in the abdominal cavity is necessary for detection, and intra-abdominal injuries must be associated with the presence of this much free fluid for a positive finding. Reported sensitivities range between 73% and 88%, and specificity ranges between 98% and 100%. Accuracy rates range from 96% to 98%. FAST is an inexpensive, rapid, portable, noninvasive technique that can be performed in serial fashion if there is a change in patient stability. In addition, it obviates the risk of exposing pregnant females to radiation. Positive findings in stable patients can be evaluated further with CT, whereas positive findings in unstable patients should prompt the surgeon to take the patient to the operating room for emergent exploration. Workup of a patient with a reliable abdominal examination may be complete with a negative FAST in the absence of abdominal signs or symptoms.

COMPUTED TOMOGRAPHY

Steady advances in the technology and speed of CT have continued to make CT an integral part of the diagnostic management of trauma patients. Multidetector scanners have drastically improved resolution and accuracy of these imaging studies. Negative predictive values as high as 99.63% have been reported for patients sustaining significant mechanisms of blunt trauma, allowing the use of CT as a reliable and noninvasive screening tool for patients with blunt abdominal trauma. In light of modern-day CT capabilities, prospective data have demonstrated that patients with a signinficant event and a benign abdomen can be released from the emergency department if a CT scan of the abdomen shows no evidence of visceral injury, provided that there are no other reasons for hospitalization.

CT reliably identifies injuries in solid organs such as the spleen, liver, and kidney because of the associated vascular nature demonstrating disruption of normal architecture, associated free fluid, and the so-called vascular blush. Established grading scales continue to be used for accurate classification and determination of management plan (Tables 3 to 5).

Detection of bowel injury via CT scan in patients who are intoxicated, are intubated, or have associated closed head injury or other distracting injuries can present a diagnostic challenge in the absence of a reliable abdominal examination. The incidence of blunt bowel injury varies from series to series but is generally reported in the 1% to 5% range in all blunt trauma patients admitted to level I trauma centers. A high index of suspicion is predicated on the mechanism of injury and physical examination findings, such as abdominal wall ecchymosis, tattooing, or seat belt sign. CT findings may be overt, such as extravasation of oral contrast or pneumoperitoneum, or more commonly may be subtle, such as bowel wall thickening, stranding of the mesentery, or free fluid in the absence of solid organ injury. Indirect findings may be fairly nonspecific and secondary to bowel edema from resuscitation or pre-existing ascites. Reproductive-age females may have a small amount of normal or "physiologic" pelvic fluid present, sometimes adding to the complexity of the evaluation. Patients undergoing positive pressure ventilation or with significant barotrauma may have mediastinal or subcutaneous emphysema that can track through the peritoneum or retroperitoneum and give the appearance of free air. Great care in the radiologic interpretation and close clinical correlation are necessary in such cases. The liberal use of diagnostic modalities (e.g., abdominal CT scan) in the hemodynamically normal injured patient may prevent nontherapeutic laparotomies. Obviously, when significant doubt remains, abdominal exploration may be required to confirm an injury.

The role of oral contrast in the evaluation of the acutely injured patient has come under question recently. Usually little time is available in the emergency setting to permit adequate opacification of the small bowel. Patients are further at risk for aspiration of the contrast media, and administration often requires placement of a nasogastric tube. Several reports have shown that elimination of oral contrast media does not lead to an increased incidence of missed bowel injury. Many centers have now safely eliminated the use of oral contrast media from their routine trauma protocols, expediting management and ease of patient care. Resuscitation edema may cause a hazy appearance around the head of the pancreas and duodenal C loop, raising the question of a pancreas or duodenal injury. Further clarification in this situation can be obtained, when it occasionally occurs, via repeat CT scan with the administration of oral contrast and the injection of 300 to 500 cc bolus of air down the nasogastric tube in order to make pneumoperitoneum obvious.

CT also may be of great importance in identifying patients with arterial hemorrhage related to pelvic fracture. CT imaging may demonstrate an arterial blush or large hematoma in the vicinity of a pelvic fracture, indicating the need for pelvic arteriography or pelvic external fixation. A "CT cystogram" also may be helpful and eliminate redundancy of x-ray evaluation. The Foley catheter is clamped after placement in the trauma bay. Real-time interpretation of the CT scan is performed by the evaluating physician, which may dictate further

TABLE 3: Spleen Injury Scale of the American Association for the Surgery of Trauma

	Grade*	Injury Description	ICD-9	AIS-90
I	Hematoma	Subcapsular, <10% surface area	865.01 865.11	2
	Laceration	Capsular tear, <1 cm parenchymal depth	865.02 865.12	2
II	Hematoma	Subcapsular, 10-50% surface area; intraparenchymal, <5 cm in diameter	865.01 865.11	2
	Laceration	1-3 cm parenchymal depth which does not involve a trabecular vessel	865.02 865.12	2
III	Hematoma	Subcapsular, >50% surface area or expanding; ruptured subcapsular or parenchymal hematoma Intraparenchymal hematoma >5 cm or expanding		3
	Laceration	>3 cm parenchymal depth or involving trabecular vessels	865.03 865.13	3
IV	Laceration	Laceration involving segmental or hilar vessels producing major devascularization (>25% of spleen)		4
V	Laceration	Completely shattered spleen	865.04 865.14	5
	Vascular	Hilar vascular injury which devascularizes spleen		5

From Moore EE, Cogbill TH, Jurkovich MD, et al. Organ injury scaling: spleen and liver (1994 revision). *J Trauma.* 1995;38:323.

*Advance one grade for multiple injuries, up to grade III.

AIS, Abbreviated Injury Score; *ICD,* International Classification of Diseases, 9th Revision.

TABLE 4: Liver Injury Scale of the American Association for the Surgery of Trauma

	Grade*	Injury Description	ICD-9	AIS-90
I	Hematoma	Subcapsular, <10% surface area	864.01 864.11	2
	Laceration	Capsular tear, <1 cm parenchymal depth	864.02 864.12	2
II	Hematoma	Subcapsular, 10-50% surface area; intraparenchymal, <10 cm in diameter	864.01 864.11	2
	Laceration	1-3 cm parenchymal depth, <10 cm in length	864.03 864.13	2
III	Hematoma	Subcapsular, >50% surface area or expanding; ruptured subcapsular or parenchymal hematoma Intraparenchymal hematoma >10 cm or expanding		3
	Laceration	>3 cm parenchymal depth	864.04 864.14	3
IV	Laceration	Parenchymal disruption involving 25-75% of hepatic lobe or 1-3 Couinaud's segments within a single lobe	864.04 864.14	4
V	Laceration	Parenchymal disruption involving >75% of hepatic lobe or >3 Couinaud's segments within a single lobe		5
	Vascular	Juxtahepatic venous injuries; i.e.; retrohepatic vena cava/central major hepatic veins		5
VI	Vascular	Hepatic avulsion		6

From Moore EE, Cogbill TH, Jurkovich MD, et al: Organ injury scaling: spleen and liver (1994 revision). *J Trauma.* 1995;38:323. With permission.

*Advance one grade for multiple injuries, up to grade III. *AIS,* Abbreviated Injury Score; *ICD,* International Classification of Diseases, 9th Revision.

TABLE 5: Kidney Injury Scale of the American Association for the Surgery of Trauma

	Grade*	Injury Description	ICD-9	AIS-90
I	Contusion	Microscopic or gross hematuria, urologic studies normal	866.00	2
			866.02	
	Hematoma	Subcapsular, nonexpanding without parenchymal laceration	866.11	2
II	Hematoma	Nonexpanding perirenal hematoma confined to renal retroperitoneum	866.01	2
	Laceration	Parenchymal depth of renal cortex (>1.0 cm) without urinary extravasation	866.11	2
III	Laceration	Parenchymal depth of renal cortex (>1.0 cm) without collecting system rupture or urinary extravasation	866.02	3
			866.12	
IV	Laceration	Parenchymal laceration extending through the renal cortex, medulla, and collecting system	866.02	4
	Vascular	Main renal artery or vein injury with contained hemorrhage	866.12	4
V	Laceration	Completely shattered kidney	866.03	5
	Vascular	Avulsion of renal hilum that devascularizes kidney	866.13	5

Adapted from Moore EE, Shackford SR, Pachter HL, et al. Organ injury scaling: spleen, liver, and kidney. *J Trauma.* 1989;29:1664.

*Advance one grade for bilateral injuries up to grade III. *AIS,* Abbreviated Injury Score; *ICD,* International Classification of Diseases, 9th Revision.

TABLE 6: Initial Assessment and Shock Management

Condition	Assessment (Physical Examination)	Management
Tension pneumothorax	• Tracheal deviation • Distended neck veins • Tympany • Absent breath sounds	• Needle decompression • Tube thoracostomy
Massive hemothorax	• Tracheal deviation • Flat neck veins • Percussion dullness • Absent breath sounds	• Venous access • Volume replacement • Surgical consultation/thoracotomy • Tube thoracostomy
Cardiac tamponade	• Distended neck veins • Muffled heart tones • Ultrasound	• Venous access • Volume replacement • Pericardiotomy • Thoracotomy • Pericardiocentesis
Intraabdominal hemorrhage	• Distended abdomen • Uterine lift, if pregnant • DPL/ultrasonography • Vaginal examination	• Venous access • Volume replacement • Surgical consultation • Displace uterus from vena cava
Obvious external bleeding	• Identify source of obvious external bleeding	• Direct pressure • Splints • Closure of actively bleeding scalp wounds

From American College of Surgeons, Committee on Trauma. *ATLS—Advanced Trauma Life Support: Manuals for Coordinators and Faculty.* Chicago: American College of Surgeons; 2013.

DPL, Diagnostic peritoneal lavage.

delayed images or a formal three-view (anterior/posterior, lateral, and postvoid views) cystogram.

Although CT can be an important diagnostic modality in the assessment of the trauma patient, it is contraindicated in the hemodynamically unstable patient who is in shock. Table 6 categorizes the common conditions that can cause an injured patient to be seen in a shock state.

SUGGESTED READINGS

American College of Surgeons Committee on Trauma. *Advanced Trauma Life Support®.* 6th ed. Chicago: American College of Surgeons; 1997.

Britt LD, Peitzman A, Barie P, Jurkovich GJ. *Acute Care Surgery.* Philadelphia: Wolters Kluwer Health/Lippincott Williams & Wilkins; 2012.

MacKenzie EJ, Rivara FP, Jurkovich GJ, et al. A national evaluation of the effect of trauma-center care on mortality. *N Engl J Med.* 2006;354: 366-378.

Nathens AB, Jurkovich GJ, Maier RV, et al. Relationship between trauma center volume and outcomes. *JAMA.* 2001;285:1164-1171.

Rozycki GS, et al. A prospective study of surgeon-performed ultrasound as the primary adjuvant modality for injured patient assessment. *J Trauma.* 1995;39:492-498, discussion 498-500.

PREHOSPITAL MANAGEMENT OF THE TRAUMA PATIENT

Trista Reid, MD, and David A. Spain, MD

Proper management of trauma patients in the prehospital setting is crucial to successful resuscitation and subsequent management. This chapter reviews the main tenets of prehospital trauma evaluation, discusses system processes of field triage and tiered response, and examines how military experience has shaped practice.

Mortality in trauma classically has been divided into three temporal categories. Fifty percent of deaths occur immediately and are attributable to exsanguination and head trauma. These patients can be targeted via prevention and public health measures, but they are not salvageable with the use of Advanced Trauma Life Support (ATLS) interventions. Thirty percent of deaths occur within 1 to 2 hours and are potentially avoidable through proper resuscitation and hospital efforts. Prehospital management of the trauma patient intercedes during that critical "golden hour" when intervention is possible. The final peak in mortality occurs within 1 to 2 weeks after trauma and is usually secondary to infection or organ failure.

■ PRINCIPLES OF PREHOSPITAL TRAUMA MANAGEMENT

The key principles of prehospital evaluation follow standard trauma resuscitation guidelines. After ensuring scene safety, **A**irway is addressed first, followed by **B**reathing, then **C**irculation (the ABCs).

Airway

In patients identified in the field with respiratory distress, supplemental oxygen and adjuvants such as nasal trumpets, oral airways, and bag valve mask can be used. In patients identified with severe respiratory distress or in those with an inability to protect their airway (emesis, oropharyngeal bleeding, altered mental status with a Glasgow Coma Score [GCS] ≤8), endotracheal intubation is considered. Considerable debate exists around intubating patients in the field. Although intubation may serve to protect the airway and oxygenate and ventilate the patient, time spent intubating is precious, aspiration risk during intubation may be increased, transport can dislodge properly placed tubes, and inadvertent esophageal or mainstem intubations may lead to significant hypoxia. Several retrospective and prospective studies have demonstrated an increase in morbidity and mortality in patients with traumatic brain injury (TBI) who were intubated in the field. Investigators postulate that this augmented mortality may be secondary to severe hyperventilation and hypoxia. If airway adjuncts and bag valve mask are adequate, the "scoop and run" technique without scene intubation allows for the most rapid transport to the emergency department (ED). Intubation is necessary in severely injured, hypotensive patients who are unresponsive to conventional noninvasive methods.

If the resources are available, a valuable aid in intubated patients is end-tidal capnography, which is most useful in verifying endotracheal tube (ETT) position and when the patient requires transport on a mechanical ventilator. End-tidal capnography is being incorporated more frequently in the prehospital setting and is particularly advantageous in TBI. Several studies have demonstrated that normocapnia reduces the mortality rate in patients once they reach the ED. As part of the San Diego Paramedic Rapid Sequence Intubation Trial, prospective data were collected in patients with GCSs of 3 to 8. Patients with end-tidal capnography monitoring had a lower incidence of severe hyperventilation. Those patients with significant hyperventilation had a 56% mortality rate compared with a 30% mortality rate in patients without hyperventilation.

Breathing

Prehospital personnel save lives through the timely identification of tension pneumothoraces. This diagnosis can be recognized readily and addressed in the field with needle decompression. Clinical findings include respiratory distress, unilateral decreased breath sounds, crepitus, tracheal deviation, distended neck veins, hyper-resonance to percussion, increased difficulty in bag masking, and hemodynamic instability. The affected side can be decompressed by perpendicular insertion of a large bore 12- to 14-gauge intravenous (IV) catheter in the second or third intercostal space, passed over the superior surface of the rib in the midclavicular line. Common pitfalls include late recognition of tension pneumothorax, improper placement causing lung laceration, or poor depth of placement such that the pleural space is not entered. Although the midclavicular, second intercostal space is classically taught, recent data suggest that needle decompression in the axilla might be more likely to be successful. Subsequently, a chest tube should be placed for definitive decompression.

Circulation

Just as the primary survey is conducted in the ED, prehospital providers assess circulation via vital signs and physical examination. Quick recognition of actively bleeding sites with application of direct pressure can prevent further extravasation. Frequently missed locations of injury include scalp, back, perineum, and axilla. IV access and resuscitation are two key components in ensuring adequate perfusion. Placement of two large bore IVs (16 gauge) facilitates fluid administration, but the success rate of IV access declines with each subsequent attempt and should not impinge on rapid transport to definitive care. Inability to secure venous access is associated with more serious injuries, and after two attempts at venous IV placement, further efforts yield diminishing returns.

If access is difficult to obtain but necessary secondary to clinical signs of hemorrhagic shock, the interosseous (IO) route is available and now considered the next choice. Possible locations include proximal anterior tibia (most common), sternum (used frequently in the military and may have faster flow rates), humerus, femur, distal tibia, and superior iliac crest. IO route has equivalent plasma concentrations to injected drugs, and both crystalloid and colloid infusions can be given at similar rates to IV access. Compared with central line placement, IO access has higher first attempt success rates and faster time to insertion.

Resuscitation previously focused on large-volume fluid administration in an attempt to achieve normotension. More recent data, particularly research from the military, demonstrate that controlled resuscitation with a goal systolic blood pressure (SBP) of 80 to 90 mm Hg may decrease mortality. In studies of penetrating torso trauma, patients who did not receive fluid resuscitation in the field had lower mortality compared with patients who were resuscitated with fluid. Liberal fluid resuscitation was associated with an increase in acute respiratory distress syndrome (ARDS), pneumonia, and coagulopathy. Blunt trauma studies corroborate these findings of improved mortality in "permissive hypotension." Postulated justifications for this difference include fluid administration leading to increased arterial pressure and venous dilation of hemorrhaging sites, disruption of newly established clot, and possible dilution of clotting factors. In patients with suspected head injury, decreased mean arterial pressure could decrease cerebral perfusion pressure to harmful levels; therefore in patients with TBI a SBP of 100 mm Hg is the goal.

Transfusion of blood products in rapidly deteriorating patients who are unresponsive to crystalloid should follow 1:1:1 replacement of fresh frozen plasma (FFP) to platelets to packed red blood cells (PRBCs). Numerous military and civilian investigations support these parameters. In a combat hospital setting, 19% mortality was found when the plasma to RBC ratio was 1:1.4 compared with 34% mortality when the ratio was 1:2.5 and 65% mortality when the ratio was 1:8. A similar retrospective review of 466 massive transfusion civilian trauma patients also noted improved survival, decreased intensive care unit (ICU) stay, and improved ventilator-free and hospital-free days among the high plasma and high platelet patients. Survival was most enhanced by a plasma to RBC ratio of greater than 1:2.

The recent Pragmatic, Randomized Optimal Platelet and Plasma Ratios (PROPPR) trial, which evaluated a 1:1:1 ratio versus a 1:1:2 ratio of FFP to platelets to PRBCs in civilian trauma patients, demonstrated no difference in overall mortality at 24 hours and at 30 days. However, the study did reveal that patients in the 1:1:1 group achieved hemostasis more often and had fewer deaths secondary to exsanguination. Early adherence to this ratio at the inception of massive transfusion has been shown to decrease mortality as well.

ROLE OF TRANEXAMIC ACID IN HEMORRHAGIC SHOCK

The role of the antifibrinolytic tranexamic acid (TXA) has been studied as an adjunct to control bleeding. The Military Application of Tranexamic Acid in Trauma Emergency Resuscitation (MATTERs) Study retrospectively evaluated nearly 900 casualties, demonstrating a significantly lower mortality among soldiers receiving TXA than among those receiving traditional therapy. The Clinical Randomisation of an Antifibrinolytic in Significant Haemorrhage (CRASH-2) study showed similar results in 20,000 civilian trauma patients. Multiple trials have revealed a decrease in mortality, although some have demonstrated a reduction in transfusion requirements and coagulopathy, particularly in patients requiring massive transfusion. Current recommendations for trauma patients with clinical signs of hemorrhage include a 1-g dose of TXA in the first 3 hours after injury, followed by an additional 1-g dose infused over 8 hours. The drug is more effective the earlier it is initiated; administration more than 3 hours after injury has been linked to an increased risk of death from bleeding. Secondary to reports of thrombotic complications when TXA is used in conjunction with prothrombin complex concentrate and recombinant factor VII, trauma centers generally are not administering these medications simultaneously.

PREHOSPITAL ARREST

As discussed earlier, following the standard algorithm of assessing trauma patients should identify reversible causes of cardiorespiratory collapse such as airway compromise, tension pneumothorax, cardiac tamponade, and hemorrhage. Prehospital arrest has a worse prognosis in the setting of blunt trauma when compared with penetrating trauma and has an overall bleak prognosis when it occurs during transit to the hospital by emergency medical services (EMS). Cardiopulmonary resuscitation (CPR) is futile if the victim of blunt trauma is found already in arrest by health care personnel. In penetrating trauma, if pupillary reflexes, spontaneous movement, or organized electrocardiogram activity is present, CPR should be attempted. In general, CPR for longer than 15 minutes without restoration of vitals is ineffective. In the event of hanging, drowning, hypothermia, electrocution, or arrest from a medical condition, the health care provider may continue resuscitative efforts longer than one might ordinarily.

DISABILITY: HEAD AND SPINAL TRAUMA

Trauma patients in the field, particularly those with a concerning mechanism of injury or high suspicion of spinal injury, should be immobilized with a backboard and rigid cervical collar. Debate exists about prehospital clearance of the cervical spine by properly trained EMS personnel. Several studies have demonstrated that trained EMS personnel are able to appropriately clear cervical spines in standardized patients. However, in the more chaotic and dynamic setting of the nonsimulated field patient, EMS personnel immobilize fewer patients in practice than do their physician colleagues. No data exist as to whether this discrepancy leads to adverse outcomes. In trauma systems that incorporate cervical spine clearance in the field, the two common criteria used for clearance are the National Emergency X-Radiology Utilization Study (NEXUS) and the Canadian C-Spine Rule. According to the NEXUS guidelines, clearance is achievable if the patient has no posterior midline cervical tenderness, is not intoxicated, has no alterations in mental status or focal neurologic deficits, and has no distracting painful injuries. Under the Canadian C-Spine Rule, the patient can be cleared and does not require imaging if he or she is less than 65 years old, has a low-impact mechanism, has no paresthesias in extremities, is either ambulatory or sitting upright in the ED, has no midline tenderness, and is able to rotate his or her neck 45 degrees to the left and right. Of note, this determination takes some time and may interfere with rapid transport of the patient to definitive care (Figure 1; Table 1).

DISABILITY: HYPOTHERMIA

Approximately 66% of patients in the civilian setting arrive at the ED with hypothermia. Prevention of hypothermia (body temperature less than 34 degrees Celsius) is a practice championed by the military, with the idea that instituting rewarming methods early impedes the spiral into the trauma "triad of death" of hypothermia, coagulopathy, and acidosis. Layers of blankets and modified pocket "body bags" to provide warmth are used in current combat situations. Passive rewarming can be achieved by increasing ambient temperatures, whereas active rewarming uses blankets and air or fluid circulating covers. Core rewarming uses fluid warmers to heat infusing fluid to 42 degrees Celsius. The key is to initiate prevention early in the field, as adequate rewarming is much more difficult to achieve once hypothermia occurs.

ADJUNCTS: TOURNIQUETS AND SPLINTS

Although tourniquets had fallen out of use secondary to a perceived concern for tissue loss, proper placement of the tourniquet proximal to the injury for less than 2 hours likely reduces hemorrhage and saves lives. Several studies have demonstrated that tourniquet use on the battlefield does not lead to unintended amputation or long-term disability and does reduce mortality in patients with severe blast injuries. In a study of deaths that occurred during Operation Iraqi Freedom, prehospital tourniquet use was associated with improved hemorrhage control. Of the deaths that did occur, up to 57% may have been prevented by earlier tourniquet use. When direct pressure fails, tourniquet placement should be attempted.

Another adjunct frequently used in the prehospital setting is the splint; common varieties include box, vacuum, and traction splints. In the case of obvious extremity fractures, splinting the injured extremity can stabilize the injury and potentially reduce pressure on skin and neurovascular structures, as well as decrease pain and bleeding. The splint must extend to the joints above and below the fracture to provide support.

**FOR ALERT (GCS=15) AND STABLE TRAUMA PATIENTS WHERE
CERVICAL SPINE INJURY IS A CONCERN.**

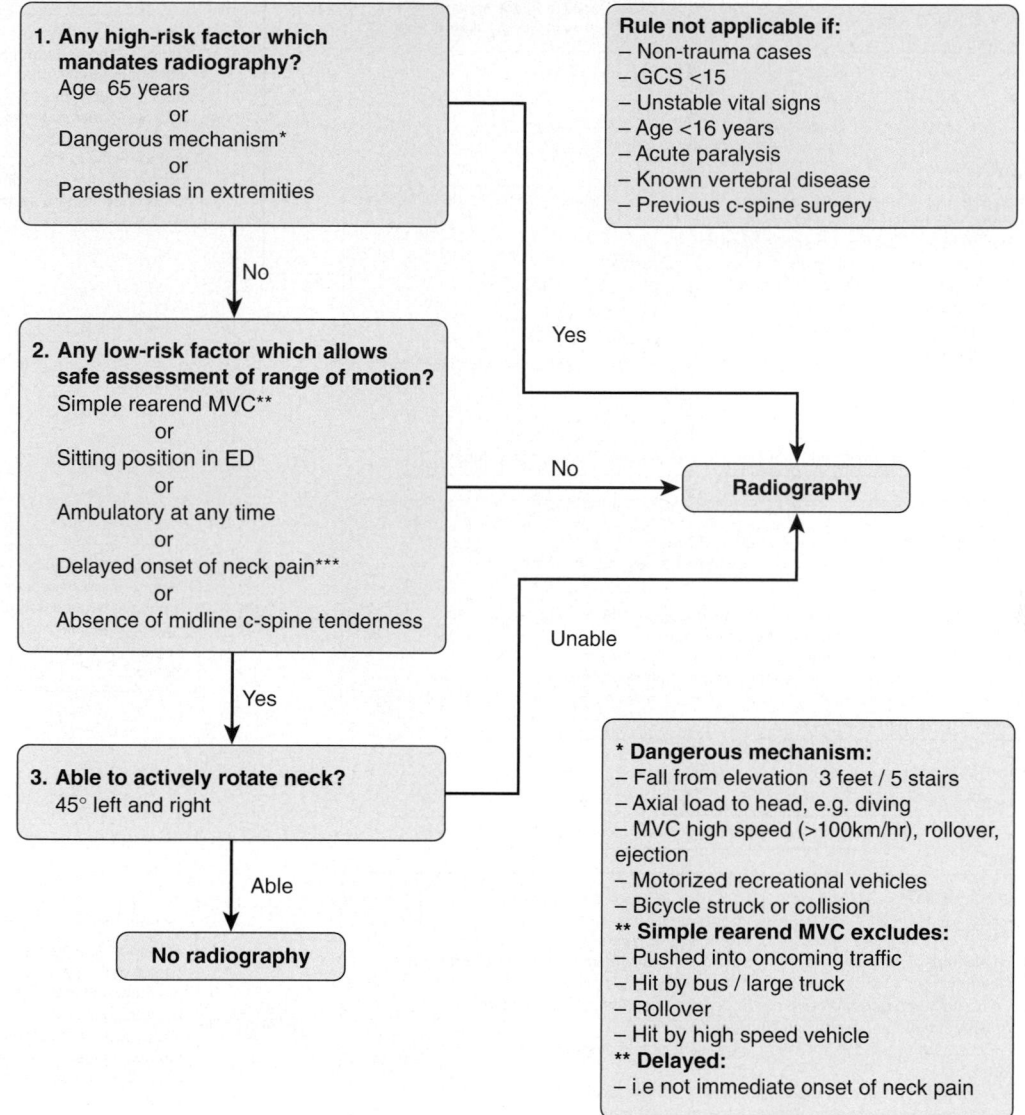

FIGURE 1 Canadian C-Spine Rule. *ED*, Emergency department; *GCS*, Glasgow Coma Score; *MVC*, motor vehicle collision.

TABLE 1: NEXUS Criteria for Low Probability C-Spine Injury

1	No midline tenderness
2	No focal neurologic deficit
3	Normal alertness
4	No intoxication
5	No painful distracting injury

NEXUS, National Emergency X-Radiology Utilization Study.

■ PREHOSPITAL TRIAGE AND TIERED RESPONSE

In the United States, in-hospital and 1-year mortality are significantly lower in trauma patients treated at trauma centers compared with those treated at nontrauma centers. Having a predetermined system in place to address injuries and triage patients saves lives. Trauma centers are divided into different tiers based on their capabilities. Level I trauma facilities have the resources for all-encompassing trauma care, including subspecialty providers, research capabilities, education, prevention, and rehabilitation. Level II trauma centers retain almost equivalent resources and can provide resuscitation and stabilization of patients but do not provide similar education and research opportunities. Level III trauma centers have more limited resources and staff. They are able to treat minor traumas and possess the capability to stabilize and transfer more severely injured patients to a higher level of care. Allocation of trauma patients into these systems requires the use of thoughtful triage parameters in the field.

Proper triage in the prehospital setting can lead to expedient transfer of the most tenuous patients to definitive care. The key is to maintain a balance between guaranteeing that the majority of critically ill patients are transported to a higher level of care facility and ensuring that these systems are not overburdened with patients who have sustained minimal injuries. A 50% overtriage rate is tolerated to attain a 5% or lower undertriage rate per the American College of Surgeons Committee on Trauma (ACS-COT).

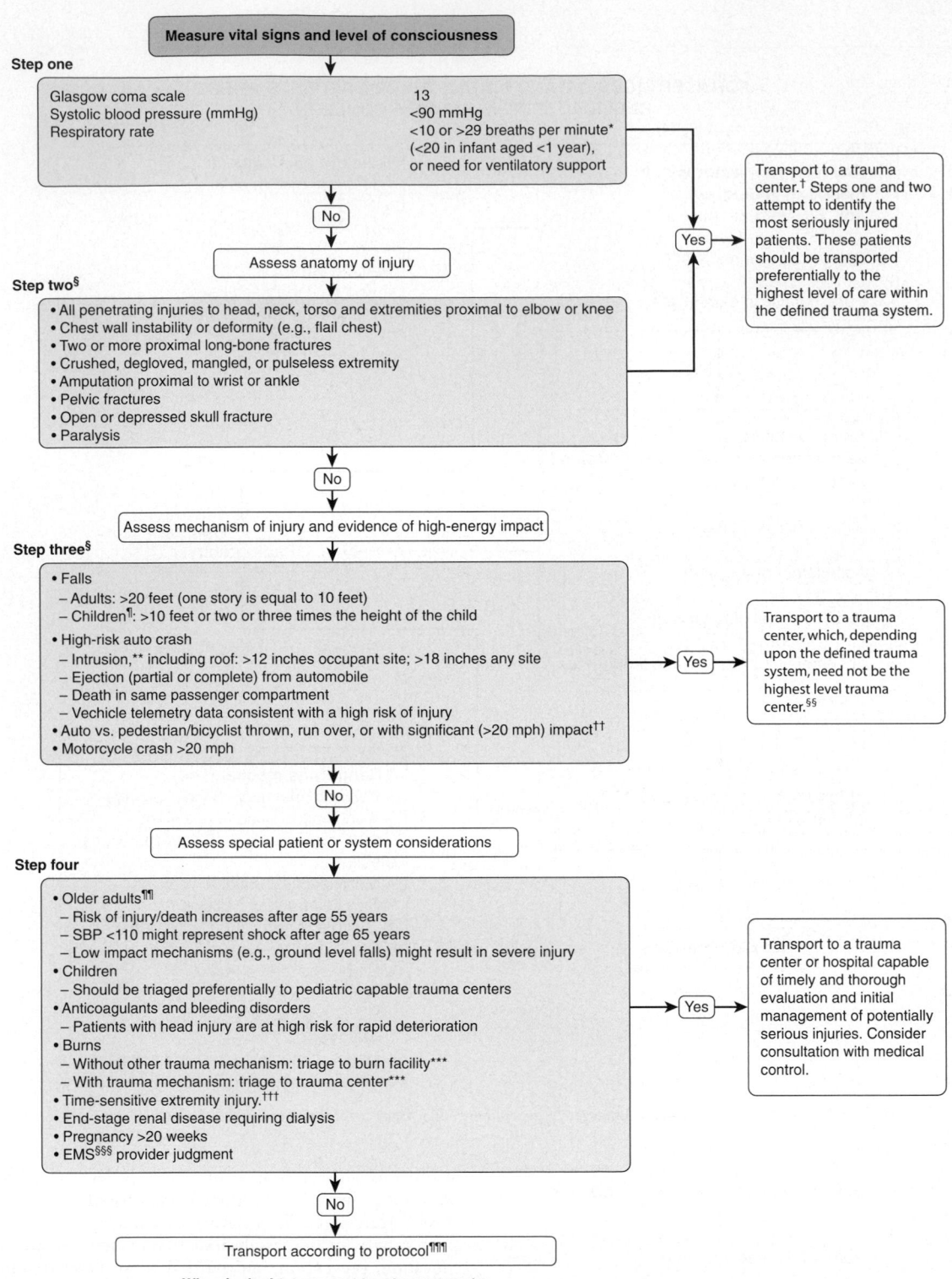

Step one

Measure vital signs and level of consciousness	

Glasgow coma scale	13
Systolic blood pressure (mmHg)	<90 mmHg
Respiratory rate	<10 or >29 breaths per minute* (<20 in infant aged <1 year), or need for ventilatory support

Transport to a trauma center.† Steps one and two attempt to identify the most seriously injured patients. These patients should be transported preferentially to the highest level of care within the defined trauma system.

Step two§

Assess anatomy of injury

- All penetrating injuries to head, neck, torso and extremities proximal to elbow or knee
- Chest wall instability or deformity (e.g., flail chest)
- Two or more proximal long-bone fractures
- Crushed, degloved, mangled, or pulseless extremity
- Amputation proximal to wrist or ankle
- Pelvic fractures
- Open or depressed skull fracture
- Paralysis

Step three§

Assess mechanism of injury and evidence of high-energy impact

- Falls
  - Adults: >20 feet (one story is equal to 10 feet)
  - Children¶: >10 feet or two or three times the height of the child
- High-risk auto crash
  - Intrusion,** including roof: >12 inches occupant site; >18 inches any site
  - Ejection (partial or complete) from automobile
  - Death in same passenger compartment
  - Vechicle telemetry data consistent with a high risk of injury
- Auto vs. pedestrian/bicyclist thrown, run over, or with significant (>20 mph) impact††
- Motorcycle crash >20 mph

Transport to a trauma center, which, depending upon the defined trauma system, need not be the highest level trauma center.§§

Step four

Assess special patient or system considerations

- Older adults¶¶
  - Risk of injury/death increases after age 55 years
  - SBP <110 might represent shock after age 65 years
  - Low impact mechanisms (e.g., ground level falls) might result in severe injury
- Children
  - Should be triaged preferentially to pediatric capable trauma centers
- Anticoagulants and bleeding disorders
  - Patients with head injury are at high risk for rapid deterioration
- Burns
  - Without other trauma mechanism: triage to burn facility***
  - With trauma mechanism: triage to trauma center***
- Time-sensitive extremity injury.†††
- End-stage renal disease requiring dialysis
- Pregnancy >20 weeks
- EMS§§§ provider judgment

Transport to a trauma center or hospital capable of timely and thorough evaluation and initial management of potentially serious injuries. Consider consultation with medical control.

Transport according to protocol¶¶¶¶

When in doubt, transport to a trauma center

Source: Adapted from American College of Surgeons. Resources for the optimal care of the injured patient. Chicago, IL: American College of Surgeons; 2006. Footnotes have been added to enhance understanding of field triage by persons outside the acute injury care field.
* The upper limit of respiratory rate in infants is >29 breaths per minute to maintain a higher level of overtriage for infants.
† Trauma centers are designated Level I–IV, with Level I representing the highest level of trauma care available.
§ Any injury noted in Steps Two and Three triggers a "yes" response.
¶ Age < 15 years.
** Intrusion refers to interior compartment intrusion, as opposed to deformation, which refers to exterior damage.
†† Includes pedestrians or bicyclists thrown or run over by a motor vehicle or those with estimated impact >20 mph with a motor vehicle.
§§ Local or regional protocols should be used to determine the most appropriate level of trauma center; appropriate center need not be Level I.
¶¶ Age >55 years.
*** Patients with both burns and concomitant trauma for whom the burn injury poses the greatest risk for morbidity and mortality should be transferred to a burn center. If the nonburn trauma presents a greater immediate risk, the patient may be stabilized in a trauma center and then transferred to a burn center.
††† Injuries such as an open fracture or fracture with neurovascular compromise.
§§§ Emergency medical services.
¶¶¶¶ Patients who do not meet any of the triage criteria in Steps One through Four should be transported to the most appropriate medical facility as outlined in local EMS protocols.

FIGURE 2 Centers for Disease Control and Prevention Guidelines for Field Triage of Injured Patients. *EMS,* Emergency medical services; *mph,* miles per hour; *SBP,* systolic blood pressure. *(From Sasser SM, Hunt RC, Faul M, et al. Guidelines for field triage of injured patients: recommendations of the National Expert Panel on Field Triage, 2011. MMWR Recomm Rep. 2012;61:1-20.)*

Prehospital triage situations can be divided into field triage and mass casualty. As per the Centers for Disease Control and Prevention (CDC) Guidelines for Field Triage of Injured Patients, a step-by-step algorithm is critical to filtering patients into appropriate avenues of treatment (Figure 2). When measuring vitals and assessing GCS, patients with a SBP of less than 90 mm Hg, a respiratory rate (RR) of less than 10 or greater than 29 (less than 20 in infants younger than 1 year of age), the need for ventilator support, or a GCS of less than 14 should be transported preferentially to the highest level of care available within the defined trauma system.

Similarly, EMS personnel assess anatomy and location of injury as well as mechanism and evidence of high impact. Specific injury patterns require evaluation in a level I trauma center or at an institution with the most advanced care within that trauma system. The particular injuries of concern include penetrating trauma to the head, neck, torso, and extremities proximal to the elbows and knees; flail chest; two or more proximal long bone fractures; crushed, degloved, or mangled extremities; amputations proximal to the wrist or ankle; pelvic fractures; open or depressed skull fractures; and paralysis.

Depending on the particular trauma system, if the patient does not have the aforementioned clinical signs or anatomic indications, he or she does not necessarily need to be transported to the highest level of care. Indications for transfer to at least a lower-level trauma center include high-impact mechanisms such as falls greater than 20 feet (2 stories) in adults or greater than 10 feet in children; intrusion greater than 12 inches in the occupant site or greater than 18 inches in any site; ejection from a vehicle; death in a compartment; speed greater than 20 miles per hour or patient thrown or run over in an automobile versus pedestrian or bicycle collision; and motorcycle collision at a speed greater than 20 miles per hour. Decisions about transport to a trauma center or hospital capable of trauma management also should consider comorbidities; age, particularly older adults and children; burns; pregnancy greater than 20 weeks; premorbid conditions such as congestive heart failure and end-stage renal disease; and patient being on anticoagulation, or be based on EMS judgment.

Type of transportation to definitive care (ground vs air) must take into consideration multiple factors, such as the patient's clinical condition, weather conditions, weight of patient and necessary equipment, location of helipads, distance to most appropriate level of care, and local emergency needs if EMS must travel far.

In mass casualty triage, principles focus on frequent evaluation of resources, with tiered appropriation of those resources. Critically ill patients are transported to definitive treatment first. One mechanism used to rapidly triage mass casualty victims is the Simple Triage and Rapid Treatment (START) method. Through this process, health professionals assess patients and assign them to triage categories with a color-coding scheme corresponding to triage tags that can be used to designate status. The walking wounded (green) have minor traumas and are ambulatory patients who can be removed from the scene. If they require care, it can be delayed for approximately 3 hours. Delayed (yellow) and immediate (red) victims are nonambulatory patients who require medical attention, with immediate patients having at least one derangement in respiration, perfusion, or mental status that requires emergent care. Therapy can be postponed for approximately 1 hour in delayed patients. Expectant (black) victims are considered deceased after one attempt to open or reposition the airway demonstrates no respirations. Comfortable, compassionate care also should be administered to these patients; the designation of expectant does not signify that no further interventions should be made.

HOSPITAL RESPONSE TO TRIAGED PATIENTS

Once the trauma center receives the field EMS call activation, the ED physician determines whether the activation is warranted. To define the extent of the ED response and determine which resources should be apportioned, similar guidelines to those in CDC triage decision scheme are followed, with health care personnel weighing physiologic and anatomic parameters. Mechanism of injury is also taken into account but is less significant. No standard criteria exist for hospital activation response, and different institutions use distinct processes. Some trauma centers use an "all or none" approach, whereas others divide patients into two or three categories by number or color scheme to classify patients as critical, less severely injured but with potential to decompensate, and minimally wounded. In patients with grave injuries, a full response from the hospital occurs with mobilization of the ED and trauma surgeons, residents, or fellows; nursing staff; respiratory therapy; the blood bank; radiology; and anesthesia made available. Partial responses require the ED attending physician, surgical residents, nursing staff, and radiology. Having a structured and controlled response system in place with predetermined trauma team activation has been shown to decrease mortality and time for resuscitation, for transport to CT scan and operating room, and to ED discharge.

LESSONS FROM THE MILITARY

Many practices in prehospital civilian resuscitation and care have been extrapolated from or reinforced by military practice, including guidelines for use of tourniquets and needle chest decompression, the practice of interosseous access, incorporation of methods for preventing hypothermia, use of TXA, and application of coagulating agents such as granular agents and hemostatic dressings. Some of these techniques were described earlier. The use of field ambulances traces back to the combat "flying ambulances" used by Dominique Jean Larrey, Napolean Bonaparte's chief physician, and helicopter transport of patients was initiated during the Korean and Vietnam wars. Resuscitation guidelines have been influenced strongly by combat trauma data, including hypotensive resuscitation to SBP of 80 to 90 mm Hg and massive transfusion protocols. The contributions from the military to this field undoubtedly will continue.

SUGGESTED READINGS

Beekley AC, Sebesta JA, Blackbourne LH, et al. Prehospital tourniquet use in Operation Iraqi Freedom: effect on hemorrhage control and outcomes. *J Trauma.* 2008;64:S28-S37.

Bickell WH, Wall MJ Jr, Pepe PE, et al. Immediate versus delayed fluid resuscitation for hypotensive patients with penetrating torso injuries. *N Engl J Med.* 1994;331:1105-1109.

Borgman MA, Spinella PC, Perkins JG, et al. The ratio of blood products transfused affects mortality in patients receiving massive transfusions at a combat support hospital. *J Trauma.* 2007;63:805-813.

Davis DP, Peay J, Sise MJ, et al. The impact of prehospital endotracheal intubation on outcome in moderate to severe traumatic brain injury. *J Trauma.* 2005;58:933-939.

Holcomb JB, Tilley BC, Baraniuk S, et al. Transfusion of plasma, platelets, and red blood cells in a 1:1:1 vs a 1:1:2 ratio and mortality in patients with severe trauma: the PROPPR randomized clinical trial. *JAMA.* 2015;313:471-482.

Morrison JJ, Dubose JJ, Rasmussen TE, Midwinter MJ. Military Application of Tranexamic Acid in Trauma Emergency Resuscitation (MATTERs) study. *Arch Surg.* 2012;147:113-119.

Sasser SM, Hunt RC, Faul M, et al. Guidelines for field triage of injured patients: recommendations of the National Expert Panel on Field Triage, 2011. *MMWR Recomm Rep.* 2012;61:1-20.

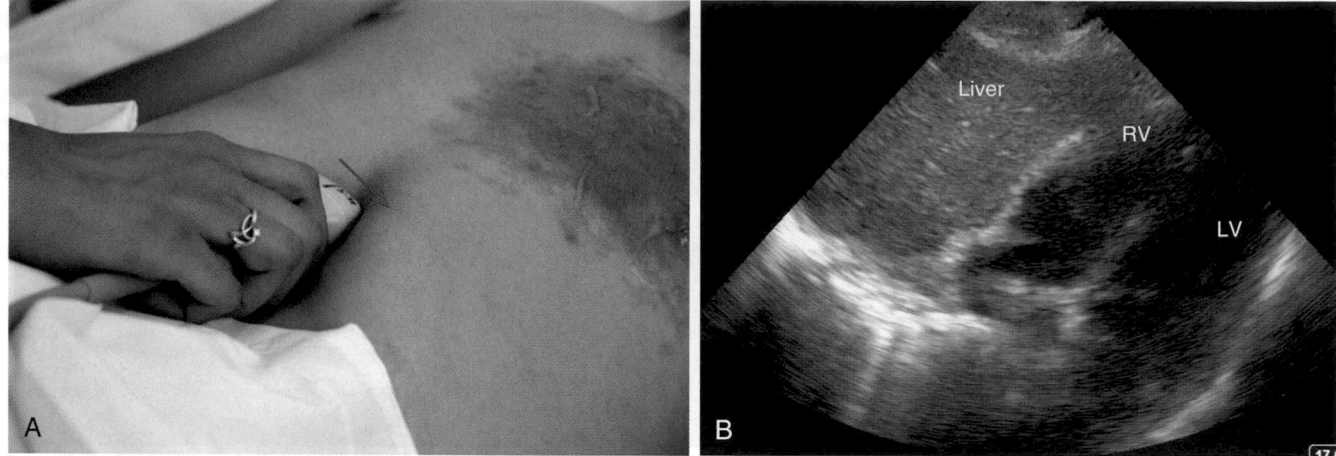

FIGURE 5 A, Probe position on the patient to obtain a subxyphoid window. Note the horizontal position of the probe. **B,** Actual SX image. *LV,* Left ventricle; *RV,* right ventricle.

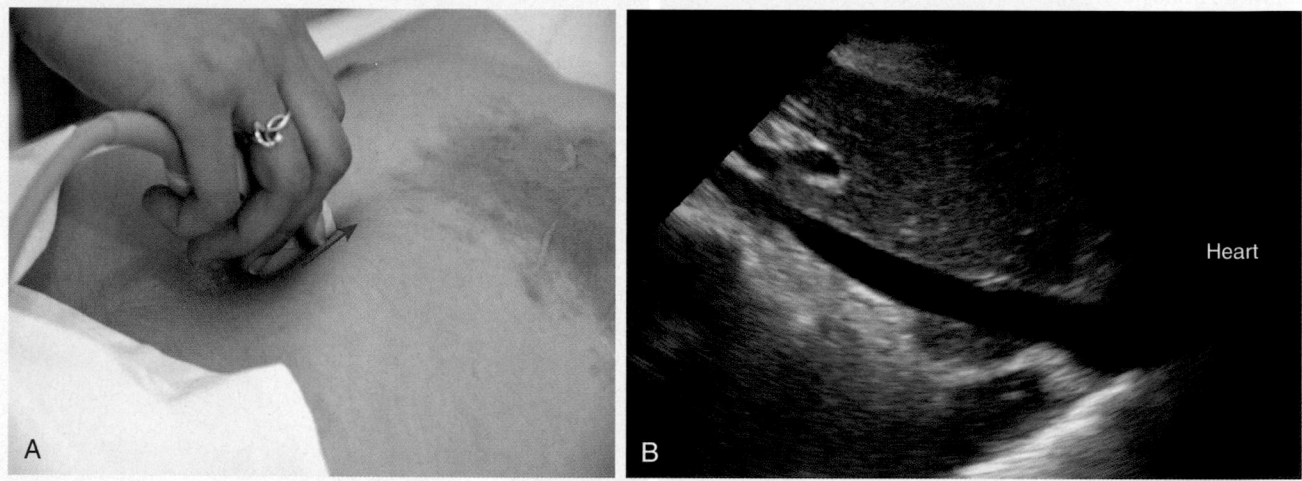

FIGURE 6 A, Probe position on the patient to obtain a longitudinal view of the inferior vena cava. The cursor is pointing up. **B,** Actual SX image.

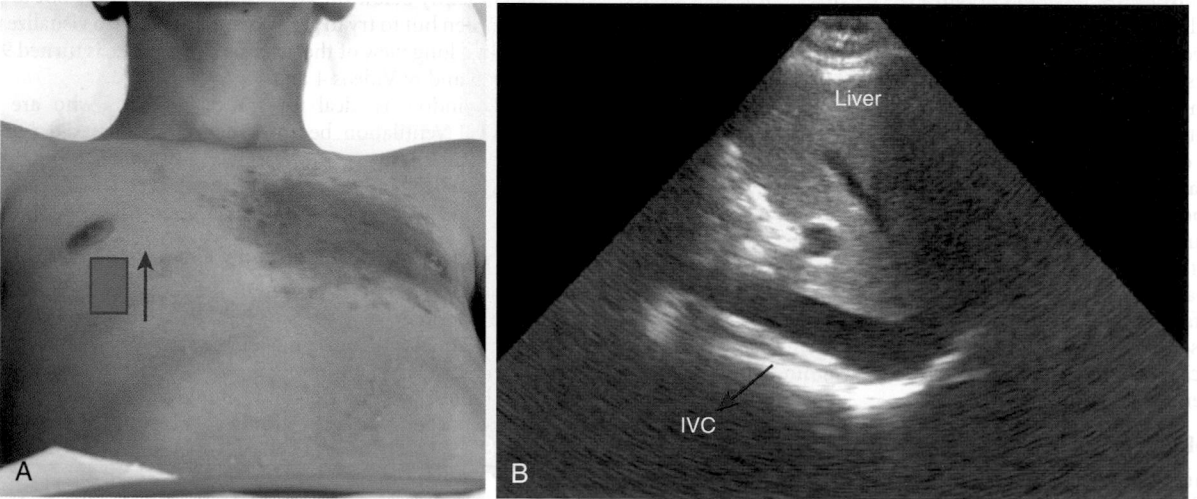

FIGURE 7 A, Probe position on the patient below the nipple. The cursor is pointing up. **B,** The view of the inferior vena cava (IVC) at this position.

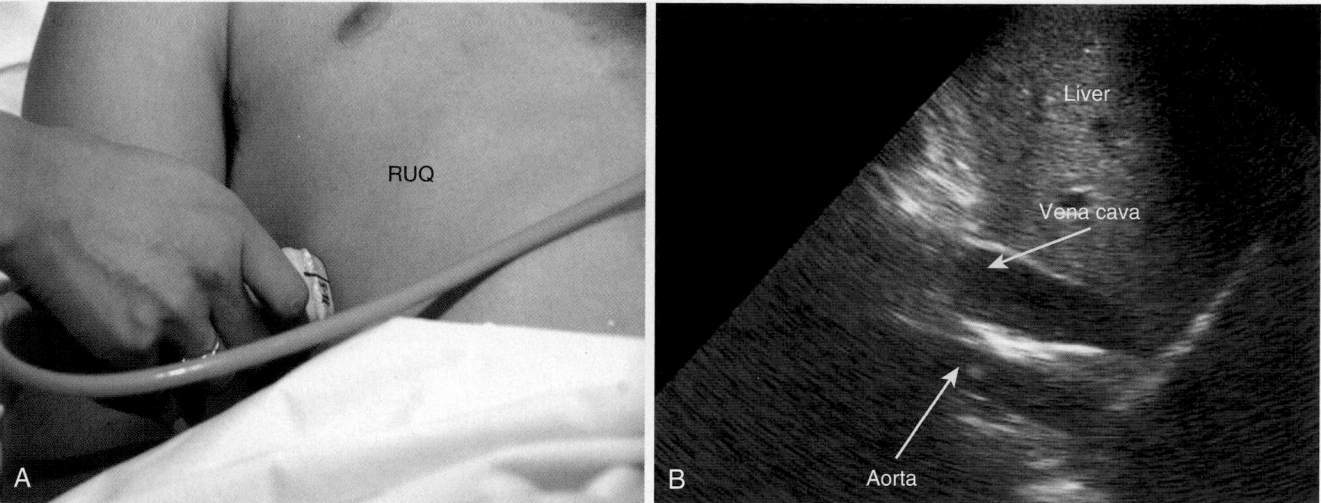

FIGURE 8 A, Probe position on the patient's right middle axillary line to visualize the inferior vena cava posteriorly. **B,** Actual image. *RUQ,* Right upper quadrant.

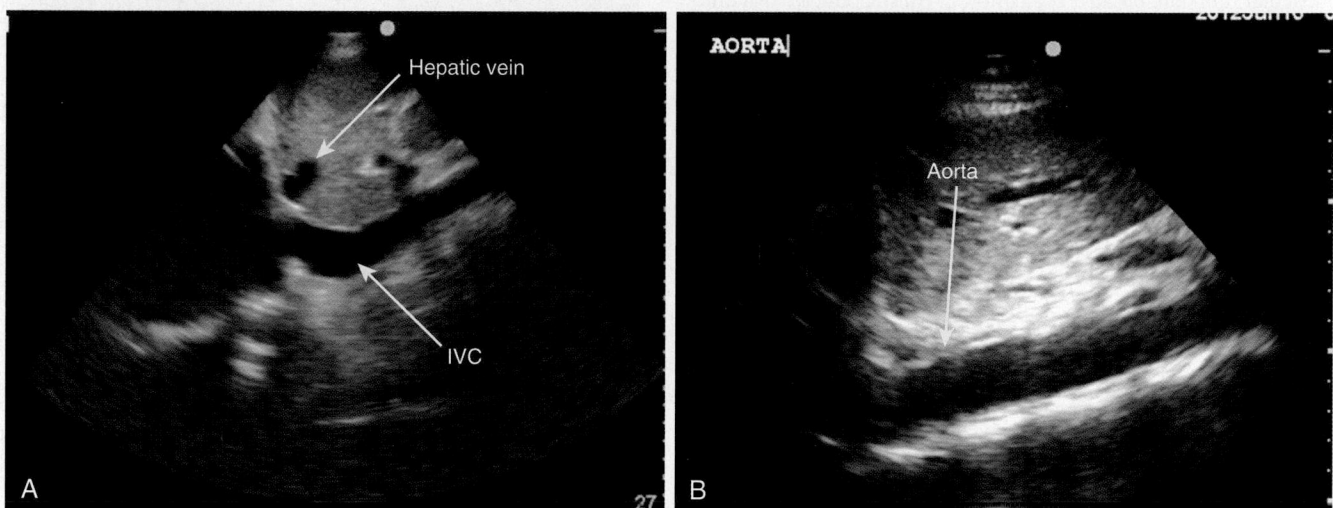

FIGURE 9 A, The inferior vena cava (IVC) looks darker and has the hepatic veins feeding into it apart to have phasic flow. **B,** This view shows the aorta more posterior, lack of hepatic veins feeding into it, as well as pulsatile flow.

IVC as well as the phasic pulsations of the IVC versus the arterial pulsatile rhythm of the aorta (Figure 9).

The Meaning of the Inferior Vena Cava

The vena cava is meaningful clinically when it is very large or completely empty. For these obvious states, measuring with numbers and calculations is unnecessary. An educated visual gestalt can differentiate between a full IVC and an empty IVC.

Mechanical ventilation increases the size of the vena cava because of the increased intrathoracic pressure. However, if a patient is ventilated and has an empty vena cava, the patient is hypovolemic until proven otherwise. In patients who are breathing spontaneously, it is important to address vena cava size in the clinical context as well as to compare the findings with the left ventricular filling. A large IVC in patients who are breathing spontaneously, however, means that the patient is not fluid responsive (Figure 10; Videos 6 and 7).

Interpreting Images

The goal of obtaining the various images through echocardiogram is to identify causes of hypotension. Volume status, pericardial effusion, and cardiac function should be identified.

Hypovolemia

In patients with hypovolemia, the vena cava will be thin and compressed. The left ventricle will be empty and hyperdynamic (the ventricle is closing nearly 100%, with almost no blood at the end of systole and little volume at the end of diastole). Video 8 shows a very large pericardial effusion on a heart that is empty and hypovolemic. As a result, the patient will be fluid responsive as well as in need of treatment for the cause of the effusion, in this case a right ventricular injury.

Contractility

Ejection fraction (EF) refers to the percentage of blood ejected from the left ventricle in systole and the amount left over inside the ventricle in diastole. EF can be measured in three ways: M-mode, Simpson's method, and visual gestalt method (by eye). There is plenty of literature indicating that the visual gestalt method is as accurate as any other measurements.

Measuring EF by the visual gestalt method is done by looking at the overall size and contractility and the inward movement and thickening of the various segments of the left ventricular wall, without having to take complicated measures. Although the accuracy of this method depends on the experience of the operator, it has been shown

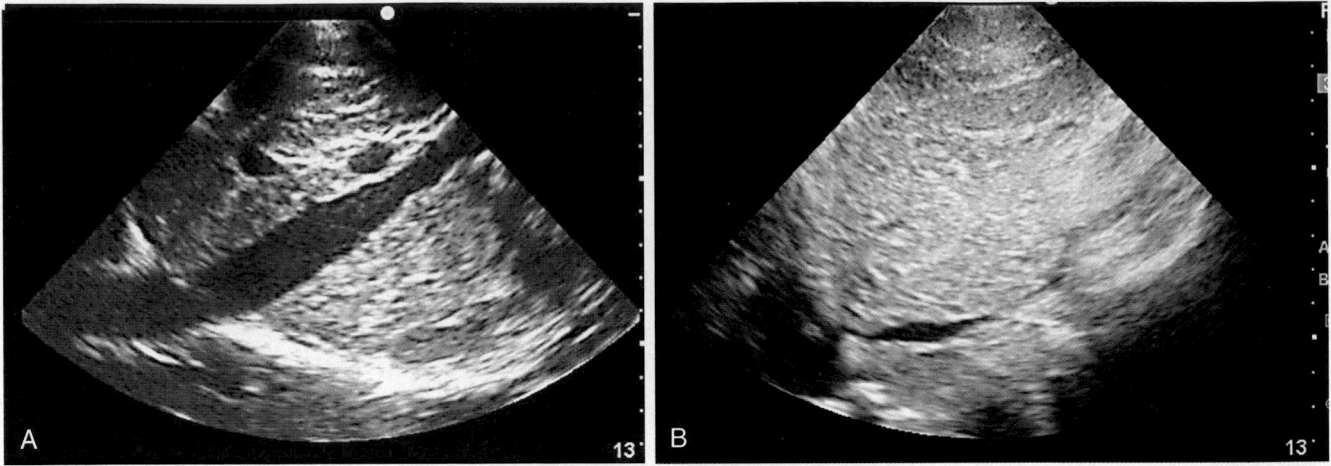

FIGURE 10 **A,** Large, full vena cava. **B,** Very thin, empty vena cava. Both images are a longitudinal view at the subxyphoid window level.

to have excellent correlation with the angiographic evaluation of ventricular function. Because evaluation of contractility is a dynamic process, it is better elucidated in Video 9, which shows a PSS window with very poor contractility. Note the minimal movement of the ventricular walls in the video.

The Heart Has Two Sides

In normal subjects, the right ventricle is about 60% of the size of the left ventricle. It is triangular in shape and has a rough inside surface on echocardiogram. The left ventricle is smoother and rounder, and in normal subjects it is larger. In patients with hypotension and a larger than usual right ventricle, right ventricular failure should be suspected. Video 10 demonstrates a very large right ventricle and right atria with a clot inside the cavity. This patient had an acute pulmonary embolism.

Pericardial Effusion

A small pericardial effusion that can be insignificant to a cardiologist is a diagnosis that means the difference between life and death in the trauma patient, especially in patients with thoracic penetrating trauma. Cardiac tamponade should be diagnosed clinically and not be a radiologic finding. However, on echocardiogram, tamponade will be seen as compression of the right atrium by a pericardial effusion.

In the limited echocardiogram, the only requirement is to evaluate the presence or absence of a pericardial effusion. Because the operator is also the clinician evaluating the patient, the clinical correlation is immediate.

It is important to differentiate between a pleural effusion and a pericardial effusion. With a pleural effusion, the aorta is bathed in this fluid; with a pericardial effusion, the pericardium separates the aorta from the fluid around the heart (Figure 11).

■ USING ULTRASOUND DURING CARDIOPULMONARY RESUSCITATION

Relying on a pulse examination to reflect cardiac activity has several limitations because the absence of a palpable pulse does not always reflect a lack of cardiac activity. The perceived "lack of pulse" caused by inefficient cardiac contractions can be the result of reversible conditions such as cardiac tamponade, pulmonary embolism, and pneumothorax. Cardiac sonography has been used successfully to evaluate patients with traumatic and nontraumatic cardiac arrest in the emergency department and prehospital arena. Lack of cardiac activity, known as "standstill heart," is associated with 100% mortality. Cardiac ultrasound can be used as a triage tool for more invasive procedures in patients with ongoing cardiopulmonary resuscitation.

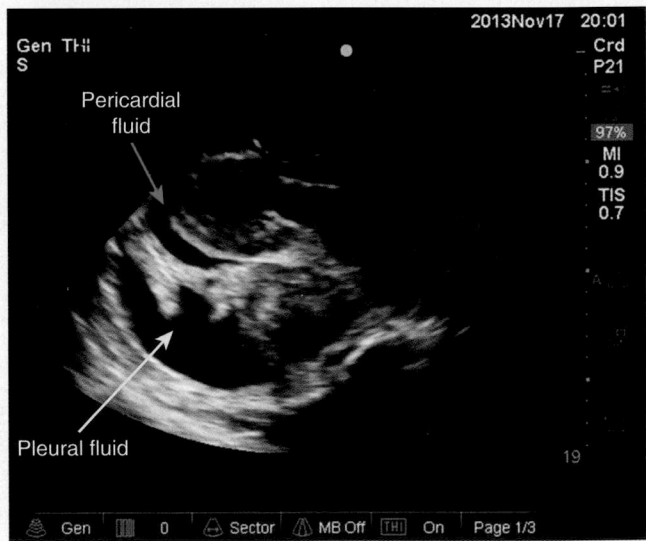

FIGURE 11 The image shows the difference between pleural effusion and pericardial effusion.

Video 11 demonstrates a standstill heart. Note that there is no movement of the ventricular walls.

■ SUMMARY AND RECOMMENDATIONS

Ultrasound is a valuable tool to guide therapy, and its applications can be extended from obtaining anatomic information to achieving a visual understanding of the patient's physiology. Many forms of focused or limited echocardiogram have been validated by noncardiologists in the past decade. Surgeons, especially those treating critically ill trauma patients, can learn and perform this test just as well as any other expert provider. When using this tool to assist with making important medical decisions, it is important to save videos and provide quality improvement to obtaining and interpreting images. Further studies regarding the sensitivity and specificity of using ultrasound to diagnose noncompressible bleeding are ongoing as a multicentric project funded by the Department of Defense (www.clinicaltrials.gov, identifier: NCT01989273).

Image-based resuscitation with ultrasound can be performed in the emergency department, operating room, or intensive care unit, or wherever the patient in need resides. In underserved areas of the world, ultrasound may be the only choice for interrogating fluid status, cardiac function, pneumothorax, and intra-abdominal or intrathoracic bleeding.

It is of critical importance that surgeons, especially those of us who are also critical care physicians, stay in the vanguard of learning, using, and teaching this technique because our patients can benefit from informed decisions.

The subxyphoid window can provide a complete visualization of all cardiac structures, allowing for an assessment of volume by visualizing the ventricles and vena cava as well as right and left ventricular function. This window is already obtained during the eFAST examination. All that is required to incorporate a hemodynamic monitoring tool in the already widely performed test is the addition of the physiologic interpretation.

SUGGESTED READINGS

Alrajhi K, Woo MY, Vaillancourt C. Test characteristics of ultrasonography for the detection of pneumothorax: a systematic review and meta-analysis. *Chest.* 2012;141:703-708.

Cotton BA, Guy JS, Morris JA Jr, Abumrad NN. The cellular, metabolic, and systemic consequences of aggressive fluid resuscitation strategies. *Shock.* 2006;26:115-121.

Ferrada P, Anand RJ, Whelan J, Aboutanos MA, Duanc T, Malhotra A, et al. Limited transthoracic echocardiogram: so easy any trauma attending can do it. *J Trauma.* 2011;71:1327-1331.

Ferrada P, Evans D, Wolfe L, Anand RJ, Vanguri P, Mayglothling J, et al. Findings of a randomized controlled trial using limited transthoracic echocardiogram (LTTE) as a hemodynamic monitoring tool in the trauma bay. *J Trauma Acute Care Surg.* 2014;76:31-37.

Ferrada P, Vanguri P, Anand RJ, Whelan J, Duane T, Aboutanos M, et al. A, B, C, D, echo: limited transthoracic echocardiogram is a useful tool to guide therapy for hypotension in the trauma bay—a pilot study. *J Trauma Acute Care Surg.* 2013;74:220-223.

Rozycki GS, Ballard RB, Feliciano DV, Schmidt JA, Pennington SD. Surgeon-performed ultrasound for the assessment of truncal injuries: lessons learned from 1540 patients. *Ann Surg.* 1998;228:557-567.

Via G, Hussain A, Wells M, Reardon R, ElBarbary M, Noble VE, et al. International evidence-based recommendations for focused cardiac ultrasound. *J Am Soc Echocardiogr.* 2014;27:683.

Volpicelli G, ElBarbary M, Blaivas M, Lichtenstein DA, Mathis G, Kirkpatrick AW, et al. International evidence-based recommendations for point-of-care lung ultrasound. *Intensive Care Med.* 2012;38:577-591.

EMERGENCY DEPARTMENT THORACOTOMY

Jay Menaker, MD, and Thomas M. Scalea, MD, FACS, MCCM

Emergency department (ED) thoracotomy is among the most dramatic procedures performed in surgery. It has the potential to be lifesaving but must be done correctly if it is to be useful. ED thoracotomy has the advantage of being relatively rapid, and it can be performed in the ED immediately after patient arrival. It requires relatively simple instrumentation. Conceptually, it is a simple procedure, and a myriad of healthcare providers can be trained to perform it.

However, ED thoracotomy is not as easy or rapid as many people think. It is a maximally invasive procedure and can cause significant morbidity or mortality if done incorrectly. Opening the chest creates another wound and patients rapidly lose blood and heat from the open thorax. The chaos that often accompanies ED thoracotomy risks direct injury to healthcare practitioners or contamination from blood that is spattered during the procedure. During a poorly performed ED thoracotomy, iatrogenic injury can occur to the intercostal vessels, heart, or even the left lung. These iatrogenic injuries then require their own repair. Despite the potential downside, the powerful emotion that makes physicians believe that they can rescue a single individual continues to make ED thoracotomy attractive. Most physicians find it difficult not to offer every effort to save a patient's life.

A number of guidelines have been published to ensure that ED thoracotomy is used correctly. However, all of these guidelines suffer from retrospective analysis of their data. None of them is truly evidence based. Clearly, a randomized prospective trial would be almost impossible to perform. However, there is substantial literature to help clinicians use this technique wisely.

ED thoracotomy is most effective when it is used to repair injuries of the heart. The heart can be accessed immediately via ED thoracotomy and repaired directly. The perfect patient for ED thoracotomy is one with recordable vital signs and a single anterior thoracic stab wound who has sustained a single chamber cardiac injury with pericardial tamponade. Such a patient who loses vital signs in front of the ED staff has lost little blood and can have a survival rate that approaches 50%. Major hemorrhage from the lung also can be temporized relatively easily and quickly via ED thoracotomy. The less likely it is that a central thoracic vascular injury exists, the less compelling the indication for ED thoracotomy is.

Virtually all of the literature defines mechanism of injury, location of injury, presence of vital signs, and signs of life as important guidelines when deciding whether it is wise to perform an ED thoracotomy. Signs of life generally are defined as electrical cardiac activity, respiratory effort, or pupillary response. Patients with cardiac injuries fare better than do patients with noncardiac injuries. Patients with penetrating trauma do better than those with blunt trauma. Stab wounds have a higher survival rate than do gunshot wounds. Patients who are seen in the ED do better if they have recordable vital signs. Finally, patients with signs of life do better than those without signs of life. Relative to the patient with a single chamber cardiac injury, a patient who has a cardiac arrest from blunt trauma without any signs of life in the field has essentially no chance of survival.

Thus most healthcare providers believe that patients with penetrating thoracic injury and some signs of life in the field are good candidates for ED thoracotomy if they did not respond to resuscitation immediately. Relative indications include patients with penetrating abdominal injury with at least signs of life in the field or patients with blunt trauma who lose signs of life in the hospital or immediately before arrival at the hospital. In the era of rapid bedside ultrasound evaluation, pericardial ultrasound can be helpful in identifying patients who have hemopericardium and those who at least have some mechanical cardiac activity.

ED thoracotomy has been described in patients with extrathoracic injury such as penetrating abdominal trauma. Theoretically, ED thoracotomy achieves inflow vascular control and stops ongoing hemorrhage in patients who are bleeding in the abdomen. Survival has been reported to be as high as 4.5%. However, it is difficult to clearly define the role for ED thoracotomy in such patients. In patients with recordable vital signs, it is hard to justify opening the chest in the ED. Those patients likely are better served with emergent laparotomy in the operating room. In patients without vital signs, it may be possible to restart cardiac activity. However, even in the best centers, transport from the ED to the operating room takes at least 15 minutes. Performing a laparotomy and gaining control of hemorrhage requires an additional 15 to 20 minutes even in the most skilled hands. Thus all such patients will have the aortic clamp in place for

Cardiac Massage

Bimanual internal cardiac massage should begin immediately if there is true cardiac arrest. The preferred method is a hinged clapping motion with the wrists apposed and ventricular compression proceeding from the apex to the base of the heart. This is best accomplished by cupping the left hand and placing it over the right ventricle. The fingers of the right hand are held tightly together to form a flat surface supporting the left ventricle (Figure 7). The right hand compresses the flat surface against the cupped surface supported by the left hand.

Controlling Noncardiac Hemorrhage

Occasionally one encounters a massive hemothorax of noncardiac origin at the time of ED thoracotomy. The chest should be evacuated, and an immediate search for the source of the hemorrhage should be undertaken. Temporary hemorrhage control is essential. If this is from a mediastinal great vessel such as the subclavian or nominate,

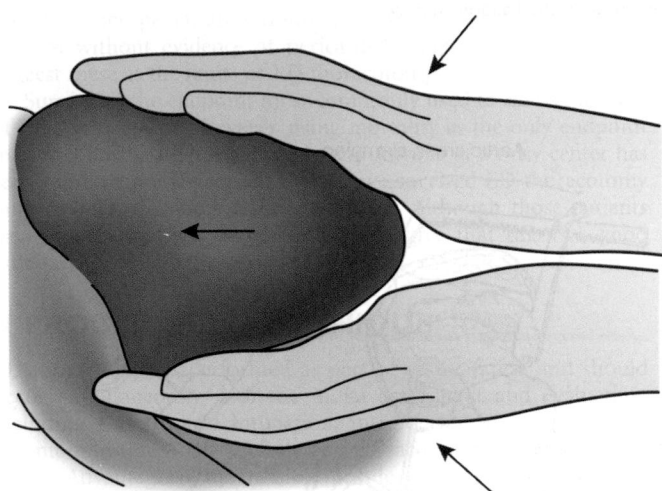

FIGURE 7 Bimanual cardiac massage. The two-handed technique provides better cardiac output and is the preferred method. The palmar surfaces of the fingers act in a clapping motion to compress the heart from the apex toward the aortic root. Fingertip pressure should be avoided at all times.

repair in the ED is almost impossible. Direct pressure, resuscitation, and transport to the operating room is the only rational course. Occasionally a very proximal aortic injury can be controlled digitally and at least temporarily repaired in the ED.

Pulmonary hemorrhage represents another potential source of bleeding. Occasionally bleeding from the lung can be controlled with either a Duval clamp or a vascular clamp. Attempts to dissect the lung out, identify injuries deep in the lung parenchyma, and perform definitive hemostasis in the ED may be dangerous.

If simple clamping does not achieve hemostasis, several other methods are available. Occluding flow of the pulmonary hilum has the advantage of achieving complete inflow control. This can be accomplished by mobilizing the inferior pulmonary ligament and simply twisting the lung on the hilum (Figure 8). This occludes blood flow and also eliminates aeration of the lung. Another method is to simply place a vascular clamp across the hilum. One should avoid dissecting the hilum structures, as this risks inadvertent injury to the bronchus or other adjacent structures. The final possibility is to pass an umbilical tape around the hilum and occlude the hilum with it.

Hilar control can provide immediate hemostasis for major hemorrhage from the lung. Unfortunately, this maneuver radically increases pulmonary vascular resistance and may produce profound right ventricular failure. This often produces significant hypotension, often leading to cardiac arrest. However, this is an important maneuver to remember if other methods fail.

■ THE FUTURE

Resuscitative endovascular balloon occlusion of the aorta (REBOA) has come back into clinical practice recently. First described in 1954, the lack of sophistication of its technology limited its use initially. Greater sophistication in the instrumentation has allowed it to become much more commonly used. REBOA can be inserted percutaneously or via a femoral artery cut down. A standard femoral arterial line is inserted, and an Amplatz guidewire is placed into the femoral artery catheter. The catheter is removed and a 12F introducer is then placed over the guidewire with the guidewire still in place. A balloon catheter is placed via the introducer and can be inserted into the lower chest to control intra-abdominal bleeding or just above the aortic bifurcation to control pelvic hemorrhage. The balloon is then inflated. Many surgeons inject contrast mixed with saline in the balloon. Balloon position can be documented with fluoroscopy, a standard kidneys, ureters, and bladder x-ray (KUB), computed tomography (CT), or ultrasound.

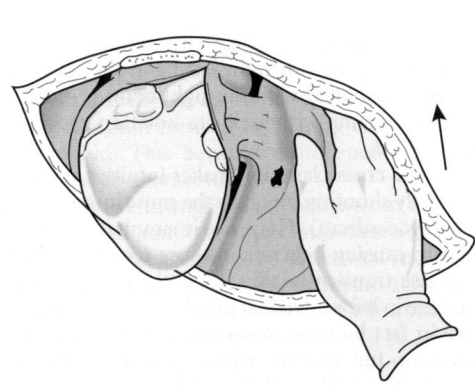
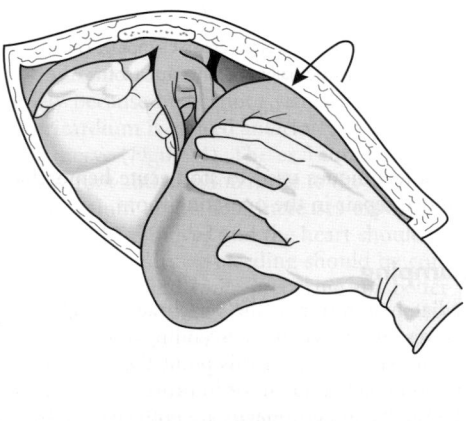

FIGURE 8 Twisting at the hilum. Isolated pulmonary hemorrhage can be controlled with either a Duval clamp or a vascular clamp. If simple clamping does not achieve hemostasis, blood flow may be occluded by twisting the lung on its hilum. This eliminates aeration of the lung as well.

A recent series by Brenner and colleagues has documented REBOA as a clinically useful tool. Several recent series have suggested that the REBOA can be deployed as quickly as aortic control obtained via ED thoracotomy. Although patients who undergo ED thoracotomy may be different than those who undergo balloon occlusion of the aorta, a recent series by Moore and colleagues has suggested that survival is much better in patients undergoing REBOA than in those undergoing ED thoracotomy. In addition, patients who were treated with ED thoracotomy were much more likely to die in the ED and more likely to die as a direct result of hemorrhage. The patients who had a REBOA placed were fundamentally different from those who had ED thoracotomy, raising a note of caution. However, the use of ED thoracotomy simply to obtain inflow control in the abdomen seems to no longer be wise. Such patients likely are much better served by placement of a REBOA.

Another rationale for ED thoracotomy has been the ability to perform open cardiac massage. Those advocating the need the thoracotomy for this indication believe that cardiac output is much better with open cardiac massage than with closed chest massage after cardiac arrest. However, recent data from our institution suggest that closed chest massage is equally efficacious as open cardiac massage. This raises questions about the use of ED thoracotomy in any patient with blunt trauma who does not have major thoracic injury or hemopericardium. In fact, in our institution, ED thoracotomy is now reserved only for patients with penetrating trauma in the central thorax or patients with blunt trauma and either hemopericardium or massive hemothorax on ultrasound. Patients with blunt trauma and cardiac arrest, those with penetrating abdominal trauma in shock, or those who have had cardiac arrest are treated with insertion of the REBOA, attempts at resuscitation, and closed chest cardiac massage.

SUGGESTED READINGS

American College of Surgeons. Thoracic trauma. In: American College of Surgeon Committee on Trauma, ed. *ATLS: Advanced Trauma Life Support for Doctors.* 9th ed. Chicago: American College of Surgeons; 2012.

Bradley M, Bonds B, Chang L, Yang S, Hu P, et al. Open chest cardiac massage offers no benefit over closed chest compressions in patients with traumatic cardiac arrest. *Quick shot presentation at: 29th Annual Eastern Association for the Surgery of Trauma Scientific Assembly;* January 2016; San Antonio, TX.

Brenner ML, Moore LJ, DuBose JJ, Tyson GH, McNutt MK, Albarado RP, Holcomb JB, Scalea TM, Rasmussen TE. A clinical series of resuscitative endovascular balloon occlusion of the aorta for hemorrhage control and resuscitation. *J Trauma Acute Care Surg.* 2013;75:506-511.

Cothren CC, Moore EE. Emergency department thoracotomy. In: Feliciano DV, Mattox KL, Moore EE, eds. *Trauma.* 6th ed. New York: McGraw-Hill; 2008.

Dubose JJ, Scalea TM, Brenner ML, Skiada D, Inaba K, et al. The AAST prospective Aortic Occlusion for Resuscitation in Trauma and Acute Care Surgery (AORTA) Registry: data on contemporary utilization and outcomes of aortic occlusion and resuscitative balloon occlusion of the aorta (REBOA). *Podium presentation at: 74th Annual Meeting of the American Association for the Surgery of Trauma and Clinical Congress of Acute Care Surgery;* September 2015; Las Vegas, NV.

Hughes CW. Use of an intra-aortic balloon catheter tamponade for controlling intra-abdominal hemorrhage in man. *Surgery.* 1954;36:65-68.

Moore EE, Knudson MM, Burlew CC, Inaba K, Dicker RA, Biffl WL, et al. Defining the limits of resuscitative emergency department thoracotomy: a contemporary Western Trauma Association perspective. *J Trauma.* 2011;70:334-339.

Moore LJ, Brenner M, Kozar RA, Pasley J, Wade C, et al. Implementation of resuscitative endovascular balloon occlusion of the aorta (REBOA) as an alternative to resuscitative thoracotomy for non compressible truncal hemorrhage. *Podium presentation at: 73rd Annual Meeting of the American Association for the Surgery of Trauma and Clinical Congress of Acute Care Surgery;* September 2014; Philadelphia, PA.

Powell DW, Moore EE, Cothren CC, Ciesla DJ, Burch JM, Moore JB, et al. Is emergency department resuscitative thoracotomy futile care for the critically injured patient requiring prehospital cardiopulmonary resuscitation? *J Am Coll Surg.* 2004;199:211-215.

Rhee PM, Acosta J, Bridgeman A, Wang D, Jordan M, Rich N. Survival after emergency department thoracotomy: review of published data from the past 25 years. *J Am Coll Surg.* 2000;190:288-298.

Working Group, Ad Hoc Subcommittee on Outcomes, American College of Surgeons, Committee on Trauma. Practice management guidelines for emergency department thoracotomy. *J Am Coll Surg.* 2001;193:303-309.

THE MANAGEMENT OF TRAUMATIC BRAIN INJURY

Carrie Sims, MD, MS, FACS, and Sarah Jean Mathew, MD, BA

When managing traumatic brain injury (TBI), the overarching objective is to preserve brain parenchyma and function by maintaining perfusion and oxygenation. Treatment strategies during the initial evaluation and subsequent medical or surgical management are all designed to meet this goal.

▪ INITIAL EVALUATION AND TREATMENT

Patients with suspected TBI should be evaluated in a standard Advanced Trauma Life Support (ATLS) fashion, with a primary survey focusing on airway, breathing, and circulation. Once stabilized, any patient with suspected TBI should receive a full trauma evaluation looking for concurrent injuries, with a particular focus on sources of hemorrhage that could compromise brain perfusion and oxygenation. Given the high likelihood of concurrent cervical spine injury, stabilization with a collar is imperative until clinical clearance is feasible or high-quality computed tomography (CT) can be performed to rule out bony injury.

Patients with TBI frequently are unable to protect their airway and require urgent intubation. Before they are sedated and paralyzed, however, it is imperative to obtain a history and a baseline neurologic examination. In addition to taking the standard history, the use of antiplatelet or anticoagulant medications should be asked about specifically. In the obtunded patient, this history should be obtained promptly from a family member or emergency medical services (EMS) provider.

A focused neurologic examination including brainstem reflexes, motor function in all extremities, and a Glasgow Coma Score (GCS; Table 1) should be obtained. The GCS is a quick and reproducible assessment of TBI severity with important prognostic implications. The GCS ranges from 3 to 15 and can be divided into mild (13 to 15), moderate (9 to 12), and severe (3 to 8) TBI.

The initial evaluation and stabilization should be performed as expeditiously as possible. Secondary imaging should include an immediate head CT without intravenous (IV) contrast in order to determine whether urgent surgical decompression is needed. The head CT should be evaluated for the presence of intracranial blood, midline shift, mass effect, herniation, and skull fractures. Once the presence of TBI has been established, the neurosurgery department should be consulted immediately. If a neurosurgery department is

TABLE 1: Glasgow Coma Scale

	Point Value
EYE OPENING	
Spontaneous	4
To speech	3
To pain	2
No response	1
MOTOR RESPONSE	
Follows commands	6
Localizes	5
Withdraws	4
Flexor posturing	3
Extensor posturing	2
No response	1
VERBAL RESPONSE	
Oriented	5
Confused conversation	4
Inappropriate words	3
Incomprehensible sounds	2
No response	1

not available, the nearest neurosurgical team should be contacted so that an early transfer can be initiated if needed. Specific criteria for surgical decompression are discussed later.

The initial treatment of patients with TBI should focus on three objectives: (1) minimizing systemic hypotension and hypoxia, (2) assessing and treating herniation, and (3) reversing antiplatelet and anticoagulant medications.

Hypotension and Hypoxia

Hypotension is independently associated with increased morbidity and mortality in patients with TBI. Hypotension is defined as a single systolic blood pressure (SBP) lower than 90 mm Hg in the prehospital or inpatient setting. Recent literature suggests that even a SBP lower than 110 or 120 mm Hg may be associated with worse outcomes. Therefore it is critical to aggressively identify and treat any concomitant traumatic injuries that could be sources of hypotension. It is important to note that patients with a traumatic mechanism serious enough to cause severe TBI often will have multiple other injuries. Interventional radiology and surgery may be required to stabilize the patient and prevent further hypotension. Normal saline is the preferred primary resuscitation fluid because it is hypertonic, thus its use minimizes hypotension while avoiding cerebral edema.

Hypoxia, defined as oxygen saturation lower than 90%, also correlates with poor neurologic function after TBI. Hypoxia is often present in the prehospital setting and during the initial evaluation. Consequently, all patients with TBI should have continuous oxygen saturation monitoring in addition to supplemental oxygen. Persistent hypoxia and a GCS of 8 or less are both indications for intubation.

Preventing Herniation

Patients with TBI may have herniation or develop it during the early stages of their evaluation. Therefore patients should be re-examined frequently after the initial baseline neurologic examination. Clinical signs of elevated intracranial pressure (ICP) include hypertension, bradycardia, and irregular respirations (Cushing's triad). Progression to transtentorial uncal herniation results in loss of consciousness, ipsilateral pupillary dilation, and contralateral hemiparesis. Any patient who develops these signs needs urgent intervention to decrease ICP. Although hyperventilation is no longer used as a long-term treatment strategy, its short-term use is appropriate while waiting for other interventions to take effect in acutely altered or herniating patients. Mannitol or hypertonic saline (HTS) should be administered for more prolonged reduction of ICP. Mannitol dosed at 1 g/kg can reduce ICP within minutes. Peak effect occurs within 15 to 120 minutes and can last up to 6 hours. Mannitol, however, is an osmotic diuretic and can be associated with profound hypotension. In patients with TBI who are hypotensive or potentially bleeding, a bolus of HTS may be a better option for reducing ICP while maintaining intravascular volume. Although recent studies have demonstrated equivalence between mannitol and HTS in terms of ICP management, the concentration and dosing of HTS has not been standardized. Bolus doses of 250 mL of 7.5% HTS, 75 mL of 10% HTS, and 30 mL of 23.4% HTS have all shown similar efficacy at reversing transtentorial herniation. If surgical decompression is indicated, the patient should be transferred expeditiously to the operating room or to an institution with a neurosurgeon.

Antiplatelet and Anticoagulant Reversal

Reversal of anticoagulants or antiplatelet agents is indicated in the setting of intracranial hemorrhage (ICH). In addition to investigating the history of anticoagulant or antiplatelet use, the trauma evaluation should include laboratory assays for prothrombin time (PT), activated partial thromboplastin time (aPTT), and platelet count. If available, thromboelastography (TEG) can be helpful in assessing the presence of newer anticoagulants such as direct thrombin and factor Xa inhibitors. Once ICH is identified on head CT, anticoagulant and antiplatelet agents should be reversed in order to prevent morbidity and mortality resulting from continued bleeding (Table 2).

■ MEDICAL MANAGEMENT

The majority of patients with TBI will be managed medically. Just as in the initial management phase, maintaining perfusion and oxygenation is paramount. In addition, the longer-term management of patients with TBI involves (1) noninvasive and invasive monitoring, (2) management of ICP, and (3) general considerations such as seizure prophylaxis, nutrition, and deep venous thrombosis (DVT) prophylaxis.

Monitoring

All patients with moderate and severe TBI should be admitted to an intensive care unit (ICU) to closely monitor vital signs, with a particular focus on blood pressure, oxygen saturation, and neurologic status. More invasive monitoring such as an arterial or central venous line may be necessary to guide resuscitation and ensure that hemodynamic targets are maintained. Serial neurologic examinations with a GCS and focused physical examinations should be performed hourly in the first 24 to 48 hours. An acute change in the neurologic examination should prompt a repeat immediate head CT to evaluate for bleeding or herniation that would require surgical management.

In addition to hypotension and hypoxia, prolonged elevation of ICP is associated with worsened outcomes. Treatment protocols that incorporate ICP monitoring and management have been shown to improve outcomes. Not all patients with TBI require invasive monitoring of ICP. In general, ICP monitoring should be considered in patients with an abnormal head CT and severe TBI (GCS of 3 to 8) and in those with a normal head CT with hypotension on admission,

TABLE 2: Reversing Anticoagulant and Antiplatelet Agents

Anticoagulant	Mechanism	Urgent Reversal Strategy
VKA (e.g., warfarin)	Epoxide reductase inhibition of thrombin	First line: PCC Second line: FFP
Oral DTI (e.g., dabigatran)	Competitive, reversible direct inhibition of thrombin	First line: PCC including FEIBA, rFVIIa Second line: hemodialysis *Pending: direct inhibitors (e.g., anti-Dabi Fab)*
Direct factor Xa inhibitor (e.g., rivaroxaban)	Competitive, reversible direct inhibition of factor Xa	First line: PCC *Poorly removed by hemodialysis*
LMWH (e.g., enoxaparin)	Potentiation of antithrombin III	First line: protamine (temporary, partial), rFVIIa
Aspirin	Cyclooxygenase-1 inhibition	First line: platelet transfusion Second line: desmopressin
Clopidogrel	Irreversible inhibition of platelet P2Y$_{12}$ ADP receptor	First line: platelet transfusion Second line: desmopressin

From McCoy CC, Lawson JH, Shapiro ML, et al. Management of anticoagulation agents in trauma patients. *Clin Lab Med.* 2014;34:567.

ADP, Adenosine diphosphate; *DTI*, direct thrombin inhibitor; *FEIBA*, factor VIII inhibitor bypassing activity; *FFP*, fresh frozen plasma; *LMWH*, low-molecular-weight heparin; *PCC*, prothrombin complex concentrate; *rFVIIa*, recombinant activated factor VII; *VKA*, vitamin K antagonist.

age older than 40 years, and posturing (decorticate or decerebrate). This decision should be made in consultation with the neurosurgical team assigned to the patient. Monitors can be placed by the neurosurgery team whenever indicated and at the bedside.

Invasive neurologic monitoring can be done in one of several ways: external ventricular drain (EVD), intraparenchymal pressure monitor, and continuous brain tissue oxygen tension (PbO$_2$) monitor. EVDs are placed in one of the lateral ventricles via a burr hole and connected to an external strain gauge. EVDs can be both diagnostic and therapeutic. In addition to measuring ICP, EVDs can be used to drain cerebrospinal fluid (CSF) in order to reduce ICP. However EVDs can be difficult to place and are associated with a rare though increased risk of infection. Intraparenchymal pressure monitors, often called bolts, are easier to place because they do not have to be positioned precisely in a ventricle. Unfortunately, once placed they cannot be recalibrated and they do not allow for CSF drainage. Measurement of PbO$_2$ can be obtained by placing a probe in the penumbra of injured parenchyma to allow for quantification of tissue oxygenation in the part of the brain that is most at risk for secondary injury. In general, it is often used in conjunction with an intraparenchymal monitoring device. Although the evidence for target brain tissue oxygenation is not as strong as targeting ICP, it is recommended that a PbO2 lower than 15 mm Hg be treated by increasing systemic oxygenation.

Once in place, ICP monitors can be used to evaluate both ICP and cerebral blood flow. Although normal ICP varies by age, it is generally lower than 10 mm Hg. ICP that is persistently higher than 20 mm Hg is considered pathologic and requires intervention. ICP also is used to calculate cerebral perfusion pressure (CPP). CPP is an approximate measure of cerebral blood flow and equals mean arterial pressure (MAP) minus ICP. It is recommended that CPP be kept between 50 and 70 mm Hg in adults with TBI. CPP lower than 50 mm Hg is associated with parenchymal ischemia, whereas CPP higher than 70 mm Hg is associated with an increased rate of acute respiratory distress syndrome (ARDS) and no improvement of outcomes.

Management of Intracranial Pressure

There are several treatment strategies to manage elevated ICP: sedation, analgesia, osmotic therapy, and normothermia. Of note, regardless of the intervention, care must be taken to avoid hypotension.

Both pain and agitation can lead to increased ICP and metabolic demand. Patients with TBI are often in pain, disoriented, and agitated. Those who are intubated also may need sedation to prevent self-extubation, resistance to ventilation, and inadvertent removal of invasive monitors or lines. In these patients, short-acting agents such as fentanyl for pain and propofol or midazolam for agitation are preferred to allow for frequent neurologic examinations. Propofol in particular must be used carefully. Although propofol can reduce cerebral metabolism and oxygen consumption, it also can cause hypotension and metabolic acidosis. In general, low-dose continuous infusions should be used instead of boluses to reduce the risk of interval rebound ICP elevation. In the setting of refractory intracranial hypertension, barbiturates such as phenobarbital can be considered. They have been shown to reduce ICP and cerebral metabolism but have not been associated with improved outcomes. The main complication of barbiturates is hypotension, which can lead to significant secondary brain injury. Therefore phenobarbital can be considered, but the patient must be hemodynamically stable and in an ICU setting with continuous monitoring.

Osmotic therapy with either mannitol or HTS can be used for both initial TBI treatment and ongoing ICP management. Repeat boluses of mannitol at 0.25 to 0.5 g/kg can be given acutely for ICP elevation greater than 20 mm Hg. Serum osmolarity should be monitored frequently and kept at less than 320 mOsm. HTS infusions or boluses also can be used to treat elevated ICP with a goal serum sodium of 160 mEq/L or less. The main contraindication for HTS is chronic hyponatremia; patients with chronically low sodium levels are susceptible to central pontine myelinolysis with rapid increases in serum sodium.

In the past, hypothermia of 33°C to 35°C was used in patients with TBI to reduce cerebral metabolism and oxygen requirements. Recent literature, however, has shown that patients who are seen with severe TBI and hypothermia (<35°C) have increased mortality. Moreover, hypothermia itself is associated with significant risks, including coagulopathy, arrhythmias, and shivering with increased ICP. As a result, the treatment paradigm has shifted from induction of hypothermia to maintaining normothermia. Because more than 80% of critically ill patients with TBI will develop fever within the first 72 hours after injury, efforts such as around-the-clock acetaminophen, ibuprofen, cooling blankets, and ice packs should be considered routinely.

When ICP elevation is refractory to medical management, including sedatives, analgesics, and osmotic therapy, a decompressive craniectomy should be considered (discussed later).

General Considerations

Patients with TBI who have ICH, depressed skull fractures, and a GCS below 10 are at risk for developing post-traumatic seizures. Post-traumatic seizures are acutely detrimental because they increase cerebral metabolic demand and may lead to increased ICP. In the long term, post-traumatic seizures may lead to chronic epilepsy. In at-risk patients, anticonvulsants should be used in the first 7 days after injury to prevent early seizures, although such prophylaxis does not change the long-term seizure risk. Although phenytoin (10 to 20 mg/kg IV bolus, 5 mg/kg/day maintenance) has been used historically for prophylaxis, levetiracetam (500 mg IV twice daily) is gaining popularity because of fewer side effects and ease of dosing without the need for monitoring serum levels.

Nutrition is vital in all injured patients but particularly important in patients with TBI. Patients with a GCS of 8 or less demonstrate significant nitrogen wasting and hypermetabolism (120% to 250% basal energy expenditure). Consequently, nutrition should be started as soon as possible after injury. Enteral feeding is preferable to parenteral nutrition, but patients should be at full nutritional support within 7 days of injury regardless.

Prevention of venous thromboembolism is a difficult topic in TBI. Patients with TBI are often at increased risk for DVT and pulmonary embolism (PE) because of recent trauma, prolonged bed rest, and multiple or prolonged surgeries. Although these are patients who would benefit from prophylactic low-molecular-weight heparin, they are also at increased risk for new or continued ICH. At a minimum, mechanical prophylaxis with sequential compression devices, passive range of motion, and early ambulation should be instituted routinely. Although the decision of when to start pharmacologic prophylaxis should be individualized and made in conjunction with the neurosurgery department, there are increasing data to suggest that starting low-molecular-weight heparin 48 hours after injury and after radiographic stability is both safe and effective.

SURGICAL MANAGEMENT

Although most TBIs are managed medically, up to 100,000 patients each year will require surgery. Criteria for operative intervention are subdivided based on the type of lesion. Epidural hematomas, subdural hematomas, and depressed skull fractures often will require emergent surgical evacuation soon after injury. Diffuse cerebral edema, intraparenchymal hematomas, and large contusions may require surgery in a more subacute fashion.

Before taking any patient with severe TBI to the operating room, the patient's age, comorbidities, neurologic status, time since injury, concomitant injuries, and prior stated wishes should be taken into consideration. Similarly, if the patient is considered an operative candidate, the prognosis and expected quality of life should be discussed with the family so they have a clear understanding of the goals and anticipated outcome of surgical management.

Epidural Hematoma

Epidural hematoma (EDH) constitutes 4% of all TBIs and is defined by the presence of blood in the potential space between the skull and the dura. Although EDHs are often arterial injuries in the setting of skull fractures, they can result from venous or sinus injuries. On head CT, EDHs have a biconvex or lens shape created by the blood pushing the dura away from the skull (Figure 1). Because of strong dural attachments at the cranial sutures, EDHs typically do not cross suture lines.

Acute EDH should be evacuated surgically in the setting of a GCS of 8 or less and anisocoria. In addition, any EDH with a volume larger than 30 cm³ should be evacuated surgically. The surgical approach typically involves a craniotomy, clot evacuation, regaining hemostasis, and then tacking the dura to the skull to obliterate the dead space. Because all of the blood is extra-axial and not associated with underlying parenchymal injury, prompt surgical evacuation is associated with excellent outcomes.

EDH may be managed nonoperatively in very select cases and under close observation. Nonoperative management should be considered only in patients without focal neurologic deficits, a GCS

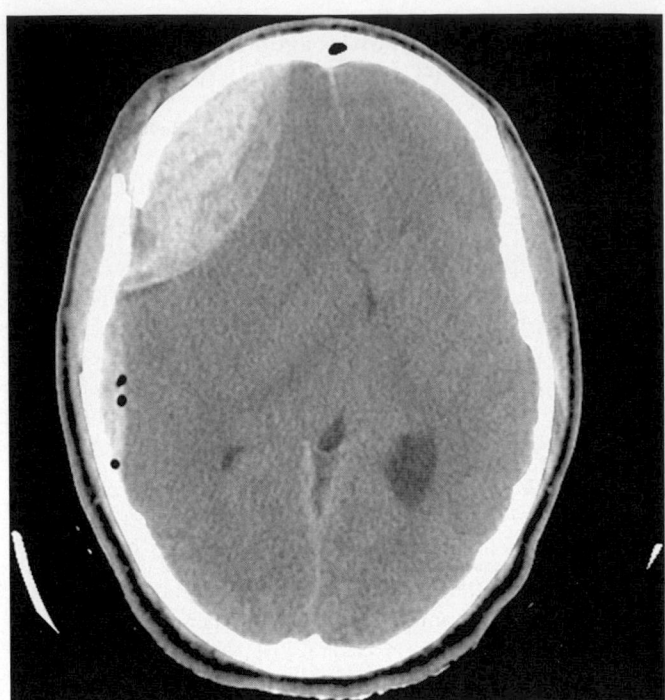

FIGURE 1 Epidural hematoma.

higher than 8, hematoma volume smaller than 30 cm³, hematoma thickness less than 15 mm, and a midline shift less than 5 mm. These patients must be watched closely in an ICU setting with serial neurologic examinations and repeat head CTs as recommended by the neurosurgery department.

Subdural Hematoma

Subdural hematoma (SDH) is found in 10% to 20% of all patients with TBI and is characterized by blood beneath the dura. SDHs usually are caused by bleeding from torn bridging veins in the subdural space and frequently are associated with parenchymal lesions. On head CT, they classically appear as crescent-shaped collections that cross sutures lines and layer along the falx (Figure 2).

An acute SDH should be evacuated, regardless of the patient's GCS, if the hematoma is more than 10 mm thick or if there is midline shift greater than 5 mm. In a patient with a SDH and a GCS of 8 or less, surgical evacuation also should occur if the patient's GCS has dropped by 2 or more points since the time of injury, the patient has anisocoria or fixed pupils, or the ICP is greater than 20 mm Hg. Depending on the size and location of the SDH, there are multiple surgical approaches ranging from craniotomy to hemicraniectomy with or without a dural patch to allow for swelling.

Patients with a GCS of 8 of less who do not meet the criteria for surgery can be managed nonoperatively but must have an ICP monitor, close observation in an ICU setting, and serial head CTs as recommended by the neurosurgery department.

Open and Depressed Skull Fractures

Skull fractures can be classified as open or closed, as well as depressed or nondepressed. All open fractures should receive antibiotics with appropriate gram-negative coverage to prevent meningitis; ceftriaxone and Unasyn are used most commonly. All open fractures with evidence of dural injury (e.g., CSF leakage, visible brain matter), depression greater than 10 mm, significant ICH, pneumocephalus, gross wound contamination, or frontal sinus involvement should be repaired surgically because of the risk of infection. Open depressed fractures that do not meet these criteria can be managed

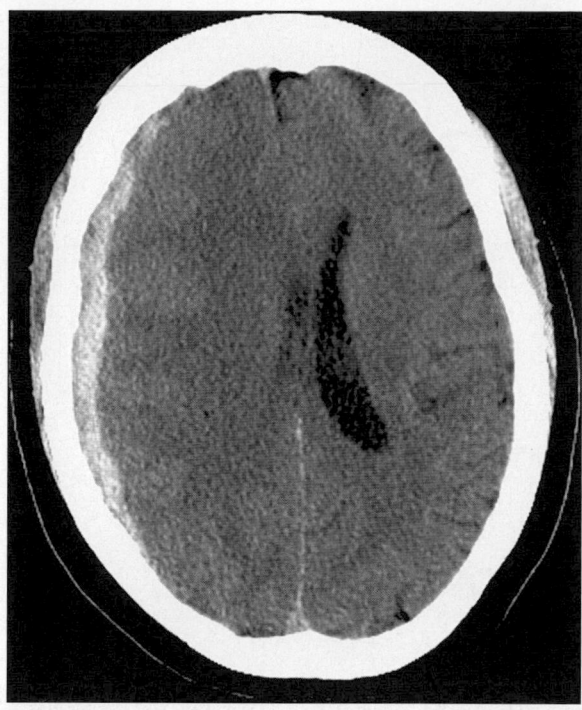

FIGURE 2 Acute subdural hematoma.

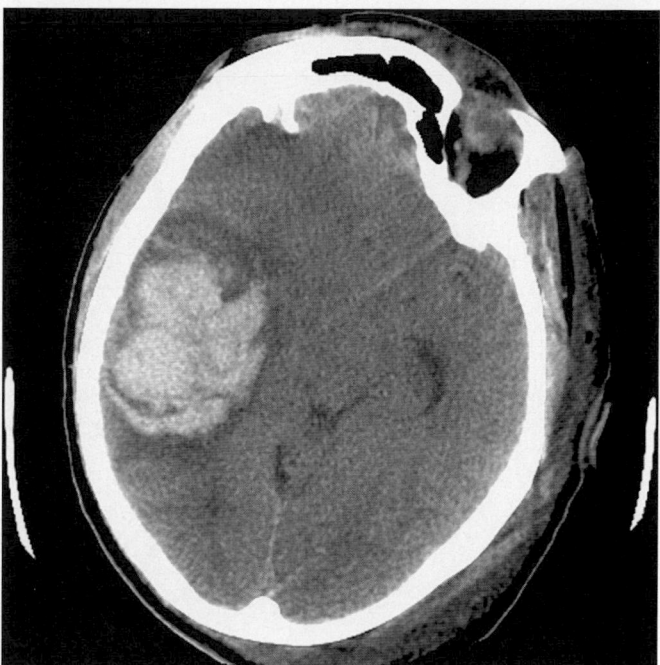

FIGURE 3 Traumatic parenchymal lesion.

nonoperatively. Closed depressed fractures displaced greater than the thickness of the skull or clearly causing a focal deficit also should undergo urgent surgical elevation and débridement. Otherwise, closed depressed skull fractures with no other TBI can be managed nonoperatively.

Parenchymal Lesions

Parenchymal lesions and contusions occur frequently and are seen in 35% of severe TBI cases. Although most are managed nonoperatively, as many as 20% require surgical intervention. On head CT, these lesions can have a coup-contrecoup pattern (Figure 3), with the "coup" lesion at the site of impact and the "contrecoup" lesion on the opposite site of the brain where it bounced off the skull. It is important to note that parenchymal hemorrhages and contusions tend to evolve and may enlarge over time. They also are associated with cerebral edema leading to significant mass effect on the surrounding parenchyma and an elevation of ICP. Even if a patient is neurologically intact on presentation, patients with parenchymal lesions should be observed closely and serially in case these lesions "blossom."

Indications for operative intervention include any signs of imminent herniation, deterioration of neurologic function attributable to the parenchymal lesions, and an elevated ICP refractory to medical management. In patients with a GCS of 6 to 8, imaging criteria for surgical intervention include any lesion with a volume larger than 50 cm^3, frontal or temporal lesions with a volume larger than 20 cm^3, midline shift greater than 5 mm, and cisternal compression. Surgical approaches can range from craniotomy with evacuation of blood to decompressive craniectomy with duraplasty for cerebral edema.

Austere Settings

Surgical management of TBI usually is performed by neurosurgeons. If no neurosurgeon is available, every effort should be made to expeditiously transfer patients with TBI who may need surgery. However, in the case of an acutely herniating patient in a rural or austere environment, general and trauma surgeons can perform a burr hole craniotomy with evacuation of extra-axial blood (EDH or SDH).

Indications for a burr hole include a GCS less than 8, unilateral pupillary dilation or hemiparesis, and no available neurosurgeon. If possible, obtain noncontrast head CT to confirm the diagnosis and guide placement of the burr hole. If CT is unavailable, the burr hole should be placed over the temporal lobe ipsilateral to the pupillary dilation and contralateral to the hemiparesis because temporal lobe decompression is the first priority in acute herniation and the temporal lobe is also the most common site of EDH secondary to middle meningeal artery injury (Figure 4).

The patient should be positioned supine with the head shaved and turned so that the side of interest is facing up. If available, use the head CT to decide which burr hole (temporal, frontal, or parietal) should be performed (see Figure 4). Make a 3-cm incision down to the bone, push the periosteum off the bone with a knife or swab, and then drill over the center of the hematoma through the skull. Evacuate the EDH. If there is an SDH, hook the dura, sharply open it, and carefully evacuate the subdural blood. If no CT is available and the initial temporal burr hole is negative, perform a burr hole in the contralateral temporal position followed by frontal and parietal burr holes. Once the blood has been evacuated, transfer the patient to a center with a neurosurgeon as soon as possible. The Committee on Trauma does not recommend that untrained surgeons perform burr holes; however, it notes that surgeons in a rural or austere environment should anticipate the need for emergent surgical management of TBI and receive the appropriate training.

■ SPECIAL TOPICS

Diffuse Axonal Injury

Patients with a normal head CT still may have significant TBI. This encompasses patients with concussions, diffuse axonal injury (DAI), and anoxic brain injury. DAI in particular is an acceleration-deceleration injury in which shearing forces on the brain stretch and damage neuronal axons, resulting in immediate unconsciousness. Though not seen on CT, DAI can be identified on magnetic resonance imaging (MRI) of the brain. Patients with mild DAI may recover with minimal deficits. In severe cases, patients may have prolonged to permanent coma.

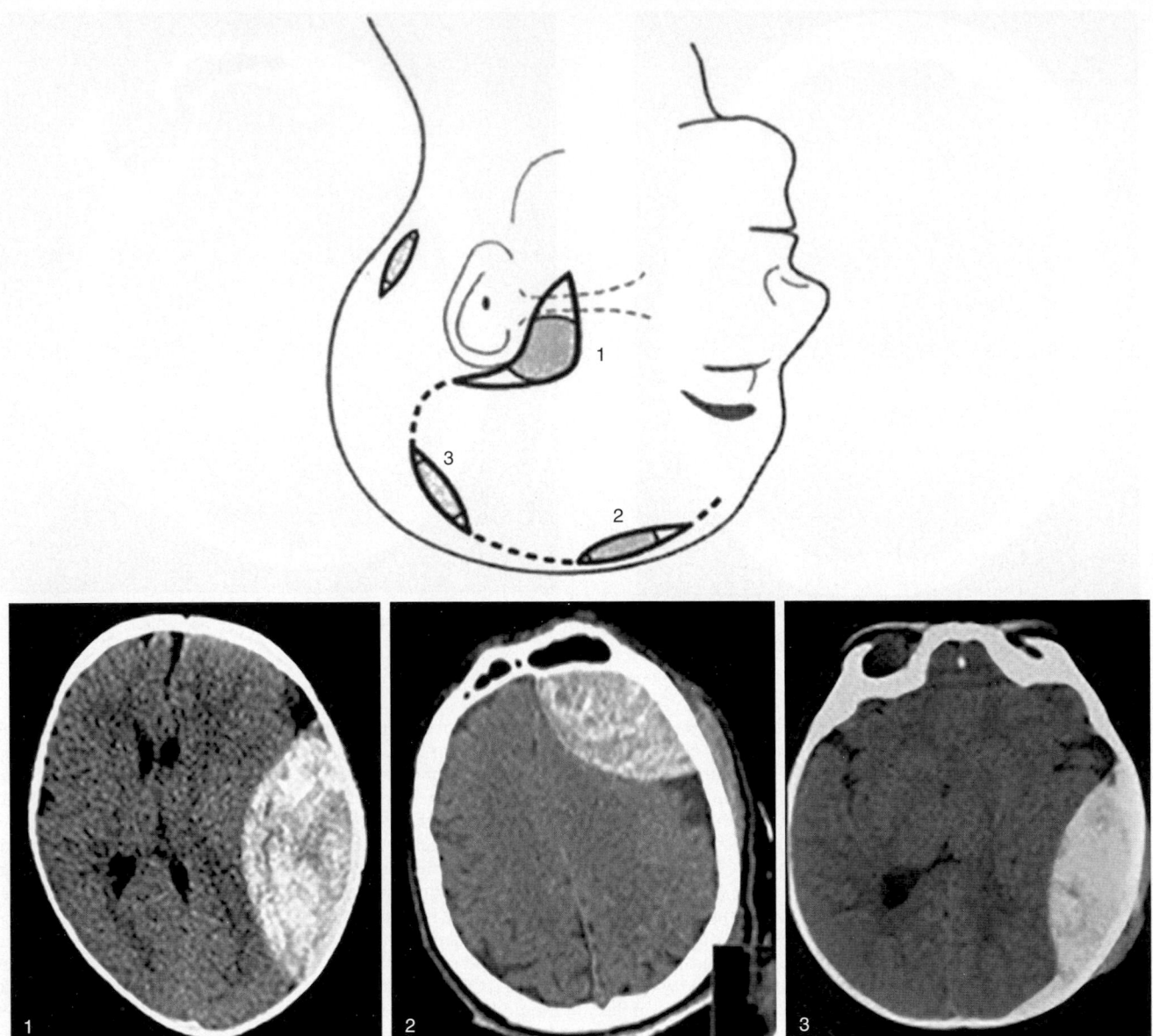

FIGURE 4 Diagram demonstrating the position of standard burr holes: *1*, temporal (above zygoma); *2*, frontal (over the coronal suture, approximately 10 cm behind and in the midpupillary line); and *3*, parietal (over the parietal eminence). Computed tomographic images correspond. A posterior fossa burr hole can be used in the extremely rare case of posterior fossa extradural haematoma. *(From Wilson MH, Wise D, Davies G, Lockey D. Emergency burr holes: "how to do it." Scan J Trauma Resusc Emerg Med. 2012;20:24.)*

Although there is no indication for surgical management of DAI, these patients can have associated cerebral edema and elevated ICP that require complex medical management. If intracranial hypertension is not a problem, the main treatment for patients with DAI is intensive rehabilitation to maximize level of function. This includes physical therapy, occupational therapy, speech therapy, adaptive equipment, and counseling.

Brain Death

Clinicians caring for patients with severe TBI will be called on to determine brain death. The American Academy of Neurology has established criteria for this process. The patient must have a core temperature higher than 36°C and SBP greater than 100 mm Hg with an irreversible and known recent cause of coma. The patient should not be sedated, paralyzed, or intoxicated. On clinical examination, the patient should be unresponsive and apneic and should have no

brainstem reflexes (pupillary, oculocephalic, oculovestibular, corneal, grimace, gag, and cough). In some states, two clinical examinations by two different clinicians are required. In addition, other confirmatory testing such as electroencephalogram (EEG), computed tomographic angiography (CTA), or magnetic resonance angiogram (MRA) may be performed as indicated or required by state law.

SUGGESTED READINGS

Bratton SL, Chestnut RM, Ghajar J, et al. Guidelines for the management of severe traumatic brain injury, 3rd ed. *J Neurotrauma.* 2007;24(suppl 1):S1-S106.

Brenner M, Stein DM, Hu PF, et al. Traditional systolic blood pressure targets underestimate hypotension-induced secondary brain injury. *J Trauma Acute Care Surg.* 2012;72:1135-1139.

Bullock MR, Chestnut R, Ghajar J, et al. Guidelines for the surgical management of traumatic brain injury. *Neurosurgery.* 2006;58(suppl 3):S2-S62.

Foreman PM, Schmalz PG, Griessenauer CJ. Chemoprophylaxis for venous thromboembolism in traumatic brain injury: a review and evidence-based protocol. *Clin Neurol Neurosurg*. 2014;123:109-116.

Konstantinidis A, Inaba K, Dubose J, et al. The impact of nontherapeutic hypothermia on outcomes after severe traumatic brain injury. *J Trauma*. 2011;71:1627-1631.

McCoy CC, Lawson JH, Shapiro ML, et al. Management of anticoagulation agents in trauma patients. *Clin Lab Med*. 2014;34:563-574.

Torre-Healy A, Marko NF, Weil RJ. Hyperosmolar therapy for intracranial hypertension. *Neurocrit Care*. 2012;17:117-130.

Wilson MH, Wise D, Davies G, Lockey D. Emergency burr holes: "how to do it." *Scan J Trauma Resusc Emerg Med*. 2012;20:24.

CHEST WALL, PNEUMOTHORAX, AND HEMOTHORAX

Scott M. Moore, MD, Fredric M. Pieracci, MD, MPH, FACS, and Gregory J. Jurkovich, MD

Although Hippocrates was the first to describe chest tube insertion for pleural drainage, this did not become the standard treatment for hemothorax and pneumothorax until the nineteenth century and was greatly facilitated by the development of the underwater seal device by Playfair. The approach to the majority of chest wall injuries in the modern era appropriately has emphasized nonoperative management. However, published reports of closed reduction and external fixation of flail chest appeared as early as the first half of the twentieth century, with the first report of internal fixation using wire suture occurring in 1950. Open reduction and plate stabilization of complex rib fractures are becoming more common as specialized plating systems have been developed.

Thoracic trauma is a major source of morbidity and mortality and is second only to head injury as a cause of death in the injured patient. Furthermore, this statistic likely underestimates the burden of thoracic injuries, which are the cause for on-scene fatalities in an estimated 50% of cases. Among those patients who reach medical attention, thoracic trauma portends an overall mortality of 8.4%, with complications from chest injuries contributing to another 25% of trauma-related deaths. Injury mechanism is a critical determinant of the pattern of thoracic injury, with chest wall injuries more often resulting from blunt mechanisms that involve crushing forces, major pulmonary and cardiac injuries resulting from penetrating trauma, and aortic injuries associated with both types of mechanisms. This chapter focuses on the management of the most commonly encountered thoracic injuries, which include chest wall injuries, pneumothorax, and hemothorax. Operative repair of cardiac, pulmonary, great vessel, and aerodigestive tract injuries are described elsewhere.

■ INITIAL APPROACH

Patients who sustain thoracic trauma are evaluated systematically according to the tenets of the Advanced Trauma Life Support (ATLS) protocol: a primary survey is conducted that prioritizes identification and correction of airway problems, then breathing abnormalities, and finally circulatory dysfunction. Endotracheal intubation or surgical airway placement, chest tube insertion, establishment of adequate intravenous access for resuscitation, and maneuvers to control hemorrhage and temperature are instituted *as soon as problems are found*. In addition, practitioners should assume the presence of a spinal cord injury and vigilantly avoid hypothermia during this stage. With specific regard to thoracic trauma, the conditions that are immediately life threatening include tension and open pneumothorax, massive hemothorax, flail chest, major pulmonary contusion, air embolism, and cardiac tamponade. Vital sign abnormalities that are accompanied by examination findings of unilateral loss of breath sounds, hyperresonance or dullness to percussion, tracheal deviation, distended or flattened neck veins, and chest wall instability or crepitus signal a life-threatening condition that requires immediate attention.

After the primary survey, a secondary survey is performed to uncover potentially life-threatening problems that were not identified initially. This is accomplished by more in-depth physical examination and diagnostic tests. In the patient with suspected thoracic trauma, the latter should include a portable chest x-ray (CXR), which has the advantage of rapidly diagnosing potentially life-threatening injuries without the need to transport the patient away from resources needed for resuscitation. It should be noted, however, that the portable supine CXR often misses intrathoracic pathology, with relatively poor sensitivity for pneumothorax (28% to 75%), hemothorax (75%), rib fractures (50%), sternal fractures (50%), pulmonary contusion (44%), and aortic injuries (41% to 88%).

Bedside ultrasound has become standard practice in the initial trauma evaluation (i.e., focused assessment with sonography for trauma, or FAST), and more recently the extended version of the FAST (i.e., eFAST) has augmented the standard pericardial, abdominal, and pelvic views with additional views of the bilateral pleural spaces. In experienced hands the eFAST has a sensitivity that surpasses portable CXR for detection of pneumothorax (86% to 98%) and can be used to identify other potentially life-threatening injuries such as hemothorax and pulmonary contusion.

Routine chest computed tomography (CT) for evaluation of thoracic trauma is costly and exposes a large patient population to harmful levels of ionizing radiation, whereas missed injuries have the potential for significant morbidity and mortality. To help guide decision making for chest imaging, the NEXUS Chest screening tools have been developed and shown to have a sensitivity greater than 99% for thoracic injuries of major clinical significance (Boxes 1 and 2). There has been recent debate about the clinical significance of injuries not identified on CXR but later seen on CT imaging. In a recent study, these so-called "occult" injuries were found to occur in 25% of all patients who undergo both CXR and CT imaging, and among injured patients the rate of occult injury identification is greater than 70%. As discussed later, many occult pneumothoraces and hemothoraces can be managed expectantly, and most rib fractures are managed nonoperatively based on their clinical sequelae (i.e., severity of pain, strength of cough) rather than on their radiologic appearance. However, clinically significant occult injuries do occur, with the aforementioned study finding that 66.2% of injuries that required major interventions (i.e., mechanical ventilation, tube thoracostomy, surgery) were occult, though it is unclear from the observational nature of this study that the CT results actually changed management. However, management of less clinically apparent injuries probably is affected by CT imaging, with 25% of occult great vessel injuries, 9.8% of occult spine fractures, and 100% of occult diaphragm ruptures in this study requiring surgery. It is also clear that CT-identified occult injuries lead to a high rate of admission, with 9 in 10 patients with occult injuries being admitted. Ongoing clinical investigations continue to try to identify the specific variants of injuries that are seen only on chest CT (vs CXR) and warrant treatment.

BOX 1: NEXUS Chest: Indications for Chest X-Ray*

Age >60 years
Rapid deceleration mechanism
Fall >20 ft
Motor vehicle collision >40 mph
Chest pain
Intoxication
Abnormal alertness or mental status
Distracting injury
Chest wall tenderness

*All criteria absent: very low risk for intrathoracic injury and chest imaging not indicated.

BOX 2: NEXUS Chest: Indications for Chest CT*

Abnormal chest x-ray
Distracting injury
Chest wall tenderness
Sternum tenderness
Thoracic spine tenderness
Scapula tenderness
Rapid deceleration injury

*All criteria absent: may forgo chest computed tomography.

■ SPECIFIC INJURIES

Rib Fractures and Flail Chest

Rib fractures are very common and have a prevalence of 10% in trauma admissions overall, making them the most common injury in patients with blunt chest trauma. The high frequency of these injuries necessitates that all surgeons caring for trauma patients be well versed in the potential complications and optimal management strategies for rib fractures. The surprisingly high mortality rate associated with chest wall injuries (10% to 20%) stems from pain-induced splinting with resultant poor pulmonary hygiene, which can lead to progressive atelectasis and pneumonia if pain is not managed aggressively. Rib fractures also commonly result in a tremendous amount of chronic pain, disability, and loss of productive life years; the majority of patients with flail chest who survive to discharge are never able to return to pre-injury levels of employment. The high incidence of associated injuries (especially pulmonary contusion and head injuries) undoubtedly contributes to the mortality rate as well. The most commonly injured ribs after blunt chest trauma are the fourth through tenth, and the specific location of rib fractures can implicate other injuries; lower rib fractures (ninth to eleventh) should direct attention to possible abdominal solid organ injury (left side spleen, kidney; right side liver, kidney), whereas upper rib fractures (first to third) are associated with injuries to the head, neck, spinal cord, and great vessels. High rib fractures have been associated with blunt cerebrovascular injury (BCVI). In addition to rib number, the total number of fractures also dictates risk, with each additional rib fracture increasing the risk of pulmonary complications and death. Fracture location within the rib also affects patient outcome. In general, lateral and subscapular fracture lines produce the most pain, whereas very posterior or anterior fracture lines usually are better tolerated. Finally, degree of displacement, overlap, and angulation of the fracture itself all contribute to alterations of pulmonary mechanics, pain, and injury to surrounding structures such as the intercostal bundle, lung, and diaphragm.

BOX 3: RibScore*

≥6 ribs fractured
≥3 bicortically displaced fractures
≥1 fracture in each anatomic area†
Flail chest
Bilateral fractures
First rib fracture

*1 point is assigned for each variable; RibScore ≥4 may benefit from surgical stabilization of rib fractures.

†Defined as anterior, lateral, and posterior.

The danger posed by chest wall injuries is compounded with increasing age, as patients over 65 years old have an overall mortality of 22% and a pneumonia rate of 33%, compared with 10% and 17%, respectively, for younger patients. Furthermore, each additional rib fracture in the older person increases the relative risk of death by 19% and that of pneumonia by 27%. The impact of age on mortality from rib fractures was reinforced by a survey of the National Trauma Data Bank (NTDB), which showed a dramatic increase in mortality with greater than six rib fractures. Even lesser extremes of age impart additional risk, as demonstrated by a study by Holcomb and colleagues that showed that patients older than 45 years have significantly increased ventilator time, intensive care unit (ICU) length of stay, and duration of hospitalization when compared with younger patients.

Flail chest is a specific rib fracture pattern that is defined by three or more adjacent ribs with fractures in two or more places. Although the most common fracture pattern that results in a flail segment is two unilateral fracture lines (lateral flail), a flail segment also can result from bilateral fractures of three or more consecutive ribs (anterior flail) or when three or more unilateral fractures are associated with a sternal fracture. In a recent multicenter retrospective study, flail chest was found in 1% of patients admitted to trauma centers with a blunt injury mechanism. Flail chest represents the most severe form of chest wall injury after blunt trauma, with more than 80% of patients needing ICU admission, more than 50% requiring mechanical ventilation, and an overall mortality of 16%. With spontaneous breathing, a paradoxical outward movement of the flail segment will be observed during expiration, followed by inward movement during inspiration. It is important to note that such paradoxical motion is eliminated during positive pressure ventilation (PPV), which may lead to initial oversight of the injury, especially in patients who are intubated before arrival in the trauma bay. Because of the large amount of force required to cause a flail chest injury, additional injuries are frequently present and can contribute greatly to patient morbidity and mortality. The most commonly associated injuries are pulmonary contusion (46% to 77%), pneumothorax and hemothorax (44% to 70%), and head injury (15%). In addition to the pain and splinting encountered with all rib fractures, flail chest imparts mechanical instability that limits thoracic volume and has a high incidence of pulmonary contusion that causes blood accumulation within the alveolar spaces.

Several scoring systems have been developed to quantify the severity of chest wall injury. We recently proposed the RibScore, which involves several detailed radiographic parameters related to rib fracture pattern (Box 3). This score has been found to be highly predictive of adverse pulmonary outcomes and is useful for predicting which patients may benefit from surgical stabilization of rib fractures (Figure 1). Other scores that incorporate nonfracture parameters (e.g., age, pulmonary contusion) include the Organ Injury Scale (OIS) Chest Wall Grade, Rib Fracture Score, Chest Trauma Score, and Pressley Score.

The treatment of rib fractures and flail chest is nonoperative in the vast majority of cases, and patients usually can be managed successfully with aggressive pain control, early and effective pulmonary

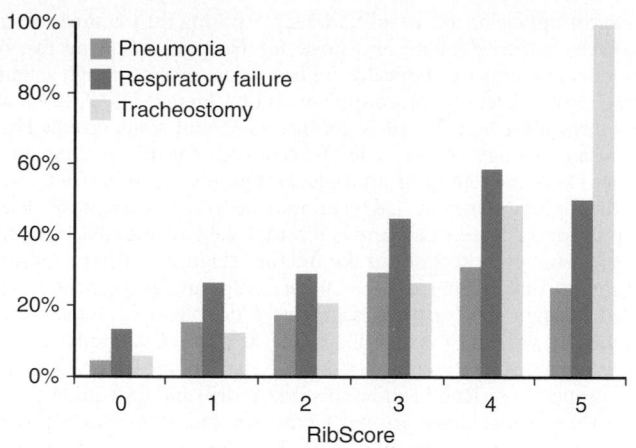

FIGURE 1 Morbidity associated with increasing RibScore. Based entirely on radiographic appearance of rib fractures, RibScore provides a prompt risk stratification for complications related to rib fractures.

BOX 4: Admission Criteria for Rib Fractures

Admission if, after pain control with oral medication, ≥2 of the following are present:
Respiratory rate >18
Incentive spirometry <75% predicted
Numeric pain score ≥6
Poor cough
Age ≥65 years
≥3 fractures

If admission criteria are met, intensive care unit (ICU) admission if ≥1 of the following are present:
Age ≥65 years
≥6 fractures
Incentive spirometry <60% predicted
Flail chest
>4 L oxygen required to maintain arterial oxygen saturation (SpO_2) >90%
Associated injury requiring ICU admission

BOX 5: Pain Management of Rib Fractures

Outpatient

Incentive spirometer
Ibuprofen 800 mg PO q6H
Gabapentin 100 mg PO TID
Diazepam 5-10 mg PO QD
Oxycodone PRN

Inpatient

Incentive spirometer
Ambulation
Ibuprofen 800 mg PO q6H
Gabapentin 100 mg PO TID
Diazepam 5-10 mg PO QD
Oxycodone PRN
Intravenous narcotics PRN
Consider epidural or paravertebral catheter
Consider surgical stabilization of rib fractures

PO, orally; *PRN*, as needed; *q6H*, every 6 hours; *QD*, daily; *TID*, three times a day.

toilet, and supportive care. For simple unilateral fractures involving no more than three ribs, young patients with adequate pain control on oral analgesics and without comorbidities can be managed successfully as outpatients. All other patients should be considered for admission, and there should be a low threshold to admit patients with high-risk features to the ICU (Box 4). Systemic analgesics with narcotic and non-narcotic agents given both orally and parenterally are necessary, as are early mobilization, aggressive use of incentive spirometry, and chest physiotherapy (Box 5). Patient-controlled analgesia (PCA) is a safe and effective method for delivering parenteral narcotics and should be implemented liberally. Whenever possible, non-narcotic analgesics such as nonsteroidal anti-inflammatory drugs (NSAIDs) and gabapentin should be prescribed to patients with rib fractures.

Epidural catheters are especially useful in patients with extensive rib fractures or flail chest, as they avoid the respiratory depression, somnolence, and gastrointestinal symptoms that accompany high-dose parenteral narcotics while providing superior pain control. Several studies have demonstrated convincingly that epidural analgesia after chest wall injuries translates into decreased ventilator days, fewer pulmonary complications, and shortened ICU and hospital length of stay, especially when used in older patients with multiple fractures. Current guidelines strongly recommend placement of an epidural for patients older than 65 years with four or more rib

fractures and suggest consideration of epidural analgesia in younger patients with four or more fractures and in older patients with lesser injuries. The most common risks associated with epidural anesthesia include hypotension and pruritus, with the more serious complications of epidural hematoma, infection, and spinal cord injury occurring very rarely. Most patients are eligible for epidural analgesia; however, some absolute contraindications that are especially relevant to the trauma population include increased intracranial pressure, localized infection or rash, and inability to maintain position for catheter placement. Relative contraindications include a history of spine surgery; spinal fracture; instability near the desired level of epidural placement; severe aortic stenosis, mitral stenosis, or pulmonary hypertension; uncorrectable coagulopathy (i.e., certain anticoagulants, antiplatelet agents, or inherited coagulopathies), and ongoing vasopressor requirement. Despite their efficacy, low complication rate, and availability at most trauma centers, recent reports from the NTDB indicate that only 8% of patients with flail chest receive epidural catheters, suggesting that this effective analgesic modality is greatly underused.

Regional analgesia also can be achieved by intercostal, intrapleural, paravertebral, and paracostal delivery of anesthetic, with the latter being an attractive option given the relative simplicity of catheter placement and encouraging efficacy in preliminary studies. Paracostal catheters (Figure 2) are placed by palpating the lower rib margin approximately 5 cm lateral to the spinous processes and passing a spinal needle to localize the rib with injection of local anesthetic in the skin, subcutaneous tissue, and paravertebral muscles. A small incision is made, and an obturator with tearaway sheath then is passed bluntly to the level of the scapula in a plane parallel and immediately superficial to the posterior rib cage. A long catheter then is exchanged for the obturator, and the sheath is removed. The catheter is secured and the incision is sealed with surgical adhesive to prevent leakage of anesthetic. The typical anesthetic regimen is a bolus dose of 0.25% bupivacaine (20 mL) followed by a continuous infusion (0.125% at 12 mL/hr) by either a pump or an elastomer reservoir.

Surgical Stabilization of Rib Fractures

Basic orthopedic principle dictates that the management of fractures involves reduction and fixation. The ribs are unique in that they move with each breath, rendering external fixation impossible. Furthermore, in the case of long bone fractures, selective immobilization

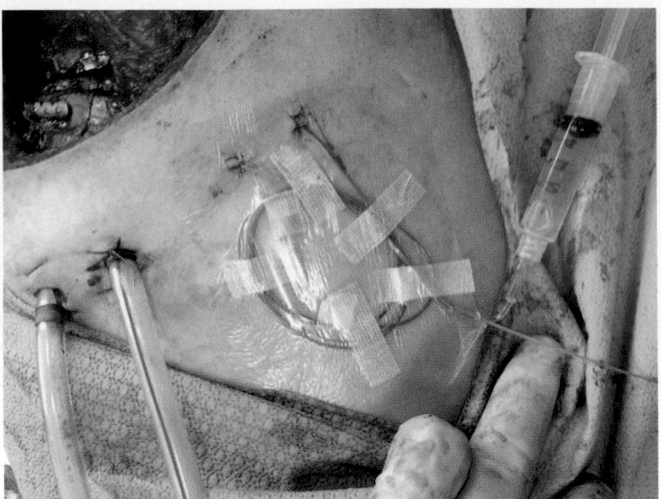

FIGURE 2 Rib fracture pain management with local-regional anesthesia. Anesthetic catheters typically are placed peri-incisional after surgical stabilization of rib fractures (SSRF). Paracostal placement can be performed at the bedside in patients not undergoing SSRF.

by patients secondary to pain is relatively inconsequential. By contrast, selective immobilization of the ribs due to pain results in atelectasis, accumulation of pulmonary secretions, pneumonia, and eventual respiratory failure. These hypothetical observations as well as the high incidence of painful nonunions from severely displaced fractures form the basis for recommending surgical stabilization of rib fractures (SSRF) in select fracture patterns.

Rib fracture repair has been performed for more than 60 years but until recently has been limited by nonspecific fixation systems, lack of efficacy data, and lack of ownership by a surgical discipline. Over the last 10 years, several prospective studies, including three randomized controlled trials and two meta-analyses, have documented the efficacy of SSRF, primarily in patients with flail chest. Specifically, reduced pneumonia rates, decreased duration of mechanical ventilation, decreased length of ICU stay, decreased need for tracheostomy, and lower medical costs have been observed. More recently, evidence suggests that certain nonflail fracture patterns, such as multiple contiguous severely displaced fractures, can progress to long-term disability and chronic pain, and SSRF potentially may abrogate this progression. We currently consider SSRF in all patients with flail chest, patients with three or more severely (bicortical) displaced fractures, and any patient who has failed maximal nonoperative management after 24 hours.

The optimal timing for SSRF is not established. Some have advocated SSRF after certain clinical variables become apparent (i.e., failed ventilator wean, intractable pain); however, earlier repair has definite advantages. Inflammation around the fractures peaks between 3 and 5 days postinjury, and pain from rib movement during respiration can cause progressive splinting, atelectasis, and potential respiratory failure. Therefore SSRF within 72 hours of patient presentation may provide the best window for technical success and prevention of complications. Ideally the patient with severe rib fractures is identified as a candidate for SSRF at the time of presentation and, assuming hemodynamic stability and the absence of competing operative priorities, is transported directly from the trauma bay to the operating room for SSRF. Choice of positioning and incision are dictated by the fracture patterns. In most cases, rib fracture repair may be accomplished without any muscle division. Anterior fractures are approached via a submammary incision in the supine position, with elevation of a pectoralis flap. For isolated lateral fractures of 3 to 5 contiguous ribs, an 8- to 10-cm longitudinal incision after the anterior border of the latissimus dorsi muscle and centered over the middle fracture usually provides adequate exposure. The serratus

anterior muscle fibers are split, thereby exposing the fractures. Alternatively, extensive lateral and posterior fractures involving five or more contiguous ribs typically are best approached through a standard posterolateral thoracotomy incision (Figure 3). Whether all fractures must be repaired is controversial, and some groups have advocated fixing only one side of a flail segment or repairing every other rib in the setting of multiple contiguous fractures. Dissection of the rib periosteum should be minimized to ensure adequate blood supply for fracture healing and is accomplished by a limited 3 to 5 cm of exposure on both sides of the fracture (Figure 4). After exposure of the fractured segments, right angle clamps and gentle traction are used to align the fractured segments ("double right angle" technique). A variety of fixation systems are currently available. For systems using plates and screws, depth gauges should be used to select the proper screw length, and a specialized drill and drill guide assists in ensuring that holes are perpendicular and at proper depth to achieve bicortical penetration. Low clearance areas (i.e., upper posterior ribs deep to the scapula) will require a specialized right angle drill and screwdriver. Newer systems use self-tapping and locking screws that eliminate the need for an additional drilling step and prevent screws from backing out. The surgeon must ensure that screws are placed perpendicular to the rib with bicortical purchase, with at least three screws on both sides of the fracture. In addition, plates should sit flush with the rib. Most commercially available plating systems have precontoured plates for each rib; however, these typically are designed for anterolateral fractures, and plate bending is often necessary for posterior fractures. SSRF also affords an opportunity to evacuate blood and fluid from the pleural space under direct visualization, perform pulmonary toilet via directed bronchoscopy, and place local-regional anesthesia catheters under direct vision and palpation. Finally, thoracoscopic SSRF has been described by our group and is currently under development.

Sternal Fractures

Once considered a major risk factor for occult thoracic injuries such as cardiac contusion or great vessel injury, the mechanism for sternal fractures has shifted over the last few decades. Before widespread implementation of three-point restraints, rapid deceleration and steering wheel impact were the most common culprits of sternal fractures; however, now they are caused most frequently by shoulder belt impingement. A recent study by Odell and colleagues found that 26.4% of sternal fractures were isolated, with the remainder being associated most commonly with extremity fractures (42.2%), head and neck injuries (39.3%), rib fractures (38.4%), spine injuries (25.7%), and pulmonary contusions (25.6%). Cardiac contusion and great vessel injury were present in only 2.3% and 1.1%, respectively. History, physical examination, basic imaging, and electrocardiography at the time of initial evaluation are adequate to rule out associated injuries. If such studies confirm that the injury is indeed isolated, fit and nongeriatric patients often can be managed on an outpatient basis. This is supported by the finding by Odell and colleagues that none of the 492 patients with isolated sternal fracture required endotracheal intubation, chest tube placement, or operative intervention. For nonisolated cases, cardiac contusion should be suspected if the electrocardiogram demonstrates unexplained tachycardia (the most common dysrhythmia), frequent premature ventricular contractions (PVCs), right bundle branch block, ST segment changes, or other arrhythmias, and such patients require admission for continuous cardiac monitoring and echocardiography. Persistent shock in the thoracic trauma patient without ongoing hemorrhage and after adequate volume resuscitation should receive echocardiography, which can detect specific pathologies such as pericardial effusion, wall motion abnormalities, septal rupture, or valvular dysfunction. Because the right ventricle underlies the sternum, wall motion abnormalities most likely are seen in this location. Cardiac biomarkers generally are not useful for the management of suspected cardiac contusion. Operative repair of sternal fractures is sometimes

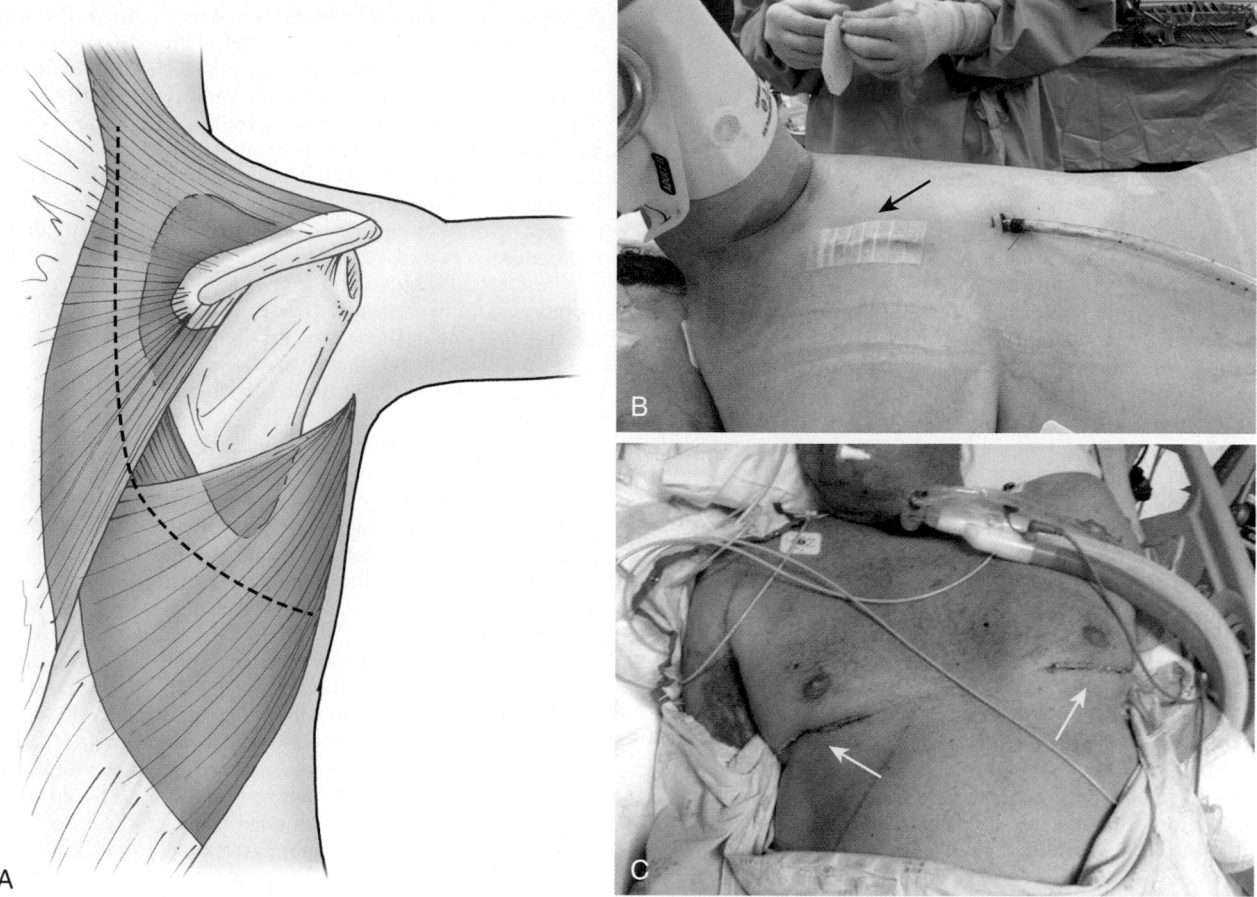

FIGURE 3 Incisions for surgical stabilization of rib fractures. **A,** Extensive posterior and lateral fractures are best exposed through a standard posterolateral thoracotomy incision. **B,** Isolated lateral fractures can be exposed through a more limited incision centered over the middle fracture (*arrow*). **C,** Anterior rib fractures are best exposed by inframammary incisions (*arrows*).

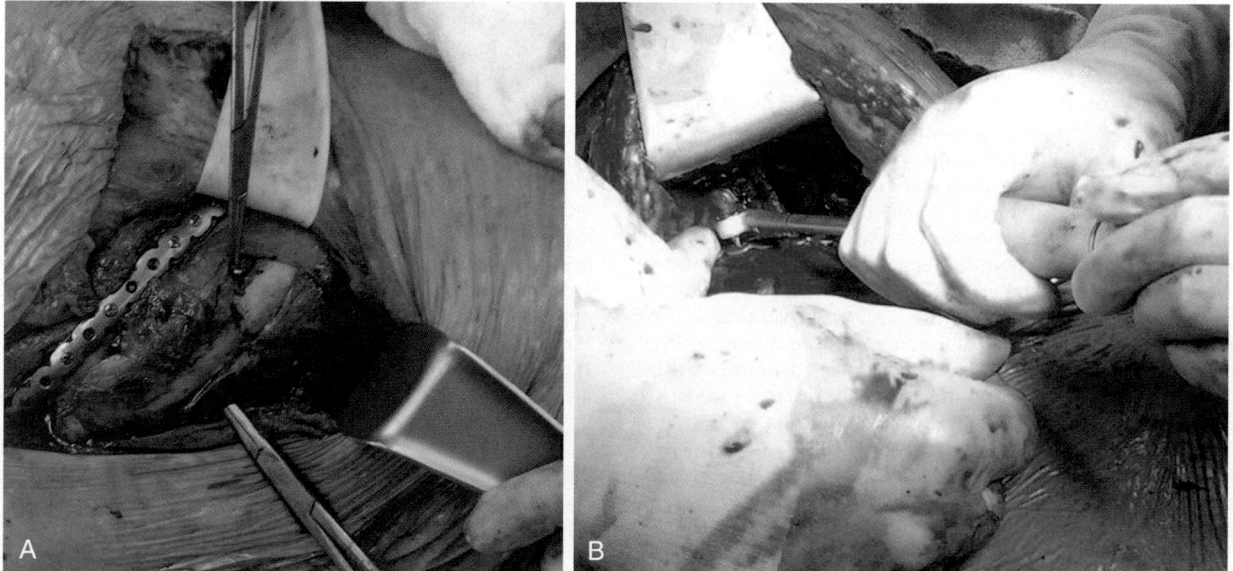

FIGURE 4 Operative technique for surgical stabilization of rib fractures. **A,** Double right angle technique aligns fracture ends before placement of rib plates. **B,** Right angle drill and screwdriver are useful for plate fixation in low-clearance areas such as the subscapular space.

indicated for significant displacement and overlap or when associated with rib fractures deemed appropriate for SSRF and can be accomplished with similar principles of exposure and fixation as SSRF.

Scapular Fractures

The scapula is uncommonly injured because of its mobility on the chest wall and protection by the rib cage anteriorly and well-developed musculature posteriorly. For this reason, fractures of the scapula typically involve high-energy transfer and are associated with other injuries in 80% to 95% of cases. Scapula fractures are considered sentinel injuries because of the relatively high rate of associated great vessel, major thoracic, abdominal, head, and spinal injuries in historical reports. A more recent study of the NTDB, which included more than 9000 scapular fractures, found that patients with scapular injuries had significantly higher rates of rib fracture (53% vs 10%), pneumothorax (33% vs 8%), spinal fracture (29% vs 12%), head injury (39% vs 26%), abdominal injury (17% vs 10%), and pelvic fracture (15 vs. 6.3%); however, there was not a significantly increased association with heart, great vessel, or brachial plexus injury, and mortality also was unaffected. After adjusting for injury severity score (ISS), fractures to the ribs, spine, and pelvis all remained independently associated with scapular fractures.

Fractures can involve the acromion, coracoid process, body, neck, or glenoid portion of the scapula, and management often is influenced by commonly encountered accompanying injuries such as acromioclavicular separation, clavicle fractures, and humeral fractures. For nondisplaced acromion, stable coracoid, and the majority of scapular body and neck fractures, several weeks in a shoulder sling followed by passive and active motion exercises usually suffice for treatment. Operative treatment may be needed for significantly displaced acromion fractures and unstable coracoid and glenoid fractures that result in instability of the superior shoulder suspensory complex. Combined fracture of the glenoid neck and clavicle can result in a "floating shoulder," which often benefits from operative stabilization in order to provide fixation with the rest of the skeleton. Especially high-energy mechanisms may result in scapulothoracic dissociation, which is a devastating injury that is defined by lateral displacement of the scapula and complete loss of the scapulothoracic articulation. These injuries are associated with a high frequency of severe brachial plexus and vascular injury (>80% to 90%), which may mandate early above-elbow amputation if the extent of nerve injury precludes a meaningful functional recovery.

Clavicle Fractures and Dislocations

The clavicle is involved in nearly half of shoulder girdle injuries, which include fractures of the proximal, middle, and distal third as well as dislocations of the acromioclavicular and sternoclavicular joints. Although historically managed nonoperatively, there has been renewed interest in operative management of distal clavicle fractures because of the recognition of increased rates of nonunion and potential for functional disability if poor fracture healing occurs. Acromioclavicular dislocation (or "shoulder separation") often is managed nonoperatively, although higher-energy mechanisms can result in concomitant coracoclavicular disruption and may require operative reduction. Sternoclavicular dislocation requires considerable force and should prompt a diligent search for associated injuries in the neck, chest wall, and shoulder. Although anterior fractures are much more common, posterior sternoclavicular dislocations can be especially troublesome if the displaced clavicular head causes injury to the underlying trachea, lung, great vessels, or esophagus. For this reason, reductions of these dislocations should be performed only with appropriate surgical expertise immediately on hand.

Pneumothorax

Pneumothorax is defined by entry of air into the pleural space, which is usually a result of parenchymal lung injury and occurs with both blunt and penetrating mechanisms. For blunt injuries, the most common cause is lung lacerations caused by fractured ribs, although increases in intrathoracic pressure and pulmonary contusions as a result of sudden deceleration mechanisms can lead to pneumothorax in the absence of rib fractures. Recent studies estimate the prevalence of pneumothorax at 29% for blunt trauma, at 20% for penetrating mechanisms, and as high as 64% in intubated patients who sustained major chest trauma (ISS >30). Undoubtedly the frequency of detection has increased with the increased use of CT imaging of trauma patients, with a recent study reporting that 67.8% of diagnosed pneumothoraces were occult (i.e., not apparent on initial CXR but later seen on CT). Although the clinical significance of occult pneumothorax is controversial (discussed later), there is no debate concerning the importance of early recognition and treatment of clinically overt pneumothorax, as these injuries continue to be a major source of preventable death in both adult and pediatric trauma populations.

Pneumothorax should be suspected in all blunt trauma patients and especially in those with evidence of thoracic trauma. As mentioned, penetrating trauma also carries a significant risk for pneumothorax and often is suggested by the offending object's trajectory. On examination, pneumothorax can be seen with crepitus, unequal chest rise, unilateral breath sounds, and hyperresonance, though the last two may be difficult to ascertain in the noisy trauma bay. Indeed, the sensitivity of physical examination for pneumothorax after trauma is 50% to 58%, with a specificity of 97% to 98%, suggesting that examination findings should be acted on when present but not relied on to rule out the condition. The anteroposterior (AP) supine CXR is used most commonly as the initial imaging test in trauma patients, and any pneumothorax large enough to be visible on plain x-ray or accompanied by respiratory compromise should be treated by tube thoracostomy. As mentioned earlier, plain x-ray is notoriously inaccurate at diagnosing pneumothorax, which has prompted interest in bedside ultrasound as an initial screening test for pneumothorax. Normally, ultrasound of the pleural space will reveal characteristic sliding between the parietal and visceral pleura as well as comet tail artifacts and B-lines, all of which are absent in the setting of pneumothorax. A recent meta-analysis comparing supine CXR with bedside ultrasound found the latter to have superior sensitivity (49.7% vs 85.3%) and equivalent specificity (99.3% vs 98.4%). Despite the evidence for its superior accuracy, pleural ultrasound has not been applied universally as a standard part of the initial trauma evaluation, which is likely because of a lack of necessary equipment and training, its high dependence on operator experience and skill, and a scarcity of high-quality studies evaluating any advantage.

Tension pneumothorax is an immediately life-threatening condition that occurs when a one-way valve leads to progressive air trapping in the pleural space. The high pressure that develops leads to total collapse of the ipsilateral lung and shifting of the mediastinal structures, which causes kinking of the superior and inferior vena cava and loss of venous return to the heart. Examination findings include the typical findings of pneumothorax (absent breath sounds, hyperresonance) with the addition of distended neck veins, elevated hemithorax on the affected side, hypotension, and cyanosis. Respiratory and cardiovascular collapse occurs rapidly, and pleural decompression can be lifesaving. Diagnostic imaging delays treatment and should be avoided. Needle decompression (second intercostal space at the midclavicular line) is rapid and the recommended initial treatment, especially for providers who are less experienced with tube thoracostomy; however, individuals with thick chest walls may not be decompressible by traditional length angiocatheters (5 cm) and may be better served by initial tube thoracostomy. Alternatively, needle decompression through the fifth intercostal space at the midaxillary line offers a shorter distance to the pleural space and is an option. Needle decompression only converts a tension pneumothorax into a simple pneumothorax and always should be followed by tube thoracostomy for definitive treatment.

Open pneumothorax results when a large chest wall defect leads to direct communication between the pleural space and the surrounding environment. If the wound is greater than two thirds the diameter of the trachea, air will preferentially enter the wound instead of the airway during inspiration. Such injuries require prompt treatment to prevent respiratory decompensation and are treated initially by placement of a three-sided occlusive dressing, which creates a flap valve that occludes the wound on inspiration but allows egress of air on expiration. Immediate tube thoracostomy should be performed after placement of the dressing. The chest wall defect then can be repaired primarily for smaller wounds or may require rotational or free flaps for extensive injuries.

The management of *occult pneumothorax* has been a subject of debate. Given that the majority of pneumothoraces diagnosed in contemporary practice are occult and up to 22% of tube thoracostomies have complications (i.e., lung injury, intercostal artery laceration, empyema, malpositioning, postremoval recurrence), the decision of whether to perform tube thoracostomy for occult pneumothoraces is not trivial. Historically, the chest tube insertion rate for occult pneumothorax is widely variable (12% to 82%), which is in contrast to the consistently high rate of tube thoracostomy for overt pneumothoraces (65% to 95%). One possible explanation for this variability is that occult pneumothoraces typically are assumed to be smaller than overt ones, although several studies have found no significant difference in the measured size of occult and overt pneumothoraces. Because of this variability and uncertainty regarding management, the American Association for the Surgery of Trauma (AAST) sponsored a multi-institutional prospective study that examined the safety of an observation strategy for occult pneumothorax. The authors followed 569 patients with occult pneumothorax, 21% of whom had chest tubes placed; the remaining patients were observed. Only 6% of patients failed observation, and none of the patients that failed observation developed a tension pneumothorax or any other adverse events related to delayed tube thoracostomy. Average size of the pneumothorax greater than 7 mm, presence of hemothorax, and PPV all were associated with higher rates of observation failure. In addition, respiratory distress was associated with 6 times higher risk for failure, and interval increase in size of the pneumothorax was associated with 70 times the risk for failure; on multivariate analysis, these were the only factors that independently predicted observation failure. The conclusion from this study was that occult pneumothoraces can be observed safely with interval CXRs, and that this strategy can be extended to patients who are undergoing PPV. The safety of withholding chest tube placement for occult pneumothoraces among ventilated patients was reproduced in a recent study of pediatric patients that reported findings similar to those of the AAST study.

Hemothorax

Accumulation of blood within the pleural space is a common occurrence in both blunt and penetrating trauma patients. For blunt injuries, the source of blood is most commonly fractured ribs and adjacent lung laceration, though intercostal artery, great vessel, pulmonary hilar, and cardiac injuries also may be implicated. In rare instances, a combination of abdominal hemorrhage and diaphragm injury can cause hemothorax. For penetrating injuries, direct injury to the lung, intercostal arteries, heart, or major intrathoracic vessels is the most common source. Bleeding from fracture-associated lung lacerations typically resolves spontaneously on re-expansion of the lung; however, high pressure sources (i.e., intercostal artery) are less likely to resolve on their own and may require operative or endovascular control. Because pulmonary parenchymal injury is the usual source for blood, air often accompanies blood within the pleural space and is referred to as a hemopneumothorax. On examination, hemothorax is signaled by absent or decreased breath sounds, dullness to percussion (unless a hemopneumothorax, which may be hyperresonant), and tracheal deviation away from the affected side. Large quantities of blood within the pleural space can cause complete lung collapse and mediastinal shift with kinking of the venous inflow to the heart, resulting in tension physiology. However, in contrast to

tension pneumothorax, such cases usually are not seen with distended neck veins because of the accompanying hypovolemia. Depending on the quantity of blood, upright AP CXR may reveal blunting of the costophrenic angle or complete opacification of the hemothorax. In general, the minimum amount of blood needed to produce plain x-ray findings is 200 to 500 mL, although much larger volumes may not be apparent if the film is taken in the semi-upright or supine position, as is often the case with the blunt trauma patient. Indeed, pleural volumes as high as 1000 mL may be missed with the supine CXR and may produce just a subtle haziness that easily can be overlooked. In general, CT imaging is much more sensitive than CXR for hemothorax, which was demonstrated in a recent multicenter study in which 80% of hemothoraces were visible on CT but not on CXR.

The management of these *occult hemothoraces* is not clear, as the size of hemothorax that warrants drainage has been a matter of debate. Proponents of drainage for all hemothoraces cite the difficulty in achieving adequate drainage if delayed and the subsequent risk of developing fibrothorax when blood is left in the pleural space. Advocates for selective drainage highlight the increased risk of infection and empyema by introducing a foreign body into the pleural space as well as the overall 20% complication rate associated with tube thoracostomy. Several small studies have attempted to provide guidance on this question and, although they are limited by observational design and lack of long-term follow-up, generally show that hemothoraces less than 1.5 cm in maximal cross-sectional diameter on CT can be observed safely. Our practice has been to selectively drain all hemothoraces that appear to be more than 500 mL.

Massive hemothorax is defined by more than 1500 mL of blood within the pleural space and is an indication for operative exploration. In contrast to smaller hemothoraces, massive hemothorax is usually the result of a major pulmonary vascular or arterial source, neither of which is likely to spontaneously stop bleeding without operative control. Ongoing blood loss (more than 200 mL/hr for 2 to 4 hours) also should prompt operation. Because of the higher risk of major vascular disruption, we have a lower threshold (>1000 mL initial drainage) for operative exploration after penetrating trauma. Though generally useful, these guidelines should be used with caution under certain circumstances. Blunt trauma patients with a delayed presentation (i.e., those in rural areas with long transport times) may be better served by placing more emphasis on ongoing losses than on initial output. Patients on anticoagulation therapy also warrant careful clinical judgment before operative exploration, as chest wall and pulmonary parenchymal injuries can cause substantial bleeding in these patients that often responds well to correction of coagulopathy rather than to immediate attempts at operative control.

Retained hemothorax is defined as a residual hemothorax despite attempted evacuation by tube thoracostomy and is estimated to occur in 10% to 20% of cases. The diagnosis should be suspected when there is a persistent opacity on CXR after tube thoracostomy and is best confirmed by noncontrast chest CT. In addition to its deleterious effects on pulmonary function, retained hemothorax is a major risk factor for development of empyema. A recent study revealed a 26.8% risk of empyema with retained hemothorax, compared with only 2% of patients who had complete evacuation. Other independent risk factors for empyema identified by this study were rib fractures (odds ratio [OR] 2.3), ISS of 25 or more (OR 2.4), and the need for additional procedures to treat the hemothorax (OR 28.8). Overall, 50% of patients who developed empyema ultimately required thoracotomy. Because of the morbidity associated with thoracotomy, there has been great interest in identifying management strategies that avoid this outcome. Options include initial observation, placement of additional chest tubes, image-guided chest drainage, instillation of fibrinolytics through the existing chest tube, and video-assisted thoracoscopic surgery (VATS). The AAST sponsored a multicenter observational study to help elucidate which of these approaches offers the most favorable patient outcomes. This study found that observation alone was associated with an 83.2% success rate (defined as not needing additional interventions) in selected patients, especially if the residual hemothorax volume was estimated to be less than 300 mL. For larger volumes (300 to 900 mL), VATS was associated with a high success rate; however, it was less successful when there was an associated diaphragm injury. Additional interventions were required in 63.9% of patients who underwent a second chest tube placement, in 41.2% who underwent image-guided chest drainage, and in 66.6% who underwent fibrinolytic therapy. On the basis of these outcomes, observation is recommended for retained hemothoraces that are less than 300 mL, whereas VATS should be performed for larger collections, with the understanding that retained hemothoraces greater than 900 mL, especially when associated with diaphragm injury, are at higher risk for needing eventual thoracotomy. Fibrinolytics, additional tube thoracostomies, and image-guided procedures are often ineffective in this setting and therefore are discouraged for treatment of retained hemothorax. In addition, there are data to support VATS within the first 3 to 7 days of hospitalization to minimize risk for infection and need for thoracotomy.

Tube Thoracostomy

Preparation for tube thoracostomy should include skin preparation with an alcohol-based 2% chlorhexidine solution and wide draping, with the surgeon wearing sterile gloves, cap, gown, and face mask. Unstable patients (i.e., those with tension pneumothorax) may require abbreviated skin preparation and draping. Use of prophylactic antibiotics before chest tube insertion is debated. This is exemplified by guidelines from the Eastern Association for the Surgery of Trauma (EAST), which initially recommended presumptive antibiotics when released in 2002; the updated guidelines in 2012 retracted this recommendation based on poor quality and conflicting data.

The optimal site is typically at the fifth intercostal space (nipple level in males) just anterior to the midaxillary line. Local anesthetic should be infiltrated liberally into the skin, subcutaneous tissues, intercostal muscles, and pleura. A 2- to 3-cm horizontal incision is made, and a Kelly clamp is used to dissect through the tissues in the direction of the intended interspace, taking care to dissect immediately on top of the rib. Once the pleura is reached, it should be bluntly punctured forcefully but in a controlled fashion so as to avoid injury to underlying lung. Generous spreading of the tract with the Kelly clamp at this point will greatly facilitate tube placement. A gloved finger then should be inserted into the pleural space. This maneuver should be done carefully or not at all in patients with multiple rib fractures, which can cause injury to the provider's finger. However, finger palpation can provide several pieces of useful information, including confirmation of intrapleural placement, diagnosis of cardiac tamponade (left side), diagnosis of diaphragmatic rupture, and sweeping away of any adhesions. The chest tube then is clamped

at its tip and directed through the tract and into the pleural space. Because trauma patients often will have a combination of fluid and air in the pleural space (i.e., hemopneumothorax), the tube should be directed along the posterior chest wall toward the apex. Spinning the tube during advancement helps to prevent lodgment into the fissure, and fogging of the tube confirms intrapleural placement. The tube then is secured with heavy suture, attached to a water seal drainage device, and covered with an occlusive and sterile dressing. Authorities historically have recommended large bore chest tubes (36F to 40F) for treatment of hemothorax, although no studies have supported this assertion and studies have shown no difference between small (28F to 32F) and large (36F to 40F) tubes for successful evacuation of hemothorax.

SUGGESTED READINGS

Bulger EM, Arneson MA, Mock CN, Jurkovich GJ. Rib fractures in the elderly. *J Trauma*. 2000;48:1040-1046, discussion 1046-1047.

Chapman BC, Herbert B, Rodil M, Salotto J, Stovall RT, Biffl W, Johnson J, Burlew CC, Barnett C, Fox C, Moore EE, Jurkovich GJ, Pieracci FM. Rib-Score. *J Trauma Acute Care Surg*. 2016;80:95-101.

Fabricant L, Ham B, Mullins R, Mayberry J. Prolonged pain and disability are common after rib fractures. *Am J Surg*. 2013;205:511-515, discusssion 515-516.

Marasco SF, Davies AR, Cooper J, Varma D, Bennett V, Nevill R, Lee G, Bailey M, Fitzgerald M. Prospective randomized controlled trial of operative rib fixation in traumatic flail chest. *J Am Coll Surg*. 2013;216:924-932.

Moore FO, Goslar PW, Coimbra R, Velmahos G, Brown CVR, Coopwood TB, Lottenberg L, Phelan HA, Bruns BR, Sherck JP, Norwood SH, Barnes SL, Matthews MR, Hoff WS, de Moya MA, Bansal V, Hu CKC, Karmy-Jones RC, Vinces F, Pembaur K, Notrica DM, Haan JM. Blunt traumatic occult pneumothorax: is observation safe?—results of a prospective, AAST multicenter study. *J Trauma*. 2011;70:1019-1023, discussion 1023-1025.

Pieracci FM, Johnson JL, Stovall RT, Jurkovich GJ. Completely thoracoscopic, intra-pleural reduction and fixation of severe rib fractures. *Trauma Case Reports*. 2015;1:39-43.

Pieracci FM, Lin Y, Rodil M, Synder M, Herbert B, Tran DK, Stoval RT, Johnson JL, Biffl WL, Barnett CC, Cothren-Burlew C, Fox C, Jurkovich GJ, Moore EE. A prospective, controlled clinical evaluation of surgical stabilization of severe rib fractures. *J Trauma Acute Care Surg*. 2016;80: 187-194.

Pieracci FM, Rodil M, Stovall RT, Johnson JL, Biffl WL, Mauffrey C, Moore EE, Jurkovich GJ. Surgical stabilization of severe rib fractures. *J Trauma Acute Care Surg*. 2015;78:883-887.

Rodriguez RM, Anglin D, Langdorf MI, Baumann BM, Hendey GW, Bradley RN, Medak AJ, Raja AS, Juhn P, Fortman J, Mulkerin W, Mower WR. NEXUS chest: validation of a decision instrument for selective chest imaging in blunt trauma. *JAMA Surg*. 2013;148:940-946.

Simon BJ, Cushman J, Barraco R, Lane V, Luchette FA, Miglietta M, Roccaforte DJ, Spector R. Pain management guidelines for blunt thoracic trauma. *J Trauma*. 2005;59:1256-1267.

BLUNT ABDOMINAL TRAUMA

Anna M. Ledgerwood, MD, and Charles E. Lucas, MD

Patients who are seen acutely with a mechanism of injury from motor vehicle crash, motorcycle collision, falls, or assaults and pedestrians struck by motor vehicles should be considered to have a blunt abdominal injury. Patients with symptoms such as abdominal pain hours to days after a blow to the abdomen often have blunt abdominal organ injury. Any delay to definitive treatment increases

morbidity and/or mortality. It is imperative that early diagnosis and definitive therapy be provided.

■ MECHANISMS OF INJURY

Blunt abdominal injury most commonly occurs from motor vehicle crashes, motorcycle or bicycle crashes, all-terrain vehicle mishaps, falls from heights greater than 10 feet, and assaults with blows to the abdomen or stomping while lying on the ground or pedestrians struck by a vehicle. The history of the mechanism of injury obtained by either the patient or a prehospital provider is essential. Most patients restrained with a seatbelt who have a motor vehicle crash at speeds less than 60 miles per hour sustain no intra-abdominal injury; however, an unrestrained victim of a motor vehicle crash who is ejected and thrown 10 feet, striking a fixed object, has a significant chance of having an intra-abdominal injury. Likewise, pedestrians and motorcycle or bicycle riders who are struck by a vehicle or thrown from their device are more susceptible to total body and/or abdominal trauma. Injuries sustained from a fall greater than a second story depend on the type of surface struck and the position of the patient on impact. Those patients who land on their back are more apt to have retroperitoneal or solid organ injuries. Those patients who are assaulted and struck in the abdomen may have rupture of a hollow viscous or, as those with stomping, may have injury to a retroperitoneal organ such as the pancreas.

■ INITIAL ASSESSMENT

The initial assessment of the patient with blunt abdominal trauma often is compromised by the patient's inability to provide an accurate history of the mechanism of injury or participate in the physical examination. Such patients may be compromised by the presence of mind-altering drugs or alcohol, a psychiatric illness, associated acute head injury, hypoxia from associated thoracic injury, or hypotension from bleeding either externally from lacerations or internally from associated thoracic or fracture blood loss and even occasionally from intra-abdominal bleeding. These patients are compromised and unable to participate in obtaining an accurate history as well as a physical examination. However, the patients who are alert, oriented, communicative, and cooperative and who have no substances in their system, no pain or tenderness in their abdomen, and a normal FAST (focused assessment with sonography for trauma) examination rarely have an intra-abdominal or retroperitoneal injury and do not require further abdominal imaging.

Patients who have distracting injuries, such as an extremity fracture, may not appreciate pain in the abdomen. Fortunately, nearly all of these patients who require operative intervention for intra-abdominal injury will demonstrate a sign or symptom within 1 hour of arrival. Patients with associated injuries should be treated for their injuries but continue to be observed for possible delayed presentation of blunt abdominal injury. A general surgeon who is serving as a trauma surgeon should admit these patients and continue to observe them for possible intra-abdominal injury while their associated extremity fractures, facial fractures, or head injury is being treated.

■ HYPOTENSIVE OR UNSTABLE PATIENT

Patients with a systolic blood pressure less than 90 mm of mercury or who develop hypotension after arrival should receive at least 2 L of intravenous fluid followed by a blood transfusion if they remain hypotensive. The rapid cursory examination is helpful in determining the cause of hypotension. The examination should begin at the neck. The hypotensive patient with neck vein distension has either a tension pneumothorax or a pericardial tamponade. Deviation of the trachea is indicative of a tension pneumothorax. An ultrasound of the pericardium would detect a pericardial effusion or a pericardial tamponade. A focused ultrasound examination of the abdomen would indicate if there were free blood in the peritoneal cavity. In our experience, it is rare to have hypotension from bleeding in the abdomen without some distension and without a positive FAST examination. The third reason for hypotension would be spinal cord injury. These patients often have bradycardia or a normal pulse in the presence of hypotension. If the patients are awake and alert, they are unable to move their legs on command. The patient who is compromised and/or unresponsive should have a rectal examination before drugs given for intubation, to determine if the patient has absent rectal tone and a spinal cord injury as a reason for their hypotension. External blood loss can be a fourth reason for hypotension. This is obvious but often not appreciated. Communication with pre-hospital providers can provide this information because they would have noted a significant blood loss at the scene. Last, there may be internal blood loss from associated fractures. A fractured rib results in one fourth of a unit of blood loss; a fractured humerus, one

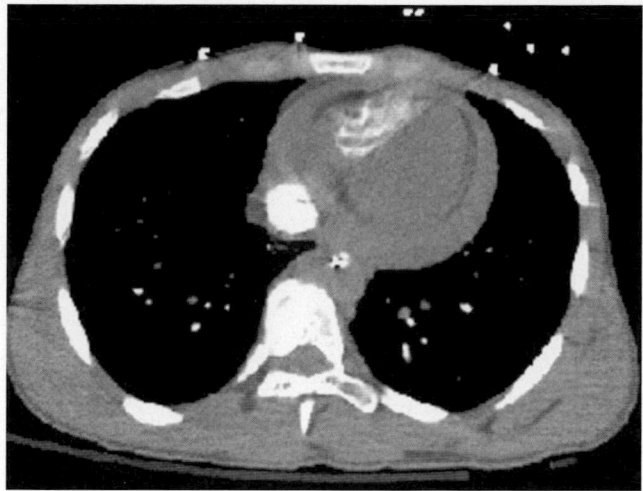

FIGURE 1 This 22-year-old victim of a motor vehicle crash was hypotensive with neck vein distension. FAST examination showed some fluid in the pericardium as well as in the abdomen. Computed tomography scan shows fluid with a density of blood in the pericardial sac. Laparotomy was performed for suspected hemoperitoneum and revealed an enlarged purple liver with edema and ascites. A midline sternotomy revealed a hemopericardium resulting from rupture of the atrial appendage.

quarter of a unit of blood loss; a fracture of the tibia/fibula, one half of a unit of blood loss; a fracture of the femur, 2 units of blood loss, and a fracture of the pelvis, approximately 4 units of blood loss. External and internal blood loss should be replaced as one is considering the abdomen as the source of bleeding. A tension pneumothorax should be treated with a chest tube, and associated fractures should be splinted and a pelvic binder applied for an unstable pelvic fracture. A pericardial tamponade should be treated with a left anterior thoracotomy and pericardiotomy with evacuation of blood (Figure 1). There may be an associated atrial rupture, and the surgeon should be prepared to treat this injury. Once hypotension is controlled, the patient needs an abdominal evaluation, which depends on the treatment provided for the other conditions. If blood pressure can be corrected in the emergency department after placement of a chest tube for a tension pneumothorax or blood transfusion for associated external blood loss or fracture bleeding and the patient has an acceptable blood pressure, a computed tomography (CT) scan of the involved areas, including the abdomen, can further evaluate the patient for intra-abdominal injury.

■ STABLE, COMPROMISED PATIENT

The patient with stable vital signs who is unable to participate in examination is considered to be compromised. This may be due to head injury, drugs or alcohol, or mental status. If the patient is breathing adequately, there is no need for intubation. A routine chest x-ray should be obtained. The patient should provide urine for examination, or a Foley catheter should be placed. The surgeon is evaluating this patient to detect any injury that would indicate the need for immediate laparotomy. Such injuries include a rupture of the diaphragm, which can be detected on chest x-ray (Figure 2). Gross blood on urination or on placement of a Foley catheter may indicate injury to the urinary bladder. If gross blood is returned on placement of the Foley catheter, a cystogram can be done in the resuscitation room by insertion of 400 mL of contrast via the Foley catheter and obtaining a pelvic film. The bladder is then emptied, and another roentgenogram is obtained (Figure 3). Intraperitoneal rupture is evident by contrast extravasation into the free peritoneal cavity. Blunt rupture of the diaphragm and intraperitoneal rupture of the urinary bladder should lead to immediate laparotomy, where all other injuries of the

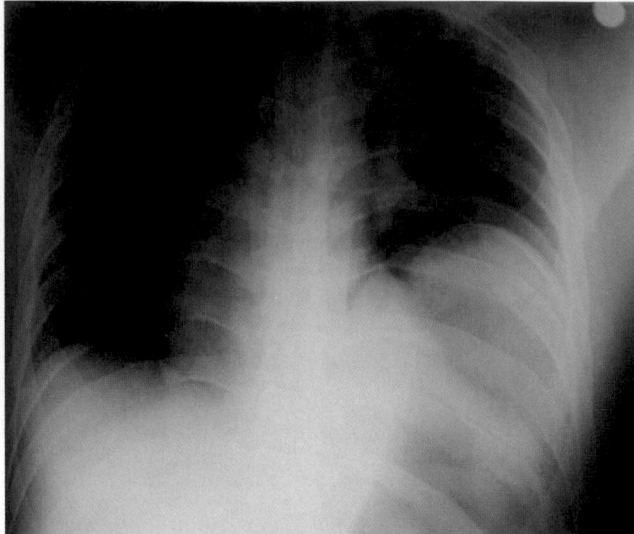

FIGURE 2 Chest x-ray in this 32-year-old victim of a motor vehicle crash shows rupture of the left hemidiaphragm. He also had three left rib fractures and a left femur fracture. Immediate laparotomy was done for repair of the diaphragm.

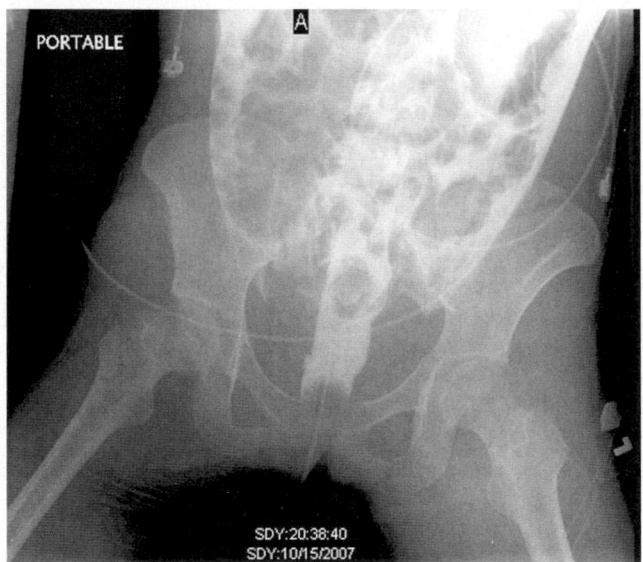

FIGURE 3 This 56-year-old victim of a motor vehicle crash had pubic rami fracture. He was unresponsive with a head injury. Foley catheter returned gross blood. The cystogram showed extravasation of dye throughout the peritoneal cavity, and he had immediate laparotomy for an intraperitoneal rupture of the urinary bladder.

abdomen can be assessed. In the absence of diaphragm rupture or intraperitoneal bladder rupture, an ultrasound could be helpful in detecting free fluid. The definitive test would be a CT scan of the abdomen to evaluate for organ injury. Although an ultrasound may have been positive, it is not definitive in knowing the organ injured. There rarely is free air in the peritoneal cavity indicating bowel rupture. The CT scan of the abdomen should be done with intravenous contrast, which assists in assessment of abdominal vasculature and perfusion of organs. A Foley catheter should be occluded to allow the bladder to fill with contrast to detect any extravasation from a bladder rupture. The surgeon must continue to remember that significant intra-abdominal injuries can and do occur without evidence of injury on CT scan; however, nearly all patients with

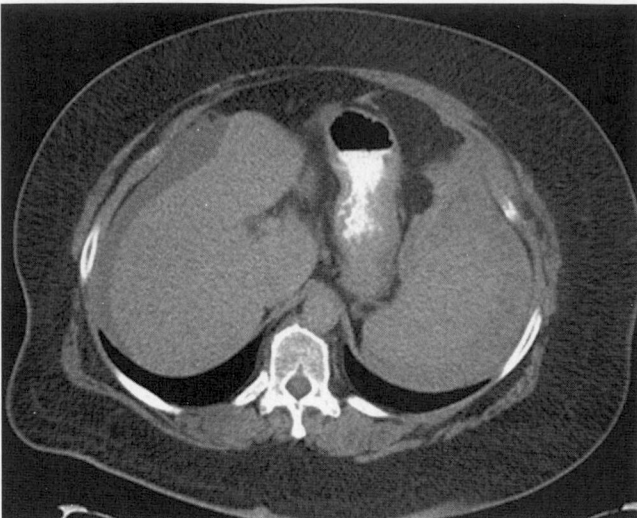

FIGURE 4 Computed tomography scan shows blood surrounding the liver and the spleen and a grade 2 splenic injury. The scan was done 7 days after a motor vehicle crash when she complained of abdominal and chest pain, weakness, and ecchymosis of the left chest. Hemoglobin was 7.8 g percent.

intra-abdominal injury will manifest some sign or symptom within 12 hours of arrival at the hospital.

■ NONOPERATIVE THERAPY OF ABDOMINAL ORGAN INJURY

The majority of patients with a positive FAST and/or CT scan of the abdomen showing free fluid do not require a therapeutic laparotomy. Even major injuries to the liver, spleen, or kidney can be treated nonoperatively if vital signs remain stable and no red blood cell replacement is necessary. The presence of free fluid in the abdomen without evidence of liver or spleen injury suggests mesenteric injury. The patient needs to be carefully observed for development of increased abdominal pain, tenderness, or tachycardia, indicating bowel ischemia. Likewise, patients with evidence of splenic or liver injury who are stable initially do not require angiographic embolization, including those patients who demonstrate a "blush" on CT scan. Even patients with grade 3 and 4 injury can be observed successfully if they remain stable and do not require blood transfusion. These patients can be observed successfully on an acute care ward, given diet on the second hospital day and discharged by the third day if they remain stable and without peritoneal signs.

There should be heightened concern for intra-abdominal injury in those patients with documented injury to surrounding structures, such as the lower ribs, pubic rami, or hematuria of renal origin. These patients have had significant impact and may have pain or tenderness from the surrounding structures. An intercostal rib block proximal to the rib fracture will alleviate pain and confirm that the pain is of somatic origin. This facilitates the abdominal examination. The subset of patients with coagulopathy from antiplatelet medications or anticoagulants should receive 2 units of fresh frozen plasma and further correction of coagulopathy as indicated by the international normalized ratio (INR).

Any patient who develops increased abdominal pain and/or tenderness or a fall in hemoglobin during observation needs prompt laparotomy. Most likely, the patient has an expanding hematoma that has ruptured (Figures 4 and 5).

■ INDICATIONS FOR OPERATION

The patient who has a period of transient hypotension that responds to fluid, an associated head, chest, or pelvic injury, which makes

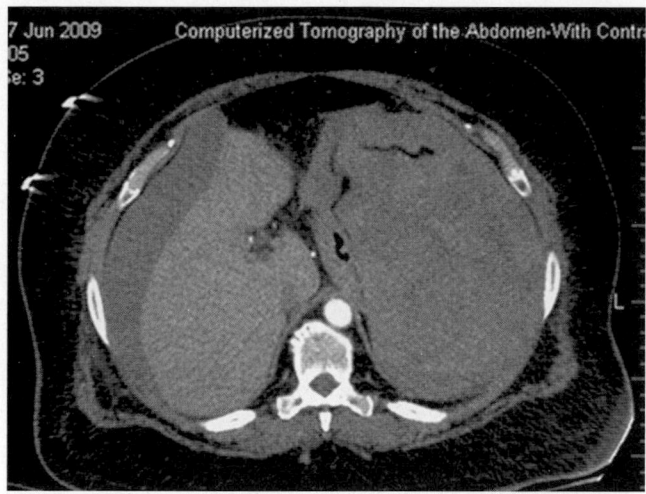

FIGURE 5 Computed tomography scan was done 24 hours later when the patient complained of increased pain and required blood for hypotension. There is an enlargement of the splenic hematoma, which was treated with splenectomy.

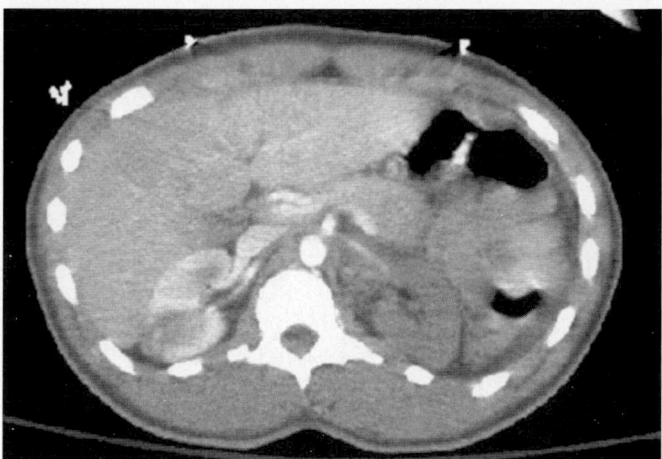

FIGURE 6 Computed tomography (CT) scan of the abdomen was done in a 24-year-old pedestrian struck by a motor vehicle and thrown into the air. There is a left kidney present with no evidence of perfusion, indicating renal artery occlusion. She had hematuria. The scan was obtained 4 hours after injury. She was observed and had normal renal function. A repeat CT scan 3 months later showed perfusion of that left kidney, and she never developed hypertension.

examination difficult, and the presence of some free fluid in the abdomen on CT scan or FAST examination, complicates decision making. A prolonged period of observation before a therapeutic laparotomy is done potentiates the development of multiorgan failure. Furthermore, a patient undergoing operative therapy of head or extremity injury cannot be observed for the development of peritoneal signs. A laparoscopic evaluation of the intra-abdominal organs while the patient is under anesthesia for associated injuries could detect a rupture of the diaphragm or identify fluid in the abdomen that is suspicious for bowel or gallbladder injury. It rarely will add anything to the CT examination and is of no value in evaluating retroperitoneal organs.

Retroperitoneal Organ Injury

Kidney Injury

The kidneys are the most common retroperitoneal solid organ injured. The kidney is the source of hematuria if the bladder is intact. This hematuria usually resolves within the first 48 hours. Rarely, there is total disruption of the kidney, and the patient has abdominal distension and hypotension, indicating the need for an immediate laparotomy. A retroperitoneal bleed from a ruptured kidney with a hematoma that approaches the level of the anterior abdominal wall requires exploration and almost always a nephrectomy to control bleeding and correct hypotension. The contrast CT scan is best at assessing renal injury in the stable patient who usually has hematuria. Even patients with severe injuries, including grades 3 and 4 renal disruption and with contrast extravasation, can be treated nonoperatively. Occasionally, a CT scan will show the presence of a kidney but no perfusion, indicating renal artery occlusion (Figure 6). We have observed a number of these patients for whom this diagnosis has been made several hours after injury, and the patients were treated nonoperatively; late hypertension did not develop, and late imaging studies usually showed extensive collateralization with preserved renal perfusion. Extraperitoneal bladder injuries with contrast extravasation can be treated with catheter drainage.

Pancreatic and Duodenal Injury

Injuries to the pancreas and duodenum are more apt to occur after crushing injury to the epigastric area, such as stomping. The CT scan is the best means of detecting such injuries to the duodenum by the presence of retroperitoneal air and hematoma. The CT scan is less helpful with pancreatic injuries. If there is a suspicion of pancreatic

injury, a serum amylase may be helpful if a progressive rise is seen at 6 and 12 hours after injury. If the CT scan suggests a pancreatic injury in a patient with no abdominal symptoms, an endoscopic retrograde cholangiopancreatography (ERCP) should be obtained to define duct anatomy. If the ERCP is normal, then no further treatment is necessary. If there is extravasation on ERCP, then operative therapy is required. The patient who has abdominal pain and tenderness and a diagnosis of pancreatic injury on CT scan also should be explored. The pancreatic injury is almost always at the body of the pancreas, where it was compressed between the anterior abdominal wall and the spine. Complete disruption of the pancreas at this level is treated best with distal pancreatectomy and usually splenectomy with oversewing of the proximal pancreas and drainage. Contusions to other areas of the pancreas without obvious total pancreatic disruption should be treated with drainage and placement of a feeding jejunostomy.

Aorta and Iliac Artery Injury

Injuries to retroperitoneal vascular structures are rare but can occur with blunt trauma. Stretching of the iliac arteries with pelvic fracture can lead to an intimal flap and thrombosis, which will be seen with pelvic hematoma and absent pulse. Angiography with stenting of the aorta and iliac vessels would be the preferred management for these injuries.

Intraperitoneal Solid Organ Injury

Liver and Spleen

Injuries to the liver and spleen almost always are treated nonoperatively. The patient who remains hypotensive with abdominal distension and requires blood transfusion for liver or spleen bleeding is treated best with immediate laparotomy. A bleeding liver wound would be treated with immediate packing, whereas a bleeding spleen would be treated with splenectomy. There is no place for attempts at splenic salvage in the hypotensive patient undergoing laparotomy for splenic bleeding. The bleeding liver wound is assessed after blood pressure has been restored by anesthesia with blood replacement. Devascularized segments of the liver are removed. If bleeding from the liver can be controlled by approximating the injured liver, then sutures are placed with a blunt needle and 2-0 chromic suture to hold the liver in place. We have found that occasional packing alone will

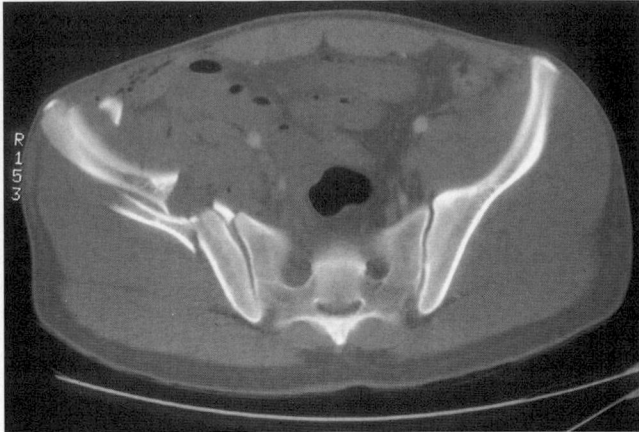

FIGURE 7 The computed tomography scan was obtained 2 hours after injury in a 24-year-old male crushed between two vehicles. There is a right pelvic fracture. There is no evidence of bowel injury. He developed tachycardia and lower abdominal tenderness over the next 12 hours.

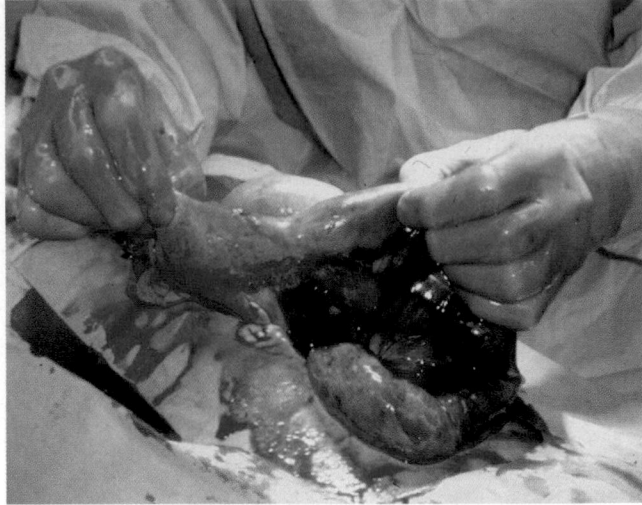

FIGURE 8 Laparotomy revealed free blood in the peritoneal cavity with disruption of the mesentery of the terminal ileum with necrosis of one foot of distal small bowel.

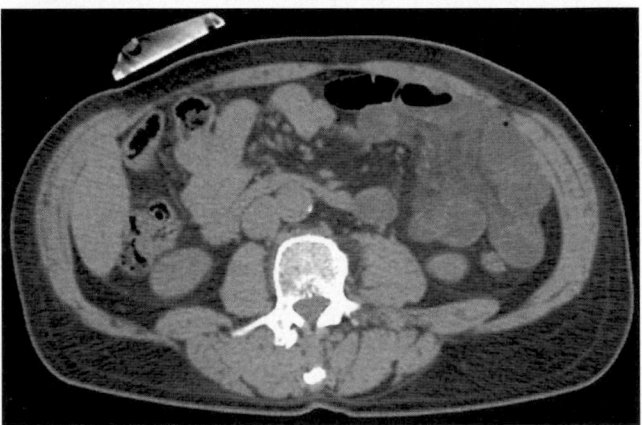

FIGURE 9 This computed tomography scan was done in a 58-year-old male with a fairly sudden onset of severe left upper quadrant abdominal pain. He had a bruise on his left anterior abdominal wall from a door that fell on him 4 days previously. CT scan shows some peculiar fat stranding in the left upper quadrant.

control liver bleeding. In such cases, the packs are left in place with temporary abdominal wound closure and correction of hypothermia and coagulopathy performed in a critical care unit. The abdomen is reopened in 36 to 48 hours and the packs removed. Almost always, bleeding is controlled, although the liver can be repacked. Hepatic artery ligation should be considered if arterial bleeding can be controlled with temporary artery occlusion. Angiography with embolization may be of help if arterial bleeding is identified. A drain always should be placed for possible bile extravasation in patients with large liver wounds. Although most patients with blunt injury to the liver or spleen do not require laparotomy or angiographic embolization, they do require careful observation. If there has been any hypotension, the patient is observed in the critical care unit. Coagulopathy from medications must be corrected. Stable patients can be observed on the acute care ward. Any patient who develops increased abdominal pain, hypotension, or the need for transfusion should have laparotomy for ongoing bleeding.

Hollow Viscus Injury

Blunt rupture of the small intestine most commonly occurs just distal to the ligament of Treitz or proximal to the ileocecal valve, although it can occur anywhere within the small intestine. Most often, there is a rent in the mesentery of the small intestine with minimal fluid in the abdomen, which leads to bowel necrosis from ischemia (Figure 7). These patients develop intense pain, tenderness, and tachycardia by 36 hours after injury. Laparotomy and/or laparoscopy is indicated, even though the CT scan done on admission may not have identified an injury (Figure 8). A mesenteric hematoma can occur after a blow to the abdomen, and the patient may have a normal or equivocal CT scan on admission (Figure 9). This hematoma can cause bowel wall necrosis, which may occur 24 to 72 hours after injury (Figure 10). Full-thickness gastric perforations are rare but usually have free fluid and a significant amount of free air on the CT scan.

Blunt injury to the colon mesentery, or partial thickness rupture of the colon wall, can lead to subsequent colon wall necrosis. These patients usually have associated injuries but will experience delayed pain, tenderness, and tachycardia. We strongly support trauma surgeon involvement and care of these patients with blunt injury until they have return of bowel function and are able to tolerate diet.

Cryptic Injuries

Certain injuries to intra-abdominal organs are rare. These include liver injury with late hemobilia, contusion of the fundus of the gallbladder wall with ischemia, and delayed rupture and extrahepatic bile duct rupture. Hemobilia usually occurs when a major liver injury

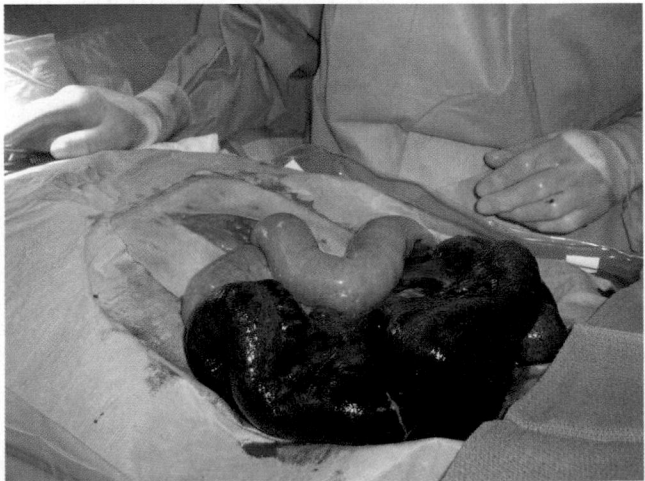

FIGURE 10 Laparotomy revealed 3 feet of dead small bowel because of a mesenteric hematoma. This was treated with resection and end-to-end anastomosis.

develops a contained hematoma that decompresses approximately 4 to 14 days after abdominal injury into the biliary system, leading to pain and hematemesis. The diagnosis is made by hepatic angiography, and treatment can be provided with angiographic embolization.

Although most gallbladder injuries have rupture of the dome with early peritonitis or avulsion from the hepatic fossa and hemoperitoneum, some patients develop an ischemic contusion of the fundus, which ruptures 2 to 4 days later when the intraluminal pressure rises after diet is reinstituted. The patient develops bilious ascites, tenderness, and jaundice. There may be extrahepatic bile duct rupture. Some patients have an isolated bile duct rupture, especially to the left hepatic duct with no associated injuries. Minimal findings are present initially. Later, jaundice and bilious ascites may occur. An ERCP will define the injury and guide treatment. Any bile staining of the retroperitoneal structures in the area of the bile duct should be evaluated carefully at the time of laparotomy for other intra-abdominal injuries.

■ ADJUNCTS TO MANAGEMENT OF BLUNT ABDOMINAL INJURY

The trauma surgeon performing a laparotomy for blunt organ injury should be aware of all other injuries. We often place a feeding jejunostomy in any patient with associated head, spinal cord, or thoracic injury who undergoes a laparotomy for abdominal injury (Figure 11). Likewise, the patient with extensive perineal laceration and associated pelvic fractures will have a colostomy performed at the initial laparotomy. If the liver is packed for bleeding or if the abdominal organs are very edematous, the abdominal wall can be closed with a temporary pack (Figure 12). We prefer to place #2 nylon sutures 2 inches apart and 2 inches from the wound edge (Figure 13). The viscera are covered with parachute silk or rayon cloth and Kerlix gauze placed over the cloth and secured in place by tying the sutures (Figure 14). This keeps the viscera below the peritoneum (Figure 15). Once diuresis occurs and edema resolves, the abdominal wall pack can be removed and the fascia closed primarily without tension.

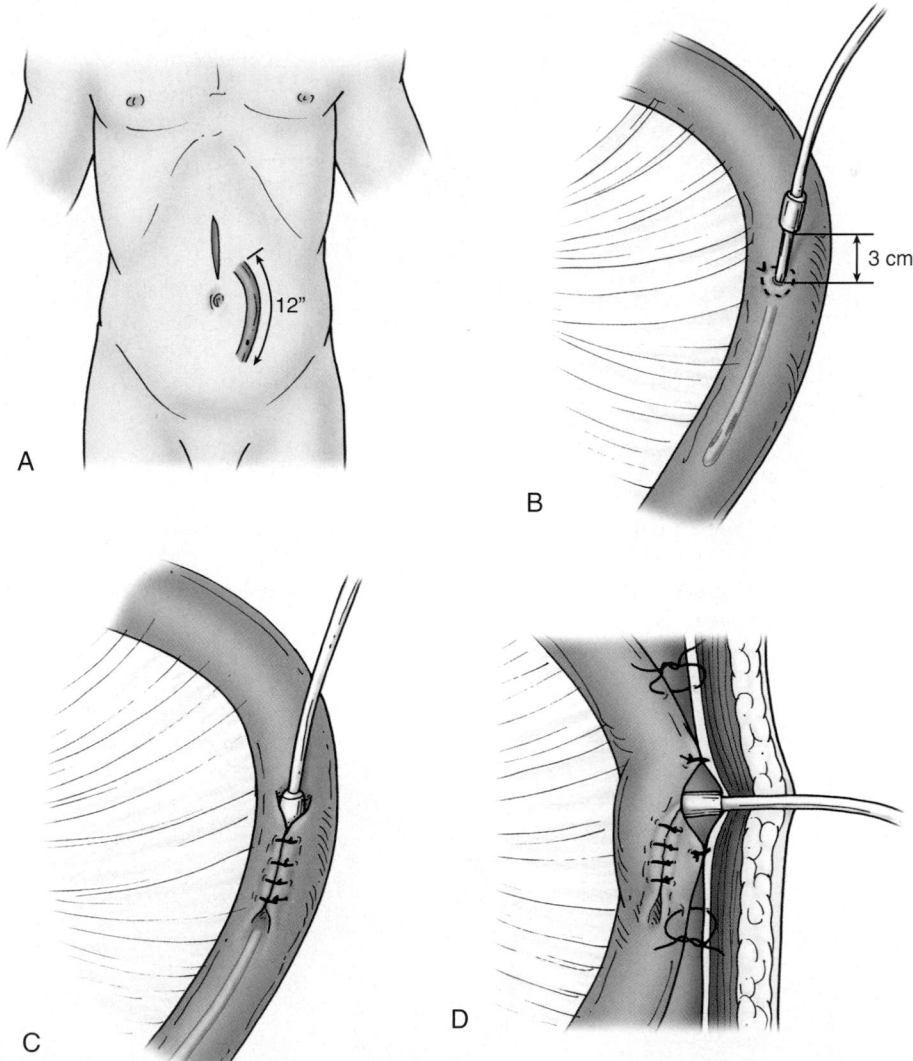

FIGURE 11 A feeding jejunostomy is placed at the time of laparotomy for blunt abdominal injury in any patient with severe associated head, spinal cord, or thoracic injury in whom prolonged ventilatory support is anticipated. We prefer to use a Tenckhoff (Quinton Instrument Company, Seattle, WA) catheter with extra holes placed about 12 inches distal to the ligament of Treitz. A 3-0 chromic suture secures the catheter 3 cm from the cuff. A Witzel tunnel is performed, and the tube is placed through the anterior abdominal wall with a number 14 Cook Catheter introducer set. The cuff is placed between the bowel wall and the peritoneum.

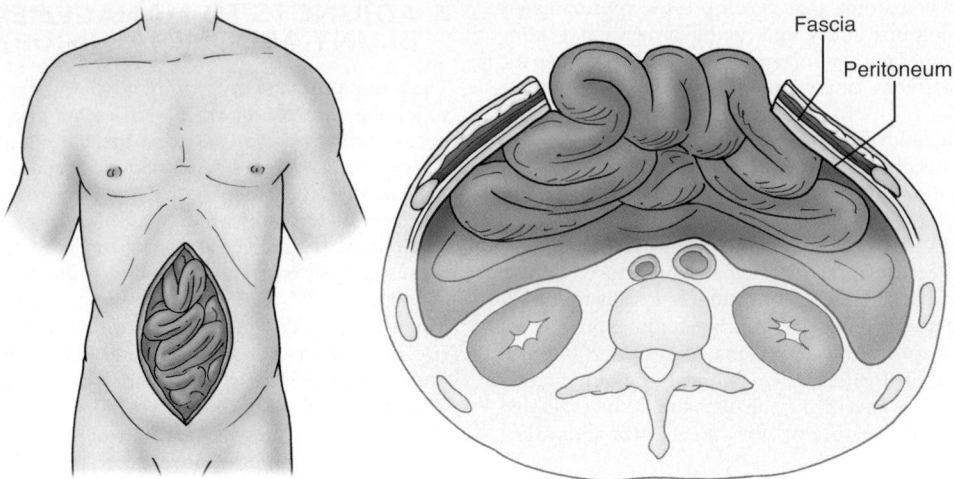

FIGURE 12 Damage control laparotomy is done when there is the need to pack intra-abdominal organs to control hemostasis or when the bowel is too edematous to provide primary closure without tension.

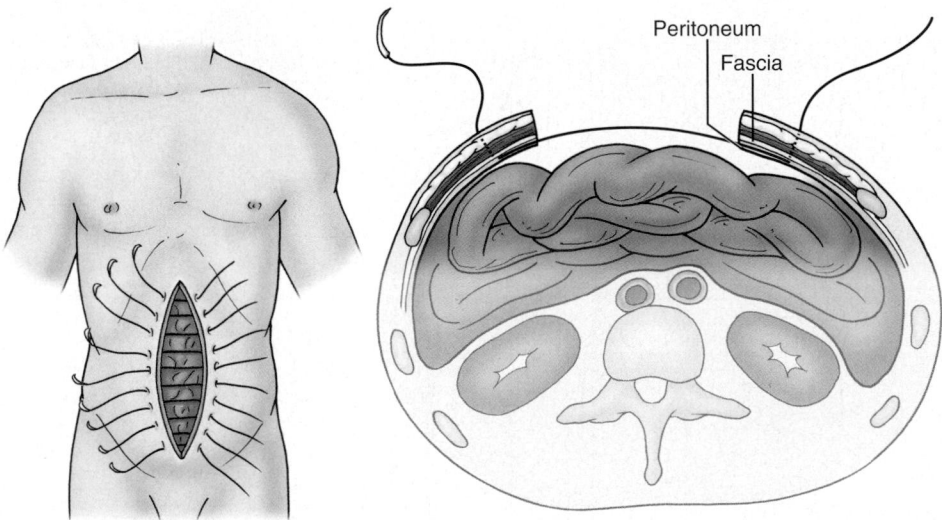

FIGURE 13 #2 nylon retention sutures are placed 1 inch from the wound margin, full thickness through skin fat fascia but staying anterior to the peritoneum. The sutures are placed 2 inches apart.

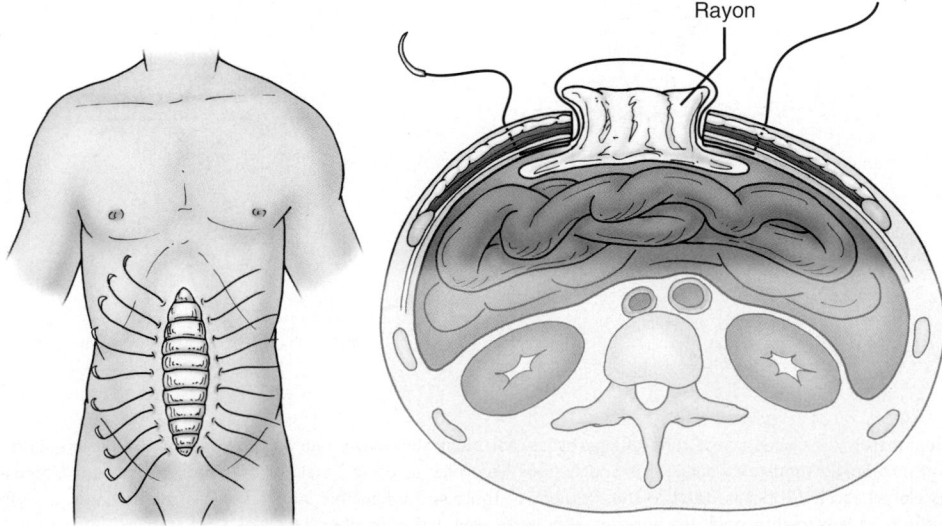

FIGURE 14 Rayon cloth or parachute silk is placed over the viscera and beneath the abdominal wall, extending 2.5 cm underneath the peritoneum to protect the bowels from the sutures. Kerlix or fluff gauze is placed over the rayon cloth, and the sutures are tied so that the abdominal wall pack acts as a tamponade.

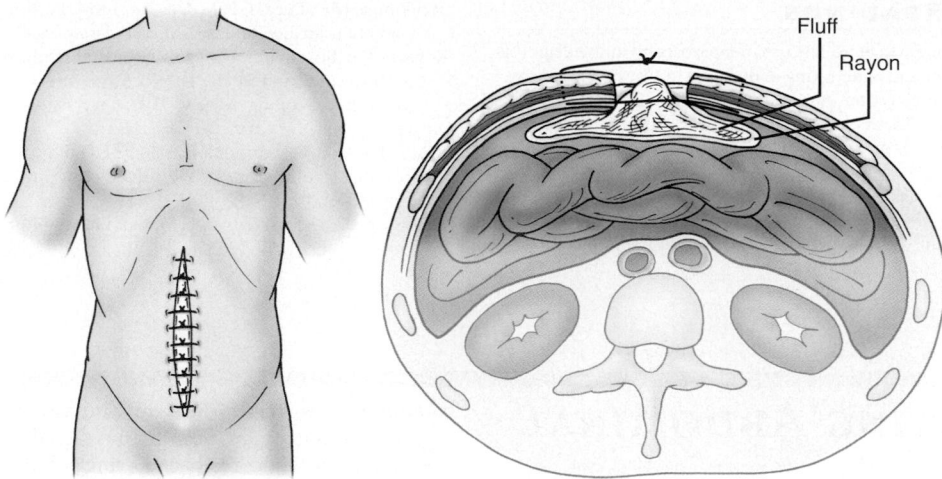

Fluff

Rayon

FIGURE 15 The wound margins may be widely separated, but it is important to keep the viscera below the level of the peritoneum. This technique can be performed rapidly and is inexpensive.

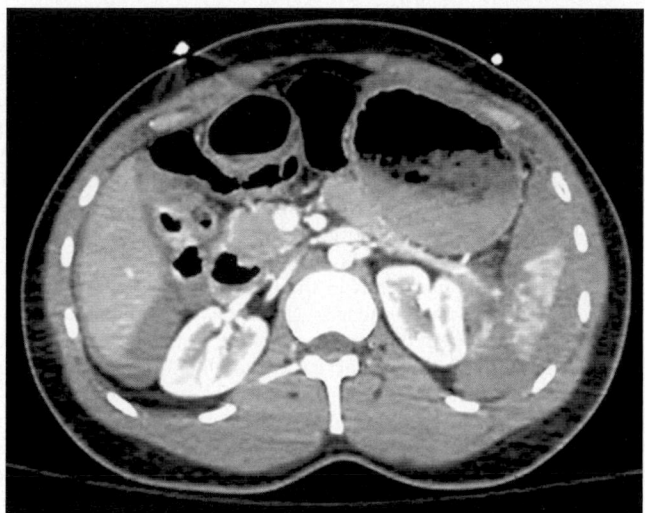

FIGURE 16 Computed tomography scan was done for a patient in a motor vehicle crash showing active extravasation of blood from a splenic injury. He had angiographic embolization. After embolization, he developed fever, tachycardia, and left upper quadrant pain.

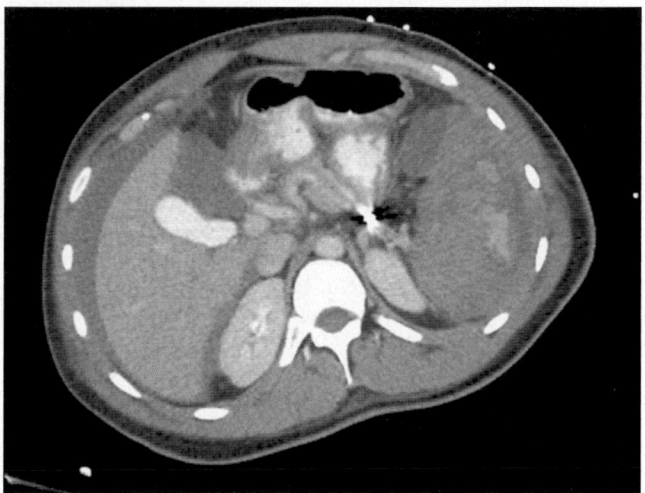

FIGURE 17 A repeat computed tomography scan done on day 6 for fever and tachycardia showed marked enlargement of the spleen with necrosis. He later formed an abscess, which grew proteus.

■ COMPLICATIONS ASSOCIATED WITH BLUNT ABDOMINAL INJURY

Nonoperative management of blunt liver injury with associated hemoperitoneum can lead to a systemic inflammatory response if the extravasated blood is mixed with bile. This is totally unpredictable but should be considered if the patient develops fever, tachycardia, and progressive ileus. This usually is manifested 3 to 4 days after the initial injury. Treatment consists of a laparotomy with evacuation of clots, irrigation of the peritoneal cavity, and placement of subhepatic drains. Any bile fistula will close in 2 to 3 weeks. This entity will occur in less than 10% of the patients with blunt liver injury. We have become disenchanted with the use of angiography and embolization for blunt splenic injury. The stable patient who has a "blush" or a false aneurysm noted on CT scan of the abdomen often is referred for angiographic embolization (Figure 16). Unfortunately, embolization can lead to necrosis of the spleen (Figure 17). This usually occurs between 2 and 4 days after embolization and results in fever, tachy-

cardia, and increased abdominal pain. When this occurs, splenectomy should be performed.

Missed injuries of solid organs as well as hollow viscus organs can occur, particularly in those patients with associated injuries that are more obvious. The abdomen can never be "cleared" with a CT scan of the abdomen but requires repeated evaluations and is never cleared completely until the patient has stable vital signs and is able to tolerate diet with normal bowel function.

Necrotizing fasciitis with wound dehiscence and possible evisceration can occur after laparotomy for blunt abdominal injury. Often the viscera are edematous and distended. The abdominal wound is closed with tension. This leads to ischemia of the fascia, necrosis, dehiscence, and possible evisceration. The temporary abdominal pack is recommended for those patients who fit the description of distended, edematous bowel with loss of compliance of the abdominal wall. These patients require a damage control procedure with correction of hypothermia and coagulopathy and acidosis. Once diuresis has occurred, the abdomen easily can be closed.

SUGGESTED READINGS

Johnson JJ, Garwe T, Raines AR, et al. The use of laparoscopy in the diagnosis and treatment of blunt and penetrating abdominal injuries: 10-year experience at a level 1 trauma center. *Am J Surg.* 2013;205:317-321.

Jones EL, Stovall RT, Jones TS, et al. Intra-abdominal injury following blunt trauma becomes clinically apparent within 9 hours. *J Trauma Acute Care Surg.* 2014;76:1020-1023.

Ledgerwood AM, Lucas CE. Postoperative complications of abdominal trauma. *Surg Clin North Am.* 1990;70:715-731.

Lucas CE. 21st century approach to splenic injury. *Panam J Trauma Crit Care Emerg Surg.* 2013;2:116-125.

McGonigal MD, Lucas CE, Ledgerwood AM. Feeding jejunostomy in patients who are critically ill. *Surg Gynecol Obstet.* 1989;168:275-277.

Roberts DJ, Bobrovitz N, Zygun DA, et al. Indications for use of damage control surgery and damage control interventions in civilian trauma patients: a scoping review. *J Trauma Acute Care Surg.* 2015;78:1187-1196.

Rostas J, Cason B, Simmons J, et al. The validity of abdominal examination in blunt trauma patients with distracting injuries. *J Trauma Acute Care Surg.* 2015;78:1095-1101.

Shalhub S, Starnes BW, Tran NT, et al. Blunt abdominal aortic injury. *J Vasc Surg.* 2012;55:1277-1285.

PENETRATING ABDOMINAL TRAUMA

Patricia Ayoung-Chee, MD, MPH, and H. Leon Pachter, MD, FACS

Historically, the initial management of penetrating abdominal trauma was nonoperative. Not surprising, this standard of care was associated with a high mortality rate, and a change in practice mandated emergent exploratory laparotomy. However, the negative laparotomy rate has been reported to be as high as 70% and associated complications (including iatrogenic injuries, postoperative ileus, evisceration, small bowel obstruction, surgical site infections, incisional hernias, and death) occurred in 8% to 41% of those receiving unnecessary laparotomy. With increasing experience in nonoperative management or "selective conservatism" (first published in 1960) and the emergence of improved imaging technology and more widespread use of bedside ultrasound, mandatory exploration is no longer the standard of care.

INITIAL MANAGEMENT

As for all patients with traumatic injuries, treatment begins with the primary survey, ABCDE—airway, breathing, circulation, disability, and exposure (Advanced Trauma Life Support protocol). For patients with penetrating injuries to the abdomen, circulation and exposure are particularly important. The unstable patient or the patient who has peritonitis should be taken directly to the operating room, as the probability of significant organ injury is high. For patients with penetrating thoracoabdominal injury, life-threatening injuries such as tension pneumothorax or pericardial tamponade may occur. A high index of suspicion is necessary, and these injuries must be diagnosed and addressed immediately in the unstable patient. In addition, patients with missile injuries (including gunshot wounds) may have simultaneous spinal cord injuries, depending on bullet trajectory. These patients may be diagnosed on initial neurologic examination and may have a component of neurogenic shock. However, in the trauma patient, hemorrhage always should be the presumed cause of hemodynamic instability until proven otherwise. The stable patient, especially when asymptomatic, can be observed and imaging modalities can be used in order to determine the need for further invasive procedures.

Suspicion for injury plays an important role in the use of the selective conservatism strategy. The likelihood of intra-abdominal injury after a gunshot wound is greater than if the patient was stabbed with a small pocket knife. Gunshot wounds are associated with a 90% incidence of intra-abdominal injury requiring operative intervention. However, depending on the caliber of the bullet and the patient's abdominal girth, there is a possibility of a tangential trajectory and no intra-abdominal injury. Other considerations with gunshot wound injuries include the significant associated blast effect, resulting in injuries to organs near but not directly in the bullet's path, and the multiple pellets contained in a single shotgun round, with varying degrees of spread or scatter resulting in multiple injuries.

In contrast, fewer than 50% of stab wounds are associated with intra-abdominal injuries that require operative intervention. If hemodynamically normal, many of these patients can be managed with initial contrast-enhanced computed tomographic (CT) scan or observation and serial abdominal examinations. Although details of the object used to injure the patient are helpful in assessing the likelihood of intra-abdominal injury, such data are not always readily available at the time of presentation. Local wound exploration with local anesthetic can be performed in the emergency department and can be helpful in determining if the anterior abdominal fascia was violated; however, this requires a co-operative patient and may require a substantial lengthening of the wound in the obese patient. The location of the stab wound is important in determining the likelihood of injury and the organs involved. Anterior abdominal stab wounds have the highest likelihood of resulting in intra-abdominal injury. For wounds in the right upper quadrant, within the thoracoabdominal boundaries (Figure 1), the highest risk of injury is to the liver and diaphragm, which in a stable patient can be managed with observation. For back and flank wounds, there is further decrease in risk for intra-abdominal injury, and imaging modalities can be used to evaluate for injuries and the need for operative intervention. Stab wounds to the left upper quadrant place the stomach, spleen, and diaphragm at high risk for injury. Of these three, a diaphragmatic injury is the most difficult to diagnose, even on CT, and a diagnostic laparoscopy may be indicated.

As previously mentioned, nonoperative management is appropriate in specific clinical scenarios. Stable patients with abdominal stab wounds and no peritoneal signs can be observed for 24 hours with serial abdominal examinations. This treatment algorithm has been found to be reliable in detecting significant intra-abdominal injuries without increased mortality or morbidity. In published series, 3% to 10% of patients initially managed nonoperatively required operative intervention, but all developed signs and symptoms within 24 hours, underwent exploration, and had uneventful recoveries. Patients who do not develop any concerning findings can be discharged with a much shorter length of stay than if they had undergone a nontherapeutic laparotomy (24 hours vs 5 days on average).

For patients with abdominal gunshot wounds with tangential trajectories and no peritoneal signs, nonoperative management can be used as well. The incidence of patients with abdominal gunshot wounds and no intra-abdominal injuries ranges from 14% to 33% in published studies. The largest study to date was published by Velmahos and colleagues, with 792 patients treated nonoperatively from 1993 to 2000. Seven percent required delayed therapeutic laparotomy and five patients had complications thought to be secondary to the delay in diagnosis and treatment. The sensitivity of initial physical examination in identifying patients without intra-abdominal injury requiring surgery was 92.8%. Projecting bullet trajectories can be difficult, and patients who are stable with minimal abdominal

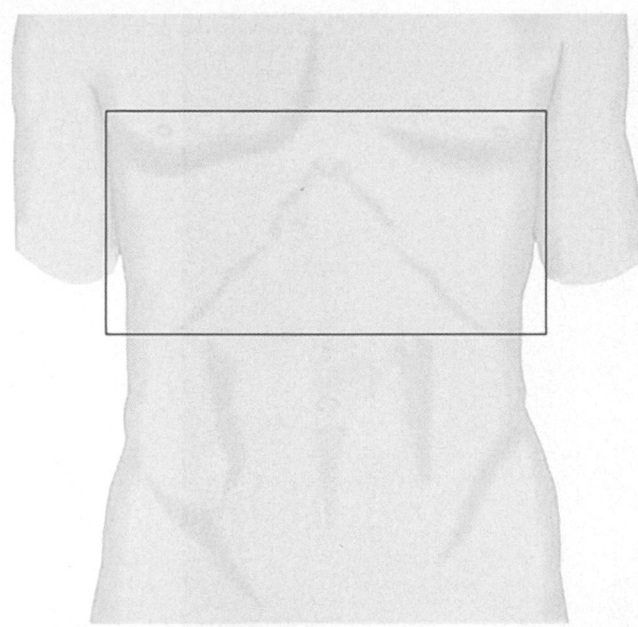

FIGURE 1 Anterior boundaries of the thoracoabdominal region.

BOX 1: Indications for Nonoperative Management in Penetrating Abdominal Trauma

1. Hemodynamically stable
2. Minimal or no abdominal tenderness
3. No neurologic deficits
   Patients who are unstable or have peritoneal signs on physical examination should undergo laparotomy.

From Como JJ, Bokhari F, Chiu WC, et al. Practice management guidelines for selective nonoperative management of penetrating abdominal trauma. *J Trauma.* 2010;68:721-733.

---

injuries can undergo further imaging to assist in proper patient selection for nonoperative management (Box 1).

CT imaging is highly recommended as a part of nonoperative management in penetrating abdominal trauma, especially in patients with gunshot wounds, altered mental status due to traumatic brain injury or intoxication, and otherwise unreliable examinations (e.g., spinal cord injury, intoxicated, or sedated). If CT findings confirm that the stab wound or bullet trajectory was completely extraperitoneal, the patient can be discharged from the emergency department (Figure 2). In one series that evaluated patients with abdominal gunshot wounds selected for initial nonoperative management, CT had a 90.5% sensitivity and a 96.0% specificity for intra-abdominal injury requiring surgical intervention. One downside of nonoperative management is the need for an experienced clinician and improved sensitivity with the same clinical team examining the patient over 24 hours. However, the benefits of this management plan are not insignificant and Dr. Shaftan's conclusions from 1960 are still appropriate today: "The application of trained surgical judgment rather than dogma is the more rational and intelligent approach to the management of abdominal injury."

In trauma patients, hemorrhagic shock still is considered the leading cause of preventable death. Recent paradigm changes promote early transfusion of red blood cells and an increased ratio of plasma and platelets to red blood cells, resulting in decreased mortality. Many trauma centers have instituted a massive transfusion protocol to help with implementation of these practices. However, modern definitions of massive transfusion are in flux and the optimal ratio of products to be transfused is still being studied. The addition of tranexamic acid (TXA) to the protocol can further reduce the number of units transfused and the risk of death in trauma patients with hemorrhagic shock. TXA is a synthetic amino acid that inhibits fibrinolysis by blocking lysine receptors on plasminogen. However, TXA is associated with thrombotic complications, which are increased in patients who receive the initial transfusion more than 3 hours after injury.

Fluid-restricted or hypotensive resuscitation is the practice of minimizing infusion of intravenous (IV) fluid (either crystalloid or blood products) in bleeding patients until hemostasis is achieved. Although the main goal of resuscitation in hemorrhagic shock is to maintain tissue perfusion, elevated blood pressures may worsen bleeding. Some studies demonstrate decreased morbidity and complications (e.g., acute renal failure, acute respiratory distress syndrome) with delayed fluid administration, and some data only show noninferiority. It is also unclear if the intervention should be a goal fluid volume or if resuscitation to a target systolic blood pressure (typically 70 to 90 mm Hg) is better. Further studies are underway and hopefully will answer some of these questions.

■ DIAGNOSTIC ADJUNCTS

Focused assessment with sonography for trauma (FAST) uses point-of-care ultrasound to look for free fluid in the abdomen and pericardium. It requires a portable ultrasound machine, which is usually readily available, and can be performed rapidly. Recently, the FAST examination has been expanded to include evaluation of the thoracic cavity for hemothorax or pneumothorax (eFAST). Like all ultrasound technology, it is a user-dependent test with excellent sensitivity in the pleural and pericardial views but only 20% to 60% sensitivity in the abdominal views. Depending on the experience of the examiner, the amount of free fluid required for a positive abdominal FAST can range from as little as 130 mL to more than 500 mL. Its true added benefit is seen in the unstable patient with a penetrating thoracoabdominal wound; it can help to diagnose life-threatening injuries in the thoracic cavity, such as pericardial tamponade or tension pneumothorax.

Chest and abdominal x-rays are useful in identifying the location of bullet fragments in relation to external wounds in order to identify possible trajectories. Radiopaque markers should be used to identify all bullet and stab wounds on the radiograph. However, x-ray evaluation should never delay progress to the operating room for an unstable patient. The sensitivity and diagnostic accuracy of x-ray evaluation has improved greatly with the introduction and widespread use of the 64-slice CT scan. All patients receive IV contrast unless a patient has known anaphylactic or angioedema reactions. Careful communication with the radiologist and technician is important, as the timing of IV contrast and obtaining delayed imaging may be crucial to diagnostic accuracy. Oral contrast is not usually indicated. However, if there is concern for a duodenal or pancreatic injury, approximately 200 mL of Gastrografin oral contrast can be administered either per ora or via an orogastric tube to look for signs of contrast extravasation. For patients with stab wounds to the back or flank, CT imaging is particularly useful because injury to retroperitoneal organs can be difficult to diagnose on the basis of symptoms, physical examination, and FAST. These patients should receive rectal contrast as well (Figure 3). Traditionally, CT has not been particularly sensitive for diagnosing intestinal or diaphragmatic injuries, but with thinner cuts on imaging this is changing. In addition, signs such as peritoneal free fluid without evidence of solid organ injury can indicate injury to the intestines even if the exact injury is not identified on CT.

When findings from FAST or abdominal CT scan are equivocal for hollow viscus or diaphragmatic injury but the patient has a concerning abdominal examination or when the findings are concerning for injury but the patient has a benign abdominal examination, laparoscopy is a useful diagnostic and sometimes therapeutic adjunct. Diagnostic laparoscopy also can be used to confirm or rule

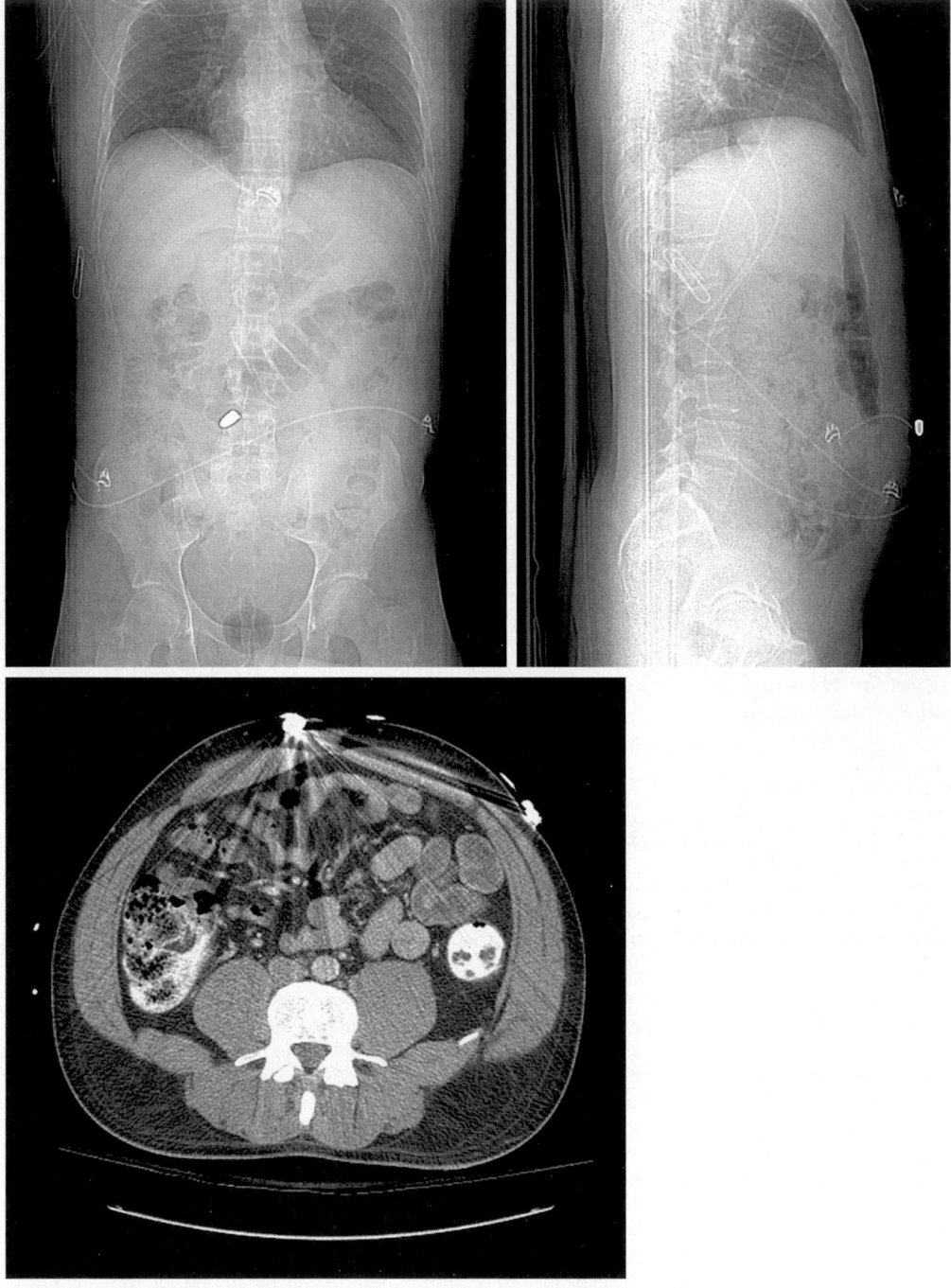

FIGURE 2 Gunshot wound to the abdomen. Computed tomographic images show a superficial trajectory.

out peritoneal violation when CT scan is not obtained. Surgical technique and familiarity have improved such that the ability to examine the entire small bowel or to identify and repair left-sided diaphragmatic injuries is a skill that many graduating surgical residents possess.

■ THERAPEUTIC CONSIDERATIONS

Drs. Hirshberg and Mattox discuss the three-dimensional (3D) trauma surgeon in *Top Knife: The Art & Craft of Trauma Surgery.* This concept refers to the trauma surgeon as operative technician, strategist, and team leader. Operative tactics are what we spend our surgical training learning, and many surgeons draw from elective techniques to inform emergency procedures. Strategy requires

constant reassessment of the patient's overall clinical picture and constant adaptation of the goals and priorities of the procedure. As team leader, communication and coordination are required to ensure that the operative team is aware of the goals and remains focused on them. Mastery of these three roles is essential to an effective trauma laparotomy.

For the traditional trauma laparotomy, the patient should be supine with both arms out and prepped from the chin to just above the knees and to both posterior axillary lines. A midline incision is made through skin and subcutaneous tissue with a scalpel, and the peritoneum can be entered bluntly with a finger just superior to the umbilicus. A pair of heavy Mayo scissors can be used to complete the peritoneal incision, as electrocautery often does not work in a wet field. Next, eviscerate the small bowel and evacuate the

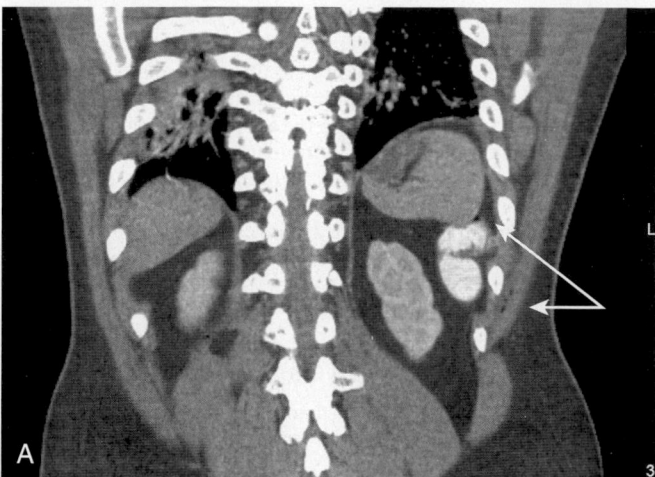

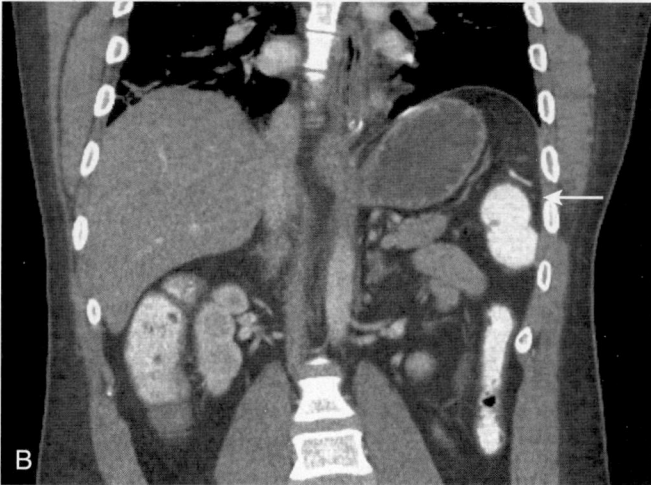

FIGURE 3 Stab wound to the left upper quadrant. **A,** Computed tomographic (CT) image with air bubbles indicating fascial violation and possible intra-abdominal injury. **B,** CT image with extravasation of rectal contrast indicating colon injury at the splenic flexure.

hemoperitoneum to determine the source of the bleeding. The first step is temporary hemorrhage control, by either manual pressure or packing. Achieving initial hemostasis allows the anesthesiology team time to catch up with resuscitation. The second step is to control contamination, and for this the peritoneal cavity must be explored and the entire length of small bowel and colon inspected. A complete inventory of injuries must be obtained in order to decide between proceeding with definitive repair and performing damage control procedures.

A damage control procedure involves the use of temporary control measures for hemorrhage and spillage, with temporary closure of the abdomen and planned return to the operating room when the patient has been resuscitated and is more hemodynamically stable. When deciding whether to adopt a damage control approach, key factors include injury pattern and physiology. Specifically, the "lethal triad" of hypothermia, coagulopathy, and acidosis are physiologic markers that, when seen together, represent irreversible shock. The goal of a damage control procedure is to avoid this lethal triad and plan to be out of the operating room before it starts.

Perioperative antibiotics have long been accepted as the standard of care for preventing surgical site infections in elective procedures. This practice is based on the science that infection is best prevented if therapeutic doses of antimicrobials are present before or at the time of bacterial contamination. For trauma patients, this is not possible. However, published studies still support the use of perioperative

antibiotics for these patients, with the first dose given as soon as possible. The antibiotic of choice should have broad aerobic and anaerobic coverage and should be discontinued if no hollow viscus injury is found and continued for no longer than 24 hours if an injury is identified. There are no studies that specifically address the role of continued antibiotics in patients with an open abdomen, but our current practice is 24 hours of antibiotics after the initial laparotomy and an additional perioperative dose for each return to the operating room.

Unlike laparotomy for blunt trauma, all retroperitoneal hematomas, even those that are nonexpanding, must be explored in patients with penetrating trauma. The major principle of proximal and distal control always must be adopted. Supraceliac control of the aorta at the diaphragmatic hiatus is the most rapid means of controlling inflow and allows time for adequate resuscitation but does result in global ischemia to intra-abdominal organs. For zone I (central) and left zone II (paracolic gutter) hematomas, left-sided medial visceral rotation provides better exposure for vascular repair, when time permits. For right zone II hematomas, access to the renal hilum and inferior vena cava (IVC) is provided by a right-sided medial visceral rotation. Retrohepatic hematomas should be approached with caution, as the tamponade effect provided by a contained hematoma is often lifesaving. If the hematoma is expanding, there are not many options; use of atriocaval shunts has been described, but successful repair of a retrohepatic IVC injury is difficult to accomplish. For nonexpanding hematomas, the associated injury is likely from a small branch off the hepatic veins, and low filling pressures along with tamponade are the best treatment options. Zone III (pelvic) hematomas require exposure of the distal aorta at the root of the mesentery for proximal control and exposure of the external iliac arteries at the femoral canal for distal control. If injury to the internal iliac artery is suspected, ligation instead of repair is a therapeutic option; if ligation is not technically feasible, pelvic packing and angioembolization can be considered.

For liver injuries, compressing the liver between two hands, reapproximating disrupted tissue planes, is a quick and effective way to achieve temporary hemostasis. If manual compression is inadequate, a Pringle's maneuver (compression of the porta hepatis) can be performed and will help to control any arterial bleeding. Coagulation devices, large hemostatic sutures, and tractotomy to identify and ligate visible bleeding vessels are all therapeutic options for obtaining surgical hemostasis. However, if all of these options are unsuccessful, the surgeon then must pack the liver and consider angioembolization. The transport of an unstable patient can be difficult at best, but with the propagation of hybrid suites this technique is becoming logistically easier. For patients in extremis because of a splenic injury, a splenectomy can be performed to rapidly gain hemorrhage control. For patients who are more hemodynamically stable, splenorrhaphy can be attempted with many of the same techniques applied for liver injuries. For stable patients found to have isolated solid organ injury (liver, spleen, or kidney) on CT, laparotomy may be avoided and angiography with angioembolization can be used if active contrast extravasation is seen or there is a significant drop in hemoglobin on serial laboratory tests.

A thorough inspection of all surfaces of the stomach, small bowel, and colon is required to avoid missed injures, especially in patients with gunshot wounds. In particular, the lesser curve of the stomach, gastroesophageal junction, ligament of Treitz, mesenteric border of the small bowel, posterior wall of the stomach, and transverse colon and extraperitoneal rectum can hide injuries if one does not inspect these areas carefully. Always reconstruct the trajectory of the wound, keeping in mind that it must be linear, and explore all subserosal hematomas. If a damage control approach is indicated, once control of hemorrhage and spillage is achieved, the operation is completed. However, if definitive repair is indicated, decisions must be made regarding type of repair and resection with anastomosis or ostomy. If there are multiple bowel injuries and resection is required, be sure to preserve bowel length while minimizing the number of suture

BOX 2: Indications for Repair or Resection and Anastomosis of Colon Injuries

1. <50% of bowel wall
2. Hemodynamically stable
3. No significant underlying disease
4. Minimal associated injuries
5. No signs of peritonitis
   All other patients, especially if evidence of shock, should be managed with resection and colostomy.

From Cayten CG, Fabien TC, Garcia VF, Ivatury RR, Morris JA. *Patient Management Guidelines for Penetrating Intraperitoneal Colon Injuries.* Chicago: Eastern Association for the Surgery of Trauma; 1998.

lines. For colon injuries, when deciding whether to anastomose bowel or to create an ostomy, consider the location of injury and overall clinical picture. Ascending and transverse colon injuries are considered "safe," and primary pair or resection and primary anastomosis is recommended. For descending colon injuries, management has evolved, and resection with colostomy is no longer mandatory (Box 2). Initial studies by Brundage and colleagues showed a trend toward increased risk of anastomotic leak and intra-abdominal abscess formation with stapled anastomoses (13%) compared with those that were hand sewn (5%) (relative risk [RR] 2.08; 95% confidence interval [CI] 0.89-4.86). However, subsequent studies, including meta-analyses, have shown more equivocal results with respect to colon-related complications. In general, we recommend that surgeons use the technique they are most comfortable with and know how to do best.

SUMMARY

Patients with penetrating abdominal trauma require immediate attention, with rapid diagnosis of injuries and therapeutic decisions. These patients have benefited from the adoption of selective conservatism, as well as from damage control laparotomy and advances in resuscitative practices. Serial physical examination by experienced clinicians remains the cornerstone of selective conservatism, but FAST, abdominal CT scans, and diagnostic laparoscopy all aid in appropriate patient selection and avoidance of nontherapeutic laparotomies.

SUGGESTED READINGS

Bickell WH, Wall MJ Jr, Pepe PE, et al. Immediate versus delayed fluid resuscitation for hypotensive patients with penetrating torso injuries. *N Engl J Med.* 1994;331:1105-1109.

CRASH-2 trial collaborators, Shakur H, Roberts I, et al. Effects of tranexamic acid on death, vascular occlusive events, and blood transfusion in trauma patients with significant haemorrhage (CRASH-2): a randomised, placebo-controlled trial. *Lancet.* 2010;376:23-32.

Holcomb JB, del Junco DJ, Fox EE, et al. The prospective, observational, multicenter, major trauma transfusion (PROMMTT) study: comparative effectiveness of a time-varying treatment with competing risks. *JAMA Surg.* 2013;148:127-136.

Kwan I, Bunn F, Chinnock P, Roberts I. Timing and volume of fluid administration for patients with bleeding. *Cochrane Database Syst Rev.* 2014;(3): CD002245.

Velmahos GC, Demetriades D, Toutouzas KG, et al. Selective nonoperative management in 1,856 patients with abdominal gunshot wounds: should routine laparotomy still be the standard of care? *Ann Surg.* 2001;234:395-402, discussion 402-403.

THE MANAGEMENT OF DIAPHRAGMATIC INJURIES

Philip T. Ramsay, MD, and David V. Feliciano, MD

Diaphragmatic injuries always have been a diagnostic challenge for the surgeon. A high index of suspicion is necessary to avoid delays in diagnosis and missed injuries with resultant visceral herniation and strangulation. The objectives of this chapter are to review the incidence and mechanisms of diaphragmatic injury and the anatomy of the diaphragm as it pertains to surgical repair and to provide an approach to diagnosis and treatment.

EPIDEMIOLOGY

Diaphragmatic injuries are infrequent, but the true incidence is difficult to estimate because an unknown number are occult or overlooked. The reported incidence rate of acute diaphragmatic injury in the literature varies and ranges from 0.8% to 8% after thoracoabdominal trauma. The incidence rate of penetrating injury is higher than blunt injury with a ratio of 2 to 3 to 1.

The most common mechanisms for blunt injuries to the diaphragm are motor vehicle crashes and falls from a height. In these patients, a transfer of kinetic energy to the diaphragm occurs through an acute increase in intra-abdominal pressure. Because blunt diaphragmatic injuries are more common on the left than the right in a ratio of 2.3 to 1 in two recent large reviews (a marked change from the 9 to 1 reported in the past), the general consensus is that the acute

increase in intra-abdominal pressure is absorbed by the liver, which partially protects the right hemidiaphragm. The liver also prevents herniation, which may lead to an underdiagnosis of this uncommon injury. Autopsy studies show an equal incidence of right and left injuries to the diaphragm after blunt trauma. In such patients, the most common associated injuries are to the lung, ribs, liver, and spleen.

The location of the diaphragmatic injury after penetrating trauma is dependent on the trajectory, but most injuries from stab wounds are to the left hemidiaphragm. This is believed to result from most assailants being right hand dominant. In contrast, gunshot wounds to the abdomen had a left to right ratio of approximately 1.25 to 1 in the aforementioned two reviews. Stab wounds to the thoracoabdominal area (nipple to costal margin medial to anterior axillary line) cause an injury to the diaphragm 15% of the time, and this increases to 45% when a gunshot wound is the mechanism of injury.

ANATOMY

The diaphragm is a dome-shaped musculotendinous partition that separates the abdominal cavity from the thoracic cavity (Figure 1). The muscle fibers of the diaphragm originate peripherally from the lower ribs, upper lumbar vertebrae, and sternum and insert into the central tendon. The diaphragm has separate hiatuses for the esophagus, aorta, and inferior vena cava. The esophagus and vagus nerves pass through the esophageal hiatus; the aorta, thoracic duct, and azygous vein pass through the aortic hiatus; and the only structure that passes through the caval hiatus is the inferior vena cava.

The arterial blood supply to the diaphragm comes from the phrenic arteries, branches of the abdominal aorta, and intercostal arteries, and venous drainage is to the inferior vena cava. Motor

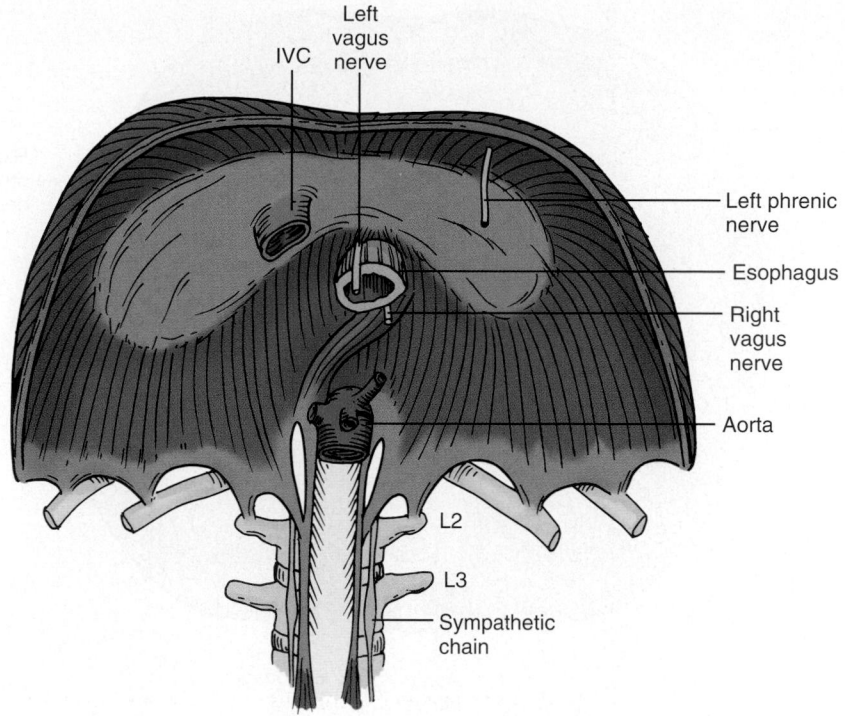

FIGURE 1 Anatomy of the diaphragm, including the central tendon and structures that pass through the three hiatuses. *IVC,* Inferior vena cava. *(From Davis JW, Eghbalieh B. Injury to the diaphragm. In Feliciano DV, Mattox KL, Moore EE, eds. Trauma. 6th ed. New York: McGraw-Hill; 2008, 624.)*

innervation to the diaphragm comes from the phrenic nerves. Sensory innervation to the central tendon and peritoneum is carried by the phrenic nerves as well, and sensory innervation to the periphery is carried by the intercostal nerves. The left and right phrenic nerves divide into a varying number of branches above the diaphragm (Figure 2). They most commonly branch anteriorly, posteromedially, and laterally. These branches enter the medial portion of the diaphragm and run obliquely, resulting in a pattern that often is described as a "double handcuff." Knowledge of this pattern is important because injury to the phrenic nerve should be avoided, if at all possible, during repair of the diaphragm.

■ DIAGNOSIS

The goal of early diagnosis of diaphragmatic injuries is to avoid the added morbidity and potential mortality of herniation of an abdominal viscus and strangulation. Diagnosis is especially difficult in patients without indications for an emergency laparotomy for other associated intra-abdominal injuries. The mechanism of injury and the location of impact can raise the index of suspicion.

A diaphragmatic injury can cause thoracic or abdominal symptoms and signs. Thoracic symptoms include dyspnea, respiratory distress, orthopnea, chest pain, and referred pain to the ipsilateral shoulder, whereas thoracic signs include dullness to percussion, decreased breath sounds, bowel sounds in the chest, crepitus, and chest wall movement from associated rib fractures. Abdominal symptoms range from mild upper abdominal pain on one side of the abdomen to severe diffuse abdominal pain, whereas abdominal signs include tenderness and a scaphoid abdomen from herniated abdominal viscera.

The surgeon-performed focused assessment with sonography for trauma (FAST) examination with a 3.5-MHz ultrasound probe is the first screening test used in most adult patients with blunt trauma to the thorax or abdomen. A break in or the absence of the usual hyperechoic curved line characteristic of a hemidiaphragm above the liver or spleen is presumptive evidence that a large blunt rupture has

occurred. The FAST examination usually does not detect small perforations that occur with stab or gunshot wounds.

A chest x-ray can still be part of the initial workup of the trauma patient and is the next screening modality used to detect injuries to the diaphragm; however, the initial study in the trauma room may be normal or inconclusive and miss 20% to 50% of diaphragmatic injuries. The accuracy of the chest x-ray is lower in penetrating injuries to the right hemidiaphragm as compared with the left because the liver may prevent herniation of abdominal contents into the right hemithorax through a small hole as previously noted. In contrast, the liver may herniate into the chest with a large blunt tear of the right hemidiaphragm (Figure 3). On the left side, gastric, small bowel, or colonic air fluid levels may be visualized in the thorax on the admission chest x-ray. Other findings on a chest x-ray include elevation of a hemidiaphragm, obscured diaphragmatic silhouette (Figure 4), failure of a hemothorax to clear after insertion of a thoracostomy tube, and associated rib and sternal fractures. In a patient with a "suspicious" chest x-ray, a nasogastric tube may be seen coiled in the left hemithorax on a repeat film if the stomach has herniated through a blunt rupture (Figures 5 and 6). If the patient is intubated in the trauma room, positive airway pressure from mechanical ventilation may, however, prevent herniation. On rare occasions, an injury to a hemidiaphragm can be diagnosed with finger palpation during insertion of an ipsilateral chest tube.

Contrast upper and lower gastrointestinal series with fluoroscopy were performed routinely in the past when the diagnosis was suspected on the admission chest x-ray but have been replaced with multidetector computed tomography (CT) scans. With reformatted images, diagnostic sensitivities of 71% to 100% and specificities of 75% to 100% have been reported with multidetector CT over the past 10 years. CT findings include discontinuity of the diaphragm, intrathoracic herniation of abdominal contents, and the "dangling" diaphragm sign from a free floating diaphragm flap. The "collar sign" is a constriction of a herniated viscus through the diaphragmatic defect, and the "dependent viscera sign" is the abnormal dependent position of the viscera against the posterior ribs. Magnetic resonance

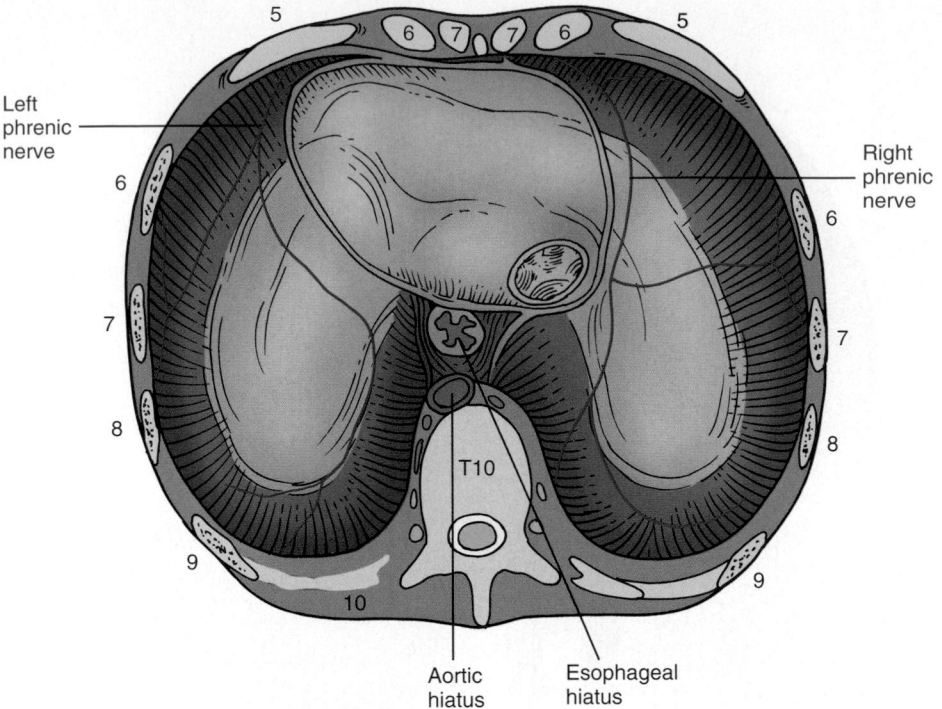

FIGURE 2 Anatomic distribution and branching pattern of the phrenic nerves. *(From Davis, JW, Eghbalieh B. Injury to the diaphragm. In Feliciano DV, Mattox KL, Moore EE, eds. Trauma. 6th ed, New York: McGraw-Hill; 2008, 625.)*

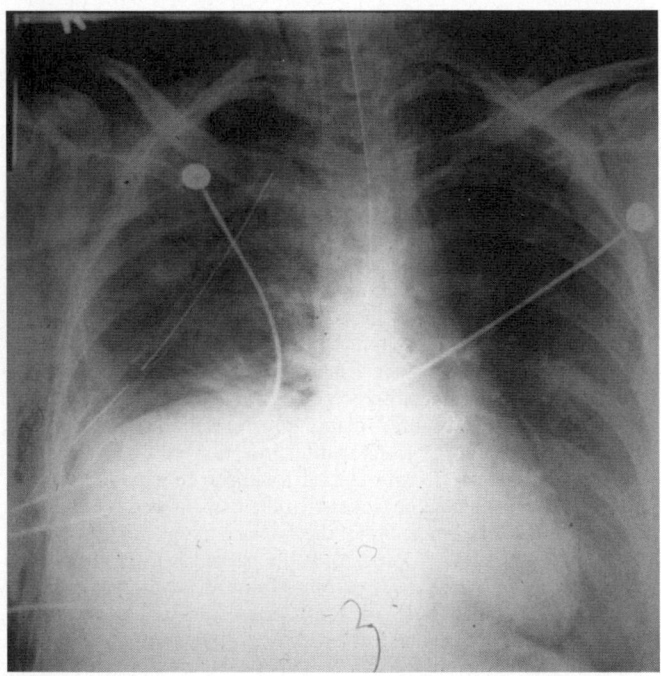

FIGURE 3 A suspicious admission chest x-ray of a 41-year-old woman who was a front-seat passenger in a right lateral impact motor vehicle collision. Computed tomographic scan confirmed a large blunt rupture of the right hemidiaphragm.

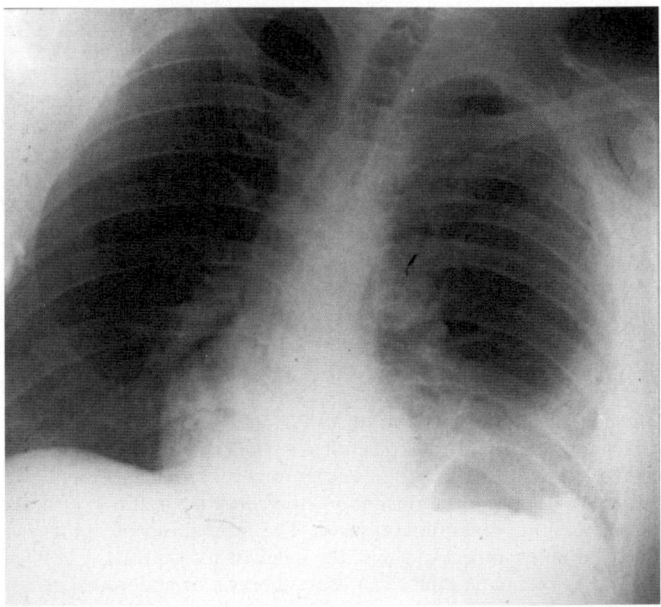

FIGURE 4 A 34-year-old man with a gunshot wound through the diaphragm and gastric fundus had an abnormal chest x-ray on admission, but the diagnosis was delayed for 4 days. *(From Feliciano DV, Cruse PA, Mattox KL, et al. Delayed diagnosis of injuries to the diaphragm after penetrating wounds, J Trauma. 1988;28:1135-1144.)*

imaging is impractical in the acute setting but may be useful in the evaluation of a possible chronic diaphragmatic hernia.

Laparoscopy with general anesthesia in the operating room is indicated in patients in whom concern still exists about a possible diaphragmatic injury after the usual imaging studies. It is indicated particularly in patients whose conditions are hemodynamically stable with no other indications for laparotomy. The use of a 30-degree or 45-degree telescope aids in evaluation of the entire diaphragm, and a risk of a tension pneumothorax exists when the pneumoperitoneum is introduced. If thoracoscopy is necessary to evacuate a clotted hemothorax, the ipsilateral hemidiaphragm always should be evaluated.

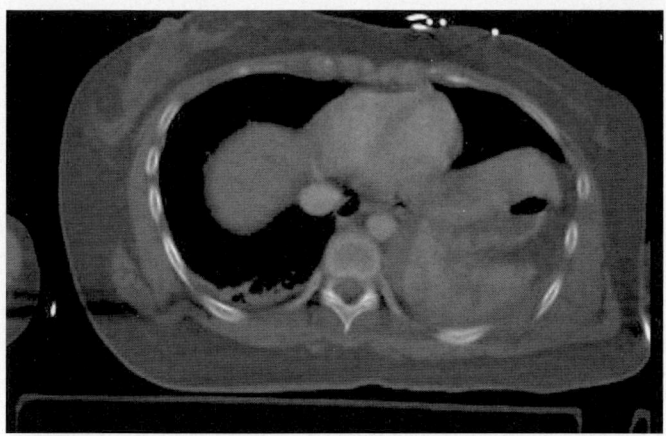

FIGURE 5 CT of patient with left-sided blunt diaphragmatic rupture.

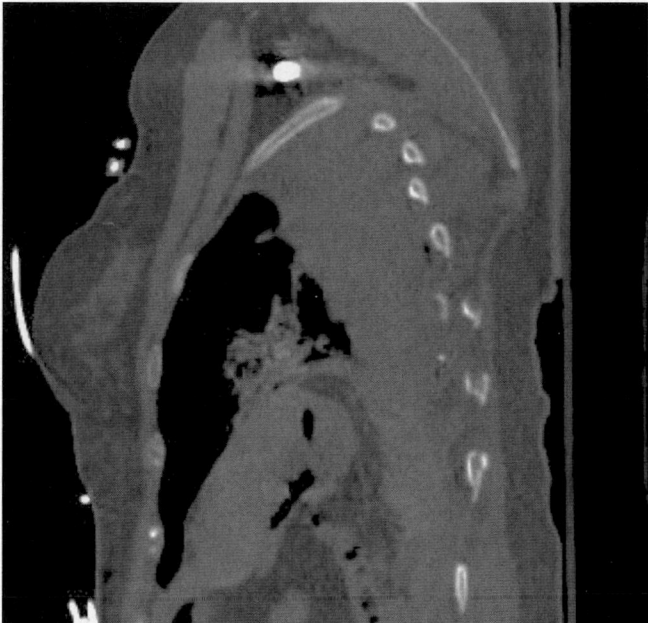

FIGURE 6 Lateral CT view of patient with left-sided diaphragmatic rupture.

■ ACUTE MANAGEMENT

Diaphragmatic injuries are graded on a scale of I to V in the Organ Injury Scale developed by the American Association for the Surgery of Trauma in 1994 (Table 1). Injuries from blunt trauma tend to be of a higher grade (III to V) and occur in the posterolateral hemidiaphragm. Penetrating injuries are typically of a lower grade (I to II) and can occur anywhere in the diaphragm. Almost all diaphragmatic perforations and lacerations, regardless of size, should be repaired to reduce the risk of herniation of intra-abdominal viscera and strangulation. The one exception is an isolated injury to the right hemidiaphragm from a penetrating wound where a subsequent CT scan documents that there is no bleeding from an associated hepatic or renal injury and that there is not an injury to the gastrointestinal tract.

Several operative approaches are used for the treatment of diaphragmatic injuries. The operative approach is determined by whether the diaphragmatic injury is acute or chronic (see subsequently), by the hemodynamic stability of the patient, the presence or absence of associated injuries, and by the surgeon's comfort level with the particular approach. For acute diaphragmatic injuries,

TABLE 1: AAST Organ Injury Scale

Grade	Injury Description
I	Contusion
II	Laceration ≤ 2 cm
III	Laceration 2-10 cm
IV	Laceration > 10 cm with tissue loss ≤ 25 cm^2
V	Laceration with tissue loss > 25 cm^2

AAST, American Association for the Surgery of Trauma.

From Moore EE, Malangoni MA, Cogbill TH, et al. Organ injury scaling. IV: Thoracic vascular, lung, cardiac, and diaphragm, *J Trauma*. 1994;36:299-300, 1994.

laparotomy is the preferred method. After the patient is placed on the operating table in the supine position, the operative field is prepared and draped, with the chest included. A nasogastric or orogastric tube should be placed carefully to allow for decompression of the stomach, but this may be difficult in the patient with gastric herniation. A midline laparotomy incision is made and, after control of bleeding and contamination, the entire abdominal cavity should be explored. Any abdominal viscus that has herniated through a diaphragmatic defect should be reduced carefully. The thoracic cavity should be inspected through the diaphragmatic defect for any ongoing bleeding or contamination from spillage of gastrointestinal contents. If any thoracic contamination has occurred, the thoracic cavity should be irrigated thoroughly with normal saline solution containing antibiotics until returns through the suction device are clear. *This often mandates enlargement of the diaphragmatic defect.*

The left side of the diaphragm is exposed fully by mobilizing and retracting the spleen, splenic flexure of the colon, stomach, and left lobe of the liver inferiorly and medially. The left triangular ligament of the liver may have to be divided to allow for adequate exposure as well. The right side of the diaphragm is exposed fully by dividing the falciform ligament and the right triangular ligament and retracting the right lobe of the liver inferiorly and medially.

For most injuries, primary closure can be achieved. Long Allis clamps are placed on the edges of the perforation or laceration to allow for elevation of the defect and easier visualization. After nonviable tissue is débrided, a #0 or #1 permanent suture is placed in a continuous locking fashion or multiple interrupted simple sutures (our preference) are used to repair large defects. Interrupted simple or vertical mattress sutures can be used to repair small defects as well. Because the diaphragm is highly vascular, the repair is inspected at completion to rule out continuing hemorrhage. If intrapleural contamination, a concomitant injury to the lung, or concern about a hemothorax related to a coagulopathy is present, then a large ipsilateral thoracostomy tube should be placed. If no injury to the lung or a hemothorax is found, there is no need to place a tube. A catheter may be inserted through the diaphragmatic defect to evacuate any air as anesthesia hyperventilates the patient just before the final diaphragmatic suture is tied down.

In patients undergoing a "damage control" trauma laparotomy, diaphragmatic repair is unnecessary. Any smaller defect can be covered with folded laparotomy pads used as packs. A larger defect can be covered with opened laparotomy pads held in place with staples or packs.

For acute diaphragmatic injuries in patients who are hemodynamically stable and have no other indication for laparotomy, laparoscopy can be used to perform the repair. The decision is dependent on the individual surgeon's comfort level with laparoscopic techniques of suturing. The risk of a tension pneumothorax with laparoscopy is significant as previously noted, and the patient must be monitored carefully during insufflation of CO_2.

■ SPECIAL SITUATIONS

Diaphragmatic Detachment From Chest Wall

In cases that involve detachment of the diaphragm from its postero-lateral attachments, any devascularized diaphragmatic muscle is débrided. The diaphragm is reattached to the body wall with placement of interrupted #1 polypropylene sutures through the edge of the detached diaphragm, around the adjacent rib, and then through the edge of the diaphragm again before tying. Visualization is improved by placing all sutures before tying the knots.

Loss of Diaphragmatic Tissue

In cases of massive diaphragmatic destruction, the insertion of the remaining hemidiaphragm may be translocated to a more superior rib level to allow a tension-free repair. The technique involves dividing anterior, lateral, and posterior attachments of the hemidiaphragm to the chest wall as needed to decrease tension as the hemidiaphragm is sutured around a more superior rib. In addition, nonporous synthetic mesh can be used as a bridge. In cases of contamination, a significant risk of infection exists if synthetic mesh is inserted, and biologic mesh may be used to provide temporary repair. Once the infection has been treated adequately, biologic mesh can be replaced by synthetic mesh if there is evidence of a diaphragmatic hernia on serial chest x-rays. Alternatively, autologous tissue such as omentum, tensor fascia lata, or a latissimus dorsi flap may be used.

Loss of Chest Wall

In patients with large open defects of the chest wall from a thoracoabdominal shotgun wound, any perforations of the hemidiaphragm are repaired before it is translocated to a more superior rib level (Figure 7). The defect in the chest wall then essentially is converted to an abdominal wall defect that can be managed with local wound care. This includes covering the defect with absorbable mesh,

performing daily gauze dressing changes above this, and applying a split-thickness skin graft after granulation tissue appears.

Injury to the Central Tendon

Rupture of the central tendon involving the pericardium is a rare event. The heart may herniate inferiorly into the peritoneal cavity or abdominal viscera may herniate superiorly into the pericardium and cause cardiac tamponade. The heart must be inspected for associated injuries, and careful attention must be given during suture repair of the rupture to avoid injury to the myocardium.

Injury to the Esophageal Hiatus

In cases of injury to the esophageal hiatus, the esophagus should be visualized clearly before suture repair is performed. If any concern exists that the repair may narrow the esophagus, a Maloney dilator should be passed down the esophagus to confirm that the lumen is patent.

■ MANAGEMENT OF THE CHRONIC POSTTRAUMATIC HERNIA

Missed diaphragmatic injuries can appear years after injury as chronic diaphragmatic hernias (Figure 8). Patients may be asymptomatic or report worsening respiratory compromise from progressive visceral herniation. Some patients may have signs and symptoms of obstruction, strangulation, or perforation of the stomach or colon. All chronic posttraumatic hernias should be repaired in patients at reasonable risk to avoid these secondary gastrointestinal complications. With time, adhesions develop between the herniated abdominal viscera and the pleural cavity. Also, the diaphragm retracts and atrophies, making reduction of herniated viscera and repair more difficult. Therefore a thoracic approach is preferred because this allows for easier division of chronic adhesions. The decision between thoracotomy and thoracoscopy is dependent on the individual surgeon's comfort level and experience with thoracoscopy. A small hernia into the pleural cavity, however, still can be approached through a laparotomy. In some patients, prosthetic mesh may be required to cover a chronic rigid defect (see previous). Occasionally,

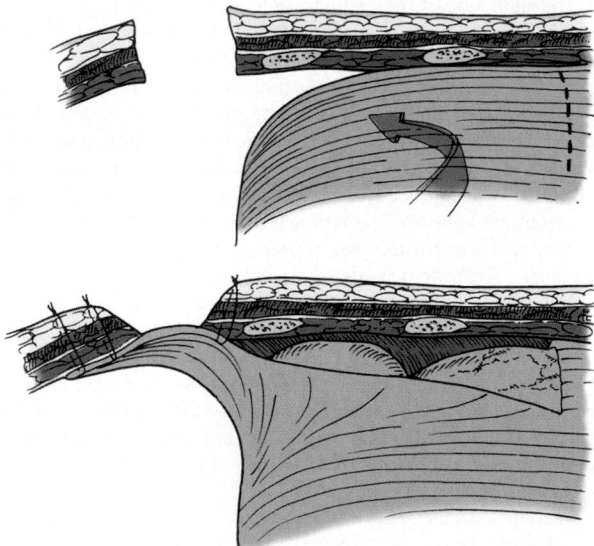

FIGURE 7 Immediate reconstruction of the chest wall after destructive types of injury may be accomplished by detaching the affected hemidiaphragm anteriorly, laterally, and posteriorly. The diaphragm is then resutured to the muscle of a higher intercostal space, thus effectively translocating it to a position above the full-thickness chest wall defect and converting such a defect functionally into an abdominal wall defect. The abdominal wall defect then is managed with local wound care in anticipation of further reconstruction with either split-thickness grafts or myocutaneous flaps at a later date. *(Courtesy Asensio JA, Demetriades D.)*

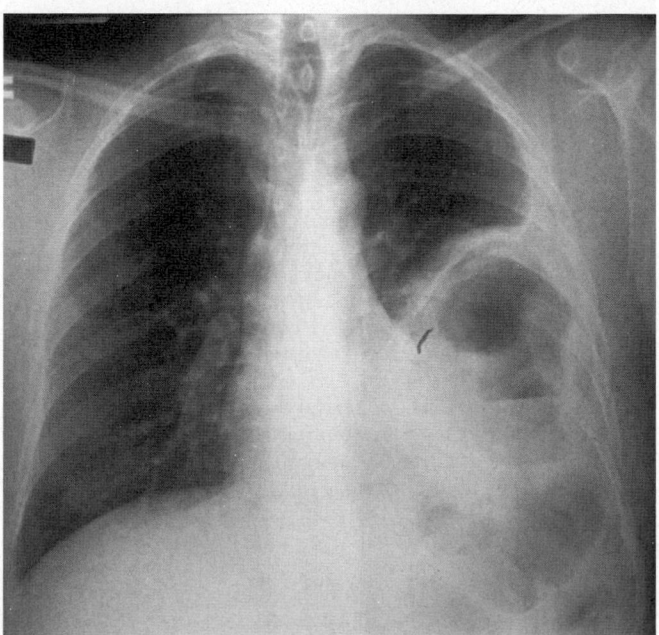

FIGURE 8 A 28-year-old man with a chronic posttraumatic diaphragmatic hernia 1 year after a stab wound to the left chest.

reduction of a giant chronic hernia has the potential to cause a secondary abdominal compartment syndrome from loss of abdominal domain. The technique of creating and gradually increasing a pneumoperitoneum before surgery is appropriate in such a patient. If the surgeon is unwilling or uncomfortable to use this uncommon approach, insertion of a permanent prosthesis into the abdominal wall may be necessary at the time of the reduction and repair to expand the volume of the peritoneal cavity.

■ MORBIDITY AND MORTALITY

The morbidity and mortality from diaphragmatic injury depends on several factors, including the mechanism of injury, the severity of injury to the diaphragm, the presence or absence of associated injuries, and the extent of surgery required to repair the injury and associated injuries. Most complications and deaths are caused by injuries to other organs. The reported mortality rate has ranged from 4.3% to 41%, with a higher mortality rate in patients with blunt injuries as opposed to those with penetrating trauma. Early complications from repair of the diaphragm include breakdown of the repair, paralysis of the hemidiaphragm from injury to the phrenic nerve, and respiratory embarrassment.

On rare occasions, a patient with a penetrating wound to the right lower lobe of the lung, right hemidiaphragm, and liver develops a bronchopleural fistula after surgical repair. This results from a biliary fistula eroding through the repair of the diaphragm and connecting to the hole in the lung. The patient has respiratory distress, may cough up bile, and has a worsening appearance of the right lower lobe on chest x-ray. Any delay in transabdominal drainage of the biliary leak, repair or re-repair of the right hemidiaphragm, and débridement or excision of the right lower lobe leads to progressive necrosis of the lung.

As previously noted, patients with chronic posttraumatic diaphragmatic hernias can have complications develop from visceral obstruction, strangulation, and perforation. Delays in treatment can lead to postoperative empyema, subdiaphragmatic abscesses, sepsis, and multiple organ failure.

SUGGESTED READINGS

Feliciano DV, Cruse PA, Mattox KL, et al. Delayed diagnosis of injuries to the diaphragm after penetrating wounds. *J Trauma*. 1988;28:1135-1144.

Hanna WC, Ferri LE, Fata P, et al. The current status of traumatic diaphragmatic injury: lessons learned from 105 patients over 13 years. *Ann Thorac Surg*. 2008;85:1044-1048.

Kemp CD, Yang SC. Thoracic trauma. In: Sellke FW, del Nido PJ, Swanson SJ, eds. *Sabiston and Spencer: Surgery of the Chest*. 8th ed. Philadelphia, PA: Elsevier; 2010:96-97 103-105.

Schuster KM, Davis KA. Diaphragm. In: Moore EE, Feliciano DV, Mattox KL, eds. *Trauma*. 8th ed. New York: McGraw-Hill; 2017 in press.

Ties JS, Peschman JR, Moreno A, et al. Evolution in the management of traumatic diaphragmatic injuries: a multicenter review. *J Trauma Acute Care Surg*. 2014;76:1024-1028.

Zarour AM, El-Menyar A, Al-Thani H, et al. Presentations and outcomes in patients with traumatic diaphragmatic injury: a 15-year experience. *J Trauma Acute Care Surg*. 2013;74:1392-1398.

THE MANAGEMENT OF LIVER INJURIES

Mario Rueda, MD, and David T. Efron, MD

The liver is the most commonly injured intra-abdominal organ. Its size and location make it vulnerable to both penetrating and nonpenetrating trauma. About 6% of trauma patients will have a liver injury on evaluation, and about 20% of those patients will need an operative intervention. It is therefore essential that a surgeon taking care of patients with these injuries understands the different treatment modalities.

In the past few decades, the approach to liver injuries has changed, especially for nonpenetrating trauma. There has been a shift from strictly operative intervention to a selective nonoperative approach. This has been made possible by improvements in the management of critically ill patients, better and faster imaging of the liver, and improvements in angiography and embolization techniques.

A significant number of patients will need operative intervention either because of failure of nonoperative management or because they are considered inappropriate candidates for nonoperative management, such as patients with grade VI liver lacerations or hemodynamic instability. It is therefore important that the surgeon is familiar with different operative techniques and approaches. Maintaining hemodynamic stability by controlling hemorrhage and providing appropriate balanced resuscitation are pillars of the operative treatment. Direct liver compression, total hepatic vascular occlusion, portal triad occlusion, finger fracture, balloon tamponade, omental packing, and suture hepatorrhaphy are some of the surgical methods used to stabilize patients and address penetrating liver trauma. Severe injuries may necessitate assistance from experienced hepatobiliary surgeons.

Although there clearly has been an improvement in the management of liver injuries, fundamentals of treatment still rely on thorough evaluation of the trauma victim and identification of the extent of hepatic injuries. Understanding the different treatment options and when to implement each strategy will help the patient to recover successfully. Close follow-up and monitoring also will help the surgeon to identify deterioration and treatment failure that can lead to a change in strategy.

■ INITIAL EVALUATION AND MANAGEMENT

All trauma patients should have an initial evaluation according to Advanced Trauma Life Support (ATLS) protocols. A thorough evaluation should be performed, as liver injuries can be associated with trauma to other abdominal organs as well as to the chest and extremities. For those patients who have had motor vehicle, motorcycle, and pedestrian versus car collisions, there should be a high level of suspicion for blunt liver injury, as the majority of blunt liver trauma described occurs after these events. The location of trajectories of penetrating injuries can provide clues as to what organs are involved.

Immediately after primary survey and resuscitation, further evaluation to diagnose a liver injury should be performed in appropriate patients (Figure 1). The method of evaluation depends on the hemodynamic stability of the trauma victim. For unstable patients, a focused assessment with sonography for trauma (FAST) should be performed as part of the primary survey. The intent is to identify hemoperitoneum that can explain the hemodynamic instability and can be a consequence of intra-abdominal trauma (and potentially a liver injury). The sensitivity and specificity of the FAST to detect intra-abdominal fluid and hemoperitoneum range from 85% to 97%. At least 400 mL of fluids needs to accumulate in order to be able to detect injury. A liver injury usually cannot be identified reliably with FAST, but evidence of intra-abdominal fluid in combination with hemodynamic instability warrants an emergent laparotomy, as it is very likely that a solid organ injury will be identified.

Another method of evaluation for hemoperitoneum is the diagnostic peritoneal lavage (DPL). In the past DPL was seen as

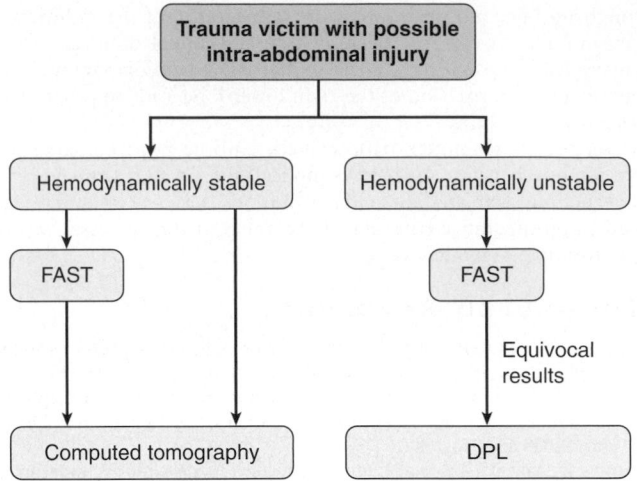

FIGURE 1 Evaluation approach to the trauma patient with possible liver injury. *DPL*, Diagnostic peritoneal lavage; *FAST*, focused assessment with sonography for trauma.

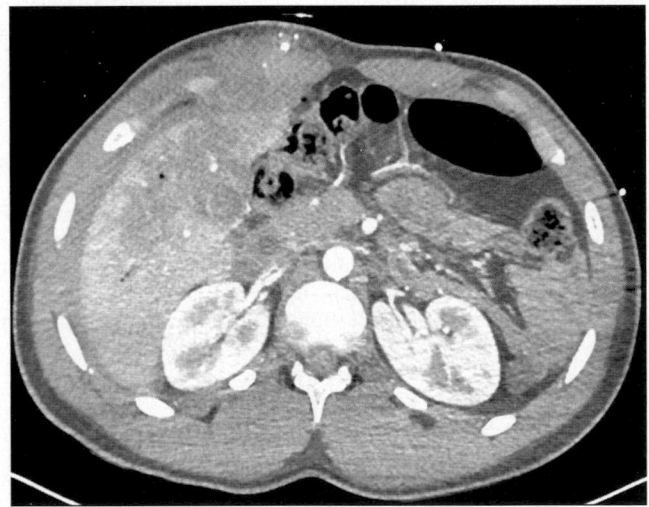

FIGURE 2 Computed tomographic scan of the abdomen obtained on a hemodynamically stable patient who had sustained a gunshot wound to the abdomen. Note the extravasation and hemoperitoneum.

an alternative to the FAST, as it has comparable sensitivities and specificities. However, it has fallen out of favor and usually is performed during the evaluation of unstable victims who had equivocal FAST results, such as those patients whose body habitus precludes appropriate sonographic interpretation. During DPL, if 10 mL of blood are aspirated before any infusion or if more than 100,000 red blood cells (RBCs) per μL are detected in the peritoneal lavage, the DPL is considered positive and transfer to the operating room should follow.

In those patients who are hemodynamically stable and in which there is a suspicion for intra-abdominal injury, a computed tomographic (CT) scan with intravenous contrast should be performed (Figure 2). Contrary to the FAST and the DPL, which identify secondary signs of hepatic trauma such as hemoperitoneum, an evaluation of the actual liver parenchyma is performed with CT scan, and liver injuries are identified more readily and can be characterized for severity and presence of active bleeding. CT scan also evaluates the presence of other intra-abdominal, vascular, and musculoskeletal

TABLE 1: American Association for the Surgery of Trauma Liver Injury Scale

Grade	Injury	Description
I	Hematoma	Subcapsular, <10% surface area
	Laceration	Capsular tear, <1 cm parenchymal depth
II	Hematoma	Subcapsular, 10%-50% surface area
		Intraparenchymal, <10 cm diameter
	Laceration	1-3 cm parenchymal depth, <10 cm length
III	Hematoma	Subcapsular, >50% surface area or expanding. Ruptured subcapsular or parenchymal hematoma
	Laceration	>3 cm parenchymal depth
IV	Laceration	Parenchymal disruption involving 25%-75% of hepatic lobe or 1-3 Couinaud's segments in a single lobe
V	Laceration	Parenchymal disruption involving >75% of hepatic lobe or >3 Couinaud's segments within a single lobe
	Vascular	Juxtahepatic venous injuries (i.e., retrohepatic vena cava/central major hepatic veins)
VI	Vascular	Hepatic avulsion

From Moore EE, Cogbill TH, et al. Organ injury scaling: spleen and liver (1994 revision). *J Trauma.* 1995;38:323-324.

injuries. Its sensitivity approaches 99%. It should be noted that liver trauma not associated with hemoperitoneum can be missed in up to 50% of cases where FAST is used alone.

The American Association for the Surgery of Trauma has published a trauma liver injury scale that determines the extent of trauma to the liver (Table 1). This scale should serve as an additional tool to complete a clinical evaluation and not as the only guide to treatment.

■ NONOPERATIVE MANAGEMENT

Blunt Injury

Initial approach to treatment of a liver injury depends on the hemodynamic status of the trauma patient. Except for grade VI lacerations, patients with any grade of liver injury have the potential to be managed with a nonoperative approach, with a success rate as high as 80% to 90%. To qualify, the trauma victim should have no evidence of peritonitis on physical examination, and there should be no other abdominal injuries that mandate a laparotomy.

Admission to a monitored unit is imperative. Patients should have frequent assessments and physical examinations. Hemoglobin and hematocrit should be checked periodically. If during initial evaluation the patient is found to have an elevated international normalized ratio (INR), active normalization of coagulation factors is essential and follow-up laboratory tests are performed. Transfer to a nonmonitored setting usually can be done after 24 hours for patients with grade I and II liver injuries; those with higher-grade injuries will require longer periods of monitoring, ranging from 2 to 3 days.

Chemical deep venous thrombosis (DVT) prophylaxis should be held initially in patients with liver injuries who are undergoing nonoperative management. Because the risk for this complication is high, trauma patients have mechanical DVT prophylaxis devices. Once the patient shows evidence of recovery and if the patient's hemoglobin remains stable, starting anticoagulation should be considered.

Mandatory bed rest remains controversial, and we prefer to reserve it for those with severe-grade injuries. If the liver injury is grade III or higher, assessment of the overall clinical status should be performed in order to determine when the patient can ambulate safely (usually 2 days after injury). After 1 to 3 months of recovery and evaluation in clinic, patients can return to full activity with no restrictions.

Failure of nonoperative management can occur and is marked by hemodynamic instability. Any deterioration requires immediate assessment, balanced resuscitation, and ultimately hemostatic intervention. It is important that the surgeon identifies these critical signs early. Risk factors for failure of nonoperative management include injury to spleen and kidney, positive FAST, hemoperitoneum in excess of 300 mL, and need for transfusion.

Successful nonoperative management has resulted in decreased lengths of hospital stay and decreased intra-abdominal infections. Liver injury grade does play a role in failure of nonoperative management: Low-grade injuries (grades I and II) have a failure rate of 3% to 7.5%, whereas high-grade injuries (grades IV and V) have a failure rate of 14% to 23%.

A falling hematocrit mistakenly can be considered failure of nonoperative management; however, in the setting of polytrauma and with no other signs or symptom of bleeding, it may be a reflection of resuscitation. For these cases, re-evaluation is very important and should include additional or repeat imaging and possible angiography with intervention. The improvements in selective embolization make it an attractive adjunct to nonoperative management because arterial bleeding within the liver parenchyma can be controlled, increasing the chances of successful outcome. If the patient becomes unstable or if active bleeding cannot be controlled with interventional procedures, an operative intervention is warranted. Angiography remains a vital adjunct to nonoperative management.

Penetrating Injury

The conservative approach to any penetrating injury to the abdomen should include an abdominal exploration. However, for highly selected patients treated at specialized trauma centers who are seen with right upper quadrant wounds and isolated liver injuries, a nonoperative approach can be considered. If the patient is hemodynamically stable, has a reliable physical examination, and has a CT scan that shows no evidence of any other injury, the patient is a candidate for nonoperative management. If patients are selected properly, the success rate of nonoperative management can be as high as 90%.

Location of the entrance and, if present, exit wounds as well as possible trajectories of bullets or stab wounds can help to determine which patients initially can be observed and followed. Most patients who are deemed inappropriate candidates have injuries to other intra-abdominal organs, including bowel; injuries to the diaphragm and lung parenchymal injuries also may prevent nonoperative management.

Approaches to treatment are the same as those for nonpenetrating liver injury and involve repeat imaging as deemed necessary, laboratory follow-up, admission to a monitored bed, use of mechanical DVT prophylaxis only, and bed rest.

■ OPERATIVE MANAGEMENT

Any patient who is hemodynamically unstable and those patients who do not qualify for nonoperative management should have an exploratory laparotomy as part of their treatment. Preparation before the procedure, assurance of bleeding control, and management of other injuries are key elements in the operative management of patients with liver injuries.

Immediately after the decision to operate has been made, an organized treatment approach should be planned, including preoperative considerations, possible intraoperative needs and approach, and postoperative placement in a monitored bed.

Preoperative Considerations

Early consideration should be given to calling an experienced hepatobiliary surgeon for assistance when there is concern for a complex injury. The operating room should be warmed, and a balanced resuscitation with warm products should continue. The institution's massive transfusion protocol should be activated immediately. Rapid infusers and fluid warmers should remain available and be used as indicated. If there is no evidence of enteric spillage and if immediately available, a cell saver unit can be set up and used. Two Yankauer suction tips also should be ready for immediate use. A self-retaining retractor such as a Thompson, Omni, or Bookwalter retractor should be available in order to optimize exposure. An argon beam coagulator and topical hemostatic agents should be requested and available for use. Appropriate preoperative antibiotics with gram-negative and anaerobic coverage should be started and redosed according to blood loss and length of case. Continuous communication with anesthesia providers will facilitate resuscitation and keep the team informed of improvements in or worsening of clinical condition.

Initial Operative Approach

The patient should be prepared widely from chin to knees. The typical approach for a patient with traumatic injury to the abdomen is a wide laparotomy incision from xiphoid to symphysis pubis. When vascular control of the suprahepatic inferior vena cava (IVC) is needed, extension of the celiotomy to a sternotomy or right thoracotomy is indicated.

Once the peritoneum is opened, massive hemorrhage may be encountered as the tamponade effect exerted by the abdominal cavity is released. It is important to alert the anesthesia providers to entrance into the abdomen. The abdomen should be packed with laparotomy pads in all four quadrants. It is important to place laparotomy pads on the anterior and posterior surface of the liver, as this may create tamponade that minimizes bleeding from the liver parenchyma. Care must be taken to avoid compressing the IVC with packing, as this will compromise venous return to the heart. While the pads are in place, the self-retaining retractor should be placed and resuscitation should continue.

To minimize contamination, enteric sources of spillage should be controlled rapidly. Vascular injuries should be addressed immediately. After examination of the left upper and the lower quadrants, attention should focus on the liver injury. The grade of injury should be assessed, and management depends on the examination and clinical condition.

Interventional Radiologic Adjuncts

Interventional radiologic (IR) techniques, including selective angiography and embolization, can be very useful in the management of liver injuries. In patients who remain hemodynamically stable and have a contrast blush, radiographic-guided intervention may improve the chances of success of nonoperative management (Figure 3).

Patients who are initially unstable and have a damage control procedure may benefit from selective angiography and embolization after resuscitation in the intensive care unit (ICU). This may facilitate re-exploration and minimizes bleeding during take back. Patients who remain hemodynamically stable should be treated in the operating room.

Venous bleeding from the liver parenchyma cannot be controlled with percutaneous techniques. Compression, either with laparotomy pads or from the developing hematoma, minimizes venous bleeding. Arterial bleeding requires surgical control or endovascular treatment.

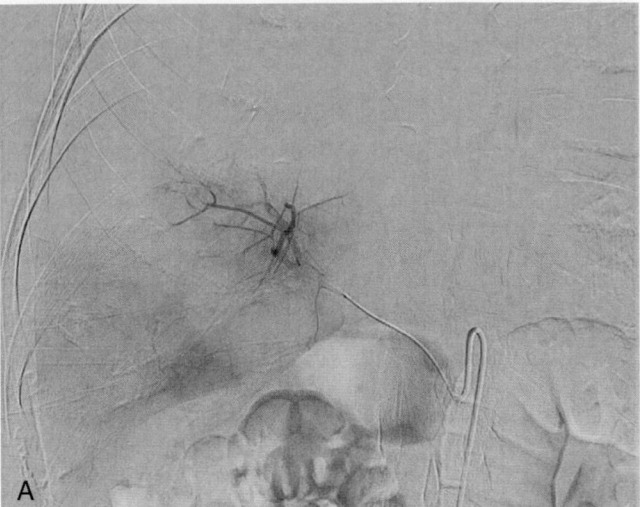
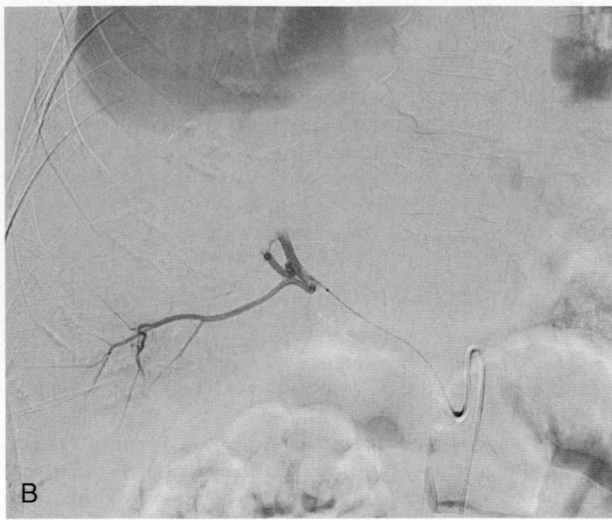

FIGURE 3 A, Active extravasation from the right lobe can be appreciated in this patient who underwent surgical packing. **B,** After successful embolization there is no evidence of bleeding on subsequent angiogram.

Blunt Trauma

Treatment of Minor Injuries

Minor injuries include capsule disruption and superficial lacerations. The raw surface of liver that is exposed after the capsule is compromised can cause significant bleeding. Direct compression for 5 to 10 minutes usually can control it. If unsuccessful, topical agents, electrocautery, and the argon beam coagulator can be used. Fibrin glue, hemostatic fabric, and topical collagen can be applied to the compromised surface. The liver then should be compressed for 5 to 10 minutes and reassessed. Clear inspection for possible bile leaks should be done. If there is no evidence of bleeding or bile leak, no further treatment is needed.

Similar to capsule disruptions, superficial lacerations initially can be treated with compression and adjuvant techniques, including hemostatic agents. If unsuccessful, suture hepatorrhaphy can be performed. Transcapsular #0 chromic sutures with blunt-nosed needles should be performed. If there is no evidence of enteric spillage, pledgets can be used to tie these sutures; if there is enteric spillage, Surgicel (Johnson & Johnson, New Brunswick, NJ) can be used as pledgets. Care should be taken to minimize necrosis of viable liver by placing sutures close to the edge of the injury. The hepatic veins, portal vein, and hepatic arteries as well as biliary structures can be injured with wide sutures; careful planning of the approach to perform hepatorrhaphy can minimize these complications.

Treatment of Moderate to Severe Injuries

Deep liver lacerations should be explored in order to identify defects in the bile system and vascular structures. With the use of 5-0 Prolene suture, figure-of-eight stitches are placed to control spillage and bleeding. A tongue of vascularized omentum can be prepared, packed into the laceration, and secured with transcapsular sutures.

If the bleeding is significant and there is concern for injury of larger vascular branches deep within the laceration, the finger fracture technique should be the initial approach. The liver injury is enlarged by pinching the parenchyma between the thumb and the index finger. The hepatic parenchyma without distinct major vascular or biliary duct structures then may be ligated. Expansion of the wound allows the identification of the larger branches that are usually on the deep aspect of the wound. Suture ligation and clips then are used to control the bleeding. Omental packing also can be performed.

In those patients in whom there is massive bleeding after release of hepatic packing, a different approach should be taken. Packing should be re-established immediately. The liver's vascular inflow should be controlled rapidly by performing Pringle's maneuver. The surgeon's left index finger should be placed through the foramen of Winslow and compression applied between the thumb and index finger. This will control the hepatic artery and the portal vein. The gastrohepatic ligament should be opened with electrocautery, being careful not to injure a replaced or accessory left hepatic artery. A vascular clamp, Penrose drain, or Rummel's tourniquet can be applied. Control of bleeding will be achieved in the majority of liver injuries by performing this maneuver. If there is control, the hepatic artery or the portal vein may be injured and causing the bleeding. Pringle's maneuver can be applied for 20 minutes, followed by 5 minutes of reperfusion. Longer application can result in ischemic liver injury. If there is overt bleeding, even after Pringle's maneuver, there should be concern for hepatic venous injury.

Once the inflow has been controlled, the liver must be mobilized in order to allow identification of injury. The falciform ligament and the ligamentum teres should be divided and followed back to the suprahepatic vena cava. The right and left triangular ligaments are divided, followed by the coronary ligaments. If during mobilization a hematoma is identified in the triangular ligaments, no attempts should be made at entering this area, as rapid exsanguination may ensue.

Once the liver is mobilized, the injury should be evaluated carefully. If intrahepatic vessels are identified as sources, suture ligation or clipping should be performed. Any visualized bile ducts should be ligated. The surgeon constantly should be assessing whether to continue efforts to surgically control the bleeding or to pack the liver, as most of its venous components can be controlled with packing and compression.

If there is evidence of bright red blood, the surgeon should be concerned for arterial bleeding. Consideration of adjunctive percutaneous embolization may be beneficial in this case. Extrahepatic suture ligation of the right or left hepatic artery can be used as an attempt to control bleeding. If the right hepatic artery is ligated, consideration should be given to performing cholecystectomy immediately or at a later date. Common hepatic artery ligation is the ultimate damage control maneuver; however, it carries high risk for liver and biliary duct ischemia.

In cases in which there is devascularization of a segment or lobe of the liver, a hepatectomy can be performed; however, this is rare, as traumatic injuries usually occur in a nonanatomic distribution and may involve central vessels. The goal of operative management of liver injuries should revolve around control of bleeding and not around resection of the injured segment. A partial hepatectomy should be performed only in the rare case where doing so will result in complete vascular control.

After mobilization, the surgeon can pack the liver more effectively. By rotating the left lobe toward the right, laparotomy pads can be placed posteriorly and in between the diaphragm and the liver. The right lobe then can be rotated medially and laparotomy pads placed along the vena cava posteriorly and also between the liver and the diaphragm. Anterior laparotomy pads then complete the packing and create effective compression and tamponade of bleeding. The abdomen then is closed with a temporary dressing and the patient is transported to the ICU for close monitoring, resuscitation, and warming. Angiography is an important adjunct if the patient may be taken to interventional radiology after packing of the liver for selective angioembolization to control arterial bleeding. The patient should return to the operating room within 24 to 72 hours, and the packs are removed. Most venous bleeding will have stopped. The decision to replace packs should be made by assessing the clinical situation of each patient. Premature removal may cause rebleeding, whereas prolonged packing is associated with onset of sepsis.

Once the decision to close the abdomen has been made, thorough evaluation for the presence of bile and identification of additional injuries should be performed. The surgeon should consider leaving closed suction drains for identification of biliary leaks and possible detection of bleeding. It is important to understand that both rebleeding and bile leaks can occur with no evidence of drain output changes.

Penetrating Trauma

Penetrating trauma tends to create long and narrow wounds with bleeding from deep vascular structures. If tangential or superficial, the previously described techniques should be implemented. However, if directly into the liver parenchyma, some additional techniques may prove to be useful.

With the use of a Penrose drain and a red rubber catheter, a balloon can be created to tamponade deep wounds. The red rubber catheter is prepared by cutting holes in the distal portion of the catheter. The catheter then is advanced through the Penrose drain and secured to the catheter with silk ties (Figure 4). The device then is inserted into the wound and, using saline, the balloon is inflated. It is important that the balloon portion of the device is long enough to "dumbbell" at the entrance and exit holes of the liver parenchyma. This can help to tamponade and control bleeding. Mobilizing the liver and packing it with laparotomy pads assists in further controlling any additional injuries. A temporary abdominal closure system can be used, and the patient then is transported to the ICU for further resuscitation and treatment (Figure 5). Within 24 to 72 hours the patient should be taken back to the operating room and the balloon is deflated (Figure 6). If there is additional bleeding, the balloon can be reinflated. It this occurs, it is likely that the patient will need a hepatectomy for definitive control.

Extrahepatic biliary and vascular structures are injured more frequently with penetrating injuries. Before performing any repair to these structures, Kocher's maneuver should be performed in order to have better exposure of the portal structures and to avoid further injury.

If the portal vein is injured, primary repair should be attempted with a lateral venorrhaphy technique and 5-0 Prolene sutures. If the patient is in critical condition and the portal vein is not amenable to primary repair, ligation can be performed, although survivability varies in the literature. Extensive resuscitation should be continued, and a second-look laparotomy should be performed to assess liver and bowel viability.

If any of the arteries are injured, primary repair should be attempted. The right and left hepatic arteries can be isolated and ligated. The common hepatic artery also can be ligated, especially if the portal vein remains intact. Follow-up of liver enzymes and coagulation parameters is needed in order to determine viability and

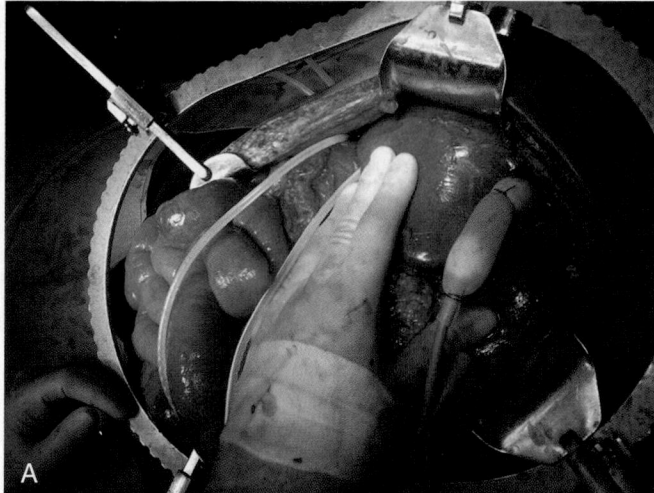

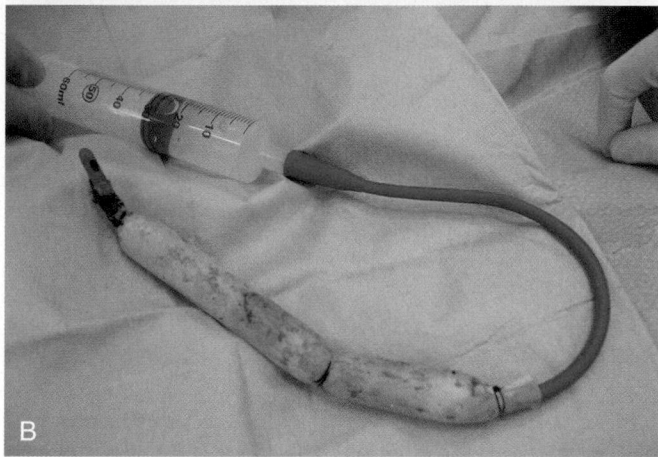

FIGURE 4 Intrahepatic balloon tamponade (**A**) constructed with a Penrose drain and a red rubber catheter (**B**).

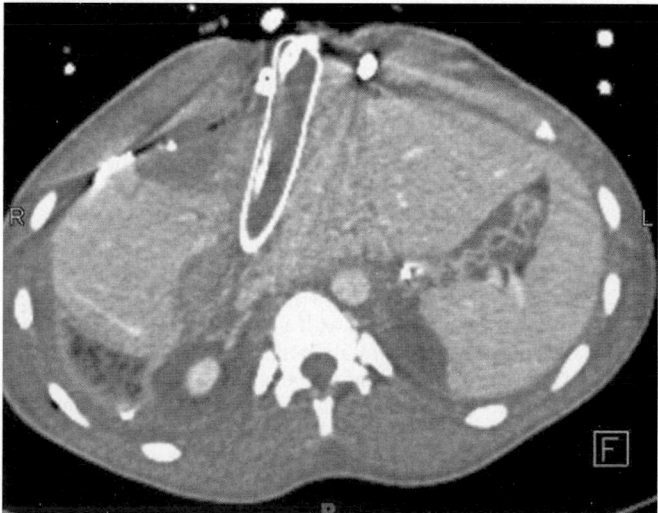

FIGURE 5 Balloon tamponade reflected on imaging.

provide necessary support during the recovery period. These patients will have a lifelong risk of biliary strictures and require long-term follow-up.

Extrahepatic injuries also occur more frequently with penetrating trauma. They should be addressed only if the patient is stabilized. Leaving drains in the area of biliary injury for evacuation of the

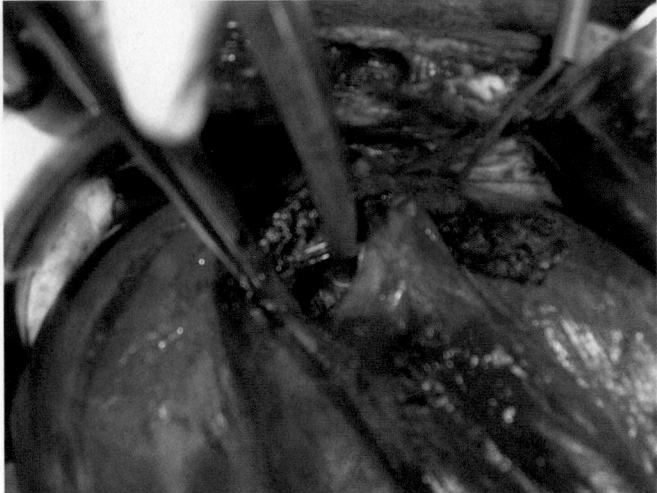

FIGURE 6 Gunshot track at 60 hours, after deflation and removal of the tamponade device. Complete hemostasis is noted.

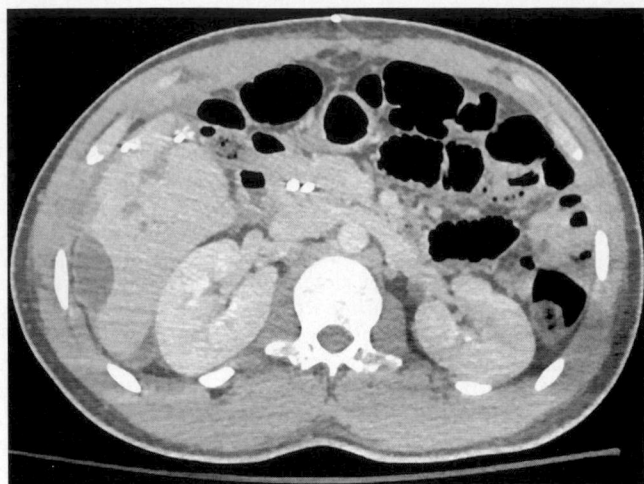

FIGURE 7 Liver abscess after operative management of a gunshot wound to the liver.

irritating bile can be used as a temporizing measure in unstable patients. If there is a minor injury, primary repair or placement of a T-tube should be attempted. However, if there is extensive injury, closed suction drains should be placed and plans should be made to perform a Roux-en-Y biliary-enteric anastomosis at a later time. Adjunctive drainage procedures, such as percutaneous transhepatic cholangiography (PTC) drains, can help to temporize patients.

Retrohepatic Caval Injury

Retrohepatic caval injury is very difficult to manage and carries significant mortality. The most conservative method of management involves liver packing, with favorable results reported. As mentioned previously, if a hematoma is seen when mobilizing the triangular ligament, the dissection should stop. Perihepatic packing with laparotomy pads and intraparenchymal packing with omentum should be used. Resuscitation is continued in the ICU and, if indicated, adjunctive radiologic techniques can be considered. Otherwise, vascular liver isolation should be considered in an attempt to repair the injured structures.

Atriocaval shunting has been abandoned because of reported mortality rates as high as 90%. However, if is to be attempted, it should be considered very early in the decision process in order to prevent exsanguination. A 36F chest tube is prepared by creating a hole in its proximal end. It is important to place the distal holes of the chest tube below the renal veins in the IVC. The chest is opened and a clamp is placed on the proximal end of the tube. The tube then is inserted through the right atrium down into the infrahepatic vena cava so that the proximal hole that was created is in the right atrium. It is secured to the right atrium with a purse-string suture and with umbilical tape around the intra-abdominal vena cava, above the renal veins. This allows return of blood by bypassing the injured area.

Hepatectomy and liver transplantation also can be performed but should be reserved for extreme situations in which no additional life-threatening injuries are present. It is not widely available, and the morbidity and mortality associated with it are high.

Adjunctive Techniques and Alternative Approaches

Venovenous Bypass

Used mainly during liver transplantation and extracorporeal oxygenation, venovenous bypass (VVB) has been used in the treatment of severe liver injuries. Rapid cannulation of the portal, common femoral, and axillary veins is performed, and bypass is established. A

clamp should be applied at the level of the infrahepatic vena cava, suprahepatic vena cava, and proximal portal vein.

The theoretical advantage of this approach is that the surgical procedure can be performed in a relatively dry field. Perfusion to the rest of the body is performed while the critically injured structure is completely controlled and isolated. The major limitation of this technique is that a perfusion therapist should be immediately available; also, the surgeon should be familiar with the placement of these cannulas in order to minimize instability.

Explantation and Autotransplantation

There have been reports of successful treatment of liver injuries by performing an explantation, repairing the injury, and then performing an autotransplantation. The patient usually undergoes rapid clamping of the suprahepatic and infrahepatic cava, portal vein, and hepatic artery. Then the liver is mobilized carefully. The common bile duct is transected and the liver is explanted. Back table repair is performed, and the liver then is autotransplanted. Patients are rarely candidates for this treatment strategy, as their hemodynamic compromise may limit the possibility of applying a suprahepatic caval clamp.

■ COMPLICATIONS

Operative as well as nonoperative management can result in complications, even after an initial favorable recovery. A patient with known liver injuries who develops abdominal pain, fever, leukocytosis, hypotension, tachycardia, or jaundice should have a thorough evaluation, including a repeat CT scan. The findings may be helpful in identifying complications.

Abscess

Patients with extensive parenchymal injuries, enteric injuries, inappropriate débridement, and large transfusion requirements are at risk for developing intra-abdominal abscesses (Figure 7). They can develop abdominal pain, fever, nausea, and decreased oral intake. Hypotension and tachycardia may accompany these symptoms. Laboratory studies may show leukocytosis.

CT scan of the abdomen will show a fluid collection that may be associated with the liver injury. Treatment includes intravenous antibiotics with gram-negative and anaerobic coverage as well as source control with imaging-guided percutaneous drainage. Four days of antibiotics after source control should provide appropriate coverage.

Operative drainage and débridement may be necessary if there is no improvement.

Pseudoaneurysm

Abdominal pain, hypotension, and anemia may suggest the presence of a vascular abnormality. If CT scan of the abdomen reveals a pseudoaneurysm, angiographic evaluation and embolization should be performed. If the abnormality is found at the level of the common hepatic artery, stent placement or open ligation and bypass should be considered.

Bile Leaks

Injury to the biliary track may result in bile leak. The patient may develop abdominal pain, fever, decreased oral intake, and liver function test (LFT) abnormality. CT scan should be obtained and if a fluid collection is identified, percutaneous drainage should follow. The presence of bile is diagnostic of a biliary leak.

Monitoring of output after drainage is necessary. If drainage decreases and eventually stops, no further treatment is necessary. If the drainage is greater than 50 mL/day for 14 days, further assessment should be pursued: cholangiographic evaluation of the biliary tree should be performed with endoscopic retrograde cholangiopancreatography (ERCP) or magnetic resonance cholangiopancreatography (MRCP). The former test is favored, as sphincterotomy and stent placement can be performed in an attempt to minimize the bile leak. PTC and percutaneous biliary drainage also can be attempted for treatment if cannulation of the sphincter of Oddi proves difficult.

Hemobilia

A patient who develops upper gastrointestinal bleeding, right upper quadrant pain, and jaundice after the management of a hepatic injury should be evaluated carefully for hemobilia. The frequency of presentation has decreased with the advent of nonoperative management because iatrogenic connections between liver parenchyma and blood vessels have been minimized. However, abnormal connections between vessels and the biliary tree still can occur in these patients. They usually result from arteriobiliary fistulae; therefore hepatic angiography, embolization, and resuscitation in the ICU are the pillars of treatment.

Necrosis

It is not uncommon to cause ischemia and necrosis of a portion of the liver after management of an injury, as vascular control may necessitate the ligation or embolization of an artery or vein that leads to necrosis (Figure 8). Patients can develop abdominal pain, LFT abnormalities, and signs and symptoms of sepsis. Repeat CT scan reveals a devascularized liver segment. It can resolve with no additional intervention, but débridement may be performed if it fails to improve. It is important to note that superimposed infections are common.

Rebleeding

Patients with liver injuries are at risk for rebleeding at any point during their management. Management is based on hemodynamic

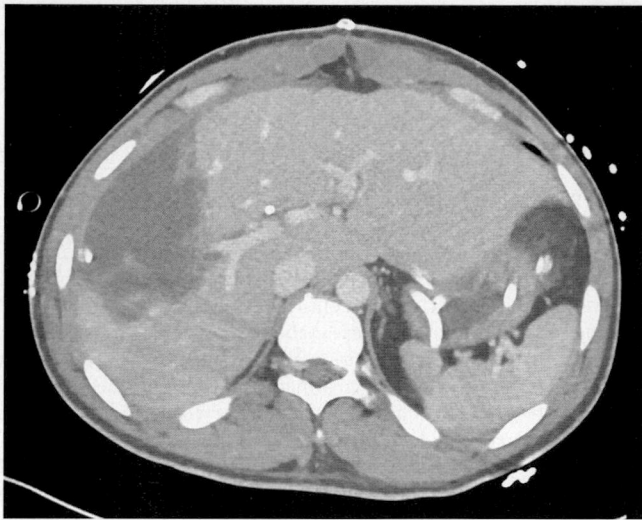

FIGURE 8 Liver necrosis after a gunshot wound to the right upper quadrant.

status: unstable patients require emergent surgical intervention, whereas stable patients can continue to be observed or treated with adjunctive radiologic interventions in order to increase the chances of successful nonoperative management.

■ CONCLUSION

The liver is the most commonly injured solid organ in patients with abdominal trauma. Approach to management depends on a patient's overall condition: for the unstable patient, immediate exploration should ensue; for stable patients, CT scans may be beneficial in determining the extent of injury and establishing a plan for nonoperative management. Operative management may require complete vascular control of the liver and ligation of named vessels. Nonoperative management may be attempted in any grade of injury (except grade VI), and adjunctive angiography and embolization may be used to control bleeding. Reimaging is a key component in the management of complications from these injuries.

SUGGESTED READINGS

Asensio JA, Demetriades D, Chahwan S, et al. Approach to the management of complex hepatic injuries. *J Trauma*. 2000;48:66-69.

Ball CG, Wyrzykowski AD, Nicholas JM, et al. A decade's experience with balloon catheter tamponade for the emergency control of hemorrhage. *J Trauma*. 2011;70:330-333.

Kozar RA, Moore JB, Niles SE, et al. Complications of nonoperative management of high-grade blunt hepatic injuries. *J Trauma*. 2005;59:1066-1071.

Polanco PM, Brown JB, Puyana JC, et al. The swinging pendulum: a national perspective of nonoperative management in severe blunt liver injury. *J Trauma Acute Care Surg*. 2013;75:590-595.

Stassen NA, Bhullar I, Cheng JD, et al. Nonoperative management of blunt hepatic injury: an Eastern Association for the Surgery of Trauma practice management guideline. *J Trauma Acute Care Surg*. 2012;73:S288-S293.

PANCREATIC AND DUODENAL INJURIES

Michael F. Rotondo, MD, FACS,
and Mark L. Gestring, MD, FACS

Injuries to the pancreas and duodenum are not common, occurring in less than 5% of patients with abdominal trauma. These injuries, however, can be difficult to identify and challenging to manage. Although both organs are reasonably well protected within the abdomen, their anatomic location can confound diagnosis, delay presentation, and complicate treatment. In addition, their location in a densely populated anatomic region adjacent to major solid organs (liver, spleen, kidney), major hollow organs (stomach, colon), and major blood vessels (inferior vena cava, superior mesenteric vessels, portal vein) accounts for the high risk of associated injuries to surrounding structures (Figure 1). These factors also contribute to the technical challenges related to management and the increased morbidity and mortality that is observed when injuries to the pancreas and duodenum occur.

■ DIAGNOSIS

Injury to the pancreas and/or duodenum can be caused by blunt or penetrating mechanisms, and a high index of suspicion is necessary to make the diagnosis in either case. Furthermore, injury to these organs can by identified by conventional imaging in the stable patient or during operation in the patient requiring urgent laparotomy. Both the mechanism of injury and the path to injury identification will affect the plan for management. A nonoperative approach, for example, may be used if a low-grade pancreatic injury is identified on computed tomography (CT) after blunt abdominal trauma in a stable patient. This would not be the case, however, if a combined injury to the pancreas and duodenum were identified during laparotomy after a gunshot wound. In either case, a stepwise approach to diagnosis in these varied settings will help to clarify subsequent management options.

Certain injury patterns should prompt suspicion for the potential of pancreatic or duodenal trauma. Significant blunt force to the epigastrium, as may be seen after sudden abdominal compression with a bicycle handlebar or a seatbelt during rapid deceleration, should trigger concern for this injury. Although the retroperitoneal location of these organs may limit physical examination findings, persistent abdominal pain and tenderness in the setting of blunt abdominal trauma should prompt concern and encourage further evaluation.

Focused assessment with sonography for trauma (FAST) is used commonly to evaluate the abdomen after trauma, but it contributes little to the diagnosis of pancreaticoduodenal injury because of the retroperitoneal location of these structures. CT, by comparison, is more helpful in this setting. CT scan allows visualization of the retroperitoneum and is the most effective way to image the pancreas and duodenum. On CT, injury to the pancreas is suggested by parenchymal laceration, intrapancreatic or retroperitoneal hematoma, peripancreatic fluid, phlegmon, or fluid between the pancreas and splenic vein. Bowel wall thickening, extraluminal gas, and contrast extravasation on CT suggest duodenal injury.

Endoscopic retrograde cholangiopancreatography (ERCP) is sensitive and specific for delineating pancreatic duct injury. Its role in the early diagnostic period may be limited, but the ability to identify an injury and potentially intervene during the same procedure with placement of a stent when necessary make this a valuable adjunct in the diagnosis and management of injury involving the pancreatic duct. Magnetic resonance cholangiopancreatography (MRCP), a noninvasive means of determining duct integrity, is useful for evaluation of the anatomy and integrity of the pancreatic duct but rarely is used in the acute setting.

Analysis of serum amylase and lipase also can be helpful in the diagnosis of pancreatic and duodenal injuries, but by themselves, they are not diagnostic. An elevated amylase level can occur after trauma without injury to the pancreas or duodenum. Conversely, injury to the pancreas or duodenum may be present in the setting of a normal amylase, especially if analyzed less than 3 hours after injury. Although a single result may be of limited value, the overall trend in amylase and lipase levels may suggest injury. Elevated amylase levels ultimately develop in nearly all patients with pancreaticoduodenal trauma, so repeated measurements increase the sensitivity and specificity of this diagnostic modality.

In the patient with indications for emergent laparotomy, the diagnosis of injury to the pancreas and duodenum should be made during surgery. This is frequently the case after penetrating injury to the abdomen. Techniques for exposure and mobilization of these organs are described later in this chapter. Findings suggestive of injury during exploration include central retroperitoneal hematoma, bile staining, or air in the surrounding tissue planes.

The likelihood of associated injuries, especially to major vascular structures, is high in patients with penetrating pancreaticoduodenal trauma. Control of hemorrhage and contamination are priorities and should come before any effort to definitively address an injury to the pancreas or duodenum identified in this scenario. A damage control approach to management may be more appropriate in such a setting with definitive repair of identified injuries deferred to subsequent laparotomies.

Increased morbidity and mortality are associated with delayed diagnosis of injuries to the pancreas and duodenum. As mentioned earlier, a high index of suspicion is required to identify these injuries with minimal delay.

■ MANAGEMENT

Duodenal Injury

Duodenal injuries can be identified with imaging, usually CT, or during laparotomy. When suspected during exploration, complete exposure and mobilization of the duodenum are required to properly exclude or assess injury to this organ. Dissection of the hepatic flexure medially away from its retroperitoneal attachments allows for the anterolateral aspects of the duodenum to be visualized. The lateral attachments of the duodenum are dissected both sharply and bluntly in the Kocher maneuver, allowing for upward and medial mobilization of the first and second portions of the duodenum. This facilitates evaluation of the anterior and posterior aspects of these segments. Division of the gastroduodenal artery sometimes may be required to fully evaluate this area. The Cattell-Braasch maneuver facilitates the exposure of the second, third, and fourth portions of the duodenum by mobilizing the posterior parietal attachments of the ascending colon and small bowel medially while rotating the viscera en bloc to the midline. Division of the ligament of Treitz with rotation of the duodenum allows the anterior and posterior surfaces of the fourth portion to be examined. Once full exposure of the duodenum has been achieved, the organ can be assessed adequately for injury. The American Association for the Surgery of Trauma-Organ Injury Scale (AAST-OIS) classifies injury to the duodenum on the basis of a grading scale from I to V (Table 1).

Duodenal hematoma (grades I and II) can be identified during surgical exploration but is identified more commonly on CT scan after blunt abdominal trauma. Duodenal hematoma can be responsible for obstruction of the gastric outlet and can be associated with vomiting and electrolyte abnormalities. In the absence of any other indications for surgery, supportive care consisting of IV hydration, nasogastric decompression, and parenteral nutrition is usually a successful treatment approach. Most duodenal hematomas will resolve spontaneously within 3 to 4 weeks. For patients who

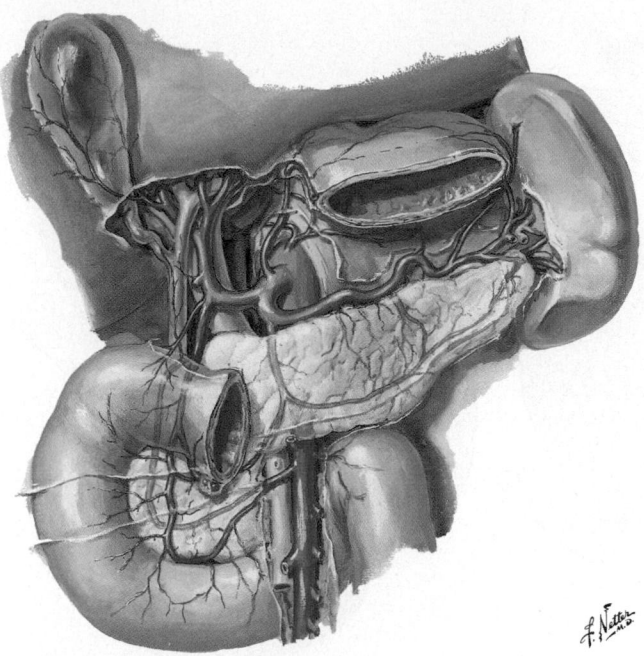

FIGURE 1 Relationship of the pancreas and duodenum to surrounding structures within the upper abdomen. *(From Netter FH.* Atlas of Human Anatomy. *5th ed. Philadelphia: Saunders; 2011.)*

TABLE 1: American Association for the Surgery of Trauma—Organ Injury Scale (AAST-OIS): Duodenal Injury Scaling

		Duodenum Injury Scale
Grade*	**Type of Injury**	**Description of Injury**
I	Hematoma	Involving single portion of duodenum
	Laceration	Partial thickness, no perforation
II	Hematoma	Involving more than one portion
	Laceration	Disruption <50% of circumference
III	Laceration	Disruption 50%-75% of circumference of D2
		Disruption 50%-100% of circumference of D1, D3, D4
IV	Laceration	Disruption >75% of circumference of D2
		Involving ampulla or distal common bile duct
V	Laceration	Massive disruption of duodenopancreatic complex
	Vascular	Devascularization of duodenum

From: Moore EE, Cogbill TH, Malangoni MA, et al. Organ injury scaling II: pancreas, duodenum, small bowel, colon and rectum. *J Trauma.* 1990; 30: 1427-1429.

*Advance one grade for multiple injuries up to grade III.

D1, First position of duodenum; *D2,* second portion of duodenum; *D3,* third portion of duodenum; *D4,* fourth portion of duodenum.

fail to improve, repeat imaging should be considered to reevaluate the obstructive process, and operative intervention may be necessary. If the diagnosis of significant duodenal hematoma is made during laparotomy, however, intervention usually is indicated at the time of discovery. In this case, the serosa should be incised

carefully over the hematoma to allow for evacuation of the contained blood. The resulting partial-thickness defect should be repaired primarily. Closed-suction drainage and nasojejunal feeding are recommended.

The majority of all full-thickness injuries to the duodenum can be repaired primarily with careful alignment of the breach. Repair consists of débridement of devitalized tissue and a two-layer closure of the defect. The closure generally should be oriented in a transverse direction, but a longitudinal repair would be acceptable in cases in which transverse repair would narrow significantly the remaining bowel lumen. Whenever possible, omentum should be used to buttress the repair.

Many adjuncts to primary repair of the duodenum have been described to reduce the incidence of suture line dehiscence and duodenal fistula formation. Pyloric exclusion, a technique described for temporary diversion of gastric contents, can be performed by oversewing the pylorus through a gastrostomy or by stapling the pylorus. A gastrojejunostomy is added for diversion until the pylorus reopens, usually within 3 months (Figure 2). Pyloric exclusion is reserved generally for protection of the most complex repairs of the duodenum or for combined injuries to both the duodenum and pancreas. Tube duodenostomy, whether antegrade or retrograde, also has been described. Neither pyloric exclusion nor tube duodenostomy have been proven to enhance the integrity of a primary duodenal repair. For tenuous repairs, however, omental buttressing or peritoneal flap reinforcement can be protective, and the placement of closed-suction drains adjacent to but not directly abutting any duodenal repair also is recommended.

A minority of duodenal injuries may not be amenable to primary repair because of the inability to bring the wound edges together without tension. Large proximal and distal duodenal injuries may be repaired by resection and primary duodenoduodenostomy. The second and third portions of the duodenum, because of their intimate relationship with the ampulla and pancreas, may not allow for the mobilization necessary to complete primary repair or duodenoduodenostomy. These injuries can be repaired with a Roux-en-Y duodenojejunostomy if the ampulla or common bile duct are not involved, although this technique is rarely necessary and should not be attempted by inexperienced hands.

Duodenal injuries that involve the ampulla, common bile duct, or pancreas are more complex and present additional management challenges. Damage to these structures should be suspected whenever injury is identified near the second and third portion of the duodenum. The ampulla is located on the posteromedial wall of the second portion of the duodenum. If the ampulla is injured, it may be repaired primarily or reimplanted into the duodenum or Roux loop of the jejunum. Any injury that cannot be reconstructed may necessitate pancreaticoduodenectomy.

Injuries to the distal common bile duct also complicate the management of duodenal trauma. Exploration of the posterior pancreatic head enhances visualization of the injury. Smaller injuries to the common bile duct (less than 50% of the circumference) can be repaired over a stent. Larger defects or involvement of the intrapancreatic or intraduodenal common bile duct require reimplantation of the duct or pancreaticoduodenectomy.

Pancreatic Injury

The Western Trauma Association (WTA) recently published an algorithm to help guide the diagnosis and management of pancreatic trauma. Because of the lack of prospective randomized clinical trials, this work was based largely on published observational studies and expert opinion. Nevertheless, it provides an excellent overview of the topic for those faced with the management of this injury (Figure 3).

The diagnosis of pancreatic injury can be made by imaging in the emergency room or during laparotomy in the operating room. As with trauma to the duodenum, the AAST-OIS classifies injury to the pancreas on the basis of a grading scale from I to V (Table 2). Injury to the

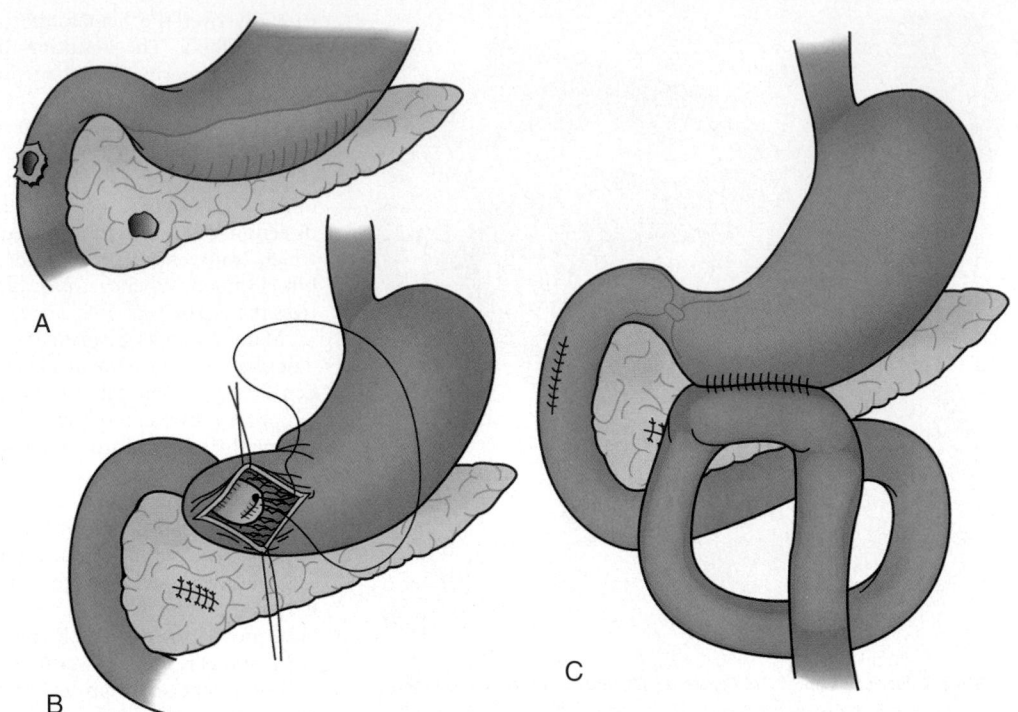

FIGURE 2 A, Pyloric exclusion is generally reserved for protection of complex duodenal repairs or for combined injuries to both the duodenum and the pancreas. **B,** The pylorus is generally closed with absorbable suture or staples. **C,** A gastrojejunostomy is added for diversion until the pylorus reopens (usually within 3 months). *(From Greenfield's Surgery: Scientific Principles and Practice. 5th ed. Baltimore, MD: Lippincott Williams and Wilkins; 2010.)*

TABLE 2: American Association for the Surgery of Trauma—Organ Injury Scale (AAST-OIS): Pancreatic Injury Scaling

	Pancreas Injury Scale	
Grade*	Type of Injury	Description of Injury
I	Hematoma	Minor contusion without duct injury
	Laceration	Superficial laceration without duct injury
II	Hematoma	Major contusion without duct injury or tissue loss
	Laceration	Major laceration without duct injury or tissue loss
III	Laceration	Distal transection or parenchymal injury with duct injury
IV	Laceration	Proximal transection or parenchymal injury involving ampulla
V	Laceration	Massive disruption of pancreatic head

From: Moore EE, Cogbill TH, Malangoni MA, et al. Organ injury scaling II: pancreas, duodenum, small bowel, colon and rectum. *J Trauma.* 1990;30:1427-1429.

*Advance one grade for multiple injuries up to grade III.

Proximal pancreas is to the patients' right of the superior mesenteric vein.

pancreatic duct is a major determinant of morbidity and becomes a concern when dealing with higher-grade pancreatic injuries.

As outlined in the WTA algorithm, abdominal imaging after trauma may demonstrate various degrees of pancreatic injury. Although CT is the preferred imaging modality, findings consistent with pancreatic injury may be subtle. This may be the case when the CT is performed shortly after injury. Findings consistent with or concerning for pancreatic injury on CT are outlined in Table 3. If concern for pancreatic injury persists despite a normal CT interpretation, the CT should be repeated to see whether additional time helps to visualize the suspected injury.

Low-grade pancreatic injuries identified on CT scan usually can be treated safely with a nonoperative approach. A surgical approach usually is recommended, however, if injury to the pancreatic duct is identified because these injuries are associated with higher complication rates. Endoscopic transpapillary pancreatic duct stenting also has been described in this setting and may be an option if this treatment modality is available. Although CT scan is very helpful in the diagnosis of pancreatic injury, it is not completely accurate in identifying injuries to the pancreatic duct. Because higher-grade pancreatic injuries are associated with greater morbidity and mortality and delays to intervention complicate outcomes further, it is recommended strongly that early evaluation of the pancreatic duct be conducted to exclude injury in patients with more than minimal pancreatic trauma.

Most ductal injuries can be identified by either preoperative studies in the stable patient (ERCP or MRCP) or during laparotomy. Full exposure and careful inspection of the pancreas during exploration are key to injury identification. In patients without significant intra-abdominal fat, the pancreas can be visualized through the transverse mesocolon. Dissection of the lesser sac through the greater and lesser omentum provides another opportunity for inspection of the pancreas. The Cattell-Braasch maneuver is used for visualizing the pancreatic head, and the Mattox maneuver is used to visualize the tail of the pancreas. Exposure of the pancreas is incomplete without mobilizing the superior and inferior borders, making sure that the posterior aspect of the pancreas is palpated for defects.

Drainage, resection, and reconstruction are the three main management options when pancreatic injury is identified during laparotomy. The degree of injury, usually based on AAST-OIS injury grade, helps to determine which management approach would be most appropriate. When grades I and II injuries to the pancreas are discovered at laparotomy, most can be treated with simple hemostasis and closed suction drainage. Drainage is used liberally because many

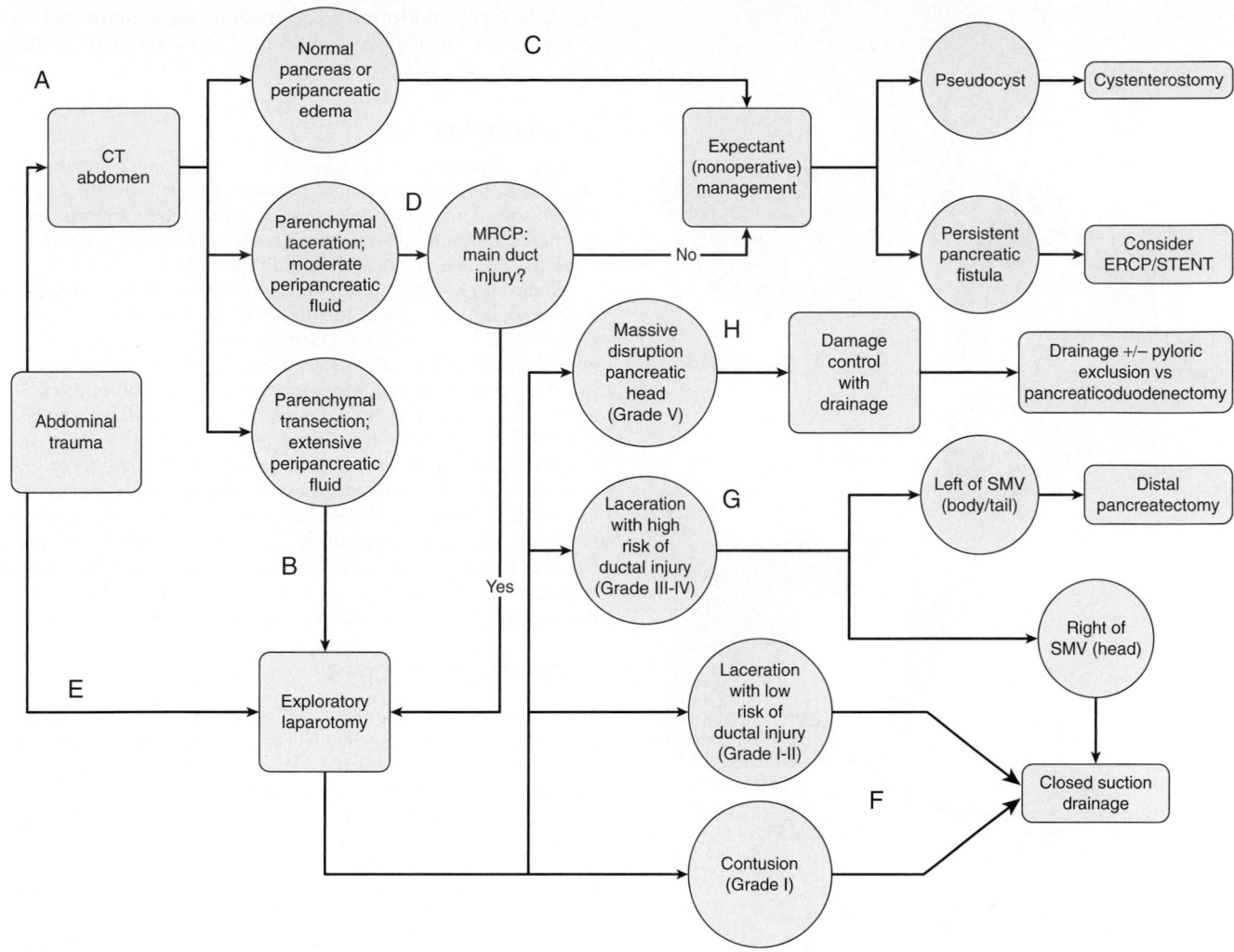

FIGURE 3 Western Trauma Association management algorithm for pancreatic injuries. *(From Biffl WL, Moore EE, Croce M, et al. Western Trauma Association critical decisions in trauma: management of pancreatic injuries. J Trauma Acute Care Surg. 2013;75:941-946.)*

TABLE 3: Contrast-Enhanced Computed Tomographic Scan Findings Suggestive and Diagnostic of Pancreatic Injury

Contrast-Enhanced CT Findings in Pancreatic Injury	
Suggestive Findings	**Diagnostic Findings**
Transverse mesocolon hematoma	Parenchymal laceration or hematoma
Fluid in the lesser sac/posterior to pancreas (between pancreas and splenic vein)	Transection of the parenchyma, with fluid in the lesser sac
Duodenal laceration or hematoma	Disruption of the head of the pancreas
Injury to left kidney, adrenal gland, or spleen	Diffuse swelling consistent with post-traumatic pancreatitis
Thickening of the left anterior renal fascia	
Lumbar spine transverse fracture (chance fracture)	

apparently minor injuries will drain for several days. Drains placed at laparotomy in these situations usually are removed within a few days, as long as the amylase concentration in the drain is less than that of serum. If amylase levels remain elevated, drainage is continued until there is no further evidence of pancreatic leak.

Major and minor injuries to the pancreas are differentiated by the integrity of the main pancreatic duct. Grade III injuries are associated with ductal injury and are best managed operatively to prevent pancreatic ascites or fistula. The anatomic division between the head and body of the pancreas is the neck, where the superior mesenteric artery and superior mesenteric vein pass behind the pancreas. Ductal injuries at or distal to the neck of the pancreas are best treated definitively with distal pancreatectomy (Figure 4). The spleen may or may not be preserved, depending on hemodynamic stability and other associated injuries. When undertaken, however, splenic salvage with distal pancreatectomy usually is reserved for children. Patients at high risk of ductal disruption should undergo distal pancreatectomy, whereas those at low risk usually are managed with closed suction drains. Ductal injuries proximal to the neck of the pancreas may be treated similarly with distal pancreatectomy. However, given the amount of pancreatic tissue loss, the likelihood of pancreatic insufficiency with the resection of greater than 80% of the pancreas is significant. In this situation, wide external drainage is recommended when there has not been complete destruction or massive devascularization of the pancreatic head.

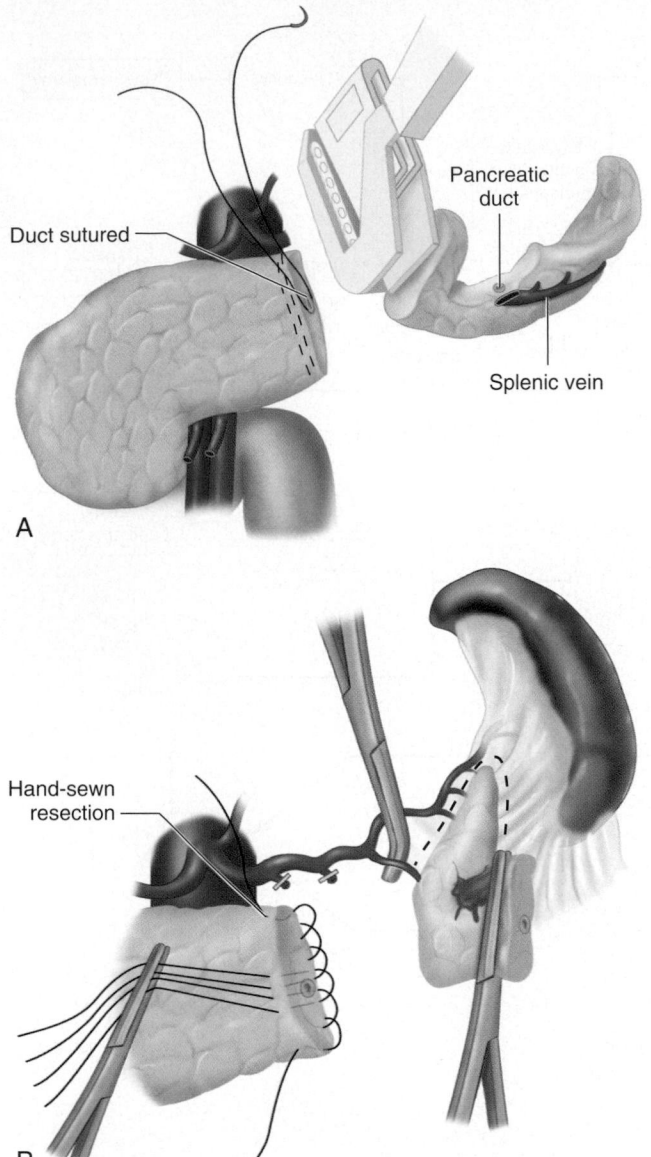

FIGURE 4 Ductal injuries at or distal to the neck of the pancreas are best treated with distal pancreatectomy. This can be done with a stapler (**A**), or the pancreas can be divided and oversewn with nonabsorbable, interrupted horizontal mattress sutures (**B**). In either case, the duct should be ligated with nonabsorbable suture if it can be identified and closed-suction drains should be used. The spleen can be preserved if indicated. *(From Cioffi W, ed. Atlas of Trauma/Emergency Surgical Techniques. Philadelphia, PA: Elsevier/Saunders; 2014.)*

High-grade injuries to the pancreas (grades IV and V) thankfully are rare but may require pancreaticoduodenectomy. Major disruption of the pancreatic head, significant injury to the intrapancreatic bile duct and proximal main pancreatic duct, and avulsion of the ampulla from the duodenum with destruction of the second portion of the duodenum may be indications for such an approach. Although pancreaticoduodenectomy may be well tolerated in the elective setting, trauma patients requiring such surgery on an emergent basis are frequently critically ill and not candidates for a prolonged surgical reconstruction. In such cases, hemostasis and control of contamination with liberal use of packing and a damage control approach should be used. More formal reconstruction can be considered when hemodynamic stability has been restored and appropriate resources are more readily available.

Combined Injuries

Although pancreatic and duodenal injuries are not common, these organs may be injured together because of their intimate anatomic relationship. This is especially true in cases of penetrating trauma. Morbidity and mortality rates are significantly higher when the pancreas and duodenum are injured at the same time.

When combined injuries occur, they should be managed as individual injuries unless the head of the pancreas is involved. Duodenal injuries without extensive tissue loss associated with nonductal pancreatic injuries are treated with primary repair and closed-suction drainage. More extensive duodenal injuries with major pancreatic duct injury may require duodenal repair, as described earlier, along with distal pancreatectomy. Pyloric exclusion frequently is described as an effective technique for temporarily diverting the gastric contents away from the injured pancreaticoduodenal complex in these situations and omental buttressing combined with closed-suction drainage of any repairs is recommended strongly. Because of the shared blood supply to the pancreas and duodenum, massive destruction or devascularization of these organs necessitates pancreaticoduodenectomy.

■ COMPLICATIONS

The majority of deaths associated with pancreatic and duodenal trauma occur within the first 48 hours of injury. The morbidity related to duodenal injuries varies with grade, ranging from 10% to 55%, whereas the morbidity related to pancreatic injuries is consistently higher. The risk of complications can be predicated on the basis of injury grade (AAST-OIS), associated injuries, the presence of combined pancreaticoduodenal injury, hypothermia, and packing without drainage during initial damage control laparotomy.

Development of pancreatic pseudocyst and persistent pancreatic fistula is the most common complication after pancreatic injury. As outlined in the WTA algorithm, large pancreatic pseudocysts may be treated with endoscopic stenting or cyst enterostomy. Pancreatic fistulae require drainage. Duodenal fistula, by comparison, generally results from failure of the surgical repair due to suture line dehiscence. Although the incidence of duodenal fistula is generally low, diversion of gastric flow from the repair while it heals through pyloric exclusion has been recommended for complex repairs of the duodenum. The establishment of enteral access in high-risk patients is also advisable.

SUGGESTED READINGS

Asensio J, Demetriades D, Berne J, et al. A unified approach to the surgical exposure of pancreatic and duodenal injuries. *Am J Surg*. 1997;174: 54-60.

Biffl WL, Moore EE, Croce M, et al. Western Trauma Association Critical Decisions in Trauma: management of pancreatic injuries. *J Trauma Acute Care Surg*. 2013;75:941-946.

Hirshberg A, Mattox KL. *Top Knife: The Art and Craft of Trauma Surgery*. Shrewsbury: TFM; 2005:115-130.

Moore EE, Cogbill TH, Malangoni MA, et al. Organ injury scaling II: pancreas, duodenum, small bowel, colon and rectum. *J Trauma*. 1990;30: 1427-1429.

Seamon MJ, Kim PK, Stawicki P, et al. Pancreatic injury in damage control laparotomies: is pancreatic resection safe during the initial laparotomy. *Injury*. 2009;40:61-65.

Sharpe JP, Magnotti LJ, Weinberg JA, et al. Impact of a defined management algorithm on outcome after traumatic pancreatic injury. *J Trauma Acute Care Surg*. 2012;72:100-105.

Injuries to the Small and Large Bowel

Leonard L. Mason III, MD, and Timothy C. Fabian, MD

Many trauma surgeons firmly believe that an operation is mandated for gunshot wounds of the abdomen. This is because gastrointestinal injuries occur in more than 80% of patients with these wounds. The incidence of hollow viscus injury after stab wounds to the abdomen is approximately 20%. The most frequently injured organs are the small bowel and colon in penetrating abdominal trauma. This is in stark contrast to blunt trauma, where the incidence of bowel injuries is between 1% and 5% in most recent series. It is easy to understand how a high-velocity missile or knife can injure a hollow viscus easily, but multiple mechanisms have been proposed for small bowel injury or rupture. Whereas in the past traffic casualties died at the scene or sustained rapidly fatal central nervous injuries, road safety efforts have reduced traffic fatalities and created different patterns of injury, one of which is small bowel rupture. The risk for small bowel rupture has increased significantly because of the increased use of seatbelts. Three possible mechanisms of blunt small bowel rupture have been postulated: (1) crush injury between the vertebrae and anterior abdominal wall, (2) sudden increase in the intraluminal pressure of the bowel, and (3) rapid deceleration causing tangential tears at relatively fixed points along the bowel.

The diagnosis of these injuries after penetrating trauma is relatively straightforward, as the injuries usually are diagnosed during exploratory laparotomy. It remains a challenge to identify small bowel and colon injuries after blunt trauma, even after the helical computed tomography (CT) became widely available in the mid-1990s. Regardless of the specific injury mechanism, the principles and techniques of operative management are similar.

■ DIAGNOSIS OF BLUNT INJURIES

Because blunt viscus injury is an infrequent diagnosis, experience with this injury is limited and a widely accepted diagnostic approach to blunt small or colon injury has not been formulated. This is evidenced by significant variation in diagnostic approaches among experienced trauma surgeons at multiple level I trauma centers. Physical examination is still an important tool in the clinical evaluation of trauma patients with intra-abdominal injury. The finding of tachycardia or abdominal tenderness may suggest the presence of hollow viscus injury. However, reliability of the examination may be compromised by obtunded patients with closed head injury, spinal cord injury, or intoxication. If the patient can participate in the abdominal examination, other associated injuries, including rib or pelvic fractures or abdominal wall hematomas, can mimic abdominal pain or peritonitis falsely, leading to diagnosis of blunt small bowel or colon injury. In addition, it is not uncommon for blunt bowel injury to occur later in the patient's hospital course, whereby the expected signs and symptoms of such injuries take some time to develop.

Laboratory abnormalities, including elevations in the white blood cell (WBC) count, amylase, and lactic acid, may point to the presence of hollow viscus injury but are relatively nonspecific.

A sign on the abdominal examination that has been shown to be one of the most significant risk factors for blunt small injuries is abdominal wall ecchymosis, also known as *seatbelt sign*. In the 2003 multi-institutional study report by Fakhry and colleagues, a seatbelt mark was associated with an increased risk of perforated small bowel injury. Also occurring with these injuries can be flexion compression fractures to the lumbar spine, called Chance fractures. Because these signs are rare and nonoperative management is becoming the standard of care for many solid organ injuries, various diagnostic methods or adjuncts are required to help aid in the diagnosis of blunt intestinal injuries.

Before the abdominal CT scan was used as the primary diagnostic modality in the evaluation of blunt abdominal trauma, diagnostic peritoneal lavage (DPL) was the most commonly used method for evaluating hemodynamically stable patients suspected of having these injuries. DPL was more sensitive than CT for identifying blunt small bowel injury, but the goal was to move toward a noninvasive approach in the management of these injuries. Late-generation scanners allow for high-resolution imaging of the bowel and mesentery, enabling successful nonoperative management of solid organ injury in more than 90% of patients in some series. Preoperative diagnosis of blunt intestinal injury was made relatively infrequently before CT was introduced because it was an incidental finding during exploratory laparotomy for hemoperitoneum and solid organ injuries. Along with CT scanning, ultrasonography and laparoscopy began to play a major role in the algorithm of identifying blunt small bowel or colon injury.

In the hemodynamically stable patient with blunt trauma, CT is the most commonly used diagnostic modality. Newer-generation CT scanning techniques have improved and become helpful in identifying patients with a possible bowel injury. The dilemma with using only CT as a method of diagnosing blunt intestinal injury is that it has a high false-negative rate. A recent study demonstrated a 15% false-negative rate for patients who had small bowel or mesenteric injuries with a negative scan. The false-negative rate in that study paralleled the 2003 study by the Eastern Association for the Surgery of Trauma (EAST), which showed a 13% false-negative rate for CT in the diagnosis of small bowel injury. Findings of free intraperitoneal fluid without solid organ injury, pneumoperitoneum, bowel wall thickening, oral or rectal contrast extravasation, mesenteric hematoma, or vascular blush have been shown to be predictive of small bowel or large bowel injury. Even though these findings are predictive of blunt intestinal injury, they occur in less than 50% of cases in some series. Reliance on a "negative" CT scan to exclude blunt intestinal or mesenteric injury is highly discouraged and not recommended. Missed blunt mesenteric injuries can be catastrophic for the critically injured trauma patient. Delay in diagnosis can result in ischemia to the bowel wall leading to bowel perforation, especially if not diagnosed within 24 hours. In "bucket handle" injuries, the mesentery is stripped away from the bowel, causing bleeding and eventually an ischemic piece of bowel. If the index of suspicion is low for this type of injury, the patient will be seen with peritonitis secondary to perforated blunt intestinal injury days later. We believe that if the patient has a CT scan with any of the previous listed abnormalities, especially the finding of free fluid without solid organ injury, an exploratory laparotomy should be strongly considered. When the physical examination is reliable, repeated examinations combined with CT should lead to accurate diagnostic results. Diagnostic laparoscopy usually is reserved for patients with subtle CT findings who are unable to participate in an abdominal examination. The risk of increased morbidity or mortality is significant with prolonged delay in diagnosis.

Focused assessment with sonography for trauma (FAST) has been a useful tool in evaluating the patient with blunt abdominal trauma. It is highly specific and moderately sensitive in identifying intra-abdominal fluid, the presence of which in a hemodynamically unstable patient is an indication for laparotomy. However, FAST does not reliably distinguish between solid organ injury and hollow viscus injury. The decision for operative intervention for suspected blunt bowel injury should not be based solely on the results of FAST.

Even though trauma surgeons have used DPL less frequently, it is still a valuable tool in the algorithm for blunt abdominal trauma patients. DPL usually begins with decompression of the stomach and urinary bladder with a nasogastric tube and Foley catheter. A supraumbilical or infraumbilical incision is made. A catheter is placed intraperitoneally after the fascia and peritoneum have been incised.

It then is directed in the upper quadrants and pelvis. A 10-mL syringe is attached to the catheter, and if there is return of blood, the patient is taken to the operating room. If this test is negative for hemoperitoneum, 1 L of saline is infused via the catheter as quickly as possible. The intravenous (IV) bag is dropped to the floor, and return of at least 300 mL is adequate for analysis. The fluid is sent to the laboratory for analysis and is considered positive if 100,000/mm³ or more red blood cells, 500/mm³ or more WBCs, bile, or fecal or vegetable matter is found. The presence of enteric content is highly predictive of blunt bowel injury, but this is a rare finding. Because of the high sensitivity and low specificity of DPL for small bowel injuries, patients with blunt abdominal trauma previously underwent laparotomy more frequently than they do now. The high nontherapeutic laparotomy rate relegated its use to specific clinical situations. These include evaluating the blunt trauma patient with a depressed level of consciousness who has free fluid without evidence of solid organ injury.

■ PENETRATING INJURIES

Gunshot wounds usually require an exploratory laparotomy or at least a diagnostic laparoscopy given the high incidence of intra-abdominal injury. Most firearms used in civilian scenarios today have moderate to high velocity, and even if peritoneal violation can be excluded, bowel perforation from blast effect occasionally occurs. Stab wounds are associated with a lower incidence of intra-abdominal injury than gunshot wounds. Approximately one third of patients with stab wounds to the anterior abdominal wall (i.e., those anterior to the midaxillary line) will have peritoneal violation with intra-abdominal injury, usually of the small bowel. These patients have high likelihood of hollow viscus injury and should undergo exploration emergently.

If the gunshot wound is considered to have taken a tangential trajectory or if the stab wound appears to be superficial, selective management algorithms can be used that rely on diagnostic tests (CT scan, diagnostic laparoscopy, and local wound exploration), serial abdominal examinations, or a combination of the two. Hemodynamic instability or peritonitis excludes the patient from taking this approach. If local wound exploration is chosen, it usually is performed in the emergency department with sterile technique and local anesthesia. The wound is extended sharply to gain better visualization of the anterior fascia. If the fascia has been violated, we proceed with laparotomy.

Because of the emergence of trauma surgeons skilled in minimally invasive surgery, laparoscopy now is being used as a therapeutic tool. Some centers have reported favorable experiences with exploratory laparoscopy and treating selected injuries (mostly small or large bowel injuries). The use of laparoscopy has been reported to result in shorter hospitalizations, fewer postoperative wound infections and ileus complications, and no missed injuries. However, the trauma community is still hesitant to embrace it. Laparoscopic bowel repair is not practiced routinely at our trauma center. It is time consuming, and we are concerned about accurate definition and repair when multiple injuries or hemorrhage is present. If the peritoneum or an injury has been visualized during diagnostic laparoscopy, we generally convert to an exploratory laparotomy.

Stab wounds to the lower back or flank (posterior to the midaxillary line) carry a lower risk of intra-abdominal injury and are evaluated by CT. These wounds potentially could result in retroperitoneal injuries. Detection of these injuries with laparoscopy is difficult even with the most experienced minimally invasive surgeon. Triple-contrast CT (oral, intravenous, and rectal contrast) is accurate for the assessment of colon and intraperitoneal and extraperitoneal rectal injuries. Some authors have argued that it should be part of the algorithm to evaluate penetrating torso trauma. We do not believe that the benefits of using oral contrast outweigh the risks (i.e., aspiration) in a trauma patient with penetrating injury who most likely will be explored surgically.

■ SURGICAL MANAGEMENT OF SMALL BOWEL

A thorough and systemic approach is necessary in managing patients with small bowel injuries. They can be evaluated intraoperatively by "running the bowel": the small bowel and its mesentery are inspected in a comprehensive fashion between at least two sets of hands from the ligament of Treitz caudal to the ileocecal valve. Management of each wound is determined by its severity according to the American Association for the Surgery of Trauma (AAST) grading system (Table 1). If a grade I small bowel injury (partial thickness or contusion/bruising on AAST injury scale; Figure 1) is encountered, the seromuscular layers are reapproximated in a single layer with 3-0 nonabsorbable Lembert suture. This increase in intraluminal pressure can lead to increased wall tension and possibly rupture (Laplace's law). There are no data to support this notion, but repair is simple and relatively risk free. Small full-thickness (grade II) and larger full-thickness (grade III) injuries are repaired with limited débridement and closure. Closure can be performed in either one or two layers. Transverse closure is preferred, to avoid luminal narrowing. Full-thickness injuries that are closely opposed should be converted to a single defect and primarily repaired. If multiple perforations are present within the same segment, they are best treated with resection and anastomosis. More extensive wounds and wounds associated with devascularization (grades IV and V) require resection with anastomosis. Intraoperative factors like hemodynamic instability, significant ongoing blood loss requiring multiple blood transfusions,

---

TABLE 1: Small Bowel Injury Scale

Grade*	Type of Injury	Description of Injury	ICD-9	AIS-90
I	Hematoma	Contusion or hematoma without devascularization	863.20	2
	Laceration	Partial thickness, no perforation	863.20	2
II	Laceration	Laceration <50% of circumference	863.30	3
III	Laceration	Laceration ≥50% of circumference without transection	863.30	3
IV	Laceration	Transection of the small bowel	863.30	4
V	Laceration	Transection of the small bowel with segmental tissue loss	863.30	4
	Vascular	Devascularized segment	863.30	4

From Moore E, Cogbill T, Malangoni M, Jurkovich G, Champion H. Scaling system for organ specific injuries. *Curr Opin Crit Care.* 1996;2:450-462.

*Advance one grade for multiple injuries up to grade III.

AIS-90, Abbreviated Injury Scale–1990 Revision; *ICD-9,* International Classification of Diseases, Ninth Revision.

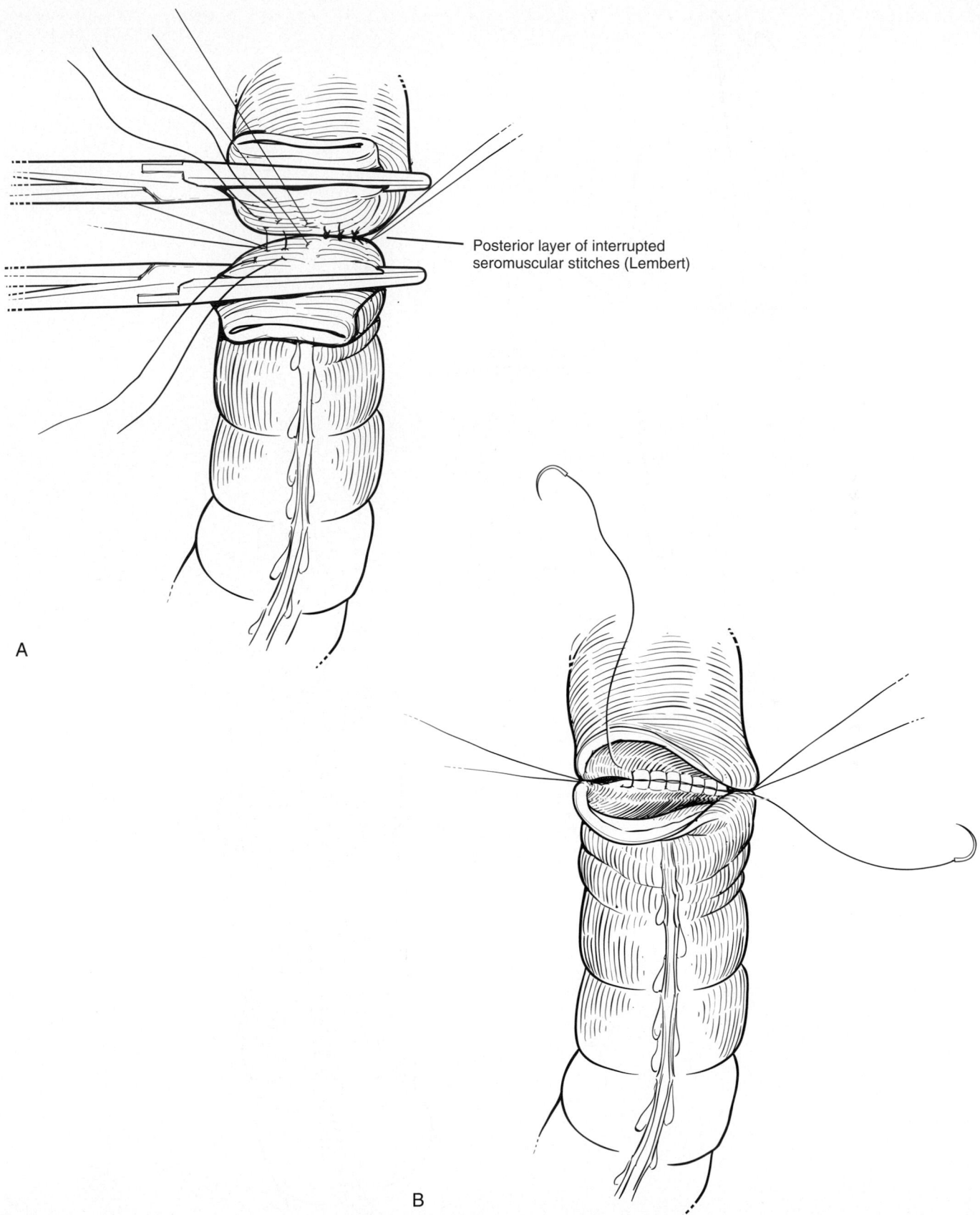

Posterior layer of interrupted
seromuscular stitches (Lembert)

A

B

FIGURE 1 Handsewn end-to-end anastomosis. **A,** After noncrushing bowel clamps are applied proximal to the bowel ends, the staple lines are cut with electrocautery or Metzenbaum scissors. In a standard two-layer anastomosis, the posterior (outer) layer of the transverse colon and proximal rectum are reapproximated with 3-0 silk interrupted (Lembert) sutures. **B,** Two continuous absorbable sutures are used in the posterior inner row, and each is brought anteriorly,

Continued

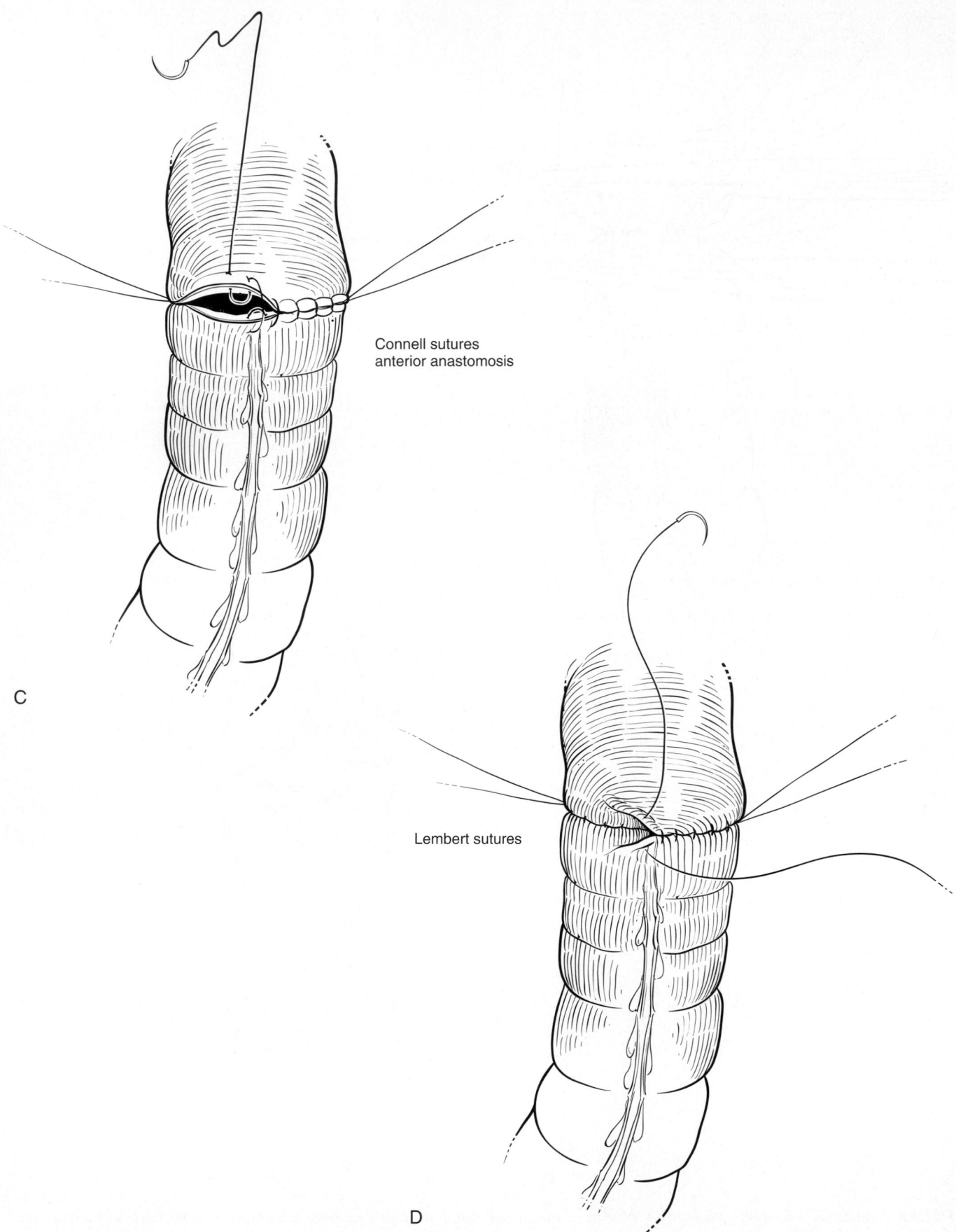

C

Connell sutures
anterior anastomosis

Lembert sutures

D

FIGURE 1, cont'd (C) where the transition to Connell sutures is made **(D)**. *(From Townsend C, Evers BM.* Atlas of General Surgical Techniques. *Philadelphia: Elsevier; 2010:Figures 60-8 through 60-11.)*

acidosis, coagulopathy, or hypothermia may influence the surgeon to forgo an anastomosis at the initial operation, perform a damage control laparotomy, and consider resection with delayed anastomosis or creation of an ileostomy.

Mesenteric injuries may be encountered without an associated small bowel injury. This segment of small bowel should be inspected closely for vascular compromise. Determination of intestinal viability begins with assessment of the bowel's appearance. Adjunctive measures, such as Doppler or fluorescein Wood's lamp illumination, may facilitate assessment of perfusion in segments where viability is questionable. If the bowel is viable with adequate blood flow, the defect in the mesentery should be reapproximated to prevent an internal hernia. Bleeding can arise from the mesenteric vessels with the rent; therefore individual vessels should be ligated as opposed to performing mass ligation, which may produce ischemia. We generally do not explore small nonexpanding mesenteric hematomas except when the mesenteric border of the small bowel wall is obscured by it. Bowel wall injury or perforation has to be excluded. Expanding hematomas should be opened and bleeding vessels oversewn.

Historically, small bowel anastomoses in trauma patients usually were performed handsewn in one or two layers. There has been recent controversy over whether stapled small bowel anastomoses have a higher rate of complications. Many trauma surgeons believe that these critically injured patients require excessive volumes of fluid resuscitation, which leads to generalized bowel edema. The bowel wall edema is likely a contributor to staple line failure. A multi-institutional study in 2001 demonstrated increased anastomotic leaks and intra-abdominal abscesses in stapled bowel anastomosis in the trauma patient. Conversely, a Minnesota group in 2000 reviewed their complication rate of just stapled small bowel anastomoses and concluded that there was no difference versus handsewn anastomoses. If bowel wall edema is evident or anticipated, we believe it is prudent to perform a sutured anastomosis.

■ MANAGEMENT OF COLONIC INJURIES

The management of traumatic colon injuries has undergone major changes since World War II. A colostomy was mandated for all colonic injuries sustained in combat because of the significant morbidity associated with anastomotic leak in the critically injured patient. Fecal diversion became the standard of care until surgeons in the 1970s started to realize that civilian wounds were different from military wounds. Experience with primary repair in the civilian setting suggested it could be performed safely and without the morbidity of a colostomy in selected patients. High-risk patients (i.e., those with shock, major blood loss, fecal contamination, destructive wounds of the colon, or delayed presentation) were excluded from

earlier studies and still treated with a colostomy. Even in these high-risk patients, primary repair became accepted, especially in managing less destructive injuries.

Operative management should be directed according to the classification of penetrating colonic injuries as either destructive or nondestructive. Nondestructive colonic injuries are defined as wounds that involve less than 50% of the bowel wall without devascularization (Table 2). Partial-thickness lacerations or serosal tears (grade I) can be repaired with interrupted nonabsorbable Lembert sutures. Full-thickness lacerations (grade II) may be closed in one or two layers; however, we prefer the latter. Destructive colonic injuries are defined as wounds that completely transect the colon (grade IV) or involve tissue loss and devascularized segments. These injuries generally require fecal diversion with a colostomy or resection with anastomosis. Management of complex colon injuries is based on grade as well as anatomic location. In right-sided injuries (grades III to V), the majority receive a total right colectomy with reconstruction using an ileocolostomy. Complex left-sided injuries undergo resection with colocolostomy (see Figure 1).

Optimal management of destructive injuries also should be based on the physiologic state of the patient. The lethal triad of coagulopathy, acidosis, and hypothermia may not allow the critically injured patient to receive a successful anastomosis. Damage control laparotomy is indicated to control fecal contamination from destructive wounds by resecting them with a gastrointestinal anastomosis (GIA) stapler and leaving the patient in discontinuity. A question arises in patients with a damage control laparotomy: Is it safe to restore bowel continuity in the subsequent operation via a colonic anastomosis versus performing diversion via end colostomy or loop ileostomy? Some studies have shown that the delayed anastomotic leak rate is reasonably high (12%). Recently we reviewed our 17-year experience with delayed anastomosis and observed that our clinical pathway (Figure 2) can be applied successfully in these patients with a significant reduction in suture line failure (4% vs 32%, $P = 0.03$) and colon-related morbidity. Risk factors for suture line failure also were identified. Similar to previous studies, the data demonstrated that patients with destructive colonic injuries who had comorbid medical conditions or transfusion requirements greater than 6 units of blood were at significantly higher risk for suture line breakdown. It is highly recommended that these patients receive an ostomy.

Even when prudent, colostomy construction has its own postoperative complications. Stomal ischemia or necrosis, obstruction, retraction, parastomal hernia, and subcutaneous abscess can occur in up to 15% of patients. Given these risks, colostomy reversal should be done in a timely manner. It usually is performed around 3 to 6 months after hospital discharge. Before closure, a contrast enema is obtained to rule out the presence of a distal stricture. There has been

TABLE 2: Colon Injury Scale

Grade*	Type of Injury	Description of Injury	ICD-9	AIS-90
I	Hematoma	Contusion or hematoma without devascularization	863.40-863.44	2
	Laceration	Partial thickness, no perforation	863.40-863.44	2
II	Laceration	Laceration <50% of circumference	86.50-863.54	3
III	Laceration	Laceration ≥50% of circumference without transection	86.50-863.54	3
IV	Laceration	Transection of the colon	86.50-863.54	4
V	Laceration	Transection of the colon with segmental tissue loss	86.50-863.54	4
	Vascular	Devascularized segment	86.50-863.54	4

From Moore E, Cogbill T, Malangoni M, Jurkovich G, Champion H. Scaling system for organ specific injuries. *Curr Opin Crit Care.* 1996;2:450-462.

*Advance one grade for multiple injuries up to grade III. 863.41, 863.51: ascending; 863.42, 863.52: transverse; 863.45, 863.53: descending; 863.44, 863.54: rectum.

AIS-90, Abbreviated Injury Scale; *ICD-9*, International Classification of Diseases, Ninth Revision.

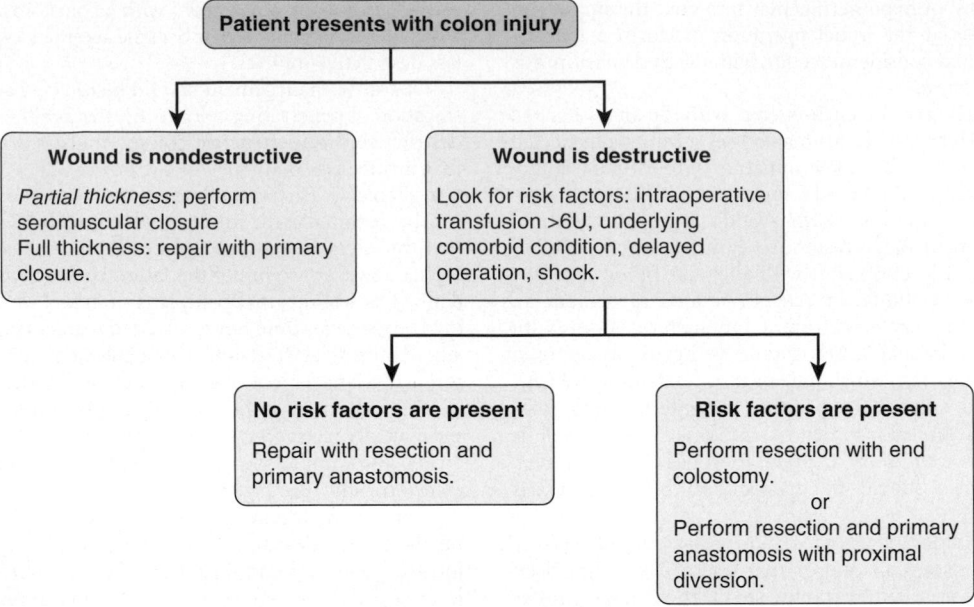

FIGURE 2 Algorithm outlines the treatment of colon injury.

argument among some surgeons that early closure (within 2 weeks) is just as safe as the traditional late closure. A study in 1995 found no significant difference in morbidity between both groups; however, there was shorter operating time and less intraoperative blood loss with early closure. To date, this practice is not widely accepted and traditional late closure has remained the gold standard.

SUGGESTED READINGS

Barnett RE, Love KM, Sepulveda EA, et al. Small bowel trauma: current approach to diagnosis and management. *Am Surg.* 2014;80:1183-1191.

Brundage SI, Jurkovich GJ, Hoyt DB, et al. Stapled versus sutured gastrointestinal anastomoses in the trauma patient: a multicenter trial. *J Trauma.* 2001;51:1054-1061.

Fakhry SM, Watts DD, Luchette FA, et al. Current diagnostic approaches lack sensitivity in the diagnosis of perforated blunt small bowel injury: analysis from 275,557 trauma admissions from the EAST multi-institutional HVI trial. *J Trauma.* 2003;54:295-306.

Greer LT, Gillern SM, Vertrees AE. Evolving colon injury management: a review. *Am Surg.* 2013;79:119-127.

Miller PR, Fabian TC, Croce MA, et al. Improving outcomes following penetrating colon wounds: application of a clinical pathway. *Ann Surg.* 2002;235:775-781.

Sharpe JP, Magnotti LJ, Weinberg JA, et al. Applicability of an established management algorithm for destructive colon injuries after abbreviated laparotomy: a 17-year experience. *J Am Coll Surg.* 2014;218:636-643.

Witzke JD, Kraatz JJ, Morken JM, et al. Stapled versus hand sewn anastomoses in patients with small bowel injury: a changing perspective. *J Trauma.* 2000;49:660-666.

THE MANAGEMENT OF RECTAL INJURIES

Mark L. Ryan, MD, MSPH, and Martin A. Croce, MD, FACS

The treatment of traumatic rectal injuries has evolved considerably with the military conflicts over the past 150 years. During the American Civil War, colorectal injuries were treated nonoperatively, with surgical management limited to possible manual reduction of eviscerated bowel and suturing of the fascial defect. This resulted in mortality rates greater than 90%. In World War I, treatment of rectal injuries consisted of wide local débridement and external drainage, achieving mortality rates of 70%. This was further reduced to approximately 36% in the beginning of World War II by the incorporation of proximal colostomy for all injuries to the rectum, which was eventually mandated in the treatment guidelines issued by the Department of the Army. By the end of the war, surgeons were reporting mortality rates as low as 6% with the addition of posterior drainage procedures. In the Vietnam War, the severity of high-velocity firearm and mine-related injuries led surgeons to implement débridement and primary repair to amenable injuries, along with irrigation of the distal rectum. Mortality for penetrating rectal trauma was reported as 17% for this conflict, aided in part by improvements in resuscitation and antibiotic therapy, along with increased usage of blood products.

The management of rectal injuries in the civilian population over the past 50 years has mirrored the treatment strategies used by the military. However, as trauma surgeons have become more experienced with the treatment of rectal wounds outside of the logistical and environmental limitations of the combat environment, the viability of these principles has been called into question. In this chapter, we present our approach to the treatment and management of rectal injuries.

■ ANATOMIC CLASSIFICATION OF INJURIES

The rectum is a 12- to 15-cm segment of bowel that extends from the rectosigmoid junction to the dentate line and functions as a fecal reservoir. Injuries are classified as intraperitoneal or extraperitoneal (Figure 1). The extraperitoneal rectum comprises the posterior aspect, which is adherent to the presacral soft tissues along the curvature of the sacrum, and the lower one third of the anterior portion.

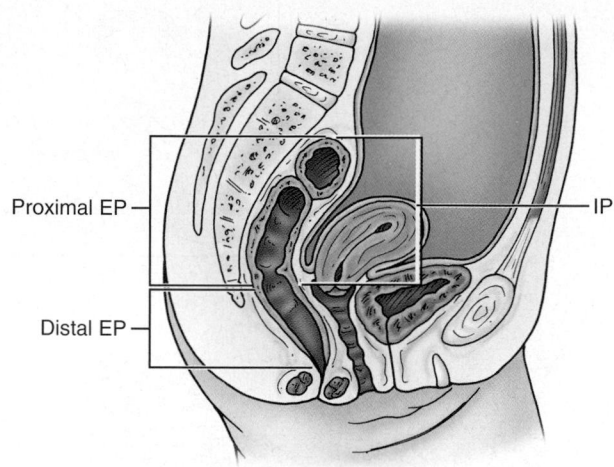

FIGURE 1 The intraperitoneal (IP) and extraperitoneal (EP) divisions of the rectum. *(From Weinberg JA, Fabian TC, Magnotti LJ, et al. Penetrating rectal trauma: management by anatomic distinction improves outcome. J Trauma. 2006;60:508-514.)*

TABLE 1: The American Association for the Surgery of Trauma Rectal Injury Grading

Grade*	Type of Injury	Description of Injury
I	Hematoma	Contusion or hematoma without devascularization
	Laceration	Partial thickness, no perforation
II	Laceration	Laceration <50% of circumference
III	Laceration	Laceration >50% of circumference
IV	Laceration	Full-thickness laceration with extension into perineum
V	Vascular	Devascularized segment

Modified from Moore EE, Cogbill TH, Malangoni MA, et al. Organ injury scaling II: pancreas, duodenum, small bowel, colon and rectum. *J Trauma.* 1990;30:1427.

*Advance one grade for multiple injuries up to grade III.

Injuries to the anterior and lateral surface of the upper two thirds of the anterior portion are classified as intraperitoneal. This is the only segment of the rectum that contains a serosal layer. Injuries are graded on the basis of whether the injury is partial or full thickness, the percentage of rectal lumen compromised, and the extension into the perineum (Table 1). The rectum is extremely well vascularized, with the upper third supplied by the superior rectal artery as it branches off the inferior mesenteric artery. The middle third is supplied by the middle rectal arteries from the internal iliac arteries, and the distal third is supplied by the internal pudendal arteries. The superior rectal veins drain into the portal system via the inferior mesenteric vein, whereas the middle and inferior rectal veins drain into the internal iliac and internal pudendal veins, respectively.

■ DIAGNOSIS

Recognition of rectal injuries requires that the surgeon maintain a high index of suspicion when evaluating any patient with a penetrating wound to the lower abdomen, pelvis, perineum, buttock, or upper thigh. After completion of the Advanced Trauma Life Support (ATLS) primary survey, complete exposure of the patient is essential

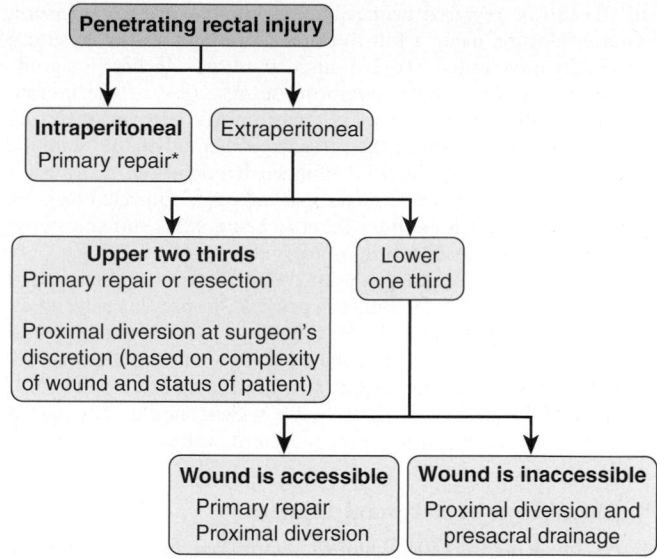

FIGURE 2 Clinical pathway for the management of penetrating rectal injury at the University of Tennessee Health Science Center, Memphis. *Primary repair is performed for nondestructive wounds or destructive wounds in the absence of blood transfusion of more than 6 units or medical comorbidities. Otherwise, resection and colostomy are performed. *(From Cameron JL, ed.* Current Surgical Therapy. *9th ed. Philadelphia: Mosby Elsevier; 2008.)*

to avoid a missed injury in the multiple folds and clefts present in this area. Digital rectal examination (DRE) is an essential tool to assess for blood within the rectal vault. However, the sensitivity of the test is not adequate to effectively rule out an injury. Proctosigmoidoscopy may reveal the location of a rectal injury, but visualization often is impaired by the presence of blood or stool. Even if the location of the injury is not identified, blood seen on rigid sigmoidoscopy has been found to have a sensitivity as high as 90% for the diagnosis of rectal injury. Computed tomography (CT) may be a useful adjunct in the stable patient to identify the missile tract and to evaluate for concomitant intra-abdominal injury. CT cystography also may be helpful for the preoperative diagnosis of an associated bladder injury if hematuria is detected during Foley catheter insertion.

■ TREATMENT

Our treatment protocol for rectal trauma is based on the anatomic classification of the injury. In addition to the anatomic distinctions noted earlier, we further characterize extraperitoneal injuries as high or low based on whether they are proximal or distal to the peritoneal reflection (Figure 2). In addition, the hemodynamic status of the patient plays an important role in determining the surgical management of these injuries. Patients should be placed on the operating table in the lithotomy position to facilitate rigid proctosigmoidoscopy and possible transanal repair of very low injuries. Before operation, broad-spectrum antibiotics with gram-negative and anaerobic coverage should be administered and continued for 24 hours postoperatively.

Intraperitoneal Injuries

Because of the anatomic and clinical similarities between the intraperitoneal rectum and the colon, the management strategies for intraperitoneal rectal injuries are similar to those used for colon wounds. Nondestructive injuries without devitalization of tissue and that do not require significant débridement (American Association for the Surgery of Trauma Organ Injury Scaling [AAST-OIS] grades

I to III) can be repaired primarily. It is our practice to perform a two-layer closure, using a full-thickness running absorbable suture followed by interrupted silk seromuscular sutures. If there is significant tissue loss or vascular compromise, resection of the injured segment is appropriate. Primary anastomosis without diverting colostomy is appropriate in the presence of hemodynamic stability. If there is evidence of shock (prolonged hypotension, transfusion requirement greater than 6 units of packed red blood cells) or multiple associated injuries (Injury Severity Score ≥25), end colostomy with closure of the rectal stump is advised.

It is important that the posterior wall of the rectum be assessed along the trajectory of the bullet if possible, to prevent missing an injury to the posterior rectum. Although it is possible that a wound to the intraperitoneal rectum is the result of a tangential injury, the possibility of a distal extraperitoneal wound must be considered. If this cannot be ruled out definitively, the patient should be managed as if a distal extraperitoneal injury is present, as described later.

Proximal Extraperitoneal Injuries

Injuries involving the extraperitoneal rectum proximal to the peritoneal reflection usually can be repaired with limited mobilization of the mesorectum. If injury is suspected, either because of extension of an anterior or lateral injury or the presence of a hematoma within the proximal mesorectum, primary repair should be attempted using the two-layer technique described previously without the need for proximal diversion or presacral drainage. As with intraperitoneal injuries, the decision to perform a diverting colostomy should be based on the patient's physiologic status, the suspicion of a more distal injury, and the complexity of the surgical repair required. Destructive rectal injuries not amenable to immediate primary repair should be treated with Hartmann's procedure.

Distal Extraperitoneal Injuries

Primary repair of extraperitoneal injuries below the peritoneal reflection often is hindered by difficult exposure, limited space (especially in males), proximity of neurovascular and genitourinary structures, and anatomic distortion secondary to associated injuries. If the wound is encountered while addressing another injury and is immediately accessible, limited dissection and repair is advised. However, only 20% of extraperitoneal wounds are amenable to repair, and extensive distal mobilization in search of a suspected wound is not indicated because of the risk for iatrogenic nerve, rectal, urologic, or vascular injury. Several authors have described forgoing laparotomy and performing laparoscopic-assisted diverting loop sigmoid colostomy in hemodynamically stable patients without signs of peritonitis. In 2006 Gonzalez and colleagues published a series of 14 patients in whom extraperitoneal rectal injury was managed without fecal diversion or presacral drainage, with no complications reported in this cohort. Our practice is to perform open evaluation and diversion of these patients, as it allows for evaluation of the mesorectum and potential repair of proximal extraperitoneal injuries. Diversion is accomplished via a loop sigmoid colostomy, making sure that the sigmoid colon is mobilized sufficiently to avoid tension and that the posterior wall of the loop is maintained above the level of the skin. A Silastic rod or red rubber catheter is placed beneath the loop to prevent retraction. If formed properly, loop colostomy is effective for diversion of the fecal stream and outcomes are equivalent to those seen with end colostomy.

For wounds to the posterior portion of the distal extraperitoneal rectum, we continue to practice proximal diversion with presacral drainage. For injuries to the anterior portion of the distal extraperitoneal rectum, we do not routinely place a presacral drain, and injuries are treated primarily with proximal diversion. However, the location of the injury is not always obvious, and if there is any concern for a posterior injury we recommend drainage of the retrorectal space. Presacral drainage is performed by making a curvilinear

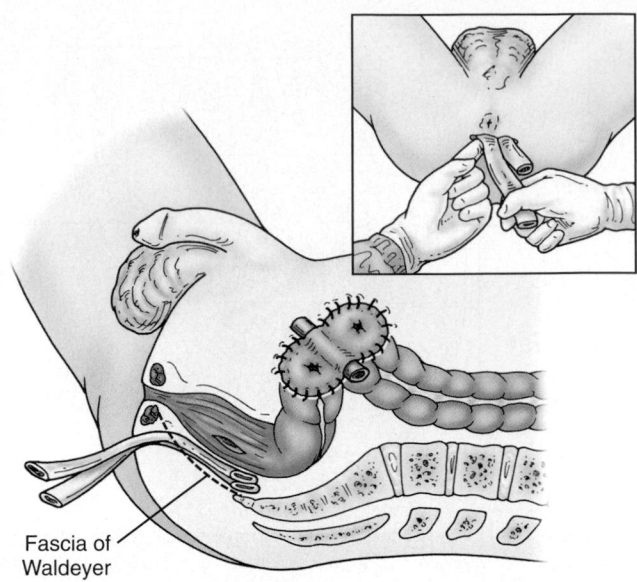

Fascia of Waldeyer

FIGURE 3 Technique for presacral drainage and proximal diversion for treatment of occult or unrepaired distal colon injuries. *(Courtesy Baylor College of Medicine, Houston.)*

incision between the coccyx and anus, followed by bluntly dissecting through Waldeyer's fascia in order to gain entry to the presacral space. A 1-inch Penrose drain is placed within the space and gradually withdrawn between postoperative days 5 and 7 (Figure 3).

The use of presacral drainage in these patients continues to be an issue of contention. In a series of 32 patients, Armstrong and colleagues demonstrated a reduction in the pelvic abscess rate from 36% to 25% with the use of presacral drainage. Burch and colleagues also were able to show a significant decrease in infections within the presacral space, and a report by McGrath in 1998 also demonstrated a reduction in morbidity when drainage was used. Several subsequent reports have failed to demonstrate a reduction in morbidity or mortality. Gonzalez and colleagues published a prospective, randomized study evaluating 48 patients with rectal injuries and failed to demonstrate a reduction in infectious complications. They postulated that the civilian injuries may be different from the high-velocity injuries encountered during combat and that violation of the presacral space actually may result in increased infectious complications. However, the sample size of the study likely was insufficient to detect a significant difference, and the report did not delineate which injuries were repaired primarily and which were treated with diversion only. We practice the selective application of presacral drainage in patients with inaccessible lesions to the distal posterior extraperitoneal rectum that are not amenable to primary repair in order to prevent the formation of pelvic and retroperitoneal abscesses. We contend that the severe consequences of infection within this space outweigh the minimal morbidity of presacral drainage. As mentioned previously, localization of these lesions is often difficult, and we prefer to err on the side of caution if the site of the injury is in question.

Distal Rectal Washout

During the Vietnam War, irrigation of the distal colon and rectum was added to the treatment regimen for these injuries in an attempt to reduce contamination and septic complications secondary to stool within the rectal vault. As the sigmoid colon is exteriorized for the creation of a diverting loop colostomy, a purse-string suture is placed on the distal segment of the sigmoid colon. A colotomy is made, a large bore Foley or red rubber catheter is inserted into the colonic lumen, and 3 to 6 L of saline is instilled via gravity drainage into the colon. As the fluid is introduced, the distal rectum is dilated digitally to facilitate drainage, and drainage is continued until the effluent becomes clear.

In 1988 Shannon and colleagues reported on their experience with distal rectal washout in a series of 27 patients, demonstrating an incidence of pelvic abscess formation in 8% of patients who received rectal irrigation versus 46% in those who did not. They reported that the greatest benefit was likely to be in patients with high-velocity gunshot wounds or other destructive injuries, such as pelvic crush injuries. Several authors have expressed concern that irrigation in patients who have not undergone primary repair may result in contamination of the surrounding soft tissues and an increased risk of pelvic abscess formation. Multiple subsequent studies have failed to demonstrate a benefit to the procedure, but rectal lavage has not been shown to actually increase the incidence of pelvic infection either. The benefit in combat situations may be related to the chronic dehydration and constipation experienced by soldiers in the field, which when combined with high-velocity, destructive injuries may increase the likelihood of contamination. We do not include this procedure as a component of our treatment algorithm, although it may have value in injuries secondary to high-caliber weaponry or explosives.

Anorectal Injuries

The majority of injuries to the anus and anal sphincters occur because of obstetric injuries due to perineal tearing or midline episiotomy. Traumatic injury to the anal sphincter complex is often secondary to sexual assault, forceful introduction of a foreign body, or blunt injury due to complex pelvic fracture or "straddle" type perineal injuries. Injuries also have been reported with insertion of enema tips or rectal thermometers and during anorectal procedures such as lateral internal sphincterotomy, hemorrhoidectomy, polypectomy, and endoscopic diathermy.

A simple laceration to the anal mucosa can be repaired primarily, but complex lesions involving the distal perineum and rectum may require diverting colostomy. In the case of foreign body insertion, it is important to perform rigid sigmoidoscopy to evaluate the patient for injury to the proximal rectum. If extensive tissue débridement is required, overlapping sphincteroplasty is the repair of choice, as simple apposition of muscle is associated with a failure rate of 40%. In the case of a complex injury to the pelvic floor with significant soft tissue defect, referral to a colorectal specialist for transposition of the gluteus or gracilis muscle with creation of a neosphincter is advised. In the event of complete destruction of the sphincter complex, abdominoperineal resection may be the most viable option.

■ TIMING OF COLOSTOMY CLOSURE

Colostomy closure is performed once the patient has recovered from the initial traumatic injury, subsequent surgeries, and associated morbidities. Resolution of inflammation, normalization of nutritional status, and proper healing of injuries are essential before performing colonic re-anastomosis. Renz and colleagues have reported on the practice of same admission colostomy closure on patients with rectal injuries, using contrast enema 5 to 10 days after injury to exclude a clinically occult leak. This was followed by closure as early as 9 days after injury without any reported complications related to leakage from the rectal wound. Although promising, this practice has not been adopted widely. We perform reversal 2 to 3 months after hospital discharge to allow for resolution of the dense inflammatory adhesions resulting from laparotomy and healing of intra-abdominal injuries.

■ MANAGEMENT OF COMPLICATIONS

Daily evaluation of the wounds, perineum, and presacral drain site (if performed) is essential to monitor the patient for possible pelvic infection or sepsis. The introduction of rectal thermometers or suppositories should be avoided. If the patient exhibits fevers, leukocytosis, and other signs of infection 4 to 5 days after surgery, CT of the abdomen and pelvis is appropriate. The most frequently occurring complication in these patients is intra-abdominal abscess. Small abscesses (<2 cm) usually can be treated with intravenous antibiotic therapy alone. Larger abscesses can be treated with percutaneous drainage if the location is favorable. If the collection is not amenable to drainage or if the patient is demonstrating signs of sepsis, re-exploration with irrigation and drainage is indicated. If feculent material is aspirated from the abscess cavity, the presence of an underlying fistula should be assumed. Distal colonic fistulas generally will resolve with time and continued adequate drainage. The catheter should be left in place and flushed twice daily with normal saline to prevent occlusion. Once drainage is minimal and there is radiographic confirmation that the abscess cavity has been obliterated, the drain can be removed slowly over the course of several days.

The complication most directly attributable to rectal injury is infection within the retrorectal space and the resulting pelvic sepsis. This may be seen as an isolated abscess within the presacral space or an extensive retroperitoneal infection tracking into the perineum and thighs. As with any necrotizing soft tissue infection, early institution of broad-spectrum antibiotics and prompt surgical débridement are the mainstays of therapy, along with admission to an intensive care unit, hemodynamic monitoring, and crystalloid resuscitation. In our experience, this complication has occurred primarily in the context of distal extraperitoneal injury managed by diversion alone. Our continued application of presacral drainage in such cases is based on the pre-emptive establishment of outflow tract before a closed-space infection can occur, with subsequent dissemination of infection throughout the surrounding soft tissues. The main potential consequence of presacral drainage is a wound infection within the drain tract, which is managed easily with Penrose drain removal, irrigation, and wound care.

Wound infections have been reported in up to 50% of patients with injuries to the colon and rectum. As such, the skin should not be reapproximated at the time of fascial closure. Either the wound can be left to heal by secondary intention or delayed primary closure can be performed after 3 to 5 days. Skin closure at the time of initial operation is feasible only in patients with minimal contamination, no evidence of shock, little subcutaneous fat, and few associated injuries. Given the contamination inherent in rectal trauma and stoma creation and the frequency of concomitant vascular, genitourinary, and orthopedic injuries, leaving the wound open is normally the preferred option.

SUGGESTED READINGS

Ahmed N, Thekkeurumbil S, Mathavan V, Janzen M, Tasse J, Chung R. Simplified management of low-energy projectile extraperitoneal rectal injuries. *J Trauma.* 2009;67:1270-1271.

Burch JM, Feliciano DV, Mattox KL. Colostomy and drainage for civilian rectal injuries: is that all? *Ann Surg.* 1989;209:600-610, discussion 610-611.

Demetriades D. Colon injuries: new perspectives. *Injury.* 2004;35:217-222.

Gonzalez RP, Falimirski ME, Holevar MR. The role of presacral drainage in the management of penetrating rectal injuries. *J Trauma.* 1998;45:656-661.

Herr MW, Wascher RA, Gagliano RA Jr. Historical perspective and current management of traumatic injury to the extraperitoneal rectum and anus. *Curr Surg.* 2005;62:625-632.

McGrath V, Fabian TC, Croce MA, Minard G, Pritchard FE. Rectal trauma: management based on anatomic distinctions. *Am Surg.* 1998;64:1136-1141.

Navsaria PH, Edu S, Nicol AJ. Civilian extraperitoneal rectal gunshot wounds: surgical management made simpler. *World J Surg.* 2007;31:1345-1351.

Renz BM, Feliciano DV, Sherman R. Same admission colostomy closure (SACC). A new approach to rectal wounds: a prospective study. *Ann Surg.* 1993;218:279-292, discussion 292-293.

Velmahos GC, Gomez H, Falabella A, Demetriades D. Operative management of civilian rectal gunshot wounds: simpler is better. *World J Surg.* 2000;24:114-118.

Weinberg JA, Fabian TC, Magnotti LJ, et al. Penetrating rectal trauma: management by anatomic distinction improves outcome. *J Trauma.* 2006;60:508-513, discussion 513-514.

INJURY TO THE SPLEEN

Paul Waltz, MD, Louis H. Alarcon, MD, and Andrew B. Peitzman, MD

The spleen is the most commonly injured organ in blunt abdominal trauma. Over the past century the management of blunt splenic injury (BSI) has evolved from expectant management in the early 1900s, to operative management for all injuries, to the current practice of selective operative and nonoperative management (NOM). The benefits of successful NOM are numerous: avoidance of general anesthesia, of a trauma laparotomy and its inherit morbidity, and of the long-term risk of incisional hernia or bowel obstruction. In addition, the important immunologic functions of the spleen are preserved. The risk for overwhelming post-splenectomy infection (OPSI) in humans was first documented in the 1950s. Although the risk for OPSI appears to be lower in patients who undergo splenectomy after trauma compared with those who undergo elective splenectomy for hematologic disorders, it remains a lifetime risk with a high associated mortality. However, because the risk for OPSI in adults is low, high risk for bleeding from the spleen is not justified in attempts to preserve the spleen. The shift toward NOM of splenic injuries may have other consequences, such as delayed splenic hemorrhage and missed associated injuries. Because computed tomography (CT) and percutaneous interventional options have improved, current debates focus on which patients should undergo splenic artery embolization (SAE) to further improve nonoperative salvage rates.

EVALUATION AND DIAGNOSIS

The evaluation of all trauma patients follows the Advanced Trauma Life Support (ATLS) guidelines. Physical examination is neither sensitive nor specific in identification of splenic injury. The symptoms of splenic injury relate to associated internal hemorrhage: patients may have tachycardia and hypotension consistent with hypovolemic shock. On secondary survey patients may exhibit tenderness in the left upper quadrant, generalized peritonitis, or referred pain to the left shoulder (Kehr's sign). Physical examination may be limited by mental status or distracting injuries. Twenty percent of patients with lower left rib fractures have associated splenic injury. Splenic injury also is associated with pelvic fractures, indicative of high-energy blunt trauma.

Because physical examination is unreliable, adjuncts are important in the diagnosis of splenic injury. The focused assessment with sonography for trauma (FAST) is an expeditious test for the evaluation of trauma patients. FAST uses three abdominal windows to evaluate for intra-abdominal fluid: sagittal views of the hepatorenal recess (Morison's pouch) and splenorenal recess and a transverse pelvic view evaluating for fluid surrounding the bladder. FAST is considered positive if fluid is identified as an anechoic band in any window. As such, FAST cannot assess solid organ injury or retroperitoneal bleeding accurately, nor can it distinguish between blood, succus, or pre-existing ascites. In general, FAST has a sensitivity of 80% and a specificity of 90%. Diagnostic peritoneal lavage (DPL) is used less frequently because of widespread adoption of FAST. Similar to FAST, DPL is not specific for solid organ injury but if positive will help to determine whether a patient should be transferred to the operating room (Figure 1).

CT has become integral in the evaluation of the stable trauma patient. The preferred protocol for evaluation for splenic injury is a CT with intravenous contrast in both the arterial and the venous phase. The arterial phase allows evaluation of early enhancement consistent with pseudoaneurysm or active hemorrhage from an arterial injury. The venous phase allows evaluation of splenic parenchymal injury. Additional CT findings include the presence and quantity of hemoperitoneum, stratified into small, moderate, and large. Small hemoperitoneum is defined as perisplenic or perihepatic blood. Moderate hemoperitoneum is blood in either pericolic gutter. Large hemoperitoneum includes free blood in the pelvis. Splenic injury is subsequently graded based on CT findings according to the American Association for the Surgery of Trauma Organ Injury Scale (AAST-OIS; Table 1).

NONOPERATIVE MANAGEMENT

NOM of BSI is appropriate only in the hemodynamically stable patient without signs of peritonitis. Patients who do not meet these criteria require urgent laparotomy. Additional considerations include adequate facilities for monitoring, serial evaluations, and the ability for rapid activation of an operative or angiographic suite should intervention become necessary. These resources typically are available at a trauma center. Specific institutional practices vary. In general, patients are admitted for serial hemoglobin measurements (every 6 to 8 hours) and a period of bed rest proportional to the severity of injury. Overall length of inpatient observation is congruent to severity of injury, with a rough guideline being the grade of BSI plus 1 for total length of stay (days). Early initiation (defined as within 48 hours) of pharmacologic venous thromboembolism (VTE) prophylaxis does not appear to affect the failure rate of NOM or the need for transfusion in retrospective reviews. Currently NOM is attempted in approximately 70% to 80% of patients with BSI, with success rates of 90% to 95%.

Sixty percent of patients who fail NOM will do so in the first 24 hours, and 90% of failures will occur within the first 4 days. Thus most failures for high-grade splenic injury should be recognized during inpatient observation. Approximately 1% of patients will have a delayed failure of NOM that occurs after discharge.

Much work has been done to try to identify risk factors associated with the failure of NOM. Risk factors for failure include age older than 40 years, high injury severity score, grade III or higher splenic injury (particularly grades IV and V), and the need for transfusion of blood product. The Eastern Association for the Surgery of Trauma (EAST) multi-institutional study evaluating BSI (published in 2000) revealed success rates of 75% for grade I, 70% for grade II, 49.3% for grade III, 16.9% for grade IV, and 1.3% for grade V. It is worth noting that this study was performed early in the acceptance of NOM and before angiography was used to a considerable degree. A more recent study from New England trauma centers evaluating severe (grades IV and V) splenic injuries found that nearly 40% of grade IV injuries and 60% of grade V injuries went immediately to the operating room. Of the patients managed nonoperatively, one third of the grade IV and one quarter of the grade V injuries failed and required splenectomy; high-grade injuries are associated with a higher rate of failure. Studies using the National Trauma Data Bank (NTDB) have corroborated that more than 50% of grade IV and V splenic injuries fail observation. The most recent guidelines put forth by the EAST

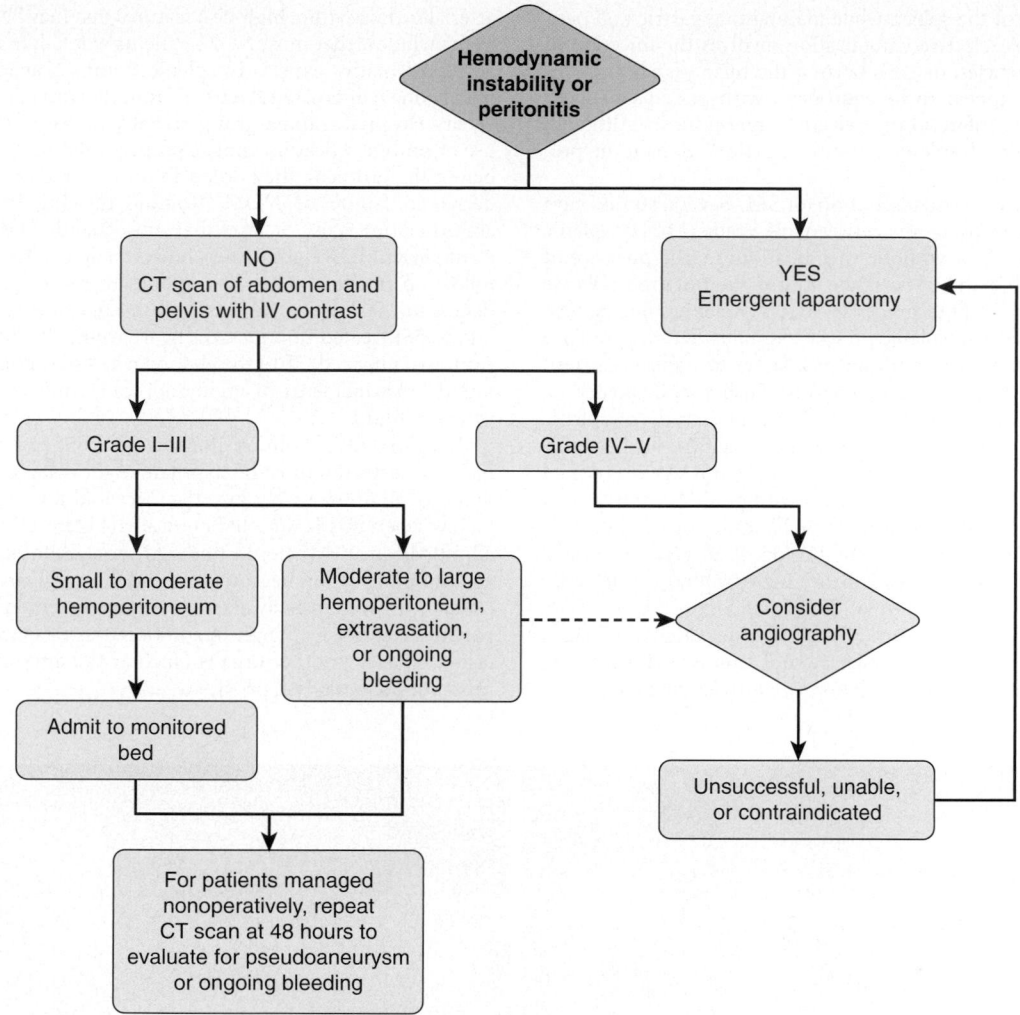

FIGURE 1 Flowchart for management of blunt splenic injury. *CT*, Computed tomography; *IV*, intravenous.

TABLE 1: Spleen Organ Injury Scale

Grade*	Injury Type	Description of Injury
I	Hematoma	Subcapsular, <10% surface area
	Laceration	Capsular tear, <1 cm parenchymal depth
II	Hematoma	Subcapsular, 10%-50% surface area
		Intraparenchymal, <5 cm in diameter
	Laceration	Capsular tear, 1-3 cm parenchyma depth that does not involve a trabecular vessel
III	Hematoma	Subcapsular, >50% surface area or expanding; ruptured subcapsular or parenchymal hematoma; intraparenchymal hematoma ≥5 cm or expanding
	Laceration	>3 cm parenchymal depth or involving trabecular vessels
IV	Laceration	Laceration involving segmental or hilar vessels producing major devascularization (>25% of spleen)
V	Laceration	Completely shattered spleen
	Vascular	Hilar vascular injury that devascularizes spleen

*Advance one grade for multiple injuries up to grade III.

underemphasize the impact of grade of injury (grades IV and V) as a contraindication to observation alone.

An adjunct to NOM for splenic injury with considerable variation between trauma centers is the use of SAE, which typically is performed through percutaneous femoral access. An angiogram is obtained, which may reveal active bleeding, pseudoaneurysm, arteriovenous fistula, or other vascular injuries. Once a lesion is identified, embolization can be performed as either proximal, selective, or a combination of both. For a proximal embolization, coils are placed distal to the dorsal pancreatic artery origin to decrease the perfusion pressure of the spleen while maintaining gastric and pancreatic collaterals. A selective embolization involves the injection of Gelfoam slurry, particles, or coils beyond the hilar vessels and collaterals. Outcomes appear to be equivalent, with perhaps a higher incidence of splenic infarction in selective embolization. Although somewhat controversial, splenic immune function seems to be preserved after SAE.

There is debate over patient selection for SAE. Several studies have shown no difference in outcome between low-grade (I to III) splenic injuries managed with or without SAE. In addition, the presence of small contrast blush in these low-grade injuries did not predict worse outcome. However, for high-grade (IV and V) splenic injuries, SAE seems to improve rates of splenic preservation. Further, the presence of blush in this cohort is a significant risk factor for failure. Current literature supports the presence of a contrast blush, pseudoaneurysm, or extravasation as an indication for SAE in any grade of splenic injury. In addition, data support routine proximal SAE for hemodynamically stable patients with grades IV and V BSI. As mentioned earlier, although the majority of patients with grade V injury and a significant proportion of those with grade IV injury proceed directly to the operating room, empiric embolization of all grade IV and V injuries (even without extravasation on angiography) significantly decreases the frequency of failure of NOM (see Figure 1).

The use of routine follow-up CT scanning in patients managed with NOM also remains controversial. Several centers perform repeat imaging at 48 hours to assess development of pseudoaneurysm or arterial extravasation, high-risk features that may be related to failure in the window that most NOM patients will fail. In a survey study of 30 representative experts in splenic trauma management, approximately one half favored the use of routine reimaging. The Oslo University Hospital trauma group recently reviewed their series in the use of routine repeat imaging. Compared with institutional controls before the protocol, they noted improved splenic salvage rates and decreased failure of NOM. Routine imaging identified vascular abnormalities in 6% of cases that subsequently underwent SAE. The most current EAST guidelines, however, do not recommend routine follow-up imaging. This also applies to postdischarge imaging to document healing. At our institution, for patients with grade II or higher BSI treated nonoperatively, we routinely obtain a dual phase contrast-enhanced CT of the abdomen 48 hours after injury and have found a 15% incidence of angiographically confirmed delayed splenic vascular injury.

Despite multiple options for interventions and reimaging, a high index of suspicion must be maintained for delayed bleed in patients managed nonoperatively, and the threshold for splenectomy should be low when this is detected clinically (Figure 2). Patients with BSI admitted for NOM should undergo serial abdominal examinations and monitoring of hemoglobin and hemodynamics at a trauma center with resources available to intervene emergently should the patient's condition change. In addition, the presence of missed associated injuries to other organs (such as the intestine) is an uncommon but potential risk of NOM.

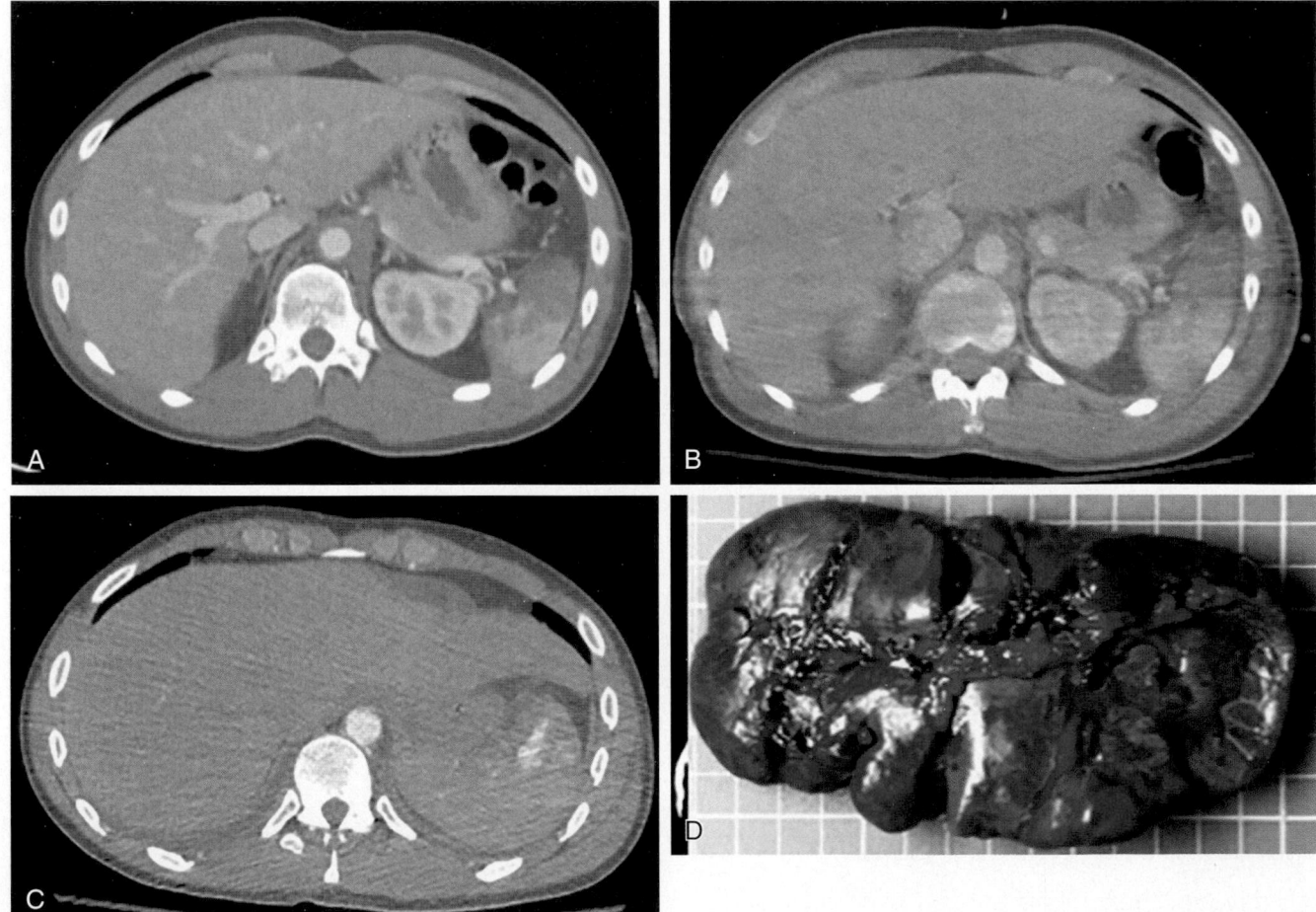

FIGURE 2 A 23-year-old male was seen after a motor vehicle accident. **A,** He was found to have a grade III splenic laceration. **B,** Repeat imaging at 48 hours revealed stable injury. **C,** On post-trauma day 5 he underwent a CT scan to evaluate for pulmonary embolism that revealed incidental parenchymal blush. **D,** He failed nonoperative management and required splenectomy. Gross pathology revealed a spleen with multiple lacerations and subcapsular hematoma.

Pediatric patients with BSI do well overall and indeed helped to change the management of adult patients toward NOM. The American Pediatric Surgical Association Trauma Committee released a set of guidelines for the management of isolated pediatric splenic or liver injury in 2000. Isolated grade V injuries were rare and not included. It was noted that children with grades I to III injuries had a transfusion rate of only 2% to 10% and an operative rate of 3%, compared with a 27% transfusion rate and 13% operative rate for grade IV injuries. This served as the basis for recommendation of admission to the intensive care unit for only grade IV injuries. No predischarge or postdischarge imaging was recommended in children, and recommended activity restrictions were 3 to 6 weeks according to grade.

■ PENETRATING SPLENIC INJURY

Most penetrating abdominal injuries require operative exploration. The principles of NOM for splenic injury are less applicable in this scenario. Although full-thickness hollow viscus injury occurs in only 0.3% of patients with blunt trauma, the incidence is much higher in those with penetrating injury. In addition, occult diaphragmatic injury must be considered with an upper abdominal penetrating wound. Nonoperative and minimally invasive options for penetrating trauma continue to evolve. Although the vast majority of patients will require laparotomy, for a small subset of patients who are hemodynamically stable, without peritonitis, and with an adequate CT evaluation revealing no other injuries, a trial of monitored nonoperative therapy may be appropriate. Failure remains high in this group, most commonly because of missed hollow viscus injury. We recommend routine laparotomy as the safest option for patients with penetrating injury to the spleen, with high risk for missing injury to the diaphragm or hollow viscus otherwise.

■ OPERATIVE MANAGEMENT

Operative management of BSI is indicated for patients who initially are seen with hemodynamic instability, peritonitis, or associated injuries that require laparotomy. Delayed operative intervention is indicated for patients with BSI who fail NOM because of delayed bleeding or missed injury. When operative intervention is necessary, the patient is prepared for a standard trauma laparotomy. Appropriate intravenous access and monitoring should be established. A type and crossmatch should be current, with blood components available and preparation for massive transfusion if necessary. An oral or nasogastric tube will decompress the stomach and facilitate exposure. The patient is placed in the supine position with the chest, abdomen, pelvis, and thighs draped sterilely.

A generous midline laparotomy is performed. On entering the abdomen, blood clots should be evacuated, and four quadrant packing is performed to control hemorrhage. Packs are removed sequentially to identify and address sources of hemorrhage. Additional injuries and gastrointestinal contamination also are controlled. The first step in evaluating an injured spleen is to mobilize it to the midline. The left costal margin is retracted superiorly for improved exposure (self-retaining retractor system). The surgeon's left hand is placed around the spleen and provides medial traction. The splenorenal and splenophrenic ligaments are generally avascular. These are approached laterally and can be divided with Metzenbaum scissors. There can be considerable variation in the baseline laxity of these ligaments. Some degree of this dissection may need to be accomplished bluntly because of bleeding or patient habitus.

Next the spleen and tail of the pancreas are mobilized to the midline together. The plane to be developed is immediately anterior to the kidney, which serves as an important tactile landmark. Being too posterior will result in mobilizing the kidney. If the tail of the pancreas is not mobilized with the spleen, the degree of midline rotation that is accomplished is limited. Packs can be placed posterior to the spleen to tamponade bleeding from the splenic fossa.

The gastrosplenic ligament can be divided next. Contained within are the short gastric vessels. These should be divided between clamps and tied, with an attempt to ligate closer to the spleen to avoid injury to the gastric wall. If there is concern for injury to the stomach during this mobilization, seromuscular stitches can be placed to minimize the chances of a gastric leak. Finally, the splenocolic ligament is transected to free the lower pole of the spleen from the colon.

The spleen now should be fully mobilized. The hilar vessels now can be ligated. Traditionally the artery and veins are ligated separately to prevent the future formation of an arteriovenous fistula. Avoidance of injury to the tail of the pancreas is critical during this procedure by division of the splenic hilar vessels immediately adjacent to the spleen.

With the specimen out, the left upper quadrant should be inspected. The diaphragm is assessed for injury. The splenic bed is assessed for hemostasis, facilitated by using a rolled lap pad and running from posterior lateral to anterior medially. The pancreas can be inspected, and if there is any concern for injury to the tail of the pancreas, a closed suction drain can be left.

The majority of the minor splenic injuries that in the past were managed with splenorrhaphy now are managed successfully with NOM. Minor splenic injuries identified at the time of trauma laparotomy in an otherwise hemodynamically stable patient may be repaired. Various methods for repair include argon beam coagulation, electrocautery, and bipolar sealers. Topical hemostatic sprays and absorbable packing also can be used. Higher-grade injuries can be managed with mesh wraps and buttressed sutures. However, if there is any doubt of a completely hemostatic repair, splenectomy should be performed.

■ VACCINATIONS

Patients who have undergone a splenectomy require vaccination against *Streptococcus pneumoniae*, *Neisseria meningitidis*, and *Haemophilus influenzae type B*. Although the optimal timing for vaccination appears to be 2 weeks after splenectomy (or preoperatively in elective cases), most institutions administer vaccinations before discharge to ensure that they are received. Further, vaccines require periodic boosters to ensure adequate titers, and thus coordination with the patient's primary physician is important. Recommendations on specific vaccinations for the anatomic asplenic patient are published by the Centers for Disease Control and Prevention Advisory Committee on Immunization Practices (CDC/ACIP). Recent additions include covering meningococcal serogroup B for patients between 10 and 55 years of age with either rLP2086 (Trumenba) or 4CMenB (Bexsero). In addition, the sequence of administration of the pneumococcal vaccinations appears to be important in immunogenicity and efficacy. These guidelines can be consulted for specific details in administration.

Daily antibiotic prophylaxis is no longer recommended for adults after splenectomy. However, patients should be provided with a prescription of amoxicillin-clavulanate, cefuroxime, or fluoroquinolone to be taken with the onset of fever or rigors. Antibiotics should be initiated immediately followed by medical evaluation. Pediatric patients receive daily penicillin or amoxicillin prophylaxis until age 5 years or for 1 year after splenectomy, as the incidence of pneumococcal bacteremia is higher in children than in adults.

■ SUMMARY

The management of splenic trauma has undergone considerable change over the past several decades. NOM is safe in appropriately selected patients. Angioembolization is appropriate empirically for grades IV and V injuries or for evidence of vascular blush, pseudoaneurysm, or extravasation in splenic injury of any grade.

SUGGESTED READINGS

Bhullar IS, Frykberg ER, Tepas JJ III, et al. At first blush: absence of computed tomography contrast extravasation in grade IV or V blunt splenic injury should not preclude angioembolization. *J Trauma Acute Care Surg.* 2013;74:105-112.

Olthof DC, van der Vlies CH, Joosse P, et al. Consensus strategies for the nonoperative management of patients with blunt splenic injury: a Delphi study. *J Trauma Acute Care Surg.* 2013;74:1567-1574.

Peitzman AB, Harbrecht BG, Rivera L, et al. Failure of observation of blunt splenic injury: variability in practice and adverse consequences. *J Am Coll Surg.* 2005;201:79-87.

Peitzman AB, Heil B, Rivera L, et al. Blunt splenic injury in adults: multi-institutional study of the Eastern Association for the Surgery of Trauma. *J Trauma Acute Care Surg.* 2000;49:177-189.

Skattum J, Naess PA, Eken T, et al. Redefining the role of splenic angiographic embolization in high grade splenic injuries. *J Trauma Acute Care Surg.* 2013;74:100-104.

Stassen NA, Bhullar I, Cheng J, et al. Selective nonoperative management of blunt splenic injury: an Eastern Association for the Surgery of Trauma practice management guideline. *J Trauma Acute Care Surg.* 2012;73: S294-S300.

Stylianos S. Evidence-based guidelines for resource utilization in children with isolated spleen or liver injury. The APSA Trauma Committee. *J Pediatr Surg.* 2000;35:164-169. doi:10.1016/S0022-3468(00)90003-4.

Velmahos GC, Zacharis N, Emhoff A, et al. Management of the most severely injured spleen: a multicenter study of the research consortium of New England Centers for Trauma. *JAMA Surg.* 2010;145:456-460.

Zarzaur BL, Savage SA, Croce MA, et al. Trauma center angiography use in high grade splenic injuries: timing is everything. *J Trauma Acute Care Surg.* 2014;77:666-673.

RETROPERITONEAL INJURIES: KIDNEY AND URETER

Marc A. Bjurlin, DO, MSc, FACOS, and Richard J. Fantus, MD, FACS

■ KIDNEY

The kidney is the most commonly injured genitourinary organ. Kidney injury occurs in 5% of all trauma patients and accounts for nearly 25% of traumatic abdominal solid organ injuries. Blunt traumatic injuries as a result of motor vehicle collisions (MVCs), falls, or blows to the abdomen may cause significant damage to the kidney and represent 80% of all renal injuries, whereas penetrating injuries account for the remaining 20%. These injuries generally occur in urban areas and are a result of gunshot wounds and stab wounds.

Although renal injury can lead to considerable morbidity and mortality, advances in imaging and treatment strategies have led to increased renal salvage and a decreased need for surgery in the majority of renal trauma cases. Increasing evidence suggests that patients who are hemodynamically stable and well staged and have sustained renal trauma, both blunt and penetrating, can be managed nonoperatively. Nonetheless, certain severely injured kidneys are best managed by exploration and reconstruction, with nephrectomy reserved for life-threatening hemorrhage or injuries that are beyond repair. Advances in angiographic embolization techniques have allowed for a minimally invasive approach to the diagnosis and management of kidney injuries. The primary objective in the management of renal trauma is to halt life-threatening hemorrhage while sparing renal function to avoid end-stage renal disease. The secondary objective is a reduction in post-traumatic renal complications.

Initial Evaluation

The initial management of any injured patient starts with rapid assessment of the injuries and resuscitation according to priorities established by the American College of Surgeons' Advanced Trauma Life Support program. The primary survey algorithm includes airway, breathing, circulation (external bleeding control), disability (neurologic status), and exposure (undress) and environment (temperature control).

Vital signs recorded in the field and on arrival at the hospital are of primary importance in managing renal trauma. Heart rate, systolic blood pressure, and respiratory rate can be used to estimate the amount of blood that may have been lost already. The lowest recorded systolic blood pressure also is used in conjunction with other information to determine whether renal imaging is indicated. Renal injuries may be seen in the primary survey as hypovolemic shock; however, most will be identified in the secondary survey after imaging. The abdomen, flank, and back should be examined carefully. Patients with trauma to the flank, abdomen, or lower chest; flank ecchymosis or tenderness; low posterior rib fractures, or lumbar transverse process fractures are at increased risk for a renal injury. In penetrating injuries, the entry and exit sites may reveal a transrenal course. If there are no abnormal physical findings, a urine sample should be obtained to evaluate for microscopic or gross hematuria. Blunt and penetrating trauma to the genitourinary tract commonly results in hematuria, but its presence or degree does not necessarily correlate with injury location or severity. The first voided or catheterized specimen should be analyzed, as hematuria may clear rapidly. Up to 40% of renal pedicle injuries are seen without hematuria. The management of polytrauma patients with an associated renal injury should be prioritized on the basis of the most significant injury.

Blunt Trauma

The suspected blunt renal trauma algorithm is shown in Figure 1. Blunt renal injuries are usually secondary to high-energy collisions such as MVCs, falls from a height, contact sports, and assaults. Nearly 70% of blunt renal trauma in the United States is secondary to MVCs. Falls, pedestrian versus motor vehicle collisions, assaults, and recreational injuries such as bicycling account for the remainder. In most trauma centers, blunt trauma is the more prevalent mechanism of injury, with blunt renal injuries as much as nine times more common than penetrating injuries. Both kidneys are at equal risk for injury. In blunt renal injuries, direct transmission of kinetic energy and rapid deceleration forces place the kidneys at risk. Major renovascular injuries, although exceedingly rare, occur at retroperitoneal points of fixation such as the renal hilum or ureteropelvic junction, resulting in renal artery thrombosis, renal vein disruption, and renal pedicle avulsion. Patients who are involved in mechanisms of injury that generate enough force to injure the kidney have concomitant injuries nearly 50% of the time.

Penetrating Trauma

The algorithm for suspected penetrating renal trauma is shown in Figure 2. Penetrating renal injuries most often are a result of gunshot or stab wounds. A large population-based review demonstrated that 16% of renal injuries in the United States are penetrating. Firearms

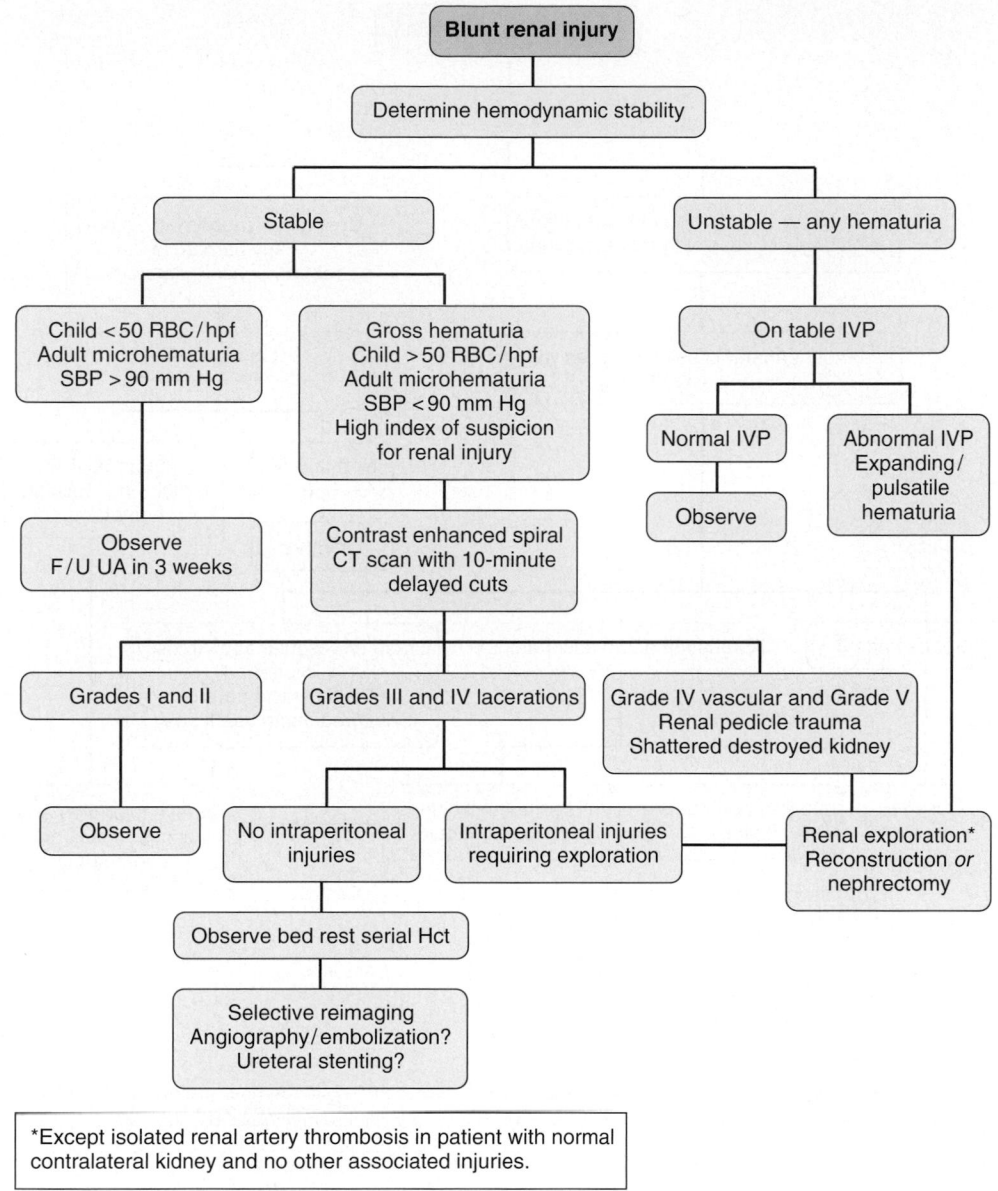

FIGURE 1 Blunt renal trauma algorithm. *CT*, Computed tomographic; *F/U*, follow-up; *Hct*, hematocrit; *hpf*, high-power field; *IVP*, intravenous pyelogram; *RBC*, red blood count; *SBP*, systolic blood pressure; *UA*, urinalysis. *(From Santucci RA, Wessells H, Bartsch G, et al. Evaluation and management of renal injuries: consensus statement of the renal trauma subcommittee. BJU Int. 2004;93:937-954.)*

account for 58% and stab wounds for 42%. Injuries to the upper abdomen or lower chest should alert the physician immediately to potential renal injury. Often associated with a more advanced grade of injury than falls or MVCs, penetrating mechanisms have a higher likelihood of renal injury that requires surgical exploration.

Initial assessment of gunshot wounds involves gathering important information about weapon characteristics, including caliber and type. Bullet size and velocity have the greatest effect on soft tissue damage. High-velocity weapons (e.g., rifle projectiles: 2600 to 3200 ft/sec) inflict greater damage because the bullets transmit large amounts of energy to the tissues, resulting in damage to a much larger area then the projectile tract itself. In lower-velocity injuries (e.g., knife stab), the damage is usually confined to the track of the stabbing implement. Stab wounds from assaults or self-inflicted injuries can cause both renovascular and parenchymal injuries. High-velocity injuries can cause substantial injury to tissue adjacent to the bullet path as a result of blast injury, often resulting in delayed tissue necrosis. For this reason, care should be taken to débride any devitalized tissue adjacent to the path of a high-velocity bullet.

Children

Children younger than 16 years require a higher index of suspicion for renal injury because of their unique anatomic and physiologic characteristics. Children are more likely to sustain a kidney injury because of the relatively larger size of the kidney in relation to the abdomen and pelvis, scant perirenal fat, underdeveloped Gerota's fascia, and incomplete rib ossification. The grand majority (80%) of pediatric renal injuries are low grade, with blunt mechanisms accounting for 90% of these. Children have a high catecholamine output after trauma, which maintains blood pressure until approximately 50% of blood volume has been lost. As a result, shock is an unreliable indicator of the extent of injury in this population.

Geriatrics

Geriatric trauma patients most commonly sustain renal injuries as a result of a fall rather than an MVC (the primary mechanism of kidney injury in the nongeriatric population). In our review of 9470

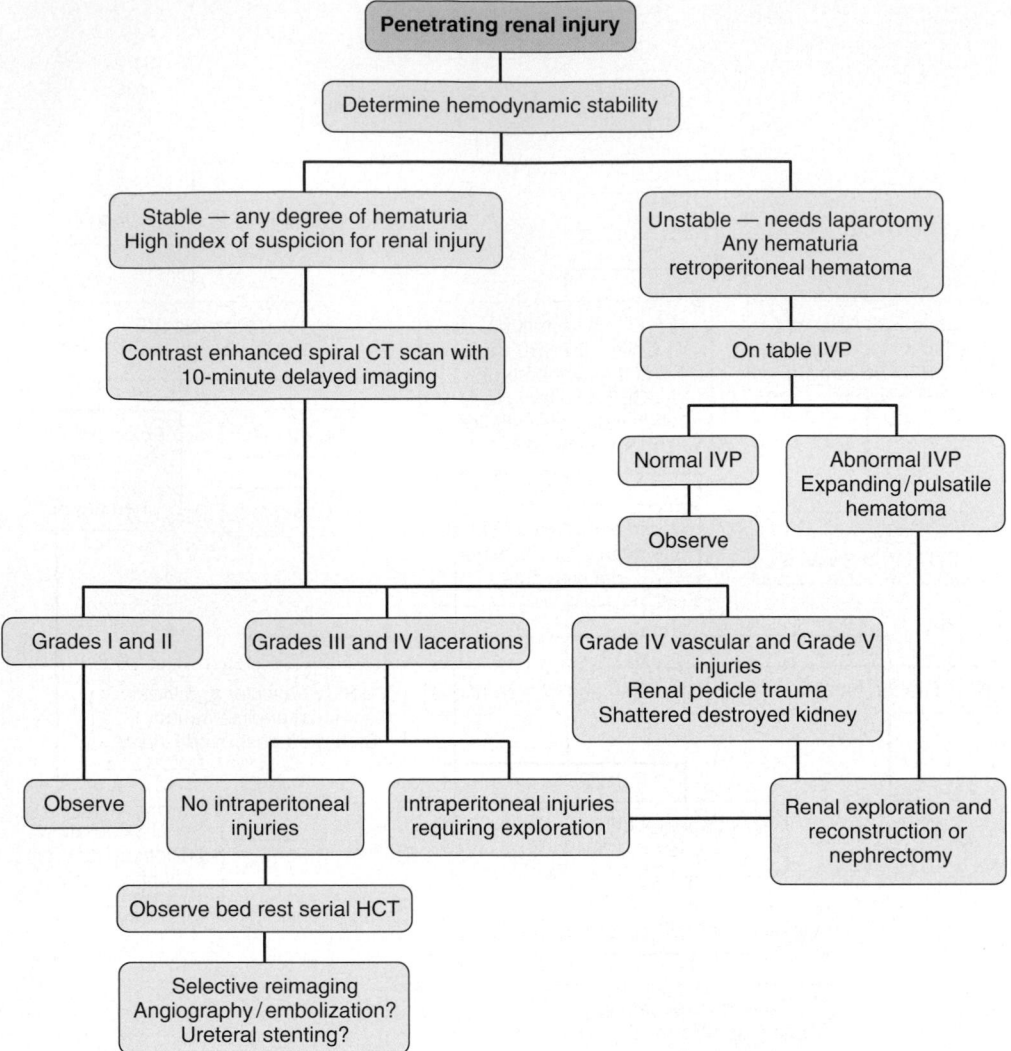

FIGURE 2 Penetrating renal trauma algorithm. *CT,* Computed tomographic; *HCT,* hematocrit; *IVP,* intravenous pyelogram. *(From Santucci RA, Wessells H, Bartsch G, et al. Evaluation and management of renal injuries: consensus statement of the renal trauma subcommittee. BJU Int. 2004;93:937-954.)*

patients with genitourinary trauma, we found that renal injuries occurred at similar rates in geriatric (67.5%) and nongeriatric (65.9%) patients. Despite a similar degree of injury severity, the geriatric patients with genitourinary trauma more commonly required admission to a higher level of care, required longer stays in the intensive care unit, and had nearly twice the mortality.

Indications for Renal Imaging

The decision to image the patient with a suspected renal injury depends on the severity and mechanism of injury and the presence of hematuria (gross or microscopic) and shock (systolic blood pressure <90 mm Hg). Diagnostic imaging with intravenous (IV) contrast-enhanced computed tomography (CT) should be performed in stable blunt trauma patients with gross hematuria or microscopic hematuria (≥3 to 5 red blood cells/high-power field) in the presence of shock. Significant deceleration or acceleration injuries (falls from a great height or high-speed MVCs) or physical examination findings concerning for renal injury (lower rib fractures; significant flank ecchymosis; penetrating injury of abdomen, flank, or lower chest) also should prompt CT imaging. Patients with blunt mechanisms and microscopic hematuria without shock can be observed clinically without imaging studies. Hemodynamically stable children with blunt trauma should undergo radiographic evaluation

if they have gross hematuria or 50 or more red blood cells/high-power field on microscopic urine analysis. In addition, any child with a significant associated injury or a suspicious mechanism of injury, such as a rapid deceleration, high-velocity strike, fall from more than 15 feet, or direct blow to the abdomen or flank, should be imaged regardless of the presence or absence of hematuria. Patients who are hemodynamically unstable after initial resuscitation require surgical intervention.

One should perform follow-up CT imaging for renal trauma patients who have either (1) deep lacerations (American Association for the Surgery of Trauma [AAST] grades IV and V) or (2) clinical signs of complications (e.g., fever, worsening flank pain, ongoing blood loss, abdominal distension). Repeat abdominal CT with IV contrast medium and delayed scan is recommended 36 to 48 hours after initial scanning for grades IV and V lacerations that are managed expectantly.

Imaging Studies
Computed Tomography

CT can define the location of the injury, identify renal contusions and devitalized segments, and allow visualization of the entire retroperitoneum and abdominal organs. Arterial phase scanning (typically 60 to 70 seconds after contrast administration) provides visualization of the kidneys in the corticomedullary phase of contrast excretion and is necessary to detect active contrast extravasation or other evidence of vascular injury. Injury to the renal collecting system may be missed, as contrast material has not had time to be excreted into the renal collecting system. Repeated or delayed scanning of the kidneys 3 to 5 minutes after injection of contrast is therefore helpful to identify urinary extravasation and other evidence of collecting system injury. Both phases should be assessed for lacerations and other renal parenchymal injuries. A pedicle injury is diagnosed by the lack of contrast enhancement of the kidney or the presence of a central parahilar hematoma. A large medial hematoma displacing the renal vasculature suggests a venous injury. CT angiography provides assessment of the renal vasculature. Images taken at a 10- to 15-minute delay will allow visualization of the renal collecting system and diagnosis of renal pelvis and ureteral injuries. Renal pelvis injuries may be indicated by contrast extravasation just medial to the renal hilum. Renal artery occlusion and renal infarct are noted by lack of parenchymal enhancement or by a cortical rim sign. Delayed films may be omitted when the kidneys are deemed normal and no perinephric, retroperitoneal, pelvic, or perivesical fluid is present.

Ultrasound

The FAST (focused assessment with sonography for trauma) is being used with greater frequency in the immediate evaluation of injuries and can facilitate the rapid diagnosis of intra-abdominal injuries (i.e., hemoperitoneum). However, the study cannot clearly delineate parenchymal lacerations, vascular disruptions, collecting system injuries, or urinary extravasation in the acute setting. Furthermore, it cannot differentiate between fresh blood and extravasated urine. If necessary, sonography can confirm the presence of two kidneys and can define a retroperitoneal hematoma. Currently it is best used for serial evaluation of stable renal injuries or after urinoma or retroperitoneal hematoma.

Intravenous Pyelography

Intravenous pyelography (IVP) is no longer the preferred modality in renal trauma patients and has been replaced by abdominal CT. In unstable patients who require immediate exploration, a one-shot intraoperative IVP on the operating room table can be performed. A single plain film is taken 10 minutes after injection of 2 mL/kg contrast medium. An IVP can establish the presence or absence of the kidneys, define the parenchyma, and outline the collecting system. Nonvisualization or nonfunction of a kidney usually indicates severe trauma to the kidney, such as pedicle injury or shattered kidney. Extravasation implies trauma involving the capsule, parenchyma, or collecting system. Practically, however, the IVP is often difficult to interpret. Although the one-shot IVP is advocated by urologists, trauma surgeons more commonly palpate the contralateral kidney to confirm its presence, administer IV methylene blue or indigo carmine, and temporarily occlude the ipsilateral kidney. A functional kidney is confirmed by noting blue urine in the urinary catheter bag. Intraoperative color Doppler ultrasound to confirm flow in the renal pedicle of the unaffected kidney is another method for intraoperative assessment.

Angiography

Selective renal artery embolization for managing bleeding in stable patients after blunt and penetrating renal trauma has been performed with increasing success. Technical success requires an experienced angiography team that is readily available for emergency intervention. Success rates for embolization of isolated renal artery branch injuries are 70% to 80%. Indications for angioembolization are not agreed on uniformly but generally include active extravasation after failed conservative management. Superselective embolization therapy for renal trauma now provides an effective and minimally invasive technique to potentially avoid unnecessary exploration that could otherwise result in a nephrectomy.

TABLE 1: American Association for the Surgery of Trauma: Injury Scale for the Kidney

Grade*	Type	Description
I	Contusion	Microscopic or gross hematuria, urologic studies normal
	Hematoma	Subcapsular, nonexpanding, and without parenchymal laceration
II	Hematoma	Nonexpanding perirenal hematoma confirmed to renal retroperitoneum
	Laceration	<1 cm parenchymal depth of renal cortex without urinary extravasation
III	Laceration	<1 cm parenchymal depth of renal cortex without collecting system rupture or urinary extravasation
IV	Laceration	Parenchymal laceration extending through renal cortex, medulla, and collecting system
	Vascular	Main renal artery or vein injury with contained hemorrhage
V	Laceration	Completely shattered kidney
	Vascular	Avulsion of renal hilum, which devascularizes kidney

Modified from Moore EE, Shackford SR, Pachter HL, et al. Organ injury scaling: spleen, liver, and kidney. *J Trauma.* 1989;29:1664-1666.

*Advance one grade for bilateral injuries up to grade III.

Injury Scale for the Kidney

The AAST renal organ injury scale is shown in Table 1. The accurate and reproducible classification of injury severity is critical to standardizing trauma research. The AAST scale for renal injury consistently has predicted worse outcomes (nephrectomy, dialysis, and mortality) with increasing grade of injury and is the strongest single predictor of the need for surgical repair. Grades I and II injuries are minor, grade III injuries are intermediate, and grades IV and V injuries are severe. Recent proposed modifications to the AAST grading system to better reflect clinical outcomes with severe injuries and predict injuries that require urgent hemostatic intervention may allow for refinement in renal staging.

Management

Nonoperative Management

In addition to nonoperative treatment of minor grade I and II injuries, hemodynamically stable, well-staged patients with grades III and IV lesions may be treated nonoperatively, regardless of mechanism. Nonoperative management has a low failure rate and ultimately may save kidneys that otherwise might have required nephrectomy as a result of attempted operative repair. Even patients with urinary extravasation can be managed expectantly, with a resolution rate of more than 90%. Patients with grades IV and V injuries more often require surgical exploration, but even grade V injuries have been managed nonoperatively with a more than 50% success rate at experienced centers. Although this success rate is substantial, surgical exploration for grade V renal injuries remains the initial management choice.

Conservative management of renal trauma requires strict bed rest until the urine visibly clears, frequent hemoglobin and hematocrit blood draws, and potential reimaging in high-grade injuries. Once the gross hematuria clears, ambulation is allowed; should gross hematuria recur, bed rest is reinstated. Ambulation without any sequelae allows hospital discharge with close clinical follow-up. Persistent bleeding requires repeat imaging, arteriography, or surgical exploration. Patients who are managed conservatively should be watched for and warned about the possibility of developing renovascular hypertension (Page kidney) and delayed bleeding. Patients with concomitant injuries should be evaluated and managed on the basis of the most significant injury.

Indications for Angioembolization

Angiography and embolization are recommended for (1) patients with persistent bleeding from a segmental renal artery, (2) unstable patients (hypotension or shock that does not respond to fluid resuscitation) with a grade III or IV renal injury, (3) treating a pseudoaneurysm or arteriovenous malformation, (4) cases of persistent gross hematuria, and (5) a rapidly declining hematocrit requiring 2 units of blood.

Indications for Renal Exploration

Absolute indications for renal exploration are (1) persistent, life-threatening hemorrhage believed to stem from renal injury, (2) renal pedicle avulsion (grade V injury), and (3) expanding, pulsatile, or uncontained retroperitoneal hematoma (thought to indicate renal pedicle avulsion). Relative indications for renal exploration include incomplete radiographic staging with concurrent traumatic injuries that require repair or exploration, extensive devitalized renal parenchyma (>50%), or vascular injury. Although urinary extravasation alone does not warrant surgical exploration, ureteropelvic junction avulsion injuries are best managed with prompt surgical repair.

Surgical Management

Retroperitoneal Exploration

Although there has been a paradigm shift to the conservative management of most renal injuries, operative exploration, with the aim of hemorrhage control and renal salvage, is required in a minority of renal trauma patients. Surgery is performed with a midline transperitoneal approach. Historically, all renal injuries were explored and early vascular control was achieved before opening Gerota's fascia, which resulted in a decreased rate of nephrectomy. Over the years, lower-grade injuries became amenable to direct lateral exposure of the kidney with a more selective approach to renal pedicle vascular control. With fewer surgeons operating on the kidney for traumatic injuries along with the paradigm shift to operating only on the most severely injured kidneys, a return to isolation of the renal hilar vessels before opening Gerota's fascia is recommended. The renal vasculature is accessed through the posterior parietal peritoneum, incising over the aorta and medial to the inferior mesenteric vein.

A midline incision from the xiphoid to the pubic symphysis allows for access to all other concomitant intra-abdominal injuries before renal exploration. The incision should be extended to the xiphoid, if this has not been done already, to gain exposure to the renal hilum. Adequate retraction and exposure are essential. The transverse colon is wrapped in a moist laparotomy sponge and placed on the chest. The small intestine is protected with moist laparotomy sponges, retracted superiorly, and placed on the chest to the right. This maneuver exposes the root of the mesentery, the ligament of Treitz, and the underlying great vessels. The retroperitoneum is incised over the aorta superior to the inferior mesenteric artery, and the incision is extended to the ligament of Treitz. Occasionally a retroperitoneal hematoma can prevent distinct palpation of the aorta. An incision can be made medial to the inferior mesenteric vein because it runs a few centimeters to the left of the aorta and is easily identifiable. March along the anterior surface of the aorta until the left renal vein is encountered at its crossing. Rarely (less than 5%), the left renal vein will be retroaortic. A vessel loop should be placed around the left renal vein, and this vessel can be used as a guide to help find the remaining renal vasculature, each of which is then encircled with a vessel loop but not clamped. The vast majority of

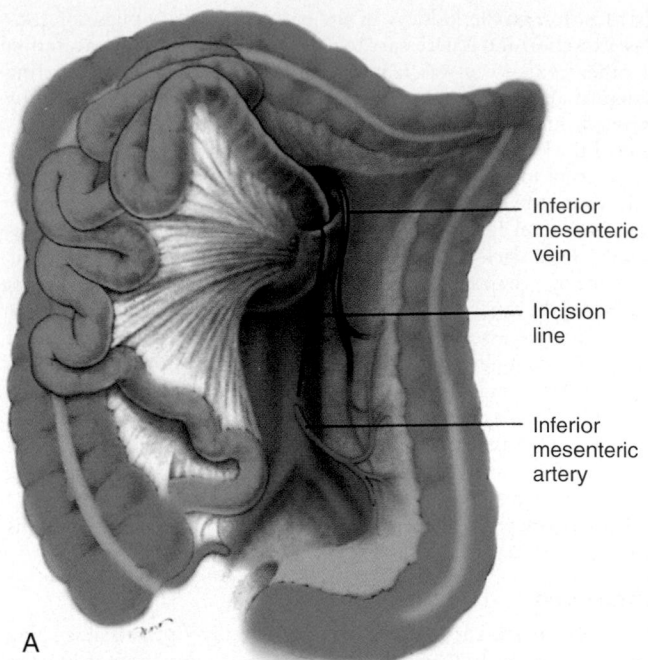

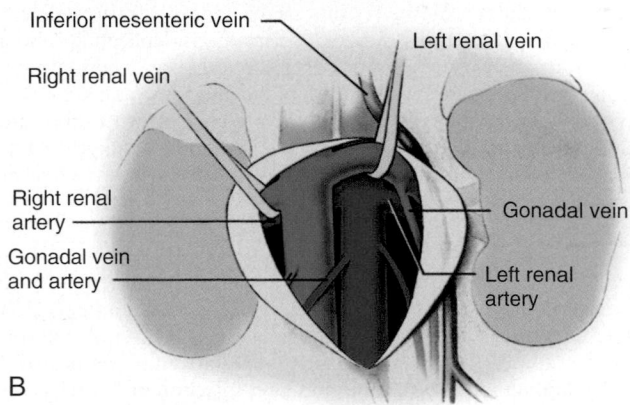

FIGURE 3 Technique to obtain vascular control. **A,** Exposure of the major vessels. **B,** Relationship of the renal vasculature after incision of the posterior peritoneum over the aorta. *(From McAninch JW. Surgery for renal trauma. In: Novick AC, Streem SB, Pontes JE, eds. Stewart's Operative Urology. Baltimore: Williams & Wilkins; 1989.)*

bleeding can be controlled during repair with manual compression of the kidney; rarely will vessel occlusion be necessary (Figure 3). After vascular control has been achieved, for an injury to the right kidney, perform a right medial visceral rotation, which includes a Kocher's maneuver of the duodenum. The surgeon must keep in mind that the right renal artery runs posterior to the inferior vena cava. For a left kidney injury, a left medial visceral rotation (Mattox's maneuver) including the descending colon, splenic flexure, spleen, and distal pancreas is performed. Gerota's fascia then is incised along its lateral aspect. A lateral incision is important because it avoids accidentally dissecting the kidney subcapsularly, avoids ureter injury, and preserves perinephric fat for reconstruction. Preserving the renal capsule is important because this fascia is a strength layer needed during reconstruction, and tearing it can result in more bleeding.

Renovascular Injuries

The incidence of renovascular injuries involves up to 25% of all major renal trauma. The diagnosis of renal vascular injuries is often delayed, as clinical signs are usually absent; up to one third of patients

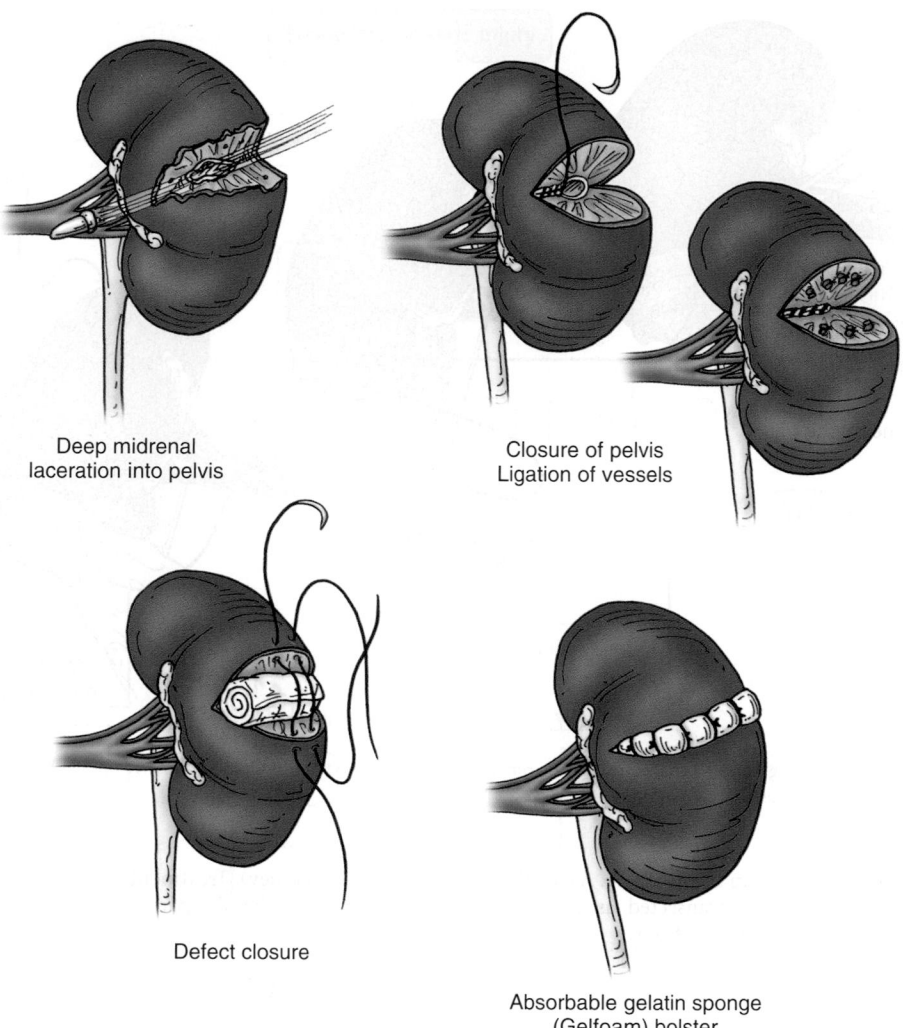

Deep midrenal
laceration into pelvis

Closure of pelvis
Ligation of vessels

Defect closure

Absorbable gelatin sponge
(Gelfoam) bolster

FIGURE 4 Example of renal repair after penetrating trauma. *(Adapted from Armenakas NA, McAninch JW. Genitourinary tract. In: Ivatury RR, Cayten CG, eds. The Textbook of Penetrating Trauma. Media, PA: Williams & Wilkins; 1996.)*

will have no hematuria. Despite advances in trauma care, successful renal salvage after renovascular injury occurs in less than half of cases, frequently resulting in nephrectomy. Proximal vascular control is of paramount importance in the surgical management of vascular injuries. Significant main renal vein bleeding may require ligation, whereas partial lacerations may be repaired with 5-0 polypropylene after careful dissection and control. Injury to the left renal vein can be treated safely with ligation near the inferior vena cava provided the adrenal and gonadal collaterals have been preserved. The right renal vein lacks collateral outflow, and nephrectomy is indicated if repair of the renal vein is not possible. Attempted renal artery repair or revascularization is associated with poor results and therefore often reserved for patients with a solitary kidney or bilaterally injured kidneys.

Renal artery thrombosis in patients who are hemodynamically stable and possess a normal contralateral kidney can be managed expectantly in most cases, occasionally warranting an attempt at immediate thrombectomy and revascularization. Successful endovascular stenting and thrombolysis has been reported.

Renal Reconstruction

Renal salvage by renorrhaphy or partial nephrectomy should be performed in hemodynamically stable patients and requires complete exposure of the injured kidney, sharp débridement of nonviable tissue, suture ligation of bleeding arterial vessels, watertight repair of the collecting system injury, and closure of parenchymal defects. Polar injuries can be amputated, with placement of an omental flap, whereas lacerations to the middle of the kidney require renorrhaphy (Figures 4 and 5). Hemostasis is obtained by figure-of-8 suture ligature of the bleeding vessels with fine, absorbable suture, or in some instances by coagulation. The collecting system should be closed in a watertight fashion with a slowly absorbable suture. An antegrade ureteral stent can be placed in the bladder over a guidewire for significant collecting system reconstructions. Defects in the renal parenchyma may be reconstructed closed, primarily in many cases with renal capsule, with a hemostatic agent such as Surgicel Nu-Knit or thrombin-soaked Gelfoam as a renal repair bolster.

Damage Control

During damage control, the wound and area around the injured kidney are packed with laparotomy pads to control bleeding, with a planned return in 24 hours once the patient has been resuscitated and returned to near normal physiology to explore and re-evaluate the extent of injury. This approach is commonly used for patients with extensive injuries and is useful in managing complex renal injuries while avoiding total nephrectomy. In unstable patients where the kidney is shattered or major vascular injury with hemorrhage is

renal pelvis or ureter and injecting methylene blue or indigo carmine dye. Extravasation of dye or staining of the sponge or adjacent tissues will aid in the diagnosis and injury location.

Delayed diagnosis of a missed ureteral injury may result in significant complications, including abscess, sepsis, ileus, urinary obstruction, and flank pain. Leakage from an abdominal drain site of yellow fluid with a creatinine level consistent with urine is a sign of missed ureteral injury. Percutaneous nephrostomy tube placement allows for urinary diversion; a drain may be placed percutaneously in the fluid collection if needed.

Imaging

Intravenous Urography

Imaging of the ureter by a one-shot IV urogram is inconsistent, unreliable, and frequently nondiagnostic and has been replaced by CT for appropriate staging of ureteral injuries. Occasionally in the unstaged patient in an acute trauma setting, an IV urogram can provide data suggestive of a ureteral injury, but the findings are often subtle, including delayed function, mild ureteral dilation, or deviation. Given the lack of sensitivity and specificity and the variability of intravenous urography, these findings do not obviate the need for direct inspection.

Computed Tomography

Clinicians should perform IV contrast-enhanced abdominal or pelvic CT with delayed imaging (urogram) for stable trauma patients with suspected ureteral injuries, as this is the staging method of choice. Medial perirenal extravasation of contrast material is the most common finding of injury to the ureteropelvic junction collecting system. To evaluate the distal ureter, delayed imaging must be obtained, typically 15 to 20 minutes after the initial scan, to assess ureteral filling. The ipsilateral ureter will not fill if a complete avulsion has occurred, whereas a partial tear may show distal ureteral filling. If results of a CT are inconclusive, a retrograde urogram may be performed.

Retrograde Pyelography

Retrograde pyelography is accurate in demonstrating the presence and location of ureteral extravasation, but the procedure has limited utility in the acute trauma setting, as it both time consuming and cumbersome. In patients who have equivocal CT imaging and are stable, retrograde pyelography both may provide the diagnosis of ureteral injury and may allow for treatment with ureteral stent placement.

Injury Scale of the Ureter

Ureteral injuries are classified according to the AAST injury scale for the ureter (Table 2). Injury severity is defined by degree of transection and length of devitalized tissue.

Management

Selection of the appropriate management of ureteral injuries depends on the patient's condition, concomitant injuries, promptness in recognition of the injury, and location and injury grade. Most patients with grades I and II injuries can be managed with placement of a ureteral stent or nephrostomy tubes. Stenting allows secure drainage of the kidney and provides canalization and stabilization of the injury.

Grades III and IV injuries should be repaired directly, with the following principles (Figure 7):

1. Minimal handling of the ureteral adventitia and careful periureteral dissection are paramount to preserve the ureteral vasculature and minimize stricture
2. Judicious débridement of ureteral ends to healthy bleeding tissue

TABLE 2: American Association for the Surgery of Trauma: Injury Scale for the Ureter

Grade*	Type	Description
I	Hematoma	Contusion or hematoma without devascularization
II	Laceration	Transection <50%
III	Laceration	Transection ≥50%
IV	Laceration	Complete transection with <2 cm of devascularization
V	Laceration	Avulsion with >2 cm of devascularization

Modified from Moore EE, Shackford SR, Pachter HL, et al. Organ injury scaling: spleen, liver, and kidney. *J Trauma.* 1989;29:1664-1668.

Note: Injury severity is defined by degree of transection and length of devitalized tissue.

*Advance one grade for bilateral injuries up to grade III.

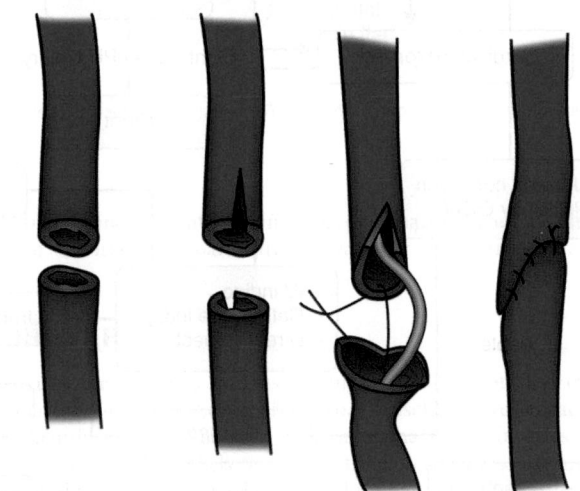

FIGURE 7 Ureteroureterostomy with débridement, spatulation, stenting, and anastomosis. *(From Peterson NE. Genitourinary trauma. In: Feliciano DV, Moore EE, Mattox KL, eds. Trauma. 3rd ed. Stamford, CT: Appleton & Lange; 1996.)*

3. Spatulation of ureteral ends and repair with 5-0 absorbable suture under magnification
4. The repair should be a tension-free, watertight, ureteral mucosa-to-mucosa anastomosis with absorbable interrupted suture
5. Placement of an internal ureteral stent over a guidewire
6. Protection of the repair with peritoneum or omental wrapping
7. Placement of an external drain adjacent to the repair to prevent urinoma

Associated bowel injury or fecal contamination neither increases the complication rate nor compromises ureteral repair success. Ureteral injuries in patients who are too unstable to tolerate surgery should be repaired in a staged fashion. If a staged repair is chosen, the damaged ureter initially is tied off with long silk ties to aid in visualization of the ureter during the second stage of the repair. The kidney is drained percutaneously, preferably in the immediate postoperative period. Some surgeons have placed an 8F feeding tube into the ureter and exteriorized it until the repair can be completed.

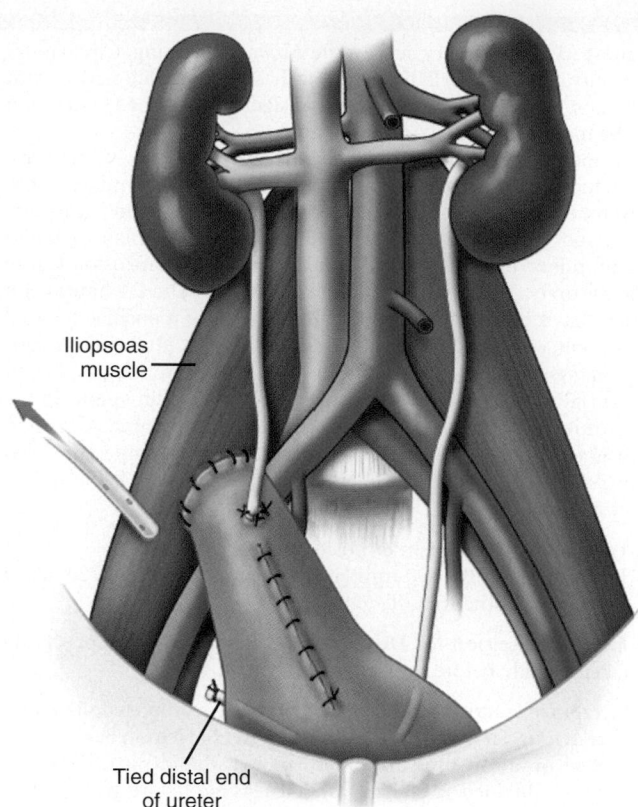

Iliopsoas muscle

Tied distal end of ureter

FIGURE 8 Use of the psoas hitch for treatment of distal ureteral injuries. *(From Maker KV, Guzman-Arrieta ED. Cognitive Pearls in General Surgery. New York: Springer Sciences+Business Media; 2015:Figure 20.7.)*

Lower Ureteral Injuries

Surgeons should repair ureteral injuries located distal to the iliac vessels with ureteral reimplantation or primary repair over a ureteral stent, when possible. The principles of repair include débridement and spatulation of the ureter and tunneling in the bladder wall toward the bladder neck. In adults with normal bladders, unobstructed urethras, and no urinary tract infection, reflux does not impair renal function and therefore a nonrefluxing ureteroneocystostomy does not need to be performed. A stent should be left in for 3 to 6 weeks.

Psoas Hitch and Boari Flap

The psoas hitch procedure is a mainstay in the treatment of injuries to the lower third of the ureter and has a high success rate, ranging from 95% to 100%. It is preferred to ureteroureterostomy in this area because the tenuous independent blood supply might not survive transection. The psoas hitch procedure is performed by suturing the bladder to the ipsilateral psoas minor tendon. Sutures should be placed in the tendon or muscle parallel to the course of its fibers to avoid entrapment of the genitofemoral nerve, which can lead to chronic pain (Figure 8). A ureteral stent and urethral catheter are left in place. Typically a cystogram is obtained before removing the urethral catheter. For longer injuries to the lower two thirds of the ureter, a Boari flap can be performed. The bladder pedicle is swung cephalad, pexed to the psoas to relieve tension, and tubularized to bridge the gap to the injured ureter.

Midureteral Injuries

Surgeons should repair ureteral injuries located proximal to the iliac vessels with primary repair in a ureteroureterostomy fashion over

a ureteral stent. In situations where the ureter loss is more significant, a transureteroureterostomy may be performed. Several contraindications to a transureteroureterostomy must be kept in mind, including recurrent nephrolithiasis, urothelial carcinoma of the upper tract, genitourinary tuberculosis, retroperitoneal fibrosis, and an abnormal contralateral kidney. In the setting of damage to a large segment of ureter that requires complex reconstruction, damage control and repair in a delayed setting is recommended. The urine can be diverted by placing a ureteral stent brought out through the abdominal wall. Future reconstruction options include ileal interposition (small bowel used as a ureteral replacement), renal displacement, autotransplantation into the pelvis, and urinary conduit diversion or neobladder.

Upper Ureteral Injuries

Repair of injuries to the upper third of the ureter should be performed by a ureteroureterostomy over a ureteral stent along with placement of a retroperitoneal drain. Avulsion of the ureteropelvic junction frequently requires acute surgical management, most commonly with a primary anastomosis. In unstable patients, a percutaneous nephrostomy tube may be placed with delayed repair.

Complications

Vigilance for delayed presentation of ureteral injuries allows detection of missed injuries, which occur in more than 50% of cases. Fever, leukocytosis, and local peritoneal irritation are the most common signs and symptoms of missed ureteral injury and should prompt CT imaging. In addition, an unrecognized ureteral injury can lead to significant complications, including urinoma, abscess, ureteral stricture, hydronephrosis, urinary fistula, and potential loss of an ipsilateral renal unit. Missed injuries that are discovered more than 48 hours after injury are best delineated with retrograde ureterography and stented if feasible. Large fluid collections should be drained percutaneously.

Delayed Treatment

The interval from injury to recognition of such is important and should guide management. If the injury is diagnosed within the first 7 days without a concomitant significant infection, surgical exploration and repair may be performed. Attempting repair after 10 to 14 days may be difficult secondary to a marked inflammatory response. In addition, the presence of an abscess, urinoma, or fistula should delay any attempt at definitive operative repair. For patients in whom recognition of a ureteral injury is delayed beyond 2 weeks, an initial endourologic approach may be attempted; if such an approach is not possible, a temporizing nephrostomy tube may be placed until the time of delayed reconstruction.

SUGGESTED READINGS

Bjurlin MA, Goble SM, Fantus RJ, et al. Outcomes in geriatric genitourinary trauma. *J Am Coll Surg.* 2011;213:415-421.

Bjurlin MA, Jeng EI, Goble SM, et al. Comparison of nonoperative management with renorrhaphy and nephrectomy in penetrating renal injuries. *J Trauma.* 2011;71:554-558.

Brandes S, Coburn M, Armenakas N, et al. Diagnosis and management of ureteric injury: an evidence-based analysis. *BJU Int.* 2004;94:277-289.

Breyer BN, McAninch JW, Elliott SP, et al. Minimally invasive endovascular techniques to treat acute renal hemorrhage. *J Urol.* 2008;179:2248-2252.

Santucci RA, Fisher MB. The literature increasingly supports expectant (conservative) management of renal trauma—a systematic review. *J Trauma.* 2005;59:493-503.

Santucci RA, Wessells H, Bartsch G, et al. Evaluation and management of renal injuries: consensus statement of the renal trauma subcommittee. *BJU Int.* 2004;93:937-954.

DAMAGE CONTROL OPERATION

Aurelio Rodriguez, MD, FACS, and David Elliott, MD

Damage control operation (DCO) modifies traditional surgical care by expediting lifesaving measures, abbreviating prolonged procedures, and postponing nonessential surgery, so that those patients most at risk for lethal physiologic deterioration from injury can have a greater chance of surviving. Most often, DCO is used to reverse or prevent the development of the "lethal triad" of hypothermia, metabolic acidosis, and coagulopathy that occurs in advanced stages of post-traumatic physiologic decompensation and that carries a mortality rate in excess of 90% when approached with traditional treatment paradigms of normotensive crystalloid resuscitation and exhaustive, protracted definitive surgery. The guiding principles of DCO are "Normal physiology is more important than normal anatomy" and "A live patient above all else."

DCO uses a strategy of staged therapeutic interventions, initially limited to essential lifesaving measures of hemorrhage cessation, contamination control, and perfusion of vital organs, followed by intensive care unit (ICU) resuscitation and then delayed definitive surgery once normal physiology is restored. The most common indicated scenarios for using DCO include:

- Complex upper abdominal or pelvic injuries
- Complex multisystem injuries
- A "stable" trauma patient with two or more of the "lethal triad": hypothermia, metabolic acidosis, coagulopathy
- A hypotensive trauma patient with one or more of the "lethal triad"
- Mass casualties
- Projected need for massive transfusion
- Projected shortage in blood product supply

The DCO strategy is resource intensive. Compared with traditional approaches to trauma surgery, DCO results in ongoing consumption of significant quantities of operating room (OR) and ICU supplies and blood products, as well as substantial use of OR and ICU personnel assets. The International Committee of the Red Cross (ICRC), which has extensive experience in operating war-zone casualty receiving hospitals in austere environments, emphasizes three factors necessary for successful implementation of the DCO strategy:

1. Early recognition of altered physiology and use of DCO
2. ICU capacity
3. Blood availability

This chapter discusses DCO in four phases:

- Phase 1: Emergency department (ED) assessment, DCO decision, begin damage control resuscitation (DCR)
- Phase 2: Damage control surgery
- Phase 3: ICU resuscitation
- Phase 4: Definitive surgery

PHASE 1: EMERGENCY DEPARTMENT ASSESSMENT

Although only a small percentage of trauma patients—perhaps 5% of civilian casualties and 8% of combat casualties—arriving in an ED will benefit from a damage control approach, they must be identified early and the proper steps must be implemented quickly in order to optimize chances of survival. The initial Advanced Trauma Life

Support (ATLS) primary survey, the Airway, Breathing, Circulation, Disability, Exposure (ABCDE) approach, should be followed as with any trauma patient, but once the vital signs are obtained, a decision can be made regarding damage control.

Numerous trauma scoring systems and laboratory values have been studied to predict the need for DCO; the easiest, quickest, and most reliable appear to be three vital signs: blood pressure, heart rate (HR), and temperature (T). The ABC score (assessment of blood consumption) predicts an 85% need for massive transfusion (more than 10 units of packed red blood cells [PRBCs] in 24 hours) if a patient has a penetrating trauma mechanism (or a positive focused assessment with sonography for trauma [FAST]) plus either hypotension (systolic blood pressure [SBP] less than 90 mm Hg) or tachycardia (HR greater than 120 beats per minute) on admission. On the basis of its experience, the ICRC asserts that any trauma admission with grade II or higher hypothermia (core body temperature less than 34°C) warrants DCO. Therefore a simple and reliable test to determine the need for DCO includes:

- Penetrating mechanism *or* positive FAST, *plus*
- Hypotension (SBP <90 mm Hg) *or* tachycardia (HR >120 beats/min), *or* hypothermia (T <34°C).

Once the decision for DCO is made, the following steps should be taken quickly before the patient is taken to the OR.

1. A rapid primary and secondary survey is completed, and life-threatening injuries are addressed per ATLS. Hemorrhage is controlled by direct pressure or tourniquet. Rapid portable x-rays may be obtained if essential and if feasible before transport to the OR.
2. DCR is initiated: intravenous (IV) access is assured, but crystalloid fluids are minimized. Preferentially, PRBCs and fresh frozen plasma (FFP) at a ratio of 1:1 are given as resuscitative fluids. The massive transfusion protocol is activated, in accordance with hospital policy. Target SBP before surgical intervention is 70 to 80 mm Hg, with patient mentation.
3. Although important for all trauma patients, warming measures for DCO patients are essential: all IV fluids are warmed; wet clothing is removed and warm blankets are applied, as is a "space" blanket or forced-air warming device if available; and supplemental oxygen is warmed if possible.
4. For the patient with multisystem injuries, or in a mass casualty situation, rapid prioritization of surgical interventions is done by the surgeon and communicated to the anesthesia and OR team, and the patient is transported to the OR.

Certain special situations mandate a modified approach to decisions about using DCO.

- *Mass casualties.* To provide "the greatest good for the greatest number," surgeons may adopt a lower threshold to use DCO, even when patients otherwise would not seem to be candidates for this strategy. When resources (e.g., OR space, blood) are limited and multiple patients require lifesaving surgery, abbreviated procedures to stop hemorrhage, ischemia, and contamination can result in more lives saved, postponing definitive procedures until time and resources are less critical.
- *Combat casualties.* The triad of (1) delayed access to surgical care in hostile conditions; (2) the extensive wounding effect of modern explosive munitions and high-energy weaponry; and (3) military policy of evacuating battlefield casualties through multiple escalating echelons of care creates unique challenges in providing optimal care of the wounded. Regarding DCO, (1) delay in care results in a high likelihood of hypothermia and prolonged hypoperfusion from shock, vascular disruption, and tourniquet use, making DCO and the need for blood products and vascular expedients like shunts more likely; (2) massive tissue destruction and contamination warrants innovative approaches to "damage

control débridement," stopping hemorrhage and removing dead tissue, dirt, and debris rapidly in large nonanatomic wounds; (3) multiechelon evacuation mandates precise communication, particularly regarding vascular shunts, abdominal packing, clamped or ligated vessels, stapled bowel, and temporary abdominal closure.

- *Austere environments.* A surgeon caring for the severely injured in a location that lacks modern medical "essentials," such as a well-stocked blood bank, ICU, fluid warmers, negative-pressure wound therapy, and laboratory capability, nonetheless can use damage control strategy modified to the context. This may imply a markedly curtailed operative intervention, with definitive surgery postponed until blood can be obtained from friends or relatives. The ICRC points out that when faced with mass casualties in an austere environment where blood is scarce and ICU care is lacking, the clinician sometimes must make difficult decisions about whether to use DCO for the questionably salvageable patient or to save those resources for a patient more likely to survive.

PHASE 2: DAMAGE CONTROL SURGERY

DCO strategies and techniques have been published for injuries to most areas of the body. This section focuses on DCO application for abdominal, thoracic, vascular, orthopedic, and soft tissue injuries. Keys to success for the surgeon include the following:

- *Preoperative* identification that DCO will be used, rather than making the decision to use DCO 3 hours into a difficult operation with the patient already in extremis from acidosis, hypothermia, coagulopathy, and hypotension.
- In the patient with multisystem injuries, strategic determination of the order of intervention. For example, in a patient with both abdominal and femoral artery injury hemorrhage, abdominal packing or arterial shunting should take priority in whichever site is bleeding the most.
- Communication with the OR team, particularly the anesthesiologist, who should be familiar and comfortable with using an ongoing DCR strategy during the operation. Permissive hypotension with end organ perfusion is achieved through IV anesthetic titration at reduced dosages, with concomitant balanced blood product resuscitation, PRBCs and FFP at a 1:1 ratio (Figure 1).
- Hypothermia is prevented or addressed by elevating the OR thermostat; replacing surgical drapes when they become wet with blood or fluids; keeping all nonoperated body parts wrapped and preferably warmed with forced-air heat; and ensuring that all gases, IV fluids, and irrigating fluids are warmed.

Damage Control Laparotomy

A stepwise approach to abdominal exploration is followed.

1. First, blood and clots are evacuated. If it wells up quickly again, the aorta can be occluded at the diaphragm with a sponge-stick.
2. Targeted abdominal packs are placed around the liver and spleen and in the pelvis.
3. The priority is control of ongoing hemorrhage. Packs are withdrawn serially, and sites of major bleeding are identified. Strategy by the source of bleeding is as follows:
   - *Liver.* (1) Discrete visible vessels are clamped and ligated. (2) Diffuse bleeding from small projectile holes can be controlled with balloon tamponade; a Foley catheter is inserted into the track and inflated. For persistent bleeding or larger tracks, a Penrose drain, cut to length, is secured at both ends with suture to a red rubber catheter passing within, inserted into the track, and the catheter is inflated with saline until the bleeding stops. (3) Diffuse, deep, ill-defined, or uncontrollable bleeding is controlled first by Pringle's maneuver. If time

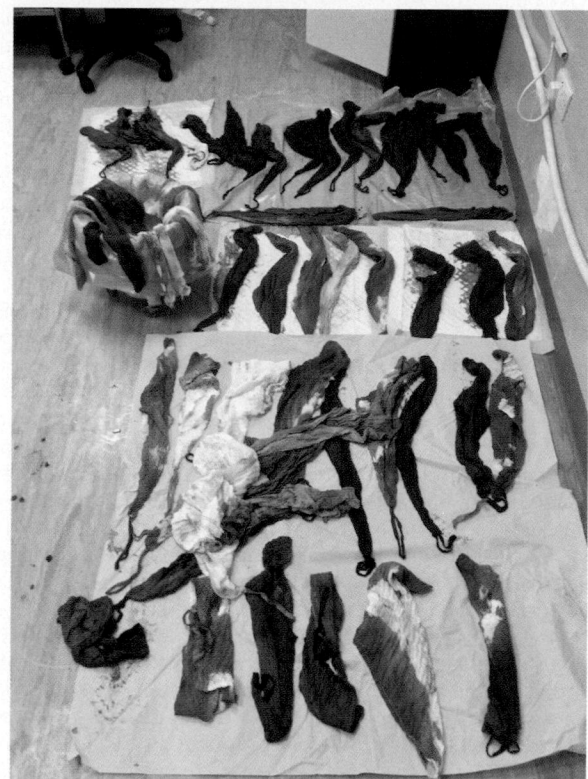

FIGURE 1 Communication with the anesthesiologist during damage control operation is critical for assessing blood loss and blood products requirement during surgery.

permits, an attempt at hepatorrhaphy with #0 or 0-0 chromic suture on a large, blunt-tipped needle is acceptable. If this is not feasible, the surgeon should use targeted packing with abdominal sponges placed concentrically around the liver to approximate a compressed, normal anatomy; of note, sponges should be placed adjacent to the retrohepatic vena cava to prevent compression and reduction of venous return to the heart. (4) Nonbleeding, contained hematomata around the retrohepatic vena cava are packed similarly and left unopened. Damage control measures for the patient in extremis because of hemorrhage from the retrohepatic vena cava, suggested by hepatic bleeding despite Pringle's maneuver, include an attempt at primary suture repair and, if unsuccessful, packing.

- *Spleen.* Splenectomy.
- *Kidney.* Small, nonpulsatile, nonexpansile hematomata are left alone; active bleeding is addressed with nephrectomy after assurance is made that the contralateral kidney is of normal size and uninjured. The Gerota's fascia is entered laterally, the kidney is brought up into the wound with a compressing hand, and the hilar vessels and ureter are clamped.
- *Vascular structures.* Smaller vessels such as those in the mesentery are clamped and ligated; this also applies to the inferior mesenteric artery, arteries of the celiac axis, the hypogastric vessels, and the infrarenal inferior vena cava. Certain important vessels—superior mesenteric artery (SMA), superior mesenteric vein (SMV), portal vein, suprarenal inferior vena cava, and iliac arteries—cannot be ligated and require either rapid suture repair or a temporary shunt (for up to 3 days; see "Damage Control Vascular Surgery" later in the chapter for technique). The abdominal aorta requires repair, although reports on using a chest tube as a temporary shunt have been published. Intact pelvic hematomata should be left alone, but if a hematoma overlying an iliac artery is bleeding or expanding, it requires opening and control.

- *Pancreas.* (1) The priority is to control hemorrhage through ligation of the SMA and SMV branches and repair or shunting of the SMA or SMV main trunks as discussed earlier. (2) A second priority is control of pancreatic ductal injury through targeted abdominal sponge packing and closed suction drainage.

4. A second priority is to control contamination from hollow visceral structures. The source of any gross spillage is identified and first sealed with a Babcock or similar clamp. Then simple lacerations of the stomach, duodenum, small intestine, and colon of up to 50% circumference are sutured using single-layer, running or interrupted, stitches as long as the sutured tissue is healthy. More destructive injuries or multiple intestinal injuries closely approximate within a limited length of bowel are resected using an intestinal stapler; neither anastomosis nor stoma formation is necessary during DCO but can be accomplished in 1 to 3 days at definitive surgery. The ends of resected bowel are left in place. For complex duodenal injuries that cannot be resected easily, suture repair should be reinforced with a loop of small intestine, suturing seromuscular bites as a buttressing ring around the repair (Thal patch), plus wide drainage for control of potential leaks. In austere environments or extreme circumstances, bowel clamps controlling visceral spillage can be left in situ until definitive surgery.

5. Another consideration during damage control laparotomy is removing dead tissue and gross external contamination (e.g., dirt, clothing, foreign bodies). Grossly necrotic bowel is resected with the stapler; solid organs and retroperitoneal muscles are assessed individually for viability. Not every speck of dirt requires removal during DCO, but large amounts of dirt, foreign material, and dead tissue should be removed or débrided to prevent sepsis.

6. Before closure, the surgeon should talk with the anesthesiologist. Occasionally the initial assessment of physiologic instability may have proven unwarranted, and the anesthesiologist may relate that the patient is stable and normothermic with acceptable pH, hematologic, and coagulation parameters. If so, consensus may justify proceeding with definitive surgical repair of injuries (with the option to resume DCO strategy should deterioration occur).

7. Damage control laparotomy warrants a temporary closure because return to the operating theater in 1 to 3 days is obligatory if the patient survives. The goals are (1) to prevent abdominal compartment syndrome from excessive closure pressure, and (2) to preserve fascia so that the surgeon has a chance to provide ultimate closure once resuscitation and definitive surgery are complete. In the past, techniques such as towel clip skin closure and plastic bag abdominal skin silo ("Bogota bag") were used for this purpose. Currently most surgeons favor some variety of negative-pressure wound dressings, as these remove excess abdominal fluids, reduce abdominal pressure, keep the fascia approximated, seal off the abdominal cavity from infecting micro-organisms, and keep the patient's external skin dry (Figure 2). Commercial products are available for this purpose, such as the V.A.C. ABThera system (KCI, San Antonio, TX); however, the surgeon can create a simple, inexpensive, and effective negative-pressure closure by:
   - Fashioning and placing a sterile, fenestrated, nonadherent layer (e.g., IV bag, Mayo stand cover) atop the bowel and tucked well under the anterior abdominal wall on all sides
   - Placing sterile gauze or towels atop the nonadherent layer, followed by two or more large fenestrated closed suction tubes, followed by more sterile gauze or towels to rise to skin level
   - Sealing the anterior abdominal wall and dressing with a sterile occlusive adhesive drape (e.g., Ioban antimicrobial incise drape; 3M, St. Paul, MN)
   - Attaching the drains to 125 mm Hg closed suction

Damage Control Thoracic Surgery

Two scenarios warrant consideration of a damage control approach to thoracotomy: (1) witnessed cardiac arrest due to penetrating

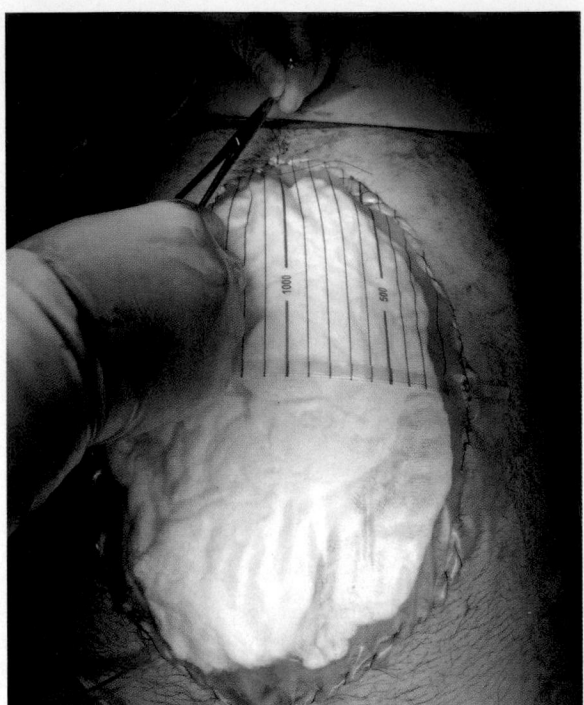

FIGURE 2 Temporary abdominal closure in an austere environment after damage control laparotomy. Expedient use of sterile urine bag in the field for both bowel-contact layer and skin-sealing layer. Urine bag tubing is cut and used for two suction drains to create vacuum.

injury to the chest; less commonly due to penetrating injury to the abdomen, pelvis, or extremities; or due to blunt trauma; and (2) massive hemorrhage from tube thoracostomy in a patient who meets the criteria for DCO (discussed earlier). In both situations, a common approach serves to identify and address most injuries rapidly.

- The patient is anesthetized in the supine position with a single-lumen endotracheal tube and with large IV lines placed above and below the diaphragm, transfusing warmed blood products (FFP to PRBC ratio 1:1) to keep SBP at 70 to 80 mm Hg.
- A left anterolateral thoracotomy is made (unless the hemorrhage obviously is coming from the right chest) and a contralateral chest tube is placed. The incision can be extended across the sternum into the other chest, clamshell-style, if necessary.
- If the patient is in arrest or near arrest, the descending aorta is palpated just above the diaphragm and a large vascular clamp is applied to occlude it.
- The pericardium is opened parallel and anterior to the phrenic nerve, any blood or tamponade is evacuated, and cardiac massage is begun if arrest is present. Cardiac injuries are addressed using pledgeted 2-0 or 3-0 polypropylene (small half [SH] needle for the atria, medium half [MH] needle for the ventricles) or, in dire circumstances, skin staples, taking care in all cases to avoid the coronary arteries. Hemorrhage from larger cardiac lesions is temporarily controlled with finger occlusion or Foley catheter tamponade.
- Pulmonary hemorrhage is addressed with clamping and suture ligation or with nonanatomic wedge resections by linear stapling. Initially massive hemorrhage can be controlled with a "hilar twist," rotating the lung 180 degrees at the hilum to occlude hilar blood flow, after careful incision of the inferior pulmonary ligament (Figure 3). Alternatively, the hilar vessels can be occluded with a vascular clamp via intrapericardial access. Bleeding from projectile tracks is approached by opening the track with a linear stapler and controlling individual vessels. Mass closure of the pulmonary surface generally is not advised, as communication

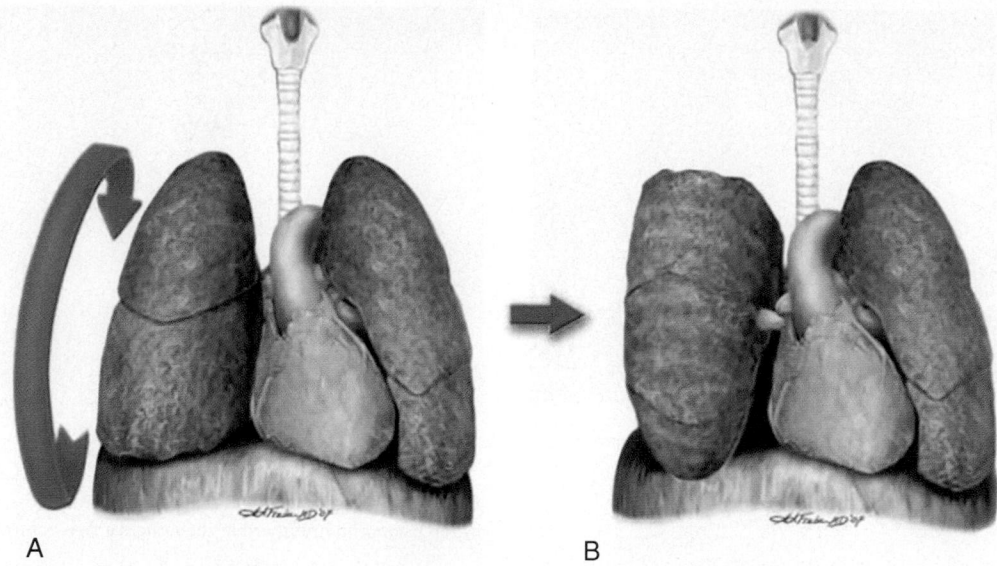

FIGURE 3 Hilar twist of 180 degrees for control of massive pulmonary hemorrhage. **A,** Before hilar twist. **B,** After hilar twist. *(Courtesy Combat Casualty Care: Lessons Learned from OEF and OIF. Fort Detrick, MD: Borden Institute, U.S. Army Office of the Surgeon General; 2012:180. Illustrator: Aletta Frazier, MD.)*

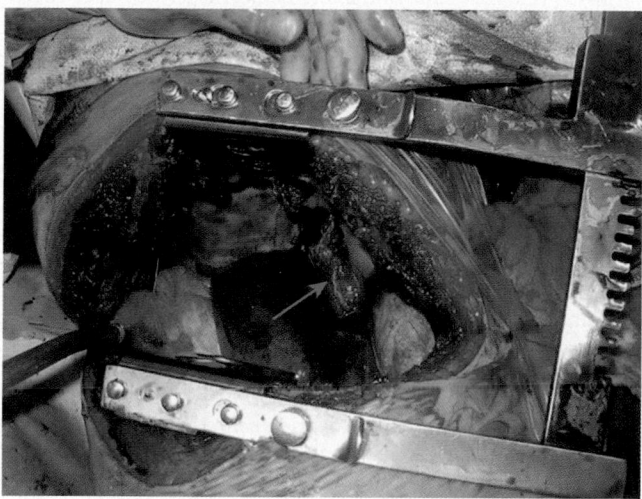

FIGURE 4 Right thoracotomy with upper and middle stapled lobectomy for hemorrhage. *(Courtesy Nessen SC, Lounsbury DE, Hetz SP, eds. War Surgery in Afghanistan and Iraq: A Series of Cases, 2003–2007. Washington, DC: Borden Institute, U.S. Army Office of the Surgeon General, Walter Reed Army Medical Center; 2008:149.)*

between the underlying open vessels and bronchi can result in air embolism.

- Hemorrhage from thoracic vascular structures is controlled with suture ligation or repair, depending on the size and importance of the vessel and the simplicity of repair, or with a temporary shunt for more complex injuries. Balloon catheter occlusion can be used for temporary control. Innominate and subclavian vessel injuries usually require additional incisions, such as supraclavicular or median sternotomy.
- Tracheobronchial injuries are repaired with suture, but if the injuries are large or proximal, stapled lobectomy may prove the most effective and expedient means of control (two firings of the stapler are preferred on the proximal side for security; Figure 4). Pneumonectomy in the trauma patient in extremis is rarely survived.

- Esophageal injuries are best repaired with suture primarily, widely drained, and buttressed with muscle or pleura, time permitting.
- Thoracotomy closure is accomplished in one layer, incorporating pleura, adjacent ribs, and muscle, using large interrupted sutures. The skin is left open for possible delayed closure, and two chest tubes are placed for suction.

Damage Control Vascular Surgery

Vascular injuries to the neck and extremities create the double risk of exsanguination and ischemia of the distal organ or extremity. The more destructive soft tissue injuries, such as those caused by explosive munitions and high-energy small arms on the battlefield, create particular challenges for the treating surgeon, who often must identify and control multiple contracted, constricted vessels within a large complex wound of distorted anatomy, contamination, and diffuse hemorrhage. On the basis of many decades of battlefield experience treating vascular injuries under austere conditions, the ICRC recommends a conservative, stepwise approach.

- For suspected extremity vascular injuries, field tourniquets and dressings should be left in place and not removed until the patient is in the OR, anesthetized, and resuscitated and a proximal pneumatic tourniquet is emplaced and inflated.
- The site of injury is cleansed and draped broadly for proximal and distal control, as is an uninvolved lower extremity for possible use of greater saphenous vein for repair.
- The wound is explored to confirm vascular injury, and then proximal and distal control is obtained, sometimes with separate incisions. Certain vessels, such as the external carotid artery, internal jugular vein, and infrageniculate and forearm arteries and veins, can be ligated preferentially rather than repaired. Most other vessels should be shunted during DCO, unless the injury to the vessel is small (less than 50% circumference) and the surgeon can rapidly apply suture for repair.
- If the decision is made to shunt, the injured ends of the transected vessels are left alone and not débrided until later definitive repair. Shunt tubing is selected; commercial Argyle or Javid shunts come in variable sizes, but any pliable sterile tubing (e.g., pediatric feeding catheter, IV infusion line) is acceptable. The appropriate-size shunt is dipped in heparin solution before use.

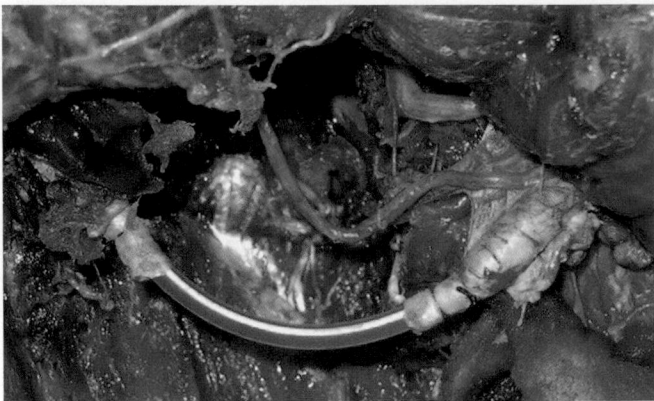

FIGURE 5 Temporary shunt placed in the superficial femoral artery. *(Courtesy Nessen SC, Lounsbury DE, Hetz SP, eds. War Surgery in Afghanistan and Iraq: A Series of Cases, 2003–2007. Washington, DC: Borden Institute, U.S. Army Office of the Surgeon General, Walter Reed Army Medical Center; 2008:21.)*

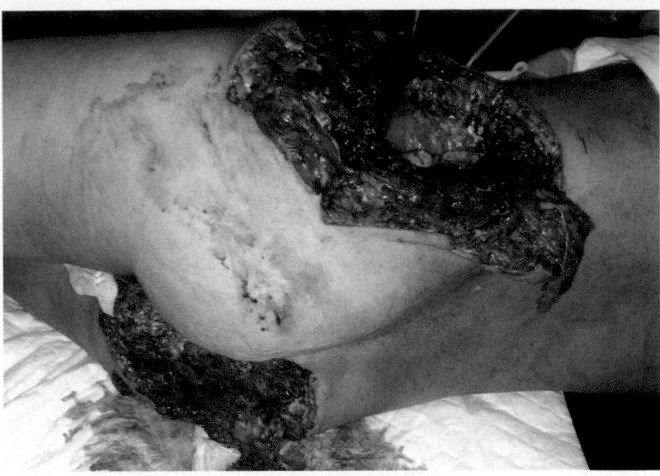

FIGURE 6 Blast wound with massive soft tissue loss, hemorrhage, hypotension, and hypothermia requiring damage control débridement.

- *Before* shunt placement, the surgeon should perform three maneuvers: (1) test for backbleeding in the distal artery; if inadequate, a balloon embolectomy catheter is passed to clear the distal clot; (2) instill 20 mL of heparinized saline, 20 IU/mL, into both the proximal and the distal limbs of transected vessels, then occlude with a vessel loop or Rumel tourniquet; systemic heparin is *not* administered; (3) because patency of vascular repair or shunting depends heavily on adequate outflow within the injured or ischemic distal extremity, it is highly recommended that distal fasciotomy *precede* shunt placement in all cases of extremity vascular injury when flow cannot be restored within 2 hours of injury.
- Shunt placement: (1) appropriate-diameter shunting material is selected and cut to a length adequate for securing in proximal and distal vessel ends; (2) blood flow is re-established as each end of the shunt is placed within the vessel; (3) 0-silk or similar ties are used to secure the shunt within the ends of the vessel (Figure 5); for shunts longer than 5 to 6 cm, a silk ligature securing the middle of the shunt to surrounding tissue is recommended, to enhance stability.
- Before wound closure, the surgeon should talk with the anesthesiologist. Occasionally the initial assessment of physiologic instability may have proven unwarranted, and the anesthesiologist may relate that the patient is stable and normothermic with acceptable pH, hematologic, and coagulation parameters. If so, consensus may justify proceeding with definitive repair of vascular injuries (with the option to resume DCO strategy should deterioration occur).
- Regardless of DCO or definitive repair, the surgeon should ensure that gross contamination, foreign bodies, and necrotic tissue are débrided quickly and then cover the shunted or repaired vessels with healthy soft tissue. With DCO, the skin is left open. Whenever a shunt is placed, the dressing should be marked with "SHUNT" in large, bold, indelible letters.
- Distal perfusion is assessed with Doppler, ultrasonography, or pulse oximetry; arteriographic assessment is reserved for questionable perfusion after definitive repair. For the unstable patient with DCO shunt or repair and fasciotomy in whom distal perfusion is questionable, the surgeon must use judgment in deciding whether to re-explore the injured vessels or take the patient to the ICU for continued resuscitation and reassessment of distal perfusion once temperature and hemodynamics are normalized.
- Definitive vascular repair typically is performed 24 hours after DCO, once ICU resuscitation is complete; however, vascular shunts can be left in for 48 to 72 hours if necessary.

Damage Control Orthopedic and Soft Tissue Surgery

In the patient with multisystem trauma or in whom orthopedic or soft tissue trauma results in massive hemorrhage, a damage control approach may be warranted. The same indications for DCO discussed earlier apply. Damage control débridement involves rapid removal of gross contamination, foreign bodies, and dead soft tissue (Figure 6). Specific injuries that require special approaches include the following:

1. *Amputations.* A pneumatic tourniquet is placed if a field tourniquet was not used at the scene. Damage control débridement is performed, saving as much viable soft tissue as possible for later bone coverage. Vessels are identified and ligated, transected nerves are cut cleanly well away from the stump, bone end is sawed cleanly and smoothed with a rasp, and then the tourniquet is released. After hemostasis, the wound is dressed loosely and closed in 4 to 5 days (delayed primary closure).
2. *Open fractures.* After assurance of vascular integrity, the surgeon performs damage control débridement, which also includes removal of loose bony fragments, then irrigation, gross reduction of the fracture, and stabilization with plaster splint, external fixation, or skeletal traction (femur fracture). For severely mangled extremities with questionable distal viability, the surgeon should consider amputation if hemostasis cannot be attained rapidly otherwise.
3. *Pelvic fracture.* Unless a laparotomy is required for other indications, the surgeon should use a stepwise approach to pelvic exsanguination control: (1) pelvic binder or sheet wrap, circumferentially incorporating and compressing the space between the anterior superior iliac spines and the femoral greater trochanters; (2) pelvic external fixation; (3) resuscitative endovascular balloon occlusion of the aorta (REBOA) with angioembolization, if a clinician with the requisite endovascular expertise is present, or extraperitoneal packing via the space of Retzius into the space of Bogros. For this last maneuver, a lower abdominal midline incision is made and carried down to the peritoneum, which is left intact. Prevesical blood is evacuated, the bladder is pressed posteriorly, and then three laparotomy sponges are introduced into each side of the perivesical space between the pelvic side wall and the bladder, downward toward the sacrum (Figure 7).
4. *Soft tissue injuries,* especially large degloving injuries, mangled extremities, and blast wounds. The surgeon should use damage control débridement; rapid identification, clamping, and ligation of obvious hemorrhaging vessels; and packing.

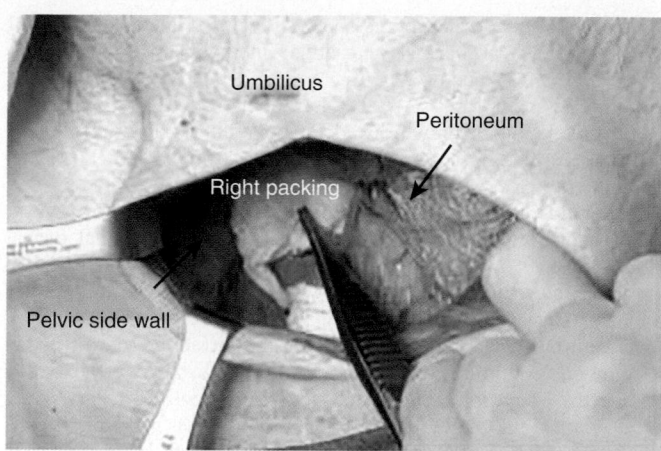

FIGURE 7 Extraperitoneal packing in the space of Retzius for pelvic hemorrhage. *(Courtesy Demetriades D, Inaba K, Vemahos G, eds.* Atlas of Surgical Techniques in Trauma. *New York: Cambridge University Press; 2015:277.)*

PHASE 3: INTENSIVE CARE UNIT RESUSCITATION

After DCO, the intensivist must use both an aggressive approach to resuscitation and cautious monitoring for signs that could necessitate early return to the OR.

The resuscitation priority is to reverse the components of the "lethal triad." Normothermia is achieved with active and passive warming via blankets, forced-air heaters, warmed IV fluids, and supplemental oxygen. Acidosis is treated with fluid resuscitation, not bicarbonate, with the goal of a normal blood lactate and base deficit less than 2. On the basis of hemoglobin and coagulation assays, blood products are the preferred resuscitative fluids. Vasopressors should be avoided for hypotension due to hypovolemia, although they have a role if sepsis develops.

If the patient underwent DCO laparotomy and has a temporary abdominal closure, adequate analgesia and sedation are imperative to prevent agitation and disruption of the dressing. Not infrequently this requires use of mechanical ventilation with neuromuscular blockade.

If lactic acidosis, hypotension, or coagulopathy worsens despite vigorous resuscitation, the intensivist should confer with the surgeon about the probability of ongoing hemorrhage, contamination, or gangrenous necrosis. This could warrant early return to the OR before ICU resuscitation is complete. The intensivist also must monitor for abdominal compartment syndrome, whether or not a temporary abdominal closure has been placed. Oliguria and elevation of peak airway pressure are early signs of abdominal compartment syndrome, which can be confirmed with bladder pressure. Normally zero, a bladder pressure exceeding 20 to 25 mm Hg warrants return to the OR.

PHASE 4: DEFINITIVE SURGERY

Once ICU resuscitation has achieved normal and stable parameters as discussed earlier, the surgeon can return the patient to the OR for definitive repair of injuries. Beyond the usual challenges inherent in the optimal treatment of complex injuries, the surgeon returning the DCO patient to the OR for definitive surgery must be aware of additional factors related to the prior surgery.

■ Regardless of who performed the DCO and any report that may accompany the patient, the surgeon must presume missed injuries because of the hurried nature of the initial lifesaving intervention. Therefore it is essential that an unhurried, meticulous, and comprehensive re-exploration is performed.

■ DCO packing to stop hemorrhage must be removed at the second operation. The surgeon should perform this gently, as adherent gauze torn from friable tissue such as injured liver can produce fresh hemorrhage that requires repacking. Therefore "underwater" packing removal, soaking the packing with sufficient warm saline to immerse all gauze before attempting removal, seems most prudent. If, despite careful removal, hemorrhage recurs, repacking with abdominal gauze sponges is occasionally necessary, followed by more ICU resuscitation and repeat laparotomy.

■ If all gauze sponges and instruments are removed from a body cavity (such as the abdomen) at the end of definitive surgery, radiographs should be obtained to ensure that none are inadvertently retained. Sponge counts from DCO are notoriously inaccurate and should not be trusted.

■ If a DCO shunt is placed for a vascular injury associated with an open fracture, it is generally prudent to ensure optimal fracture fixation (external or internal) *before* replacing the shunt with a definitive repair (such as with saphenous vein), as the additional bony manipulation could disrupt the repair.

■ EFFECTIVENESS

Despite widespread practice of DCO as a lifesaving strategy for the most critically injured and irrespective of the large volume of peer-reviewed literature published on its efficacy (at least 2551 articles), repeated Cochrane Collaboration reviews attempting to assess DCO by comparing it with traditional surgical treatment have concluded that "evidence that supports the efficacy of damage control surgery with respect to traditional laparotomy in patients with major abdominal trauma is limited" (Cirocchi et al., 2013). This study's authors point to the lack of any randomized controlled trials as the basis for their conclusion. However, until such a study is published, surgeons will have to rely on retrospective and historically controlled published studies to guide their decision making.

Compared with older studies quoting mortality rates of 90% for injured patients with elements of the "lethal triad" undergoing definitive surgery, more recent studies show markedly improved survival, particularly those that combined DCO and DCR, an approach that emphasizes permissive hypotension, limitation of crystalloid infusion, and blood component resuscitation with balanced ratios of packed cells, plasma, and platelets. Whereas initial DCO studies proclaimed a 50% survival rate as a significant step forward, the last 5 years have seen published data with comparably injured patients achieving 73% to 86% survival using this combined strategy (Cotton et al, 2011; Duchesne et al, 2010).

■ UNRESOLVED ISSUES

Other than lack of a randomized controlled trial to definitively establish DCO as superior to traditional approaches for injured patients in extremis, the surgical literature reflects that a number of other issues associated with use of DCO remain unresolved.

1. The optimum ratio of blood products for DCR and the utility of hemostatic adjuncts. Consensus seems to have emerged that a PRBC to FFP ratio less than 2:1 is superior to ratios greater than that. The importance of early platelet use is unquestioned, but whether similar ratios (1:1 or 2:1) must be adhered to for optimal survival is undetermined. The utility of such adjuncts as cryoprecipitate, recombinant factor VIIa, tranexamic acid, and vasopressin is still debatable. However, recent published studies indicate that rotational thromboelastometry (ROTEM; Figure 8) in assessing the severity and cause of acute trauma coagulopathy and therefore in directing appropriate blood component therapy appears superior to traditional assays of coagulation (prothrombin time, activated partial thromboplastin time, international normalized ratio, platelet count).

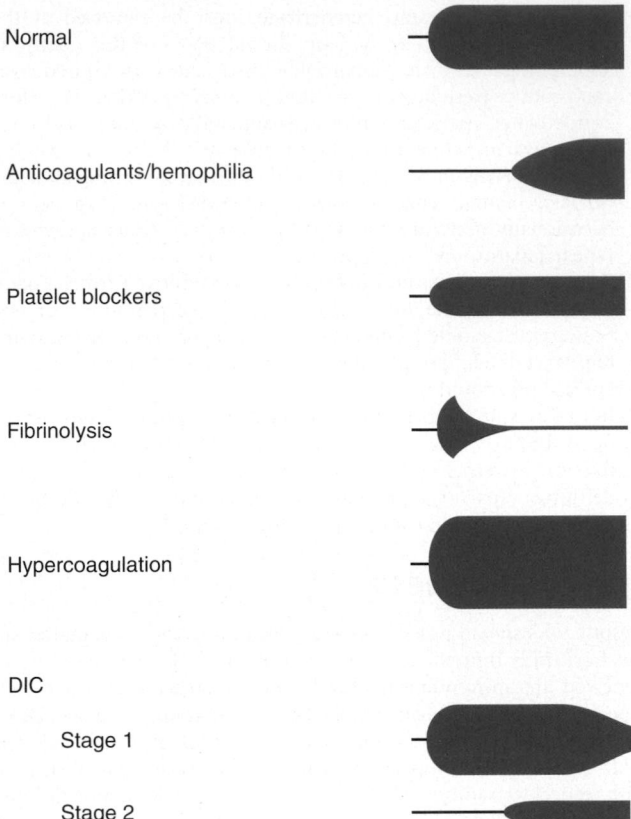

Normal

Anticoagulants/hemophilia

Platelet blockers

Fibrinolysis

Hypercoagulation

DIC

    Stage 1

    Stage 2

FIGURE 8 Typical rotational thromboelastometry (ROTEM) patterns. *DIC,* Disseminated intravascular coagulation. *(Courtesy Combat Casualty Care: Lessons Learned from OEF and OIF. Fort Detrick, MD: Borden Institute, U.S. Army Office of the Surgeon General; 2012:139.)*

2. The use of REBOA in the management of uncontrolled torso hemorrhage. Although a number of recently published case series illustrate successful use of REBOA, there are insufficient data to warrant its adoption as an equivalent or superior standard of care, especially when comparing its safety and timeliness with that of resuscitative thoracotomy and laparotomy (Biffl et al., 2015). Currently the primary utility of REBOA seems to be as an adjunct to hemorrhage control with pelvic fractures.

3. The use of DCO for conditions other than trauma. At least one study (Weber et al, 2014) asserts that damage control laparotomy has utility in nontrauma situations such as peritonitis with septic shock, hemorrhage during elective surgery, and mesenteric ischemia. This study reviewed 15 published series with more than 450 patients who underwent DCO for such reasons. Whether this results in a survival advantage has yet to be determined.

4. The place of therapeutically induced hypothermia in the care of the trauma patient. Whereas accidental, uncontrolled hypothermia potentiates acidosis and coagulopathy as part of the "lethal triad," animal experiments have shown a beneficial effect of controlled hypothermia on cellular metabolism, inflammatory response, and hemodynamic function, with a concomitant decrease in mortality. We feel confident that, in the foreseeable future, therapeutically induced controlled hypothermia will have widespread utility and success in the treatment of the critically injured.

5. An increase in expected mortality rate when DCO is overused. At least one study of 532 patients (Higa, 2010) noted that over a 2-year period, as the rate of DCO decreased from 36% to 8.8%, mortality also decreased (22% to 13%), even though the number of patients requiring trauma laparotomy increased. The authors attributed this to better preoperative and intraoperative resuscitation and communication with anesthesiologists, thereby expanding the pool of candidates for early, initial definitive care. They also noted that DCO results in marked increases in hospital costs, resource use (blood products, ICU beds), length of hospital stay, and development of postoperative ventral hernia and enteroatmospheric fistula.

In conclusion, for optimal results from a damage control strategy, (1) the decision for DCO must be made early and for appropriate indications; (2) DCR (permissive hypotension, crystalloid limitation, early and balanced blood product administration) is started immediately and continued through the OR and into the ICU; (3) good communication between the surgeon and the anesthesiologist and intensivist is essential; (4) the surgeon follows a stepwise approach to address the life-threatening injuries encountered at DCO; and (5) normothermia is assured.

SUGGESTED READINGS

Biffl WL, Fox CJ, Moore EE. The role of REBOA in the control of exsanguinating torso hemorrhage. *J Trauma Acute Care Surg.* 2015;78:1054-1058.

Cirocchi R, et al. Damage control surgery for abdominal trauma. *Cochrane Database Syst Rev.* 2013;(3):CD007438.

Cothren CC, Osborn PM, Moore EE, et al. Preperitoneal pelvic packing for hemodynamically unstable pelvic fractures: a paradigm shift. *J Trauma.* 2007;62:839-842.

Cotton BA, et al. Damage control resuscitation is associated with a reduction in resuscitation volumes and improvement in survival in 390 damage control laparotomy patients. *Ann Surg.* 2011;254:598-605.

Duchesne JC, et al. Damage control resuscitation in combination with damage control laparotomy: a survival advantage. *J Trauma.* 2010;69: 46-52.

Emergency War Surgery. 4th U.S. revision. Fort Sam Houston, TX: Borden Institute, U.S. Army Medical Department Center and School; 2013.

Higa G, et al. Damage control laparotomy: a vital tool once overused. *J Trauma.* 2010;69:53-59.

Lenhart MK, Savitsky E, Eastridge B, eds. *Combat Casualty Care: Lessons Learned From OEF and OIF.* Fort Detrick, MD: Borden Institute, U.S. Army Office of the Surgeon General; 2012.

Nunez TC, Voskresensky IV, Dossett LA, et al. Early prediction of massive transfusion in trauma: simple as ABC (assessment of blood consumption)? *J Trauma.* 2009;66:346-352.

War Surgery: Working With Limited Resources in Armed Conflict and Other Situations of Violence. Geneva: International Committee of the Red Cross; 2009.

Weber DG, et al. Damage control surgery for abdominal emergencies. *Br J Surg.* 2014;101:e109-e118.

UROLOGIC COMPLICATIONS OF PELVIC FRACTURE

Gladys Ng, MD, MPH, and H. Gill Cryer, MD, PhD

Pelvic fractures can be severely debilitating because of the enormous amount of force associated with these injuries and often occur with multiple organ injury. There is a strong association between pelvic fractures and bladder injuries, such that pelvic fractures are estimated to be present in 70% of all bladder ruptures. Most pelvic fractures are a result of high-energy blunt trauma from motor vehicle accidents, pedestrian versus automobile collisions, falls, or crush injuries, with an overall male predominance.

The estimated direct costs are more than $1 billion per year to the healthcare system and even higher when accounting for disability and loss of quality of life. To minimize these costs, essential components of the management of these severely injured patients are an expeditious assessment with accurate diagnosis and a combined multidisciplinary approach. This chapter provides an overview of the management of urogenital injuries in these patients in the acute setting.

■ INITIAL EVALUATION OF THE PATIENT WITH PELVIC FRACTURE

More than 90% of bladder injuries after blunt trauma are associated with pelvic fractures, whereas up to 20% of pelvic fractures are associated with bladder injury. Similarly, pelvic fracture urethral injuries (PFUIs) complicate pelvic fractures in up to a quarter of these patients. The determination of these patients depends on a complete history, full physical examination, urine analysis, and appropriate imaging. The history with the type, degree, and force of impact is revealing because there is often a substantial force of impact such as in motor vehicle accidents, pedestrians hit by motor vehicles, high-level falls, and pelvic crush injuries.

On examination, the pelvis and lower extremities should be inspected for signs of rotation, instability, displacement, lower extremity length disparities, ecchymosis, edema, or bleeding. In the male, a digital rectal examination should be performed to assess the prostate position, with a high-riding prostate combined with blood at the urethral meatus highly suggestive for urethral injury. The rectum also should be assessed for injury, including perforation, foreign bodies, nerve sensation, and the bulbocavernous reflex. In the female, if there is gross blood or difficulty in placing a catheter, a vaginal examination with a speculum is warranted to identify lacerations or foreign bodies.

Pelvic radiographs typically are obtained during a trauma admission, and when a pelvic fracture is seen on plain film radiography, a computed tomographic (CT) scan of the pelvis is necessary to further delineate the location and type of fractures. Studies have shown that there is positive correlation of concomitant bladder and urethral injury when the pelvic CT scan shows fractures in the inferior pubic rami or diathesis of the pubic symphysis; there is less correlation of urogenital injuries to acetabular fractures.

■ BLADDER INJURY DUE TO BLUNT TRAUMA

Gross hematuria is the diagnostic sign of bladder injury, and the combination of gross hematuria and pelvic fracture should warrant cystography. Microscopic hematuria without signs of pelvic trauma likely is not associated with bladder injury, but studies have shown that if the urine analysis shows greater than 30 red blood cells (RBCs) per high-power field in the setting of an associated injury, cystography still should be pursued.

Bladder injuries are staged according to the American Association for the Surgery of Trauma (AAST) injury scoring scale (Table 1). The decision for operative management depends on the presence of bladder rupture, the location of the rupture, the degree of rupture, and associated findings or injury. The best diagnostic test to evaluate for blunt traumatic bladder injury is a CT cystogram. Its availability, ease of acquisition, and high sensitivity and specificity (100% and 95%, respectively) make this the preferred study. A CT scan also can determine if there is any foreign body or bladder neck injury, both of which would require immediate surgical intervention. The alternative is a plain film cystography with several views needed: the scout, anterior-posterior, oblique view, and a postemptying film. Both studies require filling the bladder with diluted contrast until capacity under gravity or with at least 200 to 350 mL infused.

The hallmark of bladder rupture is extravasation of the contrast. The location, intraperitoneal versus extraperitoneal, and the degree of extravasation are key pieces of information to be noted from the studies. In general, isolated intraperitoneal bladder ruptures occur at the dome of a fully distended bladder and are associated with pelvic fractures less frequently, whereas extraperitoneal ruptures occur more often with pelvic fractures.

An intraperitoneal rupture is an indication for operative management, whereas an extraperitoneal rupture may be managed nonoperatively with proper catheter drainage. However, proper patient selection for nonoperative repair of extraperitoneal ruptures is important. Studies have shown significant complications of delayed healing, continued extravasation, development of bladder calculi, and sepsis with just catheter drainage. Strong consideration of operative management is recommended if there are other associated injuries and if the rupture is large. Other absolute indications for operative management regardless of peritoneal cavity involvement are concomitant vaginal and rectal injury, injury to the bladder neck, foreign body or bone fragments involved in the injury, inability to maintain bladder drainage from clot retention, and a patient who is already undergoing operative management for abdominal injury or orthopedic repairs.

Operative Management

Formal repair of the bladder can be approached from a lower midline incision for adequate exposure and also to allow inspection of any other related visceral organ injuries. A Pfannenstiel incision may be used as well. The bladder should be mobilized fully and inspected because there often can be multiple sites of injury. Therefore proper exposure, including the intraperitoneal and extraperitoneal portions of the bladder, is necessary. Intraperitoneal ruptures are usually large and visible at the dome. These can be extended and repaired primarily in two layers using 3-0 absorbable suture, with the first layer comprising the mucosa and muscularis and the second layer being a 2-0 absorbable suture approximating the muscularis and the serosa.

If there is no suspected injury to the ureters on the basis of preoperative imaging, a longitudinal midline incision is made onto the anterior surface of the bladder. The bladder then is inspected for injuries, including the bladder neck for tears, bone fragments, and foreign bodies. The ureteral orifices also should be inspected for efflux of clear urine seen from both orifices; alternatively, they can be intubated with a 5F feeding tube for evaluation. If there is any suspicion of injury, a retrograde pyelogram should be obtained. Small lacerations in the bladder can be repaired intravesically with a one-layer closure using a 2-0 polydioxanone (PDS) suture. The bladder then can be closed with a two-layer closure as described earlier.

Bladder drainage should be large bore and can be done with either a Foley catheter or a suprapubic cystotomy tube. There is no evidence

TABLE 1: Bladder Injury Scale

Grade*	Injury Type	Description of Injury	ICD-9	AIS-90
I	Hematoma	Contusion, intramural hematoma	867.0/867.1	2
	Laceration	Partial thickness		3
II	Laceration	Extraperitoneal bladder wall laceration <2 cm	867.0/867.1	4
III	Laceration	Extraperitoneal (≥2 cm) or intraperitoneal (<2 cm) bladder wall laceration	867.0/867.1	4
IV	Laceration	Intraperitoneal bladder wall laceration ≥2 cm	867.0/867.1	4
V	Laceration	Intraperitoneal or extraperitoneal bladder wall laceration extending into the bladder neck or ureteral orifice (trigone)	867.0/867.1	4

From Moore EE, Cogbill TH, et al. Organ injury scaling III: chest wall, abdominal vascular, ureter, bladder and urethra. *J Trauma*. 1992;29:337-339.

*Advance one grade for multiple lesions up to grade III.

AIS-90, Abbreviated Injury Scale–1990 Revision; *ICD-9*, International Classification of Diseases, Ninth Revision.

supporting which method is superior, although orthopedic studies favor a Foley catheter to avoid contamination of wounds from leakage around the suprapubic catheter. A drain may be left in place after bladder repair for concerns of urine leak.

The catheter should be indwelling for 10 to 14 days after repair or injury. In both operative management and nonoperative management for bladder rupture, the patient should undergo a plain film cystogram before catheter removal. If extravasation is seen at the time of cystography, the catheter is left in place and cystography is repeated in 1- to 2-week intervals until there is no extravasation. Persistent leakage is rare and should warrant further evaluation.

POSTERIOR URETHRAL INJURY: MALE

The posterior urethra is protected by the pelvic bone, and injuries are not common. However, if present, injuries are associated with an enormous force. As such, there can be significant long-term genitourinary morbidity that can involve urethral strictures, urinary incontinence, erectile dysfunction, and chronic pelvic pain.

The typical presentation is urinary retention, blood at the meatus, and a high-riding prostate on digital rectal examination, with or without a butterfly perineal hematoma in the setting of probable mechanistic injury. On imaging, injuries to the pelvic bone causing diathesis and inferior pubic rami fractures are highly associated with posterior urethral injuries.

Retrograde urethrogram (RUG) is the best study to delineate male urethral injury when suspected. This study determines identification, location, and degree of injury. The patient is placed lying with his hips rotated obliquely to a slight 30- to 45-degree angle with x-ray or fluoroscopy. Contrast is injected via the urethral meatus with the penis on stretch using a 12F catheter with the balloon inflated with 1 to 2 cc of fluid or a 60-cc catheter-tip syringe with a tapered adapter until the entire urethra can be visualized. Alternatively, cystoscopy can be used to visualize and evaluate the urethra; however, it is not suggested as a primary diagnostic study.

Grading of urethral trauma is classified according to the AAST injury score (Table 2). Grades I and II or injury due to stretching and contusion can be managed with catheter drainage until the patient is mobile. Grade III or a partial disruption can be managed with catheter realignment, and grades IV and V can be managed with endoscopic realignment or suprapubic cystotomy tube.

The management of these injuries is debatable, with either endoscopic realignment or delayed repair and immediate suprapubic cystotomy tube drainage. Studies have shown that stricture rates requiring further operation are greater than 90% in those managed with immediate suprapubic cystotomy tube drainage, whereas stricture rates requiring operation range from 14% to 45% in those managed with endoscopic alignment. However, the choice of management really depends on the stability of the patient, with the goal of providing the most efficient, safest, and most reliable method of urinary drainage to avoid complications of urine extravasation and delay in controlling other associated traumatic injuries.

Placement of a suprapubic cystotomy tube can be done at the same time as any other required abdominal or orthopedic surgery. Endoscopic alignment should be performed by skilled urologists using fluoroscopy and endoscopy in a retrograde and antegrade approach. Alignment can be done up to 1 week after injury when the patient is better stabilized, and the catheter is left indwelling for 4 to 8 weeks. A voiding cystourethrogram (VCUG) is performed to assess for urine extravasation, and the catheter remains removed if there is no evidence of extravasation. If there is leakage, the catheter is replaced and further workup, including cystourethroscopy to assess for the reasons for delayed healing, should be performed. Regardless, close surveillance of these patients is needed to assess for development of urethral stricture, incontinence, and erectile dysfunction.

URETHRAL INJURY: FEMALE

Injuries to the female urethra are even rarer than to the male urethra and should be suspected in patients with pelvic ring fractures, gross hematuria, and blood at the vaginal introitus. A full examination with a speculum examination, urethroscopy, and proctoscopy for associated rectal injuries should be performed to determine the degree of injury and identify foreign bodies and bone fragments. Bladder neck injuries should be repaired and a suprapubic tube placed for drainage. Vaginal lacerations at the anterior wall should be reapproximated over the urethra to prevent stenosis and potential fistula formation. There are no set guidelines for these injuries, but the principles of providing early and effective drainage and repair are consistent.

CONCLUSIONS

Associated genitourinary injuries after traumatic pelvic fractures are significant injuries with potential long-term sequelae, including urinary strictures, urinary fistula, incontinence, chronic pelvic pain, and sexual dysfunction. Expeditious identification and proper management are essential to avoid complications and morbidity. Collaboration with the trauma team and other specialists helps to put individual treatment decisions in context and may drive optimal care for the patient, with the primary urologic objective being to repair and provide adequate urinary drainage. Close follow-up of these patients is recommended to monitor for urologic morbidity.

TABLE 2: Urethra Injury Scale

Grade*	Injury Type	Description of Injury	ICD-9	AIS-90
I	Contusion	Blood at urethral meatus; retrography normal	867.0/867.1	2
II	Stretch injury	Elongation or urethra without extravasation on urethrography	867.0/867.1	2
III	Partial disruption	Extravasation of urethrography contrast at injury site with visualization in the bladder	867.0/867.1	2
IV	Complete disruption	Extravasation of urethrography contrast at injury site without visualization in the bladder; <2 cm of urethra separation	867.0/867.1	3
V	Complete disruption	Complete transaction with >2 cm urethral separation, or extension into the prostate or vagina	867.0/867.1	4

From Moore EE, Cogbill TH, et al. Organ injury scaling III: chest wall, abdominal vascular, ureter, bladder and urethra. *J Trauma*. 1992;29:337-339.

*Advance one grade for bilateral injuries up to grade III.

AIS-90, Abbreviated Injury Scale–1990 Revision; *ICD-9*, International Classification of Diseases, Ninth Revision.

SUGGESTED READINGS

Avery G, Blackmore CC, Wessells H, et al. Radiographic and clinical predictors of bladder rupture in blunt trauma patients with pelvic fracture. *Acad Radiol*. 2006;13:573-579.

Black PC, Miller EA, Porter JR, Wessells H. Urethral and bladder neck injury associated with pelvic fracture in 25 female patients. *J Urol*. 2006;175:2140-2145.

Blaschko SD, Sanford MT, Schlomer BJ, et al. The incidence of erectile dysfunction after pelvic fracture urethral injury: a systematic review and meta-analysis. *Arab J Urol*. 2015;13:68-74.

Figler B, Hoffler CE, Reisman W, et al. Multi-disciplinary update on pelvic fracture associated bladder and urethral injuries. *Injury*. 2012;43:1242-1249.

Gomez RG, Mundy T, Dubey D, et al. SIU/ICUD consultation on urethral strictures: pelvic fracture urethral injuries. *Urology*. 2014;83:S48-S58.

Johnsen NV, Young JB, Reynolds S, et al. Evaluating the role for operative repair of extraperitoneal bladder rupture following blunt pelvic trauma. *J Urol*. 2016;195:661-665.

McGeady JB, Breyer BN. Current epidemiology of genitourinary trauma. *Urol Clin North Am*. 2013;40:323-334.

Warner JN, Santucci RA. The management of the acute setting of pelvic fracture urethral injury (realignment vs suprapubic cystostomy alone). *Arab J Urol*. 2015;13:7-12.

SPINE AND SPINAL CORD INJURIES

Nilesh A. Vyas, MD, FAANS, Erik J. Teicher, MD, FACS, and Margaret M. Griffen, MD, FACS

The incidence of spinal cord injury (SCI) is approximately 11,000 new cases each year with 95% of patients surviving their initial hospitalization. In blunt trauma, cervical SCI is reported at 3% to 4% and 6% for thoracolumbar regions. The majority of SCI occurs in patients aged 16 to 30 years; the average age is 33, which is an increase since the 1970s. The majority of patients with SCI are male, and the three leading causes are motor vehicle crash (MVC), falls, and gunshot wounds. It is estimated that 3% to 25% of SCI occur after the initial insult. Involvement of noncontinuous vertebral levels can occur in up to 20% of SCI, and the entire spinal column is potentially at risk. Cervical spine level for SCI is most prevalent followed by thoracic and then lumbar. Incomplete quadriplegia (38%) is the most common SCI on discharge from the hospital, and complete quadriplegia is the least common (17%).

■ INITIAL EVALUATION, DIAGNOSIS, AND MANAGEMENT

The management of the patient with a potential SCI begins at the scene. A principal concern during the initial management of patients with potential SCI is that neurologic function may worsen with pathologic motion of injured vertebrae. Since the introduction of cervical and spinal immobilization there has been a substantial improvement in the neurologic condition of patients arriving at emergency departments with SCI over the past 30 years. Recently, the use of full spinal immobilization in all trauma patients has been questioned because it seems that many patients will be treated with full spinal immobilization, but few will sustain injuries. It has been demonstrated that spinal immobilization techniques cause increased pain and discomfort along the occipital scalp, mandible, back, and sacrum, which can lead to unnecessary testing, increased respiratory effort, and skin ischemia. Guidelines based on clinical criteria such as altered mental status, evidence of drug use or intoxication, spinal tenderness or pain, focal neurologic deficit, or suspected extremity fracture have been developed for full spinal immobilization and are being used currently in certain regions.

The initial management of the SCI patient is identical to all other trauma patients. A primary survey to evaluate airway, breathing, and circulation is completed followed by a full assessment in the secondary survey. The specific management of spinal injuries should be deferred until life-threatening injuries are identified and treated. Physiologic consequences of SCI include airway compromise, inadequate oxygenation and ventilation, bradycardia, and hypotension that may require immediate attention during the primary survey. Patients with complete SCI above the C5 level with respiratory distress, hypoxia, and severe respiratory acidosis from hypoventilation should have their airway secured immediately. Patients with high cervical and thoracic SCI may develop airway compromise resulting from localized edema or neck hematoma. These patients must be observed even without immediate indication for endotracheal intubation because there may be progression of the injury and worsening of the patient's respiratory condition.

After completion of a primary and secondary survey any evidence for potential spine or SCI should be identified. As detailed by the National Emergency X-Radiography Utilization Study Group (NEXUS), awake and nonintoxicated patients without cervical pain or tenderness, neurologic symptoms, or distracting injury do not require imaging or continued cervical immobilization. In awake and symptomatic patients, imaging of the cervical spine should be obtained. The evaluation for spine fracture and SCI in the obtunded patient should include full imaging. There are many algorithms that exist for clearance of the cervical collar after imaging in awake and symptomatic patients and the obtunded patient and will not be discussed further.

During the secondary survey a careful examination should be performed to identify motor and sensory deficits that help localize the injury, are predictive of complications, and have prognostic value. The preferred examination method used for classification of SCI was developed by the American Spinal Injury Association (ASIA) as detailed in Figure 1. The neurologic examination focuses on motor, sensory, rectal tone, and rectal sensation findings. ASIA uses a 0 to 5 scale for assessment of motor strength of 10 muscle groups on each side of the body. The scores for all 20 muscle groups are added, providing the total ASIA motor score. Sensation is evaluated as absent (0 points), altered (1 point), normal (2 points), or untestable. The ASIA impairment scale (AIS) then is used to classify the lesion as complete or incomplete. AIS uses a letter to signify the description of the neurologic status being a complete SCI (A), sensory incomplete (B), motor incomplete (C and D), and normal (E). The combination of the ASIA impairment scale with the ASIA motor score comprises the best description of a patient's neurologic status after SCI.

In addition to the SCI that can be elucidated with the ASIA classification, there are a number of discrete syndromes of SCI that have been described. Central cord syndrome is the most common syndrome, accounting for about 9% of SCI. It represents an incomplete injury to the cervical spine, resulting in more extensive motor weakness in the upper extremities than the lower extremities and distal more than proximal. The mechanism of injury occurs from forceful hyperextension of the neck. Commonly in older patients, there is usually no obvious associated fracture or evidence of spinal instability but rather with prior existence of degenerative

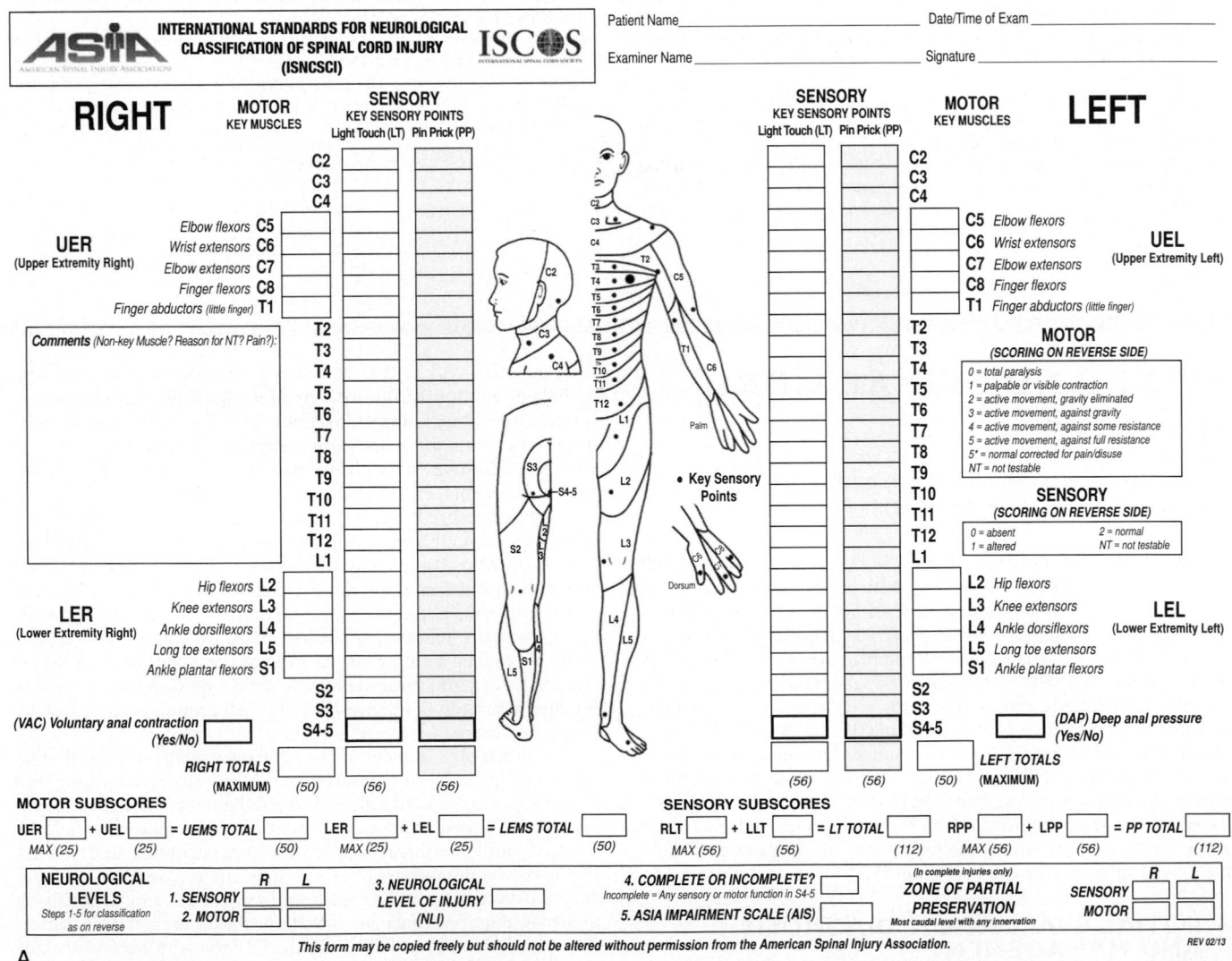

FIGURE 1 A and **B,** The American Spinal Injury Association (ASIA) classification of spinal cord injury. A tool to standardize spinal cord injury assessment. *(Copyright 2016 American Spinal Injury Association, www.asia-spinalinjury.org. Accessed March 25, 2016.)*

Muscle Function Grading

0 = total paralysis

1 = palpable or visible contraction

2 = active movement, full range of motion (ROM) with gravity eliminated

3 = active movement, full ROM against gravity

4 = active movement, full ROM against gravity and moderate resistance in a muscle specific position

5 = (normal) active movement, full ROM against gravity and full resistance in a functional muscle position expected from an otherwise unimpaired person

5* = (normal) active movement, full ROM against gravity and sufficient resistance to be considered normal if identified inhibiting factors (i.e. pain, disuse) were not present

NT = not testable (i.e. due to immobilization, severe pain such that the patient cannot be graded, amputation of limb, or contracture of > 50% of the normal range of motion)

Sensory Grading

0 = Absent

1 = Altered, either decreased/impaired sensation or hypersensitivity

2 = Normal

NT = Not testable

Non Key Muscle Functions (optional)

May be used to assign a motor level to differentiate AIS B vs. C

Movement	Root level
Shoulder: Flexion, extension, abduction,adduction, internal and external rotation **Elbow:** Supination	C5
Elbow: Pronation **Wrist:** Flexion	C6
Finger: Flexion at proximal joint, extension. **Thumb:** Flexion, extension and abduction in plane of thumb	C7
Finger: Flexion at MCP joint **Thumb:** Opposition, adduction and abduction perpendicular to palm	C8
Finger: Abduction of the index finger	T1
Hip: Adduction	L2
Hip: External rotation	L3
Hip: Extension, abduction, internal rotation **Knee:** Flexion **Ankle:** Inversion and eversion **Toe:** MP and IP extension	L4
Hallux and Toe: DIP and PIP flexion and abduction	L5
Hallux: Adduction	S1

ASIA Impairment Scale (AIS)

A = Complete No sensory or motor function is preserved in the sacral segments S4-5

B = Sensory Incomplete Sensory but not motor function is preserved below the neurological level and includes the sacral segments S4-5 (light touch or pin prick at S4-5 or deep anal pressure) AND no motor function is preserved more than three levels below the motor level on either side of the body

C = Motor Incomplete Motor function is preserved below the neurological level**, and more than half of key muscle functions below the neurological level of injury (NLI) have a muscle grade less than 3 (Grades 0-2)

D = Motor Incomplete Motor function is preserved below the neurological level**, and at least half (half or more) of key muscle functions below the NLI have a muscle grade ≥ 3

E = Normal If sensation and motor function as tested with the ISNCSCI are graded as normal in all segments, and the patient had prior deficits, then the AIS grade is E. Someone without an initial SCI does not receive an AIS grade

** For an individual to receive a grade of C or D, i.e. motor incomplete status, they must have either (1) voluntary anal sphincter contraction or (2) sacral sensory sparing with sparing of motor funtion more than three levels below the motor level for that side of the body. The International Standards at this time allows even non-key muscle function more than 3 levels below the motor level to be used in determining motor incomplete status (AIS B versus C)

NOTE: When assessing the extent of motor sparing below the level for distinguishing between AIS B and C, the **motor level** on each side is used; whereas to differentiate between AIS C and D (based on proportion of key muscle functions with strength grade 3 or greater) the **neurological level of injury** is used

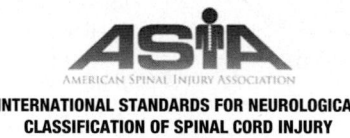

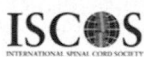

INTERNATIONAL STANDARDS FOR NEUROLOGICAL CLASSIFICATION OF SPINAL CORD INJURY

Steps in Classification

The following order is recommended for determining the classification of individuals with SCI

1. Determine sensory levels for right and left sides.
The sensory level is the most caudal, intact dermatome for both pin prick and light touch sensation

2. Determine motor levels for right and left sides.
Defined by the lowest key muscle function that has a grade of at least 3 (on supine testing), providing the key muscle functions represented by segments above that level are judged to be intact (graded as a 5)
Note: In regions where there is no myotome to test, the motor level is presumed to be the same as the sensory level, if testable motor function above that level is also normal

3. Determine the neurological level of injury (NLI)
This refers to the most caudal segment of the cord with intact sensation and antigravity (3 or more) muscle function strength, provided that there is normal (intact) sensory and motor function rostrally respectively
The NLI is the most cephalad of the sensory and motor levels determined in steps 1 and 2

4. Determine whether the injury is Complete or Incomplete.
(i.e. absence or presence of sacral sparing)
If voluntary anal contraction = **No** AND all S4-5 sensory scores = **0** AND deep anal pressure = **No**, then injury is **Complete**
Otherwise, injury is **Incomplete**

5. Determine ASIA Impairment Scale (AIS) Grade:

Is injury **Complete?**   If YES, AIS=**A** and can record
NO ↓   ZPP (lowest dermatome or myotome on each side with some preservation)

Is injury Motor **Complete?**   If YES, AIS=**B**
NO ↓   (No=voluntary anal contraction OR motor function more than three levels below the motor level on a given side, if the patient has sensory incomplete classification)

Are **at least** half (half or more) of the key muscles below the neurological level of injury graded 3 or better?

NO ↓   **YES** ↓

AIS=**C**   AIS=**D**

If sensation and motor function is normal in all segments, AIS=**E**
Note: AIS E is used in follow-up testing when an individual with a documented SCI has recovered normal function. If at initial testing no deficits are found, the individual is neurologically intact; the ASIA Impairment Scale does not apply

B

FIGURE 1, cont'd

ligamentous and osteophytic spinal column disease. In younger patients there is often evidence of fracture and spinal instability. The injury occurs as a result of anterior and posterior compression of the spinal cord, leading to edema, hemorrhage, or ischemia to the central portion of the spinal cord. Because of the anatomic lamination of the corticospinal tract with the upper extremity fibers medially and the lower extremity fibers laterally, the arms are affected more so than the legs, resulting in a disproportionate motor impairment. The site of most injuries is in the mid to lower cervical cord. Brown-Séquard syndrome is less common and characterized by ipsilateral disruption of the corticospinal tract, resulting in hemiplegia, and the posterior column–medial lemniscus tract, resulting in loss of fine touch and proprioception, and contralateral disruption of the spinothalamic tract, resulting in loss of pain and temperature sensation. The most common cause of this is a penetrating injury to the spinal cord. Anterior cord syndrome is a relatively rare SCI and commonly follows an ischemic event from the anterior spinal artery. It is characterized by loss of motor function below the level of injury, loss of pain and temperature sensation carried by the spinothalamic tract of the spinal cord, and preservation of fine touch and proprioception sensation carried by the posterior column-medial lemniscus tract. Posterior cord syndrome is another rare SCI that is characterized by loss of fine touch and proprioception sensation carried by the posterior column–medial lemniscus tract below

the level of injury. This usually follows an ischemic insult to the spinal cord and is uncommon in trauma. Cauda equina syndrome can follow damage to the cauda equina, resulting in loss of function of the lumbar plexus of the spinal canal below the conus medullaris. This may result in severe back pain, a saddle-type paresthesia involving perineum, external genitalia, and anus, bladder, and bowel dysfunction, weakness of lower extremities, and sexual dysfunction. Figure 2 demonstrates the areas of injury for the discrete SCI discussed earlier.

■ IMAGING

Imaging of the spine traditionally has been performed with plain radiographs, but computed tomography (CT) scan has become almost entirely the initial imaging modality for evaluation of the spine. NEXUS and the Eastern Association for the Surgery of Trauma (EAST) guidelines for imaging of the cervical and thoracolumbar spine include back pain, point tenderness, neurologic deficit, altered mental status, or distraction. Patients with alterations in sensorium from traumatic head injury, shock, or intoxication may not have a reliable clinical examination and require imaging. It is important to image the entire spinal column in the setting of a known segment injury because 10% to 40% of patients may show a noncontiguous injury.

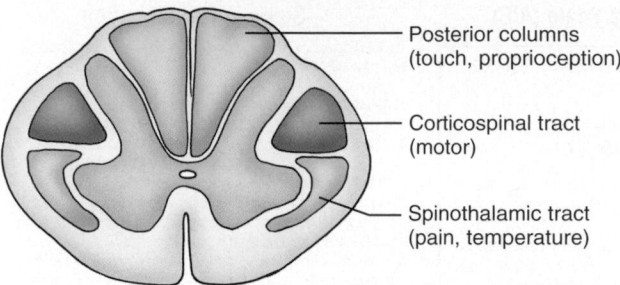

Posterior columns
(touch, proprioception)

Corticospinal tract
(motor)

Spinothalamic tract
(pain, temperature)

Normal spinal cord with major tracts

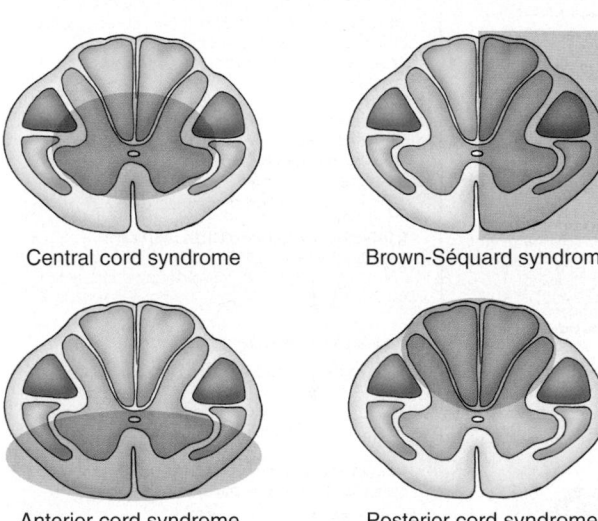

Central cord syndrome

Brown-Séquard syndrome

Anterior cord syndrome

Posterior cord syndrome

FIGURE 2 Drawings of the spinal cord with identification of the areas of damage resulting in specific spinal cord injuries.

SCI without radiographic abnormalities (SCIWORA) typically is described in children because of the elasticity of the pediatric spinal column, allowing for displacement of the spinal cord without disruption of the bony and ligamentous support. SCIWORA can be seen in adults as well. The cervical or upper thoracic spine usually is affected. This was characterized classically by an absence of radiographic findings and may be seen as complete or incomplete injury patterns. Since the widespread use of magnetic resonance imaging (MRI), specific abnormalities of the spinal cord have been documented increasingly, and so the term has evolved to only those injuries not seen on plain radiograph or CT scan. The application of MRI is important in the early diagnosis of SCIWORA in children and adults. Spinal cord concussions have been described and are transient spinal cord dysfunction without radiographic abnormalities of the spinal cord. Typical symptoms include paresthesia, numbness, and tingling.

■ INTENSIVE CARE UNIT MANAGEMENT

Those patients with high cervical fractures and those with SCI should be managed in an intensive care unit (ICU). Respiratory dysfunction can occur in greater than 85% of patients with cervical SCI. The SCI patient should be maintained with a combination of chest physiotherapy, secretion clearance mechanisms, bronchodilators, and respiratory muscle training. Weaning patients from mechanical ventilation may be challenging, and many patients will require long-term ventilation. Many will eventually require tracheostomy, and although the ideal timing of tracheostomy is unknown, studies have shown reduc-

tion in duration of ventilation and ICU length of stay with early tracheostomy.

Up to 90% of patients with cervical SCI develop cardiovascular dysfunction. Aggressive management of hypotension is recommended and may be associated with an improved neurologic outcome. Treatment of hypotension after SCI initially involves volume resuscitation followed by vasopressors. Cervical and upper thoracic injuries above the T6 level should receive a vasopressor with vasoconstrictive, inotropic, and chronotropic properties such as norepinephrine or dopamine. Lower thoracic injuries below the T6 level should receive a vasopressor with vasoconstrictive effects such as phenylephrine. In general, patients with cervical cord injuries require vasopressors more often than those with thoracolumbar injuries, and those with complete SCI require vasopressors more often than those with incomplete SCI.

Current recommendations are to maintain mean arterial blood pressure between 85 and 90 mm Hg for 7 days after injury. This is based on several studies documenting neurologic improvements with this aggressive hemodynamic management. A recent study demonstrated improved outcome measures when blood pressure was maintained at or above 85 mm Hg for 2 to 3 days after injury. Oral vasopressor agents such as midodrine and pseudoephedrine have been used with success when there is a continued intravenous vasopressor requirement. In many patients this hemodynamic abnormality will resolve 2 to 6 weeks after injury, whereas others may have long-term hemodynamic alterations. Bradycardia may lead to other dysrhythmias and even asystole. Symptomatic bradycardia should be treated up front with atropine, or other chronotropic agents such as dopamine or isoproterenol, to ensure adequate cardiac output. Bradycardia that is refractory to medical therapy should be considered for temporary cardiac pacing.

For many years, the administration of methylprednisolone has been used for the treatment of acute SCI. The National Spinal Cord Injury Study (NASCIS) has conducted three trials on early steroid usage after SCI. Conclusions from these trials have been questioned in recent years because of relatively modest neurologic improvements compared with risks of high-dose steroids. Despite its administration to patients with SCI at many institutions, evidence of deleterious effects continues to accumulate, which include immunosuppression with increased susceptibility to infections such as pneumonia and sepsis, increased risk of gastrointestinal disturbances including peptic ulceration, bleeding, and ileus, adult respiratory distress syndrome (ARDS), hyperglycemia, deep venous thrombosis (DVT), and pulmonary embolism. Available guidelines now recommend against the use of methylprednisolone in the treatment of SCI.

Preliminary studies have demonstrated a possible beneficial therapeutic effect of systemic hypothermia in acute management of SCI. Smaller series of patients with isolated complete SCI were treated with systemic moderate hypothermia after injury or surgical stabilization, maintained for 24 to 48 hours, and then underwent slow rewarming with many patients showing improved outcome scores.

Cervical Spine Injury: Initial Management

Once a cervical spine injury (CSI) is identified, strict immobilization with a rigid cervical collar is critical especially while managing airway issues. Because CSI commonly is associated with SCI, spinal cord perfusion must be maintained by avoiding hypotension and hypoxia. If there is an incomplete neurologic injury, then early reduction of any fracture or dislocation should be strongly considered. Timing of reduction in the setting of a complete injury (ASIA A) varies widely. Definitive treatment of the CSI can involve no immobilization for minor fractures, rigid cervical collar, or Halo-vest immobilization, or surgical fusion with instrumentation with or without decompression. In general, use of Halo has decreased dramatically as the outcomes and complications of cervical instrumentation have improved. Often in cases in which Halo was the standard this has been replaced

TABLE 1: Craniocervical Fracture Locations and Treatment Recommendations

Craniocervical Fracture Location	Treatment Recommendation
Atlanto-occipital dislocation	Occiput to cervical fusion
Unilateral occipital condyle fracture	Cervical collar 6-12 weeks
C1 fracture (unstable)	Halo vest 6-12 weeks
Odontoid (type I): stable	Brace only
Odontoid (type II): >5 mm displacement	Surgical stabilization + Halo
Odontoid (type III): stable	Rigid cervical collar
Hangman's (type I): <4 mm subluxation - stable	Rigid cervical collar
Hangman's (type II): >11 mm angulation or >4 mm subluxation - unstable	Surgical stabilization: C1-3 posterior fusion
Hangman's (type III): C2-3 joint disruption	Surgical stabilization

TABLE 2: Subaxial Cervical Spine Injury Classification System (SLICS)

The Subaxial Cervical Spine Injury Classification System (SLICS) is a classification system for subaxial cervical spine trauma that helps determine information about injury pattern and severity, in addition to treatment considerations and prognosis.

Characteristic	Points
MORPHOLOGY	
No abnormality	0
Compression	1
Burst	+1=2
Distraction (e.g., facet perch, hyperextension)	3
Rotation/translation (e.g., facet dislocation, unstable teardrop or advanced-stage flexion compression injury)	4
DISCOLIGAMENTOUS COMPLEX (DLC)	
Intact	0
Indeterminate (e.g., isolated interspinous widening, MRI signal change only)	1
Disrupted (e.g., widening of disk space, facet perch or dislocation)	2
NEUROLOGIC STATUS	
Intact	0
Root injury	1
Complete cord injury	2
Incomplete cord injury	3
Continuous cord compression in setting of neurodeficit (Neuro Modifier)	+1

Score	Interpretation
<4	Nonoperative treatment
4	Operative versus nonoperative
>5	Operative treatment

by surgical instrumentation with good results. The following section describes the more traditional recommendations, but surgeons should recognize this trend and understand that surgery may be appropriate treatment in these cases.

Cervical Spine Injury: Surgical Management

Cervical spine injuries fall into two subdivisions: craniocervical junction (occiput to C2) and subaxial (C3-T1) injuries. The location of the fracture, stability of the spine, and neurologic status affect the decision making for treatment. Atlanto-occipital dislocations typically result in patient fatality because of SCI, vertebral artery or carotid injuries, or other associated polytrauma. Cases in which the patient survives require occiput to cervical fusion. Unilateral occipital condyle fractures will heal with cervical collar in 6 to 12 weeks. Lower cranial nerve injury with atlanto-occipital injuries infrequently may require decompression of the damaged nerve. C1 fractures are typified by the Jefferson fracture that is a four-part fracture of the C1 ring. Variations with two or three fractures in C1 are similar and require the same treatment, namely Halo-vest immobilization for 6 to 12 weeks. C2 fractures involve either the odontoid process or the rest of the vertebra. Type 1 odontoid fractures are stable and require no surgical treatment. Type 2 odontoid fractures with greater than 5 mm of displacement require surgical treatment or realignment followed by Halo placement. Age older than 55years and nicotine use increases the risk of nonunion and need for surgery. Type 3 odontoid fractures heal well without surgery and a rigid cervical collar alone. Hangman's fractures (HF), classically bilateral C2 pars interarticularis fractures, vary based on degree of subluxation of C2 on C3 and angulation. A patient with a type 1 HF has less than 4 mm of subluxation and heals without surgery but requires cervical collar. Type 2 HF with more than 11 degrees of angulation or 4 mm or greater of subluxation are unstable and require C1-3 posterior cervical fusion with instrumentation. Type 3 HF have greater disruption of the C2-3 joint and require surgical stabilization (Table 1).

Subaxial cervical spine fractures can be identified with classifications systems AO (Arbeitsgemeinschaft für Osteosynthesefragen), SLICS (subaxial cervical spine injury classification system), and Allen and Ferguson (Table 2). Common features among these systems are few but include a grading based on clinical as well as radiographic features. Each has unique components as well, which leads to variation in treatment options. Neurologic examination will be the initial determining factor for urgent or emergent decompression and reduction of C3-7 spine fractures. Current data suggest patients with incomplete cord injuries should be decompressed or at least reduced as soon as possible to maximize recovery. Subaxial fractures with complete SCI can be addressed less urgently. The plan for only external orthosis versus internal stabilization will be based on severity of injury and extent of structural element damage. Surgical approaches include anterior cervical discectomy and fusion with instrumentation as well as posterior lateral mass instrumentation and fusion. As a general guideline the location of injury will dictate the approach—anterior spinal element injury anterior approach, posterior injury posterior approach. Severe cases may best be treated with a combined anterior and posterior fusion in either a single trip to the operating room or in staged fashion.

Thoracolumbar Fractures

Thoracic and lumbar spine fractures can be considered together. Injuries to the upper thoracic spine (T1-9) constitute a minor fraction because of the additional structural rigidity supplied by the ribs and sternum in this less mobile spinal region. Injuries in this area therefore are associated with greater forces and also commonly with neurologic compromise. Most thoracic spine injuries are at the thoracolumbar junction because of the lack of additional structural stabilization. Because the spinal cord commonly ends in this region, neurologic injury is less common.

Treatment of thoracolumbar spine fractures relies on the stability of the injury. Stability can be judged on the basis of the three-column model of the spine. The anterior column includes the anterior longitudinal ligament, the anterior two thirds of the vertebral body, and disc. The middle column includes the posterior one third of the vertebral body and disc and the posterior longitudinal ligament. The posterior column includes the pedicles, facets joints, laminae, spinous processes, and posterior ligamentous complex. Injury of one column typically can be treated with thoracic-lumbar-sacral orthotic (TLSO) brace alone, whereas two- and three-column injuries will more commonly, but not always, dictate operative management.

Stable fractures may be treated with TLSO braces and followed with radiographic imaging over months to ensure bony union across the fracture site. Progressive kyphosis, loss of height, or failed bony union may indicate failure of nonoperative treatment. Compression fractures of less than 50% loss of height, less than 2.5 mm of sagittal listhesis, or less than 20 degrees of kyphosis may be managed with TLSO. Burst fractures (compression fracture plus vertebral body fragment retropulsion into canal) with less than 30% canal compromise also may be considered for TLSO use, although this is variable with burst fractures.

Unstable fractures require surgical stabilization, and location will determine the operative approach. A posterior approach with pedicle screw instrumentation allows for rigid fixation and can be highly effective. Anterior approaches are increasing in frequency with improving surgical skill of the spine surgeon and the approach surgeon, as well as with improvements in spinal instrumentation and implants. Significant deformity and kyphosis may be treated best by an anterior or combined anterior and posterior approach. As with cervical spine fractures the urgency of the surgery for T-L fractures is based on the neurologic examination. Incomplete spinal cord injuries should be treated urgently within 48 hours. Similar to CSI, reduction and decompression done as soon as possible theoretically can produce the best chance of neurologic recovery. Use of a postoperative external orthosis in addition to the internal fixation at the time of surgery is common. Partial stress-shielding of the instrumented area to optimize fusion across the fracture can improve surgical outcomes in the long term.

■ COMPLICATIONS

Patients with spine fracture and SCI can develop acute and chronic complications. The potential for development of complications will be related to many factors, including comorbidities, multisystem trauma, neurologic injury associated with fractures, level of paralysis, and need for operative intervention.

In the acute setting, as already discussed, the patient with cervical spine fracture and paralysis may have respiratory failure requiring intubation with necessity for a tracheostomy and prolonged ventilator management. Infectious complications such as urinary tract infection and pneumonia can occur, and noninfectious complications include venous thromboembolic events, neuropathic pain, delirium and pressure ulcers. The acute management of this population of patients must include care to all of these potential complications. Deep venous thrombosis (DVT) occurs nearly 100% of the time in patients with SCI but remains asymptomatic and is detected by ultrasound. Use of vena cava filters has evolved and now retrievable filters are recommended because of a 40% incidence of inferior vena cava thrombosis with permanent filters. Also controversial is the duration of chemical prophylaxis for DVT, but consensus seems to be only until completion of inpatient rehabilitation.

Those patients requiring operative intervention have the potential for development of complications directly related to the intervention along with those already mentioned earlier. Technical concerns resulting in SCI and ischemia may occur and with an anterior approach a potential pneumothorax, hemothorax, or chylothorax may develop. Wound issues may occur with multiple contributing factors, including age, nutritional status, multisystem trauma, technical, and body habitus. Optimization of care postoperatively to minimize these potential complications is a must.

■ OUTCOMES

Mortality for the first year after injury is 6%, and advanced age, male gender, C4 or above level of SCI, vent dependency, complete neurologic injury, and violent cause affect the mortality. The cost for care of the SCI patient varies based on level. CSI is estimated to cost $700,000 in the first year after injury with an annual cost after that of $150,000 per year. Yearly cost in the United States for SCI is estimated to be close to $10 billion. To affect the incidence of SCI requires prevention strategies. In the event of such an injury, organized care with up-to-date treatment methods to avoid potential secondary injury will help maximize the patient's recovery.

SUGGESTED READINGS

Eastern Association for the Surgery of Trauma Practice Management Guidelines for Cervical and Thoracolumbar Trauma. 2009, 2015.

Guidelines for Management of Acute Cervical Spine and Spinal Cord Injuries. Section of Disorders of the Spine and Peripheral Nerves: American Association of Neurologic Surgeons and the Congress of Neurological Surgeons, 2001.

Vaccaro AR, Hulbert RJ, Patel AA, et al. The subaxial cervical spine injury classification system: a novel approach to recognize the importance of morphology, neurology, and integrity of the disco-ligamentous complex. *Spine.* 2007;32:2365-2374.

Vaccaro AR, Oner C, Kepler CK, et al. AOSpine thoracolumbar spine injury classification system: fracture description, neurological status, and key modifiers. *Spine.* 2013;38:2028-2037.

EVALUATION AND MANAGEMENT OF THE PATIENT WITH CRANIOMAXILLOFACIAL TRAUMA

Justin M. Sacks, MD, MBA, FACS, and Srinivas M. Susarla, MD, DMD, MPH

The maxillofacial skeleton is composed of three distinct regions: the upper face, midface, and lower face (Figure 1). The upper facial skeleton predominately is made up of the frontal bone, supraorbital rims, and lateral orbital elements. The midface includes the medial, inferior, and inferolateral orbits as well as the nasal complex, zygomata, and maxilla. The lower facial skeleton is represented by the mandible and its associated temporomandibular joints. It is helpful to consider these facial skeletal thirds when discussing the evaluation and management of craniomaxillofacial injuries, as injuries may involve a single portion of the facial skeleton (e.g., isolated frontal sinus fracture) or may involve all portions of the facial skeleton (e.g., panfacial fracture).

The bones that comprise the upper, middle, and lower thirds of the facial skeleton are supported by vertical and horizontal skeletal buttresses (Figures 2 and 3). These buttresses assist with the dispersion of forces such that energy is dissipated before being transmitted to the intracranial structures or cervical spine. The vertical buttresses of the facial skeleton include the nasomaxillary, zygomaticomaxillary, pterygomaxillary, and posterior mandibular. These points of skeletal fusion support the bones of the midface and lower face. The horizontal buttresses of the facial skeleton include the frontal, zygomatic, maxillary, and mandibular and offer support to the associated bones and their articulations.

The surgeon managing acutely injured patients would be well served to know the regions of the face and the associated buttress. Although the finer anatomy of the facial bones is relevant for operative management of these injuries, an understanding of the regional gross anatomy and biomechanical principles can assist the trauma surgeon with recognizing patterns of injury and effectively communicating the types of injuries to the maxillofacial surgeon.

The discussion that follows focuses on the constituent parts of each third of the facial skeleton, the patterns of injury that commonly occur within each, and the clinical signs and symptoms associated with injuries to these regions, whether in isolation or concomitantly with other fractures.

■ UPPER FACIAL INJURIES

The frontal bone, which comprises the upper facial skeleton and provides the contour of the forehead, superior orbital rim, and orbital roof, is a prominent feature of the facial skeleton, particularly in children. The frontal bone has a central, air-filled cavity known as the frontal sinus, which is bounded anteriorly and posteriorly by thin pieces of frontal bone. Sinus pneumatization is not complete until late childhood, which influences the patterns of frontal injuries seen in children (e.g., linear bone fractures) versus those seen in adults (frontal sinus fractures). Frontal sinus fractures may involve the anterior wall of the sinus (anterior table fractures), the posterior wall of the sinus (posterior table fractures), or both. Patients with frontal bone injuries often have lacerations over the forehead or eyebrows with associated edema. Isolated upper eyelid ecchymosis may be consistent with an orbital roof injury (the orbital roof represents a

portion of the floor of the frontal sinus and is composed of the orbital plate of the frontal bone). Rhinorrhea is a worrisome clinical finding in these patients, as it suggests a complex injury that involves the posterior table of the frontal sinus with associated dural injury.

Evaluation should include a careful inspection of the forehead and scalp; examination of the eyes, particularly to assess visual acuity and extraocular movements; and inspection of the nose to identify rhinorrhea. Relevant consultations should include maxillofacial surgery and possibly neurosurgery and ophthalmology.

Isolated anterior table fractures of the frontal sinus without significant displacement or comminution rarely require operative intervention. In contrast, displaced injuries of the anterior table (Figure 4), particularly those that violate the integrity of the nasofrontal outflow tracts (which allow for sinus drainage into the nose), or displaced posterior table fractures are complex injuries that often require multidisciplinary management (e.g., maxillofacial surgery and neurosurgery). In patients with posterior table injuries, the evaluating clinician should consider the likelihood of intracranial vascular injury and cerebrospinal fluid leak. Pneumocephalus on computed tomography (CT) is one sign suggestive of a posterior table injury and may be helpful for diagnosis in situations where a nondisplaced fracture exists.

■ MIDFACIAL INJURIES

The midface is arguably the most complex bony anatomy of the facial skeleton, as it is composed of many small bones with important soft tissue structures. The nasal, orbital, zygomatic, and maxillary regions are components of the midface, and midfacial injuries often include multiple regions. Patients with midfacial injuries often have a clinical history of direct trauma to the midface or eyes. Clinical symptoms may include double vision, decreased vision, periorbital edema and ecchymosis (Figure 5), nasal bleeding or congestion, cheek or upper lip swelling, facial asymmetry due to loss of nasal or zygomatic projection, malocclusion, and paresthesia to the lower eyelid, cheeks, and upper lip.

Clinical evaluation of patients with midfacial injuries should systematically assess four distinct areas: the nasal complex, the orbit, the zygoma, and the maxilla. Evaluation of each area should focus on assessment of soft tissue injury (frequently with associated lacerations to the nose, eyelids, or cheeks) as well as distinct findings associated with specific bony injuries. Nasal bone fractures often are seen with swelling and tenderness to palpation over the nasal root, with associated crepitus. An intranasal examination is important to assess the position of the septum, identify any sources of intranasal bleeding (which may require packing or urgent airway management), and identify a septal hematoma. Orbital examination should focus on palpation of the external orbital rim, which is composed of the frontal bone, zygomatic bone, and maxilla, to assess for discontinuities or step-offs. Close evaluation of the eye (vision, extraocular movements, etc.) is paramount, as many patients with orbital fractures will have altered vision or injuries to the ocular adnexa. Patients with zygomatic injuries may complain of cheek swelling, loss of cheek projection, cheek numbness, or difficulty opening their mouth (trismus). The latter finding suggests impingement of the zygomatic arch on the temporalis muscle or coronoid process of the mandible, consistent with a displaced zygomatic arch fracture or displaced zygomaticomaxillary complex (ZMC) injury. Patients with maxillary fractures often have associated intranasal and/or intraoral bleeding, malocclusion, dental and/or dentoalveolar injury, or facial asymmetry.

Radiographic assessment of midfacial injuries should be systematic and focus on identifying patterns of injury rather than on specifying which particular bones are fractured. Given the complex interbony connections within the midface, it is more useful to know the patterns of injury that are commonly seen than it is to describe each bone or portion thereof that is injured. Fortunately there are well-established classifications for complex injuries of the midface

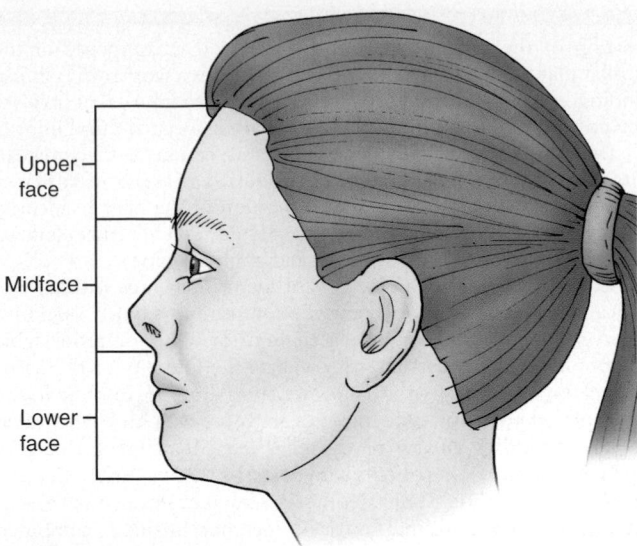

FIGURE 1 Regions of the maxillofacial skeleton. (*Adapted from Avery LL, Susarla SM, Novelline RA. Multidetector and three-dimensional CT evaluation of the patient with maxillofacial injury. Radiol Clin North Am. 2011;49:183-203.*)

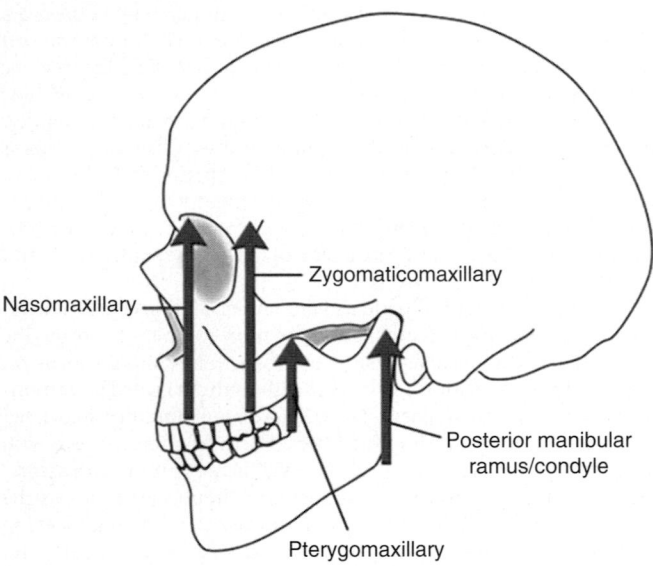

FIGURE 2 Vertical skeletal buttresses.

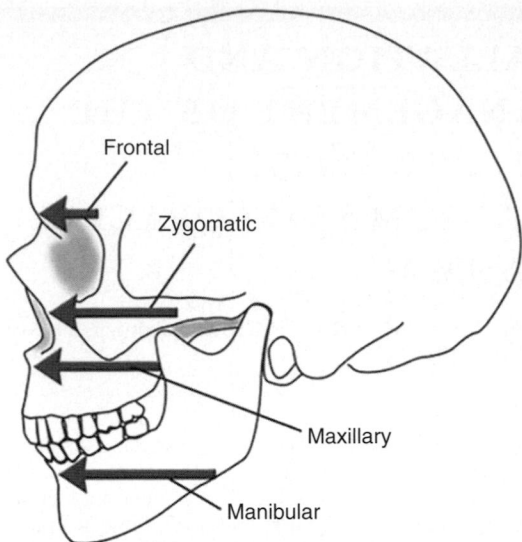

FIGURE 3 Horizontal skeletal buttresses. (*Adapted from Avery LL, Susarla SM, Novelline RA. Multidetector and three-dimensional CT evaluation of the patient with maxillofacial injury. Radiol Clin North Am. 2011;49:183-203.*)

that can aid the trauma surgeon with communicating the findings to the facial trauma specialist.

Injuries of the nasal region commonly can be classified as isolated nasal bone or septal fractures and the more complex naso-orbitoethmoid (NOE) fractures. Nasal bone fractures are very common because of the thin bony support and prominent position of the nasal complex as a central component of the face. Radiographically, nasal bone fractures can be identified by the degree of displacement, laterality, and associated soft tissue swelling (Figure 6). Deviation of the septum or septal hematoma also should be considered as one reviews the relevant imaging. Higher-energy injuries will cause greater displacement or comminution. The highest-energy injuries will include the medial orbit, resulting in NOE complex fractures. These fractures involve the nasal bones, inferior medial orbital rim, and medial orbital wall, which is composed of the ethmoid bones. Damage to the medial canthal tendons can cause increased distance between the medial canthi (telecanthus)

and has important implications for management. The classification system is based on the integrity of the medial canthal tendon complex (Figure 7).

Orbital injuries are encountered frequently in patients of all ages and may occur in conjunction with nasal injuries, frontal bone injuries, and zygomaticomaxillary injuries. Isolated orbital fractures can involve any of the four walls of the orbit (roof, floor, medial, or lateral) but most frequently involve the orbital floor and medial wall (Figure 8). These injuries may be associated with entrapment of the extraocular muscles, herniation of the periorbital soft tissues into the adjacent air-filled spaces (ethmoid or maxillary sinuses), and globe injuries.

Zygomatic injuries often are described as injuries to the different articulations of the zygoma. However, the trauma surgeon should be cognizant of the regional anatomy and should recognize the components of a ZMC injury. The zygoma articulates with the frontal bone, maxilla, lateral wing of the sphenoid bone, and temporal bone via the zygomatic arch. In a complete ZMC fracture, all four articulations are disrupted, which may result in varying degrees of displacement of the zygoma, loss of cheek projection, or facial widening. Incomplete fractures of the ZMC will involve one or more articulations but not all. A simple classification scheme for ZMC fractures is based on the degree of injury to the various articulations, with minor injuries being those with involvement of only one articulation and major injuries involving all four articulations (Figure 9), with or without comminution of the zygoma proper.

Maxillary injuries classically have been characterized by Le Fort designation (Figure 10). Le Fort I injuries (see Figure 10, *A*) are those that separate the maxilla from the remainder of the midface. Le Fort II injuries (see Figure 10, *B*), or "pyramidal fractures," separate the maxilla and nasal complex from the surrounding midfacial structures. Le Fort III fractures (see Figure 10, *C*), or "craniofacial dysjunctions," separate the midface from the skull base in its entirety. Regardless of the level of injury, patients with maxillary fractures commonly have midfacial swelling, pain, and subjective complaint of malocclusion. Physical findings will include malocclusion, intraoral or midfacial ecchymoses, maxillary mobility, and facial paresthesia related to the infraorbital or nasopalatine nerves. Characteristic imaging findings are associated with the level of injury, but strictly speaking all Le Fort fractures will involve injury to the pterygoid plates. It should be noted that, although classically described as bilateral injuries, Le Fort fractures can occur unilaterally or asymmetrically (e.g., Le Fort I injury on one side, Le Fort II injury on the other

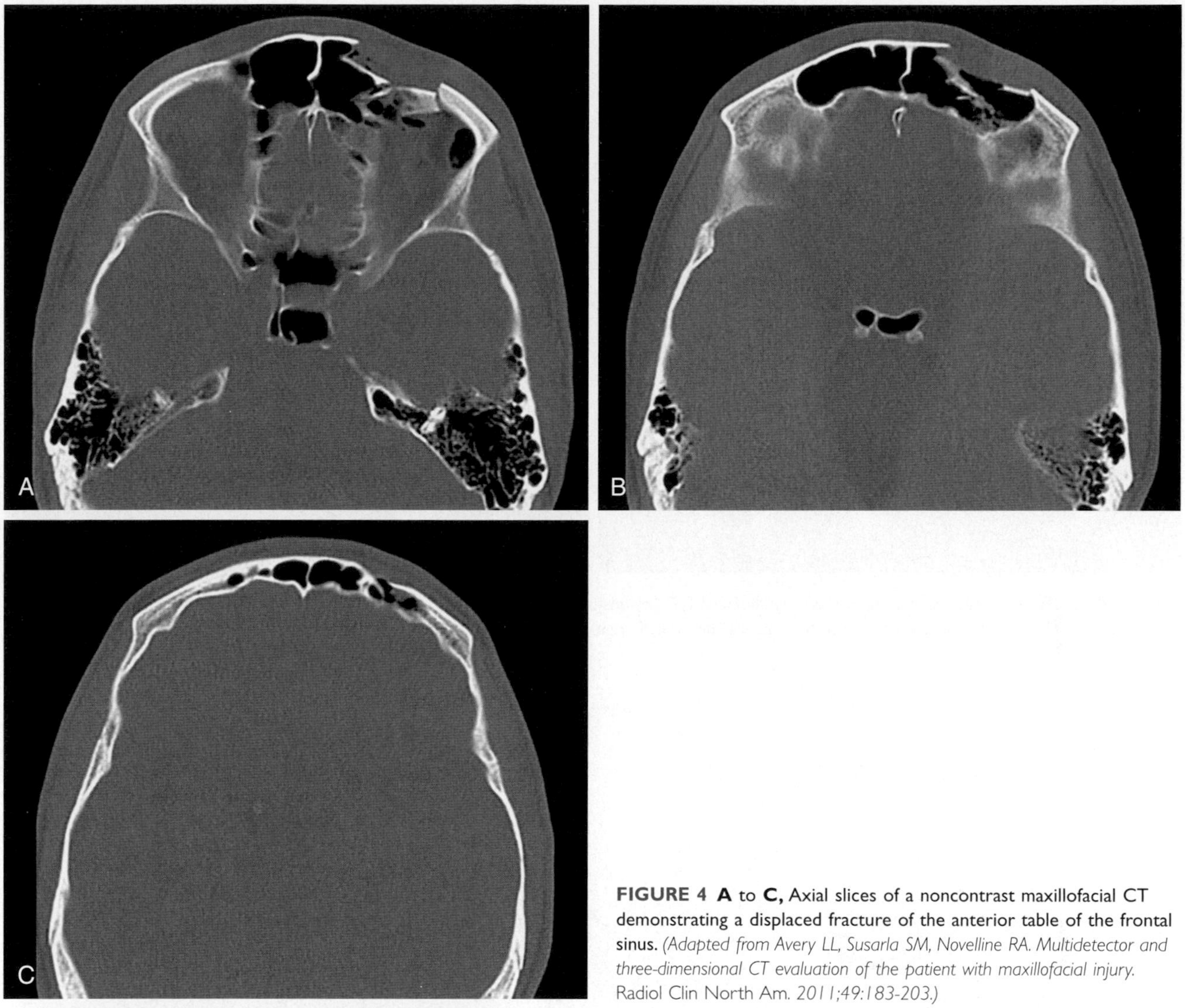

FIGURE 4 **A** to **C,** Axial slices of a noncontrast maxillofacial CT demonstrating a displaced fracture of the anterior table of the frontal sinus. *(Adapted from Avery LL, Susarla SM, Novelline RA. Multidetector and three-dimensional CT evaluation of the patient with maxillofacial injury.* Radiol Clin North Am. *2011;49:183-203.)*

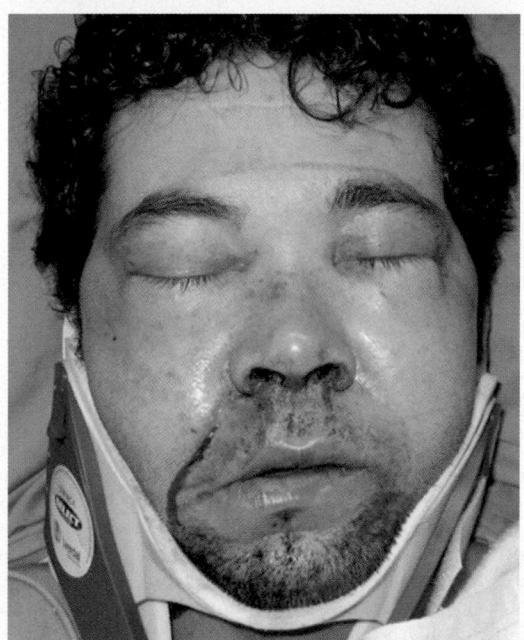

FIGURE 5 Clinical appearance of a midfacial injury.

side). In addition, patients with high-energy mechanisms may have multilevel Le Fort injuries (Figure 11).

■ LOWER FACIAL INJURIES

Lower facial skeletal injuries involve the mandible and its associated alveolar housing. As the only mobile bone within the face, the mandible is, arguably, the most complex bone and presents a unique reconstructive challenge when injured. The most common causes of mandibular fractures are motor vehicle accidents, assaults, and falls. The clinical history is often diagnostic, as patients will relate an injury mechanism whereby their chin or lower face was struck directly and will complain of an altered bite, intraoral bleeding, and lower lip or tongue paresthesia.

Physical examination of the patient with mandibular trauma often reveals an intraoral laceration or fractured teeth (Figure 12). Sublingual hematoma often is associated with injuries of the dentate mandible. Patients with subcondylar fractures may have deviation of the mandible to the side of the fracture when opening their mouth. Patients with bilateral subcondylar fractures often have an anterior open bite (i.e., the maxillary and mandibular incisors do not occlude). When evaluating patients with mandibular injuries (or maxillary injuries), it behooves the practitioner to ask the patients if their bite feels different and how so. Patients often can provide a description of how their teeth fit together before the injury.

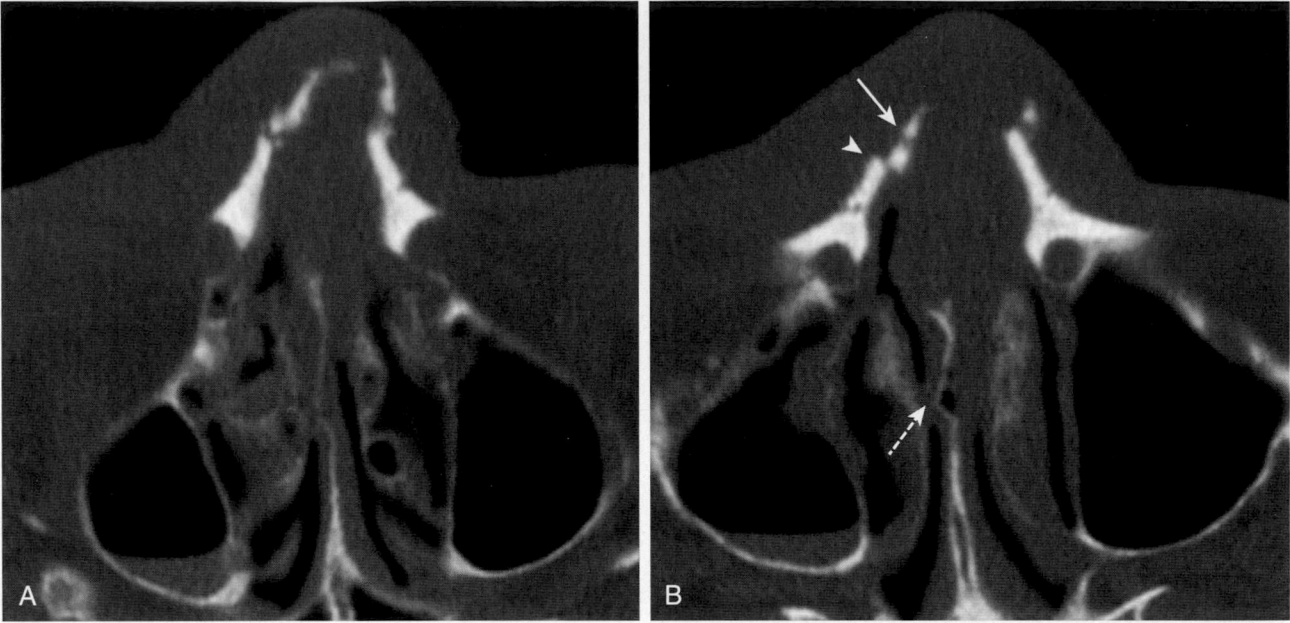

FIGURE 6 **A** and **B,** Axial slices of a noncontrast maxillofacial CT demonstrated displaced nasal bone fractures. Panel **B** demonstrates the significant displacement of both the right frontal process of the maxilla (*arrowhead*), right nasal bone (*solid arrow*), and bony nasal septum (*dashed arrow*).

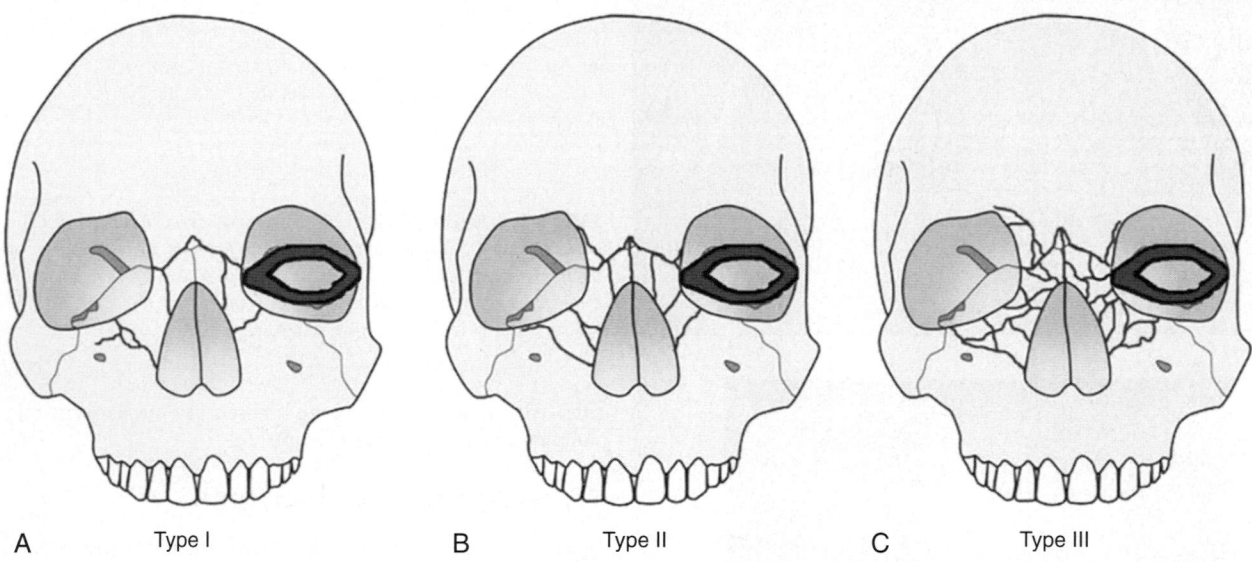

| A | Type I | B | Type II | C | Type III |

FIGURE 7 The Markowitz classification of nasoorbitoethmoid (NOE) fractures. This classification scheme is based on the integrity of the medial canthal tendon (MCT) attachment to the NOE complex. **A,** In type I injuries, the tendon remains attached to a large central NOE fragment. **B,** In type II injuries, there is a higher degree of comminution of the central fragment, but the MCT remains attached to the bone. **C,** In type III injuries, there is a high degree of comminution, and the MCT attachment to the bone needs to be reestablished during reconstruction.

Although many plain film imaging techniques historically have been described for imaging of mandibular injuries, multidetector CT scans largely have replaced plain films as the technique of choice for evaluation. Three-dimensional reformations of maxillofacial CT scans are often helpful for demonstrating the fracture with the affected dentition in the same image. Finally, because the mandible is a single, contiguous bone connecting two joints, forces distributed at the site of injury may result in coup or contrecoup injuries, with bilateral fractures. These often are not immediately evident on clinical examination but should be ruled out carefully on imaging (Figure 13).

■ SOFT TISSUE INJURIES

Facial skin defects secondary to trauma can be several centimeters wide and involve regions in which obtaining appropriate aesthetic and functional results can be challenging. For example, lesions in the lower eyelid need to be reconstructed appropriately so as not to cause ectropion, or pulling down, of the lower eyelid. The blood supply to the face is robust, and all tissues should be preserved for potential soft tissue closure after a traumatic injury. The wound should be cleaned of all debris and irrigated. All tissue should be handled meticulously and closed loosely with monofilament sutures if there is concern for ischemia or infection.

Small superficial defects of the facial skin often can be closed primarily after an elliptical incision. Such an incision must be short and made in the direction of the facial skin tension lines. If the wound cannot be closed primarily, the next option is a local tissue flap based on a random blood supply, such as a transposition or rhomboid flap. Full-thickness skin grafts can be used instead if they match the thickness and color of the skin at the wound site. The best skin graft donor site for facial reconstruction is the region above the clavicle, as both the color and the texture of the skin there match that of the facial skin. Defects in the face greater than 5 cm often require large fasciocutaneous rotation flaps from the cervical and deltopectoral region. In rare instances in which local or regional tissue cannot cover exposed critical neurovascular or bony structures, reconstruction with free tissue transfer may be necessary.

■ CERVICAL SPINE AND INTRACRANIAL INJURIES

In addition to assessment of the upper, middle, and lower facial skeletons, the traumatologist should have a high suspicion for cervical spine or intracranial injury in the patient with maxillofacial trauma. Among patients evaluated with craniomaxillofacial trauma, 5% to 10% have a concomitant cervical spine injury and up to 50% have an intracranial injury. Upper facial injuries are associated with lower cervical spine and intracranial injuries. Midfacial injuries, particularly unilateral injuries, are associated with basilar skull fractures and intracranial injuries. Upper cervical spine injuries often are seen with mandibular fractures.

■ CONCLUSION

The evaluation and management of the patient with craniomaxillofacial trauma are based on a fundamental understanding anatomy. It is the interaction of the bones of the facial skeleton with the overlying soft tissue envelope that creates an interesting dynamic for the reconstructive surgeon in the setting of trauma. Adherence to basic surgical principles regarding bone stabilization and soft tissue handling will assist the reconstructive surgeon to optimize clinical outcomes in the treatment of patients who have experienced craniomaxillofacial trauma.

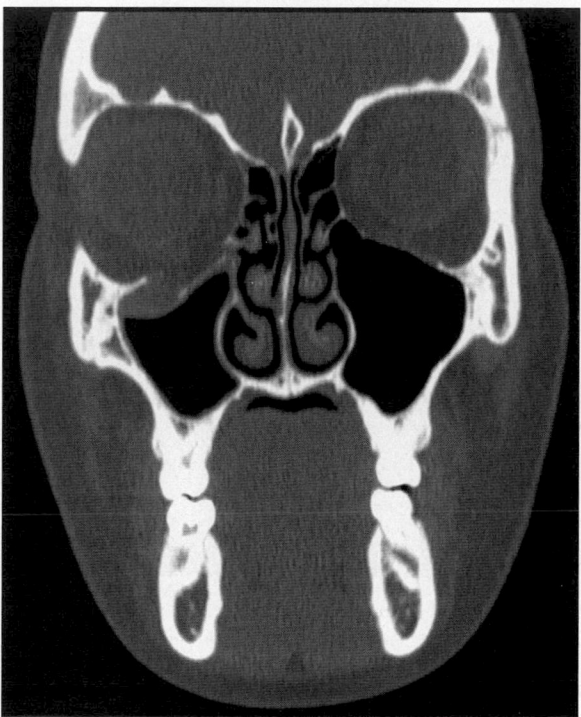

FIGURE 8 Orbital injury.

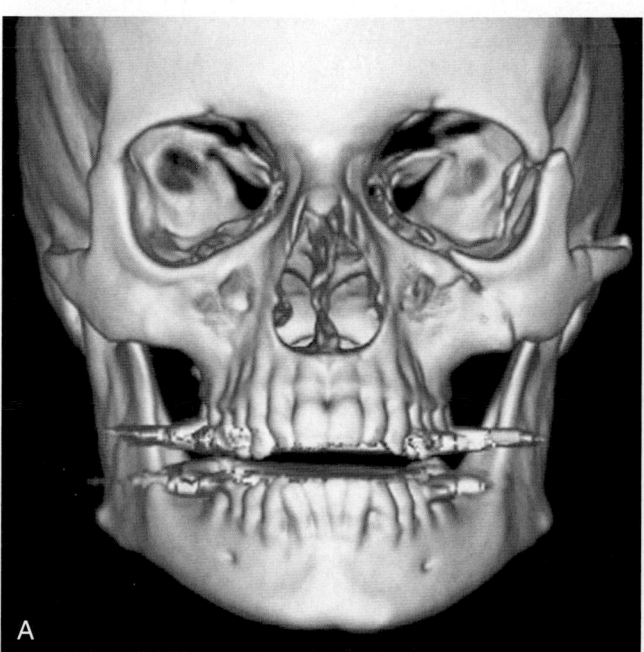

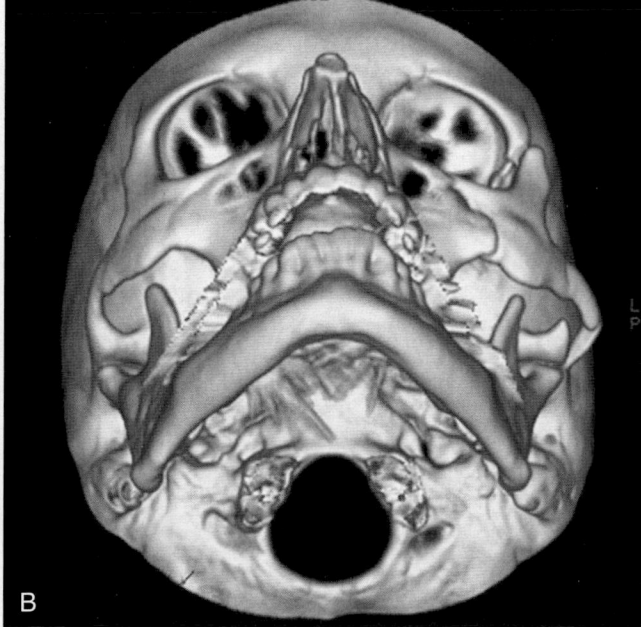

FIGURE 9 Three-dimensional computed tomographic reconstructions of a patient with a displaced left zygomaticomaxillary complex (sometimes referred to as an orbitozygomatic) fracture. Panel **A** demonstrates the displacement in the frontal plane, most notably at the inferior orbital rim and frontozygomatic suture. Panel **B** demonstrates the displacement at the zygomaticomaxillary buttress and zygomatic arch, as viewed from below.

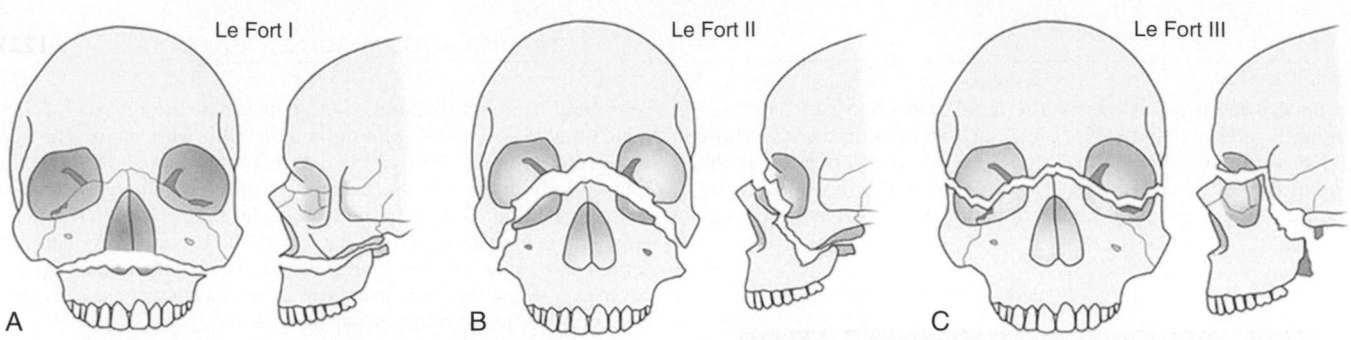

FIGURE 10 **A** to **C,** Le Fort classification of maxillary injuries.

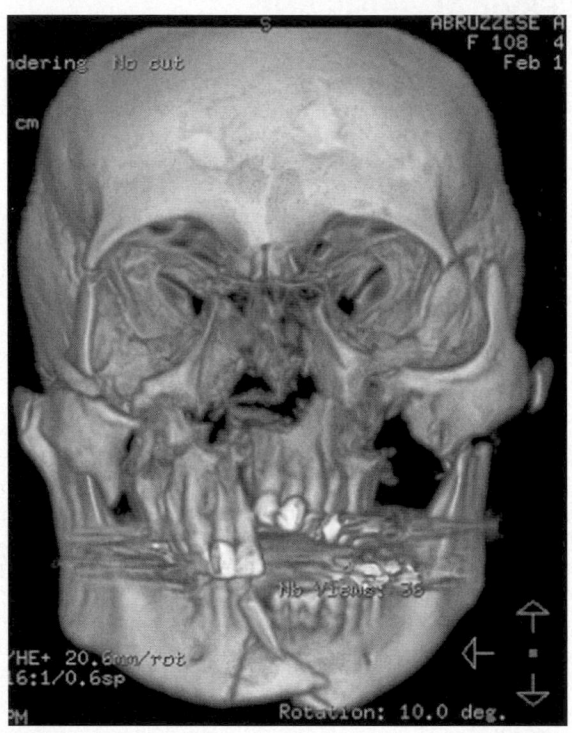

FIGURE 11 Multilevel Le Fort injury. *(Adapted from Avery LL, Susarla SM, Novelline RA. Multidetector and three-dimensional CT evaluation of the patient with maxillofacial injury. Radiol Clin North Am. 2011;49:183-203.)*

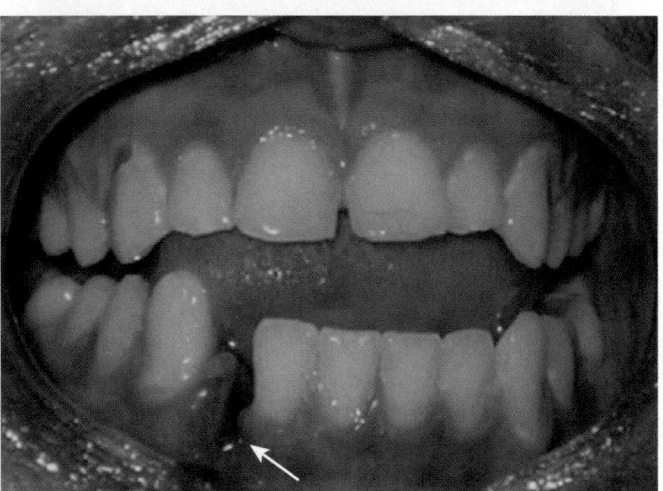

FIGURE 12 Clinical photograph of a patient with a right mandibular parasymphysis fracture. The fracture extends through the dentoalveolar segment, with a visible laceration and stepoff in the occlusal plane between the right mandibular lateral incisor and canine *(arrow).*

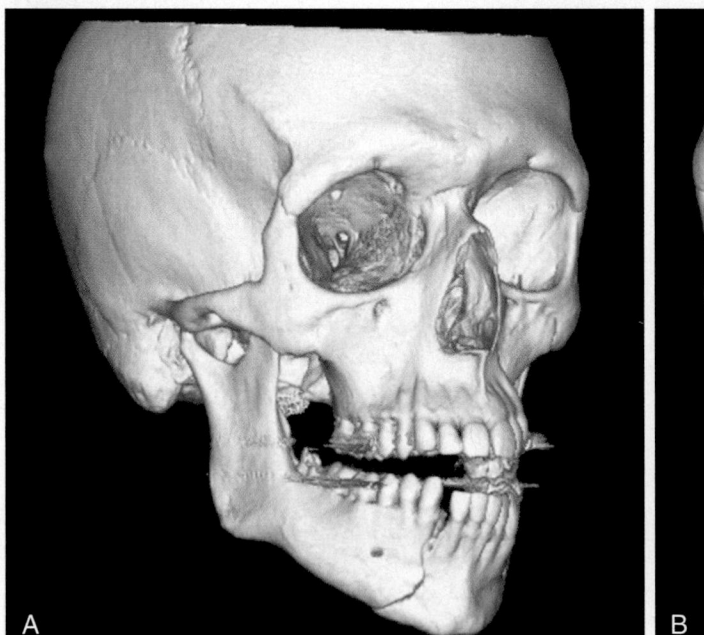

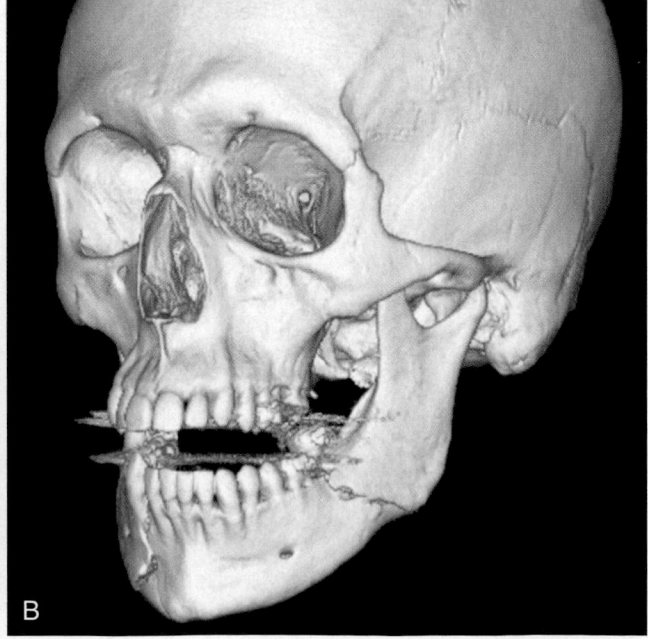

FIGURE 13 **A** and **B,** Three-dimensional reformations of maxillofacial computed tomographic scans for mandibular injury. *(Adapted from Avery LL, Susarla SM, Novelline RA. Multidetector and three-dimensional CT evaluation of the patient with maxillofacial injury. Radiol Clin North Am. 2011;49:183-203.)*

SUGGESTED READINGS

Avery LL, Susarla SM, Novelline RA. Multidetector and three-dimensional CT evaluation of the patient with maxillofacial injury. *Radiol Clin North Am.* 2011;49:183-203.

Holmgren EP, Bagheri S, Bell RB, Bobek S, Dierks EJ. Utilization of tracheostomy in craniomaxillofacial trauma at a level-1 trauma center. *J Oral Maxillofac Surg.* 2007;65:2005-2010.

Kellman RM, Tatum SA. Pediatric craniomaxillofacial trauma. *Facial Plast Surg Clin North Am.* 2014;22:559-572.

Mithani SK, St-Hilaire H, Brooke BS, Smith IM, Bluebond-Langner R, Rodriguez ED. Predictable patterns of intracranial and cervical spine injury in craniomaxillofacial trauma: analysis of 4786 patients. *Plast Reconstr Surg.* 2009;123:1293-1301.

Patel R, Reid RR, Poon CS. Multidetector computed tomography of maxillofacial fractures: the key to high-impact radiological reporting. *Semin Ultrasound CT MR.* 2012;33:410-417.

Ricketts S, Gill HS, Fialkov JA, Matic DB, Antonyshyn OM. Facial fractures. *Plast Reconstr Surg.* 2016;137:424e-444e.

PENETRATING NECK TRAUMA

Charles E. Lucas, MD, and Anna M. Ledgerwood, MD

The neck may be divided into bilateral anterior and posterior triangles by the sternocleidomastoid muscle (SCM). Wounds to the posterior cervical triangles require operative management only for the control of bleeding and repair of wounds; there are no hidden structures that lead to late complications when not treated promptly.

Consequently, the challenges regarding care of penetrating neck wounds relate to injuries in the anterior triangles. These include (1) emergent airway control; (2) prompt control of active bleeding; (3) urgent operative treatment of major injuries not causing acute airway compromise or life-threatening bleeding; (4) timely diagnostic investigations for patients not requiring emergent or urgent operation; (5) the decision whether to explore or observe stable patients; (6) optimal exposure for patients requiring operation; and (7) care of specific injuries.

EMERGENT AIRWAY PROBLEMS

Potentially life-threatening airway injuries may be caused by tracheal or cartilaginous rupture, soft tissue compression of the airway from adjacent arterial injury, or active hemorrhage into the tracheobronchial tree resulting from a vascular airway fistula. Air escape through the skin wound, dyspnea, stridor, hoarseness, or significant subcutaneous emphysema points toward airway disruption. The stable patient with hemoptysis wishes to sit up and lean forward in order to efficiently expectorate blood that enters the airway. Forcing the patient to lie down should be avoided until all preparations for a rapid sequence intubation (RSI) have been made. Ideally the intubation is performed in the operating room (OR) by experienced anesthesia personnel. When excessive bleeding into the oral cavity is not present, an oral intubation should be successful; when bleeding obscures the passages, a fiber optic nasotracheal intubation may be accomplished by experienced personnel. Although a coniotomy (cricothyroidotomy) usually is not needed in this circumstance, the resuscitation team should be prepared mentally to use this approach in patients suspected of having airway rupture. Significant hemoptysis portends an arterial tracheal fistula; when the endotracheal tube is inserted, the balloon should be inflated at or below the site where the fistula most likely is located. Likewise, when a coniotomy is needed, the tracheostomy tube balloon should be positioned to occlude the fistula. After airway control, immediate neck exploration is performed.

EXTERNAL BLEEDING

Major external bleeding or a pulsatile hematoma is indicative of an artery injury. Direct digital pressure with the gloved finger is the optimal way to provide temporary control of bleeding while the patient is taken to the OR. Wraps and compression dressings are ineffective and potentially dangerous. The digital control of bleeding is maintained during RSI and preoperative preparation of the operative field.

URGENT OPERATION

Patients without life-threatening signs of airway injury or compromise and without uncontrolled external bleeding require urgent operation when there are hard signs indicative of major injury. These signs include a large hematoma, pulsatile hematoma, continued oozing, cervical crepitus, hoarseness, dyspnea, and large wounds with severance of soft tissues that need reapproximation. They should go directly to the OR without diagnostic tests.

URGENT DIAGNOSTIC INVESTIGATION

Patients without the hard signs that require emergent or urgent operative intervention (discussed in the previous section) need to have diagnostic studies performed to exclude a subtle injury to important structures. These patients may have soft signs, such as superficial bleeding from the skin or subcutaneous tissue, a history of bleeding before arrival, hoarseness, a bruit, dysphagia, blood-streaked sputum, or mild neck swelling, after a penetrating wound in the midportion of the neck. The first component of this urgent investigation is a thorough physical examination of the neck, including an intraoral examination looking for blood in the oral cavity or the hypopharynx. Chest auscultation and examination for trachea deviation help to identify a pneumothorax from a thoracic outlet injury. Chest x-ray will confirm or rule out a pneumothorax or hemothorax. Tracheal or esophageal penetration may be identified by combined endoscopy of the trachea and esophagus. However, small injuries may be missed with these procedures. Barium swallow, which is potentially hazardous and fails to identify some injuries, is not recommended. Computed tomographic angiography (CTA), formal angiography, or color flow duplex ultrasound will help to identify arterial injury. All of these procedures should be available in the trauma center providing care for patients with penetrating neck wounds.

NECK EXPLORATION VERSUS OBSERVATION

The decision to explore a penetrating neck wound in a stable patient without the so-called hard signs depends on the diagnostic findings and the zone in which the injury occurred (Figure 1). The anterior cervical triangles can be divided into three zones (see Figure 1). Zone I is sometimes referred to as the "thoracic outlet" and extends from the clavicle to the cricoid cartilage. The decision to explore zone I injuries would be made on the basis of confirmed injury to the named vessels, trachea, or esophagus. Zone II of the anterior triangles extends from the cricoid cartilage to the angle of the mandible. Formerly, all patients who had penetration of the platysma muscle in zone II underwent mandatory exploration. Most surgeons now explore zone II injuries only for patients who have evidence of organ injury, hematoma, continued bleeding, or high suspicion for tracheal or esophageal injury. Zone III of the anterior triangles extends from the mandible to the base of the skull. The decision to explore zone III injuries would be based on angiographic evidence of arterial injury.

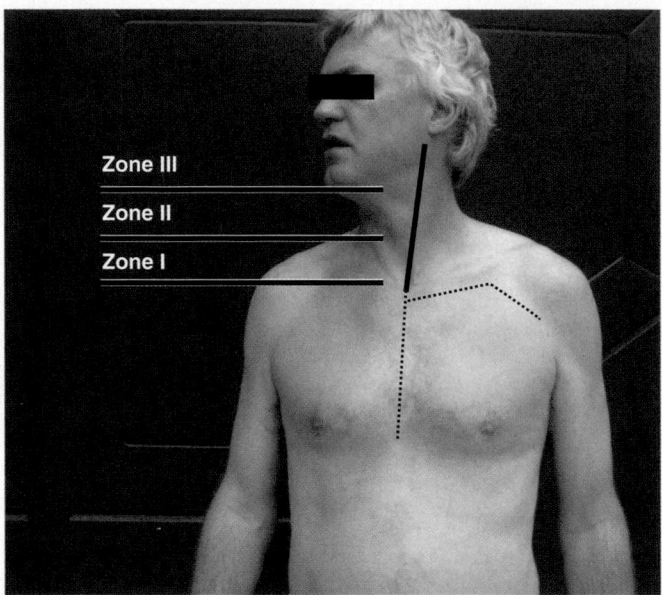

FIGURE 1 Zones of the neck and optimal exposures. An incision along the anterior border of the sternocleidomastoid muscle provides access to zone I and zone II injuries. Extension of this incision inferiorly as a median sternotomy exposes anterior mediastinal injury. A lateral extension along the medial half of the clavicle and then over the cephalic vein gives access to the subclavian vessels.

■ OPERATIVE EXPOSURE

Most penetrating cervical wounds are best explored through an ipsilateral incision along the anterior border of the SCM (see Figure 2). The incision is extended through the platysma into the deeper planes; the trachea and thyroid gland are retracted anteriorly and the neurovascular bundle and esophagus are retracted posteriorly. This exposes the tracheoesophageal groove and allows the operator to dissect anteriorly or posteriorly as determined by operative findings. Superficial crossing veins are divided and ligated along with the omohyoid muscle, thus facilitating deeper dissection. When a zone III injury requires repair of the internal carotid artery at the base of the skull, the mandible can be detached posterior to the angle and subluxated anteriorly to facilitate a direct primary repair. When the injury involves zone I structures in the thoracic outlet, the incision can be extended as a median sternotomy, thereby providing excellent exposure of the thymus, trachea, innominate artery, left common carotid artery, subclavian artery, subclavian veins, innominate vein, and superior vena cava. When the injury involves the subclavian vessels as they pass laterally, the incision can be teed off over the medial half of the clavicle and then laterally and inferiorly toward the groove between the anterior and posterior arm muscles (see Figure 1). Resection of the medial head of the clavicle facilitates exposure, control, and repair of the subclavian arteries and subclavian veins. Rarely, a bilateral incision along the anterior border of the SCM is required for bilateral injuries. We prefer not to combine bilateral incisions by joining them just superior to the manubrium.

■ REPAIR OF SPECIFIC INJURIES

Venous Injuries

Venous injuries are the most common cause of non–life-threatening hemorrhage from penetrating neck wounds. Small veins, including the external jugular vein, are best ligated. The internal jugular vein often can be repaired primarily with a running nonabsorbable fine suture. When there are large through-and-through wounds to the

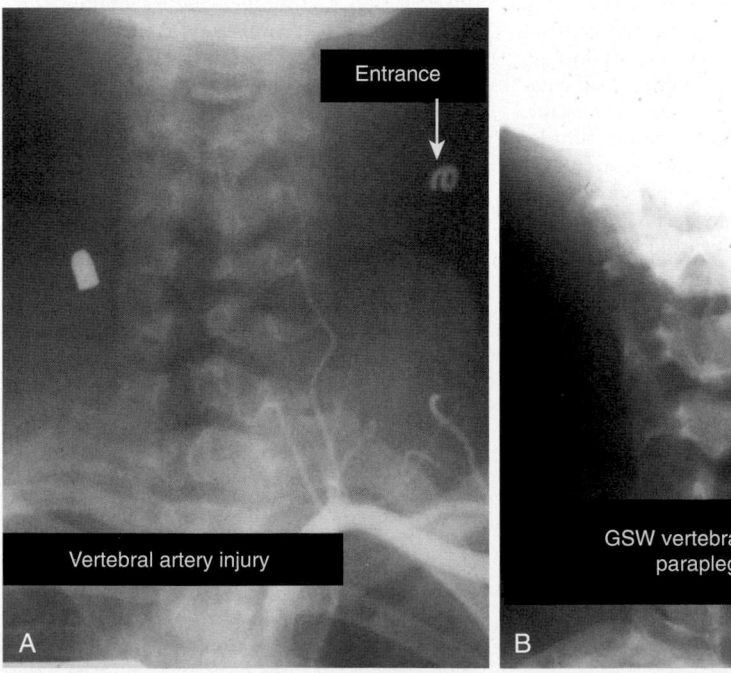

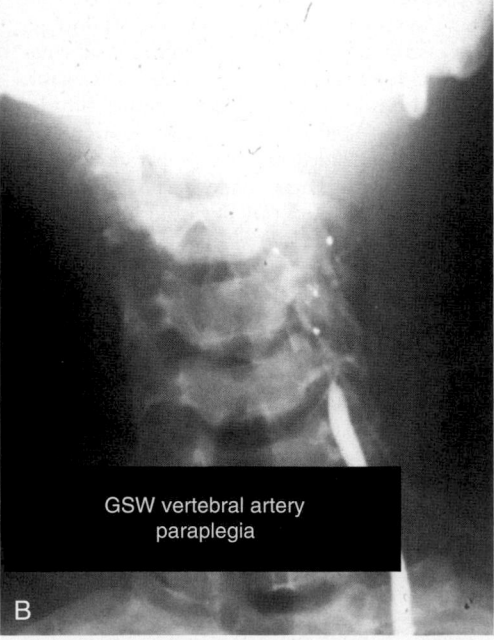

FIGURE 2 A, This patient was seen with a gunshot wound (GSW) of the posterior lateral neck. The missile passed anterior and medially to involve the internal carotid artery at the base of the skull, causing an extending hematoma with swelling. **B,** Once exposed, proximal ligation was associated with pulsatile backbleeding, therefore justifying distal ligation without repair. There were no postoperative neurologic sequelae.

internal jugular vein, the vein should be ligated; this is well tolerated.

Thoracic Duct Injuries

The thoracic duct courses superiorly through the mediastinum and enters the neck, where it drains posteriorly and laterally into the junction of the innominate and internal jugular veins. When the patient has eaten immediately before injury, drainage of a whitish fluid into the wound portends a thoracic duct injury that is unidentified and ligated. When there are no chylomicrons in the leaking fluid, identification is more difficult and the operator needs to seek out the thoracic duct to confirm integrity or ligate if an injury is present. When such injuries are missed, there will be lymphatic drainage out of the wound or through the drain. This annoying complication can be treated expectedly because the drainage eventually will cease.

Arterial Injuries

Active bleeding from the carotid arteries during operation usually can be controlled by digital pressure over the point of injury. Dissection should begin just above the clavicle and proceed distally after proximal control is obtained. Digital pressure of the area of injury is maintained while distal control is obtained. Once exposure is obtained, most arterial injuries can be treated by a primary lateral repair with a running 5-0 nonabsorbable suture. When there is more extensive arterial injury from a gunshot wound, the segment is resected. When the gap is 1 cm long or less, an end-to-end anastomosis can be accomplished. Resection of longer segments requires a reversed saphenous vein graft interposition. Prosthetic grafts should be avoided unless the patient has no saphenous vein. Local instillation of a heparin solution proximally and distally precludes the need for systemic heparinization. A temporary arterial shunt should be used when the arterial repair cannot be performed promptly (within 30 minutes) because of higher treatment priorities to other organs.

For zone II injuries, the branches of the external carotid artery can be ligated safely. When there is disruption at the carotid bifurcation, the intact external carotid artery can be anastomosed to the internal carotid artery distal to the area of irreparable damage. The distal stump of the external carotid artery is ligated.

Primary carotid arterial repair in patients with a neurologic neural deficit is controversial. This concern, in part, reflects the fear that a primary repair will convert an ischemic stroke into a hemorrhagic stroke. We recommend repair in this setting because patients who subsequently succumb have diffuse cerebral edema without hemorrhage at the time of postmortem examination. Maintenance of intracerebral pressure in these patients may facilitate survival.

The vertebral artery arises from the subclavian artery in zone I of the neck, where proximal ligation can be achieved, and ascends superiorly within the cervical foramen from C6 to C1, where it is relatively inaccessible except between C1 and C2 where a 2-cm segment of the artery can be ligated. Ligation proximal to C1 may be associated with uncontrollable venous bleeding (Figure 3). When the injury involves the internal carotid artery at the base of the skull and there is excellent backbleeding after proximal control, proximal and distal ligation may be performed without fear of neurologic swelling (see Figure 2).

Esophageal Injuries

Exposure of the esophagus through the anterior SCM approach permits the esophagus to be freed from the trachea anteriorly and the prevertebral fascia posteriorly and then surrounded with a Penrose drain. The presence of a nasogastric tube facilitates identification and safe digital mobilization of the esophagus (Figure 4). Once mobilized, most unilateral stab wounds can be repaired in two layers, being certain to incorporate the full-thickness mucosal and muscular wall in the inverted inner layer with an absorbable suture. The second layer of the muscular esophagus can be closed with interrupted 4-0

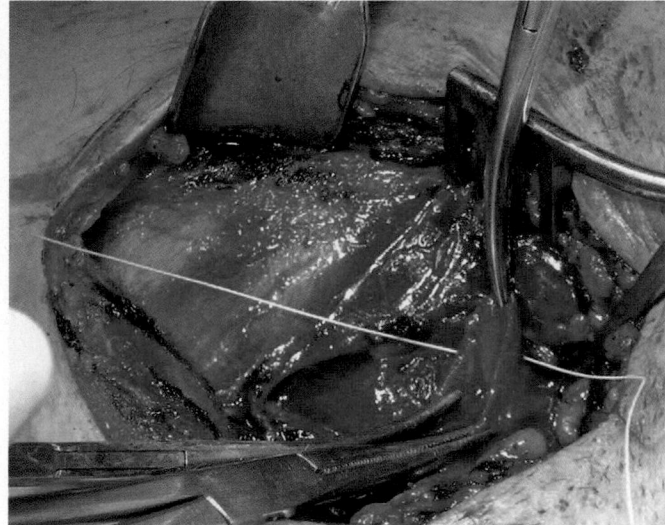

FIGURE 3 Using the intraesophageal nasogastric tube as a "handle," one can easily identify the esophagus through a lateral anterior sternocleidomastoid muscle incision as it lies between the trachea and anterior vertebral ligaments, thus permitting easy mobilization and exposure to permit primary repair.

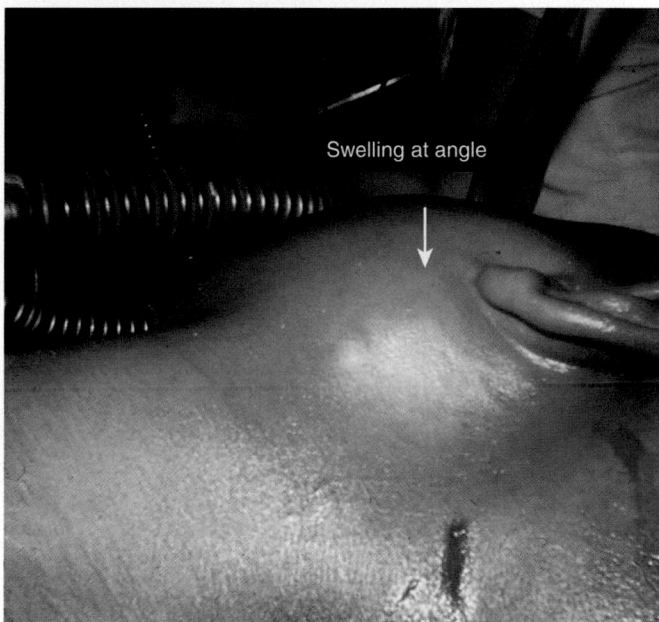

FIGURE 4 This patient sustained a gunshot wound to the neck that caused spinal cord injury and a vertebral artery injury, which were treated by proximal and distal ligation as described in the text.

permanent sutures. With bilateral injury, the esophagus can be rotated to facilitate bilateral simple repair. Alternatively, the injury on the ipsilateral side of the esophagus can be extended slightly to permit the contralateral wound to be closed from the intraluminal approach. The ipsilateral wound then can be closed as described previously. It is essential to identify all injuries to prevent an esophageal cutaneous fistula resulting from a missed injury.

After closure, a paraesophageal drain should be left in place. If any drainage exudes, it should be monitored for amylase. The likelihood of an esophageal cutaneous fistula is low for patients who have early operative intervention. Once a fistula is confirmed, nasogastric tube feedings are instituted while the fistula closes within the ensuing 3 weeks. The nasogastric tube is left in place to allow immediate feeding postoperatively. A gastrostomy tube also can be used for feeding as the fistula closes.

Pharyngeal Injuries

Perforations of the pharynx and hypopharynx often are suspected when blood is seen on the deep oral examination and may be confirmed at operation by following the penetrating wound tract to the perforation. Primary closure with full-thickness inverted bites of tissue with absorbable suture provides both hemostasis and a secure closure.

Laryngeal Injuries

Penetrating wounds may cause contusion with edema, hematoma, mucosal penetration, cartilaginous fracture, or, rarely, separation between the larynx and the trachea. Most of these injuries not involving cartilage or without laryngotracheal separation will heal with time, but the airway needs to be protected by way of a tracheostomy. Complete separation of the larynx and trachea requires suturing, which can be achieved with interrupted absorbable sutures followed by protection of the airway by a tracheostomy.

Tracheal and Cartilaginous Injuries

Through the anterior SCM approach, the trachea is freed posteriorly by blunt dissection in the tracheoesophageal groove. Perforations of the posterior wall can be repaired with running or interrupted 3-0 absorbable sutures, with the knots tied on the outside. Identification of a posterior wound is essential to be certain that there is no adjacent esophageal injury. Closure of perforations of the anterior wall often require that sutures be placed in the inner space above the superior tracheal ring and below the inferior tracheal ring at the site of injury; the knots are tied on the outside. Likewise, cartilaginous injuries can be repaired with sutures heavy enough to go through the cartilage and to provide apposition. Some cartilaginous injuries are best left alone. Significant tracheal ring injuries often require a formal tracheostomy to ensure airway control and circumvent airway resistance from the glottis. High tracheostomy insertion at the second tracheal ring is preferred even when the actual injury is located more distally. This prevents erosion into the innominate artery, a highly lethal complication.

Thyroid Injuries

Most wounds that cause tracheal injury also will cause injury to the thyroid. When the injured thyroid gland is not directly over the tracheal injury it may be made hemostatic with simple sutures or electrocoagulation. When the thyroid injury occurs in the absence of tracheal injury, simple hemostasis by the previously described techniques is required. When the injury goes through the thyroid gland into the trachea, that portion of the thyroid is best resected. Alternatively, the thyroid may be divided at the isthmus and rotated laterally in order to facilitate a primary tracheal repair.

Nerve Injuries

Injuries to the recurrent laryngeal nerve from a penetrating neck wound are rare. If the injury is the result of a gunshot wound, the nerve is unlikely to be severed completely and is best left alone. If one identifies a stab wound with complete severance of the recurrent laryngeal nerve, a primary approximation is indicated with fine sutures. The results of such repairs are unknown.

Vagus nerve injuries are also rare but should be repaired primarily. When the nerve is severed partially because of a stab wound, the divided portion of the nerve should be reapproximated with interrupted fine (5-0) nonabsorbable sutures placed on both ends of the divided perineuron. The portion that is not divided should be left alone in order to avoid complete Wallerian degeneration. Gunshot wounds to the vagus nerve typically cause severe contusion without total nerve division; these wounds should be left alone because complete division of the nerve with an end-to-end primary anastomosis causes Wallerian degeneration; the alignment of the severely contused but undivided nerve is much better than that which can be achieved surgically. When the nerve has been divided completely by a missile, the two ends should be minimally (1 mm) débrided followed by an end-to-end repair with fine nonabsorbable sutures to the perineuron.

SUGGESTED READINGS

Azuaje RE, Jacobson LE, Glover J, Gomez GA, Rodman GH, Broadie TA, Simons CJ, Bjerke HS. Reliability of physical examination as a predictor of vascular injury after penetrating neck trauma. *Am Surg.* 2003;69: 804-807.

Demetriades D, Theodorou D, Cornwell E, Berne TV, Ascensio J, Belzberg H, Velmahos G, Weaver F, Yellin A. Evaluation of penetrating injuries of the neck: prospective study of 223 patients. *World J Surg.* 1997;21:41-48.

Ledgerwood AM, Mullins RJ, Lucas CE. Primary repair vs ligation for carotid artery injuries. *Arch Surg.* 1980;115:488-493.

Meyer JP, Barrett JA, Schuler JJ, Flanigan DP. Mandatory vs selective exploration for penetrating neck wounds: a prospective assessment. *Arch Surg.* 1987;122:592-597.

Weireter LJ, Britt LD. Penetrating neck injuries: diagnosis and current management. In: Ascension JA, Trunkey DD, eds. *Current Therapy of Trauma and Surgical Critical Care.* 2nd ed. St. Louis: Elsevier; 2016:179-185.

BLUNT CARDIAC INJURY

Nishant Patel, MD, David Lehenbauer, MD, and Christopher Sciortino, MD, PhD

Blunt cardiac injury (BCI) refers to a spectrum of injury resulting from blunt trauma to the heart. Patients with BCI may be asymptomatic, have a silent or subclinical pathology, or be seen with a range of pathologies from arrhythmias to ventricular free wall rupture and sudden death.

BCI can be classified according to the mechanism of injury and symptomatology: (1) arrhythmia; (2) minor electrocardiogram abnormalities or cardiac enzyme leakage; (3) cardiogenic shock; (4) coronary artery dissection or thrombosis; and (5) septal or ventricular free wall rupture.

BCI can be challenging to diagnose. Although many patients with BCI are already admitted to critical care settings because of other or associated injuries, there is much debate about how to manage the hemodynamically stable patient who does not otherwise require intensive monitoring. All patients with significant blunt trauma to the chest should be evaluated for BCI. It is critical to rule out BCI and identify those patients who are safe for discharge or who can be observed in a nonmonitored setting.

■ INCIDENCE

The true incidence of BCI is unknown because of the wide spectrum of injury. Reports in the literature show incidence rates ranging from 8% to 71% among patients who have blunt thoracoabdominal trauma. Overall, the incidence of BCI is likely underestimated because many patients with BCI die in the field from cardiac or other traumatic injuries. In addition, the lack of consensus regarding the appropriate workup for patients with suspected BCI further complicates management.

In a 2004 study by Schultz and colleagues, the most common BCI reported was myocardial contusion in 60% to 100% of cases. Given their anterior position in the chest, the right ventricle (17% to 32%) and right atrium (8% to 65%) are injured more commonly than the left ventricle (8% to 15%) and left atrium (0% to 31%). Valvular and coronary artery injuries are even rarer, with autopsy studies reporting an incidence of 3% to 5% after blunt trauma.

■ MECHANISM OF INJURY

The heart must encounter significant force in order to cause BCI because it is well protected in the thorax by the ribs and sternum. Motor vehicle accidents and pedestrians struck by vehicles historically have been the most frequent causes of BCI. Blast injuries, sports injuries, crush injuries, and assault are other potential mechanisms for BCI. Diagnosing BCI requires a high degree of clinical suspicion, and BCI should be considered in patients with thoracic bruising, sternal fracture, multiple rib fractures, pneumothorax, hemothorax, cardiac murmur, jugular venous distension, and cardiogenic shock. Table 1 lists the American Association for the Surgery of Trauma scale for quantifying the extent of BCI.

Myocardial contusion is the most common and usually the most innocuous form of BCI. Myocardial contusion is poorly defined but involves direct injury to the myocardium. This direct injury often results in electrocardiographic (ECG) abnormalities, such as nonspecific ST changes, ST elevation or depression, and premature atrial or ventricular contractions. Although not clinically useful, these patients often will manifest elevations in cardiac enzymes. All patients who have persistent arrhythmias, exhibit ECG abnormalities, or demonstrate hemodynamic compromise after blunt thoracic trauma should undergo transthoracic echocardiography to exclude functional and structural abnormalities.

Pericardial injury after blunt thoracic trauma results from high-energy forces or dramatic increases in intra-abdominal pressure. The pericardial sac usually will rupture parallel to the phrenic nerve along the pleural surface or on the diaphragmatic surface. Acute pericardial rupture may manifest as cardiac herniation and torsion, which may result in hemodynamic instability or even cardiac arrest. Patients with pericardial rupture may show displacement of the cardiac silhouette on chest x-ray or pneumopericardium. A focused assessment with sonography for trauma (FAST) may help to make the diagnosis. Treatment is surgical and is best approached via median sternotomy.

Valvular injuries are rare entities in BCI. Regardless, their sequelae can be significant. Therefore valvular injury should be suspected in the presence of cardiac murmur, thrill, left ventricular dysfunction, pulmonary edema, or cardiogenic shock. The aortic valve is the most common valve involved in BCI, followed by the mitral and tricuspid valves. Aortic valve injuries usually manifest as a new diastolic murmur in the setting of a torn noncoronary leaflet. Stable patients with this pattern of injury can be managed conservatively and then repaired electively. However, in those patients who develop dyspnea, arrhythmias, and heart failure, acute aortic insufficiency must be considered. If acute aortic insufficiency is diagnosed, it is unlikely that the valve can be salvaged, and urgent aortic valve replacement should be performed. Atrial and ventricular septal injury appears to be rare, may involve tears or rupture, and may occur in isolation or be associated with valvular injuries.

TABLE 1: American Association for the Surgery of Trauma Organ Injury Scale: Cardiac Injuries

Grade	Cardiac Injury
I	BCI with minor ECG abnormality (nonspecific ST or T wave changes, premature atrial or ventricular contraction, or persistent sinus tachycardia). Blunt or penetrating pericardial wound without cardiac injury, cardiac tamponade, or cardiac herniation.
II	BCI with heart block or ischemic changes without cardiac failure. Penetrating tangential cardiac wound, up to but not extending through endocardium, without tamponade.
III	BCI with sustained or multifocal ventricular contractions. Blunt or penetrating cardiac injury with septal rupture, pulmonary or tricuspid incompetence, papillary muscle dysfunction, or distal coronary artery occlusion without cardiac failure. Blunt pericardial laceration with cardiac herniation. BCI with cardiac failure. Penetrating tangential myocardial wound, up to but not through endocardium, with tamponade.
IV	Blunt or penetrating cardiac injury with septal rupture, pulmonary or tricuspid incompetence, papillary muscle dysfunction, or distal coronary artery occlusion producing cardiac failure. Blunt or penetrating cardiac injury with aortic or mitral incompetence. Blunt or penetrating cardiac injury of the right ventricle, right or left atrium.
V	Blunt or penetrating cardiac injury with proximal coronary artery occlusion. Blunt or penetrating left ventricular perforation. Stellate injuries, less than 50% tissue loss of the right ventricle, right or left atrium.
VI	Blunt avulsion of the heart. Penetrating wound producing more than 50% tissue loss of a chamber.

BCI, Blunt cardiac injury; *ECG,* electrocardiographic.

Cardiac rupture with tamponade is probably the most dramatic presentation of BCI. Patients who develop free wall rupture at the time of injury usually do not survive. For patients that do survive to hospital presentation, tamponade usually is found. It is important to note that these patients may not have all of the findings associated with Beck's triad: hypotension, muffled heart sounds, and jugular venous distension. Trauma patients who have had major hemorrhage are not likely to manifest distended neck veins. Prompt diagnosis and treatment are critical. Ventricular rupture is more common than atrial rupture, and right-sided chambers are more often involved than left-sided structures. Management requires resuscitation and surgery, which is achieved through median sternotomy and primary repair. Cardiopulmonary bypass may be necessary for more complex repairs.

Coronary artery injury secondary to BCI is a rare entity. The left anterior descending coronary artery is the most common vessel injured. BCI may lead to intimal disruption and dissection, which can result in decreased coronary perfusion or vessel thrombosis. Myocardial infarction, aneurysm, heart failure, and malignant arrhythmias may result. Coronary artery laceration or rupture with pericardial tamponade also has been reported. Asymptomatic patients with coronary artery injury after BCI can be managed medically with antiplatelet therapy. Those with proximal to midvessel injuries can be treated with percutaneous coronary intervention (balloon angioplasty or stenting). Those with injuries that cannot be managed percutaneously will require coronary artery bypass grafting.

Ventricular aneurysm formation may develop in a delayed fashion after BCI. Myocardial injury with subsequent necrosis and scar formation may lead to a ventricular aneurysm, most often of the anterolateral wall of the left ventricle. These patients may develop arrhythmias, heart failure, or thrombus in the left ventricle with subsequent embolization. Surgical management of ventricular aneurysm may involve aneurysm resection or plication of the aneurysmal wall.

BCI is often a part of multisystem trauma, and more than three quarters of patients will have associated thoracic injuries. These injuries include rib fractures, sternal fractures, pneumothorax, hemothorax, pulmonary contusions, and great vessel injury. Extrathoracic injuries are also common and include closed head, extremity, solid abdominal organ, and spinal injuries.

■ DIAGNOSIS

The initial evaluation of BCI should proceed according to the standard Advanced Trauma Life Support (ATLS) algorithm. An ECG should be the initial screening test performed on hemodynamically stable patients with suspicion for BCI. The ECG may show sinus tachycardia (most common), atrial fibrillation, other arrhythmias, bundle branch block, or ST changes. It is challenging for the provider to determine whether the ECG changes are related to the stress of trauma or caused by direct injury. In experienced hands, a FAST can be instrumental in providing the initial sonographic evaluation of the heart. FAST may determine the presence of pericardial effusion and tamponade as well as evaluate overall ventricular function. In the absence of findings that require urgent operative intervention, abnormalities on FAST should be evaluated further with formal echocardiography.

Once cardiac tamponade has been ruled out, transthoracic echocardiography may be useful in trauma patients with persistent cardiac dysfunction and may help to identify other injury, the potential need for inotropic support, and the need for further volume resuscitation. Transesophageal echocardiography is superior to the transthoracic approach and offers improved sensitivity for valvular injuries and wall motion abnormalities but at the risk of increased invasiveness. Cervical spine and esophageal injuries should be ruled out before proceeding with transesophageal echocardiography.

The Eastern Association for the Surgery of Trauma (EAST) guidelines for the evaluation and management of BCI are shown in Box 1. The EAST guidelines encourage the use of ECG as an important screening test for hemodynamically stable patients with possible BCI. Transthoracic echocardiography and admission with continuous cardiac monitoring should be reserved for those patients who either are unstable or have ECG abnormalities on admission. The EAST guidelines also argue against the routine use of cardiac biomarkers and nuclear medicine tests because these rarely alter management. Patients who are found to have arrhythmias or ECG changes while on continuous monitoring or are found to have abnormal echocardiograms (wall motion abnormalities, valvular abnormalities, effusion) require cardiology and cardiac surgery consultation. Cardiac catheterization, initiation of antiarrhythmic agents, antiplatelet therapy, and cardiac surgery may be required for both preventative and definitive management.

■ TREATMENT

Management of patients with suspected BCI depends on the presumed injury and the stability of the patient (Figure 1). All trauma patients should be evaluated according to the ATLS guidelines.

BOX 1: EAST Practice Management Guidelines for Blunt Cardiac Injury Workup

Recommendation Level 1

1. An admission ECG should be performed on all patients in whom BCI is suspected.

Recommendation Level 2

1. If the admission ECG reveals a new abnormality (arrhythmia, ST changes, ischemia, heart block, and unexplained ST changes), the patient should be admitted for continuous ECG monitoring. For patients with preexisting abnormalities, comparison should be made to a previous ECG to determine need for monitoring.
2. In patients with a normal ECG result and normal troponin I level, BCI is ruled out. The optimal timing of these measurements, however, has yet to be determined. Conversely, patients with normal ECG results but elevated troponin I level should be admitted to a monitored setting.
3. For patients with hemodynamic instability or persistent new arrhythmia, an echocardiogram should be obtained. If an optimal transthoracic echocardiogram cannot be performed, the patient should have a transesophageal echocardiogram.
4. The presence of a sternal fracture alone does not predict the presence of BCI and thus should not prompt monitoring in the setting of normal ECG result and troponin I level.
5. Creatinine phosphokinase with isoenzyme analysis should not be performed because it is not useful in predicting which patients have or will have complications related to BCI.
6. Nuclear medicine studies add little when compared with echocardiography and should not be routinely performed.

Recommendation Level 3

1. Elderly patients with known cardiac disease, unstable patients, and those with an abnormal admission ECG result can safely undergo surgery provided that they are appropriately monitored. Consideration should be given to placement of a pulmonary artery catheter in such cases.
2. Troponin I should be measured routinely for patients with suspected BCI; if elevated, patients should be admitted to a monitored setting and troponin I should be followed up serially, although the optimal timing is unknown.
3. Cardiac computed tomography (CT) or magnetic resonance imaging (MRI) can be used to help differentiate acute myocardial infarction (AMI) from BCI in trauma patients with abnormal ECG result, cardiac enzymes, and/or abnormal echo to determine need for cardiac catheterization and/or anticoagulation.

From Clancy K, et al. Screening for blunt cardiac injury: an Eastern Association for the Surgery of Trauma practice management guideline. *J Trauma Acute Care Surg.* 2012;73:S301-S306.

BCI, Blunt cardiac injury; *ECG,* electrocardiogram.

Hemodynamically unstable patients require prompt resuscitation with diagnosis and treatment of the underlying problem (e.g., shock, pneumothorax, tamponade). In hemodynamically stable patients with evidence of pericardial effusion on FAST or echocardiography, definitive management with pericardial window should be performed, with subsequent median sternotomy, if necessary. Pericardiocentesis can be performed while awaiting definitive pericardial window or sternotomy. Hemodynamically stable patients with normal FASTs and normal ECGs have no evidence of BCI. However, in patients older than 55 years or those with a history of cardiac disease, admission to a monitored unit may be warranted despite a normal ECG. Hemodynamically stable patients who are seen with

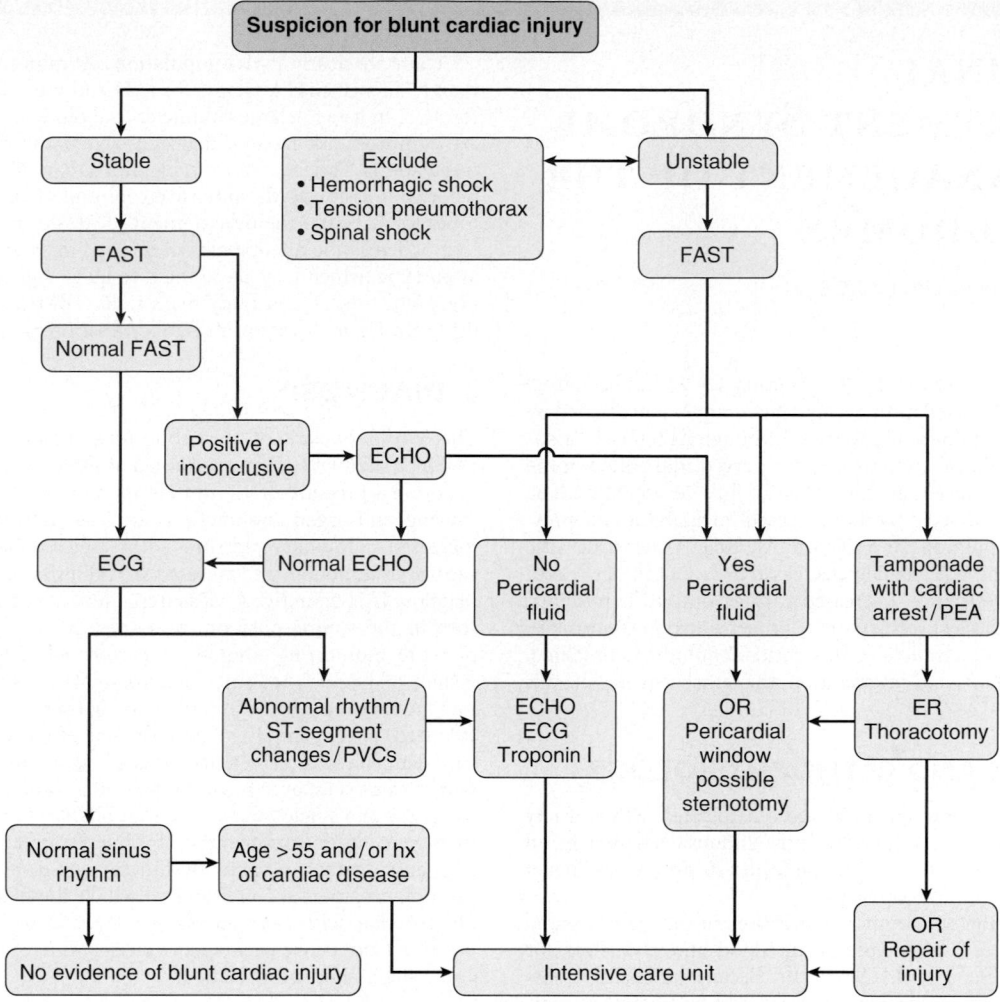

FIGURE 1 Algorithm for blunt cardiac injury. *ECG*, Electrocardiogram; *ECHO*, echocardiogram; *ER*, emergency room; *FAST*, Focused assessment with sonography for trauma; *hx*, history; *OR*, operating room; *PEA*, pulseless electrical activity; *PVC*, premature ventricular contraction. *(Adapted from Shah A, Balsara K. Blunt cardiac injury. In: Cameron J, Cameron A, eds. Current Surgical Therapy. 11th ed. Philadelphia: Elsevier; 2013:1085-1087.)*

ECG changes or arrhythmias should be admitted to a continuous monitoring unit for at least 24 hours because of the risk for life-threatening ventricular arrhythmias. Echocardiography should be performed to investigate valvular and wall motion abnormalities, and serial ECGs should be performed to monitor for persistent arrhythmias. Defibrillation for ventricular fibrillation is the treatment of choice and should be performed expeditiously.

According to the EAST guidelines, patients with blunt trauma who arrive at the emergency department pulseless and with no signs of life should *not* undergo resuscitative thoracotomy. However, the EAST guidelines conditionally recommend that patients who have tamponade and witnessed cardiac arrest or pulseless electrical activity in the emergency department may undergo resuscitative left anterolateral thoracotomy with subsequent evacuation of pericardial fluid until definitive therapy can be performed. Hemodynamically stable patients with pericardial effusion on FAST should proceed to the operating room for pericardial window and possible median sternotomy. BCI patients with complex coronary or valvular injuries warrant cardiology and cardiac surgery consultation. These patients with complex injuries likely will require surgical repair in the operating room via median sternotomy and the use of cardiopulmonary bypass.

Long-term outcomes for patients with BCI are highly variable, and longitudinal studies are lacking. Patients with myocardial contusion and those with mild or transient arrhythmias or ECG changes often fully recover. Anecdotally, some patients at our institution who have required surgical management for BCI have had good long-term outcomes without residual effects, provided their other injuries were not life threatening. In conclusion, activation of appropriate ATLS protocol, prompt diagnosis, and early definitive intervention are paramount for patient survival after BCI.

SUGGESTED READINGS

Becker A, Elias M, Mizrahi H, et al. Blunt heart trauma. *J Trauma.* 2011;71:261.

Clancy K, Velopulos C, Bilaniuk J, et al. Screening for blunt cardiac injury: an Eastern Association for the Surgery of Trauma practice management guideline. *J Trauma Acute Care Surg.* 2012;73:S301-S306.

Mattox K, Flint L, Carrico C, et al. Blunt cardiac injury. *J Trauma.* 1992;33: 649-650.

Moore EE, Malangoni MA, Cogbill TH, et al. Organ injury scaling. IV: thoracic, vascular, lung, cardiac, and diaphragm. *J Trauma.* 1994;36: 299-300.

Schultz JM, Trunkey DD. Blunt cardiac injury. *Crit Care Clin.* 2004;20: 57-70.

ABDOMINAL COMPARTMENT SYNDROME AND MANAGEMENT OF THE OPEN ABDOMEN

Clay Cothren Burlew, MD, FACS

The term *abdominal compartment syndrome* (ACS) has been used to describe the constellation of physical derangements caused by an acute increase in abdominal pressure. Although ACS may be associated with many clinical scenarios, it is observed most often in the multiply injured trauma patient after massive fluid resuscitation. The organ systems most affected by the increased intra-abdominal pressure are the renal, pulmonary, and cardiovascular systems. Because the manifestations of ACS (namely decreased urine output, increased systemic vascular resistance, decreased cardiac output, hypoxemia, and elevated peak airway pressures) may be attributed to the primary injury, a heightened awareness of this entity should be maintained. With prompt diagnosis and intervention, the lethal sequelae of ACS may be avoided.

ETIOLOGY AND PATHOPHYSIOLOGY

The etiology of ACS is multifactorial and is associated with a variety of clinical scenarios. ACS is typified by intra-abdominal hypertension (IAH) due to either an intra-abdominal injury or process (primary) or massive resuscitation (secondary).

The most common scenario for ACS is the critically ill or injured patient who requires a large volume of blood and crystalloid for resuscitation. In these patients IAH occurs because of resuscitation-associated bowel edema, retroperitoneal edema, and large amounts of ascites. Patients who require lengthy operative procedures often develop the triad of hypothermia, acidosis, and coagulopathy; abbreviating the laparotomy permits physiologic restoration in the surgical intensive care unit (SICU) before definitive closure. This subset of patients is particularly at risk for ACS and therefore the abdomen is often purposefully "left open," with temporary closure techniques utilized.

Increased intra-abdominal pressure affects multiple organ systems (Figure 1). The intra-abdominal pressure causes direct compression of the retroperitoneal vascular structures, resulting in decreased venous return to the heart; this decrease in preload results in a decrease in cardiac output. The upward displacement of the diaphragm results in elevated intrathoracic pressures and decreased compliance of the thorax; this restrictive process is manifested clinically by elevated airway pressures and hypoxemia. Increased intra-thoracic pressure also magnifies the decrease in venous return and further compromises cardiac function with decreased ventricular end diastolic volumes. Stroke volume also is affected by the increase in systematic vascular resistance. Effects on the renal system are the result of both a direct compressive effect causing increased renal vascular resistance and a relative obstruction of external venous drainage. The overall result is a significant decrease in blood flow and a marked decrease in urine output. Similar phenomena in hepatic and intestinal perfusion have been documented. ACS also may result in elevated intracranial pressure (ICP). Because many trauma patients have associated traumatic brain injuries, this association should be appreciated to avoid intracranial hypertension in the multiply injured patient. Polycompartment syndrome, in which two or more anatomic compartments have elevated pressures, also is recognized.

There are clearly at-risk populations. At minimum, there are more than 30 identified risk factors for IAH and more than 20 risk factors for ACS. In general, large volume crystalloid resuscitation and shock are common risk factors identified across the diversity of patient populations. Patients who receive more than 7500 cc of crystalloid before admission to the intensive care unit (ICU) should be monitored for IAH and the development of ACS. It is interesting to note that patients who are obese have elevated intra-abdominal pressures at baseline, which may cause them to be at higher risk for IAH. For every unit increase in body mass index (BMI), there is a reported 0.14 mm Hg increase in intra-abdominal pressure.

DIAGNOSIS

The World Society of the Abdominal Compartment Syndrome (WSACS) defines IAH as a sustained or pathologic elevation of intra-abdominal pressure of 12 mm Hg or more. ACS is defined by IAH causing end-organ dysfunction such as decreased urine output, increased pulmonary pressures, decreased preload and subsequent cardiac dysfunction, and elevated ICP. Physical examination cannot diagnose IAH definitively. Measurement of the patient's bladder pressure in the supine position, by either manometry or continuous pressure monitoring, should be performed. The original grading system of bladder pressure measurements is presented in Table 1; measurements are listed in both mm Hg (current WSACS definition standard) and in cm H_2O (the value one obtains with bedside measurement via central venous pressure water manometers). Organ failure can occur over a wide range of recorded bladder pressures. There is not a single measurement of bladder pressure that prompts therapeutic intervention; rather it is the combination of clinical findings and degree of organ dysfunction associated with IAH that prompts treatment. Conditions in which the bladder pressure may not correlate with intra-abdominal pressure include external compression from pelvic packing, bladder rupture, significant adhesions, and a small neurogenic bladder.

THERAPY

Management of Intra-abdominal Hypertension

After the identification of IAH in a patient, strategies should be implemented to reduce intra-abdominal pressure and prevent the progression of IAH to overt ACS. Suggested interventions before the onset of ACS include brief trials of neuromuscular blockade and nasogastric decompression of the stomach. Enteral decompression also may be accomplished with rectal tubes or neostigmine if colonic dilatation or Ogilvie's syndrome is identified. Body position may affect intra-abdominal pressure. Elevation of the head of the bed 30 degrees or more, often performed as part of a ventilatory care protocol, is associated with an increase in intra-abdominal pressures.

Although perhaps counterintuitive in the acute resuscitation phase, early use of vasopressors to limit crystalloid infusion may be a therapeutic alternative. In patients with oliguric acute renal failure, judicious fluid administration, early use of pressors, and institution of renal replacement therapy before fluid overload also may be warranted. Positive fluid balance due to uncontrolled crystalloid resuscitation clearly promulgates the development of IAH and ACS; modification of the patient's resuscitation to use massive transfusion protocols when appropriate and aggressive attempts to achieve a negative fluid balance once physiologic restoration is accomplished is recommended. There are minimal to no available data on the specific role of diuretic therapy, renal replacement therapy, or hypertonic saline administration in these patients. However, often a "biphasic approach" is touted in the literature, particularly in patients with septic shock, to provide early fluid resuscitation followed by a focus on negative fluid balance.

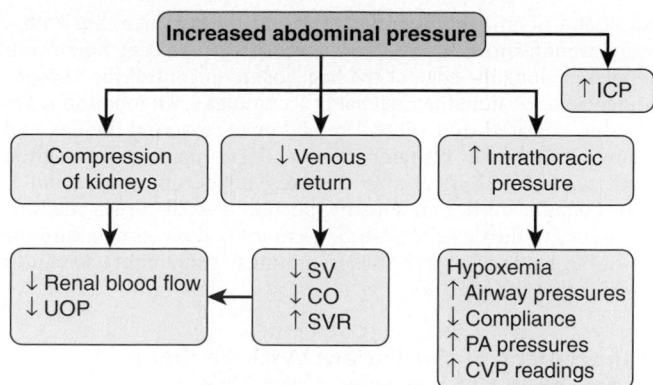

FIGURE I Clinical manifestations of increased abdominal pressure and resultant abdominal compartment syndrome. *CO*, Cardiac output; *CVP*, central venous pressure; *ICP*, intracranial pressure; *PA*, pulmonary artery; *SV*, stroke volume; *SVR*, systemic vascular resistance; *UOP*, urine output.

TABLE I: Grading System of Bladder Pressure Measurements

	Bladder Pressure	
ACS Grade	**mm Hg**	**cm H$_2$O**
I	10-15	13-20
II	16-25	21-35
III	26-35	36-47
IV	>35	>48

ACS, Abdominal compartment syndrome.

Intervention for Abdominal Compartment Syndrome

Patients with sustained intra-abdominal pressure of 20 mm Hg or more and organ dysfunction warrant abdominal decompression. Patients with a significant ascitic component of their ACS may be candidates for decompression with a percutaneous drain. Bedside ultrasound should determine those who are amenable, hence potentially obviating a trip to the operating room and the morbidity of an open abdomen. If the reduction in intra-abdominal pressure after drainage of intraperitoneal fluid or blood is not sufficient to reverse the organ dysfunction, operative decompression still can be performed. Recent investigations support that the abdominal pressure–volume curve demonstrates an exponential function above an intra-abdominal pressure of 15 mm Hg; thus removing only a small volume may affect the patient's IAH and clinical condition markedly. Another potentially less invasive option for decompression that has been described in patients with ACS due to pancreatitis is linea alba fasciotomy.

Operative decompression via midline laparotomy remains the definitive treatment for ACS. Opening the midline fascia often results in the rapid extrusion of the abdominal viscera and egress of peritoneal fluid (Figure 2). With equalization of intra-abdominal pressure and ambient pressure, there is typically prompt resolution of elevated airway pressures and hypoxemia as well as an increase in cardiac and urinary output. The midline incision does not need to extend from the xyphoid to the pubis for effective decompression; the length of the abdominal incision may be individualized. For example, trauma patients who undergo preperitoneal pelvic packing for unstable pelvic fractures can be decompressed effectively with just an upper midline abdominal incision (Figure 3). In patients with

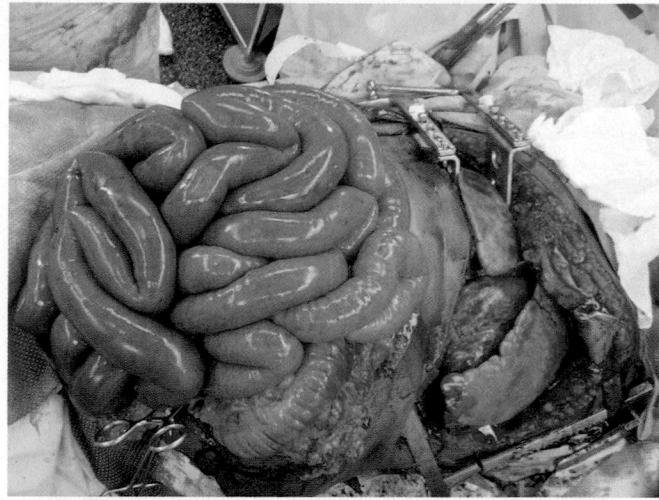

FIGURE 2 Operative decompression via midline laparotomy permits extrusion of the markedly swollen viscera and egress of peritoneal fluid.

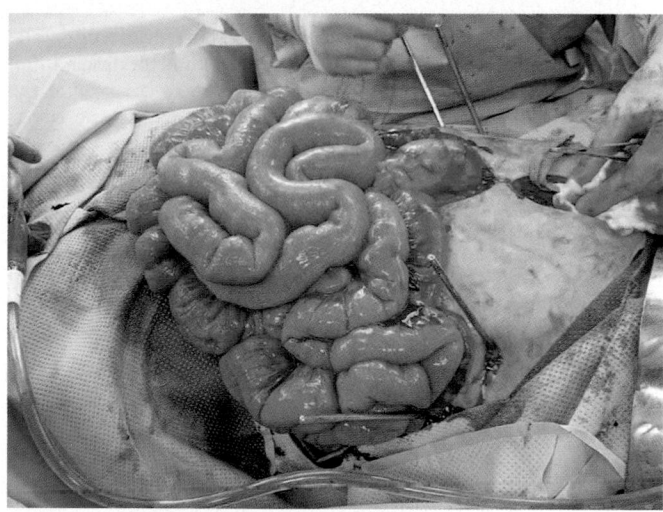

FIGURE 3 Laparotomy incisions for abdominal compartment syndrome may be individualized; effective decompression is possible with just an upper midline abdominal incision. The lower midline incision evident in the photo was used for preperitoneal pelvic packing for an unstable pelvic fracture.

hemodynamic instability mandating multiple pressors, transport to the operating room may be precarious. With minimal equipment required (scalpel, suction, cautery, and abdominal temporary closure dressings), the operating room can be "transported" to the ICU and bedside decompressive laparotomy performed (Figure 4).

After decompressive laparotomy, the abdominal viscera must be contained while preventing recurrent IAH or ACS. There are several temporary closure options. Our preferred option is the "10-10 Ioban" closure (Figure 5). One begins by fenestrating a 1010 Steri-Drape (3M Health Care, St. Paul, MN), with a scalpel to cut small holes (approximately 1 to 2 cm in length) in the plastic drape (see Figure 5, *A*). These holes permit resuscitation-associated ascitic fluid to pass through the drape while not allowing the Ioban to stick to the extruded bowel. If the apertures in the plastic drape are too big, which can occur if they are cut with scissors, the applied Ioban can stick to the surface of the bowel. A towel or laparotomy pad can be placed over the plastic drape and under the Ioban to prevent this (see Figure 5, *B* and *C*); however, this obscures the view of the bowel,

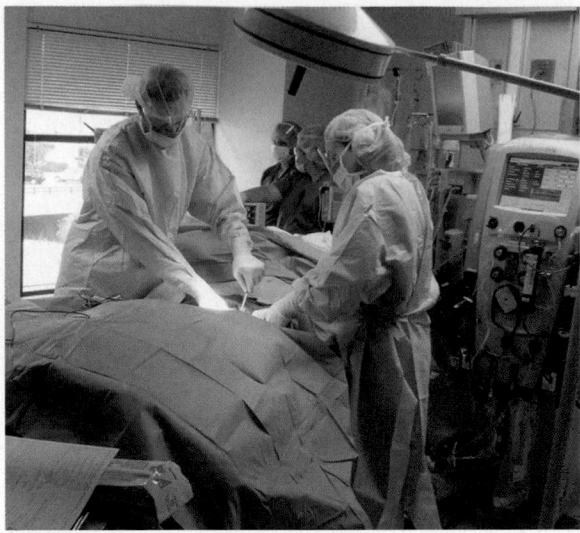

FIGURE 4 Bedside decompressive laparotomy can be performed in the intensive care unit.

preventing evaluation for either ischemia or recurrent bleeding. The plastic drape covers the bowel and is tucked under the fascia in all directions. Occasionally two drapes are necessary to cover all of the viscera and still permit subfascial placement of the plastic edges. Then two Jackson-Pratt (JP) drains are placed along the incisional subcutaneous space with the tubing running cephalad (see Figure 5, D). These do not have to be sutured to the adjacent tissue. The JP drains will control the egress of fluid from the abdomen, which may be more than 1 L/day. A large Ioban dressing (3M Health Care, St. Paul, MN) covers the entire surface, including the adjacent skin of the chest, pelvis, and lateral abdominal wall. When applying the Ioban, observe two points of caution: (1) incorporate the JP drain tubing into the Ioban folds rather than allowing it to remain on the skin surface above the incisional opening (see Figure 5, E), and (2) when pulling the Ioban over the top of the viscera, do not pull it tight; rather, leave some "expansion" space for ongoing bowel swelling so the patient does not develop recurrent ACS (see Figure 5, F and G). Commercially available vacuum-assisted devices are a similar option but may be more expensive and require appropriate resources. If such a device is used, one must ensure that recurrent ACS does not occur because of the application of suction-related pressure on the abdominal viscera. These devices may be best utilized after physiologic stabilization during subsequent operative attempts at fascial closure.

Other options for temporary closure are of more historical interest but may have the occasional practical application. Towel clip closure of only the patient's skin was one of the original methods of closing the abdomen after damage control surgery (DCS). Penetrating towel clips are used to reapproximate the abdominal wall by placing these through the skin, 2 to 4 cm apart (Figure 6). Although this results in some additional intra-abdominal volume and hence some reduction in pressure, it is often not sufficient. An additional downside should be considered; the metal clamps may obstruct radiographs and fluoroscopy images (Figure 7). "Towel clipping" the abdomen can be advantageous on return to the operating room for abdominal closure. Temporary reapproximation of the abdominal wall allows one to determine whether the abdomen can be closed without an increase in peak airway pressures or return of hemodynamic compromise.

Bogota bag closure, named for the Colombian surgeons who popularized the technique, is another temporary closure option. This temporary silo consists of a sterile, open 3-L urologic irrigation bag. Although an x-ray cassette cover also may be used, the irrigation bag is made of more durable plastic. The irrigation bag silo contains the bowel and is sutured circumferentially to the patient's skin with a heavy monofilament nylon suture (Figure 8). Closed suction drains are placed along the edge of the bag closure to control the serosanguineous ascitic fluid that inevitably accumulates. An Ioban adhesive covering is placed over the entire abdomen, covering the bag and drains to minimize contamination and maintain closed suction drainage. This technique provides excellent decompression but is labor intensive during the suturing portion; as well, it risks inadvertent injury to the bowel (it can be technically difficult to suture the plastic bag to the skin while also attempting to contain the edematous bowel within the bag).

Management of the Patient With an Open Abdomen in the Intensive Care Unit

In general, management of the patient with an open abdomen is not markedly different from the care of any other critically ill patient. Techniques previously illustrated for the management of IAH should be used. Adverse physiology, including acidosis, hypothermia, and coagulopathy, is corrected. Fluid resuscitation, an original contributor to the development of ACS, must be judicious and vasopressor support used wisely. Antibiotic use is not warranted for the mere presence of the open abdomen and should be limited to the perioperative period unless treatment of associated conditions (e.g., open fractures, documented infection) is indicated. The specifics of abdominal effluent, nutrition support, and directed peritoneal resuscitation, however, do deserve comment.

On arrival to the ICU, the JP drains placed during temporary abdominal closure should be attached to wall suction; bulb suction will not be effective for the 500 to 2500 mL/day of abdominal effluent produced. Appropriate volume compensation for this albumin-rich fluid remains controversial, both in the amount administered (replacement based on clinical indices vs routine 0.5- to 1-mL replacement for every milliliter lost) and in the type of replacement (crystalloid vs colloid and blood products). This abdominal effluent is a significant source of nitrogen loss, hence potentially accelerating the catabolic response and placing these patients at risk for protein malnutrition. Timely nutritional support is a logical priority.

Patients with an open abdomen are among the sickest patients in the ICU and hence could benefit from early nutritional support. However, the exposed and edematous abdominal viscera understandably can create anxiety about the initiation of enteral nutrition (EN) (Figure 9). The use of EN in the patient with an open abdomen has been discussed in the surgical literature for more than a decade. Seven studies to date, the majority incorporating postinjury patients requiring DCS, support the feasibility of EN in patients with an open abdomen. The largest trial to date on EN in patients with an open abdomen was performed by the Western Trauma Association (WTA) multicenter trials group. They demonstrated higher abdominal closure rates (albeit with a longer time until closure) and a reduction in mortality for patients who received EN compared with those who were kept nil per os (nothing by mouth). Therefore, after resolution of shock, EN should be considered in all patients with an open abdomen.

Specifics of optimal EN formulation, delivery location, and quantity administered for patients with an open abdomen remain to be defined. In the WTA study, patients receiving EN were predominantly fed in the stomach (60%); the remainder were fed distal to the pylorus. The amount of EN delivered was not quantified, although the authors reported that 38% of patients tolerated full goal tube feeds and 62% had tube feeds held at a constant rate of 20 mL/hr or less. There are no data on the use of standardized or specialized EN formulas that are specific to the open abdomen population. One consideration for specific components of nutrition support in these patients is the addition of up to 2 g of nitrogen to the patient's daily protein requirement for every liter of abdominal fluid output. This suggestion is based on a single institution's direct measurement of the albumin-rich abdominal effluent; the effect of additional protein

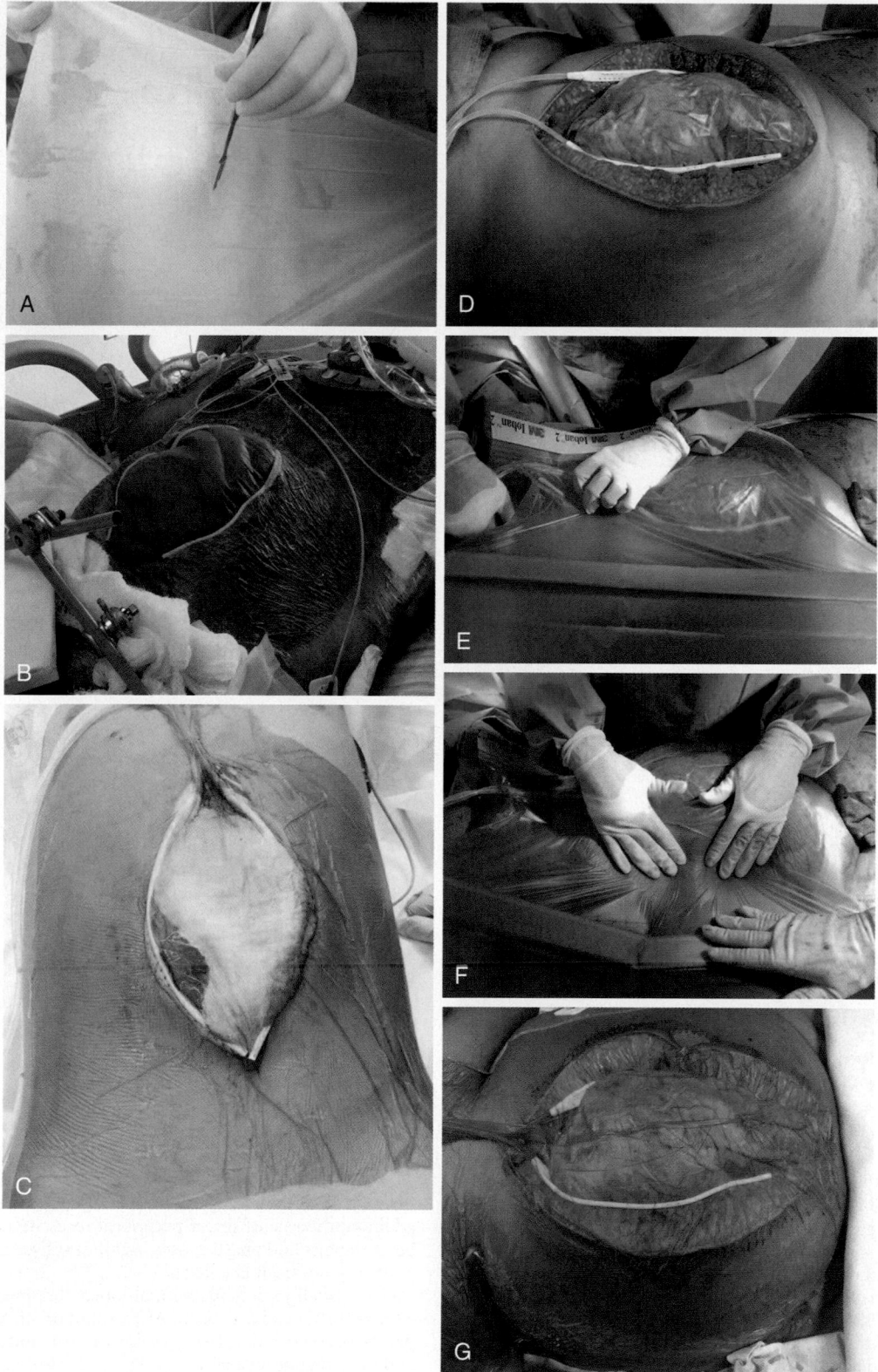

FIGURE 5 A, The "10-10 Ioban" closure begins with fenestrating a 1010 Steri-Drape with a scalpel. **B** and **C,** The plastic drape covers the bowel and is tucked under the fascia in all directions; a towel or laparotomy pad may be used to cover the plastic drape. **D,** Two Jackson-Pratt (JP) drains then are placed along the incisional subcutaneous space with the tubing running cephalad. **E,** When applying the Ioban, the JP drain tubing is incorporated into the Ioban folds rather than allowing it to remain on the skin surface above the incisional opening. **F** and **G,** A large Ioban covers the entire surface, including the adjacent skin of the chest, pelvis, and lateral abdominal wall.

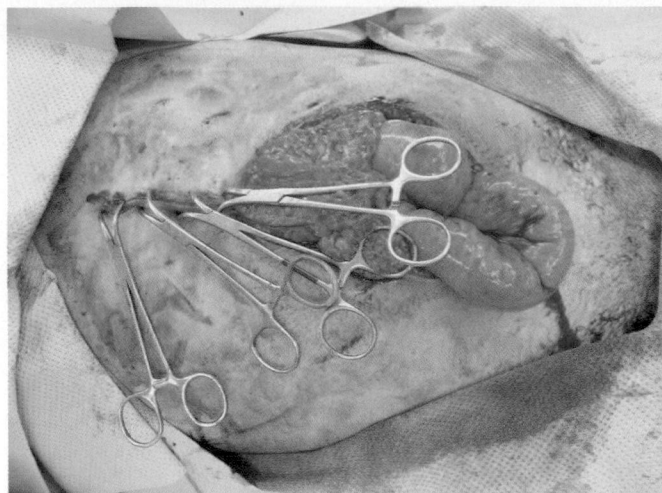

FIGURE 6 Towel clip closure of the abdomen uses penetrating towel clips to reapproximate the abdominal skin.

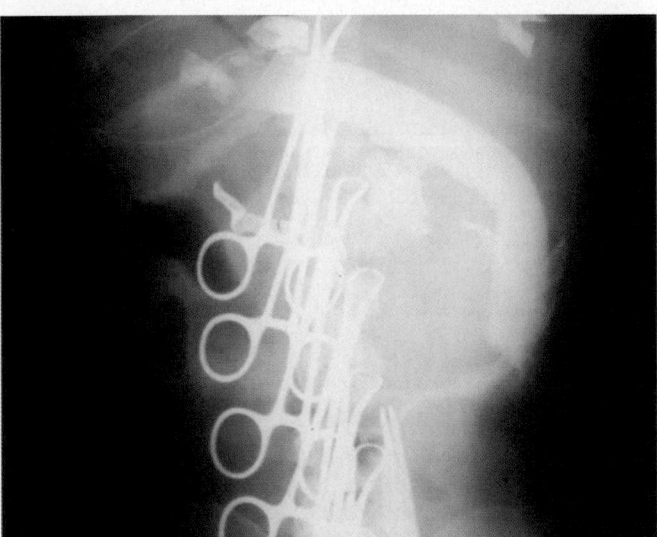

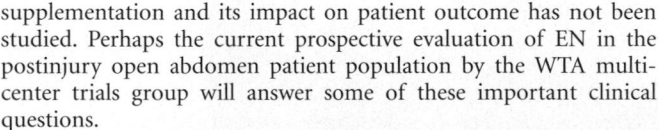

FIGURE 7 Towel clip closure of the abdomen may obstruct radiographs and fluoroscopy images.

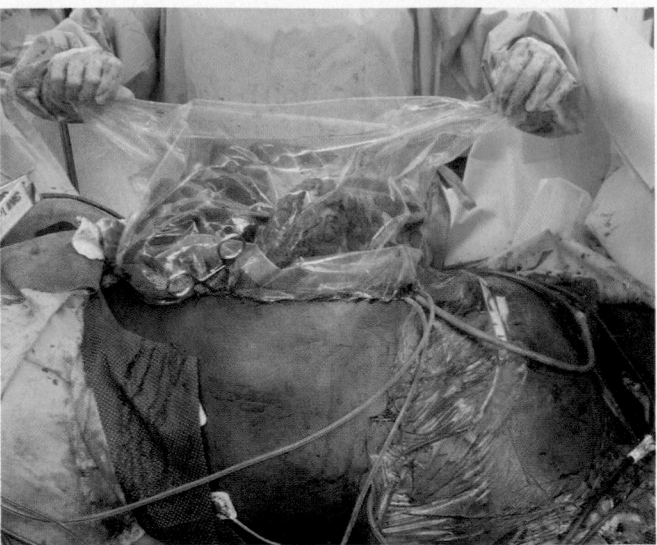

FIGURE 8 Bogota bag closure with an x-ray cassette cover just before Ioban placement.

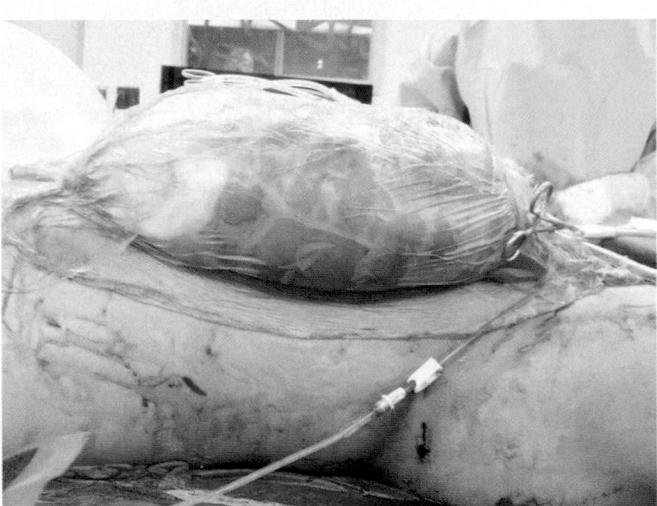

FIGURE 9 The marked visceral swelling understandably can create anxiety about the initiation of enteral nutrition.

supplementation and its impact on patient outcome has not been studied. Perhaps the current prospective evaluation of EN in the postinjury open abdomen patient population by the WTA multi-center trials group will answer some of these important clinical questions.

A recent technique that has added significantly to the surgeon's armamentarium in dealing with the impressive bowel edema encountered with ACS is direct peritoneal resuscitation. A 2.5% hypertonic glucose-based peritoneal dialysis solution (Delflex; Fresenius USA, Waltham, MA) is infused continuously into the abdomen. At the time of temporary closure, one or two 19F round Blake drains are placed in the abdomen through lateral stab incisions; the drains are placed either in the paracolic gutters bilaterally or along the root of the mesentery (Figure 10). The drains are used to continuously infuse the dialysate at a rate of 1.5 mL/kg/hr. The JP drains placed on top of the 1010 plastic drape evacuate the dialysate. In our experience, bathing the viscera with dialysate can result in a profound reduction in edema in is little as 24 to 48 hours. Fascial closure rates with this technique are reported to be higher, with a faster time to closure and fewer abdominal complications. One important caveat: Standard

wound vacuum-assisted closure (VAC) sponges, particularly the white sponge often used on top of exposed viscera, do not allow egress of the fluid and should not be used during this technique. In addition, the role of direct peritoneal resuscitation in patients with bowel repairs and anastomoses, significant liver injuries, or vascular grafts has not been elucidated.

One pitfall in patients with an open abdomen is to assume that recurrent IAH and associated ACS cannot occur. Monitoring bladder pressures ensures that IAH despite an open abdomen is recognized and treated appropriately.

Closure of the Open Abdomen

Coverage of the enteric contents is the most critical step in management of the patient with an open abdomen. Leaving the bowel exposed to the atmosphere can result in enteroatmospheric fistulas, which are notoriously problematic. After physiologic restoration, the patient is returned to the operating room 24 to 48 hours after the initial decompressive laparotomy. The occlusive Ioban covering should be trimmed to within 5 to 8 cm of the edge of the incision.

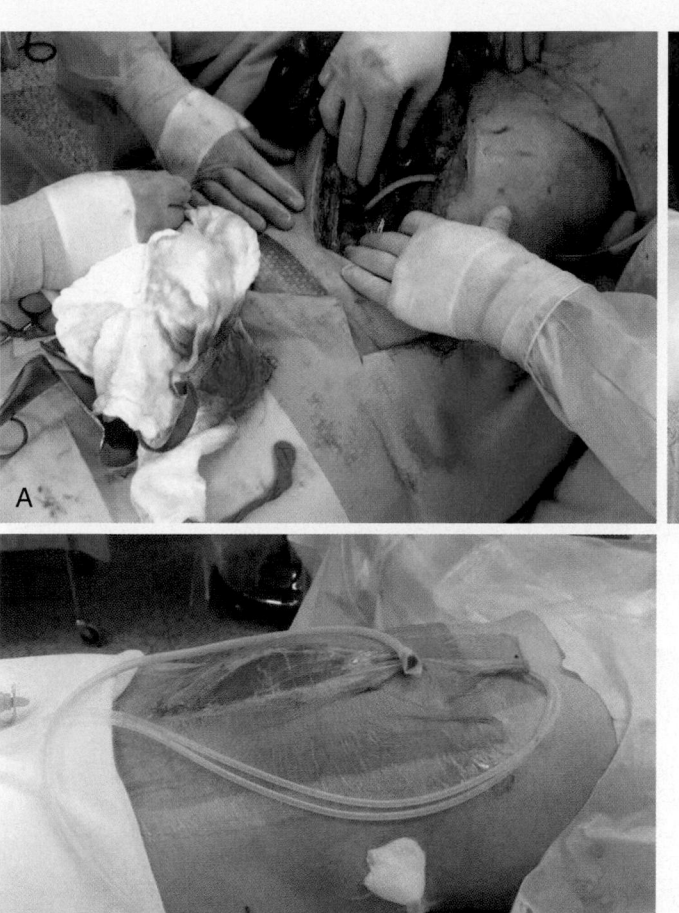

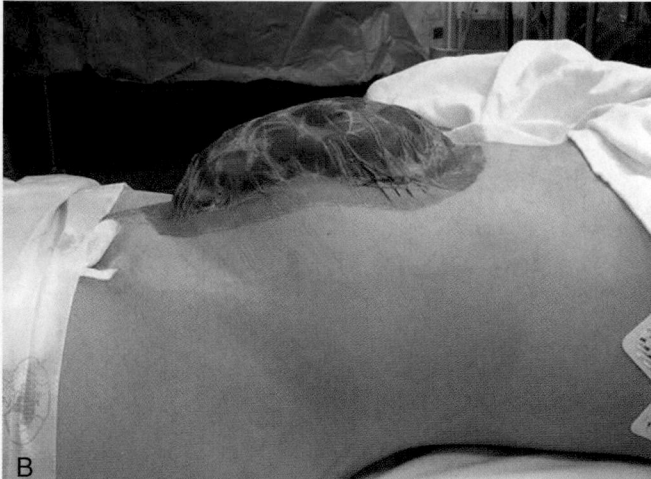

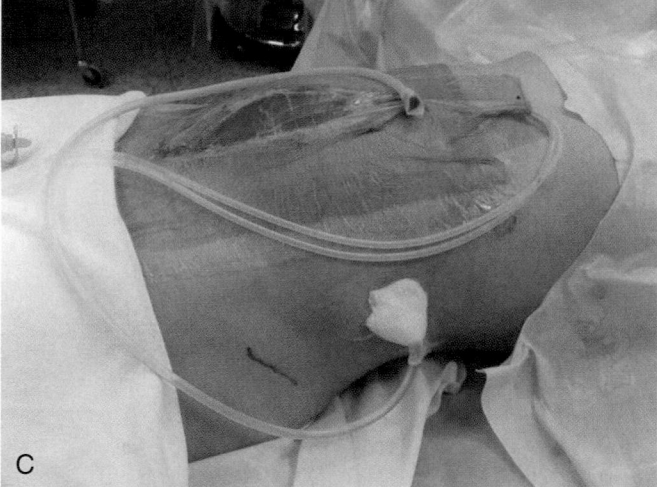

FIGURE 10 A, Direct peritoneal resuscitation utilizes one or two 19F round Blake drains to continuously infuse hypertonic glucose-based peritoneal dialysis solution. **B** and **C,** Within 24 to 48 hours there can be a profound reduction in bowel edema.

The entire covering is then prepared (Figure 11). Removing the Ioban covering before preparation makes the process unnecessarily difficult. Primary closure is the goal, with either early fascial closure or sequential fascial closure techniques.

Our preferred approach for patients who are not closed at second laparotomy is a sequential fascial closure technique. There are three key components of the closure: (1) constant fascial tension toward the midline to prevent lateralization of the abdominal wall musculature, (2) Wound VAC application, and (3) diligent return to the operating room every other day for fascial closure and replacement of the VAC sponges and fascial sutures. The technique described later is just one method used to accomplish sequential closure. There are multiple techniques to maintain fascial traction, which include but are not limited to commercially available products such as the Wittmann patch or bridging devices. Likewise, use of the Wound VAC system can use a variety of sponge options, with or without Silastic draping to protect the viscera and prevent adhesions to the undersurface of the abdominal wall.

In the Denver technique of sequential fascial closure, multiple white VAC sponges are overlapped to cover the small bowel and omentum. If more than one white sponge is necessary, which is true in the vast majority of cases, the sponges are lined up and stapled together along their edges with a skin stapler; this prevents the bowel from extruding between the sponges. The patchwork of white sponges covers the bowel and extends out under the fascial edges of the midline laparotomy incision. To prevent lateral fascial retraction, 1-PDS sutures then are placed with full-thickness fascial bites (2 cm back from the fascial edge), approximately 5 cm apart, in an interrupted fashion. These spaced "retention" sutures are tied down over

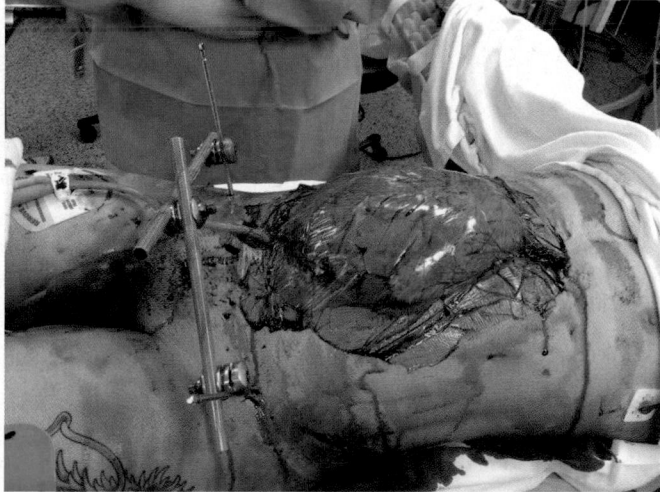

FIGURE 11 When returning to the operating room for repeat laparotomy, sterile preparation of the abdomen is done most effectively with the Ioban still covering the bowel.

the white sponges, pulling the fascia toward the midline and placing it under moderate tension (Figure 12, *A*). One or two large black VAC sponges are placed on top of the white sponges and affixed with an occlusive dressing, and standard suction is applied. Patients are returned to the operating room in less than 48 hours for repeated

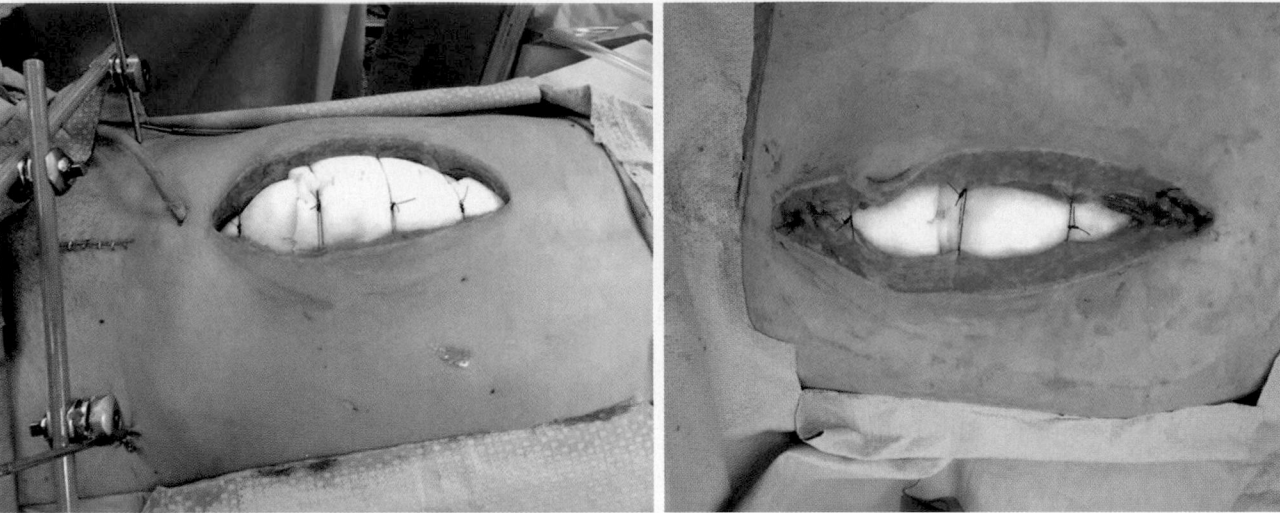

FIGURE 12 The Denver technique of sequential fascial closure.

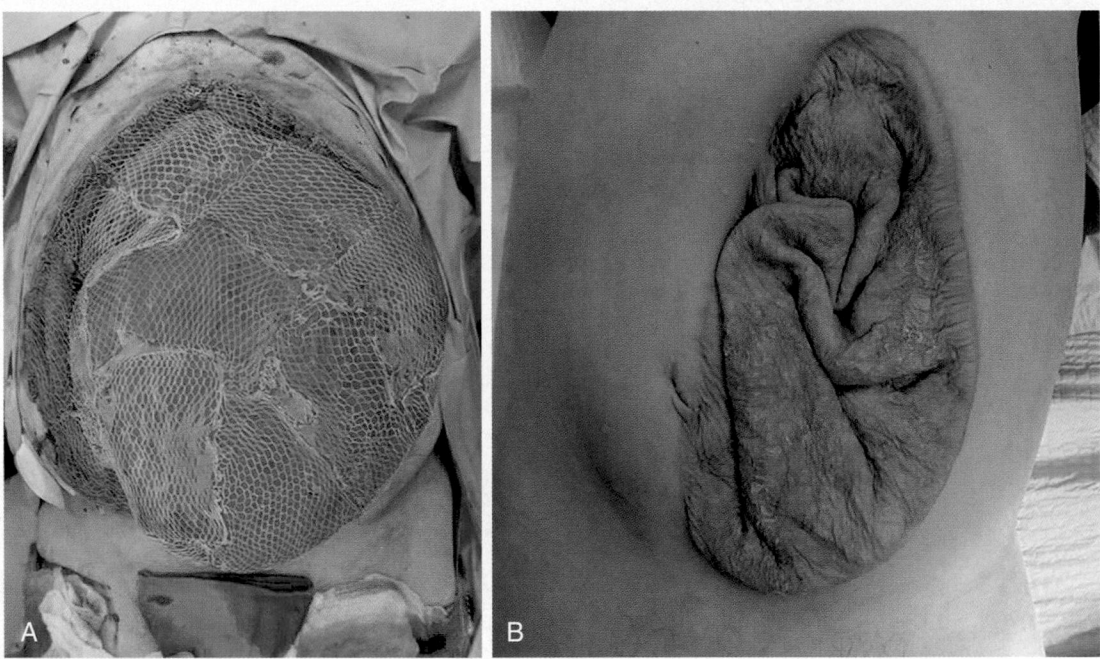

FIGURE 13 A, Split-thickness skin grafts can be placed directly on the bowel. Despite the awkward appearance, healing is reliable and the percentage of graft that survives is usually nearly 100%. **B,** The healed skin graft will separate from the underlying bowel; this is the indication that one can excise the skin graft operatively and perform herniorrhaphy, typically 9 to 12 months after the original insult.

attempts at fascial closure. If complete closure is possible, a running monofilament suture may be used. If not, interrupted fascial sutures are placed from both superior and inferior directions until tension precludes further closure; skin also may be closed over the fascial closure with skin staples. If the entire length of the fascial incision cannot be closed, replacement of the sponge sandwich and retention sutures occurs. As the fascial defect closes, the number of white sponges used diminishes and fascial separation decreases (Figure 12, *B*). Of note, the abdomen does not need to be re-explored nor the bowel eviscerated during each trip to the operating room. Only if there is concern for an intra-abdominal complication should a thorough exploration be performed.

Enteral access and nutrition should be considered early in these patients' hospital course. Gastrostomy and jejunostomy tubes may be placed before complete abdominal closure. Because of concerns about manipulation of access sites, with subsequent leak or fistula, operatively placed feeding tubes usually are not placed until that section of the fascia is closed completely; for example, if placing a Stamm gastrostomy tube, the upper abdominal fascia should be closed at the same operation. Placement of jejunostomy tubes in edematous bowel in the postinjury abdomen has been shown to be feasible. Alternatively, nasogastric or nasojejunal access for enteral feeding is a viable option for early nutrition support.

Other options for bowel coverage include prosthetic fascial closure with either polyglycolic acid (Vicryl) mesh or biologics and simple skin closure over the viscera. These options should be chosen only if further fascial closure despite all medical and surgical interventions is halted. There is no specific postinjury day that mandates abandoning attempts at sequential fascial closure. Rather, experienced surgical judgment should be used when changing course to use prosthetic or skin closure. For the few patients truly relegated to an open abdomen, another option for bowel coverage is split-thickness skin grafts (STSGs) and a planned ventral hernia (Figure 13). STSGs can be placed either directly on the bowel or on granulated polyglycolic acid (Vicryl) mesh. VAC placement will hold the STSGs in place for the first 5 postoperative days for optimal healing. Approximately 9 to 12 months later, once the healed skin graft has separated from the underlying bowel, one can excise the skin graft operatively and perform herniorrhaphy.

Complications

Complications in this patient population can be extremely morbid. Although any patient with an open abdomen and temporary abdominal covering can develop an enteroatmospheric fistula, they most commonly are seen in patients with significant delay to abdominal closure (>7 days) or in those who undergo skin grafting to the small bowel. They often materialize once the abdomen is "frozen," preventing proximal diversion or repair. Management of enteroatmospheric fistulas requires diligence and innovation. Primary repair of the fistula with fibrin glue or acellular dermal matrix has been reported. Failure of this repair results in persistent fistula output in the midst of an adhesed small bowel mass. Control of the fistula effluent is the first component of care, to prevent contamination of the rest of the abdomen. The fistula may be isolated using a small silo sewn to the opening of the bowel or Silastic tubing adjacent to the opening followed by negative pressure therapy to the remaining area of the abdomen. Once granulation tissue has developed around the fistula site, SPSGs can be used to close the open wound.

Intra-abdominal infection rates in patients with secondary ACS without other intra-abdominal pathology are low but not unreported. With the performance of sequential washouts, patients may not develop significant purulence. Therefore clinical suspicion should mandate intraoperative abdominal cultures in the febrile patient with an unexplained leukocytosis.

■ SUMMARY

Management of the open abdomen is an essential component in the care of critically ill and injured patients. Recognizing the potential etiologies and the at-risk patient population will enable the clinician to effectively diagnose IAH and ACS. Effective strategies after operative decompression combine medical management and operative techniques. Successful fascial closure of the open abdomen often hinges on the commitment and innovation of the surgeons who are managing these complex patients.

SUGGESTED READINGS

Balogh ZJ, Lumsdaine W, Moore EE, Moore FA. Postinjury abdominal compartment syndrome: from recognition to prevention. *Lancet.* 2014; 384:1466-1475.

Burlew CC, Moore EE, Cuschieri J, et al. Who should we feed? A Western Trauma Association multi-institutional study of enteral nutrition in the post-injury open abdomen. *J Trauma Acute Care Surg.* 2012;73: 1380-1388.

Burlew CC, Moore EE, Johnson JL, et al. 100% Fascial approximation can be achieved in the post-injury open abdomen. *J Trauma.* 2012;72:235-241.

Holodinsky JK, Roberts DJ, Ball CG, et al. Risk factors for intra-abdominal hypertension and abdominal compartment syndrome among adult intensive care unit patients: a systematic review and meta-analysis. *Crit Care.* 2013;17:R249.

Kirkpatrick AW, Roberts DJ, De Waele J, et al. Intra-abdominal hypertension and the abdominal compartment syndrome: updated consensus definitions and clinical practice guidelines from the World Society of the Abdominal Compartment Syndrome. *Intensive Care Med.* 2013;39: 1190-1206.

Smith JW, Garrison RN, Matheson PJ, et al. Direct peritoneal resuscitation accelerates primary abdominal wall closure after damage control surgery. *J Am Coll Surg.* 2010;210:658-664.

BLOOD TRANSFUSION THERAPY IN TRAUMA

Bryce R. H. Robinson, MD, MS, FACS, FCCM

Significant advances in trauma surgery throughout the ages can be traced to the necessity for innovation during times of military conflict. Modern, civilian transfusion practices parallel methods developed during conflicts of the last century, beginning with whole blood transfusions by the British Expeditionary Force because of recently developed ABO typing and citrate anticoagulation. The United Kingdom entered World War II with an active blood transfusion system; however, the United States, because of known complexities and assumed danger, instead utilized plasma and later albumin for the reversal of hemorrhage shock. U.S. medical officers quickly realized the benefits of whole blood transfusion and changed their transfusion practices after working in British field hospitals in North Africa, India, and the South Pacific. By 1945 a national blood program was established in the United States, leading to the collection of more than 13 million whole blood pints for military use. The Korean War led to improvements in the shelf life of whole blood and the introduction of plastic storage bags to mitigate deterioration of product secondary to extended supply lines. During the conflict in Vietnam, individual component therapy became available, leading to the delivery of universal donor, type O packed red blood cells (PRBCs), fresh frozen plasma (FFP), and platelets (from in-country whole blood).

Recent conflicts in Southwest Asia have led to paradigm shifts in the acute delivery of blood to reverse the "lethal triad" of hypothermia, acidosis, and coagulopathy. Termed *damage control resuscitation* or *hemostatic resuscitation*, these resuscitation methods aim to (1) identify those with emergent resuscitative needs early by the repetitive use of point-of-care testing, (2) allow for permissive hypotension until surgical bleeding is controlled, (3) rapidly deliver whole blood (when available) or component therapy in ratios that mimic whole blood, the so-called 1:1:1 blood transfusion, where each unit of PRBCs is accompanied by a unit of plasma and a unit of platelets, (4) minimize exposure to intravenous crystalloid solutions, and (5) utilize adjunct hemostatic pharmacotherapy, specifically tranexamic acid (TXA) and factor VII or IX, when indicated. The application of damage control resuscitation has been associated with improved mortality and morbidity as well as with decreased resource utilization in both military and civilian settings.

■ BLOOD COMPONENTS

The current civilian practice of fractionating whole blood into its separate components traces back to the post–World War II hypothesis of increasing blood efficiency by transfusing only the component that was needed. Civilian blood banks fractionate a unit of blood into PRBCs and plasma; the plasma is subsequently frozen and designated as FFP, platelets, and cryoprecipitate (Figure 1). Specific component therapy can be highly effective for nonemergent disorders that

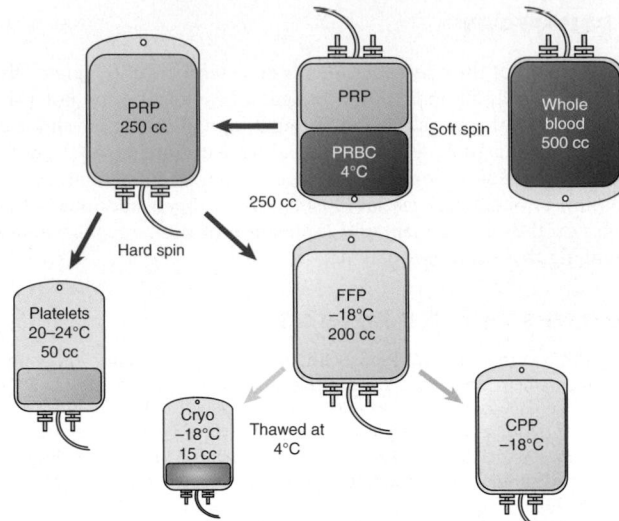

FIGURE 1 Fractionation of whole blood into its components for storage. *CPP*, Cryoprecipitate-poor plasma; *Cryo*, cryoprecipitate; *FFP*, fresh frozen plasma; *PRBC*, packed red blood cell; *PRP*, platelet-rich plasma. *(Courtesy Dr. Ravi Sarode, Blood Bank Director, Department of Pathology, UT Southwestern Medical Center, Dallas, TX.)*

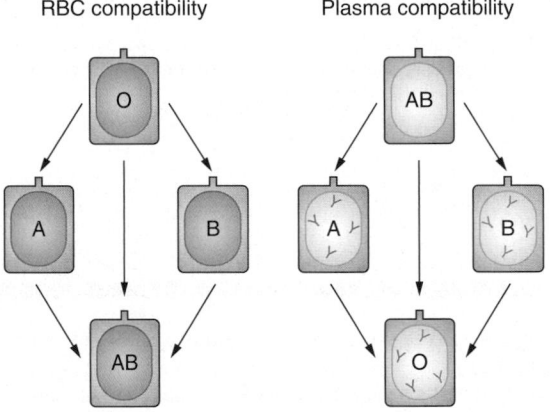

FIGURE 2 Blood matching by ABO type between donors and recipients. *RBC*, Red blood cell. *(From Hemmings H, Egan T. Pharmacology and Physiology for Anesthesia: Foundations and Clinical Application. Philadelphia: Elsevier; 2012.)*

require a specific product for correction or reversal. For example, most patients with anemia do not have a clinical coagulopathy and therefore can be treated solely with PRBCs. Conversely, patients with iatrogenic coagulopathy from warfarin do not require PRBCs but rather benefit from reversal by the transfusion of FFP if anemia or active bleeding is not present.

Universal to any elective component transfusion is the need for proper ABO typing and the identification of Rh factor, if present. The four blood types—A, B, AB, and O—are based on the presence of three cell wall antigens, A, B, or O. Furthermore, an additional antigen called the Rh factor may or may not be present (+ or −). The proportion of individual blood types within any given population varies by ethnicity; however, O+ is the most common blood type in the United States. Individuals with type O− blood are referred to as "universal red cell donors" because PRBCs from these individuals lack A or B antigens on the cell walls (Figure 2). Those with type AB plasma are referred to as "universal plasma donors" because they lack anti-A and anti-B antibodies within their plasma. However, because

of the relatively low availability of AB plasma for emergent, untyped transfusions, some institutions are promoting the use of A plasma as the universal plasma product in order to conserve AB plasma when indicated. The presence of Rh typing becomes especially important in females of reproductive age. Rh− individuals may develop antibodies to Rh factor if they are exposed to Rh+ blood. In pregnant females these antibodies have the potential to cross the placenta and cause hemolytic reactions within an Rh+ fetus.

PRBCs are stored at 4°C in a variety of citrated buffers and have a shelf life of either 35 days if buffered in citrate phosphate dextrose adenine solution or 42 days if commercial additive solution storage systems are used. PRBCs lose their oxygen-carrying capacity during storage because of the decreasing concentrations of 2,3-diphosphoglycerate (2,3-DPG). Stored blood units also are associated with increasing concentrations of potassium, the potential for bacterial overgrowth, and resultant immunomodulation from cell wall debris containing membrane ligands and lipids. Retrospective evaluations of trauma patients with PRBC transfusions have found a linear association between the age of PRBCs and mortality. These concerns have led to debated recommendations that patients with critical conditions, such as hypoxemia, or the need for large volume transfusions after trauma receive only "fresh" blood (i.e., <7 days old). Recent prospective randomized controlled trials examining the effects of newer (stored 7 to 10 days) versus older blood (stored up to 22 days) in both critically ill adults and patients undergoing cardiac surgery failed to show benefit of newer blood in terms of 90-day mortality and the rate of multiorgan failure, respectively. Future trials examining the effects of blood age will need to focus on trauma patients and, more specifically, those who require blood for hemorrhagic shock reversal.

In most U.S. blood banks, the practice of leukoreduction of PRBCs before storage has become the standard of care. Because donor leukocytes have been implicated as having potential immunosuppressive effects, additional blood processing aims for their removal. Prior meta-analyses in heterogeneous surgical populations point to a potential reduction in infectious complications, and mortality benefit through large prospective work focusing on trauma patients continues to be lacking.

The average unit (approximately 300 mL) of PRBCs has a hematocrit of approximately 80%, which will raise the hemoglobin level by 1 g/dL or the hematocrit by 3% in nonbleeding patients. Trauma patients who need red blood cell transfusions must be separated clearly into two groups: (1) those who are actively bleeding and (2) those who are no longer bleeding but remain critically ill. For patients who are actively bleeding, the principles of damage control resuscitation are critically important to understand and apply. PRBC transfusion criteria for critically ill patients who are no longer bleeding but have anemia appear to be clearer. The randomized controlled Transfusion Requirements in Critical Care (TRICC) trial, which compared a restrictive transfusion strategy (maintaining hemoglobin levels between 7 and 9 g/dL) with a more liberal strategy (10 to 12 g/dL), demonstrated safety with a more restrictive strategy in critically ill adults. The two strategies were equivalent in terms of overall survival, although improved survival was found in younger patients (<55 years old) and in those with lower Acute Physiology and Chronic Health Evaluation–II (APACHE II) scores (<20) who were exposed to the restrictive strategy. These findings have led to institutional lowering of transfusion triggers and to a general abandonment of the arbitrary "10/30 rule" (i.e., transfusing patients to 10 g/dL or to a hematocrit of 30%). Although a lower threshold for PRBC transfusion appears to be safe, even in patients with a history of cardiovascular disease, a higher threshold is warranted in those with active acute myocardial infarction and unstable angina.

FFP can be stored at −18°C for up to 1 year. However, after thawing FFP has a shelf life of only 5 days. Thawed plasma contains varying amounts of fibrinogen, von Willebrand factor, and coagulation factors I, VII, VIII, IX, X, and XIII. To extend the safe and useful interval for plasma transfusions, some have looked to utilize plasma

TABLE 1: Platelet Transfusion Triggers

Clinical Condition	Platelet Count per Microliter
Stable hematology and oncology	10,000
Complicated oncology	>20,000
Minor surgery	25,000-50,000
Major surgery	>50,000
Neurosurgery	100,000
Platelet dysfunction: congenital or acquired	As clinically indicated

separated from whole blood that has never been frozen. Termed liquid plasma, it can be stored at 1°C to 6°C for up to 26 days. Small ex vivo studies have demonstrated improved hemostatic profiles in comparison with sex- and blood group–matched FFP, although local blood bank logistics may make this product inaccessible, particularly for centers with a reduced need for plasma transfusions. Regardless of the type of product utilized, plasma transfusions are indicated for the reversal of either acquired or congenital coagulation defects as well as for the reversal of warfarin. For stable, nonbleeding patients, plasma should never be used to correct abnormal coagulation tests alone (e.g., per the international normalized ratio [INR]).

Platelets are stored at room temperature (20°C to 24°C) on a gentle shaker and must be discarded after 5 days because of concerns for bacterial contamination. Because of the inability to store platelets, they are a precious commodity and should be used judiciously. Nonetheless, for those requiring large volume blood resuscitations after injury, the platelet to PRBC ratio transfused appears to be related to survival in a stepwise fashion. Platelets can be collected in two ways: (1) from random donors, yielding a volume of about 50 mL—that is, 5×10^{10} platelets; or (2) from a single donor by apheresis, yielding a volume of 200 to 250 mL, equivalent to 5 to 8 random units—that is, a minimum of 3×10^{11} platelets. Accepted transfusion triggers for platelet transfusion are shown in Table 1.

Cryoprecipitate is so named because it is the cold-insoluble portion of plasma that precipitates out of solution when FFP is slowly thawed at 1°C to 6°C. It contains clotting factors from a single donor that then are suspended in 10 to 15 mL of plasma. Each unit contains a minimum of 80 IU of factor VIII and at least 150 mg of fibrinogen, in addition to significant amounts of von Willebrand factor, factor XIII, and fibronectin. Cryoprecipitate is available in prepooled concentrates of 5 units. Each unit is from a separate donor and is suspended in 15 mL plasma before pooling. Cryoprecipitate is stored at −18°C. It is thawed to room temperature when needed and must be transfused within 6 hours after thawing or after 4 hours if pooled. Cryoprecipitate is indicated for bleeding or immediately before an invasive procedure in patients with significant hypofibrinogenemia (<100 mg/dL). The inclusion of cryoprecipitate into massive transfusion protocols is controversial and institutionally specific.

The re-emergence of whole blood transfusions for those in hemorrhagic shock is gaining popularity in both military and civilian centers because of the improved outcomes seen with the application of damage control resuscitation techniques. During the recent conflicts in Southwest Asia, fresh whole blood has been used successfully by the U.S. military to acutely treat hemorrhagic shock. The ability for high volume, damage control resuscitative component therapy in austere environments is at times impossible. Whole blood transfusions became a feasible alternative because of the military's ability to access a "walking blood bank" (i.e., obtaining fresh donations from a previously screened group of individuals whose blood type is already known). Use of fresh whole blood has been credited with helping to reduce the incidence of mortality from the serious,

simultaneous penetrating injuries that have been characteristic of these conflicts.

Whole blood is rarely used in civilian settings because of the inactivation of platelets by refrigeration and the assumed delay in obtaining type-specific whole blood over emergency release universal donor PRBCs and plasma. In a recent randomized controlled pilot trial comparing traditional component therapy with whole blood in trauma patients, those randomized to whole blood experienced an additional 5 to 10 minutes of delay in obtaining product because of the need for cross-matching. However, when patients with severe head injury were excluded, the whole blood cohort received fewer red blood cells, plasma, platelets, and total products during the first 24 hours after admission.

ACUTE COAGULOPATHY OF TRAUMA

Twenty-five percent of trauma patients arrive at the emergency department with a clinically significant coagulopathy. These patients with coagulopathy have a threefold to fourfold increase in mortality and an eightfold increase in intraoperative death within the first 24 hours of injury. Traditional teachings for the causes of acute coagulopathy of trauma have implicated dilution, hypothermia, acid-associated dysfunction, or consumption of coagulation factors. However, recent evidence now suggests that a combination of shock-induced activation of the protein C pathway and increased hyperfibrinolysis due to direct endothelial damage may lead to systemic anticoagulation. As such, common tests for acute coagulopathy after injury may lack the precision to identify these newly implicated mechanisms.

DIAGNOSIS OF ACUTE COAGULOPATHY OF TRAUMA

Traditional testing for coagulopathy after injury has used elevations of the prothrombin time (PT) and partial thromboplastin time (PTT). PTT has been associated with a higher specificity for predicting outcomes and correlating to low protein C levels compared with PT. PT presented as the INR, although originally developed to monitor patients who require warfarin therapy, has been implicated as a strong early predictor of the need for substantial resuscitation and mortality. Nonetheless, there are problems with measures of clotting time. Most centers require between 15 and 60 minutes for analyses of these tests. Point-of-care testing may reduce wait time to less than 10 minutes; however, the use of these tests, specifically INR, to predict the need for large volume PRBC transfusions is based on retrospective work with a propensity for selection bias. Furthermore, these tests reflect only the first 20 to 60 seconds of clot formation, which is a process that evolves over 15 to 30 minutes. These tests also lack information pertaining to clot strength, hyperfibrinolysis, or platelet function.

Thromboelastography (TEG) has been promoted within the trauma community to address the known shortcomings of PT, PTT, and INR. The test is conducted by placing a thin wire into a rotating cup that contains a small whole blood sample. The timing and strength of clot formation on the wire is measured directly, and the various components of coagulation and fibrinolysis are represented visually in a computer-generated tracing (Figure 3). TEG helps to assess multiple arms of the clotting cascade simultaneously, including platelet function, and therefore may represent higher accuracy for diagnosing in vivo clot dysfunction. Its downsides include the need for dedicated equipment, the requirement of frequent and accurate calibration, and appropriate provider interpretation of the tracings. Kaolin-activated (traditional) TEG requires 30 to 60 minutes for completion of the tracing, contradicting its practicality for acute coagulopathy diagnoses. Rapid TEG using tissue factor to accelerate clot formation does require noncitrated whole blood samples to be run within 4 minutes of acquisition but provides useful measures within 5 to 10 minutes. Finally, standard and rapid TEG is not

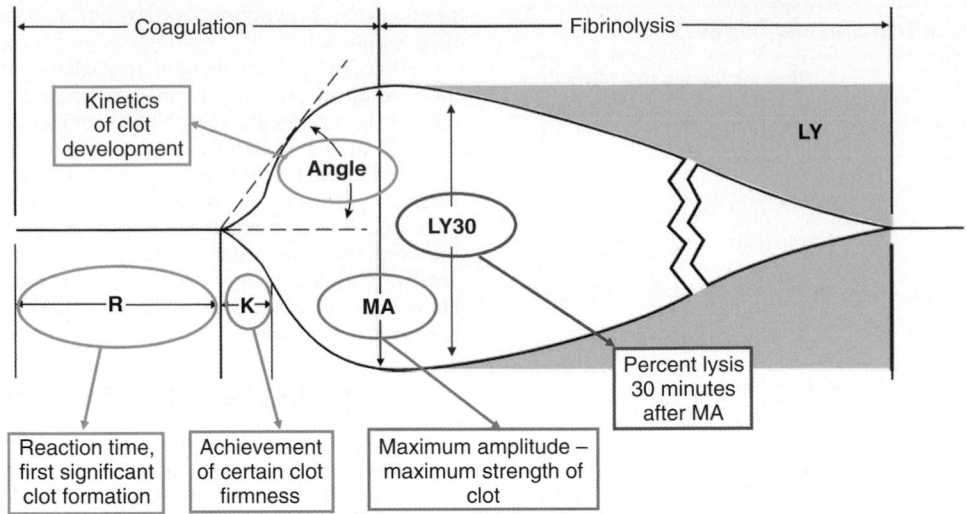

FIGURE 3 Sample of thromboelastography tracing with associated values of clot formation. *(From Anderson L, Quasim I, Steven M, et al. Interoperator and intraoperator variability of whole blood coagulation assays: a comparison of thromboelastography and rotational thromboelastometry. J Cardiothorac Vasc Anesth. 2014;28:1550-1557.)*

sensitive to aspirin or clopidogrel and will remain normal despite adequate platelet inhibition by these medications. TEG-based platelet mapping to assess functionality in the presence of these antiplatelet agents is possible but requires proprietary reagents.

Devices that directly measure platelet function and reactivity (e.g., VerifyNow; Accriva Diagnostics, San Diego, CA) are becoming more popular because of reduced cost and maintenance. These types of devices may play a role in more accurately assessing the impact of antiplatelet therapy and the adequacy of platelet transfusions for reversal than standard coagulation testing or platelet counting. Regardless of how platelet functionality is measured, a growing need for assessment is anticipated because of the aging trauma population using antiplatelet agents.

MASSIVE TRANSFUSION AND MASSIVE TRANSFUSION PROTOCOLS

After injury, hemorrhage is responsible for 50% of deaths occurring within the first 24 hours of care and up to 80% of intraoperative trauma deaths. It is becoming clear that the rapid and aggressive diagnosis and treatment of trauma-associated coagulopathy has beneficial effects. In those with hemorrhagic shock and ongoing blood loss, the activation of a massive transfusion (MT) via an institutional massive transfusion protocol (MTP) is mandated. Delays in obtaining the results of coagulation testing can lead to undertreatment in those patients with active hemorrhage, so most MTPs use fixed ratios of blood products until coagulation testing can be obtained, so as not to delay treatment.

MT has been defined generally, but the two most common and useful definitions are as follows: (1) transfusion of 10 units or more of PRBCs in a 24-hour period or (2) transfusion equivalent to patient's blood volume in 6 to 24 hours. Both definitions have been criticized as arbitrary and flawed because of concerns for survival bias (e.g., patients with significant hemorrhage that die before meeting predefined transfusion criteria would be excluded). Defining validated indicators for acute blood loss and rates of ongoing, active hemorrhage is a challenge for bedside practitioners and transfusion research. To account for these concerns, others have proposed using the "critical administration threshold," which is the transfusion of 3 units or more of PRBCs within a single hour, as a more rapid tool for categorizing those who may require an MT. Others advocate for the early identification of "substantial bleeders," which is defined as receiving the first PRBCs within 2 hours of arrival at the emergency

department and the subsequent use of 5 units or more of PRBCs within 4 hours. Regardless of the way those at risk for MT are acutely identified, this subgroup of severely injured patients, equivalent to 3% to 5% of the total civilian trauma population, represents a separate clinical entity with immense physiologic disarrangement and associated mortality.

Much of the impetus for the 1:1:1 ratio came from recent retrospective military data that pioneered work on MTs because of the considerable injuries sustained by combatants in Southwest Asia. The preponderance of improvised explosive device injuries with multiple amputations and severe blood loss led to the in-theater implementation of both fresh whole blood and MTPs. With the return of military surgeons to civilian centers, the use of MTPs has promulgated civilian practice for the most severely injured.

The essential components of an MTP are as follows: (1) its automaticity (i.e., blood products are prepared without being specifically requested); (2) its ability to be activated 24 hours a day, 7 days a week, and in locations as diverse as the emergency department, intensive care unit, operating room, and angiography suite; (3) its lack of requirements for blood testing; (4) its delivery of blood products in predefined ratios; and (5) its automatic continuation until stopped by a physician. The protocol's precise form, components, ratio, and timing depend on the individual institution, with the vast majority of level I and level II trauma centers now having an MTP. An example of MTP ratios is given in Table 2. Finally, damage control resuscitation is an example of an MTP where the delivery of balanced blood products is provided pre-emptively in the context of permissive hypotension, reduced exposure to crystalloids, repetitive point-of-care testing for resuscitation endpoint and coagulopathy, and adjunct hemostatic pharmacotherapy.

A thawed plasma protocol can be an adjunct to an institutional MTP. Once thawed, FFP can be kept refrigerated for up to 5 days with minimal loss (roughly 20%) of functional activity. Having prethawed plasma readily available can reduce the time for emergent patient delivery by approximately 30 to 60 minutes. With careful attention to institutional inventory, thawed plasma also can be used for nontrauma purposes, thus preventing waste and improving efficiency for emergent delivery.

The optimal ratio for blood product delivery during MTPs is becoming clearer. The Pragmatic Randomized Optimal Platelet and Plasma Ratios (PROPPR) trial at 12 civilian trauma centers compared the effectiveness of transfusing patients with severe trauma and major bleeding using plasma, platelets, and PRBCs in a 1:1:1 ratio

TABLE 2: Contents of Container Cycles for Each Ratio Group

		Container 1	Container 2
Group 1*	Platelets	1	1
1:1:1	Plasma	6	6
	RBCs	6	6
Group 2†	Platelets	0	1
1:1:2	Plasma	3	3
	RBCs	6	6

From Baraniuk S, Tilley BC, del Junco DJ, et al. Pragmatic Randomized Optimal Platelet and Plasma Ratios (PROPPR) Trial: design, rationale and implementation. *Injury*. 2014;45:1287-1295.

*Group 1: Platelets first, then alternate RBCs and Plasma, as clinically required.

†Group 2: Platelets first (if available), then alternate 2 RBCs and 1 Plasma, as clinically required.

The container cycles were repeated until hemostasis was achieved and resuscitation completed.

RBCs, Red blood cells.

versus a 1:1:2 ratio. With approximately 340 patients per group, no significant differences were detected in mortality at 24 hours or at 30 days. Those in the 1:1:1 cohort achieved hemostasis and experienced less exsanguination at 24 hours. Complication rates were equal between the ratio groups. Previous work from the Prospective, Observational, Multicenter, Major Trauma Transfusion (PROMMTT) study demonstrated the benefit of early and higher amounts of plasma and platelets to reduce mortality during the first 6 hours after admission. Together these two studies establish safety equipoise between the two ratio groups, while favoring the early use of a 1:1:1 strategy because of improved early hemostasis and reduced exsanguination leading to death.

■ HEMOSTATIC ADJUNCTS

Factor VIIa generated much interest as an adjunct for bleeding trauma patients in the early 2000s after its military use in Southwest Asia. However, two recent randomized controlled trials did not reveal a survival benefit and demonstrated only a reduction in PRBCs transfused in those with blunt trauma. Furthermore, factor VIIa is prohibitively expensive to support widespread use in MTPs, as each dose is estimated to cost $4000 to $5000. Although this drug has fallen out of favor, others have come to the forefront, such as prothrombin complex concentrates (PCCs) and, more recently, TXA.

PCC is a pooled plasma product containing a mixture of vitamin K–dependent proteins. Four-factor PCCs (factors II, VII, IX, and X) have received more attention because of perceived superiority versus three-factor (II, IX, and X) products. Although originally designed as a therapeutic option for bleeding in those with hemophilia B, traumatic intracranial hemorrhage secondary to anticoagulation with vitamin K antagonists (warfarin) appears to be the primary indication for use in recent guidelines. In comparison with FFP, PCCs can be stored at room temperature as a lyophilized powder and reconstituted in approximately 80 mL of sterile water, allowing for rapid bolus therapy over a shorter period of time. These characteristics are especially beneficial in older populations that require rapid reversal of anticoagulation but may not be able to tolerate an equivalent dosing of FFP with a volume in excess of 800 mL. Although the majority of research on this topic is retrospective, a recent prospective randomized controlled trial demonstrated superiority in comparison with plasma for rapid and effective hemostasis in those with

vitamin K–antagonist anticoagulation requiring urgent surgical or invasive procedures. Patients who needed a procedure in which an accurate estimate of blood loss could not be obtained (e.g., trauma) were excluded from this trial. Future work with PCCs will need to focus on those with extracranial injuries and those without a history of vitamin K antagonists but with markers for the acute coagulopathy of trauma.

In contrast, strong evidence exists for the use of TXA in bleeding trauma patients. The pragmatic Clinical Randomisation of an Antifibrinolytic in Significant Haemorrhage (CRASH-2) trial randomized 17,000 patients with or at risk for significant bleeding in 40 countries to receive either TXA or placebo. Those who received TXA experienced a significant drop in mortality from 16% to 14.5%. However, a prespecified subgroup analysis showed increased mortality in patients given TXA 3 or more hours after injury. Because of the significant benefit, a strong safety profile, and low cost with easy delivery, many U.S. trauma centers have incorporated the use of TXA in their MTPs but restrict its use to those patients in whom infusions can begin before the 3-hour postinjury mark.

■ COMPLICATIONS FROM TRANSFUSION THERAPY

In the United States, blood transfusion is one of the most common medical procedures performed during hospitalization, although it is not without risk and clinicians need to be aware of the sequelae discussed here.

Nonhemolytic Febrile Reactions

Approximately 1 in 100 to 200 patients will develop a nonhemolytic febrile reaction during or after blood transfusion. This is thought to result from the formation of complexes of donor leukocyte antigens reacting with plasma antibodies of the recipient that later activate complementary and inflammatory cytokine release. A decrease in nonhemolytic febrile reactions has occurred since the widespread use of leukoreduced PRBCs. Constitutional symptoms include fever, chills, headache, myalgia, and general malaise. Only in rare circumstances do these symptoms progress to nausea, vomiting, or hypotension. A direct antiglobulin test (Coombs test) will be negative in these individuals because of the lack of attachment of recipient plasma antibodies to donor red blood cells. Ceasing the transfusion is controversial and dependent on the clinical need for blood. However, it is recommended to reduce the rate of transfusion if a febrile reaction occurs and to stop the transfusion if a more serious hemolytic reaction is suspected. Supportive therapy for nonhemolytic febrile reactions includes acetaminophen and diphenhydramine.

Hypothermia

PRBCs are stored at 4°C. Patients who undergo multiple transfusions can progress rapidly to hypothermia with deleterious consequences for global hemostasis. A number of commercially available warming devices (e.g., Level 1 and Hotline, Smiths Medical, Rockland, MA; Belmont, Belmont Instrument, Billerica, MA; enFlow, Vital Signs, Totowa, NJ) can be used to allow for the warming of fluids during infusion (usually to 40°C). Such devices should be used whenever more than 2 units of blood products are to be rapidly transfused.

Electrolyte Disturbances

During storage the cell wall integrity of PRBCs diminishes, leading to a gradual leak of potassium into the supernatant. Patients who receive multiple units of older PRBCs are at risk for hyperkalemia. In clinical practice this is rarely an issue in those with normal renal function. Even in patients who undergo MTs, data suggest that potassium levels rarely rise to become clinically significant. A more significant concern is hypocalcemia associated with multiple transfusions because of the accumulation of calcium-binding citrate. Hypocalcemia can lead to myocardial depression resulting in hypotension, reduced pulse pressure, and electrocardiogram abnormalities. Patients who undergo multiple transfusions should have their ionized calcium level checked regularly. If the level is low, supplementation with calcium gluconate should occur.

Transfusion-Associated Circulatory Overload

Transfusion-associated circulatory overload (TACO) is the constellation of circulatory overload symptoms that may occur after transfusion of blood products. Currently there is no universal definition of TACO, although symptoms may include the development of respiratory distress, hypoxemia, orthopnea, and hypotension during or within several hours of transfusion. Chest radiography may reveal cardiomegaly and pulmonary infiltrates. The incidence of TACO is difficult to quantify, but it may occur in up to 8% of all transfusions in high-risk populations to include those younger than 3 years and older than 60 years with underlying cardiac failure. Treatment of TACO is supportive and begins with reducing intravenous fluid exposures and stopping the blood transfusion. If acute hypoxic respiratory failure is encountered, aggressive diuresis should be started. The best strategy is prevention by the judicious administration of blood products.

Transfusion-Related Acute Lung Injury

Transfusion-related acute lung injury (TRALI) is the leading cause of transfusion-related deaths in the United States. The incidence of TRALI is approximately 1 per 1300 transfusions, with a death rate of 1 per 1700 to 5000 confirmed cases. It is defined by acute onset of hypoxemia with bilateral infiltrates on chest radiograph that occurs during or within 6 hours of transfusion without alternative causes for acute hypoxemia. The term *possible TRALI* is used when a clear temporal relationship to an alternative etiology for hypoxemia is present. Patients with circulatory overload or TACO should not be defined as having TRALI (Box 1).

TRALI is thought to result from the interaction of leukocyte antibodies in the donor plasma of transfused blood products to recipient leukocytes and neutrophils. A nonimmune form of TRALI may exist, resulting from the interaction of lipid membranes of donor blood cells with recipient neutrophils. Common to both of these processes is a neutrophil-mediated inflammatory cascade with associated neutrophil aggregation, complement activation with subsequent pulmonary endothelial damage, capillary leak, alveolar fluid and protein accumulation, and clinical pulmonary edema.

Treatment of TRALI is supportive and focuses on the use of supplemental oxygen when needed. If TRALI is associated with acute respiratory failure and the need for mechanical ventilation, care plans should mimic those implemented for acute respiratory distress syndrome, with an emphasis on low tidal volume ventilation. Among patients who develop TRALI, 80% will survive with normal lung

function. The diagnosis of TRALI does not affect the ability to receive blood transfusions in the future. The risk of TRALI is highest among recipients of FFP, particularly from multiparous women, but other blood products have been implicated. It is of utmost importance to inform the blood bank of any case of TRALI or "possible TRALI" so that both the donor and the recipient can be tested for the presence of antibodies. Such testing is usually not of immediate clinical importance, although the identification of human leukocyte antigen (HLA) and neutrophil antibodies in donors may prevent future donations. Because of the high risk associated with plasma from multiparous females, the American Association of Blood Banks in 2014 recommended the transfusion of plasma and whole blood from males, females who have not been pregnant, or females who have been found to be negative of HLA antibodies since their most recent pregnancy. Nonetheless, because of shortages of AB plasma (the universal donor), female plasma has been accepted by some regional blood centers.

Hemolytic Reactions

Hemolytic reactions can be either acute or delayed. Patients can develop different symptomatic patterns, depending on the timing of the presentation of the reaction. Acute hemolytic reactions typically occur within 24 hours after a transfusion with intravascular symptoms. Delayed hemolytic reactions more commonly occur 1 to 10 days after a transfusion with extravascular manifestations (Table 3). The incidence of hemolytic reactions is 1 in 12,000 to 25,000 patients, but the mortality rate is as low as 1 in 650,000 patients. Reactions are caused by the immune-mediated lysis of red blood cells. Acute hemolytic reactions usually are related to preformed antibodies within the recipient's plasma to surface antigens on donated blood. If a hemolytic reaction is suspected, the transfusion should be stopped immediately, the reaction reported to the blood bank with return of the blood products, and a confirmatory direct antiglobulin test (Coombs test) performed. Treatment consists of increasing levels of supportive care with fluid resuscitation to ensure adequate renal perfusion. If renal failure should occur because of hemoglobin deposition in the distal renal tubule and renal microvascular thrombosis, hemofiltration should be initiated.

Infectious Risk

Bacterial contamination of blood products is exceptionally rare in developed countries. Contamination can occur during venipuncture for collection or if the donor has bacteremia. During storage of

BOX 1: Criteria for Transfusion-Related Acute Lung Injury

- Acute onset: during or within 6 hours of transfusion
- Hypoxemia
  - Oxygen saturation <90% at room air
  - Ratio of partial pressure of oxygen to fraction of inspired oxygen <300 mm Hg
- Bilateral infiltrates on chest x-ray
- No evidence of left atrial hypertension
- No pre-existing acute lung injury before transfusion
- No temporal relationship to alternative risks for acute lung injury

TABLE 3: Incidence of Symptoms in Hemolytic Reactions

Symptom	Acute (Intravascular)	Delayed (Extravascular)
Fever, chills	80%	55%
Renal failure	35%	5%
Pain	15%	2.5%
Nausea, vomiting	10%	–
Hypotension, tachycardia	12%	–
Disseminated intravascular coagulation	10%	5%
Jaundice	–	10%

TABLE 4: Risk of Exposure to an Infectious Agent per Unit of Blood Component Therapy

Infectious Agent	Risk per Unit
HIV	1 : 1,860,000
Hepatitis B	1 : 365,000
Hepatitis C	1 : 1,650,000
HTLV	1 : 3,390,000
Bacterial contamination	1 : 1000 to 1 : 100,000 for platelets 1 : 100,000 to 1 : 1,000,000 for red blood cells
NvCJD	Unknown, not yet described
Rabies	Unknown
Dengue, West Nile virus	Possible, risk unknown

HIV, Human immunodeficiency virus; *HTLV*, human T-cell lymphotropic virus; *NvCJD*, new variant Creutzfeldt-Jakob disease.

PRBCs, gram-negative bacteria, specifically *Yersinia* and *Pseudomonas* species, have the potential to proliferate. Gram-positive bacteria, to include *Staphylococcus* and *Bacillus*, have the potential to grow at room temperatures and are the primary pathogens found in platelet contamination. Because there are no screening tests for bacterial contamination, visual inspection of the product before infusion is important.

Viral contamination of blood products has been reduced significantly by the introduction of pre-donation questionnaires in the 1980s and rapid serology and nucleic acid testing in the 1990s. Currently the American Red Cross tests every unit of blood for hepatitis B, hepatitis C, human immunodeficiency virus–1 (HIV-1) and HIV-2, human T-cell lymphotropic virus 1 and 2, syphilis, Chagas disease, and West Nile virus. Estimates of the current incidence of various infections per unit of donated blood are shown in Table 4. These numbers represent the risk of exposure; however, the actual rates of seroconversion are multifactorial.

■ NOVEL ANTICOAGULANTS

Novel anticoagulants that directly inhibit thrombin (dabigatran, argatroban) or factor Xa (rivaroxaban, apixaban) are becoming more common for the prevention of thromboembolism with atrial fibrillation or after joint replacement. These drugs have a perceived favorable safety profile and improved efficacy in comparison with warfarin. Although they have a short half-life of 9 to 14 hours, they currently lack reversible agents when life-threatening bleeding occurs. Furthermore, traditional coagulation testing is ineffective in monitoring the presence or extent of anticoagulation that may be present with these therapies. Holding these medications for at least 24 hours before an elective procedure with standard bleeding risk (uncomplicated laparoscopy, colonoscopy with polyp removal) is recommended. For those having major surgery with a higher risk of bleeding (cardiac surgery, spinal surgery or anesthesia, neurosurgery), holding these drugs for at least 2 to 6 days is recommended. These longer recommendations also apply to those with impaired renal function.

For those with life-threatening bleeding and direct thrombin inhibitor use, enteral activated charcoal may be beneficial if the medication has been taken within the last 2 to 3 hours. Emergent hemodialysis can be initiated for drug removal in these patients because of the high amounts of free drug in the plasma. Currently an antidote is in phase III trials for the reversal of dabigatran before emergent surgery. Produced by the manufacturer of dabigatran, idarucizumab is a monoclonal antibody to the drug. The results of using PCCs and factor VII have been contradictory, so their use is reserved for life-threatening bleeding. The manufacturers of argatroban suggest the use of PRBCs, FFP, and even factor VII but with minimal human data to support this recommendation.

The reversal of factor Xa inhibitors is even more worrisome. Both charcoal and hemodialysis are ineffective. The use of PCCs appears to have some benefit in the context of emergent bleeding, although the impact of factor VII is unknown. An antibody antidote for these medications, andexanet alfa, is being developed and is currently in phase III trials with healthy volunteers.

■ FUTURE DIRECTIONS

Most new directions have a foundation in past experiences, both good and bad. Lyophilized "freeze-dried" plasma continues to gain interest, especially after its military application in recent conflicts. First introduced during World War II, the process of lyophilization uses low pressure, temperature, and humidity to convert liquid plasma into a fine powder. This formulation is compatible to all recipients, can be stored at room temperature for up to 2 years, is reconstituted with sterile water within 6 minutes, and has minimal degradation of clotting factors. Because of modern methods of serology and nucleic acid testing preprocessing, viral contamination risk of this product is minimal. Currently this product is not approved by the Food and Drug Administration (FDA) for use in the United States, but military forces in Israel and France utilize lyophilized plasma as a resuscitation adjunct. Recent literature from Norway reports its use for civilian trauma during prehospital rotary wing transport in an effort to begin damage control resuscitation before hospital arrival. Although large animal studies with lyophilized plasma continue in the United States, the status of future clinical trials or regulatory approval is unclear.

Cryopreservation of PRBCs with glycerol, first introduced in the 1950s, is again gaining interest. Such processes allow for the storage of blood at –80°C for up to 10 years. After thawing, automated deglycerolization, and cell washing, PRBCs must be used within 14 days. These cells may be advantageous in that they contain less anticoagulation, cell debris, platelets, leukocytes, anti-A and anti-B isoagglutinins, and biologically active mediators that have been implicated in post-transfusion inflammation. Cryopreserved blood allows for storage by small or remote blood banks for disaster scenarios with little risk of wastage and without compromising efficacy or safety. Nonetheless, the processing of cryopreserved blood for use takes approximately 90 minutes, and these units can be three times more expensive compared with traditional PRBCs.

The promise of a blood substitute with oxygen-carrying capacity continues to elude the trauma community. Theoretically, such substitutes would provide the benefits of transfusion, reduce the risks of infection, obviate the need for blood donation, and ideally cost less. PolyHeme (Northfield Laboratories, Evanston, IL) underwent a controversial multi-institutional, phase III, prospective, randomized controlled (with crystalloid) trial with an exemption from informed consent. Unfortunately this blood substitute did not meet the pre-specified primary efficacy endpoint and may place patients at a higher risk for adverse events. As a result, the trauma community continues to wait for a safe and efficacious universally compatible oxygen carrier for patients with life-threatening hemorrhage.

SUGGESTED READINGS

Brohi K, Cohen MJ, Davenport RA. Acute coagulopathy of trauma: mechanism, identification and effect. *Curr Opin Crit Care.* 2007;13:680-685.

CRASH-2 collaborators, Roberts I, Shakur H, et al. The importance of early treatment with tranexamic acid in bleeding trauma patients: an exploratory analysis of the CRASH-2 randomised controlled trial. *Lancet.* 2011;377:1096-1101.

Hébert PC, Wells G, Blajchman MA, et al. A multicenter, randomized, controlled clinical trial of transfusion requirements in critical care. *N Engl J Med.* 1999;340:409-417.

Holcomb JB, del Junco DL, Fox EE, et al. The prospective, observational, multicenter, major trauma transfusion (PROMMTT) study: comparative effectiveness of a time-varying treatment with competing risks. *JAMA Surg.* 2013;148:127-136.

Holcomb JB, Jenkins D, Rhee P, et al. Damage control resuscitation: directly addressing the early coagulopathy of trauma. *J Trauma.* 2007;62: 307-310.

Holcomb JB, Tilley BC, Baraniuk S, et al. Transfusion of plasma, platelets, and red blood cells in a 1:1:1 vs a 1:1:2 ratio and mortality in patients with

severe trauma: the PROPPR randomized clinical trial. *JAMA.* 2015;313: 471-482.

Lacroix J, Hebert PC, Fergusso DA, et al. Age of transfused blood in critically ill adults. *N Engl J Med.* 2015;372:1410-1418.

Maxwell MJ, Wilson MJ. Complications of blood transfusion. *Contin Educ Anaesth Crit Care Pain.* 2006;6:225-229.

Steiner ME, Ness PM, Assmann SF, et al. Effects of red-cell storage duration on patients undergoing cardiac surgery. *N Engl J Med.* 2015;372: 1419-1429.

COAGULATION ISSUES AND THE TRAUMA PATIENT

Michael B. Streiff, MD, and Nadia Ijaz, MD

Each year more than 5 million people die as a result of major trauma. Trauma is the fifth leading cause of death worldwide and the number one cause of death in individuals 5 to 44 years of age. Among trauma-related deaths, hemorrhage is responsible for 30% to 40% of fatalities. Over the last decade multiple advances have been made in the understanding of trauma-induced bleeding. In this chapter we review the current theories on the pathogenesis of traumatic hemorrhage and the current approaches to diagnosis and treatment.

■ OVERVIEW OF NORMAL HEMOSTASIS

Normal hemostasis involves the coordinated, synergistic, and balanced interactions of the vascular system, platelets, procoagulant and anticoagulant proteins, and the fibrinolytic system. In the absence of vascular injury, each component exists in a quiescent state such that the blood remains fluid but has the potential to rapidly form an insoluble coagulum and platelet plug. In the event of injury, exposed subendothelial collagen binds to platelets via von Willebrand factor, and tissue factor activates the coagulation cascade to form fibrin clot. The vessel wall simultaneously contracts to reduce blood loss and shunts blood to intact vessels.

The prothrombotic potential of platelets and the coagulation proteins is tempered by platelet inhibitors such as prostacyclin and nitric oxide and by endogenous anticoagulants such as antithrombin, protein C, and protein S that downregulate thrombin generation and fibrin formation. In addition, the fibrinolytic system digests fibrin clot, preventing its dissemination beyond the breached vessel (Figure 1).

In major trauma, severe tissue injury and hypoperfusion precipitate massive activation of hemostatic and inflammatory responses that are maladaptive and can lead to a fatal hemorrhagic diathesis. The following section describes the current theories on the pathogenesis of trauma-induced coagulopathy (TIC).

■ TRAUMA-INDUCED COAGULOPATHY

Historically, the coagulopathy associated with trauma has been attributed to massive tissue factor release triggering disseminated intravascular coagulation (DIC) with consumption of platelets and coagulation factors leading to a bleeding diathesis; a dilutional coagulopathy resulting from intravenous (IV) fluids used in resuscitation; and the negative impact of acidosis, hypothermia, and hypocalcemia on coagulation protein function. In the past 10 years Brohi and colleagues have demonstrated that the coagulopathy of trauma is not an iatrogenic insult induced by resuscitation but a consequence of the traumatic injury. Brohi has called this entity trauma-induced

coagulopathy (TIC). Brohi and colleagues have noted that acute tissue injury and hypoperfusion activate protein C, leading to degradation of factors V, Va (activated factor V), and VIIIa (activated factor VIII). The auto-anticoagulant phenotype of TIC also may result from endothelial damage and degradation of endothelial glycocalyx, which has anticoagulant properties similar to heparin. Thrombocytopenia and platelet dysfunction also contribute to the pathogenesis of TIC and are strong predictors of mortality. Hyperfibrinolysis also has been demonstrated in patients with TIC, which Brohi and colleagues propose is because of degradation of plasminogen activator inhibitor-1, the principal endogenous negative regulator of tissue plasminogen activator (tPA), by activated protein C. Gando and colleagues have attributed TIC to thrombin activation and factor and platelet consumption as seen in DIC accentuated by secondary fibrinolysis (Figure 2).

The acute coagulopathy of trauma can be compounded further by hypothermia, acidosis, hemodilution, and hypocalcemia. The coagulation cascade is a series of enzymatic reactions. Enzymatic reactions are temperature sensitive. Hypothermia can be classified as mild (temperature <32°C to 35°C), moderate (28°C to 32°C), or severe (20°C to 28°C). There is a 10% reduction in coagulation factor activity for each 1°C drop in body temperature. Temperatures below 33°C have been shown to reduce coagulation factor activity below 33% and alter fibrin kinetics. Hypothermia also affects platelet function by reducing the rate of thromboxane B2 production and the interaction of platelet surface glycoproteins with von Willebrand factor. Hypothermia also may cause hepatic sequestration of platelets. Core body temperatures above 34°C adjusted for other variables have a mortality rate of 7%, which increases to 40% with core body temperatures below 34°C. To reduce iatrogenic hypothermia, cold wet clothing should be removed; patients should be covered with warming blankets; and IV fluids, blood products, and operating rooms should be kept warm.

Massive injury and prolonged hypotension can cause acidosis, which in conjunction with hypothermia can significantly impair hemostasis. Acidosis significantly impairs coagulation protease function at a pH below 7.1. Activation of thrombin is reduced by 50% at a pH of 7.2 and by 90% at a pH of 6.8. Acidosis impairs the propagation phase of clot formation and promotes accelerated degradation of fibrin by a factor of 1.8. Platelet aggregation is impaired by 50% at a pH of 7.1 or less because of changes in platelet structure. Although bicarbonate and Tris(hydroxymethyl)aminomethane (THAM) have both been shown to increase pH, there is no evidence that these medications can significantly improve hemostasis in trauma patients.

After trauma injury the body attempts to correct hypotension by shifting extravascular fluid into the intravascular space. This adaptive response is compounded by administration of crystalloids during routine resuscitation. The result can be a dilutional coagulopathy that reduces coagulation factor levels and platelets. Among trauma patients who receive more than 2 L of fluid, more than 40% develop a coagulopathy. The incidence of coagulopathy increases to more than 50% among patients who receive more than 3 L of fluid and to more than 70% among patients who receive more than 4 L of fluid. Crystalloids also lead to tissue edema and compartment syndrome and promote inflammation. Therefore current trauma resuscitation

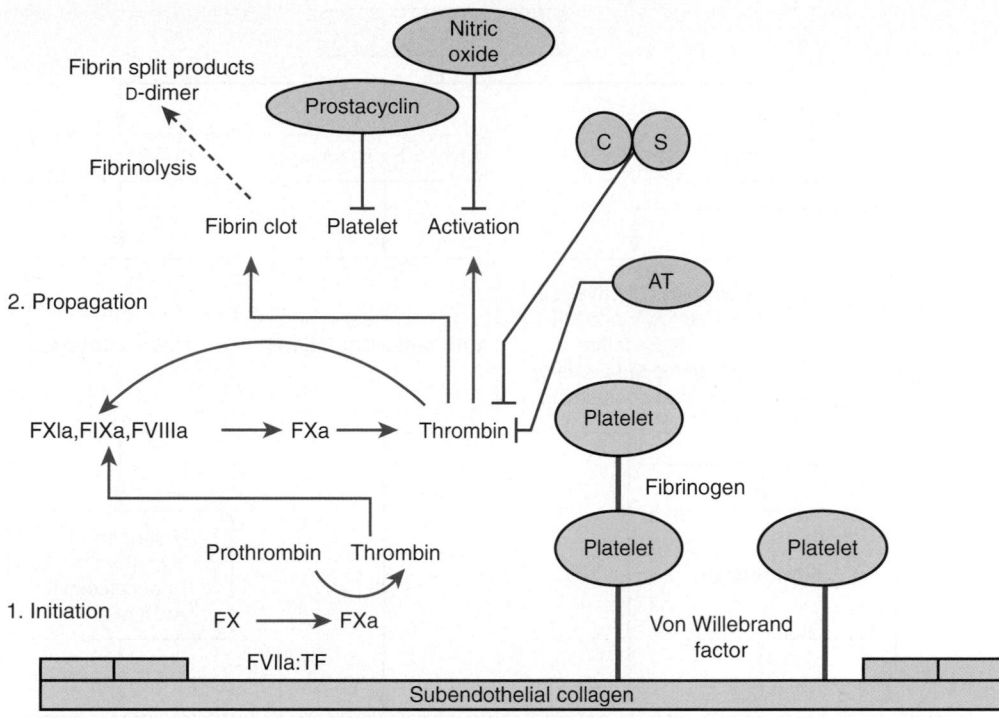

FIGURE 1 Diagram of normal hemostasis. Hemostasis is initiated by the exposure of subendothelial collagen, which initiates activation of the coagulation cascade through tissue factor (TF) and factor VIIa (FVIIa). Subsequent production of small amounts of thrombin results in propagation and amplification of the coagulation response, leading to fibrin clot formation and platelet activation. Collagen exposure also triggers platelet adhesion and aggregation through interactions with von Willebrand factor (adhesion) and fibrinogen (aggregation). The endogenous anticoagulant proteins, antithrombin (AT) and the protein C (C)/protein S (S) complex, inhibit thrombin activity and generation, and prostacyclin and nitric oxide inhibit platelet function. The fibrinolytic system degrades fibrin clot into fibrin degradation products such as D-dimers. *FIXa*, Activated factor IX; *FVIIIa*, activated factor VIII; *FX*, factor X; *FXa*, activated factor X; *FXIa*, activated factor XI.

guidelines recommend permissive hypotension with a mean arterial pressure (MAP) of 50 mm Hg. Hypotensive resuscitation (MAP ≥50 mm Hg) is associated with lower blood product use, a decreased incidence of coagulopathy, and lower mortality compared with standard resuscitation goals (mean MAP of 65 mm Hg). An exception is made for patients with severe traumatic brain injury (Glasgow Coma Scale score ≤8) or spinal injury where a MAP of 80 mm Hg or higher is recommended to maintain tissue perfusion.

Calcium is essential for normal coagulation. About 55% of calcium is bound to albumin, and the rest is ionized calcium. Calcium ions are essential for the vitamin K–dependent coagulation factors II (prothrombin), VII, IX, and X to bind to the phospholipid-rich membranes of activated platelets. Calcium is also necessary for fibrin polymerization, clot stabilization, and platelet aggregation and activity. For optimal functioning of the hemostatic system, the ionized calcium concentration should be maintained above 0.9 mmol/L. Infusion of IV fluids and citrated blood products such as plasma and packed red blood cells can cause hypocalcemia, so close monitoring of calcium levels should be performed in all trauma patients.

The incidence of TIC also is influenced by the type of traumatic injury. Patients with severe blunt force trauma experience more widespread tissue damage than those with penetrating trauma, where damage is more localized, so victims of blunt force trauma are more prone to TIC. In patients with traumatic brain injury (TBI), local release of tissue factor, which activates the coagulation cascade, may potentiate TIC and cause greater coagulation abnormalities. Nonetheless, hypotension and decreased tissue perfusion appear to be the biggest drivers of TIC.

The presence of concomitant disease states and drug therapy also can influence TIC adversely. Patients with diseases of the bone marrow, kidney, and liver can have hemostatic aberrations because of decreased blood counts, platelet function, and coagulation factor activity. Patients on antiplatelet medications, such as aspirin, clopidogrel, and prasugrel, and on anticoagulants, such as warfarin, low-molecular-weight heparin (LMWH), and direct oral anticoagulants, will present additional challenges to hemostatic management.

Clinical Assessment of Trauma-Induced Coagulopathy

Clinical examination of the trauma patient focuses on vital signs and vital sign trends as well as signs and symptoms of bleeding, including changes in mental status, urine output, abdominal distension, evidence of penetrating wounds, and intra-abdominal hemorrhage, including Cullen's sign (ecchymosis around the umbilicus or over the left upper quadrant reflecting intra-abdominal bleeding or splenic rupture) and Grey Turner's sign (flank bruising reflecting retroperitoneal hemorrhage) (Tables 1 and 2). Thoracic trauma should prompt investigation for pneumothorax and hemothorax as well as rib and sternal fracture and rupture of the thoracic aorta. Clinical examination is supplemented with imaging techniques, including chest and abdominal radiographs, ultrasonography (including bedside), computed tomography, and angiography.

Laboratory testing in the diagnosis of TIC relies on standard laboratory studies, including complete blood cell (CBC) count, activated partial thromboplastin time (aPTT), prothrombin time (PT), fibrinogen, arterial blood gas analysis, and lactate, as well as on point-of-care (POC) testing with thromboelastography (TEG) or rotational thromboelastometry (ROTEM). Serial monitoring of the laboratory tests is essential to monitor the patient for ongoing bleeding and progressive coagulopathy. Standard laboratory testing has a number of limitations. The CBC count assesses only platelet numbers, not platelet function. Similarly, the PT, aPTT, and fibrinogen do not provide the most accurate picture of hemostasis in vivo, as they are

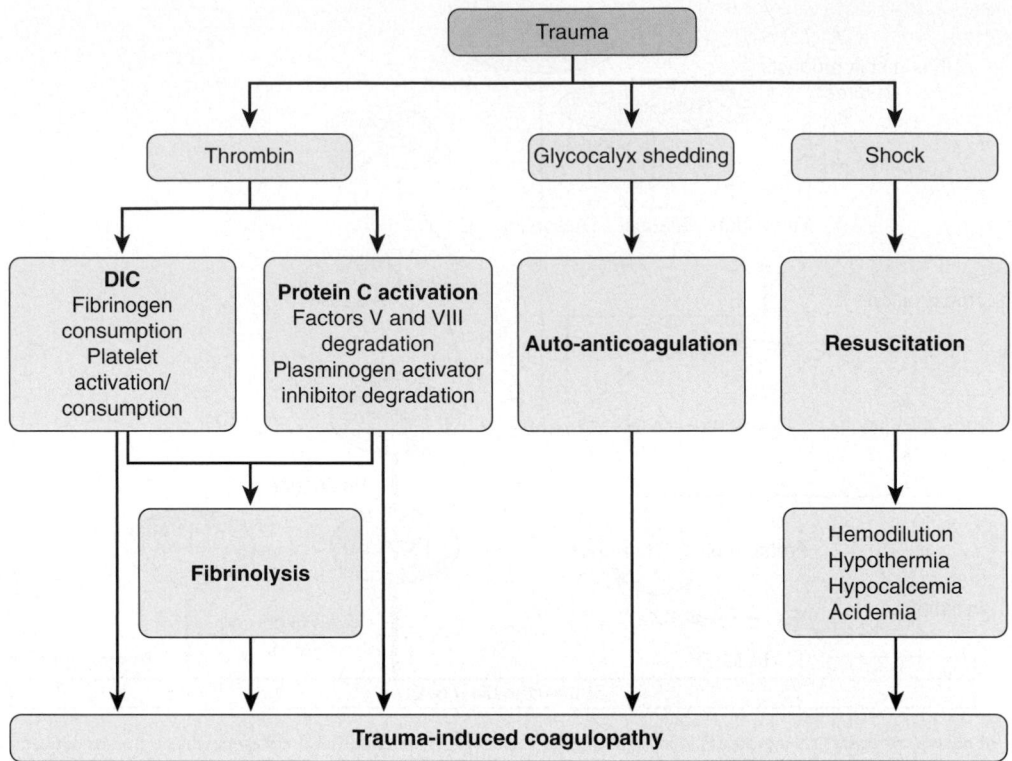

FIGURE 2 The pathogenesis of trauma-induced coagulopathy (TIC). TIC is multifactorial. Trauma results in thrombin generation, which may induce a coagulopathy by activation of the coagulation cascade and fibrinogen as well as platelets, leading to a consumptive coagulopathy akin to disseminated intravascular coagulation (DIC). Secondary fibrinolysis can result in clot lysis and microvascular bleeding. Alternatively, the coagulopathy of trauma may result from the formation of thrombin-thrombomodulin complexes, which activate protein C and degrade factors V and VIII and plasminogen activator inhibitor-1. Some evidence suggests that endothelial injury may trigger shedding of the endothelial glycocalyx, which contains endogenous glycosaminoglycan anticoagulants that lead to a coagulopathic state. Hypotension and fluid resuscitation contribute to the coagulopathy of trauma by leading to hypothermia, hypocalcemia, acidosis, and a dilutional coagulopathy.

TABLE 1: Advanced Trauma Life Support Classification of Blood Loss Based on Initial Patient Presentation

Parameter	Class I	Class II	Class III	Class IV
Estimated blood loss	Up to 750 mL	750-1500 mL	1500 to 2000 mL	More than 2000 mL
Estimated blood loss	Up to 15% blood volume	15% to 30% blood volume	30% to 40% blood volume	More than 40% blood volume
Pulse rate	<100	100 to 120	120 to 140	More than 140
Systolic blood pressure	Normal	Normal	Decreased	Decreased
Pulse pressure	Normal or increased	Decreased	Decreased	Decreased
Respiratory rate	14 to 20	20 to 30	30 to 40	More than 35
Urine output	More than 30 mL/hr	20 to 30 mL/hr	5 to 15 mL/hr	Negligible
Mental status	Slightly anxious	Mildly anxious	Anxious, confused	Confused, lethargic
Initial fluid replacement	Crystalloid	Crystalloid	Crystalloid and blood	Crystalloid and blood

Adapted from Spahn DR, Bouillon B, Cerny V, et al. Management of bleeding and coagulopathy following major trauma: an updated European guideline. *Crit Care.* 2013;17:R76.

performed at 37°C and at a normal pH and thus do not reflect the true extent of the coagulopathy in vivo. The PT and aPTT are relatively insensitive to reduced factor levels until they decline below 30%. In addition, conventional laboratory testing takes a median of 80 minutes to perform and does not provide information on clot strength and fibrinolysis.

The shortcomings of conventional laboratory testing have stimulated interest in POC tests. The i-STAT critical care analyzer (Abbott Point of Care Inc., Princeton, NJ) is a handheld POC hemoglobin analyzer that can provide results within minutes. Although excellent agreement with the central laboratory CBC count was obtained in cardiac surgery patients, moderate concordance with the CBC count

TABLE 2: Advanced Trauma Life Support Responses to Initial Fluid Resuscitation

Parameter	Rapid Response	Transient Response	Minimal or No Response
Vital signs	Return to normal	Transient improvement; recurrence of hypotension, tachycardia	Remain abnormal
Estimated blood loss	Minimal (10% to 20% blood volume)	Moderate and ongoing (20% to 40% blood volume)	Severe (more than 40% blood volume)
Need for more crystalloid	Low	Low to moderate	Moderate as bridge to blood transfusion
Need for blood	Low	Moderate to high	Immediate
Blood preparation	Type and crossmatch	Type-specific	Emergency blood release
Need for surgery	Possible	Likely	Highly likely
Early presence of surgeon	Yes	Yes	Yes

Adapted from Spahn DR, Bouillon B, Cerny V, et al. Management of bleeding and coagulopathy following major trauma: an updated European guideline. *Crit Care*. 2013;17:R76.

was noted in trauma patients. A meta-analysis of 32 studies of non-invasive hemoglobin testing in 4425 patients using co-oximetry and spectroscopy devices recommended caution when using these devices for decision making regarding transfusions. More positive results have been noted with POC viscoelastic hemostatic tests such as thromboelastography (TEG 5000 Thrombelastograph Hemostasis Analyzer, Haemoscope Inc., Niles, IL) and rotational thromboelastometry (ROTEM, Tem Systems Inc., Durham, NC). Unlike central laboratory coagulation tests, these viscoelastic POC tests provide a rapid assessment of whole blood coagulation as well as platelet and fibrinogen function and fibrinolysis. In the TEG system, the whole blood sample is placed in a sample cup in which a pin is suspended. The cup rotates back and forth through an arc of 4 degrees 45 minutes every 5 seconds, which recreates the low-shear environment of venous blood flow. As fibrin strands are formed, they cause the pin to deviate toward the side of the sample cup. With the onset of fibrinolysis, the pin deviates back toward the center of the sample cup. The process of clot formation, contraction, and fibrinolysis is measured and graphically displayed by a transducer or electromagnetic sensing system attached to the pin, which sends the information to a computer for analysis and graphing. In rapid TEG (rTEG) activators of coagulation such as kaolin or kaolin and tissue factor can be used to accelerate the clotting process, so results on activated clotting time are available within 5 minutes.

In ROTEM, the pin rather than the cup oscillates through an angle of 4 degrees 75 minutes every 6 seconds, and clot formation is detected by an optical transducer. Both tests measure the time to onset of clot formation (in TEG, r time for reaction time; in ROTEM, clotting time or CT). In both TEG and ROTEM, the alpha angle represents the burst of thrombin generation that results in rapid fibrin formation and pin deviation. The coagulation time or k time (TEG) or clot formation time (ROTEM) represents the kinetics of clot formation. The maximal amplitude (MA) with TEG or the maximal clot formation (MCF) with ROTEM represents the maximal strength of the clot, reflecting the joint contributions of fibrin and platelets. Addition of antibodies directed against glycoprotein IIb/IIIa (abciximab) and inhibitors of platelet cytoskeletal proteins (cytochalasin D) can be used with ROTEM to focus exclusively on the contribution of fibrinogen to clot strength, the so-called FIBTEM. The FIBTEM has been demonstrated to be a predictive parameter of coagulopathic bleeding in trauma, cardiac surgery, and massive postpartum hemorrhage. Excessive fibrinolysis or hyperfibrinolysis has

been associated with poor outcomes. Measurement of hyerfibrinolysis with TEG and ROTEM has been shown to be associated with increased mortality in trauma patients. FIBTEM and MCF have been shown to predict the need for massive transfusion more accurately than PT. Goal-directed transfusion therapy based on point-of-care ROTEM testing protocols has been shown to be associated with lower than expected mortality and reduced need for blood products. However, a Cochrane systematic review found that although TEG- or ROTEM-guided transfusion protocols were associated with reduced bleeding, they had no impact on morbidity or mortality. Therefore prospective management trials assessing the benefits of POC viscoelastic testing protocols are needed.

The limitations of TEG and ROTEM include long testing times (clotting time within 5 minutes, but full hemostatic analysis with fibrinolysis requires 30 to 40 minutes) and the need for testing at 37°C (although testing algorithms can be adjusted to 32°C and 39°C). Normal results have been seen in patients with von Willebrand disease and platelet dysfunction associated with antiplatelet medications. In addition, POC testing requires daily calibration to ensure quality control and ongoing training to ensure that testing is performed correctly.

The 2014 update of the European practice guideline on management of trauma-associated coagulopathy recommended that early and repeated measurements of PT, aPTT, fibrinogen, and platelets and POC viscoelastic testing (TEG, ROTEM) be used to characterize TIC and guide hemostatic therapy.

Management of Trauma-Induced Coagulopathy

The recent evolution of understanding of TIC has led to a shift in clinical management to damage control resuscitation (Figure 3). This approach involves management of the "lethal triad" by addressing hypothermia, correcting acidosis, and restricting resuscitative fluids to avoid dilutional coagulopathy and allow permissive hypotension, early correction of coagulopathy, and hemostatic management. The damage control strategy involves a "grab and run" approach in the field involving temporary cessation of bleeding by direct pressure, use of tourniquets, and bandaging. There is minimal fluid resuscitation followed by in-hospital control of bleeding or damage control surgery to control hemorrhage. This is followed by further stabilization of the patient in the intensive care unit (ICU) and then finally by plans for definitive surgery.

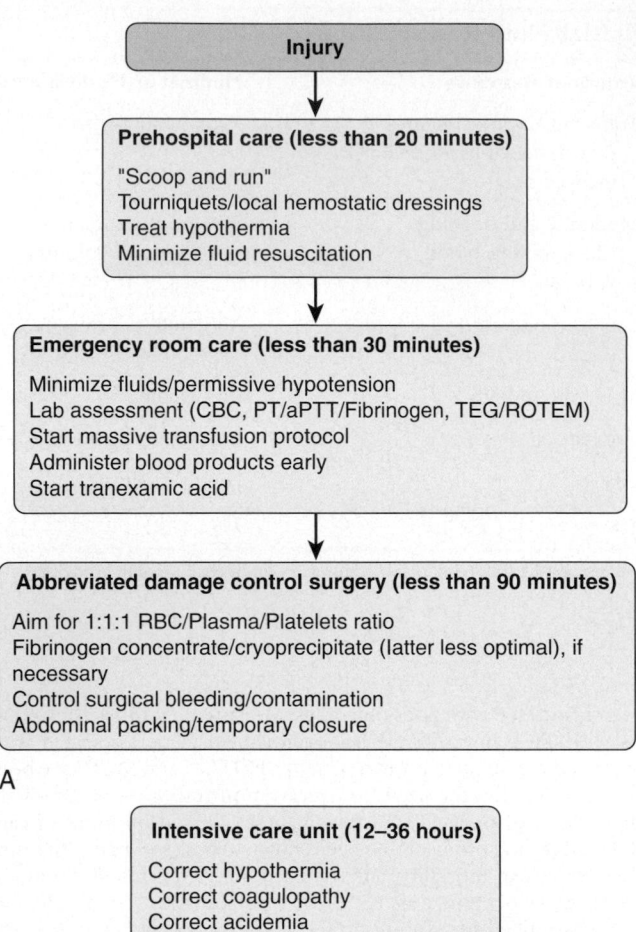

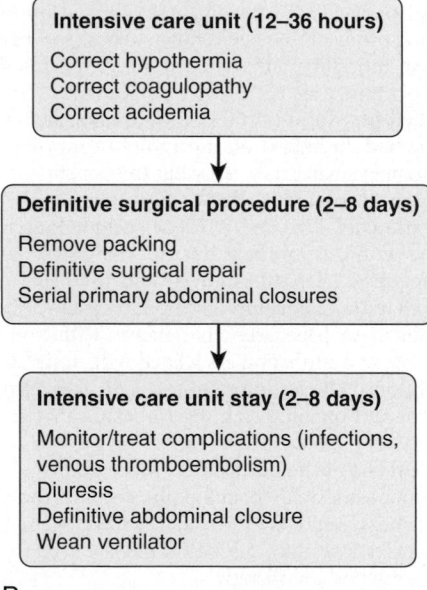

FIGURE 3 A and **B,** Contemporary approach to traumatic injury management. *aPTT,* Activated partial thromboplastin time; *CBC,* complete blood cell count; *PT,* prothrombin time; *RBC,* red blood cells; *ROTEM,* rotational thromboelastometry; *TEG,* thromboelastography. *(Adapted from Kaafarani HM, Velmahos GC. Damage control resuscitation in trauma. Scand J Surg. 2014;103:81-88.)*

Permissive Hypotension

Instead of the traditional approach to restoring near normal blood pressure, permissive hypotension aims to maintain a MAP of 50 mm Hg, limiting systolic blood pressure to 80 to 100 mm Hg. This strategy is supported by animal trauma models, which demonstrated that restoration of systolic blood pressure above 90 mm Hg was associated with disruption of hemostatic plugs, rebleeding, and worse

outcomes. These results have been confirmed in trauma patients. Patients whose MAP was maintained above 50 mm Hg required less IV fluids and fewer blood products and had lower mortality than patients with a MAP target of 65 mm Hg. One exception to this rule is patients with TBI, where maintenance of intracranial perfusion pressure is of paramount importance to limit neurologic injury. Therefore maintenance of a MAP of 80 mm Hg is recommended for patients with TBI.

Targeting a lower mean arterial blood pressure limits administration of IV crystalloid, reducing the likelihood of dilutional coagulopathy. If IV fluids are used in resuscitation, a randomized controlled trial in ICU patients found no advantage to colloid (albumin) versus crystalloid. Albumin was associated with worse survival in patients with TBI. Use of hypertonic saline is not associated with benefit in TBI or hypovolemic shock and may increase nosocomial infections in patients with TBI. Hypotonic solutions should be avoided in TBI, as they can increase intracerebral edema.

Hypothermia, Acidosis, and Hypocalcemia

Hypothermia is a key component of the lethal triad. Passive warming (warm ambient temperature, blankets, removal of wet or cold clothing) and active warming (forced hot air warming devices, warmed IV fluids and blood products) techniques should be used. Acidosis can contribute to TIC, but there is no evidence that use of IV bicarbonate or THAM is beneficial. Instead, aggressive blood product support and surgical control of bleeding should be emphasized. If reversal of severe acidosis is necessary, experts have recommended THAM over bicarbonate because it does not result in excess sodium administration or carbon dioxide production.

Calcium is necessary for normal function of vitamin K–dependent coagulation factors II (prothrombin), VII, IX, and X. Therefore maintenance of normal calcium concentrations is necessary for normal hemostasis. Blood products contain large amounts of sodium citrate as an anticoagulant, which can result in systemic hypocalcemia. Because citrate is metabolized by the liver, patients with hypotensive shock liver are at especially high risk for hypocalcemia. Hypocalcemia has been associated with increased mortality. Therefore the 2014 European trauma guidelines recommend regular monitoring of ionized calcium during massive transfusion and calcium supplementation as needed to maintain calcium levels in the normal range.

Blood Product Management

Transfusional management of traumatic injuries has been influenced profoundly by advances made in the treatment of combat injuries. Experience in the Iraq War suggested that a transfusion ratio of 1:1:1 for red blood cells, platelets, and plasma was associated with improved outcomes for patients with massive bleeding. It is important to note that these studies and subsequent civilian studies are observational and mostly retrospective in nature. No randomized controlled studies have been conducted. Many of the studies suffer from survivorship bias such that patients who survived longer were more likely to live long enough to receive more plasma, which requires time to thaw. A meta-analysis demonstrated that a plasma to red blood cell ratio of 1:1 to 1:2.5 was associated with a 62% reduction in the risk for death, although the authors underscored that the level of supporting evidence was low. A recent prospective study that measured hemostatic parameters after every 4 units of blood found that plasma to red blood cell ratios of 1:2 to 3:4 were associated with optimal hemostasis by laboratory testing. Nevertheless, the ideal ratio of blood products to treat TIC remains to be defined. The current European trauma guidelines recommend that plasma be administered in a ratio of at least 1:2 with red blood cells in patients with massive hemorrhage. A target hemoglobin of 7 to 9 g/dL should be maintained.

Fresh Whole Blood

The military has been using fresh whole blood (FWB) since World War I. A single 500-mL unit of FWB has a hematocrit (Hct) of 38%

to 50%, 15 to 40 × 10^5 platelets, and 100% clotting factor activity. This makes FWB an attractive replacement product, especially in combat settings where there is a large and ready supply of available donors. The use of whole blood (WB) in civilian trauma patients is uncommon. A civilian trial conducted by Cotton and colleagues reported that use of WB was not superior to use of individual blood components in severely injured patients predicted to receive massive transfusion.

Packed Red Blood Cells

Most patients who are actively bleeding receive packed red blood cells (PRBCs) instead of WB. Red blood cells not only improve tissue perfusion and oxygenation, but PRBCs also express phosphatidylserine on their surface and so actively participate in thrombin generation and hence assist in coagulation. PRBCs also augment hemostasis via a phenomenon called "margination" where PRBCs cause platelets to shift toward the periphery, increasing their proximity to injured vessel walls and facilitating adhesion during trauma. Anemia is associated with a reduction in platelet aggregation and activation. A drop in the Hct from 40% to 10% decreases platelet function fivefold. The loss of as little as 2 units of blood is associated with a 60% increase in the bleeding time.

PRBC transfusions are not without risks. Acute reactions include acute febrile or hemolytic transfusion reactions and hypocalcemia due to the acid citrate dextrose used as an anticoagulant in PRBC units. The delayed effects of PRBCs include transfusion-transmitted infections, delayed immunologic transfusion reactions, multiorgan failure, systemic inflammatory response syndrome, and sepsis. Mortality is increased in trauma patients transfused with PRBCs and is further increased with the use of blood products more than 14 days old. Strategies to minimize the need for PRBCs include intraoperative salvage of spent red blood cells, permissive hypotension, and ICU protocols with lower transfusion triggers. Regarding the logistics, group O PRBCs and AB plasma are used as universal donor products, and they are available immediately for transfusion. Type-specific blood usually is available in 5 to 10 minutes, and crossmatched blood usually takes 40 minutes to 1 hour to prepare.

Plasma

Plasma is an excellent source of albumin and all of the coagulation factors, including fibrinogen. Plasma is collected from WB or by apheresis and is termed fresh frozen plasma (FFP) if it is frozen within 8 hours of collection or called FP24 if frozen within 24 hours. FFP is stored at −25°C and keeps for 1 year. It requires thawing before use and should be compatible with the recipient ABO type. Because FFP must be thawed before use and thawing plasma can take time, major trauma centers usually have thawed plasma on hand. In addition, they have rapid thawing devices that can thaw 2 units of plasma in about 2 minutes. Once thawed, plasma should be transfused within 24 hours. Thawed plasma can be kept refrigerated for 5 days. A 250-mL unit of plasma provides about 500 mg of fibrinogen. There is some loss of factors V and VIII, but most coagulation factors are still available at satisfactory levels.

Another type of plasma called liquid plasma or never frozen plasma keeps for 26 days and can be used in settings where availability of thawed plasma may be problematic. Lyophilized or freeze dried plasma initially was used by the U.S. Army in World War II for rapid resuscitation of war casualties. This plasma is compatible with all blood groups and does not contain ABO antibodies. It is leukocyte depleted and attenuated to reduce the risk for infection and transfusion-related reactions. It can be stored at room temperature for 2 years and reconstituted within minutes. Some studies have examined its use for prehospital treatment of hemorrhagic shock in the civilian population, but so far this is not routine practice. Disadvantages of plasma include its greater product volume (although this can be an advantage during resuscitation), transfusion-associated infectious diseases (less for solvent/detergent-treated plasma), transfusion-related acute lung injury (TRALI), and allergic reactions.

Fibrinogen Replacement

Fibrinogen is the precursor to fibrin clot and the principal mediator of platelet aggregation. Hypofibrinogenemia is common in patients with massive blood loss and independently associated with severe bleeding in patients with postpartum hemorrhage. In a multicenter trial, fibrinogen values below 229 mg/dL were associated with significantly increased mortality. Fibrinogen function can be monitored using conventional laboratory assays such as the Clauss fibrinogen assay or with POC tests such as TEG or ROTEM. Retrospective studies suggest that the use of TEG and ROTEM for blood product management is associated with reduced mortality and blood product usage, although confirmatory prospective studies are needed. Fibrinogen can be administered via FFP, cryoprecipitate, or fibrinogen concentrate (Table 3).

A prospective study of 517 trauma patients found that cryoprecipitate or fibrinogen concentrate, but not plasma, was able to maintain fibrinogen concentrations and that patients with fibrinogen supplementation had better outcomes. Cryoprecipitate, the precipitate harvested after thawing FFP slowly at 4°C, contains 150 to 250 mg of fibrinogen per 15- to 20-mL unit. In an average-size adult (80 kg), each unit of cryoprecipitate should raise the fibrinogen level 10 mg/dL. An advantage of cryoprecipitate is that it allows infusion of larger amounts of fibrinogen (2500 mg in one 10-unit transfusion) in a smaller fluid volume (200 mL), avoiding the larger volumes required for FFP and allowing for more rapid administration of fibrinogen. Disadvantages of cryoprecipitate include the risk for transfusion-associated infectious diseases (10 donor exposures for one 10-unit cryoprecipitate transfusion), TRALI, and allergic reactions.

Fibrinogen concentrates such as RiaSTAP (CSL Behring, Kankakee, IL) are virally inactivated concentrates of human fibrinogen that have been approved by the U.S. Food and Drug Administration (FDA) for the treatment of congenital afibrinogenemia and hypofibrinogenemia. Fibrinogen concentrates afford the advantages of a more rapid preparation time, larger fibrinogen concentrations in smaller infusion volumes, and lower risks for transfusion-related infectious diseases. The European trauma guidelines recommend close monitoring of fibrinogen levels with TEG or ROTEM and replacement with fibrinogen concentrate (3 to 4 grams for a 70-kg adult) or cryoprecipitate (15 to 20 units for a 70-kg adult). Repeat doses should be guided by serial TEG or ROTEM monitoring.

Platelets

Platelets are a critical component of the hemostatic plug. Platelet counts less than 100,000/μL and 50,000/μL have been identified as thresholds below which diffuse bleeding and microvascular bleeding, respectively, ensue. Therefore expert panels have recommended that platelet counts should not be allowed to decline below 50,000/μL in patients with traumatic injuries and that platelet counts should be maintained above 100,000/μL for patients with massive bleeding or TBI. The standard dose of platelets is 1 platelet concentrate (60 to 80 × 10^9 platelets) per 10 kg body weight. This dose should increase the platelet count by 30,000 to 50,000/μL (see Table 3).

Antiplatelet Medications

It is important to note that platelet count does not measure platelet function and that severe injury is associated with platelet dysfunction. In addition, use of antiplatelet medications is common in the general public. Pretrauma use of antiplatelet medications has been associated with an increased risk of intracranial hemorrhage in patients with head trauma. However, viscoelastic POC tests do not appear to be sensitive to platelet dysfunction. Platelet function testing with whole blood platelet aggregometry is the gold standard. For reversing platelet dysfunction associated with aspirin, transfusion of 5 units of platelets is recommended. For patients on dual antiplatelet regimens (i.e., aspirin and clopidogrel), 10 to 25 units of platelets are recommended (see Table 3).

Anticoagulant Medications

Use of anticoagulant medications is widespread in the general public given the prevalence of thromboembolic disorders such as atrial fibrillation and venous thromboembolism. In patients taking warfarin, a four-factor prothrombin complex concentrate (Kcentra, CSL Behring, King of Prussia, PA) that contains all of the vitamin K–dependent factors is superior to FFP for rapid reversal of warfarin. IV vitamin K (infuse no faster than 1 mg/min) should be administered to ensure sustained reversal. Protamine should be used for reversal of unfractionated heparin and LMWH, although protamine only partially reverses LMWH (dalteparin 80% reversal, enoxaparin 60% reversal). There is growing use of direct oral anticoagulants such as the oral direct thrombin inhibitor dabigatran and the oral direct factor Xa inhibitors apixaban, edoxaban, and rivaroxaban. Idarucizumab (Praxbind, Boehringer Ingelheim, Ridgefield, CT), a humanized mouse monoclonal antibody against dabigatran, has been demonstrated to rapidly reverse dabigatran and should be administered in any trauma patient on dabigatran. Andexanet alfa, a recombinant modified inactive form of factor Xa, has been demonstrated in phase II trials to rapidly reverse the anticoagulant effects of apixaban and rivaroxaban. It has been granted fast track designation by the FDA and is expected to be approved in the next 12 months. Until it is available for reversal of oral direct factor Xa inhibitors, prothrombin complex concentrates (Kcentra) or activated prothrombin complex concentrates (FEIBA NF, Baxter Healthcare Corporation, Westlake Village, CA) should be used for the reversal of these anticoagulants in the setting of life-threatening bleeding (dose of 25 to 50 units/kg; see Table 3).

Recombinant Activated Factor VII

Recombinant activated factor VII (rfVIIa) (Novoseven RT, Novo Nordisk, Plainsboro, NJ) is a recombinant concentrate of activated factor VII that was developed initially for treatment of hemophilia with factor VIII inhibitors. It since has been applied to a broad array of patients with refractory bleeding, including trauma patients. In two parallel randomized placebo-controlled trials involving 301 severely injured trauma patients, Bofford and colleagues found that rFVIIa reduced RBC transfusion and the need for massive transfusion in patients with blunt but not penetrating trauma. In the CONTROL trial, Hauser and colleagues randomized major trauma patients who had bled 4 to 8 units of blood within 12 hours of surgery and were still bleeding despite damage control resuscitation and operative management. The trial was terminated early because of futility after enrolling 573 of 1502 patients. The authors found that rFVIIa reduced blood product use but did not improve mortality.

TABLE 3: Hemostatic Agents for Management of Traumatic Bleeding

Hemostatic Agent	Indication	Mechanism of Action	Dose
Tranexamic acid	Active bleeding or significant risk of bleeding	Inhibits plasmin-mediated fibrinolysis	1 g IV over 10 minutes followed by 1 g over 8 hours
Cryoprecipitate	Fibrinogen deficit (fibrinogen <150-200 mg/dL or fibrinogen deficit by TEG or ROTEM)	Corrects fibrinogen deficit	15-20 single-donor units in 70-kg adult
Fibrinogen concentrate	Fibrinogen deficit (fibrinogen <150-200 mg/dL or fibrinogen deficit by TEG or ROTEM)	Corrects fibrinogen deficit	3-4 g in 70-kg adult
Recombinant activated factor VII	Persistent major bleeding despite conventional hemostatic measures	Induces burst of thrombin generation, triggering platelet activation, fibrin clot formation	Initial dose of 200 μg/kg IV followed by 100 μg/kg at 1 and 3 hours later
Platelets	Thrombocytopenia	Restores adequate functional platelet mass for hemostasis	1 platelet concentrate per 10 kg (increases platelets 30,000-50,000/μL)
Platelets	Reversal of antiplatelet medications	Restores adequate functional platelet mass for hemostasis	For reversal of aspirin: 5-10 platelet concentrates. For reversal of dual antiplatelet agents: 10-25 platelet concentrates
Vitamin K	Warfarin reversal	Bypass warfarin inhibition of vitamin K–dependent coagulation factor synthesis	10 mg of vitamin K IV (slow infusion no faster than 1 mg/min)
Prothrombin complex concentrate	Warfarin reversal	Replaces vitamin K–dependent coagulation factors	INR 2-3.9: dose 25 units/kg (not to exceed 2500 units). INR 4-6: dose 35 units/kg (not to exceed 3500 units). INR >6: dose 50 units/kg (not to exceed 5000 units)
Idarucizumab	Dabigatran reversal	Antibody binds and inactivates dabigatran	5 g IV (administered as two 2.5-g IV 50 mL infusions)

INR, International normalized ratio; *IV*, intravenously; *ROTEM*, rotational thromboelastometry; *TEG*, thromboelastography.

A case-control study of rFVIIa in patients with TBI was associated with higher mortality. In light of these results, the European trauma guidelines suggested that rFVIIa be considered if major bleeding and traumatic coagulopathy persist despite conventional therapy. The recommended dose is 200 µg/kg for the first dose and 100 µg/kg for doses 2 and 3, administered 1 and 3 hours after the first dose (see Table 3). Studies have suggested that rFVIIa is ineffective in patients with a pH of 7.2 or less, platelet counts less than 100,000/µL, hypothermia, and hypocalcemia, so these conditions should be corrected before therapy. The guidelines do not support the use of rFVIIa in patients with TBI.

Tranexamic Acid

Tranexamic acid (Cyklokapron, Pfizer, New York, NY) is a lysine analogue that inhibits fibrinolysis because of its activity as a competitive inhibitor of plasminogen activation and at high doses as a noncompetitive inhibitor of plasmin. In the CRASH-2 trial, tranexamic acid (1-g loading dose over 10 minutes followed by 1 g over 8 hours) significantly reduced all-cause mortality (14.5% vs 16%; relative risk [RR] 0.91 [95% confidence interval: 0.85 to 0.97]) and the risk for death due to bleeding (4.9% vs 5.7%; RR 0.85 [95% confidence interval: 0.76 to 0.96]). Further analysis found that early administration of tranexamic acid (within 1 hour and 1 to 3 hours of trauma) was associated with reduced death due to bleeding but that administration after 3 hours increased the risk for death due to bleeding (4.4% vs 3.1%; RR 1.44 [95% confidence interval: 1.12 to 1.84]). The European trauma guidelines recommend that tranexamic acid be administered as early as possible (within 3 hours) after injury. Clinical data regarding the use of other antifibrinolytic agents such as aminocaproic acid and aprotinin are still lacking (see Table 3).

Desmopressin

Desmopressin (DDAVP; 1-desamino-8-D-arginine vasopressin) is a vasopressin analogue that induces the release of preformed stores of von Willebrand factor and factor VIII from the endothelium. Desmopressin is used in the treatment of mild von Willebrand disease, hemophilia A, and platelet dysfunction disorders. There are no studies documenting the efficacy of desmopressin in trauma patients.

Local Hemostatic Agents and Dressings

Local hemostatic agents and dressings are important adjuncts to blood products in achieving hemostasis in trauma patients. Collagen-based hemostatic agents induce platelet aggregation. They often are combined with thrombin to activate fibrin clot formation. Gelatin-based products swell when in contact with blood, resulting in local compression of bleeding vessels. These products often contain thrombin to activate the coagulation cascade. Fibrin sealants have been used extensively in cardiac and vascular surgery, neurosurgery, and orthopedic surgery for local hemostasis. Zeolite, a mineral that absorbs fluid-concentrating coagulation factors and platelets at the site of injury, has been used for control of hemorrhage from external wounds. Zeolite generates significant heat, so it should be used only for hemostasis of external injuries. Newer versions that are less exothermic have been developed. Chitosan is a chemically modified form of chitin, the structural constituent of the exoskeleton of crustaceans. It is thought to augment platelet aggregation and adhesion. Poly-N-acetyl glucosamine is a polysaccharide derived from marine algae that triggers vasoconstriction and platelet activation. It has been FDA approved as a hemostatic agent (Rapid Deployment Hemostat

[RDH], Marine Polymer Technologies Inc., Danvers, MA) and a bandage (mRDH Bandage) for the treatment of trauma patients. The European trauma guidelines have recommended the use of local hemostatic agents in combination with conventional surgical management in the treatment of traumatic injury–associated bleeding.

Recommended Approach to Trauma-Associated Bleeding

In the field, trauma patients should be stabilized quickly for rapid transport to the nearest trauma center. Bleeding should be controlled with local hemostatic measures such as hemostatic dressing and tourniquets (see Figure 3). Hypothermia should be treated. IV crystalloid resuscitation should be minimized consistent with the paired goals of permissive hypotension and limiting dilution coagulopathy. Upon arrival in the emergency department, the initial clinical trauma evaluation should proceed while laboratory studies, including screening coagulation studies, CBC counts, and a type and crossmatch, are being drawn and radiographic studies are ordered. Until a type and crossmatch is available, type O blood and AB plasma can be used for replacement. Maintenance of a ready pool of thawed plasma in the blood bank facilitates rapid replacement therapy. Satellite blood banks in the emergency department also can speed blood product transfusion. To limit dilution of coagulation factors and platelets, PRBCs, FFP, and platelets should be transfused in a 1:1:1 ratio while damage control surgery proceeds. Tranexamic acid should be administered as early as possible (within 3 hours) in all trauma patients who are actively bleeding or at risk for significant hemorrhage. Hypothermia should be limited by administering warmed fluids and blood products and keeping the patient in a warm environment. Serial laboratory testing can assist in tailoring blood product component therapy to the patient's clinical situation. POC testing such as TEG or ROTEM increasingly is being used to complement conventional laboratory testing, although prospective studies demonstrating improved clinical outcomes are needed. Fibrinogen concentrates or cryoprecipitate should be considered for patients with hypofibrinogenemia (fibrinogen less than 229 mg/dL). rFVIIa can be considered in patients with bleeding unresponsive to conventional blood product support. For trauma patients who are taking antiplatelet agents or anticoagulants, reversal strategies, including platelet transfusions (for antiplatelet agents), IV vitamin K and prothrombin complex concentrates (for warfarin), and activated prothrombin complex concentrates (for the oral factor Xa inhibitors apixaban, edoxaban, and rivaroxaban), should be used early in treatment. Idarucizumab should be used for reversal of dabigatran. Local hemostatic therapies (fibrin sealants, collagen hemostats, etc.) can be used to complement damage control surgery.

SUGGESTED READINGS

Davenport RA, Brohi K. Cause of trauma-induced coagulopathy. *Curr Opin Anaesthesiol.* 2016;29:212-219.

Kaafarani HM, Velmahos GC. Damage control resuscitation in trauma. *Scand J Surg.* 2014;103:81-88.

Noel P, Cashen S, Patel B. Trauma-induced coagulopathy: from biology to therapy. *Semin Hematol.* 2013;50:259-269.

Spahn DR, Bouillon B, Cerny V, et al. Management of bleeding and coagulopathy following major trauma: an updated European guideline. *Crit Care.* 2013;17:R76.

White NJ. Mechanisms of trauma-induced coagulopathy. *Hematology Am Soc Hematol Educ Program.* 2013;2013:660-663.

THE ABDOMEN THAT WILL NOT CLOSE

**W. Robert Leeper, MD, BSc, FRCSC, FACS,
and Elliott R. Haut, MD, PhD**

The principle of damage control has changed the practice of surgery dramatically over the past 2 decades and has become one of the central and dominant dogmas of trauma and acute care surgery. As a result, the morbidity and mortality associated with abdominal compartment syndrome (ACS), dilutional coagulopathy, hypothermia, acidosis, and myriad other resuscitative complications have been reduced dramatically. However, with all significant advances come new challenges. As surgeons have embraced completely the concept of damage control surgery (DCS) and abbreviated laparotomy, a new epidemic has been created in surgical intensive care units (ICUs) across the United States: the abdomen that will not close.

This chapter aims to define the terms and conditions of the present epidemic of the open abdomen, to examine the causes of and solutions to the problem, and to propose a rational framework for management. Although no one strategy will fit all varieties of difficult abdominal closures, we believe that it is important for each surgical service to develop an agreed-upon approach to this issue and to adhere to similar management principles across the service. This chapter presents the tools and techniques that should make up any comprehensive approach to the challenging open abdomen.

■ INDICATIONS FOR LEAVING THE ABDOMEN OPEN

Appropriate indications for a truncated laparotomy with temporary abdominal closure (TAC) essentially fall into one of three categories:

1. **Too** dirty
   - Severe contamination requiring repeated irrigation and débridement
   - Necrotizing soft tissue infection of the abdominal wall
2. **Too** much tension
   - Patients at high risk of ACS
   - Patients with loss of domain in whom primary closure is mechanically impossible
3. Need **to** look again
   - Questionable viability of residual hollow viscus
   - Intentional retention of foreign bodies (e.g., sponges for liver packing)
   - After DCS when definitive repairs are to be completed at a later date (discussed in detail in other chapters)

Indications outside of these three broad domains should be examined carefully for validity. Simple expediency is rarely if ever a sufficient, isolated reason for TAC. It is rare that a patient cannot tolerate physiologically the additional short period of time required for closure of the otherwise closeable abdomen. Several recent studies point to the pendulum having swung too far in the direction of DCS, with reports of patients being left open inappropriately as a result.

■ INITIAL TEMPORARY ABDOMINAL CLOSURE

Once it has been decided that an appropriate indication exists for truncated laparotomy and TAC, a standard initial dressing should be applied immediately. Attributes of the ideal TAC dressing include the following:

- Ease of application, reliability, and durability
- Ability to manage abdominal fluid losses and drainage
- Avoidance of trauma to the abdominal fascia
- Relatively tension-free closure to avoid secondary ACS
- Maintenance of abdominal domain

In the 20-plus years since Rotondo and Schwab coined the term *damage control surgery* there have been a huge number of techniques used by surgeons in an attempt to identify the ideal method of initial TAC. Inventive techniques, including the use of various types of synthetic mesh, the Bogota bag, penetrating towel clip skin closures, and all varieties of homemade closed suction or vacuum devices, have been described and utilized for TAC. Although these improvised techniques share the benefit of being inexpensive, none has clearly demonstrated superiority over the others, nor has any achieved the reliability and reproducibility of the commercially available open abdomen vacuum-assisted closure (VAC) devices now in wide use across North America.

■ VACUUM-ASSISTED CLOSURE DEVICES FOR INITIAL TEMPORARY ABDOMINAL CLOSURE

In the contemporary practice of surgery the dominant modality for initial TAC is one of the commercially available VAC devices. VAC dressings address all desirable attributes of TAC and are the preferred method of initial TAC. The components of a typical VAC dressing include the following:

1. *Semipermeable (fenestrated), nonadherent inner membrane.* The innermost layer of fenestrated plastic or sponge acts to protect the viscera from the overlying suction device and simultaneously permit evacuation of intra-abdominal fluid.
2. *Sponge inlay.* The middle layer of the VAC device consists of a porous sponge, often made of polyurethane, placed in an inlay position between the fascial edges and flush with the level of the skin. This layer transmits the suction effect onto the inner membrane to remove intra-abdominal fluid. Suction effect on the inlay sponge also produces wound contraction and gentle fascial edge reapposition over time.
3. *Adhesive impermeable outer layer.* The outer layer of the VAC dressing is an adhesive, impermeable layer utilized to create a seal around the edges of the wound and to anchor the dressing to the periwound skin and allow gentle tension or wound contraction over time.
4. *Suction device or machine.* Finally, the suction device or machine typically connects to the dressing via an adapter placed overtop an intentionally created defect in the impermeable outer layer to allow transmission of negative pressure directly onto the middle sponge layer (Figure 1).

■ PRACTICAL TIPS FOR USE OF VACUUM-ASSISTED CLOSURE DRESSING AS TEMPORARY ABDOMINAL CLOSURE

Maximally lateralize the inner, visceral protective layer. To prevent viscera from sneaking out at the edges of the inlay sponge it is important to maximally lateralize the inner, visceral protective layer. This also prevents adhesions of the viscera to the undersurface of the abdominal wall, which may make eventual abdominal closure more difficult. To do this we find it helpful to universally take down the falciform ligament as well as any secondary adhesions to the anterior abdominal wall. During placement of the inner layer we prefer to wet both the dorsal and the volar aspects of the surgical gloves to permit deep placement of the inner layer and then smooth removal of the placing hand without removing the inner layer. We also often leave

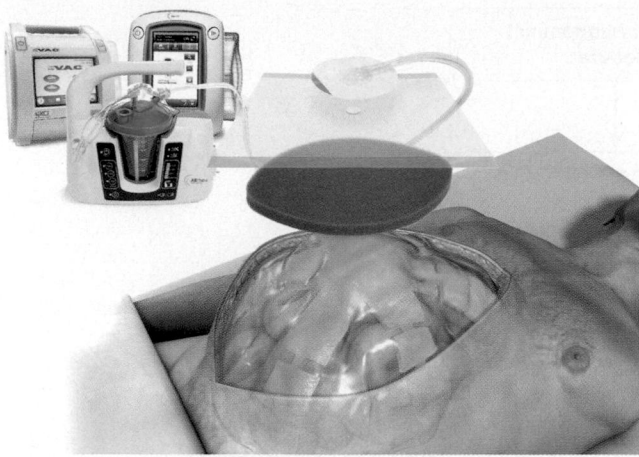

FIGURE 1 The various components and application of one commercially available vacuum-assisted closure (VAC) dressing, the ABThera VAC device (Kinetic Concepts Inc., San Antonio, TX). *(Reproduced with permission from KCI/Acelity, http://www.kci1.com/KCI1/vactherapy.)*

■ OPEN ABDOMEN POSTOPERATIVE CARE

Resuscitative Phase

In the early postoperative period, an appropriate and balanced resuscitation must be undertaken. Rewarming, repletion of blood and coagulation factors, and administration of warmed crystalloid solution to reverse metabolic derangements are critical. Antibiotics are appropriate for a 24-hour perioperative period at most but are not mandated simply by virtue of an open abdomen for any period beyond this. During this early, so-called "fluid-seeking" phase, patients should not be restricted in terms of fluid administration because of concerns about bowel edema and ultimate fascial closure. Resuscitation trumps reconstitution of the abdominal wall as a priority at this time. However, we do find it helpful to utilize hypertonic crystalloid solutions for both infusion and bolus therapy during the resuscitative phase, as these agents may provide durable volume expansion while restricting edema to a certain degree. Further goals for this phase are well delineated in the DCS literature as well as in the chapter Damage Control Operation. In brief, we believe that patients should receive judicious sedation and return to the operating room every 24 to 48 hours for abdominal washout and decontamination.

Reconstructive Phase

The most important and challenging phase in the postoperative care of patients with an open abdomen is the reconstructive phase. The first challenge is to recognize when patients have entered this phase. One hallmark of the reconstructive phase is the cessation of "fluid seeking," when shock has resolved and the patient now can be largely weaned from vasopressors and begin either diuresis or aggressive fluid removal via renal replacement therapy. In addition, the patient should have source control and no signs of ongoing sepsis within the abdomen. Some patients complete their resuscitation and reach the reconstructive phase before the first operative takeback. Others may never truly enter the reconstructive phase.

It is in this phase that a critical decision must be made about the general approach to abdominal closure. Ideally primary fascial closure will be possible in many patients. If not, the decision tree involves the choice of (1) a tension-bearing transfascial abdominal wall closure technique or (2) more immediate surgical closure methods with a willingness to accept one of several mesh, with or without skin graft, bailout techniques if primary closure ultimately cannot be obtained. In general, this decision is based on local practice and individual surgeon preference. Descriptions of successful use of each technique are provided later, and an algorithm for the management of the open abdomen is presented in Figure 2.

■ STANDARD CLOSURE TECHNIQUES

Although no gold standard technique for closure of the difficult abdomen is agreed upon, our preferred "standard" closure technique is to return to the operating room every 24 to 48 hours and gradually attempt to close more of the abdominal fascia in the upper and lower portions of the wound using heavy, interrupted, nonabsorbable (i.e., 2-0 nylon) sutures in figure-of-8 fashion. Achieving a negative fluid balance before each subsequent closure technique can assist with fascial closure. In addition, lipocutaneous flaps can be raised by retracting the linea alba using two Kocher clamps and dissecting the fat and abdominal wall tissue off the anterior surface of the most superficial fascial layer. These flaps disarticulate the fascia from the overlying abdominal wall soft tissue and often give a further few inches of relaxation toward midline closure when raised bilaterally. Limited component release also can be considered judiciously by identifying the lateral border of the rectus abdominis and incising over a short distance along the external oblique fascia. This allows further laxity on each side as the rectus musculature is pulled toward midline. It should be pointed out that at this stage of reconstruction

the self-retaining retractor (i.e., Bookwalter) in place, holding the abdominal wall up while placing the inner layer.

Avoid leaks. Air leaks, typically at the edges of the wound or at skin creases and ostomy sites, are the Achilles heel of VAC therapy. Utilizing an appropriate overlap of adhesive is important, as is intraoperative leak testing before leaving the operating room. The use of ancillary liquid adhesives, such as tincture of benzoin or Mastisol, is absolutely critical, especially in hair-bearing or other difficult areas for adhesion.

Staples for skin-sponge apposition. Polyurethane sponge damages the epidermis when direct contact is made under negative pressure. However, the inlay sponge must come to a flush apposition with the skin edge to maximize the effectiveness of the dressing. One solution that we have found successful is the use of skin staples to temporarily affix the inlay sponge to the edges of the wound during dressing application and initial suction, although this is not necessary in all cases. These staples then are removed at the next VAC dressing change.

Overlap ostomies with adhesive outer layer. VAC therapy in the presence of an ostomy creates a very difficult problem for wound management. Ideally a new ostomy is placed far enough from the midline to make wound coverage as easy as possible. However, if the ostomy is close to the wound or if the patient has an enteroatmospheric fistula in the middle of the wound, there are possible makeshift solutions. To avoid peristomal VAC leaks we prefer to remove the ostomy appliance and place the adhesive outer layer over the stoma. With the ostomy appliance off, a sheet of adhesive outer layer can be used to completely cover and widely overlap the stoma site, with a small hole cut to allow the stoma to pass through. The ostomy appliance then is reapplied on top of the adhesive layer and simply changed every 48 hours with the dressing.

Gradually contract wound and sponge size. With each sequential application of the VAC dressing, an attempt should be made to perform minimal tension fascial closure at both the superior and the inferior aspects of the wound using interrupted sutures. Simultaneously the inlay sponge should be cut smaller and smaller to promote wound contraction and fascial edge re-apposition. During this early phase of TAC, no suprafascial flaps are raised, and as such the skin, subcutaneous layer, and fascia move and behave as one myofasciocutaneous unit, influenced similarly by the negative pressure therapy.

Appropriate hole for vacuum device. Although simple, the use of an appropriately sized hole in the outer adhesive layer is a critical step. At least a 2- × 2-cm hole is appropriate and allows efficient transmission of negative pressure.

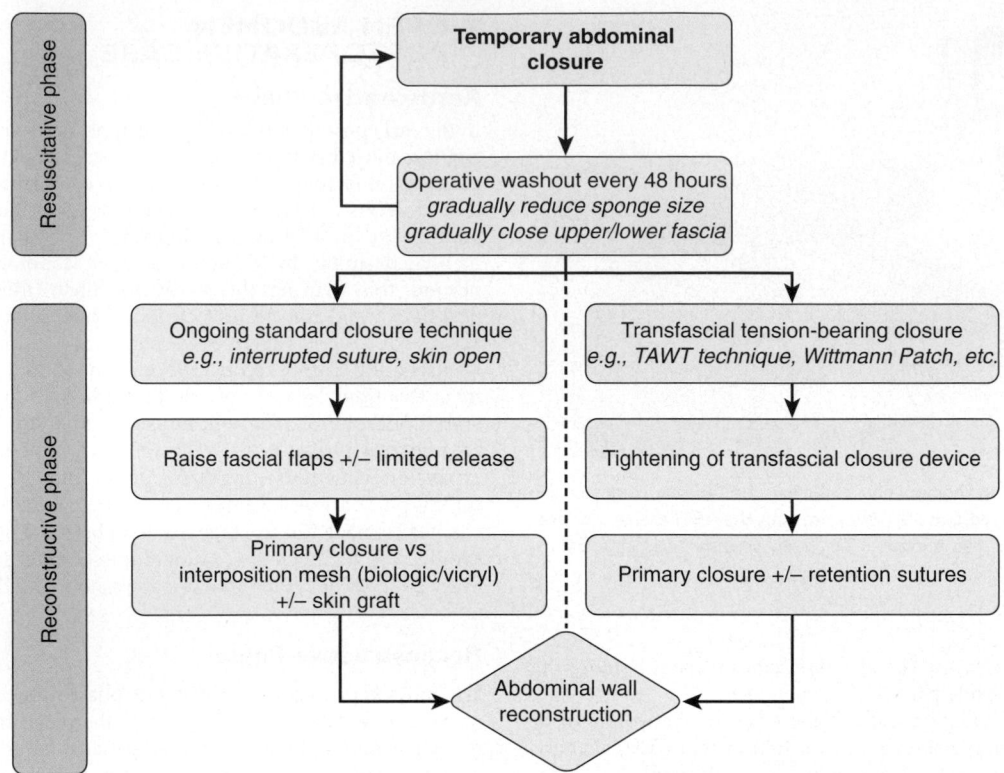

FIGURE 2 Flow diagram of standard (left column) or tension-bearing (right column) technique for abdominal closure. *TAWT*, Transabdominal wall traction.

it is ill advised to perform a full component separation, and even partial component releases are controversial both in the literature and among surgeons with a high volume of such cases. Bilateral component separation with myofascial advancement flap closure is one of the most useful and versatile methods of achieving durable long-term abdominal wall reconstruction. Preserving this technique for the convalescent phase so that it can be utilized for ultimate hernia repair or ostomy takedown is critical, and the choice to utilize component release in the acute setting should not be taken lightly.

Figure 3 shows the standard closure technique being applied in a patient who underwent trauma laparotomy and required venovenous extracorporeal membrane oxygenation (VV-ECMO) for pulmonary support in the immediate postoperative period. This patient required massive resuscitation and suffered from severe edema and concern for ACS, leading to the choice of TAC. Despite her resuscitative requirements, the patient was able to achieve definitive closure, while remaining on VV-ECMO, after only three trips to the operating room. This case highlights the fact that regaining abdominal domain and success with vacuum-assisted TAC and standard closure techniques are often more achievable than they may initially appear.

■ BAILOUT OPTIONS

If closure of all patients with an open abdomen could be achieved through patience and standard fascial closure techniques, this would be a rather short and unimportant chapter. The reality, however, is that a subset of patients will never achieve primary midline closure during their index hospitalization. Indeed, our practice is that if patients are not imminently closeable within about 1 week, consideration must be given to a "bailout" option for peritoneal coverage. Although we recognize that this cut-off is somewhat arbitrary, the logic behind limiting the number of takebacks that a given patient should be subjected to is sound. Ultimately, as time progresses and the number of operations increases, so too does the risk of inadvertent injury to the now fused conglomerate of intestines, also known as the "bowel ball." Enterocutaneous and enteroatmospheric fistulae

are lethal adversaries in difficult abdominal closures, and prevention of these is the key to success. We prefer to utilize one of two techniques at this stage.

Where the skin of the abdominal wall is lax enough to achieve midline closure, we prefer to place an underlay biologic mesh to bridge the fascial defect and bring the overlying skin as close as possible to midline so that it can act as the ideal native tissue coverage for the mesh. In this situation the method of skin closure or reapproximation typically is assisted by some form of VAC therapy. The underlay of biologic mesh typically is placed in an intraperitoneal position and affixed to the abdominal wall using transfascial suture techniques that permit a minimum of 5 cm overlap from the fascial edges. Biologic mesh is preferred in this setting, as it inevitably will have direct contact with the viscera. Although we typically utilize a bovine product (because this is what our institution has decided to stock), other available human and porcine products likely produce similar clinical results.

Where neither fascia nor skin has the capacity for midline closure, we routinely default to a temporary Vicryl (polyglactin) mesh closure with delayed placement of a split-thickness skin graft. For such patients, a sheet of vicryl (polyglactin) is quilted over on itself two to three times to produce a slightly thicker, absorbable mesh. This temporary absorbable mesh then is placed in an underlay, intraperitoneal position and tacked to the underside of the abdominal wall with a minimum of 5 cm overlap. Standard saline-soaked gauze dressings are used twice daily for about 2 to 4 weeks until satisfactory granulation tissue has appeared in the wound bed. At this time a split-thickness skin graft can be placed to cover the wound. We routinely suggest external support via an abdominal binder and physical limitations relating to strenuous activity and heavy lifting during the several months of convalescence. Although this technique is neither novel nor aesthetically or functionally appealing, it is a time-tested strategy to extricate a patient from the most dire of open abdomen catastrophes. With the advent of modern abdominal wall reconstruction techniques, these patients now can be offered a genuine and fairly reliable opportunity for restoration of abdominal

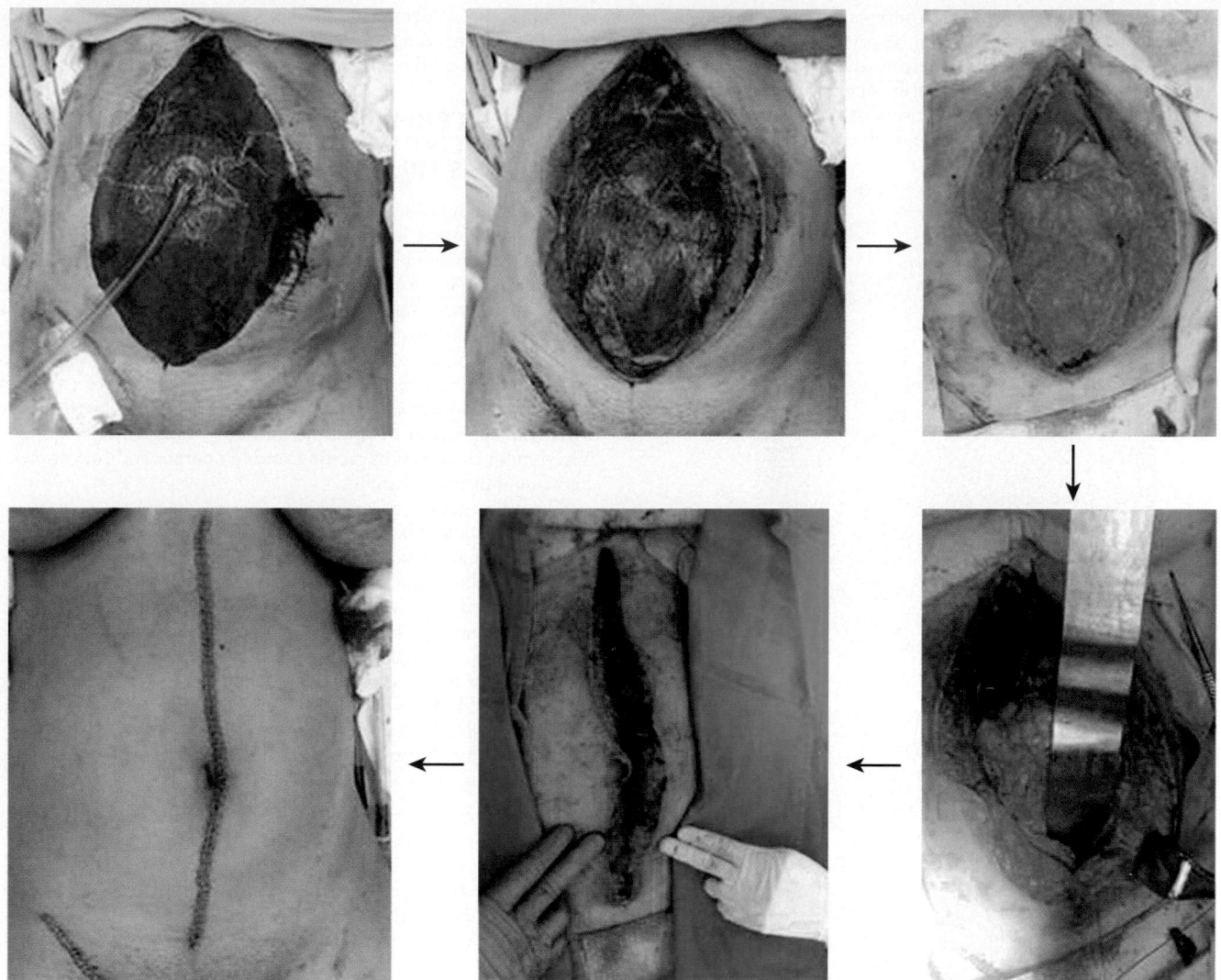

FIGURE 3 Standard closure technique with gradual recovery of abdominal domain by serial closure of upper and lower aspects of fascia. Note that in this case, closure was achieved after only three trips to the operating room, myocutaneous flaps were not required, and skin was closed because of a limited degree of contamination.

wall continuity, albeit at a later date once they have completed convalescence for their acute illness. Usually this is accomplished after a minimum of 9 to 12 months, allowing for softening of intra-abdominal adhesions and recovery from what is likely an extended stay in the ICU, hospital, and rehabilitation center. The benefit of this approach is that the native abdominal wall musculature is not violated and remains intact, allowing a number of possible delayed definitive closure techniques. Figure 4 shows a polyglactin bailout technique during the granulation phase before skin grafting and the ultimate hernia defect after skin grafting.

■ TRANSFASCIAL TENSION-BEARING CLOSURE TECHNIQUES

A distinct alternative to standard closure for management of the open abdomen is a group of techniques that we collectively refer to as transfascial tension-bearing closure techniques. Typical examples of such closures include the standard Wittmann Patch of hook and loop (Velcro) sheets and the commercially available Canica ABRA system (Figure 5). The guiding principle in all such techniques is to redistribute the tension to a position lateral to the rectus sheath rather than in the medial portion of the abdominal wound, where the tension is highest in a standard closure. In doing so, these techniques are postulated to produce myofascial release by gradually lengthening the retracted oblique and transversus abdominis myofascial groups to regain abdominal domain.

The most recently described application of this technique has been popularized by the trauma and acute care surgical group at Cook County Hospital in Chicago and is known as the transabdominal wall traction (TAWT) method (http://www.starsurgical.com). The TAWT technique takes advantage of a variation on the original Wittmann Patch whereby the same hook and loop (Velcro) sheets are utilized but are affixed lateral to the rectus sheath using heavy sutures passed through all layers of the abdominal wall and fixed externally over heavy plastic bolsters. The skin beneath the bolsters is protected by a hydrocolloid layer, and the viscera beneath the hook and loop sheets are protected by a semipermeable plastic adhesion barrier. This system, shown in Figure 6, then can be tightened gradually during serial abdominal washouts and adhesion barrier changes every 48 hours. The group at Cook County Hospital reports great success with this technique and has a near 100% rate of eventual abdominal closure, with only a relatively small number of tightening and washout procedures required. A standard vacuum suction dressing is applied on top of the wound between tightening procedures.

Once a midline, tension-free closure can be obtained with the TAWT system, a layered closure can be performed either primarily or via a retrorectus approach. The retrorectus space is developed and the posterior sheath is closed primarily. Then a mesh can be placed in the retrorectus position before closure of the anterior sheath and vacuum-assisted management of the open cutaneous portion of the wound. Figure 7 demonstrates this sequence of definitive closure steps in a patient who required use of retention sutures over external bolsters to unload the ultimate midline closure.

■ LONG-TERM MANAGEMENT AND DEFINITIVE ABDOMINAL WALL RECONSTRUCTION

The development of significant ventral hernia in long-term survivors of an open abdomen is a common phenomenon. When a Vicryl mesh "bailout" option has been used, the need for eventual abdominal wall reconstruction is a foregone conclusion. However, even when standard or transfascial tension-bearing techniques have been successful at achieving midline closure, there is still a significant rate of hernia formation. Although entire chapters and textbooks have been written on abdominal wall reconstruction, we describe our preferred technique for abdominal wall reconstruction as illustrated by the case of a 25-year-old victim of multiple gunshot wounds who required a Vicryl mesh closure, skin grafting, and temporary end colostomy for his acute injuries (Figure 8).

During a period of outpatient convalescence, typically several months, the patient achieves optimal nutrition status and completes rehabilitation and resolution of all physiologic abnormalities. Sufficient remodeling time is permitted such that the overlying skin graft can be pinched easily and lifted off the underlying viscera. This indicates that adhesions have softened and will be more favorable for dissection. In particularly large defects, we have our plastic and reconstructive surgeons place tissue expanders to ensure that enough skin is available for final closure. In the case presented, no tissue expanders or plastic surgical consultation was required. The series of photographs in Figure 9 illustrates our preferred repair and reconstructive sequence.

1. Excision of skin graft and extensive lysis of adhesions to release all abdominal viscera
2. Takedown of any intestinal stoma or fistula and, in this case, a handsewn two-layer colo-colonic anastomosis to restore gastrointestinal continuity
3. Reapproximation or as near as possible reapproximation of fascia utilizing:
   a. Large skin flaps dissected off the anterior fascia out to the anterior superior iliac spines and well beyond the costal margins
   b. Component separations, in this case involving the incision of the aponeuroses of the bilateral external oblique myofascial units longitudinally. The incision is made approximately 1 cm

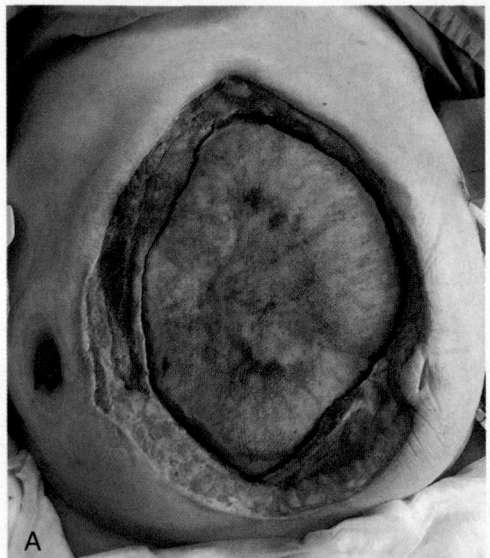
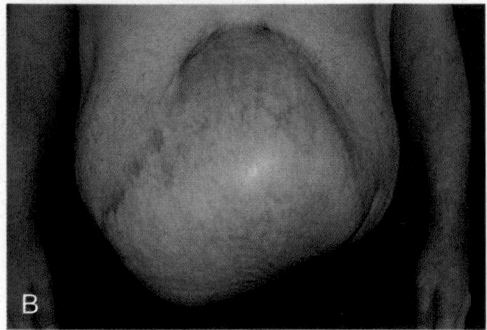

FIGURE 4 A, Polyglactin interposition during granulation phase. **B,** The ultimate hernia defect after skin graft closure. This hernia was managed with tissue expanders and composite repair after appropriate convalescence.

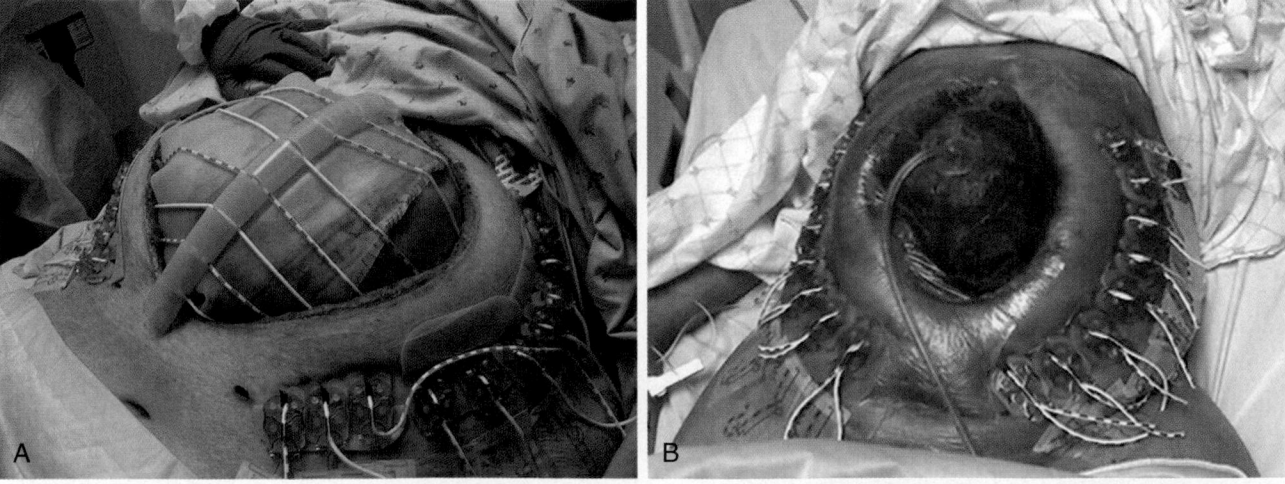

FIGURE 5 A and **B,** Canica ABRA system used in two cases of difficult abdominal closure. Progressive tension is applied across the wound using button elastomers and button anchors placed lateral to the rectus myofascial complex.

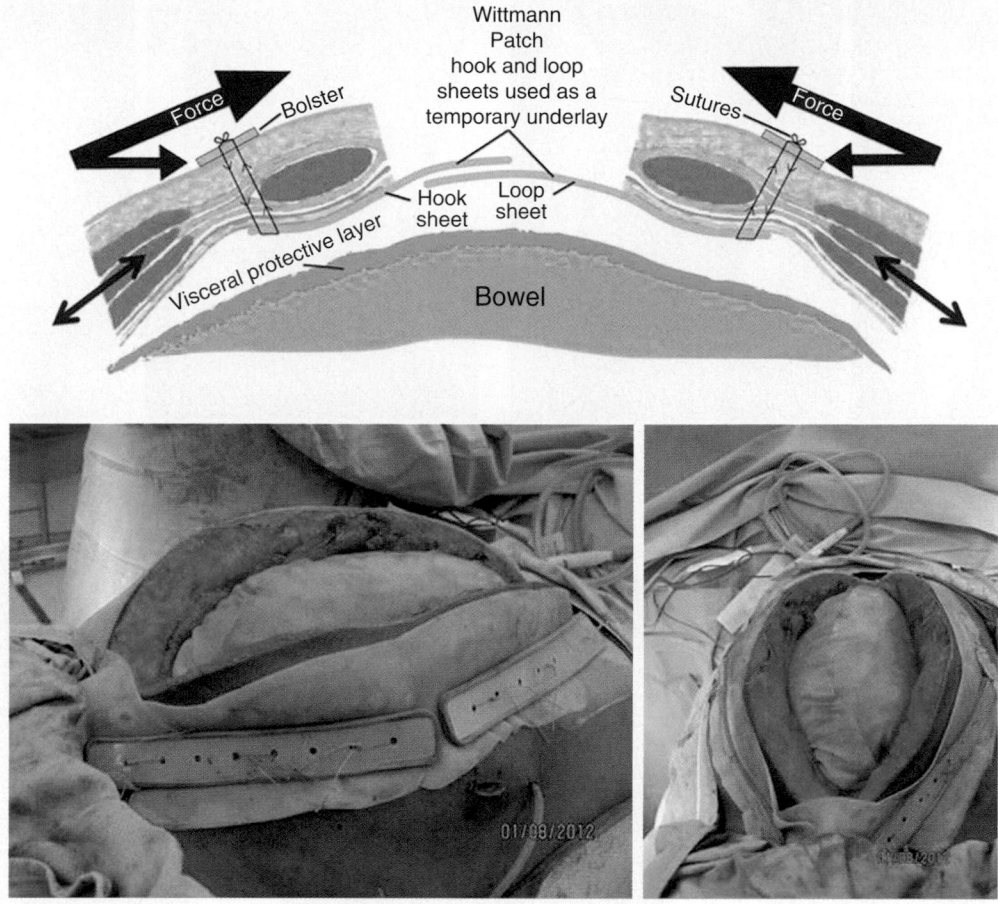

FIGURE 6 Transabdominal wall traction (TAWT) utilizes laterally anchored hook and loop patches anchored to progressively recreated midline closure and regains abdominal domain *(Photos courtesy Michael Deutsche, Chicago, IL.)*

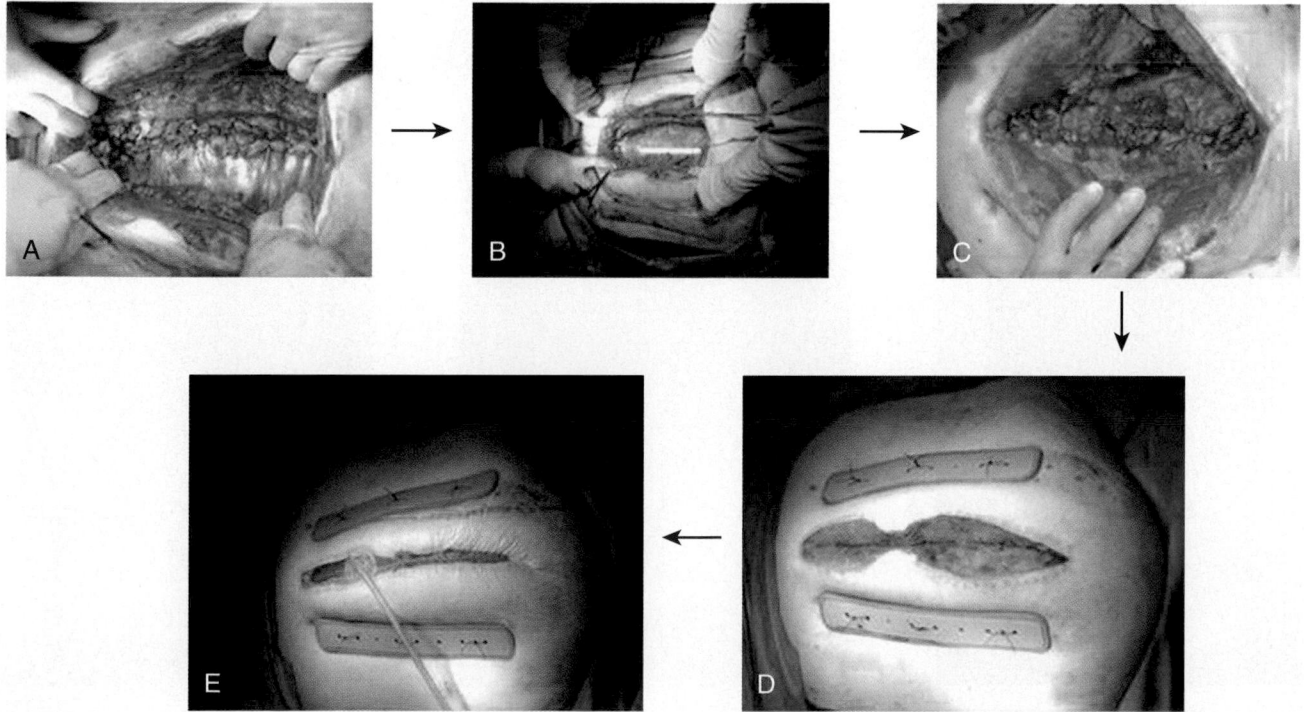

FIGURE 7 Closure sequence once midline closure has been facilitated using the transabdominal wall traction (TAWT) system. **A,** Posterior sheath is closed. **B,** Retrorectus biologic mesh implant with retention sutures. **C,** Anterior fascia closed. **D,** Retention sutures with bolsters. **E,** Vacuum-assisted skin closure device. *(Photos courtesy Michael Deutsche, Chicago, IL.)*

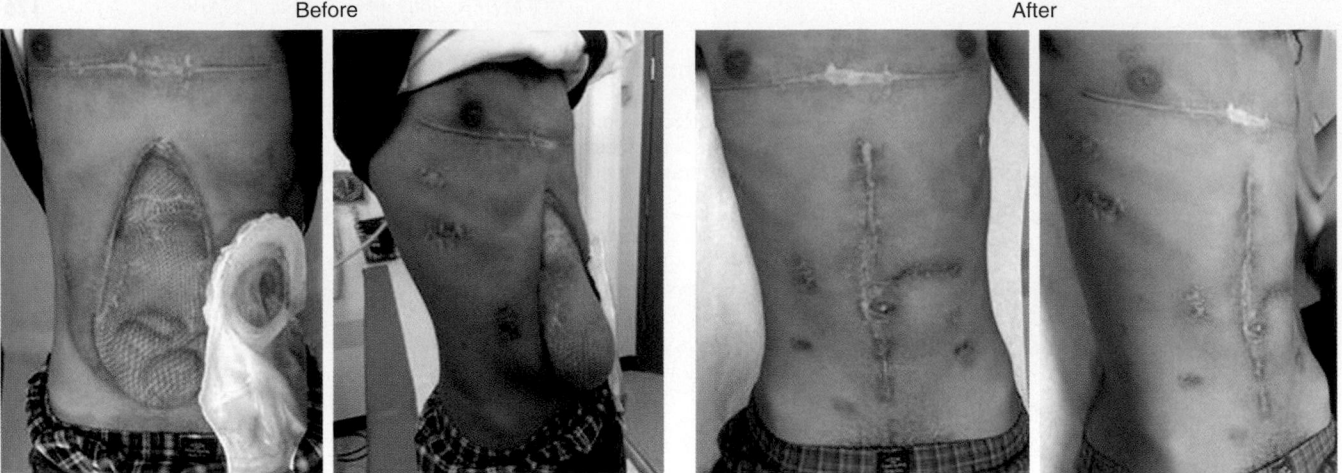

FIGURE 8 Before and after images of a patient with prior colostomy and polyglactin and skin graft closure who went on to receive abdominal wall reconstruction and restoration of intestinal continuity.

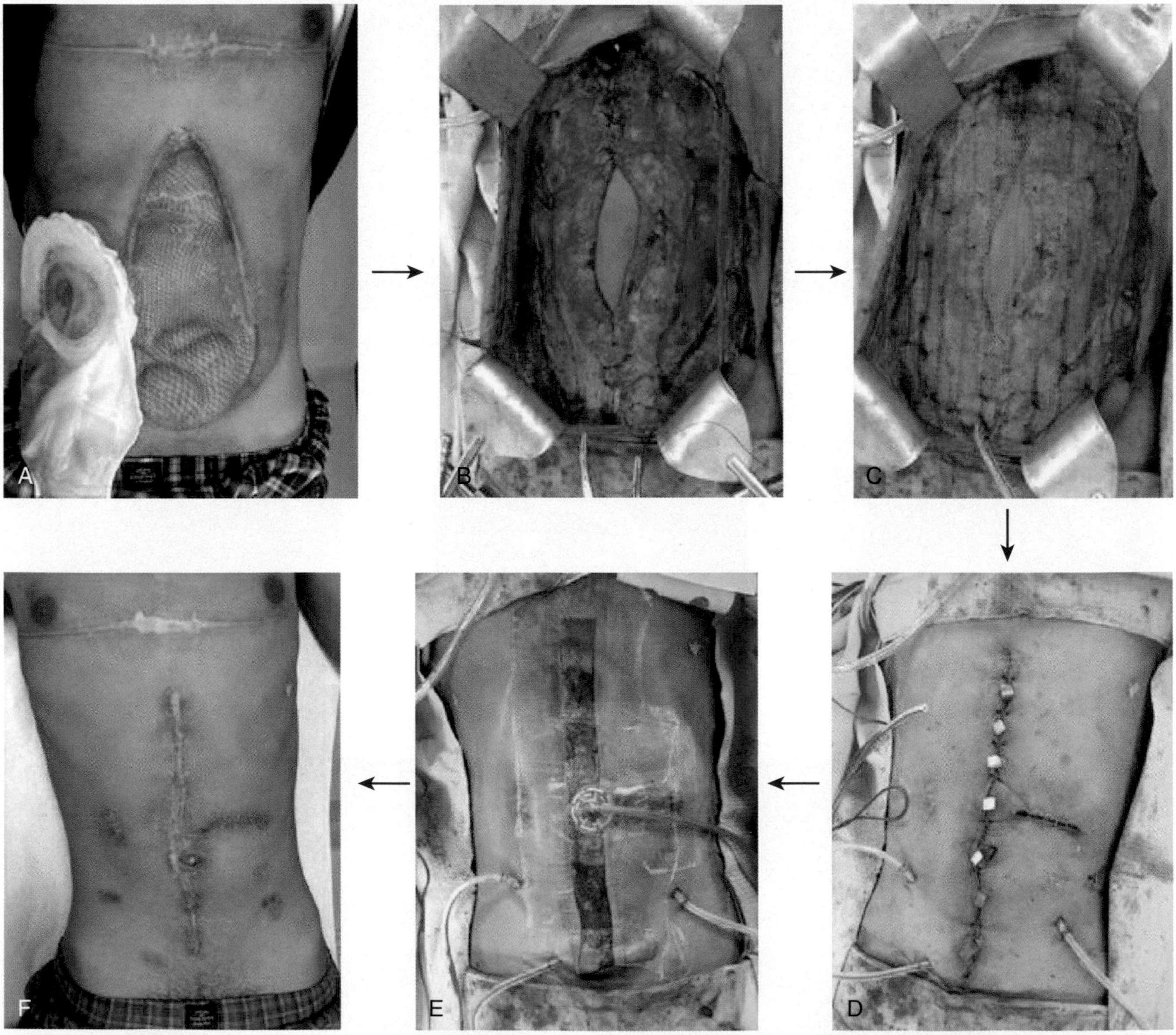

FIGURE 9 Reconstructive sequence for complex abdominal wall reconstruction. **A,** Preoperative image with skin graft and end colostomy in place. **B,** Intraoperative photo after extensive component separation and underlay of biologic graft, anchored laterally beyond the edges of the component release. **C,** Onlay soft polypropylene graft anchored laterally with same transfascial nonabsorbable sutures used to affix underlay graft. **D,** Wound closure with polyvinyl chloride "feet" every 2 to 3 cm. **E,** Skin protective barrier layer and polyurethane sponge with vacuum applied overtop wound. **F,** Ultimate result at 3 months postoperative.

lateral to the rectus sheet and is carried as far superiorly as the muscular portion of the thoracic wall, up to 5 to 7 cm above the costal margin.

   c. Selective use of posterior rectus sheath or transversus abdominis muscle releases (not used in this case)

4. Underlay biologic mesh of thick (2 to 3 mm) acellular dermal matrix with minimum 5-cm overlap
5. Onlay of soft polypropylene "sandwich" mesh extending laterally beyond the edges of the component separation and affixed to the underlay biologic mesh using the same transfascial nonabsorbable suture (or alternatively can be affixed with glue, tacks, or skin staples)
6. Placement of three surgical drains (one below polypropylene mesh, two above)
7. Skin closure utilizing a hybrid skin VAC system. Skin is closed near completely with absorbable deep dermal suture, with small gaps left every 2 to 3 cm. Polyvinyl chloride (PVC) sponge "feet" are placed in each gap, skin is protected with a hydrocolloid layer, and a polyurethane sponge is placed overtop the wound to distribute suction across all PVC feet. Alternatively, a standard primary skin closure with staples is another reasonable option.

Changes of the modified skin VAC system are performed every 48 hours, and PVC feet are removed gradually with each subsequent VAC change until only a polyurethane sponge is applied over an otherwise closed wound. Long-term results of this technique have been favorable in some series and may decrease wound complication rates, although definite data on this method are still lacking.

■ SUMMARY

In the appropriately selected patient, an open abdomen will serve as a lifesaving component of an overall damage control strategy.

Techniques to achieve eventual closure of the open abdomen should include balanced resuscitation with crystalloid minimization, regular returns to the operating room, and a carefully selected approach to closure based on patient, surgeon, and institutional factors. Rapid advances in surgical management of abdominal wall reconstruction have been made with disruptive technologies such as DCS, VAC therapy, and biologic mesh. Surgical techniques also have grown and likely will continue to do so such that vascularized abdominal wall composite tissue allotransplantation likely will be a more routinely utilized option within the next 1 to 2 decades. Ongoing improvement in abdominal wall reconstructive techniques will allow survivors of the open abdomen epidemic to regain functional reconstitution of their abdominal wall and salvage not only mortality but also morbidity from what previously may have been a lethal or disabling abdominal catastrophe.

SUGGESTED READINGS

Campbell A, Chang M, Fabian T, et al. Management of the open abdomen: from initial operation to definitive closure. *Am Surg.* 2009;75(suppl 11):S1-S22.

Diaz JJ Jr, Cullinane DC, Khwaja KA, et al. Eastern Association for the Surgery of Trauma: management of the open abdomen, part III—review of abdominal wall reconstruction. *J Trauma Acute Care Surg.* 2013;75: 376-386.

Kirkpatrick AW, Roberts DJ, De Waele J, et al. Intra-abdominal hypertension and the abdominal compartment syndrome: updated consensus definitions and clinical practice guidelines from the World Society of the Abdominal Compartment Syndrome. *Intensive Care Med.* 2013;39: 1190-1206.

Soares KC, Baltodano PA, Hicks CW, et al. Novel wound management system reduction of surgical site morbidity after ventral hernia repairs: a critical analysis. *Am J Surg.* 2015;209:324-332.

THE MANAGEMENT OF VASCULAR INJURIES

Patrick E. Georgoff, MD, and Meghan A. Arnold, MD

Vascular injuries are associated with high morbidity and mortality. Management can be complex, especially in the multiply injured patient who is in hemorrhagic shock. Failure to recognize and triage injuries in a timely fashion can have devastating consequences. To effectively treat these patients, a thorough understanding of vascular anatomy, exposure techniques, and methods for obtaining control of bleeding vessels is imperative. Unstable patients should proceed to the operating room without delay. However, those that are stable after initial resuscitation may undergo computed tomographic angiography (CTA), which provides rapid and accurate diagnosis of vascular injuries. Increasingly, these injuries are being managed successfully with endovascular techniques. Hybrid operating rooms are now widely available and allow for the combined use of open and endovascular techniques. This chapter reviews the evaluation and treatment of vascular injuries to the neck, chest, abdomen, pelvis, and extremities.

■ INITIAL EVALUATION AND MANAGEMENT

The clinical presentation of vascular injury is broad and depends on the mechanism, anatomic areas involved, and associated injuries.

Diagnosis is based on a thorough history and physical examination in addition to selective imaging. Hard or diagnostic physical examination findings of significant vascular injury include pulsatile bleeding, expanding hematoma, the presence of a bruit or thrill, and evidence of ischemia. The signs and symptoms of ischemia (the six "Ps") include pain, pallor, paresthesia, paralysis, poikilothermia, and pulselessness. Hard findings are diagnostic of severe vascular injury and in most settings mandate immediate operative intervention. Soft or suggestive signs of vascular injury include a history of moderate hemorrhage, nonexpanding hematoma, present but diminished pulses, and injury in proximity to a name vessel (Box 1). In these patients, vascular imaging can help to determine the need for intervention. It is good practice to obtain as much information as possible from first providers, including the mechanism of injury, time of injury, and amount of blood loss at the scene. Overall, less than 10% of injured patients will be seen with hard signs. The rest will be asymptomatic, have a delayed presentation, or be seen with soft signs of injury.

Vascular injuries are often associated with trauma to local musculoskeletal structures. Table 1 lists these associations, which can be used to recognize patterns of injury and facilitate expedient diagnosis. For most patients, physical examination alone is sufficient for diagnosing a vascular injury. This is especially true in the case of vascular injury to the extremities, where ankle-brachial or wrist-brachial indices enhance diagnostic accuracy. Although arteriography remains the gold standard for diagnosing vascular injuries, its implementation can be logistically challenging and may be inappropriate in the multiply injured patient. CTA can be obtained quickly, is noninvasive, and is highly sensitive and specific for diagnosing vascular injuries. Although CTA has been shown to be a viable

BOX 1: Findings of Vascular Injury

Hard Findings

- Pulsatile bleeding
- Expanding hematoma
- Bruit or thrill
- Evidence of ischemia (pain, pallor, paresthesia, paralysis, poikilothermia, and pulselessness)

Soft Findings

- History of moderate hemorrhage
- Nonexpanding, nonpulsatile hematoma
- Present but diminished pulses
- Injury in proximity to a name vessel

alternative to formal arteriography, consideration must be given to the associated risks, including intravenous (IV) contrast dye complications, radiation exposure, and the identification of "occult" injuries of unclear significance. Despite identification on imaging, not all vascular injuries require operative management.

In the setting of a normal physical examination, asymptomatic patients found on imaging to have minor injuries, such as nonocclusive intimal flaps, small false aneurysms (<2 cm), or segmental arterial narrowing, can be managed conservatively with close observation and follow-up. Ultimately, less than 10% of these patients require operative intervention, and those who do tend to have good outcomes. Additional diagnostic information can be obtained from duplex ultrasound (DUS), which can be performed at the bedside or in the operating room without the associated risks of contrast complications or radiation exposure. DUS is a quick and accurate method for initial evaluation of extremity injuries and may help to avoid

TABLE 1: Patterns of Associated Musculoskeletal and Other Structures With Specific Vessel Injury

Vessel	Musculoskeletal	Other
Carotid artery	Cervical spine Mandible, Le Fort II/III facial fracture Skull base	Vertebral vein Carotid artery Trachea, esophagus
Vertebral artery	Cervical spine (vertebral foramina) Skull base	Jugular vein Carotid artery
Subclavian artery or vein	Clavicle Sternum, manubrium	Thoracic duct (left) Brachial plexus, recurrent laryngeal nerve
Axillary artery or vein	Shoulder, proximal humerus	Brachial plexus, axillary nerve
Brachial artery	Midhumerus Biceps, triceps	Ulnar nerve Median nerve
Radial or ulnar artery	Elbow fracture or dislocation Radius, ulna, wrist Forearm and hand flexor tendons	Distal radial nerve (sensation only) Ulnar nerve
Thoracic great vessels	Sternum, manubrium	Innominate vein, recurrent laryngeal nerve
Descending aorta	Thoracic spine Posterior rib fracture or dislocation Diaphragm	Esophagus Lung Left subclavian vein (blunt)
Abdominal aorta or vena cava Suprarenal Infrarenal	Thoracic or lumbar spine T12-L2 (with or without spinal cord injury) L2-sacral fractures	Zone 1 retroperitoneal hematoma Stomach, transverse colon, pancreas Duodenum, small bowel
Portal vein or superior mesenteric vein	Lumbar spine fracture or ligament injury Rib fractures	Zone 4 retroperitoneal hematoma Duodenum (second or third portion), head of pancreas Portal triad (hepatic artery, common bile duct)
Renal artery or vein	Lumbar spine Posterior rib fracture or dislocation	Zone 2 retroperitoneal hematoma Kidney, proximal ureter, adrenal or gonadal vessels
Iliac vessels	Pelvic fracture Sacral fracture Sacroiliac joint disruption	Zone 3 retroperitoneal hematoma Cecum (right), sigmoid colon (left) Bladder, ureters
Femoral artery or vein	Pelvic fracture Acetabulum Proximal to mid-femur	Femoral nerve, sciatic nerve (rare) Inguinal ligament Spermatic cord
Popliteal artery or vein	Dislocated or "floating" knee Distal femur, proximal tibia	Tibial nerve Calf compartment syndrome
Tibioperoneal vessels	Tibia, fibula Ankle fracture or dislocation	Tibial nerve, peroneal nerve (footdrop) Calf compartment syndrome

From Cronenwett JL, Johnston KW. *Rutherford's Vascular Surgery.* 8th ed. Philadelphia: Saunders; 2014:2427.

unnecessary arteriography, CTA, or operative intervention. However, it is highly operator dependent.

Uncontrolled hemorrhage is the leading cause of preventable death in trauma patients. Severe hemorrhage can lead to the "lethal triad" of hypothermia, coagulopathy, and acidosis. Historically, resuscitation consisted primarily of crystalloid fluids. However, excessive crystalloid-based resuscitation has been shown to exacerbate the lethal triad and worsen outcomes. Damage control resuscitation (DCR) is a strategy that emphasizes permissive hypotension, the use of blood products over isotonic fluid for volume replacement, and the rapid and early correction of coagulopathy with blood component therapy for severely injured patients who are in hemorrhagic shock. The goal of permissive hypotension is to keep the blood pressure low enough to avoid exsanguination while simultaneously maintaining perfusion to end organs (a systolic blood pressure of approximately 80 to 90 mm Hg). Although no evidence-based recommendations currently exist, available literature suggests that patients with ongoing hemorrhage should have limited increase in blood pressure until definitive surgical control can be obtained. One important caveat to this rule may be patients with traumatic brain injury, for whom maintenance of cerebral perfusion pressure is paramount.

With regards to blood products, results from observational studies suggest that patients who require massive transfusion (e.g., >10 units of packed red blood cells [PRBCs]) have improved survival when the ratio of PRBCs (in units) to fresh frozen plasma (FFP, in units) to platelets (in 5-packs) approaches 1:1:1. This is likely because of a decreased incidence of coagulopathy as well as improved oxygen delivery. Ongoing resuscitation can be directed using thromboelastography (TEG), which can identify specific clotting deficiencies. Although more research is required to determine its efficacy, safety, and optimal dosing, recombinant factor VIIa may be beneficial in the coagulopathic patient. Providers also should familiarize themselves with the proper use of tourniquets and topical hemostatic agents such as QuickClot Hemostatic Bandage (kaolin-impregnated gauze; Z-Medica, Wallingford, CT), both of which are effective adjuncts in the primary control of hemorrhage. Unquestionably, the most important determination in the initial evaluation and management of patients with vascular injury is recognizing whether the patient is stable or unstable. Patients with persistent hypotension (systolic blood pressure <80 mm Hg) despite adequate resuscitation are likely to have uncontrolled hemorrhage and require immediate intervention.

■ PRINCIPLES OF MANAGEMENT

A systematic approach to managing patients with vascular injuries is necessary. If there is any possibility that the injured patient may require surgical intervention, an operating room and the appropriate support staff should be readied immediately. If available, consideration should be given as to whether an operating suite outfitted for both endovascular and open procedures will be needed. If specific expertise is required to effectively treat the patient, care should be coordinated carefully. Before starting any surgical procedure, it is imperative that the patient has adequate vascular access and that an adequate supply of blood products is readily available. If the patient meets criteria (at our institution, >4 units of PRBCs in <4 hours with ongoing uncontrolled bleeding), the institution's massive transfusion protocol should be activated.

In the severely injured patient, definitive repair of vascular injuries may not be indicated in the immediate period. In the context of vascular surgery, the term *damage control* refers to hemorrhage control and the expedient restoration of blood flow to ischemic tissue in order to avoid further injury. This process prioritizes short-term physiologic recovery over anatomic reconstruction in the multiply injured patient. In the damage control setting, definitive repair of extremity injuries may not be feasible. Instead, vessels may be ligated or shunted while life-threatening issues are managed and the patient's

physiologic abnormalities are addressed. This is especially relevant in patients with injuries to both the torso and limbs. In the most extreme cases, amputation may be required.

Over the past 3 decades catheter-based therapy has evolved from a diagnostic entity to both a primary and an adjunctive treatment for vascular injuries. In carefully selected patients, endovascular treatment can be highly effective. However, open surgery remains the primary treatment modality for unstable patients with hard signs of vascular injury. In general, endovascular treatments should be considered for vascular injuries to the neck, proximal extremities, and torso (e.g., retroperitoneal hemorrhage, blunt aortic injury). A hybrid approach, in which open and endovascular techniques are used in concert, can be used to obtain rapid control of vessels that are difficult to expose. A prime example of this technique is resuscitative endovascular balloon occlusion of the aorta (REBOA), which allows for perfusion of vital organs while the patient is resuscitated and definitive control of the hemorrhage is obtained. Specific applications of endovascular therapy are discussed in detail in later sections of this chapter.

There are a number of operative considerations to address when treating patients with vascular trauma. Before starting any case, the neurological status of an affected extremity should be documented. This allows postoperative neurologic deficits to be put into the appropriate context. In general, patients should be prepped widely and after options for autologous reconstructive conduit have been reviewed. For example, in the patient with penetrating neck trauma, the chest and at least one lower extremity should be prepped to allow for prompt sternotomy and greater saphenous vein harvest. In most situations, autologous saphenous vein contralateral to the injured extremity is the preferred conduit for reconstruction. If saphenous vein is not available, polytetrafluoroethylene (PTFE) can be used with the knowledge that patency rates are lower and the risk of graft infection is relatively high. It is also important to obtain generous surgical exposure of the affected area. This is best achieved with a longitudinal incision over named vessels. Proximal and distal control should be obtained as quickly and as safely as possible, and heparinization should be performed only in stable patients with extremity injuries that are at low risk for further bleeding. Patients with multiple injuries, traumatic brain injury, or severe torso trauma should not be heparinized, although local heparinization at the repair site may be used to prevent local thrombotic complications. In grossly contaminated areas, aggressive débridement and temporary shunting may be indicated to avoid infection, which can occur in up to 50% of traumatic vascular repairs. One way to decrease the rate of infection in patients with extensive soft tissue loss is to ensure adequate soft tissue coverage with a regional skin or muscle flap or skin grafting. Finally, failure to perform fasciotomy after revascularization of an ischemic extremity may result in neuropathy or limb loss due to compartment syndrome (discussed in more detail in the "Extremities" section).

■ OPERATIVE TREATMENT BY BODY REGION

Neck and Thoracic Outlet

The three zones of the neck dictate the treatment of penetrating injuries to this area. Zone I is located below the cricoid cartilage, zone II extends between the cricoid cartilage and the angle of the mandible, and zone III is above the angle of the mandible (Figure 1). Most injuries (47%) occur in zone II, 19% occur in zone III, and 18% occur in zone I. Patients with hard signs of vascular trauma or evidence of injury to the aerodigestive tract (e.g., respiratory distress, bubbling from the wound) should obtain a chest x-ray and proceed directly to the operating room. Zone II injuries are best addressed via a cervical incision (along the anterior border of the sternocleidomastoid) with direct repair. Depending on their location, zone I injuries may require a median sternotomy or anterolateral thoracotomy, whereas zone III injuries are approached via a high cervical incision with subluxation

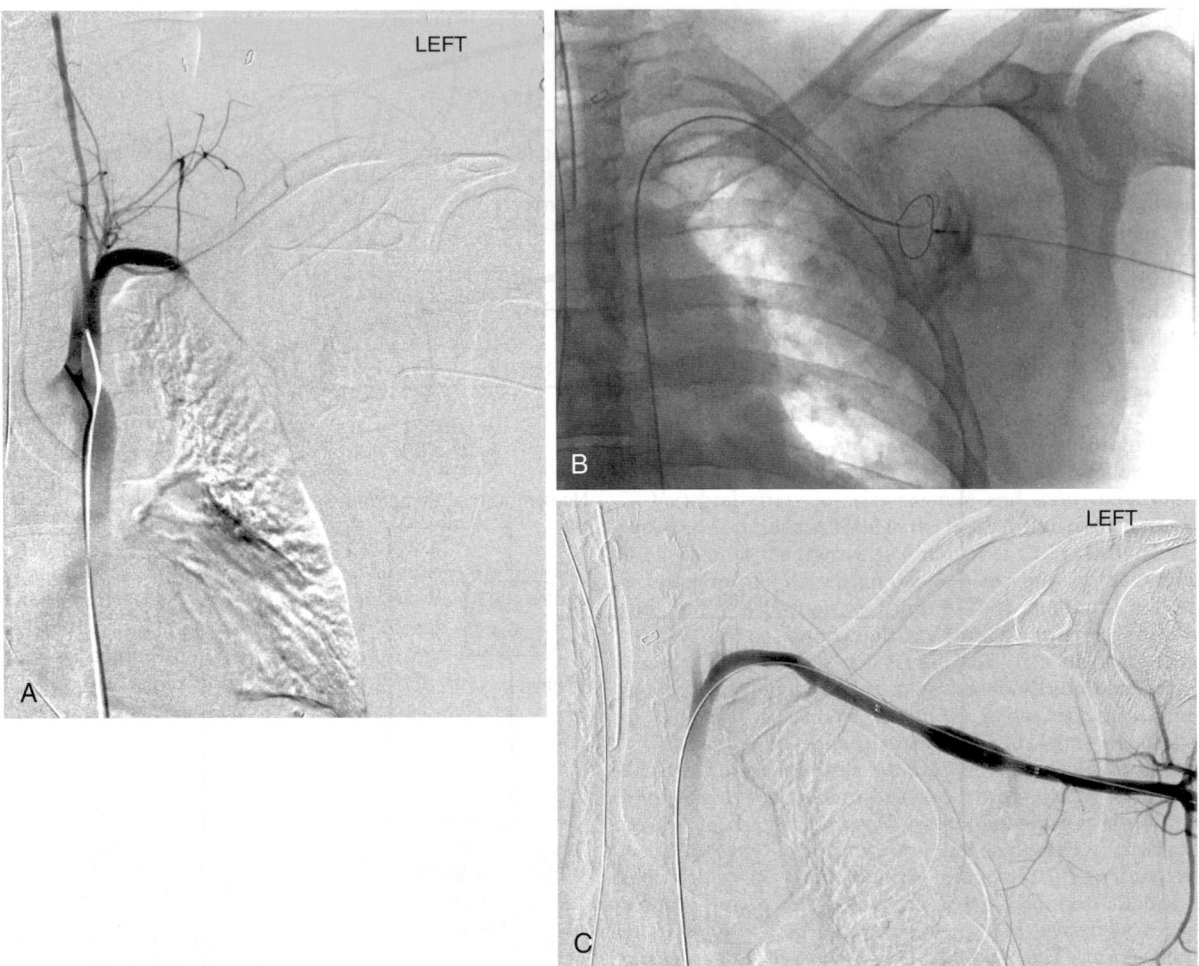

FIGURE 4 A, Left subclavian artery selection via right femoral artery access to traumatic disruption of the left subclavian artery after a stab injury. **B,** Through-and-through brachial-femoral wire technique used to traverse the vascular defect. **C,** Covered stent placement with re-establishment of continuity and antegrade flow. *(Courtesy Dr. Jonathan Eliason, University of Michigan, Ann Arbor, MI.)*

rhythm, intracardiac injection of 1 mg of epinephrine and direct defibrillation may be attempted. Aggressive resuscitation with blood products via large-bore catheters in the neck or upper extremity should be initiated as quickly as possible. In appropriately selected patients, survival after RT for penetrating injury is 8% to 21% (Figure 6).

Blunt aortic injury (BAI) is similarly devastating. Approximately 80% of patients expire at the scene of injury, and of those that survive, half die within 24 hours. BAI is a rare event and typically the result of deceleration injuries that occur during motor vehicle accidents. The most commonly injured area is the aortic isthmus just distal to the origin of the left subclavian artery. CTA is the preferred diagnostic modality for BAI, which can be seen as a small intimal tear (grade I), intramural hematoma (grade II), pseudoaneurysm (grade III), or frank rupture (grade IV). Most patients who reach the hospital alive have contained aortic injuries at risk for rupture. This risk for rupture can be reduced from 12% to 1.5% with aggressive control of blood pressure and heart rate. Most vascular surgeons target a systolic blood pressure lower than 100 mm Hg and a heart rate less than 100 beats per minute using an IV beta-blocker such as esmolol. Treatment of grades II to IV injuries should occur urgently (<24 hours) but only after the patient has been resuscitated adequately, the blood pressure and heart rate have been controlled, and other injuries have been evaluated. Patients with concomitant traumatic brain injury require greater brain perfusion pressure and should be repaired immediately.

Thoracic endovascular aortic repair (TEVAR) is the recommended treatment for BAI in anatomically suitable candidates. Conventional treatment via an open approach (thoracotomy/sternotomy with distal aortic perfusion) is associated with higher morbidity and mortality when compared with TEVAR. The AAST-2 (American Association for the Surgery of Trauma) trial showed a decrease in mortality from 23.5% to 7.2% when comparing open repair with endovascular stent-graft placement. Other studies confirm reduced mortality and have shown that paraplegia, stroke, renal injury, and pulmonary complications are decreased with TEVAR. One of the most important technical aspects of stent-graft placement involves the adequacy of the proximal landing zone. Although most stent-grafts require a 2-cm seal zone, the average distance from the left subclavian artery to traumatic tears is approximately 6 mm. As such, the left subclavian artery may need to be covered to ensure adequate seal. Revascularization is selective and based on vertebral artery anatomy, the condition of the patient, and local expertise. Complications of TEVAR occur in up to 20% of patients and include stroke, paraplegia, endoleak, and stent migration. Long-term follow-up with serial CTA is standard practice to evaluate for late complications (Figure 7).

Abdomen

The vast majority of abdominal vascular injuries are caused by penetrating trauma. Half of patients will die from their injuries, and the

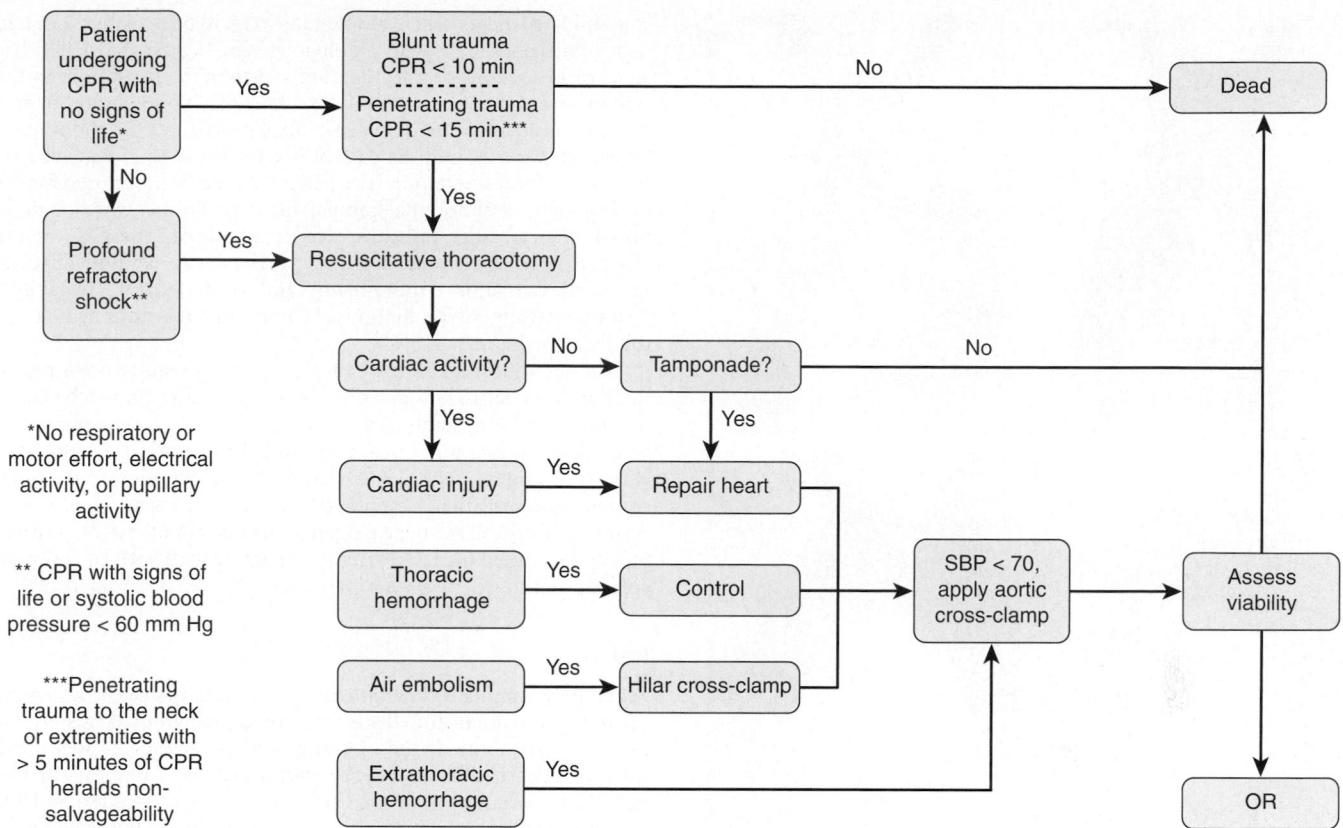

FIGURE 5 Algorithm for resuscitative thoracotomy (Western Trauma Association, 2012). *CPR*, Cardiopulmonary resuscitation; *OR*, operating room; *SBP*, systolic blood pressure. *(From Burlew CC, et al. Western Trauma Association critical decisions in trauma: resuscitative thoracotomy. J Trauma Acute Care Surg. 2012;73:1359-1364.)*

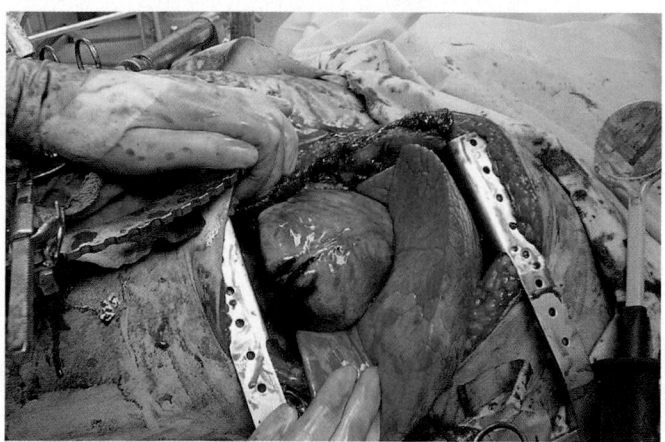

FIGURE 6 Resuscitative thoracotomy performed via left anterolateral thoracotomy. *(Courtesy Dr. Jonathan Eliason, University of Michigan, Ann Arbor, MI.)*

majority will suffer concomitant trauma to gastrointestinal organs. The treatment of these injuries is challenging and hinges on early surgical intervention and a thorough knowledge of abdominal anatomy. The most commonly injured vessels are the inferior vena cava (IVC; 25% of injuries), aorta (21%), iliac arteries (20%), iliac veins (17%), superior mesenteric vein (SMV; 11%), and superior mesenteric artery (SMA; 10%). Patients in extremis may require RT, as discussed in the prior section. Another option to temporarily

control noncompressible subdiaphragmatic bleeding is REBOA, which involves placement of an occlusive balloon in the distal thoracic aorta via the femoral artery (Figure 8). In most cases of penetrating abdominal trauma, definitive endovascular treatment does not play a role.

The abdominal vasculature is divided into three anatomic areas, as shown in Figure 9. Zone 1 is central, zone 2 is lateral, and zone 3 is pelvic. Unstable patients require immediate surgical intervention via a midline laparotomy extending from the xiphoid to the pubis. Active bleeding is controlled by direct compression, packing, and/or compression of the aorta at the hiatus. For proximal abdominal aortic injuries, control of the aorta may require a left-sided thoracotomy. Exploration of the abdomen then proceeds systematically. Bleeding from the aorta, celiac axis, SMA, and left renal vessels is best approached via a left medial visceral rotation (the Mattox maneuver; Figure 10). Because of rich collateralization, ligation of the celiac artery and inferior mesenteric artery (IMA) typically is well tolerated. In contrast, ligation of the proximal SMA may result in ischemic necrosis of the small bowel and right colon. As such, all attempts should be made to maintain SMA continuity. Bleeding from the IVC and right renal vessels is best approached via a right medial viscera rotation (the Cattell-Braasch maneuver; Figure 11). Most IVC injuries can be repaired primarily. Posterior injuries can be exposed by twisting the IVC or through an anterior wall incision. Ligation, although morbid, can be considered in damage control situations.

Depending on the severity of injury and the patient's overall physiologic status, a damage control approach may be indicated. In this setting, bleeding should be controlled with gauze packing and selective vessel ligation. Major arterial structures are shunted, and gross contamination is minimized. Of note, PTFE may be used in

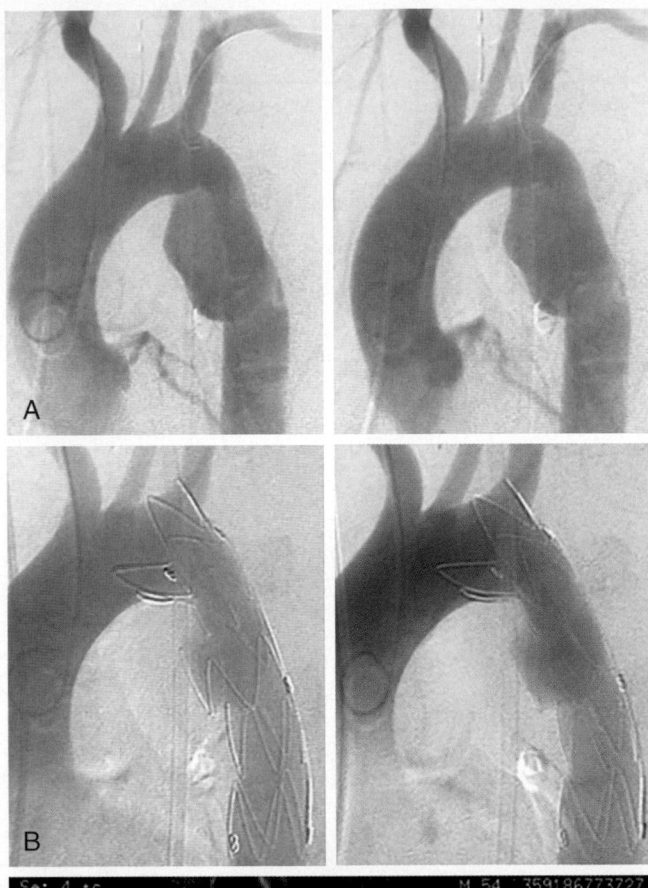

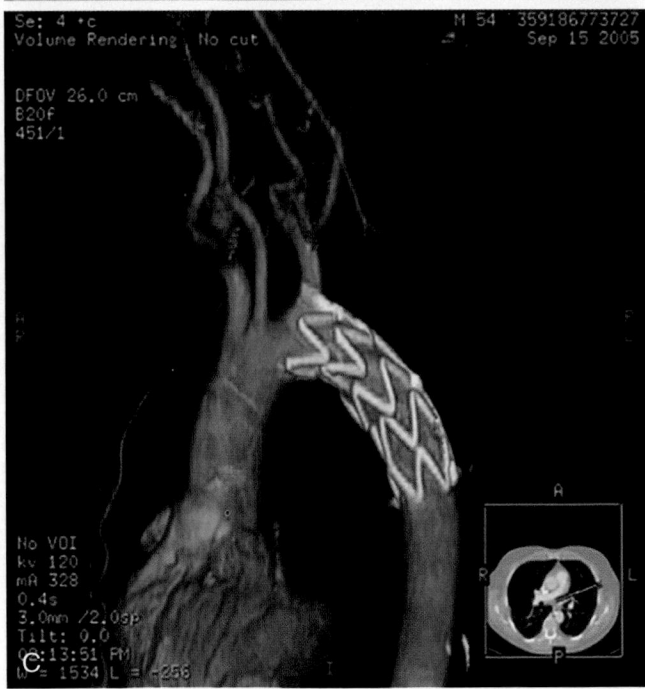

FIGURE 7 A, Angiogram showing traumatic disruption of the aorta with pseudoaneurysm formation after high-speed motor vehicle crash. **B,** Completion angiogram after stent-graft deployment showing complete exclusion of the injury. **C,** Five-year computed tomographic angiography follow-up with three-dimensional volume rendering reconstruction. *(From Rousseau H, et al. The role of stent-grafts in the management of aortic trauma.* Cardiovasc Intervent Radiol. 2012;35:2-14.)

contaminated fields when autologous vein is unavailable. Limited data comparing PTFE with autologous vein suggest that PTFE has equal or lower rates of infection and anastomotic disruption. In the case of severe enteric contamination, however, axillofemoral bypass may be considered. After damage control procedures the abdomen is closed temporarily, and the patient is returned to the intensive care unit (ICU) for resuscitation. The patient should be monitored for the development of abdominal compartment syndrome, which is diagnosed when bladder pressure exceeds 20 mm Hg. Because of the elevated intra-abdominal pressure, patients may develop oliguria, increased ventilator requirements, and hemodynamic instability. Definitive treatment for abdominal compartment syndrome is surgical decompression.

Although most abdominal vascular injuries require open repair, there are some situations in which the endovascular approach should be considered. In stable patients with contained retroperitoneal hematoma, endoluminal treatment avoids the morbidity associated with open surgery, aortic cross-clamping, and exposure to potential contamination. Patients found to have intimal flaps, pseudoaneurysms, or fistulae also can be treated with endovascular stent grafting. Finally, injuries to the renal arteries are best treated with an endovascular approach whenever feasible.

Pelvis

Penetrating trauma to the iliofemoral vessels is managed by rapidly obtaining proximal and distal control of the injured vessels via midline laparotomy. If the bleeding vessel(s) cannot be identified, total vascular exclusion may be performed by clamping (in this order) the aorta, the right and left common iliac arteries, and the IVC. All efforts should be made to restore continuity to the common iliac and external iliac arteries in order to avoid leg ischemia. In patients with severe injuries or significant enteric contamination, delayed extra-anatomic bypass (e.g., axillofemoral bypass) may be warranted. In contrast, complex reconstruction of the hypogastric arteries and pelvic veins is not recommended, as these vessels can be ligated safely.

Blunt injury to the pelvis from high-energy traumas such as motor vehicle accidents or falls can result in pelvic fractures and uncontrolled retroperitoneal hemorrhage. Although normally a "closed" space, the retroperitoneum expands in the setting of unstable fractures (displacement of more than 0.5 cm), allowing for high-volume blood loss. More than 90% of bleeding results from the shearing of pelvic veins. Early hemorrhage is controlled by stabilizing the pelvic ring and reducing the available volume in the retroperitoneal space. This can be accomplished using a sheet, pelvic binder, or external fixator. Angioembolization is recommended over surgery for these injuries, as open exploration results in unacceptably poor outcomes. Angioembolization can control arterial bleeding but is less effective in the setting of diffuse venous oozing. In centers without endovascular capabilities, preperitoneal packing may be performed in an attempt to slow bleeding. Preperitoneal packing is performed by opening the anterior fascia beneath the umbilicus, retracting the rectus muscles laterally, and placing three laparotomy sponges on each side of the bladder without opening the peritoneum (Figure 12).

Extremities

The accuracy of physical examination and Doppler-derived blood pressure measurements in extremity vascular injury is excellent. Patients with hard signs of vascular injury should proceed to the operating room immediately. Whenever possible, procedures should take place in a hybrid operating room to allow for fluoroscopy-based diagnosis and treatment of vascular and orthopedic injuries. In general, all fractures and dislocations should be reduced before vascular reconstruction. A temporary shunt may be required to allow for reduction, in which case adequate redundancy of the shunt should be ensured to allow for manipulation of the extremity.

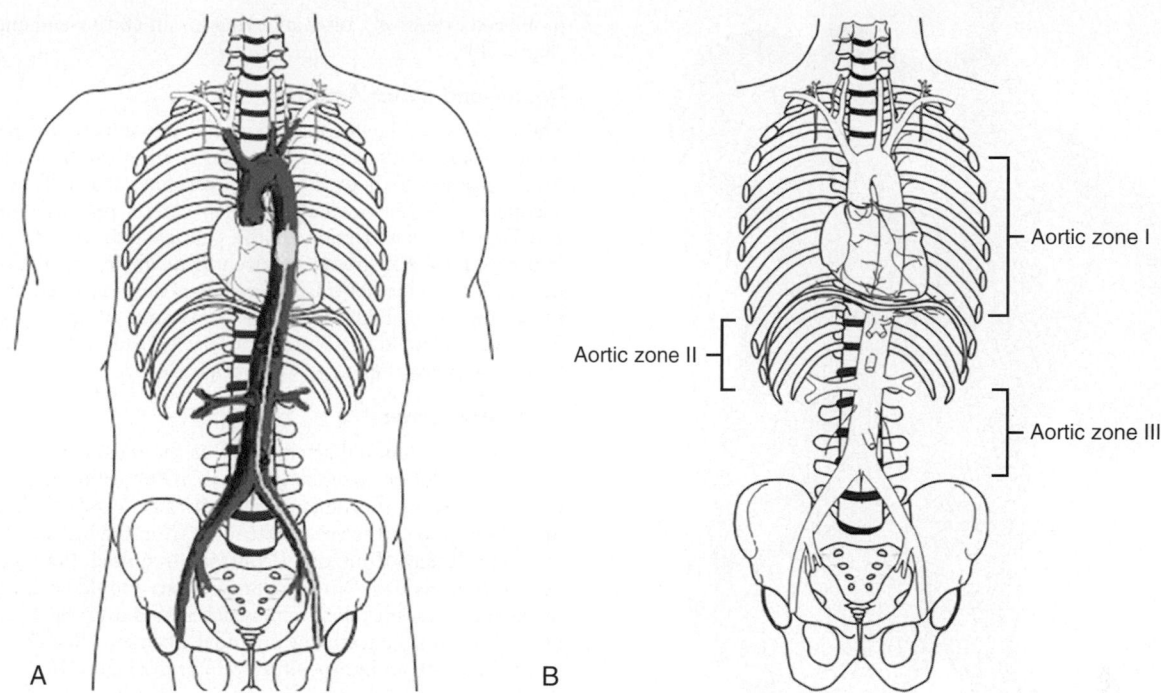

FIGURE 8 A, Resuscitative endovascular balloon occlusion of the aorta (REBOA). **B,** Aorta occlusion zones. Occlusion of zone I (left subclavian artery to the celiac trunk) is used to control abdominal hemorrhage. Occlusion of zone III (lowest renal artery to aortic bifurcation) is used to control pelvic hemorrhage. Zone II (celiac trunk to lower renal artery) is a no occlusion zone. (**A,** *Courtesy Dr. Lena Napolitano, University of Michigan, Ann Arbor, MI;* **B,** *From Stannard A, et al. Resuscitative endovascular balloon occlusion of the aorta (REBOA) as an adjunct for hemorrhagic shock.* J Trauma. *2011;71:1869-1872.)*

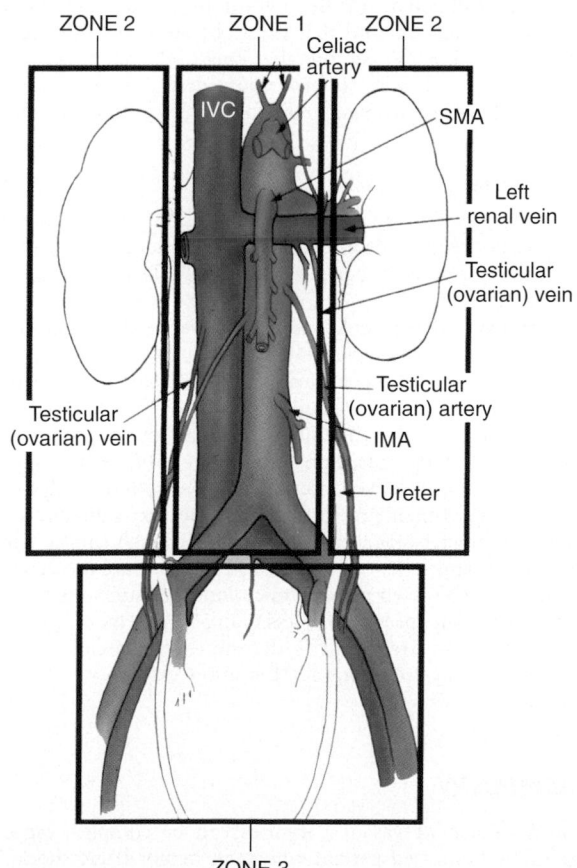

FIGURE 9 The retroperitoneal zones. Zone 1 is central. Zone 2 is lateral. Zone 3 is pelvic. *IMA,* Inferior mesenteric artery; *IVC,* inferior vena cava; *SMA,* superior mesenteric artery.

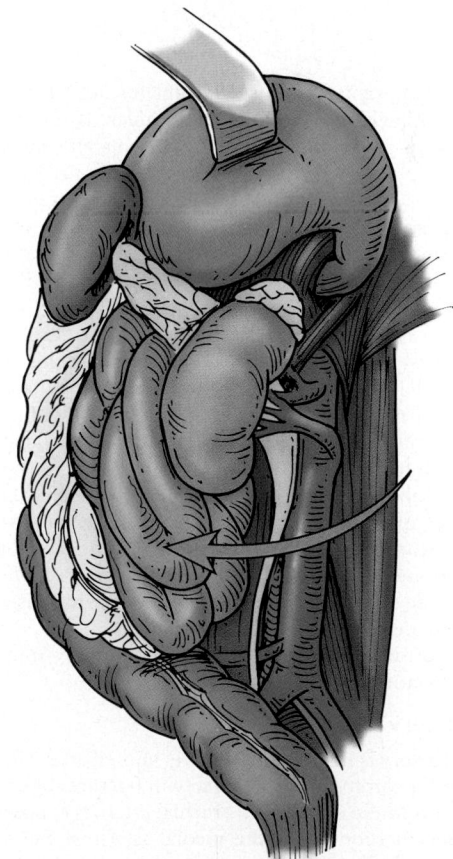

FIGURE 10 Medial rotation of the left-sided viscera. This will expose the aorta from the diaphragm to the aortic bifurcation.

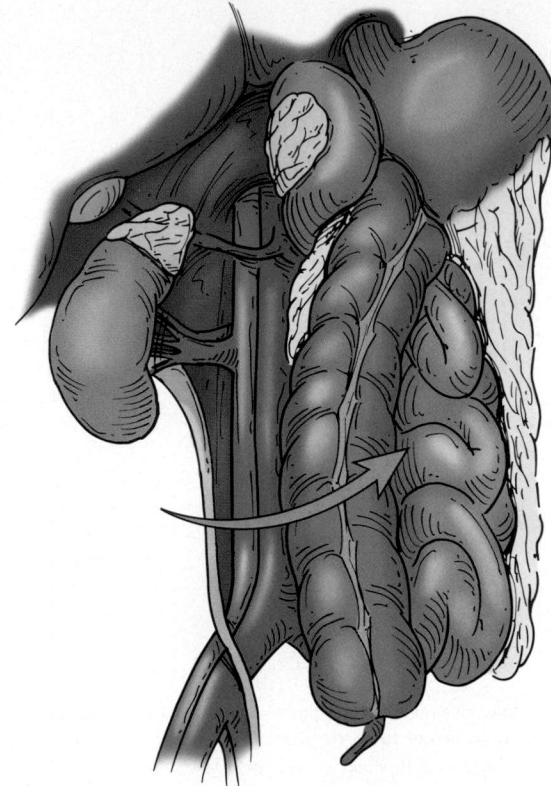

FIGURE 11 Medial rotation of the right-sided viscera. This will expose the right renal artery, right common iliac artery and vein, and inferior vena cava.

Patients with soft signs of injury warrant further workup, starting with an ankle-brachial or wrist-brachial index. If the index is less than 1.0, CTA is recommended. Many patients already will have a tourniquet in place. When properly applied, tourniquets can be highly effective. However, improper application paradoxically can increase bleeding by occluding venous outflow while inadequately occluding arterial inflow. Although timely repair is essential, the extremities can withstand 4 to 6 hours of ischemia without permanent injury.

Extremity vascular injuries can be repaired primarily, with vein patch angioplasty or with interposition grafting using autologous vein conduit. PTFE has lower patency than autologous vein and should be used only when the latter is not available. Endovascular treatment is limited to areas in which exposure is challenging and is associated with high morbidity. The use of endoluminal stent-grafts in axillary and iliofemoral vessels has proven successful. Endovascular techniques are also useful in obtaining proximal control with balloon occlusion in these critical areas. All extremity venous injuries can be ligated safely, but large veins should be repaired when feasible to avoid the development of limb edema and increased rates of venous thromboembolism.

Surgical considerations for the most commonly injured upper and lower extremity arteries are as follows.

Brachial Artery

The brachial artery is the most frequently injured artery in the upper extremity and is commonly associated with fractures of the humerus and dislocation of the elbow. The brachial artery is exposed through a longitudinal incision along the medial aspect of the arm in the groove between the biceps and triceps muscles. Care is taken to avoid the median nerve, which is immediately adjacent to the brachial artery within the brachial sheath. The brachial artery can be mobilized extensively, often allowing for an end-to-end anastomosis (Figure 13).

Radial and Ulnar Arteries

The arteries of the forearm typically are injured by penetrating trauma. Isolated ulnar or radial artery injuries can be managed with simple ligation if there is absolute certainty that collateral flow is adequate. This can be determined by careful physical examination and Doppler interrogation of the palmar arch. If both vessels are injured, preference should be given to repair of the ulnar artery, as this tends to be the dominant vessel. Exposure is gained by performing a longitudinal incision over the course of the vessels in the forearm. Similar to the brachial artery, end-to-end anastomoses of these vessels are often achievable (Figure 14).

Femoral Arteries

The superficial femoral artery (SFA) is the most commonly injured artery of the lower extremity. More than 90% of injuries to the SFA will have hard signs. The femoral arteries are exposed via a longitudinal incision over the vessel extending from the inguinal ligament 8 to 12 cm distally. If proximal control is required, the inguinal ligament can be divided. During exposure, care should be taken to avoid the lateral circumflex iliac vein, which passes over the distal external iliac artery and beneath the inguinal ligament. Repair typically is performed with an interposition vein graft (Figure 15).

Popliteal Artery

The popliteal artery is the second most commonly injured artery of the lower extremity. Unlike other lower extremity vascular injuries, the cause is typically blunt trauma resulting in a fracture and dislocation of the tibial plateau. Exposure is obtained via separate above-knee and below-knee medial incisions. This exposure allows proximal and distal control and avoids the division of the semimembranosus and semitendinosus tendons that would be required with exposure of the artery directly behind the knee. All popliteal injuries should be repaired with interposition graft or above-knee to below-knee popliteal bypass, preferably with contralateral greater saphenous vein.

Tibial Arteries

Unless there are clinical signs of ischemia, injury to a single tibial artery does not require reconstruction. However, in the case of multiple injuries or known peripheral arterial disease, tibial vessels should be repaired.

Patients who suffer vascular extremity injuries are at high risk for developing compartment syndrome because of ischemia-reperfusion injury. If not diagnosed and treated in a timely fashion, compartment syndrome can result in permanent disability or limb loss. The most common findings on examination include pain out of proportion to injury, tense compartments, pain with passive stretch (early finding), paresthesia (30 minutes to 2 hours after onset), and paralysis (late finding). Compartment pressures can be measured directly with a portable manometer (e.g., Stryker needle), although clinical context and physical examination are often sufficient to make the diagnosis. If the difference between the diastolic blood pressure and compartment pressure (delta pressure) is less than 30 mm Hg, compartment syndrome is likely. Treatment is decompressive fasciotomy. Two-incision fasciotomy technique for the lower extremity is shown in Figure 16.

■ SUMMARY

The management of vascular injuries can be complex, especially in the multiply injured patient who is in hemorrhagic shock. The first priority in these patients is to determine whether the patient is stable. If the patient is unstable, he or she should be taken to the operating room without delay. Those who are stable may undergo

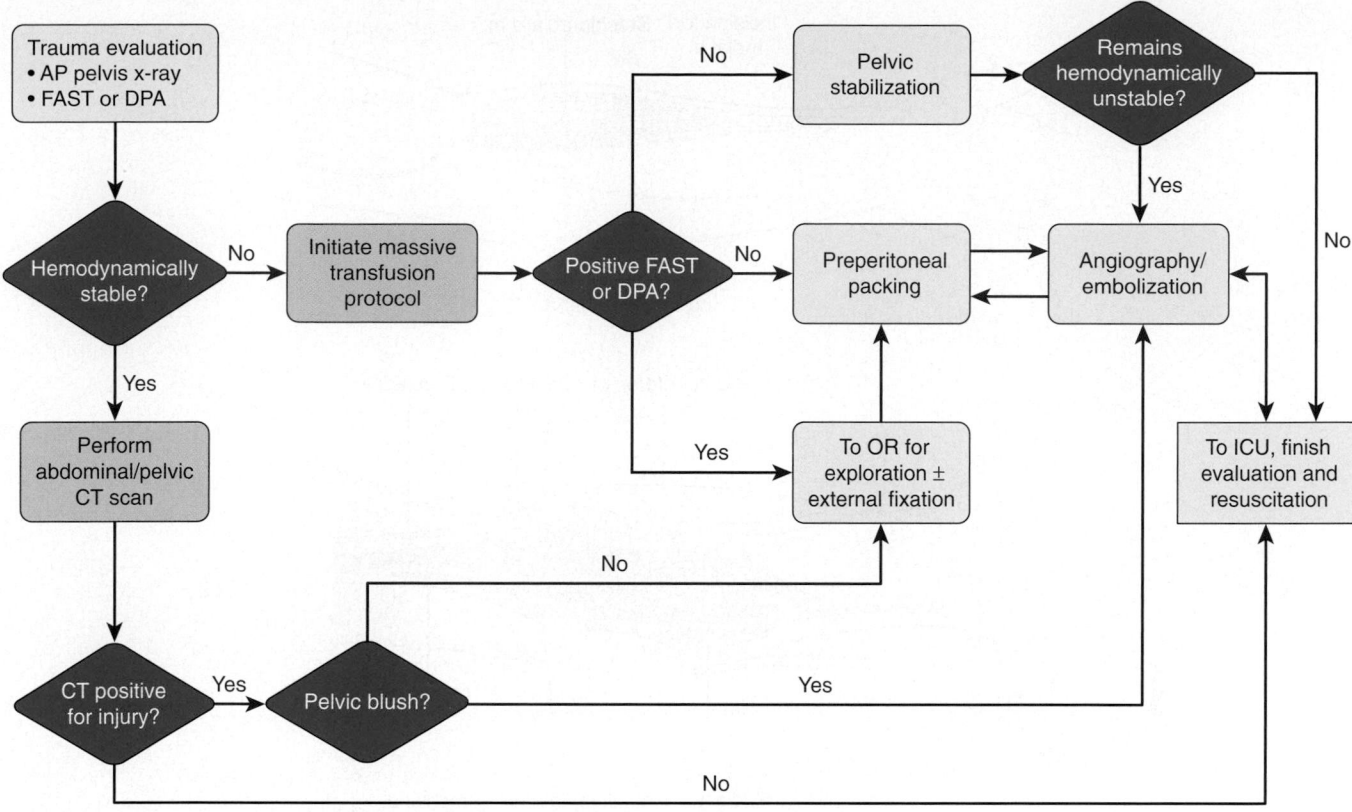

FIGURE 12 Algorithm for the management of pelvic fracture with hemodynamic instability (Western Trauma Association, 2008). *AP*, Anteroposterior; *CT*, computed tomography; *DPA*, diagnostic peritoneal aspiration; *FAST*, focused assessment with sonography for trauma; *ICU*, intensive care unit; *OR*, operating room. *(From Davis JW, Moore FA, McIntyre RC, Cocanour CS, Moore EE. Western Trauma Association critical decisions in trauma: pelvic fracture with hemodynamic instability. J Trauma. 2008;65:1012-1015.)*

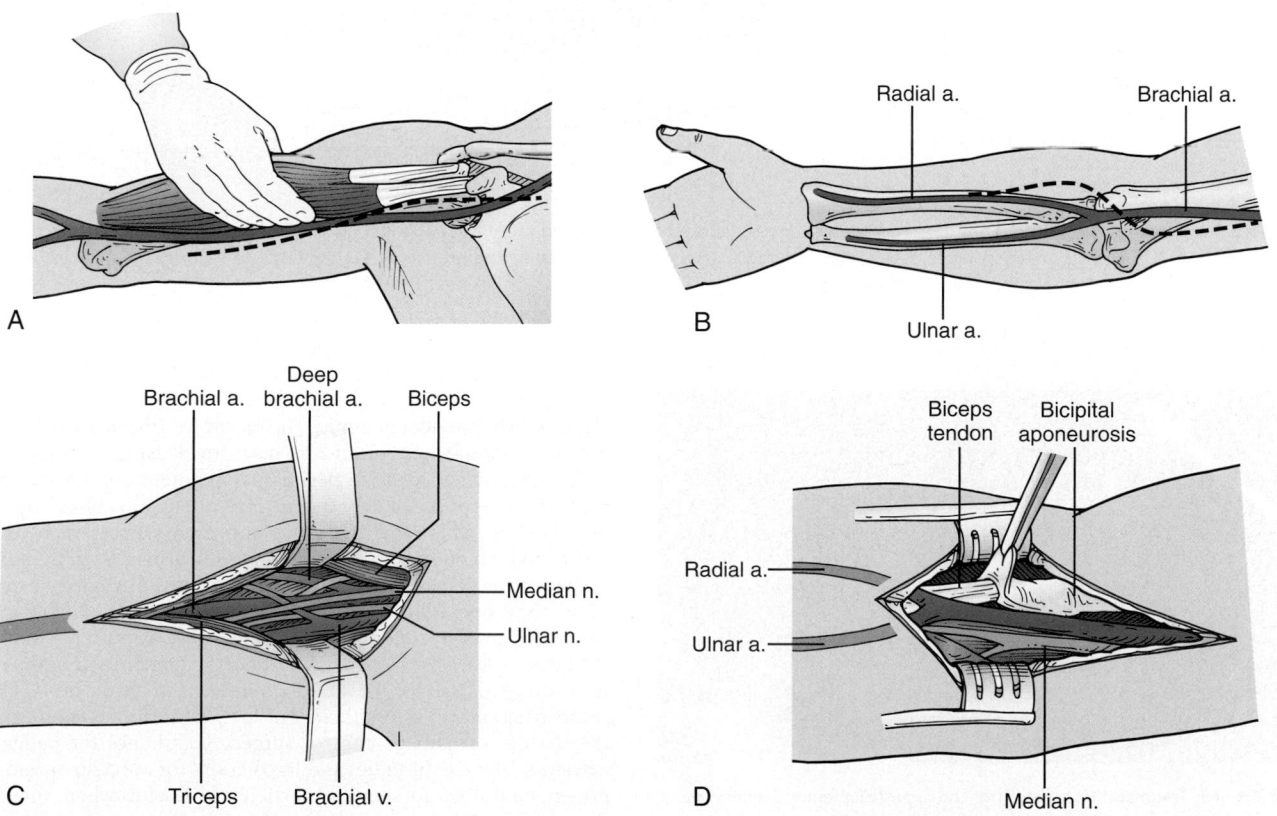

FIGURE 13 Exposure of the brachial artery. **A,** The incision for the brachial artery should lie just inferior to the biceps muscle. **B,** A "lazy S" incision can be used to traverse the antecubital fossa. **C** and **D,** Note the close association between the brachial artery and the median nerve. *a.*, Artery; *n.*, nerve; *v.*, vein. *(From Cronenwett JL, Johnston KW. Rutherford's Vascular Surgery. 8th ed. Philadelphia: Saunders; 2014:2493.)*

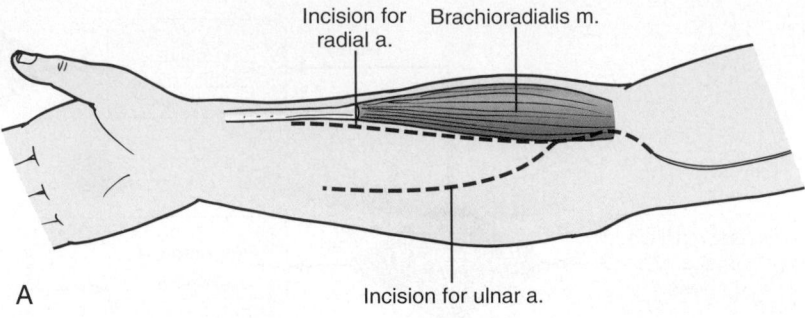

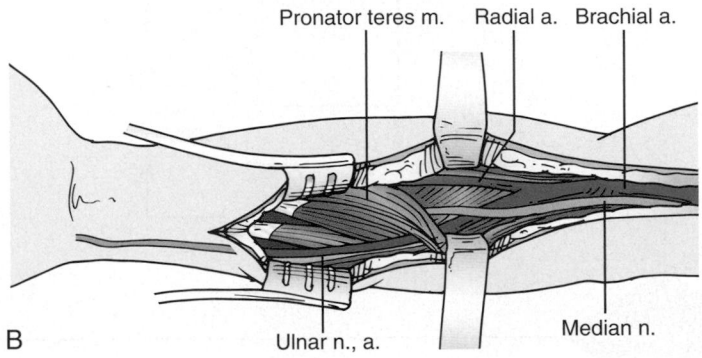

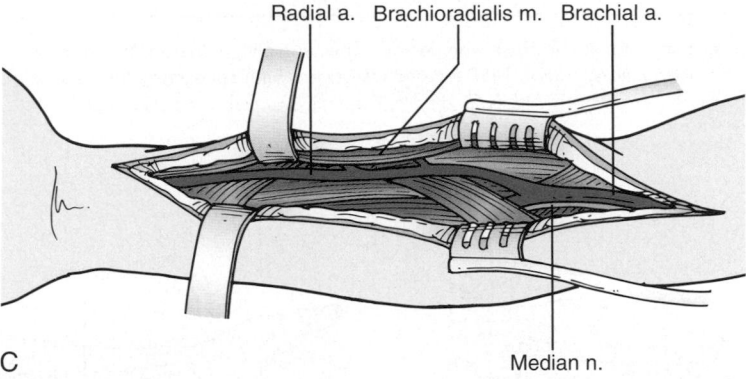

FIGURE 14 Exposure of the radial and ulnar arteries. **A,** Incisions for the brachial and radial artery should overlie the course of the vessels in the forearm. **B** and **C,** The ulnar artery courses deeper than the radial artery and is crossed by the median nerve just distal to its origin. *a.,* Artery; *m.,* muscle; *n.,* nerve. *(From Cronenwett JL, Johnston KW. Rutherford's Vascular Surgery. 8th ed. Philadelphia: Saunders; 2014:2494.)*

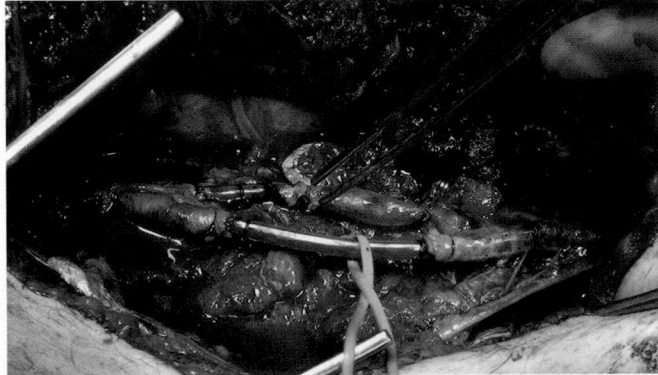

FIGURE 15 Traumatic transection of the superficial femoral artery and femoral vein requiring temporary shunting. *(Courtesy Dr. Jonathan Eliason, University of Michigan, Ann Arbor, MI.)*

CTA, which provides a rapid and accurate diagnosis of vascular injuries. Resuscitation should be performed using damage control techniques that emphasize permissive hypotension (systolic blood pressure of approximately 80 mm Hg), the use of blood products over isotonic fluid, and the rapid and early correction of coagulopathy with blood component therapy. Key principles of the surgical management of patients with vascular injuries include (1) the use of a hybrid operating room when available, (2) adequate IV access, (3) readily available blood products, (4) wide skin preparation that includes at least one lower extremity, (5) generous intraoperative exposure, (6) the use of autologous vein in favor of PTFE for reconstruction, (7) a low threshold for performing fasciotomy, and (8) the use of damage control surgery techniques for patients in extremis. The use of endovascular therapy for vascular trauma has grown, and this therapy is particularly useful when managing difficult-to-expose vessels, such as those in the neck, thoracic outlet, or groin.

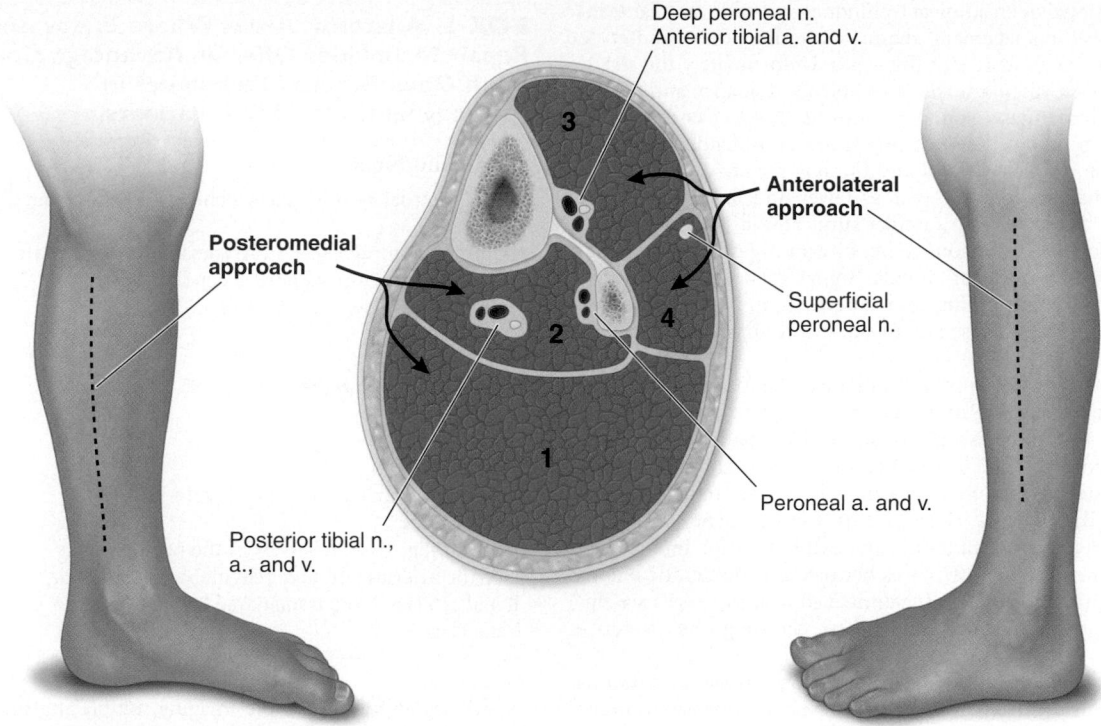

FIGURE 16 Two-incision technique for four-compartment fasciotomy of the leg. *Left,* Posteromedial incision for decompression of the superficial and deep posterior compartments. This incision must extend far enough distally to allow complete decompression of the entire deep posterior compartment. *Right,* Anterolateral incision for release of the anterior and lateral compartments. Care should be taken to identify and protect the superficial peroneal nerve. This incision must extend far enough proximally to ensure complete decompression of the muscles near their origin. *a.,* Artery; *n.,* nerve; *v.,* vein. *(From Herring JA. Tachdjian's Pediatric Orthopaedics: From the Texas Scottish Rite Hospital for Children. 5th ed. Philadelphia: Elsevier; 2013.)*

SUGGESTED READINGS

Avery LE, Stahlfield KR, Corcos AC, et al. Evolving role of endovascular techniques for traumatic vascular injury: a changing landscape? *J Trauma.* 2012;72:41-46.

Biffl WL, Moore EE, Ryu RK, et al. The unrecognized epidemic of blunt carotid arterial injuries: early diagnosis improves neurologic outcome. *Ann Surg.* 1998;228:462-470.

Demetriades D, Velmahos GC, Scalea TM, et al. Operative repair or endovascular stent graft in blunt traumatic thoracic aortic injuries: results of an American Association for the Surgery of Trauma Multicenter Study. *J Trauma.* 2008;64:561-570.

Duchesne JC, McSwain NE, Cotton BA, et al. Damage control resuscitation: the new face of damage control. *J Trauma.* 2010;69:976-990.

Fabian TC, Richardson JD, Croce MA, et al. Prospective study of blunt aortic injury: Multicenter Trial of the American Association for the Surgery of Trauma. *J Trauma.* 1997;42:374-380.

Holcomb JB, del Junco DJ, Fox EE, et al. The prospective, observational, multicenter, major trauma transfusion (PROMMTT) study: comparative effectiveness of a time-varying treatment with competing risks. *JAMA Surg.* 2013;148:127-136.

Lee WA, Matsumura JS, Mitchell RS. Endovascular repair of traumatic thoracic aortic injury: clinical practice guidelines of the Society for Vascular Surgery. *J Vasc Surg.* 2011;52:187-192.

Seamon MJ, Smoger D, Torres DM. A prospective validation of a current practice: the detection of extremity vascular injury with CT angiography. *J Trauma.* 2009;67:238-244.

Stannard A, Eliason JL, Rasmussen T. Resuscitative endovascular balloon occlusion of the aorta (REBOA) as an adjunct for hemorrhagic shock. *J Trauma.* 2011;71:1869-1872.

ENDOVASCULAR MANAGEMENT OF ARTERIAL INJURY

Michael Sise, MD, and Matthew J. Wall, Jr., MD

Vascular injuries fall into three distinct categories of clinical presentation and management priorities. First, injuries with life-threatening hemorrhage require immediate vascular control, prompt diagnosis, and restoration of vascular continuity. If appropriate, damage control measures or ligation may be required. Second, vascular injuries with contained hemorrhage, ischemia, or threatened hematoma rupture require urgent intervention. Third, occult vascular injuries without the presence or threat of hemorrhage may require timely intervention to avoid the risk of hemorrhage or ischemia. Endovascular techniques have an important role in each of these categories of vascular injury.

Despite the rapid advances in endovascular therapy, it cannot be the only approach available and is not sufficient for many vascular injuries. The ideal approach to vascular trauma management is a blend of traditional open surgical techniques and endovascular techniques. Optimal management requires avoiding the mindset to choose one at the exclusion of the other. Unfortunately the steady reduction in open vascular experience during residency and fellowship training leads many younger surgeons to select endovascular techniques even though an open procedure or a blended approach would result in more successful and durable repairs. This problem increases in magnitude every year as fewer and fewer graduating surgeons have adequate open vascular surgical skills and more older and more experienced surgeons retire. Integrating endovascular and open surgical techniques for vascular injury management requires adequate preparation, training, and experience in both approaches. Each of these skill sets is essential to successful management of vascular trauma.

Surgical specialists with little trauma experience must avoid the pitfalls of using the elective surgical case approach when dealing with injuries. The anatomic disruption, surgical exposure, and trauma management priorities are distinctly different from those of elective procedures. This has become increasingly important in the management of vascular injuries. There is a growing tendency to pursue elective endovascular techniques in the extremities for trauma that are not appropriate. The differences between atherosclerotic lesions and the anatomic disruption of traumatized healthy vessels are significant and must be considered when choosing the operative approach.

Iatrogenic vascular injuries are a unique type of vascular trauma with special considerations. Many are the result of catheterization site or close proximity vessel injuries during diagnostic or endovascular procedures for either cardiac or peripheral vascular lesions. The surgeon, radiologist, or cardiologist performing the procedure usually is able to treat this lesion promptly with stent deployment at the lesion site. Pseudoaneurysms at catheter access sites may be treated with thrombin injection while preserving adequate luminal flow. This chapter does not focus on these lesions. There are, however, unique vascular injuries that occur during open or laparoscopic procedures. These challenging lesions require skills similar to those required for trauma patients with vascular injuries. The management principles discussed in this chapter also apply to these injuries.

At the time of this writing, there is a paucity of outcome data for endovascular management of vascular injuries. In this brief chapter we attempt to provide a balanced approach that integrates open surgical techniques and endovascular approaches to give the best possible outcome for trauma patients. We indicate where there is a lack of adequate outcome data to assess long-term success rates. However, we also include promising if not yet proven approaches. We attempt to give our readers the best advice at this time by describing what we do for our patients. Vascular trauma cases that illustrate endovascular management decision making are included at the end of this chapter.

■ CREATING ENDOVASCULAR CAPABILITY FOR VASCULAR TRAUMA MANAGEMENT

There are a variety of vascular injuries that do not require the capability to perform an open procedure for associated injuries or hematoma drainage and that can be managed in the interventional radiology suite. However, successful management of the full spectrum of vascular injuries using endovascular techniques requires a variety of special skills, equipment, and operating room (OR) capabilities. This includes endovascular catheter skills; the proper imaging capability; an adequate and immediately available inventory of catheters, wires, and endovascular stents; and an OR capable of supporting both percutaneous and open surgical approaches. Most trauma centers do not have a 24-hour, immediately available, fully equipped and staffed hybrid OR with all of the advanced imaging modalities for elective procedures. However, all trauma centers have an OR immediately available to support orthopedic trauma surgical

---

BOX 1: Anatomic Areas Where Endovascular Repair Techniques Offer an Advantage Compared With Open Surgical Techniques in Hemodynamically Stable Patients

Head and Neck

Distal internal carotid artery behind and above the digastric muscle
Common carotid artery from the arch to the low neck
Vertebral artery throughout its course
Subclavian and axillary arteries

Chest

Thoracic aorta and the arch vessels
Superior vena cava

Abdomen

Aorta and proximal mesenteric arteries
Iliac arteries
Internal iliac branch vessels in the pelvis
Hepatic arteries and parenchymal branch vessels
Renal arteries and parenchymal branch vessels
Vena cava

---

techniques with fluoroscopic imaging. By placing the patient on a fluoroscopy-capable OR table, using a high-resolution C-arm with digital subtraction angiography, and adding the proper prestaged catheters, wires, and stents, trauma centers can create a "hybrid OR of opportunity" (Figure 1).

There are a myriad of catheters, wires, and stents available for endovascular techniques. It would not be financially sustainable to stock all of them for emergency vascular trauma management. Choosing what to stock in rolling equipment cabinets that can be moved into an available OR requires a balance of both anticipating difficult technical challenges and limiting supplies to only what is necessary. Box 1 is an example of such an inventory from a trauma center with experience in endovascular techniques for vascular trauma. This center does not use a hybrid suite and moves equipment by rolling carts to a variety of available ORs for trauma.

A key principle to understand is that endovascular tools are used to achieve the same goals as those for open surgery. Rather than obtaining access to the injury externally by making a skin incision, percutaneous access is achieved intravascularly with a wire. Rather than dissecting externally and identifying the outside of the vascular structures, dissection occurs intravascularly with the wire getting intraluminal access to the area of injury. Instead of placing an external retractor so that the area of concern is readily available, a sheath is placed intravascularly so that ready access to the injury is obtained from inside the vessel. Rather than external repair, placing a graft or vascular structure externally, the injuries are addressed intravascularly with a covered stent or coils. This is just like in open surgery, only a limited number of endovascular tools and instruments are commonly needed.

For trauma cases, we try to keep our setup as simple as possible. Ultrasound is used routinely for vascular access because trauma patients often have spasm in small-diameter arteries. Access is obtained with a micropuncture kit, and a 0.035-inch wire system is commonly used. A 4F or 5F access sheath is placed initially. Access to the area of concern typically is achieved with a directable catheter, such as a Bern or KMP, with either a stiff or a floppy angled tip wire. For diagnostic procedures, a pigtail catheter with radiopaque markers is used to help size the diameter and needed length of the vessel. When access to the area of concern is achieved, an appropriate size working sheath, based on the needed diameter of the anticipated device, is placed. For smaller vessels, devices typically can be delivered over the stiff wire. For areas that are more angulated, a Rosen wire

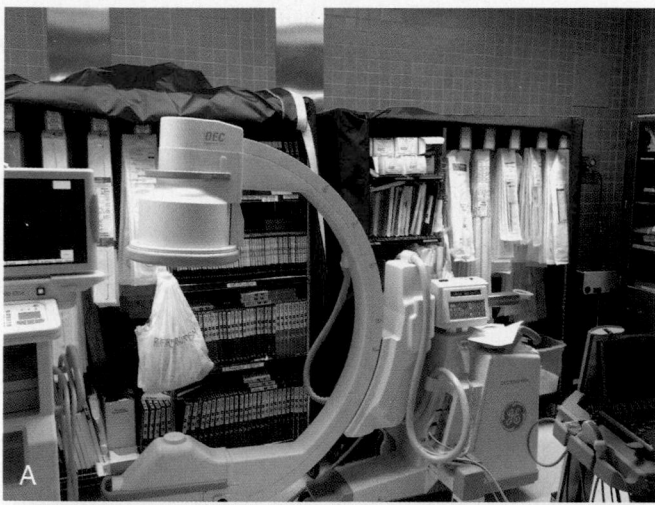

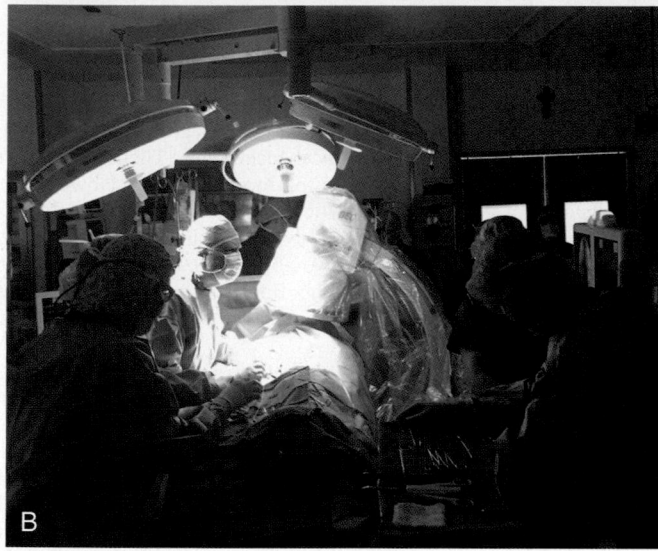
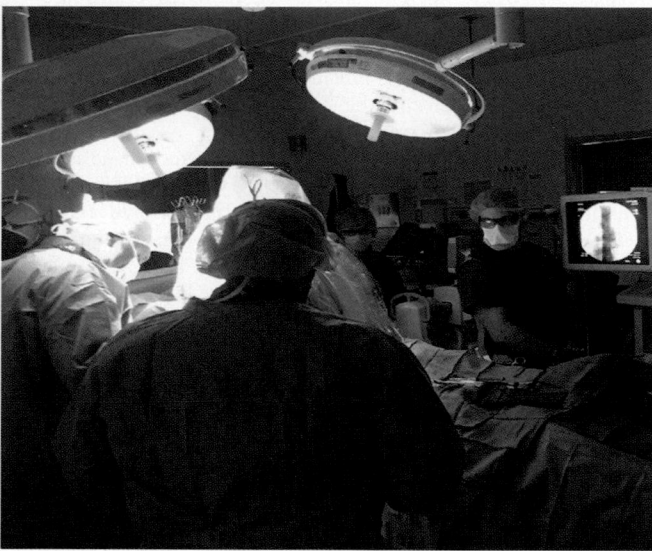

FIGURE 1 A, Digital fluoroscopy C-arm and equipment carts ready to be moved to transform any standard sized operating room with a fluoroscopy-capable table into a hybrid suite. **B,** Endovascular repair of a traumatic thoracic aortic pseudoaneurysm in a standard operating room.

sometimes is used to achieve distal purchase to prevent migration before delivering the device. For the larger aortic devices, a Lunder-quist wire is used as a delivery wire.

Ninety percent of procedures can be done with this relatively simple setup. For injuries that are more difficult to access, specialty catheters such as double recurve catheters may be needed. We have been using intravascular ultrasound to interrogate many injuries. Based on our experience with dealing with ruptured aneurysms, intravascular ultrasound can provide additional information to define the injury, presence of side branches, and sizing and lengths of needed devices for patients who could not be evaluated preoperatively because of instability.

Each trauma center needs to identify who is both qualified in endovascular techniques and immediately available. This varies from center to center. Successful management of vascular injuries requires that the most qualified person perform the indicated intervention in the appropriate patient in the appropriate place at the appropriate time. Endovascular surgery is an operative procedure and, like all operations, should be performed by readily available trained clinicians who are not only cognizant of the technical aspects of a procedure, but also knowledgeable about the disease for which the procedure is being performed. In many centers this person is the interventional radiologist. Other centers have catheter-trained vascular surgeons, and a few others have trauma surgeons who are capable of performing endovascular procedures.

Vascular surgeons, interventional radiologists, and cardiologists all perform elective endovascular techniques. Endovascular management of vascular trauma requires not only continuous and immediately available physicians with catheter skills, but also a thorough understanding of the unique aspects of vascular injuries. Most centers have interventional radiologists or vascular surgeons with this capability who provide emergency coverage for trauma. At the time of this writing, a growing number of trauma surgeons are gaining endovascular skills in short, highly focused courses such as ESTARS (Endovascular Skills for Trauma and Resuscitative Surgery). Others are completing vascular surgery fellowships to become capable to manage both vascular trauma and acute care vascular surgery.

No trauma center can provide successful endovascular management of vascular injuries without the capability to perform open vascular repairs when needed. The reduced volume of open cases has affected vascular fellowship training. The decrease in open case volume during training and the significant rise in endovascular experience have produced a generation of vascular fellowship graduates who are more comfortable with closed techniques than open techniques in many areas. This translates to a reluctance to convert to open technique and an inability to effectively treat vascular trauma where endovascular techniques may not be an option. Each center must identify surgeons with open vascular skills who are available when needed for the management of vascular injuries.

MANAGEMENT OF TORSO ARTERIAL INJURIES

Endovascular techniques offer a variety of options for both hemorrhage control in the torso and definitive arterial repair. Intra-arterial catheter-directed embolization has become a mainstay of the management of solid organ hemorrhage in the abdomen. Whether used as the sole treatment or in combination with open procedures, this approach has been very effective in liver, spleen, and kidney injuries. Less commonly used, resuscitative endovascular balloon occlusion of the aorta (REBOA) for proximal control is another adjunct for hemorrhage control. Initial reports of its use are promising but also have revealed a significant risk for complications. REBOA is only an adjunct to successful management and has yet to be adopted at most centers.

At the time of this writing, catheter introduction site complications and large catheter size with the need for fluoroscopy have somewhat limited its adoption. These techniques are theoretically quick and easily performed. The major obstacle to widespread popularity has been the reluctance of surgeons to either adopt catheter skills or partner with vascular surgeons or interventional radiologists to bring these techniques to the trauma OR. A fully built-out endovascular suite is not required to perform these techniques. A digital C-arm and the proper catheters transform any OR into an endovascular-capable room.

The early use of catheter-directed control of hemorrhage associated with pelvic fracture is an effective method of limiting blood loss and improving outcome. This approach is well tolerated and has proven to be superior to open attempts at hemorrhage control by packing in most patients. Unstable patients benefit from an immediate trip to the OR. If endovascular OR capability is present, a combined approach may offer the best results. Some have placed these patients on a vascular-capable bed. While laparotomy or pelvic packing is occurring, the trauma surgeon can get femoral access. By that time a vascular surgeon or interventional radiologist is available to perform the embolization.

Enthusiasm for stent-graft management of great vessel injuries in the chest has grown steadily. The placement of stent-grafts in the infrarenal aorta has been a very promising development in managing aneurysms. There is great enthusiasm for using similar devices in the thoracic aorta for blunt rupture, and thoracic endovascular aortic repair (TEVAR) has become the first choice for management of trauma aortic injuries. Short-term results indicate fewer immediate complications with TEVAR. Lifelong computed tomographic (CT) imaging and the risk for aortic enlargement and the loss of device fixation are serious considerations.

There is a growing experience in the use of covered stents in the intrathoracic and intra-abdominal proximal branches of the aorta. In stable injuries at risk for delayed hemorrhage or thrombosis, carefully placed stents may offer significant advantages over open procedures that require extensive dissection for exposure and control. However, these techniques are not to be tried by the unskilled or unprepared interventional radiologist or surgeon. They should be used only in centers with an active elective endovascular practice.

In unstable patients who require immediate exploratory laparotomy for active hemorrhage, there is a role for a combined approach to vascular injuries. Creating this approach requires always using a fluoroscopy-capable OR table and having an active endovascular vascular trauma management program with equipment and personnel immediately available. Direct manual control and clamp placement followed by femoral vessel access and catheter-directed embolization or stent-graft placement can augment the open approach effectively, with improved outcomes. However, this combined approach must be planned for carefully and guided by the appropriate preparation.

CEREBROVASCULAR ARTERIAL INJURIES

Endovascular techniques offer advantages in areas that are difficult to reach in the OR. Hemorrhage at the base of the skull from carotid injury or vertebral canal hemorrhage is difficult to control and repair. Catheter-directed coil, balloon, or hemostatic agent placement is an important tool in managing these injuries. Managing carotid artery injury with covered stent placement should be reserved only for those injuries that are inaccessible and associated with significant hemorrhage. Stent placement has proven inferior to anticoagulation in partial occlusion injuries without associated hemorrhage. Thrombotic strokes have resulted in a significant number of patients treated with covered stents in the injured carotid artery.

Vertebral artery injuries not associated with hemorrhage also are best treated with anticoagulation. In the presence of active bleeding, endovascular occlusion with coils, balloons, or stents offers an advantage in lesions within the vertebral canal or at the base of the skull. Endovascular treatment of intracranial traumatic pseudoaneurysms has proven to be safe and effective. However, this area of intervention requires the highest level of training and experience.

EXTREMITY ARTERIAL VASCULAR INJURY

Extremity vascular injury resulting in hemorrhage is best treated with promptly performed open surgical techniques. The use of stent-grafts in the extremities is becoming more common. However, the results are not yet well documented. Caution may well be the best approach. Covered stents are easily placed in partially occluded vessels, and although they have favorable early patency rates, they are prone to occlusion. Autologous vein interposition grafts have excellent long-term patency rates and remain the most durable choice for vascular repairs in the extremities.

Catheter-directed therapies for hemorrhage from large branch vessels in the extremities are often both effective and sufficient to manage these injuries successfully. Although these measures in addition to ultrasound-guided thrombin injection are effective in iatrogenic acute pseudoaneurysms after invasive procedures, this approach is not effective in most vascular trauma. The small hole in the artery after removal of an arterial sheath is usually very different from the larger defects seen with vascular trauma. The risk for complete arterial thrombosis or distal emboli is high with this approach.

VENOUS INJURIES

The role of endovascular management in venous injuries is limited to the great vein and proximal extremity veins. Venous stent-graft placement is an important adjunct to hemorrhage control in the great veins of the chest and abdomen. However, the patency of stent-grafts is dependent on both adequate width of the prosthesis and high flow. Superior and inferior vena cava stent-grafts have a very good patency rate. Femoral, iliac, subclavian, and axillary vein stent-grafts do not share the same success rate because of small diameter and lower blood flow rates.

The main advantage of great vein stent-graft placement is hemorrhage control without extensive surgical dissection and clamp placement. This is especially true in superior vena cava and distal inferior vena cava penetrating injuries. In both the chest and the abdomen, there is a role for a blend of open and endovascular technique in patients who have a contained hematoma at the site of a great vein injury. Superior vena cava injuries in the chest often involve significant hemorrhage that requires direct open control and repair. Inferior vena cava wounds in the retroperitoneum often are seen as large contained hematomas.

Once other thoracic or abdominal injuries have been identified, the hematoma surrounding the vena cava can be imaged with jugular or femoral venous catheterization and fluoroscopy, and an occluding balloon can be placed to augment proximal and distal vascular control. If appropriate, a sufficiently large stent-graft may be deployed or open repair may be performed.

■ ENDOVASCULAR TRAUMA CASE MANAGEMENT

Case I

History. A 20-year-old man with a gunshot wound of the left cheek is seen with active nasal hemorrhage and right hemiparesis. He requires immediate intubation and placement of nasal balloons for hemorrhage control. A CT scan of the head and neck reveals active extravasation from the left external maxillary artery and the left internal carotid artery at the base of the skull.

Decision making. The site of hemorrhage is extremely difficult to manage with open technique, and carotid ligation almost certainly will be required. The catheter-based endovascular approach will allow for hemorrhage control and possible stent-graft placement. Hemorrhage is controlled, and no open procedure is currently needed.

Management. The patient is taken to an interventional radiology suite. Percutaneous femoral access is used to place a wire into the left common carotid artery, and an angiogram is obtained. Active extravasation at the base of the skull is confirmed (Figure 2, A). The carotid lesion is crossed with a guidewire, and distal angiogram reveals a patent distal internal carotid artery (Figure 2, B). A polytetrafluoroethylene (PTFE) covered stent is deployed successfully (Figure 2, C). The external branch of the maxillary artery is occluded with Gelfoam and coils.

Outcome. Postprocedure, the right hemiparesis rapidly resolves. The patient has severe difficulty swallowing from a suspected injury to cranial nerve IX. He is discharged with a feeding tube on postinjury day 5. Swallowing ability gradually returns over 6 months. Carotid duplex scan is normal at 6 months. The patient is lost to follow-up at 9 months.

Case 2

History. A 22-year-old man is chased into the street by two assailants and struck by a truck. He is seen with stable vital signs and tender abdomen, back, pelvis, and chest. Torso CT reveals a distal thoracic aorta pseudoaneurysm and T10 fracture, grade III liver and grade III spleen injuries, and a left renal infarct in addition to a left acetabular fracture without pelvic hematoma (Figure 3, A). There is minimal intra-abdominal hemorrhage.

Decision making. The patient is hemodynamically stable but severely injured and requires prompt intervention. The thoracic aortic injury and the abdominal visceral injuries are amenable to endovascular management. However, the ability to perform prompt exploratory laparotomy in the event of instability due to abdominal hemorrhage is essential to successful management.

Management. The patient is taken to the OR for endovascular repair of the aorta and embolization of the spleen. Percutaneous femoral access is used to selectively catheterize the splenic artery and place coils and Gelfoam. The thoracic aortic pseudoaneurysm (Figure 3, B) is repaired with overlapping AneuRx cuffs (Figure 3, C). The patient undergoes staged fixation of the acetabular fracture 72 hours later.

Outcome. The patient recovers uneventfully. However, he is lost to follow-up despite efforts to contact both him and his family.

Case 3

History. A 46-year-old man is seen with stab wound of the left upper chest. There is a small hematoma at the site but no active hemorrhage. The left arm neurovascular examination is normal and a chest x-ray is normal. A CT scan of the chest reveals a pseudoaneurysm of the proximal left axillary artery just distal to the clavicle.

Decision making. The site of injury is amenable to treatment with a stent-graft that should have excellent long-term patency because of vessel size and high flow. The pseudoaneurysm is contained and there is no current need to perform an open procedure.

Management. The patient is taken to an interventional radiology suite. Percutaneous femoral access is used to place a wire into the left subclavian artery, and an angiogram demonstrates the site of the lacerated axillary artery (Figure 4, A). A covered stent is placed (Figure 4, B).

Outcome. The patient has a normal left arm neurovascular examination postprocedure, recovers uneventfully, and is discharged the next day. His left arm vascular examination remains normal during 2 years of follow-up.

Case 4

History. A 33-year-old man is seen with an epigastric gunshot wound left of the midline and hypotension. Focused assessment with sonography for trauma (FAST) of the abdomen is grossly positive, and the patient is taken directly to the OR.

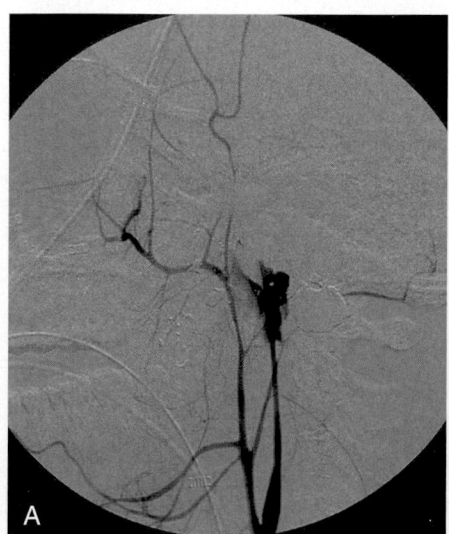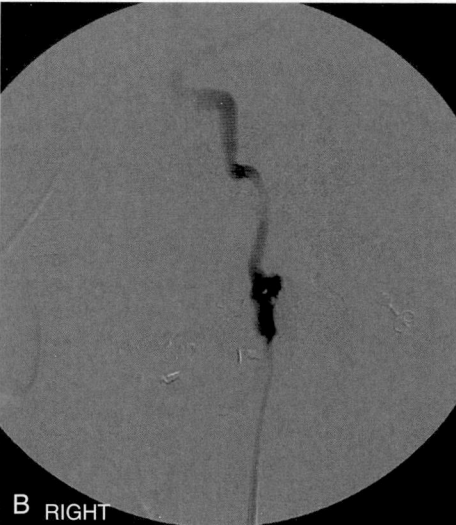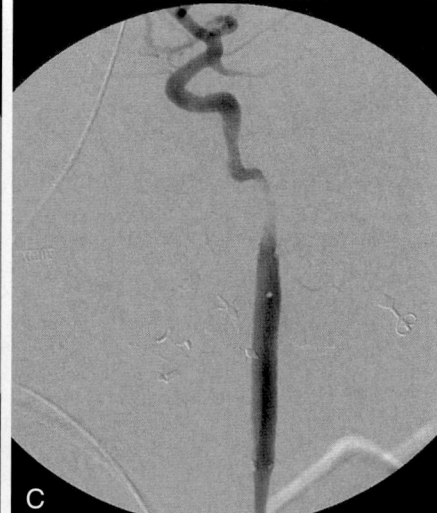

FIGURE 2 A, Laceration of internal carotid artery just below the skull with acute pseudoaneurysm. **B,** Catheter across the area of injury with demonstration of patent distal carotid artery. **C,** Covered stent repair of internal carotid artery with distal vessels patent.

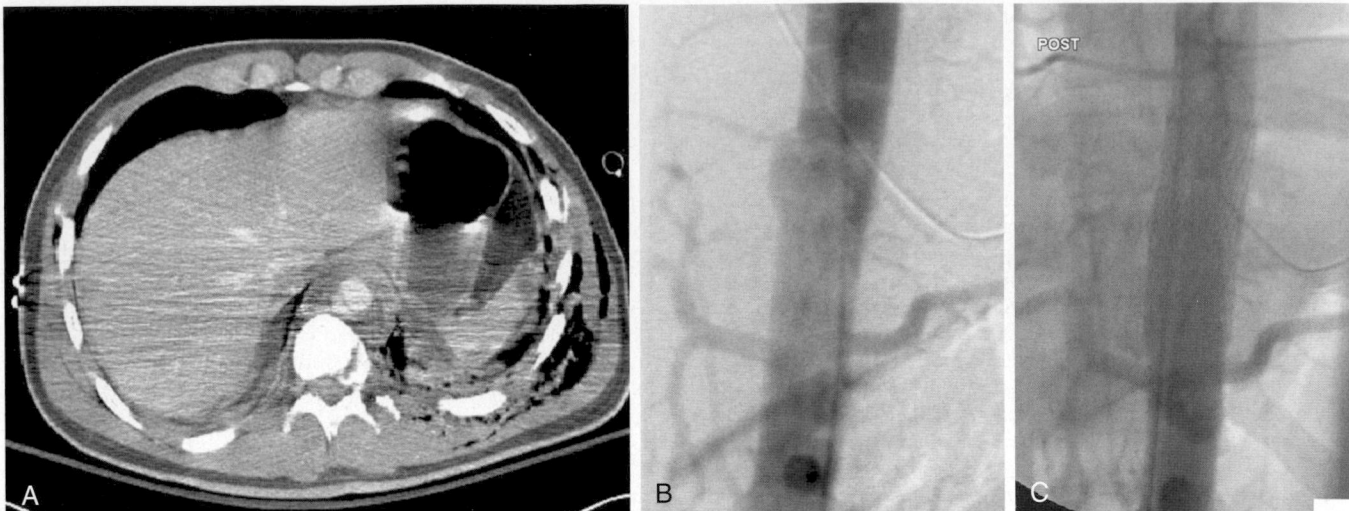

FIGURE 3 A, Torso computed tomographic scan revealing distal thoracic aortic injury with pseudoaneurysm and splenic injury. **B,** Catheter angiogram documenting distal thoracic aortic injury. **C,** Endovascular stent-graft repair with overlapping graft segments just above the origin of the celiac axis.

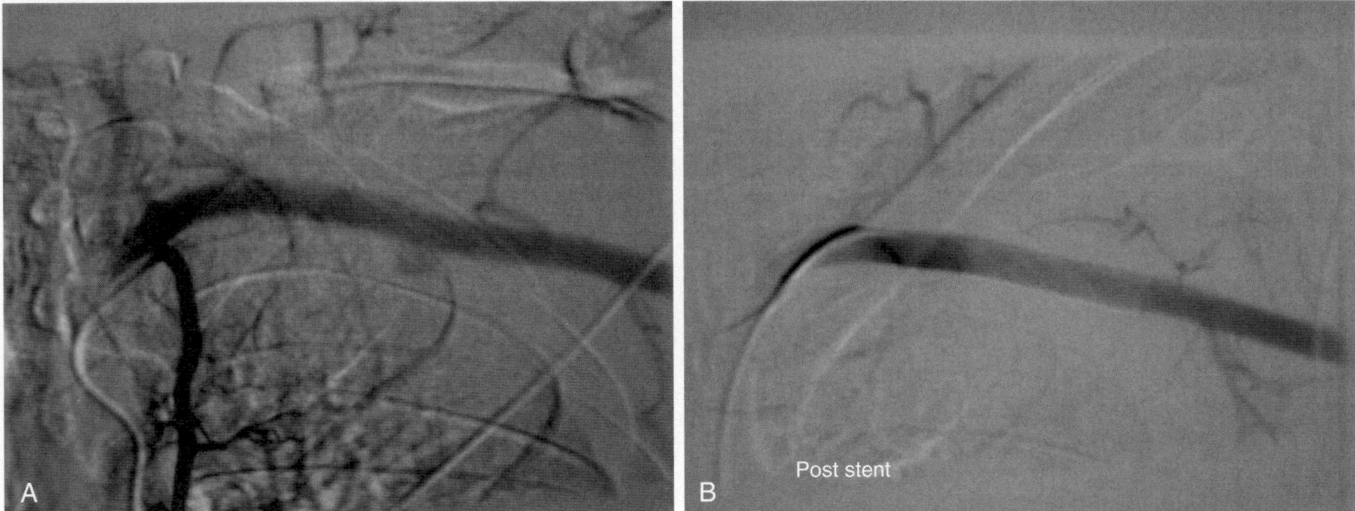

FIGURE 4 A, Left axillary artery pseudoaneurysm from a stab wound with partial transection. **B,** Endovascular repair with a covered stent.

An exploratory laparotomy reveals a through-and-through injury to the stomach and a large pulsatile retroperitoneal mass in the midline just inferior to the body of the pancreas. The bleeding is contained and the patient's blood pressure is 110/60 mm Hg with a heart rate of 100 beats per minute.

Decision making. The patient appears to have an injury of the aorta. Proximal aortic control must be obtained before opening the hematoma. This can be accomplished in one of two ways. First, a clamp can be placed at the supraceliac aorta after bluntly dissecting through the lesser sac and crura of the diaphragm to expose an aortic segment for clamp placement. Second, the femoral artery can be cannulated and an occluding aortic balloon can be advanced to the aorta above the level of injury for proximal control. By either means, hemorrhage is controlled.

Management. The gastric injury site is packed off, and digital subtraction angiography via femoral artery catheterization reveals an aortic injury below the renal arteries. An appropriate size aortic cuff stent-graft is deployed to repair the aorta. The hematoma is opened to explore the area of injury, confirm adequate hemorrhage control, and evaluate the area for other injuries. An omental pedicle flap is mobilized and placed in the retroperitoneum to cover the injury site

and exposed stent-graft. The stomach injury is repaired, the abdomen is closed, and the patient is transferred to the surgical intensive care unit (ICU).

Outcome. The patient has normal postoperative lower extremity pulses and recovers uneventfully. Abdominal CT scan before discharge on hospital day 5 reveals an appropriate repair. Follow-up aortic ultrasound is done at 1 month and 6 months and demonstrates a stable repair. Yearly follow-up ultrasound of the aorta is planned.

Case 5

History. The patient sustains a stab wound to the supraclavicular fossa with a decreased right radial pulse. The patient is brought to the OR by the trauma surgeon and placed on a fluoroscopic OR table. Arteriography reveals a likely transection of the right subclavian artery with a large pseudoaneurysm (Figure 5, *A*).

Decision making. Proximal control of this injury requires median sternotomy with supraclavicular extension. Alternatively, proximal control can be obtained with a balloon catheter in the proximal subclavian artery.

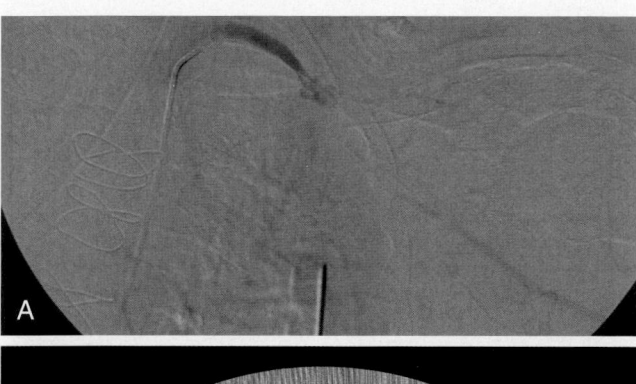

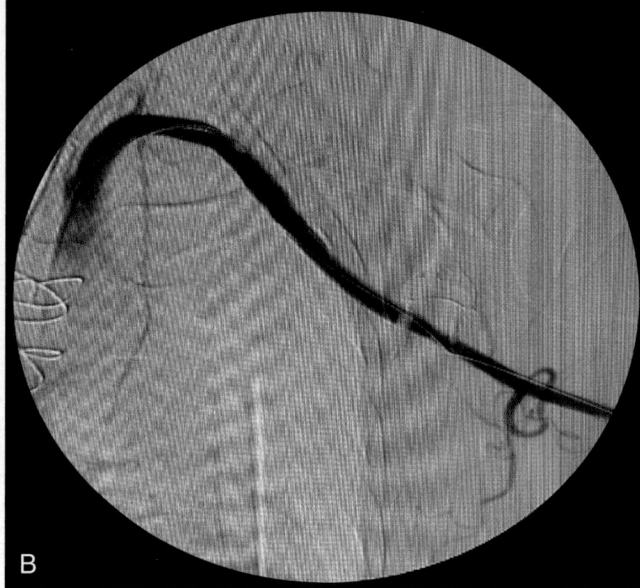

FIGURE 5 A, Transected left subclavian artery with extravasation. **B,** Repaired site of subclavian artery injury with covered stent-graft.

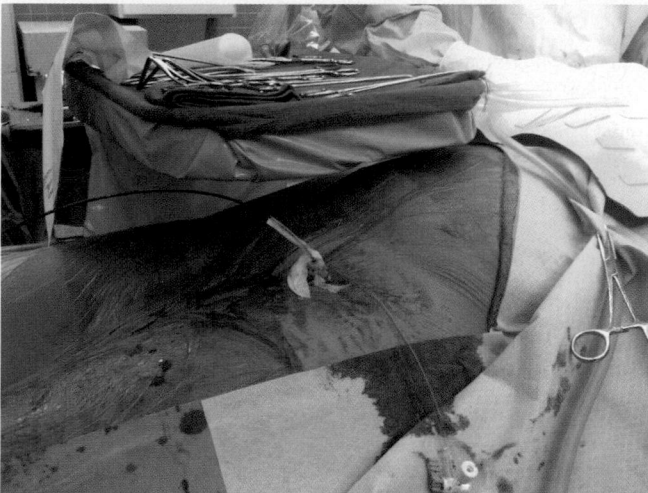

FIGURE 6 Left femoral access with occluding balloon placed across the bifurcation to achieve proximal right iliac control before open exploration of a right groin stab wound with large hematoma.

Management. The brachial artery is accessed. A wire is able to traverse the injury, and proximal luminal placement is confirmed. A Viabahn self-expanding covered stent is deployed successfully (Figure 5, *B*).

Outcome. Postoperatively, the patient has a normal radial pulse. He recovers uneventfully. The repair remains patent at the follow-up visit 1 year later.

Case 6

History. Patient is a chef, and when bringing a box of knives down from the top shelf, a knife lodges in the left supraclavicular fossa. The patient is initially hypotensive with brisk bleeding from the wound. Bleeding is controlled with a Foley catheter and direct pressure. The patient also is noted to have a median sternotomy scar. There are wires and an aortic valve prosthesis on chest x-ray. In addition, the patient is on Coumadin.

Decision making. In a hypotensive patient on Coumadin with previous thoracic surgery, proximal control via chest incision potentially can be very difficult.

Management. The patient is taken to the OR by the thoracic surgeon and placed on a portable vascular bed. Access is achieved via the common femoral artery, and a diagnostic selected subclavian arteriogram is obtained. A cutdown is performed over the left brachial artery in the upper arm and achieves access across the transected subclavian artery with a tri-lobe snare (see Figure 5, *A*). A Viabahn self-expanding covered stent is used to transverse the injury (see Figure 5, *B*).

Outcome. Postoperatively, the patient has a normal radial pulse and normal neurologic examination. The repair remains patent at follow-up 1 year later.

Case 7

History. The patient is involved in a high-speed motor vehicle accident. The patient is hypotensive and is brought stat to the OR. The patient undergoes small bowel and colon resection for a significant mesenteric injury with significant enteric spillage throughout the abdomen. The patient undergoes damage control, is closed temporarily, and is resuscitated in the ICU. The patient is noted to lose the left femoral pulse in the ICU.

Decision making. The patient has a common iliac artery injury, with concomitant significant enteric spillage. An endolumenal approach is considered to avoid placing a vascular graft on an infected field.

Management. The patient is returned to the OR. Bilateral femoral access is obtained with one wire going over the aortic bifurcation. It is noted that there is a complex intimal flap when the area is interrogated with intravascular ultrasound (IVUS). IVUS is used to ensure that true lumen to lumen wire placement is obtained. The injury is bridged with the Viabahn self-expanding covered stent.

Outcome. The patient has a normal distal pulse postoperatively and recovers uneventfully.

Case 8

History. A male patient who is obese sustains a stab wound to the right groin with expanding hematoma.

Decision making. Open surgical proximal control for this injury would require an abdominal incision or a retroperitoneal exposure incision to gain proximal control of the external iliac artery. An endovascular approach would require placement of an occluding balloon via the contralateral femoral artery (Figure 6).

Management. The patient is brought to the OR, and contralateral femoral access is obtained. Access to the external iliac artery above the injury is obtained by going up and over the aortic bifurcation, and an occluding balloon is placed, achieving proximal control. A groin incision then is made to address a proximal common femoral artery injury.

Outcome. The patient recovers uneventfully.

SUGGESTED READINGS

Arthurs ZM, Sohn VY, Starnes BW. Vascular trauma: endovascular management and techniques. *Surg Clin North Am.* 2007;87:1179-1192.

Avery LE, Stahfield KR, Corcos AC, et al. Evolving role of endovascular techniques for traumatic vascular injury: a changing landscape? *J Trauma Acute Care Surg.* 2012;72:41-47.

Brenner M, Hoehn M, Pasley J, et al. Basic endovascular skills for trauma course: bridging the gap between endovascular techniques and the acute care surgeon. *J Trauma Acute Care Surg.* 2014;77:286-291.

Brenner ML, Moore LJ, DuBose JJ, et al. A clinical series of resuscitative endovascular balloon occlusion of the aorta for hemorrhage control and resuscitation. *J Trauma Acute Care Surg.* 2013;75:506-511.

Calcutt RA, Mell MW. Modern advances in vascular trauma. *Surg Clin North Am.* 2013;93:941-961.

Desai SS, DuBose JJ, Parham CS, et al. Outcomes after endovascular repair of arterial trauma. *J Vasc Surg.* 2014;60:1309-1314.

Gilani R, Saucedo-Crespo H, Scott BG, et al. Endovascular therapy for overcoming challenges presented with blunt abdominal aortic injury. *Vasc Endovascular Surg.* 2012;46:329-331.

Gilani R, Tsai PA, Wall MJ Jr, Mattox KL. Overcoming challenges of endovascular treatment of complex subclavian and axillary artery injuries in hypotensive patients. *J Trauma Acute Care Surg.* 2012;73:771-773.

Jack R, Degiannis E. Endovascular therapy and controversies in the management of vascular trauma. *Scand J Surg.* 2014;103:149-153.

Johnson CA. Endovascular management of peripheral vascular trauma. *Semin Intervent Radiol.* 2010;27:38-43.

Lee WA, Matsumare JS, Michell RS, et al. Endovascular repair of traumatic thoracic aortic injury: clinical practice guidelines for the Society for Vascular Surgery. *J Vasc Surg.* 2011;53:187-192.

Moore LJ, Brenner ML, Kozar RA, et al. Implementation of resuscitative endovascular balloon occlusion of the aorta as an alternative to resuscitative thoracotomy for noncompressible truncal hemorrhage. *J Trauma Acute Care Surg.* 2015;79:523-532.

Sinha S, Patterson BO, Ma J, et al. Systemic review and meta-analysis of open surgical and endovascular management of thoracic outlet vascular injuries. *J Vasc Surg.* 2013;57:547-567.

Villamaria VY, Eliason JL, Napolitano LM, et al. Endovascular skills for trauma and resuscitative surgery (ESTARS) course: curriculum development, content validation and program assessment. *J Trauma Acute Care Surg.* 2014;76:929-936.

THE MANAGEMENT OF EXTREMITY COMPARTMENT SYNDROME

Greg Osgood, MD

The ability to diagnose and perform emergency treatment of compartment syndrome is one of the most important aspects of extremity care. Compartment syndrome is the excessive swelling of tissue within a closed space, to the degree that the pressure exceeds the capillary bed perfusion pressure and effective blood flow is cut off. This phenomenon occurs most commonly in the setting of trauma and crush injury but also is seen in burn patients, coagulopathic patients who bleed into an enclosed space, insect and snake bites, constrictive dressings and casts, prolonged immobilization during surgery (e.g., lithotomy), and reperfusion after repair of vascular injury. Missed compartment syndrome is one of the leading causes of litigation in trauma cases.

First described in World War II, compartment syndrome was recognized as a complex injury pattern that was limb and life threatening. The high volume of extremity injury associated with combat injuries in the past 2 decades has again increased our awareness of the evolving nature of compartment syndrome resulting from blast mechanism. Soldiers injured in the field who were initially evaluated and débrided were found to have increased tissue pressures 8 to 12 hours after injury, necessitating compartment releases at later intervals. Ongoing tissue necrosis and edema from the primary injury are thought to be causative.

Regardless of the injury that causes compartment syndrome, the complex physiology involves increased tissue pressure, impeded venous and lymphatic outflow, and increased interstitial and intracellular pressure. The end product is capillary hypoperfusion, tissue ischemia, and necrosis. Early recognition of the predisposing conditions and early diagnosis of compartment syndrome are essential in minimizing the limb morbidity and mortality associated with this diagnosis.

■ DIAGNOSIS

Compartment syndrome is a clinical diagnosis that may be supported by objective measurements (Box 1). The affected extremity is not always tensely swollen. The most sensitive examination findings associated with compartment syndrome include pain with passive stretch of the muscles within the compartment and pain out of proportion to the injury to the extremity. These are the earliest and most important symptoms to detect. The other examination findings in compartment syndrome—pallor, poikilothermia, pulselessness, and paresis—are late findings that should not be waited for to make the diagnosis. It must be noted that distal pulses and digital capillary refill often are preserved during compartment syndrome.

Most surgeons use clinical findings and injury mechanism to diagnose compartment syndrome. Objective pressure measurements also can be made to support or refute the diagnosis. This is especially helpful in patients who are difficult to examine, children in whom there are distracting injuries, substance abuse, the obtunded patient, or the background of sedation. In any setting in which the classic physical examination findings may be difficult to obtain, compartment syndrome monitoring is recommended. The Stryker pressure transducer is the most common method of measuring compartment pressures, but the Whitesides needle manometer method may be used if a Stryker device is not available. The needle is placed into the affected compartment and flushed. A pressure reading is then taken. Pressure measurements should be taken at the site of fracture because elevated pressures are identified most reliably at the injury location (Figures 1 and 2).

Adequate tissue perfusion is achieved when the measured pressure is well below the patient's diastolic pressure. Delta P is the most accurate way to determine compartment syndrome. Delta P greater than 30 mm Hg indicates adequate perfusion. Delta P less than 30 mm Hg indicates compartment syndrome. Other pressure thresholds are not sensitive or specific enough in diagnosing compartment syndrome. Emerging research supports the use of continuous pressure monitoring in patients with threatened compartment syndrome, but this is not available at many hospital centers.

■ EXTREMITY COMPARTMENT SYNDROME: TREATMENT PRINCIPLES

Unlike escharotomy for burn injury, fasciotomy involves incision through the skin and also through the deep investing fascia that contains and constricts the expanding volume within the specific compartment. Incisions are made through the full thickness of the skin until fascia is identified. The fascia then is incised along the entire length of the compartment to allow expansion of the edematous tissue beneath. The surgeon must confirm that the proximal and

BOX 1: Objective Measurement of Compartment Syndrome

Delta P = Diastolic Pressure – Measured Pressure
Delta P <30 mm Hg indicates compartment syndrome

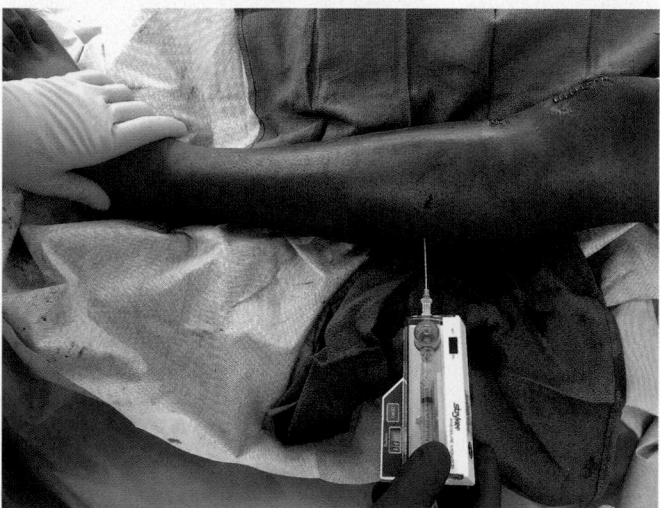

FIGURE 1 After intramedullary nailing, the compartment pressures are measured in this left leg. The lateral compartment is being measured. The drop of blood anterior to the needle marks the location where the anterior compartment pressure was measured.

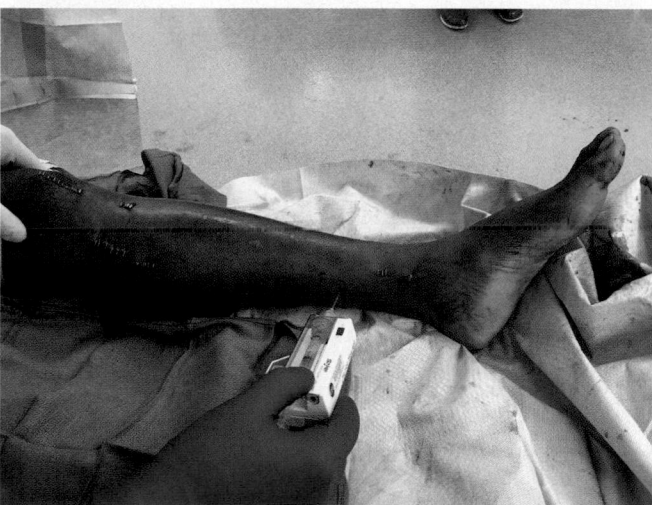

FIGURE 2 The deep posterior compartment pressure is measured just posterior to the posteromedial border of the tibia distally.

distal ends of the incision through the fascia are not constricting the tissue beneath, in order to determine that the fasciotomy is complete and that tissue compression and necrosis will not continue postoperatively. Incomplete fasciotomy is a common reason to return to the operating room (OR).

When a fasciotomy is performed, the edematous tissue expands into the opening created by the fascial incision. The surgeon inspects the tissue to assess its viability. It is difficult to assess the viability of nerve tissue, the most susceptible to compartment syndrome; however, the surrounding muscle is used as a surrogate to assess the viability of the entire compartment. Muscle viability is determined based on the color of the tissue and its contractility, consistency, and

capacity to bleed (the 4 Cs). Nonviable muscle must be débrided to minimize the risk for infection.

Normal red muscle that contracts when stimulated by touch or light electrocautery is not débrided. Muscle in emerging compartment syndrome often has a pink or brown contused appearance; with continued ischemia, this tissue loses its properties of contractility and brisk arterial flow. Late compartment syndrome is characterized by friable muscle tissue with a dusky gray appearance that does not respond to external stimulation. In patients with excessive bleeding during surgery, a tourniquet may be inflated judiciously. However, use of the tourniquet may obscure accurate diagnosis of viable tissue.

In an evolving compartment syndrome, surgical discretion must be used when evaluating contused muscle tissue that remains pink or tissue that is minimally contractile. Often this tissue responds to reperfusion and regains circulation, contractility, and long-term function. For this reason, a "second look" in 24 to 48 hours is recommended to reassess the tissue bed. A more aggressive débridement can be performed during this second look; this optimizes the patient's prognosis for functional return and minimizes the risk of late infection resulting from remaining necrotic tissue.

It is not recommended that the skin be closed immediately after the fasciotomy. On initial suspicion of acute traumatic compartment syndrome, it is most prudent to leave the skin open, dressed with either wet-to-dry dressings or a vacuum-assisted closure dressing. This allows the sterile environment to be protected and continued swelling of the lower leg period the patient can return in 24 to 48 hours for re-inspection of the tissues, redébridement of ongoing or more clearly defined necrotic tissue, and possible delayed primary closure of one of the wounds. If only one incision can be closed in the lower leg at the second look procedure, the medial incision should be closed first. This causes the lateral incision to gap slightly, but there is usually adequate lateral soft tissue overlying the bone to support later closure with a skin graft if necessary.

■ LOWER LEG COMPARTMENT SYNDROME

Compartment syndrome of the lower leg is the most common compartment syndrome diagnosis. The lower leg contains four discrete muscular compartments. A patient rarely may develop isolated compartment syndrome in only one compartment, but usually all four compartments are affected. A four-compartment fasciotomy of the lower leg is performed most often when the diagnosis of lower leg compartment syndrome is made, to ensure that the risk for leg compartment is minimized.

In the lower leg, compartments are measured individually with individual pricks of the Stryker monitor. The anterior compartment is measured anterior to the usual skin incision on the lateral leg for compartment release, and the lateral compartment is measured posterior to the planned incision. In the medial lower leg, the superficial posterior compartment is entered in the calf overlying the gastrocnemius medial head. However, the deep posterior compartment should be measured by placing the needle immediately posterior to the medial metaphyseal border of the distal tibia. This allows the needle to pass directly into the deep posterior compartment most easily. The needles passed through the skin can be felt to pop through the fascia in the compartment that is being measured. Surgeons should practice using the monitoring device well in advance of having to measure pressure in the acute setting.

When performing a four-compartment release in the lower leg, surgical preparation and draping of the patient should allow complete access to the entire affected lower extremity from the groin to the toes. Surgical incisions are made on both the medial and the lateral aspects of the lower leg. On the medial side, the 20-cm incision is made approximately 1 cm posterior to the palpable posterior medial tibia diaphysis (Figure 3). The incision is carried directly down to the fascia without elevating skin flaps. The saphenous vein and saphenous nerve must be protected. The superficial posterior

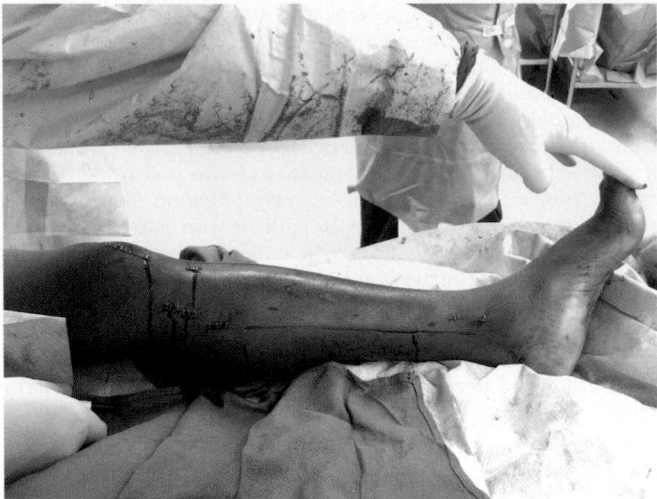

FIGURE 3 The medial incision is made 1 cm posterior to the palpable tibia.

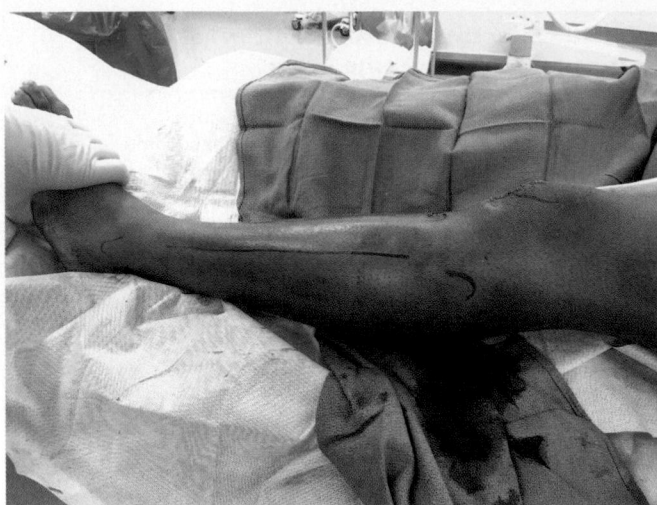

FIGURE 4 The lateral incision is centered between the tibial crest and the fibula.

compartment contains the gastrocnemius muscle and the soleus muscle. The fascia overlying the gastrocnemius-soleus complex is incised along its entire length, thereby releasing the superficial posterior compartment. A fascial incision that extends down to the musculotendinous junction at the Achilles tendon will ensure that both the soleus and the gastrocnemius muscles are visualized and adequately released. Next, a separate fascial incision is made at the most distal extent of the surgical incision, directly onto the posterior medial border of the distal tibia. Below this fascia, the tendons of the deep posterior compartment are identified. The incision through the fascia of the deep posterior compartment is then carried proximally along the posterior medial border of the tibia. To adequately visualize and release the deep posterior compartment of the lower leg, the origin of the soleus muscle must be elevated off of the metaphyseal proximal tibia. In doing so, significant bleeding from the venous plexus in this area should be anticipated by the surgeon and cauterized appropriately. The muscular origin of the tibialis posterior should be released from the posterior metaphyseal tibia in order to confirm that a thorough release of the deep posterior compartment has been performed; some surgeons believe that the tibialis posterior muscle is contained within a separate fascial compartment and that this increases the risk of residual deep posterior compartment dysfunction after inadequate fasciotomy. Once the viability of the superficial and deep posterior compartment musculature elements has been confirmed and débridement of necrotic fascia and muscle has been completed in these areas, attention can be turned to the lateral lower leg.

On the lateral side, a 20-cm incision is made centered midway between the anterior tibial crest and the fibular shaft (Figure 4). The longitudinal incision is then carried down to the fascia. Full-thickness flaps generally are not created; soft tissue elevation at the middle of the wound allows identification of the anterior and lateral compartments. The most critical step in performing the lateral approach, that of identifying both compartments, is simplified by performing a *transverse* incision with the scalpel only through the fascia at the middle of the incision, in the middle of the leg. At the middle lower leg, more than 10 cm above the ankle joint, it is very unlikely that the superficial branch of the peroneal nerve will be injured by this maneuver. In making this important transverse fascial incision, the longitudinal fascia between the anterior and lateral compartments is identified easily just beneath the transverse incision (Figure 5). This longitudinal fascial layer separates the large anterior compartment and the smaller lateral compartment containing the peroneal muscles.

Large scissors, such as curved Mayo scissors, can be used to pass deep to the fascia of the anterior and lateral compartments

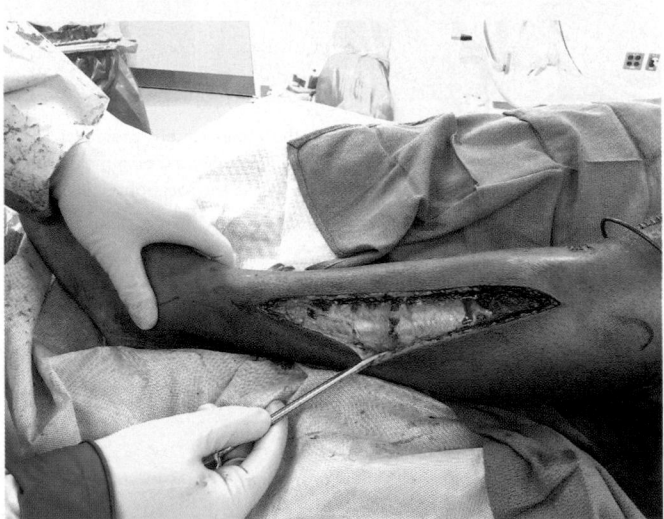

FIGURE 5 Using a transverse incision through the fascia, a distinct deep fascial layer is found separating the anterior and lateral compartments.

proximally and distally both anteriorly and posteriorly to the fascial division between the anterior and lateral compartments. Then incisions are made proximal to the transverse incision in both the anterior and the lateral compartments. When making the distal incisions, the surgeon must be very careful because the superficial branch of the peroneal nerve exits the lateral compartment and enters the superficial tissues anterior to the anterior compartment. It is this area, 8 to 10 cm proximal to the ankle joint, where the superficial branch of the peroneal nerve is most vulnerable. Once this H-type incision is made through the fascia, the muscle needs to be inspected, débrided, and irrigated. By making a transverse incision across both the anterior and the lateral compartments in the lateral approach, the surgeon can be assured that both compartments have been identified and released adequately. Lastly, before dressing application the surgeon must inspect the proximal and distal extents of the fascial incisions. A sharp edge of the fascia can continue to impair blood flow locally at the fascial edge or throughout the limb.

Although compartment syndrome is best studied and most easily identified in the lower leg, it can occur in any enclosed fascia. In the lower extremity this includes gluteal compartment syndrome, thigh compartment syndrome, and foot compartment syndrome.

■ GLUTEAL COMPARTMENT SYNDROME

Pressure in the gluteus maximus and gluteus medius can be increased, causing gluteal compartment syndrome. This can occur when a patient is in a prolonged position, lying on the affected extremity gluteal region. It can be possible also in the intensive care setting when the patient lies recumbent in the supine position for an extended admission. Like any compartment syndrome, its diagnosis is made by severe pain on passive stretch of the compartment musculature, pain out of proportion to the injury, and paresthesias or paresis in the affected extremity caused by compression on the sciatic nerve. In the impaired patient, or in order to confirm suspicion of this diagnosis, pressure measurements can be obtained by needle insertion in the superolateral buttock. Delta P less than 30 mm Hg indicates compartment syndrome.

Treatment of compartment syndrome in the gluteal region requires exposure of the entire compartment. This is done through a Kocher-Langenbeck approach or through a modified Gibson approach. The incision is made through the skin and the fascia of the thigh, and the tensor fascia latae is incised longitudinally. The fascia of the gluteus maximus then is incised overlying the muscle, and the fibers of the gluteus maximus muscle can be split bluntly to expose the deeper tissues. The gluteus medius can be identified inserting discretely onto the proximal greater trochanter. A retractor placed beneath the gluteus medius will identify the gluteus minimus on its origin at the posterior column of the acetabulum and iliac wing. The short external rotators also should be inspected for their viability.

■ THIGH COMPARTMENT SYNDROME

Compartment syndrome of the thigh most commonly occurs with blunt or ballistic trauma involving fracture of the femur; however, a spontaneous hematoma in the hypocoagulable patient also may cause compartment syndrome. The diagnosis should be suspected in high-energy injuries involving comminuted diaphyseal fractures.

The upper leg has three compartments: an anterior compartment containing the quadriceps muscles, a posterior muscular compartment containing the hamstrings, and a medial compartment containing the adductor musculature. Each of these compartments can be affected individually by increased pressure. Delta P less than 30 mm Hg indicates compartment syndrome. A single lateral incision on the midlateral thigh is made to evaluate the anterior and posterior compartments; this is followed by a separate medial incision overlying the adductor compartment if the surgeon finds the medial pressure is elevated after lateral release.

The lateral incision is made approximately 20 cm in length along the midlateral thigh. The incision is carried down to the fascia of the lateral upper leg. In the setting of compartment syndrome, the muscles of the quadriceps expand through the fascial incision. Care should be taken to ensure that there is not a sharp proximal or distal fascial edge in the lateral thigh. The musculature of the anterior compartment can be evaluated and débrided. Blunt deep retractors then are placed deep to the vastus lateralis to expose the lateral intermuscular septum. In doing so, crossing vascular branches of the profunda femoris are encountered and must be cauterized or ligated. A longitudinal incision is made under direct visualization through the intermuscular septum. This allows inspection and débridement of the posterior hamstring compartment (Figure 6).

Once the anterior and posterior compartments have been released, inspected, and débrided, the surgeon turns attention to the medial side of the thigh. It is very common to find that once the anterior and posterior compartments of the thigh have been released, the medial compartment is under substantially less pressure. In this situation a medial compartment release usually is not performed. If the medial thigh remains palpably tense, a separate incision is made extending from the proximal thigh crease over the adductor compartment approximately halfway down the thigh. Blunt dissection is carried down to the fascia overlying the adductor compartment. The

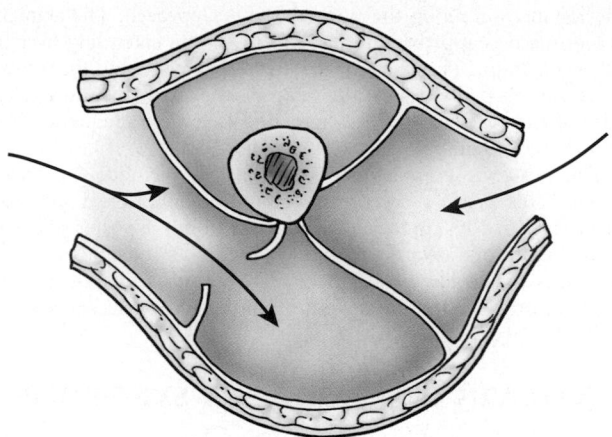

FIGURE 6 Right thigh line drawing depicting the lateral incision used to approach anterior and posterior compartments and the medial incision used to release the adductor compartment. The lateral intermuscular septum must be incised through the lateral approach to access the posterior compartment.

fascia of the adductor compartment then is released under direct visualization with an incision through only the fascia. Finger dissection beneath the medial compartment fascia then can be performed, delivering hematoma and allowing assessment of the medial compartment tissues. Blunt retractors will allow evaluation of the viability of the medial compartment structures.

■ FOOT COMPARTMENT SYNDROME

Patients are at significant risk of foot compartment syndrome after crush injury, burns, and calcaneus fractures and their treatment. Surgical release of the 10 compartments in the foot can be done through an open approach or percutaneous technique. To perform an open fasciotomy, two incisions are made on the dorsal midfoot, parallel to the metatarsals between the first and second rays and overlying the fourth metatarsal, extending from the cuneiforms distally to the metatarsal neck. The fascia of the foot is less robust than in other areas of the lower extremity. Sharp débridement of necrotic interosseous muscles is performed. A third 10- to 12-cm incision then is made, centered at the tarsometatarsal joint on the medial foot just plantar to the palpable first metatarsal base. The deep plantar compartments of the foot are dissected from the medial side, accessing the deeper tissues that could not be excised through the dorsal incisions. Care should be taken when dissecting to protect the neurovascular structures, especially branches of the tibial nerve in the plantar foot.

Using the pie-crusting technique, the surgeon makes 1-cm incisions separated by 1-cm skin bridges in the same area as the open approach on the dorsal and medial foot. Additional 1-cm stab incisions can be interspersed between the three major incision areas to allow complete access to the deep layers throughout the foot. Blunt dissection then can be used to enter the fascia at multiple points, releasing the tissue edema. It should be noted that in using the pie-crusting technique the surgeon has very limited capability to inspect, evaluate, and débride muscle. For this reason, if the surgeon expects to find necrotic tissue, a direct open approach should be performed or the surgeon can extend the pie-crusting incisions to make complete incisions.

■ UPPER EXTREMITY COMPARTMENT SYNDROME

The upper arm has two compartments, anterior and posterior. The anterior compartment of the upper arm is released through an anterior incision along the normal Henry approach. The standard incision used is approximately 15 cm in length, extending over the biceps brachium. The fascia of the biceps is incised and this muscle is retracted medially or laterally to access the brachialis muscle. The fascia of the brachialis muscle is incised to ensure adequate release of the anterior compartment of the upper arm.

The posterior compartment of the arm includes the triceps muscle. This can be accessed easily through a direct posterior approach with a 15-cm incision line made from the posterior corner of the acromion toward the olecranon tip. A full-thickness skin incision is made down to and through the posterior fascia of the triceps muscle. This allows inspection of the entire triceps muscle at its three heads.

■ FOREARM COMPARTMENT SYNDROME

Crushing injuries, ballistic injuries to the forearm, and comminuted diaphyseal fractures are the most common cause of compartment syndrome in the forearm. Three compartments need to be evaluated in the forearm: the mobile wad of three (extensor carpi radialis longus [ECRL], extensor carpi radialis brevis [ECRB], brachioradialis), the anterior, and the posterior compartments. One or two dorsal incisions and one volar incision may be used to release all three compartments. The deep volar musculature must be evaluated completely in the forearm to ensure complete release. The deep fascia is incised along the course of the superficial skin incision or longitudinally between the proximal and distal extents of the incision. Care must be taken to inspect each of the muscle bellies, as individual muscular compartment syndrome has been described in both the dorsal and the volar forearm. Unlike the incisions that are made for other components of the extremities, the incision on the volar forearm should extend from very close to the antecubital fossa crease to the distal wrist crease. This allows adequate exposure of all muscles in the forearm for inspection and débridement.

On the dorsal side of the forearm, a longitudinal incision can be made centered between the landmarks of Lister's tubercle and the lateral upper condyle. Through a 15-cm incision, adequate exposure of the dorsal compartment can be performed. It should be noted that isolated compartment syndrome of individual muscles within the dorsal and volar compartments also has been described; for this reason the individual muscles must be inspected and deeper fascial incisions may be necessary in order to allow tissue perfusion.

■ HAND COMPARTMENT SYNDROME

There are 10 compartments in the hand. These include the thenar and hypothenar compartments, four dorsal interossei, and three palmar interossei muscles. These compartments can be released through two dorsal incisions centered on the second and fourth metacarpals and radial thenar and ulnar hypothenar incisions. A carpal tunnel release often is performed at the time of release to prevent median nerve pressure injury.

■ LATE DIAGNOSIS OF COMPARTMENT SYNDROME

The late diagnosis of compartment syndrome is a clinical challenge that usually involves prolonged immobilization in the intensive care

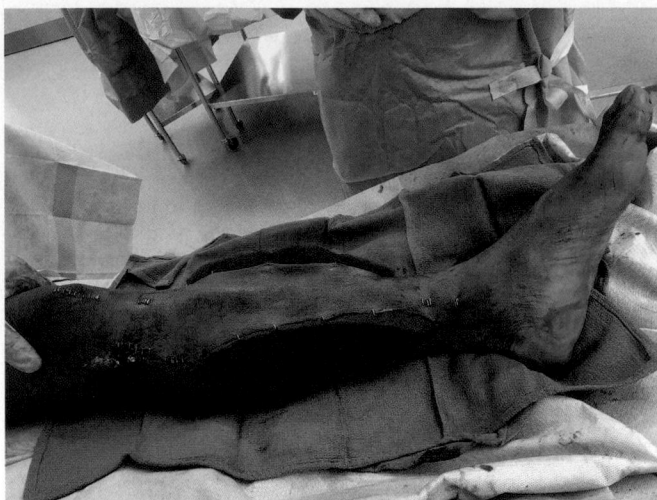

FIGURE 7 The wounds are covered with vacuum-assisted dressings to decrease edema and maintain a clean environment between débridements.

unit (ICU) or patients who are found down for extended periods. In the ICU the compromised extremity usually is identified after extended lifesaving measures, during which limb viability is secondary. Shiny-appearing skin that is stretched to its capacity is usually the clinical finding that alerts the physician to underlying compartment syndrome in the obtunded patient. Pallor, pulselessness, paresthesias, and paresis also are commonly identified in the delayed diagnosis.

When the diagnosis of compartment syndrome is made in a delayed fashion, there is debate about whether the compartments should be released. Magnetic resonance imaging (MRI) may be useful in identifying underperfused necrotic tissue. Release of compartment syndrome when it has been present for more than 48 hours should be discouraged. In this setting, compartment release exposes the underlying necrotic tissue to increased rates of infection through large surgical exposures. Although the surgeon may be compelled to open and débride the dead tissue, this provides a fertile environment for infection; the postoperative complication rate is high. Decompression and débridement of the compartment are unlikely to improve patient function. Supportive measures include hydration to prevent renal complications of rhabdomyolysis and splinting of contractures.

■ POSTOPERATIVE MANAGEMENT

After compartment syndrome release, even in the setting of compartments that appear normal, fascial and skin closure is not recommended. The wounds should be dressed with vacuum-assisted dressings (Figure 7) or wet-to-dry dressings. Patients return to the OR for dressing changes and repeat débridement. When the wounds appear stable, they may be closed with delayed primary closure or with skin grafts. Splinting through all phases of wound management allows soft tissue to rest and decreases pain.

BURN WOUND MANAGEMENT

James J. Gallagher, MD, FACS, and Philip S. Barie, MD, MBA, Master CCM, FIDSA, FACS

A broad area of damaged or lost skin resulting in a wound without the capacity to heal is the subject of this chapter. Burn injury is a common mechanism, but the principles apply to care for wounds from other causes. Scar from burn injury is commonly not a line that can be hidden in a natural crease, under hair, or in the umbilicus but rather it is often broad and visible. Mechanism of injury varies; understanding the unique characteristics of flame, scald, cold, chemical exposure, radiation, crush, and conductive electrical current provides guidance to achieve the best care. Surgical excellence is facilitated by an appreciation of surgical burn care goals: closure, function, and cosmesis. These goals are interdependent, yet individual; maximization of each simultaneously is the path to the best result. An understanding of when to recommend surgery, meshing of split-thickness skin grafts, position of graft seams, and selection of donor sites are some of the considerations that, approached thoughtfully, improve the long-term result. The surgeon should not accept a poor cosmetic and functional outcome as an unavoidable result of the injury.

After wound closure, the subsequent weeks and months often bring dramatic changes. Knowledge of scar behavior and indications for interventions, from compression to early reconstruction, is important for best results. Untreated scar can lead to deterioration of appearance, loss of range of motion, new wounds, and joint dislocation with loss of function. The behavior of scar during maturation is multifactorial but strongly influenced by early care. Close surgical follow-up and coordination with a rehabilitation therapist are needed in all burns of consequence.

Burn care attempts to preserve what was not destroyed, close the wound, and return the patient to his or her preinjury state. The degree to which the patient reintegrates into society is a measure of success in burn care. The spectrum of possible long-term problems associated with the care of the burn patient is best avoided through close and complete follow-up. This chapter focuses on the unique problems associated with the evaluation and treatment of burn wounds and is aimed at the surgeon whose practice is not burn focused.

■ EVALUATION

Assessing the Patient and the Burn

The drama of burn injury and its relative infrequency when compared with other traumatic injuries may lead to distraction from a thorough and complete evaluation. The systematic principles of modern trauma care should be applied in the care of the burn patient. Early in the evaluation and treatment of a burn patient, consideration must be given to whether providing care locally with a surgeon who is not part of a burn team is preferable to a referral to a burn center. This decision is made easier by a review of the burn center transfer criteria published by the American Burn Association. These criteria have been developed to aid physicians in identifying patients who need the specialized multidisciplinary care that is routine at a burn center (Box 1).

The estimate of burn size and depth is foundational to the care of the patient. All subsequent decisions about patient treatment are affected by these estimates. The calculation of percent total body surface area (TBSA) burned is best done with assistance of an experienced practitioner. Multiple studies have demonstrated a lack of congruity between the estimates of burn size at a referring institution and the burn center. It is often helpful with larger and scattered burns to write down each of the body area estimates and sum them when complete. The "rule of nines" is used commonly to estimate burn size (Figure 1). In children, especially toddlers, the standard rule of nines does not work well. At that age, the child's head is proportionately larger and the lower extremities are smaller. Another helpful standard is that the patient's palm represents approximately 1% of the body surface area in patients of all ages. Tips for burn wound assessment are provided in Box 2.

No proved, widely accepted diagnostic tool is available currently to guide the clinician in assessing the depth of the burn and therefore the ability of the wound to heal versus the need for surgery. Work is ongoing to find a reliable, objective, and practical method for determination of burn depth. The clinical examination of burn depth by an experienced clinician remains the standard for determining the need for surgery.

The importance and impact of early, accurate decision making and treatment planning by an experienced surgeon in achieving best results must not be underestimated. The benefit of early wound excision and grafting is proved to reduce catabolism, pain, psychologic stress, scarring/contracture, and the risk of infection. Allowing a wound to declare its healing potential over weeks before operating leads to several substantial problems that are better avoided. Painful daily dressing changes lead to excessive pain medication and their attendant complications, as well as a psychologic pain syndrome and post-traumatic stress disorder. A wound that remains incompletely healed for more than 21 days is at greater risk of hypertrophy and contracture formation. Conversely, an inexperienced surgeon who performs surgery on a wound that would have healed, had it been left in place, removes viable tissue that has natural regenerative capacity. It is therefore the challenge to be simultaneously aggressive and conservative with the burn wound in decision making, wound care, and surgical treatment. Most areas of the body that heal within 17 days should be left to do so in most patients. This guideline is modified by comorbidity, age, and body area involved.

Burn wound evaluation should be done after light cleaning and before any topical treatment is placed. The surgical team should evaluate and determine the treatment for the wound. If burn center transfer is indicated, contact the burn center for directives about wound care in transit. Topical salves may preclude the use of dressings designed to adhere to wounds until closed. Typically, receiving burn centers will ask that smaller wounds be kept in a clean, moist dressing and the larger wounds in dry dressings to prevent excessive loss of heat. Often mixed-depth wounds are observed for a time for final evaluation and surgical recommendation. The need for formal burn resuscitation is present with a burn of more than 15% to 20%. Larger burns stimulate a systemic inflammatory response, which is treated with fluid to prevent hypovolemia, hypoperfusion, and the sequelae of tissue ischemia from shock. Lesser but substantial burns may need increased fluid as a result of evaporative fluid loss, particularly in children. Burn fluid formulas are designed as a guide for the inception volume of resuscitation. The true volume and rate of administration of fluid required is dictated by an assessment of the endpoints of resuscitation and the condition of the patient.

Large burns have an absolute need for nutritional supplementation, preferably with tube feedings. Speed of epithelialization, formation of granulation tissue, and immunocompetence depend on adequate nutrition. When to intervene with smaller and medium-size burns is best guided by admission status, clear caloric goals, and an accounting of intake.

Assessing the Need for Decompression

After burn injury, the identification and treatment of elevated tissue pressure can avoid the loss of deeper tissues and eliminate a profound cause of morbidity. Tissue that has suffered burn injury forms edema because of loss of microvascular integrity and the movement of fluid from the intravascular compartment to the injured tissue interstitium. The larger the burn the greater the edema, which forms even

BOX 1: Criteria for Specialized Multidisciplinary Care at a Burn Center

Partial-thickness burn greater than 10% TBSA
Burns involving the face, hands, feet, genitalia, perineum, or major joints
Third-degree burns
Electric burns (including lightning)
Chemical burns
Inhalation injury
Burn injury with pre-existing medical conditions that may potentially complicate patient management, prolong recovery, or affect mortality
Burn injury with concomitant trauma, in which the burn injury poses a greatest risk of morbidity or mortality (if the trauma poses the greater immediate risk, the patient should first be stabilized in the trauma center before transfer to the burn facility). Decisions should be made according to regional medical control plans and triage protocols
Children with burns in hospitals without personnel or equipment qualified for care of children
Burn injuries in patients who will require special social, emotional, or long-term rehabilitative treatment

From Sood R, Achauer B. *Achauer and Sood's Burn Surgery, Reconstruction and Rehabilitation.* Philadelphia: Saunders; 2006.

TBSA, Total body surface area.

BOX 2: Estimating Burn Size

Do not include first-degree burns in the estimate.
Second-degree burns blister and lose the epidermis.
It is possible to estimate burn size before thorough cleaning of wounds.
It is often difficult to assess burn depth before thorough cleaning of wounds.
Superficial second-degree burns are moist, with blanching redness, and painful.
Deeper burns are less sensitive; they may be red but will not blanch with pressure.
Dryness and hair that is easily removed are signs of a deep wound.
Third-degree burns are dry, leathery, and insensate.

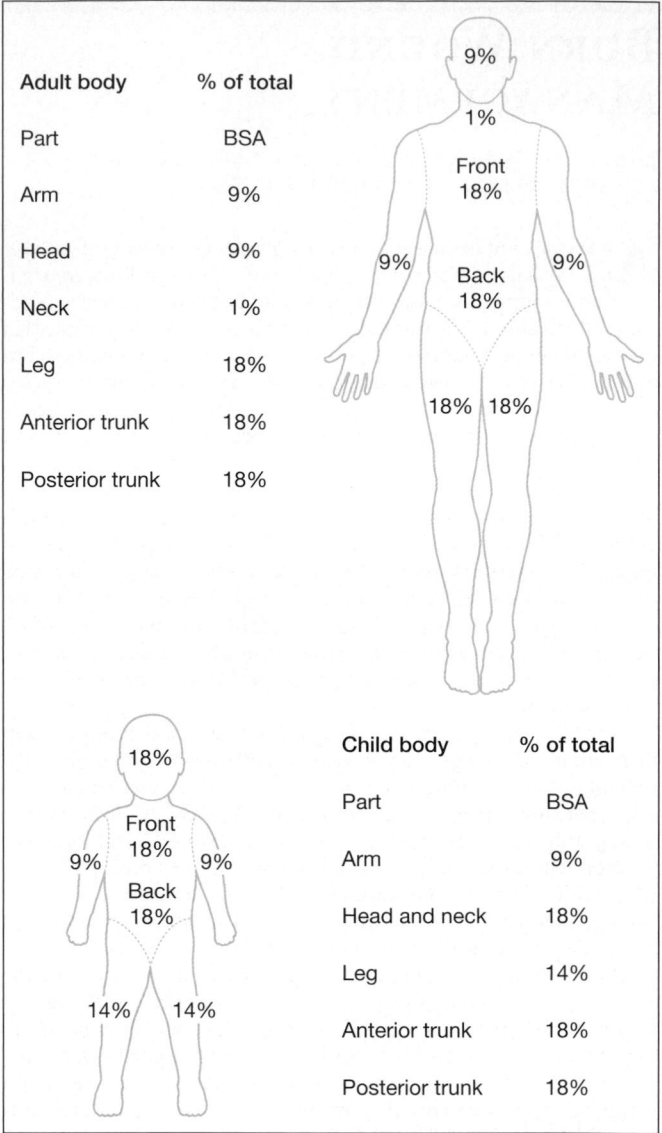

Adult body	% of total
Part	BSA
Arm	9%
Head	9%
Neck	1%
Leg	18%
Anterior trunk	18%
Posterior trunk	18%

Child body	% of total
Part	BSA
Arm	9%
Head and neck	18%
Leg	14%
Anterior trunk	18%
Posterior trunk	18%

FIGURE 1 Diagram of the rule of nines. *(From Herndon D. Total Burn Care. 4th ed. Philadelphia: Saunders; 2012.)*

in unburned tissues, owing to the systemic effects of inflammation. In unburned areas, edema formation usually does not cause problems. However, after burning, skin is less compliant than normal. Edema and decreased skin compliance in a circumferential extremity burn can result in high levels of tissue pressure and ischemic deep tissue loss similar to a classic compartment syndrome. Releasing the increased tissue pressure from burn injury normally does not require the decompression of the deep fascial compartments, as in classic compartment syndrome. In burn injury the constriction is at the level of the burned skin. Full-thickness incision of the burned skin or eschar (i.e., "escharotomy") to an edge of normal skin results in resolution of the increased pressure. Figures 2 and 3 give the recommended locations of decompressive escharotomies on the hands and body.

Circumferential burns often are considered for decompression; however, the presence of a circumferential burn is not an automatic indication for decompression. In patients with partial-thickness burns, the incisions for decompression can be a cosmetic issue. In a cooperative, communicating patient with a small-to-medium size burn, a safe option is careful fluid administration with elevation as

possible, coupled with serial examinations for increased tissue pressure. By contrast, larger burns almost universally require decompression of circumferential burns and possibly deep fascial decompression as well. Subeschar and deep fascial compartment pressure monitoring is useful and encouraged; although there is no standard, tissue pressures exceeding 20 mm Hg should prompt consideration for decompression. Escharotomy performed with electrocautery should be painless and near bloodless through a full-thickness burn.

Electrical Injury

Burn injury from a conductive electrical source is a particularly difficult clinical problem requiring a rapid, aggressive surgical approach. Routine physical examination can be misleading by underestimating the extent of damage because the amount of tissue damage to deep structures can be severe but hidden by intact overlying skin. This dead tissue can lead to compartment syndrome with further tissue loss. In addition, pigment (principally myoglobin) from dead or damaged muscle can produce acute kidney injury, which increases mortality. Dead muscle in situ is an excellent medium for bacterial colonization and sepsis. The multiple possible long-term sequelae of

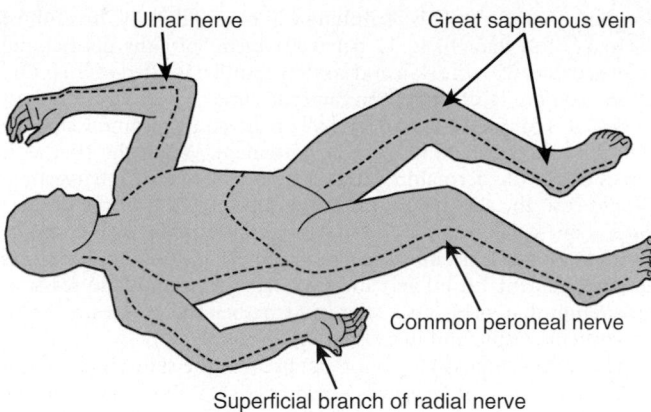

FIGURE 2 Locations for escharotomy placement on the hands.

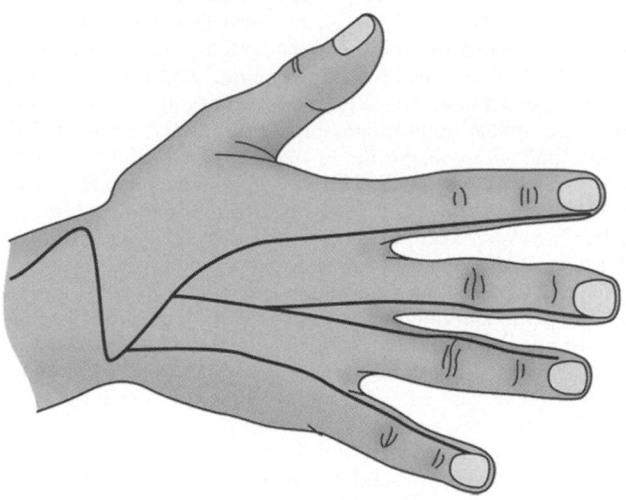

FIGURE 3 Locations for escharotomy placement on the body. *(From Wolfe S, et al. Green's Operative Hand Surgery. 7th ed. Philadelphia: Elsevier; 2016.)*

BOX 3: Warning Signs for Child Abuse

Lack of splash marks in scald injury
Straight-line distribution of skin injury with immersion
Contact burns that are evenly injured
A halo of scaled buttocks skin around unburned area, indicating
    the child was held down with force during the immersion
Unburned adults
A previous history of burn injury

conductive electrical injury and the complexity of the care required dictate that once a patient with such an injury is identified, transfer to a burn center should be prompt.

Child Abuse

Intentionally inflicted burn injury is a method used frequently for direct child abuse or to cover up other manifestations of child abuse. The surgeon caring for a burned child must remain vigilant to the possibility and obtain an absolutely clear understanding of the circumstances surrounding the burn injury (Box 3). It is usual practice to have multiple practitioners interview the involved adults and child separately, then discuss as a group the circumstances reported by the adults and the child before the injury is attributed to an accidental cause.

OPERATIVE CARE OF THE BURN WOUND

General

Meticulous preoperative planning will dictate the steps of the procedure. This will decrease operative delays and optimize results. Intraoperative patient positioning and draping is undertaken based on the wound location and the proposed donor site. To address the entire wound adequately one must identify any areas that have retained the ability to heal spontaneously with wound care versus those that will require surgery to achieve closure. All wounds, including those not planned for surgery, are cleaned and dressed as part of the procedure. This affords the opportunity for the surgeon to clean and examine thoroughly, under anesthesia, in a way that may not be otherwise possible. For burns of area greater than 40% TBSA, rapid wound closure is the prime directive to save the patient's life. Wound closure is the best defense against ongoing risk of sepsis, catabolism, and death. During the early period when the focus is necessarily on closure, some consideration of the two remaining goals, function and cosmesis, greatly improve the complete result long term. The operative discussion that follows will focus on less extensive burns.

Preparing the Wound Bed

The basic principles of burn care involve the efficient removal of all dead tissue, without damaging or sacrificing living tissue, while minimizing blood loss. Small wounds may be excised completely and closed either primarily or with a flap. Areas that will require grafting on an extremity can be excised under tourniquet safely and confidently; this technique minimizes blood loss associated with débridement. The determination of living versus dead tissue is best made with complete exsanguination of the extremity followed by inflation of the tourniquet. The remaining red to purple staining after complete exsanguination is a reliable marker for compromise. Healthy dermis is characterized by a pearly white appearance. Fat tissue that is compromised is a dull yellow to orange color; the yellow of healthy fat is bright. Care must be taken when using this technique; experience is required. In a chronic burn wound and in lower extremities with clinical evidence of venous stasis, the dermal coloration may be misleading and lead to overaggressive surgery.

Tangential excision is the most common method for removal of dead tissue. Specially made tangential excision knives are used, including the dermatome, which may be used as a tool for débridement. It is important to complete the excision to the surgeon's satisfaction in one stage and then to achieve hemostasis because this will shorten the procedure and limit blood loss. Very large areas can be excised in stages. To achieve hemostasis of a large surface area after tangential excision, use clamps or cautery on vessels with pulsatile blood flow. Do not spend excessive time before application of a moist dressing with epinephrine and light manual compression. The majority of bleeding points do not require direct attention, and compressive dressings may be left in place for 10 to 15 minutes before removal. Thrombogenic products (e.g., topical bovine thrombin) can be applied in saline solution to the wound bed in an effort to minimize blood loss further; however, the cost must be considered.

On the trunk, tourniquet excision is not possible, and blood loss can be substantial. The bleeding pattern and tissue appearance is used to determine tissue viability and completeness of excision. Tangential excision that removed dead tissue to a depth that remains within the dermis is characterized by diffuse bleeding from the entire cut surface. When it is necessary to remove the full thickness of skin to reach a viable tissue bed, bleeding is often pulsatile from the perforating branches to the skin. Tumescent fluid administration beneath the wound will limit blood loss, but reading the wound requires more experience. Burn wounds of great depth over a large area may require excision at the level of the fascia; this can limit blood loss greatly and increases efficiency, but the resulting marked functional and cosmetic impact must be considered with this approach. Small wounds may be excised completely and closed primarily or with a local tissue flap.

Special Considerations

Exposed vital structures such as bone, periosteum, tendon, peritenon, and nerve require special consideration. These structures are often poor beds for a skin graft to "take" onto, which may lead to graft failure. Worse still, the resulting wound will leave these delicate structures at risk of further compromise. Consider use of homograft or moist dressings until granulation tissue has formed. Dermal templates have been used to temporize the wound as well. However, there is little evidence that they can bridge gaps in the wound bed at sites without vascularized tissue coverage, such as peritenon. The dermal template can provide a layer between the skin graft and the structure below to allow smooth and separate movements of each until a viable bed for grafting is attained. Dermal templates are used for covering the aforementioned delicate structures, as well as more broadly in burn surgery to close wounds. Disadvantages associated with the use of dermal templates include the 2 weeks or more for templates to mature, the requirement for a second procedure for skin graft overlay after they mature, and the careful handling necessary to prevent infection. The putative benefits of decreased scarring and improved function in the long-term have not been not proved. Technical points to consider in skin graft placement are listed in Box 4.

Donor Sites

The creation of a donor site wound is necessary in burn wounds that require a skin graft. The goal of donor site location selection is to minimize the impact of the harvest. Factors to consider in choosing a donor site are (1) cosmesis; (2) healing potential; (3) intraoperative positioning and draping; (4) pain; and (5) practical postoperative positioning to facilitate graft maturation but also protect the donor site. It is important to counsel the patient that the harvest site will create an additional permanent scar. When approaching the donor site, remember to never trust the dermatome calibration: inspect the gap created by the chosen setting visually. Routinely the gap is set at 6 per 0.001 inch to 12 per 0.001 inch. It can be useful to attempt to pass a #15 scalpel blade tip into the gap as confirmation. The blade should enter partially and glide the length of the dermatome without

dropping in entirely. This technique will ensure that the breadth of the gap is less than 10 to 12 per 0.001 inch. Start the dermatome before contact with the skin and continue until it is lifted off the skin. Good positioning of the patient and the surgeon will yield the best harvest. It is routine to use mineral oil on the skin to promote smooth gliding of the dermatome with advancement. Watch the skin as it comes out of the dermatome to be sure of what you are harvesting. Do not rush the skin harvest: if the skin coming out of the dermatome is not satisfactory, keep the dermatome running and communicate with your assistants to try to improve the situation. If there is no improvement, lift off and abort the harvest attempt and reassess. An attempt that yields poor skin will lengthen the procedure, harm the cosmetic result, and increase morbidity.

The scalp is a possible donor site because the skin obtained is a good color match for face, neck, and upper chest. It can be a reliable donor site in patients with poor healing potential as a result of other chronic disease. When done properly in an individual with hair, the donor site is invisible just weeks after the procedure. The scalp tissue typically yields 3% to 4% of the body surface area before meshing. Late pain with the scalp donor site is usually less than with other donor sites. When the skin is taken carefully, healing is rapid and reliable but with minimal risk of postsurgical alopecia with standard harvest depth. Harvesting a graft from the scalp should never be attempted unless appropriate tumescent infiltration with 0.25% bupivacaine with epinephrine in a balanced salt solution has been done beforehand. Attempting harvest without having placed appropriate tumescent fluid will result in excessive blood loss from the scalp, which is difficult to control. Approximately 500 mL of tumescent fluid is routine for a complete adult scalp harvest. To harvest a scalp graft, remove the hair from the area with clippers before entering the operating room; shave the scalp with a razor after the patient is under anesthesia, and instill the tumescent fluid with a 14-g spinal needle moving about the area. The appropriate depth is recognized by the relative ease of infiltration. Tending to the burn wound débridement at this point will allow the 10 to 15 minutes required for the epinephrine to have effect to pass without adding to the operative time. When wound-bed preparation of the burn is complete, return to the head, and harvest the needed skin based on the open wound area. The principle of wound bed preparation followed by skin harvest is used broadly because this approach often minimizes excessive harvest and decreases operative time.

Dressings

A grafted wound bed requires a period free of shear forces during which attachment of the skin graft to the wound bed can take place. In addition, the skin graft requires a moist environment free from overt bacterial contamination. The creation of a dressing to address these goals is as crucial to success as the other aspects of burn surgical care. Postoperative position, nursing care, and patient compliance, especially in children, can be major issues. A grafted extremity is dressed easily with petrolatum-based fine gauze, a clean gauze overdressing, and a splint; however, the task becomes more difficult with grafting that involves the anterior shoulder and lateral neck. Options include a tie-on bolster in conjunction with a neck collar and axillary splint. A negative-pressure dressing (see earlier) can be considered if a good circumferential seal can be obtained with or without splinting, depending on the mobility of the wound.

Special problems are encountered with small children and their ability to work their way free of a dressing, so consider this as you plan the procedure. When the grafted areas require a complex dressing, it is good practice to discuss postoperative plans with nursing, rehabilitation staff, and with the patient—or in the case of a child, with the patient's parents—to increase the likelihood of success. For example, postoperative prone positioning may be an excellent choice for grafts placed on the back; however, such a plan is unlikely to succeed if it is not discussed with nursing, rehabilitation, and the patient, and agreed on. An unusual position can be tried with the

---

BOX 4: Placing the Skin: Technical Points to Consider

Place the skin under mild stretch, aided by attaching one edge then pulling toward the other edge.

Trim the skin carefully so that it is fitted to the wound; a 1- to 2-mm gap from wound edge to graft is ideal.

The skin graft should contact the wound bed completely. This can be difficult with deep contours and can be aided by dressings. Placement of a vacuum-assisted wound closure device is a protective and promoted contact of the graft with the wound bed.

Avoid meshing skin whenever possible, particularly on exposed areas such as hands and face.

Anticipate that seams between grafts will become visible scars and areas of more intense contraction. Plan orientation of the grafts appropriately.

Staples, sutures, glues, and other adjuncts may all be used, depending on the need. For children, consider fixation that is absorbable or sutures that are removed easily to minimize the burden of aftercare.

patient before surgery, and bed modifications can be made to prepare for the patient after surgery. Innovative dressings are possible if the goals are understood, and open communication takes place with everyone involved. A dressing failure may lead to graft loss and a return to the operating room.

■ SUMMARY

This chapter on burn wound management is offered to assist primarily the surgeon whose practice is not burn focused. An effort has been made to offer advice to avoid problems and treat burns that do not require a burn center in the judgment of the treating physician. For a more complete discussion of burn care see the resources listed in Suggested Readings. Burn centers can be contacted for advice on burns not believed to need the burn center. Use of a burn center as a source of education on best practices as well as for tertiary referral is to be encouraged.

SUGGESTED READINGS

Janzekovic Z. A new concept in the early excision and immediate grafting of burns. *J Trauma*. 1970;10:1103-1108.

Klein MB, Heimbach DM, Gibran NS. Management of the burn wound. In: Souba WW, Fink MP, Jurkovich GJ, et al. *ACS Surgery: Principles & Practice*. 6th ed. Hamilton, Ontario: B.C. Decker; 2010.

Mosier MJ, Gibran NS. Surgical excision of the burn wound. *Clin Plast Surg*. 2009;36:617-625.

Tompkins RG, Remensnyder JP, Burke JF, et al. Significant reduction in mortality for children with burn injuries through the use of prompt eschar excision. *Ann Surg*. 1988;208:577-585.

MEDICAL MANAGEMENT OF THE BURN PATIENT

Stephen M. Milner, MS, BS, BDS, DSc, FRCS(Ed), and Julie Caffrey, DO, MS

■ INITIAL RESUSCITATION

First Aid

The initial treatment of burns begins at the scene. The patient must be removed from the source of injury as quickly as possible. Flames can be extinguished, chemical injuries can be irrigated with water, and patients with electrical injuries can be removed from contact with the source. Prolonged cooling of the wound should be avoided. The patient should be kept warm and covered with a clean, dry sheet. Blisters and wounds should be left undisturbed and application of ointments delayed, as this inhibits subsequent wound assessment by the burn team.

Emergency Department

Endotracheal intubation is not performed routinely in all patients with suspected inhalation injury; however, it should be considered in patients with deep burns to the face, hoarseness, and stridor and in those with burns to more than 40% of their total body surface area (TBSA), where large volume resuscitation is necessary. We administer 100% oxygen for 6 hours after burn casualties with inhalation injury despite falling carboxyhemoglobin levels to protect against central nervous system (CNS) effects of carbon monoxide. Other injuries should not be overlooked. Control of hemorrhage and stabilization of fractures are mandatory. Burned patients lose heat rapidly and must continue to be kept warm. If possible, a detailed history should be obtained from the patient before intubation, and family and emergency medical services (EMS) staff should be questioned. It is important to ascertain the mechanism of injury, initial neurologic status, extrication time, tetanus immunization status, and any medications and fluids received in transport to the hospital. Careful examination of the eyes should be carried out with fluorescein staining, and an ophthalmology consultation should be requested if injection, periocular burns, or clouded cornea is present.

An estimate of burn size should be calculated using the Lund and Browder chart. Fluid is administered through large bore peripheral intravenous catheters, preferably inserted through nonburned skin. Fluid resuscitation is initiated using the Parkland formula estimated from the time of the burn (Figure 1).

■ BURN INTENSIVE CARE UNIT

Fluid Resuscitation

After burn injury there is a massive release of chemical mediators, leading to an increase in vascular permeability that results in the extravasation of fluid and electrolytes. This capillary leak lasts 18 to 24 hours after injury. Failure to correct fluid losses leads to hypovolemia, renal failure, and burn shock. Intravenous fluid resuscitation is required for all patients younger than 10 years or older than 50 years who have second- and third-degree burns greater than 10% TBSA; in all other age groups, intravenous fluid resuscitation is required for patients who have second- and third-degree burns greater than 20% TBSA.

There are no prospective randomized studies comparing the numerous resuscitation protocols; however, we prefer the Parkland formula, which provides both burn and maintenance fluid requirements. Quality resuscitation is dependent on hourly evaluation of urine output, titrated to a urine output of 0.5 to 1 mL/hr, with subsequent adjustments of infusions (Figure 2). Increased fluid requirements may be seen in patients with inhalation injury or high-voltage electrical injuries and in children. Today the complication of renal failure largely has been replaced by a host of compartment syndromes resulting from excessive resuscitation. The role of colloid in burn resuscitation may mitigate the excessive volumes of crystalloid required. Our routine practice is to initiate 5% albumin for most patients with burns in excess of 40% TBSA at 8 hours postinjury. Resuscitation endpoints include return of normal vital signs, adequate urine output, and good peripheral perfusion.

Escharotomy

Decreased chest compliance and elevated peak airway pressures may indicate compartment syndrome, which may necessitate immediate escharotomy (Figure 3). With circumferential deep burns, the extremities should be assessed for perfusion and tense compartments should be decompressed. Classically, incisions are placed along the medial and lateral aspect of the limbs. In the upper extremity, care is taken to avoid injury to the ulnar nerve behind the medial epicondyle and the superficial radial nerve in the anatomic snuff box. Similarly, one must avoid injury to the common peroneal nerve as it winds around the neck of the fibula (Figure 4). Escharotomies of the hand are best performed by incisions between the metacarpals decompressing the interossei. The utility of finger escharotomies is controversial (Figure 5).

Care of the Burn Wound

Débridement should be delayed until the patient is warmed adequately to a temperature of 37°C. Loose skin and blisters are removed, and the depth and size of the injury are charted. Superficial burns are treated with a nonadherent dressing such as Xeroform and bacitracin, whereas deeper burns are dressed preferentially with silver sulfadiazine cream because more potent antibacterial cover is required.

■ BURN CRITICAL CARE

Neurologic Issues

Pain management can be variable given the patient's tolerance, the size and depth of the burn, and the need for mechanical ventilation. Opioids are used commonly, along with anxiolytics. Intravenous opioids are reserved for the acute period and for procedures, whereas oral medications are used for background pain.

Prevalence of delirium in ventilated burn patients has been reported to be as high as 77% (Agarwal et al. 2010). Delirium may be hyperactive, hypoactive, or mixed. Characteristic features include impaired memory and attention and disorientation, developed over a short period of time with a fluctuating course.

Treatment first should be aimed at nonpharmacologic therapies, including prevention of sleep deprivation and restoration of the sleep-wake cycle by reducing noise, exposing patients to natural light during the day, and minimizing artificial light at night. Pharmacologic therapy should focus on limiting sedatives.

Inhalation Injury

Inhalation injury is a major contributor to mortality in the burn patient. The exposure time, concentration of gases, toxic substances, and degree of concomitant cutaneous burns are critical to the mortality risk. Noninvasive monitoring may be misleading, and therefore laboratory adjuncts, including arterial blood gas and carboxyhemoglobin levels, should be performed. Fiber optic bronchoscopy is the gold standard for diagnosis and allows for quantification of hyperemia, edema, and carbonaceous material.

Carbon Monoxide and Cyanide Toxicity

Carbon monoxide toxicity is a leading cause of death in house fires. Carbon monoxide is transported across the alveolar membrane and preferentially binds to hemoglobin, causing a left shift of the oxygen-hemoglobin dissociation curve and preventing unloading of oxygen to the tissues. Symptoms of toxicity are present when carboxyhemoglobin levels exceed 15%. The initial manifestations are neurologic. The diagnosis is suggested by persistence of metabolic acidosis despite adequate fluid resuscitation and cardiac output. A low carboxyhemoglobin level does not always indicate minimal exposure. Treatment consists of administration of 100% oxygen, which reduces the half-life of carboxyhemoglobin from 120-200 minutes to 30 minutes. Hyperbaric oxygen produces a more rapid displacement and may be helpful in cases of prolonged exposure. The use of hyperbaric oxygen in burn therapy, however, is hampered by the need to rapidly treat a patient who is in a critical time of potential hemodynamic and pulmonary instability.

Hydrocyanide is produced with burning of polyurethane and is a well-recognized cause of mortality. It is absorbed rapidly and inhibits production of adenosine triphosphate (ATP). Cyanide metabolism and clearance is impaired in the presence of hypovolemia, putting patients with concomitant cutaneous injury at greater risk. Clinical symptoms resemble those caused by carbon monoxide poisoning, with severe metabolic acidosis and obtundation. Current treatment involves the use of the "hydroxocobalamin kit."

Upper Airway Obstruction From Tissue Edema

Direct heat injury caused by inhalation of air with a temperature higher than 150°C results in burns to the face, oropharynx, and upper airway. Heat produces an immediate injury to the airway mucosa, resulting in edema, erythema, and ulceration. Mucosal changes may be present immediately; however, physiologic alterations usually are not apparent until the edema can produce clinical symptoms, which may not occur until 12 to 18 hours after injury. The presence of a large cutaneous burn compounds the issue because of massive fluid resuscitation. Deep facial burns contribute to airway obstruction by

PARKLAND FORMULA

> **4 cc x weight (kg) x %TBSA burned = volume of Lactated Ringer's solution**

- Give ½ total solution over first 8 hours
- Give ½ total solution over second 16 hours

FIGURE 1 Parkland formula. *TBSA,* Total body surface area.

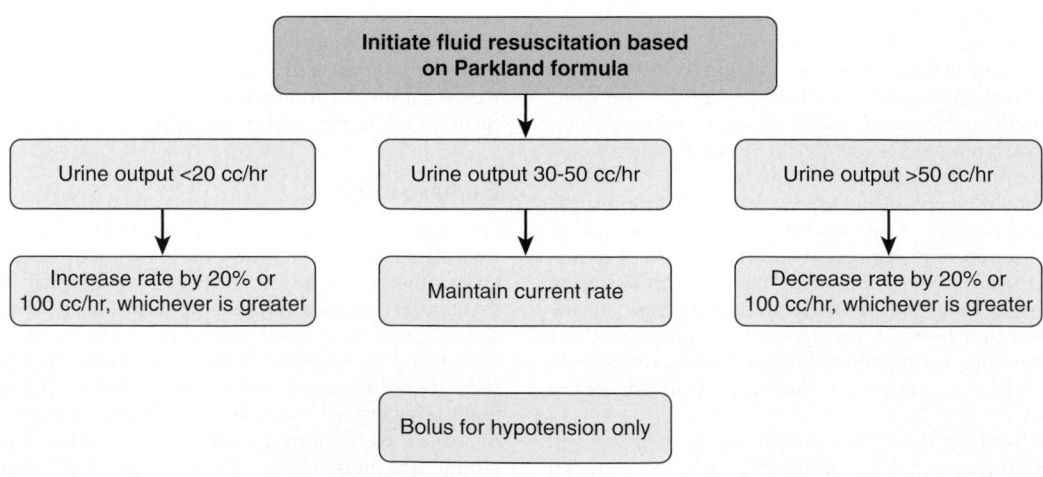

Initiate fluid resuscitation based on Parkland formula

| Urine output <20 cc/hr | Urine output 30-50 cc/hr | Urine output >50 cc/hr |
| Increase rate by 20% or 100 cc/hr, whichever is greater | Maintain current rate | Decrease rate by 20% or 100 cc/hr, whichever is greater |

Bolus for hypotension only

FIGURE 2 Proposed resuscitation protocol.

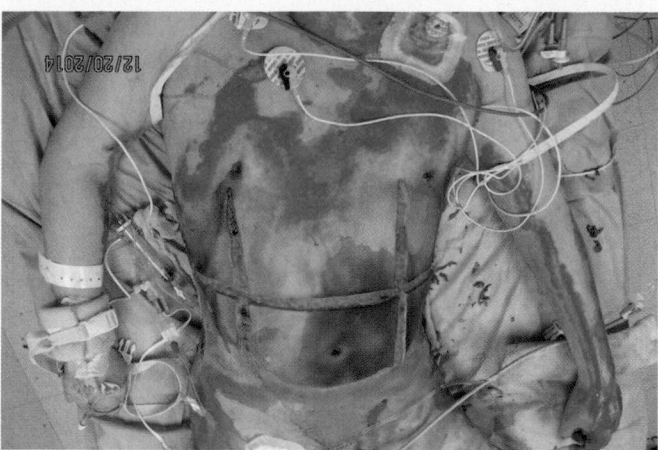

FIGURE 3 Escharotomies of the chest.

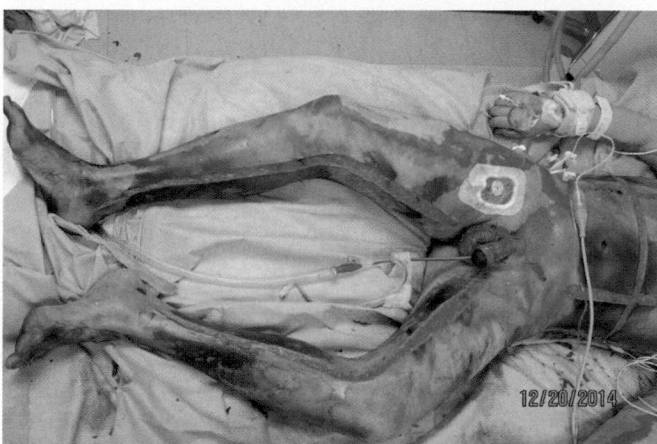

FIGURE 4 Escharotomies of the lower extremities.

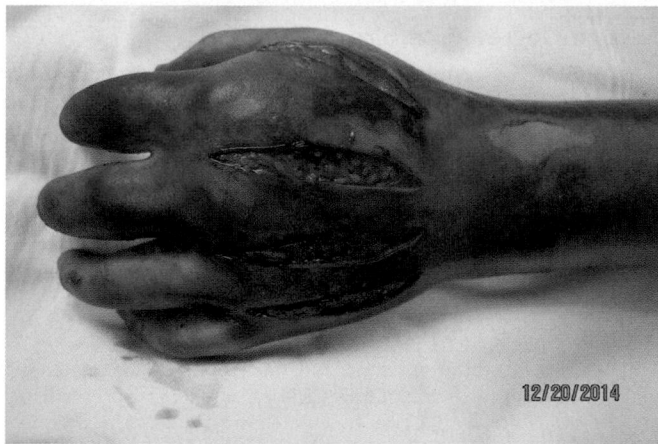

FIGURE 5 Escharotomies of the hand.

intraoral and laryngeal edema, anatomic distortion, decreased clearance of secretions, and impaired protection of the airway from aspiration.

Adjunctive Therapies

Aggressive pulmonary toilet, nebulized heparin, N-acetyl cysteine, and bronchodilators all have been recommended (Desai et al, 1998).

Nebulized heparin prevents fibrin deposition, maintains alveolar structure, and reduces the likelihood of obstruction in patients with inhalation injury. Inhaled bronchodilators, such as β2-agonists, cause preferential bronchodilation and attenuation of lung inflammation and improve clearance without affecting the cardiovascular system. The use of corticosteroids has not been shown to improve acute pulmonary inflammation (Miller et al, 2014).

Nutrition and Metabolism

Patients who sustain large burns are in a continuous catabolic state that may last up to 1 year after injury. Initiation of nutritional supplementation by enteral feeding is essential in the first 24 to 48 hours in order to preserve gut mucosal integrity, prevent bacterial translocation, and achieve nutritional goals. A marked increase in energy expenditure, which may be 2 to 3 times normal in a patient with burns to more than 30% TBSA, leads to mobilization of amino acids and protein catabolism. This results in proportional loss of muscle and proteins necessary for organ structure and cellular function. The hypermetabolic response is amplified by fever, pain, presence of burn eschar, multiple surgical procedures, and recurrent infections. The goals are to provide adequate energy to minimize the stress response, maximize immune competence, minimize loss of lean body mass, and facilitate wound healing. Numerous tube feeding formulations are commercially available. In the majority of cases, a calorie-dense, high-protein formula containing less than 30% total calories as fat is ideal. Parenteral nutrition should be avoided if possible because of its associated high mortality.

The most effective anabolic strategies for patients with severe burns are early excision and grafting (Williams et al, 2009); prompt treatment of sepsis; maintenance of adequate core temperature; continuous feeding of high-protein, high-carbohydrate diet; and early institution of exercise programs

Beta-blockers have been shown to diminish thermogenesis, cardiac work, and resting energy expenditure. The dose should be titrated to reduce heart rate by 20% in order to decrease cardiac workload. Treatment with anabolic steroids such as oxandrolone, a testosterone analogue, improves muscle protein catabolism and reduces weight loss. It has low levels of virilizing androgenic effects.

Renal Issues

Early-onset renal failure results from reduced cardiac output. Causes include hypovolemia, myocardial depression, stress-related hormones, inflammatory mediators, nephrotoxins, and denatured proteins. This results in increased vascular permeability and production of microthrombi in the capillaries of the glomeruli and renal tubule. There follows a reduction of renal flow and tubular necrosis. Late renal failure is usually a consequence of sepsis and multiorgan failure.

Sepsis and Antibiotics

Burn sepsis is a major cause of mortality. The presence of open wounds, lung injury, central venous catheters, and urinary catheters place the patient at risk. Altered physiology and a hyperdynamic state complicate early diagnosis. Overuse of antibiotics leads to resistant organisms and opportunistic infections. Wound infections generally are treated with early débridement and daily dressing changes with antimicrobial topical agents and frequent inspection of wounds. Antibiotics are reserved for proven infections in patients with systemic symptoms.

SUGGESTED READINGS

Agarwal V, O'Neill PJ, Cotton BA, Pun BT, et al. Prevalence and risk factors for development of delirium in burn intensive care unit patients. *J Burn Care Res.* 2010;31:706-715.

Barr J, Fraser GL, Puntillo K, Ely EW, Gelinas C, et al. Clinical practice guidelines for the management of pain, agitation and delirium in adult patients in the intensive care unit. *Crit Care Med*. 2013;41:263-306.

Desai MH, Mlcak R, Richardson J, Nichols R, Herndon DN. Reduction in mortality in pediatric patients with inhalation injury with aerosolized heparin/acetylcysteine therapy. *J Burn Care Rehabil*. 1998;19:210-212.

Miller AC, Elamin EM, Suffredini AF. Inhaled anticoagulation regimens for the treatment of smoke inhalation–associated acute lung injury: a systematic review. *Crit Care Med*. 2014;42:413-419.

Price LA, Milner SM. The totality of burn care. *Trauma*. 2012;15:16-28.

Williams FN, Herndon DN, Jeschke MG. The hypermetabolic response to burn injury and interventions to modify this response. *Clin Plast Surg*. 2009;36:583-596.

The Management of Frostbite, Hypothermia, and Cold Injuries

Paul N. Manson, MD

The several types of localized cold injuries may be classified according to the temperature that produces them: (1) nonfreezing or (2) freezing temperatures. *Trench foot, immersion hand and foot,* and *chilblains* are produced by cold but not freezing temperatures. *Frostbite* is produced by freezing temperatures. Trench foot and immersion foot and hand are seen principally in military populations, whereas chilblains and frostbite are seen more commonly in civilian populations.

Further, cold injuries may be divided into:

1. Localized cold injuries (i.e., frostbite)
2. Generalized cold injuries (i.e., hypothermia)

Frequently, localized cold injuries such as frostbite do not co-exist with systemic hypothermia.

Localized cold injuries have in common the fact that they are produced by exposure to cold stimuli and that they occur at the extremities of circulation. Localized cold injuries may be seen in the cheeks, nose, ears, and face but are seen primarily in the hands and feet. Cold injuries in the face tend to be superficial because of the blood supply. Serious cold injuries are confined almost exclusively to the extremities, where there is a small margin of difference between the injuries that produce superficial versus deep injury.

■ TRENCH FOOT

Trench foot usually is seen in military populations and occurs with exposure to above-freezing temperatures, generally over a prolonged period of time. The presence of moisture is very important in its pathogenesis. Chronic symptoms produced after recovery from the acute injury are those of pain, paresthesia, and a particular susceptibility to further cold injury.

■ IMMERSION FOOT AND HAND

Immersion foot and hand are seen after prolonged exposure to cold but not freezing water. After recovery from the acute episode, major nerve paralysis may be seen in addition to chronic vasospastic cold sensitivity and pain. Pain in the affected area and paresthesias commonly are seen after all types of cold injury.

■ CHILBLAINS

Chilblains represent the mildest form of cold injury and occur after prolonged exposure to cold and wet conditions. The symptoms consist of burning and itching and are associated with a mild dermatitis. Vesicles and hemorrhagic lesions may be seen in the acute period.

The chronic condition is characterized by cold sensitivity, itching, paresthesias, and skin eruptions, which may be reddish lesions, vesicles, or superficial ulcers. The chronic condition may be treated by protection from cold and heat to avoid production of dermatitis symptoms and pain. The role of sympathetic denervation in the management of the chronic condition has been suggested but not established. Some feel it may be helpful in chronic, well-established symptoms that require treatment. Chilblains do not produce tissue loss, and thus they require no reconstruction.

■ FROSTBITE

Frostbite occurs from exposure to freezing temperatures. The period of exposure required for its production may be short or long, depending on environmental conditions, wind, and protection. Frostbite has been classified into degrees of injury depending on the depth of damage. Often several degrees of injury will be seen in the same extremity, with the damage increasing as injury progresses from proximal to distal.

First-Degree Frostbite

First-degree frostbite is a superficial skin injury characterized by numbness, edema, and erythema. The injury is similar to a first-degree burn in that it heals spontaneously (in terms of the epithelium) in 1 to 2 weeks. Superficial desquamation may occur and regeneration is usually complete with decreased but adequate skin appendages (Figure 1).

Second-Degree Frostbite

In second-degree frostbite, partial-thickness skin injury occurs that is characterized by numbness, edema, erythema, and vesiculation. The vesicles may be filled with either clear or bloody fluid. The partial-thickness skin injury heals in 2 to 4 weeks (Figure 2). The quality of the regenerated skin depends on the depth of the injury to the dermis and parallels thermal burn injuries in that deep second-degree injuries heal with thin atrophic skin that has a reduced number of skin appendages.

Third-Degree Frostbite

Third-degree frostbite represents full-thickness skin loss. After the injury a nonviable segment of full-thickness skin loss is observed; this may be seen initially as a gray-blue patch, or death of the skin may follow an initial period of reactive hyperemia after 24 to 72 hours. Eventually a black eschar forms, which generally separates slowly in 1 to 3 months unless infection occurs (Figure 3).

Fourth-Degree Frostbite

Fourth-degree frostbite signifies necrosis of all deep tissue parts down to and sometimes including bone. Black, mummified tissues are present with the initial episode. If the mummified area becomes infected, it softens and becomes swollen and macerated at the margin with viable tissue.

Pathophysiology of Frostbite

There are two pathophysiologic mechanisms that account for the production of frostbite injury. One is vasoconstriction and damage to the microcirculation in the "zone of vascular stasis," which results in progressive vascular thrombosis. The second is direct damage to the cells or cellular toxicity from freezing. Experts disagree on the importance of these two mechanisms, and the importance of each mechanism varies according to the amount of tissue freezing that occurs and the local conditions, such as circulation.

The "Hunting" Reaction

The body responds to cold with an alternating cycle of vasoconstriction and vasodilatation (called the hunting reaction) in an attempt to conserve heat loss from the skin. As the injury becomes worse, the cycle may involve actual freezing and thawing of tissue. Circulation virtually ceases as the vasoconstriction increases, creating marked ischemia of the tissue.

Direct (Freezing) Damage to Cells

Freezing produces extracellular and then intracellular ice crystals. Extracellular ice crystals produce direct damage to cell walls and also cause a "leaching out" of electrolytes and water from the intracellular compartment, resulting in intracellular dehydration followed by cell

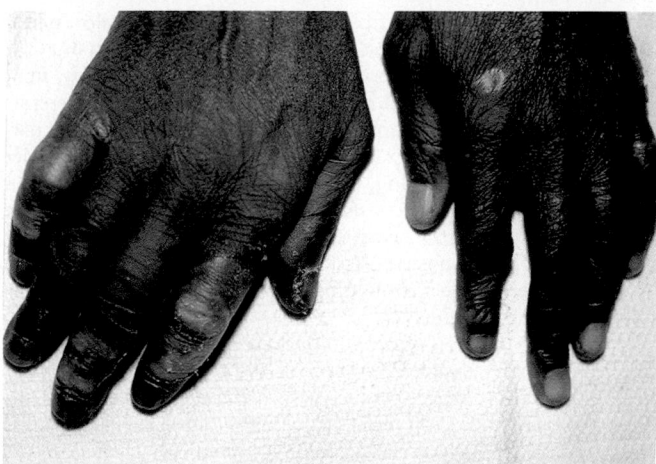

FIGURE 1 First- and second-degree frostbite. Epidermal skin loss and peeling are seen.

death. Intracellular ice crystals produce direct damage to important cell structures.

Progressive Vascular Thrombosis

Frostbite produces progressive dermal ischemia, similar to the process seen in thermal burns or in the "no-reflow" phenomenon. The role of edema and endothelial injury in the subsequent arrest of dermal blood flow has implicated various inflammatory mediators such as thromboxanes, prostaglandins, histamine, and bradykinin; these observations have led to the use of inhibitors of these mediators, in an attempt to ameliorate the harmful tissue reaction and improve tissue survival.

Tissue injury occurs both from direct damage to cells and from the vasoconstriction anoxia, which results in vascular stasis and thrombosis. After the state of decreased circulation, a state of "reactive hyperemia" occurs, which may or may not be associated with a "no-reflow" phenomenon, where capillary thrombosis occurs in the "zone of stasis." The pathology of tissue repair is similar to that of burn injuries in that epithelium migrates to cover the wound from the surviving remnants of sweat glands, hair follicles, and margins of the living wound. The quality of the skin produced is inversely proportional to the depth of damage. Deep injuries have necrotic nerve, muscle, and bone and are healed by scar after the shedding of dead tissue. Frequently, autoamputation occurs after ischemic necrosis and gangrene. Left untreated, the process is generally dry and progresses to autoamputation without infection over several months.

Environmental Influences

A number of behavioral and environmental factors may influence the production of cold injuries. Two of the most significant environmental factors are the ambient temperature and the wind.

The effects of temperature may be modified by wearing protective clothing, which provides insulation proportional to its thickness and weight. The effects of temperature are modified by the presence of wind and wet conditions, which accelerate heat loss. Wet conditions increase heat conduction to the environmental air, whereas wind accelerates the loss of heat in the air. Siple has developed a "wind chill index" (WCI) to reflect the magnitude of the contribution of wind in heat loss. The heat loss would be the same at 20°F with a wind of 45 miles/hour as at −40°F with a wind of 2 miles/hour.

The mean outdoor temperature recorded in frostbite injury series is −29°C. Frostbite is seen isolated to the upper extremities in 19% of cases, isolated to the lower extremities in 47% of cases, in both upper and lower extremities in 31% of cases, and with no extremity involvement in only 3% of cases.

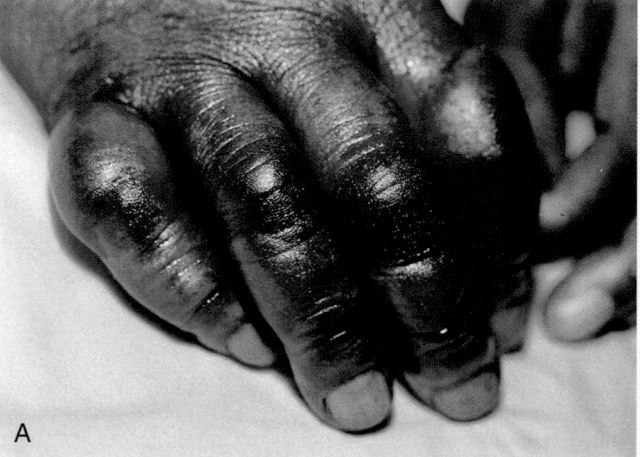

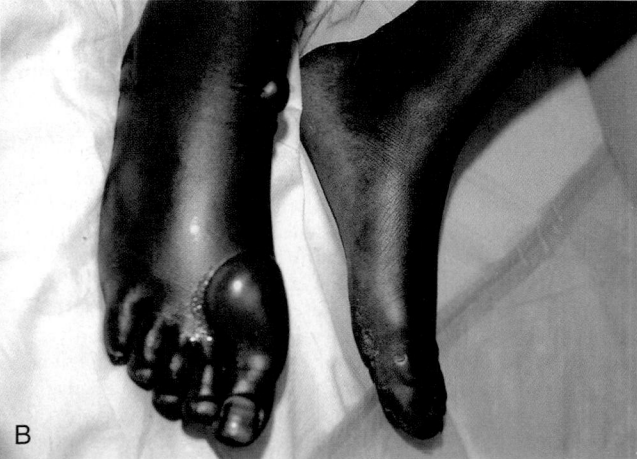

FIGURE 2 A, Second-degree frostbite in the fingers. Vesicles and swelling are seen. **B,** Second-degree frostbite in the feet. Vesicles and swelling are seen.

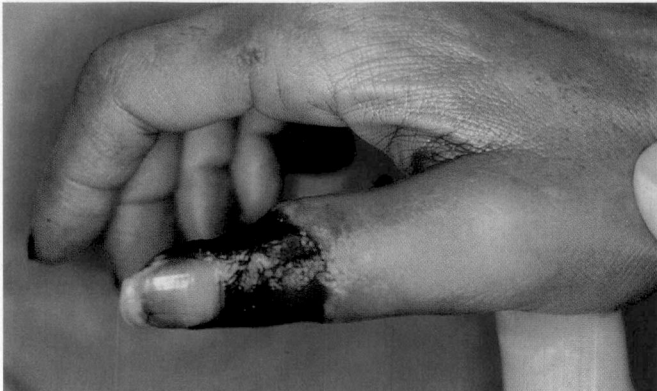

FIGURE 3 Third- and fourth-degree frostbite with tissue death and demarcation beyond the interphalangeal joint.

Clothes provide insulation proportional to their thickness (one quarter of an inch equals one clothing unit) and weight. They should be light to allow activity and trap air in multiple layers to be effective. Sweating wets the clothing, reducing the insulation value. The importance of light clothing permitting work (heat production) is emphasized. The proper use of protective clothing is important. In one study, 65% of those who suffered frostbite had inadequate protective clothing, whereas 20% had adequate clothing but were wearing it improperly. Only 15% of frostbite victims had adequate clothing and were wearing it properly. Moisture accelerates heat loss.

Behavioral factors also predispose to cold injuries. Alcohol and drug intoxication; smoking; accidents such as car, plane, skiing, and vehicular failure; homelessness; high altitude; and outdoor pursuits predispose to frostbite, as does a previous cold weather injury. Medical conditions that decrease circulation (peripheral arterial disease), neuropathy, and diabetes all decrease the body's ability to adapt to colder temperatures; psychiatric illness is observed much more frequently in patients who suffer frostbite. The average age of a frostbite victim is 30 to 49 years, with men outnumbering females by 10 to 1.

Prevention of Frostbite

There are two ways to prevent cold injury: (1) by increasing heat production; and (2) by decreasing heat loss. Heat loss may be decreased by avoiding wetness or contact with metal (which accelerates heat loss) and by wearing adequate protective clothing. The extremities have a large surface-to-mass ratio and thus represent prime sites for heat loss. Other factors may affect the circulation to extremities, such as the presence of arterial occlusive disease (some feel that the presence of a frostbite injury should prompt an examination for an arterial occlusive lesion or conditions such as diabetic neuropathy, which do not permit reflex vasoconstriction and vasodilatation). The importance of inactivity and immobility in reducing heat production, producing orthostatic edema, and decreasing circulation has been emphasized in studies on military frostbite. Malnutrition, hemorrhage, anemia, and the use of tobacco and alcohol all have been implicated in the increased susceptibility to frostbite injuries. Acclimatization and cold tolerance probably occur. African Americans have increased susceptibility to cold injuries, probably because of less frequent waves of cold-induced vasodilatation and thus less effective skin warming. Military experience has emphasized the importance of working and keeping active so as to increase heat production. The importance of avoiding sweating to avoid wetness and replacing wet with dry clothing also is emphasized.

Superficial Versus Deep Frostbite

Frostbite in the head and neck area is generally superficial. The face is not subject to the same vasoconstrictive phenomena as are the extremities. The drying potential of cold in the facial area is manifested in chapped lips, nose tip, ears, and mucous membranes. Facial frostbite is generally superficial, whereas serious frostbite usually is confined to the extremities.

Mills believes that the differentiation of frostbite into first-, second-, third-, and fourth-degree injuries is cumbersome and not clinically useful. He believes that one can only classify frostbite as superficial (tissue remains soft) or deep (tissue is hard). It is initially difficult to tell the depth of the injury, and differentiation can be accomplished only after rewarming and a period of observation. Cauchy (2001) feels that the extent of the initial lesion and the result of three-phase bone scanning can predict the ultimate result: If the initial lesion is confined to the distal digit, the probability of amputation is 1%; the probability increases to 31% for the middle digit, 67% for the proximal phalanx, 98% for the metacarpal and metatarsal, and 100% for the carpal and tarsal areas. In the face, a small white patch of tissue may be seen, and this clears over the course of a week.

Medically, frostbite heals with no therapy, therapy with dressings alone, or surgical débridement amputation and dressings. Twenty-five percent of patients with frostbite are seen more than 48 hours after the injury.

In the extremities, mild frostbite is manifested by pallor, paresthesias, and a dull yellow color of the skin. Ice crystals may be observed. The area is numb, and after rewarming a prickly, itchy sensation or aching pain occurs. After rewarming, reactive hyperemia is observed superficially; in deeper injuries, hypersensitivity and paresthesias are observed. Deep frostbite is differentiated by the absence of circulation; on rewarming, the progression (progressive vascular thrombosis) to full-thickness tissue loss (eschar formation) occurs. The tissue may remain insensitive after rewarming, presenting as a blue-gray patch with absent circulation. Burning pain, paresthesias, and thick-walled blisters containing blood may follow rewarming in full-thickness tissue injury.

The history of the injury is important in predicting tissue loss. Important factors include duration of the exposure, temperature, protective clothing worn, contact with metal or moisture, and the presence of previous symptoms that would indicate reduced arterial circulation. These include claudication, Raynaud's phenomenon, and superficial phlebitis. It is important to assess if there is any contribution of underlying vascular disease in patients with frostbite.

Diagnosis of Hypothermia

Hypothermia must be excluded, and the management of frostbite should include general and specific measures (Box 1). Management of frostbite must include restoration of core body temperature. In patients with hypothermia (temperature <35°C), the hypothermic condition must be corrected before specific treatment of frostbite begins. Death may occur at a body temperature of 28°C.

Hypothermia is defined as a core body temperature below 35°C or 95°F; it is seen principally in the military or secondary to outdoor recreation, homelessness, or substance abuse. Hypothermia has been classified as the following:

1. Mild (90°F to 94°F)
2. Moderate (80°F to 89°F)
3. Severe (less than 80°F).

In mild hypothermia, the patient is shivering, complains of being cold, and has mental confusion but is normotensive. In moderate hypothermia, the patient becomes more confused and is often agitated, delirious, or combative, and the shivering ceases. There are muscle spasticity, dilated pupils, and slow respirations. At this stage,

BOX 1: Therapy for Frostbite

Correct systemic hypothermia (temperature <35°C)
General measures (includes detection of other injuries)
Rapid rewarming of frozen extremities (15-30 minutes until a
    digital flush is observed) in a 104°F-108°F agitated water bath
    and topical antiseptic
Tetanus immunization
    ± Antibiotics
    Aspirin: 325 mg every 6 hours for 72 hours (Robson)
Open or light dressings
    Clear blebs: débride
    Hemorrhagic blebs: keep intact
    Topical aloe vera (Robson) and antithromboxanes
    Infected blisters: débride, antibiotics, antiseptics
Functional splinting, elevation
    Twice daily cleanse with antiseptics
    Avoid macerating dressings
Surgery
    Await clear demarcation
    Access spontaneous epithelialization
    If within the first 24-48 hours:
1. Consider regional sympathectomy in those with troublesome,
    persistent symptoms; normal or low vascular response after
    rewarming; arteriogram of magnetic resonance imaging or
    magnetic resonance angiogram evidence of vascular spasm
    and lack of complete flow (Rakower)
2. Hyperbaric oxygen
3. Intra-arterial tissue plasminogen activator, initially 0.5 mg/hr,
    then decreasing daily
4. Heparin therapy
5. Steroids

mild myocardial irritability is encountered. In severe hypothermia, the patient becomes comatose, has a flaccid paralysis, and begins to develop apnea; eventually this progresses to ventricular fibrillation and death.

The body physiologically responds to lowered temperatures by increasing cardiac output with tachycardia. Hypotension then follows, with apnea, bradycardia, and an increase in total peripheral vascular resistance with decreased cardiac output and an increase in mean arterial pressure. Cardiac arrhythmias and sudden death occur in this sequence and follow ventricular ectopy and atrial fibrillation. Cardiac standstill occurs with temperature decrease below 21°C. The blood becomes more viscous with each drop in temperature, and hemoconcentration is seen related to cold diuresis. Sludging occurs in the peripheral vessels, and respiratory depression follows. Pulmonary edema accompanies rewarming. There is a decrease in the ability to clear bronchial secretions and a diminished cough reflex resulting in "cold bronchorrhea." Metabolic acidosis follows rewarming. The "cold diuresis" results in hypovolemia.

Treatment of Hypothermia

When the victim is identified in the prehospital setting, removal of wet clothing and replacement with dry clothing should be performed. No massage, friction rubbing, or manipulation should be performed. Patients who have sustained cardiopulmonary arrest should undergo resuscitation according to standard protocols. Patients have been salvaged followed rewarming. In the field, only passive warming is undertaken because active rewarming can lead to myocardial arrhythmia and hypotension and can be managed only by precise, "in hospital" monitoring.

In the hospital, accurate recording of temperature and vital signs is imperative. Complete examinations of the blood, including complete blood cell count (CBC), electrolytes, liver function tests, coagulation, and arterial blood gas analyses, are performed urgently. The workup should include toxicology screens to assess the effect of alcohol or other sedatives. A Foley catheter is inserted with urimeter, and urine volumes are monitored. Several large bore intravenous cannulas are inserted to combat the inevitable hypotension that occurs after rewarming. Continuous electrocardiographic monitoring and a chest x-ray or appropriate extremity x-rays for trauma are obtained. The intensive care setting is mandatory, with serial blood testing. Hypoglycemia should be excluded, as should narcotic overdose. Passive rewarming at the rate of 0.5°C to 2°C hourly results in a slow increase in body temperature. Oxygen that is warm and humidified is provided.

Therapy of Frostbite After Hypothermia Has Been Resolved

There is no place for vigorous rubbing of frostbitten tissue or the application of snow (treatments mentioned in the lay literature). This merely accelerates damage to skin. There is no place for slow thawing, rubbing the area, and especially application of snow or other measures that would increase tissue damage. A frozen part should not be thawed if refreezing is likely to occur.

The management of frostbite is divided into the following phases:

1. Pre-thaw field care phase
2. Acute hospital rewarming phase
3. Post-thaw care phase

Before reaching the hospital, the frostbitten part should be protected from mechanical trauma and splinted. Warming should not be attempted if refreezing is likely.

Management of frostbite is carried out in accordance with the guidelines popularized by Mills. The patient's general condition should be assessed and other injuries detected and managed. Shelter should be obtained, wet garments removed, and the part wrapped in warm, dry covers or blankets, being careful to avoid trauma. The benefit of antibiotics has been difficult to establish; although some prescribe them as for burn injuries, others believe that they are not appropriate. Cultures should be done so that appropriate antibiotic treatment can be instituted if infection occurs. Long-term care includes physical therapy, neurologic rehabilitation, psychological support, and counseling for management of specific localized injuries.

Patients with serious frostbite (i.e., frostbite of the extremities) should be hospitalized. On admission, the frozen areas should be rewarmed properly in an agitated water bath whose temperature is controlled precisely from 104°F to 108°F (40°C to 44°C) for 15 to 30 minutes. Rewarming should be continued for 15 minutes beyond recirculation.

The rewarming may be stopped soon after the digital flush signifying a hyperemic state of perfusion is observed. Rewarming is often painful, implying that a free radical reaction is present on reperfusion. Excessive rewarming results in further tissue damage. The temperature is critical, as excessive temperatures (>44°C) cause heat damage and lesser temperatures (<38°C) are ineffective. Rewarming should be continued for 15 minutes beyond thawing. Rewarming may be painful, and narcotic analgesics may need to be given. The pain associated with rewarming is felt to be a reperfusion injury and secondary to free radical generation.

In general, it has been recommended that open treatment or light dressings be utilized, keeping the blisters intact and bathing (hydrotherapy) the affected area once or twice daily in an antiseptic solution.

Most affected areas heal spontaneously if infection is prevented. Compression dressings are not necessary.

Hands should be splinted in a functional position, as should feet. Nonadherent (petrolatum or Xeroform) dressings assist with gentle treatment of the skin areas. It has been our experience that ointments macerate the areas and may contribute to increased infection. Dry treatment is preferred where possible. The value of prophylactic antibiotics has not been shown, and they should be used only prophylactically for short durations, such as 48 to 72 hours.

Robson has shown that blisters contain increased amounts of thromboxane derivatives, which can accelerate production of progressive vascular thrombosis and dermal ischemia, similar to that observed in thermal injury. Therefore therapeutic advantage may be obtained from débriding the blisters. Robson differentiates between white and hemorrhagic blisters, débriding only the white blisters. Robson recommends treatment of affected frostbite areas with topical aloe vera (Dermaide Aloe), aspirin, and antibiotics. The effectiveness of this treatment has not been shown clearly.

Daily cleansing of affected areas should be performed in a 40°C water bath, using antiseptic skin cleansers. Photographic records of progress should be taken at 2-day intervals. Tetanus prophylaxis is recommended on admission.

It is important that the affected part be elevated and splinted in a position of function according to the usual principles of treatment of significant extremity injuries. Gentle exercise and range of motion are important, as is physical therapy. Elevation decreases edema, which is part of the vicious cycle that contributes to decreased capillary circulation.

Surgical Intervention for Frostbite

There are two options for surgical treatment of frostbite:

1. Early surgical intervention
2. Delayed (observation) treatment

Early surgical intervention is not necessary in the typical frostbite injury but may be necessary if acute progressive infection occurs. Full demarcation of dead tissue may take several weeks or 2 to 3 months, and the general recommendation is that the process of separation of tissue be allowed to progress spontaneously. Some feel that surgery may be appropriate at 3 weeks if the demarcation is clear. Escharotomy may be necessary when circumferential extremity constriction causes impaired circulation and occurs because of an unyielding third-degree eschar.

Assessing the Circulatory System and Early Surgical Intervention

There has been considerable interest in assessing the circulation, which has been done by arteriography but mostly by technetium imaging (three-phase bone scans) done on admission. This assessment results in the ability to predict tissue loss, which accurately reflects the ultimate degree of tissue loss. These scans should be done on the first day after injury.

The efficacy of magnetic resonance imaging (MRI) and magnetic resonance angiography (MRA) examinations for the same purpose also have been suggested. The hope that earlier surgical intervention could lead to earlier resolution of the injury for many patients after the use of these circulatory assessments generally has not been realized. Gotleib and colleagues used this to aggressively débride the soft tissue and ultimately probably salvaged digits that otherwise would have been lost with aggressive microsurgical reconstruction of digits destined to be amputated.

Therapy of Microcirculation

The damage to the microcirculation has been treated with anticoagulation, hyperbaric oxygen, and free radical scavengers. Agents such as heparin have been shown to slightly increase tissue survival in experimental frostbite tissue injury, as have free radical scavengers. Clinical experience has not confirmed a definite advantage of these medications, obviously because of the critical time window in which they must be administered. It has been difficult to demonstrate

the clinical effectiveness of agents such as low-molecular-weight dextran in preventing sludging, and although steroids have been recommended for the vasculitis, the evidence for their beneficial effect has not been confirmed clinically. Heparin and anticoagulants have not been show to influence the ultimate degree of tissue loss. Ultrasound treatments have been suspected of increasing tissue damage.

Robson's recommendations have been used by some to limit the progressive vascular thrombosis and include prostacyclin and thrombolytics such as recombinant tissue plasminogen activator (rtPA). Hyperbaric oxygen may be of limited value but must be begun within 24 to 48 hours to be effective. Although many question its effectiveness, several experimental studies demonstrate improved tissue salvage when hyperbaric oxygen is begun promptly; a number of case reports since 1997 suggest some effectiveness, but a true trial has not been conducted. Hyperbaric oxygen increases tissue oxygen concentrations; stimulates angiogenesis; reduces edema, improving the microcirculation; stimulates anti-inflammatory proteins and antioxidant enzymes; and stimulates several wound healing mediators such as basic fibroblast growth factor, transforming growth factor beta 1, and platelet-derived growth factor.

Tissue plasminogen activator (tPA) has shown some progress in ameliorating the microcirculatory injury and in improving circulation and tissue loss (30% compared with historical controls) of lesions destined to be amputated that did not receive treatment (Bruen et al, 2007; Twomey et al, 2005).

rtPA must be administered intra-arterially within 24 hours after the injury, the earlier the better; therapy salvaged and the clinical reports are supported by some laboratory studies. The treatment must begin within the first 24 hours to be effective and is continued for several days if effective.

Sympathectomy

Regional sympathetic blockade has been utilized to decrease the pathologic vasoconstriction and sympathetic response. Based on the theory of the importance of progressive vascular damage in serious frostbite, several authors have advocated early surgical or chemical sympathectomy. At one time we used intra-arterial reserpine to regionally block the sympathetic nervous system (chemical sympathectomy). Arteriograms have demonstrated significant proximal vasospasm a considerable distance proximal to the clinically obvious area of frostbite (Figure 4). Recently Rakower has attempted to define the patient populations that benefited from sympathectomy according to Doppler ultrasound and digital plethysmographic examinations after rewarming. Patients had digital plethysmograms and Doppler ultrasound mapping of digital vessels, and three degrees of vascular response to cold were found. Most common was the hyperdynamic response, implying patent digital vessels; this response was clinically apparent as warm, red digital tissue. Regional sympathectomy was troublesome in these patients. Patients with a normal or hypodynamic response had evidence of vascular compromise at the digital, palmar, or pedal arch level and benefitted from regional sympathectomy with chemical mechanisms. Patients with the hyperdynamic response did not have severe pain, whereas patients with a normal or decreased vascular response had ischemic pain, stiffness, and coldness in the digital areas. It thus seems possible that sympathectomy may be utilized for a group of patients who could most benefit from it.

Those who support regional sympathectomy claim that it provides earlier cessation of pain, more rapid decrease of tissue inflammation and edema, tissue salvage, quicker demarcation, and earlier healing. In addition, there is some evidence that regional sympathectomy provides significant diminution of the late sequelae of frostbite: impaired circulation, hyperhidrosis, pallor, and vasospastic and pain symptoms. It is claimed that extremities that have been subjected to a cold injury are able to perceive repeated significant cold injuries more accurately than extremities without sympathectomy.

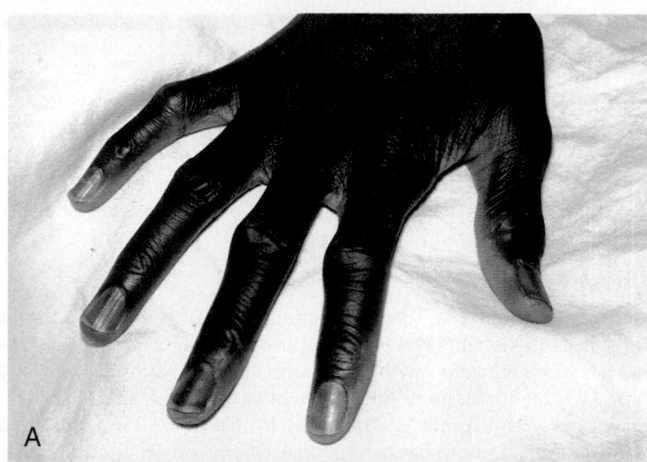

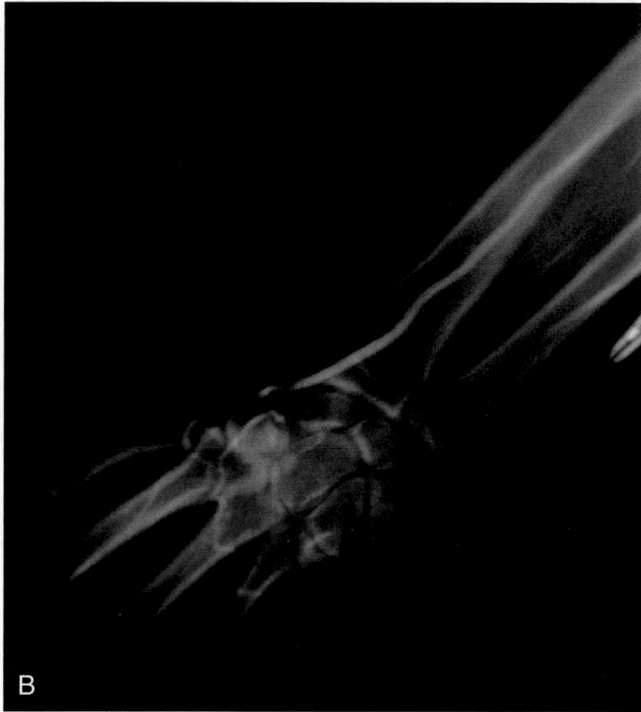

FIGURE 4 A, Second-degree frostbite. Note the poor capillary perfusion of the nail bed of the middle finger. **B,** Arteriogram of the patient in part A demonstrating loss of distal circulation secondary to intense vasoconstriction. The ulnar artery flow ceases in the forearm, and the palmar arch and digital vessels are not seen.

Chronic Changes

The chronic sequelae of frostbite may benefit from sympathectomy in that sympathetic overactivity (hyperhidrosis and vasoconstriction) and cold sensitivity are reduced. The symptoms represent diminished circulation and reflect pallor and vasospastic and pain symptoms. Lubrication of atrophic skin and protection from extreme temperatures are important. It is important that the parts affected be prevented from further cold exposure, as they are unusually more susceptible to cold injury. Flatt has advocated digital artery sympathectomy for patients with troublesome digital symptoms.

Radiographic and Joint Changes

Degenerative joint disease may be seen in severe cases of frostbite, and stiff, painful joints with fibrosis may be a sequela of moderately severe frostbite.

Intrinsic Muscle Atrophy

Flatt has described intrinsic muscle atrophy and fibrosis in severe frostbite. It may be possible to minimize the intrinsic muscle damage of contracture with proper physiotherapy, splinting, and appropriate exercise.

■ INJURIES IN CHILDREN

Injuries to epiphyseal growth centers may result from even minor cases of frostbite in children, with joint changes being radiographically demonstrable even 6 months after injury. These changes may result in short digits, deviation of the digits, and osteoarthritis. Parents should be advised that these sequelae are possible despite appropriate therapy of frostbite during the period of injury.

SUGGESTED READINGS

Brown DJ, Brugger H, Boyd J, Paal P. Accidental hypothermia. *N Engl J Med.* 2013;368:394.

Bruen KJ, Ballard JR, Morris SE, Cochran A, Edelman LS, Saffle JR. Reduction of the incidence of amputation in frostbite injury with thrombolytic therapy. *Arch Surg.* 2007;142:546-553.

Heggers JP, Robson MD, Manavalen K, et al. Experimental and clinical observations on frostbite. *Ann Emerg Med.* 1987;16:1056-1062.

Higdon B, Youngman L, Regehr M, Chiou A. Deep frostbite treated with hyperbaric oxygen and hyperbaric therapies. *Wounds.* 2015;27:215-223.

Imray C, Grieve A, Dhillon S, Caudwell Xtreme Everest Research Group. Cold damage to the extremities: frostbite and non-freezing cold injuries. *Postgrad Med J.* 2009;85:481-488.

Koljonen V, Andersson K, Mikkonen K, Vuola J. Frostbite injuries treated in the Helsinki area 1995 to 2002. *J Trauma.* 2004;57:1315-1320.

Manson PN, Jesudass R, Marzella L, et al. Evidence for an early free radical-medicated reperfusion injury in frostbite. *Free Radic Biol Med.* 1991;10:7-11.

Marzella L, Jesdass RR, Manson PN, et al. Morphologic characterization of acute injury to vascular endothelium of skin after frostbite. *Plast Recon Surg.* 1989;83:67-75.

McCauley RI, Hing DN, Martin RD, Heggers JP. Frostbite injuries: a rational approach based on the pathophysiology. *J Trauma.* 1983;23:143-147.

McCrary BF, Hursh TA. Hyperbaric oxygen therapy for a delayed frostbite injury. *Wounds.* 2005;17:327-331.

Mekjavic IB, Gorjanc J, Mekjavic PJ, Bajrovic F, Milcinski M. Hyperbaric oxygen as an adjunct treatment of freezing cold injury. *Prev Cold Injuries.* 2005;16:1-4.

Murphy JV, Benwell PE, Roberts AH, McGrouther DA. Frostbite: pathogenesis and treatment. *J Trauma.* 2000;48:171-178.

Singh NK. Frostbite. In: Cameron J, ed. *Current Surgical Therapy.* 8th ed. St. Louis: Elsevier Mosby; 2001:887-889.

Twomey JA, Peltier GL, Zera RT. An open-label study to evaluate the safety and efficacy of tissue plasminogen activator in treatment of severe frostbite. *J Trauma.* 2005;59:1350-1355.

Urschel JD. Frostbite: predisposing factors and predictors of poor outcome. *J Trauma.* 1990;30:340-342.

Uygur F, Noyan N, Sever C, Gümüs T. The current analysis of the effect of hyperbaric oxygen therapy on the frostbitten tissue: experimental study in rabbits. *Cent Eur J Med.* 2009;4:198-202.

Valnicek SM, Chasmar LR, Clapson JB. Frostbite in the prairies: a 12-year review. *Plast Reconstr Surg.* 1993;92:633-641.

ELECTRICAL AND LIGHTNING INJURY

Leigh Ann Price, MD, and Laurie A. Loiacono, MD, FCCP

Electrical injury is one of the most destructive and disfiguring traumatic events a human can sustain. The injury complex is typically a combination of electric shock, thermal injury, and blunt trauma, involving potentially devastating associated multisystem damage with high morbidity and mortality. Overall incidence of these injuries is low compared with other multisystem trauma injuries in the United States. Because of this, most healthcare teams have limited experience with this mechanism of injury, which adds to the complexity of developing an effective medical and surgical care plan.

Optimal management of electrical and lightning injury victims necessitates (1) basic understanding of electrical injury mechanisms and their associated patterns of disease, (2) timely and appropriate resuscitation, (3) aggressive surgical and critical care medical management, and (4) implementation of coordinated multidisciplinary care for these patients from onset of injury through injury recovery and rehabilitation.

■ EPIDEMIOLOGY

The term *electrocution*, originally defined as death caused by the passage of electrical current through the body, was derived from the combination of *electro* and *execution* and coined in the late nineteenth century after the implementation of the first electric chair in 1890. With the implementation and advancement of commercial applications for electricity throughout the nineteenth and twentieth centuries, the word *electrocution* commonly has been applied to circumstances of accidental death after exposure to electrical current. The first recorded nonjudicial fatality from accidental exposure to electricity (other than lightning strikes) occurred in France in 1879.

Electrical burns and lightning injuries result in approximately 6000 injuries per year in the United States. Electrical burn survivors make up approximately 5% of total admissions to major burn centers, and a bimodal distribution exists with respect to age. In the majority of cases, non–lightning-related electrical injuries to children are accidental in nature and occur in the home; similar injuries to adults generally occur in the workplace. About two thirds of all non–lightning-related electrical injuries occur in the workplace, and the majority of the remaining injuries occur in the home.

Electrical injuries account for 2% to 3% of all burns in children, and the majority of these injuries in children are associated with transient, low-voltage exposure to household electrical and extension cords and wall outlets. Older children are exposed to life-threatening high-voltage injury through climbing activities. More than 200 household-related electrocutions (i.e., death by electricity) occur annually and typically are associated with consumer product misuse or malfunction.

The majority of electrical injuries in construction and utility workers are related to brief, high-voltage exposure. Up to 40% of serious electrical injuries are fatal (56% of these deaths occur in the workplace). Electrocution represents 5% to 6% of all work-related traumatic mortality, accounting for more than 500 deaths per year and making it the second leading cause of occupation-related deaths in the United States. Short-term and long-term morbidity in many electrical injury survivors is typically related to significant musculoskeletal and neurologic disability.

■ ELECTRICITY BASICS

Current

Electricity is defined as the flow of electrons through a conductor. *Electrical current* (I) is the volume of electrons between two points per second. Current exists in two forms: *alternating current* (AC) and *direct current* (DC). High-voltage utility power lines may be either AC (most common, commercial) or DC.

Alternating Current

Alternating current (AC) is the directional flow of current in a circuit that constantly is being reversed back and forth in a repetitive pattern and is a more efficient way of generating and distributing electricity than DC. Standard household current is AC at a rate of 60 Hz (cycles per second) and is supported by 100 to 250 amperes (A). AC can be much more dangerous than DC in certain circumstances because it causes tetanic muscle contractions that prevent a victim from releasing the electrical source. This is known as the "let-go" threshold. The bidirectional flow of AC produces cutaneous burns known as contact points; this is in contrast to the entrance and exit wounds caused by DC current. The "let-go" current intensity varies from 3 to 9 mA depending on body size; tetany occurs at 16 to 20 mA. Although AC is generally lower voltage and produces less direct tissue injury, prolonged contact can alter the cardiac cycle, causing arrhythmias and cardiac arrest. Ventricular fibrillation occurs at 50 to 100 mA, and asystole occurs at more than 2 A. Keep in mind that although most providers speak about voltage, it is the amperage that kills.

Direct Current

Direct current (DC) means that the direction of electrical current remains constant. It is found in automobile electrical systems, railway tracks, batteries, and lightning. DC provides a vector directionality to the electrical current exposure, hence the typical entrance and exit point cutaneous wounds that identify potential current pathway. High-voltage DC injury often produces smaller cutaneous entrance and exit wounds but much more significant deep tissue injury in addition to the electrical current tissue effects. DC does not produce the same contraction of muscles that is found with AC. Although low-voltage DC is not as dangerous as the corresponding AC, contact with high-voltage DC is more likely to be fatal than contact with AC of the same voltage.

Voltage and Resistance

Voltage

The force that drives electrical current (I) across the potential difference is the voltage (V) and contributes critically to the intensity of the electrical injury. Medically speaking, electrical injuries are classified as either *high voltage* (>1000 V) or *low voltage* (<1000 V). (Note: The U.S. National Electrical Code defines the difference between low-voltage and high-voltage injury as 600 V.) Typical voltage delivered to homes in the United States and Canada is 120/240 V, providing 240 V for appliances that require high power and 120 V for general use. Low-voltage injuries tend to occur indoors and are almost exclusively AC. Our AC power system operates at 60 Hz, causing the current to reverse polarity 120 times a second. Based on this fact, the terms *entrance* and *exit* should be abandoned, and the resultant wounds from AC should be referred to as *contact points*. Voltage in high-tension power lines tends to exceed 100,000 V and is most commonly AC in developed areas. High-voltage mortality and amputation rates typically exceed low-voltage rates twofold to threefold.

Resistance

Resistance (R) is the hindrance to current flow and is measured in ohms. Resistance creates heat based on Joule's law. *Joule heating* is

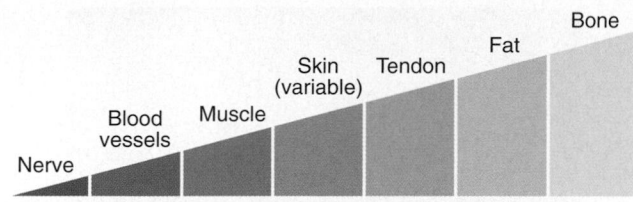

FIGURE 1 The magnitude of average electrical resistance across body tissues.

energy transfer that occurs when charged particles meet resistance and lose energy to tissues in the form of heat.

Joule's Law

$$\text{Power (J, joule)} = I^2 \text{ (Current)} \times R \text{ (Resistance)}$$

Materials that are the best conductors (meaning that they facilitate current flow) have the least resistance. With increasing resistance, more energy is expended in the form of heat and results in thermal tissue damage.

Different tissues have innately different resistances (Figure 1), and resistances vary under different conditions. Overall resistance of a tissue depends on the surface area of contact, tissues in the current's pathway, pressure applied, duration of exposure, magnitude of current flow, and absence or presence of moisture. For example, dry skin has a much greater resistance (approximately 100,000 ohms) than moist skin (<2500 ohms).

The magnitude of average electrical resistance across body tissues is as follows:

Nerve < Blood vessels < Muscle < Skin (variable) < Tendon
   < Fat < Bone

The relationship between the forces discussed is described by *Ohm's law*:

$$I = V/R$$

where the current (I) is directly proportional to voltage (V) and inversely proportional to resistance (R).

■ PHYSICS AND PATHOPHYSIOLOGY OF ELECTRICAL INJURY

All electrical injury involves both direct and indirect mechanisms. The direct damage is caused by the actual effect of electrical current on the body tissues or organs (i.e., brain or heart) or by the conversion of electrical to thermal energy resulting in burns. Indirect injuries are the result of associated tissue injury from severe muscle contraction, blunt trauma from falls or ejection, or associated multiorgan system dysfunction (i.e., renal failure from rhabdomyolysis).

Direct Injury (Electrical and Lightning)

The severity of direct electrical injury is determined by several critical factors:

1. Voltage (high or low)
2. Type of current (alternating or direct)
3. Intensity of current (amperage)
4. Pathway of the current through the body (vertical, horizontal, peripheral)

TABLE 1: Examples of Acute, Direct Electrical Injury Organ Tissue Dysfunction

Tissue	Acute Effects
Heart	Asystole, arrhythmia, cardiac tissue necrosis (myocardium, nodal tissue, conduction pathways, coronary arteries)
Central nervous system	Brainstem dysfunction, central apnea, loss of consciousness, seizure, confusion, amnesia, cranial nerve deficits, spine fracture, paralysis or keraunoparalysis, spinal cord transection, visual and hearing disturbances, tympanic membrane rupture
Muscle	Tetany: rhabdomyolysis, lactic acidosis, bone stress fracture, "locking-on" phenomenon

TABLE 2: Examples of Late Electrical Injury Organ Tissue Dysfunction

Tissue	Late Effects
Heart	Patchy cardiac tissue necrosis (myocardium, nodal tissue, conduction pathways, coronary arteries), late arrhythmias are rare
Central nervous system	Cognitive deficits, spinal cord and peripheral nerve dysfunction, cataracts
Muscle	Weakness, arthropathy, nonspecific myopathy and fibrosis, limitation of joint function
Vascular	Venous thrombosis, arterial rupture

5. Duration of current exposure
6. Area of contact on the body
7. Resistance of the body tissues involved

Injury to the affected tissue predominantly depends on the intensity and duration of electrical exposure. For example, brief exposure to current will conduct rapidly across low-resistance tissues (Ohm's law), with less heat production and structural tissue damage but more electrophysiologic derailment of end organs (i.e., heart, central nervous system [CNS], and muscle). Hence, lightning causes little if any direct tissue injury.

If contact time is brief, nonthermal direct electrical damage to tissue occurs as the current disrupts the microelectrical gradient across cell membranes via electroporation and conformational changes in membrane proteins. Electroporation results in a significant increase in the electrical conductivity and cell plasma membrane permeability, leading to tissue edema and possible cell injury. Muscle fibers and nerves are the most susceptible. It can either induce cell necrosis or permanently, partially, or reversibly affect cell membrane function in the absence of joule heating. Damage will be relatively localized to the involved tissue cell membranes and result in functional disruption of those end organs dependent on coordinated electrical activity such as heart, brain, spinal cord, and muscle (Table 1). These cell membrane effects may progress over time and partially explain some of the delayed clinical symptoms observed after electrical injury, such as vascular thrombosis and rupture, cognitive dysfunction, and late-appearing spinal cord deficits (Table 2).

Lightning primarily is thought to be a form of DC, but it can be both positively and negatively charged, taking on the form of direct

TABLE 3: Lightning Strikes Can Occur in Different Patterns

Direct strike	Lightning directly strikes the victim
Splash strike	Lightning hits another object and "splashes" onto the victim
Side flash	Individual is inside a building and exposure to current occurs through a conductive source within the structure (i.e., metal object or landline telephone)
Step voltage	Lightning strikes the ground and the current is conducted along the ground to an adjacent victim

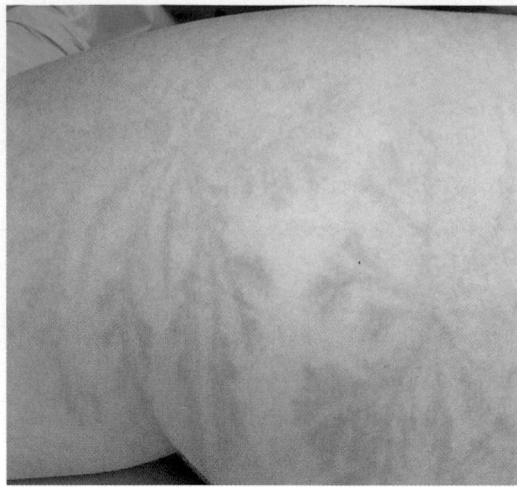

FIGURE 2 Lichtenberg figure. *(Photo courtesy Andrew R. Doben, MD, FACS.)*

and alternating current depending on the circumstance. Positively charged lightning is considered more dangerous because its electrical field is stronger, flash duration is longer, and peak charge can be much greater than that of a negative strike. The most important difference between lightning AC and electrical AC is that lightning does not cause the muscle tetany seen with AC electrical injuries. Lightning is one of the most dramatic examples of high-voltage direct electrical injury. Its injuries account for a small subset of electrical injuries, but lightning is responsible for an average of 400 injuries and approximately 50 deaths per year in the United States. The odds of being struck by lightning in a lifetime (estimated 80 years) are 1 in 3000. Estimated fatality from lightning is 30%, and 70% to 80% of survivors may have permanent disabilities. Occasionally lightning can move along a horizontal pathway and strike "out of the blue sky" 10 miles or farther from its generation point. In the United States, the Gulf Coast and Rocky Mountain states, particularly Florida and Colorado, have the highest strike densities and report the highest number of lightning-related injuries and deaths.

In addition to tissue injury related to direct contact with an electricity source, injuries noted from the various lightning strike patterns include thermal burns through clothing or other heated material, ruptured tympanic membranes caused by shock wave from a thermoacoustic phenomenon (i.e., thunder), concussive or blast-type injuries secondary to the rapidly expanding air near a lightning strike, and injury caused by a subsequent fall (Table 3).

Lightning injury can be minor, moderate, or severe.

1. *Minor:* often awake and alert, may have confusion or amnesia, dysesthesia, hearing or vision changes. Physical findings may be temporary, and complete recovery can occur.
2. *Moderate:* disorientation, combative, unconscious, paralysis, skin mottling, hypotension, respiratory failure, secondary cardiac arrest. Physical symptoms may resolve over time. Long-term sequelae such as cognitive and sleep disorders, weakness, dysesthesia, and peripheral neuropathy can develop.
3. *Severe:* serious injury or death in 30% of victims, blunt trauma, contusion from shock wave, cardiac dysrhythmias, cardiac arrest (primary or secondary), CNS dysfunction. Asystole may be transient, and spontaneous rhythm may recover because of cardiac automaticity. Hypoxia related to central apnea may lead to secondary cardiac arrest. Long-term sequelae such as cognitive and sleep disorders, weakness, dysesthesia, and peripheral neuropathy can develop without direct evidence of initial direct anatomic brain injury.

Keraunoparalysis is transient paralysis that can occur after a lightning strike and is characterized by signs and symptoms of motor and sensory loss (affecting lower limbs more than upper limbs), pulselessness, and pallor associated with vasospasm. Keraunoparalysis

typically resolves within several hours after the injury but can mimic spinal cord injury and temporarily mask underlying musculoskeletal injury.

Unlike high-voltage electrical injuries, where massive internal tissue damage may occur, lightning seldom causes substantial burns. Historically, most burns related to lightning are caused by other objects (moisture, metal on a belt, jewelry or coins in a pocket) being heated and causing a contact burn rather than by the lightning itself. The transformation of the electrical energy to heat can generate temperatures as high as 50,000°F. However, the duration of this transmission is only 1 to 2 milliseconds; as a result, the insulating properties of the skin do not have time to break down.

The two most common causes of death related to lightning injury are (1) cardiopulmonary arrest caused by an interruption of the cardiac cycle by the direct current, resulting in asystole; and (2) apnea from the direct current's interference with the brain's respiratory center, which if left untreated will result in hypoxia, arrhythmia, and secondary cardiac arrest. There is an estimated morbidity 5 to 10 times higher than for non–lightning-related electrical injury (Table 4). A pathognomonic fernlike pattern called keraunographic markings or Lichtenberg figure (Figure 2) may appear on the skin of lightning strike victims. This is not a burn and often disappears within 24 hours.

Direct Injury (Thermal)

When contact time is prolonged, heat damage will dominate as the whole cell in the pathway is compromised. Thermal burn injury caused by electricity may be classified into three categories as follows:

- *Joule heat:* Direct effect of electrical current on tissue resistance causes heating of tissue, resulting in deep and superficial burns. Extent of specific tissue injury depends on current path, Joule's law, and duration of exposure.
- *Arc:* Direct thermal injury from arcing is caused by high-voltage current passing through the air. These injuries most commonly are seen in electricians working with metal objects close to an electrical source. These injuries occur without actual current flowing *through* tissue. Electricity arcs at a temperature up to 4000°C to 5000°C generate a "flash" type injury.
- *Flame:* Thermal burns result from ignited clothing or surroundings and are managed as conventional flame burns.

Most direct injuries are a combination of both electrical current conduction and heat transfer to tissues (Figure 3). Both mechanisms should be expected and fully explored in the course of the electrically injured patient's evaluation.

TABLE 4: Comparison of Lightning, High-Voltage, and Low-Voltage Electrical Injury

	Lightning	High Voltage	Low Voltage
Voltage (V)	>100 × 10⁶	>1000	<1000
Current (A)	>200,000	Variable	240
Duration	Instantaneous	Brief	Prolonged
Type of current	Mostly DC	DC or AC	Mostly AC
Cardiac effect	Arrest: asystole	Arrest: ventricular fibrillation	Arrest: ventricular fibrillation
Respiratory effect	Respiratory arrest: direct CNS injury	Respiratory arrest: indirect trauma or tetanic contractions of respiratory muscles	Respiratory arrest: tetanic contractions of respiratory muscles
Muscle effect	Single	Contraction: DC—single AC—tetanic	Contraction: tetanic
CNS effect	Early and delayed brain injury, coma, seizures, blindness, deafness, aphasia, cerebral vein thrombosis, late spinal cord deficits, cataracts	Early and delayed brain injury, coma, seizures, blindness, deafness, aphasia, cerebral vein thrombosis, late spinal cord deficits, cataracts	Paresthesias, transient neuropathy
Burns	Rare: superficial ("flashover" diverts current around the body)	Common: superficial (less) and deep (most)	Usually superficial, can be full thickness
Rhabdomyolysis	Uncommon	Very common	Common
Blunt injury	Blast effect, shock wave	Muscle contraction, fall	Fall (uncommon)
Mortality (early)	Very high (about 30%)	Moderate (about 5%-15%)	Low

AC, Alternating current; *CNS*, central nervous system; *DC*, direct current.

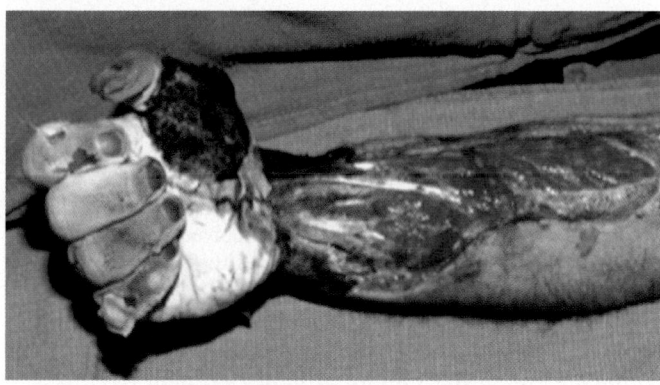

FIGURE 3 High-voltage electrical injury.

Importance of Current Pathways

Identification of contact points often helps to establish the path that the current has taken. A path parallel or "vertical" to the axis of the body (craniocaudal) is most dangerous because it may affect all vital organs. A "horizontal path" (e.g., from hand to hand) may spare the brain but still be fatal because of its effect on the heart and respiratory muscles. A path with contact points confined to a single extremity may cause extensive local damage but not be lethal (Figure 4).

Immediate cardiac arrest and life-threatening arrhythmias may occur with the conduction of current across the heart. AC tends to cause ventricular fibrillation, whereas DC tends to cause asystole. Actual injury to the heart or the metabolic effects from injury elsewhere in the body (e.g., hyperkalemia and rhabdomyolysis) may result in delayed cardiac arrhythmias and acute renal failure. Paralysis of the muscles of respiration can result in apnea. Effects on the spinal cord and brain can lead to immediate death or long-term neurologic abnormalities.

Indirect Injury

Additional tissue and organ injury not caused directly by but clearly related to the electrical insult is a significant contribution to morbidity and mortality of these patients. Many electrically injured patients fall from a height or are thrown or ejected after a blast or arc. These patients should receive a full multitrauma assessment on initial evaluation, including full spine and airway stabilization.

Respiratory failure can result from direct, blunt, or electrical lung injury; smoke or chemical inhalation; pulmonary edema; or acute lung injury (ALI). Many victims who develop muscle injury from tetany, direct electrical injury, or blunt trauma develop early acute kidney injury secondary to rhabdomyolysis or shock. CNS abnormalities can be transient, permanent, or delayed based on gross and histologic anatomic structure injury.

■ MANAGEMENT

The development of guidelines and outcome-based benchmarks requires established standards of practice; however, no specific guidelines for electrical injuries exist at this time. Because of the traumatic, multisystem nature of electrical injury (including potential associated blunt or penetrating trauma injuries), these patients should be managed according to both trauma and burn reconstruction guidelines for care. These guidelines include the following:

1. Establish safe access to the electrically injured patient.
2. Rapidly assess the patient's airway, breathing, circulation, and disability (rapid neurologic assessment) and provide in-line immobilization of the entire spine (primary survey).

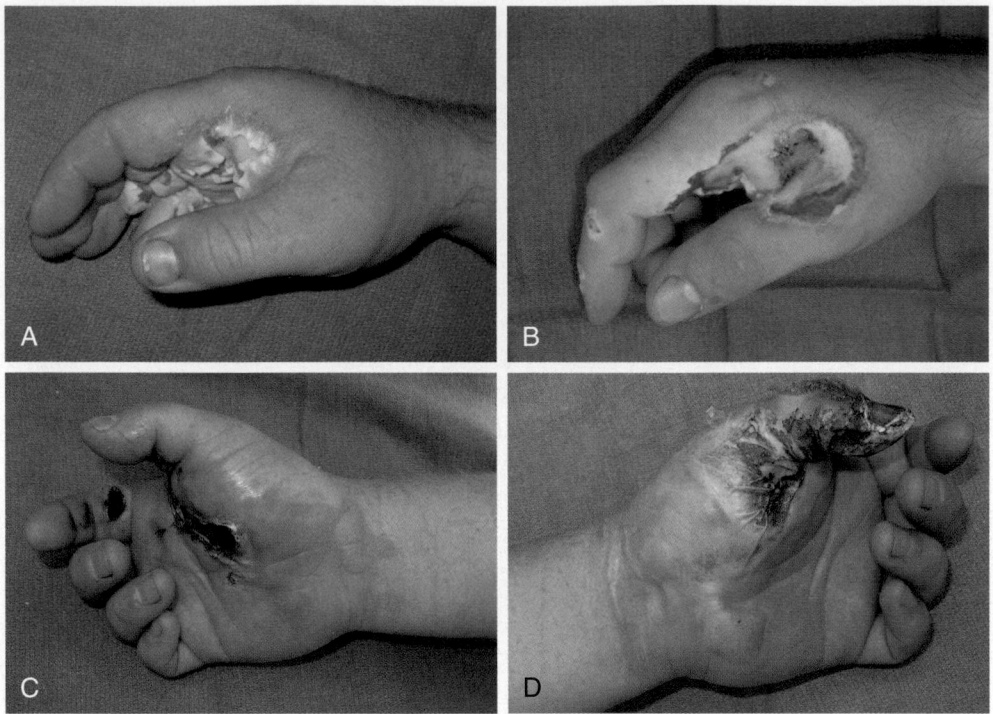

FIGURE 4 A, A farmer working in the field came in direct contact with a low-hanging wire (7000 V). **B,** An electrician grabbed a cable (270 V, alternating current) overhead to avoid falling into a ditch. **C** and **D,** A lineman touched a power line (7620 V, alternating current).

3. Treat life-threatening findings immediately: control threatened airway or ventilation, decompress tension pneumothorax or pericardial tamponade, control external hemorrhage, expose patient and manage potential core temperature heat loss (hypothermia).
4. Establish intravenous (IV)—or interosseous, if in the field—access and continuously monitor vital signs (including temperature), neurologic examination, pulse oximetry, respiratory function, electrocardiogram (ECG), urine output (urinary catheter). Consider central venous pressure monitoring.
5. Expose and cover thermal burn sites with clean, dry sheets or towels and then with appropriate topical dressing when at the hospital. Keep in mind the need for escharotomy and/or fasciotomy.
6. Initiate fluid resuscitation with warmed, isotonic crystalloid IV fluids to a target urine output (UO) of 0.5 cc/kg/hr if the patient is at low risk for rhabdomyolysis (or greater than 1.0 cc/kg/hr if the patient is at high risk for rhabdomyolysis). Monitor for the development of hyperkalemia and hyperchloremia.
7. Continuous close assessment of physiologic response to multisystem support.
8. Provide aggressive surgical and critical care support in an appropriate burn or critical care setting.
9. Implement coordinated multidisciplinary care for these patients from onset of injury through injury recovery and rehabilitation.

Prehospital Management and Special Considerations

The scene of an electrical injury is unique compared with other trauma sites. The rescuer easily can become another victim.

Be aware of:

- Victim's existing contact with the current source—"DO NOT TOUCH"; specialized nonconductive equipment is necessary to safely recover these victims

- Active live electrical sources—confirm disconnection
- Environment conductors to avoid (i.e., puddles of liquid, exposed metals and wires)

Victims of lightning injury may be treated immediately.

Critical Care Management

Early, goal-directed resuscitation; targeted multiorgan system assessment and support; and aggressive surgical management are critical in the first hour after injury and are cornerstones of optimal patient outcome (Table 5). Optimal surgical treatment varies with the severity and etiology of the electrical injury and the specific location of the injury site.

Multidisciplinary, System-Based Critical Care Management of the Electrical Injury Patient

Neurologic

Serial global and focal neurologic assessments are necessary. Full spine assessment should be completed within the first 24 hours. Attention to aggressive pain management is important to optimize respiratory mechanics and clinical response to therapy. Emphasize early mobilization; aggressive physical and occupational therapy; and cognitive, vision, and hearing assessments, and develop a comprehensive rehabilitation plan.

Complications. Neurologic complications are common sequelae of electrical injuries and can affect both the central and the peripheral nervous system. Early manifestations include varying levels of unconsciousness (including coma), sensory dysfunction, memory disturbances, autonomic dysfunction, respiratory paralysis, and motor dysfunction. Victims of lightning strikes can be seen with fixed and dilated pupils resulting from focal neuromuscular effects of the electrical injury rather than permanent brain injury. Deficits may be "patchy," with sensory deficits not coinciding to the motor findings. Clinical manifestations of neurologic injury may be delayed for days

TABLE 5: Critical Care Management of the Electrical Injury Patient (First Hour)

Concern	Action	Goal
Airway (PRIORITY) Assess for • Airway patency • Altered mental status • Facial injuries • Airway obstruction • Aspiration	1. Manual airway support as needed (i.e., clear airway, bag valve mask) 2. Intubate *early*. Diffuse edema and multisystem organ dysfunction may progress quickly (surgical airway may be necessary) 3. Clinically confirm placement with examination and end-tidal CO_2 monitor (radiologic confirmation of ETT placement ASAP); well-secure ETT in place 4. Immediate C/T/L/S spine immobilization 5. Initiate pulse oximetry	• Secure airway
Breathing Assess for • Spontaneous effort • Pneumothorax • Hemothorax • Chest wall compromise (musculoskeletal or burn) • Smoke inhalation (if associated material ignition)	1. Treat pneumothorax immediately 2. Initiate mechanical ventilation if needed 3. Correct hypoxia with supplemental O_2 (start with 100% FiO_2) 4. Check ABG 5. CXR (confirm tube placement, identify injury) 6. Consider early bronchoscopy to assess for inhalation injury if flame exposure is involved 7. Early escharotomy if needed	• *Avoid* hypoxia • SaO_2 >92% • PCO_2 35-45 mm Hg • Plateau pressure <30 mm Hg
Circulation Assess for • Shock • Distended neck veins • Cardiac tamponade • Cardiac arrhythmia • Cardiac dysfunction • Hemorrhage • Peripheral pulses	1. BLS/ACLS/ATLS algorithms 2. Treat cardiac tamponade immediately 3. Establish adequate IV access. Edema and multisystem organ dysfunction will progress quickly 4. Infuse isotonic IV fluids toward target goals 5. Continuous ECG and blood pressure monitoring 6. Place urinary catheter 7. FAST +/− focused CT to assess for hemorrhage 8. Consider central venous access for resuscitation monitoring 9. Early fasciotomy 10. Complete blood count, type and cross, cardiac enzymes, lactate	• MAP ≥60-65 mm Hg • UO ≥0.5 cc/kg/hr (if suspect rhabdomyolysis: UO >1.0 cc/kg/hr) • SvO_2 60-65 mm Hg • Lactic acid <2.0 • Closely monitor for development of pulmonary edema
Disability Assess for • Acute brain injury • Acute spine injury • Musculoskeletal deformity	1. Assess consciousness, pupillary size and response, lateralizing signs, level of spinal cord injury 2. Assess Glasgow Coma Score 3. Assess spine pain and gross function 4. Full neurologic examination when possible 5. Head and spine CT as needed	
Exposure Assess for • Core temperature • Cutaneous injury	1. Warm IV fluids 2. Warm room 3. Insulating covers (if needed) 4. Burn wound area assessment 5. Cover burn sites with dry, clean linen (pending definitive burn care) 6. Splint unstable fracture sites to avoid neurovascular compromise 7. Serial, focused neurovascular checks	• *Avoid* hypothermia • Core temperature 98.6°F (37°C)
Comprehensive evaluation Assess for • Efficacy of current treatment • Additional or missed injuries	1. Secondary and tertiary surveys per ACS trauma protocol 2. Pertinent additional studies and laboratory tests such as UA, CK-MB, troponin, ECG 3. Focused radiologic studies 4. Consider transfer to burn center	

ABG, Arterial blood gas; *ACLS*, Advanced Cardiovascular Life Support; *ACS*, American College of Surgeons; *ASAP*, as soon as possible; *ATLS*, Advanced Trauma Life Support; *BLS*, Basic Life Support; *CK-MB*, creatine kinase-MB; *CO₂*, carbon dioxide; *CT*, computed tomography; *C/T/L/S*, cervical, thoracic, lumbar, sacral; *CXR*, chest x-ray; *ECG*, electrocardiogram; *ETT*, endotracheal tube; *FAST*, focused assessment with sonography for trauma; *FiO₂*, fraction of inspired oxygen; *IV*, intravenous; *MAP*, mean arterial pressure; *O₂*, oxygen; *PCO₂*, partial pressure of carbon dioxide; *SaO₂*, saturated oxygen; *SvO₂*, mixed venous oxygen saturation; *UA*, urinalysis; *UO*, urine output.

or even months and are not consistent with the size or location of the injury.

Cardiac

After severe electrical current exposure, cardiac arrest (asystole or ventricular fibrillation) and respiratory arrest can occur simultaneously as the result of synchronous depolarization of all myocardial cells and medullary CNS paralysis. Spontaneous recovery of cardiac automaticity may facilitate return of spontaneous circulation before recovery of respiratory dysfunction, predisposing the patient to development of severe respiratory acidosis with secondary cardiac arrest. Electrocution victims without gross clinical signs of life may have occult cardiac activity, so Basic Life Support, Advanced Cardiovascular Life Support, and possibly Advanced Trauma Life Support guidelines should be the standard of care for all victims of electrical injury.

Monitoring. Continuously monitor ECG for the first 24 hours. If no acute cardiac issues or arrhythmia are identified, continuous monitoring can be stopped. Avoid hypotension and tachycardia. Check an echocardiogram if hypotension occurs or if acute myocardial injury is suggested by cardiac enzymes.

Complications. Ventricular fibrillation is the most common fatal arrhythmia, occurring in up to 60% of patients in whom the current has taken a horizontal pathway. However, virtually any cardiac dysrhythmia can be precipitated by any electrical injury. The overall estimate of arrhythmia after electrical injury is up to 15%; most of these arrhythmias are benign and occur within the first few hours of hospital admission. Recent studies have shown that new onset atrial fibrillation is the most common dysrhythmia seen in survivors; it can be managed easily with medical treatment. ECG should be performed in all patients who sustain electrical injuries, whether low or high voltage. Duration of cardiac monitoring needed is generally between 24 and 48 hours but should continue beyond that period if any underlying cardiac injury has not been ruled out completely.

Direct myocardial injury is uncommon but can be seen as a traumatic cardiac contusion. Myocardial infarction is rare.

Respiratory

Extubated patients: incentive spirometry, cough and deep breathing, early mobilization, oxygen as needed to maintain oxygen saturation (SaO_2) greater than 92%.

Intubated patients: use a "lung protective ventilator strategy" in the presence of ALI or acute respiratory distress syndrome (ARDS), develop a weaning plan, consider the value of early tracheostomy, maintain head of bed at 30 degrees or higher, provide venous thromboembolism (VTE) and ulcer prophylaxis, perform a daily sedation holiday and ventilator weaning assessment.

Gastrointestinal

Early enteral feeds, twice-weekly acute phase protein assessment, daily bowel assessment and regimen.

Renal

Goal UO is 0.5 cc/kg/hr (adjusted goal for rhabdomyolysis is UO >1.0 cc/kg/hr).

Complications. Rhabdomyolysis-induced acute renal failure is a feared complication that results from massive tissue necrosis and can be complicated by pigment-induced kidney injury. Myoglobin plays a dominant role in the pathogenesis of rhabdomyolysis-induced acute renal failure. These mechanisms involve (1) renal constriction and ischemia from hypovolemia due to extravascular extravasation of fluid, (2) direct cytotoxic action of myoglobin on the proximal convoluted tubules due to tissue and muscle breakdown, and (3) myoglobin cast formation in the distal convoluted tubules.

The most essential components used to avoid and potentially treat these complications are adequate fluid resuscitation and increased UO by maintaining a urine output of approximately 100 mL/hr until the urine visibly appears clear. Osmotic diuresis with mannitol and alkalinization of urine have been proposed as adjunct strategies but currently are not supported by level I evidence.

Infectious Disease

Tetanus administration should be considered where appropriate. Systemic inflammatory response syndrome (SIRS) criteria should be monitored closely for needed sepsis workup.

Musculoskeletal

Obtain radiologic studies of suspicious areas as necessary to evaluate for fractures, and perform frequent neurovascular checks of affected extremities to monitor for evolving tissue injury. Early fasciotomy is required for compartment syndrome. Early carpal tunnel release may be necessary for clinical signs of tissue entrapment. Early aggressive débridement of nonviable tissue should include splinting the affected extremity in a position of function.

Complications. Bone has the highest resistance of any body tissue, thus generating the greatest amount of heat when exposed to an electrical current. This then causes the greatest amount of thermal damage to tissue adjacent to long bone structures and manifests as periosteal burns and possible osteonecrosis. Tetanic muscular contractions induced by AC may result in fractures or dislocation of bone or joint.

In addition, traumatic injuries resulting in fractures from blast injuries, falls, or repetitive forceful muscle contractions have been reported. Patients with significant electrical injuries or altered mental status should have imaging studies of their cervical spine to rule out any evolving pathology.

Unfortunately, escharotomy is not of much use in electrical burn patients because of the depth of the injury. Fasciotomies and carpal tunnel releases should be performed immediately in the operating room when the circulation is presumed to be impaired. Initial fasciotomy should be performed in the areas of contact and conduction; for instance, the carpal tunnel may be released if the injury occurs in the wrist. The injury may be confined to the digits or hand, but if the patient has a considerable amount of pain, it may be advisable to complete a carpal tunnel release because the canal may become narrow secondary to swelling from the recent trauma and deep tissue, leading to early signs of compression. Fasciotomy plays a major role in the early management of electrical burns and can dramatically improve the salvage of tissue, including the limb. Splinting extremities in positions of function must be accomplished for preservation of joint use in the extremities.

Skin Complications

By far, the most common manifestations of electrical injuries can be attributed to the thermal damage caused to exposed skin. Although we often refer to entry (more tissue damage) and exit wounds, with AC there is no such thing as current entering or leaving. Instead, injuries are labeled as contact points.

Superficial, partial-thickness, and full-thickness burns can occur from any electrical injury. Estimates have shown that exposure to only 20 to 35 mA per mm^2 of skin surface for 20 seconds raises the skin temperature to 50°C, causing denaturing of protein, which leads to blistering and swelling. A crucial point to remember is that the degree of external injury cannot be used to determine the extent of the internal damage, regardless of voltage. Minor superficial burns may co-exist with massive muscle coagulation and necrosis.

Of note, the incidence of superficial surface burns is high in victims of lightning injury, but deep burns are uncommon.

■ SURGICAL MANAGEMENT

Low-Voltage Injury Management

Low-voltage injuries (<1000 V; see Figure 2, *B* and even Figure 2, *A*, although considered a high-voltage injury) are less devastating but can remain just as debilitating. These injuries often require close monitoring for the first few hours of admission in order to rule out evolving vascular sequelae to the limb or potential complications of myoglobin clearance. The first elective operative procedure is sharp excision of the eschar, often completed using a tourniquet, followed by initial placement of meshed allograft. The allograft is placed during the first excision even if the wound bed appears healthy and completely viable; this allows metabolic changes to alter the tissue beneath. In general, after the second débridement, sheet (non-meshed) autograft is applied to wounds on the face, neck, and hands; otherwise, meshed autograft can be used at the surgeon's discretion. Again, splinting the extremity in a position of function must be accomplished for preservation of joints use in the extremity. Early intervention by a rehabilitation therapist (occupational therapy and physical therapy) will optimize patient outcome and advance function with better range of motion and strengthening. It is considered good practice to educate patients that they may require additional surgical therapy in the distant future for burn contracture release, which may include placement of a full-thickness skin graft.

High-Voltage Injury Management

Most electrical injuries cause damage to limb tissue by generation of heat causing thermal insult and by endothelial damage with progressive tissue necrosis. These injuries often are associated with limb loss via amputation at various levels and carry a high rate of morbidity. Limb salvage and appropriate, aggressive initial resuscitation are challenging from the moment these injuries are first encountered. The American Burn Association referral criteria recommend that patients with high-voltage electrical trauma to the upper extremity be referred to specialized burn centers that are experienced with these injuries.

Most high-voltage (>1000 V) injuries are associated with deep tissue injury that often is underappreciated and more extensive than initially apparent. The initial management of the limb involves immediate (within 6 to 8 hours after injury) surgical exploration and decompressive fasciotomies. Fasciotomy plays a major role in the early management of electrical burns and can dramatically improve the salvage of tissue, including the limb. Escharotomy alone (incision is made into the subcutaneous fat just beyond the eschar) is of limited benefit. Although escharotomies often may be performed at the bedside, fasciotomies and carpal tunnel release should be performed in the operating room.

Indications for surgical decompression include progressive neurologic dysfunction, vascular compromise, increased compartment pressure, and systemic clinical deterioration from suspected ongoing myonecrosis. Decompression includes forearm fasciotomy and assessment of muscle compartment integrity. The decision to include a carpal tunnel release should be made on a case-by-case basis. Initial fasciotomy should be performed in the areas of contact and conduction; for instance, the carpal tunnel may be released if the injury occurs in the wrist. Delayed exploration and decompression in the compromised extremity may result in increased amputation rates as well as increased organ failure and mortality. To date, no definitive data exist to illustrate that immediate surgical decompression reduces the need for amputation in any series.

As shown in Figure 3, lack of opportunity for limb salvage may be obvious early regardless of the number of surgical débridements because of the extent of devitalized tissue noted on presentation. However, one important consideration regarding amputation is the length of tissue able to be retained and the remaining length required to fit a prosthesis. Do not confuse nonviable tissue with minimally bleeding tissue. As a general surgical principle, we are not trained to "leave behind" nonviable tissue because there is increased risk for infection; however, there is evidence to suggest that keeping some (minimally bleeding) tissue in question with multiple serial débridements, under a watchful eye, may improve the overall outcome.

Always start with débridement of devitalized tissue and continue every 48 hours until sustainably viable tissue is apparent and the source is controlled. Superficial muscle may be found viable and even appear uninjured by color and electrical stimulation with cautery. However, the muscle located deeply along the bone may be severely injured. Any questionably viable tissue is not débrided at the first exploration. Leaving a tendon that lacks its peritenon intact may be of use in long-term limb salvage, as there may be regeneration along the intact, viable tissue. Open wounds remaining at the end of the initial and subsequent débridements are closed with sheet (unmeshed) skin allograft to provide the most optimal environment for the marginally viable tissues and to prevent bacterial contamination in the sterile wounds. Serial débridements and re-exploration of the wounds should be performed and continued until no further necrotic tissue is present and the wound has stabilized (6 to 8 days), making the final preparations for definitive reconstruction or formal amputation possible. Splinting the extremity in a position of function must be accomplished for preservation of joint use in the extremity, and this should be commenced even before the first surgery.

Significant advances in extremity reconstruction have been made through the development of high-quality, functional prostheses and advances in tissue engineering such as vascularized composite allotransplantation (VCA). VCA is an option held in reserve after all other attempts have been exhausted and the patient has survived the initial injury, as the immunosuppression necessary for graft survival can harm the patient in the acute phase as we continue to await chimerism.

In addition to basic general surgical principles such as débridement of nonviable tissue, protection of tissue perfusion, nutritional optimization, and control of infection, reconstructive surgery follows basic principles of the reconstructive ladder: healing by secondary intention, primary closure, delayed primary closure, grafts (split thickness, full thickness), tissue expansion, and flaps (random, axial, and free). This provides a systematic approach to wound closure by emphasizing simple to complex techniques based on local wound requirements and complexity.

In burn surgery, rarely are the first few rungs of the ladder helpful because of the nature of the injury; we often jump to the rung of grafting secondary to tissue loss. There must be a healthy, vascularized wound bed for a split-thickness graft to take (i.e., if the peritenon or periosteum is lacking, the graft will not take). Allograft versus autograft is a very important tissue choice and ultimately the surgeon's decision (keep in mind that if the allograft does not adhere, neither will the autograft). Use of allografting preserves the patient's tissue until the wound bed is ready and allows the surgeon to return to the operating theatre for redébridement of areas where microscopic changes at the cellular level are noted.

Full-thickness skin grafting is often susceptible to infection if nonviable tissue is left behind because of lack of adequate vascular blood supply. Rarely is tissue expansion even considered in the acute burn injury. Random and axial flaps are used when appropriate and often the preferred method of reconstruction, especially in the acutely injured patient. However, the operating surgeon must keep in mind that during an electrical injury, significant vessel damage may occur to the media or endothelium of the vessel in which the flap is based.

Other vascular abnormalities such as vascular occlusions, arteritis and aneurysm formation, thrombosis and segmental narrowing of major extremity vessels, and a marked decrease in the density of small nutrient vessels have been described after electrical injuries. As a rule of thumb, the ideal tissue to be used is outside the zone of injury; this principle also should be respected and strongly adhered to during free tissue transfer. Free flap reconstruction is rarely indicated in an acute burn injury because the versatility and variability of free flaps have evolved, as has their applicability to tissue reconstruction. Timing of the reconstructive procedure in relation to the injury, age of patient, existing medical comorbidities, length of the operative

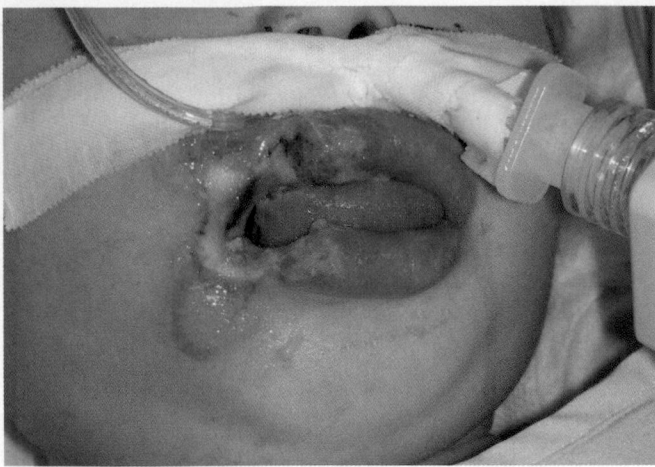

FIGURE 5 Oral commissure burn resulting from contact with a household electrical wire. Associated complication: labial artery rupture may occur 7 days after burn.

procedure, and extent of the zone of injury has a significant impact on the success rate of a free flap reconstruction. The importance of these issues should not be minimized because free flaps may be necessary for coverage of exposed joint, bone, vessels, tendons, and so on. The failure of free tissue transplantation postinjury is well documented to range from postoperative day 5 to 6 weeks. Therefore it is critical to optimize the burn patient's treatment from its onset, as the outcome of these types of injuries will be life altering.

Commissure Injuries

The American College of Surgeons has recommended that all facial burns be triaged to an American Burn Association burn center. Commissure burns typically occur in the young patient and commonly result from biting or teething on a household appliance cord. Although it is considered a relatively low-voltage (120 to 240 V) injury, the soft tissue injury can be devastating and lead to significant tissue loss (Figure 5). The burn is a result of saliva permitting the local conduction and arcing of electricity. The electrical energy generally is concentrated to the oral commissure and the anterior tongue. As with any trauma, the initial management, according to the Advanced Trauma Life Support guidelines, involves a thorough assessment from head to toe. Rarely do these isolated injuries require intubation.

The contact burn wound, often a grayish-white eschar, should be cleaned gently and dressed with an ointment of choice. On examination of the vestibule of the mouth, digital palpation may reveal a "woody," indurated buccal mucosa as far posterior as the tonsillar pillars. Early surgical intervention can lead to loss of potentially salvageable tissue that may be necessary for the reconstructive surgery and thus should be avoided. The goal is to maintain a clean, moist

environment that allows the tissue to heal. The child should be encouraged to continue to eat and drink. Involvement of a speech pathologist can be of significant help from the outset. The use of a custom-made splint can help to reduce scar formation and should be initiated between 10 and 14 days postinjury. The eschar will continue to demarcate and slough within 7 to 21 days. Based on the proximity of the labial artery to the oral commissure, vessel rupture can be expected to occur in approximately 10% of patients. Parents and caregivers should be educated that if labial artery rupture bleeding occurs, compression of the site between the index finger and thumb should be performed to minimize the hemorrhage and that they should return immediately to the hospital. Seldom do these ruptures need surgical intervention for ligation.

The continued healing from the burn can result in tissue scarring and contracture. Contracture can interfere with normal vocalization, facial expression, eating, and oral hygiene (including dental care), not to mention the psychologic sequelae of the trauma. Long-term burns to the mouth can be associated with microstomia. Contracture of the angle of the mouth generally is treated approximately 1 year after burn injury, as it takes at least 1 year for the burn to become stable because of the sphincteral action of the orbicularis oris muscle. Late effects of burn reconstructive surgery may include Z-plasty, tongue advancement flap, or commissuroplasty. Of note, the tongue advancement flap, often the only choice based on initial injury, may give a less aesthetically pleasing appearance because the tongue papilla are transferred to the external orifice.

■ LATE COMPLICATIONS

A multitude of late complications from electrical injuries include cataracts, increased cholelithiasis causing cholecystitis, delayed hemorrhage from blood vessel rupture, skeletal complications of fibrosis, and limitation of joint function.

Although there have been significant advances in both burn management and critical care management of these specialized patients, prevention and safety remain the best way to avoid or minimize the occurrence and severity of electrical injury. With the exception of lightning, electrical injuries are almost always preventable.

SUGGESTED READINGS

Arnoldo BD, Purdue GF, Kowalske K, Helm PA, Burris A, Hunt JL. Electrical injuries: a 20-year review. *J Burn Care Rehabil*. 2004;25:479-484.

Davis C, Engeln A, Johnson EL, et al. Winderness Medical Society practice guidelines for the prevention and treatment of lightning injuries: 2014 update. *Wilderness Environ Med*. 2014;25(suppl 4):S86-S95.

Hunt JL, Mason AD, Masterson TS, Pruitt BA. The pathophysiology of acute electric burns. *J Trauma*. 1976;16:335-340.

Koumbourlis AC. Electrical injuries. *Crit Care Med*. 2002;30(suppl 11): S424-S430.

Lee R. Injury by electrical forces: pathophysiology, manifestations and therapy. *Curr Prob Surg*. 1997;34:677-764.

Luce EA. Electrical burns. *Clin Plast Surg*. 2000;27:133-143.

Purdue GF, Arnoldo BD, Hunt JL. Electrical injuries. In: Herndon D, ed. *Total Burn Care*. 3rd ed. St. Louis: Saunders Elsevier; 2007:513-520.

PREOPERATIVE AND POSTOPERATIVE CARE

FLUID AND ELECTROLYTE THERAPY

Nathan Kugler, MD, and Jasmeet Singh Paul, MD, FACS

Fluid and electrolyte management is vital to patient care in both medical and surgical disease states. Surgeons must understand fluid and electrolyte balance at the cellular and systems level in order to anticipate the clinical implications of resuscitative and maintenance therapy. This chapter discusses the fluid and electrolyte distribution in the setting of normal physiology as well as resuscitation and corrective therapies for fluid and electrolyte abnormalities.

■ FLUID COMPARTMENTS, DYNAMICS, AND OSMOLALITY

Water accounts for 50% to 60% of an individual's total body weight. As a result of the decreased water content in fat compared with muscle, total body water (TBW) as a percentage of total body weight is lower in obese individuals. In addition, males tend to have a greater lean muscle mass as a percentage of total body weight, resulting in TBW accounting for approximately 60% of total body weight compared with 50% to 55% in females.

TBW is distributed throughout multiple compartments, with the majority residing within the intracellular compartment, as shown in Figure 1. In normal, healthy subjects, approximately two thirds of fluid resides intracellular, with the remainder constituting the extracellular space. The extracellular compartment is subdivided into interstitial and intravascular or plasma compartments, with two thirds of fluid within the interstitial compartment. Thus a 70-kg male would be predicted to have a TBW content of 42 L (60% of total body weight), with 28 L (two thirds of TBW) intracellular volume and 14 L extracellular (one third of TBW), of which 4.7 L (one third of extracellular volume) would be the circulating blood volume (packed red cells and plasma).

To understand TBW balance, one must take into consideration water movement between different compartments and the factors that determine the volume of TBW. Membranes separating intracellular and extracellular compartments are freely permeable to water, such that the osmolality of the intracellular, interstitial, and intravascular compartments remains equal. However, membrane permeability to different solutes varies, resulting in a nonequal distribution of solutes. As a result, effective osmoles are solutes that have the ability to direct osmotic forces, resulting in water movement across a membrane. The shifting of water, via intercellular junctions or transcellular routes, from areas of lower osmolality to higher osmolality results in osmotic equilibration. Lipid-rich cell membranes result in simple diffusion of water whereas fenestrations or water channels known as aquaporins embedded in cell membranes allow alternative routes for movement.

Capillary membranes are permeable to most small solutes, including sodium, potassium, glucose, and low-molecular-weight proteins (less than 50,000 kDa). These small solutes have no role as effective osmoles in the setting of capillary fluid movement. Movement of water across the capillary membranes is the result of oncotic pressure and hydrostatic pressure from blood flow. Oncotic pressure is generated by plasma proteins too large to cross the capillary wall. Starling's forces are the result of the combined oncotic and hydrostatic pressures. Starling's law states that net filtration is the difference between the hydrostatic and oncotic pressures of both the interstitial and the capillary fluids. Plasma proteins provide oncotic pressure that holds fluid intravascular whereas the hydrostatic pressure of blood flow tends to force fluid into the interstitial space. On the arteriolar end of a capillary bed, intravascular hydrostatic pressure exceeds oncotic pressure, resulting in net efflux of fluid. However, this situation reverses as hydrostatic pressures drop along the length of the capillary bed, resulting in net fluid influx into the intravascular compartment near the venous side.

Although small solutes do not contribute to water movement across capillary membranes, they do function as effective osmoles that direct water movement between the intracellular and extracellular spaces across cell membranes. Sodium (Na^+) and potassium (K^+) are the principal determinants of extracellular osmolality and intracellular osmolality, respectively. Na^+ and K^+ are unable to passively diffuse across the lipid-rich membrane with a gradient generated and maintained by the Na^+/K^+ adenosine triphosphatase (ATPase) mechanism. This transmembrane transporter exchanges three Na^+ molecules for two K^+ molecules, generating a net negative cell membrane potential. Manipulation of either of these ions results in water movement from lower to higher osmolality in order to re-establish equilibrium. For example, administration of hypotonic solution (e.g., 0.45% sodium chloride normal saline solution) results in decreased extracellular osmolality, so water moves from the extracellular space to the intracellular space, resulting in cellular swelling. In contrast, administration of a hypertonic solution (e.g., 3% sodium chloride normal saline solution) results in increased extracellular osmolality, so water moves from the intracellular space to the extracellular space, resulting in cellular dehydration.

Serum osmolality is maintained within a narrow range through osmoregulation and is calculated using the following formula:

$$mOsm/kg = 2 \times (Na + K) + (BUN/2.8) + (Glucose/18)$$

where *BUN* is blood urea nitrogen and *mOsm/kg* is serum osmolality. Normal serum osmolality ranges from 275 to 290 mOsm/kg, with a threshold of 1% to 2% variation before activation of osmoregulatory processes. Osmoreceptors within the hypothalamus detect elevations in plasma osmolality, resulting in stimulation of thirst along with antidiuretic hormone (ADH) secretion from the posterior pituitary gland. ADH release results in upregulation of aquaporin channels in the basolateral membrane of distal collecting tubules in the kidney, promoting free water resorption down an established gradient. As a result of increased aquaporin insertion, urine osmolality increases, with variations from 100 to 1200 mOsm/kg depending on the serum

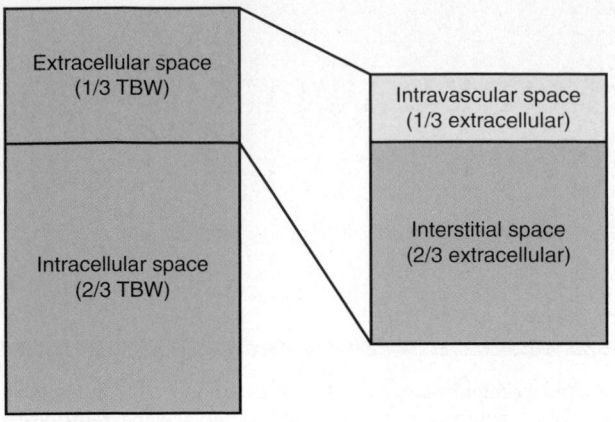

FIGURE 1 Body fluid distribution. *TBW,* Total body water.

osmolality. Patients who demonstrate an elevated serum osmolality and have intact renal function often demonstrate urine osmolalities greater than 500 mOsm/kg. Aside from hypothalamic activation, activation of central baroreceptors through decreased plasma volume triggers increased ADH secretion, albeit a less potent stimulus than plasma osmolality.

Osmoregulation can be viewed as a separate process from volume regulation; however, changes in osmoregulation result in volume shifts. Hormones that influence total body sodium content are the principal mediators of volume regulation. The renin-angiotensin-aldosterone (RAA) axis promotes volume expansion. Renin is secreted by the juxtaglomerular cells in response to renal hypoperfusion or low sodium concentration in the macula densa region of the distal tubule. Renin secretion promotes formation of angiotensin from angiotensinogen and the eventual production of aldosterone, which promotes sodium reabsorption. Contrary to the RAA axis, atrial natriuretic peptide (ANP) results in net diuresis. ANP is a systemic hormone released in response to cardiac atrial stretch and results in increased renal blood flow through dilation of the afferent glomerular arteriole and inhibition of sodium reabsorption in the kidney.

■ FLUID STATUS AND THE MANAGEMENT OF VOLUME REPLETION AND MAINTENANCE

Assessment of Fluid Status

In the immediate postoperative period, patients may have fluid deficits resulting from preoperative or intraoperative fluid losses. Continued fluid losses in the extended postoperative period from urine, skin, and the gastrointestinal (GI) tract are common. Fluid management requires close assessment of fluid status and selection of an appropriate type and rate of fluid replacement.

Inflammatory states, commonly seen in the postoperative period, result in a low effective intravascular volume despite an overall positive fluid balance due to cytokine-induced permeability. Common signs and symptoms of low effective circulatory volume include abnormal mentation, excessive thirst, dry mucous membranes, poor skin turgor, tachycardia, hypotension, orthostatic changes in heart rate and blood pressure, and oliguria. Daily weights, serum and urine electrolyte levels, acid-base balance, and invasive monitoring can be used to assess a patient's volume status and the adequacy of resuscitation. Urine output is an excellent measure of volume status; adults should produce at least 0.5 mL/kg/hr whereas small children should produce nearly 1 to 2 mL/kg/hr. However, in the setting of renal insufficiency, those receiving diuretics, or those in hyperglycemic states, urine output may be an inaccurate measure of volume status and resuscitation. Elevated urine osmolality may suggest intravascular hypovolemia, but in the setting of renal insufficiency or use of

diuretics it is often an inaccurate measure. Other indicators of intravascular depletion include an elevated hematocrit, a low serum bicarbonate level with associated base deficit, a BUN/creatinine (Cr) ratio greater than 20:1 (prerenal azotemia), or a fractional excretion of sodium (FENa) of less than 1%.

$$FENa = [(Urine\ Na \times Plasma\ Cr)/(Plasma\ Na \times Urine\ Cr)] \times 100$$

Similar to urine output and urine osmolality assessments, in the setting of renal dysfunction or use of diuretics FENa is not a useful indicator of volume status. Instead, fractional excretion of urea (FEUrea) provides a useful tool. FEUrea is calculated in the same fashion as FENa.

$$FEUrea = [(Urine\ urea \times Plasma\ Cr)/(Plasma\ urea \times Urine\ Cr)] \times 100$$

FEUrea less than 35% is suggestive of a prerenal condition.

Resuscitative Fluids

The rate of fluid administration is determined by the severity of the existing deficit, presence of ongoing losses, and comorbidities. Resuscitation should be accomplished utilizing isotonic fluids. Severe fluid losses resulting in hemodynamic instability should be replaced with intravenous (IV) fluid boluses of 0.9% sodium chloride (normal saline solution [NS]) or Lactated Ringer's solution (LR) at volumes of 10 to 20 mL/kg, with boluses repeated until adequate resuscitation is reached. The composition of various replacement fluids is shown in Table 1. NS and LR best approximate the composition of extracellular fluid and therefore are used as replacement fluid most often. LR has a pH of 6.5 and provides 28 mEq of bicarbonate (HCO_3^-) per liter, making it preferential in the setting of acidosis. NS, at a pH of 4.5, does not contain HCO_3^- but has a greater concentration of Na^+ and Cl^- (154 mEq), making it preferential in patients with a metabolic alkalosis. However, it can create hyperchloremic metabolic acidosis in the setting of high volume resuscitation. Colloid solutions, such as 5% albumin, theoretically provide an advantage when restoring intravascular volume because of the oncotic pressure afforded by the protein content. However, liberal use of colloid solutions has not demonstrated improved patient outcomes in randomized studies.

Type of fluid resuscitation should take into account the source of fluid loss. The electrolyte compositions of different GI fluids are listed in Table 2. Optimal replacement for gastric losses is 5% dextrose in 0.45% normal saline (D5 1/2 NS) with 20 mEq/L potassium chloride (KCl); for pancreatic, biliary, or small intestinal losses it is LR; and for large intestinal losses it is LR with 20 mEq/L KCl. Persistent or substantial GI losses should be replaced on a milliliter-for-milliliter basis with the appropriate fluid on a schedule to prevent the need for large volume replacements.

Daily Electrolyte Requirements and Maintenance Fluids

Maintenance fluids replace normal sensible and insensible losses. Sensible losses can be quantified and occur primarily in urine (~800 to 1500 mL daily) and stool (~250 mL daily). Insensible losses are unable to be quantified and include cutaneous losses from the skin (75%) and upper respiratory tract (25%). Insensible losses often are quantified roughly at 8 to 12 mL/kg/day. Sensible and insensible losses vary greatly in different physiologic states and pathologic conditions, including fever, hyperventilation, burns, tachycardia, and other hypermetabolic states. Cutaneous insensible losses increase by 10% per day for each 1°C increase in body temperature above 37.1°C. Laparotomy and thoracostomy increase sensible losses from the operative site at rates that approach nearly 1 L/hr.

Daily maintenance fluid administration in both pediatric and adult populations can be calculated for a 24-hour period utilizing the

TABLE 1: Electrolyte Composition (mEq) of Parenteral Fluids

Fluid	Na$^+$	K$^+$	Cl$^-$	Ca^{2+}	HCO$_3^-$	Dextrose	pH	Osmolality
Extracellular fluid	142	4	103	5	27	0	7.4	280
Lactated Ringer's solution	130	4	109	2.7	28	0	6.5	275
Normal saline (0.9% NaCl)	154	0	154	0	0	0	4.5	308
1/2 Normal saline (0.45% NaCl)	77	0	77	0	0	0	4.5	154
1/4 Normal saline (0.22% NaCl)	34	0	34	0	0	0	4.5	77
3% Saline	513	0	513	0	0	0	4.5	1026
5% Dextrose in water	0	0	0	0	0	50 g	5.0	278
5% Albumin	145	0	0	0	0	0	7.4	290
Normosol®	140	5	98	0	0	0	6.6	294
Plasma-Lyte®	140	5	98	0	0	0	7.4	294

Ca^{2+}, Calcium; Cl^-, chloride; HCO_3^-, bicarbonate; K^+, potassium; Na^+, sodium; $NaCl$, sodium chloride.

TABLE 2: Electrolyte Composition (mEq) of Gastrointestinal Fluids

Source	Daily Production (mL)	Na+	K+	Cl$^-$	HCO$_3^-$
Saliva	1000	30-80	20	70	30
Gastric	1000-2000	60-80	15	100	0
Pancreas	1000	140	5-10	60-90	40-100
Bile	1000	140	5-10	100	40
Small bowel	2000-5000	140	20	100	25-50
Large bowel	200-1500	75	30	30	0

Cl^-, Chloride; HCO_3^-, bicarbonate; K^+, potassium; Na^+, sodium.

TABLE 3: Maintenance Fluid Requirements

Body Mass (kg)	Fluid Volume (mL/kg/hr)	Fluid Volume (mL/kg/day)
First 10 kg	4	100
Second 10 kg (11-20 kg)	2	50
Each kg >20 kg	1	20
70 kg	110	2500

Note: Calculated utilizing the 4-2-1 rule and the 100-50-20 rule. See text for details.

100-50-20 rule or hourly utilizing the 4-2-1 rule (Table 3). The electrolyte composition of maintenance fluids is dependent on perceived sensible and insensible losses. Electrolyte and carbohydrate requirements vary with the clinical situation and require close monitoring in critically ill patients. In general, in the postoperative period sodium requirements range between 1 and 2 mEq/kg/day and potassium requirements range between 0.5 and 1 mEq/kg/day. Maintenance fluids most often include dextrose to maintain plasma osmolality and reduce risk of short-term proteolysis. The usual postoperative maintenance fluid for adults consists of D5 1/2 NS with 20 mEq/L KCl. Children older than 2 years can receive the same maintenance fluids as adults. Until age 2 years, the kidney has a glomerular filtration rate (GFR) that is one quarter the adult level, and the distal nephrons are unable to effectively concentrate the urine, leading to a difficulty in excreting high sodium loads. Therefore children younger than 2 years usually receive D5 in 0.22% normal saline (1/4 NS) with 20 mEq/L. When administering maintenance fluids, utilizing a 4-2-1 dosing regimen in a 70-kg male (110 mL/hr) results in a total sodium load of 203 mEq in a 24-hour period, which is greater than the required 1 to 2 mEq/kg/day. Although patients with normal kidney function are able to excrete the excess sodium load, caution should be utilized in patients with underlying renal dysfunction, cardiac failure, or other serious comorbidities. In general, maintenance fluids should be reassessed at least daily to ensure that correct electrolyte and fluid volume needs are met but not exceeded.

DIAGNOSIS AND TREATMENT OF ELECTROLYTE DISORDERS

Sodium

Homeostasis and Clinical Significance

Sodium is the principal determinant of serum osmolality and free water balance. Thus abnormalities in serum sodium levels occur at all osmolar and volume states. Sodium predominates in the extracellular space and is an effective osmole, stimulating free water movement across cellular membranes secondary to cell wall impermeability to sodium. Evaluation of both volume status and osmolarity is vital to the safe, effective treatment of sodium abnormalities.

Hypernatremia

Hypernatremia is defined as a serum sodium concentration greater than 145 mEq/L. It can be subdivided further into mild, moderate, and severe (>160 mEq/L). Symptoms of severe hypernatremia are related primarily to central nervous system depression as a result of cellular dehydration and include muscle weakness, restlessness, insomnia, lethargy, and coma. Unlike hyponatremia, in which multiple osmolar states can exist, hypernatremia is always associated with a hypertonic state but can be seen in hypervolemic, euvolemic, and hypovolemic states. Assessment of volume status is the key to successful management of hypernatremia.

The most common cause of hypernatremia is a *hypovolemic* state seen in patients in dehydrated states and with uncontrolled fluid losses. Older patients and patients with end-stage liver disease are particularly vulnerable. Patients with GI losses from nasogastric suction, vomiting, diarrhea, or lactulose administration are particularly at risk and can become dehydrated quickly. Individuals who demonstrate *euvolemic* hypernatremia most often exhibit inappropriate urinary loss of free water (inappropriate low urine osmolality) seen with neurogenic or nephrogenic diabetes insipidus (DI). In the setting of head injury, pituitary surgery, or cerebral hemorrhage, neurogenic DI should be suspected for patients who exhibit euvolemic hypernatremia. A significant response (50% increase in urine osmolality) after administration of desmopressin (DDAVP) in the setting of DI suggests a neurogenic origin. Treatment of nephrogenic DI simply requires replacement utilizing desmopressin. Finally, *hypervolemic* hypernatremia is usually iatrogenic in nature, resulting from fluid resuscitation with hypertonic solutions. Other medical causes include mineralocorticoid excess, such as with Conn's or Cushing's syndrome.

Treatment of hypernatremia begins with calculation of the free water deficit.

$$\text{Free water deficit (L)} = [(\text{Serum Na} - 140)/140] \times 0.6 \times \text{Weight (kg)}$$

Patients with severe hypernatremia or symptomatic hypernatremia should undergo treatment with D5 water replacements. Those with mild or moderate hypernatremia can be corrected utilizing isotonic NS. Rate of replacement for hypernatremia is dependent on the development time frame. Those with acute development (<24 hours) should be replaced more rapidly whereas those with chronic hypernatremia (>48 hours) should be approached cautiously. Acute hypernatremia should be corrected at an initial rate of 2 to 3 mEq/L/hr but should not exceed a maximum correction of 12 mEq/L/day. Chronic hypernatremia should be corrected at a rate not to exceed 0.5 mEq/L/hr, with a total change of 8 to 10 mEq/L/day. In patients with neurologic abnormalities, serum sodium measurements should be obtained every 2 hours until the patient is neurologically stable. In cases of extreme hypernatremia (>170 mEq/L), patients should not be corrected to below 150 mEq/L for the first 48 to 72 hours.

Hyponatremia

A commonly accepted definition of hyponatremia is a serum sodium concentration lower than 135 mEq/L. Hyponatremia can be subdivided further into mild (130 to 135 mEq/L), moderate (120 to 130 mEq/L), or severe (<120 mEq/L). It is estimated that approximately 1% of postoperative patients develop hyponatremia with serum sodium concentration lower than 130 mEq/L, with upward of 20% of these cases deemed clinically significant. Severe cases or acute changes in serum sodium concentrations can result in cellular edema and cerebral swelling, leading to clinical manifestation as headaches, lethargy, seizures, and coma. Clinical manifestations of hyponatremia are mainly secondary to cerebral edema. Significant hyponatremia can remain asymptomatic, as in the case of cirrhosis or heart failure, as the nervous system can adapt. Conversely, patients with mild hyponatremia may manifest with severe symptoms. However, some acute changes do not result in symptoms. These facts suggest that although the time course for development of hyponatremia plays a role, multiple other factors affect the clinical manifestation of hyponatremia. Previous work has demonstrated the roles of gender (females worse than males), age (young worse than old), and the presence of hypoxia (worse with hypoxia) to be of greater importance when assessing clinical outcomes than the rate of development or severity of hyponatremia alone.

To guide corrective therapy, calculation of the sodium deficit is required utilizing the patient's TBW estimate.

$$\text{Na deficit} = (140 - \text{Serum Na}) \times \text{TBW}$$

TBW is estimated utilizing 0.6 times total body weight for males and 0.55 times total body weight for females. When correcting hyponatremia, the rate of correction is important, as rapid correction can lead to central pontine myelinolysis (CPM) with potential for permanent spastic quadriparesis and pseudobulbar palsy. Patients with liver disease are particularly susceptible to demyelination. In patients with severe liver disease, the upper limit for a safe rate of correction is unknown. In the majority of patients, serum sodium correction should not exceed 0.25 mEq/L/hr or 9 mEq/L/day. Severe manifestations of hyponatremia (active seizures, respiratory failure, etc.) require immediate treatment with the goal of raising the serum sodium by 2 to 4 mEq/L through a 100 mL bolus of 3% saline over a 10-minute period. If the clinical manifestations do not improve, repeat bolus is indicated. For those patients with less severe manifestations of hyponatremia but who demonstrate hyponatremic encephalopathy (recent seizure, altered mental status, headache, nausea, emesis, etc.), infusion of 3% saline given at a rate of 1 mL/kg/hr is recommended. As a general rule, infusion of 3% saline at a dose of 1 mL/kg provides a serum sodium increase of 1 mEq/L. However, patients receiving hypertonic saline require frequent testing of serum sodium levels, often every 2 hours, until serum levels are stable, as predicting free water loss is difficult in critically ill patients.

In the setting of asymptomatic hyponatremia or as an adjunct to hypertonic saline, furosemide-induced diuresis can aid in more gradual correction of serum sodium. Treatment of asymptomatic hyponatremia requires assessment of serum osmolality, as it can occur in high, normal, or low serum osmolality states. Aside from osmotic variations, hyponatremia can be present in hypovolemic, euvolemic, or hypervolemic states. Assessment of serum osmolality and volume status is extremely important when determining the appropriate corrective therapy. In the postoperative period, abnormalities in volume status are most common.

Hypovolemic hypotonic hyponatremia is the most common form of hyponatremia in the postoperative setting. When hypovolemia is suspected, urine sodium levels less than 20 mmol/L suggest hyponatremia secondary to sequestration of isotonic fluids in the extravascular space or loss from the GI tract or skin. Contrary to treatment of hypervolemic or euvolemic hyponatremia, fluid restriction in the setting of hypovolemia will worsen the clinical picture. Thus mild to moderate cases are treated utilizing isotonic saline solution. Treatment of hypovolemic hyponatremia with hypertonic saline is unnecessary unless severe symptoms are present.

Less common postoperative causes of hyponatremia include hypervolemic and euvolemic states. *Hypervolemic* hyponatremia is the least common type in the postoperative period, as it is most commonly the iatrogenic result of excessive hypotonic fluid administration. To avoid hypervolemic hyponatremia, hypotonic fluid administration should be reserved primarily for correction of free water deficits in the setting of hypernatremia. Treatment for hypervolemic hypernatremia can be accomplished easily with a combination of water restriction and gentle diuresis. *Euvolemic* hyponatremia is uncommon in the postoperative period, as it is often the result of syndrome of inappropriate ADH secretion (SIADH), hypothyroidism, or excessive water intake (psychogenic polydipsia). In the postoperative period, transient increases in ADH as the result of pain, stress, narcotic medications, and volume depletion promote free water reabsorption, but not typically at a level sufficient to create a hyponatremic state. SIADH occurs in the setting of traumatic brain injury, pulmonary malignancies (carcinoid and small cell), and lung infections. Diagnosis of SIADH usually is made on findings of high urine osmolality (>150 mmol/kg) and high urine sodium (>25 mmol/L). The absence of hypokalemia helps to differentiate SIADH from adrenal insufficiency. In the setting of SIADH, administration of isotonic saline often worsens hyponatremia, as the sodium is filtered out with reabsorption of free water. Treatment for euvolemic hyponatremia consists of fluid restriction (~1 L/day) for gradual correction of serum sodium levels.

Assessment of osmolality in addition to volume status is important. *Hypertonic* states can occur in the setting of hypovolemia; however, in the setting of hypertonic hyponatremia it is important to evaluate serum BUN and glucose levels. Elevations in BUN or glucose create increased extracellular oncotic pressure, resulting in an influx of water into the extracellular space, resulting in a relative hypervolemic state. The first step in assessment of hypertonic hyponatremia is to determine the true serum sodium level. In the setting of hyperglycemia, for every 100 mg/dL increase in glucose over 100 mg/dL, 2 mEq/L should be added to the reported sodium. *Isotonic* hyponatremia is rarely seen anymore, as it is now often corrected for by most laboratories. It is caused by elevated elements such as proteins and triglycerides, resulting in a false lowering of the serum sodium measurement. Finally, *hypotonic* hyponatremia occurs most commonly in the setting of a hypervolemic state resulting from expanded extracellular and interstitial volumes with relative intravascular depletion resulting in ADH release. This is seen most commonly in the settings of congestive heart failure, chronic renal insufficiency, nephrotic syndrome, cirrhosis (often in the setting of hepatorenal syndrome), and hypoalbuminemia. Treatment of hypotonic hyponatremia most commonly includes sodium (1500 to 200 mg/day) and fluid (~1 L/day) restriction.

Potassium

Homeostasis and Clinical Significance

Approximately 98% of potassium is sequestered within the intracellular compartment secondary to the action of the Na^+/K^+-ATPase pump, with a total body store of approximately 4000 mEq. Given the relative lack of potassium in the extracellular space, transcellular shifts in potassium are the primary culprit for the development of potassium abnormalities. Metabolic acidosis, and less commonly lactic acidosis, results in efflux of potassium into the extracellular space in exchange for intracellular movement of hydrogen (H^+) in an attempt to buffer serum pH. On the contrary, insulin and beta-2 receptor stimulation result in an influx of potassium intracellular.

Serum potassium levels are maintained in a narrow range (3.5 to 5 mmol/L) via tight regulation at the level of the kidney. Within the distal nephron, filtrate movement leads to potassium movement into the filtrate via epithelial potassium channels. The main stimulus for potassium efflux via this mechanism is the effect of epithelial sodium channels (ENaCs) on the apical membrane of the distal tubules and the resulting potassium excretion seen in an attempt to increase sodium retention. Activation of the RAA system ultimately results in potassium efflux via ENaC activation by aldosterone.

Hyperkalemia

Hyperkalemia is cardiotoxic and can lead to ventricular arrhythmias. Electrocardiographic (ECG) findings include, in order of progression, peaked T waves, QRS widening, shortened QT intervals, and ventricular ectopy. Hyperkalemia develops through two distinct mechanisms: total body excess or translocation of intracellular potassium into the extracellular space. In the setting of renal failure, the body typically is capable of excreting potassium unless the GFR falls below 15 mL/min. Acute hyperkalemia, often seen with acute renal failure, is not tolerated to the extent that hyperkalemia is in patients with chronic renal failure. Notable causes of acute hyperkalemia include heparin administration, acidosis, rhabdomyolysis, cell lysis, and insulin deficiency. Because of the instability of red blood cells (RBCs) in an in vitro environment, pseudohyperkalemia occurs with RBC lysis before laboratory measurements. A unique surgical cause includes ischemia-reperfusion injuries, where after revascularization after 4 to 6 hours of ischemia, severe systemic hyperkalemia may occur. Many surgeons utilize prophylactic bicarbonate administration before reperfusion. Additional patients in whom the risk of hyperkalemia is increased include those with profuse atrophy (often secondary to prolonged bed rest), neurologic denervation syndromes, severe burns, or muscular trauma.

Treatment of hyperkalemia is differentiated by presence or lack of symptoms. Treatment consists of promoting either intracellular shift of potassium or excretion of potassium by the kidneys. For patients in whom cardiac instability is detected, administration of intravascular calcium gluconate 1000 mg over 2 to 3 minutes with continuous cardiac monitoring stabilizes cardiac membranes with no effect on serum potassium levels. If ECG changes remain, calcium bolus may be repeated. To quickly affect serum potassium concentration, intracellular shift of potassium can be achieved by administering 10 units of regular insulin with 1 ampule of 50% dextrose (D50) to prevent hypoglycemia or administering an ampule of sodium bicarbonate ($NaHCO_3$). Intracellular shifts temporize the situation; ultimately excretion of excess potassium is accomplished with administration of loop diuretics or cation exchange resins (kayexalate). Exchange resins can be given orally or as a retention enema (contraindicated with immunosuppression) with sorbitol. They act via exchange of a single K^+ for two Na^+, creating an osmotic diarrhea. In critically ill patients, hemodialysis can be utilized to reduce serum potassium.

Hypokalemia

Hypokalemia is commonly encountered in the postoperative period. Signs and symptoms of hypokalemia include generalized fatigue and weakness, atrial arrhythmias, and ileus. ECG findings include flattening of T waves or the formation of prominent U waves. Common causes of hypokalemia seen in surgical patients include large losses from the kidney or GI tract via nasogastric suctioning, vomiting, or diarrhea; alkalosis; catecholamine secretion; and insulin administration. As 98% of total body potassium is stored within the intracellular compartment, small changes in serum K^+ reflect large changes in total body stores. Low potassium frequently is associated with hypomagnesemia and acidemia. Magnesium first must be replenished before K^+ corrects in response to exogenous administration. In patients who are both hypokalemic and acidemic, potassium administration should precede correction of acidemia with bicarbonate because of the intracellular shift of potassium seen with increases in pH. Potassium can be replenished via oral or IV routes. Treatment of mild hypokalemia should be accomplished via oral replacement; however, oral therapy often is not well tolerated. Given the high oral bioavailability of KCl, IV administration should be reserved for patients who do not tolerate the oral form or for those who have severe hypokalemia. Severe hypokalemia should be treated utilizing IV KCl at a rate of 10 to 20 mEq/hr with simultaneous replacement of any magnesium deficits. Given the large total body deficit reflected by serum abnormalities, serial replacements often will be necessary.

Calcium

Homeostasis and Clinical Significance

Calcium is the most abundant electrolyte in the body, with the vast majority found in bone stores. Serum concentrations are tightly regulated by processes that promote calcium extracellular influx via bone demineralization and interstitial absorption and efflux via urinary excretion and bone formation. Calcium concentrations are regulated through complex hormonal regulation, with the majority via parathyroid hormone and calcitriol. Nearly 50% of calcium exists in a biologically active ionized state; the other 50% exists in a nonionized inactive state bound to albumin. With such a large portion of circulating calcium bound to albumin, serum calcium measurements must be adjusted for serum albumin levels; calcium levels fall by 0.8 mEq/L for every 1 g/dL reduction in serum albumin. Although this correction generally is utilized, measurement of ionized calcium in critically ill patients is necessary for patient care and is readily available in all laboratories.

Hypercalcemia

Hypercalcemia is defined by total calcium level greater than 10.4 mg/dL or ionized concentration greater than 5.6 mg/dL. It most commonly is seen with malignancy (breast cancer most common) or in hyperparathyroidism. Other causes include thiazide diuretics, lithium, familial hypocalciuric hypercalcemia, excess intake, vitamin A and D overdose, and immobilization. Symptoms of hypercalcemia include headache, nausea, emesis, altered mental status, lethargy, myalgias, arthralgias, polyuria, and abdominal flank pain secondary to renal stones.

Treatment should be sought for all individuals with total serum concentration greater than 14 mg/dL or those with symptoms. Treatment goals include volume expansion with normal saline (rate of 200 to 300 mL/hr) to dilute concentration and increase renal excretion of fluid (urine output of 100 to 150 mL/hr) and calcium-utilizing furosemide, but only after appropriate volume resuscitation. Treatment with calcitonin (4 IU/kg) can be a useful adjunct for fluid resuscitation with repeat ionized calcium several hours after administration. Calcitonin often is administered along with a bisphosphonate. Bisphosphonates, such as zoledronic acid (4 mg IV over 15 minutes) and pamidronate (60 to 90 mg IV over 2 hours), inhibit osteoclast-induced bone resorption, providing prolonged control with onset of action between 24 and 48 hours. Bisphosphonates are the best choice for long-term calcium control and for hypercalcemia from enhanced bone resorption.

Hypocalcemia

Causes of hypocalcemia are broken into two broad categories: increased efflux from the extracellular space or decreased influx into the extracellular space. Common causes include hypoparathyroidism and vitamin D deficiency. Acid-base disturbances alter protein binding: alkalosis increases albumin affinity for calcium. Severe pancreatitis results in saponification of calcium intravascular, resulting in a hypocalcemic state. Hyperphosphatemia and hypomagnesemia alter calcium homeostasis. In the postoperative period, large volume resuscitation or rapid transfusion of blood products before removal of citrate from blood can result in hypocalcemia.

Symptoms of hypocalcemia include perioral numbness and tingling, hyperreflexia when mechanically stimulating the facial nerve (Chvostek's sign), muscle spasms of the hand and forearm with inflation of a blood pressure cuff proximally (Trousseau's sign), and prolonged QT and arrhythmias on ECG. Treatment should be pursued in the setting of symptoms, total serum calcium below 7.0 mg/dL, or ionized calcium below 3.0 mg/dL. Reflexively treating hypocalcemia regardless of cause can have serious implications; for example, replacement for hypocalcemia caused by hyperphosphatemic precipitation can result in severe vascular calcification formation. Treatment with IV calcium gluconate or calcium chloride should be reserved for cases of severe hypocalcemia or cases with serious symptoms, including overt tetany, laryngospasm, and seizures. Treatment with 10% calcium chloride (27.3 mg Ca^{2+} per mL) provides three times as much elemental calcium as 10% calcium gluconate (9.3 mg Ca^{2+} per mL). Calcium should not be administered at a rate greater than 2.5 to 5 mmol in 20 minutes because of arrhythmia risk. In addition, administration of calcium chloride requires central venous access and a monitored setting to avoid associated bradycardia or hypotension. Oral replacement of calcium can be done through either calcium carbonate (399 mg Ca^{2+} per g) or calcium gluconate (93 mg Ca^{2+} per g). It is important to monitor calcium levels after administration, as certain causes can create ongoing calcium loss and the need for continued replacements. Resistant or severe hypocalcemia may require concurrent vitamin D_3 supplementation. Replacement of magnesium is important, as magnesium deficiency may help to normalize serum calcium levels.

Magnesium

Homeostasis and Clinical Significance

Magnesium is essential for energy metabolism, protein synthesis, and calcium and potassium homeostasis. Magnesium primarily is stored intracellular, with less than 1% contained in the extracellular compartment.

Hypermagnesemia

Hypermagnesemia is a rare event usually seen with burns, trauma, or long-term hemodialysis. Symptoms are uncommon unless serum magnesium levels reach 4.0 mg/dL or greater, with the most common symptom being lethargy. Treatment usually consists of normal saline to expand plasma volume and decrease serum concentration with loop diuretics to induce renal excretion. Severe hypermagnesemia is treated with IV 10% calcium gluconate (10 to 20 mL given over 10 minutes).

Hypomagnesemia

Hypomagnesemia often is seen in the postoperative period secondary to dilution. Patients at high risk for hypomagnesemia include alcoholics and critically ill patients. Alternatively, hypomagnesemia may occur as a result of poor intake or GI losses, including diarrhea and biliary and enteric fistulas. Signs and symptoms rarely occur unless serum levels are below 1.0 mEq/dL. Postoperative monitoring is necessary, as severe hypomagnesemia may cause ventricular arrhythmias such as torsades de pointes. IV therapy with magnesium sulfate ($MgSO_4$) typically is reserved for patients unable to take oral medications, those with severe hypomagnesemia (<1.2 mg/dL), or those with associated arrhythmias.

Magnesium is easily replenished with oral or IV $MgSO_4$. Patients who develop ventricular arrhythmias are treated acutely with bolus doses of IV $MgSO_4$, 1 to 2 g over 3 to 5 minutes.

Phosphorus

Homeostasis and Clinical Significance

Phosphate is important in many of the basic cellular processes within the body. Phosphate levels often are altered in critically ill individuals and in the postoperative setting, given phosphate's role in cellular metabolism. Individuals who have a poor nutritional status, including critically ill individuals, may experience deficient phosphate levels. Approximately 80% of body stores for phosphate reside within bone, with less than 1% within the intravascular compartment. However, the renal system is crucial in homeostasis, as thyroid hormone and insulin favor reabsorption of phosphate whereas parathyroid hormone plays a role in the excretion of excess phosphate. Reabsorption is principally at the proximal tubule through *NPT2* sodium/phosphate transporters.

Hyperphosphatemia

Hyperphosphatemia rarely occurs in the postoperative period. Typically hyperphosphatemia is seen in patients with renal insufficiency and is the result of a deficiency in 1,25-dihydroxyvitamin D production. Typically these patients also experience hypocalcemia from increased precipitation resulting from the elevated phosphate levels. The predominant symptoms associated with hyperphosphatemia are mostly those associated with the hypocalcemic state. Treatment of hyperphosphatemia includes plasma volume expansion with normal saline followed by renal stimulation with acetazolamide. In patients with extremely poor renal function or in severe cases, hemodialysis provides corrective therapy. For those with chronic renal failure with chronic hyperphosphatemia, treatment with phosphate binders such as aluminum hydroxide is standard.

Hypophosphatemia

Symptoms of hypophosphatemia, defined by serum concentrations below 2.5 mg/dL, include left shift in oxygen dissociation, arrhythmias, platelet dysfunction, abnormal glucose metabolism, and respiratory and cardiac failure. Hypophosphatemia is much more common in the postoperative period and among individuals in the intensive care unit. Causes of hypophosphatemia include internal redistribution, deficient intake, or excessive loss. Internal redistribution is the result of increased insulin secretion, epinephrine, acute respiratory alkalosis, or bone hunger. Deficient intake can result from intestinal malabsorption (phosphate-binding medications, GI tract surgery), vitamin D deficiency, or steatorrhea and chronic diarrhea. Increased excretion can result from diuretic therapy (acetazolamide), hyperparathyroidism, and major hepatic resection. Refeeding syndrome occurs with nutritionally depleted individuals after insulin surge resulting from carbohydrate administration. Insulin surges result in redistribution of phosphate intracellular, further lowering serum phosphate levels. Emerging evidence suggests that hypophosphatemia in the setting of liver resection is not the result of increased use but rather a transient hyperphosphaturia secondary to deranged hepatorenal signaling.

Appropriate treatment should include assessment of the cause of hypophosphatemia. The cause is often clinically apparent. However, in cases where the cause is unknown, measurement of urinary phosphate excretion can narrow possible causes. Renal phosphate wasting is suggested by 24-hour urine phosphate of 100 mg or more or iron (III) phosphate ($FePO_4$) of 5% or more. Fractional excretion of phosphate (FEPO4) is calculated as:

$$FEPO4 = ([P]u \times [Cr]pl)/([P]pl \times [Cr]u)$$

where P is phosphorus level, u is urine, pl is plasma, and Cr is creatinine level. Treatment of hypophosphatemia includes either IV or oral replacement with goal serum levels above 2.0 mg/dL. For cases of symptomatic or severe hypophosphatemia (<1.0 mg/dL), treatment with IV phosphate should be utilized until serum levels exceed 1.5 mg/dL, followed by oral therapy. One millimole (mmol) of phosphate equals 31 mg of phosphorus. IV dosing varies, but for most cases 0.25 to 0.50 mmol/kg given over 8 to 12 hours with a maximum dose of 80 mmol is recommended. Oral therapy, administered as a sodium or potassium salt, usually is dosed at 1 mmol/kg of elemental phosphorus (maximum dose of 80 mmol) divided into three doses over 24 hours. In cases where serum phosphate levels are between 1.0 and 1.9 mg/dL, treatment with oral therapy alone is sufficient. Given that only 1% of total body phosphate resides in the intravascular compartment, continuous therapy with phosphate for 5 to 7 days is often indicated. Replacement in patients with renal failure should be done judiciously given the significant risk for development of hyperphosphatemia.

■ SUMMARY

Fluid status and electrolyte disorders (Table 4) are complex clinical problems that require frequent assessment and correction in critically ill patients. Stable postoperative patients do not mandate frequent electrolyte measurements and small corrections, as this provides no overall clinical benefit. Each patient is unique, with different factors playing a central role in appropriate resuscitation and maintenance. Resuscitation often results in excess sodium loads that can be troublesome for patients with comorbid conditions. Therefore every patient deserves daily reassessment to develop an appropriate fluid and electrolyte plan with adjustments as clinically necessary.

TABLE 4: Signs, Symptoms, and Treatment of Electrolyte Disorders

Disorder	Neurologic	Cardiovascular	Gastrointestinal	Renal	Therapy
Hyponatremia	Confusion, seizures, coma	Hypotension, hypertension	Salivation	Oliguria	Fluid resuscitation 0.9% NaCl Hypertonic saline + diuretic
Hypernatremia	Confusion, seizures, coma	Fluid overload	Thirst		Free water 0.45% NaCl
Hypokalemia	Fatigue, weakness	Atrial arrhythmias, flat T waves or U waves	Ileus	Nephrotoxicity	Oral/IV potassium Magnesium replacement
Hyperkalemia	Confusion, paralysis, areflexia	Ventricular arrhythmias, peaked T wave, prolonged PT, wide QRS	Nausea, vomiting, abdominal pain		Insulin + 50% dextrose 10% Calcium gluconate
Hypocalcemia	Paresthesia, perioral tingling, carpopedal spasms, Chvostek's sign	Ventricular arrhythmias, prolonged QT interval			IV calcium gluconate 1,25-Dihydroxyvitamin D
Hypercalcemia	Confusion, fatigue, coma	Shortened QT	Abdominal pain	Renal stones, nephrogenic DI (long term)	0.9% NaCl Furosemide
Hypomagnesemia	Weakness, cramping, hyperreflexia	Atrial ventricular arrhythmias (torsades de pointes)	Dysphagia		IV magnesium Magnesium sulfate
Hypermagnesemia	Sedation, paralysis, areflexia	Atrial, ventricular arrhythmias	Diarrhea		0.9% NaCl Furosemide
Hypophosphatemia	Confusion, seizures, weakness	Heart failure, respiratory failure			Sodium or potassium phosphate
Hyperphosphatemia	Symptoms of hypocalcemia				0.9% NaCl Diuretics Acetazolamide

DI, Diabetes insipidus; *IV,* intravenous; *NaCl,* sodium chloride.

SUGGESTED READINGS

Gumz ML, Rabinowitz L, Wingo CS. An integrated view of potassium homeostasis. *N Engl J Med.* 2015;373:60-72.

Jacob M, Chappell D, Rehm M. Clinical update: perioperative fluid management. *Lancet.* 2007;369:1984-1986.

Myburgh JA, Mythen MG. Resuscitation fluids. *N Engl J Med.* 2013;369:1243-1251.

Seifter JL. Integration of acid-base and electrolyte disorders. *N Engl J Med.* 2014;371:1821-1831.

Sterns RH. Disorders of plasma sodium—causes, consequences, and correction. *N Engl J Med.* 2015;372:55-65.

FRAILTY AND THE SURGICAL CARE OF THE OLDER ADULT

Thomas N. Robinson, MD, MS,
and Michael E. Zenilman, MD

Surgical decision making and care for the oldest-old patient requires surgeons to abandon the traditional framework in which operative care is delivered. Long-term survival as a primary goal of undergoing an operation may be superseded by the desire to palliate symptoms. Similarly, the 30-day morbidity and mortality risk may be less significant than the risk of loss of functional independence requiring long-term or permanent stay at a nursing home. Given that nearly 40% of all inpatient operations in the United States are performed on patients aged 65 years or older, understanding the unique preoperative decision making and postoperative management of older adults is vital to providing optimal surgical care.

Older adults are vulnerable to poor surgical outcomes because of frailty. Traditional preoperative evaluation and management focuses on single end organ dysfunction, most notably represented by the American Heart Association guidelines for perioperative cardiovascular evaluation (cardiac risk in noncardiac surgery). Although this strategy is equally important for the oldest old, the additional step of quantifying frailty is imperative because it defines the need for unique preoperative decision making and identifies patients who will benefit from postoperative geriatric specialized care pathways.

The clinical assessment of frailty used for preoperative risk stratification of the geriatric patient should supplement but not replace traditional assessment of critical end organs. For example, an older patient with unstable coronary disease or uncompensated liver disease has high operative risk irrespective of the presence of frailty. The remainder of this chapter focuses on the clinical characteristics unique to the geriatric patient that are useful in preoperative risk stratification (Figure 1).

The purpose of this chapter is twofold: (1) to understand frailty and the measurement of frailty in the surgical context, and (2) to describe preoperative and postoperative geriatric specialty care beneficial to the frail older adult.

■ IMPORTANCE OF FRAILTY

Older adults with baseline preoperative frailty have poor surgical outcomes. By definition, frail older adults have poor healthcare outcomes, and this fact is particularly profound in the postoperative setting. Multiple studies across a range of surgical disciplines consistently relate baseline preoperative frailty to poor surgical outcomes, including increased serious complications, prolonged length of stay, need for discharge to an institutional care facility, hospital readmission, 30-day mortality, and 1-year mortality.

■ CONCEPTUALIZING FRAILTY

Frailty is defined as a state of reduced physiologic reserve associated with increased susceptibility to disability. Frailty is conceptualized in two different ways, as follows:

1. The muscle-based definition of frailty, so-called "phenotypic frailty," views frailty as a biologic syndrome that can be quantified by measuring unintentional weight loss, poor grip strength weakness, slow walking speed, self-reported exhaustion, and low activity levels. Phenotypic frailty is used most commonly by gerontologists in research.
2. The accumulation of deficits definition of frailty, the so-called "frailty index," views frailty as a nonspecific age-associated vulnerability that is reflected in an accumulation of medical, social, and functional deficits. Accumulation of deficits frailty is measured by counting an individual's health problems or deficits. Although the Canadian Study of Health and Aging is the most widely recognized frailty index, many frailty indexes are used in the surgical populations. Frailty indexes are used in the clinical setting.

Because the accumulation of deficits or "frailty index" is clinically accessible, this chapter focuses on describing this conceptualization in the context of surgery.

■ MEASURING FRAILTY

To move from a qualitative appreciation of frailty to a calculated quantitative determination of frailty, the surgeon must measure individual frailty characteristics in preoperative clinic and then sum the total number of frailty traits present in an older patient. A higher number of frailty deficits correlates with decreased physiologic reserve to withstand the operative stress and poor surgical outcomes. Typical frailty assessment strategies define the presence of frailty when a threshold number of deficits, usually three or more, are present. "Pre-frail" or "relative frailty" occurs when frailty traits are present but do not reach the threshold required for the diagnosis of frailty (e.g., two frailty deficits are present and three are required for the diagnosis). Both pre-frail and frail patients are predisposed to adverse outcomes in comparison with the nonfrail population.

Frailty traits useful in the preoperative risk stratification of older surgical patients include markers of (1) disability (function), (2) comorbidity burden, (3) nutrition, (4) mobility, (5) cognition, (6) exhaustion, and (7) social vulnerability. The subsequent text describing each marker of frailty is meant to supplement Table 1, which provides a practical, "hands-on" guide on how to administer and score the frailty assessment tools recommended for implementation in a surgeon's practice.

1. *Disability* is defined as difficulty or dependence in one or more activities of daily living. Activities of daily living (often referred to as ADL) describe six tasks necessary for independent living: bathing, dressing, transferring, walking, toileting, and feeding. Disability has emerged as an important risk for mortality, need for postoperative institutionalization, and ultimately higher healthcare costs. Bathing is typically the first activity of daily living that requires assistance. Excellent tools to assess functional

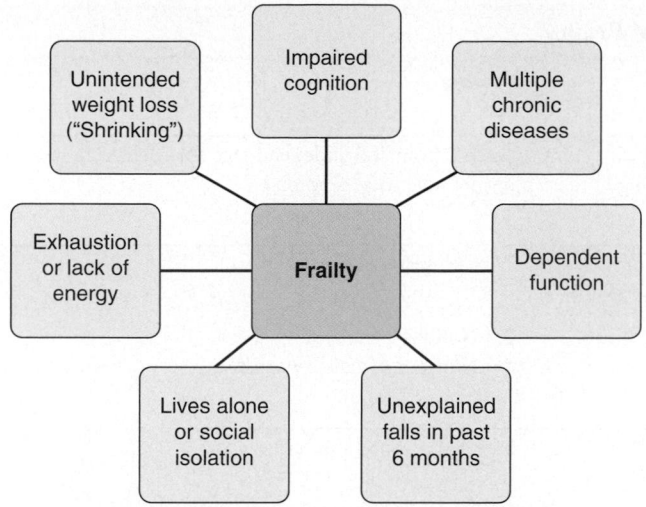

FIGURE 1 Characteristics of the frail older adult.

dependence include the Katz Index of Independence in Activities of Daily Living and the Barthel Index of Activities of Daily Living.

2. *Chronic disease burden* is a recognized characteristic of frailty. Multimorbidity is defined as the presence of two or more disease processes. Review of Medicare databases reveals that two thirds of individuals in the United States 65 years and older have two or more chronic diseases, and that one third have four or more chronic diseases. The Charlson Comorbidity Index quantifies burden of chronic disease by addressing 19 categories of comorbidity and assigning a weighted value to each comorbidity based on risk of 1-year mortality. The Charlson Index has proven utility for risk stratifying older patients preoperatively.

3. *Malnutrition* occurs in the oldest old because of the physiologic anorexia of aging and the associated sarcopenia. An older individual's unexplained weight loss therefore can be a result of a medical illness and lack of interest in eating or even failure to feed. Weight loss of 10 lb in the previous 6 months is used to measure malnutrition. A low preoperative albumin level is a well-recognized predictive factor of adverse postoperative outcomes in surgical patients. Results from the National Veterans Affairs Surgical Risk Study found that low albumin level was the most important preoperative predictor for 30-day postoperative mortality.

4. *Mobility* can be measured by a recent history of falls and the Timed Up and Go Test. Timed Up and Go allows the surgeon to observe an older patient's mobility while the patient performs tasks of standing, walking, and turning. This test reliably determines functional mobility and has prognostic validity for predicting falls. A time of 15 seconds has been found to be predictive of increased complications and higher 1-year mortality. As a single test, Timed Up and Go predicts phenotypic frailty with high accuracy. A recent history of unexplained falls signals frailty because falling represents the expression of a multifactorial geriatric syndrome relating to loss of sensory input, central proprioception, and musculoskeletal function. A study has linked the presence of one or more unexplained falls in the 6 months before an operation to both postdischarge institutionalization and 6-month mortality.

5. *Cognition* is a term that describes "process of thought." Dementia is the progressive, long-term cognitive decline that is a normal part of aging and affects areas of memory, attention, language, and problem solving. Dementia must be distinguished from delirium, which is an acute-onset confusional state that occurs after a physiologic stress and must be worked up in the postoperative state. Dementia screening should be performed before elective surgery to obtain accurate baseline assessment. Dementia screening cannot be performed accurately in a patient who is stressed

(e.g., an individual who is having emergent surgery or an individual after a surgical intervention). Multiple screening tools exist for cognitive dysfunction, most notably the Mini-Mental State Examination and the Mini-Cog test.

6. *Exhaustion*, or fatigue, describes an individual's motivation and effort. Question the patient as to whether he or she agrees with these statements: "I felt that everything I did was an effort" and "I could not get going." If the patient agrees with these statements, the characteristic of exhaustion is present. The rate of developing exhaustion is thought to increase as frailty progresses.

7. *Social vulnerability* refers to an individual's inability to withstand a stressor from a social standpoint. Factors composing social vulnerability include social support (e.g., marital status, living alone) and social engagement (e.g., frequency of contact with family and friends, pets). Although surgeons commonly do not think about the relationship of social vulnerability and adverse outcomes, greater social vulnerability is associated with increased 5-year mortality in community-based geriatric studies. Intuitively, social vulnerability likely affects the need to change immediate postdischarge care plans, whether by requiring home health care or temporary institutional care.

IMPLEMENTING FRAILTY ASSESSMENT IN A SURGICAL PRACTICE

The goal of implementing a preoperative frailty scoring system in a surgeon's office is to discriminate the highly vulnerable aged patient from the older patient with average risk. Defining an older adult as frail should change the perioperative care. Table 1 reviews simple clinical tools that assess, score, and quantify the various clinical characteristics necessary to diagnose frailty. These frailty characteristic tests can be administered and interpreted by nonspecialists.

The practicing surgeon can implement preoperative frailty screening in their practice without excessive burden. The healthcare professional who takes vital signs should perform and record the assessment of frailty characteristics in every preoperative patient aged 65 years and older. The time to complete a frailty assessment can range from less than 10 minutes to longer than 30 minutes, depending on the frailty tool used. We recommend creating a template scoring sheet that allows the assessor to rapidly mark or circle the score achieved for each test. Immediately before the preoperative consultation, the surgeon reviews this scoring sheet by glancing at each frailty measurement and summing the total number of frailty deficits present. The total number of frailty deficits present in an individual older patient is determined by the total number of positive test scores achieved. By understanding that higher numbers of positive frailty deficits correspond to increasing physiologic compromise, this frailty assessment provides the surgeon with prognostic information about the older patient just before the preoperative consultation during which the decision to operate or not is made.

MODIFYING MANAGEMENT OF THE FRAIL PATIENT

Establishing the diagnosis of frailty in an older adult who is considering surgery must result in changes to the preoperative, intraoperative and postoperative care of the high-risk patient. Frailty establishes an older adult's increased vulnerability to adverse surgical outcomes. This increased risk for poor outcomes includes not only higher 30-day morbidity to traditional surgical complications, but also increased susceptibility to adverse outcomes that are specific to the geriatric population, such as functional decline. The goals of interventions for frail older adults shift from the traditional ones of minimizing short-term morbidity and maximizing long-term survival (Figure 2). Instead, the goals of undergoing an operation for a frail older adult may focus on preserving quality of life in the setting of limited life expectancy and minimizing the risk of catastrophic complications.

TABLE 1: Simple Tools to Measure the Characteristics of Frailty

	How to Administer Test	Scoring
FUNCTION		
Katz ADL score	Ask about dependence in each of six ADL: bathing, grooming, feeding, toileting, dressing, transferring	Score 1 point for independence for each ADL (possible total 6 points)
MOBILITY		
Timed Up and Go	Timed activity: rise from hard chair (without use of arms), walk 10 feet, turn, and return to sitting in chair	Time in seconds
Falls	Ask: "How many times have you fallen in the previous 6 months?"	0 = No falls # = Number of falls reported
COMORBIDITY		
Charlson Index	Record conditions with assigned values: Myocardial infarction (1) Heart failure (1) Peripheral vascular disease (1) Cerebrovascular disease (1) Dementia (1) COPD (1) Connective tissue disease (1) Ulcer disease (1) Mild liver disease (1) Diabetes (1) Hemiplegia (2) Moderate to severe renal disease (2) Diabetes with end organ damage (2) Any tumor (2) Leukemia (2) Lymphoma (2) Moderate to severe liver disease (3) Metastatic solid tumor (6) AIDS (6)	Sum values to obtain point score
NUTRITION		
Recent weight loss	Review weight over time for unexplained weight loss	Calculate weight differential over previous 6 months
Albumin	Serum albumin	Laboratory value (g/dL)
COGNITION		
Mini-Cog test	1. Ask to remember three words: "apple, table, penny" 2. Ask to draw clock, with all numbers and hands at 11:10 3. Ask to recall three words	Three-item recall: 1 point per word (possible total 3 points) Clock draw: 2 = accurate clock 0 = abnormal clock
SOCIAL VULNERABILITY		
Social isolation	Does patient live alone? Does patient regularly interact with other people? Does the patient have someone to count on when he or she gets sick?	Yes/No
EXHAUSTION		
Fatigue	Everything is an effort. Could not get going.	Yes/No

ADL, Activities of daily living; *AIDS*, acquired immunodeficiency syndrome; *COPD*, chronic obstructive pulmonary disease.

Prehabilitation

Prehabilitation describes an intervention designed to increase physiologic reserve before an operation with the goal of allowing the patient to better tolerate the operative stress. The most common strategy is preoperative exercise therapy consisting of strength training, endurance training, or a combination of both. Although this approach intuitively makes sense, the results of clinical trials have not consistently shown clinical benefit of preoperative exercise therapy compared with usual care. Reasons for the lack of efficacy may include the limited window of time before the operation and improper patient inclusion criteria. The one exercise training

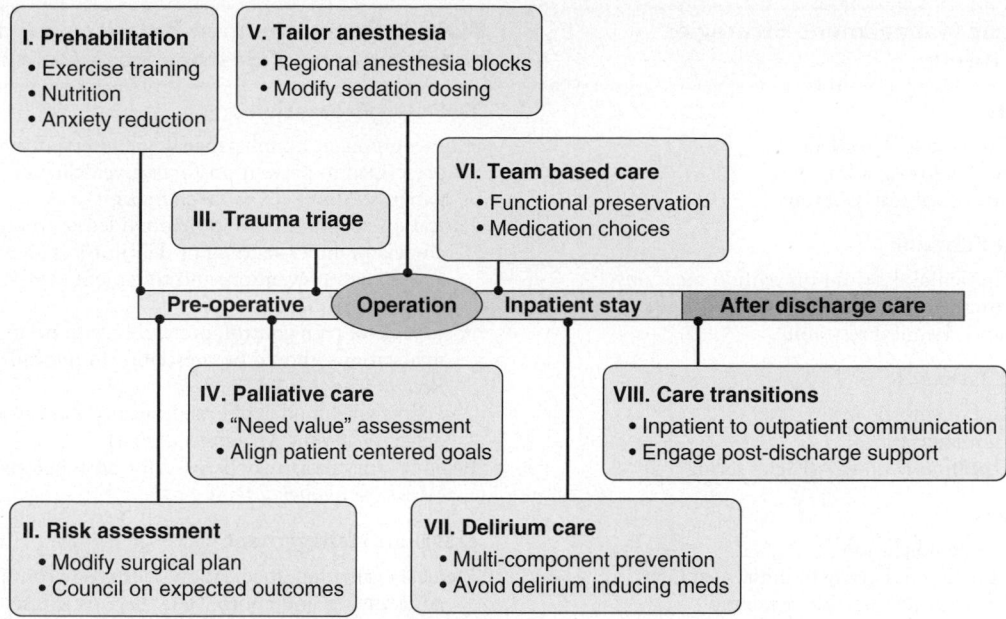

FIGURE 2 Interventions to improve surgical outcomes in frail older adults.

intervention shown to decrease postoperative complications is daily incentive spirometry for at least 2 weeks, which has been shown to decrease pulmonary complications.

In addition to single-modal physical training, multimodal strategies for prehabilitation have been proposed. Common interventions include nutritional supplementation, anxiety reduction, smoking cessation, and medication reconciliation. A critical factor perceived as vital to making any prehabilitation protocol work is selecting patients with depleted physiologic reserve at baseline that is amenable to improvement who are not so compromised that they cannot tolerate a prehabilitation protocol.

Trauma Triage

Geriatric trauma accounts for a major percentage of all trauma consultations. The specific mechanism of an unexpected fall from standing height is of particular importance to the frail population. A fall is one of the five described geriatric syndromes. The importance of a geriatric syndrome is that it is a clinical symptom that commonly is seen in the physiologically vulnerable frail older adult preceding death. A trauma-specific frailty assessment that uses the accumulation of deficits conceptualization exists and is performed on initial examination of older adult trauma victims. This baseline trauma frailty assessment is able to forecast which patients require discharge to an institutional care setting.

Risk Assessment

Risk assessment using frailty is best established before elective operations. A positive preoperative frailty assessment predicts poor surgical outcomes, including complications, mortality, length of stay, and need for discharge to a facility other than home. There are two ways in which measuring frailty before an operation can modify preoperative care: (1) Accurate counseling on poor expected postoperative outcomes can be provided. Instead of focusing solely on postoperative morbidity and mortality, clinicians can counsel older adults on postoperative functional and quality of life outcomes. Knowledge of the need for a postdischarge nursing home stay and increased risk of complications prepares patients and families for the postoperative course. (2) The presence of baseline frailty can modify the surgeon's decision about the extent of the planned operative procedure. Tailoring of surgical recommendations to the actual physiologic capacity of the patient is important. Offering frail patients less extensive

operations (e.g., minimally invasive, endoscopic or endovascular) may allow preservation of postprocedure function while still affording palliation of the main symptoms.

Palliative Care Approaches

Assessment of the "need value" of an operation is important for frail older adults. Palliative care takes a multidisciplinary approach to helping patients define their care goals, with a primary focus on improving quality of life. The palliative care approach does not have the intention to cure as the most important factor in determining whether an operation is in the best interest of the patient. This mindset is a significant departure from the traditional approach of counseling patients solely on 30-day morbidity. The proactive use of palliative care in the preoperative setting to help the patient decide whether to proceed with an operation is useful. Allowing palliative care to help align the patient's surgical decision with his or her patient-centered goals provides insight that supplements the surgeon's consultation.

Tailored Anesthesia Regimen

There currently is no established evidence-based anesthesia regimen for frail older adults. However, the intraoperative time point is clearly a major event. Using adjuvant regional anesthesia and minimizing overall doses of sedative medications are widely thought to be beneficial in vulnerable older adults. Light sedation intraoperatively may provide benefit by reducing postoperative delirium, but the risks versus benefits of this approach have not been established fully. Minimizing intraoperative total fluid intake is another strategy of potential benefit to the older adult in the operating room.

Team-Based Care Pathways

Interdisciplinary team-based inpatient care for older adults improves outcomes. For inpatients, the Acute Care for Elders (ACE) model and the Hospital Elder Life Program (HELP) are both recognized to improve hospital outcomes for older adult medical patients. The ACE model uses a unit-based geriatric ward, with the main emphasis on preserving function during the hospital stay. Proven benefits of ACE units include fewer falls, decreased delirium, functional preservation, and shorter hospital stays in comparison with usual care. The HELP involves a skilled interdisciplinary team with geriatric expertise to

BOX 1: Inpatient Management Strategies for Frail Older Adults

Preserve Mobility

- Prescribe mandatory activity orders
- Consult physical therapy on admission
- Avoid physical and chemical restraint

Preserve Mental Function

- Prescribe environmental delirium prevention measures
- Avoid precipitating delirium
- Avoid physical and chemical restraint

Avoid Iatrogenic Issues

- Minimize invasive diagnostic testing
- Remove excess lines and tubes
- Avoid Beers medication (rational drug ordering)

Preserve Function

- Evaluate function on admission
- Link inpatient functional therapy to initial evaluation
- Provide handrails and walking aids as needed

Address Nutrition

- Evaluate nutritional status on admission
- Prescribe nutritional supplements
- Order swallow evaluation

Manage Depression and Anxiety

- Assess mood and anxiety on admission
- Implement behavioral and environmental interventions
- Encourage family socialization

BOX 2: Recommended Practices for the Prevention and Treatment of Postoperative Delirium

Delirium Prevention

Multicomponent nonpharmacologic intervention should be prescribed to prevent postoperative delirium in at-risk patients (*Strong Recommendation*)

Education programs should be provided to improve the clinician's understanding of delirium's epidemiology, assessment, prevention, and treatment (*Strong Recommendation*)

Postoperative pain control, preferably with nonopioid pain medications, should be prescribed to minimize pain (*Strong Recommendation*)

The clinician should avoid medications that cause postoperative delirium (*Strong Recommendation*)

Regional anesthesia may be used for postoperative pain control (*Weak Recommendation*)

Delirium Management

Medical evaluation, medication and/or environmental adjustments, and appropriate diagnostic tests and consultations should be performed in patients with delirium (*Strong Recommendation*)

Benzodiazepines should not be prescribed as first-line pharmacologic treatment choice for delirium (*Strong Recommendation*)

Pharmacologic treatment with antipsychotics or benzodiazepine medications should be reserved only for patients with severe agitation at risk for harm to self or others (*Strong Recommendation*)

Antipsychotics at the lowest effective dose for the shortest possible duration may be used to treat patients who have failed behavioral interventions, who are severely agitated or distressed, and who are threatening substantial harm to self or others (*Weak Recommendation*)

Data from American Geriatrics Society Clinical Practice Guideline for Postoperative Delirium in Older Adults. Publisher: American Geriatrics Society. 2014.

implement protocols focusing on early mobilization, sleep enhancement, therapeutic cognitive and physical activities, and provider education. Benefits of the program include delirium prevention, functional preservation, fewer falls, and decreased nursing home placement at discharge. Multicomponent, multidisciplinary geriatric care pathways will become commonplace given the demographics of hospitalization required by older adults (Box 1).

Delirium Prevention and Treatment

Baseline preoperative frailty is associated with the development of postoperative delirium. The presentation of delirium, particularly the hypoactive delirium motor subtype, is the most common postoperative complication in frail older adults. Delirium is an important outcome in older persons because of its close association with increased postoperative complications, prolonged length of stay, increased need for discharge to a skilled nursing facility or nursing home, and death. Risk factors for delirium are essentially the same as the clinical characteristics of the frail patient. Delirium risk factors include advanced age, dementia, high burden of chronic diseases, poor nutrition, functional dependence, and polypharmacy. Delirium is important to understand because one third of all hospitalized delirium is preventable. A recent high-quality guideline statement outlined multiple strong recommendations for both the prevention and the treatment of postoperative delirium (Box 2).

Care Transition

Careful discharge planning for older adults minimizes readmissions and suboptimal outpatient care after discharge. Approximately 20% of all Medicare beneficiaries require readmission within 30 days after hospital discharge. Poor communication between inpatient and outpatient caregivers, changes in medication regimen, and new care responsibilities all account for readmissions. Frail older adults are at particularly high risk for readmission. Strategies to optimize postdischarge care and minimize readmissions include effective education regarding medication prescriptions, communication between inpatient and outpatient clinicians, engagement of social support, and close medical follow-up.

■ SUMMARY

As surgeons, we must embrace the aging population as a demographic inevitability and recognize the unique vulnerabilities of the older adult patient to improve our surgical care of the oldest old. Measuring frailty during the preoperative assessment provides evidence of global loss of physiologic reserve for the vulnerable older adult. The diagnosis of frailty should lead to specific management strategies aimed to improve the surgical care of frail geriatric patients.

SUGGESTED READINGS

American Geriatrics Society Expert Panel on Postoperative Delirium in Older Adults. American Geriatrics Society abstracted clinical practice guideline for postoperative delirium in older adults. *J Am Geriatr Soc.* 2015;63: 142-150.

Fried LP, Tangen CM, Walston J, Newman AB, Hirsch C, Gottdiener J, Seeman T, Tracy R, Kop WJ, Burke G, McBurnie MA, Cardiovascular Health Study Collaborative Research Group. Frailty in older adults: evidence for a phenotype. *J Gerontol A Biol Sci Med Sci.* 2001;56:M146-M156.

Inouye SK, Bogardus ST Jr, Baker DI, Leo-Summers L, Cooney LM Jr. The Hospital Elder Life Program: a model of care to prevent cognitive and functional decline in older hospitalized patients. Hospital Elder Life Program. *J Am Geriatr Soc.* 2000;48:1697-1706.

Landefeld CS, Palmer RM, Kresevic DM, Fortinsky RH, Kowal J. A randomized trial of care in a hospital medical unit especially designed to improve the functional outcomes of acutely ill older patients. *N Engl J Med.* 1995;332:1338-1344.

Robinson TN, Eiseman B, Wallace JI, Church SD, McFann KK, Pfister SM, Sharp TJ, Moss M. Redefining geriatric preoperative assessment using frailty, disability and co-morbidity. *Ann Surg.* 2009;250: 449-455.

PREOPERATIVE PREPARATION OF THE SURGICAL PATIENT

Jerry Stonemetz, MD

Health care is striving towards value-based purchasing rather than volume based under the assumption that this will result in better outcomes for patients. Various methodologies have been devised to revise reimbursement to achieve better focus on outcomes, including accountable care organizations (ACOs), bundled payments, and the medical home. One of the basic tenets of these activities is to make individual health care more patient centered rather than provider or facility centered.

There is likely no better example of how to make this transition than the standardized form letters that surgical patients receive from their surgeons. Examples of adverse patient events originate from these instructions when the patient has cardiac stents but has been advised to stop aspirin 7 to 10 days before surgery; or the ubiquitous nil per os (NPO) after midnight when the patient has insulin-dependent diabetes. Specific patient instructions taking into account the patient's comorbidities and medication list are needed; however, they represent a significant change from current workflow.

■ PERIOPERATIVE SURGICAL HOME

In this chapter we discuss an approach to converting your preoperative routine to being more patient centered and more aligned with better postoperative outcomes. One concept we discuss is the perioperative surgical home. This approach has been described in detail by the national society for anesthesiologists, the American Society of Anesthesiology (ASA). Essentially, this "home" is similar in design to the medical home in that it calls for a patient advocate to collate and manage the preoperative, intraoperative, and postoperative course for the patient. These advocates may be anesthesiologists, surgeons, or even physician-extenders such as nurse practitioners or physician assistants. These individuals oversee a process that is more proactive in the preparation of the patient for surgery as well as more focused on outcomes during surgery and postoperative care (Figure 1).

A perfect example of how this may work is the development of protocols such as enhanced recovery after surgery (ERAS), originally designed by colorectal surgeons, and now being spread to other surgical specialties (Table 1). These patients are prescribed a very standard protocol involving things such as consumption of clear liquids and a carbohydrate load 2 hours before surgery. Frequently, they are given instructions to consume 20 ounces of Gatorade in the parking garage before they enter the hospital on the day of surgery. This obviously will be confusing when the patient has been given instructions to remain NPO after midnight.

Development of ERAS protocols also typically use standardized anesthetic pathways, such as regional blocks for postoperative pain management with the reduction or elimination of opiates for pain control. At Johns Hopkins, we have deployed these protocols for our colorectal patients and seen a significant improvement in length of stay as well as other adverse outcomes. We now are deploying these same protocols to hepatobiliary, urology, plastics, and other specialties. Clearly, even standardized protocols may need revisions or alterations depending upon the patient's medical condition. For example, some patients may not be appropriate candidates for an epidural despite the advantage of using this regional block for pain management. What is essential is that every patient must be managed appropriately for his or her condition and functional capability. Possibly the most important aspect of management should address the postoperative care. Do your patients have the social support necessary to ensure adequate management after discharge, or will they become a readmission secondary to surgical infections, DVT/PE, or cardiac events? Too many patients suffer adverse events because they have not resumed their antiplatelet therapies, DVT prophylaxis, or normal medication regimens. Not infrequently, patients return to the primary care providers on different medications, and no indications as to why they are now on something different.

Even without a surgical home, there are steps that can be implemented to make the preoperative preparation more patient centered. Ideally, all surgical patients should receive contact in some manner to allow customization of their preoperative instructions. In many facilities this involves a phone call. This call should be attempted within 48 hours of scheduling, which allows more time to define how to optimize the patient. The call or some other method of capturing a subset of clinical information, such as medications, allergies, and functional capacity, allows for appropriate triage of these patients. Many will be able to come directly to surgery after obtaining specific lab tests or studies, whereas others will require a more involved approach, such as an appointment with a preoperative clinic if one exists in your facility. Figure 2 provides a graphical triage approach to scheduling preoperative clinic visits.

■ ONLINE PRESURGICAL QUESTIONNAIRE

In reality, most facilities are not prepared to staff enough nurses or similar providers to make all these calls. Fortunately, we now have technology to facilitate the collection of clinical data during the preoperative period. Most electronic health records contain patient portals, such as Epic's My Chart or Cerner's Patient Portal, which can be used to attempt to collect some of this information from the patient. This would require some extensive development by your hospital or facility IT staff and may not be feasible in your practice. Other vendors exist that specialize in the preoperative questionnaire and are easier to deploy, albeit at a cost to the facility. Table 2 outlines several of the more notable vendors in this space.

These questionnaires typically are initiated once a patient is scheduled for surgery. The patient receives either a link to log into via e-mail or a text message on their phones. If the online form is not completed within a specific period of time, the patient is sent reminders. Obviously, it will be important to capture e-mail and cell phone numbers for patients for this to occur. There has been concern that not all patients will be capable of answering these online questionnaires, but data seem to suggest that it is infrequent that patients are not able to complete the questionnaire, or at least procure help to complete them.

Conceptually, once patients complete this questionnaire, it is feasible to rank patients according to a rating system that defines how

PERIOPERATIVE SURGICAL HOME OVERVIEW*

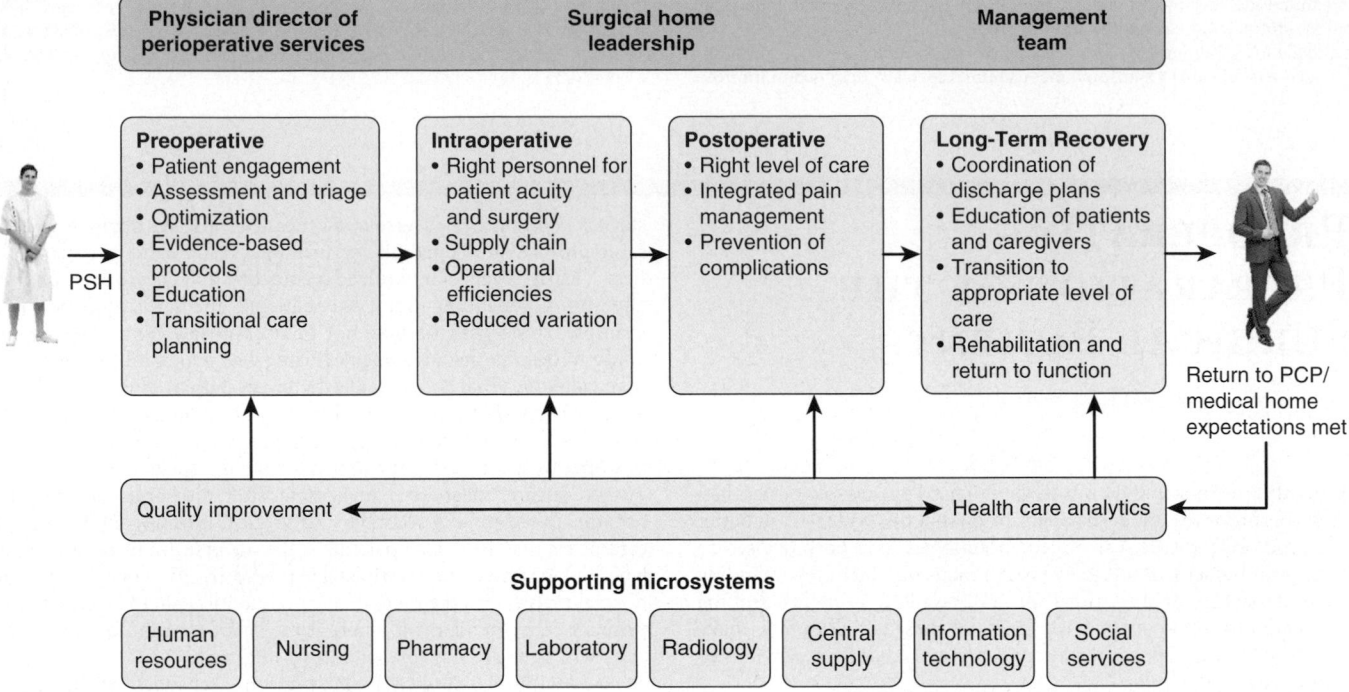

In the PSH model, the patient's experience of care is coordinated by a director of perioperative services, additional surgical home leadership and supportive personnel, which constitutes an interdisciplinary team. The expected metrics include improved operational efficiencies, decreased resource utilization, a reduction in length of stay and readmission, and a decrease in complications and mortality—resulting in a better patient experience of care.

*Figure developed by Daniel J. Cole, M.D.

FIGURE 1 Perioperative surgical home overview chart. *(Used with permission from the American Society of Anesthesiologists.)*

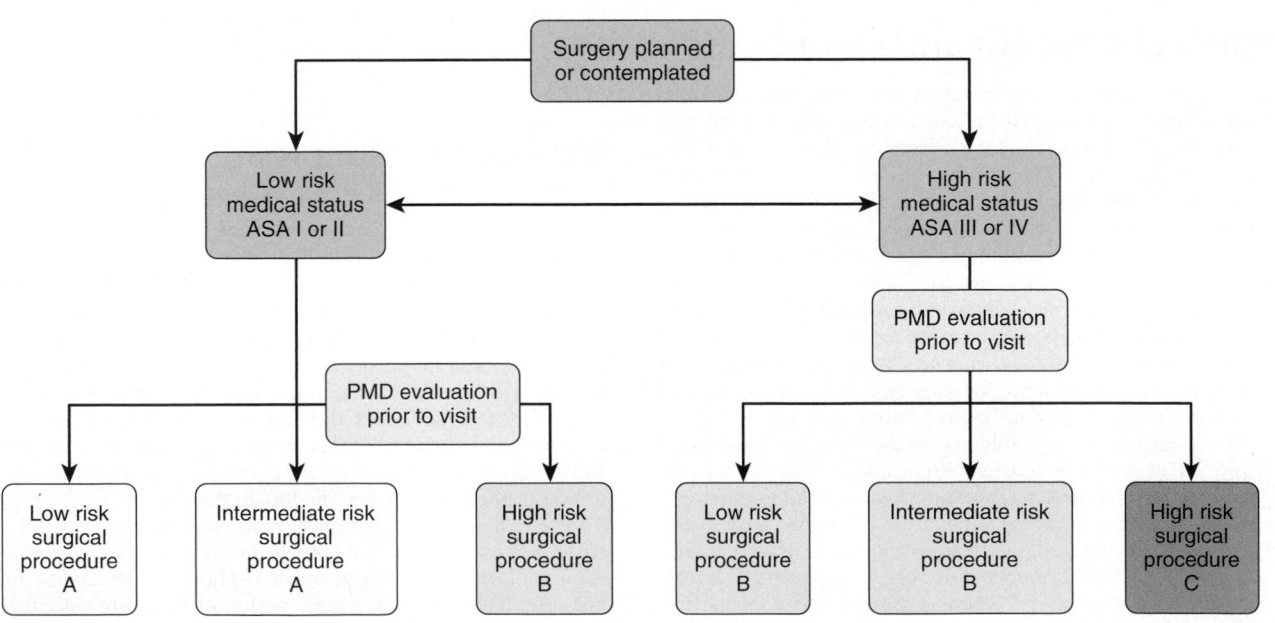

A A – May have preanesthesia assessment done day of surgery

B B – Recommend preanesthesia assessment with PEC visit at least 24 hours preoperatively. Should have an evaluation done prior to PEC visit by PMD.

C C – Recommend Preanesthesia Consult scheduled in PEC at least 48 hours preoperatively. Should have an evaluation done prior to anesthesia consult by PMD.

FIGURE 2 Preoperative triage of surgical patients.

TABLE 1: Integrative Pathways for Enhanced Recovery After Surgery

Before Surgery	Day of Surgery	Inpatient Recovery	Outpatient Recovery
Preoperative counseling about surgery, anesthesia, pain management and recovery plan	Preoperative multimodal analgesia and postoperative nausea and vomiting prevention	Early ambulation protocol	Phone call from hospital nurse to review discharge instructions 2 days after hospital discharge
Facilitate smoking cessation if appropriate (SSI prevention)	Preoperative VTE prophylaxis (before incision or 1 hour after epidural placement if applicable) (VTE prevention)	Urinary catheter removal on postoperative day 1 if no epidural; removal on day 2 if epidural or pelvic procedure (CAUTI prevention)	Referral to home health care agency for transition to home if new ostomy
Preoperative visiting with enterostomal therapist if ostomy planned for procedure	Maintenance of normothermia by preoperative and intraoperative forced air warming devices (SSI prevention)	Discontinue intravenous fluids	Return office visit in 10-14 days with surgeon and enterostomal therapist (if applicable)
Mechanical bowel preparation with oral antibiotics (SSI prevention)	Prophylactic antibiotic administration (cefotetan 2 gm or clindamycin 600 mg and gentamicin 5 mg/kg) before incision and redosed per recommendations during procedure (SSI prevention)	Rapid resumption of regular oral intake	
Chlorhexidine bathing (SSI prevention)	Intraoperative anesthesia management protocol (epidural anesthesia, total intravenous anesthesia, colloid and crystalloid protocol to reduce total intravenous fluids, avoid immunosuppressive agents)	Multimodal analgesia (with or without epidural analgesia) delivered by acute pain team (physicians and nurses)	
Continue oral intake until 2 hr before surgery (anesthesia guidelines)	Avoidance of urinary catheter placement for procedures less than 2 hours (CAUTI prevention) Mobilization to a chair and resumption of oral intake	Risk-stratified VTE prophylaxis (VTE prevention) Education by enterostomal therapist about ostomy (if applicable)	

Courtesy Johns Hopkins Colorectal Surgery.

CAUTI, Catheter-associated urinary tract infection; *SSI*, surgical site infection; *VTE*, venous thromboembolism.

TABLE 2: Vendors of Preoperative Questionnaires

Vendors	URL	Costs
ePreop	http://epreop.com/	Typically a "per click" cost. May be able to arrange for volume discounting
One Medical Passport	https://www.onemedicalpassport.com/	Typically a "per click" cost. May be able to arrange for volume discounting
My Medical File	https://www.mmf.com/	Usually free if subscribed to indexing service
Medsleuth	http://www.medsleuth.com/	Typically a "per click" cost. May be able to arrange for volume discounting
HealthQuest, Cleveland Clinic	https://eweb4.ccf.org/HQCQSurvey/PTLogin.aspx	Not commercially available

URL, Uniform resource locator.

to triage patients. Healthy patients with low-risk surgical procedures should be able to bypass further evaluations by the team. Sicker patients should be cued up for evaluation to allow patient-specific testing and instructions. Obviously this still requires personnel, but the evaluation process is much more streamlined with the clinical data already collected by the online questionnaire.

■ PERIOPERATIVE ROADMAP

For those who cannot convince their facilities to adopt an online questionnaire, a manual process can be put into place. Again, we should endeavor to contact 100% of all surgical patients in some format. One option is to have a brief questionnaire completed at the time of surgical posting that provides enough clinical information to allow effective triage of patients. Attached to the end of this chapter are appendixes that come from our perioperative roadmap that could be customized to your facility with input from anesthesia, nursing, and surgery. This roadmap provides guidance on how to manage surgical patients with specific focus on particular issues that may affect patient's outcomes, such as diabetic management, blood product administration, cardiac stents, and NPO instructions.

Special considerations should be given to the following areas.

Preoperative Roadmap   10

Appendix A: Patient Evaluation Screening Form

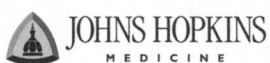

PATIENT IDENTIFICATION INFORMATION

DATE: _____   **Patient Evaluation Screening Form**

Please answer the following questions:		
1. Do you have sleep apnea; use CPAP or Bi-PAP and or told you need a "sleep study"?	□YES	□NO
2. Do you have difficulty climbing stairs or walking 4 blocks? ➤ If YES, what stops you? *(Check all that apply)*	□YES	□NO
Chest pain □YES Shortness of breath □YES Pain □YES Other:		
3. Do you have high blood pressure that requires three or more medications to manage?	□YES	□NO
4. Have you ever had a blood clot, stroke, carotid blockage or TIA (mini stroke)?	□YES	□NO
5. Are you currently taking blood thinners, such as Aspirin, Coumadin, Plavix, etc.?	□YES	□NO
6. Do you have problems with bleeding after surgical or dental procedures?	□YES	□NO
7. Do you have a history of liver disease or cirrhosis?	□YES	□NO
8. Have you ever had a heart attack, or problems with your heart?	□YES	□NO
9. Do you have diabetes that requires insulin treatment?	□YES	□NO
10. Have you had any problems with anesthesia other than nausea or vomiting? For example, difficult airway or awareness during surgery.	□YES	□NO
11. Do you have kidney problems (except for kidney stones or recurrent infections) that require treatment by a kidney specialist or are you on dialysis?	□YES	□NO
12. Are you pregnant or is there a chance you are pregnant?	□YES	□NO
13. Do you have or have you had any Implantable devices? ➤ If yes identify which device(s) below:	□YES	□NO
□ Pacemaker/Defibrillator □ Cardiac Stent Year: □ Ventricular Assist Device Year: □ Insulin Pump		
14. Currently smoking 1 pack per day or more?	□YES	□NO
15. Current Alcohol: More than 2 drinks a day?	□YES	□NO
16. Current Recreational Drug use?	□YES	□NO

To be completed by clinical staff:

Any YES answers to the questions above indicate a patient requires a PEC visit;
All NO answers to the questions above indicate no PEC visit is required.

If the surgeon requires a PEC visit for another reason, please fill in the information below.

Surgeon Request:

Patient to be scheduled for: □ Anesthesiologist Consult   □ Pre Evaluation Center visit

REASON:_____

Please indicate reason when requesting consult with anesthesiologist and or Pre Evaluation Center Appointment

Surgeon/Designee: Name: _____ Date_____

(Please Print Clearly)

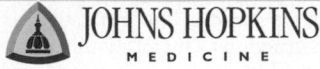

APPENDIX A Preoperative Screening Questionnaire.

NPO Status

As alluded to earlier, it is no longer appropriate to simply indicate "NPO after midnight." Data are strong that fasting 2 to 4 hours results in lower gastric volume and better acidity than more than 4 hours. In addition, adoption of an ERAS protocol will require consumption of clear liquids and a carbohydrate load 2 hours before surgery. Patients with insulin-dependent diabetes are now routinely taking long-acting insulin in the morning, and new diabetic guidelines require 50% of these doses to be given in the morning before any procedures. These patients should not be NPO and potentially will need sugar-containing fluids before surgery (Appendix C). Finally, it

---

Preoperative Roadmap 8

NPO Guidelines

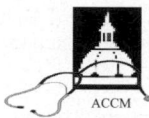

ADULT FASTING INSTRUCTIONS

PLEASE READ BEFORE THE DAY OF PROCEDURE

If you have end stage renal disease, gastroparesis (slow emptying of the stomach), are receiving dialysis, or if you are pregnant, **DO NOT** eat or drink anything for **6** hours before you are told to arrive at the hospital.

Type of food	Examples	Latest time you can eat or drink
Clear Liquids	Liquids you can see through: water, apple juice (no pulp), Gatorade®, black coffee or tea (with or without sugar or sweetener), NO MILK, CREAM OR ALCOHOL	1 hour before you are told to arrive at the hospital

* **You may only have a total of 20 ounces of clear liquids between midnight and 1 hour prior to your arrival**
** **You may only have 8 ounces of clear liquids in the last hour you are allowed to drink****

ALL other foods and liquids	NO! All solid food, all liquids you are unable to see through, all candy, chewing gum and mints 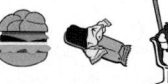	6 hours before you are told to arrive at the hospital

Please note, patients are normally told to arrive **2** hours prior to their surgery start time. If you have not yet been given your surgery start time, please contact your surgeon's office.

If you are having surgery under the **E**nhanced **R**ecovery **A**fter **S**urgery **(ERAS)** protocol, please disregard these instructions and follow the instructions given to you by your surgeon.

If you have any questions, call the Preoperative Evaluation Center at 410-955-8533; Monday-Friday 7:30AM- 4:00PM

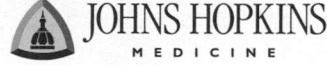

APPENDIX B NPO Guidelines.

is not very patient centered to have patients NPO for hours before afternoon surgery.

Antiplatelet Therapy

Patients who have cardiac stents must be maintained on ASA up to the time of surgery except for very few select types of cases, such as neurosurgery, major spine, retinal, and some bladder surgery. Appendix D highlights an appropriate set of guidelines for these patients. Again, using form letters informing patients to stop all aspirin 7 to 10 days before surgery is not warranted.

Better outcomes and lower readmissions are related directly to individualizing patient instructions and preparations.

Preoperative Roadmap   13

Appendix D: Diabetic Management

General Considerations for the Diabetic Patient:

Schedule insulin-dependent diabetic patients early in the day (by noon). If unable to schedule by noon, please have patient arrive at hospital by 9 am regardless of the time of their surgery.

Have patients bring insulin medications to the facility.

Preoperative evaluation may include the level of glycemic control, i.e. by blood glucose (BG) levels and glycosylated hemoglobin A1c. Patient's with an A1c >8.5% may benefit from further evaluation prior to elective surgery in an attempt to reduce surgical site infections.

Optimal intraoperative BG level: 180 mg/dL or less.

Have the patient take BG at bedtime; if > 180 mg/dL take insulin according to patient's individualized instructions[2].

Elective cases should be postponed in patients with fasting BG>400 mg/dl or in patients with significant complications of hyperglycemia such as severe dehydration, ketoacidosis, and hyperosmolar non-ketotic states[1]. Postponing elective cases is always up to the discretion of the provider.

Table 1 Pre-Operative Antidiabetic Guidelines* [1,2,3]

Type of Medication	DAY & EVENING BEFORE Surgery	MORNING of Surgery
Oral Agents	Continue all oral agents. *If the patient has renal dysfunction or is likely to receive IV contrast, you may want to discontinue metformin 24-48 hours prior to surgery. Hold metformin if undergoing bowel preparation.	Hold.
Non-insulin injectable Examples: Byetta (exenatide), Victoza (liraglutide)	Continue.	Hold.
Short/rapid-acting Insulin Examples: Novolog (Aspart), Humalog (Lispro), Apidra (Glulisine), Novolin R or Humulin R (Regular)	Maintain usual meal plan & insulin dose.	Hold.
Intermediate-Acting Insulin (taken twice daily) Examples: Novolin-N, Humulin-N (NPH)	Take usual morning dose and 75% of the usual evening dose.	Take 50% of the usual morning dose.
Long-Acting Insulin Examples: Lantus (Glargine), Levemir (Determir)		
➤ **Taken once daily in the morning**	Take usual morning dose.	Take 50% of the usual morning dose.
➤ **Taken once daily in the evening**	Take 75% of the usual evening dose.	Do not take any insulin.
➤ **Taken twice daily**	Take usual morning dose and 75% of the usual evening dose.	Take 50% of the usual morning dose.
Pre-Mixed Insulins (e.g. 70/30; 75/25; 50/50) (taken twice daily)	Take usual morning dose and 75% of evening dose.	Take 50% of the usual morning dose.
Insulin Pump	Maintain usual meal plan & basal rate.	Maintain basal rate.

***Developed in Conjunction with the Johns Hopkins Inpatient Diabetes Management Service**

[1] Joshi GP, Chung F, Vann MA, et al. Society for Ambulatory Anesthesia consensus statement on perioperative blood glucose management in diabetic patients undergoing surgery. *Anesth Analg*; 2010; 111:1378-87.

[2] Joslin Diabetes Center and Joslin Clinic. Guideline for inpatient management of surgical and ICU patients (pre-, peri and postoperative care). 2009. Available at: http://www.joslin.org/docs/Inpatient_Guideline_10-02-09.pdf

[3] Sara M. Alexanian, Marie E. McDonnell, and Shamsuddin Akhtar. Creating a Perioperative Glycemic Control Program. *Anesthesiology Research and Practice*; Vol. 2011, Article ID 465974, 9 pages, 2011.

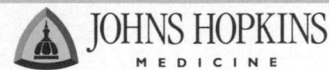
JOHNS HOPKINS MEDICINE

APPENDIX C Diabetic Management Guidelines.

Preoperative Roadmap   16

Appendix G: Patients with Cardiac Stents

The Johns Hopkins Hospital
Antiplatelet Bridging for Patients with Cardiac Stents

Cardiac stent patients on dual antiplatelet therapy (DAP -aspirin & antiplatelet agents) pose a clinical challenge during surgeries or invasive procedures. The risk of uncontrolled bleeding if DAP therapy is continued versus acute stent thrombosis if DAP is discontinued in the perioperative period presents a clinical dilemma. To help guide perioperative DAP therapy and improve clinical outcomes for patients with coronary stents, a JHH multidisciplinary task force has developed the following one-page decision support tool (please see below).

In addition, the Pre-operative Evaluation Center (PEC) has agreed to assist the attending providers with perioperative management of patients on DAP therapy. A mandatory field in ORMIS for documenting whether the patient has a coronary stent will be used to help facilitate the scheduling of pre-operative/pre-procedural PEC appointments for these patients. If the scheduled case will occur within one week of the posting, the PEC clinic coordinator should be called (410-283-3510) to facilitate a stent patient appointment.

If you would like someone from the task force to present the program goals and assist with staff education, please contact the task force chair, Sean Berenholtz, MD, MHS at sberenho@jhmi.edu. If you have questions regarding this information, please contact Steven Jones, MD, Cardiology (sjones64@jhmi.edu); Michael Streiff, MD, Hematology (mstreif@jhmi.edu), or Sean Berenholtz, MD, Anesthesiology and Critical Care Medicine (sberenho@jhmi.edu).

Antiplatelet Bridging Tool for Patients with Cardiac Stents

1. <u>Postpone</u> Elective Procedures until minimum duration of dual antiplatelet therapy (DAP) is complete, unless DAP can be continued without interruption throughout the periprocedure period.

Minimum Duration Stent Implantation	
Bare Metal Stent (BMS)	1 month
Drug Eluting Stent (DES)	12 months

2. High Risk Stent Thrombosis: <u>Consult cardiology and refer to PEC.</u>

Consult Cardiology and Refer to PEC 14 days prior to procedure for antiplatelet management for:
Surgery required prior to minimum DAP (Bare Metal Stent < 1 month, Drug eluting stent < 12 months)
Any episodes of stent thrombosis

3. For <u>urgent surgery or patient deemed high risk of thrombosis</u>, consider intravenous antiplatelet bridge therapy (IV IIb/IIIb inhibitor) with Cardiology Consult.

4. If minimum antiplatelet duration met <u>and</u> patient does not have high risk factors above, stop antiplatelet according to the table below:

Antiplatelet	Maximum Holding Time
Clopidogrel	5 days
Prasugrel	7 days
Ticagrelor	5 days

5. Continue low-dose aspirin (81 mg) throughout the periprocedure period for all patients, <u>except</u> patients <u>at high risk for bleeding.</u>

High Bleed Risk- Aspirin may be held for <u>maximum of 5 days</u>
Intracranial Procedures
Posterior Chamber of eye
Spinal Canal
TURP, Cystoprostatectomy

6. <u>Post-operative</u> initiation of antiplatelet therapy should begin as soon as adequate hemostasis is achieved. Patients can be restarted on their home dual antiplatelet therapy. A loading dose of their antiplatelet can be considered.

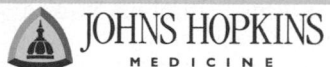

APPENDIX D Patients with Cardiac Stents.

SUGGESTED READINGS

Adamina M, et al. Enhanced recovery pathways optimize health outcomes and resource utilization: a meta-analysis of randomized controlled trials in colorectal surgery. *Surgery.* 2011;149:830-840.

Joshi GP, Chung F, Vann MA, et al. Society of Ambulatory Anesthesia consensus statement on perioperative blood glucose management in diabetic patients undergoing surgery. *Anesth Analg.* 2010;111:1378-1387.

Perioperative Surgical Home. <http://www.asahq.org/psh.> Accessed 2.11.15.

Practice guidelines for preoperative fasting and use of pharmacologic agents to reduce risk of pulmonary aspiration. *Anesthesiology.* 2011;114:495-511.

Wu CL, Benson A, Hobson D, et al. Initiation of an Enhanced Recovery Pathway Program; An Anesthesiology Department's Perspective. *Jt Comm J Qual Patient Saf.* 2015;41:447-456.

IS A NASOGASTRIC TUBE NECESSARY AFTER ALIMENTARY TRACT SURGERY?

Cynthia E. Weber, MD, MS, Gerard J. Abood, MD, and Sam G. Pappas, MD

The nasogastric tube (NGT) historically has been used in the postoperative period for patients undergoing abdominal surgery. The long-standing belief held by many surgeons is that nasogastric decompression allows the bowel to rest; prevents air and fluid accumulation; decreases postoperative nausea and vomiting; prevents abdominal distension; and protects the patient from aspiration, pneumonia, anastomotic leak, and fascial dehiscence. It also has been part of surgical dogma that NGTs promote earlier return of bowel function and thus a shorter hospital length of stay (LOS). Pervasive use of NGTs coincided with significant advances in the administration of anesthesia, the development of germ theory and aseptic technique, and improvements in hemostasis that revolutionized surgery at the turn of the twentieth century and allowed surgeons to successfully operate in the abdomen. More recent evidence, however, has shown that prophylactic NGT use after alimentary tract surgery is not necessary and may contribute to increased morbidity and LOS. Despite these data, though, many surgeons have been hesitant to abandon routine NGT use.

■ HISTORICAL PERSPECTIVE

Originally described by John Hunter in the eighteenth century as eel skin wrapped around whalebone, the NGT initially was used to feed liquid nutrients to the sick. The first description of a flexible tube (Levin tube) used to decompress the gastrointestinal (GI) tract after surgery was in 1921 by American gastroenterologist Dr. Abraham Louis Levin. In 1926 McIver hypothesized that postoperative abdominal distension resulted from swallowed air, which could be prevented by an indwelling NGT. Despite the lack of scientific evidence to support the benefit of routine prophylactic NGT use after GI tract and abdominal surgery, it has remained common practice even into the twenty-first century. Gerber and colleagues were the first to challenge prophylactic NGT use in 1958 when they published results showing that in their cohort of 600 patients with postoperative ileus, the half managed without an NGT had lower morbidity and mortality as well as fewer respiratory tract complications. Their data were nonrandomized but started the conversation that perhaps NGTs were not mandatory postoperatively. The first prospective randomized trial comparing patients with enteric anastomoses was published in 1984, and although it showed no difference in complication rates between patients with and without NGTs, it was limited by small sample size and too much heterogeneity.

Cheatham and colleagues published the first meta-analysis on the topic in 1995. Their study included 26 clinical trials (3964 patients) that compared the use of selective versus routine NGT decompression after elective laparotomy. Routine use was defined as an NGT placed preoperatively or intraoperatively that remained in place until an unspecified point in the patient's postoperative course (usually return of bowel function, flatus, or decreased output). Selective use was defined as either no NGT used or an NGT placed intraoperatively but removed in the operating room or in the recovery room and replaced only if the patient developed the need for decompression clinically in the postoperative course. The authors demonstrated a significantly lower rate of total complications as well as a decreased incidence of postoperative pneumonia, aspiration, and fever. There was no significant difference between groups in the incidence of anastomotic leak, wound infection, wound dehiscence, or LOS. The authors reported that 30.5 patients could be spared nasogastric decompression for every 1 patient who required NGT reinsertion postoperatively. The main limitation of their meta-analysis was that it included a large number of nonrandomized studies.

In the 20 years since that first meta-analysis there have been numerous randomized controlled trials and subsequent meta-analyses that have repeatedly shown that prophylactic NGT decompression after elective surgery on the alimentary tract does not afford the benefits ascribed to it by surgical dogma. In fact, the majority of studies indicate that the liberal use of an NGT prolongs hospital postoperative LOS and perhaps actually increases the risk of certain complications, especially respiratory complications. A 2010 Cochrane review that examined 37 studies (5711 patients) showed that prophylactic NGT decompression is ineffective at (1) hastening return of bowel function, (2) decreasing risk of aspiration and subsequent pulmonary complications, (3) improving patient comfort by lessening abdominal distension, (4) protecting intestinal anastomoses from leakage, and (5) shortening hospital LOS. The use of NGTs also is associated with significant morbidity related to both placement and prolonged use, not to mention the significant patient discomfort experienced.

Evidence-based medicine has transformed all aspects of patient care, including surgical decision making, which traditionally was highly subjective, individualized, and primarily emulated the practice of prior master surgeons. The conservative dogma that focused on prolonged bed rest, NGT decompression, and delay of oral intake in order to allow the alimentary tract time to heal and recover and thus prevent postoperative complications has been refuted repeatedly in the scientific literature. The 1980s and 1990s saw significant advances in perioperative pain control and minimally invasive surgical techniques that aimed at either outpatient or reduced LOS surgery. The Danish surgeon Henrik Kehlet pioneered the idea of "fast-track surgery" in the 1990s, with the intent of developing a multidisciplinary approach to reduce surgical stress and achieve a smoother and faster recovery. One of the major tenets of surgery to be eliminated by "fast-track" pathways was the prophylactic use of NGTs.

■ COLORECTAL SURGERY AND ENHANCED RECOVERY AFTER SURGERY

"Fast-track surgery," as described by Kehlet, perhaps has been integrated most successfully into colorectal surgery, specifically elective surgery for colorectal cancer (CRC). Enhanced recovery after surgery (ERAS) pathways have been shown to significantly reduce postoperative morbidity and decrease LOS and healthcare expenditure. Consensus ERAS Society guidelines were developed in 2005 and updated in 2009 and 2012, and have become the standard of care for colorectal surgery. These guidelines center around 20 items in the preoperative, intraoperative, and postoperative arenas. The elements included in ERAS focus on ensuring adequate preadmission counseling, avoiding prolonged fasting and unnecessary bowel preparations, using appropriate antibiotic and thromboembolic prophylaxis, using short-acting anesthetic agents and epidural analgesia, maintaining normothermia and euvolemia, preventing nausea and vomiting, and using postoperative early mobilization and nonopioid analgesia. In addition, the use of laparoscopic or laparoscopic-assisted technique should be the first choice when appropriate.

Another important element in ERAS is early oral nutrition, often within 2 hours of surgery, which is made possible by either the avoidance of NGTs or the removal of NGTs in the operating room upon awakening. A 2013 publication titled "The Evidence Against Prophylactic Nasogastric Intubation and Oral Restriction" reviews the current literature surrounding prophylactic NGT decompression in colorectal surgery. The study provides evidence that prophylactic NGT decompression (1) does not improve time to return of bowel function or LOS (in some studies it prolongs time to flatus and LOS); (2) does not reduce the incidence of anastomotic leak, wound infection, dehiscence, or incisional hernia; (3) does not prevent pulmonary complications of fever, atelectasis, or aspiration pneumonia and likely promotes pharyngolaryngitis; and (4) does not prevent abdominal discomfort as measured by nausea, vomiting, or distension (and NGT reinsertion rates are low). The study also argues that early feeding, which is tolerated by 80% to 90% of patients within 24 hours after colorectal surgery, (1) enhances recovery time and decreases LOS; (2) reduces the risk for any type of postoperative infection; (3) decreases the risk for hyperglycemia; and (4) results in no difference in duration of ileus, although it does increase risk for vomiting.

For ERAS pathways to confer the expected benefits on patient outcomes, there has to be significant collaboration, buy-in, and communication between all members of the healthcare team: surgeon, anesthesiologist, patient, nurses, and others. Compliance with the steps of the pathway cannot be assumed, and studies have found that adherence rates drop over time without repetitive education of staff. On the other hand, installation of a dedicated midlevel provider and teaching sessions on the surgical wards can increase adherence. A web-based survey of colorectal and general surgeons found that only about 30% were actively following a perioperative protocol for elective bowel resections. With regard to NGT removal, 61% reported avoidance of NGT completely and 15% reported removal of NGT on postoperative day zero. Another study found that despite the development of a multidisciplinary fast-track protocol and training sessions for all staff, only 3 of the 7 key elements of the pathway met 80% compliance after implementation. The authors hypothesized that more time is needed to overcome the deep-seated beliefs taught by tradition. This study and others highlight the need for continued monitoring of compliance with ERAS pathways.

■ FOREGUT AND PANCREATIC SURGERY

Whereas ERAS pathways after colorectal surgery have been in place for 10 years, the introduction of "fast-track" protocols for upper GI tract and pancreatic surgery has just begun. As expected, there is often hesitation by surgeons regarding early removal of NGTs and earlier oral feeding after an esophagectomy, gastrectomy, or pancreaticoduodenectomy (Whipple's procedure). This is because of concern over the integrity of the more proximal anastomoses as well as the duodenal stump and, especially in the case of pancreaticoduodenectomy, the fact that multiple enteric anastomoses are involved. Traditional surgical training has taught that an NGT is necessary after an esophagectomy to prevent overdistension of the gastric conduit, protect the esophagogastric anastomosis from dehiscence, and prevent vomiting and aspiration. Surgeons also harbor concern that feeding too early after a pancreaticoduodenectomy will increase the risk of pancreatic leak and fistula formation.

In the last few years, a number of studies examining ERAS programs after elective esophagectomy have been published. In most of these studies the NGT is removed on postoperative day 2, and some studies forego NGTs altogether. One study found no difference in complication rate or readmission rate when comparing an ERAS study group of 103 patients, in which the NGT was removed on postoperative day 2, with a historical control group of 78 patients. Another study that compared early removal (postoperative day 2) with delayed removal (postoperative day 6 to 10) also found no difference in pulmonary complications, anastomotic leak rates, need for reintubation, mortality, or LOS between groups. The authors did note that patient discomfort scores were higher in the delayed removal group and that only about 30% of patients required NGT reinsertion for postoperative ileus, with no complications from reinsertion despite the fresh anastomosis. They concluded that early

removal is safe and affords two thirds of patients relief of NGT discomfort early in the postoperative course.

The ERAS Society has published official consensus guidelines for "fast-track" care after gastrectomy for gastric cancer (2012) and after pancreaticoduodenectomy (2014). The guidelines after gastrectomy are based on nine randomized controlled trials and two meta-analyses and present strong evidence against the routine use of NGTs. The cited studies repeatedly have shown no difference in time to flatus, anastomotic leaks, pulmonary complications, morbidity, or mortality, and many demonstrated a longer LOS in patients with routine NGT decompression compared with those without an NGT postoperatively. The guidelines after pancreaticoduodenectomy also recommend against routine NGT decompression. The most common complication after a pancreaticoduodenectomy is delayed gastric emptying (DGE), which occurs in up to 30% of patients. Multiple studies comparing a "fast-track" program with historical controls actually have demonstrated that DGE rates are higher when routine NGT decompression is used.

■ EMERGENCY SURGERY AND NASOGASTRIC TUBES

The data for "fast-track" protocols in emergency abdominal surgery are very sparse. One single-institution study randomized approximately 170 patients to early oral feeding, which meant that a soft diet was given within 24 hours postoperatively. The other half of the patients were stratified as high risk (evidence of peritonitis, GI tract obstruction or perforation, or an anastomosis) and placed on nothing by mouth (NPO) status for 3 days postoperatively or as low risk (none of the high-risk criteria) and given liquids and then a soft diet once they passed either flatus or stool. The authors found no difference in complication rate, LOS, or need for reoperation. However, a large proportion of the operations (63%) were for appendicitis, which typically is not associated with a prolonged hospital course or an inability to tolerate diet.

Another institution performed a prospective randomized trial to evaluate the safety and efficacy of ERAS pathways after emergency laparoscopic surgery for perforated peptic ulcer disease (excluded if ulcer >10 mm). The 21 patients assigned to the ERAS group had their NGT removed in the operating room and were given liquids on postoperative day 1. The control group had their NGT removed only after the output was less than 300 mL a day. The study demonstrated no difference in morbidity or mortality and a significantly shorter LOS for the ERAS group (3.8 vs 6.9 days). However, the exclusion criteria were numerous—American Society of Anesthesiologists (ASA) class 3 or 4, evidence of septic shock, conversion to an open procedure, and others—which limits the generalizability of the results. Finally, a study in Nepal randomized 115 patients after emergency laparotomy for perforation peritonitis, intestinal obstruction, or abdominal trauma to two groups: with or without an NGT postoperatively. The authors found no difference in the rate of wound complications, gastric upset, respiratory complications, anastomotic leaks, or NGT reinsertions. Similarly, they demonstrated a shorter LOS in the group managed without an NGT.

■ COMPLICATIONS OF NASOGASTRIC TUBES

Avoiding unnecessary morbidity from NGT complications is another motive to forgo routine NGT decompression. Complications can occur during the placement of an NGT or as a result of prolonged NGT use. Some adverse effects, such as patient pain and discomfort, sinusitis, epistaxis, and pharyngolaryngitis, are likely underrecognized and possibly even regarded as worth enduring to prevent the more severe complications that surgical tradition has taught are more likely to occur without prolonged NGT decompression. Despite the seemingly simple technique for insertion, serious

TABLE 1: Criteria for Defining a Surgical Site Infection (SSI)

SUPERFICIAL INCISIONAL SSI

Infection occurs within 30 days after the operation

and

infection involves only skin or subcutaneous tissue of the incision

and at least one of the following:

1. Purulent drainage, with or without laboratory confirmation, from the superficial incision.
2. Organisms isolated from an aseptically obtained culture of fluid or tissue from the superficial incision.
3. At least one of the following signs or symptoms of infection: pain or tenderness, localized swelling, redness, or heat and superficial incision is deliberately opened by surgeon, unless incision is culture-negative.
4. Diagnosis of superficial incisional SSI by the surgeon or attending physician.

Do not report the following conditions as SSI:

1. Stitch abscess (minimal inflammation and discharge confined to the points of suture penetration).
2. Infection of an episiotomy or newborn circumcision site.
3. Infected burn wound.
4. Incisional SSI that extends into the fascial and muscle layers (see deep incisional SSI).

Note: Specific criteria are used for identifying infected episiotomy and circumcision sites and burn wounds.

DEEP INCISIONAL SSI

Infection occurs within 30 days after the operation if no implant† is left in place or within 1 year if implant is in place and the infection appears to be related to the operation

and

infection involves deep soft tissues (e.g., fascial and muscle layers) of the incision

and at least one of the following:

1. Purulent drainage from the deep incision but not from the organ/space component of the surgical site.
2. A deep incision spontaneously dehisces or is deliberately opened by a surgeon when the patient has at least one of the following signs or symptoms: fever (>38°C), localized pain, or tenderness, unless site is culture-negative.
3. An abscess or other evidence of infection involving the deep incision is found on direct examination, during reoperation, or by histopathologic or radiologic examination.
4. Diagnosis of a deep incisional SSI by a surgeon or attending physician.

Notes:

1. Report infection that involves both superficial and deep incision sites as deep incisional SSI.
2. Report an organ/space SSI that drains through the incision as a deep incisional SSI.

ORGAN/SPACE SSI

Infection occurs within 30 days after the operation if no implant† is left in place or within 1 year if implant is in place and the infection appears to be related to the operation

and

infection involves any part of the anatomy (e.g., organs or spaces), other than the incision, which was opened or manipulated during an operation

and at least one of the following:

1. Purulent drainage from a drain that is placed through a stab wound† into the organ/space.
2. Organisms isolated from an aseptically obtained culture of fluid or tissue in the organ/space.
3. An abscess or other evidence of infection involving the organ/space that is found on direct examination, during reoperation, or by histopathologic or radiologic examination.
4. Diagnosis of an organ/space SSI by a surgeon or attending physician.

From Horan TC, Gaynes RP, Martone WJ, Jarvis WR, Emori TG. CDC definitions of nosocomial surgical site infections, 1992: a modification of CDC definitions of surgical wound infections. *Infect Control Hosp Epidemiol.* 1992;13:606-608.

†National Nosocomial Infection Surveillance definition: a nonhuman-derived implantable foreign body (e.g., prosthetic heart valve, nonhuman vascular graft, mechanical heart, or hip prosthesis) that is permanently placed in a patient during surgery.

‡If the area around a stab wound becomes infected, it is not an SSI. It is considered a skin or soft tissue infection, depending on its depth.

controlled study demonstrated no benefit in treating peritonitis managed surgically with appropriate source control for more than 4 days of postoperative antibiotics compared with longer courses based on clinical findings. Extending the length of antibiotic administration only increases costs as well as the risk of drug resistance and secondary infections, such as *Clostridium difficile*–related disease, without decreasing the risk of SSI.

■ APPROPRIATE HAIR REMOVAL

The method of hair removal used in the preoperative period has been related to the incidence of SSIs. A large prospective trial randomized 2000 patients to either electrical clipping or manual shaving with a razor for hair removal before open heart surgery. The patients who were electrically clipped had a significantly lower rate of mediastinitis

TABLE 2: Surgical Wound Classifications

Surgical Wound Classification	Description
Class I, clean	An uninfected operative wound in which no inflammation is encountered and the respiratory, alimentary, genital, or uninfected urinary tract is not entered. In addition, clean wounds are primarily closed and, if necessary, drained with closed drainage.
Class II, clean-contaminated	An operative wound in which the respiratory, alimentary, genital, or urinary tracts are entered under controlled conditions and without unusual contamination. Specifically, operations involving the biliary tract, appendix, vagina, and oropharynx are included in this category, provided that no evidence of infection or major break in technique is encountered.
Class III, contaminated	Open, fresh, accidental wounds. In addition, operations with major breaks in sterile technique (e.g., open cardiac massage) or gross spillage from the gastrointestinal tract and incisions in which acute, nonpurulent inflammation is encountered are included in this category.
Class IV, dirty/infected	Old traumatic wounds with retained devitalized tissue and those that involve existing clinical infection or perforated viscera. This definition suggests that the organisms causing postoperative infection were present in the operative field before the operation.

Modified from Mangram AJ, Horan TC, Pearson ML, et al. Guideline for prevention of surgical site infection. *Infect Control Hosp Epidemiol.* 1999;20:247-278.

TABLE 3: Patient and Operative Characteristics That May Influence the Risk of Surgical Site Infection

Patient Factors	Environmental Factors	Treatment Factors
Ascites	Contaminated medications	Emergency procedure
Chronic inflammation	Inadequate disinfection and sterilization	Failure to obliterate dead space
Coexistent remote infection	Inadequate skin antisepsis	Hypothermia
Colonization with micro-organisms	Inadequate ventilation	Inadequate antibiotic prophylaxis
Corticosteroid therapy		Intraoperative blood transfusion
Diabetes		Oxygenation
Extended preoperative admission		Poor hemostasis
Hypocholesterolemia		Prolonged operative time
Hypoxemia		Surgical drains
Malnutrition		Tissue trauma
Obesity		
Peripheral vascular disease		
Perioperative anemia		
Perioperative shaving		
Prior site irradiation		
Recent operation		
Skin disease in the area of infection (e.g., psoriasis)		

Modified from National Nosocomial Infections Surveillance (NNIS) system report: data summary from January 1992–June 2001. *Am J Infect Control.* 2001;29:404-421; and Mangram AJ, Horan TC, Pearson ML, et al. Guideline for prevention of surgical site infection. *Infect Control Hosp Epidemiol.* 1999;20:247-278.

compared with the manually shaved group ($P = 0.024$). A Cochrane systematic review confirmed these findings, revealing three randomized trials that compared shaving with clipping. Statistically more SSIs occurred with shaving than with clipping. The same Cochrane review failed to demonstrate a statistically significant difference in SSIs when comparing depilatory creams with shaving and when comparing shaving or clipping on the day before surgery with the same methods on the day of surgery; however, studies were small and underpowered. Given the current data, shaving with a blade is considered an inappropriate method of hair removal in the preoperative period and is not recommended.

■ POSTOPERATIVE NORMOGLYCEMIA

Appropriate glucose control in the perioperative period has been shown to reduce the incidence of SSIs. Hyperglycemia impairs the immune system, increases the risk of infection, and worsens the outcomes in sepsis. Studies have shown that tight intraoperative

TABLE 4: National Healthcare Safety Network (NHSN) Risk Index Scoring

Wound Class	NHSN Risk Index Category				
	NNIS 0	NNIS 1	NNIS 2	NNIS 3	All
I: Clean	1.0%	2.3%	5.4%	NA	2.1%
II: Clean-contaminated	2.1%	4.0%	9.5%	NA	3.3%
III: Contaminated	NA	3.4%	6.8%	13.2%	6.4%
IV: Dirty/infected	NA	3.1%	8.1%	12.8%	7.1%
All	1.5%	2.9%	6.8%	13.0%	2.8%

Data from National Nosocomial Infections Surveillance (NNIS) system report: data summary from January 1992–June 2001. *Am J Infect Control.* 2001;29:404-421.

NA, Not applicable; *NNIS,* National Nosocomial Infections Surveillance system.

TABLE 5: Surgical Care Improvement Project (SCIP) Performance Measures Applicable to the Perioperative Period

SCIP Infection (INF) Measure	Performance Measure
INF 1	Prophylactic antibiotic received within 1 hour before surgical incision
INF 2	Prophylactic antibiotic selection for surgical patients
INF 3	Prophylactic antibiotics discontinued within 24 hours after surgery end time
INF 4	Cardiac surgery patients with controlled 6:00 AM postoperative blood glucose
INF 6	Surgery patients with appropriate hair removal
INF 9	Urinary catheter removed on postoperative day 1 or postoperative day 2 (with day of surgery being day 0)
INF 10	Surgery patients with perioperative temperature management

Modified from Rosenberger LH, Politano AD, Sawyer RG. The surgical care improvement project and prevention of post-operative infection, including surgical site infection. *Surg Infect.* 2011;12:163-168.

TABLE 6: Association Between Timing and Surgical Site Infections for Antimicrobial Prophylaxis, Cephalosporins, or Antimicrobials Designated to Be Given Within 60 Minutes of Incision

Timing of Antimicrobial Prophylaxis	Infections/No. of Operations	Infection Risk
>120 min before incision	4/96	4.7%
61-120 min before incision	12/489	2.4%
31-60 min before incision	38/1558	2.4%
0-30 min before incision	22/1339	1.6%
1-30 min after incision	4/100	4.0%
>30 min after incision	5/74	6.8%

Modified from Steinberg JP, Braun BI, Hellinger WC, et al. Timing of antimicrobial prophylaxis and the risk of surgical site infections. *Ann Surg.* 2009;250:10-16.

glucose control by anesthesia personnel significantly decreases the risk of SSIs, as do implementation of a postoperative intravenous insulin therapy protocol, continuous insulin infusions (as compared with subcutaneous injections), and maintenance of a mean capillary glucose concentration below 200 mg/dL for a minimum of 48 hours after surgery.

Although early data supported strict blood glucose control (<110 mg/dL) as a means to decrease morbidity and mortality in critically ill patients, recent data show higher rates of severe hypoglycemia and adverse events with intensive insulin protocols. The Normoglycemia in Intensive Care Evaluation–Survival Using Glucose Algorithm Regulation (NICE-SUGAR) study supported conventional (<180 mg/dL), as opposed to strict, insulin control with equivalent outcomes. This was not specific to SSI outcomes, but this target (180 mg/dL) is recommended as an appropriate glucose concentration level for surgical patients in the perioperative period.

■ POSTOPERATIVE NORMOTHERMIA

Postoperative hypothermia is a common problem and has been hypothesized to increase SSIs by peripheral vasoconstriction, reduced

blood flow and oxygen tension at the tissue level, and impaired immune function in terms of decreased antibody production and reduced neutrophil function. A prospective randomized clinical trial found that an active intraoperative warming protocol resulted in significantly fewer SSIs when compared with a standard of care group ($P = 0.009$). Active warming protocols should be implemented in all surgical patients because this is a simple prevention strategy to reduce SSIs.

■ PERFORMANCE MEASURES

The SCIP quality measures have been implemented by CMS, and mandatory reporting of certain performance measures now helps to determine hospital reimbursement. Numerous organizations endorse the notion that adherence to process measures serves as a valid assessment of surgical quality, and public reporting is intended to guide patients to quality centers for surgical care. However, process measures often serve as poor proxies for overall quality of surgical care, and a number of studies have revealed that adherence to quality measures does not always result in improved outcomes. The implementation of performance measures to improve surgical outcomes is an important step to improving surgical care; however, their use as quality metrics or reimbursement standards must be viewed with caution because of limited data proving that adherence actually improves outcomes.

The inconsistent correlation between increased rates of adherence to these process measures (all based on previous positive trials) and

TABLE 7: Surgical Care Improvement Project (SCIP) Pocket Card: Prophylactic Antimicrobial Regimen Selection for Surgery

Surgical Procedure	Approved Antibiotics
Coronary artery bypass grafting, other cardiac or vascular procedures	• Cefazolin, cefuroxime, or vancomycin* • If beta-lactam allergy: • Vancomycin[†] or clindamycin[†]

Hysterectomy	• Cefotetan, cefaxolin, cefoxitin, cefuroxime, or ampicillin/sulbactam
	• If beta-lactam allergy:
	  • Clindamycin + aminoglycoside, or
	  • Clindamycin + quinolone, or
	  • Clindamycin + aztreonam
	  or
	  • Metronidazole + aminoglycoside, or
	  • Metronidazole + quinolone

Hip or knee arthroplasty	• Cefazolin, cefuroxime, or vancomycin* • If beta-lactam allergy: • Vancomycin[†] or clindamycin[†]

Colon operations	• Cefotetan, cefoxitin, ampicillin/sulbactam, or ertapenem[‡]
	or
	• Cefazolin or cefuroxime + metronidazole
	• If beta-lactam allergy:
	  • Clindamycin + aminoglycoside, or
	  • Clindamycin + quinolone, or
	  • Clindamycin + aztreonam
	  or
	  • Metronidazole + aminoglycoside, or
	  • Metronidazole + quinolone

Modified from Oklahoma Foundation of Medical Quality, the Quality Improvement Organization Support Center for Patient Safety, under contract with the Centers of Medicare & Medicaid Services (CMS), an agency of the U.S. Department of Health and Human Services. Surgical Care Improvement Project pocket card. October 2010.

This table does not necessarily reflect Centers of Medicare & Medicaid Services policy.

*Vancomycin is acceptable with a physician/APN/PA/pharmacist documented justification for its use.

[†]For cardiac, orthopedic, and vascular surgery, if the patient is allergic to β-lactam antibiotics, vancomycin or clindamycin is an acceptable substitute.

[‡]A single dose of ertapenem is recommended for colon procedures.

decreased SSI rates has two other implications. First, even with total adherence to these measures, SSIs still occur, highlighting the fact that the pathophysiology of SSI is not completely understood. More research is needed to delineate the causes of SSI and to develop new technologies that can prevent them. Second, at this point in time SSIs cannot be considered "never events" and must not be considered so by regulating agencies.

■ INTRAOPERATIVE AND POSTOPERATIVE INCISION MANAGEMENT

Sound surgical technique, including adequate hemostasis, conservation of blood supply, atraumatic tissue handling, débridement of devitalized tissue, and limited use of electrocautery, must be used. The skin may be incised with either a scalpel or electrocautery with no resultant difference in wound complications. The technique of fascial closure may have an impact on SSI. Recent data for elective abdominal surgery support the use of small bite (5 mm every 5 mm) fascial closure to decrease the risk of hernia formation, and there are limited data supporting its use to decrease the risk of SSI. Current data do not support or refute the utility of closing subcutaneous tissue or peritoneum.

Clean and clean-contaminated incisions should be closed primarily and covered with a sterile dressing for 24 to 48 hours to allow sealing of the wound by epithelialization before dressing removal. Tissue adhesives and glue, such as Dermabond (Ethicon, Somerville, NJ), an octyl cyanoacrylate, are alternatives to sterile dressings and provide an effective barrier to bacterial contamination of a sterile incision but may be associated with higher rates of wound dehiscence (though not SSI).

Management of contaminated or dirty/infected wounds continues to be a dilemma for surgeons because current data are conflicting and of high heterogeneity. The most recent meta-analysis of primary skin closure versus delayed primary closure of these wounds demonstrated that delayed primary closure may reduce the rate of SSI, but current evidence is of poor quality and more data are needed. A prudent approach is to take other patient risk factors into account in making this decision and to consider the significant morbidity of SSI when considering primary closure of high-risk wounds.

The use of drains for clean or clean-contaminated incisions is not supported because drains provide a portal for pathogen entry and have been shown to increase the rate of SSI in these wound classes. When drains are used, they should be removed as soon as possible and should not justify concomitant antimicrobial therapy.

Finally, the use of negative pressure wound therapy (NPWT) over primarily closed incisions has become more popular in recent years. However, a recent Cochrane review concluded that there are inconclusive data for its use to decrease the incidence of wound complications, including seroma, hematoma, dehiscence, and SSI. Therefore at this time the widespread or routine use of NPWT over primarily closed incisions is not supported.

■ SPECIAL CONSIDERATIONS

Hand hygiene is an important topic within infection control practices. Preoperative surgeon hand antisepsis has transformed from the historic full 10-minute hand scrubbing to quicker protocols with various alcohol rubs. A large randomized clinical trial found that a 1-minute nonantiseptic hand wash followed by an aqueous alcohol-based handrub was equivalent to the traditional hand-scrubbing protocols. Numerous additional studies have found that alcohol-based handrubs are as effective as aqueous scrubbing procedures in SSI prevention.

Controversy certainly exists regarding the ideal preoperative skin antisepsis for the surgical site. The intent of skin preparation is to cleanse the skin of any micro-organisms, by far the leading source of pathogens for postoperative SSIs. Numerous skin preparations, including various combinations of chlorhexidine, povidone-iodine, iodine povacrylex, and isopropyl alcohol, are available. The data are inconsistent, with the most recent large randomized trial concluding that chlorhexidine-alcohol is superior to povidone-iodine. Ultimately, the routine use of a skin antiseptic should be undertaken with attention to the correct application protocol for the particular agent being used. Povidone-iodine alone, without alcohol, is probably inferior and should not be used. Differences between combinations of chlorhexidine and an iodophor with alcohol are perhaps minimal, and either approach is currently acceptable.

The pendulum continues to swing in terms of bowel preparation and enteric antibiotics for elective colorectal surgery. Traditional belief was that mechanical bowel preparation would reduce SSIs and anastomotic leak. Recent data have revealed no statistically significant evidence that patients benefit from bowel preparations or enemas in terms of wound infection or anastomotic leak. Antimicrobials, however, have been shown to reduce postoperative infectious complications substantially. Data reveal that antibiotics covering aerobic and anaerobic organisms should be given both orally and intravenously before colorectal surgery. Some expert opinion continues to recommend mechanical bowel preparation before enteric antibiotics for improved efficacy; however, data are conflicting. Currently, mechanical bowel preparation is clearly indicated only when intraoperative colonoscopy is either planned or likely, and its use at other times is based on surgeon preference, not evidence.

■ TREATMENT

All clearly infected wounds should be opened, irrigated, débrided, and treated with basic wound care. Most superficial and deep incisional SSIs can be managed with these techniques. The wound should be opened sufficiently for adequate visualization of the underlying tissue to ensure that no additional processes, such as fascial dehiscence, drainage from an organ/space SSI, or enteric fistula, are occurring.

Infected incisional wounds should be irrigated with an isotonic solution such as a saline solution to remove loose, dead tissue and exudate, and mechanical débridement with sharp excision or pressure irrigation may be indicated to remove devitalized tissue. Wounds should be packed in a "wet to dry" fashion, with moistened gauze against the wound bed covered by layers of dry gauze. Daily dressing changes assist in débridement, as the wet gauze removes residual necrotic tissue and exudate. Once the wound has stabilized and most of the devitalized tissue has been removed, consideration can be given to placement of a NPWT device ("wound vac"). Although the overall outcome may not change, placement of such a device generally speeds closure and may be particularly helpful in larger wounds and those in which dressing changes are difficult, such as wounds in the distal extremities.

The need for antimicrobial therapy is determined by magnitude of the infection, evidence of systemic involvement, presence of prosthetics, and status of the patient, including comorbidities. Uncomplicated SSIs that have been managed with incision and drainage usually can be managed without antibiotics. Topical antibiotics and additional agents such as antiseptics (hydrogen peroxide, povidone-iodine) have an unclear role in the management of infected wounds. Traditionally, many antiseptics have been applied to wounds, including iodine-containing solutions and sodium hypochlorite (Dakin's solution). These compounds can inhibit fibroblast growth in vitro and are used only for a relatively short period of time. Topical antibiotics, as opposed to antiseptics, probably have no role in the management of infected wounds. In resource-poor areas, both honey and granulated sugar have been used to treat open wounds, and their effectiveness may be based on their hypertonicity. Enzymatic débridement of wounds may be beneficial when aggressive wide surgical débridement is impossible.

For moderate to severe SSIs, including those associated with systemic toxicity, significant cellulitis (>2 cm beyond the incision), purulent drainage, fascial dehiscence, and deep drainage, antibiotics should be administered empirically. Initial selection should cover gram-positive organisms and likely infecting organisms based on colonization status, operative location, and recent infections. For wounds associated with operations on the gastrointestinal or genitourinary tracts, gram-negative coverage also should be provided. Source control is imperative for organ/space SSIs, including intra-abdominal abscess, and requires either percutaneous or operative drainage.

Culture of wounds is at the discretion of the surgeon. Straightforward, uncomplicated incisional SSIs without significant cellulitis that do not require antimicrobial therapy do not need to be cultured. On the other hand, all organ/space SSIs should be cultured because the role of antibiotics is greater in this instance. In other cases, cultures should be sent only when antibiotics are planned, the culture results will be used to guide antibiotic choice, and the patient is at high risk of having resistant pathogens. Patient characteristics that suggest that culture might be indicated include history of methicillin-resistant *Staphylococcus aureus* infection or colonization, recent receipt of therapeutic antibiotics, immunosuppression, care in an intensive care unit, and an unusually aggressive infection. Ideally cultures should be sterile aspirations or tissue, but swabs are useful if cautious interpretation of the results is used.

■ SUMMARY

SSIs are a common surgical complication and represent the most common nosocomial infection among surgical patients. These infections cause significant morbidity and increase costs, making them the focus of discussion and regulation at various levels. A number of process measures have been identified to reduce the risk of SSIs, and evidence-based standards should be incorporated into all surgeons' practices.

SUGGESTED READINGS

Berger RL, et al. Development and validation of a risk-stratification score for surgical site occurrence and surgical site infection after open ventral hernia repair. *J Am Coll Surg.* 2013;217:974-982.

Bhangu A, et al. Systemic review and meta-analysis of randomized clinical trials comparing primary vs delayed primary skin closure in contaminated and dirty abdominal incisions. *JAMA Surg.* 2013;148:779-786.

Buchleitner A, et al. Perioperative glycaemic control for diabetic patients undergoing surgery. *Cochrane Database Syst Rev.* 2012;(9):CD007315. doi:10.1002/14651858.CD007315.pub2.

Deerenberg EB, et al. Small bites versus large bites for closure of abdominal midline incisions (STITCH): a double-blind, multicentre, randomised controlled trial. *Lancet.* 2015;386:1254-1260. doi:10.1016/S0140-6736(15)60459-7.

Kao LS, Meeks D, Moyer VA, Lally KP. Peri-operative glycaemic control regimens for preventing surgical site infections in adults. *Cochrane Database Syst Rev.* 2009;(3):CD006806. doi:10.1002/14651858.CD006806.pub2.

Lefebvre A, et al. Preoperative hair removal and surgical site infections: network meta-analysis of randomized controlled trials. *J Hosp Infect.* 2015;91:100-108.

Mangram PJ, et al. Guideline for prevention of surgical site infection, 1999. *Infect Control Hosp Epidemiol.* 1999;20:247-278.

McCartan DP, et al. Purse-string approximation is superior to primary skin closure following stoma reversal: a systematic review and meta-analysis. *Tech Coloproctol.* 2013;17:345-351.

Mihaljevic AL, et al. Multicenter double-blinded randomized controlled trial of standard abdominal wound edge protection with surgical dressings versus coverage with a sterile circular polyethylene drape for prevention of surgical site infections. *Ann Surg.* 2014;260:730-739.

Nguyen MT, et al. Comparison of outcomes of synthetic mesh vs suture repair of elective primary ventral herniorrhaphy: a systematic review and meta-analysis. *JAMA Surg.* 2014;149:415-421.

Pinkney TD, et al. Impact of wound edge protection devices on surgical site infection after laparotomy: multicentre randomised controlled trial (ROSSINI Trial). *BMJ.* 2013;347:f4305. doi:10.1136/bmj.f4305.

Sawyer RG, et al. Trial of short-course antimicrobial therapy for intraabdominal infection. *N Engl J Med.* 2015;372:1996-2005.

Tanner J, Swarbrook S, Stuart J. Surgical hand antisepsis to reduce surgical site infection. *Cochrane Database Syst Rev.* 2008;(1):CD004288. doi:10.1002/14651858.CD004288.pub2.

Webster J, Scuffham P, Stankiewicz M, Chaboyer WP. Negative pressure wound therapy for skin grafts and surgical wounds healing by primary intention. *Cochrane Database Syst Rev.* 2014;(10):CD009261. doi:10.1002/14651858.CD009261.pub3.

THE MANAGEMENT OF INTRA-ABDOMINAL INFECTIONS

Mario Rueda, MD, and Albert Chi, MD, MSE

Intra-abdominal infections (IAIs) result from the invasion of micro-organisms, usually gram-negative and anaerobic bacteria, into the sterile abdominal cavity. This can result in physical examination changes, including peritonitis and decompensation of the host, and require the prompt attention of the surgeon. Multiple disease processes result in IAIs, and they can be grouped into three categories: primary, secondary, and tertiary infections.

Primary IAI occurs when there is an infection of the abdominal cavity without an obvious abdominal source. It usually occurs in patients with ascites and liver disease. In the majority of cases, enteric bacteria are isolated from ascitic fluid; the exact mechanism of this migration into the fluid is not clearly defined. Secondary IAI is more common and usually seen as a result of an acute infective process such as appendicitis or as contamination by enteric content such as a perforated viscus or anastomotic leak. These infections are usually polymicrobial and require not only antibiotic therapy but also source control. Tertiary IAI usually is identified in immunosuppressed patients, such as those undergoing organ transplantation. Despite appropriate therapy, the immunosuppressed host is unable to clear the micro-organism, resulting in a chronic infection marked by resistant organisms.

■ DIAGNOSIS

Presentation

Patients can have variable symptoms, but they usually report abdominal pain and fevers. Pain can be localized to a particular quadrant in the abdomen or generalized if the infection has progressed. Patients can exhibit altered mentation secondary to bacteremia or hypotension. Presence of a subdiaphragmatic infection may result in breathing and ventilatory difficulties. If the infection is localized, vital signs may be within normal limits. However, if the infection has continued to progress, the patient may be tachycardic and hypotensive. Gastrointestinal symptoms can range from simple pain to intolerance to diet and severe nausea and diarrhea. Irritation of the bladder by surrounding infected organs or fluid collections may result in dysuria.

Early identification of IAIs and prompt therapy will result in improved outcomes. Manifestation of septic shock such as dry mucosa, respiratory difficulty, hypotension, tachycardia, and poor urine output require emergent intervention and management.

Diagnostic Workup

Obtaining a detailed history and physical examination is key to formulating the diagnostic workup that should follow the evaluation of a patient with IAI. It is important to determine whether the patient has had previous infections with similar presentations. Understanding any recent surgical interventions as well as potential anastomoses can help to determine the source of the infection.

Serum laboratory tests such as complete blood count (CBC), electrolytes, and lactate are beneficial to determine potential bleeding and metabolic derangement. Blood, urine, and any catheter cultures should be sent, but results should not prevent therapy or treatment. It is our practice to obtain sputum cultures to help identify other potential sources of infection.

Computed tomographic (CT) scan of the abdomen and pelvis with contrast can be of great assistance in identifying the potential source of infection as well as in helping to plan a potential surgical or radiologic intervention. It is important to understand that it is *not* necessary to perform this study on every patient with IAI and that different imaging modalities may be more beneficial in certain instances, such as acute biliary disease. If a CT scan is being considered and the patient appears to have acute kidney insufficiency or is known to have chronic kidney disease (CKD), intravenous (IV) contrast should be used with caution, as it may precipitate further renal insult.

In those patients with primary IAI, paracentesis, fluid cell count, and culture should be performed. A neutrophil count greater than 250 cells/μL suggests bacterial peritonitis.

In a patient with a diffusely tender abdomen, chest and abdominal x-rays may be the only tests needed before proceeding to an exploration. For those patients with right upper quadrant (RUQ) pain, workup should include a RUQ ultrasound scan (US) and a liver function test (LFT) to evaluate the gallbladder. Biliary disease may require further imaging modalities such as magnetic resonance imaging (MRI). For female patients with right lower quadrant (RLQ) pain, a pregnancy test should be added to the diagnostic tests.

■ MANAGEMENT

The management of IAI, regardless of its cause, should start with patient resuscitation and stabilization. Antimicrobial therapy and a thorough workup for identification of a potential source should follow. It is very important not to withhold antimicrobial therapy while waiting for diagnostic tests such as cultures, as this may result in worsening outcomes for the patient.

Resuscitation

This is the most critical step in the management of IAI. In those patients who appear to be decompensating or in those with multiple medical comorbidities, management should be performed in the intensive care unit. Providers should establish adequate IV lines. If necessary, central venous access should be established in order to ensure appropriate resuscitation.

After obtaining necessary laboratory tests and in the absence of hemorrhage, crystalloid should be administered to hypotensive patients or those with a lactate level higher than 4 mmol/L. The recommendation of the Surviving Sepsis Campaign is to administer 30 mL/kg within 3 hours. To monitor appropriate response, a Foley catheter should be placed in order to ensure adequate perfusion.

Nasogastric tubes may be beneficial in those patients who are at risk of aspiration or suffering from a small bowel obstruction. If there is a strong suspicion for a perforated gastric or duodenal ulcer, care should be taken when placing the tube. Although not absolutely necessary, placement of arterial lines may be helpful in patients who require active titration of vasoactive substances or those in need of serial laboratory tests.

Antimicrobial Therapy

Early administration of antibiotics has been shown to result in better outcomes. Broad coverage should be initiated within 3 hours. As results from different cultures are obtained, the antimicrobial therapy should be modified in order to ensure appropriate treatment and de-escalation of therapy if necessary.

For those patients with primary IAI, *Escherichia coli* and *Klebsiella* usually are isolated. However, gram-positive bacteria also have been isolated. Febrile or symptomatic patients as well as those with a PMN count of 250 cells/μL should start taking a third-generation cephalosporin such as cefotaxime. If the patient has been receiving nonselective beta-blocker therapy, this should be discontinued because it has been associated with worse outcomes. Antibiotic therapy for these patients should continue for 5 days. Prophylaxis with oral antibiotics can be used, as it has been associated with decreased mortality.

Secondary IAIs usually are caused by enteric gram-negative bacilli such as *E. coli* and *Klebsiella* as well as obligate anaerobes such as *Bacteroides fragilis*. As opposed to patients with primary IAIs, it is not uncommon to isolate gram-positive bacteria such as viridans streptococci and *Enterococcus faecium* from affected tissues. We therefore recommend that patients start taking broad-spectrum antimicrobials to cover both gram-positive and gram-negative pathogens. The choice of antibiotics varies depending on provider. Piperacillin/tazobactam and vancomycin are common choices for initial therapy. Ertapenem also is used, although providers should be aware that this carbapenem has poor pseudomonal coverage. For those with penicillin allergy, combination therapy with ciprofloxacin and metronidazole may offer appropriate gram-negative coverage. If intolerance to metronidazole is discovered, clindamycin provides an appropriate alternative. For vancomycin-resistant *Enterococcus* (VRE), linezolid and tigecycline can be used, although the latter has been associated with worse outcomes, especially in patients on mechanical ventilation.

The management of tertiary IAI is far more complex, as it involves multidrug-resistant (MDR) organisms. Both gram-positive and gram-negative bacteria as well as fungi are isolated. The treatment approach is similar, with broad-spectrum coverage and tailoring therapy to cover the offending organisms. It is paramount to review previous cultures, as it is common to see reinfection with similar organisms.

Empiric antifungal therapy remains controversial. We routinely provide prophylaxis with fluconazole to all critically ill patients. In terms of treatment, we empirically treat those patients with recurrent IAI (tertiary), uncontrolled diabetes, parenteral nutrition, and upper gastrointestinal (UGI) injuries or perforations.

Duration of antibiotic therapy traditionally has been provider dependent. However, recent literature suggests that after obtaining source control, antimicrobial therapy should extend only for an additional 4 days. Longer courses do not provide any additional benefit and in fact may mask further complications. Antimicrobials should not be discontinued before source control is achieved or the infection process resolves, as premature discontinuation may precipitate further infection with resistant organisms.

The surgeon should keep in mind that the goal of antibiotic therapy is to control the infective process and allow the patient to undergo further therapy for source control *or* to allow the immune system to clear the infective process. Antimicrobial therapy is not a tool to "eradicate" all bacteria.

Source Control

There are basic principles that should be followed when performing a procedure for source control. In some instances, such as primary IAI, source control is achieved with antimicrobial therapy. In most others, an intervention is needed.

Surgical Control

Regardless of the procedure, surgical intervention should ensure complete removal of affected tissue and organ and their infective burden. As mentioned earlier, the intent is not to eliminate every micro-organism but rather to reduce the load so that the patient's immune system can eradicate and control the infection.

Débridement of necrotic and infective tissue should be performed. Débridement should continue until viable tissue is encountered. Hemostasis is necessary, as blood may serve as a growth medium to different bacteria. Complete evacuation of any infected fluid collection or abscess also should be performed. In the case of anastomotic disruption, diversion should be considered. Traditionally, irrigation of affected areas has been performed. However, there are clear instances in which it should not be performed, such as washing a perforated appendix. This may result in further seeding of micro-organisms and recurrent infections.

Aggressive intervention is favored, as failure to control infection will result in further morbidity and increase mortality. If necessary, serial procedures should be planned in order to ensure source control; early and effective control leads to improved outcomes.

Interventional Radiology

Percutaneous drainage has become an important tool in helping to achieve source control for several disease processes, including perforated appendicitis, complicated diverticulitis, and even acute cholecystitis in patients unable to tolerate exploration. It can be used as the sole therapy to achieve control or in combination with other more invasive procedures.

Drainage can be achieved with CT-guided imaging or US in those too unstable to travel to an interventional radiology suite. It is important to constantly reassess the patient and establish whether additional therapy is needed; repeat imaging may show worsening collection, and further therapy should be instituted. It is also important to recognize instances in which drainage would serve only as a temporizing measure and surgery is necessary. Laparotomy is still necessary in patients in whom, despite drainage, further decompensation follows.

Drain Management

A single percutaneous (PC) needle aspiration may eradicate an abscess successfully, especially when the abscess is small and contains low viscosity fluid. However, there is evidence that PC catheter drainage is more effective than aspiration. Typically, intervention begins with a 7F sump drain that should be flushed regularly with saline to remain patent. The drain site should be monitored and cleaned. Daily output should be recorded and may be removed once the clinical sepsis is resolved and output is minimal (<20 mL minus saline injected). Clinical improvement should be seen within 72 hours after intervention. Persistent fever and leukocytosis on the fourth day after intervention is correlated with failure. Nonresponders should be reimaged, with the next appropriate course of action being either upsizing or manipulating the PC drain or operative intervention. Placement of PC drainage catheters has become first-line therapy in the treatment of appropriate patients with intra-abdominal abscesses. Catheters can be used to avoid surgical intervention as well as to improve surgical outcomes.

■ SUMMARY

IAIs occur when an infective micro-organism invades the sterile abdominal cavity. This can be the result of physiologic derangement caused by liver failure and ascites, an extension of an organ infection such as diverticulitis or appendicitis, or disruption of anatomic continuity such as a perforation or an anastomotic leak. A detailed history and physical examination can reveal the diagnosis, although further studies are necessary. Treatment should focus on resuscitation, antibiotic therapy, and source control. Early intervention results in better outcomes.

SUGGESTED READINGS

Dellinger RP, Levy MM, Rhodes A, et al. Surviving Sepsis Campaign: international guidelines for management of severe sepsis and septic shock: 2012. *Crit Care Med.* 2013;41:580-637.

Namias N, Solomkin JS, Jensen EH, et al. Randomized, multicenter, double-blind study of efficacy, safety, and tolerability of intravenous ertapenem versus piperacillin/tazobactam in treatment of complicated intra-abdominal infections in hospitalized adults. *Surg Infect.* 2007;8:15-28.

Sawyer RG, Claridge JA, Nathens AB, et al. Trial of short-course antimicrobial therapy for intraabdominal infection. *N Engl J Med.* 2015;372:1996-2005.

Occupational Exposure to Human Immunodeficiency Virus and Other Bloodborne Pathogens

Susan E. Beekmann, RN, MPH,
and David K. Henderson, MD

Healthcare workers are known to be at risk for occupational bloodborne infections, including human immunodeficiency virus (HIV), hepatitis B (HBV), and hepatitis C (HCV). HBV has the highest risk of occupational infection, with a risk between 19% and 37% after a parenteral exposure to patients known to be HBV infected and who have circulating e-antigen. The risk of developing HCV after a parenteral exposure is estimated at 1.9%, whereas the risk of acquiring HIV after a parenteral exposure from a known HIV-infected source is 0.32%.

The number of individuals infected with these bloodborne pathogens, in particular the subset of these individuals who are unaware of their infective status, also affects the risk of exposure. The pool of patients infected with these bloodborne infections is highest for HCV: an estimated 2.7 million persons in the United States have chronic HCV, and most of these individuals do not know they are infected. An estimated 29,718 cases of acute HCV infection were reported in the United States in 2013.

Currently more than 1.2 million people in the United States are living with HIV infection, and almost 1 in 8 (12.8%) are unaware of their infection. Over the past decade, the number of people living with HIV has increased, whereas the annual number of new HIV infections has remained relatively stable. Antiretroviral therapy (ART) increasingly is recognized as an effective tool to prevent HIV transmission, although more than half of persons living with HIV in the United States are estimated *not* to be virologically suppressed and are thus are capable of transmitting the virus to others.

In 2013, 3050 cases of acute HBV in the United States were reported to the Centers for Disease Control and Prevention (CDC); the overall incidence of reported acute HBV was 0.9 cases per 100,000 population. However, because many HBV infections are either asymptomatic or never reported, the actual number of new infections is estimated to be approximately tenfold higher. In 2013 an estimated 19,764 persons in the United States were newly infected with HBV. The rate of new HBV infections has declined by approximately 82% since 1991, when a national strategy to eliminate HBV infection was implemented in the United States. Nonetheless, an estimated 700,000 to 1.4 million persons in the United States have chronic HBV infection.

The most effective way to prevent occupational transmission of bloodborne infections is to prevent the initial occupational exposure or injury. Primary prevention of occupational exposures and injuries begins with effective implementation of standard precautions used with all patients. Should primary prevention fail, secondary prevention consists of postexposure prophylaxis customized for the specific exposure, including immunoprophylaxis for individuals susceptible to HBV and antiretrovirals for those exposed to HIV.

GENERAL EPIDEMIOLOGY

Occupational injuries and exposures to blood and body fluids continue to be commonplace in virtually every healthcare setting.

The CDC reported that in 2004 more than 380,000 parenteral exposures to blood occurred annually, which means that almost 1 in 10 U.S. healthcare workers have a needlestick exposure per year. Underreporting of percutaneous injuries is a significant issue. A CDC surveillance system of healthcare workers from 1995 to 2007 surveyed these workers and concluded that more than half of the total injuries that occurred were not reported to occupational health services.

Although "average risk" estimates for occupational infection after percutaneous exposures are highest for HBV, intermediate for HBC, and lowest for HIV, a number of factors are known to influence the risk associated with an individual exposure to any bloodborne pathogen. These factors include, at a minimum, characteristics of the actual exposure, the exposure inoculum, and the exposed worker's immunologic response. Characteristics of the exposure that modify risk include whether it is parenteral or mucous membrane and whether it is deep or superficial. The exposure inoculum is predicated on both the viral concentration in the material to which the healthcare worker is exposed and the volume of the exposure. In a retrospective case-control study of healthcare workers who sustained parenteral exposures to HIV, increased risk for HIV infection was associated with exposure to larger quantities of blood from the source, as indicated by a needle or other device that was visibly contaminated with the patient's blood, a procedure that involved a needle being placed directly in a vein or artery, or a deep (as compared with superficial) injury. This same study also found that a source patient with terminal HIV disease (i.e., the source patient died from HIV infection within 60 days after the exposure) also was associated with increased risk (likely reflecting the higher circulating viral burden found in advanced stages of illness).

Studies suggest that spontaneous clearance of HCV is common and estimate that at least 30% of HCV infections resolve spontaneously. Acute HCV infection is highly curable, and early therapy results in significantly higher rates of eradication. The potential for occupational exposure to HCV is increasing, as recent data suggest that use of inpatient health services is increasing among individuals who have HCV infection.

PREVENTION OF EXPOSURES

The first and primary line of defense for preventing transmission of bloodborne infections is use of standard precautions by all healthcare workers. Education of staff is vital; healthcare students, new employees, and existing employees should all receive training that includes information about both the presence and the magnitude of occupational risks, as well as methods effective in preventing exposures, the importance of prompt reporting should exposure occur, and the availability of postexposure immunoprophylaxis for HBV and chemoprophylaxis for HIV. Healthcare institutions should review occupational exposure data on a periodic and ongoing basis to determine whether any trends are occurring or if specific interventions should be implemented to decrease exposures. Healthcare institutions also have an obligation to assess and introduce engineering controls (i.e., new and/or safer devices), to prevent exposure from intrinsically risky procedures.

IMMEDIATE EVALUATION AND MANAGEMENT OF EXPOSURES

Workplace injuries should receive immediate first aid, including washing the exposed site with soap and water or flushing exposed mucous membranes with saline or water. Exposures should be reported promptly to a supervisor, and an incident report should be completed per institutional policy. The exposed healthcare worker should report immediately to the occupational health service or, if after hours, to the emergency department or other area as specified by institutional policy.

Initial assessment of the exposure should include the date and time of exposure and the procedure or task performed, including when, where, and how the exposure occurred and with what type of device, including brand name. Assessment also should include details of the exposure, including route, body substance involved, volume, and duration of contact. The exposed healthcare worker also should be evaluated for pre-existing bloodborne pathogen infection, current medication use (for potential drug interactions), and any underlying medical conditions, including pregnancy.

Information about the source person, where available, should include HBV and HCV serostatus and HIV status or risk factors for HBV, HCV, and HIV if serostatus is unknown. If testing is performed, source persons should be evaluated for hepatitis B surface antigen (HBsAg), anti-HCV, and HIV antibody (rapid testing should be used to guide decisions about postexposure prophylaxis). The CDC and other authorities have advocated "opt-out testing," which would treat HIV tests much like other tests—meaning that the patient has the opportunity to decline the test—except that there is no requirement for signed informed consent with counseling. Whether signed informed consent is required before obtaining blood from the source patient for HIV testing varies by state, and occupational health services should know all relevant laws. If the source patient is known to be infected, the stage of disease, history of ART, and viral load status for any or all of the bloodborne pathogens should be documented. Prophylaxis and follow-up should be predicated on either known testing results or the epidemiologic assessment of the risk for infection, if test results are not immediately available. Discarded needles, syringes, and other devices *are not* tested for virus contamination.

■ OCCUPATIONAL EXPOSURES TO HIV

Healthcare Worker Testing for HIV

A negative result from an enzyme-linked immunosorbent assay (ELISA) for antibodies to HIV should be documented at the time of the initial assessment of an occupational exposure. If possible, HIV antibody testing should be done with a rapid test kit approved by the Food and Drug Administration (FDA), with results available in less than an hour. Fourth-generation HIV antigen and antibody tests, which detect p24 antigen as well as conventional HIV antibodies, may be used in place of HIV antibody tests. These tests have a sensitivity and specificity of approximately 99%. Early antigen recognition with these assays reduces the window period for detection by approximately 5 days.

Initial Care After Exposure

If postexposure prophylaxis is to be offered, it should be offered as soon as possible, preferably within a few hours of exposure. It should not be delayed while waiting for test results. For example, a surgeon who sustains an occupational exposure to HIV while performing a surgical procedure should promptly scrub out of the surgical case, if possible, and seek immediate medical evaluation for the injury and postexposure prophylaxis. If initiation of postexposure prophylaxis is delayed, the likelihood increases that benefits might not outweigh the risks inherent in taking antiretroviral medications.

All women of childbearing age not known to be pregnant should be offered pregnancy testing. Expert consultation is recommended for all postexposure prophylaxis decisions, but timely initiation of such prophylaxis should not be delayed to obtain such consultation. PEPline (the National Clinicians' Postexposure Prophylaxis Hotline) is available from 9 AM to 2 AM EST daily for clinicians managing occupational exposures. PEPline can be contacted by phone at (888) 448-4911 or online at http://www.nccc.ucsf.edu/. Exposed healthcare workers should be counseled to avoid the potential for transmission of HIV to others, particularly during the first 6 to 12 weeks after exposure. Recommended practices should include either sexual abstinence or use of barrier protection, as well as avoidance of blood and organ donation.

Rationale for Postexposure Prophylaxis

Postexposure prophylaxis was first used after occupational HIV exposures in the late 1980s, with the CDC issuing the first set of guidelines that included considerations regarding the use of antiretroviral agents for postexposure prophylaxis after occupational HIV exposures in 1990. A case-control study of HIV seroconversion in healthcare workers after percutaneous exposure published in 1997 provided the first evidence in humans that postexposure prophylaxis with a single antiretroviral agent (zidovudine) appeared to be protective against infection.

Animal data suggest that antiretroviral chemoprophylaxis administered soon after an exposure, in concert with cellular immunity, may prevent or inhibit systemic HIV infection. This preventive effect theoretically is caused by limiting proliferation of the virus in dendritic cells in skin or in T cells in regional lymph nodes during the time in which the virus remains relatively localized. This effect may be bolstered by a robust cellular immune response.

In the CDC's retrospective case-control study of healthcare workers, postexposure prophylaxis with zidovudine was associated with an 81% reduction in the odds of infection after adjustment for relevant exposure risk factors. In addition, studies of prevention of mother-to-child transmission, including AIDS Clinical Trial Group Protocol 076 (which included treating the infant postpartum), indicated a protective effect of zidovudine that was not attributable solely to a reduction in maternal HIV viral load.

Finally, the number of occupational infections with HIV reported to the CDC has decreased steadily since the first use of postexposure prophylaxis in the late 1980s. Since 1999 only one confirmed case of occupationally acquired HIV has been reported. This decrease in cases is related to multiple factors, likely including better primary prevention strategies, HIV treatment as prevention with decreased viral burden in source patients infected with HIV, fewer hospitalizations of patients infected with HIV, fewer exposure-prone procedures performed on these patients, and perhaps the use of postexposure prophylaxis for occupational exposures.

Postexposure Prophylaxis Regimen

The U.S. Public Health Service (USPHS) recommendations for prophylaxis after exposure to HIV were updated in 2013 and no longer recommend attempting to characterize the level of risk for HIV transmission when selecting regimens for postexposure prophylaxis. Postexposure prophylaxis should be continued for 4 weeks. The CDC now recommends the combination of raltegravir, tenofovir, and emtricitabine as the "preferred" regimen for postexposure prophylaxis (Table 1); these guidelines will be updated continually online as newer options become available. For example, additional integrase inhibitors (e.g., dolutegravir) have been marketed that might offer the potential for once-daily therapy (in combination with tenofovir-emtricitabine). For alternative regimens, the 2013 guidelines recommend use of three agents (e.g., two nucleoside reverse transcriptase inhibitors and an integrase strand transfer inhibitor, a "ritonavir-boosted" protease inhibitor, or a non-nucleoside reverse transcriptase inhibitor; see Table 1).

The risks of postexposure prophylaxis should be considered very carefully before an exposed healthcare worker starts taking medication, as the great majority of these exposures will not result in infection. HIV resistance is an increasing concern, with resistance to all antiretroviral drugs and transmission of resistant strains reported. If the source patient's resistance pattern for currently circulating virus is known, that information should guide selection of the postexposure prophylaxis regimen. Those most knowledgeable about the drugs, their efficacy, and their side effects (i.e., HIV physician team, infectious disease consultants) should be

TABLE 1: Recommended Postexposure Prophylaxis (PEP) for All Occupational Exposures to Human Immunodeficiency Virus (HIV)

PREFERRED HIV PEP REGIMEN

Raltegravir (Isentress) 400 mg PO (by mouth) twice daily
plus
Tenofovir DF (Viread) 300 mg + emtricitabine (Emtriva) 200 mg; available as Truvada, PO once daily

ALTERNATIVE REGIMENS

May combine one drug or drug pair from the left column with one pair of nucleoside/nucleotide reverse transcriptase inhibitors from the right column

Dolutegravir (Tivicay)	Tenofovir DF (Viread) + emtricitabine (Emtriva); available as Truvada
Raltegravir (Isentress)	Tenofovir DF (Viread) + emtricitabine (Emtriva); available as Truvada
Darunavir (Prezista) + ritonavir (Norvir)	Tenofovir DF (Viread) + lamivudine (Epivir)
Etravirine (Intelence)	Zidovudine (Retrovir) + lamivudine (Epivir); available as Combivir
Rilpivirine (Edurant)	Zidovudine (Retrovir) + emtricitabine (Emtriva)
Atazanavir (Reyataz) + ritonavir (Norvir)	
Lopinavir/ritonavir (Kaletra)	

Stribild (elvitegravir, cobicistat, tenofovir DF, emtricitabine); a complete fixed-dose combination regimen with no additional antiretrovirals needed

ALTERNATIVE ANTIRETROVIRAL AGENTS FOR USE AS PEP *ONLY* WITH EXPERT CONSULTATION

Abacavir (Ziagen)

Efavirenz (Sustiva)

Enfuvirtide (Fuzeon)

Fosamprenavir (Lexiva)

Maraviroc (Selzentry)

Saquinavir (Invirase)

Stavudine (Zerit)

ANTIRETROVIRAL AGENTS GENERALLY NOT RECOMMENDED FOR USE AS PEP

Didanosine (Videx EC)

Nelfinavir (Viracept)

Tipranavir (Aptivus)

ANTIRETROVIRAL AGENTS CONTRAINDICATED AS PEP

Nevirapine (Viramune)

Adapted from Kuhar DT, Henderson DK, Struble KA, Panlilio AL, Heneine W, Thomas V, Cheever LW, Gomaa A. Updated U.S. Public Health Service guidelines for the management of occupational exposures to HIV and recommendations for postexposure prophylaxis. *Infect Control Hosp Epidemiol.* 2013;34:875-892.

consulted to determine an optimal regimen for known exposures to resistant HIV.

Recommended Monitoring and Follow-up

All healthcare workers who start taking postexposure prophylaxis should be re-evaluated within 72 hours. The exposed worker should have the opportunity to ask additional questions, and management of associated symptoms and side effects should be discussed along with the need for adherence to the medication regimen. Follow-up HIV testing should occur at 6 weeks, 12 weeks, and 6 months after exposure. The 2013 CDC guidelines indicate that if a fourth-generation immunoassay for HIV is used, HIV follow-up testing could be concluded at 4 months after exposure. Testing for more than 6 months is not routinely recommended, although individuals who become infected with HCV after exposure to a source who is coinfected with HIV and HCV should be tested again at 12 months.

Symptoms of acute retroviral infection (e.g., fever, lymphadenopathy, pharyngitis, rash, headache, profound fatigue) have been associated with approximately 80% of reported occupational infections, even when postexposure prophylaxis was administered. Exposed workers should be encouraged to seek evaluation should any of these symptoms occur.

Workers on postexposure prophylaxis should return for evaluation at least every 2 weeks for the first 6 weeks after exposure, and weekly visits for the first month may be indicated. Evaluation should include a careful history (focusing on the potential for acute infection and the potential for drug toxicity), a focused physical examination, and relevant laboratory tests appropriate to the drug regimen. As a general rule, a complete blood cell count and renal and hepatic chemical function tests are indicated. A random blood glucose measurement and a lipid profile should be considered whenever a protease inhibitor is included in the regimen.

OCCUPATIONAL EXPOSURES TO HBV

The three intramuscular doses of hepatitis B vaccine that all healthcare workers should receive at time of entry to patient care induce a protective antibody response in more than 90% of healthy recipients. Once an individual has a protective antibody response, protection from clinical disease and chronic infection should be lifelong. No follow-up is required for healthcare workers who are known to be vaccinated with a protective antibody response (Table 2). Persons who previously have been infected with HBV are immune to reinfection and do not require postexposure prophylaxis.

The option of giving one dose of hepatitis B immune globulin (HBIG) and reinitiating the vaccine series is preferred for nonresponders who have not completed a second three-dose vaccine series. For persons who previously completed a second vaccine series but failed to respond, two doses of HBIG (the second dose administered 4 weeks after the first) are preferred. Vaccinated healthcare workers whose antibody response is unknown should have their level of serum antibody to HBsAg (anti-HBs) checked to determine whether HBIG should be administered. Follow-up for susceptible healthcare workers should include HBsAg, hepatitis B surface antibody (HBsAb), and hepatitis B core antigen (anti-HBc) plus a liver enzyme panel 6 months after exposure and at the time of the third dose of vaccine. Anti-HBs levels typically peak 1 week after injection of HBIG, and the mean half-life of HBIG is 22 days. Anti-HBs should not be tested for any sooner than 4 to 6 months after HBIG administration.

OCCUPATIONAL EXPOSURES TO HCV

No marketed vaccine prevents HCV infection; the mainstay of preventing HCV infection in healthcare workers is primary prevention of exposure to the virus. Healthcare workers who have been exposed to HCV should be tested at the time of exposure for antibody to HCV

TABLE 2: Recommended Postexposure Prophylaxis for Exposure to HBV

Vaccination and Antibody Response Status of Exposed Workers	Treatment		
	Source HBsAg Positive	Source HBsAg Negative	Source Unknown or Not Available for Testing
Unvaccinated	HBIG* × 1 and initiate HBV vaccine series	Initiate HBV vaccine series	Initiate HBV vaccine series
Previously vaccinated			
a. Known responder†	No treatment	No treatment	No treatment
b. Known nonresponder‡	HBIG × 1 and initiate revaccination or HBIG × 2§	No treatment	If known high-risk source, treat as if source were HBsAg positive
c. Antibody response unknown	Test exposed person for anti-HBs 1. If adequate,† no treatment is necessary 2. If inadequate,‡ administer HBIG × 1 and vaccine booster	No treatment	Test exposed person for anti-HBs 1. If adequate,† no treatment is necessary 2. If inadequate,‡ administer vaccine booster and recheck titer in 1-2 mo

Adapted from Centers for Disease Control and Prevention. Updated U.S. Public Health Service guidelines for the management of occupational exposures to HBV, HCV, and HIV and recommendations for postexposure prophylaxis. *MMWR Morb Mortal Wkly Rep.* 2001;50:1-42.

*Dose is 0.06 mL/kg intramuscularly, given as soon as possible after exposure and within 24 hours, if possible.

†A responder is a person with adequate levels of serum antibody to HBsAg (i.e., anti-HBs ≥10 mIU/mL).

‡A nonresponder is a person with inadequate response to vaccination (i.e., serum anti-HBs <10 mIU/mL).

§The option of giving one dose of HBIG and reinitiating the vaccine series is preferred for nonresponders who have not completed a second three-dose vaccine series. For persons who previously completed a second vaccine series but failed to respond, two doses of HBIG are preferred.

Anti-HBs, Hepatitis B surface antigen antibody; *HBIG,* hepatitis B immune globulin; *HBsAg,* hepatitis B surface antigen; *HBV,* hepatitis B.

and for HCV RNA by qualitative polymerase chain reaction (PCR). These tests should be monitored no earlier than 2 weeks after exposure and then periodically at least every 2 months until 6 months after exposure.

Even if the HCV PCR or the anti-HCV serology becomes positive, a high rate (30% to 40%) of spontaneous viral clearance occurs within 12 weeks after the onset of symptomatic disease. "Watchful waiting" for 12 weeks after seroconversion likely will result in avoiding unnecessary treatment and does not alter the likelihood of successful treatment of HCV infection. Repeatedly reactive anti-HCV assays should be confirmed with supplemental tests, and the patient referred for consideration of treatment for early acute infection.

Current guidelines do not support the administration of postexposure prophylaxis for HCV exposures, and the likelihood of a cure is very good if infection is treated in the acute phase (3 to 6 months after infection), although this tenet may change as more experience is gained with the use of newer direct-acting anti-HCV antivirals. Unlike the case for HBV infection, immunoglobulin prophylaxis should not be used in managing occupational exposures to HCV.

Direct-acting anti-HCV antivirals that inhibit HCV protease, polymerase, and nonstructural protein 5A are changing the landscape for successful therapy of HCV. These agents ultimately may be shown to have a role in postexposure chemoprophylaxis for occupational exposures to HCV, though to our knowledge no data yet exist that support their use in this setting. In addition, the concept of genotype-specific monoclonal antibodies is being investigated aggressively and, if successful, may offer potential for postexposure immunoprophylaxis.

■ SOURCE-UNKNOWN EXPOSURES

Current USPHS guidelines are based on exposures to blood or other potentially infectious materials known to contain HIV, not materials of uncertain HIV status. When the source material is not known to contain HIV, decisions about treatment should be predicated on the probability of HIV infection in the source patient, as well as the type of exposure and the associated risk of HIV transmission with such an exposure, if HIV were in fact present. Any risks associated with treatment for the exposed individual also should be considered, as treatment should not be undertaken unless the risk of HIV transmission outweighs the risk of treatment. In many "source-unknown" exposures, the risk of transmission is negligible, and treatment simply is not indicated.

SUGGESTED READINGS

Cardo DM, Culver DH, Ciesielski CA, et al. A case-control study of HIV seroconversion in health care workers after percutaneous exposure. Centers for Disease Control and Prevention Needlestick Surveillance Group. *N Engl J Med.* 1997;337:1485-1490.

Henderson DK. Management of needlestick injuries: a house officer who has a needlestick. *JAMA.* 2012;307:75-84.

Joyce MP, Kuhar D, Brooks JT. Occupationally acquired HIV infection among health care workers—United States, 1985-2013. *MMWR Morb Mortal Wkly Rep.* 2015;64:1245-1246.

Kuhar DT, Henderson DK, Struble KA, et al. Updated US Public Health Service guidelines for the management of occupational exposures to human immunodeficiency virus and recommendations for postexposure prophylaxis. *Infect Control Hosp Epidemiol.* 2013;34:875-892.

ANTIFUNGAL THERAPY IN THE SURGICAL PATIENT

Mark A. Malangoni, MD, Jeffrey A. Claridge, MD, and Brenda M. Zosa, MD

Fungal infections are an increasing problem in hospitalized surgical patients. The most commonly seen infections are caused by a variety of *Candida* species, most notably *C. albicans*. Aspergillosis and mucormycosis are other significant fungal pathogens. Superficial fungal infections are rarely dangerous, but invasive fungal infections continue to be associated with serious complications and a high mortality. The reasons for this are related to both host and fungal factors. Risk factors for developing invasive fungal infections include critical illness, recent abdominal surgery often complicated by an anastomotic leak, solid organ transplantation, prolonged exposure to broad-spectrum antibiotics, and additional immunocompromised states. Moreover, diagnosis of infection can be difficult, and often implementation of appropriate antifungal therapy is delayed.

In addition to antifungal chemotherapy, surgical management of invasive fungal infections often plays a critical role. These interventions can range from removal of a potentially infected intravascular catheter, to drainage of infected fluid collections, to débridement of invasive tissue disease. This chapter summarizes fungal infections typically encountered in a surgical practice, with special emphasis on the use of antifungal therapy as treatment (Table 1).

■ SPECIFIC FUNGI

Candida

Candida species are the most common fungal pathogens in surgical patients. These fungi are commensals of the human gastrointestinal (GI) tract, genital tracts, and skin. Infections are almost always of endogenous origin, but cross-contamination can occur between colonized patients or from healthcare workers' unwashed hands to patients. Invasion occurs when host defenses break down or are breached. Patients with a central venous catheter, with prolonged exposure to broad-spectrum antibiotics, or who have had a recent operation, particularly when there has been GI contamination, are at greater risk for candidiasis.

C. albicans is the most common colonizing and infecting species and represents about half of all fungal isolates. The other important species include *C. parapsilosis, C. glabrata, C. tropicalis,* and *C. krusei.* The most virulent of these species are *C. albicans, C. glabrata,* and *C. tropicalis.* Exposure to antifungal agents and transfer of the yeast among patients via healthcare workers' hands can alter fungal colonization patterns and subsequent infecting species.

Infection due to *Candida* can be broadly divided into mucosal and systemic disease. Oropharyngeal candidiasis tends to occur in patients with abnormal cell-mediated immunity (as in those with advanced human immunodeficiency virus [HIV] and those receiving corticosteroids). Cutaneous and vulvovaginal candidiasis sometimes are triggered by antimicrobial use and poor glycemic control but also can occur spontaneously. The majority of women with candidal vaginitis are not immunocompromised. Invasive candidiasis tends to occur in patients with breached anatomic barriers due to surgery, cytotoxic chemotherapy, or vascular access catheters and in those with abnormalities in neutrophil quantity or function.

Filamentous Fungi

Infections due to filamentous fungi most commonly are caused by *Aspergillus* and to a lesser extent by the zygomycetes *Fusarium* and *Scedosporium.* These fungi are present in the environment, and infection can develop after inhalation or direct inoculation from external sources. Patients with abnormal lung anatomy or function may be chronically colonized with *Aspergillus* or other molds, which then can progress to invasive or saprophytic disease. Risk factors for these infections include profound neutrophil dysfunction and use of corticosteroids and other immunosuppressive drugs. Because the respiratory tract is the main site of contact with *Aspergillus* spores, patients with significant abnormalities of respiratory tract structure and function, such as cystic fibrosis, chronic lung diseases, lung transplantation, and prolonged mechanical ventilation, are also at risk for aspergillosis. Rarely, infection occurs because of direct inoculation of a surgical site or after traumatic injury. *A. fumigatus* is the most common filamentous species involved in human disease.

Invasive aspergillosis most commonly manifests as a progressive, cavitary pulmonary infection that can result in hemoptysis. These cavitary lesions usually are seen on chest radiograph or computed tomography of the chest. Cutaneous infections may occur after a break in the skin barrier, either because of burn injury or after an operation in a severely immunocompromised patient.

■ ANTIFUNGAL AGENTS

Azoles

The azoles are a commonly used class of antifungal agents with activity against a broad range of fungi. These drugs inhibit ergosterol biosynthesis, thereby impairing formation of the fungal cell membrane. Azoles are available in oral, intravenous (IV), or topical forms depending on the specific agent. Azoles have the potential for multiple drug interactions via the cytochrome P450 system, and care must be taken when they are administered at the same time as other drugs metabolized by these isoenzymes. Azoles are preferred to treat *Candida* urinary tract infections.

Fluconazole

Fluconazole is the predominant azole used to treat fungal infections in surgical patients. It is effective against most species of *Candida* and is used often as first-line therapy. It is available in oral and IV formulations and is generally well tolerated. Fluconazole has excellent activity against *C. albicans* but has variable activity against *C. glabrata,* which can account for up to 25% of candidal infections. It is inactive against *C. krusei.* Fluconazole is a first-line agent for oropharyngeal and esophageal candidiasis as well as for urinary tract infections due to *Candida.* It also has a role in cases of invasive candidiasis in moderately ill, non-neutropenic patients, although dosing needs to be significantly higher (400 to 800 mg/day). Dose adjustment is required with renal dysfunction. The use of fluconazole has been associated with hepatic toxicity, GI upset, rashes, and drug interactions.

Voriconazole

Voriconazole is effective against most species of *Candida* and *Aspergillus* and multiple other filamentous fungi. It is available in oral and IV formulations. Voriconazole is the first-line treatment for invasive aspergillosis and can be used in cases of invasive candidiasis. It has excellent bioavailability, allowing for oral administration. Steady-state levels are reached more rapidly with IV loading doses of 6 mg/kg every 12 hours for 2 doses, followed by 4 mg/kg IV every 12 hours or 200 mg orally every 12 hours. Patients with renal dysfunction should receive the oral form of voriconazole for maintenance, as the cyclodextrin carrier used in the IV formulation can accumulate and may damage the kidneys. Patients with hepatic impairment should receive the standard loading dose, but the maintenance dose should be decreased by 50%.

Voriconazole is associated with multiple adverse reactions, most commonly visual changes such as photophobia, reduction in visual acuity, and blurred vision. Routine monitoring of drug levels is not recommended; however, monitoring can be helpful when there are

TABLE 1: Patient Types and Treatment Options for Fungal Infections

Infection	Patient Type	Primary and Alternative Treatments	Duration of Therapy	Comments
Candidemia	Critically ill, abdominal surgery, cancer chemotherapy, vascular access, burns, parenteral nutrition	**Primary** Caspofungin 70 mg × 1, then 50 mg/day IV Anidulafungin 200 mg × 1, then 100 mg/day IV Micafungin 100 mg/day IV Fluconazole 800 mg × 1, then 400 mg/day IV or PO **Alternative** Deoxycholate AmB 0.7-1.0 mg/kg/day IV Lipid AmB 3-5 mg/kg/day IV Voriconazole 6 mg/kg BID × 2 doses, then 4 mg/kg BID	14 days after clearance of blood cultures Longer if ocular involvement. If possible, can switch to oral agent to complete therapy once patient has stabilized.	Remove vascular access devices, if possible. Do not use fluconazole for critically ill patients. Evaluate for ocular involvement with fundoscopic examination.
Candiduria/UTI	Urinary catheter, DM, kidney transplant recipients	**Primary** Fluconazole 200-400 mg/day IV or PO **Alternative** Deoxycholate AmB 0.3-0.6 mg/kg/day IV Flucytosine 25 mg/kg QID PO	14 days 1-7 days 7-10 days	Patients with asymptomatic candiduria do not routinely need to be treated. Exceptions are neutropenia or planned instrumentation.
Oropharyngeal candidiasis	Immunocompromised, radiotherapy, ill-fitting dentures	**Primary** Clotrimazole 10 mg 5 times/day PO Nystatin suspension (100,000 U/mL) 4-6 mL QID PO Fluconazole 100-200 mg/day PO **Alternative** Itraconazole solution 200 mg/day PO Posaconazole 400 mg BID × 3 days, then 400 mg/day BID PO Voriconazole 200 mg BID PO Caspofungin 70 mg × 1, then 50 mg/day IV Anidulafungin 200 mg × 1, then 100 mg/day IV Micafungin 100 mg/day IV Deoxycholate AmB oral suspension 100 mg/mL QID PO or 0.3 mg/kg IV daily	7-14 days	Use topical therapy for mild disease; relapses more common with echinocandins.
Esophageal candidiasis	Immunocompromised	**Primary** Fluconazole 200-400 mg/day PO or 400 mg/day IV **Alternative** Micafungin 150 mg/day IV Caspofungin 70 mg × 1, then 50 mg/day IV Anidulafungin 200 mg/day IV Deoxycholate AmB 0.3-0.7 mg/kg/day IV Itraconazole 200 mg/day PO Voriconazole 200 mg BID IV or PO Posaconazole 400 mg BID PO	14-21 days	Relapses may be more common with echinocandins.
Vulvovaginal candidiasis	Antibacterial therapy, DM	Topical therapy (e.g., clotrimazole, nystatin, miconazole) Fluconazole 150 mg × 1 PO	Schedules vary by agent	Vulvovaginal candidiasis, even if recurrent, usually does not result from an immunocompromised state.

TABLE 1: Patient Types and Treatment Options for Fungal Infections—cont'd

Infection	Patient Type	Primary and Alternative Treatments	Duration of Therapy	Comments
Aspergillosis	Abnormalities of neutrophil number or function, structural lung abnormalities, burns	**Primary** Voriconazole 6 mg/kg BID × 2, then 4 mg/kg/day +/− echinocandin **Alternative** Lipid AmB 3-5 mg/kg/day Caspofungin 70 mg × 1, then 50 mg/day IV Posaconazole 800 mg/day in 2-4 divided doses IV or PO	Length of treatment not clear	Consider monitoring voriconazole and posaconazole levels to help guide therapy.
Mucormycosis	Systemic immunosuppression, burns, trauma, near drowning, uncontrolled DM, deferoxamine use	**Primary** Lipid AmB 5-7.5 mg/kg/day +/− posaconazole	Length of treatment not clear	Débridement and excision are often needed. If patient is stable, consider switching to posaconazole after 3 weeks AmB.

AmB, Amphotericin B; *BID,* twice daily; *DM,* diabetes mellitus; *IV,* intravenously; *PO,* orally; *QID,* four times daily; *UTI,* urinary tract infection.

concerns about efficacy or toxicity. Like fluconazole, voriconazole is associated with multiple drug interactions.

Posaconazole

Posaconazole is effective against a broad range of fungi, including most species of *Candida* and *Aspergillus* and many filamentous fungi, including the zygomycetes. It is available in oral suspension, delayed-release tablets, and IV formulations. Oral suspension or delayed-release tablets are indicated for prophylaxis of invasive *Aspergillus* and *Candida* infections in patients at high risk of developing these infections because of being severely immunocompromised (e.g., recipients of hematopoietic stem cell transplant with graft vs. host disease, those with hematologic malignancies with prolonged neutropenia from chemotherapy). Attainment of steady-state levels can take a week or longer, and for this reason it generally is not recommended as first-line therapy for established infections. The dose for invasive fungal infections varies depending on the formulation used, and it is imperative that this be taken into account. Like voriconazole, IV dosing should be reduced in patients with renal impairment because of toxicity from accumulation of the associated vehicle. Side effects of posaconazole are common and include fever, nausea, diarrhea, headache, hypokalemia, and thrombocytopenia. Long QT syndrome and hepatotoxicity are less common but serious complications. Posaconazole also is associated with multiple drug interactions similar to those with other azoles.

Itraconazole

Itraconazole's spectrum of activity is similar to that of fluconazole. It is active against *Candida* but also against some filamentous and dimorphic fungi, including *Aspergillus, Blastomyces,* and *Histoplasma.* It also can be used to treat onychomycosis. Itraconazole has been of limited use in surgical patients. The use of itraconazole has been limited by erratic bioavailability of the oral capsule, which has improved with the oral cyclodextrin solution. In some countries itraconazole also is available for IV therapy. Several factors limit its use, including erratic gut absorption, need for drug level monitoring, GI upset (particularly with the cyclodextrin solution), hepatic toxicity, and negative inotropic cardiac effects that can lead to congestive heart failure.

Echinocandins

The echinocandins (caspofungin, micafungin, and anidulafungin) are an important class of antifungal agents, and they have emerged as a preferred treatment class for many fungal infections. They act by inhibiting fungal cell wall formation and have fungicidal activity against almost all *Candida* species. Echinocandins are used widely for the treatment of invasive candidiasis, especially in critically ill and neutropenic patients. They also are used for empiric antifungal therapy in immunocompromised patients with neutropenic fever. The major advantages of echinocandins relative to other antifungal agents are their fungicidal activity against a variety of *Candida* species, including fluconazole-resistant *C. glabrata* and *C. krusei.* Treatment failures have been reported with *C. parapsilosis,* which has some innate resistance to the echinocandins. Under selective pressure, other species of *Candida* also can become resistant because of mutations. The echinocandins also can inhibit growth of *Aspergillus,* but they are not fungicidal. There may be a role for their use in nonresponsive *Aspergillus* infections. Experience suggests that this class is among the safest and best tolerated of the antifungals available. They are available only via the IV route. Echinocandins are first-line therapy against invasive candidiasis and also may be used but are not ideal for cases of oropharyngeal and esophageal candidiasis.

Polyenes

Polyene antibiotics are a class of antimicrobial compounds that bind to ergosterol, the main sterol in the fungal cell membrane, and cause depolarization. This increases membrane permeability and leads to leakage of intracellular cations causing cell death. Amphotericin B and nystatin are examples of polyene antimycotics. Amphotericin B deoxycholate, which was the standard drug for the treatment of candidiasis for decades, demonstrates rapidly fungicidal in vitro activity against most species of *Candida* but is associated with significant nephrotoxicity. Because of this adverse effect, it is rarely used. Instead, most physicians use a lipid-based amphotericin B formulation, either liposomal amphotericin B or amphotericin B lipid complex, when selecting a polyene agent. These lipid-based compounds have much less toxicity than amphotericin deoxycholate but are significantly more expensive. Polyenes have been relegated to situations in which other antifungals are ineffective.

■ MUCOCUTANEOUS DISEASE

Mucocutaneous fungal infections are very common, and their risk factors (e.g., diabetes mellitus, antibiotic exposure, corticosteroids) are found frequently in surgical patients. These infections can cause significant discomfort but are rarely dangerous. Typical sites of infection include the skin, oropharynx (thrush), genitalia, and esophagus.

Patients with symptomatic superficial infection should be treated, but because *Candida* species normally exist on the skin and mucosal surfaces as commensals, culturing the organism from a superficial surface in the absence of symptoms is not an indication for treatment.

Cutaneous Candidiasis

Cutaneous infections can occur anywhere on the body but typically involve intertriginous areas (candidal intertrigo). Warm, moist, and macerated skin sites, such as inframammary and large abdominal folds, the axillae, or the groin, are common sites of involvement and must be examined. Cutaneous candidiasis is almost always caused by *C. albicans* and tends to occur around open incisions, wounds, or decubitus ulcers being treated with moist dressings. Diabetes mellitus, obesity, treatment with antibiotics or steroids, and inflammatory skin diseases are risk factors for these infections. The affected area may be itchy, red, and moist. The skin can be eroded with whitish scaling at the borders. Satellite lesions just beyond the border of the grossly affected area are common.

Diagnosis generally is based on clinical appearance. Superficial candidiasis can be treated with topical therapy. For moist macerated skin, an antifungal powder formulation is preferable because of its drying properties. Nystatin (100,000 units/g) and miconazole (2%) are available as either a powder or a cream. A variety of other antifungal creams are also available, such as ketoconazole (2%) and clotrimazole (1%). More extensive infections may require oral azole drugs in conjunction with topical treatments.

Vulvovaginal Candidiasis

Candidal vulvovaginitis is common, and most women will have at least one attack during their lifetime. Most infections are caused by *C. albicans* and represent a patient's own organisms. Risk factors include antibiotics, diabetes mellitus, and pregnancy. Vulvovaginitis may be seen with local irritation, itching, erythema, vaginal discharge, dysuria, and dyspareunia. Patients often make a self-diagnosis of "yeast" vaginitis. This can be confirmed by identifying candidal elements (pseudohyphae and blastoconidia) on microscopic evaluation of a 10% KOH treated sample. Fungal cultures are usually neither necessary nor helpful.

There are multiple intravaginal treatment options, including nystatin tablets (100,000 units/tablet), various azole creams and vaginal suppositories (e.g., miconazole 2%, butoconazole 2%, clotrimazole 1%, terconazole 0.4% and 0.8%, tioconazole 6.5%, miconazole cream 2% and 4% or suppositories at 100 and 200 mg), and oral fluconazole (150 mg as a single dose). The duration of treatment varies with different agents and concentrations. Most infections can be treated with a single dose of oral medication or a 1- to 3-day course of topical therapy. Some patients with recurrent or severe disease require longer treatment with either 7 to 14 days of topical azole or 150 mg of fluconazole in two sequential oral doses (second dose 72 hours after initial dose).

Oropharyngeal and Esophageal Candidiasis

Oropharyngeal candidiasis is mainly a problem in immunosuppressed patients, particularly after organ transplantation and in those with advanced HIV. Additional risk factors include extremes in age, poorly controlled diabetes mellitus, nutritional deficiencies, inadequately fitting dentures, systemic or inhaled steroids, radiotherapy, and cytotoxic chemotherapy. Clinical manifestations include thrush, which is characterized by curdlike, white patches on multiple surfaces of the oral mucosa, and erythematous candidiasis (acute atrophic candidiasis), which occurs by itself or in association with the white patches. Symptoms include local pain, burning, and changes in taste perception. Microscopic examination of scrapings of the involved area may help with the diagnosis if in doubt.

Oropharyngeal candidiasis is almost always caused by *C. albicans* and usually responds to topical treatments such as clotrimazole troches, 10 mg 5 times daily, or nystatin suspension (nystatin "swish and swallow"). Systemic antifungal medication such as fluconazole, 100 to 200 mg daily, or itraconazole, 200 mg daily, may be necessary for oropharyngeal infections that do not respond to these treatments. Treatment is typically for 7 to 14 days but may need to be extended, depending on response to therapy.

Esophageal candidiasis usually occurs in patients with a highly compromised immune system. Additional risk factors include advanced liver disease and inhaled steroids. Usual symptoms include odynophagia, dysphagia, and retrosternal pain. Concurrent oropharyngeal candidiasis is common but not always present. Infection is generally limited to the mucosa. Complications include dehydration and malnutrition resulting from poor oral intake, esophageal strictures, and even esophageal perforation.

Treatment is with oral fluconazole, 200 to 400 mg daily. If the patient is unable to tolerate oral therapy, fluconazole should be given intravenously, 400 mg daily. Therapy is typically for 14 to 21 days, depending on patient response. Oropharyngeal and esophageal candidiasis refractory to fluconazole occasionally can develop in patients who are highly immunosuppressed or those previously treated with an azole. Alternative oral options include itraconazole solution 200 mg/day, voriconazole 200 mg BID (twice daily), and posaconazole 400 mg BID. These regimens cost more and are potentially more toxic than fluconazole. Furthermore, they may be ineffective because of resistance across the entire azole class. IV antifungal therapy with echinocandins (micafungin 150 mg daily; caspofungin 70 mg loading dose, then 50 mg daily; and anidulafungin 200 mg daily) can be effective, but their use is associated with higher relapses; therefore recommended dosages are higher. Systemic amphotericin B deoxycholate or lipid formulations are another option but can be associated with substantial toxicity.

Patients at significant risk for oropharyngeal and esophageal candidiasis, such as those receiving cytotoxic chemotherapy or high-intensity immunosuppression or those who have advanced HIV, should be considered for prophylaxis. Topical agents such as nystatin or clotrimazole are generally effective. Systemic fluconazole 400 mg PO or IV daily also may be effective as suppressive therapy in cases of recurrent infection.

Candiduria

Candiduria is a common finding in hospitalized surgical patients. Candiduria can represent a spectrum of clinical scenarios, such as colonization and cystitis and more serious conditions such as upper urinary tract infection or disseminated disease. It is often difficult to distinguish true urinary infection from mere colonization, particularly in patients with indwelling urinary catheters. The decision to treat should be based on the clinical scenario and not solely on the presence of yeast in urine cultures.

Treatment is indicated in patients who are symptomatic or neutropenic or who have planned urinary instrumentation. Removal or exchange of urinary catheters may be helpful in clearing candiduria. Oral fluconazole (200 mg or 3 mg/kg daily) for 2 weeks is recommended for the treatment of cystitis due to *Candida*. Alternatives include systemic amphotericin B deoxycholate or oral flucytosine. Bladder irrigation with amphotericin B deoxycholate may be useful in cases of refractory cystitis due to azole-resistant strains. Lipid formulations of amphotericin B should be avoided because they do not achieve adequate concentrations in the urinary system. Patients with persistent candiduria and additional risk factors should be evaluated for presence of a fungus ball or renal parenchymal disease.

■ FUNGAL PULMONARY INFECTIONS

Fungi represent only a small fraction of pathogens responsible for pulmonary infections, but they are important to recognize in light of the growing population of immunosuppressed patients. Fungal pneumonias most commonly are caused by opportunistic organisms, whereas pulmonary infections due to endemic fungi are rare in surgical patients.

Candida Pneumonia

Candida pneumonia is very rare, yet it is a common organism found in respiratory secretions. Most cases are related to disseminated *Candida* infection arising from distant sites and usually occur among patients with additional risk factors, such as prolonged antibiotic use, hematologic malignancies, and other immunocompromised states. Definitive diagnosis of *Candida* pneumonia is based on isolating the organism from lung tissue samples. There are no clear guidelines for treatment of primary *Candida* pneumonia. Most cases have been treated with amphotericin B deoxycholate or lipid formulations, although milder cases have been treated successfully with fluconazole. Disseminated disease should be treated similarly to candidemia.

Aspergillus Pneumonia

Invasive aspergillosis is an increasingly important problem in surgical patients. It remains an uncommon disease but carries significant mortality. Early epidemiologic studies in the United States have estimated its incidence to be 12 cases per 1 million people per year.

Invasive aspergillosis most commonly is seen as a progressive, cavitary pulmonary infection that can result in hemoptysis. Common symptoms include fever, dyspnea, cough, and pleuritic chest pain. However, one third of patients are asymptomatic initially. Cavitary lesions usually are identified on plain radiographs or computed tomography of the chest. Other radiologic findings such as the "halo" sign and "air crescent" sign are highly suggestive of *Aspergillus* pneumonia but nonspecific. Diagnosis can be difficult because of the relative insensitivity of microscopy and culture to detect *Aspergillus*. A definitive diagnosis requires both histopathologic evidence of infection and culture of the organism from a sterile site. Galactomannan antigen detection, beta-D-glucan detection, and polymerase chain reaction (PCR) are additional laboratory studies that may improve detection. Voriconazole remains the treatment of choice. Amphotericin B is another option, and caspofungin is reserved as salvage therapy.

Mucormycosis

Mucormycosis, also referred to as zygomycosis, is another very rare infection caused by one of the organisms belonging to the order Mucorales, most commonly *Rhizopus spp.* or *Mucor spp.* It has an incidence of less than 2 per 1 million people per year. Although this infection typically affects immunocompromised patients, it also may be seen after traumatic injuries, near drownings, or burns. Additional risk factors include poorly controlled diabetes mellitus, malignancy, and treatment with the iron chelator deferoxamine. This infection carries significant morbidity, with mortality rates greater than 50%.

The most common sites of mucormycosis include the sinuses, respiratory tract, and skin. Less commonly, the GI tract may be involved. Infection may extend locally to adjacent structures such as the orbits, brain, and blood vessels, which can lead to extensive tissue destruction. Vascular invasion can lead to serious complications such as massive hemoptysis. Pulmonary mucormycosis is characterized by angioinvasion and a high degree of tissue necrosis leading to rapidly progressive pneumonia and development of cavitations. Reversed halo sign may be an early radiographic finding but is nonspecific and also may be seen in aspergillosis. Symptoms of pulmonary infection are nonspecific, with patients typically having fever and hemoptysis. Definitive diagnosis of mucormycosis requires histologic evidence of tissue invasion, but bronchoalveolar lavage is helpful in making a diagnosis.

Management of this disease requires a multidisciplinary approach. This includes correction of metabolic abnormalities, reduction of immunosuppression medications, and excision or débridement of infected tissues. This is particularly important if there is angioinvasion or necrosis. Liposomal amphotericin B at doses of at least 5 mg/kg/day is recommended. Posaconazole may be used in combination with liposomal amphotericin B in refractory cases. Echinocandins have not been shown to have in vitro activity against this species and therefore are not recommended.

■ FUNGAL BLOODSTREAM INFECTIONS

Fungi are the fourth most common pathogen isolated in bloodstream infections overall and the third most common pathogen in intensive care units in the United States. The majority of cases are attributed to *Candida spp.*, in particular *C. albicans, C. glabrata, C. parapsilosis, C. tropicalis,* and *C. krusei.* Candidemia occurs more commonly at the two extremes of age (<1 and ≥65 years old). Risk factors include receiving prolonged therapy with multiple antibiotics, total parenteral nutrition, neutropenia, immunosuppression, hemodialysis, previous fungal colonization, presence of an intravascular catheter, major surgery, and burns. Fungal bloodstream infections are associated with a high mortality, despite advances in pharmacologic agents.

Blood cultures remain the gold standard for diagnosis; however, poor sensitivity rates have been reported. Newer diagnostic assays, including PCR, beta-D-glucan, and T2Candida, may facilitate the diagnosis. The associated mortality rates for candidemia are between 40% and 60%. Candidemia due to *C. glabrata* has been increasing recently, and this organism now comprises about one fourth of isolates. This is important to note because of this organism's increased likelihood of resistance to azoles and emerging multidrug resistance.

Treatment recommendations vary for specific patient populations, taking into consideration recent drug exposure and risk factors for infection due to resistant strains. Fluconazole remains a reasonable option for stable patients who have no previous exposure to azoles and lack additional risk factors for *C. glabrata* (e.g., advanced age, malignancy, diabetes mellitus). Fluconazole should be given with an initial loading dose of 800 mg (12 mg/kg), followed by 400 mg (6 mg/kg) daily. Echinocandins are preferred for treatment of patients with greater risk factors, including neutropenic patients, and those at risk for infection with *C. glabrata* or *C. krusei* isolates. Echinocandin dosing recommendations are caspofungin, loading dose of 70 mg, then 50 mg daily; micafungin, 100 mg daily; or anidulafungin, loading dose of 200 mg, then 100 mg daily. Liposomal amphotericin B formulations (3 to 5 mg/kg daily) also may be used as a first-line therapy in neutropenic patients. Patients should have blood cultures drawn every 1 to 2 days. Treatment should continue for 2 weeks after the first documented negative blood culture.

As a general rule, central venous catheters should be removed in patients with candidemia because it is not always possible to determine whether the catheter is the primary source of infection, became infected secondarily, or is not infected at all. Retention of the catheter can be considered in patients with implanted access devices and candidemia in the setting of cytotoxic chemotherapy and neutropenia. All patients with candidemia should have a dilated funduscopic examination within the first week after initiation of treatment to evaluate for chorioretinitis or endophthalmitis.

■ FUNGAL INTRA-ABDOMINAL INFECTIONS

Intra-abdominal fungal infections can occur as a result of a complication of an intra-abdominal operation or less commonly from disseminated disease. Risk factors for *Candida* intra-abdominal infections include recurrent abdominal operation, bowel perforation, anastomotic breakdown, and multifocal colonization. Patients undergoing an operation to manage pancreatic necrosis are at particularly high risk. Disseminated candidiasis and rarely aspergillosis have been known to spread to the GI tract, usually in the setting of immunocompromised states. Diagnosis of an intra-abdominal fungal infection should be based on culture results from samples obtained intraoperatively or by percutaneous aspiration. The presence of yeast in samples obtained from an existing surgical drain may represent simply colonization and not necessarily an intra-abdominal infection.

Early source control is essential in managing these infections. Antifungal treatment with fluconazole is appropriate for most patients with infection due to *C. albicans*. An echinocandin should be used for critically ill patients and those with isolates likely to be resistant to the azoles. The optimal duration of treatment is unclear. A recent multinational expert panel recommended treatment for 10 to 14 days for intra-abdominal *Candida* infections. However, the Surgical Infection Society's Study to Optimize Peritoneal Infection Therapy (STOP-IT) evaluated the duration of treatment for patients with complicated intra-abdominal infections and demonstrated that 4 days of treatment along with adequate source control resulted in similar outcomes compared with patients who received a longer course of therapy. Although patients with fungal infections were included in that study, it is unclear whether these recommendations apply to this group. The current Infectious Diseases Society of America guideline for management of candidiasis recommends that duration of treatment be determined by the adequacy of source control and clinical response.

■ FUNGAL SURGICAL SITE INFECTIONS

Fungi account for approximately 3% of surgical site infections (SSIs), with *C. albicans* being the most common fungal pathogen. Although infrequent, these infections are important to recognize, as there have been case reports of *C. albicans* causing necrotizing infections at a surgical or central line site. Certain patient populations, such as those suffering from traumatic injuries, burns, or secondary or tertiary peritonitis, are at higher risk of developing fungal SSIs. Burn patients are at particularly high risk, with fungi reported to contribute to approximately 20% to 25% of burn wound infections, often as one isolate of a polymicrobial infection. Fungal wound infections in this population typically occur about 2 weeks after burn injury and have been associated with a greater mortality. It is unclear if fungal SSIs are the direct cause of death or simply represent a more severe disease state in these patients. Diagnosis of a fungal wound infection in burn wounds requires histopathologic evidence of fungal invasion into viable tissue. The presence of fungi in necrotic tissue is considered to represent colonization. These patients require both surgical débridement and systemic antifungal therapy.

Both *Candida* and *Aspergillus* have infrequently been implicated in poststernotomy infections (e.g., osteomyelitis and mediastinitis), with most patients requiring surgical débridement and several months of antifungal therapy.

SUGGESTED READINGS

Azie N, Neofytos D, Pfaller M, Meier-Kriesche HU, et al. The PATH (Prospective Antifungal Therapy) Alliance® registry and invasive fungal infections: update 2012. *Diagn Microbiol Infect Dis.* 2012;73:293-300.

Bassetti M, Marchetti M, Chakrabarti A, et al. A research agenda on the management of intra-abdominal candidiasis: results from a consensus of multinational experts. *Intensive Care Med.* 2013;39:2092-2106.

Fridkin SK, Jarvis WR. Epidemiology of nosocomial fungal infections. *Clin Microbiol Rev.* 1996;9:499-511.

Pappas PG, Kauffman CA, Andes DR, et al. Clinical practice guideline for the management of candidiasis: 2016 update by the Infectious Diseases Society of America. *Clin Infect Dis.* 2016;62:e1-e50.

Sawyer RG, Claridge JA, Nathens AB, et al. Trial of short-course antimicrobial therapy for intraabdominal infection. *N Engl J Med.* 2015;372:1996-2005.

Walsh TJ, Anaissie EJ, Denning DW. Treatment of aspergillosis: clinical practice guidelines of the Infectious Diseases Society of America. *Clin Infect Dis.* 2008;46:327-360.

MEASURING OUTCOMES OF SURGERY

Justin B. Dimick, MD, MPH

Outcomes of surgery are determined in large part based on where and by whom a procedure is performed. Seminal studies in pancreatic surgery, conducted nearly 2 decades ago, documented wide gaps in clinical outcomes between high-volume and low-volume hospitals. More recent studies using large, detailed clinical databases suggest similar differences in outcomes for nearly all surgical procedures. These studies suggest substantial opportunities for improving the outcomes of surgical care.

Reducing these variations, however, has proven more difficult than finding them. Two key challenges need to be addressed before we can use outcomes measures to reduce these disparities. First, we need to be able to accurately determine when differences in outcomes truly result from gaps in quality. Second, we need to understand the strengths and limitations of outcomes measures as applied in the "real world." This chapter offers a brief overview of these two challenges and then closes with a discussion of emerging strategies for addressing them.

■ UNDERSTANDING VARIATION IN OUTCOMES

Surgeons often view variations in *outcomes* as synonymous with variations in *quality*. Traditional morbidity and mortality conferences often encourage this view by expecting surgeons to accept blame for all adverse outcomes. However, surgical outcomes can vary for reasons other than quality. In any outcomes measurement program, it is important to consider—and account for—other determinants of adverse events. In a more complete conceptual model, it should be recognized that variation in surgical outcomes results from three contributing factors: *chance, case mix* (i.e., patient factors), and *quality of care*. Although the main themes of this chapter apply to all surgical outcomes, the focus is on surgical mortality, reflecting the predominance of this measure in the literature and ongoing quality measurement activities.

Chance

Outcomes can vary across hospitals and surgeons simply because of good or bad luck. Provider-specific outcome measures often are based on small numbers of adverse events and surgical cases, resulting in "noisy"—that is, statistically imprecise—estimates of performance. Chance is particularly important when the event rate is low (e.g., mortality rate after cholecystectomy) or the procedure is uncommon (e.g., pancreatectomy).

Chance can cause two types of errors in quality measurement. First, extreme outcomes may be attributed to quality when they actually result from chance alone; this is a type 1 error. In many quality measurement platforms, for example, hospitals are labeled as "outliers" if their outcomes are statistically different from those expected, such as when the 95% confidence intervals around their outcome rates fail to overlap the average. Depending on where the statistical threshold for outliers is set, some hospitals will be labeled outliers based on chance alone.

A conceptual type 1 error is made often when evaluating a provider with no deaths: the so-called *zero mortality paradox*. Although having no deaths is considered a sign of superior quality, it is also possible that such providers have no deaths simply because of chance (i.e., good luck), especially if they perform a low number of cases. In a recent study that used national Medicare data for five surgical procedures, we demonstrated that *zero mortality hospitals*, defined as hospitals with no deaths during 3 years, had the same or higher mortality rates in the subsequent year. Pancreatic resection showed the most striking zero mortality paradox. For this operation, a history of zero mortality—that is, no deaths over a 3-year period—was associated with a 30% increased risk of death in the subsequent year; therefore hospitals with no deaths for this operation are more likely to be lucky than good. This paradoxical finding, that hospitals with no deaths are actually lower quality, is explained by the well-known relationship between low volume and high mortality for pancreatic resection.

Type 2 errors occur when chance obscures real differences in quality. Widely recognized in clinical trials as an underpowered study, this type of error often is overlooked in quality measurement programs. One recent study by our group examined seven surgical procedures for which hospital mortality rates had been recommended as quality indicators by the Agency for Healthcare Quality and Research. For only one operation, coronary artery bypass grafting (CABG), did the majority of U.S. hospitals perform enough cases over a 3-year period to detect with statistical confidence mortality rates at least twice that of the national average (Figure 1). For most procedures, only a minority of hospitals had sufficient caseloads to meet this low bar of statistical power.

Case Mix

Differences in patient characteristics such as comorbidities, functional status, indications for surgery, and so on also contribute to variation in outcomes. Some providers may have worse outcomes because they treat sicker, higher-risk patients than do other hospitals. When measuring provider quality, these differences in patient factors are adjusted for using statistical techniques that are now fairly standard. Although risk adjustment in comparisons of provider performance is obviously important, the evidence that differences in patient factors explain variations in surgical outcomes is mixed.

The importance of risk adjustment is a function of the population being studied. In intensive care, for example, the physiologic status of the patient—as evidenced by the Acute Physiology and Chronic Health Evaluation II (APACHE II) score, for example—is an important driver of outcomes, and this may vary extensively across hospitals. In contrast, with elective surgery patients tend to be very homogenous with respect to physiologic status; in other words, these patients all walk through the door. However, types of procedures performed at different hospitals may vary extensively. Large teaching hospitals may perform more complex, higher-risk procedures than small community hospitals. Even within otherwise comparable hospitals, procedure mix varies according to the specific practices of the surgeons operating there. For this reason, adjusting for procedure mix is crucial for fair comparisons of hospitals' overall surgical morbidity and mortality rates, such as those offered by provider-driven quality improvement programs such as the American College of Surgeons National Surgical Quality Improvement Program (ACS NSQIP).

In contrast, the importance of risk adjustment may be overstated for interpreting procedure-specific comparisons, largely because case mix varies much less across hospitals among patients undergoing the same operation. For example, we examined publicly reported

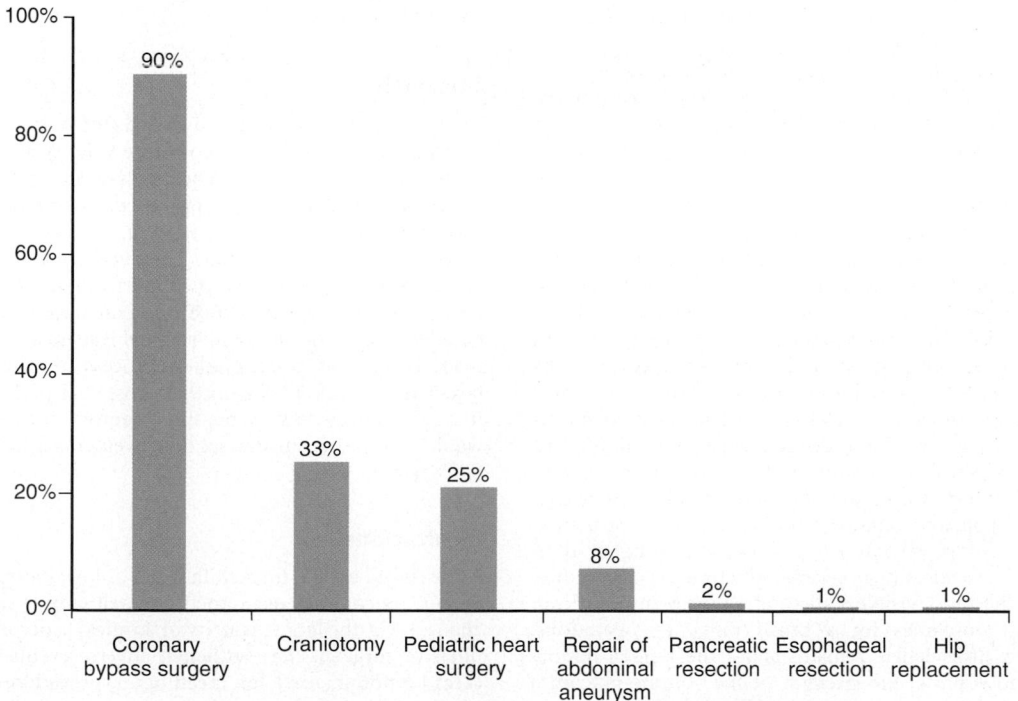

FIGURE 1 Big problems with small samples. The proportion of hospitals in the United States with sufficient caseloads (sample size) to reliably use mortality rates to measure quality.

mortality rates for 35 hospitals performing isolated CABG surgery in New York state in 2000 and 2001, as derived from their state-mandated clinical registries. Observed mortality rates varied considerably, from less than 1% to more than 4%. However, risk adjustment had a negligible impact in reducing apparent variation in outcomes: unadjusted and adjusted hospital mortality rates were nearly identical (correlation 0.95). We conducted similar analyses of noncardiac procedures based on more recent NSQIP data and reached similar conclusions.

These data are not meant to imply that patient factors are not important determinants of surgical risk. Rather, they suggest that such factors may contribute less to variations in procedure-specific outcomes than we previously thought, perhaps leading to more efficient and equally robust risk adjustment algorithms. Nonetheless, rigorous risk adjustment is important to account for those variables that do matter. Perhaps equally important, surgeons and health system leaders must accept the risk adjustment as adequate, or they will not implement improvement efforts in response to outcomes monitoring programs.

Quality of Care

Variation in surgical outcomes that is a result of neither chance nor case mix can be attributed reasonably to differences in the quality of care. For the purpose of this discussion, we consider "good quality" to comprise the details of clinical care that lead to optimal outcomes. These details often are referred to as *processes of care*. Some processes that lead to good outcomes are known and relatively easy to measure. However, many other processes are either unknown or much more difficult to measure (e.g., those related to intraoperative surgical skill and technique).

Although a list of known processes of care that potentially link to outcomes would be extensive, payers and policymakers currently are focusing on a narrow set of perioperative care practices in their ongoing quality measurement initiatives. These include measures aimed at reducing the risks of surgical site infection (e.g., prophylactic antibiotic administration within 60 minutes before surgery), venous thromboembolism, cardiac events, and ventilator-acquired pneumonia. However, recent evidence questions whether increasing compliance with this narrow set of processes will reduce variation in surgical outcomes substantially.

Based on the national Medicare population, Nicholas and colleagues (2010) noted wide variation in hospital compliance with the process measures of the Surgical Care Improvement Project (SCIP), ranging from 54% in the lowest third of hospitals to 91% in the highest third. However, compliance with these processes was not associated with risk-adjusted mortality for any of six procedures studied. Moreover, compliance with specific processes of care was not associated with lower rates of the adverse events that each process was designed to minimize; for example, hospitals with higher rates of prophylaxis did not have lower rates of venous thromboembolism. Such data do not imply that processes of care are unimportant in understanding and improving surgical mortality; instead, they underscore the *complexity* of clinical care and the innumerable unmeasured processes of care that collectively determine good outcomes after surgery. For many procedures, focusing on a limited set of individual processes will not be sufficient for improving outcomes.

In surgery, we often rely on structural measures to act as proxies for these unmeasurable and unknown processes of care. Structural variables are hospital-level resources (e.g., hospital volume) or attributes of individual providers (e.g., subspecialty training). Procedure volume is by far the most visible structural variable and has been linked to surgical outcomes for a broad range of operations. Although relatively little debate remains about the general importance of procedure volume, the strength of the volume-outcomes relationship varies widely by procedure. Hospital volume is most important for high-risk but relatively uncommon procedures, such as esophagectomy and pancreatectomy. For other operations (e.g.,

CABG), hospital volume has a much weaker relationship to important outcomes. Other structural variables, such as surgeon volume and surgeon specialty, are correlated tightly with outcomes.

Although these structural variables are useful for a narrow set of policy applications, such as selective referral, we ultimately need to understand the processes of care that explain differences in outcomes across hospitals. Once these "high-leverage" processes of care are known, they can be promoted as best practices to improve care at all hospitals. Future research should use the tools of clinical epidemiology to isolate the root causes of variation in outcomes. For example, a study by Ghaferi and colleagues (2009) shed light on the mechanisms underlying variations in surgical mortality rates. Using detailed, clinically rich data from the NSQIP, they ranked hospitals according to risk-adjusted mortality. When comparing the "best" and "worst" hospitals, they found no significant differences in overall (24.6% vs 26.9%) or major (18.2% vs 16.2%) complication rates. However, so-called *failure to rescue*—that is, death after major complications—was almost twice as high in hospitals with very high mortality as in those with very low mortality (21.4% vs 12.5%, $P < 0.001$). This study highlights the need to focus on processes of care related to the timely recognition and management of complications and aimed at eliminating failure to rescue and reducing variations in surgical mortality.

■ USING OUTCOMES TO MEASURE QUALITY

Outcome measures reflect the end result of care, either from a clinical perspective or as judged by the patient. Although mortality rate is by far the most commonly used measure in surgery, other outcomes that could be used as quality indicators include complications, hospital readmission, and a variety of patient-centered measures of quality of life or satisfaction. One great example of this type of measurement is found in the ACS NSQIP, a surgeon-led, clinical registry that provides feedback on risk-adjusted morbidity and mortality rates to participating hospitals. After its successful implementation in Veterans Affairs (VA) hospitals, it was introduced in the private sector with good results. Under the guidance of the ACS, hospital participation in the program continues to grow, with more than 240 hospitals currently participating.

Strengths

There are at least two key advantages of outcome measures. First, outcome measures have obvious face validity and thus are likely to get the greatest "buy in" from hospitals and surgeons. Surgeon enthusiasm for the NSQIP and the continued dissemination of the program clearly underline this point. Second, the act of simply measuring outcomes may lead to better performance (the Hawthorne effect). For example, surgical morbidity and mortality rates in VA hospitals have fallen dramatically since implementation of the NSQIP two decades ago. No doubt many surgical leaders at individual hospitals made specific organizational or process improvements after they began receiving feedback on their hospital's performance. However, it is very unlikely that even a full inventory of these specific changes would explain the substantial improvements in morbidity and mortality rates.

Limitations

As discussed earlier, the Achilles heel of hospital-specific or surgeon-specific outcomes measurement is small sample size (i.e., the role of chance). For the large majority of surgical procedures, very few hospitals or surgeons have sufficient adverse events (numerators) and cases (denominators) for meaningful, procedure-specific measures of morbidity or mortality. For example, as discussed earlier, a very small proportion of U.S. hospitals have adequate caseloads to reliably detect quality problems (see Figure 1). Although identifying poor quality outliers is an important function of outcomes measurement, focusing on this goal alone significantly underestimates problems associated with small sample sizes. Discriminating among individual hospitals with intermediate levels of performance is even more difficult.

This lack of discrimination among providers (type 2 errors) has important practical implications. When reporting outcomes in a hospital report card, we often use historical data from 2 to 3 years before to make inferences about how a hospital is currently performing. However, some empirical data show that outcome measures are inferior to other measures, such as hospital volume, in predicting future performance (Figure 2). Using national Medicare data, we examined the ability of historical data on hospital volume and risk-adjusted mortality (2003 to 2004) to discriminate future performance (2005 to 2006). We found that hospital volume was much better at reliably predicting future performance for less common operations, such as pancreatic resection (see Figure 2). These findings can be explained by the role of chance, as discussed earlier. Later in this chapter, we discuss new tools that will help us to sort out the true quality "signal" from this statistical "noise."

Another significant limitation of outcomes assessment is the expense of data collection. Reporting outcomes requires the costly collection of detailed clinical data for risk adjustment. For example, it costs more than $100,000 annually for a private sector hospital to

participate in the NSQIP. Because of the expense of data collection, the program currently collects data on only a sample of patients undergoing surgery at each hospital. Although this sampling strategy decreases the cost of data collection, it exacerbates the problem of small sample size with individual procedures. As discussed later in this chapter, changes in the ACS NSQIP and other clinical registries are focusing on reducing the expense of data collection without compromising the rigor of risk adjustment.

Improving Outcomes Measurement

Although great progress has been made in measuring outcomes, the science is still in early stages of development. Nonetheless, there are solutions on the horizon for many of the limitations discussed earlier.

Addressing Small Sample Size With Reliability Adjustment

One of the biggest limitations of surgical quality measurement is the statistical "noise" from the small sample sizes at most hospitals. This problem of limited numbers is even more of a problem when outcomes are measured for individual surgeons. Small sample size—and the resulting imprecision—makes it difficult to isolate the quality "signal" from the background statistical "noise." In other words, it is often hard to know whether a surgeon or a hospital has poor performance because it provides low quality care or because it was unlucky. For obvious reasons, labeling surgeons and hospitals correctly is extremely important.

An emerging technique, *reliability adjustment*, directly addresses the problem of statistical noise. This technique, based on hierarchical modeling, quantifies and subtracts noise from the measurement process. Essentially, it "shrinks" a provider's performance back toward average, unless it deviates to such an extreme that it is safe to assume that the performance is truly different. In this way, reliability adjustment gives providers the benefit of the doubt. For example, Figure 3 shows the risk-adjusted mortality rates for pancreatic cancer resection in 20 hospitals before and after reliability adjustment. Before reliability adjustment, the mortality rates varied from 0% to 100%. After reliability adjustment, the mortality rates only varied from 2% to 22%, yielding a range of performance that is clinically more realistic. These reliability-adjusted mortality rates are much more accurate in terms of capturing true performance, as assessed by their ability to predict future performance.

Despite its increasing use in other fields, such as ambulatory care, reliability adjustment is only beginning to find applications in surgery. Perhaps the most prominent example is the Massachusetts

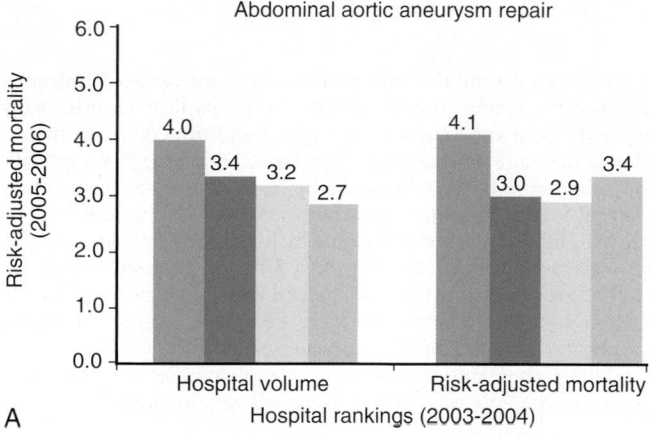

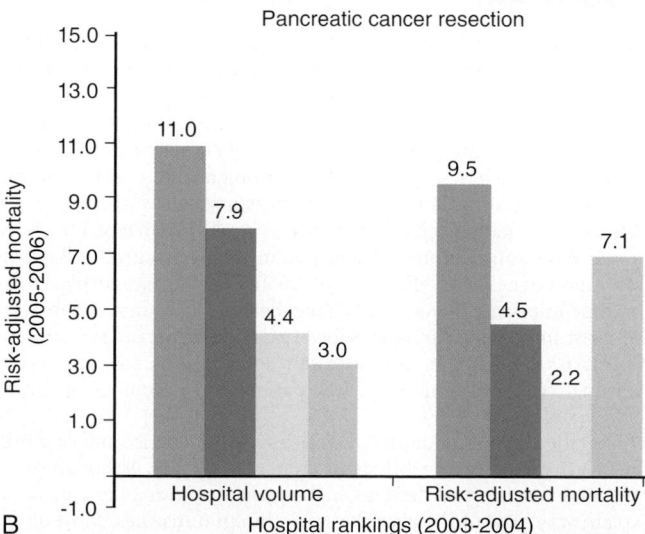

FIGURE 2 Ability of hospital rankings based on 2003 to 2004 mortality rates and hospital volume to predict risk-adjusted mortality in 2005 to 2006. **A,** Data for abdominal aortic aneurysm repair. **B,** Data for pancreatic cancer resection. *(Data from national Medicare database, 2003-2006.)*

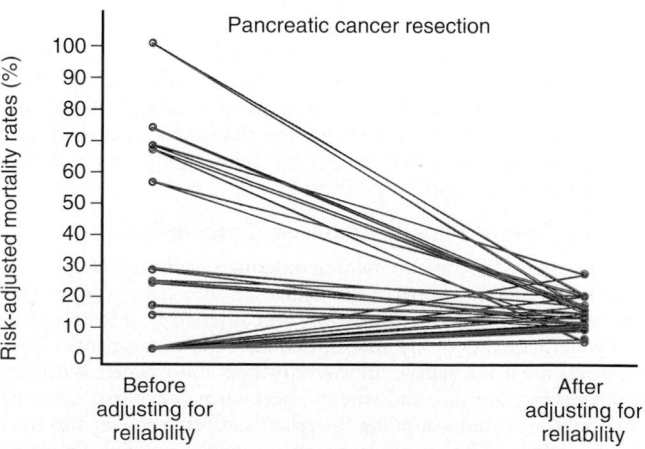

FIGURE 3 Variation in hospital mortality rates before and after adjusting for reliability. Twenty randomly sampled hospitals are shown for pancreatic cancer resection. *(Data from national Medicare database, 2003-2004.)*

cardiac surgery report card, which publishes reliability-adjusted mortality rates for each hospital in the state. This approach likely will be applied to other clinical registries as the "gold standard" for profiling hospital and surgeon performance. Reliability adjustment is not a panacea, however, and has certain limitations. The biggest disadvantage of this approach is that it may obscure poor performance by assuming that small hospitals have average performance—that is, it does not address type 2 errors. Because of the well-known volume-outcomes relationship for many operations, the assumption that small hospitals have average outcomes may not be true.

Even with reliability adjustment, careful consideration should be given to sample size when designing outcomes measurement programs. Outcome measures should be pursued only when there will be a sample size sufficient to make meaningful comparisons across hospitals and surgeons. How does one know if sample sizes are sufficient? There is no single cut-off that determines when there will be enough "signal" to make outcome measures worthwhile. However, a general rule of thumb is that outcome measures will be useful for common operations with relatively high rates of adverse outcomes (e.g., mortality after cardiac surgery, morbidity after bariatric surgery or colectomy). Even for these common procedures there likely will not be enough cases to measure surgeon-specific outcomes for the majority of procedures.

For rare procedures, such as pancreatic or esophageal resection, caseloads will never be high enough to reliably measure hospital-specific outcomes. A variable that is correlated with outcomes, such as hospital volume, may be the best available measure for these less common operations.

Developing More Efficient Risk Adjustment Models

Improvements in risk adjustment modeling are also imminent. For example, the NSQIP recently has undergone several changes that will affect risk adjustment. One major organization change is the shift from an overall (all procedures combined) morbidity and mortality measure to procedure-specific measurement. This change will have a significant impact on the risk adjustment strategy. As discussed earlier, patients undergoing the same procedure tend to be a more homogenous group. As a result, it is likely that fewer variables will be necessary for risk adjustment.

To test this hypothesis, we evaluated a more limited model that used 5 variables, rather than the "full" model of up to 30 variables, for the 5 procedures—colectomy, pancreatectomy, bariatric surgery, cholecystectomy, and ventral hernia repair—targeted by the procedure-specific general surgery NSQIP module. In assessing hospital-specific outcomes, results from the limited and full risk models were highly correlated for both mortality (0.94 to 0.99 across the five operations) and morbidity (0.96 to 0.99). Figure 4 shows the tight correlation (0.97) of hospital risk-adjusted morbidity (O/E ratios) for all five procedures combined.

Based on these data, we believe that procedure-specific hospital quality measures can be risk adjusted adequately with a limited number of variables. In the context of the clinical registries, such as ACS NSQIP, moving to a more limited risk adjustment model will reduce the burden of data collection dramatically and make risk adjustment much more cost effective.

Moving Toward Patient-Centered Outcomes

In recent years, the measurement of outcomes has begun to shift away from traditional measures of morbidity and mortality toward rigorous assessment of patient-centered outcomes (e.g., disease-specific and generic quality of life and functional status assessments). These measures are particularly important for operations where morbidity and mortality are rare and where longer-term functional outcomes are essential to understanding the relative effectiveness of two treatment options. The creation of the Patient-Centered Outcomes Research Institute (PCORI) in 2010 has greatly accelerated scientific development and understanding of the patient perspective in outcomes measurement.

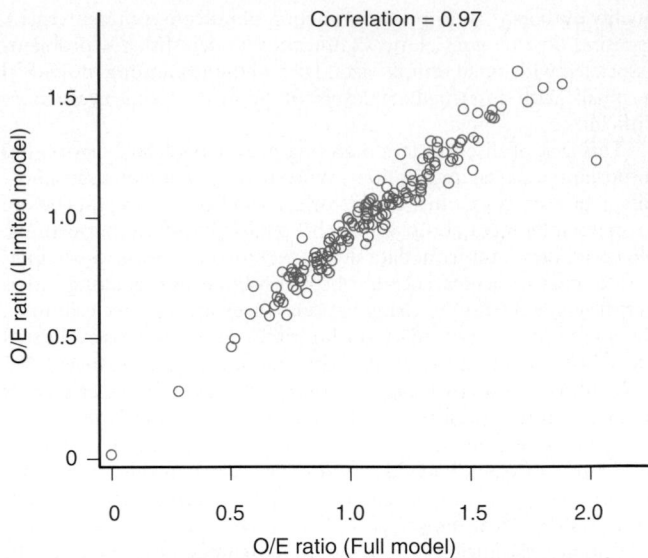

FIGURE 4 Comparison of hospital O/E ratios created using the full (up to 30 variables) and limited (5 variables) models for morbidity after 5 common general surgery procedures. (*Data from American College of Surgeons National Surgical Quality Improvement Program.*)

However, despite the enthusiasm for patient-centered outcomes in comparative effectiveness, there has been very little scientific work exploring their use for assessing hospital and surgeon performance. This is therefore an important area for scientific inquiry, especially for those procedures where quality is best assessed using these metrics. Several important questions need to be addressed. First, we need to understand the extent to which patient-centered outcomes vary across hospitals and surgeons. Second, we need to develop methods for risk adjustment of patient-centered outcomes. Finally, we need to understand whether these are unique measures of quality or whether they are tightly correlated with traditional metrics of morbidity. These questions need to be evaluated for each candidate procedure, because the answers likely will vary by procedure.

■ SUMMARY

Although quality is a key driver of outcomes, it is also important to consider the roles of chance and patient case mix. Chance is particularly important when the number of cases per hospital is small. New techniques, such as reliability adjustment, can be used to minimize statistical "noise" and prevent mislabeling of surgeons and hospitals. Nonetheless, the best way to avoid this problem is to select common, high-risk procedures for outcomes measurement. Adjustment for differences in patient risk factors is obviously important but likely can be done much more efficiently than with our current "kitchen sink" approaches. The efficiency of quality measurement platforms could be improved by focusing data collection on a smaller subset of the most important variables. However, it is important to maintain robust risk adjustment to ensure fair comparisons and to prevent "gaming" (e.g., avoiding the sickest patients) of outcomes measurement systems.

Variation in outcomes that are not a result of chance and case mix can be attributed reasonably to differences in quality. Although some processes of care that lead to high-quality care are known, these explain very little of the observed variation in outcomes. Most of the processes of care that explain variations in outcomes, so-called high-leverage processes, are either unknown or unmeasurable with current methods. Using outcomes measurement to improve quality ultimately will require the use of clinical epidemiology to isolate these unknown and unmeasurable processes of care.

SUGGESTED READINGS

Birkmeyer JD, Dimick JB, Birkmeyer NJ. Measuring the quality of surgical care: structure, process, or outcomes? *J Am Coll Surg.* 2004;198:626-632.

Birkmeyer JD, Shahian DM, Dimick JB, et al. Blueprint for a new American College of Surgeons: National Surgical Quality Improvement Program. *J Am Coll Surg.* 2008;207:777-782.

Dimick JB, Ghaferi AA, Osborne NH, et al. Reliability adjustment for reporting hospital outcomes with surgery. *Ann Surg.* 2012;255:703-707.

Dimick JB, Osborne NH, Hall BL, et al. Risk adjustment for comparing hospital quality with surgery: how many variables are needed? *J Am Coll Surg.* 2010;210:503-508.

Dimick JB, Welch HG. The zero-mortality paradox in surgery. *J Am Coll Surg.* 2008;206:13-16.

Dimick JB, Welch HG, Birkmeyer JD. Surgical mortality as an indicator of hospital quality: the problem with small sample size. *JAMA.* 2004;292:847-851.

Ghaferi AA, Birkmeyer JD, Dimick JB. Variation in hospital mortality associated with inpatient surgery. *N Engl J Med.* 2009;361:1368-1375.

Khuri SF, Daley J, Henderson WG. The comparative assessment and improvement of quality of surgical care in the Department of Veterans Affairs. *Arch Surg.* 2002;137:20-27.

Krell RW, Hozain A, Kao LS, et al. Reliability of risk-adjusted outcomes for profiling hospital surgical quality. *JAMA Surg.* 2014;149:467-474.

Nicholas LH, Osborne NH, Birkmeyer JD, Dimick JB. Hospital process compliance and surgical outcomes among Medicare patients. *Arch Surg.* 2010;145:999-1004.

Osborne NH, Nicholas LH, Ryan AM, et al. Association of hospital participation in a quality reporting program with surgical outcomes and expenditures for Medicare beneficiaries. *JAMA.* 2015;313:496-504.

COMPARATIVE EFFECTIVENESS RESEARCH IN SURGERY

Karl Y. Bilimoria, MD, MS, and Jonah J. Stulberg, MD, PhD, MPH

We all want to provide the optimal treatment for our patients, and comparative effectiveness research (CER) is the methodology by which we can achieve that goal. CER encompasses evidence generation and evidence synthesis, allowing us to move from knowing what works in a clinical trial to knowing what works in practice. It is this pursuit of effectiveness, rather than efficacy, that separates CER from other forms of research, and there has been unprecedented interest in CER methods in the last decade. This increased interest has been reflected in a marked increase in PubMed-indexed, peer-reviewed articles using CER (Figure 1). Politicians, and in particular the White House, have started to realize the value of CER for curbing the costs of health care and have pushed through multiple efforts that bring CER to the forefront of decision making.

Probably the biggest shift we are seeing is from a fee-for-service (FFS) model to a value-based purchasing (VBP) model for physician reimbursement. With our physician-level and hospital-level reimbursement models moving toward VBP, now more than ever surgeons need to be familiar with the concepts of CER and how they apply to their practice.

WHAT IS COMPARATIVE EFFECTIVENESS RESEARCH?

CER is any research study that is designed to compare the benefits and harms of multiple treatments in order to inform healthcare decisions. This can take the form of prospective trials or retrospective analyses of existing data sources. The pursuit of the right treatment for the right patient at the right time is at the heart of evidence-based medicine, and CER is the constellation of tools that we use to generate that evidence and put it into practice. At its core, CER should involve generating new information quickly in order to produce timely results for clinicians, patients, policymakers, health plans, hospitals, and any other healthcare stakeholders. The research study can compare medical devices, drugs, laboratory or radiologic tests, new surgeries, or even the way in which we deliver health care, but it must be timely and relevant and provide evidence on the effectiveness of the given treatment in a real-world setting.

EFFECTIVENESS VERSUS EFFICACY

Evidence-based medicine has become a common phrase among practicing physicians in the twenty-first century. It now stands without debate that we all must strive to use the best available evidence to treat our patients, which means that our practices are constantly evolving as our evidence base grows. There are scoring standards to grade the level of evidence on which we are basing treatment decisions; for individual studies, randomized controlled trials (RCTs) are at the top of this data quality pyramid (Table 1). RCTs are considered the gold standard for the evaluation of new surgical treatments, devices, or drugs because they control for both known and unknown confounders and ideally measure efficacy. Then why is it that so many new interventions seem to work wonderfully in the setting of an RCT but have disappointing results in clinical practice? The answer is that RCTs typically are designed to measure efficacy and not effectiveness.

Although the evidence pyramid topped by RCTs is focused on measuring efficacy, perhaps more important to our daily clinical practice is whether the intervention of interest is effective. Effectiveness of a clinical intervention can be defined as the likelihood that the intervention will be successful in producing the desired effect in clinical practice. Studies of comparative effectiveness give up some of the control that often leads to better isolation of effect in order to gain an understanding of the true effect in clinical practice.

METHODS USED IN COMPARATIVE EFFECTIVENESS RESEARCH

A broad array of tools is available to researchers who are interested in conducting CER. Here we provide a brief overview of many of these methods, organized by category. Choosing the type of study design should be based on sound scientific principles, just as in other disciplines. The researcher must first develop a compelling question before going through the process of determining the best way to answer that question given the available tools, resources, and expertise.

Experimental Studies

By definition, experimental studies involve manipulation of the environment by some means and are designed to provide insight into the cause and effect relationship between an intervention and a given outcome. They do this by demonstrating that the outcome varies as the particular intervention is manipulated. Experimental study designs allow for the manipulation of dose, timing, rate, and other factors that collectively can build convincing evidence of a cause and effect relationship.

In clinical research, RCTs stand out as the typical experimental study design that most clinicians would recognize. However, as

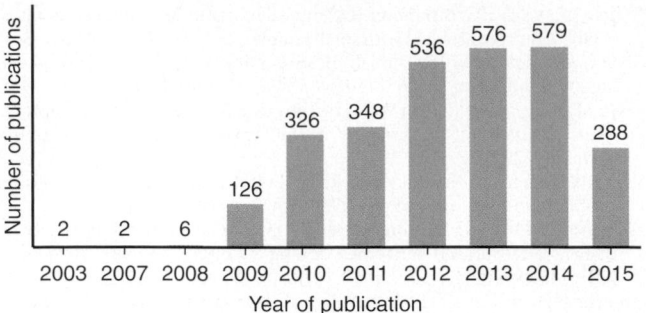

FIGURE 1 Comparative effectiveness research in PubMed.

TABLE 1: Levels of Evidence

Level	Type of Evidence
Ia	Evidence from meta-analysis of randomized controlled trials
Ib	Evidence from at least one randomized controlled trial
IIa	Evidence from at least one controlled study without randomization
IIb	Evidence from at least one other type of quasi-experimental study
III	Evidence from nonexperimental descriptive studies, such as comparative studies, correlation studies, and case-control studies
IV	Evidence from expert committee reports or opinions or clinical experience of respected authorities

described earlier, classic RCTs are designed to measure the efficacy of an intervention and not its effectiveness. Therefore researchers interested in addressing the clinical effectiveness of a given intervention manipulate RCTs in subtle ways to better address their research question. The most prominent examples of this are pragmatic trials, cluster randomized trials, and adaptive trials.

Pragmatic trials attempt to improve the external validity of RCTs through relaxation of varying degrees of control. This relaxation often leads to decreased effect sizes, which in turn may result in the need for a larger sample size in order to show a statistically significant effect, but the amount of relaxation can vary greatly. The amount of pragmatism a researcher builds into the RCT design must be carefully considered and matched to the research question. Examples of ways in which researchers can build pragmatism into their study design in order to estimate effectiveness over efficacy include performing an intention-to-treat analysis, relaxing inclusion and exclusion criteria, relaxing the study setting, and not blinding the treatment arm.

Intention-to-treat analysis is an attractive first step in estimations of effectiveness, as it can be introduced in the analysis phase only; however, it typically underestimates the regression to the mean that will be seen when the intervention is introduced into practice. RCTs typically have stringent inclusion and exclusion criteria in order to decrease study group heterogeneity and improve the likelihood of estimating a treatment effect. Therefore if a researcher chooses to relax the inclusion and exclusion criteria in order to better estimate an intervention's effect for a broader treatment population, another way must be found to overcome this heterogeneity. Finally, by not blinding the treatment arm, researchers inadvertently may introduce bias.

Cluster randomized trials are trials in which the randomization is performed on groups of study subjects rather than on individual study subjects. This can have many practical applications; for example, randomly assigning an entire practice to the intervention or control arm rather than requiring the practice to treat each patient differently according to a random allocation at the time of treatment may be much easier for a practice to implement. It also may help to minimize inadvertent contamination of the intervention and control groups. This type of study design is ideally suited for interventions that involve changes in the process of care, educational interventions, or procedural assessments.

Adaptive trials are prospective trials that intentionally plan to use interim analyses to modify their trial methodology. This could introduce bias if the data were not blinded for these analyses or if the plan to make these adjustments was not stated before trial initiation. Therefore modifying a trial at an interim time point must be approached carefully and with specific safety measures to avoid introducing bias. Adjustments to the trial may include changing or relaxing inclusion and exclusion criteria, modifying treatment settings, increasing or decreasing a dose, or building in oversampling of certain groups to help answer a secondary research question.

Observational Studies

In theory, observational studies also seek to understand the cause and effect relationship between an intervention and a given outcome, but they lack the ability to control how subjects are assigned to groups or which treatment a group receives. Because of this, they lack the ability to introduce randomization into their intervention assignment, and they therefore always can be criticized for their inability to control for confounding of unknown variables. For this reason, they are often seen as hypothesis generating rather than conclusively defining a cause and effect relationship. However, certain research questions would never be suitable for randomization, either because randomization would be unethical or because it simply would be impossible. For these questions, observational studies are necessary to determine cause and effect. Observational study designs are the foundation of epidemiology and include cohort studies, case-control studies, and cross-sectional studies.

Cohort studies are considered the gold standard of observational study design and are able to estimate risk. They start by identifying one or several large groups of individuals at risk for a problem of interest. A carefully documented investigation into the exposures is carried out, and then these individuals are followed over time until the outcome of interest occurs. It is important to note that in a cohort study the population at risk is identified first and then followed until the outcome of interest occurs, which is in stark contrast to a case-control study design, which identifies the outcome of interest first. The classic example of a well-designed and well-implemented cohort study that has helped to change clinical practice is the Nurses' Health Study (www.channing.harvard.edu/nhs/).

Case-control studies are observational studies that compare a group of patients that has an exposure of interest (cases) with a group of patients that does not (controls). They can be used to compare drugs, devices, procedures, or environmental exposures. They are often smaller and less expensive than cohort studies, and they often can provide faster results. They are also particularly well suited for the study of rare outcomes.

Cross-sectional studies are retrospective analyses of a data set that is representative of a single point in time. They lack the longitudinal aspects of cohort studies and therefore cannot be used for risk estimation. However, because they are snapshots in time, using data that have been collected already, researchers can obtain results much more expediently. Often the data are readily available, and with improved computing power a researcher can now analyze thousands or even millions of records using advanced statistical methodology and get results quickly. This study design is therefore excellent for hypothesis generation, early investigation of a new or unique research area, or generating background data to build an argument for the need for a larger study.

TABLE 2: Large Databases Available for Surgical Research

Name	Description	Website
ACS NSQIP	The American College of Surgeons National Surgical Quality Improvement Program (ACS NSQIP) is a hospital-based nationally validated, risk-adjusted, outcomes-based program to measure and improve the quality of surgical care in the private sector.	https://www.facs.org/quality-programs/acs-nsqip
VASQIP	The Veterans Affairs Surgical Quality Improvement Program (VASQIP) collects and reports risk-adjusted morbidity and mortality rates after major surgery to the 123 Veterans Affairs Medical Centers (VAMCs) performing major surgery, and uses risk-adjusted outcomes to monitor and improve the quality of surgical care to all veterans.	Accessible through Veterans Health Administration only
HCUP NIS HCUP SID	The Nationwide Inpatient Sample (NIS) and the State Inpatient Databases (SIDs) are part of a family of databases and software tools developed by the Agency for Healthcare Research and Quality (AHRQ) for the Healthcare Cost and Utilization Project (HCUP). The NIS is the largest publicly available all-payer inpatient healthcare database in the United States.	https://www.hcup-us.ahrq.gov/nisoverview.jsp https://www.hcup-us.ahrq.gov/sidoverview.jsp
Medicare LDS	The Centers for Medicare and Medicaid Services (CMS) collects information about Medicare beneficiaries, Medicare claims, Medicare providers, clinical data, and Medicaid eligibility and claims and then includes these data in a publicly available file stripped of beneficiary identifiers. These are known as the Limited Data Set (LDS) files.	https://www.cms.gov/Research-Statistics-Data-and-Systems/Files-for-Order/LimitedDataSets/
NCDB	The nationally recognized National Cancer Data Base (NCDB), jointly sponsored by the American College of Surgeons and the American Cancer Society, is a clinical oncology database sourced from hospital registry data that are collected in more than 1500 Commission on Cancer (CoC)-accredited facilities.	https://www.facs.org/quality%20programs/cancer/ncdb
SEER	The Surveillance, Epidemiology, and End Results (SEER) Program of the National Cancer Institute (NCI) collects and publishes cancer incidence and survival data from population-based cancer registries covering approximately 30% of the U.S. population.	http://seer.cancer.gov/about/overview.html

Observational studies can be conducted prospectively or retrospectively. Several large databases are available to researchers to enable retrospective evaluations of data for comparative effectiveness research. Table 2 lists a few of the largest and most well-known data sets and provides references to learn more.

Systematic Reviews

Given the unprecedented rate at which new medical knowledge is being generated, systematic reviews are an essential tool for all medical professionals. Formal systematic reviews are designed to provide an objective appraisal of the evidence from original research. They follow well-described steps to identify and avoid bias and to produce reliable results and inform decision making. They are distinctly different from narrative reviews, which represent an informal summary of the current literature and the opinion of the author.

A systematic review starts with an exhaustive and methodical exploration of the current literature pertaining to a single research question. The literature search typically spans several bibliographic databases (e.g., MEDLINE, Embase, CINAHL) and is based on prespecified search terms. Once all articles felt to be related to the specified research question have been identified, they are screened further based on prespecified inclusion and exclusion criteria. This process of exclusion is specified before starting the review and should be transparent in order to avoid bias in the findings. Then the review summarizes not only the results of each included study but also the quality of evidence produced by the study given the study design. This is often provided to the reader in the form of a table.

Many systematic reviews also will include a meta-analysis when appropriate. A meta-analysis is the pooling of data from prior independent analyses for the purpose of performing a statistical analysis and generating an estimate of treatment effect. Merging the data from prior studies improves the power of the researcher's estimate. Results from multiple prior studies may have trended toward a specified treatment effect but lacked the power to demonstrate a statistically significant effect. By aggregating the results of these trials, a meta-analysis could help to provide a more definitive answer to the underlying question.

It is important to note that the primary limitation of a systematic review is that it does not generate new data. Because of this, the quality of a systematic review with or without a meta-analysis is limited by the quality of the underlying studies. If systematic bias exists in the underlying studies, there may be little a researcher can do to overcome that bias, and hence the results of the systematic review also will be biased. For this reason, a large, well-designed RCT may get a very different result from the aggregation of many smaller RCTs.

Decision Analysis

In contrast to the research methods already described, decision analysis compares different treatment options through modeling rather than primary analysis of prospective or retrospective groups of individuals. These modeling techniques are based on a decision tree. A decision tree uses discrete points of division at which a researcher must input two or more branch points, applying a probability weight to each branch. Depending on the research question, the decision tree can become complex and terminate in two to many discrete endpoints. These endpoints then represent the possible outcomes for the patient and are inherently reflective of different benefits and disadvantages.

Decision analysis attempts to estimate the downstream benefits or disadvantages of multiple treatment options using the current literature. Much like with a meta-analysis, these data are generated through the synthesis of data from prior studies, and therefore the value of a formal decision analysis is based in the quality of data available to the researcher. If there are very few data to guide a researcher in the probability of a given event or the value of a given decision, the decision analysis may not be possible until further primary research is undertaken. As the research base becomes more robust, decision analysis techniques are becoming more important in guiding medical and political decision making.

Cost-Effectiveness Analysis

With medical expenses in the United States continuing to grow at speeds that substantially outpace the growth of the country's economy, cost-effectiveness analyses are becoming increasingly popular and important. Cost-effectiveness analyses attempt to apply standardized values to the costs and benefits of various treatment options and provide insight into the relative value of various treatments in terms of cost-benefit ratios. How a researcher defines costs is of critical importance and often can vary greatly from one study to another, making comparison of these studies difficult. Some analyses choose to reflect only economic costs, such as the direct costs of a given drug, whereas others take into account more intangible costs, such as pain, suffering, or the loss of productive years of life. Benefits, on the other hand, mostly are reflected in quality-adjusted life years (QALYs). Then treatments are compared with respect to a cost-benefit ratio, and the treatment with the lowest cost per QALY benefit is deemed the most cost effective. These studies are becoming a critical component of medical decision making on a national level but are often misunderstood and dismissed by practicing clinicians. Their nontraditional description of an outcome in terms of QALYs can be off-putting, but we contend that physicians need to work to understand this important analytic methodology, as these studies are starting to shape our current practice already and will play a greater role in our future.

■ THE GROWING ROLE OF COMPARATIVE EFFECTIVENESS RESEARCH IN SURGICAL PRACTICE

The growing role of CER in surgical practice is evident all around us. From increased publications using CER methodology to increased attention in new health policies such as the Affordable Care Act, CER is changing the surgical practice environment. New computing power made large databases accessible to more researchers, and this has led to a rapid rise in publications. The surgical literature and statistical methodology are becoming increasingly complex. Systematic reviews and meta-analyses therefore are becoming more important. As VBP becomes our reality, an understanding of CER methodology will be imperative for clinicians. Cost-effectiveness analysis and decision analysis also will become more popular as the evidence base from primary studies grows to enable these more complex decision support tools. Previously we stated that the era of CER was coming. It is now here.

■ CONCLUSIONS

Not only do surgeons need to understand CER, but we all need to be champions of CER and integrate findings appropriately into our practices. The first step is to understand the common terminology and methodology laid out in this chapter, but to be fully informed we recommend starting with the suggested reading list provided. CER is becoming an integral part of our surgical literature and our political climate, and doing the best for our patients means integrating these research findings appropriately into our clinical practices.

SUGGESTED READINGS

Agency for Healthcare Research and Quality. *What is comparative effectiveness research?* <http://effectivehealthcare.ahrq.gov.>.

Bilimoria KY, Minami CA, Mahvi DM, eds. *Comparative Effectiveness in Surgical Oncology.* New York: Springer; 2015.

FIRST Trial – pending publication, will update reference soon.

Health Services Research Information Central (HSRIC). *Comparative effectiveness research (CER).* <https://www.nlm.nih.gov/hsrinfo/cer.html.>.

Patient Protection and Affordable Care Act, 42 U.S.C. § 18001. 2010.

SURGICAL PALLIATIVE CARE

Elizabeth J. Lilley, MD, MPH, and Zara Cooper, MD, MSc

Palliative care is a specialized, multidisciplinary approach to managing patients with serious, life-limiting illness. This model of medical care acknowledges the global impact of illness on quality of life and aims to reduce suffering by addressing patients' physical, emotional, social, and spiritual needs. Numerous studies have demonstrated benefits of providing palliative care to hospitalized patients. These benefits include improved symptom management, fewer burdensome health care transitions, and reduced end-of-life health care use without an increase in mortality rates. In 2005 the American College of Surgeons Task Force on Surgical Palliative Care and the Committee on Ethics endorsed a Statement of Principles of Palliative Care (Box 1). This statement emphasized the appropriateness of palliative care for a broad range of patients receiving surgical treatment, noting that its life-affirming approach to relieving pain and suffering should not be limited only to those patients who are nearing death. Despite efforts to promote early palliative care, many patients and clinicians continue to mistakenly believe that palliative care is analogous to end-of-life care after curative treatment options have been exhausted. On the contrary, palliative care can be understood as an added layer of supportive care for patients and their families that is provided appropriately alongside disease-directed treatment.

The need for palliation is well defined at the end of life, and palliation is sometimes confused with *hospice*, which is an insurance benefit exclusively for patients who choose to forgo cure-directed treatment. Unlike palliative care, hospice is reserved for patients with a life expectancy of 6 months or less (Box 2). This benefit provides patients with health care coverage for physician and nursing services, medical equipment and supplies, medications for pain and symptom management, physical and occupational therapy, home health aide services, social work services, and bereavement support services. Treatment of unrelated diagnoses is still available under regular Medicare coverage. Despite the benefits of hospice care, the majority of Americans do not receive any hospice before death, and those who do are frequently referred late, enrolling within days of death. Timely and appropriate discussion about hospice is an important task of all physicians who manage patients with serious illness.

■ PRIMARY PALLIATIVE CARE FOR SURGEONS

Increasing life expectancy, improvements in chronic disease management, and advances in surgical safety have led to an increase in the proportion of operations performed on older and sicker patients. As such, there is an expanding need for palliative care among surgical patients. In response to the high cost and low quality of health care for patients nearing the end of life, the Institute of Medicine released a 2014 report, *Dying in America*, which declared providing palliative care a national priority and called for physicians managing seriously ill patients to ensure appropriate and timely access to palliative care. As providers for patients with critical illness and those nearing the end of life, surgeons must be proficient in *primary palliative care*, the basic skills and competencies required of all physicians, which includes management of physical symptoms, management of nonphysical symptoms (i.e., depression and anxiety), and communication about prognosis, goals of treatment, suffering, and code status. These elements of primary palliative care, as they relate to surgical practice, are described later.

Symptom Management

Serious illness may be manifested in a variety of symptoms. As such, surgeons managing complex patients must be prepared to treat any number of physical and emotional complaints. Surgeons are very familiar with managing acute, postoperative pain. However, patients may have other types of acute and chronic nonsurgical pain, which surgeons encounter less frequently (Table 1). Determining the type and origin of a patient's pain is essential for designing an effective treatment regimen. Somatic pain, including surgical, bone, and musculoskeletal pain, is typically a well-localized, dull or aching pain and is treated with nonsteroidal anti-inflammatory drugs (NSAIDs) and opiates. Visceral pain tends to be dull or colicky and diffuse and is treated with opiates. Neuropathic pain often is described as having a burning or itching quality and should be treated with gabapentin. Severe pain should be managed with a combination of long-acting and short-acting medications. In addition, it is important to recognize that pain is multidimensional and may have a psychological component. When pain is refractory to appropriate pharmacologic regimens, behavioral interventions or spiritual support should be considered.

Other common physical symptoms in surgical patients include chronic nausea, vomiting, delirium, diarrhea, constipation, xerostomia, and insomnia. Select physical symptoms and approaches to their treatment are described in Table 2. When these symptoms are identified, they should be managed aggressively. Under-recognition and undertreatment of symptoms remains a persistent problem in medicine. Established approaches to screening and evaluating these symptoms are available and may aid in diagnosis. Validated symptom inventories, such as the Edmonton Symptom Assessment Scale (ESAS), can be useful for routinely assessing symptoms in patients at high risk for unmet palliative needs. The ESAS can be completed by a patient or caregiver and asks the respondent to rate the severity of nine common symptoms on a scale of 0 to 10: pain, tiredness, nausea, depression, anxiety, drowsiness, appetite, feeling of well-being, and shortness of breath.

In addition to physical symptoms, coping with serious illness or injury affects patients' quality of life in emotional, social, and spiritual domains. Psychological distress, including anxiety and depression, may manifest as physical symptoms in patients who are navigating major illness, unexpected complications, or poor prognoses. Inquiring about patients' emotional well-being and

BOX 1: Statement of Principles of Palliative Care

- Respect the dignity and autonomy of patients, patients' surrogates, and caregivers.
- Honor the right of the competent patient or surrogate to choose among treatments, including those that may or may not prolong life.
- Communicate effectively and empathically with patients, their families, and caregivers.
- Identify the primary goals of care from the patient's perspective, and address how the surgeon's care can achieve the patient's objectives.
- Strive to alleviate pain and other burdensome physical and nonphysical symptoms.
- Recognize, assess, discuss, and offer access to services for psychological, social, and spiritual issues.
- Provide access to therapeutic support, encompassing the spectrum from life-prolonging treatments through hospice care, when they can realistically be expected to improve the quality of life as perceived by the patient.
- Recognize the physician's responsibility to discourage treatments that are unlikely to achieve the patient's goals, and encourage patients and families to consider hospice care when the prognosis for survival is likely to be less than a half-year.
- Arrange for continuity of care by the patient's primary and/or specialist physician, alleviating the sense of abandonment patients may feel when "curative" therapies are no longer useful.
- Maintain a collegial and supportive attitude toward others entrusted with care of the patient.

From Task Force on Surgical Palliative Care. Statement of principles of palliative care. *Bull Am Coll Surg.* 2005;90:34-35.

BOX 2: Medicare Hospice Benefit: Eligibility and Coverage as of 2015

Hospice Eligibility

- Enrolled in Medicare Part A
- Two physicians certify terminally ill status with life expectancy ≤6 months
- Patient opts for comfort-directed care only; forgoes curative treatments for the terminal illness and related conditions

Services Covered by Hospice

- Physician and nursing care
- Medical equipment and supplies
- Medications prescribed for symptom control (copayment ≤$5)
- Hospice aide and home care services
- Physical therapy, occupational therapy, and speech-language pathology services
- Social work services
- Dietary counseling
- Short-term inpatient care for management of symptoms
- Short-term respite care in nursing home, hospice inpatient facility, or hospital (copayment 5% of Medicare-approved rate)
- Bereavement support
- Other treatments or services recommended by hospice provider for management of pain and symptoms related to terminal disease

Services Not Covered by Hospice

- Treatments and medications intended to cure the terminal illness or related conditions
- Room and board; short-term inpatient respite care may be covered if arranged through the hospice team
- Emergency room and inpatient care or ambulance transportation is not covered unless it is arranged by the hospice provider or it is unrelated to the terminal illness (covered under Medicare Part A)

Adapted from *Centers for Medicare and Medicaid Services.* Hospice & respite care. <https://www.medicare.gov/coverage/hospice-and-respite-care.html.> Accessed 17.11.15.

acknowledging the validity of their nonphysical concerns helps to build trust with patients and families and hastens their recovery. As with physical symptoms, emotional suffering should be managed aggressively and appropriately. The interdisciplinary care team–based approach of palliative care is particularly valuable for attending to nonphysical symptoms. A request for assistance from colleagues in psychotherapy or psychiatry may be helpful to the surgeon and welcomed by the patient and family. When patients are coping with spiritual distress, visitation from the hospital chaplain or religious leaders in the community may provide comfort and fulfill patients' spiritual needs.

Palliative Procedures

Surgical care is sometimes considered as a means of reducing symptom burden. Palliative procedures aim to alleviate suffering and improve quality of life, without the expectation of prolonging it. Examples of palliative surgical procedures are described in Table 3. These include both procedures performed near the end of life for patients with incurable conditions and procedures performed to relieve chronic suffering for patients without terminal prognoses. In these situations, high-quality communication is crucial to ensure that the treatment goals of the patient, family, and surgical team are aligned.

The Palliative Triangle, a communication model for shared decision making about palliative procedures, has been shown to improve patient selection and be satisfactory to patients and families (Figure 1). In this model, the patient, family, and surgeon discuss the patient's symptoms and the goals of the intervention from each of their unique perspectives. Although the risks and treatment burdens are weighed against the potential benefits of surgical and nonsurgical treatment options, the surgeon shares what outcomes can and cannot

be attained. Patients and families may harbor unrealistic beliefs about the outcomes from intervention. This approach allows surgeons to temper expectations and direct the focus toward achievable palliative goals.

Palliative care strives to improve quality of life from the patient's perspective; therefore benchmarks for success of palliative treatments diverge from traditional outcome measurement. Optimal symptom management is an iterative process and requires frequently reassessing symptoms and refining the care plan as directed by response to treatment. Patient-reported outcomes are the gold standard for assessing outcomes of palliative treatment. Symptom screening tools can help to identify whether symptom burden has been affected appreciably by different interventions. Measuring health-related quality of life can provide further information on how treatment has affected the patient's lived experience. Frequently used health-related quality of life instruments include the Functional Assessment of Cancer Therapy–General (FACT-G), the McGill Quality of Life Questionnaire (MQOL), and the European Organization for Research and Treatment of Cancer Quality of Life Questionnaire–Core 30. In addition, several validated condition-specific or procedure-specific quality of life measures also exist. However, measures for quality of life are rarely used at the bedside. Eliciting patient-reported health might be a good proxy.

TABLE 1: An Overview of Pain Symptoms

Symptoms	Assessment and Considerations	Treatment Strategy
Somatic pain	• Easily localized; includes acute postsurgical pain • Prescribe standing regimen with immediate release rescue doses available for breakthrough or uncontrolled pain • Unless contraindicated, a bowel regimen should be administered with opioids for prophylaxis against constipation • Symptomatic control should be assessed frequently to guide evaluation and refinement of the treatment regimen	• Mild pain: acetaminophen or nonsteroidal anti-inflammatory drugs (NSAIDs) • Moderate pain: titrate short-acting opioids • Severe pain: titrate short-acting opioids until adequately controlled, then transition to long-acting opioids of equivalent potency and rescue doses
Bone pain	• Type of somatic pain from highly sensitive nociceptors of periosteum • Can be caused by fractures or irritation from underlying metastases found on radiographs and isotope bone scans • Bone metastases in the spine may lead to spinal cord compression and neurologic deficits • To decrease risk of NSAID-induced gastropathy with chronic NSAID use, selective COX-2 inhibitors and coadministration with a gastroprotective agent (i.e., proton pump inhibitors) is advisable	• A regimen combining NSAIDs and opioids may alleviate generalized bone pain • Radiotherapy is effective for isolated metastases • Orthopedic interventions can be considered to stabilize pathologic fractures
Muscle spasm	• Prolonged, forceful, or sustained involuntary muscle contraction • Can be iatrogenic from medication side effects or because of electrolyte imbalances or dehydration	• Pharmacologic therapeutics to include anticonvulsants (e.g., diazepam) and muscle relaxants (e.g., baclofen) • Manipulations to relax the muscle include stretching and massage • Physiotherapy treatments include electrical stimulation of the nerves or ultrasound thermotherapy
Neuropathic pain	• Common examples include postthoracotomy pain, phantom limb pain after amputation, ischemic limb pain, and pain from tumor invasion of nerves (i.e., pancreatic cancer pain) • May be accompanied by altered sensation	• Tricyclic antidepressants (e.g., amitriptyline) and anticonvulsant medications (e.g., gabapentin) may be helpful in combination with opioids • Pancreatic cancer pain may be alleviated temporarily by local neuroanesthetics (celiac axis blockade) or permanently by celiac axis neurolysis procedures • Anti-inflammatory properties of corticosteroids may reduce peritumoral edema
Visceral pain	• Often diffuse and poorly localized • Can be caused by distension, ischemia, and inflammation of the thoracic, pelvic, or abdominal organs • Solid organ tumor burden may cause stretch or irritation of peritoneal surfaces	• Treatment options are tailored to the site and etiology, and may include anti-inflammatory medications, corticosteroids, and opioids
Intestinal colic	• Distension of the small intestine and colon cause visceral pain • Common examples include paralytic ileus, malignant obstruction, and intestinal pseudo-obstruction	• Treatment begins with addressing any reversible causes of distension • Nonobstructive distension pain can be treated with antispasmodic agents (e.g., hyoscine butylbromide) and opioids

Communication

Communicating a poor prognosis is perhaps the most technically challenging situation that physicians encounter. As with any complex procedure, surgeons achieve poise, dexterity, and mastery through thoughtful preparation and training. Studies show that patients and families value communication about prognosis with their physicians, even when outcomes are uncertain. Furthermore, when patients and families possess an accurate understanding of poor prognosis, they are more likely to forgo life-prolonging measures in favor of comfort-directed care. This leads to reduced intensity of treatment near the end of life without increased mortality. Useful tools, such as the American College of Surgeons National Surgical Quality Improvement Program (ACS NSQIP) Surgical Risk Calculator (http://riskcalculator.facs.org/) and ePrognosis (http://eprognosis.ucsf.edu/default.php), provide evidence-based prognostic information, which can inform treatment decision making and provide context to these conversations.

Determining and documenting existing advance directives should occur on hospital admission and be confirmed by the critical care

TABLE 2: Nonpain Physical Symptoms Commonly Encountered in the Surgical Intensive Care Unit

Symptoms	Assessment and Considerations	Treatment Strategy
Nausea/vomiting	• Rule out reversible causes such as hypercalcemia and infection. Treat underlying cause if nausea and vomiting results from intestinal obstruction or intracranial processes (i.e., increased intracranial pressure from space-occupying lesion or hemorrhage) • Toxins and medications can act centrally to stimulate the chemoreceptor trigger zone of the brain, inducing nausea and vomiting • Upper gut dysmotility from ineffective and delayed gastric emptying results in gastric distension, nausea, and vomiting	• Antiemetics target different receptors and may be combined • Dopamine antagonists (e.g., prochlorperazine, haloperidol) are effective for vomiting related to the chemoreceptor trigger zone • Antihistamines (e.g., meclizine) and anticholinergics (e.g., scopolamine) act centrally on receptors in the vomiting center of the vestibular system. They can be combined with dopamine antagonists • Serotonin antagonists (e.g., ondansetron) have diffuse inhibitory effects on serotonin receptors of the small bowel, vagus nerve, and chemoreceptor trigger zone. They are indicated for chemotherapy-induced nausea and vomiting • Nausea from dysmotility can be treated with prokinetics (e.g., metoclopramide, domperidone)
Delirium/agitation	• May be caused by electrolyte imbalances and accumulation of toxic metabolites • Can be produced or worsened by certain medications (e.g., opioids, benzodiazepines)	• Identify underlying causes • Frequent reorientation • Antipsychotics are first-line pharmacotherapy (e.g., haloperidol, chlorpromazine) for moderate symptoms • For severe symptoms, benzodiazepines (e.g., lorazepam, midazolam) can be combined with antipsychotics to achieve sedation
Diarrhea	• First consider infectious (e.g., *Clostridium difficile*) and iatrogenic (e.g., laxatives, medication side effect) causes • Diarrhea may be caused by chemotherapy or radiation enteritis • Patients may have altered anatomy (e.g., extensive bowel resection, high output from a proximal ostomy, enteric fistulae)	• Dietary modification, electrolyte repletion and adequate hydration • If infectious and reversible causes are ruled out, antidiarrheals can be used (e.g., loperamide, kaolin and pectin) • Patients with steatorrhea from pancreatic insufficiency should receive pancrelipase • Octreotide can be given to patients with secretory diarrhea, high-output stoma, or gastrointestinal fistula • Aspirin or nonsteroidal anti-inflammatory drugs (NSAIDs), cholestyramine, and psyllium may be helpful for patients with radiation enteritis
Constipation	• Commonly associated with poor fluid intake, weak or debilitated patients, and those on opioid analgesics • Fecal impaction can cause partial or complete obstruction	• Stimulant laxatives (e.g., senna, bisacodyl) are indicated for patients without complete obstruction and should be given in combination with stool softeners (e.g., docusate sodium, polyethylene glycol, lactulose)
Dyspnea	• Several acute processes may cause dyspnea in surgical patients, including pneumothorax, atelectasis, and uncontrolled pain • The physiologic stressors of surgical treatment may exacerbate chronic conditions, including congestive heart failure and chronic obstructive pulmonary disease • When physical causes of dyspnea have been ruled out, emotional or situational etiologies should be considered (i.e., anxiety)	• Reversible causes of dyspnea should be assessed quickly and treated appropriately. This may include management of fluid overload for congestive heart failure and administration of bronchodilators or steroids for obstructive airway disease • Administration of supplemental oxygen using face masks should be avoided in the terminal setting • "Air hunger" is palliated with opioids and anxiolytics • Particularly when impending respiratory failure is a concern, an immediate conversation about preferences for invasive and noninvasive ventilation should occur with the patient or surrogate, with appropriate documentation in the medical record

TABLE 3: Examples of Palliative Procedures Performed Near the End of Life

Nature of Procedure	Examples
Symptom relief for incurable benign disease	Excision of large condylomata Procedures (e.g., banding of esophageal varices or shunt procedures) for end-stage liver disease
Symptom relief for incurable malignant disease: nonresectional	Biliary and/or gastric bypass for unresectable, obstructing periampullary cancers Chemical splanchnicectomy for intractable pain (e.g., locoregionally advanced pancreatic cancer) Intestinal bypass or ostomy for malignant bowel obstruction Decompressing gastrostomy tube placement for malignant bowel obstruction Peritoneal dialysis catheter for drainage of recurrent malignant ascites
Symptom relief for incurable malignant disease: resectional/debulking (cytoreductive) procedure	Resection of primary tumor or metastatic lesion(s) for pain, obstruction, and/or bleeding in setting of unresectable distant disease (e.g., palliative mastectomy, resection of primary tumor in stage IV colorectal cancer) Resection/debulking of symptomatic carcinoid tumor
Intended prolongation of survival	Debulking of advanced ovarian cancer resectional/debulking procedure Metastasectomy or ablation of advanced cancer with incomplete or suboptimal treatment (e.g., R2 – gross disease remaining)

From Mosca PJ, Blazer DG 3rd, Wheeler JL, Abernethy AP. When a chance to cut is not a chance to cure: a future for palliative surgery? *Ann Surg Oncol.* 2011;18:3235-3239, Table 1.

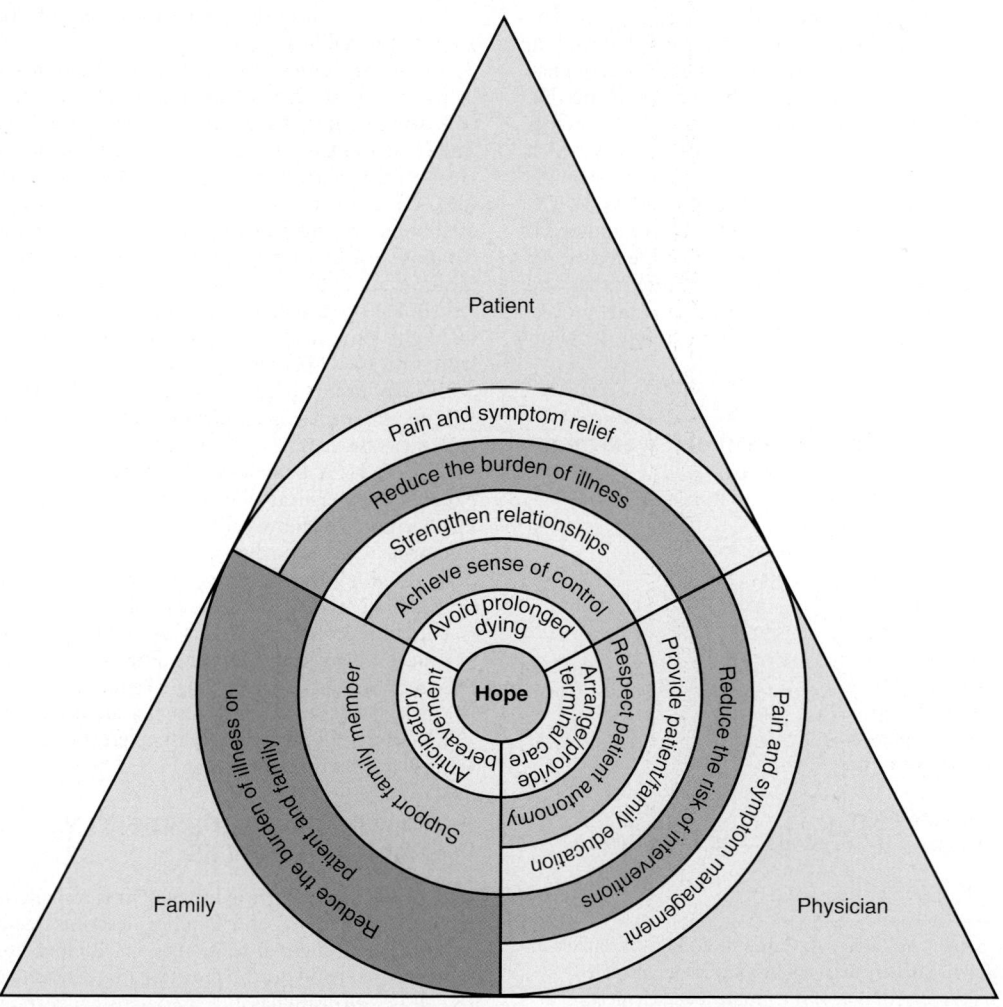

FIGURE 1 The Palliative Triangle. Interactions among the patient, the family, and the surgeon guide individual decisions regarding palliative care. Hope for achievable goals is advanced as each participant of the Palliative Triangle fulfills specific obligations. *(From Thomay AA, Jaques DP, Miner TJ. Surgical palliation: getting back to our roots. Surg Clin North Am. 2009;89:27-41, vii-viii, Figure 4.)*

team. Advance directives allow patients to document their wishes for future health care and are used if patients become incapacitated and cannot speak for themselves. The broad language of most advance directives complicates their interpretation in specific clinical circumstances. However, when available, they can provide clinicians and families with insight into the patient's values and preferences regarding the intensity of care at the end of life and use of life-sustaining treatments. Surgical patients in the surgical intensive care unit (ICU) are at high risk for impairment due to delirium, mechanical ventilation, pharmacologic sedation, and acute critical illness. When this happens, family members are asked to serve as surrogate decision makers. Whenever possible, patients should be asked to identify who they want to make medical decisions for them should they become unable to speak for themselves. In addition to coping with a critically ill family member, the burden of making medical decisions can be a source of anxiety and social tension for surrogates. The clinician team can support surrogates through high-quality communication about the patient's health status and care plan. Social work involvement and spiritual support also may be of comfort to families.

Shared decision making is the preferred method for health care choices with high-risk and uncertain outcomes, including life-sustaining treatments or emergency interventions for patients with poor prognosis. This collaborative model is an entirely distinct process from informed consent. Patients share their goals for treatment and priorities for quality of life in the context of serious illness, and clinicians share the best available scientific evidence to describe how different therapies align with the patients' stated goals. The risks, benefits, and burdens of all treatments are described, including aggressive comfort-directed care in lieu of life-sustaining treatments. During these conversations, clinicians elicit the aspects of life that are most important to the patient, including anniversaries or events that would affect treatment decisions. Patients also identify which trade-offs they are willing to accept in order to achieve a favorable outcome and which outcomes would be unacceptable (Box 3). The clinician then must synthesize this into a treatment recommendation, based on the prognosis, values, and priorities of the individual patient. This recommendation may include time-limited trials and plans to revisit the decision at a later date. Engaging in this process allows the patient and clinician to collaboratively reach decisions about life-sustaining treatments that best reflect the patient's wishes for intensity of care.

Family meetings facilitate communication about the goals of care and are most effective when they occur early during the ICU stay, within the first 5 days of admission. All members of the care team may participate in the meeting and should be encouraged to attend. Social workers and nurses, who are frequently the family's primary in-hospital contact, can help coordinate a meeting and notify physicians of social tensions or specific concerns to be addressed. The results of the family meeting should be documented in the medical record, including the content of the discussion, plan of care, and participants involved.

■ MODELS OF PALLIATIVE CARE DELIVERY IN THE INTENSIVE CARE UNIT

Delivery of palliative care can be accomplished through a consultative model or an integrative model. The consultative model uses triggers to prompt palliative care consultation. The success of this system hinges on the ability of screening criteria to detect those who would benefit from palliative care consultation. Some studies have found that triggers, based on signs of critical illness, create too high a threshold. Therefore few patients meet criteria for palliative care, and those who do are identified late in their course as they are nearing the end of life. Others have found that triggers increase palliative care consultation and decrease hospital use. Palliative care referral criteria from the Center to Advance Palliative Care (CAPC) are listed in Table 4.

In the integrative model, the critical care team provides primary palliative care to all patients. This model incorporates principles of palliative care unto usual care. This may be aided by using protocols. The Care and Communication Bundle, introduced by the Veterans Health Administration and the Society of Critical Care Medicine (SCCM) in their efforts to transform ICU care, is a collection of quality metrics for palliative care quality in the ICU. This bundle is composed of benchmarks for patient and family-centered communication in the ICU. The nine process measures, developed through stakeholder engagement, are outlined in Table 5. These measures highlight time-triggered strategies for improved communication with critically ill patients and their families.

Incorporating palliative care principles into the standards of ICU treatment has been demonstrated to improve communication and decrease length of stay without increasing mortality in the surgical ICU. A benefit of this model is that it ensures that all patients with critical illness receive the benefits of palliative care. Furthermore, it allows allocation of specialty palliative care consultation, which is a limited resource in most hospitals, to those patients with refractory symptoms or complex needs. In an integrative palliative care model, specialty palliative care consultation is still indicated for patients with (1) progressive deterioration; (2) life-limiting conditions leading to declines in quality of life, functional status, or cognition; (3) suboptimal symptomatic control; (4) lack of clarity or disagreement surrounding goals of care; and (5) decisions to forgo disease-directed treatment and transfer focus toward comfort-directed care.

■ MANAGING IMMINENTLY DYING PATIENTS

Care of the imminently dying patient is a challenging phase of treatment. Most patients and families describe freedom from suffering and time to strengthen relationships with loved ones as critical components of a "good death." However, the intensity of care that patients receive before death has increased in recent years, and a rising number of patient deaths occur during or immediately after an ICU stay. Physicians should do their best to provide comfort to actively dying

---

BOX 3: Postoperative Outcomes Where Treatment Burdens May Outweigh the Benefits

- Permanent nursing home residence
- Prolonged hospitalization or ICU course
- Dependence on life-sustaining therapies
  - Mechanical ventilation
  - Hemodialysis
  - Feeding tubes
  - Total parenteral nutrition
- Severe cognitive impairment
- Complete functional dependence
- Burden to family or loved ones
- Intractable pain
- No time to get affairs in order
- Inability to enjoy a personal milestone (birthday, wedding, anniversary)
- Death away from home

From Cooper Z, Courtwright A, Karlage A, Gawande A, Block S. Pitfalls in communication that lead to nonbeneficial emergency surgery in elderly patients with serious illness: description of the problem and elements of a solution. *Ann Surg.* 2014;260:949-957, Table 2.

ICU, Intensive care unit.

TABLE 4: Referral Criteria for Specialty Palliative Care

General referral criteria *Presence of a serious illness and one or more of the following:*	• New diagnosis of life-limiting illness for symptom control, patient/family support • Declining ability to complete activities of daily living • Weight loss • Progressive metastatic cancer • Admission from long-term care facility (nursing home or assisted living) • Two or more hospitalizations for illness within 3 months • Difficult-to-control physical or emotional symptoms • Patient, family, or physician uncertainty regarding prognosis • Patient, family, or physician uncertainty regarding appropriateness of treatment options • Patient or family requests for futile care • DNR order conflicts • Conflicts or uncertainty regarding the use of nonoral feeding or hydration in cognitively impaired, seriously ill, or dying patients • Limited social support in setting of a serious illness (e.g., homeless, no family or friends, chronic mental illness, overwhelmed family caregivers) • Patient, family, or physician request for information regarding hospice appropriateness • Patient or family psychologic or spiritual/existential distress
Intensive care unit criteria *Presence of a serious illness, any of the above, and one or more of the following:*	• Admission from a nursing home • Two or more ICU admissions within the same hospitalization • Prolonged or failed attempt to wean from ventilator • Multiorgan failure • Consideration of ventilator withdrawal with expected death • Metastatic cancer • Anoxic encephalopathy • Consideration of patient transfer to a long-term ventilator facility • Family distress impairing surrogate decision making
Cancer criteria *Presence of any of the above, and/or:*	• Metastatic or locally advanced cancer progressing despite systemic treatments • Karnofsky <50 or ECOG >3 • Brain metastases, spinal cord compression, or neoplastic meningitis • Malignant hypercalcemia • Progressive pleural/peritoneal or pericardial effusions
Neurologic criteria *Presence of any of the above, and/or:*	• Folstein Mini Mental State score <20 • Feeding tube is being considered for any neurologic condition • Status epilepticus >24 hr • ALS or other neuromuscular disease considering mechanical ventilation • Any recurrent brain neoplasm • Parkinson's disease with poor functional status or dementia • Advanced dementia with dependence in all activities of daily living

Adapted from *Center to Advance Palliative Care.* Policies and tools for hospital palliative care programs, page 45. <https://media.capc.org/filer_public/88/06/8806cedd-f78a-4d14-a90e-aca688147a18/nqfcrosswalk.pdf.>

ALS, Amyotrophic lateral sclerosis; *DNR,* do not resuscitate; *ECOG,* Eastern Cooperative Oncology Group; *ICU,* intensive care unit.

patients and their families, which includes allowing families to spend time in the room with their loved ones. Efforts should be made to grant families privacy by minimizing interruptions, and unnecessary monitors, restraints, and medical devices should be silenced or removed.

The physician's goals in terminal care are to protect the patient's dignity and reassure grieving family members of continued dedication to the patient (Box 4). As death approaches, dyspnea (air hunger), upper airway secretions (death rattle), altered sensorium (delirium, loss of consciousness, agitation), incontinence, and pain are common symptoms and should be managed aggressively. Opioids are administered to treat both dyspnea and pain. Positioning patients on their side or elevating the head of the bed may reduce noisy respirations, and antisecretory drugs, such as glycopyrrolate or scopolamine, also should be given. Witnessing these symptoms may be distressing to family members. If family members are present at the bedside, it is important to prepare them for the dying process by describing what death will look like.

The majority of patient deaths in the ICU follow decisions to withdraw or withhold life-sustaining treatment. Involvement of the attending physician and the patient or legal surrogate decision maker is obligatory, and other family members, the primary nurse, social worker, and chaplain should be included unless the patient or surrogate requests otherwise. When patients are conscious and competent, they should participate in these conversations. However, in the surgical ICU, where delirium or impairment is prevalent and advanced medical technology is ubiquitous, patients often are unable to make these decisions. The difficult task of decision making in this context is emotionally and mentally burdensome for surrogates and can be associated with post-traumatic stress disorder or a prolonged bereavement period. The team-based approach of palliative care can again be helpful here: Palliative care clinicians, social workers, and

TABLE 5: Care and Communication Bundle of the Intensive Care Unit Palliative Care Quality Measures

Day 1	Day 3	Day 5
Identify medical decision maker	Offer social work support	Conduct interdisciplinary family meeting
Investigate advance directive status	Offer spiritual support	
Address cardiopulmonary resuscitation preference		
Distribute family information leaflet		
Assess pain regularly		
Manage pain optimally		

Adapted from Nelson JE, Mulkerin CM, Adams LL, Pronovost PJ. Improving comfort and communication in the ICU: a practical new tool for palliative care performance measurement and feedback. *Qual Saf Health Care.* 2006;15:264-271, Table 1.

BOX 4: American College of Surgeons Statement on the Principles Guiding Care at the End of Life

- Respect the dignity of both patient and caregivers.
- Be sensitive to and respectful of the patient's and family's wishes.
- Use the most appropriate measures that are consistent with the choices of the patient or the patient's legal surrogate.
- Ensure alleviation of pain and management of other physical symptoms.
- Recognize, assess, and address psychological, social, and spiritual problems.
- Ensure appropriate continuity of care by the patient's primary and/or specialist physician.
- Provide access to therapies that may realistically be expected to improve the patient's quality of life.
- Provide access to appropriate palliative care and hospice care.
- Respect the patient's right to refuse treatment.
- Recognize the physician's responsibility to forego treatments that are futile.

From American College of Surgeons' Committee on Ethics. Statement on principles guiding care at the end of life. *Bull Am Coll Surg.* 1998;83:46.

---

chaplains are able to offer further emotional, social, and spiritual support to patients' families.

In addition to discussing removal of mechanical ventilation, the conversation should cover withdrawal of the endotracheal tube, antibiotics, artificial feeding, fluid products, blood pressure support, and orogastric or nasogastric tubes. A do not resuscitate and do not intubate code status should be ordered and signed. The agreed-upon plan must be documented in the medical record, by the attending physician, when the appropriate orders are placed. The physician should convey information about the process of discontinuing life-sustaining treatments and share prognostic expectations of when death will occur. In addition, physicians have to prepare the family that timing of death frequently is uncertain and offer reassurance when death does not happen quickly.

Before ventilator withdrawal, paralytics should be discontinued, allowing time for neuromuscular function to return. The patient must be premedicated adequately for sedation with opioids and benzodiazepines to prevent dyspnea and anxiety. Additional medications may be required and should be drawn and available at the bedside for immediate administration. After the respiratory therapist silences all alarms, reduces fraction of inspired oxygen (FiO_2) to 21%, and removes positive end-expiratory pressure (PEEP), the physician observes for signs of respiratory distress. If present, medications should be adjusted to alleviate symptoms before continuing. Over the next 5 to 15 minutes, the inspiratory rate is reduced to 4 and pressure support is decreased to 6. When there are no signs of respiratory distress symptoms, the endotracheal tube can be removed. A T-piece can be used if the family wants to continue intubation. If the patient remains stable for more than 2 hours, transfer to inpatient palliative care or another non-ICU bed may be appropriate. After death occurs, the family should be given adequate time to say goodbye and grieve at the bedside. Condolences and bereavement support should be offered to family members.

This chapter provides an overview of how the major tenets of palliative care can be incorporated into routine surgical practice in order to achieve optimal patient management. The basic competencies summarized previously are required of all surgeons providing care for seriously ill patients. Fellowships to obtain board certification as well as palliative care skills workshops from the American College of Surgeons are available to surgeons who are interested in further training.

SUGGESTED READINGS

Cooper Z, Courtwright A, Karlage A, et al. Pitfalls in communication that lead to nonbeneficial emergency surgery in elderly patients with serious illness: description of the problem and elements of a solution. *Ann Surg.* 2014;260:949-957.

Cooper Z, Koritsanszky LA, Cauley CE, et al. Recommendations for best communication practices to facilitate goal-concordant care for seriously ill older patients with emergency surgical conditions. *Ann Surg.* 2016;263: 1-6.

Dunn GP, Johnson AG, eds. *Surgical Palliative Care.* Chicago: Oxford University Press; 2004.

Dunn GP, Martensen R, Weissman D. *Surgical Palliative Care: A Resident's Guide.* Chicago: American College of Surgeons; 2009.

Lilley EJ, Khan KT, Johnston FM, et al. Palliative care interventions for surgical patients: a systematic review. *JAMA Surg.* 2016;151:172-183.

CARDIOVASCULAR PHARMACOLOGY

Emily Miraflor, MD, and Alden H. Harken, MD, FACS

■ WE HOLD THE FOLLOWING TRUTHS TO BE SELF-EVIDENT:

A. Sinus tachycardia is not a dysrhythmia but a healthy response to another problem.
B. Cardioversion is a logical therapeutic response for any patient who is deemed "unstable" by virtue of a cardiac dysrhythmia.
C. A patient who is in trouble but who exhibits a ventricular rate between 60 and 100 does not have a cardiac rhythm problem—look somewhere else.
D. For each hour of delay in infusing antibiotics into a patient in septic shock, there is a 4% increase in mortality.

■ DYSRHYTHMIAS

At a Glance

See Table 1 for the treatments for different types of tachyarrhythmias.

Cardioversion

An electrical shock should depolarize all cardiomyocytes that are not in an absolute refractory period. Then the myocardium should repolarize synchronously, restoring a regular rhythm.

Wide Complex Tachycardia

Wide complex tachycardia is almost always ventricular in origin and will respond to cardioversion.

Narrow Complex Tachycardia

If the QRS complex is narrow (0.08 second, or 2 little boxes on the electrocardiogram [ECG] paper), the impulse must have originated above the atrioventricular (AV) node. Block the AV node with diltiazem—20 mg intravenously (IV) over 2 minutes. For different durations of AV nodal blockade, see Table 2.

A Deeper Look

Cardioversion

Optimally, cardioversion should be accomplished with a biphasic waveform defibrillator in a synchronized fashion. The biphasic waveform typically cardioverts successfully with half the transmitted energy. In the synchronized mode, the defibrillator requires 4 to 5 seconds to calculate the RR interval so that the shock does not occur during repolarization of ventricular tachycardia (VT), resulting in further destabilization into ventricular fibrillation (VF). Although it is frightening if VF occurs, simply cardiovert again. Remember, in the synchronized mode the machine requires 4 to 5 long seconds (seconds come in different lengths, and when you are waiting for the defibrillator to charge, they are long seconds) in order to time the RR interval.

After successful cardioversion, infuse amiodarone (see Table 2). For patients who previously received digoxin, the amiodarone infusion should be cut in half (0.25 mg/min IV over 18 hours).

Wide Complex Tachycardia

An impulse derived above and via the AV node travels down the Purkinje fibers at 3 meters per second. This impulse activates the entire ventricle very rapidly, in 0.08 second (or 80 milliseconds, or 2

little boxes on the ECG paper). When an impulse originates in the ventricle (ventricle origin beat), it takes longer to access the Purkinje fibers and therefore longer to activate the entire ventricle (a long duration or "wide" QRS complex). If all QRS complexes appear the same (monomorphic VT; Figure 1), the ventricular activation typically derives from a single electrophysiologically unstable locus at the edge of a prior ischemic scar (Figure 2). If the QRS complexes exhibit differing morphology (different patterns of ventricular activation; Figure 3), the entire myocardium is hyperexcitable.

There are five appropriate therapeutic responses to the five causes of polymorphic ventricular ectopy (Box 1), as follows:

1. Local myocardial hypoxia: Augment inhaled oxygen.
2. Hypokalemia: Infuse potassium chloride. Although the total body deficit may be huge, never infuse more than 20 mEq/hr.
3. Hypomagnesemia: Infuse 2 g magnesium over 1 minute, and possibly repeat in 10 minutes.
4. Excess catecholamines: Decrease exogenous infusion of catecholamines; however, frequently the catechols are derived endogenously as a result of pain. Morphine can be an effective antidysrhythmic drug.
5. Drugs: One of the classic manifestations of digitoxicity is polymorphic ventricular ectopy/tachycardia (see Figure 3). Discontinue digoxin.

In a patient with previous myocardial ischemic damage (the characteristic pattern is a right or left bundle branch block, but any deviation in QRS activation can cause it), an impulse originating above the AV node will still produce a wide QRS ventricular complex. Ninety percent of wide complex tachycardias are ventricular in origin. However, 10% are not. These are supraventricular with aberrancy. Electrical cardioversion will still be successful, and cardioversion is never wrong, especially in an unstable patient.

Narrow Complex Tachycardia

These rhythm disorders have many different aliases (atrial fibrillation, atrial flutter, supraventricular tachycardia [SVT], ectopic atrial tachycardia, accelerated junctional rhythms), but for the surgeon who is interested in ending up with a live patient, the treatments are all the same. The problem is that too many supraventricular impulses are being conducted into the ventricles; they travel rapidly down the Purkinje fibers and activate the entire ventricle quickly, so the QRS complex is narrow (Figure 4). For the unstable patient, the therapy is always electrical cardioversion. For the stable patient, the logical therapeutic response is pharmacologic AV nodal blockade. There are several effective AV node blockers (diltiazem, verapamil, and nifedipine) whose mechanisms are calcium-channel blockade. Pick one and get comfortable with it. Diltiazem is the current favorite (see Table 2). Remember that the calcium-channel blockers initially were developed as antihypertensive agents, so until the supraventricular rhythm "breaks," the patient's blood pressure (BP) will drift down a little.

It is possible to make antidysrhythmic therapy much more complicated, but when you and your patient are in a difficult situation, it is always permissible to resort to the treatments outlined in Table 1.

Treatment for All Bradydysrhythmias

Many elite distance runners and swimmers sport a resting heart rate in the 30s. Therefore heart rate alone is not the whole package. Typically, if your patient's ventricular rate is between 60 and 100 and your patient is in trouble, the heart rate is not the problem. When you are confronted with what you believe is a symptomatic or dangerous bradycardia, there are three logical and effective steps:

1. Atropine: 0.5 mg IV push (may be repeated once).
2. Isoproterenol (beta-1 adrenergic receptor agonist) is the most positively chronotropic catecholamine.

TABLE 1: Treatment for Tachyarrhythmias

Unstable	Cardioversion
Wide complex	Cardioversion
Narrow complex	Diltiazem (20 mg intravenously over 2 minutes)

TABLE 2: Treatment Duration of Atrioventricular Nodal Blockade

Seconds	Adenosine (12 mg intravenous [IV] push)
Minutes	Diltiazem (20 mg IV over 2 minutes)
Hours	Digitalis (0.5 mg IV over 30 minutes)
Days	Amiodarone (150 mg IV push followed by 0.5 mg/min over next 18 hours)

BOX 1: Five Causes of Polymorphic Ventricular Ectopy

1. Local myocardial hypoxia and ischemia
2. Hypokalemia
3. Hypomagnesemia
4. Excess endogenous or exogenous catecholamines
5. Drugs (typically digitalis)

3. External cardiac pacemaker: Place the posterior patch just to the right of the spine and the anterior patch just below the left nipple. Begin with the highest energy output and decrease output until you lose capture; then go up a little. You will stimulate thoracic skeletal muscle, but that is a small price to pay until you accomplish transvenous pacing (which always takes longer to establish than you think it will).

Antidysrhythmic Drugs

Adenosine

Adenosine is a very rapid AV nodal blocker that is metabolized by the red cell adenosine deaminase in seconds. You may begin with 6 mg IV push, but you eventually will infuse a repeat dose, so we recommend giving 12 mg as an initial dose. It is worthwhile to warn the patient and the nurses that successful AV nodal block with adenosine typically results in a frightening 8- to 10-second asystolic pause before resumption of sinus rhythm. Adenosine is also useful when you cannot tell whether the QRS complex looks narrow or wide. Give 12 mg adenosine; if the tachycardia does not "break," it is ventricular in origin; if it does "break," proceed to diltiazem.

Diltiazem

Again, there are several effective AV nodal blockers that work via calcium-channel blockade (like diltiazem) (see Table 2).

Beta-Blockers

Beta-blockers are very effective in preventing perioperative dysrhythmias. When a patient arrives for surgery on a beta-blocker, do not discontinue it. Metoprolol may be infused 15 mg IV every 4 hours.

Amiodarone

Amiodarone is a very effective antidysrhythmic and electrophysiologically stabilizing agent. It functions as both an alpha and a beta adrenergic blocker with a half-life of several weeks.

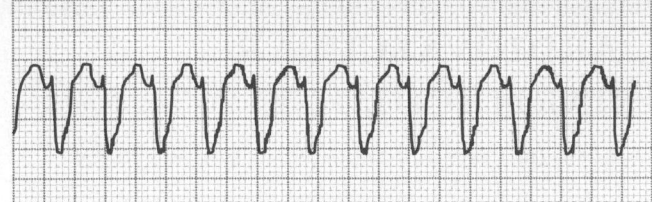

FIGURE 1 Monomorphic ventricular tachycardia. All QRS complexes take a long time (wide complex) to traverse the ventricles. Treatment: Cardioversion.

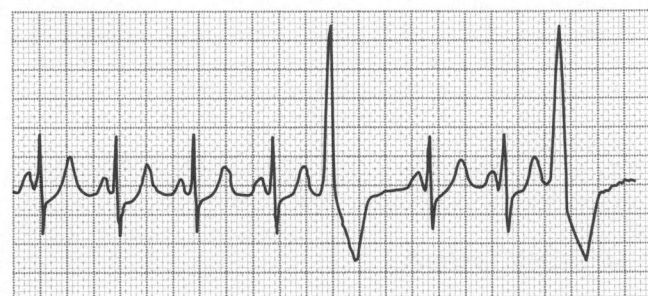

FIGURE 2 Monomorphic ventricular ectopy. The premature ventricular contractions (PVCs) exhibited here all look the same. They derive from a single irritable focus in the border zone of a prior myocardial infarction. Single PVCs are not dangerous (couplets are more ominous). Treatment: See Table 1, or give 100 mg lidocaine intravenous push plus a 2 mg/min drip (maximum total dose 500 mg per 24 hours).

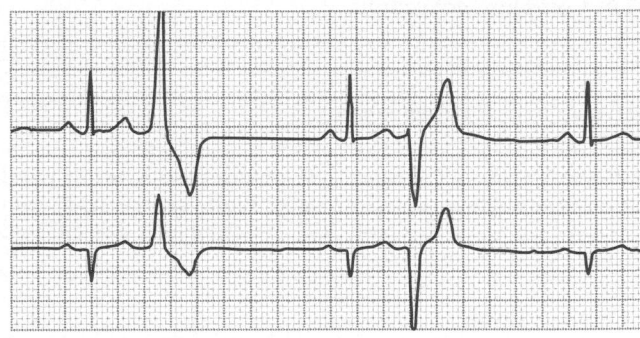

FIGURE 3 Polymorphic ventricular ectopy. The premature ventricular contractions derive from different loci in the ventricles and therefore produce different QRS complexes (or "morphologies"). This patient's myocardium is globally hyperexcitable and should respond to the five interventions delineated in Box 1.

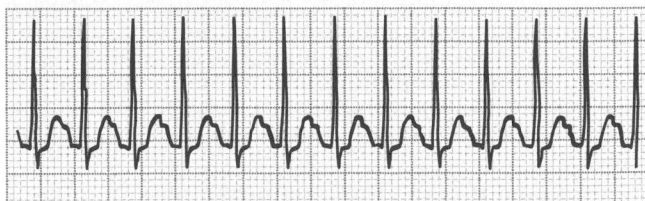

FIGURE 4 Supraventricular tachyarrhythmias. You do not need to name this dysrhythmia in order to treat it. For the ventricles to be activated very rapidly (less than 0.08 second—narrow complex), the initial impulses must have initiated above the atrioventricular node and have traveled down the high-velocity Purkinje fibers. Treatment: Block the node with diltiazem 20 mg intravenously over 2 minutes.

■ MYOCARDIAL FUNCTION

At a Glance

Step I: Increase preload with crystalloid until the patient's ventricles are at the top of the Frank-Starling curve (central venous pressure [CVP] of at least 12 cm H_2O).

Step II: Enhance ventricular contractility with a cardiotonic agent up to the point of electrophysiologic irritability (dobutamine: start at 0.05 to 0.1 μg/kg/min; or epinephrine: start with 0.05 to 0.1 μg/kg/min and titrate)

Step III: With adequate cardiac output and systemic hypotension (mean arterial pressure [MAP] <65 mm Hg), infuse norepinephrine (start with 0.1 μg/min and titrate).

Step IV: It is safe to permit a critically ill patient's hemoglobin (Hgb) to drift down to 7 gms% before transfusion unless you are worried about myocardial ischemia; otherwise, keep the Hgb above 10 gms%.

Step V: After the diagnosis of septic shock, every hour of delay before infusing antibiotics increases mortality by 4%.

A Deeper Look

The circulatory system is governed by Ohm's law: To increase the blood flow (current), you must either increase ventricular contractility (voltage) or decrease the BP (peripheral vascular resistance). More than 2 decades ago, Shoemaker's group in Los Angeles recognized three distinguishable patterns of insufficient systemic oxygen delivery (shock). Each has a well-defined therapeutic response; the problem is that some patients have several of these patterns simultaneously. The patterns are distinguishable by virtue of their filling pressure (CVP) or pulmonary capillary wedge pressure (PCWP), their cardiac output (CO), and their systemic vascular resistance (SVR). These patterns are related by the following equation:

$$SVR = \frac{80 \times (MAP - CVP)}{CO}$$

Pattern 1: Hypovolemia Shock

$$BP = 85/65; MAP = 72; CVP = 2; CO = 4 \text{ L/min}$$

$$SVR = \frac{80 \times (72 - 2)}{4} = 1400 \text{ dynes/sec/cm}^{-5}$$

Pattern 2: Cardiogenic Shock

$$BP = 85/50; MAP = 62; CVP = 12; CO = 4 \text{ L/min}$$

$$SVR = \frac{80 \times (62 - 12)}{4} = 1000 \text{ dynes/sec/cm}^{-5}$$

Pattern 3: Distributive or Septic Shock

$$BP = 85/50; MAP = 62; CVP = 12; CO = 8 \text{ L/min}$$

$$SVR = \frac{80 \times (62 - 12)}{8} = 500 \text{ dynes/sec/cm}^{-5}$$

Notice that, in some instances, the diagnostic parameters are similar for each of these patterns.

In 2001 Rivers and colleagues promoted a sequence of steps (early goal-directed therapy [EGDT]) for septic shock, but their algorithm works beautifully for all three patterns of shock. This group proposed infusing 500 mL of lactated Ringer's solution every 30 minutes (most of us infuse faster than that), until the CVP is 12 mm Hg. If the MAP is lower than 65 mm Hg, infuse dobutamine (start at 0.05 to 0.1 μg/kg/min) or epinephrine (start with 0.05 to 0.1 μg/min) and titrate. Then, if the mixed venous oxygen saturation (blood taken from the central venous line) is less than 70%, transfuse to a hematocrit of 30%. Investigators from the Surviving Sepsis Campaign added norepinephrine (5 μg/min) as the "first choice" vasopressor for patients in a high-output (pattern 3) state, to maintain a MAP greater than 65 mm Hg.

This sequential therapeutic strategy of responding to the various patterns of shock was adopted rapidly by the surgical critical care community, but one group had already challenged the necessity of transfusing to a hematocrit of 30%. The Canadian Transfusion Requirements in Critical Care (TRICC) trial had previously documented the safety and, indeed, benefit of permitting a critically ill patient's Hgb to drift down to 7 gms% before transfusion. Admittedly, the patients studied were different:

EGDT trial: Patients were treated within 6 hours of arrival in an emergency department.

TRICC trial: Patients were euvolemic in an intensive care unit (ICU) for at least 3 days.

However, most of us believe that the transfusion threshold of Hgb of 7 gms% is safe unless the patient has coronary artery disease, and then it is probably wise to increase oxygen-carrying capacity by transfusing to a Hgb of 10 gms% (very soft data).

Enthusiasm for EGDT swept the surgical critical care community, and almost all ICUs had incorporated it when EGDT was challenged again. In 2014 both the Protocol-Based Care for Early Septic Shock (ProCESS) and the Australasian Resuscitation in Sepsis Evaluation (ARISE) trials questioned the necessity of a mandatory central venous line. Both trials compared rigid EGDT with "usual care." The "usual care" therapy was guided by the experience and wisdom of a seasoned "team leader." To everyone's surprise, at 60 and 90 days after randomization, both prospective randomized trials identified no difference in mortality as a result of the mandatory insertion of a central venous line. Appropriately, however, a closer look at these data was revealing. The team leader who directed the "usual care" was permitted to place a central venous line if he or she was uncertain as to the volume and oxygen delivery status of the patient. In addition, more than a decade after publication of the initial EGDT study, it looked as if the team leaders had all incorporated similar EGDT strategies. Both groups infused almost the same volume of crystalloid and used the same frequency of pressors, but the "usual care" intensivists did transfuse less blood.

Finally, as soon as you recognize sepsis, give antibiotics. There are good data indicating that every hour of delay in the initiation of antibiotics results in a 4% increase in mortality.

SUGGESTED READINGS

ARISE Investigators. Goal-directed resuscitation for patients with early septic shock. *N Eng J Med*. 2014;371:1496.

Hebert PC, Wells G, Blajchman MA, et al. A randomized, controlled, clinical trial of transfusion requirements in critical care: Transfusion Requirements in Critical Care investigators, Canadian Critical Care Trials Group. *N Eng J Med*. 1999;340:1056.

ProCESS Investigators. A randomized trial of protocol based care for early septic shock. *N Eng J Med*. 2014;370:1683.

Rivers E, Nguyen B, Havstad S, et al. Early goal directed therapy in the treatment of severe sepsis and septic shock. *N Eng J Med*. 2001;345:1368.

Shoemaker WC, Appel PL, Kram HB, Bishop MH, Abraham E. Temporal, hemodynamic and oxygen transport patterns in medical patients: septic shock. *Chest*. 1993;104:1529.

Glucose Control in the Postoperative Period

Shaina Schaetzel, MD, and Krista L. Kaups, MD, MSc

Hyperglycemia in the inpatient setting is both a quality of care and patient safety issue. In 2012 29.1 million Americans, or 9.3% of the population, had diabetes. An additional 86 million had prediabetes. Although postoperative glucose control in this population is essential, it is becoming increasingly evident that hyperglycemia in nondiabetic patients is associated with an even greater risk of complications when compared with hyperglycemia in diabetics. It is estimated that hyperglycemia occurs in up to two thirds of surgical patients not known to have diabetes. Elevated blood glucose also has been associated with postoperative complications in a wide variety of surgical patients. Elective general surgery patients have a twofold higher risk of infection with hyperglycemia, and the risk of postoperative infection in patients undergoing noncardiac general surgery is estimated to increase by 30% for every 40 mg/dL increase in hyperglycemia. Postoperative hyperglycemia, and the resultant increases in cost, morbidity, and mortality, must be recognized and addressed while avoiding hypoglycemia.

■ INDICATIONS

Postoperative hyperglycemia occurs in three categories of patients: those with a known diagnosis of diabetes, those with unrecognized diabetes, and those experiencing stress-induced hyperglycemia. Patients with unrecognized diabetes are those with perioperative hyperglycemia that persists after discharge, whereas those with stress-induced hyperglycemia will normalize their glucose levels after resolution of the proinflammatory state.

Stress-induced hyperglycemia seen in the postoperative period results from the release of counter-regulatory hormones, including epinephrine and cortisol, as well as proinflammatory cytokines, resulting in a state of impaired insulin release and sensitivity. Glucose production is also increased because of stimulation of gluconeogenesis and glycogenolysis. Medical treatments, such as dextrose infusions and corticosteroids, that promote hyperglycemia may exacerbate the problem further. The resultant acute hyperglycemia limits vascular reactivity by the angiotensin II and nitric oxide synthase pathways. Immune suppression also occurs by inactivation of immunoglobulins and inhibition of neutrophil chemotaxis and phagocytosis. Vascular permeability and leukocyte and platelet activation are also enhanced. The result of these pathways is an increased risk of stroke, myocardial infarction, surgical site infections, and impaired wound healing. Stress-induced hyperglycemia is particularly challenging to manage, as it is often unanticipated and unrecognized. Its prevalence and history are poorly understood and therefore optimal management is yet to be fully defined.

It is becoming increasingly evident that nondiabetic patients with postoperative hyperglycemia have an equal, if not greater, risk of complications to patients with diabetes. In a study of elective general surgical patients, Kwon found a nearly twofold risk of infection, in-hospital mortality, and operative complications in both diabetics and nondiabetics with hyperglycemia, but with the greatest risk of infection among patients without diabetes. Kotagal evaluated the effect of perioperative hyperglycemia in diabetic and nondiabetic patients undergoing general surgery, bariatric surgery, vascular surgery, and spine procedures. A dose-response relationship between hyperglycemia and adverse events was found among nondiabetic patients experiencing postoperative hyperglycemia, which was not found among diabetic patients.

■ MANAGEMENT

Hyperglycemia in the surgical patient occurs frequently, and the management of inpatient hyperglycemia may be challenging. The strongest evidence for the benefit of postoperative glycemic control is in cardiac surgery patients. In this group of patients, glucose levels greater than 200 mg/dL in the immediate postoperative period contribute to an increased risk of surgical site infections. In addition, higher perioperative glucose levels are an independent predictor of mortality in both diabetic and nondiabetic patients. Recent randomized controlled trials have shown that cardiac surgery patients who are managed with more liberal glycemic control (121 to 180 mg/dL) have fewer hypoglycemic episodes and equivalent outcomes when compared with those managed with strict glycemic control (90 to 120 mg/dL). The Society of Thoracic Surgeons clinical practice guideline recommends that diabetics undergoing cardiac surgery maintain serum blood glucose no higher than 180 mg/dL for at least 24 hours postoperatively and that all patients maintain this level through the duration of their stay in the intensive care unit (ICU). The use of an intravenous (IV) insulin infusion is recommended.

Although it is clear that perioperative hyperglycemia (glucose >180 mg/dL) is associated with increased risks of infection, need for reoperative surgery, and death in surgical patients, efforts at more rigorous glucose management have not been shown to improve outcomes. Preoperative hyperglycemia is associated with increased 1-year mortality, with patients without diabetes showing higher mortality at similar preoperative glucose levels. A Cochrane review by Kao and colleagues evaluated perioperative glycemic control and its effects on outcomes including surgical site infections, hypoglycemia, and mortality. The rate of surgical site infections did not differ between strict and conventional glucose control groups. More episodes of hypoglycemia occurred in strict glucose control groups; however, no study reported adverse outcomes due to hypoglycemia, and short-term, all-cause mortality was not different between the treatment groups. More stringent glucose control also has been examined in the management of critically ill patients. In a randomized controlled trial by Van den Bergh in 2001, patients in the ICU were randomized to either conventional insulin therapy (blood glucose levels 180 to 200 mg/dL) or intensive insulin therapy (blood glucose levels 80 to 110 mg/dL). Irrespective of diabetes status, patients in the intensive therapy group had decreased morbidity and mortality. However, the emphasis on tight glucose control in critically ill patients was challenged in 2009 with the NICE-SUGAR (Normoglycemia in Intensive Care Evaluation–Survival Using Glucose Algorithm Regulation) study. This study randomized 6104 critically ill patients, including surgical patients, to conventional glucose control (<180 mg/dL) or intensive glucose control (81 to 108 mg/dL) using IV insulin infusions to achieve target blood glucose levels. The intensive glucose control group had an increased risk of death ($P = 0.02$) and severe hypoglycemic events (blood glucose ≤40 mg/dL; $P < 0.001$); no increase in morbidity was seen in the conventional glucose control group. The 2015 American Diabetes Association clinical practice guidelines recommend that an IV insulin infusion be used in critically ill patients to achieve a blood glucose goal of 140 to 180 mg/dL.

Beyond concerns of hypoglycemia and hyperglycemia in critically ill patients, glycemic variability also must be managed. At present, there is no universally accepted definition of glycemic variability; however, wide swings in blood glucose levels have an independent effect on mortality. This effect is additive when it occurs with hypoglycemia and is more pronounced in patients without diabetes. It is suggested that glycemic variability impairs endothelial function, causes oxidative stress, and enhances cell apoptosis. Iatrogenic swings in blood glucose levels can occur with overly aggressive correction of dysglycemia. The optimal management strategy to minimize variability remains unclear. Krinsley performed a multicenter cohort analysis of 44,964 critically ill patients evaluating hypoglycemia, hyperglycemia, and glycemic variability and their association with mortality. The occurrence of hypoglycemia, defined as blood glucose lower than 80 mg/dL, was independently associated with mortality regardless of diabetes status. However, diabetic patients tolerated higher levels of glucose better. Diabetics with blood glucose of 110 to 180 mg/dL had a decreased risk of mortality, and in these patients increasing glycemic variability was not associated with an increased risk of mortality. Conversely, in patients without diabetes, the lowest mortality occurred in patients with mean blood glucose of 80 to 140 mg/dL, and in this group increasing glycemic variability was associated with increased risk of mortality. Finally, in the entire cohort of patients, diabetes was independently associated with a decreased risk of mortality. Other studies also have shown that the in-hospital death rate in surgical patients is higher with greater glucose variability.

Insulin, administered either subcutaneously (SQ) or intravenously (IV), is the indicated agent for inpatient glucose control. The use of oral agents in the acutely ill and hospitalized patient is challenging and associated with hazards. Sliding scale insulin regimens, in which administration of a predetermined amount of regular insulin is given in response to hyperglycemia, should not be used. This reactive, rather than proactive, strategy results in suboptimal glucose control. An IV insulin infusion with frequent blood glucose checks should be used for management in critically ill patients. In the non-ICU setting, SQ insulin is the preferred agent. A combination of basal, bolus, and correction SQ insulin regimens should be tailored to individual patients with consideration of their nutritional status and overall condition. Basal, long-acting insulin with a duration of action of 20 to 24 hours given once or twice daily provides the coverage necessary in the fasting state. Rapid-acting insulin for pre-meal or corrective administration is given for postprandial glucose elevations. This combination strategy optimally simulates normal physiologic insulin secretion patterns. Recent randomized trials have shown a strategy of basal-bolus insulin in both medical and surgical patients to be superior to sliding scale insulin regimens, with improved glucose control, decreased complications, and overall low rates of hypoglycemia.

Protocols and order sets for insulin and hypoglycemia management should be established, and recommendations are available from various sources. When transitioning from an insulin infusion to SQ administration, the most recent insulin infusion rate is used to estimate daily insulin needs. Approximately 50% of the calculated dose can be administered as basal insulin and the remaining 50% as prandial insulin administered in divided doses with meals. Initial basal doses of insulin in non–critically ill patients are generally between 0.4 U/kg/day and 0.5 U/kg/day. This scheduled dose should be adjusted daily based on blood glucose response, the total amount of insulin administered on the previous day, and the overall condition of the patient. The 2015 American Diabetes Association clinical practice guidelines recommend random glucose goals of lower than180 mg/dL in non–critically ill patients, with pre-meal glucose lower than 140 mg/dL, as long as these levels can be achieved safely.

Beyond acute perioperative hyperglycemia, poor long-term glucose control, as measured by hemoglobin A_{1c} (HbA_{1c}), has been associated with worse surgical outcomes. HbA_{1c} indicates average glucose levels over the preceding 120 days, so it is a better indicator of overall status than an isolated blood glucose level. According to the American Diabetes Association, prediabetes is defined as HbA_{1c} of 5.7% to 6.4%, diabetes as HbA_{1c} greater than 6.4%, and poorly controlled diabetes as HbA_{1c} greater than 7.0%. In a prospective observational study of abdominal surgery patients, Goodenough and colleagues evaluated the relationship between HbA_{1c} obtained within 3 months of surgery and 30-day major complications. Patients were included whether or not they had a preoperative diagnosis of diabetes. On univariate analysis, patients who experienced major complications were more likely to have elevated perioperative glucose and HbA_{1c} but were not more likely to be diabetic. On multivariate analysis, HbA_{1c} greater than 6.4% predicted major complications. Others have identified HbA_{1c} greater than 8.0% as associated with a prolonged postoperative hospital length of stay. The current recommendation from the American Diabetes Association is for diabetes screening to be performed in asymptomatic individuals who are overweight or obese and have one additional risk factor for diabetes. Any individual, particularly if overweight or obese, should begin testing at age 45. Preoperative workup for elective surgical procedures is an ideal time to screen patients for diabetes and identify those at higher risk of hyperglycemia-related postoperative complications. Measuring HbA_{1c} during hospitalization also allows differentiation between stress-induced hyperglycemia and undiagnosed diabetes. However, the optimal preoperative HbA_{1c} and whether lowering HbA_{1c} will improve surgical outcomes are unknown. Routine preoperative HbA_{1c} testing beyond current American Diabetes Associated recommendations is not indicated.

■ CONCLUSION

Postoperative hyperglycemia is associated with increased morbidity and mortality in both diabetic and nondiabetic patients. The deleterious effects of hyperglycemia, including perioperative complications and mortality, are even greater in nondiabetic patients. Routine postoperative glucose monitoring should be strongly considered in all patients and is mandatory for all critically ill patients. Aggressive regimens for tight glucose control increase the risk of hypoglycemia and mortality risk and are not indicated. The target range for glucose control in critically ill patients is 140 to 180 mg/dL, which should be managed via an insulin infusion. Non–critically ill patients should have a target pre-meal blood glucose lower than 140 mg/dL, with any random blood glucose level lower than 180 mg/dL. These patients should be managed with a basal, bolus, and correction SQ insulin administration strategy, with abandonment of sliding scale insulin protocols.

SUGGESTED READINGS

Kotagol M, et al. Perioperative hyperglycemia and risk of adverse events among patients with and without diabetes. *Ann Surg*. 2015;261:97-103.

Krinsley JS, et al. Diabetic status and the relation of the three domains of glycemic control to mortality in critically ill patients: an international multicenter cohort study. *Crit Care*. 2013;17:R37.

Kwon S, et al. Importance of perioperative glycemic control in general surgery: a report from the Surgical Care and Outcomes Assessment Program. *Ann Surg*. 2013;257:8-14.

The NICE-SUGAR Study Investigators, Finfer S, Chittock DR, et al. Intensive versus conventional glucose control in critically ill patients. *N Engl J Med*. 2009;360:1283-1297.

POSTOPERATIVE RESPIRATORY FAILURE

Nicole L. Werner, MD, MS, and Pauline K. Park, MD

Pulmonary complications are among the most frequent and costly events after surgery. Increases in morbidity, mortality, and length of stay observed after development of pulmonary complications are similar to those seen after cardiac complications. This chapter focuses on management of postoperative respiratory failure, including classification, risk assessment, prevention, and noninvasive and mechanical ventilation.

POSTOPERATIVE RESPIRATORY FAILURE

Acute respiratory failure (ARF) can be classified as either hypoxemic or hypercapnic. Hypoxemic failure is the most common form of respiratory failure and is a major immediate threat to organ function.

Hypoxemic respiratory failure (type I) is defined as arterial partial pressure of oxygen (PaO_2) less than 60 mm Hg on room air. Hypoxemia most commonly is related to increases in dead space ventilation (ventilation of unperfused lung or increases in ventilation-perfusion mismatch) and shunt (perfusion of unventilated lung).

Hypercapnic respiratory failure (type II) is defined as arterial partial pressure of carbon dioxide ($PaCO_2$) greater than 50 mm Hg on room air.

Common causes of respiratory failure in surgical patients include pneumonia, atelectasis, aspiration, pulmonary edema, and pulmonary embolus (Figure 1).

Acute respiratory distress syndrome (ARDS) is a form of acute hypoxemic respiratory failure in which direct or indirect insults induce diffuse pulmonary inflammation and damage to the alveolar-capillary interfaces. It may occur after surgery, trauma, multiple transfusions, or sepsis. ARDS is defined according to the Berlin Definition. Overall mortality varies with degree of baseline hypoxemia, quantified by the ratio of the PaO_2 to the fraction of inspired oxygen (FiO_2) (P/F ratio). A P/F ratio of 100 or less defines the most severe disease.

RISK ASSESSMENT

The goal of risk stratification is to identify opportunities for prevention of complications. Preoperative pulmonary risk assessment includes consideration of patient-related and procedure-related factors. Age-related diminution of pulmonary function and increasing age are independent risk factors for postoperative pulmonary complications.

The surgeon should be diligent in using specific interventions to reduce the risk of developing postsurgical pulmonary complications. Preoperatively, this includes smoking cessation 6 to 8 weeks before surgery and optimization of chronic pulmonary diseases. Intraoperative strategies include use of a minimally invasive approach when possible, consideration of adjunctive regional anesthesia and analgesia, and use of short-acting neuromuscular blockade. Postoperative prevention strategies focus on adequacy of pain control, lung expansion maneuvers (incentive spirometry, deep-breathing exercises, and positive airway pressure therapies), pulmonary toilet, and preventing aspiration using selective gastric decompression. Of all interventions, postoperative lung expansion maneuvers have the strongest evidence for significant risk reduction.

NONINVASIVE VENTILATION

Noninvasive ventilation (NIV) provides positive pressure ventilator support without the need for an invasive airway. It can be administered via face mask or nasal mask. The patient breathes spontaneously while being supported with continuous positive airway pressure (CPAP) or bilevel positive airway pressure (BiPAP).

NIV is considered first-line therapy in ARF because of chronic obstructive pulmonary disease exacerbation and acute cardiogenic pulmonary edema. In these applications, it is associated with decreased mortality rates, decreased need for intubation, decreased complications, and reduced length of hospital stay. There are encouraging data evaluating NIV use in postoperative respiratory failure and in preoxygenation of patients with hypoxemic respiratory failure before intubation in the intensive care unit (ICU). There is conflicting evidence on the role of NIV in hypoxemia from other causes, and disparate data on its superiority to high-flow nasal oxygen.

NIV is not indicated in patients with cardiopulmonary arrest or uncontrolled cardiac ischemia or arrhythmias, or in situations where a definitive airway is needed. Patients with copious secretions, frequent vomiting, or upper airway obstruction are not candidates for NIV. Agitated patients and those with claustrophobia are unlikely to tolerate an NIV mask.

INTUBATION

Intubation is a secure airway in which a tube is advanced past the upper airway into the trachea. Use of a cuffed tube allows positive pressure mechanical ventilation to be performed. Indications for intubation are shown in Box 1.

The recommended technique for intubation is orotracheally with direct or video-assisted laryngoscopy (i.e., GlideScope, C-MAC). Short-acting sedatives or hypnotics with neuromuscular blockade are required for induction. Caution should be used with propofol, which can cause significant hypotension, and with etomidate, which is associated with adrenal insufficiency, particularly in older patients and in patients with hypotension or hemodynamic instability. Awake fiberoptic intubation may be used for patients with a potentially difficult airway. The endotracheal tube should be inserted to approximately 23 cm in men and 21 cm in women, measured at the incisor. Chest radiograph should be obtained to confirm position. The tip of the tube should be positioned 2 to 4 cm from the carina.

Sedation usually is required for tolerance of an endotracheal tube and mechanical ventilation. Intravenous infusions of short-acting narcotics and sedatives are most commonly used for this purpose. A validated sedation scale should be used to assess sedation levels, and drugs should be titrated to the least amount required. Daily awakening trials, in which sedation is paused to allow assessment of mental status, have been associated with reduced number of ventilator days, duration in the ICU, and length of hospital stay. Benzodiazepines are associated with increased delirium; thus caution should be used with these agents, particularly in older patients and in critically ill patients with organ dysfunction or failure.

PREVENTION OF VENTILATOR-ASSOCIATED PNEUMONIA

Efforts to prevent ventilator-associated pneumonia (VAP) should be implemented immediately after intubation and initiation of mechanical ventilation. The key components of the ventilator bundle for VAP prevention are (1) elevation of the head of the bed, (2) daily oral care with chlorhexidine gluconate, (3) peptic ulcer disease prophylaxis, and (4) deep venous thrombosis prophylaxis. Other strategies for VAP prevention can be considered in ICUs with a high prevalence of VAP. These can include use of endotracheal tubes permitting continuous aspiration of subglottic secretions, the use of silver-coated endotracheal tubes, and selective oral or digestive tract decontamination.

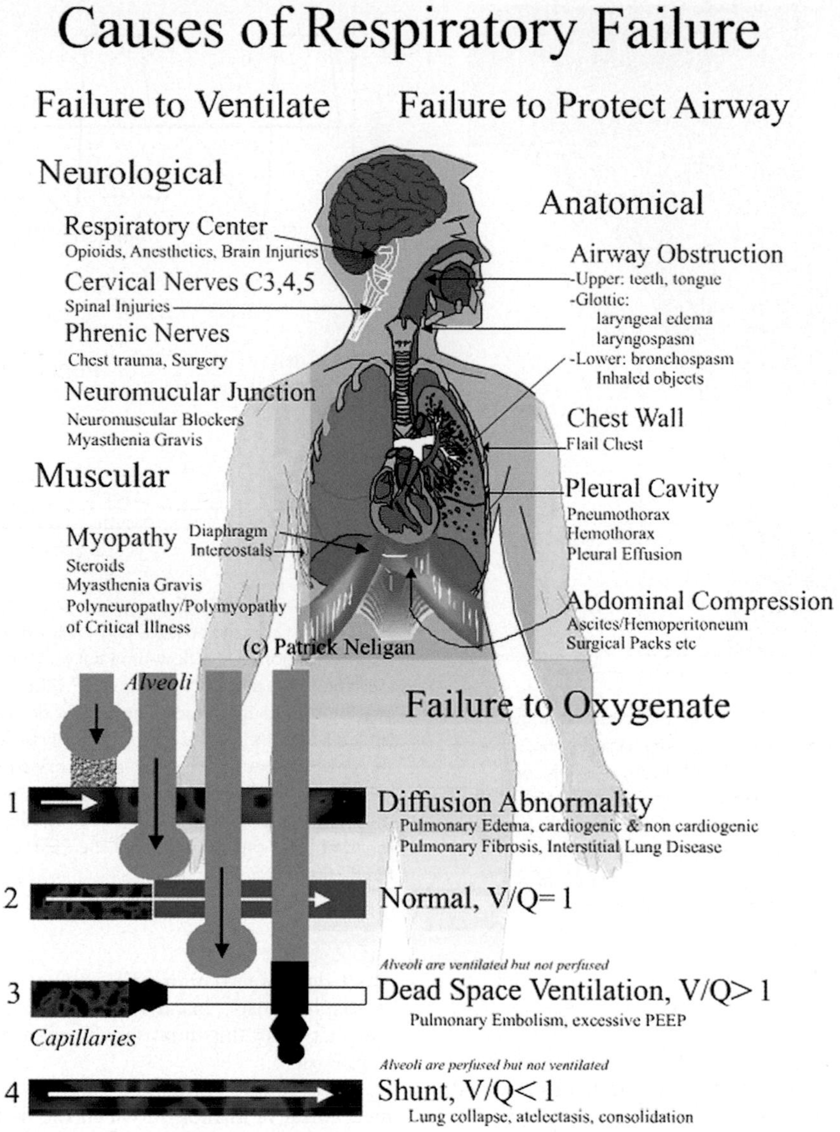

Causes of Respiratory Failure

Failure to Ventilate

Neurological

Respiratory Center
Opioids, Anesthetics, Brain Injuries

Cervical Nerves C3,4,5
Spinal Injuries

Phrenic Nerves
Chest trauma, Surgery

Neuromucular Junction
Neuromuscular Blockers
Myasthenia Gravis

Muscular

Myopathy   Diaphragm
                Intercostals
Steroids
Myasthenia Gravis
Polyneuropathy/Polymyopathy
of Critical Illness

(c) Patrick Neligan

Failure to Protect Airway

Anatomical

Airway Obstruction
-Upper: teeth, tongue
-Glottic:
    laryngeal edema
    laryngospasm
-Lower: bronchospasm
    Inhaled objects

Chest Wall
Flail Chest

Pleural Cavity
Pneumothorax
Hemothorax
Pleural Effusion

Abdominal Compression
Ascites/Hemoperitoneum
Surgical Packs etc

Failure to Oxygenate

Alveoli

1 **Diffusion Abnormality**
Pulmonary Edema, cardiogenic & non cardiogenic
Pulmonary Fibrosis, Interstitial Lung Disease

2 **Normal, V/Q= 1**

Alveoli are ventilated but not perfused
3 **Dead Space Ventilation, V/Q> 1**
Pulmonary Embolism, excessive PEEP

Capillaries

Alveoli are perfused but not ventilated
4 **Shunt, V/Q< 1**
Lung collapse, atelectasis, consolidation

FIGURE 1 Causes of respiratory failure. *PEEP,* Positive end-expiratory pressure; *V/Q,* ventilation/perfusion. *(From Sachdev G, Napolitano LM. Postoperative pulmonary complications: pneumonia and acute respiratory failure. Surg Clin North Am. 2012;92:321-344.)*

BOX 1: Indications for Intubation and Mechanical Ventilation

Airway protection
Hypoxemia
Hypercarbia
Apnea or respiratory arrest
Tachypnea (respiratory rate >30 breaths/minute)
Vital capacity <15 mL/kg, <1.0 L, or <30% predicted
Minute ventilation >10 L/minute

■ MECHANICAL VENTILATION

The goal of mechanical ventilation is to ensure adequate oxygenation and ventilation while reducing the work of breathing.

Oxygen uptake via the lungs is dependent on both the partial pressure of oxygen and ventilation-perfusion matching. To improve oxygenation, three main strategies are utilized:

1. *Increase FiO_2.* Systemic oxygen delivery varies with cardiac output and oxygen carrying capacity; increasing the FiO_2 increases the amount oxygen available for transport by hemoglobin. High FiO_2 levels (>50%) are generally well tolerated but may be associated with oxygen toxicity and absorptive atelectasis.

2. *Increase pressure gradient at the alveolar level.* This is accomplished most efficiently by increasing the mean airway pressure, most commonly either by increasing positive end-expiratory pressure (PEEP) or by adjusting the inspiratory time to increase the inspiratory-to-expiratory (I:E) ratio. Care must be taken to limit increases in inspiratory plateau pressure to minimize the risk of barotrauma and ventilator-induced lung injury.

3. *Recruitment maneuvers.* The goal of these maneuvers is to increase the fraction of lung recruited for gas exchange by applying transient increases in airway pressure. After recruitment, increased PEEP may be necessary to prevent recurrent alveolar collapse.

Ventilation is determined by carbon dioxide elimination via the lungs and is largely dependent on alveolar ventilation. Alveolar ventilation is equal to the respiratory rate × (tidal volume – dead space). To improve ventilation, the tidal volume or the respiratory rate should be increased.

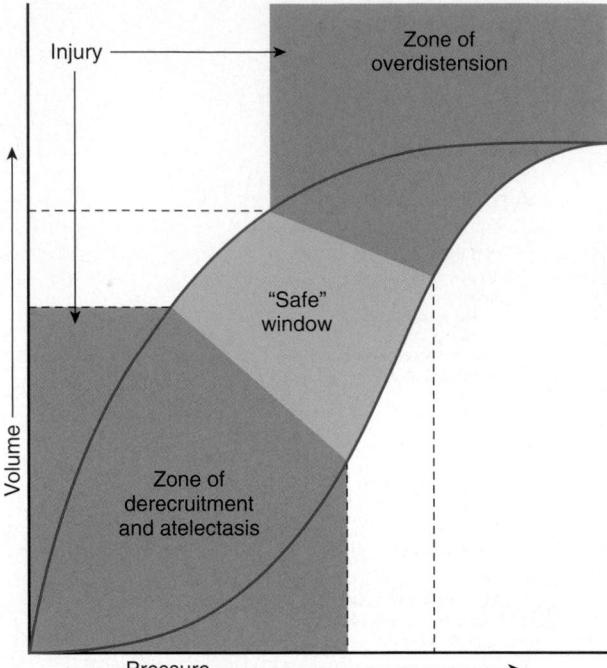

FIGURE 2 Pressure-volume curve of a moderately diseased lung, such as in acute respiratory distress syndrome. Two hazard zones exist: overdistension and derecruitment/atelectasis. Higher end-expiratory pressures and small tidal volumes are needed to stay in the "safe" window. Open lung ventilation may have a larger margin of safety in keeping the lung open within the desired target range and avoiding alveolar overdistension. *(Reprinted with permission from Imai Y, Slutsky AS. High-frequency oscillatory ventilation and ventilator-induced lung injury. Crit Care Med. 2005;33 Suppl 3:S129-S134.)*

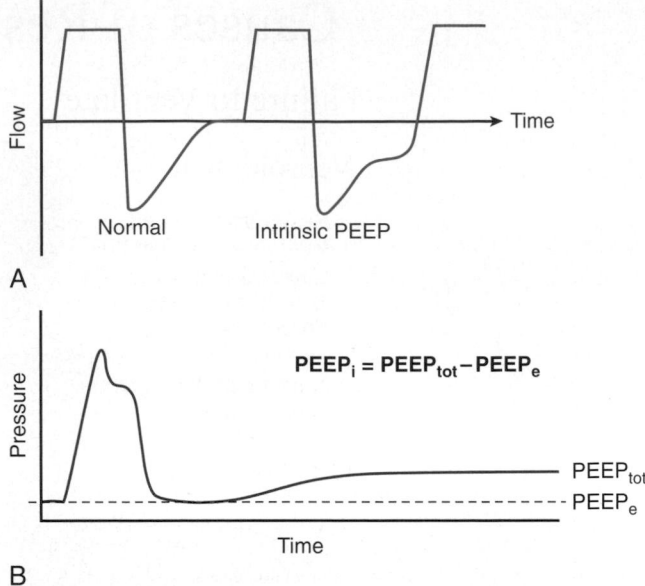

FIGURE 3 Intrinsic positive end-expiratory pressure (PEEP). **A,** Examination of the flow-time curve from the ventilator gives an indication that there is intrinsic PEEP ($PEEP_i$) but does not give an indication of its magnitude. The patient does not need to be apneic. **B,** A quantitative measurement of intrinsic PEEP can be obtained in an apneic patient by using the expiratory pause hold control on the ventilator. This allows equilibration of pressures between the alveoli and the ventilator, allowing the total PEEP ($PEEP_{tot}$) to be measured. The value for total PEEP can be read from the PEEP display. Intrinsic PEEP = Total PEEP − Set PEEP ($PEEP_e$).

Mechanical ventilation can lead to additional lung injury known as ventilator-induced lung injury (VILI). VILI mechanisms include barotrauma, volutrauma (diffuse alveolar injury resulting from overdistension; Figure 2), or atelectrauma (injury caused by repeated cycles of recruitment and derecruitment; see Figure 2). Injury also can be related to the release of local mediators in the lung, referred to as biotrauma.

Modes of Mechanical Ventilation

No single mode of mechanical ventilation for ARF is superior in terms of clinical outcomes. Mechanical positive pressure ventilation can be delivered via a volume or pressure target. Using either mode, plateau pressure (measured during a ventilator inspiratory pause) should be monitored; plateau pressures greater than 30 cm H_2O are associated with lung injury. In addition, when insufficient time is allowed for exhalation, intrinsic PEEP, also known as auto-PEEP, can develop (Figure 3). Intrinsic PEEP (measured during a ventilator expiratory pause) is equivalent to total PEEP minus the set PEEP.

Volume Modes

In volume modes, tidal volume is set and the airway pressure is variable. The airway pressure will vary based on the rate of delivery of the tidal volume, pulmonary compliance, and airway resistance. Barotrauma may occur if high peak airway pressures are required to reach the preset volume; close monitoring of airway pressures is required.

Controlled mechanical ventilation (CMV). Respiratory rate and tidal volume are set to achieve an exact minute ventilation. This mode does not accommodate patient interaction. CMV may result in diaphragmatic inactivity, promoting atrophy and contractility dysfunction in this important inspiratory muscle, so it is not commonly used.

Assist-control ventilation (ACV). A commonly used mode of mechanical ventilation in which the tidal volume of each delivered breath is the same, whether triggered by the patient or by the ventilator. When patient triggered, the ventilator delivers breaths in coordination with the respiratory effort of the patient. If a patient-initiated triggering event does not occur in a set time interval, the ventilator will deliver a controlled breath. This allows for patient participation. ACV is associated with low work of breathing, as every breath is supported and tidal volume is guaranteed.

Synchronized intermittent mandatory ventilation (SIMV). The ventilator delivers mandatory breaths, with set rate and tidal volume, delivered in coordination with the respiratory effort of the patient, as well as pressure-supported breaths for additional patient-initiated breaths above the mandatory rate. Most SIMV modes will default to a control-mode setting in the event that the patient does not trigger the ventilator in the time interval mandated by the preset respiratory rate. Synchronization of the tidal volume delivery with the patient's inspiratory effort attempts to minimize the barotrauma that may occur with nonsynchronized ventilation—that is, it avoids delivery of a preset breath to a patient who is already inhaling maximally (breath stacking) or is exhaling forcefully.

Pressure Modes

In pressure modes, the airway pressure is set and tidal volume is variable. The tidal volume will be affected by any factor that changes the airway pressure, including thoracic compliance, pulmonary resistance, and inspiratory time. A sudden decrease in pulmonary compliance can cause a rapid reduction in tidal volume and minute ventilation, resulting in acute respiratory acidosis; thus close monitoring of minute ventilation is necessary.

Pressure control ventilation (PCV). Inspiratory pressure and inspiratory time are set. The resultant tidal volume is dependent on both these values and the patient's compliance or resistance. Changing from a volume control mode to a pressure control mode may result in lower peak airway pressures and possibly less VILI.

Pressure support ventilation (PSV). Breaths are assisted by a set inspiratory pressure, which is delivered until inspiratory flow drops below a predetermined threshold (e.g., 25% of peak flow). Respiratory rate is determined by the patient. PSV can be a stand-alone mode or can be incorporated with SIMV, where PSV is used for spontaneous breaths. PSV has been advocated to limit barotrauma and decrease the work of breathing. Because this is a patient-triggered mode, apnea alarms are required to ensure patient safety. Some ventilators may allow a backup intermittent mechanical ventilation rate to be set in the event that spontaneous triggering ceases.

Pressure-regulated volume control (PRVC) or volume control plus (VC+). This mode automatically adjusts inspiratory pressure in response to dynamic changes in patient mechanics to guarantee a set tidal volume during a pressure control breath. Constant pressure is applied throughout inspiration as in pressure control, but the ventilator will adjust the inspiratory pressure with each breath, compensating for changes in airway resistance and compliance, in order to deliver the set tidal volume. PRVC is a patient-triggered or time-triggered, pressure-limited mode.

Airway pressure release ventilation (APRV). This is an inverse-ratio pressure mode of mechanical ventilation that alternates between high PEEP, generally set between 25 and 30 cm H_2O, and low PEEP, usually 0 cm H_2O. It has a longer inspiratory time (time of high PEEP, time-high), with an I:E ratio of commonly 7:1 to 10:1, and a very short expiratory time or "release" (time low). Tidal volume is determined by the difference between high PEEP and low PEEP. Spontaneous breathing at the higher pressure is encouraged, and this mode is well tolerated hemodynamically and in terms of patient comfort with minimal sedation. APRV has been advocated for use in the treatment for severe hypoxemia, as it achieves high mean airway pressures, resulting in improved alveolar recruitment.

Bilevel or biphasic ventilation. This mode is similar to APRV in that high and low PEEP levels are set; however, the time of low PEEP is generally longer. Spontaneous breathing can occur at both time-high and time low (Figure 4) and may be pressure supported.

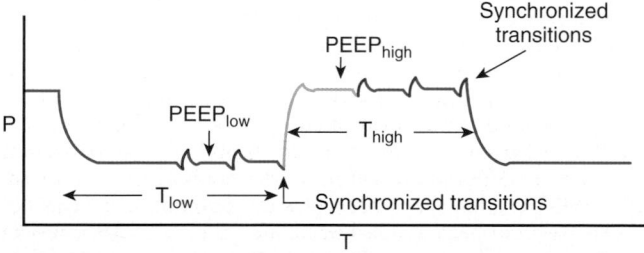

FIGURE 4 Bilevel ventilation uses two pressure levels (PEEP_low and PEEP_high) for two time periods (time low [T_low] and time high [T_high]), with spontaneous breathing at PEEP_low or PEEP_high. *P*, Pressure; *PEEP*, positive end-expiratory pressure; *T*, time.

Mechanical Ventilation Strategies for Acute Respiratory Distress Syndrome

Several multicenter randomized controlled trials have been performed to develop effective mechanical ventilation strategies for patients with ARDS. These strategies include lung protective ventilation, open lung strategy, neuromuscular blockade, prone positioning, and fluid restriction. A number of salvage adjuncts are also available, based on less robust evidence, including recruitment maneuvers, inhaled nitric oxide, and extracorporeal membrane oxygenation. Figure 5 illustrates evidence-based and salvage treatment options for ARDS.

Evidence-Based Therapies

Lung protective ventilation. Lung protective ventilation remains the standard of care in ARDS. It involves administering low tidal volume (6 mL/kg) ventilation to prevent excessive alveolar distension that may result in VILI and an exaggerated alveolar and systemic inflammatory response. The ARDS Network's landmark, multicenter randomized controlled trial, ARMA, documented that lower tidal volume (6 mL/kg) versus higher tidal volume (12 mL/kg) ventilation in patients with ARDS was associated with a significantly decreased mortality rate. Initiation of low tidal volume ventilation should start at 6 to 8 mL/kg of predicted body weight based on height (in men: 50 kg + 2.3 kg/inch for each inch over 5 feet; in women: 45.5 kg + 2.3 kg/inch for each inch over 5 feet). Tidal volumes should be reduced by 1 mL/kg at intervals of 2 hours until the tidal volume is set at 6 mL/kg. Plateau pressure should be maintained at less than 30 cm H_2O. Oxygenation goals include PaO_2 of 55 to 80 mm Hg or SpO_2 of 88% to 95% while using the lowest FiO_2 possible.

Permissive hypercapnia. Permissive hypercapnia accepts the consequences of deliberate hypoventilation in order to prioritize reduction of alveolar overdistension and airway pressures in patients with poor lung compliance. Avoiding volutrauma in this fashion can lead to decreases in minute ventilation to well below normal levels. The resultant hypercarbia and respiratory acidosis are managed medically with sodium bicarbonate or tromethamine. Hypercapnia may worsen intracranial pressure, and this strategy should be avoided in patients with traumatic brain injury.

Open lung strategy. An open lung strategy uses increased levels of PEEP to support oxygenation in combination with the low tidal volume strategy. Increased levels of PEEP lead to recruitment of collapsed alveoli, reduced ventilation-perfusion mismatch, improved arterial oxygenation, and increased functional residual lung capacity. By maintaining an elevated PEEP, alveoli that are unstable and prone to collapse will remain open. Table 1 is an example of an open lung FiO_2/PEEP table that may guide PEEP setting.

The optimal PEEP level is difficult to determine, as both underdistension and overdistension of the alveoli can lead to VILI. Variations in chest wall compliance may influence the "best" level of PEEP. Measurements of transpulmonary pressure and driving pressure (ΔP) may permit more individualized PEEP titration. *Transpulmonary pressure* can be calculated by subtracting the transpleural pressure, estimated by esophageal balloon manometry, from the measured airway pressure. Ventilator pressures are set to avoid negative transpulmonary pressure. *Driving pressure* is defined as the change in tidal volume divided by respiratory system compliance, which effectively normalizes tidal volume to functional lung size. In patients receiving

TABLE 1: Example of an Open Lung Strategy FiO₂/PEEP Table											
FiO₂	0.3	0.3	0.3	0.3	0.4	0.4	0.5	0.5	0.5-0.8	0.8	0.9	1.0
PEEP (cm H₂O)	8	10	12	14	14	16	16	18	20	22	22	22-24

FiO₂, Fraction of inspired oxygen; *PEEP,* positive end-expiratory pressure.

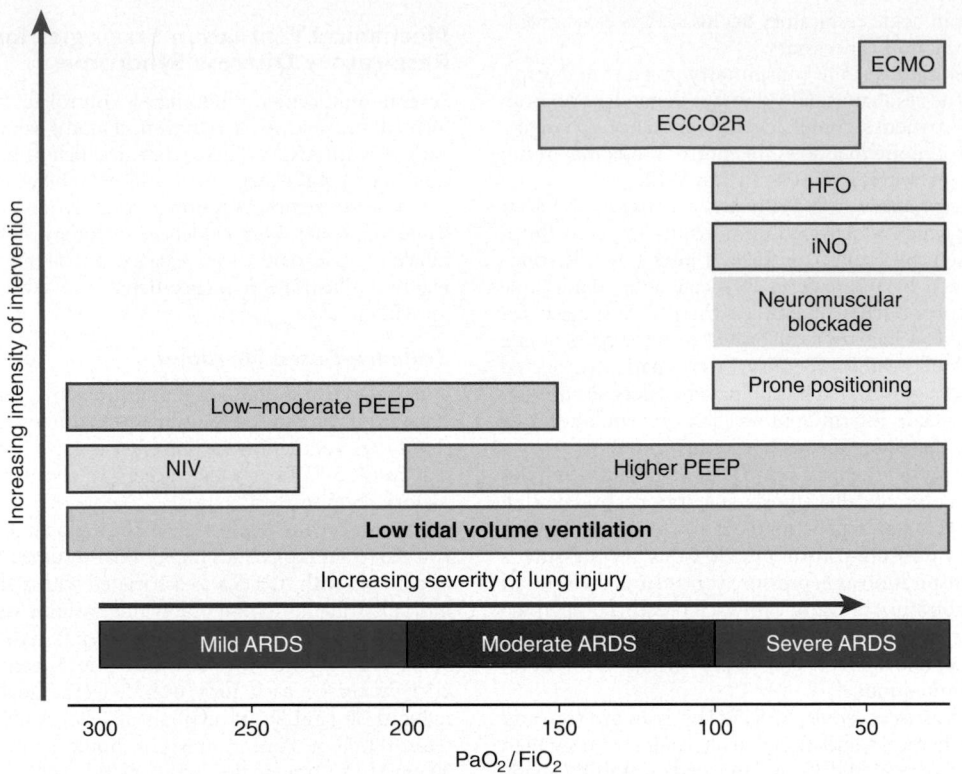

FIGURE 5 Increasing intensity of treatment intervention for increasing severity of acute respiratory distress syndrome (ARDS), with all treatment strategies, including extracorporeal membrane oxygenation (ECMO), available at an ARDS Referral Center. Blue shading indicates current evidence-based strategies associated with decreased mortality; yellow shading indicates salvage strategies requiring confirmation in prospective clinical trials. *ECCO2R*, Extracorporeal carbon dioxide removal; *FiO₂*, fraction of inspired oxygen; *HFO*, high frequency oscillation; *iNO*, inhaled nitric oxide; *NIV*, noninvasive ventilation; *PaO₂*, arterial partial pressure of oxygen; *PEEP*, positive end-expiratory pressure. *(Modified from Ferguson ND, Fan E, Camporota L, et al. The Berlin definition of ARDS: an expanded rationale, justification, and supplementary material. Intensive Care Med. 2012;38:1573-1582.)*

controlled ventilation (without spontaneous breathing), this can be calculated as plateau pressure minus the PEEP level. Initial studies suggest that even when patients are receiving "protective" plateau pressures and tidal volumes, increased ΔP may be associated with increased mortality. Ventilator titration using both of these approaches is being evaluated in clinical trials.

Neuromuscular blockade. A neuromuscular blocking agent, such as cisatracurium, may be considered for early, moderate-to-severe ARDS (P/F ratio ≤150, <36 hours after intubation). A multicenter double-blind trial of 340 patients with severe ARDS confirmed that early administration of a neuromuscular blocking agent improved 90-day survival and increased time off mechanical ventilation without increasing muscle weakness compared with placebo. A confirmatory trial is under way. Enthusiasm for this approach must be tempered with concern for associated critical illness polyneuropathy.

Prone position. Placing a patient in a prone position can result in a dramatic improvement in oxygenation and ventilation in patients with severe ARDS. Improvements in oxygenation typically are seen within the first hour after position change. The distribution of perfusion to ventilated lung regions may be improved, decreasing intrapulmonary shunt and improving oxygenation. Prone positioning also has the benefit of recruiting the dependent lung regions. Careful planning and execution is necessary to avoid unplanned extubation and inadvertent removal of indwelling lines and tubes while transitioning between supine and prone positions.

Conservative fluid management. A conservative fluid management strategy is recommended in patients with ARDS. Avoiding excess volume administration decreases duration of mechanical ventilation and ICU stay. Diuretic therapy should be considered in patients with hypoxemia and a central venous pressure (CVP) greater than 4. A

careful assessment of adequacy of perfusion and cardiac performance should be completed before initiation of diuresis, and reassessment should be continued while diuresis is ongoing.

Adjuncts for Severe Hypoxemia

Recruitment maneuvers (RMs). Recruitment maneuvers refer to the dynamic process of reopening unstable, airless alveoli to improve pulmonary gas exchange and prevent VILI and atelectasis. This is accomplished through an intentional transient increase in transpulmonary pressure, either by hand bagging or by altering ventilator settings. Common ventilator methods include a 2-minute period at high PEEP of 40 cm H_2O, low PEEP of 20 cm H_2O, respiratory rate of 10 to 20, and I:E ratio of 1:1 or shorter holds at a set, consistent high PEEP. The optimal approach, pressure, duration, and frequency of RMs have not been established in large clinical trials. Transient hypotension and desaturation during RMs is common but usually is self-limited.

Inhaled nitric oxide. Nitric oxide and prostacyclin are selective pulmonary vasodilators that decrease pulmonary vascular resistance, pulmonary arterial pressure, and right ventricular afterload. In clinical trials, the use of low-dose inhaled pulmonary vasodilators has been shown to improve short-term oxygenation in patients with ARDS but has not reduced duration of mechanical ventilation or mortality rate. Inhaled nitric oxide and prostacycline should be considered as salvage therapy in patients who continue to have life-threatening hypoxemia despite optimization of all other treatment strategies.

High-frequency oscillatory ventilation. High-frequency oscillatory ventilation uses a piston-driven ventilator that delivers small tidal volumes at frequencies of 3 to 15 Hz to maintain ventilation at

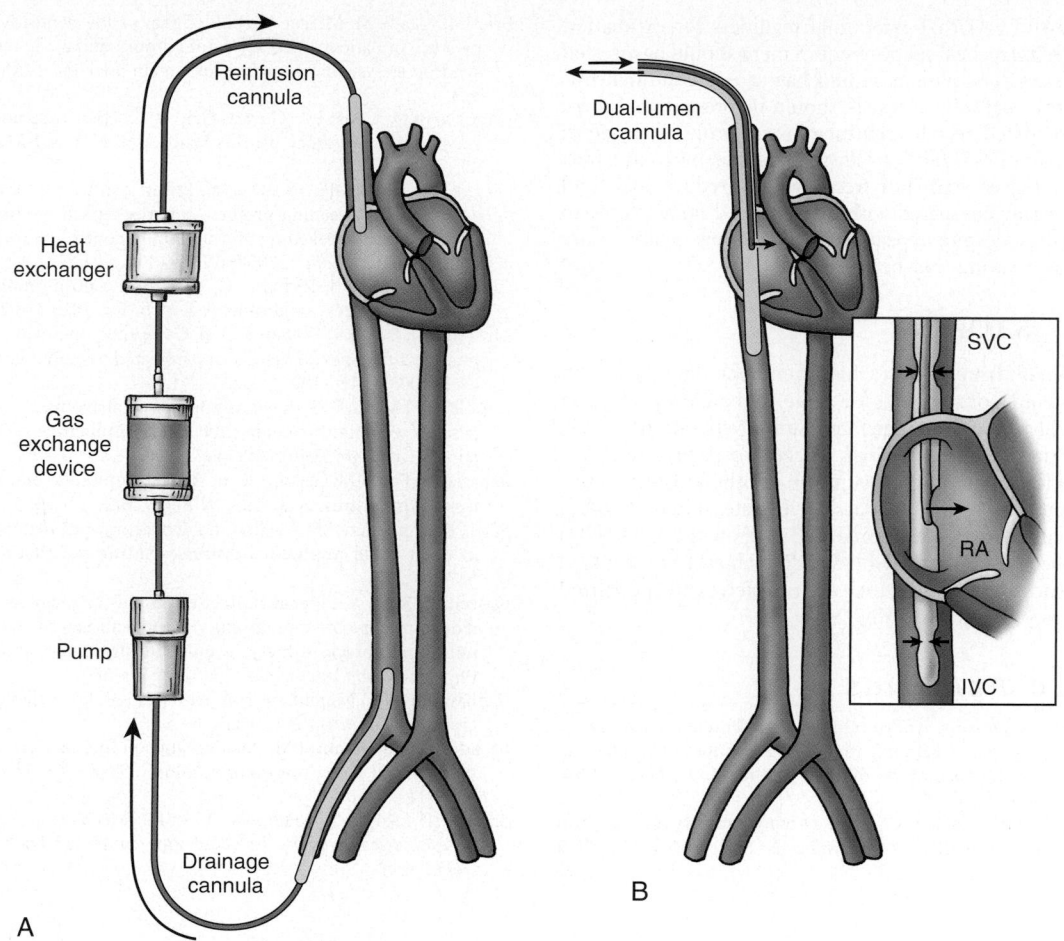

FIGURE 6 Venovenous extracorporeal membrane oxygenation. **A,** Dual-site configuration. Blood is drained from the femoral vein and then passes through a pump, gas exchange device, and heat exchanger before reinfusing into the internal jugular vein. **B,** Single-cannula configuration using a dual-lumen cannula. Blood is drained from the superior vena cava (SVC) and inferior vena cava (IVC) and reinfused to the right atrium (RA).

higher mean airway pressure. It commonly is used in neonatal respiratory failure. Although initial trials in adults were favorable, two recent randomized trials showed no mortality benefit, and this mode cannot be recommended routinely outside salvage situations.

Extracorporeal membrane oxygenation (ECMO). ECMO is extended-duration cardiopulmonary bypass, which may be considered in patients with reversible lung disease who have failed other rescue strategies. ECMO provides oxygenation and ventilation support until endogenous lung function improves. It also permits use of reduced ventilator settings ("lung rest") in order to minimize further barotrauma to already injured lungs. Cannulation is performed with percutaneously placed 21F to 31F venous catheters (Figure 6), either in a dual site or a single-site, dual-lumen venovenous configuration. Anticoagulation is necessary to prevent circuit thrombosis. Potential complications resulting from the use of ECMO include mechanical complications and bleeding complications, including intracranial hemorrhage, coagulopathy, and thrombosis. Modern evidence for ECMO as an ARDS salvage therapy is promising but controversial, and further randomized controlled studies are currently under way.

Weaning and Liberation From Mechanical Ventilation

Mechanical ventilation has significant potential risks such that efforts should be focused on liberation from mechanical ventilation as soon

as adequate lung recovery has occurred. Nearly half of the time spent on mechanical ventilation is spent weaning the patient. Continuous protocols for weaning directed by respiratory therapists are associated with shorter duration of ventilation and shorter ICU length of stay.

One evidence-based approach to ventilator liberation involves a daily spontaneous awakening trial (SAT) followed by a spontaneous breathing trial (SBT). SAT involves a complete interruption in sedation. In a successful trial, the patient is without sustained anxiety, agitation, or pain; keeps a normal respiratory rate; and maintains oxygen saturation. An SBT should be performed only after the SAT is successful.

The SBT is performed with CPAP at a low pressure support (5 cm H_2O), automatic tube compensation settings, or T-piece for 30 minutes. Trial failure is determined by tachypnea or apnea, desaturation, or signs of respiratory distress. Otherwise, a rapid shallow breathing index (RSBI), the ratio of respiratory frequency to tidal volume in liters (f/VT), should be calculated. As an example, a patient who has a respiratory rate of 25 breaths/minute and a tidal volume of 250 mL/breath has an RSBI of (25 breaths/minute) ÷ (0.25 L/breath) = 100 breaths/minute/L. An RSBI less than 105 is associated with 80% wean success. An RSBI that is 105 or higher is associated with 95% wean failure. An arterial blood gas also may be obtained to evaluate for associated hypercarbia.

Patients who fail an SAT/SBT trial are returned to their previous ventilator settings and placed on reduced sedation, with plans to repeat the SAT/SBT trial in 24 hours.

After a successful SAT/SBT trial, final readiness for extubation should be evaluated. Tracheal suction requirement should be assessed and not be excessive. The patient should have a good spontaneous cough. An endotracheal tube cuff leak should be present, and there should be no anticipated need for reintubation for bronchial hygiene.

The use of paired SAT/SBT trials reduces the mortality rate, increases the number of ventilator-free days, and reduces ICU and hospital length of stay compared with SBT alone. If failure to wean or extubate persists despite repeated trials, prolonged and more gradual ventilator weaning may be required.

■ TRACHEOSTOMY

Some patients benefit from early tracheostomy, including those with traumatic brain injury or the need for prolonged airway protection and those who will require prolonged mechanical ventilation. Timing of tracheostomy may be individualized; a large, prospective, randomized clinical trial found no difference in VAP or other outcome measures when comparing early (4 days) with late (after 10 days) tracheostomy. Data from observational studies show that up to 60% of ventilator-dependent patients who are discharged from the ICU can be weaned successfully when they are transferred to specialized units dedicated to ventilator weaning.

SUGGESTED READINGS

The Acute Respiratory Distress Syndrome Network. Ventilation with lower tidal volumes as compared with traditional tidal volumes for acute lung injury and the acute respiratory distress syndrome. *N Engl J Med*. 2000;342:1301-1308.

Amato MBP, Meade MO, Slutsky SA, et al. Driving pressure and survival in the acute respiratory distress syndrome. *N Engl J Med*. 2015;372: 747-755.

Briel M, Meade M, Mercat A, et al. Higher vs lower positive end-expiratory pressure in patients with acute lung injury and acute respiratory distress syndrome: systematic review and meta-analysis. *JAMA*. 2010;303:865-873.

Ferguson ND, Cook DJ, Guyatt GH, et al. High-frequency oscillation in early acute respiratory distress syndrome. *N Engl J Med*. 2013;368:795-805.

Girard TD, Kress JP, Fuchs BD, et al. Efficacy and safety of a paired sedation and ventilator weaning protocol for mechanically ventilated patients in intensive care (awakening and breathing controlled trial): a randomised controlled trial. *Lancet*. 2008;371:126-134.

Guerin C, Reignier J, Richard JC, et al. Prone positioning in severe acute respiratory distress syndrome. *N Engl J Med*. 2013;368:2159-2168.

Muscedere J, Dodek P, Keenan S, et al. Comprehensive evidence-based clinical practice guidelines for ventilator-associated pneumonia: prevention. *J Crit Care*. 2008;23:126-137.

Napolitano LM, Park PK, Raghavendran K, et al. Nonventilatory strategies for patients with life-threatening 2009 H1N1 influenza and severe respiratory failure. *Crit Care Med*. 2010;38:e74-e90.

Papazian L, Forel JM, Gacouin A, et al. Neuromuscular blockers in early acute respiratory distress syndrome. *N Engl J Med*. 2010;363:1107-1116.

Park PK, Napolitano LM, Bartlett RH. Extracorporeal membrane oxygenation in adult acute respiratory distress syndrome. *Crit Care Clin*. 2011;27: 627-646.

Qaseem A, Snow V, Fitterman N, et al. Risk assessment for and strategies to reduce perioperative pulmonary complications for patients undergoing noncardiothoracic surgery: a guideline from the American College of Physicians. *Ann Intern Med*. 2006;144:575-580.

Raghavendran K, Napolitano LM. ALI and ARDS: challenges and advances. *Crit Care Clin*. 2011;27:xiii-xiv.

Sachdev G, Napolitano LM. Postoperative pulmonary complications: pneumonia and acute respiratory failure. *Surg Clin North Am*. 2012;92: 321-344.

Talmor D, Sarge T, Malhotra A, et al. Mechanical ventilation guided by esophageal pressure in acute lung injury. *N Engl J Med*. 2008;359: 2095-2104.

VENTILATOR-ASSOCIATED PNEUMONIA

Jacob Swann, MD, and Forrest O'dell Moore, MD

Pneumonia continues to be a vexing disease pathology for the healthcare practitioner. Controversies exist in diagnostic criteria, empirical treatment algorithms, and methods to prevent this pathology in the various clinical settings in which it is encountered. In the community setting, pneumonia accounts for 0.4% of primary care physician visits annually. Although these visits carry a significant societal burden, hospital-acquired pneumonia (HAP) and healthcare-associated pneumonia (HCAP) are estimated to cost the United States healthcare system more than $7 billion annually. When diagnosed in the intensive care unit (ICU) for patients who are on a ventilator, HAP is a herald of a significantly difficult hospital course. Ventilator-associated pneumonia (VAP) continues to consume a large portion of healthcare dollars, prolongs time on a ventilator, lengthens a patient's hospital stay, and contributes to significant mortality. Certainly, any steps that can be taken to prevent a VAP would mitigate the issues above. Moreover, the Centers for Medicare and Medicaid Services now have made any VAP diagnosis a measure in the National Quality Forum's list of Serious Reportable Events—so-called "never events"—and tied access to public funds and reimbursement for hospital systems; preventing VAP is a major goal in ICUs today.

Although preventing VAP is critical, the definitions and treatment regimens for VAP frequently are changing. Providers have different thresholds for treating suspected cases of VAP. Some providers have a low threshold such that any new infiltrate may be treated with a course of antibiotics; others may require a culture diagnosis before treatment. This leads to problems in which providers may treat suspected cases of VAP that, in fact, are not of an infectious cause. For example, a multisystem trauma patient who is ventilated with a new pulmonary infiltrate could be developing adult respiratory distress syndrome (ARDS) without any infectious component. As such, these patients would not require antibiotic treatment. Similarly, in a patient with a proven VAP, different providers may have an antibiotic regimen that they prefer to use based on their clinical experience. However, this regimen may promote antibiotic resistance because of length of therapy or inadequate coverage for the infecting organism. With these imprecise definitions, nonuniform reporting standards, and varying treatment regimens, there is significant variability between practitioners, hospital systems, and patient outcomes (Michetti et al, 2012). This variability is the impetus for a new categorization by the Centers for Disease Control and Prevention (CDC) under the umbrella definition of ventilator-associated events (VAE), of which VAP is considered. Given the confusing clinical management of VAP, the goals of this chapter are to define VAE, review current diagnostic and empirical treatment regimens for VAP, and discuss current regimens to prevent VAP (colloquially known as "VAP bundles").

■ DEFINITIONS AND DIAGNOSTIC WORKUP

As previously mentioned, VAP does not have a uniform definition that is accepted universally. Moreover, the various definitions are often confusing, and the differences between these pathologic entities can be subtle. The veritable alphabet soup of definitions for various pneumonias and associated conditions—CAP, HAP, HCAP, VAE, VAC, IVAC, PVAP, and VAP—makes it critical to clearly establish what defines each so that appropriate diagnosis and treatment regimens can be instituted. The CDC 2015 guidelines on VAE are a good reference to refer to throughout this discussion (Figure 1).

HAP is defined as a pneumonia that occurs after a patient has been admitted for 48 hours or longer. HCAP is a pneumonia that develops in a nonhospitalized patient who is exposed frequently to the bacteriologic milieu of healthcare institutions. These patients are at risk for being exposed to multidrug-resistant (MDR) organisms, may be in an immunocompromised state, or live in a location that has a propensity for more virulent (and less common) organisms—such as *Legionella* species. HCAP is defined specifically as one or more of the following: admission to a hospital for 48 hours or more within the past 90 days, residing in a long-term nursing facility, using dialysis, or receiving IV antibiotics, chemotherapy, or wound care in the prior 30 days. Any pneumonia that does not meet the above criteria is community-acquired pneumonia (CAP) and is treated as such. The discussion in this chapter does not address CAP nor its management. For purposes of our discussion, VAP is considered a subset of HAP, and both should be treated in the same manner.

VAP initially exhibits symptoms or clinical signs similar to many infectious and noninfectious pathologies. These symptoms are both objective clinical signs, such as progressive worsening ventilator settings, along with subjective clinical signs, such as a new infiltrate on chest radiography. Multiple noninfectious causes can be the source of those findings above (e.g., pulmonary embolism). Similarly, ventilator-associated tracheobronchitis—a bacterial infection of the trachea and mainstem bronchi—can show signs and symptoms of inflammation and infection without being a VAP. To prevent every infectious cause from being labeled as a VAP but to include VAP in the initial differential diagnosis of a concerning clinical indicator, the term *ventilator-associated events* was used as an umbrella to consider all of these issues. From this overarching definition, subgroups within this umbrella define specific patient populations, namely, ventilator-associated conditions, infection-related ventilator-associated complications, and possible ventilator-associated pneumonia.

Ventilator-associated conditions (VACs) are the first diagnostic definition under the umbrella of VAE. VACs are defined by objective clinical criteria, specifically deterioration in respiratory status after a period of stability. Deterioration in respiratory status is defined broadly by worsening ventilator settings after a 2-day period of stability. The ventilator settings of concern are positive end-expiratory pressure (PEEP) and the fraction of inspired oxygen (FiO$_2$). PEEP settings that increase by 3 cm H$_2$O or an FiO$_2$ increase by greater than or equal to 20% are the two criteria used for deterioration. Remember, these must include a 48-hour period of stability on the ventilator with unchanged ventilator settings during this time period to be considered a VAC. Any progressive worsening of PEEP/FiO$_2$ that is within 48 hours of the prior ventilator settings does not qualify as a VAC. Once a VAC is diagnosed, the next decision point in diagnosis depends on whether this is an infectious or inflammatory process.

If signs or symptoms of infection/inflammation are present, then an infection-related ventilator-associated complication (IVAC) has occurred. This is defined by the following two criteria: systemic signs of infection/inflammation and treatment of this process with a new antimicrobial agent. Moreover, there is a time course associated with this definition. Both of these criteria must be present on ventilator day 3, and both must occur within 2 days of the VAC event above. The two clinical signs that are applicable for systemic signs are fever greater than 38° C or hypothermia to less than 36° C, or a white blood cell count (WBC) of greater than or equal to 12,000 cells/mm^3 or less than 4,000 cells/mm^3. New antimicrobial agents must be started within the 48-hour VAC window, and they must be started after at least 3 days of ventilator therapy. Moreover, they must be continued for 4 days to qualify the underlying disease process as an IVAC.

BOX 1: Excluded Organisms From the Diagnosis of a Possible Ventilator-Associated Pneumonia

Normal respiratory/oral flora
Mixed respiratory/oral flora or equivalent
Candida species or yeast not otherwise specified
Coagulase-negative *Staphylococcus* species
Enterococcus species
Blastomyces species
Histoplasma species
Coccidioides species
Paracoccidioides species
Cryptococcus species
Pneumocystis species

From Centers for Disease Control Ventilator-Associated Events guidelines: Device-associated module, pp 10-1, January 2015 (Modified April 2015).

Once an IVAC is diagnosed, the final determination of a possible ventilator-associated pneumonia (PVAP) must occur. The determination of a PVAP depends on three criteria: a high number of colony-forming units (CFU) on a quantitative or semiquantitative culture of the airway in a patient without purulent secretions, purulent secretions with a lower CFU threshold on quantitative or semiquantitative culture of the airway, or one of several diagnostic tests/culture results. A caveat does exist, however: certain culture results do not qualify as positive results because these organisms are either universally viewed as nonpathologic, are indeterminate results because of contamination, are fungal infections that will not respond to antibiotics, or are associated with CAP because these pathogens do not need the empirical, broad-spectrum antibiotics that HAP and VAP require (Box 1). Certainly, purulent secretions from a patient's endotracheal tube suction should raise the clinical index of suspicion for pneumonia. However, PVAP can occur without the presence of purulent sputum. In that regard, the following are the requirements based on culture assay to diagnose a PVAP without purulent sputum:

1. Endotracheal aspirate: ≥10^5 CFU/mL
2. Bronchoalveolar lavage (BAL): ≥10^4 CFU/mL
3. Lung tissue: ≥10^4 CFU/mL
4. Protected specimen brush: ≥10^3 CFU/mL

If the patient does have purulent sputum—defined as a sputum sample with at least 25 neutrophils and 10 or fewer squamous epithelial cells per low-power field—then a lower CFU threshold is needed for the above sampling techniques. Specifically, any positive result—regardless of the CFUs obtained—by the above collection techniques in the presence of purulent sputum is diagnostic of a PVAP. Finally, other special tests may be obtained in ventilated patients who require a provider to treat a patient aggressively. These include the following:

1. Pleural fluid culture in which the fluid culture is taken during thoracentesis or on initial chest tube insertion (indwelling chest tubes do not qualify)
2. Positive *Legionella pneumophila* testing
3. Respiratory secretions positive for influenza virus, respiratory syncytial virus, adenovirus, parainfluenza virus, rhinovirus, coronavirus, or human metapneumovirus
4. Lung histopathology with the following criteria:
   a. Abscess formation/consolidation/intense neutrophil presence in the bronchioles/alveoli
   b. Evidence of fungal invasion of the parenchyma
   c. Evidence of viral invasion of the parenchyma by the above mentioned viruses

Once a provider has gone through this algorithm and a PVAP is diagnosed, it remains for the physician to determine if a VAP has

Patient has a baseline period of stability or improvement on the ventilator, defined by ≥2 calendar days of stable or decreasing daily minimum* FiO_2 or PEEP values. The baseline period is defined as the 2 calendar days immediately preceding the first day of increased daily minimum PEEP or FiO_2.
*Daily minimum defined by lowest value of FiO_2 or PEEP during a calendar day that is maintained for at least 1 hour.

After a period of stability or improvement on the ventilator, the patient has at least one of the following indicators of worsening oxygenation:
1) Increase in daily minimum* FiO_2 of ≥0.20 (20 points) over the daily minimum FiO_2 in the baseline period, sustained for ≥2 calendar days.
2) Increase in daily minimum* PEEP values of ≥3 cm H_2O over the daily minimum PEEP in the baseline period,[†] sustained for ≥2 calendar days.
*Daily minimum defined by lowest value of FiO_2 or PEEP during a calendar day that is maintained for at least 1 hour.
[†] Daily minimum PEEP values of 0–5 cm H_2O are considered equivalent for the purposes of VAE surveillance.

Ventilator-Associated Condition (VAC)

On or after calendar day 3 of mechanical ventilation and within 2 calendar days before or after the onset of worsening oxygenation, the patient meets *both* of the following criteria:

1) Temperature >38°C or <36°C, **OR** white blood cell count ≥12,000 cells/mm^3 or ≤4,000 cells/mm^3.
AND
2) A new antimicrobial agent(s) is started, and is continued for ≥4 calendar days.

Infection-related Ventilator-Associated Complication (IVAC)

On or after calendar day 3 of mechanical ventilation and within 2 calendar days before or after the onset of worsening oxygenation, ONE of the following criteria is met (**taking into account organism exclusions specified in the protocol**):

1) Criterion 1: Positive culture of one of the following specimens, meeting quantitative or semiquantitative thresholds as outlined in protocol, *without* requirement for purulent respiratory secretions:
   - Endotracheal aspirate, ≥10^5 CFU/mL or corresponding semiquantitative result
   - Bronchoalveolar lavage, ≥10^4 CFU/mL or corresponding semiquantitative result
   - Lung tissue, ≥10^4 CFU/g or corresponding semiquantitative result
   - Protected specimen brush, ≥10^3 CFU/mL or corresponding semiquantitative result

2) Criterion 2: Purulent respiratory secretions (defined as secretions from the lungs, bronchi, or trachea that contain ≥25 neutrophils and ≤10 squamous epithelial cells per low power field [lpf, ×100])[†] *plus* a positive culture of one of the following specimens (qualitative culture, or quantitative/semiquantitative culture without sufficient growth to meet criterion #1):
   - Sputum
   - Endotracheal aspirate
   - Bronchoalveolar lavage
   - Lung tissue
   - Protected specimen brush

   [†] If the laboratory reports semiquantitative results, those results must correspond to the above quantitative thresholds. See additional instructions for using the purulent respiratory secretions criterion in the VAE Protocol.

3) Criterion 3: One of the following positive tests:
   - Pleural fluid culture (where specimen was obtained during thoracentesis or initial placement of chest tube and NOT from an indwelling chest tube)
   - Lung histopathology, defined as: 1) abscess formation or foci of consolidation with intense neutrophil accumulation in bronchioles and alveoli; 2) evidence of lung parenchyma invasion by fungi (hyphae, pseudohyphae, or yeast forms); 3) evidence of infection with the viral pathogens listed below based on results of immunohistochemical assays, cytology, or microscopy performed on lung tissue
   - Diagnostic test for *Legionella* species
   - Diagnostic test on respiratory secretions for influenza virus, respiratory syncytial virus, adenovirus, parainfluenza virus, rhinovirus human metapneumovirus coronavirus

January 2015   (Modified April 2015)

Possible Ventilator-Associated Pneumonia (PVAP)

FIGURE 1 Ventilator-associated events surveillance algorithm. *(From The Centers for Disease Control and Prevention. Ventilator-Associated Event [VAE], Device-Associated Module. NHSN Patient Safety Component Manual, pp 10-1–10-46, January 2015 [modified April 2015]. <http://www.cdc.gov/nhsn/pdfs/pscmanual/pcsmanual_current.pdf> Accessed December 2015.)*

TABLE 1: Clinical Pulmonary Infection Score

Diagnostic Feature	0	1	2
Tracheal secretions	Rare	Abundant	Abundant and purulent
CXR infiltrate	None	Diffuse	Localized
Temperature (°C)	≥ 36.5 and ≤ 38.4	≥ 38.5 and ≤ 38.9	≥ 39.0 or ≤ 36.5
White blood cells ($\times 10^9$/L)	≥ 4.0 and ≤ 11.0	< 4.0 or > 11.0	< 4.0 or > 11.0 + bands ≥ 0.5
PaO_2/FiO_2 (mm Hg)	> 240 or ARDS	–	< 240 or no ARDS

From Pugin J. Clinical signs and scores for the diagnosis of ventilator-associated pneumonia. *Minerva Anestesiol.* 2002;68:261-265.

ARDS, Adult respiratory distress syndrome; *CXR,* chest x-ray; *PaO_2/FiO_2,* partial pressure of oxygen in arterial blood/fractional concentration of oxygen in inspired gas.

occurred. Unfortunately, the definition of VAP has not been universally accepted. Therefore scoring systems have been created to help define what constitutes a VAP. Some providers feel that the definition of VAP should have subjective criteria included in the definition, such as new consolidations noted on portable or formal chest radiographs. Others feel that, because of the varied diseases that can occur with new chest radiographic findings (e.g., ARDS, pulmonary contusions, atelectasis, or pulmonary edema) including radiographs in the diagnosis of VAP is of limited value because these other disease processes can occur independently of an infectious process. However, most accepted criteria use a combination of subjective and objective measurements. An example of this is the Clinical Pulmonary Infection Score (CPIS) published by Pugin.

This scoring system accounted for subjective findings (tracheal secretions and chest x-ray infiltrate) and objective findings (temperature, WBC, and PaO_2/FiO_2) (Table 1). A score of six or more correlated with a 100% sensitivity and 93% specificity in the cohort studied. However, like other scoring systems, these results are not universally applicable as a subsequent study found that the CPIS had a sensitivity and specificity of 77% and 42%, respectively. That being said, a universally accepted definition as to what clinical criteria should be used to define which patients have VAP is hard to achieve because these scoring systems have inadequate sensitivity and specificity to be applied universally. If fewer criteria are required to diagnose VAP (i.e., too many patients are being treated empirically), then too many patients will receive a diagnosis of pneumonia, causing the number of MDR organisms to increase in a patient population and specificity plummets. The converse is also true in that the application of too many criteria causes many cases of pneumonia to not be diagnosed, antibiotics to be held, and worse patient outcomes to occur. CPIS and other grading systems, although imprecise, are relevant to apply to VAP because no better metrics exist currently. Developing a working scoring system with a high sensitivity and specificity that can be applied universally to ventilated patients remains a critical area of clinical research.

■ TREATMENT

One of the main goals of therapy for VAP is starting early, appropriate, broad-spectrum antibiotics. Although guidelines exist for the type of empirical antibiotics to use, it cannot be emphasized enough that antibiotic therapy must be tailored to the infective pathogen causing the VAP as quickly as possible. This means that empirical antibiotics must be decelerated once a bacterial species is identified—for example, withdrawing antipseudomonal antibiotics if *Pseudomonas aeruginosa* is not isolated—with further tailoring of the antibiotics once bacterial sensitivities are established—for example, by discontinuing vancomycin in methicillin-sensitive *Staphylococcus aureus* isolates. This fine line must be followed diligently; to err in not starting appropriate, broad-spectrum antibiotics early in a patient's hospital course places patients at an increased risk of high morbidity

outcomes or increased mortality risks. Similarly, if broad-spectrum antibiotics are maintained for too long of a period of time without appropriate tailoring, then this will promulgate resistance. Finally, it is important to ensure that any institution's antibiogram be used in antibiotic planning for patients with VAP. If an ICU has a high rate of an uncommon bacteria, frequent MDR organisms, uncommon opportunistic organisms, or if a critical care surgeon is taking care of a significant number of patients with altered immune systems (e.g., AIDS patients; oncology patients; patients on chronic, high-dose steroids; or patients on antirejection medications after organ transplantation), then these empirical guidelines may not apply. It is incumbent upon the critical care surgeon to be aware not only of the macroscopic recommendations for antibiotic control applied nationally but also of the bacterial demographics of the unique environment in which the surgeon operates.

Empirical antibiotic coverage for VAP is started based on one of two clinical scenarios. For suspected VAP in a patient who has been hospitalized for less than 5 days or who has zero risk factors for MDR pathogens, these patients are treated with limited-spectrum empirical therapy. If, however, a patient has been hospitalized for 5 or more days or has risk factors for MDR organisms, these patients are started on broad-spectrum empirical antibiotics. These risk factors include the following:

1. Antimicrobial therapy in the preceding 90 days
2. Current hospitalization of 5 days or more
3. High frequency of antibiotic resistance in the community or hospital unit
4. Immunosuppressive disease or therapy
5. Presence of risk factors for HCAP (see Definitions earlier in chapter)

In the low-risk group, the main pathogens to consider are *Streptococcus pneumoniae, Haemophilus influenzae,* methicillin-sensitive *S. aureus,* and non-MDR enterics, such as *Escherichia coli, Klebsiella pneumoniae, Enterobacter* spp., *Proteus* spp., or *Serratia marcescens.* These bacteria require monotherapy with one of the agents in Table 2. These antibiotics are targeted at both gram-positive and gram-negative organisms with enteric coverage. Current literature does not support the use of combination therapy in this population of patients because of the general susceptibility of the inoculates to limited-spectrum antibiotics.

In the high-risk group, these patients are at risk of infection with more virulent strains of the common bacteria mentioned above as well as other, new groups of bacteria that require stronger antibiotics. *P. aeruginosa,* MDR *K. pneumoniae, Acinetobacter* spp., methicillin-resistant *S. aureus* (MRSA), and *L. pneumophila* must be covered empirically in this higher risk group. As such, empirical coverage requires an antipseudomonal cephalosporin or carbapenem or a β-lactam with a β-lactamase inhibitor for primary coverage of *P. aeruginosa.* Moreover, because of *P. aeruginosa*'s propensity to be an MDR organism, an aminoglycoside or antipseudomonal

TABLE 2: Initial Empirical Antibiotic Therapy for Hospital-Acquired Pneumonia or Ventilator-Associated Pneumonia in Patients With No Known Risk Factors for Multidrug-Resistant Pathogens, Early Onset, and Any Disease Severity

Potential Pathogen	Recommended Antibiotic
*Streptococcus pneumoniae** *Haemophilus influenza* Methicillin-sensitive *Staphylococcus aureus* Antibiotic-sensitive enteric gram-negative bacilli *Escherichia coli* *Klebsiella pneumonia* *Enterobacter* species *Proteus* species *Serratia marcescens*	Ceftriaxone *or* Levofloxacin, moxifloxacin, or ciprofloxacin *or* Ampicillin/sulbactam *or* Ertapenem

From Guidelines for the management of adults with hospital-acquired, ventilator-associated, and healthcare-associated pneumonia. *Am J Respir Crit Care Med.* 2005;171:388-416.

*The frequency of penicillin-resistant *S. pneumoniae* and multidrug-resistant *S. pneumoniae* is increasing; levofloxacin or moxifloxacin is preferred to ciprofloxacin and the role of other new quinolones, such as gatifloxacin, has not been established.

TABLE 3: Initial Intravenous, Adult Doses of Antibiotics for Empirical Therapy of Hospital-Acquired Pneumonia, Including Ventilator-Associated Pneumonia, and Healthcare-Associated Pneumonia in Patients With Late-Onset Disease or Risk Factors for Multidrug-Resistant Pathogens

Antibiotic	Dosage*
Antipseudomonal cephalosporin	
Cefepime	1-2 g every 8-12 hr
Ceftazidime	2 g every 8 hr
Carbapenems	
Imipenem	500 mg every 6 hr or 1 g every 8 hr
Meropenem	1 g every 8 hr
β-Lactam/β-lactamase inhibitor	
Piperacillin–tazobactam	4.5 g every 6 hr
Aminoglycosides	
Gentamicin	7 mg/kg per day†
Tobramycin	7 mg/kg per day†
Amikacin	20 mg/kg per day†
Antipseudomonal quinolones	
Levofloxacin	750 mg every day
Ciprofloxacin	400 mg every 8 hr
Vancomycin	15 mg/kg every 12 hr‡
Linezolid	600 mg every 12 hr

From Guidelines for the management of adults with hospital-acquired, ventilator-associated, and healthcare-associated pneumonia. *Am J Respir Crit Care Med.* 2005;171:388-416.

*Dosages are based on normal renal and hepatic function.

†Trough levels for gentamicin and tobramycin should be less than 1 μg/mL and for amikacin they should be less than 4 to 5 μg/mL.

‡Trough levels for vancomycin should be 15 to 20 μg/mL.

fluoroquinolone should be considered strongly in association with the primary agent above. Last, vancomycin or linezolid should be started for MRSA and *L. pneumophila* coverage. Treatment dosing and length of treatment are listed in Table 3.

During recent years, investigations have attempted to assess what the optimal duration of therapy is for VAP. For low-risk patients, some studies have shown that tracheal aspirates are cleared of the pathogen within 72 hours of antibiotic therapy for most organisms; however, some isolates are still present at 6 days. Other studies have shown that some pathogens—namely, *P. aeruginosa* and some enterics—may persist for much longer in tracheal secretions. However, prolonged treatment regimens over greater than 8 days may put the patient at risk for repeat infection with an MDR isolate of the original bacterial pathogen or promote an environment in which superinfection with a novel bacterial species (which will likely be an MDR organism) can occur. As such, significant research has been turned to this field.

Recent work by Magnotti et al has attempted to solve the issue of when to discontinue antibiotics for hardier forms of organisms causing VAP. In their recent work (see Suggested Readings), the authors developed a novel system for assessing the dynamic bacterial environment of the respiratory tract during treatment. Namely, they performed a screening BAL on day 4 of treatment for VAP, and—if the BAL demonstrated growth of less than 10,000 CFU/mL—then appropriately tailored antibiotics were continued for a total of 7 days. However, if the BAL demonstrated more than 10,000 CFU/mL on day 4 of treatment, then patients were given 10 to 14 days of therapy. Using this schema, this study showed no difference between patients treated for the shorter course of antibiotics compared with the longer course for the following parameters: length of stay (LOS), number of ventilator days, length of ICU stay, number of recurrent VAP, and mortality. This novel strategy provides an example of how providers can incorporate screening BAL to help define when a patient no longer needs antibiotic therapy for these more resilient organisms.

The Infectious Disease Society of America (IDSA) in association with the American Thoracic Society (ATS) has incorporated the use of CPIS scores into their algorithm to guide the evaluation and treatment of patients with VAP (Figure 2). Once a patient has developed

an IVAC, a lower respiratory tract culture is obtained via BAL or one of the tests mentioned above, and the patient is risk stratified using the CPIS score. If both a low clinical suspicion of VAP exists (as evidenced by a CPIS of less than 6) and the initial BAL results show no evidence of pathogens, then antibiotics are not started for VAP with a plan to reassess in 24 to 48 hours. If, however, clinical concern exists because of an elevated CPIS or if the culture shows bacteria on Gram stain, then empirical antibiotics are started per the appropriate regimen above. After 48 to 72 hours of antibiotic therapy, the patient is reassessed using the CPIS, and the culture results are analyzed. This groups patients into four populations. If the patient has clinically improved (e.g., they have remained afebrile, they have a normalized WBC, and their ventilator settings have improved) and the culture results are negative, then the antibiotics are discontinued. If the patient has improved clinically and the culture results are positive, then the antibiotics are de-escalated depending on speciation and sensitivities of the isolated pathogens with a short course of antibiotics (typically 7 to 8 days). If the patient has not clinically improved and the culture results are negative, then the patient is assessed for either an occult pathogen in the lungs or a separate source of their ongoing infectious process. Finally, if a patient has not clinically improved and the culture results are positive, then the patient's antibiotics are adjusted based on speciation and sensitivities (to include broadening, if necessary) as well as a repeat assessment of an occult infectious process.

In summary, studies have shown that shortening the antibiotic period has not shown worse outcomes when curtailing from 14 days

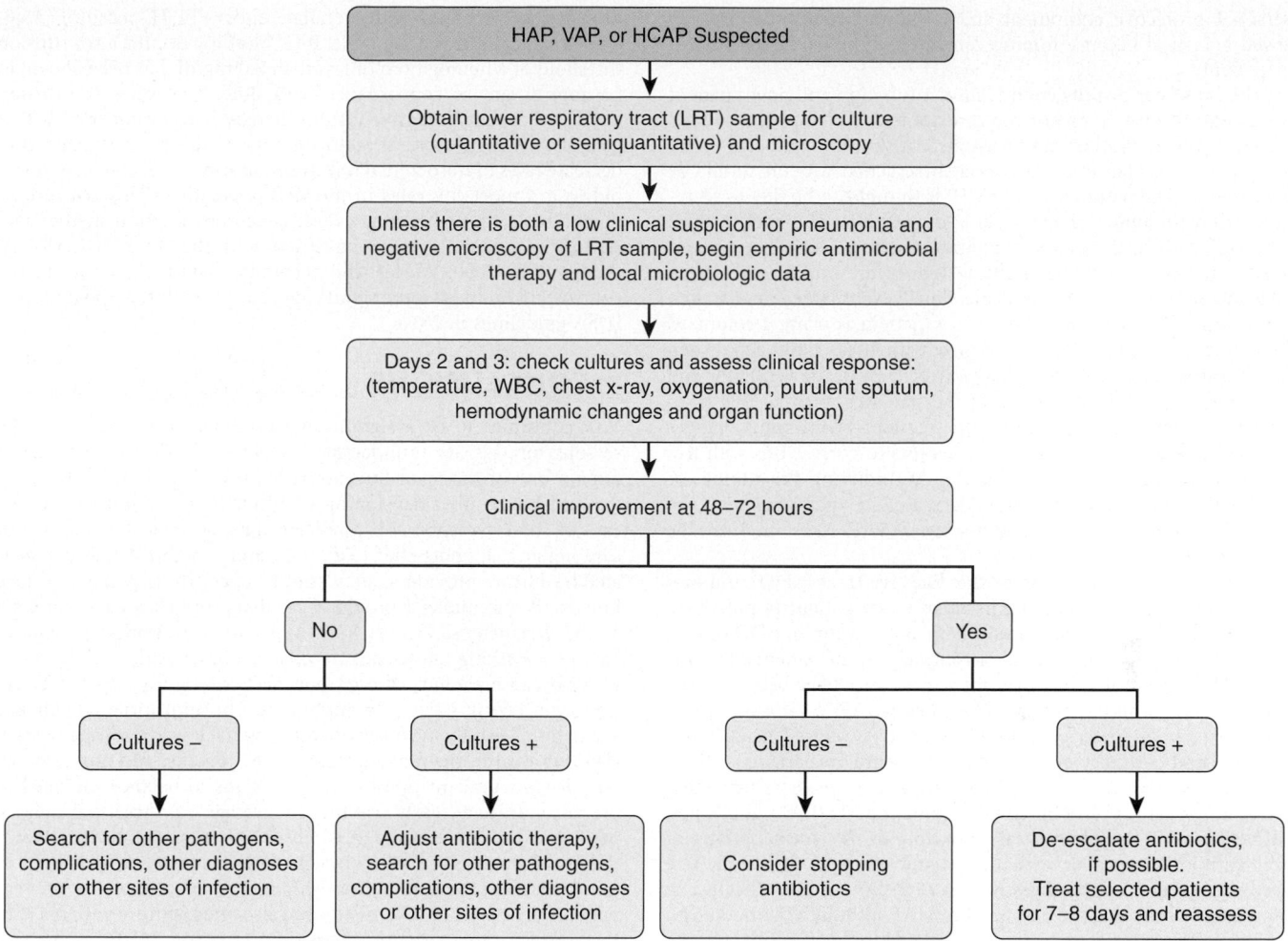

FIGURE 2 Summary of the management strategies for a patient with suspected hospital-acquired pneumonia (HAP), ventilator-associated pneumonia (VAP), or healthcare-associated pneumonia (HCAP). The decision about antibiotic discontinuation may differ depending on the type of sample collected (protected specimen brush, bronchoalveolar lavage, or endotracheal aspirate), and whether the results are reported in quantitative or semiquantitative terms. *(From Guidelines for the management of adults with hospital-acquired, ventilator-associated, and healthcare-associated pneumonia. Am J Respir Crit Care Med. 2005;171:388-416.)*

to 8 days. Current ATS/IDSA guidelines recommend shortening the dogmatic period of 14 to 21 days as clinically able with treatment periods as low as 7 days being reasonable. Longer periods of antibiotic coverage should be used only in patients who have not shown clinical improvement (evidenced by persistent fever, leukocytosis, progressive infiltrates on chest radiography, or purulent sputum).

■ PREVENTION

In an effort to help define, prevent, and treat the problem of VAPs, the CDC's National Health Safety Network and the IDSA, in collaboration with the ATS, have issued definitions for what constitutes the diagnosis of a VAP and empirical antibiotic regimens to treat VAP as noted above. However, prevention remains the mainstay of treating VAP. As such, a discussion on the management of VAP cannot be conducted fully without a word on how best to prevent this disease process from occurring. What follows are the level I recommendations from the current ATS/IDSA guidelines. Of note, the ATS/IDSA guidelines were last published in 2004; however, the updated guidelines are expected to be published in spring of 2016. For a full review of all of the level I through III recommendations, refer to the suggested reading list at the end of the chapter.

Multiple investigators have assessed prophylactic interventions— the so-called VAP bundle—to prevent VAP formation in ICU

settings. These issues originally were addressed by the Institute for Healthcare Improvement Ventilator Bundle. The bundle originally consisted of head of bed (HOB) elevation at least 45 degrees above horizontal, daily sedation holidays with an evaluation on whether extubation could occur, daily oral care with chlorhexidine, proton pump inhibitor (PPI) or histamine (H_2) receptor antagonist therapy to prevent stress gastritis and stress ulceration, and mechanical and chemical venous thromboembolism (VTE) prophylaxis. Using this bundle as a starting point, multiple researchers have investigated new techniques and procedures to assist in VAP prophylaxis. The ATS/IDSA has issued level I through III recommendations on these latest techniques which primarily revolve around five areas: infection prevention and control, endotracheal intubation and mechanical ventilation, modulation of oropharyngeal and gastric colonization, prevention of aspiration of oropharyngeal and gastric contents, and other general critical care interventions for ventilated patients. The following paragraphs summarize the level I recommendations published by the ATS/IDSA.

Infection prevention and control goes back to the basics of infection control practices in ICUs. It is critical that an alcohol-based hand sanitizer is used liberally by all members of the hospital care team (physicians, midlevel providers, and nursing staff) as well as ancillary staff and patient visitors. Moreover, following the guidance of infectious disease services by ensuring that appropriate personal protective equipment and isolation precautions are followed is critical because fomites can carry pathogens from patient to patient.

The act of performing endotracheal intubation and how a patient is maintained on a ventilator can contribute to development of VAP. Obviously, if intubation can be avoided, it should be; liberal use of noninvasive ventilation in appropriately screened patients should be used if able. The pathogenesis of VAP is thought to be due to secretions from the upper airway leaking down below the endotracheal tube cuff. Subglottic secretion aspiration devices have been developed that have shown the ability to reduce the rate of early onset VAP and should be used if available. Finally, ventilator circuits often are colonized by bacteria. When a new patient is using a colonized ventilator, the patient can be infected with these pathogens when condensation from the patient's airway collects in the ventilator and this condensate refluxes back into the patient's airway. This is an especially common occurrence with frequent positioning changes seen in these critically ill patients. Attempts to correct this with frequent ventilator tubing exchanges, de-humidifying the tubing, or heating the airway were thought to decrease VAP incidence; however, these interventions have failed to lower VAP rates and can be disregarded.

Selective decontamination of the digestive tract (SDD) and oral hygiene have been investigated in a variety of patient populations; however, the data are sparse and general application of SDD or oral hygiene cannot be recommended routinely to all patients. Specifically, SDD with oral and intravenous antibiotics have been assessed and—although this has decreased the rates of VAP in various populations (e.g., MDR pathogen outbreaks in units, closed head injury patients, and coronary artery bypass graft surgery patients)—there are multiple studies that show less efficacious results when these interventions are applied broadly. To quote the ATS/IDSA guidelines, "Modulation of oropharyngeal colonization—by combinations of oral antibiotics, with or without systemic therapy, or by selective decontamination of the digestive tract (SDD)—is also effective in significantly reducing the frequency of HAP, although methodologic study quality appeared to be inversely related to the magnitude of the preventative effects." Clearly, more research is needed in this field before universal recommendations for or against flora modulation can be applied.

Lying supine is associated with markedly increased rates of VAP. As mentioned above, upper airway secretions leaking into the lower airway past the endotracheal tube are thought to be the pathogenesis of VAP cases. Enteral feedings in these patients is preferred over parenteral feedings because of the multiple risks of parenteral access. However, enteral feedings pose their own risk for reflux of gastric contents into the upper airway with subsequent inoculation of the lower airway. As such, HOB elevation assists in decreasing this rate when the HOB is elevated between 30 and 45 degrees. Prepyloric or postpyloric feedings have failed to show statistically significant differences, but a trend toward lower VAP rates with postpyloric feedings has been demonstrated.

Although it is not an infection prevention issue, VTE prevention, bleeding prophylaxis, transfusion thresholds, and treatment of hyperglycemia also have been assessed in patients with VAP to assess what are appropriate therapies for these conditions. Currently, VTE prophylaxis with sequential compression devices and chemical prophylaxis with unfractionated heparin or low-molecular-weight heparins are critical in the VAP patient. Similarly, bleeding prophylaxis with a PPI or H_2-receptor antagonist typically is used to prevent stress gastritis and stress ulcers. However, a hypothetical risk of gastrointestinal (GI) flora overgrowth in the relatively lower pH of the stomach with these agents has given some providers pause to not treat their patients. This has lead to some proponents to use sucralfate for GI bleeding prophylaxis. Although a trend toward lower VAP

rates has been achieved with sucralfate, either PPI, H_2-receptor antagonist, or sucralfate is acceptable. If GI bleeding occurs, a transfusion threshold of a hemoglobin of less than 7.0 mg/dL has been shown to be appropriate in concordance with other restrictive transfusion strategies. Finally, intensive insulin therapy is recommended with a goal of a serum glucose of 80 to 110 mg/dL; this has been shown to decrease rates of nosocomial infections, shorten LOS, and lower morbidity and mortality rates in the VAP population. This last recommendation, although being a level I recommendation in the 2004 ATS/IDSA guidelines, is not consistent with the NICE-SUGAR trial published in 2009. We feel this recommendation for tight glucose control will undergo some significant changes with the updated ATS/IDSA guidelines in 2016.

■ CONCLUSIONS

VAP continues to be a significant pathologic entity in ICUs. The reasons for this are multifactorial; however, critical care surgeons remain one of the front-line stewards for caring for these patients. Stewardship requires developing a multidisciplinary approach to the care of these patients with physician-directed education of critical care nursing, support staff (e.g., respiratory therapists), and associated healthcare providers (such as other specialty providers, surgical housestaff, and midlevel providers) so that prophylactic measures act as the first defense against VAP. Appropriate stewardship requires having a working knowledge of what defines a patient as having a PVAP because patients who do not meet criteria for a PVAP should not begin taking started on antibiotics. The appropriate diagnostic evaluation, with the primacy of culturing the lower respiratory tract, also is critical in the management of VAP. Finally, and most important, it is incumbent upon these physicians to balance the need to provide adequate, early antibiotic coverage to these critically ill patients with the need to aggressively decelerate antibiotics to steward the hospital course of patients with VAP. It is necessary to keep in mind that appropriate stewardship not only affects the current patients in an ICU on a ventilator but also affects future patients with VAP because of the ever-increasing rates of MDR organisms. Although many clinical questions persist for all of the areas mentioned—namely, defining VAP, diagnosing VAP, treating VAP, and creating better prophylactic methods—these remain ripe fields for novel research and continued guidelines refinement to provide optimal care for these critically ill patients.

SUGGESTED READINGS

American Thoracic Society and the Infectious Disease Society of America. Guidelines for the management of adults with hospital-acquired, ventilator-associated, and healthcare-associated pneumonia. *Am J Respir Crit Care Med.* 2005;171:388-416.

The Centers for Disease Control and Prevention. *Ventilator-Associated Event (VAE), Device-associated Module. NHSN Patient Safety Component Manual,* pp 10-1–10-46, January 2015 (modified April 2015). Available at: <http://www.cdc.gov/nhsn/pdfs/pscmanual/pcsmanual_current.pdf>; Accessed December 2015.

Magnotti LJ, Croce MA, Zarzaur BL, et al. Causative pathogen dictates optimal duration of antimicrobial therapy for ventilator-associated pneumonia in trauma patients. *J Am Coll Surg.* 2011;212:476-484.

Michetti CP, Fakhry SM, Ferguson PL, et al. Ventilator-associated pneumonia rates at major trauma centers compared with a national benchmark: a multi-institutional study of the AAST. *J Trauma Acute Care Surg.* 2012;72: 1165-1173.

Pugin J. Clinical signs and scores for the diagnosis of ventilator-associated pneumonia. *Minerva Anestesiol.* 2002;68:261-265.

Sharpe JP, Magnotti LJ, Weinberg JA, et al. Impact of pathogen-directed antimicrobial therapy for ventilator-associated pneumonia in trauma patients on charges and recurrence. *J Am Coll Surg.* 2015;220:489-495.

EXTRACORPOREAL LIFE SUPPORT FOR RESPIRATORY FAILURE

Seth Goldstein, MD, MPhil, and Fizan Abdullah, MD, PhD

Acute respiratory failure is a major contributor to morbidity and mortality, as well as an important component of resource consumption, in adult and pediatric intensive care units. Acute respiratory distress syndrome, commonly known as *ARDS*, is the most serious manifestation of acute lung disease causing respiratory failure and is initiated by a broad spectrum of causes. Causes include intrinsic pulmonary (e.g., infection, aspiration, inhalation, congenital hypoplasia, persistent pulmonary hypertension of the newborn) and extrapulmonary (e.g., sepsis, circulatory shock, cardiac disease) processes. Conventional management revolves around mechanical ventilation with minimization of barotrauma and attempted mitigation of hypoxemia. However, survival after ARDS remains low despite new developments in optimizing ventilator strategies.

■ EXTRACORPOREAL MEMBRANE OXYGENATION

Extracorporeal membrane oxygenation (ECMO) is a form of partial cardiopulmonary bypass that is indicated for reversible causes of acute respiratory failure. First successfully implemented in the 1970s, within a decade ECMO became a standard of care in infants with respiratory distress syndrome. Wide adoption for adults has been slower but is progressively increasing. Figure 1 depicts the cumulative number of cases reported to the Extracorporeal Life Support Organization since its inception in 1990, as well as the most contemporary statistics regarding cannulation strategy.

Indications

The crux of appropriate ECMO patient selection is the identification of a reversible disease process that can be treated with either specific therapy or general lung healing. ECMO can offer a period of pulmonary "rest" or can be a bridge to definitive therapy such as surgery or transplant but is not a destination therapy. Both the CESAR trial in adults and the U.K. Collaborative trial in children prospectively have shown benefit regarding survival and quality of life in favor of ECMO over conventional ventilator management for severe reversible respiratory failure.

Clinical indications include the presence of potentially reversible pulmonary disease that is progressively severe despite maximal conventional ventilation with 100% inspired oxygen. In neonates, a commonly used objective measure is the oxygenation index (OI), calculated as

$$OI = [\text{Mean arterial pressure} \times \text{Fraction of inspired oxygen} \times 100] \div \text{Arterial partial pressure of oxygen}$$

Sequential multiple measurement OI of greater than 40 on maximal ventilation is a commonly used criteria to initiate ECMO. In adults, a Murray score of greater than 3 (Table 1) may trigger ECMO consideration. Box 1 lists the minimum studies to obtain acutely before cannulation when active ECMO referral is made.

Contraindications

Absolute contraindication for ECMO are active hemorrhage, preexisting intracranial hemorrhage, irreversible pulmonary disease, or uncorrectable lethal extrapulmonary anomaly. Relative contraindications include prolonged mechanical ventilation greater than 10 days (signifying nonreversible injury), malignancy with poor prognosis, and multiorgan system failure. Baseline comorbidities should be evaluated on a case-by-case basis with attention to premorbid function, duration of current illness, and overall prognosis. For neonates, a gestational age of less than 34 weeks puts patients at prohibitively high risk of intracranial hemorrhage because of the systemic anticoagulation. Weight under 2 kg also can be problematic because of the inability to achieve sufficient flows through the pump circuit.

System Components and Cannulation Strategy

The goal of ECMO for respiratory failure is to oxygenate venous blood and recirculate to the patient's systemic vasculature. A typical system, depicted in Figure 2, comprises a bladder, a pump, an oxygenator, a heat exchanger, circuit tubing, and catheters appropriate to the mode of access. Heparin-bonded components are used where possible to decrease anticoagulation requirements and reduce the systemic inflammatory response to the circuit.

A bladder, or volume capacitance reservoir, is placed at the lowest point on the drainage side of the circuit. This is required to ensure a constant supply of blood for the pump that follows. The ECMO circuit contains a fixed volume, and flow rates are controlled tightly to deliver a sufficient amount of oxygenated blood. However, drainage from the patient can vary with cardiac output, venous tone, and third-space edema; thus the bladder exists to regulate stability in the circuit.

The pump is the active component of the ECMO system and can be roller or centrifugal. Roller pumps work by squeezing the tubing forward; they are not dependent on inlet or outlet pressure, but the mechanical pressure can damage tubing and may hemolyze red blood cells. Centrifugal pumps are theoretically capable of more constant flow but must be real-time regulated because of dependence on pump preload/afterload as well as the risk of generating high negative pressures leading to air embolus if flow falls too rapidly. The pump is used to pressurize the blood to return to the patient, either simply to overcome resistance of the tubing in a venovenous circuit or all the way to mean arterial pressure in a venoarterial system.

Following the pump is an oxygenator. These are constructed using a variety of semipermeable membranes or hollow fibers that expose blood to as high surface area as possible for gas exchange. Regulated inputs are the fraction of oxygen and the flow, or sweep rate, of the gas through the oxygenator. Just as in the case of mechanical ventilation, carbon dioxide is more soluble and is transferred across the membrane more efficiently. Thus oxygenation of circuit blood is proportional to the oxygen fraction in the sweep gas, whereas carbon dioxide removal is determined by the flow rate.

The heat exchanger can be separate or be incorporated into the oxygenator. It generally consists of a water bath, through which the ECMO tubing passes and is modulated to achieved the desired patient temperature. The maximum temperature of the bath itself is 42° C to prevent bubble formation or hemolysis resulting from overheating.

The bridge is a connection between the drainage and the return tubing at points near the patient. It is generally closed or clamped. In the event that the patient is to be temporarily isolated from ECMO but not decannulated (e.g., a weaning trial), the cannulae are clamped and the bridge opened to preserve flow and avoid clots in the circuit.

The two principal modes of ECMO are venovenous (VV) and venoarterial (VA), which refer to the areas of circulation from which deoxygenated blood is drained and oxygenated blood is returned (Figure 3). For VV ECMO in the most typical fashion, venous cannulae are inserted into the right internal jugular vein with the tip in the right atrium, and right femoral vein with tip near the cavoatrial junction. In children, blood is drained from right atrium, run through the ECMO circuit, and reinfused into the right femoral vein

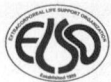

ECLS registry report
International summary
January, 2016

Extracorporeal life support organization
2800 Plymouth Road
Building 300, room 303
Ann Arbor, MI 48109

Neonatal respiratory runs by diagnosis

	Total runs	Avg run time	Longest run time	Survived	% Survived
CDH	7,584	256	2549	3,865	51%
MAS	8,915	133	1327	8,345	94%
PPHN/PFC	5,011	156	1908	3,862	77%
RDS	1,556	136	1093	1,307	84%
Sepsis	2,884	143	1200	2,101	73%
Pneumonia	385	249	1002	223	58%
Air leak syndrome	135	169	979	100	74%
Other	2,669	185	1843	1,623	61%

2015 cannulation strategies

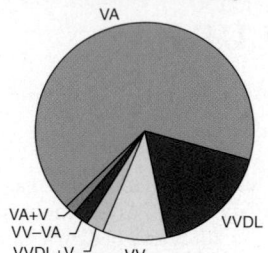

Pediatric respiratory runs by diagnosis

	Total runs	Avg run time	Longest run time	Survived	% Survived
Viral pneumonia	1,564	317	2968	1,021	65%
Bacterial pneumonia	736	284	1411	435	59%
Pneumocystis pneumonia	35	373	1144	18	51%
Aspiration pneumonia	322	242	2437	220	68%
ARDS, postop/trauma	191	247	935	119	62%
ARDS, not postop/trauma	571	305	3086	310	54%
Acute resp failure, non-ARDS	1,331	259	2718	738	55%
Other	2,605	223	2465	1,357	52%

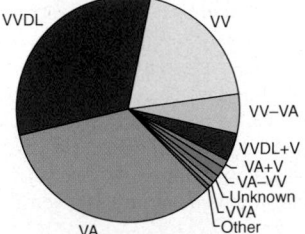

Adult respiratory runs by diagnosis

	Total runs	Avg run time	Longest run time	Survived	% Survived
Viral pneumonia	751	321	3208	495	66%
Bacterial pneumonia	1,239	257	3288	760	61%
Aspiration pneumonia	190	239	2634	122	64%
ARDS, postop/trauma	445	253	1993	251	56%
ARDS, not postop/trauma	778	311	6248	420	54%
Acute resp failure, non-ARDS	1,597	269	4527	897	56%
Other	4,331	239	6745	2,407	56%

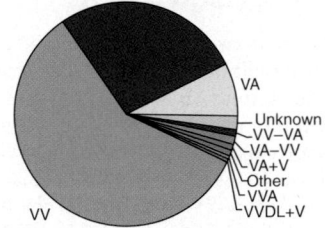

Run time in hours. survived = survival to discharge or transfer based on number of runs

FIGURE 1 Cumulative number of cases reported to the Extracorporeal Life Support Organization (ELSO) since its inception in 1990, as well as the most contemporary statistics regarding cannulation strategy. *ARDS,* Acute respiratory distress syndrome; *CDH,* congenital diaphragmatic hernia; *MAS,* meconium aspiration syndrome; *PFC,* persistent fetal circulation; *PPHN,* persistent pulmonary hypertension of the newborn; *VA,* venoarterial; *VV,* venovenous; *VVDL,* venovenous with double-lumen catheter. *(From ECMO Registry of the Extracorporeal Life Support Organization [ELSO], Ann Arbor, Michigan, January 2016.)*

TABLE 1: Murray Score Is Calculated as the Average of All Four Parameters

Parameter / Score	0	1	2	3	4
PaO$_2$/FIO$_2$ (on 100% oxygen)	≥300 mm Hg	225-299	175-224	100-174	<100
	≥40 kPa	30-40	23-30	13-23	<13
CXR	Normal		1 point per quadrant infiltrated		
PEEP	≤5	6-8	9-11	12-14	≥15
Compliance (mL/cm H$_2$O)	≥80	60-79	40-59	20-39	≤19

CXR, Chest x-ray; *PEEP,* positive end-expiratory pressure.

---

catheter. This often is reversed in adults, with the femoral catheter acting as the drainage cannula. Although these are the most common arrangements for VV circuits, theoretically any combination of two large-bore central catheters can be used as patient factors or as extenuating circumstances require and as previously mentioned can be placed in a variety of techniques. The venous cannulae should be as large as the target vessel will accommodate to ensure adequate flow; sizes range from 12F in a newborn to 29F in adults. Tables exist of maximum flows for a given catheter size and should be consulted.

Catheters may be placed either by direct cutdown or using percutaneous Seldinger technique. The choice of site to use for venous drainage as mentioned above is made with the knowledge that flow of deoxygenated blood into the pump circuit is the rate-limiting step to achieve sufficient volume though the system because the ability of the pump to pressurize the oxygenated blood makes it easier to return to the patient. In addition, the resistance of any fluid in a vessel or catheter is proportional to its length and inversely proportional to the fourth power of its radius. Thus, although the femoral vein of a patient is often slightly larger than the internal jugular and can accommodate a larger catheter, the length of femoral cannulae is longer; this is the typical tradeoff that must be considered on an individual basis.

Alternatively, use of a double-lumen cannula with channels for both drainage and return is possible if the target vessel can accommodate a larger catheter size; these range from 13F to 31F. A major limitation of VV ECMO is recirculation, which is the amount of oxygenated blood that is immediately redrained before circulating

because of the proximity of the catheter tips. This is particularly prominent at high pump flows. In the commercially available double-lumen venous cannulae, the drainage and infusion ports have been engineered to minimize recirculation by relying on bicaval drainage and a side infusion port that is directed towards the tricuspid valve.

VA ECMO uses the same components as VV and additionally offers cardiac support by pressurizing blood to mean arterial pressures and returning it into arterial circulation. In children the cannulation strategy uses ipsilateral internal jugular vein and carotid artery, whereas in adults the femoral vessels often are used. The choice of VA cannulation is based on the patient's native cardiac function as well as current vasoactive support. Some fraction of cardiac dysfunction resulting from hypoxia will be mitigated by VV ECMO alone, but if there is question regarding ability to maintain cardiac output based on the pre-ECMO echocardiogram or clinical parameters, a VA strategy should be considered.

BOX 1: Recommended Studies Before Extracorporeal Membrane Oxygenation Cannulation

Pre-ECMO Recommended Studies

Serum chemistry
Complete blood count
Coagulation studies
Arterial blood gas
Blood bank crossmatch
Chest radiograph
Echocardiogram
Head ultrasound (neonates)

ECMO, Extracorporeal membrane oxygenation.

Circuit Management

Neurologic

Regular neurologic exams should be performed while on ECMO. Paralysis and sedation should be used only to the extent necessary to avoid catheter dislodgement. Some adult units have recently reported patients' ability to fully ambulate even while on the ECMO circuit. If feasible, head ultrasonography should be performed before ECMO initiation in neonates (Box 2). Intracerebral hemorrhage should be

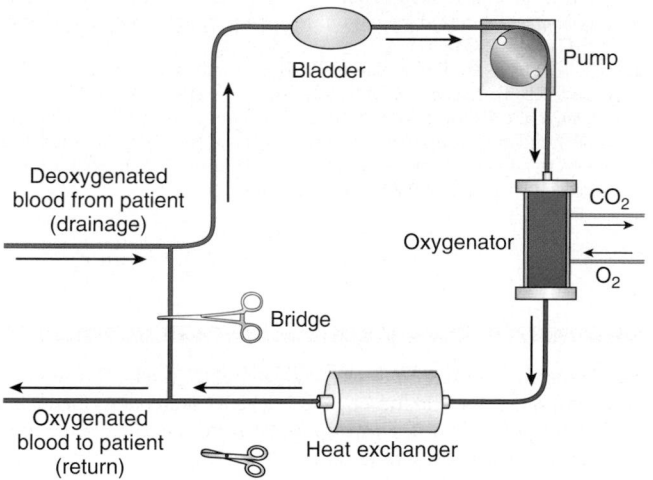

FIGURE 2 ECMO circuit components.

BOX 2: Recommended Studies After Extracorporeal Membrane Oxygenation Cannulation

Intra-ECMO Recommended Studies

Serum chemistry
Complete blood count
Coagulation studies
Patient arterial blood gas
Preoxygenator circuit blood gas
Postoxygenator circuit blood gas
Activated clotting time
Fibrinogen
Chest radiograph
Interval head ultrasound (neonates)

ECMO, Extracorporeal membrane oxygenation.

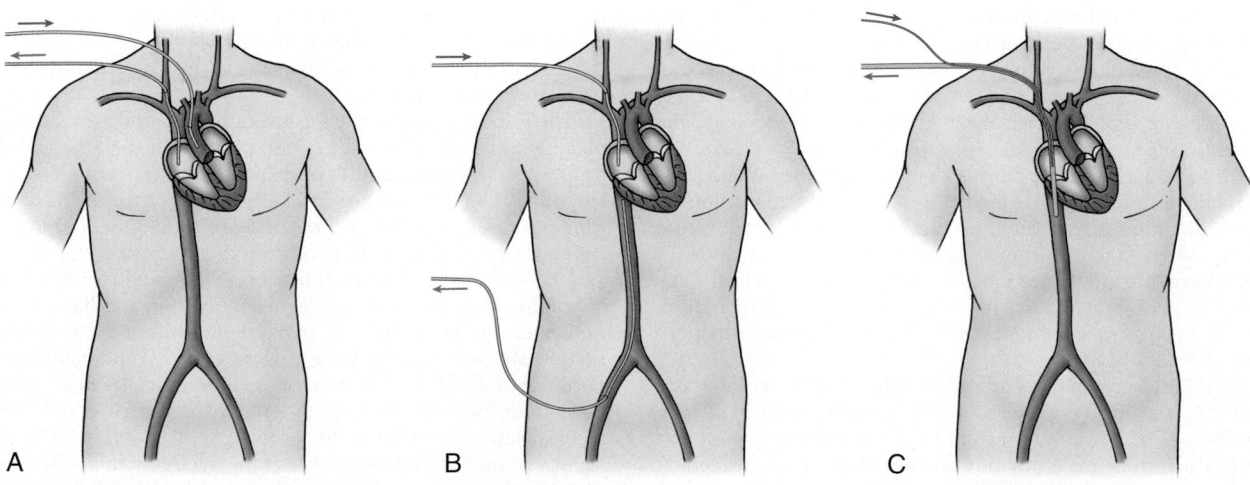

FIGURE 3 Cannulation strategies. **A,** Venoarterial; **B,** venovenous; **C,** double-lumen venovenous.

suspected if focal deficits in neurologic status develop in the absence of hypoxemia.

Cardiovascular

Precannulation echocardiography will reveal baseline cardiac function. Normal intravascular volume should be maintained and can be assessed by urine output and patient-side venous and arterial pressures as appropriate. Subsequent to cannulation, the initiation of ECMO begins by first unclamping the arterial or oxygenated line, followed by clamping of the bridge and unclamping of the venous line. The flow is increased gradually to the desired flow that will achieve patient cardiac output and oxygenation. Inotropes are tapered off gradually and should be avoided whenever possible on a VA circuit.

Respiratory

Ventilator settings during ECMO are adjusted to minimize barotrauma. Relatively low peak pressure, end-expiratory pressure, rate, and fraction of oxygen are employed. A daily chest radiograph should be obtained. Pulmonary hygiene is of utmost importance when considering that the entire goal of ECMO for respiratory failure is lung recovery and should include frequent endotracheal suctioning with periodic position changes.

Gastrointestinal

Patients can be fed enterally via various routes or parenterally directly into the circuit. As a general principle, enteral feeds should be avoided in the presence of hypotension or vasoactive pressor to avoid intestinal ischemia.

Fluid Management

A strict recording of intake and output from the patient and the circuit should be maintained. ECMO can initiate an inflammatory reaction that may lead to oliguria and fluid sequestration. Adding fluid or blood to the circuit is not difficult to maintain volume or

blood counts, but subsequent reduction in the total fluid requires diuresis, hemofiltration, or actually removing blood from the circuit. Dialysis can be initiated in parallel to the circuit, usually preoxygenator. Electrolytes should be maintained in the normal range and may be checked from the patient or the circuit.

Hematologic

Immediately before cannulation the patient should be heparinized systemically with a bolus dose if possible. Continued anticoagulation is critical to avoid the formation of clots in the circuit. Heparin infusion is used typically to maintain the partial thromboplastin time at a value greater than two times normal. Thrombocytopenia is a common problem, and platelet transfusions may be necessary to decrease the risk of spontaneous bleeding. If heparin-induced thrombocytopenia occurs, alternative anticoagulant such as argatroban or bivalirudin is required.

Infectious

A first-generation cephalosporin may be used as empirical prophylaxis. Routine blood cultures should be obtained, and all catheter sites inspected regularly. Infection and sepsis should be promptly identified and treated appropriately.

SUGGESTED READINGS

McNally H, Bennett CC, Elbourne D, Field DJ, UK Collaborative ECMO Trial Group. United Kingdom collaborative randomized trial of neonatal extracorporeal membrane oxygenation: follow-up to age 7 years. *Pediatrics.* 2006;117:e845-e854.

Peek GJ, Mugford M, Tiruvoipati R, Wilson A, Allen E, Thalanany MM, Hibbert CL, Truesdale A, Clemens F, Cooper N, Firmin RK, Elbourne D, CESAR trial collaboration. Efficacy and economic assessment of conventional ventilatory support versus extracorporeal membrane oxygenation for severe adult respiratory failure (CESAR): a multicentre randomised controlled trial. *Lancet.* 2009;374:1351-1363.

TRACHEOSTOMY, PART ONE

Roy Semaan, MD, and David Feller-Kopman, MD

Tracheostomy is a common procedure performed by otolaryngologists, trauma surgeons, pulmonologists, and intensivists. It has increased gradually in frequency because of a rise in critical care and the need for prolonged mechanical ventilation. Tracheostomy is one of the oldest surgical procedures performed with the first record of an open tracheostomy recorded more than 3500 years ago on stone slabs during the first Egyptian dynasty. Fabricius is credited with being the first to describe a tracheal cannula in 1617 with another Italian surgeon, Sanctorio Sanctorius, documenting the first percutaneous tracheotomy in 1626. He used a "ripping needle" to introduce a silver cannula into the tracheal lumen and then removed the needle. The first cuffed tracheostomy tube was developed in 1869 by Trendelenburg, but it was not until the early twentieth century that tracheotomy became a popular procedure because of the standardization of open surgical tracheotomy by the famous American surgeon Chevalier Jackson.

In the 1930s, tracheotomy use increased because it was advocated as an effective means to provide bronchopulmonary toilet in patients with poliomyelitis. However, not until the increasingly widespread use of positive pressure ventilation in the 1950s was considerable energy focused on the development of tracheostomy tubes as a means of providing long-term ventilatory support. In the late 1960s, Toye

and Weinstein used a Seldinger guidewire to safely introduce a cannula into the tracheal lumen, and in 1985, Ciaglia described what has now become one of the most popular techniques for percutaneous dilational tracheostomy (PDT).

■ TRACHEAL ANATOMY

As with any procedure, knowledge of relevant anatomy is essential. For tracheostomy, this includes airway anatomy, as well as an understanding of the surrounding structures such as the thyroid gland and vasculature of the neck.

The trachea is a centrally located unpaired organ extending in an oblique fashion from the superficial position of the neck and diving deeper into the mediastinum once in the thoracic cavity. The average length of the adult trachea is 11 cm with a range of 10 to 13 cm. Along the course of the trachea there are 18 to 22 incomplete cartilaginous rings with an anteroposterior diameter on average of 1.8 cm and 2.3 cm in the lateral dimension. The cricoid cartilage in the larynx has the only complete cartilaginous ring and has a membranous attachment to the first tracheal ring inferiorly as well as the thyroid cartilage superiorly forming the cricothyroid membrane. The posterior wall of the trachea or membranous trachea comprises fibroelastic tissue between the ends of the tracheal rings and abuts the anterior-lateral portion of the esophagus. The combination of the rigidity of the anterior two thirds of the trachea with the flexibility of the posterior one third allows for a wide range of flexibility and stability.

There are several structures that lie anterior to the trachea that should be identified before tracheostomy. The thyroid isthmus typically is located between the second and third tracheal rings; the innominate artery most often crosses the anterior trachea in an oblique fashion distal to the third tracheal ring. Although the blood supply to the cervical trachea enters posteriolaterally from the inferior thyroid artery, the inferior thyroidal artery and vein and the anterior jugular vein may lie between the skin and trachea, and the operator must be aware of these vessels.

■ INDICATIONS, CONTRAINDICATIONS, AND TIMING

The major indication for surgical tracheostomy and PDT is chronic ventilator dependence. This includes chronic hypoxic or hypercapnic respiratory failure because of a multitude of respiratory, cardiac, or systemic conditions as well as airway protection after neurologic events such as cerebrovascular accidents, intracranial hemorrhage, or traumatic brain injury. Chronic debilitating neuromuscular diseases that require airway protection or chronic ventilator support are also common indications for tracheostomy. Tracheostomy also can be indicated in cases of inherited or acquired airway obstruction such as high-tracheal or subglottic stenosis, central airway obstruction from neoplasm, stricture from radiation therapy, angioedema, burn injury, trauma, and obstructive sleep apnea. Finally, tracheostomy along with cricothyrotomy can be used as an adjunct in emergency situations in which an airway cannot be established through endotracheal intubation and a patient cannot be ventilated.

There are few absolute contraindications for tracheostomy, including cellulitis/deeper infection at the insertion site and operator inexperience. Relative contraindications to both surgical tracheostomy and PDT include coagulopathy/thrombocytopenia, and worsening acute critical illness (i.e., septic shock, acute respiratory distress syndrome [ARDS]). In terms of ventilator setting the most important variable to note is the positive end-expiratory pressure (PEEP) as for PDT the stoma is created distal to the endotracheal tube cuff with resultant derecruitment. We recommend that oxygenation be assessed with PEEP below 12 cm H_2O, increasing FiO_2 as needed to maintain oxygenation. Relative contraindications to PDT include inability to palpate relevant tracheal anatomy, overlying vessels, and emergent airways.

The timing of tracheostomy remains a controversial issue with set guidelines difficult to establish as the decision to perform a tracheostomy is still an individualized process taking into account the current clinical scenario, likely future need of a tracheostomy, daily weaning attempts, risk of continued endotracheal intubation and the risk of the tracheostomy procedure itself. Prolonged translaryngeal endotracheal intubation has been thought to contribute to several complications, including laryngeal injury, subglottic and tracheal stenosis, tracheomalacia, ventilator-associated pneumonia, as well as the need for higher levels of sedation and the associated morbidity. Several studies have been performed looking at the above complications and the optimal timing of tracheostomy with mixed outcomes. Late tracheostomy was defined classically as tracheotomy performed after 3 weeks; however, more recently the cutoff has been moved up to as soon as 1 to 2 weeks, or even 48 to 96 hours of mechanical ventilation. There has been a general paradigm shift in critical care medicine toward early tracheostomy, but it is unclear whether this is actually supported by data because no clear benefit has been shown in recent trials. In a multicenter trial of 1032 patients at 57 sites who were randomized to early (within 4 days) versus late (greater than 10 days) tracheostomy, no difference was seen in 30-day or 2-year mortality as well as length of mechanical ventilation, antibiotic use, and sedative use. More than half of the subjects randomized to the late tracheostomy arm did not end up getting the procedure, indicating that possibly delaying significantly reduces the need for tracheostomy. A recent Cochrane database systematic review also did not find significant evidence of benefit from early versus late tracheostomy.

Another recent meta-analysis of 13 published studies on the topic also did not find evidence of reduced mortality with early tracheostomy but did find a reduction in ventilator-associated pneumonia with early tracheostomy. These data emphasize the timing of tracheostomy remains a clinically based decision that should be made on a case-by-case basis.

■ SURGICAL TRACHEOSTOMY

Surgical tracheostomy generally is performed under general anesthesia but theoretically can be done under conscious sedation if an airway cannot be established orally. It can be performed in the operating room (OR) or at the bedside with all the appropriate equipment being brought to the ICU, including adequate lighting, electrocautery, and surgical tools. The patient is supine on the table, and the neck is extended moderately with a shoulder roll to improve anatomic landmarks (Figure 1). The head of the bed should be elevated slightly either through flexion at the hip or through reverse Trendelenburg to reduce pressure in the cervical veins. Before prepping the skin proper identification of the appropriate anatomic landmarks including the thyroid cartilage, the cricothyroid membrane, the cricoid cartilage, and the tracheal rings should be completed.

After appropriate prepping and draping from the nipple line to above the thyroid cartilage a transverse incision is preferred in a controlled setting with a stable airway because this follows Langer's lines and is more cosmetically appealing. A 3- to 4-cm incision should be made 1 cm below the cricoid cartilage and not based on the sternal notch as the trachea and larynx move independently of the sternum (Figure 2). The subcutaneous tissue and platysma can be dissected with electrocautery, at which point the sternohyoid and sternothyroid muscles are encountered and retracted laterally. Deep to the strap muscles lies the thyroid isthmus, which then can be ligated using sutures or electrocautery and then retracted laterally. The pretracheal fascia then should be dissected sharply exposing the trachea anteriorly from just below the cricoid cartilage to the fourth tracheal ring. A cricoid hook then can be used to elevate the tracheal rings and facilitate the tracheal incision. This incision can be made using a #11 blade horizontally between the

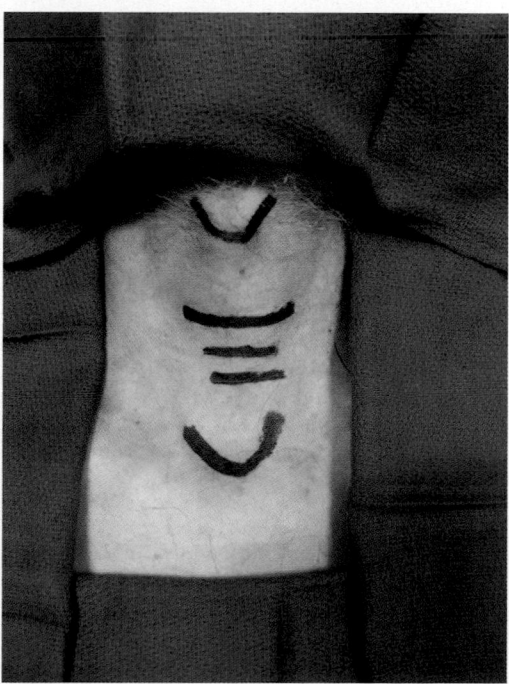

FIGURE 1 Preoperative landmarks from top to bottom: thyroid cartilage, cricoid cartilage, first tracheal ring, second tracheal ring, sternal notch.

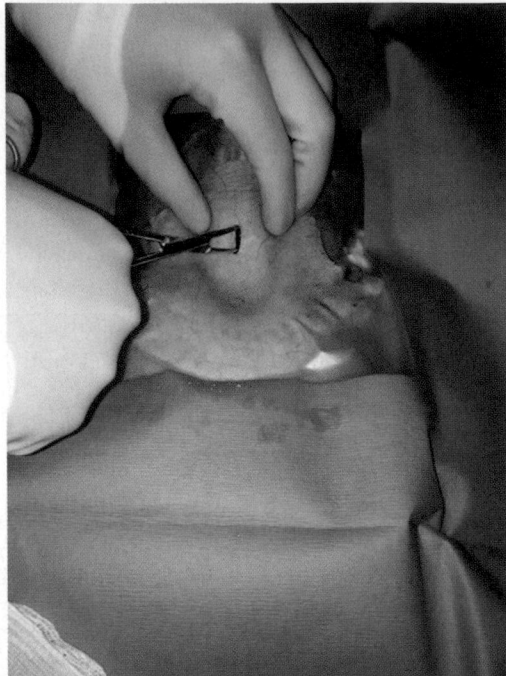

FIGURE 2 I cm vertical incision during initial Kelly forceps dilation.

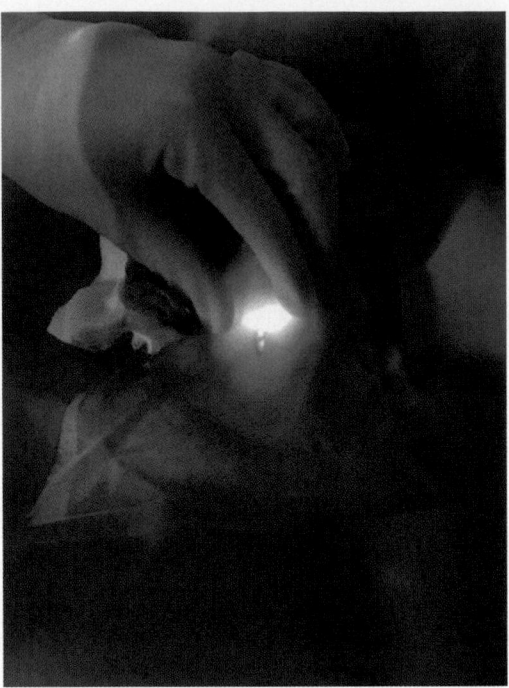

FIGURE 3 Transillumination using bronchoscope during percutaneous dilational tracheostomy.

second and third tracheal rings or vertically dividing the second and third rings. Once the tracheal lumen has been exposed, the endotracheal tube should be retracted just proximal to the lumen at which point the surgeon can insert the tracheostomy tube under direct visualization. The tube should then be connected to a ventilator circuit with adequate placement and ventilation ensured using auscultation, CO_2 detectors and adequate return of tidal volume without a significant leak. The endotracheal tube can then be removed, and 3-0 Prolene sutures can be used to secure the tracheostomy neck plate.

■ PERCUTANEOUS DILATIONAL TRACHEOSTOMY

PDT generally is performed at the bedside in the intensive care unit (ICU). Preprocedure evaluation includes a careful review of the history and respiratory status of the patient, as well as a careful physical examination that is focused on the neck and tracheal structures. Especially when starting PDT, patients should have ideal anatomy with an easily palpable thyroid cartilage, cricoid cartilage, and first and third tracheal rings, with no underlying vessels. Pertinent lab studies include a platelet count, PT, PTT, as well as blood urea nitrogen (BUN) to evaluate for uremia.

PDT can be performed safely in patients with uremia; however, pretreatment of these patients with DDAVP should be considered and a PT/PTT below 1.5 times control and a platelet count above 50,000/mm is ideal. Generally high-risk patients or those with difficult anatomy or significantly noncorrectable coagulopathy should be referred for surgical tracheotomy.

Optimal staffing includes an anesthesiologist or a physician who is trained in airway management and basic bronchoscopy positioned at the head of the bed to control the endotracheal tube, perform the bronchoscopy, and administer anesthetic medication. Sedation, analgesia, and short-acting paralysis is preferred to minimize patient discomfort and coughing as well as optimize the first attempt success. A nurse familiar with the procedure should be available to assist with monitoring of vital signs, administer medications, and act as a nonsterile circulator if supplies or tools are needed during the case. As with surgical tracheostomy (ST) a shoulder roll is placed the skin is prepped with chlorhexidine and draped, the patient's FiO_2 is increased

to 1.0, and a mode of ventilation is selected to ensure adequate minute ventilation.

Just as with ST, anatomic landmarks should be identified. It is also important to palpate and inspect for overlying vessels because ligation and electrocautery control of bleeding is generally not performed in PDT as it is during ST. Ultrasound also has been used to identify vasculature anterior to the trachea. The ideal entry site is between the first and second, or second or third tracheal rings. Some data suggest a higher incidence of tracheal stenosis if the cricothyroid membrane is involved. The risk of tracheoinnominate artery fistula increases if the tracheostomy tube is placed too inferiorly or in the setting of a high-riding innominate artery. The skin and subcutaneous tissues are infiltrated with up to 10 cc of 1.5% lidocaine with epinephrine, mostly for the vasoconstrictive properties. After an initial 1 to 1.5 cm horizontal or vertical incision through the skin and subcutaneous fascia, the soft tissue is dissected bluntly and the tracheal rings are palpated. At this time the bronchoscope is withdrawn and transillumination through the anterior neck incision is visualized giving the bronchoscopist an estimation of how far to pull back the ETT after the cuff has been deflated (Figure 3). After the ETT has been pulled back, the operator can then insert the 14-gauge needle under direct bronchoscopic visualization optimally in the midline of the trachea, avoiding the posterior membrane. Aspiration of air and direct visualization confirms the proper location of the needle in the lumen of the trachea. Holding the needle in place, the syringe is removed and a J-tipped guidewire is advanced in the direction of the carina (Figure 4). The tract initially is dilated with the short 14F dilating catheter followed by a single tapered dilator. The tracheostomy tube then is inserted on a separate obturator over the wire with the cuff inflated once in the tracheal lumen (Figure 5). Adequate position is confirmed via bronchoscopy through the tracheostomy tube in addition to observing return of tidal volume from the ventilator once the circuit is connected to the tracheostomy tube (Figure 6). The tracheostomy tube is secured with a strap such that one finger can be placed between the strap and the skin, and the neck plate is either sutured or stapled to the neck. It is crucial that one operator always hold the tracheostomy tube as it is being secured. If accidental decannulation occurs, the patient should be reintubated with a translaryngeal endotracheal tube with the cuff of the tube distal to the

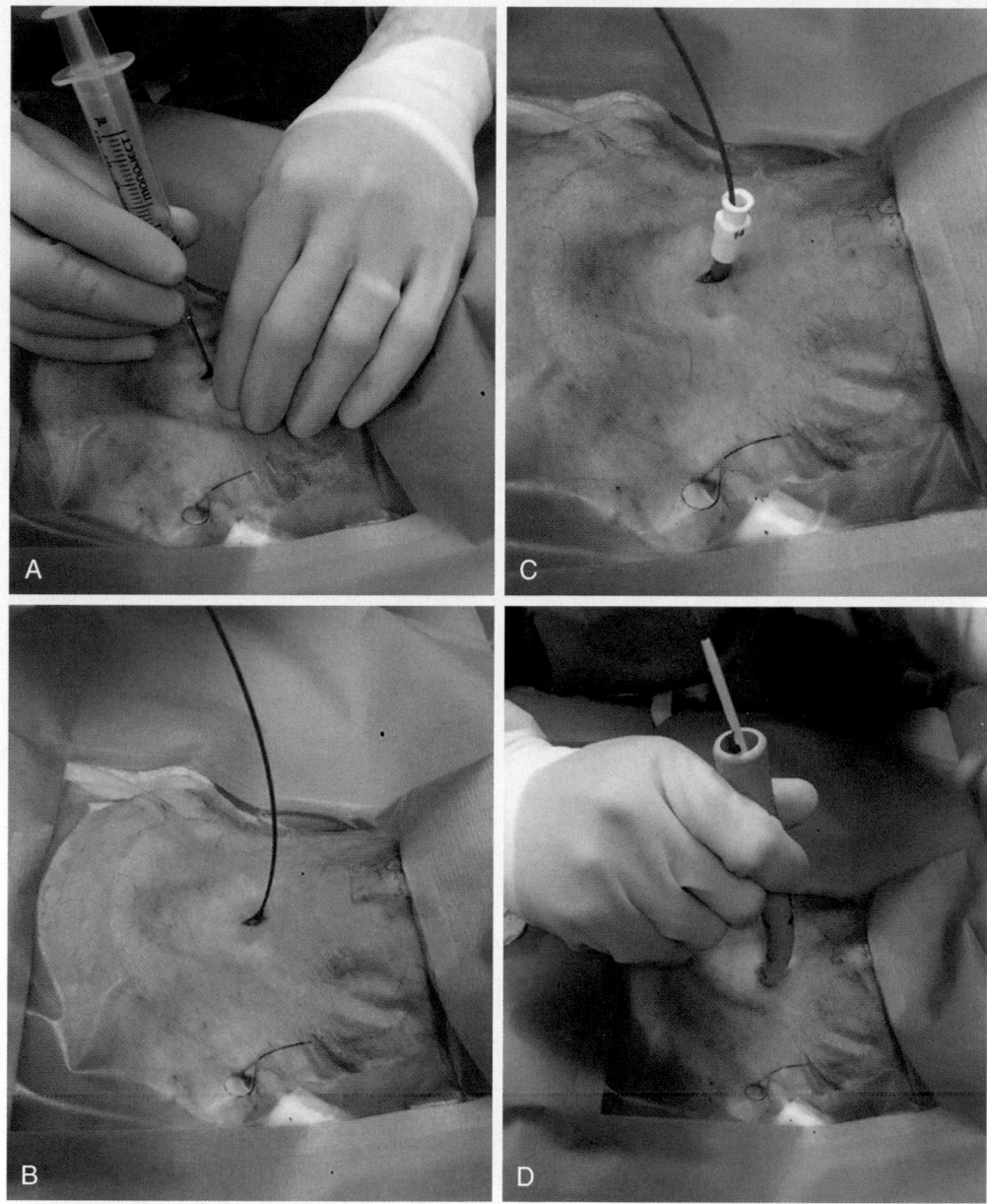

FIGURE 4 A, Insertion of wire through finder needle. **B,** Wire in place. **C,** 14F dilator over wire. **D,** Rhino dilator.

stoma. Attempts at reinserting the tracheostomy tube should be done only when the airway is secure, and as the tract is immature, the introducer needle and guidewire should be used to avoid misplacement into the mediastinum.

■ COMPLICATIONS

In general, the complications of surgical and percutaneous dilational tracheotomy are small, comparable between the two methods, and can be divided into early or late complications. Early complications for PDT include bleeding, infection, inadvertent decannulation, paratracheal insertion, injury to the posterior tracheal membrane, pneumothorax, pneumomediastinum, and tracheal ring fracture. Overall, the rate of these complications is low, with subcutaneous emphysema and pneumothorax being cited at 1.4% and 0.85%, respectively. Significant hemorrhage is also extremely low with one retrospective study of 3162 bedside PDT citing only one significant bleeding event requiring surgical intervention. Early complications for ST are similar, including hemorrhage, pneumothorax, pneumomediastinum accidental decannulation, and airway

fire as electrocautery is used frequently in ST while generally not in PDT. However, tracheal ring fractures and posterior tracheal wall injury or paratracheal insertions are very rare in ST as the tracheostomy tube is placed in the tracheal lumen under direct visualization.

Most complications of ST and PDT can be managed easily. Almost all bleeding around the tracheostomy stoma can be stopped with simple maneuvers including tightening the tracheostomy collar or placing a hemostatic agent such as Surgicel (Ethicon, Somerville, NJ) or Quick Clot (ZMedica, Wallinford, CT) circumferentially around the stoma. Infections should be treated with antibiotics and rarely require surgical intervention unless a paratracheal abscess develops. If accidental decannulation occurs before a mature tract has developed (typically approximately 7 days), orotracheal intubation should be performed and the cuff of the tube placed distal to the tracheal stoma. Reinsertion of the tracheostomy tube through an immature stoma can result in generation of a false tract into the subcutaneous tissue or mediastinum with disastrous consequences. After a secure airway has been established, the stoma can then be redilated and the tracheostomy replaced under more controlled circumstances.

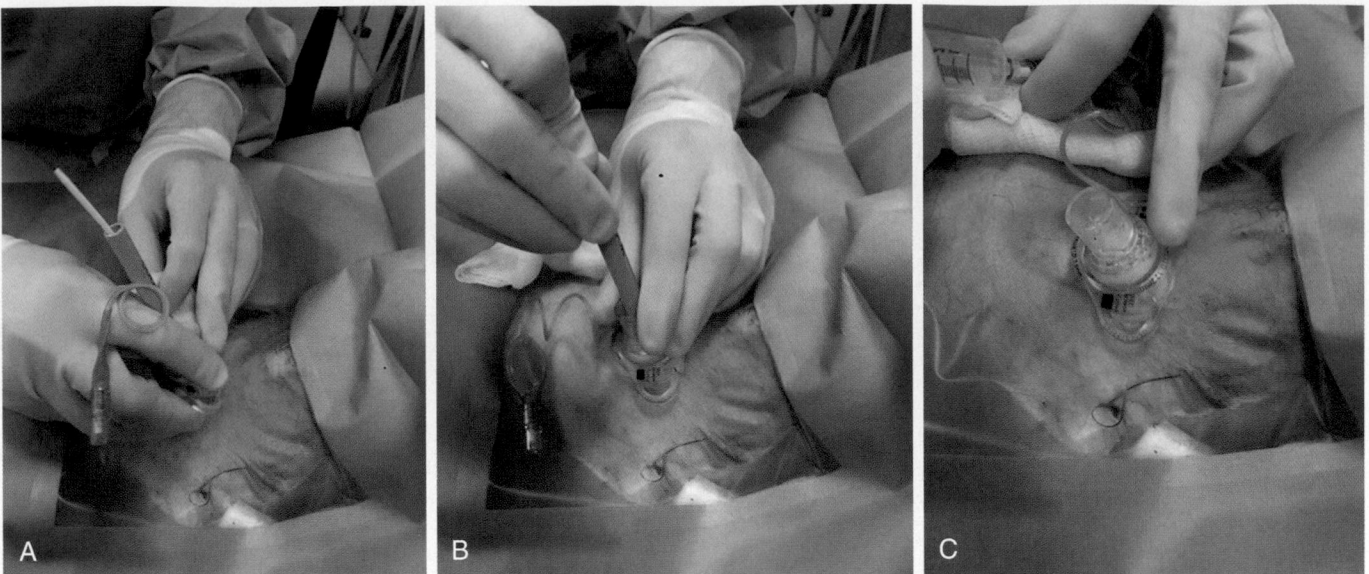

FIGURE 5 A, Tracheostomy being inserted over introducer. **B,** Introducer being pulled out of tracheostomy. **C,** Tracheostomy complete.

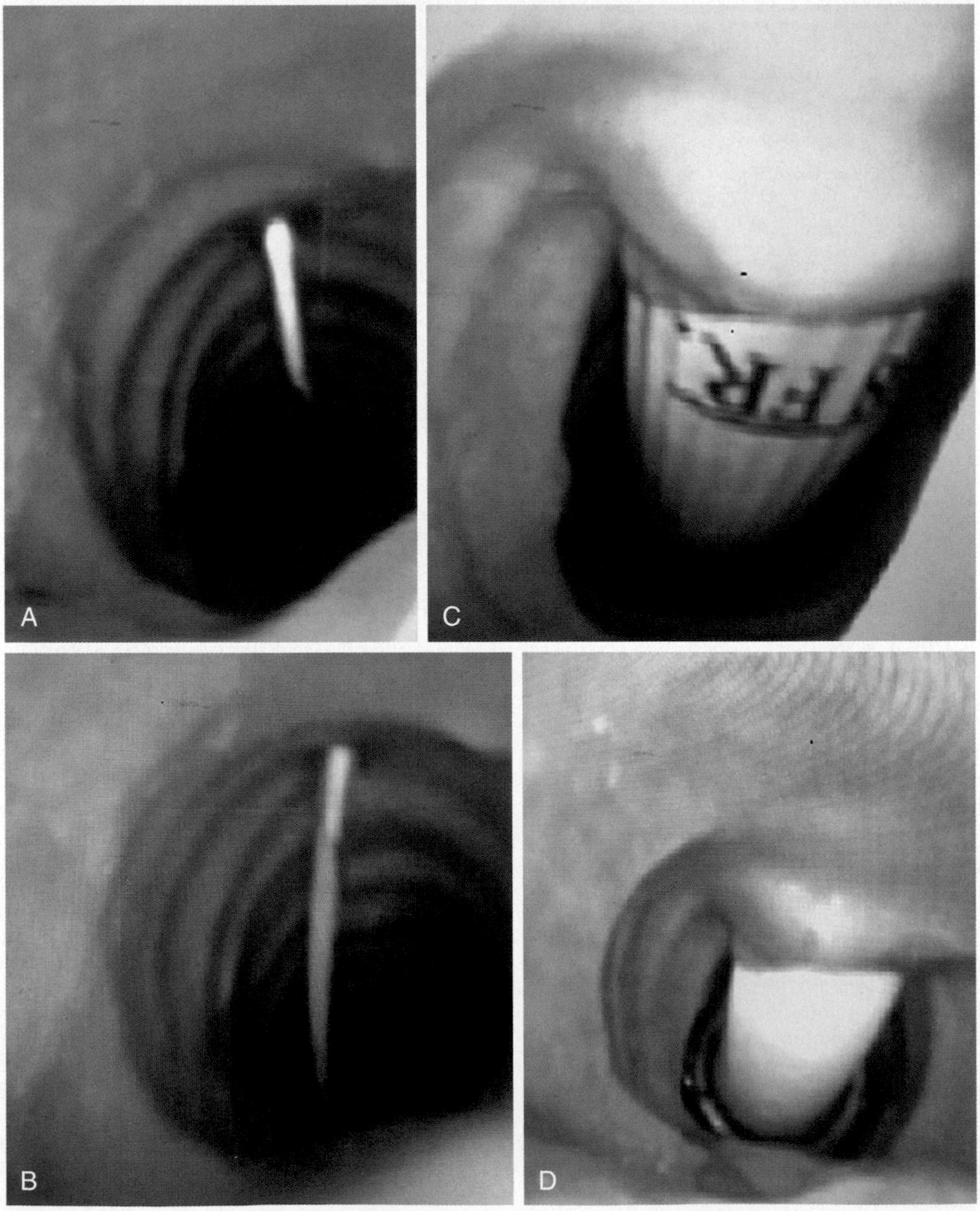

FIGURE 6 Bronchoscopic view during PDT. **A,** Needle below first tracheal ring. **B,** Wire visualized descending toward carina. **C,** Rhino dilator. **D,** Tracheostomy confirmed in place.

Pneumomediastinum and pneumothorax after ST and PDT generally can be managed conservatively unless the patient is unstable or the pneumothorax is expanding, at which point tube thoracostomy would be indicated. Finally, airway fire is a serious complication that should be avoided by careful collaboration between anesthesiology and the surgeon during ST, keeping the FiO_2 below 0.4 during the use of electrocautery. If an airway fire does occur, the FiO_2 should be lowered, the inciting stimulant must be stopped, and if any foreign bodies are in the airway including a bronchoscope, ETT or tracheostomy tube, they must be removed as they can further propagate a fire. The patient then can be bag masked and reintubated to re-establish a secure airway.

Late complications of ST and PDT are similar and include laryngotracheal stenosis, tracheomalacia, delayed stomal closure after prolonged cannulation and most seriously tracheoinnominate artery fistula formation. Tracheal stenosis can occur after both translaryngeal intubation and tracheotomy. The stenosis can occur in the subglottic space, at the level of the tracheal stoma, or at the level of the cuff of the endotracheal or tracheostomy tube. Because almost all patients with tracheostomy tubes have had orotracheal tubes, it can be difficult to identify the causal factor. With this in mind, the overall incidence of clinically significant tracheal stenosis is low and cited to be anywhere from as low as 0.16% in a large meta-analysis of more than 3000 patients undergoing PDT to as high as at 23.8% in a smaller retrospective study of 105 patients who underwent PDT and then were admitted to a long-term care facility because of the need for prolonged mechanical ventilation or poor neurologic outcomes. The much higher rate of tracheal stenosis in the second article is likely the result of the patient population that is selected for placement at a long-term care facility, which is not likely representative of all patients undergoing PDT. Overall there has been a marked decrease since the 1960s and is due in part to the development of high-volume, low-pressure cuffs. It is also important to understand that tracheal stenosis is generally not clinically significant until there is a 75% reduction in luminal diameter, and that stridor will not develop until the luminal diameter is less than 5 mm.

Tracheoinnominate artery fistula (TIF) formation is a more feared complication that can be fatal if not recognized early. TIF is a rare complication generally occurring in less than 1% of all ST and PDT and can occur 48 hours after insertion but is most common 7 to 14 days postoperatively. The mortality associated with TIF is extremely high with survival being cited around 14.3%. If a patient is suspected to have a TIF but is stable, computed tomography scanning of the neck can be obtained with contrast to visualize the relationship of the tracheostomy cuff to the innominate and if a fistulous tract is forming (Figure 1). If that is the case, the patient should be taken to the operating room (OR) for immediate repair before any further significant bleeding occurs. If a patient is actively hemorrhaging, the tracheostomy tube should be replaced with an endotracheal tube through the vocal cords with the cuff inflated distal to the bleeding source, and digital pressure with one finger should be applied in the stoma applying force anteriorly and the patient taken emergently to the OR for surgical repair. The best way to avoid a TIF is to place tracheostomy tubes above the third tracheal ring, ideally between the second and third rings, and as with endotracheal tubes, tracheostomy tube cuff pressures should be monitored and kept below 25 mm Hg to avoid focal ischemic necrosis. Once ventilation is no longer required, thought should be given toward changing the tube to an uncuffed tube and/or proceeding with downsizing and decannulation.

■ COMPARISON BETWEEN SURGICAL AND PERCUTANEOUS DILATIONAL TRACHEOSTOMY

PDT does offer advantages over ST because it is generally a quicker procedure and is performed sooner because the surgical or critical

care team does not have to wait for scheduled OR time and staff. PDT is also generally more cost effective than ST because the procedure does not take up OR time and staff. In terms of complications, numerous studies have been completed comparing ST and PDT, some indicating a higher incidence of bleeding and infection with ST as compared with PDT, with others reporting no significant difference. There also have been several meta-analyses published comparing complication rates between ST and PDT, generally with equivalent results. A recent meta-analysis of 17 randomized controlled trials containing a total of 1212 patients found PDT was associated with fewer infections and less bleeding as compared with surgical tracheostomy completed either in the OR or at the bedside. Another meta-analysis of five prospective studies performed by Freeman and colleagues involving 115 patients receiving PDT (via the Ciaglia technique) and 121 STs found no significant difference in the overall operative complication rate. PDT was associated with a reduction in operative bleeding, and postoperative complications were significantly less common in the PDT group.

However, not all meta-analyses have shown complication rates in favor of PDT. An earlier meta-analysis of 65 observational, retrospective and prospective trials published by Dulguerov and colleagues examined serious perioperative complications, including death, cardiorespiratory arrest, pneumothorax and pneumomediastinum, which were significantly less common in the ST group as compared with the PDT group (86 vs 149 per 10,000 cases, respectively). Intermediate perioperative complications such as desaturation, hypotension, and injury to the posterior tracheal wall were also less common in the ST group. However, the incidence of these complications is small: injury to the posterior tracheal wall occurs in 6 out of 10,000 patients in the ST group as compared with 50/10,000 in the PDT group. The rates of serious postoperative complications (death, tracheoesophageal fistula, mediastinitis, sepsis, postoperative cannula obstruction or displacement, and tracheal stenosis) were similar in the ST and PDT groups. Minor hemorrhage and wound infections were less common in the PDT group.

■ SUMMARY

Tracheostomy is an extremely common procedure that can be performed safely both in the OR and at the bedside in the ICU using a surgical technique or PDT. As with any procedure, tracheostomy should be performed by experienced personnel with additional expertise in airway management. Benefits to PDT over ST include cost savings compared with ST performed in the OR, but minimal savings when compared with ST performed at the bedside. However, PDT may be associated with less delay once the decision to perform tracheotomy is made. There are still various circumstances when ST is preferred and the safer option over PDT, making it important for intensivists and surgeons to understand the relative benefits and risks of both techniques.

SUGGESTED READINGS

Delaney A, Bagshaw SM, Nalos M. Percutaneous dilatational tracheostomy versus surgical tracheostomy in critically ill patients: a systematic review and meta-analysis. *Crit Care (London, England)*. 2006;10:R55.

Dennis BM, Eckert MJ, Gunter OL, Morris JA Jr, May AK. Safety of bedside percutaneous tracheostomy in the critically ill: evaluation of more than 3,000 procedures. *Journal of the Am Coll Surgeons*. 2013;216:858-865, discussion 865-857.

Siempos II, Ntaidou TK, Filippidis FT, Choi AM. Effect of early versus late or no tracheostomy on mortality and pneumonia of critically ill patients receiving mechanical ventilation: a systematic review and meta-analysis. *Lancet Respir Med*. 2015;3:150-158.

Young D, Harrison DA, Cuthbertson BH, Rowan K. Effect of early vs late tracheostomy placement on survival in patients receiving mechanical ventilation: the TracMan randomized trial. *J Am Med Assoc*. 2013;309: 2121-2129.

TRACHEOSTOMY, PART TWO

Lena M. Napolitano, MD, FACS, FCCP, FCCM

Acute respiratory failure requiring mechanical ventilation is common in critical illness. Progressive advancements in technologies for the care of the critically ill have resulted in an increase in the number of patients who remain dependent on mechanical ventilation. Prolonged translaryngeal endotracheal intubation (TEI) increases the risk of ventilator-associated pneumonia (VAP) by bypassing and disabling the laryngeal mechanisms promoting oropharyngeal contamination of the bronchial tree and lung. Prolonged TEI also is associated with the development of sinusitis and may cause severe laryngeal and tracheal damage. Placement of a tracheostomy is a viable alternative to prolonged TEI, with the benefits of improving patient comfort, reduced need for sedation, lowering airway resistance, and allowing for easier airway care. The indications, technique, timing, and selection of critically ill patients for tracheostomy have been topics of considerable debate that are addressed in this chapter.

■ EPIDEMIOLOGY

In a study of the National Inpatient Sample from 1993 to 2012, 9.1% of mechanical ventilation patients (1,352,432 adults) underwent tracheostomy, and tracheostomy was more common in surgical patients. The average number of tracheostomies performed annually in the United States now is more than 100,000.

■ INDICATIONS FOR TRACHEOSTOMY

General indications for the placement of tracheostomy include acute respiratory failure with the expected need for prolonged mechanical ventilation, failure to wean from mechanical ventilation, upper airway obstruction, difficult airway, and copious secretions (Box 1). The most common indications for tracheostomy are (1) acute respiratory failure necessitating prolonged mechanical ventilation (representing two thirds of all cases) and (2) traumatic or catastrophic neurologic insult requiring either airway protection or mechanical ventilation or both. Upper airway obstruction is a less common indication for tracheostomy.

■ COMPLICATIONS OF TRACHEOSTOMY

Tracheostomy complications can be considered in three time frames: immediate, early, and late complications (Table 1). Complications related to tracheostomies include pneumothorax, bleeding, subglottic stenosis, tracheoesophageal fistula, vocal cord dysfunction, stomal granulation, persistent tracheal fistula, and scarring. In the most recent prospective randomized tracheostomy trials, adverse events associated with tracheostomy were common, especially bleeding, but were not life threatening. All clinicians who are credentialed to perform tracheostomy should be familiar with the proper methods of managing complications associated with tracheostomy.

■ OUTCOMES OF TRACHEOSTOMY

Because the main indication for tracheostomy is in patients with acute respiratory failure requiring mechanical ventilation, it is no surprise that the mortality rates in tracheostomy patients are high. A recent systematic review reported pooled mortality at hospital discharge was 29%, 1-year mortality was 59%, only 19% were discharged to home, and only 50% were successfully liberated from mechanical ventilation.

■ TIMING OF TRACHEOSTOMY

Optimal timing for tracheostomy has remained controversial. The question of early versus late tracheostomy is complex and requires a two-part assessment: first, we must predict which patients will require prolonged ventilation, and second, we must make a decision about when the tracheostomy should be performed. If prediction of prolonged ventilation is imperfect, then a strategy of early tracheostomy will lead to some patients undergoing tracheostomy unnecessarily, whereas a strategy of late tracheostomy will result in other patients facing unnecessarily prolonged TEI and potentially prolonged weaning from mechanical ventilation.

The definition of "early" tracheostomy differs between studies. Of the trials from the past decade, "early" was generally defined as within 3 to 10 days of mechanical ventilation, whereas "late" was variously defined as any time outside the "early" period, such as in 7 to 14 days, 14 to 28 days, or greater than 28 days after initiation of mechanical ventilation.

2010 Early Versus Late Tracheotomy Study, Italian Multicenter Prospective Randomized Trial

The 2010 Early Versus Late Tracheotomy Study Italian Multicenter Prospective Randomized trial was performed in 12 Italian ICUs from June 2004 to June 2008 and enrolled 600 adult patients without pneumonia (estimated by a Clinical Pulmonary Infection Score, CPIS, of <6) who had been ventilated for 24 hours, had a Simplified Acute Physiology score II between 35 and 65, and a Sequential Organ Failure Assessment (SOFA) score of 5 or greater. These patients were monitored for 48 hours, and those with worsening respiratory failure, unchanged or worse SOFA score, and no pneumonia then were randomized to early (after 6 to 8 days of laryngeal intubation, n = 209) or late (after 13 to 15 days of laryngeal intubation, n = 210) tracheostomy.

The primary outcome measure was VAP, with secondary endpoints of 28-day assessment of ventilator-free days, intensive care unit (ICU)–free days, and survival. The presence of VAP was defined using the simplified CPIS, with CPIS score greater than 6 indicative of VAP, calculated at study entry, at randomization, and every 72 hours until study day 28.

This study included both medical and surgical patients with no difference in early (40% medical, 8% scheduled surgery, 41% unscheduled surgery, 11% trauma) versus late (36% medical, 10% scheduled surgery, 45% unscheduled surgery, 9% trauma) tracheostomy groups. Many of the randomized patients did not undergo tracheostomy (31% early and 43% late) related to proximity to either extubation or death. In the early group, 145 of 209 patients (69%) underwent tracheostomy compared with 119 of 210 patients (57%) in the late group.

All tracheostomies were performed bedside using percutaneous techniques (Griggs technique in 72% early and 73% late; PercuTwist technique in 25% early and 22% late groups). Adverse events occurred in 39% of early and late tracheostomy groups, with postoperative stoma inflammation most common, occurring in 15% of each group.

VAP, defined by CPIS, developed in 30 (14%) of early versus 44 (21%) of late tracheostomy patients (P = 0.07). Although the number of ICU-free and ventilator-free days was higher in the early tracheostomy group, the long-term outcome endpoint of 28-day survival (154/209, 74% early vs 144/210, 68% late, P = 0.25) did not differ. The use of CPIS for VAP diagnosis is a significant limitation in this study. The diagnostic accuracy of CPIS is limited in surgical, trauma, and burn patients as CPIS was unable to differentiate VAP from systemic inflammatory response syndrome. Furthermore, the utility of the modified CPIS to diagnose VAP was assessed in 740 patients enrolled in a multicenter randomized trial, and no CPIS threshold was clinically useful (ROC AUC [receiver

BOX 1: Indications for Tracheostomy

Prolonged intubation
Facilitation of ventilation support/ventilator weaning
More efficient pulmonary hygiene (i.e., managing secretions)
Upper airway obstruction with any of the following:
- Stridor, air hunger, retractions
- Obstructive sleep apnea with documented arterial desaturation
- Bilateral vocal cord paralysis
Inability to intubate
Adjunct to major head and neck surgery/trauma management
Airway protection (neurologic diseases, traumatic brain injury)

TABLE 1: Complications of Tracheostomy

Immediate Complications	Early Complications	Late Complications
Hemorrhage	Hemorrhage	Tracheal stenosis
Structure damage to trachea	Tube displacement	Granulation tissue
	Pneumothorax	Tracheomalacia
Failure of procedure	Pneumomediastinum	Pneumonia
	Subcutaneous emphysema	Aspiration event
Aspiration event		Tracheoarterial fistula
Air embolism	Stomal infection	
Loss of airway	Stomal ulceration	Tracheoesophageal fistula
Death	Accidental decannulation	
Hypoxemia, hypercarbia	Dysphagia	Accidental decannulation
		Dysphagia

operator characteristic/area under curve] 0.47, 95% confidence interval [CI]: 0.42-0.53).

Early tracheostomy (performed after 6 to 8 days of endotracheal intubation) did not result in significant reduction in the incidence of VAP compared with late tracheostomy (performed after 13 to 15 days of endotracheal intubation) and was associated with an adverse event related to the tracheostomy procedure in more than one third of patients. These data suggest that tracheostomy should not be performed earlier than after 13 to 15 days of intubation.

2013 TracMan: Largest Multicenter Prospective Randomized Trial, United Kingdom

The TracMan trial was an open multicenter randomized controlled trial conducted from 2004 through 2011 in 70 adult general and 2 cardiothoracic ICUs in 13 university and 59 nonuniversity hospitals in the United Kingdom. Of 1032 eligible patients, 909 patients were enrolled. Inclusion criteria were mechanically ventilated patients in adult ICUs who were identified by the treating clinician in the first 4 days after admission as likely to require at least 7 more days of ventilator support. Exclusion criteria included those in whom immediate tracheostomy was needed, contraindicated because of anatomic or other reasons, or respiratory failure because of chronic neurologic diseases since study centers indicated those patients receive early tracheostomies.

Patients were randomized to early (within 4 days after intubation, n = 455) or late (after 10 days if still indicated, n = 454) tracheostomy. Most patients were medical (n = 712, 79.2% of study cohort) with respiratory failure as the primary admission diagnosis (n = 515, 59.5%).

In the early tracheostomy group 91.9% of the patients received tracheostomy as planned; in contrast, in the late tracheostomy group, only 45.5% of patients required tracheostomy. Many patients in the late tracheostomy group were liberated from mechanical ventilation without requiring tracheostomy. Percutaneous tracheostomy technique was used in 90%, with 88.7% performed in the ICU at the bedside, and the majority (n = 426, 77.3%) used a single-tapered dilator technique. Complications related to tracheostomy occurred in 6.3% of patients with the majority (3.1%) related to bleeding, and no difference between the early group (5.5%) versus the late group (7.8%).

No differences in 30-day mortality (30.8% early vs 31.5% late), 2-year mortality (51.0% early vs 53.7% late), or median ICU length of stay in survivors (13.0 days early vs 13.1 days late) were identified. No difference in hospital length of stay or duration of mechanical ventilation was identified. Early tracheostomy was associated with significantly decreased sedation use. In survivors at 30 days after randomization, the median number of days on which any sedatives were received was 5 (interquartile range [IQR], 3 to 9) days in the early group and 8 (IQR, 4 to 12) days in the late group ($P = 0.001$), with a mean difference between the groups of 2.4 (95% CI: 1.6-3.6) days. No specific assessment of VAP was performed in this study, but antibiotic use to 30 days after randomization was the same in both groups.

This study confirmed that tracheostomy within 4 days of ICU admission was not associated with an improvement in 30-day mortality or other important secondary outcome. This study also documented that the ability of clinicians to predict which patients required extended ventilator support was limited. At the study's presentation at the Twenty-Ninth International Symposium of Intensive Care and Emergency Medicine, the lead author stated the following: "If you had 100 patients requiring tracheostomy, doing it early results in 2.4 days less sedation overall, but you would perform 48 more, with 3 more procedural complications and no effect on mortality or ICU length of stay."

Limitations of European Tracheostomy Timing Studies

There are significant limitations of the recent large randomized controlled trials regarding tracheostomy timing:

- Small number of trauma and surgical patients
- Different outcomes measures: all-cause mortality versus VAP versus ICU/ventilator-free days
- VAP was not measured in the TracMan trial
- VAP definition was problematic in Italian trial (CPIS > 6 not valid in surgical and trauma patients)
- Italian trial controlled for weaning and sedative/analgesic use, but TracMan did not
- No standardization of tracheostomy technique (open or percutaneous in TracMan; Griggs vs PercTwist in Italian multicenter trial)
- No large U.S. randomized controlled trial to date

2015 Meta-Analysis

Analyses of 13 trials (n = 2434 patients) confirmed no difference in all-cause ICU mortality in patients who received early tracheostomy versus the late or no tracheostomy cohort (Figure 1). There was also no evidence of a difference in 1-year mortality (RR 0.93, 95% CI: 0.85-1.02, $P = 0.14$, 3 trials with 1529 patients). The incidence of VAP was lower in the early tracheostomy group (OR 0.60, 95% CI: 0.41-0.90, $P = 0.01$; 13 trials with 1599 patients), but the VAP definitions used in these studies was not rigorous.

The recent large randomized trials (Italian multicenter trial and TracMan U.K. multicenter trial) are consistent in the findings that earlier tracheostomy was not associated with improved survival and that clinicians cannot predict accurately which patients will require

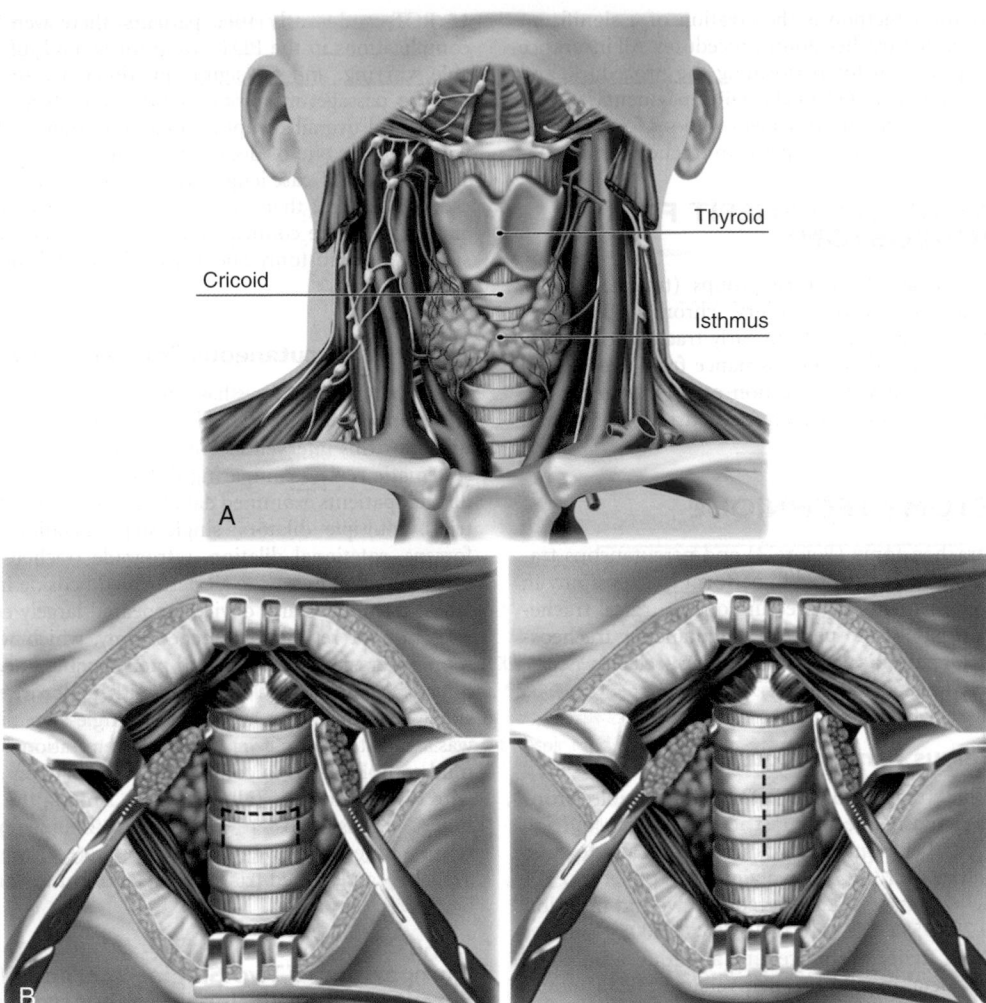

FIGURE 3 A, Surgical open tracheostomy requires knowledge of neck anatomy. **B,** Optimal surgical technique includes a vertical skin incision below the inferior cricoid cartilage, retraction of strap muscles bilaterally, and retraction of the thyroid isthmus either superiorly or inferiorly or divided for anterior tracheal exposure. An anterior tracheal incision (horizontal [*left*] or vertical [*right*]) is created at the first or second tracheal rings. A sideways "H" incision is ideal and provides an "open book" exposure without resection.

TABLE 3: Specific Techniques for Percutaneous Tracheostomy Procedure

Methodology	Year	Technique
Sequential dilators, Ciaglia	1985	Multistep dilation with sequential dilators, antegrade
Dilating forceps, Griggs	1990	Dilation with specific forceps, antegrade
Translaryngeal tracheostomy, Fantoni	1997	Retrograde passage; specific cannula acts as dilator and tracheostomy tube
Single-step dilator, Ciaglia Blue Rhino	1999	Single-step dilation with a curved dilator and loading dilator, antegrade
Dilating screw, Frova/Quintel	2002	Self-trapping screw, antegrade
T-Dagger, Ambesh	2005	Single-step dilation with a curved, T-shaped dilator, elliptical in cross section, antegrade
Balloon-facilitated dilational tracheostomy, Ciaglia Blue Dolphin	2005	Single-step dilation with balloon and loading dilator assembly, antegrade

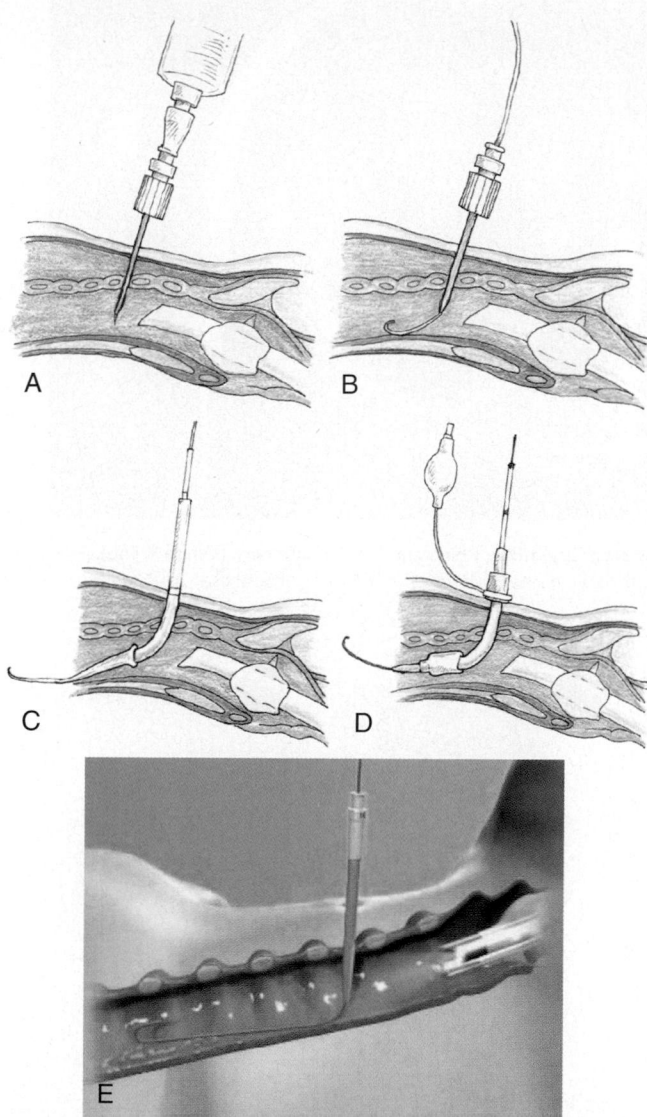

FIGURE 4 Percutaneous dilational tracheostomy (PDT). PDT should be performed with flexible bronchoscopy guidance to visualize the anterior entry site of the needle, to avoid posterior tracheal injury, and to ensure that the guidewire and dilator are advanced distally. The single graded dilator technique is optimal. Advantages of PDT include the following: (1) time required for bedside PDT is shorter than for open tracheostomy; (2) scheduling difficulty associated with operating room (OR) and anesthesiology for intensive care unit patients is eliminated; (3) PDT expedites performance of the procedure because critically ill patients who would require intensive monitoring to and from the OR need not be transported; (4) cost of performing PDT is roughly half that of open surgical tracheostomy because of the savings in OR charges and anesthesiology fees. (*From Kong MS, Brietzke SE, Schindler JS, Bliznikas D, Baredes S. Percutaneous tracheotomy treatment and management. Medscape. <http://emedicine.medscape.com/article/866567-treatment#a1133>.*)

have been established: Size 8 Shiley tracheostomy with the 28F loading dilator; size 8 Bivona Hyperflex and Portex Blue Line Adjustable flange with 24F loading dilator. There is no gap between the loading dilator and tracheostomy tube with these combinations.

New Longer Tapered Tip and Low-Profile Tracheostomy Tubes for Percutaneous Dilational Tracheostomy

A simple solution to the poor fit of regular tracheostomy tubes and loading dilators in the PDT kit is to use tracheostomy tube that are made specifically for PDT with a longer distal tapered tip and a low profile cuff (Table 4). This reduces the force required for tracheostomy insertion with PDT and allows a safer and more rapid procedure to be performed.

Need for Proximal or Distal Extension Tracheostomy

Proximal extension tracheostomy may be required with thick neck anatomy and in obese patients, and distal extension tracheostomy may be required in patients with long tracheal anatomy, tracheal obstruction (to get tip distal to the obstruction), or tracheomalacia (Figure 7). PDT has been contraindicated in these patients, but the recent development and availability of new longer percutaneous tracheostomy tubes (VersaTube) has provided additional PDT options for these challenging patients who require distal extension tracheostomy.

Two New Percutaneous Tracheostomy Procedures

Ciaglia Blue Dolphin

The new balloon dilation PDT technique uses primarily radial force to widen the tracheostomy (Ciaglia Blue Dolphin system, Figure 8). The initial experience with this method reported that tracheostomy surgery time averaged 3.3 ± 1.9 minutes with minimal complications. Another single-center study randomized trial (n = 70) comparing single-step (Rhino) and balloon (Dolphin) dilational tracheostomy in ICU patients reported that median procedure time was significantly shorter in the Rhino group compared with the Dolphin group (1.5 vs 4 minutes, $P = 0.035$), and the presence of limited intratracheal bleeding at bronchoscopy 6 hours postprocedure was more frequent in the Dolphin group (68.6% vs 34.3%, $P = 0.008$). Although the Blue Dolphin technique is feasible, the PDT Rhino technique had a shorter execution time and was associated with fewer tracheal injuries. Additional studies are warranted to validate these disparate findings.

PercuTwist

The controlled rotating dilatation method (PercuTwist) is a relatively new technique and was used in the ELTS Italian Multicenter early versus later tracheostomy trial (Figure 9). A recent study compared techniques (n = 130) of PDT: guidewire dilating forceps technique (Griggs) and PercuTwist technique. The duration of the procedure was significantly shorter in the PercuTwist group compared with each of the other groups. It was easy to perform, was associated with minimal complications, and is a practical alternative to the PDT technique, which is performed most commonly. Limitations to this study include the small sample size; use of the Ciaglia multiple dilator kit for PDT, which is inferior to the single dilator kit; and comparison with a technique that is not used frequently, the guidewire-dilating forceps technique.

High-Risk Patients and Percutaneous Dilational Tracheostomy

Potentially high-risk patients for PDT include those with coagulopathy, thrombocytopenia, and other bleeding diatheses, or obesity. The largest study examining this reported a single-center prospective analysis of 1000 PDT procedures (2001 to 2009) in ICU patients with increased bleeding risk or obesity. They identified that increased international normalized ratio (INR) was the most important risk factor for bleeding (OR 2.99, 95% CI: 1.26-7.08) followed by thrombocytopenia with platelet count less than 100,000 (OR 1.99, 95% CI: 0.99-3.95). Interestingly, platelet dysfunction associated with continuous renal replacement therapy was not associated with increased bleeding risk (OR 1.02, 95% CI: 0.39-2.66). The rate of complications in patients with high body mass index was not increased. The decision to perform percutaneous tracheostomy in a patient with obesity or coagulopathy should take into account factors

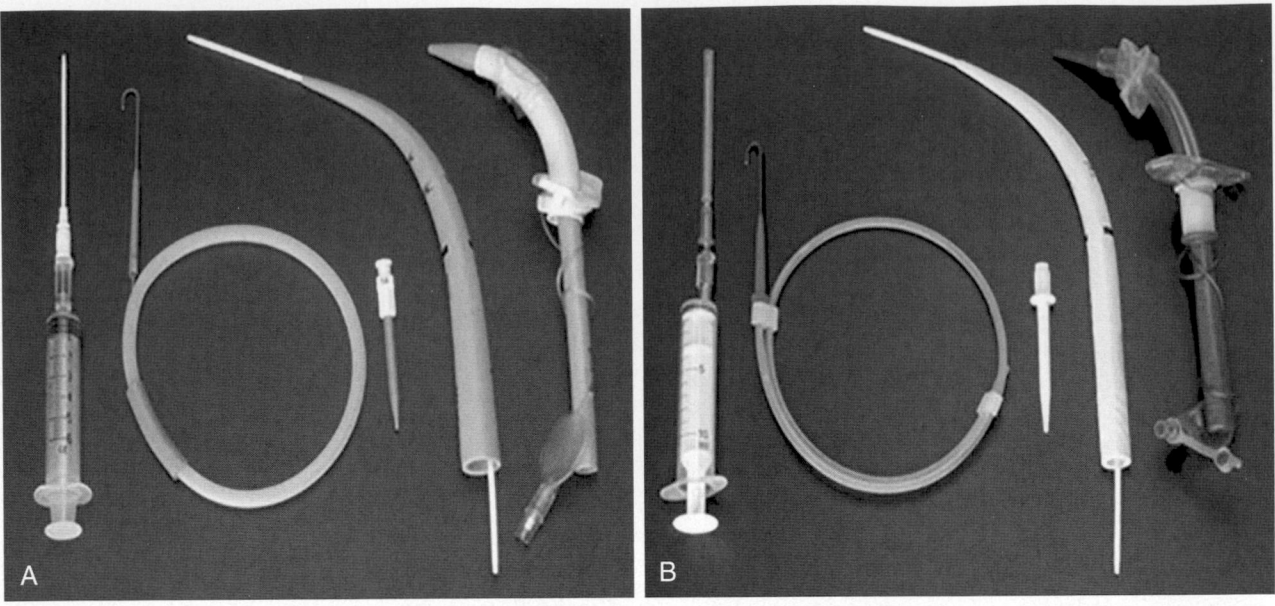

FIGURE 5 Comparison of two single tapered dilator percutaneous tracheostomy sets: Ciaglia Blue Rhino and Portex Ultraperc (White Rhino). *(From Patel PB, Ferguson C, Patel A. A comparison of two single dilator percutaneous tracheostomy sets: the Blue Rhino and the Ultraperc. Anaesthesia. 2006;61:182-186.)*

Shiley 10 Dilator 28F   Shiley 8 Dilator 28F   Bivona 8 Dilator 24F   Blueline 8 Dilator 24F

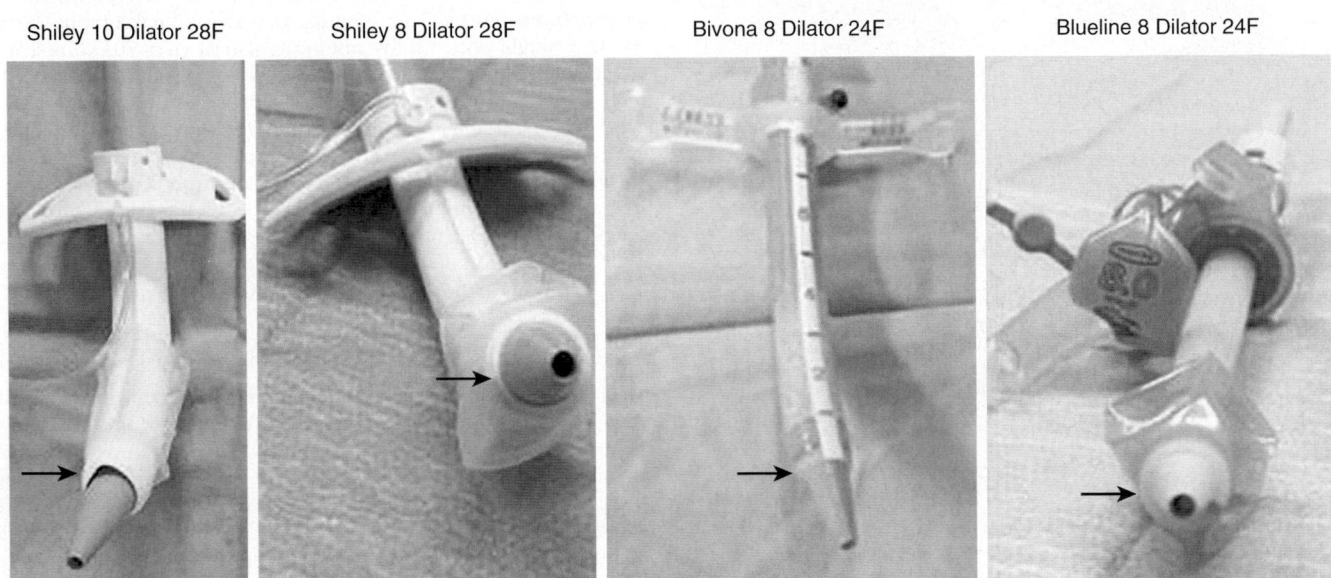

FIGURE 6 Diametrical differences between PDT loading dilators and percutaneous tracheostomy tubes. Size 10 Shiley loaded over 28F loading dilator leaves an "escalated step." Note the deformity (Black Arrow) caused by the "step" during the process of insertion of the tube. Best fit combinations: size Shiley 8 and 28F loading dilator; size 8 of both Bivona Hyperflex and Portex Blueline adjustable flange with 24F loading dilator. There is no gap between the loading dilator and the tube *(arrows)*. *(From Majeed A, Kannan S. Diametrical differences between Blue-Rhino kit loading dilators and percutaneous tracheostomy tubes. <http://www.apicareonline.com/?p=892>.)*

TABLE 4: Tapered Tracheostomy Tubes for Use With Percutaneous Dilational Tracheostomy

Tube	Inner Diameter (mm)	Outer Diameter (mm)	Length (mm)
Portex Per-fit 7	7.0 (6.0 with IC)	9.6	82
Portex Per-fit 8	8.0 (7.0 with IC)	10.9	86
Portex Per-fit 9	9.0 (8.0 with IC)	12.3	93
Shiley PERC 6	6.4	10.8	74
Shiley PERC 8	7.6	12.2	79
VersaTube 7	7.0 (6.0 with IC)	10.0	78
VersaTube 8	8.0 (7.0 with IC)	11.0	86
VersaTube 9	9.0 (8.0 with IC)	12.0	97

Courtesy Cook Medical: https://www.cookmedical.com/data/resources/CC-BM-VTQRC-EN-201102.pdf. Courtesy Smith's Medical: http://www.smiths-medical.com/catalog/portex-percutaneous-tracheostomy-kits/pdt/perfit/per-fit-percutaneous-tracheostomy.html.

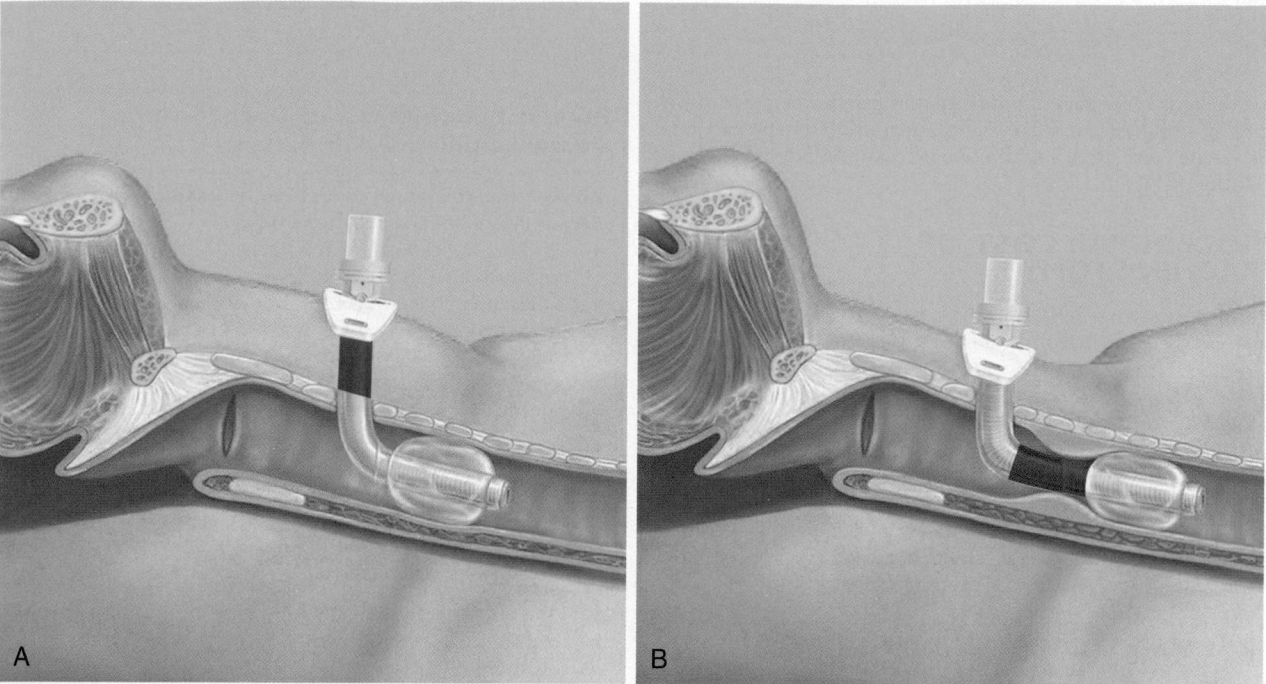

FIGURE 7 Percutaneous dilational tracheostomy limitations: need for proximal extension (**A**) or distal extension (**B**) tracheostomy. Black section indicates additional length. *Proximal extension*: For full or thick neck. *Distal extension*: For long tracheal anatomy, tracheal stenosis, or tracheomalacia.

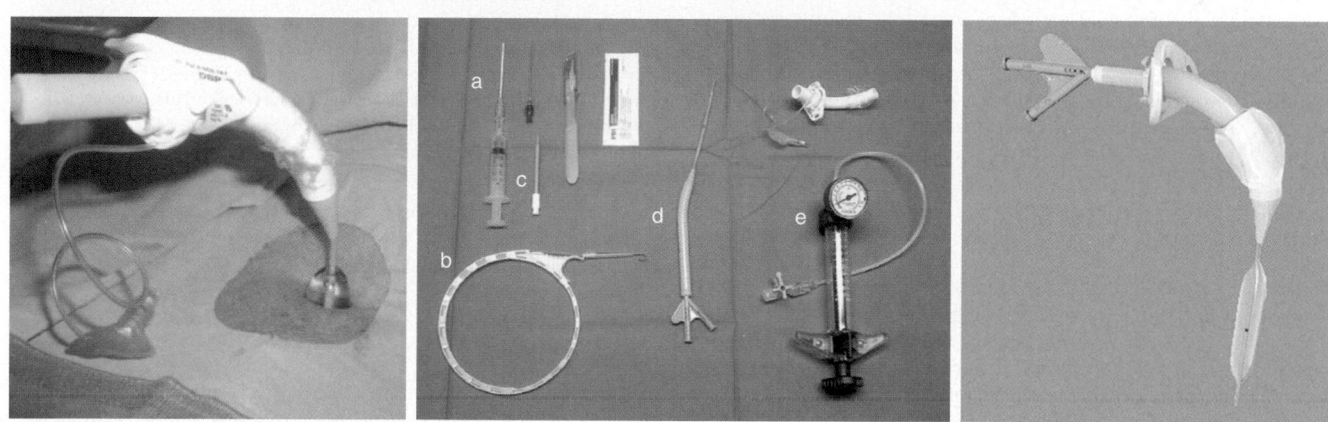

FIGURE 8 Ciaglia Blue Dolphin percutaneous technique. This is a safe and effective percutaneous tracheostomy technique that uses radial outward dilation to minimize bleeding and injury to tracheal rings. Tracheostomy surgery time averaged 3.3 ± 1.9 minutes. No evidence of increased complications. *(From Gromann TW, et al. Anesth Analg. 2009;108:1862-1866.)*

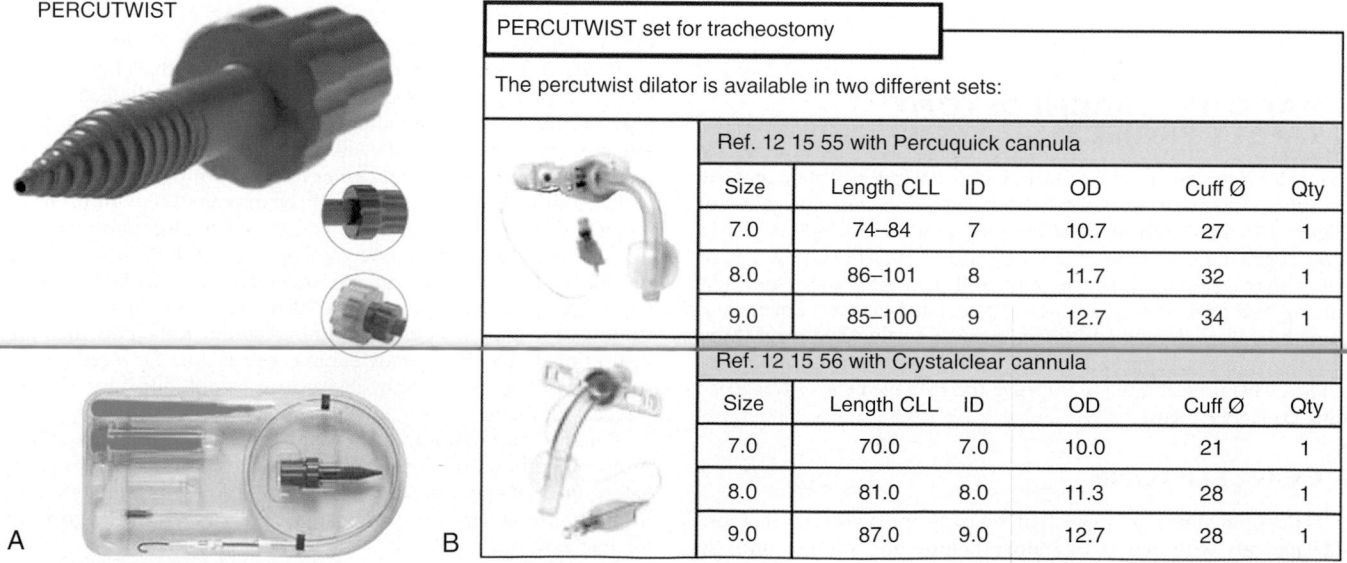

PERCUTWIST

PERCUTWIST set for tracheostomy

The percutwist dilator is available in two different sets:

Ref. 12 15 55 with Percuquick cannula					
Size	Length CLL	ID	OD	Cuff Ø	Qty
7.0	74–84	7	10.7	27	1
8.0	86–101	8	11.7	32	1
9.0	85–100	9	12.7	34	1

Ref. 12 15 56 with Crystalclear cannula					
Size	Length CLL	ID	OD	Cuff Ø	Qty
7.0	70.0	7.0	10.0	21	1
8.0	81.0	8.0	11.3	28	1
9.0	87.0	9.0	12.7	28	1

FIGURE 9 PercuTwist Technique of percutaneous tracheostomy. *(Courtesy Teleflex: <http://www.teleflex.com/emea/documentLibrary/documents/939940-000011_Tracheostomy_1305.pdf>.)*

such as the individual patient's neck anatomy and experience of the performing physician, and the practitioner must be prepared to convert to the open surgical technique if complications are encountered during PDT.

■ PROCEDURAL COST OF TRACHEOSTOMY

Significant cost savings related to PDT versus surgical open tracheostomy have been reported (see Figure 2). On average, procedural costs for PDT are approximately 50% less than open surgical tracheostomy, and the reduced cost is related mostly to lack of use of the operating room and anesthesia teams. The cost difference does depend, however, on whether the open surgical tracheostomy is performed in the operating room or bedside in the ICU. We have the capability to perform open tracheostomy in the ICU bedside and have all appropriate equipment, including headlights, operating room portable light, fine-point electrocautery, and surgical tracheostomy trays for all appropriate surgical equipment.

■ TRACHEOSTOMY DECANNULATION

Decisions regarding optimal timing for tracheostomy decannulation require clinical judgment, particularly with determination that the indication for tracheostomy has resolved. A recent clinical consensus statement on tracheostomy care achieved consensus on 77 statements with the goal to reduce variations in practice when managing tracheostomy patients to minimize complications. A list of prerequisites for consideration for tracheostomy decannulation in adults is provided (Box 3), and we strongly recommend consideration of type/quantity of secretions and suctioning frequency required.

■ MULTIDISCIPLINARY TRACHEOSTOMY TEAM

Tracheostomy teams enhance consistency of patient care and implementation of standardized protocols of care. The use of an intensivist-led tracheostomy team was associated with shorter decannulation time and length of stay. Additional studies have reported that use of a dedicated multidisciplinary team designed to streamline tracheostomy practice was associated with increased PDT, decreased procedural complications, reduced procedure time, and improved efficiency. The implementation of a multidisciplinary percutaneous tracheostomy team documented a significant reduction in airway injury (6.8% vs 1.1%, $P = 0.006$), hypoxemia (13.6% vs 3.3%, $P = 0.005$), loss of airway (5.1% vs 0.5%, $P = 0.039$), and overall complication rate (25.4% vs. 4.9%, $P < 0.001$). No difference in stoma infection or mortality was identified.

■ NATIONAL TRACHEOSTOMY SAFETY PROJECT

The U.K. National Tracheostomy Safety Project has standardized resources for education of both healthcare providers and patients (Figure 10). Three self-directed learning modules include (1) basic knowledge (anatomy, physiology, indications, procedures); (2) emergency management (tracheostomy and laryngectomy), and (3) nursing and general care, including associated devices. Emergency algorithms were developed by consensus, and the final algorithms describe a universal approach to management of tracheostomy emergencies. This project aims to improve the management of tracheostomy critical incidents.

■ CONCLUSIONS

In conclusion, there is no benefit to early tracheostomy in most ICU patients with acute respiratory failure, and waiting until at

---

BOX 3: Prerequisites for Tracheostomy Decannulation in Adult Patients*

Answer the following to determine readiness of patient for decannulation of tracheostomy tube:

- Have the indications for the tracheostomy placement resolved or significantly improved?
- Is the patient tolerating a decannulation cap on an appropriately sized uncuffed tracheostomy tube without stridor?
- Does fiberoptic laryngoscopy confirm airway patency to the level of the glottis and immediate subglottis?
- Does the patient have an adequate level of consciousness and laryngopharyngeal function to protect the lower airway from aspiration?
- Does the patient have an effective cough while the tracheostomy tube is capped?
- Have all procedures that require general endotracheal anesthesia been completed?

If yes to all, proceed with the following decannulation process:

- Remove the tracheostomy tube
- Clean the site
- Cover the site with a dry gauze dressing
- Instruct the patient to apply pressure over the dressing with fingers when talking or coughing
- Change dressing daily and as needed if moist with secretions until the site has healed
- Monitor for decannulation failure

From Mitchell RB, Hussey HM, Setzen G, Jacobs IN, Nussenbaum B, Dawson C, Brown CA 3rd, Brandt C, Deakins K, Hartnick C, Merati A. Clinical consensus statement: tracheostomy care. *Otolaryngol Head Neck Surg.* 2013;148:6-20.

*In addition to the factors listed above, consider the type and amount of tracheal secretions, and the frequency of tracheal suctioning required prior to consideration of decannulation.

---

least 10 to 14 days of intubation and mechanical ventilation is recommended to determine whether ongoing respiratory support is required. There may be special patient populations that may benefit from early tracheostomy, including the following: (1) patients with a high likelihood of prolonged mechanical ventilation (ARDS, COPD, failed primary extubation), (2) patients with spinal cord injury or chronic neurologic disorders, and (3) traumatic brain injury patients and other patients with need for airway.

Recent large randomized trials have confirmed that clinicians and intensivists are poor at predicting who will need prolonged intubation and mechanical ventilation. There is a need for tools to accurately predict which patients will require prolonged intubation and therefore could benefit from earlier tracheostomy.

The optimal technique for tracheostomy is PDT with bronchoscopic guidance, except in those patients with contraindications to PDT (coagulopathy, thrombocytopenia, other risk factors for bleeding, inadequate surface landmarks, inability to tolerate hypoxemia or hypercarbia, need for proximal or distal extension tracheostomy). Choice of technique must take into account both individual and institutional experience, body habitus, risk factors for bleeding, and pathophysiology (i.e., airway obstruction or not, difficulty of endotracheal intubation).

Finally, "tracheostomy teams" are associated with standardized protocols and improved outcomes. The U.K. National Tracheostomy Safety Project has standardized resources for education for both healthcare providers and patients, including emergency algorithms for tracheostomy incidents.

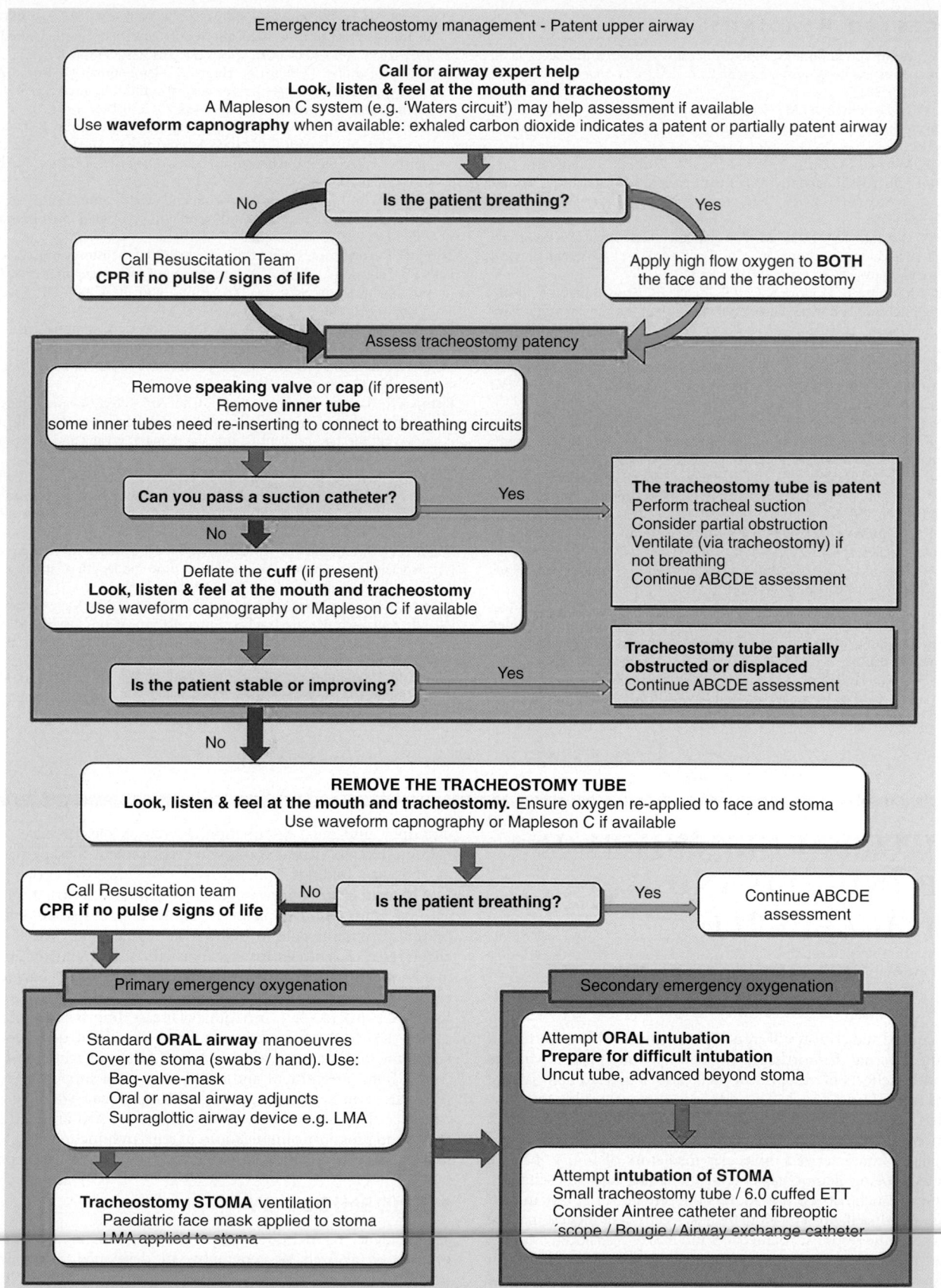

FIGURE 10 UK National Tracheostomy Safety Project algorithm. *(From National Safety Tracheostomy Project <www.tracheostomy.org.uk>. Reproduced from McGrath BA, Bates L, Atkinson D, Moore JA. Multidisciplinary guidelines for the management of tracheostomy and laryngectomy airway emergencies. Anaesthesia. 2012;67:1025-1041, with permission from the Association of Anaesthetists of Great Britain & Ireland/Blackwell Publishing Ltd.)*

SUGGESTED READINGS

Cabrini L, Monti G, Landoni G, Biondi-Zoccai G, Boroli F, Mamo D, et al. Percutaneous tracheostomy, a systematic review. *Acta Anaesthesiol Scand.* 2012;56:270-281.

Cheung NH, Napolitano LM. Tracheostomy: epidemiology, indications, timing, technique and outcomes. *Respir Care.* 2014;59:895-915, discussion 916-919.

Damuth E, Mitchell JA, Bartock JL, Roberts BW, Trzeciak S. Long-term survival of critically ill patients treated with prolonged mechanical ventilation: a systematic review and meta-analysis. *Lancet Respir Med.* 2015;3:544-553.

Delaney A, Bagshaw SM, Nalos M. Percutaneous dilatational tracheostomy versus surgical tracheostomy in critically ill patients: a systematic review and meta-analysis. *Crit Care.* 2006;10:R55.

Fartoukh M, Maitre B, Honore S, Cerf C, Zahar JR, Brun-Buisson C. Diagnosing pneumonia during mechanical ventilation: the clinical pulmonary infection score revisited. *Am J Respir Crit Care Med.* 2003;168:173-179.

Frova G, Quintel M. A new simple method for percutaneous tracheostomy: controlled rotating dilation: a preliminary report. *Intens Care Med.* 2002;28:299-303.

Griggs WM, Myburgh JA, Worthley LI. A prospective comparison of a percutaneous tracheostomy technique with standard surgical tracheostomy. *Intens Care Med.* 1991;17:261-263.

Gromann TW, Birkelbach O, Hetzer R. Balloon dilatational tracheostomy: initial experience with the Ciaglia Blue Dolphin method. *Anesth Analg.* 2009;108:1862-1866.

Higgins KM, Punthakee X. Meta-analysis comparison of open versus percutaneous tracheostomy. *Laryngoscope.* 2007;117:447-454.

Johns Hopkins Medical Institutes. *Tracheostomy.* <http://www.hopkinsmedicine.org/tracheostomy/>.

Lauzier F, Cook D, Heyland D, Dodek P, Albert M, Shorr AF, et al. Canadian Critical Care Trials Group. The value of pretest probability and modified clinical pulmonary infection score to diagnose ventilator-associated pneumonia. *J Crit Care.* 2008;23:50-57.

McGrath BA, Bates L, Atkinson D, Moore JA. Multidisciplinary guidelines for the management of tracheostomy and laryngectomy airway emergencies. *Anaesthesia.* 2012;67:1025-1041.

Mehta AB, Syeda SN, Bajpayee L, Cooke CR, Walkey AJ, Wiener RS. Trends in Tracheostomy for Mechanically Ventilated Patients in the United States, 1993-2012. *Am J Respir Crit Care Med.* 2015;192:446-454.

Mirski MA, Pandian V, Bhatti N, Haut E, Feller-Kopman D, Morad A, et al. Safety, efficacy, and cost-effectiveness of a ultidisciplinary percutaneous tracheostomy program. *Crit Care Med.* 2012;40:1827-1834.

Mitchell RB, Hussey HM, Setzen G, Jacobs IN, Nussenbaum B, Dawson C, Brown CA 3rd, Brandt C, Deakins K, Hartnick C, Merati A. Clinical consensus statement: tracheostomy care. *Otolaryngol Head Neck Surg.* 2013;148:6-20.

Napolitano LM. Use of severity scoring and stratification factors in clinical trials of hospital-acquired and ventilator-associated pneumonia. *Clin Infect Dis.* 2010;51:S67-S80.

National Tracheostomy Safety Project. <http://tracheostomy.org.uk/>.

Patel PB, Ferguson C, Patel A. A comparison of two single dilator percutaneous tracheostomy sets: the Blue Rhino and the Ultraperc. *Anaesthesia.* 2006;61:182-186.

Rosseland LA, Laake JH, Stubhaug A. Percutaneous dilatational tracheotomy in intensive care unit patients with increased bleeding risk or obesity. A prospective analysis of 1000 procedures. *Acta Anaesthesiol Scand.* 2011;55:835-841.

Siempos II, Ntaidou TK, Filippidis FT, Choi AM. Effect of early versus late or no tracheostomy on mortality and pneumonia of critically ill patients receiving mechanical ventilation: a systematic review and meta-analysis. *Lancet Respir Med.* 2015;3:150-158.

Terragni PP, Antonelli M, Fumagalli R, Faggiano C, Berardino M, Pallavicini FB, et al. Early vs late tracheotomy for prevention of pneumonia in mechanically ventilated adult ICU patients: a randomized controlled trial. *JAMA.* 2010;303:1483-1489.

Tobin AE, Santamaria JD. An intensivist-led tracheostomy review team is associated with shorter decannulation time and length of stay: a prospective cohort study. *Crit Care.* 2008;12:R48.

Young D, Harrison DA, Cuthbertson BH, Rowan K. TracMan Collaborators. Effect of early vs late tracheostomy placement on survival in patients receiving mechanical ventilation: the TracMan randomized trial. *JAMA.* 2013;309:2121-2129.

Yurtseven N, Aydemir B, Karaca P, Aksoy T, Komurcu G, Kurt M, et al. PercuTwist: A new alternative to Griggs and Ciaglia's techniques. *Eur J Anaesthesiol.* 2007;24:492-497.

ACUTE KIDNEY INJURY IN THE INJURED AND CRITICALLY ILL

Priya Prakash, MD, and Lewis J. Kaplan, MD

The injured and critically ill are at high risk for renal hypoperfusion from external hemorrhage, vasoconstriction, plasma volume loss, and the effects of vasopressor medications used to help salvage patients in profound shock. The kidney is also susceptible to toxin-mediated injury from myoglobin, therapeutic medications, illicit substances, toxic oxygen metabolites, invasive pathogens, and incompletely characterized molecular mediators of injury that are elaborated during hemorrhagic or septic shock and resuscitation. Importantly, such lists do not address the genetic variability in host response to nonself-protein. Nonetheless, recent data suggest that the human genomic response to infection and injury is strikingly similar.

Clinical care of patients with abnormal renal function hinges on identifying the degree of renal dysfunction compared with the patient's baseline. As a result, several classification systems categorize the degree of departure from baseline. In the absence of well-defined criteria, a host of terms with disparate criteria denote renal dysfunction, including but not limited to acute, chronic, and acute-on-chronic renal failure, renal insufficiency, renal impairment, renal dystrophy, and renal dysfunction. Moreover, the presence of renal failure often was tied to using renal replacement therapy regardless of laboratory findings.

The term *kidney injury* previously was limited to structural injury and was not used for impaired renal function. Disparate definitions prevent combining data to improve knowledge and clinical care, or enable research ventures. Instead, a structured and validated approach to identifying and treating renal dysfunction would enable these goals. The Acute Dialysis Quality Initiative (ADQI), the Acute Kidney Injury Network (AKIN), and Kidney Disease: Improving Global Outcomes (KDIGO) have each articulated structured definitions and taxonomy for both acute kidney injury (AKI) and acute renal failure (ARF). Both intermittent and continuous renal support techniques (RST) are used to manage acutely inadequate renal water and solute clearance. This review explores the criteria for AKI and ARF, therapeutic and prognostic implications of renal dysfunction, and support techniques and outcomes in injured and critically ill surgical patients.

EPIDEMIOLOGY

The incidence of AKI differs depending on patient age, time frame of inquiry, as well as geography. In developed countries, AKI primarily affects the elderly (mean = 23.8 cases/1000 discharges). Less severe AKI appears to affect 2000 to 3000/million population, whereas AKI requiring RST occurs with one tenth of that frequency. In developing nations, AKI afflicts the young with widely varying incidences spanning 4.8 cases/100,000 population/year to 20 cases/1000 discharges to 20 cases/year/million population. In developed nations, non–fluid-responsive AKI predominates, whereas fluid-mediated AKI occurs more frequently in developing nations from malaria, obstetric hemorrhage, infections, toxins, and hemolytic uremic syndrome.

AKI peak incidence varies by season in developing nations and often leads to critical medical, resource, and nursing shortages. Reported mortality spans 30% to 40% in developed and 40% to 50% in developing nations. In comparison, ARF has been estimated to affect 1% to 25% of intensive care unit (ICU) patients with a mortality of 15% to 60%. Alarmingly, the incidence of ARF in hospitalized patients appears to be increasing at approximately 11% per year and cannot be ascribed to enhanced reporting or recognition because the data preceded modern taxonomy and reporting structures. This finding has been confirmed in later studies of general hospital and ICU patients.

Prior Definitions of Renal Dysfunction

Cardinal signs of renal failure include both azotemia (elevated blood urea nitrogen, BUN) and reduced urine flow; both elements provide insight into the more difficult to measure glomerular filtration rate (GFR). Accordingly, the majority of renal dysfunction definitions rely on three elements: urine flow as a function of time and weight, BUN, and serum creatinine (Scr). As of 2008, there were more than 35 reported ARF definitions. Unfortunately, azotemia and oliguria can represent AKI as well as an appropriate and adaptive response to reduced plasma volume or cardiac performance and may represent "acute renal success."

Nonetheless, Scr is a problematic isolated measure because it reflects lean body mass and may be low in the elderly or malnourished. Oliguria (urine flow <0.5 cc/kg/hr) is a frequent component of prior ARF definitions but was generally without a time metric (duration of oliguria in hours). In addition, oliguria may be more profound with intact renal tubular function because the tubules can respond to vasopressin increases and maximally concentrate urine. Renal tubular dysfunction may be accompanied by *normal* urine flow because impaired tubules may be unable to respond to hormonal stimuli to resorb salt and water. Furthermore, excess urine flow may accompany later AKI phases (i.e., high output renal failure) because tubules can neither concentrate nor dilute urine (Uspg = 1.010, also known as *isosthenuria*), reducing the sensitivity and specificity of urine flow as a guide. Moreover, normal urine indices may accompany impaired renal function in patients with sepsis, the condition most commonly linked with AKI in the ICU.

Prior Definitions of Acute Renal Failure

ARF definitions have focused on Scr as an absolute value, a multiple of, or a percent increase from baseline. Most commonly a doubled Scr, or an absolute value of 2.0 gm%, has been used to denote ARF. AKI was not an established diagnosis during the time that these definitions were used. Although using changes in Scr makes some physiologic sense, defining ARF on the basis of using renal replacement therapy (RRT) does not because the indications for initiating therapy as well as the applied modality are not uniform, creating substantial definition, allocation, and treatment biases.

The Acute Dialysis Quality Initiative

In 2004 the ADQI established data-driven definitions of renal dysfunction and articulated a structured approach to defining renal dysfunction termed *RIFLE*, standing for three increasing severity classes (Risk, Injury, Failure) as well as two outcome states (Loss and End-stage disease) (Figure 1). The severity classes are driven by either Scr or urine output (Uop), using the worst of each criterion to establish severity, whereas the outcome states are defined by time. Accordingly, the term *AKI* encompasses the entire spectrum of disease spanning minor perturbations in renal function to the need for

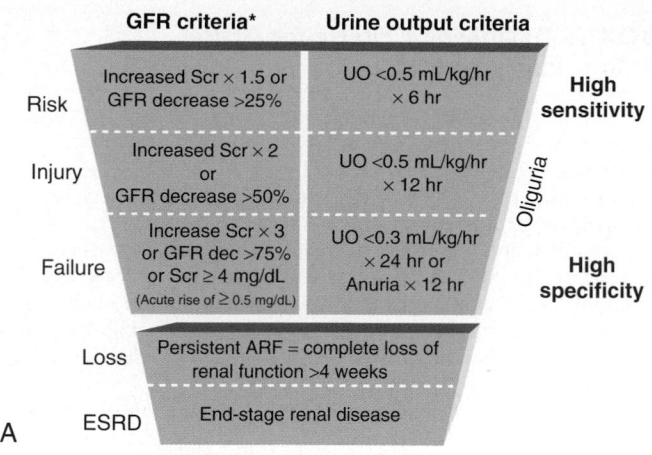

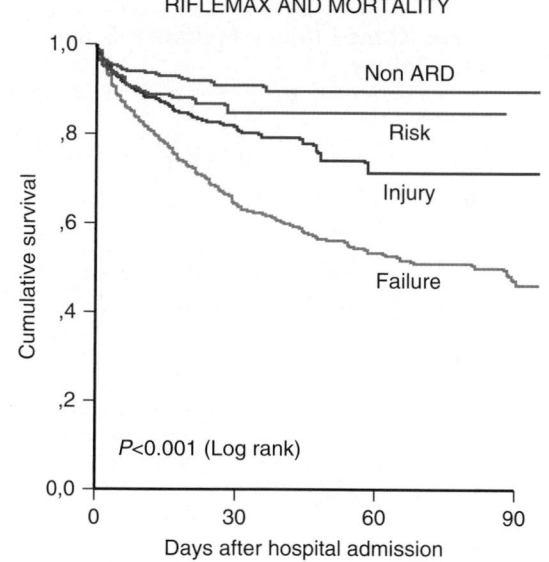

FIGURE 1 RIFLE criteria for acute kidney injury. *ARF,* Acute renal failure; *GFR,* glomerular filtration rate; *SCr,* serum creatinine; *UO,* urine output.

lifelong dialysis. *Therefore the term ARF need no longer be separately used because it is part of the spectrum of AKI.*

RIFLE metrics have been applied across medical, surgical, and specialty ICUs. In a seminal study in more than 5000 patients, the maximum RIFLE category reached during an ICU stay strongly correlated with mortality with two thirds of all ICU patients having some form of AKI falling into a maximal RIFLE class of R (12%), I (27%), and F (28%). Slightly more than half of R patients progressed into I or F categories. This study has been replicated and ascribes an attributable mortality to AKI based on maximal RIFLE class: R (8.8%), I (11.4%) and F (26.3%); patients without AKI establish a comparator mortality rate of 5.5%.

Modifications by the Acute Kidney Injury Network and Kidney Disease: Improving Global Outcomes

RIFLE laid the groundwork for classifying AKI into severity classes and outcome states. The AKIN further refined the diagnostic criteria (Box 1) and expanded the injury state into three stages (Table 1). Stages 1 through 3 rely on either Uop or Scr criteria and represent consensus modifications of RIFLE. KDIGO has collapsed the AKI diagnostic criteria to any of the following three elements: (1) Scr increase ≥0.03 mg/dL within 48 hr, (2) Scr increase ≥1.5 Xs baseline,

BOX 1: Diagnostic Criteria for Acute Kidney Injury (AKIN)

Reduction in kidney function occurring within 48 hours defined as:

- Increase in Scr ≥ 0.3 mg/dL, *or*
- Increase in Scr by ≥ 50% (baseline Scr × 1.5 or greater), *or*
- Reduced urine output (<0.5 mL/kg/hr for >6 hr)

Note that at least two Scr are required and reduces the need for a baseline Scr. Also, the absolute and percentage increase criteria account for variations related to age, gender, and lean body mass. Using the Uop criteria requires that lower urinary tract obstruction, as well as other common causes of low Uop are excluded, including inadequate plasma volume resuscitation.

Scr, Serum creatinine.

TABLE 1: Acute Kidney Injury Network Stages of Acute Kidney Injury

Stage	Scr Increase	Uop
1	>0.03 mg/dL *or* 150%-200% of baseline	<0.5 mL/kg/hr for >6 hr
2	>200%-300% of baseline	<0.5 mL/kg/hr for >12 hr
3	>300% baseline *or* Scr ≥ 4.0 mg/dL plus an acute increase of at least 0.5 mg/dL	<0.3 mL/kg/hr for 24 hr *or* anuria for 12 hr

Note: Only one criterion must be met to qualify for a stage, and any patient who is receiving renal replacement therapy is considered to be at Stage 3 regardless of what stage they are in at the time they begin RRT.

Scr, Serum creatinine; *Uop,* urine output.

which is known or suspected to have occurred within the prior 7 days, or (3) Uop <0.5 mL/kg/hr for 6 hr. KDIGO, the only group that incorporates estimated glomerular filtration rate (eGFR), defines stage 3 as an eGFR <35 mL/min/1.73 m^2 body surface area (BSA) for patients younger than 18 years of age.

■ ACUTE KIDNEY INJURY PREVENTION

Current evidence-based strategies to prevent AKI include ensuring adequate plasma volume and avoiding dehydration, hypotension, or known nephrotoxins. Although a host of pharmacologic agents (fenoldopam, dopamine, N-acetyl cysteine [NAC], calcium-channel antagonists, and loop diuretics) have been explored, none reliably reduces AKI incidence in ICU patients. Patients requiring radiocontrast administration for emergency cardiac procedures who cannot be plasma volume expanded may derive benefit from NAC; such an effect is not evident in patients who can undergo plasma volume expansion, including the injured elderly.

Loop diuretics have exerted no impact on AKI incidence, RRT requirement, or in-hospital mortality in two large meta-analyses. However, an increase rate of temporary auditory dysfunction and tinnitus was noted in those receiving high-dose furosemide. Loop diuretics instead may exert a deleterious effect on recovery from AKI. One observational study noted an increased risk of death as well as nonrecovery of renal function with diuretic use (OR 1.77; 95% CI 1.14 to 2.76). A larger multinational study assessed loop diuretic use and outcome using three different multivariable models. Although this trial could not statistically associate mortality and loop diuretic use, the odds ratio for death (1.2) repeatedly fell to the side of harm

in all model iterations. Therefore the advisability of loop diuretic use remains unclear.

The ADQI investigated fluids that initiate, mitigate, or prevent AKI noting that there were no data that any normotonic crystalloid fluid or hypo-oncotic albumin initiated or mitigated AKI when used as part of a multiple fluid resuscitation strategy. The group, however, noted that induced hyperchloremia created a likely undesirable acidosis (hyperchloremic metabolic acidosis [HCMA]), can lead to additional fluid administration and longer time to normalized pH. An Australian multidisciplinary ICU study (760 chloride-liberal vs 773 chloride-restrictive) demonstrated that chloride restriction was associated with less Scr change ($P = 0.03$), a reduced incidence of RIFLE I and F class patients (8.4 vs 14%, $P < 0.001$), and reduced RRT requirement (6.3 vs 10%, $P = 0.005$). After covariate adjustment, the association of low chloride management and reduced RIFLE I and F classes persisted (OR 0.52; 95% CI: 0.37-0.75) as did reduced RRT need (OR 0.52; 95% CI: 0.33-0.81, $P = 0.004$). Therefore AKI incidence may be affected directly by controlling chloride administration.

Although a definitive review of hydroxyethyl starch (HES) for plasma volume expansion is beyond this review's scope, certain elements of this controversial fluid merit discussion. Starch administration is associated with molecule retention within and vacuolization of renal tubular cells and is implicated in AKI genesis. Intervention studies comparing starch-based resuscitation to other volume expanders have nearly uniformly incorporated a major methodologic flaw: the absence of maintenance fluid and the inadvertent creation of hyperoncoticity because starch solutions provide very little free water. One study comparing hypo- to hyper-oncotic fluids noted that all renally relevant events, including RST and mortality, occurred exclusively in those receiving hyperoncotic fluids.

Starch-based resuscitation often is not compared with equivalent volumes of crystalloid solutions. It is apparent that the presumed 3:1 ratio of crystalloid to colloid is not accurate for septic patients but is instead approximately 1.4:1. Starch trials typically deliver equal volumes of crystalloid and colloid, leading to over-resuscitation, decreased hemoglobin, and therefore increased transfusion in the colloid arm. Moreover, the starch trial doses commonly exceed U.S. Food and Drug Administration (FDA) recommendations. As part of multimodality fluid management, the European SOAP trial noted that starch at approximately 1500 mL/day had no impact on Uop, Scr, or renal function, reflecting that this strategy likely avoided hyperoncoticity.

The most recent trial investigating this question is the 6S (Scandinavian Starch in Severe Sepsis and Septic Shock) trial, which compared 6% HES in Ringer's acetate (n = 398) with Ringer's acetate (n = 400). This trial coupled the same crystalloid in both arms and avoided hyperoncoticity; starch was limited to 33 mL/kg/24 hr and follow-up spanned 90 days. Starch resuscitation established increased mortality (51% vs 43%; relative risk, 1.17; 95% CI, 1.01-1.36; $P = 0.03$), and RRT need (22% vs 16%; relative risk, 1.35; 95% CI, 1.01-1.80; $P = 0.04$); no differences were noted in end-stage renal disease (one patient per arm) nor bleeding (10% vs 6%; $P = 0.09$). It is not clear whether the data represent a threshold event or an all-or-none phenomenon. However, the 6S trial provides the strongest data linking starch, AKI, and mortality risk in patients with severe sepsis.

The working group for nephrology of the European Society of Intensive Care Medicine created an expert opinion document that articulates GRADE-based recommendations for AKI prevention and renal function protection using data spanning 1966 to 2009 (Box 2). There were no grade 1A recommendations *supporting* the use of specific agents or interventions.

■ ABDOMINAL COMPARTMENT SYNDROME

Oliguria as the representation of an attributable organ failure in the setting of intra-abdominal hypertension that exceeds 20 cm H$_2$O

BOX 2: Selected ESICM Consensus Recommendations for Acute Kidney Injury Prevention

Plasma Volume Expansion

Recommendations:
1. Fluid resuscitation for volume depletion (**1C**)
   Note: No fluid or fluid type was identified as ideal, provided electrolyte derangements were avoided during or after administration.
2. Prophylactic PVE with isotonic fluids in those at risk of RCN (**1B**)
   Note: NaHCO$_3$-based isotonic fluid was *suggested*.
3. AVOID 10% HES 250/0.5 (**1B**) and higher molecular weight HES and dextrans in sepsis (**2C**)

Suggestions:
1. Prophylactic PVE with crystalloids to prevent AKI by certain medications (**2C**)
   Note: amphotericin B, intravenous antivirals, medications associated with crystal nephropathy

Diuretics

Recommendations:
1. AVOID loop diuretics to prevent or ameliorate AKI (1B)

Vasopressors and Inotropes

Recommendations:
1. MAP should be maintained >60-65 mm Hg (1C); individualize when possible if premorbid blood pressure is known
2. Norepinephrine or dopamine (plus PVE) are first-line agents for vasodilatory shock (1C)
3. AVOID low-dose dopamine to protect against AKI (1A)

Vasodilators

Suggestions:
1. Vasodilators may be useful for renal protection after resuscitation and with hemodynamic monitoring (2C)
2. Fenoldopam may be useful in cardiovascular surgery patients at risk of AKI (2B)
3. AVOID fenoldopam for RCN prophylaxis (1A)
4. Theophylline to mitigate RCN risk in those who cannot undergo PVE (2C)
5. AVOID natriuretic peptides as protective agents against AKI in general ICU patients (2B) but may be considered in cardiovascular surgery patients (2B)

Metabolic Interventions

Recommendations:
1. AVOID routine selenium supplementation as an AKI preventative (1B).

Suggestions:
1. Enteral nutrition is preferred for patients at risk of AKI (2C).
2. AVOID N-acetyl cysteine as prophylaxis against RCN or other forms of AKI (2B).

AKI, Acute kidney injury; *ESCIM*, European Society of Intensive Care Medicine; *HES*, hydroxyethyl starch; *PVE*, portal vein embolization; *RCN*, renal cortical necrosis.

---

pressure establishes the abdominal compartment syndrome (ACS). Although relieving the ACS by laparotomy (hemorrhage, visceral edema) or percutaneous drainage (massive ascites) may correct hemodynamics, it less reliably improves renal function despite reducing or eliminating renal venous hypertension and improving arterial hypotension. Moreover, abdominal decompression does not address intrarenal hypertension because of organ edema, or contained

subcapsular hematoma; incising Gerota's fascia to correct intrarenal hypertension can improve renal function. This effect could not be modeled using extrinsic renal compression but could be recreated with imposed and then relieved renal vein hypertension. Using a "crystalloid cap" fluid-management strategy (2 L in the ED and 4 L total pre-ICU) decreased pre-ICU fluid volumes by 0.8 L and reduced intra-abdominal hypertension, open abdomen rate, and ICU length of stay.

■ SEPTIC ACUTE KIDNEY INJURY

Septic AKI may be profoundly different from other forms of AKI in that with resuscitation, renal blood flow may become hyperemic, and as such is a unique form of AKI. Similarly, nonhemodynamic mechanisms of renal injury are likely involved in the evolution and progression of this form of AKI. Immune-mediated, toxin-derived, and inflammatory mechanisms are likely more important in understanding septic AKI than are systemic hemodynamics. Of key importance would be accurate and reproducible measurements of renal blood flow to track septic AKI progression and resolution. A related novel form of AKI is one that is clinically inapparent.

■ SUBCLINICAL ACUTE KIDNEY INJURY

There is a time frame in which the kidney has sustained injury, but it is not yet apparent when evaluating Uop or Scr. Therefore another tool must be used to identify the injured kidney before traditional markers become apparent. Urinary or serum biomarkers may fill this role. The three most reliable biomarkers are urinary neutrophil gelatinase-associated lipocalin, kidney injury molecule-1, and cystatin-C. Each of these detect renal injury before a Scr rise and are therefore useful in shaping definitions, evaluating incidence, and perhaps directing therapy to improve outcome. The present challenge is to determine what to do for the patient who is biomarker positive but Scr and/or Uop negative.

■ IMPACT OF ACUTE KIDNEY INJURY ON OUTCOME

AKI increases ICU length of stay by 2 to 10 days and generally relates to RIFLE class as well as the need for RST. RST outcomes have improved over time, reflecting changes in technology and delivery. Overall outcome for those with RRT requiring AKI also is influenced heavily by concomitant organ failure, leading to a mortality rate of 50% to 60%. Recovery from RST requiring AKI is generally good in that the majority of survivors regain renal function by hospital discharge (Figure 2). However, between 13% and 22% of AKI patients require chronic RRT. Chronic kidney disease before developing AKI led to a 53% incidence of postdischarge RST requirement versus 13% in those with baseline normal renal function.

■ RECOVERY FROM ACUTE KIDNEY INJURY

The impact of dialysis modality has been elucidated by two large multinational trials (Acute Renal Failure Trial Network [ATN] and Randomized Evaluation of Normal versus Augmented Level Renal Replacement Therapy [RENAL]). The ATN trial evaluated the impact of more than 5000 intermittent hemodialysis events on renal recovery documenting day-28 dialysis dependence in 45.2% of survivors.

The RENAL trial used intermittent dialysis much less frequently (314 events) and was associated with reduced day-28 dialysis dependence (13.3% of survivors). Lack of delay in recovery is associated with a net positive fluid balance. The Sepsis Occurrence in Acutely Ill Patients (SOAP) trial (1120 patients with septic AKI) found that survivors had a lower daily fluid balance and that fluid balance was independently associated with death (Cox hazard ratio = 1.21;

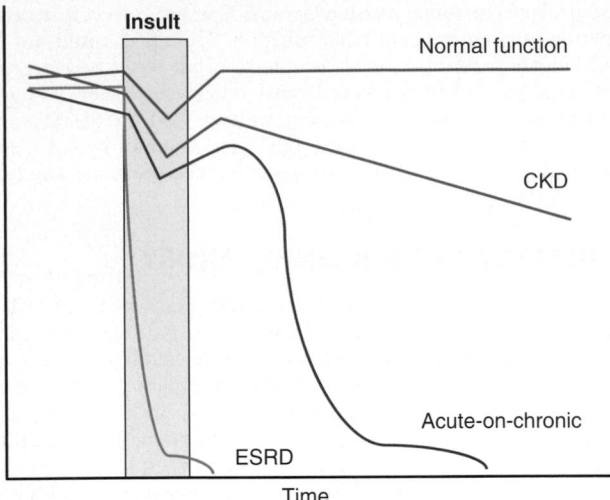

FIGURE 2 Natural history of acute kidney injury. *CKD,* Chronic kidney disease; *ESRD,* end-stage renal disease; *KD,* kidney disease.

95% CI 1.13-1.28). Nonetheless, not all patients require RRT for management, and the "answer" to improving renal outcomes is not as simple as selecting continuous RST as opposed to intermittent RST, or avoiding positive fluid balance. One must explore how to manage AKI that requires RST when renal clearance is inadequate to meet demand.

RENAL SUPPORT THERAPY

Once a patient has suffered sufficient kidney injury to establish inadequate water and solute clearance to meet the demand placed on the remaining functional nephrons, one must consider how best to support the failing renal function. The technology that has been applied to do so comes in two general formats: intermittent and continuous. However, the optimal use of these modalities has been plagued by questions of initiation, ideal modality, duration of therapy, dose of therapy, cost of care, method and timing of termination, and impact on renal recovery. Although these techniques have been termed *renal replacement therapy (RRT),* they only manage deficient water and solute clearance, rather than addressing vascular tone, oxygen utilization, and paracrine or autocrine functions; instead, the dialytic techniques may be more properly termed *renal support techniques (RST).*

Furthermore, recent controversy surrounds ownership of the required devices, and therapy prescriptional capacity much in the same way that characterized the early emergency department use of ultrasound for the FAST (focused assessment with sonography for trauma) examination. Instead of radiology ownership, RST generally is viewed as being the sole purview of nephrology regardless of intensivist training or experience with RST. In a related fashion, RST is one of the very few ICU therapies applied in an on/off fashion instead of being titrated to a physiologic endpoint; virtually all others are titrated to a target that may be serially monitored in real time. As a result, current RST use is to salvage nephron failure rather than as a deliberate means of offloading renal work during a high-stress period when work may be maladaptive. The following sections explore basic RST concepts, practical applications, and comparative outcomes between intermittent and continuous RST modes.

Basic Concepts and Terms

Although an in-depth review of all of the mechanisms that underpin dialysis modes is beyond the scope of this review, certain elements are essential to understanding and interpreting clinical and basic science data on this topic. Intermittent hemodialysis (IHD) is a technique that is not continuous, generally spans 4 hours, clears water and solute at a high rate using a countercurrent mechanism (parallel to native renal function), requires a dialysis nurse, and typically is applied three to four times per week. IHD also can be used for short period of time with high flow rates for ultrafiltration (e.g., volume overload, hyperkalemia, drug overdose) instead of metabolic clearance of waste and byproducts of metabolism (e.g., uremia, acidosis). The mechanisms by which hemodialysis works is passive solute transport along a concentration gradient across a semipermeable membrane separating two unique compartments. A related process is hemofiltration.

Hemofiltration describes the use of a hydrostatic pressure gradient to establish convective clearance of plasma water across a semipermeable membrane that separates two unique compartments. Based on the hydrostatic pressure gradient, friction is generated between water and solutes, termed *solvent drag.* Solvent drag is the process responsible for the convective clearance of small and middle molecules (<50 kDa) along with water movement. Small solutes such as anionic and cationic electrolytes as well as urea are cleared in the same concentration as plasma, and therefore hemofiltration is not expected to effect changes in their concentrations. Therefore changes in these substances while using hemofiltration are achieved by delivering diluting fluids (i.e., crystalloids) containing substances of lower concentration than already exist in plasma. In contradistinction, hemodialysis with its countercurrent flow does alter these concentrations efficiently. Both hemodialysis and hemofiltration may be combined as hemodiafiltration, in which the overwhelming majority of solute clearance occurs via diffusion (dialysis), but some convective clearance does contribute to total solute loss.

Continuous techniques are available in multiple formats, including arteriovenous and venovenous; since venovenous modes predominate, the discussion will focus on those. Continuous venovenous hemofiltration (CVVH) is similar to its related modes, CVVH dialysis, (CVVH-D) and CVVH diafiltration (CVVH-DF). All run continuously as their name implies, but only the latter two incorporate a countercurrent mechanism. Of necessity, the three modalities will have different efficacies at clearing water and solutes. In particular, solute clearance will differ based upon the molecular size as well as whether clearance is occurring by convection (water movement-based transport; ultrafiltration, CVVH) or by diffusion (concentration-gradient driven; CVVH-D); similar to the intermittent mode described above, CVVH-DF includes both convective and diffusive clearance mechanisms. Although convection more effectively clears larger molecular weight substances (5 to 50 kDa, also known as "middle molecules"), diffusion more effectively clears small molecules (<1 kDa). Thus modality selection may be influenced by the target that is to be cleared.

By way of example, CVVH is predicted to be more efficacious at clearing inflammatory mediators than would CVVH-D, and mediator clearance in patients receiving CVVH is well documented. Continuous modes establish a constant GFR that may enable therapeutic drug dosing and allows for instant regulation of net fluid volume to accommodate medication and nutritional prescription volumes. Furthermore, because the rate of fluid exchange is less than with IHD, continuous modes are used almost exclusively in those with hemodynamic instability supported by pressor agents in the United States. Other countries, Australia, for example, uniformly provide CRST in their critical care units; IHD is reserved for those on the general ward and the outpatient setting. The advantages and disadvantages of IHD versus continuous techniques are presented in Table 2.

There are also hybrid techniques (prolonged intermittent renal replacement therapy, PIRRT). The most notable of these is slow low-efficiency (daily) dialysis (SLEDD), which uses a lower rate of dialysis, leading to reduced efficiency and requiring a longer therapy time. SLEDD is associated with fewer side effects because rapid fluid and electrolyte shifts are reduced. Longer dialysis times with slower rates are called *extended dialysis,* and when applied on a daily basis, *extended daily dialysis.* PIRRT is much less common than IHD in U.S.

TABLE 2: Comparison of Dialysis Modes

Element	Intermittent	Continuous
Time	3-4 hours	24 hours
Flow rate	High	Low
Specialty nurse required	Yes	No (ICU nurse run)
Cost	Lower	Higher
Constant glomerular filtration rate	No	Yes
Real-time volume management	Only during session	Continuous
Recirculation	Higher	Lower
Pressor-dependent patient use	No	Yes
Membrane clotting during therapy	Uncommon	Occasional
Suitable for intraoperative use	No	Yes
Reduced renal blood flow during therapy	Yes	No
Nutritional support	More difficult to manage volume	Easier to manage volume

critical care units but is gaining in practice in the European Union. SLEDD is a hybrid of intermittent and continuous techniques and serves as a "middle ground" that capitalizes on the most advantageous elements of each technique; regardless, hemodialyzer clotting remains a problem with this mode. Instead, it is appropriate to explore when the commonly used techniques should be applied in the surgical ICU.

Indications for Initiating Renal Support Techniques in the Intensive Care Unit

Standard indications for starting dialysis in the outpatient setting as well as for the noncritically ill inpatient have been well articulated. Earlier dialysis at lower BUN values has been associated with improved outcome in several studies. However, the larger studies were retrospective and targeted BUN values of approximately 90 to 160 versus 160 to 200 as initiation breakpoints, targets far greater than modern starting points. Modern data interrogating the utility of early versus later initiation of CRST suggest an outcome advantage in the early groups, including trauma, cardiac surgery, and mixed medical and surgical patients. Nonetheless, there are not universally agreed upon indications for starting either IHD or CRST in the critically ill and injured surgical patient. Often institutional preference as well as device and technician availability influences these decisions.

Renal Support Techniques Outcomes

Several proponents have touted the superiority of CRST for the critically ill and injured patient compared with intermittent techniques with regard to hemodynamic stability, ease of medication management, lack of limitation of nutrition support volume, and survival and recovery of renal function (dialysis independence). Instead, current data support equivalent outcome regardless of which mode is selected after adjusting for severity of illness (IHD is generally not applied in patients who require pressor support). Although initial studies were observational or retrospective, prospective randomized data have become available that also support this conclusion and are based on data from patients with AKI who were randomized to IHD or CRST, as well as meta-analyses that reached the same conclusion: there is no discernible benefit to CRST compared with IHD. Similarly, CRST fails to provide enhanced recovery of renal function compared with IHD. As a matter of perspective, one must consider whether the putative benefits of CRST remain clinically relevant in the face of similar outcome as that obtained using IHD.

Dosing

One must be conversant with the tools used to analyze the effectiveness of a dialysis dose. The two main tools are urea reduction ratio (URR) and Kt/V. URR represents the cleared urea as a percent of the starting urea. Thus, if the starting urea were 75 and the ending were 50, the removed urea would be 20 and the URR would be 25 (removed)/75 (starting), or 33.3%. A typical target URR is more than 65%. URR generally is measured every 12 to 14 treatments and principally applies to outpatient IHD. Kt/V is a different but related measure of dialysis adequacy that may be applied in all circumstances.

K represents dialyzer clearance in milliliters per minute and is the rate at which blood passes through the dialyzer. The t stands for the time that the dialysis session lasts in minutes. Thus Kt stands for the volume of blood that is cleared completely of urea during a single treatment in liters. V represents the volume of water in a patient's body, using an average value of 60% water multiplied times the patient's actual or adjusted body weight. Thus a dialyzer with a clearance rate of 350 mL/min applied on a dialysis session spanning 240 minutes in an 80-kg patient would have a Kt/V of (350 mL/min × 240 min) × (1/1000) / (80 kg × 0.60) = 1.75. Therefore Kt/V compares the amount of fluid that passes through the dialyzer to the patient's total body water volume. A target Kt/V of more than 1.2 is believed appropriate in most circumstances. Kt/V and URR are related, but Kt/V is more accurate because it takes into account urea that is generated during the dialysis session as well as any extra urea removed during dialysis along with extra fluid.

A higher dose of dialysis may result in improved outcome. This hypothesis has been multiply tested with conflicting outcomes dependent on included patient population, timing of initiation, actual delivered dose, and a host of related factors, including the main outcome measure (principally survival). The two largest and best-designed trials that investigated dialysis dosing in both intermittent and continuous support techniques are the U.S. VA/NIH Acute Renal Failure Trial Network study (ATN; 1124 patients) and the Australia and New Zealand Intensive Care Society Randomized Evaluation of Normal versus Augmented Level of RRT study (RENAL; 1508 patients). Both of these studies determined that more intense dialysis did not achieve improved survival when compared with standard dosing regimens. These findings were supplemented by two meta-analyses that arrived at identical conclusions. However, often the prescribed dose and the delivered dose were not identical with delivery, not achieving that which was prescribed because of dialyzer clotting and time off dialysis for interventions. Thus the present recommendation for CRST is an effluent flow rate of 20 to 25 mL/kg per hour.

Cessation of Therapy

The vast majority of ICU therapies are titrated optimally to a physiologic endpoint, including analgesics, sedative, and vasoactive agents. RST are not often discontinued on the basis of such endpoints. Instead, empirical evidence predominates, including reestablishment of urine flow or a progressive decrease in Scr. Urine flow is less robust in those who are not initially oliguric, and Scr as a marker of renal recovery requires that the dialysis dose is held constant. A more precise measure would be creatinine clearance. Although a definitive level that should prompt cessation of RST has not been established, and the measured creatinine clearance must be assessed in light of nutritional support and other therapeutics, at least one trial (ATN) stopped renal support when the creatinine clearance exceeded 20 mL/min with lesser values left to clinician discretion. It is unlikely that clearance less than 20 mL/min will be sufficient to achieve solute and water clearance in a highly catabolic critically ill or injured surgical patient.

NEW CONCEPTS AND THE MOLECULAR UNDERPINNINGS OF ACUTE KIDNEY INJURY

Although the preceding discussion has explored identifying, categorizing, and managing AKI/ARF in the critically ill and injured patient population, it has not described events at the cellular or subcellular level. New information has arisen that integrates observations from sepsis with intercellular and intracellular signaling that directly affects renal tubular cell function. This recently articulated paradigm links the elaboration, infiltration, circulation, and filtration of pathogen-associated molecular patterns (PAMPs) or damage-associated molecular patterns (DAMPs) with local events leading to what we recognize as decreases in renal function, most notably as oliguria, elevated serum creatinine, rising BUN, and solute and acid clearance failure. Filtered DAMPs and PAMPs initiate inflammatory cascades that lead to reactive oxygen species, endothelial activation, neutrophil recruitment, and retarded microvascular flow. This concentrates inflammation and increases the length of exposure to cytokines as well as signaling molecules that act in a paracrine fashion. Such molecules initiate intracellular pathways that lead to mitophagy and cell cycle arrest, effectively crafting a bioenergetically downregulated cell. These adaptations to AKI triggers appear to be focused on enhancing cell survival. Understanding such events in the context of septic AKI, the most common form in the United States, may help understand other forms of AKI and perhaps identify suitable molecular targets. One should note that at least in one animal model, typical phenotypic changes of AKI are associated with enhanced overall renal blood flow at the same time that microvascular flow is reduced, effectively functioning akin to an intrapulmonary shunt supporting the septic AKI is likely a functional event rather than a structural one.

CONCLUSIONS

The precision with which we define increasing degrees of renal impairment has increased substantially in the last decade. These advances have relied upon investigating proscribed definitions of changes in urine flow, serum creatinine, and glomerular filtration rate using a boundaried time metric. As a result, the correct term to describe reduction in renal function is *acute kidney injury (AKI)*. AKI encompasses the entire spectrum of renal impairment that includes renal failure and its management with extracorporeal therapies. It is clear that AKI cause and prevalence vary by region, season, and an individual country's degree of socioeconomic development. Current data do not support an outcome advantage to continuous versus intermittent renal support therapies, although one should note that intermittent techniques are infrequently used in those requiring pressor support. A uniform reporting format to assess renal dysfunction and management techniques is one opportunity to powerfully investigate elements that affect renal outcomes in critically ill and injured patients because controversy persists regarding the optimal method of management to best promote renal recovery.

SUGGESTED READINGS

Bellomo R, Cass A, Cole L, Finfer S, Gallagher M, Lo S, McArthur C, McGuinness S, Myburgh J, Norton R, RENAL Replacement Therapy Study Investigators. Intensity of continuous renal-replacement therapy in critically ill patients. *N Engl J Med*. 2009;361:1627-1638.

Bellomo R, Ronco C, Kellum JA, et al. Acute renal failure–definition, outcome measures, animal models, fluid therapy and information technology needs: the Second International Consensus Conference of the Acute Dialysis Quality Initiative (ADQI) Group. *Crit Care*. 2004;8:R204-R212.

Gomez H, Ince C, De Bakker D, et al. A unified theory of sepsis-induced acute kidney injury: inflammation, microcirculatory dysfunction, bioenergetics, and the tubular cell adaptation to injury. *Shock*. 2014;41:3-11.

Kaplan LJ, Cheung NH, Maerz L, et al. A physiochemical approach to acid-base balance in critically ill trauma patients minimizes errors and reduces inappropriate plasma volume expansion. *J Trauma*. 2009;66:1045-1051.

Kellum JA, Cerda J, Kaplan LJ, Nadim MK, Palevsky PM. Fluids for prevention and management of acute kidney injury. *Int J Artif Organs*. 2008;31:96-110.

Kellum JA, Lameire N, KDIGO Working Group. KDIGO Clinical Practice Guideline for Acute Kidney Injury. *Kidney Int Suppl*. 2012;2:8-12. doi:10.1038/kisup.2012.7.

Langenberg C, Gobe G, Hood S, et al. Renal histopathology during experimental septic acute kidney injury and recovery. *Crit Care Med*. 2014;42:e58-e67.

Palevsky PM, Zhang JH, O'Connor TZ, et al. VA/NIH Acute Renal Failure Trial Network. Intensity of renal support in critically ill patients with acute kidney injury. *N Engl J Med*. 2008;359:7-20.

Perner A, Haase N, Guttormsen AB, et al. Hydroxyethyl starch 130/0.42 versus Ringer's acetate in severe sepsis. *N Engl J Med*. 2012;367:124-134.

ELECTROLYTE DISORDERS

Scott M. Moore, MD, and Anthony A. Meyer, PhD

Claude Bernard, the father of modern experimental physiology, wrote in 1878 of "the organic liquid that circulates and bathes all the anatomic elements of the tissues" in describing the distribution of body fluid and its constituents. One of his great accomplishments was his demonstration of the critical role that fluid compartments play in whole body homeostasis. The physiologic stress imposed by surgery, trauma, and critical illness often leads to major alterations in the balance between fluid compartments and their principal electrolytes. A thorough understanding of the physiologic mechanisms governing electrolyte distribution and how this balance may be altered under conditions of critical illness is fundamental to the care of the surgical patient.

COMPARTMENTAL DISTRIBUTION OF BODY FLUID AND ELECTROLYTES

The adult human body is composed of approximately 50% to 60% water by weight (Figure 1). This proportion of total body water (TBW) varies based on the percent body fat of an individual, with a 10% to 20% relative decrease in TBW seen among obese patients. The majority of fluid is contained within the intracellular fluid (ICF) compartment, which accounts for two thirds of TBW, with the remainder contained within the extracellular fluid (ECF) compartment. The main components of the ECF include the interstitial and

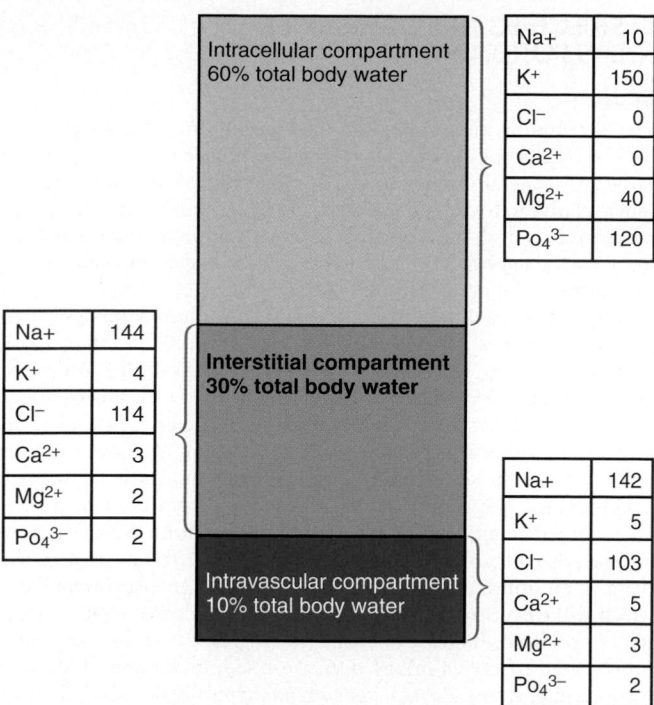

Na+	10	
K+	150	
Cl⁻	0	
Ca²⁺	0	
Mg²⁺	40	
Po₄³⁻	120	

Na+	144
K+	4
Cl⁻	114
Ca²⁺	3
Mg²⁺	2
Po₄³⁻	2

Na+	142
K+	5
Cl⁻	103
Ca²⁺	5
Mg²⁺	3
Po₄³⁻	2

FIGURE 1 Distribution and composition (mEq/L) of total body water. *Ca²⁺*, Calcium; *Cl⁻*, chloride; *K⁺*, potassium; *Mg²⁺*, magnesium; *Na⁺*, sodium; *Po₄³⁻*, phosphate.

intravascular compartments, which account for approximately 10% and 30% of TBW, respectively. The transcellular space occupies the remaining portion of the ECF compartment and includes the cerebrospinal, synovial, and ocular fluids as well as water contained within the lumen of the gastrointestinal (GI) tract. Actual blood volume (~5 L) is significantly higher than intravascular fluid volume (~3.5 L) because of the presence of blood cells, with red blood cells (RBCs) contributing approximately 40% of the total blood volume (TBV).

The composition of the ICF and ECF compartments vary considerably in terms of their predominant ions (see Figure 1). The major cations of the intracellular space are K⁺ (potassium; 150 mEq/L) and Mg⁺ (magnesium; 40 mEq/L), which are electrically balanced by anionic intracellular proteins and organic phosphates. The chief cation of the extracellular space is Na⁺ (sodium; 142 mEq/L), which is balanced by the anions Cl⁻ (chloride; 103 mEq/L) and HCO₃⁻ (bicarbonate; 24 mEq/L), with minor contributions by sulfates, phosphates, and anionic proteins. Within the ECF compartment itself, the interstitial and intravascular fluids have similar concentrations of anions and cations, with the only major difference being the relatively lower concentration of protein within interstitial fluid (1 g/dL) compared with plasma (7 g/dL). The barrier between the ICF and ECF is a highly selective lipid bilayer that is intrinsically impermeable to charged solutes and large molecules. The maintenance of high extracellular sodium and intracellular potassium concentrations is performed by the membrane bound Na⁺-K⁺ pump, which utilizes energy from adenosine triphosphate (ATP) hydrolysis to generate a greater than tenfold difference in Na⁺ and K⁺ concentrations across the plasma membrane. Strict maintenance of these concentrations expends substantial energy and is the driving force for nutrient and ion movement into cells, in addition to providing the substrate for signal propagation within the nervous, cardiovascular, and GI systems.

Osmolality and Tonicity

Any molecule that does not freely traverse a semipermeable membrane that separates two fluid compartments is considered an *osmole*, and the concentration of osmoles within a solution is the *osmolarity* (mOsm/L). The osmolarity of human plasma can be calculated using readily available laboratory values and the following formula.

$$P_{osm}(mOsm/L) = 2 \times [Na^+] + [glucose]/18 + BUN/2.8$$

Water freely moves between the extracellular and intracellular space; therefore determination of the plasma osmolarity also provides the osmolarity of the ICF compartment. Most modern laboratories can measure osmole concentration directly using methods such as freezing point depression osmometry, which determines the number of osmoles per *weight* of solution, in which case the term *osmolality* (mOsm/kg) is more appropriate. Osmolality has the theoretical advantage of independence from temperature and pressure, although the influence of these factors is small and usually not clinically significant. *Tonicity* is a similar property to osmolality in that both denote the concentration of osmotic substances within a solution. However, tonicity differs from osmolality in that it is influenced only by solutes that are impermeable to cell membranes (i.e., *effective osmoles*), whereas osmolality includes both impermeable molecules (i.e., Na⁺, glucose) and freely permeable solutes (i.e., urea, ethanol). An isotonic solution, such as 0.9% NaCl (sodium chloride), contains approximately the same concentration of effective osmoles as the ICF, and cells neither shrink nor swell when exposed to such a solution. In contrast, a hypertonic solution (i.e., 3% NaCl) contains a higher concentration of effective osmoles than the ICF and will result in cell shrinkage due to an osmotic force that leads to efflux of water from the cells. Conversely, a hypotonic solution (i.e., 0.45% NaCl) has a lower concentration of effective osmoles than the ICF, leading to free water influx and cellular swelling.

Extracellular Volume Shifts Due to Changes in Ultrafiltration

Though a major determinant of fluid distribution between the ICF and ECF, tonicity has little effect on the distribution of fluids between the intravascular and interstitial compartments, which is instead determined by hydrostatic pressures that tend to favor fluid movement out of the vasculature and into the interstitium and by colloid osmotic forces that act in the reverse direction. The latter results from the relative impermeability of the capillary wall to proteins, which causes high protein concentrations within the vasculature and low protein concentrations within the interstitium. Accordingly, any process that leads to an increase in the permeability of the capillary wall will lead to protein leakage and a decrease in intravascular protein concentration and colloid osmotic forces, which will favor fluid movement into the interstitial space. Mathematically, this relationship is represented by Starling's equation:

$$J_v \approx K_f \times (P_c - P_{if} - \pi_c + \pi_{if})$$

Under normal conditions, where capillary permeability (K_f) is low and the net hydrostatic pressure ($P_c - P_{if}$) is counterbalanced equally by the net colloid osmotic pressure ($\pi_c + \pi_{if}$), ingested and reabsorbed fluid and electrolytes are distributed rapidly and proportionately between the intravascular and interstitial spaces. However, movement of fluid into the interstitium, or edema, can occur with increased capillary hydrostatic pressure (P_c), decreased plasma colloid osmotic pressure (π_c), increased capillary permeability (K_f), or obstruction of lymphatic vessels.

Control of Osmolality

Plasma osmolality is normally maintained between 285 and 295 mOsm/L, and the primary means for achieving this tight control is through regulation of the thirst mechanism and secretion of *antidiuretic hormone* (ADH). When plasma osmolality rises above the normal range, osmoreceptors in the anterior hypothalamus are stimulated and lead to increased thirst as well as increased ADH secretion by the posterior pituitary. As water intake increases, ADH simultaneously acts on the distal tubule and collecting duct to increase water reabsorption, thereby returning plasma osmolality to the physiologic range. Conversely, a decrease in plasma osmolality to below 280 mOsm/L leads to decreased thirst and inhibition of ADH secretion, accompanied by decreased water intake, excretion of a dilute urine, and correction of the hypo-osmolar state. Urine osmolality can be as low as 50 mOsm/L when ADH secretion is minimal but can be as high as 1200 to 1400 mOsm/L when plasma osmolality is elevated and ADH levels are at their peak. Remarkably, the ADH feedback mechanism accomplishes this wide range in water resorption and osmolality regulation without significant effects on solute excretion. Although plasma osmolality is the most potent regulator of ADH secretion, major decreases (>10% to 20%) in blood volume and blood pressure are detected by cardiopulmonary and arterial baroreceptors, respectively, whose signaling can potentiate the ADH feedback mechanism and cause massive release of ADH in an effort to correct the volume deficit.

Syndrome of Inappropriate Antidiuretic Hormone Secretion

In contrast to the normal situation in which plasma osmolality and volume status are tightly coupled to ADH production, conditions exist that can cause this feedback loop to be disrupted. The syndrome of inappropriate antidiuretic hormone secretion (SIADH) is characterized by excessive ADH secretion that is autonomous from plasma osmolality or volume status. Among surgical patients, hypersecretion of ADH is common in the postoperative period and likely is related to increased afferent pain signals. Other causes seen among surgical patients include head trauma, neurosurgical interventions (especially pituitary surgery), alcohol withdrawal, drugs (including haloperidol, ciprofloxacin, amiodarone, nonsteroidal anti-inflammatory drug [NSAIDs], and opiates), malignancies (especially small cell lung cancer), and pulmonary and central nervous system (CNS) disturbances. The diagnosis is confirmed by demonstrating decreased plasma osmolarity (<270 mOsm/kg), high urinary concentration (>100 mOsm/kg), and elevated urinary sodium concentration (>40 mEq/L) with normal salt and water intake. The diagnosis also requires that the patient is euvolemic; not receiving diuretics; and has no evidence of adrenal, thyroid, or pituitary insufficiency. Treatment of SIADH includes fluid restriction (less than 1 L/day) and avoidance of intravenous fluid (IVF) infusions, as even isotonic saline (IS) can result in worsening of hyponatremia because of ADH-induced excretion of sodium and reabsorption of free water.

Diabetes Insipidus

In contrast to SIADH, deficient ADH signaling can lead to marked increases in urinary free water losses independent of plasma osmolality or volume status, a condition known as diabetes insipidus (DI). With central DI, which can be encountered among surgical patients after neurosurgical operations and head trauma, ADH secretion by the posterior pituitary is deficient and leads to excretion of large volumes (3 to 6 L/day) of dilute urine (<200 mOsm/kg). It is notable that urinary losses in severe central DI can be greater than 10 L/day and are characteristically hypo-osmolar, which leads to increased plasma osmolality (>290 mOsm/kg) and contraction of the ECF and ICF compartments. Nephrogenic DI is characterized by intact ADH secretion centrally and instead a deficiency in the response of the distal tubules and collecting ducts to ADH. Lithium toxicity is the most common cause for nephrogenic DI in the adult population. Exogenous administration of the synthetic vasopressin analogue DDAVP (desmopressin) helps to differentiate central and nephrogenic DI, as urine output osmolality is at least partially normalized in the former condition but not in the latter one.

■ SPECIFIC ELECTROLYTE DISTURBANCES

Sodium

The distribution and regulation of sodium balance throughout the ECF and ICF is linked closely to tonicity and fluid balance as described earlier. In general, hyponatremia is the result of an excess of free water relative to total body sodium, and hypernatremia is the reverse scenario. For all dysnatremias, a systematic approach is needed for the correct diagnosis of the underlying cause and subsequent choice of treatment (Figure 2).

Hyponatremia is defined as a plasma sodium level less than 135 mEq/L and is further classified as mild (130 to 134 mEq/L), moderate (120 to 130 mEq/L), or severe (<120 mEq/L). Although most cases of hyponatremia are associated with low plasma osmolality, hypertonic hyponatremia can be encountered when glucose, mannitol, or other aqueous solutes are present at high concentrations in the ECF. As the solute levels in the ECF rise and cause an increase in osmolality, free water moves from the ICF compartment to the ECF compartment, leading to a fall in ECF sodium concentration. For every 100 mg/dL increase in glucose above the normal range, there is an approximately 1.6 mEq/L decrease in plasma sodium, which will correct without further treatment once the hyperosmolar state is resolved. Increases beyond 400 mg/dL cause an even more pronounced effect (2.4 mEq/L decrease in sodium for every 100 mg/L increase in glucose). *Pseudohyponatremia* typically occurs under isotonic conditions and arises when there are abnormally high plasma protein or lipid levels. It is not a "true" hyponatremia and is instead a result of older measurement methods that used total plasma volume rather than the aqueous portion when measuring sodium concentration. Aside from these conditions, hyponatremia is almost always accompanied by hypotonicity, as described later.

Hypervolemic hyponatremia is encountered among patients with high ECF volume but low effective circulating volume, which may be seen with congestive heart failure, cirrhosis, and hypoalbuminemia. Nonosmotic release of ADH occurs, leading to retention of free water that tends to parallel the severity of the underlying disease process. Aggressive attempts to correct mild to moderate hyponatremia in this setting are unnecessary, as the disturbance is usually asymptomatic and chronic in nature; furthermore, correction of hyponatremia in patients with heart failure and cirrhosis has not been shown to improve outcomes. The mainstay of treatment for these patients is fluid restriction. Other treatment options beyond fluid restriction include correction of hypokalemia and use of vasopressin receptor antagonists such as tolvaptan. Hypervolemic hyponatremia also can be caused by prolonged transurethral procedures in which the bladder is irrigated continuously by glycine-buffered water. Hysteroscopy uses similar irrigants and can lead to similar electrolyte disturbances. *Euvolemic hyponatremia* is the most common sodium disturbance among hospitalized patients and is characteristic of both SIADH (discussed earlier) and conditions that lead to excessive free water intake, such as psychogenic polydipsia. Hypothyroidism and adrenal insufficiency also can lead to euvolemic hyponatremia.

Hypovolemic hyponatremia is the most common form of hyponatremia in the postoperative period and is usually the consequence either of sequestration of isotonic fluids (i.e., "third spacing") or of GI losses, wound leakage, or bleeding. Each of these conditions leads to the nonosmotic release of ADH in response to intravascular volume depletion. As a consequence of the volume contraction, the kidneys maximize sodium and chloride retention and excrete a concentrated urine with low sodium concentration (<10 mEq/L). An exception to this occurs in the setting of metabolic alkalosis due to excessive vomiting or nasogastric suctioning, in which case the need to eliminate bicarbonate mandates simultaneous sodium excretion with resultant increases in urine sodium (>20 mEq/L). Renal loss also can cause hypovolemic hyponatremia and is differentiated by a urine sodium of more than 20 mEq/L. Finally, a syndrome known as *cerebral salt wasting* is sometimes encountered

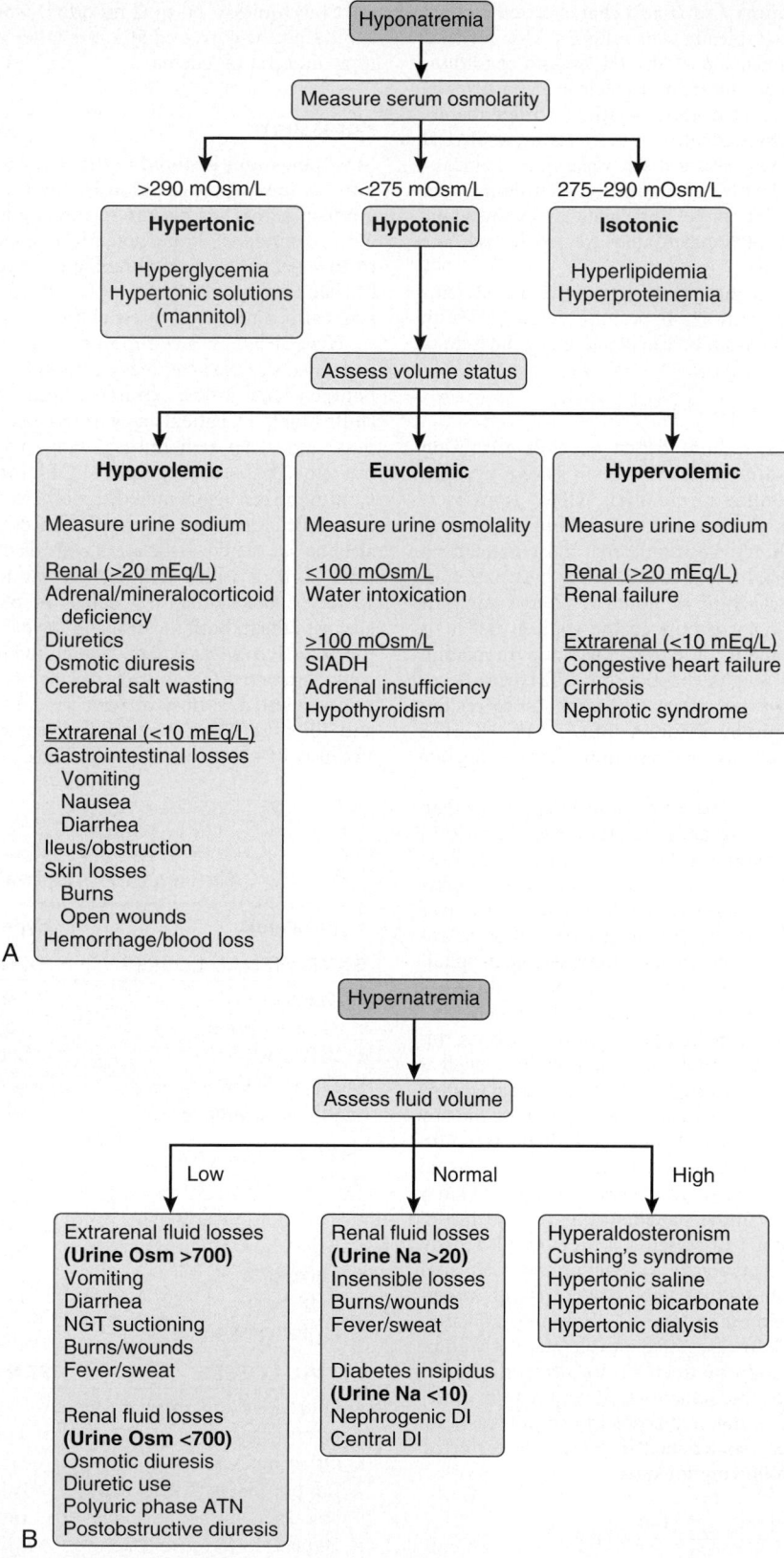

FIGURE 2 A, Hyponatremia. **B,** Hypernatremia. *ATN,* Acute tubular necrosis; *DI,* diabetes incipitus; *Na,* sodium; *NGT,* nasogastric tube; *Osm,* osmolality; *SIADH,* syndrome of inappropriate antidiuretic hormone secretion.

in patients suffering head trauma and is also characterized by high urine sodium concentration (typically >40 mEq/L). This form of hyponatremia may be easily mistaken as SIADH, as both conditions can occur in patients after head injury, and result in hyponatremia associated with high urine sodium concentration. Differentiating these conditions requires an assessment of volume status, as SIADH is defined by euvolemia, whereas cerebral salt wasting is characterized by hypovolemia. Unlike the other forms of hyponatremia, water restriction will worsen the electrolyte imbalance in hypovolemic hyponatremia, which is instead appropriately treated by isotonic volume replacement.

In severe (<120 mEq/L) or symptomatic hyponatremia, patients should be treated aggressively with 3% hypertonic saline (HTS) to correct the sodium deficit, which can be calculated using the following formula:

$$Na\ deficit = (140 - plasma\ Na) \times TBW$$

The rate of correction of the sodium deficit depends greatly on the chronicity of the hyponatremia. With chronic severe hyponatremia, the risk of central pontine myelinolysis (CPM) from overzealous correction outweighs the risks of continued hyponatremia, and plasma sodium levels should be monitored and corrected no faster than 0.25 to 0.5 mEq/L/hr. For acute severe hyponatremia, which is characterized by onset within 48 hours or severe symptoms such as seizures, more rapid correction of the sodium deficit is better tolerated. In these patients, the risk for brain herniation from the sodium deficit outweighs the risk for CPM because of rapid correction, and a more aggressive approach to correction should be pursued. This typically includes infusion of 3% HTS over a 2- to 4-hour period to achieve a maximum correction rate of 1 to 2 mEq/L/hr.

Hypernatremia is defined as a plasma sodium level greater than 145 mEq/L and is categorized further as moderate (146 to 159 mEq/L) or severe (≥160 mEq/L). Symptoms include muscle weakness, restlessness, insomnia, and with severe elevations, lethargy and coma. CPM may result from abrupt increases in plasma sodium and is characterized by paralysis, dysarthria, dysphagia, and other neurologic symptoms. *Hypovolemic hypernatremia* can be seen in hospitalized patients where uncontrolled losses of hypotonic fluid are occurring (i.e., evaporative losses from respiratory tract, skin, and wounds) and access to water is limited. In postoperative patients, this condition should be suspected when GI losses are ongoing—such as with nasogastric suctioning, vomiting, or diarrhea—and volume replacement has been inadequate. Renal losses from diuretic therapy or severe hyperglycemia can result in hypovolemic hypernatremia, which can be differentiated from the aforementioned causes by an elevated urinary sodium (>20 mEq/L). *Euvolemic hypernatremia* may be seen among surgical and trauma patients as a consequence of increased insensible losses or DI (as discussed previously). Finally, *hypervolemic hypernatremia* is typically iatrogenic and seen after resuscitation with IS or HTS but also may be associated with mineralocorticoid and glucocorticoid excess (Conn's syndrome and Cushing's syndrome, respectively). In cases of hypovolemia, the volume deficit should be restored in addition to efforts to correct the hypernatremia; conversely, hypervolemic patients often will require diuresis simultaneous with free water replacement. In all cases of hypernatremia, there is a free water deficit that must be corrected. This is calculated using the following formula:

$$FW\ deficit = \frac{[Na_{plasma}] - 140}{140} \times TBW$$

In general, one half of the calculated deficit is replaced in the first 24 hours, and the remaining half is replaced in the following 24 hours. Moderate hypernatremia should be corrected with 0.45% NaCl, whereas severe cases should be corrected with 5% dextrose. The rate of correction depends on the chronicity of the sodium disturbance. Acute hypernatremia (<48 hours) can be corrected relatively quickly (1 to 2 mEq/hr), whereas chronic disturbances should not be corrected at a rate faster than 0.5 mEq/L/hr in order to avoid cerebral edema.

Potassium

Most potassium is stored in the ICF, with ECF levels maintained at a much lower concentration by the Na^+-K^+ pump. The potassium gradient across the plasma membrane is the principal determinant of the resting membrane potential in most cells, and the maintenance of this electrochemical potential is essential for nerve, muscle, and cardiac function. In addition to cellular uptake, potassium homeostasis also is regulated by renal excretion.

Hypokalemia is a common problem in the postoperative period; is defined as a plasma potassium less than 3.5 mEq/L; and is divided between renal losses, extrarenal losses, and intracellular potassium shifts (Table 1). Patients may experience symptoms of fatigue, weakness, and atrial arrhythmias, with characteristic flattened T or U waves on electrocardiography (ECG). Intestinal ileus also may occur. Common risk factors include renal (i.e., diuretics) and GI losses (i.e., nasogastric drainage, diarrhea, high ostomy output). Hypokalemia also may be seen in association with alkalosis and insulin administration, both of which increase cellular uptake of K^+. To effectively correct hypokalemia, any deficit in plasma magnesium must be addressed first. Both the oral and the parenteral route can be utilized for potassium replacement, though the intravenous (IV) route typically is reserved for severe hypokalemia or inability to tolerate oral replacement. The dose of replacement typically ranges between 40 and 100 mEq/L and typically is given in two to four divided doses. Because of the risk of arrhythmias, cardiac monitoring should

TABLE 1: Causes of Abnormal Potassium Levels

Hypokalemia	Hyperkalemia
EXTRARENAL LOSSES	**EXTRARENAL CAUSES**
• Diarrhea	• Pseudohyperkalemia
• Malabsorption	• Metabolic acidosis
• VIPomas	• Succinylcholine
• ZE syndrome	• Beta-2 adrenergic antagonists
• Villous adenomas	• Digoxin
	• Rhabdomyolysis
INTRACELLULAR POTASSIUM SHIFT	• Tumor lysis syndrome
	• Ethanol or methanol
• Metabolic alkalosis	• Salicylates
• Beta-2 adrenergic agonists	• Insulin deficiency
• Theophylline	
• Caffeine	
• Hyperthyroidism	
RENAL LOSSES	**RENAL ETIOLOGIES**
• Diuretics (loop, thiazide, and osmotic agents)	• Renal failure
• Other medications (amphotericin B, cisplatin, foscarnet, aminoglycosides)	• Mineralocorticoid deficiency (1° hypoaldosteronism, Addison's disease, ACE inhibitors, ARBs, NSAIDs)
• Hyperaldosteronism (Conn's syndrome, Cushing's syndrome, dehydration)	• Mineralocorticoid resistance (spironolactone, trimethoprim, cyclosporine, tacrolimus)
• Magnesium deficiency	
• Delirium tremens	

ACE, Angiotensin-converting enzyme; *ARBs*, angiotensin receptor blockers; *NSAIDs*, nonsteroidal anti-inflammatory drugs; *ZE*, Zollinger-Ellison.

be used when replacement exceeds 10 mEq/hr. The majority of potassium stores are intracellular, and full repletion often takes several days. It is important that patients with compromised renal function receive smaller doses for potassium replacement because of their reduced capacity for potassium excretion, and electrolyte replacement protocols generally are not appropriate for these patients (Table 2).

Hyperkalemia is defined as a plasma potassium level exceeding 5.5 mEq/L and typically is divided into extrarenal and renal origins (see Table 1). Pseudohyperkalemia is encountered commonly in hospitalized patients and is a spurious result that results from hemolysis during venipuncture or sample handling. The most important toxicity associated with hyperkalemia is ventricular arrhythmias. Before the onset of such arrhythmias, the ECG will demonstrate peaked T waves, widened QRS complexes, shortened QT intervals, and ventricular ectopy. Common causes of hyperkalemia include acute renal failure, acidosis, rhabdomyolysis, cell lysis, and insulin deficiency (see Table 1). The depolarizing neuromuscular blocker succinylcholine also is known to cause hyperkalemia, which can be exacerbated in patients with severe muscle atrophy, major trauma, or burn injury. Significant hyperkalemia also can be seen with ischemia-reperfusion events that can occur after revascularization of an ischemic limb, especially if the duration of ischemia is in the range of 4 to 6 hours. Mineralocorticoid deficiency or resistance (i.e., hypoaldosteronism) also is associated with elevated potassium levels and can be accompanied by renal tubular acidosis. Treatment of hyperkalemia typically involves an initial dose of calcium gluconate (1 g) that helps to stabilize cardiac myocytes from potassium-induced depolarization. Plasma levels can be reduced by driving potassium into the ICF compartment and increasing elimination. Intracellular movement is promoted by giving 25 g of IV dextrose along with 10 U of insulin, as well as 50 mEq of bicarbonate. Beta-2 adrenergic agonists such as albuterol (10 to 20 mg in 4 mL nebulized saline) also may be used to increase cellular uptake of potassium. Although these measures will cause a transient decrease in plasma potassium levels, elimination is accomplished either by increasing renal or GI excretion or by hemodialysis. Sodium polystyrene is a Na-K exchange resin that facilitates GI elimination of potassium and can be given by either the oral or the rectal route at a usual dosage of 40 g. Caution must be used with the rectal route in immunosuppressed patients, as intestinal perforation has been reported. Loop diuretics such as furosemide can be used to increase renal elimination of potassium, but this route depends on intact kidney function. Finally, patients with hypoaldosteronism due to mineralocorticoid deficiency can be treated with fludrocortisone (0.05 to 0.2 mg/day).

Calcium

Calcium is the most abundant electrolyte in the body, although the vast majority is in the mineralized state within bone and only 1% resides in the ECF compartment. Within the ECF fraction, 40% is bound to albumin and other proteins, 15% is complexed with anions such as phosphate and citrate, and the remaining 45% is in the biologically active ionized form. Because a large portion of the total ECF calcium is bound to albumin, any decrease in plasma albumin also will lead to a decrease in the measured total plasma calcium (approximately 0.8 mEq/L for every 1 g/dL decrease in albumin). Plasma calcium levels are controlled principally by parathyroid hormone (PTH) and vitamin D levels under normal conditions. Figure 3 illustrates the feedback mechanisms that control calcium and phosphate hemostasis under normal conditions. Decreases in plasma ionized calcium levels stimulate PTH secretion by chief cells in the parathyroid glands. Magnesium levels influence this feedback loop by increasing PTH secretion when plasma Mg^{2+} levels are mildly decreased but inhibiting PTH secretion when Mg^{2+} levels are severely decreased. Increases in PTH lead to an overall increase in ECF calcium concentration and a decrease in phosphate levels. PTH accomplishes this by stimulating osteoclasts to increase resorption of

TABLE 2: Example of Electrolyte Replacement Protocol*

Potassium	
Serum Level (mg/dL)	**Replacement Dose[†]**
3.3-3.9	40 mEq KCl PO/IV
3.0-3.2	60 mEq KCl PO/IV
2.6-2.9	80 mEq KCl IV
<2.6	100 mEq IV

[†]IV KCl infusion rate should not exceed 10 mEq/hr through peripheral line or 40 mEq/hr using central line and continuous cardiac monitoring.

Magnesium	
Serum Level (mg/dL)	**Replacement Dose[†]**
1.6-1.9	4 g MgSO₄ IV or 250 mg MgO PO × 2 doses[‡]
1.0-1.5	6 g MgSO₄ IV
<1.0	8 g MgSO₄ IV

[†]IV MgSO₄ infusion rate should not exceed 2 g/hr.
[‡]Oral magnesium replacement should be avoided in patients with poor oral tolerance or GI disturbance.

Phosphorus	
Serum Level (mg/dL)	**Replacement Dose[†]**
2-2.5	20 mmol Na-Phos or K-Phos (provides ~30 mEq K⁺)
1.6-1.9	30 mmol Na-Phos or K-Phos (provides ~44 mEq K⁺)
<1.6	40 mmol Na-Phos or K-Phos (provides ~60 mEq K⁺)

[†]For simultaneous K⁺ replacement, subtract the amount given with K-Phos and give remainder as KCl.

Calcium	
Serum Level (mg/dL)[†]	**Replacement Dose[‡]**
3.5-3.9	2 g IV Ca-gluconate
3.0-3.4	4 g IV Ca-gluconate
<2.9	6 g IV Ca-gluconate

[†]Ionized calcium, 1 mg/dL = 0.25 mmol/dL.
[‡]IV Ca-gluconate infusion rate should not exceed 2 g/hr; for CaCl, give one-third dose using central line and continuous cardiac monitoring.

*Excludes patients on dialysis or with creatinine clearance <20 mL/min.

CaCl, Calcium chloride; *Ca-gluconate*, calcium gluconate; *GI*, gastrointestinal; *IV*, intravenous; *K⁺*, potassium; *KCl*, potassium chloride; *K-Phos*, potassium phosphate; *MgO*, magnesium oxide; *MgSO₄*, magnesium sulfate; *Na-Phos*, sodium phosphate; *PO*, per os (oral).

bone, thereby liberating mineralized calcium into the ECF compartment, and to increase phosphate excretion by the kidney, which permits the calcium liberated from bone to remain in the ionized form. PTH further regulates calcium levels by its effects on the kidney, where it increases tubular reabsorption of calcium and

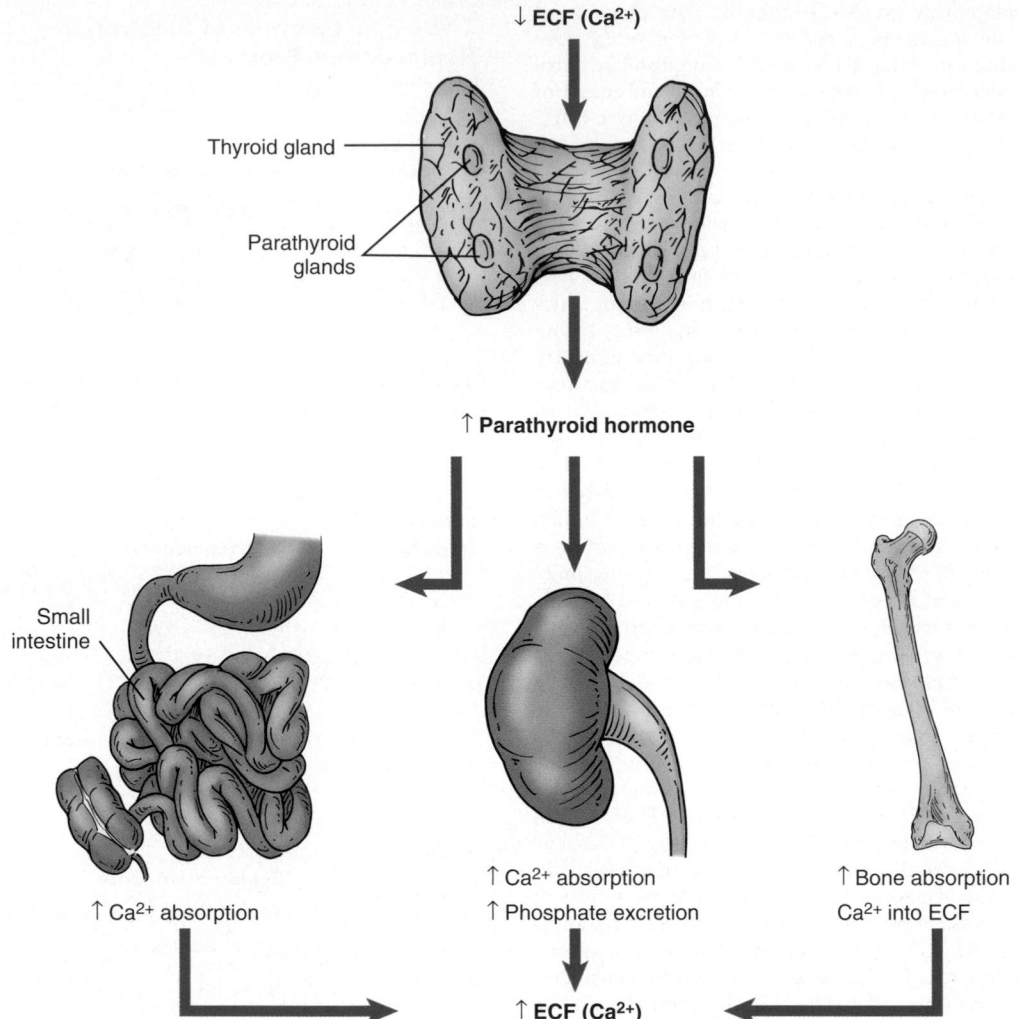

↓ ECF (Ca²⁺)

Thyroid gland

Parathyroid glands

↑ **Parathyroid hormone**

Small intestine

↑ Ca²⁺ absorption

↑ Ca²⁺ absorption
↑ Phosphate excretion

↑ Bone absorption
Ca²⁺ into ECF

↑ ECF (Ca²⁺)

FIGURE 3 Calcium homeostasis. *Ca²⁺*, Calcium; *ECF*, extracellular fluid.

stimulates production of calcitriol (1,25-dihydroxycholecalciferol). Calcitriol plays an important role in calcium and phosphate homeostasis, and its secretion by the kidney leads to increased intestinal and renal absorption of Ca²⁺ and phosphate as well as increased bone resorption and remodeling. Calcitonin, produced by the parafollicular cells of the thyroid gland, also is involved in regulation of plasma calcium levels and functions to lower calcium levels primarily by inhibiting bone resorption.

Hypocalcemia is defined as an ionized calcium level less than 4.5 mEq/L or a total plasma level less than 8.4 mEq/L. Symptoms of hypocalcemia tend to be fairly conspicuous and include perioral numbness, tingling, and twitching of facial muscles upon tapping of the facial nerve (Chvostek's sign). Inflation of a blood pressure cuff on the arm causes a characteristic tetany of the muscles of the hand and forearm (Trousseau's sign). Typical ECG findings include a prolonged QT interval and arrhythmias. More severe disturbances include overt tetany, laryngospasm, and seizures. Hypocalcemia can arise acutely after parathyroid or thyroid surgery and also is seen with severe acute pancreatitis, vitamin D deficiency, hyperphosphatemia, hypomagnesemia, malnutrition, rhabdomyolysis, large fluid resuscitations, or rapid blood transfusions. Treatment for hypocalcemia should be undertaken with total adjusted plasma levels less than 7.0 mEq/L, ionized levels less than 3.0 mg/dL, or symptoms. For acute disturbances, IV forms should be utilized and include both calcium gluconate and calcium chloride. The latter contains three

times as much elemental calcium as the former; therefore calcium chloride should be administered only through a central line and in a monitored setting because of concerns for bradycardia and hypotension. Oral forms include calcium carbonate and calcium gluconate, which typically are used in the chronic or mildly symptomatic setting (see Table 2). Supplementation with vitamin D₂ (ergocalciferol) or D₃ (cholecalciferol) also may be considered with vitamin D deficiency or hypoparathyroidism and often permits a lower dose of calcium supplementation.

Hypercalcemia is defined as total plasma calcium greater than 10.4 mEq/L or an ionized level greater than 5.6 mEq/L. Symptoms include nausea, vomiting, altered mental status, depression, lethargy, myalgias, arthralgias, constipation, and symptoms related to kidney stones. Hypercalcemic crisis is characterized by oliguria or anuria, somnolence, and coma and can be seen with plasma calcium levels greater than 14 mEq/L. Severe calcium elevations leading to crisis are seen most commonly with hyperparathyroidism, although they have been described with malignant causes for hypercalcemia. Hyperparathyroidism is the most common cause for hypercalcemia in nonhospitalized patients, whereas underlying malignancies (especially breast, lung, and multiple myeloma) are the most common cause among inpatients. Other less common causes include vitamin A and D overdose, thyrotoxicosis, immobilization, excess calcium supplementation, granulomatous diseases, familial hypocalcemic hypercalciuria, and medications such as thiazide diuretics and lithium. Treatment for hypercalcemia depends on the degree of elevation and presence of symptoms. For mild to moderate increases (10.4 to 14 mEq/L), no immediate treatment is needed unless the rise is sudden or symptoms are present. For severe elevations (>14 mEq/L), aggressive hydration with IS in order to maintain urine output above 100 to 150 mL/hr is undertaken, along with loop diuretics, which help to promote calcium excretion and prevent volume overload. Bisphosphonates such as pamidronate or zoledronic acid, which decrease osteoclast-mediated resorption of bone, also can be utilized. Finally, calcitonin also should be considered with severe hypercalcemia, with the usual dose being 4 IU/kg, repeated every 6 to 12 hours if the first dose is effective.

Phosphorus

Eighty percent of phosphorus is contained within bone, and plasma levels are regulated by PTH and vitamin D as described earlier and illustrated in Figure 3. *Hypophosphatemia* (<2.5 mg/dL) is seen frequently in the postoperative setting and can lead to heart and respiratory failure if severe and left untreated. Major hepatic resections are one of the more common postsurgical conditions associated with hypophosphatemia; however, it also can be seen with intestinal malabsorption, diuretic medications, vitamin D deficiency, hyperparathyroidism, and refeeding syndrome. Treatment should commence when plasma phosphorus is less than 2.0 mg/dL and can be accomplished by the parenteral route using either potassium or sodium phosphate (see Table 2). Adequate repletion of phosphorus may require several days of therapy. *Hyperphosphatemia* (>5 mg/dL) can be seen postoperatively after parathyroid or thyroid surgery, and symptoms are related mostly to concomitant hypocalcemia, with the treatment being volume expansion. Chronic hyperphosphatemia is common in patients with chronic renal insufficiency and can be treated with phosphate binders.

Magnesium

The majority of magnesium is found in the ICF compartment, with less than 1% found extracellularly. *Hypomagnesemia* (<1.6 mg/dL) is common among surgical patients and is usually a consequence of dilution, poor oral intake, and GI losses (i.e., diarrhea, high ostomy output, entcrocutancous fistulae). Symptoms rarely develop until levels drop below 1 mg/dL and include tetany, involuntary movements, seizures, and ventricular arrhythmias (i.e., torsades de pointes). Treatment can be attempted by both the oral and the IV route, although the former is often limited in efficacy because of the development of diarrhea with most commonly available oral supplements. The parenteral route is usually effective but also can present challenges in severe hypomagnesemia because of inhibition of magnesium reabsorption in the kidney as plasma levels acutely increase on initiation of the infusion. For this reason, severe hypomagnesemia should be treated by a long infusion time (6 to 12 hours). For acute treatment of arrhythmias, magnesium sulfate should be given over 3 to 5 minutes (see Table 2). *Hypermagnesemia* is rare and defined as a magnesium level greater than 2.8 mg/dL, although symptoms (lethargy, decreased deep tendon reflexes, cardiac conduction abnormalities) rarely develop until levels are significantly higher (>4 mg/dL). The treatment is similar to that for hypercalcemia and includes IS infusion and loop diuretics. Calcium gluconate should be used if arrhythmias develop.

Chloride

Chloride is the second most abundant electrolyte in the ECF and is the principal plasma anion. In addition to its contribution to osmolality, as noted earlier, chloride plays important roles in muscular function, control of GI and pulmonary secretions, and urine concentration by the kidney.

The normal range for plasma chloride is typically 97 to 107 mEq/L, although this range may vary slightly based on measurement methodology. *Hypochloremia* in surgical patients most commonly results from GI losses from either vomiting or nasogastric suctioning but also may be seen with certain forms of secretory diarrhea such as congenital chloridorrhea or giant rectal villous adenoma (often also accompanied by hypokalemia). High ileostomy output also is encountered commonly among surgical patients and may lead to hypochloremia. Other than GI losses, renal loss is the other main cause for hypochloremia and can be secondary to prolonged diuretic therapy, renal failure, or physiologic chloriduria associated with respiratory acidosis. In the latter, a compensatory metabolic alkalosis is generated by the kidneys, which is accomplished by reabsorption of bicarbonate in exchange for chloride excretion. Dilution also can be a cause of hypochloremia, which can be seen with infusions of hypotonic solutions as well as with pathologic conditions where the ECF is expanded abnormally (i.e., congestive heart failure [CHF]), and typically is accompanied by hyponatremia.

Hyperchloremia may be seen in conditions that cause contraction of the ECF and typically is accompanied by hypernatremia in such cases. High plasma chloride also can be seen with severe diarrhea during which large amounts of bicarbonate are lost in the stool. Other surgically relevant causes for hyperchloremia include pancreatic and biliary fistulas and urinary diversion into the sigmoid colon, which causes prolonged colonic exposure to urine with resultant hypokalemic hyperchloremic acidosis. Probably the most common cause of hyperchloremia among surgical patients is excessive administration of IS, which has a significantly higher chloride concentration (154 mEq/L) than human plasma (typically <110 mEq/L). As in other cases of hyperchloremia, the elevation in plasma chloride is accompanied by a drop in plasma bicarbonate and metabolic acidosis.

Abnormal chloride levels historically have been viewed as clinically insignificant when compared with the other major electrolyte disturbances and only relevant to the extent that they assist in diagnosing acid-base disorders and can signify disturbances in overall fluid balance. Recent work has questioned this dictum, with high chloride levels shown experimentally to be associated with increased circulating inflammatory factors, decreased renal and splanchnic perfusion, and coagulopathy. Clinical studies have demonstrated that septic patients with hyperchloremia have higher rates of mortality and that chloride-restricted fluids associate with less acute kidney injury.

■ BALANCED VERSUS NONBALANCED CRYSTALLOIDS

The term *strong ion difference* (SID) describes the net charge of all fully dissociated cations and anions in a solution. Plasma cationic charge is represented almost exclusively by the strong ion Na^+, whereas anionic charge is contributed mostly by Cl^-, HCO_3^-, and organic anions. Of these, only Cl^- is considered a strong anion, which leads to a calculated SID of approximately 40 mEq/L for plasma. Infusion of an electrolyte solution that causes a decrease in the SID would be expected to cause an increase in H^+ (hydrogen) concentration in order to preserve electroneutrality, with the result being a decrease in plasma pH. The SID of IS is zero because of equimolar concentrations of Na^+ and Cl^-. Conversely, lactated Ringer's solution (LR) has a SID of 28 mEq/L because of unequal concentrations of Na^+ and Cl^- (130 vs 109 mEq/L), with the difference in anionic charge made up by lactate (not a strong ion).

Because the SID of LR is fairly close to that of plasma, it has been categorized as a *balanced* fluid, in contrast to IS, which is considered *nonbalanced*. Consequently, large volume infusions of IS would be expected to decrease plasma SID and lead to acidosis, in addition to the hyperchloremia that occurs with large infusions of IS. Because of these biochemical properties, some investigators have hypothesized that resuscitation with nonbalanced crystalloid solutions has potentially harmful effects when compared with resuscitation with balanced solutions. Supporting this theory, retrospective studies have demonstrated that use of balanced crystalloids results not only in less acidosis, but also fewer perioperative infections, less incidence of dialysis-requiring renal failure, fewer blood transfusions, and decreased overall complications when compared with more traditional resuscitation strategies that utilize predominantly IS. In a recent retrospective study by Raghunathan and colleagues, which included more than 3000 patients in the final matched cohort, the authors found that a higher risk of mortality was seen among septic patients who received a larger proportion of nonbalanced crystalloids for resuscitation. Controlled comparison in a large prospective trial is needed to further investigate the potential benefits of balanced fluids in resuscitation of the critically ill.

■ SUMMARY

The management of electrolyte disturbances requires the modern surgical specialist to combine the fundamentals of physiology with sound clinical judgment and evidence. A systematic approach to these disorders allows for a measured and safe response that can improve efficiency in daily practice and occasionally is lifesaving when severe electrolyte disturbances arise. Recent evidence suggests that electrolytes such as chloride, which previously was thought to be rather mundane from a physiologic standpoint, may warrant closer attention in the setting of resuscitation from critical illness.

SUGGESTED READINGS

Adrogue HJ, Madias NE. The challenge of hyponatremia. *J Am Soc Nephrol.* 2012;23:1140-1148.

Berend K, van Hulsteijn LH, Gans ROB. Chloride: the queen of electrolytes? *Eur J Intern Med.* 2012;23:203-211.

Handy JM, Soni N. Physiological effects of hyperchloraemia and acidosis. *Br J Anaesth.* 2008;101:141-150.

Lindner G, Funk G-C. Hypernatremia in critically ill patients. *J Crit Care.* 2013;28:216.e11-216.e20.

Morgan TJ. The ideal crystalloid—what is "balanced"? *Curr Opin Crit Care.* 2013;19:299-307.

Piper GL, Kaplan LJ. Fluid and electrolyte management for the surgical patient. *Surg Clin North Am.* 2012;92:189-205.

Raghunathan K, Shaw A, Nathanson B, et al. Association between the choice of IV crystalloid and in-hospital mortality among critically ill adults with sepsis. *Crit Care Med.* 2014;42:1585-1591.

ACID-BASE PROBLEMS

Kathleen M. O'Connell, MD, and Ronald V. Maier, MD, FACS, FRCS Ed (Hon)

The human body attempts to maintain the pH of its fluids between 7.35 and 7.45 in order to optimize enzymatic function. Different theories exist to explain acid-base physiology, the most prominent of which are the traditional and the physiochemical models.

The *traditional model* characterizes acids as hydrogen ion (H^+) donors and bases as H^+ acceptors. It is based on the notion that any change in concentration of H^+ in body fluid results in a compensatory response to restore the pH into normal range. The direction of equilibrium between carbon dioxide (CO_2) and bicarbonate (HCO_3^-) is demonstrated in the following equation.

$$CO_2 (gas) \leftrightarrow CO_2 (aqueous) + H_2O \leftrightarrow H_2CO_3 \leftrightarrow H^+ + HCO_3^-$$

The traditional model uses measured concentrations of plasma CO_2 and HCO_3^- to determine the pH of the blood and is based on the Henderson-Hasselbalch equation. As demonstrated by the Henderson-Hasselbach equation, HCO_3^- is a hydrogen ion acceptor, and CO_2, by its association with H_2CO_3 (carbonic acid), is a hydrogen ion donor. In this equation, the pK is the acid dissociation constant, 0.03 is the solubility constant of CO_2 in the blood, and $PaCO_2$ is the partial pressure of carbon dioxide in the arterial blood.

$$pH = pK + \log_{10}\{HCO_3^-/0.03(PaCO_2)\}$$

The *physiochemical model*, also known as Stewart's strong ion approach, defines acid-base balance according to the laws of electroneutrality. H^+ and HCO_3^- concentrations are dependent on other ion variables, with the preservation of mass balance as the driving force of equilibrium. The physiochemical model accounts for the fact that the same cellular mechanisms that control acid-base physiology also regulate electrolyte homeostasis and therefore are not mutually exclusive.

A combined approach using both models offers a more complete understanding of acid-base physiology. Recent literature focusing on this expanded view of acid-base physiology is referenced in the suggested readings. This chapter focuses more on the traditional approach of categorizing acid-base disorders.

■ ACID-BASE HOMEOSTASIS

The pH range that is compatible with life is 6.8 to 7.8. Acid-base homeostasis is maintained by a combination of alveolar ventilation, renal processes, and various buffering systems (extracellular and intracellular).

Respiratory system: In patients with normal gas exchange, CO_2 diffuses 20 times faster than oxygen, allowing for rapid changes in partial pressure of carbon dioxide ($PaCO_2$). Medullary chemoreceptors monitor changes in cerebral spinal fluid pH and initiate compensatory changes to alveolar ventilation.

Renal system: The proximal tubule functions to reabsorb 85% of the filtered HCO_3^-. Carbonic anhydrase inhibitors such as acetazolamide act in the proximal tubule by preventing HCO_3^- reabsorption. The distal tubule functions to excrete H^+, either in exchange for sodium ions (Na^+), or in combination with ammonia as ammonium chloride (NH_4Cl).

Extracellular buffers: The bicarbonate–carbon dioxide buffer is the most prominent extracellular buffer. Plasma proteins such as albumin and inorganic phosphates contribute to a lesser extent. Bone, although not an acute buffer, absorbs H^+ in exchange for Na^+ and potassium (K^+) and releases calcium, HCO_3^-, carbonate, and phosphates.

Intracellular buffers: The main intracellular buffers are proteins and phosphates. Hemoglobin is the main buffer within red blood cells, with histidine moieties acting as H^+ binding sites.

■ DISORDERS OF ACID-BASE METABOLISM

Acidemia is defined as a plasma pH less than 7.35, and alkalemia is defined as a plasma pH greater than 7.45. These definitions are simply a reflection of the serum pH; they are not a reflection of the acid-base disorders that collectively may or may not lead to pH alteration. Acid-base disorders can be either metabolic or respiratory. An acidosis is any process, metabolic or respiratory, that lowers the pH. An alkalosis is any process, metabolic or respiratory, that

TABLE 1: Expected Compensation for Primary Acid-Base Disturbance

Metabolic acidosis	$PaCO_2 = (1.5 \times [HCO_3^-]) + 8$
Metabolic alkalosis	$PaCO_2 = (0.6 \times [HCO_3^-]) + 40$
Acute respiratory acidosis	$\uparrow HCO_3^- = \Delta PaCO_2/10$
Acute respiratory alkalosis	$\downarrow HCO_3^- = 2(\Delta PaCO_2/10)$
Chronic respiratory acidosis	$\uparrow HCO_3^- = 3.5(\Delta PaCO_2/10)$
Chronic respiratory alkalosis	$\downarrow HCO_3^- = 5(\Delta PaCO_2/10)$

$\Delta PaCO_2$ is calculated from the normal value of 40.

HCO_3^-, Bicarbonate; *$PaCO_2$*, partial pressure of carbon dioxide.

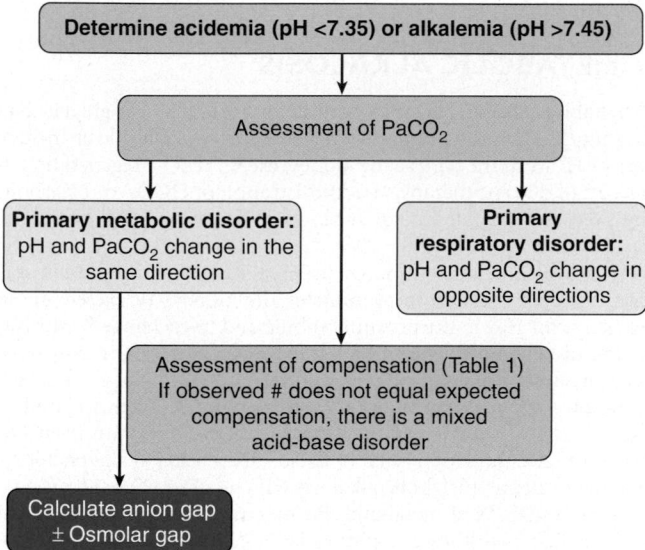

FIGURE 1 Systematic approach to interpreting arterial blood gas. *$PaCO_2$*, Partial pressure of carbon dioxide.

increases the pH. Multiple acid-base disorders can exist at one time (Table 1).

ARTERIAL BLOOD GAS INTERPRETATION

The arterial blood gas (ABG) sample is the clinical tool most commonly used to evaluate acid-base physiology at the bedside. The pH, arterial partial pressure of oxygen (PaO_2), and $PaCO_2$ are measured directly. The derived components include arterial oxygen saturation (SaO_2), HCO_3^- (using the Henderson-Hasselbalch equation), and the base excess (BE).

The BE is the amount of acid measured in mmol/L required to titrate 1 liter of blood to a pH of 7.4 at 37°C; normal values are between −3 and 3. When the BE is a positive value, there is a lack of acid, resulting in a component of metabolic alkalosis. A negative BE value indicates an excess amount of acid, with a contributing metabolic acidosis. Therefore the BE reflects the pure metabolic component of the acid-base disorder and is not affected by acute changes in respiratory variation (Figure 1).

VENOUS BLOOD GAS INTERPRETATION

Although ABG analysis is the gold standard for determining arterial metabolic milieu in critically ill patients, access to arterial blood may

BOX 1: Anion Gap Metabolic Acidosis

Methanol, metformin, muscle injury (rhabdomyolysis)
Uremia (renal failure), uncoupling oxidative phosphorylation (cyanide)
Diabetic ketoacidosis
Propofol infusion syndrome, paraldehyde, propylene glycol (pentobarbital, lorazepam)
Isoniazid
Lactic acidosis
Ethanol, ethylene glycol (antifreeze)
Salicylates, short gut (D-lactate with bacterial overgrowth)

be difficult at times. Studies have demonstrated acceptable correlation of venous blood gas (VBG) samples for pH, $PaCO_2$ (in normocapnia), HCO_3^-, BE, and lactate (when less than 2). Hypercapnia is a clinical situation in which an ABG, not a VBG, should be utilized.

PaO_2 has significant variability and is typically 37 mm Hg lower in venous samples drawn from large central veins than in arterial blood samples. Although this difference is much smaller when the blood sample is drawn from a peripheral vein, the difference is not reliable. Central venous blood gases offer the additional benefit of providing an assessment of global oxygen consumption simply by measuring the central venous oxygen saturation ($ScvO_2$).

ANION GAP METABOLIC ACIDOSIS

Metabolic acidosis occurs when the plasma HCO_3^- is less than 22 mEq/L. The differential diagnosis depends on the presence or absence of an anion gap (AG). The actual AG represents unmeasured serum anions, predominantly albumin, and to a lesser extent phosphates, sulfates, and lactic acid. The AG is calculated by subtracting the measured serum anions (chloride [Cl^-] and HCO_3^-) from the cations (Na^+ and K^+). Because K^+ has such a low concentration in the serum, it generally is negated from the equation.

$$AG = Na^+ - (Cl^- + HCO_3^-)$$

The normal range for AG without potassium is 8 ± 4; however, with various measurement techniques, each institution reports its own expected normal AG. An elevated AG indicates an increase in unmeasured anions. The drawback of the AG is that its validity is dependent on normal circulating levels of albumin. Because most critically ill patients have hypoalbuminemia, the AG is lower than expected. Thus a critically ill patient with low serum albumin may have a metabolic acidosis with a "normal" AG. To correct for this, 2.5 mEq is added to the AG for every 1 g/dL decrease in serum albumin below 4.4 g/dL.

The mnemonic MUDPILES indicates the differential diagnosis of an AG metabolic acidosis (Box 1).

The osmolar gap (OG) is the difference between the measured plasma osmolarity and the calculated plasma osmolarity. Elevation in the OG indicates the presence of unidentified osmotically active substances in the plasma, typically ingested agents such as methanol or ethylene glycol. The OG should be calculated in patients with an AG metabolic acidosis not explained by common causes (i.e., lactic acidosis, renal failure, diabetic ketoacidosis) and when toxic ingestion is suspected. The normal OG is less than 10 mOsm/kg.

$$OG = \text{Measured plasma osmolarity} - \text{Calculated plasma osmolarity}$$

$$\text{Calculated plasma osmolarity} = 2[Na^+] + [(\text{glucose mg/dL})/18] + [(\text{BUN mg/dL})/2.8]$$

where *BUN* is blood urea nitrogen.

■ LACTIC ACIDOSIS

Lactic acidosis results from accumulation of lactate and H⁺ in body fluids and accounts for approximately half of all AG metabolic acidoses. The vast majority of cases of lactic acidosis are caused by sepsis, shock (cardiogenic and hypovolemic), trauma, or severe heart failure. Hypoperfusion leading to tissue hypoxia and anaerobic metabolism results in lactate production that exceeds clearance rates. Mortality is increased by a factor of three when lactic acidosis is secondary to hypoperfusion or sepsis, and a dose-response correlation between lactate levels and mortality has been demonstrated. However, not all cases of lactic acidosis are associated with tissue hypoxia (e.g., liver disease, poisoning with salicylates, cyanide, toxic alcohols).

Pyruvate is a normal end product of glycolysis. During an anaerobic state, pyruvate is not recycled into the Krebs cycle and instead is converted to lactate. Conversion of pyruvate to lactate is catalyzed by lactate dehydrogenase (LDH) and depends on the ratio of reduced to oxidized nicotinamide adenine dinucleotide (NADH/NAD⁺).

$$\text{Pyruvate} + \text{NADH} + \text{H}^+ \underset{(\text{PDH} + \text{thiamine})}{\overset{(\text{LDH})}{\rightleftarrows}} \text{lactate} + \text{NAD}^+$$

The majority of lactic acid is cleared by the liver; however, up to 20% is eliminated renally. Pyruvate dehydrogenase (PDH) is the enzyme responsible for the breakdown of lactate. Deficiency of thiamine, a cofactor of PDH, is a cause of persistent lactic acidosis. Monitoring of lactic acidosis with serum lactate levels, using either arterial or venous samples, is appropriate every 2 to 6 hours until resolution. Restoration of tissue perfusion with fluid resuscitation and optimization of oxygen delivery are the mainstays of treatment. Again, resolution of lactic acidosis is variably dependent on the impact of cellular injury.

■ NORMAL ANION GAP METABOLIC ACIDOSIS

A metabolic acidosis with a normal AG results from a loss of HCO_3^- and a compensatory increase in Cl^- reabsorption by the kidneys (hyperchloremic metabolic acidosis). Common causes of normal AG metabolic acidosis are listed in Box 2.

The most common iatrogenic cause of normal AG metabolic acidosis is rapid normal saline infusion. The normal plasma Na^+ to Cl^- ratio of 140:100 is decreased with aggressive normal saline infusion, as there is a relative increase in the Cl^- concentration. Increased serum Cl^- results in decreased renal HCO_3^- reabsorption.

When HCO_3^- is lost and H^+ secretion is impaired from the kidneys, as in renal tubular acidosis, there is either dysfunction of

---

BOX 2: Normal Anion Gap Metabolic Acidosis

1. Iatrogenic
   - Rapid administration of 0.9% normal saline
   - Total parenteral nutrition with insufficient acetate
2. Kidneys
   - Renal tubular acidosis
   - Carbonic anhydrase inhibitors
   - Spironolactone
   - Ureteral diversion
3. Gastrointestinal tract
   - Diarrhea
   - Duodenal, biliary, or pancreatic diversion

HCO_3^- absorption in the proximal kidney or inability to secrete H^+ as ammonium in the distal kidney. The urinary pH will be alkaline, usually greater than 6 in patients with renal tubular acidosis.

A normal AG metabolic acidosis can result from loss of bicarbonate-rich fluid from the gastrointestinal (GI) tract (duodenal, biliary, and pancreatic fluid and diarrhea). Normal kidneys will compensate by increasing H^+ excretion and HCO_3^- regeneration. As a result, urinary pH will be low (<5) in normal AG metabolic acidosis secondary to a GI source.

Treatment of Severe Metabolic Acidosis

Severe metabolic acidosis occurs at a pH less than 7.2. At this pH, catecholamine resistance dominates, resulting in loss of vasomotor tone and decreased myocardial contractility. Sodium bicarbonate infusion may be warranted in cases of vasopressor resistance, with caution to monitor for increased CO_2 production and excess volume expansion.

■ METABOLIC ALKALOSIS

A metabolic alkalosis occurs when the plasma HCO_3^- is greater than 26 mEq/L. The most common causes of metabolic alkalosis include loss of H^+ from the GI tract or kidney, excess HCO_3^- regeneration as a result of diuretic therapy, or administration of HCO_3^- or bicarbonate precursor (citrate in stored blood or acetate in total parenteral nutrition).

Hypovolemia is a common cause of aldosterone secretion in surgical patients. Aldosterone stimulates the kidneys to excrete H^+ in exchange for Na^+ in the proximal tubule and to exchange K^+ for Na^+ in the distal tubule. The overall effect of aldosterone is avid renal reabsorption of filtered Na^+, Cl^-, and HCO_3^-, with a loss of K^+. Furthermore, hypochloremia (vomiting, nasogastric suction) inhibits the Cl^-/HCO_3^- exchanger in collecting ducts, preventing HCO_3^- excretion. Accumulation of all of these effects leads to a hypochloremic hypokalemic metabolic alkalosis with a paradoxic aciduria.

Manifestations of metabolic alkalosis are mainly neuromuscular and include paresthesias, lightheadedness, and carpopedal spasm from an associated hypocalcemia. Treatment depends on whether the alkalosis is chloride responsive (most common) or chloride resistant. A urinary chloride less than 25 mmol/L is suggestive of chloride-responsive metabolic alkalosis, which can be treated simply with intravenous sodium chloride with potassium supplementation. A urinary chloride concentration greater than 40 mmol/L is often indicative of mineralocorticoid excess, in which case the treatment is directed toward the underlying cause.

■ RESPIRATORY ACIDOSIS

Respiratory acidosis occurs when the $PaCO_2$ is greater than 40 mm Hg secondary to a failure of ventilation to remove all CO_2 produced by cellular metabolism. Acute respiratory acidosis results from central nervous system (CNS) depression (narcotics, sedatives, stroke, trauma), residual paralysis after general anesthesia causing weakness of respiratory muscles, or exacerbation of obstructive lung disease. Chronic respiratory acidosis can be caused by long-standing chronic obstructive pulmonary disease (COPD), pulmonary fibrosis, sarcoidosis, and neuromuscular diseases.

Respiratory acidosis is usually a problem of CO_2 excretion as opposed to overproduction. CO_2 excretion can be altered by the centrally mediated respiratory drive, mechanical components of respiration (myopathies, neuropathies, and obstruction), and alveolar gas exchange (pleural effusions, pulmonary embolism, restrictive or end-stage lung disease).

Symptoms that develop at CO_2 levels greater than 70 mm Hg are known collectively as CO_2 narcosis, which develops as cerebral vasodilation leads to cerebral edema. The syndrome manifests as headache, blurred vision, restlessness, depressed consciousness, and potentially coma. Treatment is directed at reversal of the underlying cause in acute respiratory acidosis, which may include reversal agents (naloxone or flumazenil), bronchodilators, and mechanical ventilation. Caution should be exercised in treating patients with acute or chronic respiratory acidosis, in that correcting the CO_2 level to normal values will lead to a difficult wean from the ventilator as well as cerebral ischemia from vasoconstriction.

■ RESPIRATORY ALKALOSIS

Respiratory alkalosis occurs when the $PaCO_2$ is less than 40 mm Hg. It develops when alveolar ventilation exceeds the rate necessary to eliminate CO_2 produced by the body's metabolism. Stimulation of the central respiratory center arises with pain, fever, CNS lesions, salicylates, and pregnancy. Activation of peripheral chemoreceptors by hypoxemia and stimulation of pulmonary receptors by pneumonia, pulmonary edema, or pulmonary embolism also lead to hyperventilation.

Manifestations are secondary to hypocalcemia, as alkalosis stimulates the binding of calcium to albumin. An abrupt decrease in CO_2 to less than 20 mm Hg causes cerebral vasoconstriction and altered level of consciousness. As with the other acid-base disorders, treatment focuses on correcting the underlying cause.

SUGGESTED READINGS

Berend K, de Vries AP, Gans R. Physiological approach to assessment of acid-base disturbances. *N Engl J Med.* 2014;371:1434-1445.

Juern J, Khatri V, Weigelt J. Base excess: a review. *J Trauma Acute Care Surg.* 2012;73:27-32.

Kellum JA. Clinical review: reunification of acid-base physiology. *Crit Care.* 2005;9:500-507.

Middleton P, Kelly A-M, Brown J, et al. Agreement between arterial and central venous values for pH, bicarbonate, base excess, and lactate. *Emerg Med J.* 2006;23:622-624.

Seifter J. Integration of acid-base and electrolyte disorders. *N Engl J Med.* 2014;371:1821-1831.

CATHETER SEPSIS IN THE INTENSIVE CARE UNIT

Kathleen M. O'Connell, MD, and Heather L. Evans, MD, MS, FACS

It is estimated that 4% of hospitalized patients will develop a healthcare-associated infection (HAI), costing the United States $10 to $30 billion annually. The HAIs with the greatest impact on the healthcare system include surgical site infections, ventilator-associated pneumonia, catheter-associated urinary tract infections, *Clostridium difficile* infections, and central line–associated bloodstream infections (CLABSIs). Although CLABSIs now account for less than 9% of HAIs, they are the most costly HAI on a per case basis, requiring up to an additional $45,000 per infection from payers. Thus in October 2008, when the Centers for Medicare and Medicaid Services (CMS) deemed CLABSI a "never event" and ceased reimbursement for treatment of these infections, a nationwide prevention-focused initiative commenced.

The Centers for Disease Control and Prevention's (CDC's) National Healthcare Safety Network (NHSN), the nation's healthcare-associated infection surveillance system, publishes an annual HAI progress report that includes CLABSI data on the state and national levels. The 2015 report, based on 2013 data, predicted 30,000 CLABSIs, with 18,000 occurring in intensive care units (ICUs) and 12,000 occurring on inpatient wards. With implementation of preventative clinical practice guidelines, mostly in ICUs, there was a 46% decrease in CLABSI rates from 2008 to 2013.

Standardized surveillance definitions are used to describe intravascular catheter-related infections in order to allow consistent identification and monitoring. The CDC defines a CLABSI as a laboratory-confirmed bloodstream infection that develops in a patient with a central venous catheter (CVC) in place for at least 48 hours before onset of the bloodstream infection. The bloodstream infection cannot be related to infection at another site. A *catheter-related bloodstream infection* (CRBSI) requires specific laboratory testing, either a culture-positive catheter tip or a differential time to positivity of blood cultures, to identify the catheter as the source of the bloodstream infection. With a national focus on eradication of CLABSI, this chapter outlines the multidisciplinary preventative measures and treatment guidelines that pertain specifically to surgical intensive care patients.

■ INFECTIOUS DISEASES SOCIETY OF AMERICA'S CLINICAL PRACTICE GUIDELINES, 2011

Implementation of evidence-based catheter care bundles have reduced rates of CLABSI by more than 70%. The bundles are based on the Infectious Diseases Society of America's (IDSA's) clinical practice guidelines, a portion of which are highlighted later. The foundation of these guidelines is education of healthcare personnel, with periodic knowledge assessments, regarding the proper procedures for insertion and maintenance of CVCs.

Selection of Catheter Site

According to a recently published study, subclavian vein catheterization is associated with the lowest risk of CRBSI (0.5%) compared with internal jugular (1.4%) or femoral (1.2%) catheterization sites. Potential explanations for this observation include a longer subcutaneous course before vein entry, the area with lowest bacterial bioburden, and the location with the least dressing disruptions. However, mechanical complications (namely pneumothorax) are highest with subclavian vein catheterization. In patients with advanced kidney disease, the subclavian vein should be avoided to prevent central vein stenosis.

Preparation

Despite the obvious benefits of hand hygiene, cleansing the hands with soap and water or alcohol-based washes before CVC insertion is the most frequently overlooked method to prevent CLABSI. The use of sterile gloves for the insertion of all arterial, central, and midline catheters is recommended. In addition, when guidewire exchanges are performed, new sterile gloves should be worn before handling the new catheter. Maximal sterile barrier precautions (cap, mask, sterile gown, sterile gloves, and sterile full body drape) should be used routinely during CVC insertion. To cleanse the skin, a greater than 0.5% chlorhexidine preparation with alcohol should be used before CVC and peripheral arterial catheter insertion.

Prophylaxis

The use of impregnated catheters, chlorhexidine–silver sulfadiazine or minocycline-rifampin, is recommended for patients whose catheter is expected to remain in place for more than 5 days in facilities where the CLABSI rate is not decreasing despite adherence to basic prevention measures. A recent Cochrane review found that although there was a reduction in the absolute risk of CLABSI and CVC colonization with impregnated catheters, there was no difference in clinically diagnosed sepsis or mortality. Currently, the guidelines recommend the use of chlorhexidine-impregnated sponge dressings if the CLABSI rate is not decreasing despite adherence to basic prevention measures. Another 2015 Cochrane review found that chlorhexidine gluconate or silver-impregnated dressings reduce CLABSI rates compared with all other dressing types. Antibiotic lock solution is recommended for use only in patients with long-term catheters and a history of multiple CRBSIs despite adherence to aseptic maintenance technique. Lastly, routine replacement of CVCs to prevent CLABSI is not supported.

■ INFECTIOUS DISEASES SOCIETY OF AMERICA'S CLINICAL PRACTICE GUIDELINES, 2009: DIAGNOSIS AND MANAGEMENT OF INTRAVASCULAR CATHETER-RELATED INFECTIONS

Diagnosis

In patients with suspected catheter-related infections, paired blood samples from a peripheral vein and the catheter should be cultured before initiation of antibiotic therapy. If a peripheral blood sample cannot be obtained, at least two blood samples should be drawn from multiple lumens on the catheter. If the CVC is removed because of suspected CRBSI, the catheter tip should be sent for culture. Catheter colonization is characterized by growth of more than 15 colony-forming units (CFU) from a 5-cm segment of the catheter tip by semiquantitative culture or by growth of more than 10^2 CFU from a catheter by quantitative broth culture. Two laboratory methods are used to analyze blood samples: quantitative blood cultures and differential time to positivity. A quantitative blood culture is positive for CRBSI when the colony count from the catheter sample is at least three times greater than the colony count from the peripheral vein sample. Quantitative blood cultures are the most accurate method for diagnosing CRBSI and should be used especially in the evaluation of long-term catheters. Differential time to positivity has comparable accuracy and uses continuous blood culture monitoring to detect onset of bacterial growth. Differential time to positivity is confirmatory for CRBSI when microbes grow from the catheter sample at least 2 hours before microbial growth is detected from a peripheral vein sample. Depending on the origin of the sample sent for culture, different criteria are required for the diagnosis of CRBSI (Box 1).

Management

The management of CRBSI depends on several factors, including removal or retention of the catheter and uncomplicated or complicated CRBSI (suppurative thrombophlebitis, osteomyelitis, endocarditis, and metastatic seeding).

BOX 1: Diagnosis of Catheter-Related Bloodstream Infections

1. Peripheral blood sample and catheter tip grow the same organism.
2. Peripheral blood sample and catheter-derived blood sample both meet criteria for quantitative blood culture or differential time to positivity.
3. Catheter-derived blood samples (different lumens): one blood sample has a colony count at least three times greater than the colony count grown from the second blood sample.

Pathogen-Specific Treatment Recommendations

Staphylococcus aureus. Because of a 25% to 30% incidence of infectious complications, traditional treatment for uncomplicated *S. aureus* CRBSI includes removal of the infected catheter and 4 to 6 weeks of antibiotics. Methicillin-susceptible organisms should be treated with nafcillin or oxacillin, with reservation of vancomycin for methicillin-resistant *S. aureus*. Selected patients, including immunocompetent nondiabetics without prosthetic intravascular devices, may be considered for a short course of antibiotic therapy (minimum 14 days). A transesophageal echocardiograph (TEE) should be completed 5 to 7 days after onset of bacteremia if the duration of antibiotics is less than 4 weeks. Concern for a hematogenous complication arises if bloodstream infection and fevers persist for 72 hours or longer after initiation of antibiotic therapy, and a TEE should be performed. Lastly, a catheter tip that grows *S. aureus* with negative peripheral blood cultures should be treated with 5 to 7 days of antibiotics.

Coagulase-negative staphylococci. This is the most common causative organism of catheter-related infections. Colonization of the skin with staphylococci leads to high rates of contamination; however, positive cultures from multiple sites are highly suggestive of coagulase-negative staphylococci CRBSI. In uncomplicated CRBSI, in which the catheter is removed, antibiotic therapy should continue for 5 to 7 days. If catheter retention is desired, antibiotic treatment should extend to 10 to 14 days in combination with antibiotic lock therapy. First-line antibiotics include nafcillin, oxacillin, or vancomycin if methicillin resistance is present. Uncomplicated CRBSI also may be treated without systemic antibiotics if the catheter is removed, the patient is without orthopedic or vascular hardware, and subsequent blood cultures are negative.

Enterococcus. The risk of endocarditis with *E. faecium* and *E. faecalis* bloodstream infection is lower than with *S. aureus*. Treatment includes catheter removal and a 7- to 14-day course of ampicillin, or vancomycin if the organism is ampicillin resistant. Of all *Enterococcus* bloodstream infections, at least 28% are resistant to vancomycin. Vancomycin-resistant *Enterococcus* (VRE) infections should be treated with linezolid or daptomycin. Combination therapy with a cell wall–active antibiotic and an aminoglycoside is not recommended currently as first-line therapy. If the catheter is retained, duration of antibiotics is the same, but antibiotic lock should be utilized.

Gram-negative bacilli. The most common CRBSI organisms include *Escherichia coli*, *Klebsiella*, *Enterobacter*, *Serratia*, *Acinetobacter*, and *Pseudomonas* spp. Critically ill patients with recent infection involving multidrug-resistant gram-negative bacteria should be treated initially with two antibiotics of different classes, followed by de-escalation with final culture and sensitivity results. Catheter removal may not be necessary, even with biofilm-producing organisms, if antibiotic lock therapy is utilized. The choice of antibiotics depends on the cultured organism, but the therapeutic course is 7 to 14 days.

Candida. Catheters with CRBSI due to *Candida* spp. should be removed, and the tip should be sent for culture. Choice of antifungal therapy and duration of treatment depends on the *Candida* species, as susceptibilities vary. *C. albicans* is treated with fluconazole for 14 days, whereas *C. glabrata* is more susceptible to caspofungin, micafungin, or amphotericin B.

■ SUMMARY

Central line catheters are necessary devices in the care of critically ill patients. CLABSIs are a common type of HAI, although their incidence has decreased notably after implementation of evidence-based preventative measures. The mainstay of treatment includes timely recognition and diagnosis, removal of the catheter, and prompt initiation of antimicrobial agents with de-escalation as finalized cultures and sensitivities become available.

SUGGESTED READINGS

Centers for Disease Control and Prevention. *National and state healthcare associated infections progress report.* 2016. <http://www.cdc.gov/hai/progress-report/.>.

Mermel LA, Allon M, Bouza E, et al. Clinical practice guidelines for the diagnosis and management of intravascular catheter infection: 2009 update by the Infectious Diseases Society of America. *Clin Infect Dis.* 2009;49:1-45.

O'Grady NP, Alexander M, Burns LA, et al. Guidelines for the prevention of intravascular catheter-related infections. *Am J Infect Control.* 2011;39(suppl 1):S1-S34.

Parienti JJ, Mongardon N, Megarbane B, et al. Intravascular complications of central venous catheterization by insertion site. *N Engl J Med.* 2015;373: 1220-1229.

Pronovost P, Needham D, Berenholtz S, et al. An intervention to decrease catheter-related bloodstream infections in the ICU. *N Engl J Med.* 2006;355:2725-2732.

THE SEPTIC RESPONSE AND MANAGEMENT

Donald H. Jenkins, MD, and Erica Loomis, MD

Sepsis is a systemic and dysregulated inflammatory response caused by infection and remains one of the most common causes for intensive care unit (ICU) admission. Septic shock resulting in multiple organ dysfunction syndrome is the most catastrophic manifestation of sepsis. Mortality rates of approximately 30% in severe sepsis and approximately 50% in septic shock, combined with a frequency of 2.4 to 3.0 per 1000 population, make sepsis a leading cause of death in noncardiac ICUs. Despite significant clinical advances, the incidence of sepsis continues to increase; with more than 750,000 cases documented in the United States each year, this amounts to $17 billion in health costs annually. In the setting of ongoing basic science and clinical research, treatment of severe sepsis and septic shock remains a challenge for practitioners.

■ DEFINITION

Sepsis and the continuum of severe sepsis and septic shock were defined during a consensus conference in 1991. The definitions were revised further during the International Sepsis Definitions Conference in 2001 and published in 2003, sponsored by multiple international critical care and infection societies. These definitions were created to assist clinicians in recognizing sepsis at a patient's bedside and to more clearly define sepsis for future research.

■ Systemic inflammatory response syndrome (SIRS) is the dysregulated inflammatory response to a variety of noninfectious stimuli, such as trauma, burns, pancreatitis, surgery, and autoimmune disorders. SIRS is considered present when two or more of the following conditions exist.
1. Temperature greater than 38°C or less than 36°C.
2. Heart rate greater than 90 beats/minute.
3. Hyperventilation, demonstrated by respiratory rate of more than 20 breaths/minute or partial pressure of carbon dioxide ($PaCO_2$) lower than 32 mm Hg.
4. White blood cell count greater than 12,000 cells/mm^3, less than 4000 cells/mm^3, or consisting of more than 10% immature forms (bands).
■ Sepsis is defined as at least two SIRS criteria in the setting of confirmed infection (Table 1).
■ Severe sepsis is defined as sepsis resulting in tissue hypoperfusion or end organ dysfunction (Table 2).
■ Septic shock is defined as sepsis with persistent hypotension despite adequate fluid resuscitation. Sepsis-induced hypotension is defined as a systolic blood pressure (SBP) lower than 90 mm Hg, a mean arterial pressure (MAP) lower than 70 mm Hg, or a SBP decrease greater than 40 mm Hg or less than two standard deviations below normal for age.

■ DIAGNOSIS

The diagnosis of sepsis requires a high index of suspicion, thorough documentation of the patient's history, and a careful physical examination to identify possible sites of infection. Then laboratory and imaging studies are ordered as appropriate to assess for evidence of infection or organ dysfunction. Routine laboratory testing should include complete blood cell count, serum electrolyte measurements, liver function testing, lactate measurement, arterial blood gas measurements, blood cultures, urinalysis and urine culture, and culture of potential sites of infection when indicated. Radiographic imaging is often valuable in localizing the site of infection and usually includes plain radiography, ultrasonography, or computed tomographic (CT) scan.

Despite myriad potential indicators for sepsis, no single test guarantees a diagnosis of sepsis; therefore clinician judgment and clinical evidence of systemic inflammation (see Table 1) are necessary to identify patients with sepsis. The use of biomarkers is being investigated and eventually may improve diagnostic accuracy. The 2001 update to the definition of sepsis stresses that documentation of infection may not be required for the diagnosis of sepsis if strong suspicion exists. Additional criteria, such as altered mental status, edema, and hyperglycemia in the absence of diabetes, are also included. Several markers other than lactate levels and white blood cell count are commonly available, including C-reactive protein (CRP), procalcitonin (PCT), interleukin-6 (IL-6), and angiopoietin-1 and angiopoietin-2. Research suggests that these, either individually or in combination, may be useful to determine infectious versus noninfectious SIRS and the risk of mortality and to aid in deciding on antibiotic duration. However, research in this area remains inconclusive, and at this point traditional biomarker strategies have not yielded a gold standard marker for sepsis. Some focus is shifting toward novel strategies such as genomics that improve assessment capabilities, but research in this area at this time is immature in its clinical relativity.

■ TREATMENT

Background

Early and aggressive treatment of patients with sepsis is crucial to improving outcomes. Rivers and colleagues demonstrated that early goal-directed therapy (EGDT) could dramatically improve outcomes for patients arriving at the emergency department with evidence of sepsis. EGDT focuses on completing a series of tasks within the first 6 hours of the patient's arrival, including placing a central venous catheter to monitor hemodynamic variables during fluid resuscitation and titrating the patient's resuscitation to specific targets of central venous pressure (CVP), MAP, and central venous oxygen saturation (ScvO$_2$). In 2004 this approach was adopted by the international Surviving Sepsis Campaign (SSC). In an effort to meet some of the EGDT directives, many institutions have put sepsis resuscitation bundles into place and have demonstrated a decrease in morbidity and mortality with high compliance. Recently three large randomized controlled trials—the Protocolized Care for Early Septic Shock (ProCESS) trial in the United States, the Australasian Resuscitation

TABLE 1: Clinical Signs and Symptoms of Sepsis

Infection	General	Inflammatory	Hemodynamic	Organ Dysfunction	Tissue Perfusion
Documented or suspected	Temperature: >38°C or <36°C Heart rate: >90 beats/min or more than two SDs above the normal value for age Respiratory rate: ≥20 breaths/min Altered mental status Hyperglycemia (plasma glucose >140 mg/dL in the absence of diabetes) Third spacing of fluid (significant edema or positive fluid balance >20 mL/kg over 24 hours)	WBC count: <4000 or >12,000 cells/µL or normal WBC count with ≥10% bands	Hypotension: systolic blood pressure <90 mm Hg MAP: <65 mm Hg or an SBP decrease >40 mm Hg SvO_2: <65%	Hypoxemia (PaO_2/FiO_2 <250) Acute oliguria (urine output <0.5 mL/kg/hr × 2 hr) Coagulopathy (INR >1.5) Platelet count: <100,000 cells/µL Hyperbilirubinemia; ileus	Lactic acidosis Skin mottling StO_2 <70%

FiO_2, Fraction of inspired oxygen; *INR*, international normalized ratio; *MAP*, mean arterial pressure; PaO_2, partial pressure of oxygen; *SBP*, systolic blood pressure; *SD*, standard deviation; StO_2, tissue oxygen saturation; SvO_2, mixed venous oxygen saturation; *WBC*, white blood cell.

TABLE 2: Signs of Organ Dysfunction and Failure

Central nervous system	Encephalopathy Polyneuropathy and myopathy
Cardiac function	Hypotension Tachycardia Tachyarrhythmias Myocardial depression
Pulmonary system	Acute respiratory failure Acute lung injury Acute respiratory distress syndrome PaO_2/FiO_2 <250 in the absence of pneumonia (<200 in the presence of pneumonia)
Renal function	Acute renal failure
Gastrointestinal system	Ileus pseudo-obstruction Gastritis Pancreatitis Gut ischemia
Hepatobiliary	Acalculous cholecystitis Cholestasis Ischemic hepatitis
Metabolic function	Hyperglycemia Hyperlipidemia Lactic acidosis
Hematologic function	Disseminated intravascular coagulation (DIC) Thrombocytopenia
Immunologic function	Immune dysfunction
Endocrine system	Pituitary, adrenal, and thyroid dysfunction

FiO_2, Fraction of inspired oxygen; PaO_2, partial pressure of oxygen.

in Sepsis Evaluation (ARISE) trial, and the Protocolised Management in Sepsis (ProMISe) trial in England—have been completed to re-examine the effect of early goal-directed resuscitation on patient outcomes. Each trial used inclusion criteria similar to the original study by Rivers and colleagues and was powered to detect a 6% to

8% absolute mortality reduction. These trials did not show a significant difference in mortality between groups treated with EGDT and those treated with standard care, which has called into question many of the EGDT guidelines and "sepsis bundles." On further review, however, the ProCESS, ARISE, and ProMISe trials reported control group mortality rates that were markedly lower compared with the original trial by Rivers and colleagues, which likely reflects gradual improvements in intensive care since the 1990s, including the adoption of SSC guidelines that support early identification of sepsis and prompt initiation of antibiotics. The majority of patients assigned to standard care in these trials received fluid boluses within the first 6 hours and antibiotics before randomization; therefore although there may be some moderation to the EGDT guidelines, which is highlighted in this chapter, the general principles appear to have withstood the test of time and thus will be reviewed.

Initial Management Approach

Patients should be assessed quickly for adequacy of the airway and breathing, appropriate intravenous access should be obtained, and fluids should be administered. Patients should be triaged to the appropriate level of care, which is frequently the ICU, but initial therapy should be started immediately and not reserved until the patient reaches the ICU (Tables 3 and 4).

Initial Resuscitation

Immediate resuscitation with isotonic fluid boluses should be started. In patients with evidence of hypoperfusion and hypovolemia, an initial fluid challenge of 30 mL/kg is recommended. After the initial fluid bolus, the patient's response to the fluid challenge is determined; if the response is inadequate, further fluid boluses should be administered as needed. Adequacy of response is determined by both clinical factors and measured endpoints of resuscitation. The initial goal should be a MAP of 65 mm Hg or higher or a urine output of 0.5 mL/kg/hr or higher. If the patient does not respond to the second fluid bolus, the clinician should consider placing a central venous catheter to measure CVP and either $ScvO_2$ or mixed venous oxygen saturation (SvO_2). Resuscitation then should continue to achieve a CVP of 8 to 12 mm Hg (12 to 15 mm Hg in patients with known pre-existing decreased ventricular compliance or in mechanically ventilated patients) and either an $ScvO_2$ of 70% or an SvO_2 of 65%. $ScvO_2$ can be monitored continuously through a commercially available triple-lumen central venous catheter or can be checked intermittently with laboratory draw. An emerging alternative to $ScvO_2$ is tissue oxygen saturation (StO_2) monitoring, wherein a commercially available sensor is placed on the patient's thenar eminence. This provides a direct, noninvasive, and continuous monitor of oxygen

TABLE 3: Summary of Recommendations and Goals of Care for the Patient With Sepsis

Initial resuscitation diagnostics	History and physical examination, cultures, radiographic studies MAP: >65 mm Hg CVP: 8-12 mm Hg $ScvO_2$: ≥70% UOP: >0.5 mL/kg/hr Hgb: >10 g/dL
Antibiotics	Broad-spectrum antibiotics against likely pathogens; adjust therapy when culture results are available
Source control	Surgical repair, resection, or drainage of source of contamination; evacuation of infectious material
Vasopressors	Goal MAP: >65; fluid resuscitation and arterial catheter required
Inotropes	Goal is to meet physiologic cardiac output; fluid resuscitation required, echocardiography should be considered
Steroids	For septic shock unresponsive to fluid resuscitation and vasopressors, consider low-dose steroid therapy
Blood transfusion	Hgb of 7-9 g/dL unless persistent lactic acidosis, hemorrhage, coronary ischemia, or severe hypoxemia
Ventilation	Tidal volume of 6 mL/kg and plateau pressure <30 cm H_2O; use PEEP to prevent alveolar collapse
Glucose control	Target serum glucose: 140-180 mg/dL; insulin infusion and frequent blood glucose monitoring may be required
Renal replacement therapy	Intermittent hemodialysis for hemodynamically stable patients; consider continuous hemodialysis for patients with unstable hemodynamics
Prophylaxis	VTE: mechanical compression devices and heparin or low-molecular-weight heparin; use cautiously in patients at risk for bleeding Stress ulcer: histamine blocker or proton pump inhibitor VAP: maintain head of bed ≥30 degrees; use oral chlorhexidine glucontate as a form of oropharyngeal decontamination

CVP, Central venous pressure; *Hgb,* hemoglobin; *MAP,* mean arterial pressure; *PEEP,* positive end-expiratory pressure; *ScvO$_2$,* central venous oxygen saturation; *UOP,* urine output; *VAP,* ventilator-associated pneumonia; *VTE,* venous thromboembolism.

content at the tissue level using near infrared spectroscopy. Levels less than 70% indicate significant tissue hypoperfusion, and abnormal values less than 70% or greater than 90% have been correlated to increased ICU length of stay. Patients with sepsis have been documented to have lower StO_2 levels than healthy controls, and sepsis survivors have been shown to have higher StO_2 levels than nonsurvivors.

In patients in whom lactate levels are elevated as a result of tissue hypoperfusion, resuscitation to a normal lactate level also may be used as an adequate endpoint of resuscitation. The use of sodium bicarbonate therapy in the treatment of hypoperfusion-induced lactic acidemia associated with sepsis is not supported for patients with a pH of 7.15 or greater. The fluid of choice during initial resuscitation should be an isotonic crystalloid. Hydroxyethyl starches should not be used because they have not been shown to improve mortality rates and have been shown to increase risk for acute kidney injury. In patients who require a large volume of resuscitative measures, albumin supplementation may be considered. Although the initial description of EGDT recommended transfusing to a hemoglobin level of 10 g/dL or higher, current recommendations support restricting blood transfusion to patients with a hemoglobin level lower than 7 g/dL with a goal hemoglobin range of 7 to 9 g/dL except in extenuating circumstances such as active hemorrhage, myocardial ischemia, and persistent and severe hypoxemia.

Antimicrobial Therapy

Broad-spectrum antimicrobial therapy targeting all likely pathogens should be administered as soon as possible, ideally within 1 hour, after the diagnosis of severe sepsis or septic shock. If possible, cultures of blood, urine, and other fluids, if necessary, should be obtained before administration of antibiotics, but the need for these specimens should not delay antibiotic therapy. Multiple studies have shown increased rates of mortality with each hour that antibiotic therapy is delayed in septic shock. When selecting an appropriate antimicrobial regimen, practitioners must be aware of the antimicrobial resistance patterns at their institutions and the most likely causative organisms. The most common pathogens that cause septic shock in hospitalized patients are gram-positive bacteria, followed by gram-negative and mixed bacterial micro-organisms. Patients with prior exposure to antibiotics, prolonged history of hospitalization, or history of colonization or infection with resistant organisms are at the greatest risk for sepsis from resistant organisms. Empiric antifungal therapy should be started in patients who are immunocompromised, including those receiving chemotherapy, chronic steroids, or immunomodulators and those who have received organ transplants. Empiric antifungal therapy also should be considered in patients on long-standing total parenteral nutrition (TPN). Recent Infectious Diseases Society of America (IDSA) guidelines recommend either fluconazole or an echinocandin. The initial selection of antimicrobial therapy should be broad enough to cover all likely pathogens. Empiric therapy should not be continued for more than 3 to 5 days, and the antimicrobial regimen should be assessed daily to determine whether de-escalation of therapy can be achieved safely. De-escalation as soon as clinically reasonable limits organism resistance, reduces toxicity, and decreases the cost of therapy. The duration of therapy is typically 7 to 10 days, although longer courses may be appropriate in patients who have a slow clinical response, undrainable focus of infection, bacteremia with *Staphylococcus aureus,* some fungal and viral infections, or immunologic deficiencies (neutropenia). Low PCT levels may be used as a marker for discontinuation of empiric antibiotics.

TABLE 4: Timeline of Implementation of Recommended Diagnostic and Therapeutic Goals

Time	Resuscitation	Antimicrobials	Vasopressors and Inotropes	Monitoring	Specific Therapy	Supportive Therapy
Within 3 hours (preferably within 1 hour)	Obtain IV access, initiate crystalloid fluid resuscitation (30 mL/kg)	Initiate empiric broad-spectrum antimicrobials (preferably after cultures have been obtained)	N/A	Telemetry, blood pressure, oxygen saturation, urine output	Send cultures, obtain labs (CBC, electrolytes, liver function tests, ABG, lactate), order imaging	Oxygen support, consider intubation and mechanical ventilation before overt respiratory distress
Within 6 hours	Consider albumin if patient has received a substantial amount of crystalloid, consider blood transfusion if Hgb <7 or if extenuating circumstances exist (myocardial ischemia or severe hypoxemia)	Continue and obtain source control once source has been identified	Start vasopressors (norepinephrine) if hypotension persists despite initial fluid resuscitation to maintain MAP ≥65 mm Hg	In the event of persistent hypotension, place arterial line, place central line to measure CVP (goal ≥8 mm Hg) and ScvO$_2$ (goal ≥70%), initiate StO$_2$ monitoring if available	Remeasure lactate if initial was elevated and adjust resuscitation as needed to normalize lactate, follow up on imaging and plan for intervention based on results	ICU admission, consider low-dose steroid therapy (200 mg/day) if shock state persists
Hours 6-24	Ongoing dynamic evaluation of resuscitative goals based on clinical and invasive monitoring endpoints		Consider vasopressin if shock is refractory to norepinephrine	If pressor dependence persists after 3-5 L crystalloid infusion and CVP ≥8, suspect intravascular volume depletion or limited cardiovascular reserves, consider bedside TEE	Follow blood glucose	Initiate enteral feeding, initiate insulin if blood glucose higher than 180 mg/dL on two consecutive readings
>24 hours		Narrow antimicrobial regimen depending on isolation of pathogenic organisms or clinical improvement, reassess necessity for or efficacy of source control				Intensive hemodialysis therapy for renal failure, advance tube feedings to goal over the next 5-7 days as patient tolerates, follow renal function and urine output and initiate hemodialysis for renal failure and low-pressure, volume-limited ventilation for ARDS

Modified from Kumar A, Kumar A: Sepsis and septic shock. In: Gabrielli A, Layon AJ, Yu M, eds. *Critical Care*. 4th ed. Philadelphia: Lippincott Williams & Wilkins; 2009.

ABG, Arterial blood gas; *ARDS*, acute respiratory distress syndrome; *CBC*, complete blood count; *CVP*, central venous pressure; *Hgb*, hemoglobin; *ICU*, intensive care unit; *IV*, intravenous; *MAP*, mean arterial pressure; *N/A*, not applicable; *ScvO$_2$*, central venous oxygen saturation; *StO$_2$*, tissue oxygen saturation; *TEE*, transesophageal echocardiography.

Monitoring

In patients with severe sepsis and septic shock, vital signs and other markers of resuscitation must be monitored frequently. All patients should be monitored with simple noninvasive measures such as telemetry, pulse oximetry, and blood pressure cuff measurements. As discussed earlier, StO_2 monitoring is an emerging noninvasive therapy used to continuously monitor oxygen content at the tissue level. With levels less than 70% or greater than 90% considered abnormal, this measure can serve as an additional resuscitation guide.

Depending on the patient's condition, a number of invasive monitors may be indicated and added in a stepwise manner as the patient's condition warrants. A Foley catheter should be placed in all septic patients, except in those who have pre-existing anuria. Arterial catheterization should be performed in patients who require prolonged vasopressor therapy, in order to more accurately measure blood pressure. Although these two interventions carry risk for serious complications, their benefit outweighs their risk in the short term. EGDT and the guidelines for surviving sepsis advocate for placement of a central venous catheter as a protocol for resuscitation in patients with evidence of tissue hypoperfusion. This catheter is used to reach a target CVP of 8 to 12 mm Hg and a target $ScvO_2$ of 70% or higher. Unfortunately, the value of CVP measurements in determining a patient's intravascular volume status remains controversial. A low CVP is probably indicative of a favorable response to volume resuscitation; however, in patients with normal to high CVP and in those with abnormal cardiac function or pulmonary hypertension, CVP is likely to be an unreliable indicator of volume status. A pulmonary artery catheter can provide more information about cardiac function than a central venous catheter, but its use has not been shown to improve outcomes in septic patients and in fact may worsen outcomes. The use of more dynamic indices of resuscitation is becoming more common, but none has been standardized yet in sepsis management.

Ultrasonography has become ubiquitous in the ICU, and it can be useful in determining a patient's volume status (measuring inferior vena cava [IVC] distensibility) and cardiac function. Ultrasonography has the advantage of being noninvasive, but it is a static measure and therefore necessitates serial imaging. Interpreting images is prone to variability in user skill.

Bedside echocardiography is emerging as a promising tool for continuous hemodynamic management in patients with sepsis. Transesophageal echocardiography provides direct cardiac visualization; left ventricular filling and function and right ventricular function and fluid responsiveness can be evaluated by obtaining three primary views. Current research suggests that this can be done by critical care physicians with no formal training in echocardiography. Previously, probe size made repeat examinations difficult and costly; a miniaturized, disposable probe has been developed that can be left in place for up to 72 hours, allowing the intensivist to optimize cardiac performance during resuscitation of the intubated patient with septic shock.

Hemodynamic Support

Vasopressor support should be instituted when patients continue to demonstrate hypotension or tissue hypoperfusion despite fluid resuscitation. The initial goal for MAP should be at least 65 mm Hg because this pressure has been shown to preserve tissue perfusion. However, the optimal MAP then may be individualized to the patient on the basis of response to resuscitation. Norepinephrine is the initial vasopressor of choice. Epinephrine should be considered in addition to norepinephrine or in place of norepinephrine when an additional agent is needed to maintain adequate blood pressure. Vasopressin should be added as the second vasopressor when patients fail to respond adequately to norepinephrine or in an effort to decrease norepinephrine dosing. Patients with septic shock have been shown to have relatively low vasopressin levels, and the addition of vasopressin has been shown to improve blood pressure and decrease norepinephrine requirements. However, vasopressin should not be used as a single agent and should be used only at low doses (up to 0.03 to 0.04 U/min); higher doses should be considered salvage therapy. Although vasopressin appears to be effective at supporting blood pressure in septic shock, studies have failed to show any survival benefit. Dopamine may be considered an alternative vasopressor agent to norepinephrine only in highly selected patients because of the increased risk for tachyarrhythmias seen with dopamine use. Low-dose dopamine should not be used for renal protection. In patients with continued hypoperfusion despite adequate fluid resuscitation and blood pressure augmentation, the addition of an inotrope should be considered. Dobutamine is recommended as the first choice for inotropic therapy in patients with measured or suspected low cardiac output in the presence of adequate left ventricular filling pressures (or clinical assessment of adequate fluid resuscitation) and adequate MAP. Milrinone could be considered as an alternative agent. Both dobutamine and milrinone can increase the cardiac output but have a high incidence of causing hypotension. Using inotropes in an attempt to increase cardiac function to supranormal levels is not recommended.

Source Control

Rapid diagnosis and treatment of septic patients is crucial for a good outcome, but early resuscitation and supportive therapy must be accompanied by early identification of the source of infection. Failure to quickly identify a surgically correctable source of sepsis frequently leads to worsening sepsis and death. Implanted devices that are the potential source of sepsis should be removed if this is feasible. Patients with surgically correctable sources of infection (e.g., necrotizing soft tissue infections, peritonitis) should be taken to the operating room as soon as possible for eradication of the infectious source. One caveat to consider is peripancreatic necrosis in the setting of severe pancreatitis. When this is identified as a potential source of infection, definitive intervention is best delayed until adequate demarcation of viable and nonviable tissues has occurred. Other infections may be amenable to percutaneous or endoscopic therapies (abdominal abscess, cholangitis, etc.). The most effective intervention associated with the least physiologic insult should be used when seeking source control in a severely septic patient.

■ SUPPORTIVE CARE

Ventilatory Support

Patients with sepsis frequently require mechanical ventilation because the sepsis increases the work of breathing or because mental status changes caused by infection can compromise the airway. Septic patients are at risk for developing acute respiratory distress syndrome (ARDS); therefore ventilation of septic patients should follow the volume- and pressure-limited strategies used in patients with ARDS.

Patients should be ventilated with a low tidal volume (6 mL/kg) and peak plateau pressures of 30 cm H_2O or lower. Positive end-expiratory pressure (PEEP) should be maintained to minimize alveolar damage from alveolar collapse at the end of expiration, and a high PEEP strategy may need to be considered to prevent or treat ARDS. Sepsis frequently progresses to severe ARDS, which may necessitate additional strategies such as recruitment maneuvers, prone positioning, advanced ventilator modes, and extracorporeal membrane oxygenation. Oral chlorhexidine gluconate should be used as a form of oropharyngeal decontamination to reduce the risk of ventilator-associated pneumonia in ICU patients with severe sepsis. In addition, ventilated patients should be kept with the head of the bed elevated to 30 to 45 degrees to limit aspiration risk. Patients should be assessed daily at a minimum for spontaneous breathing trial and extubation.

Blood Products

Red blood cell transfusions during active resuscitation for sepsis-induced hypoperfusion are still a consideration during EGDT, but a more restrictive approach to transfusion is required once hypoperfusion has been corrected. Transfusion should be reserved for patients with hemoglobin levels lower than 7.0 g/dL, those with active cardiac ischemia, or those with evidence of poor oxygen delivery. Large studies have demonstrated that with more restrictive transfusion practices, outcomes have been similar or improved, even in patients with a history of cardiac disease. The reasons for improved outcomes appear to depend on the multiple complications associated with transfusions, such as immunosuppression, acute lung injury, and transfusion reactions.

Corticosteroids

The adrenal glands and cortisol production are vital to the patient's response to stress and critical illness. Multiple investigators have evaluated the use of glucocorticoid supplementation during sepsis with mixed results; however, patients who remain in shock despite adequate fluid resuscitation and vasopressors appear to be the best candidates for hydrocortisone therapy. Hydrocortisone therapy (200 mg/day) should be started in patients with septic shock refractory to fluids and vasopressors. Corticosteroids are not recommended in septic patients who are not in shock and should be tapered when vasopressors are no longer required.

Glycemic Control

Hyperglycemia is associated with poor outcomes in critically ill patients; however, tight glucose control does not improve mortality rates and results in increased episodes of hypoglycemia. Blood glucose levels of 140 to 180 mg/dL should be the target of therapy, with insulin therapy started when two consecutive blood glucose levels are higher than 180 mg/dL.

Renal Replacement Therapy

The incidence of acute kidney injury and renal failure in patients with sepsis remains high. The timing and intensity of renal replacement therapy have not been shown to affect patient outcome consistently, but early and intensive renal replacement may be helpful. In addition, no clear benefit of continuous renal replacement over intermittent hemodialysis has been shown. Therefore recommendations for acute renal replacement therapy in septic patients should be similar to those in nonseptic patients.

Nutrition

In patients without contraindications to enteral nutrition (bowel obstruction, ileus, peritonitis, etc.), feedings should be started within 48 hours of diagnosis. Enteral delivery is preferred to parenteral nutrition when possible to decrease the risk of infection. Glutamine levels are reduced during critical illness, and exogenous supplementation was once thought to enhance immune cell function and decrease proinflammatory cytokine production; however, a large multicenter randomized trial has shown no benefit and some deleterious effects from glutamine supplementation. No large, reproducible findings suggest a clear benefit in the use of immunomodulating nutritional supplements in sepsis, although trials are ongoing.

Chemical Prophylaxis

Patients with sepsis are at high risk for thromboembolic events as a result of the inflammatory response and immobility. Chemoprophylaxis should be administered with daily subcutaneous low-molecular-weight heparin along with intermittent pneumatic compression devices. Patients with decreased creatinine clearance should receive unfractionated heparin in place of low-molecular-weight heparin. Prophylaxis of stress ulcers in vulnerable patients in the ICU has been shown to decrease gastrointestinal bleeding; therefore septic patients with coagulopathy-related need for mechanical ventilation longer than 48 hours, with traumatic brain or spinal cord injury, with burns, or with recent upper gastrointestinal bleeding should receive prophylaxis gastric ulcer prophylaxis. Once the patient's risk factors have been eliminated, stress ulcer prophylaxis should be discontinued.

Activated Protein C

Recombinant human activated protein C (rhAPC) was introduced in 2001 after a large trial showed decreased rates of mortality among septic patients; however, more recent trials have failed to show a mortality benefit, and the drug has been withdrawn from the market.

Goals of Care

Sepsis is a significant disease process with a high rate of morbidity and mortality despite our best management strategies. Goals of care and prognosis should be discussed with patients and families as early as possible after hospital admission and preferably within 72 hours of admission. Palliative care principles, along with end-of-life care planning when appropriate, should be incorporated in this discussion.

SUGGESTED READINGS

Dellinger RP, Levy MM, Rhodes A, Annane D, Gerlach H, Opal SM, Sevransky JE, Sprung CL, Douglas IS, Jaeschke R, Osborn TM, Nunnally ME, Townsend SR, Reinhart K, Kleinpell RM, Angus DC, Deutschman CS, Machado FR, Rubenfeld GD, Webb SA, Beale RJ, Vincent JL, Moreno R, Surviving Sepsis Campaign Guidelines Committee including the Pediatric Subgroup. Surviving sepsis campaign: international guidelines for management of severe sepsis and septic shock: 2012. *Crit Care Med.* 2013;41:580-637.

Holst LB, Haase N, Wetterslev J, Wernerman J, Guttormsen AB, Karlsson S, Johansson PI, Aneman A, Vang ML, Winding R, Nebrich L, Nibro HL, Rasmussen BS, Lauridsen JR, Nielsen JS, Oldner A, Pettilä V, Cronhjort MB, Andersen LH, Pedersen UG, Reiter N, Wiis J, White JO, Russell L, Thornberg KJ, Hjortrup PB, Müller RG, Møller MH, Steensen M, Tjäder I, Kilsand K, Odeberg-Wernerman S, Sjøbø B, Bundgaard H, Thyø MA, Lodahl D, Mærkedahl R, Albeck C, Illum D, Kruse M, Winkel P, Perner A, TRISS Trial Group, Scandinavian Critical Care Trials Group. Lower versus higher hemoglobin threshold for transfusion in septic shock. *N Engl J Med.* 2014;371:1381-1391.

Mouncey PR, Osborn TM, Power GS, Harrison DA, Sadique MZ, Grieve RD, Jahan R, Harvey SE, Bell D, Bion JF, Coats TJ, Singer M, Young JD, Rowan KM, ProMISe Trial Investigators. Trial of early, goal-directed resuscitation for septic shock. *N Engl J Med.* 2015;372:1301-1311.

Peake SL, Delaney A, Bailey M, Bellomo R, Cameron PA, Cooper DJ, Higgins AM, Holdgate A, Howe BD, Webb SA, Williams P, ARISE Investigators, ANZICS Clinical Trials Group. Goal-directed resuscitation for patients with early septic shock. *N Engl J Med.* 2014;371:1496-1506.

Rivers E, Nguyen B, Havstad S, Ressler J, Muzzin A, Knoblich B, Peterson E, Tomlanovich M, Early Goal-Directed Therapy Collaborative Group. Early goal-directed therapy in the treatment of severe sepsis and septic shock. *N Engl J Med.* 2001;345:1368-1377.

Yealy DM, Kellum JA, Huang DT, Barnato AE, Weissfeld LA, Pike F, Terndrup T, Wang HE, Hou PC, LoVecchio F, Filbin MR, Shapiro NI, Angus DC, ProCESS Investigators. A randomized trial of protocol-based care for early septic shock. *N Engl J Med.* 2014;370:1683-1693.

MULTIPLE ORGAN DYSFUNCTION SYNDROME

Nathaniel McQuay, Jr., MD

Multiple organ dysfunction syndrome (MODS) is defined as a systemic, dysfunctional imbalance of the immunologic response to critical illness. Clinically this imbalance of both the inflammatory and the anti-inflammatory responses is associated with dysregulation of coagulation, mitochondrial dysfunction with subsequent cellular failure, and dysregulated apoptosis (programmed cell death). MODS remains the leading cause of death in the critical care population, with associated mortality rates ranging from 27% to 100%. This wide range in mortality is directly proportional to the number of organ systems involved (Figure 1). Several studies have shown that patients who develops MODS (compared with those who do not) have a higher mortality rate, thereby emphasizing the importance of its development. Historically, sepsis was thought to be the causes of the uncontrolled response. However, subsequent investigations have shown that the body's dysregulated response results from various other stimuli, including infection, injury, and shock. Also noted was a bimodal time-sensitive pattern of MODS with an early and late phase based on the presence of both modifiable and nonmodifiable factors. Recognition of these factors has resulted in changes in the management of these critically ill patients, with a resulting decreasing mortality. The results of evidence-based changes in clinical practice, advancements in organ support, and measures aimed at preventive organ failure are the focus of this chapter.

■ PATHOPHYSIOLOGY AND RISK FACTORS

MODS was thought to result from the nondiscriminatory response to various stimuli, resulting in the inability of the host's defenses to combat the insult. The hyperinflammatory response by neutrophils, lymphocytes, monocytes and macrophages, cytokines, and endothelial cells leads to tissue damage and cellular death via several mechanisms, including ischemia-reperfusion, inflammatory mediators, and the toxic effects of free radicals. This deregulated response is the genesis of MODS. All of these effects have been shown to occur in both injury- and non–injury-induced MODS. The development of MODS is not an "all or nothing" phenomenon but more accurately represents a continuum of varying levels of organ function. Several identified risk factors, serving as either the one-hit or the two-hit insult in the initiation of MODS, serve as the ignitor. Time-sensitive patient profiles based on the immunologic response and etiology categorizes patients into either early or late MODS (Figure 2). The recognition of this continuous process has led to the development of scoring systems to more accurately describe the patient's clinical status as it relates to severity of organ dysfunction. Although no gold standard scoring system currently exists, various systems perform well, with the two commonly used being the Marshall MODS Score (Table 1) and the Sequential Organ Failure Assessment (SOFA) Score (Table 2).

Early diagnosis and intervention appear to be the key in preventing progression of a disease process. Early identification based on risk stratification assists in accomplishing the goal. Previous studies have demonstrated that with each organ dysfunction and eventual failure there is an associated 11% to 23% increased risk of death. The organ system most commonly involved is the respiratory system (hypoxemia), followed by the cardiovascular (shock), renal (oliguria, anuria) and hematologic (coagulopathy, thrombocytopenia) systems in descending order. Sepsis and shock represent the most common risk factors for the development of MODS in the critical care population. In the trauma population, several independent risk factors for the development of MODS have been identified: high injury severity score (ISS), age of transfused red blood cells (RBCs), amount of RBCs transfused, age greater than 55 years, elevated base deficit, male gender, and abdominal compartment syndrome (ACS). These along with other patient injury– and treatment-specific factors serve as causes of the initiation of the unregulated cascade that leads to MODS.

■ SYSTEMIC INFLAMMATORY RESPONSE SYNDROME AND SEPSIS

Originally defined in 1992, with subsequent inception of the Surviving Sepsis Campaign guidelines in 2004, several updates to include the most recent in 2012 have been published. Along with improvements in understanding of the disease process, sepsis has been better defined and classified based on the progression of the disease to include evidence of tissue hypoperfusion or development of organ system dysfunction. Systemic inflammatory response syndrome (SIRS) is defined as a nonspecific clinical response to infection, trauma, burn, or any inflammatory process. The responses include hyperthermia or hypothermia, tachycardia, tachypnea, leukocytosis, or leukopenia. Sepsis is defined as SIRS in the setting of a presumed or documented infection source. Severe sepsis is defined as sepsis-induced tissue hypoperfusion (hypotension persisting after initial fluid challenge or blood lactate concentration ≥ 4 mmol/L) or organ dysfunction. Septic shock is defined as sepsis-induced hypotension persisting despite adequate fluid resuscitation (Table 3).

Recent reports have documented an increase in the rate of severe sepsis in the United States, with more than 750,000 cases per year and rising (projected incidence increase of 1.5% per year) and half of these cases requiring critical care admission. Although severe sepsis mostly is associated with the medical population, critically ill surgical patients are not immune. A recent report by Moore and colleagues at Houston Methodist Hospital looking at 364,000 patient records from the American College of Surgeons National Surgical Quality Improvement Program (ACS NSQIP) database demonstrated a 4% postoperative incidence of sepsis and septic shock. Risk factors identified included age greater than 60 years, emergency surgery, and one or more comorbid conditions. Historically, sepsis has been associated with a high mortality in excess of 80%. With advancements in critical care, improved surveillance, and prompt initiation of evidence-based therapeutic and supportive care, mortality rates have been documented as being closer to 20% to 30% in more recent series.

Sepsis may result from either community-acquired or nosocomial infections. Sepsis management consists of two phases of care: initial resuscitation phase and the critical care phase. Upon identification of sepsis-induced hypoperfusion, a resuscitation protocol following endpoints with the goal of normalizing lactate is recommended, as this approach has demonstrated a significant reduction in mortality in various studies. Crystalloids are the recommended fluid of choice during the initial resuscitation phase, as several trials have failed to show a benefit of colloids during this phase. These resuscitation management goals, along with infectious source management, should occur during the first 3 hours. The second phase of care representing monitoring, organ function support, complication prevention, and appropriate de-escalation of care should occur during the first 6 hours in the critical care setting (Box 1).

Central to the management of the critically ill patient with severe sepsis or septic shock is the early identification of the source of infection and adequate source control. Source control may be achieved via drainage of abscesses, débridement of infected tissue, control of contamination, or the excision of an infected organ. Vascular access devices may serve as a source of sepsis and when

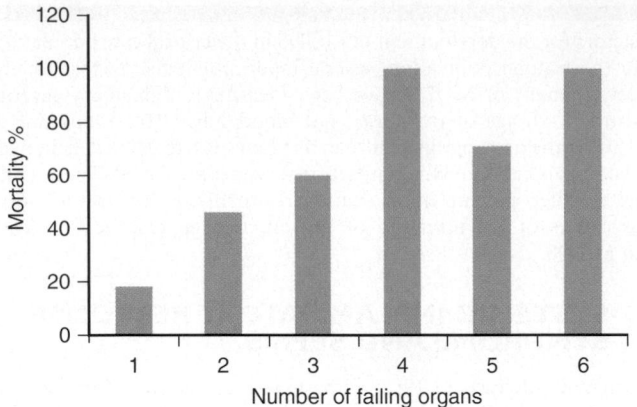

FIGURE 1 Increasing mortality associated with increasing number of organ system failures. *(Adapted from Bilevicius E, Dragosavac D, Dragosavac S, Araújo S, Falcão ALE, Terzi RGG. Multiple organ failure in septic patients. Braz J Infect Dis. 2001;5:103-110. Copyright © 2001 by The Brazilian Journal of Infectious Diseases. All rights reserved.)*

suspected should be removed after placement of additional access. Systemic antibiotic therapy is a crucial adjunct in the management of the septic patient. Clinical outcomes are associated not only with the choice of the appropriate agent, but also with the timing of initiation of therapy. Evidence demonstrates an incremental increase in sepsis-related mortality with each hour delay of antibiotic therapy from time of diagnosis. Thus the initiation of empiric broad-spectrum antibiotics with adequate coverage for the most likely organism is essential for optimal outcomes. The result of time-sensitive infection-related outcomes has resulted in the guideline-recommended initiation of antibiotics within 1 hour of recognition of sepsis. Upon speciation of the causative pathogen, the antibiotics spectrum should be narrowed based on sensitivities. This management practice assists in the reduction of resistance, agent-associated toxicity, and cost.

■ RESPIRATORY SYSTEM

Ventilator-associated pneumonia (VAP) is the most commonly encountered nosocomial infection in the critical care unit. Evidence-based guidelines for the prevention of VAP have been associated with

FIGURE 2 Causes, mechanisms, and types of multiple organ dysfunction syndrome (MODS). *IL*, Interleukin; *MOF*, multiple organ failure; *PMN*, polymorphonuclear leukocyte; *RBCs*, red blood cells. *(Adapted from El-Menyar A, et al. Multiple organ dysfunction syndrome (MODS): is it preventable or inevitable? Int J Clin Med. 2012;3:722-730.)*

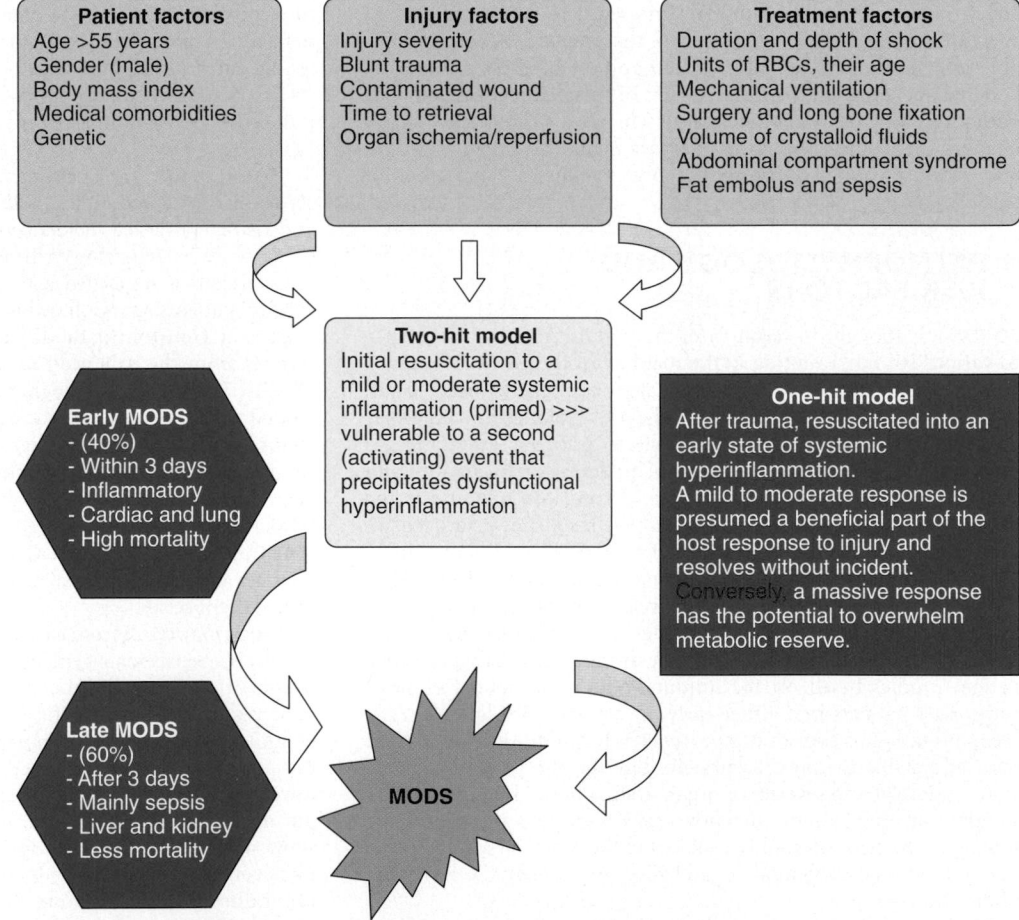

TABLE 1: Marshall Multiple Organ Dysfunction Score

Variable	0	1	2	3	4
Respiratory PaO$_2$/FiO$_2$	>300	226-300	151-225	76-150	≤75
Renal Serum creatinine	≤100	101-200	201-350	351-500	>500
Hepatic Serum bilirubin	≤20	21-60	61-120	121-240	>240
Cardiovascular Pulse-adjusted HR	≤10.0	10.1-15.0	15.1-20.0	20.1-30.0	>30.0
Hematologic Platelet count	>120	81-120	51-80	21-50	≤20
Neurologic	15	13-14	10-12	7-9	≤6

FiO$_2$, Fraction of inspired oxygen; HR, heart rate; PaO$_2$, partial pressure of oxygen.

TABLE 2: Sequential Organ Failure Assessment (SOFA) Score

Variable	1	2	3	4
Respiration PaO$_2$/FiO$_2$	<400	<300	<200	<100
Coagulation Platelets, 10^3/mm^2	<150	<100	<50	<20
Liver Bilirubin mg/dL	1.2-1.9	2.0-5.9	6.0-11.9	≥12.0
Cardiovascular Hypotension	MAP <70 mm Hg	Dopamine ≤5, or dobutamine any dose	Dopamine >5, or epinephrine ≤0.1, or norepinephrine ≤0.1	Dopamine >15, or epinephrine >0.1, or norepinephrine >0.1
Central nervous system Glasgow Coma Scale	13-14	10-12	6-9	<6
Renal	1.2-1.9	2.0-3.4	3.5-4.9	≥5

FiO$_2$, Fraction of inspired oxygen; MAP, mean arterial pressure; PaO$_2$, partial pressure of oxygen.

TABLE 3: Definition of SIRS, Sepsis, Severe Sepsis, and Septic Shock

Term	Definition
SIRS (at least two are needed to meet criteria for SIRS)	Body temperature ≥38°C or <36°C Heart rate >90/min Respirations >20/min or PaCO$_2$ <32 mm Hg
Sepsis	SIRS plus infection
Severe sepsis	Sepsis associated with organ dysfunction, systemic hypoperfusion, or hypotension
Septic shock	Sepsis with arterial hypotension despite adequate fluid replacement

PaCO$_2$, Partial pressure of carbon dioxide; SIRS, systemic inflammatory response syndrome.

BOX 1: Sepsis Management Bundles

To Be Completed Within 3 Hours of Time of Presentation

1. Measure lactate level.
2. Obtain blood cultures before administration of antibiotics.
3. Administer broad-spectrum antibiotics.
4. Administer 30 mL/kg crystalloid for hypotension or lactate ≥4 mmol/L.

To Be Completed Within 6 Hours of Time of Presentation

5. Apply vasopressors (for hypotension that does not respond to initial fluid resuscitation) to maintain a mean arterial pressure (MAP) ≥65 mm Hg.
6. In the event of persistent hypotension after initial fluid administration (MAP <65 mm Hg) or if initial lactate was ≥4 mmol/L, reassess volume status and tissue perfusion and document findings according to Table 1.
7. Remeasure lactate if initial lactate was elevated.

its decreased incidence as well as a decrease in ventilator days and length of stay in the intensive care unit (ICU). VAP is one of several well-described risk factors for the development of acute respiratory distress syndrome (ARDS). These risk factors are categorized into two main groups: direct and indirect (Box 2).

First described in 1967 and defined in 1994, further understanding of ARDS has led to the proposal of several management revisions. The acute and heterogeneous inflammatory-induced lung damage results in atelectatic areas in the dependent regions and aerated areas in the nondependent regions. Various levels of hypoxemia are the predominant clinical manifestation. The majority of patients require ventilator support, although noninvasive ventilator management has been described. Although intuitively it appears benign, mechanical ventilation has been shown to be detrimental because inadvertent lung damage may result. These unintended effects may exacerbate the inflammatory process, thereby contributing to the development of MODS. As a result of further understanding of these and other findings, the landmark ARDS Network study was performed and a survival benefit was demonstrated when comparing ventilator strategies of 10 cc/kg predicted body weight and 6 cc/kg predicted body weight with the aim of preventing alveolar overdistension. This finding has led to the incorporation of the low tidal volume strategy as the standard of care for the management of these patients. The study's authors also recommended targets of plateau pressure of 30 cm H_2O or less, hypercapnia with accepting of pH 7.15, and higher levels of positive end-expiratory pressure (PEEP) with or without recruitment maneuvers. Recently the definition has been refined further with the publication of the Berlin Definition in 2012. Three categories of ARDS based on hypoxemia severity were proposed, and clarity in the diagnostic criteria was given (Table 4). Applying the classification-based definition to a patient-level meta-analysis of 4188 patients, the new definition was able to demonstrate better predictive validity for mortality. With increasing severity, various therapeutic management options have been proposed (Figure 3).

BOX 2: Risk Factors for the Development of Acute Respiratory Distress Syndrome

Direct Risk Factors

Pneumonia
Aspiration of gastric contents
Inhalation injury
Pulmonary contusion
Near drowning

Indirect Risk Factors

Nonpulmonary sepsis
Major trauma
Multiple transfusions
Major burns
Pancreatitis
Noncardiogenic shock

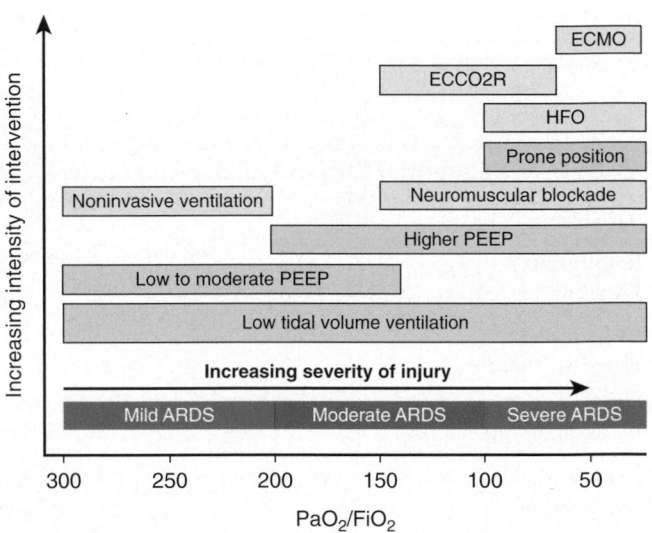

FIGURE 3 Therapeutic options in acute respiratory distress syndrome (ARDS). *ECCO2R,* Extracorporeal carbon dioxide removal; *ECMO,* extracorporeal membrane oxygenation; *FiO₂,* fraction of inspired oxygen; *HFO,* high-frequency oscillation; *PaO₂,* partial pressure of oxygen; *PEEP,* positive end-expiratory pressure.

TABLE 4: Berlin Definition of Acute Respiratory Distress Syndrome (ARDS)

	ARDS		
	Mild	**Moderate**	**Severe**
Timing	Acute onset within 1 week of a known clinical insult or new or worsening symptoms		
Hypoxemia	PaO₂/FiO₂ 201-300 with PEEP/ CPAP ≥5	PaO₂/FiO₂ ≤200 with PEEP ≥5	PaO₂/FiO₂ ≤100 with PEEP ≥10
Origin of edema	Respiratory failure associated with known risk factors and not fully explained by cardiac failure or fluid overload. Need objective assessment of cardiac failure or fluid overload if no risk factors are present.		
Radiologic abnormalities	Bilateral opacities*	Bilateral opacities*	Opacities involving at least 3 quadrants*
Additional psychologic derangement	N/A	N/A	V_E Corr >10 L/min or C_RS <40 mL/cm H₂O

*Not fully explained by effusions, nodules, masses, or lobar/lung collapse; use training set of chest x-rays.

CPAP, Continuous positive airway pressure; *C_RS,* compliance; *FiO₂,* fraction of inspired oxygen; *PaCO₂,* partial pressure of carbon dioxide; *PaO₂,* partial pressure of oxygen; *PEEP,* positive end-expiratory pressure; *V_E,* respiratory minute volume; *V_E Corr,* V_E × PaCO₂/40 (corrected for body surface area).

TABLE 5: Child-Turcotte Pugh Classification System and Liver Disease Severity

Clinical and Laboratory Criteria	Points		
	1	2	3
Encephalopathy	None	Mild to moderate (grade 1 or 2)	Severe (grade 3 or 4)
Ascites	None	Mild to moderate (diuretic responsive)	Severe (diuretic refractory)
Bilirubin (mg/dL)	<2	2-3	>3
Albumin (g/dL)	>3.5	2.8-3.5	<2.8
Prothrombin time			
Seconds prolonged	<4	4-6	>6
International normalized ratio	<1.7	1.7-2.3	>2.3

Child-Turcotte-Pugh class obtained by totaling the scores for each parameter (total points).

Class A = 5 to 6 points (least severe liver disease).

Class B = 7 to 9 points (moderately severe liver disease).

Class C = 10 to 15 points (most severe liver disease).

■ HEPATIC SYSTEM

The patient with cirrhosis presents various challenges to the intensivist. One must first differentiate compensated from decompensated cirrhosis. Patients with compensated cirrhosis lack cirrhosis-related symptoms, whereas those with decompensated cirrhosis have symptomatic complications (jaundice, ascites, variceal hemorrhage, hepatic encephalopathy) and an overall poor survival. Previous studies have demonstrated the direct relationship between increasing hepatic disease–specific severity and mortality. Disease classification is therefore important. Classification systems such as the Child-Turcotte-Pugh score (Table 5) and more recently the Model for End-Stage Liver Disease (MELD) score (Table 6) are good indicators of survival. The management of patients with varying degrees of hepatic disease is not uncommon in the critically ill population and presents various challenges. The European Association for the Study of the Liver guidelines published in 2010 offer evidence-based recommendations for the management of this high-risk population.

Spontaneous bacterial peritonitis (SBP) is the most common infection in patients with cirrhosis. SBP is associated with both an in-hospital mortality rate of 10% to 20% and a high rate of recurrence. Diagnosis is via paracentesis demonstrating a neutrophil count greater than 250/mm³. Although ascetic fluid cultures should be obtained, a positive culture is not required for the diagnosis. The mainstay of management is empiric antibiotic therapy, with third-generation cephalosporins being the agent of choice because gram-negative aerobic bacteria are the most common causative organisms. Antibiotic management is successful in 90% of cases. Treatment failures often result from resistant organisms or secondary peritonitis. Ascites should be graded (grade 1, 2, or 3) and managed accordingly.

Hepatic encephalopathy (HE) is a brain dysfunction caused by liver insufficiency or portosystemic shunting. HE should be classified based on underlying disease, severity of manifestations, time course, and precipitating factors. Known causative factors should be sought and treated accordingly (Box 3).

The diagnosis of HE is that of exclusion of other causes based on clinical examination and laboratory and radiologic studies. Only HE that is recurrent or persistent requires intervention. Lactulose is the first-line treatment of HE. Rifaximin is an effective add-on therapy to lactulose for prevention of HE recurrence. Other alternatives include oral branched-chain amino acid (BCAA)–enriched enteral feedings, intravenous L-ornithine-L-aspartate, neomycin, and metronidazole. Refractory HE in the setting of liver failure is an indication for liver transplantation.

TABLE 6: Model for End-Stage Liver Disease (MELD) Scoring System and Associated 3-Month Mortality

MELD score	≤9	10-19	20-29	30-39	≥40
Hospitalized patient	4%	27%	76%	83%	100%
Outpatient with cirrhosis	2%	6%	50%		

MELD score = $10 \times [0.957 \times \log e \, (\text{creatinine}) + \log e \, (\text{bilirubin}) + 1.12 \times \log 2 \, (\text{INR})] + 6.43$.

INR, International normalized ratio.

BOX 3: Precipitating Factors for Hepatic Encephalopathy

Episodic

Infections
Gastrointestinal (GI) bleeding
Diuretic overdose
Electrolyte disorder
Constipation
Unidentified

Recurrent

Electrolyte disorder
Infections
Unidentified
Constipation
Diuretic overdose
GI bleeding

Hepatorenal syndrome (HRS) is defined as the development of renal failure in the setting of advanced liver disease with no identifiable cause for the renal failure. The reduction in the effective circulating blood volume resulting in hypoperfusion of the kidney is the basic underlying mechanism for HRS development. HRS usually develops in patients with cirrhosis after a septic insult such as SBP

BOX 4: Criteria for Diagnosis of Hepatorenal Syndrome in Cirrhosis

Cirrhosis with ascites
Serum creatinine >1.5 mg/dL (133 μmol/L)
Absence of shock
Absence of hypovolemia as defined by no sustained improvement of renal function (creatinine decreasing to <133 μmol/L) after at least 2 days of diuretic withdrawal (if on diuretics) and volume expansion with albumin at 1 g/kg/day up to a maximum of 100 g/day
No current or recent treatment with nephrotoxic drugs
Absence of parenchymal renal disease as defined by proteinuria <0.5 g/day, no microhematuria (<50 red blood cells/high-powered field), and normal renal ultrasonography

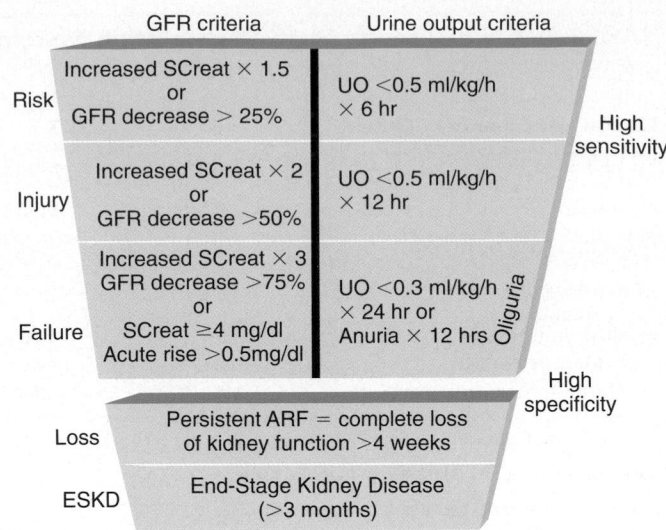

FIGURE 4 RIFLE classification scheme for acute kidney injury. *ARF*, Acute renal failure; *GFR*, glomerular filtration rate; *SCreat*, serum creatinine; *UO*, urine output. *(From Bellomo R, Ronco C, Kellum JA, et al. Acute renal failure—definition, outcome measures, animal models, fluid therapy and information technology needs: the Second International Consensus Conference of the Acute Dialysis Quality Initiative (ADQI) Group. Crit Care Med. 2004;8:R204-R212.)*

or other infective processes. The pathogenesis of HRS involves four factors: splanchnic vasodilation development, activation of the sympathetic and renin-angiotensin-aldosterone system, cardiac impairment as a result of cirrhotic cardiomyopathy, and increased synthesis of vasoactive mediators that affect renal hemodynamics. The diagnostic criteria were initially defined in 1994 and subsequently updated in 2007 (Box 4). HRS is classified into types 1 and 2. Type 1 HRS is characterized by a rapid increase in serum creatinine of more than 100% compared with baseline to a level greater than 2.5 mg/dL in less than a 2-week period. Type 2 HRS renal impairment is less progressive. Treatment includes initiation of a vasoconstrictor, more specifically a vasopressin analogue. Large studies have demonstrated that terlipressin, a vasopressin analogue, in combination with albumin as first-line therapy resulted in improved renal function and survival in patients with Type 1 HRS. The role of renal replacement therapy (RRT) in the management of HRS currently is not definitive. Liver transplantation is the treatment of choice, and patients who respond to vasopressor therapy should be referred appropriately.

■ RENAL SYSTEM

Acute renal failure generally has been defined as an abrupt and sustained decrease in renal function. This vague definition, combined with many variations described in the literature, has led to a wide range of reported incidence (1% to 31%) and attributed mortality (19% to 83%). The Acute Dialysis Quality Initiative established the Risk, Injury, Failure, Loss, and End-Stage Kidney Disease (RIFLE) multilevel classification system in 2004. The RIFLE classification system categorizes renal dysfunction into three classes based on increasing severity of disease (Figure 4). Subsequent studies have documented the association of increased mortality with increasing severity of renal dysfunction across both medical and surgical critical care populations based on the RIFLE classification. Even with the development of renal dysfunction at the risk level, an increased in-hospital mortality has been demonstrated when compared with patients who did not develop renal dysfunction. To date, there are no pharmacologic therapies to treat acute kidney injury (AKI). Therapeutic agents such as dopamine, fenoldopam, and diuretics are not central in the management of AKI and in fact may be harmful for the patient. Randomized controlled trials have not demonstrated a benefit in terms of renal function and overall outcome, and the routine use of dopamine is not supported. There is a paucity of clinical data to support the use of diuretics in the management of AKI, and recent studies have either correlated the use of diuretics to increased mortality or shown no benefit.

The use of diuretics to convert oliguric to nonoliguric renal failure previously has been recommended. However, this management approach does not appear to affect eventual need for dialysis or overall mortality and therefore is not recommended based on recent studies.

Management of renal dysfunction is mainly supportive. Priorities include preventing further insult (avoidance of contrast media), treating any life-threatening features (hyperkalemia, metabolic acidosis), attempting to halt or reverse the decline in renal function, and providing support by RRT with the anticipated goal of renal recovery. First, one should review the patient's medication regimen to assess for renal toxic agents that should be discontinued. Renally excreted agents that are necessary should have the dosage appropriately adjusted. Prerenal causes mostly result from hypovolemia, which should be corrected with isotonic fluid resuscitation with the goal of achieving euvolemia. AKI in the setting of hypervolemia requires diuresis, but hypovolemia must be prevented. Patients who are not responsive to medical management are potential candidates for RRT. The two modalities commonly used are intermittent hemodialysis (IHD) and continuous hemofiltration and hemodialysis (CHH). The outcomes of patients receiving either IHD or CHH are equivalent. The choice of the mode utilized is based mainly on the advantages and disadvantages of each. IHD is more effective in solute and fluid removal but is associated with hypotension. CHH is better tolerated in the hemodynamically unstable patient but requires greater critical care resources and anticoagulation.

■ CARDIOVASCULAR SYSTEM

Hypoperfusion in the form of hypovolemic shock is a common cause in the development of MODS. The initial approach includes early, aggressive fluid resuscitation guided by endpoints. Isotonic fluid resuscitation is preferred, as multiple studies have failed to show a benefit of colloid (albumin) resuscitation on the development of MODS or improved survival. Once adequate fluid resuscitation is ensured and the patient continues to show evidence of decreased end organ perfusion, vasopressor therapy is indicated, with the goal of mean arterial pressure (MAP) of 65 mm Hg. The optimal MAP should be individualized, as patients with hypertension or atherosclerotic disease may require a higher targeted goal in order to preserve tissue perfusion. Various agents such as dopamine, epinephrine, vasopressin, and norepinephrine are effective in achieving this goal. Choice of agents should be guided by desired effect and side effect profile. Guidelines for the management of sepsis-induced hypotension recommend against the routine use of phenylephrine and dopamine. For patients with septic shock, norepinephrine is the preferred first-line agent. Additional agents such as epinephrine and low dose vasopressin (0.03 to 0.04 U/min) are suggested, as multiple agents often are required in order to achieve desired goals. It should be reiterated that vasopressor management should not be used in place of volume resuscitation but used only after adequate resuscitation or during ongoing resuscitation. Septic patients with hypotension also may demonstrate evidence of cardiac dysfunction requiring ionotropic support. Dobutamine is the recommended first-line agent for patients with evidence of low cardiac output in the presence of adequate mean arterial and left ventricular filling pressures. Also, patients who require the initiation of vasopressors should have either invasive or noninvasive hemodynamic monitoring placed.

ENDOCRINE SYSTEM

Patients with sepsis and septic shock often develop adrenal insufficiency (AI). Both functional and relative forms of AI have been shown to occur in the critically ill population. The patient with ongoing evidence of shock despite adequate fluid resuscitation and high vasopressor requirement should raise suspicion for AI. Diagnosis of AI in the critically ill population has been challenging because of lack of consensus and varying cortisol levels used for diagnosis. Clinical trials have produced conflicting results on corticotrophin test–confirmed diagnosis and hydrocortisone treatment dosage.

Current recommendations suggest forgoing the adrenocorticotropic hormone (ACTH) stimulation test and proceeding with empirical treatment of the adult septic shock patient with hemodynamic lability despite adequate fluid resuscitation and vasopressor therapy. Hydrocortisone at physiologic dosage (200 to 300 mg/day) for a 5- to 7-day course is recommended, as evidence has demonstrated a benefit in survival and reversal of shock with lower complications when compared with higher dose usage.

Vasopressin deficiency represents another endocrinopathy that occurs in the critically ill. Early in the shock state, vasopressin levels are appropriately elevated. However, as shock persists, levels have been demonstrated to decline, contributing to refractory hypotension. Vasopressin at physiologic dosage (0.01 to 0.04 U) has been shown to have a pressor effect. Higher doses are associated with excessive vasoconstriction resulting in end organ ischemia. When used in conjunction with other vasopressors, lower doses of these agents are required to maintain end organ perfusion. Current recommendations are for the use of vasopressin at physiologic dosage (0.04 U) in addition to vasopressor therapy as a continuous infusion for the management of sepsis-induced shock requiring high levels of vasopressors.

In conclusion, MODS remains a leading cause of death in the critically ill. Survival is directly proportional to the number of organ systems involved. Many precipitating factors have been identified, with infection being the most common cause. Severe sepsis and septic shock represent common causes contributing to the development of MODS. The principles of early diagnosis, aggressive resuscitation, timely initiation of broad-spectrum antibiotics, and end organ support guided by evidence-based medicine (Table 7) has had a positive effect on survival.

TABLE 7: Guidelines for the Treatment of Severe Sepsis and Septic Shock From the Surviving Sepsis Campaign

Element of Care	Grade
RESUSCITATION	
Begin goal-directed resuscitation during first 6 hr after recognition	1C
Begin initial fluid resuscitation with crystalloid and consider the addition of albumin	1B
Consider the addition of albumin when substantial amounts of crystalloid are required to maintain adequate arterial pressure	2C
Avoid hetastarch formulations	1C
Begin initial fluid challenge in patients with tissue hypoperfusion and suspected hypovolemia to achieve ≥30 mL of crystalloids per kg body weight	1C
Continue fluid challenge technique as long as there is hemodynamic improvement	UG
Use norepinephrine as the first-choice vasopressor to maintain MAP ≥65 mm Hg	1B
Use epinephrine when an additional agent is needed to maintain adequate blood pressure	2B
Add vasopressin (at a dose of 0.03 units/min) with weaning of norepinephrine, if tolerated	UG
Avoid the use of dopamine except in carefully selected patients (e.g., patients with a low risk of arrhythmias and either known marked ventricular systolic dysfunction or low heart rate)	2C
Infuse dobutamine or add it to vasopressor therapy in the presence of myocardial dysfunction (e.g., elevated cardiac filling pressures or low cardiac output) or ongoing hypoperfusion despite adequate intravascular volume and MAP	1C
Avoid the use of intravenous hydrocortisone if adequate fluid resuscitation and vasopressor therapy restore hemodynamic stability; if hydrocortisone is used, administer at a dose of 200 mg/day	2C
Target a hemoglobin level of 7 to 9 g/dL in patients without hypoperfusion, critical coronary artery disease or myocardial ischemia, or acute hemorrhage	1B

Continued

TABLE 7: Guidelines for the Treatment of Severe Sepsis and Septic Shock From the Surviving Sepsis Campaign—cont'd

Element of Care	Grade
INFECTION CONTROL	
Obtain blood cultures before antibiotic therapy is administered	1C
Perform imaging studies promptly to confirm source of infection	UG
Administer broad-spectrum antibiotic therapy within 1 hr after diagnosis of either severe sepsis or septic shock	1B/1C
Reassess antibiotic therapy daily for de-escalation when appropriate	1B
Perform source control with attention to risks and benefits of the chosen method within 12 hr after diagnosis	1C
RESPIRATORY SUPPORT	
Use a low tidal volume and imitation of inspiratory plateau pressure strategy for ARDS	1A/1B
Apply a minimal amount of PEEP in ARDS	1B
Administer higher rather than lower PEEP for patients with sepsis-induced ARDS	2C
Use recruitment maneuvers in patients with severe refractory hypoxemia due to ARDS	2C
Use prone positioning in patients with sepsis-induced ARDS and a ratio of the partial pressure of arterial oxygen (mm Hg) to the fraction of inspired oxygen of <100, in facilities that have experience with such practice	2C
Elevate the head of the bed in patients undergoing mechanical ventilation, unless contraindicated	1B
Use a conservative fluid strategy for established acute lung injury or ARDS with no evidence of tissue hypoperfusion	1C
Use weaning protocols	1A
CENTRAL NERVOUS SYSTEM SUPPORT	
Use sedation protocols, targeting specific dose escalation endpoints	1B
Avoid neuromuscular blockers if possible in patients without ARDS	1C
Administer a short course of a neuromuscular blocker (<48 hr) for patients with early, severe ARDS	1C
GENERAL SUPPORTIVE CARE	
Use a protocol-specified approach to blood glucose management, with the initiation of insulin after 2 consecutive blood glucose levels >180 mg/dL (10 mmol/L) targeting a blood glucose level <180 mg/dL	1A
Use the equivalent of continuous venovenous hemofiltration or intermittent hemodialysis as needed for renal failure or fluid overload	2B
Administer prophylaxis for deep vein thrombosis	1B
Administer stress ulcer prophylaxis to prevent upper gastrointestinal bleeding	1B
Administer oral or enteral feedings, as tolerated, rather than either complete fasting or provision of only intravenous glucose within the first 48 hr after a diagnosis of severe sepsis or septic shock	2C
Address goals of care, including treatment plans and end-of-life planning as appropriate	1B

Data adapted from Dellinger RP, Surviving Sepsis Campaign Guidelines Committee including the Pediatric Subgroup, et al. Surviving Sepsis Campaign: international guidelines for management of severe sepsis and septic shock: 2012. *Crit Care Med.* 2013;41:580-637.

ARDS, Acute respiratory distress syndrome; *ICU,* intensive care unit; *MAP,* mean arterial pressure; *PEEP,* positive end-expiratory pressure; *UG,* ungraded.

SUGGESTED READINGS

Acute Respiratory Distress Syndrome Network. Ventilation with lower tidal volumes as compared with traditional tidal volumes for acute lung injury and acute respiratory distress syndrome. *N Engl J Med.* 2000;342:1301-1308.

ARDS Definition Task Force, et al. Acute respiratory distress syndrome: the Berlin Definition. *JAMA.* 2012;307:2526-2533.

Bellomo R, Ronco C, Kellum JA, Mehta RL, Palevsky P, ADQI workgroup. Acute renal failure—definition, outcome measures, needs: the Second International Consensus Conference of the Acute Dialysis Quality Initiative (ADQI) Group. *Crit Care Med.* 2004;8:R204-R212.

Dellinger RP, et al. Surviving Sepsis Campaign: international guidelines for management of severe sepsis and septic shock. *Crit Care Med.* 2013;41:580-637.

El-Menyar A, Al Thani H, Zakaria ER, et al. Multiple organ dysfunction syndrome (MODS): is it preventable or inevitable? *Int J Clin Med.* 2012;3:722-730.

European Association for the Study of the Liver. EASL clinical practice guidelines on the management of ascites, spontaneous bacterial peritonitis, and hepatorenal syndrome in cirrhosis. *J Hepatol.* 2010;53:397-417.

MULTIPLE ORGAN DYSFUNCTION AND FAILURE

Damon Clark, MD, and Heidi Frankel, MD, FACS, FCCM

Multiple organ dysfunction syndrome (MODS), culminating in multiple organ failure (MOF), is the constellation of signs and symptoms that results from a patient's adaptive response to a physiologic insult and therapy thereof. Although the triggers that drive MODS are highly variable and include toxin ingestion and inhalation, the most common causes in a surgical intensive care unit (ICU) are sepsis and injury with resuscitation. Sepsis is the most frequent cause in operative and nonoperative patients. These insults and therapies appear to cause MODS by promoting microvascular thrombosis, endothelial leak, ischemia, and reperfusion.

MODS is the potentially reversible presence of altered organ function in two or more systems that requires medical intervention to achieve homeostasis. As such, the clinical condition of MODS owes its existence to the development of the ICU and is the most common cause (or end presentation) of death there. Strictly speaking, dysfunction need not affect an organ but rather a system (such as hematologic or endocrine).

The term MOF was coined in an editorial by Arthur Baue in 1975. In subsequent years, attempts have been made to ascribe an etiology to this entity and to recognize that organ systems may suffer dysfunction short of absolute failure (i.e., MODS). Much early attention focused on hemodynamic monitoring, recognition of impaired oxygen delivery, and efforts to modify this deficit. However, attempts at providing so-called supranormal levels of oxygen did not result in improved outcomes.

■ PATHOPHYSIOLOGY

A definitive unifying pathophysiology for MODS has not been identified. Local and systemic responses are initiated by tissue damage that in the past has been described by several hypotheses. The gut hypothesis of Edward Deitch posits that splanchnic hypoperfusion causes increased gut permeability, promoting bacterial translocation that activates an immunologic response. This has engendered work on the role of immunonutrition and selective decontamination to prevent MODS. The endotoxin hypothesis postulates that inflammatory cytokines are released in response to endotoxin in gramnegative infections. However, attempts to block the effects of endotoxin have not been successful in treating sepsis and MODS. Alternatively, tissue hypoxia resulting from injury promoting mitochondrial DNA release has been incriminated. Therapies targeting this deficit have not been tested extensively. Likely, a combination of all of these hypotheses promotes the development and sustenance of MODS.

Sepsis, the most common cause of MODS and MOF in surgical and all ICUs, is a significant cause of hospital morbidity and mortality and contributor to cost, as noted elsewhere in this text. Much national and regulatory attention has focused on the prompt diagnosis and treatment of sepsis. Sepsis recently has been reclassified by a panel of experts, and treatment continues to evolve. In the past, sepsis was defined as the presence of systemic inflammatory response syndrome (SIRS) in a patient with a suspected or documented infection. SIRS criteria included elevated or depressed white blood cell count, respiratory rate, heart rate, and temperature. Severe sepsis referred to infected patients with hypotension or hypoperfusion (generally expressed as an elevated lactate level) with MODS (manifested by oliguria, acute mental status change, new coagulopathy or

thrombocytopenia, or acute lung injury). Septic shock referred to those patients who remained septic despite adequate volume resuscitation and who thus required vasopressors. However, a majority of patients in the ICU are seen with SIRS in the absence of infection, challenging the established diagnosis of sepsis. The new definition of sepsis is "life-threatening organ dysfunction due to a dysregulated host response to infection where organ dysfunction is represented by an increase of ≥2 total SOFA [Sequential Organ Failure Assessment] points." The term *severe sepsis* is now considered redundant. Septic shock is "the subset of sepsis identified by a vasopressor requirement to maintain MAP [mean arterial pressure] ≥65 mm Hg and lactate <2 mmol/L in the absence of other causes, particularly hypovolemia." These new definitions appear to focus attention on those at the greatest risk of death by including those with MODS.

Mechanisms other than sepsis may cause MODS in surgical patients. Common causes include acute pancreatitis and trauma. Apparent with these two causes is that both exuberant and inadequate resuscitation may be as much or more of a culprit than the underlying disease in promoting MODS. The impact of limiting excessive crystalloid administration on mitigating against the development of abdominal compartment syndrome and acute respiratory distress syndrome (ARDS) is discussed further later in the chapter.

Despite the myriad advancements in the care of the critically ill patient, few specifically address MODS, whose therapy is largely supportive. The therapy for sepsis, as noted elsewhere in this text, has been established by a series of evidence-based care guidelines, as described in the 2004 Surviving Sepsis Campaign guidelines and two subsequent revisions. All versions focus on the rapid identification of patients with sepsis, early invasive monitoring, and resuscitation targeted to specified endpoints. However, three recent randomized controlled trials challenged the notion of early goal-directed therapy, instead pointing to the efficacy of clinical judgment guiding resuscitation. Perhaps greater attention should be given to rapid identification of the source of sepsis and source control and targeted empiric antibiotic therapy, particularly in surgical patients. In the past, in our zeal to invasively monitor and resuscitate patients to predetermined endpoints, we unwittingly caused MODS through reperfusion injury.

In addition, as our resuscitation knowledge and capabilities expand and as our population ages, newer forms of MODS have come to the fore. Persistent inflammation, immunosuppression, and catabolism syndrome (PICS) and compensatory anti-inflammatory response syndrome (CARS) describe a novel patient population in many ICUs, consisting of older, comorbid, and chronically critically ill patients. This cohort is characterized by a smoldering inflammatory state with catabolism, sarcopenia, poor wound healing, and multiple recurrent infections (many iatrogenic) and eventual progression to disability and death. Inherent to the understanding of PICS is the progression from an innate, polymorphonuclear leukocytes (PMN)–driven, proinflammatory state to one of adaptive, lymphocyte-driven CARS.

■ SCORING AND PROGNOSIS

Organ dysfunction in the critically ill patient can be described by the native systemic physiologic derangement that mandates clinical intervention or by the degree and extent of the intervention necessary (e.g., mechanical ventilation, renal replacement therapy, cardiovascular support agents). Several scales to characterize MODS have been developed using the following organ systems: respiratory, cardiovascular, renal, hepatic, neurologic, and hematologic. The Sequential Organ Failure Assessment (SOFA) score was described by J.L. Vincent and colleagues in 1996 and assigns a score of 0 to 4 in six organ system categories, with higher scores indicating a greater severity of disease (Table 1). The Marshall MODS score, developed in 1995, assigns a score of 0 to 4 in six organ system categories (Table 2). With each of these scoring systems, the risk of ICU death increases as the severity of organ dysfunction and number of failing organs increase.

TABLE 1: Sequential Organ Failure Assessment (SOFA) Score

Organ System	0	1	2	3	4
Respiratory: PaO_2/FiO_2	>400	<400	<300	<200 with ventilator support	<100 with ventilator support
Cardiovascular: Hypotension (mm Hg)	MAP >70 No pressors	MAP <70 No pressors	Dopamine <5	Dopamine >5 or epinephrine <0.1 or norepinephrine <0.1	Dopamine >15 or epinephrine >0.1 or norepinephrine >0.1
Hepatic: Bilirubin (mg/dL)	<1.2	1.2-1.9	2.0-3.4	3.5-4.9	>5.0
Coagulation: Platelet count ($\times 10^3/mm^3$)	>150	<150	<100	<50	<20
Neurologic: GCS	15	13-14	10-12	6-9	<6
Renal: Creatinine (mg/dL) or urine output (mL/day)	<1.2	1.2-1.9	2.0-3.4	3.5-4.9 or Urine <500	>5.0 or Urine <200

Vasopressor doses in µg/kg/min.

FiO$_2$, Fraction of inspired oxygen; *GCS*, Glascow Coma Scale score; *MAP*, mean arterial pressure; *PaO$_2$*, partial pressure of oxygen.

TABLE 2: Marshall Multiple Organ Dysfunction Score

Organ System	0	1	2	3	4
Respiratory: PaO_2/FiO_2	>300	226-300	151-225	76-150	≤75
Cardiovascular: HR × CVP/MAP	≤10	10.1-15	15.1-20	20.1-30	>30
Hepatic: Bilirubin (mg/dL)	<1.2	1.2-3.5	3.5-7.0	7.0-14	>14
Hematologic: Platelet count ($\times 10^3/mm^3$)	>120	81-120	51-80	21-50	≤20
Neurologic: GCS	15	13-14	10-12	7-9	≤6
Renal: Creatinine (mg/dL)	<1.1	1.1-2.3	2.3-4.0	4.0-5.7	>5.7

CVP, Central venous pressure; *FiO$_2$*, fraction of inspired oxygen; *GCS*, Glasgow Coma Scale score; *HR*, heart rate; *MAP*, mean arterial pressure; *PaO$_2$*, partial pressure of oxygen.

Other scoring systems, described elsewhere in this text, define single organ system dysfunction and failure, including those for the pulmonary, renal, and hematologic systems.

MODS generally develops within 48 hours of an inciting insult. Subtle neurologic disturbances are noted first, followed more dramatically by respiratory dysfunction, followed by hepatic and gastrointestinal (GI) dysfunction and then renal dysfunction. New-onset renal failure portends the worst outcome. Long-term disability and delayed risk of death in long-term acute care hospitals are common.

■ PHYSIOLOGIC DERANGEMENTS

Central Nervous System Dysfunction

Neurologic manifestations of sepsis—specifically delirium and cognitive disorders—often are seen as the first component of MODS. These mental status changes may be subtle, and when present the patient should be evaluated for possible causes of MODS. This is particularly true of pediatric and geriatric patients, whose cerebral perfusion is affected rapidly by systemic perturbations, especially older patients with pre-existing cognitive deficits. In addition, although not necessarily overt, neurologic derangements of MODS may be the most long-lasting and most contributory to long-term disability. Nonetheless, these deficits often are overlooked or ascribed to the consequences of therapy for MODS—namely sedation and

narcotic-based analgesia to afford cardiopulmonary support and other treatments. Over the past decade it has become clear that these neurologic disorders can be attenuated by paying attention to minimizing sedation (particularly by avoidance of benzodiazepines), use of analgesic-only sedation, atypical antipsychotics, maintenance of the sleep-wake cycle, and daily mobilization and physical therapy to preserve pre-illness fitness and mental states.

Pulmonary System Dysfunction

The characteristic abnormality of the lung in MODS is a failure of normal gas exchange, reflected predominantly in arterial hypoxemia. Multiple pathologic factors contribute to impaired gas exchange. Atelectasis and altered regional flow contribute to ventilation-perfusion mismatch early on, whereas increased capillary permeability leads to alveolar flooding and impaired diffusion later. Finally, tissue repair results in fibrosis and hyaline membrane formation, pathologic features of late ARDS. In the past, MODS patients universally developed severe ARDS and often died of an inability to oxygenate. As the prompt diagnosis of MODS triggers (infection, ongoing bleeding) has been prioritized and the therapy of ARDS has evolved, both its incidence and lethality have markedly decreased in surgical ICUs. Rapid diagnosis of bleeding or sepsis affords prompt source control and the ability to minimize overly aggressive resuscitation, particularly with crystalloid. Moreover, the willingness to (appropriately) provide pressor support earlier may minimize fluid administration later and the development of ARDS. At least as important in ARDS mitigation is the avoidance of barotrauma by use of so-called "low stretch" ventilation that limits tidal volume to 6 cc/kg and plateau pressure to less than 30 cm H_2O. It is also clear that the use of low stretch ventilation should be initiated in all patients, not just in those who have already developed ARDS. The use of modes involving patient-controlled physiologic variables, as is possible in pressure-supported or limited ventilation, may be an alternative strategy to prevent barotrauma. Finally, it is important to recognize that a very small subset of MODS patients will develop severe acute lung injury with the potential to die of, not just with, ARDS. The care of these patients is best provided by regional referral centers that possess all of the possible tools for management of ARDS, including extracorporeal membrane oxygenation (ECMO). Although only brief use of neuromuscular blockade and rotational therapy has shown a mortality benefit across a population of patients with ARDS, whereas all other therapies have not, it is clear that other advanced modalities may save individual patients. Substantial experience with the use of alternative ventilatory modes, inhaled pulmonary vasodilators, and ECMO at selected centers by around-the-clock expert staff, once proning and neuromuscular blockade have failed, may provide the most rational use of limited resources.

Cardiovascular System Dysfunction

The hallmark of MOF, and certainly the most frequent indication for ICU admission, is cardiovascular system collapse where systemic vasodilation causes hypotension. In addition, generalized increase in capillary permeability produces edema that along with diminished regional blood flow and microvascular thrombosis further drives other organ dysfunction. Classically, there is a concomitant increase in cardiac output, and the extremities are warm (so-called warm sepsis). Before adequate resuscitation patients may have the cold, clammy extremities noted in "cold sepsis." Cardiac depression may persist because of the presence of circulating inflammatory factors and metabolic acidosis. Furthermore, regional wall motion abnormalities and right-sided as well as left-sided dysfunction may be present. For this reason, the use of bedside echocardiography performed by the treating clinician may be particularly helpful to understand the pathophysiologic presentation to guide therapy. Of course, as previously noted, resuscitation to pre-established endpoints has not been proven beneficial to survival to date. On the other hand, use of bedside echocardiography can provide data on volume responsiveness, both diastolic and systolic cardiac function, right-sided morphology and function, and lung water that may allow for more precise titration of fluids and pressors. Finally, the use of norepinephrine followed by epinephrine is now favored as the front-line pressor and inotrope/pressor. Norepinephrine leads to an increase in blood pressure, cardiac output, and renal and cerebral blood flow with minimal increase in the heart rate. Compared with dopamine, norepinephrine may have less arrhythmogenicity (tachycardia) and immune suppression and may promote renal preservation by more selective vasoconstriction of the efferent arteriole of the glomerular apparatus. In addition, several large studies have noted improved overall clinical outcome when using norepinephrine versus dopamine. As such, norepinephrine has supplanted dopamine as the pressor of choice in the Surviving Sepsis Campaign guidelines. In patients who remain hypotensive on norepinephrine and in whom ventricular dysfunction has been ruled out, the addition of vasopressin has been recommended in patients with sepsis.

Hepatic System Dysfunction

The liver is frequently involved as a component of MODS. Dysfunction includes "shock liver" transaminitis, coagulation abnormalities, and hyperbilirubinemia. Shock liver is a result of hypoperfusion, ischemia, and cellular hypoxia. Eventually patients with shock liver develop coagulopathy and hyperbilirubinemia as well. Patients may progress to acute liver failure. Treatment is supportive and includes the management of encephalopathy and bleeding due to coagulopathy. Enteral nutrition is generally tolerated and recommended in these patients. There are little data on the use of extracorporeal liver support devices in this situation. Transplantation is rarely possible because of ongoing infection and other organ dysfunction. In pure hyperbilirubinemia, hepatic synthetic function is not affected. It is important to exclude other causes of hyperbilirubinemia such as acalculous cholecystitis, biliary obstruction, and pancreatitis that may be treated.

Gastrointestinal System Dysfunction

GI dysfunction as a component of MODS results from reduced local blood flow, impaired motility, and alterations in normal microbial flora. The "stress bleeding" and ulceration of the past largely has been eliminated, well before the introduction of nearly universal use of histamine H_2 or proton pump inhibitors. Ileus manifested by intolerance of enteral feeding, bloating, and diarrhea is a common component of MODS. Nonetheless, it is often possible to provide enteral nutrition, as will be discussed in detail later in the chapter.

Renal System Dysfunction

Acute kidney injury (AKI) describes the spectrum of renal dysfunction from insufficiency to outright failure that necessitates renal replacement therapy (RRT), most often in the form of hemodialysis in ICU patients with MOF. Acute renal failure complicates at least 5% and as many as 30% of all surgical ICU admissions with a mortality of more than 50%. AKI has been described as the most prognostic component of MOF. AKI can be graded along a spectrum as described by the RIFLE classification (Risk, Injury, Failure, Loss of kidney function, and End-stage kidney disease), as defined by the Acute Dialysis Quality Initiative (ADQI), and may be oliguric or nonoliguric (urine output <400 mL/day or >400 mL/day, respectively, in adults). Oliguric renal failure and higher grades of injury portend a greater mortality. There are two additional classification systems, including one developed by the Acute Kidney Injury Network (AKIN) that is also composed of urine output and serum creatinine criteria. The Kidney Disease Improving Global Outcomes (KDIGO) work group recently proposed a hybrid definition as well (Table 3).

Attention must be directed toward management of electrolyte disturbances, metabolic derangements, and hypervolemia in patients with AKI. Diuretics are not successful in either preventing or ameliorating AKI and have a significant risk of morbidity and even mortality in some. RRT is indicated for intractable fluid overload, hyperkalemia (potassium concentration >6.5 mmol/L or >5.5 mmol/L with electrocardiogram [ECG] changes), severe metabolic acidosis (pH <7.1), uremic encephalopathy, and pericarditis. There is no benefit from increasing the intensity of RRT beyond 20 to 25 mL/kg/hr of effluent flow, even in those with sepsis. The use of continuous RRT may be preferred in patients with brain edema, persistent metabolic acidosis, large fluid removal requirements, and severe hemodynamic instability. However, intermittent hemodialysis is not contraindicated absolutely in those with hemodynamic instability; special adaptations can be utilized to promote safety, or hybrid modes such as slow low-efficiency dialysis (SLED) can be substituted. Sufficient data do not exist to determine which dialysis mode—intermittent or continuous—is optimal in promoting eventual renal recovery.

Hematologic and Immune System Dysfunction

Thrombocytopenia, with multifactorial etiology, is the most common hematologic manifestation of MODS. Mild anemia, resulting from bone marrow suppression or iatrogenic causes, is also common. The immunologic dysfunction of MODS is most apparent in the

TABLE 3: RIFLE, AKIN, and KDIGO Classifications of Renal Failure

RIFLE Classification of Renal Failure		
Stage	**GFR**	**Urine Output**
R—Risk for renal injury	Baseline Cr × 1.5 Decrease GFR >25%	<0.5 mL/kg/hr × 6 hr
I—Injury to kidney	Baseline Cr × 2 Decease GFR >50%	<0.5 mL/kg/hr × 12 hr
F—Renal failure	Baseline Cr × 3 Cr >4 mg/dL with increase of 0.0 mg/dL Decrease GFR >75%	<0.3 mL/kg/hr × 24 hr Anuric × 12 hr
L—Loss of renal function	Persistent renal failure Loss of renal function >4 weeks	
E—ESRD	Renal failure >3 months	
Acute Kidney Injury Network (AKIN) Classification of AKI		
Stage	**GFR**	**Urine Output**
1	Baseline Cr × 1.5-2 Increase >0.3 mg/dL in 48 hr	<0.5 mL/kg/hr × 6 hr
2	Baseline Cr × 2-3	<0.5 mL/kg/hr × 12 hr
3	Baseline Cr × 3 Cr >4 mg/dL with acute increase 0.5 mg/dL Renal replacement therapy	<0.3 mL/kg/hr × 24 hr Anuric × 12 hr
Kidney Disease Improving Global Outcomes (KDIGO) Staging of AKI		
Stage	**Serum Creatinine**	**Urine Output**
1	Baseline × 1.5-1.9 Increase >0.3 mg/dL	<0.5 mL/kg/hr for 6-12 hr
2	Baseline × 2-2.9	< 0.5 mL/kg/hr for > 12 hr
3	Baseline × 3 Increase >4 mg/dL Initiation of renal replacement therapy <18 years old decreased GFR <35 mL/min per 1.73 m^2	<0.3 mL/kg/hr for 24 hr Anuria >12 hr

AKI, Acute kidney injury; *Cr*, creatinine; *ESRD*, end-stage renal disease; *GFR*, glomerular filtration rate.

development of nosocomial infections with usually avirulent commensal organisms such as *Staphylococcus, Enterococcus, Candida,* and *Pseudomonas.*

Endocrine System Dysfunction

Critically ill patients with MODS are hypermetabolic because of elevated cortisol, growth hormone, and catecholamines, leading to increased hepatic gluconeogenesis, insulin resistance, and hyperglycemia. Because critically ill patients with hyperglycemia have increased mortality and complications, including infection and worse neurologic outcomes, assiduous glucose control has been practiced in critically ill hyperglycemic patients. Current guidelines recommend moderate blood glucose control of 144 to 180 mg/dL for critically ill patients to avoid both marked hyperglycemia and iatrogenic hypoglycemia.

Relative adrenal insufficiency, manifested by hypotension and fever (and rarely by electrolyte abnormalities), is common in ICU patients and associated with worse outcomes. Although total levels of cortisol may be normal, they may not respond appropriately to stress situations. Current recommendations advise administration of low-dose "replacement" steroids (glucocorticoids) to septic patients

who remain hypotensive despite adequate volume resuscitation and vasopressor therapy, particularly those whose serum cortisol levels are below 20 μg/dL. A parallel to the relative insufficiency of cortisol seen in ICU patients with septic shock is that of arginine vasopressin. Therapy with low replacement doses of vasopressin might be considered analogous to that with glucocorticoids and may, in fact, be complementary to this therapy.

Finally, there is an entity of pseudohypothyroidism, the so-called sick euthyroid syndrome, that occurs in ICU patients who have normal thyroid function but low levels of triiodothyronine (T3), free thyroxine (T4), and T4, as T3 is converted to its isomer reverse T3. No treatment is required. Similarly, replacement of growth hormone or androgens is not beneficial in patients with MODS.

■ THERAPY

Sepsis

The therapy of sepsis is eloquently described in the 2012 Surviving Sepsis Campaign international guidelines for management of severe sepsis and septic shock. These guidelines focus on the identification of eligible patients by assaying lactate levels, obtaining blood and appropriate cultures, and undertaking invasive monitoring (via central venous and arterial catheters) and goal-directed resuscitation in those deemed at risk for poor outcomes. However, it is vital to note that in the surgical patient cohort not specifically addressed in the guidelines—that is, those with intra-abdominal, intrathoracic, or soft tissue infections—attention to rapid source identification and control is as important. Further, three large, recent well-conducted studies questioned the value of resuscitative therapy targeted to a specific goal. Thus, in order to prevent and lessen the severity of MOF in patients with severe sepsis and septic shock, the surgeon should strive to drain or excise the septic source as quickly as possible once antibiotics have been administered and resuscitation has been initiated. In the surgical patient who has severe sepsis and requires source control, the therapy with the least physiologic insult should be used (percutaneous drainage vs surgical drainage). The optimal timing for surgical (or catheter-based) therapy, surprisingly, has not been established in these patients.

Supportive Therapy

Nutrition

Specifics of nutritional therapy are discussed elsewhere in this text. It is important to note here that the type and intensity of nutritional therapy can alter the outcome of MOF. In general, providing enteral nutrition, within 24 hours if possible, is preferred. This should result in amelioration of translocation and gut-derived inflammation to fuel MODS. There does not appear to be a benefit of decreased aspiration rates or improved nutrition tolerance by delivering nutrients into the small intestine rather than the stomach. Nutrition should be delivered at goal rather than in a hypocaloric manner. In general, nutrition should provide 25 to 30 kcal/kg/day and 2.0 g/kg/day of protein in those with MOF. If a patient is unable to tolerate goal enteral nutrition, the use of trophic enteral nutrition (8 to 10 kcal/kg/day) may be beneficial. Patients in MOF often require vasopressor agents to maintain MAP greater than 65 mm Hg, and these agents should not discourage from the use of enteral nutrition therapy.

Certain elements of immunonutrition may be beneficial to deliver to septic patients, whereas others, such as arginine and glutamine, likely are not. Contemporary supplemental nutrition contains sufficient trace elements and vitamins to make deficiency in ICU patients a thing of the past in most instances. Finally, the surgeon must decide what course of action to take if, in the midst of MOF, the GI tract is not functional. There is evidence to suggest that riding out a temporary ileus is preferred over early initiation of parenteral alimentation.

Ventilation

Respiratory failure is the most resource-intensive component of MOF, and its management profoundly affects outcome. For both the prevention (intraoperatively) and the management of ARDS, one should use low stretch ventilation, as described earlier, to prevent secondary pulmonary injury from barotrauma. Inevitably, a small subset of patients with MOF will require therapy beyond this standard. It is important to note that although proning and brief use of neuromuscular blockade have been shown to be successful in randomized trials, no specific ventilatory modality for rescue ventilation has been proven to improve mortality. Whether airway pressure release ventilation (APRV), high-frequency modalities, or early use of ECMO are used will depend largely on local resources. The specifics of each of these modalities are discussed elsewhere in this text. Equally as important as selecting the appropriate ventilator mode and prescription is to regularly assess the patient's ability to be liberated from support.

Fluids, Blood Products, and Vasopressors

Increased attention is being given to limiting undisciplined crystalloid resuscitation of septic shock to mitigate the consequences of reperfusion injury and volume overload. There are no data to suggest that large volume fluid resuscitation reliably improves hemodynamics or end organ perfusion. In truth, those with a greater positive fluid balance invariably experience worse outcomes, including mortality. Unfortunately, data do not support the use of colloids as a viable alternative. Certainly synthetic starch-containing preparations should be avoided in the context of MOF because of the association with worsening renal function. However, use of albumin has not been associated with improved outcomes in MOF because of associated sepsis. There is evidence that a restrictive transfusion trigger (hemoglobin value of 7.0 g/dL) is appropriate in the resuscitation of septic shock. Liberal transfusion with packed red blood cells is associated with increased risk of secondary infections, worsening MODS, and increased mortality. Finally, norepinephrine, with renal sparing properties in its therapeutic range, has emerged as the pressor of choice in septic shock. Low dose vasopressin, steroids, and inotropes such as epinephrine are second-line agents. The optimal time to start a vasopressor agent in patients with sepsis has not been well studied.

Abdominal Compartment Syndrome

Secondary abdominal compartment syndrome (ACS) may result as a consequence of exuberant fluid and blood resuscitation of septic shock. Although its management in the context of trauma generally involves decompressive laparotomy (in part to exclude bleeding as a cause), it may be appropriate to use other methods to treat abdominal hypertension in the context of septic shock resuscitation. These include use of neuromuscular blockade, paracentesis if significant ascites are present, and diuresis, if possible. Once end organ manifestation, such as respiratory embarrassment and renal failure, of abdominal hypertension occurs (i.e., ACS develops), decompressive laparotomy is appropriate. Of course, in the context of pre-existing MOF, it may be difficult to attribute organ dysfunction to ACS. For this reason, it is imperative to routinely measure abdominal compartment pressures in patients with shock who are undergoing high volume resuscitation. Whether minimizing crystalloid resuscitation through the use of hypertonic saline, colloid, or pressors can minimize the development of ACS remains to be determined.

Palliative Care

Finally, it is vital to consider just what therapies should be offered and for how long, particularly as the population ages and supportive technology increases in scope and possibility. In an ICU setting the critical care provider unfortunately often cannot query the patient as to his or her wishes. The family acts as the surrogate best able to interpret these desires. Surgeons and ICU providers must interpret honestly and realistically how various therapies will affect outcome and define what "success" truly means. Discharging a patient to a long-term acute care hospital after a long ventilator stay in the ICU results in death at 1 year more often than not. Further, surgeons must be forthcoming and address the panoply of disorders encountered in the post–intensive care syndrome (a different PICS than that described earlier). What quality of life would the patient accept after a long, complicated ICU stay to warrant aggressive therapy? Hopefully, primary care physicians will begin to have conversations about end-of-life wishes more frequently with their patients before these patients are in the ICU and cannot participate in key healthcare decisions.

■ SUMMARY

MODS is a common and morbid inflammatory response to injury, illness, and resuscitation thereof. Despite advances in supportive care, MODS results in high mortality and long-term disability for survivors. A focus on early recognition and treatment of surgical sources of sepsis and trauma is vital to abrogate the effects of MODS.

SUGGESTED READINGS

Baue AE. Multiple, progressive or sequential systems failure. *Arch Surg.* 1975;110:779-781.

Deitch EA. Multiple organ failure: pathophysiology and potential future therapy. *Ann Surg.* 1992;216:117-134.

Dellinger RP, Levy MM, Rhodes A, Annane D, et al. Surviving Sepsis Campaign: international guidelines for management of severe sepsis and septic shock, 2012. *Crit Care Med.* 2013;41:580-637.

Marik PE. Early management of severe sepsis: concepts and controversies. *Chest.* 2014;145:1407-1418.

Marshall JC, Cook DJ, Christou NV, et al. Multiple organ dysfunction score: a reliable descriptor of a complex clinical outcome. *Crit Care Med.* 1995;23:1638-1652.

Rosenthal MD, Moore FA. Persistent inflammatory, immunosuppressed, catabolic syndrome (PICS): a new phenotype of multiple organ failure. *J Adv Nutr Hum Metab.* 2015;2:e784.

Vincent JL, Moreno R, Takala J, et al. The sepsis-related organ failure assessment (SOFA) score to describe organ dysfunction/failure. *Intensive Care Med.* 1996;22:707-710.

ANTIBIOTICS FOR CRITICALLY ILL PATIENTS

Shea C. Gregg, MD, FACS, and Walter Cholewczynski, MD

Infection continues to be a source of significant morbidity and mortality in the intensive care unit (ICU). With such initiatives as the Surviving Sepsis Campaign, hospitals have become more focused on efficiently diagnosing and managing septic conditions. Although such strategies have been shown to improve outcomes, the most fundamental tenet in the management of the septic patient is source control. In surgical patients, procedural interventions should remain a mainstay for achieving source control in the appropriate clinical setting. To complement this, proper antibiotic choice and duration has the ability to augment surgical control through local and systemic effects (Tables 1 and 2).

■ APPROACH TO ANTIBIOTIC USE IN THE CRITICALLY ILL

Surgical intensivists face several challenges when managing septic patients with antibiotics. First, defining the source of infection remains a priority. Taking a history and performing a thorough physical examination should always guide one's decisions for which laboratory tests, imaging studies, or interventions are necessary. Traditional practices such as "panculturing" or starting antibiotics empirically on all patients who have such commonplace findings as "fever" have been brought into question because of concerns about both cost and evolving resistance patterns of organisms. Once potential sources are identified, directed culturing has the ability to capture organisms to allow for tailored therapy. Depending on the site of infection and its contributions to physiologic disruption, empiric antibiotics may be beneficial while cultures are being incubated or other interventions are being arranged. It is imperative that every practitioner who is faced with the decision to start antibiotics approaches this responsibility with good clinical stewardship. This means starting appropriate broad-spectrum antibiotics with the discipline to narrow the spectrum when culture data return and the clinical situation allows. The evolving evidence that is produced continually through clinical trials should guide duration of use. If such an approach is used in conjunction with adequate source control and management of alterations in physiology, optimal outcomes hopefully will result.

■ PATHOGENS ENCOUNTERED IN CRITICALLY ILL PATIENTS

Patients who are admitted to the ICU early in a hospital stay are more likely to have a wild-type spectrum of pathogens, including gram-positive cocci and gram-negative bacilli; however, resistance to antibiotics is increasing, and newly hospitalized patients as well as those who have had recent encounters with illness are at a higher risk of falling ill to more resistant strains.

Community-Acquired Pathogens

Among gram-positive cocci, *Staphylococcus* spp. and *Streptococcus* spp. are common causes of skin and skin structure infections. Methicillin-susceptible *Staphylococcus aureus* (MSSA) is very sensitive to the penicillinase-resistant penicillins, oxacillin and nafcillin, and to cefazolin, a first-generation cephalosporin. Community-acquired methicillin-resistant *Staphylococcus aureus* (CA-MRSA) is becoming more common and is genetically distinct from hospital-acquired MRSA (HA-MRSA). CA-MRSA strains include several clonal groups, including USA300 and USA400, that contain the genetic package staphylococcal cassette chromosome mec (SCCmec) type IV. This is a smaller genetic package than HA-MRSA strains contain and is thought to explain why CA-MRSA is less resistant than HA-MRSA. Characteristics of patients with CA-MRSA are that they tend to be younger and healthier, may live in crowded conditions, or may be athletes. CA-MRSA is more prevalent in injection drug abusers and in children under 2 years of age. It usually is seen as cutaneous abscesses or boils. Most strains of CA-MRSA are susceptible to clindamycin, trimethoprim-sulfamethoxazole (TMP/SMX), or a tetracycline and are usually resistant to macrolides and fluoroquinolones.

Beta-hemolytic *Streptococcus*, groups A, B, C, and G, are responsible for many cases of cellulitis. Group A *S. pyogenes* is often the causative agent of streptococcal necrotizing fasciitis. These organisms may be virulent but are susceptible to penicillin G, cefazolin, or ceftriaxone.

Gram-negative bacilli and anaerobes causing intra-abdominal infections in the community usually are susceptible to cephalosporins with metronidazole and to extended-spectrum penicillins with a beta-lactamase inhibitor. A notable exception is *Escherichia coli*, which more commonly is resistant to ampicillin/sulbactam. For this reason, ampicillin/sulbactam no longer is recommended as initial empirical therapy for intra-abdominal infections.

Nosocomial Pathogens

Gram-positive cocci in the hospitalized or other healthcare-associated patient include HA-MRSA, methicillin-resistant *Staphylococcus epidermidis* (MRSE), and vancomycin-resistant *Enterococcus* spp. (VRE). HA-MRSA includes the USA100 and USA200 strains, which have larger genetic packages and greater resistance. MRSE and other coagulase-negative *Staphylococci* are common skin flora and frequently are infecting agents in implanted devices, such as central venous catheters. VRE overgrowth results from the selective pressure from broad-spectrum antibiotic therapy. VRE contains plasmids that

TABLE I: Antibiotic Classes and Agents Clinically Important in the Critically Ill: Beta-Lactam Antibiotics

Beta-lactam antibiotics	Attach to penicillin-binding proteins in the cell membrane, interfering with peptide chain crosslinkages in the bacterial cell wall peptidoglycan, leading to cell lysis

PENICILLINS

Groups	Examples	Comments
Natural penicillins	Penicillin G	• Very effective against *Streptococcus* spp., nonresistant *Enterococcus faecalis*, and *Clostridium perfringens*
Penicillinase-resistant penicillins	Oxacillin Nafcillin	• Very effective against MSSA and *Streptococcus* spp.
Aminopenicillins	Ampicillin Ampicillin-sulbactam	• Active against *Streptococcus* spp., MSSA, *E. faecalis*; variable activity against VRE • Adding BLI extends activity against gram-negative bacilli and *Bacteroides fragilis* • *Pseudomonas* is resistant and *Escherichia coli* resistance is rising
Ureidopenicillins	Piperacillin-tazobactam	• Broad-spectrum activity including against *Pseudomonas* and anaerobes

CEPHALOSPORINS

Groups	Examples	Comments
First generation	Cefazolin	• Active against MSSA, *Streptococcus* spp., *E. coli*, *Klebsiella*, *Proteus mirabilis*
Second generation	Cefuroxime	• Increased aerobic gram-negative activity, including against *Haemophilus influenzae*
Second generation (cephamycins)	Cefoxitin Cefotetan	• Extended activity against *B. fragilis*; resistance increasing • Methylthiotetrazole side chain inhibits vitamin K activation, resulting in rise in international normalized ratio
Third generation	Cefotaxime Ceftizoxime Ceftriaxone	• Increased spectrum of activity against aerobic gram-negative bacilli • Very susceptible to extended-spectrum beta-lactamases and AmpC cephalosporinases
Third generation antipseudomonal	Ceftazidime Ceftazidime-avibactam Ceftolozane-tazobactam	• Active against *Pseudomonas*, less active against *Staphylococcus* • Adding BLI extends activity against resistant aerobic gram-negative bacilli
Fourth generation	Cefepime	• Very effective against aerobic gram-negative bacilli, including *Pseudomonas* • Able to avoid destruction by beta-lactamases by rapid penetration through the cell wall • Maintains activity against *Staphylococcus* and *Streptococcus*
Fifth generation	Ceftaroline	• Broad-spectrum activity, including against MRSA and aerobic gram-negative bacilli • Inactive against *Pseudomonas*

OTHER BETA-LACTAMS

Groups	Examples	Comments
Carbapenems	Ertapenem	• Broad-spectrum activity against gram-positive cocci, gram-negative bacilli, and anaerobes; readily penetrate cell membranes of gram-negative bacilli, have high affinity for penicillin-binding proteins, and are resistant to hydrolysis by beta-lactamases • Ertapenem is not active against *Pseudomonas*
AP carbapenems	Imipenem-cilastatin Doripenem Meropenem	• Seizure risk is greater than with other beta-lactam antibiotics • Doripenem is indicated for complicated intra-abdominal infections and urinary tract infections but not for pneumonia
Monobactam	Aztreonam	• Active against aerobic gram-negative bacilli, including *Pseudomonas*

BLI, Beta-lactamase inhibitor; *MRSA*, methicillin-resistant *Staphylococcus aureus*; *MSSA*, methicillin-susceptible *Staphylococcus aureus*; *VRE*, vancomycin-resistant *Enterococcus*.

TABLE 2: Antibiotic Classes and Agents Clinically Important in the Critically Ill: Non–Beta-Lactam Antibiotics

Groups	Examples	Comments
Glyco-lipopeptides	Vancomycin Telavancin Oritavancin Dalbavancin	• Disrupts bacterial cell wall synthesis by impairing peptidoglycan synthesis • Active against gram-positive cocci, including MRSA • Daptomycin and oritavancin active against VRE • Oral vancomycin effective against *Clostridium difficile* • Oritavancin and dalbavancin have very long half-lives, allowing single dosing (oritavancin) or weekly × 2 dosing (dalbavancin) • Daptomycin is inactivated by surfactant, not used for pneumonia; also associated with myopathy; statins should be stopped; check CPK weekly
Polymyxins	Polymyxin B Colistin (polymyxin E)	• Cationic polypeptides that act as detergents to disrupt the bacterial cell membrane • Active against Enterobacteriaceae, *Acinetobacter*, *Pseudomonas*, and *Stenotrophomonas* • Cause significant renal toxicity
Aminoglycosides	Gentamicin Tobramycin Amikacin	• Inhibit bacterial protein synthesis by binding irreversibly to the 30S ribosomal subunit • Active against gram-negative bacilli, including *Pseudomonas* • Synergistic activity with penicillins and vancomycin against *Enterococcus* and *Staphylococcus* • Exhibit concentration-dependent activity and a significant postantibiotic effect • Significant incidence of renal toxicity and ototoxicity (auditory and vestibular) • Once-daily dosing improves effectiveness and reduces toxicity • Limiting usage to 5 days reduces toxicity
Tetracyclines	Doxycycline Minocycline	• Inhibit bacterial protein synthesis by binding to the 30S ribosomal subunit • Active against *Staphylococcus,* including MRSA; variable activity against VRE and *Streptococcus*
Glycylcycline	Tigecycline	• Broad-spectrum agent active against gram-positive cocci (MRSA and VRE), gram-negative bacilli, and anaerobes • Inactive against *Pseudomonas*
Macrolides, lincosamides, chloramphenicol	Erythromycin Clarithromycin Azithromycin Fidaxomicin Clindamycin Chloramphenicol	• Inhibit bacterial protein synthesis by reversibly binding to 50S ribosomal subunit at overlapping sites; use of 2 or more of these classes results in antagonism • Variable activity against MSSA and *Streptococcus* spp.; active against atypical bacterial • Fidaxomicin only active against *C. difficile* • Azithromycin and clarithromycin active against *Haemophilus influenzae* • Active against *Staphylococcus* and *Streptococcus*, 66% to 75% of *Bacteroides fragilis* • Potentially additive in clostridial and streptococcal gangrene for its ability to inhibit toxin production • Active against *Staphylococcus* (MRSA), *Streptococcus*, *Escherichia coli*, *Klebsiella*, *H. influenzae*, anaerobes • Variable activity against VRE • Limited use because of bone marrow suppression and rare aplastic anemia
Streptogramins	Quinupristin-dalfopristin	• Inhibits bacterial protein synthesis by binding to 50S ribosomal subunit • Active against gram-positive cocci, including MRSA and VRE • Inactive against *Enterococcus faecalis* • Causes severe phlebitis; infuse through central line
Oxazolidinones	Linezolid Tedizolid	• Inhibit bacterial protein synthesis by binding to the 23S ribosomal RNA of the 50S subunit • Active against gram-positive cocci. including MRSA and VRE • High bioavailability: oral is as effective as IV • Bone marrow suppression with thrombocytopenia may occur after 14 days of treatment with linezolid, reversible after cessation • Tedizolid indicated for acute bacterial skin and skin structure infections for 6 days • Weak monoamine oxidase inhibitors, 1% to 3% incidence of serotonin syndrome when given with monoamine oxidase inhibitors or selective serotonin reuptake inhibitors

TABLE 2: Antibiotic Classes and Agents Clinically Important in the Critically Ill: Non–Beta-Lactam Antibiotics—cont'd

Groups	Examples	Comments
Fluoroquinolones	Ciprofloxacin Levofloxacin Moxifloxacin	• Inhibit DNA gyrase and topoisomerase IV • Active against broad spectrum of nonresistant gram-positive cocci and gram-negative bacilli, including *Pseudomonas* (not moxifloxacin) • Moxifloxacin active against 85% of *B. fragilis* • Concentration-dependent antibacterial effect • High bioavailability: oral is as effective as IV • Not approved for children <16 years, associated with joint and tendon injuries
Nitroimidazoles	Metronidazole	• Chemically reduced in the bacterial cell and disrupts the DNA helix, causing strand breakage • Active against *Bacteroides* and *Clostridium, Entamoeba histolytica* • Often combined with cephalosporins and fluoroquinolones for intra-abdominal infections • One of the main therapies for *C. difficile* colitis • Disulfiram-like reaction occurs with alcohol consumption
Rifamycins	Rifampin	• Inhibits DNA-dependent RNA polymerase • Active against MRSA and VRE • Always used in combination with other agents, may reduce development of resistance • Has many drug interactions and may be hepatotoxic
Sulfonamides	Trimethoprim- sulfamethoxazole (TMP/SMX)	• SMX inhibits dihydropteroate synthase, TMP inhibits dihydrofolate reductase: 2 steps in bacterial folate pathway • Active against MSSA, MRSA, coagulase-negative *Staphylococcus; Stenotrophomonas, Enterobacter, Serratia* • Inactive against *Enterococcus* (despite in vitro sensitivity)
Other	Nitrofurantoin	• Inhibits bacterial enzymes, leading to cell death • Active against VRE, *E. coli, Klebsiella* • Oral antibiotic, used in urinary tract infection • Macrocrystal form causes less nausea • Do not use if creatinine clearance <50 mL/min

CPK, Creatine phosphokinase; *IV*, intravenous; *MRSA*, methicillin-resistant *Staphylococcus aureus*; *MSSA*, methicillin-susceptible *Staphylococcus aureus*; *VRE*, vancomycin-resistant *Enterococcus*.

confer resistance, and the VanA plasmid has been transferred to MRSA, conferring vancomycin resistance.

Clinically important members of the Enterobacteriaceae family include *E. coli, Klebsiella pneumoniae, Proteus* spp., *Enterobacter* spp., *Serratia* spp., and *Citrobacter* spp. These organisms often are referred to as aerobic, but they are facultative anaerobes, which means that they are able to make adenosine triphosphate (ATP) by aerobic respiration as well as by fermenting sugars to produce lactic acid (lactose fermenters) in anaerobic environments. Other important gram-negative rods are *Pseudomonas* spp., *Acinetobacter* spp., and *Stenotrophomonas* spp. Many of these organisms have developed resistance by producing extended-spectrum beta-lactamases (ESBLs), which hydrolyze penicillins and cephalosporins. AmpC beta-lactamase hydrolyzes first-, second-, and third-generation cephalosporins. Carbapenemases that hydrolyze penicillins, cephalosporins, and carbapenems, but not aztreonam (a monobactam), are now being observed. Some of these organisms contain plasmids that confer aminoglycoside resistance.

Clostridium difficile can be selected out by broad-spectrum antibiotic therapy, especially by fluoroquinolones, and can result in a mild to severe colitis. The NAP1 strain is particularly virulent: 40% demonstrate in vitro resistance to vancomycin but remain sensitive to metronidazole.

Multidrug resistance is a worsening problem, especially among the ESKAPE organisms: *E. faecium, S. aureus, K. pneumoniae, A. baumannii, P. aeruginosa*, and *Enterobacter* spp. The Infectious Diseases Society of America (IDSA) launched the 10 × '20 Initiative in 2010 to encourage greater research and development of antibiotic therapies to combat these organisms, with the goal of developing 10 new antibiotics by 2020. Since 2010 the U.S. Food and Drug Administration (FDA) has approved eight new antibiotics.

■ COMMON CONDITIONS

The following is a review of common conditions encountered in surgical ICUs. Treatment descriptions are based on general recommendations and should be tailored based on institutional antibiogram resistance patterns.

Pneumonia

Background

Pulmonary complications after surgery have been shown to contribute significantly to postoperative morbidity and mortality. Pneumonia is one of the three most common postoperative infections and may account for almost half of nosocomial infections in ICU patients. The foci for developing postoperative pneumonia tend to revolve around the use of endotracheal intubation and the occurrence of aspiration in the perioperative period. As such, prevention efforts should be multidisciplinary among anesthesia providers and surgical care providers at all levels. Specific strategies for reduction of pneumonia in the immediate operative time period include preoperative chlorhexidine mouthwashes, expert technique in endotracheal tube placement, and appropriate timing of tube removal. If a tube is necessary postoperatively, patients remain at risk for ventilator-associated pneumonia (VAP). Means of mitigating VAP have included upright positioning of patients, proper circuit maintenance, reduced sedation levels, and effective mouth care. Other strategies that may provide benefit include the use of selective decontamination of the digestive tract and antiseptic-coated endotracheal tubes. Hand hygiene remains a pillar of good management and a primary means of reducing possible postoperative pneumonia. Like most devices, removal of endotracheal tubes as early as clinically possible will allow patients with appropriate mental status to utilize their own means of secretion expulsion for the purposes of pneumonia reduction.

Treatment

Early-onset pneumonia, in which there is low risk for multidrug-resistant organisms, can be treated with ceftriaxone, a fluoroquinolone, ampicillin/sulbactam, or ertapenem. Late-onset pneumonias, in which multidrug-resistant organisms are likely, need to be treated more aggressively with empirical combination therapy to minimize the chance of coverage gaps and to decrease mortality. Cefepime, piperacillin-tazobactam, or meropenem should be combined with either a fluoroquinolone or an aminoglycoside. If MRSA is also a risk, vancomycin or linezolid should be added. Once culture and sensitivity results are available, the antibiotic regimen can be refined further. Combination therapy for *Pseudomonas* spp. remains controversial. Ampicillin/sulbactam, a carbapenem, or a polymyxin may be necessary for *Acinetobacter* spp. Avoid third-generation cephalosporins for ESBL-producing Enterobacteriaceae. Carbapenems are better choices. Vancomycin and linezolid are appropriate choices for MRSA. Inhaled aminoglycosides or colistin may play a role in difficult-to-treat pneumonias, but the results of trials are not conclusive.

Catheter-Associated Urinary Tract Infections

Background

Urinary catheter insertion is another common practice used with critically ill patients for the purposes of bladder drainage and urinary output monitoring. With the incidence of catheter-associated bacteriuria developing at 3% to 8% a day, catheter-associated urinary tract infections (CA-UTIs) in the United States are estimated to total more than 500,000. In addition, increases in hospital length of stay have been associated with CA-UTI. Preventative measures to help reduce the incidence of CA-UTI focus on sterile technique on insertion, the use of nonobstructed closed drainage systems, hand hygiene, early removal, and the avoidance of catheter use altogether. Alternatives to catheterization, including the use of diapers, condom catheters, and bladder scan–driven intermittent catheterization, may have benefits, but data are limited. In addition, certain silver alloy catheters and antibiotic-impregnated catheters have decreased the incidence of bacteriuria in short-term catheterized patients (<7 days); however, ultimate reductions in CA-UTI remain unclear.

Treatment

Uncomplicated UTIs are usually susceptible to TMP/SMX. Nitrofurantoin is effective against VRE and *E. coli* but should not be used in end-stage renal failure. Ciprofloxacin and levofloxacin are very effective agents and concentrate in the urine. Because complicated UTIs, including CA-UTIs, are caused primarily by Enterobacteriaceae, *Pseudomonas* spp., and *Enterococcus* spp., ampicillin and gentamicin,

piperacillin-tazobactam, a carbapenem, or a fluoroquinolone can be used. If the risk of *Enterococcus* is low, ceftazidime, ceftazidime-avibactam, ceftolozane-tazobactam, or cefepime is an appropriate choice. De-escalation or change of antibiotic should be based on culture and sensitivity results.

Surgical Site Infections

Background

Surgical site infections are one of the most commonly encountered postoperative complications. The risks for developing such infections have been associated with the perioperative care of the patient, surgical technique, intraoperative anesthetic management, and a wide range of host conditions. Risk for infection at surgical sites has been associated with entry into contaminated luminal organs or pre-existing infection at or near the operative site. This risk is captured through the levels of wound classification: clean, clean-contaminated, contaminated, and dirty. Should an infection arise at the surgical site, the classification of actual infections is delineated by the depth of the process:

- *Superficial:* Involves skin and subcutaneous tissue
- *Deep:* Involves the deep soft tissues of the incision (fascia and muscle layer)
- *Organ/space:* Involves any part of the body deeper than the fascia or muscle layer that was opened or manipulated during the operative procedure

Such infections should be suspected when abnormalities arise in baseline physiologic parameters and should be assessed by a combination of thorough examination of the surgical sites followed by appropriate imaging. Antibiotic therapy should be considered only once the decision has been made about whether to perform instrumentation of the site to ensure proper source control.

Treatment

Antibiotic therapy for surgical site infections involving "clean cases" (those not involving the gastrointestinal [GI] or genitourinary [GU] tract) is directed against skin flora. Mild infections that require only oral therapy can be treated with cephalexin or dicloxacillin. If there is concern for MRSA, TMP/SMX, clindamycin, minocycline, or doxycycline can be used. More severe infections should be treated with cefazolin or vancomycin for MRSA. Daptomycin, telavancin, ceftaroline, linezolid, or tedizolid also may be used. Oritavancin and dalbavancin are long-acting lipoproteins that may be used for outpatient therapy.

Surgical site infections in clean-contaminated, contaminated, or dirty cases involving the GI or GU tract may be caused by skin flora and/or coliforms and anaerobes. Treatment choices against aerobic gram-negative bacilli and *Bacteroides fragilis* include ceftazidime, ceftazidime-avibactam, ceftolozane-tazobactam, cefepime, or a fluoroquinolone with metronidazole. Piperacillin-tazobactam and antipseudomonal carbapenems can be used as single agents. Vancomycin should be used if MRSA is likely. De-escalation or change in antibiotic therapy should be based on the results of culture and sensitivity.

Vascular Access Device–Related Infections

Background

Vascular access for the purposes of monitoring, fluid resuscitation, nutrition, and therapeutic administration of medications is necessary in critically ill patients. Unfortunately, significant infectious morbidity and mortality can result from its use. One of the most popular types of access, the central venous catheter, has become more ubiquitous since its earliest development in the 1950s. With its increased use, the number of central line–associated bloodstream infections is estimated to be more than 80,000 per year in the United States, and its use is thought to increase length of hospital stay up to about 7 days. Two types of catheters are typically used in the ICU population: noncuffed, nontunneled central venous catheters (NTCVCs) and peripherally inserted central catheters (PICCs). The first type has evolved with such technology as increasing number of lumens, larger bore, antibiotic versus antiseptic coatings, and variable lengths to accommodate placement in a variety of patients. Infection rates have been reported to be around 1.5 to 2.1 per 1000 central line days; however, this rate can be reduced significantly based on the use of broad-reaching infection control efforts. The other type of common device, PICCs, maintains the potential benefit of patient comfort while allowing for multilumen administration of various medications. Regarding infectious rates, studies show variability when comparing PICCs with NTCVCs. In summary, there may be equal to increased rates of infection when PICCs are used in ICU populations, whereas there may be lower rates of infection when using them in non-ICU settings. Regardless of device, best practice strategies that aim to reduce infectious complications associated with insertion and maintenance of the device should be utilized. These strategies generally involve proper hand hygiene, skin antisepsis, full barrier precautions at insertion, proper catheter site maintenance, and removal of the device as early as the clinical situation allows. Once removed, nontunneled peripheral venous access devices may be used to continue therapy; however, these devices have their own infection risks that tend to be more local rather than systemic.

Treatment

The majority of catheter-associated infections are caused by *S. aureus* and *S. epidermidis*. Vancomycin is the primary agent used for empiric treatment. If there is concern for aerobic gram-negative bacilli, as in immunocompromised or burn patients, cefepime, piperacillin-tazobactam, or an antipseudomonal carbapenem should be added. Femoral catheters and catheters used for parenteral alimentation and in immunocompromised patients may be infected with *Candida* spp. Fluconazole should be added. If fluconazole has been used in the previous 3 months or there is a known high prevalence of resistant species, use an echinocandin. De-escalation is appropriate once culture and sensitivity results are available.

Abdominal Sepsis

Gastrointestinal Tract

Conditions associated with perforation, inflammation, and ischemic processes of the GI tract continue to provide surgeons with diagnostic and therapeutic challenges despite being commonly encountered disease processes. When operative management is chosen, appropriate preoperative and postoperative antibiotics are imperative not only to treat the primary process, but also hopefully reduce the incidence of postoperative surgical site infections. When nonoperative management is chosen, source control through minimally invasive or percutaneous means may be indicated in addition to antibiotic therapy.

Treatment

Infections of mild to moderate severity, including perforated appendicitis and diverticulitis in which there is no physiologic impairment, can be treated with first-, second-, or third-generation cephalosporins or fluoroquinolones with metronidazole. Appropriate single agents include cefoxitin, moxifloxacin, ertapenem, and tigecycline. Ampicillin/sulbactam should not be used as empiric therapy because of the high rate of resistance of *E. coli*. Severe infections with physiologic compromise should be treated with ceftazidime, ceftazidime-avibactam, ceftolozane-tazobactam, cefepime, or a fluoroquinolone with metronidazole. Piperacillin-tazobactam and antipseudomonal carbapenems are appropriate single agents. Add an aminoglycoside when there is a high rate of resistant *Pseudomonas* spp. and ESBL-producing Enterobacteriaceae in hospitalized patients. If MRSA is considered, add vancomycin to the regimen. De-escalation or change

in antibiotic therapy is appropriate based on culture and sensitivity reports. *B. fragilis* may not grow but should be expected and treated.

Infections of the Biliary Tree

The biliary tree remains an important source of sepsis among the critically ill. Whether from primary infections of the ductal structures (cholangitis) or infections arising from stasis with or without obstructive causes (i.e., acute cholecystitis, acalculous cholecystitis, choledocholithiasis), significant morbidity and mortality can arise unless early diagnosis is achieved, appropriate instrumentation is performed, and effective antibiotic therapy is started.

Treatment

Cholecystitis of mild to moderate severity can be treated with a first-, second-, or third-generation cephalosporin. More severe infections, including those in patients with biliary obstruction, bilioenteric anastomosis, recent hospitalization(s), or are immunocompromised are more likely to be drug resistant and/or anerobic. Piperacillin-tazobactam and carbapenems are effective against gram-negative aerobes and *B. fragilis*. Fluoroquinolones, cefepime, ceftolozane-tazobactam, and ceftazidime-avibactam all should be combined with metronidazole.

Clostridium Difficile *Colitis*

Although accounting for less than 25% of antibiotic-associated diarrhea, *C. difficile* infections are an important pathogen to monitor for in the ICU setting. Given the 30-day overall mortality of around 40% among ICU patients with *C. difficile* colitis and its ability to spread via direct contact, infection control strategies include strict hand hygiene, contact precautions, and antibiotic stewardship to combat this potentially fatal pathogen. Given that fulminant *C. difficile* colitis accounts for less than 5% of patients and the need for surgery is around 1% of all hospitalized patients, antibiotics remain the mainstay of treatment.

Treatment

Oral metronidazole is the mainstay of treatment of *C. difficile* colitis. More severe infections and those that do not respond to initial oral metronidazole should be treated with oral vancomycin or fidaxomicin. Vancomycin enemas should be considered when there is an impairment in the GI tract, either ileus or interruption, and oral administration would not reach the colon or rectum effectively. Fidaxomicin results in fewer recurrences unless the NAP1 strain, which has a recurrence rate similar to vancomycin, is involved. Toxic megacolon often is treated with subtotal colectomy. An alternative approach is to create a loop ileostomy, perform intraoperative colonic lavage with polyethylene glycol 3350–electrolyte solution, and then provide antegrade vancomycin instillations postoperatively. Recurrence often is treated with vancomycin. Evidence for probiotics is mixed, with some reports showing benefit in prevention and others showing no benefit. Fecal transplant has been shown to be an effective therapy for antibiotic treatment–resistant cases.

Necrotizing Soft Tissue Infections

Aggressive infections ultimately leading to necrosis of one or more layers of the skin, subcutaneous tissues, fascia, or muscle have been shown to have high morbidity and mortality. These infections tend to be extremely painful on palpation and can be accompanied by signs of septic shock. When suspected, early antibiotic therapy, resuscitation, and surgical débridement should be sought immediately.

Treatment

Empiric therapy should consider the likelihood of polymicrobial infections versus those caused by a single organism. Antibiotic regimens initially should be broad spectrum. ESBLs with beta-lactamase inhibitors (piperacillin-tazobactam), fourth-generation (cefepime) or fifth-generation (ceftaroline) cephalosporins with metronidazole, carbapenems, and tigecycline are appropriate initial choices. If MRSA is a possible pathogen, add vancomycin or daptomycin. Clindamycin is often added, as it is potentially effective in blocking the toxins responsible for toxic shock syndrome.

De-escalation of antibiotics may be appropriate as culture results become available. Anaerobes are difficult to isolate, and therapy against them is often continued. If clostridial or streptococcal gangrene is identified, high-dose penicillin G with clindamycin is effective. Staphylococcal infections are treated with vancomycin or daptomycin with clindamycin (for toxin inhibition). Linezolid inhibits toxin production and can be used alone. MSSA infections can be treated with an antistaphylococcal penicillin (oxacillin or nafcillin) with clindamycin.

Fungal Infections

Candida spp. may be causative agents in catheter infections, especially if the catheter is used for hyperalimentation. *Candida* peritonitis may complicate perforated viscus. *C. albicans* is susceptible to fluconazole. *C. krusei* and *C. glabrata* are resistant to fluconazole and should be treated with an echinocandin. For this reason, echinocandins are recommended as initial empiric therapy and can be altered based on culture results. *Candida* rarely causes pneumonia or cystitis unless the patient is immunocompromised. *Aspergillus* may infect burn wounds and can be found as pulmonary "fungus balls." Voriconazole is effective for *Aspergillus*. Amphotericin B is used less frequently. The lipid formulations are as effective as the standard formulation but often are better tolerated and less toxic to the renal system.

SUGGESTED READINGS

Cohen SH, Gerding DN, Johnson S, Kelly CP, Loo VG, McDonald LC, Pepin J, Wilcox MH, Society for Healthcare Epidemiology of America, Infectious Diseases Society of America. Clinical practice guidelines for *Clostridium difficile* infection in adults: 2010 update by the Society for Healthcare Epidemiology of America (SHEA) and the Infectious Diseases Society of America (IDSA). *Infect Control Hosp Epidemiol.* 2010;31:431-455. doi:10.1086/651706.

Gould IM, David MZ, Esposito S, Garau J, Lina G, Mazzei T, Peters G. New insights into methicillin-resistant *Staphylococcus aureus* (MRSA) pathogenesis, treatment and resistance. *Int J Antimicrob Agents.* 2012;39:96-104. doi:10.1016/j.ijantimicag.2011.09.028.

Kusminsky RE. Complications of central venous catheterization. *J Am Coll Surg.* 2007;204:681-696.

Neal MD, Alverdy JC, Hall DE, et al. Diverting loop ileostomy and colonic lavage: an alternative to total abdominal colectomy for the treatment of severe complicated *Clostridium difficile* associated disease. *Ann Surg.* 2011;254:423-429. doi:10.1097/SLA.0b013e31822ade48.

Saint S, Kaufman SR, Rogers MA, Baker PD, Ossenkop K, Lipsky BA. Condom versus indwelling urinary catheters: a randomized trial. *J Am Geriatr Soc.* 2006;54:1055-1061.

Sawyer RG, Claridge JA, Nathens AB, Rotstein OD, Duane TM, Evans HL, Cook CH, O'Neill PJ, Mazuski JE, Askari R, Wilson MA, Napolitano LM, Namias N, Miller PR, Dellinger EP, Watson CM, Coimbra R, Dent DL, Lowry SF, Cocanour CS, West MA, Banton KL, Cheadle WG, Lipsett PA, Guidry CA, Popovsky K. Trial of short-course antimicrobial therapy for intraabdominal infection. *N Engl J Med.* 2015;372:1996-2005. doi:10.1056/NEJMoa1411162.

Solomkin JS, Mazuski JE, Bradley JS, et al. Diagnosis and management of complicated intra-abdominal infection in adults and children: guidelines by the Surgical Infection Society and the Infectious Diseases Society of America. *Clin Infect Dis.* 2010;50:133-164. doi:10.1086/649554.

Stevens DL, Bisno AL, Chambers HF, et al. Practice guidelines for the diagnosis and management of skin and soft tissue infections: 2014 update by the Infectious Diseases Society of America. *Clin Infect Dis.* 2014;59:147-159. doi:10.1093/cid/ciu296.

To KB, Napolitano LM. Common complications in the critically ill patient. *Surg Clin North Am.* 2012;92:1519-1557. doi:10.1016/j.suc.2012.08.018.

ENDOCRINE CHANGES IN CRITICAL ILLNESS

Christopher J. Goodenough, MD, MPH, and Lillian S. Kao, MD, MS, FACS

Critical illness results in changes in both the hypothalamic-pituitary-adrenal (HPA) and the hypothalamic-pituitary-thyroid (HPT) axes. These endocrine changes have been postulated to be adaptive responses to stress, and therefore it is controversial whether interventions to restore these axes to their normal state are necessary or beneficial. This chapter reviews the changes in endocrine function resulting from critical illness and the evidence for interventions to address these changes.

■ ADRENAL INSUFFICIENCY

During stress, activation of the HPA axis results in release of corticotrophin-releasing hormone (CRH) and arginine vasopressin from the hypothalamus, which stimulate the anterior pituitary gland to secrete adrenocorticotropic hormone (ACTH). In turn, ACTH activates the adrenal cortex to synthesize and release glucocorticoids, mainly cortisol, into the circulation. Regulation of the HPA axis occurs through a feedback loop; elevated circulating cortisol levels provide negative feedback to suppress CRH and ACTH production (Figure 1). Cortisol acts on the adrenal medulla to stimulate secretion of epinephrine and norepinephrine, resulting in the "fight-or-flight" response to stress and acute illness. Increased cortisol levels result in metabolic, cardiovascular, and immune effects. Cortisol mobilizes glucose for use by the brain and heart by increasing liver gluconeogenesis and decreasing glucose uptake by muscle and other tissues, improves hemodynamics by maintaining the responsiveness of vascular smooth muscle to catecholamines, inhibits the inflammatory response to injury, and suppresses the immune response.

Normally, more than 90% of cortisol is bound to corticosteroid-binding globulin (CBG). However, during acute illness CBG decreases, resulting in a rise in the percentage of free cortisol. In addition, there is an increase in cortisol production as a result of stimulation of the HPA axis, although this increase is likely more modest than originally believed. Recent studies have demonstrated decreased ACTH levels in critical illness, which is opposite that expected if stimulation of the HPA axis is the primary mechanism resulting in elevated cortisol levels. Alternative mechanisms include decreased cortisol breakdown during critical illness; the resulting increased serum cortisol levels feed back and inhibit CRH and ACTH production. For example, elevated circulating bile acids during critical illness, which may result from decreased transport from the blood into the bile canaliculi, may increase suppression of cortisol metabolizing enzymes in the liver (see Figure 1). Despite elevated circulating cortisol levels, the downstream effects may not be augmented during critical illness because of increased tissue resistance (i.e., because of

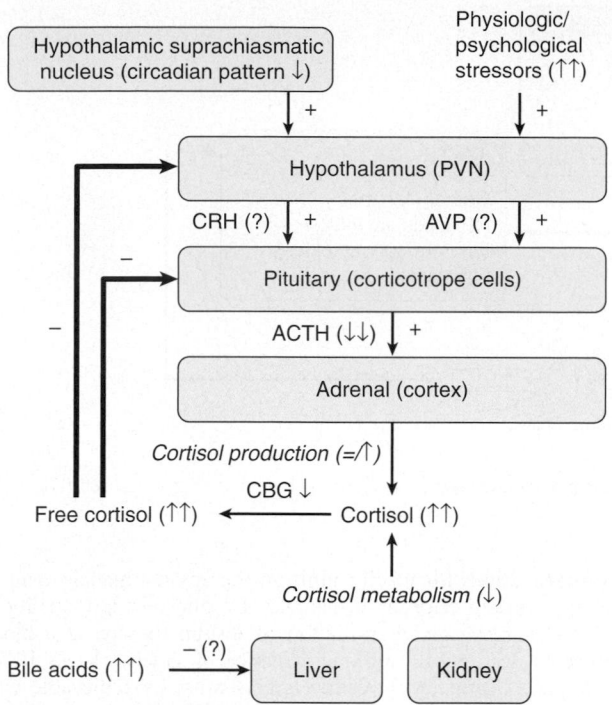

FIGURE 1 Simplified overview of the regulation of the hypothalamus-pituitary-adrenal axis and cortisol metabolism during critical illness. ↑, Elevated plasma concentrations; ↓, decreased plasma concentrations; ?, uncertain; +, stimulates; −, inhibits; *ACTH*, adrenocorticotropic hormone; *AVP*, arginine vasopressin; *CBG*, corticosteroid-binding globulin; *CRH*, corticotrophin-releasing hormone; *PVN*, paraventricular nucleus. *(Modified from Peeters B, Boonen E, Langouche L, Van den Berghe G. The HPA axis response to critical illness: new study results with diagnostic and therapeutic implications. Mol Cell Endocrinol. 2015;408:235-240.)*

alterations in the concentration or affinity of tissue glucocorticoid receptors).

Both high and low circulating cortisol levels in acute critical illness have been associated with increased mortality. The concept of an inadequate response of the HPA axis to stress has been termed relative adrenal insufficiency or critical illness–related corticosteroid insufficiency (CIRCI). Significant controversy exists regarding the diagnostic criteria and indications for treatment of CIRCI.

Symptoms and signs of adrenal insufficiency are often vague and nonspecific, particularly in critically ill patients; examples include weakness and fatigue; anorexia, nausea, and vomiting; abdominal pain; fever; and tachycardia. In critically ill patients, consideration for adrenal insufficiency should be triggered by the presence of hemodynamic instability refractory to adequate fluid resuscitation and vasopressor administration. Unfortunately there is no consensus on the diagnostic criteria for CIRCI. Traditionally, random total serum cortisol level (<10 µg/dL) has been considered diagnostic of CIRCI. However, measurement of total cortisol is problematic in that there is lack of uniformity in the accuracy of the tests; measurement of total serum cortisol levels does not reflect free, biologically active cortisol levels; and there is variability in the hourly secretion of cortisol. Another test measures the change in cortisol in response to 250 µg of synthetic ACTH (corticotropin or cosyntropin) after 30 and 60 minutes; a change in delta cortisol less than 9 µg/dL was considered diagnostic of CIRCI. However, in a large multicenter randomized trial of glucocorticoids in septic shock, the results of this test did not predict responsiveness to glucocorticoid treatment. Other tests that have been considered include stimulation with low-dose synthetic ACTH, at 1 µg, and measurement of salivary cortisol. However, neither of these tests has been studied extensively in critically ill patients.

Trials have had conflicting results regarding the effects of treating CIRCI with "low-dose" glucocorticoids. Although termed low dose, 200 to 300 mg per day of hydrocortisone typically is administered, which is six times higher than normal daily cortisol production. Although multiple trials and meta-analyses have been performed, two main trials form the cornerstone of the debate about low-dose corticosteroids. In 2002 Annane and colleagues reported a 28-day mortality benefit among patients with septic shock who did not respond to the corticotropin stimulation test and who received hydrocortisone (50 mg intravenously every 6 hours for 7 days) and fludrocortisone (50 µg orally per day for 7 days) as compared with placebo. Subsequently, in 2008 Sprung and colleagues reported the results of a multicenter trial (CORTICUS) of hydrocortisone (50 mg intravenously every 6 hours for 5 days, followed by a 6-day taper) versus placebo. Patients receiving hydrocortisone had a faster time to shock reversal, but there was no significant difference in mortality. Postulated reasons for the differing results included that the latter trial included less severely ill patients, allowed enrollment up to 72 hours after shock onset (as compared with up to 8 hours), treated for a longer duration of time, and did not administer fludrocortisone. A subsequent 2 × 2 factorial randomized trial demonstrated that the addition of fludrocortisone did not improve mortality when used with hydrocortisone in patients with septic shock.

Although the use of steroids in critically ill patients with septic shock or severe sepsis remains controversial, there is consensus regarding the lack of benefit of high-dose corticosteroids (i.e., 30 mg/kg methylprednisolone) in these patients and the lack of utility of the corticotropin stimulation test in predicting response to corticosteroids. Dexamethasone, which used to be administered during the corticotropin stimulation test, is also no longer used given its suppressive effects on the HPA axis. Rather, for patients with septic shock refractory to adequate fluid resuscitation and vasopressor administration, a trial of intravenous hydrocortisone (200 mg/day) can be considered. A recent systematic review suggested that there may be benefits on short-term mortality with longer course, low-dose glucocorticoid treatment in septic shock. The Surviving Sepsis Campaign guidelines consider this to be a weak recommendation supported by low quality of evidence. Institution of therapy should not be based on biochemical testing. Furthermore, the guidelines recommend tapering the steroid therapy after restoration of hemodynamic status, again as a weak recommendation with very low evidence supporting it. This recommendation is based on observed rebound shock in several studies and postulated rebound production of proinflammatory mediators with abrupt cessation of corticosteroids.

■ HYPERGLYCEMIA

Under normal physiologic conditions, blood glucose is maintained by a balance of pancreatic secretion of insulin and glucagon, hepatic gluconeogenesis, and peripheral uptake of available glucose. Insulin functions globally to upregulate glucose uptake and downregulate gluconeogenesis and other fasting responses. Insulin is produced by pancreatic beta cells as preproinsulin, which is cleaved to proinsulin and finally to active insulin, which consists of an alpha and beta chain bound together by sulfide bonds. Glucose stimulates insulin release by facilitated transport via a glucose transporter expressed on the surface of pancreatic beta cells. Glucose stimulates insulin release by facilitated transport via glucose transporter 1 (GLUT1), expressed on the surface of pancreatic beta cells. Insulin is released in a pulsatile pattern of 10 minutes, with larger amplitude releases occurring every 80 to 150 minutes. Gut-derived incretins potently upregulate the insulin release and augment the effect of glucose on pancreatic beta cells after a normal meal. Beta cells secrete insulin into the portal venous system, of which 50% is metabolized in the liver. Remaining insulin enters the circulation and binds to receptors on target cells, which stimulates multiple downstream effects. In skeletal muscles,

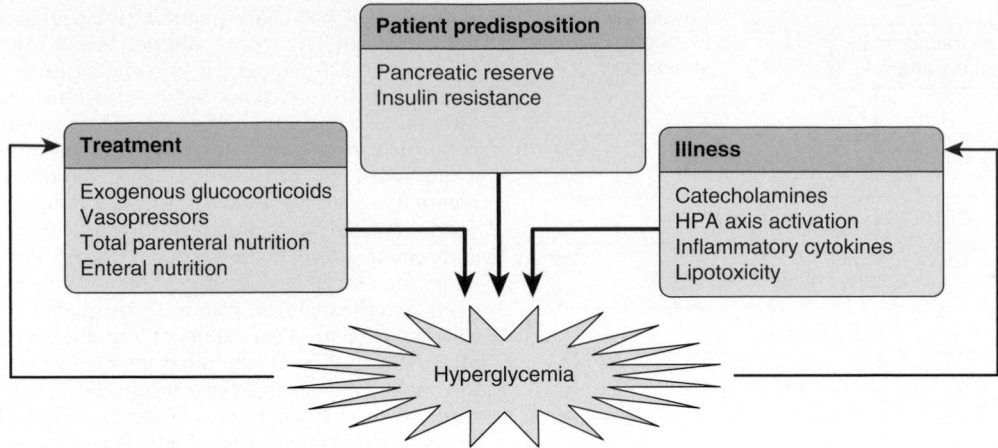

FIGURE 2 Multifactorial causes of hospital-related hyperglycemia. *HPA*, Hypothalamic-pituitary-adrenal. *(Reproduced with permission from Dungan KM, Braithwaite SS, Preiser JC. Stress hyperglcaemia. Lancet. 2009;373:1798-1807.)*

for example, insulin triggers the expression of glucose transporter 4 (GLUT4), which facilitates the intracellular transfer of glucose.

Disruption of multiple steps described earlier can result in dysfunctional glycemic control. Chronic causes of dysfunctional glucose metabolism, such as those that lead to type 2 diabetes mellitus, should be distinguished from the physiologic response to trauma or surgical stress, which includes a sympathetic response that often results in transient hyperglycemia. This response is termed stress hyperglycemia and results from a combination of factors, including patient-, illness-, and treatment-related factors (Figure 2). Glucagon, catecholamines, cytokines, and other upregulated hormones act on downstream targets to increase glucose production in the liver and decrease insulin and non–insulin-mediated peripheral glucose uptake via upregulation and downregulation of glucose transporters (Figure 3). Hyperglycemia subsequently activates proinflammatory mediators and augments the catabolic state of illness. Subsequently, stress hyperglycemia improves with resolution of the underlying insult.

Multiple studies published over the past two decades have reported an association between uncontrolled stress hyperglycemia in hospitalized patients and poorer clinical outcomes, such as increased surgical site infections and healthcare-acquired infections. In 2001 a landmark single-center randomized trial, the Leuven trial, reported that tight glycemic control with an insulin infusion to target glucose levels of 80 to 110 mg/dL resulted in improved outcomes as compared with conventional control to target glucose levels of 180 to 200 mg/dL. Although the most significant benefit of tight glycemic control was a reduction in mortality due to multiple organ failure in septic patients, other benefits included decreases in bloodstream infections, acute renal failure requiring dialysis or hemofiltration, median number of red blood cell transfusions, and critical illness polyneuropathy. Although tight glycemic control with intensive insulin therapy was adopted widely, its benefit has not been substantiated in subsequent trials. Furthermore, in 2009 a multicenter randomized trial, the NICE-SUGAR (Normoglycemia in Intensive Care Evaluation–Survival Using Glucose Algorithm Regulation) trial, demonstrated increased mortality in patients receiving tight glycemic control. Multiple explanations have been offered for the differences between these studies, with regard to both biologic mechanisms and clinical trial methodology. In particular, the NICE-SUGAR trial had less risk of bias and more generalizability given its heterogeneous patient population and pragmatic trial design.

Although current glycemic targets are debated, several societies have advanced recommendations based on best available evidence. Across societies, the recommended glucose target range for critically ill patients is less than 180 to 200 mg/dL. In addition, the Society of Critical Care Medicine convened a task force regarding recommendations for insulin infusion therapy for management of hyperglycemia in critically ill patients. Despite very low quality of evidence, it recommends initiation of insulin therapy at a blood glucose of 150 mg/dL and maintenance of glucose levels below 180 mg/dL. Ultimately, glycemic targets must be achievable with low rates of hypoglycemia (less than 70 mg/dL) given the association between hypoglycemia and increased mortality. Therefore individual intensive care units need to carefully evaluate their insulin protocols and monitoring processes to ensure reasonable rates of hyperglycemia and hypoglycemia. Furthermore, patients on insulin infusions should be transitioned off using basal and bolus insulin rather than sliding scale insulin regimens. Basal-bolus insulin regimens based on long-acting insulin (i.e., glargine) have been associated with improved glycemic control and reduced surgical site infections in non–critically ill surgery patients.

Additional strategies are under investigation in terms of their impact on glycemic control and clinical outcomes. Glucose-insulin therapy, whereby high glucose and high insulin infusions are administered simultaneously, has metabolic and immune effects that theoretically could improve outcomes. It has been evaluated in multiple randomized trials in cardiac surgery, but the results are mixed, and it is not currently recommended for routine use. Nutritional strategies for improving glycemic control, such as diabetic formulas (i.e., low in carbohydrates and high in monounsaturated fatty acids), hypocaloric feeds, and glutamine supplementation, have been studied as well. Although diabetic formulas and glutamine show promise in terms of intermediate outcomes such as rates of hypoglycemia and hyperglycemia, none of these therapies has been demonstrated to improve clinical outcomes. Improved strategies for delivering insulin therapy, such as use of short-acting insulin infusions, continuous glucose monitoring in the inpatient and intensive care setting, and development of closed-loop control systems, are also promising, although further study is needed.

THYROID DYSFUNCTION

In healthy patients, serum levels of thyroid hormones are regulated by the HPT axis through a feedback loop. Neurons in the paraventricular nucleus of the hypothalamus synthesize thyrotropin-releasing hormone (TRH), which in turn stimulates the anterior pituitary gland to synthesize and release thyroid-stimulating hormone (TSH or thyrotropin) in a diurnal and pulsatile manner. Binding of TSH to receptors on thyroid follicular cells results in the release of thyroid hormones into the circulation, 90% as tetraiodothyronine (thyroxine or T4) and 10% as triiodothyronine (T3). Free thyroid hormone makes up less than 1% of total circulating T4 and T3; the rest is bound to thyroxine-binding globulin, transthyretin, and albumin, in

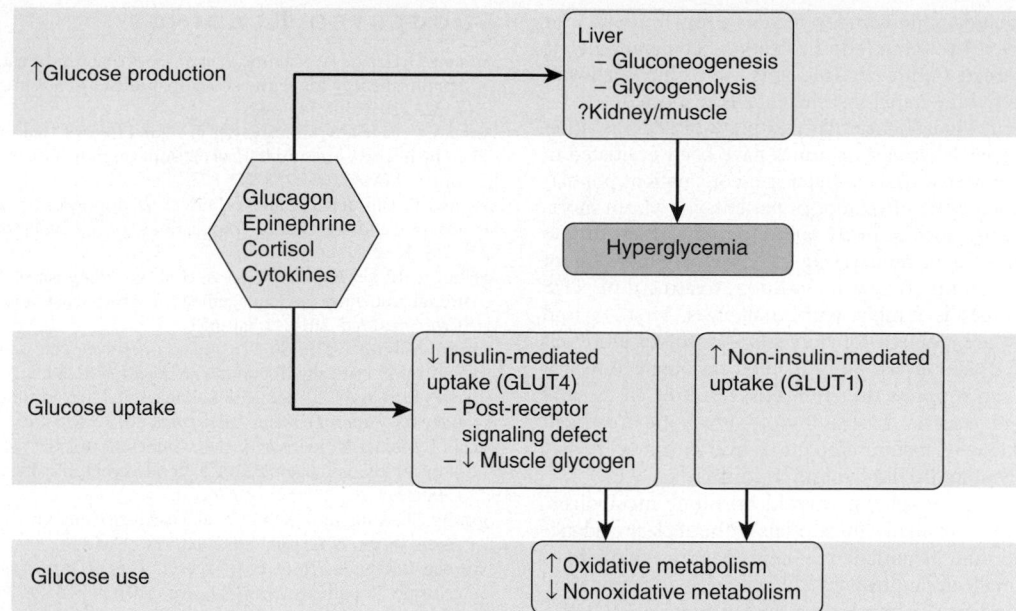

FIGURE 3 Glucose metabolism in stress hyperglycemia. *GLUT1*, glucose transporter 1; *GLUT4*, glucose transporter 4. *(Reproduced with permission from Dungan KM, Braithwaite SS, Preiser JC. Stress hyperglcaemia. Lancet. 2009;373:1798-1807.)*

that order. Once taken up by the target tissues, T4, which acts as the prohormone, is acted on by deiodinases (D1, D2, and D3). Depending on the location of the iodine that is removed, T4 can be converted either to its active form, T3, or to an inactive form, reverse T3 (rT3). Serum thyroid hormones provide negative feedback to the hypothalamus and pituitary, which regulate TSH secretion (Figure 4).

In acute critical illness, total and free T3 levels decrease because of inhibition of peripheral activation of T4, and rT3 levels increase within a few hours of the inciting event. Concomitantly, both T4 and TSH increase. These are believed to be adaptive changes to stress that do not require intervention. In prolonged critical illness, T3 levels remain low and rT3 levels remain elevated. Total and free T4 levels decrease, and TSH is no longer secreted diurnally or with as elevated a pulse amplitude. These changes during critical illness are referred to by several interchangeable terms, including nonthyroidal illness syndrome (NTIS), euthyroid sick syndrome, and low T3 syndrome.

Because of the changes that occur in the HPT axis, newly diagnosing primary thyroid disorders can be difficult in critically ill patients. Both primary hypothyroidism and NTIS can result in elevated TSH levels. Although a normal TSH level rules out primary hypothyroidism in healthy patients, TSH may be low in patients with primary hypothyroidism and NTIS. Furthermore, drugs may contribute to a paradoxically low TSH level. Primary hypothyroidism usually is accompanied by decreased T3 and T4 levels, which also can be seen in patients with prolonged critical illness or during recovery from NTIS. A high serum T3 to T4 ratio, a low serum rT3, and a low thyroid hormone-binding ratio may be more suggestive of primary hypothyroidism, but the diagnostic accuracy of these tests is limited. Longitudinal follow-up with repeated testing after recovery from critical illness is necessary to confirm the diagnosis. Primary hyperthyroidism should be considered in patients with elevated serum T3 and T4 levels, given the rarity of this finding because of critical illness.

The management of thyroid dysfunction in the setting of known or suspected underlying disease is different from that for NTIS. If a patient is known to have pre-existing primary hypothyroidism, the previous dose of thyroid replacement medication is continued. If a patient has myxedema coma, treatment consists of thyroid hormone replacement, treatment of the underlying condition, and supportive care such as passive rewarming, vasopressor therapy, and antibiotics. Intravenous glucocorticoids are recommended because of the possibility of concomitant adrenal insufficiency. If a patient has thyroid

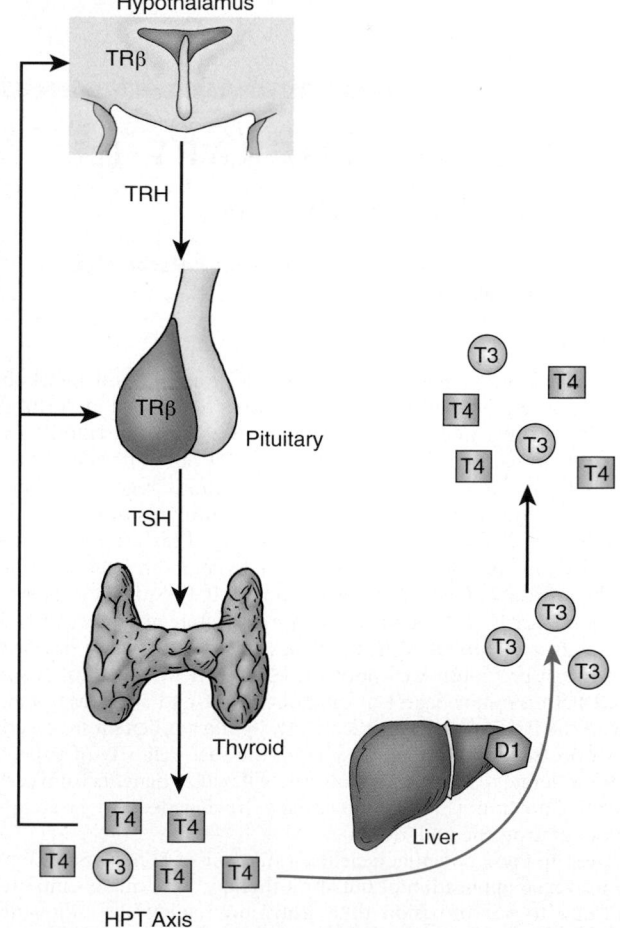

FIGURE 4 The hypothalamic-pituitary-thyroid (HPT) axis. *D1*, Deiodinase 1; *T3*, triiodothyronine; *T4*, thyroxine; *TRβ*, thyroid hormone receptor beta; *TRH*, thyrotropin-releasing hormone; *TSH*, thyrotropin. *(Reproduced with permission from Waung JA, Bassett JH, Williams GR. Thyroid hormone metabolism in skeletal development and adult bone maintenance. Trends Endocrinol Metab. 2012;23:155-162.)*

storm, treatment includes thionamides such as propylthiouracil or methimazole followed by iodine administration. Hyperadrenergic symptoms can be treated with beta-blockers, and glucocorticoids should be administered if adrenal insufficiency is suspected.

There is no convincing evidence that treatment of NTIS is either warranted or beneficial. Thyroid hormones have been evaluated in several small, underpowered trials in heterogeneous patient populations. Although there may be subgroups of patients for whom short-term benefits may exist, such as heart failure patients, there are no long-term outcome data demonstrating clear benefit in terms of long-term morbidity and mortality. In addition, treatment of NTIS with thyroid hormones is fraught with challenges. First, thyroid hormone doses that are required for normalization of serum levels may result in high tissue levels. Second, pharmacologic doses of thyroid hormones can suppress the HPT axis, resulting in use and depletion of thyroid reserves. Lastly, thyroid hormone treatment must be monitored closely, as simultaneous recovery from NTIS may result in overtreatment and acute hyperthyroidism.

Selenium, which is necessary for thyroid hormone metabolism, has been evaluated in a few small clinical trials without clear evidence for benefit. In addition, hypothalamic neuropeptides have been studied in a few small, underpowered clinical trials. Combination therapy (i.e., TRH and growth hormone releasing peptide-2 [GHRP-2]) has been shown to improve surrogate outcomes such as circulating thyroid hormone levels and markers of metabolism, but no impact on morbidity or mortality has been demonstrated.

SUGGESTED READINGS

Annane D, Cariou A, Maxime V, et al. Corticosteroid treatment and intensive insulin therapy for septic shock in adults: a randomized controlled trial. *JAMA.* 2010;303:341-348.

Annane D, Sebille V, Charpentier C, et al. Effect of treatment with low doses of hydrocortisone and fludrocortisone on mortality in patients with septic shock. *JAMA.* 2002;288:862-871.

Boonen E, Van den Berghe G. Endocrine responses to critical illness: novel insights and therapeutic implications. *J Clin Endocrinol Metab.* 2014;99: 1569-1582.

Dellinger RP, Levy MM, Rhodes A, et al. Surviving Sepsis Campaign: international guidelines for management of severe sepsis and septic shock: 2012. *Crit Care Med.* 2013;41:580-637.

Finfer S, Chittock DR, Su SY-S, et al. Intensive versus conventional glucose control in critically ill patients. *N Engl J Med.* 2009;360:1283-1297.

Fliers E, Bianco AC, Langouche L, Boelen A. Thyroid function in critically ill patients. *Lancet Diabetes Endocrinol.* 2015;3:816-825.

Jacobi J, Bircher N, Krinsley J, et al. Guidelines for the use of an insulin infusion for the management of hyperglycemia in critically ill patients. *Crit Care Med.* 2012;40:3251-3276.

Sprung CL, Annane D, Keh D, et al. Hydrocortisone therapy for patients with septic shock. *N Engl J Med.* 2008;358:111-124.

Van den Berghe G, Wouters P, Weekers F, et al. Intensive insulin therapy in critically ill patients. *N Engl J Med.* 2001;345:1359-1367.

NUTRITION THERAPY IN CRITICAL ILLNESS

Robert G. Martindale, MD, PhD, Jayshil J. Patel, MD, and Laszlo Kiraly, MD

Critical illness leads to highly variable immune and metabolic responses. Nutrition support is now considered a form of primary therapy in critically ill patients, with both nutritional and non-nutritional benefits. Virtually every critically ill patient has a metabolic or immune response to injury or illness, regardless of pre-existing malnutrition, that may be attenuated by appropriate nutrition therapy. In fact, nutrition therapy provided early in a stay in the intensive care unit (ICU) has been shown to favorably alter outcomes for the critically ill patient. However, not all ICU patients will derive a similar benefit from nutrition therapy or tolerate prolonged periods of energy and protein deficit. Using risk scores, it now has been shown that previously well-nourished ICU patients (medical or surgical) with a minor degree of catabolic insult and a relatively short stay in the ICU may derive little, if any, significant benefit from early nutrition therapy. On the other hand, the vast majority of patients with moderate to severe nutrition risk will realize benefits from early enteral nutrition (EN) or potentially be harmed by prolonged ongoing iatrogenic underfeeding.

Despite these potential benefits, a number of controversies limit the universal application of nutrition therapy. First, many clinicians continue to see provision of a nutrition regimen as adjunctive support and not true primary therapy. Second, recent studies on trophic feeding have been misinterpreted to imply that nutrition therapy is not important in the first week of hospitalization after admission to the ICU. Third, many practitioners have the misconception that ICU patients who are obese do not require nutrition therapy, when in fact these may be some of the patients at highest risk. Fourth, some ICUs continue to over-rely on use of parenteral nutrition (PN)

when the enteral route remains feasible. Trying to define malnutrition using surrogate parameters such as visceral proteins is essentially useless in severe catabolic illness, and identifying degree of nutrition risk has become a more attainable goal. Whether a benefit from nutrition therapy can be expected depends on factors such as route, dosing, timing, content of nutrient substrate, interruptions in delivery, and efforts to promote patient mobility.

Nonetheless, artificial nutrition support (delivered by feeding tube or parenterally) has evolved into a primary therapeutic intervention that has both nutritional and non-nutritional benefits. It should be delivered early to achieve metabolic optimization and attenuation of catabolic response while maintaining the ideal immune responses, rather than simply providing nutrients to prevent "malnutrition" or loss of lean body tissue. This chapter reviews such therapy in the critically ill adult patient in a surgical, trauma, or medical ICU who is expected to be in the ICU for more than 48 to 72 hours.

■ PHYSIOLOGIC BASIS FOR NUTRITION SUPPORT

In 1930 David Paton Cuthbertson described three successive phases of the metabolic response to critical illness. First is the ebb phase, in which basal metabolism is reduced. Second is a hypercatabolic phase, in which protein catabolism leads to a negative nitrogen balance. Third is an anabolic phase, which leads to muscle mass reconstruction and progression toward homeostasis.

The metabolic response to critical illness and surgical stress involves activation of neuroendocrine, inflammatory and immune, adipose tissue hormones, and gastrointestinal (GI) hormone components. The neuroendocrine component begins within seconds to minutes after stress, activating the sympathetic nervous system and hypothalamic-pituitary axis. The inflammatory and immune components are activated within hours and lead to release of cytokines and inflammatory mediators. Trauma and surgery induce a predominant T helper 2 (Th2) response, leading to an increase in interleukin-4 (IL-4), IL-10, and IL-13. On the contrary, septic shock leads to a predominant T helper 1 (Th1) response with IL-1, tumor necrosis factor (TNF) alpha, and interferon gamma expression. Consequences of the inflammatory response lead to impaired wound healing, immune dysfunction, muscle mass loss with negative nitrogen balance, and immobility. Clinically, the uncontrolled catabolism and subsequent cumulative caloric deficit are associated with an increased risk for infections, occurrence of acute respiratory distress syndrome (ARDS), renal dysfunction, need for surgery, and pressure sores. Indeed, both enteral and parenteral routes can provide the nutritional benefits. Both routes can provide calories, protein, micronutrients, and antioxidants for energy substrate repletion to mitigate cumulative caloric deficit. However, only EN can provide the non-nutritional benefits associated with nutrition therapy.

■ THE VALUE OF EARLY ENTERAL NUTRITION

The value of early EN is derived from physiologic effects that provide both non-nutritional and nutritional benefits to the critically ill patient (Box 1). In the absence of luminal nutrients, enterocyte mass and function are lost. In addition, gut contractility is reduced, promoting bacterial overgrowth and virulence and leading to contact-dependent programmed enterocyte apoptosis. The ensuing enterocyte death leads to structural defects, increasing gut permeability, and accentuation of the systemic inflammatory response syndrome (SIRS).

Therefore EN should be started as soon as possible after admission to the ICU in order to achieve the non-nutritional benefits of early enteral therapy and minimize the development of a protein-calorie debt that frequently occurs during the first week of critical illness. The non-nutritional benefits are derived from physiologic mechanisms that maintain structural and functional gut integrity, thus preventing increases in intestinal permeability. Immune mechanisms elicited by EN result in attenuation of oxidative stress and SIRS and support of the humoral immune system. Enteral feeding modulates metabolic responses that help decrease insulin resistance. In contrast, the nutritional benefits are derived from delivery of exogenous nutrients, which provide sufficient protein and calories, deliver micronutrients and antioxidants, and maintain lean body mass.

Distinct bodies of evidence exist in recent literature to support the value of early EN in the critically ill medical and surgical patient: (1) Randomized controlled trials (RCTs) of early versus delayed EN have shown that feedings started within the first 24 to 48 hours reduce infections, hospital and ICU length of stay, and mortality compared with similar feeding regimens started after the first 24 to 48 hours. (2) Studies comparing EN with standard therapy (STD) where no specialized nutrition therapy is provided, conducted in the setting of elective surgery and surgical ICU, have shown that EN initiated on postoperative day 1 reduced infection, hospital length of stay, and mortality compared with controls where patients were started on an oral diet when the patient requested it. (3) Large and small observational cohort studies in critically ill patients evaluating the concept of caloric deficit acquired in the first week of ICU stay have shown that delays in initiation of EN or processes that interrupt feedings create a caloric deficit between calories expended (i.e., caloric requirements) and actual calories delivered by the nutrition regimen. A caloric deficit in the first week that exceeds 4000 to 10,000 calories has been associated with increased incidence of organ failure and an increase in ICU infections, hospital and ICU length of stay, and total associated complications. (4) Finally, prospective studies on the impact of nurse-driven enteral feeding protocols (both RCTs and studies evaluating patients before and after protocol implementation) have shown that patients placed on an EN protocol experience increased delivery of EN, which subsequently decreases infection, hospital length of stay, and mortality compared with patients not placed on such protocol.

When initiating early EN, issues of dose, composition, and level of infusion within the gastrointestinal tract are less important than

BOX 1: Reported Benefits of Early Enteral Nutrition

Advantages Independent of Caloric and Energy Supply

Gastrointestinal Benefits

Maintains gut integrity
Reduces gut-lung axis of inflammation
Enhances motility and contractility
Maintains absorptive capacity
Maintains gut-associated lymphoid tissue and mucosa-associated lymphoid tissue (MALT)
Enhances production of secretory immunoglobulin A
Has trophic effect on epithelial cells
Helps to maintain variability of commensal bacteria
Reduces virulent transformation to pathogen phenotype of endogenous organisms

Immune and Metabolic Responses

Promotes dominance of anti-inflammatory T helper 2 over proinflammatory T helper 1 responses
Supports oral tolerance
Influences anti-inflammatory nutrient receptors in the gastrointestinal tract (duodenal vagal, colonic)
Maintains MALT at all epithelial surfaces (lung, liver, lacrimal, genitourinary, and pulmonary)
Modulates adhesion molecules to attenuate transendothelial migration of macrophages and neutrophils

Metabolic Responses

Promotes insulin secretion through the stimulation of incretins
Reduces hyperglycemia (advanced glycation end products [AGEs]), muscle and tissue glycosylation
Attenuates stress metabolism to enhance more physiologic fuel use
Reduces insulin resistance

Advantages of the Nutrient Load

Provides sufficient protein and calories for cell metabolism
Provides micronutrients and antioxidants
Maintains lean body mass by providing substrate for optimal protein synthesis
Supports cellular and subcellular (mitochondria) function
Stimulates protein synthesis to meet metabolic demand of the host

simply getting EN started. Subsequent assessment within 24 to 72 hours helps to identify the patient at high nutrition risk, when a more sophisticated and tailored nutrition prescription can be provided. High risk is defined by disease severity (which reflects inflammation and SIRS), pre-existing deterioration of nutritional status (reduced nutrient intake before admission, low body mass index [BMI], or recent weight loss before admission), and anticipated prolonged length of stay in the ICU. A patient identified to be at high risk needs more aggressive, more complete nutrition therapy, with an attempt to reach target goals for both calories and protein. More recent data suggest that reaching protein goals may be a higher priority than energy. Such patients may benefit from prokinetic agents, small bowel feeding tubes, or even early supplemental PN if EN is insufficient in reaching target goals. A key point is that adequate feeding to target goal protein and calories becomes more important as risk and length of stay increases.

Not all ICU patients are candidates or will benefit from nutrition therapy. It is not appropriate to provide EN to a patient with sufficient oral intake (or who is expected to achieve adequate intake within a few days), low stress, and minimal risk; to one who is pre-terminal or hemodynamically unstable; or to one in whom there is bowel discontinuity.

■ APPROPRIATE ASSESSMENT WITH INITIATION OF NUTRITION THERAPY FOR THE INTENSIVE CARE UNIT

The pre-existing nutritional status and metabolic stress response predispose the critically ill patient to nutritional risk. Nutritional risk is the risk of acquiring complications and other forms of adverse outcomes that may have been prevented by timely and adequate nutritional therapy. Classic variables such as BMI and recent weight loss take into account only pre-existing nutritional status, and traditional nutrition assessment tools such as serum albumin and prealbumin have not been validated for critical illness. Therefore a number of published scoring systems have been developed for nutritional assessment. The Nutritional Risk Score (NRS) 2002 and the NUTRIC Score 2015 assess both disease severity and pre-existing nutritional status and have been either derived from randomized trials in critical care or validated in the ICU setting. Other systems such as the Mini Nutritional Assessment (MNA), Malnutrition Universal Screening Tool (MUST), Nutritional Risk Index (NRI), and Subjective Global Assessment (SGA), which focus only on nutritional status, are of limited value for patients in the ICU setting.

The goal of nutrition therapy should be defined clearly by determining caloric requirements and protein needs. Weight-based equations to predict energy expenditure such as 25 kcal/kg/day are appropriate for use in most critically ill patients. Published predictive equations have not been proven to be more beneficial than the weight-based equations. However, at extremes of BMI, estimates are less accurate and may benefit from the use of indirect calorimetry (IC). Recent studies have emphasized the need to not only meet caloric requirements, but also provide sufficient formula to meet daily protein requirements. Protein requirements, which tend to be more difficult to estimate than caloric requirements, may be approximated by using weight-based equations.

■ CONTROVERSIES IN CRITICAL CARE NUTRITION THERAPY

Several issues in the literature can complicate nutrition optimization. First, studies of permissive underfeeding and trophic feeding have suggested that less EN is better. Second, the obesity epidemic has raised questions of optimal nutrition timing and dose in this population. Third, despite the paucity of data to suggest harm, practitioners often withhold EN in critically ill patients who are in shock.

Intentional or "permissive" underfeeding for the nonobese patient on EN is thought to be a simpler, safer strategy with better tolerance and lower risk for aspiration or hyperglycemia. The supporting literature for this concept has numerous flaws in methodologic design and directly contradicts the four bodies of evidence mentioned earlier in the section titled "The Value of Early Enteral Nutrition" that support the value of EN. Four RCTs published previously have provided evidence to suggest that less feeding has better outcomes than full feeds. In an early study by Ibraham, patients were randomized to 20% of goal feeding in the first week of hospitalization to the ICU versus full feeds at 100%. Patients were fed by bolus infusion into the stomach; unfortunately, intolerance issues resulted in the study group getting 7% of goal calories and the control group (which was supposed to get full feeds) getting only 27%. In a single-center RCT, Arabi randomized patients to full feeds or 70% of goal feeds. At the end of the study, the underfeeding study group received 59% of goal calories, whereas the full feeding control group received only 71%. A statistically significant greater 90-day mortality was seen in the group randomized to full feeds (42.5% vs 30.0%, $P < 0.05$). That a 12% difference in percent of goal calories delivered accounted for the difference in mortality is somewhat implausible, and the likelihood of a type 1 (alpha) error is high (because this same group of researchers in a subsequent larger multicenter trial of similar design showed no difference in outcomes between underfeeding and full feeding).

Trophic feeding in patients with acute respiratory therapy, where patients received 10 to 20 mL/hr for the first 6 days before advancing to goal, was shown to have similar outcome to patients randomized to full feeds. Such limited delivery should not be the initial goal for nutrition therapy in any ICU patient. Similar short-term outcomes in the trophic feeding group (compared with controls who received full feeds) may be explained by the fact that study patients were younger than average ICU patients (mean 52 years), had a normal or slightly elevated BMI (mean 29.9 to 30.4), had a relatively short ICU stay (average length of stay 5 days), and thus were at low nutritional risk. The long-term outcome effects of such a strategy are not known with regard to muscle mass and function, ambulation, and return to baseline functional status after discharge from the ICU (in the single-center trial, study patients on trophic feeds were less likely to go home after discharge from the hospital). Results of these studies on trophic feeding in patients with acute lung injury should not be extrapolated to other ICU patient populations in which considerable erosion of lean muscle mass may result in impaired recovery and worse clinical outcomes.

The impact of obesity on assessment parameters requires appropriate adjustments. Calorie and protein goals for the critically ill patient who is obese have not been standardized, possibly reflecting the controversy as to whether obesity is a risk or a benefit with respect to mortality. Patients at the extremes of BMI (thin, cachectic patients with BMI <20 or those patients with severe obesity and a BMI >40) have been shown clearly to be at high risk, with increased morbidity and mortality compared with normal weight controls. The curve for mortality versus BMI in the critically ill patient may be U-shaped, suggesting that those patients in the nadir of the curve (who are overweight or have class 1 or class 2 obesity) actually may be protected by their obesity. Such findings may be misleading in these patients, as risk may be better defined by the presence or absence of metabolic syndrome and other comorbidities. Sarcopenia and reduced functional status at any range of BMI are additional factors that identify the ICU patient at increased risk.

Based on limited data from retrospective cohort studies and small prospective randomized trials, a reasonable strategy for the critically ill patient who is obese and on either EN or PN is to provide high-protein, hypocaloric feedings (where patients receive 2.0 to 2.5 g protein/kg ideal body weight/day and 65% to 70% of caloric requirements) to maintain lean body mass, promote loss of fat mass, and still improve clinical outcome.

For EN to be delivered safely and nutrients utilized, there must be sufficient mesenteric blood flow. Critically ill patients are often hemodynamically unstable and require vasoactive support, putting them at risk for gut hypoperfusion and subsequent EN intolerance. Human studies have shown tolerance to EN in shock. Ischemic bowel in the patient on enteral feeding occurs very rarely, unpredictably, and often later in hospitalization (i.e., not during the acute resuscitative phase). It is appropriate and safe to provide EN on vasopressor agents in the stable patient after full volume resuscitation. Once EN is initiated, the assessment strategy should focus on ensuring that resuscitation goals continue to be met, that risk for aspiration is minimized, that the rate of delivery is advanced quickly to goal, and that the patient appears to be well tolerating the feeding regimen. Gastric feeding is successful and usually well tolerated in the vast majority of ICU patients when it is started early. Decisions on enteral access device, the level of infusion within the gastrointestinal tract, and whether simultaneous aspiration of the stomach is required are all predicated on the degree of tolerance of gastric feeding.

■ FORMULA SELECTION

Although the majority of patients in the critical care setting will tolerate a standard enteral formula (polymeric at 1.0 to 1.5 kcal/mL), it is appropriate to consider limited use of various specialty formulas in the individual patient under specific circumstances. The formulations designed for pulmonary compromise, hepatic failure, and renal failure are rarely, if ever, needed in the acute ICU setting. Clinical trials and multiple meta-analyses, as well as physiologic studies in animal models, support the use of pharmaconutrition formulas in some critically ill surgical populations. Provision of arginine to an ICU patient with sepsis has been shown to be safe from a hemodynamic standpoint. Formulas with arginine, fish oil, and nucleotides have proven effective in reducing infection and hospital length of stay in the elective major surgery patient, but probably do not change outcome in the medical ICU setting. Data to support the use of a formula specifically designed for ARDS with an anti-inflammatory lipid profile delivered by continuous infusion in patients with acute lung injury, or for ARDS on mechanical ventilation, have not shown it to be consistently beneficial, and therefore it cannot be recommended routinely. Provision of fish oil by bolus infusion does not appear to achieve the same physiologic effects or outcome benefits. Although use of fish oil traditionally has been thought to reduce or limit the inflammatory process in the critically ill, a new class of endogenously produced, highly active lipid mediators derived from arachidonic acid and omega-3 fatty acids (lipoxins, resolvins, protectins, and maresins) has been shown to actively enhance resolution of inflammation. These specialized proresolving molecules (SPMs) stimulate the cardinal signs of resolution of inflammation, which include cessation of leukocytic infiltration, countering of the effects of proinflammatory mediators, stimulation of the uptake of apoptotic neutrophils, promotion of the clearance of necrotic cellular debris, and enhancement of the host's ability to eliminate microbial invasion. As SPMs are incorporated in ICU studies, exact mechanisms and benefits will be better understood.

Glutamine is a nonessential amino acid that in times of trauma and severe critical illness is believed to become essential. Since the first descriptions of the benefits of glutamine in critical illness, multiple papers have reported benefit. Not until the REDOX trial was any potential harm believed to result from delivering glutamine in the critically ill patients. Since that publication, the MetaPlus study has once again questioned the safety of glutamine in the critically ill. In both of these trials, a higher mortality was noted in the glutamine groups. That being said, it does appear that only those patients with renal or multiple organ failure suffered from the glutamine supplementation. Based on these trials, the American Society for Parenteral and Enteral Nutrition and the Society of Critical Care Medicine guidelines for the provision of nutrition to the critically ill have not recommended the use of supplemental parenteral glutamine in critically ill patients.

Many disease-specific enteral formulas are designed with sound physiologic rationale for specific disease and patient populations, but outcome benefits in the ICU are not reported consistently and use should be on an individual, case-by-case basis. Such formulations include small peptide, medium chain triglyceride formulas to promote more efficient nitrogen absorption in patients with gut dysfunction; a high-protein, low-calorie formula for obese patients; and organ failure formulas for patients with liver disease or acute kidney injury. The physiologic basis for provision of pulmonary or glucose control formulas does not apply to the current critical care setting, and use of these formulas is not supported by appropriate outcome data in ICU patients.

Numerous trials have shown a benefit from the provision of antioxidant cocktails to ICU patients on continuous feeding. The most effective cocktails appear to contain selenium at higher doses, but the optimal combination and method of administration (bolus vs continuous infusion) are not clear. In the most recent large RCT, combination therapy did not report any positive effects on outcome.

Use of probiotics has shown benefit in the ICU setting when commercially available products are given per the nasogastric tube and swabbed throughout the oropharynx, reducing ventilator-associated pneumonia, likelihood to acquire antibiotic-associated diarrhea, pseudomembranous colitis, and possibly overall infections. Probiotic benefits appear to be species specific, which should be taken into account when deciding which product to use.

A number of metabolically active ancillary agents have been proposed for use in the critically ill patient in hopes of controlling the extremes of catabolic illness. Beta-blockers decrease the hyperdynamic response, statins have a general pleiotropic effect, and anabolic agents such as insulin, recombinant human growth hormone, glucagon-like peptide 2, and anabolic steroids have been shown to have trophic effects on the gut and/or to build lean body mass. Leucine stimulates protein synthesis, citrulline serves as a substrate for arginine synthesis and subsequent nitric oxide production, and carnitine may be beneficial in transporting long-chain fatty acids into the mitochondria for oxidation. Use of all of these agents in this manner in the ICU setting may be considered experimental and should be neither used outside a research protocol setting nor extrapolated for use in the general heterogeneous ICU patient population.

■ WHY IS IT DIFFICULT TO DELIVER ENTERAL NUTRITION THERAPY?

Because many factors impede delivery of early EN in the ICU setting, patients routinely get approximately 50% of the calories and protein that are required. Reluctance to initiate early feeds arises from the difficulties in defining full resuscitation and stabilization. Keeping patients NPO (nothing by mouth) for diagnostic tests or surgical procedures, holding EN for inappropriately low gastric residual volumes, stopping feeds for perceived intolerance, tube dislodgement arising from poorly secured access devices, and holding feeds for routine nursing care are notorious causes that result in persistent iatrogenic underfeeding by EN alone. Cessation of delivery of EN for these reasons is estimated to be inappropriate 66% of the time. It is important for intensivists to understand gut dysfunction in critical illness, which involves segmental dysmotility, reduced villous height and absorptive surface, and alterations in gut microbiota. The key point is that patients usually can be fed through the gut dysfunction, with the feeding itself leading to restored gut integrity, contractility, increase in brush border enzymes, and restoration of the commensal bacteria. Intensivists should attempt to determine the etiology of ileus in the ICU and be more attentive as feeds are initiated, but it is appropriate to use more aggressive strategies than normally would be used to deliver EN with ileus in the postoperative setting.

Intensivists should avoid the misconception that feeding is inappropriate in the setting of high gastric residual volumes (up to 500 mL), stable hypotension on pressor therapy, or hypoactive bowel sounds without evidence of ileus. Eliminating use of gastric residual volume as a clinical monitor surprisingly promotes increased EN delivery without adverse sequelae. Based on the four bodies of evidence supporting the value of early EN mentioned earlier, withholding EN to avoid suppression of autophagy would not seem appropriate, and such a strategy would not be expected to improve outcome.

Challenging traditional dogma is just the beginning of overcoming barriers that prevent change in practice. Barriers to implementation of EN protocols and aggressive early feeding derive from perceived lack of supporting evidence, poor implementation processes, systems characteristics (financial regulations, organizational structure, lack of resources), individual provider behavior, and patient complexity. Moving forward, strategies designed to reduce the barriers likely will improve our ability to provide adequate nutrition to critically ill patients.

■ STRATEGIES TO ENHANCE SUCCESSFUL DELIVERY OF ENTERAL NUTRITION

Institutional practice can be changed by adopting specific strategies to promote delivery of EN. Routine underdelivery of prescribed calories can be countered successfully by simply setting a higher than needed goal, assuming that patients receive only a portion of what is actually ordered, and overordering calories (prescribe goal calories at 120%, such that patients end up getting 100% of requirements). Traditional rate-based feeding is calculated from a total 24-hour goal volume of enteral feeding divided into an appropriate hourly rate delivered throughout the day. Interruptions in delivery because of diagnostic tests and operative or bedside procedures result in significant lost nutrition delivery, as patients are restarted at the same rate when they return to the floor. Volume-based or top-down feeding is a strategy that identifies the total volume of EN based on goal target calories that needs to be delivered over the entire 24 hours. After any period of cessation, nurses are empowered via protocols to increase the rate to make up for lost volume, such that the rest of the entire volume is delivered over the period of time remaining. Rather than waiting for patients to demonstrate intolerance (a reactive approach), a number of strategies can be initiated proactively and simultaneously at the start of feeds to promote tolerance. Such strategies include starting at goal rate with the use of prokinetic therapy, elevating the head of the bed, not measuring gastric residual volumes or setting a higher cut-off value for gastric residual volume (400 to 500 mL), incorporating post-pyloric infusion when gastric intolerance is noted with a small peptide formula, and adding supplemental protein during the first few days of feeding. Development and implementation of a nurse-driven enteral feeding protocol (containing set orders to initiate feeds, set the goal and ramp-up rate, determine appropriate gastric residual volumes, etc.) have been shown to increase delivery of EN. Such protocols should be modified by the individual institution depending on local expertise, culture of the ICU, and nursing practice to enhance use.

Although not yet available for critical care nutrition, the concept of a nutrition bundle ties together key elements from societal guidelines, identifying those few most important action items for recommendation that when performed together are most likely to affect outcome (see Box 2 for potential bundle elements). Large-scale prospective databases are a new concept that provides audit and feedback to programs, allowing comparison with other ICUs and institutions. The international audit and feedback system database (www.criticalcarenutrition.com) is based on compliance with the Canadian clinical practice guidelines and shows that greater compliance is associated with greater delivery of EN.

■ ROLE OF PARENTERAL NUTRITION IN THE INTENSIVE CARE UNIT SETTING

Because PN has a dramatically narrower risk/benefit ratio than EN in the critical care setting, identifying the appropriate candidate and choosing the optimal timing of initiation for PN is very often difficult. In the malnourished critically ill patient for whom EN is not feasible, exclusive PN should be initiated on admission during the

---

BOX 2: Approaches to Maximizing Gut Function in Critical Illness

Correction of acidosis and electrolyte abnormality
Prokinetic agents
Glycemic control
Maintain visceral perfusion
Early nutrition support
    Enteral preferred
    <48 hours (<24 hours may be even better)
    Specific nutrients to attenuate metabolic response
Minimize medications that alter gastrointestinal function
    Anticholinergics
    Narcotics
    Pressors
Support gut microbiome

---

first week of hospitalization. If the patient is previously well nourished on admission to the ICU (and EN is not feasible), exclusive PN should be initiated after the first 7 days of hospitalization. Adding supplemental PN to hypocaloric EN should be considered in the nutritionally high-risk patient at about 72 hours if EN feeds are providing less than 60% of caloric and protein goal requirements (the optimal timing is not clear). There may be little if any role for supplemental PN in the low-risk patient who is receiving hypocaloric EN. Refer to the 2016 American Society for Parenteral and Enteral Nutrition and Society of Critical Care Medicine nutrition guidelines for a detailed outline of the use of PN in the ICU.

In the appropriate candidate, additional factors that may help to maximize the benefit from PN in the ICU setting have been published recently. RCTs in nonobese patients on PN have shown that permissive underfeeding, in which 80% of caloric requirements are provided, reduces insulin resistance, avoids the potential for overfeeding, and improves ICU outcome. In the United States, the only lipid formulations currently routinely available are soy based. It has been hypothesized that the soy-based lipid emulsions can exacerbate a hyperdynamic response; as such, strategies to withhold soy-based lipid emulsions over the first week of hospitalization may improve outcome. New types of parenteral lipids—olive oil, fish oil, and the combination SMOF (soy, medium-chain triglycerides, olive oil, and fish oil)—are on the horizon and widely available around the globe (i.e., outside the United States). These newer emulsions show promise in reducing the inflammatory profile of parenteral lipids. Adding supplemental parenteral glutamine to the PN regimen has shown some benefit in the past. More recent randomized trials have questioned the benefit of supplemental parenteral glutamine in both medical and surgical ICU patients, with two studies showing net harm (increased mortality) in patients with multiorgan failure and several studies showing no benefit. Parenteral glutamine should be reserved for specific indications or study protocols.

■ FUTURE TRENDS

Nutritional therapy in the ICU has continued to evolve, and recent literature has made decisions on nutritional therapy and specialized metabolic care even more critical. Combining early EN with early aggressive resistance exercise and early mobilization in the ICU has been shown to promote the uptake and use of delivered protein with maintenance of muscle mass and enhancement of functional outcome. Prospective randomized trials on the effect of resistance exercise in the ICU have shown reduced ICU and hospital length of stay, duration of mechanical ventilation, and post-ICU need for skilled nursing facilities. Greater use of the concept of gut microbiome manipulation with probiotics in the ICU should be expected, as manipulation of intestinal microbiota already has been shown to reduce ventilator-associated pneumonia, likelihood of acquiring antibiotic-associated diarrhea or *Clostridium difficile*, and risk for colonization with vancomycin-resistant *Enterococcus*. A recently described persistent inflammation, immunosuppression, and catabolism syndrome (PICS) highlights the long-term adverse metabolic and immune sequelae of a prolonged ICU length of stay where a patient goes on to develop a pattern of chronic inflammation, catabolism, loss of lean body mass, and a shift in immune responses with bone marrow production of ineffective myeloid-derived suppressor cells. This patient population often is transferred from the ICU to a ward to a long-term acute care facility yet never returns to baseline function and often dies after a prolonged need for healthcare facilities. It is likely that aggressive early nutritional therapy may prevent the PICS progression, but this hypothesis needs confirmation.

■ CONCLUSION

A major paradigm shift has occurred in the importance of nutrition therapy, as intensivists understand that early EN represents a primary therapeutic intervention designed to achieve metabolic manipulation rather than a supportive therapy designed to prevent the ravages of malnutrition. Nutrition therapy should be considered as part of the initial resuscitative efforts, which immediately follow acute lifesaving maneuvers to restore oxygenation and circulatory status. Emphasis should focus on nutrition strategies that improve outcome. Although other areas of critical care are becoming more consistent, the appropriate standardization of nutrition therapy has not yet been achieved. Protocol-driven nutrition therapy adapted for each institution based on local expertise, culture, and resource availability is vital to ensure that each patient is provided the opportunity to receive optimal evidence-based nutrition therapy.

SUGGESTED READINGS

Allingstrup MJ, Esmailzadeh N, Wilkens Knudsen A, et al. Provision of protein and energy in relation to measured requirements in intensive care patients. *Clin Nutr.* 2012;31:462-468.

Gentile LF, Cuenca AG, Efron PA, et al. Persistent inflammation and immunosuppression: a common syndrome and new horizon for surgical intensive care. *J Trauma Acute Care Surg.* 2012;72:1491-1501.

Heidegger CP, Berger MM, Graf S, et al. Optimisation of energy provision with supplemental parenteral nutrition in critically ill patients: a randomised controlled clinical trial. *Lancet.* 2013;381:385-393.

Heyland DK. Critical care nutrition support research: lessons learned from recent trials. *Curr Opin Clin Nutr Metab Care.* 2013;16:176-181.

Heyland DK, Muscedere J, Wischmeyer P, et al. A randomized trial of glutamine and antioxidants in critically ill patients (REDOXS). *N Engl J Med.* 2013;368:1489-1497.

Martindale RG, Deveney CW. Preoperative risk reduction: strategies to optimize outcomes. *Surg Clin North Am.* 2013;93:1041-1055.

McClave SA, Heyland DK. The physiologic response and associated clinical benefits from provision of early enteral nutrition. *Nutr Clin Pract.* 2009;24:305-315.

Reignier J, Mercier E, Le Gouge A, et al. Clinical Research in Intensive Care and Sepsis (CRICS) Group: effect of not monitoring residual gastric volume on risk of ventilator-associated pneumonia in adults receiving mechanical ventilation and early enteral feeding: a randomized controlled trial. *JAMA.* 2013;309:249-256.

Taylor BE, McClave SA, Martindale RG, et al. Guidelines for the provision and assessment of nutrition support therapy in the adult critically ill patient: Society of Critical Care Medicine (SCCM) and American Society for Parenteral and Enteral Nutrition (A.S.P.E.N.). *Crit Care Med.* 2016;44: 390-438.

COAGULOPATHY IN THE CRITICALLY ILL PATIENT

Terence O'Keeffe, MBChB, FACS, FCCM, and Bellal Joseph, MD, FACS

Coagulopathy remains a significant challenge in critically ill patients in both the intensive care unit (ICU) and the emergency room, with hemorrhage related to coagulopathy being a leading cause of death worldwide. The clotting cascade is a complex interaction between multiple proteins, enzymes, and platelets, with abnormalities in any of the complex interactions having potentially life-threatening consequences. Given that the definition of coagulopathy is "a condition in which the blood's ability to clot is impaired," it is clear that many parts of the pathway can be affected, leading to impaired clot formation. We do not discuss these complex pathways exhaustively in this chapter but rather provide some practical tools that allow the clinician to both recognize and treat these conditions.

■ CAUSES OF COAGULOPATHY

One broad classification of coagulopathy is congenital versus acquired, as outlined in Table 1. Most of the congenital causes of coagulopathy are rare and usually do not present a problem for the practicing surgeon. In contrast, in the twenty-first century, medically induced "coagulopathy" is by far the most commonly seen type because of the increasing number of patients on antiplatelet drugs for stents or on anticoagulation therapy for stroke prevention in atrial fibrillation (AF). An estimated 2 million Americans have AF, and it is anticipated that 1 in 4 people will develop AF in his or her lifetime. Clearly, chemical anticoagulation is only going to become more frequent with time and with the "graying" of the population. The so-called novel anticoagulants have provided a new source of concern, as these drugs have been prescribed widely before effective antidotes are available, although these antidotes are now starting to appear on the market. There are many other specific disease conditions (see Table 1) that also can lead to significant coagulation disturbances, and the practicing intensivist needs to look for bleeding manifestations related to these conditions.

■ TESTS OF COAGULOPATHY

It has been recognized for some time that none of the blood tests available to the clinician tell the complete picture when it comes to coagulopathy, especially as many of the tests required are not rapidly available. Table 2 lists the blood tests currently available, as well as the parts of the coagulation cascade to which they correspond. It should be noted that the most commonly used test, international normalized ratio (INR), was developed to test for nothing other than the effect of warfarin on the coagulation cascade; however, it has become the de facto surrogate of coagulopathy for both trauma patients and many chronic conditions, such as liver disease (e.g., it forms part of the Model for End-Stage Liver Disease score).

Platelets require their own form of testing, separate from the standard battery of coagulation tests, although none of these tests are used commonly in most hospitals. The bleeding time may be the most specific test of overall coagulation, but this test is impractical to perform in all but the most clinical settings and generally has been abandoned. Thromboelastography (TEG) testing has become a widely used method to assess multiple aspects of coagulation, including platelet function and fibrinolysis, and may hold promise in developing more sophisticated ways to evaluate and treat coagulopathy, particularly in the acute setting, such as in trauma patients. We discuss this test separately, as it requires more detailed discussion because of the relative complexity of interpreting its results.

■ ACUTE COAGULOPATHY OF TRAUMA

Our understanding of trauma-associated coagulopathy has improved significantly over the last several years. Previously it was believed that large volume crystalloid resuscitation, hypothermia, and acidosis were responsible for the coagulopathy seen in trauma patients, but it is now well known that acute traumatic coagulopathy (ATC) is a distinct entity that sets in even before the initiation of resuscitation. ATC is observed in up to 25% of trauma patients, is associated with the severity of injury, and increases post-traumatic hemorrhage and mortality. ATC has been identified in patients as early as 25 minutes after trauma. Severe tissue injury and systemic hypoxia are the prerequisites for the production of ATC, and the absence of either of these two variables prevents its development. Systemic hypoxia secondary to hemorrhagic shock seems to be the primary driver for

TABLE 1: Congenital and Acquired Causes of Coagulopathy

Type of Coagulation Disorder	Effect on Clotting	Notes
Congenital		
Hemophilia A	Increased bleeding	1 in 10,000, mostly males
Hemophilia B	Increased bleeding	1 in 50,000, mostly males
Antithrombin II deficiency	Hypercoagulability	1 in 2000, increased VTE risk
Antiphospholipid syndrome/lupus anticoagulants	Hypercoagulability	2-4 in 100, increased VTE risk in some patients
Von Willebrand factor disease	Increased bleeding	Usually mild, no spontaneous bleeding
Protein C deficiency	Hypercoagulability	2-5 in 1000, increased VTE risk
Protein S deficiency	Hypercoagulability	1 in 700, increased VTE risk, often asymptomatic
Factor V Leiden	Increased bleeding	Rare, affects 1/million
Congenital fibrinogen deficiency	Increased bleeding	Rare, affects 1-2/million
Congenital prothrombin deficiency (factor II)	Increased bleeding	Rare; symptoms include easy bruising, epistaxis
Congenital factor deficiencies—VII, X, XIII	Increased bleeding	Rare; symptoms include easy bruising, epistaxis, joint bleeding
Acquired		
Medication induced	Increased bleeding and/or prothrombotic	See Table 6 for specific drugs
Traumatic brain injury	Increased bleeding	Possibly because of release of brain thromboplastin
Obstetric emergencies	Increased bleeding	Dilutional coagulopathy from blood loss or DIC
Sepsis/infection	Increased bleeding and/or prothrombotic	Proinflammatory cytokines cause activation of clotting cascade, DIC also present
Pancreatitis	Increased bleeding and/or prothrombotic	Proinflammatory cytokines activate clotting cascade and platelets, also DIC
Burns	Increased bleeding	Dilutional coagulopathy from resuscitation, DIC
Disseminated intravascular coagulation	Increased bleeding	Multiple precipitating conditions
Hepatic disease	Increased bleeding	Prolonged PT
Renal disease	Increased bleeding	Platelet dysfunction from chronic uremia
Vitamin K deficiency	Increased bleeding	Most common in infants, in adults related to chronic conditions or medications

DIC, Disseminated intravascular coagulation; *PT*, prothrombin time; *VTE*, venous thromboembolism.

ATC, but some degree of tissue damage is necessary for the development of ATC.

The devastating effects of ATC on the clinical outcome of trauma patients have been well studied. The presence of ATC in trauma patients at the time of arrival is independently associated with four times higher odds of mortality and increased transfusion requirements. ATC results in prolonged partial thromboplastin time (PTT) and prothrombin time (PT). However, in patients with ATC, PTT is a better predictor of mortality compared with PT. The effects of ATC are even observed in survivors. These patients are known to have a higher incidence of acute kidney injury, acute lung injury, and multiple organ failure (MOF). Trauma patients who require massive transfusions are known to have a higher incidence of sepsis. All of these factors lead to higher ventilator need and longer ICU and hospital length of stay. Of interest, trauma also induces a late hypercoagulable state, which leads to an increased risk for deep venous thrombosis (DVT) and pulmonary embolism (PE). The exact reason for this is unclear, but it is possible that early widespread activation

of protein C may lead to its depletion, ultimately resulting in a hypercoagulable state.

ATC can be described as a loss of normal equilibrium between the procoagulant and anticoagulant factors, and several theories exist that describe its mechanism of development. Studies have described it as a phenotypic variant of disseminated intravascular coagulation (DIC) resulting from widespread endothelial damage inducing a state of consumptive coagulopathy. Systemic anticoagulation and activation of the protein C pathway also have been proposed as mechanisms for this coagulopathy. Severe tissue hypoperfusion increases the expression of thrombomodulin on the endothelial surface, which cleaves thrombin from a procoagulant molecule into an anticoagulant molecule. Thrombin then leads to activation of protein C, which inhibits coagulation factors (V and VIII) of the extrinsic pathway, leading to widespread anticoagulation. Hyperfibrinolysis is a well-recognized component of ATC and is seen in up to 10% of trauma patients. Widespread tissue damage from trauma leads to a large release of tissue plasminogen activator (tPA) from the

TABLE 2: Blood Tests of Clotting

Name of Blood Test	Measures	Comments
PT	Extrinsic pathway of coagulation	Useful in liver disease, warfarin effect, vitamin K deficiency
PTT	Intrinsic pathway of coagulation	Mostly used to measure efficacy of heparin infusions
INR	Standardized test of PT for patients on warfarin	Often used (incorrectly as a measure of coagulopathy)
Platelet count	Absolute platelet count	Does not measure platelet activity (e.g., if on medications)
Fibrinogen level	Levels of plasma fibrinogen	Can be useful if other tests are normal in the face of continued bleeding
D-Dimer	Degradation product of fibrin	Used in diagnosing PE and also DIC
Fibrin split products	Degradation products of fibrin	Used in diagnosing DIC
Thrombin time	Bleeding disorders, in evaluating levels and function of fibrinogen	Superseded by functional fibrinogen assay
ACT	High doses of heparin therapy	Mostly used during cardiopulmonary bypass or cardiac device anticoagulation
Bleeding time	Mostly platelet function	Rarely used
TEG	All facets of coagulation	See discussion in chapter
Platelet function tests	Platelet function either native or postmedication	Not often used routinely, controversial
Factor assay	Specific factors associated with a condition	Often used to investigate clotting protein deficiencies
Reptilase test	Conversion of fibrinogen to fibrin	Used where heparin is present, as reptilase is insensitive to it

ACT, Activated whole blood clotting time; *DIC*, disseminated intravascular coagulation; *INR*, international normalized ratio; *PE*, pulmonary embolism; *PT*, prothrombin time; *PTT*, partial thromboplastin time; *TEG*, thromboelastography.

damaged endothelium. This release is a physiologic phenomenon that reduces the propagation of clot; however, it becomes pathologic when tPA is activated in large quantities. The significance of this phenomenon is evident in the survival benefit associated with the use of antifibrinolytic drugs such as tranexamic acid in severely injured trauma patients.

Factors such as large volume resuscitation, crystalloid use, hypothermia, and acidosis are all known to exacerbate trauma-associated coagulopathy; however, they are not primarily responsible for it. Although rarely used in current trauma centers, colloidal solutions such as hetastarches and dextran also have been associated with worsening of coagulopathy and should be avoided. Clinically significant effects of hypothermia and acidosis are observed only below a temperature of 33°C and pH of 7.2. Hypothermia results from the combination of a multitude of factors, the most important of which is shock itself. Adenosine triphosphate (ATP) is the energy currency for the body that is used for all metabolic processes, including maintaining the body temperature at 37°C. Shock induces a state of generalized ischemia, and ATP production falls dramatically. Other factors such as failure of shivering response, tissue hypoxia, anesthetic use, use of cold resuscitation fluids, and intraoperative heat losses all contribute to hypothermia in trauma patients. Acidosis results from lactic acidemia secondary to hemorrhagic shock. Coagulation factor activity, fibrinogen crosslinking, thrombin generation, and platelet aggregation are affected by both hypothermia and acidosis, leading to a state of ineffective coagulation. The combination of hypothermia, acidosis, and coagulopathy is called the "lethal triad" and is highly associated with mortality.

■ THROMBOELASTOGRAPHY OR VISCOELASTIC TESTING

Coagulopathy of trauma is a dynamic phenomenon, rather than a static phase, that goes through stages of hypocoagulability,

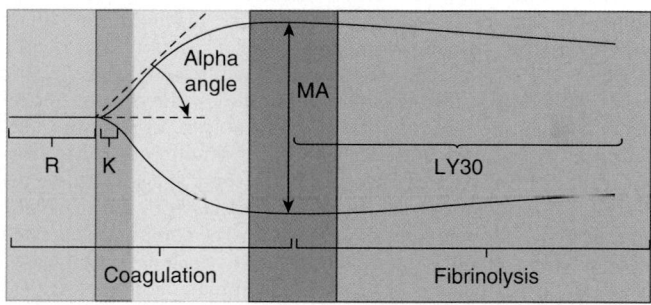

FIGURE 1 Thromboelastography tracing. *K*, Interval between reaction time and fixed value of clot firmness; *LY30*, degree of clot lysis at 30 minutes; *MA*, maximum amplitude; *R*, reaction time.

hypercoagulability, and fibrinolysis. The viscoelastic test is the only method currently available that is able to evaluate thrombosis and lysis simultaneously. PT is a measure limited only to the extrinsic clotting system (factors VIIa, Xa, and IIa), and PTT is limited to intrinsic clotting reactions (factors XIIa, XIa, IXa, and IIa). TEG, however, allows the assessment of the whole process from initiation of coagulation to fibrinolysis and clot degradation. Conventional assays (PT, INR) are performed in the laboratory under optimal temperature and pH, so they fail to take into account the in vivo effects of hypothermia and acidosis on the coagulation cascade. In contrast, viscoelastic tests are performed on a whole blood sample that takes into account the effects of complex pathologic processes affecting the coagulation cascade. Rapid TEG (rTEG) is a technique that involves the addition of tissue factor to the blood sample to speed up the process, reducing the time from 45 minutes for normal TEG to 30 minutes for rTEG, especially important for trauma patients. TEG is a graphic representation (Figure 1) of the complete timeline of the evolving blood clot generated using a transducer,

TABLE 3: Thromboelastography-Directed Resuscitation Guidelines

TEG Parameters	Blood Product Transfusion
ACT >128	PRBCs and plasma
Reaction time >10 min	PRBCs and plasma
K >2.5 min	Cryoprecipitate/fibrinogen/plasma
Alpha angle <55	Cryoprecipitate/fibrinogen/plasma
MA <55	Platelets/cryoprecipitate/fibrinogen
LY30 >3%	Tranexamic acid

TEG-based resuscitation guidelines. (Reference: Annals of surgery 2012 based on experience with 1974 consecutive trauma patients using TEG as point of care test.)

ACT, Activated clotting time; *K,* interval between reaction time and fixed value of clot firmness; *MA,* maximum amplitude, *LY30,* degree of clot lysis at 30 minutes; *PRBCs,* packed red blood cells; *TEG,* thromboelastography.

which detects resistance to motion of a microprobe placed in a rotating blood sample. The reaction time, or *R* in Figure 1 (TEG-ACT [activated clotting time] in rTEG), represents the time taken for the first measurable clot formation and is a reflection of enzymatic clotting activation. *K* in Figure 1 is the interval measured from the reaction time to the fixed value of clot firmness, or the point at which the amplitude of tracing reaches 20 mm; this reflects thrombin's ability to cleave soluble fibrinogen into insoluble fibrin strands. The *alpha angle* is the angle between the tangent line drawn from the base horizontal line to the beginning of the crosslinking process, measured in degrees, and primarily reflects the speed at which fibrin builds up and crosslinking takes place. The maximum amplitude (*MA*) measures the result of maximal platelet and fibrin interaction, reflecting the ultimate clot strength. The final reading of the tracing is *LY30,* the degree of clot lysis at 30 minutes of the tracing. Above-normal values are indicative of hyperfibrinolysis. In addition, TEG can measure (G), which is a logarithmic derivation of the MA, representing the clot strength in dynes per second, suggested to be the best measure of clot strength because it reflects both the enzymatic and the platelet components of hemostasis. The computer-generated tracing reflects component deficits, if any, in coagulation proteases, platelets, fibrinogen, and fibrinolysis. The unique ability of TEG to assess the component-specific functionality of clotting blood provides a road map that can guide goal-directed therapy for ATC, as described later in the chapter (Table 3).

THROMBOELASTOGRAPHY AND PLATELET MAPPING

Platelet function plays a pivotal role in hemostasis. Substantial evidence exists to suggest that platelet dysfunction is one of the major contributors to ATC independent of fluid or blood transfusion. Early recognition of platelet dysfunction is challenging, as conventional plasma-based tests (activated partial thromboplastin time [aPTT], INR) are unable to determine platelet function and are insensitive to coagulopathy unless severely deranged. Platelet mapping currently is used most commonly in patients undergoing cardiac surgery, with preoperative inhibition of adenosine diphosphate (ADP) predicting the development of microvascular bleeding in patients on clopidogrel. TEG assays measure ultimate clot strength as maximum amplitude, which is 80% dependent on platelet function and 20% dependent on fibrin activity. Platelet mapping is a focused technique to assess the independent contribution of platelets in clot formation by measuring the reactivity of platelet activators such as arachidonic acid (AA) and ADP with glycoprotein IIb/IIIa (GPIIb/IIIa) and ADP

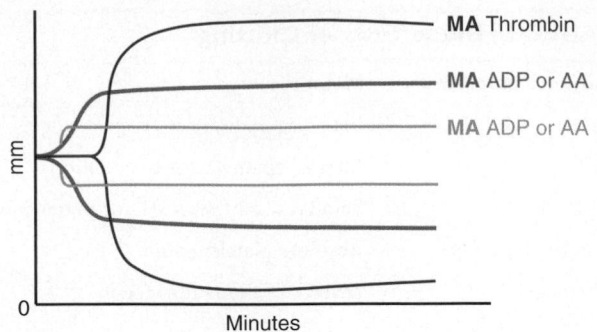

FIGURE 2 Thromboelastography platelet mapping traces. *AA,* Arachidonic acid; *ADP,* adenosine diphosphate; *MA,* maximum amplitude.

receptors. The whole blood TEG platelet mapping assay measures maximum hemostatic activity and also detects independent platelet response to either the ADP or AA agonist (Figure 2). Platelet mapping assay is a revolutionary technique for rapid assessment of platelet dysfunction early in the course of traumatic coagulopathy and hence can guide timely platelet transfusions for immediate reversal of life-threatening coagulopathy.

GOAL-DIRECTED THERAPY OF COAGULOPATHY OF TRAUMA

Transfusion therapy guided by viscoelastic testing has become a common practice in many institutions across United States and Europe. Because of the rapid availability of results, versatility of information, and point of care, this technology has allowed for evolution of goal-directed therapy for specific coagulation deficits identified during early resuscitation of trauma patients. Such an approach has allowed for accurate, stepwise correction of coagulation dysfunction with comparative analysis of various tracings generated (Figure 3).

Institutional experience with these techniques is increasing; however, TEG-guided resuscitation strategies to revert coagulopathy and to resuscitate severely injured patients have shown improved survival compared with resuscitation strategies guided by conventional coagulation assays. TEG-guided resuscitation strategies also have been shown to reduce the use of plasma and platelet transfusions during the early phase of resuscitation.

DILUTIONAL COAGULOPATHY AND MASSIVE TRANSFUSION PROTOCOLS

In contrast to supranormal resuscitation, which was popularized in the 1970s and 1980s and focused on using increased doses of crystalloid to drive oxygen delivery, resuscitation in the twenty-first century has focused on a more balanced approach, particularly the early use of blood and blood products. This has led to a decrease in the incidence of dilutional coagulopathy, which historically has been one of the more common causes of coagulopathy, present in up to 50% of patients who received 3 L of fluid or more in a study examining more than 8000 patients in the German Trauma Registry. However, in ICU patients receiving large amounts of crystalloid fluids as part of their resuscitation (e.g., patients with burns), it is important to continue to monitor coagulation parameters to detect changes early.

Massive transfusion protocols ostensibly were developed for trauma patients, and there are minimal data supporting their efficacy in the bleeding nontrauma patient (e.g., obstetric hemorrhage, massive gastrointestinal bleeding). Intuitively, it makes sense that a similar balanced resuscitation strategy would be effective, and based on level III data it does at least appear to be safe in these circumstances. The nature of most protocols, with their inherent

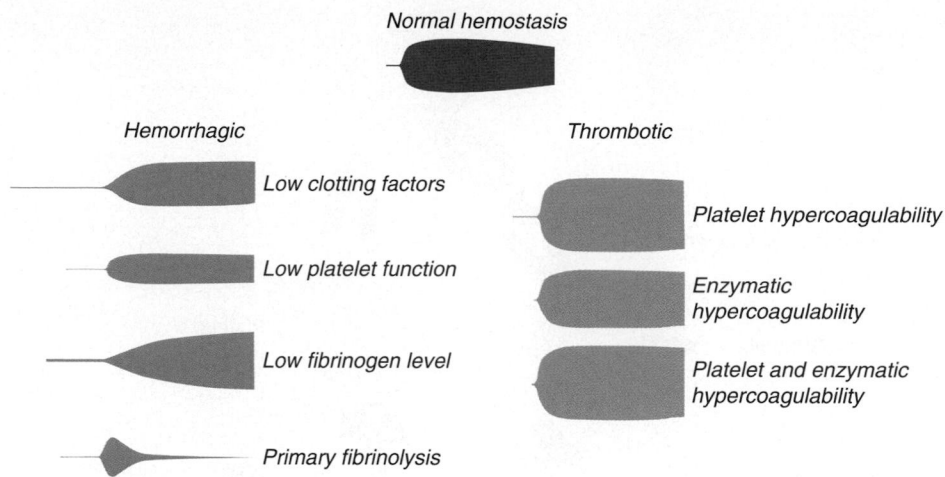

FIGURE 3 Thromboelastography tracings for different coagulation disorders.

automaticity of blood products and rapid availability of the products at the bedside, may be the most important feature for these cases, as opposed to an actual 1 : 1 or other ratio of fresh frozen plasma (FFP) to packed red blood cells (PRBCs). Massive transfusion protocols for trauma is discussed elsewhere in this text.

DISSEMINATED INTRAVASCULAR COAGULATION

DIC is a complex clinical condition that is characterized by systemic intravascular activation of coagulation that results in the generation and deposition of fibrin, leading to microvascular thrombi in various organs and contributing to multiple organ dysfunction syndrome (MODS). It usually is seen with hemorrhage because of the consumption and subsequent exhaustion of coagulation proteins and platelets, although 5% to 10% of the time it can be seen with microthrombi. DIC is highly lethal, with mortality rates as high as 60%, depending on the underlying condition. It is most commonly caused by sepsis, although it can be caused by trauma, pancreatitis, transfusion reactions, malignancy, obstetric complications, and severe toxic reactions, to name just a few precipitating factors. The Japanese Association for Acute Medicine DIC criteria have been validated prospectively as both an aid in the diagnosis of DIC and being useful in predicting MODS and 28-day mortality. This simple score uses the presence of systemic inflammatory response syndrome (SIRS) criteria, platelet count, and PT to make the diagnosis. Of interest, this score does not use testing for fibrin degradation products, which has been used as part of the International Society of Haemostasis and Thrombosis (ISTH) overt DIC scoring criteria. These blood tests may be useful in differentiating DIC from other conditions, such as chronic liver disease, that also exhibit thrombocytopenia and prolonged PTs.

Treatment of DIC by necessity is focused on the underlying clinical disorder, which should be managed aggressively, while also supporting the patient's coagulopathy. Platelet transfusion may be necessary if the platelet count falls significantly, although this count may be allowed to drop as low as $20,000 \times 10^6/mm^3$ if the patient is not bleeding, even though higher levels will be necessary in cases of active hemorrhage. Other blood products may be necessary but should be directed by blood testing (e.g., giving cryoprecipitate to correct fibrinogen levels). FFP may be necessary in patients with excessively prolonged clotting tests. Other treatments for DIC such as heparin, antifibrinolytics, or antithrombin, although intuitively attractive, have not been shown to affect outcomes and remain controversial. In severe cases, early consultation with a hematologist may be prudent to help address specific factor deficiencies.

TABLE 4: Transfusion Triggers for Platelets

Condition	Desired Platelet Count
Stable hematology/oncology patient	≥10,000
Complicated hematology/oncology patient	≥20,000
Minor surgery/procedure	25,000-50,000
Major surgery/procedure	≥50,000
Neurosurgery	≥100,000
Acquired platelet dysfunction (e.g., medications, uremia)	Unknown if transfusion is effective
Congenital platelet dysfunction (e.g., von Willebrand factor, Glanzmann's thrombasthenia)	Unknown

THROMBOCYTOPENIA

It has been estimated that between 35% and 45% of patients admitted to an ICU will develop thrombocytopenia during their stay (defined as a platelet count of less than $100,000 \times 10^6/mm^3$). After dilution (most commonly from massive transfusion), the most common causes are sepsis and heparin-induced thrombocytopenia (HIT). Sepsis can exert its effects by increased platelet consumption, increased platelet destruction, or decreased platelet function due to suppression of the bone marrow. A rarer cause is pseudothrombocytopenia, in which patients develop immunoglobulin G antibodies to EDTA and so the test is inaccurate, as the platelets clump together and cannot be properly appreciated.

Platelets are critical to the body's response to bleeding, as they form the initial "plug" at the site of injury even before the deposition of fibrin and thrombin crosslinking (Figure 4). The critical nature of platelets in the clotting process has led to their inclusion early in massive transfusion protocols. Table 4 demonstrates generally accepted platelet transfusion triggers under various circumstances.

Heparin-Induced Thrombocytopenia

HIT merits some discussion, as it is often misunderstood and frequently overdiagnosed. HIT is a complication of heparin therapy that

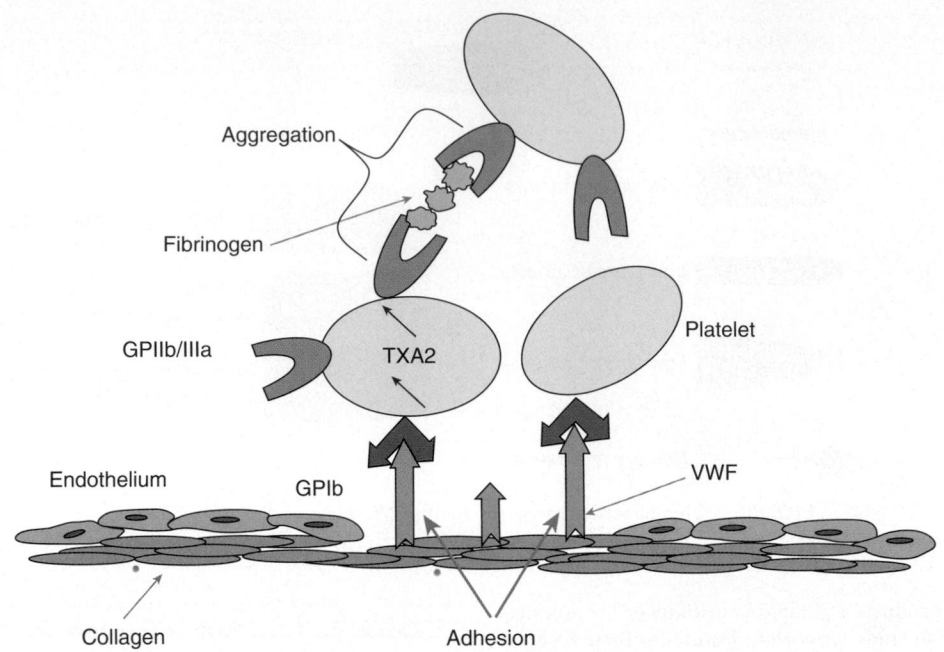

FIGURE 4 Platelet activation diagram. *GPIb*, Glycoprotein Ib; *GPIIb/IIIa*, glycoprotein IIb/IIIa; *TXA2*, thromboxane A2; *VWF*, von Willebrand factor.

may manifest in one of two ways. Type 1 HIT is a nonimmune disorder that results from the direct effect of heparin on platelet activation. It usually is seen within the first 2 days of heparin exposure and resolves with continued heparin therapy. Type 2 HIT is an immune-mediated prothrombotic disorder caused by antibodies to complexes of platelet factor 4 (PF4) and heparin. The antibodies bind to the PF4-heparin complexes on the platelet surface and induce platelet activation. This usually occurs 4 to 10 days after exposure to heparin and has life- and limb-threatening thrombotic complications. In general, the term *HIT* refers to type 2 HIT. The overall risk of HIT is thought to be approximately 0.2% in all heparin-exposed patients.

HIT should be suspected when any patient who is receiving heparin has a drop in platelet count below 50% of baseline. Clinical findings may include skin lesions at heparin injection sites or acute systemic reactions, including fever or chills, after administration of an intravenous bolus of heparin. Venous thromboembolism is the most common complication of HIT, although arterial thrombosis also may occur.

The diagnosis of HIT is based on clinical findings, thrombocytopenia characteristics, timing of the platelet drop, and laboratory studies of HIT antibodies. The Warkentin score, or 4Ts score, is used often as a clinical pretest screening tool to guide in the diagnosis of HIT (Table 5). The heparin/PF4 ELISA is a widely available immunoassay that has high sensitivity but low specificity in the diagnosis of HIT. A serotonin release assay is a functional study often used to confirm a positive heparin/PF4 ELISA result.

The treatment of HIT begins with the discontinuation of all heparin products, including heparin flushes of intravenous catheters. It also should be remembered that some catheters may have heparin bonded on their surface, and these need to be removed. There are multiple recommended alternative anticoagulants to heparin in a patient with HIT: a direct thrombin inhibitor such as lepirudin (recombinant hirudin), bivalirudin, argatroban, and fondaparinux. In practice, the exact agent used will depend on whether the patient has normal renal and hepatic function, as well as on what is available on the hospital formulary. Anticoagulation should be continued for at least 3 months (longer if thrombosis occurred), with the patient transitioned to warfarin once stable and with a normal platelet count ($>150,000 \times 10^6/mm^3$).

PROCEDURES IN COAGULOPATHIC PATIENTS

There are very few data regarding (1) which procedures are safe to perform in patients with coagulopathy and (2) what levels of clotting function are necessary to mitigate risk. In general, it seems that INR is the most universally used coagulation test for decision making, and a level somewhere between 1.4 and 1.6 seems to be acceptable for most anesthesiologists (e.g., for epidural placement) or for neurosurgeons looking to place an intracranial pressure monitor. Less invasive procedures such as central line or arterial line placement may be performed with higher INRs, particularly if the lines are placed in locations where pressure can be applied in the case of an unsuccessful attempt. There is almost no evidence in the current literature of effectiveness of the prophylactic use of FFP.

There is a similar issue with platelet transfusion, which is of even greater importance given the usual issues with platelet storage and lack of supply. Recent clinical practice guidelines from the American Association of Blood Banks suggest a platelet transfusion trigger of $20,000 \times 10^6/mm^3$ for central venous catheter placement and of $50,000 \times 10^6/mm^3$ for lumbar puncture; the organization did not feel that it could make any recommendations regarding traumatic intracranial hemorrhage. There are retrospective studies in trauma patients that suggest that patients with severe traumatic brain injury should have their platelet count maintained above $100,000 \times 10^6/mm^3$, but this remains controversial without data to suggest that correcting this thrombocytopenia by platelet transfusion can improve outcomes.

ANTICOAGULANT MEDICATIONS

At least brief mention should be made of anticoagulant drugs, as some circumstances in the critically ill may lead to inadvertent overanticoagulation and subsequent spontaneous hemorrhage in patients. Of particular concern is the development of acute kidney injury in the patient on low-molecular-weight heparin. Because this drug is cleared renally, in a patient with normal renal function who subsequently develops acute kidney injury due to sepsis, for example, there is a tendency for excessive buildup that may not be

TABLE 5: Estimating the Pretest Probability of Heparin-Induced Thrombocytopenia (HIT): The 4Ts

Category	2	1	0
Thrombocytopenia	>50% platelet fall and platelet nadir ≥20	Platelet count fall by 30%-50% or nadir 10-19	Platelet count fall by <30% or nadir <10
Timing of onset of platelet fall (or other sequelae of HIT)	Clear onset days 5-10 or platelet fall ≤day 1 with recent heparin in past 30 days	Consistent with days 5-10 fall, but not clear, onset after day 10; or fall <day 1 with recent heparin (past 31-100 days)	Platelet count fall <day 4 without recent exposure
Thrombosis or other sequelae	Confirmed new thrombosis, skin necrosis, or acute systemic reaction after intravenous unfractionated heparin bolus	Progressive or recurrent thrombosis, erythematous skin lesions, suspected thrombosis (not proven)	None
Other cause(s) of platelet fall	None evident	Possible	Definite

Points (0, 1, or 2 for each of 4 categories: maximum possible score = 8)

Pretest probability score: 6-8 indicates high; 4-5, intermediate; and 0-3, low.

TABLE 6: Anticoagulants and Reversal Agents

Therapeutic Agent	Target	Comments
FFP	Warfarin Hepatic coagulopathy Traumatic coagulopathy	Rapid reversal for warfarin INR of FFP itself is 1.3-1.4 Risk of TRALI
Cryoprecipitate	Low fibrinogen levels	Stored frozen, requires preparation time
Platelets	Clopidogrel, prasugrel aspirin	Risk of new platelets being inhibited by drug still present
Prothrombin complex Concentrates Kcentra, Beriplex	Warfarin ? Rivaroxaban/apixaban/edoxaban	Rapid reversal, needs vitamin K in addition for warfarin
Factor VIIa	Warfarin Fondaparinux ? Dabigatran	Rapid reversal, needs vitamin K in addition for warfarin Acute trauma coagulopathy
FEIBA (anti-inhibitor coagulant complex)	Direct thrombin inhibitors Anti factor Xa inhibitors Fondaparinux	Activated PCC Factors II, VIIa, IX, X
Protamine	Heparin, dalteparin, enoxaparin	Risk for hypotension, anaphylaxis
Desmopressin (DDAVP)	Uremic platelet dysfunction ? Clopidrogel, prasugrel	Rapid onset Lasts 4-8 hours Unclear if effective for drugs
Vitamin K	Warfarin Vitamin K deficiency	Relatively slow onset IV vs PO equivalent at 24 hours
Aminocaproic acid	Hyperfibrinolysis	Often used post–cardiac bypass, decreases blood loss
Tranexamic acid	Hyperfibrinolysis	Used in trauma patients (CRASH-2 study) and post–cardiac bypass
Praxbind (idarucizumab)	Dabigatran (Pradaxa)	Direct thrombin inhibitor antidote, antibody fragment
Andexanet	Rivaroxaban Apixaban Edoxaban	Factor Xa inhibitor antidote, awaiting final FDA clearance in 2016

FDA, U.S. Food and Drug Administration; *FFP*, fresh frozen plasma; *INR*, international normalized ratio; *IV*, intravenous; *PCC*, prothrombin complex concentrate; *PO*, per os (by mouth); *TRALI*, transfusion-related acute lung injury.

appreciated initially, as it does not demonstrate prolongation of clotting on standard laboratory testing. Although the "packet insert" discusses renal dosing, we suggest that in any patient who does not have stable renal function, this drug should be held or the patient should be transitioned to another medication, as there have been reports of significant bleeding episodes in patients with kidney disease.

In addition, there are many drug-drug interactions that can play havoc with the metabolism of warfarin, which is difficult enough to dose correctly at the best of times. Clinicians need to be aware of these interactions, especially when new medications have been started in the hospital and the patient is then transitioned back to his or her home anticoagulation.

Table 6 lists the currently available anticoagulants, where they exert their effects, and the currently recommended antidote, where available. Special mention should be made of the novel anticoagulants, which until recently did not have any specific reversal agents. The previous recommendation for reversal of dabigatran, for example, was to use dialysis to remove the drug, with 70% to 80% of the effect of the drug apparently removed by dialysis in 2 to 3 hours. Clearly, this is not a strategy that will be rapidly effective for the bleeding patient. Luckily, an antidote called Praxbind was introduced in 2015. It is a recombinant immunoprotein that has high affinity for the dabigatran molecule and can neutralize the anticoagulant effect of this drug effectively. A reversal agent for factor Xa inhibitors (apixaban, rivaroxaban, edoxaban) called Andexanet likely will become available in the United States within 6 months of this writing, providing another useful tool for the

clinician to treat life-threatening bleeds in these patients. Factor VIIa and prothrombin complex concentrates have been suggested as potential reversal agents for both classes of these novel anticoagulants, but there are limited data (either from animals or healthy volunteers) for their efficacy.

SUGGESTED READINGS

Brohi K, Cohen MJ, Davenport RA. Acute coagulopathy of trauma: mechanism, identification and effect. *Curr Opin Crit Care.* 2007;13:680-685.

Ganter MT, Pittet JF. New insights into acute coagulopathy in trauma patients. *Best Pract Res Clin Anaesthesiol.* 2010;24:15-25.

Gonzalez E, Moore EE, Moore HB, et al. Goal-directed hemostatic resuscitation of trauma-induced coagulopathy: a pragmatic randomized clinical trial comparing a viscoelastic assay to conventional coagulation assays. *Ann Surg.* 2016;263:1051-1059.

Holcomb JB, Minei KM, Scerbo ML, et al. Admission rapid thrombelastography can replace conventional coagulation tests in the emergency department: experience with 1974 consecutive trauma patients. *Ann Surg.* 2012;256:476-486.

Hunt BJ. Bleeding and coagulopathies in critical care. *N Engl J Med.* 2014;370:2153.

Hunt H, Stanworth S, Curry N, et al. Thromboelastography (TEG) and rotational thromboelastometry (ROTEM) for trauma induced coagulopathy in adult trauma patients with bleeding. *Cochrane Database Syst Rev.* 2015;(2):CD010438.

Joseph B, Aziz H, Pandit V, et al. Prothrombin complex concentrate versus fresh-frozen plasma for reversal of coagulopathy of trauma: is there a difference? *World J Surg.* 2014;38:1875-1881.

Kaufman RM, Djulbegovic B, Gernsheimer T, et al. Platelet transfusion: a clinical practice guideline from the AABB. *Ann Intern Med.* 2015;162:205-213.

LAPAROSCOPIC CHOLECYSTECTOMY

Jin He, MD, PhD

Laparoscopic cholecystectomy has been the standard treatment of choice for removal of the gallbladder since the 1990s. It is considered the basic laparoscopic procedure in the Fundamentals of Laparoscopic Surgery (FLS), which is required by the American Board of Surgery for general surgery certification. Compared with open cholecystectomy, the laparoscopic approach results in less incisional pain and fewer complications, shorter length of hospital stay, decreased overall costs in the health system, and improved patient satisfaction. With these advantages of the minimally invasive laparoscopic approach, new technology such as robotic single-site cholecystectomy has been developed recently and utilized for selected patients to achieve better outcomes. This chapter reviews the indications for and technique of laparoscopic cholecystectomy, with emphasis on avoiding biliary injury.

■ INDICATIONS

The indications for laparoscopic cholecystectomy do not differ from those for open cholecystectomy.

Asymptomatic Disease

Asymptomatic cholelithiasis or gallbladder polyps are usually incidental findings of imaging studies. Prophylactic cholecystectomy is not justified for asymptomatic cholelithiasis, as only 2% to 3% of healthy persons with asymptomatic cholelithiasis become symptomatic per year. Patients with a higher risk of developing complications, such as those with sickle cell disease or immunodeficiency disorders, should be considered for cholecystectomy. Prophylactic cholecystectomy is not recommended in the setting of diabetes. Gallbladder polyps larger than 1 cm or imaging findings of a calcified or "porcelain" gallbladder indicate cholecystectomy.

Symptomatic Disease

Patients with biliary colic have intermittent, colicky, right upper quadrant or epigastric abdominal pain radiating to the right upper back and shoulder, often triggered by a fatty meal. Because these symptoms are not specific to underlying gallbladder disease, other causes such as angina, myocardial infarction, kidney stones, and inflammatory bowel disease need to be ruled out. Biliary dyskinesia is another common reason for right upper quadrant discomfort. This can be diagnosed with a gallbladder ejection fraction less than 35% at 20 minutes on hepatobiliary iminodiacetic acid (HIDA) scan when dysfunction of the sphincter of Oddi or other periampullary pathology is ruled out.

When fever and leukocytosis are present with biliary colic, acute cholecystitis is suspected and needs to be confirmed with either ultrasound or computed tomography (CT). Patients with acute cholecystitis within 72 hours from the onset of symptoms often can be treated safely with laparoscopic cholecystectomy. Surgery for acute cholecystitis more than 72 hours from the onset of symptoms is related to a higher rate of conversion to open cholecystectomy and a higher incidence of complications. Therefore conservative management with bowel rest and intravenous antibiotics is recommended. Laparoscopic cholecystectomy then can be performed 4 to 6 weeks after the patient has recovered from the acute cholecystitis.

■ CONTRAINDICATIONS

Previous abdominal surgery is not a contraindication to a laparoscopic approach, as laparoscopic adhesiolysis is feasible in most patients. Conditions that favor use of an open rather than laparoscopic cholecystectomy include severe liver cirrhosis with portal hypertension, biliary-enteric fistulae (e.g., gallstone ileus), Mirizzi's syndrome, and suspicion of advanced gallbladder cancer.

Pregnancy is not a contraindication to laparoscopic cholecystectomy, but the operation should be deferred until after delivery when possible. If operation is necessary, the second trimester is preferred because of a lower risk of spontaneous abortion.

■ PREOPERATIVE PREPARATION

Preoperative laboratory tests should include a complete blood count, renal function and electrolytes, hepatic enzymes, coagulation parameters, amylase, and lipase.

When patients with cholelithiasis also have elevated total bilirubin, further workup is necessary to rule out choledocholithiasis, cholangitis, or Mirizzi's syndrome.

When patients are hospitalized with gallstone pancreatitis with elevated amylase or lipase, they should undergo cholecystectomy before discharge after their pancreatitis has resolved. Delay in cholecystectomy has been shown to increase the risk of recurrent pancreatitis by 30% over the 6 to 8 weeks after discharge. If choledocholithiasis is present, endoscopic retrograde cholangiopancreatography (ERCP) either before or after cholecystectomy is indicated to clean the stones from the common bile duct. We prefer to use an endoloop or endostapler to close the cystic duct to avoid any potential leakage if ERCP is necessary after cholecystectomy. If cholangitis is present, ERCP should be performed first to decompress the common bile duct. Laparoscopic cholecystectomy with common bile duct exploration is necessary if ERCP is unsuccessful.

Imaging of the gallbladder and biliary tract with ultrasound or a CT scan is necessary to confirm the cholecystitis and to rule out the presence of choledocholithiasis. Anomalous anatomy of the biliary tract and hepatic artery sometimes can be delineated on CT with contrast. The majority of patients with choledocholithiasis currently are managed by preoperative ERCP and sphincterotomy and stone extraction.

When preoperative ultrasound or CT scan shows a possible choledochocyst, a magnetic resonance cholangiopancreatography (MRCP) or ERCP is indicated to confirm the diagnosis.

■ PATIENT POSITIONING AND SURGICAL TECHNIQUES

The patient is placed in the supine position. A footboard may be used to prevent the patient from slipping off the end of the bed during the procedure. This is especially useful for obese patients. Because the length of surgery is difficult to predict, a Foley catheter is recommended before surgery. It can be removed before the extubation if no complications occurred during the surgery. If an intraoperative cholangiogram is planned, the patient should be placed on a fluoroscopy-compatible table, with one arm tucked to facilitate positioning of C-arm fluoroscopy. The operating surgeon stands on the left side of the patient with the main viewing monitor on the patient's right at the level of the operator's shoulder. The assistant can be on either side depending on different surgical approaches.

We favor the Hasson technique to place the first trocar into the abdomen. A curved 1-cm skin incision is made just above the edge of the umbilicus. After blunt dissection of the subcutaneous tissue, the fascia is grasped and divided longitudinally in the midline. The peritoneum can be entered either bluntly or sharply. The 10-mm blunt Hasson trocar is inserted. Anchoring sutures are not necessary if a balloon trocar is used. The 10-mm trocar is preferred because this first trocar site will be the extraction site of the specimen. Initial insufflation should be done at low-flow settings to avoid vasovagal responses. After establishing pneumoperitoneum safely, a 30-degree rigid laparoscope is used to explore the abdominal cavity to ensure that no iatrogenic injury occurred during placement of the Hasson trocar. Then two or three accessory ports (5 mm) are inserted under direct visualization. The position of these accessory ports may vary based on the patient's body habitus and the surgeon's preference. In general, two 5-mm ports are placed approximately two fingerbreadths below the right costal margin, one in the anterior axillary line and the other in the midclavicular line. Should it be necessary to convert to an open procedure, these trocar incisions can be connected. The last 5-mm port for the dissection instrument generally is placed in the left upper quadrant, around the subxiphoid to the right, or through the falciform ligament. After all trocars are placed, the patient should be positioned in reverse Trendelenburg with a slight lift on the right side to improve exposure of the gallbladder.

Some authors have proposed using needle-type 2-mm trocars as the accessory ports because of the potential advantage of less postoperative pain. One prospective study compared various trocar sizes, including the use of only 2-mm and 5-mm trocars for the procedure. The study concluded that there was no overall difference in cosmetic satisfaction, incidence of complications, or postoperative pain score.

Whether patients have acute inflammation or chronic inflammation, laparoscopic adhesiolysis is often necessary to expose the gallbladder. Often a combination of sharp and blunt dissection using laparoscopic scissors or a suction irrigator can successfully take down the omentum around the gallbladder. Electrocautery can be used safely as long as the surgeon is clear about the anatomy and the dissection plane. Blind application of the cautery without delineating the anatomy is dangerous. The surgeon should ensure that no cautery application takes place outside the visual field.

Once the gallbladder fundus has been exposed, the dissection should remain close to the gallbladder wall. The duodenum and the transverse colon often can be dissected bluntly off the gallbladder.

Patients with acute cholecystitis often have a tense gallbladder. If the grasping of a tense gallbladder is difficult, decompression is necessary. We often use a laparoscopic 14-gauge needle (Figure 1) to decompress under direct visualization.

Regardless of what technique is used, the key to a safe and successful laparoscopic cholecystectomy is to achieve the critical view

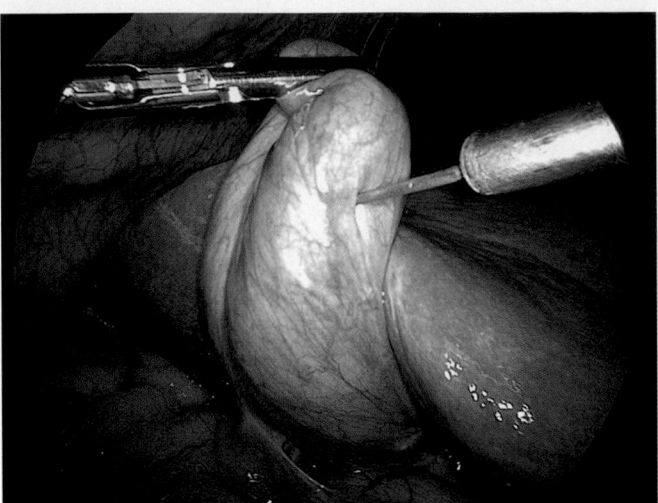

FIGURE 1 Technique of needle aspiration of a distended gallbladder. This approach is useful in the setting of a tense, distended gallbladder to avoid perforation from a grasper and spillage of bile and stones. *(From Cameron JL, Cameron AM. Current Surgical Therapy. 11th ed. Philadelphia: Saunders; 2013. Figure 4, page 1308.)*

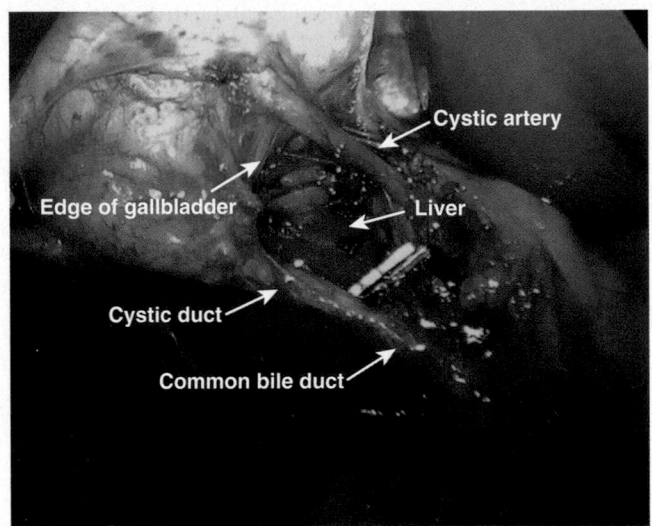

FIGURE 2 Calot's triangle, defined superiorly by the inferior border of the liver, inferolaterally by the cystic duct, and medially by the common bile duct, is clearly identified. *(From Cameron JL. Current Surgical Therapy. 9th ed. St. Louis: Mosby; 2007. Figure 2a, page 1274.)*

(Figure 2). This critical view means that before any structures are clipped or divided, the cystic duct and artery are the only tubular structures entering the gallbladder, with the infundibulum retracted laterally and the liver visible posteriorly through the window developed between those structures.

Several anatomic landmarks that help to attain this view have been described, including Calot's triangle, Calot's node, and Rouvière's sulcus.

Next, a few commonly used techniques of cholecystectomy are described.

One-Handed Technique

The assistant grasps the fundus of the gallbladder with a left hand grasper, retracting in a superior and lateral position over the liver.

The assistant then grasps the infundibulum with a grasper in the right hand, retracting in an inferolateral direction. Thereby the Calot's triangle between the cystic duct and the common bile duct is exposed. The surgeon on the patient's left side operates the camera with the left hand while performing a circumferential dissection of the cystic duct and cystic artery with the right hand. Staying close to the gallbladder neck during dissection of Calot's node will help to define the cystic artery, which invariably stays behind the lymph node. After the gallbladder–cystic duct junction has been identified, all fatty tissue in the Calot's triangle (the inferior border of the liver superiorly, the cystic duct inferolaterally, and the common hepatic duct medially) needs to be dissected out to achieve the critical view.

Two-Handed Technique

The assistant controls the camera. The surgeon uses the left hand to grasp the infundibulum and provide traction inferolaterally to expose the Calot's triangle. Dissection begins by opening the visceral peritoneum in the triangle. After teasing away the loose fatty tissue and the Calot's node, the cystic duct and artery will be identified in the triangle. Once the critical view is achieved, clips are applied on the cystic duct and artery. Usually two clips are placed on the stay side of the cystic duct or artery and one clip is placed as close to the gallbladder as possible, leaving enough space between the clips for division with sharp scissors. If the cystic duct is too large for a 5-mm clip, we use a 5-mm camera through the subxiphoid port and a 10-mm clip through the umbilical port. Another alternative for a large, inflamed, thickened cystic duct is to use an endostapler or endoloop.

The gallbladder is dissected away from the cystic plate on the liver bed using the hook electrocautery. The hook is very useful, allowing the operator's pulling, hooking, sweeping, and teasing motions before the cautery application.

The Endo Catch Pouch (Covidien, Norwalk, CT) is inserted through the umbilical port (10 mm), and the gallbladder is removed in the bag under direct visualization. During the specimen extraction, we usually decompress the gallbladder in the bag if necessary. Any large stone also can be crushed in the bag. Almost all specimens can be removed using these techniques without enlarging the umbilical incision. The umbilical trocar is then replaced and pneumoperitoneum is re-established to confirm hemostasis and no bile leakage. After removing the accessory ports under direct visualization, the abdomen is then desufflated. We recommend closing any accessory trocar site larger than 8 mm in diameter using a Carter-Thomason needle and #0 monofilament synthetic absorbable sutures. The umbilical trocar site can be closed with #0 or #1 monofilament synthetic absorbable sutures using a GU or UR needle. Although the incidence of trocar site hernia is low after using a noncutting trocar, closing the trocar site correctly will decrease the hernia rate further.

■ PREVENTION OF BILE DUCT INJURY

Correct interpretation of the anatomy is the key in preventing bile duct injury. Most bile duct injuries are not recognized at the time of injury, suggesting that anatomic orientation is a major problem. To facilitate orientation before starting dissection, Hugh and colleagues recommend identifying Rouvière's sulcus as the anatomic landmark. Rouvière's sulcus runs to the right of the liver hilum anterior to the caudate process and usually containing the right portal pedicle. Dissection on the visceral peritoneum on the gallbladder ventral to this sulcus will help to avoid major injury to hilar structures with the gallbladder being retracted to the inferolateral position. Extending this dissection along the gallbladder fossa both posteriorly and anteriorly allows Calot's triangle to be fully exposed. This ensures no unexpected anatomy and confirms the correct anatomic position before any significant tubular structure is divided. Dome-down technique also can be useful when chronic

inflammation in Calot's triangle renders dissection unsafe. No dissection is necessary in the hepatoduodenal ligament at the base of segment IV, as the left hepatic duct often lies extrahepatically within this tissue. The electrocautery should be used only on tissue that can be seen through. Avoidance of electrocautery close to the common hepatic duct and dissection close to the gallbladder–cystic duct junction are helpful.

When dissection of the gallbladder off the cystic plate is impossible because of severe inflammation, it is safe to leave a portion of the posterior wall of the gallbladder on the liver. The residual mucosa of the gallbladder should be cauterized. A drain should be left using the trocar site in the right upper quadrant to evacuate fluid and monitor for low-grade bile leaks from the liver bed area after difficult dissections.

■ COMPLICATIONS

With careful and meticulous dissection technique, complications such as bowel injuries can be avoided. Bleeding complications can be from the trocar site during the insertion or the removal. If active bleeding happens after trocar removal under direct visualization, the use of the electrocautery or a suture using the Carter-Thomason needle is usually sufficient to achieve hemostasis. Bleeding during dissection in Calot's triangle can be from the cyst artery or its posterior branch. Often this can be controlled with precise grasp of the bleeding site and then electrocautery or clips. Bleeding from the liver bed is common when inflammation obliterates the plane between the gallbladder and the cystic plate. Using electrocautery in the spray mode will help to control the liver bleeding. In cases in which hemorrhage cannot be controlled, pushing the gallbladder to tamponade the bleeding site and conversion to an open procedure in a controlled fashion are necessary.

Bile duct injuries are the most devastating complication of laparoscopic cholecystectomy. It is best to avoid bile duct injury by following the steps outlined previously. If an isolated bile duct injury happens and is recognized during surgery, seeking help from another experienced biliary surgeon is highly recommended. If experienced help is not available, a drain should be left in the operative field whether the gallbladder is removed or not. The patient should be extubated and transferred to a tertiary hospital with experience in hepato-pancreato-biliary (HPB) surgery. Attempting to repair the bile duct injury either laparoscopically or by conversion to open surgery is not recommended. Most bile duct injuries are not recognized during surgery. Injuries recognized in the early postoperative period, manifested by jaundice or biloma formation, should be investigated with ERCP or percutaneous cholangiography. For low-volume leaks, sphincterotomy or stenting may help to control the leak. For advanced injuries such as complete ductal division, obstruction, or combined vascular injuries, if recognized within 7 days of surgery, the best option is hepaticojejunostomy reconstruction by a highly experienced biliary surgeon after control of the septic response. Otherwise, a delayed repair 2 to 3 months after injury is recommended. During this period, the biliary system should be decompressed with an ERCP stent or percutaneous drain and catheter. If a bile duct injury occurs with a vascular injury, the goal is to control bleeding and stabilize the patient. Seeking help from another experienced biliary surgeon or transfer to a tertiary hospital with experience in HPB surgery is highly recommended.

■ SUMMARY

Laparoscopic cholecystectomy can be performed safely, and is the procedure of choice for removal of the gallbladder when indicated. The principles and experiences gained in performing laparoscopic cholecystectomy form the foundation of the general surgeon's laparoscopic skills. All residents should master the principles of laparoscopic cholecystectomy during their residency training.

SUGGESTED READINGS

Hugh TB, Kelly MD, Mekisic A. Rouviere's sulcus: a useful landmark in laparoscopic cholecystectomy. *Br J Surg.* 1997;84:1253-1254.

Novitsky YW, Kercher KW, Czerniach DR, et al. Advantages of minilaparoscopic vs conventional laparoscopic cholecystectomy. *Arch Surg.* 2005;140:1178-1183.

Strasberg SM, Brunt LM. Rationale and use of the critical view of safety in laparoscopic cholecystectomy. *J Am Coll Surg.* 2010;211:133-138.

Strasberg SM, Gouma DJ. "Extreme" vasculobiliary injuries: association with fundus-down cholecystectomy in severely inflamed gallbladders. *HPB (Oxford).* 2012;14:1-8.

Winslow ER, Fialkowski EA, Linehan DC, et al. "Sideways": results of repair of biliary injuries using a policy of side-to-side hepatico-jejunostomy. *Ann Surg.* 2009;249:426-434.

LAPAROSCOPIC COMMON BILE DUCT EXPLORATION

Ezra N. Teitelbaum, MD, and Eric S. Hungness, MD

Symptomatic gallstone disease is extremely common both in the United States and worldwide, and laparoscopic cholecystectomy, the gold-standard treatment, is the most common intra-abdominal operation performed by general surgeons, with more than 700,000 operations performed annually in the United States alone. Choledocholithiasis, or migration of stones from the gallbladder into the common bile duct (CBD), is a common complication, occurring in 3% to 17% of patients who undergo laparoscopic cholecystectomy for symptomatic cholelithiasis.

During the open surgery era, choledocholithiasis typically was treated with a CBD exploration performed at the time of open cholecystectomy. A dramatic shift in the approach to treating CBD stones occurred with the introduction and rapid proliferation of laparoscopic cholecystectomy in the late 1980s and early 1990s. As surgeons were grappling with safely incorporating laparoscopy into their practices, the surgical management of CBD stones fell by the wayside. Increasingly, choledocholithiasis was treated using a two-stage approach: endoscopic retrograde cholangiopancreatography (ERCP) to remove the CBD stones and then laparoscopic cholecystectomy to remove the gallbladder in order to prevent recurrence of biliary colic and choledocholithiasis. In a recent analysis of the National Inpatient Sample, 93% of patients with CBD stones were treated using this two-stage approach and only 7% were treated using a single-stage strategy of laparoscopic common bile duct exploration (LCBDE) performed at the time of laparoscopic cholecystectomy.

Although the two-stage approach of ERCP and laparoscopic cholecystectomy has become the dominant treatment modality, there is robust evidence that the single-stage approach of LCBDE and laparoscopic cholecystectomy results in superior patient outcomes. This is most notable in terms of reductions in hospital length of stay and hospital costs, as well as possible reductions in procedure-related complications. The reasons for the underutilization of LCBDE despite these clinical advantages are multifocal, but lack of exposure to the procedure during surgical residency likely is largely responsible. A study of the case logs of graduating general surgery residents showed that they had performed a mean of only 0.7 LCBDEs throughout the course of their entire training.

This chapter describes the indications for and use of intraoperative imaging to identify choledocholithiasis. It also will detail the technical steps of LCBDE, utilizing both transcystic and transcholedochal approaches. Lastly, the evidence comparing outcomes of LCBDE with those resulting from the two-stage approach of ERCP and laparoscopic cholecystectomy is discussed. It is our hope that if practicing surgeons are able to develop an increased familiarity with LCBDE and training in the procedure during residency is expanded, the clinical use of LCBDE will increase, with resulting improvement in clinical outcomes for patients with choledocholithiasis.

■ OPERATIVE TECHNIQUE

Preoperative Setup and Planning

Patient undergoing laparoscopic cholecystectomy should all have a thorough medical history and physical examination. Liver function tests and a transabdominal ultrasound should be performed in all patients preoperatively to help predict the presence of CBD stones. Preoperative magnetic resonance cholangiopancreatography (MRCP) is rarely, if ever, required.

When planning for a laparoscopic cholecystectomy in a patient with suspected choledocholithiasis, preparations should be made to perform intraoperative imaging (with either intraoperative cholangiography [IOC] or laparoscopic ultrasonography [LUS]) to confirm the presence of CBD stones and then to perform an LCBDE. These elements of the procedure should be discussed with the patient preoperatively and added to the operative consent form. The necessary equipment to perform imaging and LCBDE should be assembled well ahead of time, as searching for these instruments intraoperatively adds unnecessary anesthetic time and risk to the procedure. If IOC is to be performed, the operating table should be checked to ensure that it can accommodate the fluoroscopy C-arm, as this requires reversing the head-foot orientation of some operating table models. The patient is positioned supine with the left arm tucked at the side to facilitate introduction of the C-arm. Appropriate intravenous (IV) antibiotics should be administered preoperatively, and sequential compression devices should be applied before induction of anesthesia as prophylaxis against venous thrombus formation.

Port Placement and Initial Dissection to Achieve a "Critical View of Safety"

Either an open Hasson trocar or a closed Veress needle technique can be used in a periumbilical location to create an initial pneumoperitoneum. The patient is placed in steep reverse Trendelenburg and left side down position. A diagnostic laparoscopy is then performed and the remaining laparoscopic trocars are placed under direct vision. We prefer the "American" port arrangement, utilizing a total of four trocars: the periumbilical camera port, a lateral right subcostal port along the anterior axillary line to retract the gallbladder fundus, a more medial right subcostal port along the midclavicular line to serve as the surgeon's left hand for retracting the gallbladder infundibulum, and a subxiphoid port for the surgeon's right hand to perform the dissection.

Once the trocars are placed, the assistant uses a grasper inserted through the lateral subcostal port to elevate the gallbladder fundus up and over the liver edge. This should expose the gallbladder infundibulum and allow for subsequent dissection. The surgeon then uses a two-handed technique to retract the gallbladder infundibulum (left hand grasper) and uses a combination of blunt and careful electrocautery dissection (right hand Maryland-type dissector or L-hook cautery) to clear the undersurface of the gallbladder of fibrous and fatty tissue. This is done until a "critical view of safety" has been achieved. The critical view is composed of three essential elements: (1) all fibrous and fatty tissue has been cleared from the undersurface of the gallbladder to completely expose Calot's triangle; (2) the

TABLE 1: Indications for Intraoperative Imaging of the Common Bile Duct to Assess for Choledocholithiasis

History	Pancreatitis
	Jaundice
	Clay-colored stools
	Dark urine
Physical examination	Jaundice
	Scleral icterus
Laboratory tests	Elevated bilirubin
	Elevated transaminases
	Elevated alkaline phosphatase
	Elevated lipase or amylase
Transabdominal ultrasound	Common bile duct diameter greater than 6 mm
	Stones visualized in the common bile duct
Intraoperative findings	Dilated cystic duct or common bile duct
	Stones within the cystic duct

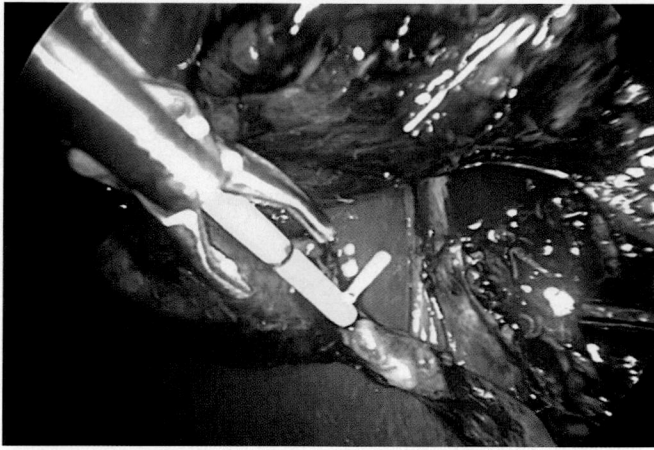

FIGURE 1 A cholangiogram catheter is inserted into the cystic ductotomy using an Olsen fixation clamp. The catheter is inserted through the midclavicular subcostal trocar (i.e., the surgeon's left hand) to facilitate introduction of the catheter and subsequent instruments for the common bile duct exploration.

gallbladder has been dissected off of the liver bed (i.e., cystic plate) at least one third of the way up its wall; and (3) only two structures (cystic duct and cystic artery) are seen coursing through Calot's triangle and entering the gallbladder. Completing a careful and meticulous dissection to achieve this critical view is the most effective way to prevent CBD injuries.

Intraoperative Imaging for Choledocholithiasis

Once the critical view of safety has been achieved, the surgeon can proceed with intraoperative imaging to confirm the presence of CBD stones. The indication for utilizing such imaging is any preoperative or intraoperative suspicion for choledocholithiasis, based on the patient's history, physical examination, laboratory values, preoperative imaging, or intraoperative findings (Table 1). Intraoperative imaging can be performed with either IOC or LUS. Although IOC is the more common modality utilized in the United States, both modalities have shown excellent sensitivity and specificity for detecting CBD stones.

IOC is performed by first placing a clip on the gallbladder-infundibulum junction to prevent subsequent spillage and migration of gallstones. A small ductotomy is then made in the cystic duct, staying high toward the gallbladder. It is important to keep this ductotomy small in order to prevent avulsion of the cystic duct during subsequent LCBDE. Once the ductotomy is made, a cholangiogram catheter is passed through it. If an LCBDE is planned, we prefer to use a 5F open tip catheter passed through an Olsen-type fixation clamp. This clamp should be inserted through the more medial subcostal trocar (i.e., the surgeon's left hand port) to facilitate passage of the catheter through the ductotomy and then introduction of LCBDE instruments (Figure 1). Once the clamp is secured, the C-arm is brought into position. A mixture of 50% saline and 50% contrast should be used, as a more concentrated contrast solution can obscure small CBD stones. It is imperative to ensure that all air has been flushed from the catheter system before injection, as air bubbles can appear as filling defects similar to stones on cholangiogram. Once the system is ready, the anesthesiologist holds ventilator respirations and the contrast is injected while fluoroscopic images are recorded. The cholangiogram recording is then examined for evidence of CBD stones, which typically appear as filling defects, a meniscus sign in the distal CBD, or a lack of duodenal filling with contrast (Figure 2).

LUS is performed using a specialized laparoscopic ultrasound probe that is inserted through the subxiphoid trocar. The probe first

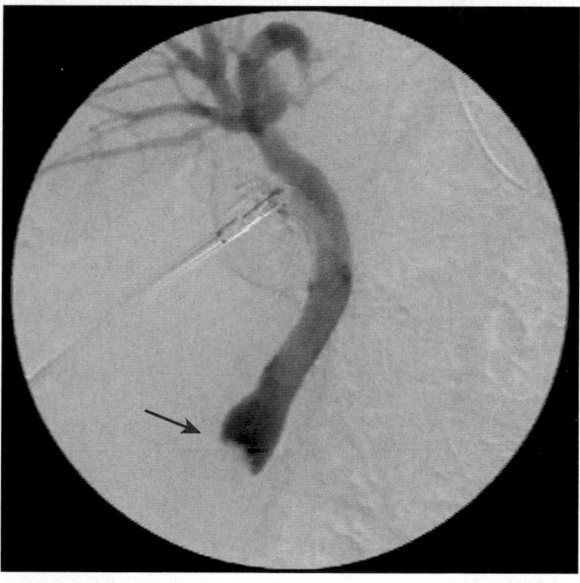

FIGURE 2 An intraoperative cholangiogram showing a clear meniscus sign (*arrow*) created by an obstructing stone in the distal common bile duct.

is positioned over the gallbladder to calibrate ultrasonic gain and depth and then moved over the porta hepatis to scan through the CBD. With the probe positioned over the porta hepatis, the CBD, hepatic artery, and portal vein can be seen simultaneously in cross-section. Stones in the CBD appear echogenic, or white on the ultrasound monitor, and create black "shadow" deep to their location, just as is the case in transabdominal ultrasound. One weakness of LUS is scanning the distal CBD intrapancreatic portion for stones. This is because the pancreatic parenchyma often has a similar echogenicity to stones and therefore can obscure ultrasonic visualization of the distal CBD.

Determination of the Optimal Approach for LCBDE

Once CBD stones have been confirmed on imaging, the surgeon can attempt to flush them through the ampulla of Vater and into the

TABLE 2: Indications and Contraindications for Transcystic and Transcholedochal Approaches for LCBDE

Transcystic LCBDE	Transcholedochal LCBDE
INDICATION	**INDICATION**
Stone(s) in the common bile duct	Stone(s) in the common bile duct or hepatic ducts
CONTRAINDICATIONS	**CONTRAINDICATIONS**
Stone greater than 10 mm in diameter	Common bile duct diameter less than 8 mm
Common hepatic duct stones (relative contraindication)	Surgeon not experienced with advanced laparoscopic dissection and suturing techniques
Five or more stones (relative contraindication)	

LCBDE, Laparoscopic common bile duct exploration.

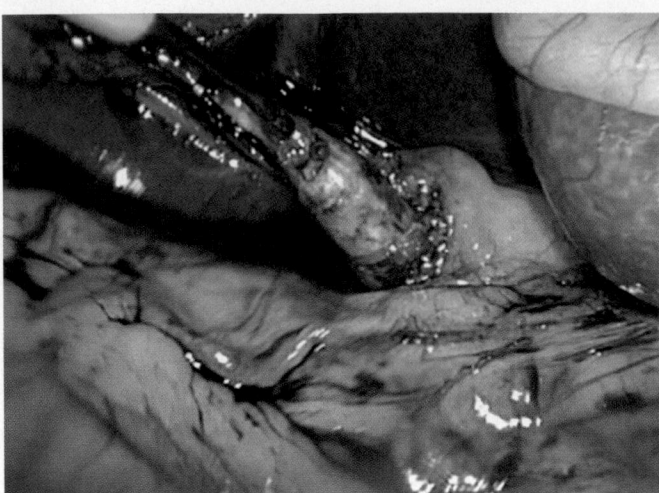

FIGURE 3 A balloon is used to dilate the cystic duct in order to facilitate choledochoscope insertion and subsequent stone extraction.

duodenum. This is done by first giving 1 or 2 mg of glucagon IV in order to relax the sphincter of Oddi. Several hundred milliliters of saline are then flushed through the cholangiogram catheter, and a repeat cholangiogram is performed to assess for stone clearance. This technique can be successful for sludge and very small stones, but generally is not effective for stones larger than 2 to 3 mm.

While attempting flushing, preparations should be made to perform an LCBDE. The first step in this process is to determine which approach should be used: transcystic, in which instruments are passed through the cystic ductotomy created for IOC, or transcholedochal, in which a longitudinal ductotomy in made in the CBD in order to access it (Table 2). Because the transcholedochal approach requires making an incision in the CBD, it is more invasive and involves greater risk of CBD injury and stricture, it therefore is generally reserved for clinical situations in which there is a contraindication to a transcystic approach. The main contraindications to transcystic LCBDE are CBD stones greater than 10 mm in diameter (because extraction of such stones through the cystic duct risks avulsion at the cystic duct–common duct junction) and stones in the common hepatic duct (because the acute angle between the cystic and common hepatic ducts makes transcystic introduction of instruments difficult). The presence of five or more CBD stones is a relative contraindication to a transcystic approach because it is faster to extract multiple stones through a choledochotomy. The one important contraindication to a transcholedochal approach is a CBD diameter of less than 8 mm. Closure of the choledochotomy in a duct narrower than 8 mm will lead to high rates of CBD stricture postoperatively.

■ TRANSCYSTIC LCBDE

Wire Access

Although transcystic LCBDE can be performed by passing wire baskets under purely fluoroscopic guidance, we prefer a direct visualization approach using a flexible choledochoscope. The first step of the procedure is to gain wire access to the CBD. An angled-tip hydrophilic 0.035-inch guidewire is passed through the cholangiogram catheter under fluoroscopic visualization. Difficulty in wire passage is often encountered at two locations: at the spiral valves of the cystic duct and at a CBD stone impacted at the ampulla. These obstructions generally can be overcome by gently manipulating the wire forward and backward, as well as by applying torque to the wire to change the direction of its angled tip. The wire should be passed well into the duodenum in order to prevent retrograde migration out of the cystic duct during subsequent instrument exchanges.

Balloon Dilation

We routinely perform a balloon dilation of the cystic duct in order to facilitate both choledochoscope insertion and subsequent stone extraction. To accomplish this, the cholangiogram catheter and Olsen clamp are removed while the guidewire is held in position simultaneously using a laparoscopic grasper. A balloon dilator is then passed over the wire and through the cystic ductotomy (Figure 3). We use a balloon with a 4-cm length and an 8-mm diameter. The balloon is inflated using a pressure injector filled with contrast, so that its expansion can be viewed fluoroscopically. The balloon should be kept at maximum inflation (2 to 5 atm, depending on balloon model) for more than 3 minutes to ensure complete obliteration of cystic duct tortuosity and valves.

Choledochoscope Insertion

After dilation is complete, the balloon is removed and once again the guidewire is held in position using a grasper. The choledochoscope is then set up (Figure 4). This involves bringing in a second video tower if the operating room contains only one laparoscopic camera box and light source. A source of continuous saline irrigation (such as a 3-L bag typically used for cystoscopy) is attached to a side port in the working channel of the choledochoscope. It is important to ensure that this irrigation is flowing continuously as the scope is introduced into the cystic and common bile ducts or the ducts will collapse and visualization will be lost. The laparoscopic camera and light source are then attached to the scope, and the white balance and focus are checked. If the operating room contains two laparoscopic monitors, we prefer to position them side by side over the patient's head and place the laparoscopic image on one monitor and import the choledochoscopic image into the second monitor.

The choledochoscope is then inserted over the guidewire and slowly advanced through the cystic ductotomy (Figure 5). During this step it is important to keep the guidewire straight, with a small amount of tension applied to its end outside the patient. This will prevent the choledochoscope from looping and coiling inside the abdomen. Once the scope is within the cystic duct, the ductal lumen should be kept centered in the scope image using a combination of scope flexion and torque. The scope alone occasionally can be manipulated external to the patient, but often a laparoscopic grasper will be needed to gently advance the scope shaft forward. It is important to use a padded grasper for this purpose, to avoid damaging the choledochoscope shaft and internal fiber optics. Maintaining the ductal lumen in the middle of the screen, the scope is advanced through the cystic duct and into the CBD. Once within the CBD, the guidewire is

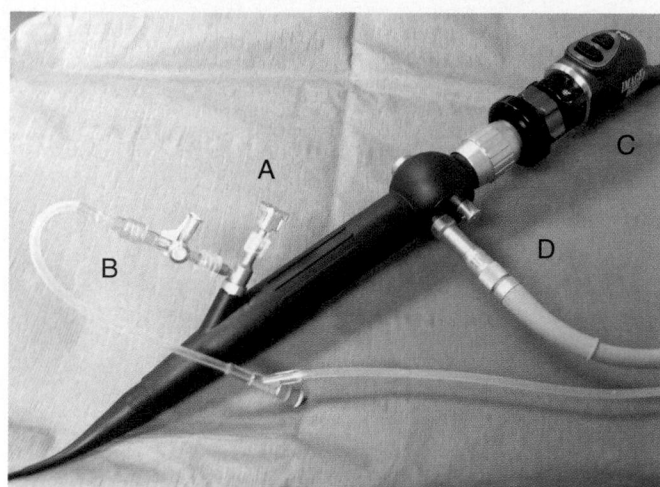

FIGURE 4 The choledochoscope has a working channel (**A**) for insertion of endoscopic instruments, such as the guidewire and wire basket. Continuous irrigation flows through tubing that is connected to a side port in the working channel (**B**). A laparoscopic camera (**C**) and light cable (**D**) are attached to the choledochoscope and plugged into a standard laparoscopic tower in order to project images onto a monitor.

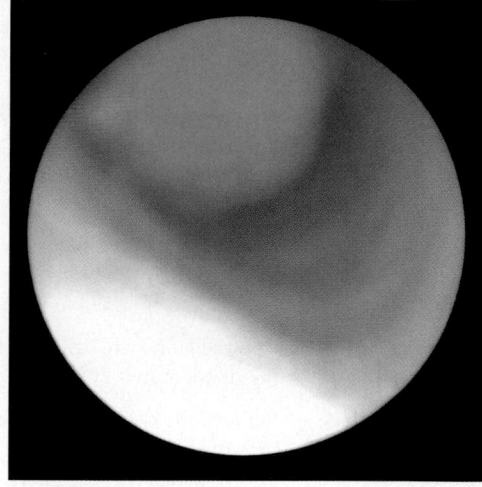

FIGURE 6 A large distal common bile duct stone is visualized through the choledochoscope.

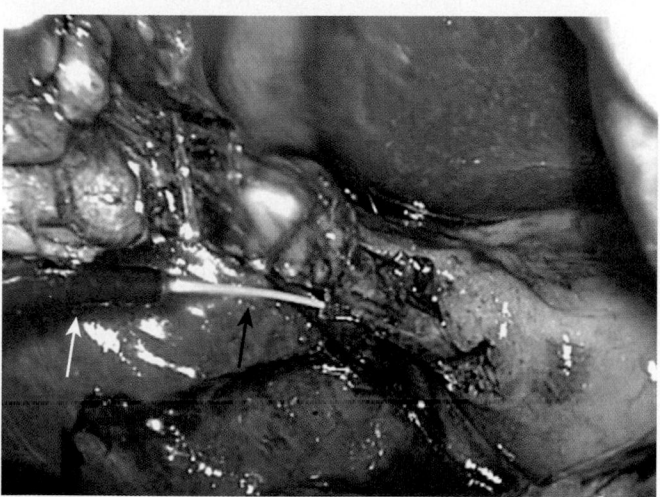

FIGURE 5 Using a Seldinger-type technique, the choledochoscope (*white arrow*) is passed over the guidewire (*black arrow*) into the cystic ductotomy.

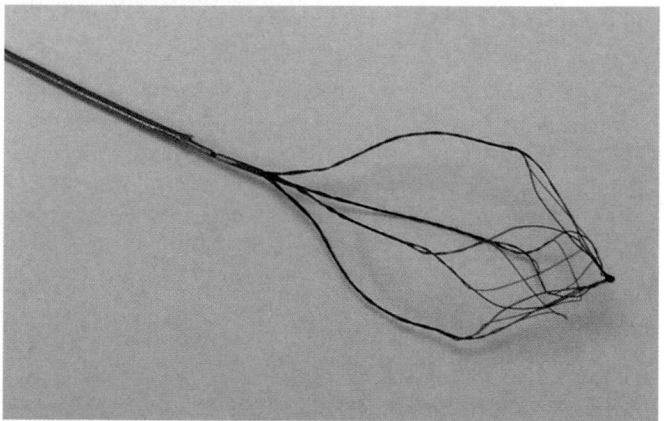

FIGURE 7 An example of a wire basket that is passed through the working channel of the choledochoscope and used to capture the common bile duct stone.

removed, which improves visualization. The scope is then advanced until the stone or stones are visualized (Figure 6; Table 3).

Stone Retrieval and Extraction

Once the CBD stone is visualized, a wire basket is passed through the choledochoscope's working channel (Figure 7). The basket is advanced past the stone in the closed position and then opened once it is distal to the stone. Care should be taken to perform these maneuvers under direct choledochoscopic visualization. After the basket is opened, it is slowly pulled backward in order to trawl and capture the stone within its tines (Figure 8). Often this requires jiggling the basket back and forth when the stone is alongside it, until the stone falls within the center of the tines. Once this occurs, the basket is closed in order to capture the stone.

The basket is then withdrawn so that the stone is pinned against the face of the scope, and the scope and basket are removed as a single unit. Resistance can occur as the stone passes through the cystic duct,

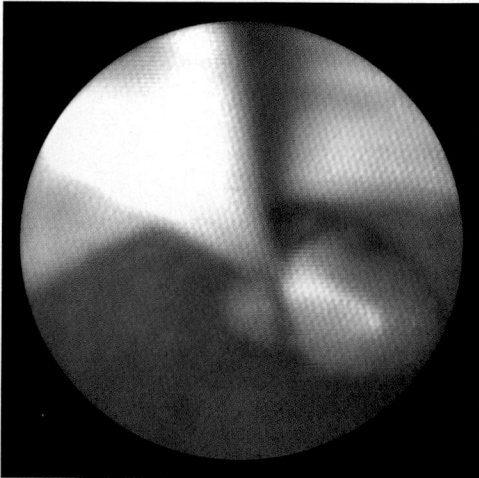

FIGURE 8 The wire basket is closed, capturing a common bile duct stone.

TABLE 3: Procedure Steps and Required Equipment for Transcystic LCBDE

Procedural Step	Key Points	Instruments
1. Cholangiogram	• Perform the IOC through the midclavicular subcostal trocar (rather than the epigastric trocar) • Perform the cystic ductotomy high towards the gallbladder side of the duct	5F open tip cholangiogram catheter Olsen clamp
2. Use adjuncts to clear common duct	• Give IV glucagon and wait several minutes, then flush with several hundred mL of saline • Repeat IOC to assess for clearance	1 or 2 mg IV glucagon
3. Guidewire access	• Pass the guidewire through the cholangiogram catheter and advance into the duodenum	0.035-inch flexible tip guidewire
4. Cystic duct dilation	• Remove the cholangiogram catheter, holding the guidewire in place • Pass the balloon dilator over the guidewire and confirm position fluoroscopically • Inflate the balloon and hold for at least 3 min	Balloon dilator Pressure injector
5. Choledochoscope insertion and maneuvering	• Remove the balloon dilator and pass the scope over the guidewire • Start continuous irrigation through the scope's working channel • Once the scope is within the common duct, the guidewire can be removed • Use only a padded grasper to manipulate the scope to avoid damaging it	Choledochoscope Saline irrigation (3-L bag or 1-L pressure bag) Second laparoscopic tower with camera and light cable Padded grasper
6. Stone capture and extraction	• Pass the wire basket through the scope channel • Advance the basket in a closed position past the stone, then open it and "trawl" backward with the basket open to capture the stone • Close the basket around the stone, and slowly remove the scope and stone as a single unit	Endoscopic wire basket
7. Completion IOC	• Regardless of findings on LCBDE, perform a final IOC to confirm stone clearance and flow of contrast into the duodenum	Same as initial IOC
8. Cystic duct ligation	• If the cystic duct was balloon dilated, use a suture loop rather than clips to ligate it	Suture loop

IOC, Intraoperative cholangiography; *IV,* intravenous; *LCBDE,* laparoscopic common bile duct exploration.

but as long as an adequate dilation was performed and the stone is no greater than 10 mm in diameter, this resistance can be overcome with gentle and persistent traction. Once the stone is removed from the cystic duct, it is released from the wire basket and can be removed using a stone grasper. Unfortunately, only one stone at a time can be captured with the wire basket, so if more than one CBD stones are present, the choledochoscope must be reinserted and the capture and extraction process repeated. However, usually at this point the cystic duct is dilated enough that the scope can be inserted directly into the ductotomy and regaining guidewire access is not necessary.

Completion Cholangiogram and Cystic Duct Ligation

Even after all stones are removed and the CBD appears clear choledochoscopically, a completion cholangiogram should always be performed to document that no residual filling defects exist and that there is brisk flow of contrast into the duodenum. Stones that migrated proximally into the hepatic ducts can be easy to miss on choledochoscopy but are seen on completion IOC. If the completion IOC is clear, the LCBDE portion of the operation is complete and the cystic duct can be ligated. Because the duct was balloon dilated, a pretied suture loop rather than clips is used for duct ligation (Figure 9). The gallbladder is then dissected off of the liver bed and removed as in a normal laparoscopic cholecystectomy. It generally is not necessary to leave an intra-abdominal drain, unless there is concern regarding the security of the cystic duct closure.

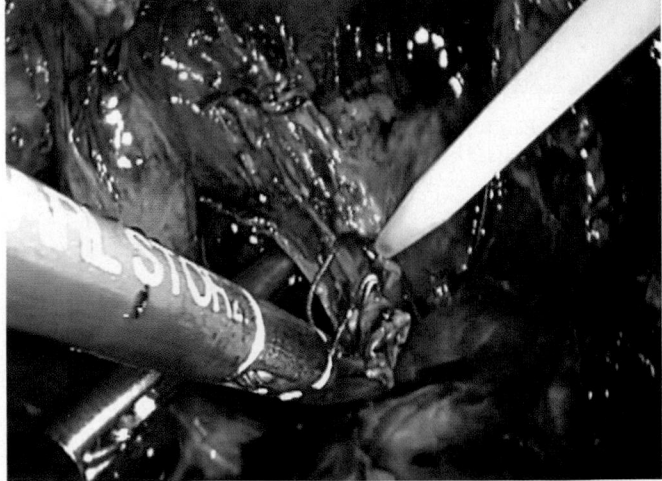

FIGURE 9 A pretied laparoscopic suture loop is used to ligate the cystic duct. It is necessary to ligate the cystic duct with a suture rather than clips because the duct has been dilated to at least 8 mm in diameter.

■ TRANSCHOLEDOCHAL LCBDE

Common Bile Duct Exposure

It should be emphasized that transcholedochal LCBDE is a more complex procedure requiring advanced laparoscopic dissection and suturing skills. Therefore it should be used only if one of the contraindications to the transcystic approach discussed previously exists and be attempted only by surgeons comfortable with the requisite techniques.

After intraoperative imaging confirms both the presence of choledocholithiasis and that the CBD is dilated to at least 8 mm, the first step is to clear an area of the anterior CBD in order to then create a common ductotomy. In patients with a largely dilated CBD and little intra-abdominal fat, this often requires little or no dissection. However, in patients with more fatty tissue overlying the porta hepatis, this dissection can be difficult and has the potential to cause CBD injury or bleeding. The dissection should be kept immediately anterior to the CBD in order to avoid disrupting the blood supply to the CBD, which comes from small vessels from the proper hepatic artery, which is medial to the patient's left. An area large enough to make an adequate ductotomy should be cleared. The ductotomy need only be slightly larger than the largest CBD stone seen on intraoperative imaging. There is usually enough CBD length superior to the duodenum to create this area for the ductotomy, and performing Kocher's maneuver to mobilize the duodenum generally is not necessary.

Choledochotomy Creation

To gain access to the CBD, a longitudinal incision is made in its anterior surface. This can be done using laparoscopic scissors (either curved or straight Potts-type, if available) or a #11 blade scalpel controlled with a locking laparoscopic grasper. If there is any question as to the location of the CBD after initial dissection, a fine needle can be used to aspirate the structure and confirm return of bile before ductotomy. The ductotomy is carefully extended superiorly until it is 2 to 3 mm larger than the estimated size of the largest CBD stone.

Stone Extraction

Because the choledochoscope does not need to traverse the cystic duct during a transcholedochal LCBDE, it is not necessary to gain wire access to the CBD. Rather, the scope simply can be inserted directly through the CBD ductotomy using a laparoscopic padded grasper. Once the choledochoscope is within the CBD, stone capture and extraction using a wire basket is performed in a manner identical to the one used during the transcystic approach (Table 4).

Choledochotomy Closure

Once all stones have been extracted successfully, the choledochotomy is closed. This is done using intracorporeal suturing and knot-tying techniques with 4-0 monofilament absorbable sutures. It is

---

TABLE 4: Procedure Steps and Required Equipment for Transcholedochal LCBDE

Procedural Step	Key Points	Instruments
1. Cholangiogram	• Perform IOC and determine that a transcystic LCBDE approach is not feasible based on either stone size (>10 mm), stone location (hepatic ducts), or number of stones (>5) • After IOC, ligate the cystic duct with clips	5F open tip cholangiogram catheter Olsen clamp
2. Choledochotomy	• Create a longitudinal incision in the CBD at least 1 cm in length and longer than the largest stone	Laparoscopic scissors (Potts, straight, or microcurved) *or* #11 blade scalpel held with a locking grasper
3. Choledochoscope insertion and maneuvering	• Use only a padded grasper to manipulate the scope to avoid damaging it • Insert the scope through the ductotomy • Start continuous irrigation through the scope's working channel	Choledochoscope Second laparoscopic tower with camera and light cable Saline irrigation (3-L bag or 1-L pressure bag) Padded grasper
4. Stone capture and extraction	• Pass the wire basket through the scope channel • Advance the basket in a closed position past the stone, then open it and "trawl" backward with the basket open to capture the stone • Close the basket around the stone, and slowly remove the scope and stone as a single unit	Endoscopic wire basket
5. Choledochotomy closure	• If the ductal system is clear of stones and sludge, the choledochotomy can be closed primarily using interrupted sutures • If any stones remain or if the CBD will need to be accessed later, a T-tube is positioned in the choledochotomy before closure around it	4-0 monofilament **absorbable** suture Laparoscopic needle drivers T-tube (10F to 14F)
6. Completion IOC	• Regardless of findings on LCBDE, perform a final IOC to confirm stone clearance and flow of contrast into the duodenum • If a T-tube was inserted, perform IOC through it. If not, remove the cystic duct clips to perform it	Same as initial IOC

CBD, Common bile duct; *IOC*, intraoperative cholangiography; *LCBDE*, laparoscopic common bile duct exploration.

important that permanent sutures not be used, as this will create a nidus for future primary CBD stone and stricture formation. We use interrupted sutures placed sequentially from superior to inferior to close the choledochotomy. Traditionally, surgeons placed a T-tube in the ductotomy closure for postoperative biliary drainage and in case subsequent cholangiogram or repeat access to the biliary tree was required. However, more recent evidence has shown that T-tube drainage does not improve postoperative morbidity, such as bile leak, cholangitis, or stricture, but it does result in longer operative time and hospital length of stay. For these reasons, we do not routinely place a T-tube during choledochotomy closure but reserve its use for cases in which there are retained stones in the CBD or we anticipate another reason that the CBD will need to be accessed postoperatively. After the choledochotomy has been closed, a completion IOC through the cystic duct is repeated to check for residual stones, ensure filling of the duodenum, and check for any leak from the choledochotomy closure. We generally leave an intraperitoneal drain after transcholedochal LCBDE to assess for and potentially control a bile leak, but this is not absolutely necessary if the surgeon is confident in the choledochotomy closure.

■ POSTOPERATIVE MANAGEMENT

After either transcystic or transcholedochal LCBDE, patients are managed similarly to those undergoing standard laparoscopic cholecystectomy. A liquid diet can be initiated immediately after surgery, and the patient can be advanced to solids as tolerated. We generally keep patients in the hospital for observation overnight and check liver function tests the morning after surgery to ensure a downward trend in their bilirubin level, but it is possible to perform LCBDE on an outpatient basis if the completion IOC is normal. Aside from a standard postoperative clinic visit, no additional specific follow-up or surveillance testing is necessary after LCBDE.

■ RESULTS

Morbidity and Mortality

LCBDE, whether performed via a transcystic or transcholedochal approach, is safe, with low rates of both postoperative morbidity and mortality. A Cochrane meta-analysis pooled data from five randomized controlled trials comparing one-stage LCBDE with two-stage ERCP plus laparoscopic cholecystectomy approaches and found no difference in terms of mortality, with both groups at or slightly below 1%. In that analysis, total morbidity was also similar in the two groups. Major complications, such as CBD injury and hemorrhage requiring return to the operating room, are extremely uncommon after LCBDE, occurring in approximately 1% of patients. Other complications, such as bile leak, wound infection, and those resulting from general anesthesia, occur in 10% to 15% of patients. One advantage of LCBDE over ERCP is lower rates of postprocedure pancreatitis, a potentially serious and even lethal complication that can occur in up to 5% of patients undergoing ERCP. After transcholedochal LCBDE, more serious bile leaks can occur if a T-tube drain is placed and becomes dislodged postoperatively. This can result in bile peritonitis, necessitating a return to the operating room. For this reason, we generally avoid the use of a T-tube, unless mandated because of one of the reasons described previously.

LCBDE fails to clear the CBD, resulting in retained stones postoperatively in 5% to 20% of patients. Again, this rate appears similar in LCBDE and an ERCP-based approach. However, one must keep in mind that if LCBDE initially fails to clear the CBD, the patient can then undergo a postoperative ERCP. The result is that the patient requires two procedures, the same as if ERCP had been utilized preoperatively before laparoscopic cholecystectomy.

Length of Stay and Hospital Costs

LCBDE has demonstrated a clear advantage over ERCP with respect to reducing overall hospital length of stay and costs. A population-based study by Poulose and colleagues showed an average reduction of almost 1 day in hospital stay, and randomized trials similarly have shown reductions in length of stay between 1 and 3 days. A mean overall savings of $4500 was determined in the population-based study, which after being adjusted for inflation would equate to $5290 in 2015 dollars.

■ SUMMARY

Although encountered frequently, choledocholithiasis is currently outside the purview of diseases typically treated by the general surgeon. This treatment pattern has evolved despite the fact that there is good evidence that LCBDE at the time of cholecystectomy results in improved patient outcomes and decreased costs when compared with a two-stage approach that includes ERCP for the clearance of the CBD. It is therefore incumbent on general surgeons to incorporate LCBDE into their armamentarium of treatment options for patients with gallstone disease and to make LCBDE a standard part of general surgery residency training. If general surgeons can "reclaim" the CBD as part of their standard practice, outcomes for tens of thousands of patients with choledocholithiasis in the United States each year could be improved.

SUGGESTED READINGS

Berci G, Hunter J, Morgenstern L, et al. Laparoscopic cholecystectomy: first, do no harm; second, take care of bile duct stones. *Surg Endosc*. 2013;27:1051-1054.

Crawford DL, Phillips EH. Laparoscopic common bile duct exploration. *World J Surg*. 1999;23:343-349.

Cuschieri A, Lezoche E, Morino M, et al. E.A.E.S. multicenter prospective randomized trial comparing two-stage vs single-stage management of patients with gallstone disease and ductal calculi. *Surg Endosc*. 1999;13:952-957.

Dasari BV, Tan CJ, Gurusamy KS, et al. Surgical versus endoscopic treatment of bile duct stones. *Cochrane Database Syst Rev*. 2013;(9):CD003327.

Helling TS, Khandelwal A. The challenges of resident training in complex hepatic, pancreatic, and biliary procedures. *J Gastrointest Surg*. 2008;12:153-158.

Houdart R, Perniceni T, Darne B, et al. Predicting common bile duct lithiasis: determination and prospective validation of a model predicting low risk. *Am J Surg*. 1995;170:38-43.

Noble H, Tranter S, Chesworth T, et al. A randomized, clinical trial to compare endoscopic sphincterotomy and subsequent laparoscopic cholecystectomy with primary laparoscopic bile duct exploration during cholecystectomy in higher risk patients with choledocholithiasis. *J Laparoendosc Adv Surg Tech A*. 2009;19:713-720.

Poulose BK, Arbogast PG, Holzman MD. National analysis of in-hospital resource utilization in choledocholithiasis management using propensity scores. *Surg Endosc*. 2006;20:186-190.

Rogers SJ, Cello JP, Horn JK, et al. Prospective randomized trial of LC+LCBDE vs ERCP/S+LC for common bile duct stone disease. *Arch Surg*. 2010;145:28-33.

Strasberg SM, Hertl M, Soper NJ. An analysis of the problem of biliary injury during laparoscopic cholecystectomy. *J Am Coll Surg*. 1995;180:101-125.

LAPAROSCOPIC 360-DEGREE FUNDOPLICATION

Daniel Boyett, MD, and Anne Lidor, MD, MPH

Gastroesophageal reflux disease (GERD) is defined as a condition that develops when the reflux of stomach contents causes troublesome symptoms or complications. GERD is one of the most common disease processes seen by both primary care physicians and gastroenterologists and accounts for 4 to 5 million office visits per year. An estimated 20% of the Western population suffers from GERD-related symptoms at least once per week.

■ SYMPTOMS AND COMPLICATIONS

Symptoms of GERD can be classified as typical, atypical, or extra-esophageal (Box 1). The cardinal symptom, heartburn (defined as a retrosternal burning sensation), is reported by 80% of patients and has high specificity but low sensitivity for the disease. Regurgitation is defined as the perception of refluxed gastric content into the mouth or hypopharynx. Extraesophageal symptoms are thought to be either caused by microaspiration of refluxate or a vagally mediated reflex (esophagobronchial reflex) triggered by exposure of the distal esophagus to acid. The shared vagal innervation of the cough reflex and the esophagus is believed to act as the pathway to GERD-related coughing. Complications of GERD can be classified as esophageal or extraesophageal (Box 2). Left untreated, these complications can progress to life-threatening conditions, including esophageal adenocarcinoma. Although no causal link has been shown, GERD has been associated with syndromes of dyspepsia and irritable bowel syndrome in up to 50% of patients.

■ DIAGNOSTIC WORKUP

Empiric Medical Therapy

The first step in the diagnosis of GERD in symptomatic patients is pharmacotherapy with proton pump inhibitors (PPIs) for the presumptive diagnosis of GERD. Resolution of symptoms after initiation of PPI therapy is considered confirmatory of the diagnosis. PPIs provide the most rapid symptomatic relief and heal esophagitis in the highest percentage of patients. Typical GERD symptoms recur within 1 year in more than 90% of patients after cessation of PPI therapy. Between 10% and 30% of patients with heartburn remain symptomatic on standard and even high-dose PPI treatment. Patients who have persistence of symptoms, additional signs of complex disease, or alarm symptoms (dysphagia, vomiting, anemia, involuntary weight loss) should prompt further workup. Likewise, patients with atypical symptoms or noncardiac chest pain as their primary complaint also should receive further diagnostic evaluation before empiric therapy.

Endoscopy

The first test of choice to either confirm the diagnosis of GERD or rule out other conditions is flexible esophagogastroduodenoscopy (EGD). It allows visualization of mucosal surfaces and diagnosis of complications of reflux disease, including ulcers, strictures, and Barrett's esophagus. This provides objective evidence of GERD. Ulcers, strictures, and polyps should undergo biopsy testing to rule out malignant disease.

Based on the findings at the time of endoscopy, patients can be classified further as having reflux symptoms without mucosal erosions (nonerosive reflux disease [NERD]) or reflux symptoms with mucosal breaks (erosive reflux disease [ERD]). ERD is found in up to 20% of patients with GERD and should be regarded as the most common complication of GERD. Barrett's esophagus is a condition in which the stratified squamous esophageal epithelium has been replaced by endoscopically detectable columnar metaplasia. This worrisome complication is present in 2% of the adult population and predisposes to esophageal adenocarcinoma. The results of large cohort studies suggest that the annual cancer risk for patients with nondysplastic Barrett's esophagus is 0.12% to 0.40%. Dysplasia within Barrett's esophagus lesions signals a marked increase in cancer risk and raises the annual risk to approximately 1% for patients with low-grade dysplasia and to more than 5% for patients with high-grade dysplasia.

pH and Impedance Testing

When unable to confirm the diagnosis of GERD by EGD, direct monitoring of the esophageal environment and correlation to subjective symptoms of reflux should be performed over a 24- to 48-hour period. This can be achieved via either a transnasally placed wired catheter or an endoscopically placed wireless device. Each method has its advantages and disadvantages. With the wireless method, a radiotelemetric pH-sensing capsule is secured to the mucosa of the distal esophagus approximately 6 cm proximal to the squamocolumnar junction and transmits data to a receiver worn on the patient's belt. The wireless method allows for greater patient comfort and longer recording times but requires endoscopy for placement and only allows for pH monitoring without impedance testing. The transnasal catheter method has multiple electrodes along the course of the catheter, which allows for detection of reflux into the upper esophagus as well as impedance testing. Impedance monitoring detects changes in the resistance to electrical current across adjacent electrodes, allowing it to differentiate the antegrade and retrograde bolus transit of both liquids and gas. This allows detection of both acid and nonacid reflux and is thus the test of choice for patients on PPI therapy. Impedance–pH monitoring has greater sensitivity than pH monitoring alone in the detection of GERD; however, catheter-based monitoring is less well tolerated, usually is limited to 24 hours, and makes it more difficult for patients to resume normal activity and eating habits while the catheter is in place. Regardless of the method used, a correlation between symptoms of reflux and objective signs of reflux is used to calculate a statistical measurement of the strength of the association between reflux events and symptoms. This helps to provide evidence that symptoms are being caused by GERD.

Barium Esophagram

The information provided by barium esophagram (or barium swallow) is insufficient to evaluate abnormal degrees of acid reflux but can be a good screening study, as severe reflux often can be noted during the examination. Esophagram is useful in defining patient anatomy (evaluation of hiatal hernia, shortened esophagus, etc.) and characterizing gastroesophageal motility. It is therefore useful before any surgical intervention is undertaken to better plan the surgery.

■ SURGICAL THERAPY

Indications for Surgery

GERD is a mechanical disorder that results from one or more of the following: an incompetent lower esophageal sphincter (LES; anatomically or functionally), impaired gastric emptying, or ineffective esophageal peristalsis. Although numerous treatment options exist for GERD, laparoscopic 360-degree fundoplication is the gold standard for reconstruction of a functioning LES. However, objective evidence of GERD is essential before any surgical intervention takes place. Once the diagnosis of GERD has been confirmed objectively, surgical intervention should be considered under certain

BOX 1: Symptoms of Gastroesophageal Reflux Disease

Typical

Heartburn, regurgitation

Atypical

Dysphagia, epigastric or chest pain, epigastric fullness, epigastric pressure, dyspepsia, nausea, bloating, belching

Extraesophageal

Chronic cough, bronchospasm, wheezing, hoarseness, sore throat, asthma, laryngitis, dental erosions

BOX 2: Complications of Gastroesophageal Reflux Disease

Esophageal

Barrett's esophagus, erosive esophagitis, esophageal ulcers, peptic strictures, esophageal adenocarcinoma

Extraesophageal

Laryngitis, laryngeal cancer, laryngeal nodules, globus, chronic bronchitis, pulmonary fibrosis, pneumonitis

BOX 3: Indications for Antireflux Surgery

- Patients who have failed medical management (inadequate symptom control, severe regurgitation not controlled with acid suppression, or medication side effects)
- Patients who opt for surgery despite successful medical management (because of quality of life considerations, lifelong need for medication intake, expense of medications, etc.)
- Patients who have complications of gastroesophageal reflux disease (e.g., erosive esophagitis, peptic stricture)
- Patients who have extraesophageal manifestations (asthma, hoarseness, cough, chest pain, aspiration)

BOX 4: Key Components of a Standardized Technique for Nissen Fundoplication

- The phrenoesophageal ligament is opened from left to right to approach the hiatus and distal esophagus.
- All attempts should be made to preserve the hepatic branch of the anterior vagus nerve.
- Complete dissection of both left and right crura.
- Generous transhiatal mobilization of the esophagus to allow approximately 3 cm of distal esophagus to rest within the abdominal cavity without tension.
- Division of all short gastric vessels to ensure a tension-free wrap.
- Posterior crural repair with nonabsorbable sutures.
- Creation of a 1.5- to 2-cm wrap of the mobile fundus around the intra-abdominal distal esophagus using nonabsorbable sutures. The sutures should be placed anteriorly, and the most distal suture should incorporate the anterior musculature of the esophagus.
- Large bougie placement at the time of wrap construction.

Technique

One criticism of laparoscopic 360-degree (Nissen) fundoplication is the lack of a standardized surgical technique leading to a perceived inability to see reproducible results from surgeon to surgeon. This lack of standardization has made it difficult to scientifically study surgical versus medical management strategies for GERD. The LOTUS (Long-Term Usage of Acid Suppression Medication with Surgery) trial included standardization of surgical technique in its design, and this standardization has been adopted by the SAGES guidelines (Box 4).

Positioning

At our institution, the patient is given general anesthesia and a Foley catheter is placed. The patient is then positioned supine, with arms extended and with a footboard. Appropriate padding is needed to allow for steep reverse Trendelenburg positioning. The surgeon stands to the patient's right, and the assistant stands to the patient's left. In addition, a camera holder and liver retractor device are secured to the bed. Some institutions prefer a split leg approach with the surgeon positioned between the patient's legs.

Port Placement

Laparoscopic access is gained with an optical trocar in the left subcostal (Palmer's point) region. The abdomen is insufflated and additional trocars are placed under direct visualization. A 12-mm camera port is placed at the dome of the abdomen, typically at the inferior edge of the falciform ligament. A 5-mm working port is placed in the right subcostal region, and a 12-mm second working port is placed approximately 10 cm inferiorly. A subxiphoid stab incision is used to introduce a Nathanson liver retractor. Both 30-degree and 45-degree laparoscopes can be used for the procedure

Early Gastric Mobilization and Left Crus Dissection

We begin with mobilization of the greater curve of the stomach by dividing the anterior and posterior short gastric vessels with an advanced energy device (bipolar or ultrasonic). This is carried up the greater curve, through the gastrosplenic ligament, until the left crus is identified (Figure 1). The angle of His is mobilized and the phrenoesophageal ligament is incised. The mediastinum is entered and the anterior surface of the esophagus is mobilized. Care is taken to identify and keep free from injury the anterior vagus nerve. The peritoneum is reflected off the esophagus from the patient's left to right. At this time any adherent fibers to the posterior portion of the left crus are also mobilized to facilitate the posterior dissection at a later time.

circumstances according to the SAGES (Society of American Gastrointestinal and Endoscopic Surgeons) guidelines (Box 3).

Patient Selection and Predictors of Success

Studies within the literature have shown that patients' symptomatic response to preoperative PPI treatment can be directly correlated to resolution of symptoms after fundoplication. Furthermore, patients who have poor compliance with preoperative PPI therapy are likely to have worse outcomes after surgery. Older age should not be considered a contraindication for surgical intervention, as long as the patient is otherwise an acceptable candidate for surgery. Outcomes in patients older than 65 years of age have been shown to be on par with those in younger patients. For patients with GERD and a body mass index (BMI) of more than 35 kg/m^2, gastric bypass, not fundoplication, should be considered if the patient is otherwise appropriate for bariatric surgery. Not only does fundoplication have a high failure rate in morbidly obese patients, but the procedure does not adequately address the underlying problem (obesity) that causes GERD, nor does it address a number of other medical conditions related to obesity for which there is opportunity for resolution.

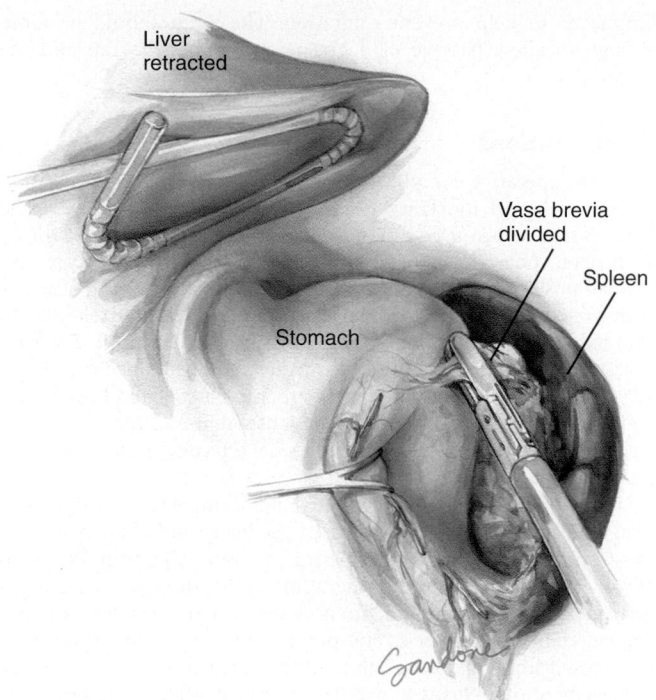

FIGURE 1 Early gastric mobilization with division of the short gastric vessels to allow visualization and dissection of the left crus.

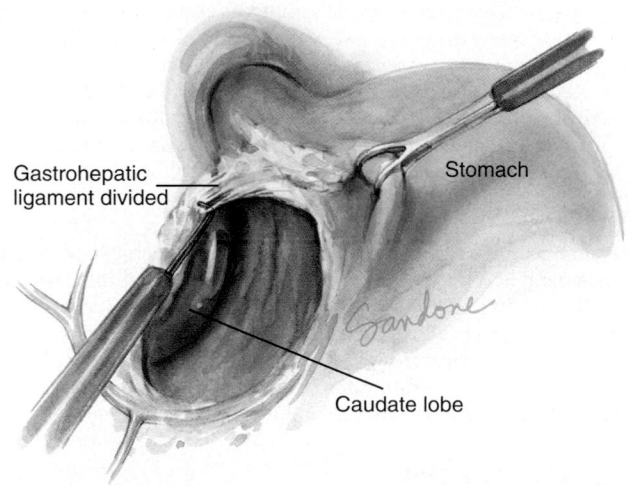

FIGURE 2 Division of the gastrohepatic ligament and dissection of the right crus.

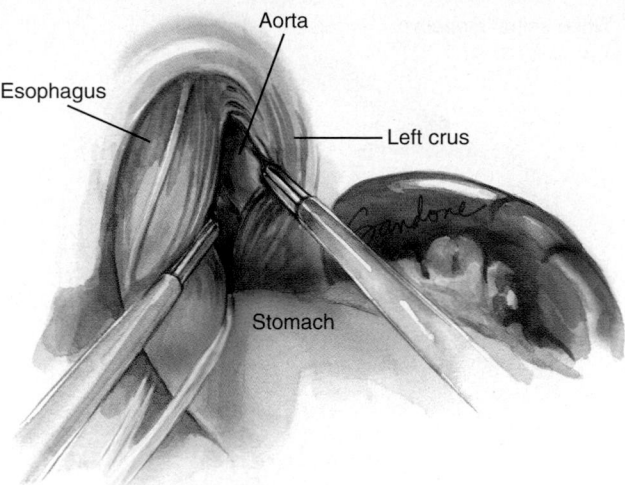

FIGURE 3 Circumferential mobilization of the esophagus using a Penrose drain for intra-abdominal retraction.

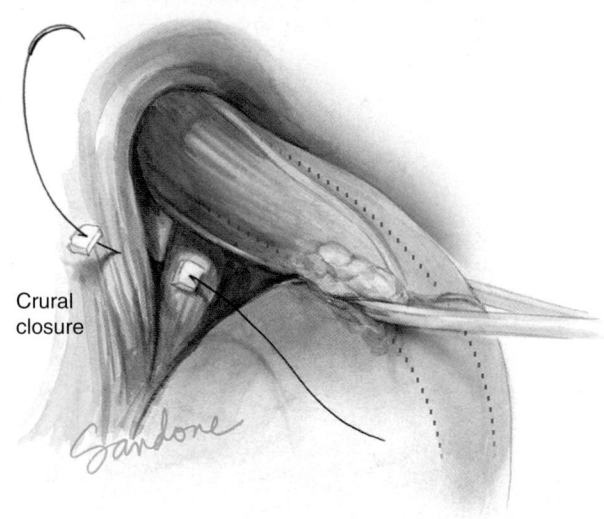

FIGURE 4 Tension-free interrupted posterior crural repair around a 52F bougie with preservation of the vagus nerve and 3 to 4 cm of intra-abdominal esophagus.

Right Crus Dissection

The gastrohepatic ligament is then divided through the avascular pars flaccida, revealing the caudate lobe of the liver and vena cava (Figure 2). Care should be taken at this time to preserve the hepatic branch of the anterior vagus nerve and to watch for aberrant anatomy such as a replaced left hepatic artery. This window is opened to expose the peritoneum overlying the right crus, which is incised. Then blunt dissection is utilized to mobilize the peritoneum anteriorly to connect with the previous anterior dissection and posteriorly along the right crus. This is continued until the posterior dissection connects with the previously mobilized left crus. Care needs to be taken during this dissection to protect the esophagus and posterior vagus nerves. A Penrose drain then is passed through this newly created window behind the esophagus at the level of the gastroesophageal junction and secured with a clip. Then this can be used as gentle retraction by the assistant. The esophagus then is further mobilized from the mediastinum using careful blunt dissection circumferentially to allow 3 to 4 cm of intra-abdominal length without traction or tension (Figure 3).

Crural Repair

The Penrose drain should be removed, and a 52F bougie is then carefully inserted through the mouth and into the esophagus and stomach. The crura are reapproximated posteriorly using interrupted nonabsorbable sutures. If the tissue quality of the crura is poor, bioabsorbable pledgets can be used to help reinforce these sutures (Figure 4). Typically a mesh is not needed in the absence of a large hiatal hernia, but if mesh is used, again a bioabsorbable option is recommended. This crural closure should be without tension and there should be 3 to 4 cm of esophagus freely within the abdominal cavity.

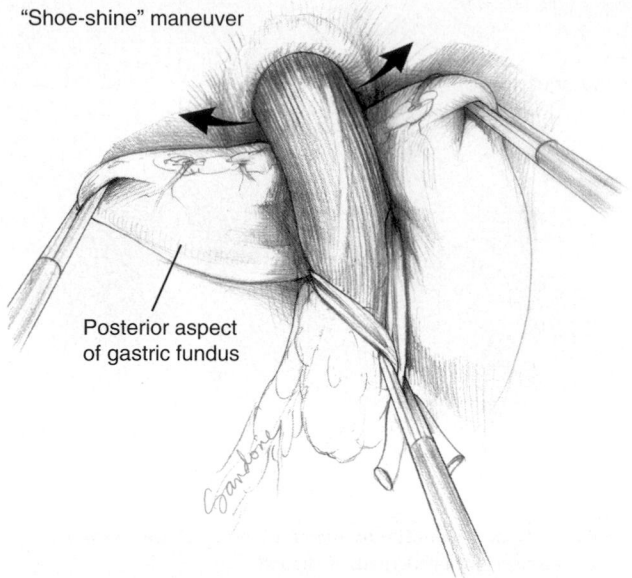

"Shoe-shine" maneuver

Posterior aspect
of gastric fundus

FIGURE 5 "Shoe-shine" maneuver helps to verify that the same portion of the fundus is being used for the edges of the wrap.

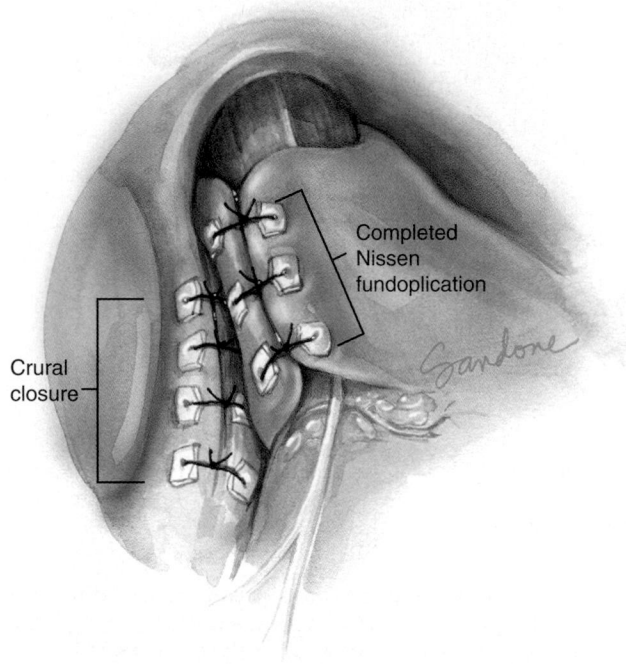

Crural
closure

Completed
Nissen
fundoplication

FIGURE 6 Completed 360-degree fundoplication with posterior crural repair.

Creation of Short and Floppy Fundoplication

The mobilized fundus then can be grasped through the posterior window and brought to the patient's right. It should lie without tension and be oriented to avoid any twisting. A "shoe-shine" maneuver (Figure 5) is done to ensure that the wrap is being done with the same part of the fundus. The wrap should lie over the distal esophagus above the Z-line and should stay in place without retraction. It then is secured using three interrupted nonabsorbable sutures, each placed 1 cm apart to create a short (2-cm) wrap (Figure 6). The inferiormost suture also should incorporate longitudinal fibers of the esophagus to help prevent migration. The wrap should be loose enough to allow passage of a grasper between the wrap and the esophagus.

Complications

Early postoperative complications after laparoscopic fundoplication are unusual, and mortality is rare (usually reported as 0%). The LOTUS trial, which used a standardized surgical approach, reported a 2% open conversion rate, 3% postoperative complication rate, and median postoperative length of stay of 2 days. Severe complications such as gastric or esophageal perforation are reported rarely (0% to 4%) but are more common in redo operations. Pneumothorax from aggressive dissection within the mediastinum can occur (0% to 1.5%) but is typically limited, as there is no associated lung injury and the pneumothorax arose from transabdominal thoracic insufflation through a pleural injury. These typically resolve without intervention.

Late complications include wrap migration, wrap slippage, dysphagia, recurrent reflux, post-Nissen gas bloat, and chest pain. The most common anatomic recurrence is wrap migration (0.8% to 26%). To help prevent this migration, some surgeons advocate a gastropexy to the diaphragm, but no reduction in migration rates has been demonstrated. Recurrent preoperative signs and symptoms often result from anatomic failure of the repair or wrap, but medical management often leads to excellent results in affected patients.

Most notable complications from fundoplication occur in the longer term. Wrap migration is the most common form of anatomic recurrence and occurs in approximately 10% of cases. Other forms of anatomic failure include slippage of the wrap onto the cardia of the stomach and twisting of the wrap. Any of these failures can lead to recurrent symptoms, most notably recurrent reflux symptoms, dysphagia, or chest pain. Atypical symptoms also may occur. Studies show that as many as 60% of patients are again placed on PPIs in the long term, but in most cases these treatments are not given based on objective evidence of recurrent reflux. In most of these patients, objective testing actually shows that pathologic reflux is not present. Approximately 3% to 4% of patients require revision.

Outcomes

Overall, outcomes for medical and surgical management of GERD are comparable. The LOTUS trial found no statistical difference in mortality or in GERD remission between medical and surgical groups but did find a lower prevalence of acid regurgitation in the surgical group. Surgical treatment also may result in better quality of life, with patient satisfaction rates ranging from 80% to 96%; 81% to 95% of patients state that they would undergo surgery again.

■ CONCLUSION

Laparoscopic Nissen fundoplication is an effective treatment option for correctly selected patients for the treatment of GERD. Careful preoperative planning is required to choose the most appropriate treatment for each patient.

SUGGESTED READINGS

Attwood S, Lundell L, Ell C, et al. Standardization of surgical technique in antireflux surgery: the LOTUS trial experience. *World J Surg.* 2008;32: 995-998.

Badillo R, Francis D. Diagnosis and treatment of gastroesophageal reflux disease. *World J Gastrointest Pharmacol Ther.* 2014;5:105-112.

Frazzoni M, Piccoli M, Conigliaro R, et al. Laparoscopic fundoplication for gastroesophageal reflux disease. *World J Gastroenterol.* 2014;20:14272-14279.

Rickenbacher N, Kötter T, Kochen MM, et al. Fundoplication versus medical management of gastroesophageal reflux disease: systematic review and meta-analysis. *Surg Endosc.* 2014;28:143-155.

LAPAROSCOPIC APPENDECTOMY

David Earle, MD, FACS

Surgical removal of the appendix is performed most commonly for acute appendicitis. However, it also can be performed for chronic appendicitis, incidentally or prophylactically, or for tumor. Although this chapter focuses on laparoscopic appendectomy related to acute appendicitis, many of the technical aspects may be applied to appendectomy for other conditions. Since the first description of a laparoscopic approach to appendectomy by German gynecologist Kurt Semm in 1983, there has been significant discussion about the technical details of the operation. Once the decision to perform an appendectomy has been made with the patient, it is of vital importance to note that the fundamental principles of appendectomy are the same regardless of approach. These principles include clear identification of the anatomy in order to completely remove the appendix, avoid injury to surrounding structures, and minimize the risk of short-term and long-term postoperative complications. Similar to the "critical view of safety" during cholecystectomy, appendectomy also has such a critical view. This view includes the base of the appendix, the mesoappendix, and the terminal ileum.

■ PATIENT SELECTION

The only absolute contraindication to a laparoscopic approach to appendectomy for appendicitis is a patient who is not a candidate for a surgical procedure. Otherwise, even in the most difficult cases, a laparoscopic approach still can be helpful. For example, a 55-year-old female patient is seen with 5 days of symptom duration, has diffuse peritonitis, and has a computed tomographic (CT) finding of intraperitoneal fluid with a right lower quadrant phlegmon or mass. For this patient, a laparoscopic approach would be expected to be extraordinarily difficult for an appendectomy, or for a proper right colon resection in an emergency scenario, but may reveal a perforated periappendiceal abscess amenable to laparoscopic drainage and peritoneal lavage rather than open laparotomy and right colon resection. This would allow achievement of the goal of treating the patient's sepsis due to a ruptured abscess and allow many diagnostic and therapeutic options for the future.

Obesity, formerly a relative contraindication to laparoscopy, has become an excellent indication for laparoscopy. This allows for excellent visibility to explore the entire peritoneal cavity through very small incisions and significantly lowers the risk of wound and intraperitoneal infectious complications compared with open approaches.

Even in the event of conversion to an open technique (which should be considered good judgment rather than a failure to complete the case laparoscopically), a laparoscopic approach can guide the surgeon to the appropriate location for the incision in the event that the appendix cannot be reached with the typical right lower quadrant incision.

A laparoscopic approach is also an excellent way to explore the abdomen in cases where the diagnosis is less clear, even during pregnancy. The likelihood of acute appendicitis can be ascertained by utilizing the clinical information at hand and is presented as a point system in Table 1.

■ SURGICAL TECHNIQUE

Equipment and Supplies

Once you have made the decision to proceed with a laparoscopic appendectomy, the operating room staff will anticipate efficient answers to their questions about what needs to be prepared. In addition to determining what you will need, you also must plan where the laparoscopic equipment will be placed. Informing your operating room team members in advance can improve the preparation process significantly. The ports required will be somewhat dependent on what instruments you will be using. In general, you will need a 10- to 12-mm port to remove the appendix and two 5-mm ports for the instruments and laparoscope. One of these may need to be a 10- to 12-mm port if a 10-mm scope is used, unless you are able to deploy a retrieval sac into the peritoneal cavity or are planning to remove the appendix without a retrieval sac, which will be described later. You will need a human or mechanical assistant to hold the laparoscope. The laparoscopic hand instruments necessary for this operation include two bowel graspers, one dissector, and one pair of scissors. Depending on your planned method of dividing the mesoappendix and ligating the appendiceal stump, you will need additional tools. The variable strategies for equipment are listed in Table 2. It is important to note, however, that there is no "best" method for division of the mesoappendix and appendix. The decision should be based on the patient's clinical scenario. Cases with minimal to no inflammation or adipose tissue generally will be more amenable to the less expensive options. Selective use of the more expensive options usually is reserved for cases with significant inflammatory reaction involving the mesoappendix and appendiceal base. In addition to the patient's clinical scenario, the availability and comfort level of the surgeon with the variety of techniques should be considered, along with other clinical needs that demand the time of the surgeon or operating room.

Room Setup

The operating room should be set up such that the monitor will be placed near the right hip of the patient. Only one monitor is necessary; however, if more than one monitor is available, their positions can be tailored to the local environment. Because the operative field is in the right lower quadrant, it is usually best for the surgeon and assistant to stand on the left side of the patient, necessitating that the left arm be placed at the patient's side, taking all appropriate precautions for proper positioning. The laparoscopy and suction and irrigation equipment can be placed at any location that does not interfere with the placement of the monitor or the location of all team members caring for the patient.

Urinary Bladder Decompression

The decision on whether or not to place a urinary bladder catheter is based on the clinical scenario and occasionally requires input from other team members. It is typically based on the anticipated length of the operation, with operations expected to last more than 3 hours having a catheter placed routinely. It is important to note that for laparoscopic appendectomy, a port is often placed in the midline suprapubic position, which in some patients will put the bladder at risk for injury. Placing a bladder catheter actually may increase the risk of injury because it will be more difficult to discern where the edge of the bladder is located if it is decompressed. For example, during some laparoscopic ventral hernia repairs, it is common to place a three-way bladder catheter in order to fill up the bladder to more easily discern its borders and thus minimize the risk of injury during dissection.

Port Placement

Port placement for any laparoscopic procedure should follow the same process. This includes making the incisions and placing the ports along an imaginary set of concentric rings surrounding the operative field. This is in contradistinction to an open operation, where the incision typically is placed directly over the operative field. The most common number of ports placed for a laparoscopic appendectomy is three, and they generally should be placed along the concentric lines surrounding the operative field in such a manner that the surgeon and assistant can work in an ergonomically favorable position. A typical port placement is shown in Figure 1. Advantages of this port placement include straightforward open access at the umbilicus to place a 10- to 12-mm port and the ability to easily extend the incision as needed for specimen extraction, then accurately close the fascia to avoid incisional hernia. A 5-mm port typically is used in the midline suprapubic region, but care must be taken to avoid injury to the bladder. It is a common misconception that decompressing the urinary bladder will help to avoid injury to it. On the contrary, the borders of a decompressed urinary bladder are more difficult to see, and thus decompression actually may increase the risk of bladder injury in some cases.

An alternative port placement may be used for patients with a less clear diagnosis of appendicitis and a need for exploration of the entire peritoneal cavity. Not only does this setup allow for better exploration of the entire peritoneal cavity, it also allows for appendectomy (Figure 2). The reason this setup is not used routinely for appendectomy is that the left upper quadrant extraction site is somewhat more difficult to expand if necessary and close the fascia compared with the periumbilical location.

The method of placement of the first port can be accomplished using an open or closed technique. Typically, at the periumbilical location an open technique is used, which allows placement of fascia closure sutures at the time of placement of the blunt tip trocar. If placing a Veress needle or optical port at the umbilicus, it is imperative to lift the abdominal wall because the great vessels are located in the midline. If using a left upper quadrant first trocar placement, an optical entry trocar with or without Veress needle can be used depending on the surgeon's training, experience, and equipment available. No single method has been shown to be superior to another, and the method the surgeon is most familiar with is generally the best option.

Single-port appendectomy consistently has shown no clinical advantage over multiport appendectomy. That does not mean the technique has no merit, but it should raise questions about the preoperative discussion with the patient, particularly because of the relatively increased risk of incisional hernia and the possibility that the operative field will not be seen as well because of the angle of view.

Ergonomics

The surgeon and assistant should be operating and assisting in an ergonomically favorable position. This will allow the best fine motor control of the instruments for the longest period of time. The ideal position is with the spine upright, the elbows adjacent to the trunk and flexed at 90 degrees, and the wrists straight at 180 degrees. Factors involved in maximizing the ability to work in an ergonomically favorable position include table height, patient position, surgeon height (with and without step stools), port placement, and how the instruments are held in the hand (Figure 3). Regarding patient position and table height, the left arm generally should be tucked at the patient's side, and the table should be placed in a left side down,

TABLE 1: A Practical Score for the Diagnosis of Appendicitis (Alvarado Score)

Symptoms	Migration of abdominal pain to the RLQ	1
	Anorexia (or acetone in the urine)	1
	Nausea or vomiting	1
Signs	Tenderness in the RLQ	2
	Rebound pain	1
	Elevated temperature (≥37.3°C)	1
Laboratory	Leukocytosis (>10,000)	2
	Shift to the left (in a differentiated WBC count) (e.g., neutrophilia >75%)	1

Cumulative Score

5-6 compatible with acute appendicitis

7-8 probable for acute appendicitis

9-10 very probable for acute appendicitis

A score of 5 or 6 may be observed. A score of 7 or higher should proceed to appendectomy. In the original 1986 monograph, MANTRELS was the mnemonic proposed by Dr. Alvarado to remember the components of the score.

Adapted from Alvarado A. A practical score for the early diagnosis of acute appendicitis. *Ann Emerg Med.* 1986;15:557-564.

RLQ, Right lower quadrant; *WBC,* white blood cell.

FIGURE 1 Operative set-up for laparoscopic appendectomy. The left arm is tucked to allow the assistant to stand adjacent to the patient. The 10-12 mm port site is typically used for the scope and specimen extraction. The two 5-mm ports are typically used for the surgeon's working ports and allow for an ergonomically favorable working position. The monitor is in line with the operative field.

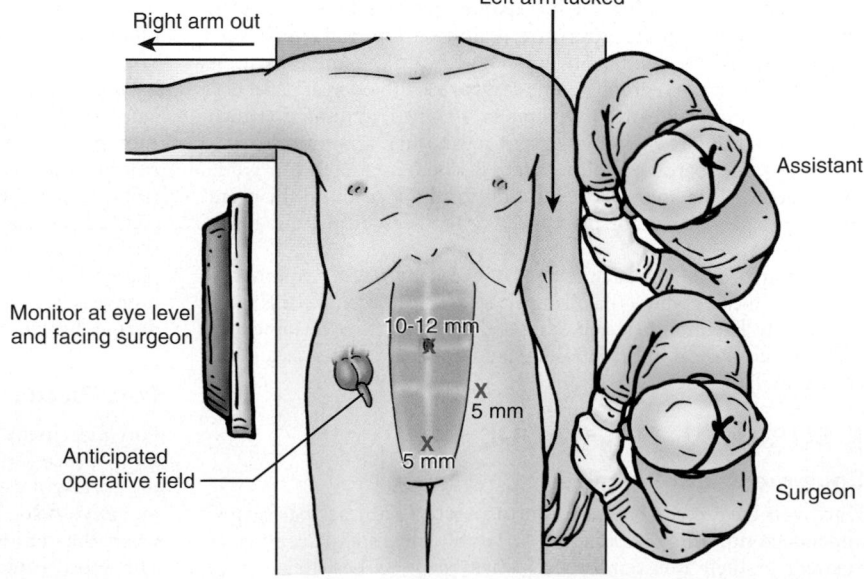

Right arm out

Left arm tucked

Assistant

Monitor at eye level and facing surgeon

10-12 mm

X 5 mm

X 5 mm

Anticipated operative field

Surgeon

TABLE 2: Details of Equipment Options for Laparoscopic Appendectomy

Method	Instruments	Advantages	Disadvantages	Comments
Suture ligation	Suture, knot pusher, pretied ligating loop ("endoloop"), dissector	Can be used for mesoappendix and appendix, commonly available, inexpensive	Requires skill not possessed by many surgeons, takes slightly more time to perform, separate tools needed for dissection	This skill is not often practiced by surgeons but can easily be performed with minimal training in a simulation environment.
Vascular clips	Vascular clip applier	Easy to use, quick, no assembly required for disposable instruments	Clips do not hold well with inflamed tissue surrounding mesoappendix, not applicable for most appendices because of size of appendix, some assembly required for reusable instruments	The term *vascular* is used to note the small size of these clips, which were not specifically designed to use for the appendiceal stump.
Appendectomy clips (metal or plastic)	Clip applier, clips	Easy to use, quick application, lower cost than disposable staplers and some energy sources	Not generally effective if appendiceal base is inflamed and/or indurated	Not widely available, relatively new to market
Monopolar energy	Hook, scissors, dissector	Commonly available, can be used for some dissection, requires 5-mm port, inexpensive	Wider thermal spread, worse for hemostasis on inflamed tissue and larger vessels, appropriate for mesoappendix only	It can be more difficult for novices to avoid adjacent tissue injury when using this method.
Bipolar energy	Bipolar forceps	Minimal thermal spread, effective on larger vessels compared with monopolar energy, works well in aqueous environment, typically reusable, inexpensive	Unfamiliarity with use among general surgeons, requires some assembly, relatively poor performance reliability compared with single-use instruments, appropriate for mesoappendix only	Performance reliability is affected by local instrument handling practices.
Advanced bipolar energy	Advanced bipolar generator and handpiece	Works well with vessels up to 7 mm in diameter, minimal thermal spread, no assembly required	Jaws not designed for dissection, usually only used on mesoappendix, expensive	There are a number of reports of safe use for the appendiceal stump; however, this is not commonly used clinically.
Ultrasonic energy	Ultrasonic generator and handpiece	Works well with vessels up to 5 mm in diameter, requires 5-mm port, can be used for dissecting and vessel ligation, less thermal spread compared with monopolar energy, quick hemostasis, easy to use	Despite minimal thermal spread, tip remains hot for a few seconds after use; requires some assembly; typically disposable; expensive; appropriate for mesoappendix only	Ultrasonic energy handpiece refers to a dissector-type device.
Stapler	Laparoscopic stapler handle, replaceable stapler cartridges	Quick, can be used for mesoappendix and appendix with separate cartridges	Requires some assembly, typically requires 10- to 12-mm port, does not work as well for hemostasis in inflamed tissue, cannot be used for dissection, expensive	Setup requires some dissection to separate the appendix and mesoappendix.

Of note, no significant clinical advantage of one technique over another has been shown consistently. Much of the literature advocates using the easiest, least expensive approach in easier cases and using more expensive technology selectively, such as with significant inflammation at the base of the appendix or within the mesoappendix.

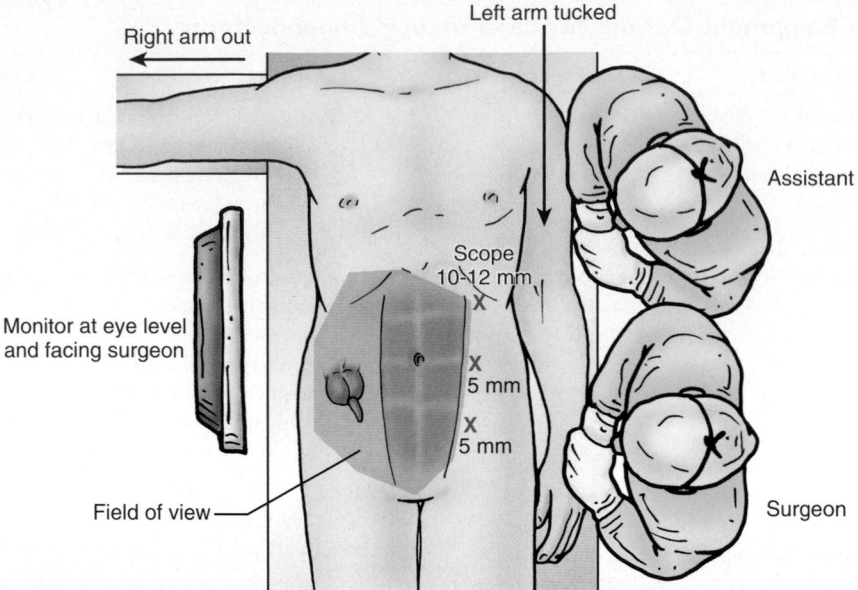

FIGURE 2 Alternative port placement for laparoscopic appendectomy. This is typically used when there is diagnostic uncertainty or a suspicion of increased technical difficulty.

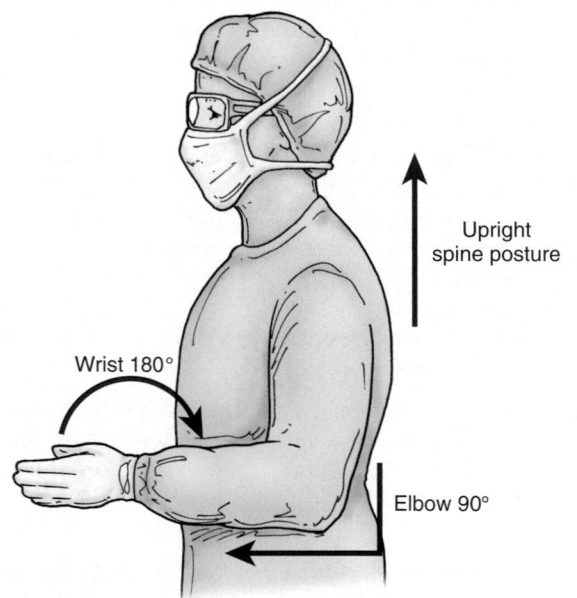

FIGURE 3 Ergonomically favorable position of the surgeon during laparoscopic appendectomy.

Trendelenburg position. This will help to expose the operative field and tilt the ports toward the surgeon and assistant, which will help to keep their elbows closer to their trunks. It occasionally may be necessary to hold the instrument without placing the thumb and middle finger through the loops of the handle. This frequently is referred to as "palming" and requires some practice, but it is readily incorporated into one's armamentarium in a short period of time.

Operative Steps and the Critical View of Safety

Once the ports are in, the patient is placed in the left side down, Trendelenburg position. The surgeon's first job is to locate the appendix. This should be done by carefully manipulating the small bowel or omentum out of the right lower quadrant in order to identify the cecum. Once the cecum is identified, find the terminal ileum. The appendiceal base is located on the cecum, just distal to the terminal

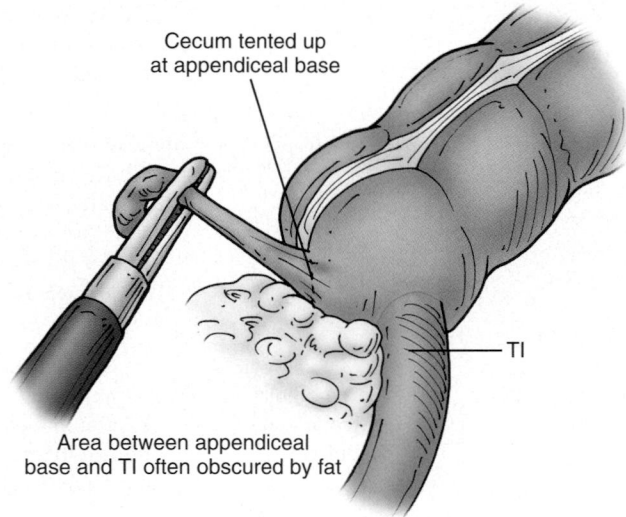

FIGURE 4 Visualization of the appendix before removal. *TI*, Terminal ileum.

ileum. This sequence of events usually takes less than 5 minutes. Once the base of the appendix has been identified, it can be used to follow toward the tip of the appendix. Depending on the individual anatomy, the entire appendix may be visible straight away or, if it occupies a retrocecal position, will need to be dissected out. In any case, finding the base first is usually easiest and will lead to the remainder of the appendix. It is important to avoid injury to the iliac vessels and ureter, both of which are not visible but at risk for injury in cases where the appendix is stuck to the retroperitoneum.

Once the appendix has been identified and dissected free, it can be removed from the mesoappendix and cecum. Methods and techniques for this procedure are outlined in Table 2. Regardless of the specific technique used, it is important to obtain the critical view of safety before removing the appendix from the cecum. In this view, the surgeon should be able to identify the appendiceal base, with a small portion of the cecum tented up, as well as the space between the appendiceal base and the terminal ileum (Figure 4). The mesoappendix usually is divided first, but it can be divided before or after this view is obtained. Division of the mesoappendix will depend on the clinical scenario and anatomy. The development of this critical anatomic view allows the surgeon to avoid ligating too close to the terminal ileum, which can cause obstruction, and avoid leaving a long stump of the appendix, which can lead to the entity known as "stump appendicitis."

Specimen Removal

Once the appendix had been excised, it needs to be removed from the peritoneal cavity. Although there are no data to support one technique of specimen removal over another for laparoscopic appendectomy, it can be inferred from other types of specimen extraction data that removing the appendix without allowing it to drag unprotected through the subcutaneous tissue and skin is the most common and logical technique. This can be accomplished with a variety of commercially available or "homemade" specimen retrieval sacs or simply by pulling the unprotected specimen through the lumen of the port if the size is appropriate.

Exiting the Abdomen

It is generally also a good idea to irrigate the area with plain saline solution. Our technique utilizes small amounts of irrigation that are frequently suctioned out. This will avoid the irrigation fluid mixed with contaminated peritoneal fluid from being spread to parts of the peritoneal cavity that cannot be accessed readily with the laparoscopic suction device. Once the operative field has been irrigated and inspected for bleeding and the appendiceal stump has been checked for complete excision and integrity, it is wise to look in the pelvis and upper abdomen briefly to ensure that there are no major collections of contaminated fluid or blood. Finally, laparoscopically observe the removal of the ports and make sure the fascia is closed properly for midline 10- to 12-mm ports. Closure of left upper quadrant 10- to 12-mm ports is performed at the surgeon's discretion based on training and experience as well as specific circumstances of the case. The skin is routinely closed, even for perforated appendicitis.

■ POSTOPERATIVE CARE

Antibiotics are not routinely given postoperatively. If there is residual indurated mesenteric inflammation, a longer course of antibiotics is utilized. Diet and activity are advanced as tolerated by the patient, with no specific restrictions. Appropriate postoperative laboratory work and imaging are performed based on the clinical scenario, and neither of these is performed as a matter of routine. Patients are discharged from the hospital when their pain is adequately controlled, they are able to maintain hydration without intravenous fluid, and they feel comfortable with being discharged to their living environment. Although the diagnosis of acute appendicitis in the pathologic specimen is common, and definitively treated with appendectomy, there is a less than 1% to 14% chance of unexpected disease, some of which would prompt additional investigation and treatment. Although the incidence of this is low, the potential morbidity for the individual is high; therefore we routinely perform histopathologic examination and inform the patient of the findings.

■ LAPAROSCOPIC APPENDECTOMY DURING PREGNANCY

Although there are conflicting data about the use of laparoscopic appendectomy versus open appendectomy during pregnancy, a laparoscopic approach is generally considered to have a number of advantages over open approaches for nonpregnant patients, namely, less overall stress, less pain, fewer wound complications, and shorter hospital stay. There is no evidence to suggest that these advantages are lost during pregnancy. It also has been shown that laparoscopy can be performed safely during any trimester, and thus necessary surgical intervention should not be delayed because of the stage of fetal development. With regard to fetal loss and preterm labor, successful treatment of the mother remains the primary goal because delayed treatment may lead to worse outcomes. There are some logical and necessary modifications to a standard laparoscopic approach for appendectomy in pregnant patients. These include medication choices, patient positioning (left side down preferred), initial and secondary trocar placement (to avoid injury to the gravid uterus), and the use of the lowest insufflation pressure possible that still maintains adequate exposure of the operative field (usually around 12 mm Hg). Intraoperative capnography is sufficient to monitor and adjust hypercarbia. Intraoperative and postoperative pneumatic compression stockings are sufficient for deep venous thrombosis (DVT) prophylaxis. Obstetrical consultation preoperatively and preoperative and postoperative fetal heart monitoring should be strongly considered, unless the clinical circumstances dictate otherwise. Tocolytics should not be used as a matter of routine but should be used when signs of preterm labor are present.

■ ALTERNATIVE MINIMALLY INVASIVE TECHNIQUES

It is beyond the scope of this chapter to discuss the details of newer methods of performing a minimally invasive appendectomy, but they are mentioned here briefly. Novel methods that currently exist but are not commonly utilized for a variety of reasons include (1) use of robotically assisted surgical devices, (2) use of natural orifice transluminal endoscopic surgery (NOTES) methods with rigid laparoscopic instruments and/or a flexible endoscope, and (3) inversion appendectomy performed with a flexible colonoscope.

SUGGESTED READINGS

Drake FT, Flum DR. Improvement on the diagnosis of appendicitis. *Adv Surg.* 2013;47:299-328.

Emre A, Akbulut S, Bozdag Z, et al. Routine histopathologic examination of appendectomy specimens: retrospective analysis of 1255 patients. *Int Surg.* 2013;98:354-362.

Gomes CA, Nunes TA, Soares C, et al. The appendiceal stump closure during laparoscopy: historical, surgical, and future perspectives. *Surg Endosc Endosc Percutan Tech.* 2012;22:1-4.

Gorter RR, et al. Diagnosis and management of acute appendicitis. EAES consensus development conference 2015. *Surg Endosc.* 2016;30:4668-4690.

Korndorffer JR Jr, Fellinger E, Reed W. SAGES guideline for laparoscopic appendectomy. *Surg Endosc.* 2010;24:757-761.

Markar SR, Penna M, Harris A. Laparoscopic approach to appendectomy reduces the incidence of short- and long-term post-operative bowel obstruction: systematic review and pooled analysis. *J Gastrointest Surg.* 2014;18:1683-1692.

Pearl J, Price R, Richardson W, et al. Guidelines for diagnosis, treatment, and use of laparoscopy for surgical problems during pregnancy. *Surg Endosc.* 2011;25:3479-3492. <http://www.sages.org/publications/guidelines/guidelines-for-diagnosis-treatment-and-use-of-laparoscopy-for-surgical-problems-during-pregnancy/>.

Shogilev DJ, Duus N, Odom SR, et al. Diagnosing appendicitis: evidence-based review of the diagnostic approach in 2014. *West J Emerg Med.* 2014;15:859-871.

Swank HA, van Rossem CC, van Geloven AA, et al. Endostapler or endoloops for securing the appendiceal stump in laparoscopic appendectomy: a retrospective cohort study. *Surg Endosc.* 2014;28:576-583.

LAPAROSCOPIC INGUINAL HERNIORRHAPHY

Andrew Bates, MD, and Aurora D. Pryor, MD

More than 750,000 inguinal herniorrhaphies are performed yearly in the United States, making it the most common general surgery procedure performed. The yearly cost of these procedures is $2.5 billion. Men have a 27% risk of developing an inguinal hernia in their lifetime, whereas women have a 3% risk. The cause is multifactorial, including repeated abdominal straining, hereditary collagen diseases, and increased intra-abdominal pressure. In men, the migration of the testes through the inguinal canal may result in a patent processus vaginalis, thus leading to the increased indirect hernia rates in men. Direct hernias are caused by attenuated transversalis fascia lateral to the rectus abdominis muscle above the inguinal ligament. Femoral hernias, which often are mistaken for inguinal hernias and occur more commonly in females, occur medial to the femoral vein in the femoral canal and carry a higher rate of incarceration and strangulation.

Although there are a few therapies aimed at symptomatic control of inguinal hernias, the only definitive therapy is surgical repair. A patient may wear a hernia truss to prevent the protrusion of the hernia and the associated pain, although this is palliative and some suggest it may increase the rate of bowel injury if used long term.

There are many benefits of laparoscopic repair over the traditional open approach, including the ability to examine the entirety of the myopectineal orifice, the ability to visualize and repair all types of hernias originating in the inguinal region, and the ability to repair bilateral inguinal hernias through the same incisions. In addition, by incorporating an underlay mesh technique, the laparoscopic approach avoids the level of mesh fixation and related pain required during an open onlay technique and requires fewer postoperative activity restrictions than typically advised after open repair. Patients have been shown to require less analgesia after laparoscopic repair and have quicker return to their normal activities. Perhaps most important, recurrence rates after laparoscopic repair have been shown to be equivalent to recurrence rates after open repair in most studies.

Many surgeons suggest that it is more difficult to achieve proficiency in the laparoscopic approach, which can influence complication rates and cost. The complication rate improves after a surgeon has performed about 250 cases. Because of this learning curve, the procedure may take longer to perform and may lead to increased operative costs in early cases. However, these costs cannot be viewed in a vacuum. According to the LEVEL-Trial, the direct surgical costs for inguinal herniorrhaphy were higher for the laparoscopic approach, although the social costs of missed work days and extended convalescence conferred a cost savings for the technique when compared with open herniorrhaphy. Subsequent studies have shown cost equivalence when including both social and medical costs. The laparoscopic technique remains an attractive option for patients when it is used by a proficient surgeon.

■ PATIENT ASSESSMENT

Patients with symptomatic inguinal hernias, whether secondary to pain, incarceration, or functional limitation, are candidates for surgical repair unless the patient cannot tolerate a surgical procedure because of comorbidity. According to Fitzgibbons and colleagues, asymptomatic or minimally symptomatic men have the option of "watchful waiting," or observation, of their hernia with a low risk of incarceration or need for emergent repair. However, this study noted a crossover rate of 23% from the observation group to the surgical group, mostly because of increasing pain and symptoms.

Although patients typically have detailed descriptions of their hernias, numerous details should be ascertained during the patient evaluation. The timing and chronicity of the symptoms, the presence of any visible or palpable bulge, and the relation of symptoms to certain activities is of particular importance. The patient should be asked to relay any symptoms suggestive of bowel obstruction. Comorbidities that may increase intra-abdominal pressure, such as pulmonary disease (coughing), liver disease (ascites), constipation, or obesity, should be assessed. The patient should be asked to describe typical daily activities and primary occupation to help identify sources of muscle straining and possible risk factors for hernia recurrence.

Physical examination for inguinal hernias should be performed both standing and supine. Initial inspection should note any obvious bulge, tenderness, or skin changes at the site. If the hernia is protruding at the time of examination, reduction of hernia contents should be attempted (unless there is significant suspicion for compromised bowel). Examination of the inguinal canal is performed by invaginating the redundant skin of the scrotum with the index finger superiorly and laterally to the level of the pubic tubercle. At this level, the external inguinal ring can be palpated. The patient then can be asked to perform a Valsalva maneuver either by cough or by abdominal strain. Indirect hernias can be palpated as originating from the inguinal canal, whereas direct hernias are palpated as external compression on the external inguinal ring.

One of the traditional indications for a laparoscopic repair instead of an open repair is the presence of bilateral hernias. However, Griffin and colleagues noted that 22% of patients with an inguinal hernia have an occult hernia on the other side. Laparoscopic repair offers the ability to detect and repair these missed hernias in the same surgical procedure without additional incisions. Moreover, recent data have shown that 6% of patients who undergo a unilateral hernia repair subsequently will develop symptoms and require repair of a contralateral, previously asymptomatic inguinal hernia.

■ INDICATIONS AND CONTRAINDICATIONS

The indications for laparoscopic inguinal herniorrhaphy are typically the same as those for open repair, with a few nuances. Previously, the presence of an inguinal hernia was an indication for repair given the risk of incarceration and strangulation. However, after multiple studies showed this risk to be less than 1% over time, this strategy was largely abandoned in favor of "watchful waiting" for asymptomatic or minimally symptomatic hernias. Symptomatic hernias remain an indication for repair. Observation of asymptomatic hernias does not appear to alter the complication rate if surgery is performed later, and there appears to be no increase in hernia-related symptoms. However, at least one large randomized trial has shown that a large percentage of patients who originally elected to observe their asymptomatic hernia subsequently required repair because of the onset of symptoms. This crossover rate has led some surgeons to abandon watchful waiting if the patient wishes to proceed with repair.

Traditionally, the indications for a laparoscopic approach instead of an open procedure include bilateral hernias or recurrent hernias after an open repair. The nature of the laparoscopic technique allows for the repair of bilateral defects using the same incisions, and the use of a fresh dissection plane makes it ideally suited for recurrent repair.

Laparoscopic repair confers increased operating room and hospital costs, which originally led surgeons and policymakers to preferentially recommend open repair as cost-effective care. The added cost associated with laparoscopic repair results from added time in the operating room, the need for laparoscopic equipment, and the prosthetic material. However, subsequent outcomes data showed that patients who underwent laparoscopic repair had a quicker return to their daily activities, including a quicker return to work. Given this difference in workforce productivity, additional economic data showed cost equivalence when including both medical and societal costs.

The choice between transabdominal preperitoneal (TAPP) and total extraperitoneal (TEP) approaches for laparoscopic repair usually is made based on surgeon proficiency and the patient's physical examination and surgical history. If the patient has had a previous surgery that violated the preperitoneal space, such as a prostatectomy, or a previous infraumbilical midline incision, TAPP repair may be easier because of scarring and disruption of the surgical planes. Higher degrees of scarring may make dissection more difficult, increasing the chance of peritoneal tears. Patients with a large amount of abdominal contents in their hernia or incarceration also may be better served by a TAPP repair given the greater ease in reducing the contents back into the abdomen.

Contraindications to TEP or TAPP repair include severe illness that precludes general anesthesia, significant coagulopathy, and active infection. An acutely incarcerated hernia poses a greater risk of bowel injury via laparoscopic repair, although more surgeons are gaining comfort at performing this procedure. Sliding hernias, large scrotal hernias, and the presence of ascites are also relative contraindications to laparoscopic repair.

■ ANATOMY

Both TEP and TAPP repairs utilize the preperitoneal space (Figure 1). The preperitoneal space is defined as the space between the peritoneum and the transversalis fascia. The space of Retzius is defined as the retropubic preperitoneal space between the bladder posteriorly and between the two medial umbilical ligaments. The entry into this space is particularly important in TEP repair. Laterally, the space of Bogros continues in the same preperitoneal plane toward the anterior superior iliac spine (ASIS). The spaces of Retzius and Bogros are both completely dissected in order to reduce the hernia sac, define the proper inguinal anatomy, and place the mesh.

The midline in the surgical space is marked by the pubic symphysis, which is the cartilaginous connection between the pubic rami. Just lateral to the symphysis in either direction is the pubic tubercle, which is important in mesh fixation. Cooper's ligaments are a lateral extension of the lacunar ligament and form the periosteum of the superior pubic rami. Cooper's ligaments are important

in proper definition of anatomy and also serve as a point of fixation for the mesh.

All inguinal hernias originate through the myopectineal orifice of Fruchaud. The boundaries include the rectus abdominis medially, the iliopsoas laterally, the arch of the transversus abdominis superiorly, and the pectineal (Cooper's) ligaments inferiorly. The iliopubic tract, or inguinal ligament, divides inguinal hernias from femoral hernias and divides the myopectineal orifice into superior and inferior regions. The tract is a thickened fold of transversalis fascia, running from the ASIS to the pubic tubercle. The femoral space contains the external iliac vessels; any potential femoral hernia typically is located medial to the vessels.

The inferior region of the myopectineal orifice can be subdivided into two clinically significant areas (Figure 2). The "Triangle of Doom" is so named for the potentially catastrophic vascular injuries that can occur. Its borders include the vas deferens medially and the spermatic vessels laterally, coming to its apex at the inguinal ring. The "Triangle of Pain" is lateral to the spermatic vessels and below and lateral to the inguinal ligament. It is so named for the

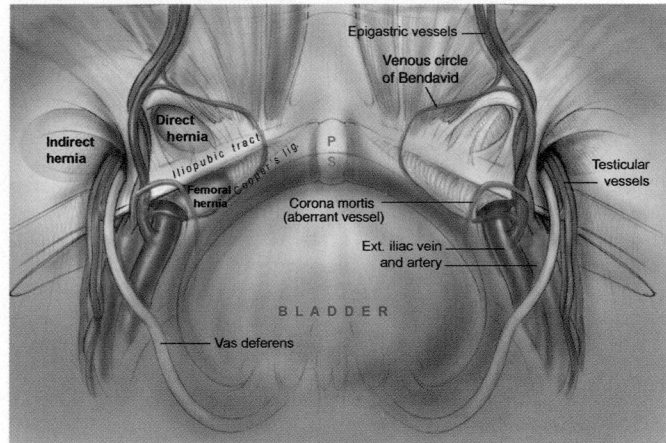

FIGURE 1 Groin defects and vasculature. This illustrates the laparoscopic total extraperitoneal view looking inferiorly in the preperitoneal space, noting the possible vascular anatomy that should be identified and avoided.

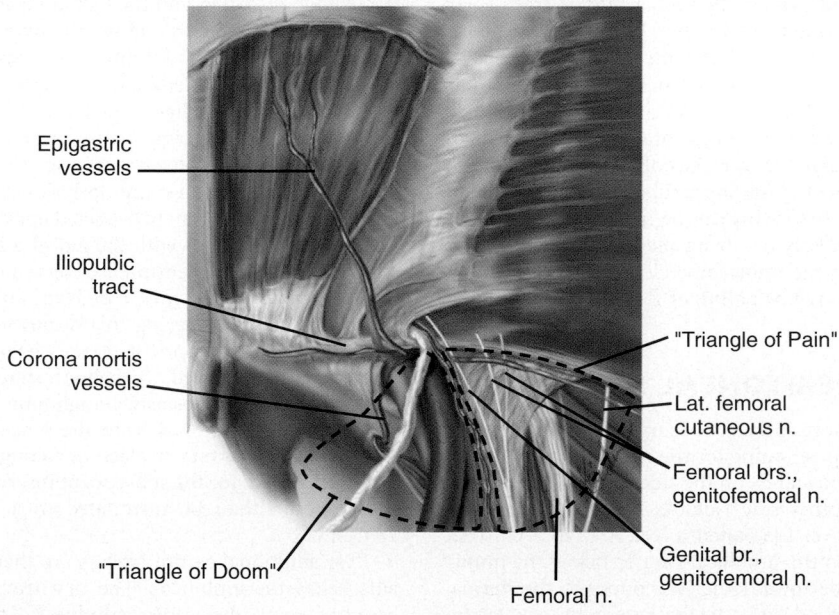

FIGURE 2 Clinical anatomy of the myopectineal orifice, defining the "Triangle of Pain" and "Triangle of Doom" to be identified during blunt dissection.

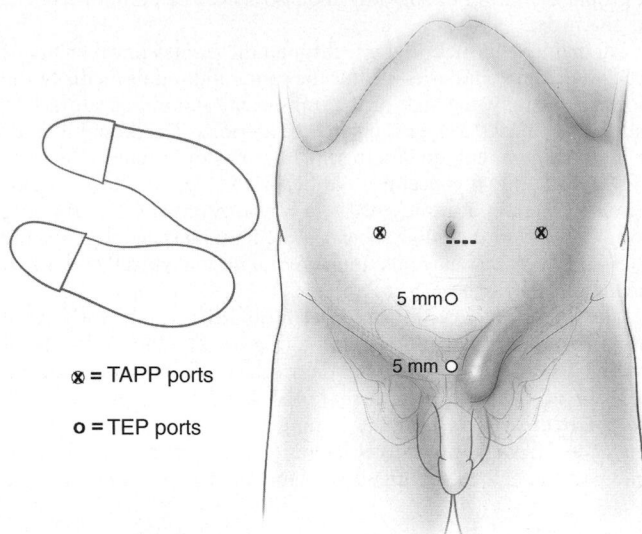

FIGURE 3 Proper patient and trocar positioning for total extraperitoneal (TEP) and transabdominal preperitoneal (TAPP) repair. Trocars should be positioned with sufficient space between them to allow for adequate hand motion.

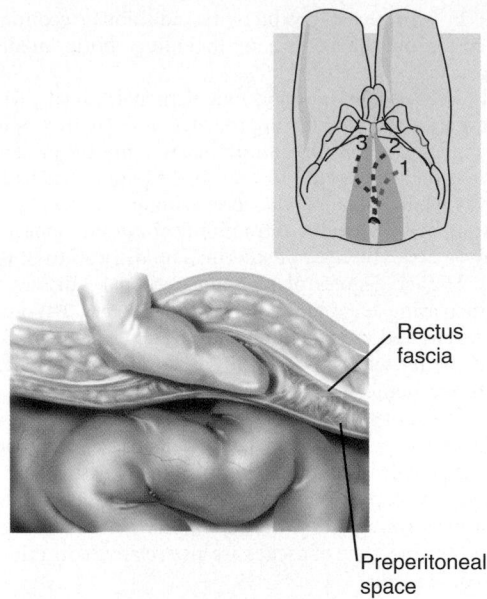

FIGURE 4 Blunt dissection of the preperitoneal space. The medial border of the rectus muscle should be retracted laterally to enter the space with minimal bleeding.

numerous nerves that cross this space and the potential for nerve injury or irritation, thus producing inguinodynia. The lateral femoral cutaneous nerve, femoral branch of the genitofemoral nerve, and inferior branch of the femoral nerve all run through this space.

Inguinal hernias are subdivided into direct and indirect defects. Direct defects occur within Hesselbach's triangle, which is defined as the space between the inferior epigastric vessels, rectus muscles, and Cooper's ligaments inferiorly. Indirect hernias protrude through the inguinal canal, which is lateral to Hesselbach's triangle. Indirect defects are more likely to be congenital in nature, often representing a failure of the processus vaginalis to close, although they can grow over time because of environmental factors. Direct defects are more likely to represent attenuated abdominal fascia.

During dissection of the preperitoneal space, knowledge of normal and aberrant circulation can help to avoid unnecessary bleeding and prevent postoperative hematoma formation. The inferior epigastric vessels ascend toward the rectus muscle from their origin off the external iliac vessels. About 20% of patients will have a corona mortis vessel, which runs from the inferior epigastric artery to the obturator artery, coursing across Cooper's ligaments and medial to the femoral canal. If this vessel is injured, it can produce significant and stubborn bleeding. The vessel often retracts if divided, making prompt control crucial. A rich plexus of veins also lies in the preperitoneal space, composed of the suprapubic, retropubic, rectal, and deep epigastric veins. These veins can be injured on blunt dissection of the space, particularly overlying the pubic tubercle. The veins lying just posterior to the pubic tubercle are also difficult to control once injured, and rough palpation of the tubercle should be avoided.

■ TOTAL EXTRAPERITONEAL REPAIR

The patient should void before surgery. Urinary catheter placement is unnecessary. The correct positioning for the patient is supine with the arms tucked. The surgeon stands on the side opposite the hernia with the assistant on the other side (Figure 3). The laparoscopic monitor should be placed over the patient's feet. A 1- to 2-cm skin incision is then made within the umbilical ring or below the umbilicus slightly off the midline toward the side opposite the hernia. Blunt dissection is then carried down to the anterior rectus fascia. The fascia is then incised sharply in a transverse fashion, taking care

not to cut the underlying rectus abdominis in order to maintain hemostasis and exposure. The medial border of the rectus abdominis is then retracted laterally to expose the posterior sheath of the rectus abdominis and enter the space of Retzius. This space can be developed bluntly with a finger or a retractor (Figure 4) down to the level of the arcuate line, where the posterior sheath is composed solely of thin peritoneum. The surgeon may elect to insert a balloon trocar into the space and complete the blunt dissection using the laparoscope. This can be facilitated with an S-shaped retractor.

Many surgeons use a balloon dissection device to develop the preperitoneal space below the arcuate line (Figure 5). The balloon dissector should be inserted into the space of Retzius and directed inferiorly, keeping as shallow an insertion angle as possible, over the symphysis pubis. This trajectory prevents injury to the urinary bladder. A palpable release should be felt as the dissector passes through the arcuate line. A 10-mm laparoscope is then inserted into the balloon dissector, and the balloon is inflated under direct visualization. The surgeon should see the peritoneum separating posteriorly with the rectus abdominis anteriorly. The surgeon also should observe the inferior epigastric vessels running along the rectus abdominis laterally. These vessels can be found as originating near the internal inguinal ring and appear as a purple stripe running superiorly. If these vessels are dissecting posteriorly, the balloon should be repositioned more posterior in order to direct the vessels anteriorly. Inappropriately dissected epigastric vessels can be secured after trocar placement with the aid of a temporary transabdominal suture. If bowel or omentum is observed posteriorly, the peritoneum has been violated and the procedure can be converted to the TAPP or open approach. Barring this occurrence, the balloon should be inflated until a portion of Cooper's ligaments can be visualized. If bleeding is encountered, the balloon should be kept inflated temporarily to provide hemostasis though tamponade. The balloon is then desufflated and removed from the space, either keeping the trocar portion of the system in place or taking care to use a retractor to reserve the space for the subsequent insertion of a 10-mm trocar. The space should then be insufflated to a pressure between 12 and 15 mm Hg.

Two additional 5-mm trocars are then placed through the linea alba below the umbilicus. The first trocar is placed 2 to 3 fingerbreadths above the pubic symphysis. The second is placed at the midpoint between the lower trocar and umbilicus. Placing these

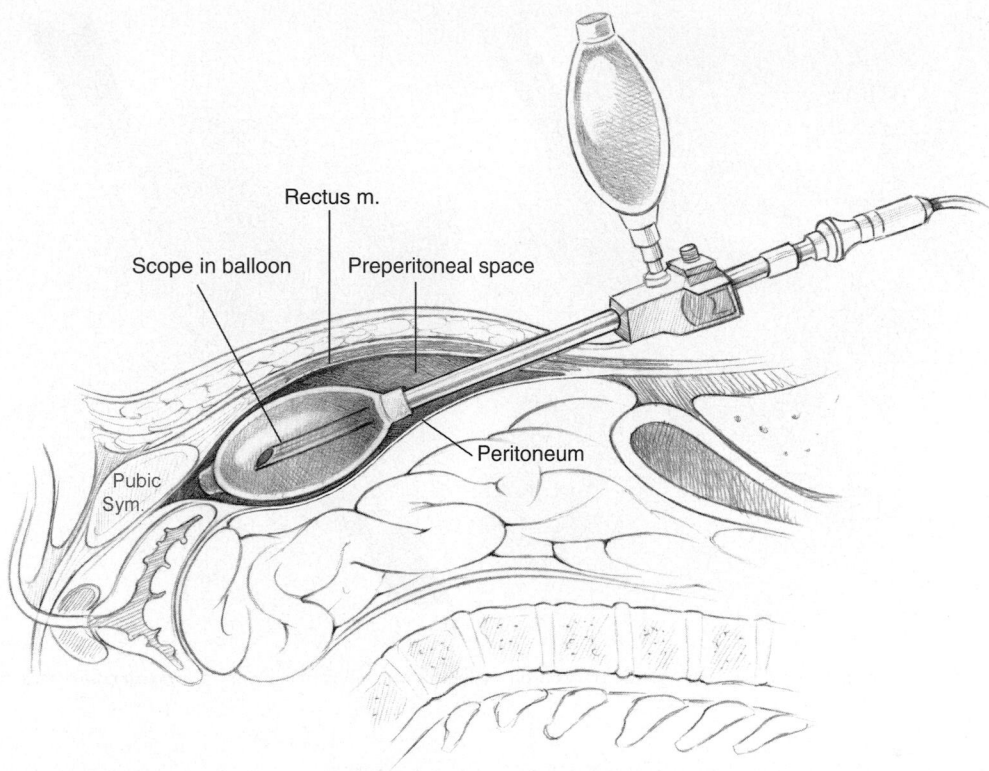

FIGURE 5 Insertion of the balloon dissector. The trajectory should remain shallow to avoid peritoneal tears.

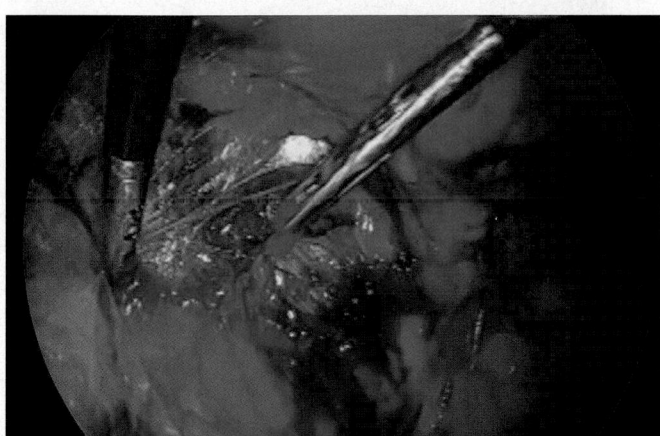

FIGURE 6 Lateral dissection of the space of Bogros. This space can be entered more easily just posterior to the origin of the epigastric vessels.

trocars as high as possible facilitates subsequent mesh placement. Trocars also can be placed off midline, away from the hernia in unilateral cases. If greater visualization is needed, the patient can be placed in Trendelenburg position.

The dissection is started at the midline, clearly identifying the pubic symphysis and clearing it of areolar tissue (Figure 6). When doing this, the surgeon should try to avoid scraping the periosteum, as this can produce stubborn bleeding that can be difficult to control. The areolar tissue is then continued laterally to expose Cooper's ligaments to the level of the femoral canal. It is in this area that the aberrant corona mortis may be found, which if injured must be grasped immediately and controlled before it retracts. This vessel lies close to the external iliac vein, which can be threatened after brisk

bleeding produces decreased visualization. It also can be cauterized prophylactically. After the medial dissection is completed, attention is directed to the lateral side wall, developing the alveolar space between the peritoneum and transversus abdominis. This dissection should be completed in a "sweeping" motion, with care being taken not to injure the peritoneum.

If a tear is made is the peritoneum, the abdominal cavity can insufflate quickly and greatly decrease the preperitoneal working space. Many peritoneal defects can be controlled quickly using a laparoscopic clip applier or an endoloop. Suturing also may be used. The abdominal insufflation also can be released via placement of an angiocatheter or Veress needle above the umbilicus through the abdominal wall. If these maneuvers are inadequate, the procedure can be transitioned to TAPP repair.

At this time, the surgeon should be able to visualize an indirect defect as the peritoneum tracks along the spermatic cord toward the internal ring. The next step in the dissection is the inspection of the direct space medial to the epigastric vessels as well as the femoral canal. The contents of a direct hernia should be pulled posteriorly out of the defect until the white edge of attenuated transversalis fascia can be seen. This fascia acts as a pseudosac and can be fixed to the rectus abdominis if the hernia is large and postoperative seroma formation or mesh migration is likely. The examination of the femoral canal should be performed delicately in order to avoid tearing braches of the iliac vein, which can be difficult to control. Dissection of the fat pad overlying the iliac vein should be avoided, as tension to this fat may tear the vessel wall.

Attention is then directed to the dissection of the spermatic cord and indirect hernia sac (Figure 7). The spermatic cord is positioned in a triangular configuration with the vas deferens and testicular vessels converging at the internal ring. The spermatic cord traces posteriorly to form the medial border and the vessels form the lateral border. The hernia sac and cord structures then should be separated from the iliac vessels using graspers. Some surgeons elect to perform

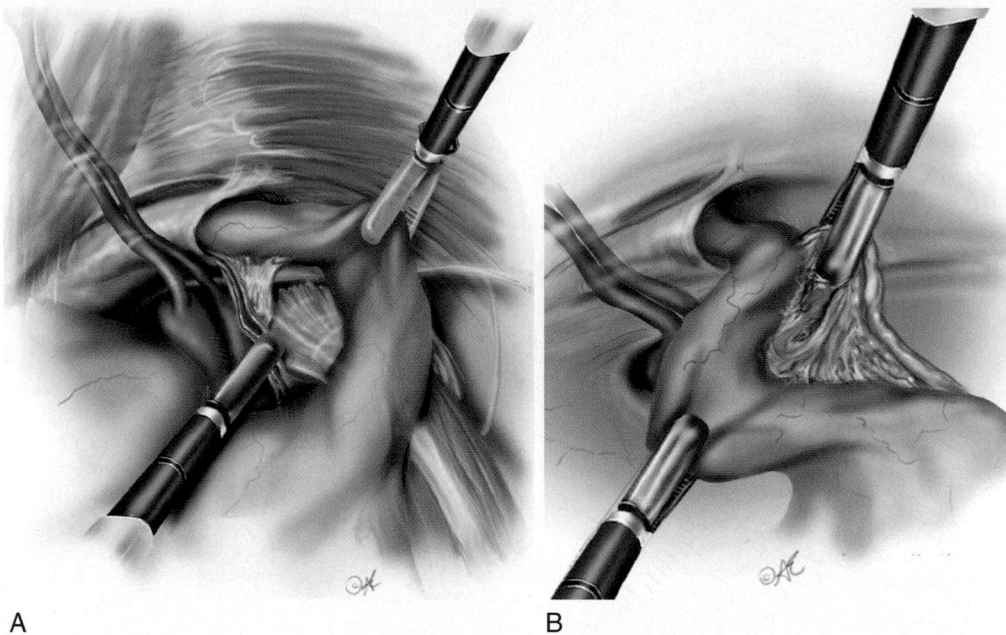

A   B

FIGURE 7 A and **B,** Dissection of the hernia sac. Apply gentle traction on the hernia sac and carefully dissect away all cremasteric fibers and spermatic structures.

this maneuver using laparoscopic Kittner dissectors and others use graspers, with or without cautery. The safest point for the separation is the internal ring. Once the structures are separated from the iliac vessels, the hernia sac should be grasped and pulled laterally and superiorly. The cord structures then should be dissected carefully off the hernia sac, taking care not to tear the thin-walled sac. This step often will require alternating between the medial and lateral sides until a sufficient window is created. Once a window has been created between cord structures and hernia sac, this window should be extended distally while providing up-and-out tension on the hernia sac. All cremasteric muscle fibers should be peeled carefully off the hernia sac until the edge of the sac is reached. Once all cremasteric attachments have been divided, the edge of the hernia sac should be peeled down carefully and separated from all attachments to the base of the spermatic cord. It is important to separate the sac well down to the posterior peritoneum to allow adequate space for mesh placement.

Once the dissection of the hernia sac has been completed, the surgeon is ready to place the prosthetic mesh. The selection of mesh and its fixation is discussed in a later section. The mesh is grasped outside the body and inserted through the umbilical trocar inferiorly toward the pubis and slightly toward the side of the hernia. A 5-mm laparoscope can be placed in one of the trocars to visualize this insertion. The camera is then reinserted into the umbilical trocar; the mesh likely is partially within the trocar and can be pushed out by the camera. Using the graspers through the 5-mm ports, the mesh should be directed into place so that it overlaps the midline by 1 to 2 cm, extends superior to the hernia defect by at least 4 cm, and reaches the anterior superior iliac spine laterally (Figure 8). The inferior border of the mesh should be lying on the cord structures. Of particular importance is the distance of the mesh border from the peritoneal edge, as any remaining strands of attachment can function as a lead point for subsequent recurrence. The mesh is then fixated according to surgeon preference and should be held in place as the space is desufflated under direct visualization (Figure 9). The inferior edge of the mesh should not move as the peritoneum rises. The trocars are then removed, and the anterior fascia is closed at the umbilical trocar site. After closure of the port sites, the testicles should be palpated and confirmed to be sitting in their usual scrotal position.

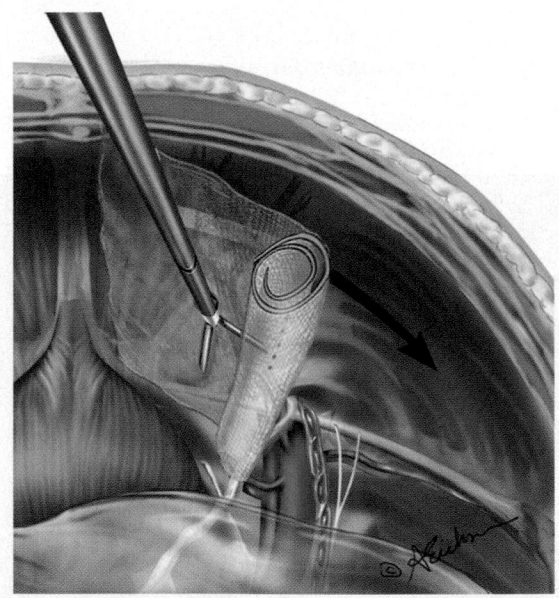

FIGURE 8 Prosthetic mesh coverage of the defects. The mesh should cross the midline and cover all three potential groin defects.

■ TRANSABDOMINAL PREPERITONEAL REPAIR

The positioning of the patient, surgeon, assistant, and laparoscopic monitors in TAPP repair is identical to that in TEP. Peritoneal access is obtained at the umbilicus, and two 5-mm ports are inserted to either side. If a unilateral defect is confirmed, the two trocars also can be placed together on the side opposite the hernia. The peritoneum is then incised about 2 cm superior to the inguinal defect using electrocautery. This incision may be performed in a "lazy S" or transverse linear fashion. The peritoneum is then dissected bluntly away from the rectus abdominis to completely develop the same preperitoneal space as in the TEP repair. As in TEP repair, the pubic tubercle,

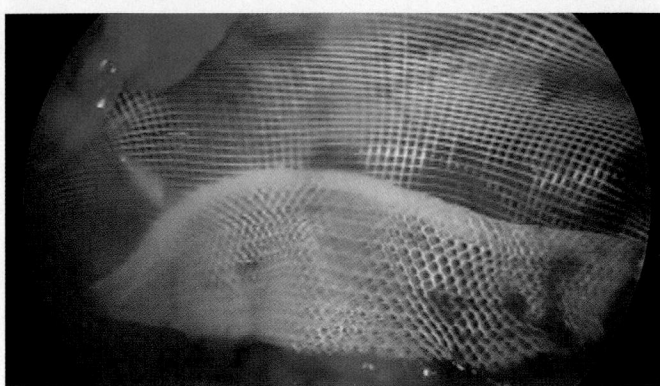

FIGURE 9 Proper orientation of the prosthetic mesh.

Cooper's ligaments, inferior epigastric vessels, and iliopubic tract are all identified. A TAPP approach may make identification of a sac easier, as the peritoneum can be manipulated to verify anatomy. It is also helpful in difficult reoperative cases, as peritoneal injuries do not limit exposure as they would in a TEP repair.

Typically, a direct hernia sac is reduced easily during the development of the preperitoneal space. An indirect hernia sac is dissected carefully away from the spermatic cord after identification of the cord structures in order to avoid injury. The femoral space should be explored gently to identify potential defects and reduce any hernia contents. A large mesh prosthesis is then placed overlying the entire myopectineal orifice, taking care to ensure adequate midline overlap of 1 to 2 cm and coverage of all potential defects. Mesh fixation is performed similar to in the TEP approach.

After mesh fixation, the peritoneal flap is closed to provide coverage of the mesh. This step is essential to protect the abdominal viscera and prevent erosion of the polypropylene or polyester mesh into the bowel. The peritoneal closure can be performed with suture or can be completed with tacks. Regardless of technique, adequate closure to prevent bowel herniation and exposed mesh is essential. If complete peritoneal exposure cannot be accomplished, a coated mesh to prevent bowel adhesions should be used and the edges of the defect secured as possible.

■ INTRAPERITONEAL ONLAY MESH PROCEDURE

The intraperitoneal onlay mesh (IPOM) procedure for inguinal hernias is a transabdominal approach that covers inguinal defects in a manner similar to that used for laparoscopic ventral hernia repairs. Because of its placement, no retroperitoneal dissection is required in this technique. The visceral contact requires the selection of coated mesh or polytetrafluoroethylene (PTFE) to avoid bowel adherence and fistulization.

The patient positioning, operative setup, and trocar positioning in IPOM are the same as in TAPP repair. Many surgeons will place a urinary catheter or instruct the patient to urinate immediately before surgery to decompress the bladder in order to avoid injury and technical difficulty. After the insertion of trocars, the entire myopectineal surface is examined. The indirect and direct hernia sacs are inverted gently and then excised about 1 to 2 cm outside the ring of fascia. The excision of the hernia sac also allows for removal of cord lipomas. After dissection is complete, a large coated mesh, approximately 12 × 15 cm in dimension, is inserted into the abdomen, laid over the groin defects, and secured in place using a combination of transfascial sutures, staples, and tacks. The mesh overlap should be at least 3 cm. The medial edge should be tacked to Cooper's ligaments and the lateral edge should be fixed anterior to the anterior superior iliac spine. The placement of transfascial sutures along the superior border adds security to the fixation as

well as stability during the tack fixation. Because of the difficulty with posterior fixation, this repair is rarely used or is used in a combination IPOM/TAPP approach, with the inferior mesh border secured extraperitoneally.

■ MESH SELECTION AND FIXATION

The ideal mesh material for laparoscopic inguinal hernia repair needs to be able to withstand the burst pressures created with abdominal flexion and strain. It needs to be resistant to infection, hypoallergenic, and chemically inert so as not to cause a foreign body reaction. The most important therapeutic feature of any hernia mesh is the ease with which it incorporates into the abdominal wall. Polypropylene mesh has been available since the late 1950s and is safe and effective. Polyester and ePTFE mesh are also available, although polypropylene mesh remains the most commonly studied material by far. Because of the peritoneal layer between the mesh and the abdominal viscera, uncoated polypropylene and polyester meshes can be used in most laparoscopic inguinal hernia repairs. If the surgeon is concerned about visceral contact, ePTFE mesh or one of many coated mesh configurations, usually containing a protective cellulose, collagen, omega-3 fatty acid, or hyaluronic acid coating on the visceral side, can be used.

Although strength is an important factor in mesh selection, increasing strength may be unnecessary and may contribute to the bulk of the mesh itself. Most meshes, except for some variations of lightweight polypropylene and woven PTFE, have a tear resistance above 20 N, the tear strength of the abdominal wall. However, heavier and thicker meshes can lead to the sensation of a foreign body for the patient, producing significant discomfort. This sensation is augmented in thin individuals with little subcutaneous fat.

The cost of hernia mesh has become more pertinent as medical centers increasingly stress cost-effective care. This has led to a focus on materials that provide adequate repair and minimize intraoperative cost. For example, after the development of biologic meshes, proponents stressed that the material eventually is replaced by the patient's native collagen. No studies have demonstrated any clear benefit in inguinal repair, however. Multiple studies have shown that low-cost materials such as mosquito netting in underdeveloped regions can be used with similar outcomes to standard mesh. This glaring example should serve to remind the surgeon that improved mesh performance needs to justify any increased cost of the material used.

The need for mesh fixation is controversial and has led to considerable variability in how surgeons place and secure the prosthesis. The mesh is secured primarily to prevent early migration and subsequent hernia recurrence. However, multiple studies have shown that the mechanism of recurrence is related to dissection technique, particularly with incomplete dissection of the hernia sac, missed cord lipomas, or inadequate dissection of the preperitoneal space relative to the size of mesh used. Further studies have shown no increased risk of early recurrence with no fixation used at all. Proponents of limited fixation stress the theoretical risk of inguinodynia that comes with tacks or other fixation materials. As a result, numerous techniques have been developed for minimizing tack use or for alternative fixation, including the use of fibrin glue or self-adhering mesh materials that replace tack fixation. Of note, the largest randomized studies completed to date mostly have examined recurrence rates after TEP repair in smaller hernias, thus highlighting that fixation still may be of benefit in larger hernias and in patients with significantly attenuated fascia.

For those surgeons who use tack fixation, the most common sites of fixation are the pubic tubercle and Cooper's ligaments medially, the rectus muscle superior to the hernia defect, and laterally into the transversus abdominis, taking care to avoid the epigastric vessels and to tack anterior to the ASIS in order to avoid injuring the lateral femoral cutaneous nerve. Absorbable tacks frequently are used to avoid any concerns about long-term pain.

CONSIDERATIONS FOR COMPLICATED REPAIRS

Complicated hernias present a technical challenge to the surgeon. Recurrent hernias, large scrotal hernias, incarcerated hernias, and repairs subsequent to previous preperitoneal dissection (e.g., prostatectomy) are examples. A general rule of thumb is to utilize a different surgical plane than that which was previously violated.

Recurrent hernias constitute up to 17% of herniorrhaphies performed in the United States, according to national databases. Because the most common open technique is an anterior repair, the TEP or TAPP approach is usually well suited for recurrences. During surgical planning for these repairs, it is important to note the number and type of previous repairs, the previous use of mesh, any perioperative complications encountered, the number and size of the defects, and the presence of a sac. The presence of significant scarring in the preperitoneal space, either by previous mesh placement or by dissection, greatly increases the risk of tearing the peritoneum and makes laparoscopic repair, particularly a TEP approach, less feasible.

Acutely incarcerated or strangulated hernias provide a challenge because of the need to reduce all abdominal contents before repair. Typically, a TAPP approach is well suited for this scenario because the surgeon is able to manually reduce the hernia contents back into the abdomen. A combination of external pressure and gentle internal traction should be used to reduce all visceral contents. Because of the risk of contamination, a permanent mesh repair may be contraindicated if there is concern for bowel integrity. After reduction, a temporary bridging mesh, such as Vicryl, can be placed to allow for sterilization of the space, with a plan to perform a definitive repair in the near future. Another alternative is to perform a tissue repair via the anterior approach. If contamination is not a concern, TAPP repair can proceed as usual with permanent mesh.

Large scrotal hernias pose a technical challenge because of the difficulty in reducing the entire hernia sac, which typically is chronically incarcerated. An experienced surgeon may be able to perform these repairs via the TEP approach, although the TAPP approach may be more feasible. If complete reduction is not possible, an option is to ligate and divide the hernia sac as distally as possible. However, this increases the risk of postoperative seroma. Scrotal hernias may pose greater risk to the cord structures and testicles because of increased traction held on the sac during reduction. The surgeon should be mindful of limiting tension on the cord whenever possible.

POSTOPERATIVE COMPLICATIONS AND FOLLOW-UP

Every technique for inguinal hernia repair carries a risk of bleeding and hematoma, infection, hernia recurrence, postoperative pain, and urinary complications. However, laparoscopic approaches also introduce the risk of trocar injuries, visceral injury secondary to abdominal entry, port site hernias, and hemodynamic instability after abdominal insufflation. Because of its transabdominal approach, TAPP repair carries a higher risk is these complications. The TAPP repair also has a higher postoperative risk of bowel obstruction because of the formation of postoperative adhesions and the potential herniation through an incomplete peritoneal closure. This risk can be minimized through careful closure, but the procedure carries about a 0.1% to 0.8% risk of small bowel obstruction postoperatively when the peritoneum is closed with sutures versus tacks, respectively. TAPP repair, however, is considered easier to learn and is useful if a peritoneal injury occurs during the TEP approach.

Urologic complications after TAPP or TEP repair are uncommon and can be divided into short-term and long-term complications. Short-term complications include bladder injury, obstructive azoospermia, and testicular ischemia secondary to vascular trauma. The urinary bladder can be injured during placement of the balloon dissector, during blunt dissection, or during trocar placement. Although there is little consensus regarding the placement of urinary catheters, most surgeons either will drain the bladder or instruct the patient to void immediately before surgery. If an injury has occurred or is suspected, methylene blue can be instilled through a catheter to help localize the injury. The injury then should be repaired immediately to prevent further extravasation of urine and possible mesh contamination. Longer-term issues such as mesh erosion into the bladder also have been reported.

Obstructive azoospermia is relatively uncommon but requires a discussion with all male patients of childbearing age. Typically, the cause of the complication is vigorous dissection of the spermatic cord leading to ischemia of the vas deferens, and obstructive azoospermia occurs afterward in 0.3% to 7.2% of cases. However, the vas deferens also can be cut or aggressively manipulated, resulting in scarring and obstruction. Testicular atrophy and ischemic orchitis also are typically caused by overly aggressive cord dissection and desvascularization of the spermatic cord. The gentle handling of tissues and preservation of the vascular structures of the cord typically can prevent these complications.

Persistent inguinodynia after laparoscopic inguinal herniorrhaphy is a difficult complication and may be difficult to manage. As many as 10% of patients report some degree of chronic postoperative pain. Typically, these pain syndromes are caused by injury, irritation, or entrapment of the nerves running through the surgical space. Although careful dissection and avoidance of the nerves while placing tacks can minimize the risk of inguinodynia, the risk cannot be eliminated fully, as the presence of the mesh itself can produce nerve irritation and pain. The type of mesh used does not appear to affect the rate of inguinodynia in the long term, although lightweight mesh does have improved patient comfort scores in the immediate postoperative period.

Hernia recurrence is the most obvious complication after laparoscopic repair. Numerous studies have demonstrated that the primary predictors of hernia recurrence are the experience of the surgeon and the size of the mesh used. A recent meta-analysis of 41 trials from the EU Hernia Trialists Collaboration showed equivalent recurrence rates between open repair and TAPP repair. Other authors with large series of laparoscopic inguinal hernia repairs have noted that the majority of recurrences occurred early in surgeons' procedural experience, with one group reporting a "matured" recurrence rate of 0.16%.

SUMMARY

The laparoscopic approach to repair inguinal hernias offers many advantages over the traditional open procedure, provided that the surgeon is proficient in the technique and the patient has been selected properly. These advantages include improved postoperative pain and shorter convalescence. The operation requires mostly blunt dissection, and the cost of surgical devices can be minimized by good surgical technique.

SUGGESTED READINGS

Jacob BP, Ramshaw B, eds. *The SAGES Manual of Hernia Repair.* New York: Springer Science & Business Media; 2012.

McKernan JB, Laws HL. Laparoscopic repair of inguinal hernias using a totally extraperitoneal prosthetic approach. *Surg Endosc.* 1993;7:26-28.

Memon MA, Cooper NJ, Memon B, Memon MI, Abrams KR. Meta-analysis of randomized clinical trials comparing open and laparoscopic inguinal hernia repair. *Br J Surg.* 2003;90:1479-1492.

LAPAROSCOPIC REPAIR OF RECURRENT INGUINAL HERNIAS

Matthew M. Hutter, MD, MPH, and Elan R. Witkowski, MD, MS

Surgical repairs of groin hernias are some of the most commonly performed operations worldwide. Although hernia surgery is extremely safe and effective, an inherent risk of any repair is the possibility of developing a recurrent hernia. This chapter focuses on recurrent inguinal hernias in adults. The management and repair of primary groin hernias are discussed in a separate chapter. Management of recurrent hernias can be technically demanding and presents unique challenges when compared with primary repair.

Recurrence can be defined as a repeat herniation of intraabdominal contents through a previously repaired defect. There may be instances of initially unappreciated hernias that later become apparent, as in the case of open inguinal hernia repair if the femoral space is not explored. This is an unsatisfactory outcome but not a true recurrence.

■ RATE OF RECURRENCE

The actual rate of hernia recurrence is uncertain, but reports generally have ranged from 1% to 15%. The best data available come from large clinical trials and population-based longitudinal studies. Unfortunately, long-term follow-up in most trials has been limited to several years. Therefore rates of reoperation have been used to estimate the frequency of hernia recurrence. This rate usually is multiplied by an arbitrary correction factor to account for patients with recurrences who do not undergo reoperation.

From 1996 to 1998, data from the Swedish Hernia Register revealed that 15% of hernia repairs were performed for recurrence. However, the majority of these patients with recurrent hernias initially had received nonmesh repairs (Haapaniemi et al., 2001). The same study showed a 1.7% chance of repeat operation within 24 months after a primary repair and a 4.6% chance of reoperation after a repair for recurrence.

In a large Danish cohort study, rates of reoperation within 30 months after primary repair were 2.4% after Lichtenstein repair, 3.6% after primary mesh (non-Lichtenstein) repair, 3.3% after primary laparoscopic repair, and 6.2% after primary nonmesh repair (Bay-Nielsen et al., 2001).

A large randomized trial comparing open hernia repair with laparoscopic hernia repair in U.S. Veterans Affairs medical centers reported recurrence rates of 10.1% and 4% after primary repair for laparoscopic and open mesh repairs, respectively, at 2-year follow-up (Neumayer et al., 2004). Rates of recurrence after a second operation were higher, but no significant difference between approaches was seen (10% vs 14.1%). The results of the laparoscopic arm in this trial have been criticized by many who believe the true rate to be lower with adequate surgeon experience.

Ultimately, the development of a recurrence depends on a number of factors, including the type of hernia, technique, surgeon experience, patient factors, and the indication for initial operation (e.g., emergent vs elective). The use of prosthetic mesh has reduced the overall risk of recurrence drastically and should be considered mandatory in adult patients unless contraindicated.

■ CLINICAL PRESENTATION, CAUSES, AND TIMING

Patients with recurrent groin hernias may have a variety of symptoms and signs, which are similar to those seen with a primary hernia. Symptoms range from acute bowel obstruction to nonspecific chronic discomfort, and signs range from an obvious bulge to a hernia appreciated only by an experienced clinician with provocative maneuvers. Careful physical examination is critical.

Recurrent hernia must be differentiated from other acute postoperative complications or chronic inguinodynia (groin pain). Patients with chronic inguinodynia will provide a history of discomfort or pain persisting longer than 3 to 6 months. Pain, paresthesia, hyperesthesia, or hypoesthesia can occur around the incision or in the distribution of the sensory nerves. These can be intermittent or constant and in some cases disabling. Examination will reveal no recurrence, but point tenderness is common.

A palpable defect with a reducible bulge may confirm the diagnosis of recurrent hernia. However, the presence of inflammation, scar, and mesh sometimes can lead to indeterminate findings. In these cases, imaging may be required to secure a diagnosis. Although imaging can be helpful, there are several limitations. Imaging can miss hernias that are reduced or apparent only during a Valsalva maneuver. In addition, fat along the spermatic cord (without a true hernia) may be confused with fat-containing inguinal hernias.

Recurrent groin hernias may be seen at any time after surgery. There is no formal definition of time periods, but recurrences generally can be described as early and late. Some authors and clinical trials have used a time frame of 5 years to differentiate early recurrences from late recurrences. The factors contributing to these failures are not mutually exclusive.

Early Recurrence

Shortly after a primary repair, it is not uncommon for patients to complain of a bulge, foreign body sensation, or discomfort. A palpable irreducible bulge frequently results from seroma, hematoma, lipoma, or postoperative tissue inflammation. With time, these usually will subside. Signs of infection, including erythema, purulence, and fever, should be noted. The treatment of common postoperative issues or suspected mesh infection is described elsewhere in this book.

An immediate or early recurrence represents a technical or biomechanical failure. This involves disruption of the repaired tissue or synthetic material (suture or mesh) and may be attributable to technical error, inappropriate tissue tension, weakened tissue, or excessive intra-abdominal pressure.

Patients may have a reducible bulge, as they did preoperatively. Mesh can be displaced completely into the space from which the hernia was dissected previously. Patients with a missed femoral hernia will be seen similarly, although these are not true recurrences. Mechanical bowel obstruction is uncommon after hernia repair and generally requires immediate reoperation.

Rates of recurrence are higher for inexperienced surgeons, particularly for laparoscopic repairs. Careful surgical technique, tension-free repair, and the use of appropriately sized and placed prosthetic mesh can reduce the incidence of early recurrence greatly.

Patient factors also may contribute to early recurrence. Associated risk factors include obesity, older age, chronic obstructive pulmonary disease (COPD), increased intra-abdominal pressure, smoking, malnutrition, diabetes, chemotherapy, use of corticosteroids, and peritoneal dialysis. Patients with connective tissue disorders and matrix metalloproteinase (MMP) abnormalities such as Ehlers-Danlos and Marfan's syndromes are also at increased risk. When possible, addressing modifiable risk factors preoperatively should be attempted to reduce the risk of recurrence.

Late Recurrence

Late recurrences are less common than early recurrences, but they do occur. The change in rate of recurrence over time is still not clear. There is no formal definition of a late recurrence, but 5 years after surgery often has been used to describe this cohort. These recurrences are more likely to be caused by ongoing biomechanical stress and patient factors rather than by technical issues. Exacerbating factors such as the development of abdominal ascites may precipitate these changes later in life. Mesh contraction or folding has been observed and described in some cases, but the frequency and clinical significance of this are unknown.

■ DIAGNOSTIC WORKUP

Recurrence can happen in many locations, including through the internal ring, in areas of the inguinal floor, and alongside the edges of prior mesh. After one or several operations, the standard anatomy can become extremely distorted. After anterior repair, recurrences are often direct defects found in the inferomedial portion of the inguinal floor near the pubic tubercle. With laparoscopic repairs, this pattern is less typical.

All patients with suspicion for a recurrent hernia should be referred to a surgeon for evaluation. A careful physical examination may be all that is required to diagnose a recurrence. The Valsalva maneuver, standing, coughing, and straining can be useful. In cases of uncertainty, surgeons should have a low threshold to re-examine the patient in the future or to obtain additional imaging.

Commonly, ultrasound, magnetic resonance imaging (MRI), and computed tomography (CT) are performed. Herniography (radiographic imaging after injection of contrast into the peritoneal cavity) has a good sensitivity and specificity for occult hernia but is frequently unavailable (Robinson et al., 2013). Ultrasound is readily available, inexpensive, and a good first-line diagnostic test in experienced hands. However, such experience is not common in the United States, and findings are not as convincing for the surgeon or patient reviewing the studies. MRI provides excellent cross-sectional detail and has the benefit of evaluating for other causes of groin pathology without ionizing radiation; thus it is a good choice for difficult cases. CT also can delineate the anatomy, is more easily understood by the patient and surgeon, and can be done with the Valsalva maneuver because of the rapid nature of today's multidetector CT. Laparoscopy also can be used in challenging cases to confirm anatomy at the time of repair.

■ MANAGEMENT

Once a diagnosis of recurrence is confirmed, several management strategies are available. These include immediate or delayed reoperation and watchful waiting.

Recurrent hernias may be more likely to require emergent repair for incarceration or strangulation, but overall this remains an uncommon occurrence (Fitzgibbons et al., 2006; Hernández-Irizarry et al., 2012).

Emergent Repair of Recurrent Hernias

Patients with strangulation should undergo emergent reoperation. Bowel should be inspected carefully through the groin incision, laparotomy, or laparoscopy. In contaminated cases, use of permanent synthetic mesh is contraindicated. The risk of re-recurrence is therefore extremely high. Tissue reapproximation should be performed, with the understanding that the patient very likely will need future definitive repair. Some data suggest that biologic or biosynthetic meshes could have a role in these scenarios (for both open and laparoscopic repairs), but long-term efficacy is unknown (Bellows et al., 2014; Bochicchio et al., 2014).

For patients with acute symptomatic incarceration, reduction should be attempted. If that is unsuccessful, repair should be performed urgently. The technical considerations are similar to those in elective repair. The involved bowel should be inspected carefully (through the groin incision, transinguinal laparoscopy, transabdominal laparoscopy, or laparotomy if necessary).

Elective Repair of Recurrent Hernias

Most patients do not have a surgical emergency that requires operation. The approach to these patients should begin with appropriate counseling. Rates of complications after reoperation are higher than for primary hernia repair, including nerve injury and chronic pain, damage to the cord structures, and testicular atrophy. Orchiectomy is rarely necessary. Furthermore, the risk of re-recurrence is higher than after primary repair. Patients should have a good understanding of these facts before operation.

For patients with asymptomatic disease, watchful waiting is a viable strategy. The rate of strangulation is low, although many asymptomatic patients ultimately are referred for surgery after becoming symptomatic. An important exception is patients with a femoral hernia. These patients have a much higher risk of strangulation and should undergo reoperation. There should be a higher level of suspicion of a femoral hernia for female patients and for male patients who did not undergo exploration of the femoral space during their first operation.

Every effort should be made to optimize preoperative risk factors. Weight loss or nutritional supplementation when appropriate, temporary discontinuation of peritoneal dialysis, tapering of steroids, smoking cessation, preventing constipation, and treatment of a chronic cough or other modifiable risk factors should be attempted when feasible.

Technical Considerations

There is no clearly demonstrated superiority of laparoscopic or open approaches to primary inguinal hernia repairs. The choice of procedure for recurrent hernias should be based on the type of initial repair. In cases of recurrence, it is generally preferable to approach the hernia through a fresh, previously undissected tissue plane. For patients with a prior mesh repair via an anterior approach, a posterior approach should be considered. Conversely, patients with prior posterior repairs should be considered for an anterior approach.

Within these categories, the choice of specific operation should be based on surgeon experience and training. The learning curve for inguinal hernia repair takes significant time to move to proficiency and then mastery, particularly for laparoscopic repair, and surgeons should be comfortable with primary repair before using a technique for a recurrent hernia. Operative reports from prior repairs may provide helpful information if they are available.

Synthetic mesh greatly reduces the risk of recurrence and should be used unless there is a contraindication. For patients who have had a previous mesh repair, well-incorporated, noninfected mesh usually should be left in place.

Understanding the inguinal anatomy and the concept of the myopectineal orifice is critical in these operations (Figure 1). First described by Dr. Henri Fruchaud, the myopectineal orifice describes a distinct area of weakness in the pelvic region. It is bordered superiorly by the transversus abdominis and internal oblique, inferiorly by the pectineal line, medially by the rectus abdominis, and laterally by the iliopsoas and iliopectineal arch. It is divided into a superior and inferior region by the inguinal ligament. The defect in the myopectineal orifice should be identified and definitively repaired.

Posterior Repair

For patients who underwent a prior anterior approach, a posterior repair is recommended. There are several options, including open and laparoscopic.

Open posterior repairs are performed less commonly but may be useful in selected cases. A large piece of mesh is placed in the preperitoneal space behind the transversalis fascia to cover the myopectineal orifice. Mesh can be inserted transinguinally (Rives' technique), through a lower midline incision (Stoppa procedure), or through the abdominal muscles (Kugel technique). Multiple variations have been

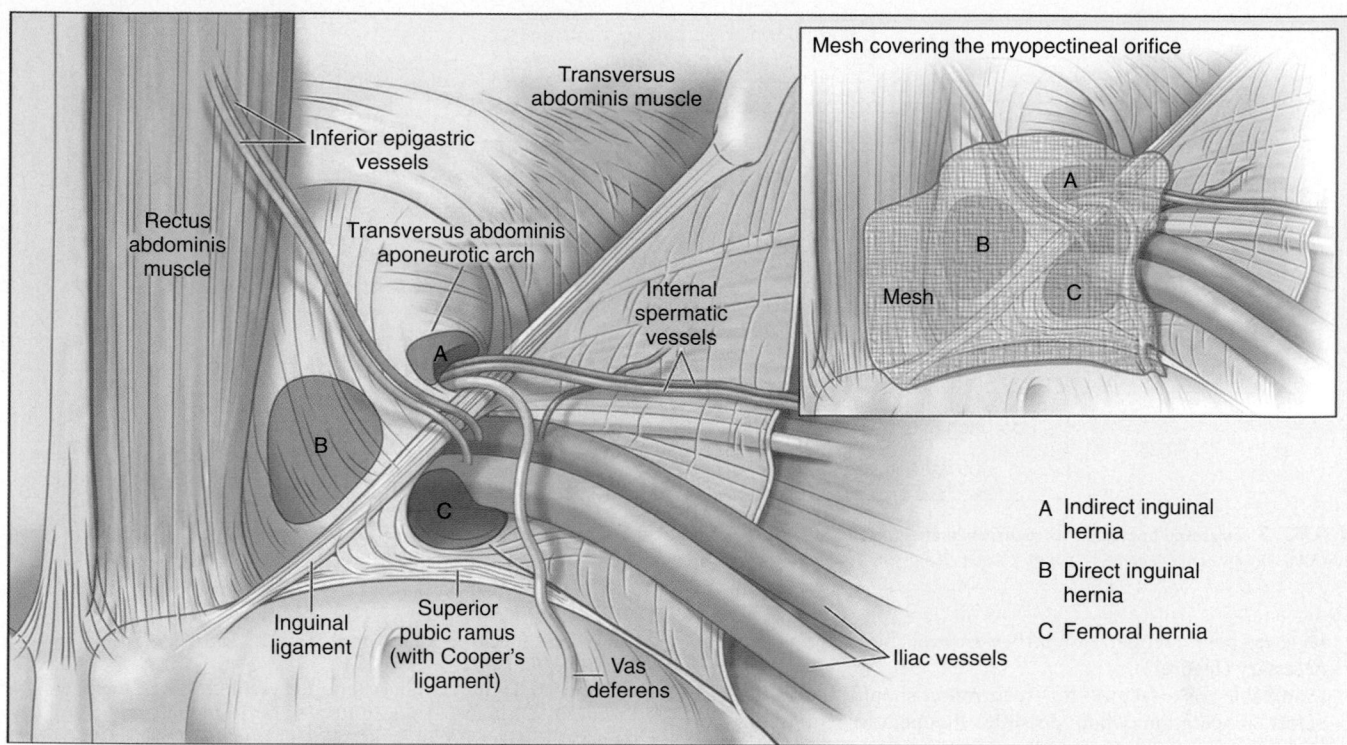

FIGURE 1 Anatomy of the groin from an intra-abdominal perspective. Groin hernias occur through the myopectineal orifice, which is bordered by the arch formed by the termination of the aponeurotic fibers of the transversus abdominis muscle cranially, the rectus abdominis muscle medially, the iliopsoas muscle laterally, and the superior pubic ramus with attached Cooper's ligament inferiorly. In the inset, a mesh prosthesis is shown covering the entire myopectineal orifice, as one would see in a laparoscopic inguinal herniorrhaphy. *(From Fitzgibbons RJ, Forse RA. Clinical practice: groin hernias in adults. N Engl J Med. 2015;372:756-763.)*

described, and these techniques still may have a role in expert hands for large or complex recurrent hernias.

The vast majority of posterior repairs are now performed laparoscopically. Both total extraperitoneal (TEP) repair and transabdominal preperitoneal (TAPP) repair should provide wide coverage of the entire myopectineal orifice. The mesh should be large enough to cover the entire myopectineal orifice, with ample medial extension. There are no strong data to suggest that medial fixation is mandatory, but it is commonly performed and may be prudent in these cases. Previously placed mesh usually can be left in place. TAPP and TEP repair have comparable outcomes, and procedure selection should be based on surgeon experience and judgment. The contraindications to each of these repairs are the same as in primary repair.

Anterior Repair

For patients with prior posterior repair, anterior repair generally is recommended. However, the data supporting this recommendation are limited. As more patients undergo primary laparoscopic repair, this scenario will become increasingly common. A tension-free mesh operation should be performed. The femoral space should be explored if a femoral hernia is suspected. The principles outlined by Lichtenstein and colleagues (1993) remain applicable:

1. Do not depend on fascial structures to close or reinforce the defect.
2. Reinforce the entire inguinal floor irrespective of the type of hernia.
3. Avoid all tension on suture lines.
4. Avoid use of scarred or devascularized tissue in the repair of recurrent hernias.
5. Use a large prosthetic material to reinforce the entire inguinal floor permanently.

The choice of anterior technique should be dictated by surgeon experience, with variations of the Lichtenstein repair being most common. Several mesh systems have been developed with the goal of providing posterior reinforcement with a traditional anterior approach. These techniques are usually straightforward in primary repairs and involve reducing the hernia sac through an anterior approach and isolating the cord structures in the standard fashion. Then a finger is used to bluntly dissect the preperitoneal space, where a nonabsorbable mesh is placed. In recurrent hernias where the preperitoneal space has been dissected previously, this blunt dissection can be challenging.

This mesh can come as a single unit, with a small central disc connecting the posterior sheet of mesh to a similar anterior portion, or it can be two units, a plug and patch. Once the posterior component is seated, the operation proceeds similar to Lichtenstein repair: a slit in the mesh is closed around the cord to recreate the internal ring, followed by circumferential or intermittent suture fixation of the mesh to the conjoined tendon and shelving edge of the inguinal ligament.

These systems have not been well studied in recurrent hernias. By placing mesh in both the preperitoneal and the anterior space, dissection may be more difficult; however, these techniques can provide robust tissue reinforcement when performed successfully.

■ SUMMARY

■ Unless contraindicated, mesh should be used in all repairs to reduce the risk of recurrence in adults.

■ Patients should be evaluated for a missed indirect or femoral hernia, particularly women with previous anterior repairs.

■ Patients with suspected recurrence should be evaluated and examined carefully, and previous operative notes should be

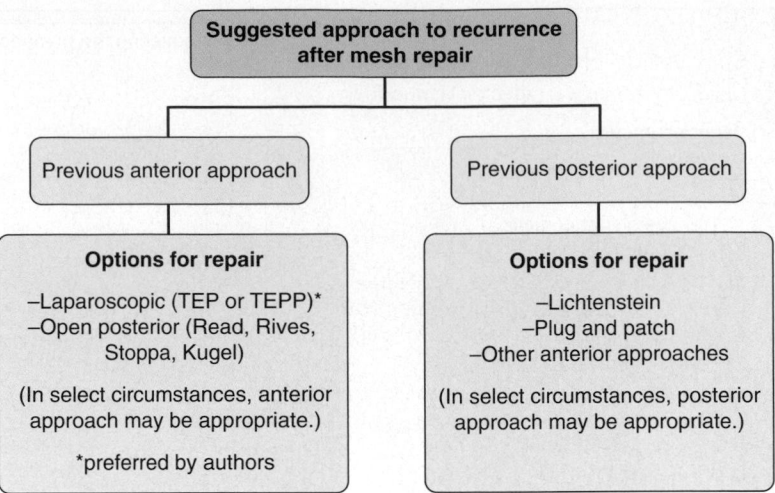

FIGURE 2 Suggested approach to recurrence after mesh repair. *TAPP,* Transabdominal preperitoneal repair; *TEP,* total extraperitoneal repair. *(Modified from Itani KMF, Fitzgibbons R, Awad SS, Duh Q-Y, Ferzli GS. Management of recurrent inguinal hernias. J Am Coll Surg. 2009;209:653-658.)*

reviewed before reoperation if they are available. Imaging may be necessary (Figure 2).

■ Modifiable risk factors for recurrence should be addressed before reoperation when possible. Preoperative counseling is important.

■ There are limited data on the repair of recurrent hernias after posterior repairs, but anterior repair may be advisable.

■ Patients with prior anterior mesh repairs should preferentially undergo posterior repair, generally laparoscopic. TEP and TAPP repair are both acceptable in experienced hands.

■ The choice of specific operation should be based on surgeon experience and training. Surgeons should be comfortable with primary repair before using a technique for a recurrent hernia, particularly for laparoscopic approaches.

SUGGESTED READINGS

Bay-Nielsen M, Kehlet H, Strand L, Malmstrøm J, Andersen FH, Wara P, Juul P, Callesen T, Danish Hernia Database Collaboration. Quality assessment of 26,304 herniorrhaphies in Denmark: a prospective nationwide study. *Lancet.* 2001;358:1124-1128. doi:10.1016/S0140-6736(01)06251-1.

Bellows CF, Shadduck P, Helton WS, Martindale R, Stouch BC, Fitzgibbons R. Early report of a randomized comparative clinical trial of Strattice™ reconstructive tissue matrix to lightweight synthetic mesh in the repair of inguinal hernias. *Hernia.* 2014;18:221-230. doi:10.1007/s10029-013-1076-9.

Bisgaard T, Bay-Nielsen M, Kehlet H. Re-recurrence after operation for recurrent inguinal hernia: a nationwide 8-year follow-up study on the role of type of repair. *Ann Surg.* 2008;247:707-711. doi:10.1097/SLA.0b013e31816b18e3.

Bochicchio GV, Jain A, McGonigal K, Turner D, Ilahi O, Reese S, Bochicchio K. Biologic vs synthetic inguinal hernia repair: 1-year results of a randomized double-blinded trial. *J Am Coll Surg.* 2014;218:751-757. doi:10.1016/j.jamcollsurg.2014.01.043.

Deysine M, Deysine GR, Reed WP. Groin pain in the absence of hernia: a new syndrome. *Hernia.* 2002;6:64-67.

Eker HH, Langeveld HR, Klitsie PJ, van't Riet M, Stassen LPS, Weidema WF, Steyerberg EW, Lange JF, Bonjer HJ, Jeekel J. Randomized clinical trial of total extraperitoneal inguinal hernioplasty vs Lichtenstein repair: a long-term follow-up study. *Arch Surg.* 2012;147:256-260. doi:10.1001/archsurg.2011.2023.

Fitzgibbons RJ, Forse RA. Clinical practice: groin hernias in adults. *N Engl J Med.* 2015;372:756-763. doi:10.1056/NEJMcp1404068.

Fitzgibbons RJ, Giobbie-Hurder A, Gibbs JO, Dunlop DD, Reda DJ, McCarthy M, Neumayer LA, Barkun JST, Hoehn JL, Murphy JT, Sarosi GA, Syme WC, Thompson JS, Wang J, Jonasson O. Watchful waiting vs repair of inguinal hernia in minimally symptomatic men: a randomized clinical trial. *JAMA.* 2006;295:285-292. doi:10.1001/jama.295.3.285.

Haapaniemi S, Gunnarsson U, Nordin P, Nilsson E. Reoperation after recurrent groin hernia repair. *Ann Surg.* 2001;234:122-126.

Hernández-Irizarry R, Zendejas B, Ramirez T, Moreno M, Ali SM, Lohse CM, Farley DR. Trends in emergent inguinal hernia surgery in Olmsted County, MN: a population-based study. *Hernia.* 2012;16:397-403. doi:10.1007/s10029-012-0926-1.

Itani KMF, Fitzgibbons R, Awad SS, Duh Q-Y, Ferzli GS. Management of recurrent inguinal hernias. *J Am Coll Surg.* 2009;209:653-658. doi:10.1016/j.jamcollsurg.2009.07.015.

Junge K, Rosch R, Klinge U, Schwab R, Peiper C, Binnebösel M, Schenten F, Schumpelick V. Risk factors related to recurrence in inguinal hernia repair: a retrospective analysis. *Hernia.* 2006;10:309-315. doi:10.1007/s10029-006-0096-0.

Lichtenstein IL, Shulman AG, Amid PK. The cause, prevention, and treatment of recurrent groin hernia. *Surg Clin North Am.* 1993;73:529-544.

Neumayer L, Giobbie-Hurder A, Jonasson O, Fitzgibbons R, Dunlop D, Gibbs J, Reda D, Henderson W, Veterans Affairs Cooperative Studies Program 456 Investigators. Open mesh versus laparoscopic mesh repair of inguinal hernia. *N Engl J Med.* 2004;350:1819-1827. doi:10.1056/NEJMoa040093.

Robbins AW, Rutkow IM. The mesh-plug hernioplasty. *Surg Clin North Am.* 1993;73:501-512.

Robinson A, Light D, Kasim A, Nice C. A systematic review and meta-analysis of the role of radiology in the diagnosis of occult inguinal hernia. *Surg Endosc.* 2013;27:11-18. doi:10.1007/s00464-012-2412-3.

Sevonius D, Gunnarsson U, Nordin P, Nilsson E, Sandblom G. Repeated groin hernia recurrences. *Ann Surg.* 2009;249:516-518. doi:10.1097/SLA.0b013e318199f21c.

Sevonius D, Gunnarsson U, Nordin P, Nilsson E, Sandblom G. Recurrent groin hernia surgery. *Br J Surg.* 2011;98:1489-1494. doi:10.1002/bjs.7559.

Treadwell J, Tipton K, Oyesanmi O, Sun F, Schoelles K. *Surgical Options for Inguinal Hernia: Comparative Effectiveness Review.* Rockville, MD: Agency for Healthcare Research and Quality; 2012.

Laparoscopic Ventral and Incisional Hernia Repair

Michael J. Rosen, MD

Ventral hernia repair is one of the most common procedures performed by general surgeons. Ventral hernias can be defined as primary or acquired. Primary hernias include epigastric, umbilical, spigelian (lateral), and rare hypogastric hernias. Acquired hernias can occur after traumatic events but most commonly are related to a prior surgical incision. The incidence rate of incisional hernia formation after a midline laparotomy is estimated at 10% to 20%, depending on the patient population at risk. With almost 2 million laparotomies performed annually, somewhere between 100,000 and 200,000 ventral hernia repairs are performed annually in the United States. Despite the prevalence of this disease, no universally accepted classification system exists. As a result, there is a wide spectrum of patients who develop ventral hernias, and significant variability is found in the complexity of ventral hernia defects. This spectrum includes those patients with small asymptomatic defects to patients with massive hernias, loss of domain, and concomitant contamination present during repair. As a result of this diversity, no single repair technique is likely to take care of all patients with ventral hernias. Therefore surgeons repairing abdominal wall defects should be familiar with both laparoscopic and open approaches to ventral hernias to offer the patient the most appropriate repair technique on the basis of unique patient factors and hernia defect characteristics (Table 1).

The laparoscopic approach to ventral/incisional hernia repair has gained widespread acceptance by the surgical community as a safe and effective approach. It borrows from the principles of abdominal wall reconstruction espoused by Rives and Stoppa of placement of a large sublay prosthetic deep to the hernia defect to provide wide coverage. Unlike the open counterpart, the laparoscopic approach requires the mesh to be placed within the peritoneal cavity. This mandates the use of appropriate tissue-separating prosthetics with a visceral side that prevents bowel ingrowth and an abdominal side that promotes tissue integration. The prosthetic should be fixed with full-thickness transfascial fixation sutures and spiral tacks. Given the absence of subcutaneous soft tissue dissection, a predictably lower rate of wound and mesh infections is seen, which is a major advantage of the laparoscopic approach. The laparoscopic repair also allows for full visualization of the entire anterior abdominal wall to avoid missing small Swiss cheese–type defects.

INDICATIONS

The natural history of an asymptomatic ventral/incisional hernia is largely unknown. Because surgical teaching has always suggested that these hernias pose significant risk for bowel incarceration or strangulation, most surgeons advocate repair on diagnosis of an incisional hernia. No large cohort of patients who have undergone nonoperative management is available, so the natural history remains largely unknown. However, given the increases in intra-abdominal pressures with activities of daily living, a ventral hernia tends to grow over time, which makes repair increasing difficult once the hernias become very large. Incisional hernias can also result in unsightly bulges that affect quality of life. In addition, the thin skin overlying a large hernia can become ischemic, ulcerate, and even result in an ascitic leak. The three general indications for operation are: (1) a hernia that is symptomatic and causes pain, discomfort, surrounding cutaneous ulcerations, or changes in bowel habits; (2) a hernia that results in an unsightly bulge and affects the patient's quality of life; and (3) a hernia that poses a significant risk of bowel obstruction (e.g., a large hernia with a narrow neck). In consideration of operative intervention, an individualized approach is important, with patient comorbidities, defect characteristics, and the presence of contamination taken into account. Because a wide spectrum of patients develop a variety of hernias, one single technique is not able to address all patients. Few absolute contraindications are found for a laparoscopic ventral hernia repair, other than inability to tolerate general anesthesia or the presence of active contamination. However, several relative contraindications deserve mention. The ability to perform safe adhesiolysis is paramount to a successful laparoscopic ventral hernia repair; therefore patients at risk for severe adhesions should likely not undergo a laparoscopic approach. Examples include patients with multiple reoperative abdomens, in particular with multiple intraperitoneal prosthetic meshes. Patients who have undergone prior intraperitoneal dialysis are at high risk for an obliterated peritoneal cavity. Surgery for patients with massive defects and loss of domain can be successfully completed laparoscopically, but an advanced laparoscopic skill set is needed, which generally involves multiple pieces of mesh sewn together and a poor functional and cosmetic result. Patients with excessive scars that need revision should undergo an open repair. Patients with inflammatory bowel disease, in particular Crohn's disease, should likely not have intraperitoneal mesh placed given the likelihood of reoperations and potential fistulas. Patients with larger defects of more than 10 to 12 cm in width are better served with an open formal abdominal wall reconstruction. The ideal candidate for a laparoscopic ventral hernia repair is an obese or elderly patient with a small to medium-sized defect. Thin, active, manual laborer patients are offered a formal abdominal wall reconstruction either laparoscopically with defect closure as described subsequently or open.

PREOPERATIVE WORKUP

A complete history and physical examination is important in ventral hernia cases. These patients often have significant comorbidities, and consideration of optimizing preoperative glucose control, nutritional parameters, smoking cessation, and weight reduction is key to a successful outcome. In addition, particular attention should be paid to the anterior abdominal wall skin for ulcerations or nonhealing wounds that might preclude a laparoscopic approach. Incarcerated hernias that cannot be reduced can be difficult laparoscopically and should be discerned before surgery. Locations of all prior surgical incisions are noted, and all prior operative reports are reviewed. Important information as to the type and location of prior prosthetic mesh and the history of upper quadrant surgery that could alter the initial access port is critical. A computed tomographic (CT) scan of the abdomen is performed in all but the smallest hernias in my practice. This image can provide valuable information as to the size of the defect, the contents of the hernia sac, the presence of occult hernias that might not be palpable in an obese patient, and the presence of prior synthetic mesh. In addition, the integrity of the rectus muscles and lateral abdominal wall musculature can be assessed for reconstructive options. Preoperative counseling is also important for patients undergoing laparoscopic ventral hernia repair. Despite the minimally invasive nature of laparoscopic ventral hernia repair, postoperative pain is often similar to the open procedure. Because the hernia sac is often not excised, a postoperative seroma is almost universally present and the patient should be aware. The possibility of an enterotomy and the appropriate management, including the need to convert to an open procedure, should be clarified.

OPERATIVE TECHNIQUE

Patient Positioning

For patients with midline incisional hernias, patients are placed in the supine position with their arms tucked to the sides. Having the arms tucked facilitates the surgeon standing on the same side of the

TABLE 1: Results of Prospective Randomized Studies That Compare Laparoscopic With Open Ventral Hernia Repairs

Study	No. of Patients	Mesh Used	Complication Rate	Recurrence Rate
Itani (2010)				
Laparoscopic	73	PTFE	32%	13%
Open	73	Polypropylene	48%	8%
Olmi (2007)				
Laparoscopic	85	Polyester/collagen	17%	2%
Open	85	Polypropylene	29%	4%
Pring (2008)				
Laparoscopic	31	PTFE	33%	3%
Open	27	PTFE	49%	4%
Asencio (2009)				
Laparoscopic	45	PTFE/polypropylene	5%	10%
Open	39	Polypropylene	33%	8%

PTFE, Polytetrafluoroethylene.

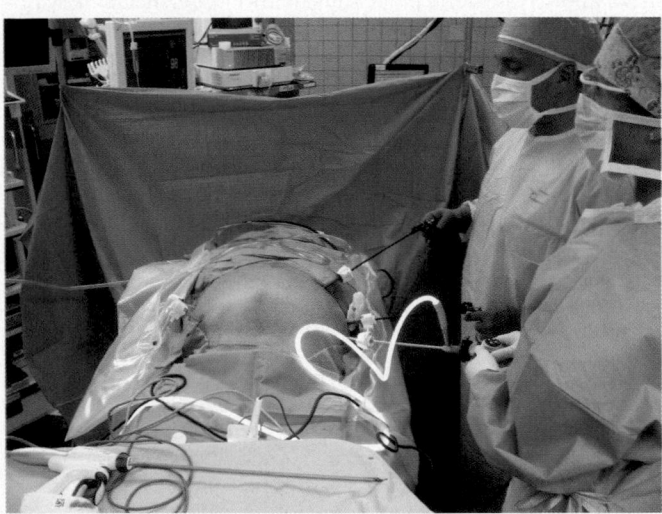

FIGURE 1 Intraoperative view of surgeon and camera operator standing on the same side of patient for adhesiolysis. Patient's arms are abducted and an iodine-impregnated drape covers the abdomen.

table as the camera operator (Figure 1). An iodine-impregnated adhesive drape is applied to the skin to protect the mesh from skin flora and facilitate marking the patient during mesh placement. A first-generation cephalosporin is given, orogastric tube is placed, and a three-way Foley catheter is placed for any defect below the umbilicus to aid in identification of the bladder during dissection. Pneumatic compression devices are applied, and subcutaneous heparin is administered before surgery.

Access of the Reoperative Abdomen and Trocar Positioning

Gaining access to the reoperative abdomen can be the most treacherous step of a laparoscopic ventral hernia repair. Typically, the upper quadrants are free of adhesions, and the tip of the 11th rib provides a good access point. Attention to prior surgical incisions and intraabdominal procedures can provide clues as to the most appropriate side. For instance, patients who have had their splenic flexure mobilized should be approached through the right upper quadrant. Several methods have been described for access, including an open cut down approach, utilization of optical viewing trocars, and the use

of a Veress needle. In skilled hands, each of these approaches is safe and effective and can be used. In general, this access point should be as far lateral as possible to avoid being covered during mesh placement. Once the abdomen is accessed and insufflated, two additional 5-mm ports are placed ipsilateral to this trocar. This facilitates two-handed technique during adhesiolysis and avoids working in reverse to the camera during dissection. Once the adhesions are completely lysed, at least 1 or 2 additional 5-mm ports are placed on the contralateral side to position and secure the mesh. A 5-mm 30-degree laparoscope is helpful to allow placement through any of the trocars during adhesiolysis, and the angled scope provides superior vision around adhesions and up to the anterior abdominal wall.

Adhesiolysis

The most dangerous part of a laparoscopic ventral hernia repair is safe adhesiolysis. This can be the most time-consuming portion of the case and requires patience and meticulous technique. In general, no electrocautery should be used during adhesiolysis. In particular, vessel-sealing devices such as the ultrasonic dissector or Ligasure (Covidien, Boulder, CO) should be avoided because they can create a sealed full-thickness injury to the bowel wall that does not leak for several days. If bleeding occurs, liberal use of 5-mm clips is warranted, or the surgeon should convert to an open approach. If prior intraperitoneal mesh is present, avoid blunt sweeping movements because the bowel will likely give way before the mesh. In cases in which the mesh is densely adherent to the intestines, the surgeon can perform a small incision and complete the adhesiolysis open and place the mesh laparoscopically or, rarely, remove the mesh off the abdominal wall and leave some adherent to the bowel if no obstruction or fistula was present before surgery. In cases of serve adhesions to mesh, an open bowel resection can be necessary. In obese patients with incarcerated hernias, bimanual palpation of the abdominal wall can help identify the dissection plane during adhesiolysis. It is imperative to clear the entire anterior abdominal wall of adhesions all the way to the pericolic gutters. This avoids missing occult Swiss cheese–type defects and allows a large prosthetic mesh to be placed. Hernias above the umbilicus often require division of the falciform ligament to adequately adhere the mesh to the abdominal wall.

Sizing the Hernia Defect

An accurate measurement of the hernia defect is critical to appropriately size the mesh for adequate overlap and position the mesh for maximal coverage of the defect. Oversizing of the mesh can result in

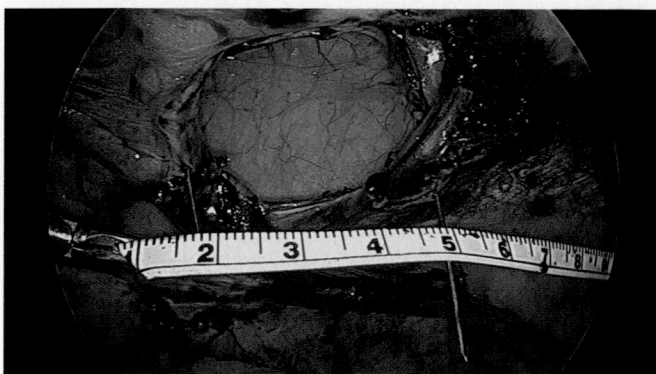

FIGURE 2 Intraperitoneal view of spinal needles placed at the edge of the defect and measured with a 15-cm plastic ruler.

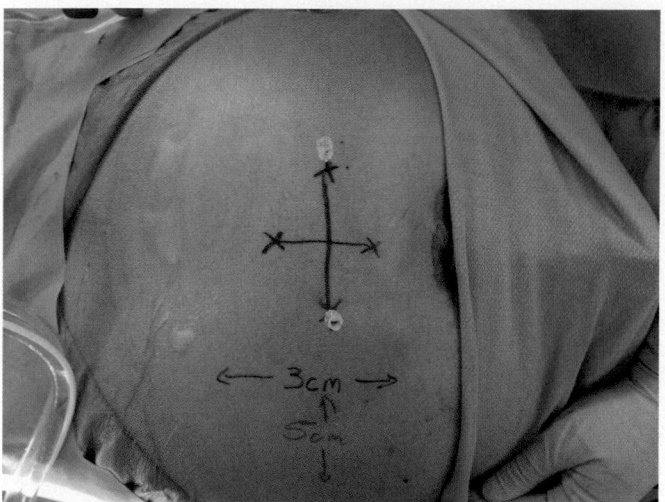

FIGURE 3 External lines mark maximal width and length of hernia defect measured internally with spinal needles.

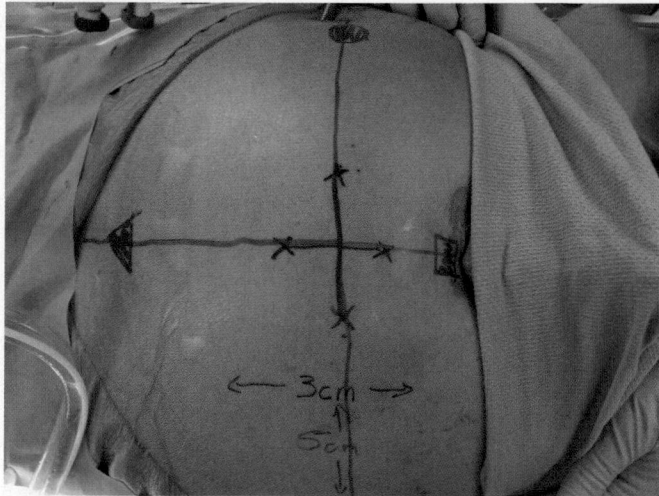

FIGURE 4 Center point of the lines marked externally is measured, which correlates to the center point of the hernia defect.

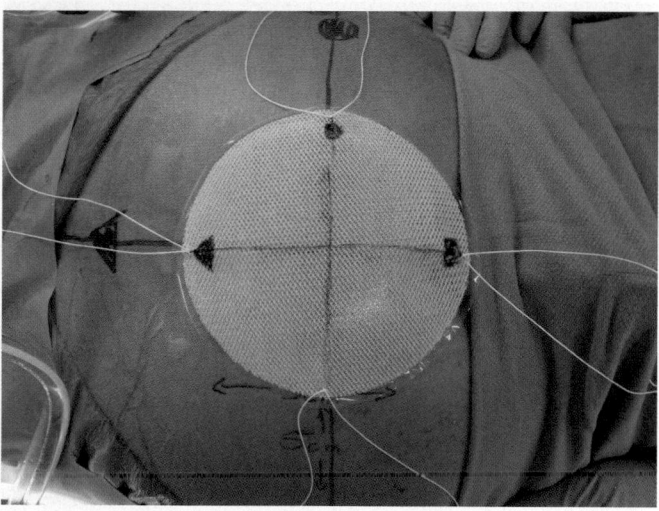

FIGURE 5 Center point of the mesh is identified, and on these lines four transfascial sutures are placed that correlate with the external center point lines previously measured.

significant technical challenges in accurate positioning of the prosthetic without buckling. In obese patients, external palpation of the hernia defects can be difficult and inaccurate. I prefer to use a 3½-inch, 20-gauge spinal needle to appropriately localize the hernia defect. Intracorporeal measurement of the defect is important because that is the location of the mesh. In obese patients with excessive subcutaneous tissue, a significant discrepancy between internal and external measurement can result in oversizing the hernia defect.

Two spinal needles are placed at the cranial and caudal limits of the hernia (Figure 2). In Swiss cheese defects, the maximal distance is used. A 15-cm plastic ruler is placed intracorporeally, and the distance between the spinal needles is recorded. The location of the spinal needles is also marked externally with a line. Next, the maximal width of the hernia defect is localized with spinal needles and measured internally and marked externally (Figure 3). Once the maximal width and length are calculated, 8 cm (4 cm of overlap on each side) is added to appropriately size the prosthetic material. Multiple different prosthetics are available for intraperitoneal placement. However, I do advocate use of a tissue-separating mesh of some type.

Because all hernias are not perfect circles, identification of the center of the hernia is important to adequately center the mesh. The center point of the hernia can be identified externally. The surgeon measures the distance of the prior lines marked on the patient that indicate the length of the hernia. A transverse line is drawn across the patient at this point to indicate the x-axis. Next, the middle of the line marking the maximal width of the hernia is measured, and

a longitudinal line is drawn across the patient's abdomen to indicate the y-axis. Where these two lines intersect is the center point of the hernia (Figure 4). In preparation of the mesh, the prosthetic is folded in half lengthwise, and a line is drawn, and in half along the width as well. Transfascial sutures are secured to the mesh at the edge of each of these lines. If done correctly, these sutures are retrieved on the labeled x-axis and y-axis on the patient to appropriately center the mesh (Figure 5).

Mesh Positioning

The four cardinal sutures are tucked into the mesh, and it is rolled tightly to fit through a trocar. Larger sheets of mesh sometimes require removal of the trocar. This can be facilitated by passing a 5-mm grasper across the abdomen, out the larger trocar; the trocar is removed, and the mesh is grasped and pulled into the abdomen. Once inside the abdomen, the mesh is unfurled and the sutures are identified.

The initial cardinal suture should be brought up at the site with the least amount of potential coverage. This may be near the xiphoid

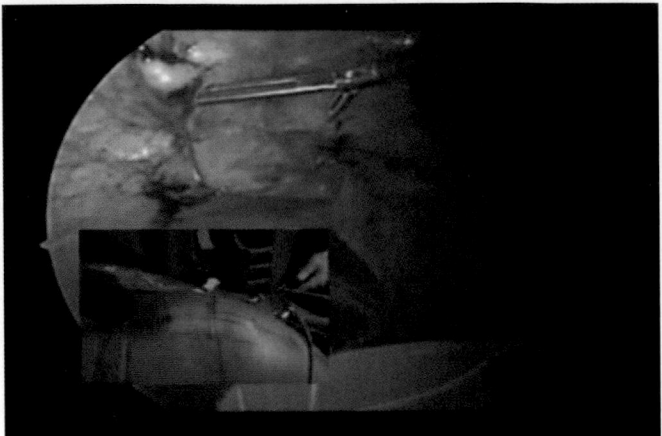

FIGURE 6 A spinal needle is placed at the edge of the defect on the external center line, and a 4-cm grasper is used to measure the overlap of the mesh and marked with another spinal needle. The skin is incised, and the transfascial suture retrieved at this site.

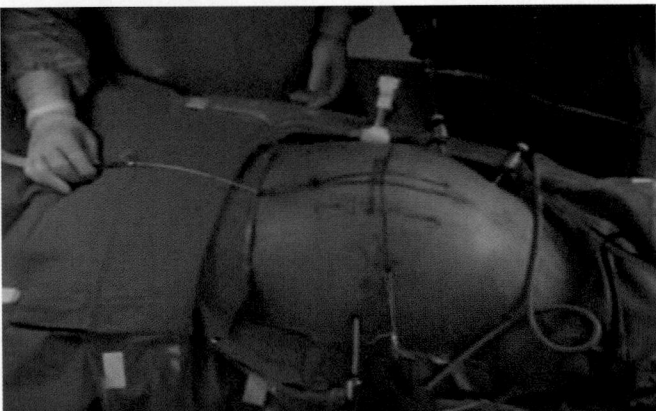

FIGURE 7 Cephalad and lateral suture retrieved through prior center point lines drawn externally on patient's abdomen.

or above the pubis. Regardless of how the mesh is measured, some excess mesh is common; to keep the mesh taut, more overlap might be necessary. The area at the edge of the hernia defect is localized on the prior y-axis line drawn on the patient with a spinal needle. With a grasper used for measurements, the next spinal needle is placed on the y-axis line 4 cm past the original spinal needle (Figure 6). A small incision is made, and a suture passer is used to retrieve each tail through separate fascial punctures. These sutures are tagged and left untied.

The lateral suture furthest from the camera is retrieved next. Again, a spinal needle is placed at the edge of the hernia defect on the prior externally marked x-axis. With use of a grasper, 4 cm is measured, and another spinal needle is placed. Another stab incision is made, and the two tails are retrieved (Figure 7). In laparoscopic ventral hernia repair, the mesh is placed under insufflation, and it is important to be taut. If the mesh is not taut, the prosthetic buckles once the abdomen is desufflated and prolapses into the hernia sac. To avoid this problem, the two sutures that were placed before are pulled tightly by an assistant, while the surgeon grasps the mesh with a Maryland grasper near the remaining longitudinal knot and pulls the mesh along the externally marked y-axis. Once the mesh is taut, the point on the y-axis is marked with a spinal needle. A skin incision is made, and the tails are retrieved. The three sutures are then secured. The final transfascial suture is then pulled taut, the point on the x-axis is identified with a spinal needle, and the tails are retrieved.

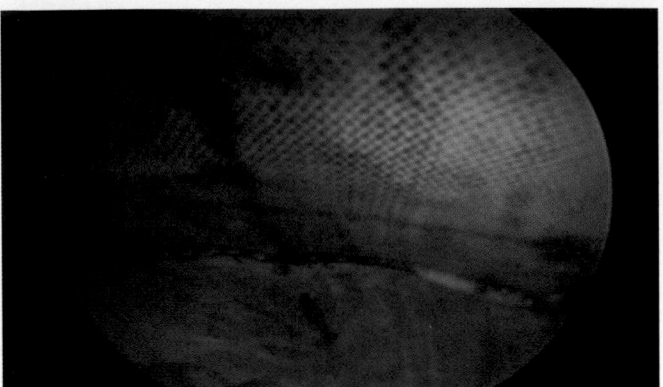

FIGURE 8 Final view of mesh taut across the abdominal cavity with tacks and transfascial sutures in place.

The four sutures are secured, and the mesh is then secured to the remainder of the peritoneum with a tacking device (Figure 8). Multiple varieties of tacking devices are available, of both a permanent and an absorbable variety. No data are found to suggest the superiority of one tacking device over another at this time. These tacks do not provide strength to the repair. However, they do prevent bowel from slipping above the mesh for the first few weeks until the mesh is reperitonealized. The integrity of the repair is maintained by the transfascial sutures. The exact number of transfascial sutures required for a durable repair is unknown. The author uses an individualized approach. In patients with small defects or Swiss cheese–type defects, a large mesh with four sutures is sufficient. However, in obese patients, or those with large defects, 12 transfascial sutures are typically used. All ports over 5-mm should have the fascia closed particularly in hernia cases.

■ POSTOPERATIVE CARE

In highly selected cases, laparoscopic ventral hernia repair can be performed on an outpatient basis. However, postoperative discomfort can be significant, and most patients benefit from at least overnight observation and a patient-controlled analgesic device. Routine administration of ketorolac or muscle relaxants can also be helpful. Patients who need extensive adhesiolysis are kept on nothing by mouth status until flatus. Routine hospital admission can also aid in detection of a missed enterotomy. This can be a life-threatening complication if diagnosis is delayed. Although radiographic evaluation can occasionally be helpful in the early postoperative period, if unexplained tachycardia or signs of sepsis persist, the patient should return to the operating room for a diagnostic laparoscopy.

■ SPECIAL CIRCUMSTANCES

Subxiphoid Hernia

Subxiphoid hernias are common after median sternotomies. They present particular challenges because the close proximity of body structures (ribs, costal margin) and major vascular structures (heart, aorta) can limit mesh fixation options. The procedure is carried out similarly to a standard laparoscopic ventral hernia repair, although the falciform ligament must be taken down completely. The defect is measured as previously described, and the mesh is sized appropriately. However, the most cranial suture is backed off at least 4 to 5 cm from the edge of the mesh. This suture can be retrieved at the xiphoid process, and the mesh is allowed to drape over the diaphragm and pericardium. To prevent buckling, the mesh can be fixated to the diaphragm with fibrin sealant. Tacking devices should not be used above the costal margin or xiphoid process to avoid injury to the pericardium.

Suprapubic Hernia

Suprapubic hernias pose challenges in obtaining adequate overlap while avoiding the bladder and major neurovascular structures. In reoperative cases, accurate identification of the superior extent of the bladder can be difficult. To facilitate identification, a three-way Foley catheter is helpful. After the intra-abdominal adhesions are mobilized fully, the Foley catheter is clamped and 300 mL of normal saline solution is instilled through the irrigation port. With the bladder clearly visible, it is mobilized to expose the pubis and space of Retzius. The inferior sutures are backed off the edge of the mesh for several centimeters. These sutures can be retrieved at the pubis or Cooper's ligament, and the tail of the mesh can be tucked into the space of Retzius to maximize overlap. With placement of tacks to secure the periphery of the mesh, the tip of the tacker must be palpated externally. Like a laparoscopic inguinal hernia repair, if the tacker is below the iliopubic tract, major vascular and neurologic injuries can occur.

Defect Closure

With renewed interest in creation of a functional dynamic abdominal wall, some surgeons advocate closure of defects laparoscopically. The theoretic advantage of closing the defect is that it restores the abdominal wall integrity, may equalize pressure across the abdominal wall and mesh, reduces seroma rates, and might refunctionalize the abdominal wall. Several techniques have been described. The basic approach involves the use of a suture passing device, placed through a small stab incision over the hernia defect. A suture is brought into the abdomen through one side of the fascia, and the device is then placed through the opposite fascia and the suture retrieved through the same skin incision. This can be repeated to form a figure of 8 suture. This is the same technique used to close laparoscopic port sites. Once these sutures are placed, they can be tied, and the mesh is secured in a similar fashion. The mesh must be sized as if the defect were open, so if the midline repair were to break down, the hernia would not recur. Although this approach has an intuitive advantage, no comparative data at this time suggest it results in a superior outcome to a standard laparoscopic ventral hernia repair. In addition, it should be limited to defects less than 8 to 10 cm in maximal width because excessive tension can result.

■ COMPLICATIONS

Nearly all patients who undergo laparoscopic ventral hernia repair have development of a seroma. These seromas are mostly clinically insignificant and resolve without interventions. Patients must be counseled as to the likelihood of having an early persistent bulge, so as to avoid confusing it with a recurrence. Indications for aspiration are limited and include significant symptoms, impending skin ischemia, and failure to resolve after 6 months. The risk of contaminating the mesh must be weighed against the advantage of removing the fluid.

An enterotomy during laparoscopic ventral hernia repair is a serious, potentially life-threatening complication if not dealt with appropriately. No steadfast rule exists for management of an enterotomy during laparoscopic ventral hernia repair, but some basic surgery principles can be applied. Most important, this complication must be recognized when it occurs. If surgeons identify an enterotomy, they must realize that this has the potential to be life threatening. Although several authors have described unique approaches to laparoscopic repair of the enterotomy and fixing the hernia with a biologic graft, or returning to the operating room in 3 to 5 days, this approach is not advocated by my group. Instead, if this complication

occurs, at a minimum, the segment of bowel is exteriorized through a small incision and adequate repair is confirmed. At that time, the hernia can be left alone, with a return several months later for another attempt at repair. Alternatively, the procedure can be converted to open, with either primary closure of the defect or use of a biologic mesh to repair the hernia. Regardless of which approach is chosen, one should not let being a minimally invasive surgeon get in the way of the right operation for the patient. All patients should clearly understand what will happen if an enterotomy is encountered and that they may wake up with their hernia.

Unlike most laparoscopic procedures, laparoscopic ventral hernia can result in significant postoperative discomfort. The exact cause of postoperative discomfort is likely multifactorial and includes peritoneal irritation from tacks, mesh, and transfascial sutures. Persistent pain beyond 6 weeks is rare and is often related to a transfascial sutures. These can be successfully managed with percutaneous injection of 30 mL of bupivacaine in most cases. Rarely, the offending suture must be removed.

The major advantage of a laparoscopic ventral hernia repair is that mesh infections are extremely rare. In fact, if the surgeon suspects a mesh infection after a laparoscopic ventral hernia repair, serious consideration should be given to an unrecognized bowel injury. Occasionally, laparoscopic mesh can become contaminated with skin flora during introduction into the abdomen. These patients present with erythema overlying the seroma cavity. The seroma should be aspirated and cultured. Rare cases of mesh salvage with percutaneous drainage, antibiotic irrigation, and lifetime suppression with antibiotics have been described. However, most patients need excision of the mesh and reconstruction.

■ OUTCOMES

Laparoscopic ventral hernia repair has gained widespread acceptance. Several prospective randomized trials have shown the safety and efficacy of laparoscopic ventral hernia repair when compared with open ventral hernia repair. The one common finding of all series is a significant reduction in wound-related morbidity associated with the laparoscopic repair. Most of these series have included a highly selected group of patients with relatively small defects, and whether the laparoscopic approach is appropriate for larger, more complex hernias is unclear. In summary, the laparoscopic repair of ventral hernias is a valuable approach for the repair of abdominal wall defects. In skilled hands, performed appropriately with safe adhesiolysis and adequate mesh placement, excellent long-term results are possible.

SUGGESTED READINGS

Asencio F, Aguiló J, Peiró S, et al. Open randomized clinical trial of laparoscopic versus open incisional hernia repair. *Surg Endosc.* 2009;23:1441-1448.

Itani KM, Hur K, Kim LT, et al. Comparison of laparoscopic and open repair with mesh for the treatment of ventral incisional hernia: a randomized trial. *Arch Surg.* 2010;145:322-328.

Olmi S, Scaubu A, Cesana GC, et al. Laparoscopic versus open incisional hernia repair: an open randomized controlled study. *Surg Endosc.* 2007;21:555-559.

Orenstein SB, Dumeer JL, Monteagudo J, et al. Outcomes of laparoscopic ventral hernia repair with routine defect closure using "shoelacing" technique. *Surg Endosc.* 2011;25:1452-1457.

Pring CM, Tran V, O'Rourke N, et al. Laparoscopic versus open ventral hernia repair: a randomized controlled trial. *ANZ J Surg.* 2008;78:903-906.

Rosen MJ, Fatima J, Sarr MG. Repair of abdominal wall hernias with restoration of abdominal wall function. *J Gastrointest Surg.* 2010;14:175-185.

LAPAROSCOPIC REPAIR OF PARASTOMAL HERNIAS

Dimitrios Stefanidis, MD, PhD

More than 750,000 Americans have an ostomy, and approximately 130,000 new enterostomies are created each year in the United States, of which more than 40% are permanent. The defect created in the abdominal wall during ostomy construction, the trephine, produces a weakness that is subject to the continuous tangential forces applied by the increased intra-abdominal pressure as compared with the atmosphere. It is therefore not surprising that hernias form next to the ostomy in up to 50% of patients.

Patient risk factors for parastomal hernia formation include advanced age, prior wound infection, malnutrition, chronic or recurrent increases in intra-abdominal pressure, chronic obstructive pulmonary disease, obesity, weight gain after ostomy construction, glucocorticoids, immunosuppression, malignancy, and inflammatory bowel disease. Technical factors that influence hernia rates include emergency surgery, the ostomy defect size (higher risk with ostomy diameter >2.5 cm; ileostomies have a significantly lower reported hernia rate compared with colostomies), and the actual surgical technique used.

Most hernias occur within the first 2 years after stomal construction, but the risk is lifelong. Although most parastomal hernias are seen as bulges and are easy to diagnose by physical examination, a computed tomographic (CT) scan of the abdomen can be useful in cases where the patient's symptoms are suggestive but the diagnosis is not obvious on examination. It should be noted that several parastomal hernia classification schemes have been proposed, but these do not affect the management of these hernias and therefore they will not be discussed in this chapter.

■ INDICATIONS AND CONTRAINDICATIONS

Indications for urgent and emergent repair include acute bowel obstruction with incarceration to avoid the risk of strangulation and bowel necrosis. Given that most patients have chronic bothersome symptoms, indications for elective repair typically include chronic abdominal or occasionally back pain related to the parastomal hernia, recurrent partial small bowel obstructions, enlargement of the hernia to the point where it interferes with appliance wear and leads to frequent leakage not amenable to conservative measures, skin breakdown around the stoma related to thinning from pressure by the enlarging hernia, or psychologic distress related to the presence of the hernia. These indications apply to permanent stomas; for temporary stomas, takedown of the ostomy and closure of the ostomy site with reinforcement is the preferred approach when appropriate. Although laparoscopic repair of parastomal hernias can be achieved in the majority of cases, relative contraindications may include extensive intra-abdominal adhesions or very large hernias (>8 to 12 cm) that may make it difficult to obtain adequate mesh overlap. The need for a concomitant open procedure may necessitate an open approach, and the surgeon's skill level and comfort with laparoscopic techniques also should be taken into consideration when repairing these hernias. Prior experience with laparoscopic ventral incisional hernia repair is important, and for optimal outcomes smaller parastomal hernias should be chosen for laparoscopic repair during the surgeon's early experience with these hernias. In high-risk patients and those with multiple prior recurrences, conservative management may be the better approach.

■ PREOPERATIVE PLANNING

Preoperative Preparation

An evidence-based approach to preoperative preparation of the patient is advised. Bowel preparation is typically not necessary, perhaps with the exception of patients with known incarceration where the risk of enterotomy during reduction may be higher. Intravenous (IV) broad-spectrum antibiotics are administered within 1 hour of skin incision as per institutional protocol. Deep vein prophylaxis also should be ordered to minimize risk of venous thromboembolism (VTE). Informed consent should include the potential for conversion to an open procedure, risk for enterotomy, mesh infection, bowel obstruction, and hernia recurrence.

Patient Positioning and Preparation

The patient is placed in supine position with all pressure points appropriately padded. The arm on the opposite side of the hernia and stoma should be tucked to prevent interference with surgeon positioning during the procedure. The arm on the same side as the hernia typically does not need to be tucked, allowing anesthesia staff access to the arm during the case if needed. A slight tilt of the table with the side of the hernia up can be useful to allow additional lateral access to the hernia side.

The patient is secured to the table with straps or tape, and an orogastric tube and indwelling urinary bladder catheter are placed. The skin is prepared with antiseptic solution; wide preparation laterally, especially on the side of the hernia, is imperative. To avoid contamination of the sterile field during the procedure, the ostomy needs to be covered securely. This can be accomplished either by suturing it closed with a suture that incorporates the submucosa or by packing a sponge into it. A sterile sponge is placed on top and covered with a healthy margin with a moderate-sized Tegaderm. Both of these approaches will isolate the ostomy and maintain sterility during the case. The use of an adhesive drape (such as Ioban) can be considered but has not been shown to decrease the rate of wound infection.

Surgeon and Monitor Positioning and Instrument Selection

The surgeon and assistant will stand on the patient's side opposite the stoma (Figure 1). The primary monitor is placed on the side of the stoma in an ergonomic position at the surgeon's eye level. Additional monitors can be used but typically are not needed.

A good-quality 30-degree, 5-mm laparoscope is recommended for optimal visualization through all ports. If this is not available, a 10-mm camera and trocar may be needed. A fixation device is needed for this procedure, and spinal needles can be very useful when measuring the hernia defect.

Port Selection and Placement

A 5-mm optical entry port is used to access the abdominal cavity under direct visualization on the surgeon's side (opposite to the hernia) in the mid-distance between the rib cage and iliac crest. If the surgeon is unfamiliar with optical entry, an open Hasson or Veress needle technique can be used. Balloon tip trocars can be considered but are not mandatory. Initial inspection of the peritoneal cavity provides clues about the feasibility of the procedure using laparoscopy and rules out unsuspected pathology. One additional 5-mm trocar is placed inferiorly, and one 11- or 12-mm trocar is placed superiorly, as shown in Figure 1, under direct vision to avoid injury of intra-abdominal organs. The latter trocar is placed directly under the costal margin to minimize postoperative hernia risk. An important point to consider when placing these trocars is that if the

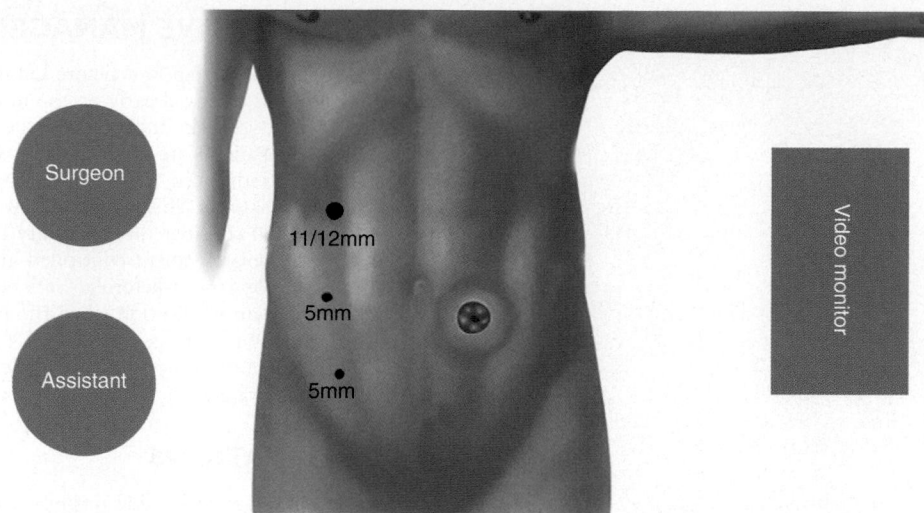

FIGURE 1 Patient positioning and trocar placement for laparoscopic parastomal hernia repair.

patient also has a midline hernia (not an unusual scenario given that many stomas are created via midline incisions), the trocars should be placed laterally enough to enable attachment of the near side of the mesh so that it appropriately covers the midline defect and the parastomal hernia defect. Ports should be spaced adequately (approximately a handwidth apart) to avoid instrument conflicts. The angle of trocar placement to the abdominal wall should be considered carefully, as perpendicular placement to slight angulation toward the target (5 to 10 degrees) generally will work best, whereas angulation away from the target will increase the difficulty of the procedure, especially in the obese patient with a thick abdominal wall.

■ OPERATIVE TECHNIQUE

Division of Adhesions and Reduction of Hernia

Omental and intestinal adhesions to the anterior abdominal wall are divided with sharp dissection (cold scissors) and appropriate traction by the nondominant hand for optimal exposure. Alternative energy–based devices, such as Harmonic scalpel or Enseal (Ethicon Endo-Surgery, Cincinnati, OH) or LigaSure (Covidien, Mansfield, MA), may be helpful, especially when faced with multiple vascular adhesions, but should be used cautiously because they increase the risk for burn injury to the intestines that may go undetected. The potential for bowel injury is real, especially when adhesions are very dense, such as in the case of a previous mesh repair. The surgeon should not hesitate to convert to an open procedure if adhesiolysis cannot be achieved safely using the laparoscopic approach. When bowel loops are incarcerated in the hernia sac, they should be reduced gently using appropriate traction and safe division of adhesions. To prevent injury to the bowel leading to the ostomy, the surgeon should inspect and follow the bowel loops carefully until it is clear which bowel leads to the ostomy and which is incarcerated in the hernia. In addition, it is important to identify the location of the mesentery of the bowel leading to the ostomy to avoid its injury; in general, the mesentery is positioned medially, but exceptions exist. The ostomy bowel also is freed from any adhesions to the hernia sac and pulled intra-abdominally to reduce any existing prolapse.

The peritoneal sac typically is not reduced. After all of the bowel has been reduced, it should be inspected carefully to ascertain that no enterotomy or deserosalization occurred during adhesiolysis.

Repair of Hernia

When a Sugarbaker approach (my preferred approach) is used to repair the hernia, the bowel leading to the stoma should have adequate laxity to allow it to fold against the lateral abdominal wall. Although adequate laxity often will exist after hernia reduction, occasionally mobilization of the bowel may be necessary to allow adequate lateralization of the bowel without tension. Next, the hernia defect size should be measured; this step is important in determining the needed mesh size. The size can be measured with the use of a suture or a flexible ruler introduced intra-abdominally and spinal needles placed transabdominally. When the defect is too large, approximating it with transfascial sutures (shoe-lace technique) can be considered using a suture passer. The size of the selected piece of mesh should provide wide coverage of the hernia defect with at least a 5-cm overlap in all directions. Although no high-level evidence exists to define the optimal mesh overlap, most experts agree that a 5-cm overlap is adequate to minimize the rate of recurrence.

A variety of mesh types can be used for the repair; I prefer to use a nonabsorbable mesh to minimize risk for recurrence. Similar to laparoscopic repair of incisional hernias, an expanded polytetrafluoroethylene (ePTFE)–based mesh or a polypropylene-polyester composite mesh with a protective nonadherent layer can be used. When using a nonabsorbable mesh, it is important to consider that the "rough" side of the mesh, which promotes ingrowth into the posterior abdominal wall, also will be in contact with the lateralized bowel when using the Sugarbaker technique. This can increase the risk for mesh erosion into the bowel; to minimize this risk, a mesh that is less adherent, such as the Gore Dualmesh (Gore Medical, Flagstaff, AZ), or a combination of a biologic-bioabsorbable mesh over the bowel and a nonabsorbable mesh on top may work best. The use of a mesh that incorporates a positioning system, such as the Ventralight ST Mesh with Echo PS Positioning System (Davol Inc, Providence, RI), may simplify mesh placement and expedite the procedure.

Sutures are preplaced on the mesh as shown in Figure 2, and the mesh is folded and introduced into the abdominal cavity via the 11- or 12-mm trocar. The mesh then is unfolded intra-abdominally and oriented appropriately, and the lateral sutures are exteriorized first through the abdominal wall via stab incisions using a laparoscopic suture passer, taking care to fold the ostomy bowel laterally on top of the mesh (see Figure 2). The surgeon should pay close attention to the location of these sutures because besides ensuring that the mesh covers the ostomy bowel and defect with excellent margins, the sutures need to be close enough to each other to appose the bowel to the abdominal wall without leaving gaps next to the bowel but loose enough to not obstruct the intestinal lumen. Some surgeons recommend not cutting the excess sutures after tying the knots down

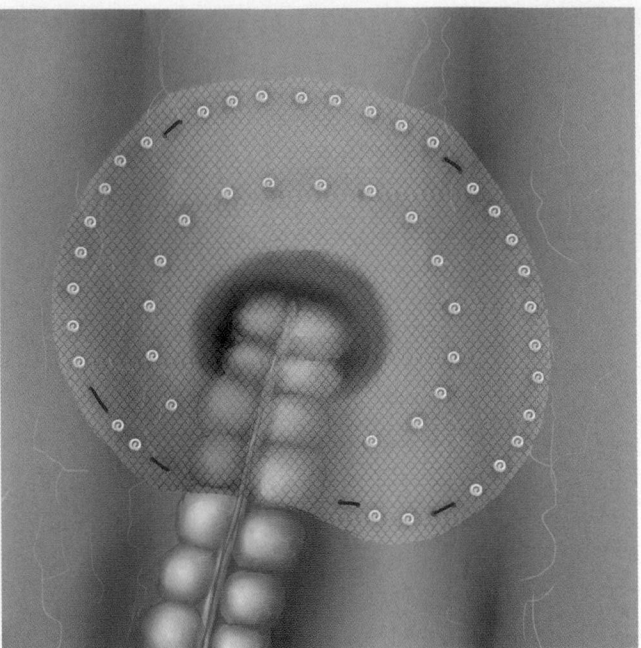

FIGURE 2 Mesh placement during laparoscopic parastomal hernia repair (Sugarbaker technique).

and taping them to the skin so that they can be removed later if the mesh proves to be too tight against the bowel (obstructing) in the postoperative period; I have not found this approach to be necessary. After the mesh has been attached laterally, the medial sutures are exteriorized, ensuring adequate coverage by the mesh of all defects (parastomal and midline), and a tacker is used at 1- to 2-cm intervals to securely attach the periphery of the mesh to the abdominal wall. The number of sutures used varies depending on surgeon preference; I typically use 4 to 6 sutures (see Figure 2). Suturing the mesh to the mesenteric peritoneum of the ostomy bowel or suturing the ostomy to the lateral abdominal wall with absorbable sutures also can be considered.

When tacking or placing extra sutures, care is advised to avoid injuring the ostomy bowel or mesentery, which is usually not easy to see once the mesh has been approximated to the abdominal wall. After mesh fixation, the bowel should be inspected a final time to exclude any unsuspected injury or bowel compression.

The keyhole technique also has been used for parastomal hernia repair. During this technique the ostomy bowel traverses the mesh through a central or slightly off-center opening, and a slit is created by the surgeon. Given that recent evidence suggests that the Sugarbaker technique has superior outcomes compared with the keyhole technique (outlined later), the latter technique will not be described in detail.

The fascia defect at the larger trocar sites is closed with absorbable sutures, and all trocar sites and the area around the mesh can be infiltrated with a long-lasting local anesthetic (Exparel [bupivacaine liposome injectable suspension]; Pacira Pharmaceuticals, Parsippany, NJ) to aid with postoperative analgesia.

■ POSTOPERATIVE MANAGEMENT

The orogastric tube is removed before extubation, and the Foley catheter typically is removed early on the next morning. Dextrose-containing IV fluids are administered until the patient is able to tolerate liquids orally. Patients are offered liquids when they are hungry, and their diet is advanced as tolerated, typically when flatus is expressed from the stoma. This may take a few days, but if prolonged, the surgeon should consider the possibility of the mesh being too tight against the bowel. Patient-controlled analgesia supplemented with IV acetaminophen or ketorolac can be used as needed and switched to oral pain medication when the patient is tolerating an oral diet. Early ambulation is encouraged. Patients are discharged when they are tolerating a diet and have evidence of bowel function; recovery is usually rapid.

■ COMPLICATIONS

Early complications may include unsuspected bowel injury, infection, or obstruction of the intestine, all of which are rare in experienced hands. Longer-term complications may include hernia recurrence, mesh erosion into the bowel, and chronic pain.

■ POSTOPERATIVE OUTCOMES

A systematic review and a meta-analysis of the literature have been published recently, examining the outcomes of laparoscopic parastomal hernia repair in several hundred patients. Overall postoperative morbidity is low; surgical site infections have been seen in 3.8% (95% confidence interval [CI]: 2.3 to 5.7) of patients, and infected mesh was observed in 1.7% to 3%. Obstruction requiring reoperation occurred in 1.7% (95% CI: 0.7 to 3.0) of patients. Other complications such as ileus, pneumonia, or urinary tract infection were noted in 16.6% (95% CI: 11.9 to 22.1) of patients. No intraoperative mortalities have been reported, but six postoperative mortalities have occurred.

The overall recurrence rate with laparoscopic parastomal hernia mesh repair was 17.4% (95% CI: 9.5 to 26.9); however, recurrence rate was significantly lower with the modified laparoscopic Sugarbaker approach (10.2% recurrence rate; 95% CI: 3.9 to 19.0) compared with the keyhole approach (27.9% recurrence rate; 95% CI: 12.3 to 46.9). The systematic review found an odds ratio [OR] of 2.3 (95% CI: 1.2 to 4.6; $P = 0.016$) for recurrence after keyhole repair versus Sugarbaker repair. It further concluded that suture repair should be abandoned, as it was associated with an OR of 8.9 (95% CI: 5.2 to 15.0) for hernia recurrence compared with mesh repair. A systematic review of open parastomal hernia repair came to the same conclusion, advocating the abandonment of suture repair.

Suggested Readings

Al Shakarchi J, Williams JG. Systematic review of open techniques for parastomal hernia repair. *Tech Coloproctol.* 2014;18:427-432.

DeAsis FJ, Lapin B, Gitelis ME, Ujiki MB. Current state of laparoscopic parastomal hernia repair: a meta-analysis. *World J Gastroenterol.* 2015;21: 8670-8677.

Hansson BM, Slater NJ, van der Velden AS, Groenewoud HM, Buyne OR, de Hingh IH, Bleichrodt RP. Surgical techniques for parastomal hernia repair: a systematic review of the literature. *Ann Surg.* 2012;255:685-695.

LAPAROSCOPIC SPLENECTOMY

Fernando Mier, MD, and John G. Hunter, MD, FRCS Edin (hon)

Splenectomy is performed as either definitive or symptomatic therapy for numerous indications. Patients with benign hematologic conditions obtain the most benefit from this procedure. Since its introduction in the 1990s, laparoscopic splenectomy has become the standard approach for elective splenectomy. It presents the special challenge of removing a fragile organ that is relatively inaccessible, tucked high and posterior beneath the left costal margin and behind the greater omentum, adjacent to the left hemidiaphragm. It is surrounded by important organs such as the stomach, pancreas, kidney, and colon. Because of its size, removal of the spleen from the abdomen challenges the small incision principles of minimally invasive surgery. Although only one randomized controlled trial has compared open splenectomy with laparoscopic splenectomy, the minimally invasive approach has become the most popular approach worldwide for elective splenectomy of the normal-sized spleen.

■ INDICATIONS

Laparoscopic splenectomy is recommended for both benign and malignant disease. In cases of benign hematologic disorders, idiopathic thrombocytopenic purpura (ITP) is by far the most common indication, responsible for 50% to 80% of splenectomies. Other less common benign hematologic indications include hemolytic anemias such as hereditary spherocytosis, major and intermediate thalassemia with secondary hypersplenism, and refractory autoimmune hemolytic anemia. In all cases of autoimmune thrombocytopenia or hemolytic anemia, it is highly recommended to search for accessory spleens at the time of the operation. Splenectomy also is indicated for diagnostic or staging purposes for malignant hematologic diseases, including myeloproliferative and lymphoproliferative disorders with splenomegaly, hairy cell leukemia, and splenic lymphoma. In these diseases, removal of the intact organ for pathologic examination may be necessary; therefore a hand-assisted laparoscopic splenectomy is recommended. Relative contraindications to the laparoscopic approach include splenomegaly, portal hypertension, obesity, and pregnancy. The primary absolute contraindications to the laparoscopic approach are emergency situations such as traumatic or spontaneous splenic rupture and the inability to tolerate pneumoperitoneum.

■ SURGICAL ANATOMY

An understanding of splenic anatomy, vasculature, and surrounding organs is essential for performing a safe laparoscopic splenectomy.

The spleen is a convex organ located beneath the ninth, tenth, and eleventh ribs in the left upper quadrant. Its medial surface is surrounded by the stomach, pancreas, kidney, and splenic flexure of the colon, all of which leave an impression on the spleen.

The spleen is surrounded by many ligamentous attachments that are formed by fused duplications of the peritoneum. Two ligaments contain vascular structures, and the remainder are usually avascular except in patients with portal hypertension. Anteriorly, the gastrosplenic ligament contains the short gastric and gastroepiploic vessels. Posteriorly, the lienorenal ligament contains the tail of the pancreas and the splenic hilar vessels. The longest ligament is the phrenocolic ligament, which courses laterally from the diaphragm to the splenic flexure of the colon.

There are two major configurations of splenic artery topography: the distributed type and the bundled type (Figures 1 and 2). The former is the most common type, found in almost 70% of anatomic specimens. The splenic trunk is short and its branches originate between 3 and 13 cm from the splenic hilum. The bundled type is present in the remaining 30% of anatomic dissections. This type is characterized by a long splenic artery that divides into short terminal branches as it approaches the hilum. There are up to six short gastric vessels that originate from the fundus of the stomach, but only the ones supplying the superior polar vessels need to be dissected during a laparoscopic splenectomy.

■ PREOPERATIVE PREPARATION

All patients should receive preoperative vaccinations 2 weeks before an elective laparoscopic splenectomy. Current recommendations include vaccination against encapsulated organisms such as meningococcus, pneumococcus, and *Haemophilus influenzae*. Booster shots usually are offered every 5 years, and an annual influenza vaccination is recommended for patients who have undergone splenectomy.

Patients with hematologic diseases should undergo the same preoperative optimization of their disease as for any other surgery. This may include administration of steroids, intravenous immunoglobulin G (IV IgG), and plasmapheresis. Chemotherapy of hematologic malignancy should be timed to optimize circulating cell counts before splenectomy. Patients on chronic or high doses of steroids should receive a stress dose of 100 mg of hydrocortisone preoperatively and tapered doses postoperatively.

Preoperative ultrasonography or computed tomographic (CT) scans will determine the spleen size accurately as well as its relation to the surrounding organs. CT scanning may be superior to ultrasound for localizing accessory spleens. For these reasons we recommend a CT scan before performing laparoscopic splenectomy in most patients.

■ OPERATIVE TECHNIQUES

The original surgical approaches to laparoscopic splenectomy were lateral and anterior. Both of these approaches had limitations for removing the normal-sized spleen. With the anterior approach, the lesser sac dissection is facile, but the retrosplenic dissection is difficult. With the lateral approach, the anterior dissection of the short gastric vessels and tail of the pancreas are unfamiliar, and an urgent conversion to open splenectomy is more difficult. Hence the most common technique is halfway between these two approaches, the 45-degree tilt, otherwise known as the "leaning spleen."

Positioning

After induction of general anesthesia, an orogastric tube and Foley catheter are placed. To achieve the 45-degree approach, a bean bag is placed on the table and a foam wedge or pillow is placed behind it to achieve the desired tilt. The hips are tilted 45 degrees, and the knees are bent and padded. A right axillary roll is placed, and the left arm is placed in an arm cradle. Before applying suction to the bean bag, the table is flexed to bend the spine and open the space between the costal margin and the left iliac wing (Figure 3). The anterior approach is used rarely but is of value for large spleens, hand-assisted cases, pediatric cases, and when a concomitant surgery such as cholecystectomy is planned.

The surgeon and first assistant should stand on the right side of the patient. The patient is tilted to the left to nearly flatten the abdomen, allowing preparation and draping from beyond the posterior axillary line on the left to the anterior axillary line on the right. An open laparotomy set should be readily available for potential conversion.

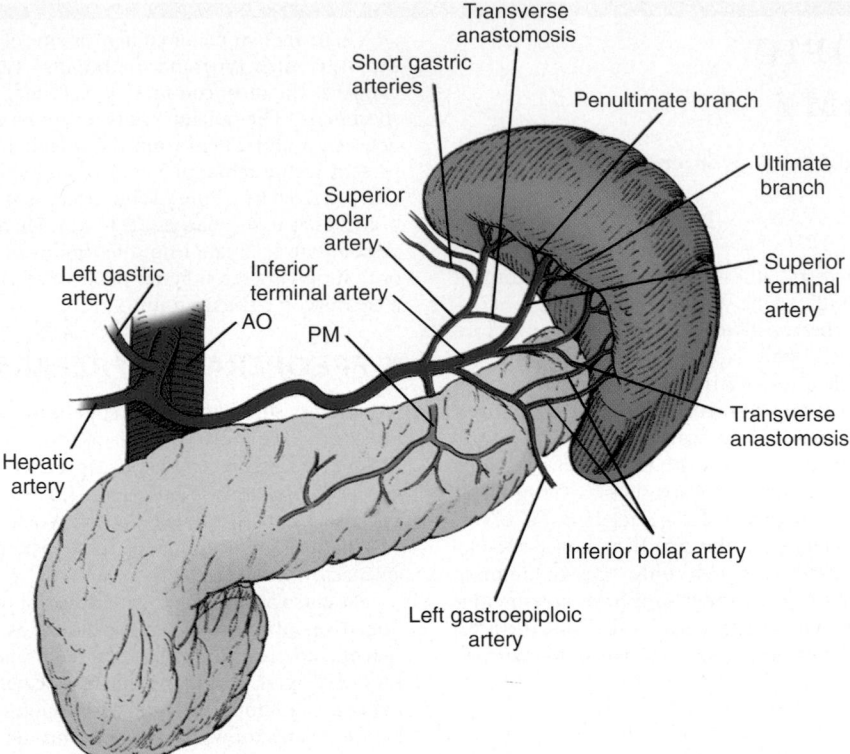

FIGURE 1 Distributed vascularization. By definition, the splenic trunk is short, and many long branches (6 to 12) enter over three fourths of the medial surface of the spleen. The branches originate between 3 and 13 cm from the hilum. Outside the spleen, the arteries also present frequent transverse anastomoses with each other, which according to Testud arise at a right angle between the involved arteries, as with most collaterals. Thus the application of hemostatic clips on or the embolization of coils occluding a branch of the splenic artery before such an anastomosis may fail to devascularize the corresponding splenic segment. *AO*, Aorta; *PM*, pancreatic magna. *(From Poulin EC, Thibault C. The anatomical basis for laparoscopic splenectomy. Can J Surg. 1993;36:485-488.)*

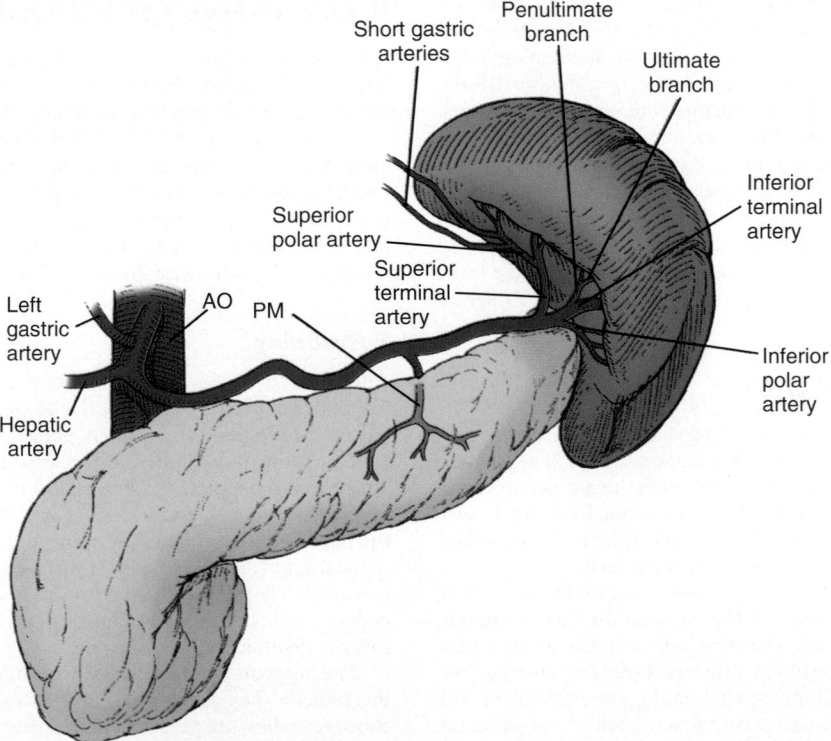

FIGURE 2 Bundled vascularization. The bundled type is characterized by the presence of a long main splenic artery that divides into short terminal branches near the hilum. In this type, the splenic branches enter over only a fourth to a third of the medial surface of the spleen. These branches are large, few (three to four), originate an average of 3.5 cm from the spleen, and reach the center of the organ as a compact bundle. *AO*, Aorta; *PM*, pancreatic magna. *(From Poulin EC, Thibault C. The anatomical basis for laparoscopic splenectomy. Can J Surg. 1993;36:485-488.)*

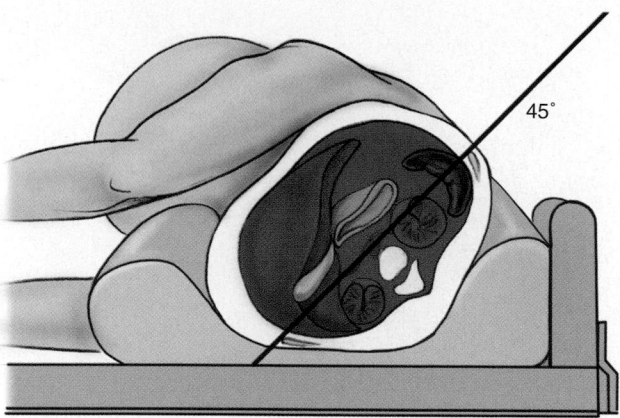

FIGURE 3 The "leaning spleen" technique requires a 45-degree tilt with a bean bag or jelly roll positioning pad.

Access and Port Placement

A pneumoperitoneum is achieved with either a closed technique with the Veress needle or an open (Hassan) technique. The Veress needle is placed through a stab incision just below the costal margin and just medial to the anterior axillary line (Palmer's point) or through the umbilicus. Once the pneumoperitoneum is created, the first trocar is inserted approximately 10 cm medial to the anterior axillary line in a line from the umbilicus to the costal margin. A 5- or 10-mm 30-degree angled laparoscope is used. The remaining trocars are placed under direct visualization. A 5-mm trocar is placed in the subxiphoid location for the surgeon's left hand. A 12-mm trocar is placed between the costal margin and the iliac crest at the anterior axillary line for the surgeon's right hand, the insertion of a surgical stapler, and to be used as the extraction port. Finally a 5-mm trocar is placed over the posterior axillary line for the assistant's left hand. Exact sites of port insertion and access may vary depending on the patient's body habitus and spleen size (Figure 4).

Dissection

Initial exploration of the abdomen should begin with a search for accessory spleens. The most frequent location for accessory spleens is the hilum of the spleen, followed by the gastrosplenic ligament, splenorenal ligament, and greater omentum. For dissection, we prefer to use the ultrasonic dissector, but other energy devices can be used as well. To begin the operation, the table is tipped to the left to nearly flatten the abdomen. In this position we take down the gastrosplenic ligament and divide the short gastric vessels. For additional exposure of the superior pole of the spleen, the patient is placed in reverse Trendelenburg position, and medial retraction of the greater curvature is required with the surgeon's left hand (Figure 5). Then we mobilize the splenic flexure of the colon by incising the inferior portion of the phrenocolic ligament (Figure 6). This will help with exposure of the posterior aspect of the splenic hilum. Then the table is rolled to the right to expose the splenorenal ligament and the phrenosplenic ligament. In most cases the weight of the spleen, now falling forward, provides adequate retraction to visualize the retrosplenic attachments, but it may be necessary for the first assistant to elevate the spleen, rolling it anteriorly. At this point the hilar vessels should be visualized easily, and cautious mobilization of the tail of the pancreas may be needed for better visualization. By lifting the spleen, the hilum is exposed and a linear surgical stapler is used to divide the vessels en masse. In the case of the distributed type of vasculature, several loads may need to be used, and the larger branches should be isolated and divided separately (Figures 7 and 8).

In cases of splenomegaly, we recommend entering the lesser sac through the gastrocolic ligament followed by identification and

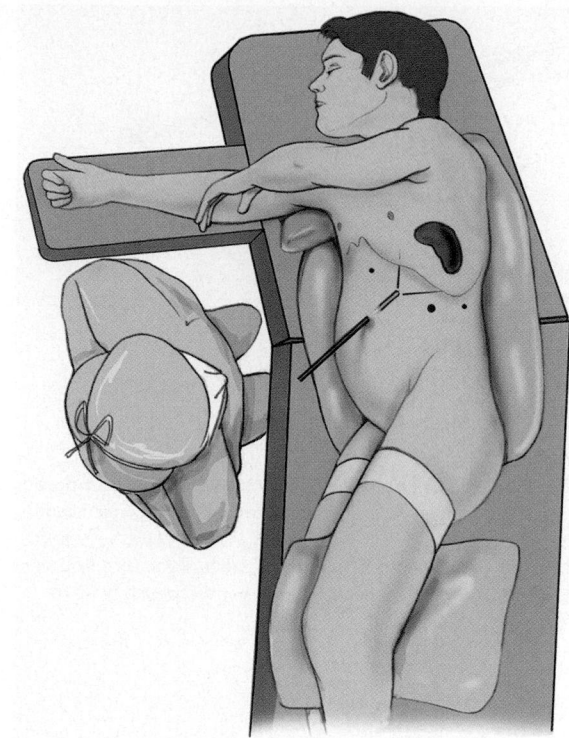

FIGURE 4 Patient, port, and laparoscope positions for the "leaning spleen" technique.

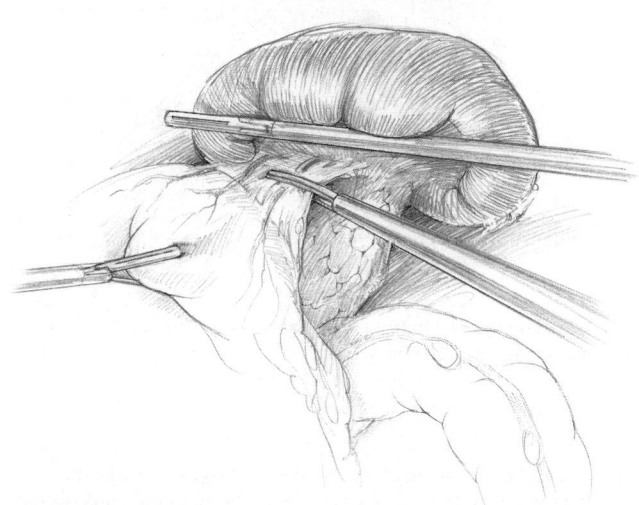

FIGURE 5 Short gastric dissection. For additional exposure of the superior pole of the spleen, the patient is placed in reverse Trendelenburg position, and medial retraction of the greater curvature is required with the surgeon's left hand. *(From Hunter JG et al, eds. Atlas of Minimally Invasive Surgical Operations [in press]. New York: McGraw Hill; 2016. Illustrations by Corinne Sandone © Art as Applied to Medicine, Johns Hopkins University, 2016.)*

posteroinferior mobilization of the tail of the pancreas to expose the splenic artery. Ligation and control of the splenic artery at the beginning will prevent hemorrhage during hilar dissection.

Once the spleen is detached it is placed in a heavy duty bag. The bag is then extracted through the 12- to 15-mm port site. The spleen is fragmented and removed from the neck of the bag in a piecemeal fashion with finger fracture or ringed forceps (Figure 9). Care should be taken to avoid spilling splenic contents, to prevent splenosis and

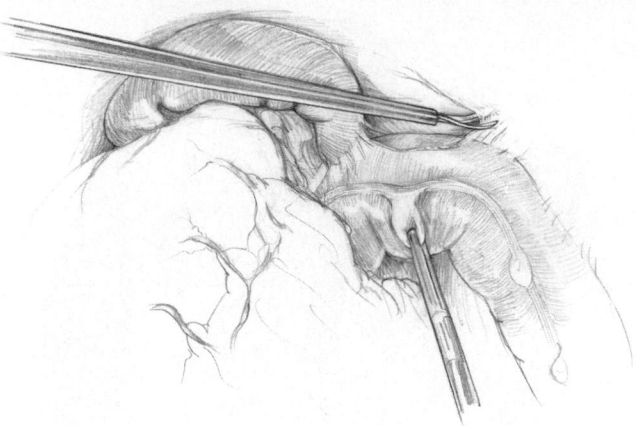

FIGURE 6 Splenic flexure dissection. By incising the inferior portion of the phrenocolic ligament, the posterior aspect of the splenic hilum is exposed. *(From Hunter JG et al, eds. Atlas of Minimally Invasive Surgical Operations [in press]. New York: McGraw Hill; 2016. Illustrations by Corinne Sandone © Art as Applied to Medicine, Johns Hopkins University, 2016.)*

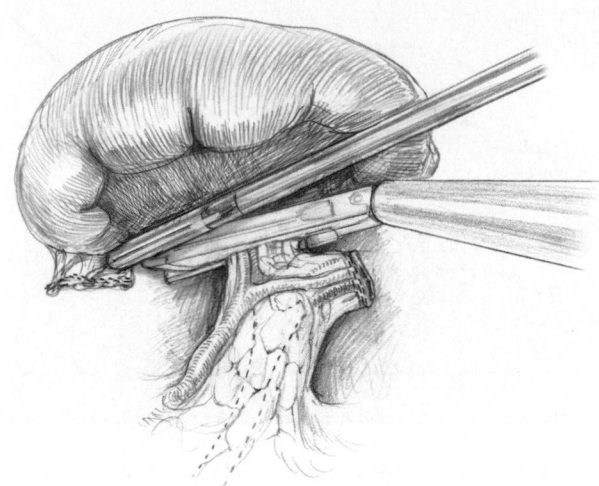

FIGURE 8 In the case of the distributed type of vasculature, several loads may need to be used, and the larger branches should be isolated and divided separately. *(From Hunter JG et al, eds. Atlas of Minimally Invasive Surgical Operations [in press]. New York: McGraw Hill; 2016. Illustrations by Corinne Sandone © Art as Applied to Medicine, Johns Hopkins University, 2016.)*

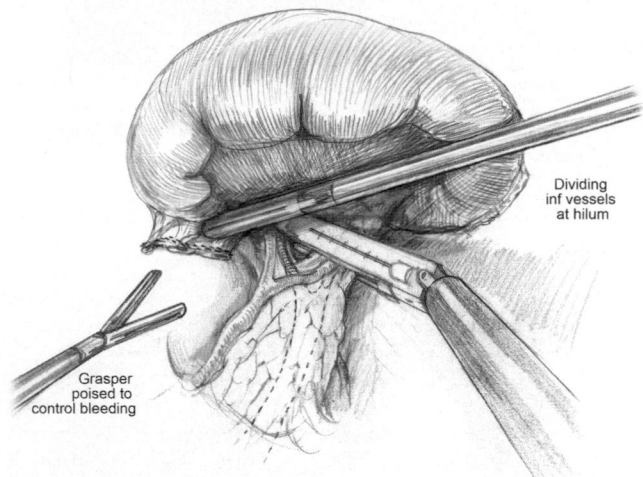

FIGURE 7 The splenic blood supply is controlled in the splenic hilum with a linear cutting stapler. *(From Hunter JG et al, eds. Atlas of Minimally Invasive Surgical Operations [in press]. New York: McGraw Hill; 2016. Illustrations by Corinne Sandone © Art as Applied to Medicine, Johns Hopkins University, 2016.)*

lose the benefit of splenectomy. We do not leave surgical drains routinely. The fascia of the extraction port is closed in the usual fashion, and the skin is closed with subcuticular sutures.

■ POSTOPERATIVE CARE

Postoperative recovery is quicker after laparoscopic splenectomy than after open splenectomy, and postoperative analgesic use is minimal after the first few days. The diet is advanced, and most patients are discharged within 2 postoperative days. All patients should be instructed of their increased risk for infection from encapsulated bacteria, warranting prophylactic antibiotics for dental procedures and vigilance should they develop an unexplained fever.

■ OUTCOMES AND COMPLICATIONS

Intraoperative hemorrhage is the most common complication of splenectomy. Bleeding is caused mainly by laceration of the hilar or short gastric vessels. If brisk bleeding cannot be controlled

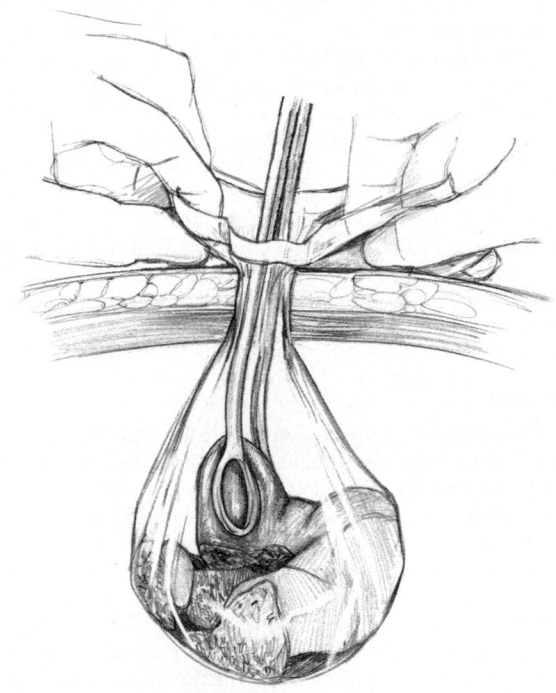

FIGURE 9 Extraction of the spleen. Once the spleen is detached, it is placed in a heavy duty bag. The spleen is fragmented and removed from the neck of the bag in a piecemeal fashion with finger fracture or ringed forceps. Care should be taken to avoid spilling splenic contents. *(From Hunter JG et al, eds. Atlas of Minimally Invasive Surgical Operations [in press]. New York: McGraw Hill; 2016. Illustrations by Corinne Sandone © Art as Applied to Medicine, Johns Hopkins University, 2016.)*

immediately laparoscopically, rapid conversion to laparotomy must occur. Resulting from their proximity, injury to the tail of the pancreas and the gastric fundus also can occur. Injuries to the stomach should be repaired with sutures or a surgical stapler. A 19F round drain should be left in place in cases where transection includes the tail of the pancreas. The incidence of pancreatic injury has been reported as 15% in some series. In the hands of experienced laparoscopists, this incidence should be approximately 1%. Although rare, overwhelming postsplenectomy sepsis carries an extremely high mortality rate, reported as up to 40% to 50%. Patients have the highest risk during the first 2 years after splenectomy. Patients with thalassemia and sickle cell anemia are at the highest risk. All patients should be counseled on this lifetime risk. Over the long term, laparoscopic splenectomy is effective in resolving hematologic diseases, especially if the preoperative indication is thrombocytopenia.

SUGGESTED READINGS

Casaccia M, Torelli P, Pasa A, et al. Putative predictive parameters for the outcome of laparoscopic splenectomy: a multicenter analysis performed on the Italian Registry of Laparoscopic Surgery of the Spleen. *Ann Surg.* 2010;251:287-291.

Feldman LS. Laparoscopic splenectomy: standardized approach. *World J Surg.* 2011;54:189-193.

Habermalz B, Sauerland S, Decker G, et al. Laparoscopic splenectomy: the clinical practice guidelines of the European Association of Endoscopic Surgery (EAES). *Surg Endosc.* 2008;22:821-848.

Kojouri K, Vesely S, Deirdra R, et al. Splenectomy for adult patient with idiopathic thrombocytopenic purpura: a systematic review to assess long-term platelet count responses, prediction of response and surgical comlications. *Blood.* 2004;104:2623-2634.

Konstadoulakis MM, Lagoundakis E, Antonakis PT, et al. Laparoscopic versus open splenectomy in patients with beta thalassemia major. *J Laparoendosc Adv Surg Tech A.* 2006;16:5-8.

Marcus CF, Schäfer M, Müller MK, et al. Laparoscopic versus open splenectomy for nontraumatic diseases. *World J Surg.* 2008;32:2444-2449.

Richardson WS, Smith CD, Braunum GD, Hunter JG. Leaning spleen: a new approach to laparoscopic splenectomy. *J Am Coll Surg.* 1997;185: 412-415.

Rubin LG, Schaffner W. Clinical practice: care of the asplenic patient. *N Engl J Med.* 2014;371:349-356.

Sampath S, Meneghetti AT, MacFarlane JK, et al. An 18-year review of open and laparoscopic splenectomy for patient with idiopathic thrombocytopenic purpura. *Am J Surg.* 2007;193:580-584.

LAPAROSCOPIC GASTRIC SURGERY

Erin M. Garvey, MD, and B. Todd Heniford, MD

Operative treatment of gastric pathology has changed dramatically since Theodore Billroth performed the first successful gastrectomy in the 1880s. Its evolution includes dramatic surgical and technological progress, such as the description of various types of anastomoses, the development of surgical staplers, the use of naso-enteric sump tubes, and as important as any advancement, the invention of the flexible endoscope and the skill set necessary to perform diagnostic and therapeutic upper endoscopy. Medical progress also has had an impact on gastric surgery; the advent of selective histamine receptor blockers and proton pump inhibitors and the description and treatment strategies for *Helicobacter pylori* all have contributed to dramatically reducing the surgical management of peptic ulcer disease.

However, because of the technical innovations of minimally invasive surgery, surgeons have generated renewed interest in upper gastrointestinal surgery. There is little doubt that laparoscopy, with its resultant reduction in morbidity and time necessary for patient recovery, has been responsible for a dramatic growth in gastric surgery since the early 1990s. Patients who previously were palliated with medications or observed for a variety of lesions are now seeking definitive surgical therapy. Few areas in all of surgery have seen the growth that has been documented in the area of the lower esophagus and stomach. The number of antireflux procedures and bariatric operations performed has grown exponentially because of the nearly systematic conversion to a laparoscopic approach. The applicability of laparoscopic gastric resection and other procedures stems from the accessibility of the stomach both laparoscopically and endoscopically, the abundance of experience with other gastric operations (e.g., antireflux surgery), the availability and reliability of laparoscopic staplers, and the fact that many gastric tumors require only simple negative margins without lymphadenectomy for curative resection. Although the indications and the expected end result for laparoscopic gastric surgery are the same as those for laparotomy, the stepwise performance of the procedure and the skill set are somewhat different.

■ INDICATIONS

Peptic Ulcer Disease

With the improved medical agents to control gastric acid secretion and eradicate *H. pylori* infection, few patients require surgical intervention for peptic ulcer disease today. More often, surgical therapy is relegated to those patients who fail medical therapy with pain, obstruction, perforation, or concern for malignancy. Medical therapy has affected even the operations performed. Omental patch closure followed by medical therapy to eradicate *H. pylori* and reduce acid production is considered by many to be the standard of care for perforations caused by peptic ulcer disease. Common minimally invasive antiulcer procedures include truncal vagotomy and antrectomy with Billroth I or Billroth II reconstruction, vagotomy and pyloroplasty, and proximal gastric vagotomy. Several series from Europe report success with posterior truncal vagotomy combined with either an anterior seromyotomy or an anterior linear gastrectomy. For patients with gastric outlet obstruction, a laparoscopic truncal vagotomy with pyloroplasty or vagotomy with antrectomy is a valid surgical option. In the setting of an acute perforation, a laparoscopic omental patch with simple closure followed by peritoneal lavage is often straightforward and frequently preferred. A more definitive antiulcer procedure with or without resection may be performed if there is minimal contamination, the patient has chronic symptoms or has failed medical management, and the condition of the patient allows for a more extensive procedure.

Gastric Masses

Many gastric tumors can be managed with local resection only. Given that a minimal negative margin without formal lymphadenectomy is all that is required, these tumors are especially amenable to a laparoscopic wedge resection. Gastrointestinal stromal tumors (GISTs), most carcinoids, pancreatic rests, and adenomyomas fall into this category. These lesions previously were described as rare; however, with the rise in the number of upper endoscopies performed, we have seen a remarkable increase in referrals for what is often an asymptomatic tumor.

The cellular origin of GISTs previously was recognized to be smooth muscle. Benign tumors were characterized as leiomyomas and malignant tumors as leiomyosarcomas. Identification of the interstitial cell of Cajal as the cell of origin of smooth muscle tumors led to the change in nomenclature for GISTs. The interstitial cell of Cajal is a pacemaker cell of the gastrointestinal tract and is found within the myenteric plexus, submucosa, and muscularis propria. Immunohistochemistry established the derivation of GISTs from the interstitial cell of Cajal by demonstrating the expression of cellular markers such as CD117, a marker of the c-Kit gene product, and CD34, a human progenitor cell antigen.

Significant effort has been expended to predict the biologic nature of GISTs. Unfortunately, distant metastasis or local invasion may not be seen until many years after diagnosis of the primary tumor and is not affected by the extent of the resection. A combination of prognostic factors (patient age, histologic grade, mitotic rate, tumor size, and DNA analysis) has been used to predict the biologic behavior of GISTs. The most significant clinical predictors of malignant behavior are tumor size (>5 cm) and mitotic activity (≥5 mitoses per 50 high-power fields). However, GISTs with completely benign characteristics have recurred or metastasized (or both). The only absolute signs of malignancy are metastasis or invasion into adjacent organs.

Gastric carcinoid (neuroendocrine) tumors typically are divided into three types, based on pathogenesis and histomorphologic characteristics, which differ in biologic behavior and prognosis. Type I, as seen in pernicious anemia (type I) or chronic atrophic gastritis, and type II, often associated with gastrin-producing neoplasms such as Zollinger-Ellison syndrome in multiple endocrine neoplasia I, characteristically are localized to the gastric body or fundus and usually are considered benign with a low risk of malignancy. Treatment of these lesions is simple excision. Type III gastric carcinoids are composed of poorly differentiated endocrine and exocrine cells that grow sporadically, irrespective of gastrin hypersecretion. Most of these tumors show a low-grade to high-grade malignant transformation and are treated much more aggressively, as for an adenocarcinoma.

Gastric Cancer

Surgical resection is the only cure for gastric cancer. In North America, most patients are seen with an advanced stage of disease at the time of diagnosis, precluding a curative resection. The surgical objectives for treating patients with gastric cancer include maximizing the probability for cure in patients with localized tumor and providing safe and effective palliation to patients with metastatic disease.

The crucial point in the decision for or against limited surgery for gastric cancer is the preoperative differentiation between mucosal and submucosal extension of the carcinoma. Endoscopic ultrasound is essential to make this decision. Lymphatic spread from early gastric cancer occurs at variable rates and appears most reliant on the grade, size, and depth of invasion of the tumor. Gastric cancers that measure less than 3 cm, are limited to the mucosa, and are nonscirrhous can be treated by local, full-thickness resection with a negative margin. This is true because lymph node metastasis is rare (1% to 3%) in these cases. Essentially, all other lesions should be treated with an extended resection. Although resections of virtually any extent can be performed using minimally invasive techniques, the more extensive resections are difficult and lengthy when performed laparoscopically. The time/cost versus benefit conundrum that surgeons face must be examined carefully when a procedure of this extent is to be undertaken. The gastric resections described in this chapter are limited to nonmetastatic lesions or those intended for palliation.

■ OPERATIVE TECHNIQUES

The operative approach to gastric resection depends on the indication for surgery (ulcer disease vs tumor), tumor size, location, and growth morphology. Laparoscopic wedge, transgastric, intragastric, and limited segmental resections all have been used to treat a variety of gastric lesions. Before the resection, a formal abdominal exploration is performed to rule out peritoneal seeding or hepatic metastasis. The diaphragm, peritoneum, and surface of the liver are examined. Intraoperative ultrasound provides distinctive anatomic detail of the

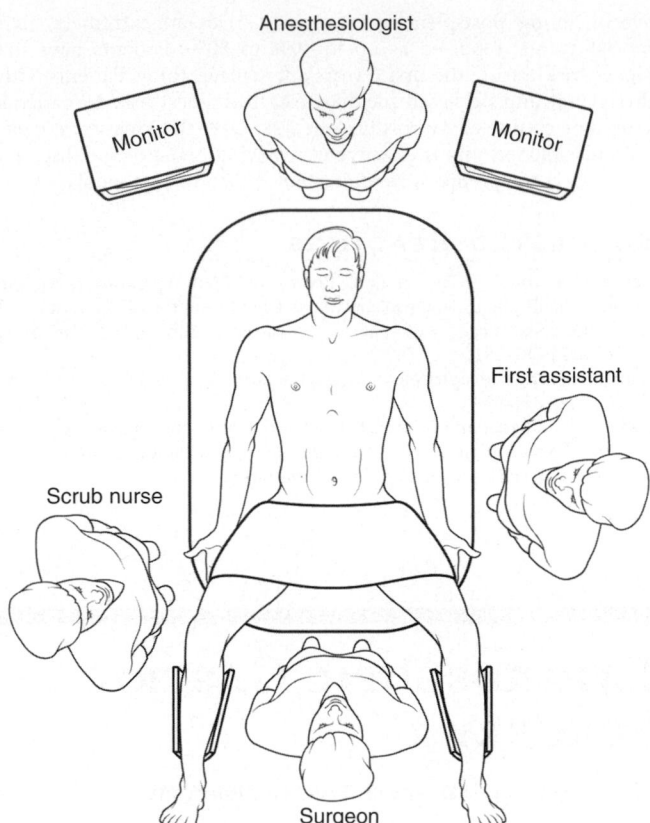

FIGURE 1 Operative positioning for gastric resection.

liver for evaluation of metastatic deposits. During a laparoscopic procedure in which tactile feedback is not available, a concomitant gastric endoscopy allows for a coordinated examination of both the inside and the outside of the stomach, which we find remarkably valuable.

The operating room setup is the same for most foregut surgeries. The patient is placed in the supine position with arms abducted on arm boards or tucked at the patient's side. We use a split leg table in nearly all circumstances, allowing the surgeon to stand between the patient's legs and directly face the epigastrium. Monitors are placed over each of the patient's shoulders (Figure 1). The typical size and locations of the ports are demonstrated in Figure 2. The upper midline and left midabdominal ports are the two main operative ports used by the operating surgeon. The camera is placed through the lower midline port. A liver retractor is placed via the right abdominal port. The assistant on the patient's left side uses the left lateral accessory port to provide retraction. An endoscopic linear stapler usually is introduced through the surgeon's right-hand port, although any port can be replaced with a 12-mm sleeve to allow for a better angle for gastric transection. The first port placed is usually in the midline, one quarter to one third of the distance between the umbilicus and the xiphoid, and is used for the camera. Periumbilical placement of the camera may be appropriate for lesions in the distal half of the stomach. In our experience, an umbilical port tends to be too low when the dissection is focused on the proximal stomach. Similarly, when the lesion is in the distal portion of the stomach, all of the trocar positions can be moved slightly inferiorly to keep the ports from being directly over the operative site.

After insertion of the initial ports and peritoneal exploration, the patient is placed in a steep reverse Trendelenburg position. Intraoperative endoscopy is crucial for localizing small lesions and assisting in the evaluation of both the extent of resection and the integrity of the staple and suture lines. An experienced endoscopist and the judicious use of air insufflation are important in avoiding troublesome

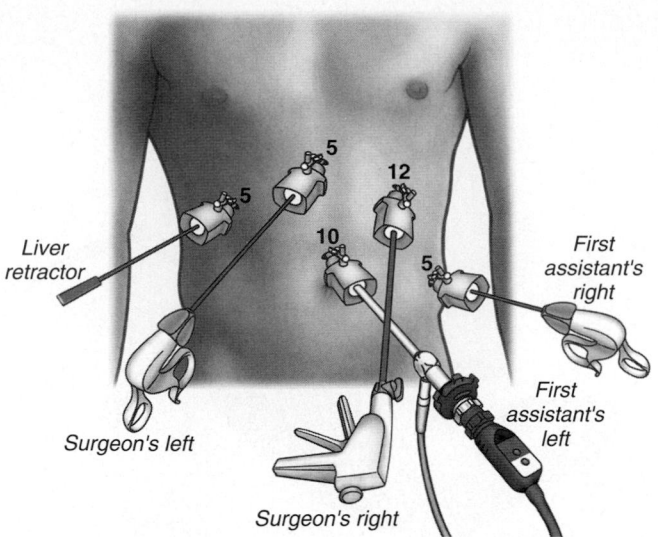

FIGURE 2 Port placement for laparoscopic gastric resection (numerals indicate port size in millimeters).

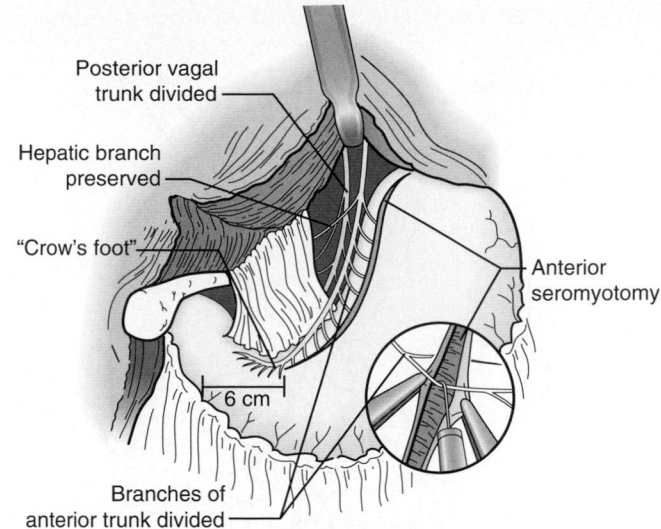

FIGURE 3 Anterior lesser curvature seromyotomy. *(From Kathouda N, Mouiel J. Laparoscopic vagotomy for treatment of peptic ulcer. In: Zucker KA, ed. Surgical Laparoscopy. 2nd ed. Philadelphia: Lippincott Williams & Wilkins; 2001. Used with permission.)*

insufflation of the small intestine with a resultant loss of an intra-abdominal working space. In all cases, specimens are placed in an impervious retrieval bag before extraction to prevent tumor spread within the abdomen and trocar sites and to decrease bacterial contamination of the abdomen and the extraction site.

Laparoscopic Treatment of Gastric Perforation

Several techniques have been described for laparoscopic treatment of perforated peptic ulcer. Following the principle of conventional open repair, ulcer closure may be performed by simple or running suture techniques incorporating omental patches. Gastroscopic-guided techniques for creating plugs of omentum of the ligamentum teres hepatis have been described. Sutureless techniques, including plugs of gelatin sponges or fibrin glue, have been used but are associated with higher leak rates, particularly if the perforation is larger than 5 mm in diameter. We prefer a simple, interrupted suture technique incorporating an omental patch and not using any additional foreign body.

Laparoscopic Highly Selective Vagotomy

Denervation of the parietal cell mass via a true highly selective vagotomy is an exigent operation. When approached laparoscopically, it most often is performed by combining a posterior truncal vagotomy with an anterior seromyotomy. After the truncal vagotomy, the seromyotomy is started at the level of the first branch of the crow's foot, which usually is found approximately 6 cm proximal to the pylorus. The superficial gastric incision proceeds along the lesser curvature, crosses over the anterior aspect of the cardia to the angle of His, and extends as far posteriorly as the lateral aspect of the left crus (Figure 3). The seromyotomy is closed with a running stitch of 2-0 silk or Vicryl (Ethicon, Somerville, NJ) (Figure 4). Essentially, the same anterior disruption of the vagus nerve can be carried out with an endomechanical stapler, as seen in Figure 5. The outcomes of this procedure are not well documented. A few series have demonstrated a 5% failure rate; however, the majority of reports show a 15% to 20% rate of recidivism.

Laparoscopic Wedge Resections

Anterior Gastric Wall Lesions

Masses within the anterior wall of the stomach are amenable to wedge resection with a linear endoscopic gastrointestinal anastomosis (GIA) stapler. After identifying the lesion laparoscopically and

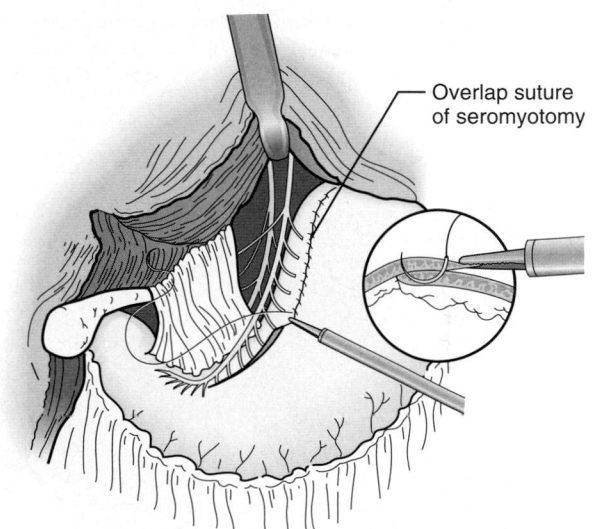

FIGURE 4 Oversewing of lesser curvature seromyotomy. *(From Kathouda N, Mouiel J. Laparoscopic vagotomy for treatment of peptic ulcer. In: Zucker KA, ed. Surgical Laparoscopy. 2nd ed. Philadelphia: Lippincott Williams & Wilkins; 2001. Used with permission.)*

endoscopically, the short gastric and gastroepiploic vessels are ligated and divided as needed. Typically this maneuver is performed with the assistant on the left retracting the omentum and gastrosplenic ligament toward the patient's left side while the surgeon retracts the stomach medially or superiorly and transects the vessels with ultrasonic coagulating shears (Harmonic scalpel; Johnson & Johnson Gateway, Piscataway, NJ). Laparoscopic gastric wedge resection is accomplished by elevating the gastric wall using two seromuscular sutures placed opposite each other 1 to 2 cm beyond the mass or ulcer. The lesion and a small cuff of the normal stomach then are divided by an endoscopic linear stapler placed just under the sutures (Figure 6) with intraluminal guidance of the endoscope. Alternatively, a lesion and surrounding rim of normal tissue may be excised using ultrasonic coagulating shears. The latter technique allows for a more precise excision of the normal tissue at the margin. The gastrotomy can be closed by laparoscopic intracorporeal suturing or by

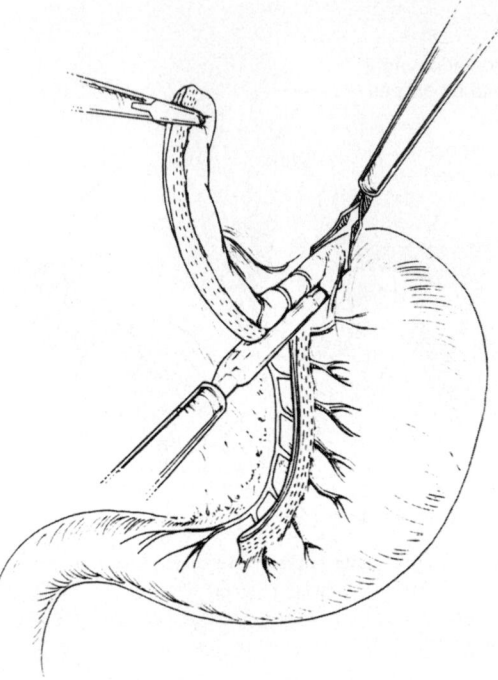

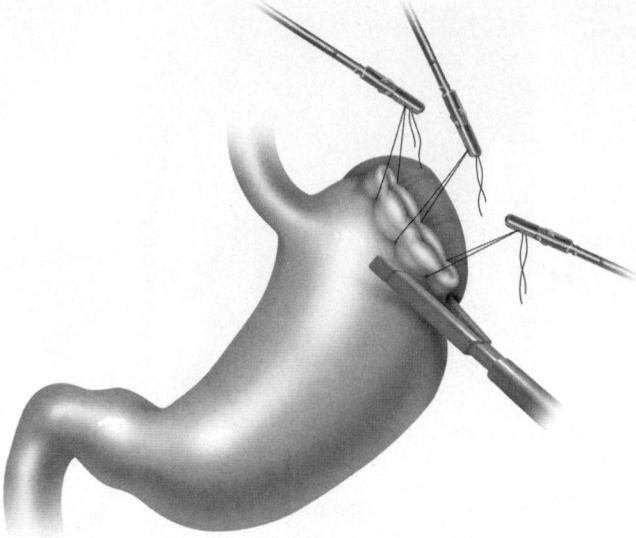

FIGURE 7 Linear stapler closure after laparoscopic anterior wall gastric wedge resection with Harmonic scalpel (Johnson & Johnson Gateway, Piscataway, NJ).

FIGURE 5 Linear gastrectomy is carried up the lesser curvature. *(From Bailey RW. Abdominal vagotomy. In: MacFadyen BV, Ponsky JL, eds. Operative Laparoscopy and Thoracoscopy. Philadelphia: Lippincott-Raven; 1996. Used with permission.)*

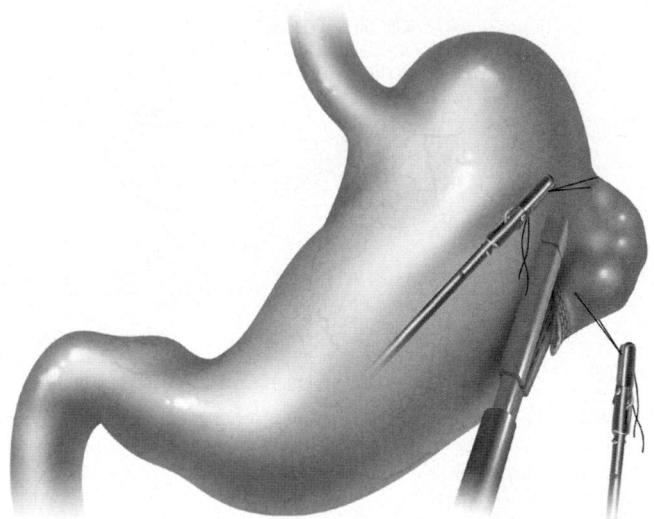

FIGURE 6 Laparoscopic anterior wall gastric wedge resection with linear stapler.

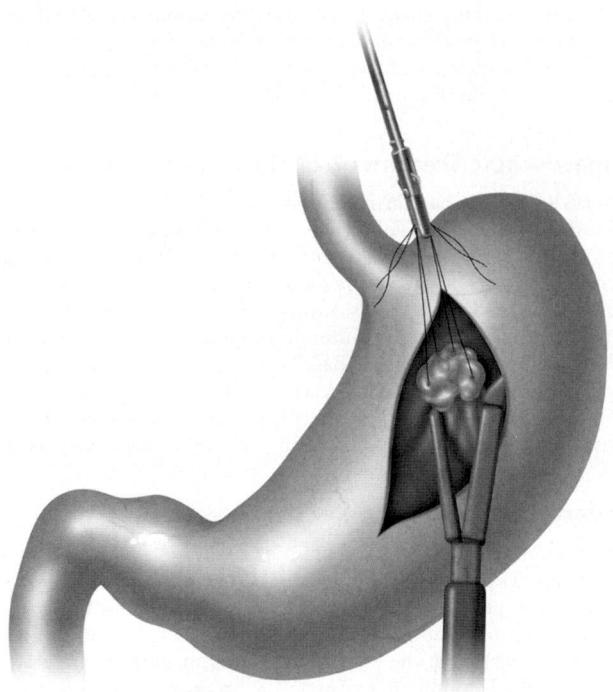

FIGURE 8 Laparoscopic posterior wall gastric wedge resection with linear stapler.

placing two to four full-thickness traction sutures along the cut edge of the gastrotomy to elevate the cut edges of the stomach so that it can be closed effectively using an endoscopic linear stapler (Figure 7).

Posterior Gastric Wall Lesions

Subserosal posterior wall lesions can be approached through the lesser sac. After the division of the gastrocolic omentum, the greater curvature is grasped to expose the posterior surface of the stomach. The lesion then is resected using a technique similar to one described earlier. We commonly perform two alternative approaches to intraluminal posterior wall ulcers or larger posterior gastric wall tumors.

One method entails creation of an anterior gastrotomy over the lesion after it is localized endoscopically within the stomach. Normal gastric tissue adjacent to the lesion is grasped with laparoscopic bowel graspers or, alternatively, traction sutures are placed 1 to 2 cm from the lesion or ulcer on opposite sides, and the lesion is elevated through the gastrotomy (Figure 8). A margin of normal tissue also is resected with the lesion using an endoscopic linear stapler. The staple line is examined for bleeding through the gastrotomy using the laparoscope, and any bleeding points are oversewn. The anterior gastrotomy is closed as described previously.

Intraluminal posterior wall lesions that are not amenable to endoscopic treatment can be approached via a percutaneous intragastric resection. Laparoscopic intragastric or "endoluminal" surgery involves the placement of balloon-tipped laparoscopic trocars (2, 5, or 10 mm) percutaneously into the stomach (insufflated by a flexible endoscope), similar to the placement of a percutaneous endoscopic gastrostomy tube (Figures 9 and 10). Our preference is to perform transperitoneal laparoscopy via a single port at the umbilicus before inserting transgastric ports. This allows for assessment of the peritoneal cavity and the serosal surface of the stomach and provides for visualization of the stomach and adjacent organs during placement of percutaneous, transgastric ports. The laparoscope is directed through one of the trocars and into the insufflated stomach. A dilute epinephrine solution (1 : 100,000) is injected circumferentially around the stromal tumor as a tumescent to aid in dissection of the submucosal plane and to limit bleeding. The lesion is enucleated from the submucosal-muscular junction using an electrocautery

hook. The mucosal defect is left open to heal or can be closed with intragastric suturing. The tumor is placed in a retrieval bag and removed transorally with the flexible endoscope. Despite the novelty of this technique, there is some concern about the adequacy of the resection. To date, we have noted no local or systemic recurrence.

Lesions of the Greater and Lesser Curvatures

Lesions of the greater and lesser curvatures are typically amenable to simple wedge resection with an endoscopic linear stapler. The greater omentum is mobilized for tumors located on the greater curvature tumors, and the lesser omentum and gastrohepatic ligament are mobilized for lesions located on the lesser curvature. The Harmonic scalpel, LigaSure (Valleylab, Boulder, CO), or laparoscopic clip ligation (or a combination of these) allows for a safe division of the short gastric vessels on the greater curvature and branches of the left gastric artery and coronary vein on the lesser curvature. Rotating the stomach so that the lesion faces anteriorly facilitates the resection. Lesions are resected using an endoscopic linear stapler and removed in an impermeable extraction bag through an enlarged 12-mm trocar site.

Lesions Near the Gastroesophageal Junction

We previously have described the technique for minilaparoscopic intragastric resection for gastroesophageal junction stromal tumors using a flexible endoscope as the "camera" and insufflator. Working ports are provided by two 2-mm mushroom-tipped trocars or 5-mm trocars placed percutaneously into the gastric lumen as described earlier (Figure 11). Hook electrocautery is used to enucleate the gastroesophageal junction tumor after a submucosal injection of dilute epinephrine. To avoid directly handling the tumor and possibly fracturing it, we frequently endoloop the lesion after the dissection is begun. The mass is removed transorally with the flexible endoscope with the aid of an endoscopic snare.

Laparoscopic Gastrectomy

Partial Gastrectomy

The trocar strategy used for the laparoscopic local resection of anterior, posterior, and greater and lesser curvature gastric masses is

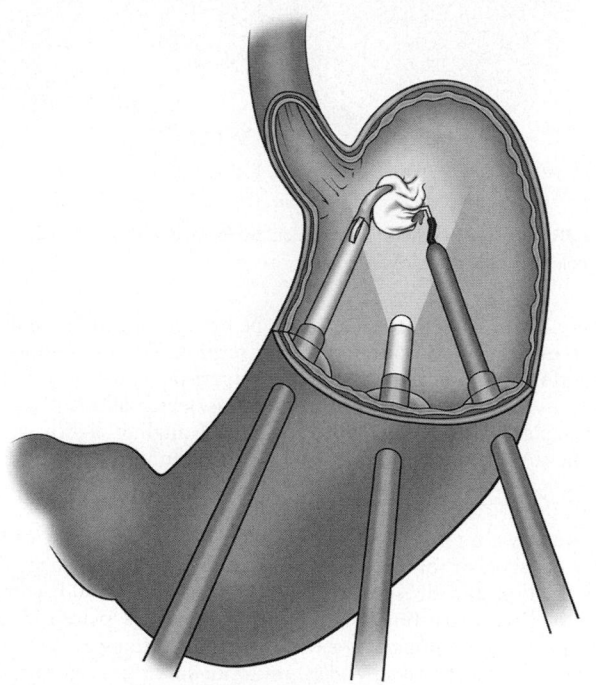

FIGURE 9 Transgastric laparoscopic resection of posterior gastric tumor.

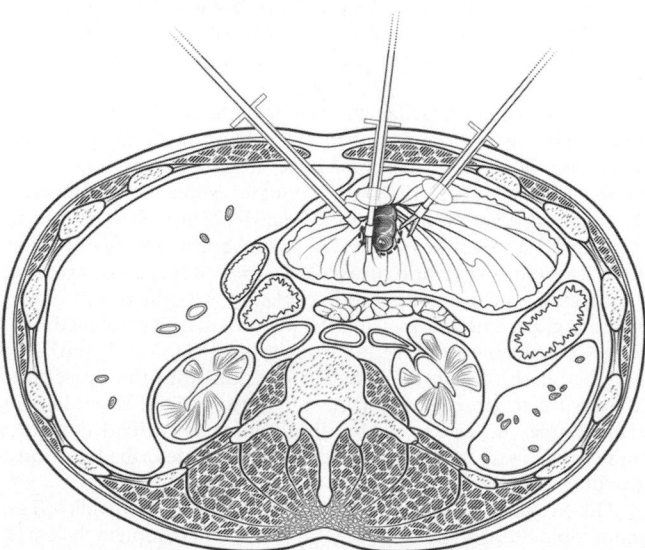

FIGURE 10 Sagittal view of transgastric laparoscopic resection of posterior gastric tumor.

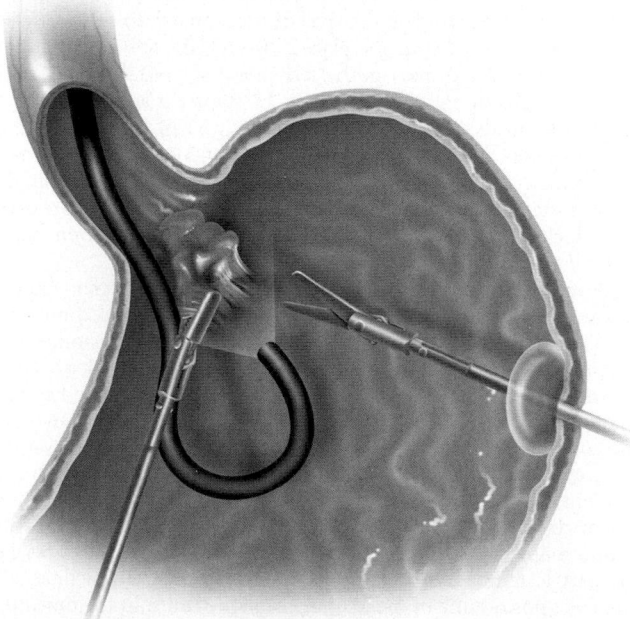

FIGURE 11 Endoscopic-assisted transgastric laparoscopic resection of gastroesophageal junction tumor.

essentially the same for minimally invasive techniques to perform a subtotal gastrectomy. We frequently move our trocars just slightly inferior while maintaining their position in a medial-to-lateral location. For a gastric adenocarcinoma in particular, examination of the peritoneal surfaces, visual inspection of the liver (laparoscopic and intra-abdominal ultrasound), and exploration of the lesser sac are critical when the resection will be performed for curative intent. In approximately 25% of patients, laparoscopic exploration detects metastasis that precludes curative resection despite the tumor appearing to be resectable with standard preoperative radiographic examinations.

The first steps in performing a gastric resection are initiated during the general exploration. The gastrocolic omentum—or, when the procedure is performed for curative resection, the omentum—is taken off the transverse colon to the end of the lesser sac. The assistant, on the patient's left side, elevates the omentum and reflects it up and over the stomach. The surgeon, retracting downward on the colon with the left hand, can divide the thin attachments between the omentum and colon using ultrasonic coagulating shears. When the resection is for palliation, the surgeon holds the stomach with his or her left hand while the assistant retracts the colon inferiorly to "tent up" the gastrocolic ligament. The gastrocolic ligament is divided, and the lesser sac is entered as the dissection proceeds from the midstomach upward along the greater curvature of the stomach toward the spleen. The gastroepiploic vessel branches then are ligated by the Harmonic scalpel or LigaSure. Distal mobilization of the stomach is continued beyond the pylorus, which is identified by its muscular rings or the vein of Mayo. The small vessels surrounding the duodenum are coagulated and transected with a 45- or 60-mm endoscopic stapler (3.5-mm staple load). The duodenal staple line frequently is fortified with staple line reinforcement (Seamguard; W. L. Gore & Associates, Newark, DE) or imbricated with 2-0 silk sutures. After transecting the duodenum, the distal part of the stomach can be rotated toward the patient's left flank, significantly facilitating transection of the posterior attachments of the stomach. The plane between the stomach and the liver also can be transected with the LigaSure or Harmonic scalpel. After deciding the level at which the stomach will be transected, additional short gastric vessels or branches of the descending left gastric artery can be divided as needed. If there is any concern about the level of transection of the stomach, an intraoperative endoscopy, as well as laparoscopic visual and palpable cues, should be able to plot the course of the gastric transection. Depending on the level of the stomach to be transected, the endoscopic stapler can be placed through the left subcostal port or through a 12-mm port in the left lateral subcostal position. The stomach is placed on some stretch as the stapler is applied. Three or four staple loads (3.5- or 4.8-mm cartridges) of a 45- to 60-mm stapler usually are required, depending on the level of the stomach to be transected. In the more proximal stomach, we have found a 3.5-mm stapler to work well and to reduce bleeding. The more distal and thicker portions of the stomach require a 4.8-mm staple cartridge.

Several techniques are used for reconstruction after a subtotal gastrectomy. We typically prefer a standard loop jejunostomy or, if the gastric pouch is small, a Roux-en-Y gastrojejunostomy. This portion of the operation is initiated by taking the patient out of reverse Trendelenburg position and maintaining him or her in a more neutral orientation. The omentum is rolled upward and over the colon, and a colonic epiploica is grasped and pulled upward to expose the full undersurface of the transverse colon mesentery and to identify the ligament of Treitz. We measure approximately 20 to 35 cm distal to the ligament of Treitz and roll this portion of the jejunum upward to the gastric remnant. If the intestine easily reaches the gastric remnant, an antecolic route is chosen. To facilitate the antecolic positioning of the jejunal limb, one can split the omentum midline in a caudal-cranial fashion using the ultrasonic coagulating shears. Otherwise a small window can be made in the avascular area of the transverse mesocolon just above and lateral to the ligament of

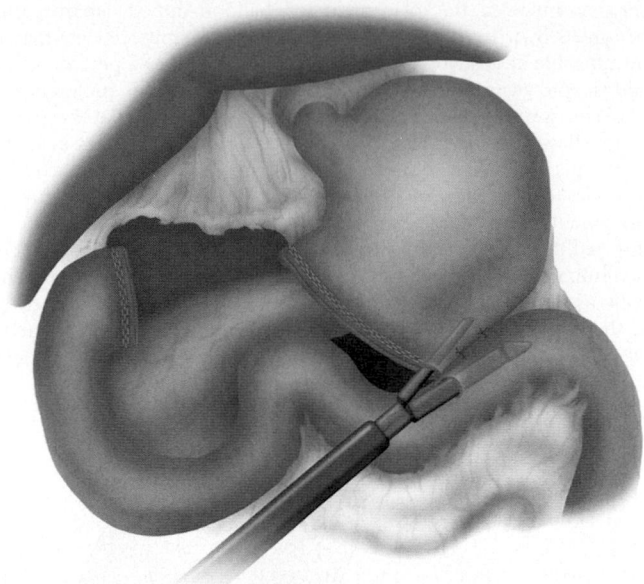

FIGURE 12 Gastrojejunal anastomosis performed with laparoscopic gastrointestinal anastomosis stapler.

Treitz. The loop of the jejunum can be brought through the mesocolon easily in a retrocolic, retrogastric fashion. The anastomosis can be performed in an isoperistaltic or antiperistaltic manner. We typically choose an antiperistaltic anastomosis, which allows placement of a stapler from the cut edge of the stomach angling slightly upward on the stomach and distally on the small intestine (Figure 12).

Total Gastrectomy

Laparoscopic total gastrectomy is performed in a method comparable to partial or subtotal gastrectomy, except for the more proximal mobilization and division of the esophagus and a more complex intestinal reconstruction. Several 12-mm ports are placed to allow for versatility in using the endoscopic linear stapler from many angles. The short gastric vessels, posterior lesser curvature attachments, and phrenoesophageal ligament are divided with ultrasonic coagulating shears, and the distal esophagus is mobilized well into the mediastinum. The division of the phrenoesophageal ligament, as well as the mediastinal dissection, is facilitated by an assistant who retracts the stomach in a caudal direction with a Penrose drain placed around the gastroesophageal junction. The posterior dissection of the stomach and anterolateral dissection of the esophageal hiatus are relatively avascular and can be performed with blunt techniques. The distal esophagus is mobilized by "pushing" the left and right crura away from the esophagus. In general, any tubes in the esophagus (orogastric, nasogastric, bougie, esophageal stethoscope) are removed before initiating the hiatal dissection. Posterior to the esophagus, segmental arteries from the aorta are divided with the ultrasonic coagulating shears. After the esophagus is mobilized, the anterior and posterior vagal trunks are identified and divided between clips. The left gastric artery is isolated and divided using an endoscopic linear stapler and vascular load (2.0 to 2.5 mm). After complete mobilization and vascular division from the celiac trunk (left gastric artery), the esophagus is transected with an endoscopic linear stapler or LigaSure. The distal stomach is divided with an endoscopic linear stapler beyond the pylorus, as described previously for subtotal gastrectomy.

The circular, flip-top EEA stapler (U.S. Surgical, Norwalk, CT) or endoscopic linear stapling device can be used to complete the esophagojejunostomy. The technique of using a 25-mm flip-top EEA stapler to perform a Roux-en-Y gastrojejunostomy for laparoscopic gastric bypass is the same technique used for reconstruction by a

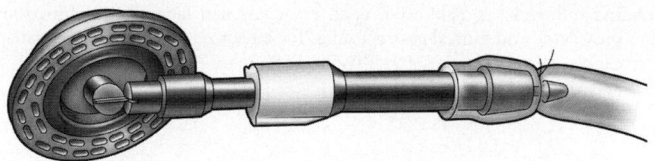

FIGURE 13 Orogastric tube secured to a flipped, 25-mm anvil.

Roux-en-Y esophagojejunostomy after laparoscopic total gastrectomy. Before performing an esophagojejunostomy, the ligament of Treitz is identified and the proximal jejunum is divided approximately 30 to 45 cm distal to the ligament of Treitz with the endoscopic linear stapler. The biliary (proximal) limb subsequently is anastomosed to the more distal jejunum, approximately 30 to 40 cm distal to the staple line on the proximal Roux limb.

To complete a circular-stapled anastomosis, the anvil has to be brought out of the distal esophagus. This is facilitated by securing a flipped, 25-mm anvil with a suture to the distal end of a 16F orogastric tube that previously has been transected proximal to the sump airport (Figure 13). The proximal end of the orogastric tube with the flipped anvil secured to the distal end is passed transorally and guided down the esophagus. The proximal end of the orogastric tube is pulled gently into the abdomen and out one of the trocar sites. As the tube is pulled through the esophagotomy, the anvil is guided through the oropharynx by the anesthesiologist. After the anvil tip emerges from the esophagotomy, the orogastric tube is cut free of the anvil and removed. The EEA stapler is placed directly through the abdominal wall via an enlarged trocar site in the left upper quadrant and advanced into an enterotomy created along the staple line on the proximal jejunal Roux limb. The EEA stapler is advanced antegrade through the Roux limb, and the spike of the EEA stapler is advanced through the antimesenteric border of the jejunum. The anvil protruding through the esophagotomy is united with the EEA stapler, and the stapler is tightened and fired. The enterotomy in the proximal Roux limb is closed with an endoscopic linear stapler.

Robotic Gastrectomy

The first robot-assisted gastrectomy for early gastric cancer was reported by Hashizume and colleagues in 2003. The indications for robot-assisted gastrectomy are similar to those for the laparoscopic approach. The use of the robot in gastric surgery has both benefits and drawbacks. With robot-assisted gastrectomy, there can be less intraoperative blood loss, more lymph nodes retrieved during lymphadenectomy, similar length of hospital stay, and a shorter learning curve of 11 to 25 cases compared with 40 to 60 cases for laparoscopic gastrectomy. On the other hand, the operating time is longer and the cost is greater with the robot. However, most of the studies from which these comparisons come are limited case series and nonrandomized comparative studies. Kim and colleagues recently analyzed more than 400 patients in a prospective multicenter study comparing robotic and laparoscopic gastrectomy for gastric adenocarcinoma and found no difference in overall or major complications, estimated blood loss, rates of conversion to open resection, or length of stay. There were no mortalities in either group. The robotic procedure was longer and had higher costs. Well-designed prospective studies with long-term follow-up would help to better delineate the role of robot-assisted gastrectomy.

Lymphadenectomy

The regional lymph nodes of the stomach are divided into stations numbered 1 through 20 and 110, 111, and 112. The extent of lymphadenectomy (D1 vs D1+ vs D2) depends on the severity of the disease (early vs advanced gastric cancer) and the type of resection performed (distal gastrectomy vs total gastrectomy). In general, D1+ is utilized for early gastric cancer and D2 is standard for advanced

gastric cancer. In early studies there was concern regarding the number of lymph nodes harvested during laparoscopic gastrectomy, but more recent studies, including Greenleaf and colleagues' review of the American experience, have shown a higher likelihood of adequate lymphadenectomy (at least 15 lymph nodes) with laparoscopic and robotic resection when compared with open resection. The role of laparoscopic gastrectomy and D2 lymphadenectomy for the treatment of advanced gastric cancer is still controversial, and a number of prospective studies evaluating short-term and long-term outcomes are pending (KLASS-02, CLASS-01, JLSSG 0901). Precise knowledge of the foregut vasculature is required for safe lymphadenectomy, and one Korean study suggested that the learning curve for laparoscopic lymphadenectomy is 42 cases.

■ CONTRAINDICATIONS

There are few absolute contraindications to laparoscopy; most often surgeon experience and disease state dictate the relative feasibility and possible advantages of laparoscopic therapy. Absolute contraindications might include uncorrected coagulopathy, a patient who is unable to tolerate a laparotomy, and a surgeon's true lack of experience with this or similar procedures. Relative contraindications include extensive previous surgery, previous peritonitis, severe cardiopulmonary disease, and a tumor of a size that would preclude safe handling. As mentioned earlier, the use of minimally invasive surgery for advanced gastric cancer is controversial.

■ POSTOPERATIVE CARE AND COMPLICATIONS

Postoperative care after laparoscopic gastric surgery is similar to that after open surgery, with the potential benefit of shorter hospitalization. Anastomotic leak is the most feared complication, with rates ranging from 1% to 5% (similar to open procedures) depending on the type of gastric resection performed. Anastomotic leak usually occurs early, within the first 7 days after surgery. Risk factors include diabetes, immunosuppressed state, older age, longer operative times, and amount of blood loss. Diagnosis is via water-soluble contrast swallow study or computed tomographic (CT) scan. Treatment should be expeditious, including antibiotics, nasogastric drainage, percutaneous drainage, endoscopic stenting, or repeat surgical intervention. Duodenal stump blow-out after total gastrectomy can be a devastating complication resulting in severe sepsis. Elevated liver function tests and leukocytosis frequently are seen, and stump leak can be confirmed with CT findings. Treatment includes antibiotics and percutaneous drainage but often may require surgical washout with duodenal and intraperitoneal drainage.

SUGGESTED READINGS

Cuschieri A. Laparoscopic gastric resection. *Surg Clin North Am.* 2000;80:1269-1284.

Degiuli M, De Manzoni G, Di Leo A. Gastric cancer: current status of lymph node dissection. *World J Gastroenterol.* 2016;22:2875-2893.

Greenleaf EK, Sun SX, Hollenbeak CS. Minimally invasive surgery for gastric cancer: the American experience. *Gastric Cancer.* 2016;PMID 26961133.

Katai H, Sasako M, Fukada H. Safety and feasibility of laparoscopy-assisted distal gastrectomy with suprapancreatic nodal dissection for clinical stage I gastric cancer: a multicenter phase II trial (JCOG 0703). *Gastric Cancer.* 2010;13:238-244.

Kim W, Kim HH, Han SU. Decreased morbidity of laparoscopic distal gastrectomy compared with open distal gastrectomy for stage I gastric cancer: short-term outcomes from a multicenter randomized controlled trial (KLASS-01). *Ann Surg.* 2010;251:417-420.

Kitano S, Shiraishi N, Fujii K, et al. A randomized controlled trial comparing open vs laparoscopy-assisted distal gastrectomy for the treatment of early gastric cancer: an interim report. *Surgery.* 2002;131(suppl 1):S306-S311.

Novitsky YW, Kercher KW, Sing RF, et al. Long-term outcomes of laparoscopic resection of gastric gastrointestinal stromal tumors. *Ann Surg.* 2006;243:738-745, discussion 745-747.

Shen W, Xi H, Chen L. A meta-analysis of robotic versus laparoscopic gastrectomy for gastric cancer. *Surg Endosc.* 2014;28:2795-2802.

Son S, Kim H. Minimally invasive surgery in gastric cancer. *World J Gastroenterol.* 2014;20:14132-14141.

Uyama I, Sugioka A, Sakurai Y, et al. Hand-assisted laparoscopic function: preserving and radical gastrectomies for advanced-stage proximal gastric cancer. *J Am Coll Surg.* 2004;199:508-515.

LAPAROSCOPIC TREATMENT OF CROHN'S DISEASE

Sharon Stein, MD

Laparoscopic treatment of Crohn's disease improves postoperative outcomes by decreasing pain scores, reducing complications, promoting earlier return of bowel function, and minimizing length of stay. Fifty percent or more of Crohn's patients will require reoperation at some point; this unique patient population may benefit from decreased adhesions and hernias and improved cosmetic outcomes associated with minimally invasive surgery. However, even experienced surgeons hesitate to use laparoscopy for patients with Crohn's disease. Concerns about the ability to handle multifocal disease, thickened mesentery, fistulas, and abscesses laparoscopically may discourage some surgeons. Successful completion of laparoscopic surgery in complex Crohn's patients requires thorough preoperative preparation, knowledge of patient disease, and mastery of advanced techniques.

■ PREOPERATIVE EVALUATION

Preoperative planning is vitally important for the treatment of patients with Crohn's disease. Laparoscopy provides a restricted view of the abdomen at any one time. Preoperative appreciation of the extent and severity of the individual patient's disease helps to focus the laparoscopic surgeon. Preoperative assessment can provide a road map for the operation and create unified goals between the patient, the gastroenterologist, and the surgeon.

Goals of surgery for Crohn's disease are identical when using either laparoscopic or open techniques. The surgeon should seek to treat complications of Crohn's disease while minimizing resection. Resection with extensive disease-free margins has never been shown to improve outcomes. The surgeon, in conjunction with the gastroenterologist and patient, must determine if disease can be resected completely, if strictureplasty is most appropriate, or if medical treatment should be pursued (Figure 1). These decisions should be based on extent of disease, remaining normal bowel, ability to restore intestinal continuity, and preoperative absorptive function.

Preoperative assessment of nutrition, immunosuppression, and bowel function are critical to surgical decision making. Patients with malnutrition can be assessed for enteric or parental supplementation to reverse catabolic state before surgery. Although data are mixed on whether the use of immunosuppressants, including biologics, increases the risk for perioperative complications, caution should be taken in these patients. The surgeon should consider a lower threshold for diversion in patients who are immunosuppressed or malnourished.

Bowel function should be assessed. The number and quality of bowel movements may improve after resection of diseased portions of the bowel, but the surgeon should be cognizant of the total length of remaining small bowel before resection. Both bowel movements and fecal incontinence may affect the decision to perform an anastomosis or to consider stoma, and these factors should be discussed with the patient before surgery.

Special mention should be made of patients with preoperative infection or abscess. The situation is analogous to patients with complex diverticulitis. Attempts should be made to control sepsis before surgery, as rates of conversion to open surgery and the length of bowel resected are decreased when inflammation has resolved. If patients are acutely septic and unstable, they should be taken to surgery immediately. If the patient is stable and an abscess is noted, drainage by interventional radiology can be considered. Long-term or short-term antibiotics are administered as appropriate. Surgery can be planned after resolution of an acute episode, generally 6 weeks or longer after the index event.

If the patient has a history of prior abdominal surgery, obtain the operative reports, records, and imaging from the prior surgery. Understanding the pre-existing anatomy, length of remaining bowel, and anastomotic configurations can prevent complications and undesired outcomes. During lysis of adhesions, knowing the configuration of a prior small bowel to small bowel anastomosis (side to end versus end to end) may prevent inadvertent bowel injury during the surgery or misinterpretation of disease on imaging.

Preoperative evaluation can help to determine whether diversion or stoma may be necessary. This is important for both informed consent and psychological preparation of the patient. Preoperative education and marking have been shown to have significant effects on postoperative quality of life.

■ PREOPERATIVE IMAGING

Most patients undergo a computed tomographic (CT) examination of the abdomen and pelvis. Ideally this should be performed with oral and intravenous (IV) contrast. Oral and IV contrast allow for optimal interpretation of obstruction, fistulization, and abscesses. Without contrast, bowel may be difficult to distinguish from an abscess, fistulization may be harder to detect, and inflammation may be less distinct. Although CT scans have high sensitivity for extralumenal findings and obstructive disease, specificity for intralumenal disease, small bowel disease, and inflammation is suboptimal. When used in isolation, there is a significant rate of unexpected intraoperative findings, such as undiagnosed fistula or small bowel involvement.

To decrease the rate of unexpected findings, a CT enterography or magnetic resonance enterography can be performed (Figures 2 and 3). Either of these examinations provides greater sensitivity for intralumenal and extralumenal disease assessment. Areas of fistulization, stenosis, and inflammation can be identified preoperatively and are key to preoperative surgical planning. Fluoroscopy studies such as small bowel follow-through can be performed, but they may be more cumbersome to perform and interpret (Figure 4). As fluoroscopy studies are ordered less frequently, finding skilled radiologists to interpret the subtle findings becomes increasingly difficult.

■ PREOPERATIVE ENDOSCOPY

Patients should have a recent colonoscopy. The extent of disease should be noted. The colonoscopy is of particular interest in patients with colonic disease. Healthy and diseased colon should be assessed carefully, as these patients have a high rate of recurrence of colonic disease. To perform a segmental colectomy, the surgeon should identify a healthy "landing area" in the colon with normal mucosa and architectural features (haustra, folds). If no normal mucosa is found, it is difficult to consider creating an anastomosis, and higher risk is involved.

If a fistula to the colon or small bowel is noted preoperatively, the area may be evaluated endoscopically for signs of primary or

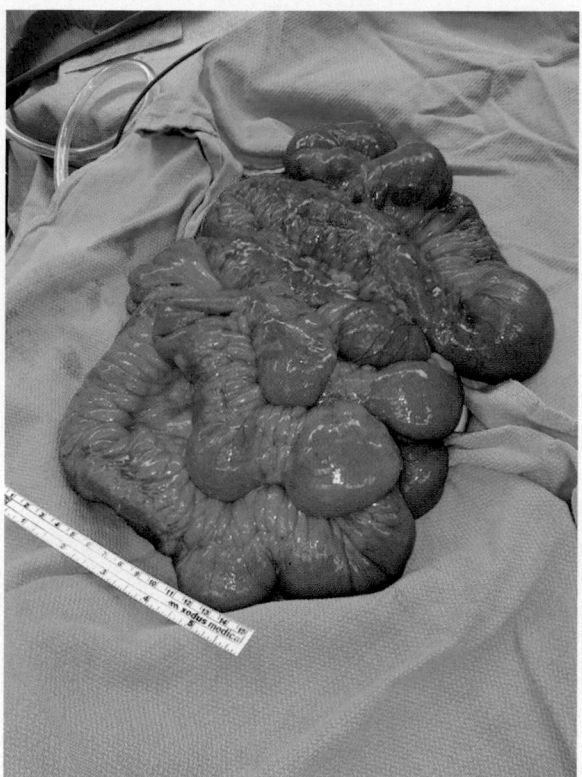

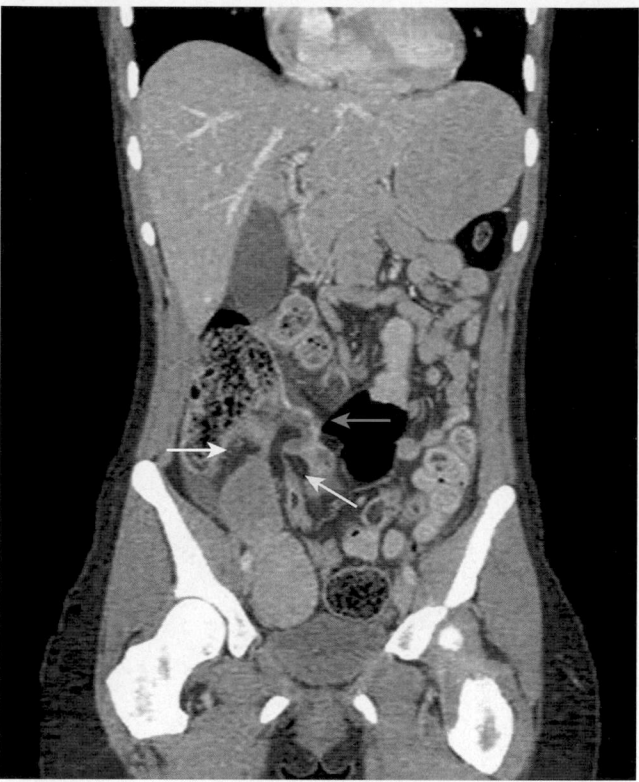

FIGURE 1 Small bowel Crohn's disease. Although this patient initially was explored laparoscopically, the decision was made for sphincteroplasty to save as much small bowel as possible. After mobilizing any adhesions, the sphincteroplasty was performed through a midline incision using open technique. Decisions on technique of surgery always should center on optimizing long-term patient outcomes rather than on sacrificing the ideal operation for a minimally invasive technique.

FIGURE 3 Computed tomographic enterography in a patient with ileocolic disease. The image demonstrates a narrow stream of contrast traversing the terminal ileum (*blue arrow*), with signs of a fistula to the sigmoid colon (*white arrow*) and proximal loop of small bowel (*yellow arrow*).

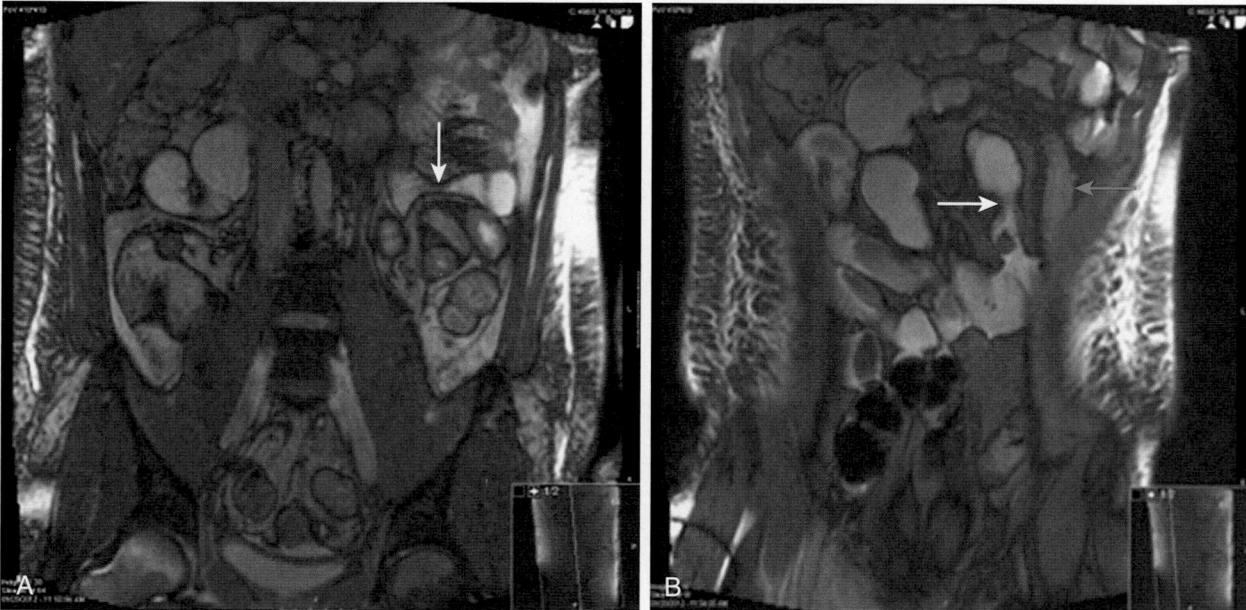

FIGURE 2 A, Magnetic resonance enterography of a patient with extensive small bowel disease. Areas of small bowel Crohn's disease are demonstrated by stenosis and dilation (*white arrows*). **B,** Inflamed, thickened, diseased segments of small bowel also can be seen (*blue arrow*).

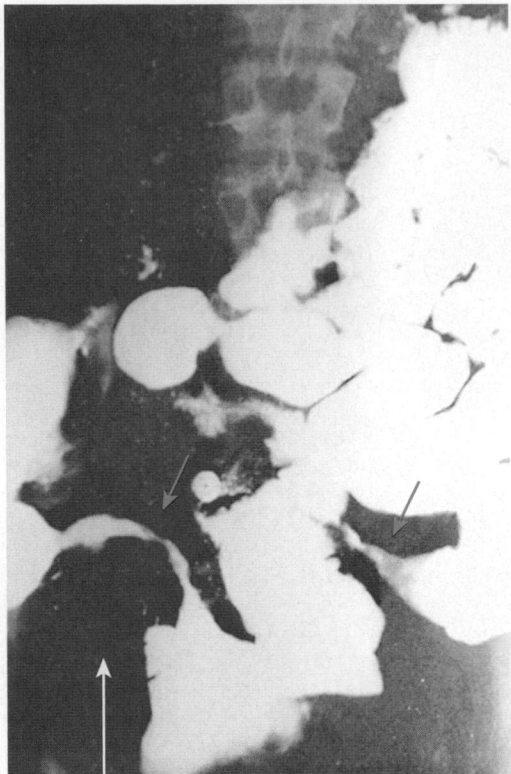

FIGURE 4 Fluoroscopy study. Although expertise in fluoroscopic studies is decreasing, these studies are still able to provide significant amounts of information about disease location and severity. The image demonstrates sections of dilation and narrowing (*blue arrows*). Spaces between radio-opaque loops of bowel are indicative of thickened mesentery causing a separation between small intestines (*yellow arrow*).

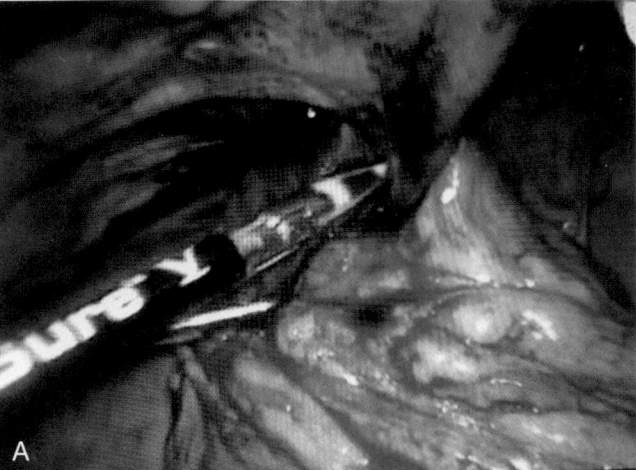

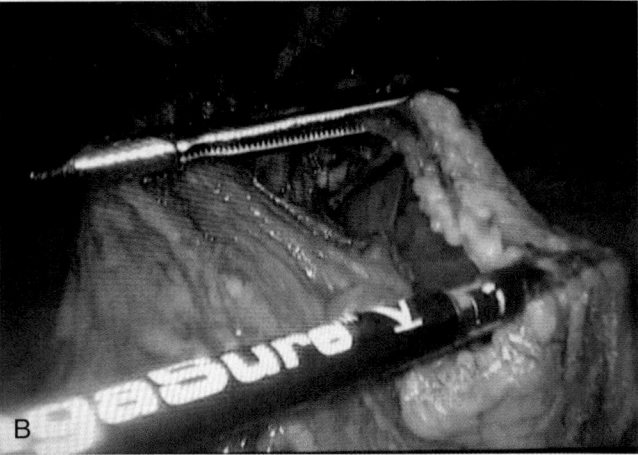

FIGURE 5 A, Takedown of fistula in a patient with history of Crohn's disease and fistula to the anterior abdominal wall at the umbilicus. Upon entry to the abdomen, the camera port was moved to the left upper quadrant port to provide better visualization of the fistula. **B,** To treat the fistula, adhesed portions of the omentum were isolated slowly and transected until the fistula was identified. This was ligated and the proximal end of the fistula and diseased segment of the bowel were resected.

secondary disease. Ileocolic disease that has not been treated surgically often fistulizes to the sigmoid colon, whereas recurrent ileocolic disease commonly fistulizes to the duodenum after a prior anastomosis. Fistulas generally have two sides, referred to as primary and secondary disease. Primary disease is the initial source or origin of fistulization and has mucosal and transmural inflammation; this portion of the disease must be resected, as repair is likely to recur. In secondary disease, the colon wall may be inflamed, but mucosa surrounding the fistula is generally normal. A wedge resection of the actual fistula and primary closure of the enterotomy is often sufficient if the bowel is not affected primarily.

Patients with long-standing Crohn's disease are also at increased risk for malignancy compared with the general population. A colonoscopy helps to rule out undiagnosed malignancy preoperatively. Random screening biopsies are recommended in patients with long-standing Crohn's disease to rule out nonpolypoid neoplasia.

Esophagogastroduodenoscopy can be performed to evaluate for upper gastrointestinal disease but is not always necessary. Patients on steroids may have signs of gastritis, and primary gastroduodenal disease may occur. In the case of duodenal fistula or suspected fistulization, this may be useful.

■ INTRAOPERATIVE PLANNING

The location of port placement will depend on the operation planned. In general, a supraumbilical camera port with 2 to 3 side ports is adequate for most operations. Two ports generally are placed across from the anatomy of interest (on the left side for ileocolic disease), and if needed an additional port is placed on the side of the anatomy. A 5-mm good-quality laparoscope allows the surgeon to move the

camera from port to port if needed. This becomes extremely important in patients with prior surgery, adhesions, or even abscesses and fistulas. Changing the camera port can help the surgeon to gain perspective on the lesion (Figure 5).

Although prior surgery is not a contraindication to surgery, it may require a variation in approach. The surgeon can avoid inadvertent injury to adhesions by entering the abdomen using an open Hasson technique and placing an initial entry point distal from prior incisions. If the patient has a phlegmon to the abdominal wall, the initial access should be distant to the phlegmon.

■ EVALUATION OF THE SMALL BOWEL

After safe entry into the abdomen, the surgeon should evaluate for general signs of disease. Adhesions are noted, and lysis of adhesions can be performed. In patients with Crohn's disease, the small bowel should be run from the ligament of Treitz to the ileocecal valve.

The bowel is run to (1) identify diseased segments that may not have been noted on imaging and may require intraoperative treatment; (2) assess the length of healthy small bowel, to determine the risk for short gut or nutritional concerns going forward; (3) determine the need for postoperative immunoprophylaxis for untreated small bowel disease; (4) localize any fistulizing disease or abscess and the location of involvement; and (5) treat any adhesions.

As in open surgery, dilation, creeping fat, inflammation, and corkscrew vessels are signs of Crohn's disease. If disease is noted, the distance from the ligament of Treitz and the length and characteristics of the disease are noted and should be dictated into the operative report. In cases of clinically significant disease, the area can be marked with a suture for later identification and surgical intervention.

If the surgeon is unsure of the clinical significance of the disease, the area can be marked and externalized through a small incision. The area of concern can be palpated. Upstream dilation is generally a sign of clinically significant disease. Alternatively, a small enterotomy can be made at the site, and a 5-mL Foley balloon can be pulled through questionable segments of bowel to determine whether resection or strictureplasty is warranted. Resection can be done intracorporeally or through the extraction site. If a strictureplasty is to be performed, this will be done through the extraction incision.

■ THICKENED MESENTERY

One concern for laparoscopy in a patient with Crohn's disease is the thickened mesentery. Creeping fat not only covers the wall of the intestines, but also creates a profound lymphatic response, which surrounds and complicates dissection of the major blood vessels. This can affect small bowel mesentery but is often most notable at the ileocolic artery, where exposure of the artery itself can be difficult.

For an ileocecectomy, approach the vessels using general laparoscopic technique. A medial to lateral approach allows for early assessment. A decision is made about the level of inflammation. If involvement is minimal, the vessel may be approached with a medial to lateral approach, scoring the mesentery, isolating the vessel, and transecting with an energy device. Before transection, ensure that a backup ligation technique, such as endoloop, is available in the operating room in case of device failure.

If the area is considerably thickened, one may have better success by moving more proximally on the vessel, at the takeoff of the superior mesenteric artery. At the proximal margin, the lymphatic response is generally minimal. This may allow for successful vessel ligation with either a stapler or an energy device; however, this approach does have potential concerns. A high ligation transects more of the vascular supply and may require a more significant bowel resection than initially planned. Also, if bleeding does occur, it can be more difficult to control. Some surgeons have success with stapling rather than bipolar ligation, but the surgeon should be prepared for possible backbleeding and have either endoloop or clips available if this occurs.

Other surgeons have advocated a retromesenteric approach, taking the ileocolic vessels at the border of the colon and mobilizing the entire right colon from a posterior approach. This may have decreased inflammation compared with a midmesenteric approach, where Crohn's mesentery tends to be thickest.

Alternatively, in "bad" Crohn's mesentery, the surgeon can decide to perform a lateral to medial approach to the resection and leave the mesentery for an open approach. The thickened Crohn's mesentery is taken with clamps and suture ligation through the extraction incision at the end of the surgery, before creation of the anastomosis. This may provide better security that hemostasis has been achieved in severely thickened disease.

■ FISTULA OR ABSCESS CAVITY

Fistulas can occur between two loops of small bowel to the abdominal wall, colon, or intra-abdominal organs, such as the uterus or bladder. Initial evaluation of a fistula or abscess cavity should determine the extent of disease and involvement. Often, blunt dissection is used to free an abscess or fistula from surrounding structures. This

is analogous to inflammation in diverticulitis. Several tools are helpful: A 30-degree scope allows the surgeon to visualize the fistula or abscess from multiple directions without changing port sites. Working from multiple angles often can be very helpful. A suction irrigator is available in case of entry into an abscess cavity or the bowel. Immediate evacuation of purulence or feculent material decreases the risk for contamination. Laparoscopic peanuts can be used to push or separate tissues. Blunt dissection is generally very useful in inflamed tissues.

When approaching the fistula, push solid organs, such as the uterus or side wall, away from the bowel. Working from several directions may help to determine the easiest course of dissection. An energy instrument or cautery can be used to remove omentum or epiploic fat that is adhered to the bowel, but the surgeon should be careful to prevent cautery injury to surrounding intestines (Figure 6).

In an enteroenteric fistula, a decision should be made about how much viable small bowel is present between the two ends of the fistula. If less than 10 cm separates the ends of the fistula and the patient does not have concerns about malabsorption, consider an en bloc resection of the fistula. If both ends of bowel appear to be involved primarily (signs of primary Crohn's disease such as creeping fat, thickened bowel, or intralumenal Crohn's disease), both sides

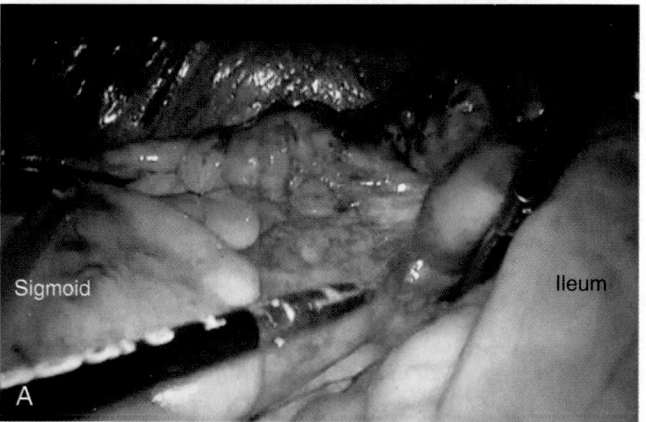

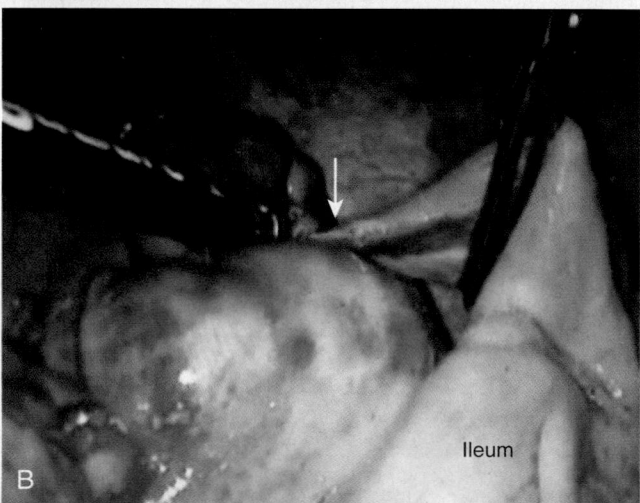

FIGURE 6 A, Intraoperative photos of a patient with ileal sigmoid fistula. Initially the area of the fistula is evaluated using blunt dissection. After removing omentum and inflammatory tissue, a clear fistula from the terminal ileum to the sigmoid was noted. **B,** This was transected using an energy device. Both ends of the fistula, the sigmoid and small bowel, were evaluated for primary versus secondary disease, and then areas of primary Crohn's disease were resected.

should be resected. If a segment is involved secondarily only, with normal mucosa and surrounding bowel, a wedge resection or repair can be considered. For colonic disease, preoperative colonoscopy with intralumenal visualization of the fistula helps to determine whether the disease is primary or secondary. If the colonoscopy was not performed preoperatively, consider intraoperative carbon dioxide endoscopy to evaluate the segment of colon.

Fistulas may need to be "taken down" intra-abdominally. Intra-loop fistulas may impede extraction of the specimen. Enterocutaneous and enterovesical fistulas should be divided if possible. Although there may be concern that fistula takedown could lead to intra-abdominal soilage, the amount of soilage is generally minimal. Always have suction irrigation available in case of soilage.

The technique used to repair the colon or bladder depends on surgeon comfort and experience. A two-layer bladder repair generally can be performed intracorporeally with absorbable suture. A two-layer repair of the colon may be performed laparoscopically, but many surgeons are more comfortable with an open repair. If this is the case, consider strategic placement of the extraction incision. In the case of sigmoid or bladder repair, this generally can be reached easily through a small Pfannenstiel incision. In either case, after a fistula has been repaired, the surgeon should consider mobilization of the omentum off the right or left side of the transverse colon and placement of an omental pedicle flap between the repaired end of the fistula and the new anastomosis.

EMERGENCY SURGERY

Emergent surgery in Crohn's disease is rare. Because of the chronic nature of inflammation, patients often wall off fistulas and abscesses rather than being seen with acute perforation. Bleeding is not as common as in ulcerative colitis. In the rare care of emergent need for surgery, laparoscopic evaluation is feasible. Determination of the etiology of disease, extent of disease, and surgeon's skill and comfort level will dictate whether laparoscopic treatment is possible.

EXTRACTION INCISIONS

One benefit of laparoscopic surgery is the ability to decrease hernia rates by selecting an extraction site away from the midline. Data have demonstrated that paramedian, transverse, and Pfannenstiel incisions have lower hernia rates than midline incisions. This must be balanced with the risk for recurrent operation and the ease of a midline incision. In addition, if open repair of the sigmoid colon or bladder is needed, the incision should be placed strategically to allow best access to this quadrant of the abdomen.

Depending on the extraction site chosen, the surgeon can perform extracorporeal anastomoses, evaluate loops of questionable small bowel, and repair bladder or colonic fistula sites. In addition,

mesentery can be taken through the extraction incision in cases of severely inflamed Crohn's mesentery.

A wound protector decreases the risk for wound infections and should be used during all colon surgery. This is particularly important in immunosuppressed patients.

■ CONVERSION

With any laparoscopic surgery, there is risk for conversion. Risk for conversion is increased in patients with complex, multifocal disease; fistulizing disease; abscesses; and prior surgeries. In addition, some studies demonstrate that malnutrition, smoking, and steroid use may increase the risk for conversion in patients with Crohn's disease. Conversion increases the rate of complications, hospital stays, and the costs associated with treatment of Crohn's disease. As with any surgery, the purpose of the surgery is to provide good, safe, and result-oriented care. If the safety, purpose, or success of the operation is limited by technique for any reason, conversion to open surgery may be prudent and necessary. Proactive conversion, before a complication or error, rather than retroactive conversion is always preferred.

■ CONCLUSION

Although laparoscopic surgery for Crohn's disease may be difficult, patients can achieve significant benefits from minimally invasive techniques. Careful preoperative planning, understanding of patient anatomy, and advanced laparoscopic tools can guide surgeons through successful laparoscopic surgery.

SUGGESTED READINGS

Alves A, Panis Y, Bouhnik Y. Factors that predict conversion in 69 consecutive patients undergoing laparoscopic ileocecal resection for Crohn's disease: a prospective study. *Dis Colon Rectum.* 2005;48:2302-2308.

Antoniou SA, Antoniou GA, Koch OO. Is laparocopic ileocecal resection a safe option for Crohn's disease? Best evidence topic. *Int J Surg.* 2014;12: 22-25.

Chebbi F, Ayadi MS, Rhaiem R. Laparoscopic ileo-cecal resection: the total retro-mesenteric approach. *Surg Endosc.* 2015;29:245-251.

Keller D, Katz J, Stein SL. Surgical cost of care in Crohn's disease. *Pol Przegl Chir.* 2013;85:511-516.

Kunitake H, Hodin R, Shellito PC. Perioperative treatment with infliximab in patients with Crohn's disease and ulcerative colitis is not associated with increased postoperative complications. *J Gastrointest Surg.* 2008;12: 1730-1737.

Samia H, Lawrence J, Nobel T. Extraction site location and incisional hernias after laparoscopic colorectal surgery: should we be avoiding the midline. *Am J Surg.* 2013;205:264-267.

Tan JJ, Tjandra JJ. Laparoscopic surgery for Crohn's disease: a meta-analysis. *Dis Colon Rectum.* 2007;50:576-585.

LAPAROSCOPIC COLON AND RECTAL SURGERY

Justin T. Brady, MD, Alison R. Althans, BA, and Conor P. Delaney, MD, MCh, PhD

Since the first laparoscopic colon resection was performed more than 2 decades ago, a multitude of studies have shown that laparoscopic colectomy is both safe and feasible, leading to its

increasing use by colorectal and general surgeons. Laparoscopic procedures for both benign and malignant diseases have been shown to have many advantages compared with open colon surgery approaches, including accelerated return of bowel function, decreased need for analgesics postoperatively, shorter hospital stay, decreased rate of wound infection, and improved cosmesis. Although laparoscopic surgery tends to have increased operating room costs because of the required instrumentation and operating room time, this is offset by a decreased length of stay, which tends to make the overall costs of laparoscopic and open techniques for colon surgery equivalent. As surgeons become more proficient at laparoscopic procedures, it is possible that laparoscopy will become even more cost effective.

■ PREOPERATIVE IMAGING AND EVALUATION

It is important that patients undergo appropriate cross-sectional imaging to evaluate for potential involvement of adjacent structures, such as fistula formation or tumor invasion. Some of these patients may remain candidates for laparoscopic resection. For patients with invasion of the abdominal wall, retroperitoneum, stomach, liver, small bowel, bladder, vagina, or prostate, we recommend an open approach unless the surgeon is comfortable with the necessary laparoscopic dissection. For laparoscopic colectomy, because of the complexities involved and the need for en bloc resection, invasion of the kidney or ureter and the superior mesenteric vein is an absolute contraindication to laparoscopic resection. For laparoscopic low anterior resection (LAR) with total mesorectal excision (TME), absolute contraindications include tumor invasion of the sacrum, bladder, or pelvic side wall because of en bloc specimen size. Of note, specimens greater than 10 cm in diameter will require a small laparotomy for removal, effectively negating the benefits of laparoscopy.

As surgical technical skills and experience have improved, the absolute contraindications to laparoscopic colorectal surgery have decreased and, conversely, the relative contraindications have increased. Physiologic limitations of severe cardiopulmonary disease such that patients will not be able to tolerate pneumoperitoneum or the Trendelenburg position on the operative table are absolute contraindications, albeit extremely rare. More commonly, medical comorbidities make a laparoscopic approach even more important to help frail patients in their postoperative recovery.

Patients who have undergone multiple previous open abdominal procedures may present particular difficulty during laparoscopy because of the presence of extensive adhesions; we generally start with an exploratory laparoscopy, as in many cases a laparoscopic adhesiolysis can permit minimally invasive surgery to be completed.

The question of open versus laparoscopic approach also must be carefully contemplated with respect to patients who are obese. Their large body habitus can limit insufflation of the abdomen. The excessive mesenteric fat present in patients who are morbidly obese can obscure visualization of major vessels and make tissue dissection and retraction more difficult, as there is less space, and the mesentery may tear easily if it is soft fat. This may require conversion for cancer cases so that the specimen is not disrupted. It is obviously much more important to have a complete and intact specimen than a laparoscopically completed case. Relative to colonic procedures, patients who undergo rectal procedures must have lower body mass indices (BMIs)—45 versus 55—because of the bulkiness of the mesentery, although this is a relative limit and very much gender dependent. Higher BMI is more tolerable in females because of the presence of less severe visceral adiposity than seen in men as well as a wider pelvis. When there is doubt regarding the feasibility of proceeding with a laparoscopic resection, one can always start with a laparoscopic inspection before converting to an open procedure if needed; however, in most cases these challenges can be superseded.

Although there are no other populations for which laparoscopic colorectal surgery has been deemed unsafe, there are some relative contraindications that are mostly dependent on the experience and skill set of the surgeon. Although laparoscopy can manage most types of fistulas, operating on enterocutaneous fistulas generally is not possible because of the extensive adhesions that are often involved. Duodenal fistulas also may be very challenging. Enteroenteric, enterocolic, colovesical, and colovaginal fistulas usually can be managed laparoscopically. The bigger challenge usually occurs when patients have two or three of the factors discussed in this section (obesity, fistula, adhesions, abscess).

For emergency cases, we pursue a laparoscopic approach if the patient is stable and the procedure appears technically possible.

■ OPERATIVE PRINCIPLES

Laparoscopic Right Hemicolectomy

Patients are placed in supine position on a bean bag with both arms tucked in lithotomy position. The bean bag and stirrups prevent the patient from sliding on the operating table and allow increased table angulation. This uses gravity to retract the small bowel, decreasing bowel manipulation and possible inadvertent injury. If the patient's body habitus prevents tucking both arms, only the left arm is tucked. Using a Hasson technique, a 10-mm infraumbilical port is placed and the abdomen is insufflated with carbon dioxide to a pressure of 12 mm Hg. The laparoscope is inserted and the abdomen is inspected carefully, especially for patients with known malignancy, with close evaluation of the liver, small bowel, and peritoneum for evidence of metastatic disease. A 5-mm port is placed lateral to the inferior epigastric vessels in the left lower quadrant, 2 to 3 cm medial and superior to the anterior superior iliac spine. This is followed by a 5-mm port in the left upper quadrant, at least 1 handwidth from the left lower quadrant port. It can be advantageous in teaching cases or difficult dissections to also place a 5-mm port in the right lower quadrant.

The surgeon stands on the patient's left side. After port placement, the assistant stands behind the surgeon, also on the left. The patient is placed in slight Trendelenburg position, and the table is angled right side up to facilitate the retraction of the omentum superiorly over the stomach and the small bowel away from the right colon.

For a medial to lateral approach, an atraumatic bowel clamp is used to tent the mesentery at the ileocecal junction toward the right lower quadrant abdominal wall, elevating the ileocolic vessels off the retroperitoneum (Figure 1, A, and Figure 2, A). Medial to the vessels, the peritoneum is opened with cautery close to and parallel to the superior mesenteric vessels, so that a complete en bloc mesocolic excision is performed (Figure 1, B, and Figure 2, B). The ileocolic vessel is dissected sharply away from the retroperitoneum. The dissection is continued proximally to the origin of the ileocolic artery on the superior mesenteric artery (SMA). This plane of dissection is anterior to Toldt's fascia, the peritoneal layer over the duodenum and ureter and the congenital peritoneum of the retroperitoneum. Then a window in the mesentery is made lateral to the origin of the ileocolic artery, allowing division of the vessels. The divided vessel is lifted, allowing continued medial to lateral dissection behind the colon and out to the white line of Toldt. Dissection continues superiorly past the duodenum and pancreas up to the liver, often opening through into the subhepatic space, or Morison's pouch (Figure 1, C, and Figure 2, C).

The dissection now turns to mobilizing the hepatic flexure. With the assistant retracting the ascending colon inferiorly and the surgeon retracting the transverse colon medially and inferiorly, the gastrocolic ligament may be divided (Figure 1, D and E). One must be cautious with dissection so as not to injure the adjacent gallbladder or duodenum. For cancers of the cecum, the greater omentum can be preserved. For cancers near the flexure or in the right transverse colon, the omentum is taken en bloc, dissecting it at its origin at the duodenum and gastroepiploic arcade. Once the hepatic flexure has been mobilized, the dissection continues laterally along the white line of Toldt inferiorly to the cecum. If it has not been seen easily and divided earlier, the dissection then returns to the transverse colon mesentery where the right branch of the middle colic is divided to allow easier specimen extraction and anastomosis (Figure 2, D).

To facilitate easy specimen extraction and anastomosis, the terminal ileum must be freed from its retroperitoneal attachments, which was started during the initial part of the procedure (Figure 2, E). Using the left hand instrument, the surgeon retracts the terminal ileum superiorly and medially; if needed, the assistant also may help to lift the terminal ileum. The mesentery should be mobilized off the retroperitoneum toward the SMA until the third portion of the duodenum can be visualized (Figure 2, F). This should be carried out in the same avascular plane that leaves a thin layer of parietal

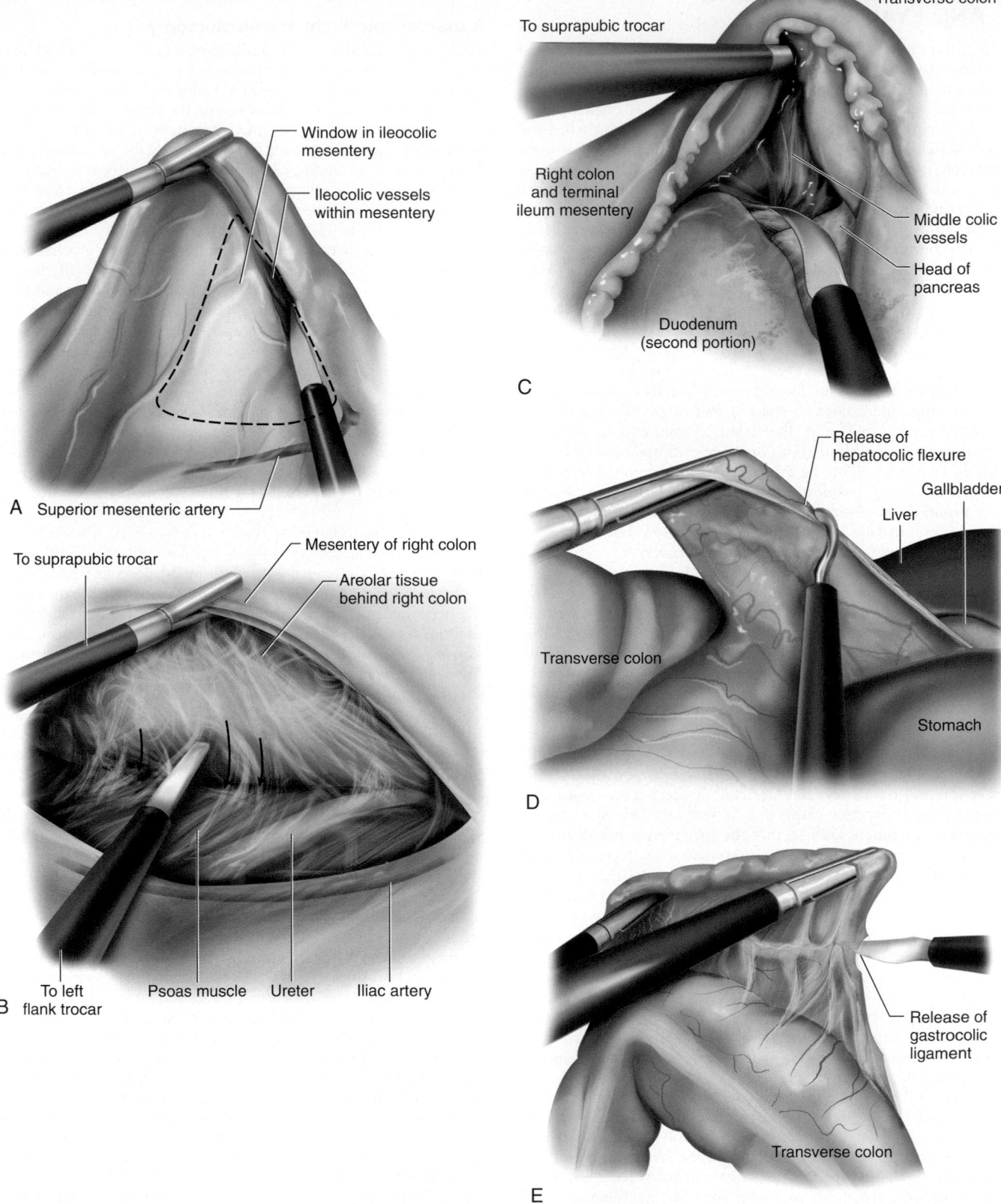

FIGURE 1 A to E, Laparoscopic posterior medial-to-lateral approach in the right colectomy: schematic views. *(From Fleshman JW, Birnbaum EH, Hunt SR, et al [eds]. Atlas of Surgical Techniques for Colon, Rectum, and Anus. Philadelphia: WB Saunders; 2012.)*

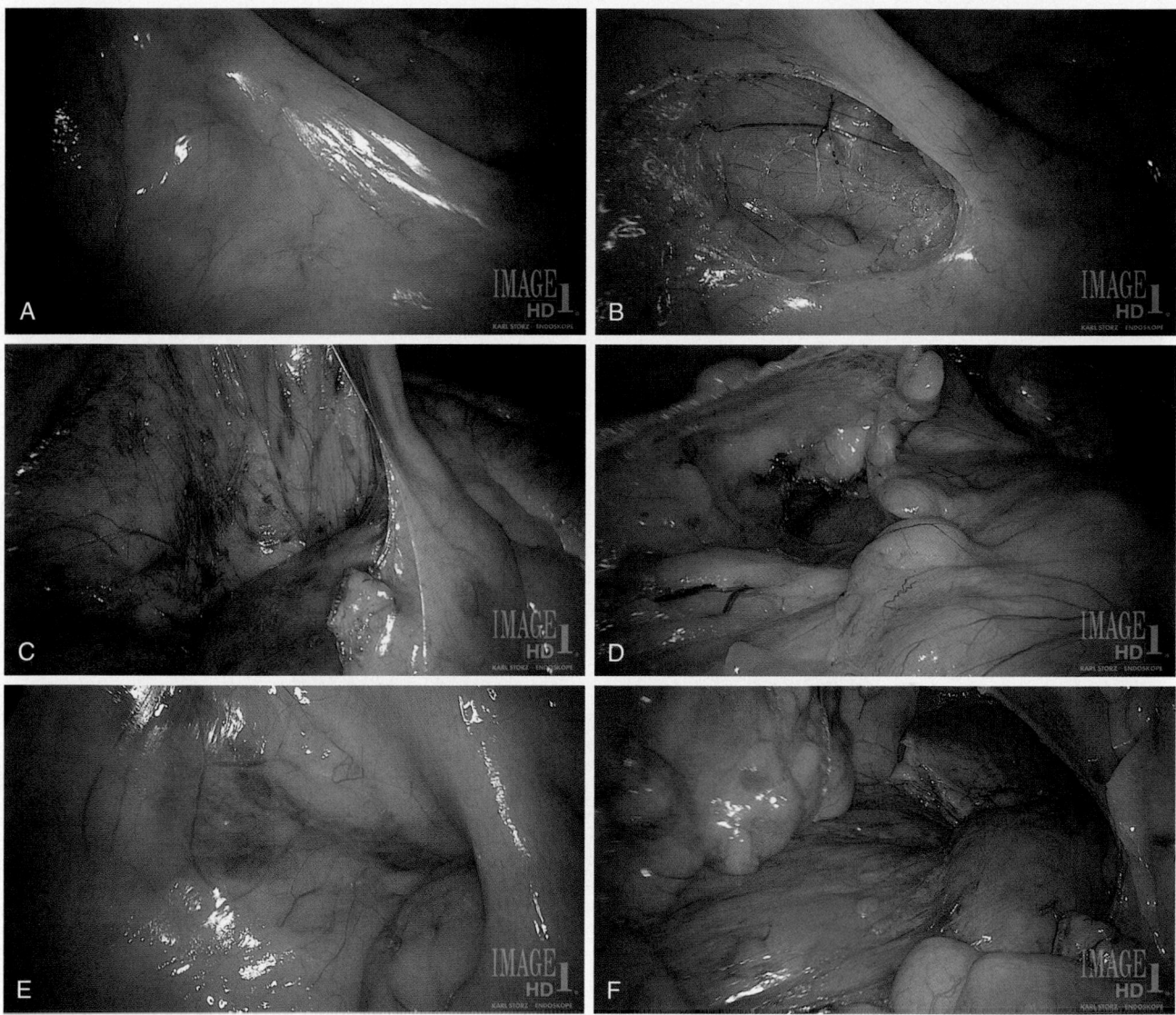

FIGURE 2 Laparoscopic right hemicolectomy with medial to lateral approach. **A,** Elevation of the ileocolic vessels. **B,** Window in the mesentery on the medial aspect of the ileocolic vessels. **C,** Medial to lateral mobilization of the right colon extending superior to the duodenum. **D,** Window in the superior aspect of the mesocolon. **E,** Elevation of the small bowel mesentery of the retroperitoneum. **F,** Right colon completely mobilized with intact retroperitoneum.

peritoneum with underlying ureter and iliac vessels undisturbed. At this point the specimen should be completely mobilized and ready for extraction. This is an opportune time to inspect for hemostasis.

The infraumbilical incision is extended to a total length of 3 to 4 cm (or more depending on tumor size) to allow for specimen removal. A wound protector is put in place, and the right colon is exteriorized. The small bowel mesentery is divided, followed by the division of the bowel with a stapling device. The assistant maintains a clamp on the proximal ileum to prevent it from returning to the abdomen. Alternatively, in the obese patient the terminal ileum may be divided intracorporeally and the specimen brought out "end first" to allow for a smaller extraction incision compared with exteriorizing a loop of intestine. The colon mesentery then is divided and inspected for adequate perfusion followed by division with a stapling device. After removal from the field, the right colon should be inspected to ensure adequate margins and intactness of the mesocolon. An ileocolic side-to-side anastomosis is then created using a gastrointestinal anastomosis (GIA) and transverse anastomosis (TA) stapling device. After ensuring adequate hemostasis, the intestine is returned to the abdomen with the mesenteric window left open. The fascial defect is closed with absorbable sutures, followed by wound irrigation and closure of the skin with staples or subcuticular sutures.

Lateral to Medial Approach

This approach may be necessary because of adhesions, inflammation of the mesentery, or bulky disease that precludes safe identification of the ileocolic vasculature. Surgeons who are more comfortable with open surgery will find this dissection similar to an open approach. The disadvantage to this dissection is that the specimen is being mobilized medially, toward the camera, which can obscure the view of the area of dissection. It is important to identify and avoid injury to the duodenum.

Superior Approach

In cases of a large cecal tumor or inflammation, it may be safer and easier to start the dissection at the gastrocolic ligament. With the patient in reverse Trendelenburg position and the omentum draped inferiorly, the assistant provides traction inferiorly on the ascending colon and the surgeon provides inferomedial traction on the transverse colon to allow division of the gastrocolic ligament. The dissection continues inferiorly with mobilization of the colon, ensuring identification of the retroperitoneal duodenum.

Laparoscopic Left Hemicolectomy and Sigmoid Colectomy

Patients are placed in the lithotomy position on a bean bag with both arms tucked. For patients with a large body habitus, the left arm may be left out, but the right must always be tucked. The surgeon and assistant stand on the patient's right side, and it is sometimes useful for them to also be able to stand between the patient's legs for splenic flexure mobilization.

Port placement starts with a 10-mm infraumbilical port using the Hasson technique. This is followed by a 12-mm right lower quadrant port approximately 2 to 3 cm medial and superior to the anterior superior iliac spine, making sure it is lateral to the epigastric vessels. At least 1 handwidth superior to this is the third port, 5 mm in size and also lateral to the epigastric vessels. A 5-mm port is placed in the left lower quadrant, 2 to 3 cm medial and lateral to

the anterior superior iliac spine at a site that will become the specimen extraction site.

The table is placed in Trendelenburg position and rotated left side up and right side down. This helps to move the small bowel away from the area of dissection and keeps the omentum reflected over the stomach.

We prefer a medial to lateral approach. At the midpoint of the bowel wall and sacral promontory, using an atraumatic bowel clamp, the rectosigmoid mesentery is tented toward the left lower quadrant port (Figure 3, A). This elevates the inferior mesenteric vessels anteriorly to reveal a sulcus between the medial aspect of the inferior mesenteric vessels and the retroperitoneum. The peritoneum is dissected sharply along this sulcus to elevate the vessels away from the retroperitoneum and presacral nerves (Figure 3, B). By staying close to the inferior mesenteric vessels, a complete mesocolic excision can be performed while safely avoiding the retroperitoneal structures. If the dissection is in the correct plane, the ureter should be visualized deep to the parietal peritoneum and adjacent to the gonadal vessels, in the same plane as the autonomic nerves.

It is easy for the initial dissection to be too deep, particularly in a surgeon's early experience, and the ureter may have been elevated

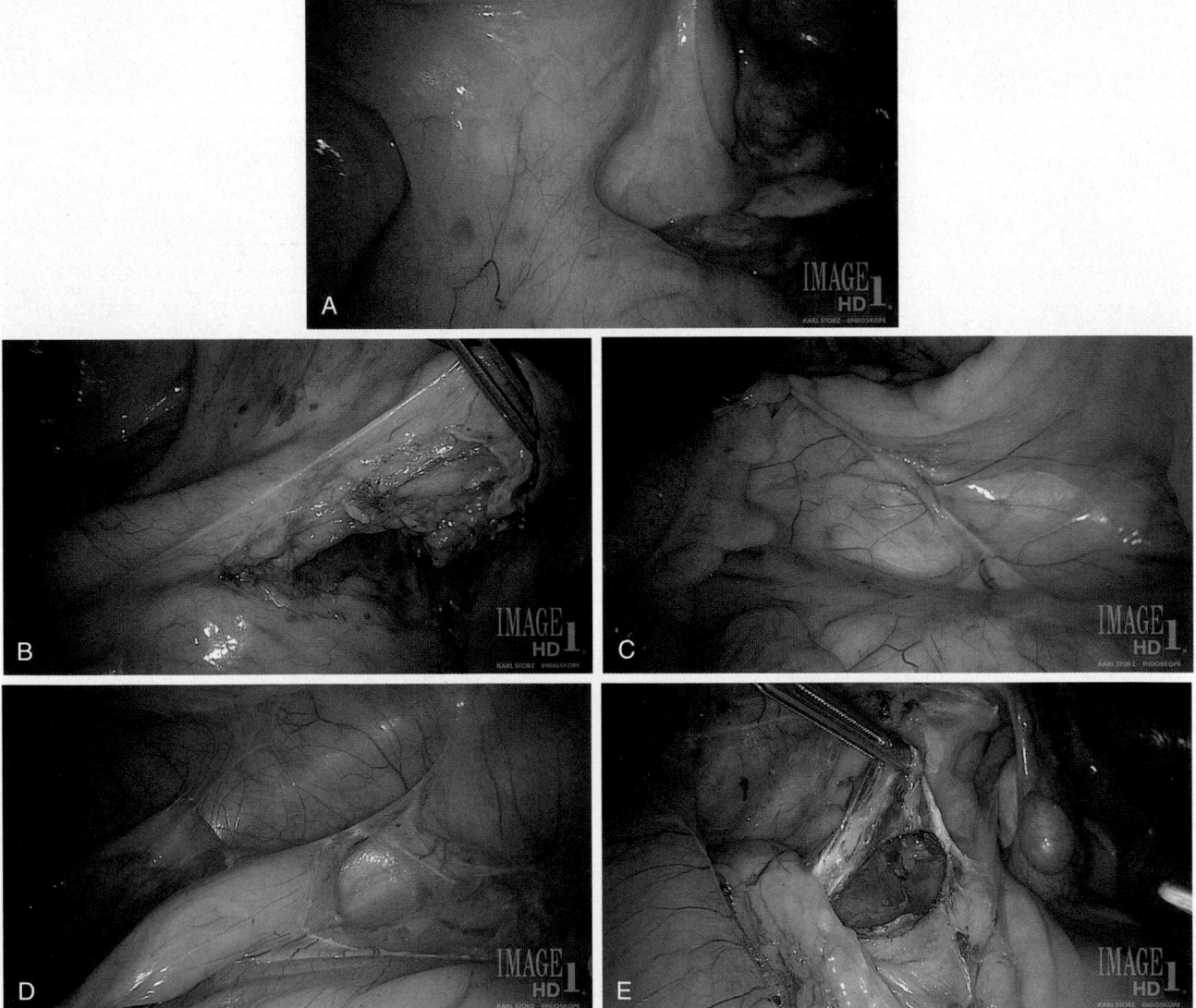

FIGURE 3 Laparoscopic proctosigmoidectomy. **A,** Elevation of the inferior mesenteric vessels. **B,** Mobilization of the inferior mesenteric vessels off the retroperitoneum. **C,** Visualization of the inferior mesenteric vein. **D,** Dissection of the lateral attachments of the left colon. **E,** Opening of the peritoneum on the left side of the rectosigmoid to display the space previously dissected by the medial to lateral dissection.

accidentally with the inferior mesenteric vessels. The ureter must be swept down off the vessels with the autonomic presacral nerves. If the planes are challenging because of inflammation or obesity, one also may dissect out the inferior mesenteric vein, cephalad to the inferior mesenteric artery (IMA) origin, which can permit the surgeon to identify the correct plane and isolate the mesenteric vessels. If this is unsuccessful, we recommend trying a lateral to medial approach (discussed later). If the surgeon is still unable to identify the ureter, one may try placement of ureteric stents, which may facilitate identification, or convert to open; however, such options are rarely necessary.

After adequate medial exposure of the mesenteric vessels, a window on the lateral aspect of the vessels is opened using cautery. Perform high ligation of the artery for malignant disease or low ligation for benign disease using energy sources or an Endo GIA stapler. With the vessel ligated, dissection between the retroperitoneum and colonic mesentery plane continues to the lateral colon attachments and superiorly to the tail of the pancreas. This superior dissection will expose the inferior mesenteric vein as it passes inferior to the pancreas, where a high ligation may be performed on the vein to increase reach of the proximal bowel for anastomosis in lower rectal cases (Figure 3, C).

Retracting the sigmoid colon medially with the bowel grasper in the left hand, the lateral attachments are divided using cautery, which will expose the previously defined retroperitoneal plane (Figure 3, D and E). Dissection continues along the white line of Toldt cranially, with the surgeon moving the atraumatic bowel grasper to maintain adequate traction.

We do not routinely mobilize the splenic flexure for benign disease, but will do so with the slightest concern of anastomotic tension. This dissection may be especially challenging in the patient who is obese or in those with prior surgery.

Dissection returns to the rectosigmoid colon. Making sure to protect the ureter, the upper left mesorectum is dissected free using cautery to permit an adequate distal margin. The assistant then uses an atraumatic bowel grasper through the left lower quadrant port to retract the distal rectosigmoid colon cranially out of the pelvis, with and without anterior or posterior movement to allow the surgeon to evaluate whether the extent of dissection is adequate. In procedures for malignancy, if the area of concern was not tattooed preoperatively, a flexible endoscopy may need to be performed to confirm adequate margins.

The peritoneal reflection is scored, and the plane between the rectum and mesorectum is developed with gentle blunt dissection using the jaws of the bowel grasper in an anterior-posterior direction. The assistant continues to retract the upper rectum cranially and anteriorly, allowing the surgeon to divide the mesorectum using an energy source. Before insertion of the stapler device, thoroughly inspect the mesorectum for any evidence of inadequate hemostasis. An Endo GIA stapler is inserted through the right lower quadrant 12-mm port and the rectum is divided. This may require more than one firing of the stapler. Before specimen extraction, inspect the site of planned proximal anastomosis to ensure adequate reach and blood supply.

The specimen can be exteriorized through the left lower quadrant port or infraumbilical port or through a suprapubic incision, 3 to 4 cm in length with a wound protector in place. However, we favor a left lower quadrant muscle splitting incision. The bowel is divided at the proximal margin and good blood supply is confirmed by visualizing pulsatile flow in the marginal artery. A size 28 anvil is secured in place with a purse-string suture. The bowel is returned to the abdomen, and the fascial defect is closed.

After the abdomen is reinsufflated, the proximal colon with anvil in place is positioned in the pelvis to evaluate for a tension-free anastomosis. If the colon lies in the pelvis without retracting to the abdomen, further mobilization of the splenic flexure or transverse colon is not needed. It is important to confirm proper colon orientation by looking at the mesenteric side of the colon. The circular stapling device is inserted into the rectum and advanced to the staple line under laparoscopic visualization. The end-to-end anastomosis is performed, followed by inspection for two complete "donuts." A leak test is performed by filling the pelvis with enough irrigating fluid to submerge the anastomosis and then distending the anastomosis with air.

If the air leak test is positive, there are two options for repair. If there is a small isolated defect that can be visualized clearly, this may be repaired with interrupted intracorporeal sutures. If the defect is larger or not amenable to suture repair, the bowel is divided distal to the anastomosis, the anastomosis is resected, and a new anvil is placed for an end-to-end anastomosis. Regardless of the type of repair used, a repeat leak test must be performed. A positive leak happens in less than 1% of cases in our experience.

After inspecting for hemostasis, the port sites and skin are closed as described previously.

Lateral to Medial Approach

There are some patients in whom a medial to lateral approach is not safe to perform for retroperitoneal dissection. This can be because of extensive inflammation that obscures the planes medially, which can be seen in Crohn's disease or sigmoid diverticulitis. Alternatively, in patients with a very high BMI with thick mesentery, it may not be possible to visualize the inferior mesenteric vessels. Starting laterally can give an easier view of the lateral side of the IMA and mesocolon and allow protection of the presacral autonomic nerves. Similar to the lateral to medial approach in a right colon dissection, the specimen is mobilized toward the camera, which may partially obscure visualization.

Proximal Left Colon Tumors

For tumors that are closer to the splenic flexure or in the distal transverse colon, the inferior mesenteric vessels may be preserved if there is an adequate distal margin. In this scenario, the inferior mesenteric vessels are identified and dissected as described earlier. They are followed proximally to allow identification of the left colic vessels. A high ligation of the left colic vessels is performed. Similar to a right colon resection, the left colon is exteriorized and a side-to-side anastomosis is performed between the transverse and sigmoid colons.

Laparoscopic Low Anterior Resection

Patient positioning, port placement, and initial steps are nearly identical to those in a sigmoid or left colon resection. Patients are placed on a bean bag in lithotomy position. With the surgeon standing on the patient's right and the assistant on the patient's left, a 10-mm infraumbilical port is placed, followed by a 12-mm right lower quadrant port and left lower quadrant port, each 2 to 3 cm medial and superior to the anterior superior iliac spines. For LAR requiring a temporary ileostomy, the right lower quadrant port is placed at the ostomy site, and this likely will be used as the specimen extraction site. A 5-mm port is placed in the right upper quadrant, at least 1 handwidth away from the infraumbilical and right lower quadrant ports.

After thorough inspection of the abdomen for evidence of metastatic disease for oncologic resections, the patient is placed in the Trendelenburg position with the left side up. Using a medial to lateral approach, the mesentery over the inferior mesenteric vessels is tented and dissected sharply as described earlier for a sigmoid resection, making sure to preserve the left ureter and autonomic presacral nerves. High ligation of the IMA for a complete mesocolic resection is performed for oncologic resections. Dissection continues in the retroperitoneal plane superiorly, leaving Gerota's fascia intact. The inferior mesenteric vein is ligated just inferior to the pancreas.

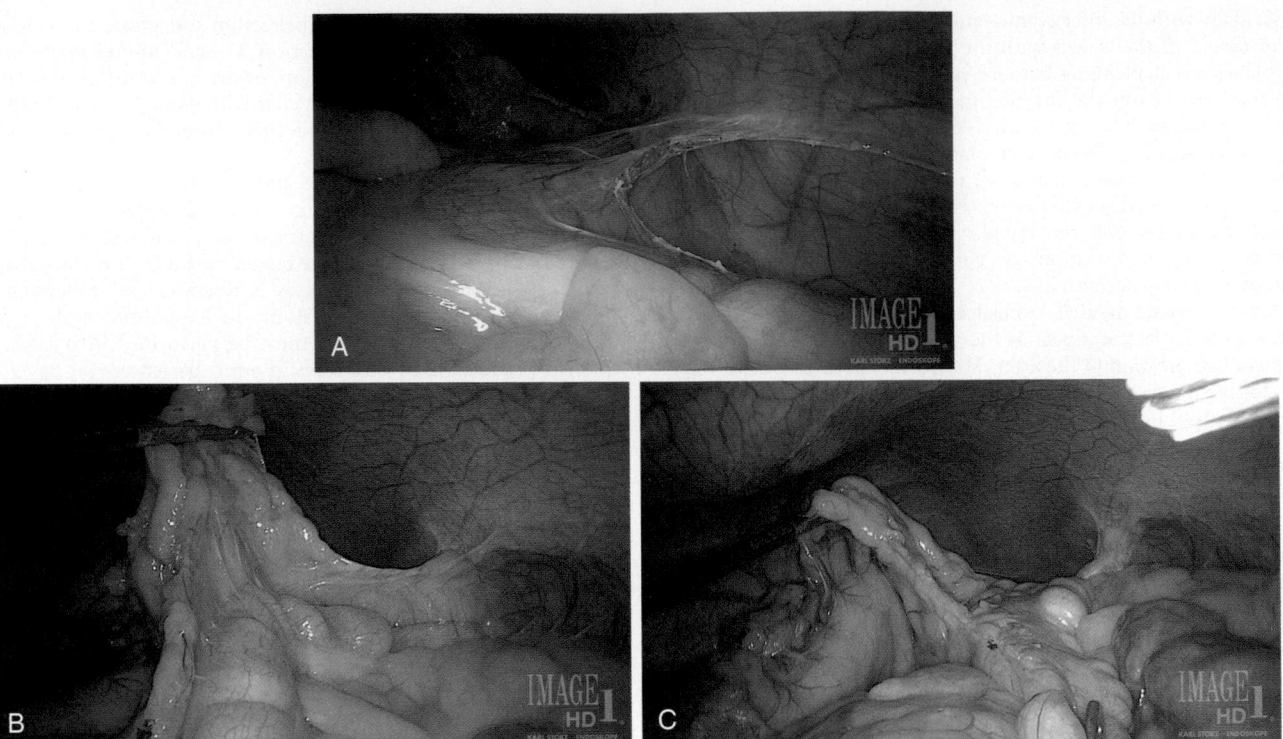

FIGURE 4 Laparoscopic splenic flexure mobilization. **A,** Lateral mobilization. **B,** Dissection in the plane between the greater omentum and colon. **C,** Demonstration of the lesser sac.

After lateral dissection along the white line of Toldt, splenic flexure mobilization is performed. At this point, placing the patient in reverse Trendelenburg position may facilitate an easier dissection.

The splenocolic, renocolic, and gastrocolic attachments are the three attachments of the splenic flexure. The renocolic attachments generally are dissected with the retroperitoneal colon mobilization from earlier in the procedure. The surgeon continues with gentle inferomedial traction, to prevent tearing of the splenic capsule, while continuing dissection with cautery close to the colon in a left to right fashion (Figure 4, *A*). Moving medially, the surgeon then enters the lesser sac by releasing the greater omentum off the transverse colon without entering the transverse mesocolon (Figure 4, *B* and *C*). Great effort is made to ensure that the entire left colon and its mesentery are brought to the midline. An additional 5-mm port in the left upper quadrant or the surgeon moving from the patient's right side to between the patient's legs may be helpful for this part of the dissection in particularly challenging cases.

The mesorectal dissection is the next part of the procedure. The patient is returned to Trendelenburg position, and the small bowel is swept away from the pelvis. With the assistant retracting the rectosigmoid junction cranially and slightly anteriorly, the avascular presacral mesorectal plane is identified. Dissection starts posteriorly and is carried out using cautery, between the presacral fascia and the fascia propria of the mesorectum, thereby preserving the autonomic nerves posteriorly (Figure 5, *A*). As dissection continues inferiorly, Waldeyer's fascia is divided and dissection follows the anterior curve of the sacrum. The right and left sides of the mesorectum then are mobilized, taking great care to observe the fascia of the pelvic side wall, thereby protecting the iliac vessels, ureters, and autonomic nerve plexi in the pelvic side wall.

Dissection then moves anteriorly between the rectovaginal septum in women and along Denonvilliers' fascia in men. These dissections are started several millimeters anterior to the lowest point of the pouch of Douglas, leaving the surgeon nicely in the correct plane and preserving the entire anterior mesorectum. Denonvilliers' fascia may need to be included in anterior tumors, thus exposing

the seminal vesicles and making the plane of dissection very close to the anterolateral nerve bundles. Usually once the anterior dissection is completed, further posterior dissection is required. The distal extent of dissection is determined by the tumor location to allow for adequate margins. This may need to be re-examined intraoperatively with rigid proctoscopy but more commonly with digital examination.

The dissection concludes where the rectum narrows into the anal canal and where the levators curve down into the anal canal. When an adequate margin can be obtained, the bowel can be divided with an Endo GIA stapler inserted through the right lower quadrant (ostomy site) port (Figure 5, *B* to *D*). It is particularly important to ensure that the plane of rectal transection is perpendicular to the bowel lumen and that the distal margin is not compromised for lower tumors. This may not be possible in patients with a deep, narrow pelvis or with a very low dissection, thus necessitating a transanal intersphincteric dissection with perineal specimen extraction and handsewn coloanal anastomosis, usually required for tumors within 2 cm of the dentate line. For patients able to undergo stapled resection, the distal end of the specimen may be brought out through the infraumbilical or lower quadrant port sites with a wound protector in place. In patients with a temporary ileostomy, the wound can be extended superiorly into a "keyhole," and this can be used for extraction. Similar to a sigmoid resection, the proximal bowel is divided, ensuring adequate blood supply before placement of a size 28 anvil and anastomosis with a circular stapling device (Figure 5, *E*). A leak test is performed as described earlier. A diverting loop ileostomy is created in the right lower quadrant, the site having been marked preoperatively by an enterostomal therapist.

Laparoscopic Abdominoperineal Resection

The abdomen and perineum are prepared and draped appropriately. Patient positioning and port placement are similar to that described earlier for the LAR and sigmoid resection. The left colon is mobilized to allow for creation of a tension-free end colostomy at the site

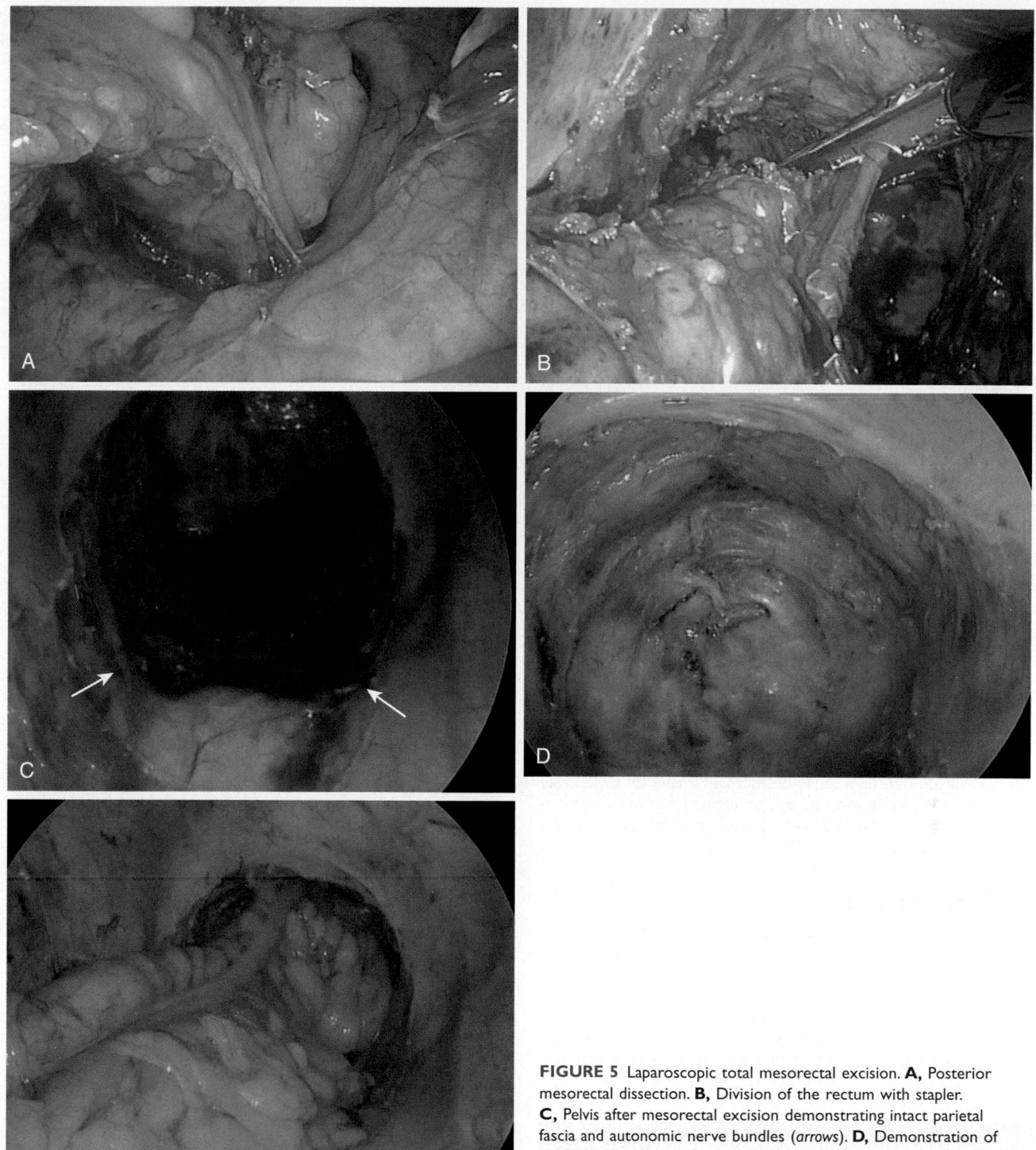

FIGURE 5 Laparoscopic total mesorectal excision. **A,** Posterior mesorectal dissection. **B,** Division of the rectum with stapler. **C,** Pelvis after mesorectal excision demonstrating intact parietal fascia and autonomic nerve bundles (*arrows*). **D,** Demonstration of staple line at anorectal junction. **E,** Tension-free side-to-end coloanal anastomosis.

marked preoperatively, and splenic flexure mobilization is rarely necessary. The rectal dissection is performed in a similar fashion as described earlier for LAR. Once the dissection has reached the levator ani, the surgeon will change from the transabdominal portion to the perineal approach.

The patient is placed in a high lithotomy position with the surgeon seated between the patient's legs. The anus is sutured closed. An elliptical incision is made around the anus to ensure adequate resection margins. Dissection proceeds with electrocautery lateral to the external anal sphincter in the ischiorectal fossa. Continuing in

the lateral and posterior aspects, dissection is deepened to the tip of the coccyx posteriorly and the levator ani muscles laterally. Starting anterior to the coccyx, the anococcygeal ligament is divided to allow entry into the pelvis. In our hands, the coccyx is removed only for locally invasive tumors. The levator ani muscles are dissected free and divided on the underlying finger, moving from posterior to lateral to anterior. The levators generally are taken laterally, close to their origin, but can be taken in a somewhat tumor-specific fashion. The anterior dissection is completed last, ensuring protection of the prostate and urethra or posterior vaginal wall. The specimen is extracted through the perineum. After inspection for hemostasis and irrigation, the perineum is closed in layers with absorbable sutures. The port sites then are closed, and the colostomy is matured.

Total Abdominal Colectomy, Proctocolectomy, and Extended Right Colectomy

Laparoscopic total abdominal colectomy or restorative proctocolectomy with ileal pouch–anal anastomosis (IPAA) is the procedure performed most commonly for inflammatory bowel disease (IBD) or hereditary polyposis syndromes such as familial adenomatous polyposis. An extended right colectomy may be required for a right or midtransverse colon cancer. Many of the same principles apply.

The total abdominal colectomy or proctocolectomy can be thought of as a combination of the previously described right hemicolectomy, left hemicolectomy, and LAR or abdominoperineal resection; the difference is obviously that the transverse colon now requires mobilization. Part of this mobilization is performed with the surgeon standing between the patient's legs. A decision must be made whether the greater omentum will be preserved and the dissection stay in the avascular plane between the transverse colon and omentum, or the omentum will be taken for oncologic reasons, when the dissection is close to the gastroepiploic vessels.

Once the planes have been defined and the omentum and transverse colon have been mobilized, the superior aspect of the transverse colon is identified to permit safe dissection and division of the middle colic vessels (Figure 6). Depending on the patient's individual anatomy, the vessels can be mobilized from a superior or inferior perspective, generally opening the mesentery to the left of the middle colic vessels. The right side already has been opened with mobilization of the ileocolic pedicle and right colon. The middle colic vessels are divided close to their origin, carefully protecting the superior mesenteric vessels, or divided more distally in benign cases.

The rectum is divided at the rectosigmoid junction for total colectomy cases, and specimen removal and anastomosis are performed as described earlier for sigmoid colectomy. For proctocolectomy, the rectum is divided in the anal canal as described earlier for LAR. Once again, usually a stapled anastomosis is performed, but mucosectomy and handsewn anastomosis may be required for colitic patients with distal rectal dysplasia.

Short-Term Recovery

The short-term benefits of laparoscopic colon and rectal surgery are well demonstrated in multiple randomized controlled trials. Patients who undergo laparoscopic surgery have decreased rates of surgical site infections, decreased narcotic usage, and accelerated return of bowel function, which contribute to an overall decreased length of stay of 2 to 3 days compared with open surgery. Patient hospital stay has been further reduced to less than 4 days at our institution with

the adoption of enhanced recovery pathway (ERP) protocols, which include patient education, intraoperative goal-directed fluid therapy, early postoperative nasogastric tube removal and enteral feeding, opioid-sparing analgesia, and early ambulation. Currently, 38% of our patients are discharged within 48 hours after laparoscopic colorectal resection. Studies have shown that this decrease in length of hospital stay with ERP protocols is not associated with an increase in readmission rate.

■ SPECIAL CONSIDERATIONS

Diverticulitis

In the elective setting, laparoscopic surgery for acute diverticulitis has been shown to have longer operative times compared with open surgery, but also decreased postoperative pain, reduced complications, a shorter duration to return of bowel function, decreased hospital length of stay, and comparable long-term outcomes. Because of the presence of inflammation, adhesions, and fistulas, laparoscopic surgery for diverticulitis may be challenging. It is important that both the proximal and the distal resection margins be free of inflamed and thickened tissue and that the distal margin is at or below the rectosigmoid junction and confluence of the taenia coli. Retrospective data have shown that a colosigmoid anastomosis has a fourfold higher rate of recurrent disease compared with a colorectal anastomosis. There is ongoing debate regarding the safety of primary anastomosis with or without proximal diversion in complicated diverticulitis; this is beyond the scope of this chapter. Performing laparoscopic lavage for Hinchey grade III or IV acute diverticulitis currently is not supported in the literature. In unstable patients, especially those with extensive comorbidities, performing a washout, resection of the diseased segment of bowel, and creation of an end colostomy (Hartmann's procedure) may be the safest option, with the acknowledgment that many of these patients will not undergo reversal. These emergency operations can be performed laparoscopically in many cases. A study of 94 patients by Stulberg and colleagues in 2009, which our group published, showed fewer complications and decreased intensive care unit length of stay, although these were not significant. Length of stay was reduced from 11 to 8 days.

Data regarding fistulas in diverticular disease are limited to small retrospective studies but indicate that laparoscopic resection is feasible and safe, with low recurrence rates. For colovesical fistulas, after resection of the affected segment of diseased bowel, only large, full-thickness bladder fistula defects are repaired laparoscopically in one or two layers with absorbable sutures. A Foley catheter usually is left in place for 7 to 14 days postoperatively for bladder decompression for sutured repairs but may be removed on day 2 after a cystogram in smaller fistulas. A cystogram is performed routinely before catheter removal. For colovaginal fistulas, suture repair typically is performed only for larger defects from the fistula tract, with smaller defects being left open. These cases are challenging because there is often a large phlegmon in the pelvis, which can be difficult to work around laparoscopically.

Colon Cancer

Before considering laparoscopic resection of a colon cancer, it is important to review the staging imaging to ensure that the tumor size, location, or invasion of adjacent structures would not preclude laparoscopic resection. In addition, reviewing the colonoscopy report for details of tumor localization and to learn whether tattooing was performed will help to guide the surgeon regarding bowel preparation and planning for an intraoperative colonoscopy. When in doubt, it is better to err on the side of caution and have the patient complete a bowel preparation to allow for intraoperative colonoscopy. Current guidelines recommend careful handling of the bowel with atraumatic graspers to avoid perforation and tumor contamination. Oncologic principles of a good dissection include high ligation of the vascular supply to the cancer, negative margins (proximal, distal,

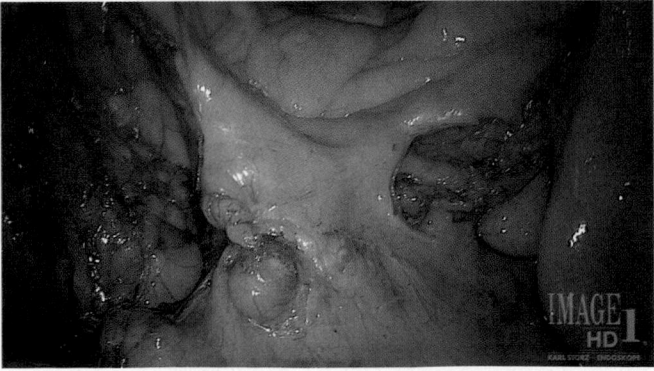

FIGURE 6 Isolated middle colic vessels.

and circumferential), and adequate lymphadenectomy with en bloc resection.

Initial results for laparoscopic resections for colon cancer reflected the technical challenges that the procedures presented. Laparoscopic bowel surgery was technically more difficult than laparoscopic cholecystectomy, and initial studies showed an increase in port site cancer recurrences. However, many randomized trials and meta-analyses show that minimally invasive approaches are at least as good as open surgery. Lacy and colleagues demonstrated improved recurrence rates overall and disease-free survival in laparoscopic compared with open colectomy, even for more advanced stage III disease. A meta-analysis of 12 randomized controlled trials with a total of 3346 patients conducted by Kuhry and colleagues in 2008 showed similar local recurrence rates (5.2% vs 5.6%) and distant recurrence rates (13.2% vs 12.6%) for colon cancer. In addition, laparoscopy can be used to obtain an equally good mesocolic excision to open surgery, with all of the short-term benefits provided by the minimally invasive approach.

Rectal Cancer

Similar to with laparoscopic colon resection, thorough review of patient imaging and endoscopy reports combined with physical examination findings allows for proper selection of patients amenable to laparoscopic resection. Preoperative magnetic resonance imaging is our preferred imaging modality to evaluate the circumferential tumor margins. Despite the predicted difficulty of dissection in some cases, initial laparoscopic inspection still can be beneficial.

Many authors feel that laparoscopy provides for better visualization in pelvic dissection and is associated with better TME quality; however, oncologic results are less mature than for colon cancer. Although the TME quality looks slightly worse for laparoscopic cases, the rectal cancer cohort from the CLASICC, COLOR II, and COREAN trials showed equivalent oncologic outcomes. Initial data from the ACOSOG Z6051 and Australasian Laparoscopic Cancer of the Rectum Trial (A La CaRT) trials also report that laparoscopic TME quality is inferior to that of open resection. Of interest, the COLOR II trial suggests that although outcomes are identical for all rectal cancer cases, laparoscopy performs slightly better for low rectal cancer, and open surgery performs slightly better for midrectal cancers.

Obviously the key is to pick the correct platform to perform as good a TME as possible for every patient. It will be interesting to see how transanal TME changes perspective and outcomes in the future, but in the interim we await the long-term oncologic data from the ACOSOG Z6051 and A La CaRT studies to add to the existing results.

Inflammatory Bowel Disease

Patients with IBD often undergo multiple procedures in their lifetime and stand to benefit from the decreased adhesion formation from laparoscopic surgery.

For patients with Crohn's disease, after laparoscopic inspection, areas of concern for stricture or fistula of the small bowel can be marked with a stitch. These areas can be exteriorized through an extended laparoscopic port site for extracorporeal inspection, resection with anastomosis, or strictureplasty. For patients with abscess formation who fail to improve with computed tomography–guided drainage and medical therapy, laparoscopic drainage and resection of the diseased portion of the bowel is a safe option. It is important to preserve as much bowel as possible but also to carefully inspect the areas for anastomosis after the specimen is exteriorized. Identical procedures can be performed laparoscopically as can be performed with open approaches. Duodenal or gastric fistulas from recurrent Crohn's disease may be the most difficult to handle, and at least in our hands have a higher chance of conversion.

Laparoscopic total colectomy or proctocolectomy with ileoanal pouch remains a complex procedure because of the many steps involved, but it is feasible in most patients. We prefer to perform a two-step procedure of total proctocolectomy with IPAA and diverting loop ileostomy. The colon generally is extracted through the ileostomy site. It is important to discuss the goals of care preoperatively, as patients with poor sphincter function or mobility may be better served by an end ileostomy than by continuity restoration. Function and outcomes are similar to open surgery, although hospital stay, cosmesis, adhesions, and hernia rates likely improve. Fertility may be improved in females because of the fewer adhesions that are formed.

Single Incision Laparoscopy

Single incision approaches were popular in the late 2000s as hand-assisted approaches faded out of practice. Many authors thought that patient recovery would be facilitated with surgery through a single site. In our hands results were essentially identical to the multiport approach, with similar rates of conversion to an open procedure, complications, and reoperation. In addition, the surgeon must hold the instruments in a more awkward position when using these approaches, and teaching is significantly more challenging. We now rarely use this approach.

■ AREAS FOR FUTURE STUDY

Robotic Surgery

Robot-assisted surgery is an area of growing interest in colorectal surgery. The technique for resection remains similar between laparoscopic and robotic colorectal surgery, with some differences in port placement. Advocates for robotic surgery tout the three-dimensional imaging, tenfold magnification, and articulating instruments with tremor reduction. Early studies have shown robotic surgery to be comparable with laparoscopy for complications and oncologic resection. However, results clearly show that robotic surgery is associated with increased operative times and hospital costs, with a similar length of stay compared with laparoscopy. Using a national inpatient database, Keller and colleagues found that robotic colorectal surgery had longer operating times by 39 minutes, higher total hospital costs by more than $5000, and a comparable length of stay. The recent Robotic versus Laparoscopic Resection for Rectal Cancer (ROLARR) randomized trial comparing robotic with laparoscopic rectal cancer surgery showed a nonsignificant trend to a reduced conversion rate with robotics. In addition, no other benefits were noted.

Transanal Total Mesorectal Excision

In the last few years, some authors have described a transanal total mesorectal excision (TaTME). This recent development may offer an exciting new approach for rectal cancer resection, as laparoscopic TME is especially challenging in patients who are obese or have midrectal and low rectal tumors (<10 cm from the anal verge), a narrow pelvis, or bulky tumors. We have used TaTME in several patients and the procedure requires further evaluation, but it may be a promising way to deal with low rectal cancers, particularly in obese males where a laparoscopic distal rectal mobilization can be challenging. In TaTME an initial distal intersphincteric dissection is performed, or the rectum is closed distal to the tumor with a purse-string suture. The rectal wall is then transected and a transanal port is inserted, which permits insufflation and laparoscopic equipment to be used to do a "reverse" TME, dissecting upward from below. The dissection then joins the abdominal dissection, and the procedure is completed laparoscopically in standard fashion.

Finding the correct plan in this retrograde approach is challenging, and early in the learning curve there is a high risk for injury to the urethra, prostate, vagina, pelvic nerves, and iliac vessels. Current data from retrospective studies are promising, but further study is needed.

SUGGESTED READINGS

Bonjer HJ, Deijen CL, Haglind E, et al. A randomized trial of laparoscopic versus open surgery for rectal cancer. *N Engl J Med.* 2015;373:194.

Delaney CP. *Operative Techniques in Laparoscopic Colorectal Surgery.* Philadelphia: Lippincott Williams & Wilkins; 2007.

Delaney CP, Brady K, Woconish D, et al. Towards optimizing perioperative colorectal care: outcomes for 1,000 consecutive laparoscopic colon procedures using enhanced recovery pathways. *Am J Surg.* 2012;203:353-355, discussion 355-356.

Miskovic D, Foster J, Agha A, et al. Standardization of laparoscopic total mesorectal excision for rectal cancer: a structured international expert consensus. *Ann Surg.* 2015;261:716-722.

Senagore AJ, Delaney CP, Brady KM, et al. Standardized approach to laparoscopic right colectomy: outcomes in 70 consecutive cases. *J Am Coll Surg.* 2004;199:675-679.

Senagore AJ, Duepree HJ, Delaney CP, et al. Results of a standardized technique and postoperative care plan for laparoscopic sigmoid colectomy: a 30-month experience. *Dis Colon Rectum.* 2003;46:503-509.

Theophilus M, Platell C, Spilsbury K. Long-term survival following laparoscopic and open colectomy for colon cancer: a meta-analysis of randomized controlled trials. *Colorectal Dis.* 2014;16:O75-O81.

MINIMALLY INVASIVE ESOPHAGECTOMY

James Donahue, MD, and Shamus R. Carr, MD

Despite significant reductions in perioperative mortality, morbidity after open esophagectomy remains considerable, ranging from approximately 30% to 50% at experienced centers. In an effort to reduce morbidity, especially from pulmonary complications, many surgeons have adopted minimally invasive approaches to esophagectomy. Experience with procedures such as laparoscopic Nissen fundoplication and thoracoscopic mediastinal lymph node dissection led to the development of minimally invasive techniques for the management of complex esophageal disorders such as achalasia and giant paraesophageal hernias. Initial attempts at minimally invasive esophagectomy (MIE) were hybrid procedures in which a portion of the procedure was performed open and another portion was performed in a minimally invasive fashion. For example, Collard and colleagues first described the use of thoracoscopy for esophageal mobilization in an attempt to decrease morbidity associated with thoracotomy. This approach still required an open midline laparotomy and cervical incision for completion of the McKeown procedure. Similarly, laparoscopy was used for creation of the gastric conduit in combination with a thoracotomy for completion of the Ivor Lewis procedure. It is important to note that no significant differences were found in terms of morbidity between hybrid and completely open approaches. In 1995 DePaula and colleagues published their experience with a totally laparoscopic transhiatal esophagectomy. In 1998 Luketich described a minimally invasive McKeown esophagectomy with thoracoscopic esophageal mobilization, followed by laparoscopic construction of the gastric conduit, and concluding with a neck incision for creation of the anastomosis. In 1999 Watson described a minimally invasive Ivor Lewis procedure with intrathoracic fashioning of the esophagogastric anastomosis.

■ CURRENT RESULTS

Several single institution reports have demonstrated lower rates of pulmonary complications and decreased length of stay with minimally invasive approaches compared with open procedures. Most striking is a report demonstrating a 21% incidence of pneumonia in 76 patients undergoing an open Ivor Lewis esophagectomy, with no cases of pneumonia in 38 patients who underwent a minimally invasive Ivor Lewis procedure. In the University of Pittsburgh experience of 1011 patients who underwent MIE, 481 patients had a McKeown procedure, whereas 530 patients had an Ivor Lewis esophagectomy. In this cohort, the median length of stay was 8 days. Pulmonary complications, defined as acute respiratory distress syndrome (ARDS) or empyema, occurred at a rate of 3% and 6%, respectively.

Recent meta-analyses also have demonstrated an advantage for MIE over open esophagectomy in terms of decreased morbidity and length of stay.

Accumulating data from multicenter studies also support the use of MIE techniques. A randomized multicenter European study assigned 56 patients to open esophagectomy and 59 to MIE. The primary endpoint of this study was the development of pulmonary infection, which developed during hospitalization in 34% of patients in the open group and 12% of those in the MIE group. In this study, mean length of stay was 14 days in the open group and 11 days in the MIE group. In the United States, a multicenter phase II feasibility study of MIE has been completed. Of the 104 patients enrolled in the study, 91% underwent successful MIE. Pulmonary complications, defined as pneumonia or ARDS, developed at a rate of 3.8% and 5.7%, respectively. Despite these encouraging results, a recent analysis of the STS database comparing open esophagectomies and MIE found no difference in the incidence of pulmonary complications between the groups. Although this finding may represent the learning curve in this technically demanding procedure, more study, ideally in the setting of a large randomized trial, is required to demonstrate a decrease in morbidity with the MIE approach.

In terms of oncologic efficacy, both retrospective and prospective studies comparing open esophagectomy with MIE show no significant differences in the median number of lymph nodes harvested or the rates of achieving an R0 resection. Although some have questioned the ability to safely perform MIE after neoadjuvant chemoradiotherapy, several reports have demonstrated the safety and efficacy of MIE in this setting. In fact, more than 90% of the patients in the randomized European study received neoadjuvant therapy.

■ MINIMALLY INVASIVE ESOPHAGECTOMY TECHNIQUES

Currently, there are no specific contraindications to the performance of an MIE, although training and experience in advanced minimally invasive esophageal procedures are necessary. Obesity, previous abdominal or thoracic surgical procedures, and the use of neoadjuvant chemoradiotherapy are factors that may increase the technical difficulty of MIE but are not absolute contraindications. Because patient safety is the ultimate goal, surgeons should not hesitate to convert to an open procedure if necessary.

There are reports of minimally invasive and robot-assisted esophagectomy techniques that mirror nearly every traditional open approach. Although the robot-assisted minimally invasive esophagectomy (RAMIE) has been described by a few groups, it has not yet been adopted widely and is still in evolution. The description that follows details a combined laparoscopic and thoracoscopic approach to MIE. Both the McKeown approach with a neck anastomosis and an Ivor Lewis esophagectomy with an intrathoracic anastomosis can be performed as minimally invasive procedures. The choice is based primarily on surgeon experience and preference, but tumor location is also an important consideration. Because we prefer an Ivor Lewis

MIE, we describe this first, with two options for anastomosis, and then highlight the differences with the McKeown approach. No matter the approach, we begin with an upper endoscopy before any incision. Because there is diminished haptic feedback in all minimally invasive approaches, this allows for evaluation of the esophagus and the stomach to determine the extent of resection necessary to achieve an adequate margin.

■ IVOR LEWIS MINIMALLY INVASIVE ESOPHAGECTOMY

Abdomen

The patient initially is positioned supine with a footboard in place and the arms extended to the sides. A double-lumen tube is placed, but the bronchial balloon is left deflated until the chest portion of the procedure. Pneumoperitoneum is established with the Veress needle technique in the right upper quadrant. Then a 5-mm port is placed through this site, and a laparoscope is inserted. A full exploration is done to evaluate for peritoneal spread or metastatic disease. Four additional ports then are placed under direct visualization, angled toward the hiatus (Figure 1). A liver retractor (Diamond Flex, Snowden-Pencer, Tucker, GA) is used from the 5-mm port at the right anterior axillary line to reflect the left lobe of the liver anteriorly to better expose the esophageal hiatus.

First, the gastrohepatic ligament is divided to expose the right crus of the diaphragm. The dissection then is carried anteriorly over the esophagus. The phrenoesophageal ligament can be divided and entry into the mediastinum can be made at this point, but care must be taken to ensure that entry into the mediastinum does not violate either pleural space, which can result in loss of pneumoperitoneum and increase the difficulty of the remaining abdominal portion of the operation. Attention then is turned to the greater curvature of the stomach, and entry is gained into the lesser sac, allowing the gastrocolic omentum to be separated from the greater curve (Figure 2). It cannot be emphasized enough that great care must be taken during this step to preserve the right gastroepiploic arcade, which will provide the blood supply to the tubularized stomach. This plane is followed toward the spleen, and the short gastric vessels then are divided, allowing the spleen to fall away. A communication between the right and left gastroepiploic arcades sometimes can be seen and should be preserved. Eventually the left crus of the diaphragm are visualized. The retroesophageal space is dissected, and the esophagus can be separated from the left crus. The stomach then is retracted medially and superiorly. This allows for dissection of the stomach from any posterior attachments and begins the mobilization of the tissue from the celiac trunk. All tissue around the celiac trunk is swept toward the specimen, and clear identification of the left gastric artery and vein is accomplished. The left gastric vessels then are divided with a single firing of an endovascular gastrointestinal anastomosis (GIA) stapler outfitted with a vascular load.

If the surgeon chooses to perform a gastric emptying procedure, either a pyloroplasty or a pyloromyotomy can be done at this point. To perform a pyloroplasty, a harmonic scalpel is used to open the pylorus from the stomach to the bulb of the duodenum longitudinally. Stay stitches then are placed at the 12:00 and 6:00 positions with the Endo360° device (EndoEvolution, Raynham, MA). This aids in retraction while the pyloroplasty is closed in the classic Heineke-Mikulicz fashion with interrupted 2-0 sutures using the Endo360° device. A small tongue of omentum can be used to cover the pyloroplasty stitches.

At this point, attention turns to creation of the gastric tube. This begins at the incisura on the lesser curve (Figure 3). The first firing of the stapler also will divide the right gastric arcade and therefore

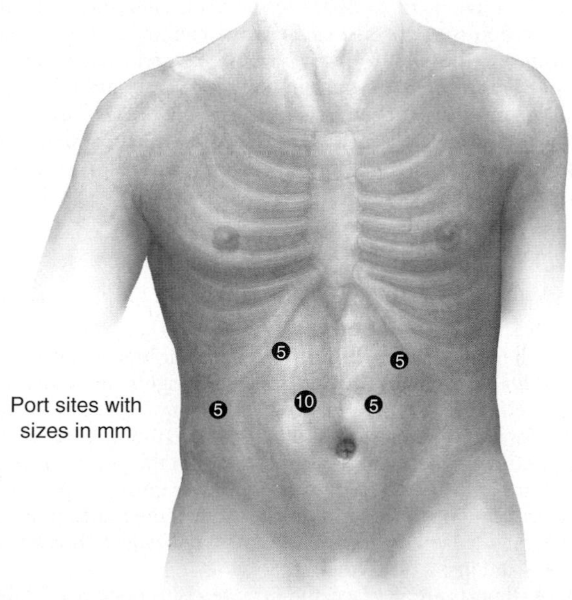

FIGURE 1 The patient initially is positioned in the supine position, and a double-lumen endotracheal tube is placed in preparation for the thoracoscopic mobilization of the esophagus. Five abdominal ports are used for the gastric mobilization. A marking pen is used to trace the midline from the xiphoid to the umbilicus, and this line is divided further into thirds. The two midclavicular ports are placed on the lower third of the marked line to assist with gastric mobilization. *(From Tsai WS, Levy RM, Luketich JD. Technique of minimally invasive Ivor Lewis esophagectomy. Op Tech Thorac Cardiovasc Surg. 2009;14:177.)*

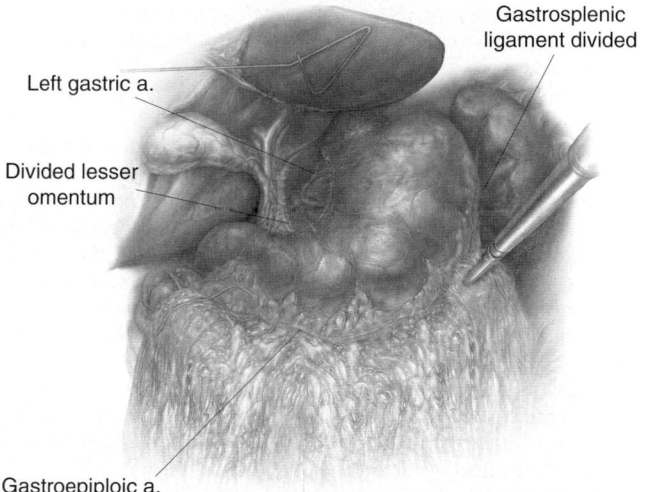

FIGURE 2 After an initial inspection of the peritoneal surfaces and the liver to rule out any metastatic disease, the gastrohepatic omentum is opened. After entry to the lesser sac is gained, the gastrocolic omentum is separated from the greater curve, taking care to preserve the right gastroepiploic artery. The short gastric arteries are divided, and the left gastric artery/vein pedicle is identified. By tracing its course proximally, the celiac lymph nodes are examined. A complete lymph node dissection is performed to include the celiac nodes, sweeping all nodal and fatty tissue with the specimen; the nodal dissection is continued along the splenic artery and the superior border of the pancreas. This plane continues cephalad toward the right and left crus, continuous with the preaortic dissection plane into the lower thoracic cavity. Dissection of the right crus is initiated to mobilize the lateral aspect of the esophagus. *a.,* Artery. *(From Tsai WS, Levy RM, Luketich JD. Technique of minimally invasive Ivor Lewis esophagectomy. Op Tech Thorac Cardiovasc. 2009;14:178.)*

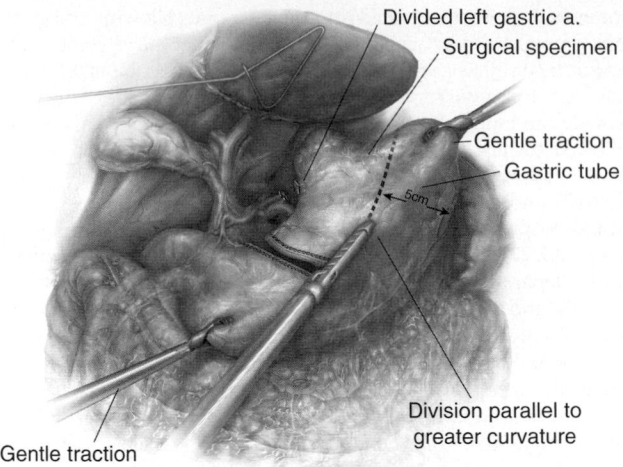

FIGURE 3 caption labels:
- Divided left gastric a.
- Surgical specimen
- Gentle traction
- Gastric tube
- Gentle traction
- Division parallel to greater curvature

FIGURE 3 Once the stomach and celiac lymph nodes are mobilized completely, the left gastric artery and vein are divided with a vascular load on the Endo GIA stapler (Covidien, Mansfield, MA). This is done by approaching the pedicle from the lesser curve. The pedicle must be dissected completely clean, with all celiac nodes swept up into the specimen. Once the pedicle is divided, the distal esophagus, gastric fundus, and antrum should be mobilized completely. The first stapler used to create the gastric conduit contains a vascular load to control bleeding from the adipose tissue and vessels along the lesser curve. The stapler is placed just up to but not onto the gastric antrum, which is usually thick and requires staples appropriate for thick tissue. The initial 5- to 12-mm right midclavicular port is changed to a 15-mm port to allow for the placement of a 4.8-mm Endo GIA stapler. An additional 12-mm port may be placed in the right lower quadrant to assist with the creation of the gastric tube. *a.*, Artery. *(From Tsai WS, Levy RM, Luketich JD. Technique of minimally invasive Ivor Lewis esophagectomy. Op Tech Thorac Cardiovasc Surg. 2009;14:181.)*

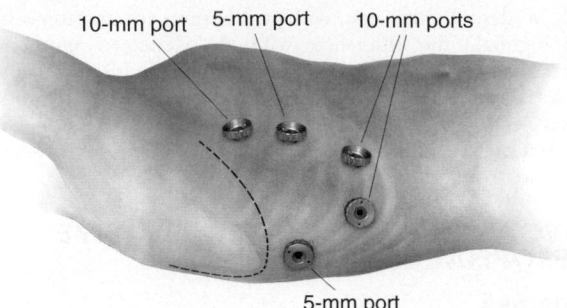

FIGURE 4 labels:
- 10-mm port
- 5-mm port
- 10-mm ports
- 5-mm port

FIGURE 4 The patient is turned to the left lateral decubitus position for the thoracoscopic mobilization of the esophagus and creation of the intrathoracic anastomosis. Five thoracoscopic ports are used. A 10-mm camera port is placed in the seventh or eighth intercostal space, just anterior to the midaxillary line. The working port is a 10-mm port that is placed at the eighth or ninth intercostal space, posterior to the posterior axillary line. Another 10-mm port is placed in the anterior axillary line at the fourth intercostal space, through which a fan-shaped retractor aids in retracting the lung to expose the esophagus. A 5-mm port is placed just inferior to the tip of the scapula, and this is used by the surgeon's left hand for countertraction. A final port is placed at the sixth rib, at the anterior axillary line for suction, and is important in the creation of the anastomosis. *(From Tsai WS, Levy RM, Luketich JD. Technique of minimally invasive Ivor Lewis esophagectomy. Op Tech Thorac Cardiovasc Surg. 2009;14:187.)*

requires a vascular staple load. Of note, the starting point can be adjusted based on the distal extent of the tumor that was determined by endoscopy at the start of the procedure. We strive to create a conduit that is 4 to 5 cm in diameter and oriented parallel to the greater curve. It is extremely important to ensure that the conduit does not spiral during stapling. Judicious use of appropriate traction helps to maintain the proper orientation. The stomach is divided with stapler loads appropriate for its thickness. Some surgeons fully separate the conduit from the specimen and then secure them together with interrupted 2-0 stitches. We prefer to leave a 3-cm area on the greater curve intact between the specimen and the conduit. This helps to ensure that the conduit does not spiral and twist while being delivered into the chest.

We advocate the placement of a jejunal feeding tube at the time of the initial operation. There are numerous kits that can be utilized for this purpose. We use a Halyard (formerly Kimberly-Clark) 14F MIC jejunostomy feeding tube (Halyard Health, Alpharetta, GA). First, the colon is retracted superiorly and the ligament of Treitz is identified. The jejunum then is followed for 40 cm distally. At this point, there is usually a portion that easily reaches the anterior abdominal wall without tension. An interrupted Ethibond stitch is used to tack the small bowel to the anterior abdominal wall with the Endo360° device. Then a second tacking stitch is placed. To place the feeding tube percutaneously, a finder needle is placed under direct laparoscopic visualization through the abdominal wall and into the jejunum that is tacked to the abdominal wall. A small amount of air is injected to confirm that the needle is intraluminal. A guidewire then is advanced into the jejunum using a modified Seldinger technique. Then the dilator and introducer sheath are passed over the wire. Once the dilator and wire are removed, the jejunal feeding tube

is placed via the introducer sheath, which is then removed, leaving the tube in place. Instilling a small amount of air via the tube again confirms intraluminal placement. Two additional stitches are used to seal the small bowel around the insertion site to the anterior abdominal wall. Finally, about 5 to 8 cm distally, an "anti-torsion" stitch is placed.

Attention then is turned back to the hiatus, and further mediastinal dissection is performed to allow the conduit and specimen to pass easily into the chest. For this purpose, we perform circumferential dissection around the esophagus in the mediastinum at least 5 cm into the chest. Retractors are removed, and the fascia of the 10-mm port site is closed with a Carter-Thomason device and a single interrupted 0 Vicryl stitch. Only skin closure is required for the 5-mm port site incisions.

Chest

The patient is placed in the left lateral decubitus position. Bronchoscopy is performed to confirm that the double-lumen endotracheal tube is still in the correct position and the right lung is isolated. The first port is a 10-mm port that is placed in the eighth intercostal space in the anterior axillary line (Figure 4). A 10-mm 30-degree thoracoscope is inserted. After exploration, a second 10-mm port is placed in the ninth intercostal space just posterior to the posterior axillary line. A 5-mm port is placed at the tip of the scapula. Then a 10-mm port is placed along the anterior axillary line in the fourth intercostal space. Finally, a 5-mm port is placed halfway between the two anterior ports and just a bit farther anterior.

Once all ports are in place, the first step is to place a 0-Ethibond stitch into the central tendon of the diaphragm using the Endo360° device to retract it inferiorly in order to aid with the exposure of the distal esophagus and the hiatus. The lung is retracted anteriorly and the inferior pulmonary ligament is divided to the level of the inferior pulmonary vein with the Harmonic scalpel. Lymph nodes that are encountered are resected and submitted for pathologic analysis. Next, we open the posterior mediastinal pleura over the esophagus, staying close to the esophagus so as not to injure the thoracic duct. If there is any concern for ductal injury, we give heavy cream mixed with methylene blue through the jejunal feeding tube to evaluate for injury to the thoracic duct. This plane is continued to the level of the azygos vein. The azygos vein is isolated and divided with the endovascular GIA stapler with a vascular load. Above the level of the azygos vein, the dissection plane switches to being on the esophagus in order to decrease the risk of recurrent laryngeal nerve injury.

Attention then turns back to the hiatus. The pleura is dissected off the pericardium, and this plane is carried superiorly along the bronchus toward the subcarinal lymph nodes. The subcarinal lymph nodes are resected en bloc when possible. During this portion of the dissection, careful attention to the membranous portion of the bronchus needs to be maintained to avoid injury. This plane eventually connects to the dissection that already has been done at the level of the azygos vein. At this point, just superior to the azygos vein, circumferential dissection of the esophagus is performed and a Penrose drain is placed around it to aid with retraction. The esophagus then is retracted anteriorly and laterally. Lymphatic and aortoesophageal vessels are identified, clipped, and then divided. This is continued all the way to the hiatus. Once the esophagus is mobilized completely, the specimen is delivered into the chest with the attached conduit.

Depending on the original site of the tumor, a point on the esophagus is chosen for the creation of the esophagogastric anastomosis that is at least 5 cm above the proximal extent of the tumor. However, even for tumors of the distal third of the esophagus, the anastomosis should not be below the level of the azygos vein in order

to minimize reflux. Once the site is identified above the tumor, an endovascular GIA stapler is used to divide the esophagus. The specimen is retracted and confirmed to be free of all tissue except the conduit, to which it is still attached. Then the specimen is disconnected from the conduit with shears, leaving a gastrostomy. This allows for evaluation of the blood supply to the distal conduit. The 10-mm port site near the posterior axillary line then is enlarged to about 4 cm. An Alexis wound protector (Applied Medical, Rancho Santa Margarita, CA) is placed and the specimen removed.

We prefer to use a 28-mm OrVil anvil (Medtronic Minimally Invasive Therapies, Minneapolis, MN) to create the anastomosis. It is passed via the mouth, and a small hole is made in the esophagus posterior to the staple line. The delivery tube is pulled into the chest and separated from the anvil. Then the stapler is placed into the chest via the enlarged incision and fed into the conduit via the gastrostomy that was created when the conduit was separated from the specimen. An appropriate site is chosen to create the anastomosis as close as possible to the gastroepiploic arcade. This creates a functional end-to-end anastomosis. Another option involves creation of a true end-to-end anastomosis. When this technique is used, the anvil of the end-to-end anastomosis (EEA) stapler is placed into the cut end of the esophagus. Sometimes the esophagus needs to be dilated to allow passage of the 28-mm anvil. If this is not possible, a 25-mm anvil is used. Using a suturing device such as the Endo360°, two purse-string sutures are placed to secure the anvil in the esophagus. The gastric conduit then is brought farther into the chest, making sure not to twist it. The distal end is opened and the handle of the EEA stapler is placed into the conduit (Figure 5). At a site near the gastroepiploic arcade, the spike on the stapler is deployed and attached to the anvil. Firing the stapler will create the end-to-end anastomosis.

After completion of the anastomosis, the nasogastric tube is passed, and then the gastrostomy and excess conduit are resected with an endovascular GIA stapler (Figure 6). If there is preserved omentum along the greater curvature, it can be used to buttress the anastomosis and serve as an interposition layer between the airway and the conduit. The parietal pleura above the azygos vein should be

Gastroesophageal anastomosis with EEA stapler

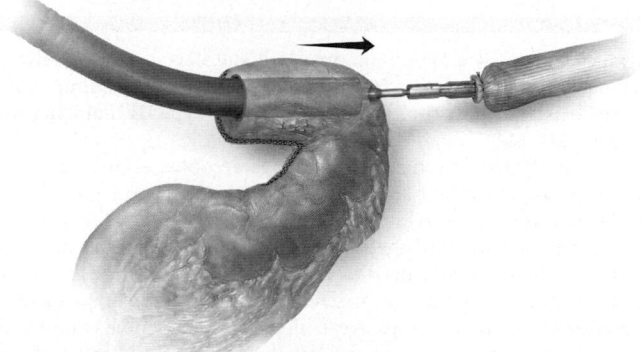

FIGURE 5 The anvil of a 28-mm end-to-end anastomosis (EEA) stapler is placed in the proximal esophagus and a 2-0 Endo Stitch purse-string suture is placed and tied (intracorporeal technique) to secure the anvil in position. It is technically challenging to make this first stitch perfect because the anvil has a tendency to migrate out of the open end of the proximal esophagus. For this reason, a second purse-string suture is placed to further secure the anvil and pull in any mucosal defects, thereby ensuring complete rings after EEA stapler firing. Ordinarily, a 28-mm EEA stapler is used in an attempt to minimize the risk for stricture and decrease the need for postoperative dilations. In most cases, the 28-mm anvil is secured without difficulty. On rare occasions, a Foley balloon catheter must be used to dilate the proximal esophagus. Should the Foley balloon catheter fail, a 25-mm stapler is used. The gastric conduit then is pulled to the apex of the chest, and the ultrasonic shears are used to open the tip of the gastric conduit along the staple line. The EEA stapler is placed through the posterior-inferior port, which had been enlarged, and positioned in the conduit. The stapler tip is brought out along the greater curve of the gastric conduit to join the anvil. Before creating the anastomosis, the amount of conduit that will lie in the chest is estimated carefully. A common mistake is to bring an excess amount of stomach into the chest in an effort to minimize tension on the anastomosis. This excess conduit often assumes a sigmoid conformation above the diaphragm and may lead to significant problems with gastric emptying. In addition, ensuring proper orientation of the stomach is critical to prevent twisting. *(From Tsai WS, Levy RM, Luketich JD. Technique of minimally invasive Ivor Lewis esophagectomy. Op Tech Thorac Cardiovasc Surg. 2009;14:189.)*

Removal of excess gastric tube

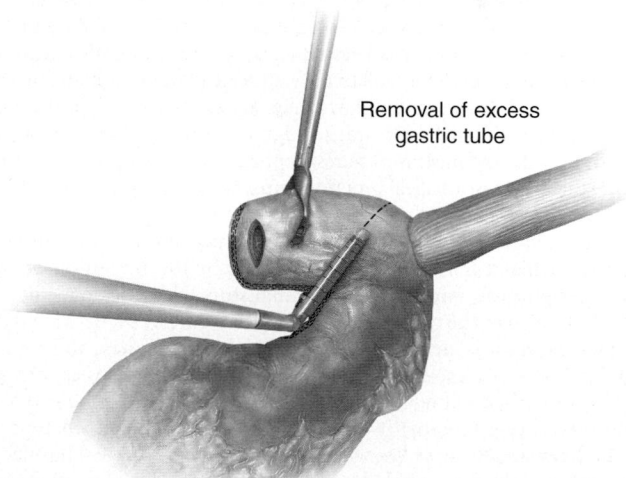

FIGURE 6 The tip of the stapler and the anvil are docked, and the stapler is fired, creating a circular esophagogastric anastomosis, joining the side of the gastric conduit to the end of esophagus, at approximately the level of the azygos vein. The excess gastric tip (the gastrostomy through which the stapler was placed) is trimmed with several loads of an articulating linear stapler, with care taken not to injure the omental pedical wrap that was mobilized along the greater curvature. Endoscopy is not routinely performed to evaluate the anastomosis. *(From Tsai WS, Levy RM, Luketich JD. Technique of minimally invasive Ivor Lewis esophagectomy. Op Tech Thorac Cardiovasc Surg. 2009;14:190.)*

preserved, as this also buttresses the anastomosis and maintains its position in the posterior mediastinum, which may help to contain, and possibly seal, any leak that may develop.

A 24F chest tube and a 10-mm flat Jackson-Pratt drain are placed into the chest. The Jackson-Pratt drain is placed into the posterior mediastinum behind the gastric conduit, with the end at least 2 cm away from the anastomosis. Finally, one or two interrupted stitches are used to tack the conduit to the diaphragm at the level of the hiatus. This is done to prevent delayed herniation of the conduit into the chest. All ports are removed and closed in the usual manner.

■ MCKEOWN MINIMALLY INVASIVE ESOPHAGECTOMY

The overall steps of the McKeown MIE are very similar to what is described earlier, except that the operation begins in the chest, where the esophagus is mobilized; moves to the abdomen, where the gastric conduit is created; and finishes in the neck. To begin the neck portion of the procedure, a 5-cm incision is made parallel to the anterior border of the sternocleidomastoid muscle (SCM) and terminates about 2 cm above the sternal notch. The SCM is retracted laterally and the omohyoid is divided. The plane between the carotid sheath and the trachea is opened. The dissection continues directly onto the anterior border of the vertebral body, and blunt dissection continues on the posterior wall of the esophagus and connects into the previous plane in the chest. A Penrose drain can be placed around the esophagus to aid in retraction. Once the dissection is complete, this should allow delivery of the specimen through the neck. While this is being done, a laparoscope should be utilized in the abdomen to confirm that the conduit is not twisted as it is delivered into the thorax. The proximal esophagus is divided and preparations are made for an anastomosis. This anastomosis can be handsewn, stapled, or a combination of the two. We prefer to use the method popularized by Dr. Orringer, which involves a combined handsewn and stapled technique. This technique is described elsewhere in the text.

SUGGESTED READINGS

Luketich JD, et al. Outcomes after minimally invasive esophagectomy: review of over 1000 patients. *Ann Surg.* 2012;256:95-103.

Sihag S, et al. Minimally invasive versus open esophagectomy for esophageal cancer: a comparison of early surgical outcomes from the Society of Thoracic Surgeons National Database. *Ann Thorac Surg.* 2016;101: 1281-1288.

Yerokun BA, et al. Minimally invasive versus open esophagectomy for esophageal cancer: a population-based analysis. *Ann Thorac Surg.* 2016;102: 416-423.

PARAESOPHAGEAL HERNIA

Alexander S. Rosemurgy II, MD

A hiatal hernia is a protrusion of the stomach into the mediastinum through a defect in the esophageal hiatus of the diaphragm. There are basically two types of hiatal hernias— sliding hiatal hernias and paraesophageal hiatal hernias—although these hernias are graded specifically from type I to type IV (Figure 1). A sliding hiatal hernia occurs when the gastroesophageal junction migrates into the mediastinum to rest cephalad to the esophageal diaphragmatic hiatus (see Figure 1, *B*). A paraesophageal hernia exists when a portion of the stomach, usually the fundus, migrates through the esophageal hiatus into the mediastinum to rest cephalad to the esophageal hiatus while the gastroesophageal junction remains normally situated below the hiatus (see Figure 1, *C*).

A type I hiatal hernia (a sliding hiatal hernia) is the most common variety of hiatal hernia. It is characterized by the migration of the gastroesophageal junction and proximal stomach into the mediastinum cephalad to the esophageal hiatus (see Figure 1, *B*). Because type I hiatal hernias occur so frequently, some consider these to be anatomically normal, especially in Americans older than 50 years of age. In and of itself, a sliding hiatal hernia is not considered to be a condition warranting therapy; it does *not* represent pathology. A type II hiatal hernia, otherwise known as a classic paraesophageal hernia, is characterized by the cephalad migration of the fundus of the stomach into the mediastinum, coming to rest cephalad to the esophageal hiatus (see Figure 1, *C*). The distinguishing characteristic between the type I and type II hiatal hernia is that in the latter, the gastroesophageal junction and consequently the lower esophageal sphincter mechanism remains in the normal anatomic position caudad to the diaphragmatic hiatus (i.e., the gastroesophageal junction resides in the peritoneal cavity). As a consequence of their distortion of normal anatomy, a type I hiatal hernia greatly reduces the acuteness of the angle of His, whereas a type II hiatal hernia increases or maintains a normal angle of His; this has implications for how these hernias (i.e., sliding hiatal hernias) promote gastroesophageal reflux. A very advanced form of a type I or type II hiatal hernia may involve a majority or even the entire stomach residing in the mediastinum with the pylorus at or near the esophageal hiatus (a type III hiatal hernia; see Figure 1, *D*).

A Type III hiatal hernia, or a mixed paraesophageal hernia, is the combination of a type I and type II hiatal hernia (see Figure 1, *D*). In other words, a type III hiatal hernia involves both a sliding hiatal hernia and a paraesophageal hernia. Type III hiatal hernias are similar to type I hiatal hernias in that both the gastroesophageal junction and the proximal stomach and fundus have been protruded cephalad through the esophageal hiatus into the mediastinum. A hiatal hernia is graded as a type IV when at least one third of the stomach has herniated into the chest, thus often giving rise to the term *giant hiatal hernia* (see Figure 1, *E*). Giant hiatal hernias may be extensive, with possibly the entire stomach herniating through the hiatus, possibly along with additional organs such as the small bowel, colon, omentum, and potentially even the pancreas and spleen (see Figure 1, *E*).

■ WHY IS IT IMPORTANT TO DIAGNOSE A HIATAL HERNIA?

A sliding hiatal hernia (i.e., a type I hiatal hernia) is generally asymptomatic and not part of a particular disease or disorder. Rather, sliding hiatal hernias are generally of no consequence and are common, particularly in older Americans. In contrast, a generation ago a paraesophageal hernia was thought to impose an urgent need for correction because of the potential loss of gastric viability. In other words, a paraesophageal hernia was thought to carry a high risk of gastric strangulation. Today, a generation later, paraesophageal hernias are not thought to require this same urgency.

Advances in medical imaging over the past 35 years have led to our greater understanding of hiatal hernias and their frequency of occurrence. Although sliding hiatal hernias (type I) are very common, particularly in older patients, paraesophageal hernias occur less frequently. However, paraesophageal hernias are not uncommon and more often are associated with a sliding hiatal hernia (type III hiatal hernia). In general, only the most extreme paraesophageal hernias pose immediate risk of strangulation and loss of gastric viability; the

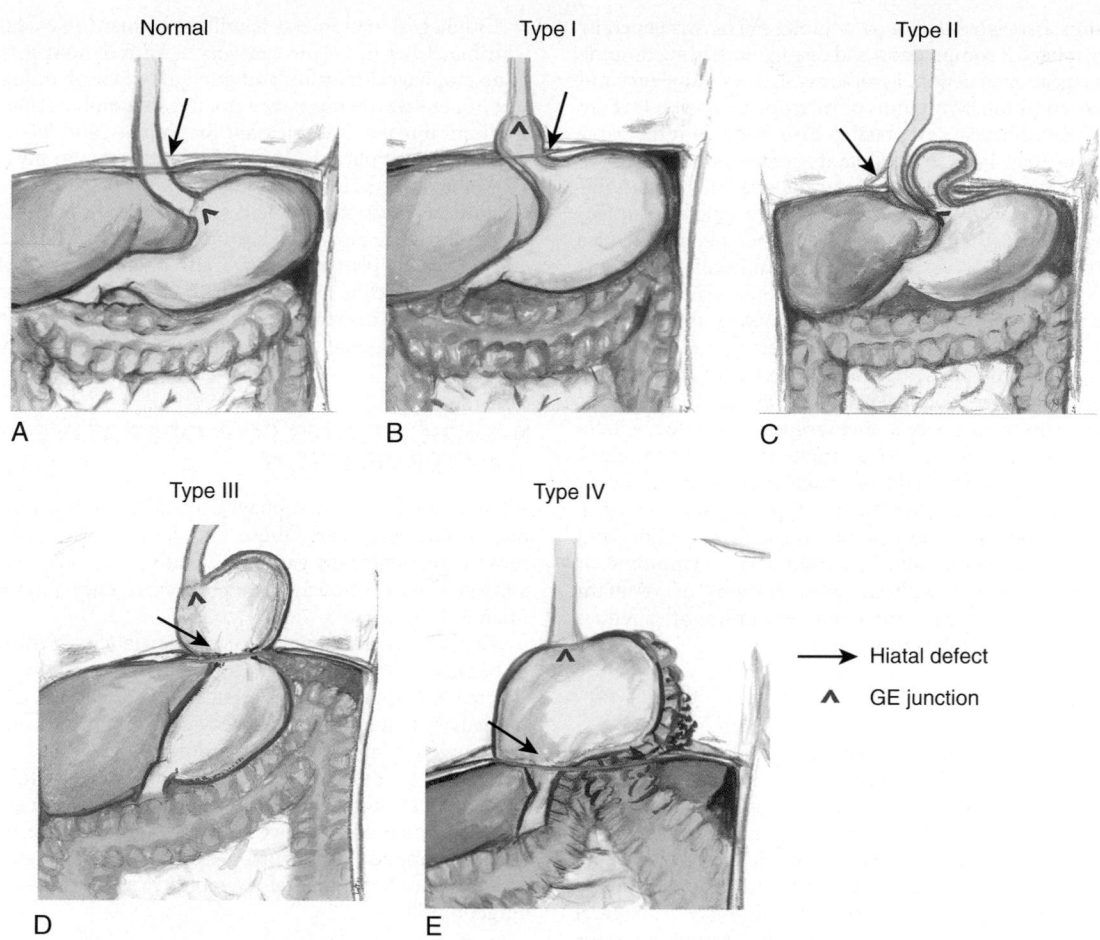

Normal   Type I   Type II

A   B   C

Type III   Type IV

D   E

→ Hiatal defect

∧ GE junction

FIGURE 1 Anatomy of the esophagus, gastroesophageal (GE) junction, and stomach displaying normal anatomy and depictions of the four types of hiatal hernias. **A,** Normal. **B,** Sliding or type I hiatal hernia. **C,** Paraesophageal or type II hiatal hernia. **D,** Type III hiatal hernia. **E,** Type IV hiatal hernia (note colon to the left of the herniated gastric fundus). *(Illustrations by Lindsay Agema and Christian B. Rodriguez.)*

risk for this occurring is multifactorial, and reduction and repair of a paraesophageal hernia should be temporized by size, accompanying symptoms, complexity, contents of the hernia, patient comorbidities, body mass index (BMI), operative history, and available resources, to mention but a few factors. Therefore patients with hiatal hernias can be evaluated in a thoughtful manner without a particular sense of immediacy in almost all instances.

Some patients do require more immediate attention. Those patients will have significant dysphagia, complications of esophageal obstruction, extraesophageal manifestations of gastroesophageal reflux (e.g., aspiration with recurring pneumonia), or other complications such as obstruction of bowel in a type IV hernia. Patients with dysphagia warrant particular attention, as their dysphagia may be a symptom of esophageal cancer; early endoscopy certainly is warranted for those complaining of dysphagia or symptoms related to esophageal outlet obstruction. Patients with esophageal obstruction may note weight loss or complications of regurgitation and aspiration. These issues should hasten evaluation and operative correction.

It would be remiss not to point out that hiatal hernias do not heal themselves. Even with significant and necessary changes in lifestyle, such as weight loss, a hiatal hernia will only get bigger with time, and its symptoms and associated risks will only become more profound. However, this is not meant to denigrate preparation before any proposed operation, given the time. I believe that weight loss to a BMI of 26 kg/m^2 or less before operative correction is particularly important.

■ HOW IS A HIATAL HERNIA DIAGNOSED?

A hiatal hernia may be detected through serendipity or through evaluation of patient symptoms. Hiatal hernias often are noted incidentally when reviewing imaging studies for disassociated problems, such as lung cancer. A systematic review of symptoms may lead to the suspicion of a hiatal hernia and can lead to further evaluation. Complaints of heartburn or dysphagia, for example, may lead to an evaluation to determine the type and extent of a hiatal hernia.

■ WHAT SYMPTOMS ARE ASSOCIATED WITH A HIATAL HERNIA?

Hiatal hernias may be asymptomatic. This is particularly true for sliding hiatal hernias. Paraesophageal hernias, particularly smaller ones (e.g., less than 2 cm), are also generally asymptomatic and generally are detected through serendipity in the course of evaluating other problems. It is difficult to make an asymptomatic patient better, and evaluation of an asymptomatic hiatal hernia should focus on the potential complications associated with it, such as gastroesophageal reflux or incarceration and strangulation (seen only with paraesophageal hernias). A hiatal hernia is not synonymous with gastroesophageal reflux, or close to it, although their association is generally assumed and the terms generally and inappropriately are used interchangeably by the uninformed.

The symptoms associated with a paraesophageal hernia generally are related to esophageal compression and distortion leading to some degree of esophageal obstruction. Symptoms such as dysphagia and regurgitation are common. Symptoms of gastroesophageal reflux are not common; the esophageal compression associated with the paraesophageal hernia may limit concomitant gastroesophageal reflux and its associated symptoms. Also, symptoms related to regurgitation, such as recurring aspiration pneumonia, recurring sinus infections, recurring and persistent cough, asthma, and changes in voice quality and strength may occur. A paraesophageal hernia with compromise of blood flow to or from the fundus could lead to chronic blood loss and anemia. Symptoms of gastroesophageal acid reflux can occur with a paraesophageal hernia, but this is not because of the paraesophageal hernia per se but rather because of the loss of a functional lower esophageal sphincter mechanism due to the loss of integrity of the phrenoesophageal membranes associated with a sliding hiatal hernia and the less acute angle of His. For example, gastroesophageal acid reflux would be much more likely to occur with a type IV hiatal hernia than with a type II paraesophageal hernia. Relief of esophageal obstruction through reduction and repair of the paraesophageal hernia should abate symptoms of esophageal obstruction, but without considerations of resultant reflux patients might have new troublesome symptoms after reduction and repair of a paraesophageal hernia.

■ WORKUP

The first step in the diagnosis and evaluation of a paraesophageal hernia is to recognize its presence. This can occur serendipitously through the evaluation of other unrelated problems or after evaluation of a patient's symptoms. Because paraesophageal hernias often are associated with dysphagia, endoscopy should be an early step in their evaluation. With esophageal cancer reaching near epidemic levels in the United States, it is important to eliminate esophageal cancer in the differential diagnosis of obstructive symptoms. This is especially true for patients who have been on proton pump inhibitor therapy for an extended period of time. Endoscopy can diagnose complications of reflux, such as esophagitis and Barrett's esophagus.

Upper gastrointestinal contrast (i.e., barium) radiography (an upper GI) is very helpful in establishing the diagnosis and extent of a paraesophageal hernia. Such a contrast study also will be helpful in evaluating the integrity and function of the esophagus. For example, an upper GI contrast study undertaken with the patient swallowing a barium-laden bite of marshmallow or bagel in a 15-degree Trendelenburg position can document the degree of esophageal motility (or dysmotility) and predict how the patient will handle a food bolus after operative reduction and correction of a paraesophageal hernia. Patients with normal esophageal motility will clear such a food bolus with one or two stripping motions of the esophagus. Dysmotility can be graded by the number of stripping motions beyond two needed to clear the food bolus. In my opinion, the best clinical predictor of how someone will handle a food bolus postoperatively is how they handle it preoperatively. With this in mind, patients who exhibit normal motility with the type of upper GI contrast study outlined here can undergo construction of a 360-degree fundoplication (i.e., Nissen fundoplication) with the confidence that notable dysphagia will not plague the patient postoperatively. Some purport that an upper GI contrast study will detect and prepare the surgeon for a short esophagus. I have not found that to be an issue in more than 200 antireflux operations. The length of the esophagus is dependent on how far it is mobilized in the mediastinum; however, I recognize that to others this is an issue.

Computed tomographic (CT) scanning and magnetic resonance imaging (MRI) have no real role in evaluating a hiatal hernia beyond that they may be the vehicle by which diagnosis is made through serendipity. Such scans will aid in detailing the organs other than the stomach involved in a type IV hernia.

Esophageal manometry is utilized by many in evaluating patients with hiatal hernias. This can very sensitively and accurately determine esophageal motility and strength when planning intervention (e.g., operative therapy), but to me its cumbersome and difficult application makes it unpleasant for patients, and its results often are not clinically applicable. It is not a routine test in my practice.

Ambulatory pH testing is something I am more likely to use. Because gastroesophageal acid reflux may be a significant concomitant problem for any hiatal hernia, ambulatory pH testing is strongly encouraged to plan an appropriate operative intervention and to establish a baseline of acid reflux for what may become lifelong follow-up. For this reason and other reasons already stated, I utilize it for almost all patients who will undergo operative correction of a hiatal hernia.

■ INDICATIONS FOR OPERATIVE INTERVENTION

All symptomatic paraesophageal hiatal hernias should be repaired operatively, particularly those that cause obstructive symptoms or those with significant gastric distortion (e.g., an associated gastric volvulus). As previously stated, an emergency intervention is not often indicated.

Concerns of pending loss of gastric viability (through endoscopy or because of the complex nature of the paraesophageal hernia discovered on upper GI, CT scan, or MRI) should raise a sense of immediacy that must be balanced against a patient's preparedness for an emergency operation (e.g., comorbidities, BMI).

Operative intervention for a completely asymptomatic paraesophageal hernia must be balanced against patient age, comorbidities, BMI, operative history, size and nature of the paraesophageal hernia, complicating factors (e.g., concomitant gastroesophageal reflux disease), esophageal dysmotility, institutional resources, and surgeon skill.

■ OPERATIVE INTERVENTION

In general, all operative interventions for paraesophageal hernias should be performed using minimally invasive surgery techniques, specifically laparoscopy. My choice is laparoendoscopic single-site (LESS) surgery for a number of reasons. Although it provides an optimal cosmetic outcome, I believe it also is associated with less pain and a quicker return to functional activities. My experience with LESS surgery involves more than 350 fundoplications and is based on a laparoscopic experience of more than 2000 fundoplications.

Occasionally it is necessary to undertake the repair of a hiatal hernia through an open approach, but this should be very uncommon and represent only near 1% of all operations for hiatal hernias. There should be no routine application of open surgery, including thoracotomy, for hiatal hernias. When open surgery for hiatal hernia correction occurs, there should be a good reason as to why the open approach was necessary. Patients who undergo open operations for the correction of a hiatal hernia often have complex histories that involve previous fundoplications, often undertaken with mesh.

In the treatment of hiatal hernia, both nonoperative and operative approaches are considered.

Nonoperative Approach

One may choose to do nothing immediately and monitor the asymptomatic patient while working to improve existing comorbidities for possible future intervention. The size and configuration of the paraesophageal hernia determines the frequency with which it is associated with symptoms. If a patient has a small paraesophageal hernia that is completely asymptomatic, it probably warrants no immediate intervention. Intervention can be expectant. In this scenario, existing comorbidities, such as diabetes and obesity, can be focused on, such that intervention in the future, if necessary, can be undertaken more safely and with a higher probability of long-term success. A nonoperative approach is predicated on the small size of a paraesophageal hernia, the lack of associated symptoms, and the presence of other factors that would make a patient a less than ideal operative candidate. The point is that not all paraesophageal hernias, by their presence alone, mandate repair. In this scenario, follow-up should be undertaken to ensure that the patient's comorbidities are treated and that the paraesophageal hernia remains small and asymptomatic. Onset of dysphagia, chest pain, regurgitation, or other symptoms should lead to re-evaluation of a nonoperative approach.

In considering whether the paraesophageal hernia is causing symptoms, consider that common complaints and findings with paraesophageal hernias include heartburn, early satiety, chest pain, dyspnea, dysphagia, regurgitation, anemia, and myriad other symptoms and signs. Most symptomatic patients are seen with more than one symptom or sign (median number of four symptoms). Symptoms that are subjectively most improved after repair of a paraesophageal hernia are, in order, heartburn, regurgitation, dysphagia, early satiety, chest pain, and dyspnea.

Although paraesophageal hernias may be asymptomatic, larger and more pronounced paraesophageal hernias are more likely to be associated with symptoms. Thus it isn't a surprise that type III paraesophageal hernias are most common in patients who undergo surgery, with type IV and then type II following in order of frequency. Most patients who undergo operative repair have more than 50% of their stomach in an intrathoracic position.

Planning and Undertaking an Operative Approach

One must identify the anatomy (i.e., the type of hiatal hernia and the size of the diaphragmatic defect) and the esophageal function before undertaking operative intervention. It is of paramount importance to establish the type of hernia and the nature of the paraesophageal hernia to ensure that you have the skills and experience required for the operative intervention. Once the paraesophageal hernia has been defined in its extent and an operative plan for reduction has been made, consideration of a concomitant fundoplication is necessary. Determination of esophageal function is required to ensure adequate esophageal function (i.e., motility) to overcome the relative resistance to esophageal emptying provided by the fundoplication and thereby to avoid complicating postoperative symptoms of esophageal obstruction (e.g., dysphagia). For me, this means obtaining an esophagram with the patient in a 15-degree Trendelenburg position utilizing a bagel or marshmallow, as mentioned previously. With normal esophageal motility, patients can clear a barium-laden bite of marshmallow or bagel with two or fewer stripping motions. These patients do well with a Nissen fundoplication. Patients with lesser function need to be addressed individually. With only modest dysmotility (i.e., clearance with three or four stripping waves), a Toupet fundoplication is recommended. Although there may be situations that contraindicate the use of a fundoplication, I have cared for few such patients in my extensive experience.

Although some authors recommend doing so, I would not reduce a paraesophageal hernia and leave the patient without an adjunctive antireflux mechanism, such as fundoplication. In the course of developing a paraesophageal hernia and its operative reduction, many or all of the antireflux means inherent to the lower esophageal sphincter mechanism are lost, leaving the patient with inadequate antireflux mechanisms after repair and a near certainty of developing profound gastroesophageal acid reflux. To my knowledge, there are no randomized controlled trials with long-term follow-up that compare operations to reduce paraesophageal hernias with esophageal hiatoplasties with or without fundoplication.

Furthermore, in cases of operative correction of a paraesophageal hernia repair, I see no purpose in utilizing a gastrostomy tube to tether the stomach in position. A gastrostomy tube does not tether

the stomach effectively, and its use for any purpose other than gastric decompression is passé.

When undertaking a laparoscopic operation, the sequence of events should be to:

1. Reduce the paraesophageal hernia (and sliding hiatal hernia, if present) to allow 6 to 8 cm of esophagus to lay in the high pressure abdominal cavity
2. Dissect the hernia sac away from the hernia and excise of it what can be excised
3. Reconstruct the esophageal hiatus snugly but not tightly about the esophagus
4. Construct an antireflux fundoplication
5. Secure the fundoplication to the crura so that the fundoplication and gastroesophageal junction are established securely below the esophageal hiatus (anchoring the fundoplication to the crura also functions to reduce tension on the wrap, making it more difficult for the wrap to come undone or to twist the esophagus, which would lead to postoperative dysphagia)

I begin the operation by opening the gastrohepatic omentum in a stellate fashion and carrying the dissection cephalad to the left gastric artery and to the right crus. The dissection then is carried up and down the right crus and into the mediastinum. It is important to be careful to not enter the right pleural space. The stomach is rolled to the right as the paraesophageal hernia is further reduced. Short gastric vessels are divided, and the dissection is carried to the left crus and into the mediastinum. Once the hernia sac is reduced, it and the gastroesophageal fat pad are removed, with great care being taken to not injure either vagal trunk. The hernia reduction should be continued until 6 to 8 cm of esophagus is delivered into the abdominal cavity. The hiatal reconstruction then is undertaken with either interrupted or running sutures. The hiatus is reconstructed to be snug but not tight about the esophagus. It is important not to remove overlying peritoneum from the left and right crura during the dissection. The peritoneal covering helps to promote the crural reconstruction and limit the dependency of the crural reconstruction on sutures alone (i.e., without healing) for long-term approximation. An antireflux fundoplication consistent with the preoperative esophageal motility is constructed. The antireflux fundoplication is constructed over a 52F to 54F bougie passed per os into the stomach for women and over a 56F to 60F bougie for men.

Although there is great debate about the need for mesh reinforcement of the reconstruction of the esophageal hiatus, it is not something I normally apply. I seldom have used mesh to reinforce the reconstruction of the esophageal hiatus because I have found it to be superfluous and not without risk. My experience with mesh and esophageal hiatus reconstruction primarily has centered around revisional operations on patients who have had hiatoplasties with mesh. Freeing the mesh from the esophagus and stomach during revisional operations is extremely difficult, risky, and time consuming. Furthermore, I have not seen the need for it in studying the outcomes of my patients, particularly those who have had type III and type IV hiatal hernias. Although I admit that there is some role for mesh in reconstructing the esophageal hiatus, I believe that this role is limited and that mesh should be applied with great caution. Mesh may be considered only in patients for whom the reconstruction is under considerable tension, in which case a biologic mesh (never a polypropylene or polytetrafluoroethylene [PTFE] mesh) may be appropriate. Although the complications associated with mesh hiatoplasties are infrequent, they are potentially catastrophic. I have encountered and reported esophageal stenosis and erosions, arterial erosions, and dense fibrosis. When undergoing revisional operations for complications or failure, patients with mesh tend to have a much more difficult operation and may require partial gastrectomy or partial esophagectomy with repair. Because the recurrence rate after paraesophageal hernia repair is high (some report up to 50% recurrence at 5 years), some surgeons have sought alternatives to biologic mesh, including diaphragmatic relaxing incisions to minimize tension.

There are a few studies with only small sample sizes detailing outcomes with alternatives to biologic mesh. Virtually all studies involving biologic mesh are noncontrolled studies.

Other authors disagree with my negative feelings about biologic mesh. It has been noted that biologic mesh does not increase postoperative dysphagia after paraesophageal hernia repair. However, utilizing biologic mesh leads to longer operations with similar hospital stays.

Although some studies have purported favorable outcomes with the use of mesh with early follow-up, 5-year follow-up shows no significant differences in recurrence rates between hiatoplasties constructed with biologic mesh or without mesh. In considering recurrence rates after paraesophageal hernia repairs, it is notable that recurrence rates increase with time.

LONG-TERM OUTCOMES WITH TREATMENT

Patients who have symptoms associated with paraesophageal hernias show significant resolution of symptoms after laparoscopic repair of their hernias, despite high radiologic recurrence rates. Symptoms that are subjectively most improved after repair of a paraesophageal hernia are, in order, heartburn, regurgitation, dysphagia, early satiety, chest pain, and dyspnea. Despite frequent radiologic recurrences after laparoscopic hiatal hernia repair, preoperative symptoms are well abated; recurrent, persistent, and new symptoms are infrequent and well controlled; patient satisfaction is high; and reoperation for recurrent paraesophageal hernia is uncommon. It seems there are no significant differences in the frequency and severity of postoperative symptoms between patients with or without radiologic recurrences of their paraesophageal hernia.

Diagnostic imaging can overstate paraesophageal hernia recurrence because very small recurrent paraesophageal hernias may be apparent on one study (e.g., esophagram) but not on another (e.g., esophagoscopy). As well, it seems that very small recurrent paraesophageal hernias may not be apparent from one day to the next. It may be that recurrent paraesophageal hernias on esophagography are significant only when they are greater than 2 cm, as they are then more likely to be associated with symptoms.

ACKNOWLEDGMENT

I gratefully acknowledge the contributions of Lindsay Agema, Darrell J. Downs, and Christian B. Rodriguez.

SUGGESTED READINGS

D'Alessio MJ, Rakita S, Bloomston M, Chambers CM, Zervos EE, Goldin SB, Poklepovic J, Boyce HW, Rosemurgy AS. Esophagography predicts favorable outcome after laparoscopic Nissen fundoplication for patients with esophageal dysmotility. *J Am Coll Surg.* 2005;201:335-342.

Kohn GP, Price RP, Demeester SR, Zehetner J, Muensterer OJ, Awad ZT, Mittal SK, Richardson WS, Stefanidis D, Fanelli RD, SAGES Guidelines Committee. *Guidelines for the management of hiatal hernia.* <http://www.sages.org/publications/guidelines/guidelines-for-the-management-of-hiatal-hernia/>.

Oelschlager BK, Pellegrini CA, Hunter JG, Brunt ML, Soper NJ, Sheppard BC, Polissar NL, et al. Biologic prosthesis to prevent recurrence after laparoscopic paraesophageal hernia repair: long-term follow-up from a multicenter, prospective, randomized trial. *J Am Coll Surg.* 2011;213:461-468.

Oelschlager BK, Petersen RP, Brunt LM, Soper NJ, Sheppard BC, Mitsumori L, Rohrmann C, Swanstrom LL, Pellegrini CA. Laparoscopic paraesophageal hernia repair: defining long-term clinical and anatomic outcomes. *J Gastrointest Surg.* 2012;16:453-459.

Sukharamwala P, Teta AF, Ross SB, Co F, Alvarez-Calderon G, Luberice K, Rosemurgy AS. Over 250 laparo-endoscopic single site (less) fundoplications: lessons learned. *Am Surg.* 2015;81:870-875.

LAPAROSCOPIC TREATMENT OF ESOPHAGEAL MOTILITY DISORDERS

Brendan M. Finnerty, MD, Cheguevara Afaneh, MD, and Rasa Zarnegar, MD

Esophageal motility disorders occur when there is an aberration in the peristaltic mechanism that propagates food from the oropharynx through the esophagus and into the stomach. They can be seen as an isolated *primary* disorder, such as achalasia or diffuse esophageal spasm, or as a *secondary* disorder associated with another esophageal disease, such as gastroesophageal reflux disease (GERD), Chagas' disease, or systemic sclerosis. Primary disorders subsequently are classified based on type of peristaltic defect ranging from complete absence of peristalsis (achalasia) to various abnormal motility patterns, including uncoordinated motility (diffuse esophageal spasm), hypercontractile peristalsis ("nutcracker esophagus"), hypocontractile peristalsis (e.g., hypotensive lower esophageal sphincter), and other states such as retrograde or triple-peaked contractions. Hypercontractile states are thought to be caused by either impaired inhibitory innervation, as in diffuse esophageal spasm, or increased activation of excitatory innervation and smooth muscle contraction, as in nutcracker esophagus and hypertensive lower esophageal sphincter (LES). Unfortunately, most of these disorders do not have definitive cures and typically are temporized by multidisciplinary medical management between gastroenterologists and surgeons. Achalasia, which is the most common type of esophageal motility disorder, typically is treated with surgery (i.e., Heller myotomy) because resolution of dysphagia symptoms can occur in more than 80% of patients.

A high degree of suspicion for esophageal dysmotility, particularly achalasia, should be maintained in patients with dysphagia to solids or liquids, noncardiac retrosternal chest pain, regurgitation, or weight loss. These symptoms comprise the Eckardt score, a staging scheme that can be used to monitor disease progression after therapeutic intervention for achalasia (Table 1). The gold standard for diagnosis of esophageal dysmotility is high-resolution manometry (HRM). Pressure topography metrics measured during HRM (i.e., contractile deceleration point, distal contractile integral, distal latency, and integrated relaxation pressure) should be analyzed using the Chicago Classification to accurately categorize the type of dysmotility. Classical findings of achalasia include failure of LES relaxation, esophageal aperistalsis, and elevated LES resting pressure. Notably, three achalasia subtypes exist based on HRM: type I, "classic" absence of esophageal pressurization with 100% failed contractions; type II, panesophageal pressurization without peristaltic contraction; and type III, presence of more than 20% preserved fragments of premature or spastic contractions. Although treatment outcomes based on subtype are currently a subject of debate, several studies have suggested that the success rate of Heller myotomy may be higher in patients with type II achalasia (93% to 100%) compared with those with type I (67% to 85%) or type III (70% to 86%) achalasia. Classical findings of diffuse esophageal spasm (DES) include increased simultaneous esophageal contractions, characterized on HRM as 20% or higher premature contractions with a distal latency

TABLE 1: Eckardt Scoring System and Staging

	Scoring System				Staging		
Score	Weight Loss (kg)	Dysphagia	Retrosternal Chest Pain	Regurgitation	Total Score	Stage	Treatment Response
0	0	No	No	No	0-1	0	Remission
1	<5	Occasional	Occasional	Occasional	2-3	I	Remission
2	5-10	Daily	Daily	Daily	4-6	II	Failure
3	>10	Every meal	Every meal	Every meal	7+	III	Failure

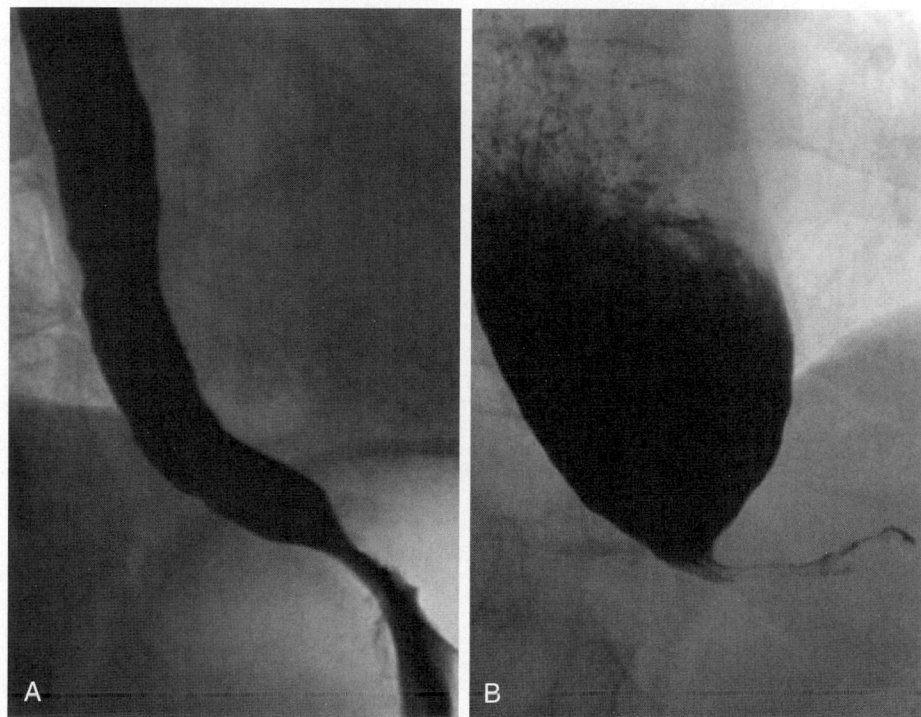

FIGURE 1 Barium swallow with (**A**) normal esophagus and (**B**) achalasia with severely dilated esophagus.

less than 4.5 seconds. Some authors have demonstrated better chest pain and dysphagia resolution rates using thoracoscopic extended Heller myotomy (to the level of the aortic arch) compared with pharmacologic (e.g., proton pump inhibitors [PPIs], smooth muscle relaxants, antidepressants) or endoscopic pneumatic balloon dilatation therapies.

Additional testing for patients with symptoms suspicious of esophageal dysmotility includes upper endoscopy with biopsy to assess for mucosal and structural abnormalities such as esophagitis, cancer, strictures, or candidiasis. Esophageal pH testing should be performed to evaluate for GERD if manometry studies are not consistent with achalasia. Finally, barium swallow is an important test to assess gastroesophageal anatomy; in addition, it can assist with operative planning by differentiating a classic "bird-beak" sign (Figure 1) from a sigmoid esophagus secondary to long-standing achalasia.

In this chapter we describe the perioperative and technical considerations of minimally invasive Heller myotomy as treatment for achalasia and hypertensive LES. We further describe aspects encountered during revisional operations after initial myotomy, treatment for end-stage achalasia, operative considerations for epiphrenic diverticula, the incorporation of the robotic-assisted platform, and recent advancements in endoscopic therapy.

■ MINIMALLY INVASIVE HELLER MYOTOMY AND PARTIAL FUNDOPLICATION FOR ACHALASIA

The most effective surgical option to treat achalasia is the Heller myotomy, which involves dividing the muscle fibers from the gastric cardia proximally onto the anterior distal esophagus, followed by either an anterior (Dor) or posterior (Toupet) wrap. The laparoscopic approach is the current standard of care; however, our group routinely uses the robotic platform for several perceived advantages, such as higher-quality visualization of the intricate muscle fibers and improved wrist articulation and visualization for proximal mediastinal dissection. Regardless of approach, both the laparoscopic and the robotic methods apply the same core principles of dissection and operative management, which are discussed here.

Preoperatively, antibiotic prophylaxis with a first-generation cephalosporin (or clindamycin if the patient is allergic to penicillin) is administered within 30 minutes of incision. Deep vein thrombosis prophylaxis with 5000 units of subcutaneous heparin is given before induction, and sequential compression devices are placed on bilateral lower extremities. When general anesthesia is induced, the patient is intubated in slight reverse Trendelenburg position to reduce the

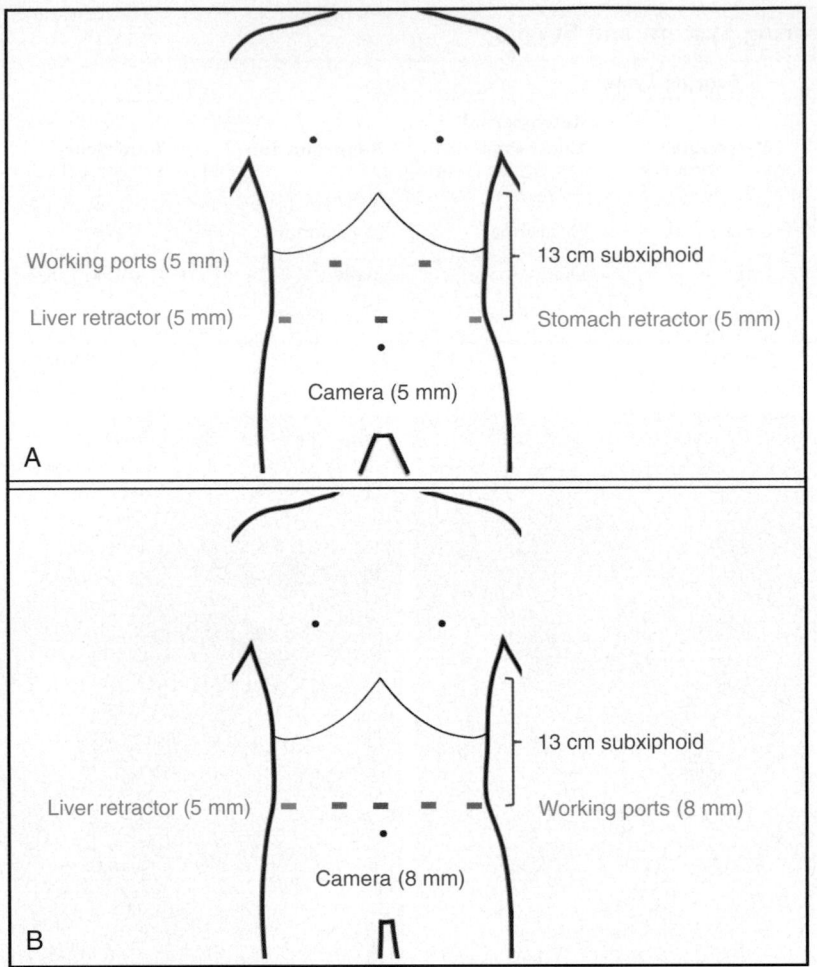

FIGURE 2 Port placement for (**A**) laparoscopic and (**B**) robotic Heller myotomy.

risk of aspiration from potential retained food particles in the dilated esophagus. A Foley catheter generally is not indicated for these procedures but can be placed at the discretion of the operating surgeon.

For the laparoscopic approach (Figure 2, *A*), the patient is placed supine on the operating table with arms tucked and footboards placed to prevent the patient from sliding during steep reverse Trendelenburg positioning. The legs then are split to 45 degrees, and the patient is prepared and draped in sterile fashion. Using Veress needle technique, intra-abdominal access and pneumoperitoneum is established 12 to 13 cm inferior to the xiphoid process in the midline. A 5-mm port is placed at the site of the Veress needle; this is designated for the 30-degree scope. Two 5-mm working ports for grasping and dissecting instruments are placed in the right and left midclavicular lines, 2 fingerbreadths below the costal margin. Two additional 5-mm ports are placed at the bilateral anterior axillary lines at the level on the umbilicus for retraction of the liver using a self-retaining retractor (right) and manipulation of the stomach using a grasper (left). The surgeon stands between the patient's split legs, manipulating the working ports; the first assistant stands on the left, controlling the camera and stomach retraction; and the scrub technician stands on the right.

For the robotic approach (Figure 2, *B*), the patient is placed supine on the operating table with arms tucked and footboards placed to prevent sliding in steep reverse Trendelenburg position, similar to the laparoscopic setup. However, the legs are kept together, as there is no need for the surgeon or assistant to work between the patient's legs. The patient is prepared and draped in sterile fashion. An 8-mm

robotic port is placed at the site of the Veress needle 12 to 13 cm below the xiphoid; this is designated for the robotic camera. Along the same horizontal plane, three additional stab incisions are made at the left anterior axillary line, left midclavicular line, and right midclavicular line; these are designated for the 8-mm robotic arm ports. Finally, a 5-mm port site is made at the right anterior axillary line for placement of a Diamond-Flex liver retractor (Snowden-Pencer, Tucker, GA). Then the patient is placed in steep reverse Trendelenburg position, and the da Vinci Xi platform is docked over the right side of the patient for the robotic approach (Figure 3). Note that if using the da Vinci Si platform, docking occurs over the head of the patient.

Dissection begins by dividing the gastrohepatic ligament, being mindful to preserve a potential aberrant left hepatic artery seen in 3% to 25% of patients. The right crus is identified (Figure 4, *A*), and the esophagus is dissected circumferentially anteriorly toward the left crus. The gastric fundus then is mobilized along the greater curvature to the gastroesophageal junction (GEJ). The stomach is retracted medial-inferiorly with a fenestrated grasper, and the superior branches of the short gastric vessels are ligated. Dissection proceeds along the angle of His until the left crus is identified and the prior right-sided dissection is encountered (Figure 4, *B*); the anterior vagus nerve must be identified and protected during this part of the operation. Then, using careful blunt dissection and bipolar electrocautery, the distal esophagus is mobilized for approximately 8 cm into the mediastinum. All remaining tissue, including the anterior gastric fat pad, is cleared from the GEJ and anterior cardia of the stomach to provide adequate exposure for the Heller myotomy.

An esophageal myotomy is created preferably at the 11 o'clock position approximately 2 to 3 cm above the GEJ but can be performed at the 2 or 3 o'clock position as well. If the latter is performed, a longer myotomy is warranted. Bipolar dissectors are used to grasp and separate the longitudinal and circular muscle fibers via a gentle "tear" technique until the submucosal plane is entered (Figure 5, A and B). The esophageal myotomy is extended to 6 to 8 cm proximal to the GEJ while ensuring 50% circumferential exposure of the esophageal mucosa. The gastric myotomy then is initiated with monopolar hook electrocautery 3 cm distal to the GEJ on the anterior cardia (Figure 5, C) and extended proximally to join the esophageal myotomy, again using the "tear" technique (Figure 5, D). Prior studies have demonstrated that a gastric myotomy of 3 cm is associated with less postoperative dysphagia and lower reoperation rates compared with a gastric myotomy of 2 cm. Of note, the anterior vagus nerve should be retracted left laterally to avoid injury during this part of the dissection. The total myotomy length should be at least 9 cm to ensure adequate release of the muscle fibers spanning

the GEJ (Figure 6). Notably, most hemostasis can be controlled with direct pressure using a sponge. If mucosal perforation is encountered during dissection, it should be repaired primarily using 4-0 interrupted absorbable sutures.

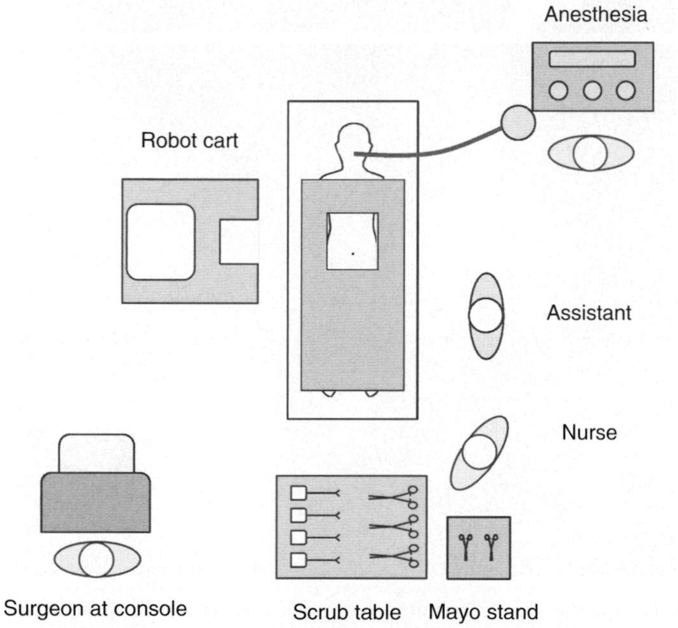

After the myotomy is complete, an antireflux procedure should be performed to reduce the likelihood of GERD postoperatively. Because a 360-degree wrap has been clearly associated with higher rates of dysphagia in achalasia patients postoperatively, we routinely perform a Dor fundoplication, which has the added benefit of covering the fresh myotomy site, especially if the mucosa was perforated inadvertently. The Toupet fundoplication is another viable option, as both fundoplication techniques have demonstrated similar improvement of dysphagia and regurgitation scores as well as similar reflux rates at 1 year after surgery in a prospective randomized control trial. The only situation where we would not perform a fundoplication is in patients with severe achalasia (sigmoid esophagus) because of the high likelihood of postoperative dysphagia; these patients can have reflux postoperatively and may require PPIs. Nevertheless, before suture fixation of the Dor fundoplication, the gastric fundus is draped across the myotomy to ensure adequate length of coverage to the right crus. Then the superior-anterior gastric fundus is anchored to the left crus and left esophageal myotomy edge with interrupted 3-0 silk sutures (Figure 7, A). Then the remaining fundus is laid across the myotomy, and the lateral edge is anchored to the right crus and right esophageal myotomy edge with interrupted 3-0 silk sutures (Figure 7, B). These crural and esophageal anchors ultimately help to prevent torsion and hiatal migration of the wrap. Instruments then are removed under direct visualization, and the skin is closed with 4-0 absorbable subcuticular sutures. We do not routinely perform esophagogastroduodenoscopy (EGD) at the end of the procedure.

On postoperative day 0, patients are given a clear liquid diet, liquid pain medications orally, and antiemetics intravenously as needed. We remain vigilant about preventing emesis and retching in order to avoid a postoperative mucosal perforation or fundoplication disruption from increased intra-abdominal pressure. Of note, we do not routinely obtain barium swallow studies postoperatively; these are obtained only if there is clinical suspicion of gastroesophageal leak or obstruction. The patient's diet is advanced to a soft food or full liquid diet on postoperative day 1. If tolerated, the patient is discharged home with the instruction to continue this diet until outpatient evaluation at 2 weeks. If there are no signs of dysphagia, we gradually transition the patient to a regular diet over the course of 4 weeks while avoiding bulky foods such as raw vegetables and thick meats.

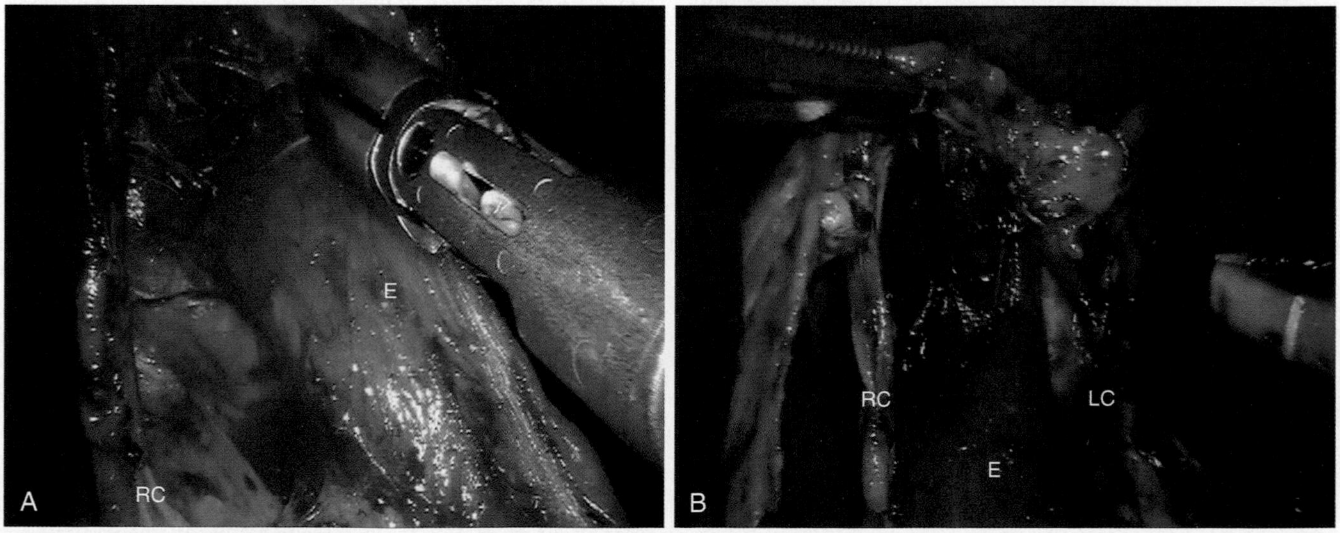

FIGURE 3 Operating room setup for robotic Heller myotomy.

FIGURE 4 Hiatal dissection: (**A**) right and (**B**) left crural exposure. *E,* Esophagus; *LC,* left crus; *RC,* right crus.

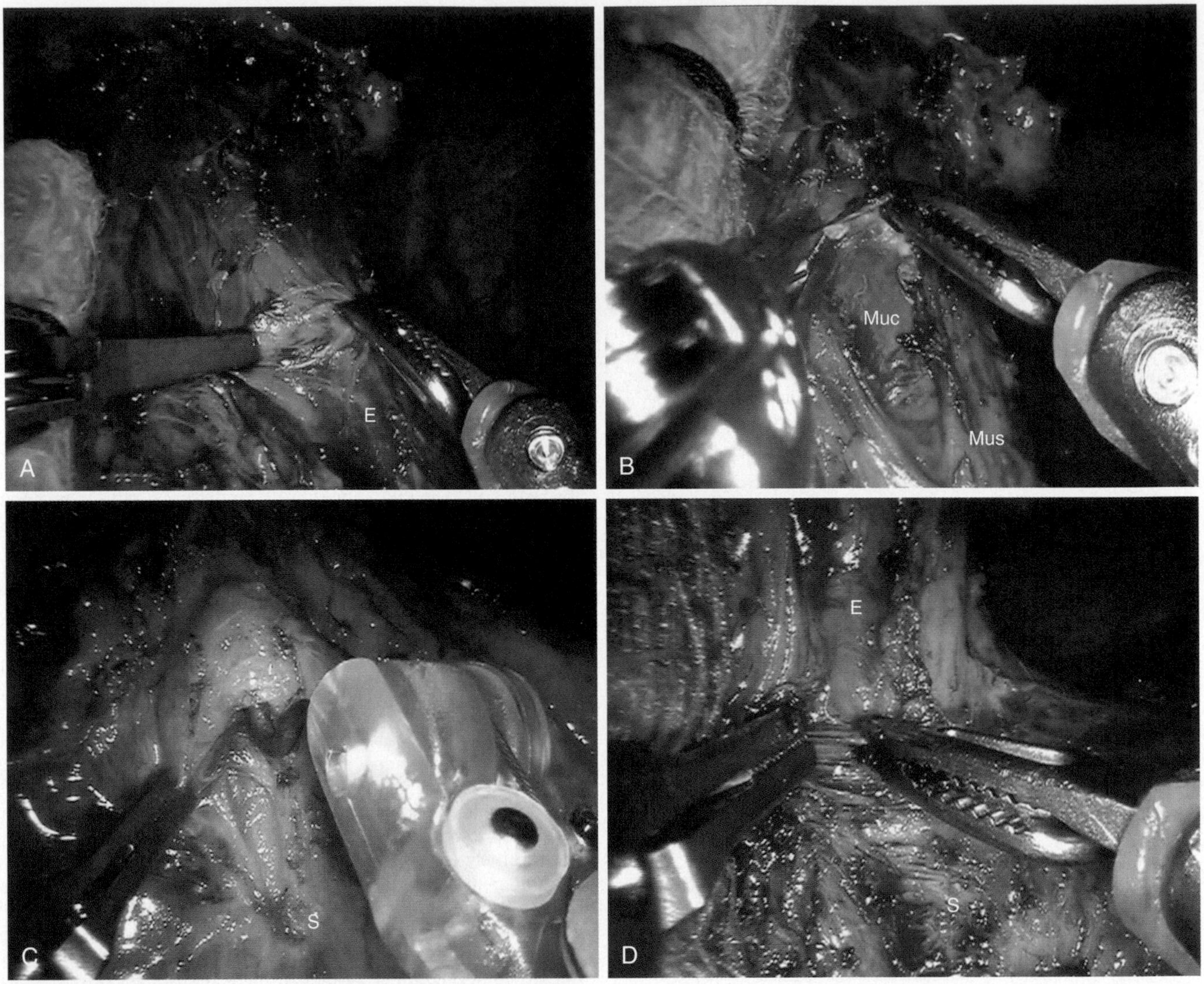

FIGURE 5 "Tear" technique during myotomy. **A,** Entering the esophageal submucosal plane. **B,** Exposing the esophageal mucosa proximally. **C,** Initiating gastric myotomy. **D,** Continuing gastric myotomy. *E,* Esophagus; *Muc,* mucosa; *Mus,* muscle layer; *S,* stomach.

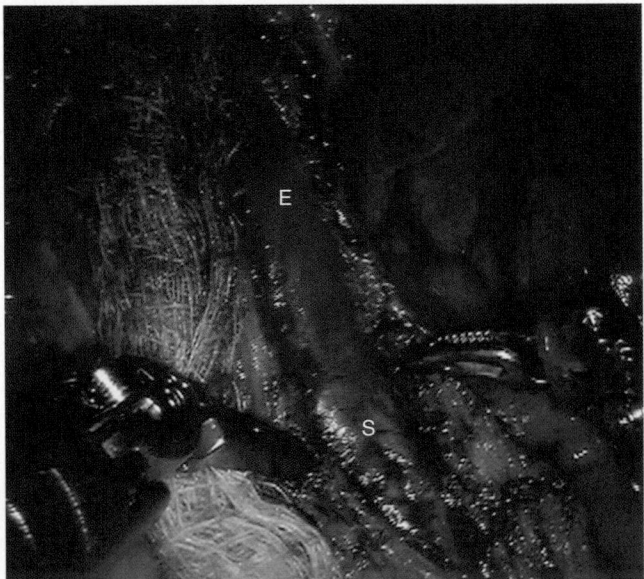

FIGURE 6 Completion of esophageal and gastric myotomy. *E,* Esophagus; *S,* stomach.

Relief of dysphagia is perhaps the most important sign of clinical success, with reduction of the Eckardt score to less than 4 marking a successful operation (see Table 1). Minimally invasive Heller myotomy with fundoplication has a symptom resolution rate of 90% at a median follow-up of 3 years. The long-term (>5 years) dysphagia resolution rate ranges from 70% to 80% without difference between laparoscopic or robotic approaches. Postoperative GERD typically occurs in less than 10% of patients undergoing minimally invasive Heller myotomy with fundoplication; this rate increases to 30% if fundoplication is not performed. The most severe surgery-specific complication after Heller myotomy is perioperative perforation; this occurs in approximately 2% of cases and requires operative intervention in about 33% of those cases.

■ REVISIONAL SURGERY AFTER HELLER MYOTOMY

Patients with even minor improvement of dysphagia postoperatively will experience great relief subjectively; however, patients with recurrence of symptoms are difficult to manage. Dysphagia is the most common recurrent symptom, and clinicians should use the Eckardt scoring system to objectively measure treatment response and help guide further interventions. It is important that clinicians determine whether symptoms postoperatively are related to disease recurrence

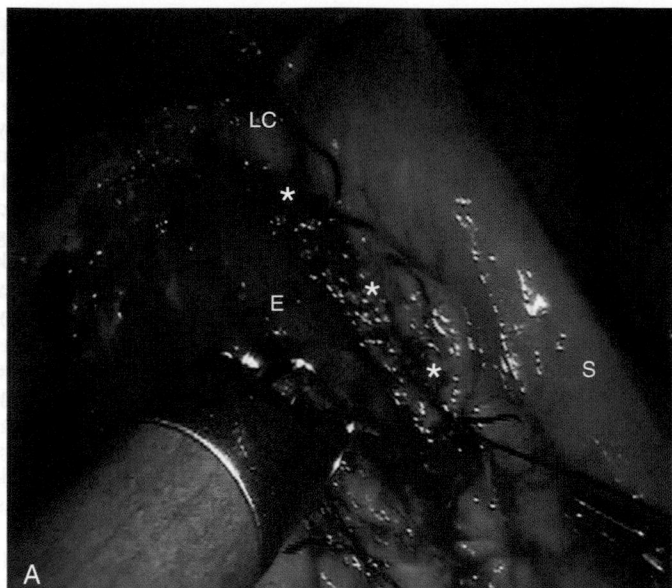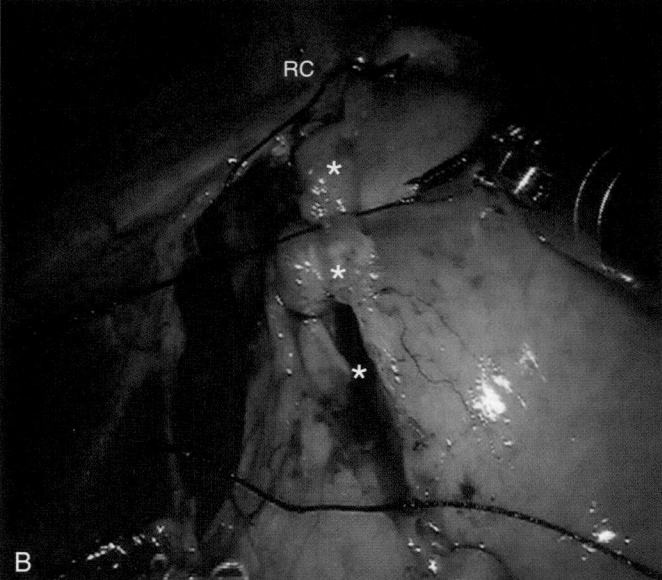

FIGURE 7 Dor fundoplication with crural and myotomy anchors on the (**A**) left and (**B**) right. *, Myotomy edge; *E*, esophagus; *LC*, left crus; *RC*, right crus; *S*, stomach.

(i.e., failed myotomy) or possible GERD. To provide insight, one should assess the exact types of symptoms, specifically dysphagia (solid or liquid), regurgitation, chest pain, heartburn, response to PPIs or H2 blockers, and atypical symptoms such as cough, postnasal drip, and hoarseness.

In addition, a careful review of preoperative endoscopy, manometry, and imaging studies should be performed to confirm that the patient had an accurate diagnosis of achalasia on initial presentation. The operative report should be reviewed for complications, length of myotomy, type of fundoplication, and anatomic abnormalities such as fibrosis at the GEJ resulting from prior botulinum toxin injections or pneumatic dilatations (thus precluding adequate myotomy). This should be supplemented by a detailed timeline to delineate either persistence or recurrence of symptoms and ultimately to determine the efficacy of the index myotomy (failure rates can range from 3% to 15%). It has been proposed that the best sign of successful myotomy is postoperative weight gain, which if present would suggest an accurate initial diagnosis and successful operation. Other causes of recurrence then would need to be elucidated.

Potential causes of postoperative dysphagia include error in the initial diagnosis, incomplete myotomy during index operation, tight fundoplication, stricture formation at the myotomy site secondary to reflux, and obstructive malignancy (i.e., squamous cell carcinoma). The first three causes result in persistent or early dysphagia postoperatively. The final two causes typically are seen more than 6 months postoperatively. It should be noted that patients with end-stage achalasia have an increased postoperative dysphagia rate, which should be considered during re-evaluation.

Diagnostic studies warranted include barium swallow, endoscopy, HRM, and pH monitoring. A barium swallow study provides insight into contrast retention of the esophagus and can pinpoint an area of obstruction, such as from a slipped fundoplication or incomplete myotomy. Endoscopy should be performed to assess for strictures, esophagitis, ulcers, tumors, diverticuli, and retained food in the distal esophagus. Most patients also will require repeat HRM to measure the mean LES pressure, which should be less than 10 mm Hg after complete myotomy; patients with elevated LES pressures should be considered for redo myotomy. Finally, pH monitoring should be used to evaluate for GERD if endoscopy and HRM show no evidence of retained food or elevated LES pressures. However, clinicians should review the pH results carefully, as prolonged periods of pH higher than 4 can signify a retained food bolus in the esophagus that is partially digested, which can increase the esophageal acid content.

Simply put, this is a sign of severe dysphagia warranting reoperation, not of reflux. Moreover, if the pH study indicates true reflux, initiation of a PPI should be considered. However, if all of these studies are negative, other causes for the patient's symptoms must be explored fully.

Management of patients with a recurrence or failed myotomy requires a multidisciplinary evaluation. The teams should consider endoscopic options, including pneumatic balloon dilatation and peroral endoscopic myotomy (POEM; described later), as well as surgical options such as minimally invasive Heller myotomy or esophagectomy. At our institution, we treat an early failed myotomy (i.e., persistence) with reoperative Heller myotomy. For a recurrence, our first-line approach is balloon dilatation; if there is an inadequate response, a repeat Heller myotomy is indicated. We typically reserve POEM for failed reoperative surgery; however, this algorithm should be tailored specifically to each center's expertise.

When performing a repeat Heller myotomy, our group prefers the robotic approach, as these are complex cases with severe adhesions that complicate the hiatal dissection. We recommend performing the myotomy at least 90 degrees away from the prior myotomy site, as this ensures entering virgin, nonfibrotic tissue to access the submucosal plane. It is important to clearly identify the right and left crura during the dissection; otherwise the risk of inadvertent esophageal injury increases. An extended myotomy—4 cm on the gastric side and 8 cm on the esophageal side—typically is warranted in these cases, and a partial fundoplication should be fashioned similar to the index operation. If a mucosal injury is encountered intraoperatively, it should be repaired primarily with 3-0 or 4-0 absorbable sutures and covered with a wrap. These patients typically require a postoperative barium swallow to ensure that there is no leak before beginning oral intake.

■ MINIMALLY INVASIVE TREATMENT OF END-STAGE ACHALASIA

End-stage achalasia is identified as a sigmoid-shaped tortuous megaesophagus (>6 cm) as seen on barium swallow, resulting in extremely poor esophageal function. Despite the severity of esophageal dysfunction associated with this disease, several studies suggest that Heller myotomy is successful in improving dysphagia symptoms and decreasing postoperative LES pressure and esophageal width in these patients. Therefore we advocate for minimally invasive Heller myotomy as an initial therapy for end-stage achalasia; however, we

Relative contraindications for a laparoscopic approach include those for any laparoscopic procedure, such as severe carbon dioxide retention, pulmonary hypertension, or a hostile abdomen because of scar tissue from prior surgeries, infection, or trauma.

■ PREPARATION

Patients with hormonally active tumors can have significant metabolic abnormalities (e.g., hypokalemia, metabolic alkalosis, and hyperglycemia) and severe hypertension, both of which need to be corrected before surgery. This is especially true for patients with pheochromocytoma, as major fluctuations in blood pressure can occur intraoperatively. The most widely used regimen for preparing patients with pheochromocytoma for surgery is for them to start taking an alpha-blocker (e.g., phenoxybenzamine, prazosin, or doxazosin) 3 to 4 weeks before surgery and titrate to normotension. If tachycardia develops after blood pressure is controlled, a beta-blocker can be added. Patients should increase their salt and fluid intake a few days before surgery so that they are well hydrated, and an experienced anesthesia team should be well prepared for potentially dramatic intraoperative hemodynamic fluctuations. Good communication with the anesthesia team is vital so that they are aware when the tumor is being manipulated and before clipping the adrenal vein. Patients with Cushing's syndrome should receive perioperative stress-dose steroids. All patients should undergo routine preoperative antibiotics and antithrombotic prophylaxis.

■ OPERATIVE TECHNIQUE

There are three basic approaches to laparoscopic adrenalectomy—anterior, lateral, and posterior—the last of which is actually a "retroperitoneoscopic" approach. There are pros and cons to each approach; however, the lateral approach is used most commonly because of a large working space, familiar anatomy, and patient positioning that helps to retract organs by gravity. The posterior approach also is used routinely and may be preferred for patients with previous abdominal surgery or obesity, as it avoids entering the peritoneal cavity altogether. In addition, the posterior approach allows for a bilateral adrenalectomy without the patient repositioning required with the lateral approach. Some drawbacks to the posterior approach are a limited working space, especially with large tumors; less familiar anatomic view; and potential for difficulty in controlling bleeding from the vena cava should it occur. The anterior laparoscopic approach provides a conventional view of the anatomy and also allows for bilateral adrenalectomy without patient repositioning; however, it is used rarely because retraction is more difficult and requires additional ports. Each of these approaches can be performed with the addition of robotic assistance; however, we have not found that this provides much advantage over the standard laparoscopic approaches. In small series, single-incision laparoscopic surgery (SILS) approaches have been reported to be equivalent in safety to the standard laparoscopic approaches, but they are technically and ergonomically more challenging.

Lateral Approach

The patient is positioned on a gel-padded bean bag in nearly full lateral decubitus position (i.e., slightly rotated toward supine) with the operative side facing up and the umbilicus centered over the break in the table. An axillary roll is placed, and arms and legs are padded carefully and positioned to avoid neurapraxia. The table is flexed to open the angle between the costal margin and the iliac crest. In addition, the table can be placed in slight reverse Trendelenburg position and rotated slightly toward dorsal (Figure 1). Using either a Veress needle or the Hasson technique, an initial 10-mm port is placed about 5 cm below the costal margin at the lateral edge of the rectus (between anterior axillary and midclavicular lines). A 30-degree laparoscope is used, and two to four additional ports (5 mm) are

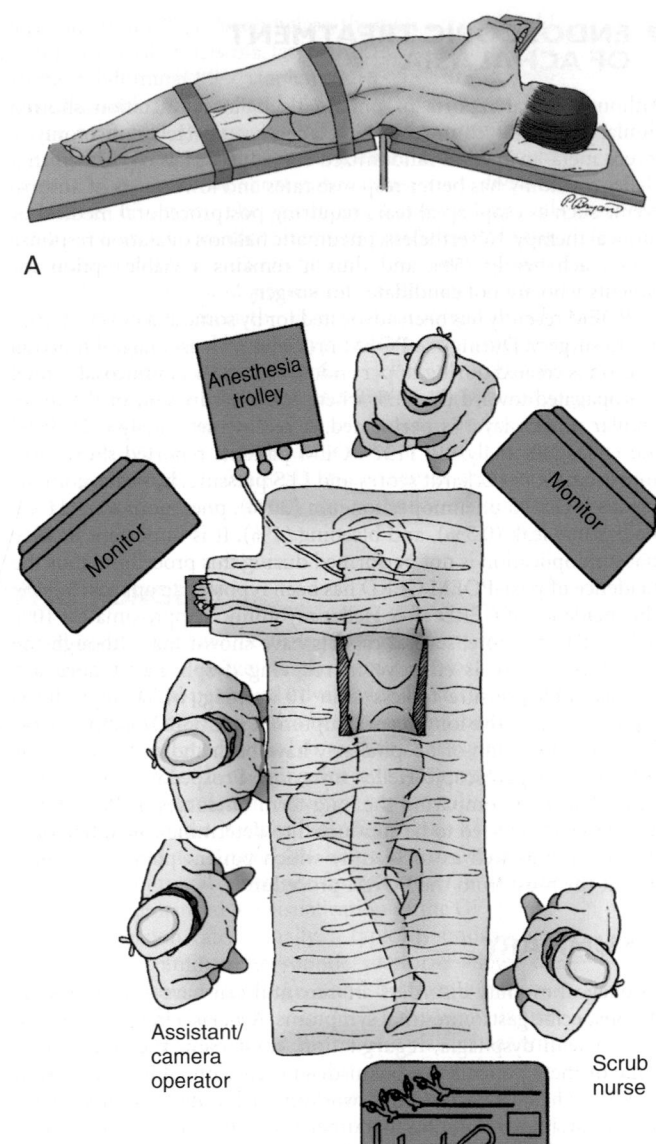

FIGURE 1 A, Patient positioning for the lateral approach to left laparoscopic adrenalectomy. **B,** Operating room setup and patient positioning for laparoscopic adrenalectomy. *(Modified from Smith CD, Weber CJ, Amerson JR. Laparoscopic adrenalectomy: new gold standard. World J Surg. 1999;23:389-396.)*

placed under direct vision at least 2 cm below the costal margin and separated by at least 5 cm (Figure 2). The surgeon and assistant both stand on the same side of the patient, facing the abdomen.

For left adrenalectomy, a total of three or four ports are used. To expose the left adrenal gland, the colon, spleen, distal pancreas, and stomach must be mobilized. An advantage of the lateral approach is that gravity aids in the retraction of these structures as the dissection plane is developed. Dissection begins by mobilizing the splenic flexure and left colon using either ultrasonic shears or a thermal-based device. Once the lateral peritoneal attachment of the colon is incised, much of the dissection of the colon and its mesentery can be performed with gentle blunt dissection using a grasper or suction device. Care should be taken to stay right on Gerota's fascia anterior to the kidney (Figure 3, *A*) rather than dissecting posterolateral to the kidney, as this can cause the kidney to fall anteromedial and compromise the exposure of the adrenal gland.

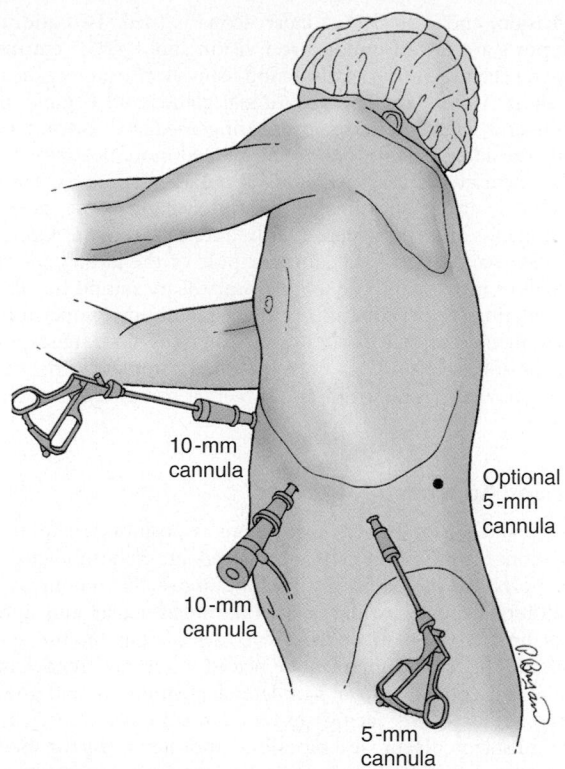

FIGURE 2 Trocar placement and instrument placement for left laparoscopic adrenalectomy. *(Modified from Smith CD, Weber CJ, Amerson JR. Laparoscopic adrenalectomy: new gold standard. World J Surg. 1999;23: 389-396.)*

Once the inferior pole of the spleen is reached, the lateral and retroperitoneal attachments of the spleen are divided, and the spleen and tail of the pancreas are dissected slowly off of the adrenal bed. Initially this can be a somewhat elusive plane to find, especially in obese patients with a large amount of retroperitoneal fat or in those with small adrenal tumors that are not evident immediately. In these cases, laparoscopic ultrasound can sometimes aid in defining the anatomy and guiding the dissection. The exposure of the left adrenal gland has been analogized to slowly opening a book with the right page being the kidney and adrenal gland and the left page being the colon (and its mesentery), spleen, and distal pancreas. As this plane is developed, gravity helps to keep the "book" open. The plane is opened sufficiently when the medial edge of the adrenal gland is visible and manual retraction is no longer needed to keep the spleen and pancreas from falling back over the adrenal. This is a relatively avascular plane (Figure 3, *B*), so any bleeding should prompt a re-evaluation of the anatomy to ensure that dissection is proceeding in the proper plane.

Dissection of the adrenal gland begins along its inferolateral aspect. The superior pole of the kidney is identified by "palpation" with a grasper, Gerota's fascia is opened, and electrocautery or ultrasonic shears are used to dissect through the perinephric fat until the adrenal gland itself is identified by its bright yellow color. Caution is exercised to avoid tearing the delicate capsule of the adrenal gland by grasping the surrounding fat instead of the gland itself or by using a blunt instrument such as a grasper or suction device to push or maneuver the adrenal gland without actually grasping it. Ideally the adrenal vein is isolated and ligated early during surgery to prevent injuring it during mobilization of the rest of the gland; however, in some cases the size of the tumor prohibits ligation of the vein until the superior and medial sides of the gland are mobilized. It is not necessary to trace the left adrenal vein to its junction with the left renal vein as long as it is clearly observed to enter the substance of

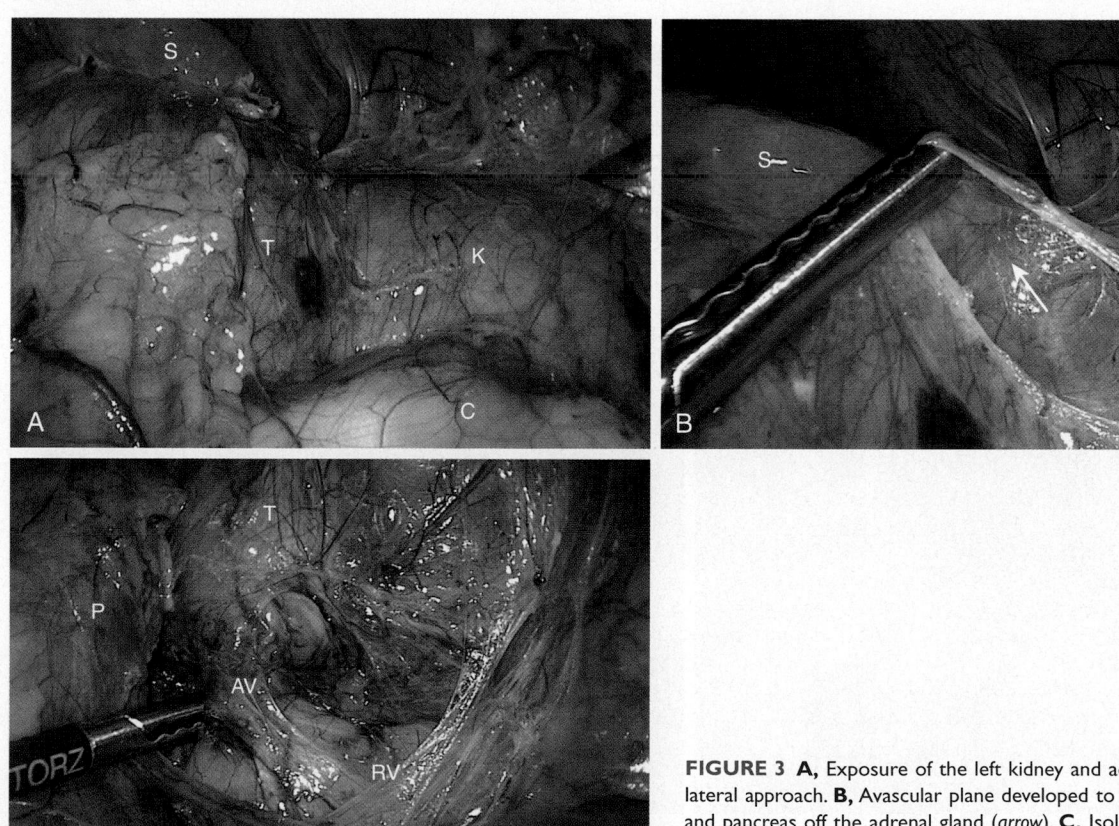

FIGURE 3 A, Exposure of the left kidney and adrenal during the lateral approach. **B,** Avascular plane developed to mobilize the spleen and pancreas off the adrenal gland *(arrow)*. **C,** Isolation of the left adrenal vein. *AV,* Adrenal vein; *C,* colon; *K,* kidney; *P,* pancreas; *RV,* renal vein; *S,* spleen; *T,* tumor.

the gland (Figure 3, *C*). We prefer to ligate the vein with clips before dividing; however, bipolar or ultrasonic shears also are commonly used to divide the left adrenal vein. The rest of the gland is dissected off the diaphragm, placed in an endoscopic bag, and removed by extending the 10-mm port incision a bit. Attempts should be made to keep the specimen intact (i.e., do not morcellate it) for pathologic review. After ensuring hemostasis, the fascia at the extraction site is closed with absorbable suture.

For right adrenalectomy, four ports are usually sufficient, with placement mirroring that for left adrenalectomy. A fan-shaped or "snake" retractor is placed in the most medial port to retract the liver, and the laparoscope usually is placed in the second-most medial port. Dissection begins by taking down the right triangular ligament of the liver to mobilize it off of the adrenal gland. As the liver is mobilized, the liver retractor is progressively advanced manually until the superior edge of the adrenal gland is visible, at which point the retractor can be fixed to the table. Dissection of the adrenal gland begins as described for left adrenalectomy and should proceed along the superior surface of the gland from lateral to medial until the vena cava is reached. Caution is used when elevating and retracting the liver medially, as there are occasionally small hepatic veins draining to the vena cava that if torn will bleed vigorously. The medial aspect of the adrenal gland then is dissected carefully away from the vena cava to expose its junction with the right adrenal vein (Figure 4, *A*). Occasionally the adrenal tumor may extend quite far posterior to the vena cava, in which case it may be helpful to insert a fifth port so that a blunt instrument can be used to gently retract the vena cava medially as the tumor is dissected from behind it. The right adrenal vein is often short and broad, so two or three clips should be left on the vena cava side (Figure 4, *B*). Rarely, the right adrenal vein must be ligated with an endovascular stapler. When the gland has been dissected completely free, surgery is completed as described for left adrenalectomy.

Posterior Approach

For the posterior approach, the patient is placed in a prone jack-knife position, and the surgeon stands on the side of the patient from which the adrenal gland is to be removed. An incision is made just inferior to the tip of the twelfth rib, and blunt dissection is used through the flank muscles until the retroperitoneum is entered. The retroperitoneal space is developed first with a finger and then with a balloon dissector, and carbon dioxide insufflation is used to maintain it. A standard 10-mm balloon-tipped laparoscopic port is placed by

this incision, and a 30-degree laparoscope is used. Two additional 5-mm ports are placed under direct vision about 4 to 5 cm medial and lateral (Figure 5). Initial dissection using electrocautery or ultrasonic shears is similar for both adrenal glands and begins on the superior and lateral surfaces, proceeding medially and anteriorly. Because the adrenal veins tend to be situated more posteriorly, they may be encountered early with this approach (Figure 6). They are ligated as described for the lateral approach. In some cases, the adrenal glands may be situated fairly anteriorly on the kidney, in which case retraction of the superior pole of the kidney inferiorly with a blunt instrument may be necessary. Care should be taken to avoid violating the peritoneum, as the resultant pneumoperitoneum may compress the retroperitoneal space, thus limiting exposure. When the adrenal gland has been dissected completely free of surrounding tissues, it is removed, and surgery is completed as described previously.

Anterior Approach

With the anterior approach, the patient is positioned supine, and insufflation of the abdomen is achieved at the umbilicus. Two 5-mm ports are placed in the midline above the umbilicus, and two additional ports are placed in the midclavicular and anterior axillary lines 3 to 4 cm below the costal margin on the side of the tumor. The patient then can be placed in reverse Trendelenburg position and rotated into a hemilateral position so that the side undergoing surgery is facing up. For left adrenalectomy, the left colon and splenic flexure are mobilized and then retracted medially to reveal the left kidney and adrenal gland. The spleen and distal pancreas are mobilized as necessary to expose the superior and medial borders of the adrenal gland. It is often necessary to use a fan retractor via one of the medial ports to maintain the retraction of the colon and spleen. The left renal vein is identified, and its superior border is dissected until the left adrenal vein is identified and clipped as described for the lateral approach. The gland is removed, and surgery is completed as described for the lateral approach. For right adrenalectomy, the hepatic flexure may need to be mobilized to expose the upper pole of the right kidney, adrenal gland, and inferior vena cava. The liver is mobilized off the adrenal gland as described for the lateral approach. The lateral border of the inferior vena cava is traced until the right adrenal vein is identified, dissected carefully, and ligated as previously described. The gland then is removed by dissecting it free from the surrounding adipose tissue.

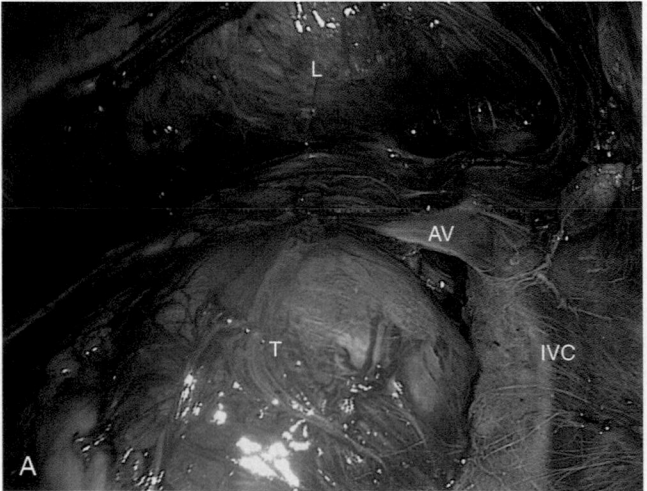
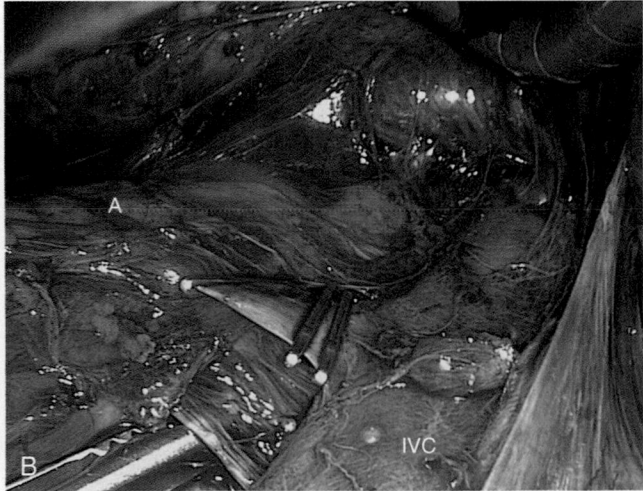

FIGURE 4 A, Exposure of the right adrenal vein during the lateral approach. **B,** Clipping of the right adrenal vein. *A,* Adrenal gland; *AV,* adrenal vein; *IVC,* inferior vena cava; *L,* liver; *T,* tumor.

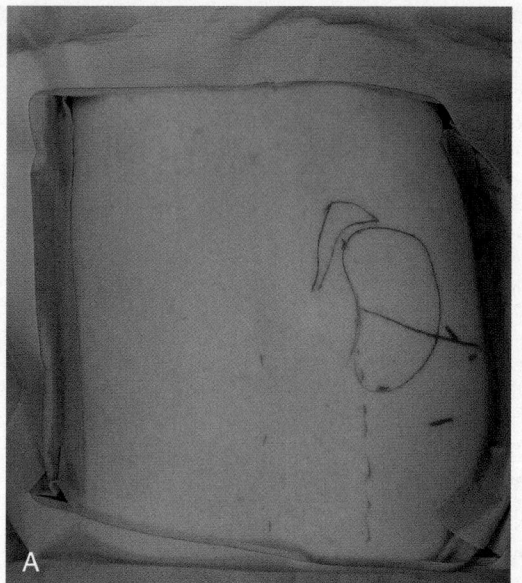 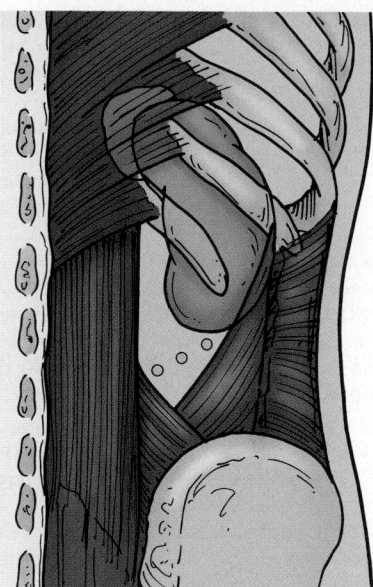

FIGURE 5 A, Posterior port placement has to be done carefully because there is limited space for placement. **B,** Underlying structures.

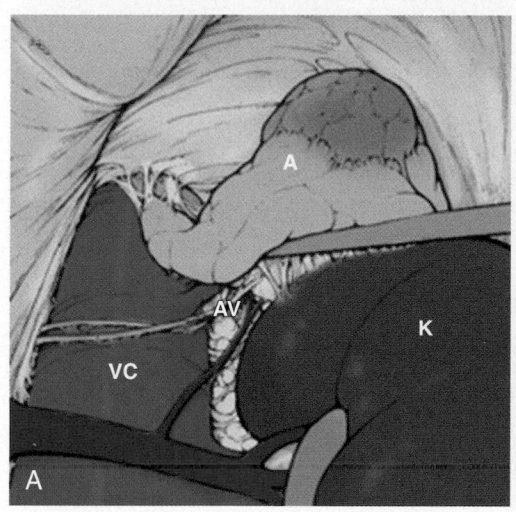 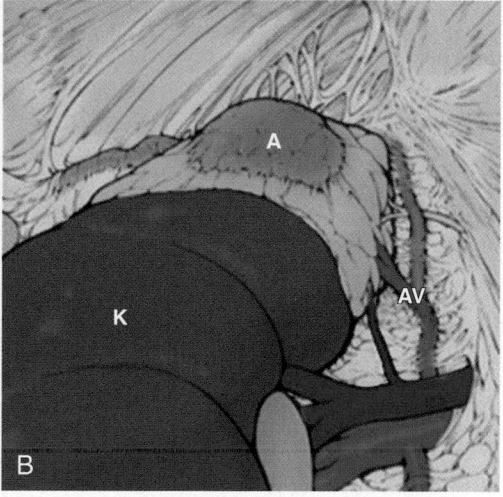

FIGURE 6 Posterior retroperitoneal endoscopic adrenalectomy. **A,** Right. **B,** Left. *A,* Adrenal; *AV,* adrenal vein; *K,* kidney; *VC,* vena cava. *(Modified from Walz MK. Minimally invasive adrenal gland surgery [in German]. Chirurg. 1998;69:613-620.)*

■ COMPLICATIONS

Overall complication rates are low (5%) and equivalent across the different minimally invasive approaches. Major complications associated with laparoscopic adrenalectomy are rare (1% to 2%) and include significant bleeding or injury to adjacent organs (e.g., spleen, pancreas, liver, colon) during exposure or retraction. Bleeding from the vena cava or left renal vein can be dramatic but in many cases can be controlled by gentle tamponade with a blunt grasper or suction tip followed by careful clip placement or suture repair. In these situations, it is important for the surgeon to remain calm but also communicate clearly to the anesthesia team and nursing staff that significant bleeding has occurred, so that preparations can be made for resuscitation or conversion to open adrenalectomy should it become necessary. Overall, conversion to an open procedure is necessary in less than 5% of cases and should not in and of itself be considered a complication, especially when used to avoid disrupting the tumor capsule.

■ POSTOPERATIVE RECOVERY

Laparoscopic adrenalectomy is very well tolerated. Postoperative pain is typically mild to moderate, and patients usually spend only 1 or 2 nights in the hospital, with return to full activity within a couple of weeks. Patients with pheochromocytoma who experience any significant intraoperative hemodynamic instability should be monitored in an intensive care unit overnight. Fluid and electrolytes should be monitored for patients with functional tumors, especially those with hyperaldosteronism. Adrenal hormone replacement is necessary only in patients with Cushing's syndrome, in which case it may take several months for the other adrenal gland to resume normal function.

SUGGESTED READINGS

Lal G, Duh QY. Laparoscopic adrenalectomy—indications and technique. *Surg Oncol.* 2003;12:105-123.

Raeburn CD, McIntyre RC Jr. Laparoscopic approach to adrenal and endocrine pancreatic tumors. *Surg Clin North Am.* 2000;80:1427-1441.

Smith CD, et al. Laparoscopic adrenalectomy: new gold standard. *World J Surg.* 1999;23:389-396.

Walz MK, et al. Posterior retroperitoneoscopic adrenalectomy—results of 560 procedures in 520 patients. *Surgery.* 2006;140:943-948.

MINIMALLY INVASIVE PARATHYROIDECTOMY

Jacob Moalem, MD, FACS

Primary hyperparathyroidism (PHPT), the most common cause of hypercalcemia, is a condition caused by autonomous function of a parathyroid gland or glands. In classical PHPT, both the calcium and the parathyroid hormone (PTH) levels are elevated. In many patients with PHPT, though, at least one of these values is within the "normal" reference range. In some patients, both the calcium and the PTH levels are "normal." These patients still have PHPT because in the context of high-normal serum calcium, PTH should be nearly undetectable, and therefore a nonsuppressed (but still "normal") PTH level represents an abnormal response. In 80% to 85% of patients with PHPT, the condition is caused by a single adenoma. Parathyroid hyperplasia accounts for most of the remaining cases, followed by multiple adenomas, which are uncommon. Parathyroid carcinoma is rare and affects less than 0.1% of patients with PHPT.

Although most patients who are diagnosed with PHPT are asymptomatic and are found to have hypercalcemia incidentally, this disorder can be associated with a variety of signs and symptoms. These include nephrolithiasis, accelerated bone loss leading to osteoporosis or osteitis fibrosa cystica, impaired renal function, and a variety of constitutional symptoms such as fatigue; decreased clarity of thought; muscle, bone, or joint pains; constipation; and urinary frequency.

Although the indications for surgery in symptomatic patients are clear, the indications for surgery in asymptomatic patients have been a subject of significant controversy. Some surgeons and endocrinologists consider the presence of PHPT to be an indication for surgery, but four consensus conferences have described a more restricted set of criteria for parathyroidectomy. Current criteria include serum calcium elevation more than 1 mg/dL above the upper limit of normal, T score less than −2.5 or a history of vertebral fracture, creatinine clearance less than 60 cc/min or 24-hour urine calcium greater than 400 mg, history or presence of nephrolithiasis or nephrocalcinosis, or age less than 50 years.

Acknowledging both that most patients fall outside of these criteria and the benefits of parathyroidectomy even in asymptomatic patients, the authors of the most recent consensus statement also have stated that parathyroidectomy is indicated for any patient with PHPT for whom surveillance is either not desired or impossible.

Recent advances in preoperative localization, as well as the widespread availability of rapid intraoperative PTH measurement, have led to a fundamental change in the operative approach to most patients with PHPT. Before these advances, parathyroidectomy often consisted of the identification of all four glands and the removal of a single adenoma. Surgeons currently attempt to identify an abnormal parathyroid gland before making a smaller incision and removing the adenoma after a more limited, unilateral exploration. Although there is no consensus on the definition of minimally invasive parathyroidectomy (MIP), this approach is thought to be associated with a reduced risk of perioperative complications. Certainly, using this limited exposure and unilateral dissection, there should be no risk of permanent hypoparathyroidism or bilateral recurrent laryngeal nerve paralysis in a patient who has not had prior neck surgery.

Although the advent of MIP has resulted in an increased number of referrals for parathyroidectomy and has simplified the procedure in many cases, it is critical that surgeons are aware of the relative contraindications to this approach and of the limitations of preoperative imaging and intraoperative PTH measurements. The evidence is very clear that the best opportunity to cure a patient with PHPT is during the first operation and that re-explorations are considerably more difficult and associated with higher risk of recurrent laryngeal nerve injury. In experienced hands, the added risk for a contralateral exploration should be very low. Therefore surgeons should have a low threshold to "convert" from a MIP and explore the remaining glands in cases where there is any uncertainty about the completeness of the minimally invasive approach.

This chapter discusses the indications for MIP, with particular emphasis on patient populations that should not be considered for this approach. In addition, the imaging studies that are the backbone of MIP are discussed, with particular attention to the causes of false-positive results. Finally, the technique of MIP along with some variations on the traditional approach, such as radioguidance or video assistance, are discussed.

■ INDICATIONS FOR MINIMALLY INVASIVE PARATHYROIDECTOMY

In general, most patients with sporadic PHPT should be considered as potential candidates for MIP, with some notable exceptions, all of whom are more likely to have multigland disease. Patients with multiple endocrine neoplasia types 1 and 2A, as well as those with isolated familial PHPT, nearly always have parathyroid hyperplasia and should not be considered for MIP. Patients with lithium-associated PHPT have a higher than average likelihood for parathyroid hyperplasia and are considered by many to require bilateral exploration. Patients with radiation-associated PHPT appear to have a similar distribution of parathyroid adenomas versus multigland disease as patients with sporadic disease and are therefore good candidates for MIP. Patients who have had imaging studies that suggest multigland disease and patients whose imaging studies have discordant findings should not be considered for MIP.

Preoperative Preparation: Imaging

Once the biochemical diagnosis of PHPT is confirmed and the patient is considered to be a good candidate for surgery, most surgeons obtain localizing studies. Of note, imaging studies should be used only to localize a tumor and guide a planned surgical exploration. These studies have no role in making or rejecting the diagnosis of PHPT and should not be used to clarify an uncertain diagnosis. Similarly, negative scans (which occur in about 30%) should not discourage parathyroidectomy in patients who have been determined to require parathyroidectomy. Most commonly, ultrasound and sestamibi scans are utilized. Both of these studies are associated with significant false-positive and false-negative rates and therefore should be interpreted with caution.

Thyroid and parathyroid ultrasound is highly user dependent but is positive in approximately 60% to 70% of patients with PHPT. Parathyroid adenomas appear as oval, hypoechoic masses, often with an associated feeding blood vessel. Commonly these are located medial to the carotid artery, on the posterior surface of the thyroid gland (Figure 1). Lower adenomas, which are located more anteriorly, are more likely to be seen on ultrasound than upper glands, which are deeper. Exophytic thyroid nodules, lymph nodes, and the cervical portion of the thymus gland all can be confused with parathyroid adenomas and contribute to false-positive examinations. It is important to note that neck ultrasound commonly identifies nonpalpable thyroid pathology, which should be evaluated formally before surgery.

Sestamibi scans rely on the high avidity of oxyphil cell parathyroid adenomas for sestamibi and are positive in 60% to 70% of patients with PHPT (Figure 2). On the other hand, chief cell parathyroid adenomas have almost no affinity for sestamibi and cannot be imaged using this technique. Thyroid nodules are a common cause of false-positive sestamibi results, and thus sestamibi scans are best interpreted in comparison with an ultrasound examination of the neck.

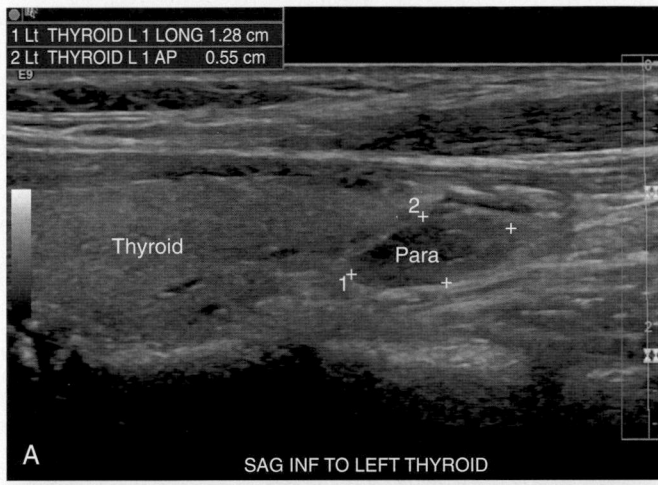

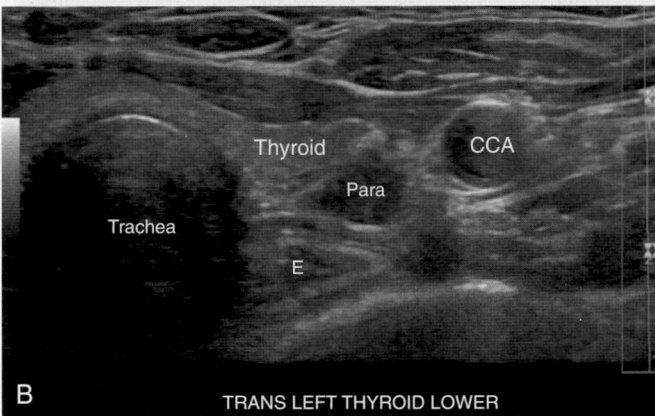

FIGURE 1 Sagittal (**A**) and transverse (**B**) ultrasound images reveal a left lower parathyroid adenoma (*Para*). *CCA*, Common carotid artery; *E*, esophagus.

Four-dimensional (4D) computed tomographic (CT) scanning is an emerging modality that combines anatomic and functional data by imaging the neck sequentially at four time periods: precontrast, immediate postcontrast, early postcontrast, and delayed postcontrast. Differences in uptake and washout characteristics of the contrast allow for distinction of adenomas from thyroid tissue and lymph nodes. Computer-generated reconstructions can provide exquisite anatomic detail that is very useful for intraoperative planning (Figure 3). Reportedly, 4D CT has a higher accuracy than sestamibi or ultrasound, although this modality is also operator dependent, as it requires an experienced radiologist to correctly interpret the images. 4D CT is used most commonly in planning for reoperative surgery but is used increasingly as a primary imaging modality.

■ MINIMALLY INVASIVE PARATHYROIDECTOMY TECHNIQUE

General Principles

MIP is based on the high likelihood that a patient with PHPT has a single adenoma as the cause of his or her disease and on our ability to frequently localize the adenoma preoperatively. Intraoperative PTH monitoring, which is meant to confirm curative resection, relies on the rapid (3- to 5-minute) half-life of PTH. It assumes that in a patient who has a single parathyroid adenoma, the remaining (normal) parathyroid glands are suppressed and therefore produce little to no PTH. Thus after the removal of the adenoma, a precipitous decline in the patient's PTH is anticipated and is highly predictive of cure. Failure of the PTH to decline can suggest the persistence of autonomous PTH release, either because of parathyroid hyperplasia or because the removed specimen was something other than a parathyroid adenoma.

Anesthetic Considerations

Although MIP can be accomplished safely under local anesthesia with sedation, many surgeons prefer general anesthesia. Supplemental cervical nerve block can decrease the narcotic and antiemetic requirements. By injecting 30 cc of a 50-50 blend of lidocaine and bupivacaine in divided portions into the area of the incision and into the anterior border of the sternocleidomastoid muscles (SCMs) bilaterally, the transverse cervical, supraclavicular, and great auricular nerves effectively are blocked. If nerve monitoring is planned, an endotracheal tube with surface electrodes should be placed to facilitate this. Because this is a clean case, antibiotics are not required, but experienced endocrine surgeons worldwide differ in their use of antimicrobial prophylaxis.

Patient Positioning and Preparation

The patient is positioned supine with the neck gently extended, arms tucked, and thumbs facing up. A shoulder roll is used to achieve neck extension, but care should be taken to avoid hyperextension, which can contribute to postoperative neck pain and migraines. It is helpful to have the operating bed's head attachment moved to the foot of the bed, thus eliminating a potential gap in the table into which the shoulder roll can slip during the operation. The head should be well supported and stabilized in a foam or gel donut.

Although most surgeons prefer the supine position with perhaps slight reverse Trendelenburg tilt, some prefer to refashion the bed into a "modified beach chair" position by tilting it fully into Trendelenburg position and then flexing the back up and feet down. This can reduce the strain to the cervical and lumbar spine, although no comparative studies of the two positions have been published to date. In both positions, the goal is to have the head slightly elevated, thereby reducing venous congestion and potentially decreasing bleeding.

Sequential compression devices are placed; chemical thromboprophylaxis is not recommended for most patients. A recent study of thyroid and parathyroid operations demonstrated that the risk for venous thromboembolism was 10 times lower than the risk for postoperative bleeding. All joints and contact surfaces are padded carefully. Even in well-localized disease, a wide surgical field including the mandible, posterior triangles of the neck, and upper chest is prepped and draped.

Optimal visualization is of paramount importance throughout parathyroidectomy in order to minimize the risk for complications. Magnifying loupes should be worn, and the field should be illuminated brightly at all times. A bloodless surgical field should be maintained scrupulously, as blood staining can interfere with visualization. Intraoperative efforts to stop bleeding must be tempered, however, as particularly in the tracheoesophageal groove imprecise maneuvers to stop bleeding inadvertently may injure a nerve or a parathyroid gland.

Incision

An anterior cervical incision is made in a convenient skin crease close to the patient's cricoid cartilage. The length of the incision is influenced by the size of the patient, the thyroid gland, and the anticipated difficulty in finding the parathyroid gland(s). In many cases an incision 3 cm or shorter suffices. It is a fallacy that a lengthy, unsightly incision is required for a four-gland exploration; most endocrine surgeons routinely "convert" from a planned MIP to a bilateral exploration without lengthening the incision. On the other hand, good visualization should never be compromised for a shorter incision length. Poor visualization may contribute to difficulty identifying a

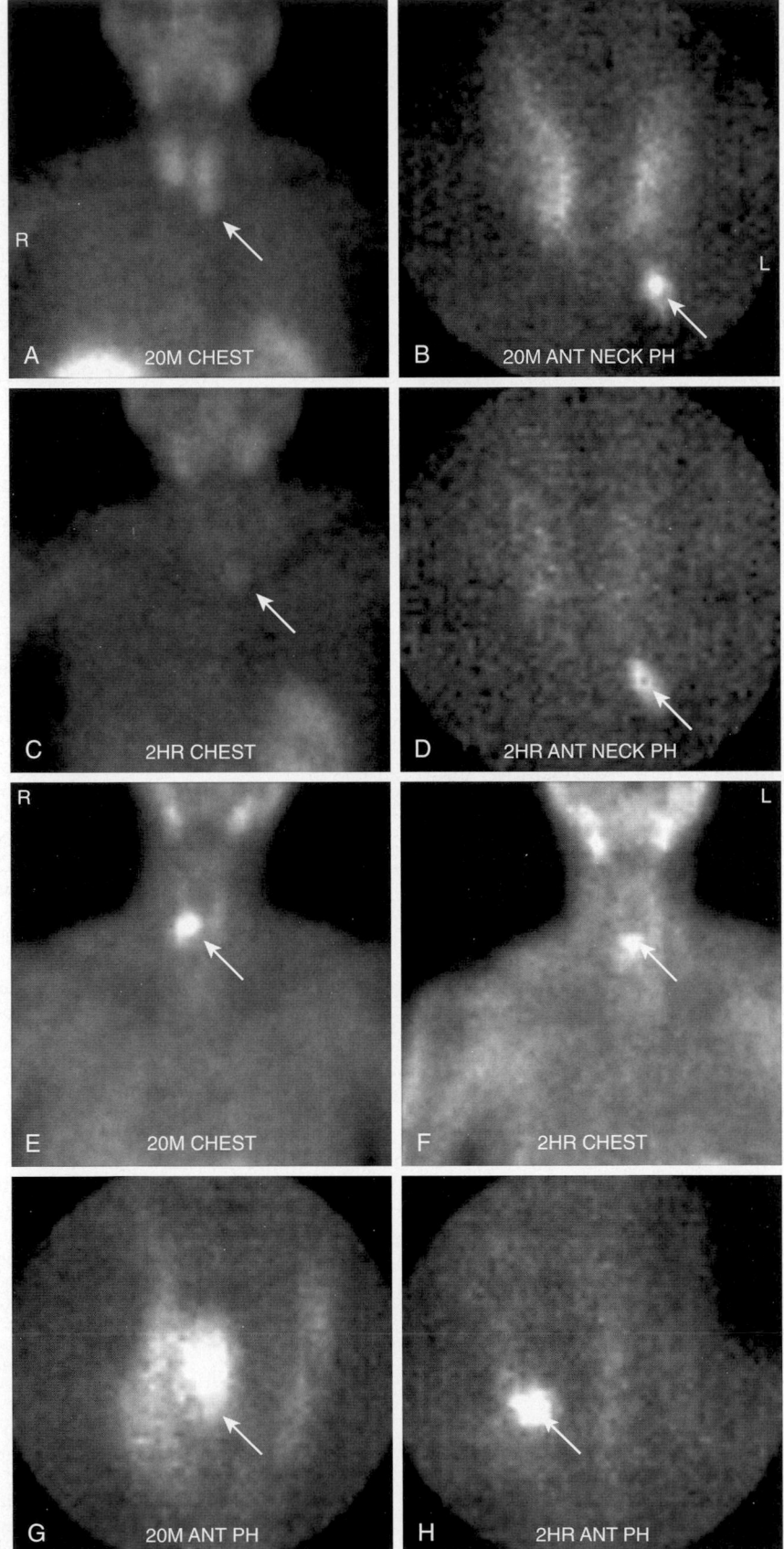

FIGURE 2 Early (**A** and **B**) and delayed (**C** and **D**) sestamibi images reveal a left lower parathyroid adenoma (*arrow*). Note the lateral position of adenoma relative to the left lobe of the thyroid. Early (**E** and **F**) and delayed (**G** and **H**) sestamibi images reveal a right upper parathyroid adenoma (*arrow*). Note the medial position of adenoma relative to the right lobe of the thyroid, best seen in **G**.

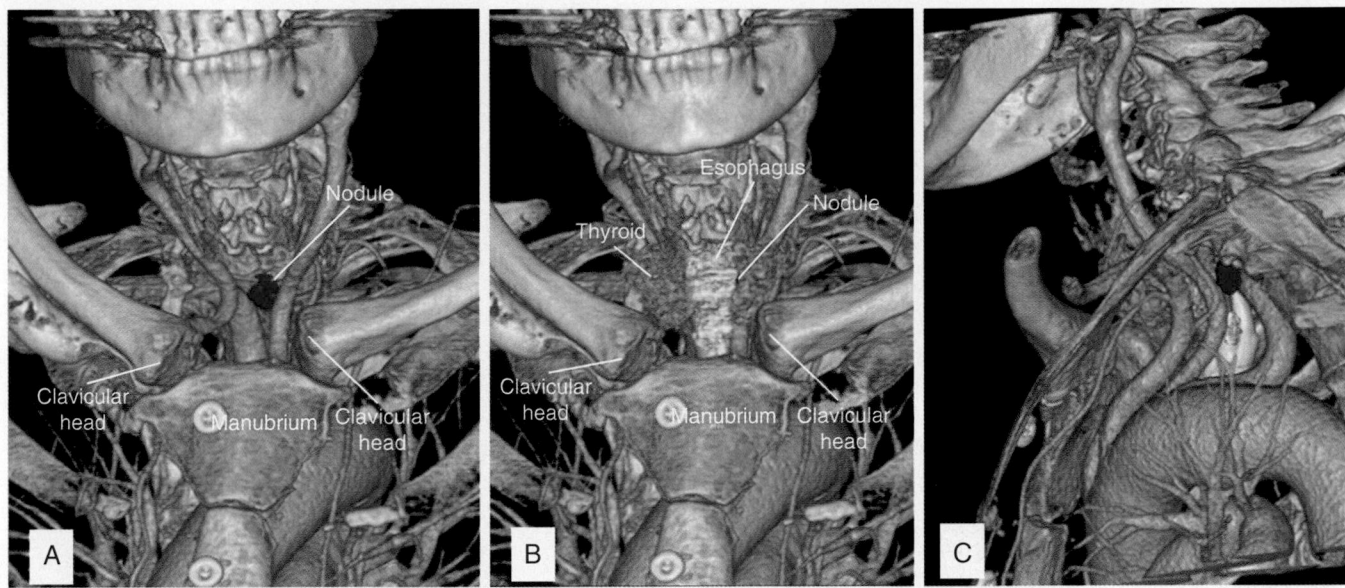

FIGURE 3 Four-dimensional computed tomographic reconstructions reveal left retroesophageal parathyroid adenoma (in blue). **A** and **B,** Anterior view. **C,** Lateral view. Thyroid lobes are in pink, and the esophagus is in yellow.

parathyroid tumor, to the diminished ability to protect surrounding structures from injury, or to the incomplete resection of a parathyroid adenoma leading to persistent or recurrent disease. In patients who do not have an optimally located skin crease, a longer incision in a skin crease is preferred over a shorter one in an area without natural folds.

Flap Elevation and Dissection of Strap Muscles

Once the skin is incised, the superior and inferior skin edges are lifted and separated with skin hooks. This facilitates the division of the platysma muscle, which is elevated easily with the skin and subcutaneous tissues from the underlying strap muscles that remain taut beneath (Figure 4, *A*). Next, the subplatysmal plane is developed, although not necessarily to the levels of the thyroid cartilage and sternal notch as is done during thyroidectomy. The skin hooks can be used to elevate the skin and platysma complex while a Kittner dissector is used to provide countertraction on the strap muscles (Figure 4, *B*). Occasionally, large anterior jugular veins are seen in this plane, and their ligation and division may facilitate the complete development of this plane.

After the subplatysmal plane is developed, a low-profile spring retractor is placed. To protect the incised skin edges from inadvertent cautery injury, the straight edge of a surgical towel is tucked under the skin edges (Figure 4, *C*). Next, the median raphe is incised. Occasionally, this is difficult to identify; it is worth noting that it is wider and therefore easier to identify caudally, near the sternal origin of the sternohyoid muscles.

The sternohyoid muscle is then dissected off of the sternothyroid in a relatively avascular plane requiring minimal or no electrocautery. When the plane between these muscles is difficult to identify, it is helpful to elevate the medial border of the sternohyoid while retracting the thyroid isthmus medially. This accentuates the groove between the two strap muscles and facilitates their separation, which should proceed laterally until the internal jugular vein is identified (Figure 4, *D*). In cases where nerve monitoring is used, the medial border of the internal jugular vein is dissected, and the vagus nerve is stimulated at this stage of the operation to ensure the baseline functional integrity of the nerve monitoring circuit and of the nerve itself.

Next, a PTH sample is obtained via direct venipuncture from the internal jugular vein using a 22-gauge needle (Figure 4, *E*). Particularly when the operation is done under local anesthesia, it is important to submerge the venipuncture site with irrigation fluid before withdrawing the needle from the vein in order to prevent air embolism. Usually this venipuncture site does not require suture repair if direct pressure is applied for a short time. Other surgeons prefer to have the levels drawn from a large bore indwelling intravenous (IV) line or an arterial line. However the sample is obtained, care should be taken to avoid hemolysis, which can result in a substantial artificial decrease in the PTH value.

Next, the sternothyroid muscle is dissected off of the thyroid gland. A Kittner dissector is used to retract the thyroid gland over the trachea while bluntly dissecting the sternothyroid muscle off of the thyroid capsule. An assistant progressively retracts the strap muscles laterally until the common carotid artery is visualized deep to the thyroid gland. Often mobilization of the sternothyroid muscle is all that is required to identify the parathyroid glands, which frequently will become apparent without any additional targeted maneuvers. Nevertheless, the discussion that follows highlights key steps in the focused identification of lower and upper parathyroid glands.

Lower Parathyroids

The lower glands are known by anatomists as the anterior parathyroids because they nearly always are located in a plane that lies anterior to the recurrent laryngeal nerve. They most commonly are located within 1 cm of the crossing of the recurrent laryngeal nerve with the inferior thyroid artery. As a result, the lower glands generally require less mobilization of the thyroid gland to identify and are sometimes visible immediately upon reflecting the sternothyroid muscle off of the thyroid gland.

Nevertheless, the lower parathyroids, derived from the third pharyngeal pouch, have a long path of descent to their final resting location. As a result of incomplete or excessive migration, ectopic "lower" glands have been identified as high as the skull base and as low as the anterior mediastinum. The most common ectopic location, accounting for 15% of all lower parathyroid adenomas, is within the cervical thymus that is also a derivative of the third pharyngeal pouch.

In cases in which a lower parathyroid is predicted and no gland is identified near the lower pole of the thyroid, the search proceeds lower in the anterior mediastinum. If thymectomy is required, the thyrothymic ligament is divided, and the cervical

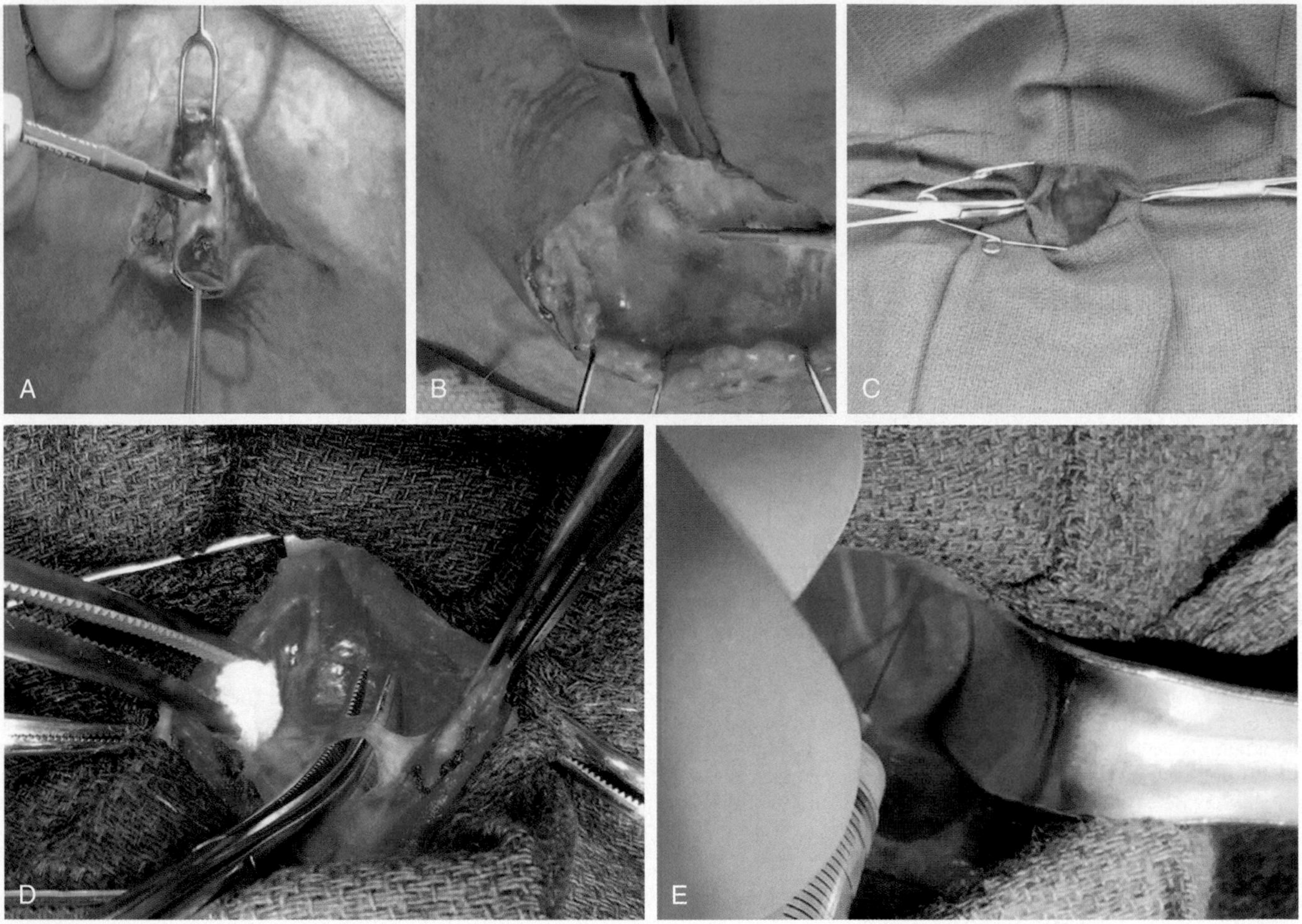

FIGURE 4 Intraoperative photographs demonstrating (**A**) deepening of incision and division of platysma and (**B**) raising the subplatysmal plane. Note the Kittner dissector pulling the strap muscle complex cephalad while dissection proceeds caudally. **C,** Placement of low-profile retractor and protection of skin edges. **D,** Separation of strap muscles. **E,** Blood draw from internal jugular vein.

portion of the thymus is grasped and retracted cephalad as the loose areolar tissues that are tethered to the thymus are pushed down. Occasional perforating vessels are clipped or divided using bipolar cautery. In this fashion, the thymus is delivered progressively, and an intrathymic parathyroid adenoma will appear as a firm, highly mobile nodule within the thymic envelope. Commonly, particularly in older patients, the cervical thymus will thin out and cleave itself. Otherwise, once sufficient thymic tissue has been mobilized to include the entire parathyroid, the cervical horn may be ligated and divided.

Upper Parathyroids

Together with the thyroid gland, the upper parathyroid glands are derived from the fourth pharyngeal pouch. These have a shorter migration path than the lower parathyroids and are therefore more consistent in their location at the posterior aspect of the thyroid gland, usually at the level of the cricoid cartilage. Anatomists refer to these as the posterior parathyroids, as they nearly always are located in a plane that is posterior to the recurrent laryngeal nerve (Figure 5). These glands are often deep behind the thyroid gland and require fairly extensive anterior mobilization of the thyroid to be identified. Rarely, the division of the middle thyroid vein or the opening of the space of Reeves between the upper pole of the thyroid and the cricothyroid muscle is necessary to mobilize the upper pole of the thyroid sufficiently to identify these glands.

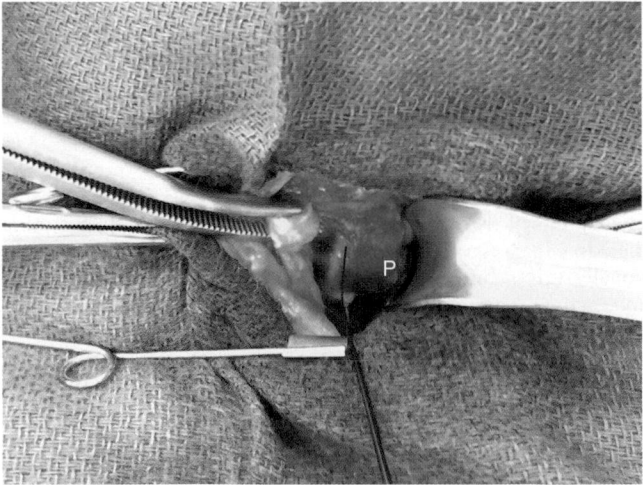

FIGURE 5 Intraoperative photo of left upper parathyroid adenoma and the left recurrent laryngeal nerve immediately overlying it, pointed to by black probe tip. The left lobe of the thyroid is being retracted by the Kittner dissector.

Enlarged upper adenomas frequently descend deep in the tracheoesophageal groove to assume a final position that is caudal and deep to the normal lower parathyroid gland. This is one potential cause for failed MIP, because in this context imaging studies easily can confuse a descended upper gland with a lower gland. Of note, on sestamibi scans, upper glands can be identified by their more medial location relative to the ipsilateral lobe of the thyroid gland, whereas lower glands assume a more lateral position. The most common ectopic locations for upper parathyroid glands include the retroesophageal region and the carotid sheath.

Intrathyroidal parathyroid adenomas occur in approximately 1% of patients with PHPT and tend to be smaller than nonintrathyroidal glands. The presence of a hypoechoic oval nodule on thyroid ultrasound should alert the surgeon to the possibility of this entity, and sestamibi scanning with single-photon emission computed tomographic (SPECT) imaging or 4D CT also may be helpful in this context. A preoperative or intraoperative fine-needle aspiration (sent for PTH level, not cytology) can confirm the diagnosis. A preoperative thyroid ultrasound that demonstrates no thyroid nodules allows the surgeon to omit thyroid lobectomy in the search for a missing gland.

Parathyroid Localization

In cases where a parathyroid gland remains elusive, it is often helpful to reflect on the gland that has been found already and its relationship with the recurrent laryngeal nerve. If the gland that was identified already is in a location anterior to the nerve, a more comprehensive search is undertaken for the upper gland, concentrating on the region of the tracheoesophageal groove, with extension of the field to include the retropharyngeal and retroesophageal spaces both above and below the thyroid gland. In cases where the lower gland is missing (i.e., the identified gland is posterior to the nerve), the search should focus on the area of thyrothymic ligament, thymus, and the accessible portion of the superior mediastinum. In all cases of a missing parathyroid, the carotid sheath is opened and explored from the root of the neck to the skull base. If thyroid nodules are present on ultrasound, thyroid lobectomy should be done. Proximal ligation of the inferior thyroid artery has not been demonstrated to be curative but could be tried. Median sternotomy is not indicated unless the operation is being performed for life-threatening hypercalcemia. In the majority of revisional parathyroidectomies, the "missing parathyroid" eventually will be found in a normal anatomic position. Therefore after this progression, even if the gland has not been found, the operation should be concluded, and the patient should be reimaged and planed for revisional surgery.

Lateral Approach

The lateral approach to the parathyroids can be taken either through a Kocher-type skin incision or through a lateral incision centered on the anterior border of the SCM. Regardless of the skin incision, the subplatysmal plane is developed, and after this the anterior border of the SCM is dissected. Then the plane between the anterior border of the SCM and the strap muscle and thyroid complex is entered, retracting the SCM and carotid artery laterally and the strap muscles and thyroid gland medially. It is imperative to keep the dissection medial to the carotid artery, which tends to slip medially from under the retractor and confuse the dissection field. This approach offers a very direct access to the tracheoesophageal groove and in my view is mostly useful in redo cases where the gland is well localized and is an upper gland. The main advantage of this approach is also its greatest weakness: The direct access to the tracheoesophageal groove means that the parathyroid can be identified more directly, but it also means that the recurrent laryngeal nerve is encountered much more rapidly than when the central approach is used. Because this approach leads so directly to the deep aspect of the tracheoesophageal groove, it takes extra effort to expose and remove a lower parathyroid, which often is located in a more anterior plane. Finally, this approach is less practical in cases where bilateral exploration may be required.

Radioguidance

Some surgeons utilize radioguidance to facilitate the intraoperative localization of parathyroid adenomas. For this technique, 10 mCi of technetium (^{99m}Tc) sestamibi is injected 1 to 3 hours before surgery. Background counts are obtained at the level of the thyroid isthmus, and then the parathyroid gland is localized and a small transverse incision is made over it. Subplatysmal planes are raised, and the straps are separated in the midline. A gamma probe can be used to guide dissection trajectory, recognizing that the heart and salivary glands also concentrate ^{99m}Tc sestamibi, which can lead to false-positive results with deep probing. When the adenoma is identified, in vivo counts are obtained; these are usually 150% above the counts at the isthmus. The adenoma then is removed and placed on the tip of the gamma probe to obtain ex vivo counts. Counts greater than 20% of background confirm the presence of parathyroid tissue in the resected specimen.

Minimally Invasive Video-Assisted Parathyroidectomy (MIVAP)

For this technique, a 15-mm incision is made in a skin crease about 2 cm above the sternal notch. Through a 12-mm trocar placed deep to the strap muscles, the field is gently insufflated to 12 mm Hg. The trocar is removed, small retractors are placed, and a 5-mm, 30-degree endoscope is used to facilitate the dissection around the thyroid, which is gasless. The dissection is done using very thin instruments, and vessels are ligated using small clips. The parathyroid is dissected circumferentially and removed.

Intraoperative Parathyroid Hormone (IOPTH) Monitoring

PTH samples should be drawn just before removing the suspected adenoma and at 5 and 10 minutes postexcision. Some surgeons also draw a sample at 15 minutes postexcision. Most surgeons are careful to restrict dissection in the tracheoesophageal groove to prevent stimulation of the remaining parathyroid glands, although theoretically manipulation of normal and suppressed glands should not result in significant release of PTH. Although there are at least six published criteria for IOPTH monitoring during parathyroidectomy, all rely on a precipitous decline in PTH after resection of a solitary adenoma. It is important to recognize that as more restrictive criteria are used, both the positive predictive value and the false-negative rates increase. In other words, if the most strict criterion is used (50% drop from baseline and normalization of PTH at 10 minutes postexcision), the chance of cure when PTH drops sufficiently is very high, but there will also be several patients whose PTH declines more slowly who would undergo unnecessary additional exploration. Conversely, looser criteria (such as a 50% drop from the highest PTH recorded intraoperatively) are associated with a lower false-negative rate, but the likelihood of persistent or recurrent disease after meeting these criteria (i.e., false positive) is higher.

It should be emphasized that the published guidelines should not be regarded as absolute requirements. The operating surgeon should consider the change in PTH as one factor in the context of the risk that the patient may have multigland disease. Other intraoperative factors should include the size and consistency of the resected parathyroid gland and whether the ipsilateral parathyroid has been identified and its size. The absolute value of the final PTH level is also a factor; a final level greater than 40 pg/mL has been suggested to be associated with a higher risk of recurrence. Preoperative risk factors for multigland disease include a family history of PHPT, a history of lithium use, and a history of multiple endocrine neoplasia.

Closure

After the extraction of the specimen and confirmation of an appropriate drop in PTH, the field is inspected for hemostasis. Topical hemostatic agents and drains have not been shown to reduce the incidence of hematoma, but these can be used at the surgeon's discretion.

The strap and platysma muscles are closed using simple interrupted absorbable suture, taking care to leave gaps between sutures so as to allow a potential hematoma a means of egress to the more superficial layers of the neck. Although some surgeons close the straps in layers, others omit reapproximating the sternothyroid muscle. Dermabond is applied as a sterile dressing, and the subcuticular stitch can be removed.

Postoperative care instructions include elevation of the head to decrease venous pooling in the neck, ice to the neck to induce vasoconstriction, and frequent examinations of the neck to ensure that no hematoma is forming. The required length of stay after parathyroidectomy remains controversial, although many patients are discharged on the day of surgery. PTH level is checked routinely 2 to 3 hours postoperatively and if undetectable may prompt the addition of Rocaltrol (calcitriol) to the discharge medications. Of note, an undetectable PTH level after a bilateral operation should prompt admission and stabilization of calcium levels on oral agents.

Postparathyroidectomy discharge instructions include routine wound care instructions, observation for hematoma, and instructions regarding the signs and symptoms of hypocalcemia, including perioral numbness and tingling and muscle cramps in the hands and feet. Most patients are prescribed calcium supplements, although there is no evidence that this accelerates or augments bone strength gains after surgery.

■ CONCLUSION

Parathyroidectomy is the second most commonly performed endocrine operation, and most procedures are done using the MIP approach. This operation is performed with excellent results and with minimal morbidity in both inpatient and outpatient settings, but failures do occur. It is worth noting that there is considerable variation among surgeons and practices in the indications for MIP, the conduct of the operation, and postoperative care. Hopefully, with high-quality data from prospectively collected, robust databases, our management of patients with PHPT will become less variable and outcomes will continue to improve.

SUGGESTED READINGS

Bilezikian JP, Brandi ML, Eastell R, Silverberg SJ, Udelsman R, Marcocci C, Potts JT Jr. Guidelines for the management of asymptomatic primary hyperparathyroidism: summary statement from the Fourth International Workshop. *J Clin Endocrinol Metab.* 2014;99:3561-3569.

Clark OH, Duh QY. Primary hyperparathyroidism: a surgical perspective. *Endocrinol Metab Clin North Am.* 1989;18:701-714.

Greene AB, Butler RS, McIntyre S, et al. National trends in parathyroid surgery from 1998 to 2008: a decade of change. *J Am Coll Surg.* 2009;209:332-343.

Iannuzzi JC, Choi DX, Farkas RL, Ruan DT, Peacock JL, Moalem J. Surgeon beware: many patients referred for parathyroidectomy are misdiagnosed with primary hyperparathyroidism. *Surgery.* 2012;152:635-642.

James BC, Kaplan EL, Grogan RH, Angelos P. What's in a name? Providing clarity in the definition of minimally invasive parathyroidectomy. *World J Surg.* 2015;39:975-980.

Miccoli P, et al. Minimally invasive video-assisted parathyroidectomy: lesson learned from 137 cases. *J Am Coll Surg.* 2000;191:613-618.

Pasieka JL, Parsons LL, Demeure MJ, et al. Patient-based surgical outcome tool demonstrating alleviation of symptoms following parathyroidectomy in patients with primary hyperparathyroidism. *World J Surg.* 2002;26:942-949.

Perrier ND, Balachandran D, Wefel JS, et al. Prospective, randomized, controlled trial of parathyroidectomy versus observation in patients with "asymptomatic" primary hyperparathyroidism. *Surgery.* 2009;146:1116-1122.

Rubin MR, Bilezikian JP, McMahon DJ, et al. The natural history of primary hyperparathyroidism with or without parathyroid surgery after 15 years. *J Clin Endocrinol Metab.* 2008;93:3462-3470.

Silberfein EJ, et al. Reoperative parathyroidectomy: location of missed glands based on a contemporary nomenclature system. *Arch Surg.* 2010;145:1065-1068.

Udelsman R, Åkerström G, Biagini C, Duh Q-Y, Miccoli P, Niederle B, Tonelli F. The surgical management of asymptomatic primary hyperparathyroidism: proceedings of the Fourth International Workshop. *J Clin Endocrinol Metab.* 2014;99:3595-3606.

LAPAROSCOPIC LIVER RESECTION

Russell C. Langan, MD, Anthony M. Villano, MD, Reena Jha, MD, Jay A. Graham, MD, and Lynt B. Johnson, MD, MBA

Minimally invasive surgery (MIS) has allowed surgeons to bridge the gap between technique and improved outcomes and as such should be in the armamentarium of the hepato-pancreato-biliary (HPB) surgeon. Understandably, since Dr. Azagra performed the first minimally invasive anatomic segmentectomy in 1993, the HPB community has remained cautious in adopting these techniques. Concerns that centered on patient safety because of a perceived lack of hemostatic control and nonadherence to accepted oncologic principles tempered initial enthusiasm. However, after 20 years of experience and excellent outcomes, minimally invasive liver surgery now has emerged as an operative alternative to the open approach, with safe short-term outcomes and comparable oncologic benefit. Moreover, although HPB surgeons were late to embrace minimally invasive techniques, there has been a paradigm shift within the field as fears regarding heightened patient morbidity largely have been dismissed.

Given the advances in minimally invasive technology and increased surgeon experience, we believe that laparoscopic liver resections, both major and minor, can be performed safely and effectively. Devices such as endostaplers and electrothermal dissectors have afforded the ability to perform parenchymal dissections with minimal blood loss. In addition, hand-assisted devices have allowed the surgeon to regain tactile feedback, haptic manipulation of the liver, and the ability to manually compress bleeding vasculature. The sum of these advances has translated to the current performance of both major and minor liver resections laparoscopically. Furthermore, certain HPB groups have published small volume series on the completion of complex resections involving the posterior segments or resections of masses encompassing major vasculature structures using minimally invasive procedures. Although currently performed only by centers that specialize in such approaches, the popularity and use of minimally invasive liver surgery likely will continue to grow. As such, it has become increasingly important for all physicians to be well versed in the techniques and nuances of this approach.

■ ADVANTAGES AND DISADVANTAGES OF THE MINIMALLY INVASIVE APPROACH

Minimally invasive HPB surgery represents one of the most advanced applications for laparoscopic surgery currently in use. Recent literature has demonstrated the safety, feasibility, and adequacy of minimally invasive HPB surgery. When performed at experienced centers, these procedures carry patient morbidity and mortality rates comparable to their open variants. Current data of more than 3000 laparoscopic hepatic resections, including both major and minor procedures, have reported morbidity rates of 10.5% and a mortality rate of 0.3%. Predictably, advantages of the minimally invasive approach mirror those afforded by other laparoscopic procedures.

First, in nearly all published studies comparing MIS with an open approach, length of stay has been found to be statistically less and at times up to half as long. Surprisingly, despite fears of an inability to control intraoperative hemorrhage, most studies have cited lower volumes of blood loss laparoscopically. This may be explained by heightened visualization with the laparoscopic camera in conjunction with the tamponade effect of pneumoperitoneum.

Return to oral intake is notably faster as well, with mean return to first meal averaging 1 to 2 days sooner than patients undergoing open resections. Postoperative pain control is a difficult metric to measure because of both the variability in the way individual patients experience pain and the difficulty in quantifying pain control. However, it has been cited often as a benefit to MIS in general. Among a small number of studies assessing this parameter in liver resections, the trend has been a lower requirement for narcotics postoperatively, as would be expected with the avoidance of a laparotomy incision.

Studies assessing operative time have generated mixed results, reporting both longer and shorter stays in the operating room (OR) with a laparoscopic approach. This may reflect both surgeon experience and the choice of instruments and technique for parenchymal dissection; the latter point refers to shorter operative times cited in those series utilizing serial firings of an endostapler rather than endothermal devices or ultrasonic surgical aspirators. Of note, when our own group assessed operative time, we found no significant difference between the hybrid and open approaches (Figure 1).

Finally, there is a large volume of data reporting similar oncologic outcomes with either approach when performed for malignant disease. To date, nearly all retrospective trials have reported no significant difference in 3-year and 5-year overall survival; disease-free survival when comparing minimally invasive with open hepatic resection for hepatocellular carcinoma or colorectal cancer metastases is also similar. Rates of positive surgical margins also have been shown to be similar among the majority of published studies, with a few groups having demonstrated fewer positive margins when utilizing a minimally invasive approach. Arguably, this finding may reflect a bias toward performing laparoscopic resections in lesions that are less complicated to resect; however, equivalence of both techniques has been illustrated clearly.

The most notable disadvantage of the laparoscopic approach is the clear requirement of advanced hepatobiliary training and minimally invasive operative experience to perform these procedures safely. The learning curve of laparoscopic liver resection approaches approximately 40 to 75 cases to become proficient in the technique. Feasibly, this is accomplished only at high-volume, specialized centers that are already well imbued with experience in HPB surgery. Increased cost also has been cited as another concern with MIS. In general, increased cost can be related to the disposable instruments and specialized devices required. That being said, although undeniably more costly in the OR, multiple groups have demonstrated comparable if not diminished total hospital costs secondary to shorter lengths of stay and fewer nonoperative costs to the patient. Other limitations are largely controversial and include difficulties with controlling catastrophic bleeding and potential for air embolism.

We believe that the hybrid technique or hand-assisted technique, as described later, is an excellent bridge between the truly laparoscopic procedure and the traditional open approach. In brief, the hybrid approach allows for hepatic mobilization and often the hilar dissection to be performed laparoscopically, and then the parenchymal division is performed in a standard fashion via a small hand-port incision. Our group, along with others, has shown that the marked advantages of purely laparoscopic abdominal procedures, such as reduced surgical pain, improved cosmesis, and shortened hospital stays, are preserved in the hand-assisted techniques, which also provide further levels of safety.

■ INDICATIONS AND CONTRAINDICATIONS

As experience has grown, the indications for MIS have broadened over the last 2 decades. Although originally performed mainly for

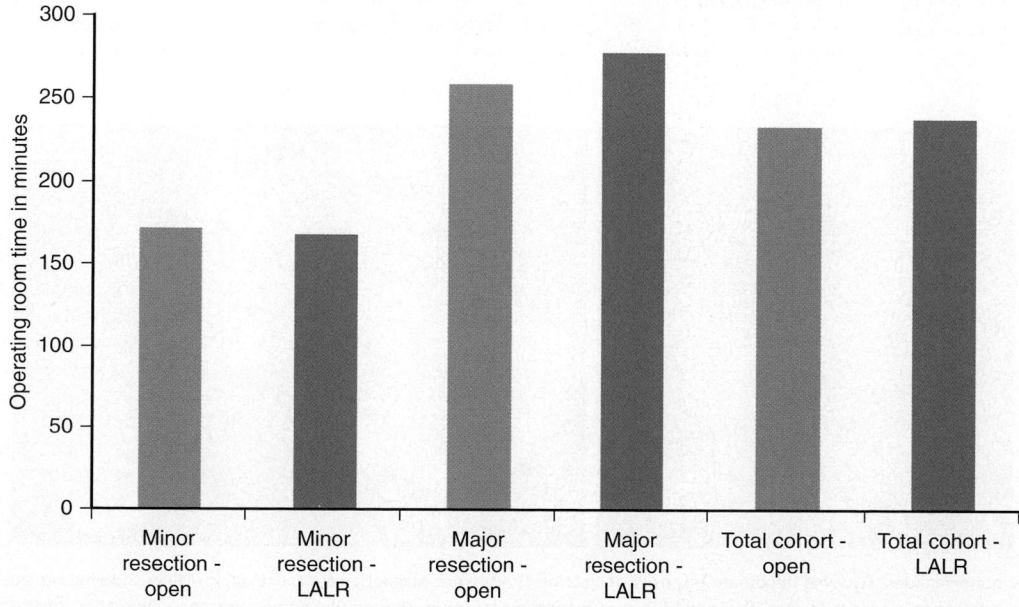

FIGURE 1 Mean operating room time, open approach versus laparoscopic-assisted liver resection (LALR).

benign and peripheral lesions, now approximately half of all laparoscopic resections are performed for malignant disease. To this effect, the pathologic indications for MIS essentially parallel those of the open approach. Lesions *most* amenable to MIS include those less than 5 cm in diameter, pedunculated lesions of any size, or lesions located in segments 2 to 6 of the liver. However, there are no absolute tumor characteristics that contraindicate the laparoscopic approach. Relative contraindications include large posterior tumors (>5 cm in diameter), lesions of the hepatic dome (i.e., segments 7 and 8), lesions located in the vicinity of major vasculature, severe portal hypertension, severe coagulopathy, poor cardiopulmonary reserve, potential need for vascular or biliary reconstruction, and prior hepatic resection or abdominal surgery (Box 1).

Particularly notable is prior hepatic resection, as several studies have demonstrated the feasibility of a minimally invasive approach after both prior laparoscopic and prior open surgeries, including prior hepatic resections. In an era in which repeat metastasectomies for colorectal cancer or various other malignant primaries have become popular, this is an increasingly common scenario. Although technically more challenging, there have been no reports of increased morbidity or worse oncologic outcomes. Conversion to open surgery in these cases should not be seen as a failure but rather as a necessary consequence of complex HPB surgery in a complex patient population.

■ PREOPERATIVE EVALUATION

Critical to the success of a minimally invasive liver resection is the careful selection of appropriate operative candidates. After a thorough history and physical examination, all patients under

BOX 1: Relative Contraindications to Laparoscopic Liver Resection

Relative Contraindications to the Pure Laparoscopic Approach

Large, nonpedunculated tumors (>5 cm in diameter)
Lesions of the hepatic dome (segments 7 or 8)
Lesions located in close proximity to major vasculature
Severe portal hypertension
Severe coagulopathy
Potential need for vascular or biliary reconstruction
Prior hepatic resection or intra-abdominal surgery
Poor cardiopulmonary reserve

consideration for liver resection should obtain basic laboratory testing. Prudent studies include a complete blood cell (CBC) count, chemistries, liver panel, coagulation panel, and blood typing. These values generate an overall idea of liver function and allow for determination of the Child-Turcotte-Pugh (CTP) score to estimate perioperative risks after a liver resection in those with cirrhosis. Thrombocytopenia, coagulopathy, renal dysfunction, and CTP class B or C are particularly concerning findings that may alter the patient's candidacy for surgery. Other studies should be tailored to the individual patient. It is important to note that patients subsequently should be risk stratified for cardiopulmonary disease and undergo appropriate workup according to the most recent American Heart Association guidelines.

■ PREOPERATIVE IMAGING

Cross-sectional imaging is of paramount importance to the hepatobiliary surgeon. Computed tomography (CT) or magnetic resonance imaging (MRI) is used to evaluate for diffuse and focal disease and assess anatomy for operative planning. CT is not only fast and reliable but also more likely than other modalities to detect extrahepatic lesions. In addition, CT offers better spatial resolution and as such is better at defining fine detail, such as vascular detail. However, MRI has better contrast resolution and enables radiologists to detect and characterize even smaller hepatic lesions that may be missed by CT. It is our practice to ensure that patients obtain either a triple-phase CT of the liver with thin cuts (a minimum of 3 mm) or an MRI with contrast (with or without Eovist depending on the pathology).

The viability of the remnant liver after resection requires adequate inflow (hepatic arteries and portal veins) and outflow (hepatic veins), all of which can be assessed using modern imaging techniques. CT or magnetic resonance angiography or venography with conventional intravenous contrast is useful in depicting variants in vascular anatomy that may alter surgical complexity (e.g., vascular reconstruction). The anatomy of the hepatic arterial and venous systems is variable, and the classic anatomy is found in only 55% and 60% of patients, respectively. Image postprocessing is used to generate three-dimensional (3D) images that are used to estimate liver volume and to map the vascular and biliary anatomy for surgical planning (Figure 2). Magnetic resonance cholangiopancreatography (MRCP) can be used to evaluate bile duct anatomy without the aid of contrast agents (Figure 3).

The detection of cirrhosis, fatty infiltration, iron deposition, or other diffuse diseases may alter the patient's management and differential diagnosis. In the setting of cirrhosis, appropriate detection and characterization of liver lesions are required to best triage the

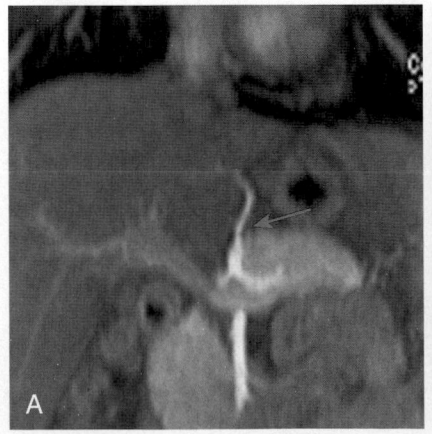 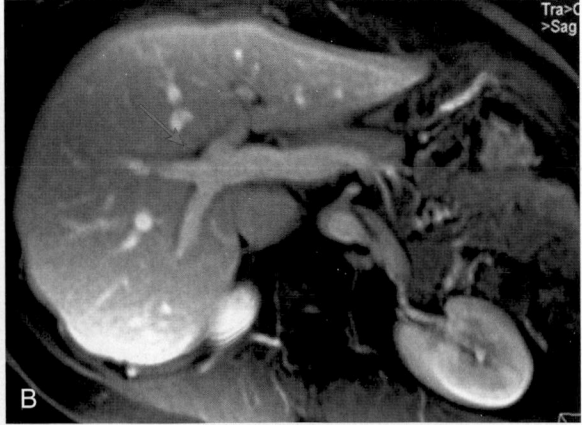

FIGURE 2 Vascular abnormalities. **A,** Axial maximum intensity projection (MIP) from magnetic resonance angiography showing replaced left hepatic artery arising from the left gastric artery (*arrow*). **B,** Axial MIP from magnetic resonance venography demonstrates a trifurcation of the main portal vein (*arrow*).

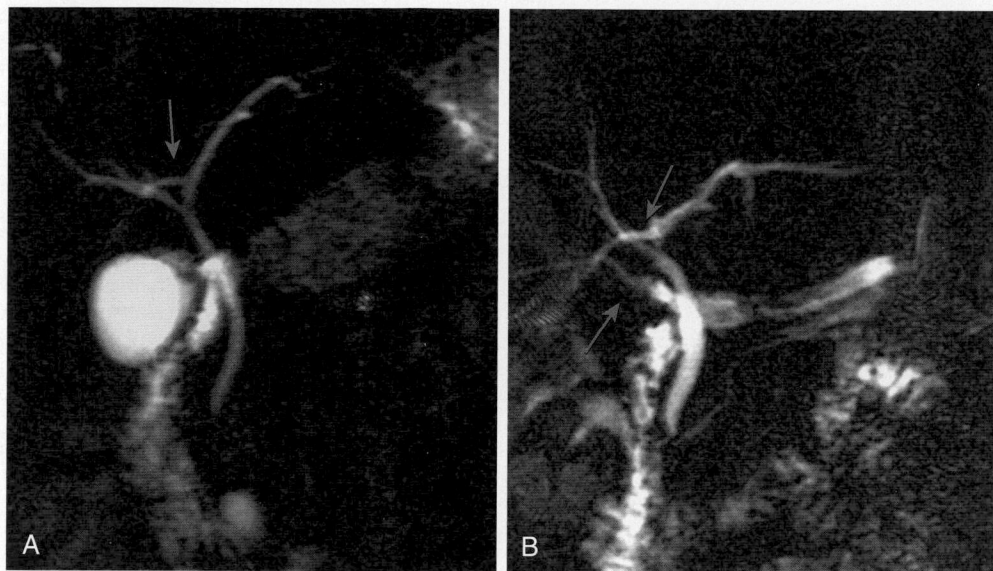

FIGURE 3 Magnetic resonance cholangiopancreatography (MRCP). **A,** Coronal projection MRCP shows an aberrant posterior right hepatic duct draining into the proximal left duct (*arrow*). **B,** Coronal projection MRCP shows an accessory right hepatic duct and aberrant right hepatic duct (*arrows*) draining into the proximal left duct.

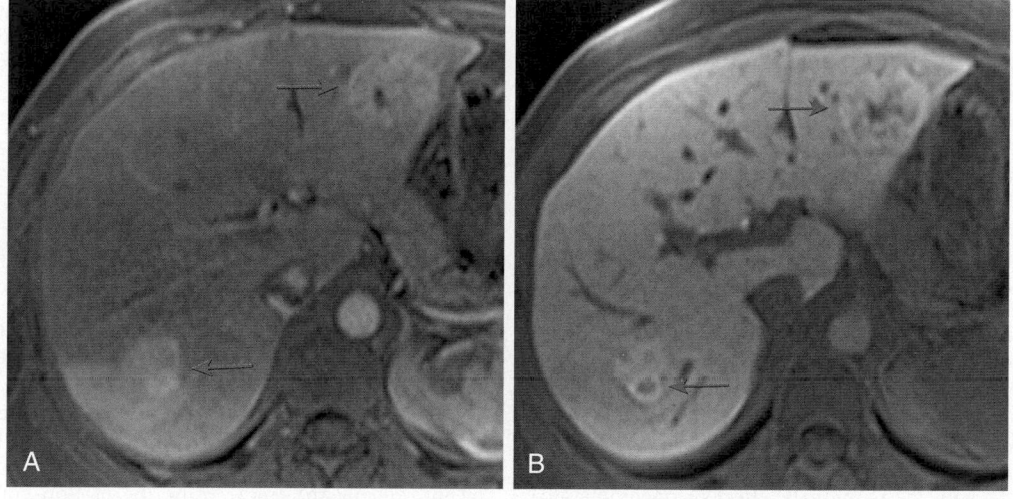

FIGURE 4 Gadoxetate disodium (Eovist) for characterization of the incidental hypervascular liver lesions. **A,** Arterial phase axial magnetic resonance image demonstrating two hypervascular liver lesions (*arrows*), one in segment 7 and the other in segments 2 and 3. **B,** On 20-minute hepatocellular phase both lesions take up contrast (*arrows*), most consistent with focal nodular hyperplasia.

patient to minimally invasive liver resection or other treatments such as ablative therapies and transplantation. The presence of portal hypertension, as demonstrated by the presence of varices, splenomegaly, and ascites, may alter both surgical approach and prognosis. The use of hepatocellular agents, such as gadolinium-ethoxybenzyl-diethylenetriamine pentaacetic acid (gadoxetate disodium), on MRI has improved the detection of focal liver lesions. Gadoxetic acid (Eovist) is specifically taken up by hepatocytes using the same molecular mechanism as bile acid. It is eliminated from the body in equal quantities by the biliary and urinary systems. This enables imaging of the hepatobiliary phase, when the normal hepatocytes and the biliary system show strong enhancement at approximately 20 minutes after the contrast media injection. MRI using gadoxetic acid increases the degree of confidence in a focal nodular hyperplasia (FNH) diagnosis (Figure 4). On the other hand, metastatic lesions do not have the ability to take up gadoxetate disodium and typically will appear hypointense during the hepatobiliary phase. Of note, there has been

a growing body of evidence showing that the use of gadoxetate disodium yields increased accuracy compared with contrast-enhanced CT in the detection of colorectal carcinoma hepatic metastases by accentuating the liver to lesion contrast.

■ INTRAOPERATIVE ANESTHESIA AND RELATED CONCERNS

Liver resection requires clear communication among the surgical and anesthesia teams. As such, operative success is built on a firm understanding of liver physiology, pathology, and systemic responses to both anesthesia and operative maneuvers.

Intraoperative monitoring should be visible to both the anesthesia and the surgical teams throughout a liver resection, whether an open or minimally invasive approach is used. Derangements in blood pressure or volumetric status may occur swiftly, especially during large volume blood loss or Pringle's maneuver. Standard monitoring for major resections should include an arterial line, a central line for central venous pressure (CVP) measurement, and a Foley catheter. CVP should be maintained at the low end of normal to minimize bleeding from the cut surface of the liver. Pringle's maneuvers are well tolerated when performed intermittently (5 to 10 minutes). Specific techniques of inflow control vary widely with surgeon preference, but 75 minutes of Pringle's maneuver after 15 minutes of ischemic preconditioning has been demonstrated to be safe, without an increase in postoperative liver injury. The most unique physiologic changes with respect to laparoscopy are those directly related to pneumoperitoneum. An intra-abdominal pressure of approximately 12 to 15 mm Hg is standard practice. Notably, this is well tolerated by most patients. Particular attention must be paid to patients who have pre-existing cardiopulmonary disease, as these individuals may not have the physiologic reserve available to tolerate the associated cardiopulmonary effects of pneumoperitoneum.

Various cardiovascular changes occur with pneumoperitoneum. Increased mean arterial pressure and systemic vascular resistance are nearly universal and occur as a result of the neuroendocrine response to intra-abdominal distension. Changes to venous return and cardiac output are variable depending on the reserve of the patient. In an otherwise healthy individual, cardiac output and ventricular filling pressures are unaffected. By contrast, a compromised ejection fraction at baseline may result in decreased cardiac output, as the diminished venous return from pneumoperitoneum is not well compensated for. There is also an increased risk of cardiac arrhythmia, which is thought to occur secondary to carbon dioxide irritation of the myocardium. It is imperative to be alert to hypotension due to pneumoperitoneum in the setting of low CVP used in liver resections. Simple release of pneumoperitoneum with infusion volume is generally all that is necessary to convert the situation. Blood pressure also can be maintained if necessary with the use of small amounts of vasoconstrictors.

Pulmonary changes also are directly related to increased abdominal pressure and decreased functional reserve capacity, which translates across the diaphragm to increased intrathoracic pressure. Reduced lung volumes equate to ventilation-perfusion mismatching and an increased alveolar-arterial oxygen gradient. These changes are well tolerated in the patient with adequate pulmonary reserve and again highlight the need for vigilant preoperative cardiopulmonary workup in those patients who may harbor underlying dysfunction.

In addition to a generalized increase in systemic vascular resistance, the HPB surgeon should be aware of the notable changes to regional blood flow. Advantageously, there is a decrease in splanchnic blood flow with concomitant decrease in portal venous inflow to the liver. In conjunction with the tamponade effect of pneumoperitoneum, hemostasis is attained more readily during parenchymal transection. Renal perfusion is similarly diminished, which puts the patient at higher risk of intraoperative and postoperative renal dysfunction. As such, a Foley catheter is always recommended to accurately gauge adequate urine output. Finally, decreased venous flow via the deep system of the lower extremities puts the patient at increased risk of venous thromboembolism (VTE). Use of mechanical VTE prophylaxis is of paramount importance for every case when possible. The decision to use chemical VTE prophylaxis must be weighed against the particular patient's risk for bleeding and the extent of the planned resection.

■ OPERATIVE TECHNIQUES

Numerous methods of laparoscopic resection have gained popularity with increased sharing and collaboration in the surgical community. Recognizing the diversity of these laparoscopic liver techniques, a panel of 45 well-known HPB surgeons worked to establish a standard classification system and summarize a unified position statement on safety and efficacy of laparoscopic liver resection. This panel of experts agreed on the terms *pure laparoscopy, hand-assisted,* and *hybrid technique* to describe the various approaches.

Pure Laparoscopy
General Principles

Pure laparoscopy commonly is used for wedge resections of anterior lesions of the liver or masses located in the left lateral segment. However, more recently it has been utilized for major lobe resections as well. Access is gained into the abdomen, depending on the surgeon's preference, and an infraumbilical trocar is placed. Safe trocar insertion is of paramount importance, and therefore our preference is a Hasson approach to entry. Viscus perforation and vasculature laceration can occur as a result of unintended and uncontrolled insertion. Although these injuries happen infrequently, significant morbidity, including death, can result. In addition, when performing liver surgery in patients with portal hypertension one must be cognizant of a patent umbilical vein, thus an infraumbilical placement avoids puncture of a recanalized umbilical vein. If using the Veress technique, the most reliable way to prevent initial trocar placement injury is macrobracing. This technique involves the use of the non-dominant hand to counter the loss of resistance as the trocar tip penetrates the fascia and peritoneum. The remaining trocars should then be inserted under direct visualization in the same manner.

After insufflation, one technique is to move the patient into reverse Trendelenburg position to enable sighting of the hilar structures and to position the small bowel in the lower abdomen and pelvis. At times, angling the OR table and patient left or right side down (depending on the target lobe) may facilitate visualization. In addition, a split leg position may be beneficial at times, with the surgeon standing between the patient's legs. Lastly, for certain right-sided lesions, placing the patient in a left lateral decubitus position may be of benefit. Trocars then are placed under direct visualization to facilitate triangulation of the intended surgery site. Here, laparoscopic ultrasound is of great use to determine the relationship of the mass to major vasculature and biliary structures. Lesions on the liver surface may be wedged out with the use of laparoscopic adaptations of the Harmonic scalpel (Ethicon Endo-Surgery, Cincinnati, OH), LigaSure (Covidien, Boulder, CO), Enseal (Ethicon Endo-Surgery, Cincinnati, OH), or any other bipolar energy or thermal devices.

Laparoscopic Left Lateral Sectionectomy

Access is gained into the abdomen, depending on the surgeon's preference, and an infraumbilical trocar is placed. Great care must be taken when inserting trocars intra-abdominally because of the inherent potential for vascular or viscus injury. The periumbilical trocar placement can be particularly risky because of its larger size and the relatively blind nature of insertion (this possibility can be minimized by introducing the trocar using the Hasson cutdown technique). After safe insufflation of the abdomen, the operation begins with mobilization of the liver after positioning the patient in slight reverse Trendelenburg. We prefer a 30-degree laparoscope. In addition, angling the OR table may facilitate visualization. In addition, some prefer to have the patient positioned in a split leg position and operate from between the legs. After port placement (Figure 5), the liver is explored with the laparoscopic ultrasound to clarify tumor characteristics (size and relation to vasculature), detect additional lesions, and assess the feasibility of continuing with a laparoscopic technique. If proceeding, the liver should be mobilized fully and the ligamentum teres, falciform, and left triangular and coronary ligaments divided using thermal energy. The falciform should be divided to the level of the diaphragm and insertion of the hepatic veins into the inferior vena cava.

Before further dissection, the porta hepatis should be encircled with Pringle's maneuver. This is accomplished after division of the gastrohepatic ligament with thermal energy. One should be mindful of arterial variances, and care should be taken during this step to assess for a replaced left hepatic artery arising from the left gastric artery traveling in the pars flaccida. After this, a Penrose drain should be placed around the porta hepatis to be used as a tourniquet. Pringle's maneuver should not yet be applied and should be implemented

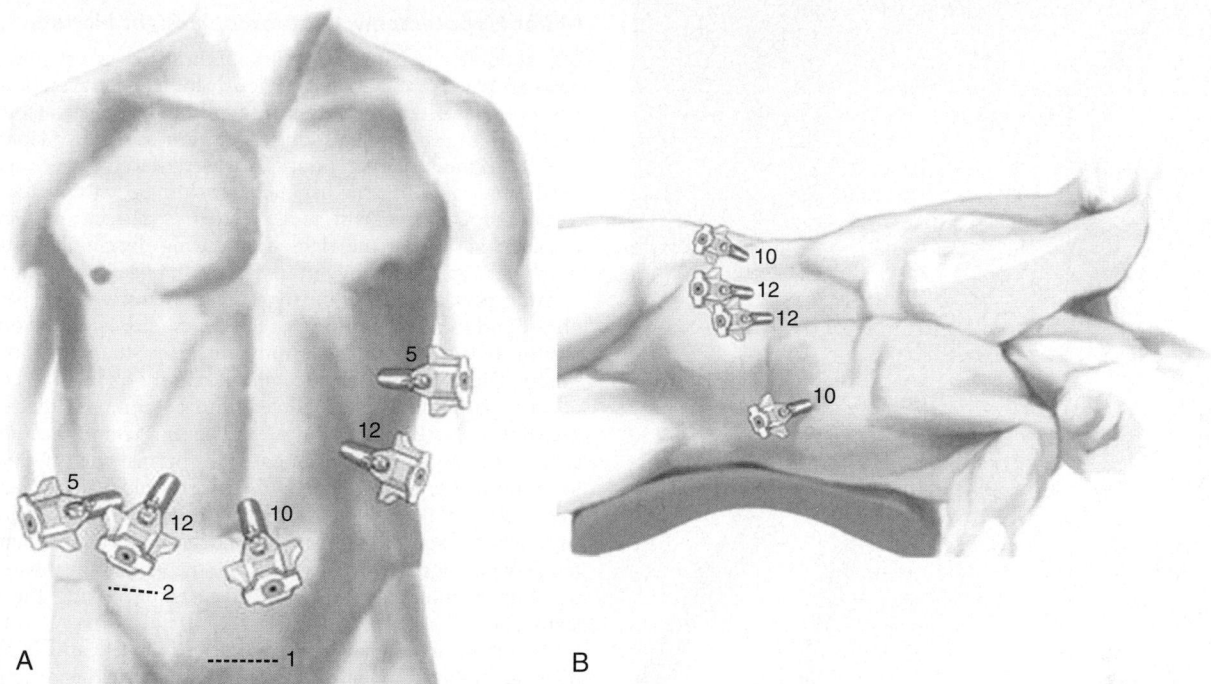

FIGURE 5 A, Pure laparoscopy port placement for resection of segments 2 through 5. Dashed lines represent options for GelPort insertion or specimen extraction. **B,** A left lateral position may be used for certain segment 6 resections *(Adapted from Cherqui D, Choulliard E. Laparoscopic liver resection. In: Clavian PA, Sarr MG, Fong Y, eds. Atlas of Upper Gastrointestinal and Hepatobiliary Surgery. 1st ed. Berlin: Springer-Verlag; 2007:393.)*

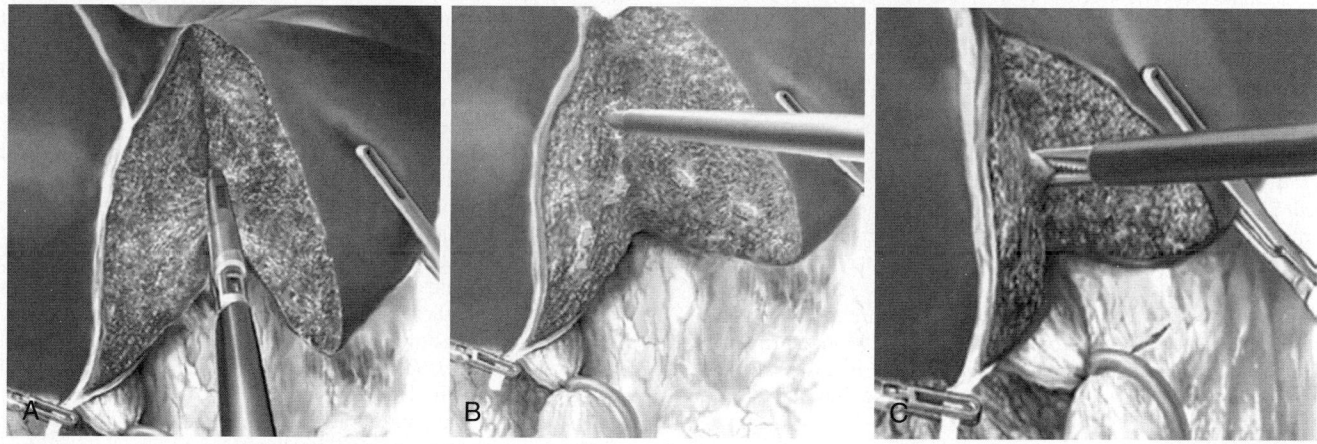

FIGURE 6 A, Parenchymal transection should proceed directly to the left of the falciform ligament using a thermal energy device and should proceed from the anterior edge caudally to the left hepatic vein. **B,** If not clipped, deeper or larger vessels can be controlled with the laparoscopic extended CUSA. **C,** The portal pedicles to segments 2 and 3 should be divided with a laparoscopic vascular loaded linear stapler, taking care to staple only to the left of the falciform ligament to avoid injury to segment 4 portal pedicles. *(Adapted from Cherqui D, Choulliard E. Laparoscopic liver resection. In: Clavian PA, Sarr MG, Fong Y, eds. Atlas of Upper Gastrointestinal and Hepatobiliary Surgery. 1st ed. Berlin: Springer-Verlag; 2007:395.)*

only to reduce bleeding during the time of transection, as needed. The segment 2 and 3 portal pedicle branches then should be dissected and incrementally stapled with a laparoscopic vascular loaded linear stapler. Note that stapling must occur to the left of the falciform ligament (Figure 6). Next, parenchymal transection begins with a combination of crushing and thermal energy and is carried out caudal to cranial directly to the left of the falciform ligament (see Figure 6). Placing traction on the ligamentum teres to the right and gentle traction on the left lateral sector with a bowel grasper can facilitate exposure. This maneuver should be carried cranially to the origin of the left hepatic vein (Figure 7). Care should be taken to remain in the same plane, directly to the left of the falciform ligament to ensure

no injury to the segment 4 portal pedicles. During transection, vessels up to 3 mm in diameter can be ligated safely with a thermal energy device. Alternatively, a CUSA energy device with a laparoscopic extender may be implemented for vessels larger than 3 mm (see Figure 7), or these vessels can be divided between clips. When the left hepatic vein is encountered, it should be stapled with the laparoscopic vascular loaded linear stapler (see Figure 7). After the completion of parenchymal transection and the stapling of the segment 2 and 3 portal pedicles and the left hepatic vein, hemostasis should be obtained in a standard fashion using a combination of the argon beam (laparoscopic extender), electrocautery, and absorbable hemostatics. Finally, the periumbilical trocar should be upsized to a 15-mm

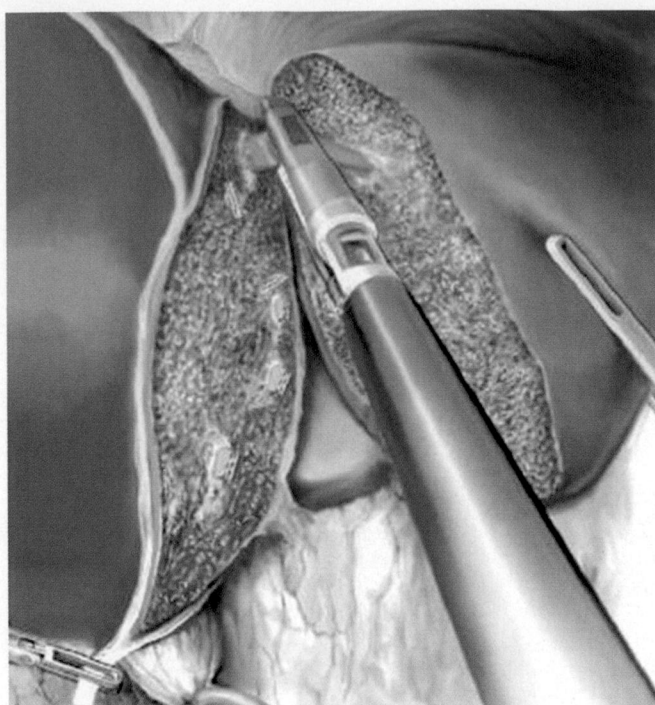

FIGURE 7 After complete parenchymal dissection and control of the segment 2 and 3 portal pedicles, the left hepatic vein should be divided with a laparoscopic vascular loaded linear stapler. *(Adapted from Cherqui D, Choulliard E. Laparoscopic liver resection. In: Clavian PA, Sarr MG, Fong Y, eds. Atlas of Upper Gastrointestinal and Hepatobiliary Surgery. 1st ed. Berlin: Springer-Verlag; 2007:396.)*

trocar inserted under direct visualization (a 5-mm camera is required for this). Next, the large specimen collection bag is inserted via this 15-mm trocar, and the specimen and trocar are removed. An approximate 5-cm incision is required for specimen removal. A final assessment for hemostasis from the cut surface of the liver should be performed after re-insufflation. A small GelPort may be beneficial during this final assessment.

Of note, the specimen must be extirpated through an extended umbilical incision (5 cm). For this reason, it is more prudent to attempt larger resections with the alternative hand-assisted and hybrid techniques, given the similarity in the incision size (as described later).

Laparoscopic Nonanatomic Wedge Resection

Nonanatomic wedge resection can be performed easily for lesions involving segments 2 to 6. However, for certain lesions in segments 7 and 8, performing a pure laparoscopic approach adds technical difficulty. Laparoscopic port positioning should be similar to that described in Figure 5. Pringle's maneuver can be used for large nonanatomic resections but typically is not required. Laparoscopic ultrasound can be quite beneficial in this setting to (1) assess for further disease and (2) assess the relationship of the target lesion to major vasculature. After ultrasonic assessment, a 1- to 2-cm margin should be marked circumferentially around malignant lesions with electrocautery. Note that this size margin is not required for benign disease. Parenchymal transection then should continue on the marked line of resection with a combination of electrocautery and a thermal energy device. Unless the lesion is a hanging or pedunculated lesion, laparoscopic staplers usually are not required. Depending on the size of the specimen, extraction can occur through a port via a laparoscopic collection bag or in a fashion similar to that described for the left lateral sectionectomy.

Major Hepatectomy: Laparoscopic Right Hepatectomy

The abdomen is entered, pneumoperitoneum is established, and ports are placed as described previously for left lateral sectionectomy. However, the left-sided 12-mm trocar should be placed closer to the midline in the epigastric region in a fashion similar to a laparoscopic cholecystectomy epigastric port. This port placement is essential for the dissection of the right hepatic artery and portal vein, for division of the coronary ligament, and in order to retract and elevate the posterior surface of the right liver during dissection of the right triangular ligament through traction on the ligamentum teres.

After port placement, the liver is explored with the laparoscopic ultrasound to clarify tumor characteristics (size and relation to vasculature), detect additional lesions, and assess the feasibility of continuing with a laparoscopic technique. Before further dissection the porta hepatis should be encircled with a Rummel's tourniquet in preparation for Pringle's maneuver. This is accomplished after division of the gastrohepatic ligament with thermal energy. One should be mindful of arterial variances, and care should be taken during this step to assess for a replaced left hepatic artery and avoid injury to this structure. Notably, Pringle's maneuver should be applied judiciously to prevent significant ischemia to the remaining parenchyma but implemented to reduce major bleeding during the time of transection.

Mobilization of the liver then is undertaken and begins with division of the ligamentum teres and falciform ligament back to the level of the hepatocaval venous confluence, until the anterior surface of the right hepatic vein is identified and dissected free. Next, the dissection should be carried laterally, dividing the anterior border of the right triangular ligament. Once visualization is impeded, the OR table should be tilted to approximately 30 degrees, right side up. The liver then is elevated using a liver retractor (multiple options exist) in order to permit dissection in the retrohepatic space. This should be carried out laterally and is achieved with a combination of blunt dissection and thermal energy down to the triangular ligament. After this, the short retrohepatic vena caval veins are skeletonized and divided between clips. The dissection is continued cranially until the right hepatic vein is encountered. The OR table then should be leveled out to complete the hilar dissection. The gallbladder then should be removed in a standard fashion, which will allow for elevation of the right liver and exposure of the portal triad for vascular dissection. Attention then should be turned to the porta hepatis and the right hepatic artery identified by placing slight traction on the cystic duct stump while countertraction is provided by pulling down on the Pringle's umbilical tape (this puts tension on the hepatoduodenal ligament without constricting the vascular inflow to the liver).

It is important to note that a thorough review of the patient's preoperative arterial phase cross-sectional imaging will provide pertinent information to the possibility of aberrant or replaced vessels. This is crucial during laparoscopy because tactile feedback is lost. Once the right hepatic artery is identified, it must be dissected using a combination of blunt dissection and electrocautery. For this we prefer the L hook cautery and an atraumatic right angle grasper. The right hepatic artery then is encircled with a vessel loop, retracted gently and laterally, and ligated between clips (two on the proximal side with a 3-mm cuff of artery). The division of the artery then will open up a plane to begin dissection of the right portal vein. This begins at the level of the extrahepatic bifurcation of the portal vein. Similar to all other vascular dissections, the right portal vein should be dissected free using a combination of blunt and thermal energy. A vessel loop or Vicryl tie (which can be left in place during stapling) then should be applied to encircle the vein for slight traction, and the vein should be stapled using a laparoscopic vascular loaded linear stapler. This is a critical step, and great care should be taken when handling the portal vein and positioning the stapler. The right hepatic duct will be divided intrahepatically during the parenchymal transection.

The parenchymal line of transection then should be confirmed with intraoperative ultrasound and marked with cautery, to the right of the vascular line of demarcation. During transection, to obtain optimal views the camera and instruments should be kept in line with the transection plane. The parenchyma is dissected using a thermal energy device and should begin on the anterior surface of the liver. Retraction can be accomplished with blunt laparoscopic graspers assisting to spread parenchyma in an open book fashion. Structures approximately 3 mm or larger should be divided between clips, stapled, or controlled with the laparoscopic CUSA device. The dissection is continued in this fashion until large middle hepatic vein branches are encountered. These venous branches should be skeletonized before division, which is accomplished by using one of the following instruments: (1) titanium clips for structures up to 5 mm in diameter, or (2) a laparoscopic articulating linear vascular loaded stapler (45 mm or 60 mm). As stated previously, the right hepatic duct is ligated intrahepatically and similar to large vessels should be stapled. Similar to the standard open approach, the dissection plane is carried posteriorly to the inferior vena cava. At the superior caval margin the right hepatic vein must be identified, dissected free, and divided with a laparoscopic vascular loaded linear stapler (this can be accomplished intrahepatically or flush on the vena cava).

The transected margin then should be irrigated lightly and inspected for bleeding or a bile leak. The transected edge is compressed with clean gauze, and any leakage of bile is controlled with 4-0 Prolene suture. Hemostasis is obtained using bipolar thermal energy for small bleeding points and clips or Prolene sutures for any substantive bleeding. The laparoscopic argon beam coagulator is used to cauterize the entirety of the transected margin (care should be taken to avoid heating any previously placed sutures). Lastly, hemostatic products such as fibrillar collagen and fibrin glue are applied.

Of note, the specimen is placed in a laparoscopic collection bag and extirpated through an extended umbilical incision or a Pfannenstiel incision. For this reason, it is more prudent to attempt larger resections with the alternative hand-assisted and hybrid techniques, given the similarity in the incision size (as described later).

Hand-Assisted Technique and the Hybrid Technique

General Principles

Although the incision that accommodates the hand port is the same for the hand-assisted and hybrid techniques, there are some differences in these two approaches. Both operative procedures use the hand as a retractor, but hand-assisted liver resection implies that the resection is performed entirely intracorporeally. Conversely, the hybrid technique uses the hand to mobilize the liver, with subsequent removal of the hand port so as to perform the liver transection in an open fashion without extending the incision. We favor the hybrid approach because we intuitively feel that this technique provides a more expeditious and practical method for mobilization, parenchymal dissection, and removal of the liver specimen without compromising the benefits of laparoscopic surgery. Nevertheless, because surgeons of great skill have been trained in both methods, the optimum procedure is the one that favors the comfort level of the practitioner. In brief, the hand-assisted technique mimics the laparoscopic approaches described previously, except that the surgeon has the option of utilizing his or her hand via the hand port. We therefore focus on and describe the hybrid approach to liver resection, the details of which are applicable to any system of laparoscopy using the hand.

In general, the hand is an optimal retractor because of its ability to conform to the contours of the liver and displace pressure to the entire organ, preventing possible parenchymal injury. Moreover, intracorporeal hand insertion during laparoscopic-assisted resection gives the surgeon enhanced tactile stabilization of the liver, allowing for more precise mobilization and dissection of the target lobe. Hand

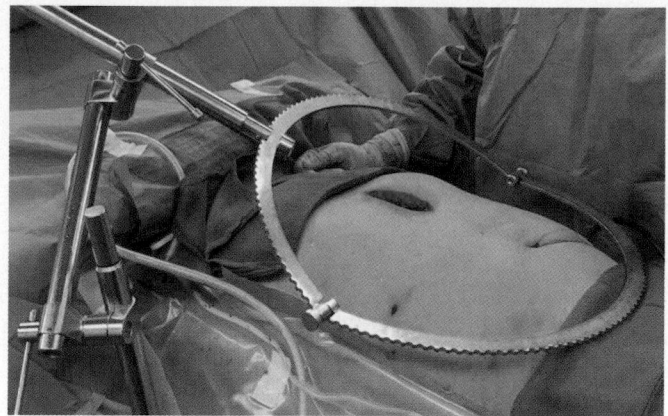

FIGURE 8 Assembly of the Bookwalter retractor system after mobilization of the liver, removal of the GelPort, and exsufflation of the abdomen.

assistance also promotes safety in providing the surgeon with an expedient method of manual control of hemorrhage during a potential vascular mishap. Furthermore, the laparoscopic camera aids in the operative procedure by enhancing acuity and magnification. Optic capture offered by laparoscopy can secondarily facilitate the identification and division of tangential structures. Angled lenses can offer an even greater advantage through visualization and ligation of the posterior medial vessels, such as the retrocaval short hepatic veins during a right hepatectomy. These retroperitoneal short vessels can be divided in the aforementioned fashion or through the hand port after exsufflation.

In the hybrid technique, once the target liver lobe has been mobilized by division of all peritoneal reflections, the abdomen is exsufflated and the hand port is removed (Figure 8). Because exposure is of paramount importance, we recommend the use of a retractor system. We prefer the segmented or split ring Bookwalter retractor system (Codman & Shurtleff, Raynham, MA), with the post on the patient's right and the extender angled at the left shoulder with a segmented ring inserted (see Figure 8). However, any variation of retractor system will do. Next, inflow and outflow vessels are controlled in a standard fashion, and the parenchymal dissection is accomplished through the hard port incision (Figure 9; technical details later). During cases of major resection, we prefer the hanging maneuver as described by Dr. Belghiti. Using this technique, an umbilical tape is passed superior to the hilum in the anterior plane above the vena cava in the space between the hepatic veins to lift the parenchyma. Draping the umbilical tape over the Bookwalter segmented ring under slight tension facilitates hepatic division. We ardently believe that the biliary ductal system should be managed during intrahepatic dissection to prevent injury to the contralateral duct. For living donor hepatectomies, the hepatic artery, portal vein, and hepatic vein branches are kept intact as the parenchymal division is completed. The patient then is heparinized before the dissection of the target vascular structures and ultimate division. Subsequently, the specimen is removed through the hand port site.

Right Hepatectomy and Posterior Sectionectomy Using the Hybrid Technique

Starting directly at the tip of the xiphoid, a 7.5-cm subxiphoid incision is made, and then a hand port (GelPort; Applied Medical, Rancho Santa Margarita, CA) is inserted for hand assistance (see Figure 9). A pneumoperitoneum is established after a standard Hasson trocar insertion infraumbilically, and a 5-mm trocar is placed obliquely in the right or left subcostal margin depending on the location of the target lobe (see Figure 9). As described previously, great care must be taken when inserting trocars intra-abdominally because of the inherent potential for vascular or viscus injury. The periumbilical trocar placement can be particularly risky because of its larger size and the relatively blind nature of insertion (this possibility can be minimized by introducing the trocar using the Hasson cutdown technique). After safe insufflation of the abdomen, the operation begins with mobilization of the liver after positioning the patient in reverse Trendelenburg. At times, angling the OR table with the patient left side down may facilitate visualization.

Liver mobilization begins with the surgeon on the patient's left inserting the left hand via the GelPort and the assistant on the patient's right inserting an electrothermal device via the 5-mm trocar

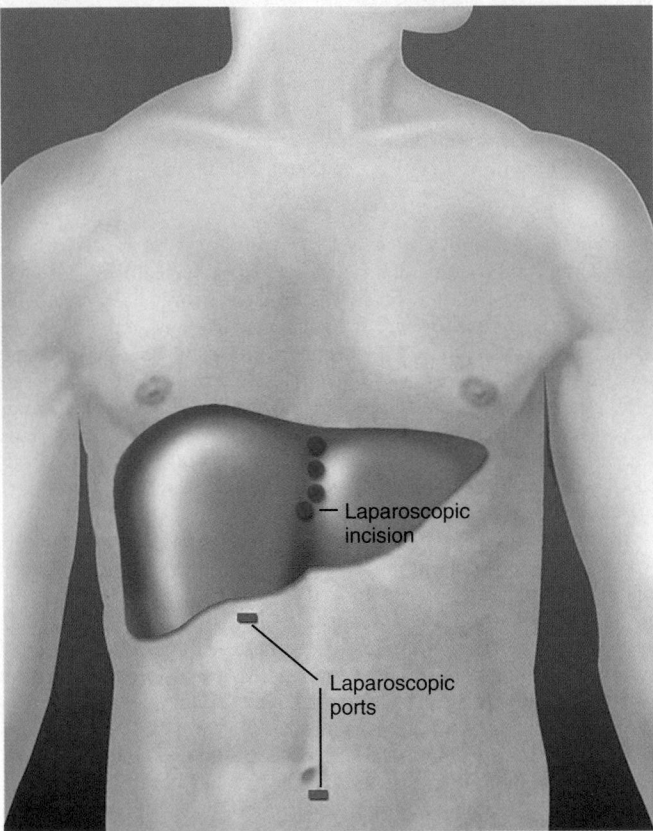

FIGURE 9 A 7.5-cm subxiphoid incision is made and a hand port (GelPort; Applied Medical, Rancho Santa Margarita, CA) is inserted for hand assistance.

(laparoscopic diathermic energy-based devices are used to divide the right triangular and coronary ligaments). A 30-degree scope is utilized via the infraumbilical port. The first maneuver is division of the falciform ligament superiorly to the level of the diaphragm (taking care to proceed with caution), as this maneuver will lead the surgeon to the insertion of the hepatic veins into the inferior vena cava. Next, the hepatorenal (Figure 10) and triangular (Figure 11) ligaments are divided with the thermal device. Note that as the mobilization is carried laterally, the surgeon must begin lifting and pulling the right lobe of the liver in an anteromedial fashion. Care should be taken during this phase to identify the inferior vena cava and right adrenal gland (Figure 12). Next, as the right hepatic lobe is continually retracted anteromedially by the surgeon's left hand, the assistant must continue to divide the triangular ligaments taking great care to avoid injury to the right hepatic vein (Figure 13). At this time, the surgeon should push the liver inferior and posterior divide the right coronary ligament with thermal energy. Care must be taken during this time to avoid inadvertent injury to the hepatic veins. In addition, during division of the triangular and coronary ligaments, the plane of division should remain on the liver capsule to avoid an inadvertent diaphragm injury. With the surgeon's left hand, the diaphragm also can be pushed away in a sweeping motion as the ligaments are divided to facilitate division and visualization.

After mobilization of the right hepatic lobe, we exsufflate the abdomen, remove the hand port, and secure the retractor system to expose the liver through the midline abdominal incision (see Figure 5). Then the remainder of the procedure is carried out in a standard open fashion via the hand port. Several laparotomy pads are placed behind the right lobe to move the liver forward into the incision. Before parenchymal transection, the liver is brought farther into the incision with the aid of the hanging maneuver, which utilizes an umbilical tape draped under the liver parenchyma, superior to the retrohepatic vena cava and draped over the Bookwalter retractor system. Note that at times the hand port incision is extended to the right with a 1-cm subcostal "J" incision. We begin by completing the mobilization of the right lobe off of the vena cava. This is accomplished with the surgeon retracting the right lobe medially. Retrohepatic caval branches then are identified individually and ligated using a combination of clips and silk ties. The caval ligament then is dissected and stapled or tied. The right hepatic vein then should be identified and encircled with a vessel loop. Next, we place lap pads behind the liver to bring the gallbladder and hilum into better view. The first maneuver is a traditional cholecystectomy when performing the right hepatectomy. Before further dissection, we methodically palpate for a replaced right hepatic artery. Given the frequency of hepatic arterial anomalies, a clear distinction of lobar inflow should

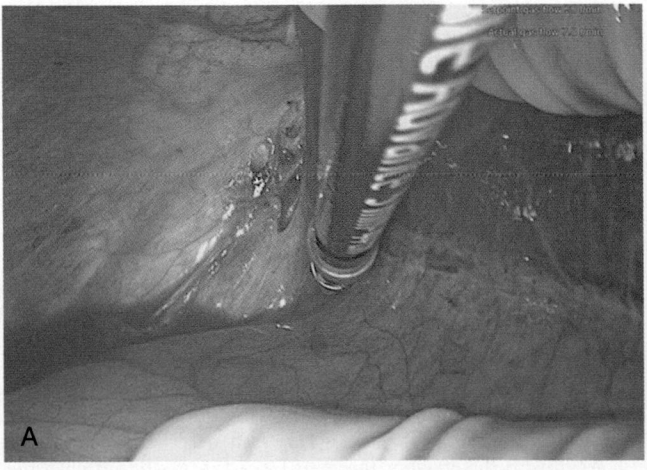
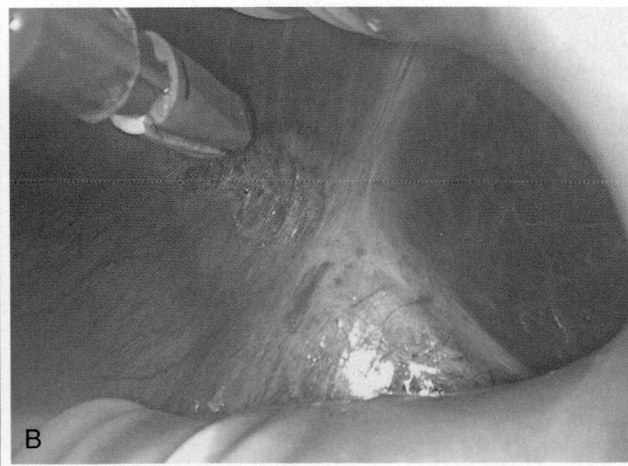

FIGURE 10 A, Hand-assisted mobilization of the right lobe of the liver. **B,** Division of hepatorenal ligament with a combination of electrocautery and bipolar energy.

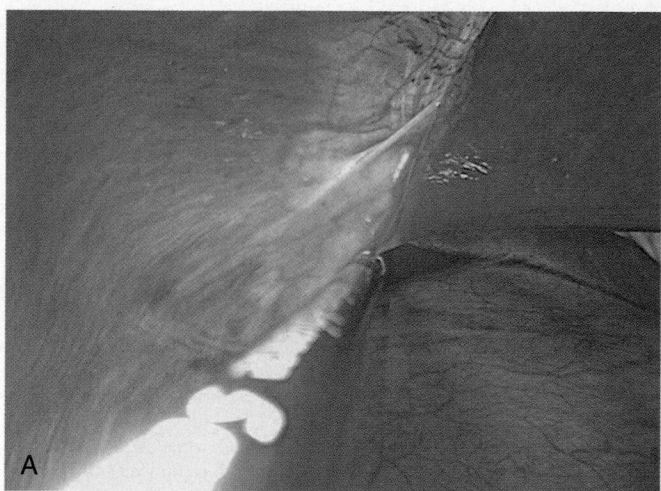 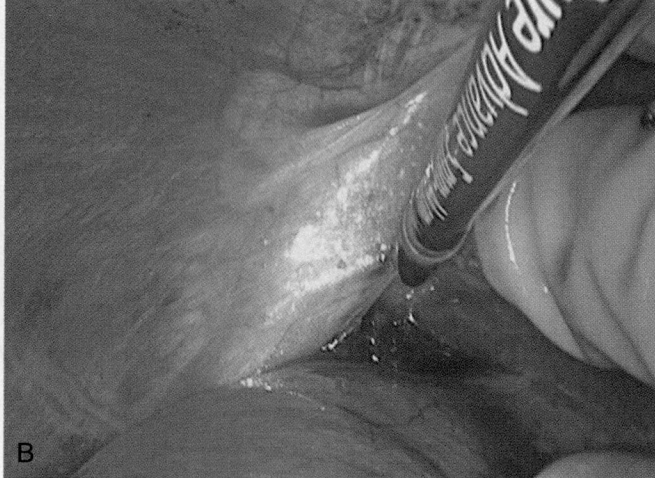

FIGURE 11 A, Hand-assisted mobilization of the right lobe of the liver. **B,** Division of the right triangular ligament using a combination of electrocautery and bipolar energy. Note that the surgeon must retract the liver medially using the hand port.

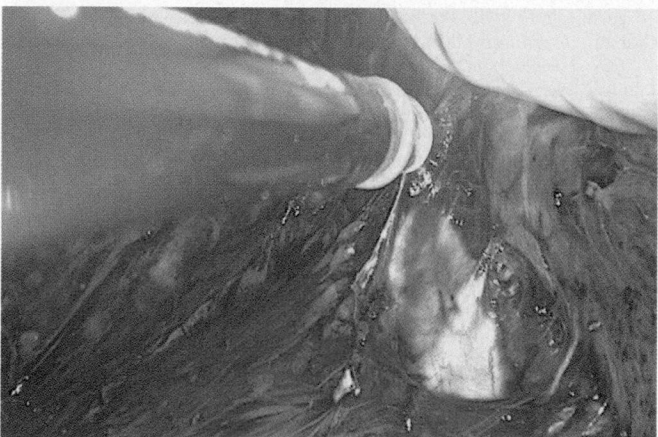

FIGURE 12 Continued mobilization of the right lobe of the liver off of the diaphragm, inferior vena cava, and adrenal gland.

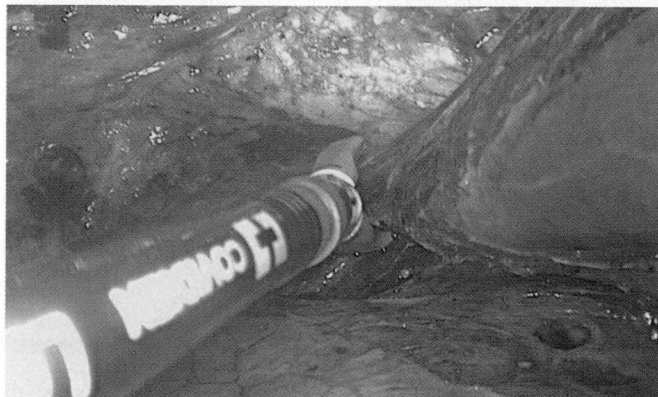

FIGURE 13 Continued retraction of the liver medial will allow for complete mobilization of the right hepatic lobe, freeing the liver from all of its right-sided attachments.

be made before ligation. Here we ligate and divide the right hepatic artery and dissect posteriorly to delineate the portal vein. Utilizing the fissure of Ganz, the extrahepatic right portal vein is mobilized circumferentially and divided. Note that if performing a posterior segmental resection, the posterior portal pedicle should be dissected

during this step and divided, taking great care to avoid injury to the anterior pedicle (this can be facilitated by utilizing intraoperative ultrasound). After division of the right lobar inflow, a clear demarcation of the right and left lobes should be identified. Then the right hepatic vein is identified on the superior aspect of the liver and divided using an articulating laparoscopic stapling device (Endopath ETS; Ethicon Endo-Surgery, Cincinnati, OH) to ensure safe control of this fragile vessel. Similar to identification of portal pedicles, we routinely use intraoperative ultrasound to characterize and mark the course of the hepatic veins, as relying on ischemic demarcation can result in injury to a slightly laterally positioned vessel during parenchymal transection. Using the aforementioned hanging maneuver, we proceed with liver division, being mindful to stay to the right of the middle hepatic vein. Parenchymal transection should be performed at the preference of the surgeon. We opt to ligate the right hepatic duct during intraparenchymal division because contralateral bile duct ischemia can occur if extrahepatic dissection is attempted. The specimen then is removed through this incision. Argon beam cauterization is utilized on the parenchymal service, taking care to avoid the stapled end of the right hepatic vein and the middle hepatic vein. Hemostasis and bile leakage is assessed for and controlled at the preference of the surgeon. Lastly, care must be taken to reapproximate the falciform ligament to the diaphragm in order to prevent torsion of the left lobe of the liver and obstruction of hepatic inflow or outflow.

Left Hepatectomy Using the Hybrid Technique

A left hepatectomy using the hybrid technique follows many of the same steps discussed previously. Liver mobilization begins with the surgeon on the patient's left, inserting the left hand via the GelPort, and the assistant on the patient's right, inserting an electrothermal device via the 5-mm trocar (laparoscopic diathermic energy-based devices are used to divide the visceral attachments and triangular and coronary ligaments). A 30-degree scope is utilized via the infraumbilical port. The first maneuver is division of the falciform ligament superiorly to the level of the diaphragm. Next, the left coronary and triangular ligaments are divided with thermal energy as the surgeon exposes the tissue utilizing his hand via the GelPort. The surgeon then utilizes his hand to expose the gastrohepatic ligament, and the assistant opens this ligament using thermal energy. Again, one should be mindful of arterial variances, and care should be taken during this step to assess for a replaced left hepatic artery arising from the left gastric artery and to avoid injury to this structure if identified.

After mobilization of the left hepatic lobe, we exsufflate the abdomen, remove the hand port, and secure the retractor system to expose the liver through the midline abdominal incision (see

Figure 9). The remainder of the procedure then is carried out in a standard open fashion via the hand port. Note that at times the hand port incision is extended 1 cm to the patient's right in a "J" formation. The first maneuver is a traditional cholecystectomy when performing the left hepatectomy. After correct identification and division of the middle and left hepatic arteries, dissection of the left portal vein begins by working posteriorly to the ligated arterial vasculature. Traditionally the caudate lobe is spared in formal left hepatic lobe resections, and therefore the surgeon should preserve the portal venous branches from the left portal vein into this segment. Next, the middle hepatic vein is characterized using intraoperative ultrasound, and its course is marked on the surface of the liver using electrocautery. Parenchymal transection then begins in the standard fashion. After completion of the parenchymal transection, the left and, if necessary, middle hepatic veins are divided in a standard fashion, as described previously.

■ OPERATIVE METRICS

In a recent study we compared our experience of conventional open liver resection with laparoscopic liver resection. As expected, in our experience the laparoscopic approach with hand assistance and parenchymal dissection through the hand port incision had equivalent operative metrics with shortened length of stay. Reports like those issued by Koffron and colleagues have shown that laparoscopic resection is less expensive because of the shortened hospital stay. This finding reflects what has already been shown conclusively with laparoscopic cholecystectomy, fundoplication, and gastric bypass surgery. As efficiency pressures continue to rise, the laparoscopic approach for liver resection likely will be embraced further. To this end, we surmise that the hybrid technique will gain favor, as it more closely assimilates the skills that hepatobiliary surgeons already possess. Moreover, this technique offers the most palatable setting of safety with the use of the hand for liver mobilization and prompt control of bleeding vasculature. Practically, the hand is the best-known liver retractor, as it is atraumatic and offers varying degrees of facile mobility. Moreover, with this approach we are able to substantially minimize the incision for an open liver resection, as the standard subcostal incision can approach 35 cm. In doing so, we believe that the potential long-term sequelae of the traditional subcostal incision, subcostal incision with midline extension, bilateral subcostal incision with midline extension (which include abdominal wall hernias), potential wound infections, and paresthesias may be lessened.

Since Dr. Jean Louis Lortat-Jacob detailed the first published hepatectomy using the road map laid out by Claude Couinaud, the field of liver surgery has seen a celebrated rise in the capability to offer resection with lower rates of morbidity and mortality. It is evident that with the arrival of the twenty-first century, the emergence of laparoscopy embodies a marriage of uncompromised surgical technique and better outcomes for our patients. Newer approaches have allowed surgeons to bridge the gap between operative technique and improved outcomes. Laparoscopy has emerged as an advancement that embodies these efforts to improve medical care and represents a significant change to the landscape of surgery. As such, we are in the renaissance of MIS, with innovation guiding a renewed operative approach to intra-abdominal pathology. Liver surgery, although initially late to embrace laparoscopy, is now gaining momentum, and an archetypal shift may be on the horizon.

SUGGESTED READINGS

Azagra JS, Goergen M, Gilbart E, et al. Laparoscopic anatomical (hepatic) left lateral segmentectomy—technical aspects. *Surg Endosc.* 1996;10:758-761.

Buell JF, Cherqui D, Geller DA, et al. World Consensus Conference on laparoscopic surgery. The international position on laparoscopic liver surgery: the Louisville Statement, 2008. *Ann Surg.* 2009;250:825-830.

Castaing D, Vibert E, Ricca L, et al. Oncologic results of laparoscopic versus open hepatectomy for colorectal liver metastases in two specialized centers. *Ann Surg.* 2009;250:849-855.

Catalano OA, Singh AH, Uppot RN, Hahn PF, Ferrone CR, Sahani DV. Vascular and biliary variants in the liver: implications for liver surgery. *Radiographics.* 2008;28:359-378.

Cherqui D, Choulliard E. Laparoscopic liver resection. In: Clavian PA, Sarr MG, Fong Y, eds. *Atlas of Upper Gastrointestinal and Hepatobiliary Surgery.* 1st ed. Berlin: Springer-Verlag; 2007.

Graham JA, Jackson PJ. Surgical pitfalls in laparoscopic surgery. In: Evans SRT, ed. *Surgical Pitfalls: Prevention and Management.* St. Louis: Elsevier; 2008.

Graham JA, Johnson LB. Right hepatectomy. In: Evans SRT, ed. *Surgical Pitfalls: Prevention and Management.* St. Louis: Elsevier; 2008.

Johnson LB, Graham JA, Weiner DA, et al. How does laparoscopic-assisted hepatic resection compare with the conventional open surgical approach? *J Am Coll Surg.* 2012;214:717-723.

Martin RC, Mbah NA, Hill RS, et al. Laparoscopic versus open hepatic resection for hepatocellular carcinoma: improvement in outcomes and similar cost. *World J Surg.* 2015;39:1519-1526.

Nguyen KT, Gamblin TC, Geller DA. World review of laparoscopic liver resections—2,804 patients. *Ann Surg.* 2009;250:831-841.

Nguyen KT, Marsh JW, Tsung A, et al. Comparative benefits of laparoscopic versus open hepatic resection. *Arch Surg.* 2010;146:348-356.

Raman SS, Leary C, et al. Improved characterization of focal liver lesions with liver-specific gadoxetic acid disodium-enhanced magnetic resonance imaging: a multicenter phase 3 clinical trial. *J Comput Assist Tomogr.* 2010;34:163-172.

Reddy SK, Tsung A, Geller DA. Laparoscopic liver resection. *World J Surg.* 2011;35:1478-1486.

Seale MK, Catalano OA, et al. Hepatobiliary-specific MR contrast agents: role in imaging the liver and biliary tree. *Radiographics.* 2009;29:1725-1748.

Steadman RH, Braunfeld MY. The liver: surgery and anesthesia. In: Barash PG, Cullen BF, Stoelting RK, et al., eds. *Clinical Anesthesia.* 7th ed. Philadelphia: Lippincott Williams & Wilkins; 2013.

Toro J, Patel AD, Lytle NW, et al. Detecting performance variance in complex surgical procedures: analysis of a step-wise technique for laparoscopic right hepatectomy. *Am J Surgery.* 2015;209:418-423.

Vanounou T, Steel JL, Nguyen KT, et al. Comparing the clinical and economic impact of laparoscopic versus open liver resection. *Ann Surg Oncol.* 2010;17:998-1009.

Vigano L, Laurent A, Tayar C, et al. The learning curve in laparoscopic liver resection: improved feasibility and reproducibility. *Ann Surg.* 2009;250:772-782.

LAPAROSCOPIC DISTAL PANCREATECTOMY

Miral Sadaria Grandhi, MD, and Martin A. Makary, MD, MPH

Are there really any benefits to doing pancreas surgery laparoscopically? If you consider the near elimination of wound infection complications, reduced pain after surgery, and reduced rates of ventral hernias and long-term bowel obstructions due to adhesions, the answer is clear. In fact, if the U.S. Food and Drug Administration (FDA) approved a medication with these four benefits, we would probably ask why every eligible patient was not getting it. Excluding the 10% to 20% of patients with vascular involvement or severe adhesive disease, where we prefer to do an open operation, laparoscopic distal pancreatectomy has become the standard of care for body and tail lesions that meet surgical criteria.

The reason for wide variation in adoption of laparoscopic pancreas surgery is largely due to the fact that the procedure can be difficult to learn. Those who have mastered the procedure generally cite having watched videos and initially teaming up with a surgeon who has advanced laparoscopic skills (e.g., bariatric surgery skills). Coaching, visiting high-volume centers, and telementoring via video (e.g., InTouch Health) to learn the procedure are increasing its adoption worldwide. We teach our fellows and residents that a surgeon should master both the open operation (first) and the laparoscopic operation.

In Martin Makary's experience of performing 500 laparoscopic pancreas operations at the Johns Hopkins Hospital, the wound infection rate is 1%, in comparison with 10% for open pancreas surgery. In addition, we observed that the laparoscopic approach is associated with decreased postoperative narcotic use, decreased time to ambulation, and increased activity level at discharge. As detailed in a systematic review (Venkat et al., 2012) conducted at the Johns Hopkins Hospital, laparoscopic distal pancreatectomy resulted in decreased postoperative complications and improvement in patient-centered outcomes. Furthermore, operative times and positive surgical margin rates using a laparoscopic approach for distal pancreas lesions were comparable to those when using an open technique, validating similar oncologic outcomes between the two approaches. Other groups have reported similar findings, also commenting on comparable pancreatic fistula rates in both approaches (Sharpe et al., 2015; Yan et al., 2015). In addition, various groups have reported significantly decreased rates of incisional hernia and postoperative bowel obstruction with a laparoscopic approach, complications that occur in as much as 20% of patients after open surgery (Yan et al., 2015). Another benefit of laparoscopy may be improved cosmesis, an outcome of particular value in young patients who classically are seen with a pancreatic cyst or neuroendocrine tumor. Finally, we have found that the 12-times magnification of newer laparoscopic, high-definition cameras allows the surgeon to visualize the anatomy better than with open surgery.

These improved patient-centered outcomes for laparoscopic distal pancreatectomy over open surgery have even greater implications than the measured outcome itself. For instance, increased wound complications with open surgery not only may delay adjuvant therapy but also is an independent predictor of hospital readmission. In addition, decreased activity with an open approach increases the patient's risk for secondary complications, such as deep venous thrombosis or pulmonary embolism. A quicker recovery with a laparoscopic approach also means an earlier start with adjuvant therapy. However, the logistics behind this require a culture change because medical oncology departments routinely schedule patients at 3 to 5 weeks after surgery, assuming that they need time to recover from open surgery. Furthermore, performing a less painful operation with laparoscopy can be of great value and of particular importance for cancer patients and their quality of life. Of note, many of these outcomes favorably influenced by laparoscopy (surgical site infection, pain level, and patient satisfaction) are metrics increasingly being used by both surgical registries and payers to measure quality in surgery. Thus these complications and their implications not only are detrimental to the patient, but also can result in increased healthcare costs.

■ PATIENT SELECTION

Most resectable distal pancreas tumors are amenable for laparoscopic resection. We offer a laparoscopic distal pancreatectomy to patients who have lesions not involving the celiac or mesenteric vessels and who are appropriate candidates for a laparoscopic procedure. Patients with a history of necrotizing pancreatitis are sometimes not amenable to laparoscopy because the stomach and colon mesentery may be densely adherent.

We have found that frail, older patients and other high-risk patients are ideal candidates for the minimally invasive approach. For such patients, we sometimes titrate the insufflation pressure (from 9 to 15 mm Hg) based on end-tidal carbon dioxide. These low pressures often allow effective visualization and can offer a suitable approach for

patients with severe lung disease and baseline hypercarbia. Using appropriate monitoring, we have observed that the recovery benefits of a laparoscopic resection are magnified in older patients who have undergone the procedure. As is true for young patients, laparoscopic distal pancreatectomy in frail, older patients is associated with less physiologic stress to the patient. Moreover, the decreased postoperative pain associated with laparoscopy reduces the need for postoperative narcotic use, which is of particular importance in older patients because they have a greater risk of narcotic-associated delirium.

■ PREOPERATIVE ENDOSCOPIC TATTOOING

Small, intraparenchymal, or posterior lesions of the pancreatic body and tail can be difficult to identify at the time of laparoscopic resection. In particular, hypervascular lesions that can be easily identified on computed tomography (CT) can be difficult to localize at surgery. We use a novel endoscopic ultrasound-guided technique to tattoo the pancreatic lesion transgastrically before surgery (Newman et al., 2010) (Figure 1). Using an endoscopic 22-gauge needle, the endoscopist injects a total of 2 to 4 mL of sterile purified carbon particles (GI Spot dye; GI Supply, Camp Hill, PA) into the pancreatic parenchyma 3 to 5 mm proximal to the tumor under direct endoscopic ultrasound visualization. Injection of the dye is continued as the needle is withdrawn from the pancreas to create an inked tract, taking great care to avoid peritoneal injection. This approach facilitates early identification of the lesion during surgery as well as identification of the dye from the posterior surface of the gland during dissection.

Preoperative marking of the pancreatic lesion enables the surgeon to quickly identify the location of the tumor at the time of laparoscopy and guides the decision of where to divide the gland. We have found that tattooing significantly decreases operative time for laparoscopic distal pancreatectomy. Furthermore, it helps to avoid the unfortunate situation of missing a subtle tumor in the resected specimen, a hazard of the decreased tactile sense in laparoscopic palpation with long instruments. Even large tumors detected on CT, which a surgeon anticipates to identify easily in the operating room, can be surprisingly difficult to find intraoperatively because of the homogeneous color of the pancreas and its retroperitoneal bed.

■ SPLENIC PRESERVATION

We routinely attempt splenic preservation when there is a low suspicion of malignancy and find that the spleen can be spared in 70% of these cases (Figure 2). Of note, in cases where malignancy is

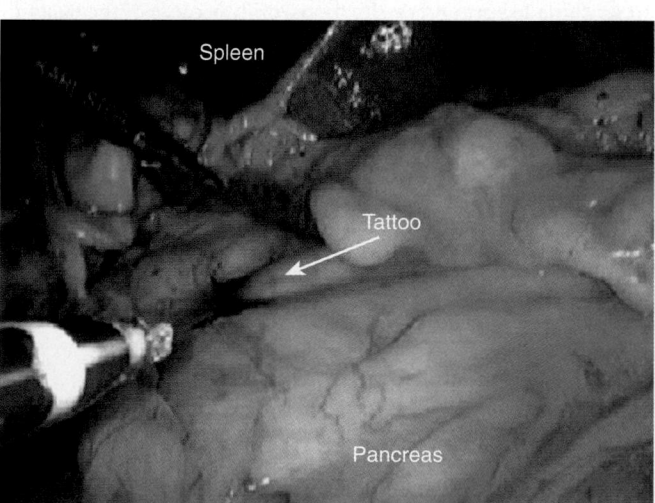

FIGURE 1 Tail of the pancreas with tattoo and spleen in background. *(© Jenny Wang, 2008.)*

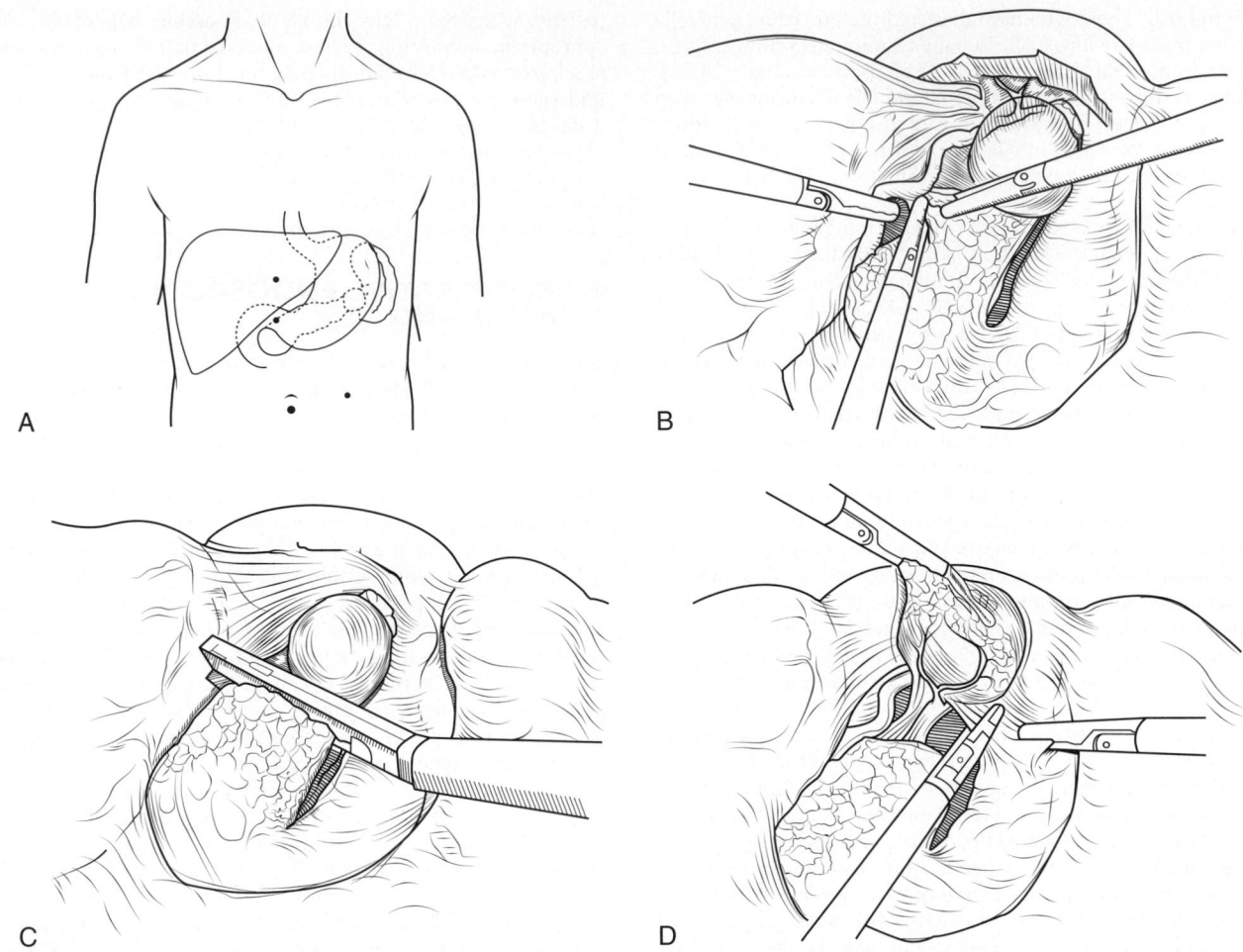

FIGURE 2 Spleen-preserving distal pancreatectomy: port site placement and vessel preserving technique. **A,** Port placement for laparoscopic distal pancreatectomy. **B,** Dissection of the inferior and superior edges of the distal pancreas laparoscopically. **C,** Transection of the pancreas with a stapler. **D,** Dissecting the tail of the pancreas and surgical specimen off of the splenic vessels for spleen preservation. (© Jenny Wang, 2008.)

suspected based on imaging studies, personal history, or family history, we remove the spleen en bloc with the tail of the pancreas to achieve a wide resection of the lymph node basin in the area of the splenic vessels and splenic hilum. In our experience, laparoscopic distal pancreatectomy can result in an increased likelihood of splenic preservation in appropriate situations, likely because of the magnification and improved visualization offered by modern equipment.

■ OPERATIVE TECHNIQUE

A Foley catheter usually is not placed, to minimize the risk of a urinary tract infection; however, we do place a Foley catheter if the patient did not void before going to the operating room, the anticipated operative time is more than 3 hours, the patient is older, or the patient is at high risk for urinary retention. The laparoscopic distal pancreatectomy steps (in order) are listed here and then described.

- Perform a staging laparoscopy.
- Open the lesser sac.
- Perform takedown of the splenic flexure of the colon.
- Distinguish the splenic vessels from the hepatic vessels.
- Divide the splenic artery unless the spleen is being preserved.
- Mobilize the distal pancreas, and divide the splenic vein unless the spleen is being preserved.
- Transect the pancreas with an appropriate sized stapler.
- Mobilize the spleen unless the spleen is being preserved.
- Extract the specimen.
- Place a drain near the cut surface of the pancreas.

We place an infraumbilical port using Hassan's method. Two ports in the upper midline (or right of midline) and one port in the left lower quadrant are inserted under direct visualization (Figure 2, A). The precise locations of these ports are dependent on the location of the tumor, the intention to preserve the spleen, and the patient's body habitus. Of note, although we prefer using the two ports in the upper midline to perform the dissection, some prefer to place a left lower quadrant and left lateral port from where they perform the pancreatic dissection. This is also a good approach. Once local landmarks are identified, the gastrocolic ligament and short gastric vessels are divided, and the splenic flexure of the colon is taken down to achieve wide visualization of the lesser sac. When surgeons struggle with visualization of the pancreas because of surrounding fat, taking down the splenic flexure of the colon can be of great help with exposure. Mobilization of the gland is easiest from the inferior border of the gland (Figure 2, B, and Figure 3). Thus beginning with the inferior approach facilitates dissection of the posterior aspect of the gland from the retroperitoneal bed. The splenic artery and vein branches can be visualized from underneath the pancreas. We alternate dissection of the splenic vessels from above and below the gland according to which exposure best offers visualization.

Laparoscopic Distal Pancreatectomy With Splenic Preservation

Once the pancreas is clear of the splenic vessels to allow for division of the gland, we attempt to dissect as much of the tail as possible, freeing the entire tail when feasible. The gland is divided with a

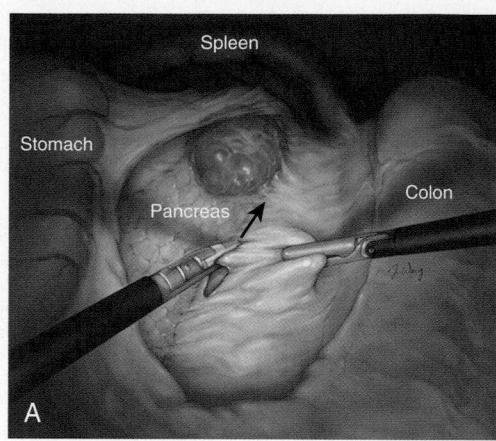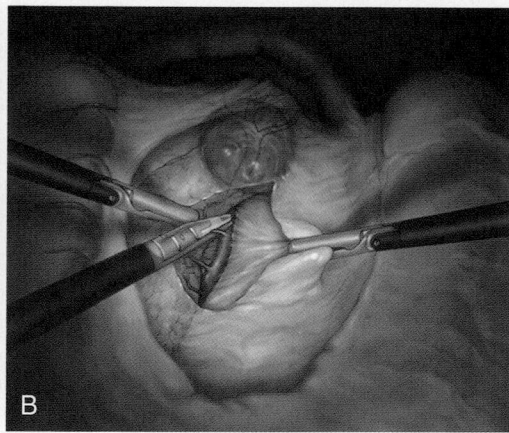

FIGURE 3 Laparoscopic distal pancreatectomy. **A,** The mobilization of the tail of the pancreas is easiest if started from the inferior edge of the pancreas. **B,** This dissection along the inferior edge of the pancreas is carried out laterally toward the tail of the pancreas and spleen. *(© Jenny Wang, 2008.)*

stapler, choosing the staple height based on the gland thickness at the site of planned transection (Figure 2, *C*). The tail of the pancreas and surgical specimen are dissected off of the splenic vessels by dividing any remaining attachments (Figure 2, *D*). The specimen is removed with an Endo Catch bag (Covidien, Minneapolis, MN), and a surgical drain is placed at the cut end of the pancreas.

Laparoscopic Distal Pancreatectomy With Splenectomy

When a malignancy is suspected or a technical reason necessitates removal of the spleen, we choose to mobilize the spleen after individual division of the splenic artery, splenic vein, and gland. Care is taken to ensure that the splenic artery is not confused with the hepatic artery. Dissection of the splenic artery toward the spleen is sometimes necessary to ensure that the splenic artery is not mistaken for the hepatic artery. The splenic artery and the splenic vein are each ligated individually, in that order, with a vascular stapler. Sometimes these vessels are approached from the posterior aspect of the gland. The spleen then is mobilized from its attachments as the last step in the operation.

When the spleen is removed for technical or anatomic (nononcologic) reasons, we divide the pancreas from the spleen to manually morcellate (liquefy) the spleen for easy extraction from the peritoneum. The intact specimen is suspended freely in the insufflated abdomen, and then the spleen is divided from the tail of the pancreas with a series of gastrointestinal anastomosis (GIA) staplers fired close to the spleen to avoid leaving residual pancreatic tissue or lymph nodes on the spleen side. This intracorporeal separation allows for removal of the pancreas intact and removal of the spleen utilizing the manual morcellation technique. A stitch or orientation via the tattoo may be necessary to identify the true pancreatic margin upon extraction. Splenic morcellation then is performed within the plastic bag, with the bag opening brought through the umbilical wound. We do not and have never used an electric morcellation device. This piecemeal extraction method is not applicable when an oncologic margin could be threatened by the intracorporeal separation of the pancreas and spleen. In the case of known or suspected malignancy, the specimen is removed en bloc. All specimens are delivered in an Endo Catch bag, which necessitates a small extension of the midline, infraumbilical 12-mm port site. A frozen section analysis is performed intraoperatively to confirm a negative and adequate pancreatic surgical margin before the operation is completed.

At all times, an Endo GIA 2.5-mm (white-matter vascular load) stapler (Covidien, Mansfield, MA) is open, loaded, and ready to use in case of injury to the splenic vessels. Clips generally are avoided because stapling devices cannot engage on a clip. As a precaution, we keep a fresh #10 blade, a clamped open suction setup, and curved heavy Mayo scissors ready at all times in case a rapid conversion to an open operation is necessary to control bleeding.

■ PATIENT OUTCOMES

Patients are admitted to the surgical unit for a typical hospital stay of 3 to 4 days after surgery. We have observed that these patients behave clinically similar to patients who have undergone laparoscopic cholecystectomy and adrenalectomy, often requiring little or no narcotic pain medication after surgery. Although wound complications are rare after the laparoscopic technique, the pancreatic leak rate for all types of laparoscopic pancreas surgery is identical to that of the open operation.

■ LAPAROSCOPIC VERSUS ROBOTIC PANCREAS SURGERY

Recently, robotic surgery has become an enabling technology for major pancreatic resections. Zureikat and colleagues (2013) reported the largest series of robotic pancreatic resections. In their experience, robotic resections had the same benefit of minimally invasive surgery. In addition, this technique can be easier to learn than straight laparoscopy. However, operative times with robotic surgery were longer, which may improve with experience and advances in robotic technology. Although these results are encouraging, we continue to favor a laparoscopic approach to pancreatic resections because it is associated with fewer incisions, shorter operative times, and haptic feedback (the ability to palpate for the purpose of sensing resistance). Robotic surgery also costs thousands of dollars more per operation than standard laparoscopic surgery. Furthermore, some argue that robot-assisted surgery may add risks for the patient if the surgeon is unfamiliar with the technique, related to the lack of haptic feedback, which can result in inadvertent injury. Moreover, the robot adds safety concerns related to the surgeon's remote position at the console, delays in emergency conversion to an open operation, and difficulty obtaining access for the anesthesiologist during emergency cardiopulmonary resuscitation. For these reasons we offer patients nonrobotic, laparoscopic distal pancreatectomy.

■ CONCLUSION

A strong foundation with open pancreas surgery is an important prerequisite for developing skills in laparoscopic pancreas surgery. In summary, when applied appropriately, laparoscopy is associated with decreased wound complications, less pain, and reduced length of hospital stay for patients. It is also associated with minimizing the risk for long-term complications such as incisional hernia and small bowel obstruction. Laparoscopy is particularly ideal for candidate patients with decreased physiologic reserve or cardiopulmonary risk factors. For small, intraparenchymal, or posterior pancreatic body or tail lesions, preoperative endoscopic tattooing of the lesion enables the surgeon to quickly identify the location of the tumor at the time of laparoscopy and guides the decision of where to divide the gland. We routinely attempt splenic preservation when there is low suspicion of malignancy. However, in the setting of suspected or known malignancy, we remove the spleen en bloc with the tail of the pancreas to achieve a wide resection of the lymph node basin in the area of the splenic vessels and splenic hilum. In the absence of a large wound postoperatively with minimal risk for wound complications, laparoscopic distal pancreatectomy for cancer allows for a shorter interval to adjuvant therapy when indicated. In the future, improved surgical techniques may decrease the learning curve and enable more patients to benefit from the decreased complications observed with laparoscopic distal pancreatectomy compared with open surgery.

■ ACKNOWLEDGMENTS

We thank Ms. Jenny Y. Wang of the Johns Hopkins University Department of Art as Applied to Medicine, who has demonstrated the procedure through the drawings presented in this chapter. The illustrations are copyrighted to Jenny Wang, 2008.

SUGGESTED READINGS

Boutros C, Ryan K, Katz S, et al. Total laparoscopic distal pancreatectomy: beyond selected patients. *Am Surg.* 2011;77:1526-1530.

Bruzoni M, Sasson AR. Open and laparoscopic spleen-preserving, splenic vessel–preserving distal pancreatectomy: indications and outcomes. *J Gastrointest Surg.* 2008;12:1202-1206.

Kooby DA, Gillespie T, Bentrem D, et al. Left-sided pancreatectomy: a multicenter comparison of laparoscopic and open approaches. *Ann Surg.* 2008;248:438-446.

Kooby DA, Hawkins WG, Schmidt CM, et al. A multicenter analysis of distal pancreatectomy for adenocarcinoma: is laparoscopic resection appropriate? *J Am Coll Surg.* 2010;210:779-785.

Newman NA, Lennon AM, Edil BH, et al. Preoperative endoscopic tattooing of pancreatic body and tail lesions decreases operative time for laparoscopic distal pancreatectomy. *Surgery.* 2010;148:371-377.

Sharpe SM, Talamonti MS, Wang E, et al. The laparoscopic approach to distal pancreatectomy for ductal adenocarcinoma results in shorter lengths of stay without compromising oncologic outcomes. *Am J Surg.* 2015;209: 557-563.

Venkat R, Edil BH, Schulick RD, et al. Laparoscopic distal pancreatectomy is associated with significantly less overall morbidity compared to the open technique: a systematic review and meta-analysis. *Ann Surg.* 2012;255: 1048-1059.

Vijan SS, Ahmed KA, Harmsen WS, et al. Laparoscopic vs. open distal pancreatectomy: a single-institution comparative study. *Arch Surg.* 2010;145: 616-621.

Yan JF, Kuang TT, Ji DY, et al. Laparoscopic versus open distal pancreatectomy for benign or premalignant pancreatic neoplasms: a two-center comparative study. *J Zhejiang Univ Sci B.* 2015;16:573-579.

Zureikat AH, Moser AJ, Boone BA, et al. 250 robotic pancreatic resections: safety and feasibility. *Ann Surg.* 2013;258:554-559.

MINIMALLY INVASIVE PANCREATIC SURGERY

Brian A. Boone, MD, Amer H. Zureikat, MD, FACS, Melissa E. Hogg, MD, MS, and Herbert J. Zeh III, MD

Minimally invasive surgery (MIS) is an operative approach, not a discrete field of surgical study. Nearly all surgical subspecialties have adopted MIS techniques in an attempt to improve patient-centered outcomes. Indeed, the overwhelming trend over the last 30 years suggests that MIS approaches do result in improved recovery, decreased length of stay, and decreased postoperative discomfort. Even to the casual observer it is obvious that operative approaches across the breadth of surgery are unlikely to devolve back to large open incisions. In fact, the opposite is true; given the ever more rapid pace of technological improvement, it is likely that even less invasive approaches to surgical management will occur.

Despite improvements over the last several decades, pancreatic surgery continues to be associated with significant morbidity and mortality. The use of minimally invasive approaches to pancreatic surgery, including laparoscopic and robotic surgery, is driven by a desire to reduce morbidity and improve postoperative recovery. It has been proposed that this high morbidity continues to prevent a large number of patients with pancreatic cancer from receiving multimodality therapy. With the availability of more effective chemotherapies in recent years, this may be a critical component to improving survival. Given the high complexity, low volume, and high morbidity associated with pancreatic surgery, it is no surprise that this subspecialty was one of the last to adopt minimally invasive approaches. However, as outlined later in the chapter, the last decade has seen a substantial increase in the use of minimally invasive pancreatic surgery, confirming its feasibility, safety, and potential advantages. Some of the renewed interest in minimally invasive pancreatic surgery is a result of robotic technology, with its perceived improvements in surgeon visualization and dexterity over traditional laparoscopic platforms. Moving forward, hepato-pancreato-biliary (HPB) surgical oncologists will focus on standardizing the approaches, patient selection, and, most important, developing appropriate training curriculum that will ensure surgeon proficiencies and optimal patient outcomes during adoption of the technology.

■ PREOPERATIVE EVALUATION

A thorough history and physical examination is performed before additional workup including patient symptoms and risk factors. A triphasic computed tomographic (CT) scan with fine cuts through the pancreas is critical for evaluation of pancreatic pathology and to evaluate resectability of pancreatic malignancy based its on relationship to the mesenteric vessels, portal vein (PV), and hepatic artery. Alternatively, magnetic resonance imaging (MRI) also may be performed. Arterial anomalies, including replaced or accessory hepatic arteries, also must be evaluated. A high-quality scan is a critically important aspect of preoperative planning because the tumor and its anatomic relationships cannot be palpated intraoperatively during minimally invasive pancreatic surgery. We routinely perform endoscopic ultrasound to further characterize pancreatic masses, evaluate the relationship to the mesenteric vessels, identify abnormal lymph nodes, and perform biopsy on masses to obtain a tissue diagnosis.

Minimally invasive pancreatic surgery is utilized for a wide variety of both benign and malignant indications but should be performed by highly trained surgeons who have extensive prior experience with laparoscopic and robotic surgery. Relative contraindications to minimally invasive pancreatic surgery include extensive prior abdominal surgery, particularly liver and foregut surgeries that promote adhesions in the upper abdomen. A high body mass index (BMI) is considered a relative contraindication; however, successful minimally invasive pancreatic surgery has been performed safely in patients who are morbidly obese, and a subset of surgeons feel that the MIS approach is preferred because of the difficulty of open surgery in patients with this body habitus and a higher rate of wound infections. Evidence of superior mesenteric or PV involvement on preoperative imaging is a relative contraindication. Although these procedures are technically more difficult and potentially increase perioperative morbidity, vein resections have been performed safely using minimally invasive platforms. Evidence of arterial involvement of the celiac trunk or common hepatic artery (CHA) is not an absolute contraindication, as modified Appleby resections also have been performed safely using minimally invasive platforms. The addition of complex arterial or vein resections should be considered carefully by the surgeon in the context of multimodal treatment of the disease being treated. Most patients with pancreatic ductal adenocarcinoma and these advanced tumors are unlikely to benefit from a purely surgical approach.

■ MINIMALLY INVASIVE DISTAL PANCREATECTOMY

Because of the less technically demanding nature of the dissection, as well as the lack of a complex anastomosis, the distal pancreatectomy was the first pancreatic resection attempted with MIS techniques. Since first being described in 1994, minimally invasive distal pancreatectomy has become the standard of care at most major academic centers. Indeed, laparoscopic distal pancreatectomy is the most frequently performed minimally invasive pancreatic surgery and has the most extensive support in the literature. Brief operative techniques utilizing the laparoscopic and robotic approaches are reviewed along with an examination of the evidence supporting the use of minimally invasive distal pancreatectomy.

Operative Approach to Laparoscopic Distal Pancreatectomy

The patient is positioned supine with a bean bag or pillow under the left flank. A footboard is utilized to provide additional support for steep reverse Trendelenburg position. The table is rotated left side up. An optical separator device in the left upper quadrant is used to gain access to the abdomen. Four additional ports are utilized: a 12-mm port just above the umbilicus, two 5-mm ports in the left upper and right upper quadrants, and an additional 5-mm port placed in the lateral right upper quadrant for the liver retractor, which will retract the left lateral segment and stomach. The lesser sac is opened with bipolar electrocautery, and the short gastric vessels are ligated. The bipolar cautery device is used to mobilize the splenic flexure, taking great care to avoid injury to the colon. The inferior border of the pancreas is dissected, and a retropancreatic tunnel is created. The splenic artery and vein are dissected individually and divided using an endovascular stapler. If a spleen-preserving approach is favored, the pancreas can be transected and the dissection is carried out along the surface of the major vessels until reaching the splenic hilum. An umbilical tape is placed to retract the pancreas anteriorly, and an endovascular stapler is used to divide the pancreas. The method of pancreatic parenchymal dissection is a matter of surgeon preference, as a recent randomized trial in Europe did not identify superiority of either stapled or cautery over sewing. It is our opinion that the thickness of the pancreas at the site of transection is critical in deciding the appropriate approach. Stapling is favored when transecting the neck, where the gland is thin, whereas more distal transections are performed with cautery and oversewing. The spleen and pancreas are placed into separate Endo Catch bags to facilitate removal through the MIS incision. The pancreas is removed through a utility incision in the left lower quadrant. The spleen is morcellated and then removed. A 19-mm Blake drain is left at the pancreatic transection margin.

Operative Approach to Robotic Distal Pancreatectomy

Our approach to robotic distal pancreatectomy is similar to that of laparoscopic distal pancreatectomy, but it takes advantage of the improved visualization and dexterity of the robotic platform. The patient is positioned supine with the left side of the table elevated and in reverse Trendelenburg position. An optical separator is placed in the left upper quadrant. The abdomen is inspected closely for evidence of metastases. Our approach utilizes a 12-mm port to the patient's left and superior to the umbilicus; two 8-mm ports, one in the lateral right upper quadrant and one in the left lower quadrant; and a 15-mm port in the left lower quadrant. This port will be enlarged to serve as the utility incision for specimen extraction. The procedure begins by entering the lesser sac. The anterior pancreas is cleared from adhesions to the stomach, and the short gastric vessels are ligated using bipolar electrocautery. Next, the dissection at the inferior and superior borders of the pancreas is performed. For malignant ductal tumors, we favor routine transection of the pancreas over the splenoportal confluence. This facilitates lymphadenectomy along the common hepatic, left gastric, and splenic arteries. After this dissection, the retropancreatic tunnel is created using a combination of blunt and sharp dissection. An umbilical tape is placed to retract the pancreas anteriorly from the superior mesenteric and portal veins, and the pancreas is divided using an endovascular stapler. The splenic artery and vein are stapled at their origins unless splenic preservation is being attempted in the case of benign disease. During the retroperitoneal dissection, care is taken to remove the fascia of Strasberg over the adrenal gland, left renal vein, and kidney with the specimen. The spleen and pancreas are removed in two separate Endo Catch bags. The specimens are removed from the left lower quadrant utility incision after morcellation of the spleen. A 19-mm Blake drain is placed near the transected pancreas before closure.

Outcomes of Minimally Invasive Distal Pancreatectomy

There have been no large randomized trials comparing minimally invasive distal pancreatectomy with open distal pancreatectomy. The data supporting minimally invasive distal pancreatectomy are based on a number of large, case-matched series that have demonstrated a reduction in blood loss, lower transfusion rates, and short postoperative stays compared with open surgery (Table 1). Meta-analyses of thousands of patients have confirmed these benefits and identified lower rates of surgical site infections after minimally invasive distal pancreatectomy.

Only a few studies have focused on the differences between laparoscopic and robotic distal pancreatic resection. A limited number of small, single-institution studies suggest that the robotic approach is associated with longer operative time and higher cost, with equivalent mortality, pancreatic fistula rate, and R0 resection rate. A few series have suggested shorter length of stay and higher rates of splenic preservation. Our own experience has suggested that the principal benefits of the robotic platform in distal pancreatectomy are decreased blood loss and lower risk for conversion to open surgery.

■ MINIMALLY INVASIVE PANCREATICODUODENECTOMY

Short of a liver transplant, there is probably no more difficult abdominal surgical procedure than the pancreaticoduodenectomy. The skill set needed to safely complete this procedure requires the surgeon to have in-depth knowledge of the retroperitoneum, be proficient in dissection and repair of sensitive vascular structures, and be able to perform complex reconstruction of the foregut. These demands are extremely difficult to master in the open surgical approach and perhaps even more difficult when using minimally invasive approaches. Indeed, the first minimally invasive pancreaticoduodenectomy performed by Gagner took more than 20 hours and was followed by a 30-day length of stay, which led the authors to question the ultimate utility of this approach at that time. However, over the last 10 years several high-volume centers across the world have developed robust minimally invasive pancreaticoduodenectomy experiences that support the safety and potential benefits of the approach

TABLE 1: Select Series Comparing Laparoscopic, Robotic, and Open Distal Pancreatectomy

Author	Journal	Year	Study Type	Patients (n)			Operation Time (min)			Splenic Preservation Rate (%)			Conversion Rate (%)			Length of Stay (days)		
				Lap	Robot	Open	Lap	Robot	Open	Lap	Robot	Open	Lap	Robot	Open	Lap	Robot	Open
Magge	*JAMA Surg*	2013	Matched cohort	28		34	317		294	–	–	–	18%		–	6*		8
Deouadi	*Ann Surg*	2013	Retrospective	94	30		371	293*		18%	7%		16%	0%*		7	6	
Chen	*Surg Endosc*	2015	Matched cohort	50	69		200	150*		26%	65%		6%	0%		15	12*	
Butturini	*Surg Endosc*	2015	Prospective	21	22		195	255*		19%	27%		4.70%	4.50%		7	7	
Lee	*J Am Coll Surg*	2015	Retrospective	131	37	637	193	213*	185	22%	8%	14%	31%	38%	–	5	5	7
Ryan	*JSLS*	2015	Prospective	16	18		254	297*		–	–		19%	11%		4	5	
Nakamura	*J Hepatobiliary Pancreat Surg*	2015	Matched cohort	729		729	319*		261	30%		13%	–	–		19*		23
De Rooij	*J Am Coll Surg*	2015	Retrospective	64		569	213		208	80%		32%	33%		–	8*		10
Shin	*J Am Coll Surg*	2015	Retrospective	70		80	239		254	–		–	–		–	9*		12

*Statistically significant, P <0.05.

and pave the way for more widespread adoption. Currently there are two important questions to be answered in this field: (1) Will the robotic platform provide additional benefit over the laparoscopic platform when performing minimally invasive pancreaticoduodenectomy? and (2) Can appropriate training centers and programs be developed to ensure adequate surgical proficiency in new trainees and adopters?

Operative Approach to Laparoscopic Pancreaticoduodenectomy

The procedure is performed with the patient in the supine position. At times, steep reverse Trendelenburg position is utilized to facilitate exposure; therefore a footboard should be placed. Seven ports—five 5-mm ports and two 12-mm ports—are placed in a crescent shape around the xiphoid process. A utility incision in the right lower quadrant is used for extraction of the specimen. After the absence of metastatic disease is confirmed by exploration of the peritoneal cavity and liver, the lesser sac is opened by dividing the gastrocolic ligament using bipolar electrocautery. The gastroepiploic vessels are preserved, and the gastroepiploic vein is followed to identify the superior mesenteric vein (SMV) and then clipped at its origin. The middle colic vein is identified and preserved if possible. The inferior border of the pancreas is dissected, and a tunnel is begun between the SMV and the pancreatic neck. This allows for early assessment of resectability by identifying involvement of the portal or superior mesenteric veins. After mobilization of the hepatic flexure, full kocherization of the duodenum to the level of the left renal vein is performed. The ligament of Treitz is divided to mobilize the third and fourth portions of the duodenum. The porta hepatis is dissected similar to the open approach. The preoperative CT scan should be reviewed carefully, and extra care is taken to visualize any replaced or aberrant hepatic arteries when dividing the common bile duct (CBD) because this area cannot be palpated using the laparoscopic approach.

Attention then is turned to the superior border of the pancreas to complete the retropancreatic tunnel. The hepatic artery is identified by dissecting the gastrohepatic ligament. The right gastric artery is divided at its origin. The distal stomach or duodenum is divided with an endovascular laparoscopic stapling device based on the surgeon's preference for pylorus preservation. The gastroduodenal artery (GDA) is stapled at its origin after a test clamp is performed and flow to the hepatic artery proper is confirmed. The superior border of the pancreas is dissected, and the tunnel behind the pancreas is completed. Bipolar electrocautery or ultrasonic shears are used to divide the pancreas. Sutures can be placed along the superior and inferior border of the pancreas to control bleeding during transection. An umbilical tape can be used to retract the pancreas anteriorly and avoid injury to the superior mesenteric and portal veins. After division of the pancreatic specimen, attention then turns to the most technically challenging portion of the procedure, the uncinate dissection. The specimen is retracted anteriorly and laterally in order to view the remaining attachments to the superior mesenteric artery (SMA) and SMV. An umbilical tape can be placed around the PV superior to the splenic vein to allow for retraction of the vein for better visualization of the SMA and to assist with control of major bleeding if it should occur. The venous tributaries to the uncinate process from the first jejunal branch are clipped and divided with bipolar electrocautery. The inferior pancreaticoduodenal artery also is clipped and divided. Careful attention is required during the uncinate dissection if the procedure is being performed for pancreatic adenocarcinoma, as this area is at high risk for positive margin. Therefore all tissues must be removed from the right side of the SMA to minimize the risk of a positive margin.

Before reconstruction the pancreatic remnant should be mobilized around 2 cm off of the splenic vein to allow it to be retracted upward and achieve better visualization of the pancreatic duct. There are two common methods of reconstruction described by surgeons performing laparoscopic pancreaticoduodenectomy: an end-to-end intussuscepting anastomosis that invaginates the pancreas into the end of the reconstructive limb of jejunum and the more traditional modified Blumgart end-to-side, duct-to-mucosa pancreaticojejunostomy. When performing the intussuscepting anastomosis, the staple line is removed from the jejunum. A double armed 4-0 polydioxanone suture is used to fashion the anastomosis. The first suture is placed on the antimesenteric border of bowel and the cephalad pancreas, then run continuously toward the mesenteric side of the bowel and the caudal pancreas to form the posterior suture line. After the first few throws are parachuted down, the assistant maintains tension on the suture line to ensure that it closely approximates bowel to the pancreas. Once the caudal pancreas is reached, the second arm of the suture is used to start the anterior suture line at the cephalad aspect of the pancreas. The jejunal mucosa is inverted, and tension is applied toward the patient's left side to facilitate invagination of the pancreas into the small bowel. Once the caudal aspect of the pancreas is reached, the two suture arms are tied.

The end-to-side, duct-to-mucosa pancreaticojejunostomy uses two layers of absorbable monofilament. The first sutures are placed full thickness through the pancreas, then a longitudinal seromuscular bite is taken on the antimesenteric border of the bowel, and the suture is taken back through the pancreas. Clips should be placed on the untied ends of suture. Approximately five of these sutures are placed along the pancreas to approximate the pancreatic parenchyma to the jejunum. After an enterotomy is made anterior to the previously placed sutures, two posterior duct-to-mucosa sutures are placed and tied. Three to five anterior duct-to-mucosa sutures then are placed and tied. The sutures that were placed full thickness through the pancreas then are tied, and the needles are left in place. The anastomosis is completed by finishing the second anterior layer using these sutures to grab seromuscular bites of jejunum anterior to the duct anastomosis.

Operative Approach to Robotic Pancreaticoduodenectomy

For purposes of teaching and analysis we find it convenient to break down the robotic pancreaticoduodenectomy into seven discrete steps. Early in our experience we often would perform step 1 laparoscopically; however, this is currently accomplished robotically. Step 1 includes mobilization of the right colon and kocherization of the duodenum (Figure 1). A near total Cattell-Braasch maneuver is performed in order to expose the SMV at the root of the small bowel mesentery. An extended Kocher's maneuver is completed in an attempt to pull the jejunum into the right upper quadrant via division of the ligament of Treitz. The jejunum is transected around 10 cm distal to the ligament of Treitz. Next, the gastrocolic omentum is divided, providing entrance into the lesser sac, followed by dissection of the posterior stomach from the anterior surface of the pancreas. The right gastric artery is ligated close to the stomach, and the right gastroepiploic artery then is ligated at the corresponding greater curvature side. The stomach is divided with a linear stapler at this time, and an automated liver retractor is inserted to facilitate exposure.

Step 2 involves dissection of the portal structures (Figure 2). Dissection often is started along the superior border of the pancreas using the robotic hook to identify the station 8a lymph node and facilitate identification of the CHA. The right gastric artery is divided again, now at its origin. Next, the GDA is identified and dissected out. The anterior surface of the PV then is identified in the anatomic triangle between the CHA, GDA, and neck of the pancreas. Dissection is carried along the PV to identify the medial wall of the CBD. Next, the dissection is moved to the lateral edge of the porta hepatis. The lymph nodes are dissected along the lateral border of the CBD, taking care to identify any aberrant right hepatic artery. After ensuring complete identification of all portal structures, the GDA and CBD are divided with vascular loads of the endovascular stapler. Step 3

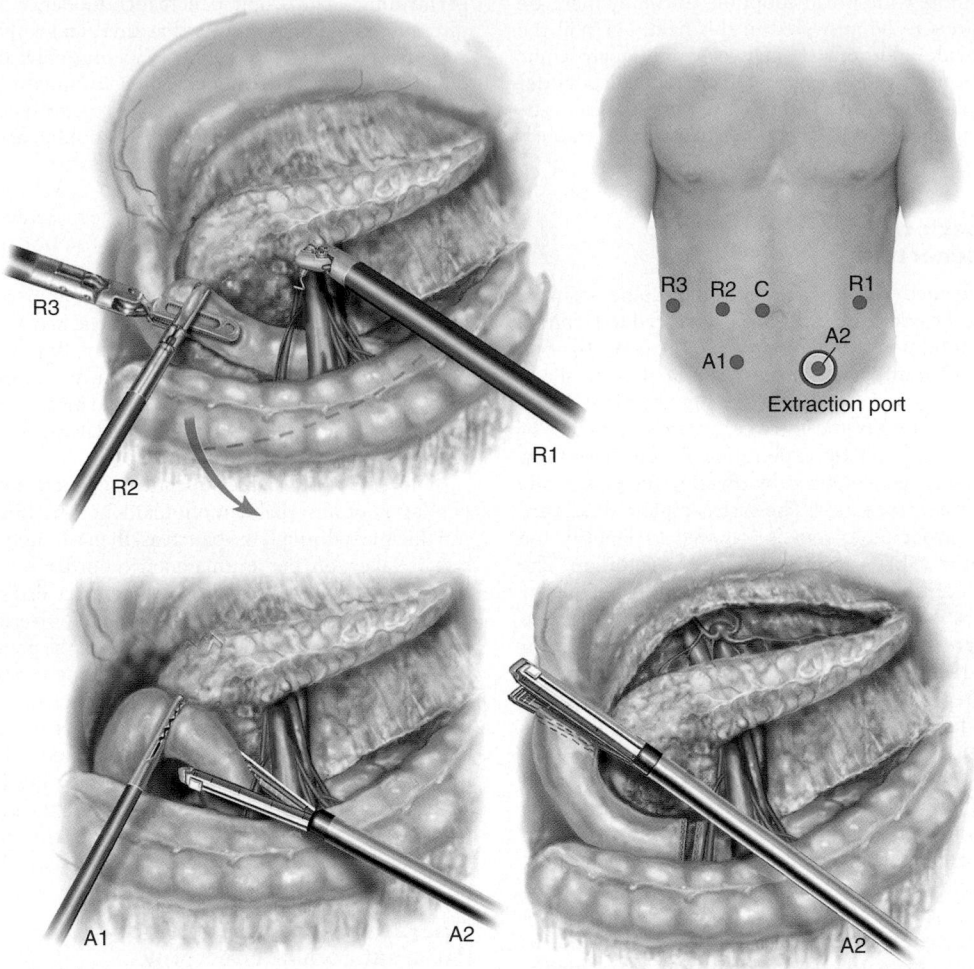

FIGURE 1 Step 1: Port placement for robotic pancreaticoduodenectomy, mobilization of the right colon, full kocherization, takedown of the ligament of Treitz, and division of the jejunum and the stomach and duodenum. *A1-2*, Assistant ports 1-2; *C*, camera port; *R1-3*, robot arm ports 1-3. *(Adapted from Zeh HJ III, et al. Robotic-assisted major pancreatic resection. Adv Surg. 2011;45:323-340. Courtesy Randal S. McKenzie, McKenzie Illustrations.)*

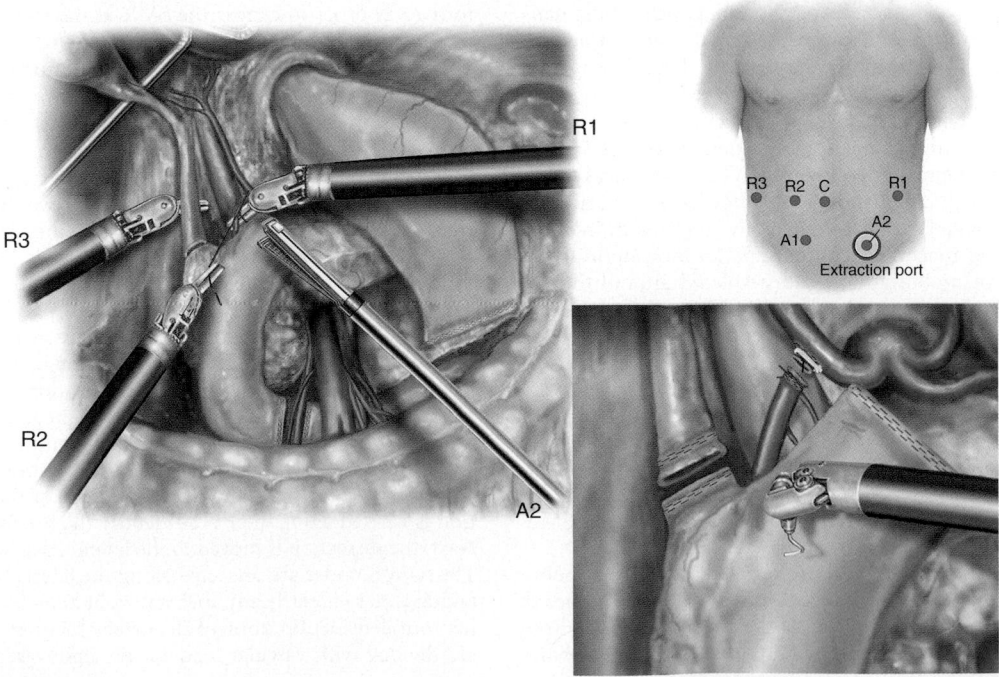

FIGURE 2 Step 2: Portal dissection during robotic pancreaticoduodenectomy. *(Adapted from Zeh HJ III, et al. Robotic-assisted major pancreatic resection. Adv Surg. 2011;45:323-340. Courtesy Randal S. McKenzie, McKenzie Illustrations.)*

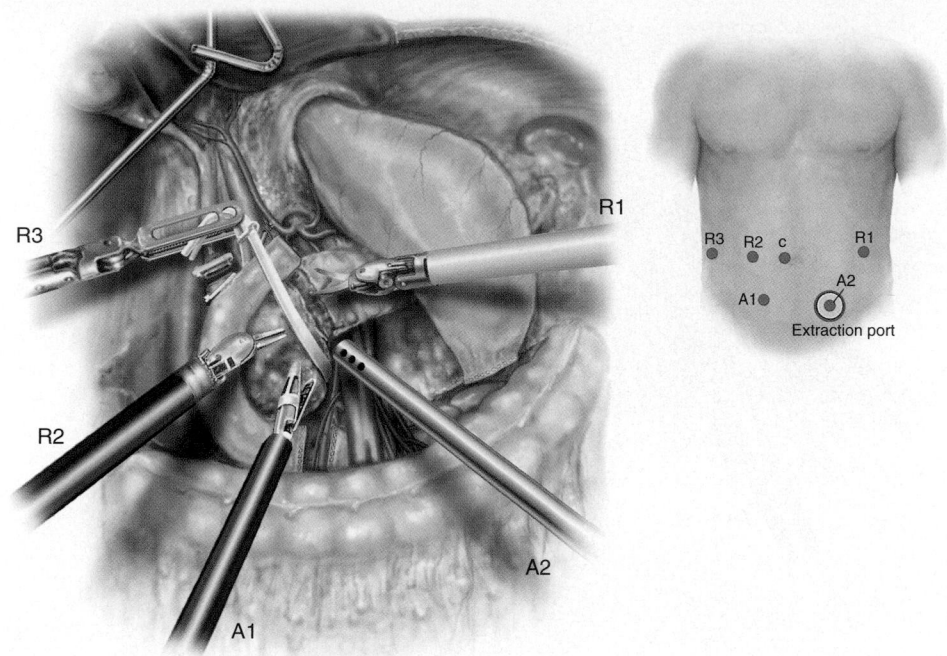

FIGURE 3 Step 3: Dissection and division of the pancreatic neck. *(Adapted from Zeh HJ III, et al. Robotic-assisted major pancreatic resection. Adv Surg. 2011;45:323-340. Courtesy Randal S. McKenzie, McKenzie Illustrations.)*

involves dissection of the infrapancreatic SMV and division of the neck of the gland (Figure 3). The right gastroepiploic vein is identified and followed to its origin to locate the SMV and middle colic vein. The gastroepiploic vein is doubly clipped, tied, or more commonly divided with the bipolar cautery device. The SMV is dissected off the inferior border of the pancreas, and a tunnel is created over the PV. The angle afforded by the robotic camera ensures safe visualization of the tunnel. After completion of the tunnel, the neck of the pancreas is divided with electrocautery, reserving sharp robotic scissor transection for the pancreatic duct. We do not routinely place stay sutures in the neck of the gland in our updated approach. Step 4 is the uncinate dissection (Figure 4). The pancreas is mobilized from the lateral border of the SMV-PV, working caudad to cephalad. The first jejunal branch is identified and the small perforating branches draining the uncinate are divided (see Figure 4, *A*). If there are tumors in this area, alternatively the first jejunal branch can be divided (see Figure 4, *B*). The SMV-PV is reflected medially, and the SMA is identified. Dissection proceeds along the SMA by clearing all tissue around the anterior, right side, and posterior surface of the SMA. Every attempt is made to identify the two named pancreatidoduodenal arteries, which are clipped and then divided with the bipolar cautery device. After removal of the specimen, the gallbladder is removed.

Step 5 starts the reconstruction with the pancreaticojejunostomy (Figure 5). We favor a two-layered, end-to-side, duct-to-mucosa pancreaticojejunostomy in a modified Blumgart fashion. Step 6 is the choledochojejunostomy, performed in a running fashion with 4-0 V-Loc braided suture. Step 7 is an antecolic Hoffmeister end-to-side gastrojejunostomy that is handsewn or stapled.

Outcomes of Minimally Invasive Pancreaticoduodenectomy

There are no randomized trials examining laparoscopic pancreaticoduodenectomy versus the open approach; however, there is a growing body of level II and III data supporting its application. There now have been a number of single-institution series that have published on more than 100 laparoscopic Whipple's procedures

(Table 2). Outcomes across these highly selected cohorts are comparable to those of historical open controls. Nonrandomized propensity controlled comparisons of open and laparoscopic Whipple's procedures demonstrate equivalent postoperative morbidity and pancreatic fistula rates, with improvement in rates of delayed gastric emptying and shorter length of stay. It is interesting to note that although there were small numbers of patients for evaluation of oncologic outcomes, there is a suggestion of a higher rate of treatment with adjuvant chemotherapy in MIS cohorts. Several meta-analyses have suggested that laparoscopic pancreacticoduodenectomy is safe with comparable oncologic outcomes and shorter length of stay.

Currently there are no randomized controlled trials comparing robotic and open or robotic and laparoscopic pancreacticoduodenectomy. The majority of the literature supporting the robotic platform is in the form of large single-institution series and several small case control analyses (see Table 2). Our group in Pittsburgh has published the largest series of minimally invasive pancreacticoduodenectomy, all performed on the DaVinci platform. Moreover, we have identified a learning curve with key inflection points corresponding to optimization of performance. Our experience suggested that it takes 20 cases to see optimization of blood loss and conversion rate, 40 cases to see optimization of pancreatic fistula rates, and 80 cases to optimize operative time. Analysis of outcomes of the robotic procedure past the learning curve, a so-called mature procedure, demonstrated median operative time of 369 minutes, 6% grades B and C fistula rate, 3% conversion rate, and 3% 90-day mortality. Median length of stay for the latter part of the cohort was 7 days.

■ OTHER MINIMALLY INVASIVE PANCREATIC OPERATIONS

The utility and diverse application of both laparoscopic and robotic approaches to pancreatic surgery has been demonstrated by the surgeons utilizing the technology. These approaches are safe and feasible for every surgery performed by an experienced pancreatic surgeon. Both laparoscopic and robotic techniques have been utilized

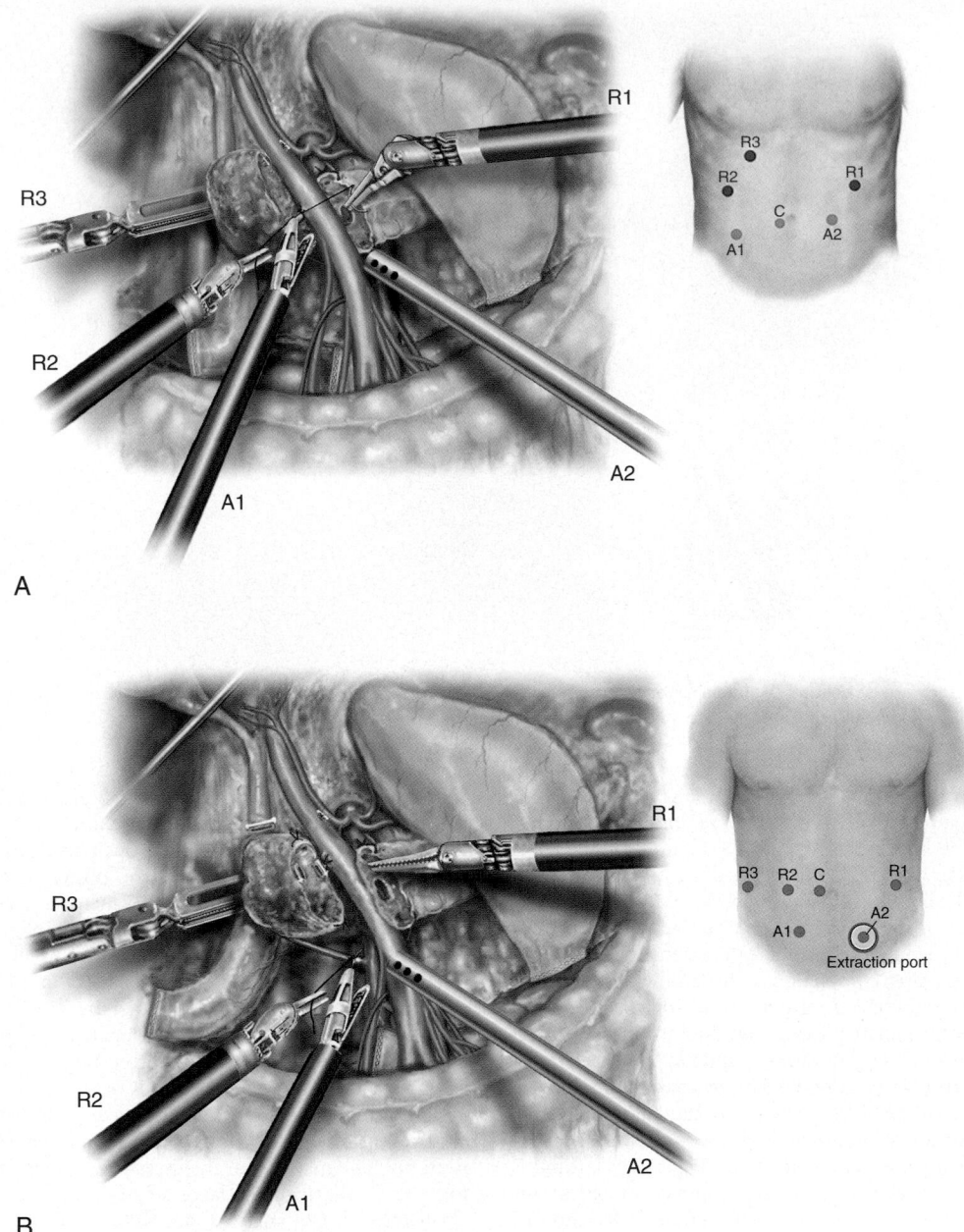

FIGURE 4 Step 4: Uncinate dissection including ligation of vein branches draining the (**A**) uncinate and (**B**) first jejunal artery. *(Adapted from Zeh HJ III, et al. Robotic-assisted major pancreatic resection. Adv Surg. 2011;45:323-340. Courtesy Randal S. McKenzie, McKenzie Illustrations.)*

for central pancreatectomy, total pancreatectomy with or without auto islet cell transplant, distal pancreatectomy with celiac axis reconstruction, and pancreatic enucleation. Minimally invasive duodenal surgery also has been performed, including periampullary resections and partial duodenal resections of D3 and D4. Surgical approaches for the management of chronic pancreatitis and its sequelae, including Frey's and Puestow procedures, and pancreatic cyst gastrostomy or enterostomy all have been performed with both the laparoscopic and the robotic approaches. Because these various procedures are performed infrequently, the data supporting their use are limited to small case series without any significant comparison of the different MIS approaches to each other or to open surgery (Table 3). The diverse array of MIS procedures performed confirms that these approaches represent a set of tools available to the surgeon that can be applied to treat patients with a variety of duodenal and pancreatic pathology.

■ REACHING PROFICIENCY IN MINIMALLY INVASIVE PANCREATIC SURGERY

Key considerations for any new surgical technology or approach are the training of future surgeons and the adoption of the new platform by mature surgeons. Pancreatic surgery in general is faced with unique challenges in this area given that it is a low-volume, highly complex specialty that is associated with high morbidity. In fact, learning curves for open pancreacticoduodenectomy and robotic pancreacticoduodenectomy are reported to be long and remarkably similar (70 to 80 cases). These numbers are daunting when one considers that the average HPB or surgical oncology fellow generally completes 20 to 30 pancreacticoduodenectomies even in their advanced training. As a specialty, we need to address how to better train pancreatic surgeons in both MIS and open procedures to ensure

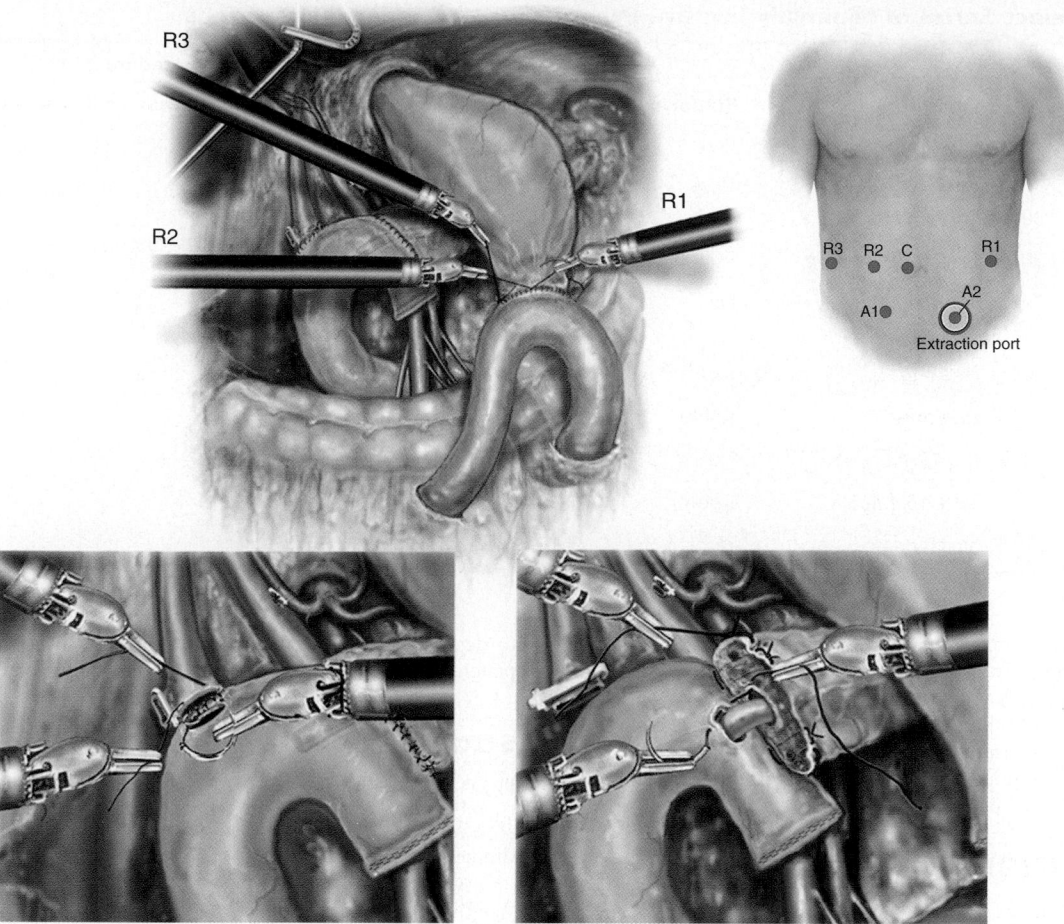

FIGURE 5 Step 5: Reconstruction including gastrojejunostomy, hepaticojejunostomy, and pancreaticojejunostomy. *(Adapted from Zeh HJ III, et al. Robotic-assisted major pancreatic resection. Adv Surg. 2011;45:323-340. Courtesy Randal S. McKenzie, McKenzie Illustrations.)*

TABLE 2: Select Series of Laparoscopic and Robotic Pancreaticoduodenectomy

Approach	Author	Journal	Year	No. of Patients	Operative Time (min)	EBL (mL)	Conversion (%)	PF Rate (%)	Mortality (%)
Total laparoscopic	Palanivelu	*J Hepatobiliary Pancreat Surg*	2009	75	357	74	0	6.67	1.33
	Kim	*Surg Endosc*	2012	100	474	NR	5	26	1
	Asbun	*J Am Coll Surg*	2012	53	541	195	22.6*	16.7	5.7
	Croome	*Ann Surg*	2014	108	379	492	6.4	11†	2
Robotic	Guilianotti	*Surg Endosc*	2010	60	421	394	18	32	3
	Buchs	*World J Surg*	2011	44	444	387	5	18	5
	Chalikonda	*Surg Endosc*	2012	30	476	486	10	7	3
	Boggi	*Br J Surg*	2013	34	597	–	0	12	3
	Boone	*JAMA Surg*	2015	120	417	250	3.3	6.9†	3.3

*Includes conversion to hand assist port.

†Includes only grades B and C pancreatic fistulas.

EBL, Estimated blood loss; *NR*, not reported; *PF*, pancreatic fistula.

optimal outcomes for our patients. Our group has developed a robotic curriculum that utilizes a combination of the robotic simulator and artificial tissue–based practice sessions, where trainees can perform anastomoses on lifelike tissue just as it would be performed during an actual robotic Whipple's procedure. Our approach gives graded responsibility in a stepwise fashion to facilitate trainee development but also to ensure efficiency of the surgical procedure.

Trainees first must complete the virtual simulator curriculum, mastering the basic skills such as instrument articulation, energy dissection, suturing, and knot tying. Once these skills have been perfected, trainees begin the artificial tissue curriculum. The enteric, biliary, and pancreatic anastomoses are performed and recorded, with feedback given at the conclusion of each session. Once the tissue curriculum has been mastered, trainees must demonstrate

TABLE 3: Select Series of Minimally Invasive Pancreatic and Duodenal Resections

| Author | Year | Journal | Platform | No. of Patients by Procedure | | | | | | | |
				Central	Total	Enucleation	Frey	Beger	Duodenal	Appleby	Uncinate
Machado	2013	*Surg Laparoscop Endosc Percutan Tech*	Lap	51							
Song	2015	*Surg Endosc*	Lap	26							
Downs-Canner	2015	*J Gastrointest Surg*	Robot						26		
Kokosis	2015	*Surg Laparoscop Endosc Percutan Tech*	Lap						12		
Stauffer	2013	*Pancreas*	Lap						10		
Zureikat	2013	*Ann Surg*	Robot	13	5	10	3			4	
Machado	2013	*Arq Gastroenterol*	Lap		2	8					5
Zhan	2013	*Int J Med Robot*	Robot	10		1	4				
Guilianotti	2010	*Surg Endosc*	Hybrid	3	1	3					

Lap, Laparoscopic.

proficiency in each step of the robotic Whipple's procedure before moving on to the next, beginning with the gastrojejunostomy, followed by the hepaticojejunostomy and the resection, and culminating with the pancreaticojejunostomy. This approach has allowed us to train fellows who are able to independently complete the entire robotic pancreaticoduodenectomy and who are capable of establishing independent MIS pancreatic programs.

■ CONCLUSION

MIS has revolutionized nearly every realm of general surgery and its subspecialties. Although the technical demands of pancreatic surgery initially slowed the adoption of MIS approaches to pancreatic resection, new technology and advancements have made minimally invasive pancreatic surgery feasible and increasingly utilized. Although the benefits of minimally invasive distal pancreatectomy have been established with large case-matched series, investigation is ongoing to demonstrate a definitive outcome benefit of minimally invasive pancreaticoduodenectomy compared with open surgery.

SUGGESTED READINGS

Boone BA, Zenati M, Hogg ME, et al. Assessment of quality outcomes for robotic pancreaticoduodenectomy: identification of the learning curve. *JAMA Surg.* 2015;150:416-422.

Croome KP, Farnell MB, Que FG, et al. Total laparoscopic pancreaticoduodenectomy for pancreatic ductal adenocarcinoma: oncologic advantages over open approaches? *Ann Surg.* 2014;260:633-638, discussion 638-640.

Kendrick ML, Cusati D. Total laparoscopic pancreaticoduodenectomy: feasibility and outcome in an early experience. *Arch Surg.* 2010;145:19-23.

Song KB, Kim SC, Park JB, et al. Single-center experience of laparoscopic left pancreatic resection in 359 consecutive patients: changing the surgical paradigm of left pancreatic resection. *Surg Endosc.* 2011;25:3364-3372.

Zureikat AH, Moser AJ, Boone BA, et al. 250 robotic pancreatic resections: safety and feasibility. *Ann Surg.* 2013;258:554-559, discussion 559-562.

LAPAROSCOPIC BYPASS FOR PANCREATIC CANCER

Ezra N. Teitelbaum, MD

Pancreatic cancer is the fourth most common cause of cancer death in the United States among both men and women. There were approximately 49,000 new diagnoses in 2015, and because of pancreatic cancer's extremely aggressive nature, almost all of those patients eventually will die from the disease. Surgical resection offers the only possibility of long-term survival; however, only 15% to 20% of patients will be resectable at the time of diagnosis because of local invasion or metastases. Median survival in patients with locally advanced disease is approximately 8 to 12 months, and those with metastatic disease have a life expectancy of only 3 to 6 months. Because of this dismal prognosis, treatment strategies should focus not only on extending the patient's life, but also on palliating symptoms and optimizing quality of life for these remaining months.

Local invasion of pancreatic cancer can cause biliary obstruction and gastric outlet obstruction (GOO). These can be present at the time of diagnosis or develop as the tumor enlarges. Both obstructions occur most commonly in patients with tumors in the head of the pancreas. Biliary obstruction leads to jaundice, which can cause intractable pruritus and lead to cholangitis and liver failure. GOO results in nausea, vomiting, and inability to tolerate any oral intake. Surgical bypass of both biliary and gastric outlet obstruction can be used to palliate these symptoms in patients with advanced pancreatic cancer. More recently, these bypass operations have been performed laparoscopically, which lessens perioperative morbidity and convalescence, helping patients to return home and to an adequate quality of life faster than after traditional open operations. However, even using minimally invasive techniques, palliative operations on patients with advanced pancreatic cancer carry significant risk for complications and mortality. This risk must be balanced with the expected benefit in terms of improvement in symptoms. In addition, endoscopic techniques for stenting of both biliary and enteric obstructions are advancing rapidly and proliferating. As a result, decision making regarding when and how to intervene in such patients is becoming increasingly complex. The optimal approach remains an area of considerable controversy and is sure to evolve as both surgical and endoscopic techniques continue to improve, and advances in radiation and chemotherapy further prolong life expectancy after initial diagnosis.

■ INDICATIONS AND CHOICE OF APPROACH

Biliary Obstruction

Half to three quarters of patients with pancreatic cancer are seen with a biliary obstruction at the time of diagnosis, and up to 80% of patients will go on to develop biliary obstruction and jaundice over the course of their disease progression. Jaundice can cause severe pruritus that is difficult to control medically and can further lead to cholangitis and eventual liver dysfunction and failure. For this reason, patients with biliary obstruction from advanced pancreatic cancer should undergo palliative drainage using either surgical bypass or stenting via endoscopic retrograde cholangiopancreatography (ERCP).

The most comprehensive randomized trial comparing surgical bypass and ERCP stenting was performed by Smith and colleagues in 1994 and compared more than 100 patients in each group. The authors found that stenting resulted in less periprocedural mortality (3% vs 14%), fewer complications (11% vs 29%), and shorter length of stay (20 vs 29 days). Conversely, there was a much higher rate of recurrent biliary obstruction in the stent group (36% vs 2%). It should be noted that the trial involved open surgical bypass and plastic biliary stents, which have lower long-term patency rates than the self-expanding metal stents that are most commonly used today. However, more recent randomized trials using metal stents have shown similar results, with ERCP stenting carrying lower upfront morbidity at the expense of high rates of recurrent biliary obstruction. Based on these results, it appears that patients with biliary obstruction from unresectable pancreatic cancer should undergo ERCP self-expanding metal stent placement as first-line therapy. If stenting is not technically possible, surgical bypass should be considered only if the patient's life expectancy is more than 4 to 6 months. In patients who are found to be unresectable at the time of diagnostic laparoscopy (or laparotomy), the surgeon should proceed with biliary bypass because much of the short-term morbidity has been incurred already by the general anesthetic and surgical exploration.

Three main options exist for surgical biliary bypass: cholecysto-enterostomy, choledoenterostomy, and hepaticojejunostomy. The bowel anastomoses can be constructed using either duodenum or jejunum, and furthermore, jejunal bypasses can be constructed using either a loop or Roux-en-Y limb. Most surgeons prefer the use of a jejunal bypass over a duodenal one because postoperatively the cancer may grow to obstruct or dehisce the duodenal anastomosis. Early studies showed adequate results from a cholecystojejunostomy; however, more recent trials have demonstrated better long-term relief of jaundice with a bile duct to bowel bypass. Based on these data, most contemporary surgeons perform either a choledochojejunostomy or a hepaticojejunostomy. When performing a bypass using jejunum, either a loop or Roux-en-Y reconstruction can be used. The loop is advantageous because it requires only one anastomosis in these already high-risk patients, whereas a Roux-en-Y reconstruction reduces the risk of cholangitis from enteric reflux into the biliary tree. In general, patients who have longer life expectancy should undergo a Roux-en-Y reconstruction in order to avoid this longer-term risk.

Gastric Outlet Obstruction

Tumor invasion or compression of the duodenum or distal stomach can lead to GOO. The resulting symptoms of nausea, vomiting, and failure to tolerate oral intake are particularly severe, and subsequent dehydration can become fatal quickly if not addressed. Fortunately, GOO is not as common as biliary obstruction, occurring in only 10% to 25% of patients with unresectable pancreatic cancer. When it occurs, GOO should be treated with either endoscopic metal stent placement or surgical bypass. Several small randomized trials have compared these two modalities for treatment of GOO, the best of which is the SUSTENT study by Jeurnink and colleagues from 2010. Similar to results for biliary obstruction, the SUSTENT trial demonstrated an earlier resumption of oral intake in the stenting group but

more delayed complications and recurrent obstruction in those patients. Based on these results the authors recommended surgical bypass if the patient has a life expectancy of more than 2 months.

If a patient is found to be unresectable upon diagnostic laparoscopy and did not have GOO preoperatively, considerable controversy exists as to whether a prophylactic gastric bypass operation should be performed. A landmark trial by Lillemoe and colleagues in 1999 randomized such patients to gastrojejunostomy or no gastric bypass operation. No patients in the bypass group went on to develop GOO, whereas late GOO occurred in 19% of patients who did not receive an initial bypass. There were no differences in perioperative complications or mortality between the two groups. Based on these data, the authors recommended prophylactic bypass in patients who are deemed to be at high risk for GOO but did not go so far as to recommend operating on patients who are known to be unresectable preoperatively. However, a study by Espat and colleagues at Memorial Sloan Kettering offers evidence to the contrary. The study followed 155 patients who were found to have unresectable disease at the time of diagnostic laparoscopy but in whom neither a biliary nor a gastric bypass procedure was performed. Of these patients, only four went on to require surgical gastric bypass, and only one required endoscopic intervention (percutaneous endoscopic gastrostomy [PEG] tube placement) for palliation of GOO. The seemingly conflicting results of these two studies paint a confusing picture regarding management of patients who do not have GOO preoperatively and are found to have unresectable disease upon diagnostic laparoscopy. Surgeons should lean toward performing a prophylactic gastric bypass in patients with longer life expectancy (more than 6 months) and in those who are more likely to go on to develop GOO (based on tumor size and location).

■ OPERATIVE TECHNIQUE

Preparation, Positioning, and Port Placement

Patients should receive preoperative antibiotics and both chemical and mechanical deep venous thrombosis (DVT) prophylaxis. Positioning can be either supine or in a split-leg position, with the surgeon standing between the patient's legs. The initial port is placed in supraumbilical position using either an open Hasson or a closed Veress needle technique. This trocar should be able to accommodate a 10-mm, 30-degree laparoscope. Working trocars then are placed in the right and left upper quadrants so that "triangulation" is achieved, with the laparoscope positioned between the surgeon's two working instruments. An additional assistant port then can be placed in a left subcostal position, and a liver retractor can be placed through a subxiphoid incision (Nathanson retractor) or right subcostal trocar (internally articulating retractor). Then a diagnostic laparoscopy is performed to assess for metastatic disease. The peritoneal surface of the anterior abdominal wall, as well as the liver, visceral peritoneal surfaces, and root of the small bowel mesentery and mesocolon, should be inspected carefully. Suspicious nodules undergo biopsy and are sent for frozen section.

Gastric Bypass

Bypass with a gastrojejunostomy can be performed with a loop or Roux limb and in an antecolic or retrocolic fashion. In the setting of advanced pancreatic cancer, a loop is preferable, as it eliminates a second anastomosis without a significant functional downside. In addition, a loop jejunostomy allows for a Roux-en-Y limb to be created further downstream for use in a biliary bypass (Figure 1). Although some surgeons prefer a retrocolic gastrojejunostomy because of theoretical advantages in gastric emptying, it is technically much easier to bring the jejunal loop up in an antecolic fashion, especially when performed laparoscopically. Functional outcomes have not been shown to be any worse with an antecolic approach, and furthermore, metastatic disease or local invasion at the root of the mesocolon can cause subsequent obstruction of a retrocolic jejunal loop.

To perform the antecolic loop gastrojejunostomy, the patient is tilted into a steep reverse Trendelenburg position. The eventual anastomosis will be in a retrogastric position to facilitate emptying of the stomach, so the lesser sac must be entered to expose this area. This is done by dividing the gastrocolic ligament adjacent to the most inferior portion of the gastric antrum. This is done using a bipolar or ultrasonic energy device and should be performed close to the stomach wall to avoid leaving excessive fat that will make visualization of the anastomosis difficult but also far enough away so as to not injure the stomach. The stomach then is freed from any posterior attachments to the body of the pancreas to create space for the anastomosis. The omentum is divided vertically from this point down to the colon wall to create space for the jejunal loop to pass up to the stomach wall with the minimum amount of tension.

The assistant then lifts the transverse colon to expose the ligament of Treitz. The small bowel is measured 60 to 100 cm distal to the ligament of Treitz, and the jejunum in that position is brought up to the stomach. The jejunum should be oriented in an isoperistaltic position, so that the proximal bowel is adjacent to the cephalad portion of the gastric antrum, just posterior to the greater curvature. To perform an anastomosis with a linear stapler, first a "back-row" running 3-0 permanent braided suture is placed between the stomach and jejunum, starting proximal and ending distal. This is done in such a way that the antimesenteric border of the jejunum is brought into alignment with the posterior gastric wall for the subsequent anastomosis and can be performed with a free needle or laparoscopic suturing device. Many surgeons place only one or two interrupted stay sutures between the stomach and bowel to achieve this alignment, but we prefer a running suture because it creates a second layer to the anastomosis, as would occur with a handsewn technique.

Once the stomach and bowel are aligned, enterotomies are made in each at the distal end of the eventual anastomosis. This can be done "cold" with scissors to nick the serosa and spread with a Maryland dissector to enter the lumen or "hot" with electrocautery or a laparoscopic energy device. If a hot method is used, extreme care must be taken to avoid "back-walling" and injuring the opposite mucosal side of the stomach and jejunum. The small end of a laparoscopic 60-mm linear stapler then is placed into the jejunotomy and rotated and slid into the gastrotomy (Figure 2). After the stapler is fired to create the anastomosis, the common enterotomy can be closed with 3-0 absorbable braided suture or with a second firing of the linear stapler. We then place a second running 3-0 permanent braided suture in a Lembert fashion as a second layer on the anterior aspect of the anastomosis.

The anastomosis also can be created in a purely handsewn fashion. This is done by making a 4- to 6-cm gastrotomy and enterotomy after aligning the stomach and bowel with a posterior running suture. Then a two-layer handsewn anastomosis is created, typically using absorbable 3-0 suture for the inner layer and permanent 3-0 suture for the outer layer. This approach takes significantly more time and has not been shown to decrease leak rates or functional outcomes, so for these reasons most surgeons prefer a linear stapler technique.

With either gastrojejunostomy technique, a leak test should be performed after completion of the anastomosis. We do this by

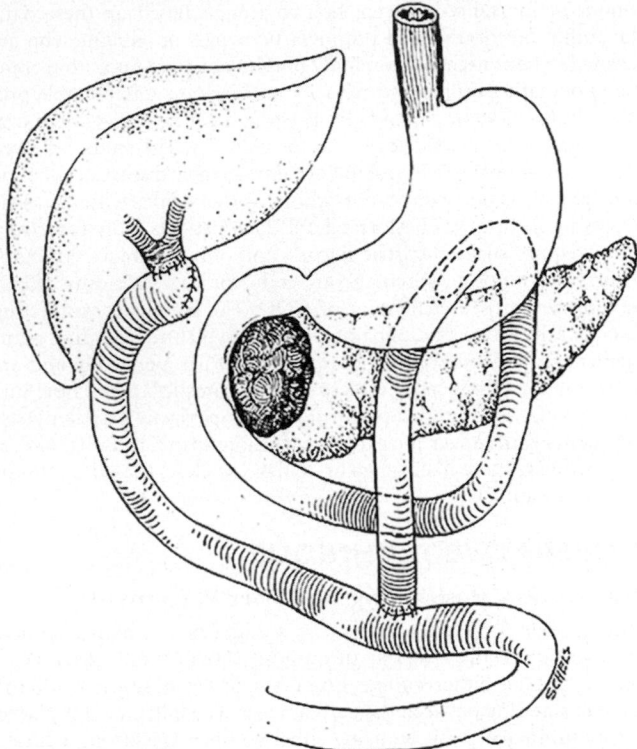

FIGURE 1 Diagram showing an isoperistaltic loop gastrojejunostomy and Roux-en-Y hepaticojejunostomy for bypass of both biliary and gastric outlet obstructions. *(From Scott EN, Garcea G, Doucas H, et al. Surgical bypass vs. endoscopic stenting for pancreatic ductal adenocarcinoma. HPB (Oxford). 2009;11:118-124.)*

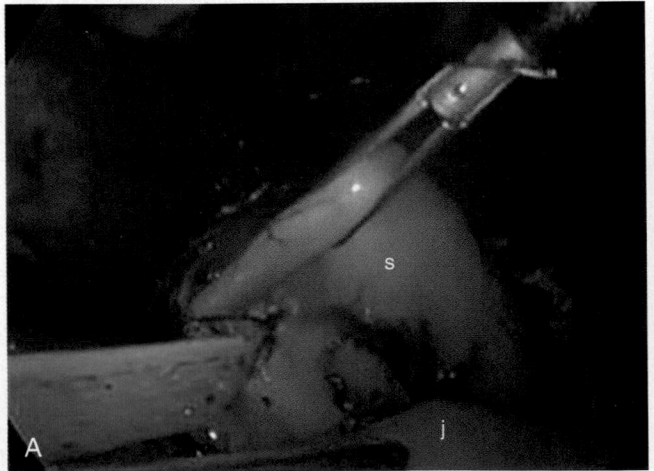 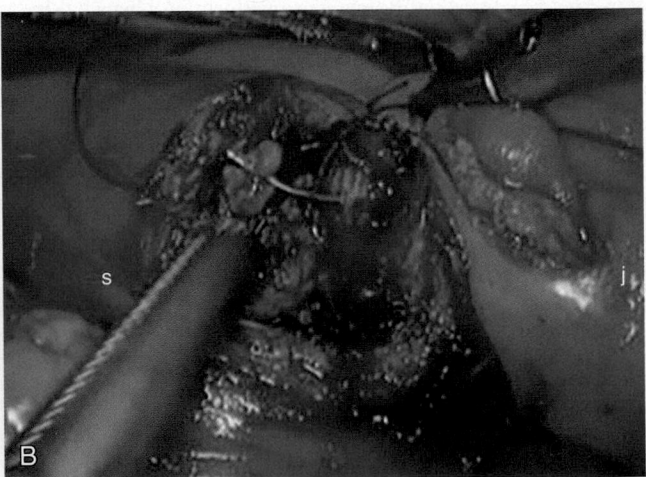

FIGURE 2 A, A stapled gastrojejunostomy is created by placing a laparoscopic linear stapler through enterotomies in the stomach (s) and jejunum (j). **B,** A handsewn gastrojejunostomy is created. *(From Kohan G, Ocampo CG, Zandalazini HI, et al. Laparoscopic hepaticojejunostomy and gastrojejunostomy for palliative treatment of pancreatic head cancer in 48 patients. Surg Endosc. 2015;29:1970-1975.)*

occluding the jejunum distal to the anastomosis and then submerging the anastomosis and performing an upper endoscopy. This checks for bubbling and allows the luminal side of the anastomosis to be inspected for bleeding. It typically is not necessary to leave a drain alongside the gastrojejunostomy. Patients who had a GOO preoperatively should have a nasogastric tube left in place, but patients in whom the gastric bypass was performed prophylactically generally do not need one. Postoperatively, the nasogastric tube can be removed once outputs have decreased, and the patient can be advanced to a liquid and then soft diet. Patients are placed on a once-daily proton pump inhibitor to prevent marginal ulcer formation at the anastomosis.

Biliary Bypass

To perform a choledochojejunostomy for biliary bypass, the patient is again placed in a steep reverse Trendelenburg position so that the viscera fall away from the portal structures. Typically, a cholecystectomy is performed first, and a liver retractor is placed in the gallbladder fossa in order to expose the porta. It is essential to first perform an adequate dissection of anterior surface of the common bile duct so that the sutures of the anastomosis are placed into the true wall of the duct and not the fatty tissue enveloping it. This is performed using mostly blunt dissection, which is kept directly anterior to the duct to avoid disrupting its blood supply, which comes in laterally from the patient's left.

After dissection of the common bile duct is performed, the jejunal Roux limb is fashioned. Alternatively, a loop of jejunum can be brought up to create the anastomosis, but as mentioned previously, this increases the patient's risk of developing cholangitis secondary to enteric reflux into the biliary tree. To create the Roux limb, the jejunum is divided 30 to 50 cm distal to the ligament of Treitz or to the gastrojejunostomy if a gastric bypass also was performed. The Roux limb then is measured to approximately 75 cm distal to this transaction, and a side-to-side jejunojejunostomy is performed at this location. This is done using a laparoscopic linear stapler, in a manner similar to the previously described gastrojejunostomy.

The Roux limb then is brought up alongside the previously dissected area of the common bile duct and held in place by the assistant. Two stay sutures are placed on the right and left side of the common bile duct and a 2-cm longitudinal ductotomy is made between them using straight scissors or a #11 blade held by a locking blunt grasper. A mirroring longitudinal enterotomy then is made in the antimesenteric border of the Roux limb. The anastomosis is performed in a single layer using an absorbable 4-0 or 5-0 suture (either braided or monofilament). A "diamond"-shaped anastomosis is created so that the right midpoint of the ductotomy is sutured to the distal apex of the Roux limb and the left midpoint is sutured to the proximal apex (Figure 3). A simple technique is to use two running sutures, the first performed on the posterior aspect of the anastomosis, running from right to left with the end left untied. Then an anterior running suture is placed, also from right to left, and the ends of the two sutures are tied together. Alternatively, interrupted sutures can be used. This can be a technically challenging anastomosis to create laparoscopically, and for this reason some surgeons have used the da Vinci robotic system (Intuitive Surgical, Sunnyvale, CA) to perform suturing for this portion of the procedure (Figure 4). A Jackson-Pratt drain is left in the hepatorenal recess, posterior to the anastomosis, to monitor for bile leak. Postoperatively, patients can have their diet advanced as tolerated.

Some authors also have described performing a hepaticojejunostomy for biliary bypass in advanced pancreatic cancer. This involves performing a complete circumferential dissection of the common hepatic duct and then transecting it with a linear stapler. The proximal staple line then is opened, and a handsewn end-to-side hepaticojejunostomy is performed. This technique adds to the complexity and potential morbidity of a circumferential ductal dissection as well as to the risk for leak from the distal bile duct

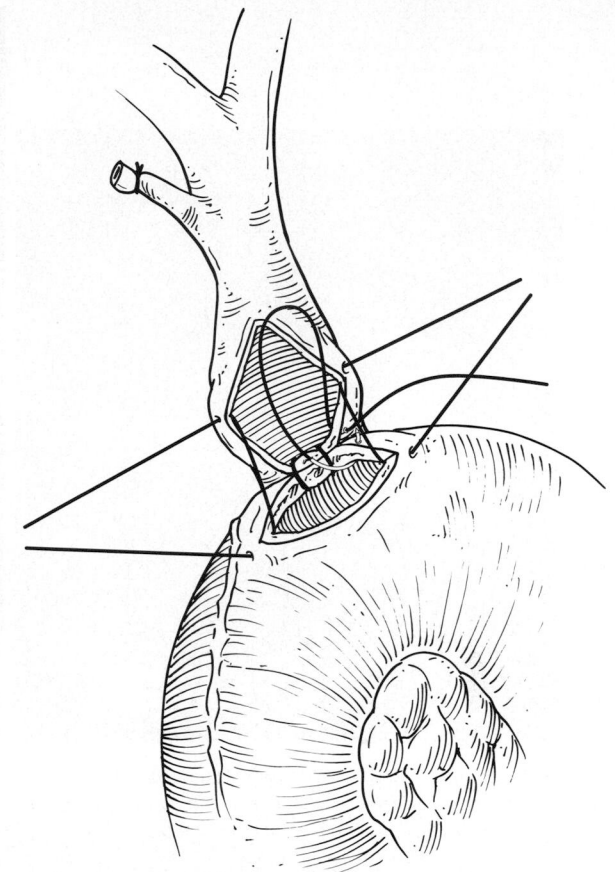

FIGURE 3 Creation of a side-to-side choledochoduodenostomy in a "diamond" configuration. The same orientation of bile duct and bowel is used when creating a choledochojejunostomy. *(From Riall TS. Choledochoduodenostomy and hepaticojejunostomy. In: Townsend CM, Evers BM, eds. Atlas of General Surgical Techniques. St. Louis: Saunders; 2010.)*

staple line. For this reason, we prefer to perform a choledochojejunostomy as previously described.

■ CONCLUSIONS

Pancreatic cancer is extremely aggressive, with average life expectancy of less than 1 year for patients with unresectable disease. For this reason, treatment decisions should focus on reducing morbidity and improving quality of life. Although surgical bypasses for both biliary and gastric outlet obstructions usually achieve good technical success, they result in considerable perioperative morbidity and mortality, even when performed laparoscopically. Surgeons need to carefully consider the risks and benefits of bypass and tailor the decision to perform one to the individual characteristics and prognosis of each patient. Patients who are known to have unresectable disease should have their biliary and gastric outlet obstructions palliated using endoscopic stenting as the initial approach. For patients who are diagnosed with unresectable disease at the time of laparoscopy, the decision of whether to proceed with bypass is more complex. Choledochojejunostomy achieves better long-term relief of biliary obstruction than ERCP stenting and generally should be performed if the patient is expected to survive for more than 4 to 6 months. Patients with GOO at the time of surgery should undergo laparoscopic gastrojejunostomy, whereas a prophylactic gastric bypass should be performed only if the patient has a life expectancy of more than 6 months and is at high risk for GOO based on tumor size and location, as the rate of GOO developing later is only approximately 20%.

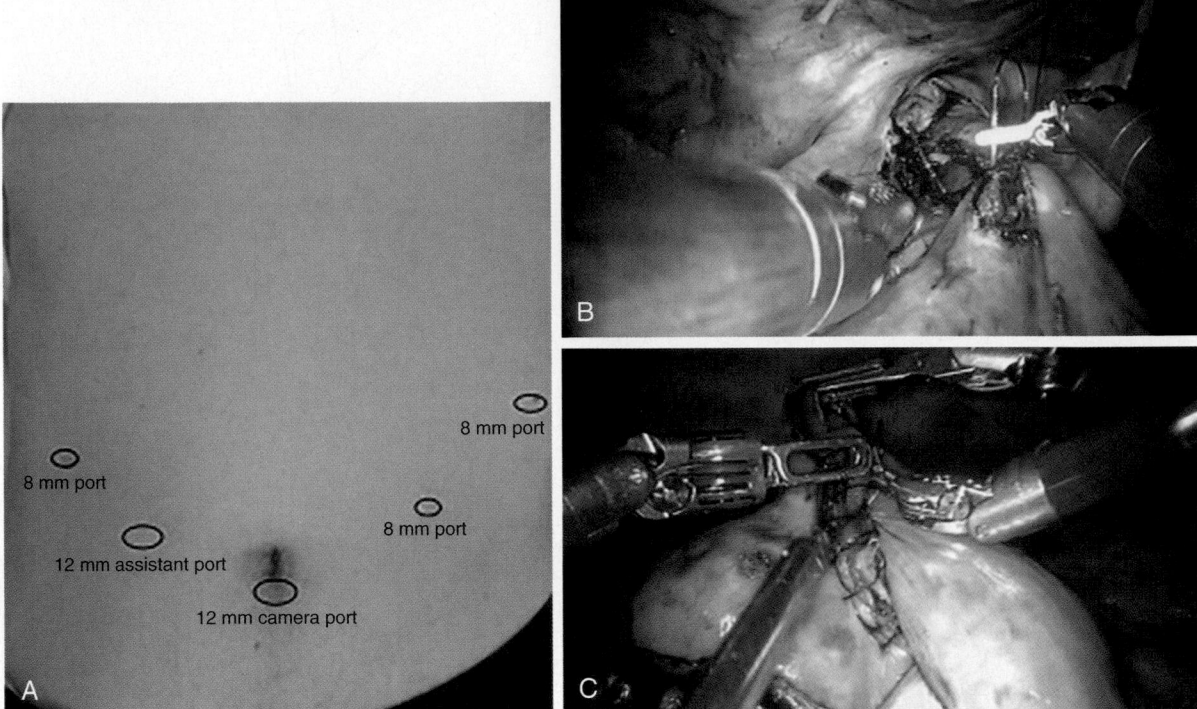

FIGURE 4 Creation of a Roux-en-Y hepaticojejunostomy using the da Vinci robotic system. **A,** Port placement is shown. **B,** A side-to-side handsewn hepaticojejunostomy is performed. **C,** A side-to-side jejunojejunostomy is performed to create the Roux limb. *(From Lai EC, Tang CN. Robot-assisted laparoscopic hepaticojejunostomy for advanced malignant biliary obstruction.* Asian J Surg. *2015;38:210-213.)*

SUGGESTED READINGS

Bartlett EK, Wachtel H, Fraker DL, et al. Surgical palliation for pancreatic malignancy: practice patterns and predictors of morbidity and mortality. *J Gastrointest Surg.* 2014;18:1292-1298.

Espat NJ, Brennan MF, Conlon KC. Patients with laparoscopically staged unresectable pancreatic adenocarcinoma do not require subsequent surgical biliary or gastric bypass. *J Am Coll Surg.* 1999;188:649-655, discussion 655-657.

Glazer ES, Hornbrook MC, Krouse RS. A meta-analysis of randomized trials: immediate stent placement vs. surgical bypass in the palliative management of malignant biliary obstruction. *J Pain Symptom Manage.* 2014;47:307-314.

Jeurnink SM, Steyerberg EW, van Hooft JE, et al. Surgical gastrojejunostomy or endoscopic stent placement for the palliation of malignant gastric outlet obstruction (SUSTENT study): a multicenter randomized trial. *Gastrointest Endosc.* 2010;71:490-499.

Kneuertz PJ, Cunningham SC, Cameron JL, et al. Palliative surgical management of patients with unresectable pancreatic adenocarcinoma: trends and lessons learned from a large, single institution experience. *J Gastrointest Surg.* 2011;15:1917-1927.

Lillemoe KD, Cameron JL, Hardacre JM, et al. Is prophylactic gastrojejunostomy indicated for unresectable periampullary cancer? A prospective randomized trial. *Ann Surg.* 1999;230:322-328, discussion 328-330.

Navarra G, Musolino C, Venneri A, et al. Palliative antecolic isoperistaltic gastrojejunostomy: a randomized controlled trial comparing open and laparoscopic approaches. *Surg Endosc.* 2006;20:1831-1834.

Siddiqui A, Spechler SJ, Huerta S. Surgical bypass versus endoscopic stenting for malignant gastroduodenal obstruction: a decision analysis. *Dig Dis Sci.* 2007;52:276-281.

Smith AC, Dowsett JF, Russell RC, et al. Randomised trial of endoscopic stenting versus surgical bypass in malignant low bile duct obstruction. *Lancet.* 1994;344:1655-1660.

Urbach DR, Bell CM, Swanstrom LL, et al. Cohort study of surgical bypass to the gallbladder or bile duct for the palliation of jaundice due to pancreatic cancer. *Ann Surg.* 2003;237:86-93.

MINIMALLY INVASIVE MANAGEMENT OF PERIPANCREATIC FLUID COLLECTIONS

Vernissia Tam, MD, and Melissa E. Hogg, MD, MS

Peripancreatic fluid collections develop when the pancreatic duct is disrupted, leading to a contained collection of pancreatic secretions within a capsule. Although the majority of cases of acute pancreatitis will resolve without intervention, 10% to 20% will progress to severe acute pancreatitis with subsequent complications such as necrotizing pancreatitis, which is associated with high rates of morbidity and mortality secondary to sepsis and multiorgan failure. Infected pancreatic necrosis is associated with a 30% mortality, which develops in 40% to 70% of cases of necrotizing pancreatitis. The traditional surgical management with open necrosectomy carries mortality and morbidity rates of 56% and 78%, respectively, prompting less invasive techniques to improve patient outcomes.

In 2012 an international consensus revised the Atlanta classification of acute pancreatitis that differentiates between different types of peripancreatic fluid collections (see Table 1). Distinguishing characteristics include clinical factors, such as duration after presentation, and morphologic features based on contrast-enhanced computed tomography (CT), such as the presence of a wall, homogeneous or heterogeneous density, and the presence of infected necrosis

TABLE 1: Definitions of Pancreatic Fluid Collections

Fluid Collection	Duration	Location	Wall	Fluid Component
Acute peripancreatic fluid collection (APFC)	<4 weeks	Extrapancreatic	No wall	Homogeneous fluid, no necrosis
Pancreatic pseudocyst	>4 weeks	Extrapancreatic	Well-defined wall	Homogeneous fluid, no necrosis
Acute necrotic collection (ANC)	<4 weeks	Extrapancreatic or intrapancreatic	No wall	Heterogeneous, solid and liquid
Walled-off pancreatic necrosis (WOPN)	>4 weeks	Extrapancreatic or intrapancreatic	Well-defined wall	Heterogeneous, solid and liquid

Adapted from the revised Atlanta classification of acute pancreatitis.

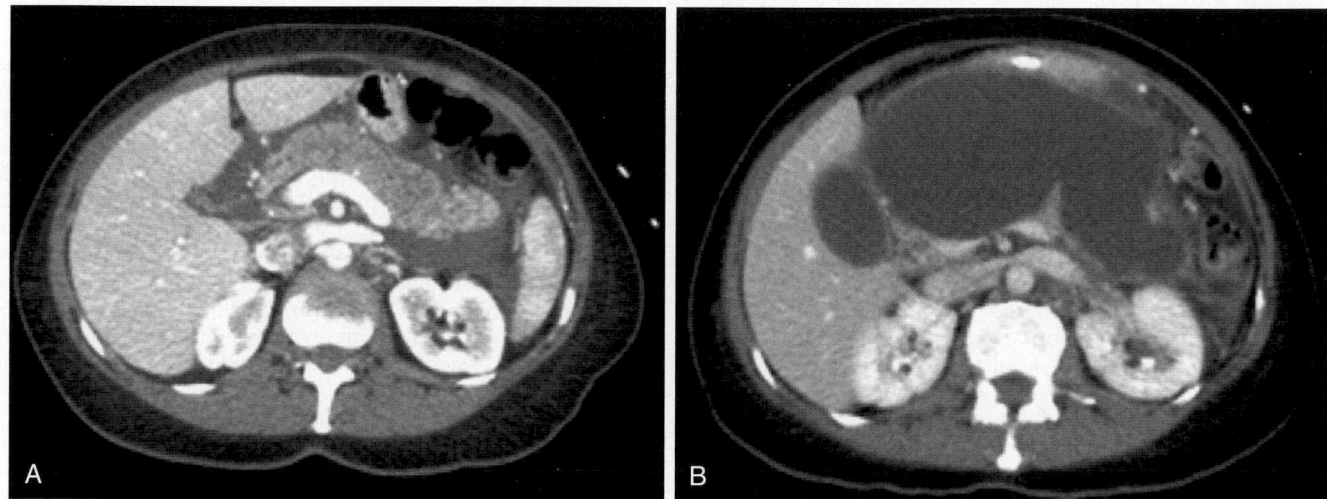

FIGURE 1 Evolution of peripancreatic fluid collections. **A,** Acute peripancreatic fluid collection. **B,** Pseudocyst in the same patient.

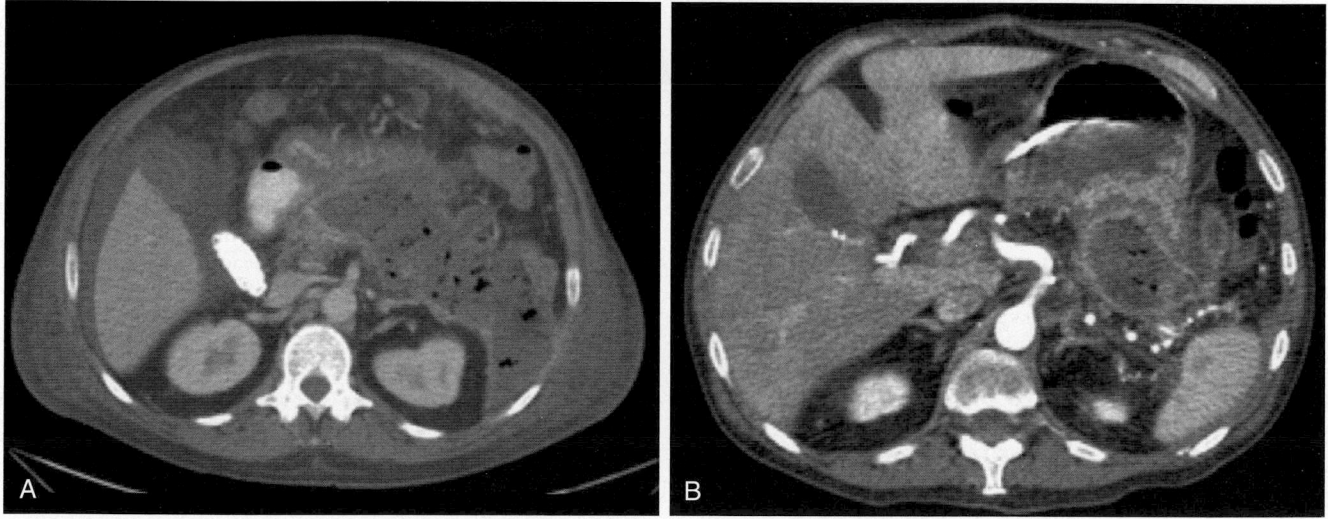

FIGURE 2 Evolution of acute necrotic collection. **A,** Acute necrotic collection. **B,** Walled-off pancreatic necrosis in the same patient.

(Figures 1 and 2). Figure 1 shows a patient with an acute peripancreatic fluid collection (APFC) that over 1 month evolved into a pancreatic pseudocyst. The patient in Figure 2 developed an acute necrotic collection (ANC) that became infected and then went on to develop walled-off pancreatic necrosis (WOPN) over a 2-month period. The definition of infected necrosis requires positive cultures from fine-needle aspiration (FNA) or evidence of gas on CT imaging. Both of these patients eventually underwent a minimally invasive cystogastrostomy.

■ INDICATIONS FOR SURGERY

At our institution we strongly advise against any procedure, surgical or otherwise, for patients with APFC (see Figure 1, *A*) or sterile necrotizing pancreatitis. Supportive therapy and postpancreatic nutrition are the treatment of choice. The presence of nasojejunal tubes (NJTs) can be seen in both patients' pancreatic protocol scans (see Figures 1, *B* and 2, *B*). In general, every stable patient is given an oral challenge of clear liquids followed by a low-fat diet. If the patient cannot tolerate or stay hydrated or nourished with oral intake, our pancreaticobiliary gastroenterologists place an NJT. For sterile necrotizing pancreatitis, supportive therapy without débridement generally is recommended.

Whether the patient has a pancreatic pseudocyst or WOPN, the major factor dictating the need for an operation is symptoms. Clinical indications for intervention on peripancreatic fluid collections include pain requiring long-term narcotics, gastric outlet or biliary obstruction, inability to tolerate oral intake, and failure to thrive. These patients either are never well enough to discharge or are readmitted to the hospital frequently with persistent symptoms. When a patient fails to improve despite best supportive therapy and NJT nutrition, an intervention is considered. In noninfected patients, considerations for surgery include time interval from initial symptoms, anatomic factors based on cross-sectional imaging, patient stability and comorbidities, and whether a cholecystectomy is indicated for pancreatitis (40% to 50% of patients).

Once infected necrotizing pancreatitis is detected, either with FNA or CT, an intervention is warranted. Surgery is often the "last resort" for treating peripancreatic fluid collections after less invasive techniques, including supportive therapy, percutaneous drainage (PCD), and endoscopic drainage, are attempted.

The PANTER trial described a "step-up approach" that begins with percutaneous or endoscopic drainage of the collection to control sepsis. If there is no clinical improvement within 72 hours, if the drains are draining inadequately, or if a new collection forms, a second drain is placed. If no clinical improvement is evident after another 72 hours, a video-assisted retroperitoneal débridement (VARD) is performed, with postoperative lavage. The study found that the step-up approach had equal rates of death compared with traditional open necrosectomy (19% vs 17%), but 35% of patients were successfully managed with drainage only, thereby avoiding an operation. In addition, step-up patients had fewer incisional hernias and less new onset diabetes and pancreatic insufficiency.

■ TIMING FOR SURGERY

For patients who are undergoing a minimally invasive cystogastrostomy, the longer surgery can be delayed, the better. A pseudocyst greater than 6 weeks is ideal, but at least 4 weeks are necessary for the cyst wall to adequately mature. There is a paradigm shift toward delaying intervention for infected pancreatic necrosis. Early interventions increase the risk of bleeding and lead to excessive resection of normal pancreatic tissue. Best outcomes are achieved when débridement is delayed for a minimum for 4 weeks after onset of symptoms, allowing liquefaction to begin. However, we prefer a delay of 3 months for minimally invasive cystogastrostomy. This interval allows the necrotic pancreatic material to wall off and become more amenable to en bloc débridement. When patients' symptoms or clinical status do not allow the pancreatic collection to reach the appropriate level of maturation for surgery, interventional gastroenterologic or radiologic procedures offer a temporizing option.

■ ANATOMIC CONSIDERATIONS FOR SURGERY

Location of the pseudocyst or WOPN and the distance between the mucosa of the stomach to inside the pancreatic collection are key components in determining whether a patient is well suited to undergo a minimally invasive cystogastrostomy. The patient in Figure 1 is an ideal candidate for a cystogastrostomy (Box 1). At 4 weeks it was apparent she would fail supportive therapy, but at that time the pseudocyst was not mature and was still evolving from multiple peripancreatic collections. Despite developing approximately 80% pancreatic necrosis and having persistent pain and nausea, the patient had not developed diabetes, pancreatic insufficiency, or a secondary infection or complication. Given her good performance status and

need for cholecystectomy secondary to biliary pancreatitis, she had a robotic cystogastrostomy with cholecystectomy at 6 weeks.

The presence of a retroperitoneal drain, preferably on the patient's left side, is one of the primary anatomic considerations for a VARD procedure. The patient in Figure 2 did not have any favorable anatomic characteristics for a cystogastrostomy. The WOPN was small, lateral, and posterior. The space between the stomach and wall, in addition to the solid necroma, made the patient ineligible for endoscopic consideration. Unfortunately there was no adequate window for a retroperitoneal drain to attempt VARD (see Figure 2, B) because of ribs, spleen, colon, and varices surrounding the collection. When the patient became infected, an anterior drain was placed through the lesser sac, but when he continued to smolder and fail NJT feeding and total parenteral nutrition (TPN), a robotic cystogastrostomy with cholecystectomy was performed.

■ PATIENT SELECTION FOR SURGERY

It is important to differentiate a pseudocyst from a WOPN; the former consists of homogeneous fluid, which simply may be drained, whereas the later contains solid necrotic debris and needs additional débridement. However, despite a scan in which the collection looks like homogeneous fluid (see Figure 1, B), a large necroma was removed from the patient in Figure 1. This is seen frequently in patients with large pseudocyst and pancreatic necrosis.

Patient-specific considerations include age, body habitus, prior surgeries, and comorbidities. Poor cardiovascular or pulmonary reserve may preclude the risks associated with general anesthesia and pneumoperitoneum. For patients who are deemed to be a poor operative candidate, endoscopic cystogastrostomy is preferable. If that is not a possibility, percutaneous drain placement with or without VARD is the best choice. Open necrosectomy is avoided if another option is viable.

Every patient with biliary pancreatitis needs a cholecystectomy. A cholecystectomy is also warranted in a patient with unknown etiology of pancreatitis after complete workup. If a patient has a known, nonbiliary etiology of pancreatitis and develops recurrent episodes despite reversal of underlying etiology, a cholecystectomy is indicated. If a patient needs a cholecystectomy and also has to address a pseudocyst or WOPN, a minimally invasive cystogastrostomy is preferred over endoscopy or VARD because cholecystectomy and cystogastrostomy can be performed simultaneously. If a patient does not have a clear indication for cholecystectomy, as discussed previously, but is undergoing a minimally invasive cystogastrostomy for symptom relief, a cholecystectomy is performed concurrently.

■ ROBOT-ASSISTED CYSTOGASTROSTOMY

At our institution, a robotic approach is preferred over a laparoscopic approach because it has more versatility for débridement of necrosis, suturing, and concomitant procedures. However, it is noted that the procedure, especially for a pseudocyst, is easily amenable to a laparoscopic approach. The patient is placed in reverse Trendelenburg position with the left side up. After port placement, as outlined in Figure 3, *A*, intraoperative ultrasound is used to confirm the location of the pancreatic collection. A 5-cm anterior gastrotomy is created with monopolar scissors, parallel to the greater curve with at least 2 cm distance. Then a 1-cm posterior gastrotomy is made. Ultrasound is performed again directly on the posterior wall within the stomach to avoid vasculature and find the best entrance site.

After the anterior wall of the collection is reached, the suction irrigator is inserted in the cavity and the effluent is suctioned until dry. The cystogastrostomy is created using either a 60-mm linear cutter stapler (Figure 3, *B*) or electrocautery, followed by plication of the posterior stomach wall to the anterior capsule using 3-0 running absorbable sutures. We recommend using a vascular stapler along the superior and lateral connection to stomach and then running suture along the inferior and medial borders, reinforcing the connection between the stomach and capsule wall opposite the staple line. Through the cystogastrostomy, the necrotic material is débrided under direct visualization. Usually a large necroma can be pulled out en bloc (Figure 3, *C*). Further débridement is approached by "scooping" and not "grabbing" with the robotic graspers and placing debris within an EndoCatch bag. Minimal manipulation of necrotic tissue posteriorly is recommended to avoid injury to the retroperitoneal vascular structures. After a judicious amount of

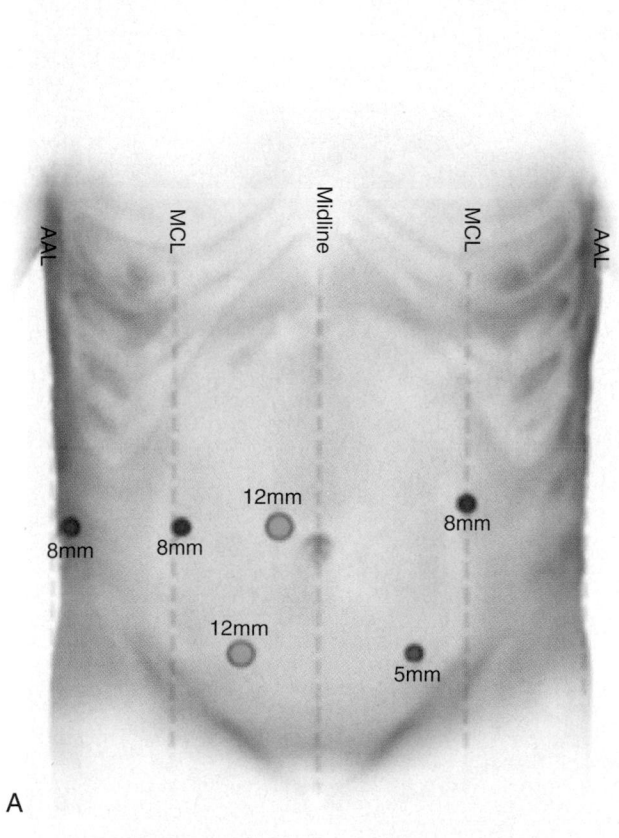

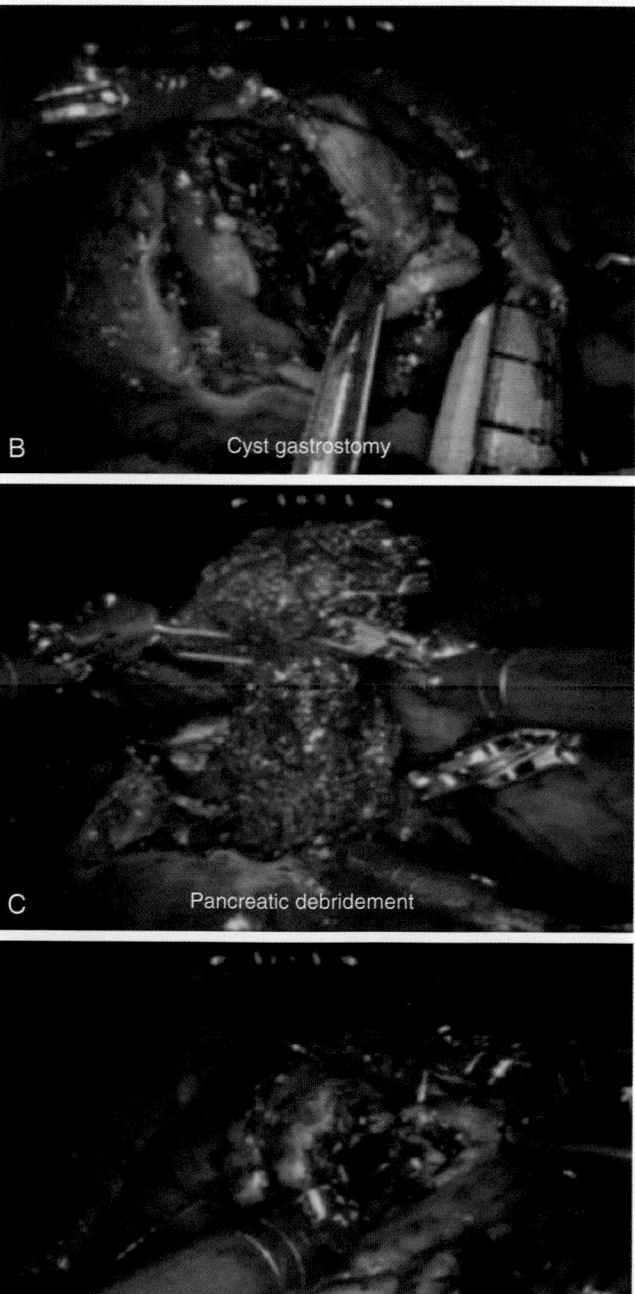

FIGURE 3 Robot-assisted cystogastrostomy. **A,** Port placement. **B,** Cystogastrostomy. **C,** Pancreatic débridement. **D,** Gastrotomy closure. *(From Khreiss M, Zenati M, Clifford A, et al. Cyst gastrostomy and necrosectomy for the management of sterile walled-off pancreatic necrosis: a comparison of minimally invasive surgical and endoscopic outcomes at a high-volume pancreatic center. J Gastrointest Surg. 2015;19:1441-1448.)*

necrotic material is removed, the cavity is irrigated. A mini laparotomy pad usually is inserted in the cavity to assist with atraumatic débridement, and the cavity can be packed to address minor bleeding while cholecystectomy is performed. The anterior gastrotomy is closed with a linear stapler or 3-0 running absorbable suture, followed by a second layer of 3-0 silk Lembert sutures (Figure 3, D). No drains are left in place.

During cholecystectomy, the robot is undocked, the patient is rotated right side up, and then the robot is redocked for better exposure. Enteral access for nutrition such as a jejunostomy tube may be placed as an adjunct procedure if continued enteral nutrition is warranted.

■ LAPAROSCOPIC VIDEO-ASSISTED RETROPERITONEAL DÉBRIDEMENT

The patient is placed in supine position, and the left side is elevated 30 to 40 degrees. A percutaneous drain, already in place, can be used as a guide into the peripancreatic collection (Figure 4, A). The fascia is dissected to enter the retroperitoneum. A flexible guidewire is inserted through the drain under fluoroscopic guidance (Figure 4, B). An introducer sheath is inserted over the wire (Figure 4, C), followed by a laparoscopic 5-mm port through the introducer (Figure 4, D). A 0-degree scope is introduced, and under direct visualization irrigation and suction is used to clear the purulent material. Under

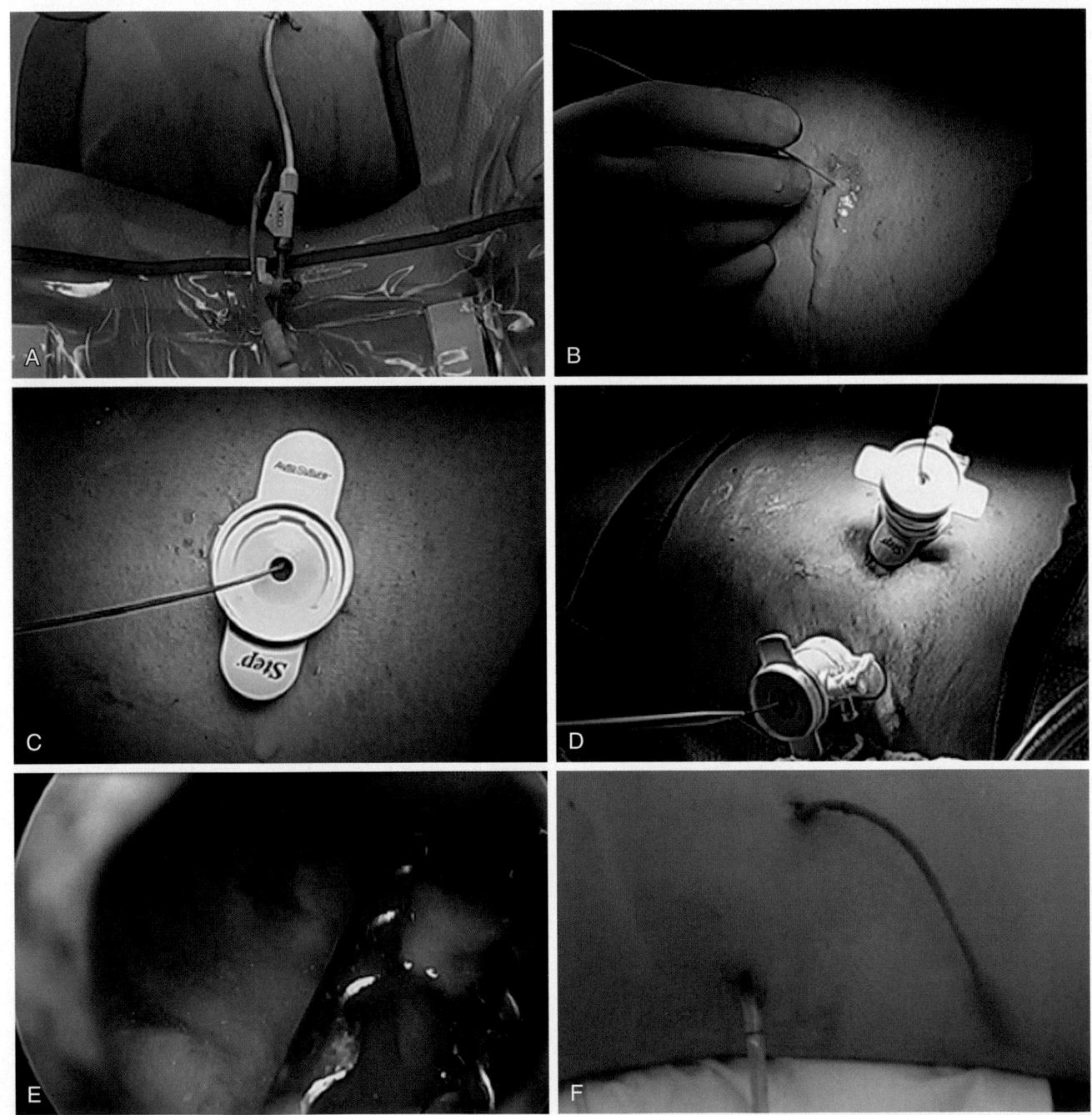

FIGURE 4 Video-assisted retroperitoneal débridement. **A,** Percutaneous drain placement prepared into sterile field. **B,** Flexible guidewire used to locate necrotic collection. **C,** Introducer sheath inserted using Seldinger technique. **D,** Insertion of laparoscopic port. **E,** Débridement under direct visualization. **F,** Drain placement. *(Photos used with permission. Courtesy Dr. Kenneth Lee.)*

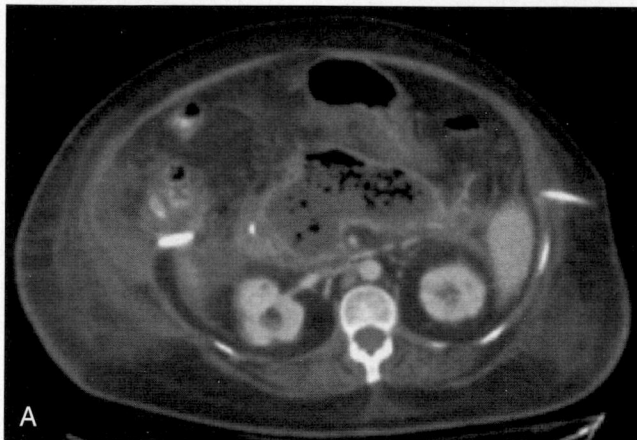

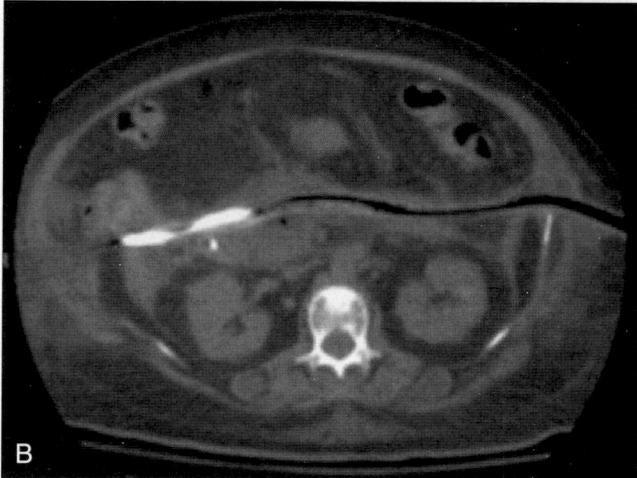

FIGURE 5 Before and after video-assisted retroperitoneal débridement (VARD) for walled-off pancreatic necrosis (WOPN). **A,** Preoperative computed tomographic scan with WOPN. **B,** Postoperative day 5 after VARD with drains in place, showing near-complete resolution of collection.

videoscopic guidance, deeper necrotic tissue retained in the cavity is further débrided using a laparoscopic alligator or empty sponge stick holder (Figure 4, *E*). Only loosely adherent pieces are removed; a complete necrosectomy is not performed. After a judicious amount of solid debris is removed, the cavity is irrigated with saline until the fluid is clear. A large sump drain is inserted into this cavity. A 0-degree scope can be inserted into the middle of the sump drain to assist with placement. The sump drain should be tested for suction and irrigation before leaving the operating room (Figure 4, *F*). Postoperatively, daily scheduled lavage through the drains with normal saline or dilute hydrogen peroxide fluid is performed until the effluent is clear. Alternatively, the irrigation can be scheduled as a continuous infusion. Examples of pre- and post-VARD CT images are shown in Figure 5.

Studies have shown that minimally invasive surgical interventions, including laparoscopic and robot-assisted cystogastrostomy and necrosectomy, have comparable mortality, failure rates, and cost compared with endoscopic approaches.

ALTERNATIVES

Most patients, even those with severe acute pancreatitis, should never undergo surgery. In patients who fail to improve despite best supportive therapy, surgical intervention should be considered only if less invasive options also have been considered. Close coordination between surgery, radiology, and gastroenterology is paramount to treating these sick patients. At our institution, a weekly pancreas conference is held and attended by these disciplines to form a mul-

tidisciplinary approach to patients who fail to improve with conservative therapy.

Endoscopic drainage may be accomplished via a transgastric, transduodenal, or transpapillary route (Figure 6). It is important to determine the relation of the peripancreatic fluid collection to the pancreatic duct. If the collection is continuous with the duct, an endoscopic retrograde cholangiopancreatography (ERCP) with sphincterotomy with or without a transpapillary stent may suffice and obviate an invasive operation. However, this can seed a sterile collection, which must be taken into consideration.

Necrosis that involves the lesser sac and is located close to the gastric or medial duodenal wall is most amenable to endoscopic drainage. The technique involves dilating the cystogastrostomy tract, débridement and irrigation under direct visualization, and deployment of stents to maintain tract patency. In addition, a drain such as a nasobiliary or jejunal tube is placed to perform scheduled irrigations after the procedure. Endoscopic necrosectomy has been shown to be safe for treating sterile or infected WOPN and more effective than endoscopic drainage alone; however, the mean number of procedures necessary to achieve resolution was four.

Surgery may be avoided in 30% to 100% of patients with necrotizing pancreatitis when they are treated with less invasive measures. In a prospective cohort of patients with ANC and WOPN, 30% of collections resolved, diminished, or completely liquefied and did not require an intervention at 6 months. Supportive therapy includes pain control, intravenous hydration, and supplemental nutrition via nasoenteric feeding. A recent meta-analysis of three randomized controlled trials found no difference between nasogastric and nasojejunal feeding on mortality, tracheal aspiration, diarrhea, exacerbation of pain, or meeting energy balance. Case series have reported reasonable survival rates for patients treated only with broad-spectrum antibiotics. When cultures and sensitivities are available, antibiotics coverage should be narrowed appropriately; positive cultures are reported to be primarily *Enterococcus*, *Pseudomonas*, and *Klebsiella*.

PCD can be a useful adjunct to surgical intervention and serve as a temporizing maneuver to control sepsis. When used as definitive treatment, disadvantages are the need for multiple procedures, the need for upsizing, and fistula and hemorrhage complications. PCD is less successful in patients with multiorgan failure and in the setting of central gland necrosis.

CONCLUSION

Severe acute pancreatitis leading to a persistently symptomatic pancreatic pseudocyst or WOPN that necessitates a surgical approach is rare. Treatment approach depends on the patient's clinical condition; timing of presentation; anatomy and location of the fluid collection; and expertise of the institution's surgeons, interventional radiologists, and gastroenterologists. With appropriate patient selection, surgical intervention via minimally invasive techniques may be the best strategy to treat a patient and avoid multiple interventions and further hospitalization.

At our institution, we recommend watchful waiting and supportive care for all peripancreatic fluid collections that are asymptomatic. We have a low threshold to place a NJT for nutritional optimization. For those patients who fail to resolve, we recommend a minimum of 4 to 6 weeks of supportive therapy to allow the collection to wall off before intervention. Carefully selected patients with an anatomically favorable collection closely adherent to the posterior wall of the stomach are good candidates for a robot-assisted cystogastrostomy. As a temporizing measure in septic patients or for poor operative candidates, PCD (or preferably endoscopic drainage) can be used to control sepsis while this period elapses. Failure to improve after endoscopic drainage or PCD is an indication for an operation. In well patients with favorable anatomy, a robotic cystogastrostomy is preferred. However, sick patients or those with infected pancreatic necrosis should undergo VARD. Finally, the indication for cholecystectomy should be a factor in decision making where appropriate.

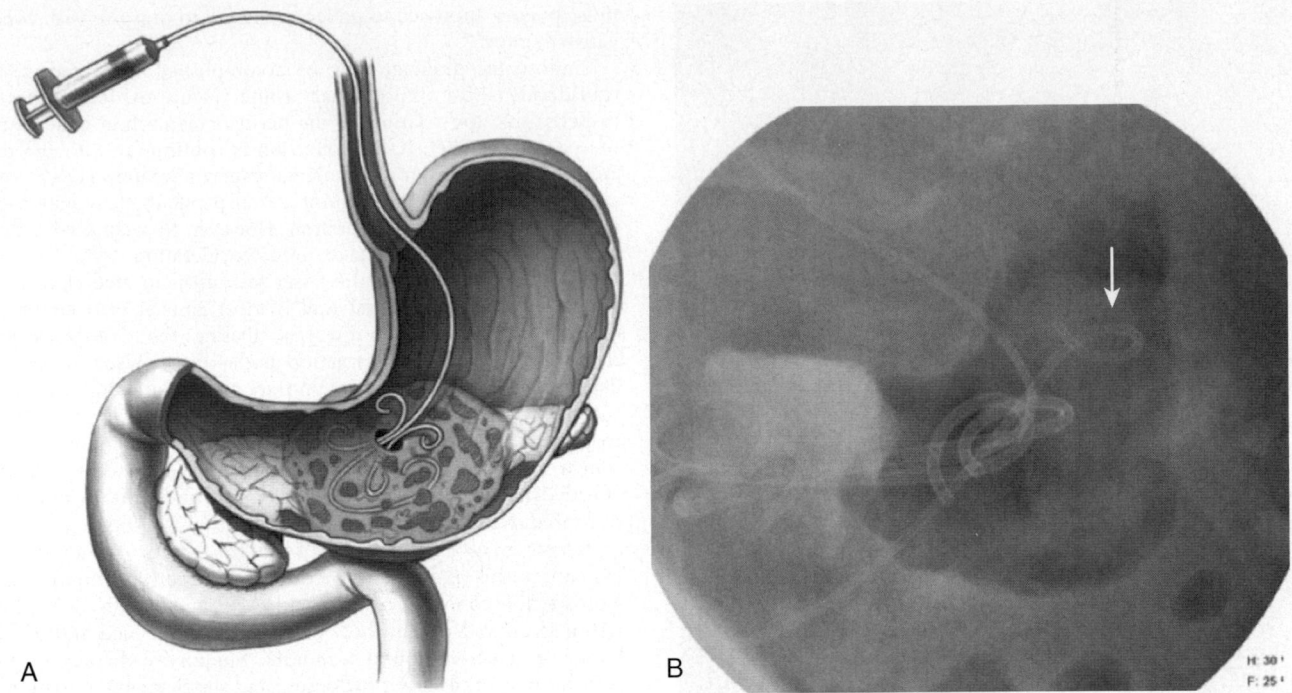

FIGURE 6 Endoscopic transgastric drainage. **A,** Schematic of transmural drainage with internal pigtail stents and nasobiliary drain. **B,** Fluoroscopic image of internal stents and nasobiliary tube. Distal tip of nasobiliary tube terminating in cavity of WOPN. *(From Papachristou GI, Takahashi N, Chahal P, Sarr MG, Baron TH. Peroral endoscopic drainage/debridement of walled-off pancreatic necrosis. Ann Surg. 2007;245:943-951.)*

SUGGESTED READINGS

Banks PA, Bollen TL, Dervenis C, et al. Classification of acute pancreatitis—2012: revision of the Atlanta classification and definitions by international consensus. *Gut.* 2013;62:102-111.

Khreiss M, Zenati M, Clifford A, et al. Cyst gastrostomy and necrosectomy for the management of sterile walled-off pancreatic necrosis: a comparison of minimally invasive surgical and endoscopic outcomes at a high-volume pancreatic center. *J Gastrointest Surg.* 2015;19:1441-1448.

Navaneethan U, Vege SS, Chari ST, Baron TH. Minimally invasive techniques in pancreatic necrosis. *Pancreas.* 2009;38:867-875.

Papachristou GI, Takahashi N, Chahal P, Sarr MG, Baron TH. Peroral endoscopic drainage/debridement of walled-off pancreatic necrosis. *Ann Surg.* 2007;245:943-951.

Spanier BW, Bruno MJ, Mathus-Vliegen EM. Enteral nutrition and acute pancreatitis: a review. *Gastroenterol Res Pract.* 2011;2011.

van Santvoort HC, Besselink MG, Bakker OJ, et al. A step-up approach or open necrosectomy for necrotizing pancreatitis. *N Engl J Med.* 2010;362:1491-1502.

van Santvoort HC, Besselink MG, Horvath KD, et al. Videoscopic assisted retroperitoneal debridement in infected necrotizing pancreatitis. *HPB (Oxford).* 2007;9:156-159.

VIDEO-ASSISTED THORACOSCOPIC SURGERY

Arjun Pennathur, MD, FACS, James D. Luketich, MD, and Peter F. Ferson, MD

The first use of thoracoscopic intervention was described by Hans Christian Jacobeus in 1910. He introduced a cystoscope into the pleural space to lyse adhesions, which encouraged the use of artificially induced pneumothorax as a treatment for tuberculosis. Currently, thoracoscopic techniques are used for most intrathoracic procedures; thus a thorough discussion of video-assisted thoracoscopic surgery (VATS) actually could involve an entire textbook of thoracic surgery. We therefore will confine our comments to several of the more commonly performed VATS operations and provide an overview for the general surgeon. Many of the basic principles with VATS are similar to the basic principles of laparoscopy, but the surgeon must be aware of the differences in anesthetic management,

positioning, and equipment. As with most minimally invasive surgical procedures, there is a significant learning curve, and VATS operations should be performed only after an adequate training period. This advanced training in thoracic surgery is essential in modern thoracic surgery because of the complexities of VATS procedures.

■ BASIC CONSIDERATIONS FOR THORACOSCOPIC PROCEDURES

Most thoracic surgical procedures can be accomplished using a VATS approach (Box 1) in the absence of relative contraindications for VATS (Box 2). Appropriate anesthesia, patient positioning, and port placement, as well as specialized instrumentation, are critical to the success of diagnostic and therapeutic VATS.

Anesthetic Management

Although VATS procedures have been performed under local anesthesia with spontaneous respiration, most interventions are performed under general anesthesia with a double-lumen endotracheal

BOX 1: Applications for Video-Assisted Thoracoscopic Surgery

1. Diagnostic thoracoscopy
2. Pleural procedures
   a. Pleural biopsy*
   b. Drainage of pleural effusions*
   c. Pleurodesis*
   d. Drainage of empyema
   e. Pleural débridement and decortication*
   f. Spontaneous pneumothorax
   g. Chylothorax
3. Pulmonary parenchymal procedures
   a. Nodule localization*
   b. Wedge resection*
   c. Segmentectomy
   d. Lobectomy*
   e. Lung volume reduction surgery
4. Mediastinal procedures
   a. Mediastinal lymph node biopsy
   b. Staging for esophageal or pulmonary malignancies
   c. Resection of mediastinal tumors and cysts*
   d. Thymectomy*
   e. Creation of a pericardial window
5. Esophageal procedures
   a. Resection of esophageal diverticulum
   b. Esophageal myotomy
   c. Resection of benign esophageal tumors
   d. Minimally invasive esophagectomy*
6. Miscellaneous
   a. Sympathectomy
   b. Repair of diaphragmatic hernia
   c. Diaphragm plication
   d. Spine procedures

*Indicates procedures detailed in this chapter.

BOX 2: Relative Contraindications to Video-Assisted Thoracoscopic Surgery

- Inability to tolerate single-lung ventilation
- Severe pulmonary hypertension
- Severe thoracic trauma
- Hemodynamic instability
- Very dense pleural adhesions
- Superior sulcus tumor
- Extensive tumor invasion of the chest wall
- Definitive chemoradiation
- Complex esophageal surgical resection when the stomach cannot be used as a conduit

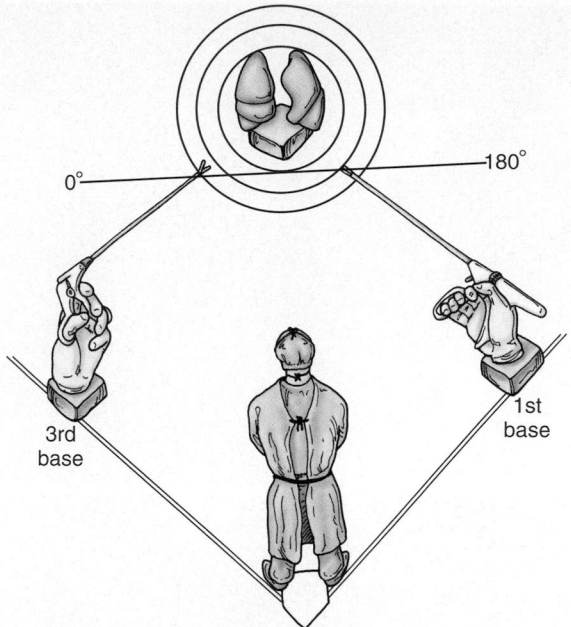

FIGURE 1 Port placement with the patient in a lateral position. The baseball diamond concept for triangulation of the instruments and thoracoscope for strategic visibility and manipulation of the target pathology is depicted. Positioning of the surgeon and assistants is noted. *(Reprinted from Landreneau RJ, et al. Video assisted thoracic surgery: basic technical concepts and intercostal approach strategies. Ann Thorac Surg. 1992;54:800.)*

tube. This allows for the use of open access ports and creates a passive pneumothorax to provide visibility. Alternatively, a single-lumen endotracheal tube can be used with airtight ports and CO_2 insufflation, although the lung collapse achieved with this method is less adequate. In addition, surgeons must be watchful of hemodynamic instability with the pneumothorax resulting from CO_2 insufflation. If a double-lumen endotracheal tube is used, clamping off the target lung during positioning and draping will result in the rapid onset of atelectasis and thus collapse of the lung once the pleura is entered with the first port.

Patient Positioning

The patient usually is placed in a lateral position with the involved side placed up, as for a standard thoracotomy. The patient is positioned and secured near the back edge of the operating table. The upper arm is supported by an overhead arm board or on blankets. A soft support is placed under the chest at the level of the axilla to prevent compression. The lower leg is bent so that the knee approaches the opposite side of the table, and the lower ankle is bent back under the upper leg, which is extended straight. This bending of the lower leg helps to support the patient and prevent rolling on the table. A pillow is placed between the legs, and all bone protuberances (iliac crest, ankle, knee, and elbow) are padded. In addition, we routinely place a sequential compression device for prophylaxis against deep vein thrombosis. A back support is placed behind the sacrum. Alternatively, some prefer a "bean bag" for positioning with a tape passed over the iliac crest and fastened to both sides of the table. The entire chest should be prepped and draped, not just the port sites.

Access Port Placement

The port placement is tailored to the procedure being performed. The placement of the ports should be planned with the strategic placement of the thoracoscope for optimal visibility and instrument manipulation relative to the target pathology (Figure 1). For most procedures performed with VATS, the operating team works best if the camera view starts low in the chest looking toward the head. Thus we usually place our viewing port in the seventh or eighth interspace in the midaxillary line. A 10-mm scope with a 30-degree angle works best for the majority of situations and permits views to both sides of the lung and hilum. Second and third ports are added as necessary, typically in the fourth or fifth intercostal space anteriorly and posteriorly. In certain situations, a single port with a straight viewing working scope is appropriate. For procedures in which removal of a mass is expected, such as lobectomy for lung cancer, a 4- to 5-cm accessory incision is made in the anterior portion of the third or fourth interspace. The interspaces are wider anteriorly, so a rib spreading retractor is rarely necessary for tumor removal. A wound

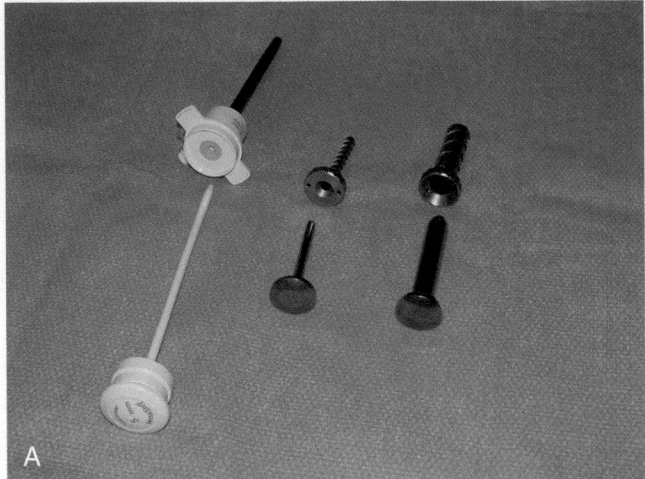

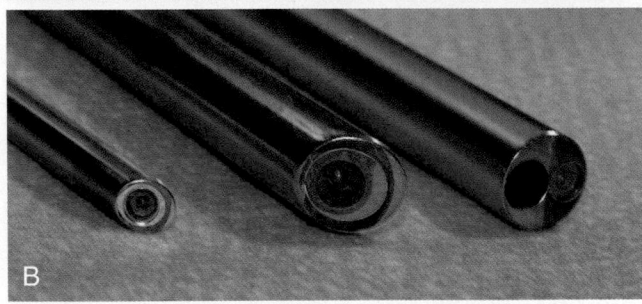

FIGURE 2 A, Trocars for video-assisted thoracoscopic surgery.
B, Thoracoscopes. The thoracoscope on the right has a working channel for endoscopic instruments.

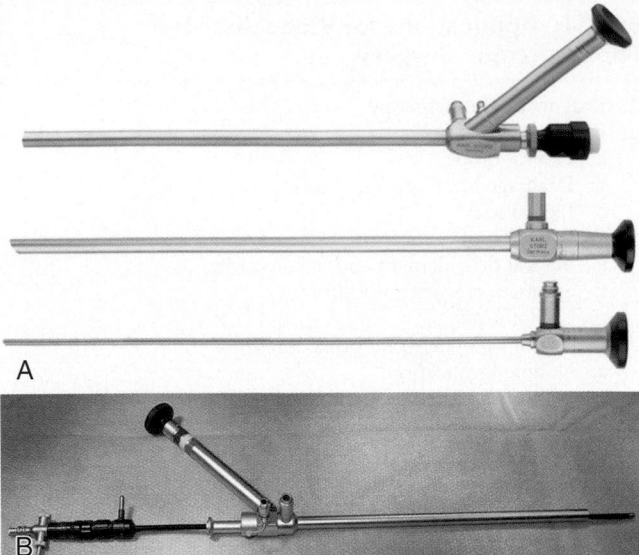

FIGURE 3 A, Operating thoracoscope with a 6-mm working channel and angled thoracoscopes. *(Courtesy Karl Storz, El Segundo, CA.)*
B, Operating thoracoscope with an instrument placed in the working channel.

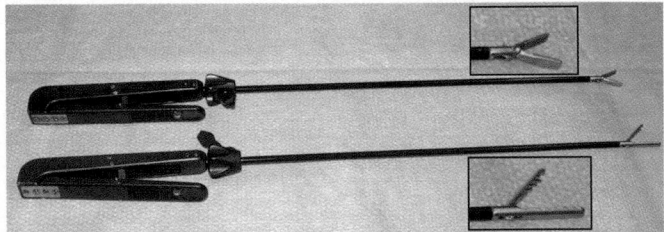

FIGURE 4 Snowden-Pencer graspers (BD-CareFusion, Franklin Lakes, NJ). Insets highlight the differences in the ends. The top instrument has a duckbill and is used for suturing. The bottom instrument has teeth and is used for manipulating tissue.

protector should be inserted to guard the incision from the potential shed of cancer cells.

Equipment

VATS requires the use of thoracic ports (Figure 2, *A*) and an endoscopic camera (Figure 2, *B*). A thoracoscope with a working channel for other instrumentation frequently is used (Figure 3). Specialized tools, including graspers and suction devices, have been developed as VATS approaches have expanded to include most thoracic surgical procedures (Figures 4 and 5).

■ VIDEO-ASSISTED THORACOSCOPIC SURGERY FOR PLEURAL DISORDERS

Most abnormalities of the pleura lend themselves well to intervention via VATS. Common disorders treated with VATS include recurring pleural effusions, empyema, hemothorax, pleural-based masses, and spontaneous pneumothorax (see Box 1).

Pleural Biopsy

Pleural exploration and biopsy is accomplished easily with a single 10-mm port placed at the seventh or eighth interspace along the midaxillary line. A working thoracoscope (which has a working channel) (see Figure 3) is introduced, and the pleura explored for evidence of masses, metastatic implants, plaque, or inflammation. Biopsy forceps introduced through the working channel can be used easily to perform multiple biopsies from both suspicious and grossly normal areas. When metastatic pleural disease is suspected and confirmed by frozen section pathologic analysis, one option is to place a second access port and proceed with chemical pleurodesis. However, if a malignant lesion of the pleura is thought to be mesothelioma,

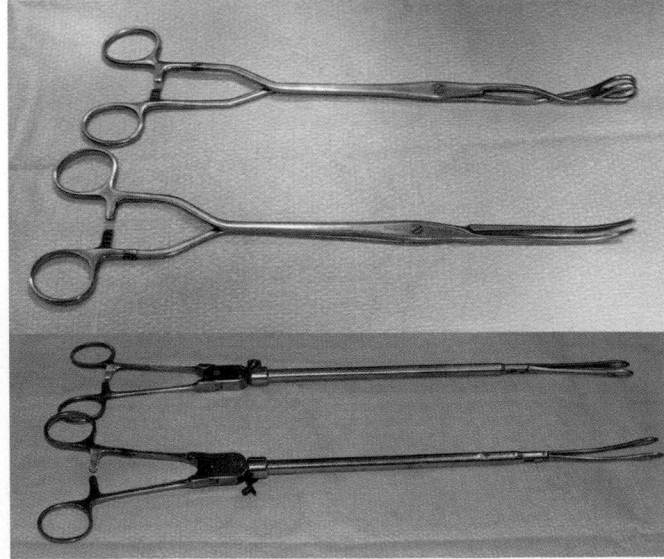

FIGURE 5 Clamps used for video-assisted thoracoscopic surgery (VATS). *From top to bottom:* VATS lung clamp, VATS tonsil clamp (Thoramet Surgical Products, Rutherford, NJ), straight lung clamp, curved lung clamp. The specialized shape of the grasping end of the lung clamps reduces trauma to the lung tissue.

surgeons can wait for the final permanent diagnosis from pathology before deciding on the course of action.

Pleural Effusions

When fluid analysis has failed to yield a cause for an idiopathic pleural effusion, a VATS procedure is indicated. VATS can be used to insert a temporary drainage tube, remove restrictive tissue around the lung, and apply therapeutics to reduce fluid accumulation. Before embarking on thoracoscopy, the initial thoracentesis should have included insertion of a small drainage catheter via a Seldinger technique or a thoracostomy tube. This will provide total drainage of the fluid and help ascertain whether the lung is capable of total expansion to fill the pleural space, or if the lung is trapped by a thickened pleural membrane. If the lung is capable of expanding, chemical pleurodesis can be performed with talc or with another sclerosing agent, such as doxycycline.

Sometimes after drainage of a pleural effusion, the lung is unable to expand because of a viscera membrane. If this is the result of a malignancy, pleurodesis cannot be performed, and the effusion should be managed with a chronic drain (PleurX catheter, Becton, Dickinson and Company, Franklin Lakes, NJ). If the membrane is from a benign effusion, then a decortication of the lung can be performed.

When the pleural fluid is infected, management will depend on the nature of the fluid. Streptococcal infections typically will have a watery, thin fluid that can be drained completely using a chest tube, or even a small diameter catheter. Thicker fluids with a fibrinopurulent quality may respond to chest tube insertion and fibrinolytic instillation. When the drainage is incomplete or when loculations have developed, thoracoscopic intervention is indicated.

Pleural Débridement and Decortication

Manual débridement and lysis of adhesions typically is accomplished with three port sites. Aggressive irrigation, in addition to physical efforts, is helpful. If the lung does not inflate completely, the fibrinous membrane and debris must be removed from the lung surface. This débridement of the lung surface is much easier in cases of the acute phase of empyema than in cases with a thick fibrotic membrane from a chronic trapped lung—a situation that usually will require an open thoracotomy and possibly hours of struggle to achieve a complete decortication. During acute phase empyema, care must be taken in débriding the parietal pleura to avoid bleeding from the inflamed surface that could lead to a hemothorax.

■ VIDEO-ASSISTED THORACOSCOPIC SURGERY PROCEDURES ON THE LUNGS

VATS is an important diagnostic and treatment tool for many pulmonary pathologies. VATS lung biopsies are common, and VATS wedge resection can be used to diagnose and remove small pulmonary nodules. VATS can be used for lung-volume reduction surgery to treat end-stage emphysema. Because VATS technology has improved, many thoracic surgeons have adopted VATS approaches for anatomic lung resections (see Box 1).

Lung Biopsy

There are two typical scenarios in which a surgical lung biopsy is indicated. In the first scenario, an outpatient has been experiencing progressive respiratory compromise, often with radiographic findings of pulmonary infiltrates. When there is no clear clinical diagnosis and when transbronchial biopsies have not provided adequate tissue, a VATS lung biopsy may help with the pathologic diagnosis. The second circumstance occurs when the patient's pulmonary status is deteriorating, often in the intensive care unit, and the response to

standard therapy has been inadequate. Although survival in such a situation is low, a VATS or an open lung biopsy may be helpful, particularly in finding an unsuspected infectious organism. In the first scenario, the VATS procedure is straightforward and gives a better chance to biopsy several areas of the lung as compared with a minithoracotomy, which gives only one edge to sample. VATS biopsies are directed anatomically by computed tomography (CT) scans to address the most involved area and also more normal locations. Unless there is a clear radiographic difference between the two sides, the right side usually is preferred. The left side is limited by the heart, and the right side has more edges for sampling. Biopsies are most easily obtained from a leading edge of a lobe or from the fissures.

Excisional Biopsy of Lung Nodules Using Video-Assisted Thoracoscopic Surgery Wedge Resection

If a patient has a lung nodule and needle biopsy has been nondiagnostic, a VATS wedge resection for diagnosis frequently can be performed, provided the nodule is relatively subpleural in location. Similarly, multiple nodules can be excised by wedge resection dependent on their locations. The excision of a nodule can be performed through a second port with a grasper through the working channel of a thoracoscope using a "2-stick" approach (Figure 6, A), or with an angled thoracoscope via a "3-stick" approach (Figure 6, B). When the nodule is near an edge of the lung, a wedge resection is performed just as for a parenchymal biopsy. More frequently, the nodule will be under a broad surface and will require a larger wedge resection for adequate clearance. The greatest challenge when performing a wedge resection of a pulmonary nodule is locating the nodule. Careful study of the CT scans will assist in general localization. If the mass is at least 1 cm wide and close to the surface, it may appear as a distinct bulge in the lung surface once the lung has become atelectatic. An instrument gently drawn across the surface over the localized region may "feel" the subpleural mass when it is not visible. When these methods fail, adding an access site over the suspected area will allow for insertion of a finger and palpating the lung. This can be assisted by enveloping a large amount of lung with a broad lung clamp and offering the suspicious area to the palpating finger. Once the nodule is located, it can be grasped with surrounding lung tissue using a sponge stick or a small Pennington clamp.

Sometimes the nodule is small or relatively deep, and localization will be difficult. In this situation, we often use localization techniques. A hook wire can be inserted under CT guidance just before the procedure, similar to localization of radiographic breast abnormalities (Figure 7). We usually instill 0.2 mL of methylene blue into the location to identify the spot if the hook wire falls out (see Figure 7). Recently, electromagnetic-navigation-bronchoscopy–guided dye marking with methylene blue has been used successfully for VATS localization of lung nodules (Figure 8).

Anatomic Lung Resection

When resecting a lung cancer, we prefer an anatomic resection over wedge resection. Using VATS gives excellent visualization of the hilar structures during anatomic lung resection. This visibility allows the procedure to progress differently than a resection performed via open thoracotomy. VATS dissection typically is performed from the hilum out so that division of the fissure is performed last. The sequence of structure division does vary depending on the involved lobe, however. For instance, a right upper lobectomy would be performed by transecting the superior pulmonary vein upper lobe branch first, then the upper lobe arteries, the bronchus, and finally the fissures. With a left upper lobectomy, the upper lobe vein is taken first, then the apical anterior artery, next the bronchus, followed by the lingular artery. The fissure is divided last. There are several excellent studies describing the VATS approach to anatomic lung resection.

FIGURE 6 Video-assisted thoracoscopic surgery approaches for wedge resection. **A,** Two-stick approach. Instruments placed through the working channel of the operating thoracoscope. **B,** Three-stick approach. Two ports are used for instrument placement, and the third port is used of an angled thoracoscope. *Insets A and B:* Excision of the lung nodule using thoracoscopic instruments. *(Modified from Ferson PF, et al. Comparison of open versus thoracoscopic lung biopsy for diffuse infiltrative pulmonary disease. J Thorac Cardiovasc Surg. 1993;106:194.)*

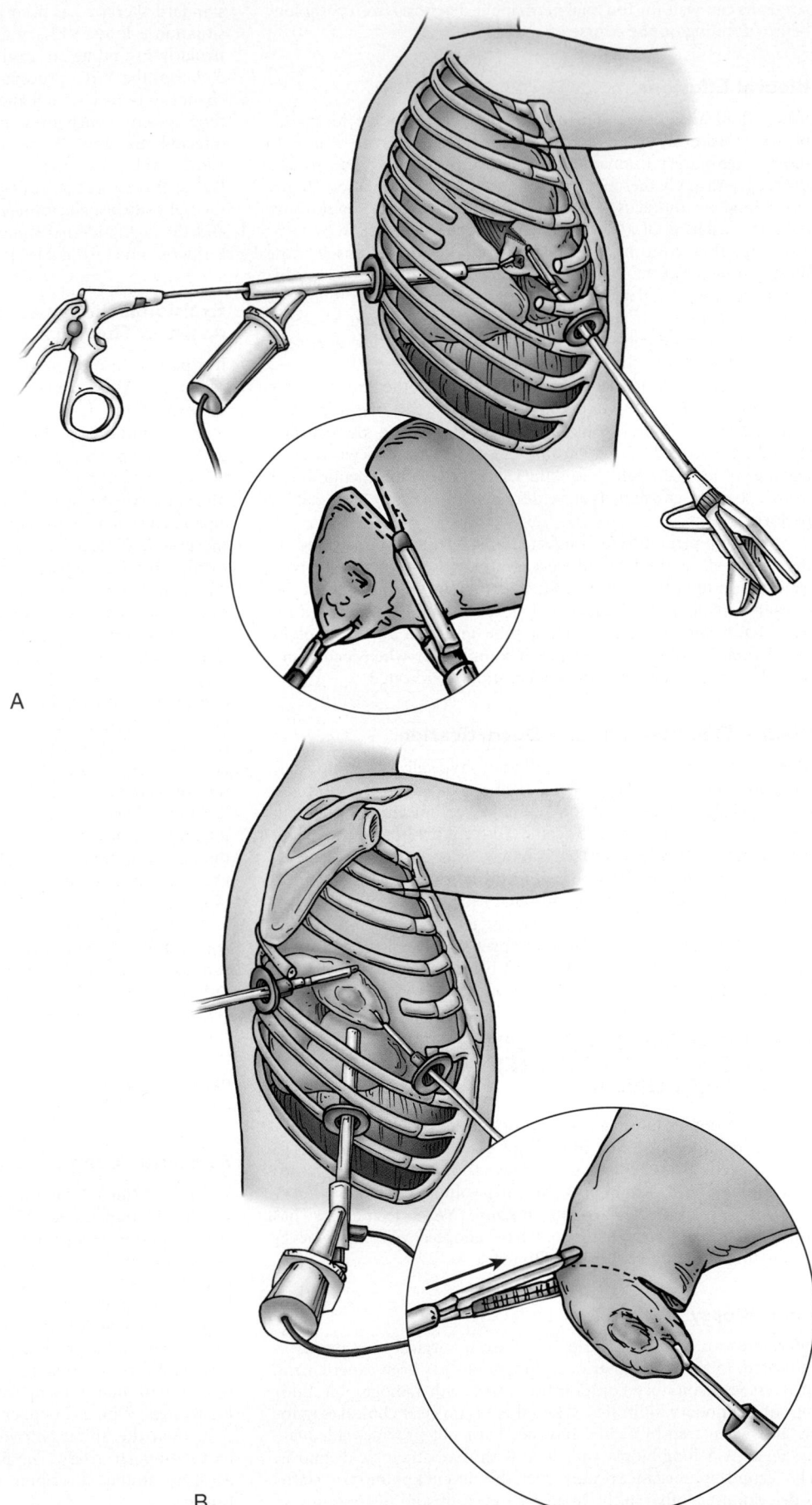

A

B

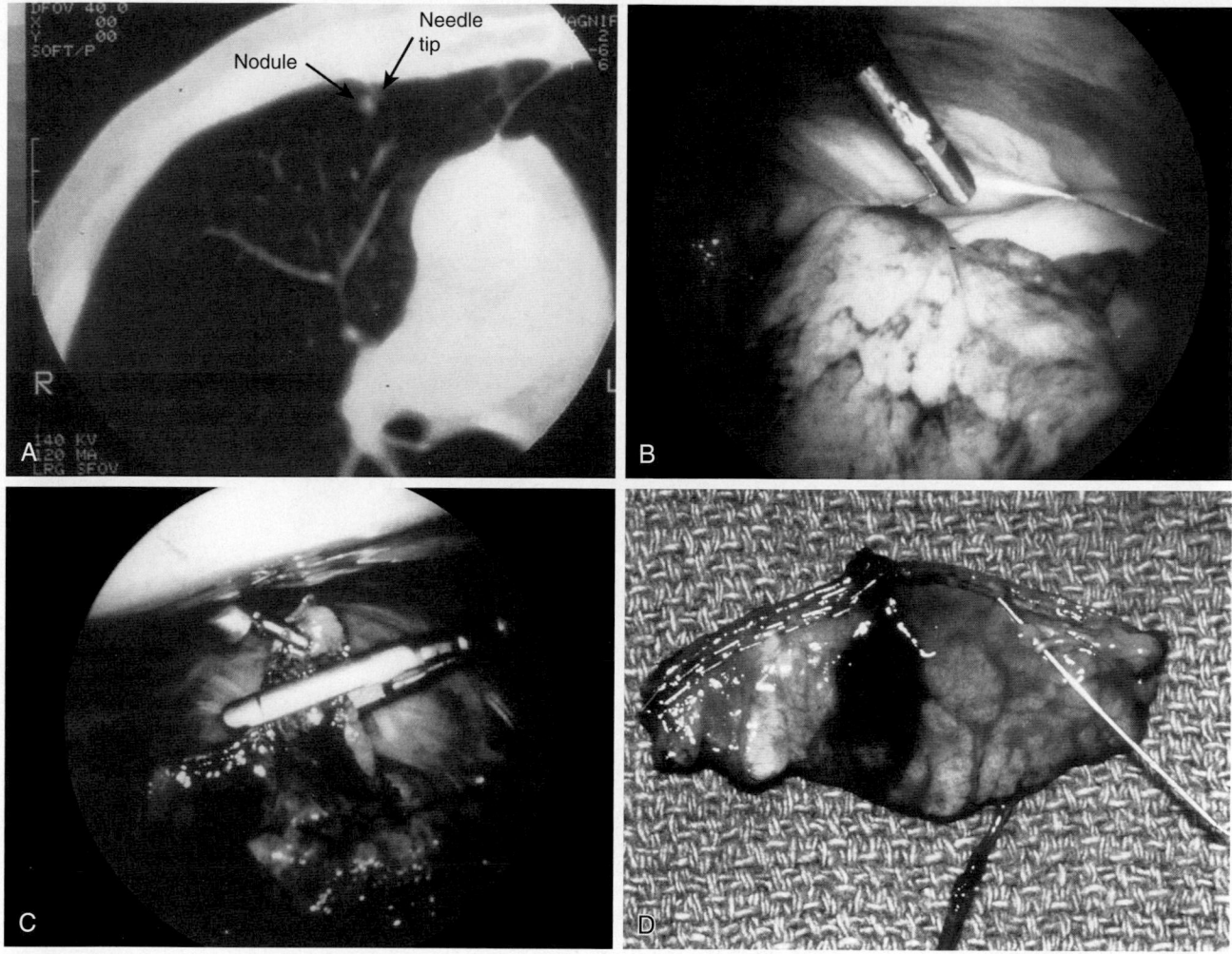

FIGURE 7 Hook-wire localization during video-assisted thoracoscopic surgery (VATS) wedge resection. **A,** Computed tomographic localization of the needle tip relative to the nodule to be resected. **B,** Endoscopic localization of the needle tip and lung nodule before VATS wedge resection. **C,** Endoscopic view of VATS wedge resection of the lung nodule. **D,** Resected specimen.

■ VIDEO-ASSISTED THORACOSCOPIC SURGERY PROCEDURES IN THE MEDIASTINUM

The indications for VATS for mediastinal pathology include the diagnosis of mediastinal masses, excision of mediastinal masses and cysts (particularly if the patient is symptomatic or malignancy is suspected), sympathectomy, and thymectomy (see Box 1).

Thoracoscopic Resection of Mediastinal Tumors

There are several reports in the literature describing the technique of VATS resection of mediastinal lesions such as thymus cysts, early stage thymoma, and posterior mediastinal tumors. VATS thymectomy for thymoma can be performed with a unilateral or bilateral approach. A double-lumen endotracheal tube or a single-lumen tube with CO_2 insufflation can be used. Currently, our favored approach for thymectomy is a bilateral VATS, because it permits better visualization of key anatomic structures and facilitates the accomplishment of a complete thymectomy. The procedure is started on the left side of the chest, and three 5-mm ports are placed in the third, fifth, and eighth interspaces. The mediastinal pleura is incised just anterior to the phrenic nerve. Dissection is started in the normal thymus, away from the tumor, with minimal manipulation of the tumor to avoid

any breaches in the capsule. It is critical that tumor manipulation is kept to a minimum and that the plane of dissection is kept beyond the capsule. Similarly, direct traction by grasping the tumor is avoided to limit capsular tears and contamination locally and in the pleural space. The dissection plane is extended cranially, taking care to preserve the integrity of the left phrenic nerve. The left portion of the thymus is mobilized free from the pericardium overlying the ascending aorta. The base of the left thymic lobe is mobilized and retracted superiorly. All thymic and perithymic fatty tissue is mobilized en bloc with the specimen, allowing exposure of the underlying pericardium and aorta. The thymus is then dissected carefully along the innominate vein, and the thymic tributaries are clipped and divided. The dissection is continued to the innominate vein–superior vena caval junction. The cervical horns are mobilized and swept inferiorly with the specimen. Once maximal mobilization is achieved on the left, the ports and instrumentation are withdrawn. The lung is re-expanded with a red-rubber catheter positioned within the pleural space to evacuate the pneumothorax, and then the catheter is removed. The procedure is repeated on the right side: three ports are placed; dissection is completed along the innominate vein–superior vena caval junction with careful avoidance of the right phrenic nerve. The venous thymic branches are clipped, any residual attachments are divided, and the specimen is removed. The VATS approach also can be utilized successfully for removal of posterior mediastinal tumors.

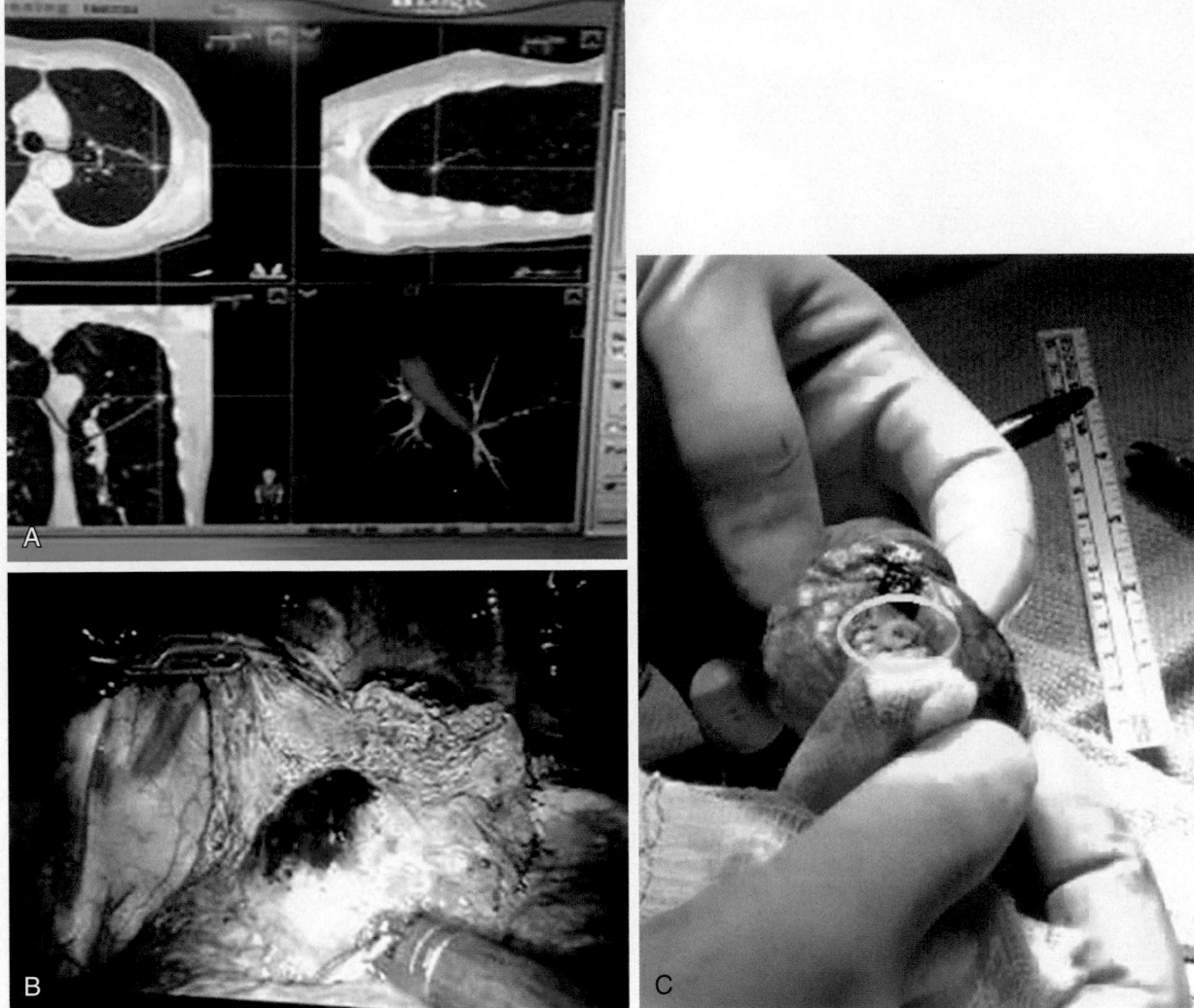

FIGURE 8 Electromagnetic-navigation-bronchoscopy–guided dye marking for localization and resection of lung nodules. **A,** CT image of lung nodule visualized in axial, coronal, and sagittal views. **B,** Focal pleural methylene blue dye visualization during VATS. **C,** Lung nodule seen beneath the surface pleural dye. All images are from a single patient. *(From Awais O et al. Electromagnetic navigation bronchoscopy-guided dye marking for thoracoscopic resection of pulmonary nodules. Ann Thorac Surg. 2016;102:223.)*

■ ESOPHAGEAL PROCEDURES USING VIDEO-ASSISTED THORACOSCOPIC SURGERY

VATS approaches have been described for many esophageal procedures, including management of thoracic esophageal diverticula, treatment of esophageal dysmotility, and complex esophageal surgeries such as minimally invasive esophagectomy (see Box 1).

Minimally Invasive Esophagectomy

We have reported our experience with minimally invasive esophagectomy in more than 1000 patients. Here, we summarize the essential steps of minimally invasive Ivor Lewis esophagectomy with an emphasis on the thoracoscopic portion of the operation. The laparoscopic portion of the surgery is performed first and includes laparoscopic gastric mobilization, formation of a gastric conduit, and lymph node dissection. We typically also perform a pyloric drainage procedure and place a feeding jejunostomy tube laparoscopically. The thoracic portion of the procedure follows and includes thoracoscopic esophageal mobilization and intrathoracic lymphadenectomy. An intrathoracic anastomosis is performed thoracoscopically through a

non–rib-spreading, mini-access incision (4 to 5 cm), typically using an end-to-end anastomotic (EEA) stapler (Covidien/Medtronics, Minneapolis, MN).

To begin the VATS portion of the procedure, the patient is placed in the left lateral decubitus position. The position of the double-lumen tube is verified, and single-lung ventilation is used. Typically, we place five thoracoscopic ports (Figure 9, *A*): a 10-mm port just anterior to the midaxillary line in the seventh or eighth intercostal space for the camera; a 10-mm port posterior to the posterior axillary line in the eighth or ninth intercostal space for the dissection instrument (ultrasonic coagulating shears, Covidien); a 10-mm port in the anterior axillary line at the fourth intercostal space for a fan-shaped retractor used to retract the lung anteriorly and allow exposure of the esophagus; a 5-mm port just posterior to the scapula tip for instruments necessary for retraction and countertraction; and a 5-mm port placed anteriorly, which is used by the second assistant intermittently for suction. Ultimately, the eighth posterior interspace port is enlarged to 4 to 5 cm to enable passage of the EEA stapler and removal of the specimen.

After thoracoscopic exploration, a retracting suture is placed near the central tendon of the diaphragm. This suture is brought out through a 1-mm skin incision in the chest wall (Figure 9, *B*). This allows us to apply downward traction on the diaphragm and improves exposure of the distal esophagus. Esophageal mobilization and lymph node dissection then is performed (see Figure 9, *B*). During the thoracoscopic mobilization of the esophagus, it is important to avoid thermal injury to the airway and the pericardium. The mediastinal pleura overlying the esophagus is divided and opened to the level of the azygos vein to expose the thoracic esophagus. The azygos vein then is divided with an endoscopic vascular stapler. The esophagus is mobilized circumferentially from the diaphragm to a level about 2 cm above the carina. Periesophageal tissue and lymph nodes are mobilized with the esophagus. We use an ultrasonic coagulating instrument for the dissection, and endoscopic clips are applied generously to larger vessels and any lymphatics. Above the azygos vein, it is important to keep the plane of dissection directly on the esophagus to prevent injury to the airway and the recurrent laryngeal nerve. A Penrose drain is placed around the esophagus to facilitate exposure

(see Figure 9, *B*). Mediastinal lymph node dissection, including a complete dissection of the subcarinal lymph nodes, is performed. Because the most common locations of esophageal tumors seen in our practice are the distal esophagus and gastroesophageal junction, we do not perform aggressive nodal dissection near the thoracic inlet. This decreases the chance of recurrent laryngeal nerve injury. In addition, the vagi are divided at the level of the azygos vein to potentially minimize traction injury.

The distal esophagus and the gastric conduit are brought up into the chest, maintaining the proper orientation of the gastric conduit and taking care not to twist the conduit. Repeat endoscopy may be required at this point to determine the site of transection if there is a concern about the proximal extent of the tumor. The port at the eighth space posteriorly is enlarged and covered with a wound protector; the specimen is removed and sent for frozen-section analysis of the margins.

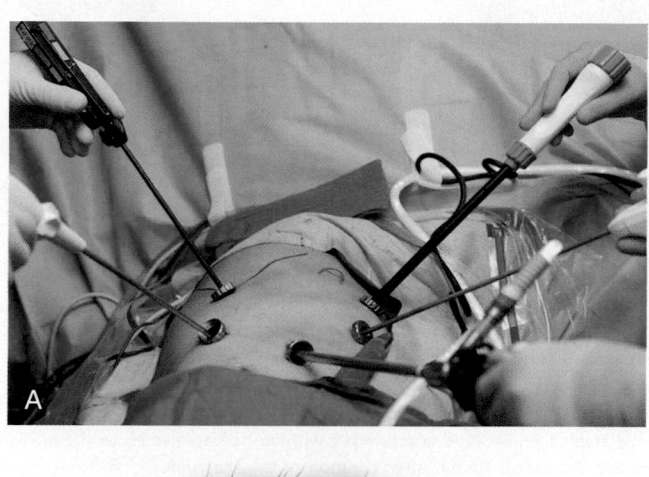

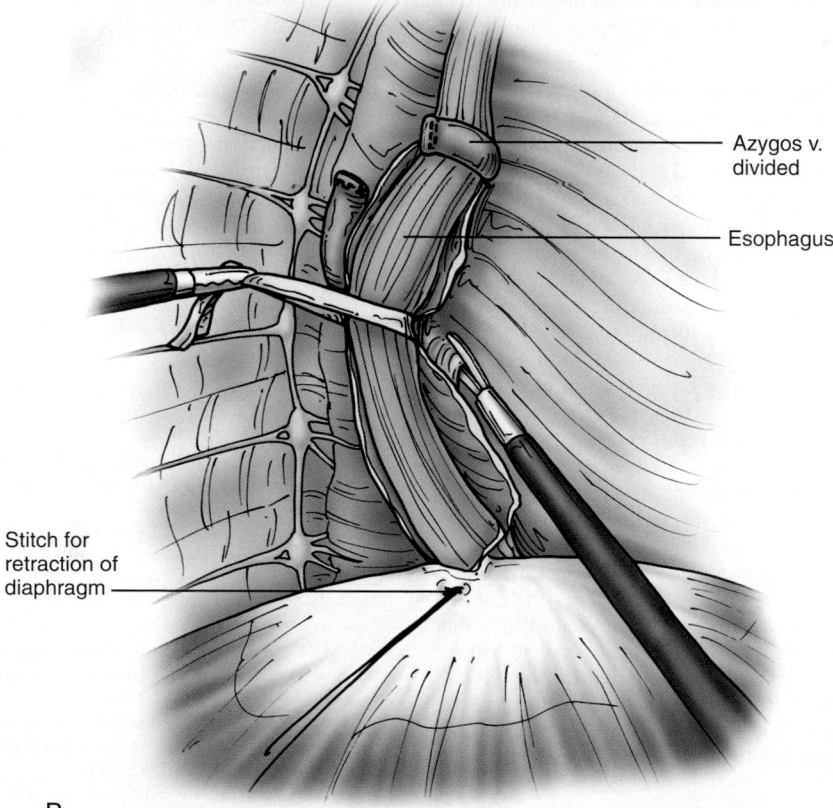

FIGURE 9 Minimally invasive esophagectomy. **A,** Thoracoscopic port placement. **B,** Mobilization of the thoracic portion of the esophagus.

Continued

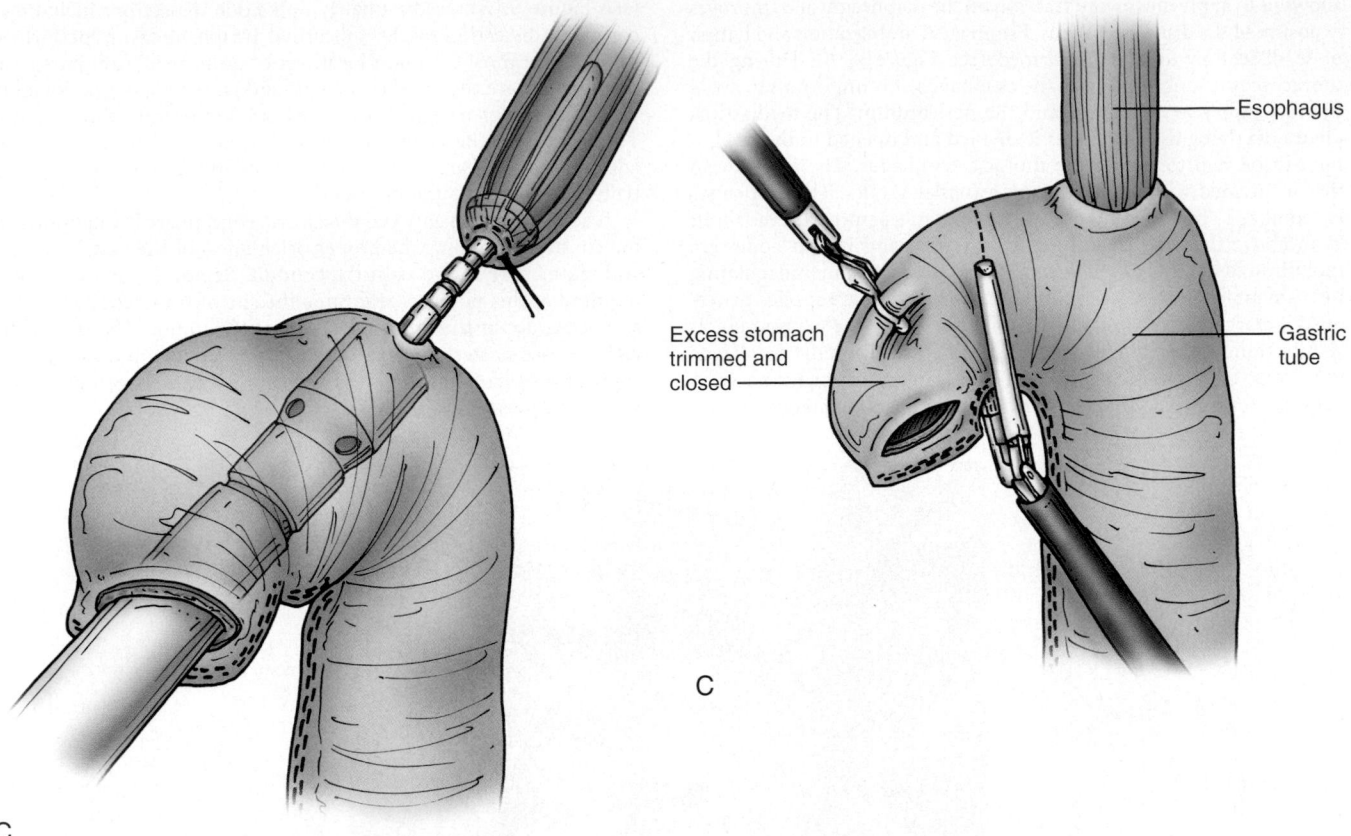

C

FIGURE 9, cont'd C, Construction of the stapled, end-to-end anastomosis with an EEA stapler. Note the anvil secured with purse-string sutures and the placement of the gastrostomy. **D,** Trimming the excess fundus after creation of the anastomosis. *(B, From Tsai WS, Levy RM, Luketich JD. Technique of minimally invasive Ivor Lewis esophagectomy. Oper Techn Thorac Cardiovasc Surg. 2009;14:176; C and D, Courtesy University of Pittsburgh Medical Center.)*

To restore continuity between the proximal esophagus and the gastric conduit, we prefer a high intrathoracic, stapled anastomosis near the thoracic inlet. The first step in creating the stapled anastomosis is the placement of a 28-mm EEA anvil in the proximal esophagus. We typically place two purse-string sutures to secure the anvil (Figure 9, C). Because the fundus of the stomach is the most ischemic portion of the conduit, we plan the anastomosis to discard the fundal tip. The tip of the fundus is opened, and the EEA stapler is advanced into the gastrostomy created in the tip of the fundus. A stapled anastomosis between the gastric conduit and the esophagus, high above the azygos vein, then is performed (see Figure 9, C). The redundant portion of the fundus is excised with a reticulating Endo-GIA stapler (Covidien) (Figure 9, D). A nasogastric tube is placed across the anastomosis and secured. The anastomosis is checked for leaks. In some patients (e.g., patients who have received neoadjuvant or definitive chemoradiation), we buttress the anastomosis with an omental flap that was mobilized during the abdominal phase of the procedure.

At the conclusion of the thoracic portion of the operation, the conduit is anchored to the right crus of the diaphragm. It is important to drain the chest well, and we place drains strategically in the chest. This is critical because if a leak occurs, a well-drained leak is easy to manage. We place a 28F chest tube posteriorly in the pleural space, and a #10 Jackson-Pratt drain posterior to the anastomosis, tracking behind the gastric conduit to the diaphragm, exiting at the costophrenic angle. It is important to secure these drains well.

■ CONCLUSIONS

VATS is currently used for a variety of thoracic surgical procedures, including complex procedures such as esophagectomy and lobectomy. The technology for VATS is evolving rapidly with improved optics, specialized instrumentation, and new imaging techniques. As with most minimally invasive surgical procedures, there is a significant learning curve for VATS. Proper advanced thoracic surgical training is essential for safe and successful performance of VATS, and a VATS approach should be attempted only after an adequate training period.

SUGGESTED READINGS

Awais O, Reidy MR, Mehta K, Bianco V, Gooding WE, Schuchert MJ, Luketich JD, Pennathur A. Electromagnetic navigation bronchoscopy-guided dye marking for thoracoscopic resection of pulmonary nodules. *Ann Thorac Surg.* 2016;102:223-229.

Landreneau RJ, Mack MJ, Hazelrigg RD, Ferson PF. Video-assisted thoracic surgery: basic technical concepts and intercostal approach strategies. *Ann Thorac Surg.* 1992;54:800.

Luketich JD, Landreneau RJ, Pennathur A. *Esophageal Surgery. Master Techniques in Surgery.* Philadelphia, PA: Wolters Kluwer Health; 2014.

Luketich JD, Pennathur A, Awais O, et al. Outcomes after minimally invasive esophagectomy: review of over 1000 patients. *Ann Surg.* 2012;256:95-103.

Mack MJ, Landreneau RJ, Yim AP, Hazelrigg SR, Scruggs G. Results of video assisted thymectomy in patients with myasthenia gravis. *J Thorac Cardiovasc Surg.* 1996;112:1352-1360.

Macke RA, Luketich JD, Pennathur A, et al. Thoracic esophageal diverticula: a 15-year experience of minimally invasive surgical management. *Ann Thorac Surg.* 2015;100:1795-1802.

Onaitis MW, Petersen RP, Balderson SS, et al. Thoracoscopic lobectomy is a safe and versatile procedure: experience with 500 consecutive patients. *Ann Surg.* 2006;244:420-425.

Pennathur A, Awais O, Luketich JD. Technique of minimally invasive Ivor Lewis esophagectomy. *Ann Thorac Surg.* 2010;89:S2159-S2162.

Pennathur A, Luketich JD. Minimally invasive esophagectomy: avoidance and treatment of complications. In: Little AG, Merrill WH, eds. *Complications in Cardiothoracic Surgery*. 2nd ed. Boston: Wiley-Blackwell; 2009:247-265.

Pennathur A, Qureshi I, Schuchert MJ, Dhupar R, Ferson PF, Gooding WE, et al. Comparison of surgical techniques for early-stage thymoma: feasibility of minimally invasive thymectomy and comparison with open resection. *J Thorac Cardiovasc Surg*. 2011;141:694-701.

LAPAROSCOPIC SURGERY FOR MORBID OBESITY

Kashif A. Zuberi, MD, Thomas Magnuson, MD, and Michael A. Schweitzer, MD

The morbid obesity epidemic continues to spread throughout industrialized nations. It is a condition with a heterogeneous origin, including genetic, psychosocial, and environmental factors. Prevention methods have currently been unable to halt the further spread of this disease. Obesity has been linked to increased healthcare costs, common physiologic derangements, reduced quality of life, and increased overall mortality. More than one third of adults and almost 17% of children in the United States are obese.

Medical therapy that can cause sustained significant weight loss may be years away. Bariatric surgery, when combined with a multidisciplinary team, continues to be the only proven method to achieve sustained weight loss in most patients. Bariatric procedures modify gastrointestinal anatomy and, in some cases, enteric hormone release to reduce caloric intake, reduce absorption, and alter metabolism to achieve weight loss. Currently, the three most common bariatric operations in the United States are Roux-en-Y gastric bypass, adjustable gastric band, and the vertical sleeve gastrectomy (Boxes 1, 2, and 3). The sleeve gastrectomy is part of a duodenal switch with biliopancreatic diversion. It has been used in patients at higher risk as a first-staged weight loss procedure, where the plan is to induce a significant weight loss and then offer patients a revision to a gastric bypass or duodenal switch with biliopancreatic diversion when they have achieved a safer weight. It is also now used as a primary bariatric operation with weight loss results that are better than adjustable gastric band but without the intestinal malabsorption issues seen after gastric bypass. Duodenal switch with biliopancreatic diversion has never been a popular weight loss surgery because of the significant malnutrition that accompanies this procedure (Box 4). All four of these operations can be performed laparoscopically in most patients.

■ PREOPERATIVE EVALUATION

The National Institutes of Health Consensus Development Conference Statement for Gastrointestinal Surgery for Severe Obesity was issued in 1991 and is still regarded as the starting point for criteria to accept patients in a surgical weight loss program. Patients are considered morbidly obese and candidates for surgery if they have a body mass index (BMI) of at least 35 kg/m^2 with an obesity-related comorbidity or greater than 40 kg/m^2. Recommendations are that patients should have tried dieting in the past before surgical therapy is considered as a treatment option (Box 5).

In evaluation of a potential patient for bariatric surgery, a multidisciplinary team should be used. This team should include a dietician and mental health professional, whose purpose is to obtain dietary and behavioral eating history, discuss postoperative dietary expectations, and decide whether the patient is appropriate for bariatric surgery. Support for the surgery from family members and friends is helpful. If the team believes that the patient is not appropriate for surgery, then consideration should be given to nonoperative medical management with appropriate counseling and surgery should be reconsidered or denied indefinitely.

Patients with severe end organ disease, such as end-stage heart failure or respiratory failure, are at higher risk for morbidity and mortality. Surgery is not necessarily contraindicated for these patients, but weight loss alone may not significantly correct end-stage heart or lung disease. Patients with cirrhosis may be at higher risk for surgery but certainly may benefit from weight loss. Patients who are morbidly obese may be rejected for heart, lung, liver, or kidney transplant and therefore may benefit from bariatric surgery–induced weight loss. Patients who are nonambulating or bedridden also should be considered at high risk for postoperative complications.

Currently, patients with type 2 diabetes with a BMI of 30 to 35 kg/m^2 are being studied for whether they would benefit from bariatric surgery. The U.S. Food and Drug Administration (FDA) has approved the adjustable gastric band for this subgroup of patients.

■ PREPARING THE PATIENT IN THE OPERATING ROOM

On the morning of surgery, the patient is injected subcutaneously with low-molecular-weight heparin to prevent venous thromboembolic complications. A peripheral intravenous (IV) line is placed, and an appropriate antibiotic is administered intravenously. The patient is placed on the operating room table in the supine position with a footboard. Appropriate padding of the patient is important because these particular patients are at increased risk for compression-related injuries. Sequential compression devices are placed on the lower extremities if they fit. General anesthesia is performed, and then a urinary catheter is inserted. The anesthetist inserts, applies suction to, and then immediately removes the orogastric tube before starting the operation. Esophageal temperature probes are not recommended because these can migrate into the stomach during stapling. The operating surgeon stands on the patient's right side, and the assistant stands on the left (Figure 1). Entering the abdomen in morbidly obese patients is safe with direct vision with a device that allows visualization of the abdominal wall layers sequentially with a 0-degree laparoscope inserted inside of it. Initial access in each procedure is through a left upper quadrant 12-mm incision.

■ TECHNIQUES

Laparoscopic Antecolic Antegastric Roux-en-Y Gastric Bypass Operative Technique

The abdomen is then insufflated with carbon dioxide to a pressure of 15 mm Hg, a 45-degree angled laparoscope is inserted, and an additional four ports are placed (a 5-mm trocar at the right subcostal margin, a 5-mm trocar inferior to the left upper quadrant 12-mm trocar, a 12-mm trocar in the right upper quadrant, and a 12-mm trocar in the upper abdominal midline). The omentum and transverse colon are retracted cephalad until the transverse colon mesentery is visualized. Anterior retraction of the mesentery allows visualization of the jejunum at the ligament of Trietz. The jejunum is then transected with a linear stapler loaded with a 60-mm–length cartridge containing variable staple sizes from 2.0 to 3.0 mm for medium-thickness tissue, approximately 40 cm to 75 cm distal to the ligament of Trietz. A long enough section of mesentery is usually found here so that the Roux limb can be placed in the antecolic antegastric position and safely reach the gastric pouch without any significant tension. The mesentery is divided with a linear stapler loaded with a 2.0-mm staple cartridge, and then the ultrasonic shears are used to extend this division as much as necessary so that the

BOX 1: Gastric Bypass

Advantages

- Proven weight loss over 5 years
- Better weight loss than restrictive-only operations
- Proven improvement in medical comorbidities
- Mortality rate less than 1% at most centers

Disadvantages

- Malabsorption
- Marginal ulcer
- Stomal stenosis
- Inability to easily access distal stomach
- Internal hernia
- Small bowel obstruction
- Iron-deficiency anemia
- Calcium and vitamin B_{12} deficiency

BOX 2: Adjustable Gastric Band

Advantages

- Reversible
- Least invasive (no stapling of the stomach)
- Lowest risk of death
- No malabsorption

Disadvantages

- Erosion
- Esophageal dilation
- Breakage
- Port problems
- Slippage or prolapse
- May worsen GERD
- Failure to lose weight
- Lower average weight loss

GERD, Gastroesophageal reflux disease.

BOX 3: Sleeve Gastrectomy

Advantages

- Better weight loss than with adjustable gastric band
- Proven improvement in medical comorbidities
- Easier to perform than gastric bypass, especially if BMI is high
- No intestinal malabsorption
- No risk of marginal ulcers
- Preserved pylorus means less risk of dumping
- Ability to convert to gastric bypass or DS-BPD
- Mortality rate less than 1% at most centers

Disadvantages

- Not reversible
- Large portion of stomach removed
- A proximal leak is difficult to treat
- Stricture (incisura angularis)

BMI, Body mass index; *DS-BPD*, duodenal switch with biliopancreatic diversion.

proximal Roux limb is able to safely reach the gastric pouch. A stay suture is placed on the proximal Roux limb, and then the bowel is run approximately 60 to 100 cm distal to the stapled off end. A stay suture is placed here to mark where the stapled side-to-side jejuno-jejunostomy will be constructed with the end of the biliopancreatic limb. The anastomosis is performed with a linear stapler loaded with

BOX 4: Duodenal Switch With Biliopancreatic Diversion

Advantages

- Excellent weight loss
- Proven improvement in medical comorbidities
- Preserved pylorus means less risk of dumping
- Less risk of marginal ulcers

Disadvantages

- Increased risk of protein malabsorption
- Increased risk of fat-soluble vitamin malabsorption (A, D, E, and K)
- Iron-deficiency anemia
- Diarrhea and excess gas more common
- Internal hernia
- Higher complication rate
- Higher risk of osteoporosis

BOX 5: Patient Requirements for Bariatric Surgery

1. Patients with a BMI of 40 kg/m² or greater are potential candidates for bariatric surgery.
2. Patients with a BMI of 35 to 40 kg/m² with significant obesity-related comorbidity are also potential candidates for bariatric surgery.
3. Patients with a history of dieting.
4. Patients with no recent substance abuse.
5. Patients should be evaluated by a multidisciplinary team that includes a dietician and psychologic evaluation before surgery.

BMI, Body mass index.

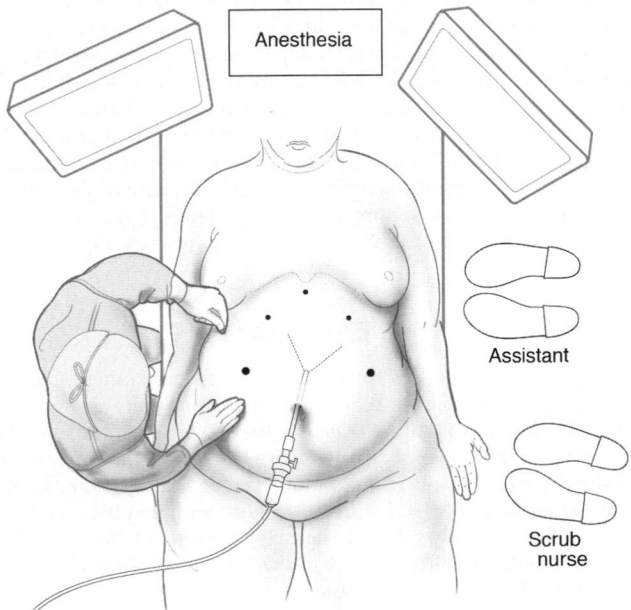

FIGURE 1 Positioning for laparoscopic gastric bypass. *(Illustration used with permission from Cameron JL, Sandone C: Atlas of Gastrointestinal Surgery, ed 2, vol II, Shelton, CT, 2014, PMPH-USA.)*

a 60-mm–length cartridge containing variable staple sizes from 2.0 to 3.0 mm that is inserted through small enterotomies made with the ultrasonic shears below the stay suture (Figure 2). The enterotomy opening is then closed with firing of a similar linear stapler that has been placed under two stay sutures at each end of the opening

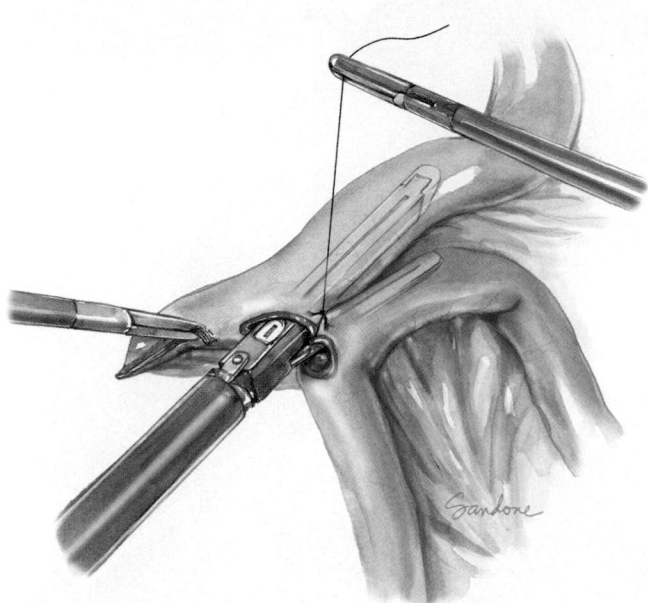

FIGURE 2 A linear stapler is used to create the jejunojejunostomy. *(Illustration used with permission from Cameron JL, Sandone C: Atlas of Gastrointestinal Surgery, ed 2, vol II, Shelton, CT, 2014, PMPH-USA.)*

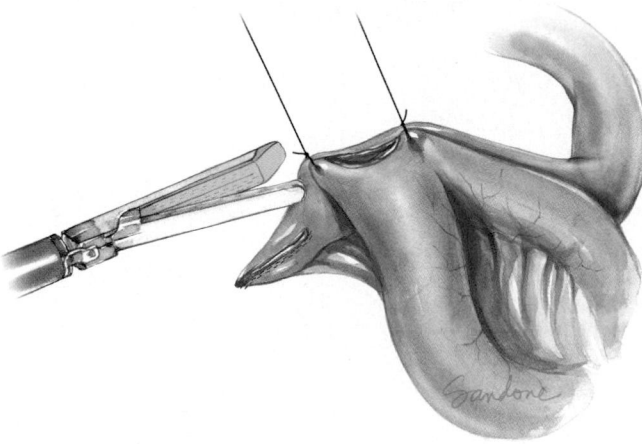

FIGURE 3 Closure of jejunojejunostomy opening. *(Illustration used with permission from Cameron JL, Sandone C: Atlas of Gastrointestinal Surgery, ed 2, vol II, Shelton, CT, 2014, PMPH-USA.)*

(Figure 3). An unzippering stitch is placed in the crotch of the stapled anastomosis, and an antiobstruction stitch is placed to keep the Roux limb from kinking at the jejunojejunostomy. The mesenteric defect is then closed with a running suture. Clips or sutures are placed on the staple line if there is any bleeding. The greater omentum is divided in half with an ultrasonic dissector or vessel-sealing device along its entire length up to the border of the transverse colon.

Next, the patient is placed into steep reverse Trendelenburg position. The legs and feet are then checked to ensure they are still straight and on the footboard. The left lateral segment of the liver is retracted with a Nathanson retractor through a subxiphoid 4-mm puncture, which is then held in position with a movable arm that attaches to the operating room table (Iron Intern with Nathanson liver retractors, Automated Medical Products Corp., Edison, NJ). The procedure then begins with dissecting the peritoneal attachments at the angle of His to expose the left crus, followed by the bare area of the gastrohepatic omentum to enter the lesser sac. Division of the neurovascular bundle on the lesser curvature side of the stomach just

distal to the left gastric vein is done with a linear stapler with a 2.0-mm staple cartridge. Next, a linear stapler loaded with a 60-mm–length cartridge containing variable staple sizes from 3.0 to 4.0 mm is first used to divide the stomach, followed by successive firings of a linear stapler containing 60-mm–length cartridges with variable staple sizes from 2.0 to 3.0 mm. The first gastric staple transection is started on the lesser curve side just below the left gastric vein and is then followed by sequential stapling until completion at the angle of His so that the proximal gastric pouch created is 15 to 20 mL in size (Figure 4). It is important to retract the posterior fundus downward and bring the stapler around the tissue at the angle of His to avoid making a large fundal pouch. This is prevented by entering the open space of the lesser sac after the first stapled division of the stomach and then dissecting through to the angle of His with an articulating dissector instrument that can then lock in place after forming a right angle. The articulating dissector can then be used to retract the fundus inferiorly while stapling sequentially to the angle of His. The stomach staple lines on both sides should be inspected for adequate staple formation, bleeding, and ischemia. Bleeding staple lines are usually easily taken care of with a clip or direct suture ligation.

The Roux limb is brought up antecolic antegastric with care to avoid a twist in the mesentery. The Roux limb is then sutured to the gastric pouch staple line approximately where the first and second gastric staple lines intersect. A small enterotomy is made below the stay suture in the Roux limb and a similar size gastrotomy in the pouch to place the linear stapler loaded with a 45-mm–length cartridge containing variable staple sizes from 3.0 to 4.0 mm to create the gastrojejunostomy where only the first 30 mm of the staple cartridge are used (Figure 5). A stay suture is placed on the lesser curve (right) side of the opening; it is then used to retract the posterior part of the anastomosis to the left and anterior, thereby exposing the entire posterior side. A running 2-0 suture is then placed starting posterior on the left side and continuously run to the stay suture on the right side, to which it is tied (Figure 6). The anesthesia team carefully passes a 32F blunt round-end bougie from the mouth and then through the gastrojejunal anastomosis and into the Roux limb. A stay suture is placed at the halfway point of the opening between the end stay sutures. This stay suture and the stay suture on the left (angle of His side) are used to elevate the tissue so that the linear stapler loaded with a 60-mm–length cartridge containing variable staple sizes from 3.0 to 4.0 mm can be used to close the openings. The stapler is brought down on top of the bougie while retracting the tissue to be transected. This firing then closes most of the opening, and the small remaining defect on the right side is easily closed with a 2-0 suture (Figure 7). Alternatively, the entire opening could be closed with a running 2-0 suture. The gastrojejunal anastomosis is then completed by running a 2-0 suture to cover the entire anterior and lateral sides in a second layer. The resultant anastomosis is approximately 12 mm in diameter and has been completely encircled by multiple continuous running 2-0 suture. An air leak test can be performed if desired to test the gastrojejunal anastomosis.

The operating room table is taken out of steep reverse Trendelenburg position, and the mesenteric defect is then closed between the Roux limb mesentery and the transverse mesocolon, up to the transverse colon with running 2-0 suture. This is to help prevent an internal hernia through Petersen's defect. The remaining jejunojejunostomy mesenteric defect is then closed with a running suture. A drain is placed in the left upper quadrant by the anastomosis, and the trocars are removed with direct vision. Long-acting local anesthetic is placed in the wound, and the sites are closed with an absorbable subcuticular suture and glue (Figure 8).

Laparoscopic Adjustable Gastric Band

The 45-degree angled viewing laparoscope is inserted, and an additional three trocars (a 12-mm trocar in the upper abdominal midline and two right upper quadrant 5-mm trocars) are placed with direct vision. The angle of His attachments are taken down with blunt dissection, and the gastrohepatic omentum in the bare area is divided

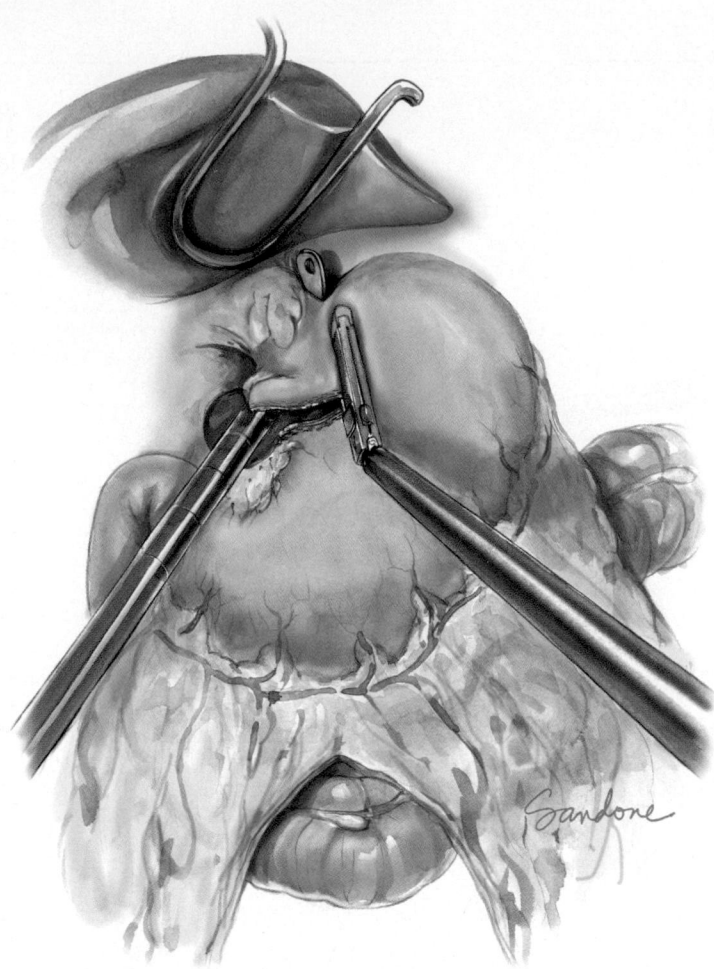

FIGURE 4 Stapled division of stomach. *(Illustration used with permission from Cameron JL, Sandone C: Atlas of Gastrointestinal Surgery, ed 2, vol II, Shelton, CT, 2014, PMPH-USA.)*

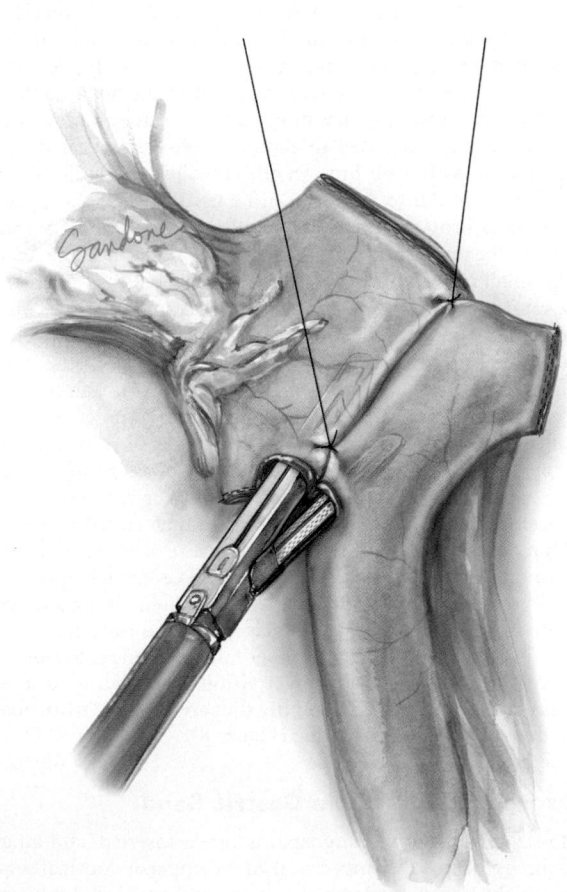

FIGURE 5 A linear stapler is used to create the gastrojejunostomy. *(Illustration used with permission from Cameron JL, Sandone C: Atlas of Gastrointestinal Surgery, ed 2, vol II, Shelton, CT, 2014, PMPH-USA.)*

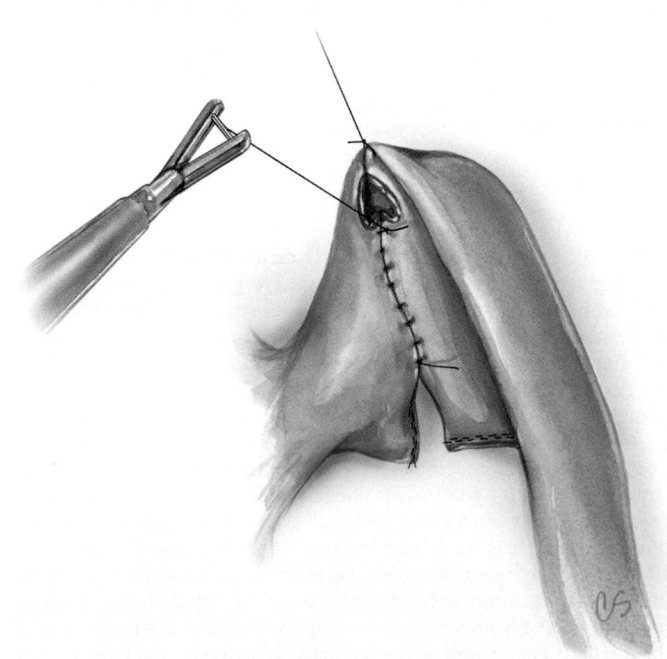

FIGURE 6 Reinforcing the posterior staple line of the gastrojejunostomy. *(Illustration used with permission from Cameron JL, Sandone C: Atlas of Gastrointestinal Surgery, ed 2, vol II, Shelton, CT, 2014, PMPH-USA.)*

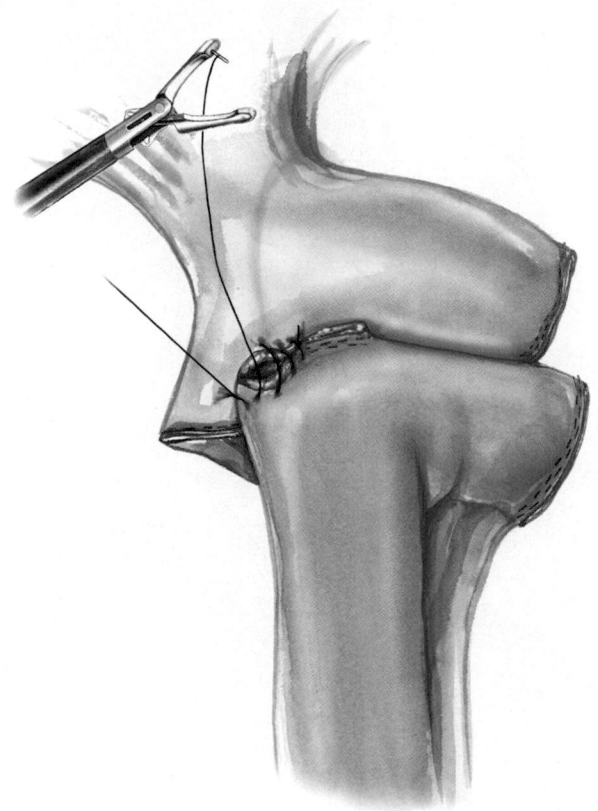

FIGURE 7 The opening used for the linear stapler is then closed with a running suture. *(Illustration used with permission from Cameron JL, Sandone C: Atlas of Gastrointestinal Surgery, ed 2, vol II, Shelton, CT, 2014, PMPH-USA.)*

with a hook electrocautery. The right crus is identified. After the hook cautery is used to divide peritoneal tissue, an articulating dissector is then placed from the right crus side to the angle of His, with gentle rotating side-to-side motion as it is advanced forward; it is then flexed into a right angle and locked. The 12-mm left upper quadrant trocar is removed, and a 15-mm trocar is placed. The adjustable band is placed into the abdomen through the 15-mm trocar. The band tubing is then placed through the opening in the articulating dissector and then brought over to the right crus side (Figure 9). The tubing is removed from the dissector and then placed through the buckle of the band. The buckle is then locked. Next, one to four interrupted 2-0 nonabsorbable sutures are placed from the fundus to the proximal stomach (superior to the band). It is easier to work closer to the angle of His side of the stomach and then sew toward the patient's right side (Figure 10). The buckle of the band should not be covered because of increased risk of erosion. The anterior fundal wrap over the band should be without tension. The tubing of the band is grasped and removed through the left upper quadrant trocar site. The trocars are then removed. A subcutaneous pocket is formed on the anterior side of the fascia, and the port is connected to the band tubing and then secured to the fascia. It is important to check the tubing and ensure it has no kinks as it enters the fascia. The site is irrigated, and then all the trocar sites are closed with subcuticular suture and glue (Figure 11).

Laparoscopic Vertical Sleeve Gastrectomy

Laparoscopic vertical sleeve gastrectomy was initially used as a first-stage operation in patients at high risk or in patients whose super morbid obesity made a laparoscopic-only approach difficult. After 12 to 24 months of weight loss, a second-stage operation could be used in those who were still at a high BMI and wanted to be revised to a

laparoscopic Roux-en-Y gastric bypass or a laparoscopic duodenal switch with biliopancreatic diversion. This staged approach is designed to reduce operative risk by improving comorbidities and reducing the technical challenges associated with super morbidly obese patients. Recent data have shown that sleeve gastrectomy is an effective operation for weight loss, resulting in 40% to 60% excess body weight loss as the primary treatment alone. It is easier to perform and has fewer complications then a Roux-en-Y gastric bypass or duodenal switch with biliopancreatic diversion. It does not involve a large foreign body that can be at risk to erode or slip as with an adjustable gastric band. It also avoids the intestinal malabsorption and small bowel obstruction risks seen with gastric bypass or duodenal switch with biliopancreatic diversion.

As previously described, entry to the abdominal cavity starts with a 12-mm trocar placed with direct vision through a left upper quadrant incision. The abdomen is then insufflated with carbon dioxide to a pressure of 15 mm Hg, a 45-degree angled laparoscope is inserted, and an additional three ports (a 5-mm trocar at the right subcostal margin, a 15-mm trocar in the right upper quadrant, and a 12-mm trocar just to the left of the upper abdominal midline) and a subxiphoid liver retractor are placed with direct vision. The operation starts with division of the stomach's greater curvature blood supply with a vessel-sealing device to divide the gastrocolic and gastrosplenic ligaments close to the stomach (Figure 12). A stay suture is placed 6 to 7 cm from the pylorus-duodenal junction. A 40F bougie is inserted transorally and brought down alongside the lesser curve until it lays against the stomach wall to the patient's right of the stay suture. Next, a narrow gastric tube is created with a linear cutting stapler starting on the patient's right side of the stay suture and sequentially stapling toward the angle of His alongside a 40F bougie. The surgeons should confirm that the bougie is on the lesser curve side of the stapler.

The stomach is first divided with two firings of the linear stapler loaded with 60-mm–length cartridges containing variable staple sizes from 4.0 to 5.0 mm for extra thick tissue. The stomach is continued to be divided with a linear stapler loaded with 60-mm–length cartridges containing variable staple sizes from 3.0 to 4.0 mm. The stomach is divided next to the bougie all the way up to the angle of His where the lateral stomach is separated (Figure 13). Care is taken not to leave any fundus behind and not to apply the stapler too close to the gastroesophageal junction. Hemostasis of the gastric staple line can be secured with running sutures or clips. The resected stomach is extracted intact through the 15-mm trocar site, after widening the fascial opening with a clamp device. If the surgeon desires, the staple line can be evaluated with an underwater leak test either with an orogastric tube or an endoscope. A drain is placed in the left upper quadrant and brought out through the 5-mm trocar site. The ports are removed with direct vision after first closing the 15-mm port site suture passing device. Long-acting local anesthetic is placed in the wounds, and the sites are closed with subcuticular sutures (Figure 14).

Laparoscopic Biliopancreatic Diversion With Duodenal Switch

The laparoscopic duodenal switch with biliopancreatic diversion (DS-BPD) is primarily a malabsorptive operation that involves preservation of the gastric pylorus and creation of a short, 100-cm ileal "common channel," where food and biliopancreatic enzymes are allowed to mix. Because of the potential for malabsorption-related nutritional deficiencies and the complexity of the operation, DS-BPD is the least common bariatric operation performed in the United States when compared with gastric bypass, sleeve gastrectomy, and adjustable gastric banding.

As previously described, entry to the abdominal cavity starts with a 12-mm trocar placed with direct vision through a left upper quadrant incision. The abdomen is then insufflated with carbon dioxide to a pressure of 15 mm Hg, a 45-degree angled laparoscope is

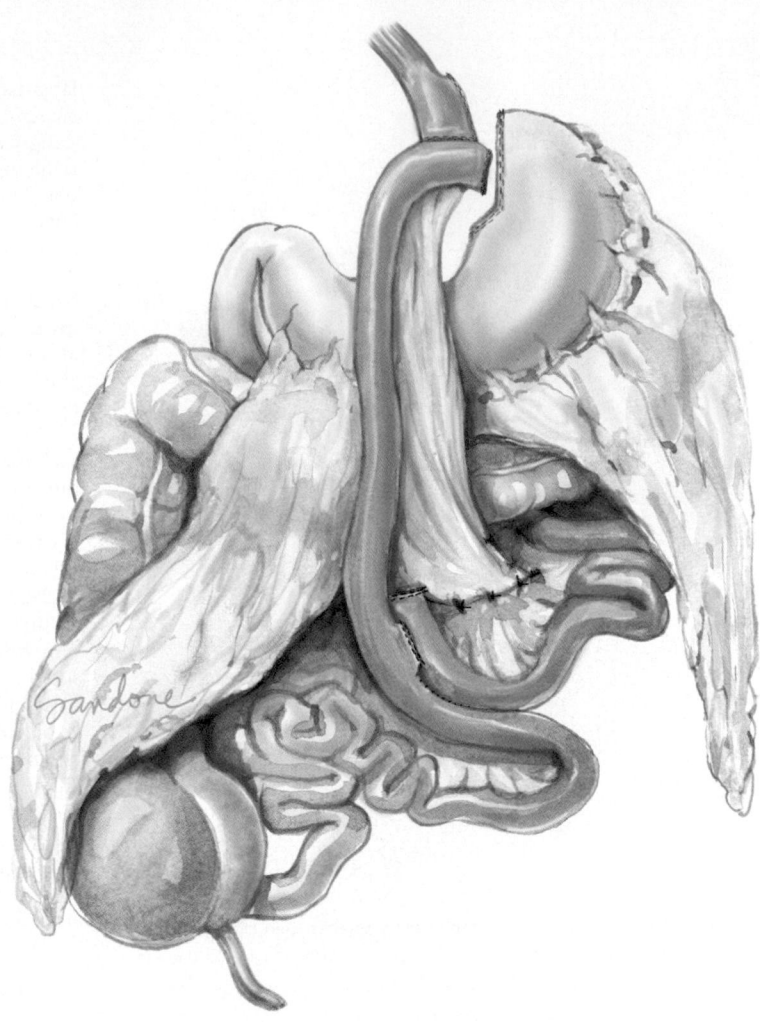

FIGURE 8 Antecolic antegastric Roux-en-Y gastric bypass. *(Illustration used with permission from Cameron JL, Sandone C: Atlas of Gastrointestinal Surgery, ed 2, vol II, Shelton, CT, 2014, PMPH-USA.)*

FIGURE 9 The band tubing attached to the articulating dissector is then brought around the posterior stomach, from patient's left to right side. *(Illustration used with permission from Cameron JL, Sandone C: Atlas of Gastrointestinal Surgery, ed 2, vol II, Shelton, CT, 2014, PMPH-USA.)*

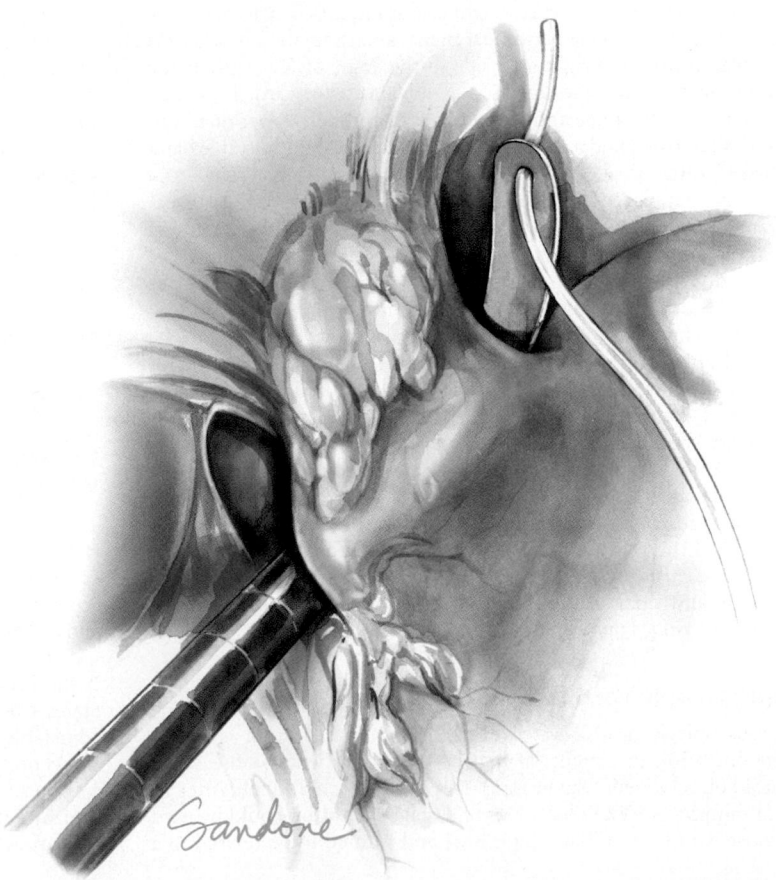

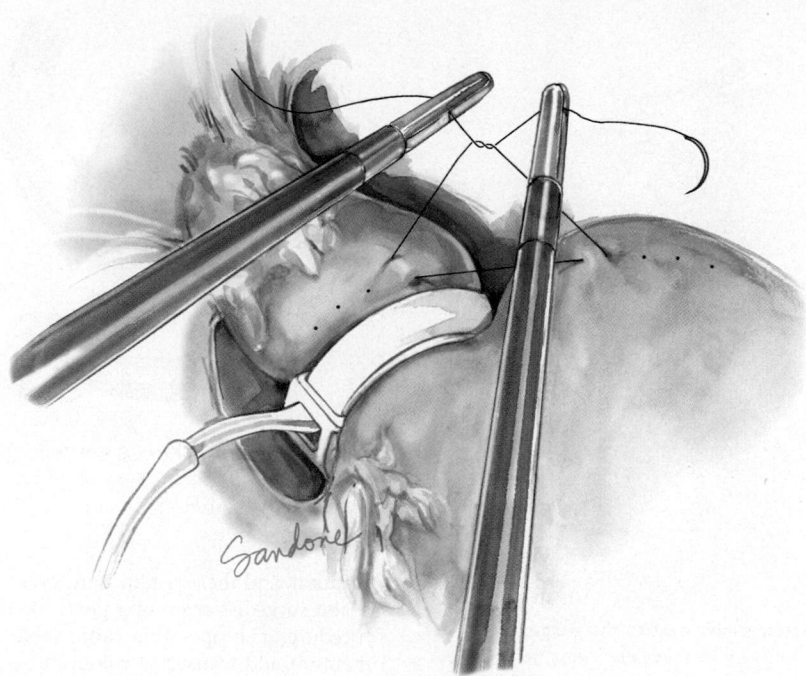

FIGURE 10 An anterior gastric wrap is performed with interrupted nonabsorbable sutures. *(Illustration used with permission from Cameron JL, Sandone C: Atlas of Gastrointestinal Surgery, ed 2, vol II, Shelton, CT, 2014, PMPH-USA.)*

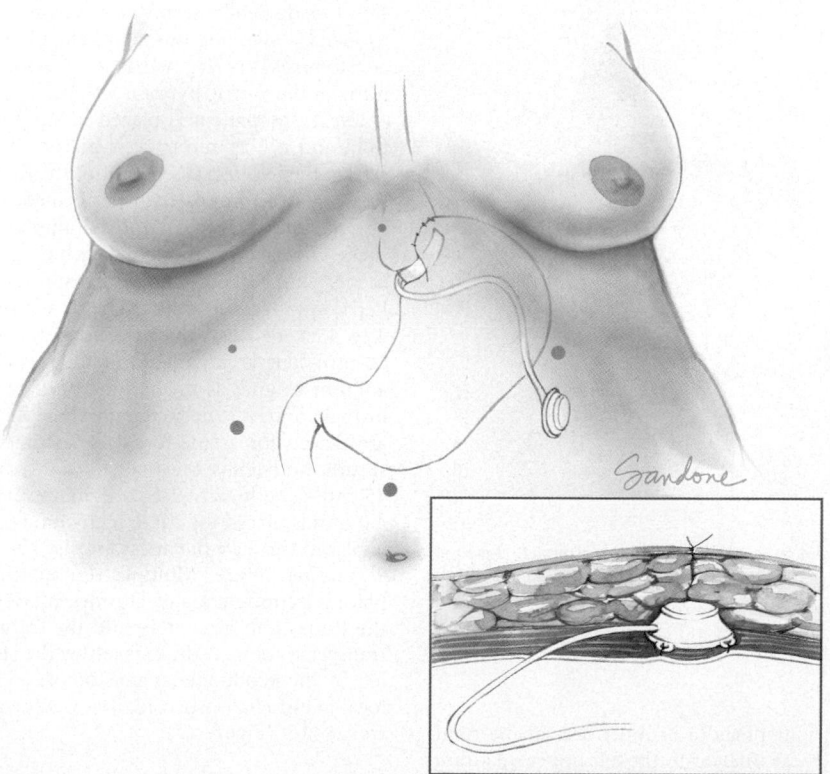

FIGURE 11 Adjustable gastric band with port placement in the left upper quadrant. *(Illustration used with permission from Cameron JL, Sandone C: Atlas of Gastrointestinal Surgery, ed 2, vol II, Shelton, CT, 2014, PMPH-USA.)*

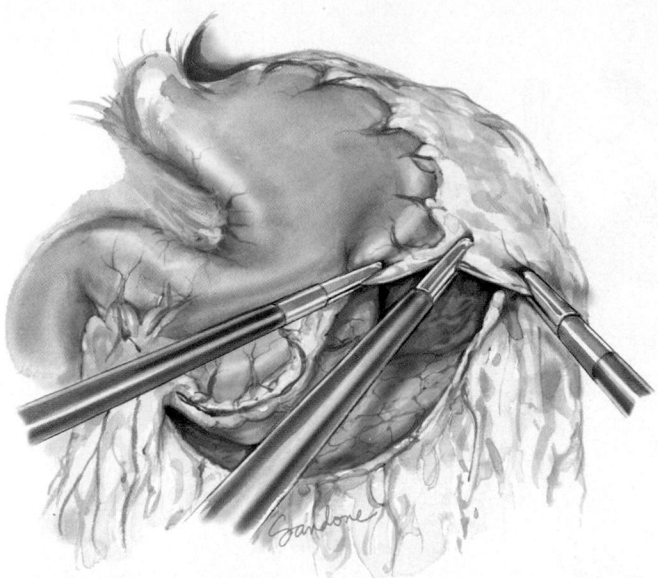

FIGURE 12 Division of the vascular supply next to the greater curvature of the stomach. *(Illustration used with permission from Cameron JL, Sandone C: Atlas of Gastrointestinal Surgery, ed 2, vol II, Shelton, CT, 2014, PMPH-USA.)*

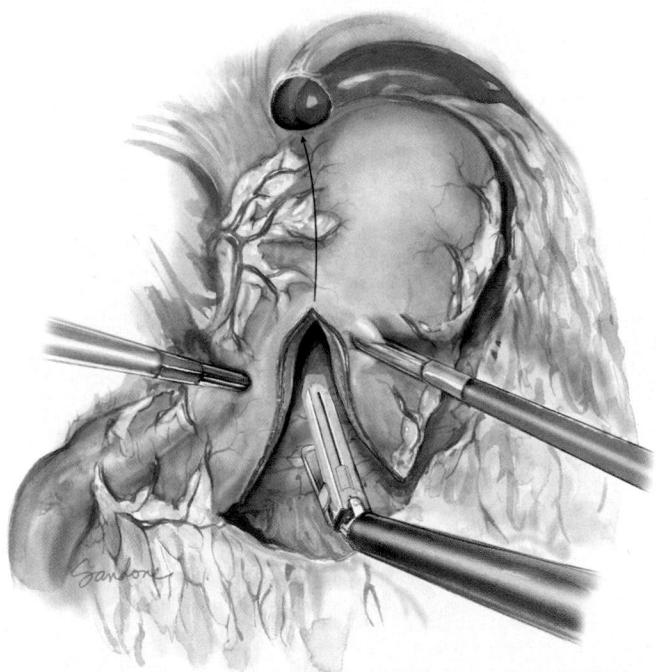

FIGURE 13 Linear stapler used to vertically divide the stomach close to the lesser curve. A 40F bougie is used to calibrate the size of the remaining stomach. *(Illustration used with permission from Cameron JL, Sandone C: Atlas of Gastrointestinal Surgery, ed 2, vol II, Shelton, CT, 2014, PMPH-USA.)*

inserted, and an additional four ports (a 5-mm trocar at the right subcostal margin, a 5-mm trocar inferior to the left upper quadrant 12-mm trocar, a 15-mm trocar in the right upper quadrant, and a 12-mm trocar in the upper abdominal midline) and a subxiphoid liver retractor are placed with direct vision. The operating surgeon stands on the patient's left side for the small intestinal part of the

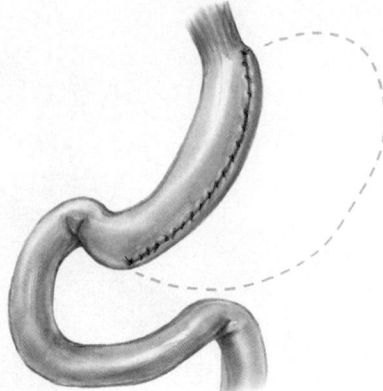

FIGURE 14 Vertical sleeve gastrectomy. *(Illustration used with permission from Cameron JL, Sandone C: Atlas of Gastrointestinal Surgery, ed 2, vol II, Shelton, CT, 2014, PMPH-USA.)*

operation, and the assistant stands on the right. The left-sided ports are the surgeon's operating ports for the ileoileostomy part of the procedure. The operating room table is then placed flat, and the omentum and transverse colon are retracted cephalad. The cecum and ileocecal valve are then identified, and the ileum is measured back 100 cm proximal to the cecum. A stay suture is placed, and then another 150 cm of ileum is measured proximal from the suture. This is where the ileum is transected with a linear stapler loaded with a 60-mm–length cartridge containing variable staple sizes from 2.0 to 3.0 mm. The mesentery is divided with the ultrasonic shears, and a stay suture is placed on the distal transected bowel to mark the Roux end that will connect to the duodenum. The proximal divided bowel is the biliopancreatic limb, which is brought down to the previous stay suture marking the ileum at 100 cm from the cecum. A stapled side-to-side ileoileostomy is then constructed. Care should be taken to avoid a twist or misalignment of the bowel at this point. The anastomosis is performed as the previously described enteroenterostomy in the gastric bypass section.

Next, the patient is placed in steep reverse Trendelenburg position, and a liver retractor is placed in the subxiphoid position to retract the left lateral segment of the liver. As previously described, a sleeve gastrectomy is then performed, with a 48F instead of a 40F bougie, and then it is removed after completion. Attention is then turned toward the duodenum, which is freed from its lateral attachments, with great care taken to not injure any of the structures in the hepatoduodenal ligament. The duodenum is divided approximately 2 to 4 cm distal to the pylorus with a linear stapler loaded with a 60-mm–length cartridge containing variable staple sizes from 3.0 to 4.0 mm (Figure 15). The omentum is split, and the Roux limb is brought antecolic up to the proximal duodenal end. Two stay sutures are placed for a side-to-side anastomosis. Under the inferior stay suture, both ends are opened and a linear stapler loaded with a 45-mm–length cartridge containing variable staple sizes from 3.0 to 4.0 mm is placed for 2.5 to 3 cm and fired (Figure 16). A 40F bougie is placed through the anastomosis. The opening is now closed with a running suture. Multiple seromuscular interrupted sutures are placed circumferentially. The mesenteric defect is then closed between the Roux limb mesentery and the transverse mesocolon, up to the transverse colon. A drain is left by the stomach, and another drain is left by the ileoduodenal anastomosis. The trocars are removed, and local anesthetic is injected, followed by a subcuticular closure of the trocar sites (Figure 17).

■ POSTOPERATIVE MANAGEMENT

Most patients are transferred after routine monitoring in the recovery room. Patients with moderate to severe obstructive sleep apnea

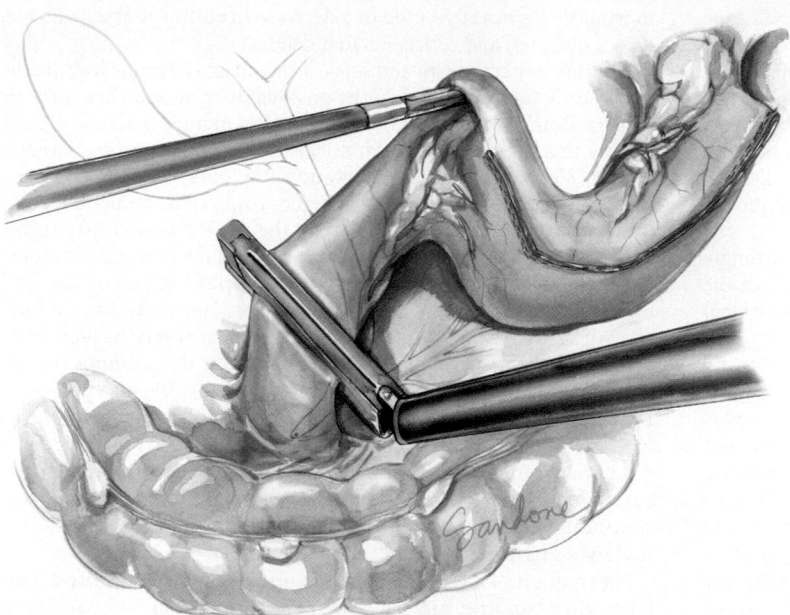

FIGURE 15 The duodenum is divided with a linear stapler. *(Illustration used with permission from Cameron JL, Sandone C: Atlas of Gastrointestinal Surgery, ed 2, vol II, Shelton, CT, 2014, PMPH-USA.)*

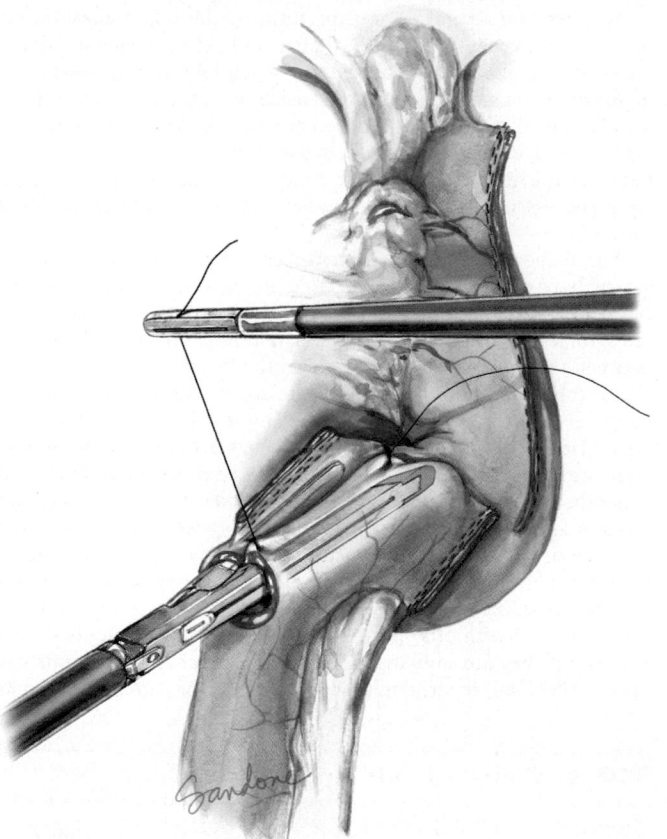

FIGURE 16 The duodenoileostomy is created with a linear stapler. *(Illustration used with permission from Cameron JL, Sandone C: Atlas of Gastrointestinal Surgery, ed 2, vol II, Shelton, CT, 2014, PMPH-USA.)*

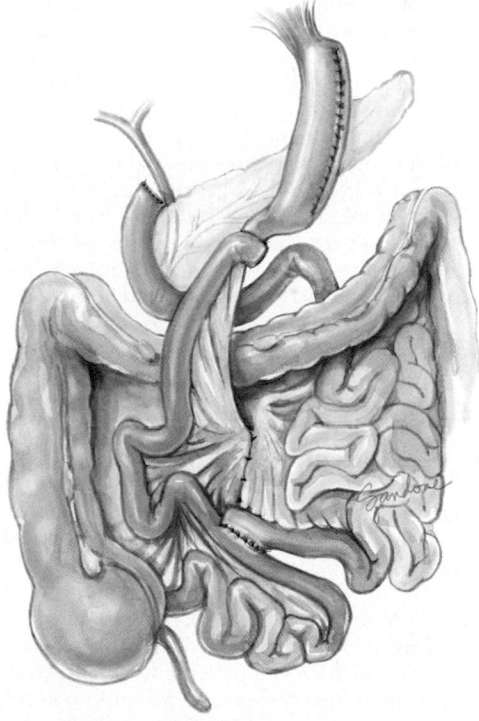

FIGURE 17 Antecolic duodenal switch with biliopancreatic diversion. *(Illustration used with permission from Cameron JL, Sandone C: Atlas of Gastrointestinal Surgery, ed 2, vol II, Shelton, CT, 2014, PMPH-USA.)*

are prescribed continuous positive airway pressure (CPAP) during sleep, if they are able to tolerate it or use it routinely at home. Low-molecular-weight heparin is continued during hospitalization for most patients, and some patients who are at higher risk for venous thromboembolism (VTE) may be treated at home for an entire month after surgery. The patient is usually in a chair or ambulating within the first 12 hours. Pain is managed with a patient-controlled analgesia delivery device for the first evening, and the patient is encouraged to use the incentive spirometer while awake.

Patients for adjustable gastric band are given a liquid diet the following morning and then discharged to home. Patients for gastric bypass and duodenal switch are started on a limited liquid diet on postoperative day 1, and then the quantity of liquids is advanced as tolerated on day 2 with discharge planned that day. Patients for sleeve gastrectomy are given a nonsugar liquid diet on postoperative day 1 and usually advanced over the course of the day, with an aim to discharge that day or the following morning. Patients after all four operations remain on a nonsugar noncarbonated liquid diet that includes protein drinks for the first week after surgery. They are then advanced to a puree diet that still includes protein drinks for the following 3 weeks, at which time they start to introduce solid foods. Selective upper gastrointestinal series radiography is used in patients who have a sustained heart rate over 120 bpm, respiratory distress, fever, increasing abdominal pain, or chest pain. The drain is removed before discharge.

Follow-up is in 2 weeks for all patients. Patients are strongly encouraged to go to monthly support group meetings and see the dietician on a routine basis, along with a mental health professional if needed or requested.

Patients for adjustable gastric band are evaluated for their first fill at the 6-week postoperative appointment. Patients who, despite making healthy food choices, have stopped losing weight, who report no "restriction" with solid foods, and who are consistently hungry between meals get a fill. Patients are then asked to follow up in 2 months. Band position and tightness can be assessed with fluoroscopy if necessary in patients who, despite repeated fills, continue to have no restriction. Patients who report continued vomiting, abdominal pain, or severe gastroesophageal reflux disease (GERD)–like symptoms should also be evaluated with an upper gastrointestinal fluoroscopic study.

All patients are placed on a multivitamin and calcium after surgery. Menstruating women are placed on iron to prevent anemia. Patients for gastric bypass are recommended to take vitamin B_{12}, and patients for duodenal switch with biliopancreatic diversion are advised to take supplements that include the fat-soluble vitamins A, D, E, and K. Patients who have not had their gallbladder previously removed are placed on ursodiol 300 mg twice a day for 6 months to reduce the risk of symptomatic cholelithiasis during the rapid weight loss phase after gastric bypass, sleeve gastrectomy, or DS-BPD surgery. Follow-up is usually around 3, 6, 12, 18, and 24 months, followed by every year thereafter. An iron panel and hematologic, electrolyte, and liver function laboratory tests are obtained at 3 months, and vitamin B_{12}, 25-hydroxy vitamin D, and parathyroid hormone levels are assessed at 1-year visits. Patients who are not taking in enough protein by diet history may need prealbumin checked along with nutritional counseling. Patients for DS-BPD may also need the additional vitamins A, E, and K tested for after surgery.

■ OUTCOMES AND COMPLICATIONS

Buchwald and colleagues conducted a meta-analysis of the bariatric literature in 2003. They found that mean excess weight losses for adjustable gastric band, Roux-en-Y gastric bypass, and biliopancreatic diversion with or without duodenal switch were 48%, 62%, and 70%, respectively. Mortality rates were 0.1%, 0.5%, and 1.1%, respectively, for the three operations. Type 2 diabetes was found overall to be completely resolved in 77% of patients and improved in an additional 9% of patients. Hyperlipidemia, hypertension, and obstructive sleep apnea were improved in 70%, 79%, and 84%, respectively. Schauer and colleagues showed in a randomized prospective trial that obese patients with uncontrolled type 2 diabetes had significant improvement in glycemic control after both Roux-en-Y gastric bypass and sleeve gastrectomy compared with medical therapy alone. The mean glycated hemoglobin was 9.2% before the study; after 12 months, the mean decreased to 7.5% in the medical therapy alone group, 6.4% in the gastric bypass group ($P < 0.001$), and 6.6% in the sleeve gastrectomy group ($P = 0.003$). Patient weight loss was only −5.4 kg in the medical therapy group as compared with the gastric bypass and sleeve gastrectomy groups (−29.4 kg and −25.1 kg, respectively; $P < 0.001$) at 12 months' follow-up. In a large retrospective cohort study comparing bariatric surgery patients matched with morbidly obese patients who did not undergo surgery, Adams and colleagues found a 40% reduction in mortality rate after 7.1 years with the surgery group. The significant decrease in the long-term

mortality rate was attributed to a decrease in coronary artery disease, type 2 diabetes, and cancer-related deaths.

Pulmonary embolism and sepsis from an anastomotic leak are the two leading causes of death in the postoperative period after bariatric surgery. Both complications are less than 1% at most bariatric surgery centers that are part of the American College of Surgeons Bariatric Surgery Center Network Accreditation Program. Perioperative measures to reduce the risk include chemoprophylaxis, sequential compression devices (if they can safely fit the patient's lower extremity), and early ambulation. Some centers go beyond the routine in-hospital prophylaxis by placing patients who may be at higher risk for VTE on low-molecular-weight heparin anywhere from 10 days to a month after discharge from the hospital. These patients may include those who have a history of pulmonary embolism or deep venous thrombosis, poor ambulation, severe venous stasis disease, and possibly a BMI of more than 70 kg/m². Inferior vena cava filters are also used in some select patients who may be at higher risk for death from pulmonary embolism. It is unclear to date whether these extra measures used to prevent VTE are helpful, because no randomized trials specifically address the morbidly obese patient population that undergoes bariatric surgery.

Prevention of a leak is one of the primary ways to decrease mortality after bariatric surgery. The most common area for a leak to occur after gastric bypass is at the gastrojejunostomy. However, a leak may also occur at the distal stomach staple line or the jejunojejunostomy. There are several ways of performing the upper anastomosis of a gastric bypass or DS-BPD that include circular stapler, linear stapler, handsewn, and a combination of stapling with an outer layer of suturing. This may account for variation in the reported rates of a leak, stomal stenosis, and marginal ulcer. At Johns Hopkins, the laparoscopic Roux-en-Y gastric bypass leak rate is less than 0.3% with the previously described technique that has an inner stapled layer and essentially an outer layer consisting of multiple running sutures.

Box 6 shows the published complication rate after laparoscopic gastric bypass. The authors have used an antecolic antegastric technique for more than 7 years, which has reduced the internal hernia rates to less than 2%. The authors continue to close the defect between the transverse mesocolon and the Roux limb mesentery up to the transverse colon along with the enteroenterostomy defect in both the gastric bypass and the DS-BPD operations. Stomal stenosis after gastric bypass most commonly occurs between 2 and 6 weeks after surgery but occasionally may be seen later in conjunction with a marginal ulcer. More than 90% of these patients respond to balloon dilation; however, late-occurring strictures are less likely to heal and may require revision of the gastrojejunostomy with or without a truncal vagotomy. A marginal ulcer after gastric bypass can occur on the jejunal side of the gastrojejunal anastomosis, and again, more than 90% heal with proton pump inhibitor therapy. Patients should be asked if they are smoking, using nonsteroidal anti-inflammatory drugs (NSAIDs), or drinking large quantities of caffeinated drinks

---

BOX 6: Complications for 251 Cases

Stomal stenosis: 10 (4%)
Marginal ulcer: 11 (4%)
Symptomatic gallstones: 8 (3%)
Internal hernia: 4 (2%)
Postoperative bleeding: 5 (2%)
Stroke (minor): 1 (0.4%)
Trocar hernia: 0 (0%)
Deep venous thrombosis: 0 (0%)
Pulmonary emboli: 0 (0%)
Wound infection: 0 (0%)
Leaks: 0 (0%)
Death: 1 (0.4%)

(coffee, tea, etc.) because these have all been attributed with marginal ulceration. The most common location of a stricture seen after sleeve gastrectomy is at the incisura angularis. These strictures may respond to balloon dilation, otherwise a revision to a gastrojejunostomy proximal to the stricture may be needed.

The laparoscopic adjustable gastric band (LAGB) operation has a lower 30-day major complication rate when compared with gastric bypass, sleeve gastrectomy, and DS-BPD. However, long-term complications after LAGB appear to be higher, with rates above 20%. Cottam and colleagues, in a case-controlled matched pair cohort study, showed excess weight loss is greater after gastric bypass when compared with LAGB (74% vs 51%, respectively; $P < 0.001$) at 3 years. Type 2 diabetes resolved more frequently after gastric bypass (78% vs 50%, respectively; $P = 0.01$). The most common complications after LAGB are port or tubing breakage, flipped port, gastric prolapse or band slippage, and GERD. Gastric prolapse or band slippage entails cephalad herniation of the stomach through the band, resulting in a larger pouch and, in some cases, near or total gastric outlet obstruction. Erosion of the band into the stomach lumen is a complication reported in approximately 1% of cases and requires removal of the band. Infection of the band system is also seen in approximately 1% of cases and again requires removal. GERD symptoms that develop when inflating the band with saline solution to increase restriction may require removal of some or all of the fluid. Patients who have an obvious hiatal hernia at the time of surgery may benefit from a crural repair at the time of gastric band placement.

■ ENDOSCOPIC APPROACHES TO THE MANAGEMENT OF OBESITY

Transoral endoluminal interventions performed entirely through the gastrointestinal tract with flexible endoscopy offer the potential for an ambulatory weight loss procedure without any incisions on the abdominal wall. The restrictive procedures include intragastric balloon treatment, endoluminal sutured gastroplasty, and transoral stapled gastroplasty. The malabsorptive procedures include duodenojejunal bypass sleeve and gastroduodenojejunal bypass sleeve. Other procedures that have been performed with varying degrees of short-term success include intragastric injection of botulinum toxin type A and gastric electrical stimulation.

The most widely studied of these therapies is the intragastric balloon. Although this device is currently not FDA approved for use in the United States, it has been used in Europe, Canada, Mexico, India, and South America with adequate short-term results. The most common complication is nausea and vomiting, but more serious complications, such as gastric erosions, ulcerations, and bowel obstructions, have been noted. There are ongoing trials looking at the use of flexible endoscopically guided staplers or suture devices to create a gastric sleeve along the lesser curvature of the stomach. Flexible endoscopic suturing devices have also been used to reduce the size of the stoma and gastric pouch in patients who have had weight regain after gastric bypass. Unfortunately, long-term weight loss has not been proven with these devices.

Malabsorptive procedures, such as the duodenojejunal bypass sleeve, use a prosthetic barrier device that intraluminally bypasses the necessary areas of absorption in the duodenum and the upper part of the jejunum. A gastroduodenojejunal bypass sleeve has also shown promise in very short-term results with regards to weight loss and glycemic control. Long-term results and safety profile studies are needed with these devices.

Endoscopic therapy for weight loss is in its infancy; newer therapies are constantly being introduced and tested. If appropriate efficacy and safety profiles can be established, these products may be introduced into the clinical mainstream practice.

■ COMMENTS

Bariatric surgery continues to be the only effective means of producing weight loss in most patients. It has been shown to reduce or even eliminate comorbidities associated with a high BMI. Mortality and leak rates less than 1% have been published by several leading surgical centers committed to bariatric surgery. Laparoscopic techniques have been shown in randomized prospective studies over open approaches to significantly reduce perioperative wound complications and incisional hernias. Appropriate attention to the risks and benefits of the procedure along with the individual patient's medical risks requires consultation and joint decision making between the physician and the patient. Center of excellence certification programs are collecting outcome data that not only will help to document in the future the beneficial long-term effects of bariatric surgery but also will define acceptable outcomes and complication rates.

SUGGESTED READINGS

Adams TD, Gress RE, Smith SC, et al. Long-term mortality after gastric bypass surgery. *N Engl J Med.* 2007;357:753-761.

Buchwald H, Avidor Y, Braunwald E, et al. Bariatric surgery: a systemic review and meta-analysis. *JAMA.* 2004;292:1724-1728.

Cottam DR, Atkinson J, Anderson A, et al. A case-controlled matched pair cohort study of laparoscopic Roux-en-Y gastric bypass and Lap-Band patients in a single US center with three-year follow-up. *Obes Surg.* 2006;16:534-540.

Schauer PR, Kashyap SR, Wolski K, et al. Bariatric surgery versus intensive medical therapy in obese patients with diabetes. *N Engl J Med.* 2012;366: 1567-1576.

Schweitzer MA, Lidor A, Magnuson TH. 251 consecutive laparoscopic gastric bypass operations using a 2 layer gastrojejunostomy technique with a zero leak rate. *J Laparoendosc Adv Surg Tech A.* 2006;16:83-87.

Steele KE, Prokopowicz GP, Magnuson T, et al. Laparoscopic antecolic Roux-en-Y gastric bypass with closure of internal defects leads to fewer internal hernias than the retrocolic approach. *Surg Endosc.* 2008;22:2056-2061.

Wittgrove AC, Clark WG. Laparoscopic gastric bypass Roux-en-Y: 500 patients: technique and results, with 3–60 month follow-up. *Obes Surg.* 2000;10:233-238.

LAPAROSCOPIC DONOR NEPHRECTOMY

Bonnie E. Lonze, MD, PhD, and Nabil N. Dagher, MD

Kidney transplantation is well established as the optimal therapy in the treatment of end-stage renal disease, but the ability to offer this therapy to the tens of thousands of patients in need is constrained by a limited supply of donor kidneys. Living donation evolved as a means to increase rates of transplantation but was hindered initially by the morbidity associated with open donor nephrectomy. The landscape of living kidney donation changed drastically in 1995 with the introduction of laparoscopic living donor nephrectomy (Ratner et al., 1995). Laparoscopy afforded donors shorter hospitalizations, substantially improved postoperative pain, improved cosmesis, and overall faster recovery with quicker return to work and daily activities. These major benefits, combined with equivalent recipient outcomes, contributed greatly to a doubling of the rate of living kidney donation in the United States within 5 years. Currently more than 6000 living donor nephrectomies are performed each year.

■ CANDIDATE SELECTION AND PREOPERATIVE EVALUATION

The evaluation for living donation can be initiated only when a candidate comes forward and volunteers to donate. An initial series of screening questions can be answered by phone or questionnaire to determine whether any absolute contraindications to donation exist (Box 1). The workup for potential donors is thorough and is performed by a donor evaluation team composed of a surgeon, nephrologist, psychologist or psychiatrist, social worker, and nurse coordinator (Davis & Delmonico, 2005). Not only must the physical health of the candidate be evaluated objectively, but the potential psychosocial and financial impact of donation also must be considered carefully and discussed frankly with the candidate before donation. It is important to note that every living donor program must have a living donor advocate. The role of this individual is to protect and promote the best interests of the potential living donor throughout the evaluation process and to ensure that the donor's decision to donate is informed and free of coercion.

A thorough medical history is taken, including a family history, with attention paid to risk factors for kidney disease. A careful surgical history is taken, and candidates who have had prior abdominal surgery must be counseled that this history may increase the difficulty of laparoscopy and increase the likelihood of conversion to an open nephrectomy. Laboratory testing includes tissue typing, blood chemistries, complete blood cell counts, coagulation studies, serologic testing for exposure to infectious diseases, urinalysis, and urine cultures. An accurate calculation of creatinine clearance and urine protein is also essential. Age-appropriate cancer screening guidelines are followed for donors as pertains to mammography, Pap smear, prostate serum antigen screening, and colonoscopy. Cardiopulmonary testing is determined on a case-by-case basis depending on the donor age, history, and risk factors.

Radiographic imaging is essential for delineating renal and vascular anatomy as well as to assess for any intra-abdominal pathology. It is our center's preference to perform computed tomographic angiography (CTA) with three-dimensional (3D) reconstruction for all donor candidates. The majority of living kidneys donated are left kidneys. Right-sided donor nephrectomy can be technically more challenging, typically requires the placement of an additional port,

and often results in shorter renal vessels; therefore left-sided nephrectomy is preferred if the two kidneys are equivalent. Occasionally, anatomic differences between two kidneys make the right kidney more appropriate for donation. These differences would include multiple arteries supplying the left kidney (three or more arteries), stones or lesions in the right kidney, or a significantly smaller size of the right kidney compared with the left.

■ OPERATIVE APPROACH

Laparoscopic donor nephrectomy is performed under general anesthesia. A nasogastric tube and urinary catheter are placed in all cases. The donor kidney ultimately is extracted through a small transverse incision in the lower pelvis, and this skin site must be marked with the patient in a supine position in order to avoid distortion incurred by lateral positioning. Thus before positioning, a 6-mm transverse incision is marked, centered 1 to 2 cm above the pubic tubercle. The patient is placed in a modified lateral decubitus position. For the sake of simplicity, we describe here the positioning and technique for a left-sided nephrectomy. Specific differences unique to right-sided nephrectomy are discussed later in this chapter.

Great care must be taken while positioning to ensure that no extremity injuries related to traction or improper padding occur and to ensure that the operating surgeon has unimpeded access to all ports. First, the supine patient is rolled gently into a right arm down position using a gel pad or shoulder roll placed longitudinally behind the left shoulder. The right arm is tucked and the left arm is extended, with the elbow flexed, across the upper chest and rested on an arm board. The arm board must be placed caudad enough to avoid traction injury to the left shoulder but cephalad enough to permit easy access to a subxiphoid dissection port. The bed then is placed in the extended position to expand the space between the anterior superior iliac spine and the costal margin, thus allowing for broader exposure. The patient must be fastened securely to the operating table, with the head and extremities well padded.

Standard skin preparation with chlorhexidine is performed, and an appropriate antibiotic for coverage of skin flora (cefazolin or substitute) is administered. A 12-mm periumbilical skin incision is made, and a Veress needle is used to access the peritoneal cavity for insufflation. The peritoneal cavity is insufflated to a pressure of 15 mm Hg. A second 12-mm skin incision is made in a transverse fashion 1 handbreadth to the left of the umbilicus. The left costal margin and the left anterior superior iliac spine are palpated, and this incision is placed midway between them, which typically is at the level of the umbilicus. A 12-mm optical trocar fitted with a 0-degree laparoscope is inserted into the insufflated peritoneum at this site. Once this left-sided port has been placed, the laparoscope is exchanged for a 45-degree angled laparoscope, which will be used for the remainder of the operation. The Veress needle at the umbilicus is removed under direct visualization and replaced with a 12-mm port. A 5-mm skin incision is made in the subxiphoid region, and a 5-mm port is introduced at this site. The trajectory for insertion of this port should be inferolateral, directed toward the left kidney.

The previously marked lower pelvic skin incision then is made, and dissection is carried down to the fascia. The eventual fascial incision for extraction of the donor kidney will be made in the midline; therefore subcutaneous flaps must be raised above and below the level of the skin incision in order to expose adequate fascial surface for vertical incision later in the operation. At this point in the case, however, the only fascial incision made here is via a 12-mm trocar, inserted under direct visualization with care taken to avoid injury to the bladder. Four ports now have been established. The umbilical site serves as the camera port for the majority of the operation. The left-sided 12-mm port and the subxiphoid 5-mm port are the two primary working ports for dissection. Through the lower pelvic port site, a laparoscopic retracting paddle is placed for medial retraction of the bowel. The operating table then is tilted fully, right side down.

BOX 1: Contraindications to Living Kidney Donation

Absolute Contraindications

Significant cardiac or vascular disease
Diabetes mellitus
Chronic kidney disease
Age <18 years
Active infection, including hepatitis B, hepatitis C, or human immunodeficiency virus
Active malignancy
Pregnancy
Significant hypercoagulable disorder
Prohibitive anatomic abnormalities
Evidence of coercion

Relative Contraindications

Hypertension
Insulin resistance or prediabetes
Decreased creatinine clearance
Morbid obesity
Intent to become pregnant within 6 months of donation
Active substance abuse
Untreated psychiatric disorder

The operation commences with mobilization of the left colon. Its attachments to the lateral abdominal wall, which can be significant or completely absent, are incised using a combination of cautery and sharp dissection with scissors. For the most part, these attachments are avascular, so sharp dissection is safe and preferred in order to minimize the risk of thermal injury to the colon. The spleen should be visualized clearly in the left upper quadrant and only rarely requires mobilization. The colon is retracted gently medially, which exposes its posterolateral peritoneal attachments. The peritoneum is incised longitudinally and parallel to the left colon, from the superior pole of the kidney toward the pelvis (Figure 1). This maneuver enables identification of the plane between the mesocolonic fat and the perinephric fat. Identification of this avascular plane is essential and ensures that the mesentery is not injured. Rents in the mesocolon can cause injury to mesenteric vessels, which can result in bleeding that is difficult to control. Any mesenteric defects must be identified and closed to eliminate the risk of internal small bowel herniation. When the proper plane is identified, the mesentery is dissected gently off of the retroperitoneal surface in a nontraumatic fashion. As mobilization of the colon and mesocolon nears completion, the gonadal vein and ureter become visible in the retroperitoneum as they course atop the psoas muscle. The ureter and its vascular pedicle are elevated bluntly off of the psoas muscle (Figure 2). With upward retraction from underneath the ureteral pedicle, this dissection is continued proximally toward the hilum of the kidney. Care must be taken to avoid skeletonizing the ureter and to identify and ligate venous branches that arise from the gonadal vein throughout its course.

The insertion of the gonadal vein into the left renal vein is identifiable as the renal hilum is approached. Lumbar branches, arising from either the proximal gonadal vein or the renal vein proper, must be identified. These can be ligated with clips, endovascular staplers, or thermal sealing devices as deemed appropriate based on their caliber. The gonadal artery, branching off the aorta, frequently will be encountered along the course of this dissection and can be ligated with clips and divided.

With the renal vein delineated, its anterior surface is carefully cleared of perivascular lymphatic tissue. This allows for identification of the adrenal vein (Figure 3), which is dissected circumferentially using a right angle. The adrenal vein is doubly clipped and divided with scissors. The adrenal gland must be dissected off of the upper pole of the kidney and mobilized medially. A plane is established between the adrenal gland and the kidney, and this is best accomplished by placing gentle lateral retraction on the kidney (Figure 4). Using a thermal dissector (LigaSure or harmonic scalpel) the tissues connecting the adrenal gland to the kidney are divided while staying as close to the adrenal gland as possible to avoid encountering upper pole renal artery branches. Care must be taken not to violate the adrenal gland, as bleeding from the gland can be cumbersome.

With the adrenal gland now fully freed from the kidney, dissection of the upper pole can be completed. Again, lateral retraction of the kidney toward the abdominal wall aids greatly in this effort. The dissection is continued cranially toward the spleen, dividing the splenorenal attachments, to complete mobilization of the upper pole.

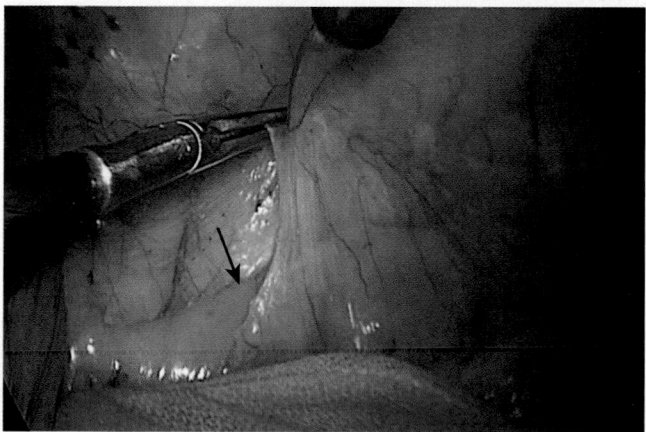

FIGURE 1 The peritoneum is incised lateral to the left colon. The arrow indicates the interface between mesenteric and retroperitoneal fat.

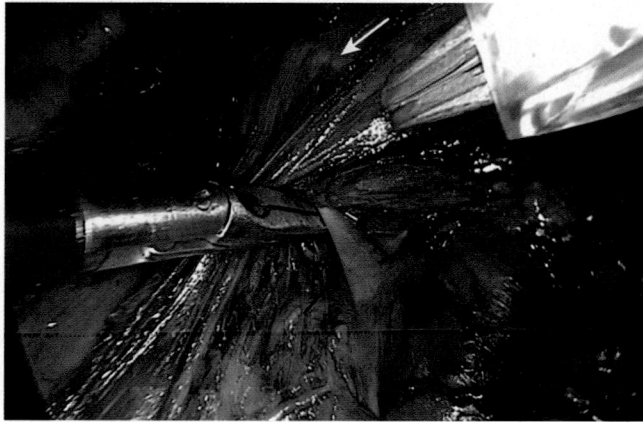

FIGURE 3 The adrenal vein (*black arrow*) is identified, clipped, and sharply divided. The yellow arrow indicates the edge of the adrenal gland.

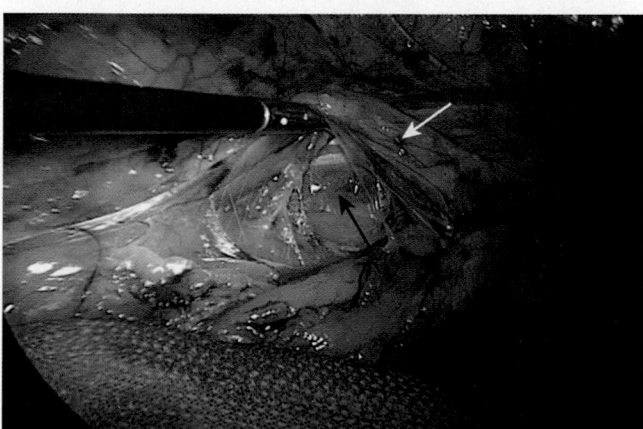

FIGURE 2 The ureteral pedicle (*yellow arrow*) is elevated off of the psoas muscle (*black arrow*).

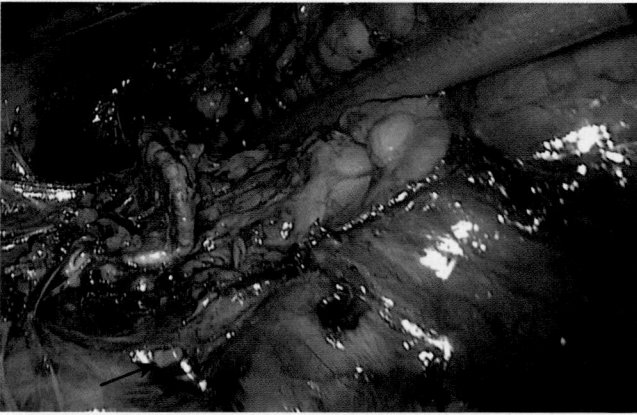

FIGURE 4 The kidney is retracted laterally, and the adrenal gland is dissected off of the upper pole. The arrow indicates the divided adrenal vein off of the renal vein.

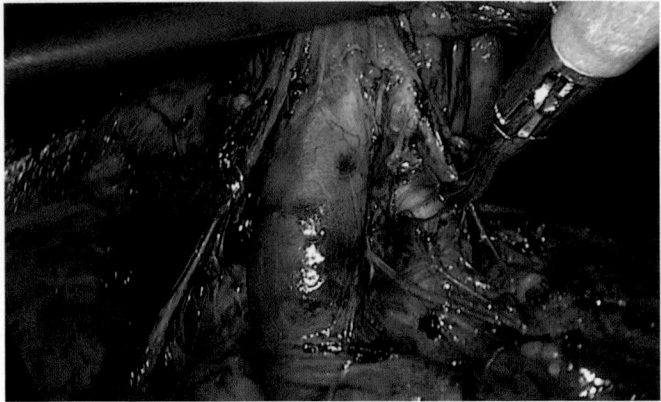

FIGURE 5 The renal artery is dissected free of investing fat and lymphatic tissues.

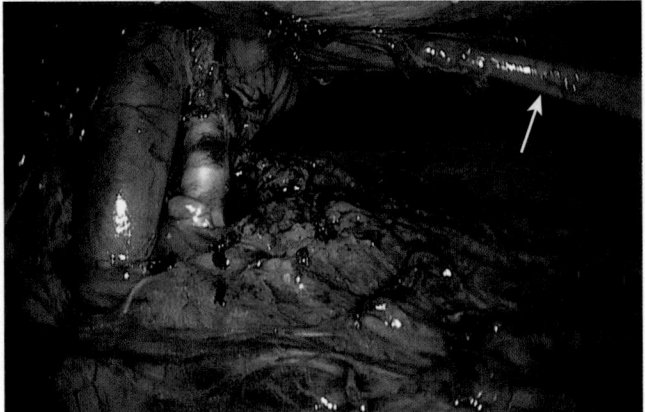

FIGURE 6 The hilar structures have been dissected, and the ureter is ready for division distally. The arrow indicates the ureteral pedicle.

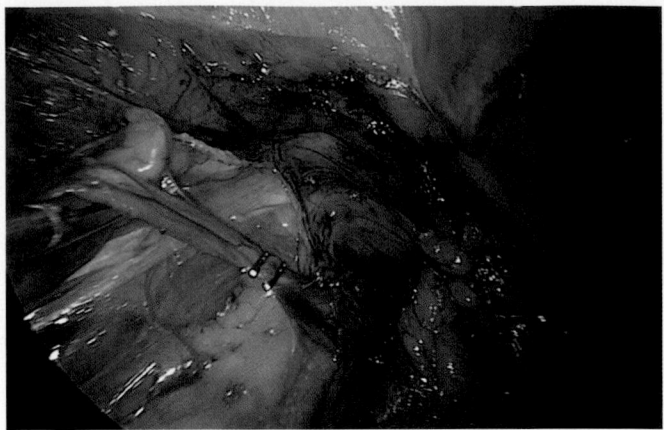

FIGURE 7 The ureter is clipped distally.

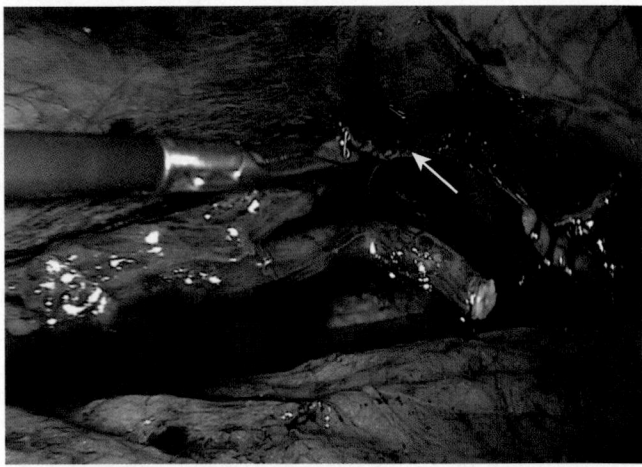

FIGURE 8 The ureter is divided sharply. The arrow indicates the proximal staple line of the divided gonadal vein.

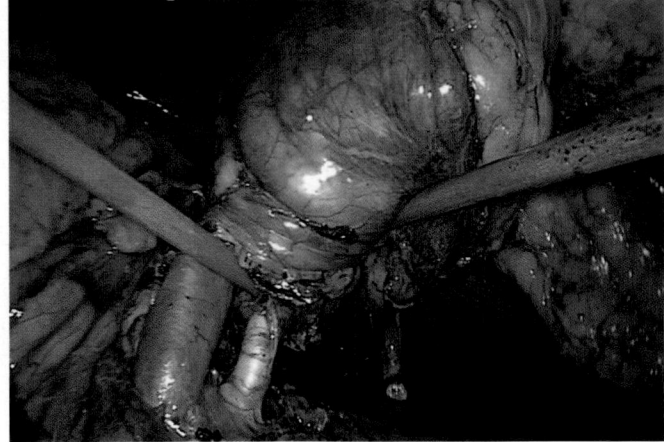

FIGURE 9 The dissection is complete, and the kidney is elevated at the hilum so that the renal vessels can be stapled and the kidney removed from the peritoneal cavity.

The hilar dissection is continued by elevating the kidney at the lower pole, which places the hilar structures under gentle traction. Great care should be taken to ensure that this is in fact gentle, as overexuberant retraction can cause vasospasm or arterial dissection that can compromise the entire allograft. The renal artery and vein are invested in perivascular lymphatics and fat, which must be dissected off of the vessels to permit safe stapling (Figure 5). Once the renal artery and vein are circumferentially free, the ureter is ready for division (Figure 6).

At this point in the operation it is important to communicate with the recipient surgical team to ensure that it is appropriate to divide the ureter. Division of the ureter is considered the point of no return in the donor operation and therefore should not be performed until it is certain that the recipient team is ready. We administer mannitol (12.5 mg) and furosemide (40 mg) before dividing the ureter to promote diuresis. It is important to ensure that adequate length on the ureter has been achieved, and occasionally additional distal mobilization of the ureteral pedicle is required. Once the site for division of the ureter is chosen, the ureter is dissected bluntly free of the gonadal pedicle. The position of the iliac vessels should be confirmed in order to avoid any iatrogenic injury. The gonadal pedicle is ligated with a stapler. The ureter is ligated with clips distally and cut with scissors proximally (Figures 7 and 8). Urine output from the transected ureter is typically brisk. The ureteral pedicle remains attached to the retroperitoneum laterally, and these attachments are taken down with a thermal ligating device, keeping safe distance from the ureter but also taking care not to encroach on the abdominal wall. This dissection is carried in a cephalad direction along the lateral aspect of the kidney toward the previous upper pole dissection plane.

Once these planes meet, the kidney has been mobilized fully and remains attached only by the renal vessels (Figure 9).

The laparoscopic retracting paddle is removed from the pelvic port and replaced with an Endo Catch device. Before deploying the bag, the Endo Catch device is used to maintain medial retraction of the colon during stapling of the vessels. The camera is moved from the umbilical port to the left-sided 12-mm port because the umbilical port affords a more favorable approach to the vessels with the stapler. Intravenous heparin is given (3000 units). The kidney is gently retracted upward at the level of the hilum, and the renal artery is ligated with an endovascular stapler. We prefer a TA stapler for two reasons. First, it allows for thorough evaluation of the arterial staple line before full transection of the vessel. Second, it does not shorten the donor renal artery by the width of an additional row of staples on the kidney side. In the setting of an early arterial bifurcation, this extra length can be crucial. We also prefer to reinforce the arterial staple line with two rows of clips. Once stapled and clipped securely, the renal artery is divided with scissors. Next, the renal vein is ligated and divided with an endovascular GIA stapler. The Endo Catch bag is deployed, and the kidney is grasped carefully and placed completely in the bag.

The kidney is ischemic at this point, and it is important to move quickly and methodically. The laparoscope is removed from the peritoneal cavity. Protamine (30 mg) is given for reversal of heparinization at this time. Through the lower pelvic incision, a vertical fascial incision is made in the midline, just large enough to permit extraction of the kidney in the Endo Catch bag. The kidney is brought immediately to the back table, where it is flushed by the recipient surgeon and prepared for implantation.

The fascial incision at the extraction site is closed by placement of simple interrupted sutures. All but the center two sutures are tied at this point. This permits replacement of a port for reinsufflation of the abdomen. The laparoscope is reintroduced into the abdomen. The colon is retracted medially using the laparoscopic retractor, and the vascular stumps are inspected for hemostasis. The ureteral pedicle stump also should be inspected for hemostasis. If there had been concern for mesenteric injury, this also must be evaluated to ensure that any mesenteric defect is closed. Once hemostasis has been ensured, the laparoscope is removed from the abdomen and insufflation is released. Fascial closure of the 12-mm port sites is important to minimize risk for trocar site incisional hernias. The skin incisions are closed with absorbable suture in a subcuticular fashion.

■ ADDITIONAL OPERATIVE CONSIDERATIONS

Right-Sided Nephrectomy

The ability to perform right-sided nephrectomy is an asset because occasionally, for reasons previously discussed, the right donor kidney is more favorable. Right-sided nephrectomy differs from left-sided nephrectomy in several key ways.

Positioning and initial port placement is essentially a mirror image to that of a left-sided nephrectomy, with two exceptions. First, it is helpful to use a 12-mm subxiphoid port rather than a 5-mm port to permit application of a clip applier or stapler from this position. Second, a fifth port usually is required for placement of a liver retractor. This is a 5-mm port placed in the subxiphoid position, cranial and to the left of the 12-mm port. A liver retractor, often simply a locking grasper, is used to retract the gallbladder and right lobe cranially for better visualization.

After mobilization of the right colon, dissection is similar to the left-sided dissection, but the vena cava is seen clearly on the right side. Care must be taken not to injure the vena cava and the second portion of the duodenum during dissection. Most surgeons preserve the right gonadal vein with the donor along its course as it drains into the vena cava and dissect it free of the ureteral pedicle. It is noteworthy that although the main renal artery usually courses posterior to the vena cava and renal vein, accessory arteries often course anteriorly. Gaining sufficient length on the retrocaval right renal artery is essential to avoid transection distal to a prehilar bifurcation leading to multiple vessels perfusing the donor graft. Significant lumbar venous branches are often absent on the right side, but the frequency of multiple renal veins is higher. The renal vein is almost always shorter on the right side. There is no adrenal vein to deal with,

as the right adrenal vein drains directly into the vena cava. In fact, the adrenal gland itself is often cranial and more easily dissected free of the upper pole. Extraction of the graft and closure are identical to left-sided nephrectomy.

Hand-Assisted Laparoscopic Nephrectomy

Rather than a fully laparoscopic approach, many have adopted a technique of hand-assisted laparoscopy. A hand port usually is placed in a periumbilical or paramedian position, and the kidney also is extracted through this incision at the completion of the operation. The benefit of tactile sensation, the ability to perform blunt finger dissection, and the ability to achieve more directed retraction are some advantages to this technique over a purely laparoscopic operation. From a cosmetic perspective, however, the hand port incision is made in a more conspicuous location compared with a low transverse pelvic incision.

Single-Incision Laparoscopic Nephrectomy

An emerging technique in minimally invasive surgery is the use of laparoendoscopic single-site (LESS) surgery, and this is now being utilized by some groups for the performance of donor nephrectomy. This technique involves the placement of a single multiadapted port, typically at the umbilicus, which is used for the introduction of all instruments and retractors and for extraction of the kidney.

■ POSTOPERATIVE MANAGEMENT AND COMPLICATIONS

The average length of stay for living kidney donors is 2 days. Donors have a Foley catheter placed before surgery, and this is removed on postoperative day 1. Blood chemistries and complete blood cell counts are checked on postoperative day 1 but not checked routinely on the following day. An increase in creatinine immediately after donation is to be expected, but within days the single-kidney glomerular filtration rate (GFR) begins to increase such that the long-term postdonation GFR returns to 70% to 80% of the predonation value. It is our practice to measure serum creatinine 1 week postdonation; 3, 6, and 12 months postdonation; and then annually for a minimum of 2 years.

Before proceeding with donation, all donors are counseled on the risks of laparoscopic nephrectomy, including the risk for mortality, the risk for subsequent renal failure, and the risks for perioperative complications. In a study of national data, which included more than 80,000 donors, the 90-day perioperative mortality rate was found to be 3.1 in 10,000 patients (Segev et al., 2010). The lifetime incidence of end-stage renal disease after donation was 90 in 10,000 patients. This risk is lower than the risk of end-stage renal disease in the general population (326 in 10,000) but is higher than that in equally healthy persons who did not donate a kidney (14 in 10,000; Muzaale et al., 2014).

Serious yet rare complications include conversion from a laparoscopic to an open operation, bleeding requiring transfusion or reoperation, injury to a solid or hollow viscus, chyle leak, pancreatitis, extremity neuropathy from improper positioning, intestinal obstruction from internal hernia, venous thromboembolism, and cardiac events. Minor complications occur more frequently but rarely prolong the hospital stay or affect overall recovery and include ileus, atelectasis, urinary retention, urinary tract infections, wound infections, and persistent abdominal pain. The overall rate of a procedure-related complication after donor nephrectomy is estimated at less than 8% (Schold et al., 2013).

■ CONCLUSIONS

Laparoscopic donor nephrectomy has increased rates of living kidney donation drastically. For appropriately selected candidates, it is a safe and well-tolerated procedure. Thousands of lives are saved each year by those who are willing to give this gift.

SUGGESTED READINGS

Davis CL, Delmonico FL. Living donor kidney transplantation: a review of the current practices for the live donor. *J Am Soc Nephrol.* 2005;16: 82098-82110.

Muzaale AD, Massie AB, Wang M-C, et al. Risk of end-stage renal disease following live kidney donation. *JAMA.* 2014;311:579-586.

Ratner LE, Cisek LJ, Moore RG, et al. Laparoscopic live donor nephrectomy. *Transplantation.* 1995;60:1047-1049.

Schold JD, Goldfarb DA, Buccini LD, et al. Comorbidity burden and perioperative complications for living kidney donors in the United States. *Clin J Am Soc Nephrol.* 2013;8:1773-1782.

Segev DL, Muzaale AD, Caffo BS, et al. Perioperative mortality and long-term survival following live kidney donation. *JAMA.* 2010;303:959-966.

LAPAROENDOSCOPIC SINGLE-SITE SURGERY AS AN EVOLVING SURGICAL APPROACH

Elan R. Witkowski, MD, MS, and David Rattner, MD

Over the last several decades, minimally invasive techniques have been developed and widely applied in surgical practice. For many operations, these produce excellent outcomes with advantages over open surgery: reduced postoperative length of stay and pain, faster recovery and earlier return to work, and improved cosmesis.

Today there are ongoing efforts to improve established minimally invasive techniques. As multiport laparoscopic and robotic surgery have become widespread, attention has been focused on making these approaches even less invasive. The goals are similar: reduce pain, improve cosmesis, and hasten recovery.

Whether single-incision surgery represents a substantial improvement over multiport techniques remains unclear. Although cosmesis may be superior with single-site surgery, the added cost and level of technical difficulty may not be worthwhile because no study to date has shown reduction in hospital length of stay, recovery time, or cost.

▪ HISTORY AND NOMENCLATURE

Moving from open surgery to multiport laparoscopy, operations were reimagined and modified in concert with technological advancements. The same process must occur in current areas of interest. These include several prominent examples.

- Single-site surgery
- Natural orifice transluminal endoscopic surgery (NOTES)
- Novel endoscopic interventions and endoluminal surgery

NOTES involves operating within a body cavity (i.e., the peritoneal cavity, mediastinum, or pleural space) after passing an operating scope and instruments through a natural orifice (e.g., mouth, anus, vagina) and through a visceral wall. Other endoluminal techniques involve performing interventions that previously could be accomplished only surgically. Prominent examples include peroral endoscopic myotomy (POEM), endoscopic submucosal dissection (ESD), endoscopic mucosal resection (EMR), transanal endoscopic microsurgery (TEM), and transanal total mesorectal excision (TaTME). The evolution of these procedures has been made possible by new techniques and specially designed tools for a flexible endoscopic platform, such as endoscopic suture devices (OverStitch; Apollo Endosurgery, Austin, TX) and multiple commercially available clips, energy devices, and dissectors.

Laparoendoscopic single-site (LESS) surgery is a logical progression from traditional laparoscopic surgery. Operations are performed through a single site with an endoscope and one or several working channels. This often results in an incision that is larger than any single laparoscopic port might require (1 to 3 cm or more) but can be placed in a cosmetically favorable location such as the umbilicus. In many cases, this leaves no visible scar.

Other terms to describe the same principle include single-port, single-site, single-access, single-incision laparoscopic surgery (SILS), and LESS surgery. These techniques were explored first in the 1990s but gained traction in the 2000s. Many operations have been performed using single-incision techniques, including appendectomy, cholecystectomy, foregut and bariatric surgery, colorectal surgery, adrenalectomy, splenectomy, and others. In the future, elements of these different techniques likely will be used in combination. Innovative methods of retraction, specimen extraction, and dissection can be applied in a variety of settings and will lead to hybrid operations.

Several collaborative efforts and organizations have been important in proposing working definitions and a framework for research in these fields. Following the model of the Natural Orifice Surgery Consortium for Assessment and Research (NOSCAR), a group called the Laparoendoscopic Single-Site Surgery Consortium for Assessment and Research (LESSCAR) was convened and published its first consensus statement in 2010. Most research in single-site surgery remains investigator and industry driven.

▪ EVIDENCE AND USAGE

In the last decade an increasing body of literature has been published. Suffice it to say that single-port surgery can be performed safely with acceptable clinical outcomes for a wide variety of operations. Whether there are substantial benefits remains a topic of research and debate.

Both appendectomy and cholecystectomy have been particularly well studied, with multiple retrospective studies and several prospective randomized controlled trials (RCTs). These generally have demonstrated acceptable safety and increased operative time. Postoperative pain has been reported as similar, mildly reduced, or mildly increased. A prospective randomized trial of single-incision versus three-port appendectomy by Carter and colleagues in 2014 was halted early because of increased postoperative pain and opiate use in the single-incision group. Little or no cosmetic improvement or other clinical benefits have been reported. The rate of wound complications may be similar or slightly lower.

Several authors have performed systematic reviews and meta-analyses of randomized trials. These remain somewhat limited by technical heterogeneity and small sample size but provide some of the best available evidence to date on the subject. Xu and colleagues published a meta-analysis of RCTs examining single-port appendectomy for appendicitis in 2015. They found that single-port appendectomy was as safe and effective as three-port appendectomy, with increased operative time and a slightly improved recovery time (Tables 1 and 2).

Single-site techniques also have been evaluated for more technically demanding cases. Many urologic and pediatric surgeons have performed complex operations with good results. For example, Zhou and colleagues published a comparison of traditional multiport versus transumbilical single-incision upper

TABLE 1: Details of Included RCTs Comparing SILA With TPLA in Meta-analysis

Authors	Year, Ethnicity	Period	Intention to Treat Analysis	Matched Factors	Sample Size
Park, et al	2010, Korea	2009.4-2009.6	NR	1, 2, 5, 6	40
St. Peter, et al	2011, America	2009.8-2010.10	Yes	1, 2, 3, 4, 5, 7	360
Teoh, et al	2012, China	2009.10-2011.3	No	1, 2, 11	200
Frutos, et al	2013, Spain	2009.9-2010.12	NR	1, 2, 3, 4, 11	184
Kye, et al	2013, Korea	2009.2-2010.4	Yes	1, 4, 5, 6, 10	102
Lee, et al	2013, Korea	2010.3-2011.9	No	1, 2, 4, 5, 6, 13	248
Perez, et al	2013, America	2009.6-2011.1	NR	1, 2, 3, 11, 12	50
Sozutek, et al	2013, Turkey	2010.9-2011.5	NR	1, 2, 4, 8, 9	50

From Xu A-M, Huang L, Li T-J. Single-incision versus three-port laparoscopic appendectomy for acute appendicitis: systematic review and meta-analysis of randomized controlled trials. *Surg Endosc.* 2015;29:822-843.

1, Age; *2,* gender; *3,* weight; *4,* body mass index; *5,* initial leucocyte count; *6,* initial C-reactive protein; *7,* admission temperature; *8,* American Society of Anesthesiologists (ASA) score; *9,* previous abdominal surgery; *10,* duration of symptoms; *11,* appendicitis type; *12,* race; *13,* erythrocyte sedimentation rate (ESR); *NR,* not reported; *RCTs,* randomized controlled trials; *SILA,* single-incision laparoscopic appendectomy; *TPLA,* three-port laparoscopic appendectomy.

TABLE 2: Analysis of Major Outcomes by Category

Category	No. RCTs	SILA	TPLA	RR	WMD	95% CI	P
Operative time (min)	8	43 (n = 616)	38 (n = 618)		5.96	2.54 to 9.38	0.0006
Hospital duration (h)	4	58 (n = 340)	59 (n = 342)		−0.96	−2.86 to 0.94	0.32
Postsurgical stay (h)	2	32 (n = 231)	32 (n = 231)		0.48	−0.86 to 1.81	0.48
Days to full activities	3	6 (n = 331)	7 (n = 331)		−0.68	−1.10 to −0.26	0.001
Overall complications	8	50/616 (8%)	49/618 (8%)	1.02		0.71-1.48	0.91
Major surgical complications	8	13/616 (2%)	9/618 (1%)	1.40		0.63-3.11	0.41
Minor surgical complications	8	33/616 (5%)	34/618 (6%)	0.97		0.62-1.54	0.91
Medical complications	8	4/616 (1%)	6/618 (1%)	0.67		0.19-2.35	0.53
Ileus	6	4/345 (1%)	6/345 (2%)	0.71		0.23-2.22	0.56
Abdominal infections	5	8/400 (2%)	4/400 (1%)	1.80		0.61-5.31	0.29
Wound infections	7	22/525 (4%)	23/525 (4%)	0.96		0.55-1.68	0.88
Reoperations	3	0/240 (0%)	2/242 (1%)	0.34		0.04-3.21	0.34

From Xu A-M, Huang L, Li T-J. Single-incision versus three-port laparoscopic appendectomy for acute appendicitis: systematic review and meta-analysis of randomized controlled trials. *Surg Endosc.* 2015;29:822-843.

Relative risks less than 1.0 favor the SILA approach.

CI, Confidence interval; *P,* probability; *RCTs,* randomized controlled trials; *RR,* risk ratio; *SILA,* single-incision laparoscopic appendectomy; *TPLA,* three-port laparoscopic appendectomy; *WMD,* weighted mean difference.

pole heminephroureterectomy for children with a duplex kidney. As illustrated in Figures 1 through 3, the latter procedure was performed through a small incision with excellent visualization. The final cosmetic result was improved subjectively compared with the multiport technique.

In the case of colectomy, a number of prospective trials have been performed. A meta-analysis published by Lujan and colleagues in 2014 identified 28 comparative studies. This analysis identified several subtle benefits, including slightly shorter length of stay, and comparable rates of complications, mortality, operative time, and lymph node harvesting (Table 3).

Robotic platforms have been adapted and specifically designed to facilitate single-port operations. Since the late 2000s a large number of early studies have demonstrated safety and feasibility using these platforms for a variety of operations. A small randomized trial of single versus multiport cholecystectomy using the da Vinci Si surgical system (Intuitive Surgical, Sunnyvale, CA) demonstrated no difference in postoperative pain but improved cosmesis with the single-site approach.

The cost of these approaches and long-term outcomes such as hernia formation have not been well described in the literature, although some trials, including one by Marks and colleagues, suggest an increased risk of incisional hernia. Given the rapid advancement of techniques and tools used for these operations, much of the innovation in LESS surgery will proceed outside of the framework of clinical trials.

TABLE 3: Variables Collected From the Studies

Study	Year	No.		Length of Incision (cm)		Operating Time (min)	
		SILS	MLC	SILS	MLC	SILS	MLC
Adair	2010	17	17	3.8	5.1	139±29.7	134±32.3
Chen	2010	18	21	4 (3-6)	4 (3-6)	175 (145-280)	165 (120-340)
Gandhi	2010	24	24	3.3±1.1	6.6±2.1	143.2±37.2	112.8±44.8
Waters	2010	16	27	2.5-4.5	2.5-4.5	106 (71-223)	100 (65-215)
Champagne	2011	29	29	3.80	4.50	103.80	134.40
Fujii	2011	23	23	3.3±1.2	5.5±2.4	174±37	179±40
Gaujoux	2011	25	50			130 (110-185)	180 (110-200)
Kim	2011	73	106			274 (105-405)	254 (80-470)
Lee	2011	46	46	5.1±1.8	6.4±2.4	135±21	134±39
Lu	2011	27	68	4.07±1.18	4.77±1.19	180 (150-205)	185 (155-230)
McNally	2011	27	46			114 (59-268)	135 (45-314)
Papaconstantinou	2011	26	26			144±24	144±51
Ramos-Valadez	2011	20	20			159.2±29.9	162.1±40.3
Rickjen	2011	20	20	3.8 (2.5-5)		137.4±28.4	166.4±37.5
Champagne	2012	165	165			135.4±45	133.2±56
Chew	2012	40	104	5 (3-12)	6 (3-25)	95 (45-180)	100 (55-190)
Costedio	2012	24	24			125.9±39.3	230±117.4
Huscher	2012	16	16			147±61	129±46
Kanakala	2012	40	78			162	170
Osborne	2012	55	327			79±37	113±44
Park	2012	37	54	3.3±0.9	9.1±1.4	118.1±41.5	140±42.2
Vasilakis	2012	20	20	4.9±1.9	5.1±1.9	175,5±40.2	178.7±50.7
Velthuis	2012	50	50			97 (60-148)	112 (70-225)
WooLim	2012	40	123	4.6±0.7	4.4±0.9	225.5±48.3	144.6±32.6
Keshava	2013	75	74	4.3 (3-6)	5 (4-9)		
Pedraza	2013	50	50			127.9±37.6	126.7±63.3
Rosati	2013	50	50			160 (115-210)*	152 (110-215)*
Yun	2013	66	93			131±27	143±54

From Luján JA, Soriano MT, Abrisqueta J, Pérez D, Parrilla P. Single-port colectomy vs multi-port laparoscopic colectomy: systematic review and meta-analysis of more than 2800 procedures. *Cir Esp*. 2015;93:307-319.

*Mean.

MLC, Multiport laparoscopic colectomy; *SILS*, single-incision laparoscopic surgery.

Conversion		Blood Loss (mL)		Lymph Nodes		Complications		Length of Hospital Stay (days)		Mortality	
SILS	MLC	SILS	MLC	SILS	MLC	SILS	MLC	SILS	MLC	SILS	MLC
0	0			20.1±11.3	18.6±4.1	5	4	3.9±3.7	4.1±2.2	1	0
1	0	75 (20-700)	50 (20-300)	19.5 (3-42)	19 (15-57)	3	2	5 (3-15)	5 (3-38)		
0	0	62.5±37.6	90.6±60.6	24.6±12.3	18.6±5.7	2	0	2.7±0.8	3.3±1.1	1	0
0	0	54 (25-120)	90 (25-300)	18 (13-22)	16 (10-21)	3	4	5 (2-24)	6 (2-28)	0	1
1	1			19.4	21.6	5	7	3.70	3.90		
0	1	9±9	109±391	19.9±5.2	23.3±11.5	3	5	8.2±3.4	12.7±12.9		
0	1	100 (50-150)	90 (50-100)			1	8	6 (6-7)	7 (6-9)	0	0
1	3	282 (105-405)	418 (100-2.600)	29.3±16	23.2±15.4	23	39	9.60	15.50	0	1
						11	12	4.6±1.6	4.3±0.8		
		35 (30-50)	50 (30-80)			2	3	7 (5-8)	7 (6-9)		
0	6	50 (5-100)	50 (5-250)	15 (3-32)	17 (0-35)	5	16	3 (2-17)	5 (2-11)	0	2
0	1	57±40	87±70	18±6	17±12			3.6±1.6	5±2.2		
0	0	58.3±34.3	98.8±52.1	20.3±3.8	18.3±6.8	2	2	3.2±1	3.8±2.1		
1	2					4	4	9±3.4	9.2±5.9		
4	8	47.20	63.50			43	48	4.3±1.6	4.6±1.4	1	0
2	7			19 (10-43)	18 (6-54)	9	21	5 (4-15)	5 (3-109)	0	1
0	2	95.8±65	241.7±135.5			11	19	6.08±4.2	6.3±3.05	0	0
		200		18±6	16±5	3	5	6±3	7±2	0	0
0	0			22.9 (11-41)	13.8 (0-28)	3	10	4 (2-11)	4 (2-20)	0	1
0	3			18 (2-34)	14 (5-53)	12	27	1 (1-8)	3 (1-24)		
0	0	92	131	14.6±6.8	23.4±11.4	3	6	5.5±2.3	7.7±4.2		
2	1	74.5±55.3	81.3±54.9			1	3	3.9±1.6	5.5±2	0	0
0	0			14 (10-28)	12.5 (10-34)	17	17	6 (2-41)	6 (2-103)	1	2
1	1	109.2±80.3	96±58.4	25.3±11.9	28.3±13.2	5	18	7.7±1.1	7.8±2.8	0	0
1	1			17.00	17.00	8	13	5 (3-43)	8 (4-33)	1	0
0	1	64.4±64.7	87.2±89.8	21.4±8.4	19.2±7.6	7	4	4.5±3.7	4±1.7		
0	1			21 (13-34)*	22 (8-38)*	4	11	6 (4-16)*	8 (4-34)*	0	1
1	5			24±11	27±13	6	14	8±4	9±5		

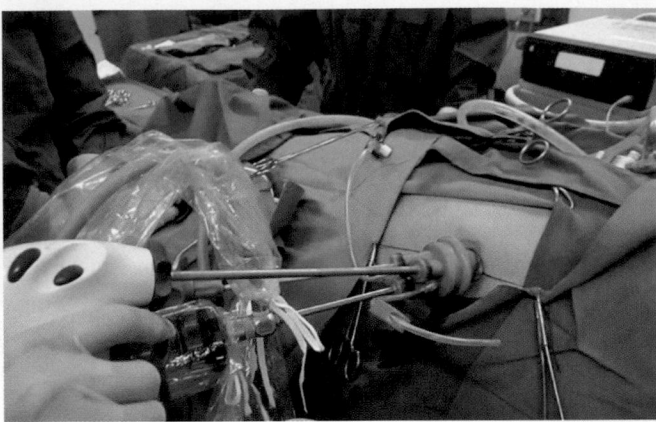

FIGURE 1 Positioning of working instruments and video laparoscope. *(From Zhou H, Ming S, Ma L, et al. Transumbilical single-incision laparoscopic versus conventional laparoscopic upper pole heminephroureterectomy for children with duplex kidney: a retrospective comparative study. Urology. 2014;84:1199-1204.)*

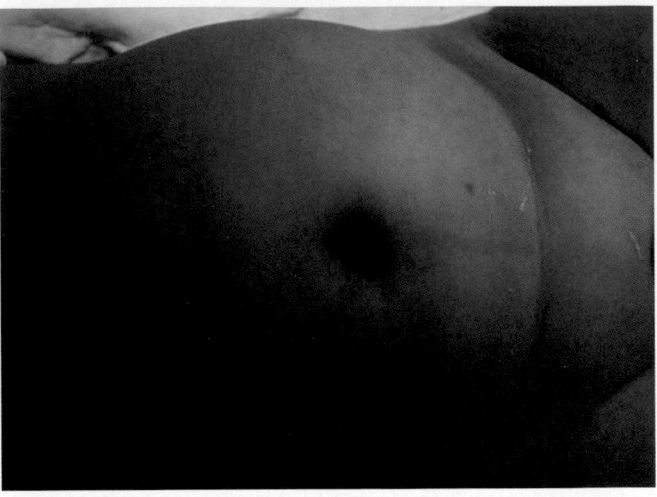

FIGURE 3 Postoperative umbilical scar 3 months after single-incision laparoscopic heminephroureterectomy. All patients made comments about their satisfaction with the cosmetic appearance. *(From Zhou H, Ming S, Ma L, et al. Transumbilical single-incision laparoscopic versus conventional laparoscopic upper pole heminephroureterectomy for children with duplex kidney: a retrospective comparative study. Urology. 2014;84:1199–1204.)*

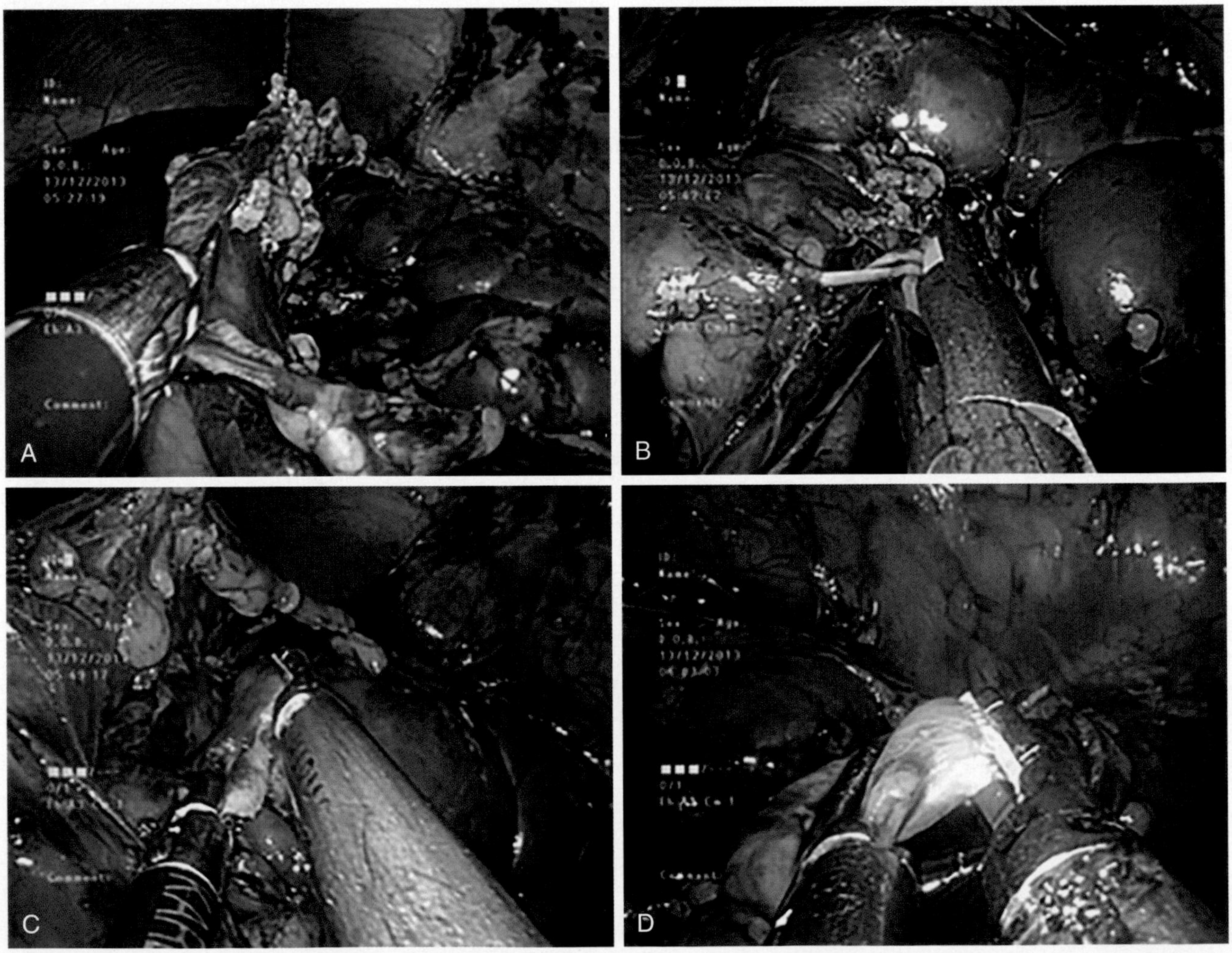

FIGURE 2 A, One 2-0 silk suture was used to hitch the Gerota's fascia to open up the space. **B,** The vessels supplying the upper pole were ligated with Hem-o-lok. **C,** Upper pole renal parenchyma was dissected with a harmonic scalpel. The surgeons made sure that urothelium of the upper pole was stripped off. **D,** The distal ureter of the upper pole was dissected as close as possible to the bladder wall. *(From Zhou H, Ming S, Ma L, et al. Transumbilical single-incision laparoscopic versus conventional laparoscopic upper pole heminephroureterectomy for children with duplex kidney: a retrospective comparative study. Urology. 2014;84:1199-1204.)*

■ TECHNICAL CONSIDERATIONS

A fundamental disadvantage of single-site surgery is that the camera and instruments are all in line with the target anatomy. Some techniques have been described using a single-lumen port with a scope and a working channel to accomplish an operation using traditional straight instruments, such as appendectomy wherein the organ is mobilized sufficiently to be delivered to the umbilicus and removed in an open fashion. Using traditional instruments and avoiding disposables can reduce the cost of these procedures. Unfortunately, the ability to perform complex operations in this manner is very limited.

More complex procedures require multiple instruments and the ability to triangulate. Several elements are necessary to perform technically complex single-site surgery. A wide variety of commercially available and improvised devices are available to satisfy the requirements of each element.

Peritoneal Access, Ports, and Endoscopes

Peritoneal access may be obtained through a single skin and fascial incision or through multiple separate fascial punctures from a single skin incision. Fascial retraction can be maintained by a simple sleeve or a soft or rigid structural component. Meanwhile, access to the peritoneum must be obtained while maintaining pneumoperitoneum. Some surgeons have fashioned a low-cost device with a surgical glove. This technique has been described by a number of authors and typically involves using an inner device to seal against the fascial incision (such as a wound protector) combined with a glove sealed against each instrument or port at the level of the finger.

Alternatively, a variety of improvised or commercially available ports can be used to allow instrument manipulation and exchange while maintaining pneumoperitoneum. These use either a gel membrane or separate channels to provide access. Most of these systems can accommodate traditional straight, angled, or flexible instruments. When using a system that requires separate port insertion, commercially available low-profile ports can be helpful to minimize crowding (Figure 4).

A variety of endoscopes have been used in LESS surgery. Standard 5-mm, 30-degree rigid scopes are used often, whereas angles of 45 or 60 degrees or higher may be helpful in certain situations. Longer scope length may bring the camera away from the surgeon's hands and reduce crowding. Some surgeons have utilized traditional flexible endoscopes, which can improve visualization but create an unstable image. Alternatively, rigid endoscopes with flexible tips are available and may offer advantages over both traditional rigid and flexible endoscopes (Figure 5).

Robotic platforms have been used to manipulate cameras as well as instruments. Simple functions such as steady camera operation and manipulation have been controlled by robot. More complex robotic platforms that incorporate both camera and instrument control also have been developed. The current market leader is the da Vinci system. A single-site platform has been developed for the da Vinci Si to allow operation of the robot's usual rigid camera and instruments through a single port. In 2014 the Sp surgical system was approved by the U.S. Food and Drug Administration (FDA) for use with the da Vinci Xi system. This allows instruments with flexible arms to be inserted through a single 25-mm cannula and controlled by a surgeon from a remote console. Several other companies have

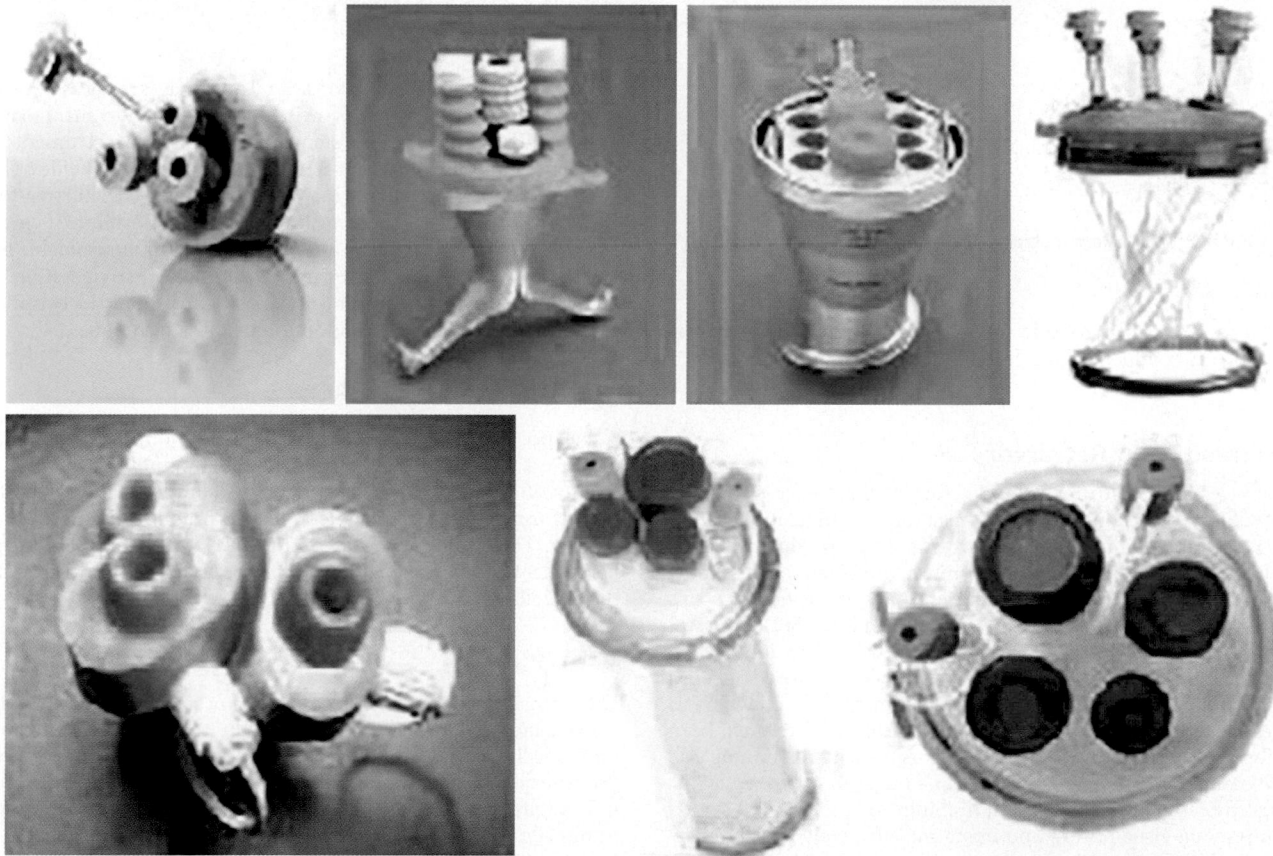

FIGURE 4 Various single-port devices. *Clockwise, from bottom left:* Dexide ports, SILSTM (both by Covidien), X-cone, Endocone (both by Karl Storz), GelPOINT (Applied Medical), Quadport, and Triport (both by Advanced Surgical). *(From Dhumane PW, Diana M, Leroy J, Marescaux J. Minimally invasive single-site surgery for the digestive system: a technological review. J Min Access Surg. 2011;7:40-51.)*

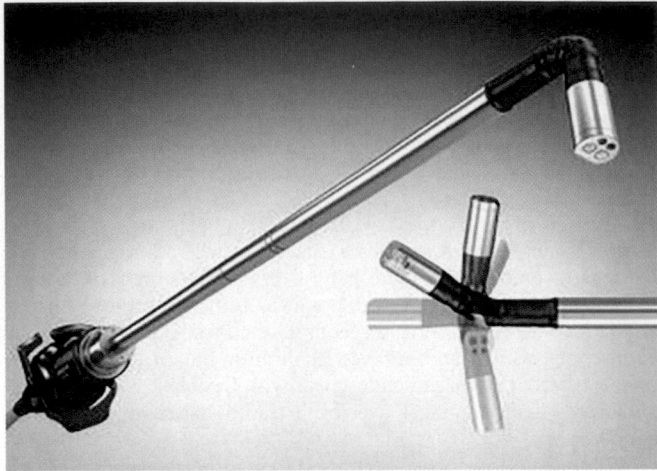

FIGURE 5 Olympus EndoEye. *(Courtesy Olympus Medical.)*

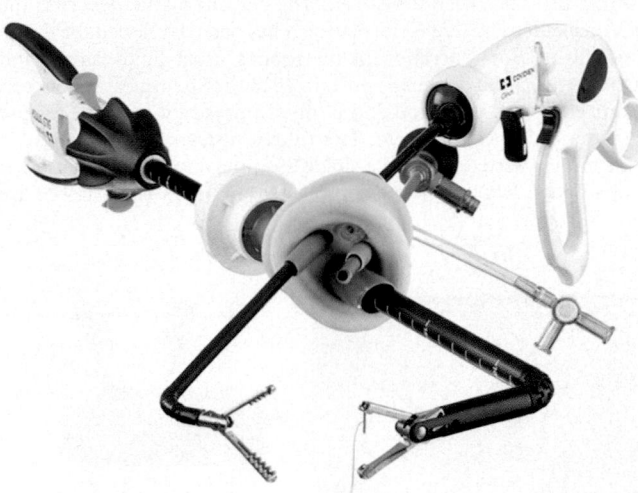

FIGURE 6 SILS Port multiple access port. *(Courtesy Covidien.)*

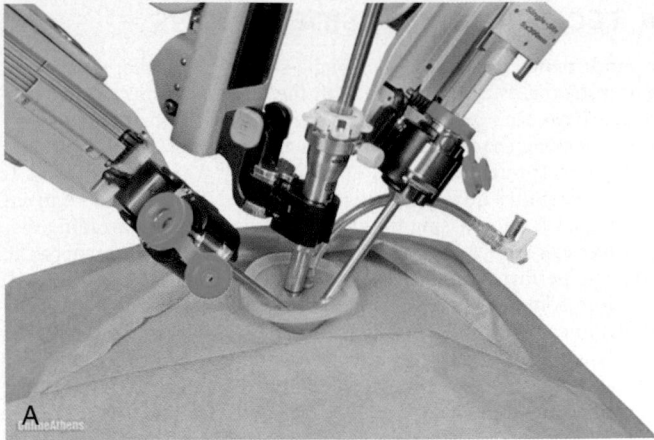

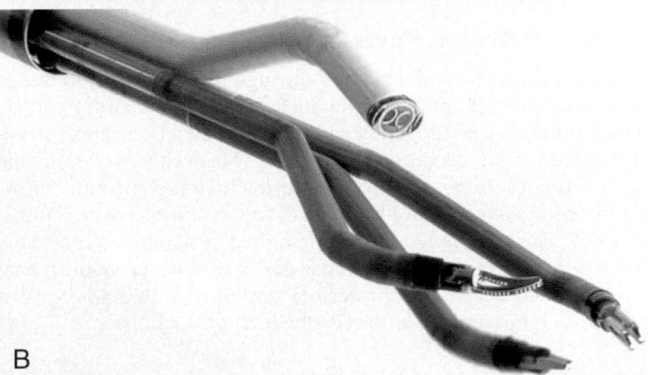

FIGURE 7 Single-port functions of the da Vinci Si (**A**) and Xi (**B**) systems. *(Courtesy Intuitive Surgical, Inc.)*

Robotic platforms may offer several advantages, such as improved ergonomics and facilitation of switching instrument control to a different hand. The da Vinci Si system is limited by rigid instruments, but the wristed instruments may facilitate complex tasks. The flexible Sp surgical system promises an increasingly versatile flexible platform, although not providing the same functional wrist flexibility (Figure 7).

The cost and complexity of these systems is an unavoidable topic of debate. The equipment used adds to the cost of an operation. The incremental benefit over multiport laparoscopy should be considered carefully before widespread adoption of these techniques.

■ RECOMMENDATIONS

A balance must be struck between innovation, safety, and cost-effective care. Of these, safety is always paramount (Box 1). The quality of an operation should never be compromised by attempts to perform it using the single-access techniques discussed in this chapter. The addition of a second 5-mm port or another "helper" instrument can be invaluable in some cases and has little impact on the overall morbidity or cosmetic result of an operation.

■ SUMMARY

LESS surgery will continue to be an area of intense research, and the convergence of flexible endoscopy with traditional surgical techniques will make the landscape all the more dynamic. Surgeons must use clinical judgment to determine the technologies that offer a significant improvement in patient outcomes over more traditional minimally invasive operations. As the number of approaches and tools grows, surgeons should remain focused on a singular purpose: improving the outcome and experience of their patients. Reducing healthcare costs (and ultimately cost to the patient) is an important secondary goal.

introduced alternative robotic and flexible endoscopic platforms with similar functions, and research in this field of computer-assisted surgery is ongoing.

Instruments and Retractors

Specially designed instruments and cameras with angled or flexible tips facilitate dissection and visualization. Triangulation is an important principle in minimally invasive surgery, which requires flexible or angled instruments when inserted through a single port (Figure 6). A number of manufacturers produce devices for this specific purpose, with a wide variety of functions. Suturing, stapling, and energy delivery all have been adapted for LESS approaches.

Innovative methods of retraction have been explored in both NOTES and LESS surgery. Novel uses of magnets, percutaneous sutures, needle-width instruments, and flexible devices have been described by a large number of investigators. Patient positioning also can be manipulated to use gravity as an adjunct to other retractors. Thoughtful retraction is important in minimizing the need for ports and improving visualization and operating efficiency. The commercial availability of these devices is changing rapidly. Ultimately, surgeons should familiarize themselves with the products currently available and previously used for each application when planning a LESS approach.

BOX 1 Common Issues Encountered During Single-Access Surgery and Potential Mitigation Strategies

Poor Visualization or Movement of Instruments

Angled or flexible endoscope; 30-degree rigid scopes are used commonly, but many options exist, including 90- and 120-degree angles.

Angled, flexible, or articulating instruments.

Retraction or "suspension" sutures or novel retraction techniques (e.g., magnetic).

Crowding and Clashing

Angled, flexible, or articulating instruments.

Instruments with double-bent design or different lengths to avoid crowding of hands.

Additional "helper" ports.

Retraction or "suspension" sutures or novel retraction techniques (e.g., magnetic).

Transmission of Movement From One Instrument to Another

Commercially available ports may better isolate movement.

Careful choice of site: umbilical may not be ideal.

Cost, Time, and Added Physical and Mental Strain

Novel tools to facilitate suturing and anastomoses (several commercially available).

Be aware of the costs of disposables and platforms (i.e., robot) used.

Consider patient preferences and clinical evidence before choosing single access over multiport.

Develop a routine and personal experience.

Collect data on personal and institutional experience.

SUGGESTED READINGS

Carter JT, Kaplan JA, Nguyen JN, et al. A prospective, randomized controlled trial of single-incision laparoscopic vs conventional 3-port laparoscopic appendectomy for treatment of acute appendicitis. *J Am Coll Surg.* 2014;218:950-959. doi:10.1016/j.jamcollsurg.2013.12.052.

Dhumane PW, Diana M, Leroy J, Marescaux J. Minimally invasive single-site surgery for the digestive system: a technological review. *J Minim Access Surg.* 2011;7:40-51. doi:10.4103/0972-9941.72381.

Gill IS, Advincula AP, Aron M, et al. Consensus statement of the consortium for laparoendoscopic single-site surgery. *Surg Endosc.* 2010;24:762-768. doi:10.1007/s00464-009-0688-8.

Luján JA, Soriano MT, Abrisqueta J, Pérez D, Parrilla P. Single-port colectomy vs multi-port laparoscopic colectomy: systematic review and meta-analysis of more than 2800 procedures. *Cir Esp.* 2015;93:307-319. doi:10.1016/j.ciresp.2014.11.009.

Marks JM, Phillips MS, Tacchino R, et al. Single-incision laparoscopic cholecystectomy is associated with improved cosmesis scoring at the cost of significantly higher hernia rates: 1-year results of a prospective randomized, multicenter, single-blinded trial of traditional multiport laparoscopic cholecystectomy vs single-incision laparoscopic cholecystectomy. *J Am Coll Surg.* 2013;216:1037-1047, discussion 1047-1048. doi:10.1016/j.jamcollsurg.2013.02.024.

Pietrabissa A, Pugliese L, Vinci A, et al. Short-term outcomes of single-site robotic cholecystectomy versus four-port laparoscopic cholecystectomy: a prospective, randomized, double-blind trial. *Surg Endosc.* 2016;30:3089-3097. doi:10.1007/s00464-015-4601-3.

Rao P, Rao P, Bhagwat S. Single-incision laparoscopic surgery: current status and controversies. *J Minim Access Surg.* 2011;6:6-16. doi:10.4103/0972-9941.72360.

Xu A-M, Huang L, Li T-J. Single-incision versus three-port laparoscopic appendectomy for acute appendicitis: systematic review and meta-analysis of randomized controlled trials. *Surg Endosc.* 2015;29:822-843. doi:10.1007/s00464-014-3735-z.

Zhou H, Ming S, Ma L, et al. Transumbilical single-incision laparoscopic versus conventional laparoscopic upper pole heminephroureterectomy for children with duplex kidney: a retrospective comparative study. *Urology.* 2014;84:1199-1204. doi:10.1016/j.urology.2014.07.040.

NOTES: WHAT IS CURRENTLY POSSIBLE?

John H. Rodriguez, MD, and Jeffrey L. Ponsky, MD

The field of minimally invasive surgery has witnessed constant surgical evolution. Progressive techniques and instrumentation have allowed and will continue to allow proceduralists to push the envelope. The evolution of flexible surgical endoscopy since the early 1950s has introduced a new level of procedures and techniques. The initial descriptions of endoscopic retrograde cholangiopancreatography in the 1970s and percutaneous endoscopic gastrostomy in the 1980s introduced the surgical community to the concept of performing advanced procedures through natural orifices.

The first published experience of natural orifice transluminal endoscopic surgery (NOTES) appeared in 2004 and was described by Dr. Kalloo from the Johns Hopkins Hospital. It involved a diagnostic peritoneoscopy and liver biopsy through a gastric wall puncture, which then was closed using standard endoscopic clips. Before this experience, there were anecdotal reports of transgastric extraction of the gallbladder after needlescopic cholecystectomy. The late 2000s witnessed NOTES gaining tremendous momentum, and new access routes were explored. The technique also expanded to other subspecialties, and reports of tubal ligations, partial hysterectomy and oophorectomy, lymphadenectomies, nephrectomies, colectomies, among other procedures, started to appear. However, as the next decade arrived, the movement seemed to fade.

In 2005 a group of experts from the American Society for Gastrointestinal Endoscopy (ASGE) in the Society of American Gastrointestinal and Endoscopic Surgeons (SAGES) met to create the Natural Orifice Surgery Consortium for Assessment and Research (NOSCAR). This group of experts recognized the obstacles to NOTES and developed a list of guidelines that needed to be followed in order to further expand this new concept. In the same fashion, our colleagues in Europe created the EURO-NOTES clinical registry as a combined effort by members of the European Association for Endoscopic Surgery (EAES) and the European Society of Gastrointestinal Endoscopy (ESGE).

There are technical and conceptual problems that still need to be addressed in order for NOTES to gain universal application and acceptance. Many of these problems are related to the limitations of currently available technology, which has further limited the application of this promising technique. So, what is currently possible?

Gastrointestinal surgery has been the field with probably the largest number of NOTES procedures. Transgastric and transvaginal cholecystectomy has been the most popular operation performed to date. There has been more limited experience with other procedures, such as splenectomy, appendectomy, liver biopsy, and even creation of gastrojejunal anastomosis. However, derivations from the original concept of NOTES have become common practice. Perhaps one of the most significant new procedures is peroral endoscopic myotomy

(POEM). Initially introduced by Dr. Inoue, POEM has established itself as a validated modality for treatment of achalasia, with multiple studies showing results comparable to Heller myotomy in well-selected patients. POEM can be performed with standard endoscopic equipment and has been mastered by many proceduralists with advanced endoscopic skills. Endoscopic submucosal dissection (ESD) is another technique that allows endoscopic management of neoplastic processes throughout the gastrointestinal tract with the use of advanced endoscopy. Colorectal surgeons also have nurtured the experience learned from early endoscopic techniques such as transanal endoscopic microsurgery (TEM), to develop more aggressive procedures such as transanal minimally invasive surgery (TAMIS). This technique was started in 2009 and allows management of rectal lesions that require full-thickness excision.

Gynecologists also have been able to use techniques learned through NOTES for clinical application. Using the vagina for access has allowed the expansion of clinical applications. There have been multiple reports of hysterectomy, oophorectomy, and NOTES-assisted ovarian cystectomy (NAOC) performed with similar success rates to the laparoscopic approach. The field of urology also has explored the vaginal route as a reproducible access site for nephrectomies with good success. However, none of these techniques has gained tremendous popularity.

In summary, the expansion of NOTES has been limited significantly by medical technology available at this time. However, we have witnessed a tremendous expansion of procedures that have derived from the original concepts of NOTES. Operations such as POEM, ESD, TAMIS, and transvaginal gynecologic surgery all have derived from the concept of natural orifice interventions. NOTES will continue to evolve and expand, and unexpected indications and applications will continue to emerge. The future of these developments will depend on advances in the technology used for suturing, tissue division, and hemostasis and on the overall application and accessibility of this technology.

SUGGESTED READINGS

Giday SA, Kantsevoy SV, Kalloo AN. Principle and history of natural orifice translumenal endoscopic surgery (NOTES). *Minim Invasive Ther Allied Technol.* 2006;15:373-377.

Rattner D, Kalloo A. ASGE/SAGES Working Group on natural orifice translumenal endoscopic surgery. *Surg Endosc.* 2006;20:329-333.

Page numbers followed by f indicate figures; t, tables; b, boxes.